MEDICINE OF THE FETUS & MOTHER

// E. ALBERT REECE, MD
The Abraham Roth Professor and Chairman of Obstetrics, Gynecology and Reproductive Sciences
Professor of Internal Medicine
Director—The Division of Maternal-Fetal Medicine
Temple University School of Medicine
Philadelphia, Pennsylvania

JOHN C. HOBBINS, MD
Professor of Obstetrics, Gynecology and Diagnostic Radiology
Yale University School of Medicine
Director of Obstetrics
Yale-New Haven Hospital
New Haven, Connecticut

MAURICE J. MAHONEY, MD
Professor of Genetics, Pediatrics and Obstetrics and Gynecology
Director of Prenatal Diagnosis Unit
Director of Clinical Affairs
Yale University School of Medicine
New Haven, Connecticut

ROY H. PETRIE, MD, ScD
Professor of Obstetrics and Gynecology
Division of Maternal-Fetal Medicine
Department of Obstetrics and Gynecology
Washington University School of Medicine
St. Louis, Missouri

MEDICINE OF THE
FETUS & MOTHER

129 contributors

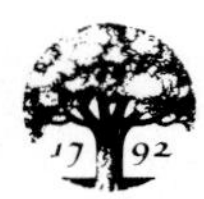

J.B. LIPPINCOTT COMPANY PHILADELPHIA

Acquisitions Editor: Lisa McAllister
Developmental Editor: Paula Callaghan
Project Editor: Elizabeth A. Durand
Indexer: Sandi Schroeder
Design Coordinator: Susan Hermansen
Interior Designer: Maria S. Karkucinski
Cover Designer: Susan Hermansen
Production Manager: Caren Erlichman
Production Coordinator: Kevin P. Johnson
Compositor: Tapsco, Incorporated
Printer/Binder: Arcata Graphics/Halliday
Color Insert Printer: Princeton Polychrome Corporation

6 5 4 3

Library of Congress Cataloging-in-Publication Data

Medicine of the fetus & mother/E. Albert Reece . . . [et al.].
p. cm.
Includes bibliographical references and index.
ISBN 0-397-51013-6
1. Pregnancy. 2. Pregnancy, Complications of. 3. Fetus—Diseases. I. Reece, E. Albert. II. Title: Medicine of the fetus and mother.
[DNLM: 1. Fetal Development. 2. Fetal Diseases. 3. Maternal-Fetal Exchange. 4. Pregnancy—physiology. 5. Pregnancy Complications. WQ 211 M489]
RG551.M43 1992
618.3—dc20
DNLM/DLC
for Library of Congress 91-42127
CIP

The authors and publisher have exerted every effort to ensure that drug selection and dosage set forth in this text are in accord with current recommendations and practice at the time of publication. However, in view of ongoing research, changes in government regulations, and the constant flow of information relating to drug therapy and drug reactions, the reader is urged to check the package insert for each drug for any change in indications and dosage and for added warnings and precautions. This is particularly important when the recommended agent is a new or infrequently employed drug.

To my wife, Sharon, and our children, Kelie, Brynne and Sharon-Andrea with love and gratitude.

E.Albert Reece

For my mother, Iona Hobbins.

John C. Hobbins

To my wife, Marjorie, and our children with love, respect and appreciation.

Maurice J. Mahoney

With appreciation to all those who lent a helping hand along the way.

Roy H. Petrie

CONTRIBUTORS

Diana Adams, MD
Assistant Professor of Obstetrics and Gynecology
Obstetrician in Gynecology
Cornell Medical College
New York Hospital
New York, New York

N. Scott Adzick, MD
Associate Professor of Surgery and Pediatrics
University of California, San Francisco
San Francisco, California

Erol Amon, MD
Associate Professor of Medicine
St. Louis University School of Medicine
St. Louis, Missouri
Attending Physician
Division of Maternal-Fetal Medicine
St. Mary's Health Center
Clayton, Missouri

Ray Bahado-Singh, MD
Post Doctoral Fellow
Section of Maternal Medicine
Department of Obstetrics and Gynecology
Yale University School of Medicine
New Haven, Connecticut

Frederick C. Battaglia, MD
Professor of Pediatrics and Obstetrics-Gynecology
University of Colorado School of Medicine
University of Colorado Health Science Campus
Denver, Colorado

David A. Beckman, PhD
Department of Pediatrics
Jefferson Medical College
Thomas Jefferson University
Philadelphia, Pennsylvania
Research Department
Developmental Biology Division
Alfred I. duPont Institute
Wilmington, Delaware

Richard L. Berkowitz, MD
Professor and Chairman
Department of Obstetrics and Gynecology —Reproductive Science
Mount Sinai Medical Center
Director, Division of Maternal-Fetal Medicine
Mount Sinai Medical Center
New York, New York

Pravit Bisalbutra, MD
Research Associate in Laboratory
Department of Dermatology
Uniformed Services University of the Health Sciences
Bethesda, Maryland

John M. Bowman, MD, OC, FRCS
Professor
Department of Pediatrics and Child Health
Professor
Department of Obstetrics, Gynecology and Reproductive Sciences
Faculty of Medicine
University of Manitoba
Director, Rh Laboratory
Section of Blood Group Serology
Department of Pediatrics and Child Health
Women's Hospital Health Science Centre
Winnipeg, Manitoba
Canada

D. Ware Branch, MD
Associate Professor of Maternal-Fetal Medicine
Department of Obstetrics and Gynecology
University of Utah
Salt Lake City, Utah

Robert L. Brent, MD
Distinguished University Professor
Louis & Bess Stein Professor of Pediatrics
Professor of Radiology
Professor of Anatomy
Chairman of Pediatrics at Jefferson Medical Center
Jefferson Medical College
Thomas Jefferson University
Philadelphia, Pennsylvania
Director, Developmental Biology Division
A. I. duPont Institute and Children's Hospital
Wilmington, Delaware

Gerard N. Burrow, MD
Vice Chancellor of the Health Sciences
Dean, School of Medicine
Professor of Medicine
Department of Medicine
University of California, San Diego School of Medicine
La Jolla, California

Tim Chard, MD, FRCOG
St. Bartholomew's Hospital Medical College
The London Hospital Medical College
Department of Reproductive Physiology
West Smithfield
London, England

Frank A. Chervenak, MD
Associate Professor of Obstetrics and Gynecology
Director of Obstetric Ultrasound and Ethics
Cornell Medical Center
New York, New York

Cecilia Y. Cheung, PhD
Associate Professor
Division of Perinatal Medicine
Department of Reproductive Medicine
School of Medicine
University of California at San Diego
La Jolla, California

David A. Clark, MD
Professor, Department of Pediatrics
Tulane Medical School, New Orleans
Children's Hospital of New Orleans
Charity Hospital of New Orleans
New Orleans, Louisiana

Steven L. Clark, MD
Professor of Obstetrics and Gynecology
University of Utah
Director of Maternal-Fetal Medicine
Intermountain Health Care Perinatal Centers
Salt Lake City, Utah

Mark J. Clinton, MD
Fellow, Pulmonary and Critical Care Medicine
Winthrop University Hospital
Mineola, New York

Wayne R. Cohen, MD
Associate Professor of Obstetrics and Gynecology
Albert Einstein College of Medicine
Director of Obstetrics and Gynecology
Bronx Municipal Hospital Center
Bronx, New York

Joshua A. Copel, MD
Director of Resident Education
Associate Professor of Obstetrics and Gynecology
Yale University School of Medicine
New Haven, Connecticut

David Cotton, MD
Professor and Chairman
Department of Obstetrics and Gynecology
Wayne State University
Chief, Obstetrics and Gynecology
Hutzel Hospital
Detroit Medical Center
Detroit, Michigan

Donald R. Coustan, MD
Professor and Chairman of Obstetrics and Gynecology
Brown University Program in Medicine
Obstetrician-Gynecologist in Chief
Women and Infants Hospital of Rhode Island
Providence, Rhode Island

Joe Craft, MD
Associate Professor of Medicine
Section of Rheumatology
Yale University School of Medicine
Attending Physician
Yale-New Haven Hospital
New Haven, Connecticut

Robert K. Creasy, MD
Emma Sue Hightower Professor and Chairman
University of Texas Medical School–Houston
Chief of Obstetrics and Gynecology Service
Hermann Hospital
Physician-in-Chief, Obstetrics and Gynecology
Lyndon Baines Johnson General Hospital
Houston, Texas

Fernand Daffos, MD
Chairman
Institut de Puericulture de Paris
Centre de Diagnostie Prénatal
Paris, France

Alan H. DeCherney, MD
Professor and Chairman
Department of Obstetrics and Gynecology
Tufts University
Northeast Medical Center
Boston, Massachusetts

Michael DeSwiet, MD, FRCP
Senior Lecturer in Medicine
Heart and Lung Institute
Consultant Physician
Queen Charlotte's Hospital
London, England

Gary A. Dildy, MD
Director of Perinatology
Utah Valley Regional Medical Center
Provo, Utah
Assistant Professor of Obstetrics and Gynecology
University Medical Center
Salt Lake City, Utah

James O. Donaldson, MD
Professor of Neurology
University of Connecticut
School of Medicine
Attending Neurologist
John Dempsey Hospital
Farmington, Connecticut

Jennifer Downey, MD
Assistant Clinical Professor
Department of Psychiatry
Consultant
Department of Obstetrics and Gynecology
Columbia University College of Physicians and Surgeons
Research Psychiatrist II
New York State Psychiatric Institute
Assistant Attending Psychiatrist
Columbia-Presbyterian Medical Center
New York, New York

Mark I. Evans, MD
Professor and Vice Chief of Obstetrics and Gynecology
Professor of Molecular Biology and Genetics
Director, Division of Reproductive Genetics
Director, Center for Fetal Diagnosis and Therapy
Hutzel Hospital/Wayne State University
Detroit, Michigan

Fiona M. Fairlie, MRCOG
Senior Registrar in Obstetrics and Gynaecology
University of Glasgow
Department of Obstetrics and Gynaecology
Glasgow Royal Maternity Hospital Rottenroh
Glasgow, Scotland
United Kingdom

Anne Ferris, PhD, RD
Associate Professor and Head
Nutritional Sciences
University of Connecticut
Storrs, Connecticut

Mieczyslaw Finster, MD
Professor of Anesthesiology, Obstetrics and Gynecology
College of Physicians and Surgeons
Columbia University
Attending Anesthesiologist
The Presbyterian Hospital
New York, New York

John C. Fletcher, PhD
Director, Center for Biomedical Ethics
Professor of Religious Studies
Professor of Internal Medicine
University of Virginia
Health Science Center
Charlottesville, Virginia

Alex Forman, MD, PhSD
Research Laboratory
Department of Obstetrics and Gynecology
University of Aarhus
Aarhus Municipal Hospital
Aarhus, Denmark

Harold Fox, MD, FRCPath, FRCOG
Professor of Reproductive Pathology
University of Manchester
Honorary Consultant Pathologist
St. Mary's Hospital, Manchester
Manchester, England

Sandro Gabrielli, MD
Attending Physician
Section of Prenatal Pathophysiology
Second Department of Obstetrics and Gynecology
University of Bologna School of Medicine
Bologna, Italy

Anne Brenda Galway, MD, FRCPC
Assistant Professor
Medicine and Obstetrics and Gynecology
Memorial University of Newfoundland
St. John's, Newfoundland
Canada

Alessandro Ghidini, MD
Fellow
Department of Obstetrics and Gynecology
Joint Fellow
Department of Pediatrics
Mt. Sinai School of Medicine
New York, NY

Ronald S. Gibbs, MD
Professor and Chair
Department of Obstetrics and Gynecology
University of Colorado Health Science Center
Denver, Colorado

J. S. Ginsberg, MD
Assistant Professor
Department of Medicine
Director of Thromboembolism Unit
Shedoka-McMaster Hospital
Hamilton, Ontario
Canada

Mitchell S. Golbus, MD
Professor of Obstetrics, Gynecology and Reproductive Sciences and of Pediatrics
University of California, San Francisco
San Francisco, California

James D. Goldberg, MD
Assistant Professor of Obstetrics and Gynecology
Department of Obstetrics, Gynecology and Reproductive Sciences
University of California, San Francisco
San Francisco, California

Ian Gross, MB
Professor of Pediatrics
Yale University School of Medicine
Director, Newborn Special Care Unit
Yale-New Haven Hospital
New Haven, Connecticut

John Henry Grossman III, MD, PhD
Professor of Obstetrics, Gynecology and Microbiology
Director, Division of Maternal-Fetal Medicine
Department of Obstetrics and Gynecology
George Washington University School of Medicine and Health Sciences
Washington, DC

James E. Haddow, MD
Associate Clinical Professor
University of Vermont School of Medicine
Courtesy Staff Maine Medical Center
Scarborough, Maine

Zion J. Hagay, MD
Director, Maternal-Fetal Medicine
Department of Obstetrics and Gynecology
Kaplan Hospital
Rehovot, Israel

Michael R. Harrison, MD, FACS
Professor of Surgery and Pediatrics
University of California, San Francisco
Chief, Division of Pediatric Surgery
Department of Surgery
Co-Director, The Fetal Treatment Program
University of California, San Francisco
San Francisco, California

Jean C. Hay, BSc(Hons), MSc
Associate Professor of Anatomy
Department of Anatomy
Faculty of Medicine
University of Manitoba
Winnipeg, Manitoba
Canada

John P. Hayslett, MD
Professor of Medicine
Department of Medicine, Section of Nephrology
Yale University School of Medicine
New Haven, Connecticut
Attending Physician
Yale-New Haven Hospital
New Haven, Connecticut

Alan Hill, MD, PhD, FRCP
Professor and Head of Neurology
Department of Pediatrics
Vancouver, British Columbia
Canada

Washington C. Hill, MD
Professor and Chairman
Department of Obstetrics and Gynecology
Meharry Medical College, School of Medicine
Chief of Obstetrics and Gynecology
George W. Hubbard Hospital of Meharry Medical College
Nashville, Tennessee

Jack Hirsh, MD, FRCP
Professor of Medicine
McMaster University
Director, Hamilton Civic Hospitals Research Centre
Hamilton, Ontario
Canada

John C. Hobbins, MD
Professor of Obstetrics, Gynecology and Diagnostic Radiology
Yale University School of Medicine
Director of Obstetrics
Yale-New Haven Hospital
New Haven, Connecticut

Angela R. Holder, LLM
Clinical Professor of Pediatrics (Law)
Yale University School of Medicine
New Haven, Connecticut

Lillian Y. F. Hsu, MD
Professor of Pediatrics
New York University School of Medicine
Director
Prenatal Diagnosis Laboratory of New York City
A Service Division of Medical and Health Research Association of New York City, Inc.
New York, New York

Karen A. Hutchinson-Williams, MD
Assistant Professor
Obstetrics and Gynecology and Medicine
Yale University
New Haven, Connecticut

Frederick R. Jelovsek, MD
Professor and Chairman
Department of Obstetrics and Gynecology
East Tennessee State University
Johnson City, Tennessee

Mark Johnson, MD
Assistant Professor of Obstetrics and Gynecology
Wayne State University School of Medicine
Assistant Professor of Obstetrics and Gynecology
Molecular Biology and Genetics
Detroit, Michigan

Ervin E. Jones, PhD, MD
Associate Professor
Division of Reproductive Endocrinology
Department of Obstetrics and Gynecology
Yale University School of Medicine
Yale-New Haven Hospital
New Haven, Connecticut

Nicholas Kadar, MD
Associate Professor
Department of Obstetrics and Gynecology
Robert Wood Johnson Medical School
University of Medicine and Dentistry of New Jersey
New Brunswick, New Jersey

Ruben Kier, MD
Assistant Professor of Radiology
Department of Diagnostic Radiology
MRI Section
Yale University School of Medicine
Yale-New Haven Hospital
New Haven, Connecticut

Charles S. Kleinman, MD
Professor of Pediatrics, Diagnostic Imaging and Obstetrics and Gynecology
Chief, Pediatric Cardiology
Yale University School of Medicine
Attending Pediatrician
Yale-New Haven Medical Center
New Haven, Connecticut

Russell K. Laros, Jr., MD
Professor and Vice Chairman
Department of Obstetrics, Gynecology and Reproductive Sciences
University of California, San Francisco
San Francisco, California

William J. Ledger, MD
Professor and Chairman
Department of Obstetrics and Gynecology
Cornell University Medical College
Obstetrician-Gynecologist in Chief
New York Hospital
New York, New York

Jean M. Lien, MD
New Port Beach, California

Charles Lockwood, MD
Assistant Professor of Obstetrics and Gynecology
Department of Obstetrics, Gynecology and Reproductive Sciences
Mount Sinai School of Medicine
Mount Sinai Medical Center
New York, New York

Barbara Luke, RD, MPH, ScD
Assistant Professor
Division of Obstetrics and Gynecology Research
Rush Medical College
Assistant Attending Scientist
Rush-Presbyterian-St. Luke's Medical Center
Chicago, Illinois

Lauren Lynch, MD
Assistant Professor of Obstetrics and Gynecology
Department of Obstetrics, Gynecology and Reproductive Science
Division of Maternal Fetal Medicine
Mount Sinai School of Medicine
Assistant Attending Physician
Mount Sinai Hospital
New York, New York

Maurice J. Mahoney, MD
Professor of Genetics, Pediatrics and Obstetrics and Gynecology
Director of Prenatal Diagnosis Unit
Director of Clinical Affairs
Yale University School of Medicine
New Haven, Connecticut

Frank A. Manning, MD
Professor and Chairman
Department of Obstetrics and Gynecology
Reproductive Sciences
University of Manitoba
Winnipeg, Manitoba
Canada

Richard Matthay, MD
Professor and Associate Chairman
Department of Internal Medicine
Yale University School of Medicine
New Haven, Connecticut

Donald R. Mattison, MD
Dean, Graduate School of Public Health
Professor of Environmental and Occupational Health Human Genetics and Obstetrics and Gynecology
University of Pittsburgh
Pittsburgh, Pennsylvania

Laurence M. McCullough, PhD
Professor of Medicine and Medical Ethics
Center for Ethics, Medicine and Public Issues
Baylor College of Medicine
Houston, Texas

James G. McNamara, MD
Assistant Professor of Pediatrics
Yale University of Medicine
Attending Physician
Yale-New Haven Hospital
New Haven, Connecticut

Philip B. Mead, MD
Clinical Professor of Obstetrics and Gynecology
University of Vermont College of Medicine
Hospital Epidemiologist
Medical Center Hospital of Vermont
Burlington, Vermont

Aubrey Milunsky, MBBCh, DSc, FRCP, DCH
Professor of Pediatrics, Obstetrics and Gynecology and Pathology
Director, Center for Human Genetics
Boston University School of Medicine
Boston, Massachusetts

Fernando R. Moya, MD
Associate Professor
Department of Pediatrics
Division of Neonatal-Perinatal Medicine
University of Texas Southwestern Medical Center at Dallas
Attending Physician
Parkland Memorial Hospital
St. Paul Medical Center
Dallas, Texas

Frederick Naftolin, MD, DPhil
Professor and Chairman
Department of Obstetrics and Gynecology
Yale University School of Medicine
Yale-New Haven Hospital
New Haven, Connecticut

Katherine V. Nichols, MD
Fellow in Pediatrics
Newborn Special Care Unit
Yale School of Medicine
New Haven, Connecticut

Jennifer R. Niebyl, MD
Professor and Head
Department of Obstetrics and Gynecology
The University of Iowa College of Medicine
Department of Obstetrics and Gynecology
The University of Iowa Hospitals and Clinics
Iowa City, Iowa

Michael S. Niederman, MD
Professor of Medicine
State University of New York, Stony Brook
Winthrop University Hospital
Mineola, New York

Barbara M. Nies, MD
Associate Professor
George Washington University
School of Medicine
Washington, DC

Carl A. Nimrod, MB, FRCSC
Professor of Obstetrics and Gynecology
University of Ottawa
Head of Division of Perinatology
University of Ottawa
Head of Division of Perinatology
Ottawa General Hospital
Ottawa, Ontario
Canada

Jose Norris, MD
Post Doctoral Fellow
Yale University
New Haven, Connecticut

Glenn E. Palomaki, BS
Director of Biometry
Foundation for Blood Research
Scarborough, Maine

Valerie M. Parisi, MD, MPH
Associate Professor
Director, Division of Maternal Fetal Medicine
Department of Obstetrics/Gynecology and Reproductive Sciences
The University of Texas Medical School
Houston, Texas

Richard H. Paul, MD
Professor of Obstetrics and Gynecology
Director, Maternal Fetal Medicine
Department of Obstetrics and Gynecology
University of Southern California School of Medicine
Women's Hospital
Los Angeles, California

Hilda Pedersen, MB, ChB, FFARCS
Professor of Clinical Anesthesia
College of Physicians and Surgeons
Columbia University
Attending Anesthesiologist
Columbia Presbyterian Hospital
New York, New York

David Peisner, MD
Assistant Professor, Obstetrics and Gynecology and Maternal-Fetal Medicine
Columbia University
Columbia Presbyterian Medical Center
New York, New York

T. V. N. Persaud, MD, PhD, DSc, FRCPath(Lond) FFPath(RCPI)
Professor and Head, Department of Anatomy
Professor of Pediatrics and Child Health
Associate Professor of Obstetrics, Gynecology and Reproductive Sciences
University of Manitoba, Faculties of Medicine and Dentistry
Consultant in Pathology and Clinical Genetics
Health Sciences Centre
Winnipeg, Manitoba
Canada

Lone K. Petersen, MD
Research Laboratory
Department of Obstetrics and Gynecology
University of Aarhus
Aarhus Municipal Hospital
Aarhus, Denmark

Roy H. Petrie, MD, ScD
Professor
Department of Obstetrics and Gynecology
Washington University School of Medicine
St. Louis Maternity Hospital
St. Louis, Missouri

Jeffrey Phelan, MD, JD
Director, Maternal-Fetal Medicine
Pomona Valley Hospital Medical Center
Pomona, California

Gianluigi Pilu, MD
Attending Physician
Cattedra Fisiopatologia Prenatale
Section of Prenatal Pathophysiology
Department of Obstetrics and Gynecology
University of Bologna
Bologna, Italy

E. J. Quilligan, MD
Professor, Obstetrics and Gynecology
University of California, Irvine
School of Medicine
Irvine, California

Christopher Redman, MD
Clinical Reader
Nuffield Department of Obstetrics and Gynecology
Consultant in Obstetric Medicine
John Radcliffe Hospital
Oxford, United Kingdom

E. Albert Reece, MD
The Abraham Roth Professor and Chairman of Obstetrics, Gynecology and Reproductive Sciences
Professor of Internal Medicine
Director—The Division of Maternal-Fetal Medicine
Temple University School of Medicine
Philadelphia, Pennsylvania

Deborah L. Reid, PhD
Assistant Professor
Department of Obstetrics and Gynecology
University of Wisconsin, Madison
Madison, Wisconsin

Carolyn Riely, MD
Professor of Medicine and Pediatrics
University of Tennessee, Memphis
College of Medicine
Memphis, Tennessee

Roberto Romero, MD
Professor and Vice Chairman
Department of Obstetrics and Gynecology
Hutzel Hospital
Detroit, Michigan

Mortimer Rosen, MD
Willard C. Rappleye Professor of Obstetrics and Gynecology and Chairman of the Department
College of Physicians and Surgeons
Columbia University
Director of Obstetrics and Gynecology
The Sloane Hospital for Women of the Presbyterian Hospital
New York, New York

Benjamin F. Sachs, MB BS, MPH
Associate Professor Obstetrics and Gynecology
Harvard Medical School and Harvard School of Public Health
Obstetrician and Gynecologist in Chief
Beth Israel Hospital
Boston, Massachusetts

Alan C. Santos, MD
Assistant Professor of Anesthesiology
Obstetrics and Gynecology
School of Medicine
State University of New York-Stony Brook
Section Chief, Obstetrical Anesthesia
University Hospital at Stony Brook
Stony Brook, New York

Ian L. Sargent, BSc, PhD
Lecturer
University of Oxford
Nuffield Department of Obstetrics and Gynaecology
John Radcliffe Hospital
Headington
Oxford, England
United Kingdom

Philip M. Sarrel, MD
Professor, Obstetrics and Gynecology and Psychiatry
Yale School of Medicine
Department of Obstetrics and Gynecology and Psychiatry
Yale-New Haven Medical Center
New Haven, Connecticut

Peter E. Schwartz, MD
Professor of Obstetrics and Gynecology
Director, Gynecologic Oncology
Yale University School of Medicine
Yale-New Haven Hospital
Department of Obstetrics and Gynecology
Yale University School of Medicine
New Haven, Connecticut

James R. Scott, MD
Professor and Chairman
Department of Obstetrics and Gynecology
University of Utah School of Medicine
Chief, Obstetrics and Gynecology
University of Utah Hospital
Salt Lake City, Utah

Ulla M. Sellgren, MD
Sex Education Therapist
Department of Obstetrics and Gynecology
Yale School of Medicine
New Haven, Connecticut

John L. Sever, MD, PhD
Professor, Department of Pediatrics and Obstetrics and Gynecology and of Microbiology and Immunology
The George Washington University
School of Medicine and Health Sciences
Washington, DC

Kathryn Shaw, MD
Assistant Professor of Obstetrics and Gynecology
University of Southern California
School of Medicine
Attending Physician Women's Hospital
Los Angeles County and University of Southern California Medical Center
Los Angeles, California

Jaye M. Shyken, MD
Instructor of Maternal Fetal Medicine
Division of Maternal Fetal Medicine
Department of Obstetrics and Gynecology
Washington University School of Medicine
St. Louis, Missouri

Baha M. Sibai, MD
Professor, Division of Maternal/Fetal Medicine
Director, Maternal/Fetal Medicine Fellowship
Director, Perinatal Research
Chief, Division of Maternal/Fetal Medicine
Department of Obstetrics and Gynecology
University of Tennessee, Memphis
Memphis, Tennessee

Joe Leigh Simpson, MD
Faculty Professor and Chairman
Department of Obstetrics and Gynecology
University of Tennessee, Memphis
Regional Medical Center, Memphis
Memphis, Tennessee

Susan L. Sipes, MD
University of Iowa College of Medicine
Department of Obstetrics and Gynecology
Fellow Associate
University of Iowa Hospitals and Clinics
Iowa City, Iowa

Kristjar Skajaa, MD, PhD
Research Laboratory
Department of Obstetrics and Gynecology
University of Aarhus
Aarhus Municipal Hospital
Aarhus, Denmark

Danny Svane, MD
Research Laboratory
Department of Obstetrics and Gynecology
University of Aarhus
Aarhus Municipal Hospital
Aarhus, Denmark

Richard L. Sweet, MD
Professor and Chairman
Department of Obstetrics, Gynecology and Reproductive Sciences
University of Pittsburgh School of Medicine
Magee-Women's Hospital
Pittsburgh, Pennsylvania

Samuel S. Thatcher III, MD, PhD
Assistant Professor
Director of Reproductive Endocrinology and Infertility
Department of Obstetrics and Gynecology
East Tennessee State University
Johnson City, Tennessee

Brian J. Trudinger, MD, FRACOG
Fetal Welfare Laboratory
The University of Sydney at Westmead Hospital
Westmead, New South Wales
Australia

Niels Uldbjerg, MD, PhD
Research Laboratory
Department of Obstetrics and Gynecology
University of Aarhus
Aarhus Municipal Hospital
Aarhus, Denmark

Linda J. Van Marter, MD, MPH
Assistant Professor
Department of Pediatrics
Harvard Medical School
Attending Neonatologist
Children's Hospital
Boston, Massachusetts

Richard R. Viscarello, MD
Assistant Professor Obstetrics and Gynecology
Director of the Women in AIDS Program
Director of Prenatal Chemical Dependence Center
Division of Maternal-Fetal Medicine
Department of Obstetrics and Gynecology
Yale University School of Medicine
New Haven, Connecticut

Joseph J. Volpe, MD
Bronson Crothers Professor of Neurology
Harvard Medical School
Neurologist-in-Chief
Children's Hospital
Boston, Massachusetts

Cheryl K. Walker, MD
Fellow, Reproductive Infectious Disease and Immunology
Department of Obstetrics, Gynecology and Reproductive Sciences
University of California, San Francisco
San Francisco, California

Carl P. Weiner, MD
Professor and Head of Maternal & Fetal Medicine Division
Department of Obstetrics and Gynecology
University of Iowa Hospitals and Clinics
Iowa City, Iowa

Agnes H. Whitaker
Assistant Professor of Clinical Psychiatry
Columbia University College of Physicians and Surgeons
New York State Psychiatric Institute
New York, New York

Kim Yancey, MD
Associate Professor
Department of Dermatology
Uniformed Service University of the Health Sciences
Consultant, Dermatology Branch
National Cancer Institute
National Institutes of Health
Bethesda, Maryland

PREFACE

The field of maternal-fetal medicine developed into a recognized subspecialty from the 1950s through the 1970s and subsequently has become the academic arm of obstetrics. With greater sophistication, the field has widened to encompass many other allied areas, including genetics, teratology, diagnostic imaging, fetal and maternal physiology, and endocrinology. In spite of these advances the fetus remained, until recently, inaccessible to the obstetrician/perinatologist. Specialized medical care was provided primarily to the mother with the hope that improving the maternal condition would benefit the fetus. In recent years, the fetus has become accessible through various technologic advances, permitting fetal disease to be diagnosed by various methods including genetics, sonographic or direct in utero testing, and treatment administered either medically or surgically.

With the fetus having emerged as a bonafide patient, the field of maternal-fetal medicine has entered a new era. It may no longer be regarded as dealing with medical complications of the mother during pregnancy, but, rather, is to be seen as embodying both normal and diseased processes of both the fetus and the mother. The editors of this textbook believe that physicians in the practice of maternal-fetal medicine need, therefore, to become familiar with the complications of pregnancy that affect the fetus and/or the mother as well as the variety of modalities that are available for diagnosis, evaluation, and treatment.

This textbook is a comprehensive treatise on maternal-fetal medicine. It discusses subjects from the time of conception to delivery, including normal processes and disease states of the fetus, as well as diagnostic and therapeutic measures that can be used. In addition, all maternal medical complications of pregnancy are discussed in detail. A separate volume consisting of a compilation of questions and answers corresponding to each chapter is available for the student of medicine who wishes to test his or her knowledge of the subject.

Although this textbook is comprehensive, it is designed in such a manner that information relating to either the fetus or the mother is readily accessible. The overall balance in scope, content and design will serve the needs of academic subspecialists, obstetricians, and house staff physicians, as well as other keen students of medicine very well.

E. Albert Reece, MD
John C. Hobbins, MD
Maurice J. Mahoney, MD
Roy H. Petrie, MD, ScD

ACKNOWLEDGMENTS

We would like to acknowledge that Dr. Philip Hamilton and Dr. Peter Grannum were each willing to contribute a chapter to this book but were precluded from doing so because of their untimely deaths. The scientific community has been robbed of two of its scholars and we mourn their passing.

We would also like to express our gratitude to our contributors, who have painstakingly written comprehensive, highly informative, and scholarly chapters. Efforts like these can only be described as labors of love. We truly appreciate as well the efforts invested in this book by Carol Homko and Susan Koch. In addition, all our secretaries collectively deserve much praise and commendation for the many hours invested in typing, reviewing, and correcting the many versions of the manuscripts. Finally, we remain indebted to the editors of J. B. Lippincott Company, especially Paula Callaghan and Lisa McAllister, whose patient yet persistent demeanor permitted the timely publication of this book.

Our lives have been greatly touched as we interact with everyone who has participated in the successful completion of this book—to you all we remain deeply grateful.

E. Albert Reece
John C. Hobbins
Maurice J. Mahoney
Roy H. Petrie

CONTENTS

III FETAL DEVELOPMENTAL BIOLOGY

IV VARIATIONS IN EMBRYONAL AND FETAL GROWTH AND DEVELOPMENT

V TERATOGENS AND TERATOGENESIS

VI FETAL INFECTIONS OF MATERNAL ORIGIN AND TREATMENT

VII FETAL DISEASES
A. Genetic Disorders

B. PRENATAL DIAGNOSIS OF CONGENITAL ANOMALIES

VIII METHODS OF EVALUATION OF FETAL DEVELOPMENT AND WELL-BEING

IX FETAL THERAPY

X MATERNAL BIOLOGIC ADAPTATIONS TO PREGNANCY

XI MATERNAL DISEASES COMPLICATING PREGNANCY

XII MEDICO-SOCIAL CONSIDERATIONS IN PREGNANCY

XIII OBSTETRIC AND PERIPARTAL EVENTS

XIV THE NEWBORN INFANT

MEDICINE OF THE FETUS & MOTHER

OVERVIEW

HISTORICAL PERSPECTIVES ON THE FETUS AS A PATIENT

Edward Quilligan

Although the fetus has been considered a patient for hundreds of years, it was considered so in the context that it was a part of the pregnancy. It was so thoroughly protected from any diagnosis or manipulation that nothing could be done to alter the course or condition of the fetus. It was a passenger, not a patient.

If we can define a patient as someone about whom we can make a diagnosis and or treat so as to alter that individual's course, then the fetus became a patient in the period between 1500 and 1600. In 1500, Jacob Nufer, a swine gelder, did the first recorded successful cesarean section on his wife. In 1588, Rousset published a book on cesarean section, and in the first Italian book on obstetrics, Mercurio advocated cesarean section for contracted pelvis.[1] Peter the Elder of the Chamberlen family invented the obstetric forcep.[2] Both of these methods of delivering the fetus, while developed primarily to assist the mother during a difficult delivery, had the potential to alter the fetal environment and thus could be said to treat the fetus, even though indirectly. The first attempts at fetal diagnosis can be attributed to Marsac who, in the 17th century, first heard the fetal heartbeat. In 1818, Mayor, a Swiss surgeon, reported the presence of fetal heart tones; three years later, Kergaradec suggested auscultation would be helpful in the diagnosis of twins and the fetal lie and position.[3] In 1833, Kennedy suggested that the fetal heart rate was indicative of fetal distress.[4] Such distress, if diagnosed late in pregnancy, could be treated using forceps for delivery; however, it wasn't until relatively recent times that cesarean section was used to treat fetal distress during the first stage of labor. Douglas and Stromme, in their 1957 text *Operative Obstetrics*, state that "fetal distress was virtually nonexistent as a cause for cesarean section on our service (New York Hospital) until 10 years ago."[1]

The next major diagnostic step forward was made by Bevis in 1952.[5] He found a good correlation between amniotic fluid non heme iron (obtained by amniocentesis) and the severity of fetal anemia. This pioneering work was amplified beautifully by Liley, who in 1961 demonstrated that the spectral peak at 450 mU reflected the severity of hemolysis.[6] This gave the obstetrician a method with which to follow the patient with Rhesus sensitization and, in some cases, deliver the fetus prematurely for fetal salvage. The next major step in the treatment of these Rhesus-sensitized fetuses was also made by Liley, who in 1963 demonstrated that one could successfully treat these anemic fetuses in utero by transfusing blood into the fetal abdomen.[7]

During this same period Hon was developing methods for continuous recording of the fetal heart rate and, more importantly, the factors acting in the fetus that altered the fetal heart rate in response to uterine contractions.[8] He identified three basic patterns: early, late, and variable decelerations, which were due to head compression, utero–placental insufficiency, and umbilical cord compression, respectively. This permitted the attending obstetrician to assign a cause for the fetal heart rate decelerations that had been described in the 1800s. It also permitted a more individualized therapy for the deceleration; change of position for the variable and maternal oxygen for the late decelerations. Baseline heart rate change and heart rate variability were also related to specific fetal or maternal conditions.

The association of late decelerations and fetal oxygen deficiency was carried into the antepartum period by Hammacher in 1966.[9] He observed that those infants who had late decelerations of their fetal heart rate in association with spontaneous uterine contractions had lower Apgar scores at birth and a higher stillbirth rate. Pose induced the contractions with oxytocin and found a similar correlation.[10] Ray, Freeman, and Pine[11] did the first prospective blind trial in the United States and confirmed the results of Hammacher and Pose.

The fetal heart rate changes are best characterized as biophysical changes. During this same period, fetal biochemical changes that related to fetal well-being were being observed. The initial biochemical change associated with fetal health was its ability to make estriol.

Although Spielman, Goldberger, and Frank[12] and Smith and Smith[13] demonstrated the association between maternal urinary estriol excretion and fetal health in 1933, the test was not used extensively until the 1950s due to the lack of a reliable and reasonably easily performed chemical assay. Brown developed such an assay, and the test was used for many years, finally succumbing to less expensive, more accurate biophysical tests.[14] Another biochemical marker of fetal distress was the acid–base balance of the fetal scalp blood introduced by Saling in 1963.[15] This is still a reasonable test to use in selected situations.

All of the above discussion of fetal monitoring has dealt primarily with the oxygenation of the fetus. The development of a method of culturing and examining the chromosomes of the fetal cells residing in the amniotic fluid of the first and early second trimester fetus permitted the diagnosis of chromosomal abnormalities when pregnancy could be safely interrupted. Barr[16] in 1949 identified the sex chromatin that allowed several investigators[17–20] to use amniotic fluid to determine whether a sex-linked genetic aberration was a possibility in a given pregnancy. Culture of amniotic fluid cells was reported by Jacobson and Barter in 1967.[21] They used available techniques to search for chromosomal abnormalities in 56 pregnancies before 20 weeks of gestation, with a greater than 90% success rate in obtaining adequate chromosomal patterns. Knowledge of chromosomal abnormalities has increased as new techniques such as banding allowed the geneticist a more detailed look at the chromosomal structure; more recently, the development of genetic probes has significantly widened the field of genetic diagnosis. Chromosomal abnormalities were not the only fetal problems that could be determined using amniotic fluid; biochemical determinations allowed the diagnosis of such inheritable diseases as Tay Sachs disease and many others. Although amniotic sac puncture to obtain fluid had relatively few risks, there were some. This, coupled with the significant work and cost associated with analyzing amniotic fluid for chromosomal abnormalities, has lead to restricting the test to those most at risk: older pregnant patients and patients who have a genetic problem in the family or had an abnormal prior pregnancy. The development of maternal blood markers for fetal abnormalities was extremely important, because using the criteria described above, one would miss a significant proportion of fetal problems. For example, although the risk of trisomy 21 is much greater in the patient over 35 years of age, screening only these patients failed to detect 75% of the trisomy 21 patients, because they occurred in patients under 35 years of age. In 1944, Pederson described a protein found only in the fetus, fetuin.[22] This was the first specific fetal protein. Bergstrand and Czar found another fetal-specific protein, which migrated between the albumen and α-1 globulin fraction.[23] This was named α-fetoprotein by Gitlin in 1966.[24] In 1972, Brock and Sutcliffe[25] reported elevated levels of α-fetoprotein in the amniotic fluid surrounding fetuses with neural tube defects, and in 1984 Merkatz and his colleagues[26] noted that pregnant patients with a trisomy 21 fetus had lower than expected maternal levels of α-fetoprotein. This marker allows all pregnant patients to be offered screening for neural tube defects and some trisomies. Placental and fetal cells enter the maternal circulation, albeit in small numbers. Investigators are currently working on methods of harvesting and culturing these cells, which would obviate the need for amniocentesis.

In 1955, Ian Donald introduced a technical innovation to obstetrics and gynecology that brought the fetus to the obstetrician's fingertips.[27,28] Ultrasound was to change the way obstetrics was practiced, because for the first time the fetus, placenta, and umbilical cord were visualized with increasing clarity. One could assess fetal position, fetal growth, fetal weight, and fetal structure for anomalies, as well as placental and umbilical cord location and vessel number. As ultrasound became technically better, it became possible to perform fetal echocardiograms and evaluate fetal blood flow through umbilical, uterine, and numerous fetal vessels. This clarity of observation allowed the obstetrician fetal access in terms of placing needles in the umbilical vessels to perform fetal diagnostic studies or therapy, such as transfusion.

Although the fetus could be very accurately visualized and treated in many instances with ultrasound, there were some conditions, such as diaphragmatic hernia, that required a surgical approach during the second trimester if pulmonary hypoplasia was to be avoided. Although removal of the fetus from the uterus had been tried since 1980, it was not successful due to premature labor or fetal death in utero. In 1990, Harrison and his colleagues reported the successful closure of a diaphragmatic hernia on a midtrimester fetus that was placed back into the uterus, the pregnancy continuing into the third trimester with delivery of a living fetus.[29]

The fetus has become a patient that the obstetrician can diagnose and treat. This is recognized in a variety of ways. The American Board of Obstetrics and Gynecology developed certification for the specialist in maternal–fetal medicine in 1974. Centers of excellence in care of the fetus have developed throughout the country, receiving referrals for difficult fetal management problems from the generalist obstetrician–gynecologist. Texts such as the one you are about to read stress fetal diagnostic and therapeutic approaches.

The saying "you've come a long way, baby" has never been so true from both the fetal and the newborn standpoints. This has been reflected in the continuing decline in perinatal mortality; however, the second portion of that statement, "you still have a long way to go," is also very true. We still do not know for certain what triggers the onset of premature labor, which is responsible for the greatest number of perinatal deaths. Research needs to continue at an accelerated pace, taking diagnosis and treatment to the molecular level. This text, while providing the known material in this field at a very high level, also accomplishes a second equally important task: asking the questions that need to be asked.

REFERENCES

1. Douglas RG, Stromme WB. Operative obstetrics. New York: Appleton-Century-Crofts, 1957:413.
2. Da KN. Obstetric forceps: its history and evolution. St. Louis: CV Mosby, 1929.
3. Goodlin R. History of fetal monitoring. Am J Obstet Gynecol 1979;33:325.
4. Kennedy E. Observations on obstetric auscultation. Dublin: Hodges and Smith, 1833.
5. Bevis DCA. The prenatal prediction of antenatal disease of the newborn. Lancet 1952;1:395.
6. Liley AW. Liquor amnii analysis in the management of the pregnancy complicated by rhesus sensitization. Am J Obstet Gynecol 1961;82:1359.
7. Liley AW. Technique of fetal transfusion in treatment of severe hemolytic disease. Am J Obstet Gynecol 1964;89:817.
8. Hon EH. The electronic evaluation of the fetal heart rate (preliminary report). Am J Obstet Gynecol 1958;75:1215.
9. Hammacher K. Fruherkennung intrauterineo gefahrenzustande durch electrophonocardiographie und focographie. In: Elert R, Hates KA, eds. Prophylaxe frunddkindicher hirnschaden. Stuttgart: Georg Theime Verlag, 1966:120.
10. Pose SV, Escarcena L. The influence of uterine contractions on the partial pressure of oxygen in the human fetus. In: Calderyo-Barcia R, ed. Effects of labor on the fetus and newborn. Oxford: Pergamon Press, 1967:48.
11. Ray M, Freeman RK, Pine S, et al. Clinical experience with the oxytocin challenge test. Am J Obstet Gynecol 1972;114:12.
12. Spielman F, Goldberger MA, Frank RT. Hormonal diagnosis of viability of pregnancy. JAMA 1933;101:266.
13. Smith GV, Smith OW. Estrogen and progestin metabolism in pregnancy: endocrine imbalance of preeclampsia and eclampsia. Summary of findings to February 1941. Endocrinology 1941;1:470.
14. Brown JB. Chemical method for determination of oestriol, oestrone, and oestradial in human urine. Biochem J 1955;60:185.
15. Saling E, Schneider D. Biochemical supervision of the fetus during labor. Br J Obstet Gynecol 1967;74:799.
16. Barr ML, Bertram LF. A morphologic distinction between neurons of the male and the female and the behavior of the nuclear satellite during accelerated nucleoprotein synthesis. Nature 1949;163:676.
17. Fuchs F, Riis P. Antenatal sex determination. Nature 1956; 177:330.
18. Serr DM, Sachs L, Danon M. Diagnosis of fetal sex before birth using cells from the amniotic fluid. Bulletin of the Research Council of Israel 1955;E5B:137.
19. Makowski EL, Prem KA, Kaiser IH. Detection of sex of fetuses by the incidence of sex chromatin body in nuclei of cells in amniotic fluid. Science 1956;123:542.
20. Shettles LB. Nuclear morphology of cells in human amniotic fluid in relation to sex of the infant. Am J Obstet Gynecol 1956;71:834.
21. Jacobson CB, Barter RH. Intrauterine diagnosis and management of genetic defects. Am J Obstet Gynecol 1967;99:796.
22. Pedersen K. Fetuin, a new globulin isolated from serum. Nature 1944;154:575.
23. Bergstrand CG, Czar B. Demonstration of a new protein fraction in the serum from the human fetus. Scand J Clin Lab Invest 1956;8:174.
24. Gitlin D, Boesman M. Serum alpha-fetoprotein albumen and gamma G-globulin in the human conceptus. J Clin Invest 1966;45:1826.
25. Brock DJH, Sutcliffe RG. Alpha-fetoprotein in the diagnosis of anencephaly and spina bifida. Lancet 1972;2:197.
26. Merkatz IR, Nitowsky HM, Macri JN, Johnson WE. An association between low serum alpha-fetoprotein and fetal chromosomal abnormalities. Am J Obstet Gynecol 1984;148:886.
27. Donald I, MacVicar J, Brown TG. Investigation of abdominal masses by pulsed ultrasound. Lancet 1958;1:1188.
28. Donald I. On launching a new diagnostic science. Am J Obstet Gynecol 1969;103:609.
29. Harrison MR, Odzick NS, Longaker MT, et al. Successful repair in-utero of a fetal diaphragmatic hernia after removal of herniated viscera from the left thorax. N Engl J Med 1990;322:1582.

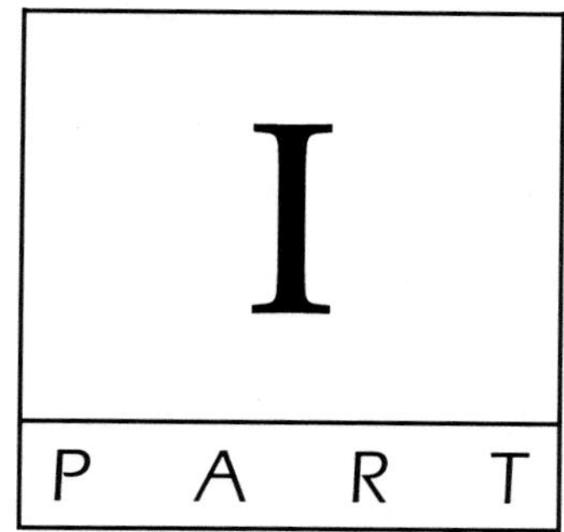

CONCEPTION AND CONCEPTUS DEVELOPMENT

1

CHAPTER

GAMETOGENESIS, FERTILIZATION, AND IMPLANTATION

Ervin E. Jones

Fertilization occurs in the distal third of the fallopian tube several hours following ovulation, and the conceptus remains in the ampulla for approximately 72 hours. The embryo is then rapidly transported through the isthmus to the uterine cavity, where it floats free for approximately 3 days. Numerous maturational events occur in the conceptus as it travels to the place where it will implant in the uterine endometrium. Implantation of the blastocyst normally occurs 6 days following ovulation in the human female. The blastocyst must be prepared to draw nutrients from the endometrium upon its arrival in the uterine cavity. Not only must the conceptus be prepared to receive nutrition from the uterus, but also the endometrium must be prepared to sustain the implanting blastocyst; therefore, endometrial preparation is essential if pregnancy is to progress successfully. This chapter elaborates on the normal developmental and physiologic events necessary for successful implantation and pregnancy.

GAMETOGENESIS

Gametogenesis, the formation and development of specialized germ cells, is a process involving chromosomes and cytoplasm that prepares these specialized cells for fertilization—the union of male and female gametes. Gametogenesis begins in utero as primordial, bipotential, germ cells migrate to the gonadal ridge from the yolk sac at approximately 5 weeks gestation. Initially, the primordial gamete possesses a diploid number of chromosomes (46). However, for survival of a species, the number of chromosomes must remain constant across generations. Meiosis, a specialized form of cell division, produces cells with a haploid number of chromosomes (23), which permits parental chromosomes to assort independently among sex cells. During gametogenesis, two sequential meiotic cell divisions occur. The first meiotic division is a process in which homologous chromosomes pair during prophase and separate during anaphase. One member of each pair of homologous chromosomes migrates to each pole of the cell; thus, the first meiotic division is a reduction division in which each new cell forms a secondary spermatocyte or secondary oocyte retaining the haploid number of chromosomes, or one half the number of chromosomes of the primary cell. The process of meiosis, the separation of paired homologous chromosomes, is the basis of segregation of allelic genes. The second meiotic division follows the first division in the absence of a normal interphase; each chromosome divides to form two chromatids and each chromatid is drawn to a different pole of the cell. Each daughter cell produced contains a haploid number of chromosomes, with one representative of each pair.

SPERMATOGENESIS

Spermatogenesis is a developmental continuum within which primitive sperm cells (spermatogonia) develop into mature sperm cells (spermatozoa). Spermatogonia developed during the fetal period lie dormant in the seminiferous tubules of the testes until puberty, when they undergo several mitotic divisions and are transformed into primary spermatocytes. The primary spermatocyte subsequently undergoes two reduction divisions. The first meiotic division results in two haploid secondary spermatocytes. The second meiotic division then occurs and the secondary spermatocyte forms four haploid spermatids. The spermatid undergoes a process of morphologic and functional differentiation, known as spermatogenesis, to form mature sperm (Fig. 1-1).

Morphologically, the mature sperm cell has three primary parts: a head, a neck, and a tail. The neck forms the junction between the head and the tail. The tail is composed of three segments: the midpiece, the principal piece, and the end piece. The head contains the nucleus bearing the haploid number of chromosomes. The anterior aspect of the nucleus is covered by the acrosome, a structure that forms a cap over the head of the sperm and contains several lytic enzymes that are believed to be involved in the dissolution of the corona radiata and the zona pellucida surrounding the oocyte, facilitating sperm penetration and fertilization of the egg.[1] The fully mature sperm cell is motile and free-swimming. The sperm tail provides motility. The middle piece contains mitochondria, which apparently provide the adenosine triphosphate (ATP) required for the generation of energy necessary for swimming.

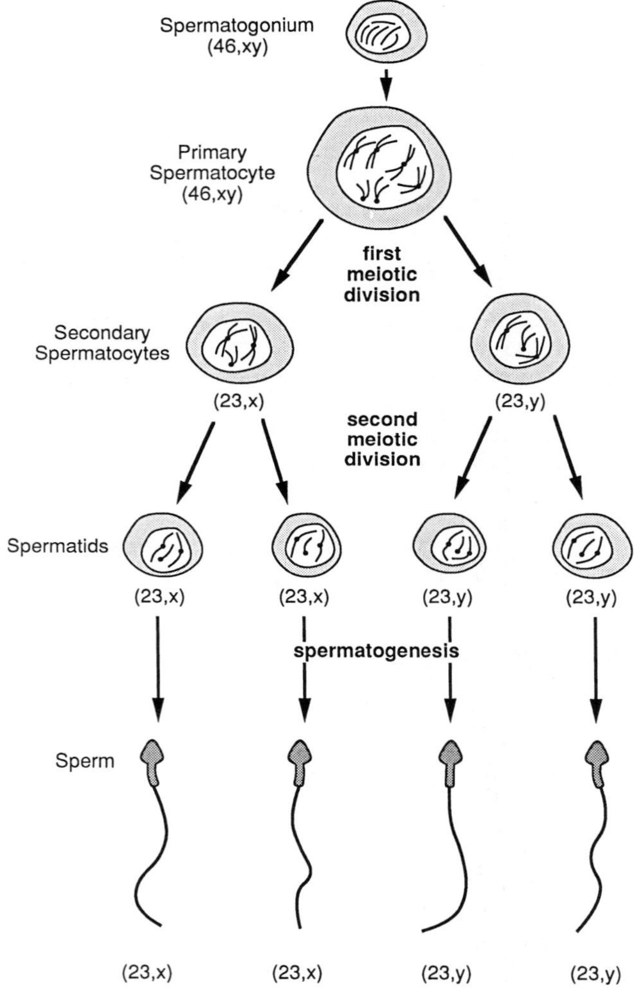

FIGURE 1–1. Spermatogenesis. Spermatogenesis normally begins at puberty. The chromosome composition of the developing sperm is shown at each stage. The total number of chromosomes, including the sex chromosomes, is shown before the comma. Following two meiotic divisions the diploid number of chromosomes, 46, is reduced to the haploid number 23. Four sperm cells form from each primary spermatocyte following each division.

OOGENESIS

Oogonia proliferate during prenatal life by mitotic division and enlarge prior to birth to form primary oocytes. Ovarian stromal cells surround the primary oocyte, forming a single flattened layer of epithelial cells. The unit thus formed constitutes the primordial follicle. At puberty, the primary oocyte enlarges, and the flattened layer of epithelial cells first becomes cuboidal and finally columnar in appearance. Thus, the primordial follicle becomes a primary follicle. The primary follicle then develops a second layer of cuboidal cells, becoming a secondary follicle, and the primary oocyte acquires an amorphous covering of intercellular material, the zona pellucida.

Although the first meiotic division of the primary oocyte begins before birth, prophase of the first meiotic division is not completed until after puberty. Therefore, primary oocytes remain suspended in prophase for several years until sexual maturity occurs and reproductive cycles are initiated. Although the mechanism of this prolonged prophase is unclear, Tsafiri and coworkers provided evidence that oocyte maturation inhibitor (OMI) keeps the meiotic process of the oocyte arrested (Fig. 1-2).[2]

As the follicle matures, the primary oocyte increases in size and, shortly before ovulation, completes the first meiotic division. During the first meiotic division, the secondary oocyte receives the majority of the cytoplasm, whereas the first polar body, a much smaller non-functional cell, receives very little. The second meiotic division begins as ovulation occurs but progresses only to metaphase when division is arrested. If a sperm cell penetrates the zona pellucida, the second meiotic division is completed, and again most of the cytoplasm is retained by the oocyte. The other cell, the second polar body, is small, and like the first polar body, rapidly degenerates. When the second polar body is extruded, ovum maturation is complete.

OVULATION

Ovulation, expulsion of the oocyte from the follicle, is the culmination of a series of hormonal and morphological events occurring in the ovary (Fig. 1-3). The ovarian cycle—recruitment of a cohort of primary follicles, selection of a dominant follicle from the cohort, maturation of the dominant follicle, ovulation and formation of the corpus luteum—is driven by the gonadotrophic hormones, follicle-stimulating hormone (FSH) and luteinizing hormone (LH).[3] At midcycle the LH surge is

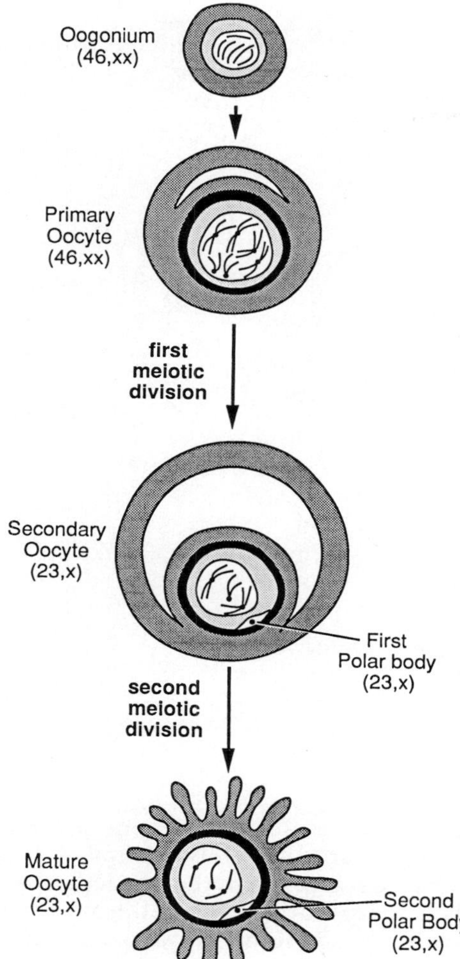

FIGURE 1–2. Oogenesis. Oogonia differentiate into primary oocytes before birth. The primary oocytes remain dormant in the ovary until puberty. The cytoplasm is conserved during oogenesis from one large cell, the mature oocyte or ovum. The polar bodies are small cells that eventually degenerate.

stimulated by rapidly rising levels of follicular estradiol, and ovulation occurs. The stigma of the follicle balloons out and forms a vesicle, which ruptures, and the oocyte is expelled, a process that is apparently facilitated by increased intrafollicular pressure and contraction of smooth muscle in the theca as a result of stimulation by prostaglandins.[4] The ovulated secondary oocyte is surrounded by the zona pellucida and one or more layers of follicular cells, the corona radiata. Prior to ovulation the granulosa and theca cells begin to undergo morphologic and functional differentiation to luteal cells, and progesterone levels begin to rise before release of the ovum under the influence of LH. Following expulsion of the oocyte, the granulosa and theca cells are thrown into folds that occupy the follicular cavity, forming the corpus luteum. The corpus luteum secretes primarily progesterone but produces estrogen as well. Luteal secretion of estrogen and progesterone is particularly important because both hormones are necessary for the development and maturation of the endometrium in preparation for implantation and support of the blastocyst.

TRANSPORT OF GAMETES

Following ovulation, the oocyte, with its investment of follicular cells, is "picked up" by the fimbria of the tube as they move over the surface of the ovary. The oocyte is then transported through the infundibulum into the ampulla, assisted by the ciliary movement of the tubal epithelium as well as the muscular contractions of the tubal muscularis. The ovum is fertilized in the ampullary portion of the fallopian tube and subsequently resides there for approximately 72 hours, followed by rapid transport through the isthmus to the uterine cavity, where it floats free for an additional 2 to 3 days prior to its attachment to the endometrium.[5] If the oocyte is not fertilized, it also passes along the tube to the uterus and then degenerates (Fig. 1-4).

Although between 200 million and 600 million sperm cells are normally deposited into the vagina during sexual intercourse, only a few viable sperm reach the distal fallopian tube where fertilization occurs. The majority of ejaculated sperm degenerate and are disposed of by the female genital tract. The swimming movements of the sperm tail propel the sperm through the mucus of the cervical canal. However, since sperm reach the tubal ampulla within five minutes of ejaculation, uterine or tubal activity must also serve a major role in sperm transport.[6] It has been suggested that prostaglandins of the seminal plasma stimulate uterine motility at the time of intercourse and that increased uterine activity facilitates sperm transport into the fallopian tube, where fertilization takes place.[7]

FERTILIZATION

Embryonic development begins with the process of fertilization. Fertilization begins with the fusion of two haploid cells, each bearing 22 autosomes and 1 of the sex chromosomes. A sperm makes contact with a secondary oocyte in the ampulla of the fallopian tube, and intermingling of maternal and paternal chromosomes occurs at the metaphase of the first meiotic division. Sperm must undergo capacitation to be able to fertilize the oocyte. Capacitated sperm show no morphological changes, but they are more active. Usually sperm cells are capacitated in the female reproductive tract—uterus or fallopian tubes—by unidentified substances.[8,9] (However, during in vitro fertilization, capacitation is induced by artificial means.[10]) When capacitated sperm make contact with the corona radiata of a secondary oocyte, perforations in the acrosome occur (acrosome reaction) and probably result in the release of hydrolytic enzymes that facilitate fertilization. Dissociation of

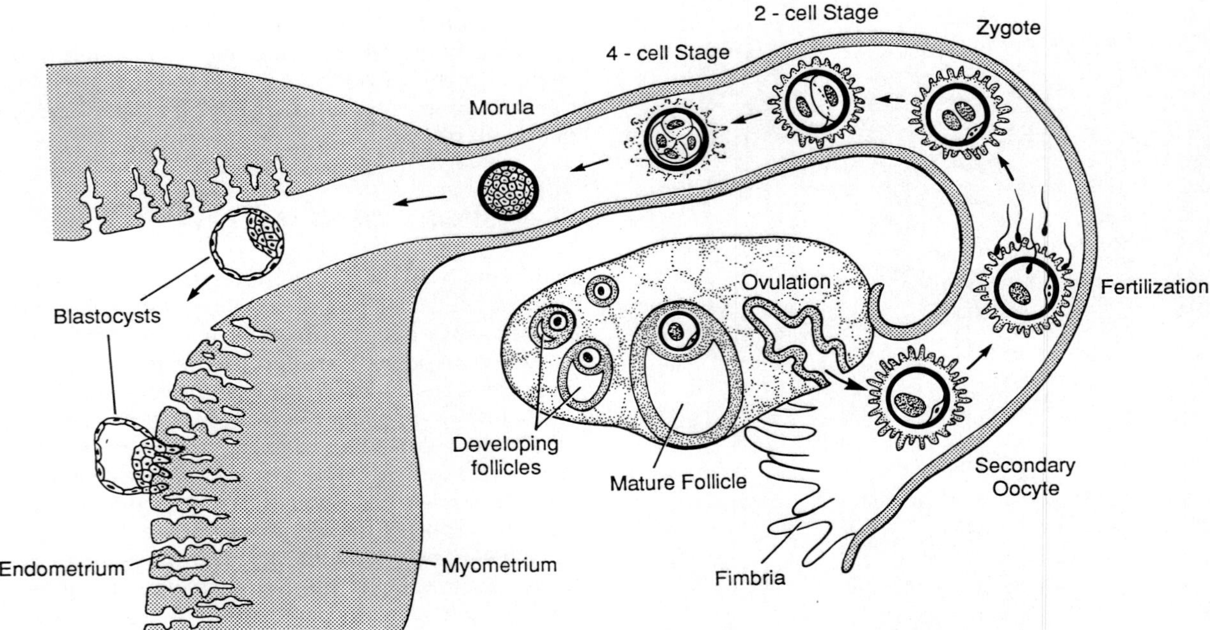

FIGURE 1–3. Ovulation and gamete transplant. Following the LH surge, the oocyte is released from the mature follicle surrounded by its cumulus oophorus. The first meiotic division occurs within the follicle. The oocyte bearing its cumulus oophorus and zona pellucida is transported by ciliary motion and tubal contractility to the ampulla, where fertilization occurs.

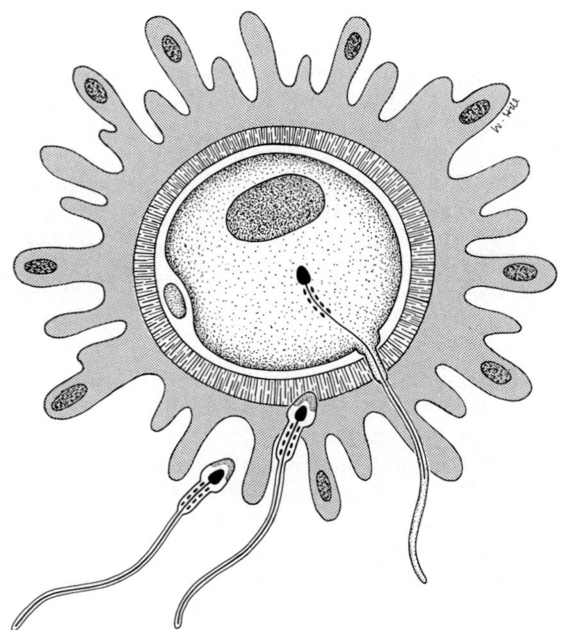

FIGURE 1–4. Fertilization. This diagram depicts penetration of an oocyte by a sperm. During the acrosome reaction perforations occur in the acrosome membrane. The sperm digests a path through the zona pellucida with enzymes released from the acrosome and enters the cytoplasm of the oocyte. The plasma membranes of the sperm and the oocyte fuse. The head and tail of the sperm enter the oocyte, leaving the sperm's plasma membrane attached to the oocyte's plasma membrane.

cells of the corona results from enzymes released from the acrosome, particularly hyaluronidase, and the sperm then passes through the corona radiata and penetrates the zona pellucida. The pathway through the zona probably results from the lytic action of acrosin and neuraminidase released from the acrosome. Once the sperm crosses the zona, a reaction that renders the zona impenetrable to other sperm occurs. This so-called zona reaction apparently prevents polyspermy and may result from a substance or substances released from cortical granules in the cytoplasm of the oocyte.[11] The sperm head attaches to the surface of the oocyte, the membranes of the sperm and egg fuse, and dissolution occurs at the area of fusion. The sperm head and tail enter the cytoplasm of the oocyte, leaving the plasma membrane behind, and the secondary oocyte completes the second meiotic division, resulting in a mature ovum and a second polar body. The nucleus of the mature ovum is known as the female pronucleus. The head of the sperm enlarges to form the male pronucleus as the tail degenerates, and the male and female pronuclei fuse, forming a new cell, the zygote. Fertilization, therefore, results in a conceptus bearing the diploid number of chromosomes, a full complement of genetic material—one half obtained from the maternal gamete and one half from the paternal gamete.

Recall that the primary spermatocyte contains two sex chromosomes—one X and one Y, whereas the primary oocyte contains two X chromosomes. Two secondary spermatocytes are produced during the first reduction division, one carrying a Y and the other carrying an X chromosome; thus, both X- and Y-bearing cell lines are established. In contrast, during oogenesis, only the X-bearing cell line is established. Thus, normal male gametes will be either X or Y, whereas normal female gametes will all be X-bearing. Fertilization of the ovum by an X-bearing sperm produces a zygote with XX sex chromosomes, which develops into a female. When the ovum is fertilized by a Y-bearing sperm, an XY zygote, which develops into a male, is produced. Therefore, chromosomal sex is established at fertilization and is usually the same as the phenotypic sex that develops during the fetal period.

THE PRE-IMPLANTATION EMBRYO

CLEAVAGE

A series of rapid mitotic divisions is activated by the process of fertilization (Fig. 1-5). Cleavage normally begins in the fallopian tube while the zygote is still enclosed in the zona pellucida, resulting in an increase in the number of cells but no increase in cytoplasmic mass.[12] Two blastomeres (daughter cells) are produced when division of the zygote occurs at about 30 hours after fertilization. Subsequent divisions follow, resulting in smaller blastomeres with each successive division. A rapid process of division continues as the conceptus makes its journey down the reproductive tract, and a berry-like mass of cells composed of 12 to 16 blastomeres known as the morula enters the uterus about three days after fertilization.

DIFFERENTIATION OF CELLS DURING CLEAVAGE

The embryo is composed of two distinct populations of cells, an enclosed mass of inner cells and the outer epithelium of trophectoderm.[13] The trophectoderm and inner cell mass apparently originate from blastomeres located outside and inside the embryo, respectively, at the time of blastocyst formation, although it remains unclear how differentiation of these two cell populations occurs during cleavage. It has been proposed that all blastomeres possess the ability to differentiate as trophectoderm cells before the eight-cell stage.[14] As an alternative hypothesis, Johnson and coworkers postulated that the embryo becomes polarized in a radial

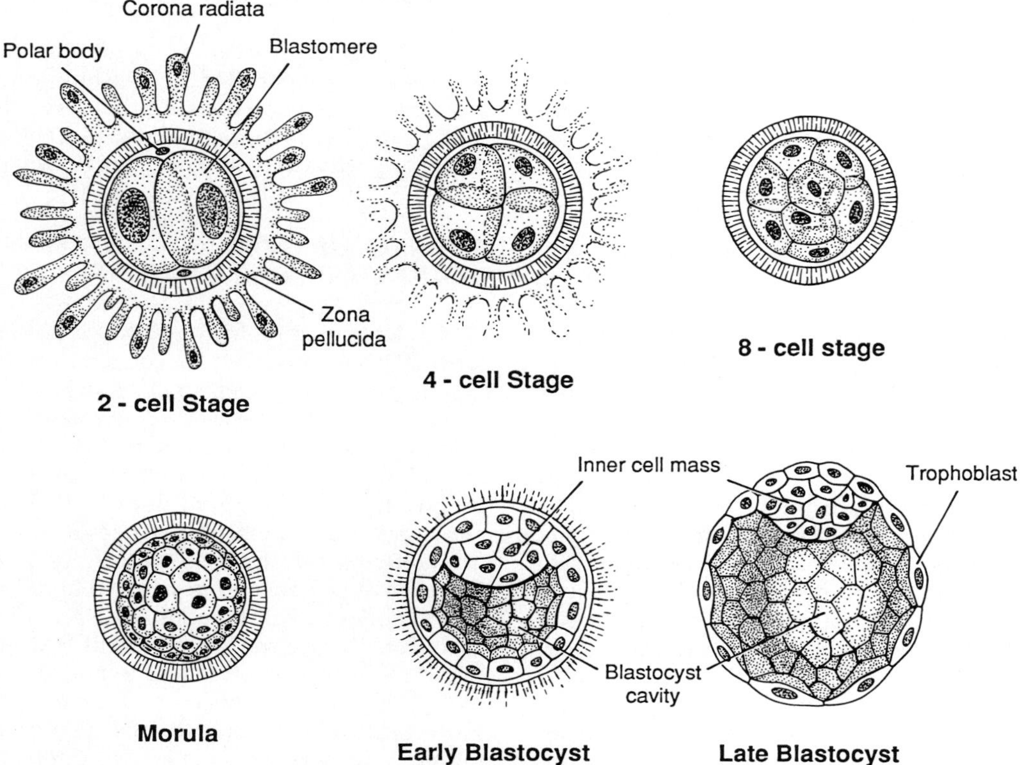

FIGURE 1–5. Cleavage and blastogenesis. Cleavage occurs in stages and results in the formation of blastomeres. The morula is composed of 12 to 16 blastomeres. The blastocyst forms when there are approximately 60 blastomeres present. Note that the zona pellucida has disappeared by the late blastocyst stage. The polar bodies are small nonfunctional cells that undergo degeneration as the zygote moves along the fallopian tube toward the uterus. Although cleavage occurs during this process, there is essentially no increase in the size of the developing embryo until the zona pellucida has been shed.

fashion at the eight-cell stage as a result of the formation of an external microvillus pole on each blastomere and that this polarity is conserved through the fourth cleavage.[15] Thus, the sixteen-cell embryo is composed of roughly nine to ten polar and six to seven apolar blastomeres resulting from a cleavage plane that bisects the microvillus pole, generating two polar daughters. The polar cells, according to this hypothesis, remain external and are assumed to give rise to trophectoderm, whereas apolar cells assume an internal location as inner cell mass precursors.

Regional differentiation of the trophectoderm and inner cell mass results in the three primitive tissue layers known as endoderm, mesoderm, and ectoderm. Differentiation within the inner cell mass results in the formation of primitive endoderm cells on the blastocelic surface, and a portion of these cells migrate laterally onto the inner surface of the mural trophectoderm to form the parietal endoderm.[16] The remainder of these cells constitute the visceral endoderm, which continues to invest the deeper cells of the inner cell mass. These cells are referred to, collectively, as primitive ectoderm. The extra-embryonic mesoderm appears to arise from primitive ectoderm, which gives rise to both allantoic and chorionic mesoderm.

FORMATION OF THE BLASTOCYST

A cystic cavity forms in the morula as cell division and differentiation occur. About 4 days after fertilization, formation of a cavity in the morula results in the formation of the blastocyst as it floats free in the endometrial cavity. First, spaces occur between the central cells of the morula and fluid passes through the zona to accumulate in these spaces. As the fluid accumulates, the cells are separated into an outer layer and an inner layer, known respectively as the outer cell mass (trophoblast) and the inner cell mass (embryoblast). The fluid-filled spaces then coalesce to form the blastocyst cavity. The blastocyst floats in the uterine cavity for approximately 2 days, during which time growth and development continue. The free-floating blastocyst obtains nourishment from the uterine contents via active and passive transport, primarily from sugars, purines, pyrimidines, and simple amino acids. Lysis of the zona occurs as the blastocyst settles into the endometrium and cell–cell contacts are formed.[17] The blastocyst implants approximately 6 days following fertilization and has completely imbedded itself within the decidua by about 9.5 days following ovulation.

When studied with ultrasound imaging, a pregnancy can be seen as early as 25 days menstrual age as an echogenic area within the thickened decidua. This intradecidual sign occurs before the appearance of the gestational sac. About 14 days later, two small bubbles (amniotic yolk sac) attach to the walls of the gestational sac, creating an ultrasonic image known as the double bleb sign. The appearance of the double bleb is the most important sign of early pregnancy (Fig. 1-6).[18]

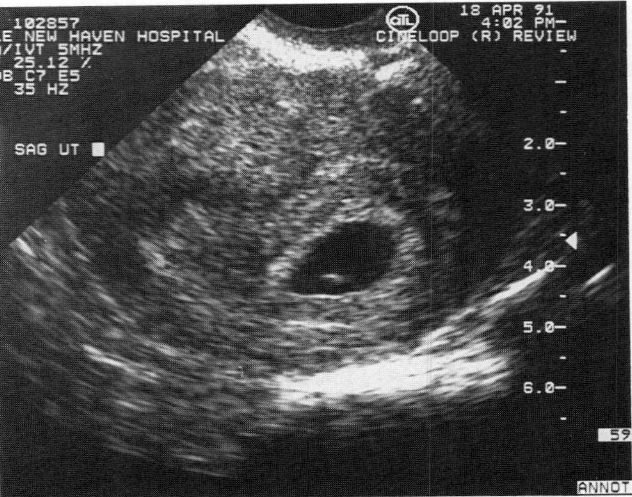

FIGURE 1–6. The double bleb sign. This ultrasound scan depicts an intrauterine pregnancy at the stage when the double ring can be visualized. The outer ring represents decidual reaction. (courtesy Dr. Ken Taylor, Department of Diagnostic Radiology, Yale University).

MOLECULAR SYNTHESIS IN THE DEVELOPING CONCEPTUS

The early conceptus exhibits a high level of metabolic activity and is capable of the synthesis and secretion of a number of macromolecules that have diverse effects on the success of implantation, placentation, maintenance of pregnancy, and future pregnancy performance.

EMBRYO DERIVED PLATELET ACTIVATING FACTOR (PAF)

A platelet activating factor with physiologically important effects is putatively secreted by the pre-implantation embryo. Early pregnancy associated thrombocytopenia has been observed in primates including the common marmoset and humans, although the extent of thrombocytopenia is variable.[19] Correlation between the production of embryo derived PAF and the pregnancy potential of embryos suggests that it may serve a fundamental role in the establishment of pregnancy. Conclusive evidence for the essential role of PAF in the establishment of pregnancy was provided by Spinks and O'Neill, who used inhibitors of PAF activity in vivo to induce implantation failure in animals.[20] Embryo derived PAF is also produced by human embryos after in vitro fertilization.[21] Culture of single pronuclear stage human embryos for 24 hours in defined medium resulted in production of detectable levels of PAF by about 40% of the embryos. Embryos that resulted in ongoing pregnancies produced detectable levels of PAF; on the other hand, embryos that failed to produce PAF failed to result in pregnancy.[22]

The mechanism of action of embryo derived PAF is

still uncertain. However, results of in vitro and in vivo experiments suggest that platelet derived products are luteotrophic. Hansel and coworkers showed that co-incubation of a dispersible line of luteal cells with bovine platelets augments basal progesterone synthesis.[23] They also obtained data suggesting that serotonin and platelet-derived growth factor appear to be major products of platelet activation responsible for luteotrophic activity. It has also been shown that the addition of platelet activating factor to media in which pre-embryos were cultured for in vitro fertilization and embryo transfer increased the subsequent implantation and pregnancy potential of these embryos.[24] The increase in the pregnancy rate after short exposure of pre-embryos to PAF in vitro suggests that PAF mediates pre-embryo development. It has also been shown that the platelet count is significantly reduced throughout the human preimplantation phase of pregnancy but returns to normal following embryo implantation.[25] Taken together, these results suggest that a direct effect of PAF on the blastocyst or PAF-dependent production of platelet derived embryonic trophic factors may be necessary for implantation in the presence of a favorable maternal environment.

CHORIONIC GONADOTROPIN

Human chorionic gonadotropin (hCG) is composed of one α and one β subunit with amino acid sequences very similar to luteinizing hormone.[26,27] Human chorionic gonadotrophin is produced by the early human trophoblast and is essential for the survival of the conceptus.[28] Whether chorionic gonadotrophin has functions other than maintenance of luteal function remains open to speculation. In the human, implantation occurs on day 6 after ovulation, and chorionic gonadotrophin is first measurable on day 9 following ovulation.[28] Embryos maintained in culture during the preimplantation period and allowed to attach to a layer of fibroblasts indicate that the embryos start secreting chorionic gonadotrophin immediately after attachment, or the equivalent of day 11 or 12 in vivo.[29] It remains unclear whether or not chorionic gonadotrophin is produced before attachment of the human embryo to the endometrium. However, the work of Haour and associates has revealed that chorionic gonadotrophin is expressed in the rabbit blastocyst prior to implantation.[30] It is not known whether chorionic gonadotrophin has a local function at the site of implantation to facilitate trophoblast invasion or embryonic differentiation. Active or passive immunization of monkeys against human chorionic gonadotrophin (hCG) β-subunit during the first six weeks of pregnancy disrupts implantation.[31] Other studies by Hearn and colleagues revealed that blastocysts cultured in the presence of antisera raised against hCG β-subunit fail to attach and continue growth, suggesting that a direct effect of chorionic gonadotrophin on the embryo is essential for normal implantation and luteal function in primates.[31]

EARLY PREGNANCY FACTOR

Early pregnancy factor (EPF) was described based on an alteration of lymphocytic reactivity in the lymphocyte rosette test, which was devised to assess the immunosuppressive characteristics of anti-lymphocyte serum in vitro.[32] Although EPF does not appear to be produced by the conceptus directly, the immunosuppressive actions of ovum factor are exerted indirectly via the production of EPF and warrant discussion here. EPF has two components, A and B. Component A is not pregnancy specific, but is instead derived from the oviduct. Component B appears to be produced by the ovary under the influence of a pituitary factor, thought to be prolactin. The oviductal component is produced in rabbits during both pregnancy and pseudopregnancy, but the ovarian component is produced only during pregnancy. Furthermore, it is necessary to combine the two components in order to express early pregnancy factor (EPF) activity.[33] The sources of stimulation of EPF production do not appear to affect component production since the activity produced by the perfused ovary and oviduct in pregnancy or in response to PAF stimulation are similar, suggesting that EPF components are produced in the ovary and oviduct individually and that the combination of the two components is necessary for expression of EPF activity.

Takimoto and coworkers, using a rosette inhibition test, demonstrated that early pregnancy factor appears in the maternal peripheral blood of mice at the pronuclear stage and concluded from their data that fertilization can be detected by EPF measurement within 48 hours after ovulation and that failure of fertilization can be distinguished from failure of implantation.[34] Passive immunization of pregnant mice against early pregnancy factor causes loss of embryonic viability, suggesting that EPF may serve as a marker for embryonic viability and that it may also be necessary for embryonic survival.[35] Other investigators have reported that EPF levels fall markedly after termination of pregnancy and that the disappearance rate of early pregnancy factor after termination of pregnancy is closely related to decreasing β-hCG concentrations.[36,37] Straube and colleagues reported data obtained from 20 patients with a tentative diagnosis of disturbed early pregnancy.[38] EPF concentrations were compared with β-hCG concentrations in serum as well as with clinical and sonographical findings. Positive EPF values were indicative of embryonic viability in intact pregnancies, whereas negative EPF values appeared to be indicative of pregnancy loss. Mesrogli and associates studied the diagnostic value of early pregnancy factor, β-hCG, progesterone, and endosonography in patients with suspected tubal pregnancy.[39,40] EPF was negative in 94% of all cases of ectopic pregnancy or disturbed intrauterine pregnancy, although all of these patients had positive β-hCG titers, suggesting that the diagnosis of ectopic pregnancy may be confirmed by negative EPF values in spite of elevated hCG levels and uncertain sonographical findings. Although the clinical utility of EPF is yet to be fully established, the data available suggest that it is potentially useful in the assessment of certain aspects of pregnancy and implantation. EPF may be useful in the evaluation of early pregnancy failure, since it becomes positive in maternal serum as early as 24 to 48 hours following conception. Therefore, disorders of menstruation may be distinguished from early spontaneous abortion. Similarly, as a test, EPF determination may be useful for studying infertile patients when defective fertilization or implantation failure is suspected.

OVUM FACTOR

Ovum factor (OF) was detected because of its ability to cause female animals to express EPF. Ovum factor is produced by mouse and sheep embryos and promotes the production of EPF by the ovary in the presence of PRL.[41,42] According to some reports, ovum factor is present in human embryo culture medium following in vitro fertilization, but others have been unable to verify this finding. Nevertheless, based on the preponderance of the data available, it appears that ovum factor may have a role in the induction of EPF expression during early gestation.

IMMUNOSUPPRESSIVE FACTOR

The human zygote produces a factor in vitro that is directly immunosuppressive.[43] Unlike the immunosuppressive actions of ovum factor, which are exerted via effects on EPF, the actions of immunosuppressive factor (IF) are direct, since the factor obtained from culture media of human embryos after in vitro fertilization suppresses mitogen induced proliferation of peripheral lymphocytes, and only those embryos producing the factor result in pregnancy. Bose studied human embryo associated immunosuppressive factors from pre- and post-implantation stages and found that the stages have some similarities.[44] Murine antibody bound to embryo-associated immunosuppressive factors purified from pregnancy sera, but not to identical fractions from control sera, indicating that these post-implantation factors possess some similarity to pre-implantation factors. The presence of embryo-associated immunosuppressive factors at various stages of gestation may play a role in suppressing maternal cellular immune responses and prevent maternal rejection of the fetal allograft.

EMBRYO-DERIVED HISTAMINE RELEASING FACTOR

Although the mechanism has not been elucidated, histamine is thought to play a role in implantation of the blastocyst. Embryo-derived histamine releasing factor (EHRF) has been identified in culture medium used to grow developing embryos.[45] EHRF induces histamine release, which is both calcium- and temperature-dependent, from sensitized basal cells. Although the role of this factor remains to be clarified, EHRF could represent a message sent by the embryo to the mother to induce histamine release at the time of implantation.

EMBRYO-ASSOCIATED PROTEASES

Experimental evidence obtained from animal studies has shown that protease systems are present in the conceptus as well as the endometrium and that they show profound changes around the time of implantation.[46–49] Proteolytic actions of proteases may be essential to the mechanisms involved in implantation. Considerable information has also been presented suggesting that maternal hormones govern the physiologic regulation of proteases. Maternal hormones apparently govern both changes in proteases and protease activities of uterine tissues or trophoblasts. Evidence that proteolysis by specific proteases forms an important element of processes such as embryo nutrition, hatching cell adhesion, and invasion has also been accumulated.[50–52]

For example, the physiologic role of the embryo-associated exopeptidase arylamidase-1 remains unknown. It is possible, however, that it participates in the conversion of proteins within the uterus, converting them into active or inactive forms. The substances produced by arylamidase-1 activity may provide fixed nitrogen in the form of amino acids or protein by the blastocysts.[53] Trophoblast-dependent blastocyst protease is a gelatin-dissolving protease found in the trophoblast at the surface of the implanting rabbit blastocyst. This enzyme is not detectable earlier than six days post-coitum but rises abruptly on the seventh day, a few hours before dissolution of the blastocyst coverings.[47] The primary physiologic function of this trophoblast-dependent protease appears to be associated with dissolution of the blastocyst coverings, suggesting that it may serve as a hatching enzyme, necessary for dissolution of the zona pellucida prior to the initiation of implantation. Specific inhibitors have been shown to block dissolution of the blastocyst covering effectively and inhibit implantation since attachment of the trophoblast to the endometrium does not occur.[53]

Another protease of potential significance to implantation is embryo-associated plasminogen activating factor (PAF). It has been reported that rat embryos contain PAF activity at all stages prior to implantation.[54] PAF is associated with embryos between the two-cell and blastocyst stage and is observed regardless of whether the embryo develops in the genital tract or in culture. Furthermore, it has been shown clearly that the PAF activity detected on pre-implantation mouse embryos is in fact associated with the zona pellucida, although it is not clear whether it is produced there or taken up from uterine secretions.[55] Evidence also exists that PAF is under the control of estrogen, progestins, or both.[56,57] Beers and coworkers demonstrated that PAF produced by rat granulosa cells was stimulated by luteinizing hormone or cyclic AMP.[58] Therefore, it appears that PAF production or secretion by the conceptus is controlled directly by hormones and that the ultimate appearance of the protease is due to exposure of the embryos to hormones. In spite of these findings, the precise origin of PAF has not been established. It is possible that the enzyme PAF functions during the invasive period of trophoblast invasion to dissolve fibrin via activation of plasminogen. Furthermore, a collagenase might be activated to break down the basement membrane of the uterine epithelium, thus facilitating implantation.[59] It appears that several proteolytic enzymes are produced during the peri-implantation period, which includes hatching from the zona pellucida, adhesion of the blastocyst to the uterine epithelium, and invasion of trophoblast cells into the uterine wall. Thus, embryo-associated proteases may have a role in the overall process of implantation.

THE PRE-IMPLANTATION ENDOMETRIUM

ENDOMETRIAL CYCLE

An orderly sequence of changes driven by ovarian steroid secretion takes place in the uterine endometrium during the ovulatory cycle. Although the endometrial cycle may be discussed in phases, it is in fact a continuum (Fig. 1-7). As estrogen secretion increases during the follicular phase, growth and reordering of the endometrium occurs. This phase of endometrial growth is known as the proliferative phase of the endometrial cycle. Marked changes occur in the glandular epithelium. Low cuboidal epithelium lines narrow tubular glands and mitoses become evident. Gland segments coalesce with their adjacent gland, the stromal component of the endometrium takes on a loose, syncytial status, and a loose capillary network is formed as a result of spiral vessels extending immediately below the epithelia basement membrane. The endometrium increases in thickness due to stromal expansion and de novo tissue growth.

The secretory phase of the cycle is dominated by progesterone but is influenced by estrogen as well. After the onset of the secretory phase relatively little growth occurs. Vacuoles move from intracellular to intraluminal locations, an event which takes place approximately one week following ovulation. The lumina become distended with secretory material, the stroma becomes edematous, and increased vascular coiling occurs. Further changes occur during the second half of the secretory phase, and the endometrium begins to differentiate into three zones: the basalis, the stratum spongiosum, and the stratum compactum. A continuous layer of stromal cells is formed as they increase in size. The subepithelial capillaries and spiral vessels become engorged and prominent. It appears that endometrial evolution represents preparation for the process of implantation and that the endometrial cycle is teleologically designed to support the early embryo.[60]

ENDOMETRIAL PREPARATION FOR IMPLANTATION

Preparation of the endometrium for implantation involves a series of coordinated events, and endometrial development depends on the appropriate sequence of

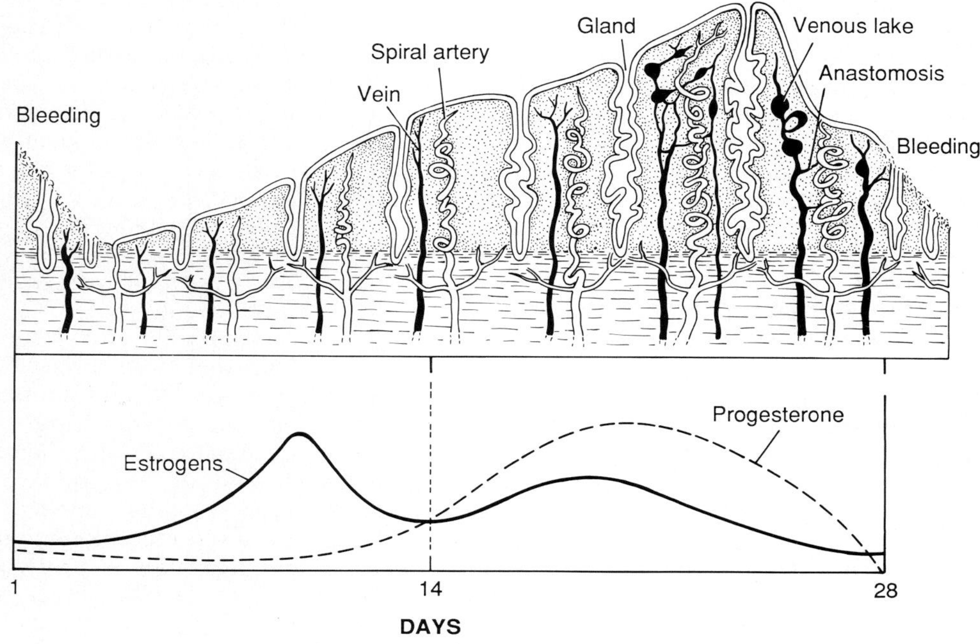

FIGURE 1–7. The endometrial cycle. The endometrium proliferates rapidly following menstruation. During the proliferative phase, the glands are straight and tubular. The blood vessels are also straight without coiling. The secretory phase of the endometrial cycle is progestin-dominated, as depicted by the branching of the endometrial glands and the coiling of the vasculature. Cellular changes occur throughout the secretory phase in preparation for arrival of the blastocyst. In response to decreasing levels of both estrogen and progesterone at the end of the luteal phase, the endometrium degenerates and sloughs as menstruation occurs.

ovarian secretion. Decidualization is a feature of the normal process of progesterone-directed endometrial differentiation during the secretory phase of the non-pregnant menstrual cycle.[61,62] In non-conception cycles, decidualization or predecidualization does not progress, presumably because of luteal demise and subsequent diminution in progesterone secretion. The major alteration involves differentiation of and alterations within the glandular epithelium. Three to four days after the initiation of the progesterone rise, subnucleolar vacuolization is maximal, followed by apocrine secretion, which peaks approximately seven days after ovulation. If conception fails to occur, a decrease in glandular secretion is followed by regression of glandular maturation eight to nine days following ovulation. Clearly, these maturational changes in the endometrium are driven by luteal progesterone secretion, and despite falling progesterone levels during the second week of the secretory phase, differentiation of the stroma together with associated vascular changes occur. The reason for this changing pattern of differentiation remains unexplained. However, it is possible that the luteal rise in estradiol redirects these progestin-dependent maturational processes from the epithelium to the endometrial stroma. Decidual cells appear first around spiral arteries and arterioles on post-ovulatory days nine to ten, and subsequently spread through the upper layer of the endometrium to form the zona compacta. As a result, the glands of the zona compacta become inconspicuous. Edema of the mid-zone also serves to delineate the compact area from the underlying zona spongiosa when the endometrial glands become localized. The other feature of decidualization is the accumulation of endometrial granulocytes, which are prominent around glands and blood vessels. When pregnancy occurs, these alterations are sustained and extended, yet there are differences in the degree of decidualization compared to a non-conception cycle, suggesting that the blastocyst itself may have effects on the process of decidualization although the endometrium undergoes predecidual change prior to the arrival of the blastocyst in preparation for implantation. Based on morphological appearance, it is not unreasonable to assume that the endometrium could accept an embryo at any time within a range of several days after ovulation.[63]

ENDOMETRIAL PROTEINS AND GLYCOPROTEINS

Cells within the decidua are secretory. Endometrial differentiation during the menstrual cycle alters the secretion of some proteins, while the synthesis of others is apparently dependent on either estrogen or progesterone and is stage-specific. The precise biologic functions of these proteins remain subject to conjecture; nevertheless, they do reflect the biosynthetic capacity of the endometrium and suggest that these proteins are involved in the process of implantation and the successful maintenance of pregnancy.

PROLACTIN

It is well established that the human decidua produces a material that is identical to pituitary prolactin.[64-67] Decidualized endometrium obtained from non-conception menstrual cycles also synthesizes and secretes prolactin in vitro and, therefore, does not require the presence of the trophoblast.[68,69] Further evidence has accumulated indicating that the decidua is a source of amniotic fluid prolactin. The capacity of decidual tissue to secrete prolactin in vitro correlates with amniotic fluid levels but not with maternal plasma levels, and the rise in maternal plasma prolactin is absent in patients hypophysectomized prior to pregnancy, although amniotic fluid prolactin levels and decidual secretion in vitro are normal.[70]

Experimental evidence indicates that prolactin synthesis in the endometrium is regulated directly by progesterone and indirectly by estradiol. During in vitro differentiation of proliferative endometrium induced by progesterone, the onset of prolactin secretion corresponds with the onset of histologically apparent decidualization, and both features are less pronounced when estradiol is included.[71] Similarly, decidualized endometrium from non-conception cycles cultured in vitro maintains prolactin secretion and histological integrity only in the presence of progesterone.[72] Short-term exposure to progesterone—as little as 3 hours—is adequate to stimulate decidual prolactin in media containing cultures of proliferative human endometrium, and the resulting pattern of prolactin production is determined by the duration of progesterone treatment.[69] Chen and coworkers investigated the effect of prolonged treatment with progestin and the anti-progestin RU-486 on the production and synthesis of prolactin.[73] Prolactin production progressively increased in stromal cells obtained from pregnant women continuously treated with medroxyprogesterone acetate, whereas RU-486 alone had no apparent effect on the production of prolactin. The production of prolactin was also increased by medroxyprogesterone acetate in stromal cells pretreated with RU-486, indicating that the effect of RU-486 is reversible. This study also demonstrates the effects of progestins on endometrial prolactin production.

Insulin-like growth factor 1 (IgF-1) stimulates the release of decidual prolactin acting through the type 1 IgF receptor.[74] Insulin stimulates de novo prolactin synthesis and secretion from monolayer cultures of human decidual cells, and the effects of insulin are relatively specific to prolactin. Collectively, these observations suggest that responses to insulin are mediated through the insulin receptor and that insulin may have a role in the regulation of prolactin synthesis and release from human decidua. Other evidence indicates that human decidual prolactin production is regulated by combined effects of estrogen and progesterone and the peptide hormone relaxin.[75] Relaxin has been immunohistochemically localized in human decidua, which lends additional support to the theory that this peptide has a role in the control of decidual prolactin secretion.[76]

Although the influence of prolactin on endometrium and the process of implantation is not completely understood, the available data suggest direct effects on decidual cells. Morphologic effects of prolactin on decidua using organ culture methodology have been reported.[77] Ultrastructurally, endometrial stromal cells and decidual stromal cells change secretory appearance when exposed to prolactin in organ culture. Ribosomes and Golgi bodies increase in number, and the cysternae of the rough endoplasmic reticulum expand. The differentiation of stromal cells into fully developed decidual cells in culture is proportional to the increase in prolactin concentrations in the medium. Explanations have been sought for the effects of decidual luteotropin on the maintenance of pregnancy, and it has been reported that prolactin increases the production of glycogen by decidual cells obtained from rats, suggesting that decidual luteotropin acts on these cells to enhance glycogen formation and that glycogen may be essential for normal implantation.[78,79]

ENDOMETRIAL SURFACE GLYCOPROTEINS

Surface glycoproteins are components of the endometrial surface glycocalyx and have also been identified in endometrial glands. Uterine secretions are modified by the changing milieu of steroids produced by the ovary throughout the menstrual cycle. The changing uterine environment that results may have a function in regulating the metabolism of the blastocyst and implantation. A significant decline in the concentration of protein occurs during the secretory phase, although little qualitative change is apparent at other stages of the menstrual cycle.[80,81] Studies performed on cultured human endometrium in vitro demonstrate the secretion of glycoproteins, and these are stimulated by the addition of estrogen and progesterone to the culture medium.[82] Stromal cells derived from proliferative or secretory phase human endometrium and cultured in the absence of steroid hormones grow as monolayers and show only occasional areas of immunoreactive fibronectin and no detectable prolactin or laminin.[83] On the other hand, treatment of these cultures with physiologic doses of estradiol and progesterone induces prolactin production and stimulates cell proliferation, resulting in multilayering with an increase of the saturation density. Electron microscopy reveals the development of gap junctions, and immunofluorescence reveals a dense pericellular matrix containing fibronectin and laminin. Immunocytochemistry studies reveal that fibronectin localizes throughout the decidual extracellular matrix. Fibronectin was also observed in fibrillar and punctate patterns in the decidual cell cytoplasm.[84] It has also been shown that decidual cells synthesize laminin, entactin, fibronectin, type 4 collagen, heparin sulfate, proteoglycan, and prolactin.[85,86] Grinnell and coworkers studied fibronectin distribution on stromal fibroblasts determined by indirect immunofluorescence staining in relationship to cell shape during decidual transformation and observed that fibroblasts of endometrial stroma were elongated cells with a fibrillar pattern of fibronectin on their surfaces.[87] During days 1 to 6 of pregnancy these elongated fibroblasts acquired a round morphology, and fibronectin first changed to a patch distribution on the cell surface, then disappeared. After implantation, fibronectin distribution in relation to the position of the conceptus in the stroma proximal to the implanting conceptus was studied. Fibronectin was absent, except around blood vessels, which may help explain how decidual tissue could act as a barrier to trophoblast invasion. Taken together, these data indicate that the production of other surface glycoproteins and secretion of fibronectin play a role in the implantation and subsequent growth in the embryo. The appearance of endometrial surface glycoproteins coincides with or precedes the time when the embryo enters the endometrial cavity.[79] Thus, a role for maternal glycoproteins in nutrition and implantation of the embryo is suggested.

PLACENTAL PROTEIN 12

Placental protein 12 (PP12) was originally isolated from soluble extracts of human placenta and its adjacent membranes. PP12 is synthesized by the human endometrium and appears in the peripheral circulation, where it can be measured using immunochemical techniques. The work of Rutanen and associates has shown that PP12 is synthesized by decidualized, secretory endometrium and not by placenta.[88] PP12 is synthesized by the epithelial cells but not by stromal cells and, reflecting the relative paucity of epithelial cells as pregnancy progresses, the levels of PP12 plateau or decline after the 20th week of gestation.

PP12 is a 34-kd glycoprotein that has an internal amino acid sequence identical to that of somatomedin binding protein purified from the amniotic fluid. PP12 also binds to IgF-1 (insulin like growth factor-1). Baboon decidua synthesizes and releases an IgF binding protein as its major secretory product.[89] Other investigators have shown that PP12 is an insulin-like growth factor binding protein that can be purified from human amniotic fluid.[90] Corroborating evidence was obtained by Julkunen and colleagues, whose studies using Southern blot analysis revealed that there is a single IgF binding protein/PP12 gene in the human genome.[91] From such studies it appears likely that a relationship exists between PP12 and IgF binding protein, the mediator of insulin-like growth factors in fetal growth.

Although the precise mechanisms controlling PP12 production and secretion have not been completely determined, experimental evidence indicates that progesterone stimulates the secretion of PP12. Olajide and coworkers induced first-trimester termination of pregnancy using RU-38486 and a prostaglandin pessary.[92] Human chorionic gonadotrophin values remained unchanged until abortion occurred. In contrast, the levels of PP12 decreased immediately following the administration of RU-38486, showing that RU-38486 has a direct inhibitory effect on tissues producing PP12, confirming the progesterone dependency of this protein. PP12 can not be induced in proliferative phase or estrogen stimulated post-menopausal endometrium and is not pregnancy-specific.[93,88]

PLACENTAL PROTEIN 14

Placental protein 14 (PP14) is a 28-kd glycoprotein that is immunologically related to the progestin associated endometrial protein (PEP), alpha-2 pregnancy associated endometrial protein (α2 PEP), and endometrial protein 15 (EP15).[94] In non-pregnant women, serum PP14 concentrations appear to reflect endometrial secretory function. This is indicated by cyclic changes in the PP14 concentration in endometrial tissue and by the rising PP14 values in the late luteal phase. In the ovulatory menstrual cycle, the concentration of PP14 increases in endometrial tissue as secretory changes advance. Serum PP14 concentrations follow the increase in circulating progesterone levels and are maintained through the first days of the next cycle. In contrast, serum PP14 levels do not increase in anovulatory cycles. PP14 appears in the endometrium approximately 4–5 days following ovulation, and it has been suggested that it may play a role in opening the implantation window.

PREGNANCY-ASSOCIATED PLACENTAL PROTEIN A

Pregnancy-associated plasma protein (PAPP-A) is a larger ($\approx$750 kd) proteoglycan originally identified in human pregnancy serum. The production of PAPP-A is low during the secretory phase and increases dramatically with the initiation of decidualization. A study reported by Sinosich and colleagues revealed that PAPP-A is under the control of progesterone when the investigator showed that the administration of the progesterone receptor antagonist RU-486 suppressed placental PAPP-A synthesis, thus supporting a role for progesterone in placental PAPP-A production and maintenance of a placental barrier against maternal phagocytic-proteolytic defenses.[95] Bishkoff and associates studied a group of spontaneous aborters and found that their levels of PAPP-A were significantly lower than those in normal pregnancies but higher than in non-pregnant controls.[96] The biologic function of PAPP-A is still open to speculation; however, it does reflect the biosynthetic capacity of decidualized endometrium and may serve as a useful marker for normal and pathologic pregnancies. The specific role of PAPP-A in implantation and pregnancy maintenance remains to be clarified.

PROGESTIN-ASSOCIATED ENDOMETRIAL PROTEIN (PEP)

Hormone dependent endometrial proteins may serve as markers of endometrial function. Joshi and coworkers reported the detection and synthesis of a protein they designated "progesterone-dependent endometrial protein" (PEP).[97] PEP is a 48-kd glycoprotein, and it appears to be the major protein synthesized in the endometrium during early pregnancy. It has been conclusively shown that PEP is secreted by endometrial glands in response to endogenous or exogenous progesterone. PEP can be detected in the peripheral blood of pregnant and non-pregnant women by specific radioimmunoassay. Late luteal phase PEP levels apparently reflect the cumulative effect of estrogen and progesterone secreted during the entire cycle on the endometrium, and low PEP levels may be associated with luteal insufficiency. Studies on pregnant women receiving progesterone support suggest that a factor of placental-embryonic origin may also stimulate PEP synthesis. PEP appears to be a specific marker of endometrial, luteal, and placental functions and may play a role in normal as well abnormal implantation.

ENDOMETRIAL PROSTAGLANDINS

Prostaglandins are produced by the endometrium and also by the conceptus itself, as demonstrated by Watson and colleagues.[98] The trophoblast secretes protein complexes that alter endometrial protein and prostaglandin secretion and induce an intracellular inhibitor of prostaglandin synthesis in vitro. The content of prostaglandins produced by the endometrium changes during the menstrual cycle, and clearly the endometrium accumulates prostaglandin precursors toward the time of menstruation.[97] Progesterone modulates prostaglandin E_2 binding sites in the rat endometrium, and it has been reported that the addition of progesterone reduces prostaglandin production in cultured monolayers of endometrial cells.[99,100] Therefore, it appears that progesterone, either directly or indirectly, modulates both the biosynthesis and the action of prostaglandins in the endometrium. The production or release of prostaglandins may be stimulated in endometrial cells by the blastocyst, leading to locally increased vascular permeability. The concentrations of prostaglandins of the E and F series, as well as prostacyclin, increase in areas of increased vascular permeability induced by blastocysts or artificial stimuli in the rat.[101] Furthermore, the administration of the prostaglandin synthesis inhibitor indomethacin, given on day five of pregnancy, transiently inhibits the endometrial vascular permeability change.[102] Other studies have revealed that endometrial receptivity for implantation and sensitivity for decidualization are controlled by the presence of receptors for PGE_2 in the endometrium.[103,104] Although much evidence exists for hormone-induced changes during the peri-implantation phase of pregnancy, the exact role(s) of prostaglandins in implantation remains to be clarified.

CONCEPTUS-ENDOMETRIAL SIGNALING

Prior to and during implantation the mother and fetus apparently "talk," via a variety of signals. The blastocyst produces several substances that send signals to the endometrium of impending implantation. The pre-implantation embryo exerts both local and systemic signals to provide a suitable environment for development and a receptive endometrium for implantation and corpus luteum function. The uterine luminal milieu assumes an essential role in the pre-implantation process. Local actions of estrogens on a progestin-primed endometrium may be required either for the release of crucial signals for blastocyst activation or to make epithelial cells sensitive to the presence of the embryo, thus inducing the decidualization reaction (Fig. 1-8).

One of the earliest indices for transmission of embryonic signals to the endometrium that surrounds the blastocyst is a marked change in capillary permeability, a phenomenon that has been demonstrated by the intravenous injection of substances such as a protamine blue or Evans dye into rats.[105] Accumulation of the blue dye in the area of the blastocyst is used as an index of increased capillary permeability. Areas in which the blue dye accumulates appear in the endometrium by the afternoon of day 5 of pregnancy, corresponding to the early attachment stage in this species. Any deciduogenic stimulus within the endometrial cavity will elicit increased capillary permeability, which precedes the decidual response in the rat endometrium. Other vasoactive substances, most notably histamine, have received some attention in past years.[106] Histamide decarboxylase, the enzyme responsible for the synthesis of histamine from histadine, when inhibited by specific inhibitors interrupts the implantation process.[107] The idea that histamine has a role in the process of implantation is supported by the fact that rabbit endometrial cells contain the H1 receptor.[108]

It is clear that the blastocyst and the endometrium communicate at the time of implantation. In order for communication between conceptus and uterus to occur, both must have achieved a specific stage of maturity. The conceptus apparently must have reached the blastocyst stage and the endometrium must be receptive. Synchronization between conceptus and endometrium is driven by the coordinated and concerted actions of estrogens and progestins secreted by the ovary during the ovulatory cycle. External signs that the mother recognizes the presence of a conceptus are cessation of menstrual function and prolongation of the life of the corpus luteum. In addition, there is considerable experimental evidence to indicate that the presence of the conceptus in the uterine cavity serves as a signal to the uterus of impending implantation. For example, it has been shown that the pig blastocyst starts to secrete estradiol at approximately ten days following coitus and that aromatase activity is present in the pig blastocyst and also in the rabbit blastocyst.[109,110] Other evidence has been obtained from rodents, showing changes in the endometrium at the potential site of implantation. Such experiments have been extended to include the hamster as well as the sheep. Based on these studies, it has been suggested that the embryo secretes a substance(s) having local effects on the endometrium in preparation for implantation. Thus, the blastocyst is metabolically active and presumably produces substances that serve as signals to the mother, either locally or peripherally, of impending implantation.

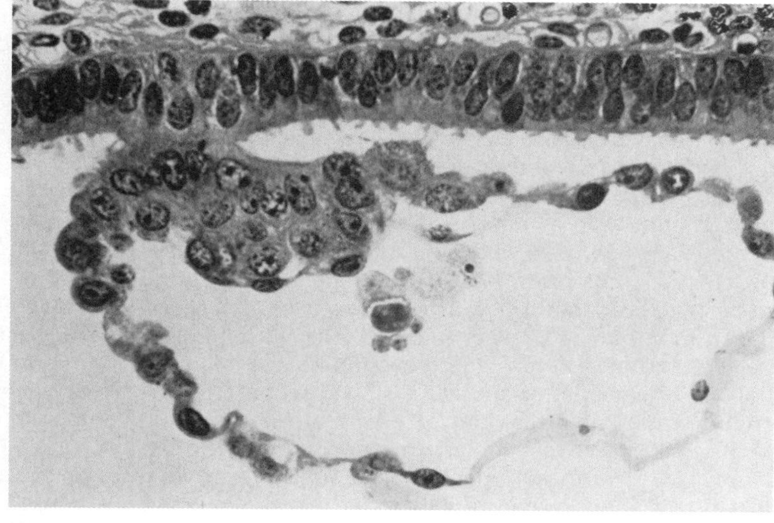

FIGURE 1–8. Early implantation. A monkey egg at approximately 9 days following ovulation. Note that the egg has attached to the uterine epithelium. There is an apparent disturbance in the arrangement of the nuclei and the cytoplasm indicating the initiation of cytolysis. (Heuser CH, Streeter GL. Development of the macaque embryo. Contributions to Embryology Carnegie Institute 1941:29:15.)

THE BLASTOCYST AND DECIDUALIZATION

The presence of the embryo appears to create three primary regions of the endometrium: the decidua basalis, which lies beneath the embryo; the decidua capsularis, which lies over the embryo; and the parietalis, which lies over the remainder of the uterine surface. The major layers of the endometrium—the upper compacta and lower spongiosa—are still apparent in the decidualized endometrium of pregnancy, termed decidua compacta and decidua spongiosa, and the glandular epithelium within the spongiosa still exhibits secretory activity during the first trimester. Some of the glands take on a hypersecretory appearance and exhibit what has been referred to as the Arias-Stella phenomenon of early pregnancy.[111] Although the decidualized endometrium is most prominent during the first trimester prior to the establishment of the definitive placenta, elements of decidualization persist throughout gestation. In the baboon and rhesus monkey, trophoblast invasion is superficial and decidualization is sparse, whereas the human appears to reflect the pattern observed in lower mammals. Since estradiol is required to sensitize the stroma to the decidualizing stimulus received via the overlying epithelium in the rat, differentiation in both the upper epithelium and stroma appear linked by dependence upon estradiol. It remains unclear whether the ability of the stroma to respond to traumatic stimuli provided by the invading trophoblast has been retained in the human over the course of evolution. The peak of luteal phase estradiol occurs during the secretory phase of the menstrual cycle, and stromal mitosis in the late secretory phase suggests that the model may be applicable to the human uterus.

THE IMPLANTATION WINDOW

The embryo's growth depends on its stage of differentiation and the conditions in the uterus. However, the window for growth is relatively small, and this is where temporal relationships assume extreme importance. The implantation window is generally believed to represent a restricted period of time when the uterus is a hospitable place for embryos to grow. However, the idea that the implantation window in the human is narrow has recently been challenged, particularly when favorable conditions exist for implantation. This challenge is based on the idea that it is possible to achieve implantation over a long period of time. A large portion of the data has been obtained in in vitro fertilization programs in which some of the pregnancies correspond to delayed implantation. Many conceptuses apparently began to implant two or even three days later than expected, and many endometria examined after stimulation are ahead of the expected normal maturation. The endometrium might be ahead of maturation in what seems a favorable case for implantation, or, on the other hand, the embryo may maintain its ability to implant for longer than previously expected. Such evidence seems to suggest that the window is quite wide, although this issue has not been completely resolved.

THE PROCESS OF IMPLANTATION

The blastocyst lies unattached in the uterine endometrial cavity for approximately 2 days before implantation. The free-floating blastocyst attains nutrition from the secretions produced by endometrial glands.

LYSIS OF THE ZONA PELLUCIDA

The zona pellucida degenerates and disappears before the initiation of implantation. The presence of a lytic factor in the endometrial cavity appears essential for dissolution of the zona pellucida in utero. The blastocyst apparently participates actively in the process of zona lysis, because unfertilized eggs under the same conditions retain their zonae intact. This may suggest that a lytic factor that is activated by the effects of a factor produced by the blastocyst is derived from a precursor within the receptive uterus. It has been suggested that the lytic factor may be plasmin produced from plasminogen, since plasmin shows a lytic effect upon the zona pellucida in vitro and inhibitors of plasmin inhibit in vitro hatching of rat blastocyst.[112] A similar situation may exist in the human uterus—while studying uterine specimens from the Carnegie collection, Larsen observed a 96-hour-old human blastocyst partially covered by zona pellucida that had completely disappeared 12 hours later (Fig. 1-9).[113]

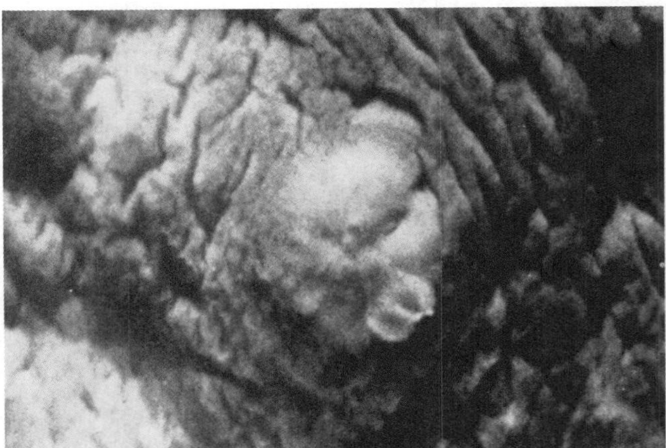

FIGURE 1-9. Implantation site of an 11-day-old ovum. The early implantation site is visible and appears to ooze a coagulum of maternal origin. Small secondary convolutions of the endometrial surface between the large fissures appear to be associated with the mouths of the endometrial glands. (Hertig AT, Rock J. Two human ova of pre-villous stage, having an ovulation age of about eleven and twelve days. Contributions to Embryology Carnegie Institute 1941;29:29.)

APPOSITION, ATTACHMENT, AND ADHESION

The process of implantation appears to involve a mutual reduction in electrostatic repulsion between the blastocyst and the epithelium, facilitating the cell surface approach.[114] Reduction in electrostatic charge may facilitate adhesion of the blastocyst to the epithelium and may be explained by surface changes in cell-surface glycoproteins and their terminal sugars on the blastocyst and epithelial cellular surfaces.[115] It has been shown that inhibitors of protein glycosylation may affect blastocyst attachment.[116] Therefore, both partners, the endometrium and the blastocyst, cooperate in the process of apposition. It is indeed interesting that unfertilized eggs and pre-blastocyst stage conceptuses surrounded by the zona pellucida show no adhesion.

The earliest contact between the blastocyst wall, trophectoderm, and endometrial epithelium is a loose connection termed apposition. The polar trophectoderm is usually in contact with the epithelial surface and the blastocyst is located in a crypt in the endometrium. The human blastocyst has a similar orientation during implantation under normal conditions.[117] It is clear that apposition necessitates direct contact between two cellular membranes, and it appears that this step takes place at a site where the zona pellucida is ruptured or lysed. Interestingly, the orientation of blastocyst at that position could be due to a lytic process of the zona occurring at the polar trophectoderm.

The role of ligand-receptor binding during adhesion and invasion of the endometrium by the blastocyst remains to be elucidated. However, the available information suggests that receptor mechanisms are involved in the process of implantation. When blastocysts spread on specific extracellular matrix component substrates composed of fibronectins, laminin, and collagen IV, receptors were identified on the blastocyst surface of these extracellular matrix components. Furthermore, Armant and coworkers were able to block blastocyst attachment and outgrowth on fibronectin using small peptides containing sequences homologous with certain sequences of fibronectin.[118]

Surface glycoproteins may contain receptors for the blastocyst since they show stage-specific changes around the time of the blastocyst implantation, and it has been suggested that heparin/heparin sulfate proteoglycans located on the surface of the blastocyst may serve as ligands to their receptors on the uterine epithelial surface.[119] It is well known that binding of ligands to cell surfaces causes changes in cytoskeleton.[120,121] Yoshinaga and associates have suggested that binding of trophoblast membrane with epithelial cell membrane via ligand-receptor interaction can modify cytoskeletal function of the epithelial cells, causing dislodgement from the basal lamina and facilitate access of the trophoblast to the basal lamina for penetration.[122]

In the rat round depressions on the surface of the trophoblast cells are observed when examined by scanning electron microscopy. In addition, there are small finger-like protrusions on the surface of the uterine epithelium.[105] It is evident that these pinopodes are involved in endocytosis of macromolecules, pinocytosis of uterine fluid, and uptake of materials from the uterine cavity for nourishment of the embryo. To further demonstrate the endocytosis feature of the pinopodes tracer such as horseradish peroxidase placed in the uterine lumen are rapidly incorporated into vacuoles formed by the pinopodes.[123] This phenomenon could reflect the possibility that specific substances diffusing from the blastocyst are picked up by the pinopodes.

THE EARLY HUMAN TROPHOBLAST

The blastocyst attaches to the endometrial epithelium at the embryonic pole 6 days after fertilization. After the trophoblast has attached to the endometrial epithelium, rapid cellular proliferation occurs and the trophoblast differentiates into two layers consisting of the inner cytotrophoblast and an outer syncytiotrophoblast, a multinucleated mass without cellular boundaries. Syncytial trophoblast processes extend through the endometrial epithelium to invade the endometrial stroma. Stromal cells surrounding the implantation site become laden with lipids and glycogen and become polyhedral in shape and are referred to as decidual cells. These decidual cells degenerate in the region of the invading syncytiotrophoblast and provide nutrition to the developing embryo. The syncytiotrophoblast apparently produces substances that erode maternal tissues and facilitate trophoblast invasion of the endometrium. The blastocyst superficially implants in the stratum compactum of the endometrium by the end of the first week and derives its nourishment from the eroded maternal tissues.[124] The trophoblast then invades the surrounding myometrium as the blastocyst becomes completely embedded in the decidua. Capillary connections are formed as the trophoblast invades and the blood supply to the developing fetus is established via which it will obtain its support until delivery occurs.

REFERENCES

1. Triana LR, Babcock DF, Lorton SP, First NL, Lardy HA. Release of acrosomal hyaluronidase follows increased membrane permeability to calcium in the presumptive capacitation sequence of spermatozoa of the bovine and other mammalian species. Biol Reprod 1980;23:47.
2. Tsafriri A. Oocyte maturation in mammals. In: Jones RA, ed. The vertebrate ovary. New York: Plenum Press, 1978:409.
3. Goodman AL, Hodgen GD. The ovarian triad of the primate menstrual cycle. Recent Prog Horm Res 1983;39:1.
4. Beck F, Moffat DB, Davies DP. Human embryology. 2nd ed. Oxford: Blackwell Scientific Publications, 1985.
5. Cheviakoff S, Diaz S, Carril M, et al. Ovum transport in women. In: Harper MJK, Pauerstein CJ, Adams CE, et al, eds. Ovum Transport and Fertility Regulation. Copenhagen: Scriptor, 1976:416
6. Settlage DSF, Motoshima M, Tredway DR. Sperm transport

from the external cervical os to the fallopian tubes in women. Fertil Steril 1973;24:655.

7. Page EW, Villee CA, Villee DB. Human reproduction: essentials of reproductive and perinatal medicine. 3rd ed. Philadelphia: WB Saunders, 1981.
8. Mastroianni L Jr, Komins J. Capacitation, ovum maturation, fertilization and preimplantation development in the oviduct. Gynecol Invest 1975;6:226.
9. Yanagimachi R, Noda YD. Physiological changes in the postnuclear cap region of mammalian spermatozoa: Necessary preliminary to the membrane fusion between sperm and egg cells. J Ultrastruct Res 1970;31:486.
10. Zaneveld LJD. Capacitation of spermatozoa. In: Ludwig H, Tauber PF, eds. Human fertilization. Stuttgart: Georg Thieme Publishers, 1978.
11. Gulyas BJ. Cortical granules of mammalian eggs. Int Rev Cytol 1980:63:357.
12. Boyd JD, Hamilton WJ. Cleavage, early development and implantation of the egg. In: Parkes AS, ed. Marshall's physiology of reproduction, vol. 2. 2nd ed. London: Longman, Green & Co, 1952:1.
13. Hensleigh HC, Weitlauf HM. Effect of delayed implantation on dry weight and lipid content of mouse blastocyst. Biol Reprod 1974;10:315.
14. Dalcq AM. Introduction to general embryology. London: Oxford University Press, 1957.
15. Johnson MH, Pratt HPM, Handyside AH. The generation and recognition of positional information in the preimplantation mouse embryo. In Glasser S, Bullock D, eds. Cellular and Molecular Aspects of Implantation. New York: Plenum Press, 1981;55–74.
16. Enders AC, Given RL, Schlafke S. Differentiation and migration of endoderm in the rat and mouse at implantation. Anat Rec 1978;190.
17. Enders AC. Embryo implantation, with emphasis on the rhesus monkey and the human. Reproduction 1981;5:163.
18. Yeh HC. Sonographic signs of early pregnancy. CRC Crit Rev Diagn Imaging 1988;28:181.
19. O'Neill C, Collier M, Ryan JP, Spinks NR. Embryo-derived platelet-activating factor. J Reprod Fertil Suppl 1989;37:19.
20. Spinks NR, O'Neill C. Embryo-derived platelet-activating factor is essential for establishment of pregnancy in the mouse. Lancet 1987;1:106.
21. O'Neill C, Saunders DM. Assessment of embryo quality. Lancet 1984;2:1035.
22. O'Neill C, Pike IL, Porter RN, Gisley-Baird AA, Sinosich MJ, Saunders DM. Maternal recognition of pregnancy prior to implantation: methods for monitoring embryonic viability in vitro and in vivo. Ann NY Acad Sci 1985:442:429.
23. Hansel W, Stock A, Battista PJ. Low molecular weight lipid-soluble luteotrophic factor(s) produced by conceptuses in cows. J Reprod Fertil Suppl 1989;37:11.
24. O'Neill C, Ryan JP, Collier M, Saunders DM, Ammit AJ, Pike IL. Supplementation of in-vitro fertilization culture medium with platelet activating factor. Lancet 1989;2:769.
25. O'Neill C, Gidley-Baird AA, Pike IL, Porter RN, Sinosich MJ, Saunders DM. Maternal blood platelet physiology and luteal-phase endocrinology as a means of monitoring pre- and post-implantation embryo viability following in vitro fertilization. J In Vitro Fert Embryo Transfer 1985;2:87.
26. Canfield RE, Morgan FJ, Kammerman S, Bell JJ, Agosto GM. Studies of human gonadotropin. Rec Prog Hormone Res 1971:27:121.
27. Pruett D. Human choriogonadotrophin. Bioessays 1986;4:70.
28. Lenton EA, Neal LM, Sulaiman R. Plasma concentrations of hCG from the time of implantation until the second week of pregnancy. Fertil Steril 1982;37:773.
29. Hearn JP, Webley GE. Regulation of the corpus luteum of early pregnancy in the marmoset monkey: local interactions of luteotrophic and luteolytic hormones in vivo and their effects on the secretion of progesterone. J Endocrinol 1987;231:231.
30. Haour F, Saxena BB. Detection of a gonadotropin in rabbit blastocyst before implantation. Science 1974;185:444.
31. Hearn JP. Immunological interference with the maternal recognition of pregnancy in primates. In: Whelan J, ed. Maternal recognition of pregnancy (Ciba Foundation Symposium No. 64). Amsterdam: Excerpta Medica, 1978:353.
32. Mehta AR, Eessalu TE, Aggarwal BB. Purification and characterization of early pregnancy factor from human pregnancy sera. J Biol Chem 1989; 264:2266.
33. Sueoka K, Dharmarajan AM, Miyazaki T, Atlas SJ, Wallach EE. In-vivo and in-vitro determination of components of rabbit early pregnancy factors. J Reprod Fertil 1989;87:47.
34. Takimoto Y, Hishinuma M, Takahashi Y, Kanagawa H. Detection of early pregnancy factor in superovulated mice. Nippon-Juigaku-Zasshi 1989;51:879.
35. Athanasas-Platsis S, Quinn KA, Wong TY, Rolfe BE, Cavanagh AC, Morton H. Passive immunization of pregnant mice against early pregnancy factor causes loss of embryonic viability. J Reprod Fertil 1989;87:495.
36. Hubel V, Straube W, Loh M, Wodrig W, Weber A, Klima F. Human early pregnancy factor and early pregnancy associated protein before and after therapeutic abortion in comparison with beta-hCG, estradiol, progesterone and 17-hydroxyprogesterone. Exp Clin Endocrinol 1989;94:171.
37. Straube W, Hubel V, Loh M, Leipe S. Human early pregnancy factor: serum concentrations before and after therapeutic abortion in comparison with beta-hCG and an early pregnancy associated protein. Arch Gynecol Obstet 1989;246:115.
38. Straube W, Loh M, Leipe S. Significance of the detection of early pregnancy factor for monitoring normal and disordered early pregnancy. Geburtshilfe Frauenheilkd 1988;48:854.
39. Mesrogli M, Degenhardt F, Maas DH, Klaus I, Busche M, Schneider J. Tubal pregnancies: early pregnancy factor, progesterone, beta-HCG and vaginal sonography as differential diagnostic parameters. Z Geburtshilfe Perinatol 1988;192:130.
40. Mesrogli M, Maas DH, Schneider J. Early abortion rate in sterility patients: early pregnancy factor as a parameter. Zentralbl Gynakol 1988;110:555.
41. Morton H. Early pregnancy factor; a link between fertilization and immunomodulation. Aust J Biol Sci 1984;37:393.
42. Smart YC, Cripps AL, Clancy RL, Roberts TK, Lopata A, Shutt D. Detection of an immunosuppressive factor in human preimplantation embryo cultures. Med J Aust 1981;I:78.
43. Daya S, Clarke DA. Immunosuppressive factor produced by human embryos in vitro. N Engl J Med 1986;315:1551.
44. Bose R. Human embryo associated immunosuppressor factor(s) from pre- and post-implantation stages share some similarities. Immunol Lett 1989;20:261.
45. Cocchiara R, DiTrapani G, Azzolina A, Albeggiani G, Geraci D. Identification of a histamine-releasing factor secreted by human pre-implantation embryos grown in vitro. J Reprod Immunol 1988;13:41.
46. Denker H-W. Interaction of proteinase inhibitors with blastocyst proteinases involved in implantation. In: Peeters H, ed. Protides of the biological fluids. Proceedings of the XXIIIrd Colloquium, Brugge 1975. Oxford: Pergamon, 1976:63.
47. Denker H-W, Fritz H. Enzymic characterization of rabbit blastocyst proteinase with synthetic substrates of trypsin-like enzymes. Hoppe-Seylers Zeitschrift fur Physiologische Chemie 1979;360:107.

48. Strickland S, Reich E, Sherman MI. Plasminogen activator in early embryogenesis: enzyme production by trophoblast and parietal endoderm. Cell 1976;9:231.
49. Pinsker MC, Sacco AG, Mintz B. Implantation-associated proteinase in mouse uterine fluid. Dev Biol 1974;38:285.
50. Ribbons DW, Brew K, eds. (1976) Proteolysis and physiological regulation. Miami Winter symposia, vol 11. New York: Academic Press, 1976.
51. Leroy F, Finn CA, Psychoyos A, Hubinont PO. Blastocyst endometrium interrelationships. Progress in Reproductive Biology, vol. 7. Basel: S Karger, 1980.
52. Denker H-W. The role of trophoblast-dependent uterine proteases in initiation of implantation. In: Ludwig H, Tauber PF, eds. Human fertilization. Proceedings of an international workshop, Essen 1976. Stuttgart: Thieme, 1978:204.
53. Denker H-W. Implantation: the role of proteinases, and blockage of implantation by proteinase inhibitors. Adv Anat Embryol Cell Biol 1977;53:5.
54. Liedholm P, Astedt B. Fibrinolytic activity of the rat ovum, appearance during tubal passage and disappearance at implantation. Int J Fertil 1975;20:24–26.
55. Sherman MI. Studies on the temporal correlation between secretion of plasminogen activator and stages of early mouse embryogenesis. Oncodevelopmental Biology and Medicine 1980;1:7.
56. Mintz B. Implantation-initiating factor from mouse uterus. In: Moghissi KS, Hafez ESE, eds. Biology of mammalian fertilization and implantation. Springfield, IL: CC Thomas, 1972:343.
57. Beier HM. Hormonal stimulation of protease inhibitor activity in endometrial secretion during early pregnancy. Acta Endocrinol (Kbh) 1970:63:141.
58. Beers WH, Strickland S, Reich E. Ovarian plasminogen activator: Relationship to ovulation and hormonal regulation. Cell 1975;6:387.
59. Potts M. The ultrastructure of egg implantation. Adv Reprod Physiol 1969;4:241.
60. Rock J, Bartlett M. Biopsy studies of human endometrium. JAMA 1937;108:2022.
61. Eichner E, Goler GG, Reed J, Gordon MB. The experimental production and prolonged maintenance of decidua in the non-pregnant woman. Am J Obstet Gynecol 1951;61:253.
62. Fishel SB, Edwards RG, Purdy JM. In vitro fertilization of human oocytes: factors associated with embryonic development in vitro, replacement of embryos and pregnancy. In Beier H, Lindner H, eds. Fertilization of the human egg in vitro, biological basis and clinical application. New York, 1983;251–270.
63. Sundstrom P, Nilsson O, Liedholm P. Scanning electron microscopy of human preimplantation endometrium in normal and clomiphene/human chorionic gonadotropin-stimulated cycles. Fertil Steril 1983;40:642.
64. Riddick DH, Luciano AA, Kusmik WF, Maslar IA. De novo synthesis of prolactin by human decidua. Life Sci 1978;23:1913.
65. Frame FT, Rogol AD, Riddick DH, Baezynski E. Gel chromatographic properties of human prolactin released from decidual tissue. Fertil Steril 1979;31:647.
66. Tomita K, McCoshen JA, Fernandez CS, Tyson JE. Immunologic and biologic characteristics of human decidual prolactin. Am J Obstet Gyn 1982;142:420.
67. Golander A, Hurley T, Barrett J, Hizi A, Handwerger S. Prolactin synthesis by chorion-decidual tissue: a possible source of prolactin in the amniotic fluid. Science 1978;202:311.
68. Maslar IA, Kaplan BM, Luciano AA, Riddick DH. Prolactin production by the endometrium of early human pregnancy. J Clin Endocrin Metab 1980;51:78.
69. Maslar IA, Riddick DH. Prolactin production by human endometrium during the normal menstrual cycle. Am J Obstet Gyn 1979;135:751.
70. Riddick DH, Luciano AA, Kusmik WF, Maslar IA. Evidence for a non-pituitary source of amniotic fluid prolactin. Fertil Steril 1979;31:35.
71. Daly DC, Maslar IA, Riddick DH. Prolactin production during in vitro decidualization of proliferative endometrium. Am J Obstet Gyn 1983;145:672.
72. Riddick DH, Daly DC. Decidual prolactin production in human gestation. Sem Perinat 1982;6:229.
73. Chen G, Huang JR, Mazella J, Tseng L. Long-term effects of progestin and RU 486 on prolactin production and synthesis in human endometrial stromal cells. Hum Reprod 1989;4:355.
74. Thrailkill KM, Golander A, Underwood LE, Richards RG, Handwerger S. Insulin stimulates the synthesis and release of prolactin from human decidual cells. Endocrinology 1989; 124:3010.
75. Huang JR, Tseng L, Bischof P, Janne OA. Regulation of prolactin production by progestin, estrogen, and relaxin in human endometrial stromal cells. Endocrinology 1987;121;2011.
76. Bryant-Greenwood GD, Rees MC, Turnbull AC. Immunohistochemical localization of relaxin, prolactin and prostaglandin synthase in human amnion, chorion and decidua. J Endocrinol 1987;114;491.
77. Morimoto Y. Ultrastructural and endocrinological study of the human endometrium and decidua using the organ culture method. Nippon Sanka Fujinka Gakkai Zasshi 1988;40:201.
78. Gibori G, Jayatilak PG, Khan I, et al. Decidual luteotropin secretion and action: its role in pregnancy maintenance in the rat. Adv Exp Med Biol 1987;219:379.
79. Jansen RP, Turner M, Johannisson E, Landgren BM, Diczfalusy E. Cyclic changes in human endometrial surface glycoproteins: a quantitative histochemical study. Fertil Steril 1985;44:85.
80. Maathuis JB, Aitken RJ. Cyclic variation in concentrations of protein hexose in human uterine flushings collected by an improved technique. J Reprod Fertil 1978;52:289.
81. Aitken RJ. The hormonal control of implantation. Maternal Recognition of Pregnancy. Amsterdam: Excerpta Medica, 1979; 53–58.
82. Shapiro SS, Forbes HH. Alterations in human endometrial protein synthesis during the menstrual cycle and in progesterone-stimulated organ culture. Fertil Steril 1978;30:175.
83. Irwin JC, Kirk D, King RJ, Quigley MM, Gwatkin RB. Hormonal regulation of human endometrial stromal cells in culture: an in vitro model for decidualization. Fertil Steril 1989;52:761.
84. Kisalus LL, Herr JC, Little CD. Immunolocalization of extracellular matrix proteins and collagen synthesis in first-trimester human decidua. Anat Rec 1987:218;402.
85. Wewer UM, Damjanov A, Weiss J, Liotta LA, Damjanov I. Mouse endometrial stromal cells produce basement-membrane components. Differentiation 1986;32:49.
86. Hochner-Celnikier D, Ron M, Eldor A, et al. Growth characteristics of human first trimester decidual cells cultured in serum-free medium: production of prolactin, prostaglandins and fibronectin. Biol Reprod 1984;31:827.
87. Grinnell F, Head JR, Hoffpauir J. Fibronectin and cell shape in vivo: studies on the endometrium during pregnancy. J Cell Biol 1982;94:597.
88. Rutanen EM, Koistinen R, Wahlstrom T, Sjoberg J, Stenman UH, Seppala M. Placental protein (PP12) in human endometrium: tissue concentration in relation in histology and serum levels of PP12, progesterone and oestradiol. Br J Obstet Gyn 1984;91:377.
89. Fazleabas AT, Verhage HG, Waites G, Bell SC. Characterization of an insulin-like growth factor binding protein, analogous to human pregnancy-associated secreted endometrial alpha

1-globulin, in decidua of the baboon (Papio anubis) placenta. Biol Reprod 1989;40:873.
90. Frauman AG, Tsuzaki S, Moses AC. The binding characteristics and biological effects in FRTL5 cells of placental protein 12, an insulin-like growth factor-binding protein purified from human amniotic fluid. Endocrinology 1989;124:2289.
91. Julkunen M, Koistenen R, Aalto-Setala K, Seppala M, Janne OA, Kontual K. Primary structure of human insulin-like growth factor-binding protein/placental protein 12 and tissue-specific expression of its mRNA. FEBS Lett 1988;236:295.
92. Olajide F, Howell RJ, Wass JA, et al. Circulating levels of placental protein 12 and chorionic gonadotropin following RU 38486 and gemeprost for termination of first trimester pregnancy. Hum Reprod 1989;4:337.
93. Wahlström T, Seppälä M. Placental protein 12 (PP12) is induced in the endometrium by progesterone. Fertil Steril 1984;41:781.
94. Julkunen M, Raikar RS, Joshi SG, Bohn H, Seppälä M. Placental protein 14 and progestagen-dependent endometrial protein are immunologically indistinguishable. Hum Reprod 1986;1:7.
95. Sinosich MJ, Lee J, Wolfe JP, Williams RF, Hodgen GD. RU 486 induced suppression of placental neutrophil elastase inhibitor levels. Placenta 1989;10:569.
96. Bischof P, Mignot TM, Cedard L. Are pregnancy-associated plasma protein-A (PAPP-A) and CA 125 measurements after IVF-ET possible predictors of early pregnancy wastage? Hum Reprod 1989;4:843.
97. Joshi SG. A progestagen-associated protein of the human endometrium: basic studies and potential clinical applications. J Steroid Biochem 1983;19:751.
98. Watson ED, Sertich PL. Prostaglandin production by horse embryos and the effect of co-culture of embryos with endometrium from pregnant mares. J Reprod Fertil 1989;87:331.
99. Martel D, Monier MN, Roche D, Psychoyos A. Effect of mifepristone (RU 486) on concentrations of prostaglandin E_2 binding sites in the rat endometrium. J Reprod Fertil 1989;85:527.
100. Nemme R, Acker GM, Papiernik E. Effect of progesterone in long-term endometrial cell culture: study of the synthesis of prostaglandins, thromboxane, prostacyclin and prolactin. Eur J Obstet Gynecol Reprod Biol 1988;28:221.
101. Kennedy TG, Zamecnik J. The concentration of 6-keto-prostaglandin F^1 alpha is markedly elevated at the site of blastocyst implantation in the rat. Prostaglandins 1978;16;599.
102. Kennedy TG. Evidence for a role for prostaglandins in the initiation of blastocyst implantation in the rat. Biol Reprod 1977;16:286.
102. Kennedy TG, Martel D, Psychoyos A. Endometrial prostaglandin E^2 binding: characterization in rats sensitized for the decidual cell reaction and changes during pseudopregnancy. Biol Reprod 1983;29:556.
104. Kennedy TG, Martel D, Psychoyos A. Endometrial prostaglandin E^2 binding during the estrous cycle and its hormonal control in ovariectomized rats. Biol Reprod 1983;29:565.
105. Psychoyos A. Hormonal control ovoimplantation. Vitam Horm 1973;31:201.
106. Shelesnyak MC. Aspects of reproduction. Some experimental studies on the mechanism of ovo-implantation in the rat. Rec Prog Horm Res 1957;13;269.
107. Dey SK, Villanueva C, Chien SM, Crist RD. The role of histamine in implantation in the rabbit. 1978;53:23.
108. Dey SK, Villanueva C, Abdou NI. Histamine receptors on rabbit blastocyst and endometrial cell membranes. Nature (London) 1979;278:648.
109. Heap RB, Perry JS, Gadsby JE, Burton RD. Endocrine activities of the blastocyst and early embryonic tissues in the pig. Biochem Trans 1975;3:1183.
110. Gadsby JE, Burton RD, Heap RB, Perry JS. Oestrogen production by blastocyst and early embryonic tissue of various species. J Reprod Fert 1980;60:409.
111. Arias-Stella J. Atypical endometrial changes associated with the presence of chorionic tissue. Arch Pathol 1954;58:112.
112. Casimiri V, Psychoyos A. Effect of Epsilon amino caproic acid on the hatching of rat preimplantation embryos in vitro. Biol Cell 1982;45:164.
113. Larsen JF. Human implantation and clinical aspects. Progr Reprod Biol 1980;7:284.
114. Morris JE, Potter SW. A comparison of developmental changes in surface charge in mouse blastocysts and uterine epithelium using DEAE beads and dextran sulfate in vitro. Develop Biol 1984;103:190.
115. Surani MAH, Fishel SB. Blastocyst-uterine interactions at implantation. Prog Reprod Biol 1980;7:14.
116. Surani MAH. Glycoprotein synthesis and inhibition of protein glycosylation by tunicamycin in preimplantation mouse embryos: compaction and trophoblast adhesion. Cell 1979; 18:217.
117. Psychoyos A (1973b). Endocrine control of egg-implantation. In: Greep RO, Astwood EB, eds. Handbook of Physiology: Endocrinology. Vol II. Baltimore: Williams & Wilkins, 1973:11.
118. Armant DR, Kaplan HA, Mover H, Lennarz WJ. The effect of hexapeptides on attachment and outgrowth of mouse embryos in vitro: Evidence for the involvement of the cell recognition tripeptide Arg-Gly-Asp. Proc Natl Acad Sci USA 1986:83:6751.
119. Farach MC, Tang JP, Decker GL, Carson DD. Heparin/heparan sulfate is involved in attachment and spreading of mouse embryos in vitro. Dev Biol 1987;123:401.
120. Lawrence TS, Ginzberg RD, Gilula NB, Beers WH. Hormonally induced cell shape changes in cultured rat ovarian granulosa cells. J Cell Biol 1979;80:21.
121. Roess DA, Niswender GD, Brisas BG. Cytochalasins and colchicine increase the lateral mobility of human chorionic gonadotropin-occupied luteinizing hormone receptors on ovine luteal cells. Endocrinology 1988;122:261.
122. Yoshinaga K. Receptor conceptive implantation research. In: Yoshinaga K, Mori T, eds. Progress in clinical and biological research. Vol 294. New York: Alan R Liss, 1988:279.
123. Parr MB. Endocytosis in the uterine epithelium during early pregnancy. Prog Reprod Biol 1980:7:81.
124. Hertig AT. Human trophoblast. Springfield, IL: CC Thomas, 1968.

2

CHAPTER

IMMUNOBIOLOGIC ADAPTATIONS OF PREGNANCY

I. L. Sargent and C. W. G. Redman

The primary role of the immune system is to protect the body from invasion by foreign organisms and their toxic products. To do this requires the ability to discriminate between self and non-self antigens, so that immune destruction can be targeted against the invading organism and not against the animal's own tissues. In pregnancy, the antigenically foreign fetus grows within its mother for 9 months unharmed by her immune system. Clearly, there must be immune adaptations in pregnancy that are central to the survival of the fetus. These adaptations must prevent immune rejection of the fetus while maintaining the mother's ability to fight infection. The aim of this chapter is to describe the immunobiologic changes of pregnancy and to determine how these seemingly conflicting requirements are satisfied.

IMMUNE RESPONSES IN GRAFT REJECTION

The fetus has frequently been compared to a transplant, and although this may not be the correct analogy, the events that govern graft rejection are nevertheless relevant to an understanding of the complexity of the immune interaction between the mother and fetus.

The ability of the immune system to discriminate between self and non-self is brought about through the products of the major histocompatibility complex (MHC)—the transplantation antigens. The genes code for two groups of cell-surface glycoproteins, some of which are highly polymorphic. The first group, or Class I antigens (HLA-A, -B, -C), are found on most adult cells and are formed from a polymorphic heavy chain and $\beta2$ microglobulin, an invariate light chain. The second group, or Class II MHC antigens (HLA-DP, -DQ, -DR), are composed of an α and β chain. They have a restricted tissue distribution, and are usually found only on immune cells such as lymphocytes, macrophages, and dendritic cells. They can be induced on other cell types, such as endothelium, in the course of an immune response.

In transplant rejection, the foreign Class II MHC antigens on the graft are recognized by the recipient's T helper cells. They respond by synthesizing and secreting interleukin-2 (IL-2), a cytokine that induces the proliferation of cytotoxic T lymphocytes (CTL). These cells recognize the graft via its foreign Class I MHC antigens and destroy it. In parallel with the production of CTL is the development of immunological memory. Thus, a second allogeneic graft from a donor is rejected more quickly than the first graft from that donor.

Although cell-mediated immunity is the major effector in graft rejection, antibodies can also be involved. Antibodies are produced by B cells with the cooperation of T helper cells and macrophages. The B cells and macrophages (antigen-presenting cells) take up antigen and process it into highly immunogenic peptides. These peptides are presented on their cell surface, in association with Class II MHC antigens, to specific T helper cells, which respond by producing IL-2 and IL-4. These cytokines cause the B cells to divide and differentiate into antibody-producing cells. The resulting antibodies may bind to the cells of the graft, which are then destroyed by macrophages or killer (K) cells binding to the antibody via their Fc receptors (antibody-dependent cell-mediated cytotoxicity—ADCC).

To understand how these destructive immune responses are controlled in pregnancy, it is necessary to determine the nature of the mother's response to the fetus. The first step is to define the areas of contact between maternal and fetal tissues and the nature of the fetal antigens to which the mother is thereby exposed.

THE MATERNAL–FETAL INTERFACE

TROPHOBLAST

The fetus itself does not come into direct contact with maternal tissue; it is the trophoblast of the placenta and fetal membranes that forms the interface between maternal and fetal tissue. This contact begins very early in pregnancy when the blastocyst invades the decidua. As the trophectoderm proliferates and invades, it differentiates into two layers: an inner cytotrophoblast layer and an outer syncytiotrophoblast layer. Spaces called lacunae develop in the syncytiotrophoblast and fill with blood from ruptured maternal capillaries. Later maternal vessels link with these lacunae, and oxygenated blood flows into them from the spiral arteries and out through the uterine veins.

At 13 to 14 days, clumps of cytotrophoblast project into the syncytiotrophoblast to form the primary chorionic villi, which develop a mesenchymal core containing blood capillaries that link with the fetal circulation. At the same time, the cytotrophoblast penetrates the syncytiotrophoblast to form the cytotrophoblast shell, which attaches the chorionic sac to the decidua. Cytotrophoblast cells infiltrate the decidua and later the myometrium, a process that continues until at least 18 weeks. The cytotrophoblast cells also invade the decidual spiral arteries as far as the myometrial segments.

Thus, two areas of contact between mother and fetus are established: a large surface area formed by the syncytiotrophoblast of the chorionic villi, bathed by maternal blood, and within the decidua extravillous trophoblast, mostly cytotrophoblast, but also syncytial elements, that mingle directly with maternal tissues.

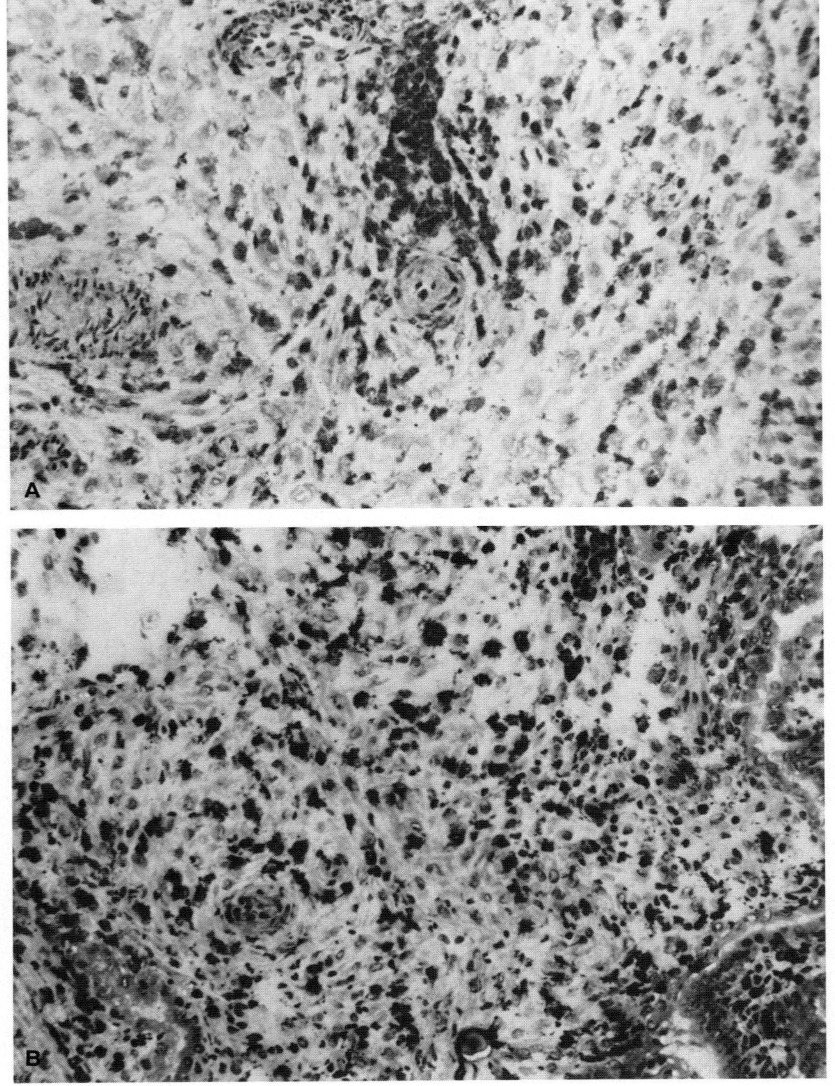

FIGURE 2–1. Immune cells in the decidua. Human first trimester decidua labelled with monoclonal antibodies using an indirect immunoperoxidase technique. (**A**) Antileukocyte common antigen: labels all bone marrow-derived cells. (**B**) Anti-CD56 antigen: labels most large granular lymphocytes. Magnification ×100 (courtesy of Dr. P. M. Starkey).

IMMUNE CELLS IN THE DECIDUA

The decidua is the tissue where immune recognition of trophoblast is most likely to occur; it is highly relevant that in the first trimester it contains many cells of bone marrow origin,[1,2] hence of potential immune function (Fig. 2-1A). The cells include macrophages, classical T cells, and an unusual lymphocyte population with the characteristics of large granular lymphocytes (LGL) (Fig. 2-1B).[3] LGL are not T or B cells, but share features with both lymphocytes and monocytes.[4] They include natural killer (NK) cells and cytolytic K cells described above, which kill targets when they are coated with antibody. NK cells attack their targets without pre-immunization, and independently of antibodies, complement or phagocytosis. They are thought to be active in the elimination of both virally infected and tumor cells, and have also been implicated in graft rejection reactions.[5]

Immune cells comprise most of the cells of the decidual stroma in the first trimester, and of these the large granular lymphocytes are the most abundant, constituting on average about 45% of all the stromal cells (Fig. 2-2).[6] They have an unusual phenotype compared to peripheral blood LGL. They are present in the endometrium throughout the menstrual cycle, but their numbers increase in the endometrium during the mid-secretory phase, suggesting that they are under hormonal control.[7] It has been suggested that their immune functions, which are as yet unknown, are important for the survival of the fetal allograft.

The second most common immune cells in the decidua are macrophages.[1,6,8] Their functions in the decidua are not well investigated, but they can present

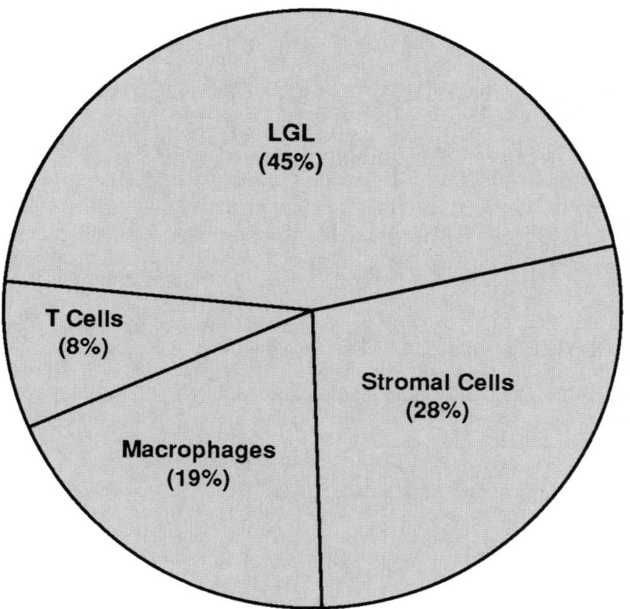

FIGURE 2–2. Immune cell populations in human first trimester decidua. LGL, large granular lymphocytes. (Courtesy of Dr. P. M. Starkey).

TABLE 2–1. CONTACT BETWEEN MATERNAL IMMUNE CELLS AND FETAL TISSUES

Local
Syncytiotrophoblast lining intervillous space
Cytotrophoblast in decidua
Systemic
Fetal red and white cell traffic
Trophoblast deportation

antigen to T cells.[9] T cells are present in the decidua—the third most common decidual immune cell—comprising about 10% of all the stromal cells. Thus, all the ingredients for a maternal immune response appear to be present.

FETAL–MATERNAL CELL TRAFFIC

The villous syncytiotrophoblast, in contact with blood, and the nonvillous cytotrophoblast, in contact with maternal decidua, are the main areas where maternal lymphocytes might be sensitized to trophoblast. The interface between mother and fetus is extended by the traffic of fetal cells into the maternal circulation, carrying fetal antigens to other parts of the maternal immune system, where priming responses could occur (Table 2-1).

Trophoblast Deportation

From early in the first trimester, trophoblast cells can be detected histologically in the myometrial and endometrial veins. These cells may embolize to the lungs, a well-documented process that is thought to be normal.[10] This process continues throughout pregnancy so that syncytial cells can be found in uterine vein blood at term, using flow cytometric techniques.[11] Most of the embolized cells lodge in the pulmonary capillaries, arouse no inflammatory changes, and are probably cleared by proteolysis.[12] It was previously thought that not all trophoblast cells were trapped in the lungs as "trophoblast cells," and that they could also be identified in the blood of 80% of normal pregnant women[13–15] by using flow cytometry and fluorescence labelling with monoclonal antibodies.[16] However, this has not been confirmed by others[17] and it is now realized that the circulating cells are not trophoblast but maternal cells, reacting in a false-positive way with the trophoblast antibody.[18,19] Embolization is usually restricted to syncytial cells, but under pathological circumstances may include villi[20] or even fragments of decidua.[21]

Traffic of Fetal Blood Cells

Fetal–maternal hemorrhage, measured by the appearance of fetal red cells in the maternal circulation, is a well-documented event. It occurs mainly at delivery, but also during pregnancy,[22] predominantly in the third trimester.[23] Rh isoimmunization may be the consequence—the best characterized disorder resulting directly from incompatibility between mother and fetus. A large transplacental hemorrhage can cause maternal transfusion reactions if there is blood group incompatibility; for example, after diagnostic amniocentesis,[24] but also as a spontaneous event.[25]

Fetal blood leukocytes have also been reported in maternal blood during pregnancy,[26–28] although some workers disagree.[29] Whether they enter the maternal circulation during fetal–maternal hemorrhages or by another process is not clear.

In summary, maternal immune cells may have contact with several different fetal tissues or cell populations. It is the nature of the antigens expressed by these cells that will determine the kinds of immune response the mother makes during pregnancy.

FETAL ANTIGENS TO WHICH THE MOTHER MAY BE EXPOSED

TROPHOBLAST ANTIGENS

As discussed above, HLA-A, -B, -C, and -D antigens have key roles in the generation and regulation of human T cell-mediated immune responses, including those involved in the rejection of foreign tissues. Their expression in the placenta, particularly on the trophoblast, must be relevant to the survival of the fetal allograft.

CLASS I TRANSPLANTATION ANTIGENS AND TROPHOBLAST

MHC antigens have not been detected on human oocytes[30,31] or preimplantation embryos,[32] but it is not yet known whether they are expressed at the morula or blastocyst stages. Later in gestation, neither the syncytiotrophoblast nor the underlying villous cytotrophoblast expresses Class I MHC antigens[33–35] or mRNA.[36] In contrast, Class I MHC antigens are present on many forms of nonvillous trophoblast throughout gestation, including the invasive trophoblast that establishes placentation and comes into direct contact with maternal decidua and myometrium (Table 2-2).[37–40] However, they do not express the specific paternal and maternal HLA-A and HLA-B haplotypes of the fetus.[38,41] The Class I MHC protein on trophoblast is a unique, nonpolymorphic glycoprotein associated with $\beta 2$ microglobulin, with a lower molecular weight of 40 kd.[42] It has recently been sequenced and shown to be almost identical to HLA-G,[43] a gene that was previously not thought to be expressed in vivo.[44] Its expression may be unique to trophoblast, but it appears to be monomorphic and is unlikely to function as a transplantation antigen.

CLASS II TRANSPLANTATION ANTIGENS AND TROPHOBLAST

The expression of Class II MHC products in the placenta is of particular interest, because these products are a major stimulus of the rejection of allografts. HLA-DR has not been found on human syncytiotrophoblast at term[45] or on immature villous trophoblast, trophoblast cell columns, or the cytotrophoblast of the amniochorion.[46]

An antibody that binds to HLA-DP labels trophoblast from the term amniochorion and first trimester chorionic villi.[46] However, the same cells do not bind other antibodies that react with epitopes common to all HLA-D molecules, including HLA-DP. This suggests that the relevant protein is either an incomplete part of HLA-DP—for example, the α chain on its own—or a cross-reactive but otherwise unrelated molecule.[46]

HLA-D positive cells, other than trophoblast, are found in the placental villous stroma and in the connective tissue underlying the amniotic epithelium in the second and third trimester, but are never found in direct contact with maternal tissue or blood.[47] These cells have been identified as macrophages.[2,48]

OTHER ANTIGENS ON TROPHOBLAST

The distribution of major histocompatibility antigens on trophoblast has been emphasized because of their relevance to maternal–fetal immune interaction. The finding that trophoblast does not express conventional transplantation antigens must be considered to be the

TABLE 2–2. MAJOR HISTOCOMPATIBILITY ANTIGEN (MHC) EXPRESSION IN HUMAN DEVELOPMENT

	CLASS 1 MHC		
	MONOMORPHIC	POLYMORPHIC	CLASS 2 MHC
Oocyte	—	—	—
Pre-implantation embryo	—	—	—
Blastocyst	?	?	?
Syncytiotrophoblast	—	—	—
Non-villous cytotrophoblast	+	—	—(?)
Fetal tissue	?	+	+

—, antigen absent; +, antigen present; ?, not yet known.

most important way in which it avoids maternal immune rejection.

Immune rejection does not depend solely on the major histocompatibility antigens. Numerous minor histocompatibility antigens can provoke rejection, although this occurs more slowly. The trophoblast surface membrane has a complex structure, associated with at least 20 to 30 protein subunits, many of which could potentially stimulate immune responses.[49] Only a few have been characterized so far.

TLX Antigens

Particular attention has been given to antigens shared by trophoblast, platelets, and lymphocytes (trophoblast/lymphocyte cross-reactive antigens—TLX),[50–52] because they might modulate maternal lymphocyte function directly or indirectly. Early studies based on the reactivities of different rabbit antisera suggested that TLX antigens are allotypic.[53] This has recently been confirmed with the demonstration that TLX antigens include the CD46 antigen, otherwise known as membrane co-factor protein, which binds C3b and C4b and acts as a co-factor for their breakdown by the I protein.[54,55] CD46 exists in several different molecular weight forms, and is physically associated with HLA Class I molecules on the membrane. Elevated levels of CD46 are found on most malignant tissues and cell lines. It is proposed that CD46 may play a role in the protection of the trophoblast from immune attack by preventing the activation of complement.

Oncotrophoblast Antigens

Some malignant tissues and cancer cell lines express surface antigens also found on trophoblast,[56–59] and trophoblast has some neoplastic characteristics, particularly invasiveness. The shared antigens are not necessarily restricted to trophoblast and tumors, but may identify cells in a particular state of differentiation or metabolic activity. They are of interest because the placenta may stimulate maternal immune responses more like those made to a tumor than to an allograft. In fact, the tumor–host rather than the host-versus-graft immune relationship may be a more appropriate model for elucidating maternal immune tolerance of the fetus. It is possible that the altered susceptibilities of parous women to certain forms of cancer[60] may result from immune reactivities induced by pregnancy. The major oncotrophoblast membrane antigen is placental alkaline phosphatase,[49,61] which has more allelic variants than any other human enzyme.[62] Its function is not defined, nor is it known if its polymorphism is important for maternal–fetal immune interactions. The transferrin receptor[56,63,64] and a 72-kd glycoprotein found on the syncytiotrophoblast membrane and various malignant cell lines, including choriocarcinoma and teratocarcinoma,[65] are other oncotrophoblast antigens.

The carbohydrate structures attached to glycoproteins and glycolipids may be what distinguish mature from immature cells, or normal from neoplastic cells.[66] Of particular interest are the glycosaminoglycans. When cells transform they tend to produce more hyaluronic acid,[67] and this may enhance their proliferation, migration, and invasion by maintaining an open, highly hydrated extracellular matrix structure.[68] Hyaluronic acid is found on the apical surface of all syncytiotrophoblast throughout gestation and around the rapidly proliferating, invasive cytotrophoblast cell columns.[69] Similar increases in hyaluronic acid around invasive carcinomas have been reported.[70]

MATERNAL IMMUNE RESPONSES TO THE FETUS

Thus, the mother is exposed to a wide variety of fetal and trophoblast antigens. Her responses to these antigens will now be considered, together with the adaptations to her immune system that may intervene to prevent rejection of the fetus.

MATERNAL RESPONSES TO PATERNAL HLA

Despite the absence of classical transplantation antigens on trophoblast, the mother is undoubtedly exposed to paternally derived HLA antigens expressed on other fetal cells.

Antibody Responses

The development of HLA antibodies is a relatively common and normal event in human pregnancy.[71–74] Because there is no HLA on trophoblast, sensitization must result either from fetal–maternal bleeding, causing maternal immunization with HLA-positive fetal leukocytes, or from breaks in the continuity of the villous trophoblast, which expose the underlying HLA-positive stromal cells. In either case, maternal exposure to fetal HLA is likely to be intermittent and random. Antibodies to HLA-A, -B, -C can develop during a first pregnancy.[72,75] They may occur after an abortion,[76] indicating that immunization is not necessarily the result of events at delivery, but they usually develop after 28 weeks[77] and their incidence increases with parity.[72] They do not develop in all pregnancies. Only about 15% of women in their first pregnancies, and never more than 60% of multiparous women, develop these antibodies.[72,78] The incidence of positive sera may decline during the third trimester for reasons that are not defined.[76,79] Antibodies to Class II MHC antigens (HLA-D) are usually associated with HLA-A, -B, and -C antibodies, but may develop independently.[74] None of these antibodies appear to cause any harm to the fetus.[78]

Cell-Mediated Immunity

T-cell and B-cell sensitization to fetal HLA should occur together. In most pregnancies there are no maternal antifetal HLA antibodies, and it is not surprising that there is only sporadic evidence for T-cell sensitization as judged by the detection of a secondary maternal–paternal (fetal) mixed lymphocyte reaction,[80–85] or paternal (fetal)-specific cytotoxic T cells.[86]

We have looked for cytotoxic T cells against paternal and unrelated control target cells in women at term.[86] Only one out of nine primiparous women gave clear evidence of cytotoxic cells specific for the father. This woman was the only one to show a secondary response in the mixed lymphocyte reaction (MLR) against the father, but not against unrelated cells. Similarly, only one of nine multiparous women showed evidence for sensitization and, in a further series of experiments, no sensitization to paternal HLA was seen in 25 normal first trimester pregnancies.[87] These results show that maternal T-cell sensitization to paternal HLA can occur, but is not a regular event in a normal pregnancy. It does not appear to be harmful to the fetus, because both women had normal pregnancies. This implies that the cytotoxic T cells cannot cross the placental barrier to gain access to the fetus. It is also further evidence of the difference between the fetal allograft and conventional allografts, where HLA immunization dominates the processes of tolerance or rejection.

MATERNAL RESPONSES TO TROPHOBLAST

Although maternal sensitization to paternal HLA antigens may occur, it is the nature of the mother's immune responses to the trophoblast that are key to the survival of the pregnancy.

Antitrophoblast Antibodies

It is probable but not certain that maternal antibodies are produced against trophoblast during normal pregnancy. Maternal alloantibodies can be detected by their binding to and cytolytic destruction of paternal lymphocytes, but not all antibodies act in this way. To investigate maternal antibodies to trophoblast-specific antigens requires binding assays using placental cells or tissues. This is difficult because the Fc receptors on trophoblast, which bind free IgG nonspecifically, render the detection of specific antitrophoblast antibodies difficult. Fc-bound antibody can be washed from the placenta, and then specifically bound antibodies can be removed by acid elution.[88–90] The specificity of the eluted antibodies and the cell types to which they bind is uncertain. Some workers have shown them to be specific for fetal (paternal) HLA[91] and trophoblast,[92] while others have found no specificity or lymphocytotoxic reactivity.[93]

Maternal IgG (and to a lesser extent IgM) antibodies to trophoblast have been detected in pregnancy sera and placental eluates using an ELISA technique,[92,94,95] with maximum levels in the first trimester that gradually decline to term.[96] Two other studies using a passive hemagglutination assay[97] and an ELISA[98,99] have failed to confirm these findings, although it is argued that this discrepancy results from the nature of the trophoblast membrane preparation used.[100]

Evidence for antitrophoblast antibodies in pathological pregnancy has come from studies in which sera from recurrent aborters has been shown to be toxic to mouse embryos in culture.[101,102] Fractionation of the serum has shown the factor to be in the IgG fraction, and the activity could be absorbed out with human trophoblast membranes.[101]

Natural Immunity

The most abundant immune cell in the first trimester decidua is the large granular lymphocyte. These cells have natural killer activity.[103,104] Natural killer (NK) cells can lyse certain tumor cells spontaneously; that is, without prior sensitization. Unlike cytotoxic T cells, they lack immunologic memory and can kill target cells that lack Class I MHC antigens. Because of their capacity to lyse tumors, NK cells may also have the potential to destroy trophoblast cells which, as discussed previously, have many characteristics of malignant cells. The cytotrophoblast seems to be resistant to both decidual and peripheral blood NK cells,[103,105] although they can be killed under special culture conditions.[106] Similarly, lysis of cultured syncytiotrophoblast by unprimed allogeneic leukocytes has been reported, but the relevance of these findings to events in vivo is unclear.[107]

If NK cells are inactive against trophoblast in normal pregnancy, it could be expected that their activity would be increased in disorders of pregnancy and placental pathology. Levels are reported to be increased in the peripheral blood LGL in preterm labor and preeclampsia. It would be more relevant to look at the activity of decidual LGL in preeclampsia or at the time of miscarriage. We have activated decidual LGL with IL-2 in vitro, and although this enhances their cytotoxic activity against tumor targets, they are still unable to kill trophoblast.[105] Natural killer activity seems to be irrelevant for trophoblast as far as the situation is understood.

Cell-Mediated Immunity

The production of lymphokines by maternal leukocytes after short-term culture with pooled placental antigens has been cited as evidence for maternal T-cell sensitization to trophoblast antigens.[108,109] It is impossible to know which component of the placenta could be the stimulating antigen, because such preparations contain stromal tissue as well as trophoblast, and so could have contained fetal Class I and Class II antigens. To study this question more rigorously requires the isolation of pure trophoblast. Syncytiotrophoblast membrane vesicles prepared from autologous placentae do not stimulate a proliferative response in maternal or unrelated donor lymphocytes.[110–112] Similarly, cytotrophoblast isolated from the chorion laeve[113] fails to stimulate a lymphocyte response directly in mixed cell culture. The trophoblast may well be immunogenic in vitro in appropriate conditions. In the mouse, maternal lymphocytes that are cytotoxic for trophoblast can be generated in culture by the addition of IL-2.[114] This bypasses the requirement for antigen-presenting cells that in vivo activate helper T cells to produce IL-2.

In summary, it is by no means certain that the maternal immune system reacts with trophoblast. T-cell effector function, which is critical to allograft survival, is certainly irrelevant to the villous (but not necessarily the extravillous) trophoblast, whereas NK and related null cell activity maybe more important. Large granular lymphocytes are numerous in the decidua in close apposition to the interstitial trophoblast, but their functions are completely unknown. B-cell function should also be considered, particularly because the decidua appears to be equipped to process and present antigen. In contrast, there is no doubt that fetal cells other than trophoblast can stimulate maternal immunization.

REGULATION OF MATERNAL–FETAL IMMUNE RESPONSIVENESS

Although the mother is exposed to many fetal and placental antigens, our present knowledge suggests that she does not regularly become sensitized to them and, even if she does, the effector responses do not appear to damage the placenta.

How are these responses controlled? The development of an immune response can be blocked at three stages: the afferent or recognition phase, the central or generation phase, and the efferent or effector phase (Fig. 2-3). These will be examined in relation to pregnancy.

BLOCKADE OF AFFERENT IMMUNE RESPONSES

Maternal recognition of the placental graft could fail in two ways: either because the placenta does not express antigens that can stimulate immune responses, or the mother's immune system could be nonspecifically suppressed. The antigenic nature of the trophoblast might constitute the primary barrier to maternal immune recognition. Because syncytiotrophoblast lacks conventional MHC antigens and nonvillous trophoblast does not express Class II MHC antigens, there may be no direct immune stimulus to the mother. It is not yet known whether the mother makes a response to the HLA-G-like Class I antigen on nonvillous trophoblast, but it may be poorly immunogenic in vivo because it lacks HLA-A and -B specificities.

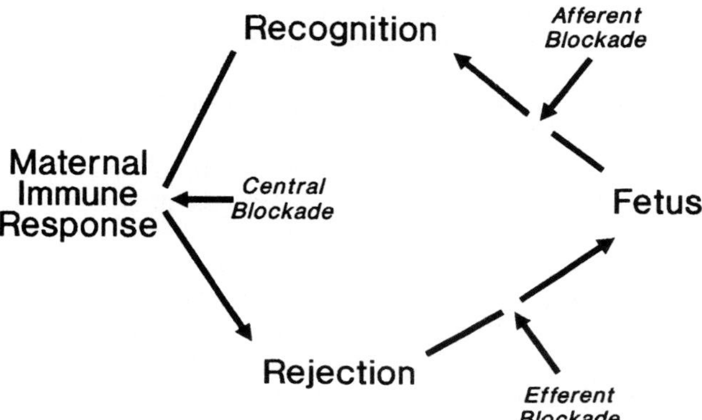

FIGURE 2–3. Regulation of maternal immune responses to the fetus.

Nonspecific Immunosuppression

It is evident from clinical observation that pregnant women are not grossly immunocompromised. However, they are more susceptible to certain infections,[115] such as hepatitis,[116] herpes simplex,[117] and Epstein-Barr virus.[118] A decrease in NK cell activity may be expected in normal pregnancy. Maternal T lymphocyte function may also be depressed. A reduction in in vitro responses to microbial and viral antigens[119,120] and mitogens[121,122] has been reported. This has lead many investigators to study the immune cell populations in the blood of pregnant women.

Natural Killer Cells

During the menstrual cycle, there is a significant fall in NK activity in the periovulatory period,[123] thought to be induced by changes in gonadotropins rather than steroid hormones; luteinizing hormone (LH) and human chorionic gonadotrophin (HCG) inhibit NK activity in vitro, whereas estradiol, progesterone, and testosterone do not.[124,125] NK activity during pregnancy is depressed from the first trimester to term,[126–130] returning to control levels between 9 to 40 weeks after delivery.[131] There is both a decrease in NK cell numbers[132] and their lytic capacity.[128,133] Consistent with this is the finding that NK activity against herpes simplex virus-infected cells is depressed in pregnancy.[134]

Antibody Dependent Cellular Cytotoxicity

In contrast to NK activity, antibody dependent cellular cytotoxicity (ADCC) appears to be unchanged in pregnancy. Studies of women during pregnancy[134] and postpartum[135] showed no differences in ADCC compared to non-pregnant controls. Therefore, NK and ADCC appear to have separate roles in pregnancy; while there may be a need to downregulate NK activity, ADCC is still available to deal with virus-infected cells.

T Cells, B Cells, and Monocytes

Although it is generally agreed that there is an increase in monocytes and little change in B cell numbers during pregnancy,[136] there is considerable variation in the results for T cells.[137,138] The underlying trend appears to be a decrease in the proportion of T helper (CD4+ve) cells.[139,140] This has lead to the conclusion that immunosuppression in pregnancy is due to a reduction in helper T cells. Consistent with this are reports that CD4+ve cells do not decrease to the same extent in women with low birthweight babies[141] or with a history of recurrent abortions,[142,143] leading to the suggestion that a failure of the immunosuppressive mechanism has exposed the fetus to immunological attack.

Thus, the numbers and function of some immune cell populations are altered during pregnancy, but not in such a way as to immunocompromise the mother. The mechanisms underlying these changes are not known, but it is very probable that they are related to the placenta.

Placental Suppressor Factors

The placenta itself can release factors that suppress lymphocyte activation. Mouse placental extracts have been shown to enhance graft survival in normal mice, possibly by promoting the activation of regulatory agents such as blocking antibodies and suppressor cells,[144] and similar factors have been demonstrated in the human placenta.[145] Microvillous preparations of syncytiotrophoblast and culture supernatants from placental cells and choriocarcinoma cell lines[146,147] nonspecifically suppress mitogen responsiveness and allogeneically stimulated lymphocytes in the MLR, as well as NK cell activity.[148] Suppressive activity may appear very early in gestation, because animal[149,150] and human preimplantation embryos[151] have been reported to produce inhibitory factors within 24 hours of fertilization. The nature of these trophoblast-derived suppressor factors is not known, but recent reports suggest that they may be related to transforming growth factor β (TGFβ).[152]

Serum Suppressor Factors

Immunosuppressive factors derived from the placenta would enter the maternal circulation, so it is not surprising that many (but not all) pregnancy sera have been shown to suppress lymphocyte responses in a nonspecific way.[153,154] Such activity appears at about 10–15 weeks of pregnancy, reaches a maximum at 20–30 weeks, declines toward the end of gestation, and disappears soon after delivery.[155] Many consider that placental hormones could explain these observations. Human chorionic gonadotrophin (HCG) at physiological levels inhibits mitogen-induced proliferation of lymphocytes, possibly by binding to accessory cells that may, in turn, release prostaglandins.[156] Likewise, physiological levels of progesterone have been shown to inhibit lymphocyte responses, and its extraction from pregnancy sera results in an 80% decrease in its suppressive activity.[157] The activity of progesterone is interrelated with prostaglandins, which are synthesized by the placenta, amniochorion, and decidua. Progesterone-treated lymphocytes release a soluble factor that inhibits the production of PGF2,[158] thus favoring synthesis of the PGE series of prostaglandins, which suppress NK cell activity and maternal T-cell responses by switching off production of IL-2. Indeed, the inhibition of the MLR by pregnancy sera can be completely restored by adding IL-2 to the cultures.[159]

Inhibitory activity is not present in all peripheral blood samples, but is found consistently in retroplacental sera.[159] This supports the idea that the activity is derived from the placenta or decidua. Indeed, the mitogen responsiveness of lymphocytes taken from uterine vein blood has been shown to be suppressed in vitro, compared to peripheral lymphocytes from the same woman.[160] The nature of the nonspecific inhibitory factor is not known, but many pregnancy-associated substances apart from hormones have been shown to be immunosuppressive. They include α-fetoprotein,[161] SP1,[162] pregnancy-associated α2-macroglobulin,[163,164] early pregnancy factor,[165] and products of the interaction between polyamine oxidase and polyamines,[166] both of which are abundant in the immediate vicinity of the placenta. Some of these are sometimes called "blocking factors," and reduced peripheral blood concentrations have been associated with pregnancy failure, particularly early in gestation.[167] These kinds of factors inhibit nonspecifically, so that the functions of all T cells, regardless of their antigen specificity, are likely to be impaired. They are detected by measuring polyclonal T-cell responses in pregnancy sera, such as those stimulated by lectins; for example, phytohemagglutinin or concanavalin-A. NK cell activity is also inhibited by pregnancy sera[168]; because NK cells do not recognize specific antigens, the inhibitory activity must be similarly nonspecific, although not necessarily due to the same factors.

Decidual Suppressor Factors

Suppressive factors released by the placenta could systemically inhibit lymphocyte responses to syncytiotrophoblast, but other mechanisms may be involved locally to prevent alloimmune recognition of extravillous cytotrophoblast that invades the decidua. In the mouse, it is thought that decidual suppressor cells are essential for the success of gestation.[169] Two cell types have been identified that nonspecifically inhibit lymphocyte responses in vitro.[170] The first is a large cell that appears in the uterine lining early in pregnancy. These are presumably hormonally activated, because short-term culture supernatants from both normal and pseudopregnancy decidua are equally inhibitory.[171,172] The second type is a small, granulated lymphocyte that lacks T-cell markers, which is localized at the implantation site and is said to be activated by trophoblast.[170]

Suppression of cell-mediated responsiveness in vitro by human decidual explants[173] and unfractionated cell populations[174,175] from first trimester human decidua has also been demonstrated. It has been proposed that, as for the mouse, suppressor activity is associated with a two populations of cells.[176] One is a large cell type that appears in the endometrium in the luteal phase and is thought to be hormone dependent. The second is a later-phase small cell, which appears to be trophoblast dependent. These cells are reported to be absent from the decidua of women who recurrently abort.[177]

Various proteins are secreted by decidual cells, which might mediate these activities. PP14, which constitutes up to 10% of the soluble protein content of decidual tissue of the first trimester, is one.[178] Other workers dispute this and say the activity is due to prostaglandins released by decidual macrophages.[179,180] Recently, a transforming growth factor β (TGFβ) has been found to be a decidua suppressor factor in murine pregnancy.[181] TGFβ is one of a group of ubiquitous cytokines which, although they stimulate growth of some cells, strongly inhibit proliferation of B cells and T cells and the cytolytic activity of NK cells.[182] It is not yet known if the same is true in human gestation, but TGFβ is present in, and has been purified from, the human placenta.[183]

Whatever the afferent blockade mechanisms are, other fetal cell populations bearing MHC antigens can immunize the mother sporadically during pregnancy, following their release into the maternal circulation. There must be a mechanism that prevents this sensitization leading to an effector cell response.

CENTRAL REGULATION OF IMMUNE RESPONSES

In contrast to the nonspecific suppressor mechanisms discussed above, which act by preventing antigen recognition or inhibiting lymphocyte proliferation, central regulation requires lymphocytes to recognize antigen and respond by the production of either blocking antibodies or suppressor cells. These specific suppressor mechanisms are directed only to the antigen in question and will not impair other immune responses.

Blocking Antibodies

Cell-mediated responses can be blocked by antibodies binding either to maternal responder lymphocytes or to the antigens that stimulate them. The production of such antibodies would depend on the recognition of fetal antigens.

As previously discussed, pregnancy sera may inhibit cell-mediated responses in a completely nonspecific way.[184–186] To demonstrate specific blocking, the proliferation or cytotoxicity of maternal cells to fetal cells and HLA dissimilar third-party cells must be tested in control and autologous maternal serum. To distinguish further the nature of the inhibitory activity, blocking antibodies are likely to persist after pregnancy, whereas placental-derived suppressor factors should disappear soon after delivery.

Maternal antifetal HLA antibodies have been extensively investigated because they block the MLR between maternal and fetal or paternal cells. The numerous reports of specific MLR inhibitory activity in pregnancy sera[187–189] can be adequately explained by the presence of these antibodies. It is not surprising that antibodies eluted from the placenta, which acts as an "antibody sponge," contain similar HLA specificities to those in maternal sera; hence, they also inhibit the MLR.[190–192]

Other pregnancy-induced antibodies may have an immunoregulatory function. Pregnancy sera contain antibodies that block the Fc receptor of B cells.[193] These are directed to an unidentified HLA determinant (not A, B, C or DR) and are present in many but not all first trimester pregnancy sera. Similar antibodies are induced by blood transfusion and allografting, and their presence correlates with enhanced renal allograft survival.[194] Other putative blocking factors have been identified in pregnancy plasmas but not in sera, implying that they are not immunoglobulins.[195]

It has been argued that blocking antibodies are essential for the success of human pregnancy. But if they are defined by their action on maternal–fetal/paternal MLR, then they are found in only about half of the sera of parous women.[196] This is a key issue. Many investigators, despite the inadequate evidence, assume that blocking antibodies are essential for normal pregnancy and that their absence causes recurrent miscarriage.[197] A more likely explanation is that they do not develop because the pregnancy fails before the time when these antibodies are normally produced.[198]

Antibodies with specificities other than for fetal (paternal) HLA may be implicated. These include anti-idiotypic antibodies that bind to the maternal T-cell receptors for paternal HLA types, and are found in the sera of parous women.[198,200] These may regulate maternal immune responses to trophoblast. Similar antibodies may also be stimulated by blood transfusions, and could be the mechanism by which renal allograft survival is enhanced after blood transfusions.[201]

None of these antibodies discussed so far is specific for trophoblast and so may not regulate maternal immune responsiveness in vivo. Because of the lack of in vitro models of maternal lymphocyte responses to trophoblast, it is not yet possible to assess the blocking activity of pregnancy serum on these responses. The role of blocking antibodies has yet to be defined; the simplest and most likely concept is that they are merely the consequence and not the cause of a successful pregnancy.

Suppressor T Cells

The activation of T lymphocytes generates not only helper and cytotoxic T cells, but suppressor T cells that can specifically downregulate responses to the immunizing antigen. Paternal-specific T cells, which totally suppressed maternal–paternal MLR, have been demonstrated in some highly parous women.[202] Others have found similar specific depression of the maternal–paternal MLR, which could be mediated by suppressor cells.[82,203] Likewise, we have found that, in highly parous women, the MLR between mother and father is significantly depressed, compared with that between the mother and an unrelated control.[86] This "suppressor cell" activity was not seen in primiparous women, and therefore its relevance to the success of pregnancy is not clear. Several studies have shown that it is possible to prime maternal lymphocytes to fetal cells to develop both secondary proliferative responses and specific cytotoxic effector cells in the normal way,[204,205] and we have confirmed this using paternal stimulator cells. Thus, there does not appear to be any fundamental impairment of maternal cell-mediated sensitization, at least in vitro.

BLOCKADE OF EFFERENT IMMUNE RESPONSES

In some pregnancies, maternal cell-mediated sensitization to fetal/paternal HLA does occur. Despite this, such pregnancies are successful. The simplest explanation for this is that the placenta functions as an antigeneically inert barrier between the mother and fetus. Cytotoxic T cells cannot lyse cells that lack HLA-A or -B antigens; thus, trophoblast would not present a suitable target (Table 2-3).

Role of the Placenta

Placental factors may also play a role. Pregnancy hormones,[206] soluble extracts, and culture supernatants from mouse trophoblast cells[207] and microvillous preparations from human syncytiotrophoblast[208] have all been shown to inhibit the cytolytic activity of cytotoxic T cells and NK cells against lymphoblast and K562 targets. It is suggested that this may be mediated by syncytiotrophoblast-derived transferrin, which blocks the transferrin receptors present on both cytotoxic lymphocytes and their targets, thereby preventing membrane interaction between the cells, or by masking the target structures in the recognition process.[209]

Alternatively, maternal antibodies could bind placental antigens,[210] or anti-idiotypic antibodies could bind directly to receptors on cytotoxic cells and prevent them from destroying their targets, although neither mechanism has yet been shown to occur in pregnancy.

Maternal cytotoxic antibodies to fetal antigens could be potentially very harmful if they crossed the placenta and entered the fetal circulation. The villous stroma contains many fetal antigens, as well as Fc receptor positive cells (these include fetal stem vessel endothelium and stromal macrophages),[211] that bind IgG, which is aggregated or complexed to antigen, but unlike syncytiotrophoblast, do not bind native IgG.[212] This binding serves to protect the fetus from immune complexes of maternal antibody and fetal antigens, which may form in situ within the placenta. This is the concept of the placental sponge. It would appear that only maternal IgG antibodies to antigens not represented within placental tissues may escape the sponge and reach the fetal circulation.[213]

The Fetal Immune System

Alloreactive cells would create a problem if they crossed the placental barrier and entered the fetal compartment. But it is disputed whether mother-to-fetus cell traffic takes place. Although maternal cells have not yet been convincingly demonstrated in the fetal circulation, cord blood contains an IgM antibody (ie, of fetal origin) that is directed against maternal alloreactive T cells,[214] to which the fetal immune system must have been exposed. These antibodies specifically inhibit the maternal MLR response and cytotoxic lymphocytes against fetal cells. Cord blood lymphocytes potently suppress the proliferation of adult lymphocytes in a nonspecific way through release of a soluble factor.[215] It can be speculated that these reactions are part of a protective mechanism that is necessary because the fetal immune system is incapable of developing full effector lymphocyte function in terms of cell-mediated lympholysis, although proliferative responses occur in the MLR with maternal cells.[216]

CONCLUSIONS

In normal pregnancy, fetal growth progresses side by side with the development of a number of maternal immune mechanisms that function at several different levels. The major factor that prevents the rejection of the fetus is undoubtedly the lack of normal HLA anti-

TABLE 2–3. IMMUNE ADAPTATIONS THAT MAY REGULATE THE MATERNAL IMMUNE RESPONSE TO THE FETUS

Afferent Blockade

1. Absence of sensitizing antigen on trophoblast
2. Nonspecific immunosuppression
   - Changes in immune cell populations
   - Suppressor factors (placenta, serum, and decidua)

Central Blockade

1. Blocking antibody (anti-fetal HLA, anti-Fc receptor, anti-idiotyopic)
2. Fetal-specific T-suppressor cells

Efferent Blockade

1. Absence of target antigen on trophoblast
2. Blocking antibodies mask fetal antigens
3. Nonspecific suppressor factors (placenta, serum, and decidua)
4. Anti-fetal cytotoxic antibodies adsorbed by placenta
5. Fetal suppressor factors

gen expression by the trophoblast. This feature protects the fetus from both maternal immune recognition and immune attack. There are both local and systemic nonspecific suppressor mechanisms, but these do not significantly impair the mother's ability to fight infection. Where sensitization to paternal HLA does occur, it appears to be a secondary event and neither it, nor the stimulation of suppressor T cells and blocking antibodies, can be regarded as essential to the success of the pregnancy. Traffic of cytotoxic cells to the fetus appears to be restricted, and cytotoxic antibodies are removed by the placenta before they reach the fetal circulation. Therefore, it is the combination of these many immune adaptations of pregnancy that ensure the success of the fetus.

REFERENCES

1. Bulmer JN, Sunderland CA. Immunohistological characterization of lymphoid cell populations in the early human placental bed. Immunology 1984;52:349.
2. Bulmer JN, Johnson PM. Macrophage populations in the human placenta and amniochorion. Clin Exp Immunol 1984; 57:393.
3. Ritson A, Bulmer JN. Endometrial granulocytes in human decidua react with a natural-killer (NK) cell marker, NKH 1. Immunology 1987;62:329.
4. Horwitz DA, Bakke AC. An Fc receptor-bearing third population of human mononuclear cells with cytotoxic and regulatory function. Immunology Today 1984;5:148.
5. Gregory CD, Atkinson ME. Large granular lymphocytes: early non-specific effector cells in allograft rejection in the mouse. Immunology 1984;53:257.
6. Starkey PM, Sargent IL, Redman CWG. Cell populations in human early pregnancy decidua: characterization and isolation of large granular lymphocytes by flow cytometry. Immunology 1988;65:129.
7. King A, Wellings V, Gardner L, Loke YW. Immunocytochemical characterization of the unusual large granular lymphocytes in human endometrium throughout the menstrual cycle. Hum Immunol 1989;24:195.
8. Nehemiah JL, Schnitzer JA, Schulman H, Novikoff AB. Human chorionic trophoblasts, decidual cells and macrophages: a histochemical and electron microscopic study. Am J Obstet Gynecol 1981;140:261.
9. Dorman PJ, Searle RF. Alloantigen presenting capacity of human decidual tissue. J Reprod Immunol 1988;191:101.
10. Douglas GW, Thomas L, Carr M, Cullen M, Morris R. Trophoblast in the circulating blood during pregnancy. Am J Obstet Gynecol 1959;78:960.
11. Kozma R, Spring J, Johnson PM, Adinolfi M. Detection of syncytiotrophoblast in maternal peripheral and uterine veins using a monoclonal antibody and flow cytometry. Hum Reprod 1986;5:335.
12. Thomas L, Douglas GW, Carr M. The continual migration of syncytial trophoblasts from the fetal placenta into the maternal circulation. Trans Assoc Am Phys 1959;72:140.
13. Luz NP, Crottogini JJ, Negrete VS. A method for identification of chorionic villi in peripheral blood of pregnant women. Am J Obstet Gynecol 1966;94:1079.
14. Goodfellow CF, Taylor PV. Extraction and identification of trophoblast cells circulating in peripheral blood during pregnancy. Br J Obstet Gynaecol 1982;89:65.
15. Goodfellow CF, Taylor PV, Jackson S. Culturing trophoblast from peripheral blood. Lancet 1984;ii:1479.
16. Covone AE, Mutton D, Johnson PM, Adinolfi M. Trophoblast cells in peripheral blood from pregnant women. Lancet 1984;ii:841.
17. Pool C, Aplin JD, Taylor GM, Boyd RDH. Trophoblast cells and maternal blood. Lancet 1987;i:804.
18. Covone AE, Kozma R, Johnson PM, Latt S, Adinolfi M. Analysis of peripheral maternal blood samples for the presence of placenta-derived cells using Y-specific probes and McAb H315. Prenat Diagn 1988;8:591.
19. Bertero MT, Camaschella C, Serra A, Bergui L, Caligaris-Cappio F. Circulating 'trophoblast' cells in pregnancy have maternal genetic markers. Prenat Diagn 1988;8:585.
20. Attwood HD, Park WW. Embolism to the lungs by trophoblast. J Obstet Gynaecol Br Commonwealth 1961;68:611.
21. Cameron HM, Park WW. Decidual tissue within the lung. J Obstet Gynaecol Br Commonwealth 1965;72:748.
22. Zipursky A, Pollock J, Neelands P, Chown B, Israels LG. The transplacental passage of foetal red blood-cells and the pathogenesis of Rh immunization during pregnancy. Lancet 1963;ii:489.
23. Woodrow JC, Finn R. Transplacental haemorrhage. Br J Haematol 1966;12:297.
24. Fairweather DVI, Walker W. Obstetrical considerations in the routine use of amniocentesis in immunized Rh negative women. J Obstet Gynaecol Br Commonwealth 1964;71:48.
25. Samet S, Bowman HS. Fetomaternal ABO incompatibility: intravascular hemolysis, fetal hemoglobinemia and fibrinogenopenia in maternal circulation. Am J Obstet Gynecol 1961;81:49.
26. Walknowska J, Conte FA, Grumbach MM. Practical and theoretical implications of fetal/maternal lymphocyte transfer. Lancet 1969;i:1119.
27. Schroder J, Tiilikainen A, de la Chapelle A. Fetal leukocytes in the maternal circulation after delivery. Transplantation 1975;17:346.
28. Herzenberg LA, Bianchi DW, Schroder J, Cann HM, Iverson GM. Fetal cells in the blood of pregnant women: detection and enrichment by fluorescence-activated cell sorting. Proc Natl Acad Sci USA 1979;76:1453.
29. Adinolfi M, Gorvette DP. The transfer of lymphocytes through the human placenta. In: Centaro A, Carretti N, eds. Immunology in obstetrics and gynaecology. London: Excerpta Medica, 1973:177.
30. Dohr GA, Motter W, Leitinger S, et al. Lack of expression of HLA class I and class II molecules on the human oocyte. J Immunol 1987;138:3766.
31. Dohr GA. HLA and TLX antigen expression on the human oocyte, zona pellucida and granulosa cells. Hum Reprod 1987;2:657.
32. Motter W, Dohr G, Desoye G, Pusch HH, Winter R, Ziegler A. Absence of HLA class I and class II antigens from human spermatozoa, oocytes and preimplantation embryos. J Reprod Immunol Suppl 1986:38.
33. Faulk WP, Temple A. Distribution of $\beta 2$ microglobulin and HLA in chorionic villi of human placentae. Nature 1976; 262:799.
34. Goodfellow PN, Barnstable CJ, Bodmer WF, Snary D, Crumpton MJ. Expression of HLA system antigens on placenta. Transplantation 1976;22:595.
35. Sunderland CA, Naiem M, Mason DY, Redman CWG, Stirrat GM. The expression of major histo-compatibility antigens by human chorionic villi. J Reprod Immunol 1981;3:323.
36. Hunt JS, Fishback JL, Andrews GK, Wood GW. Expression of class I HLA genes by trophoblast cells. Analysis by in situ hybridization. J Immunol 1988;140:1293.

37. Sunderland CA, Redman CWG, Stirrat GM. HLA A,B,C antigens are expressed on nonvillous trophoblast of the early human placenta. J Immunol 1981;127:2614.
38. Redman CWG, McMichael AJ, Stirrat GM, Sunderland CA, Ting A. Class 1 major histocompatibility antigens on human extra-villous trophoblast. Immunology 1984;52:457.
39. Hsi BL, Yeh CJ, Faulk WP. Class 1 antigens of the major histocompatibility complex on cytotrophoblast of human chorion leave. Immunology 1984;52:621.
40. Wells M, Hsi BL, Faulk WP. Class 1 antigens of the major histocompatibility complex on cytotrophoblast of the human placental basal plate. Am J Reprod Immunol 1984;6:167.
41. Hunt JS, Lessin DL, King CR. Ontogeny and distribution of cells expressing HLA-B locus-specific determinants in the placenta and extraplacental membranes. J Reprod Immunol 1989;15:21.
42. Ellis SA, Sargent IL, Redman CWG, McMichael AJ. Evidence for a novel HLA antigen on human extra-villous trophoblast and a choriocarcinoma cell line. Immunology 1986;59:595.
43. Ellis SA, Palmer MS, McMichael AJ. Human trophoblast and the choriocarcinoma cell line BeWo express a truncated HLA Class 1 molecule. J Immunol 1990;144:731.
44. Geraghty DE, Koller BH, Orr HT. A human MHC Class 1 gene that encodes a protein with a shortened cytoplasmic segment. Proc Natl Acad Sci USA 1987;84:9145.
45. Galbraith RM, Kantor RRS, Ferrara GB, Ades EW, Galbraith GMP. Differential anatomical expression of transplantation antigens within the normal human placental chorionic villus. Am J Reprod Immunol 1981;1:331.
46. Starkey PM. Reactivity of human trophoblast with and antibody to the HLA class II antigen, HLA-DP. J Reprod Immunol 1987;11:63.
47. Sutton L, Mason DY, Redman CWG. HLA-DR positive cells in the human placenta. Immunology 1983;49:103.
48. Sutton L, Gadd M, Mason DY, Redman CWG. Cells-bearing class II MHC antigens in the human placenta. Immunology 1986;58:23.
49. Johnson PM. Immunobiology of the human trophoblast. In: Crighton DB, ed. Immunological aspects of reproduction in mammals. London: Butterworths, 1984:1091.
50. Johnson PM, Cheng HM, Molloy CM, Stern CMM, Slade MB. Human trophoblast-specific surface antigens identified using monoclonal antibodies. Am J Reprod Immunol 1981;1:246.
51. Kajino T, McIntyre JA, Faulk WP. Antigens of human trophoblast: trophoblast-lymphocyte cross-reactive antigens on platelets. Am J Reprod Immunol 1987;14:70.
52. McIntyre JA. In search of trophoblast-lymphocyte crossreactive (TLX) antigens. Am J Reprod Immunol 1988;17:100.
53. McIntyre JA, Faulk WP. Allotypic trophoblast-lymphocyte cross-reactive (TLX) cell surface antigens. Hum Immunol 1982;4:27.
54. Purcell DFJ, McKenzie IFC, Johnson PM, Lublin DM, Atkinson JP, Deacon NJ. CD46 (HuLy-m5) antigen of humans includes the trophoblast-leucocyte antigen (TLX) and the membrane cofactor protein (MCP) of complement. J Reprod Immunol Suppl 1989;207.
55. Purcell DFJ, Brown MA, Russell SM, Clark GJ, McKenzie IFC, Deacon NJ. The cDNA cloning of human CD46, an antigen system incorporating TLX and MCP; existence of multiple alternative splice variants. J Reprod Immunol Suppl 1989;207.
56. Faulk WP, Yeager C, McIntyre JA, Ueda M. Oncofoetal antigens of human trophoblast. Proc R Soc Lond [Biol] 1979;206:163.
57. Hamilton TA, Wada HG, Sussman HH. Expression of human placental cell surface antigens on peripheral blood lymphocytes and lymphoblastoid cell lines. Scand J Immunol 1980;11:195.
58. Loke YW, Whyte A, Davies SP. Differential expression of trophoblast-specific membrane antigens by normal and abnormal human placentae and by neoplasms of trophoblastic and non-trophoblastic origin. Int J Cancer 1980;25:459.
59. Shah LCP, Ogbimi AO, Johnson PM. A cell membrane antigen expressed by both human breast carcinoma cells and normal human trophoblast. Placenta 1980;1:299.
60. Beral V. Parity and susceptibility to cancer. In: Fetal antigens and cancer. Ciba Foundation Symposium 96. London, Pitman, 1983:182.
61. Stirrat GM, Sunderland CA, Redman CWG. Human reproductive immunology — elucidation by monoclonal antibody techniques. Obstet Gynecol Annu 1983;12:43.
62. Harris H. Multilocus enzyme systems and the evolution of gene expression: the alkaline phosphatases as a model example. The Harvey Lectures 1982;76:95.
63. Galbraith GMP, Galbraith RM, Temple A, Faulk WP. Demonstration of transferring receptors on human placental trophoblast. Blood 1980;55:240.
64. Bulmer JN, Morrison L, Johnson PM. Expression of the proliferation markers Ki67 and transferring receptor by human trophoblast populations. J Reprod Immunol 1988;14:291.
65. Hole N, Stern PL. A 72kD trophoblast glycoprotein defined by a monoclonal antibody. Br J Cancer 1988;57:239.
66. Feizi T. Demonstration by monoclonal antibodies that carbohydrate structures of glycoproteins and glycolipids are oncodevelopmental antigens. Nature 1985;314:53.
67. Hook M, Kjellen L, Johansson S, Robinson J. Cell-surface glycosaminoglans. Ann Rev Biochem 1984;53:847.
68. Comper WD, Laurent TC. Physiological function of connective tissue polysaccharides. Physiol Rev 1978;58:255.
69. Sunderland CA, Bulmer JN, Luscombe M, Redman CWG, Stirrat GM. Immunohistological and biochemical evidence for a role for hyaluronic acid in the growth and development of the placenta. J Reprod Immunol 1986;8:197.
70. Toole BP, Biswasd C, Gross B. Hyaluronate and invasiveness of the rabbit V2 carcinoma. Proc Natl Acad Sci USA 1979;76:6299.
71. Overweg J, Engelfriet CP. Cytotoxic leucocyte iso-antibodies formed during the first pregnancy. Vox Sang 1969;16:97.
72. Ahrons S. HLA-A antibodies: influence on the human foetus. Tissue Antigens 1971;1:121.
73. Winchester RJ, Fu SM, Wernet P, Kunkel HG, Dupont B, Jersild C. Recognition by pregnancy of non-HLA alloantigens selectively expressed on B lymphocytes. J Exp Med 1975;141:924.
74. Borelli I, Amoroso A, Richiardi P, Curtoni ES. Evaluation of different technical approaches for the research of human anti-Ia alloantisera. Tissue Antigens 1982;19:380.
75. Van der Werf AJM. Are lymphocytotoxic iso-antibodies produced by the early human trophoblast? Lancet 1971;i:595.
76. Nakajima H, Mano Y, Tokunaga E, Nozue G. Influence of previous pregnancy on maternal response to foetal antigens. Tissue Antigens 1982;19:92.
77. Regan L, Braude PR. Is antipaternal cytotoxic antibody a valid marker in the management of recurrent abortion? Lancet 1987;ii:1280.
78. Van Rood GG, Eernisse G, Van Leuween A. Leucocyte antibodies in sera from pregnant women. Nature 1958;181:1735.
79. Vives J, Gelabert A, Castillo R. HLA antibodies and period of gestation: decline in frequency of positive sera during last trimester. Tissue Antigens 1976;7:209.
80. Carr MC, Stites DP, Fudenberg HH. Cellular immune aspects of the human fetal-maternal relationship. 3. Mixed lymphocyte reactivity between related maternal and cord blood lymphocytes. Cell Immunol 1974;11:332.
81. Herva E, Tiilikainen A. Mixed lymphocyte culture reactions at delivery and in the puerperium. Effects of parity, HLA antigens and maternal serum. Acta Pathol Microbiol Scand [C] 1977;85:333.

82. Moen T, Moen M, Palbo V, Thorsby E. In vitro foeto-maternal lymphocyte responses at delivery: no gross changes in MLC and PLT responsiveness. J Reprod Immunol 1980;2:213.
83. Genetet N, Genetet B, Amice V, Fauchet R. Allogenic responses in vitro induced by fetomaternal alloimmunisation. Am J Reprod Immunol 1982;2:90.
84. Sargent IL, Redman CWG, Stirrat GM. Maternal cell-mediated immunity in normal and pre-eclamptic pregnancy. Clin Exp Immunol 1982;50:601.
85. Moore MP, Sargent IL, Ting A, Redman CWG. Maternal cell-mediated immunity in pregnancy — lymphocyte responses of mothers and their non-pregnant HLA identical sisters to paternal HLA. Clin Exp Immunol 1983;54:91.
86. Sargent IL, Arenas J, Redman CWG. Maternal cell-mediated sensitization to paternal HLA may occur but is not a regular event in normal human pregnancy. J Reprod Immunol 1987;10:111.
87. Sargent IL, Wilkins T, Redman CWG. Maternal immune responses to the fetus in early pregnancy and recurrent miscarriage. Lancet 1988;ii:1099.
88. Doughty RW, Gelsthorpe K. An initial investigation of lymphocyte antibody activity through pregnancy and in eluates prepared from placental material. Tissue Antigens 1974;4:291.
89. Doughty RW, Gelsthorpe K. Some parameters of lymphocyte antibody activity through pregnancy and further eluates of placental material. Tissue Antigens 1976;8:43.
90. McCormick JN, Faulk WP, Fox H, Fudenberg HH. Immunohistological and elution studies of the human placenta. J Exp Med 1971;133:1.
91. Brochier J, Bonneau M, Robert M, Sambrut C, Revillard JP, Traeger J. Anti-HLA-DR alloantibodies eluted from human placental tissue. Transplant Proc 1979;11:779.
92. Kajino T, McIntyre JA, Faulk WP, Cai DS, Billington WD. Antibodies to trophoblast in normal pregnant and secondary aborting women. J Reprod Immunol 1988;14:267.
93. Faulk WP, Jeannet J, Creighton WS, Carbonara A. Characterization of immunoglobulins on trophoblastic basement membranes. J Clin Invest 1974;54:1011.
94. Davies M. An ELISA for the detection of maternal anti-trophoblast antibodies in human pregnancy. J Immunol Methods 1985;77:109.
95. Davies M. Antigenic analysis of immune complexes formed in normal human pregnancy. Clin Exp Immunol 1985;61:406.
96. Davies M, Browne CM. Anti-trophoblast antibody responses during normal pregnancy. J Reprod Immunol 1985;7:285.
97. Nicklin DA, Sutcliffe RG. A search for antibodies in term maternal sera to solubilized syncytiotrophoblast surface components. A passive haemagglutination assay yields negative evidence. J Reprod Immunol 1986;9:303.
98. Johnson PM, Cheng HM, Stevens VC, Matangkasombut P. Antibody reactivity against trophoblast and trophoblast products. J Reprod Immunol 1985;8:347.
99. Hole N, Cheng HM, Johnson PM. Antibody reactivity against human trophoblast membrane antigens in the context of normal pregnancy and unexplained recurrent miscarriage? In: Chaouat G, ed. Reproductive immunology: materno-fetal relationship. Paris, INSERM, 1987:213.
100. Loke YW. Human trophoblast antigens. In: Stern CMM, ed. Immunology of pregnancy and its disorders. Lancaster, UK: Kluwer, 1989:61.
101. Chavez DJ, McIntyre JA. Sera from women with histories of repeated pregnancy losses cause abnormalities in mouse preimplantation blastocysts. J Reprod Immunol 1984;6:273.
102. Oksenberg JR, Brautbar C. In vitro suppression of murine blastocysts growth by sera from women with reproductive disorders. Am J Reprod Immunol 1986;11:118.
103. King A, Birkby C, Loke YW. Early human decidual cells exhibit NK activity against the K562 cell line but not against first trimester trophoblast. Cell Immunol 1989;118:337.
104. Ferry B, Starkey PM, Sargent IL, Watt GO, Jackson M, Redman CWG. Cell populations in the human early pregnancy decidua: natural killer activity and response to interleukin-2 of NKH-positive large granular lymphocytes. Immunology 1990;70:446.
105. Ferry BL, Sargent IL, Starkey PM, Redman CWG. Cytotoxic activity against trophoblast and choriocarcinoma cells of large granular lymphocytes from human early pregnancy decidua. Cellular Immunology 1990;142:140.
106. Szerkeres Bartho J, Nemeth A, Varga P, Csernus V, Koszegi T, Paal M. Membrane fluidity of trophoblast cells and susceptibility to natural cytotoxicity. Am J Reprod Immunol 1989;19:92.
107. Paul S, Jailkhani BL. Lysis of placental syncytiotrophoblast by allogeneic leukocytes in vitro: effects of neuraminidase and chorionic gonadotrophins. Am J Reprod Immunol 1982;2:204.
108. Youtananukorn V, Matangkasombut P, Osathanondh V. Onset of human maternal cell-mediated immune reaction to placental antigens during the first pregnancy. Clin Exp Immunol 1974;16:593.
109. Stimson WH, Strachan AF, Shepherd A. Studies on the maternal immune response to placental antigens: absence of a blocking factor from the blood of abortion-prone women. Br J Obstet Gynaecol 1979;86:41.
110. Khalfoun B, Degenne D, Crouzat-Reynes G, Bardos P. Effect of human syncytiotrophoblast plasma membrane-soluble extracts on in vitro mitogen-induced lymphocyte proliferation. A possible inhibition mechanism involving the transferrin receptor. J Immunol 1986;137:1187.
111. Paul S, Jailkhani BL. Failure of placental syncytiotrophoblast to provoke allogeneic recognition by lymphocytes in vitro. Indian J Exp Biol 1982;20:248.
112. Sargent IL, Redman CWG. Maternal immune responses to the fetus in human pregnancy. In: Stern CMM, ed. Immunology of pregnancy and its disorders. Dordrecht, Kluwer, 1989:115.
113. Hunt JS, King CR, Wood GW. Evaluation of human chorionic trophoblast cells and placental macrophages as stimulators of maternal lymphocyte proliferation in vitro. J Reprod Immunol 1984;6:377.
114. Toder V, Blank M, Nebel L. Trophoblast cells do not provide the 'second' signal for CTL generation. Am J Reprod Immunol 1984;6:58.
115. Larsen B, Galask RP. Host-parasite interactions during pregnancy. Obstet Gynecol Surv 1978;33:297.
116. Khuroo MS, Teli MR, Skidmore S, Sofi MA, Khuroo MI. Incidence and severity of viral hepatitis in pregnancy. Am J Med 1981;70:252.
117. Brown ZA, Vontver LA, Benedetti J, et al. Genital herpes in pregnancy: risk factors associated with recurrences and asymptomatic viral shedding. Am J Obstet Gynecol 1985;153:24.
118. Sakamoto K, Greally J, Gilfillan RF, et al. Epstein-Barr virus in normal pregnant women. Am J Reprod Immunol 1982;2:217.
119. Gehrz RC, Christianson WR, Linner KM, Conroy, MM, McCue SA, Balfour HH. A longitudinal analysis of lymphocyte proliferative responses to mitogens and antigens during human pregnancy. Am J Obstet Gynecol 1981;140:665.
120. Gehrz RC, Christianson WR, Linner KM, Conroy, MM, McCue SA, Balfour HH. Cytomegalovirus-specific humoral and cellular immune responses in human pregnancy. J Infect Dis 1981;143:391.
121. Strelkauskas AJ, Davies IJ, Dray S. Longitudinal studies showing alterations in the levels and functional response of T and B lymphocytes in human pregnancy. Clin Exp Immunol 1978;32:531.
122. Brunham RC, Martin DH, Hubbard TW, et al. Depression of the

lymphocyte transformation response to microbial antigens and to phytohemagglutinin during pregnancy. J Clin Invest 1983;72:1629.
123. Sulke AN, Jones DB, Wood PJ. Variation in natural killer activity in peripheral blood during the menstrual cycle. Br Med J 1985;290:884.
124. Sulke AN, Jones DB, Wood PJ. Hormonal modulation of human natural killer activity in vitro. J Reprod Immunol 1985;7:105.
125. Uksila J. Human NK cell activity is not inhibited by pregnancy and cord serum factors and female steroid hormones in vitro. J Reprod Immunol 1985;7:111.
126. Baines MG, Pross HF, Millar KG. Spontaneous human lymphocyte-mediated cytotoxicity against tumour target cells. IV: the suppressive effect of normal pregnancy. Am J Obstet Gynecol 1978;130:741.
127. Toder V, Nebel L, Gleicher N. Studies of natural killer cells in pregnancy. I: analysis at the single cell level. J Clin Lab Immunol 1984;14:123.
128. Lee H, Gregory CD, Rees GB, Scott IV, Golding PR. Cytotoxic activity and phenotypic analysis of natural killer cells in early normal human pregnancy. J Reprod Immunol 1987;12:35.
129. Okamura K, Fuurukawa K, Nakakuki M, Yamada K, Suzuki M. Natural killer cell activity during pregnancy. Am J Obstet Gynecol 1984;149:396.
130. Baley JE, Schacter BZ. Mechanisms of diminished natural killer cell activity in pregnant women and neonates. J Immunol 1985;134:3042.
131. Gregory CD, Shah LP, Lee H, Scott IV, Golding PR. Cytotoxic reactivity of human natural killer (NK) cells during normal pregnancy: a longitudinal study. J Clin Lab Immunol 1985;18:175.
132. Iwatani Y, Amino N, Tachi N, et al. Changes of lymphocyte subsets in normal pregnant and postpartum women: postpartum increase of NK/K (Leu 7) cells. Am J Reprod Immunol Microbiol 1987;18:52.
133. Gregory CD, Lee H, Rees GB, Scott IV, Shah LP, Golding PR. Natural killer cells in normal pregnancy: analysis using monoclonal antibodies and single cell cytotoxicity assays. Clin Exp Immunol 1985;62:121.
134. Gonik B, Loo LS, West S, Kohl S. Natural killer cytotoxicity and antibody-dependent cellular cytotoxicity to herpes simplex virus-infected cells in human pregnancy. Am J Reprod Immunol 1987;13:23.
135. Kohl S, Shaban SS, Starr SE, Wood PA, Nahmias AJ. Human neonatal and maternal monocyte-macrophage and lymphocyte-mediated antibody-dependent cytotoxicity to cells infected with herpes simplex. J Pediatr 1978;93:206.
136. Lucivero G, Selvaggi L, Dell'osso A, et al. Mononuclear cell subpopulations during normal pregnancy. I: analysis of cell surface markers using conventional techniques and monoclonal antibodies. Am J Reprod Immunol 1983;4:142.
137. Moore MP, Carter NP, Redman CWG. Lymphocyte subsets defined by monoclonal antibodies in human pregnancy. Am J Reprod Immunol 1983;3:161.
138. Vanderbeeken Y, Vlieghe MP, Delespesse G, Duchateau J. Characterization of immunoregulatory T cells during pregnancy by monoclonal antibodies. Clin Exp Immunol 1982;48:118.
139. Sridama V, Pacini F, Yang SL, Moawad A, Reilly M, DeGroot LJ. Decreased levels of helper T cells. A possible cause of immunodeficiency in pregnancy. N Engl J Med 1982;307:352.
140. Castilla, JA, Rueda R, Vargas ML, Gonzalez-Gomez F, Garcia-Olivares E. Decreased levels of circulating CD4+ T lymphocytes during normal pregnancy. J Reprod Immunol 1989;15:103.
141. Milns NR, Gardner ID. Maternal T cells and human pregnancy outcome. J Reprod Immunol 1989;15:175.
142. Cheney RT, Tomaszewski JE, Rabb SJ, Zmijewski C, Rowlands DT. Subpopulations of lymphocytes in maternal peripheral blood during pregnancy. J Reprod Immunol 1984;6:111.
143. Virag I, Schecter E, Elgat M, Zakut H, Meyetes D. Lymphocyte subsets in habitual abortion. Am J Reprod Immunol 1986;12:7.
144. Duc HT, Masse A, Bobe P, Kinsky RG, Voisin GA. Deviation of humoral and cellular alloimmune reactions by placental extracts. J Reprod Immunol 1985;7:27.
145. Remacle-Bonnett MM, Rance RJ, Depieds RC. Non-specific immunoregulatory factors in the cytosol fraction of human trophoblast. J Reprod Immunol 1983;5:123.
146. Matsuzaki N, Okadan T, Kameda T, Negoro T, Saji F, Tanizawa O. Trophoblast-derived immunoregulatory factor: demonstration of the biological function and the physiochemical characteristics of the factor derived from choriocarcinoma cell lines. Am J Reprod Immunol Microbiol 1989;19:121.
147. Rubenstein A, Koren Z, Murphy RA. Suppression of maternal lymphocyte mitogenic responses by supernatants from short term placental cell cultures. Am J Reprod Immunol 1982;2:260.
148. Saji F, Koyama M, Kameda T, Negoro T, Nakamuro K, Tanizawa O. Effect of a soluble factor secreted from cultured human trophoblast cells on in vitro lymphocyte reactions. Am J Reprod Immunol Microbiol 1987;13:121.
149. Murray MK, Segerson EC, Hansen PJ, Bazer FW, Roberts RM. Suppression of lymphocyte activation by a high-molecular-weight glycoprotein released from preimplantation ovine and porcine conceptuses. Am J Reprod Immunol Microbiol 1987;14:38.
150. Newton GR, Vallet JL, Hansen PJ, Bazer FW. Inhibition of lymphocyte proliferation by ovine trophoblast protein-1 and a high molecular weight glycoprotein produced by the peri-implantation sheep conceptus. Am J Reprod Immunol 1989;19:99.
151. Daya S, Lee S, Underwood J, Mowbray, J, Craft I, Clark DA. Prediction of outcome following transfer of in vitro fertilized human embryos by measurement of embryo-associated suppressor factor. In: Clark DA, Croy BA. eds. Reproductive immunology 1986. Amsterdam, Elsevier, 1986:277.
152. Menu E, Chaouat G. Human placental supernatant and IL-2 and IL-4 dependent cell proliferation. J Reprod Immunol Suppl 1989;149.
153. Jha P, Talwar GP, Hingorani V. Depression of blast transformation of peripheral leucocytes by plasma from pregnant women. Am J Obstet Gynecol 1975;122:965.
154. St Hill CA, Finn P, Denye V. Depression of cellular immunity in pregnancy due to a serum factor. Br Med J 1973;3:513.
155. Davis M, Browne CM. Pregnancy associated nonspecific immunosuppression: kinetics of the generation and identification of an active factor. Am J Reprod Immunol Microbiol 1985;9:77.
156. Ricketts RM, Jones DB. Differential effect of human chorionic gonadotrophin on lymphocyte proliferation induced by mitogens. J Reprod Immunol 1985;7:225.
157. Szekeres-Bartho J, Csernus V, Pejtsik B, Emody L, Pasca AS. Progesterone as an immunologic blocking factor in pregnancy serum. J Reprod Immunol 1981;33:333.
158. Szekeres-Bartho J, Csernus V, Hadnagy J, Pacsa AS. Progesterone-prostaglandin balance influences lymphocyte function in relation to pregnancy. Am J Reprod Immunol 1983;4:139.
159. Nicholas NS, Panayi GS. Inhibition of interleukin 2 production by retroplacental sera: a possible mechanism for human fetal allograft survival. Am J Reprod Immunol Microbiol 1985;9:6.
160. Fuchs T, Hammarstrom L, Smith E, Brundi J. In vivo suppression of uterine lymphocytes during early human pregnancy. Acta Obstet Gynecol Scand 1977;56:151.
161. Lu CY, Changelian PS, Unanue ER. α-Fetoprotein inhibits macrophage expression of Ia antigens. J Immunol 1984;132:1722.
162. Harris SJ, Anthony FW, Jones DB, Masson GM. Pregnancy-

specific-β1-glycoprotein: effect on lymphocyte proliferation in vitro. J Reprod Immunol 1984;6:267.
163. Stimson WH. Immunosuppressive effect of pregnancy-associated α2-macroglobulin. Lancet 1975;ii:989.
164. Fizet D, Bousquet J, Piquet Y, Cabantous F. Identification of a factor blocking a cellular cytotoxicity reaction in pregnant serum. Clin Exp Immunol 1983;52:648.
165. Noonan FP, Halliday WJ, Morton H, Clunie GJA. Early pregnancy factor is immunosuppressive. Nature 1979;278:649.
166. Morgan DML, Illei G. Polyamine-polyamine oxidase interaction: part of maternal protective mechanism against fetal rejection. Br Med J 1980;280:1295.
167. Fizet D, Bousquet J. Absence of a factor blocking a cellular cytotoxicity reaction in the serum of women with recurrent abortions. Br J Obstet Gynaecol 1983;90:453.
168. Barrett DS, Rayfield LS, Brent L. Suppression of natural cell-mediated cytotoxicity in man by maternal and neonatal serum. Clin Exp Immunol 1982;47:742.
169. Clark DA, Slapsys AR, Chaput A, et al. Immunoregulatory molecules of trophoblast and decidual suppressor cell origin at the materno-fetal interface. Am J Reprod Immunol 1986;10:100.
170. Clark DA, Brierly J, Slapsys R, et al. Trophoblast-dependent and trophoblast independent suppressor cells of maternal origin in murine and human decidua. In: Clark DA, Croy BA, eds. Reproductive immunology 1986. Amsterdam, Elsevier, 1986:219.
171. Badet MT, Bell SC, Billington WD. Immunoregulatory activity of supernatants from short term cultures of mouse decidual tissue. J Reprod Fertil 1985;68:351.
172. Badet MT. Comparative study of biological properties of proteins synthesized in vitro by murine decidua and deciduoma. Am J Reprod Immunol Microbiol 1986;10:20.
173. Golander G, Zakuth V, Schechter Y, Spirer Z. Suppression of lymphocyte reactivity in vitro by a soluble factor secreted by explants of human decidua. Eur J Immunol 1981;11:849.
174. Nakayama E, Asano S, Kodo H, Muira S. Suppression of mixed lymphocyte reaction by cells of human first trimester pregnancy endometrium. J Reprod Immunol 1985;8:25.
175. Daya S, Clark DA, Devlin C, Jarrell J, Chaput A. Suppressor cells in human decidua. Am J Obstet Gynecol 1985;151:267.
176. Daya S, Clark DA, Devlin C, Jarrell J. Preliminary characterization of two types of suppressor cells in the human uterus. Fertil Steril 1985;44:778.
177. Clark DA, Mowbray J, Underwood J, Liddel H. Histopathologic alterations in the decidua in human spontaneous abortion: loss of cells with large cytoplasmic granules. Am J Reprod Immunol Microbiol 1987;13:19.
178. Pockley AG, Mowles EA, Stocker RJ, Westwood OMR, Chapman MG, Bolton AE. Suppression of in vitro lymphocyte reactivity to phytohemagglutinin by placental protein 14. J Reprod Immunol 1988;13:31.
179. Lala PK, Kennedy TG, Parhar RS. Suppression of lymphocyte alloreactivity by early gestational human decidua. II: characterization of the suppressor mechanisms. Cell Immunol 1988;116:411.
180. Parhar RS, Kennedy TG, Lala PK. Suppression of lymphocyte alloreactivity by early gestational human decidua. I: characterization of suppressor cells and suppressor molecules. Cell Immunol 1988;116:392.
181. Clark DA, Falbo M, Rowley RB, Banwatt D, Stedronska-Clark J. Active suppression of host-vs-graft reaction in pregnant mice. IX: soluble, suppressor activity obtained from allopregnant mouse decidua that blocks the cytolytic effector response to IL-2 is related to transforming growth factor-beta. J Immunol 1988;141:3833.
182. Sporn MB, Roberts AB, Wakefield FM, Assoian RK. Transforming growth-beta: biological function and chemical structure. Science 1986;233:532.
183. Frolik CA, Dart LL, Meyers CA, Smith DM, Sporn MB. Purification and initial characterization of a type beta transforming growth factor from human placenta. Proc Natl Acad Sci USA 1983;80:3676.
184. Bissenden JG, Ling NR, Mackintosh P. Suppression of mixed lymphocyte reactions by pregnancy serum. Clin Exp Immunol 1980;39:195.
185. Herva E, Jouppila P. Mixed lymphocyte culture reactions between parental cells in pregnancy and puerperium. Acta Pathol Microbiol Scand [C] 1977;85:99.
186. Robert M, Betuel H, Revillard JP. Inhibition of the mixed lymphocyte reaction by sera from multipara. Tissue Antigens 1973;3:39.
187. Greenberg LJ, Reinsmoen N, Yunis EJ. Dissociation of stimulation [MLR-S] in mixed leukocyte culture by serum blocking factors. Transplantation 1973;16:520.
188. Robert M, Betuel H, Revillard JP. Inhibition of the mixed lymphocyte reaction by sera from multipara. Tissue Antigens 1973;3:39.
189. Brochier J, Roitt IM, Festenstein H. Inhibition of lymphocyte proliferative responses by anti-HL-A-alloantisera. Eur J Immunol 1974;4:709.
190. Faulk WP, Jeannet M, Creighton WD, Carbonara A. Immunological studies of the human placenta. J Clin Invest 1974;54:1011.
191. Jeannet M, Werner C, Ramirez E, Vassalli P, Faulk WP. Anti-HLA, anti-human "Ia-like" and MLC blocking activity of human placental IgG. Transplant Proc 1977;9:1417.
192. Kajino T, Kanazawa K, Takeuchi S. Blocking effects of maternal serum IgG and placental eluate IgG on materno-fetal mixed lymphocyte reaction and their individual specificity. Am J Reprod Immunol 1985;4:27.
193. Power DA, Catto GRD, Mason RJ, et al. The fetus as an allograft: evidence for protective antibodies to HLA-linked paternal antigens. Lancet 1983;ii:701.
194. MacLeod AM, Mason RJ, Stewart KN, et al. Fc-receptor-blocking antibodies develop after blood transfusions and correlate with good graft outcome. Transplant Proc 1983;15:1019.
195. McIntyre JA, Faulk WP. Maternal blocking factors in human pregnancy are found in plasma not serum. Lancet 1979;ii:821.
196. Jonker M, Van Leeuwen A, Van Rood JJ. Inhibition of the mixed leukocyte reaction by alloantisera in man. II: incidence and characteristics of MLC-inhibiting antisera from multiparous women. Tissue Antigens 1977;9:246.
197. Takakuwa K, Kanazawa K, Takeuchi S. Production of blocking antibodies by vaccination with husband's lymphocytes in unexplained recurrent abortion: the role in successful pregnancy. Am J Reprod Immunol Microbiol 1986;10:1.
198. Burke J, Johnasen K. The formation of HLA antibodies in pregnancy. The antigenicity of aborted and term fetuses. J Obstet Gynaecol Br Commonwealth 1974;81:222.
199. Singal DP, Butler L, Liao SK, Joseph S. The fetus as an allograft: evidence for anti-idiotypic antibodies induced by pregnancy. Am J Reprod Immunol 1984;6:145.
200. Sucia-Foca N, Reed E, Rohowsky C, Kung P, King DW. Anti-idiotypic antibodies to anti-HLA receptors induced by pregnancy. Proc Natl Acad Sci USA 1983;80:830.
201. Singal DP, Fagnilli L, Joseph S. Blood transfusions induce anti-idiotypic antibodies in renal transplant patients. Transplant Proc 1983;15:1005.
202. McMichael AJ, Sasazuki T. A suppressor T cell in the human mixed lymphocyte reaction. J Exp Med 1977;146:368.
203. Kovithavongs T, Dossetor JB. Suppressor cells in human pregnancy. Transplantation 1978;10:911.

204. Bonnard GD, Lemos L. The cellular immunity of mother versus child at delivery: sensitization in unidirectional mixed lymphocyte culture and subsequent 51Cr release cytotoxicity test. Transplant Proc 1972;4:177.
205. Granberg C, Hirvonen T, Toivanen P. Cell-mediated lympholysis by human maternal and neonatal lymphocytes: mother's reactivity against neonatal cells and vice versa. J Immunol 1979;123:2563.
206. Szerkeres-Bartho J, Hadnagy J, Pacsa AS. The suppressive effect of progesterone on lymphocyte cytotoxicity: unique progesterone sensitivity of pregnancy lymphocytes. J Reprod Immunol 1985;7:121.
207. Kolb JP, Chaouat G, Chassoux D. Immunoactive products of placenta. III: suppression of natural killing activity. J Immunol 1984;132:2305.
208. Degenne D, Khalfoun B, Bardes P. In vitro inhibitory effect of human syncytiotrophoblast plasma membrane on the cytolytic activities of CTL and NK cells. Am J Reprod Immunol 1986;12:106.
209. Taylor PV, Hancock KW. Antigenicity of trophoblast and possible antigen masking effects during pregnancy. Immunology 1975;28:973.
210. Johnson PM, Faulk WP, Wang C. Immunological studies of human placentae: subclass and fragment specificity of binding of aggregated IgG by placental endothelial cells. Immunology 1976;31:659.
211. Wood GW, Bjerrum K, Johnson B. Detection of IgG bound within human trophoblast. J Immunol 1982;129:1479.
212. Johnson PM, Brown PJ. Fc receptors in the human placenta. Placenta 1981;2:355.
213. Tongio MM, Mayer S, Lebec A. Transfer of HLA antibodies from the mother to the child. Transplantation 1975;20:163.
214. Miyagawa Y. Further characterization of IgM antibodies against maternal alloreactive T cells produced by clonal Epstein Barr virus transformed cord B cells. J Immunol 1984;133:1270.
215. Jacoby DR, Olding LB, Oldstone MB. Immunologic regulation of fetal-maternal balance. Adv Immunol 1984;35:157.
216. Rayfield LS, Brent L, Rodeck CH. Development of cell-mediated lympholysis in human fetal blood lymphocytes. Clin Exp Immunol 1980;42:561.

3

CHAPTER

NORMAL EMBRYONIC AND FETAL DEVELOPMENT

Jean C. Hay and T. V. N. Persaud

This chapter is a synopsis of the main events in normal human development. The reader should consult the references[1–10] for a more detailed discussion of individual topics.

THE FIRST WEEK

Fertilization normally occurs in the ampulla of the uterine tube and results in the formation of a diploid cell, the zygote (Fig. 3-1). The zygote, still surrounded by the zona pellucida, undergoes cleavage or mitotic divisions to form blastomeres. Contraction of smooth muscle in the wall of the uterine tube propels the dividing zygote toward the uterine cavity. About day 3, the morula, composed of approximately 16 blastomeres, enters the uterine cavity. Fluid from the uterine cavity passes through the zona pellucida and between the blastomeres, and the cells are rearranged to form a blastocyst consisting of the outer cell mass or trophoblast, the inner cell mass or embryoblast, and the blastocyst cavity. The zona pellucida degenerates and, about day 6, the blastocyst adheres to and begins to implant in the endometrium. As the trophoblast contacts and penetrates the endometrium, it differentiates into the syncytiotrophoblast and cytotrophoblast. At the end of this week a layer of cells, the hypoblast, appears on the side of the inner cell mass facing the blastocyst cavity.

THE SECOND WEEK

This week is marked by the completion of implantation and formation of the bilaminar embryonic disc (Fig. 3-2).

The amniotic cavity develops between the inner cell mass and cytotrophoblast. The epithelial roof of this cavity is the amnion. The layer of inner cell mass cells forming the floor of the cavity constitutes the epiblast. The epiblast and hypoblast form the bilaminar embryonic disc, which will give rise to the embryo.

The exocoelomic membrane, continuous with the hypoblast, surrounds a cavity called the primary yolk sac. Cells derived from the trophoblast form the extraembryonic mesoderm, which surrounds the amnion and primary yolk sac. Fluid-filled spaces in the extraembryonic mesoderm coalesce to form the extraembryonic coelom or chorionic cavity. As the extraembryonic coelom develops, the primary yolk sac is reduced and, as hypoblast cells grow out and line it, the secondary or definitive yolk sac forms. Except for a band of tissue, the connecting or body stalk, the extraembryonic coelom splits the extraembryonic mesoderm into two layers: the extraembryonic splanchnic mesoderm covering the yolk sac, and the extraembryonic somatic mesoderm that covers the amnion and lines the trophoblast. The trophoblast and the extraembryonic mesoderm lining it form the chorion.

The prochordal plate, a midline circular thickening of the hypoblast, marks the future mouth region and the cranial end of the embryonic disc.

THE THIRD WEEK

During this week, the trilaminar embryonic disc is formed, differentiation of the germ layers begins, and a primitive circulatory system is established (Fig. 3-3).

A midline thickening of epiblast, the primitive streak, appears in the caudal region of the embryonic disc. Pro-

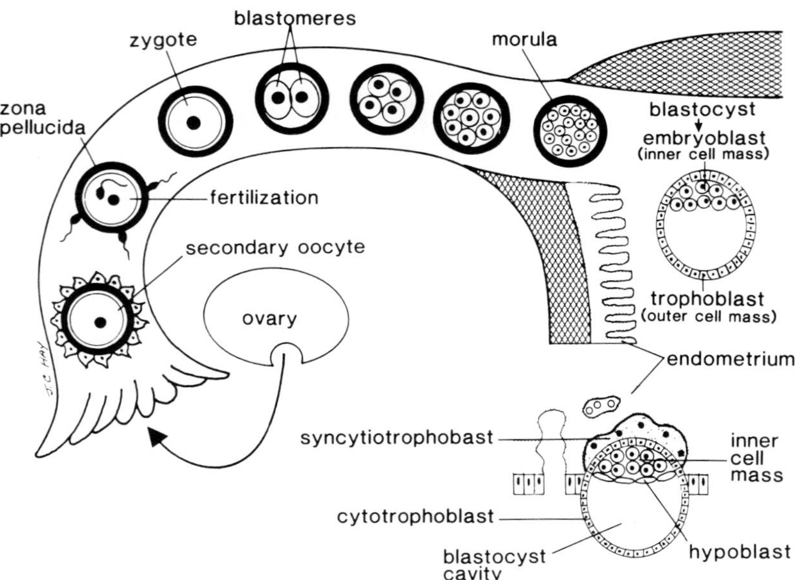

FIGURE 3–1. Diagram illustrating the first week of development.

liferation of cells at its cranial end forms the primitive node or knot. Epiblast cells move to the primitive streak, and pass laterally and cranially between the epiblast and hypoblast to form the embryonic or intraembryonic mesoderm. The epiblast is now called the embryonic ectoderm. Epiblast cells are thought to displace much of the hypoblast to form the embryonic endoderm.

Cells from the primitive node pass between the endoderm and ectoderm in the midline, and extend cranially to the prochordal plate. These cells form the notochordal process, which will give rise to the notochord.

At the cranial end of the embryonic disc, the endoderm of the prochordal plate is tightly fused to the overlying ectoderm to form the oropharyngeal membrane. Just caudal to the primitive streak is a similar midline circular area of fused ectoderm and endoderm, the cloacal membrane.

Embryonic mesoderm passes between the ectoderm and endoderm except in three places: at the oropharyngeal and cloacal membranes, and where the notochord extends in the midline. Mesoderm cranial to the oropharyngeal membrane forms the cardiogenic area. Some mesodermal cells retain their epithelial characteristics, but others give rise to mesenchyme, a primitive connective tissue. Normally, the primitive streak will regress and disappear.

Under the inductive influence of the notochord and adjacent mesoderm, the overlying ectoderm forms the neural plate, which extends from the primitive node to the oropharyngeal membrane. This ectoderm is neuroectoderm. Differential growth gives rise to a neural groove flanked by neural folds. The neural folds begin to approach each other and fuse to form the neural tube with the central neural canal. Fusion of the neural folds commences in the future cervical region and extends cranially and caudally (the anterior neuropore closes between day 25 and 26 of gestation, followed by the posterior neuropore 2 days later; Color Figure 3-1*A*). Some neuroectodermal cells are not incorporated into the neural tube and form the neural crests. The neural tube detaches from the ectoderm, and the surface ectoderm mainly forms the epidermis and the structures derived from it.

Differentiation of the mesoderm on each side of the notochord forms the paraxial mesoderm adjacent to the notochord. This becomes organized into somewhat cuboidal blocks called somites. Forty-two to 44 pairs eventually form. Each somite is composed of a dermatome, which contributes to the dermis; a myotome, which gives rises to skeletal muscle; and a sclerotome, the cells of which migrate around the neural tube and notochord to form the precursors of the vertebrae, and also the ribs. It also forms the intermediate mesoderm, a small area of mesoderm lateral to the paraxial mesoderm. It is associated with development of the urogenital system. Finally, it forms the lateral mesoderm, found at the margins of the disc. Spaces in this mesoderm coalesce to form the horseshoe-shaped intraembryonic coelom, which will form the pericardial, pleural, and peritoneal cavities. This coelom splits the lateral mesoderm into somatic and splanchnic layers. The somatopleure, the embryonic somatic mesoderm and ectoderm, will form the body walls. The splanchnopleure, the embryonic splanchnic mesoderm and endoderm, will form the primitive gut and the structures derived from it. In the cardiogenic area, mesoderm cranial to the embryonic coelom forms the septum transversum, which will form part of the diaphragm.

Concurrently, chorionic villi, consisting of a core of extraembryonic mesoderm covered with cytotrophoblast and syncytiotrophoblast, develop around the cho-

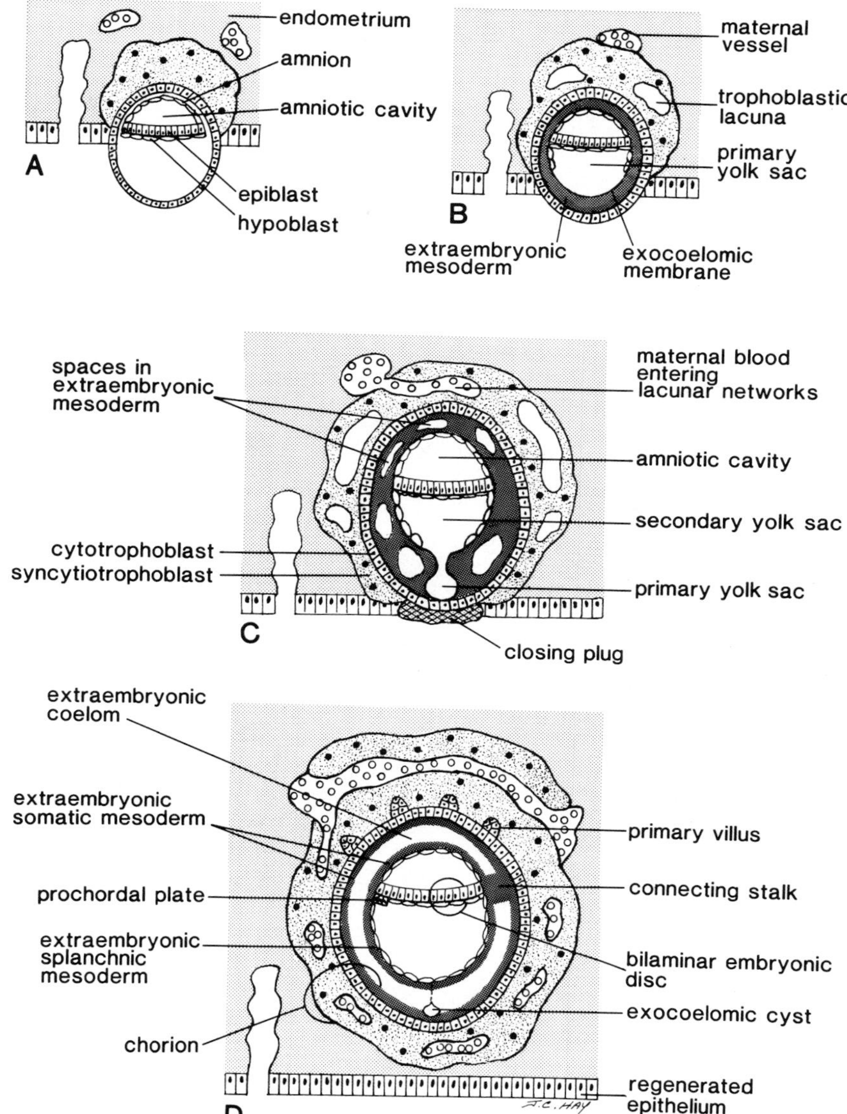

FIGURE 3–2. Diagrams illustrating the second week of development. Sections of the implanting blastocyst at approximately 8 days (**A**), 9 days (**B**), 12 days (**C**), and 14 days (**D**).

rionic sac. The allantois, a finger-like extension of endoderm from the caudal wall of the yolk sac, extends into the mesoderm of the connecting stalk.

Blood vessels first appear in the extraembryonic mesoderm (except that covering the amnion) and shortly thereafter in the embryo. Clusters of cells, the blood islands, acquire lumina. The surrounding cells form the endothelium and other layers of the vessel wall. As the vessels develop and sprout, the intra- and extraembryonic vessels are linked. Blood cells develop in association with the vessels of the yolk sac and allantois. Blood cells may arise from cells trapped within the lumen as the vessel forms, or from cells shed into the lumen (blood cells do not develop within the embryo until the second month). Paired endothelial heart tubes develop in the cardiogenic area as just described. These fuse to form a single contractile heart tube and, by the end of the third week, a primitive circulation is established between the embryo and the chorion.

THE EMBRYONIC PERIOD

The embryonic period extends from the beginning of the fourth week to the end of the eighth week. During this period, all the major internal and external structures begin their development; thus the embryo is very vulnerable to the effects of teratogens. By the end of this period, the embryo has acquired characteristic human features (Color Figures 3-1*B* and 3-2).

In the fourth week, the embryonic disc undergoes folding (Fig. 3-4) as a result of rapid elongation of midline structures (notochord, neural tube), rapid growth of midline structures (neural tube, somites) relative to

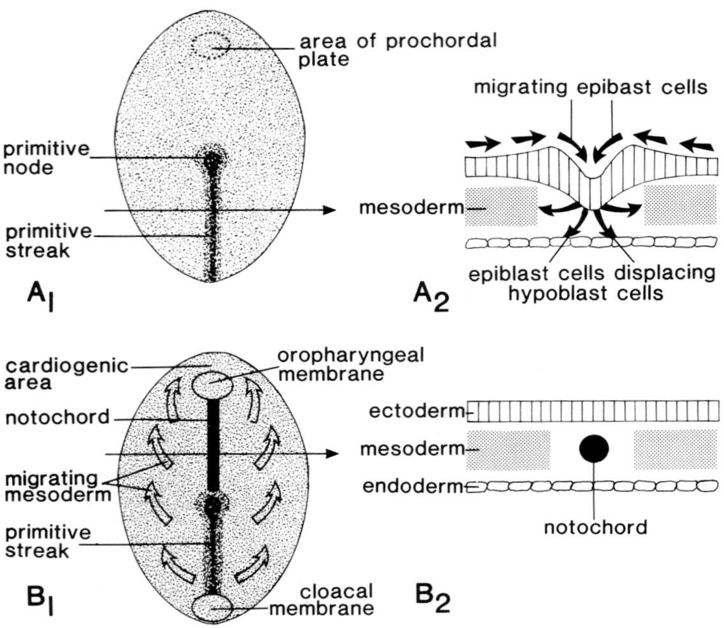

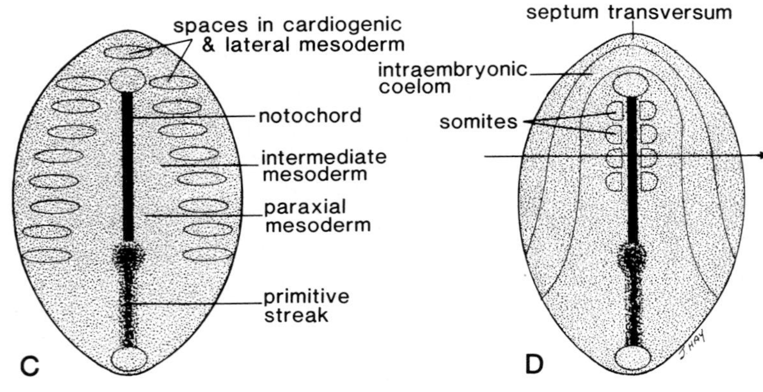

FIGURE 3–3. Diagrams illustrating some of the developmental events in the third week. (**A₁** and **B₁**) Dorsal views of the embryonic disc. (**A₂** and **B₂**) Transverse sections of the embryonic disc at the levels indicated in **A₁** and **B₁**. (**C** and **D**) Dorsal views of the embryonic disc showing differentiation of the mesoderm and formation of the intraembryonic coelom (the developing neural tube has been omitted).

those at the margins of the disc, and enlargement of the amniotic cavity. Folding converts the flat embryonic disc into a cylindrical embryo.

Folding in the longitudinal axis results in the formation of the head and tail folds. With the head fold, the developing heart and pericardial cavity are swung onto the ventral surface, and the septum transversum then lies caudal to the developing heart. The dorsal part of the yolk sac is incorporated into the embryo to form the foregut. This is separated by the oropharyngeal membrane from the stomodeum or primitive oral cavity. With the tail fold, the body or connecting stalk, the future umbilical cord, is swung onto the ventral surface and part of the allantois is incorporated into the embryo. The dorsal part of the yolk sac is incorporated into the embryo to form the hindgut. The terminal portion of the hindgut dilates to form the cloaca, which is separated from the amniotic cavity by the cloacal membrane.

Folding in the transverse axis, the lateral folds, results in the somatopleure forming the lateral and ventral body walls. As the dorsal part of the yolk sac is incorporated into the embryo, the splanchnopleure forms the primitive gut. The midgut, between the fore- and hindgut, is connected to the yolk sac by the narrow vitelline duct. The remnant of the yolk sac ultimately degenerates. As the caudal limbs of the intraembryonic coelom are moved ventrally, they are initially separated by a ventral mesentery. This mesentery disappears, except in the region of the foregut, and a single peritoneal cavity is formed. From the pericardial cavity, the pericardioperitoneal canals or future pleural cavities pass dorsally and caudally to communicate with the peritoneal cavity.

THE FETAL PERIOD

The fetal period extends from the beginning of the ninth week until birth. The main features of this period are the growth and differentiation of those tissues and organs which began their development in the embry-

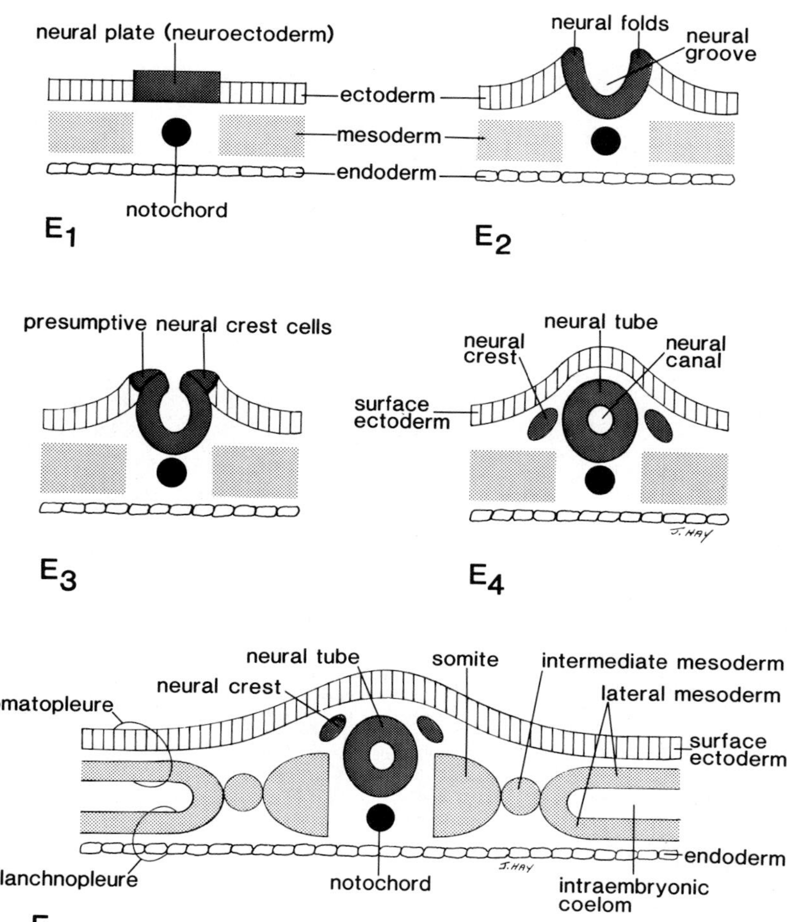

FIGURE 3–3 (Continued) (**E₁** to **E₄**) Development of the neural tube and neural crests. (**F**) Transverse section of the embryonic disc at the level indicated in **D.**

onic period. Few new structures (hairs, nails) appear. Exposure to teratogens in this period tends to result in functional defects rather than major morphological defects. During this period, fetal movement begins and the life-sustaining reflexes (sucking, swallowing, etc) are established (Color Figures 3-3, 3-4, and 3-5).

BRANCHIAL APPARATUS

In the fourth week, ridges and grooves appear in the future neck region (Fig. 3-5). These form part of the branchial apparatus (Greek *branchia* means gills), which consists of the following:

1. Six pairs of branchial or pharyngeal arches numbered in a craniocaudal sequence (in humans, the fifth and sixth pairs are rudimentary and not visible externally). Each arch consists of a core of mesoderm covered internally by endoderm and externally by ectoderm.
2. The branchial grooves or clefts. These are lined by ectoderm and occur externally between the arches.
3. The pharyngeal pouches. These are lined by endoderm and occur internally between the arches.
4. The branchial or closing membranes. These are formed by the ectoderm and endoderm between the arches (mesoderm soon penetrates between this ectoderm and endoderm).

The first or mandibular arch gives rise to the maxillary and mandibular prominences. The second or hyoid arch enlarges and grows caudally, concealing the posterior arches and creating an ectodermal depression, the cervical sinus; this arch ultimately fuses with the upper thoracic wall, giving the neck a smooth contour (remnants of the posterior grooves and the cervical sinus normally disappear). The first branchial groove, between the first and second arches, persists as the primordium of the external auditory meatus.

In the mesodermal core of each arch is a cranial nerve, a skeletal muscle element, an artery, and a rod or bar of hyaline cartilage (considered to be derived from neural crest cells). The cartilage may remain as cartilage, ossify, disappear completely, or disappear with the perichondrium persisting as ligaments. The ventral portions of the first arch or Meckel's cartilage disappear, and the mandible is derived from intramembran-

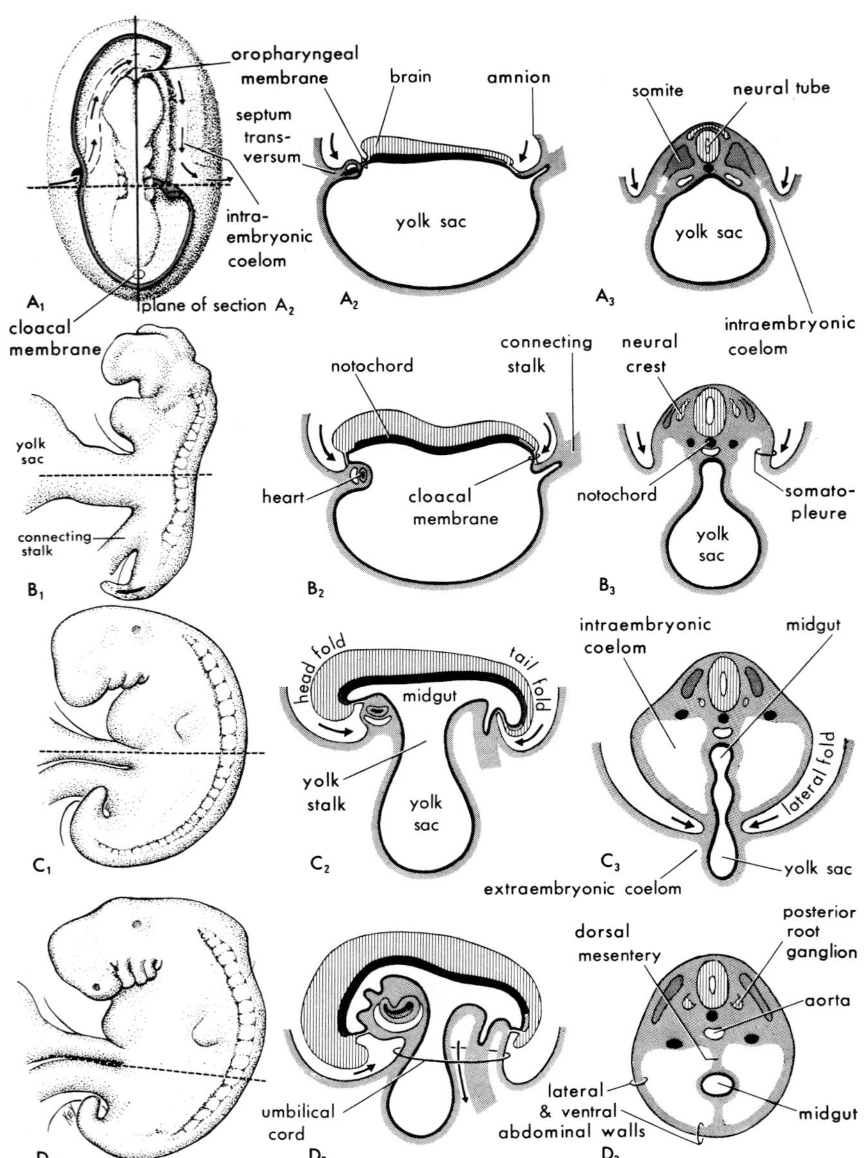

FIGURE 3–4. Diagrams illustrating folding of the embryonic disc during the fourth week. (**A_1**) Dorsal view. (**B_1** to **D_1**) Lateral views of the embryo. (**A_2** to **D_2**) Longitudinal sections at the levels shown in **A_3** to **D_1**. (From Moore KL. The developing human. 4th ed. Philadelphia: WB Saunders, 1988 with permission.)

ous ossification. The second arch cartilage is also called Reichert's cartilage.

The derivatives of the branchial arch components are summarized in Table 3-1.

PHARYNGEAL POUCHES

The first pair of pouches (between the first and second arches) forms the tympanic cavity and pharyngotympanic tube. The first branchial or closing membrane forms the tympanic membrane.

The second pair of pouches persists in part to form the tonsillar fossa. This pair is associated with development of the palatine tonsils.

The third pair of pouches develop dorsal and ventral portions, lose their connection with the pharynx, and migrate caudally and medially. The dorsal portions separate, attach to the posterior aspect of the thyroid gland, and form the inferior parathyroid glands. The ventral portions meet and fuse to form the thymus, which descends into the thorax.

The fourth pair of pouches also develop dorsal and ventral portions and lose their connection with the pharynx. The dorsal portions separate, attach to the posterior aspect of the thyroid gland, and form the superior parathyroid glands. The small ventral portions of the fourth pouches and the rudimentary fifth pouches form the ultimobranchial bodies, which are incorporated into the thyroid gland to form the parafollicular cells.

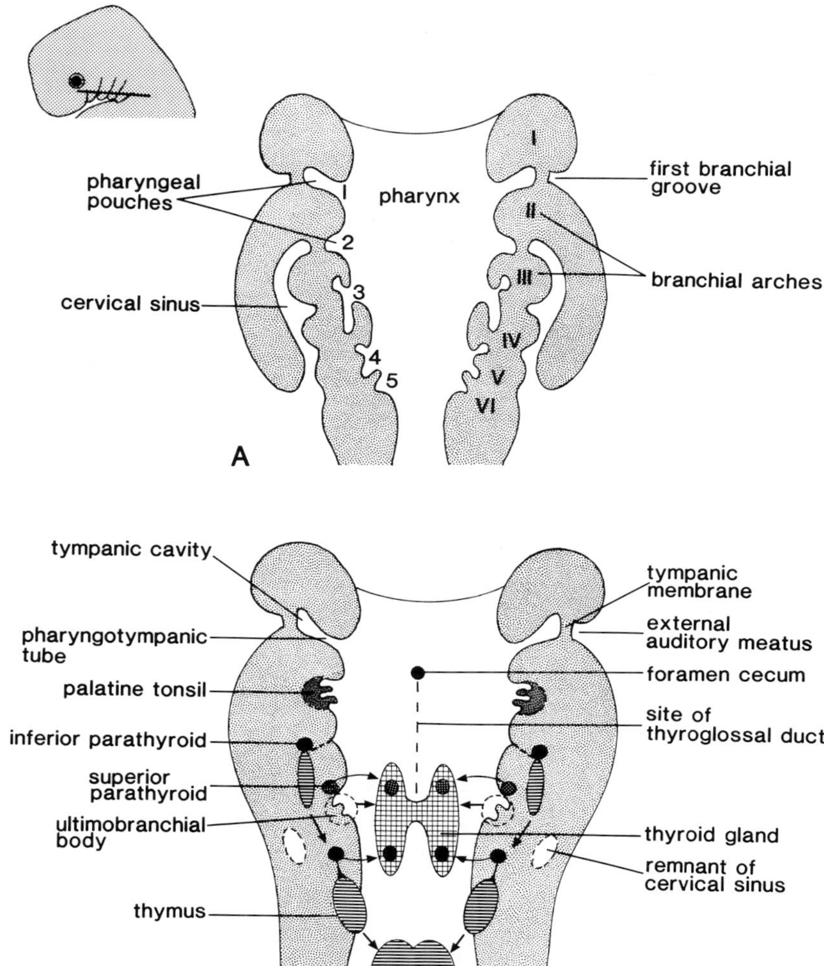

FIGURE 3-5. Diagrams illustrating the branchial apparatus. Inset indicates the level of the horizontal sections shown in **A** and **B.**

THE THYROID GLAND

In the fourth week, a thickening of endoderm appears in the floor of the pharynx; this grows downward to form the thyroid diverticulum. As it grows caudally, it becomes bilobed; the lobes are connected by the isthmus. The gland reaches its definitive position in the seventh week and is attached to its site of origin by the thyroglossal duct. This duct normally degenerates except for a small pit, the foramen cecum, in the tongue (see Fig. 3-5). (In about 50% of individuals, the caudal portion of the duct persists to form a pyramidal lobe that extends upward from the isthmus.) The endoderm becomes organized into follicles and the parafollicular cells are derived from the ultimobranchial bodies.

THE TONGUE

The primordia of the tongue appear in the floor of the pharynx in the fourth week.

The body or oral part consists of the anterior two thirds. Proliferation of mesoderm at the ventromedial ends of the first branchial arches forms the median tongue bud (tuberculum impar) just anterior to the foramen cecum. This bud is flanked by the two distal tongue buds (lateral lingual swellings). The median tongue bud is overgrown as the distal tongue buds enlarge and fuse, and the median sulcus indicates the plane of fusion.

The root or pharyngeal part consists of the posterior one third. The copula, just posterior to the foramen cecum, is formed by proliferation of mesoderm at the ventromedial ends of the second branchial arches. Posterior to the copula, the hypobranchial eminence is derived from proliferation of mesoderm at the ventromedial ends of the third and fourth branchial arches. The cranial part of this eminence overgrows the copula; the caudal portion will form the epiglottis.

The sulcus terminalis roughly demarcates the junction of the root and the body. The intrinsic muscles of the tongue are considered to be derived from cells that

TABLE 3–1. DERIVATIVES OF THE BRANCHIAL ARCH COMPONENTS*

ARCH	NERVE	MUSCLES (MAJOR GROUPS)	CARTILAGES: SKELETAL STRUCTURES	CARTILAGES: LIGAMENTS
I	Trigeminal (V)	Muscles of mastication†	Malleus, incus	Sphenomandibular, anterior ligament of malleus
II	Facial (VII)	Muscles of facial expression‡	Stapes, styloid process, part of hyoid bone	Stylohyoid
III	Glossopharyngeal (IX)	Stylopharyngeus	Remainder of hyoid bone	
IV	Vagus (X) superior laryngeal branch	Muscles of palate,§ pharynx and larynx (IV–VI)	Laryngeal cartilages (except epiglottis) (IV–VI)	
V	??			
VI	Vagus (X) recurrent laryngeal branch			

* Derivatives of the branchial arch arteries are discussed with the circulatory system.
† Also anterior belly of digastric, stylohyoid, tensor tympani, and tensor palatini.
‡ Also posterior belly of digastric, stapedius, and stylohyoid.
§ Except tensor palatini.

migrate from the occipital somites, and this explains why they are innervated by the hypoglossal nerve rather than by the branchial arch nerves.

THE FACE

The primordia of the face appear at the end of the fourth week and are related to the stomodeum or primitive oral cavity as follows: the frontonasal prominence forms the cranial boundary, the maxillary prominences form the lateral boundaries, and the mandibular prominences form the caudal boundary (see Color Figure 3-1*B*). These prominences, formed by accumulations of mesenchyme, are separated by grooves and furrows. During development, the prominences merge with one another as the grooves are smoothed out by proliferation of the underlying mesenchyme. Much of the mesenchyme in the facial region is considered to be of neural crest origin. Merging occurs mainly during the fifth to eighth weeks.

Ectodermal thickenings on the inferolateral aspects of the frontonasal prominence form the nasal placodes. Mesenchyme around the placodes proliferates to form the medial and lateral nasal prominences, and the placodes then lie in depressions, the nasal pits or future nostrils. Expansion of the back of the head moves the eyes forward and contributes to the growth of the facial components toward the midline. The maxillary prominences merge with the medial nasal prominences, and the medial nasal prominences merge with each other to form the intermaxillary segment. The mandibular prominences merge with each other in the midline.

The adult derivatives are the frontonasal prominence—the forehead, dorsum, and apex of the nose; the lateral nasal prominences—the alae of the nose; the merged medial nasal prominences (intermaxillary segment)—the columella, philtrum of the upper lip, the maxilla that bears the incisors (the premaxilla), and the primary palate; the maxillary prominences—the lateral portions of the upper lip, the upper cheeks and face, the rest of the maxilla, and the secondary palate; and the mandibular prominences—the lower lip, lower cheeks and face, and the mandible.

Myoblasts from the second branchial arch migrate into the facial region to form the muscles of facial expression. Along the nasolacrimal groove between the lateral nasal and maxillary prominences, a cord of cells sinks into the underlying mesenchyme; this canalizes to form the nasolacrimal duct.

THE PALATE

The palate develops from two primordia: the primary palate or median palatine process, a wedge-shaped mass of mesoderm from the innermost aspect of the intermaxillary segment that appears in the fifth week; and the secondary palate, which develops from the lateral palatine processes, shelf-like projections of mesoderm from the medial aspects of the maxillary prominences. These processes appear in the sixth week. As the developing tongue occupies most of the oral cavity, the lateral palatine processes are forced to assume a vertical position. As the stomodeum enlarges, the tongue drops down to the floor of the stomodeum and the lateral palatine processes elevate to a horizontal position; this elevation occurs slightly later in females.

Beginning anteriorly and proceeding posteriorly, the lateral palatine processes fuse with the posterior margin of the median palatine process, the inferior border of the nasal septum, and each other. Fusion involves epithelial contact, adhesion, and the replacement of the epithelial seam by mesoderm. Fusion begins in the ninth week and is completed by the 11th week in males and the 12th week in females. Intramembranous ossification spreads into the palate from the maxillary and palatine bones and extends to the posterior border of the nasal septum. Posterior to this, the unossified portion forms the soft palate and uvula. The palatal muscles are derived from the branchial arches.

THE RESPIRATORY SYSTEM

THE UPPER RESPIRATORY SYSTEM

The nasal pits deepen to form the nasal sacs, which grow dorsally and caudally. The oronasal membrane separating the oral and nasal cavities ruptures and the cavities communicate just posterior to the primary palate. Development of the secondary palate moves this communication posteriorly to the nasopharynx. The nasal septum, a midline downgrowth from the frontonasal prominence, separates the nasal cavities. In the late fetal period, the paranasal sinuses develop as bone is resorbed under the influence of the respiratory epithelium; most of their expansion occurs postnatally. The epithelium of the nasal placodes, now located in the roof of the nasal cavities, forms the olfactory epithelium.

THE LOWER RESPIRATORY SYSTEM

In the fourth week, the laryngotracheal groove appears in the floor of the pharynx; it deepens to form the laryngotracheal diverticulum. As it grows caudally, longitudinal folds of mesenchyme fuse to form the tracheoesophageal septum, which separates the laryngotracheal tube (ventrally) from the esophagus (dorsally). The laryngotracheal tube gives rise to the larynx and trachea. A lung bud develops at the caudal end of the tube, and this soon bifurcates to give two bronchopulmonary or lung buds. The right lung bud develops two secondary buds and the left lung bud gives rise to one secondary lung bud; these buds demarcate the future lobes of the lung. Dichotomous branching forms the air-conducting passages, the bronchi and bronchioles. Respiratory tissue—the respiratory bronchioles, alveolar ducts and sacs, and the alveoli—develops at the terminal ends of the bronchioles and continues to develop postnatally. The epithelium and structures derived from it are of endodermal origin; all other components are derived from splanchnic mesenchyme. As the lungs grow into the medial aspects of the pericardioperitoneal or pleural canals, they acquire a layer of visceral pleura.

THE DIGESTIVE SYSTEM

The primitive gut forms during the fourth week as the head, tail, and lateral folds incorporate the dorsal part of the yolk sac into the embryo (see Fig. 3-4). The endoderm of the primitive gut gives rise to the epithelium and glands of most of the digestive tract; the epithelium at the cranial and caudal ends of the tract is derived from the ectoderm of the primitive oral cavity (stomodeum) and the anal pit (proctodeum), respectively. The muscular and fibrous elements of the digestive tract and the visceral peritoneum are derived from splanchnic mesenchyme. The primitive gut is divided into three parts.

THE FOREGUT

The derivatives of the foregut are the pharynx and its derivatives; the lower respiratory tract; the esophagus; the stomach; the duodenum, proximal to the common bile duct; and the liver, biliary tract, gallbladder, and pancreas.

The esophagus develops from the cranial part of the foregut. Initially short, it elongates rapidly. The striated muscle of the esophagus is derived from the caudal branchial arches, and the smooth muscle of the lower esophagus develops locally from the surrounding splanchnic mesenchyme. The lumen of the esophagus becomes occluded by proliferation of the endodermal cells, but these cells degenerate and the lumen is recanalized (similar occlusion and recanalization occurs during development of parts of the intestines).

The stomach appears during week 4 as a fusiform dilatation of the caudal part of the foregut; this primordium soon expands and broadens dorsoventrally. The dorsal border, which grows more rapidly than the ventral border, forms the greater curvature. As the stomach enlarges and acquires its adult shape, it rotates 90° in a clockwise direction about its longitudinal axis. Thus, the ventral border (lesser curvature) moves to the right, and the dorsal border (greater curvature) moves to the left. The original left side becomes the ventral surface and the right side becomes the dorsal surface. The stomach is suspended from the dorsal wall of the abdominal cavity by the dorsal mesentery (dorsal mesogastrium). As the dorsal mesogastrium is carried to the left during rotation of the stomach, the lesser sac forms. Isolated clefts develop in the thick dorsal mesogastrium and coalesce to form a single cavity, the lesser peritoneal sac, which communicates with the main peritoneal cavity or greater peritoneal sac through a small opening, the epiploic foramen. The elongated dorsal mesogastrium, the greater omentum, hangs from the greater curvature anterior to the developing intestines. As the embryo lengthens, the caudal part of the septum transversum thins and becomes the ventral mesentery, which attaches the stomach and duodenum to the ventral wall of the abdominal cavity. The ventral mesentery persists only where it is attached to the caudal part of the foregut. The final shape and position of the stomach are influenced by the development of the liver and the omental bursa.

The duodenum has a composite origin from the most caudal part of the foregut and the most cranial part of the midgut. These parts grow rapidly and form a C-shaped loop that projects ventrally. The junction of the foregut and the midgut is at the apex of this duodenal loop, and is demarcated by the duodenal papilla.

The liver arises as an endodermal bud from the most caudal part of the foregut; this hepatic diverticulum extends into the septum transversum, enlarges rapidly, and divides into a larger cranial part, the primordium of the liver, and a smaller caudal part, which will form the gallbladder and cystic duct. The stalk connecting the hepatic and cystic ducts to the duodenum becomes the common bile duct.

The proliferating endodermal cells give rise to interlacing cords of liver cells and the epithelial lining of the intrahepatic portion of the biliary apparatus. As the liver cords invade the septum transversum, they break up the umbilical and vitelline veins to form the hepatic sinusoids. The mesenchyme of the septum transversum gives rise to the fibrous and hemopoietic tissue and the Kupffer cells. Hemopoiesis begins in the liver during the sixth week. The lobes of the liver grow extensively and soon fill most of the abdominal cavity. Initially, the lobes are about the same size, but the right lobe becomes much larger; the caudate and quadrate lobes develop as subdivisions of the left lobe.

The ventral mesentery gives rise to the lesser omentum (gastrohepatic ligament and duodenohepatic ligament), the falciform ligament (liver to the anterior abdominal wall), and the visceral peritoneum of the liver.

The pancreas develops from dorsal and ventral pancreatic buds. The ventral pancreatic bud forms as an evagination of the hepatic diverticulum, and the dorsal pancreatic bud is derived from the proximal part of the duodenum, opposite the hepatic diverticulum. As the duodenum grows and rotates to the right, the two buds come together and fuse. The ventral pancreatic bud gives rise to the main pancreatic duct, the uncinate process, and the lower part of the head of the pancreas. The rest of the pancreas and the accessory pancreatic duct are formed from the dorsal pancreatic bud. The two pancreatic ducts usually anastomose to form a single pancreatic duct.

The spleen is derived from the fusion of mesenchymal nodules located in the dorsal mesogastrium. Along the anterior border fusion is incomplete, with the result that the anterior border is notched.

THE MIDGUT

The derivatives of the midgut are the small intestines (except for the duodenum from the stomach to entry of the common bile duct); the cecum and appendix; and the ascending colon and the proximal one half to two thirds of the transverse colon.

The dorsal mesentery, which suspends the midgut from the dorsal abdominal wall, elongates rapidly. The midgut elongates during the sixth week, forming a ventral, U-shaped intestinal loop.

The midgut loop has a proximal or cranial limb, and a distal or caudal limb. The communication of the midgut with the yolk sac is reduced to the narrow yolk stalk or vitelline duct, which is attached to the apex of the loop and marks the junction between the two limbs.

The midgut loop migrates into the umbilical cord. This "herniation" of the intestines occurs because there is not enough room in the abdomen, mainly because of the relatively large size of the liver and kidneys. The proximal limb grows rapidly and forms intestinal loops, but the caudal limb undergoes very little change except for development of the cecal diverticulum. The midgut loop then rotates within the umbilical cord. During the tenth week, as the intestines return rapidly to the abdomen, they undergo further rotation. The midgut segment undergoes a total counterclockwise rotation of 270°. This so-called "reduction of the midgut hernia" is usually attributed to an increase in the size of the abdominal cavity, and a decrease in the relative size of the liver and kidneys.

The primordium of the cecum and appendix appears during the sixth week as the cecal bud, a conical pouch of the caudal limb of the midgut loop. The apex of this blind pouch does not grow as rapidly as the rest of the cecum and forms the vermiform appendix. Elongation of the proximal part of the colon results in the cecum and appendix "descending" from the upper to the lower right quadrant of the abdomen. Because of the growth, rotation, and descent of the cecum, the position of the appendix is variable, but it is usually retrocecal.

As the intestines assume their final positions, in some places the mesentery fuses with the parietal peritoneum and disappears; those parts of the midgut become retroperitoneal. The proximal part of the duodenum and the ascending colon become retroperitoneal. Other derivatives of the midgut loop retain their mesenteries. The transverse colon is attached to the greater omentum.

THE HINDGUT

The derivatives of the hindgut are the distal one third to one half of the transverse colon; the descending colon (which becomes retroperitoneal); the sigmoid (pelvic) colon; the rectum and the upper portion of the anal canal; and part of the urogenital system.

The expanded terminal part of the hindgut, the cloaca, is separated from the amniotic cavity by the cloacal membrane. The cloaca receives the allantois ventrally. A mesodermal partition, the urorectal septum, develops in the angle between the allantois and the hindgut. As it grows toward the cloacal membrane, it divides the cloaca into the rectum and upper anal canal dorsally, and the urogenital sinus ventrally. By the end of the seventh week, the urorectal septum fuses with the cloacal membrane, dividing it into a dorsal anal membrane and a larger ventral urogenital membrane.

Proliferation of mesenchymal tissue around the anal membrane elevates the surface ectoderm and forms the shallow anal pit or proctodeum. The anal membrane, now at the floor of this pit, ruptures by the end of the seventh week, forming the anal canal. The caudal part of the digestive tract is now in communication with the amniotic cavity. The proximal (upper) two thirds of this canal is derived from the hindgut; the distal (lower) one third develops from the proctodeum. The pectinate line, about the level of the anal valves, indicates the approximate former site of the anal membrane and the junction of endoderm and ectoderm. The other layers are mesenchymal in origin.

THE URINARY SYSTEM

THE KIDNEYS

At the beginning of the fourth week, the intermediate mesoderm on each side detaches from the somites and forms the nephrogenic cords. From the nephrogenic cords, three successive sets of excretory organs develop in a cranial to caudal sequence. These are the pronephros, the mesonephros, and the metanephros.

The pronephros is formed in the cervical region and is a transitory nonfunctional structure. It regresses soon after its formation, leaving the pronephric ducts, which run caudally to enter the cloaca. These ducts will become the mesonephric ducts.

The mesonephros also appears during the fourth week, caudal to the degenerating pronephros. Cell clusters in the nephrogenic cords give rise to mesonephric tubules, which drain into the mesonephric duct. The mesonephros serves as a temporary excretory organ and probably functions in urine production, but it degenerates during the latter part of the embryonic period. In the male, the mesonephric ducts will form some components of the reproductive system. In the female, the mesonephric ducts degenerate, except for vestigial remnants.

The permanent adult kidney, the metanephros, begins to develop early in the fifth week and is functional 2 to 3 weeks later. The ureteric bud develops as an outgrowth from the mesonephric duct, close to its entry into the cloaca. The ureteric bud grows dorsally and cranially to meet the metanephrogenic blastema (intermediate mesoderm). The ureteric bud forms the ureter, renal pelvis, calyces, and collecting tubules. The nephrons are derived from the metanephric blastema. At birth, all nephrons are formed, but are still short. During infancy, the nephrons complete their differentiation and increase in size until adulthood.

Initially, the metanephros is located in the sacral region of the embryo and receives its blood supply from the dorsal aorta at that level. The metanephroi gradually ascend to the abdomen, probably as a result of caudal growth of the embryo. This results in a relative change in the position of these organs, and they receive their blood supply from progressively higher levels. As the kidney ascends, it rotates and the position of the hilum changes from ventral to medial.

THE URINARY BLADDER

The urinary bladder is derived from the cranial part of the urogenital sinus. It is lined by endoderm, and the other layers are derived from the adjacent splanchnic mesenchyme. It is believed that the mucosa and musculature of the trigone area are derived from incorporation of the caudal ends of the mesonephric ducts and are therefore mesodermal in origin; possibly this mucosa is later overgrown by endodermal epithelium.

The allantois, continuous with the bladder, constricts to form the urachus. The adult derivative of the urachus is the median umbilical ligament, which passes from the apex of the bladder to the umbilicus.

THE URETHRA

In both sexes, the urethra is derived from the caudal part of the urogenital sinus. The epithelium of the entire female urethra is derived from the endoderm of the urogenital sinus. In the male, except for its most distal part, which is derived from ectoderm, the urethral epithelium has a similar origin. In both sexes, the other layers of the urethra are derived from adjacent splanchnic mesenchyme. Rupture of the urogenital membrane brings the urinary system into communication with the amniotic cavity.

THE SUPRARENAL (ADRENAL) GLANDS

Aggregates of mesenchymal cells, derived from the mesothelium lining the posterior body wall, form the cortex. The medulla is derived from cells of neural crest origin.

THE GENITAL SYSTEM

The genetic sex of the embryo is determined at fertilization by the type of spermatozoon that fertilizes the oocyte. There is no morphological indication of sexual differences until the eighth week, when the gonads begin to acquire sexual characteristics. Initially, all normal human embryos are potentially bisexual; male and female embryos have identical gonads, genital ducts, and external genitalia. This period of early genital development is referred to as the indifferent stage of the reproductive organs.

THE GONADS

The gonads first appear during the fifth week of development, as the intermediate mesoderm on the dorsal body wall forms the gonadal ridges. The coelomic epithelium grows into the underlying mesenchyme and forms the primary sex cords. A week later the cords become populated by primordial germ cells, precursors of the spermatogonia or oogonia. The Y chromosome has a strong testis-determining effect on the indifferent gonad. Under its influence, the primary sex cords differentiate into seminiferous tubules. Absence of a Y chromosome results in formation of an ovary. Thus, the type of sex chromosome complex established at fertilization determines the type of gonad that develops from the indifferent gonad. The type of gonad then determines the sexual differentiation of the genital ducts and external genitalia.

THE GENITAL DUCTS

Two pairs of genital ducts develop in both sexes: mesonephric (Wolffian) ducts and paramesonephric (Müllerian) ducts. In the male, the fetal testes produce at least two hormones: one stimulates development of the mesonephric ducts into the male genital tract, and the other suppresses development of the paramesonephric ducts. Some mesonephric tubules near the testis persist and are transformed into efferent ductules or ductuli efferentes, which connect the rete testis to the epididymis. The mesonephric duct becomes the ductus epididymis and the vas deferens. The seminal vesicles develop from paired lateral diverticula from the caudal ends of the mesonephric ducts. The part of the mesonephric duct between the duct of this gland and the urethra becomes the ejaculatory duct. The appendix of the epididymis and the paradidymis are nonfunctional rudiments of the mesonephric duct and mesonephric tubules, respectively. In the male, the paramesonephric ducts largely degenerate, except for two vestigial remnants: the appendix of the testis and the prostatic utricle.

In female embryos, the mesonephric ducts regress and the paramesonephric ducts give rise to the female genital tract. The cranial unfused ends of the paramesonephric ducts form the uterine tubes. The caudal portions of the ducts converge and fuse in the midline to form the uterovaginal primordium, which gives rise to the uterus, cervix, and possibly part of the vagina. The development of the vagina is not entirely settled. One theory is that the uterovaginal primordium induces the formation of paired, endodermally derived outgrowths from the urogenital sinus. These fuse to form a solid vaginal plate, which eventually canalizes to become the vagina. Thus, the vaginal epithelium is derived from the endoderm of the urogenital sinus, and the fibromuscular wall of the vagina develops from the mesenchymal cells of the uterovaginal primordium. Another view is that the uterus and upper third of the vagina are formed from the uterovaginal primordium and surrounding mesenchyme, while the lower two thirds of the vagina is presumed to be derived from the vaginal plate and the surrounding mesenchyme. A few blind mesonephric tubules, the epoophoron, may persist in the mesovarium. Parts of the mesonephric duct may persist as Gartner's duct in the broad ligament along the lateral wall of the uterus, or as a Gartner's cyst in the wall of the vagina.

THE EXTERNAL GENITALIA

The external genitalia also pass through an indifferent stage that is not distinguishable as male or female. Early in the fourth week, a genital tubercle develops ventral to the cloacal membrane; this elongates to form the phallus. By the sixth week, labioscrotal swellings and urogenital folds develop on each side of the future urogenital membrane.

In the male, masculinization of the indifferent external genitalia is caused by androgens produced by the testes. The phallus will form the penis. The urogenital folds fuse with each other along the ventral (under) surface of the penis and form the penile urethra. The paired labioscrotal swellings grow toward each other and fuse to form the scrotum.

In the female, because of the absence of androgens, feminization of the indifferent external genitalia occurs. The phallus elongates rapidly at first, but as its growth gradually slows, it becomes the relatively small clitoris. The unfused urogenital folds form the paired labia minora, whereas the labioscrotal swellings give rise to the labia majora. The caudal portion of the urogenital sinus gives rise to the vestibule of the vagina.

THE CARDIOVASCULAR SYSTEM

THE HEART TUBE

The development of the heart begins in the third week in the cardiogenic area (see Fig. 3-3). Splanchnic mesoderm ventral to the pericardial cavity aggregates to form a pair of elongated heart cords. By day 17 of gestation, these cords canalize to form endothelial tubes, called endocardial heart tubes. As the lateral folds develop, the heart tubes fuse to form a single median endocardial heart tube; fusion begins cranially and rapidly extends caudally. A single endocardial tube is formed by day 22. It is surrounded by a myoepicardial mantle and separated from the endothelial lining by cardiac jelly. With the development of the head fold, the cardiac tube comes to lie dorsal to the pericardial cavity and ventral to the foregut. They are now caudal to the oropharyngeal membrane (see Fig. 3-4).

As the tubular heart elongates, it differentiates into four main regions. From cranial to caudal, these are the bulbus cordis, ventricle, atrium, and the sinus venosus. The bulbus cordis represents the arterial end of the heart and consists of a proximal part, the conus, and a distal part, the truncus arteriosus. The sinus venosus represents the venous end of the heart. It receives the umbilical veins from the placenta, the vitelline veins from the yolk sac, and the common cardinal veins from the embryo. The arterial and venous ends of the heart tube are fixed by the branchial arches and the septum transversum, respectively.

Because the bulbus cordis and ventricle grow faster than the other regions, the heart tube bends upon itself, forming a U-shaped bulboventricular loop. It later becomes S-shaped. As the heart tube bends, the atrium and the sinus venosus come to lie dorsal to the bulbus cordis, truncus arteriosus, and ventricle. By this stage, the sinus venosus has developed lateral expansions, called right and left horns. The right horn of the sinus venosus subsequently becomes larger than the left. The developing heart tube now gradually invaginates into the dorsal aspect of the pericardial cavity.

THE ATRIOVENTRICULAR CANAL

Partitioning of the atrioventricular canal, the atrium, and the ventricle begins about the middle of the fourth week and is essentially complete by the end of the seventh week. Although described separately, it must be emphasized that these processes occur concurrently.

At first, the atrioventricular opening is round. In the region of the atrioventricular canal two thickenings of subendocardial tissue, the endocardial cushions, appear in the dorsal and ventral walls of the heart. During the fifth week, these cushions grow toward each other and fuse, dividing the atrioventricular canal into right and left atrioventricular canals.

THE ATRIA

The primitive atrial chamber communicates posteriorly with the sinus venosus, and inferiorly with the ventricle through the atrioventricular canal. A crescent-shaped membrane, the septum primum, grows down toward the endocardial cushions. A large gap, the foramen primum, exists between its lower free edge and the endocardial cushions. As the septum primum grows toward the endocardial cushions, the foramen primum becomes progressively smaller. Before the foramen primum is obliterated, an opening, foramen secundum, appears in the upper part of septum primum. Concurrently, the free edge of the septum primum fuses with the left side of the fused endocardial cushions and obliterates the foramen primum. At this stage, the left atrium receives most of its blood from the right atrium via the foramen secundum.

Toward the end of the fifth week, a second membrane, the septum secundum, arises from the roof of the atrium on the right side of septum primum. As this septum grows downward toward the endocardial cushions, it gradually overlaps the foramen secundum. The septum secundum forms an incomplete partition with an oblique opening, the foramen ovale, through which the two atria communicate. The upper part of the septum primum gradually degenerates, while the remaining part of the septum primum persists as the valve of the foramen ovale. Whereas the lower border of the septum secundum (crista dividens) is thick and firm, the edge of the septum primum is thin and mobile, and offers no obstruction to blood flow from the right to the left atrium. The foramen ovale persists throughout fetal life.

Initially, the sinus venosus is a separate chamber, opening into the part of the primitive atrium that will become the right atrium. The left horn of the sinus venosus and its tributaries regress, leaving the coronary sinus. After the formation of the interatrial septum, the right horn of the sinus venosus becomes incorporated into the wall of the right atrium, forming the smooth part of its wall.

Most of the wall of the left atrium is smooth and is derived from the primitive pulmonary vein. Initially, a single pulmonary vein opens into the primitive left atrium. As the atrium expands, this vein is gradually incorporated into the wall of the left atrium, and the proximal portions of its branches are progressively absorbed. This results in four pulmonary veins, which open separately into the atrium.

THE VENTRICLES

The ventricles are derived from the primitive ventricular chamber and the proximal part of the bulbus cordis, the conus. The infundibulum of the right ventricle and the aortic vestibule of the left ventricle arise from the conus. Partitioning of the primitive ventricle into right and left ventricles is first indicated by a muscular ridge, the interventricular septum, which grows upward from the floor of the bulboventricular cavity, and divides it into right and left halves. Initially, most of the growth of the interventricular septum results from dilatation of the ventricles on each side of it. This produces an external interventricular groove. Later, there is active growth of septal tissue as the muscular portion of the interventricular septum forms. The gap between the upper free edge of the interventricular septum and the endocardial cushions permits communication between the right and left ventricles until about the end of the seventh week. Proliferation of tissue from several sources forms the membranous portion of the interventricular septum, and it completes the partitioning of the ventricles.

PARTITIONING OF THE TRUNCUS ARTERIOSUS AND BULBUS CORDIS

During the fifth week, opposing ridges of subendocardial tissue, the bulbar ridges, arise in the wall of the bulbus cordis. Similar ridges also form in the truncus arteriosus and are continuous with those in the bulbus cordis. The spiral orientation of the ridges is possibly caused by the streaming of blood from the ventricles. Fusion of these ridges results in a spiral aorticopulmonary septum. The septum subdivides the bulbus cordis and the truncus arteriosus into two channels, the ascending aorta and the pulmonary trunk. Blood from the aorta now passes into the third and fourth pairs of aortic arch arteries, and blood from the pulmonary trunk flows into the sixth pair of aortic arch arteries. Because of the spiral orientation of the septum, the pulmonary trunk twists around the ascending aorta. Proximally, the pulmonary trunk lies ventral to the aorta, but distally it lies to the left of the aorta. The bulbus cordis is gradually incorporated into the walls of the ventricles.

Closure of the interventricular foramen, about the end of the seventh week, results from the fusion of subendocardial tissue from the right bulbar ridge, the left bulbar ridge, and the fused endocardial cushions. The membranous part of the interventricular septum is derived from proliferation of tissue from the right side of the fused endocardial cushions. This tissue fuses with the aorticopulmonary septum and the muscular part of the interventricular septum. Following closure of the interventricular foramen, the pulmonary trunk is in communication with the right ventricle and the aorta with the left ventricle.

Cardiac valves develop as swellings or ridges of subendocardial tissue that become hollowed out and reshaped.

THE BRANCHIAL ARCH ARTERIES

Six pairs of aortic or branchial arch arteries arise from the aortic sac, a dilated region of the truncus arteriosus, and terminate in the dorsal aorta of the corresponding side. Their derivatives are

- 1st pair: parts of the maxillary arteries
- 2nd pair: no adult derivatives
- 3rd pair: common carotid arteries and part of internal carotid arteries
- 4th pair:
  - left—part of arch of aorta
  - right—part of right subclavian artery
- 5th pair: no adult derivatives
- 6th pair:
  - left—proximal: proximal part of left pulmonary artery; distal: ductus arteriosus (acts as shunt in prenatal life)
  - right—proximal: proximal part of right pulmonary artery; distal: degenerates

FETAL CIRCULATION

Well-oxygenated blood returns from the placenta in the umbilical vein. About half of the blood passes through the hepatic sinusoids; the remainder bypasses the sinusoids by going through the ductus venosus into the inferior vena cava. This blood flow is regulated by a muscular sphincter in the ductus venosus near the umbilical vein.

After a short course in the inferior vena cava, the blood enters the right atrium. Because the inferior vena cava also receives deoxygenated blood from the lower limbs and viscera, the blood entering the right atrium is less oxygenated than that in the umbilical vein. The blood from the inferior vena cava is largely directed by the lower border of the septum secundum (the crista dividens) through the foramen ovale into the left atrium. In the left atrium it mixes with a relatively small amount of deoxygenated blood returning from the lungs via the pulmonary veins. From the left atrium, the blood passes into the left ventricle and leaves via the ascending aorta. Consequently, the vessels to the heart, head and neck, and upper limbs receive rather well-oxygenated blood.

A small stream of oxygenated blood from the inferior vena cava is diverted by the crista dividens and remains in the right atrium. This blood mixes with deoxygenated blood from the superior vena cava and coronary sinus and passes into the right ventricle. From the right ventricle, the blood enters the pulmonary trunk. Only a small amount of this blood reaches the lungs. The greater part of the blood is diverted through the ductus arteriosus into the aorta. Some of this blood circulates to the abdominal and pelvic viscera and the lower limbs and is returned to the fetal heart, but much of the blood in the aorta is transported by the umbilical arteries to the placenta.

CHANGES AT BIRTH

Changes occur in several fetal blood vessels. Muscle in the walls of the umbilical arteries contracts, occludes the lumen, and thus prevents the loss of fetal blood. When the umbilical vein is occluded and blood flow from the placenta ceases, the pressure in the right atrium is lowered. The ductus venosus also becomes occluded. Occlusion of the ductus arteriosus results in all the blood from the right ventricle going to the lungs for oxygenation. Because this increases the volume of blood returning to the left atrium from the lungs, the pressure in the left atrium is raised. As a result of the difference in pressure between the right and left atria, the valve of the foramen ovale closes.

Anatomical closure of the fetal blood vessels by fibrous tissue forms various ligamentous remnants:

Umbilical arteries: medial umbilical ligaments
Left umbilical vein: ligamentum teres of the liver
Ductus venosus: ligamentum venosum
Ductus arteriosus: ligamentum arteriosum

THE NERVOUS SYSTEM

THE CENTRAL NERVOUS SYSTEM

The neural tube (see Fig. 3-3) gives rise to the entire central nervous system, with the exception of its blood vessels and certain neuroglial cells. At first, the neural tube consists of a layer of pseudostratified columnar neuroepithelial cells. As a result of continuous cell proliferation, the walls of the neural tube become thickened and develop an inner ventricular (ependymal) layer, an intermediate (mantle) layer, and an outer marginal layer. All nerve and macroglial cells (astrocytes and oligodendrocytes) are derived from the neuroepithelial cells; the microglial cells differentiate from mesenchymal cells that have entered the central nervous system with developing blood vessels. The sulcus limit-

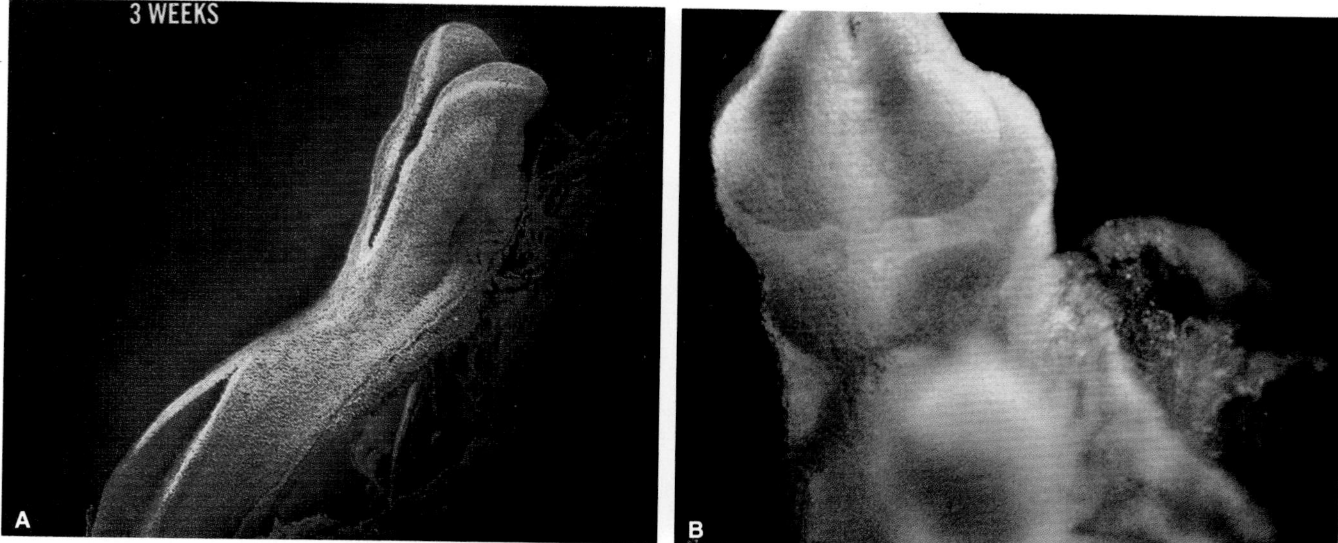

COLOR FIGURE 3–1. (**A**) Three weeks. The neural tube is forming. The anterior and posterior neuropores are still open. (**B**) Three and one-half weeks. Ventral view of the cranial region. Note the forebrain and anterior neuropore, the maxillary and mandibular prominences, the stomodeum, and the cardiac primordium.

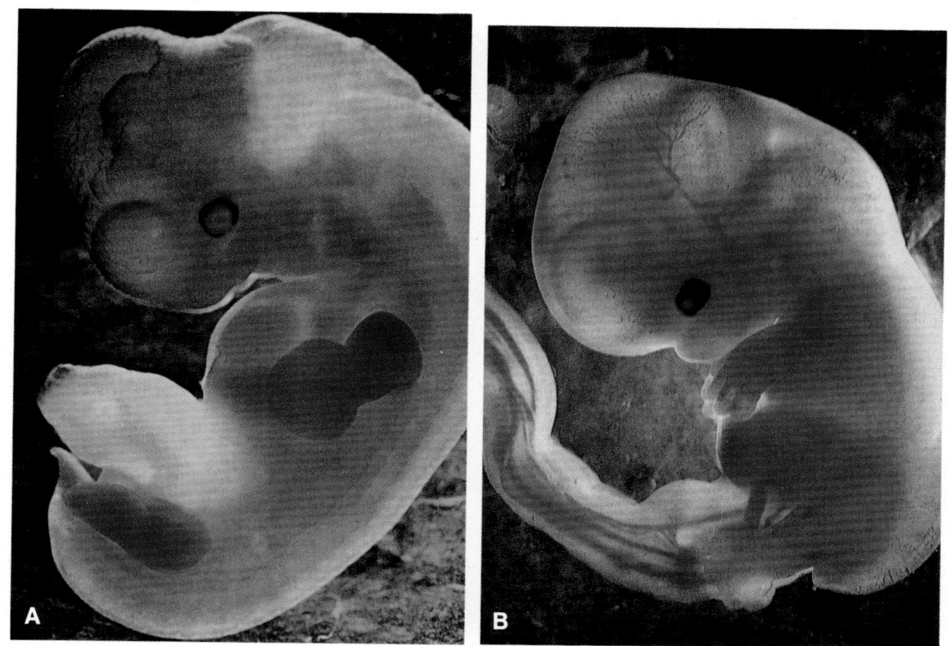

COLOR FIGURE 3–2. (**A**) Five weeks. Note development of the flexures of the brain. The eyes, the liver, and the limb buds are in early development. (**B**) Six and one-half weeks. Note the further development of the features indicated in **A**. The upper limb is always slightly more advanced in development than the lower limb. The back is becoming straighter. Note the umbilical vessels in the umbilical cord.

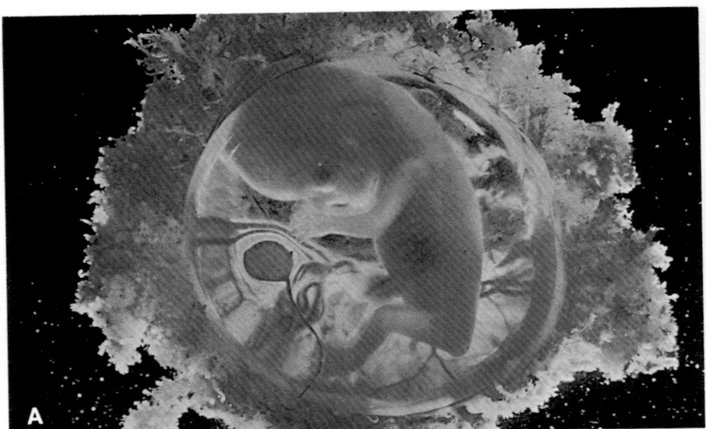

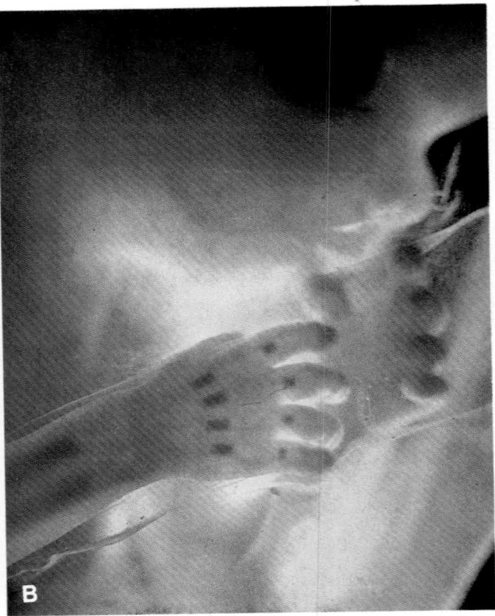

COLOR FIGURE 3–3. (**A**) Eleven weeks. The chorionic sac has been opened to reveal the fetus within the amniotic sac. Note the remnant of the yolk sac and the developing ribs. (**B**) Twelve weeks. Note the separation of the digits and ossification of the bones in the forearm and hand.

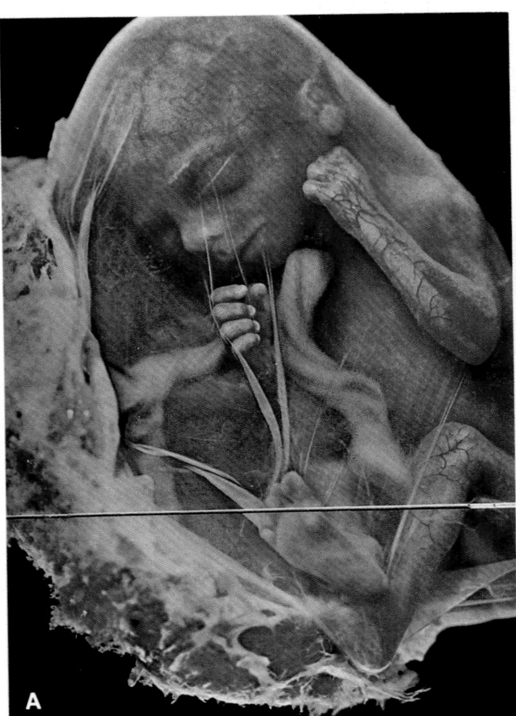

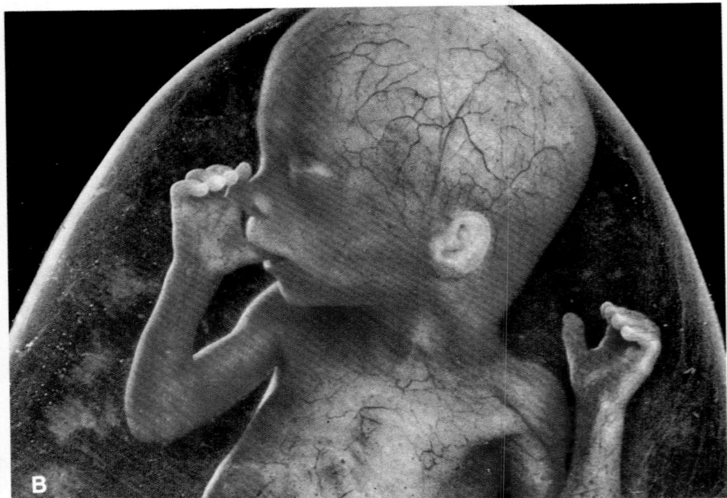

COLOR FIGURE 3–4. (**A**) Sixteen weeks. The fetus is within the amniotic sac. Note the vessels in the umbilical cord. (**B**) Eighteen weeks. The fetus is within the amniotic sac.

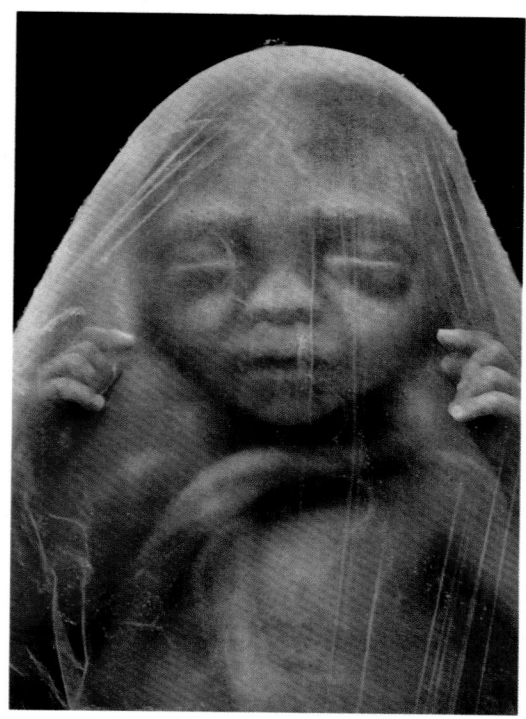

COLOR FIGURE 3–5. Twenty-eight weeks. The fetus is within the amniotic sac. Note that the umbilical cord is looped around the neck.

ans separates the dorsal alar plate (sensory) from the ventral basal plate (motor).

THE BRAIN

The cranial part of the neural tube grows rapidly to form the three primary brain vesicles: the forebrain vesicle (prosencephalon), the midbrain vesicle (mesencephalon), and the hindbrain vesicle (rhombencephalon). The lumen of the neural tube mainly forms the ventricles of the brain. The derivatives of the primary brain vesicles are summarized in Table 3-2.

The rapid growth of the brain results in the formation of two flexures, the cranial (midbrain) and caudal (cervical) flexures. Later, a third flexure, the pontine flexure, appears between the metencephalon and myelencephalon (see Color Figure 3-2*A*).

THE SPINAL CORD

The spinal cord develops from the caudal part of the neural tube. From the alar and basal plates, the posterior and anterior horns are derived, respectively. These plates contribute to the formation of the lateral horn. The neural canal becomes the central canal of the spinal cord.

THE PERIPHERAL NERVOUS SYSTEM

From the neural crest cells, the following structures differentiate: sensory ganglia of the cranial and spinal nerves, autonomic ganglia, neurilemmal (Schwann) cells, cells of the suprarenal medulla, and melanocytes. Neural crest cells probably contribute to the development of the connective tissues of the head, the meninges, and the branchial arches.

THE PITUITARY GLAND

The pituitary gland (hypophysis) develops from two sources: the neurohypophysis develops as a downgrowth from the floor of the diencephalon, and the adenohypophysis develops from an ectodermal outgrowth (Rathke's pouch) from the roof of the stomodeum.

THE MUSCULOSKELETAL SYSTEM

LIMB DEVELOPMENT

By the end of the fourth week, the limb buds appear as paddle-shaped thickenings of the somatic mesoderm at the level of the lower cervical and lumbosacral somites (see Color Figure 3-2*A*). At the apex of each limb bud, the overlying ectoderm thickens to form the apical ectodermal ridge. The apical ectodermal ridge induces proliferation of the underlying mesenchyme, some of which differentiates into cartilage.

The cartilaginous segments of the limbs are sequentially established in a proximodistal order. The flattened hand and foot plates develop five mesenchymal condensations (digital rays), which will give rise to the metacarpals, metatarsals, and phalanges. Degeneration of the loose mesenchyme between the digital rays separates the fingers and toes (interdigital clefts; see Color Figure 3-2*B*).

By the seventh week, endochondral ossification begins (see Color Figure 3-3*B*). Myoblasts differentiate in situ from the surrounding mesenchyme and, immediately following their formation, the muscles are penetrated by nerves. The muscle masses separate into extensor (dorsal) and flexor (ventral) compartments.

Between the seventh and ninth weeks, the developing limbs rotate longitudinally in opposite directions at the elbow and knee regions. Whereas the arm buds ro-

TABLE 3–2. MAIN DERIVATIVES OF THE THREE PRIMARY BRAIN VESICLES

PRIMARY VESICLES	SECONDARY VESICLES	DERIVATIVES	LUMEN
Prosencephalon	Telencephalon	Cerebral hemispheres consisting of the olfactory system, corpus striatum, cortex, and medullary center	Lateral ventricle and part of the third ventricle
	Diencephalon	Thalamus, epithalamus, hypothalamus, and subthalamus	Major part of the third ventricle
Mesencephalon	Mesencephalon	Midbrain: collicular region and cerebral peduncles	Cerebral aqueduct
Rhombencephalon	Metencephalon	Pons and cerebellum	Fourth ventricle
	Myelencephalon	Medulla oblongata	Fourth ventricle and part of the central canal

tate laterally, the limb buds rotate medially. Thus, the anterior (flexor) compartments of the arm and forearm are homologous to the posterior compartments of the thigh and leg.

SKULL DEVELOPMENT

The skull consists of the neurocranium, which surrounds the brain, and the viscerocranium or facial skeleton. The flat bones surrounding the brain form the membranous part of the neurocranium, and the cartilaginous part gives rise to the bones of the base of the skull. The skull develops from the mesenchyme surrounding the developing brain, with contributions from the first four occipital somites and the first branchial arch.

The frontal, parietal, zygomatic, palatine, nasal, and lacrimal bones, the maxilla, and the vomer are formed by intramembranous ossification. Only the ethmoid bone and the inferior nasal conchae are completely formed in cartilage. Bones formed by intramembranous and endochondral ossification include the occipital, sphenoid, and temporal bones, and the mandible.

REFERENCES

1. Arey LB. Developmental anatomy. 7th ed. Philadelphia: WB Saunders, 1974.
2. Corliss CE. Patten's human embryology. New York: McGraw-Hill, 1976.
3. England MA. Color atlas of life before birth. Chicago: Year Book Medical, 1983.
4. Gilbert SG. Pictorial human embryology. Toronto: University of Toronto Press, 1989.
5. Hamilton WJ, Boyd JD, Mossman HW. Human embryology. 3rd ed. Cambridge: W Heffer & Sons, 1964.
6. Langebartel DA. The anatomical primer. An embryological explanation of human gross morphology. Baltimore: University Park Press, 1977.
7. Moore KL. The developing human. Clinically oriented embryology. 4th ed. Philadelphia: WB Saunders, 1988.
8. Sadler TW. Langman's medical embryology. 6th ed. Baltimore: Williams & Wilkins, 1990.
9. Snell RS. Clinical embryology for medical students. 3rd ed. Boston: Little, Brown, 1983.
10. Williams PL, Warwick R, Dyson M, Bannister LH. Gray's anatomy. 37th ed. Edinburgh: Churchill Livingstone, 1989:96.

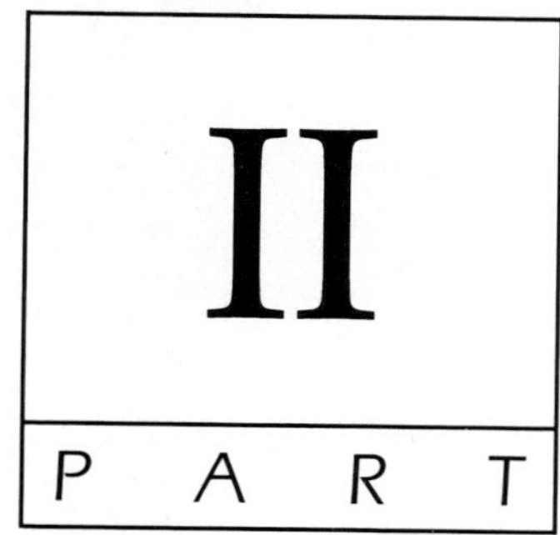

PART II

PREGNANCY AND THE FETOPLACENTAL UNIT

4

CHAPTER

NORMAL PLACENTATION AND DEVELOPMENT

Harold Fox

NORMAL PLACENTATION

The placenta as expelled from the uterus is generally regarded as a complete organ. This, the fetal placenta, is not, however, the total structure; there is also a vitally important maternal component of the placenta, which comprises the placental bed and the uteroplacental vessels.

DEVELOPMENT OF THE FETAL PLACENTA

The fertilized ovum enters the uterine cavity as a morula that rapidly converts into a blastocyst and loses its surrounding zona pellucida. The outer cell layer of the blastocyst proliferates to form the primary trophoblastic cell mass (Fig. 4-1*A*), from which cells infiltrate between those of the endometrial epithelium. The latter degenerates and the trophoblast thus comes into contact with the endometrial stroma. This process of implantation is complete by the 10th or 11th postovulatory day. In the 7-day conceptus, the trophoblast forms a peripheral circumferential plaque (Fig. 4-1*B*), which rapidly differentiates into two layers, an inner layer of large, mononuclear cytotrophoblastic cells with well-defined, limiting membranes, and an outer layer of multinucleated syncytiotrophoblast, which is a true syncytium. That the syncytiotrophoblast is derived from the cytotrophoblast, not only at this early stage but throughout gestation, is now well established. Even when trophoblast is growing rapidly, DNA synthesis and mitotic activity occur only in the nuclei of the cytotrophoblastic cells,[1,2] because the syncytiotrophoblast is a postmitotic, terminally differentiated, tissue. The syncytiotrophoblast appears to be formed by a breaking down of the limiting membrane of the cytotrophoblastic cells. Although no true intercellular membranes are present in the syncytial layer, remnants of such membranes can occasionally be found on electron microscopy.[3] Cells with a cytoplasmic complexity and nuclear structure intermediate between those of the trophoblastic layers can also be identified on electron microscopy, and these "intermediate-type" cytotrophoblastic cells appear to be ones that are beginning to differentiate into syncytiotrophoblast but have not yet lost their limiting membranes.

Between the 10th and 13th postovulatory days, a series of intercommunicating clefts, or lacunae, appear in the rapidly enlarging trophoblastic cell mass (Fig. 4-2). These are probably formed as a result of engulfment within the trophoblast of endometrial capillaries. These lacunae soon become confluent to form the precursor of the intervillous space and, as maternal vessels are progressively eroded, this becomes filled with maternal blood. At this stage the lacunae are incompletely separated from each other by trabecular columns of syncytiotrophoblast which, between the 14th and 21st postovulatory days, tend to become radially orientated and come to possess a central cellular core that is produced by proliferation of the cytotrophoblastic cells at the chorionic base. These trabeculae are not true villi but serve as the framework, or scaffolding, from which the villous tree will later develop. The placenta at this time is a labyrinthine rather than a villous organ and the trabeculae act as "primary villous stems."[4] Continued growth of the cytotrophoblast leads to its distal extension into the region of decidual attachment while, at the same time, a mesenchymal core appears within the villous stems. This is formed by a distal extension of the extraembryonic mesenchyme. Later, the villous stems become vascularized, with the vessels developing in situ from mesenchyme within the core and establishing, in

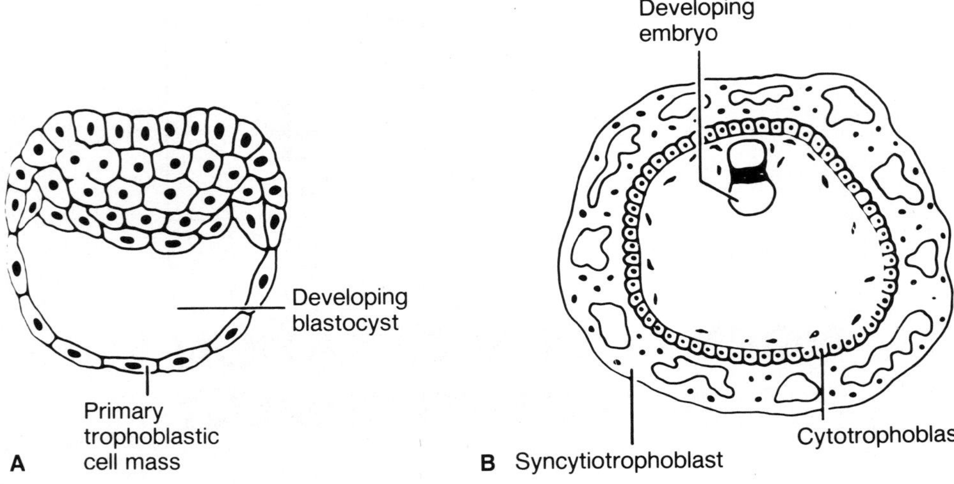

FIGURE 4–1. Diagrammatic representation of formation of primary trophoblastic cell mass (**A**) and the differentiation of this into cytotrophoblast and syncytiotrophoblast (**B**).

due course, functional continuity with others, differentiating in the body stalk and inner chorionic mesenchyme.

The distal part of the villous stems is now formed almost entirely by cytotrophoblastic cells, which form columns anchored to the decidua of the basal plate. The cells in these "cytotrophoblastic cell columns" proliferate and spread laterally to form a continuous cytotrophoblastic shell that splits the syncytiotrophoblast into two layers, the definitive syncytium on the fetal aspect of the shell and the peripheral syncytium on the maternal side. The definitive syncytium persists as the lining of the intervillous space, but the peripheral syncytium eventually degenerates and is replaced by fibrinoid material (Nitabuch's layer). The establishment of the cytotrophoblastic shell is a mechanism to allow for rapid circumferential growth of the developing placenta, and this leads to an expansion of the intervillous space, into which sprouts extend from the primary villous stems. These offshoots consist initially only of syncytiotrophoblast, but as they enlarge they pass through the stages previously seen during the development of the primary villous stems— intrusion of cytotrophoblast, formation of a mesenchymal core, and eventual vascularization. These sprouts are the primary stem villi and, as they are true villous structures, the placenta is by the 21st postovulatory day a vascularized villous organ. The primary stem villi later grow and divide to form secondary and tertiary stem villi, and these latter eventually break up into the terminal villous tree.

Between the 21st postovulatory day and the end of the fourth month of gestation, there is not only continuing growth but also considerable remodelling of the placenta. The villi orientated toward the uterine cavity degenerate and form the chorion laeve, while the thin rim of decidua covering this area gradually disappears to allow the chorion laeve to come into contact with the parietal decidua of the opposite wall of the uterus. The villi on the side of the chorion orientated toward the decidual plate proliferate and progressively arborize to

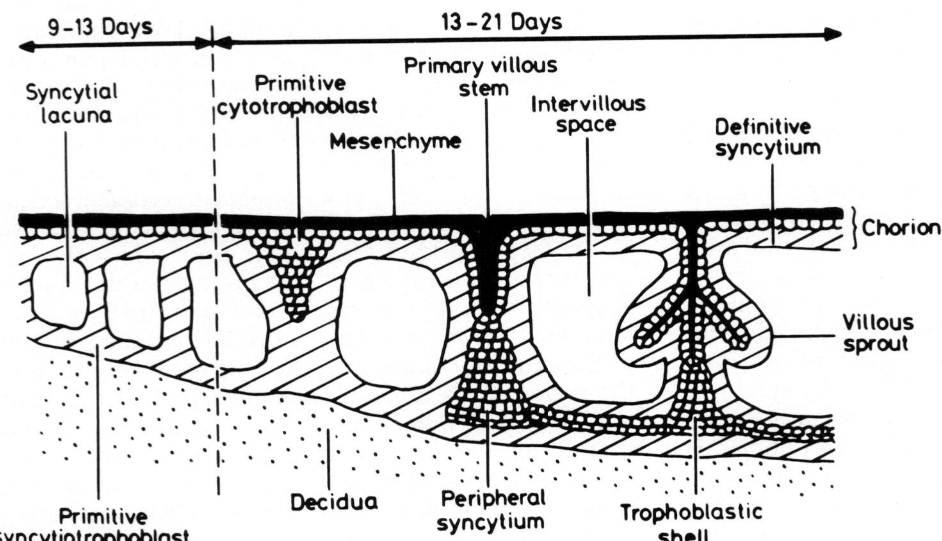

FIGURE 4–2. Diagrammatic representation of the development of the placenta during the first 21 days of gestation.

form the chorion frondosum, which develops into the definitive fetal placenta. During this period there is some regression of the cytotrophoblastic elements in the chorionic plate and in the trophoblastic shell, while the cytotrophoblastic cell columns largely degenerate and are replaced by fibrinoid material (Rohr's layer); clumps of cells persist, however, as "cytotrophoblastic cell islands."

The placental septa appear during the third month of gestation: they protrude into the intervillous space from the basal plate and divide the maternal surface of the placenta into 15 to 20 lobes. These septa are simply folds of the basal plate, formed partly as a result of regional variability in placental growth and partly by the pulling up of the basal plate by the anchoring columns, which have a poor growth rate.[4] Because the basal plate is formed principally by the remnants of the trophoblastic shell embedded in fibrinoid material, it follows that the septa are similarly constituted, although some decidual cells may also be carried up into the folds. The septa are simply an incidental byproduct of the architectural remodelling of the placenta, and have no physiological or morphological role to play.

By the end of the fourth month of gestation, the fetal placenta has achieved its definitive form and undergoes no further anatomical modification. Growth continues, however, until term and is due principally to the continuing branching of the villous tree and formation of fresh villi.

DEVELOPMENT OF THE MATERNAL PLACENTA

During the early weeks of gestation, cytotrophoblastic cells stream out from the tips of the anchoring villi, penetrate the trophoblastic shell, and extensively colonize the decidua and adjacent myometrium of the placental bed. These cells are known as the "interstitial extravillous cytotrophoblast"; in addition, trophoblastic cells stream into the lumens of the intradecidual portions of the spiral arteries of the placental bed, where they form intralumenal plugs and constitute the "intravascular extravillous cytotrophoblast." These endovascular trophoblastic cells destroy and replace the endothelium of the maternal vessels and then invade the media, with resulting destruction of the medial elastic and muscular tissue[5]: the arterial wall becomes replaced by fibrinoid material that appears to be derived partly from fibrin in the maternal blood and partly from proteins secreted by the invading trophoblastic cells.[6] This process is complete by the end of the first trimester, at which time these "physiological" changes within the spiral arteries of the placental bed extend to the myometriodecidual junction. There then appears to be a pause in this process, but between the 14th and 16th week of gestation there is a resurgence of endovascular trophoblastic migration, with a second wave of cells moving down into the intramyometrial segments of the spiral arteries, extending as far as the origin of these vessels from the radial arteries. Within the intramyometrial portion of the spiral arteries the same process that occurs in their intradecidual portion is repeated, ie, replacement of the endothelium, invasion and destruction of the medial musculo-elastic tissue, and fibrinoid change in the vessel wall. The end result of this trophoblastic invasion of, and attack on, the vessels is that the thick-walled muscular spiral arteries are converted into flaccid, sac-like uteroplacental vessels (Fig. 4-3) that can passively dilate in order to accommodate the greatly augmented blood flow through this vascular system, which is required as pregnancy progresses.

It will be apparent that the extravillous intravascular population of trophoblastic cells plays a key role in placentation, and that via these cells the placenta establishes its own low-pressure, high-conductance vascular system, thus ensuring an adequate maternal blood flow to itself and an ample supply of oxygen and nutrients to the fetus.

Although the function of the intravascular population of extravillous trophoblastic cells appears clear, that of the interstitial extravillous trophoblastic cells is obscure. The number of these cells has been seriously underestimated in the past, for it is now known that they are a major component of the placental bed.[7] The interstitial trophoblastic cells tend to aggregate around

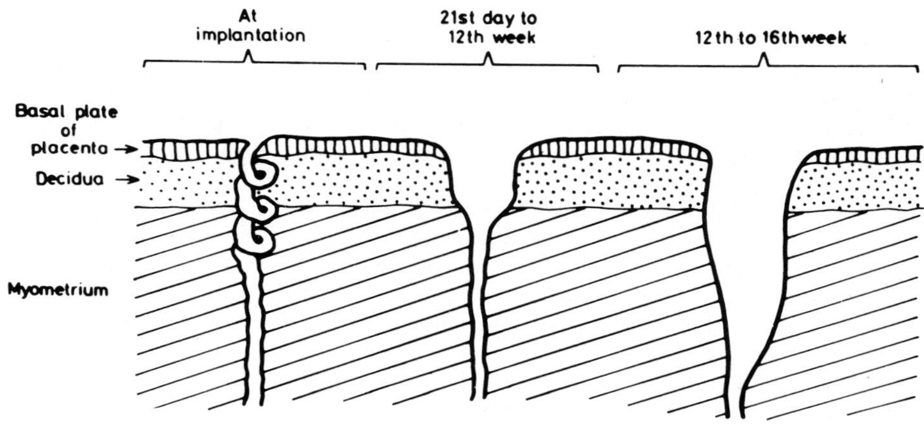

FIGURE 4–3. Diagrammatic representation of the conversion of the spiral arteries in the placental bed into uteroplacental vessels.

the spiral arteries, and it has been suggested that they prime these vessels to allow them to react to their eventual invasion by endovascular trophoblast[8]; if this is indeed the function of these cells, then their mode of action on the vessels is unknown.

The extravillous trophoblastic cells differ, as a whole, from villous trophoblast in their ability to express Class I major histocompatibility antigens[9–11] and in the fact that their principal synthetic product is hPL rather than hCG.[11–13] Studies with monoclonal antibodies have, however, shown that the apparently morphologically homogenous extravillous trophoblastic cells are actually constituted by a number of antigenically heterogenous populations.[14]

ANATOMY OF THE FETAL PLACENTA

The fetal placenta is made up of a number of subunits that are now generally known as lobules. The injection studies of Wilkin[15] have shown that the primary stem villi break up just below the chorial plate into a number of secondary stem villi which, after running parallel to the chorionic plate for a short distance, divide into a series of tertiary stem villi. The lobules are derived from these tertiary stem villi, which sweep down through the intervillous space to anchor onto the basal plate; during the course through the intervillous space they give off multiple branches that ramify into the terminal villous network. As the tertiary stem villi pass down towards the basal plate, they are arranged in a circular fashion around the periphery of an empty cylindrical space; the lobule thus forms a hollow globule (Fig. 4-4), with the bulk of the terminal villi mainly in the outer shell of this globular structure and the center of the lobule relatively empty and free of villi. The lobules are separated from each other by interlobular areas that are in continuity with the subchorial space.

There has been considerable confusion as to the meaning of the term "cotyledon" when applied to the human placenta. This name should not be used to describe the lobes seen on the maternal surface; these are merely the areas lying between the septa and lack any other morphological significance. The term cotyledon should be restricted to the functional unit of the placental villous tree, which is best defined as that part of the villous tree that is derived from a single, primary stem villus.[16] A primary stem villus can, however, give rise to a varying number of secondary stem villi and thus to a differing number of lobules, because there is no fixed relationship between cotyledons and lobules. Thus, centrally placed cotyledons may contain as many as five lobules, while those situated laterally may have only one or two lobules. The situation has, however, been made unduly complicated by the fact that some morphologists have applied the term cotyledon to the maternal surface lobes, and others have also used this name to describe the lobule. The human placenta is not really a cotyledonary structure, and there is a strong case for abandoning the term cotyledon when referring to the human placenta.

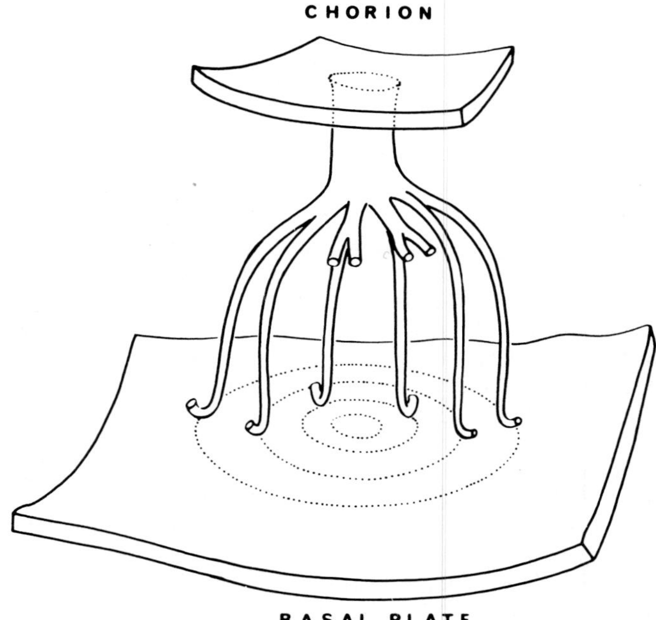

FIGURE 4–4. Diagrammatic representation of a fetal lobule. The stem villi are arranged in a circular fashion around a central hollow core.

THE MATERNAL UTEROPLACENTAL CIRCULATORY SYSTEM

Maternal blood enters the intervillous space via arterial inlets in the basal plate and is then driven by the head of maternal pressure toward the chorionic plate as a funnel-shaped stream (Fig. 4-5).[17] The driving head of maternal pressure is gradually dissipated, a process aided by the baffling effect of the villi, and lateral dispersion of the blood occurs. This forces the blood already present in the intervillous space out through basally sited wide venous outlets, into the endometrial venous network. India ink injection studies originally suggested that the maternal blood entered the intervillous space as a "jet" or "spurt," but cineangiography has shown that these terms give an undue impression of both speed and intermittency. The maternal blood enters the space "much as water from an actively flowing brook penetrates a reed-filled marsh."[18]

The physiological basis for this circulatory system is a series of pressure differentials. The pressure in the maternal arterioles is higher than the mean intervillous space pressure which, in turn, exceeds that in the maternal veins during a myometrial diastole. This entire system is, however, a low-pressure one, for whereas in most organs there is a progressive decrease in the diameter of the arteries as they approach their target tissues, the reverse is true for the placenta. The uteroplacental vessels assume an increasing diameter as they approach their entry into the intervillous space. There is, therefore, a considerable drop in pressure from the proximal to the distal portion of these vessels, and the full arterial pressure is not transmitted to the intervillous space. The

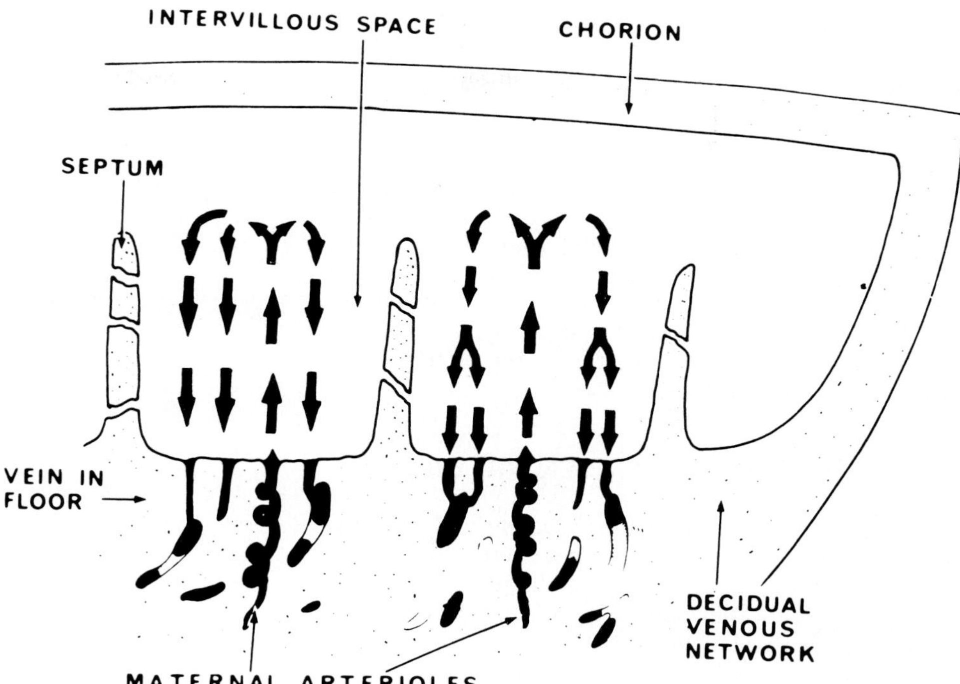

FIGURE 4–5. Diagrammatic representation of the circulation of maternal blood through the placenta.

placenta itself offers little flow resistance to maternal blood and has a high vascular conductance; there is thus very little fall in pressure across the intervillous space, and the main factor governing the rate of maternal blood flow in a normal pregnancy is the vascular resistance within the radial arteries.[19,20] Despite the fact that the pressure difference between arterial and venous sides of the intervillous space is small, it is apparently sufficient to drive arterial blood toward the chorionic plate, to stop short-cutting of the stream into adjacent venous outlets, and to prevent mixing of neighboring arterial inflows.

Cineangiography has shown that the individual uteroplacental arteries act independently of each other. They are not all patent and do not discharge blood simultaneously into the intervillous space. Furthermore, during myometrial contractions, the afferent blood flow through the intervillous space may be markedly reduced or can even cease. This is probably due to compression and occlusion of the veins draining the intervillous space,[21] but ultrasonic studies have shown that during a myometrial contraction the intervillous space distends,[22] so the fetus is not severely deprived of an oxygen supply during myometrial systole.

RELATIONSHIP OF MATERNAL CIRCULATORY SYSTEM TO FETAL LOBULE

The hemodynamic system originally proposed by Ramsey[18] postulated that the maternal blood flow into the intervillous space was through randomly situated arterial inlets, but it has since become clear that this is not the case and that a definite relationship exists between the maternal vessels and the fetal lobules. This is not coincidental, because it is probable that the lobules tend to develop preferentially around the flow from eroded maternal vessels.[23] The exact nature of this relationship is still not fully determined, and two contrasting schemes have been proposed. Some have thought that arterial inlets into the intervillous space are so situated that the inflow from each uteroplacental vessel is into the central, villous-free space of a fetal lobule,[24,25] and that the maternal blood then flows laterally through the lobule into the interlobular, area from which it is drained by basal venous outlets (Fig. 4-6). Others consider that the maternal vessels open, not into the central

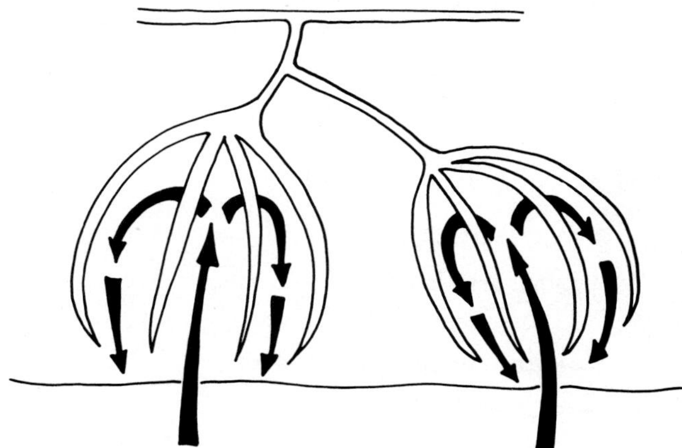

FIGURE 4–6. Diagrammatic representation of the relationship between the maternal blood flow (*black arrows*) and the fetal lobule as envisaged by Wigglesworth.

space of a lobule, but into the interlobular spaces,[26–28] and that the maternal blood then encircles the lobule in streams to form a shell around them, entering and leaving the lobule while doing this and before draining through the basal outlets (Fig. 4-7).

Whichever of these two concepts is correct, it is clear that maternal–fetal exchange takes place principally in those villi that form the shell of the lobule, and that it is only here that a true functional intervillous space, which is probably only of capillary caliber, exists; elsewhere, in the subchorial lake, the interlobular spaces and the central intralobular spaces, villi are either sparse or absent, and these areas are, in functional terms "physiological dead spaces."

HISTOLOGY OF THE PLACENTAL VILLI

In the first 2 months of pregnancy, the villi are relatively few in number, have a homogenous pattern, and measure approximately 170 μ in diameter (Fig. 4-8). Their outer surface is covered by a trophoblastic mantle, which has two layers: an outer layer of syncytiotrophoblast, and an inner layer of cytotrophoblastic cells (Langhans' cells). The latter, which form a complete layer, are cuboid, polyhedral, or ovoid, and have well-marked cell borders. No cell boundaries are visible between the nuclei of the syncytiotrophoblast, and microinjection studies have shown that substances flow freely through this layer and can pass from one villus to another, indicating that there is a continuous common cytoplasm over the entire surface of the placental villi.[29] The syncytiotrophoblast is of uniform thickness, while the syncytial nuclei are regularly spaced and are smaller and more densely staining than those of the trophoblast.

A delicate brush border is often discernible on the outer surface of the syncytium. This corresponds with the microvilli that are seen on electron microscopy, which probably have no absorptive function, but may well play a role in pinocytotic vesicle formation and

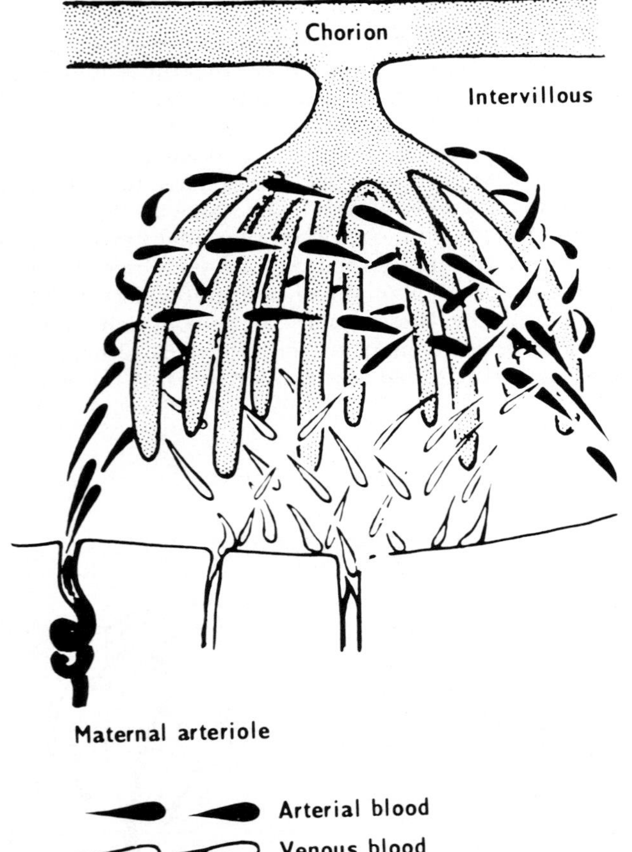

FIGURE 4–7. Diagrammatic representation of the relationship between the maternal blood flow (*black*) and the fetal lobule (*stippled*) as envisaged by Gruenwald.

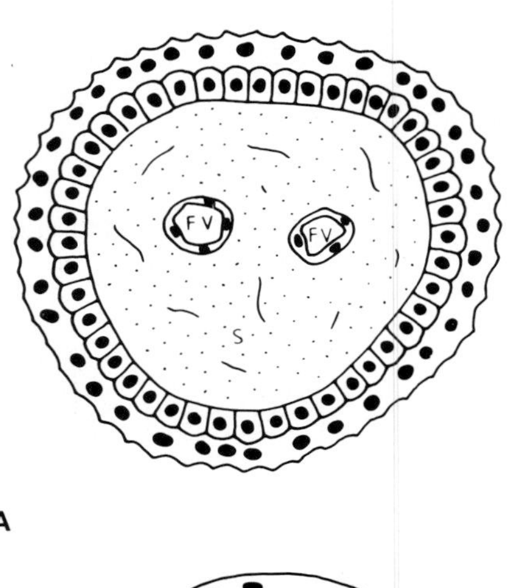

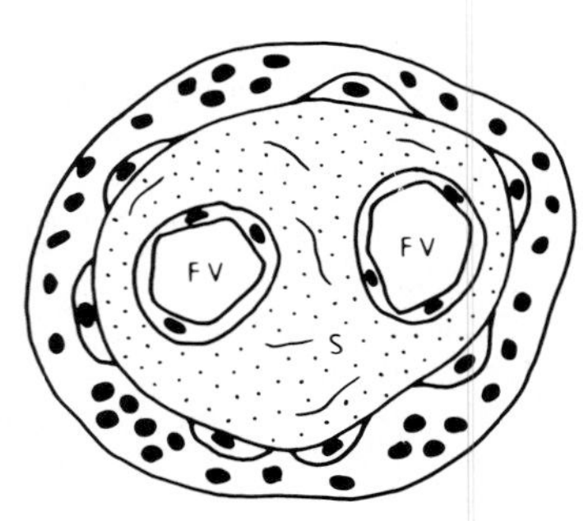

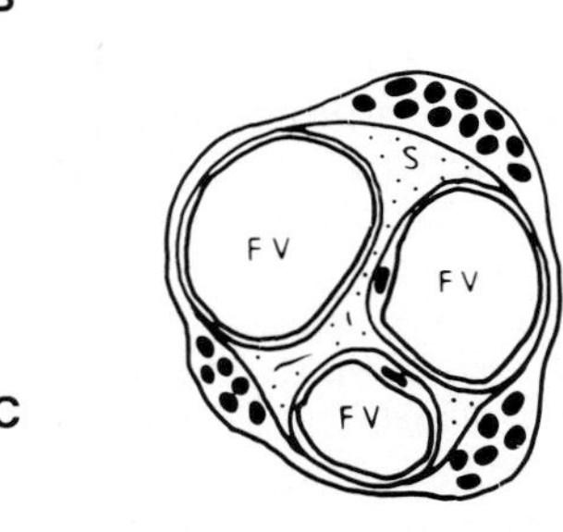

FIGURE 4–8. Diagrammatic representation of the histological appearances of the placental villi in the first trimester (**A**), second trimester (**B**), and at term (**C**).

could also serve to increase the density of specific surface receptor sites.[30] It is worth noting that the syncytiotrophoblast lines the intervillous space and thus acts as an "endothelium": the structure of the syncytiotrophoblast is quite unlike that of an endothelial cell, and hence its ability to function in this manner is something of a mystery. It is possible, however, that some of the many placental proteins secreted by the syncytiotrophoblast act to prevent coagulation, while studies with monoclonal antibodies have shown that, despite their structural dissimilarity, syncytiotrophoblast and endothelial cells do appear to share otherwise specific antigens.[31]

The villous stroma is, at this stage, formed by loose mesenchymal tissue: by the end of the second month of gestation, small, centrally placed vessels, lined by large, immature endothelial cells, are present. Hofbauer cells are a prominent feature of the villous stroma: these cells may be round, ovoid, or reniform, measure about 25 μm in diameter, and have an eccentrically placed nucleus. There is now overwhelming evidence that the Hofbauer cells are fetal tissue macrophages[32–35]; their origin is, however, obscure, for they are present in the villi before they are vascularized by fetal vessels and before hematopoiesis begins in the fetus. It has been suggested that there may be several populations of Hofbauer cells, those in early pregnancy developing from chorionic mesenchyme but later being supplemented by cells derived either from the fetal liver or bone marrow.[36] The Hofbauer cells probably play a number of roles, some related to transport mechanisms and others to immunological protection of the fetus; in this latter respect, their ability to trap maternal antibodies crossing over into the placental tissues is almost certainly of considerable importance.

Between the eighth and 30th weeks of gestation, the villi become more numerous, and the predominant form of villus has an average diameter of about 40 μm. In these villi the cytotrophoblastic cells are less prominent, while the syncytiotrophoblast is thinner and somewhat irregular: the syncytial nuclei are less evenly distributed than in the first trimester, and often show a degree of clustering. A distinct, but thin, trophoblastic basement membrane is present, separating the trophoblast from the stroma. The stroma is more compact than is the case in the villi of early gestation, and contains a variable number of fibroblasts, myofibroblasts, and delicate collagen fibers. Hofbauer cells are seen in the stromal interfibrillary spaces, but appear less numerous than in the villi of the early placental. The villous fetal capillaries are quite prominent, tend to lie more toward the villous periphery, and are lined by flattened, fully mature endothelial cells.

From about the 30th week of gestation, small terminal villi, measuring about 40 μm in diameter, begin to appear; these are the predominant form of villi seen in the term placenta. Their trophoblastic-covering layer is irregularly thinned, while cytotrophoblastic cells are few and inconspicuous.

In terminal villi, the syncytial nuclei are irregularly distributed and are often aggregated from multinucleated protrusions into the intervillous space.[37] It has been claimed that many, even most, of these knots are histological artifacts due to tangential sectioning of the villi;[38,39] nevertheless the nuclei within these knots differ considerably from those in the rest of the villous syncytiotrophoblast and show all the ultrastructural features of sensscence. It appears therefore that syncytial knots are formed of aged nuclei that become sequestrated away from the functional areas of the syncytium, their loss being made up for by the formation of fresh syncytial nuclei from the cytotrophoblast.[40]

In many terminal villi, the syncytiotrophoblast is focally attenuated and anuclear; these thinned areas commonly overlie a dilated fetal capillary vessel and form what is known as "vasculo-syncytial membranes." These membranous areas of the syncytiotrophoblast differ markedly from the nonthinned areas of the syncytium in their content of histochemically detectable enzymes,[41] in their ultrastructure,[42] and in their surface characteristics[43]; it is almost certain that they are specialized zones for the facilitation of gas transfer across the placenta.

The trophoblastic basement membrane of the terminal villi is well defined, whereas the villous stromal tissue is reduced to a thin layer between the sinusoidally dilated villous capillaries. Hofbauer cells are present in the stroma but are difficult to recognize because of their compression by vessels and collagen fibers.

In the terminal villi, there are usually between two and six fetal capillary vessels, which are characteristically situated toward the villous periphery in close approximation to the covering trophoblast. These vessels are commonly sinusoidally dilated and occupy most of the cross-sectional area of the villus. Aherne[44] thought that the dilatation of the fetal villous vessels was a mechanism for crowding flow lines, and hence increasing concentration gradients, for substances crossing from maternal to fetal blood, and was thus a mechanism for augmenting the efficiency of placental transfer mechanisms. By contrast, other have considered that the sinusoidal dilatation of these vessels was a means of decreasing blood flow resistance, for allowing an evenness of blood flow throughout the placenta, and for facilitating fetal placental perfusion.[45]

REFERENCES

1. Richart R. Studies of placental morphogenesis I: radiographic studies of human placenta utilizing tritiated thymidine. Proc Soc Exp Biol Med 1961;106:829.
2. Galton M. DNA content of placental nuclei. Cell Biol 1962;13:183.
3. Enders AC. A comparative study of the fine structure of the trophoblast in several hemochorial placentae. Am J Anat 1965;116:29.
4. Boyd JD, Hamilton WJ. The human placenta. Cambridge: Heffer, 1970.
5. Brosens I, Robertson WB, Dixon HG. The physiological response

of the vessels of the placental bed in normal pregnancy. J Pathol Bacteriol 1967;93:569.
6. de Wolf F, de Wolf-Peeters C, Brosens I. Ultrastructure of the spiral arteries in the human placental bed at the end of normal pregnancy. Am J Obstet Gynecol 1973;117:833.
7. Pijnenborg R, Bland JM, Robertson WB, Dixon G, Brosens I. The pattern of interstitial trophoblastic invasion of the myometrium in early human pregnancy. Placenta 1981;2:303.
8. Pijnenborg R, Bland JM, Robertson WB, Brosens I. Uteroplacental arterial changes related to interstitial trophoblast migration in early human pregnancy. Placenta 1983;4:397.
9. Redman CW, McMichael AJ, Stirrat GM, Sunderland CA, Ting A. Class I major histocompatibility complex antigens on human extra-villous trophoblast. Immunology 1984;52:457.
10. Bulmer J, Smith J, Morrison L, Wells M. Maternal and fetal cellular relationships in the human placental basal plate. Placenta 1988;9:237.
11. Sasagawa M, Yamazaki T, Endo M, Kanazawa K, Takeuchi S. Immunohistochemical localization of HLA antigens and placental proteins (alpha hCG, beta hCG, CTP, hPL and SP_1) in villous and extavillous trophoblast in normal human pregnancy: a distinctive pathway of differentiation of extravillous trophoblast. Placenta 1987;8:515.
12. Kurman RJ, Main CS, Chen H-H. Intermediate trophoblast: a distinctive form of trophoblast with specific morphological, biochemical and functional features. Placenta 1984;5:349.
13. Gosseye S, Fox H. An immunohistological comparison of the secretory capacity of villous and extravillous trophoblast in the human placenta. Placenta 1985;5:329.
14. Bulmer JN, Johnson PM. Antigen expression by trophoblast populations in the human placenta and their possible immunobiological relevance. Placenta 1985;6:127.
15. Wilkin P. Pathologie du placenta. Paris: Masson, 1965.
16. Ramsey EM. Circulation in the placenta. In: Villee CA, ed. Gestation: transactions of the fifth conference. New York: Macy Foundation, 1959:77.
17. Ramsey EM, Donner MW. Placenta vasculature and circulation. Philadelphia: WB Saunders, 1980.
18. Ramsey EM. Circulation of the placental. Birth Defects 1965;1:5.
19. Moll W, Zunzell W, Herburger J. Hemodynamic implications of hemochorial placentation. Eur J Obstet Gynecol Rep Biol 1975;5:67.
20. Moll W. Physiologie der maternen placentaren Durchblutung. In: Becker V, Schiebler TH, Kubli F, eds. Die Plazenta des Menschen. Stuttgart: Thieme, 1981:172.
21. Adamson K, Myers RE. Circulation in the intervillous space: obstetrical considerations in fetal deprivation. In: Gruenwald P, ed. The placenta and its maternal supply line. Lancaster: Medical and Technical Publishing, 1975:158.
22. Blecker OP, Kloosterman GJ, Mieras DJ, Oosting J, Sallé HJA. Intervillous space during uterine contractions in human subjects: an ultrasonic study. Am J Obstet Gynecol 1975;123:697.
23. Reynolds SRM. Formation of fetal cotyledons in the hemochorial placenta: a theoretical consideration of the functional implications of such an arrangement. Am J Obstet Gynecol 1966;94:425.
24. Freese UE. The fetal-maternal circulation of the placenta. I: histomorphologic, placental injection and x-ray cinematographic studies on human placenta. Am J Obstet Gynecol 1966;94:354.
25. Wigglesworth JS. Vascular organization of the human placenta. Nature 1967;216:1120.
26. Lemtis H. Physiologie der Plazenta. Fortschritte für Geburtshilfe und Gynakologie 1970;41:1.
27. Gruenwald P. Lobular structure of hemochorial primate placentas, and its relation to maternal vessels. Am J Anat 1973;136:133.
28. Schumann R. Plazenten: Begriff, Entsehung, funktionelle Anatomie. In: Becker V, Schiebler TH, Kubli F, eds. Die Plazenta des Menschen. Stuttgart: Thieme, 1981:199.
29. Gaunt M, Ockleford CD. Microinjection of human placenta. II: biological application. Placenta 1986;7:325.
30. Dearden I, Ockleford CD. Structure of the trophoblast: correlation with function. In: Loke YW, Whyte A, eds. Biology of trophoblast. Amsterdam: Elsevier, 1983:69.
31. Voland JR, Frisman DM, Baird SM. Presence of an endothelial antigen on the syncytiotrophoblast of human chorionic villi: detection by a monoclonal antibody. Am J Rep Immunol Microbiol 1986;11:24.
32. Fox H, Kharkongor NF. Enzyme histochemistry of the Hofbauer cells of the human placenta. J Obstet Gynaecol Br Commonwealth 1969;76:918.
33. Moskalewski S, Ptak W, Czernik Z. Demonstration of cells with IgG receptor in human placenta. Biol Neonate 1975;26:269.
34. Castellucci M, Zaccheo D, Pescetto G. A three-dimensional study of the normal human placental villous core. I: the Hofbauer cells. Cell Tissue Res 1980;210:235.
35. Demir R, Erbengi T. Some new findings about Hofbauer cells in the chorionic villi of the human placenta. Acta Anat 1984;119:18.
36. Castellucci M, Celona A, Bartels H, Steininger B, Benedetto V, Kaufmann P. Mitosis of the Hofbauer cell: possible implications for a fetal macrophage. Placenta 1987;8:65.
37. Fox H. Pathology of the placenta. Philadelphia: WB Saunders, 1978.
38. Küsterman W. Uber "Proliferationaknoten" und "syncytialknoten" der menschlichen plazenta. Anat Anz 1981;150:144.
39. Cantle SJ, Kaufmann P, Luckhardt M, Schweikhart G. Interpretation of syncytial sprouts and bridges in the human placenta. Placenta 1987;8:221.
40. Jones CJP, Fox H. Syncytial knots and intervillous bridges in the human placenta: an ultrastructural study. 1977;124:275.
41. Amstutz E. Beobachtungen über die Regung der Chorionzotten in der menslichen Plazenta mit beswonderer Berückichtigung der Epithelplatten. Acta Anat 1960;42:12.
42. Burgos MH, Rodriguez EM. Specialized zones in the trophoblast of the human term placenta. 1966;96:342.
43. Fox H, Agrofojo Blanco A. Scanning electron microscopy of the human placenta in normal and abnormal pregnancies. Eur J Obstet Gynecol Rep Biol 1974;4:45.
44. Aherne W. Morphometry. In: Gruenwald P, ed. The placenta and its maternal supply line. Lancaster: Medical and Technical Publishing, 1975;80.
45. Kaufmann P, Bruns U, Leiser R, Luckhardt M, Winterhager E. The fetal vascularisation of term human placenta villi. II: intermediate and terminal villi. Anat Embryol 1985;173:203.

PLACENTAL PATHOLOGY, ABNORMAL PLACENTATION, AND CLINICAL SIGNIFICANCE

Harold Fox

This chapter considers the general pattern of placental pathology, as opposed to giving a detailed account of the placental abnormalities seen in every possible complication of pregnancy. Particular attention is paid to the concept of placental insufficiency.

DEVELOPMENTAL ABNORMALITIES

The only common developmental abnormality of the placenta is extrachorial placentation, in which the chorionic plate, from which the villi arise, is smaller than the basal plate, the transition from villous to nonvillous chorion taking place not at the placental margin but at some distance inside the circumference of the fetal surface of the placenta (Fig. 5-1). If this transition is marked by a flat ring of membranes, the placenta is classed as "circummarginate," whereas if this ring has a raised, rolled edge, the placenta is "circumvallate" (Fig. 5-2). The clinical significance of extrachorial placentation has been much debated, but it is now clear that the circummarginate form is devoid of any functional importance and that, although circumvallate placentation is associated more frequently than can be explained by chance alone with a rather small baby[1,2] and, possibly, with a slight excess of congenital malformations,[3] it does not appear to be associated with any excess of perinatal mortality.[1] Other aberrant forms of placentation are either relatively common but functionally unimportant, eg, bilobate placenta and accessory lobe, or functionally important but excessively rare, eg, placenta membranacea and girdle placenta.

It has been claimed in the past that marginal or velamentous insertion of the cord is associated with a high perinatal mortality, but more modern studies have shown that the site of insertion of the cord is, in functional terms, of no importance.[4,5] Velamentous insertion does, however, present a small risk to the fetus because of the danger of trauma to, and consequent bleeding from, unprotected umbilical vessels running through the membranes.

A placenta previa is one that is implanted, either wholly or partly, in the lower uterine segment. This may result in antepartum bleeding and premature delivery, but there is no evidence that placental function is in any way impaired when the implantation site is unduly low.

GROSS LESIONS OF THE PLACENTA

A fresh placental infarct is moderately firm and dark red; as it ages, it becomes progressively harder and its color changes successively to brown, yellow, and white, so that an old infarct appears as an amorphous, hard, white plaque (Fig. 5-3). Histologically, an early infarct is characterized by aggregation of the villi with obliteration of the intervillous space and early necrotic changes in the villous syncytiotrophoblast (Fig. 5-4); with the passage of time, the infarcted villi undergo a progressive necrobiosis, so that the old infarct consists only of crowded ghost villi.

Small placental infarcts are common and of no importance, but there is general agreement that extensive infarction, ie, necrosis of more than 10% of the placental parenchyma, is accompanied by a high incidence of fetal hypoxia, growth retardation, and intrauterine death.[6] At first sight it appears obvious that these ill

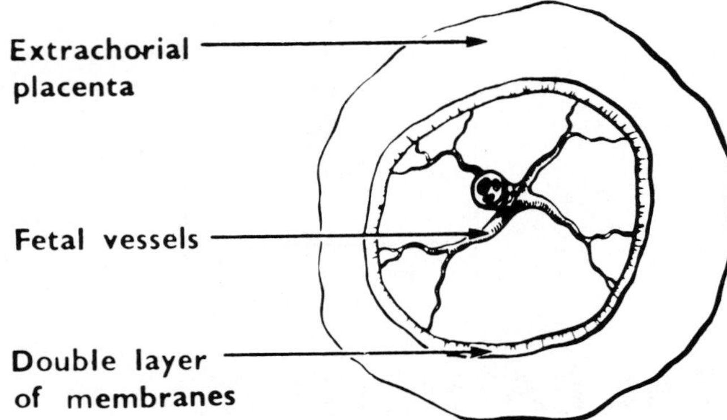

FIGURE 5–1. Diagrammatic representation of an extrachorial placenta as seen from the fetal aspect.

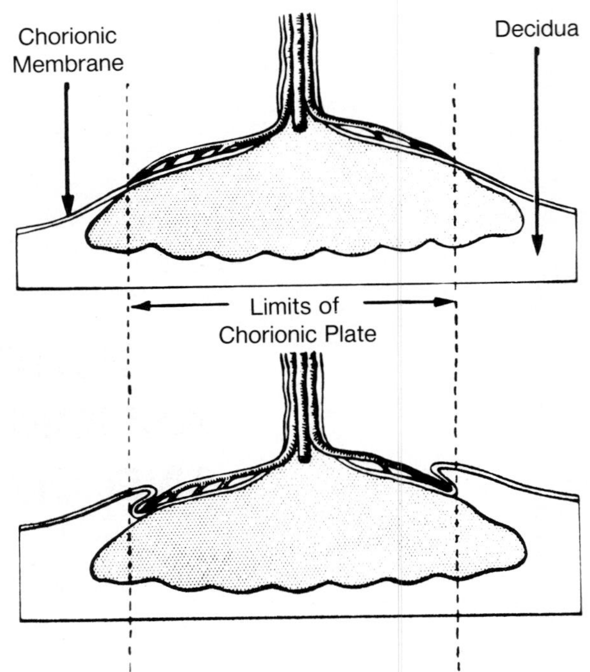

FIGURE 5–2. Diagrammatic representation of a circummarginate placenta (above) and a circumvalate placenta (below).

effects are a direct consequence of the loss of viable villous tissue. It is this finding that has led many to conclude that the placenta has little or no functional reserve capacity. This is a reasonable extension of the belief that the placenta can only withstand the loss of no more than 10% of its villous tissue without endangering the development, and even the viability, of the fetus. That this is far too simplistic a view is made apparent by consideration of another common lesion that reduces the number of functioning villi, namely, perivillous fibrin deposition. Some degree of fibrin deposition around villi occurs in all placentas, but in many this process is sufficiently extensive to result in a macroscopically visible lesion, which is seen as either a hard white plaque or an area of irregular whitish mottling (Fig. 5-5). Histologically, such lesions consist of widely separated villi that are entrapped in fibrin, which is filling in and obliterating the intervillous space (Fig. 5-6). The entrapped villi undergo a secondary sclerosis and are not in any sense of the word infarcted; nevertheless, they are effectively excluded from playing any role in maternal–fetal transfer and are just as much lost, in a physiological sense, to the fetus as they would be if they were infarcted.

Despite the fact that perivillous fibrin deposition depletes the population of functional villi, this lesion is of no clinical importance, even when it is extensive enough to functionally inactivate 30% of the villi by entrapment in fibrin.[6] The ability of the placenta to withstand the loss of one third of its functioning tissue without any discernible effect on fetal growth or development bears eloquent witness to the fact that the placenta quite obviously has a considerable functional reserve capacity, but it still leaves unexplained the apparent paradox that loss of villi due to infarction poses a grave threat to the fetus while a similar, or even greater, loss of villi due to entrapment in fibrin is of no consequence. This paradox is more real than apparent if the pathogenesis of these two lesions is considered. Perivillous fibrin deposition is due to hemodynamic turbulence within the intervillous space, with eddy stasis of maternal blood and laying down of fibrin; therefore, the greater the quantity of maternal blood entering the closed, irregular intervillous space per unit of time, the greater is the risk of turbulence and hence of perivillous fibrin deposition. This lesion tends to occur,

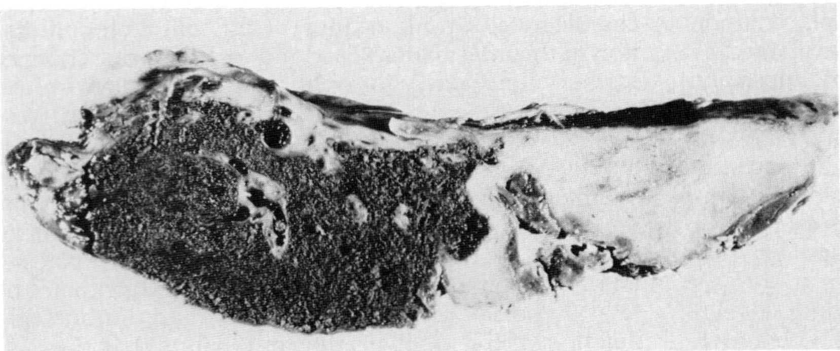

FIGURE 5–3. An old placental infarct. This is seen as a white plaque.

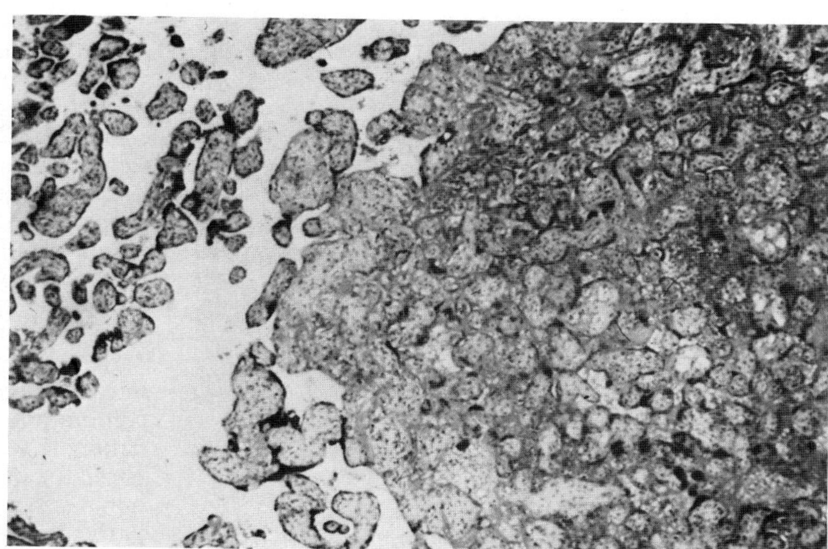

FIGURE 5–4. Histologic appearances of a fresh placental infarct. The villi are aggregated together and the intervillous space is obliterated (hematoxylin and eosin, ×50).

therefore, in placentas with a particularly good maternal uteroplacental blood flow. Infarction, however, is usually due to thrombosis of a maternal uteroplacental vessel, and therefore extensive infarction implies widespread thrombosis within the maternal vasculature. This is an event that one would not expect to occur in a healthy maternal tree, and it is therefore no coincidence that extensive infarction is virtually confined to placentae from women with preeclampsia, a condition in which an acute "atherosis" is found in the uteroplacental vessels[7] and which predisposes to thrombosis. Far more importantly, however, there is in preeclamptic women, whether thrombosis occurs or not, a severely restricted maternal blood flow to the placenta (the reasons for which are discussed later), and it is this limitation of maternal blood flow that is the real cause of the apparent complications of placental infarction.

The true significance of extensive placental infarction is therefore that it is the visible hallmark of a markedly abnormal maternal vasculature and of a severely restricted maternal uteroplacental blood flow. It is true that under these circumstances the placental infarction may further worsen the situation, but the infarction per se is not the primary cause of the fetal complications and would be of little or no importance if it occurred in a placenta with an adequate maternal blood supply.

All other macroscopic lesions of the placenta (with the sole exception of the hemangioma, which is considered later) are of no functional significance and can be ignored. The various plaques, thrombi, and cysts that can occur in the placenta lack clinical importance, and this banality extends also to gross placental calcification, a change often thought to indicate placental "degeneration" or senescence, but one that occurs most commonly in the placentas of primigravid women of high socioeconomic status delivered during the spring and summer months and which is devoid of any clinical importance.[8]

PLACENTAL WEIGHT

It is difficult, and in routine practice virtually impossible, to obtain a true estimate of placental mass and, indeed, a knowledge of placental weight is, by itself, of little value. Placental:fetal weight ratios are more meaningful, but it would not be an undue oversimplification to suggest that the only conclusion that can be drawn from the many studies of this ratio is that small babies usually have small placentas, whereas big babies have large placentas. Several findings suggest, however, that placental mass is unlikely to be a limiting factor for fetal growth. First, if fetal weight was narrowly limited by placental mass, this would imply that

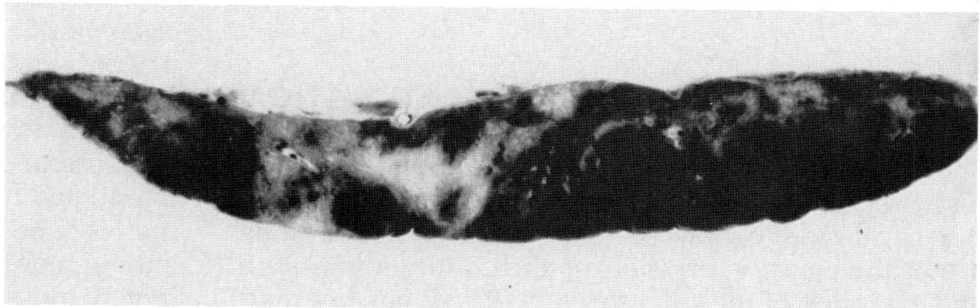

FIGURE 5–5. An irregular whitish plaque of perivillous fibrin deposition.

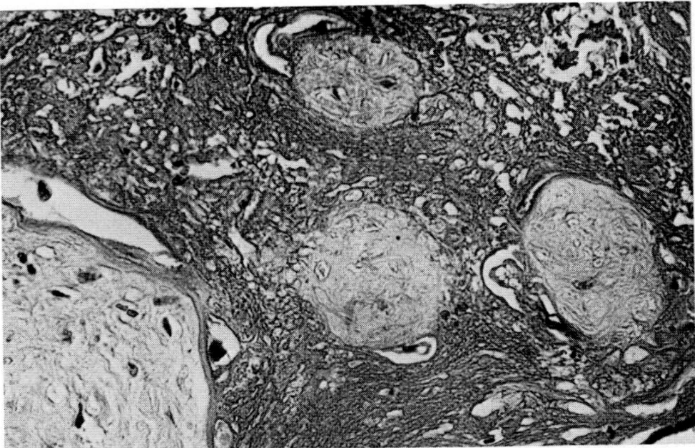

FIGURE 5–6. Villi entrapped in a plaque of perivillous fibrin.

the term placenta has no functional reserve capacity. As already remarked, simple pathologic findings indicate that this is not the case, and experimental studies involving either surgical reduction of placental mass[9] or artificially increased fetal oxygen consumption[10] have confirmed the striking functional reserve capacity of the placenta. Second, the placenta also has a normally unrealized potential for further incremental growth, as evidenced by the large placentas encountered in such conditions as pregnancy at high altitude, severe maternal anemia, and decompensated maternal heart disease.

This ability of the placenta to show a compensatory increment of growth in the face of an unfavorable maternal milieu is further evidence against limitation of fetal weight by placental mass, and it must therefore be concluded that the placenta is usually small because the baby is small, the placenta sharing in the generally reduced growth of the fetal organs, and its small size not acting as a contributory factor to fetal growth retardation.

HISTOLOGICAL ABNORMALITIES OF THE PLACENTA

It is preferable to classify villous abnormalities on a functional, rather than a purely morphological, basis. These may be grouped into (1) abnormalities of villous maturation, (2) changes secondary to a reduced maternal uteroplacental blood flow, (3) changes secondary to a reduced fetal villous blood flow, and (4) abnormalities of unknown pathogenesis.

ABNORMALITIES OF VILLOUS MATURATION

During the 9 months of a normal gestation there is, as discussed in Chapter 4, a progressive change in the predominant type of villus seen in the placenta, this being a morphological expression of the continuing growth and evolution of the villous tree.[11] This villous tree maturation is essential for fully effective functioning of the placenta. The corollary of this is that a failure of the villous tree to undergo full maturation, with a resulting paucity of terminal villi at term, will result in a decreased functional efficiency of the placenta. It is therefore not surprising that a deficiency of the terminal villi toward the end of gestation (a phenomenon usually simply classed as "villous immaturity") is associated with a high incidence of fetal growth retardation.[12]

The relatively simple concept of villous immaturity has been expanded in recent years into an elaborate subclassification based on the use of such terms as "arrested ramification," "discordant retardation," "intercalary defective ramification," "centroperipheral discontinuity of vascularization," and "concordant retardation," with the suggestion that each of these particular patterns represents a specific form of maturational arrest resulting from an insult to the placenta at a particular stage of gestation.[13] It remains to be proved, however, whether this complex classification is founded on any firm basis of fact.

Although there is a good association between inadequate maturation of the villous tree and poor fetal nutrition, most small-for-gestational age infants have fully mature placentas. It should also be noted that this association holds only if there is a generalized immaturity of the villi, because in all term placentas, a few highly immature villi are always to be found scattered among an otherwise fully mature villous population, usually in the center of a lobule. These are an indication of continuing placental growth with the formation of fresh villi.[6]

CHANGES SECONDARY TO A REDUCED MATERNAL UTEROPLACENTAL BLOOD FLOW

Villi in placentas subjected to a reduced maternal uteroplacental blood flow, eg, in severe maternal preeclampsia, show a consistent and characteristic pattern of abnormalities that is identical to that noted in villous tissue grown in vitro under conditions of low oxygen tension.[14,15] There is an undue prominence and number of the villous cytotrophoblastic cells (Fig. 5-7), together with irregular thickening of the trophoblastic basement membrane; although the syncytiotrophoblast usually appears remarkably normal on light microscopy, small focal areas of syncytial necrosis are seen on ultrastructural examination.[16]

The cytotrophoblastic cells are the trophoblastic stem cells even during rapid periods of trophoblastic growth; it is only in these cells that DNA synthesis and mitotic activity occurs. The syncytiotrophoblast is formed by a breaking down of the limiting membranes of the cytotrophoblastic cells and is a postmitotic, terminally differentiated tissue. The cytotrophoblastic stem cells can therefore be considered as forming a germinative zone, although one which, in the later stages of pregnancy, is largely quiescent, the cytotrophoblastic cells becoming

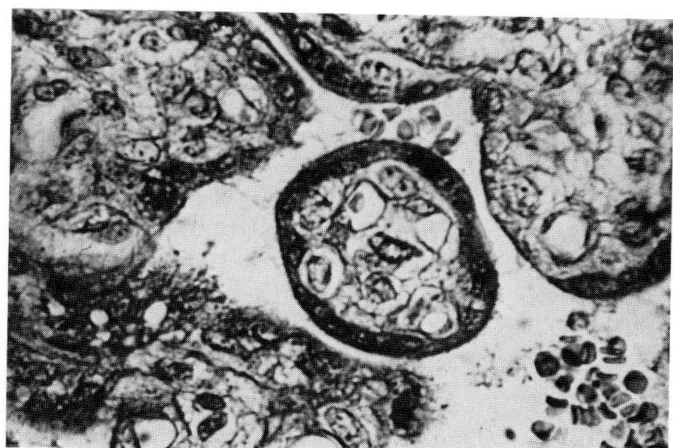

FIGURE 5–7. Placenta from a woman with severe preeclampsia. Villous cytotrophoblastic cells are numerous and conspicuous (periodic acid-Schiff, ×720).

progressively less numerous and prominent as gestation proceeds; their inactivity at term indicates that there is little need for the formation of fresh trophoblast at this time.

If, however, the necessity of forming new syncytiotrophoblast arises, as is the case when this tissue suffers ischemic damage as a result of a reduced maternal blood flow, the germinative zone will be reactivated, and the cytotrophoblastic cells proliferate in an attempt to repair and replace injured syncytial tissue; thus, the cytotrophoblastic cells become more numerous and unusually prominent, while mitotic figures are seen with modest frequency, all features suggesting a resurgence of activity. This repair process is a highly successful one, for it often requires prolonged search to detect residual focal areas of syncytial damage at the ultrastructural level.[16]

The trophoblastic basement membrane thickening that is seen in the villi of placentae subjected to ischemia is probably an incidental byproduct of the cytotrophoblastic cell hyperplasia, for basement membrane protein is almost certainly secreted, in part at least, by these cells, and an unusual degree of proliferative activity on their part would therefore be accompanied by an excessive production of basement membrane material.

The essential response of the placenta to ischemia is therefore a reparative one, with gross trophoblastic damage being efficiently repaired.

CHANGES SECONDARY TO A REDUCED FETAL BLOOD FLOW

These are seen in their purest form in the localized group of villi which, while fully oxygenated from the maternal blood, have been deprived of their fetal circulation by thrombosis of a fetal stem artery; such villi invariably show stromal fibrosis and an excess formation of syncytial knots. These changes are seen in generalized form whenever there is an overall reduction of fetal perfusion of the placenta, and are invariably found as a postmortem change in placentas from fetuses that have been dead in utero for several days or weeks before delivery.[6] Why these particular changes should result from an impairment of fetal blood flow through the placenta is unknown. The placental villi do not in any way depend on the fetal blood supply for either their oxygenation or supply of nutrients; hence there is no good reason why a reduced fetal perfusion should affect the functional activity of the placenta. It is therefore not surprising that neither stromal fibrosis nor excess syncytial knot formation can be correlated with any evidence of adverse effects, during life, on the fetus, although both are found in association with the dead fetus as postmortem changes.[6]

It should, perhaps, be noted that syncytial knots, which are focal clumps of syncytial nuclei that protrude into the intervillous space from the villous surface, are not, as is often thought to be the case, a manifestation of any degenerative change in the trophoblast or a reaction to uteroplacental ischemia: their appearance in the placenta as gestation progresses is a time-related phenomenon but is not a true aging change.

ABNORMALITIES OF UNKNOWN PATHOGENESIS

Prominent among the abnormalities of unknown pathogenesis is fibrinoid necrosis of placental villi. In this lesion, the fibrinoid material appears first in a cytotrophoblastic cell, and its presence is not due to deposition within the villus of fibrin derived from the maternal blood in the intervillous space. The lesion has been attributed to an immunological reaction within villous tissue, but this is far from proven; currently, the significance (if any) of an excess of villi showing fibrinoid change is unknown.

Villous edema is of unknown origin, although it has been attributed to the effects of prostaglandins released from inflamed membranes or to catecholamines secreted by a "stressed" fetus.[17,18] It has been suggested that the increased size of the edematous villi decreases the capacity of the intervillous space and hence restricts maternal blood flow[19] with consequent fetal hypoxia.[18,19] A recent study has, however, failed to show that villous edema is of any clinical significance.[20]

AGING OF THE PLACENTA

There is a widely and tenaciously held belief that during the course of a normal pregnancy the placenta progressively ages and that the term placenta is in, or is on the verge of, a decline into morphological and functional senescence. The villi of the term placenta are often described as showing all the morphological hallmarks of senescence, but this view is based almost entirely on a misunderstanding and misinterpretation of the histological manifestations of the normal processes of maturation of the villous tree and of trophoblastic differentiation. There are no light or electron microscopic features in the villi that can be considered indicative of an aging process.[21,22]

It is often suggested that a feature of placental aging is the cessation of DNA synthesis that has been claimed to occur at the 36th week of gestation,[23] but more recent studies have shown that total placental DNA levels continue to rise in a linear fashion until and beyond the 40th week of pregnancy.[24] This finding is in accord with histological evidence of fresh villous growth in the term placenta,[6] with autoradiographic and flow cytometric demonstration of continuing DNA synthesis[25,26] and with morphometric studies that have demonstrated a continuing expansion of the villous surface area and progressive branching of the villous tree up to and beyond term.[27]

Placental growth certainly slows during the last few weeks of gestation, although this decline in growth rate is neither invariable nor irreversible, because the placenta can continue to increase in size if faced with an unfavorable maternal environment (eg, pregnancy at high altitude, severe maternal anemia), while the potential for a recrudescence of growth is shown by the proliferative response to ischemic syncytial damage. Those arguing that a decreased placental growth rate during late pregnancy is evidence of senescence often appear to be comparing the placenta to an organ such as the gut, in which continuing viability is dependent on a constantly replicating stem cell layer producing short-lived postmitotic cells. A more apt comparison would be with an organ such as the liver, which is formed principally of long-lived postmitotic cells and which, once an optimal size has been attained to meet the metabolic demands placed on it, shows little evidence of cell proliferation while retaining a latent capacity for growth activity. There seems no good reason why the placenta, once it has reached a size sufficient to adequately meet its transfer function, should continue to grow, and the term placenta, with its considerable functional reserve capacity, has more than met this aim.

PLACENTAL INFECTION

If the placenta is taken to include the membranes, then infective agents may reach the organ either from the maternal bloodstream or from the endometrium to produce a villitis, or they may ascend from the birth canal to produce a chorioamnionitis.

A predominantly villous inflammation may be due to placental involvement in specific maternal infections, such as rubella, toxoplasmosis, listeriosis, syphilis, or cytomegalovirus disease,[28,29] but such conditions account for only a small proportion of cases of villitis, the vast majority of which are of unknown cause.[30] The reported incidence of villitis in unselected series of placentas in the United Kingdom, Australia, and the United States has varied between 6% and 14%,[28,30,31] but it has to be borne in mind that a villitis is usually discovered only by careful examination, because the villous lesions are often few and scattered. The cells participating in the inflammatory process are lymphocytes and histiocytes; these usually form a mixed villous infiltrate, with instances of purely lymphocytic or solely histiocytic villitis being uncommon.

There is a clear association between the presence of a villitis and a high incidence of fetal intrauterine growth retardation,[30] although the nature of this relationship is obscure. It is assumed, almost certainly correctly, that villitis is usually a true infection, probably with non-bacterial organisms or viruses[32]; if this is so, however, the deficit of fetal growth cannot be attributed, in the vast majority of cases, to damage inflicted on the placenta by an inflammatory process. Occasional examples of a widespread, diffuse necrotizing villitis are encountered, but lesions of this extent are exceptional; most cases of villitis are of a focal nature with only a small, widely scattered, proportion of the villous population showing any evidence of either a healed or an active inflammatory process. This degree of villous damage is unlikely to impair, let alone dissipate, the functional reserve capacity of the placenta, and it is possible that the low birth weight in such cases is due not to villous damage but to fetal infections, of which villitis simply serves as an indicator. The placenta is a much less impermeable barrier to the passage of organisms than is generally thought, and indeed virtually all known organisms are capable of breaching the placental defenses and infecting the fetus. The inhibitory effect of infection on fetal DNA synthesis could well explain the fetal growth retardation. It has been shown, however, that infants with growth retardation associated with a villitis usually have a high ponderal index, ie, show harmonic growth retardation,[33] and this suggests that the deficit of fetal growth dates from the early stages of pregnancy. This, and the fact that villitis may recur in successive pregnancies, may indicate that placental infection is secondary to a chronic endometritis, but it has also been suggested that the villitis is a hallmark not of an infection, but of an immunological reaction within placental tissue,[34,35] and that this could lead to inhibition of normal transformation of the spiral arteries into uteroplacental vessels. Currently, therefore, the nature and significance of a villitis remain debatable.

A chorioamnionitis, characterized by polymorphonuclear leukocytic infiltration of the extraplacental and placental membranes, is now generally accepted as being due to an ascending infection; it is also widely agreed that prolonged membrane rupture is complicated by a high incidence of chorioamnionitis and that chorioamnionitis is frequently found in the placentas of prematurely delivered infants.

It is widely believed that ascending infections can cause both premature onset of labor and premature rupture of the membranes, although the magnitude of the contribution of infection to preterm labor is still controversial, some regarding chorioamnionitis as the major etiological factor in preterm labor[18] and others considering infection to be a relatively minor cause of premature delivery.[36,37] The relationship between chorioamnionitis and premature onset of labor appears to be independent of the confounding factor of prolonged membrane rupture, although this clearly, when present, may contribute to an increased severity of the inflammatory process in these cases. The mechanism by which an ascending infection stimulates the premature onset of labor is still uncertain, although it has been shown that infection greatly increases the ability of amniotic cells to synthesize prostaglandins: the amniotic production of prostaglandin in the membranes, normally low in gestations of less than 35 weeks duration, is increased 30-fold if the membranes are inflamed,[38] and it is assumed that this excess production of prostaglandins is responsible for the early onset of labor. Some cases of preterm delivery associated with an ascending infection are, however, due not to premature onset of labor, but to premature rupture of the membranes.[17,39] It has been suggested that this may be the result of the release of elastases and collagenases from the neutrophil polymorphonuclear leukocytes infiltrating the membranes.[18]

TOXIC DAMAGE TO THE PLACENTA

Remarkably little is known about the possible injurious effects on the placenta of toxins, drugs, or environmental pollutants. The only example of toxic damage that has been adequately studied is that of the effects of maternal cigarette smoking, an interest stimulated by the well-established association between maternal cigarette smoking and low birth weight. Placentas from smoking mothers show evidence of ischemic damage on light microscopy; this is probably due to the vasoconstrictive effects of nicotine on the uterine vasculature, for infusion of nicotine into pregnant animals results in a sharp decrease in uterine blood flow,[40] while in the pregnant human the smoking of a single cigarette causes an acute reduction in intervillous space blood flow.[41] Electron microscopic study of placentas from smoking women shows, however, abnormalities that are not explicable on an ischemic basis, such as degenerative changes in a proportion of the villous cytotrophoblastic cells and small areas of abnormal infolding of the villous syncytiotrophoblastic plasma membrane with local loss of syncytial cytoplasm and microvilli.[42] Damage of this type could be due to any one of the several thousand chemical compounds in cigarette smoke, but suspicion has fallen particularly on cadmium: this metal, which is present is tobacco smoke and is present in high concentration in the placentas of smokers, but not of nonsmokers, has been shown experimentally to be specifically toxic for placental tissue.[43]

Irrespective of the exact manner by which the placenta is injured in cigarette smokers, it is highly unlikely that the damage inflicted could be held responsible for the increased incidence of low birth weight babies. Any ischemic lesions suffered by the placenta are efficiently repaired, most of the villous trophoblast is normal, and any presumed loss of placental functional capacity is probably compensated for by the increased placental growth that occurs in cigarette smokers.[44] Reduced fetal growth is therefore probably due partly to an inadequate maternal supply of oxygen consequent on nicotine-induced constriction of the uterine vessels and partly to the direct effects of nicotine and carbon monoxide on the fetus.

NONTROPHOBLASTIC TUMORS OF THE PLACENTA

The only common nontrophoblastic tumor of the placenta is the hemangioma or "chorangioma." Hemangiomas, usually single but occasionally multiple, are present in 1% of placentas. The vast majority are small and are not visible on external examination of the placenta; they are detected only on slicing the organ, where they are seen as well-demarcated, rounded, red, brown, tan, or white intraparenchymal nodules. The uncommon large hemangiomas, ie, measuring more than 5 cm in diameter, are seen most frequently as bulging protruberances on the fetal surface of the placenta; occasionally they are found on the maternal surface, where they often appear to replace an entire lobe (Fig. 5-8), or in the membranes attached to the main placental mass only by a vascular pedicle. Histologically, most placental hemangiomas have a microscopic appearance identical to that seen in similar tumors elsewhere in the body, but some have a predominance of the stromal component and are classed as a "fibrous" variant.

The vast majority of placental hemangiomas are of no clinical importance, but a very small minority—those measuring more than 5 cm in diameter—may be associated with a variety of complications that can affect the mother, the fetus, or the neonate.[45] There is a

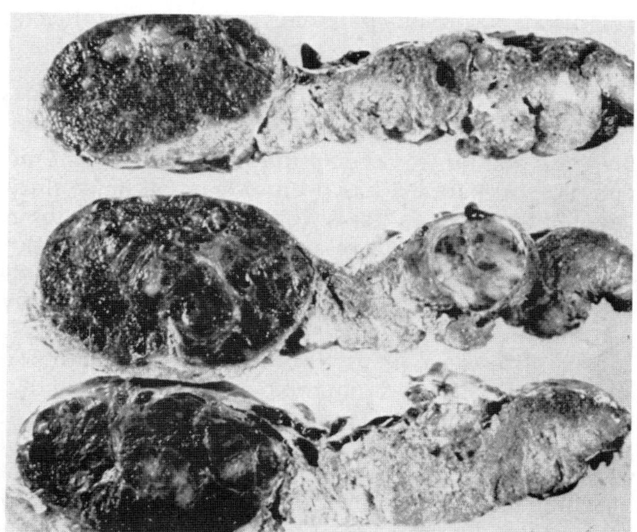

FIGURE 5–8. A large hemangioma in a placenta.

high incidence of polyhydramnios in association with large hemangiomas; the cause of this excess of fluid is obscure, but it may precipitate premature labor. Large tumors are also associated, as are multiple small tumors within a single placenta, with an increased incidence of intrauterine fetal hypoxia, intrauterine growth retardation, and intrauterine death; all these complications have been attributed to the fact that a considerable proportion of the fetal blood passes through the tumor, rather than through functional placental tissue, and is therefore returned to the fetus in an unoxygenated and nutrient-poor state. The neonate whose placenta contains a large hemangioma is also subject to a number of complications, usually of a transitory nature, which are a direct consequence of the placental tumor. Prominent among these is cardiomegaly; this is probably a result of the increased fetal cardiac output required for pumping blood through the hemangioma, which in hemodynamic terms can be considered a peripheral arteriovenous shunt. Neonatal edema is sometimes a manifestation of cardiac failure, but can also be due to hypoalbuminemia, a deficiency that may result either from transudation of protein from the surface vessels of the tumor or from chronic fetal–maternal bleeding from the hemangioma. Neonatal anemia can be a result of sequestration of fetal erythrocytes within the tumor, of a massive fetal–maternal bleed from the hemangioma, or of a microangiopathic hemolytic anemia induced by injury inflicted on fetal red blood cells as they traverse the labyrinthine vascular channels of the tumor. Neonatal thrombocytopenia can also be due to platelet injury within the tumor vessels, but is sometimes a manifestation of disseminated intravascular coagulation triggered off by a thromboplastic substance released from the hemangioma.

IMMUNOPATHOLOGY OF THE PLACENTA

The placenta contains paternal antigens and is thus an allograft; it is therefore possible that placental damage could be due to a form of graft rejection. Such a rejection would imply a breakdown of the mechanisms that allow the placenta to flourish as a graft, and although these are still far from being fully understood, this immunological paradox has been at least partially elucidated in recent years.[46] It is well established that villous trophoblast does not express antigens of the major histocompatibility complex, and it has been thought that this deficiency may protect trophoblast from recognition by maternal immunocytes and from cytotoxic immune reactions. The extravillous trophoblast in the placental bed, which is clearly in intimate contact with maternal tissues, does appear to express Type I HLA antigens; it is possible, however, that these are non-HLA Class I mixed histocompatibility antigens[47] and serve to elicit blocking antibodies against a similar antigen expressed on activated lymphocytes. Other factors possibly contributing to the placenta's privileged immunological status include the presence of suppressor T cells in the decidua, the presence in trophoblast of antigens that are shared with lymphocytes and that appear to block maternal lymphocytic immune reactions against trophoblast, and the development of blocking antigens in the sera of pregnant women that inhibit the cytotoxic effect of maternal lymphocytes against cultured trophoblastic cells. Other factors, such as the relative immunological privilege conferred by decidua or the immunosuppressive effects of placental hormones, appear to be of lesser or only transitory importance.

Evidence that these protective mechanisms sometimes fail is scant. There are certainly no grounds for believing that either premature or term labor is caused by a graft rejection process, but some women who repetitively abort do fail to develop blocking antibodies.[48] This appears to be because of an excess sharing of HLA antigens between mother and father and a resulting inability of the mother's body to recognize the trophoblast as antigenically alien. Abortion under these circumstances cannot, however, be regarded as a graft rejection, for it is the failure of the mother to recognize the placenta as a graft that results in abortion. There have, unfortunately, been no morphological or immunohistological studies of placentae from these cases of apparently immunologically mediated abortions.

Quite apart from the possibility of graft rejections, the question arises as to whether the placenta ever suffers immune-mediated damage in a fashion similar to that suffered by, for example, the kidney. There is a widespread belief that some form of immunologically mediated attack on placental tissue is an important factor in the pathogenesis of preeclampsia, but immunohistological findings to support this view are lacking. There is, in placentas from preeclamptic women, an amplification of the normal deposition of complement components in the placental tissues, but this appears to be simply a quantitative augmentation of immune processes that are normally operative in the host–graft relationship of pregnancy.[49] Electron microscopic studies have also consistently failed to demonstrate antigen-antibody formation or deposition in placentas from preeclamptic women; indeed, all the abnormalities found in such placentas are explicable on a nonimmunological basis.[16] Immunohistological findings similar to those noted in preeclampsia have also been described in placentas from diabetic women, ie, an increased deposition of complement components,[50] and again, appear to be an expression of enhanced physiological processes rather than an indication of an immunopathological process.

The high fetal wastage in women suffering from systemic lupus erythematosus (SLE) has been attributed to immune-mediated placental damage. Grennan and coworkers[51] have shown that complement-binding DNA-anti-DNA immune complexes are bound to the villous trophoblastic basement membrane in placentas from women with SLE, and have suggested that these may cause trophoblastic damage in a manner akin to the renal damage resulting from binding of similar complexes to the glomerular basement membrane in lupus nephritis. Grennan and his colleagues also noted that anti-DNA antibodies appear to penetrate into the nuclei of villous cytotrophoblastic cells, a finding confirmed by Abramowsky and associates,[52] who also described an acute vasculopathy in the vessels in the basal decidua of placentae from women with SLE. This vascular lesion was characterized by fibrinoid necrosis and lipophage infiltration of the vessel wall, a perivascular inflammatory infiltrate, and deposition of IgG and C3 in the vessel walls. Abramowsky and colleagues[52] suggested that the vasculopathy was due to immune complex deposition in the walls of the uteroplacental vessels, and that it could lead to extensive placental infarction. It has been shown that the presence of lupus anticoagulant in women suffering from SLE is frequently associated with fetal loss.[53] This factor, despite its name, is often accompanied by intravascular thrombosis, and it has therefore been proposed that the combination of an immunologically mediated vasculosis with a predisposition to thrombosis induced by lupus anticoagulant could lead to extensive placental infarction and subsequent fetal death.[54,55] This theoretical possibility has not, however, been confirmed by pathological examination of placentas from women with SLE; such placentas, including those from cases of fetal death associated with circulating lupus anticoagulant, usually show no excess of infarction[56] and appear histologically normal.[6]

It has to be concluded that there is currently no evidence that the placenta ever suffers immunologically mediated damage.

EXTRAVILLOUS TROPHOBLAST AND THE PATHOLOGY OF THE UTEROPLACENTAL VESSELS

It is difficult to accept that most cases of "placental insufficiency" are caused by intrinsic placental damage, and it is becoming increasingly clear that the common factor in most cases of presumed placental inadequacy is a reduced maternal blood flow to the fetoplacental unit. It has been previously pointed out that the placenta establishes its own blood supply as a result of invasion of the spiral arteries in the placental bed by extravillous trophoblast, with the process occurring in two stages. The factors controlling and limiting intravascular invasion by extravillous trophoblast are unknown, but the crucial importance of this process is shown by the finding that in women destined to develop preeclampsia in the later stages of pregnancy, there is a partial failure of placentation, which results in a markedly restricted blood flow to the placenta. This failure has two components. First, while in a normal pregnancy all the spiral arteries in the placental bed are invaded by trophoblast, this process occurs in only a proportion of these vessels in patients who later develop preeclampsia, a significant fraction of the placental bed arteries showing a complete absence of physiological change.[57] Second, in those arteries that are invaded by extravillous trophoblast, the first stage in this process occurs quite normally with trophoblast-evoking physiological changes in their intradecidual segments, but there is subsequently a complete failure of the second stage, with endovascular trophoblast failing to advance into the intramyometrial portion of these vessels.[58,59] Hence, in these women there is an incomplete transformation of the spiral arteries to uteroplacental vessels, and this abnormality, with its consequent restriction of maternal uteroplacental blood flow, is in itself an adequate cause for all the placental abnormalities and all the fetal complications seen in preeclampsia.

Preeclampsia is not the sole instance of the serious consequences of inadequate placentation. It is now becoming clear that a similar defective invasion of the spiral arteries by extravillous trophoblast is also a feature of many cases of normotensive intrauterine fetal growth retardation, the deficit in fetal growth being due to the reduced maternal supply of oxygen and nutrients.[60] Placentas from such cases show evidence of ischemic damage on electron microscopy.[61] Experimentally induced limitation of maternal blood flow in animals results in an unduly small fetus,[62] and hemodynamic studies have demonstrated a significantly reduced maternal blood flow to the placenta in many cases of human fetal growth retardation.[63] Although some have observed occlusive, atheroma-like lesions in the spiral vessels in cases of intrauterine growth retardation,[64] others have failed to confirm this finding.[65] There is more general agreement that in many but not all cases of intrauterine growth retardation, there is either a partial or a complete failure of cytotrophoblastic invasion and normal physiological changes in the intramyometrial segments of the spiral arteries,[60] a situation akin to that found in preeclampsia.

It is clear, therefore, that most cases of apparent placental insufficiency are in fact examples of maternal vascular insufficiency. It may appear pedantic to some to draw this distinction, but the use of the term "placental insufficiency" gives the obstetrician a false sense of having identified, or at least localized, the abnormality, induces a mood of therapeutic nihilism, and directs research along unrewarding pathways.

CONCLUSION

The placenta is a vigorous, energetic, versatile organ with a considerable physiologic reserve capacity. Most pathologic lesions of the placenta are functionally irrelevant, and it is doubtful if the placenta often, or ever, becomes "insufficient." Attention is being increasingly directed to the interaction of extravillous trophoblast and maternal tissues during placentation, and it is becoming clear that many of the ills that may beset a pregnancy have their origin in an abnormal interrelationship between fetal and maternal tissues during the early stages of gestation.

REFERENCES

1. Fox H, Sen DK. Placenta extrachorialis: a clinicopathological study. J Obstet Gynaecol Br Commonwealth 1972;79:32.
2. Galton M. DNA content of placental nuclei. J Cell Biol 1962;13:183.
3. Ladermacher DS, Vermeulen RCW, Harten JJ, et al. Circumvallate placenta and congenital malformation. Lancet 1981;2:737.
4. Uyanwah Akpom WP, Fox H. The clinical significance of marginal and velamentous insertion of the cord. Br J Obstet Gynaecol 1977;84:941.
5. Wood DL, Malan AF. The site of umbilical cord insertion and birthweight. Br J Obstet Gynaecol 1978;85:332.
6. Fox H. Pathology of the placenta. Philadelphia: WB Saunders, 1978.
7. Labarrere CA. Review article: acute atherosis: a histopathological hallmark of immune aggression? Placenta 1988;9:95.
8. Tindall VR, Scott JS. Placental calcification: a study of 3025 singleton and multiple pregnancies. J Obstet Gynaecol Br Commonwealth 1965;72:356.
9. Robinson JS, Kingstone EJ, Jones CT, Thorburn GD. Studies of experimental growth retardation in sheep: the effect of removal of endometrial caruncles on fetal size and metabolism. J Dev Physiol 1979;1:379.
10. Lorijn RHV, Longo LD. Clinical and physiologic implications of increased fetal oxygen consumption. Am J Obstet Gynecol 1980;136:451.
11. Kaufmann P. Development and differentiation of the human placental villous tree. Bibl Anat 1982;22:29.
12. Becker V. Pathologieder Aureifung der Plazenta. In: Becker V, Scheibler TH, Kubli F, eds. Die Plazenta der Menschen. Stuttgart: Thieme, 1981:266.
13. Hopker WW, Ohlendorf B. Placental insufficiency: histomorphologic diagnosis and classification. Curr Top Pathol 1979;66:57.
14. Fox H. Effects of hypoxia on trophoblast in organ culture. Am J Obstet Gynecol 1970;107:1058.
15. MacLennon AH, Sharpe F, Shaw-Dunn J. The ultrastructure of human trophoblast in spontaneous and induced hypoxia using a system of organ culture: a comparison with ultrastructural changes in pre-eclampsia and placental insufficiency. J Obstet Gynaecol Br Commonwealth 1972;79:113.
16. Jones CJP, Fox H. An ultrastructural and ultrahistochemical study of the human placenta in maternal pre-eclampsia. Placenta 1980;1:61.
17. Naeye RL, Maisels MJ, Lorenz RP, Botti JJ. The clinical significance of placental villous edema. Pediatrics 1983;71:888.
18. Naeye RL. Functionally important disorders of the placenta, umbilical cord and fetal membranes. Hum Pathol 1987;18:680.
19. Alvarez H, Salae MA, Benedetti WL. Intervillous space reduction in the edematous placenta. Am J Obstet Gynecol 1972;112:819.
20. Schen-Schwarz S, Ruchelli E, Brown D. Villous edema of the placenta: A clinicopathologic study. Placenta 1989;10:297.
21. Fox H. The placenta as a model for organ aging. In: Beaconsfield P, Villee C, eds. Placenta — a neglected experimental animal. Oxford: Pergamon, 1979:351.
22. Haigh M, Taylor CJ, Fox H. A morphometric analysis of age-related changes in villous syncytiotrophoblastic subcellular organelles in the human placenta using a computerized image analysis system. Fetus 1989;1:27.
23. Winick M, Coscia A, Noble A. Cellular growth in human placenta. I: normal cellular growth. Pediatrics 1967;39:248.
24. Sands J, Dobbing J. Continuing growth and development of the third trimester human placenta. Placenta 1985;6:13.
25. Geier G, Schuhmann R, Kraus H. Regional unterschiedliche Zellproliferation innerhalb der Plazentenone reifer menschlicher Plazenten: autoradiographische Untersuchungen. Archiv für Gynäkologie 1975;218:31.
26. Iversen DE, Farsund T. Flow cytometry in the assessment of human placental growth. Acta Obstet Gynecol Scand 1985;64:605.
27. Boyd PA. Quantitative studies of the normal human placenta from 10 weeks of gestation to term. Early Hum Dev 1984;9:297.
28. Altshuler G, Russel P. The human placental villitides: a review of chronic intrauterine infection. Curr Top Pathol 1975;60:63.
29. Fox H. Placental involvement in maternal systemic infection. Perspect Pediatr Pathol 1981;6:63.
30. Russell P. Inflammatory lesions of the human placenta. III: the histopathology of villitis of unknown aetiology. Placenta 1980;1:227.
31. Knox WF, Fox H. Villitis of unknown aetiology: its incidence in placentae from a British population. Placenta 1984;5:395.
32. Altshuler G. Placental infection and inflammation. In: Perrin EVDK, ed. Pathology of the placenta. New York: Churchill Livingstone, 1984:141.
33. Althabe O, Labarrere C. Chronic villitis of unknown aetiology and intrauterine growth-retarded infants of normal and low ponderal index. Placenta 1985;6:369.
34. Labarrere C, Althabe O, Telenta M. Chronic villitis of unknown aetiology in placentae of idiopathic small for gestational age infants. Placenta 1982;3:309.
35. Redline RW, Abramowsky CR. Clinical and pathologic aspects of recurrent placental villitis. Hum Pathol 1985;16:727.
36. Zaaijma JT, Wilkinson AR, Keeling JW, Mitchell RG, Turnbull AC. Spontaneous premature rupture of the membranes: bacteriology, histology and neonatal outcome. J Obstet Gynecol 1982;2:155.
37. Perkins RP, Zhou S-M, Butler C, Skipper BJ. Histologic chorioamnionitis in pregnancies of various gestational ages: implications in preterm rupture of the membranes. Obstet Gynecol 1987;70:856.
38. Lopez-Bernal A, Hansell DJ, Soler RC, Keeling JW, Turnbull AC. Prostaglandins chorioamnionitis and preterm labour. Br J Obstet Gynaecol 1987;94:1156.
39. Evaldson GR, Malmburg AS, Nord CA. Premature rupture of the membranes and ascending infection. Br J Obstet Gynaecol 1982;89:793.
40. Suzuki K, Minei IJ, Johnson EE. Effect of nicotine on uterine blood flow in the pregnant rhesus monkey. Am J Obstet Gynecol 1980;136:1009.
41. Lehtovirta P, Forss M. The acute effect of smoking on intervillous blood flow of the placenta. Br J Obstet Gynaecol 1978;85:720.
42. Uyanwah Akpom WP, Fox H. The clinical significance of marginal and velamentous insertion of the cord. Br J Obstet Gynaecol 1977;84:941.
43. Di Sant 'Agnese PA, Jensen KD, Levin A, et al. Placental toxicity of cadmium in the rat: an ultrastructural study. Placenta 1983;4:149.
44. Christianson RE. Gross differences observed in the placentae of smokers and non-smokers. Am J Epidemiol 1979;110:178.
45. Fox H. Nontrophoblastic tumors of the placenta. In: Perrin EVDK, ed. Pathology of the placenta. New York: Churchill-Livingstone, 1984:199.
46. Johnson PM. Immunobiology of human trophoblast. In: Crighton DB, ed. Immunological aspects of reproduction in mammals. London: Butterworth, 1984:109.
47. Bulmer JN, Johnson PM. Antigen expression by trophoblast populations in the human placenta and their possible immunobiological relevance. Placenta 1985;6:127.
48. Taylor C, Faulk WP. Prevention of recurrent abortions with leucocyte transfusions. Lancet 1981;ii:68.
49. Faulk WP, Johnson PM. Immunological studies of human placentae: basic and practical implications. In: Thompson RA, ed.

Recent advances in clinical immunology, vol 2. Edinburgh: Churchill Livingstone, 1980:1.

50. Galbraith RM, Sinha DP, Galbraith GMP, Faulk WP. Immunohistological studies of placentae from insulin-dependent diabetic women. In: Sutherland HW, Stowers JM, eds. Carbohydrate metabolism in pregnancy and the newborn. New York: Churchill-Livingstone, 1984:23.
51. Grennan DM, McCormick JN, Wojtacha P, Carty M, Behan W. Immunological studies of the placenta in systemic lupus erythematosus. Anat Rheum Dis 1979;37:129.
52. Abramowsky CR, Vegas ME, Swinehart G, Gyves MT. Decidual vasculopathy of the placenta in lupus erythematosus. N Engl J Med 1980;303:668.
53. Reece EA, Romero R, Clyne LP, Kriz NS, Hobbins JC. Lupus-like anticoagulant in pregnancy. Lancet 1984;i:344.
54. Abramowsky CR. Lupus erythematosus, the placenta and pregnancy: a natural experiment in immunologically mediated reproductive failure. Prog Clin Biol Res 1981;70:309.
55. De Wolf F, Carreras LO, Moerman P, Vermylen J, van Assche A, Renaer M. Decidual vasculopathy and extensive placental infarction in a patient with repeated thromboembolic accidents, recurrent fetal loss and a lupus anticoagulant. Am J Obstet Gynecol 1982;142:829.
56. Lockshin MD, Druzin ML, Goei S, et al. Antibody to cardiolipin as a predictor of fetal distress or death in pregnant patients with systemic lupus erythematosus. N Engl J Med 1985;313:152.
57. Khong TY, de Wolf F, Robertson WB, Brosens I. Inadequate maternal vascular response to placentation in pregnancies complicated by pre-eclampsia and by small-for-gestational-age infants. Br J Obstet Gynaecol 1986;93:1049.
58. Robertson WB, Brosens I, Dixon HG. The pathological response of the vessels of the placental bed in hypertensive pregnancy. J Pathol Bacteriol 1967;93:581.
59. Robertson WB, Brosens I, Dixon HG. Uteroplacental vascular pathology. Eur J Obstet Gynecol Rep Biol 1975;5:47.
60. Robertson WB, Brosens IA, Dixon HG. Maternal blood supply in fetal growth retardation. In: Van Assche FA, Robertson WB, eds. Fetal growth retardation. Edinburgh: Churchill-Livingstone, 1981:126.
61. van der Veen F, Fox H. The human placenta in idiopathic intrauterine growth retardation: a light and electron microscopic study. Placenta 1983;4:65.
62. O'Shaughnessy EW. Uterine blood flow and fetal growth. In: Van Assche FA, Robertson WB, eds. Fetal growth retardation. Edinburgh: Churchill-Livingstone, 1981:101.
63. Lunell NO, Sarby B, Lavender R, et al. Comparison of uteroplacental blood flow in normal and in intrauterine growth retarded pregnancy. Gynecol Obstet Invest 1979;10:106.
64. Sheppard BL, Bonnar J. The ultrastructure of the arterial supply of the human placenta in pregnancy complicated by fetal growth retardation. Br J Obstet Gynaecol 1976;83:948.
65. Brosens I, Dixon HG, Robertson WB. Fetal growth retardation and the arteries of the placental bed. Br J Obstet Gynaecol 1977;84:645.

6

CHAPTER

FETAL–PLACENTAL PERFUSION AND TRANSFER OF NUTRIENTS

Frederick C. Battaglia and John C. Hobbins

Technical advances in the tools obstetricians can use for evaluation of a pregnancy have progressed faster than our basic understanding of some of the developmental aspects of fetal and placental physiology. In this chapter we will try to bring out those aspects of perinatal physiology that are reasonably well established. Whenever possible, clinical advances in high-risk obstetrics will be presented against the backdrop of this basic science foundation.

PERFUSION AND PLACENTAL TRANSPORT

A number of concepts related to placental perfusion and transport, most of which have considerable clinical significance, have become relatively well established. One of these is the absence of autoregulation in the uterine vascular bed. This has been shown in animal studies by the absence of reactive hyperemia after uterine artery occlusion.

The clinical implication of these observations is that the uterine bed in late pregnancy may be regarded as an almost fully dilated bed. Thus, it cannot easily compensate by further vasodilatation for an abrupt fall in maternal arterial pressure. From a clinical perspective, maternal hypotension must then be regarded as a direct causal factor in producing a reduction in uterine and placental blood flow. From this perspective, maternal hypotension should be avoided, particularly in late gestation. For similar reasons, obstetrical anesthesia must have avoidance of any maternal hypotension and support of maternal oxygenation as two of its goals.

Another characteristic of the uterine vascular bed is the unresponsiveness of the uterine vascular vessels to changes in Po_2 or Pco_2. Again, this has considerable clinical significance, because it means that oxygen therapy for the mother does not carry with it the risk of increased fetal hypoxia through the mechanism of vasoconstriction of the uterine bed. It has been well demonstrated in animal studies that administration of oxygen to the mother will increase fetal oxygenation, lending support to the clinical approach of using maternal oxygen therapy when there are signs of fetal distress during labor and delivery. Unfortunately, as is true with many areas of physiology, we have much less information about the effects of chronic maternal oxygen therapy. Because this is such an important issue in clinical obstetrics, it is worth reviewing in some detail the animal studies that support the use of maternal oxygen therapy for fetal hypoxia. Figure 6-1 is taken from the first study to directly address the question of the impact of maternal oxygen administration on uterine and umbilical blood flows and fetal oxygenation.[1] In that study, the increased maternal Po_2 had no effect on uterine or umbilical blood flows and, as expected, umbilical venous Po_2, representing the most oxygenated blood of the fetus, increased significantly. In these studies, where fetal oxygen consumption was normal to begin with, no further increase in fetal oxygen consumption occurred during oxygen administration. However, in other studies, where fetal oxygen consumption was reduced before maternal oxygen therapy, there was an increase in fetal oxygen consumption to within the normal range during maternal oxygen administration.

Clinically, the first studies demonstrating an effect on fetal oxygenation by maternal oxygen administration were based on changes in fetal scalp Po_2 done by scalp sampling during labor. More recently, maternal oxygen administration has been used in pregnancies complicated by intrauterine growth retardation (IUGR), and the beneficial effect confirmed both by the changes in

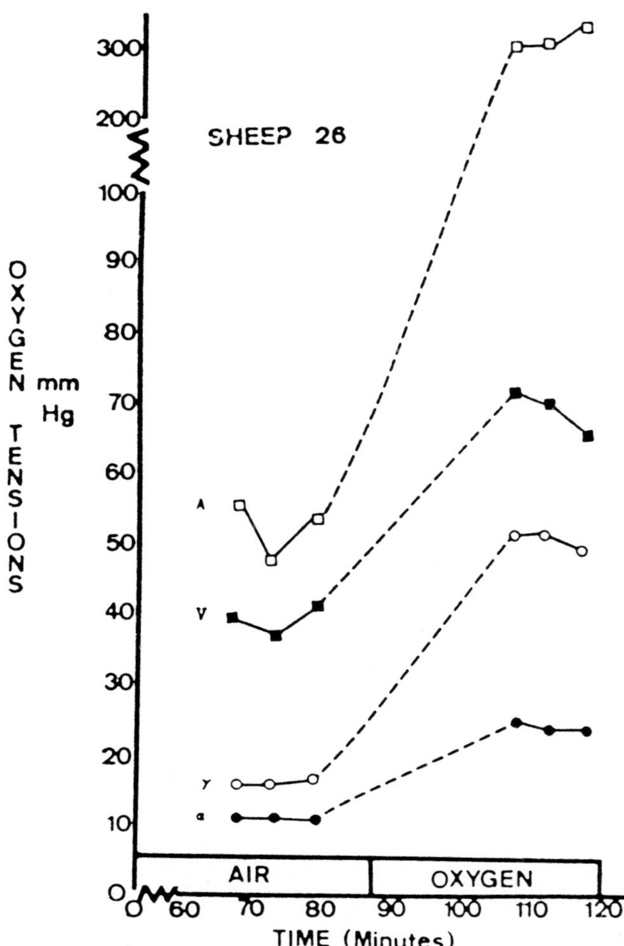

FIGURE 6–1. Oxygen tensions and saturations in maternal artery (A □), uterine vein (V ■), umbilical vein (y ○), and umbilical artery (α ●) are presented during periods of air and oxygen inhalation. (Battaglia FC, Meschia G, Makowski EL, Bowes W. The effect of maternal oxygen inhalation upon fetal oxygenation. J Clin Invest 1968;47:551.)

fetal blood Po_2 and saturation in blood obtained by cordocentesis (periumbilical blood sampling), and by an apparent improvement in velocity waveform measurements on the fetal descending aorta, suggesting a reduced placental impedance during maternal oxygen therapy.[2]

The relationship between fetal oxygenation and maternal oxygenation is complex in that a number of factors enter into determining the "normal" umbilical venous Po_2 in any species. These factors include placental oxygen consumption, uterine and umbilical blood flows, placental permeability, pattern of placental perfusion (ie, concurrent, crosscurrent, countercurrent), maternal arterial Po_2 and hemoglobin concentration, and shape of maternal and fetal oxygen dissociation curves. For a more complete discussion of the contribution of each of these factors, see Battaglia and Meschia.[3]

In humans, umbilical venous Po_2 tends to equilibrate with uterine *venous* Po_2, not arterial; that is, it simulates a concurrent exchanger. With the advent of techniques to sample umbilical venous blood transabdominally (ie, cordocentesis), data are now available describing umbilical venous Po_2 through the latter half of gestation. The umbilical venous Po_2 of the human fetus is higher in midgestation and decreases as gestation advances.[4,5] However, at any gestational age it is clear that the human fetal umbilical venous Po_2 is very low by postnatal standards. Thus, the importance of the difference in fetal versus adult whole blood oxygen affinity is apparent, because the higher affinity of fetal hemoglobin ensures that the bulk of the hemoglobin will be oxygenated even at the low Po_2 of fetal umbilical venous blood. Figure 6-2, from the studies of Bozzetti and coworkers, illustrates two features of interest in the interpretation of umbilical venous samples obtained by cordocentesis.[5] First, there is clearly a bimodal distribution of values, with the subset of low oxygen saturations reflecting the fact that occasionally one will obtain umbilical arterial rather than umbilical venous blood. Secondly, the values have a bit more scatter than similar data obtained using chronic fetal catheters in animal studies. Despite this variability, the majority of the values reflect the very high oxygen saturations found in early pregnancy in sheep. Studies in the midgestation fetal lamb have shown a higher Po_2 and oxygen saturation in fetal vessels compared to late gestation (Fig. 6-3).[6] Thus, the data for the human fetus are similar to the data in the lamb: the oxygen environment is higher in midgestation and decreases toward term.

Soothill and associates[7] have shown a relationship between fetal lactate concentration and fetal hemoglobin and oxygen concentration in Rh-isoimmunized pregnancies. Similarly, Ferrazzi and coworkers[8] and Soothill and colleagues[2] described lactic acidemia in association with abnormal velocity waveforms in the fetal descending aorta or umbilical artery. It seems likely that biochemical assessment of the high-risk fetus through application of cordocentesis combined with biophysical measurements, including velocity of flow measurements in fetal and uterine vessels, will play an increasingly important role in the evaluation of high-risk obstetrical patients.

UTERINE FLOW AND PLACENTAL TRANSPORT

Uterine blood flow increases remarkably during late gestation. Furthermore, the partition of total uterine blood flow to the placenta versus myometrium also changes. Although such data are not available in humans, it is clear that there is an increase in uterine blood flow to the pregnant uterus in all species. How the mother accommodates to this increased demand for uterine perfusion varies considerably among species. In humans and in other large mammals that have been studied, such as sheep and goats, there is a relatively large increase in maternal cardiac output. However, the

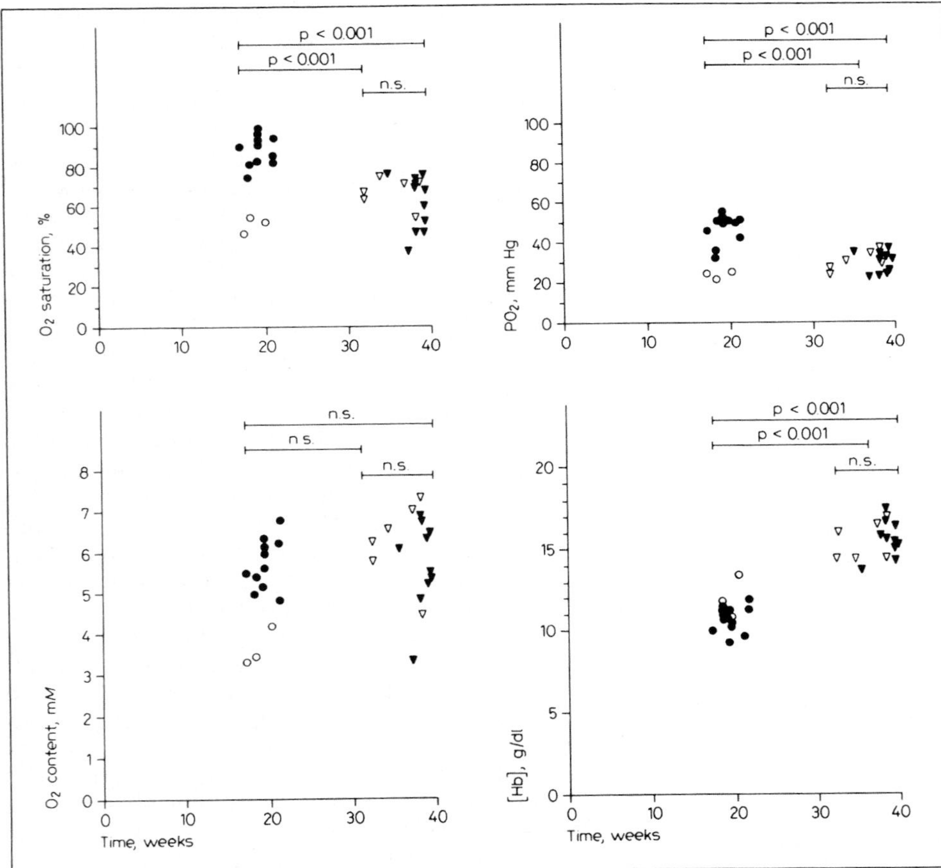

FIGURE 6–2. Oxygen saturation, PO_2, oxygen content, and hemoglobin concentrations in fetal blood obtained at fetoscopy (●), cord blood sampling (▽), and term cesarean section (▼). ○ = three fetoscopy samples with oxygen saturation values lower than the rest (<2.0 SD). (Bozzetti P, Buscaglia M, Cetin I, et al. Respiratory gases, acid-base balance and lactate concentrations in the mid-term human fetus. Biol Neonate 1987;51:190.)

increase in uterine blood flow does not keep up with the increase in uterine oxygen consumption. For this reason, the coefficient of extraction of oxygen across the uterine circulation increases. In essence, this means that the uterine venous Po_2 and oxygen content decrease with increasing gestational age. A decrease in uterine venous Po_2 in turn leads to a lower umbilical venous Po_2. The data mentioned earlier regarding umbilical venous Po_2 in human fetuses at midgestation would suggest that a similar process is involved in humans; that is, that placental uterine blood flow is relatively high in relation to the oxygen demands of the pregnant uterus in midgestation compared to that same relationship in late gestation.

One of the more important contributions in fetal physiology was made by the studies that described a nonlinear relationship between uterine blood flow and placental transport of oxygen and nutrients to the fetus. Figure 6-4, from the studies of Wilkening and coworkers[9] in pregnant sheep, illustrates the fact that uterine blood flow can decrease over a fairly wide range without any effect on oxygen transport; after that, a critical point is reached beyond which any further reduction in uterine blood flow leads to a decrease in oxygen transport. Similar data have been obtained by the same investigators for umbilical blood flow versus placental transport.[10] Although no similar study has been done for other nutrients, the transport of all nutrients should share this common characteristic: that there is a margin of safety provided by the fact that uterine blood flow can be reduced without affecting transport until a critical point, beyond which transport is affected. This has considerable clinical significance. It would appear that a critical need in obstetrics is to determine whether such inflection points—that is, critical levels of uterine perfusion beyond which reductions in uterine flow profoundly affect fetal oxygenation and fetal nutrition—exist in high-risk pregnancies; and to devise techniques to evaluate such relationships in humans. In this way, it would be possible to evaluate whether in any given pregnancy uterine blood flow is reduced to the point where there is little margin of safety for the fetus in terms of placental transport of oxygen and nutrients.

From such animal studies it has become clear that both an assessment of perfusion (that is, an evaluation of umbilical and uterine blood flows) and a biochemical assessment of the fetus are required to define such fetuses in jeopardy. In clinical medicine the group of patients that best exemplify the need for such assessment before the onset of labor are the fetuses with marked intrauterine growth retardation. It is not surprising that

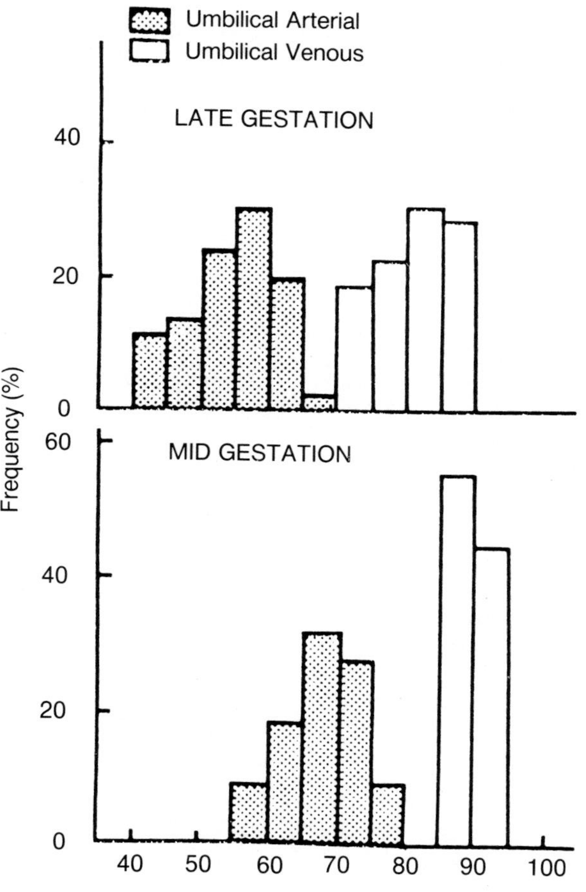

FIGURE 6–3. Frequency distributions of oxyhemoglobin saturation of umbilical arterial and venous blood in late versus midgestation in the fetal lamb. (Bell AW, Kennaugh JM, Battaglia FC, Makowski EL, Meschia G. Metabolic and circulatory studies of fetal lamb at midgestation. Am J Physiol 1986;250:E543.)

most current clinical effort in high-risk obstetrics is directed at this group, attempting to evaluate whether such monitoring techniques as velocity flow patterns and cordocentesis can help distinguish among the heterogeneous group of fetuses with intrauterine growth retardation—those that are at grave risk of fetal death in utero. Studies have suggested that an ominous velocity flow pattern in the fetal descending aorta or umbilical artery is characterized by a high systolic velocity and an absent diastolic flow.[11,12] (For further discussion, see the review by McParland and associates[13] of normal and abnormal flow velocity waveforms.) Several groups of investigators have found this pattern to be significantly associated with reduced fetal oxygenation and elevated fetal lactate concentrations, although not necessarily with acidosis or an increased base deficit.[2,4,8,14]

UTERINE VENOUS DRAINAGE

Although uterine arterial flow has been relatively well studied in animals, the venous drainage has not received such careful attention. Maternal position has been considered important in clinical obstetrics, principally through the potential to relieve inferior vena caval obstruction by the pregnant uterus and increase right-sided venous return to the heart. Alleviation of some signs of fetal distress has been reported after positioning the mother from the supine into the left lateral decubitus position.

Let us consider more carefully the issue of uterine venous drainage. Whether the blood draining the placenta mixes with blood draining the myometrium and other uterine tissues in approximately the same proportion on the left and right sides of the uterus, is very species dependent. Figure 6-5 presents a diagram of the mixing of placental and nonplacental blood in different species. In small laboratory animals where large litter sizes are the norm, the question is almost meaningless, because the uterine venous composition will be a function of the number of conceptuses in each horn.

If we compare the rhesus monkey and the sheep we find that, in late gestation, when the placenta is fully developed in both uterine horns in the sheep, the left and right uterine veins have the same proportion of placental and nonplacental drainage in each vein. This is not true in early gestation, when the placenta is not yet fully developed in the non-pregnant horn. By contrast, two laboratories have confirmed that in the rhesus monkey the drainage is not predictable. Occasionally, one vein carries essentially all of the placental drainage. This can put the fetus at risk, as shown in Figures 6-6

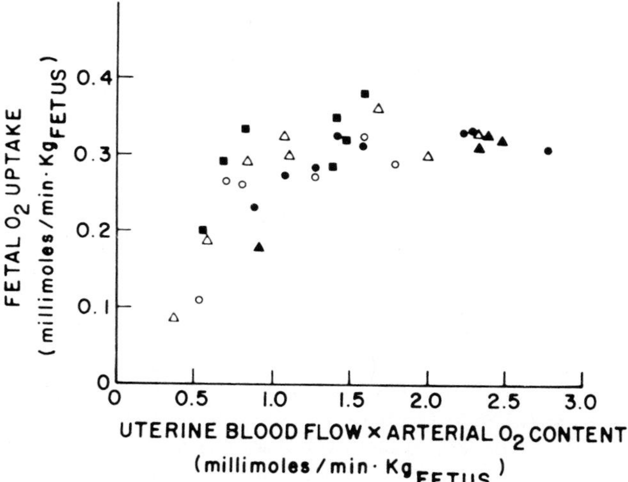

FIGURE 6–4. Relationship of fetal oxygen uptake to rate of oxygen delivery to pregnant uterus. Different symbols are used for each animal studied. (Wilkening RB, Meschia G. Fetal oxygen uptake, oxygen, and acid–base balance as a function of uterine blood flow. Am J Physiol 1983;244:H749.)

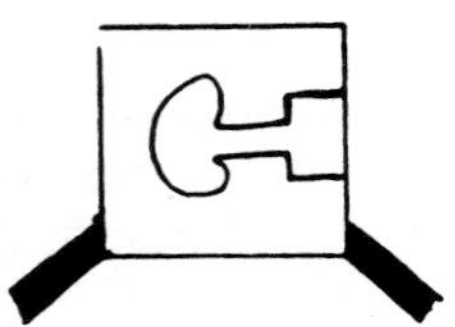

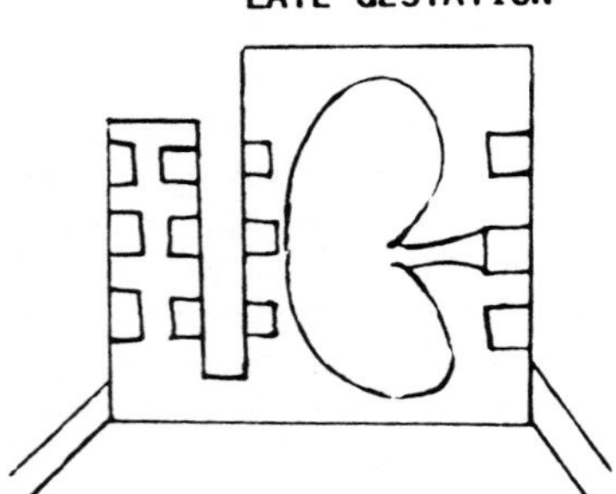

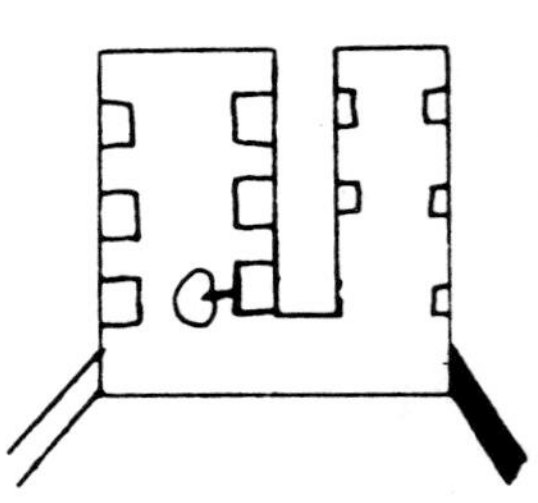

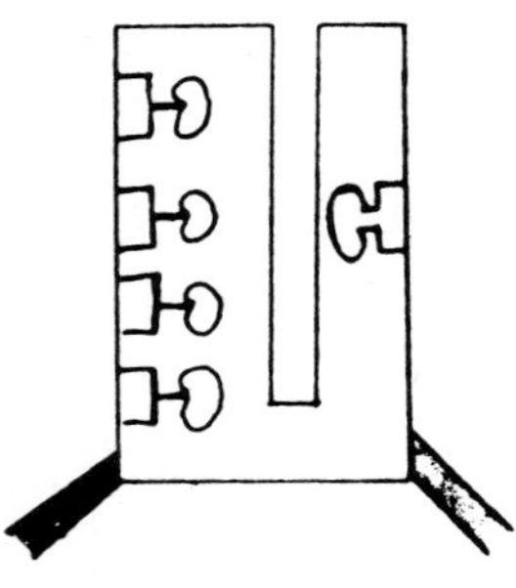

FIGURE 6–5. Diagram of different potential uterine venous drainage patterns.

and 6-7, from the study of Battaglia and coworkers.[15] Figure 6-6 illustrates that the tritiated water infused into the fetal rhesus monkey as a marker appeared in only one uterine vein. The other vein had a concentration no different from that of the maternal arterial blood. Occlusion of this latter vein would have no repercussions upon placental clearance of tritiated water. However, obstruction of the vein carrying all of the placental drainage leads to a rapid accumulation of tritiated water in the fetus because placental clearance is virtually zero, as shown in Figure 6-7. Such data are not available in humans, but there is sufficient reason to believe that the placental drainage in humans is not equally distributed to the venous drainage on the two sides of the uterus. Thus, the question of whether uterine venous obstruction contributes to the maternal positional effects on fetal well-being is an important one that needs further investigation. It may be answerable as ultrasonic visualization of the venous drainage of the uterus in humans becomes feasible.

PLACENTAL TRANSPORT AND METABOLISM

The characteristics of placental transport vary among mammals, determined largely by the placental type. The major factor that affects placental permeability as one compares one species to another is the number of tissue layers transposed between the maternal and fetal circulations. Unfortunately, most of the physiologic in vivo data on placental transport has been obtained in the sheep, which has an epitheliochorial placenta. Thus, there are two epithelial layers separating the two

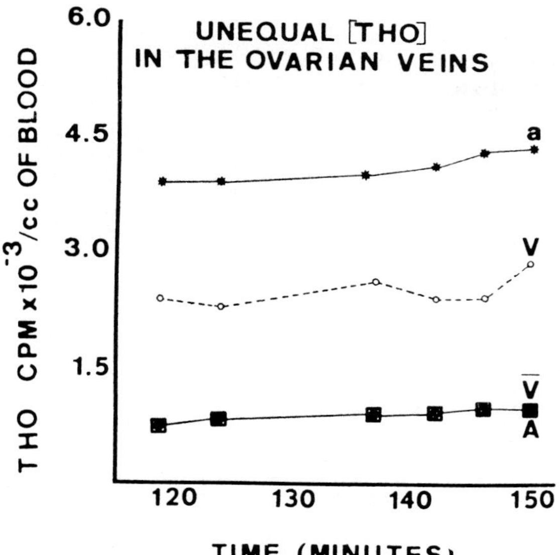

FIGURE 6–6. Tritiated water concentrations in both arteries and both ovarian veins of a rhesus monkey preparation. It is clear that only one ovarian vein was carrying blood from the placenta, whereas the other was draining nonexchange tissues within the uterus, and thus had a ^3H_2O concentration indistinguishable from the maternal artery. It should be stressed that this difference in tissue drainage cannot be detected from the gross appearance of the two veins, either in color or size of the vessels. (Battaglia FC, Makowski EL, Meschia G. Physiologic study of the uterine venous drainage of the pregnant rhesus monkey. Yale J Biol Med 1970; 42:221.)

circulations; one is the maternal endometrium and the other is trophoblast. When in vivo studies are carried out in this species, it is not clear which epithelial layer is principally responsible for the characteristics described. In general, the species with a persistent maternal uterine epithelial layer, such as the placenta of sheep and goats, is far less permeable than that of mammals with endotheliochorial or hemochorial placentas, such as that of humans and other primates. This is brought out fairly clearly by comparing placental clearance of sodium or chloride across the sheep and rhesus monkey placentas. The reason for such differences is not known, although it seems reasonable to attribute the relative impermeability of the sheep placenta to the presence of the uterine endometrial layer. Because the production of lactate and NH_3 by the pregnant uterus has been a general characteristic among species with very different placental types, it seems reasonable to hypothesize that this reflects the metabolic activity of the trophoblast, because this epithelial layer persists in all placental types.

In order to study the relative permeability of the placentas of different species, one must establish some reference point against which the permeability of other compounds can be judged, much as a measurement of glomerular filtration rate (GFR) is used in renal physiology. The flow-limited placental clearance of a compound has been used to define a maximal clearance within a placental type. It implies that the permeability of the placenta to a compound is so great that its rate of transfer is a function only of the rate of perfusion of the placenta.

The actual relationship between clearance and perfusion will depend on whether the placenta of that species functions as a concurrent or countercurrent exchanger. The ratio of placental clearance/flow has been termed "effectiveness"[16] or "transfer index."[17] At any given uterine/umbilical flow ratio, the countercurrent exchanger has a much greater effectiveness on transfer index. Although data are not available for the human placenta, work in rhesus monkeys suggests that the primate placenta simulates a concurrent exchanger. From a clinical viewpoint, compounds such as water, ethanol, anesthetic gases, and other small, lipid-soluble, nonionized molecules can be expected to cross the placenta readily with a rapid equilibration in maternal and fetal concentrations. This received clinical attention in the early descriptions of neonatal hyponatremia secondary to maternal hyponatremia. In general, the rapid movement of water across the placenta leads to equilibration of fetal and maternal plasma osmolalities. Unfortunately, the rapid placental transport and equilibration of fetal and maternal concentrations also applies to compounds such as ethanol, anesthetic gases, and local anesthetics, compounds which may affect the fetus adversely.

Differences in placental type markedly affect transport in placental transport of free fatty acids and ketone bodies. The human placenta is quite permeable to these compounds, in contrast to the sheep placenta. However, in the absence of maternal pathology, the quantities of free fatty acids transferred across the human placenta do not seem adequate to account for all of the white fat deposits that accumulate in the human infant during the latter half of gestation. The transfer of ketone bodies had been a major concern in diabetic pregnancies, because there have been some reports that have suggested neurodevelopmental delays in infants of diabetic mothers in association with episodes of maternal ketonemia.[18,19] Subsequent reports, however, have not supported this association.

The transport characteristics of the human placenta have also been studied in terms of the identification of specific carrier systems for carbohydrates and amino acids. In general, the work done thus far has tended to confirm the presence of carrier systems analogous to those found in most other tissues. Unfortunately, there has been no attempt to compare data obtained from in vitro studies of the placenta, such as those on isolated microvesicles, with in vivo data of transport characteristics, because the latter studies have been done in sheep, whereas the former studies have been carried out in the placentas of small mammals or in the human placenta. For in vivo studies in the sheep placenta, the data are consistent with carrier-mediated transport.[20,21]

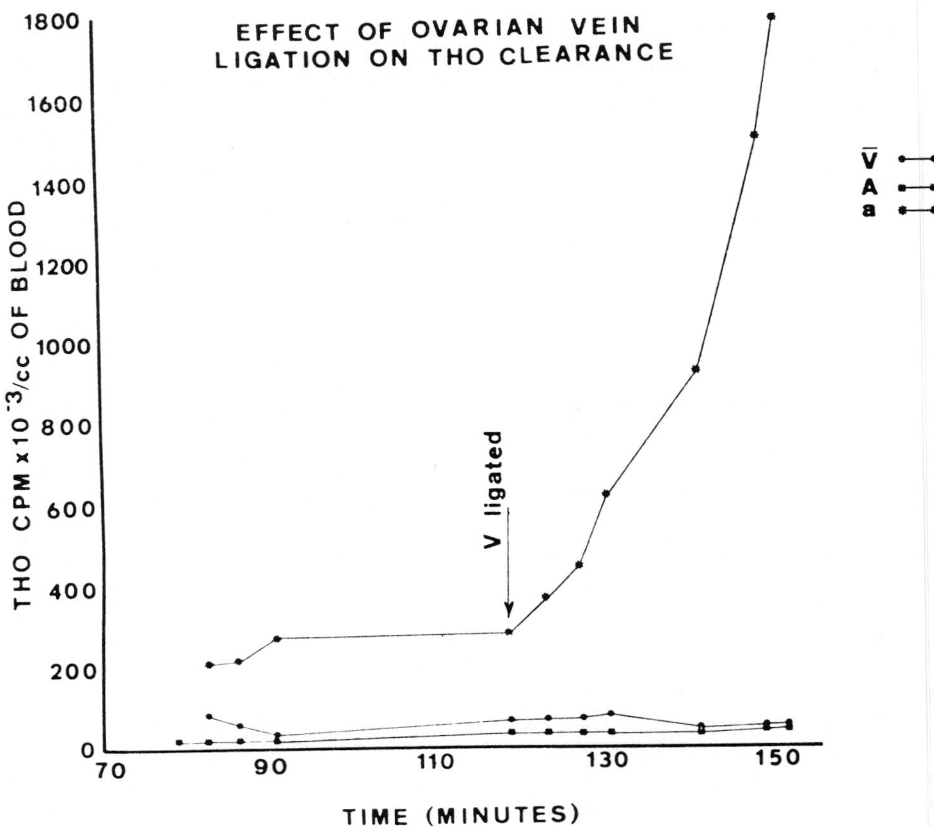

FIGURE 6–7. Assymmetric uterine venous drainage in the pregnant rhesus monkey. Obstruction of the one uterine vein draining the placenta leads to rapid accumulation of ^3H_2O in the fetus as placental clearance of ^3H_2O becomes virtually zero. (From Battaglia FC, Makowski EL, Meschia G. Physiologic study of the uterine venous drainage of the pregnant rhesus monkey. Yale J Biol Med 1970;42:225.)

In the sheep placenta, the data are more consistent with a model in which the maternal endometrium provides the major obstacle to glucose transport, compared to the fetal trophoblast. It should be emphasized that, despite the fact that placental tissue has a high concentration of insulin receptors on the maternal surface of the trophoblast, there is no evidence for a direct effect of insulin on placental glucose uptake or transport.

Amino acid transport has been studied under in vivo steady-state conditions in sheep,[22–25] as well as under a variety of in vitro conditions in small mammals and in the human placenta.[26] Although carrier systems have been identified, largely following work done in other epithelial tissues, the data have not been illuminating in terms of understanding the interrelationships among amino acids under in vivo conditions. Again, it is interesting that insulin has not been shown to affect amino acid transport. There is evidence that amino acid metabolism within the placenta may be important in understanding the factors governing the rate at which an amino acid is delivered into the fetal circulation.

The transport of free fatty acids and proteins, including lipoproteins, has been less well studied. Receptor-mediated endocytosis should play an important role in the placenta with regard to the transfer of large molecules, but less work has been done thus far in defining specific receptor systems within the placenta.

PLACENTAL METABOLISM

The high metabolic rate of the placenta has only recently been documented. The reason is that in vitro studies of the perfused human placenta and other placental types have described relatively low metabolic rates. In contrast, in vivo studies in sheep have documented very high rates of oxygen and glucose use. For example, in late gestation, approximately half of the oxygen consumption and two thirds of the glucose consumption of the uterus can be accounted for by the uteroplacental tissues, that is, by tissues other than the fetus.[27] If one assumes that the bulk of use is by placental tissues rather than by the uterine wall, the rate of oxygen and glucose consumption approaches that of brain tissue. In all species, including humans, the placenta accumulates glycogen in early gestation and decreases its glycogen content as gestation advances. However, there has been relatively little work regarding the factors controlling glycogen synthesis and mobilization within the placenta. In every species studied, data clearly demonstrate that the uterus is a site of a relatively high rate of lactate and ammonia production.[28–31] The lactate carrier system within the placenta has been fairly well studied in a number of species, including the guinea pig[32] and the human.[33] The latter studies have characterized the lactate transporter as sodium independent and stimulated by an inwardly directed hydrogen gradient; that is, it is a hydrogen-coupled transport system. However, all of these studies have tended to focus on the transport of lactate from maternal surface to the fetal surface of the placenta, whereas all in vivo data suggest that the normal process is one of lactate production by placental tissue, presumably trophoblast, and efflux of lactate into both fetal and maternal circulations. In vivo studies in sheep carried out in late gestation have found that the quantity of total amino acid nitrogen taken up from the uterine circulation was approximately equal to that delivered into the umbilical circulation, suggesting little net use by the uteroplacental tissues of amino acids.[30] However, such estimates of flux have fairly large errors. Tracer methodology is required to confirm the use of individual amino acids by the uteroplacental tissues. In addition, such studies have only been carried out in late gestation, when the placenta is no longer increasing in size.

PLACENTAL GROWTH

In all mammalian species, placental growth is much more rapid than fetal growth in early gestation, and then placental growth either stops or is at a very low rate during the later part of gestation. Fetal growth, conversely, is largely exponential throughout gestation. There is a slower rate of fetal growth in late gestation, but this still far exceeds placental growth. The outcome of these differences is that the fetal:placental ratio increases markedly as gestation advances. Although the growth rate of the placenta decreases, its maturation continues. This can be demonstrated by morphometric techniques that bring out the continued exponential increase in surface area of the placenta during late gestation, when the weight is no longer increasing.[34] Physiologic studies support the morphometric data in that there is a marked increase in the diffusing capacity of the placenta to urea in late gestation, which parallels the changes in surface area.[35] From such studies it is clear that there is an increased functional capacity per gram of placental tissue. Conversely, this cannot be regarded as a more "efficient" placenta than the midgestation placenta if the fetus to be supplied is used as a reference point because of the different growth rates of the placenta and fetus, and because midgestation placenta has a greater functional capacity per gram of fetus than the late-gestation placenta.

FETAL GROWTH

A key aspect of fetal growth is not only the rate of change in fetal body weight, but the changing body composition as gestation advances. This is particularly striking for the human fetus, which grows at approximately 1.5% per day. Accompanying this growth there is a reduction in total body water concentration, attributable largely to a decrease in extracellular fluid volume as a fraction of total body water and a large increase in white fat depots. There are a number of clinical implications of these changes in body composition. Because water represents no caloric density and fat has the highest caloric density of tissues, the human fetus has a relatively high caloric accretion rate. Because fat is nitrogen free and 78% carbon, the human fetus has a low nitrogen accretion rate in late pregnancy, but builds up large carbon stores in fat and in glycogen.[36]

The accumulation of large white fat depots in the human fetus has important nutritional implications. Fat depots are important storage sites for the fat soluble vitamins and essential fatty acids, particularly the polyunsaturated, long-chain fatty acids. Intrauterine growth retarded (IUGR) infants and very preterm infants are born with depleted fat and glycogen stores and are at risk of developing essential fatty acid deficiency relatively quickly (ie, in days) compared to term infants (ie, in weeks).[37,38] Similarly, IUGR and preterm infants are at risk of neonatal hypoglycemia.

FETAL METABOLISM

Fetal metabolism has been intensively studied in the past few years as techniques for the application of tracer methodology to fetal metabolism have become more available.

UMBILICAL UPTAKE OF NUTRIENTS

The net uptake of nutrients into the umbilical circulation from the placenta is indispensable for understanding fetal metabolism. The reason for this is that the net umbilical uptake represents the dietary supply of nutrient to the fetus. Although it is possible for the fetus to synthesize nutrients such as glucose or nonessential amino acids within the fetal tissues, such interconversions of compounds do not satisfy the absolute requirement for an exogenous (to the fetus) supply of carbon and nitrogen for growth and for oxidation (and CO_2 production).

Although some data have been collected in other species, the most complete description of the umbilical uptake of nutrients has been compiled in the fetal lamb.[3,39] These studies have brought out some unique features of fetal metabolism. The major nutrients the fetus receives include glucose, lactate, and amino acids. Glucose and the essential amino acids are derived from the maternal circulation. Lactate is produced within the placenta and transferred to the fetus. There is no information about individual nonessential amino acids. Presumably, most of the amino acid nitrogen transferred in the form of nonessential amino acids represents a direct transfer from the maternal to the fetal circulations. Because of the permeability characteristics of the sheep placenta, there is little transfer of free fatty acids or ketone bodies to the fetus in this species, with the exception of acetate, for which there is a measurable umbilical uptake. To what extent is this relatively simple fetal diet of carbohydrates (glucose and lactate) and amino acids a characteristic of other mammals, including humans? The general features of fetal metabolism would seem to be similar among fetuses of different species. In man, there is a transplacental glucose gradient from mother to fetus of approximately 15 mg/dL^{-1}.[40,41] The characteristic of this maternal–fetal concentration difference is that it is smaller in mid- than in late gestation, and also that the difference increases as maternal glucose concentration increases.[42] The latter finding of an increased transplacental glucose gradient would imply increased glucose transport to the fetus as maternal hyperglycemia develops. There is good evidence that, as the concentration difference across the placenta increases, the glucose/oxygen quotient across the umbilical circulation also increases, suggesting an increased transplacental glucose transport. We have already described the fact that lactate production by the perfused human placenta has been demonstrated. It would seem likely that the lactate produced by the placenta would be taken up by the fetus. Thus, the carbohydrates glucose and lactate would appear to provide an important source of carbon for accretion and oxidation in the human fetus.

Both glucose and lactate have been shown to have fairly high oxidation rates during fetal life. If their transport is increased, their contribution to oxidation would also increase, sparing the use of amino acids as metabolic fuels. Conversely, during maternal fasting, placental glucose transport is decreased and amino acid oxidation increased.

There is little quantitative information about amino acid and nitrogen transport to the human fetus, because it is impossible to obtain meaningful data for umbilical venous–arterial differences of amino acids either at the time of delivery or by cordocentesis. Amino acids do seem to be provided to the human fetus in amounts that exceed their net rates of accretion. The data supporting this interpretation stem from the observations of a relatively large transplacental urea gradient with fetal concentrations higher than maternal.[43] Given the large urea clearance in the primate placenta, the urea concentration difference across the placenta implies a fairly high urea production rate during fetal life. Recently, umbilical venous amino acid concentrations have been measured both in samples obtained at cordocentesis and at cesarean section.[44] These studies have demonstrated a fairly marked reduction in total amino acid concentration and specifically in branched-chain amino acids in IUGR fetuses. Because these are umbilical venous concentrations, this may reflect decreased amino acid transport in IUGR pregnancies. Very little is known about peptide transport into the fetal circulation from the placenta.

In addition to serving as fuels for the fetus, amino acids are used for protein synthesis. There are a number of conceptual problems in attempting to estimate protein synthetic rate during fetal life. However, it is clear that the protein synthetic rate expressed per gram of fetus is higher in early gestation and decreases toward term, roughly in parallel with the changes in metabolic rate.[45] The protein synthetic rate exceeds the rate of net protein accretion from growth, reflecting a relatively high rate of protein turnover during fetal life.

Fatty acids and ketone bodies cross the placenta in humans and in several other species, maintaining relatively small transplacental concentration gradients. Their fate on entering the fetal circulation has not been well studied, although it is clear that fatty acids are used largely for carbon accretion and are not oxidized to any significant extent during fetal life.[46]

CONCLUSION

Basic investigation in the laboratory animal has allowed a better understanding of the mechanisms involved in fetal hypoxia and deprivation. Recent techniques to assess waveforms nonivasively in various fetal and maternal circulations and the invasive technique of cordocentesis have provided information which, thus far, has validated most of the results from animal experiments. We now know that in the human fetus the extent of lactic acidema is a better indicator of the degree of chronic hypoxia than direct measurement of oxygen concentration or Po_2 in umbilical venous blood, and that the level of branch chain amino acids may be an excellent predictor of the severity of intrauterine growth retardation. However, only further investigation with these techniques will fully explain the complex mechanisms involved in various fetal conditions to a point where plans of management can be fashioned for the individual fetus.

REFERENCES

1. Battaglia FC, Meschia G, Makowski EL, Bowes W. The effect of maternal oxygen inhalation upon fetal oxygenation. J Clin Invest 1968;47:548.
2. Soothill PW, Nicolaides KH, Bilardo CM, Campbell S. Relation of fetal hypoxia in growth retardation to mean blood velocity in the fetal aorta. Lancet 1986;ii:1118.
3. Battaglia FC, Meschia G. An introduction to fetal physiology. Orlando, Academic Press, 1986.
4. Soothill PW, Nicolaides KH, Rodeck CH, Gamsu H. Blood gases and acid-base status of the human second-trimester fetus. Obstet Gynecol 1986;68:173.
5. Bozzetti P, Buscaglia M, Cetin I, et al. Respiratory gases, acid-base balance and lactate concentrations in the mid-term human fetus. Biol Neonate 1987;51:188.

6. Bell AW, Kennaugh JM, Battaglia FC, Makowski EL, Meschia G. Metabolic and circulatory studies of fetal lamb at midgestation. Am J Physiol 1986;250:E538.
7. Soothill PW, Nicolaides KH, Rodeck CH, Clewell WH, Lindridge J. Relationship of fetal hemoglobin and oxygen content to lactate concentration in Rh isoimmunized pregnancies. Obstet Gynecol 1987;69:268.
8. Ferrazzi E, Pardi G, Buscaglia M, et al. The correlation of biochemical monitoring versus umbilical flow velocity measurements of the human fetus. Am J Obstet Gynecol 1988;159:1081.
9. Wilkening RB, Meschia G. Fetal oxygen uptake, oxygenation, and acid-base balance as a function of uterine blood flow. Am J Physiol 1983;244:H749.
10. Wilkening RB, Meschia G. Effect of umbilical blood flow on transplacental diffusion of ethanol and oxygen. Am J Physiol 1989;256:H813.
11. Steel SA, Pearce JM, Chamberlain GV. Doppler ultrasound of the uteroplacental circulation as a screening test for severe pre-eclampsia with intra-uterine growth retardation. Eur J Obstet Gynecol Reprod Biol 1988;28:279.
12. Dempster J, Mires GJ, Taylor DJ, Patel NB. Fetal umbilical artery flow velocity waveforms: prediction of small for gestational age infants and late decelerations in labour. Eur J Obstet Gynecol Reprod Biol 1988;29:21.
13. McParland P, Pearce JM. Review article: doppler blood flow in pregnancy. Placenta 1988;9:427.
14. Pardi G, Buscaglia M, Ferrazzi E, et al. Cord sampling for the evaluation of oxygenation and acid-base balance in growth-retarded human fetuses. Am J Obstet Gynecol 1987;157:1221.
15. Battaglia FC, Makowski EL, Meschia G. Physiologic study of the uterine venous drainage of the pregnant rhesus monkey. Yale J Biol Med 1970;42:218.
16. Moll W, Kastendieck E. Transfer of N_2O, C_o and HTO in the artifically perfused guinea pig placenta. Respir Physiol 1977;29:283.
17. Faber JJ. Steady-state methods for the study of placental exchange. Federation of American Societies for Experimental Biology Proceedings 1977;36:2640.
18. Stehbens JA, Baker GL, Kitchell M. Outcome at ages 1, 3, and 5 years of children born to diabetic women. Am J Obstet Gynecol 1977;127:408.
19. Churchil JA, Berendes HW, Nemore J. Neuropsychological deficits in children of diabetic mothers: a report from the collaborative study of cerebral palsy. Am J Obstet Gynecol 1969;105:257.
20. Simmons MA, Battaglia FC, Meschia G. Placental transfer of glucose. J Dev Physiol 1979;1:227.
21. Stacey TE, Weedon AP, Haworth C, Ward RHT, Boyd RDH. Fetomaternal transfer of glucose analogues by sheep placenta. Am J Physiol 1978;234:E32.
22. Marconi A, Battaglia F, Meschia G, Spanks J. A comparison of amino acid arteriovenous differences across the placenta and liver in the fetal lamb. Submitted to Am J Physiol 1989;257:E909.
23. Lemons J, Adcock E, et al. Umbilical uptake of amino acids in the unstressed fetal lamb. J Clin Invest 1976;58:1428.
24. Lemons J, Schreiner R. Metabolic balance of the ovine fetus during the fed and fasted states. Ann Nutr Metab 1984;28:268.
25. Lemons J, Schreiner R. Amino acid metabolism in the ovine fetus. Am J Physiol 1983;244:E459.
26. Yudilevich DL, Sweiry JH. Transport of amino acids in the placenta. Biochim Biophys Acta 1985;822:169.
27. Battaglia F, Meschia G. Foetal and placental metabolisms: their interrelationship and impact upon maternal metabolism. Proc Nutr Soc 1981;40:99.
28. Block S, Johnson R, Sparks J, Battaglia F. Uterine metabolism of the pregnant guinea pig as a function of gestational age. Pediatr Res 1988;23:45.
29. Johnson R, Gilbert M, Block S, Battaglia F. Uterine metabolism of the pregnant rabbit under chronic steady-state conditions. Am J Obstet Gynecol 1986;154:1146.
30. Holzman I, Lemons J, Meschia G, Battaglia F. Uterine uptake of amino acids and placental glutamine-glutamate balance in the pregnant ewe. J Dev Physiol 1979;1:137.
31. Burd L, Jones MD, et al. Placental production and foetal utilization of lactate and pyruvate. Nature 1975;254:710.
32. Moll W, Girard H, Gros G. Facilitated diffusion of lactic acid in the guinea-pig placenta. Pflugers Arch 1980;385:229.
33. Balkoveta D, Leibach F, et al. A proton gradient is the driving force for uphill transport of lactate in human placental brush-border membrane vesicles. J Biol Chem 1988;263:13823.
34. Baur R. Morphometry of the placental exchange area. Advances in anatomy embryology and cell biology. Berlin, Springer-Verlag, 1977.
35. Kulhanek J, Meschia G, Makowski E, Battaglia FC. Changes in DNA content and urea permeability of the sheep placenta. Am J Physiol 1974;226:1257.
36. Sparks JW, Girard J, Battaglia F. An estimate of the caloric requirements of the human fetus. Biol Neonate 1980;38:113.
37. Clandinin MT, Chappell JE, Heim T, et al. Fatty acid utilization in perinatal de novo synthesis of tissues. Early Hum Dev 1981;5:355.
38. Clandinin MT, Chappell JE, Heim T, et al. Fatty acid accretion in fetal and neonatal liver: implications for fatty acid requirements. Early Hum Dev 1981;5:355.
39. Battaglia FC, Meschia G. Fetal nutrition. Ann Rev Nutr 1988;8:43.
40. Stembera ZK, Hodr JI. The relationship between the blood levels of glucose, lactic acid and pyruvic acid in the mother and in both umbilical vessels of the healthy fetus. Biol Neonate 1966;10:227.
41. Paterson P, Phillips L, Wood C. Relationship between maternal and fetal blood glucose during labor. Am J Obstet Gynecol 1967;98:938.
42. Bozzetti P, Ferrari M, Marconi M, et al. The relationship of maternal and fetal glucose concentrations in the human from midgestation until term. Metabolism 1988;37:358.
43. Gresham E, Simons P, Battaglia FC. Maternal-fetal urea concentration difference in man: metabolic significance. J Pediatr 1971;79:809.
44. Cetin I, Marconi AM, Bozzetti P, et al. Umbilical amino acid concentrations in appropriate and small for gestational age infants: a biochemical difference present in utero. Am J Obstet Gynecol 1988;158:120.
45. Kennaugh JM, Bell AW, Meschia G, Battaglia FC. Ontogenetic changes in protein synthesis rate and leucine oxidation rate during fetal life. Pediatr Res 1987;22:699.
46. Warshaw JB. Fatty acid metabolism during development. Semin Perinatol 1979;3:131.

7

CHAPTER

PLACENTAL HORMONES AND METABOLISM

Tim Chard

Pregnancy is a time of major physiological and metabolic changes (see Chapters 54 and 55). Some of these changes are so dramatic that if they occurred in the non-pregnant state, they would be considered to represent major pathology.

All of the maternal changes are assumed to be beneficial inasmuch as they represent adjustments of maternal physiology in such a way as to ensure optimal survival of the fetus. However, this assumption of "benefit" is a matter of belief rather than proven fact. For example, although it is simple to perceive the benefits to the fetus of some of the changes in maternal carbohydrate and lipid metabolism (ensuring a nutrient supply for both fetus and neonate), it is less easy to interpret the changes in renal physiology which, if anything, might appear to be counterproductive.

There are four mechanisms by which the fetoplacental unit* can influence maternal physiology and metabolism:

1. The uteroplacental circulation represents a massive arteriovenous shunt which demands major adaptations in the maternal cardiovascular system and, secondarily, in other maternal organs.
2. The fetoplacental unit consumes large quantities of nutrients to support its normal metabolism and growth, and at the same time excretes a range of waste products. With some nutrients (for example, folate), the fetus seems to exercise preferential demands over the mother.
3. The conceptus and uterus have major mechanical effects on surrounding organs and vessels. This is a consequence of upright posture and is one reason why most animal species provide a poor experimental model of the human situation.
4. The fetoplacental unit secretes a number of "specific" products that are considered to have hormonal activity in the mother.

Discussion of the physiologic and metabolic changes of pregnancy frequently places major, indeed almost exclusive, emphasis on the last of these mechanisms. However, this may not reflect the reality of the situation. As will be shown below, there are doubts about the physiological role of many of these specific products, and a serious argument can be put forward that many or most of them have no function whatsoever.

PRODUCTS OF THE HUMAN FETOPLACENTAL UNIT

The fetus itself secretes a number of specific products that are transferred to the mother and are found in significant levels in the maternal circulation. These products include α-fetoprotein and carcino-embryonic antigen. They are not considered to play any role in maternal physiology, so they will not be discussed further here.

The placenta secretes a wide range of materials that are considered to be specific to that organ (Table 7-1) and that may play a part in the physiological response to a pregnancy. The specificity of these materials may be either quantitative or qualitative. Quantitative specificity refers to the steroid hormones (estrogens and progesterone) that are secreted by the ovary in the non-pregnant state, but are secreted in much greater quantities by the placenta. Qualitative specificity refers to those placental proteins (hormones and other materials) that are associated almost exclusively with preg-

* "Fetoplacental unit" is used here as a convenient term for the ensemble of the conceptus, although to some extent fetus and placenta may behave as independent organisms.[1]

TABLE 7–1. A CLASSIFICATION OF HUMAN PLACENTAL PRODUCTS BASED ON A VARIETY OF BIOLOGICAL AND CLINICAL CHARACTERISTICS

GROUP 1	GROUP 2	GROUP 3*
Heat stable alkaline phosphatase (HSAP) Cystine aminopeptidase (CAP; oxytocinase) Estrogens (E) Progesterone (P) Human chorionic gonadotropin (hCG) Human placental lactogen (hPL) Placental growth hormone (pGH) Schwangerschaftsprotein 1 (SP1) Releasing hormones	Placental protein 5 (PP5) Pregnancy-associated plasma protein A (PAPP-A)	Placental protein 12† (PP12) Placental protein 14† (PP14)

* Group 3 products, although originally isolated from placental extracts, are synthesized by the maternal endometrium/decidua.

† There are many synonyms for these materials.

nancy. However, qualitative specificity is always relative rather than absolute, because small quantities of the placental proteins are found in sites such as seminal plasma[2] and ovarian follicular fluid.[3] Indeed, it has been suggested that these materials would be better termed "reproductive proteins" rather than "placental proteins."

The tissue of origin of the "placental" proteins (see Table 7-1) is either the placental syncytiotrophoblast (Groups 1 and 2) or the maternal decidua (Group 3).† It should be noted that the secretion of the major pregnancy estrogen, estriol (E_3), is dependent on precursors from the fetal adrenal and liver.[5] This unusual synthetic pathway has been advocated as a means by which the fetus may communicate endocrinologically with the mother. This view is probably exaggerated, because E_3, although present in vast quantities, has no recognized action in the mother, and its total absence (in placental sulfatase deficiency) has no effect on the progress or outcome of the pregnancy. It should also be noted that the trophoblast proteins (Groups 1 and 2) are secreted almost exclusively into the mother; the levels in the fetal circulation are 100-fold less.

This arises from the fact that the trophoblast cell is in direct contact with maternal blood in the intervillous space, whereas it is separated from the fetal circulation by at least a basement membrane and the endothelium of the capillaries in the chorionic villi. This anatomical relationship would tend to focus attention on a physiological role in the mother, rather than the child.

The main functional characteristics of the placental proteins are summarized in Table 7-2. It is important to emphasize that these characteristics are derived from experimental observations that cannot necessarily be extrapolated to a function of the endogenous material in a normal pregnant woman.

† The decidual proteins (PP12 and PP14) were originally isolated from the placenta, and were only subsequently recognized as being of maternal origin (endometrium/decidua).[4] As a result, the terminology is confused; until a final agreement is reached, most of the reproductive literature will probably prefer the original "PP" terminology, and this convention is followed here.

SOME PROBLEMS WITH THE ATTRIBUTION OF METABOLIC EFFECTS TO PLACENTAL PRODUCTS

The range of maternal physiological and metabolic effects that have been attributed to placental hormones and other products is extensive (see Table 7-2). However, it has proved difficult to specify the precise functional role, in a normal pregnant woman, of any one of these products. The reasons for this problem are as follows:

1. The hormonal effects of placental products are only one of a number of mechanisms that can alter maternal physiology. The cardiovascular, nutrient, and mechanical changes imposed by the presence of the conceptus can explain many of the maternal changes without the need to postulate additional factors.
2. There is a multiplicity of placental products, and some of these might have very similar effects: for example, the circulating levels of both hPL and the placental steroids correlate with various aspects of carbohydrate and lipid metabolism.[6] Thus, it is difficult to point to any one compound as having a preeminent role in any aspect of maternal physiology.
3. Most of the proposed functions of placental products (see Table 7-2) are based on experiments in which the effects of the chemically purified product are examined in animals, in non-pregnant humans, or in tissue culture. For the reasons already given, none of these can provide a satisfactory emulation of the complete pregnant woman. Nevertheless, there is a strong temptation, resisted by few workers in the field, to extrapolate from experimental effects to biological functions.

TABLE 7–2. A SUMMARY OF THE MAIN FUNCTIONAL CHARACTERISTICS OF THE THREE GROUPS OF PLACENTAL PRODUCTS

MATERIAL	FUNCTIONAL CHARACTERISTICS
Group 1	
Heat stable alkaline phosphatase (HSAP)	Unknown
Cystine aminopeptidase (CAP)	Proteolysis of oxytocin
Estrogens and progesterone	Various physiological and metabolic adjustments in the mother (see Tables 7-3 and 7-4)
Human chorionic gonadotropin (hCG)	Maintenance of corpus luteum
Human placental lactogen (hPL)	Mammotrophic. Various metabolic effects
Placental growth hormone (pGH)	Control of IGF-I levels
Schwangerschaftsprotein 1 (SP1)	Unknown
Group 2	
PAPP-A	Antiproteolytic; anticomplementary
PP5	Antithrombin
Group 3	
PP12	IGF-binding protein
PP14	Beta lactoglobulin

It should be noted that these characteristics, all or most of which have been demonstrated under experimental conditions, cannot necessarily be extrapolated to a true "function" in the normal pregnant woman. The list is not encyclopedic. A variety of minor functions have been reported for all of these materials, often in a single publication not subsequently confirmed by other workers. For example, most of these materials have at various times been ascribed immunosuppressive properties, often on the basis of very limited data.

4. There are rare pregnancies in which one or another of the placental products is completely absent. This has been described many times for hPL and estriol (the latter the result of a placental sulfatase deficiency that stops processing of the fetal precursors), or in isolated but clearcut cases for SP1, PAPP-A, pGH, and even progesterone. In all of these situations the pregnancy itself has appeared entirely normal. This "experiment of nature" may well exclude an essential function for any of the wide range of materials for which the phenomenon has been described.
5. Some of the most dramatic alterations in maternal physiology, especially those in the kidney, show the major change during the first trimester. At this time the synthesis of placental products is still relatively limited. The obvious exceptions are hCG and PP14, but neither of these is considered to have any significant effects on general maternal physiology.
6. As will be shown later, in the case of hPL, there is a notable absence of the feedback control mechanisms that characterize most classical endocrine systems. The specific control mechanisms that have been described are mostly derived from experiments under conditions (especially in respect of dose levels) that do not accurately reflect the situation in normal pregnancy. Indeed, it has been proposed that the major factors controlling the time-to-time variation in the secretion of placental products is the total mass of the trophoblast and the bloodflow in the intervillous space. This apparent lack of feedback control greatly weakens the case for specific metabolic effects of placental products. For example, it is difficult to believe that hPL plays a highly significant role in the control of maternal glucose metabolism in light of the fact that glucose has little or no short-term effect on hPL secretion[7] and that there appears to be little or no relationship between circulating hPL levels and standard glucose variables.[8]
7. Although there are random time-to-time fluctuations in the levels of placental products, there is little or no systematic change in circulating levels over a 24-hour period.[9,10]

MATERNAL METABOLIC EFFECTS OF PLACENTAL PRODUCTS

PRODUCTS THAT ARE NOT CONSIDERED TO HAVE SIGNIFICANT METABOLIC EFFECTS

Of the materials listed in Table 7-1, the following are not generally considered to have significant metabolic functions: HSAP, CAP, hCG, SP1, PAPP-A, and PP14. It should be emphasized that this statement refers to *maternal metabolic* effects. Obviously, hCG has important endocrine effects on the mother. It should also be noted there have been occasional, unconfirmed reports of metabolic functions of almost all of these products.

EFFECTS OF ESTROGENS AND PROGESTERONE

Virtually all of the maternal physiological and metabolic changes in pregnancy have at some time been attributed to either or both of estrogens and progesterone secreted by the placenta (Tables 7-3 and 7-4). However, the evidence for this suffers from most of the problems already described. In particular, a large part of the literature consists of observations of the effects of oral contraceptive agents on non-pregnant woman. The spectrum of estrogenic and progestogenic steroids in these is not necessarily representative of endogenous materials. Furthermore, orally administered estrogens have a far greater effect on metabolic functions than do parenterally administered steroids.[11] That being said, there is little doubt that the placental steroids do have highly significant effects on maternal metabolism. The main arguments concern the precise targets of such effects, and the quantum of the effects. The flavor of such arguments is nicely illustrated by the dispute as to

TABLE 7–3. METABOLIC CHANGES IN PREGNANCY THAT HAVE BEEN ATTRIBUTED TO ESTROGENS

AUTHOR	EFFECTS
Ablin et al (1974)[86]	Immunosuppression
Adams & Oakley[84]	Increased insulin response and glucose intolerance
Anderson (1974)[96]	Increase in sex hormone binding globulin (SHBG)
Cain et al (1971)[92]	Increase in renin substrate and angiotensin II
Carr and Gant[100]	Sodium diuresis and potassium retention
Davis and Hipkin (1974)[89]	Inhibition of lymphocyte transformation
Doring et al (1950)[95]	Overbreathing and reduction of pCO_2
Dowling et al (1974)[99]	Increase of thyroxine binding globulin
Gazioglu et al (1970)[91]	Decrease in pulmonary gas transfer
Marshall et al (1966)[93]	Ureteral dilatation
Reeve (1980)[90]	Increased urinary excretion of phosphate
Roth et al (1978)[97]	Increase in serum cholesterol
Song et al (1965)[88]	Liver phagocytosis increased (Kupffer cells)
Tacchi (1960)[94]	Dilatation of small vessels
Warth et al (1975)[98]	Increase in triglycerides

In some cases the observations are derived from animal studies, or from investigation of non-pregnant women receiving estrogens. This list is not encyclopedic: in many situations, especially those involving observation of changes following administration of oral contraceptive agents to non-pregnant women, there may be several dozen similar publications. A detailed review of the effects of estrogens and progesterone on lipid and carbohydrate metabolism has been published by Gaspard (1987).[85]

whether the ureteral dilatation of pregnancy can be ascribed to progesterone, or to mechanical obstruction at the pelvic brim, or to a combination of the two. Of the various metabolic changes listed in Tables 7-3 and 7-4, probably the least ambiguous in terms of attribution are the substantial gestational increase in various circulating binding proteins (thyroxine-binding globulin, cortisol-binding globulin, sex hormone-binding globulin) due to an increase in synthesis by the liver.

EFFECTS OF HUMAN PLACENTAL LACTOGEN (hPL)

Placental lactogen is the archetype of placental products considered to have metabolic effects on the mother. As a consequence, the evidence concerning this topic is more extensive than that for any of the other materials described here, and a strong case has been made that hPL plays a major role in maternal metabolism and fetal growth.[12–14] This evidence can be discussed under four headings: the effect of experimental administration of hPL, the effects of experimental manipulations on hPL levels in vivo, the relationship of maternal hPL levels to glucose metabolism, and findings in the rare cases of spontaneous deficiency of hPL.

Administration of hPL

A great variety of biological activities has been proposed for hPL, including growth promotion, lactogenesis, an effect on carbohydrate and lipid metabolism, stimulation of the corpus luteum, erythropoiesis, inhibition of fibrinolysis, and immunosuppression.

Although it is chemically similar to hGH, hPL has only weak somatotrophic activity, variously estimated

TABLE 7–4. METABOLIC CHANGES IN PREGNANCY THAT HAVE BEEN ATTRIBUTED TO PROGESTERONE

AUTHOR	EFFECTS
Cain et al (1971)[92]	Increase in renin substrate and angiotensin II
Doring et al (1950)[95]	Overbreathing and reduction of pCO_2
Ehrlich & Lindheimer (1972)[104]	Reduction of potassium secretion
Hervey (1969)[101]	Change in appetite leading to fat accumulation
Hettiaratchi and Pickford (1961)[105]	Vasodilatation
Marshall et al (1966)[93]	Ureteral dilatation
Munroe (1971)[102]	Immunosuppression
Siiteri et al (1977)[103]	Immunosuppression

In some cases the observations are derived from animal studies, or from investigation of non-pregnant women receiving estrogens.

at 0.1% to 10% of that of pituitary prolactin.[15,16] However, the growth-promoting activity of hPL may be greater than that of hGH for some fetal tissues.[17]

The extent of the lactogenic activity of hPL has been disputed. Early reports suggested that its potency was some 75% that of sheep prolactin.[18] However, later studies showed much lower activity[19,20] (1 to 5 U/mg in the pigeon crop-sac assay). The potency in the rabbit intraductal assay is greater than that in the pigeon crop-sac assay; a similar discrepancy has been observed with human growth hormone. Studies using intact animals have yielded estimates ranging from 20% to 100% of that of prolactin.[21] Thus, it is difficult to assign a potency because the apparent lactogenic activity of hPL is highly dependent on the purity of the material examined, on the type of assay, and on the animal species used for the assay. Surprisingly, substantial modification of the hPL molecule (reduction and alkylation, oxidation) does not seem to be associated with loss of lactogenic activity.[22]

Administration of hPL in animals leads to a rise in blood sugar[23,24] and free fatty acids[25]; this may be due to increased peripheral resistance to insulin action, although in hypophysectomized rats, hPL can cause an increase in insulin release in vitro from islet cells.[26]

Administration of hPL to rhesus monkeys can decrease the hypoglycemic response to exogenous insulin, without affecting glucose tolerance or the insulin response to glucose.[27] hPL can modulate insulin production by cultured human fetal pancreas, and it has been suggested that this might contribute to fetal body growth.[28] hPL can also inhibit the effect of insulin on glucose transport in fat cells in vitro.[29]

In the mouse, hPL can stimulate erythropoietin secretion and thus the incorporation of iron into red blood cells.[30] Both hPL and hCG can suppress phytohemagglutinin-induced lymphocyte transformation.[31,32] However, the suggestion that either of these compounds plays a significant role in the immune survival of a pregnancy is now largely discredited.

Experimental Manipulation of hPL Secretion

A wide variety of factors have been tested for possible effects on the secretion of hPL:

1. Releasing hormones: thyrotrophin-releasing hormone (TRH), which is a powerful stimulant for pituitary prolactin secretion, and is also found in the placenta,[33] has no effect on circulating hPL levels.[34] Gonadotrophin-releasing hormone (GnRH) has no effect in vitro,[35,36] although administration of GnRH antagonist has a delayed suppressive effect.[37] It is interesting to note that growth hormone-releasing hormone can stimulate release of pituitary growth hormone (GH) in pregnant woman, but not that of placental GH.[38] This further confirms the relative insensitivity of placental hormones to the control mechanisms that apply to their pituitary analogues.
2. Steroid hormones: in the rat, ovariectomy[39] produces an increase in hPL levels. In the sheep, there is no evidence that endogenous progesterone secretion affects hPL secretion.[40] Similarly, no effect of estradiol or progesterone has been shown on secretion of hPL by human placental cells in vitro.[41]
3. Carbohydrate and lipid metabolism: because of the close relationship to growth hormone, several groups have examined the relationship of hPL levels to alterations in carbohydrate and lipid metabolism. Blood levels of hPL decrease following intravenous administration of glucose, although Pavlou and his colleagues showed that the change is small and inconsistent, and might also be attributed to trivial mechanisms such as the osmotic expansion of plasma volume that results from injection of a hypertonic solution.[7,42–44]
4. Increases of blood hPL levels have been shown during insulin-induced hypoglycemia,[43] prolonged starvation,[45,46] and intravenous arginine,[47] but changes are small when compared with those of pituitary growth hormone under similar circumstances. Administration of high-density lipoprotein (HDL) can stimulate PL secretion in pregnant sheep.[48] Equally, a number of studies do not support a significant role of carbohydrate or lipids in the control of hPL secretion. There is no change in hPL levels after oral administration of glucose.[7] In the sheep, maternal hyperglycemia produces no change in placental lactogen levels in fetus or ewe.[46] Experimentally induced changes in circulating levels of free fatty acids do not produce any consistent change in hPL concentrations.[49] The secretion of hPL by dispersed placental cells in vitro is not influenced by changes in insulin or glucose concentrations,[41] although contrary results were obtained by Bhaumick and coworkers, who showed that both insulin and insulin-like growth factor-I (IGF-I) could stimulate hPL production by placental explants.[50]
5. Other factors: neither epidermal growth factor,[51] adrenergic beta receptor agonists or antagonists,[52] dibutyryl cyclic AMP,[53] nor corticosteroids[54] have any effect on secretion of hPL by placental cells in vitro. Prostaglandin $F_{2\alpha}$ has no direct effect on hPL secretion in vivo.[55] Dopamine reduces hPL production in vitro.[56]

THE RELATIONSHIP OF MATERNAL hPL LEVELS TO GLUCOSE METABOLISM

Despite some conflicting findings, it would now appear that there is no direct relationship between circulating hPL levels and standard parameters of glucose metabolism, such as the fasting blood glucose and the response to intravenous glucose.[8,57] In the study by Langhoff-Roos and colleagues,[8] the relationship of hPL levels to fetal weight persisted after the glucose variables were taken into account.

Spontaneous Deficiency of hPL

Pregnancies in which there is a partial or total deletion of the hPL gene have been widely documented (eg, Simon and coworkers[58]). There is universal agreement that such pregnancies are normal in every other way. Superficially, this might seem to end further discussion of a functional role for hPL. However, advocates of this role have raised questions that might cast doubt on this "experiment of nature." First, there is the possibility that the deficiency may not be complete, and that only a small amount of the hormone might suffice. But it has now been shown that many cases have a *homozygous* deletion; ie, the deficiency is total.[58] Second, it has been argued that the hormone might simply be modified so that it is undetectable in standard immunochemical assays but still retains biological activity. Specific examination of this possibility yielded negative results.[59,60] Finally, it has been suggested that the pregnancies are normal because other factors may compensate for the deficiency of hPL. But this begs the question of what is meant by an "essential role." Furthermore, it would be highly untypical of protein endocrinology in general, where total absence of a hormone is *invariably* associated with gross abnormalities.

EFFECTS OF PLACENTAL GROWTH HORMONE

Placental growth hormone (GH) is the product of the hPL-V gene, which until recently was thought to be silent.[61] The effects of pGH have yet to be fully explored, but a case has been made that it might control maternal (and even fetal levels) of IGF-I.[62,63] In addition, arguments similar to those made for hPL can be put forward in respect of maternal carbohydrate metabolism. However, the fact that a "normal" pregnancy has been described in which there was a total deletion of the hPL-V gene clearly does not support a vital role for this hormone in the mother.[58]

EFFECTS OF PLACENTAL PROTEIN 5

Placental protein 5 (PP5) has been shown to be biologically (but not chemically) analogous to antithrombin III.[64] A sharp increase in maternal blood levels is seen following administration of small doses of heparin,[65] and substantial increases may also occur in severe preeclampsia and placental abruption.[66] These observations suggest that PP5 might be involved in the extensive changes in coagulation factors seen in normal pregnancy. Equally, it has been suggested that the most likely functional effects of PP5 are *local* rather than systemic, and that it represents a natural defense of the placenta against coagulation in the intervillous space.

EFFECTS OF PLACENTAL PROTEIN 12

Placental protein 12 (PP12) was originally isolated from placental extracts,[4] then shown to be synthesized by the endometrium/decidua,[67] and finally demonstrated to be identical to the small molecular weight IGF-I binding protein (IGFBP-I).[68] The latter had already been characterized by a number of workers following isolation from other tissues, thus explaining the currently confused nomenclature.

The most obvious functions of IGFBP-I (PP12) are binding of IGF-I in the circulation and an important but not yet completely specified role in the action of IGF-I and its cell surface receptors.[69] The latter may be of considerable significance in the control of fetal growth, there being an *inverse* relationship between maternal PP12 levels and the size of the fetus.[70,71]

At the metabolic level, there is a clearcut inverse relationship between the levels of IGFBP-I and insulin.[72,73] This relationship is reflected by a dramatic diurnal rhythm of IGFBP-I levels in both pregnant and nonpregnant subjects.[74] Thus, IGFBP-I is probably an important part of the insulin-glucose homeostasis system, and the substantial rise in IGFBP-I levels during pregnancy would obviously be relevant to maternal metabolism. However, the precise source of the bulk of IGFBP-I in pregnancy has yet to be specified. It is possible that it arises mainly from the decidua, but an origin from more distant maternal tissues, especially the liver, has not been excluded. The general physiological significance is, of course, the same regardless of the source. However, if it does prove that IGFBP-I in pregnancy is primarily of placental/decidual origin, then this may be among the most significant of all placental products in terms of the adjustment of maternal physiology.

THE CLINICAL SIGNIFICANCE OF PLACENTAL PRODUCTS IN RELATION TO MATERNAL METABOLISM

At one time, measurement of Group 1 placental products, especially hPL and estriol, was widely used in the assessment of fetal well-being in late pregnancy. These "placental function tests" have now been largely superceded by the more efficient biophysical procedures.[75] Some of the more recently discovered products of Groups 2 and 3 have also been advocated as potential clinical tests (eg, PP5,[76] PP12[71]). However, the precise role of these remains to be determined. The main parameter to which the maternal circulating levels of Group 1 products relate is the weight of the fetus.[75] It would be attractive to speculate that there is a direct functional relationship between some of these products and fetal growth. However, there is no evidence for this, even in the case of hPL, which is chemically and biologically related to growth hormone.[77] As already noted, the main (indeed only) factors controlling secretion of Group 1 products are the mass of the trophoblast and uteroplacental and intervillous bloodflow. These are directly related to the size of the fetus. The relationship between fetal size and Group 1 products is therefore secondary to the relationship to both tissue mass and bloodflow.

The association between elevated levels of hPL and maternal diabetes was at one time widely discussed in the context of maternal metabolic effects of hPL. It is interesting to note that the phenomenon, which was described by virtually all of the earlier workers in the field (eg, Ursell and coworkers[78]), may have disappeared.[57,79] This can probably be attributed to the better management of diabetic pregnancy which, if well controlled, can now be considered as metabolically normal. Furthermore, it is apparent that the phenomenon has little or no functional significance, but is merely a secondary consequence of the overgrowth of the trophoblast that is (or was) characteristic of maternal diabetes.

The levels of placental hormones can also be affected by changes in maternal metabolism. For example, pregnant women with renal transplants have elevated levels of hPL,[80] even though fetal weight in this group is relatively low. The increase is attributed to decreased elimination in the renal tubules.

CONCLUSION

The dramatic changes in maternal physiology and metabolism during normal pregnancy may be attributed to four factors: the uteroplacental unit as an arteriovenous shunt, the nutrient and excretory demands of the fetus and placenta, the mechanical obstructive effects of the pregnancy, and the secretion of hormonal products by the placenta. Despite the emphasis often given to the last of these, the placental products may in reality make only a small contribution to maternal changes during pregnancy. This applies especially to hPL, which, despite much research effort and argument, appears to have little or no functional significance. Current interest is focusing on the "placental" products that are of endometrial/decidual origin, in particular IGFBP-I, which may be an essential functional component in the link between maternal insulin/carbohydrate metabolism and fetal growth.

REFERENCES

1. Gordon YB, Chard T. The specific proteins of the human placenta: some new hypotheses. In: Klopper A, Chard T, eds. Placental proteins. New York: Springer-Verlag, 1979:1.
2. Salem HT, Menabawey M, Seppala M, Shaaban MM, Chard T. Human seminal plasma contains a wide range of "trophoblast-"specific proteins. Placenta 1984;5:413.
3. Westergaard L, Sinosich MJ, Grudzinskas JG, et al. Pregnancy-associated plasma protein A (PAPP-A) in preovulatory, nonovulatory healthy, and atretic human ovarian follicles during the natural cycle. Ann N Y Acad Sci 1985;442:205.
4. Bohn H, Kraus W. Isolierung und charakterisierung eines neue plazentaspezifischen proteins. Archiv fur Gynekologie 1980;229:279.
5. Chard T, Klopper A. Placental function tests. Berlin: Springer-Verlag, 1982.
6. Desoye G, Schweditsh MO, Pfeiffer KP, Zechner R, Kostner GM. Correlation of hormones with lipid and lipoprotein levels during normal pregnancy and postpartum. J Clin Endocrinol Metab 1987;64:704.
7. Pavlou C, Chard T, Landon J, Letchworth AT. Circulating levels of hPL in late pregnancy: effect of glucose loading, smoking and exercise. Eur J Obstet Gynaecol Reprod Biol 1973;3:45.
8. Langhoff-Roos J, Wibell L, Gebre-Medhin M, Lindmark G. Placental hormones and maternal glucose metabolism. A study of fetal growth in normal pregnancy. Br J Obstet Gynaecol 1989;96:320.
9. Houghton DJ, Newnham JP, Lo K, Rice A, Chard T. Circadian variation of circulating levels of four placental proteins. Br J Obstet Gynaecol 1982;89:831.
10. Nakajima ST, McAuliffe T, Gibson M. The 24-hour pattern of the levels of serum progesterone and immunoreactive human chorionic gonadotropin in normal early pregnancy. J Clin Endocrinol Metab 1990;71:345.
11. von Schoultz B, Carlstrom K, Collste L, et al. Estrogen therapy and liver function — metabolic effects of oral and parenteral administration. Prostate 1989;14:389.
12. Handwerger S, Freemark M. Role of placental lactogen and prolactin in human pregnancy. Adv Exp Biol Med 1987;219:399.
13. Freemark M, Handwerger S. The role of placental lactogen in the regulation of fetal metabolism and growth. J Pediatr Gastroenterol Nutr 1989:8:281.
14. Freemark M, Comer M, Mularoni T, D'Ercole AJ, Grandis A, Kodack L. Nutritional regulation of placental lactogen receptor in fetal liver: implications for fetal metabolism and growth. Endocrinology 1989;125:1504.
15. Josimovich JB. Potentiation of somatotrophic and diabetogenic effects of growth hormone by human placental lactogen (hPL). Endocrinology 1966;78:707.
16. Murakawa S, Raben MS. Effect of growth hormone and placental lactogen on DNA synthesis in rat costal cartilage and adipose tissue. Endocrinology 1968;83:645.
17. Hill DJ, Crace CJ, Milner RDG. Incorporation of ^{3}H thymidine by isolated fetal myoblasts and fibroblasts in response to human placental lactogen (hPL): possible mediation of hPL action by release of immunoreactive SM-C. Br J Cell Physiol 1985;125:337.
18. Josimovich JB, Brande BL. Chemical properties and biologic effects of human placental lactogen (hPL). Trans N Y Acad Sci 1964;27:161.
19. Friesen H. Purification of a placental factor with immunological and chemical similarity to human growth hormone. Endocrinology 1965;76:369.
20. Florini JR, Tonelli G, Breuer CB, Coppola J, Ringler I, Bell PH. Characterization and biological effects of purified placental protein (human). Endocrinology 1966;79:692.
21. Handwerger S, Sherwood LM. Human placental lactogen (hPL). In: Jaffe BM, Behrman HF, eds. Methods of hormone radioimmunoassay. New York: Academic Press, 1974:427.
22. Aloj SM, Edelhoch H, Handwerger S, Sherwood LM. Correlation in the structure and function of human placental lactogen and human growth hormone. II: the effects of disulfide bond modifications on the conformation of human placental lactogen. Endocrinology 1972;91:728.
23. Burt RL, Leake NH, Pruitt AB. Observations on the metabolic activity of a human placental fraction. Am J Obstet Gynecol 1966;95:579.
24. Handwerger S, Fellows RE, Crenshaw MC, Hurley T, Barrett J, Maurer WF. Ovine lacental lactogen: acute effects on interme-

diary metabolism in pregnant and non-pregnant sheep. J Endocrinol 1976;69:133.

25. Riggi SJ, Boshart CR, Bell PH, Ringler I. Some effects of purified placental protein (human) on lipid and carbohydrate metabolism. Endocrinology 1966;79:709.
26. Martin JM, Friesen H. Effect of human placental lactogen on the isolated islets of Langerhans in vitro. Endocrinology 1969; 84:619.
27. Beck P. Reversal of progesterone-enhanced insulin production by human chorionic somatomammotropin. Endocrinology 1970;87:311.
28. Swenne I, Hill DJ, Strain AJ, Milner RDG. Effects of human placental lactogen and growth hormone on the production of insulin and somatomedin C/insulin-like growth factor I by human fetal pancreas tissue. J Endocrinol 1987;113:297.
29. Ryan EA, Enns L. Role of gestational hormones in the induction of insulin resistance. J Clin Endocrinol Metab 1988;67:341.
30. Jepson JH, Friesen HG. The mechanism of action of human placental lactogen on erythropoiesis. Br J Haematol 1968;15:465.
31. Contractor SF, Davies H. Effect of human chorionic somatomammotrophin and human chorionic gonadotrophin on phytohaemagglutinin-induced lymphocyte transformation. Nature 1973;243:284.
32. Cerni C, Tatra G, Bohn H. Immunosuppression by human placental lactogen (hPL) and the pregnancy-specific beta-1 glycoprotein (SP-1). Archiv fur Gynekologie 1977;223:1.
33. Gibbons JM, Mitnick M, Chieffo V. In vitro biosynthesis of TSH- and LH-releasing factors by the human placenta. Am J Obstet Gynecol 1975;121:127.
34. Hershman JM, Kojima A, Friesen HG. Effect of thyrotropin-releasing hormone on human pituitary thyrotropin, prolactin, placental lactogen and chorionic thyrotropin, prolactin, placental lactogen and chorionic thyrotropin. J Clin Endocrinol Metab 1973;36:497.
35. Khodr G, Siler-Khodr TM. The effect of luteinizing hormone-releasing factor on human chorionic gonadotropin secretion. Fertil Steril 1978;30:301.
36. Siler-Khodr TM, Khodr GS, Valenzuela G, Rhode J. Gonadotropin-releasing hormone effects on placental hormones during gestation. I: Alpha-human chorionic gonadotropin, human chorionic gonadotropin and human chorionic somatomammotropin. Biol Reprod 1986;34:245.
37. Siler-Khodr TM, Khodr GS, Vickery BH, Nestor JJ. Inhibition of hCG, alpha-hCG and progesterone release from human placental tissue in vitro by GnRH antagonist. Life Sci 1983;32:2741.
38. de Zegher F, Vanderschueren-Lodeweyckx M, Spitz B, et al. Perinatal growth hormone (GH) physiology: effect of GH-releasing factor on maternal and fetal secretion of pituitary and placental GH. J Endocrinol 1990;77:520.
39. Robertson MC, Owens RE, Klindt J, Friesen HG. Ovariectomy leads to a rapid increase in rat placental lactogen secretion. Endocrinology 1984;114:1805.
40. Taylor MJH, Jenkin G, Robinson JS, Thorborn GD. Regulation of ovine placental lactogen: lack of correlation with progesterone secretion. J Endocrinol 1982;95:275.
41. Zeitler P, Markoff E, Handwerger S. Characterization of the synthesis and release of human placental lactogen and human chorionic gonadotrophin by an enriched population of dispersed placental cells. J Clin Endocrinol 1983;57:812.
42. Burt RL, Leake NH, Rhyne AL. Human placental lactogen and insulin-blood glucose homeostasis. Obstet Gynecol 1970;36:233.
43. Spellacy WN, Buhi WC, Schram JD, Birk SA. Control of human chorionic somatomammotrophin levels during pregnancy. Obstet Gynecol 1971;37:567.
44. Ajabor IN, Yen SSC. Effect of sustained hyperglycemia on the levels of human chorionic somatomammotrophin in mid-pregnancy. Am J Obstet Gynecol 1971;37:77.
45. Kim YK, Felig P. Plasma chorionic somatomammotropin levels during starvation in mid-pregnancy. J Clin Endocrinol Metab 1971;32:864.
46. Brinsmead MW, Bancroft BJ, Thorburn GD, Waters J. Fetal and maternal ovine placental lactogen during hyperglycaemia, hypoglycaemia and fasting. J Endocrinol 1981;90:337.
47. Prieto JC, Cifuentes I, Cerrano-Rios M. hCS regulation during pregnancy. Obstet Gynecol 1976;48:287.
48. Grandis A, Jorgensen V, Kodack L, Quarfordt S, Handwerger S. High-density lipoproteins (HDL) stimulate placental lactogen secretion in pregnant ewes: further evidence for a role of HDL in placental lactogen secretion during pregnancy. J Endocrinol 1989;120:423.
49. Morris HHB, Cinik A, Mulvihal M. Effects of acute alterations in maternal free fatty acid concentration on human chorionic somatomammotropin secretion. Am J Obstet Gynecol 1974;119:224.
50. Bhaumick B, Dawson EP, Bala RM. The effects of insulin-like growth factor-I and insulin on placental lactogen production by human term placenta. Biochem Biophys Res Comm 1987;144:674.
51. Wilson EA, Jawad MJ, Vernon MW. Effect of epidermal growth factor on hormone secretion by term placenta in organ culture. Am J Obstet Gynecol 1984;149:579.
52. Shu-Rong Z, Bremme K, Eneroth P, Nordberg A. The regulation in vitro of placental release of human chorionic gonadotropin, placental lactogen and prolactin: effects of an adrenergic beta-receptor agonist and antagonist. Am J Obstet Gynecol 1982;143:444.
53. Winikoff J, Braunstein GD. In vitro secretory patterns of human chorionic gonadotrophin, placental lactogen and pregnancy-specific beta-1-glycoprotein. Placenta 1985;6:417.
54. Tatra G, Tempfer H, Gruber W. Influences of 16-beta-methyl-prednisone on serum concentrations of pregnancy-specific proteins SP-1 and hPL during the last trimester of pregnancy. Eur Obstet Gynecol Reprod Biol 1976;6:59.
55. Ward RHT, Whyley GA, Fairweather DVI, Allen EA, Chard T. A comparative study of plasma 17-beta-oestradiol, progesterone, placental lactogen and chorionic gonaotrophin in abortion induced with intra-amniotic prostaglandin F_2 alpha. Br J Obstet Gynaecol 1977;84:363.
56. Macaron C, Famuyiwa O, Sing SP. In vitro effect of dopamine and pimozide on human chorionic somatomammotropin (hCS) secretion. J Clin Endocrinol Metab 1978;47:168.
57. Braunstein GD, Mills JL, Reed GF, et al. Diabetes in Early Pregnancy Study Group. J Clin Endocrinol Metab 1989;68:3.
58. Simon P, Decoster C, Brocas H, Schwers J, Vassart G. Absence of human chorionic somatomammotropin during pregnancy associated with two types of gene deletion. Hum Genet 1986;74:235.
59. Sideri M, De Virgiliis G, Guidobono F, et al. Immunologically undetectable human placental lactogen in normal pregnancy. Br J Obstet Gynaecol 1983;90:771.
60. Alexander I, Anthony F, Letchworth AT. Placental protein profile and glucose studies in a normal pregnancy with extremely low levels of human placental lactogen. Br J Obstet Gynaecol 1982;89:241.
61. Hennen G, Frankenne F, Closset F, Gomez F, Pirens G, El Khayat N. A human placental GH: increasing levels during second half of pregnancy with pituitary GH suppression as re-

vealed by monoclonal antibody radioimmunoassays. Int J Fertil 1985;30:27.

62. Frankenne F, Closset J, Gomez F, Scippo ML, Smal J, Hennen G. The physiology of growth hormones (GHs) in pregnant women and partial characterization of the placental GH variant. J Clin Endocrinol Metab 1988;66:1171.
63. Caufriez A, Frankenne F, Englert Y, et al. Placental growth hormone as a potential regulator of maternal IGF-I during human pregnancy. Am J Physiol 258:E1014,1990.
64. Salem HT, Seppala M, Chard T. The effect of thrombin on serum placental protein 5 (PP5): is PP5 the naturally occurring antithrombin III of the human placenta? Placenta 1981;2:205.
65. Menabawey M, Silman R, Rice A, Chard T. Dramatic increase of placental protein 5 levels following injection of small doses of heparin. Br J Obstet Gynaecol 1985;92:207.
66. Salem HT, Westergaard JG, Hindersson P, Lee JN, Grudzinskas JG, Chard T. Maternal serum levels of placental protein 5 in complications of late pregnancy. Obstet Gynecol 1982;59:467.
67. Rutanen EM, Koistinen R, Wahlstrom T, Bohn H, Seppala M. Synthesis of placental protein 12 by decidua. Endocrinology 1985;116:1304
68. Koistinen R, Kalkkinen N, Huhtala ML, Seppala M, Bohn H, Rutanen EM. Placental protein 12 is a decidual protein that binds somatomedin and has an identical N-terminal amino acids sequence with somatomedin-binding protein from human amniotic fluid. Endocrinology 1986;118:1375.
69. Rutanen EM, Pekonen F, Makinen T. Soluble 34K binding protein inhibits the binding of insulin-like growth factor I to its cell receptors in human secretory phase endometrium: evidence for autocrine/paracrine regulation of growth factor action. J Clin Endocrinol Metab 1988;66:173.
70. Howell RJS, Perry LA, Choglay NS, Bohn H, Chard T. Placental protein 12 (PP12): a new test for the prediction of the small-for-gestational-age infant. Br J Obstet Gynaecol 1985;92:1141.
71. Chard T. Hormonal control of growth in the human fetus. J Endocrinol 1989;123:3.
72. Holly JMP, Biddlecombe RA, Dunger DB, et al. Circadian variation of GH-dependent IGF-binding protein in diabetes mellitus and its relationship to insulin. A new role for insulin. Clin Endocrinol 1988;29:667.
73. Suikkari AM, Koivisto VA, Rutanen EM, Yki-Jarvinen H, Karonen SL, Seppala M. Insulin regulates the serum levels of low molecular weight insulin-like growth factor-binding protein. J Clin Endocrinol Metab 1987;66:266.
74. Howell RJS, Kyei-Mansah A, Bohn H, Holly JMP, Wass JAH, Chard T. The circadian variation of PP12 in the second and third trimeters of pregnancy. [Submitted for publication]
75. Chard T. What is happening to placental function tests? Ann Clin Biochem 1987;24:435.
76. Salem HT, Chard T. Clinical studies on placental protein 5 (PP5). In: Grudzinskas JG, Teisner B, Seppala M, eds. Pregnancy proteins: biology, chemistry and clinical application. New York: Academic Press, 1982:271.
77. Houghton DJ, Shackleton P, Obiekwe BC, Chard T. Relationship of maternal and fetal levels of human placental lactogen to weight and sex of the fetus. Placenta 1984;5:455.
78. Ursell W, Brudenell M, Chard T. Placental lactogen levels indiabetic pregnancy. Br Med J 1973;i:80.
79. Stewart MO, Whittaker PG, Persson B, Hanson U, Lind T. A longitudinal study of circulating progesterone, oestradiol, hCG and hPL during pregnancy in type 1 diabetic mothers. Br J Obstet Gynaecol 1989;96:415.
80. Klebe JG, Marushak A, Bock J. Human placental lactogenic hormone as a parameter for placental function in renal transplanted women. Acta Obstet Gynecol Scand 1990;69:41.
81. Lewis PJ. Drug metabolism. In: Hytten F, Chamberlin G, eds. Clinical physiology in obstetrics. Oxford, London: Blackwell Scientific Publications, 1980:270.
82. Letsky E. The haematological system. In: Hytten F, Chamberlain G, eds. Clinical physiology in obstetrics. Oxford, London: Blackwell Scientific Publications, 1980:43.
83. Hytten FE. Weight gain in pregnancy. In: Hytten F, Chamberlain G, eds. Clinical physiology in obstetrics. Oxford, London: Blackwell Scientific Publications, 1980:193.
84. Adams PW, Oakley NW. Oral contraceptives and carbohydrate metabolism. 1972;3:697.
85. Gaspard UJ. Metabolic effects of oral contraceptives. Am J Obstet Gynecol 1987;157:1029.
86. Ablin RJ, Bruns GR, Guinan P, Bush IM. Oestrogenic suppression of lymphocyte blastogenesis. Transplantation Abstracts, Fifth Internat Cong Transplantation Society 1974; p 136.
87. Jacobi JM, Powell LW, Gaffney TJ. Immunochemical quantitation of human transferrin in pregnancy and during the administration of oral contraceptives. Br J Haematol 1969;17:503.
88. Song CS, Rifkind AB, Gillette PN, Kappas A. Hormones and the liver. Am J Obstet Gynecol 1969;105:813.
89. Davis JC, Hipkin LJ. Depression of lymphocyte transformation in woman taking oral contraceptives. Lancet 1974;ii:217.
90. Reeve J. Calcium metabolism 257. In: Hytten F, Chamberlain G, eds. Clinical physiology in obstetrics. Oxford, London: Blackwell Scientific Publications 1980:257.
91. Gazioglu K, Kaltreider NL, Rosen M, Yu PN. Pulmonary function during pregnancy in normal women and in patients with cardiopulmonary disease. Thorax 1979;25:445.
92. Cain MD, Walters WAS, Catt KJ. Effects of oral contraceptive therapy on renin-angiotensin system. J Clin Endocrinol Metab 1971;33:671.
93. Marshall S, Lyon RP, Minkler D. Ureteral dilatation following use of oral contraceptives. J Amer Med Assn 1966;33:671.
94. Tacchi D. The response of the bulbar conjunctival vascular bed to humoral stimuli. J Obstet Gynaec Brit Commonw 1960; 67:966.
95. Doring GK, Loescheke HH, Ochwadt B. Weitere untersuchungen uber die wirkung der sexualhormone auf die atmung. Pflugers Archiv Physiol Mensch Tiere 1950;252:216.
96. Anderson DC. Sex-hormone-binding globulin. Clin Endocrinol 1974;3:69.
97. Roth MS, Donato DM, Lansman HH, Robertson EG, Hisa SL, Lemaire WJ. Effect of steroids on serum lipids and serum cholesterol binding reserve. Am J Obstet Gynecol 1975;132:1512.
98. Warth MR, Arky RA, Knopp RH. Lipid metabolism in pregnancy. III. Altered lipid composition in intermediate, very low, low and high density lipoprotein fractions. J Clin Endocrinol Metab 1975;41:649.
99. Dowling JT, Freinkel L, Ingbar SH. Thyroxine-binding of sera of pregnancy in women, newborn infants and women with spontaneous abortion. J Clin Invest 1974;35:1263.
100. Carr BR, Gant NF. The endocrinology of pregnancy-induced hypertension. Clin Perinatol 1983;10:737.
101. Hervey GR. Regulation of energy balance. Nature 1969; 222:629.
102. Munroe JS. Progesteroids as immunosuppressive agents. J Reticuloendothelial Soc 1971;9:361.
103. Siiteri PK, Gebres F, Clemens LE. Progesterone and maintenance of pregnancy: Is progesterone nature's immunosuppressant? Ann NY Acad Sci 1977;286:384.
104. Ehrlich N, Lindheimer MD. Effect of administered mineralocorticoids on ACTH in pregnant women: Attenuation of kaliuretic influence of mineralocorticoids during pregnancy. J Clin Invest 1972;51:1301.
105. Hettiaratchi ESC, Pickford M. The effect of oestrogen and progesterone on the pressor action of angiotensin in the rat. J Physiol 1968;196:447.

THE ENDOCRINOLOGY OF PREGNANCY

Karen A. Hutchinson-Williams and Alan H. DeCherney

The endocrinology of pregnancy departs drastically in its complexity from any other endocrinologic event. Superimposed on distinct maternal and fetal systems is the extraordinary placenta, which is both dependent on and independent of the other two compartments and contributes comparatively "pharmacologic" amounts of hormones. The uniqueness of this relationship in human endocrine biology makes its study intriguing and our incomplete knowledge frustrating.

In this chapter, an overview of the role of the integrated endocrine system during pregnancy, fetal endocrine function, and the fetoplacental–maternal steroid unit will be presented. The reader is encouraged to consider other chapters in this text for additional considerations of the subject matter.

ROLE OF THE INTEGRATED ENDOCRINE SYSTEM DURING PREGNANCY

As discussed by Heinrichs and Gibbons,[1] the integrated endocrine system of the mother, placenta, and fetus serves several critical roles during pregnancy that promote gestational health. The following discussion briefly reviews these vital endocrine functions of pregnancy.

PROLONGATION OF CORPUS LUTEUM FUNCTION

In the absence of pregnancy, the functional life span of the corpus luteum is approximately 14 days. Maximal activity is attained by day 7 to 8 after the luteinizing hormone (LH) peak, and leuteolysis occurs 2 to 3 days before the onset of menses.

Maintenance of corpus luteum function is mandatory for early pregnancy continuation. Indeed, removal of the corpus luteum before 7 weeks gestation results in abortion. Human chorionic gonadotropin (hCG), a product of the syncytiotrophoblast, is luteotropic during early pregnancy: it maintains the corpus luteum of the menstrual cycle, permitting it to become the corpus luteum of pregnancy. The endocrine function of the latter is to maintain progesterone (P) production, necessary for decidual development, until the placenta is capable of doing so.

ACHIEVEMENT OF IMMUNOLOGIC COEXISTENCE

Recurrent spontaneous abortion may be secondary to an aberrant maternal response directed at antigens on placental or fetal tissues. Clearly, in normal pregnancy, the fetoplacental unit escapes immunologic rejection. Several hormones, including P, hCG, and cortisol have been suspected of playing a protective role in this process.

Current theory holds that the conceptus is immunogenic and must therefore stimulate a maternal response that allows successful implantation and growth. In a detailed review by Scott and coworkers,[2] several immunologic mechanisms are discussed as critical in the prevention of pregnancy rejection: histocompatibility, maternal antileukocytotoxic antibodies, local suppressor factors, and circulating blocking factors.

ADAPTATION OF THE MATERNAL CARDIOVASCULAR SYSTEM

Alterations in the maternal cardiovascular system are dramatic during pregnancy. Excess sodium accumulation reaches 500 to 900 mEq by parturition.[3] Maternal blood volume rises by an average of 40% above nonpregnant levels, with extremely wide individual variations.[4] Total red blood cell volume increases by 20% to

40%. This significant departure from the non-pregnant state is critical to ensure that adequate transport mechanisms are functioning, which allows for the optimal exchange of metabolic products and to provide nutrients for the growing fetus.

The increase in maternal blood volume begins in the first trimester (approximately week 6) and plateaus after the 30th week.[5] It is usually not accompanied by a significant increase in blood pressure, suggesting a concomitant decrease in peripheral vascular resistance. The latter probably reflects "shunting" of the increased cardiac output through the low resistance uteroplacental circulation and the systemic vasodilitation.[6] Both progesterone and desoxycorticosterone (DOC) play a role in this process. The former is known to cause relaxation of the arteriolar smooth muscle, and the latter has mineralocorticoid activity and therefore may be implicated in the fluid volume expansion and changes in blood pressure associated with pregnancy.

Estrogens, available in pharmacologic levels during pregnancy, are also key to these hemodynamic alterations. Hepatic production of the renin substrate angiotensinogen is increased after exposure to estrogen. This results in increasing aldosterone levels, which in turn lead to increases in blood volume. Estrogen infusions are known to increase blood flow. This effect is secondary to a rise in angiotensin II that increases uterine blood flow and local production of prostaglandin E or prostacyclin within the vessel wall, which leads to vasodilatation.[7] Prostaglandin synthetase inhibitors can block this angiotensin II effect. Speroff and Dorfman[8] have proposed a model involving estrogens, the renin-angiotensin-aldosterone system, and prostaglandins in fetoplacental vascular support (Fig. 8-1).

Vascular reactivity to circulating angiotensin II becomes blunted during pregnancy via a prostaglandin E-mediated mechanism. Indeed, by midpregnancy systolic and diastolic pressures fall by 10 to 20 mm Hg. This is a critically important adaptive response that, if defective, increases the risk for developing pregnancy-induced hypertension (PIH). The altered vascular reactivity cannot be explained on the basis of the high circulating levels of angiotensin II or the relative volume deficit of the pregnant state. One of the metabolites of progesterone, 5α-dihydropregnane-3, 20-dione, has been casually linked.[1] The administration of this compound has been noted to restore angiotensin II refractoriness in a woman with mild PIH. Moreover, infusion of 5α-dihydropregnane-3, 20-dione also counteracted the loss of refractoriness induced by the administration of a prostaglandin synthetase inhibitor in a normal pregnant woman.[1]

MAINTENANCE OF THE NUTRITIONAL SUPPORT OF THE FETUS

Pregnancy is associated with profound alterations in fetal metabolism. Circulating levels of glucose and amino acids are reduced, while levels of free fatty acids, ketones, and triglycerides are increased. Moreover, the secretion of insulin is augmented in response to a glucose load. This metabolic profile has been characterized as one of "accelerated starvation."[9]

The fuel requirements of the developing fetus are met primarily by glucose.[10,11] Glucose both provides the energy necessary for protein synthesis and serves as a precursor for the synthesis of fat and the formation of glycogen. Glucose turnover in the human neonate almost doubles that observed in the normal adult, at 4.2 mg/kg/min versus 2 to 2.5 mg/kg/min, respectively.[12,13]

Fetal blood glucose levels are generally 10 to 20 mg/100 mL below those in the maternal circulation, suggesting that diffusion favors the net movement of glucose from the mother to the fetus. However, considering the rapid rate of glucose delivery, "facilitated diffusion," a carrier-mediated but not energy-dependent process, better describes glucose transfer in this setting. In contrast, maternal insulin and glucagon fail to cross the placenta.

Amino acids are actively transported from the maternal to the fetal circulation by the placenta, and are used for protein synthesis.[14] In addition, amino acids, especially alanine, are critical precursors for glucose formation by the maternal liver in the fasting state. Therefore, the fetus "drains" not only glucose, but also glucose precursors, from the mother.[12,15,16]

Free fatty acid transfer from the maternal to the fetal

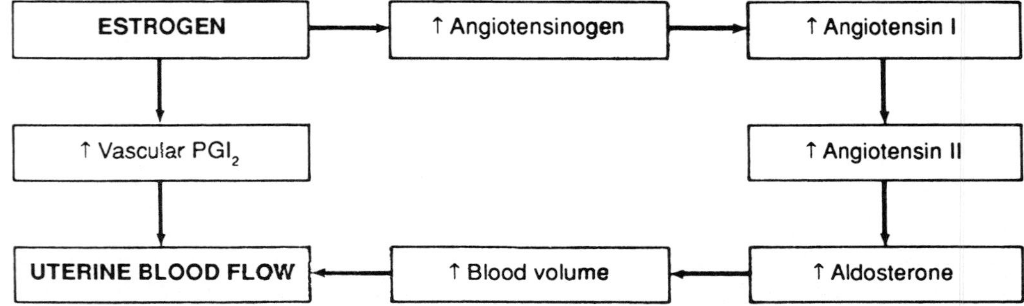

FIGURE 8–1. Schematic illustration of the proposed relationship during pregnancy between estrogens and uterine blood flow. (From Speroff L, Dorfman GS. Prostaglandins and pregnancy hypertension. Clin Obstet Gynecol 1977;4:435.)

circulation is limited, although ketones are readily transferred by diffusion. The enzymes necessary for ketone oxidation are present in fetal brain tissue, as well as in the liver.[17,18]

The fetal–maternal fuel hormone relationship (Fig. 8-2) favors glucose use by the fetus and forces the maternal tissues to increase their usage of alternative energy sources.[19] The endocrine hallmark of this hormonal environment is insulin resistance. Several hormones prevalent during pregnancy are believed to be responsible for this altered milieu: estrogens, progesterone, glucocorticoids, and human chorionic somatomammotropin (hCS).

Early in pregnancy, glucose usage increases, leading to a decrease in maternal glucose levels. Insulin secretion rises and pancreatic β-cell hyperplasia occurs, possibly under the influence of estrogen and progesterone. Glycogen storage is favored and gluconeogenesis is reduced.

hCS secretion is stimulated by the increasing energy demands of the developing fetoplacental unit late in pregnancy. hCS, like growth hormone, alters carbohydrate metabolism by diminishing the effectiveness of maternal insulin. In addition, it shares the lipolytic capabilities of growth hormone, leading to a marked increase in the mobilization of free fatty acids from peripheral fat stores.

The fasting state enhances hCS secretion, which leads to lipolysis to provide the mother with an alternative fuel source. The insulin effects of hCS on maternal glucose metabolism spare glucose and amino acids for use by the fetus. The metabolism of free fatty acids to ketones with further reduction in blood sugar provides an additional fetal energy source.

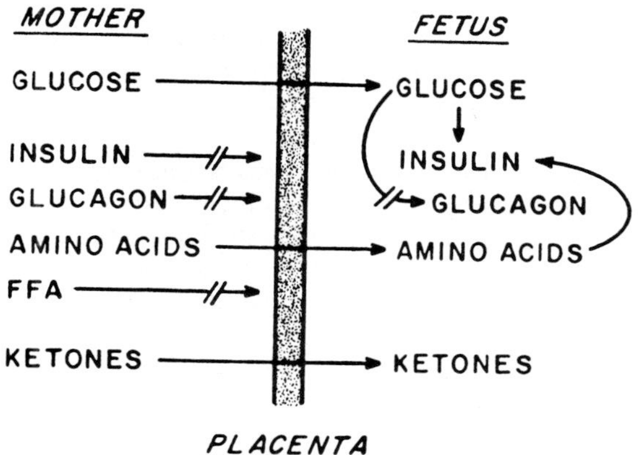

FIGURE 8–2. Maternal–fetal fuel and hormone exchange. Glucose, amino acids, and ketones are transferred from mother to fetus, whereas insulin and glucagon are not. Free fatty acids are transferred only to a very limited extent. An increase in glucose concentration in the maternal circulation results in fetal hyperglycemia, which stimulates the secretion of insulin and inhibits the secretion of glucagon by fetal islet cells. Amino acids are also potent stimuli of fetal insulin secretion. (From Felig P. Med Clin North Am 1977;61:43.)

The maternal metabolic response to feeding in pregnancy is characterized by hyperinsulinemia, hyperglycemia, and hypertriglyceridemia.[20] The plasma insulin response to glucose overcomes the contrainsulin effects of hCS. This allows restoration of hepatic glycogen and lipid stores. Moreover, the increased insulin, now acting in concert with hCS, results in increased protein synthesis.[21]

ALLOWANCE FOR OPTIMAL MECHANICAL SUPPORT

In the non-gravid state, the uterus is almost a solid structure with a cavity volume of no more than 10 mL. The term uterus achieves a capacity that is 500 to 1000 times greater; indeed, the total volume averages 5 L, but can be greater than 10 L. This transformation occurs in order to successfully accommodate the fetus, placenta, and amniotic fluid.

During the first trimester, the uterine wall hypertrophies under the influence of estrogen and probably progesterone. This early hypertrophy is not entirely the result of mechanical distention by the products of conception, because it also occurs when embryo is implanted in the fallopian tube or ovary.[22] Estrogens also influence the polymerization of acid mucopolysaccharides, which make up the ground substance of connective tissue.[23] Such alterations in the microstructure are involved in the changes that increase the distensibility of the uterine ligaments and cervix.

As the fetus develops, it is surrounded by a fluid environment that offers protection from external pressures. Moreover, optimal development of the lungs and face requires adequate amniotic fluid volumes. The endocrine basis of this homeostatic relationship is not clearly defined in humans. A number of studies in a variety of animal models have identified prolactin as a major osmoregulator.[24,25] The significant production by human decidual tissues of prolactin suggests that this hormone may be important in humans as well. Indeed, by 15 to 17 weeks gestation, amniotic fluid prolactin concentrations can reach 1000 ng/mL or more and then decline to 450 ng/mL during the latter part of pregnancy.[26] A decreased concentration of prolactin receptors has been noted in pregnancies complicated by polyhydramnios.[27]

FETAL HORMONES

HYPOTHALAMUS

The embryonic development of the brain is an early event in human gestation. The forebrain can be identified by day 22 after conception, and the primitive diencephalon by day 35. Within the ventral portion of the diencephalon (which later develops into the hypothalamus), primitive fibertracts and neuroblasts can be observed. By gestational day 42, the hypothalamus has coalesced beneath the third ventricle and contains thyroid releasing factor (TRF).

The anlage of the pituitary gland appears at about this time and is composed of ectoderm that migrates caudally from the oral cavity, joining the neurohypophysis. Secretory granules are already evident and portend the future role of this structure in human endocrine regulation.

Scant information is available on the development of the human hypophysial portal system. Capillaries appear within the mesenchymal tissue adjoining Rathke's pouch and the diencephalon by 9 weeks. Rapid vascularization begins with the development of the primary plexus of the portal system at approximately 100 days. Simultaneous development of the hypothalamus is also taking place, and all of the hypothalamic nuclei are differentiated by 14 weeks. As described by Kaplan and associates in their detailed review, the continuity of the primary and secondary plexus of the portal system is finally completed by gestational weeks 19 to 21.[28] Thus, by midgestation this integrated neuroendocrine unit is morphologically and functionally developed. Receptors for steroid hormones have been identified in vitro, and feedback mechanisms are intact.[28–31]

Gonadotropin-Releasing Hormone

Immunoreactive gonadotropin-releasing hormone (GnRH) is present in the fetal hypothalamus by 10 weeks at a concentration of 0.54 pg/mg. It is not clear whether or not this represents the entire pool of biologically active GnRH or includes a larger molecular weight precursor, pro-GnRH. Kaplan and colleagues[28] have demonstrated that there is not a significant correlation between sex or gestational age in the concentration of GnRH between 10 and 22 weeks, although the content of hormone detected varied widely (208 to 4300 pg).

Huhtaniemi and coworkers[32] have studied the response of the pituitary–gonadal axis to GnRH stimulation in fetal male monkeys. They found that when either 10 or 50 μg of GnRH was administered intravenously to catheterized fetuses in utero the LH measured was 857 ± 494% greater and the testosterone measured was 69 ± 20% greater than basal levels. These authors concluded that by the last third of gestation the pituitary–gonadal axis of male monkeys responds to GnRH stimulation, and suggest that a similar relationship probably exists in the human fetus.

Thyrotropin-Releasing Hormone

Immunoreactive thyrotropin-releasing hormone (TRH) has also been detected in significant levels in the fetal hypothalamus by 10 weeks. Working with 44 hypothalami from fetuses at 10 to 22 weeks gestation, Kaplan and colleagues found the concentration varied from 0.2 to 218 pg/mg and the content ranged from 0.64 to 184 ng.[28] As noted with GnRH, there was not an appreciable correlation between gestational age or sex.

Growth Hormone Release-Inhibiting Hormone (Somatostatin)

In contrast to GnRH and TRH, Kaplan and associates found a positive correlation between somatostatin concentration and fetal age.[28] The concentration more than tripled from 7.3 pg/mg to 28.5 pg/mg from 10 to 20 weeks gestation. The content increased from 7.8 ng to 36.6 ng during the same time. It has been theorized that the pattern of growth hormone secretion in the fetus reflects maturational changes in the secretion of growth hormone-releasing hormone and somatostatin.[29]

Corticotropin-Releasing Hormone

It has only been within the last 10 years that adult human corticotropin-releasing hormone (CRH) has been isolated and its amino acid sequence elucidated.[33] Injection of CRH in humans causes a rapid increase in ACTH release from corticotrope cells into the blood.[34] To date, although corticotropin peptides have been found in human fetal pituitary glands, CRH has yet to be identified in fetal hypothalami.

Growth Hormone-Releasing Hormone

The presence of a growth hormone-releasing hormone (GHRH)-like factor late in gestation is suggested by the elevated levels of plasma growth hormone in prematurely born neonates.[29] This peptide has yet to be identified in fetal tissues.

PITUITARY

In embryonic life, the pituitary is formed from fusion of two hollow ectodermal processes. Rathke's pouch is derived from the floor of the diencephalon and gives rise to the adenohypophysis. This process is met by a second pouching of the ventral diencephalon, which gives rise to the neurohypophysis.

Toward the end of the third gestational month, secretory granules appear in the fetal pituitary and several pituitary hormones can be detected by radioimmunoassay. The following discussion will focus on the tropic hormones of the adenohypophysis.

Growth Hormone

By 7 to 9 weeks gestation, growth hormone (GH) is present in the fetal pituitary.[29] Peak concentrations of immunoreactive GH occur between 25 and 30 weeks, and then do not change significantly for the remainder of pregnancy. Bioactive GH is present in fetal pituitaries by 18 weeks and increases progressively thereafter. "Little" or monomeric GH predominates in the fetal pituitary, with only a small amount of "big" GH present. This pattern is similar to that observed in adults.[28]

From 68 days onward, GH is detectable in fetal

plasma. Because GH does not cross the placenta, circulating GH is entirely of pituitary origin. Peak levels (119 ± 20 ng/mL) occur before 24 weeks and subsequently fall. This essential feature of fetal growth hormone secretion, high midgestational levels followed by a fall in the third trimester, coincides with maturation of hypothalamic neuroregulation (Fig. 8-3). The reader is referred to an excellent review by Gluckman and coworkers.[29]

There is little evidence that fetal GH has any significant influence on fetal growth.[29,35–37] This observation may reflect a reduced number or immaturity of GH receptors in the fetus.[29] The limited data that are available were reviewed by Gluckman and coworkers, who concluded that GH may play a role in the following physiologic settings: fetal glycogen metabolism, fetal enzyme induction, fetal brain development, and fetal adrenal function.[29]

Somatomedin

As discussed by Gluckman and colleagues, the concentration of somatomedin (SM) activity in umbilical cord blood increases during gestation from 24 weeks to term, although SM activity can be detected in fetal sera by 14 weeks.[29] A growth-promoting function for SM in fetal life is supported indirectly by the observations that cord SM concentrations correlate directly with body weight,[38,39] and infants with intrauterine growth retardation have lower SM levels than normal newborns of similar gestational age.[38,40–42] Moreover, fetal chondrocytes are responsive to the growth-promoting effects of this peptide.[44]

In the human fetus, SM secretion is not GH-dependent. Because a transient rise in neonatal SM has been observed during the first month of life when estrogen levels are declining, it has been theorized that estrogen may serve some suppressive regulatory function in utero.

Prolactin

Immunoreactive prolactin (PRL) is present in the pituitary gland in small but measurable amounts early in gestation. However, both the content and concentration rise rapidly between 20 and 30 weeks gestation. There does not appear to be any relationship between fetal sex and pituitary content of this hormone.[28]

Plasma PRL concentrations are somewhat low (19.5 ± 2.5 ng/mL) before 25 weeks, but rise to high concentrations at term (168 ± 14 ng/mL). Several authors have proposed that the major modulating force behind the late trimester climb in fetal PRL is placentally derived estrogen. It is also possible that, developmentally, the pituitary is functionally able to respond to tropic agents including TRF after 20 weeks gestation.

Cord blood from preterm infants who develop respiratory distress syndrome has been shown to have lower mean PRL levels.[44,45] Respiratory distress syndrome is a disease characterized by deficient production of pulmonary surface active phospholipids (surfactant) from Type II alveolar cells. It is not yet clear whether the lung maturation is dependent on end organ effects of estrogen only or an interaction of estrogen and PRL on surfactant synthesis. Fetal PRL may also play a role in the regulation of normal fetal osmolality.[29]

Adrenocorticotropic Hormone

Bioassayable adrenocorticotropic hormone (ACTH) is demonstrable in the fetal pituitary by 8 to 10 weeks, and its concentration rises steadily with gestational age. Kaplan and colleagues have demonstrated that at 26 weeks, the concentration of pituitary ACTH is comparable to that in the pituitary gland of the newborn.[28]

Fetal plasma ACTH concentration is elevated between 12 to 19 weeks (249 ± 65.7 pg/mL), and declines slowly throughout the third trimester. There appears to be little maternal contribution to the fetal pool of

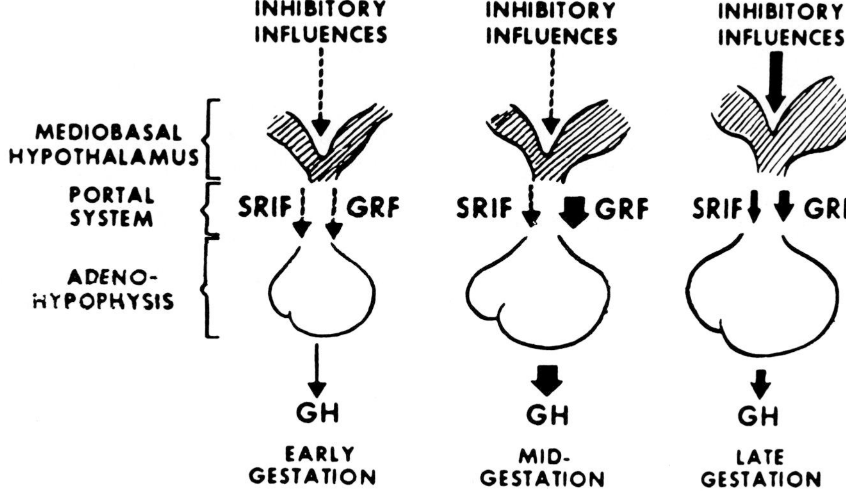

FIGURE 8–3. Schematic illustration of the proposed ontogenesis of hypothalamic neurohormonal control of fetal growth hormone (GH) secretion. (Reproduced with permission from Gluckman PD, Grumbach MM, Kaplan SL. The neuroendocrine regulation and function of growth hormone and prolactin in the mammalian fetus. Endocr Rev 1981; 2:363.)

ACTH. As discussed by Kaplan, this concept of limited transplacental passage of ACTH to the fetus is supported by the higher levels of ACTH in cord blood than maternal blood during normal pregnancy, and the marked discrepancy in the levels of ACTH in fetal and maternal circulation in cases of anencephaly and in a patient with Nelson's syndrome.[28,46]

ACTH appears to play a critical tropic role at midgestation on the developing fetal zone of the adrenal gland. However, pituitary ACTH may not provide the only stimulus for adrenal growth: placentally derived pro-opiomelanocortin (the parent compound of ACTH and β-lipotropin) may also share this activity.

Thyrotropin

The fetal thyroid gland does not require thyrotropin (TSH) secretion for its initial phase of differentiation and acquisition of secretory activity. Indeed, although the thyroid gland first appears at 16 to 17 days of gestation, thyrotropes are not demonstrable in the human fetal pituitary gland until 13 weeks. As noted in the extensive review by Kaplan and colleagues, immunoreactive TSH is present by 12 to 14 weeks in the pituitary and serum of the human fetus, during which time iodine uptake and the synthesis of iodothyronines commences.[28] Bioassayable TSH has been found in the fetal pituitary by 14 weeks.

Secretion of TSH in utero is regulated by both hypothalamic TRF as well as an intact pituitary–thyroid feedback system. The latter is probably not operational until mid- or late gestation and can be appreciated from clinical evidence of goiter formation in the fetuses of mothers treated with antithyroid drugs and other goitrogens. In addition, elevated TSH levels are found at term in infants with congenital hypothyroidism.[47] Fetal thyroid function is not affected to any significant degree by the limited transplacental passage of TSH and iodothyronines.

Gonadotropins

FSH and LH have been detected in fetal pituitary glands by 9 to 10 weeks gestation. Concentrations continue to rise to a peak at about 20 to 22 weeks, thereafter falling until term. Kaplan and associates have noted that LH concentrations are always higher than those of FSH, and female glands appear to contain more hormone than male glands.[28]

Early in gestation, the pituitary acquires the capacity to secrete these glycoproteins. In the case of both FSH and LH, there is a trend toward achieving maximum serum concentrations at midgestation; thereafter a progressive fall is observed toward term (Fig. 8-4). The same sex difference noted in terms of pituitary concentration of LH and FSH also holds for fetal plasma gonadotropin levels.

The alpha and beta subunits of FSH and LH have been found in the pituitary gland and the fetal circulation. Alpha subunits appear to dominate in both the pituitary gland and serum throughout much of pregnancy. However, the significance of this observation remains uncertain. The in vitro studies of Franchimont and Pasteels[48] show that the fetal pituitary secretes large amounts of the alpha glycoprotein hormone subunit with little of the beta subunit or intact hormone in the absence of hypothalamic stimulation.

Kaplan and coworkers have theorized that the changes in pituitary and serum FSH and LH in the human fetus throughout pregnancy can be correlated with the functional development of the central nervous system, particularly the hypothalamus and the hypophysial portal system.[28] The pattern of change in FSH and LH concentration demonstrated in both fetal sera and pituitary glands is evidence of a developing system, wherein increasing sensitivity of the hypothalamus and pituitary to the negative feedback of sex steroids becomes fully operational. As discussed by Kaplan and colleagues, the relatively high levels of gonadotropins found at midgestation reflect either autonomous LH and FSH secretion or "relatively unrestrained" secretion of GnRH into the hypothalamic–hypophysial portal system.[28] With advancing fetal development, the inhibitory feedback mechanism matures and the hypothalamus secretes less GnRH, resulting in decreased secretion of fetal gonadotropins.

THYROID

The ontogeny of fetal thyroid function and its regulation have been studied extensively. Although the capacity of the developing follicular cells to form thyroglobulin is established by the 29th day of gestation, the development necessary to concentrate iodide into synthesized thyroxine (T4) is not operational until the 11th week.[49] The major thyroid hormone-binding protein in plasma, thyroid-binding globulin (TBG), can be detected in serum by the 10th gestational week, increasing in concentrations progressively to term. The second and third trimester rise in serum thyroxine (T4) concentration reflects not only this increase in TBG, but the greater secretory capacity of the fetal thyroid gland under the influence of the maturing hypothalamic-hypophysial portal system (Fig. 8-5).[50]

The metabolism of T4 in utero differs dramatically from the situation found in adults. Not only are production and degradation rates greater in the fetus (on the basis of unit body mass), but the specific enzymatic pathway by which T4 is metabolized favors the formation of the inert iodothyronine, reverse triiodothyronine (T3) at the expense of the metabolically active product generally found in adults, T3.

Transplacental passage of TSH, T4, and T3 from mother to fetus is essentially negligible. Indeed, the human placenta appears to contain a highly active 5-monodeiodinase that converts T4 to reverse T3.[51] Somatic development in utero is not a phenomenon

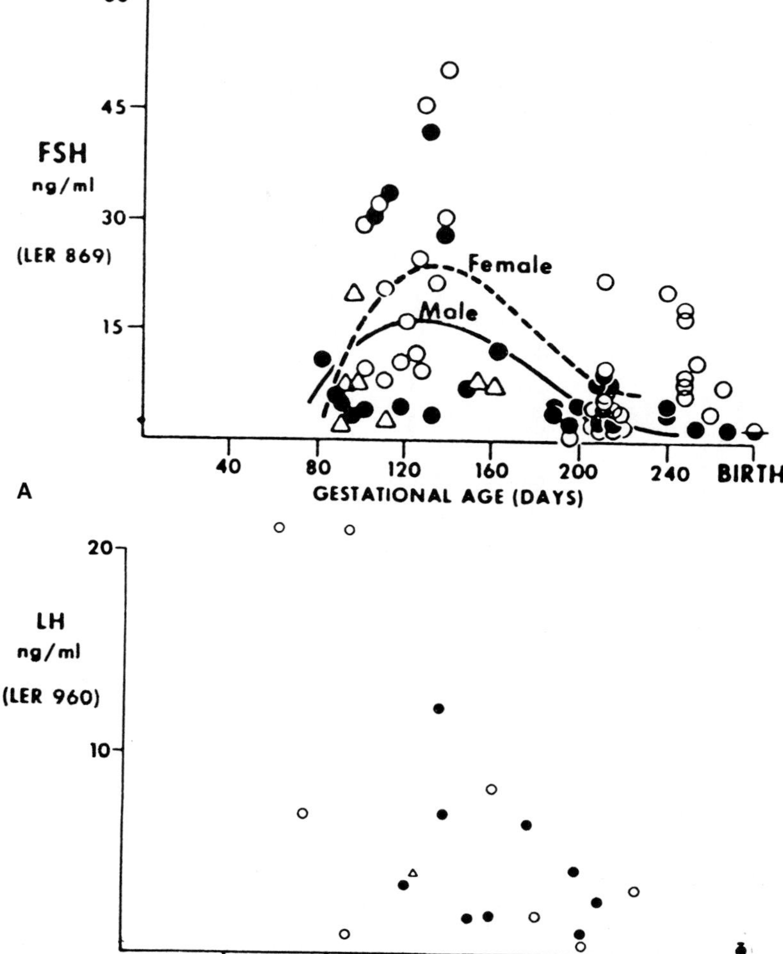

FIGURE 8–4. (**A**) The concentration of follicle-stimulating hormone (FSH) plotted as polynomial regression curves against gestational age for female (●) and male (○) fetuses. The mean (±SE) concentration of serum FSH in umbilical venous serum for 29 males and females is shown on the right. △ = sex unknown. (**B**) The concentration of luteinizing hormone (LH) measured in a specific β-LH radioimmunoassay is plotted against gestational age. The symbols are the same as in **A.** (From Kaplan FL, Grumbach MM, Aubert ML. The ontogenesis of pituitary hormones and hypothalamic factors in the human fetus: maturation of the central nervous system regulation of anterior pituitary function. Recent Prog Horm Res 1976;32:161.)

dependent on thyroid hormones. However, as discussed by Ingbar, thyroid hormones do appear to be necessary for late phase skeletal maturation and late prenatal pulmonary development, as well as the normal development of the brain and intellectual function.[49]

GONADS

At approximately gestational week 6, the structure of the fetal testis can be recognized, and within it prominent interstitial (Leydig) cells. These cells have the biosynthetic capacity to produce testosterone (T), a hormone critical for male secondary sexual development; specifically, the development of the internal genital structures. In contrast, dihydroxytestosterone (DHT), a reduced metabolite of testosterone formed in certain androgen target tissues, is the trophic hormone for the external genitalia. Testosterone also stimulates the production of two proteins within the adjacent Sertoli cells of the testes, müllerian inhibiting substance (MIS) and androgen binding protein (ABP). The former causes inhibition of müllerian duct development, and the latter binds testosterone and possibly DHT within the Wolffian duct system and may be involved in the transduction of androgens into their target tissues. Maximal human chorionic gonadotropin (hCG) production by the placenta coincides with the time of the greatest biosynthetic activity by the interstitial cells, suggesting that these events are interrelated.[31,52,53]

The fetal ovary and its function are much more enigmatic. Although it can be histologically recognized by 10 weeks gestation, the female gonad lacks the impressive biosynthetic capacity of the testis at this point in utero. In vitro studies have demonstrated that fetal ovarian tissue has the capacity to cleave pregnenolone sulfate and further metabolize pregnenolone to the C-19 steroid dehydroepiandrosterone and androstenedione. However, production of free progesterone,

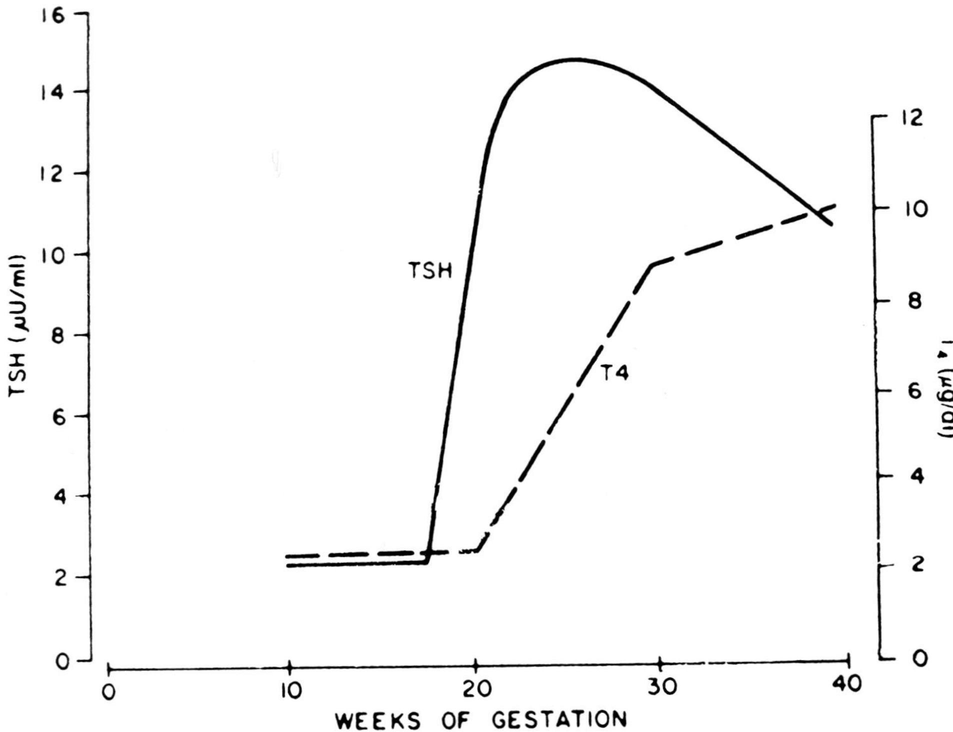

FIGURE 8–5. Patterns of maturation of serum thyroid-stimulating hormone (TSH) and thyroxin (T_4) concentrations in the human fetus. (From Fisher DA, Klein AH. Thyroid development and disorders of thyroid function in the newborn. N Engl J Med 1981;304:704.)

testosterone, estradiol, or estrone has not been documented.[54]

The role of the ovary, therefore, in directing female sexual differentiation may be minimal. This is in sharp contrast to the situation found in the male. However, there is morphologic work supporting the presence of cells within the ovary with steroid-secreting characteristics.[55] As suggested by Jaffe, the failure of earlier studies to demonstrate significant steroidogenic capabilities in the fetal ovary may have been a function of the precursor used for the study or the stage of gestation in which the studies were performed.[31] Further work is necessary to address these critical questions.

ADRENAL GLAND

The human fetal adrenal gland is a remarkable endocrine organ, due to its tremendous capacity for steroid biosynthesis in utero and because of its unique morphologic characteristics. At term, the adrenals are as large as those of adults, weighing 10 g or more. What ultimately develops into the adult adrenal cortex, the outer or definitive zone, accounts for only 15% of the fetal gland (Fig. 8-6). The unique inner or fetal zone comprises 85% of the volume of the adrenal in utero and is largely responsible for the robust secretory capacity of this organ.

Dehyroepiandrosterone sulfate (DHEAS) and cortisol are the two major steroids produced by the fetal adrenal gland (Fig. 8-7). The former is produced principally by the fetal zone and serves as a precursor for placental estrogen production, and the latter is produced by the definitive zone.

At term, the mean concentration of DHEAS in the fetal circulation is 130 mg/100 mL.[56] Cortisol concentrations range between 36 µg/100 mL in induced labor and 44 µg/100 mL in spontaneous labor.[57]

Androgens

The role of tropic hormones in fetal zone androgen production has provoked considerable investigative effort. In late gestation the fetal zone appears to be dependent on the fetal pituitary. This is indirectly supported by observations of fetal zone atrophy in anencephalic and apituitary fetuses and gland atrophy and reduced DHEAS secretion subsequent to glucocorticoid treatment.[58–60] However, prior to midgestation, the endocrine support of the pituitary appears unnecessary, because anencephalic fetuses demonstrate normal adrenal growth and development up to week 20.[1] Early tropic support was thought to be due to the action of hCG, although some investigators have been unable to confirm a regulatory role for this hormone in steroidogenesis. It has even been suggested that the "stimulatory" activity of hCG might reflect contamination of hCG preparations used in test settings with growth factors.[61] Other peptides, including prolactin, human placental lactogen, growth hormone, and α-MSH, have also been proposed to play a tropic role in adrenal development.[31] Prolactin's effect on the adrenal gland may be secondary to its promotion of cholesterol storage in endocrine tissues.[62] Growth factors such as epidermal

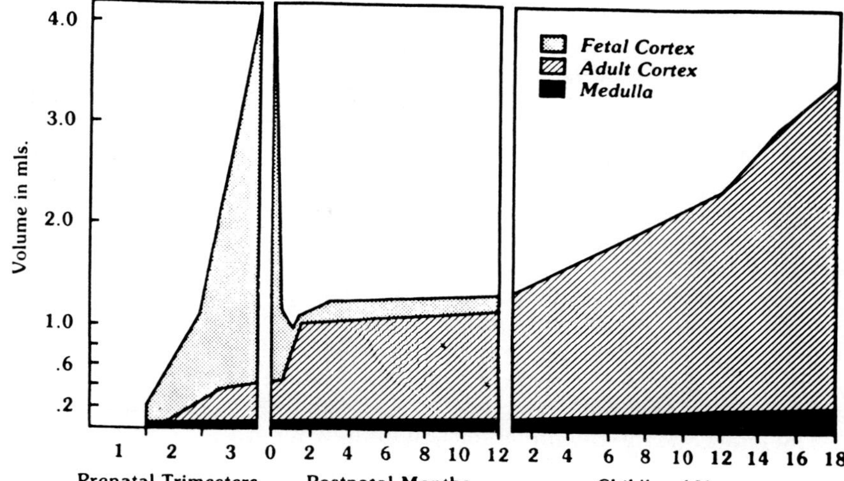

FIGURE 8–6. Size of adrenal gland and its component parts in utero, during infancy, and during childhood. (Reproduced with permission from Bethune JE. The adrenal cortex. A Scope Monograph. Kalamazoo: Upjohn, 1974:11.)

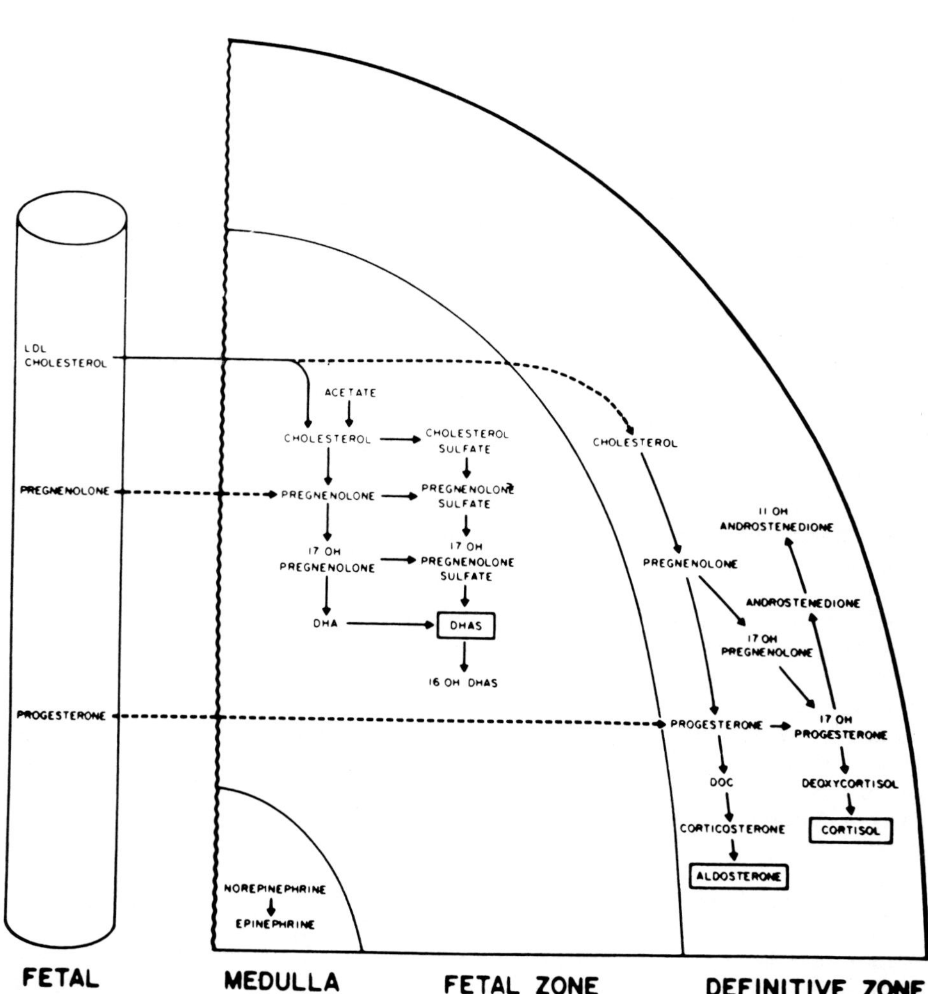

FIGURE 8–7. Schematic illustration of generalized pathways of hormone formation in the human fetal adrenal gland. (From Seron-Ferre M, Jaffe RB. The fetal adrenal gland. Ann Rev Physiol 1981;43:141.)

growth factor and fibroblast growth factor are also under investigation as potential promoters of fetal adrenal gland growth and secretory activity.[63,64]

As noted, the fetal zone produces in great quantity the biologically weak androgen DHEAS. This reflects the restricted availability of Δ, 3β-hydroxysteroid dehydrogenase and Δ 4,5 isomerase activity necessary for the biosynthesis of progesterone, cortisol, and testosterone. The high circulating levels of progesterone and estradiol found during pregnancy inhibit this enzyme complex and thereby indirectly promote DHEAS production. Maternal LDL cholesterol appears to be the major precursor of fetal adrenal DHEAS. Other steroid sulfates can also be converted to DHEAS without loss of the sulfate side chain.

The fetal zone rapidly undergoes involution at parturition, and by 1 year it has completely disappeared. Recent work in nonhuman primates suggests that the fasciculata zone of the adult adrenal gland may stem from the fetal zone.[65]

The key role that DHEAS plays as a precursor in placental estrogen production will be discussed later. Jaffe and Payne[66] have demonstrated that the human fetal testis has the capacity to use DHEAS in vitro to form active steroids.

Other Adrenal Steroids

Corticosteroids are derived primarily from the definitive zone. ACTH appears to be the only tropic hormone of significance. LDL cholesterol is used as a substrate for the synthesis of cortisol via the pathways of 17α, 21- and 11β-hydroxylation. Progesterone derived from the placental circulation can also be used within the definitive zone for the production of cortisol, deoxycorticosterone, corticosterone, and aldosterone.[1]

The functional role of cortisol during gestation is far reaching. Although fetal production of cortisol is important in initiating parturition in some species, an obligatory role for this steroid has not been established in humans.[31] However, the impact of cortisol on a number of key systems in utero is critical. In the lung, glucocorticoids induce cytodifferentiation of type II alveolar cells and stimulate synthesis of surfactant and its release into the alveolus. In addition, corticosteroids induce the development and maturation of a number of hepatic enzyme systems, including those concerned with liver glycogen synthesis, tyrosine aminotransferase, aspartate aminotransferase, arginine synthetase, and phospholenopyruvate carboxykinase. Cortisol may also play a role in the transfer from fetal to adult type hemoglobin.

Much of the work that has focused on the protean aspects of cortisol in utero has been done employing animal models. It is appropriate to be cautious regarding the extrapolation of experimental animal data to the human subject. However, there can be no doubt regarding the critical, multisystem impact of cortisol on the fetus as well as the adult. The reader is referred to an excellent review of this topic by Liggins.[67]

Medulla

Early in embryonic development, primitive sympathetic cell precursors appear in the region of the neurocrest and neurotube. These stem cells subsequently differentiate into neuroblasts, which become sympathetic ganglion cells, and pheochromoblasts, which become pheochromocytes or mature chromaffin cells. Pheochromoblasts invade the developing adrenal cortex to form the primordial adrenal medulla by 7 weeks gestation. The close proximity of the adrenal medulla to the adrenal cortex suggests an intimate functional relationship. Corticosteroids are capable of activating the biosynthetic enzymes necessary for catecholamine synthesis.[68] Catecholamine release is predominantly regulated by sympathetic nerves that secrete acetycholine.[31]

Catecholamine production by the adrenal medulla is critical for optimal regulation of the central nervous, cardiovascular, and metabolic systems. Morphologic studies in humans indicate that the adrenal medulla reaches full development only after 3 years of age.[69,70]

PARATHYROID: CALCIUM HOMEOSTASIS

Fetal parathyroid hormone appears between the 12th and 13th gestational week (Fig. 8-8). Parathyroid function, however, remains suppressed throughout most of pregnancy due to the relatively hypercalcemic state of the fetus. The latter is secondary to the considerable placental transport of calcium, which is critical for bone formation. Calcitonin levels are elevated, which enhances bone development.

At term, fetal 1,25-dihydroxyvitamin D levels are

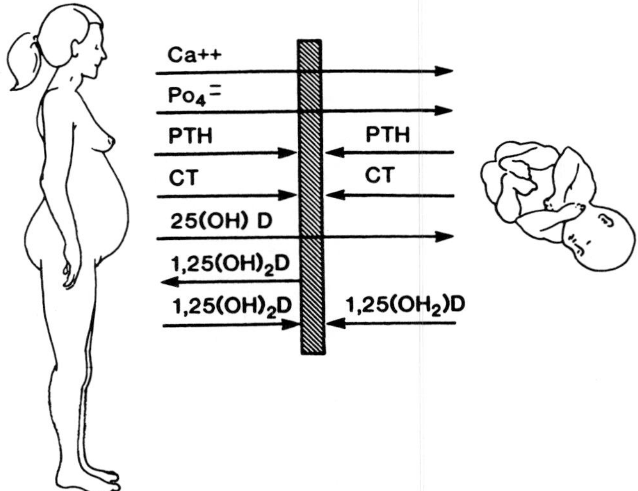

FIGURE 8-8. Schematic representation of transplacental transport of calcium (Ca^{++}), phosphorus (PO_4^-), parathyroid hormone (PTH), calcitonin (CT), and mono- and dihydroxy vitamin D (25(OH)D and 1,25$(OH)_2$D, respectively). (From Fuchs F, Klopper A, eds. Endocrinology of pregnancy. Philadelphia: Harper and Row, 1983:186.)

considerably below maternal levels, supporting the concept that 1,25-dihydroxyvitamin D does not cross the placenta, although 25-hydroxyvitamin D probably does cross it. Direct comparisons of serum concentrations of vitamin D in mother and fetus are complicated by the fact that there are estrogen-induced changes in vitamin D-binding protein. The fetal kidney can hydroxylate 25-hydroxyvitamin D, although the placenta can synthesize 1,25-dihydroxyvitamin D directly. Excellent reviews of vitamin D and vitamin D metabolism have been recently published.[71–73]

RENIN-ANGIOTENSIN SYSTEM

Renin secretion clearly doubles as early as the 8th week of gestation and increases to 32 weeks, after which time no further significant changes occur. Equally dramatic and not surprising, based on the known stimulatory effects of estrogens on liver production of plasma renin substrate, is that plasma renin substrate doubles by the 8th week of pregnancy, plateaus by the 20th week, and remains steady thereafter.[74] This concurrent stimulation of enzyme and substrate levels results in a dramatic rise in plasma renin activity. The large size (molecular weight 43,000) of renin makes it unlikely that this molecule crosses the placenta. Not surprisingly, anephric infants have been found to have undetectable renin levels.

The circulating concentrations of the octapeptide angiotensin II in the fetus are similar or greater than maternal values, both exceeding those observed in the nongravid state. Placental metabolism of angiotensin I into angiotensin II or production by the placenta of angiotensin II is suggested by the observation that venous blood from the umbilical cord has higher levels than arterial cord blood. It has been theorized that these findings support a significant role for the renin-angiotensin system in the regulation of fetoplacental blood pressure.

The pattern of aldosterone secretion as well as of plasma aldosterone levels may diverge from that of plasma renin activity in pregnancy. Although changes in plasma renin activity begin to plateau as early as 20 to 32 weeks, plasma and urine aldosterone continue to exhibit progressively greater rises throughout pregnancy. This pattern appears to closely parallel the profile of other steroid hormones, such as progesterone, estriol (E_3), and estradiol (E_2).[75]

THE FETOPLACENTAL–MATERNAL STEROIDAL UNIT

The fetoplacental–maternal unit is a uniquely interdependent endocrine system. Although individual adult steroid producing glands are capable of the formation of progestins, androgens, and estrogens, the placenta is unable to do so. Placental estrogen production mandates "contributions" by both the fetal and maternal compartments in the form of DHEAS (primarily from the fetal adrenal gland), and progesterone production cannot proceed without maternally derived cholesterol (Fig. 8-9). This mutually beneficial compartmentalization stems from certain critical enzymatic limitations. The placenta lacks 16- and 17-hydroxylase activity. Therefore, placental estrogen production is dependent on an external source of DHEAS. As previously noted, the fetal zone of the adrenal gland supplies 90% of the DHEAS needed by the placenta.

Because "fetal zone" capacity to convert Δ-5 compounds to Δ-4 compounds is reduced, progesterone cannot be converted from pregnenolone to any significant degree. As a consequence, fetal adrenal gland production of corticosteroids mandates the importation from the placenta of progesterone.

Most of the progesterone produced by the placenta is derived from maternal LDL cholesterol. This maternal contribution is required because the placenta synthesizes cholesterol from acetate in a limited fashion. As described by Henricks and Gibbons, this reflects the progesterone inhibition of cholesterol esterification secondary to blockage of acetyl CoA cholesterol acetyltransferase (ACAT).[1] The resulting increase in intercellular cholesterol inhibits the rate-limiting enzyme in cholesterol synthesis, 3-hydroxymethylgluteryl-CoA reductase (HMG-CoA), thereby inhibiting cholesterol synthesis.

A composite picture evolves wherein shared enzymatic activities allow the fetoplacental–maternal unit to produce massive amounts of estrogen and progesterone (Fig. 8-10), which are critical for gestational health. By the end of pregnancy, production of progesterone approximates 250 mg/day; plasma concentrations reach 130 ng/mL. Placental production of this hormone, however, has not always been critical to survival of the pregnancy. Under the stimulatory influence of trophoblastic hCG, the corpus luteum of pregnancy maintains progesterone production for up to 10 weeks. Indeed, removal of the corpus luteum prior to 7 weeks gestation results in pregnancy termination. Progesterone performs a number of critical functions throughout gestation: reduction in myometrial irritability, smooth muscle relaxation, and stimulation of the maternal respiratory center. In addition, interesting works have emerged proposing that progesterone is critical for pregnancy maintenance, secondary to its ability to inhibit T lymphocyte cell-mediated responses involved in tissue rejection. Work by Siiteri and colleagues has demonstrated the role of progesterone in prolonging xenogeneic graphs, preventing inflammation, and promoting the survival of human trophoblastic tissue in rodents. These authors have theorized that high intrauterine concentrations of this hormone serve to block cellular immune responses to foreign antigens, and thereby prevent early pregnancy wastage.[76]

After the first 3 to 4 weeks of human pregnancy, nearly all the estrogens produced are products of the trophoblast. Maternal concentrations of estradiol (E_2), estrone (E_1), and estriol (E_3) rise steadily throughout

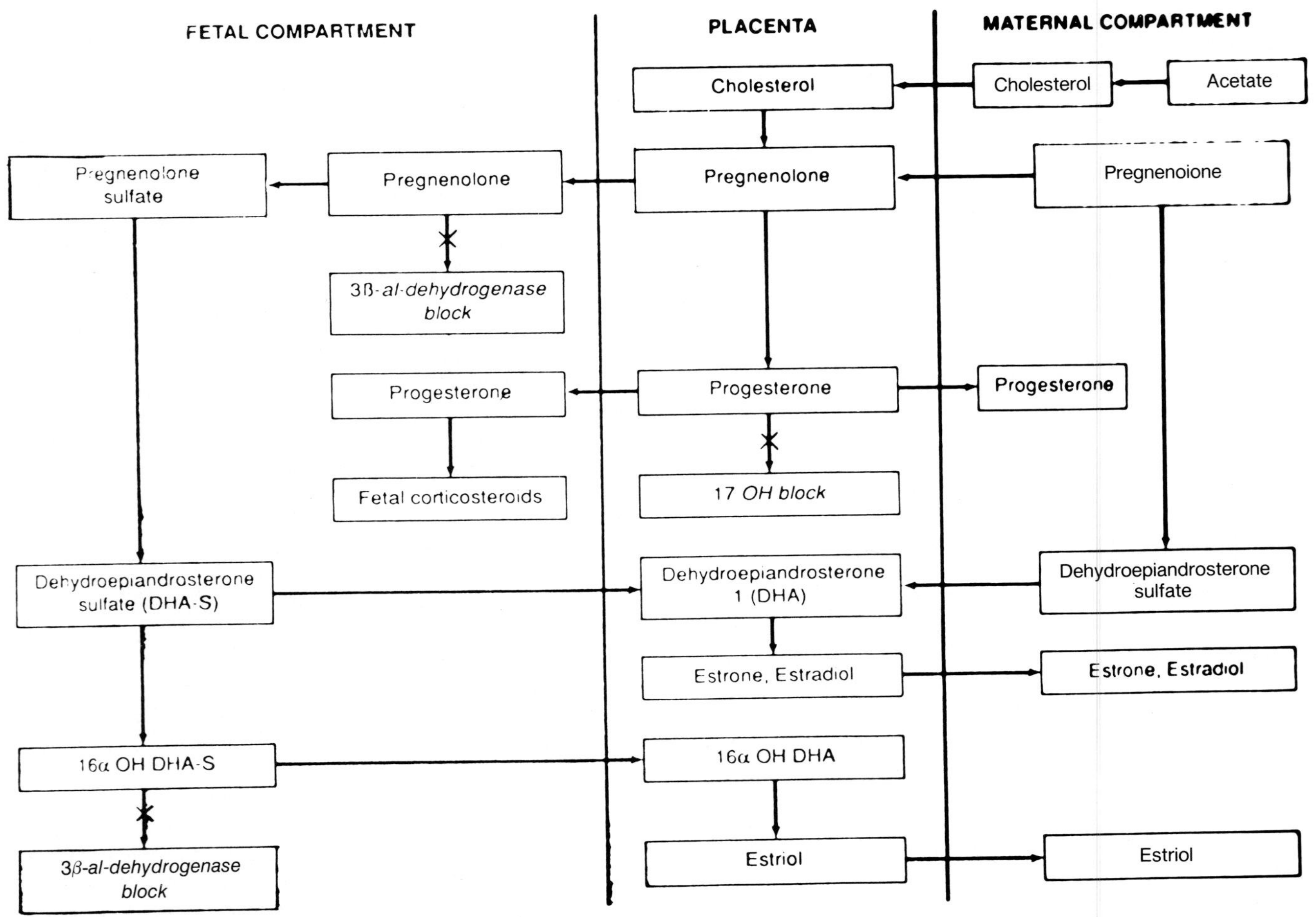

FIGURE 8–9. Maternal–fetal–placental steroid compartments. (From Brody SA, Ueland K, eds. Endocrine disorders in pregnancy. Norwalk: Appleton and Lange, 1989:68.)

pregnancy. Indeed, E_1 and E_2 production are increased 100-fold over non-pregnant levels, and estriol production increases by 1000-fold.[77–79] The mechanism by which estrogen is produced in the placenta is unique, due to the negligible steroid 17α-hydroxylase activity in this tissue. Consequently, unlike in adult steroid-producing glands, there is little if any conversion of C-21 steroids to C-19 steroids. As has been mentioned earlier, it is now clear that E_2 and E_1 are formed in the placenta from DHEAS, a C-19 steroid present in both fetal and maternal plasma (see Fig. 8-10). The product of aromatization of DHEAS that enters the maternal compartment is primarily E_2. Probably both E_2 and E_1 are secreted into fetal plasma, although, as discussed by Casey and coworkers, E_2 could also be converted to E_1 by fetal erythrocytes or other intervillous tissues before reaching the fetus.[80,81] Work by Siiteri and McDonald has demonstrated that near term, approximately 50% of the E_2 synthesized in the placenta is derived from precursors in the fetal circulation and 50% from precursors in the maternal circulation.[82] The biosynthesis of E_3 during pregnancy demonstrates clearly the interdependence of the fetus, placenta, and mother. DHEAS, of either fetal or maternal origin, is converted to E_1 and E_2 in the placenta. However, there is little placental conversion of either to E_3. Rather, some DHEAS undergoes 16α-hydroxylation in the fetal liver and adrenal. In the placenta, a sulfatase enzyme cleaves the sulfate side chain and the unconjugated 16α-hydroxy DHEAS is aromatized to form E_3. This E_3 is then secreted into the maternal circulation and ultimately reaches the liver, where it is conjugated to form E_3 sulfate, E_3 glucosiduronate, and a mixed conjugate. The bulk of these metabolites are excreted in the maternal urine.[80] Critical to this process is the tremendous steroid sulfatase activity in the placenta. As a consequence, the entry of DHEAS into the placental circulation does not present an obstacle to the use of the sulfoconjugate for the biosynthesis of estrogen.

E_3 is certainly a considerably weaker estrogen than E_1 and E_2. On a weight basis, it is approximately 0.1 times the potency of the former and 0.01 times the potency of the latter. Regardless, E_3 appears to be as effective as other estrogens in terms of stimulating uteroplacental blood flow. It has been proposed, therefore, that this may be the primary function of the massive levels of E_3

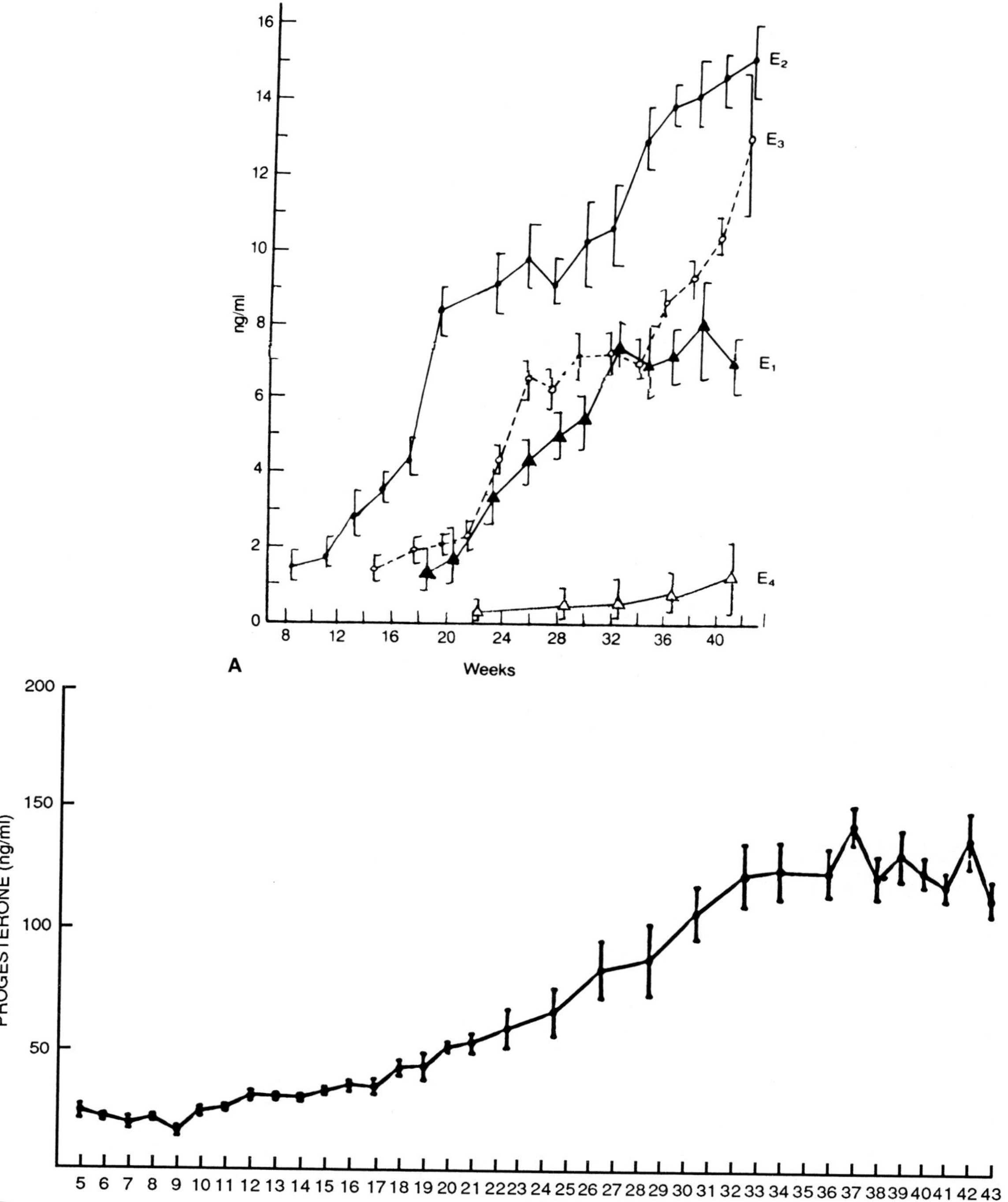

FIGURE 8–10. (**A**) Mean plasma concentrations (±SE) of unconjugated estrone (E_1), estradiol (E_2), estriol (E_3), and estetrol (E_4) during pregnancy. (From Levitz M, Young BK. Estrogens in pregnancy. Vitamins Horm 1977;35:109.) (**B**) Mean plasma concentration of progesterone (±SE) during pregnancy. (From Johansson ENB. Plasma levels of progesterone in pregnancy measured by a rapid competitive protein binding technique. Acta Endocrinol 1979;61:607.)

synthesized on a daily basis during pregnancy.[83] This effect of estrogens on blood flow appears to be mediated through prostaglandin stimulation.[84]

A placental sulfatase deficiency has been reported.[85] Failure of hydrolysis of DHEAS for 16α-hydroxy DHEAS is the hallmark of this disorder. Consequently, there is a deficiency in estrogen formation by the placenta. The clinical characteristics of this entity include low plasma and urinary estriol levels in pregnant women. Despite the fact that these low estriol levels can be associated with fetal demise, the infants born of such pregnancies usually are normal at birth. This disorder appears to occur only in male offspring and appears to represent a sex linked recessive characteristic. Many pregnancies associated with placental sulfatase deficiency have been complicated by a delay in the onset of parturition. This point remains controversial, and to date no causal relationship has been established. The characteristic clinical findings are extremely low levels of E_3 and esterol, accompanied by elevated levels of DHEAS in the amniotic fluid.

PLACENTAL PROTEIN HORMONES

Considering the totipotential nature of the trophoblast, it is not surprising that this tissue secretes a variety of substances, including several proteins that are produced very early in human pregnancy. The following discussion considers the most prominent of these and their role in gestation.

Human Chorionic Gonadotropin (hCG)

Human chorionic gonadotropin, which has a molecular weight of 36,000 to 40,000, is a glycoprotein that is biologically and immumologically similar to luteinizing hormone (LH).[86,87] However, the half-life of hCG is considerably greater than that of LH (5 to 40 hours versus 1 to 2 hours). This illustrates the fact that important differences in molecular structure exists between these two substances with similar biologic actions. All of the glycoprotein hormones—hCG, LH, follicle stimulating hormone (FSH), and TSH—share nearly identical α-subunits, which are essentially interchangeable. Indeed, these α-subunits can recombine with any of the four distinct β-subunits to form a product with the biologic activity characteristic of the β-subunit component. The α-subunits and the carbohydrate components are required for expression of the biologic activity unique to the β-subunits. When hCG and LH are compared, it is the 28 to 30 terminal amino acids on the carboxy end of the β-subunit of the former that represent its unique sequence. It is the unique immunoreactive properties of these β-subunits that permit the diagnosis of pregnancy or extrapregnancy sources of hCG (ie, gonadal tumors) with great accuracy. Even in the presence of LH, hCG is produced by the syncytiotrophoblast during pregnancy. It is also elaborated by all other types of trophoblastic tissue, including that derived from chorioadenodestuins, choriocarcinoma, and hydatidiform mole.[31]

The physiologic role of hCG in human pregnancy has yet to be fully elucidated. It is known to play a luteotropic role early in pregnancy; ie, hCG maintains the corpus luteum of the menstrual cycle and thereby promotes the continued production of progesterone necessary for decidual development until the placenta assumes this role. Late in pregnancy, hCG assumes a gonadotropic role by inducing the secretion of testosterone from the fetal testes prior to the availability of LH secretion from the fetal pituitary. Seron-Ferre and colleagues have also obtained data indicating that hCG may regulate DHEAS production by the fetal zone of the adrenal gland.[88] Another proposed role for hCG is the immunologic protection of the trophoblast. Naughton and associates, studying mixed lymphocyte cultures, have demonstrated that hCG inhibits lymphocyte function in vitro.[89] In both phytohemagglutinin-induced and mixed lymphocyte reactions, they have observed that hCG inhibits blast cell transformation of human lymphocytes. This immunosuppression was noncytotoxic and specific. These authors have postulated that hCG may play a critical immunosuppressive role in vivo by preventing the rejection of the fetal allograft by its maternal host. However, other investigators using highly purified hCG preparations were unable to demonstrate inhibition of T lymphocyte activity. On the basis of these observations and because of the supraphysiologic concentrations of hCG required for inhibition, it is not clear that hCG contributes significantly to immunologic coexistence between the fetus and its maternal host.[31,90] The relative roles of progesterone, hCG, and cortisol in this context have yet to be fully explained.

hCG can be detected in spontaneous pregnancy by the 9th day after the LH surge.[91] This initial detection in maternal blood has been found to correlate with the implantation of the blastocyst and specifically with the moment that lacunae receive maternal blood.[92,93] Concentrations of intact hCG rise to peak values by 60 to 90 days gestation. Subsequently, these levels fall to a plateau that is maintained throughout the duration of the pregnancy. Cole and coworkers studied the different occurrence of free α-subunits and β-subunits in pregnancy sera.[94] These researchers propose that β-subunit production by the trophoblast parallels that of intact hCG throughout the first trimester. During this period, free α-subunit levels are low or absent. Thereafter, the relative production of α and β reverse, and levels of the former increase until term.

Human Chorionic Somatomammotropin (hCS)

Human chorionic somatomammotropin (hCS) is a single-chain polypeptide of 190 amino acids with two disulfide bridges. It has 96% homology with growth hormone (GH). hCS is also known as human placental lactogen (hPL). Despite significant structural homology, hCS has less than 3% of the somatotrophic activity of GH. In animal studies, it has been found to display 50% of the lactogenic activity of prolactin. The half-life of hCS is 14 to 29 minutes. However, it is produced in massive amounts (grams per day) and therefore represents 10% of the total placental protein production.[95] The level of this hormone in the circulation has been correlated with fetal and placental weight, circulating levels increasing 10-fold or greater from the first to third trimester. During the last 4 weeks of gestation, hCS levels plateau, and this protein rapidly becomes undetectable in serum and urine after the delivery of the placenta or evacuation of the uterus. hCS can be detected in the urine and serum in normal and molar pregnancies, as well as in the urine of patients with trophoblastic tumors and in men with choriocarcinoma of the testes. It is a product of the syncytiotrophoblast layer of the placenta.

The major metabolic role of hCS during pregnancy is to ensure the nutritional needs of the fetus. Hypoglycemia stimulates hCS secretion. As the supply of glucose decreases during the fasting state, hCS levels rise, stimulating lipolysis. The increased ketones induced by metabolism of free fatty acids are an important energy source for the fetus. Indeed, a critical physiologic action of hCS during pregnancy appears to be shifting the pattern of energy metabolism from carbohydrates to one that is dependent on fats. During the fed state and in response to rising glucose levels, insulin secretion increases and hCS secretion decreases, leading to glucose use and lipogenesis. Because of increasing substrate requirements by the fetus as pregnancy progresses, the functional role of hCS assumes great significance in the second and third trimesters.[21]

Chorionic Corticotropin and Other Related Peptides

Several investigators have isolated an ACTH-like compound from extracts of placental tissue.[96–98] Placental ACTH or human chorionic corticotropin (hCC) is a glycoprotein of about 34,000 daltons. Its bioactivity is only one third to one fifth that of ACTH. hCC cross reacts with β-endorphin and may be a large "pro-hormone" produced by the trophoblast, similar to the ACTH/β-lipoprotein precursor produced by the hypothalamus and pituitary gland.

The ACTH-like material in human term placentas reacts with antisera raised to the end terminal,[1–24] mid-portion,[13–18] and C-terminal of ACTH.[99] Dexamethasone administration does not alter significantly the levels of ACTH in placentas as measured by bioassay or by immunoassay.[97]

Fetal and maternal ACTH do not cross the placenta. Therefore, the plasma concentrations of each reflect the secretory activity of their respective compartments. The physiologic role of hCC and its related peptides has not been elucidated, although it has been suggested that its secretion is at least partially regulated by cytotrophoblast-derived GnRH.[100] hCC may subserve placental steroidogenesis by stimulating maternal adrenal gland production of the steroid substrates cholesterol and pregnenolone.[97] Moreover, placental ACTH may contribute to the relative resistance to negative feedback suppression of pituitary ACTH by glucocorticoids during much of gestation.[101,102]

A β-endorphin-like peptide has also been demonstrated in human placental extracts. Liotta and colleagues have shown that this substance is comparable to synthetic human β-endorphin.[103] Concentrations of immunoreactive β-endorphin remain relatively low throughout pregnancy (mean levels approximate 15 pg/mL). Levels rise during late labor and even further at delivery, approaching 70 pg/mL and 113 pg/mL, respectively. Cord plasma levels at term are similar (105 pg/mL), suggesting secretion by the placenta or fetal pituitary.[31]

Pro-opiomelanocortin (POMC) or 31-K ACTH/endorphin is the parent compound of ACTH, and a number of anterior pituitary peptides, including β-endorphin, β-lipotropin, and α-MSH. Liotta and colleagues have also found a high molecular weight glycoprotein substance in placental cultures with the physical and chemical properties of POMC.[103] These observations of placental synthesis of both the 31-K parent molecule and ACTH and β-endorphin provide even more evidence of the similar biosynthetic capacities of the placenta and the pituitary. The physiologic role of β-endorphin and placental POMC has yet to be elucidated.

Human Chorionic Thyrotropin (hCT)

Human chorionic thyrotropin (hCT) has been identified in extracts of placental and hydatidiform mold tissues. This 28,000-dalton glycoprotein is immunologically distinct from human TSH, but cross reacts with antisera to the TSH from various animal species, including bovine and porcine. Injection of TRH causes an increase in human TSH but not hCT, suggesting distinct secretory control mechanisms.

The physiologic role of hCT is not clear. It has been suggested by Hennen and colleagues that hCT may play a role during pregnancy in the variations often observed in thyroid function indices and the common occurrence of thyroid enlargement.[104]

The excessive amount of thyroid-stimulating activity found in neoplastic trophoblastic tissue is not secondary to an hCT effect. Indeed, recent studies in molar pregnancies have failed to identify hCT.[31] The hyperstimulation of thyroid tissue that occurs in some women with molar pregnancy is attributed to the high circulating concentrations of hCG that have some thyrotropic activity (1/4000 of TSH).[105]

Gonadotropin-Releasing Hormone (GnRH)

Cytotrophoblast cells of the placenta elaborate several neuropeptides, including GnRH, somatostatin, TRH, and CRF. Over 15 years ago, Gibbons and associates demonstrated that GnRH could be synthesized by human placental cells in vitro.[106] Khodr and Siler-Khodr have measured the placental content of GnRH throughout gestation and found that this releasing factor is localized primarily in the cytotrophoblast layer. Moreover, additional in vitro work has demonstrated placental production of GnRH as well as enhanced hCG secretion.[106–109] Both α and β hCG subunits are secreted after GnRH administration. Because GnRH receptors have been demonstrated in human placenta, it is tempting to speculate about autoregulation of hCG production within the placenta. A complete intraplacental regulatory system can be hypothesized,wherein cytotrophoblastic GnRH stimulates the production of syncytiotrophoblastic hCG, which influences steroidogenesis.

Chorionic Somatostatin

Another cytotrophoblast product is the tetradecapeptide somatostatin. The concentration of this neuropeptide decreases with increasing gestational age, in contrast to the pattern seen with hCS production. It has been hypothesized that placental somatostatin regulates the syncyctiotrophoblastic secretion of hCS through inhibitory influences. This action mimics the inhibition of pituitary GH secretion by hypothalamic somatostatin. In addition, this relationship between a cytotropoblastic product and a syncytiotrophoblastic product is reminiscent of the regulation of hCG production by placental GnRH (although inhibitory rather than stimulatory).[110,31]

Chorionic Corticotropin-Releasing Hormone

Corticotropin-releasing hormone (CRH) activity has been identified in human placental extracts. A 600-fold increase is observed in maternal plasma from the first to the third trimester. As discussed by Heinrichs and Gibbons, this amounts to approximately 800 pg/mL of immunoreactive human chorionic corticotropin-releasing hormone (hCCRH). During labor, the concentration rises significantly; it diminishes rapidly after delivery. Maternal plasma levels correlate well with placental concentrations, although fetal cord venous blood levels are significantly greater than fetal arterial blood and maternal blood concentrations. These observations lend credence to the hypothesis that hCCRH may be an integral part of an autoregulatory system responsible for rising maternal ACTH and cortisol levels at parturition.[1,110,111]

CONCLUSION

Endocrine influences on fetal growth and development are complex. Although significant gaps in our knowledge exist, tremendous progress has been advanced. The fetoplacental–maternal unit stands as a wondrous example in human biology of interrelated systems that allow for the concurrent processes of fetal progression and maternal adaptation.

REFERENCES

1. Heinrichs WL, Gibbons WE: Endocrinology of pregnancy. In: Brody SA, Ueland K, eds. Endocrine disorders in pregnancy. Norwalk, CT: Appleton and Lange, 1989:65.
2. Scott JR, Rote NS, Branch DW. Immunologic aspects of recurrent abortion and fetal death. Obstet Gynecol 1987;70:645.
3. McAnulty JH, Metcalfe J, Ueland K. Cardiovascular disease. In: Burrow GN, Ferris TF, eds. Medical complications during pregnancy. Philadelphia: WB Saunders, 1982:145.
4. Hytten FF, Paintin DB. Increase in plasma volume during normal pregnancy. J Obstet Gynecol Br Commonwealth 1963;70:402.
5. Pritchard JA. Changes in blood volume during pregnancy and delivery. Anesthesiology 1965;26:393.
6. Kase NG, Reyniak JV. Endocrinology of pregnancy. Mt Sinai J Med 1985;52:11.
7. Resnick R. The endocrine regulation of uterine blood flow in the non-pregnant uterus: a review. Am J Obstet Gynecol 1981;140:151.
8. Speroff L, Dorfman GS. Prostaglandins and pregnancy hypertension. Clin Obstet Gynecol 1977;4:635.
9. Freinkel N. Of pregnancy and progeny. Diabetes 1980;29:1023.
10. Adam PAJ. Control of glucose metabolism in the human fetus and newborn infant. Advances in Metabolic Disorders 1971; 5:183.
11. Battaglia FC, Meschia G. Principle substrates of fetal metabolism. Physiol Rev 1978;58:499.
12. Felig P. Maternal and fetal fuel homeostasis in human pregnancy. Am J Clin Nutr 1973;26:998.
13. Kalhan SC, Savin SM, Adam PAG. Attenuated glucose production rate in newborn infants of insulin dependent diabetic mothers. N Engl J Med 1977;296:375.
14. Holzman IR, Lemons JA, Meschia G, Battaglia FC. Uterine uptake of amino acids and placental glutamine-glutamate balance in the pregnant ewe. J Dev Physiol 1979;1:137.
15. Felig P, Kim YJ, Lynch V, Hendler R. Amino acid metabolism during starvation in human pregnancy. J Clin Invest 1972;51:1195.
16. Metzger BE, Hare JW, Frenkel N. Carbohydrate metabolism in pregnancy. IX: plasma levels of gluconeogenic fuels during fasting in the rat. J Clin Endocrinol 1971;32:864.
17. Page MA, Williamson DH. Enzymes of ketone-body utilization in human brain. Lancet 1971;ii:66.
18. Shambaugh GE III, Mrozak SC, Frenkel N. Fetal fuels. I: utilization of ketones by isolated tissues at various stages of maturation and maternal nutrition during late gestation. Metabolism 1977;26:623.
19. Felig P, Coustan D. Diabetes mellitus. In: Burrow GN, Ferris TF, eds. Medical complications during pregnancy. Philadelphia: WB Saunders, 1982:36.
20. Frenkel N. Banting lecture 1980: pregnancy and progeny. Diabetes 1980;29:1023.
21. Kaplan S. The endocrine mileu of pregnancy. In: Jaffe RB, ed. Puerperium and childhood, report of the Third Roth Conference on Obstetric Research. Columbus: Roth Laboratories, 1974:77.
22. Maternal adaptation to pregnancy. In: Pritchard JA, McDonald PC, Gant NF, eds. Williams obstetrics. 17th ed. Norwalk, CT: Appleton Century Crofts, 1985:181.
23. Zacharia EF. Acid mucopolysaccharides in the female genital system and their role in the mechanism of ovulation. Copenhagen: Periodica, 1959.
24. Dons PA, Bell FR. Plasma prolactin during the body fluid and electrolyte changes of dehydration and sodium depletion in steers. Life Sci 1984;34:1683.

25. Blyss DJ, Lote CJ. Effect of prolactin on urinary excretion and renal hemodynamics in conscious rats. J Physiol 1982;322:399.
26. Clements JA, Reyes FI, Winter JSD, et al. Studies on human sexual development. IV: fetal pituitary in serum and amniotic fluid concentrations of prolactin. J Clin Endocrinol Metab 1977;44:408.
27. Healey DL, Herrington AC, O'Herlihy C. Chronic polyhydramnios is a syndrome with a lactogen receptor defect in the chorion laeve. Br J Obstet Gynaecol 1985;92:461.
28. Kaplan SL, Grumbach MM, Aubert ML. The ontogenesis of pituitary hormones and hypothalamic factors in the human fetus: maturation of central nervous system regulation of anterior pituitary function. Recent Prog Horm Res 1976;32:161.
29. Gluckman PD, Grumbach MM, Kaplan SL. The neuroendocrine regulation and function of growth hormone and prolactin in the mammalian fetus. Endocrine Rev 1981;2:363.
30. DeCherney A, Naftolin F. Hypothalamic and pituitary development in the fetus. Clin Obstet Gynecol 1980;23:749.
31. Jaffe RB. Endocrine physiology of the fetus and fetoplacental unit. In: Yen SSC, Jaffe RB, eds. Reproductive endocrinology: physiology, pathophysiology and clinical management. Philadelphia: WB Saunders, 1986:737.
32. Huhtaniemi IG, Koritnik VR, Korenbrot CC, Mennin S, Foster DB, Jaffe RB. Stimulation of pituitary testicular function with gonadotropin-releasing hormone in fetal and infant monkeys. Endocrinology 1979;105:109.
33. Vale W, Spiss J, Rivier C, et al. Characterization of a forty-one-residue ovine hypothalamic peptide that stimulates secretion of corticotropin and β-endorphin. Science 1981;213:1394.
34. Orth DN, Jackson RV, DeCherney GS, et al. Effect of synthetic ovine corticotropin releasing factor. Dose response of plasma adrenal corticotropin and cortisol. J Clin Invest 1983;71:587.
35. Jost A. Fetal hormones and fetal growth. Contrib Gynecol Obstet 1979;5:1.
36. Liggins GC. The influence of fetal hypothalamus and pituitary on growth. Ciba Foundation Symposium (new series) 1974; 27:165.
37. Cheek DB, Greystone JE, Niall M. Factors controlling fetal growth. Clin Obstet Gynecol 1977;20:925.
38. Gluckman PD, Brinsmead MW. Somatomedin in cord blood: relationship to gestational age and birth size. J Clin Endocrinol Metab 1976;43:1378.
39. Kastrup KW, Anderson HT, Lebech P. Somatomedin in newborns and the relationship to human chorionic somatotropin and fetal growth. Acta Pediatr Scand 1978;67:757.
40. Ashton IK, Vesey J. Somatomedin activity in human cord plasma and relationship to birth size, insulin, growth hormone and prolactin. Early Hum Dev 1978;2:115.
41. Heinrick UE, Schalch DS, Jawadi MH, Johnson CJ: NSILA and fetal growth. Acta Endocrinol (Copenh) 1979;90:534.
42. Foley TP, DeFilip R, Pericelli A, Miller A. Low somatomedin activity in cord serum from infants with intrauterine growth retardation. J Pediatr 1980;96:605.
43. Ashton IK, Francis MJO. Response of chondrocytes isolated from human fetal cartilage to plasma somatomedin activity. J Endocrinol 1978;76:473.
44. Hauth JC, Parker CR, McDonald PC, Porter JC, Johnston JM: A role of fetal prolactin in lung maturation. Obstet Gynecol 1978;51:81.
45. Gluckman PD, Ballard PL, Kaplan SL, Liggins GC, Grumbach MM. Prolactin in umbilical cord blood and the respiratory distress syndrome. J Pediatr 1978;93:1011.
46. Allen JP, Cooke DM, Kendall JW, McGilvra R. Maternal fetal ACTH relationship in man. J Clin Endocrinol Metab 1973;37:230.
47. Klein AH, Augustin AV, Foley TP. Successful laboratory screening for congenital hypothyroidism. Lancet 1974;ii:77.
48. Franchimont P, Pasteels JL. Secretion endependante des hormones gonadotropes a et de leurs sous-unites. Comptes Rendus de l'Academie des Sciences (Paris) 1972;275:1799.
49. Ingbar SH. The thyroid gland. In: Wilson JD, Foster DW, eds. Williams textbook of endocrinology. 7th ed. Philadelphia: WB Saunders, 1985:682.
50. Fisher DA, Klein AH. Thyroid development and disorders of thyroid function in the newborn. N Engl J Med 1981;304:702.
51. Roti E, Gnudi A, Braverman LE, et al. Human cord blood concentrations of thyrotropin, thyroglobulin and iodothyronines after maternal administration of thyrotropin-releasing hormone. J Clin Endocrinol Metab 1981;53:813.
52. Siiteri PK, Wolfson JD. Testosterone formation and metabolism during male sexual differentiation in the human embryo. J Clin Endocrinol Metab 1974;38:113.
53. Jaffe RB. Fetoplacental endocrine and metabolic physiology. Perinatal Endocrinology 1983;10:669.
54. Payne AH, Jaffe RB. Androgen formation from pregnenolone sulfate by the human fetal ovary. J Clin Endocrinol Metab 1974;39:300.
55. Gondos B, Hobel CJ. Interstitial cells in the human fetal ovary. Endocrinology 1973;93:736.
56. Easterling EW Jr, Simmer HH, Dignam WJ, Frankland MV, Naftolin F. Neutral C-19 steroids and steroid sulfates in human pregnancy. II: dehydroepiandrosterone sulfate, 16α-hydroxydehydroepiandrosterone, and 16α-hydroxydehydroepiandrosterone sulfate in maternal and fetal blood of pregnancies with anencephalic and normal fetuses. Steroids 1966;8:157.
57. Goldkrand JW, Schulte RL, Messer RH. Maternal and fetal plasma cortisol levels at partuition. Obstet Gynecol 1976;47:41.
58. Benirschke K. Adrenals in anencephaly and hydrocephaly. Obstet Gynecol 1956;8:412.
59. Ballard PL, Gluckman PD, Liggins GC, Kaplan SL, Grumbach MM. Steroid and growth hormone levels in premature infants after perinatal betamethasone therapy to prevent respiratory distress syndrome. Pediatr Res 1980;14:112.
60. Simmer HH, Tulchinsky D, Gold Em, Frankland M, Greipel M, Gold AS. On the regulation of estrogen production by cortisol and ACTH in human pregnancy at term. Am J Obstet Gynecol 1974;119:283.
61. Abu-Hakima M, Branchaud CL, Goodyear CG, et al. The effects of human chorionic gonadotropin on growth and steroidogenesis of the human fetal adrenal gland in vitro. Am J Obstet Gynecol 1987;156:681.
62. Winters AJ, Calston C, McDonald PC, Porter JC. Fetal plasma prolactin levels. J Clin Endocrinol Metab 1975;41:626.
63. Jaffe RB, Seron-Ferre M, Crickard K, Koritnik D, Mitchell BF, Huhtaniemi IT. Regulation and function of the primate fetal adrenal gland and gonad. Recent Prog Horm Res 1981;37:41.
64. Crickard K, Ill CR, Jaffe RB. Control of proliferation of human fetal adrenal cells in vitro. J Clin Endocrinol Metab 1981;53:790.
65. McNulty WP, Novy MJ, Walsh SW. Fetal and postnatal development of the adrenal glands in Macaca mulatta. Biol Reprod 1981;25:1079.
66. Jaffe RB, Payne AH. Gonadal steroid sulfates and sulfatase. IV: comparative studies on the steroid sulfokinase in the human fetal testes and adrenal. J Clin Endocrinol Metab 1971;33:592.
67. Liggins GC. Adrenocortical-related maturational events in the fetus. Am J Obstet Gynecol 1976;126:931.
68. Wurtmann RJ, Axelrod J. Adrenaline synthesis. Control by the pituitary gland and adrenal glucocorticoids. Science 1965;150:1464.
69. Seron-Ferre M, Jaffe RB. The fetal adrenal gland. Ann Rev Physiol 1981;43:141.
70. Wurtman RJ. Controlled epinephrine synthesis in the adrenal medulla by the adrenal cortex: hormonal specificity and dose response characteristics. Endocrinology 1966;79:608.

71. Gray TK, Lame W, Lester GE. Vitamin D and pregnancy: the maternal fetal metabolism of vitamin D. Endocr Rev 1981;2:264.
72. Lester GE, Gray TK, Lorenc RS. Evidence for maternal and fetal differences in vitamin D metabolism. Proc Soc Exp Biol Med 1978;159:303.
73. Reddy GS, Norman AW, Willis DM, et al. Regulation of vitamin D metabolism in normal human pregnancy. J Clin Endocrinol Metab 1983;56:363.
74. Wilson M, Morganti AG, Zervoudakis I, et al. Blood pressure, the renin aldosterone system and sex steroids throughout normal pregnancy. Am J Med 1980;68:97.
75. Resnick LM, Laragh JH. The renin-angiotensin-aldosterone system in pregnancy. In: Fuchs F, Klopper A, eds. Endocrinology of pregnancy. Philadelphia: Harper & Row, 1983:191.
76. Siiteri PK, Febre F, Clemens LE, Chang RJ, Gondos B, Stites D. Progesterone and maintenance of pregnancy: is progesterone nature's immunosuppressant? Ann NY Acad Sci 1977;286:384.
77. Levitz M, Young BK. Estrogens in pregnancy. Vitam Horm 1977;35:109.
78. Buster JE, Abraham GE. The applications of steroid hormone radioimmunoassays to clinical obstetrics. Obstet Gynecol 1975;46:489.
79. Madden JD, Gant NF, McDonald PC. Study of the kinetics of conversion of maternal plasma dehydroisoandrosterone sulfate to 16α-hydroxydehydroisoandrosterone sulfate, estradiol and estriol. Am J Obstet Gynecol 1978;132:392.
80. Casey ML, McDonald TC, Simpson ER. Endocrinological changes of pregnancy. In: Wilson JD, Foster EW, eds. Williams textbook of endocrinology. 7th ed. Philadelphia: WB Saunders, 1985:422.
81. Gurpide E, Marks C, diZiegler D, et al. Asymmetric release of estrone and estradiol derived from labeled precursors in profused human placentas. Am J Obstet Gynecol 1982;144:551.
82. Siiteri PK, McDonald PC. Placental estrogen biosynthesis during human pregnancy. J Clin Endocrinol Metab 1966;26:751.
83. Resnik R, Killam AP, Battaglia FC, Makowski EL, Meschia G. The stimulation of uterine blood flow by various estrogens. Endocrinology 1984;94:1192.
84. Resnik R, Brink GW. Modulating effects of prostaglandins on the uterine vascular bed. Gynecol Invest 1977;8:10.
85. Tabei T, Heinrichs WL. Diagnosis of placental sulfatase deficiency. Am J Obstet Gynecol 1976;124:409.
86. Midgley AR, Pierce GB. Immunohistochemical localization of human chorionic gonadotropin. J Exp Med 1962;111:289.
87. Jaffe RB. Protein hormones of the placenta, decidua and fetal membranes. In: Yen SSC, Jaffe RB, eds. Reproductive endocrinology. Philadelphia: WB Saunders, 1988:758.
88. Seron-Ferre M, Lawrence CC, Jaffe RB. Role of hCG in the regulation of the fetal zone of the human fetal adrenal gland. J Clin Endocrinol Metab 1978;46:834.
89. Teasdale F, Adcock EW III, August CS, Cox S, Battaglia FC, Naughton MA. Human chorionic gonadotropin: inhibitory effect on mixed lymphocyte cultures. Gynecol Invest 1973;4:263.
90. Carr MC, Stites DP, Fudenberg HH. Cellular aspects of human fetal maternal relationship. II: in vitro response of gravida lymphocytes to phytohemagglutin. Cell Immunol 1973;8:448.
91. Jaffe RB, Lee PA, Midgley AR Jr. Serum gonadotropin before, at the inception of, and following human pregnancy. J Clin Endocrinol Metab 1969;29:1281.
92. Lenton EA, Neal LM, Sulaimin R. Plasma concentrations of human chorionic gonadotropin from the time of implantation until the second week of pregnancy. Fertil Steril 1982;37:773.
93. Catt KJ, Dufau ML, Vaitukaitis JL. Appearance of human chorionic gonadotropin in pregnancy plasma following the initiation of implantation of the blastocyst. J Clin Endocrinol Metab 1975;40:537.
94. Cole LA, Kroll TG, Ruddon RW, et al. Differential occurrence of free β and free α subunits of human chorionic gonadotropin in pregnancy sera. J Clin Endocrinol Metab 1984;48:1200.
95. Friesen HG, Suwa S, Pare P. Synthesis and secretion of placental lactogen and other proteins by the placental. Rec Prog Horm Res 1969;25:161.
96. Rees LH, Burke CW, Chard T. Possible placental origin of ACTH in normal human pregnancy. Nature 1975;254:620.
97. Liotta A, Osathanondtt R, Ryan KJ, et al. Presence of corticotropin in human placenta: demonstration of in vitro synthesis. Endocrinology 1977;101:1552.
98. Odagiri E, Sherrell BJ, Mount CD, et al. Human placental immunoreactive corticotropin, lipotropin, and β-endorphin: evidence for a common precursor. Proc Natl Acad Sci USA 1979;76:2027.
99. Simpson ER, McDonald PC. Endocrine physiology of the placenta. Ann Rev Physiol 1981;43:163.
100. Siler-Khodr TM, Khodr GS. Production and activity of placental releasing hormones. In: Novy MJ, Resko JA, eds. Fetal endocrinology. New York: Academic Press, 1981:183.
101. Rees LH, Burcke CW, Chard T, Evans SW, Letchworth AT. Possible placental origin of ACTH in normal human pregnancy. Nature 1975;154:620.
102. Genazzani AR, Fraioli F, Hurlimann J, Fiorette P, Felber JP. Immunoreactive ACTH and cortisol plasma levels during pregnancy: detection and partial purification of corticotropin-like placental hormone: the human chorionic corticotropin (hCC). Clin Endocrinol 1975;4:1.
103. Liotta AS, Krieger DG. In vitro biosynthesis and comparative post-translational processing of immunoreactive precursor corticotropin/beta endorphin by human placental and pituitary cells. Endocrinology 1980;106:1504.
104. Hennen G, Pierce JG, Freychet P. Human chorionic thyrotropin: further characterization and study of its secretion during pregnancy. J Clin Endocrinol Metab 1969;29:581.
105. Kenimer JG, Hershman JM, Higgins HP. The thyrotropin in hydatidiform moles is human chorionic gonadotropin. J Clin Endocrinol Metab 1975;40:482.
106. Gibbons JM, Mitnick M, Chieffo V. In vitro biosynthesis of TSH- and LH-releasing factors by the human placenta. Am J Obstet Gynecol 1975;121:127.
107. Khodr GS, Siler-Khodr TM. Localization of leutinizing hormone-releasing factor in the human placenta. Fertil Steril 1978;29:523.
108. Khodr GS, Siler-Khodr TM. The effect of leutinizing hormone-releasing factor on human chorionic gonadotropin secretion. Fertil Steril 1978;30:301.
109. Khodr GS, Siler-Khodr TM. Placental leutinizing hormone-releasing factor and its synthesis. Science 1980;207:315.
110. Siler-Khodr TM. Hypothalamic like releasing hormones of the placenta. Perinatal Endocrinology 1983;10:566.
111. Shibasaki T, Odagiri E, Shizume K, et al. Corticotropin releasing factor like activity in human placental extracts. J Clin Endocrinol Metab 1982;55:384.

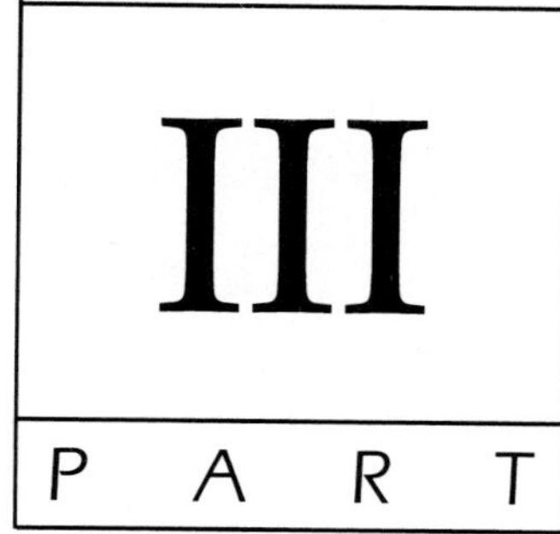

FETAL DEVELOPMENTAL BIOLOGY

9

CHAPTER

FETAL LUNG DEVELOPMENT AND AMNIOTIC FLUID PHOSPHOLIPID ANALYSIS

Katherine V. Nichols and Ian Gross

Respiratory distress syndrome (RDS) is a developmental disorder of prematurely born infants characterized by progressive atelectasis and respiratory insufficiency. It was originally called hyaline membrane disease (HMD) because microscopic membranes were found in the alveoli of the lungs of infants who died from this disorder. The pathogenesis of RDS was first developed by Avery and Mead in 1959,[1] who described the surface behavior of lung extracts from infants with hyaline membrane disease. They demonstrated that the surface tension of lung extracts from premature infants who died of RDS was higher than that of infants who died of other causes. They speculated that a lung lining material was necessary to keep alveoli open at low lung volumes, and that lack of the lining material contributed to the atelectasis seen in RDS.

That a surface active substance might be responsible for maintaining lung inflation was first suggested by a Swiss pathologist, van Neergard, in 1929,[2] when he compared pressure–volume curves in isolated lung inflated and deflated with either air or saline. The difference in the inflation and deflation curves suggested that surface tension at the air–fluid interface played a role in maintaining lung inflation, because this difference was abolished by saline inflation. In 1955 Pattle,[3] noting the stability of bubbles expressed from the cut surface of lung, suggested that the bubbles were lined with a detergent substance that maintained stability. Clements in 1957[2] isolated a surface-active substance from lung.

This lung lining has since come to be known as pulmonary surfactant. Its composition, biochemistry, ontogeny, and regulation have been studied in detail, as has its use in the prenatal assessment of lung maturity and clinical use in replacement therapy.

ANATOMIC DEVELOPMENT

The lung develops as an outpouching of the primitive foregut at about 24 days. At 26 to 28 days, this bud branches into two primary bronchi.[4] Further anatomic development can be divided into four overlapping phases. The first phase, from 28 days to 16 weeks, is termed the glandular period, because the lung is glandular in histologic appearance, with cuboidal epithelium lining the terminal airways.[5] This phase is characterized by successive branching of the bronchial tree. Pulmonary arterial branching follows that of the bronchi, and capillaries are present but separated from the terminal airways by a large amount of interstitial tissue. Extrauterine survival could not be expected at this stage due to the limited capacity for gas exchange across the large distance between the capillaries and terminal airways.

During the second phase, the canalicular phase, from 13 to 25 weeks, there is canalization of the airways. Each bronchiole gives rise to two or more respiratory bronchioles, then each of these divides into three to six alveolar ducts. The epithelium becomes flatter. Capillaries are closer to the respiratory epithelium, but there is still much interstitial tissue, limiting the potential for gas exchange and reducing lung compliance.

In the terminal sac period, from 24 weeks to birth, alveolar ducts give rise to primitive alveoli. Epithelial cells differentiate into Type I alveolar cells, which eventually cover 95% of the alveolar surface.[5] The capillaries increase in number and are closer to the Type I cells, allowing for better gas exchange. Type II alveolar cells differentiate during this period. These cells are responsible for the synthesis, storage, and secretion of surfactant.[6]

The final phase, the alveolar period, begins in later fetal life and continues through the eighth year. True alveolarization begins at about 34 to 36 weeks.[5] At birth, one eighth to one sixth of the adult number of alveoli are present. The number of alveoli increases until adult numbers are reached in the eighth year.

The lung contains 40 different cell types.[6] The alveolar lining is composed primarily of two epithelial cell types, Type I and Type II pneumocytes. The main alveolar epithelial cell, the Type I, is a thin, squamous cell, making up the alveolar wall. It is in intimate contact with the capillary endothelial cell, and it is across these cells that gas exchange takes place. Type II cells, which are smaller than the Type I cells, are located in the corners of alveoli. They are cuboidal and contain characteristic lamellar inclusions when seen by electron microscopy.[7] The lamellar bodies are the intracellular sites of storage of surfactant. Biochemical analysis of lamellar bodies has shown that they contain the same phospholipids as surfactant. Type II cells are responsible for the synthesis, storage, and secretion of surfactant.[6] They rapidly take up the precursors from which phospholipids and proteins are synthesized. Synthesis takes place in the endoplasmic reticulum. After modification in the Golgi apparatus, surfactant components are transported to and stored in lamellar bodies.[8] These bodies are secreted by exocytosis and then unfold, outside the cell, to form tubular myelin. From this is derived the surfactant monolayer, which is absorbed to the air–liquid interface. Tubular myelin appears under electron microscopy as a lattice formed of rectangular tubes.[9]

An additional function of Type II cells is proliferation in response to injury. After some types of injury, Type I cells are sloughed from the alveolar lining into the alveolar space and Type II cells proliferate to reestablish the alveolar lining. They may then develop into Type I cells.[10] There is some evidence that Type II cells differentiate into Type I cells in the process of normal development as well.

BIOCHEMICAL DEVELOPMENT

Pulmonary surfactant is a complex mixture of phospholipids and proteins. Adult surfactant is 85% to 90% phospholipid and 10% protein. Although the lipid components of surfactant are not unique to the lung, the phospholipid composition differs from that found elsewhere, such as in cell membranes.[11] The membrane phospholipids are rich in oligo- and polyunsaturated fatty acids, whereas surfactant phospholipids predominantly contain saturated palmitic acid. The major species of phospholipid in surfactant are phosphatidylcholine (PC, lecithin), which accounts for 80% to 85% of total phospholipid, and phosphatidylglycerol (PG), which accounts for 6% to 11% of total phospholipid. Approximately half of the phosphatidylcholine or about 45% to 50% of total phospholipid is in the disaturated form (DSPC).[12,13] Surfactant composition is summarized in Table 9-1.

A biochemical developmental profile has been described for several species. Fatty acid and phospholipid synthesis occur de novo in Type II cells. Preformed fatty acids supplied via the bloodstream are also used in phospholipid production.[13] Glycogen acts as a substrate and energy source for phospholipid synthesis.[8] The content of glycogen in fetal lung increases in early development, peaks in late gestation, and then rapidly decreases, coincident with an increase in phospholipid synthesis.[14] In association with the developmental increase in the rate of phosphatidylcholine synthesis, there is an increase in the activity of the rate regulatory enzyme, cholinephosphate cytidyl transferase (CYT), in late gestation.[13] There is also a developmental increase in fatty acid synthesis and a parallel increase in the enzyme fatty acid synthase.[15] At 80% to 90% of gestation, a marked increase in total lung phospholipid oc-

TABLE 9–1. SURFACTANT COMPOSITION

	% TOTAL WEIGHT
Protein	10–15
Phospholipid	85–90
	% of total phospholipid
Phospholipids	
Phosphatidlycholine (PC)	80–85
Disaturated phosphatidylcholine	45–50
Phosphatidylglycerol	6–11
Phosphatidylethanolamine	3–5
Phosphatidylinositol	2
Sphingomyelin	2

Data from Jobe A. State of the art. Surfactant for the treatment of respiratory distress syndrome. Am Rev Respir Dis 1987;136:1256.

curs, with a large increase in phosphatidylcholine accounting for most of the change.[16] An increase in the surface activity of lung extracts[17] and in lung distensibility and stability on deflation as measured by pressure–volume relationships also occurs at this time.[18]

In addition to the phospholipid components of surfactant, four surfactant-related proteins have been described and characterized. Their properties are summarized in Table 9-2. Surfactant protein A (SP-A) is a highly glycosylated protein with a molecular weight of 28 to 36 kd.[19,20] It plays a role in surfactant secretion and reuptake by Type II cells. In vitro studies have demonstrated that it inhibits secretion but enhances reuptake of surfactant, perhaps by receptor-mediated endocytosis.[21–25] It also appears to be important in the formation of tubular myelin. Two smaller proteins, SP-B and SP-C, have also been extensively studied. These hydrophobic proteins with molecular weights of 4 to 8 kd are believed to be important in the surface activity of surfactant and are present in clinically effective surfactant preparations. SP-D is a lectin-like protein, the structure and function of which have yet to be fully characterized.

A variety of physical, biochemical, and hormonal stimuli can alter lung development and phospholipid synthesis and secretion. The incidence of RDS is lower in infants delivered after labor, whether by vaginal delivery or cesarean section, than those delivered without labor at the same gestational age.[26] Animal studies have shown that labor increases the rate of surfactant secretion without altering the rate of synthesis.[27] Sex appears to play some role in lung maturation. At the same gestational age, males are more likely than females to develop RDS.[28,29] Differences in amniotic fluid phospholipids indicate that the biochemical maturity of the female lung precedes that of males by about 1 week.[30] Some animal studies suggest that this difference may be due to increased secretion rather than increased biosynthesis.[13] Maternal diabetes also influences lung maturity. Avery and Mead noted the high incidence of RDS in infants of diabetic mothers.[1] This association has been borne out by careful study and, for infants born prematurely, there is a higher incidence of RDS at all gestational ages. There is, as yet, no consensus regarding the cause of delayed lung maturation, whether hyperglycemia, hyperinsulinemia, abnormal fatty acid metabolism, or a combination of factors.

TABLE 9–2. SURFACTANT PROTEINS

SP-A (28–36 kd)
Inhibits surfactant secretion
Enchances re-uptake
Plays a role in the formation of tubular myelin
Small Lipophilic Proteins, SP-B and SP-C (4–8 kd)
Present in clinically effective surfactant preparations
Important for surface activity
SP-D
Lectin-like, function unknown.

Surfactant synthesis is stimulated by a variety of hormones, including glucocorticoids, thyroid hormone, TRH, and prolactin, and growth factors such as epidermal growth factor (EGF).[13] Of these, glucocorticoids have been most extensively studied. Administration of glucocorticoids to fetuses results in a number of morphologic changes indicative of accelerated lung maturity, including larger alveoli, thinner interalveolar septae, increased numbers of Type II cells, and increased lamellar bodies within Type II cells.[31,32] In addition, glucocorticoids enhance the biosynthesis of both lung phospholipids and surfactant proteins.[33] There is also substantial clinical evidence that antenatal steroids can accelerate lung maturation.

Surfactant secretion is stimulated by a number of agents, including β-adrenergic agonists, such as terbutaline, purinoceptor agonists, such as adenosine, and cAMP.[13]

EVALUATION OF FETAL LUNG MATURITY

Assessment of fetal lung maturity by analysis of phospholipids in amniotic fluid began in 1971, when Gluck reported gestational changes in amniotic fluid phospholipid concentrations.[34] Previous studies had shown that the phospholipids that appeared in amniotic fluid originated principally from the fetal lung. In an analysis of 302 amniocenteses from both normal and abnormal pregnancies, from 12 weeks to term, Gluck showed that total phospholipids in amniotic fluid increased throughout gestation, and that there was a sharp increase at 35 weeks. Both lecithin (phosphatidylcholine) and sphingomyelin were measured. The concentrations of lecithin and sphingomyelin were nearly equal until 35 weeks, when there was an increase in lecithin concentration to almost four times that of sphingomyelin. After 35 weeks, lecithin concentration increased while sphingomyelin declined somewhat (Fig. 9-1). From this report, the concept of the lecithin/sphingomyelin (L/S) ratio emerged. Because sphingomyelin remained fairly constant while lecithin increased, a ratio between the two was used to correct for any changes in amniotic fluid volume.

This report was followed by a number of studies on the clinical utility of the L/S ratio in predicting lung maturity. In an early report, Hobbins[35] used as a definition of maturity lecithin concentration greater than sphingomyelin concentration and found that no infant, regardless of birthweight, developed RDS if the amniotic fluid phospholipids indicated maturity. Twenty-five percent of infants with equal concentrations of lecithin and sphingomyelin developed RDS. One of these infants, with a birthweight greater than 2500 g, was the child of a diabetic mother.

As noted earlier, the original study included both

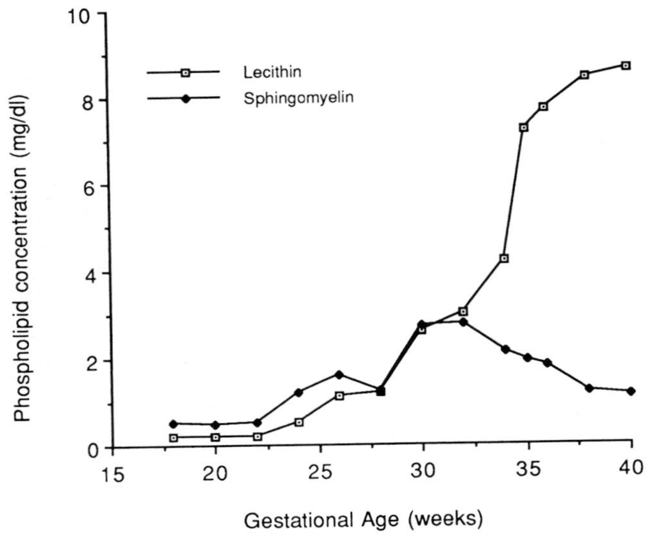

FIGURE 9-1. Amniotic fluid phospholipid concentration versus gestational age.

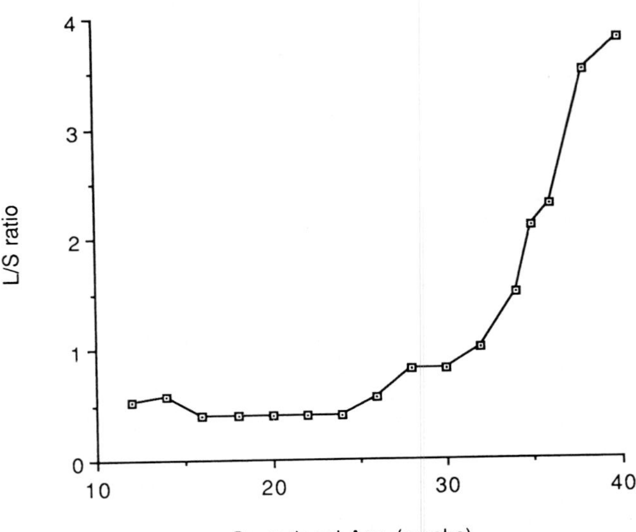

FIGURE 9-2. Lecithin/sphingomyelin (L/S) ratio versus gestational age.

normal and abnormal pregnancies. Further studies were done, separating completely normal pregnancies from those complicated by maternal or fetal disease.[36] The lecithin and sphingomyelin concentrations in normal pregnancies paralleled those previously reported. An L/S ratio of 2 occurred at 35 weeks and increased thereafter (Fig. 9-2). The L/S ratio was determined in a variety of maternal and fetal conditions. Accelerated or delayed lung maturation was found in association with a number of these conditions. Accelerated lung maturity was described as an L/S ratio of 2 or more at less than 35 weeks gestation, while delayed maturity was defined as an L/S ratio of 1 after 35 weeks. Conditions associated with accelerated lung maturation were pregnancy-induced hypertension (PIH); hypertension associated with renal or cardiovascular disease; sickle cell disease; narcotics addiction; class D, E, and F diabetes; and premature rupture of the membranes for longer than 24 hours. Conditions associated with delayed lung maturation were class A, B, and C diabetes; fetal hydrops; and nonhypertensive renal disease (Table 9-3).

In this study, all infants with an L/S ratio of less than 2 developed RDS to some degree, but none of those with an L/S ratio greater than 2 developed RDS. In later clinical studies,[37,38] RDS occurred in 2% to 3% of infants with an L/S ratio of 2 or greater. Most of the cases of RDS occurred in infants born to class A, B, or C diabetics. An L/S ratio of less than 2 was found to have a low predictive value for RDS. Almost half of the infants with a low L/S failed to develop RDS. In an effort to improve the accuracy of amniotic fluid phospholipid analysis in predicting RDS, other phospholipids such as phosphatidylinositol (PI) and phosphatidylglycerol (PG) were studied in normal and complicated pregnancies.[38,39] PI increased, then decreased, during the course of gestation. PG appeared at 34 to 35 weeks, and the concentration increased with gestational age thereafter. The appearance of PG as 3% or more of total phospho-

TABLE 9-3. CONDITIONS ASSOCIATED WITH ACCELERATED OR DELAYED LUNG MATURATION BY L/S RATIO

Accelerated Maturation	Delayed Maturation
PIH	Diabetes, Class A, B, C
Hypertensive renal disease	Nonhypertensive renal disease
Hypertensive cardiovascular disease	Hydrops fetalis
Sickle cell disease	
Narcotics addiction	
Diabetes, class D, F, FR	
Premature rupture of membranes, >24 hrs	
Placental insufficiency	
Chronic retroplacental bleeding	

Data from Gluck L, Kulovich M. Lecithin/sphingomyelin ratios in amniotic fluid in normal and abnormal pregnancy. Am J Obstet Gynecol 173;115:539; and Kulovich M, Gluck L. The lung profile. II: Complicated pregnancy Am J Obstet Gynecol 1979;135:57.

lipids was predictive of lung maturity. Combining L/S ratio and PG measurements improved both the positive and negative predictive accuracy of amniotic fluid phospholipid analysis. This was particularly important in diabetic pregnancies, where the incidence of RDS was higher despite an L/S ratio greater than 2. Class A, B, and C diabetics showed a delayed appearance of PG, until 37 to 39 weeks. Class D, F, and R diabetics had normal or early appearance of PG.[39] Patients with PIH or premature rupture of the membranes (PROM) also had earlier appearance of PG.

L/S ratio plus PG has since become the standard means of determining fetal lung maturity. A mature L/S with PG positive has a negative predictive value (a mature test = clinical maturity) of close to 100%. The positive predictive value (an immature test = clinical immaturity) of a low L/S is, however, about 70%. The L/S–PG has other drawbacks as well. The test is done by the time-consuming method of thin-layer chromatography. Blood and meconium in the amniotic fluid can greatly reduce the accuracy of the L/S ratio. As little as 0.03 mL of blood in 5 mL amniotic fluid can give a false-positive result.[35] As a result of these limitations, other methods of determining fetal lung maturity have been devised. The ideal method would be reproducible, technically simple, and have a short turnaround time. It would have both positive and negative predictive accuracy. To date, no ideal method has been developed.

In 1972, Clements[40] reported a rapid test for surfactant in amniotic fluid. The foam stability or shake test is based on the ability of surfactant to produce a stable foam in the presence of ethanol. The technique is fairly simple, requires no special equipment, and results are available rapidly. A "mature" test is the presence of foam at a 1:2 dilution of amniotic fluid. An "immature" test is absence of foam at a 1:1 dilution. When compared to the L/S ratio, the shake test is as good at predicting maturity, but it has a higher false immature rate.[41] As with the L/S ratio, the shake test is not accurate in the presence of blood or meconium.[42] Although it is easier and more rapidly performed than the L/S ratio, the shake test should only be used as a screen. An immature test should be confirmed with an L/S–PG.

The concentration of lamellar bodies in amniotic fluid is directly related to the absorbance at 650 nm,[43] and this absorbance has been used as a rapid test for fetal lung maturity.[43,44] This test is limited by a very high false immaturity rate. It is valuable only as a screen.

Amniotic fluid microviscosity as determined by fluorescence polarization has also been used a fairly rapid method of evaluating lung maturity. Amniotic fluid has a high, constant viscosity until about 30 to 32 weeks, when there is an abrupt decrease followed by a steady decline to term.[45] As with other tests, determination of microviscosity accurately predicts maturity but overestimates immaturity.[46]

A further refinement of fluorescence polarization uses a ratio of surfactant to albumin rather than microviscosity.[47] As an automated test, it is simple to perform and can be done quickly, although it does require special instrumentation. A "mature" test correlates well with clinical maturity, but an immature test is not as good a predictor of who will actually develop RDS.

Surfactant proteins in the amniotic fluid have been studied as a way of predicting lung maturity more accurately. The timing of the appearance of surfactant proteins was determined by King and coworkers.[48] Amniotic fluid from 12 weeks to term was assayed for surfactant-associated protein. From 12 to 32 weeks, there was essentially no protein found. The protein titers increased from 32 to 37 weeks and then plateaued. This parallels the gestational age-related increase in phospholipids. This developmental profile of amniotic fluid surfactant protein was confirmed by others.[49] A more specific monoclonal antibody assay for surfactant protein A was used to determine the predictive accuracy of protein assay in amniotic fluid.[50] Lit-

TABLE 9–4. PREDICTIVE VALUE OF PRENATAL TESTS FOR LUNG MATURITY

TEST	POSITIVE* ACCURACY	NEGATIVE* ACCURACY	REFERENCES
L/S	0.541	0.982	36–38, 41, 44, 46, 47, 50
L/S-PG	0.470	0.993	50, 51
Shake test	0.120	1.0	41
OD650	0.128	0.987	44
35 kd protein	0.315	1.0	50
35 kD + L/S + PG	0.714	1.0	50
FELMA	0.330	1.0	46
TDX-FLM	0.307	0.996	47

* These values were calculated using data from the references cited.

Definitions from Feinstein AR. On the sensitivity, specificity and discrimination of diagnostic tests. In: Feinstein AR, ed. Clinical biostatistics. St. Louis: CV Mosby, 1977:214. Positive test, immaturity; positive predictive accuracy, the accuracy with which an immature test predicts RDS; false-positive rate, 1-positive predictive accuracy; negative test, maturity; negative predictive accuracy, accuracy with which a mature test predicts no RDS; false-negative rate, 1-negative predictive accuracy; FELMA, microviscosity by fluorescence polarization; TDx-FLM, fluorescence polarization, Abbott Laboratories.

tle protein was found before 32 weeks. There was then a slow increase between 32 and 37 weeks, and a sharp increase after 37 weeks. When correlated with clinical outcome, a surfactant protein concentration of 3 μg/mL or greater accurately predicted maturity. The test was much less accurate in predicting immaturity, with a large false-positive rate. However, when a protein determination was combined with an L/S–PG, the ability to correctly predict immaturity increased dramatically. In this study, the accuracy of protein analysis in diabetics was not evaluated, because those patients were not delivered until they were PG positive, and none of the infants had RDS. Other studies have shown that surfactant protein levels are decreased in the amniotic fluid of diabetic pregnancies.[51] A low protein level, regardless of L/S ratio, seems a better predictor of RDS in the diabetic pregnancy and may help to reduce erroneous predictions of maturity by L/S ratio alone.

Table 9-4 summarizes the predictive accuracy of each of the methods discussed. The values in this table were calculated from the data in the references cited. All of the tests accurately predict lung maturity with a very low false-negative rate. This means that a baby with a mature test has a very low risk of developing RDS, which is of great value in determining the timing of delivery of a complicated pregnancy. Conversely, an infant with an immature test has about a 50% chance of developing RDS. False immature tests are much less risky than false mature tests. Perhaps the greatest value of these tests is in the diabetic pregnancy, where the fetal lung appears to reach biochemical maturity at a different rate than in nondiabetics. Using the presence of PG as an indicator of maturity or using protein analysis along with phospholipid analysis greatly reduces the chance of a false mature test.

CORTICOSTEROIDS AND LUNG MATURITY

The influence of glucocorticoids on lung maturation has been extensively studied both in vitro and in vivo, in human lung and in a variety of animal systems. These steroids accelerate the anatomical, biochemical, and physiologic maturation of the lung in several species, including the human. Accumulation of the phospholipid and protein components of surfactant is enhanced by glucocorticoids.

Glucocorticoid action in the lung is by the classic steroid receptor mechanism. Steroids enter cells and bind to specific cytoplasmic receptors. The receptor–steroid complex is then translocated to the nucleus, where it interacts with specific sites on DNA, resulting in transcription of messenger RNA. The RNA is then translated in the cytoplasm to protein. As shown in Table 9-5, a variety of proteins are stimulated by steroids. Surfactant proteins A, B, and C and their messenger RNAs are increased by glucocorticoids in cultured human fetal lung,[52–54] as is fatty acid synthase[55] and the structural proteins collagen and elastin.[56] Steroids modulate or regulate surfactant synthesis, but do not appear to be responsible for initiating it.[57,58]

TABLE 9-5. mRNA AND PROTEINS INCREASED BY GLUCOCORTICOIDS IN FETAL LUNG

Surfactant proteins A, B, C
Fatty acid synthase
Collagen
Elastin

Evidence from animal studies that steroids accelerated lung maturity and improved viability in prematurely born fetuses[59,60] led to clinical trials of antenatal steroids. Liggins and Howie administered betamethasone in two doses 24 hours apart to women in spontaneous preterm labor at 24 to 36 weeks gestation.[61] They found a significant reduction in the incidence of RDS in infants under 32 weeks gestation who had been treated for at least 24 hours prior to delivery. There was also a significant reduction in deaths due to RDS. In their study, there was no increased incidence of maternal or neonatal infection. A number of studies followed using other steroids, including dexamethasone and hydrocortisone.[62–66] Almost all demonstrated a reduction in the incidence of RDS with maternal steroid treatment, but with limitations. In general, antenatal steroids are most effective when administered before 32 weeks gestation. There is little benefit if infants are delivered less than 24 hours after starting treatment, and the optimal benefit appears to occur when infants are delivered at least 2 to 3 days but less than 7 to 10 days after starting treatment.[67] Male infants may derive less benefit from antenatal steroids than females, although this has not been observed in all studies.[66,68,69] The use of steroids in prolonged rupture of membranes has been controversial. In a meta-analysis of published data from this area, Romero et al found that steroids are effective in reducing the incidence of RDS in pregnancies complicated by premature rupture of the membranes.[70] There was no increased risk of neonatal infection, but there was a small increase in maternal infections.

Even with optimal steroid treatment, some infants develop RDS. This varies from about 10% in infants over 30 weeks gestation to about 35% in infants before 30 weeks. The incidence of RDS in infants not exposed to antenatal steroids is about 25% and 60%, respectively. In an effort to further reduce the incidence of RDS, combinations of hormones have been studied. Thyroid hormone (T3) is effective in stimulating surfactant synthesis in vitro, and glucocorticoids combined with T3 produce an additive or supra-additive stimulation of surfactant synthesis in vitro. T3 does not cross the placenta well, but TRH (thyrotropin releasing hormone) does; maternally administered TRH has been shown to increase TSH and T3 levels in cord blood. A multicenter trial of TRH plus steroids compared to steroids alone showed, surprisingly, that the combination did not produce a lower incidence of RDS than steroids alone, but did result in a 50% reduction in the incidence of chronic lung disease.[71] The mechanism for this effect is currently being examined.

Research efforts in the area of lung development continue in laboratory and in clinical trials. The regulation of genes involved in surfactant production and hormonal manipulation of surfactant and structural elements of the lung are under investigation and may provide even more effective treatment regimens in the future.

REFERENCES

1. Avery ME, Mead J. Surface properties in relation to atelectasis and hyaline membrane disease. Am J Dis Child 1959;97:517.
2. Clements JA. Surface tension of lung extracts. Proc Soc Exp Biol Med 1957;95:170.
3. Pattle RE. Properties, function and origin of the alveolar lining layer. Nature 1955;175:1125.
4. Moore KL. The developing human. Philadelphia: WB Saunders, 1982:216.
5. Stahlman MT, Gray ME. Anatomical development and maturation of the lungs. Clin Perinatol 1978;5:181.
6. Mason RJ, Dobbs LG, Greenleaf RD, Williams MC. Alveolar type II cells. Federation Proceedings 1977;36:2697.
7. Williams MC. Development of the alveolar structure of the fetal rat in late gestation. Federation Proceedings 1977;36:2653.
8. Kresch MJ, Gross I. The biochemistry of fetal lung development. Clin Perinatol 1987;14:481.
9. Williams MC. Conversion of lamellar body membranes into tubular myelin in alveoli of fetal rat lungs. J Cell Biol 1977;72:260.
10. Adamson IYR, Bowden DH. The type II cell as progenitor of alveolar epithelial regeneration. Lab Invest 1974;30:35.
11. Sundler R. Surface stabilizing properties of phospholipids. In: Ekelund L, Jonson B, Malm L, eds. Surfactant and the respiratory tract. Amsterdam: Elsevier Science, 1989:33.
12. Rooney SA. Lung surfactant. Environ Health Perspect 1984; 55:205.
13. Rooney SA. The surfactant system and lung phospholipid biochemistry. Am Rev Resp Dis 1985;131:439.
14. Maniscalco WM, Wilson CM, Gross I. Development of glycogen and phospholipid metabolism in fetal and newborn rat lung. Biochem Biophys Acta 1978;530:333.
15. Maniscalco WM, Finkelstein JN, Parkhurst AB. De novo fatty acid synthesis in developing rat lung. Biochem Biophys Acta 1982;711:49.
16. Rooney SA, Wai Lee TS, Gobran L, Motoyama EK. Phospholipid content, composition and biosynthesis during fetal lung development in the rabbit. Biochem Biophys Acta 1976;431:447.
17. Gluck L, Motoyama EK, Smits EL, Kulovich MV. Biochemical development of surface activity in mammalian lung. Pediatr Res 1967;1:237.
18. Kotas RV, Avery ME. Accelerated appearance of pulmonary surfactant in the fetal rabbit. J Appl Physiol 1971;30:358.
19. Whitsett JA, Weaver T, Hull W, et al. Synthesis of surfactant associated glycoprotein A by rat type II epithelial cells: primary translation products and post translational modification. Biochem Biophys Acta 1985;828:162.
20. Whitsett JA, Ross G, Weaver T, et al. Glycosylation and secretion of surfactant associated glycoprotein A. J Biol Chem 1985; 260:15273.
21. Ryan RM. Type II cells bind and internalize SP-A by receptor mediated endocytosis. J Histochem Cytochem 1989;37:429.
22. Rice WR, Ross GF, Singleton FM, Dingle S, Whitsett JA. Surfactant associated protein inhibits phospholipid secretion from type II cells. J Appl Physiol 1987;63:692.
23. Dobbs LG, Wright JR, Hawgood S, Gonzalez R, Venstrom K, Nellenbogen J. Pulmonary surfactant and its components inhibit secretion of phosphatidylcholine from cultured rat alveolar type II cells. Proc Natl Acad Sci 1987;84:1010.
24. Wright JR, Wager RE, Hamilton RL, Huang M, Clements JA. Uptake of lung surfactant subfractions into lamellar bodies of adult rabbit lungs. J Appl Physiol 1986;60:817.
25. Wright JR, Wager RE, Hawgood S, Dobbs L, Clements JA. Surfactant apoprotein Mr = 26,000–36,000 enhances uptake of liposomes by type II cells. J Biol Chem 1987;262:2888.
26. Oliver RE. Of labor and the lungs. Arch Dis Child 1981;56:659.
27. Marino PA, Rooney SA. The effect of labor on surfactant secretion in newborn rabbit lung slices. Biochem Biophys Acta 1981;664:389.
28. Naeye RL, Burt LS, Wright DL, Blane WA, Tatler D. Neonatal mortality, the male disadvantage. Pediatrics 1971;48:902.
29. Khoury MJ, Marks JS, McCarthy BJ, Zaro SM. Factors affecting sex differential in neonatal mortality: The role of RDS. Am J Gynecol Obstet 1985;151:777.
30. Torday JS, Nielson HC, Fencl MDM, Avery ME. Sex differences in fetal lung maturation. Am Rev Resp Dis 1981;123:205.
31. Kikkawa Y, Kaibara M, Motoyama EK, et al. Morphologic development of fetal rabbit lung and its acceleration with cortisol. Am J Pathol 1971;64:423.
32. Hitchcock KR. Hormones and the lung. I: thyroid hormones and glucocorticoids in lung development. Anat Rec 1979;194:15.
33. Rooney SA, Gobran LI, Marino PA, et al. Effect of betamethasone on phospholipid content, composition and biosynthesis in fetal rabbit lung. Biochem Biophys Acta 1979;572:64.
34. Gluck L, Kulovich MV, Borer, RC, et al. Diagnosis of the respiratory distress syndrome by amniocentesis. Am J Obstet Gynecol 1971;109:440.
35. Hobbins JC, Brock W, Speroff L, Anderson GG, Caldwell B. L/S ratio in predicting pulmonary maturity in utero. Obstet Gynecol 1972;39:660.
36. Gluck L, Kulovich M. Lecithin/sphingomyelin ratios in amniotic fluid in normal and abnormal pregnancy. Am J Obstet Gynecol 1973;115:539.
37. Donald IR, Freeman RK, Goebelsmann U, Chan WH, Nakamura RM. Clinical experience with the amniotic fluid lecithin/sphingomyelin ratio. I: antenatal prediction of pulmonary maturity. Am J Obstet Gynecol 1973;115:547.
38. Kulovich M, Hallman M, Gluck L. The lung profile. I: normal pregnancy. Am J Obstet Gynecol 1979;135:57.
39. Kulovich M, Gluck L. The lung profile. II: complicated pregnancy. Am J Obstet Gynecol 1979;135:64.
40. Clements JA, Platzker ACG, Tierney DF, et al. Assessment of the risk of the respiratory distress syndrome by a rapid test for surfactant in amniotic fluid. N Engl J Med 1972;286:1077.
41. Goldstein AS, Fukunaga K, Malachowski N, Johnson JD. A comparison of the lecithin/sphingomyelin ratio and shake test for estimating fetal pulmonary maturity. Am J Obstet Gynecol 1972;118:1132.
42. Keniston KC, Noland GL, Pernoll ML. The effect of blood, meconium and temperature on the rapid surfactant test. Obstet Gynecol 1976;48:442.
43. Dubin SB. Determination of lamellar body size, number density, and concentration by differential light scattering from amniotic fluid: physical significance of A_{650}. Clin Chem 1988;34:938.
44. Copeland W. Rapid assessment of fetal pulmonary maturity. Am J Obstet Gynecol 1979;135:1048.
45. Freda VJ, James LS. Amniotic fluid microviscosity determined by fluorescence polarization: methodology and relation to gestational age. Pediatrics 1979;63:213.

46. Golde SH, Mosley GH. A blind comparison study of the lung phospholipid profile, fluorescence microviscosimetry and the lecithin/sphingomyelin ratio. Am J Obstet Gynecol 1980;136:222.
47. Russell JC, Cooper CM, Ketchum CH, et al. Multicenter evaluation of TD_x test for assessing fetal lung maturity. Clin Chem 1989;35:1005.
48. King RJ, Ruch J, Gikas EG, Platzker ACG, Creasy RK. Appearance of apoproteins of pulmonary surfactant in human amniotic fluid. J Appl Physiol 1975;39:735.
49. Shelley SA, Balis JU, Paciga JE, Knuppel RA, Ruffolo EH, Bours PJ. Surfactant apoproteins in human amniotic fluid. An enzyme linked immunosorbent assay for the prenatal assessment of lung maturity. Am J Obstet Gynecol 1982;144:224.
50. Hallman M, Arjomaa P, Mizumoto M, Akino T. Surfactant proteins in the diagnosis of fetal lung maturity. I: predictive accuracy of the 35 kd protein, the lecithin/sphingomyelin ratio, and phosphatidylglycerol. Am J Obstet Gynecol 1988;198:531.
51. Katyal SL, Singn AG, Silverman JA. Deficient lung surfactant apoproteins in amniotic fluid with mature phospholipid profile from diabetic pregnancies. Am J Obstet Gynecol 1984;148:48.
52. Ballard PL, Hawgood S, Liley H, et al. Regulation of pulmonary surfactant apoprotein SP 28–36 gene in human fetal lung. Proc Natl Acad Sci USA 1986;83:9527.
53. Mendelson CR, Boggaram V, Snyder JM, Odom MJ. Glucocorticoids have a biphasic effect on surfactant apoprotein (SP-35) synthesis and mRNA levels in human fetal lung in vitro. Pediatr Res 1988;25:248A.
54. Whitsett JA, Weaver TE, Clark JC, et al. Glucocorticoid enhances proteolipid Phe and pval synthesis and mRNA in fetal lung. J Biol Chem 1987;262:15618.
55. Palayoor T, Smart DA, Rooney SA. Glucocorticoid induced expression of the fatty acid synthase gene in fetal rat lung explants. FASEB J 1988;2:A1540.
56. Jacobs HC, Lima DM, Mercurio MR, Fiascone JM. Steroid effects on lung collagen and elastin are dependent on gestational age. Pediatr Res 1987;21:216A.
57. Mescher EJ, Platzker ACG, Ballard PL, Kitterman JA, Clements JA, Tooley WH. Ontogeny of tracheal fluid, pulmonary surfactant and plasma corticoids in the fetal lamb. J Appl Physiol 1975;39:1017.
58. Kitterman JA, Liggins GC, Campos GA, et al. Prepartum maturation of the lung in fetal sheep: relation to cortisol. J Appl Physiol 1981;51:384.
59. Liggins GC. Premature delivery of fetal lambs infused with glucocorticoids. J Endocrinol 1969;45:515.
60. DeLemos RA, Shermenta DW, Knelson JH, Kotas R, Avery ME. Acceleration of appearance of pulmonary surfactant in fetal lamb by administration of corticosteroids. Am Rev Resp Dis 1970;102:459.
61. Liggins GC, Howie RN. A controlled trial of antepartum glucocorticoid treatment for prevention of the respiratory distress syndrome in premature infants. Pediatrics 1972;50:515.
62. Morrison JC, Whybrew WD, Bucorag ET, Schneider JM. Injection of corticosteroids into mother to prevent neonatal respiratory distress syndrome. Am J Obstet Gynecol 1978;131:358.
63. Taeusch HW, Frigoletto F, Kitzmiller J, et al. Risk of respiratory distress syndrome after prenatal dexamethasone treatment. Pediatrics 1979;63:64.
64. Ballard RA, Ballard PL, Granberg JP, et al. Prenatal administration of betamethasone for prevention of respiratory distress syndrome. J Pediatr 1979;94:97.
65. Block MF, Kling OR, Crosby WM. Antenatal glucocorticoid therapy for the prevention of respiratory distress syndrome in the premature infant. Obstet Gynecol 1977;50:186.
66. Collaborative group on antenatal steroid therapy. Effect of antenatal dexamethasone administration on the prevention of respiratory distress syndrome. Am J Obstet Gynecol 1981;141:276.
67. Ballard PL. Combined hormonal treatment and lung maturation. Semin Perinatol 1984;8:283.
68. Papageorgiou AN, Desgranges MF, Masson M, Colle E, Shatz R, Gelfand MM. The antenatal use of betamethasone in the prevention of respiratory distress syndrome: a controlled double blind study. Pediatrics 1979;63:736.
69. Ballard PL, Ballard RA, Granberg JP, et al. Fetal sex and prenatal betamethasone therapy. J Pediatr 1980;97:451.
70. Romero R, Oyarzun E, Mazor M, et al. Meta analysis of the effect of steroids in the prevention of respiratory distress syndrome in premature rupture of membranes. Presented at 9th Annual Meeting of the Society of Perinatal Obstetricians, New Orleans, February 1990.
71. Ballard RA, Ballard PL, Creasy R, Gross I, Padbury JF, Collaborators in the TRH Study Group. Prenatal thyrotropin releasing hormone plus corticosteroid decreases chronic lung disease in very low birth weight infants. Pediatr Res 1991;29:307A.

10
CHAPTER

FETAL CARDIOVASCULAR PHYSIOLOGY UNDER NORMAL AND STRESS CONDITIONS

Deborah L. Reid

The fetal lifeline is a simple umbilical cord containing two arteries and one vein that connect the fetal circulation to the placenta, the organ of fetal gas exchange. Via the umbilical circulation, the fetus gains the nutrients and oxygen it requires for survival while losing carbon dioxide and other waste products. The cardiovascular system provides constant perfusion of the placenta and therefore facilitates these exchanges. To survive periods of stress the healthy fetus must have mechanisms that adjust the circulation to meet the metabolic requirements of organs that cannot tolerate short periods of oxygen deprivation.

Study of the regulation of the fetal cardiovascular system is a particular challenge to investigators. Very little work can be ethically tolerated in the human fetus. The sheep fetus is one of the few animal models large enough for cardiovascular studies. Therefore, unless otherwise stated, the information presented in this chapter is based on research conducted in the fetal sheep.

Even in sheep, many confounding factors exist that must be accounted for in the critical analysis of control systems. These variables include cardiovascular oscillations that accompany the clinically recognized characteristics of fetal behavioral states; changes in regional vascular resistances of important organs such as the placenta and brain[1–4]; changes in heart rate and arterial blood pressure; alterations in the levels of plasma catecholamines[5]; and modulation of the fetal heart rate pattern by fetal breathing movements.[6–9] Thus, the control of the fetal cardiovascular system is not as clearly understood as that in the adult. Considerable progress has been made toward elucidating the mechanisms that control the fetal cardiovascular system.

To the clinician, the control of the cardiovascular system is particularly important. Fetal heart rate, heart rate variability, and acid–base status are three important parameters available to monitor fetal well-being, particularly during labor. These indices are all manifestations of the state of the fetal cardiovascular system. A thorough understanding of the regulation of the cardiovascular system should therefore extend beyond mere academic interest.

CARDIOVASCULAR PHYSIOLOGY OF THE NORMAL NEAR-TERM FETUS

The circulation of the fetus is characterized by high cardiac output and blood volume (per kilogram weight) relative to that of the adult. High regional blood flows help to provide adequate delivery of oxygen and substrates. This is especially important, because fetal blood gas tensions and pH differ markedly from those of the adult. Normal fetal oxygen tensions range from 20 to 25 mm Hg in the fetus, as opposed to 80 to 100 mm Hg in adults. Fetal arterial carbon dioxide partial pressure, which ranges from 40 to 45 mm Hg, is higher than that in maternal blood, with values of 30 to 35 mm Hg. Likewise, normal fetuses are slightly acidotic, with pH values ranging from about 7.33 to 7.38, compared to the normal adult pH of 7.40. Fetal blood pressures are also markedly different from those of the adult, which has mean pressures of about 95 mm Hg. The mean arterial blood pressure ranges from about 45 to 50 mm Hg in the fetal lamb.

In the adult an oxygen tension of 20 mm Hg would result in hemoglobin saturations of only about 35%, whereas fetal arterial blood is more than 50% oxygen saturated at the same oxygen tension. This increased oxygen affinity can be accounted for by a specialized fetal hemoglobin that is able to combine with oxygen at much lower partial pressures than those of adult hemoglobin.[10] As seen in Figure 10-1, the fetal oxygen–hemoglobin dissociation curve is shifted to the left of the adult hemoglobin curve and exhibits a much steeper relationship between oxyhemoglobin and the partial pressure of oxygen. This latter adaptation probably allows hemoglobin to exchange oxygen for carbon dioxide in the periphery in response to much smaller changes in oxygen tension and therefore facilitates the removal of carbon dioxide as well. With these basic concepts in mind it is easier to understand how the fetus can successfully grow and develop in the low-oxygen environment of the uterus. The fetus has other unique mechanisms that will be addressed in the sections that follow.

HEMODYNAMIC AND ANATOMICAL CHARACTERISTICS OF NORMAL FETAL CIRCULATION

The fetal circulatory system is uniquely arranged to permit the survival of the fetus in the intrauterine environment. The pattern of fetal blood flow can be examined in Figure 10-2.[11] Four special vascular structures allow the fetus to circulate blood to the placenta for oxygenation rather than to the lungs. These structures are:

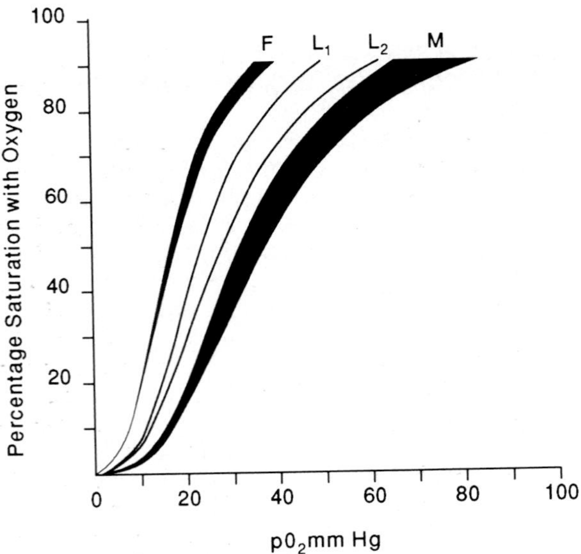

FIGURE 10–1. The oxygen hemoglobin dissociation curves for fetal (F), maternal (M), and newborn (L_1 and L_2) sheep blood. The graph depicts percentage of hemoglobin saturated with oxygen as a function of oxygen tension (Po_2). Values were adjusted for 38°C and pH 7.4. (Redrawn after Meschia G, Hellegers A, Blechner JN, Wolkoff AS, Barron DH. A comparison of the oxygen dissociation curves of the bloods of maternal, fetal and newborn sheep at various pHs. Quart J Exp Physiol 1961; 46: 95.)

1. The ductus venosus, a conduit between the umbilical vein and the inferior vena cava
2. The foramen ovale, a valvelike communication between the right and left atria of the fetus
3. The ductus arteriosus, a vessel connecting the pulmonary artery and the aorta
4. The umbilical vessels.

The anatomical arrangement of these central shunts permits the left and right ventricles to eject dissimilar stroke volumes such that fetal (biventricular) cardiac output is the sum of the outputs of the left and right ventricles.

Another characteristic that differentiates the fetal from the adult circulation is the high vascular resistance of the fetal pulmonary vascular bed. The mechanisms that maintain this high pulmonary vascular resistance are not clearly understood. The high resistance to blood flow serves to divert blood away from the relatively inactive fetal lungs, which are not needed for respiration in fetal life.

Venous Return

Of the total combined output of the fetal right and left ventricles, approximately 40% flows through the umbilical artery to perfuse the placenta.[12,13] The hemoglobin in blood flowing through the placenta acquires oxygen by diffusion and returns to the fetus through the umbilical veins 80% to 85% saturated with oxygen.

In the liver, the umbilical vein bifurcates and blood flow continues through the portal sinus and the ductus venosus, as shown in Figure 10-3.[14] About 45% of the umbilical blood flows through the portal sinus to perfuse the left, and to some degree the right, hepatic lobe. The remainder of the right hepatic blood supply is contributed by the portal vein with only 10% of the blood supplied by the hepatic artery.[15] Thus, the fetal liver is supplied with blood high in oxygen and nutrients and, in the sheep, receives more than 20% of combined biventricular cardiac output.

The remaining 55% of the umbilical blood flow is shunted through the ductus venosus into the inferior vena cava, where it joins oxygen-depleted blood returning from the fetal hindlimbs. This confluence undergoes very little mixing. Filmy, valvelike structures at the proximal orifice of the ductus venosus apparently direct the bloodstream along the perimeter of the inferior vena cava. This probably serves to minimize the turbulence that would otherwise promote a homogeneous mixture in the inferior vena cava.[16] Similar structures exist at the entrances of the right and left hepatic veins into the inferior vena caval stream. As a result of this incomplete mixing, the oxygen- and nutrient-rich blood originating from the umbilical vein continues its path within the left dorsal portion of the inferior vena cava, and the remainder of the vessel is occupied by blood returning from the lower body via the distal inferior vena cava, where hemoglobin is about 67% saturated.[17] In such fashion the inferior vena caval blood

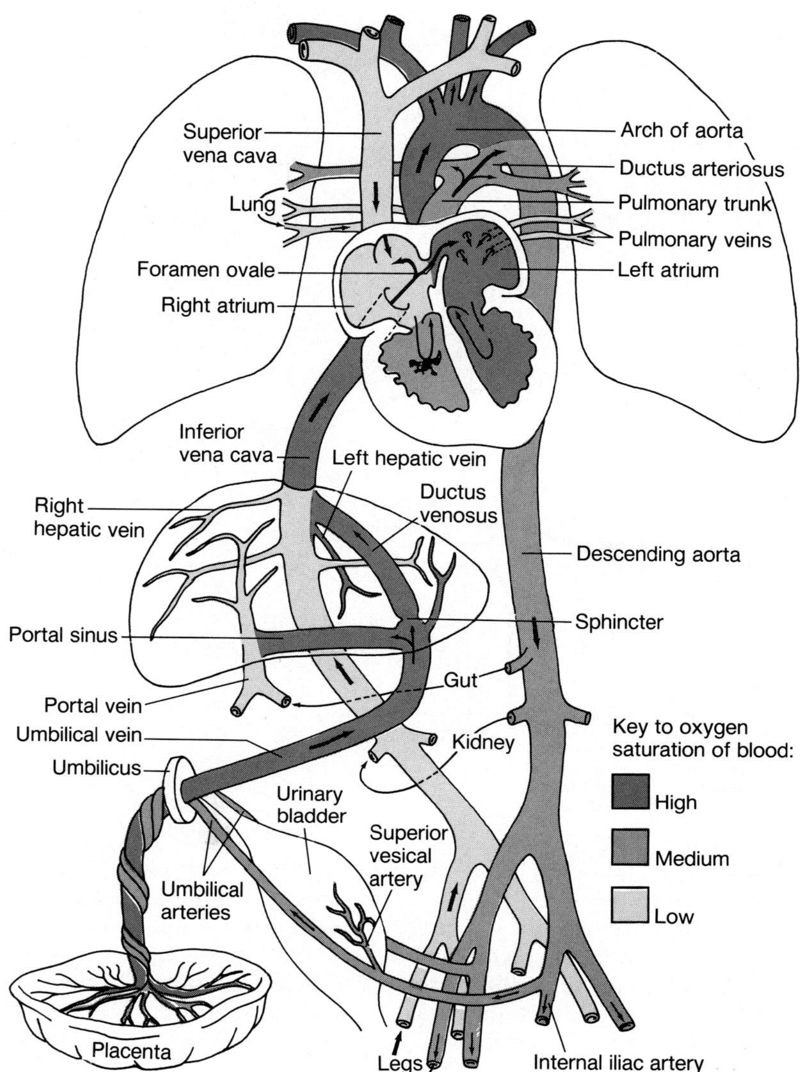

FIGURE 10–2. Schematic diagram of the human fetal circulation. The degree of oxygen saturation is indicated by shading, as explained in the figure key. (Redrawn after Moore KL. The developing human. 3rd ed. Philadelphia: WB Saunders, 1982.)

flows toward the right atrium. In addition, superior vena caval blood drains the fetal upper body toward the right atrium and is only 30% to 40% oxygen saturated. Because of the anatomical arrangement of the inflow vessels, the bloodstream entering the right atrium from the superior vena cava does not mix completely with the stream from the inferior vena cava. The physiologic importance of this phenomenon will be addressed shortly.

Central Blood Flow Patterns

Most of the oxygenated blood returning to the heart via the inferior vena cava bypasses the right atrium. Inferior vena caval blood is partitioned into two branches by the crista dividens, the lower margin of the septum secundum. The first, and major, fork is the foramen ovale; the second is termed the inferior caval inlet and leads to the right atrium.[18] The relative positions of these two branches can be better appreciated from Figure 10-4, which is a Silastic cast made from the atria of a fetal sheep.[19] The kinetic energy of the stream in the inferior vena cava propels it through the channel of the foramen ovale and into the left atrium, bypassing the right atrium.[19–21] This route through the foramen ovale represents a flow shunt, which carries about 34% of biventricular output from the right side of the circulation to the left and permits oxygenated blood to bypass the pulmonary circulation.

The physiologic importance of the streaming that occurs in the inferior vena cava becomes apparent at this point in the circulatory pattern. The bloodstream is split so that the majority of the blood of umbilical origin along with some distal venous blood traverses the foramen ovale into the left atrium.[22] The remainder is deflected through the inferior caval inlet into the right atrium and continues into the right ventricle through the tricuspid valve. Thus, the blood with the highest oxygen and nutrient content is shunted to the left atrium for distribution to the preductal circulation (ie,

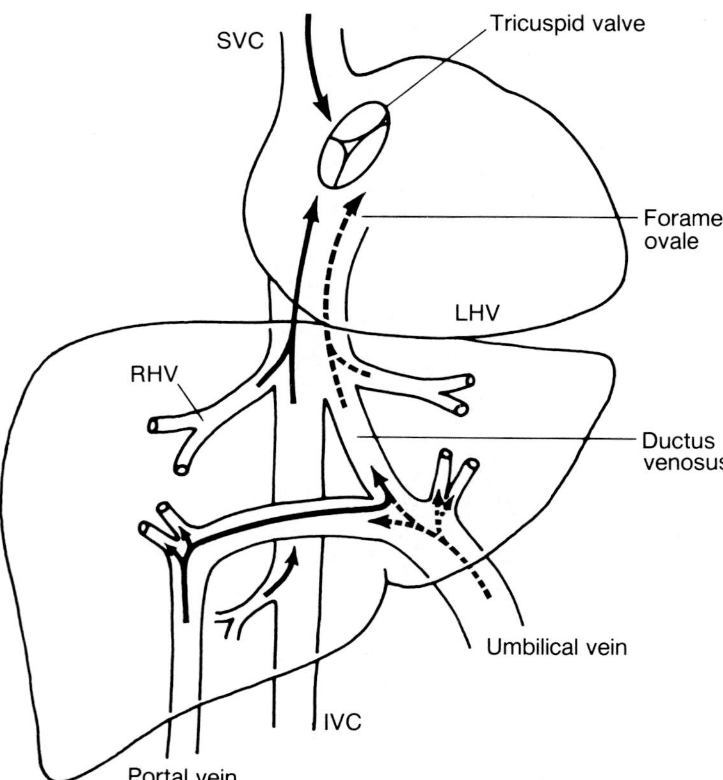

FIGURE 10–3. Diagram of venous return through the liver in the fetal lamb. Blood from the umbilical vein and left hepatic vein (LHV) flows into the proximal inferior vena cava without mixing with blood from the distal inferior vena cava (IVC) and right hepatic vein (RHV). SVC, superior vena cava. (Redrawn after Rudolph AM. Hepatic and ductus venosus blood flows during fetal life. Hepatology 1983; 3: 254.)

the aortic arch and its branches); the blood of systemic origin, with a lower oxygen content, passes through the right atrium to the right ventricle. (These differences in oxygen content are depicted schematically in Fig. 10-2.) In addition, most of the blood returning from the upper body via the superior vena cava enters the right atrium and is directed across the tricuspid valve and into the right ventricle. Blood is ejected from the right ventricle via the pulmonary artery 50% to 55% saturated with oxygen. The pulmonary artery bifurcates at the ductus arteriosus, providing a route by which blood leaving the right ventricle can flow either through the ductus arteriosus or into the pulmonary vascular bed. Since vascular resistance of the pulmonary circuit exceeds that of the systemic circuit, most of the pulmonary arterial blood is diverted through the ductus arteriosus to increase further the flow through the systemic circulation. This creates a second fetal right-to-left shunt. These two shunts permit the fetal lungs to receive only about 5% to 10% of the combined output of both ventricles, rather than the entire cardiac output (or, in fetal terms, one half of biventricular cardiac output) as in the adult circulation.

Cardiac Output and Distribution

The small volume of blood returning from the lungs flows through the pulmonary veins that empty into the left atrium. This blood mixes in the left atrium with the well-oxygenated blood entering through the foramen ovale from the right side of the circulation and is ejected from the left ventricle into the aorta. The coronary arteries branch immediately from the aorta and supply the myocardium with well-oxygenated blood. In the human, several arteries branch from the aorta at the level of the aortic arch to supply the fetal upper body. This anatomical arrangement provides blood to the fetal brain and heart that is about 60% to 65% saturated with oxygen. Thus, the liver, the myocardium, and the upper body, including the brain, receive the most highly oxygenated blood supply in the fetus. At the ductus arteriosus the less oxygenated blood (52% saturated), representing about 54% of biventricular cardiac output in the fetal sheep,[21] is shunted from the pulmonary artery and joins blood in the aorta. The rest of the body is thus perfused with blood that is about 58% saturated with oxygen. Much of this blood flows to the placenta, where oxygen and nutrients are replenished and waste products are removed.

Although the percentage of biventricular cardiac output to various organs has been determined in fetal sheep studies, these data cannot be applied accurately to the human fetal circulation. Brain blood flow is a much greater proportion of cardiac output in the primate than in the sheep fetus.[23] This distribution therefore affects the relative portion of biventricular output supplied to all other fetal organs, but the differences have not been quantitated.

Whereas blood in the adult is pumped through the systemic and pulmonary circuits in series, the fetal cir-

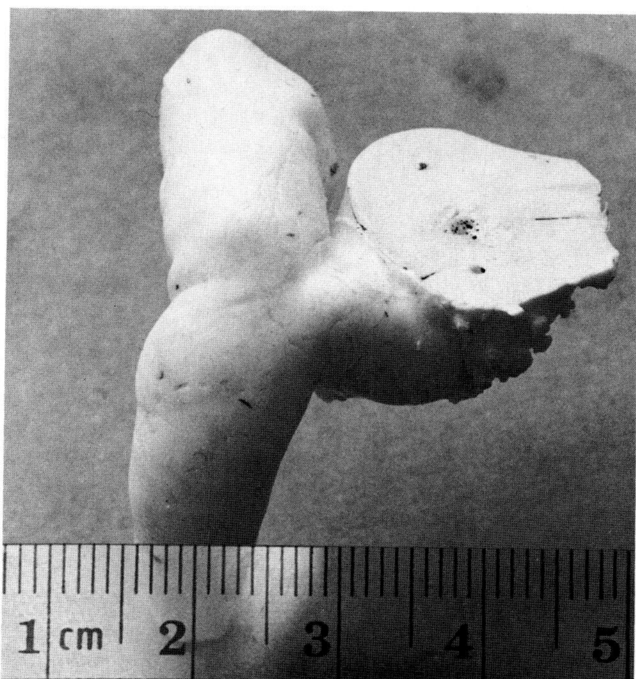

FIGURE 10–4. Silastic cast of the inferior caval inlet and foramen ovale (FO) in a fetal lamb. The inferior caval inlet is the connection between the inferior vena cava (IVC) and the right atrium (RA). The two channels are divided by the crista dividens (CD) of the atrial septum. Note that the blood that passes through the foramen ovale never enters the right atrium. (From Anderson DF, Faber JJ, Morton MJ, Parks CM, Pinson CW, Thornburg KL. Flow through the foramen ovale of the fetal and newborn lamb. J Physiol 1985; 365: 29.)

culations are arranged largely in parallel. Therefore, instead of referring to cardiac output as that from a single ventricle as in the adult, fetal cardiac output is expressed as biventricular output, the sum of the outputs of the left and right ventricles. The ovine fetal right ventricle contributes slightly more to the combined output of the heart than does the left. Estimates of right ventricular output in the ovine fetus range from 60% to 67% of biventricular output.[21,24] Despite initial reports to the contrary,[25,26] it now appears that the human fetal heart is also right-side dominant, although right ventricular output may be as little as 55% of the combined ventricular outputs.[27–31]

Although nearly all the work on fetal arterial and venous blood flows has been performed in sheep, much work has been reported on flows within the human fetal heart through the use of velocimetry and two-dimensional Doppler echocardiography. With these methods both velocity of blood flow and vessel diameter can be estimated; with proper application, the technique can yield fairly accurate measurements of the volume flow of blood through the fetal heart and great vessels.[32] Although the physical constraints of human fetal studies prevent strict adherence to these standards, the data from these studies are still valuable. These data reveal that although the peak velocities of blood flowing through the left side of the fetal heart are approximately 10% greater than those on the right side of the heart, mean velocities are similar.[29,31] The annular diameters of the atrioventricular (mitral and tricuspid) and semilunar (pulmonary and aortic) valves of each ventricle appear to differ, with the right side tracts wider than the left. This yields a dominant flow through the right ventricle compared to the left, a relationship that holds true irrespective of gestational age.[28,31,33] Mean blood flows from 18 normal human fetuses between 26 and 30 weeks gestation, presented in Figure 10-5, show that the right ventricle clearly has a greater output than the left, with a ratio of 1.33 to 1.[30] Some researchers have reported that the right ventricular to left ventricular output ratio begins to decline toward the end of gestation.[34]

As the fetus matures, both ventricular outflows rise. Increased cardiac output with fetal development is

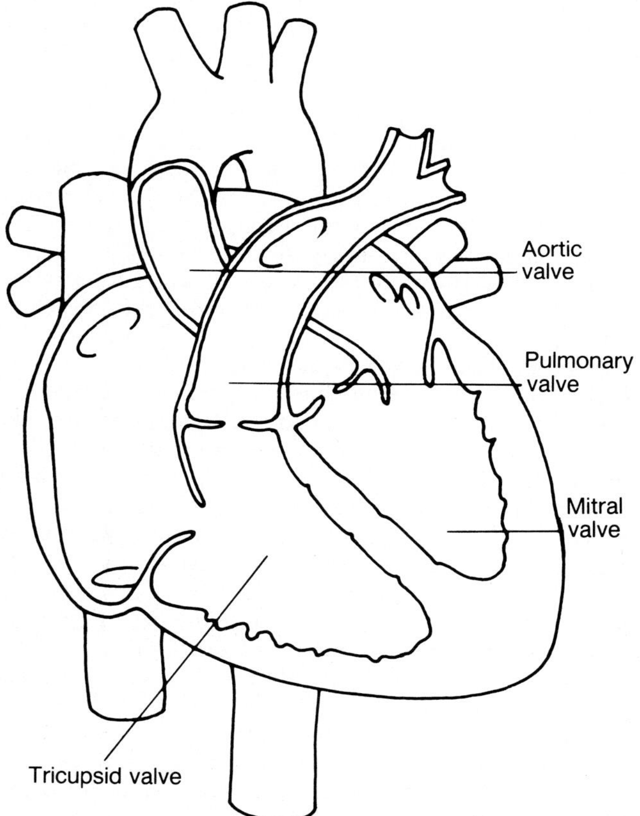

FIGURE 10–5. Schematic diagram of the human fetal heart depicting flow ($mL \cdot min^{-1} \cdot kg^{-1}$) across the tricuspid valve, pulmonary valve, mitral valve, and aortic valve. (Redrawn from Reed KL, Anderson CF, Shenker L. Changes in intracardiac Doppler blood flow velocities in fetuses with absent umbilical artery diastolic flow. Am J Obstet Gynecol 1987; 157: 774.)

probably due to growth of the ventricles and outflow tracts, rather than to an increase in mean velocity of blood flowing through the ventricles.[28,31]

CONTROL OF CARDIAC OUTPUT

The determinants of biventricular output in the fetus are essentially the same as for cardiac output in the adult: heart rate and stroke volume. In the adult it is recognized that stroke volume can be changed by alterations in any of the following:

1. Preload, the force per unit area that "stretches" the myocardium before contraction
2. Afterload, the force per unit area exerted during contraction
3. Contractility, the strength of contraction in response to a stimulus
4. Chamber size.

These factors have been investigated in the fetal sheep and in the human fetus to varying degrees.

In the heart, atrial filling pressure is considered a fairly accurate indicator of preload in the myocardium. In the adult heart there is a small amount of preload reserve; that is, when atrial pressure increases, end diastolic pressure rises and stroke volume increases. Increases in left and right atrial pressures have little effect on fetal stroke volume.[24,35–37] This is because the fetus operates at the top of the steep portion of its cardiac function (or Frank-Starling) curve, as shown in Figure 10-6.[24] From the normal operating point in the fetal heart, increases in atrial pressure cause only minimal increases in stroke volume. On the other hand, a small decrease in preload can cause a sharp fall in fetal stroke volume.

Although the left and right sides of the heart seem to have equal sensitivities to preload, this is not true for afterload. Arterial blood pressure, the major component of myocardial afterload, has dissimilar effects on the left and right ventricles. Although both respond to an increase in afterload with decreased stroke volume, left ventricular output is affected very little compared to the right ventricle, which is exquisitely sensitive to changes in arterial blood pressure.[24,36–38] Conversely, a decrease in afterload increases both left and right ventricular output but has a more powerful effect on right ventricular output.[36,37] Thus, diminished arterial blood pressure can cause increased right and, to a lesser extent, left ventricular stroke volume.

Fetal myocardial contractility has been given very little research attention, except in the immediate perinatal period; these changes will be discussed in the section on the fetus in transition. Contractility of the normal fetal lamb ventricle may increase slightly as the fetus matures, but the cause of this additional strength of contraction has not been explored.[39]

The relationship between chamber size and stroke volume in the fetal lamb has been well studied. There are no sudden changes in fetal chamber size that might

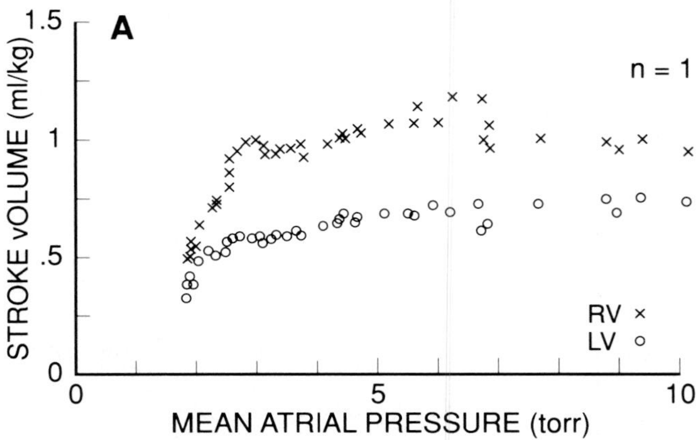

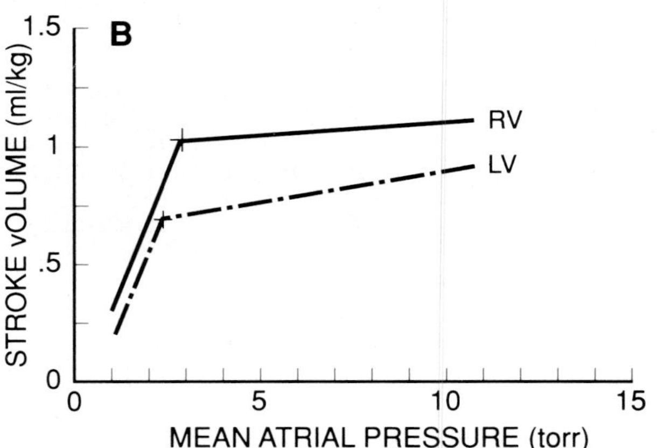

FIGURE 10-6. Average relationship between preload (mean arterial pressure) and stroke volume in the fetal sheep. (**A**) Simultaneous stroke volumes of the right (+) and left (□) ventricle are shown during simultaneous changes in mean right and left atrial pressures generated by withdrawal and reinfusion of fetal blood. (**B**) Average relationship between preload and stroke volume of the right (RV) and left (LV) ventricles in 12 fetal lambs. (Redrawn from Reller MD, Morton MJ, Reid DL, Thornburg KL. Fetal lamb ventricles respond differently to filling and arterial pressures and to in utero ventilation. Pediatr Res 1987; 22: 621.)

influence regulation of cardiac output until parturition, although there is a steady enlargement of the chambers throughout gestation.[28,31] Still, the growth of the ventricular chambers with maturity undoubtedly plays an important role in the slow increase in fetal cardiac output with advancing maturity.

It has been suggested that in the absence of a mechanism for substantial changes in fetal stroke volume, the primary regulator of cardiac output is heart rate. This issue has been studied in both human and ovine fetuses. Acceleration of human fetal heart rate by vibroacoustic stimulation has been shown to have no effect on cardiac output.[40] It is likely that the heart rate response in this study was stimulated by a rise in catecholamine levels that would simultaneously increase arterial blood pressure and might therefore decrease right ventricular stroke volume independent of the heart rate effect. The heart rate issue has also been examined in fetal sheep under natural conditions and in response to atrial pacing.[41,42] When the relationship between heart rate, stroke volume, and cardiac output was examined during spontaneous variations in fetal heart rate, heart rate was positively correlated with biventricular cardiac output and stroke volume was unaffected. When the right atrium was artificially paced, right ventricular stroke volume decreased in such a way that cardiac output remained constant. When the left atrium was paced, left ventricular stroke volume decreased to such a degree that overall cardiac output was decreased as well. Thus, although cardiac output can be affected by heart rate, it is apparently only increased within the normal range of fetal heart rate.

Heart rate demonstrates a slow decline with gestational age. As shown schematically in Figure 10-7,[43] the fetal heart rate can be considered as the sum of two components: intrinsic heart rate and the net influence of autonomic and hormonal factors. In the nonstressed fetus, hormonal factors have little or no influence on fetal heart rate. In the first 15 weeks of human gestation (developmental phase 1 portrayed in Fig. 10-7), the autonomic nervous system is immature and has no influence on heart rate.[44] Thus, the decline in heart rate at this stage in gestation is due solely to changes in the frequency of myocardial pacemaker activity. After the fifteenth week, the influence of the autonomic nervous system on the heart rate gradually increases. As in the adult, beta-stimulation by the sympathetic nervous system increases fetal heart rate, whereas the parasympathetic nervous system depresses heart rate. In the normal fetus, the parasympathetic nervous system exerts a greater influence on heart rate than the sympathetic nervous system and is therefore responsible for the gradual decrease in human fetal heart rate from about 15 weeks' gestation until term.

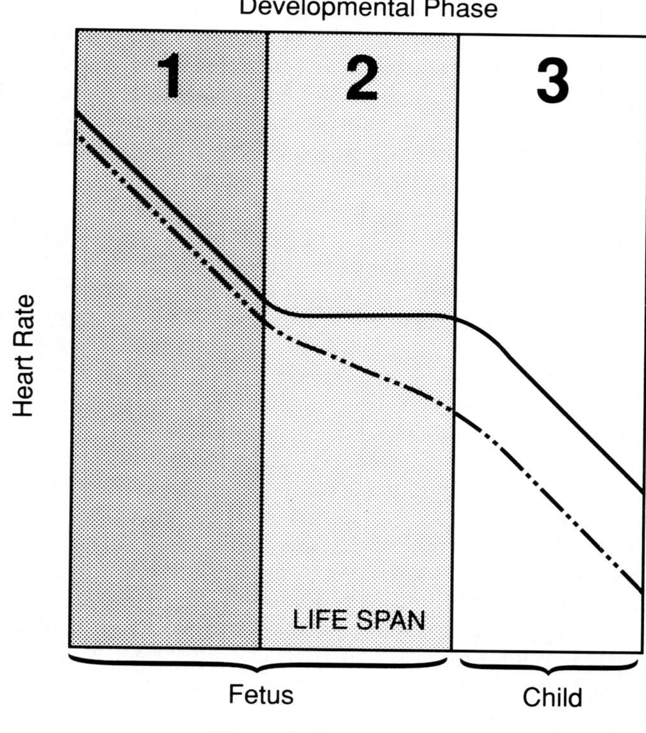

FIGURE 10–7. Changes in heart rate with fetal maturation. The intrinsic rate is the heart rate with no autonomic influence, whereas normal rate is the heart rate that exists under the influence of the autonomic nervous system. During late gestation (developmental phase 2) the normal heart rate begins to decline in response to increasing autonomic nervous input. (From Walker AM. Physiological control of the fetal cardiovascular system. In: Fetal physiology and medicine: the basis of perinatology. 2nd ed. New York: Marcel Dekker, 1984: 287.)

THE NORMAL FETUS: CONTROL OF BLOOD PRESSURE AND DISTRIBUTION OF CARDIAC OUTPUT

There are three fetal organs whose perfusion is critical for normal fetal development and survival: the brain, the heart, and the placenta. The brain and heart are capable of autoregulation to maintain adequate perfusion and oxygen delivery. The brain is able to vasodilate to an extent that maintains close to normal oxygen deliveries even under conditions of severe acute hypoxia.[45–48] The power of the cerebral response to hypotension is markedly reduced from adult levels of autoregulation.[49–51] The fetal myocardium is also capable of tremendous vasodilation in response to hypoxia.[47,48,52–54] The placenta, on the other hand, is not capable of autoregulation[55]; it appears to be totally dependent on perfusion pressure. Therefore, the regulation of arterial blood pressure is critically important to the fetus.

Baroreceptors

Carotid and Aortic Arch Baroreceptors. In the adult the baroreceptors play an important role in the short-term regulation of arterial blood pressure. Changes in blood pressure cause a change in the rate of firing in the carotid sinus or aortic arch baroreceptors. These impulses are relayed to the nucleus tractus solitarius via the carotid sinus and vagal nerves. Outgoing impulses are sent to the heart and to peripheral blood vessels to alter heart rate and vascular resistance, respectively, in compensation for the change in blood pressure sensed by the baroreceptors. The development and activity of baroreceptors in the fetus constitute an area of intense interest and great relevance to the health of the fetus. Blood pressure homeostasis may be even more important to the fetus than to the adult, as it determines the level of placental perfusion and therefore the extent to which respiratory gas exchange can occur.

The bulk of the research, which has been performed in fetal sheep, focused on the heart rate response limb of the baroreceptor reflex. An acute increase in arterial blood pressure causes an immediate fall in heart rate.[56–58] In acute surgical preparations, electrical activity of the baroreceptors has been demonstrated to coincide precisely with induced changes in blood pressure.[59,60] Denervation of the baroreceptors completely eliminates the heart rate response to changes in blood pressure in conscious, chronically instrumented fetal sheep.[59,61] Therefore, fetal baroreceptors are undoubtedly present and capable of responding to a stimulus, and the heart rate response limb appears to be operative.

The larger question, however, is whether baroreceptors play a role in the physiologic regulation of blood pressure. Studies on the fetal response to abrupt changes in blood volume suggest that the sympathetic arm of the feedback loop (which controls vascular resistance) does not function in the fetus to the degree it operates in the adult, since fetuses were unable to maintain normal blood pressure under these conditions.[62] Denervation studies have revealed that under normal conditions the fluctuations in arterial blood pressure more than double in the absence of baroreceptor control mechanisms.[59,61] Furthermore, fetuses with denervated baroreceptors were also shown to have slightly (5 mm Hg) higher mean arterial blood pressures than sham operated control animals.[59] Therefore, it appears that the baroreceptors are important in maintaining a constant blood pressure under normal conditions and that tonic activity may regulate the blood pressure at an absolute level. The baroreceptor reflex does not appear to be able to compensate for large perturbations in arterial blood pressure by way of a change in vascular resistance. This may be due to the large volume of blood that flows to the placenta, an organ that is not under autonomic control, and to the relative immaturity of the fetal sympathetic nervous system.

Renal Baroreceptor. Another major "baroreceptor" or arterial blood pressure control system of the fetus (and of the adult) is the renin–angiotensin system in the kidneys. This topic is covered in detail in Chapter 12 and is therefore only briefly summarized here. The macula densa senses a change in renal perfusion pressure and reacts by altering plasma renin secretion in the opposite direction. For example, plasma renin activity increases in logarithmic proportions in response to a decrease in renal arterial blood pressure.[63] Renin is the rate-limiting enzyme in the conversion of angiotensinogen to angiotensin I and thence to angiotensin II, a potent vasoconstrictor and pressor agent. In the sheep fetus, an isolated decrease in renal perfusion pressure can cause hypertension in the fetal upper body to a degree that serves to return renal perfusion to near-normal levels.[64] Thus, although the physiologic contribution of the carotid and aortic baroreceptors to the control of blood pressure is somewhat uncertain, the renal baroreceptor mechanism is definitely active in the mature fetal lamb.

Hormonal Control of Blood Pressure

Because of the nature of regulatory mechanisms, it is generally easier to study the contribution of a given mechanism under abnormal conditions. Such is the case with cardiovascular control in the fetus. Although a fair amount is known about the fetus under stress, very little work has been done to elucidate the control of the fetal circulation under normal conditions. Some important information has been gleaned from studies that block the effects of proposed regulators; these include angiotensin II, arginine vasopressin (or antidiuretic hormone), the parasympathetic nervous system, and beta- and alpha-adrenergic receptors. A change in cardiovascular status when a class of receptors is blocked suggests that the endogenous hormone that stimulates that receptor contributes to the regulation of the cardiovascular system in the normal fetus. In contrast, a cardiovascular response to infusion of a hormone merely suggests that it can contribute to cardiovascular control under conditions that would stimulate an endogenous increase in plasma levels of the hormone.

Blockade of the effects of angiotensin II by the drug saralasin causes a moderate fall in blood pressure of about 12%, a twofold increase in plasma renin activity, a pressure-dependent fall in placental perfusion, and redistribution of blood flow to the skin, muscle, bone, thyroid, and adrenal glands.[65] It appears that angiotensin II normally acts to maintain blood pressure, thus providing adequate blood flow to the placenta, but does not have an effect on heart rate or combined biventricular output. On the other hand, infusion of angiotensin II causes beta-adrenergic and cholinergic-independent increases in arterial blood pressure; increased placental resistance (with no associated change in blood flow); gastrointestinal, renal, and thyroid vasoconstriction; and myocardial and pulmonary vasodilation.[66,67] Dose–response curves for the effect of angiotensin II infusion lead to the conclusion that any role that angiotensin II may play in maintaining sufficient placental perfusion is working at its greatest efficiency under normal conditions; even small increases in angiotensin II levels cause no further increase in umbilical blood flow, but rather increase umbilical resistance.[68] Thus, it appears that angiotensin II plays an important role in normal cardiovascular physiology and could play a role in aberrant conditions.

The effects of arginine vasopressin on the fetus have been studied primarily by increasing plasma levels. However, a recent study reports no effect of arginine vasopressin blockade on vascular pressures, heart rate, or blood gas tensions.[69] Therefore, it is unlikely that arginine vasopressin exerts a tonic influence on the normal fetal circulation. However, arginine vasopressin infusion increases blood pressure, decreases heart rate, and has no effect on the absolute level of cardiac output.[70,71] Arginine vasopressin also causes a redistribution of blood flows to the heart, brain, and placenta while decreasing flows to peripheral organs. As will be discussed later in this chapter, this pattern of blood flow is highly reminiscent of that in the distressed fetus.

Contributions of the Adrenal Medulla and Autonomic Nervous System to Regulation of Blood Pressure

The magnitude of the parasympathetic influence on the maturing fetal cardiovascular system has been examined with antagonist studies.[72] Elimination of parasympathetic tone causes an increase in fetal heart rate that begins at about 85 days (of a 147-day) gestation in the fetal lamb. The importance of parasympathetic tone increases with age. In fetuses less than 100 days gestation, the heart rate increased only 5% of the baseline rate in response to blockade of the parasympathetic nervous system. In animals at 100 to 120 days gestation, heart rate increased slightly more than 15% when the parasympathetic influence was blocked. No further increases in response were elicited after 120 days gestation.

A cardiovascular response to blockade of the alpha-adrenergic or beta-adrenergic receptors indicates only the presence of receptor and postreceptor mechanisms. It does not necessarily indicate that the sympathetic nervous system exerts a tonic influence on the cardiovascular system. Cardiovascular alpha- and beta-receptor stimulation can occur in response to adrenal medullary release of epinephrine and norepinephrine or as a result of sympathetic stimulation. In turn, circulating catecholamine release from the adrenal medulla can be elicited by two mechanisms. Neural stimulation can cause adrenal catecholamine release in both the mature fetus and the adult; the fetal adrenal glands can also release catecholamines in response to a direct stimulus such as hypoxia.

In the fetus, the sympathetic nervous system develops sequentially. First, neurotransmitter uptake and degradation mechanisms develop; next, the response to transmitter activation of the receptor appears; and finally, the preganglionic neuronal synapse develops the ability to release neural transmitters.[73] Hence, the end organ response to catecholamines develops prior to full maturation of the autonomic nervous system, and the response to adrenal medullary release of catecholamines is of primary importance throughout most of gestation. Recent evidence suggests that the adrenal medulla itself is innervated at 0.75 gestation.[74] This innervation is probably not complete until about 130 days (0.9) gestation in the fetal lamb. At this point in gestation the adrenal medulla exhibits a diminished response to a direct stimulus and must rely primarily on neural stimulation for catecholamine release. Even when the autonomic nervous system is fully developed, fetal end organ response (in both blood vessels and the heart) is of a much smaller magnitude than the adult response. The natural role of alpha- and beta-receptors in regulation of fetal cardiovascular state can be determined by selective blockade of adrenergic receptors.

Elimination of endogenous beta-receptor stimulation causes decreases in heart rate from 85 days gestation onward in the fetal lamb.[72] The chronotropic influence of beta-receptor stimulation on fetal heart rate increases to a maximum of 15% of control heart rate as the fetus matures.

Blockade of the alpha-adrenergic receptors causes a decrease in arterial blood pressure that increases in magnitude as gestation progresses until gestational day 120, after which no further increases occur.[72,75] This indicates a fully developed fetal alpha-adrenergic receptor system at 120 days (0.80) gestation and demonstrates that the alpha-adrenergic receptor system exerts a tonic vasoconstrictive influence on the fetal vasculature.

CARDIOVASCULAR PHYSIOLOGY OF THE FETUS IN THE TRANSITION PERIOD

The period during which mammalian circulation changes from the fetal pattern to the adultlike pattern of neonatal life is termed the *transition period.* As parturition begins, several changes in the fetal circulation become characteristic of the "transitional circulation." The most readily observable of these is the loss of the placental circulation as the umbilical cord is tied or severed. Collapse and functional closure of the umbilical vessels and of the ductus venosus closely follow the events of birth. In the fetus, the placenta has a low vascular resistance. When the neonate is separated from the placenta, systemic vascular resistance rises as a result of the loss of the umbilical circuit and of active systemic vasoconstriction.

HEMODYNAMIC AND ANATOMICAL CHANGES IN THE TRANSITIONAL CIRCULATION

The most obvious feature of birth is the onset of ventilation. Since 1952, it has been known that the first breaths of air cause pulmonary vascular resistance to fall dramatically.[76] The drop in resistance is associated temporally with increased left atrial pressure, pulmonary blood flow, and volume.[77,78] Left atrial pressure increases and soon exceeds pressure in the inferior vena cava. This acts to reverse the pressure gradient across the foramen ovale, and in some species closes the septum secundum, which covers the left side of the atrial septum, and inhibits left-to-right flow through the foramen ovale. This functionally closes the foramen ovale.

The combination of decreased pulmonary vascular resistance and increased systemic resistance causes a reversal in the direction of flow through the ductus arteriosus.[79,80] Under these conditions, pulmonary blood flow (as opposed to right ventricular output) is probably more than 50% of biventricular cardiac output. The blood flowing through the pulmonary vessels exchanges gases with the gases filling the neonatal lung.

Thus, blood leaving the lungs of the neonate has a higher oxygen content and tension and lower carbon dioxide tension than ever before encountered by the fetus. Human neonates attain carotid arterial PO_2 values slightly greater than 60 mm Hg and PCO_2 values slightly below 40 mm Hg within 1 hour of birth.[81] The increased oxygen tension has several actions on the circulation. It appears to stimulate constriction of the systemic vessels, increasing systemic vascular resistance beyond that expected by the loss of the placental circulation. Second, it causes constriction of the ductus arteriosus. Thus, two major shunts of the fetal circulation close when the neonate begins to breathe, and within 24 hours the series circulation of the adult is established.

Closure of the ductus arteriosus in response to increased oxygen concentration has been studied and reviewed in detail.[82] On closure of the ductus arteriosus, pulmonary and systemic arterial pressure change in opposite directions. Pulmonary arterial pressure declines with decreasing pulmonary vascular resistance to a value still greater than normal adult pressure but substantially lower than fetal pulmonary artery pressures.[75] In contrast, aortic pressures increase as the ductus arteriosus closes. It should be noted that the closure of the ductus arteriosus appears to be due to active constriction and that the constricted condition can be reversed during the first few hours of life by decreased arterial oxygen tension.[82]

The vascular shunts unique to the parallel circulation of the fetus are no longer patent in the normal adult, but their remnants are recognizable. The ligamentum arteriosum and ligamentum venosum are fused vestiges of the ductus arteriosus and ductus venosum, respectively. The fossa ovalis is a depression in the atrial septum that replaces the foramen ovale. Likewise, the vessels of the umbilical circulation can be identified in the adult. The umbilical vein becomes the ligamentum teres and the remnants of the umbilical arteries become the lateral umbilical ligaments.

CONTROL OF CARDIAC OUTPUT IN THE PERINATAL PERIOD

A third major circulatory change that accompanies birth is an increase in cardiac output. Changes in heart rate and stroke volume both contribute to increased output at birth, but stroke volume is the primary factor. Stroke volumes increase from 1.1 and 1.4 mL · kg^{-1} for the left and right fetal ventricles, respectively, to approximately 2.0 mL · kg^{-1} with right and left ventricular output equal within 24 hours of birth.[83,84]

In the adult, the four well-recognized mechanisms that can mediate increases in ventricular stroke volume include increased sarcomere length (preload), increased strength of contraction (contractility), decreased load on the sarcomeres during contraction (afterload), and increased chamber size.[85] Mean atrial pressure is one of the more commonly used indices of preload. The relationship between mean atrial pressure and stroke volume has been studied extensively in the fetal lamb.[35,36,86] The fetus operates at a filling pressure that produces near maximal stroke volume, so that it has little preload reserve. Therefore, simultaneous increases in mean atrial pressure above the operation point cause only very small increases in stroke volume. One must conclude that increased atrial pressure is not the only mechanism that augments stroke volume at birth.

Other mechanisms that may be responsible for the birth-related increase in stroke volume have been studied by ventilating fetuses in utero. During in utero ventilation and at birth, the left ventricular function curve that relates mean atrial pressure (preload) to ventricular stroke volume is shifted upward,[84] so that stroke volume is larger at the same filling pressure. An increase in contractility could cause such a shift. To shed some light on the contractility issue, the shift in dimensions of the left ventricle during contraction has been examined in both fetal and neonatal states.[87,88] Although fractional shortening (ie, the amount the ventricle contracts with each beat) is slightly greater in neonates than in fetuses,[88] this change may not be due entirely to changes in contractility and cannot account for the magnitude of change in stroke volume at birth.

The effect of arterial pressure on stroke volume has been examined in the fetus as a method to estimate afterload sensitivity,[24,36,38] although it should be noted that the relation between arterial pressure and systolic wall tension has not been adequately studied in the fetus. These studies show that the right ventricle is very sensitive to decreases in arterial pressure, whereas the left ventricle is relatively insensitive.[24,84] Even if the left ventricle were sensitive to arterial pressure, systemic arterial pressure generally increases at birth and thus would not be a mechanism for increasing left ventricular stroke volume.

The final mechanism available to the fetus to augment stroke volume at birth is an acute increase in ventricular chamber size. Although this possibility has not yet been adequately studied, evidence from fetal and neonatal humans using echocardiographic imaging suggests that left ventricular dimension increases and right ventricular dimension decreases slightly after birth.[25,89,90] This may come about as the result of ventricular interaction with the formation of a left–right ventricular gradient. That is, the pressure in the left ventricle exceeds that in the right ventricle. This forces the interventricular septum to the right and increases left ventricular chamber size. Therefore, the mechanism for increasing right ventricular stroke volume at birth appears to be a fall in pulmonary artery pressure, whereas increased chamber size is the most likely explanation for the increase in left ventricular stroke volume.

CONTROL OF PULMONARY VASCULAR RESISTANCE IN THE PERINATAL PERIOD

The mechanisms behind the fall in pulmonary vascular resistance with the onset of ventilation constitute a subject that has generated much controversy. After several reversals in prevailing opinion, it now appears that increased pulmonary blood flow at birth is the result of a complex interplay of several basic mechanisms. It has been classically believed that the fetal pulmonary vasculature is tonically constricted due to the low oxygen environment of the fetus. It was theorized that the increase in oxygen at birth caused the pulmonary blood vessels to dilate. This theory was the so-called release from hypoxic pulmonary vasoconstriction. The concept is derived from the well-described adult phenomenon but is an oversimplification of the regulation of the fetal pulmonary vascular bed. There is evidence from several groups that the initiators of the chain of events leading to pulmonary vasodilation at birth include the separate effects of mechanical ventilation without a change in arterial blood gas tensions, increased oxygen tension, and decreased carbon dioxide tension, with its concomitant increase in pH.

The Influence of Mechanical Ventilation on Pulmonary Blood Flow

Mechanical ventilation of fetal lamb lungs with respiratory gases low in oxygen and relatively replete with carbon dioxide cause an increase in pulmonary blood flow.[77,80,91,92] These studies suggest that mechanical action alone contributes to the fall in pulmonary vascular resistance. Some caution must be used in the interpretation of these studies, as very small local changes in alveolar oxygen or carbon dioxide tensions could also be involved in these changes in vascular tone. Interestingly, mechanical ventilation has been associated with release of the pulmonary vasodilator PGI_2 by the lung.[93,94]

Mechanical ventilation may also affect more than just the resistance of the pulmonary vascular bed. In the normal sheep fetus, the downstream determinant of the driving pressure for blood flow through the lungs is a pressure exerted by the surrounding pulmonary tissues rather than the conventional left atrial pressure. This force or surrounding pressure causes the flow through the lungs to cease at very high arterial pressures, on the order of 25 mm Hg,[80] and can be viewed as an extreme of the Starling resistor,[95] which characterizes blood flow in Zone II of adult lungs. Early studies in acutely prepared fetal goats suggest that the pressure that surrounds the pulmonary blood vessels also falls in response to mechanical ventilation.[96] This has recently been confirmed in experiments in conscious fetal lambs, but changes in respiratory gas tensions with mechanical ventilation caused a more reliable fall in this pressure.[80]

The Effects of Carbon Dioxide and pH on the Lungs

Few studies have addressed the importance of carbon dioxide tension and pH as mediators of the changes that occur during the onset of ventilation. A fall in carbon dioxide tension with increased pH but no change in oxygen tension does cause decreased pulmonary vascular resistance.[80,91] However, once oxygen tensions have increased, a fall in carbon dioxide tension does not appear to produce further pulmonary vasodilation. Although it appears that changes in carbon dioxide tension and pH play a role in pulmonary vasodilation at birth, the mechanisms behind this action have not yet been determined.

The Actions of Oxygen on the Pulmonary Vessels

The effects of a change in oxygen tension on pulmonary vascular resistance and blood flow during ventilation have been studied in detail in anesthetized fetal sheep[91,97,98] and to a lesser extent in chronically catheterized fetal sheep.[80,92] As anticipated, increases in oxygen tension under almost any initial condition cause a substantial fall in the resistance to pulmonary blood flow. An increase in oxygen tension alone during ventilation causes decreased pulmonary vascular resistance.[80] Isolated increases in oxygen tension in the absence of ventilation also cause a rise in pulmonary blood flow,[99,100] but this response is not sustained in the fetal sheep.[99] Furthermore, denervation of the afferent pathway of the carotid chemoreceptors and baroreceptors completely eliminates the pulmonary vascular response to a rise in oxygen tension in the absence of mechanical ventilation.[101] Because no concurrent change occurs in arterial blood pressure, the phenomenon is probably mediated by the chemoreceptors.

Although a decrease in carbon dioxide tension causes pulmonary vasodilation, an increase in oxygen after carbon dioxide tensions have fallen causes even further pulmonary vasodilation.[80,92] As noted before, the reverse is not true; a fall in carbon dioxide tension after oxygen has been increased to maximal levels has only negligible effects on the vasculature.[80] These effects of oxygen may be mediated by a release of bradykinin, which occurs in response to elevations in oxygen tension.[102] Thus, both the chemoreceptors and bradykinin are potential mediators of the pulmonary vasodilation that occurs in response to oxygen during the transitional period.

A host of other mediators has been proposed to exert an influence on the changing pulmonary vascular tone of the neonate. These include prostaglandins D_2, E_1, and E_2; thromboxane; and leukotrienes.[103] The actual role that each plays, however, remains elusive.

Postnatal Changes in Pulmonary Vascular Resistance

Following birth, the pulmonary vascular resistance continues to decline with development, so that it is even lower in adulthood than in the neonatal period. This is due primarily to anatomical development; that is, the cross-sectional area of the vasculature increases as new capillary growth occurs in the alveolar region.[104] The decrease in pulmonary vascular resistance with maturity is also accompanied by regression of the medial muscle layer in small arteries and by increased diameter of larger arteries.[105] Recent evidence also suggests that the fall in resistance from neonatal to adult life may be accounted for in part by the physiologic effect of oxygen on the pulmonary vessels.[106]

CARDIOVASCULAR ADAPTATIONS CHARACTERISTIC OF THE FETUS IN DISTRESS

Fetal distress is a clinical term used to describe the characteristics that are generally associated with hypoxia or asphyxia. In the laboratory, fetal distress can be induced by several mechanisms. These include a reduction in maternal fractional inspired oxygen, reduction of maternal uteroplacental blood flow, occlusion of umbilical blood flow, and hemorrhage. A reduction in the maternal inspired oxygen is the most commonly studied animal model of fetal distress. This causes only hypoxemia and does not compromise the placental exchange of carbon dioxide and energy substrates. Although it is also encountered only rarely in clinical medicine, the study of hypoxemia offers basic knowledge about the contribution of oxygen to the pathophysiology of fetal distress.

A decrease in placental perfusion, from either the maternal or the fetal side, causes fetal asphyxia. The distinction between asphyxia and hypoxia is based on changes in arterial carbon dioxide levels that do not change during hypoxia and rise during asphyxia. Asphyxia is much more clinically relevant than hypoxia. For example, impaired uteroplacental circulation is commonly encountered in many medical and obstetrical complications, especially those involving renal and cardiovascular pathology, and decreased fetal placental perfusion characterizes umbilical cord compression or fetal hemorrhage in cases such as placental abruption and vasa previa.

THE CARDIOVASCULAR PROFILE OF THE FETUS IN DISTRESS

With very mild fetal distress, blood pressure and heart rate exhibit very little or no change; however, catecholamine levels begin to increase.[107] As the severity of the insult increases, hypertension develops and fetal heart rate begins to fall. In experimental models of fetal distress, cardiac output is maintained despite a decrease in heart rate. This, of course, indicates an increase in stroke volume that must be mediated primarily by increased contractility, but also by increased preload. Although this facet of fetal distress has not yet been explored, the increased contractility is most likely mediated by increased catecholamine levels.

Although cardiac output does not appear to change in response to moderate hypoxemia, the distribution of cardiac output is altered. Vascular resistance falls in the fetal brain, heart, and adrenal glands. Blood flow is thus increased and oxygen delivery to the heart, brain, and adrenal glands is maintained or increased.[47,48,52,54,108] Peripheral and splanchnic organs, such as kidneys, intestines, muscle, and skin, respond to stress with vasoconstriction and thus participate in the rise in arterial blood pressure as well as the redistribution of blood flow to vital organs. When hypoxia or asphyxia is prolonged, these blood flow patterns are maintained until severe acidemia develops.[47,109] As the severity of the stress increases and acidemia progresses, biventricular cardiac output begins to fall as a result of magnified bradycardia.[52] Recent evidence suggests that in instances of extreme acidemia (pH <6.9), oxygen consumption also falls.[100]

Thus, the general fetal response to cardiovascular distress is a redistribution of blood flow to vital organs. This response is mediated by local changes in vascular resistance and by increased perfusion pressure. The fetal heart rate pattern is an additional variable that changes in response to a stressful stimulus. These patterns are readily accessible to the clinician and have become an indispensable aid in the diagnosis of fetal distress. This subject merits separate consideration and is covered in detail in Chapter 48.

SPECIFIC FEATURES OF FETAL DISTRESS

Hypoxemia

Hypoxemia is distinguished by a fall in oxygen tension with little or no change in pH, carbon dioxide, or delivery of metabolic substrates, although late in hypoxemia, metabolic acidosis may develop. Episodes of hypoxemia are marked by elevated arginine vasopressin, cortisol, endogenous opioids, plasma renin activity, epinephrine, and norepinephrine.[111–114]

The fetal adrenal medulla responds directly to a hypoxic stimulus to release both epinephrine and norepinephrine independent of sympathetic stimulation.[115–117] Activation of the alpha-adrenergic receptors during hypoxia or asphyxia causes increased arterial blood pressure and splanchnic vasoconstriction.[118,119] Beta-adrenergic stimulation tempers the bradycardia that occurs in response to vagal stimulation during fetal distress.[118,120]

Arginine vasopressin may be important in the cardiovascular response to a stress stimulus. Plasma vasopressin levels rise in response to both hypoxia and asphyxia.[69,70,111] Fetal hypertension, bradycardia, gastrointestinal vasoconstriction, and brain vasodilation are diminished when arginine vasopressin receptors are blocked during fetal asphyxia.[121] Thus, arginine vasopressin may be one cause of the rise in blood pressure, fall in heart rate, and redistribution of blood flow that occurs during fetal distress.

Blockade of the actions of endogenous opioids during hypoxemia potentiates bradycardia and reduces both biventricular cardiac output and placental blood flow in the absence of a significant change in blood pressure.[122] Endogenous opioids may also have some role in increasing peripheral vascular resistance and blood pressure in asphyxiated fetuses.[123]

Hypoxia alone also stimulates peripheral chemoreceptor activity. This influences the fetal cardiovascular system in two ways. First, chemoreceptors act through a reflex pathway to increase vagal tone and depress fetal heart rate.[124,125] This is the mechanism behind late heart rate decelerations seen in human fetuses in distress. Second, chemoreceptor stimulation causes increased sympathetic tone and produces arterial hypertension and the redistribution of cardiac output that has been described earlier. The increase in arterial blood pressure probably potentiates the chemoreceptor-activated bradycardia by a baroreceptor mechanism.

Finally, excitation of the chemoreceptors by hypoxia has another interesting effect on the fetus. Normally, the fetus cycles through behavioral states that may be characterized by fetal breathing movements and somatic motions. However, a fall in oxygen tension causes decreased fetal breathing movements and a fall in the incidence of general body movements.[126–133] This action most likely helps the fetus to survive brief periods of stress by reducing energy expenditure and thus oxygen consumption. When hypoxemia or asphyxia is prolonged, fetal breathing movements and general body movements return to normal within 12 hours.[134]

Acidemia

A fall in pH may accompany any advanced form of fetal distress. For instance, in hypoxemia, only oxygen is restricted to the fetus, but if the hypoxia is sufficiently severe, as time progresses it will cause the fetus to shift to anaerobic metabolism, build up lactic acid, and cause metabolic acidosis. In contrast, asphyxia is associated with an immediate respiratory acidosis that is a byproduct of the hypercarbia caused by reduced placental perfusion from either the maternal or fetal side.

Hypercarbia and acidemia also cause a rightward shift in the hemoglobin–oxygen dissociation curve. This shift reduces the oxygen-carrying capabilities of the hemoglobin and further exacerbates the associated fall in oxygen tensions.

Acidemia elicits a more intense chemoreceptor response than does simple hypoxia. The combined effects of hypoxia and acidemia cause greater falls in fetal heart rate, maximize redistribution of cardiac output, and increase blood pressures above those generally seen in purely hypoxic fetuses. In addition, stimulation of the central chemoreceptors by acidemia causes a somewhat paradoxical increase in fetal breathing movements.[135] Thus, asphyxiated fetuses are subjected to the opposing forces of a hypoxia-mediated suppression of fetal breathing and an acidemia-driven stimulation of fetal breathing.

Reduced Placental Perfusion

A fall in placental blood flow from either the maternal or fetal side of the placenta causes redistribution of blood flows, hypertension, and bradycardia, as described in the previous section. These actions are potentiated by accentuated chemoreceptor action stimulated by the acidemia that is characteristic of fetal asphyxia.

The effects of fetal asphyxia are compounded by reduced placental blood flow because the fetal nutrient supply is also cut short. The fetus compensates for this during acute periods of reduced placental blood flow by mobilizing glucose stores, partially from the liver, to maintain the glucose supply.[107] Obviously, this mechanism can only function successfully over relatively short periods of time. When placental perfusion is reduced over a prolonged period of time, fetal growth rate falls.[55,136–139] This adaptive response most likely produces mature newborns with birth weights that are small for gestational age.

Hemorrhage

Fetal blood volume is much greater than adult blood volume when adjusted for body mass. In the fetal lamb, blood volume has been estimated at 110 mL · kg^{-1}.[140] Approximations of human fetal blood volume have also been made and appear to correspond well with weight-adjusted volumes in the sheep model.[141,142] For comparison, adult blood volume is more on the order of 50 to 70 mL · kg^{-1}.[143,144]

Chronic Blood Loss. The fetus has a remarkable ability to recover blood volume after substantial hemorrhage. The sheep fetus recovers from a 2-hour loss of 30% of blood volume in 3 to 5 hours. Blood volume restoration appears to be driven by the mass appearance of plasma proteins in the circulation; thus far the origin of these proteins is unknown.[145] However, the proteins exert an oncotic pressure that restores blood volume.

Several investigators have proposed that the fetus relies primarily on blood volume to maintain its arterial blood pressure.[62,146] On the surface, the results of blood volume studies seem to cloud this theory. During a 2-hour chronic hemorrhage to 70% of control volume, lamb fetuses were able to maintain arterial blood pressure.[146] As seen in Figure 10-8, during the recovery period blood pressure fell as blood volume rose. When blood volume had fully returned to control, arterial blood pressure exhibited a small (5 mm Hg) but significant depression when compared to control. Hematocrit was also below control levels at this point and did not recover during the ensuing 2-hour period.

This fall in hematocrit may be an important key to the enigmatic fall in blood pressure with normal blood volumes. Red blood cells and plasma proteins are the principal determinants of the viscosity of the blood. In turn, blood viscosity is directly proportional to vascular resistance according to the combined laws of Poiseuille and Ohm. Thus, as blood viscosity falls, resistance declines uniformly throughout the circulatory system with little or no change in cardiac output. This also causes a fall in arterial blood pressure. The increase in plasma protein content probably helps to offset the loss of viscosity caused by decreased hematocrit, and this minimizes the hypotension associated with recovery from chronic hemorrhage. To summarize, the fetal sheep has an as-

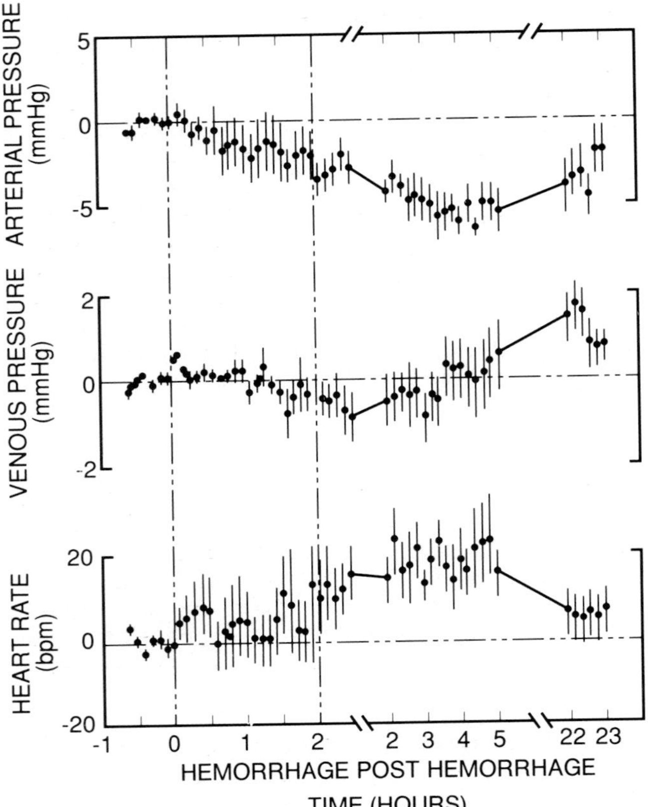

FIGURE 10–8. Changes in fetal arterial blood pressure, venous pressure, and heart rate during prolonged fetal hemorrhage and recovery (post hemorrhage). Data are expressed as absolute change from control values (mean ± SEM) for 12 sheep. (Redrawn from Brace RA, Cheung CY. Fetal cardiovascular and endocrine responses to prolonged fetal hemorrhage. Am J Physiol 1986; 251: R417.)

tounding ability to recover from a large loss of blood volume, provided it occurs over a prolonged period of time. The data from these animal studies may explain the survival of some human fetuses after fetal–maternal hemorrhages in excess of 250 mL.[147]

Acute Fetal Loss of Blood. The fetus also responds more rapidly to acute hemorrhage than does the adult. Ovine fetuses are much less apt to survive a rapid hemorrhage than a prolonged loss of the same volume of blood. Whereas it may take an adult 1 to 2 days to recover from an acute 20% loss of blood volume,[148] 50% of fetal blood volume is recovered within 30 minutes of an acute 14% hemorrhage.[149] A more recent study somewhat tempers these results.[150] Sheep were studied over a 48-hour period after an acute 20% blood loss. Full blood volume recovery took 6.5 hours. However, 24 hours after the hemorrhage, only 58% of the fetuses still survived. Those that remained were hypoxic, hypercarbic, and acidotic; had elevated levels of arginine vasopressin and norepinephrine; and had become hypovolemic in the ensuing 24 hours. In addition, fetuses that were subjected to hemorrhages that exceeded 30% of blood volume suffered immediate cardiovascular collapse.

Thus, from this one recent study,[150] it appears that acute fetal hemorrhage is not tolerated as well as a chronic loss of similar quantities of blood. In addition, blood volume recovery time is approximately twice that for slow hemorrhage and appears to increase with greater blood losses. Cautious application of these data to human fetuses would suggest that a fetus has a better chance of surviving a hemorrhage that occurs over a long period of time than one that occurs rapidly.

SUMMARY

The normal fetal cardiovascular system is characterized by three specialized shunts and the umbilical circulation. These features allow the fetus to oxygenate blood at the placenta and preferentially deliver the blood that is highest in oxygen content to the fetal upper body. This arrangement permits the heart and brain to receive the richest blood in the body. A high pulmonary vascular resistance serves to divert blood flow away from the lungs to the rest of the body and thus maximize oxygen delivery to other fetal organs. Fetal cardiac output and arterial blood pressure are controlled in a fashion very different from adult cardiovascular control mechanisms. This appears to reflect late development and maturation of sympathetic innervation.

The driving force for cardiovascular adaptation to birth is the dramatic fall in pulmonary vascular resistance as the newborn takes its first breath. This is regulated by a complex interplay of the changes in pulmonary gas tensions, mechanical forces and a large number of humoral mediators. As pulmonary vascular resistance falls, left atrial pressure rises and prevents blood flow through the foramen ovale; increasing oxygen tensions cause constriction of the ductus arteriosus. These actions functionally close the central cardiac shunts. Cardiac output also rises at birth when the central circulation pattern switches to series flow through the ventricles and pulmonary and systemic circulations. Increased cardiac output is achieved by a small increase in right ventricular stroke volume and a much larger rise in left ventricular outflow. Right ventricular output appears to increase in response to a fall in pulmonary arterial blood pressure, whereas increased left ventricular stroke volume is probably caused by an increase in chamber size as the intraventricular septum shifts toward the right ventricle.

The ability of the fetus to adapt to periods of stress depends on several mechanisms that allow it to increase blood flow to the heart and brain and thus maintain oxygen and nutrient delivery while maintaining blood flow to the placenta. This occurs through a combination of increased arterial pressure and the selective vasodilation and vasoconstriction of several vascular beds. These actions are a result of increased plasma levels of catecholamines, arginine vasopressin, plasma renin activity, and endogenous opioids in addition to chemoreceptor and baroreceptor mechanisms. Finally, hypoxia causes decreased fetal breathing activity and a fall in general body movements.

Acknowledgments

I am indebted to several people for their assistance in preparation of this chapter. Doctors CB Martin, Jr, JJ Faber, KL Thornburg, SL Pedron, and DA Carter proofread the manuscript and made many helpful suggestions; and Ruth Ledin provided her expert clerical skills in the preparation of this chapter.

REFERENCES

1. Walker AM, Fleming J, Smolich J, Stunden R, Horne R, Maloney J. Fetal oxygen consumption, umbilical circulation and electrocortical activity transitions in fetal lambs. J Dev Physiol 1984;6:267.
2. Rankin JHG, Landauer M, Tian Q, Phernetton TM. Ovine fetal electrocortical activity and regional cerebral blood flow. J Dev Physiol 1987;9:537.
3. Slotten P, Phernetton TM, Rankin JHG. Relationship between fetal electrocorticographic changes and umbilical blood flow in the near-term sheep fetus. J Dev Physiol 1989;11:19.
4. Abrams RM, Post JC, Burchfield DJ, Gomez KJ, Hutchison AA, Conlon M. Local cerebral blood flow is increased in rapid-eye-movement sleep in fetal sheep. Am J Obstet Gynecol 1990;162:278.
5. Reid DL, Jensen A, Phernetton TM, Rankin JHG. Relationship between plasma catecholamine levels and electrocortical state in the mature fetal lamb. J Dev Physiol 1990;13:75.
6. Dalton KJ, Dawes GS, Partick JE. Diurnal, respiratory, and other rhythms of fetal heart rate in lambs. Am J Obstet Gynecol 1977;127:414.
7. Wheeler T, Gennser G, Lindvall R, Murrills AJ. Changes in the fetal heart rate associated with fetal breathing and fetal movement. Br J Obstet Gynaecol 1980;87:1068.
8. Van der Wildt B. Heart rate, breathing movements and brain activity in fetal lambs. Nijmegen, Netherlands: Krips Repro Meppel, 1982.
9. Davidson SR, Reid DL, Leavitt LA, Martin CB, Rankin JHG. Power spectral analysis of fetal heart rate during high and low voltage electrocortical activity. [Abstract] Soc Gynecol Invest 37th Annual Meeting 1990:235.
10. Meschia G, Hellegers A, Blechner JN, Wolkoff AS, Barron DH. A comparison of the oxygen dissociation curves of the bloods of maternal, fetal and newborn sheep at various pHs. Quart J Exp Physiol 1961;46:95.
11. Moore KL. The developing human. 3rd ed. Philadelphia: WB Saunders, 1982.
12. Rudolph AM, Heymann MA. Circulatory changes during growth in the fetal lamb. Circ Res 1970;26:289.
13. Mott JC. Control of the foetal circulation. J Exp Biol 1982;100:129.
14. Rudolph AM. Hepatic and ductus venosus blood flows during fetal life. Hepatology 1983;3:254.
15. Edelstone DI, Rudolph AM, Heymann MA. Liver and ductus venosus blood flows in fetal lambs in utero. Circ Res 1978;42:426.
16. Bristow J, Rudolph AM, Itskovitz J. A preparation for studying liver blood flow, oxygen consumption, and metabolism in the fetal lamb *in utero*. J Dev Physiol 1981;3:255.
17. Edelstone DI, Rudolph AM. Preferential streaming of ductus venosus blood to the brain and heart in fetal lambs. Am J Physiol 1979;237:H724.
18. Amoroso EC, Barclay AE, Franklin KJ, Pritchard MML. The bifurcation of the posterior caval channel in the eutherian foetal heart. J Anat 1942;76:240.
19. Anderson DF, Faber JJ, Morton MJ, Parks CM, Pinson CW, Thornburg KL. Flow through the foramen ovale of the fetal and new-born lamb. J Physiol 1985;365:29.
20. Barcroft J. Researches on pre-natal life. Oxford: Blackwell.
21. Anderson DF, Bissonnette JM, Faber JJ, Thornburg KL. Central shunt flows and pressures in the mature fetal lamb. Am J Physiol 1981;241:H60.
22. Reuss ML, Rudolph AM, Heymann MA. Selective distribution of microspheres injected into the umbilical veins and inferior venae cavae of fetal sheep. Am J Obstet Gynecol 1981;141:427.
23. Behrman RE, Lees MH, Peterson EN, deLannoy CW, Seeds AE. Distribution of the circulation in the normal and asphyxiated fetal primate. Am J Obstet Gynecol 1970;108:956.
24. Reller MD, Morton MJ, Reid DL, Thornburg KL. Fetal lamb ventricles respond differently to filling and arterial pressures and to *in utero* ventilation. Pediatr Res 1987;22:621.
25. Wladimiroff JW, Vosters R, McGhie JS. Normal cardiac ventricular geometry and function during the last trimester of pregnancy and early neonatal period. Br J Obstet Gynecol 1982;89:839.
26. St John Sutton MG, Raichlen JS, Reichek N, Huff DS. Quantitative assessment of right and left ventricular growth in the human fetal heart: a pathoanatomic study. Circulation 1984;70:935.
27. Kleinman CS, Donnerstein RL. Ultrasonic assessment of cardiac function in the intact human fetus. J Am Coll Cardiol 1985;5:84S.
28. Kenny JF, Plappert T, Doubilet P, et al. Changes in intracardiac blood flow velocities and right and left ventricular stroke volumes with gestational age in the normal human fetus: a prospective Doppler echocardiographic study. Circulation 1986 74:1208.
29. Reed KL, Meijboom EJ, Sahn DJ, Scagnelli SA, Valdes-Cruz LM, Shenker L. Cardiac Doppler flow velocities in human fetuses. Circulation 1986;73:41.
30. Reed KL, Anderson CF, Shenker L. Changes in intracardiac Doppler blood flow velocities in fetuses with absent umbilical artery diastolic flow. Am J Obstet Gynecol 1987;157:774.
31. Reed KL, Anderson CF, Shenker L. Fetal pulmonary artery and aorta: two-dimensional Doppler echocardiography. Obstet Gynecol 1987;69:175.
32. Fisher DC, Sahn DJ, Friedman MJ, et al. The mitral valve orifice method for noninvasive two-dimensional echo Doppler determinations of cardiac output. Circulation 1983;67:872.
33. Allan LD, Chita SK, Al-Ghazali W, Crawford DC, Tynan M. Doppler echocardiographic evaluation of the normal human fetal heart. Br Heart J 1987;57:528.
34. De Smedt MCH, Visser GHA, Meijboom EJ. Fetal cardiac output estimated by doppler echocardiography during mid- and late gestation. Am J Cardiol 1987;60:338.
35. Gilbert RD. Control of fetal cardiac output during changes in blood volume. Am J Physiol 1980;238:H80.
36. Thornburg KL, Morton MJ. Filling and arterial pressures as determinants of RV stroke volume in the sheep fetus. Am J Physiol 1983;244:H656.
37. Thornburg KL, Morton MJ. Filling and arterial pressures as determinants of left ventricular stroke volume in fetal lambs. Am J Physiol 1986;251:H961.
38. Gilbert RD. Effects of afterload and baroreceptors on cardiac function in fetal sheep. J Dev Physiol 1982;4:299.
39. Anderson PAW, Glick KL, Manring A, Crenshaw C. Develop-

mental changes in cardiac contractility in fetal and postnatal sheep: in vitro and in vivo. Am J Physiol 1984;247:H371.
40. Kenny J, Plappert T, Doubilet P, Salzman D, St John Sutton MG. Effects of heart rate on ventricular size, stroke volume, and output in the normal human fetus: a prospective Doppler echocardiographic study. Circulation 1987;76:52.
41. Anderson PAW, Glick KL, Killam AP, Mainwaring RD. The effect of heart rate on *in utero* left ventricular output in the fetal sheep. J Physiol 1986;372:557.
42. Anderson PAW, Killam AP, Mainwaring RD, Oakeley AE. *In utero* right ventricular output in the fetal lamb: the effect of heart rate. J Physiol 1987;387:297.
43. Walker AM. Physiological control of the fetal cardiovascular system. In: Fetal physiology and medicine: the basis of perinatology. 2nd ed. New York: Marcel Dekker, 1984:287.
44. Schifferli P-Y, Caldeyro-Barcia R. Effects of atropine and beta-adrenergic drugs on the heart rate of the human fetus. In: Fetal pharmacology. New York: Raven Press, 1973:259.
45. Jones MD, Traystman RJ, Simmons MA, Molteni RA. Effects of changes in arterial O_2 content on cerebral blood flow in the lamb. Am J Physiol 1981;240:H209.
46. Bocking AD, Gagnon R, White SE, Homan J, Milne KM, Richardson BS. Circulatory responses to prolonged hypoxemia in fetal sheep. Am J Obstet Gynecol 1988;159:1418.
47. Rurak DW, Richardson BS, Patrick JE, Carmichael L, Homan J. Blood flow and oxygen delivery to fetal organs and tissues during sustained hypoxemia. Am J Physiol 1990;258:R1116.
48. Reid DL, Parer JT, Williams K, Darr D, Phernetton TM, Rankin JHG. Effects of severe reduction in maternal placental blood flow on blood flow distribution in the sheep fetus. J Dev Physiol 1991;15:183.
49. Tweed WA, Cote J, Wade JG, Gregory G, Mills A. Preservation of fetal brain blood flow relative to other organs during hypovolemic hypotension. Pediatr Res 1982;16:137.
50. Papile L-A, Rudolph AM, Heymann MA. Autoregulation of cerebral blood flow in the preterm fetal lamb. Pediatr Res 1985;19:159.
51. Hohimer AR, Bissonnette JM. Effects of cephalic hypotension, hypertension, and barbiturates on fetal cerebral blood flow and metabolism. Am J Obstet Gynecol 1989;161:1344.
52. Cohn HE, Sacks EJ, Heymann MA, Rudolph AM. Cardiovascular responses to hypoxemia and acidemia in fetal lambs. Am J Obstet Gynecol 1974;120:817.
53. Fisher DJ, Heymann MA, Rudolph AM. Fetal myocardial oxygen and carbohydrate consumption during acutely induced hypoxemia. Am J Physiol 1982;242:H657.
54. Yaffe H, Parer JT, Block BS, Llanos AJ. Cardiorespiratory responses to graded reductions of uterine blood flow in the sheep fetus. J Dev Physiol 1987;9:325.
55. Anderson DF, Faber JJ. Regulation of fetal placental blood flow in the lamb. Am J Physiol 1984;247:R567.
56. Brinkman CR, Ladner C, Weston P, Assali NS. Baroreceptor functions in the fetal lamb. Am J Physiol 1969;217:1346.
57. Shinebourne EA, Vapaavouri EK, Williams RL, Heymann MA, Rudolph AM. Development of baroreflex activity in unanesthetized fetal and neonatal lambs. Circ Res 1972;31:710.
58. Maloney JE, Cannata J, Dowling MH, Else W, Ritchie B. Baroreflex activity in conscious fetal and newborn lambs. Biol Neonate 1977;31:340.
59. Yardley RW, Bowes G, Wilkinson M, et al. Increased arterial pressure variability after arterial baroreceptor denervation in fetal lambs. Circ Res 1983;52:580.
60. Blanco CE, Dawes GS, Hanson MA, McCooke HB. Carotid baroreceptors in fetal and newborn sheep. Pediatr Res 1988;24:342.
61. Itskovitz J, Rudolph AM. Denervation of arterial chemoreceptors and baroreceptors in fetal lambs in utero. Am J Physiol 1982;242:H916.
62. Faber JJ, Green TJ, Thornburg KL. Arterial blood pressure in the unanaesthetized fetal lamb after changes in fetal blood volume and haematocrit. Quart J Exp Physiol 1974;59:241.
63. Anderson DF, Binder ND, Qui J, Brooks VL. Pressure dependent increases in plasma renin activity in fetal sheep. (Abstract) Society for the Study of Fetal Physiology 1990; 17th meeting, Asilomar CA:B-2.
64. Anderson DF, Parks CM, Faber JJ. Arterial pressure after chronic reductions in suprarenal aortic flow in fetal lambs. Am J Physiol 1987;253:H838.
65. Iwamoto HS, Rudolph AM. Effects of endogenous angiotensin II on the fetal circulation. J Dev Physiol 1979;1:283.
66. Iwamoto HS, Rudolph AM. Effects of angiotensin II on the blood flow and its distribution in fetal lambs. Circ Res 1981;48:183.
67. Scroop GC, Marker JD, Stankewytsch-Janusch B, Seamark RF. Angiotensin I and II in the assessment of baroreceptor function in fetal and neonatal sheep. J Dev Physiol 1986;8:123.
68. Clark KE, Irion GL, Mack CE. Differential responses of uterine and umbilical vasculatures to angiotensin II and norepinephrine. Am J Physiol 1990;259:H197.
69. Piacquadio KM, Brace RA, Cheung CY. Role of vasopressin in mediation of fetal cardiovascular responses to acute hypoxia. Am J Obstet Gynecol 1990;163:1294.
70. Rurak DW. Plasma vasopressin levels during hypoxaemia and the cardiovascular effects of exogenous vasopressin in foetal and adult sheep. J Physiol 1978;277:341.
71. Iwamoto HS, Rudolph AM, Keil LC, Heymann MA. Hemodynamic responses of the sheep fetus to vasopressin infusion. Circ Res 1979;44:430.
72. Vapaavouri EK, Shinebourne EA, Williams RL, Heymann MA, Rudolph AM. Development of cardiovascular responses to autonomic blockade in intact fetal and neonatal lambs. Biol Neonate 1973;22:177.
73. Su C, Bevan JA, Assali NS, Brinkman CR. Development of neuroeffector mechanisms in the carotid artery of the fetal lamb. Blood Vessels 1977;14:12.
74. Cheung CY. Fetal adrenal medulla catecholamine response to hypoxia-direct and neural components. Am J Physiol 1990; 258:R1340.
75. Rudolph AM, Heymann MA. Fetal and neonatal circulation and respiration. Annu Rev Physiol 1974;36:187.
76. Ardran GM, Dawes GS, Prichard MML, Reynolds SRM, Wyatt DG. The effect of ventilation of the foetal lungs upon the pulmonary circulation. J Physiol 1952;118:12.
77. Dawes GS, Mott JC, Widdicombe JG, Wyatt DG. Changes in the lungs of the new-born lamb. J Physiol 1953;121:141.
78. Walker AM, Alcorn DG, Cannata JC, Maloney JE, Ritchie BC. Effect of ventilation on pulmonary blood volume of the fetal lamb. J Appl Physiol 1975;39:969.
79. Assali NS, Sehgal N, Marable S. Pulmonary and ductus arteriosus circulation in the fetal lamb before and after birth. Am J Physiol 1962;202:536.
80. Reid DL, Thornburg KL. Pulmonary pressure-flow relationships in the fetal lamb during in utero ventilation. J Appl Physiol 1990;69:1630.
81. Oliver TK, Demis JA, Bates GD. Serial blood-gas tensions and acid-base balance during the first hour of life in human infants. Acta Paediatr 1961;50:346.
82. Clyman RI. Ductus arteriosus: current theories of prenatal and postnatal regulation. Semin Perinatol 1987;11:64.
83. Erath HG, Graham TP, Smith CW, Thompson SL, Hammon JW. Comparative right and left ventricular volumes and pump function in the newborn lamb. Am J Cardiol 1981;47:855.
84. Morton MJ, Pinson CW, Thornburg KL. *In utero* ventilation with oxygen augments left ventricular stroke volume in lambs. J Physiol 1987;383:413.

85. Braunwald E, Sonnenblick E, Ross J. Contraction of the normal heart. In: Heart disease: a textbook of cardiovascular medicine. Philadelphia: WB Saunders, 1984:409.
86. Kirkpatrick SE, Pitlick PT, Naliboff J, Friedman WF. Frank-Starling relationship as an important determinant of fetal cardiac output. Am J Physiol 1976;231:495.
87. Kirkpatrick SE, Covell JW, Friedman WF. A new technique for the continuous assessment of fetal and neonatal cardiac performance. Am J Obstet Gynecol 1973;116:963.
88. Anderson PAW, Manring A, Glick KL, Crenshaw CC. Biophysics of the developing heart. III. A comparison of the left ventricular dynamics of the fetal and neonatal lamb heart. Am J Obstet Gynecol 1982;143:195.
89. Sahn DJ, Lange LW, Allen HD, et al. Quantitative real-time cross-sectional echocardiography in the developing normal human fetus and newborn. Circulation 1980;62:588.
90. Azancot A, Caudell TP, Allen HD, et al. Analysis of ventricular shape by echocardiography in normal fetuses, newborns, and infants. Circulation 1983;68:1201.
91. Cassin S, Dawes GS, Mott JC, Ross BB, Strang LB. The vascular resistance of the foetal and newly ventilated lung of the lamb. J Physiol 1964;171:61.
92. Teitel DF, Iwamoto HS, Rudolph AM. Effects of birth-related events on central blood flow patterns. Pediatr Res 1987;22:557.
93. Leffler CW, Hessler JR, Terragno NA. Ventilation-induced release of prostaglandinlike (sic) material from fetal lungs. Am J Physiol 1980;238:H282.
94. Leffler CW, Hessler JR. Perinatal pulmonary prostaglandin production. Am J Physiol 1981;241:H756.
95. West JB. Respiratory physiology—the essentials. Baltimore: Williams & Wilkins, 1979:32.
96. Gilbert RD, Hessler JR, Eitzman DV, Cassin S. Site of pulmonary vascular resistance in fetal goats. J Appl Physiol 1972;32:47.
97. Dawes GS, Mott JC. The vascular tone of the foetal lung. J Physiol 1962;164:465.
98. Cook CD, Drinker PA, Jacobson HN, Levison H, Strang LB. Control of pulmonary blood flow in the foetal and newly born lamb. J Physiol 1963;169:10.
99. Accurso FJ, Alpert B, Wilkening RB, Petersen RG, Meschia G. Time-dependent response of fetal pulmonary blood flow to an increase in fetal oxygen tension. Respir Physiol 1986;63:43.
100. Morin FC, Egan EA, Ferguson W, Lundgren CEG. Development of pulmonary vascular response to oxygen. Am J Physiol 1988;254:H542.
101. Hanson MA, McCooke HB. Evidence for a carotid chemoreflex component of pulmonary vasodilatation during hyperoxia in unanaesthetized fetal sheep *in utero*. (Abstract) J Physiol 1988;399:30P.
102. Heymann MA, Rudolph AM, Nies AS, Melmon KL. Bradykinin production associated with oxygenation of the fetal lamb. Circ Res 1969;25:521.
103. Cassin S. Role of prostaglandins, thromboxanes, and leukotrienes in the control of the pulmonary circulation in the fetus and newborn. Semin Perinatol 1987;11:53.
104. Reid L. Structural and functional reappraisal of the pulmonary artery system. In: Scientific basis of medicine, annual reviews. London: Athlone Press, 1968:289.
105. Hislop A, Reid L. Pulmonary arterial development during childhood: branching pattern and structure. Thorax 1973;28:129.
106. Custer JR, Hales CA. Influence of alveolar oxygen on pulmonary vasoconstriction in newborn lambs versus sheep. Am Rev Respir Dis 1985;132:326.
107. Gu W, Jones CT, Parer JT. Metabolic and cardiovascular effects on fetal sheep of sustained reduction of uterine blood flow. J Physiol 1985;368:109.
108. Sheldon RE, Peeters LLH, Jones MD, Makowski EL, Meschia G. Redistribution of cardiac output and oxygen delivery in the hypoxemic fetal lamb. Am J Obstet Gynecol 1979;135:1071.
109. Bocking AD, Gagnon R, White SE, Homan J, Milne KM, Richardson BS. Circulatory responses of prolonged hypoxemia in fetal sheep. Am J Obstet Gynecol 1988;159:1418.
110. Rurak DW, Richardson BS, Patrick JE, Carmichael L, Homan J. Oxygen consumption in the fetal lamb during sustained hypoxemia with progressive acidemia. Am J Physiol 1990;258:R1108.
111. Stark RI, Wardlaw SL, Daniel SS, et al. Vasopressin secretion induced by hypoxia in sheep: developmental changes in relationship to β-endorphin release. Am J Obstet Gynecol 1982;143:204.
112. Bocking AD, Harding R. Effects of reduced uterine blood flow on electrocortical activity, breathing, and skeletal muscle activity in fetal sheep. Am J Obstet Gynecol 1986;154:655.
113. Martin AA, Kapoor R, Scroop GC. Hormonal factors in the control of heart rate in normoxaemic and hypoxaemic fetal, neonatal, and adult sheep. J Dev Physiol 1987;9:465.
114. Hooper SB, Coulter CL, Deayton JM, Harding R, Thorburn GD. Fetal endocrine responses to prolonged hypoxemia in sheep. Am J Physiol 1990;259:R703.
115. Comline RS, Silver M. Catecholamine secretion by the adrenal medulla of the foetal and new-born foal. J Physiol 1971;216:659.
116. Iwamoto HS, Rudolph AM, Mirkin BL, Keil LC. Circulatory and humoral responses of sympathectomized fetal sheep to hypoxemia. Am J Physiol 1983;245:H767.
117. Cheung CY. Direct adrenal medullary catecholamine response to hypoxia in fetal sheep. J Neurochem 1989;52:148.
118. Lewis AB, Donovan M, Platzker ACG. Cardiovascular responses to autonomic blockade in hypoxemic fetal lambs. Biol Neonate 1980;37:233.
119. Reuss ML, Parer JT, Harris JL, Krueger TR. Hemodynamic effects of alpha-adrenergic blockade during hypoxia in fetal sheep. Am J Obstet Gynecol 1982;142:410.
120. Walker AM, Cannata JP, Dowling MH, Ritchie BC, Maloney JE. Age-dependent pattern of autonomic heart rate control during hypoxia in fetal and newborn lambs. Biol Neonate 1979;35:198.
121. Perez R, Espinoza M, Riquelme R, Parer JT, LLanos AJ. Arginine vasopressin mediates cardiovascular responses to hypoxemia in fetal sheep. Am J Physiol 1989;256:R1011.
122. LaGamma EF, Itskovitz J, Rudolph AM. Effects of naloxone on fetal circulatory responses to hypoxemia. Am J Obstet Gynecol 1982;143:933.
123. Espinoza M, Riquelme R, Germain AM, Tevah J, Parer JT, LLanos AJ. Role of endogenous opioids in the cardiovascular responses to asphyxia in fetal sheep. Am J Physiol 1989; 256:R1063.
124. Parer JT, Krueger TR, Harris JL. Fetal oxygen consumption and mechanisms of heart rate response during artificially produced late decelerations of fetal heart rate in sheep. Am J Obstet Gynecol 1980;136:478.
125. Itskovitz J, Goetzman BW, Rudolph AM. The mechanism of late deceleration of the heart rate and its relationship to oxygenation in normoxemic and chronically hypoxemic fetal lambs. Am J Obstet Gynecol 1982;142:66.
126. Boddy K, Dawes GS, Fisher R, Pinter S, Robinson JS. Foetal respiratory movements, electrocortical and cardiovascular responses to hypoxaemia and hypercapnia in sheep. J Physiol 1974;243:599.
127. Natale R, Clewlow F, Dawes GS. Measurement of fetal forelimb movements in the lamb in utero. Am J Obstet Gynecol 1981;140:545.
128. Blanco CE, Dawes GS, Walker DW. Effect of hypoxia on polysynaptic hind-limb reflexes of unanaesthetized fetal and newborn lambs. J Physiol 1983;339:453.

129. Clewlow F, Dawes GS, Johnston BM, Walker DW. Changes in breathing, electrocortical and muscle activity in unanaesthetized fetal lambs with age. J Physiol 1983;341:463.
130. Dawes GS. The central control of fetal breathing and skeletal muscle movements. J Physiol 1984;346:1.
131. Bocking AD, McMillen IC, Harding R, Thorburn GD. Effect of reduced uterine blood flow on fetal and maternal cortisol. J Dev Physiol 1986;8:237.
132. Martin CB, Voermans TMG, Jongsma HW. Effect of reducing uteroplacental blood flow on movements and on electrocortical activity in fetal sheep. Gynecol Obstet Invest 1987;23:34.
133. Woudstra BR, Aarnoudse JG, de Wolf BTHM, Zijlstra WG. Nuchal muscle activity at different levels of hypoxemia in fetal sheep. Am J Obstet Gynecol 1990;162:559.
134. Bocking AD, Gagnon R, Milne KM, White SE. Behavioral activity during prolonged hypoxemia in fetal sheep. J Appl Physiol 1988;65:2420.
135. Hohimer AR, Bissonnette JM, Richardson BS, Machida CM. Central chemical regulation of breathing movements in fetal lambs. Respir Physiol 1983;52:99.
136. Creasy RK, Barrett CT, de Swiet M, Kahanpää KV, Rudolph AM. Experimental intrauterine growth retardation in the sheep. Am J Obstet Gynecol 1972;112:566.
137. Robinson JS, Kingston EJ, Jones CT, Thorburn GD. Studies on experimental growth retardation in sheep. The effect of removal of endometrial caruncles on fetal size and metabolism. J Dev Physiol 1979;1:379.
138. Clapp JF, Szeto HH, Larrow R, Hewitt J, Mann LI. Fetal metabolic response to experimental placental vascular damage. Am J Obstet Gynecol 1981;140:446.
139. Jacobs R, Robinson JS, Owens JA, Falconer J, Webster MED. The effect of prolonged hypobaric hypoxia on growth of fetal sheep. J Dev Physiol 1988;10:97.
140. Brace RA. Blood volume and its measurement in the chronically catheterized sheep fetus. Am J Physiol 1983;244:H487.
141. Nicolaides KH, Clewell WH, Rodeck CH. Measurement of human fetoplacental blood volume in erythroblastosis fetalis. Am J Obstet Gynecol 1987;157:50.
142. MacGregor SN, Socol ML, Pielet BW, Sholl JT, Minogue JP. Prediction of fetoplacental blood volume in isoimmunized pregnancy. Am J Obstet Gynecol 1988;159:1493.
143. Ueland K. Maternal cardiovascular dynamics. VII. Intrapartum blood volume changes. Am J Obstet Gynecol 1976;126:671.
144. Pritchard JA, Cunningham FG, Pritchard SA. The Parkland Memorial Hospital protocol for treatment of eclampsia: evaluation of 245 cases. Am J Obstet Gynecol 1984;148:951.
145. Brace RA. Mechanisms of fetal blood volume restoration after slow fetal hemorrhage. Am J Physiol 1989;256:R1040.
146. Brace RA, Cheung CY. Fetal cardiovascular and endocrine responses to prolonged fetal hemorrhage. Am J Physiol 1986;251:R417.
147. Sebring ES, Polesky HF. Fetomaternal hemorrhage: incidence, risk factors, time of occurrence, and clinical effects. Transfusion 1990;30:344.
148. Grimes JM, Buss LA, Brace RA. Blood volume restitution after hemorrhage in adult sheep. Am J Physiol 1987;253:R541.
149. Brace RA. Fetal blood volume responses to acute fetal hemorrhage. Circ Res 1983;52:730.
150. Brace RA, Cheung CY. Fetal blood volume restoration following rapid fetal hemorrhage. Am J Physiol 1990;259:H567.

11 CHAPTER

IMMUNOLOGY OF THE FETUS

James G. McNamara

The immune system is an integral part of the developing human fetus. Advances in cellular immunology over the past several decades have been challenging our understanding of how the immune system develops, and tremendous strides in molecular immunology have occurred in the most recent decade. It was only in 1952 that the first case of a primary immunodeficiency with agammaglobulinemia was reported. This discovery opened the door to our current awareness of a host of congenital immune defects that all share the same clinical manifestation of increased susceptibility to infections, which may be as life threatening as severe developmental defects in other organ systems.[1]

The intent of this chapter is to provide the reader with an overview of how the immune system develops in the fetus from molecular, cellular, and functional perspectives. Many questions and issues remain as yet unsolved, but it is hoped that the framework provided will communicate the message of a tightly regulated schema of development and provide a basis for understanding future insights into the ontogeny of the immune system.

The purpose of the developing immune system is to generate functionally mature B and T lymphocytes, which have the capacity to recognize virtually all foreign pathogens (that is, to have a very broad repertoire of responses) and yet not respond to normal host products (that is, not react to self). Understanding the generation of B and T lymphocyte diversity has been the subject of intense investigations that have provided a number of useful and interesting models of how the developing fetus acquires functional competence, and will be further discussed in the context of these developing systems. Before going further, a summary of some general concepts and recent advances will allow us to discuss developmental immunology issues from a common framework.

The nomenclature used in immunology can be very cumbersome and confusing. To help with one area that was particularly problematic, the naming of cell-surface markers, a series of meetings was held to establish uniform definitions for cell-surface proteins. These surface markers have now been defined as cluster designations (CD), some of which are listed in Table 11-1.[2] For example, the sheep erythrocyte rosette receptor, a pan T-cell marker, which was also called OKT11, Leu5, or LFA-2 after the monoclonal antibodies that identified it, has now been given the designation CD2. This designation is used for all species if homologous structures have been identified.

By definition, a mature B or T cell expresses a cell-surface receptor, which it uses to recognize foreign antigens. For B cells, this represents surface immunoglobulin, a protein composed of two heavy chains of a single isotype (IgA, IgG, IgM, IgD, or IgE) and two light chains (κ or λ). Immunoglobulins are able to recognize both membrane-associated or soluble antigens. T cells also have surface receptors for antigens that are composed of two glycoprotein chains (α/β or τ/δ heterodimers) that are associated with a group of nonpolymorphic proteins (CD3) involved in signal transduction. In contrast to B cells, however, T cells only recognize foreign antigens in association with a major histocompatibility antigen (MHC)-bearing cell that has "processed" the antigen. Thus, as an illustration, immunoglobulins are able to bind to circulating free antigens (bacteria, toxins), while T cells are better able to recognize cells that are infected with intracellular organisms (viruses, bacteria) which are expressing on their cell-surface peptide fragments of those organisms in association with MHC molecules. T cells can also recognize protein antigens, but not in the soluble form that immunoglobulins can. T cells require that the antigen be endocytosed by another cell (macrophage or B cell, for example), processed, and then re-expressed on the cell surface in association with MHC. At this time the antigen, which is expressed as small peptide fragments, is no longer recognizable by antigen-specific antibodies, but only by

TABLE 11-1. HUMAN LEUKOCYTE SURFACE MOLECULE CLUSTER DESIGNATIONS

	CD DESIGNATION	PREVIOUS DESIGNATIONS	ASSOCIATED REACTIVITY/FUNCTION
T-Cell Markers	CD1	Leu6	Cortical thymocytes
	CD2	T11	Pan T cell
	CD3	T3,Leu4a	Pan T cell
	CD4	T4,Leu3a	Helper/inducer subset
	CD5	T1	T/B subset
	CD6	T12	T/B subset
	CD7	3A1	Pan T cell
	CD8	T8,Leu2a	Suppressor/cytotoxic subset
	CD25	TAC	IL-2 receptor
B-Cell Markers	CD19	B4	Pan B cell
	CD20	B1	Pan B cell
	CD21	B2	Pan B cell
	CD22	HD39	B-cell subset
	CD23	Blast-2	B-cell subset
	CD24	BA-1	B-cell subset

antigen-specific T cells. It has recently become clear that soluble antigens that are picked up and processed are presented to CD4+ (helper/inflammatory) T cells in the context of Class II MHC molecules (HLA-DR, -DP, -DQ), whereas antigens derived from intracellular organisms, for example, that are not picked up exogenously are processed through a different cellular compartment. These antigens are generally characterized by CD8+ (cytotoxic/suppressor) T-cell responses that recognize antigen in association with Class I MHC molecules (HLA-A, -B, and -C). Thus, the route of antigen processing largely determines the kind of MHC association/restriction and the nature of the T-cell response. The association between antigen and MHC has been further elucidated by x-ray crystallography. Peptide fragments of antigen can reside within a cleft between the two distal extracellular domains of a Class I molecule, and by analogy to Class II molecules that share structural homology in this area of antigen binding.[3] These recent findings help to combine through a structure–function relationship the role of well-defined surface markers and their functional characteristics observed at the level of cellular interactions.

B cells and T cells can be defined in the context of their expression of receptors that recognize antigens. The study of the molecular biology of these receptors has led to an explosion of information and models of how these receptors can generate sufficient immunologic diversity to provide us with the ability to respond to virtually all antigens and successfully achieve immunologic competence. An issue central to these findings is the development of immunologic competence by the fetus and neonate, in addition to the response of the mature immune system to new antigens.

Functional immunoglobulins and T-cell receptors require the ordered rearrangement and expression of families of genes that encode the genetic message required for their production. The immunoglobulin family of genes were the first to be cloned and have become the prototype for the more recently described T-cell receptor genes. Immunoglobulin genes undergo a complex and highly organized sequence of rearrangements to produce functional antibodies. These families of genes have coding sequences (exons) for constant regions (C), variable regions (V), joining regions (J) and, in heavy chains, diversity regions (D), that are encoded in a nonrearranged form (germ-line configuration) on different chromosomes: chromosome 14 for immunoglobulin heavy chains; chromosome 2 for kappa light chains, and chromosome 22 for lambda light chains. The cascade of events leading up to a productively rearranged heavy chain can be summarized as follows. First, a D-gene exon is transposed next to a J-chain exon, with the intervening genes being deleted as a result of the rearrangement. Then a V-gene exon is similarly transposed to form a VDJ recombinant, and finally, this recombination alters nuclear regulatory genes and allows the transcription of the VDJ complex as well as the downstream C exon. Subsequently, the transcribed RNA is spliced to remove the intervening sequences to produce mature mRNA, which can be translated to produce a functional IgM heavy chain. Other immunoglobulin isotypes are produced by recombination events between the VDJ complex and sequences for switch sites further downstream, which bring the complex to the regions encoding other heavy chain exons, which again undergo RNA splicing in generating the final mRNA product. This process is termed isotype switching.

Additional points pertinent to this process of successfully creating antigen receptors are worth highlighting. Immunologic diversity is generated through several mechanisms. A combinatorial mechanism exists out of the shear number of different V, D, and J exons available for use. Junctional diversity comes from the addition or deletion of base pairs at the time of recombinations and, lastly, somatic mutations, or the mutational events that occur within genes after rearrangement has occurred, is also an important diversification mechanism. By the process known as allelic exclusion, only one chromosomal allele at a time can be productively rearranged for each heavy or light chain immunoglobulin gene. Significantly, the entire process of gene rearrangements to form immunoglobulins in immature B cells occurs as an antigen-independent event. The signals that drive the initiation of this cascade, which culminates with the production of a highly sophisticated mechanism of protection, are not known.

Within this decade, it was discovered that T-cell receptors are encoded by families of genes that undergo rearrangements to generate T-cell diversity. T-cell receptors are composed of heterodimers of α/β chains or the numerically much less common τ/δ chains, which constitute generally less than 5% of peripheral blood T cells. Studies of the genes that encode these glycoprotein subunits have revealed a striking similarity to the immunoglobulin genomic organization. Like immunoglobulin, there are constant region exons as well as VDJ rearrangements that compose the variable region of the T-cell receptor chain. Like immunoglobulin, the T-cell antigen receptor heterodimer undergoes gene rearrangements that are not driven by antigen-dependent mechanisms. Similarly, the diversity of antigen specificities is generated through combinatorial and junctional mechanisms, as in immunoglobulins; however, somatic mutations giving rise to further receptor diversity is much lower than that seen in immunoglobulins.

In summary then, although the antigen-recognizing receptors on B cells and T cells are quite different in their functional roles in the host defense network and in how they "see" foreign antigens, they do share several striking features that can be demonstrated at the genomic organizational level, as well as conserved mechanisms for gene rearrangements and receptor diversity.

THYMUS DEVELOPMENT

The development of the thymus is essential to the normal evolution of a functional immune system. This absolute requirement has been demonstrated in humans with immune deficiencies, as in some patients with the DiGeorge anomaly (triad of cardiac abnormalities, hypoparathyroidism, and absent thymus), who may develop a severe combined immunodeficiency.[4] Histologic descriptions of the developing thymus were reported over 50 years ago.[5] However, within the past decade the development of monoclonal antibodies against elements of thymic stroma, as well as the lymphocytes that populate it, has allowed for elegant and detailed studies that have greatly advanced our understanding of thymic ontogeny.

The thymus develops very early in gestation, from the third and fourth branchial pharyngeal cleft/pouches. The rudimentary thymic anlage migrates caudally and fuses at the midline at approximately the 8th week. Shortly after this, hematopoietic stem cells seed the thymus, and at 8.5 to 9.5 weeks, lymphocytes are discernible. The cortical and medullary zones of the thymus become distinct by approximately 14 weeks, and Hassall's corpuscles are identifiable at 15 to 16 weeks. Thus, at an early age in gestation, the histologic development of the thymus is complete.[5,6]

An elegant series of investigations by Haynes and his collaborators, using a panel of monoclonal antibodies against thymic epithelial cells, have given us a more precise understanding of the development of the human thymic microenvironment. The antibody TE-4 identifies thymic endocrine epithelium that reacts with the subcapsular cortical and medullary zones. These cells express Class I (HLA-A, -B, and -C) and Class II (HLA-DR, -DP, and -DQ) major histocompatibility complex (MHC) antigens, and additionally produce thymosin α-1, a thymic hormone implicated in normal T cell development. TE-4+ thymic epithelial cells are identifiable at 7 weeks gestation and evolve a postnatal pattern of reactivity by 15 weeks.[7] The reciprocal population of epithelial cells is identified by the antibody TE-3. This antibody binds to cortical, but not medullary, epithelial cells that do not contain thymosin α-1 but, like TE-4+ epithelial cells, do express MHC antigens. Thus, the histologically distinct subcapsular cortical, inner cortical, and medullary zones are also antigenically distinct between TE-3+ cortical thymic epithelium and TE-4+ endocrine medullary thymic epithelium. TE-3+ epithelial cells are recognized later than TE-4+ epithelial cells. This subset of thymic epithelial cells is first identifiable as TE-3+ at 10 weeks gestation, and achieves a postnatal pattern in 4 to 6 weeks.[8] Antibody TE-7 primarily identifies mesodermal-derived mesenchymal tissue and thus reacts with fibrous septae and vessels found in thymus. TE-7 is also identifiable at 7 weeks as a rim of connective tissue surrounding the TE-4+ thymic rudiment. At 9 to 10 weeks, TE-7+ interlobular septae are forming, which give rise to thymic lobule formation at 12 weeks gestation.[7] Hassall's corpuscles (or bodies) are keratinized epithelial cell swirls that are further identified by a series of monoclonal antibodies (TE-8, TE-15, TE-16, TE-19) that also react with other epithelial cells, particularly epidermal keratinocytes. They are first demonstrated in the thymic medullary zone at 15 to 16 weeks gestation, and are postulated to be the product of differentiated TE-4+ medullary thymic epithelium.[9]

LYMPHOCYTE DEVELOPMENT WITHIN THE THYMUS

In concert with the development of thymic epithelial elements is the populating of the thymus by lymphocyte precursors. The earliest T-cell precursors that have been identified are CD45+ (family of T-200 molecules found on all leukocytes) and CD7+. CD7 has gained a role of increased prominence since its first description as a marker on T-cell lineage malignancies. Most T-cell leukemias are CD7+, as are some rare stem-cell leukemias.[10–12] Recently, the gene for CD7 has been cloned.

It has been demonstrated that CD7 belongs to a large family of cell-surface molecules that are involved in lymphocyte activation, recognition, and adhesion called the immunoglobulin supergene family, the designation of which is based on DNA homology and deduced structurally homologous regions among family members.[13,14] CD7+ cells have been found in 7-week fetal liver and yolk sac, as well as in perithymic thoracic mesenchyme.[15] These latter cells appear in a wave at 7 to 8.5 weeks, which suggests a cellular migration to the primordial thymus prior to the vascularization of the thymus. After this time and in conjunction with a more mature vascular system and subsequent hematopoietic seeding of the thymus, perithymic CD7+ cells are no longer demonstrable.[16] In vitro assays support the ability of these cells to give rise to more mature T cells. CD7+ cells from both fetal liver and fetal thoracic tissue could both be stimulated to develop into populations of T cells expressing mature T-cell phenotypes.[14] Thus, CD7 is a marker found predominantly on T-cell lineage cells and is the only marker reported as yet to identify putative T-cell precursors prior to lymphoid colonization of the thymus.

Once lymphoid colonization of the thymus has been initiated, the identification of more mature T-cell surface markers proceeds quickly, through an orderly progression of well-characterized surface polypeptides. At 8.5 weeks of gestation, approximately 20% to 50% of CD45+, CD7+ cells also express CD2, although it remains unclear what percent is cytoplasmic versus surface CD2.[6,16] A number of earlier workers had demonstrated surface CD2 expression through the formation of sheep erythrocyte rosettes (E-rosettes) on fetal thymocytes from 11 weeks of gestation through birth.[17–20] It appears that CD2 is the second T-cell lineage marker expressed on the surface of T cells and is the first intrathymic marker. At 9.5 to 11 weeks of gestation, T lymphocytes in the thymus also express CD1, CD3, CD4, CD5, and CD8. However, the intensity and pattern of CD1 staining becomes more prominent and achieves a postnatal thymic distribution over the next several weeks of development.[16,21] At 17 weeks, the distribution of these T-cell surface markers is essentially identical to the adult (Table 11-2).[22]

Knowledge of the chronological appearance of T-cell surface markers during ontogeny is of little value without the framework of proposed models for T-cell differentiation. Because of the severe limitation of fetal tissue available for study, analogies must be made with the study of intrathymic development of pediatric and adult thymus tissue obtained at the time of cardiothoracic surgery. With the advent of the monoclonal antibodies we have been discussing, Reinherz and Schlossman were able to identify different stages of intrathymic differentiation (Table 11-3).[23,24] These stages are as follows:

I. The early thymocyte of the outer cortex, which is CD2+ and CD38+ (a lymphocyte activation marker)
II. The common thymocyte of the inner cortex, which is CD1+, CD2+, CD3+ (dim), CD4 and CD8+, as well as CD38+
III. The mature thymocyte of the thymic medulla, which is CD2+, CD3+, CD4+ or CD8+ and CD38+.

This model of thymocyte differentiation is morphologically correct, but the implied progression of differentiation has not been fully substantiated experimentally. This is true because the activation and maturation potential of the common thymocyte (CD1+, CD4+, and CD8+ "double positive") remains an enigma. It is widely accepted that the vast majority of intrathymic lymphocytes die in situ, probably as a result of tolerance induction. Some investigators have found that the double-positive common thymocyte is poorly responsive to proliferative signals.[25,26] A more recent study, using an alternate mechanism of activation through the CD2 pathway, demonstrated that this population could be induced to proliferate and express IL-2 receptors. This activity was largely dependent on the presence of accessory cells, and provides evidence that some of the double positive thymocyte population may have the potential for further differentiation to mature to CD3+, CD4+ and CD8- or CD3+, CD4-, CD8+ thymocytes.[27]

A very different model of T-cell differentiation has been advocated by Toribio and collaborators (see Table 11-3). They observed that a small percentage of thymic

TABLE 11–2. T LYMPHOCYTE DEVELOPMENT

WEEKS GESTATION	THYMUS MORPHOLOGY	INTRATHYMIC SURFACE MARKERS	FUNCTIONAL RESPONSES
6			
7		Perithymic CD7+	
8	Thymic fusion		
9	Hematopoietic seeding	CD2+ cells	
10		CD1,3,4,8+ cells	PHA
11			
12			MLR
13			
14	Cortex/medulla distinction		
15			
16	Hassall's bodies		

TABLE 11–3. MODELS OF HUMAN THYMOCYTE DIFFERENTIATION

	CD7	CD2	CD1	CD3	CD4	CD8
Thymus Morphology*						
Stage I outer cortex	+	+	−	−	−	−
Stage II inner cortex	+	+	+	dim	+	+
Stage III medulla	+	+	−	bright	+	−
	+	+	−	bright	−	+
In Vitro Differentiation Model†						
Pro-T cells	+	−	−	−	−	−
Pre-T cells	+	+	−	−	−	−
Double negatives	+	+	−	+	−	−
Mature T cells	+	+	−	+	+	−
	+	+	−	+	−	+

* Data from Reinherz EL, Schlossman SF. The differentiation and function of human T lymphocytes. Cell 1980;19:821.

† Data from Toribio ML, Alonso JM, Barcena A, et al. Human T-cell precursors: involvement of the 16-2 pathway in the generation of mature T cells. Immunol Rev 1988;104:55.

lymphocytes has the same surface phenotype as the first recognizable T-cell precursor in the fetus; that is, CD45+ and CD7+. These pro-T cells[28] can be isolated from mature thymus through a series of depletion steps, using monoclonal antibodies directed at more mature surface markers. When stimulated with interleukin 2 (IL-2), these cells differentiate into pre-T cells that now additionally express CD2. The next structure to be expressed in culture is CD3, giving rise to the CD2+, CD3+, CD4-, and CD8- ("double negative") subset. This double-negative T-cell population, which expresses CD3 and therefore a functional T-cell receptor, has been demonstrated to be able to give rise directly to reciprocal populations of CD4+ or CD8+ mature T cells. This can occur without the transition through the CD1+, CD4+, and CD8+ double positive common thymocyte intermediate in these in vitro studies.[29–32]

CD2, the first T cell-specific surface marker found on thymocytes and on all mature T cells, has been proposed as a pivotal component in thymocyte growth and differentiation; however, the experimental support for this hypothesis is still tenuous. CD2 was identified almost two decades ago as a pan T-cell marker because of the ability of sheep red blood cells to form rosettes (E-rosettes) on a subpopulation of lymphocytes.[33,34] A series of monoclonal antibodies against CD2 have been generated that recognize different antigenic regions (epitopes) on the molecule. Anti-$T11_1$ is capable of blocking E-rosette formation. Anti-$T11_2$ also recognizes a T-cell surface epitope. CD2 epitopes recognized by anti-$T11_3$ are expressed only after T cell activation and, in conjunction with anti-$T11_2$, provide a mitogenic signal to T cells.[35] This activation pathway has been termed an alternate pathway of T cell activation in deference to T-cell receptor (TCR)/CD3 complex-mediated T cell activation. Through the generation of genetic mutants of leukemia cell lines that do or do not express CD2 or CD3, important patterns of activation interrelationships have been deduced. The expression of TCR/CD3 on the cell surface is required for activation though CD2; however, the converse is not true.[36,37] Submitogenic doses of antibodies against both of these structures also can lead to cellular activation, suggesting a functional interaction between CD2 and CD3.[38] The understanding of an interrelationship between CD2 and CD3 provides some problems for the initial Reinherz and Schlossman model of intrathymic development, because the Stage II common thymocyte, which was noted to be CD2+ and CD3-, could not be activated through the CD2 pathway. However, more recent studies have demonstrated this cell population does express CD3, but at a lower level of intensity (CD3 dim).[38,39] Because monoclonal antibodies directed against CD2 can induce proliferation of mature T cells, much speculation has centered on the question of whether natural ligand binding to CD2 could initiate the intense proliferation seen in the thymus.

A paradox exists in that anti-CD2 antibodies that are mitogenic for peripheral blood T cells are not by themselves mitogenic to thymocytes, on which they first appear, although they can induce IL-2 receptor expression.[40] However, the addition of a co-mitogenic monoclonal antibody (anti-CD28) is able to induce the proliferation of mature but not immature thymocytes.[41] Recent studies have demonstrated that a molecule previously recognized for its role in cellular adhesion, lymphocyte function-associated antigen 3 (LFA-3), appears to be a major ligand for CD2 and is found ubiquitously on many cell types.[42] Thymic epithelial cells have been demonstrated to be able to act as accessory cells for mitogen-stimulated mature thymocytes. Additionally, thymocyte proliferation in this model is inhibitable by both anti-CD2 and anti-LFA-3 monoclonals.[43,44] This suggests that the CD2/LFA-3 interaction provides an important cell adhesion function between the thymic epithelial cell and the thymocyte, but leaves open the question of thymocyte activation through this interaction. More directly, purified LFA-3 has been shown to be mitogenic for mature thymocytes when used as a cofactor with other non-mitogenic stimuli.[45] CD2 plays a clear role in cell adhesion and cell activation pathways in the mature thymocyte, but what role the early appearance of CD2 in ontogeny may play in regulating the activation of precursor T cells remains unclear.

ACQUISITION OF FUNCTIONAL MATURITY

Thus far, we have examined the development of the thymus and the ordered acquisition of T-cell surface markers on pro-T cells through mature T cells, as well as their implications. In addition to defining mature T cells by their surface molecule characteristics, it is also critical to assess their ability to respond to exogenous stimuli. Because these cells are by definition naive, that is, not yet exposed to exogenous antigens, standard assays using antigens that the individual has previously been exposed to (eg, tetanus, candida, and purified protein derivative of tuberculin [PPD]) are not informative ways to assess the functional capability of fetal T cells. Allogeneic stimulation of immature populations of cells is possible and, in conjunction with nonspecific stimulation with mitogens, has been used to ascertain T cell functional maturity. A number of pioneering studies were done in the early 1970s to help answer these questions. The essence of these studies is that at the time when the thymus achieves a mature postnatal appearance by histologic definitions at approximately 15 weeks gestation, vigorous responses to both allogeneic antigens and mitogens can be demonstrated. A detectable response to the mitogen PHA is first demonstrable at 10 weeks, a time when functional T-cell receptors are also first being expressed on intrathymic lymphocytes. A mixed lymphocyte response can first be demonstrated 2 weeks later in gestation. The appearance of these proliferative activities in other organs, such as spleen and liver, generally follows by 2 to 3 weeks when they have been demonstrated in the fetal thymus.[17,46–48]

T cells proliferate in response to the autocrine (a factor produced by a cell for its own use) production of T-cell growth factors. A number of factors that have effects on T-cell proliferation have been described. However, the two principal growth factors described for mature T cells are IL-2 and IL-4. IL-2 was initially reported as a T-cell growth factor in 1976 by Gallo and his associates in landmark studies that translated into the ability to establish long-term T cell lines and clones.[49] IL-4 was first recognized for its ability to support B cell growth and differentiation and subsequently identified as another potent T-cell growth factor.[50] In murine systems, reciprocal populations of CD4+ T-cell clones make either IL-2 or IL-4; however, in most human clones, both growth factors can be demonstrated.[51,52]

These findings imply that the mitogen and mixed lymphocyte responses previously noted indicate the ability of those stimulated lymphocytes to produce growth factors. Additionally, those cells must be able to express on their cell-surface receptors for those growth factors to mediate growth factor signal transduction. Equally interesting is the deduction that because these factors play a role in cell growth and proliferation, they may also play a role in the differentiation of developing T cells.

Attempts to examine these issues critically have used studies of immature populations of lymphocytes isolated from thymic tissue obtained from children at the time of cardiothoracic surgery. The least mature T cell identifiable, a pro-T cell (CD45+7+), proliferates in response to both IL-2 and mitogenic stimulation.[26] Thymocytes additionally expressing the marker CD2 form a more mature subpopulation. This population of cells, designated as pre-T cells (CD45+7+2+), also produces IL-2 after mitogenic stimulation, as assessed by their diminished proliferation in the presence of anti-IL-2 receptor antibodies (anti-CD25), as well as by standard IL-2 bioassays.[53,54] Unlike the pro-T cell population, this CD45+7+2+ population constitutively expresses the IL-2 receptor defined by the expression of CD25.[26,54] By similar means, IL-2 production has been demonstrated for double-negative thymocytes (CD45+7+2+3+4-8-), as well as for an immature thymocyte-derived T-cell clone with the same expression of surface markers.[55]

None of these studies addressed the issue of the role of IL-4 as a T-cell growth factor for thymocytes. However, by analogy with the murine system, where IL-4 has been demonstrated to be produced and used in an autocrine fashion by immature thymocytes,[56] it seems likely that IL-4 will also play a prominent part in the development of human thymocytes.

Recent evidence does suggest that IL-2 is more than just a growth factor for thymocytes. Phenotypically, pro-T cell lymphocytes isolated from mature thymus as well as from fetal tissue have been shown to be able to differentiate to mature T cells by the addition of IL-2 to their culture media.[16,26] These findings support the concept that IL-2 is an integral factor in generating the intense proliferation seen in the thymus, as well as the accompanying differentiation to more mature thymocyte subpopulations.

The developmental regulation of other lymphokines is largely unknown. A number of reports have demonstrated that neonates have a reduced capacity to produce interferon-τ (IFN-τ) as compared to adults.[57,58] This may be secondary to regulatory controls, because irradiation of neonatal cells results in increased IFN-τ production or an intrinsic T-cell deficiency.[59,60] Clinically, the inability of the fetus and the neonate to produce adequate IFN-τ correlates with that host's increased incidence of infection with intracellular organisms such as Toxoplasma and Listeria. It is postulated that both of these infections are controlled largely by the host's ability to activate macrophages to kill these intracellular organisms with IFN-τ.[61] As the neonate's ability to produce IFN-τ increases over the first several months of life, the susceptibility to these organisms and others falls.

Another characteristic of functionally competent T cells is their ability to reject HLA disparate cells and, conversely, to induce a graft-versus-host (GvH) reaction in immunocompromised hosts. Fetal thymocytes have been used for transplantation in children with severe combined immunodeficiencies (SCID) in efforts to reconstitute the immune systems of the affected children. Thymocytes from as early as 13 weeks of gestation are capable of producing GvH in these patients, demonstrating the functional competence of at least some of these cells.[62] Unfortunately, GvH disease has been reported in infants after intrauterine transfusions for Rh incompatability, as well as in a premature infant after a transfusion of nonirradiated blood products.[63,64] These studies serve to dramatize the concept that developing cellular immunity is part of a continuum, during which functionally competent cells can exist within a functionally incompetent immune system.

ONTOGENY OF T-CELL RECEPTOR GENE EXPRESSION

As with the defining of T cell development by the expression of surface markers and functional capabilities, molecular biologists have further refined their studies to include the development of gene expression for T-cell receptors. Only limited studies have been completed with human tissues, but elegant studies in the murine system have provided new insights and much speculation about T-cell ontogeny. As a frame of reference, the mouse has a gestational period of approximately 20 days and, unlike the human species, acquires immunologic competence late in gestation. The thymic rudiment is colonized by lymphocytes at days 11 to 12, with increasing numbers of thymocytes over the remainder of gestation.[65]

The activation of TCR genes follows a highly organized sequence of rearrangements and transcription in the mouse. What has been learned from this can be summarized as follows. First, TCR τ mRNA transcripts can be detected as early as day 14, peak at day 15, and then decline until birth.[66,67] Second, TCR δ mRNA transcripts can be detected at approximately the same time, giving rise to τ/δ heterodimers about 2 days earlier than α/β heterodimers.[68,69] Third, β chain mRNA transcripts can also be detected at the same time as τ and δ transcripts, but they are usually not full-length transcripts, which generally appear later and plateau at day 17 to 18.[70] Finally, α chain transcripts are rare at the early time points in gestation, but increase in quantity until maximum levels are achieved in the adult thymocyte, during which time increasing amounts of α/β heterodimers are detected.[66,71] Thus, in the murine model, at least two waves of T-cell development have been described. An early peak population of T cells uses τ/δ heterodimers, which then diminishes over the remaining 5 days of gestation and gives way to the numerically superior α/β TCR population. The relationship, if any, between these two waves of T cells remains unclear, but likely represents the development of two completely separate T-cell lineages.

Our current understanding of the ontogeny of TCR genes in humans is derived from studies of T-cell leukemias and thymocyte populations that have been characterized on the basis of their phenotypes into different developmental stages, as was discussed earlier. As in the rodent model, τ chain transcription appears to arise very early in development, because expression of τ chain mRNA can be found in all thymic subpopulations.[26] Transcripts of TCR β chain mRNA reach a plateau in the intermediate stages of T-cell ontogeny (double positives and double negatives), whereas α chain mRNA is expressed later in ontogeny and reaches peak levels in the mature thymocyte populations.[26,72] Further studies examining these TCR genes, in addition to CD3 mRNA in similar thymocyte populations, have suggested that the controlling event in the expression of a mature α/β heterodimer T-cell receptor complex is the production of functional α chains.[71]

The availability of monoclonal antibodies against the protein products of these genes has allowed limited study of human fetal tissues. Thus, it has been confirmed in this manner that β chain products are found prior to the appearance of mature cell surface expression of α/β heterodimers in fetal liver.[73] Of considerable interest from this study was that over the range of gestational ages examined for thymus, 10.5 weeks onward, only rare τ/δ cells were demonstrated. This is in striking contrast to the murine model of ontogeny, which clearly demonstrates waves of thymocyte development, beginning with a wave of τ/δ T cells. This study clearly does not preclude this from happening at an earlier time in gestation, but serves to highlight the considerable future work that needs to be carried out at the molecular level before we can hope to claim insightful understanding to T-cell receptor ontogeny.

B-CELL ONTOGENY

As might be anticipated from the preceding sections, B lymphocyte development parallels in many ways the findings discussed with reference to T-cell ontogeny. Examples of these parallels include the observations that, like T cells, precursor B cells initially undergo a series of maturational events that occur independent of antigen stimulation, while the terminal maturation events are absolutely dependent on the presence of antigen. These changes occur as a result of remarkably similar events at the genomic level that involve the use of related gene families and combinatorial mechanisms. B-cell phenotypes mature early in fetal gestation but, as with T cells, functional maturation takes much longer to achieve.

The first recognizable cells belonging to a B-cell lineage are termed pre-B cells and are characterized by their cytoplasmic expression of μ immunoglobulin heavy chains. In the human fetus, pre-B cells can be identified as early as 7 to 8 weeks in fetal liver samples (Table 11-4).[74] These are large lymphoid cells that appear to be rapidly dividing and give rise to small, resting pre-B cells.[74,75] A population of small pre-B cells also expresses cytoplasmic immunoglobulin light chains and is considered to be the direct precursors of B cells;

TABLE 11–4. B LYMPHOCYTE DEVELOPMENT

WEEKS GESTATION	PRE-B CELLS	B CELLS	PLASMA CELLS
5			
	Cytoplasmic μ chain+		
10		sIgM+	
		sIgG+	
		sIgA+	
		sIgD+	
15			IgM
20			IgG
30			IgA

that is, lymphocytes that express immunoglobulins on surface membranes (sIg).[76,77]

B cells bearing a sIgM phenotype are first detected in fetal liver at 9 to 10 weeks gestation. Shortly after this time, B cells that also express sIgG and sIgA can be found in small numbers, and by weeks 12 to 13 sIgD+ cells can also be found. Although B cells are first observed in fetal liver, they are rapidly observed subsequently in fetal bone marrow, spleen, and blood, where they reach the numerical proportions found in umbilical cord blood and adult samples by approximately 15 weeks gestation.[19,74,78–80] During this same time period, the function of generating B-cell precursors and their progeny switches from fetal liver, where it is located early in gestation, to exclusively bone marrow during the second trimester. Bone marrow continues to be the source of pre-B cells throughout adult life.[79,80] The final step in the B-cell maturational pathway is the production of immunoglobulin by plasma cells. Plasma cells secreting IgM can first be detected at 15 weeks gestation, followed by IgG- and IgA-secreting plasma cells at approximately 20 and 30 weeks gestation, respectively.[81,82] This orderly progression of immunoglobulin isotype expression is recapitulated frequently throughout B-cell development.

A significant characteristic of immature B cells that express only sIgM is their inactivation after exposure to anti-IgM, and by inference, after exposure to self antigens during development. This critically important process has been termed clonal anergy, and provides a mechanism for the negative selection of autoreactive B cells and prevention of potentially harmful autoantibody production.[83] Another unique characteristic of B cells as they further develop is that they may express multiple immunoglobulin isotypes on their cell surface; that is, IgM and IgD alone or in combination with IgG or IgA. This is in marked contrast to mature B cells, which generally express a single isotype. This was first suggested by the observation that the total number of B cells enumerated by counting the total number of cells that were sIgA, sIgG, and sIgM positive outnumbered the light chain positive B cells in fetal liver samples. This observation has subsequently been confirmed and extended using double and triple immunofluorescence studies.[19,74,82,84] This immature B-cell phenotype of multiple immunoglobulin isotype expression is also the dominant B-cell phenotype found in cord blood, and likely is the cell surface representation of isotype switching events that are occurring at the genomic level.

DEVELOPMENT OF B-CELL SURFACE MARKERS

As we saw in T-cell development, other cell-surface molecules can be used to identify physiologically relevant and lineage-specific B-cell markers in addition to the molecules that are used for antigen recognition. Pre-B cells express HLA-DR, CD19, and CD24, although the function of the latter two surface markers remains unknown.[79,85–87] The pan B-cell marker, CD20, is detected at 14 to 16 weeks, and other markers, such as CD21 and CD22, are found shortly thereafter. CD21 has had two distinct receptor-ligand interactions identified. It is the complement cascade receptor for C3d, in addition to being the cell-surface receptor for the Epstein-Barr virus (EBV).[88] CD21 is also found on a population of pre-B cells, because they can be infected and immortalized with EBV even though they poorly stain with antibodies directed against CD21.[89] CD23 is a B-cell differentiation marker found on mature B cells. It is of particular interest because it is the low-affinity IgE receptor whose surface expression can be upregulated by IL-4.[90,91] Another cell-surface antigen found on subpopulations of both T and B cells is CD5. Although CD5 is found on 10% to 15% of adult B cells, it is the predominant phenotype on cord blood B cells; similarly, it is much more highly expressed in fetal spleen than in adult splenic tissue. The function of this phenotype of B cell is unknown; however, CD5+ cells are more highly represented in adults with autoimmune disorders and chronic lymphocytic leukemia (CLL), as well as after bone marrow transplantation. It has been suggested that CD5+ B cells produce less immunoglobulin than CD5- B cells, and may contribute to the immunologic incompetence of neonates and transplant recipients. CD5+ B cells are postulated to be a distinct lineage of B cells and not a precursor of CD5- B cells.[91–94] Many other receptors exist for B-cell growth and differentiation factors; however, their roles in ontogeny have not yet been defined.

FUNCTIONAL ASSESSMENT OF B-CELL MATURITY

Another tool used in assessing B-cell functional maturity is the ability to induce immunoglobulin production in vitro after stimulation with a variety of mitogens. Normal adult lymphocytes respond with the polyclonal production of all immunoglobulin isotypes after activation with pokeweed mitogen (PWM). Fetal samples, however, produce quantitatively less immunoglobulin, which is almost exclusively restricted to IgM. Small amounts of IgG production can be detected after 18 to 20 weeks gestation, but no IgA can be induced from fetal cells.[95,96] Identical findings have also been reported in studies of PWM-stimulated cord blood.[95–99] However, PWM activation of B cells is dependent on the presence and co-activation of T cells. Thus, the findings above could be interpreted as evidence for B-cell immaturity, a regulatory influence of developing T-cell populations, or elements of both. Studies designed to examine these questions have yielded conflicting and interesting results, and can be summarized as follows:

1. Neonatal B cells have an intrinsic defect, resulting in diminished and restricted immunoglobulin production.
2. Co-culture studies of adult and newborn T and B cells have demonstrated little to normal helper function in neonatal T cells.
3. The wide range of results appears to be related to a suppressive T cell activity of neonatal lymphocytes, which is radiosensitive.[96–100]

Activation of fetal and cord blood B cells with EBV, a T cell-independent B-cell mitogen, has been used with results similar to those found with PWM. IgM responses are much greater than IgG, which is more again than the small amounts of IgA that is produced.[101–103]

The normal fetus and neonate have only rare plasma cells and produce small amounts of detectable immunoglobulin; this is probably from the antigenic naivete of the environment, rather than from an inability to respond to antigens. This has been demonstrated in dramatic fashion by the frequently strong fetal response to congenital infections. In early studies of congenital infections with syphilis and toxoplasmosis, plasma cell responses were commonly found after 29 weeks gestation.[104] Similarly, antibody responses attributed to the fetus have been reported in congenital rubella during the second trimester. The earliest and most prominent antibody response is in both viral specific and nonspecific IgM production; however, IgG and IgA responses can be detected later in gestation or at the time of birth.[105,106]

In the normal postnatal development of the child, both specific antibody responses to new antigens and the orderly achievement of adult levels of immunoglobulins in the blood follow this same pattern of isotype progression. Adult quantities of IgM, IgG, and IgA are reached at approximately 1 year, 5 years, and 10 years, respectively.[107] Thus, although B cells expressing all immunoglobulin isotypes can be found well before birth, humoral immune responses measured in vivo and in vitro show a striking predominance of IgM antibodies in the fetus and neonate, which gradually matures over the first few years of life to the adult pattern of predominant IgG responses to foreign antigens.

CONCLUSION

The immune system develops in a highly orchestrated and integrated fashion. B and T lymphocyte development is initiated midway through the first trimester, and in many ways achieves significant maturity, equal to that seen in the term neonate, during the second trimester of pregnancy. The early stages of lymphocyte maturation occurs as the result of mechanisms that are not dependent on antigenic stimulation, and provides us with an immunologic repertoire capable of responding to virtually any antigenic challenge. Further maturation of the immune system, with the development of specific immunologic memory and more potent humoral and cellular effector mechanisms, occurs after exposure to the myriad of environmental challenges that occurs in postnatal life. Thus, the immune system is a highly responsive organ system that has its origins early in gestation, reaches maturity during the first decade of life, but continues to evolve and respond to pathogenic insults throughout life until immunologic senescence occurs.

REFERENCES

1. Bruton OC. Agammaglobulinemia. Pediatrics 1952;9:722.
2. Knapp W, Rieber P, Dorken B, Schmidt RE, Stein H, Borne AEGK. Towards a better definition of human leucocyte surface molecules. Immunol Today 1989;10:253.
3. Bjorkman PJ, Saper MA, Samraoui B, Bennett WS, Strominger JL, Wiley DC. Structure of the human class I histocompatibility antigen, HLA-A 2. Nature 1987;329:506.
4. Goldsobel AB, Haas A, Stiehm ER. Bone marrow transplantation in DiGeorge syndrome. J Pediatr 1987;111:40.
5. Weller GL Jr. Development of the thyroid, parathyroid and thymus glands in man. Contrib Embryol Carnegie Inst 1933;22:95.
6. Lobach DF, Haynes BF. Ontogeny of the human thymus during fetal development. J Clin Immunol 1987;7:81.
7. Haynes BF, Scearce RM, Lobach DF, Hensley LL. Phenotypic characterization and ontogeny of mesodermal-derived and endocrine epithelial components of the human thymic microenvironment. J Exp Med 1984;159:1149.
8. McFarland EJ, Scearce RM, Haynes BF. The human thymic microenvironment: cortical thymic epithelium is an antigenically distinct region of the thymic microenvironment. J Immunol 1984;133:1241.
9. Lobach DF, Scearce RM, Haynes BF. The human thymic microenvironment. Phenotypic characterization of Hassall's bodies with the use of monoclonal antibodies. J Immunol 1985;134:250.
10. Haynes BF, Eisenbarth GS, Fauci AS. Human lymphocyte antigens: production of a monoclonal antibody that defines functional thymus-derived lymphocyte subsets. Proc Natl Acad Sci USA 1979;76:5829.
11. Haynes BF, Metzgar RM, Bunn PA, Minna J. Phenotypic characterization of cutaneous T cell lymphoma: use of monoconal anti-

bodies to compare with other malignant T cells. N Engl J Med 1981;304:1319.

12. Kurtzberg J, Waldmann TA, Davey MP, et al. CD7+, CD4-, CD8- acute leukemia: a syndrome of malignant pluripotent lymphohematopoietic cells. Blood 1989;73:381.
13. Aruffo A, Seed B. Molecular cloning of two CD7 (T-cell leukemia antigen) cDNAs by a COS cell expression system. EMBO J 1987;6:3313.
14. Hunkapiller T, Hood L. Diversity of immunoglobulin gene superfamily. In: Dixon FJ, ed. Advances in immunology, vol 44. San Diego: Academic Press, 1989:1.
15. Lobach DF, Hensley LL, Ho W, Haynes BF. Human T cell antigen expression during the early stages of fetal thymic maturation. J Immunol 1985;135:1752.
16. Haynes BF, Martin ME, Kay HH, Kurtzberg J. Early events in human T cell ontogeny-Phenotypic characterization and immunohistologic localization of T cell precursors in early human fetal tissues. J Exp Med 1988;168:1061.
17. Stites DP, Caldwell J, Carr MC, Fudenberg HH. Ontogeny of immunity in humans. Clin Immunol Immunopathol 1975;4:519.
18. Wara DW, Golbus MS, Ammann AJ. Fetal thymus glands obtained from prostaglandin-induced abortions. Cellular immune function in vitro and evidence of in vivo thymocyte activity following transplantation. Transplantation 1974;18:387.
19. Hayward AR, Ezer G. Development of lymphocyte populations in the human foetal thymus and spleen. Clin Exp Immunol 1974;17:169.
20. Wybran J, Carr MC, Fudenberg HH. The human rosette-forming cell as a marker of a population of thymus-derived cells. J Clin Invest 1972;51:2537.
21. Kamps WA, Cooper MD. Development of lymphocyte subpopulations identified by monoclonal antibodies in human fetuses. J Clin Immunol 1984;4:36.
22. Rosenthal P, Rimm IJ, Umiel T, et al. Ontogeny of human hematopoietic cells: analysis utilizing monoclonal antibodies. J Immunol 1983;31:232.
23. Reinherz EL, Kung PC, Goldstein G, Levey RH, Schlossman SF. Discrete stages of human intrathymic differentiation: analysis of normal thymocytes and leukemic lymphoblasts of T-cell lineage. Proc Natl Acad Sci USA 1980;77:1588.
24. Reinherz EL, Schlossman SF. The differentiation and function of human T lymphocytes. Cell 1980;19:821.
25. Lopez-Botet M, Moretta L. Functional characterization of human thymocytes: a limiting dilution analysis of precursors with proliferative and cytolytic activities. J Immunol 1985;134:2299.
26. Hayward AR, Kurnick JT, Clarke DR. T cell growth factor-enhanced PHA response of human thymus cells: requirement for T3+ cells. J Immunol 1981;127:2079.
27. Blue ML, Daley JF, Levine H, Craig KA, Schlossman SF. Activation of immature cortical thymocytes through the T11 sheep erythrocyte binding protein. J Immunol 1987;138:3108.
28. Palacios R, Kiefer M, Brockhaus M, et al. Molecular, cellular, and functional properties of bone marrow T lymphocyte progenitor clones. J Exp Med 1987;66:12.
29. Toribio ML, de la Hera A, Borst J, et al. Involvement of the interleukin 2 pathway in the rearrangement and expression of both α/β and τ/δ T cell receptor genes in human T cell precursors. J Exp Med 1988;168:2231.
30. Toribio ML, Alonso JM, Barcena A, et al. Human T-cell precursors: involvement of the IL-2 pathway in the generation of mature T cells. Immunol Rev 1988;104:55.
31. Toribio ML, Martinez AC, Marcos MAR, Marquez C, Cabrero E, de la Hera A. A role for T3+4-6-8- transitional thymocytes in the differentiation of mature and functional T cells from human prothymocytes. Proc Natl Acad Sci USA 1986;83:6985.
32. de la Hera A, Toribio ML, Marquez C, Marcos MAR, Cabrero E, Martinez AC. Differentiation of human mature thymocytes: existence of a T3+4-8- intermediate stage. Eur J Immunol 1986;16:653.
33. Snodgrass HR, Dembic Z, Steinmetz M, von Boehmer H. Expression of T-cell antigen receptor genes during fetal development in the thymus. Nature 1985;315:232.
34. Howard FD, Ledbetter JA, Wong J, Bieber CP, Stinson EB, Herzenberg LA. A human T lymphocyte differentiation marker defined by monoclonal antibodies that block E-rosette formation. J Immunol 1981;126:2117.
35. Meuer SC, Hussey RE, Fabbi M, et al. An alternative pathway of T-cell activation: a functional role for the 50 kd T11 sheep erythrocyte receptor protein. Cell 1984;36:897.
36. Alcover A, Alberini C, Acuto O, et al. Interdependence of CD3-Ti and CD2 activation pathways in human T lymphocytes. EMBO J 1988;7:1973.
37. Moingeon P, Alcover A, Clayton LK, Chang HC, Transy C, Reinherz EL. Expression of a functional CD3-Ti antigen/MHC receptor in the absence of surface CD 2. J Exp Med 1988;168:2077.
38. Lanier LL, Allison JP, Phillips JH. Correlation of cell surface antigen expression on human thymocytes by multi-color flow cytometric analysis: implications for differentiation. J Immunol 1986;137:2501.
39. Blue ML, Daley JF, Levine H, Schlossman SF. Discrete stages of human thymocyte activation and maturation in vitro: correlation between phenotype and function. Eur J Immunol 1986;16:771.
40. Fox DA, Hussey RE, Fitzgerald KA, et al. Activation of human thymocytes via the 50KD T11 sheep erythrocyte binding protein induces the expression of interleukin 2 receptors on both T3+ and T3- populations. J Immunol 1985;134:330.
41. Yang SY, Denning SM, Mizuno S, Dupont B, Haynes BF. A novel activation pathway for mature thymocytes. J Exp Med 1988;168:1457.
42. Selvaraj P, Plunkett ML, Dustin M, Sanders ME, Shaw S, Springer TA. The T lymphocyte glycoprotein CD2 binds the cell surface ligand LFA-3. Nature 1987;326:400.
43. Denning SM, Tuck DT, Singer KH, Haynes BF. Human thymic epithelial cells function as accessory cells for autologous mature thymocyte activation. J Immunol 1987;138:680.
44. Denning SM, Tuck DT, Vollger LW, Springer TA, Singer KH, Haynes BF. Monoclonal antibodies to CD2 and lymphocyte function-associated antigen 3 inhibit human thymic epithelial cell-dependent mature thymocyte activation. J Immunol 1987;139:2573.
45. Denning SM, Dustin ML, Springer TA, Singer KH, Haynes BF. Purified lymphocyte function-associated antigen-3 (LFA-3) activates human thymocytes via the CD2 pathway. J Immunol 1988;141;2980.
46. Asantila T, Vahala J, Toivanen P. Response of human fetal lymphocytes in xenogeniec mixed leukocyte culture: phylogenetic and ontogenetic aspects. Immunogenetics 1974;3:272.
47. Asantila T, Vahala J, Toivanen P. Generation of functional diversity of T-cell receptors. Immunogenetics 1974;1:407.
48. Stites DP, Carr MC, Fudenberg HH. Ontogeny of cellular immunity in the human fetus. Cell Immunol 1974;11:257.
49. Morgan DA, Ruscetti FW, Gallo RC. Selective in vitro growth of T lymphocytes from normal human bone marrows. Science 1976;193:1007.
50. Mosmann TR, Cherwinski H, Bond MW, Giedlin MA, Coffman RL. Two types of murine helper T cell clone. J Immunol 1986;136:2348.
51. Mosmann TR, Coffman RL. Two types of mouse helper T-cell clone. Immunol Today 1987;8:223.

52. Maggi E, Del Prete G, Macchia D, et al. Profiles of lymphokine activities and helper function for IgE in human T cell clones. Eur J Immunol 1988;18:1045.
53. De la Hera A, Toribio ML, Marcos MAR, Marquez C, Martinez AC. Interleukin 2 pathway is autonomously activated in human T11+3-4-6-8-thymocytes. Eur J Immunol 1987;17:683.
54. Vives J, Sole J, Suarez B. Unfractionated human thymocytes have a lower proliferative capacity than CD3-4-80- ones but have a similar capacity for expression of interleukin 2 receptors and production of interleukin 2. Proc Natl Acad Sci USA 1987;84:8593.
55. Bank I, DePinho RA, Brenner MB, Cassimeris J, Alt FW, Chess L. A functional T3 molecule associated with a novel heterodimer on the surface of immature human thymocytes. Nature 1986;322:179.
56. Carding SR, Jenkinson EJ, Kingston R, Hayday AC, Bottomly K, Owen JJT. Developmental control of lymphokine gene expression in fetal thymocytes during T-cell ontogeny. Proc Natl Acad Sci USA 1989;86:3342.
57. Frenkel L, Bryson YJ. Ontogeny of phytohemagglutinin-induced gamma interferon by leukocytes of healthy infants and children: evidence for decreased production in infants younger than 2 months of age. J Pediatr 1987;111:97.
58. Wilson CB, Westall J, Johnston L, Lewis DB, Dower S, Alper A. Decreased production of interferon gamma by human neonatal cells: intrinsic and regulatory deficiencies. J Clin Invest 1986;77:860.
59. Seki H, Taga K, Matsuda A, et al. Phenotypic and functional characteristics of active suppressor cells against IFN-τ production in PHA-stimulated cord blood lymphocytes. J Immunol 1986;137:3158.
60. Lewis DB, Larsen A, Wilson CB. Reduced interferon-gamma mRNA levels in human neonates. Evidence for an intrinsic T cell deficiency independent of other genes involved in T cell activation. J Exp Med 1986;163:1018.
61. Wilson CB, Haas JE. Cellular defenses against *Toxoplasma gondii* in newborns. J Clin Invest 1984;73:1606.
62. Bortin MM, Rimm AA. Severe combined immunodeficiency disease. Characterization of the disease and results of transplantation. JAMA 1977;238:591.
63. Parkman R, Mosier D, Umansky I, Cochran W, Carpenter CB, Rosen FS. Graft-versus-host disease after intrauterine and exchange transfusions for hemolytic disease of the newborn. N Engl J Med 1974;290:359.
64. Berger RS, Dixon SL. Fulminant transfusion-associated graft-versus-host disease in a premature infant. J Am Acad Dermatol 1989;20:945.
65. Moore MAS, Owen JT. Experimental studies on the development of the thymus. J Exp Med 1967;126:715.
66. Raulet DH, Garman RD, Saito H, Tonegawa S. Developmental regulation of T-cell receptor gene expression. Nature 1985;314:103.
67. Snodgrass HR, Dembic Z, Steinmetz M, von Boehmer H. Expression of T cell antigen receptor genes during fetal development in the thymus. Nature 1985;315:232.
68. Pardoll DM, Fowlkes BJ, Bluestone JA, et al. Differential expression of two distinct T-cell receptors during thymocyte development. Nature 1987;326:79.
69. Chien YH, Iwashima M, Wettstein DA, et al. T-cell receptor δ gene rearrangements in early thymocytes. Nature 1987; 330:722.
70. Snodgrass HR, Kisielow P, Kiefer M, Steinmetz M, von Boehmer H. Ontogeny of the T-cell antigen receptor within the thymus. Nature 1985;313:592.
71. Haars R, Kronenberg M, Gallatin WM, Weissman IL, Owen FL, Hood L. Rearrangement and expression of T cell antigen receptor and τ genes during thymic development. J Exp Med 1986;164:1.
72. Royer HD, Ramarli D, Acuto O, Campen TJ, Reinherz EL. Genes encoding the T-cell receptor α and β subunits are transcribed in an ordered manner during intrathymic ontogeny. Proc Natl Acad Sci USA 1985;82:5510.
73. Campana D, Janossy G, Coustan-Smith E, et al. The expression of T cell receptor-associated proteins during T cell ontogeny in man. J Immunol 1989;142:57.
74. Gathings WE, Lawton AR, Cooper MD. Immunofluorescent studies of the development of pre-B cells, B lymphocytes and immunoglobulin isotype diversity in humans. Eur J Immunol 1977;7:804.
75. Oskos AJ, Gathings WE. Characterization of precursor B cells in human bone marrow. Fed Proc 1977;36:1294.
76. Coffman RL, Weissman IL. Immunoglobulin gene rearrangement during pre-B cell differentiation. J Mol Immunol 1983;1:31.
77. Kubagawa H, Gathings WE, Levitt D, Kearney JF, Cooper MD. Immunoglobulin isotype expression of normal pre-B cells as determined by immunofluorescence. J Clin Immunol 1982;2:264.
78. Lawton AR, Self KS, Royal SA, Cooper MD. Ontogeny of B-lymphocytes in the human fetus. Clin Immunol Immunopathol 1972;1:84.
79. Kamps WA, Cooper MD. Microenvironmental studies of pre-B and B cell development in human and mouse fetuses. J Immunol 1982;129:526.
80. Asma GEM, Langlois van den Bergh R, Vossen JM. Development of pre-B and B lymphocytes in the human fetus. Clin Exp Immunol 1984;56:407.
81. Van Furth R, Schuit HRE, Hijmans W. The immunological development of the human fetus. J Exp Med 1965;122:1173.
82. Gathings WE, Kubagawa H, Cooper MD. A distinctive pattern of B cell immaturity in perinatal humans. Immunol Rev 1981;57:107.
83. Nossal GJV. Cellular mechanisms of immunological tolerance. In: Paul WE, Fathman CG, Metzger H, eds. Annual review of immunology, vol 1. Palo Alto, Annual Reviews, 1983:1.
84. Conley ME, Kearney JF, Lawton AR, et al. Differentiation of human B cells expressing the IgA subclass as demonstrated by monoclonal hybridoma antibodies. J Immunol 1980;125:2311.
85. Stamenkovic I, Seed B. CD19, the earliest differentiation antigen of the B cell lineage, bears three extracellular immunoglobulin-like domains and an Epstein-Barr virus-related cytoplasmic tail. J Exp Med 1988;168:1205.
86. Hofman FM, Danilovs J, Husmann L, Taylor CR. Ontogeny of B cell markers in the human fetal liver. J Immunol 1984;133:1197.
87. Bofill M, Janossy G, Janossa M, et al. Human B cell development. II: subpopulations in the human fetus. J Immunol 1985;134:1531.
88. Fingeroth JD, Weiss JJ, Tedder TF, Strominger JL, Biro PA, Fearon DT. Epstein-Barr virus receptor of human B lymphocytes is the C3d receptor CR2. Proc Natl Acad Sci USA 1984;81:4510.
89. Hansson M, Falk K, Ernberg I. Epstein-Barr virus transformation of human pre-B cells. J Exp Med 1983;158:616.
90. Yukawa K, Kikutani H, Owaki H, et al. A B cell-specific differentiation antigen, CD23, is a receptor for IgE (FcϵR) on lymphocytes. J Immunol 1987;138:2576.
91. Defrance T, Aubry JP, Rousset F, et al. Human recombinant interleukin 4 induces Fcϵ receptors (CD23) on normal human B lymphocytes. J Exp Med 1987;165:1459.
92. Antin JH, Emerson SG, Martin P, Gadol N, Ault KA. Leu-1+ (CD5+) B cells. A major lymphoid subpopulation in human fetal spleen: phenotypic and functional studies. J Immunol 1986;136:505.

93. Hardy RR, Hayakawa K. Development and physiology of LY-1 B and its human homolog, LEU-1 B. Immunol Rev 1986;93:53.
94. Gadol N, Ault KA. Phenotypic and functional characterization of human LEU1 (CD5) B cells. Immunol Rev 1986;93:23.
95. Wu LYF, Blanco A, Cooper MD, Lawton AR. Ontogeny of B-lymphocyte differentiation induced by pokeweed mitogen. Clin Immunol Immunopathol 1976;5:208.
96. Hayward AR, Lawton AR. Induction of plasma cell differentiation of human fetal lymphocytes: evidence for functional immaturity of T and B cells. J Immunol 1977;119:1213.
97. Morito T, Bankhurst AD, Williams RC Jr. Studies of human cord blood and adult lymphocyte interactions with in vitro immunoglobulin production. J Clin Invest 1979;64:990.
98. Tosato G, Magrath IT, Koski IR, Dooley NJ, Blaese RM. B cell differentiation and immunoregulatory T cell function in human cord blood lymphocytes. J Clin Invest 1980;66:383.
99. Miyagawa Y, Sugita K, Komiyama A, Akabane T. Delayed in vitro immunoglobulin production by cord lymphocytes. Pediatrics 1980;65:497.
100. Hayward AR, Lydyard PM. Suppression of B lymphocyte differentiation by newborn T lymphocytes with an Fc receptor for IgM. Clin Exp Immunol 1978;34:374.
101. Pereira S, Webster D, Platts-Mills T. Immature B cells in fetal development and immunodeficiency: studies of IgM, IgG, IgA and IgD production in vitro using Epstein-Barr virus activation. Eur J Immunol 1982;12:540.
102. Miyawaki T, Moriya N, Nagaoki T, Noboru T. Maturation of B-cell differentiation ability and T-cell regulatory function in infancy and childhood. Immunol Rev 1981;57:61.
103. Andersson U, Bird AG, Britton S, Palacios R. Humoral and cellular immunity in humans studied at the cell level from birth to two years of age. Immunol Rev 1981;57:5.
104. Silverstein AM, Lukes RJ. Fetal response to antigenic stimulus. I: plasmacellular and lymphoid reactions in the human fetus to intrauterine infection. Lab Invest 1962;11:918.
105. Alford CA, Neva FA, Weller TH. Virologic and serologic studies on human products of conception after maternal rubella. N Engl J Med 1964;271:1275.
106. South MA, Alford CA Jr. The immunology of chronic intrauterine infections. In: Stiehm ER, Fulginiti VA, eds. Immunologic disorders of infants and children. 2nd ed. Philadelphia: WB Saunders, 1980:702.
107. Buckley RH, Dees SC, O'Fallon WM. Serum immunoglobulins. I: levels in normal children and in uncomplicated childhood allergy. Pediatrics 1968;41:600.

12 CHAPTER

FETAL ENDOCRINOLOGY

Cecilia Y. Cheung

An integrated understanding of the fetal endocrine systems has been progressively achieved during the past decade. Despite the limitations imposed by ethical and practical considerations on investigations in the human fetus, significant information has been gained in the developing fetus using tissues obtained from abortuses or anencephalic fetuses, and more recently using fetal blood obtained by cordocentesis. The bulk of information regarding the development of the fetal endocrine system has been derived largely from investigations using pregnant animal models. These studies form the basis of our current understanding of fetal endocrinology.

The fetus exists in a unique endocrine environment that is largely autonomous from maternal influences. Each endocrine system develops and matures at a different rate, and each component within a system may become functional at a different stage in gestation. Each system will be considered from the viewpoint of development of overall function rather than from the aspect of maturation of separate components within the system. The first part of this chapter constitutes a review of the fundamental concepts of the fetal pituitary–endocrine axis. The second part focuses on details of the fetal cardiovascular endocrine system.

FETAL HYPOTHALAMIC PITUITARY SYSTEM

DEVELOPMENT OF THE NEUROENDOCRINE AXIS

The mature neuroendocrine system is characterized by a tightly regulated hypothalamic–pituitary axis, which controls the functions of the endocrine target organs. In turn, the hypothalamic–pituitary axis is regulated by feedback loops, resulting in maintenance of homeostasis within the organism. The development of this intricate system has been recently reviewed.[1–5]

The basic anatomical units that comprise the neuroendocrine axis are the hypothalamus, the median eminence, the hypothalamo-hypophyseal portal vessels, and the pituitary gland. The classical view of the embryonic origin of the pituitary has been described as an evagination of Rathke's pouch arising from a diverticulum of the stomadeum. This comes into contact with a downgrowth from the floor of the third cerebral ventricle. Rathke's pouch, which is ectodermal in origin, gives rise to the anterior and intermediate lobes of the pituitary; and the floor of the diencephalon, which is neuroectodermal in origin, gives rise to the posterior lobe. Recent evidence has questioned this view and suggests that both the pituitary and the hypothalamus are derived from the same neuroectodermal anlage.[1,6] In this context, the progenitors of the secretory cells lining Rathke's pouch originate from the ventral neural ridge of the primitive neural tube. This region also gives rise to the diencephalon. Thus, the pituitary and the hypothalamus share a common embryonic origin. This new concept allows for important interaction between the hypothalamus and pituitary very early in development.

The human anterior pituitary differentiates very early in embryonic life.[7] At the 7th to 8th week of embryonic development, the glycoprotein containing basophils appears. By the 9th to 10th week, acidophils are present. However, at this early stage the chromophobes, or undifferentiated cells, predominate. It is not until the end of the 7th month that the cells of the anterior lobe ultimately differentiate into the different cell types resembling those of the adult gland. Classically, these are gonadotropes producing luteinizing hormone (LH) and follicle-stimulating hormone (FSH), thyrotropes producing thyroid-stimulating hormone (TSH), lactotropes producing prolactin, somatotropes producing growth hormone (GH), and corticotropes producing adrenocorticotropin (ACTH). In addition to the five classical cell types, a multipotential progenitor cell type that secretes both prolactin and GH has been described.[8] LH, FSH, and TSH are glycoproteins consisting of a common α-subunit, each with a unique β-subunit. Prolactin, GH, and ACTH are polypeptides. The first hormones to be detected in the fetal anterior pituitary are ACTH, β-endorphin, and GH.[9] These appear at 8 weeks of gestation. The α-subunit of the glycoprotein hormones can be identified at 9 weeks, while the β-subunits of these hormones appear by 12 weeks. At this age, prolactin is also present. The posterior pituitary hormones, arginine vasopressin (AVP) and oxytocin, are detected at 10 to 11 weeks of gestation.

Three distinct regions can be identified in the human fetal pituitary gland: the anterior, intermediate, and posterior lobes. As term approaches, the cells of the intermediate lobe begin to disappear. In the human adult, an intermediate lobe is no longer present. The human fetal intermediate lobe contains and secretes β-endorphin and a melanocyte stimulating hormone (MSH)-like peptide, desacetyl-αMSH.

The secretion of hormones from the anterior pituitary is under the control of the hypothalamus. This is mediated through releasing and release-inhibiting hormones produced in specific nuclei of the hypothalamus. These peptide hormones are released into the portal vessels, whose capillaries arise from the median eminence of the medial basal hypothalamus and terminate in sinusoids of the anterior pituitary. The median eminence is formed by 9 weeks, and an intact hypothalamo-hypophyseal portal vascular system can be distinguished at 12 weeks gestation. The hypothalamic nuclei and fiber tracts are identifiable at 14 to 16 weeks, and the hypophysiotropic hormones appear at about this time. Specifically, thyrotropin-releasing hormone (TRH), gonadotropin-releasing hormone (GnRH), and somatostatin have been found in the fetal hypothalamus at around 15 weeks gestation. GH- releasing hormone (GHRH) is identified at 18 weeks, corticotropinreleasing hormone (CRH) at 16 weeks, and catecholamine-containing cells at 12 to 16 weeks. Thus, by the end of the first half of gestation, the major components required for the regulation of anterior pituitary function, namely the secretory cells of the anterior pituitary, the hypophysiotropic hormones produced in the hypothalamus, and the neurovascular link connecting the hypothalamus with the anterior pituitary, are formed. The integrity of these components is essential for the normal function of the anterior pituitary. Conversely, because the differentiation of the anterior pituitary cells occurs before the appearance of the hypothalamic hormones and the vascular link, it appears that the fetal pituitary has a limited potential for differentiation in the absence of hypothalamic input.

ANTERIOR PITUITARY HORMONES

Gonadotropins (LH and FSH)

The fetal pituitary contains LH and FSH at 9 weeks of gestation. In female fetuses, pituitary LH and FSH con. tent rises at midgestation, and this is followed by a decline. In male fetuses, the content of LH and FSH increases progressively throughout gestation.[10] Pituitaries obtained from human fetuses at 5 weeks gestation can release LH and FSH when incubated in vitro.[11] In the fetal circulation, gonadotropins can be measured at 12 weeks gestation. Plasma LH and FSH concentrations rise during the first trimester to peak levels in the second trimester, and gradually decline by the third trimester. The concentrations of gonadotropins in the fetal circulation show sexual dimorphism in that their levels in the female fetus are higher than those in the male during the second half of gestation. This difference can be attributed to the presence of feedback-active gonadal steroids in the male fetus.

The primary regulators for the release of gonadotropins are GnRH and the gonadal steroids. GnRH can be detected in the human brain as early as 5 weeks gestation, and GnRH neurons in the preoptic area of the hypothalamus are identified at 10 weeks. GnRH is necessary for the normal synthesis of the β subunit of LH and FSH, because anencephalic fetuses secrete predominantly the α subunit.[12] Responsiveness of the human fetal pituitary to GnRH stimulation can be demonstrated in vitro at 10 weeks,[13] and in vivo at 15 weeks gestation. The role of the gonadal steroids in modulating pituitary gonadotropin release during the fetal period is less understood. In an in vitro study using dispersed cells from human fetal pituitaries at midgestation, estradiol augments the responsiveness to GnRH.[14] In addition, studies in the monkey fetus have shown that testosterone suppresses LH secretion, because castration in male fetuses increases LH levels in the circulation. Conversely, castration of female fetuses has no effect on circulating LH concentrations. These observations suggest an involvement of the steroids in the regulation of gonadotropin release during the fetal period. However, the exact role played by the gonadal steroids and the sites of feedback regulation of gonadotropin secretion have not been investigated in the human fetus during development.

A unique gonadotropin present in fetal life is human chorionic gonadotropin (hCG), produced by the syncytiotrophoblasts of the placenta. The concentration of hCG in the fetal circulation increases to peak levels at 12 weeks and then declines. This high concentration of hCG is largely responsible for the early development of the testes and of testosterone production before the appearance of fetal LH in the circulation. Thus, the fetal testis is a target organ for hCG. Other fetal tissues, in particular the kidney, are also capable of synthesizing hCG.[15,16]

In the male fetus, the interstitial cells of the testis begin synthesizing testosterone from low density lipoprotein cholesterol at about 8 weeks of gestation. Production rate is maximal at 17 to 21 weeks, but declines thereafter. This pattern coincides closely with the differentiation of the male urogenital tract. Estradiol synthesis in the fetal testes is negligible. In the female fetus, ovarian formation of estradiol from testosterone is detectable at 10 weeks, suggesting the presence of aromatase activity at this early age. Circulating levels of testosterone in the male fetus parallel the rise and fall of testicular testosterone production, while levels in the female fetus remain relatively low and constant throughout gestation. Estradiol concentrations in the circulation of male and female fetuses are low throughout gestation.

Gonadal development and steroidogenesis in the fetal testes is under the control of gonadotropins—placental hCG during early gestation, and fetal pituitary LH and FSH in the second half of gestation. This view is supported by the observation in anencephalic male fetuses that the testicular size is reduced but the steroid-producing capacity is normal. The fetal ovary is relatively quiescent during early pregnancy, and anencephalic female fetuses have normal ovarian development until the third trimester. The role of testosterone during the fetal period is, first, to ensure the normal development of the male gonads, and second, to serve as the feedback-active agent in the regulation of pituitary LH secretion. In the later stages of testicular maturation, events such as seminiferous tubule development and spermatogenesis are FSH dependent. FSH release from the fetal pituitary is regulated by the feedback action of inhibin, which is produced by the fetal testes and ovary. The testes appear to contain greater amounts of inhibin than the ovary. This may account for the lower plasma concentration of FSH in the male than in the female fetus.

Thyroid-Stimulating Hormone

In human fetal pituitaries, TSH can be detected at 12 weeks gestation. The content of TSH increases with advancing gestation and, by 32 weeks, fetal pituitary TSH content is about one tenth of that in the adult pituitary.[17] TSH in the fetal circulation is measurable by 11 to 18 weeks gestation. It increases thereafter to a maximum at 30 to 35 weeks, and then decreases toward term. At term, fetal plasma TSH levels are higher than those in maternal blood.[18] Concurrent with the appearance of TSH in the fetal circulation, TRH is detectable in the hypothalamus by 12 weeks gestation.[19] In humans, TRH crosses the placenta, and administration of TRH to the mother results in a rise in fetal cord plasma TSH followed by an increase in triiodothyronine (T_3) and thyroxine (T_4) levels.[20] In the adult, pituitary TSH secretion is regulated by somatostatin and dopamine in addition to TRH. However, in the fetal period, these mechanisms appear not to be operative. In addition, TSH release is modulated by the feedback action of iodothyronines. In the fetus, negative feedback inhibition of TSH by T_4 can be demonstrated by midgestation. Thus, by this age, the human fetus has developed a functional hypothalamic-pituitary-thyroid axis. However, the role of intrapituitary conversion of T_4 to T_3 in the feedback regulation of TSH during this stage of development is not known.

Anencephalic fetuses have low to normal plasma TSH levels and normal T_4 and T_3 concentrations, and can respond to TRH by an increase in TSH release.[21] These observations suggest the possibility that extrahypothalamic sources of TRH may be maintaining the secretory activity of the thyrotropes in these fetuses. The pancreas of the human newborn and the placenta are known to contain TRH or TRH-like immunoreactivity.

In the human fetus, the thyroid gland has acquired its capacity to concentrate iodine and synthesize iodothyronines by 10 to 12 weeks gestation.[19] Thyroid secretory activity is low until midgestation, when the release of T_4 begins to increase. This increase in T_4 secretion is due to two factors. First, there is a rise in TSH release from the fetal pituitary preceding the increase in T_4. Second, between 26 and 33 weeks gestation, fetal thyroid sensitivity to TSH increases.[22] Thereafter, fetal cord plasma concentrations of total T_4, free T_4, and thyroid-binding globulin increase with gestational age up to 35 weeks, and remain constant until term. In contrast, T_3 levels are very low during gestation until 30 weeks, and rise slightly toward term when the levels are below those in maternal plasma. The concentrations of reverse T_3 reach high levels in the third trimester and then decrease toward term. At birth, T_3 levels increase further to concentrations several-fold greater than that in utero, while reverse T_3 levels remain unchanged. In term human fetuses, intra-amniotic administration of T_4 increases umbilical cord T_4 concentrations and reduces TSH levels, demonstrating the feedback action of T_4 on fetal TSH release.[23] In human newborns, there is a marked stimulation of the pituitary-thyroid axis. However, at birth, umbilical cord TSH levels do not appear to be affected by the mode of delivery, sex of the newborn, or maternal administration of dexamethasone. In congenital hypothyroid newborns, thyroid hormone therapy diminishes the elevated TSH levels.[24]

Prolactin

In the anterior pituitary of the human fetus, prolactin is first detected by 10 weeks gestation. Between 10 and 15 weeks, total pituitary prolactin content is above 2 ng.[25] From 21 weeks onward, the content progressively increases and is accompanied by a rapid increase in prolactin messenger RNA in the pituitary.[26] At 25 to 29 weeks, total prolactin content reaches 550 ng and continues to increase to 2000 ng at term (approximately 15 ng/mg of tissue). Pituitary prolactin content is independent of the sex of the fetus. Secretion of prolactin can be demonstrated in vitro in pituitaries from 5-week-old human fetuses.[11] The fetal pituitary first secretes prolactin into the circulation at 10 weeks to achieve plasma levels of 5 ng/mL. Between 12 and 24 weeks, plasma prolactin levels increase to 20 to 35 ng/mL. Thereafter, prolactin levels rise sharply to 300 to 500 ng/mL in late gestation.[27–29] Because transfer of prolactin across the placenta is limited, the source of the prolactin in the fetal circulation is the fetal pituitary. In the newborn, prolactin levels fall after the first postnatal day to levels below those in the fetus. Premature, small for gestational age, and twin newborns have lower plasma prolactin concentrations, but growth-retarded infants have higher prolactin levels than normal, full-term newborns. Studies in experimental animals and observations in humans have suggested a role for prolactin in the regulation of fluid and electrolyte in the neonate.

Dopaminergic regulation of prolactin secretion develops during the perinatal period. In the midgestational fetus, prolactin secretion does not appear to be tonically inhibited. In the fetal sheep, the dopaminergic mechanism mediating the inhibition of prolactin release is not operative until the last third of gestation.[30] Similarly, in the human fetus the lactotropes do not respond to TRH stimulation until after 20 weeks of gestation. During the fetal period, plasma prolactin level is significantly affected by estrogen. The high levels of prolactin in the circulation of the near-term fetus are largely related to the concurrent increase in placental estrogen secretion. In anencephalic fetuses, plasma prolactin levels at birth are within the range of normal fetuses at delivery, and they can respond to TRH by releasing prolactin. In humans and other primates, high concentrations of prolactin are found in the amniotic fluid. The source of this amniotic prolactin is the decidua rather than the fetal pituitary.[31,32]

The function of prolactin in the fetus remains obscure. Although reproductive, behavioral, or osmoregulatory roles for prolactin have been postulated, these have not been documented. Indirect evidence suggests that prolactin may influence fetal lung maturation by facilitating surfactant synthesis.

Growth Hormone

GH is present in the human fetal pituitary as early as 7 weeks of gestation. GH content increases progressively from 45 μg at 10 weeks to 225 μg at 30 weeks, and increases further to 675 μg at term.[25] Pituitary GH messenger RNA content increases from the early midtrimester to high levels by 27 weeks.[33] Pituitaries obtained from human fetuses at 5 weeks gestation secrete GH when incubated in vitro.[11] GH is detectable in the fetal circulation at 10 weeks, reaches peak levels of 130 ng/mL at 20 weeks, and falls gradually until term to 35 ng/mL. Transfer of GH across the human placenta is minimal; thus, circulating GH is of fetal origin. Premature newborns have higher GH levels in umbilical cord blood than term newborns.

The hypothalamic factors that regulate GH secretion are primarily GHRH and somatostatin. At 12 weeks of gestation, somatostatin can be demonstrated in the hypothalamus, and its content increases until midgestation.[34] GHRH appears later, at 18 to 22 weeks gestation.[35] At this age, the somatotropes are responsive to the effect of GHRH, as well as somatostatin. Because somatostatin crosses the human placenta, administration of somatostatin into the mother can suppress fetal pituitary GH release and hence reduce GH concentration in umbilical cord blood.[36] The fall in plasma GH concentration in the latter half of gestation may be due to an increase in somatostatin release or a simultaneous decrease in GHRH release. Thus, the adult type of regulatory mechanisms for GH release are already established in the fetus by midgestation. Furthermore, the effects of the hypothalamic factors can be modified by other hormones such that T_3 suppresses while dexamethasone enhances the responsiveness of the somatotropes to GHRH. These mechanisms, although present, may not be fully mature at birth, as evidenced by the lack of a sleep-associated rise in plasma GH in the newborn. In anencephalic fetuses, pituitary GH content is low and plasma GH concentrations at term are significantly less than those in normal term fetuses. This finding is consistent with the concept that, in the term fetus, the hypothalamic influence on GH release is primarily stimulatory.

The function of GH in the fetus is unclear. Most evidence suggests that GH is not a major regulator of fetal somatic growth, and anencephalic fetuses have relatively normal birth weight. The lack of peripheral GH receptors may account for the ineffectiveness of GH in the fetus.

Adrenocorticotropin

ACTH is detectable by immunocytochemical methods in the human fetal pituitary at 10 weeks gestation.[37] Release of ACTH from cultured fetal pituitary cells can be demonstrated even earlier, at 7 weeks gestation. At 10 weeks ACTH release begins to increase, but from the second trimester on, plasma ACTH levels do not change with advancing gestation. ACTH in the fetal circulation at term is several-fold greater than that measured in normal adult.[38] Because there is no demonstrable transfer of ACTH from the mother to the fetus, fetal plasma ACTH is derived from the fetal pituitary.

Responsiveness of pituitary corticotropes to CRH can be demonstrated after the 10th week of gestation, and from 10 to 32 weeks the responses of the corticotropes are similar. Thus in the human fetal pituitary, responsiveness to CRH does not change in association with maturation. In the adult, ACTH release is regulated by AVP in addition to CRH. Glucocorticoids modulate the effects of CRH and AVP on ACTH release. Studies using pituitary cells obtained from human fetuses at 14 weeks gestation have shown that synthetic CRH can stimulate the release of ACTH, and this effect is augmented by AVP. In addition, dexamethasone treatment of these cells reduces basal ACTH release, as well as responsiveness to CRH.[39] It appears that the development of responsiveness of the corticotropes to CRH, AVP, and glucocorticoids occurs before the 14th week of gestation. This implies that, at this age, the fetal pituitary is capable of responding to stressful stimuli by releasing ACTH. However, the intricate regulatory mechanisms responsible for maintaining normal ACTH secretion appear to be immature, because factors such as catecholamines or prostaglandins do not modulate basal or stimulated ACTH release during the fetal period.

The human fetal adrenal cortex consists of two zones, the outer definitive (adult) zone, and the inner fetal zone, which comprises 80% to 85% of the volume of the fetal adrenal cortex. The human fetal adrenal grows rapidly after the 10th week of gestation and is nearly as large as the fetal kidney. The fetal adrenal cortex doubles in size between 20 and 30 weeks, and again between 30 weeks and term. This increase in size is largely due to the growth of the outer definitive zone.[40] During the first week of postnatal life, the fetal zone undergoes rapid involution and is no longer present in the adult gland. At 13 weeks gestation, the fetal adrenal is capable of synthesizing glucocorticoids from steroid precursors. In vitro studies using human fetal adrenal tissues at midgestation demonstrate that cortisol is the primary steroid produced and secreted by the definitive zone, while dehydroepiandrosterone sulfate (DHAS) is the main secretory product of the fetal zone.[41] At this age, the release of steroids from these two zones is responsive to ACTH stimulation. A distinct feature of the fetal adrenal is the absence of desensitization to its trophic hormone ACTH.[42] The physiological significance of this phenomenon may be to ensure production of high levels of steroid essential for fetal development and maturation. The fetal zone actively secretes DHAS from the first trimester through the end of pregnancy.

Maintenance of fetal adrenal cortical function after midgestation requires the fetal pituitary, and anencephalic fetuses have atrophic adrenals. The principal trophic factor for the fetal adrenal cortex is ACTH from the fetal pituitary. Placental estrogen also modulates steroid secretion from the fetal zone. Other pituitary and placental peptides have been suggested as potential regulators of the fetal adrenal cortex, but none of these have been shown to have significant effects on steroid secretion from either zone.[43] In addition to stimulation of steroid secretion, ACTH induces the activities of the enzymes 3β-hydroxysteroid dehydrogenase and $\Delta^{4,5}$-isomerase in the fetal zone leading to an increase in cortisol production. This indicates that one of the actions of ACTH in the fetal adrenal is to stimulate the acquisition of activities characteristic of the adult cell phenotype.[44] In asphyxiated newborns at birth, umbilical cord plasma cortisol concentrations are significantly higher than those in normal newborns. Thus, the fetal adrenal is capable of responding to stress by increasing the release of cortisol.

FETAL CARDIOVASCULAR HORMONES

ATRIAL NATRIURETIC FACTOR

Atrial natriuretic factor (ANF) is a hormone produced by the atrial cardiocytes of the heart. It possesses potent natriuretic, diuretic, and vasorelaxant properties. Other commonly used names for ANF include atrial natriuretic peptide (ANP), atriopeptin, and cardiodilatin.[45] Since the discovery of ANF in 1981 by de Bold and coworkers, extensive investigations have been conducted to elucidate its function in the maintenance of vascular pressures and volume in several mammalian species, including the human.[46] Because of its acute effects on body fluids and pressure homeostasis, a role for ANF in hypertension has been implicated, yet many aspects of its function remain unclear.

Physiology of ANF

Function. The best established effect of ANF is on the kidney, where it produces a diuresis and natriuresis (Fig. 12-1). This effect is mediated by an increase in glomerular filtration rate (GFR) and filtration fraction. This results from constriction of the efferent and dilation of the afferent glomerular arterioles. In addition, ANF acts directly at the distal and collecting tubules, presumably to suppress renal tubular transport mechanisms. These effects, coupled with an ANF-induced inhibition of renin release and suppression of angiotensin II-stimulated aldosterone secretion, result in a pronounced but short-lasting diuresis and natriuresis.[47] High densities of ANF receptors at the renal glomeruli and moderate densities at the collecting tubules support the suggestion that these two structures are the target organs for ANF action. At the cellular level, the action of ANF is mediated by a receptor activation of guanylate cyclase, leading to an increase in cyclic GMP levels.

In addition to its primary action at the kidney, ANF has a vasorelaxant effect on vascular smooth muscles. This effect is especially marked in vessels preconstricted with angiotensin II or norepinephrine. Other cardiovascular effects of ANF include a lowering of systolic and

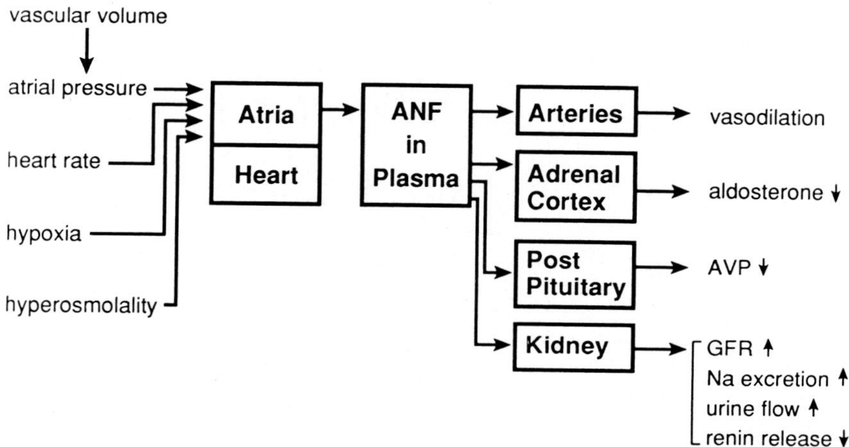

FIGURE 12–1. Regulation and function of atrial natriuretic factor (ANF).

diastolic blood pressures, with a concomitant increase in heart rate and a moderate decrease in blood volume. It interacts with other endocrine systems to inhibit renin release from the kidney, aldosterone secretion from the adrenal cortex, and stress-induced release of AVP.

Localization. In the adult mammalian heart, ANF is localized in the atria with concentrations in the left atrium greater than that in the right. Immunoreactive ANF is more abundant in the atrial epicardial myocardium than in the endocardial myocardium. High concentrations are found in areas where distentional forces are greatest, suggesting that atrial stretch stimulates ANF release. ANF is found in the adventitia of the aortic arch, but not in the endothelial surface or muscularis. In the lower thoracic or abdominal aorta, ANF is not present. ANF messenger RNA in the atria constitutes 0.8% to 3% of total atrial messenger RNA, indicating that it is a major gene transcription product. In the ventricles of the adult heart, ANF is undetectable.[48] Low levels of ANF gene expression have been observed in the ventricles and can be activated by pressure or volume load. Adults with congestive heart failure have elevated levels of ANF messenger RNA.

Regulation of Release. The ANF found in the circulation is a 28-amino acid peptide with a cystein-cystein disulfide bridge, which is essential for biological activity.[49] This molecule is derived from a prohormone of 126 amino acids, which is stored in the secretory granules of the cardiocytes. The prohormone is in turn derived from a precursor molecule of 151 amino acids (Fig. 12-2). Upon stimulation, posttranslational processing of the prohormone takes place within the cardiocyte to liberate the active 28-amino acid fragment immediately prior to release into the circulation. Stretching of the atrial cardiocytes leads to rapid release of ANF. Thus, under conditions of atrial distention such as increases in central venous pressure, plasma ANF levels are generally elevated. Expansion of vascular volume is similarly a powerful stimulus for ANF release. In addition, severe hypoxia and hyperosmolality can stimulate ANF release from atrial cardiocytes.

ANF During Human Development

In the human fetus, a functional circulation begins at 3 to 4 weeks and the four-chambered heart is formed by 8 weeks of gestation. ANF can be demonstrated in fetal atria at 10 weeks of gestation in concentrations comparable to those found in the adult atria.[48] Thus, the first appearance of ANF in the human heart is at the very early stage of cardiac development. Throughout gestation, ANF concentration in the fetal atria is greater than that in the adult atria, with little change associated with maturation. During the fetal period, ANF content is higher in the right atrium than in the left, whereas in the adult, the content is higher in the left than in the right. A unique situation occurs in the fetus in that ANF is found in the ventricles, with similar concentrations in the right and the left, but both much lower than those in the atria. Ventricular ANF concentration decreases as gestation advances and, in the adult ventricles, ANF is no longer detectable. It has been suggested that prenatal ventricular ANF is released by a constitutive rather than a regulative pathway, because the ventricular cells lack secretory granules and release ANF rapidly after synthesis.

Analysis of the molecular form of ANF in the fetal heart shows that fetal ANF is identical to that in the adult. Human fetal atria express the ANF gene at a high level throughout gestation, accruing substantial quantities of ANF and ANF messenger RNA. Atrial ANF messenger RNA levels do not change significantly with maturation. The fetal ventricles also express the ANF gene, but at levels lower than those in the atria. Ventricular ANF messenger RNA concentration decreases with advancing gestation.[50] Thus, ANF gene expression in the human heart during development parallels the appearance of ANF.[51] In addition to their presence in the heart, immunoreactive ANF and ANF messenger RNA are found in fetal lung tissues. This suggests that ANF may play a role in fetal pulmonary development.[52]

In the human fetus, the concentrations of ANF in the fetal circulation range from 23 to 283 pg/mL (Table 12-1). These levels are higher than those in the maternal circulation, and are not related to gestational age,

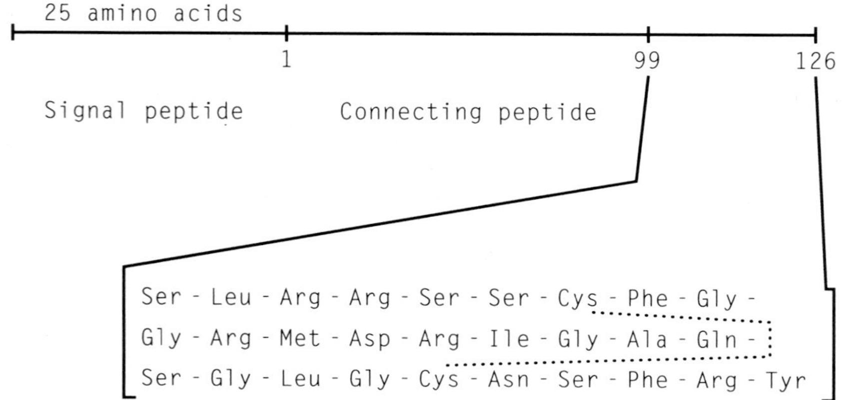

FIGURE 12–2. Amino acid sequence of atrial natriuretic factor (ANF).

TABLE 12–1. PLASMA ANF CONCENTRATIONS IN NORMAL PREGNANT WOMEN AND THEIR FETUSES

ADULT FEMALE			
NON-PREGNANT	TERM PREGNANCY	PIH	REFERENCE
44 ± 2 (SD)	98 ± 4	244 ± 6	Miyamoto et al (1988)[53]
29 ± 6 (SEM)	62 ± 7	116 ± 19	Otsuki et al (1987)[54]
38 ± 14 (SD)	43 ± 20	162 ± 95	Hirai et al (1988)[55]
–	80 ± 4 (SEM)	116 ± 13	Hatji et al (1989)[56]
FETUS			
ARTERIAL	VENOUS		REFERENCE
118 ± 13 (SD)	89 ± 12		Hatji et al (1989)[56]
–	69 ± 8 (SD)		Tulassay et al (1987)[57]
98 ± 15 (SEM)	56 ± 9		Castro et al (1989)[58]
157 ± 66 (SD)	56 ± 42		Kikuchi et al (1988)[59]
283 ± 56 (SEM)	165 ± 27		Yamaji et al (1986)[60]
–	101 ± 33* (SEM)		Weiner & Robillard (1989)[61]
–	23		Panos et al (1989)[62]
–	44		Kingdom et al (1989)[63]

The ANF concentrations are expressed as pg/mL (mean ± SEM or SD). The fetal blood samples were collected from the umbilical cord vessels at the time of normal term delivery.

* These samples were obtained by cordocentesis at 19 to 39 weeks gestation, and contained both arterial and venous samples.

sex, or fetal weight. An umbilical arterial and venous difference in ANF concentration is found, being higher in the arterial plasma (Fig. 12-3).[60] This suggests that the placenta may act as a clearance site for fetal ANF. Studies in the fetal sheep suggest that the fetal kidney may be an additional clearance site for ANF, because urinary and amniotic ANF concentrations are 5% of that measured in the fetal circulation.[64] Using the pregnant sheep as a model, the half-life of ANF in the fetal circulation has been measured and is found to be 0.4 minutes. The ANF plasma clearance rate is 115 mL/min/kg, and the endogenous release rate is 13 ng/min/kg.[65] These levels are significantly higher than those measured in the adult sheep.[66] Thus, the high release rate of ANF in the fetus is sufficient to account for the elevated ANF levels measured in the fetal circulation. This not only indicates that ANF in the fetal circulation is of fetal origin, but that ANF may be functionally important in the regulation of fetal body fluid and renal function.

In the fetus, the regulation of ANF release is presumably similar to that in the adult. Because very few studies have been conducted to investigate the control of ANF secretion in the human fetus, the bulk of information has been derived from studies using the chronically catheterized fetal sheep model. In the sheep fetus, infusion of ANF into the circulation lowers arterial pressure and reduces blood volume. This is accompanied by an increase in urine flow.[67] The fetal kidney responds to ANF by increasing glomerular filtration rate, free water clearance, and excretion of sodium and chloride.[68] These fetal responses to ANF are similar to those in the adult. The known factors that elevate plasma ANF concentrations in the fetus are hypoxia, atrial pacing, and vascular volume expansion. The latter effect can be potentiated by hyperosmotic stimuli.

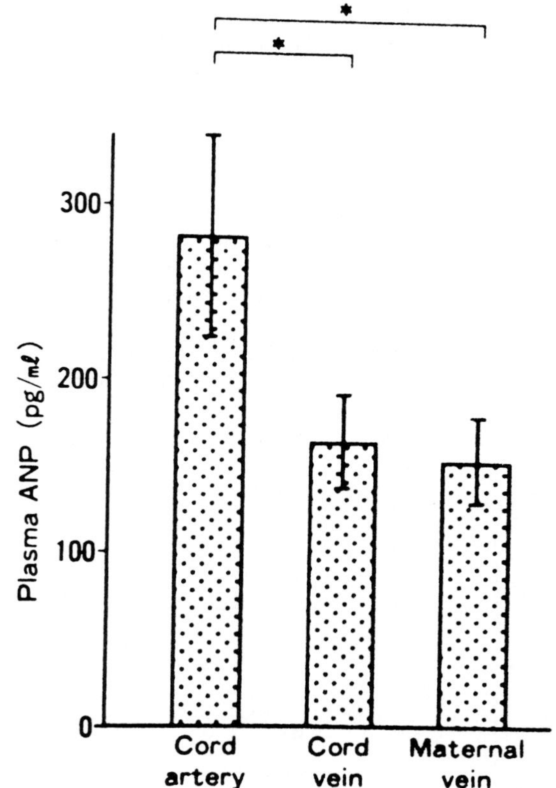

FIGURE 12–3. Concentrations of atrial natriuretic peptide (ANP) in umbilical arterial, umbilical venous, and maternal peripheral venous plasma at the time of delivery in full-term pregnancy. Each bar represents mean ± SEM ($n = 10$). *$P < 0.05$. (From Yamaji T, et al. Atrial natriuretic peptide in umbilical cord blood: evidence for a circulating hormone in the human fetus. J Clin Endocrinol Metab 1986;63:1414.)

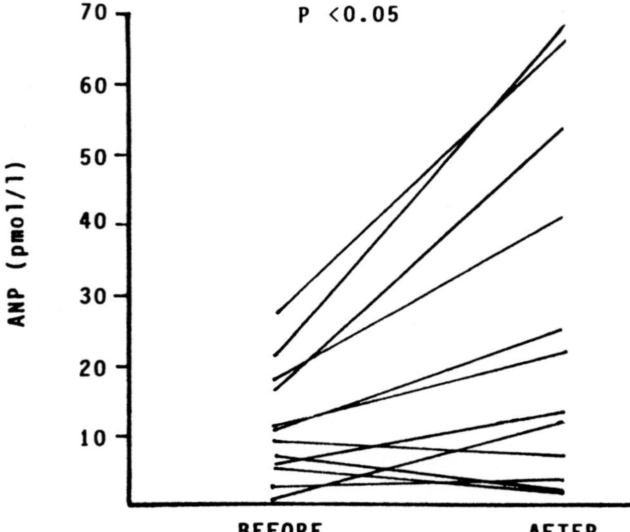

FIGURE 12–4. Plasma atrial natriuretic peptide (ANP) concentrations before and immediately after intravascular transfusion of packed blood in 12 fetuses at 21 to 35 weeks gestation with red-cell isoimmunization. The volume of blood transfused expressed as a ratio of the estimated fetoplacental volume was 0.29 to 1.37 (median, 0.76). (From Panos MZ, et al. Plasma atrial natriuretic peptide in human fetus: response to intravascular blood transfusion. Am J Obstet Gynecol 1989;161:357.)

Available evidence suggests that, in the human fetus and neonate, ANF is an important hormone in the regulation of plasma sodium concentration and fluid volume homeostasis. ANF measurements taken in umbilical cord blood obtained by cordocentesis from fetuses at 19 to 39 weeks gestation show that ANF levels are generally high in fetuses with abnormalities in body fluid regulation.[61] Isoimmune fetuses with hydrops have elevated plasma ANF concentrations, but isoimmunized fetuses without hydrops have normal ANF levels. Experimentally induced hydrops in fetal sheep have greatly elevated plasma ANF concentrations, and these high levels are reversed after resolution of the hydrops.[69] Vascular volume expansion by blood transfusions in human fetuses with immune hemolytic anemia at 21 to 35 weeks gestation elevates plasma ANF levels (Fig. 12-4).[62,70] Fetuses with renal disorders such as renal agenesis and multicystic dysplastic kidneys have lower plasma ANF concentrations than in normal fetuses. Overall, these observations indicate that there are significant interactions between ANF and the fetal vascular and extravascular fluid systems. In patients with severe preeclampsia, maternal plasma ANF concentrations are higher than those in normal pregnancies.[54,55] The fetuses of these preeclamptic mothers have elevated cord arterial and venous ANF levels at the time of delivery (Fig. 12-5).[56] These observations appear to be in conflict with the known stimulus of volume expansion for ANF release, because both maternal and fetal volumes may be contracted in these patients. One possible explanation for these findings is an increase in preload and thus in left atrial pressure, resulting in increase in ANF release. In patients with acute fetal distress as revealed by late heart rate deceleration at the time of delivery, umbilical arterial and venous ANF concentrations are elevated.[71] At term, fetal umbilical plasma ANF levels appear not to be affected by the mode of delivery or the stress of labor (Fig. 12-6).[58,72]

ANF in the Newborn

In newborn infants, plasma ANF concentrations increase during the first 24 hours and then gradually decline in the next 4 days (Fig. 12-7).[73] The initial rise in ANF is largely the result of the postnatal circulatory changes that occur at birth—that is, the closure of the ductus arteriosus and loss of placental circulation. As a consequence, in the immediate postnatal period pulmonary vascular resistance falls, pulmonary blood flow increases, and systemic vascular resistance is elevated.

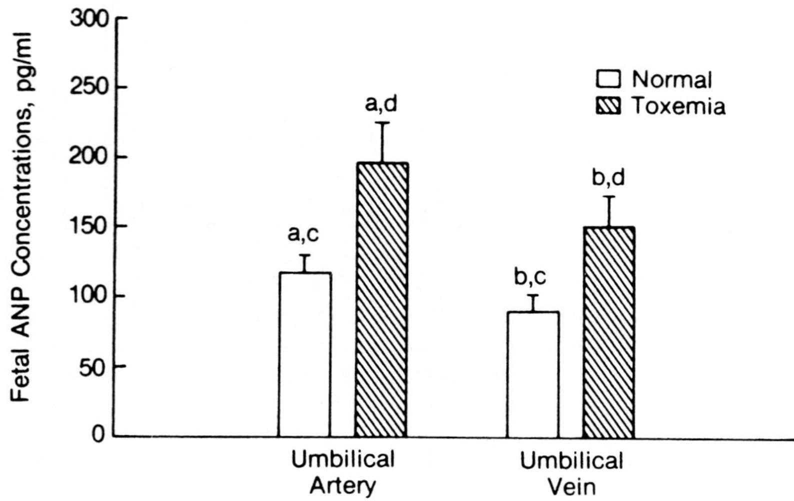

FIGURE 12–5. Plasma atrial natriuretic peptide (ANP) concentrations in umbilical artery and vein of fetuses born to women with normal pregnancy (n = 13) and patients with preeclampsia (n = 8) at the time of delivery. Each bar represents mean ± SEM. a, $P < 0.01$; b, $P < 0.02$; c, $P < 0.001$; d, $P < 0.02$. (From Hatjis CG, et al. Atrial natriuretic factor maternal and fetal concentrations in severe preeclampsia. Am J Obstet Gynecol 1989;161:1015.)

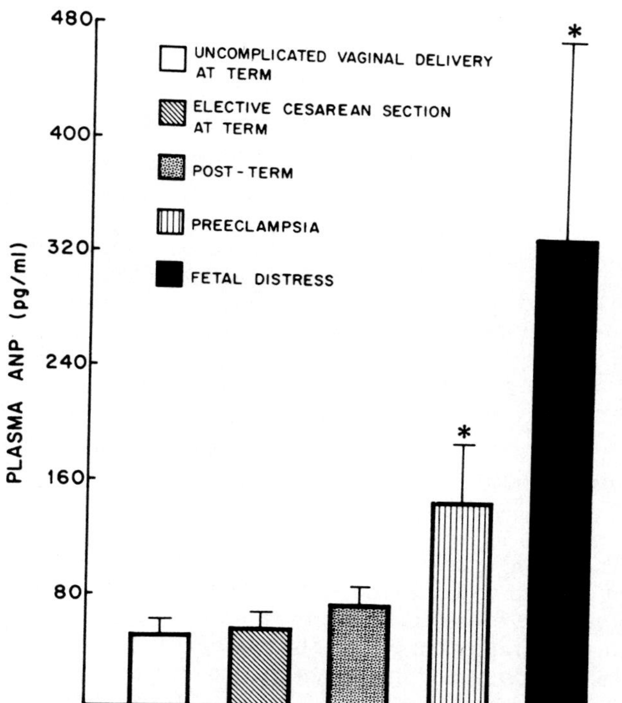

FIGURE 12-6. Plasma atrial natriuretic peptide (ANP) concentrations in umbilical artery at the time of delivery in fetuses born to women with normal term pregnancies and uncomplicated vaginal delivery (n = 19), with normal term pregnancies and elective cesarean section (n = 10), with post-term pregnancies and vaginal delivery or cesarean section (n = 21), with preeclampsia and delivered vaginally or by cesarean section (n = 8), and with fetal distress as evidenced by abnormal fetal heart rate tracing, low umbilical arterial pH, and low Apgar score. Each bar represents mean ± SEM. *$P < 0.01$ compared to uncomplicated vaginal delivery at term. (From Castro, et al., Perinatal factors influencing atrial natriuretic peptide levels in umbilical arterial plasma at the time of delivery. Am J Obstet Gynecol 1989;161:623.)

These changes are associated with increases in atrial pressure and volume, which stimulate ANF release. It has been suggested that this rise in ANF may be the cause for the postnatal diuresis and natriuresis, resulting in extracellular volume contraction and weight loss in newborns.[74]

Premature newborns with patent ductus arteriosus have distended left atria and markedly elevated plasma ANF concentration. The degree of distention is significantly correlated with the rise in ANF levels. In these patients, surgical treatment or indomethacin administration causes closure of the ductus, restores left atrial size, and returns plasma ANF levels to normal.[75] In a similar situation, premature newborns with left-to-right foramen ovale shunting have elevated plasma ANF concentrations, and the increase in ANF is correlated with the magnitude of shunting.[76] Newborns with ventricular septal defect that leads to various degrees of volume loading in the left atria have elevated plasma ANF levels. Premature infants with respiratory distress syndrome,[77] meconium aspiration syndrome, and various forms of heart failure similarly have abnormally high plasma concentrations of ANF.

These clinical observations lead to the conclusion that, under normal conditions, ANF is involved in the maintenance of body fluids in the fetus and newborn. Any deviation from normal can result in stimulation of ANF release, as manifested by increased ANF concentrations in the circulation. It is clear that further research is needed in order to elucidate the mechanisms by which ANF modulates fetal renal and cardiovascular functions, and to determine the factors that regulate the release of ANF in the perinatal period.

RENIN-ANGIOTENSIN-ALDOSTERONE SYSTEM

The renin-angiotensin-aldosterone system in the adult plays an important role in the regulation of blood pressure and vascular fluid volume, as well as in the maintenance of sodium and potassium homeostasis. In the fetal and neonatal period, the role of the renin-angiotensin system in cardiovascular regulation is less well understood. Yet very early in gestation, all the components of the system are present and the fetus is capable of producing the active hormone angiotensin II. Infusion of angiotensin II into experimental fetal animals significantly affects cardiovascular function. The following sections review our current understanding of the renin-angiotensin-aldosterone system in the human fetus.

Components of the Renin-Angiotensin System

Renin is a carboxyl-peptidase enzyme that acts on a plasma α_2 globulin, referred to as renin substrate or angiotensinogen, to produce the biologically inactive decapeptide angiotensin I. Angiotensin I is acted on by converting enzyme to liberate the octapeptide angiotensin II (Fig. 12-8). This conversion occurs primarily in pulmonary vessels, and to a lesser extent in plasma and other parts of the body, including the placenta during pregnancy. Angiotensin II is the biologically active hormone with a circulatory half-life of 1 to 2 minutes. Angiotensin I and angiotensin II are deactivated by the action of angiotensinases to form the less active peptide angiotensin III. Angiotensin II has two major actions, a potent pressor effect mediated by a strong vasoconstrictor action, and a stimulatory effect on aldosterone secretion from the adrenal cortex. Angiotensin III is less potent than angiotensin II in its presser effect, but it is equal to if not more effective than angiotensin II in stimulating aldosterone secretion.

The source of renin in the kidney is the juxtaglomerular cells located in the wall of the afferent arterioles as they enter the glomeruli. Renin is stored in secretory granules of these cells. At the point where the afferent arterioles enter and the efferent arterioles leave the glo-

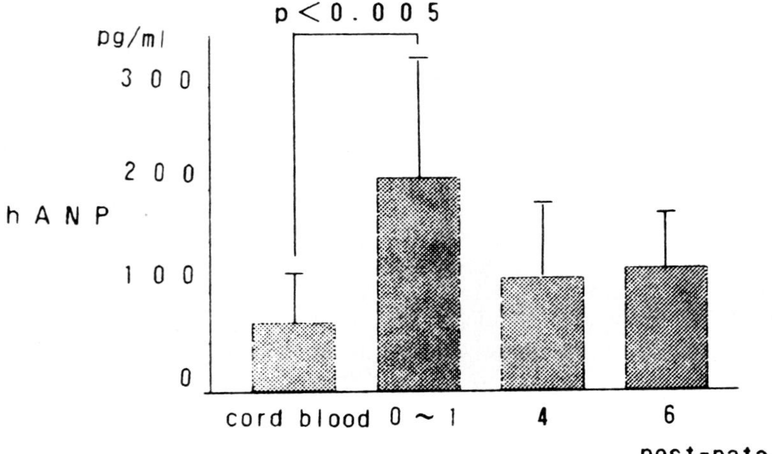

FIGURE 12–7. Fetal plasma atrial natriuretic peptide (ANP) concentration in umbilical plasma at the time of vaginal delivery at term. ANP concentrations were also measured in newborn infants on 0 to 1, 4 or 6 postnatal days. Each bar represents mean ± SD. A total of 25 newborns were studied. (From Ito Y, et al. Concentrations of human atrial natriuretic peptide in the cord blood and the plasma of the newborn. Acta Paediatr Scand 1988;77:76.)

meruli, the nephron tubule is modified to become the macula densa. This structure is involved in the regulation of renin release. Several mechanisms control the secretion of renin. One mechanism is a change in blood pressure in the renal arterioles at the level of the juxtaglomerular cells. A fall in pressure is sensed by an intrarenal baroreceptor or stretch receptor that stimulates renin release. Another mechanism is the transport of chloride or sodium across the macula densa. An increase in reabsorption of sodium and chloride across the macula densa or a decrease in delivery of electrolytes activates renin release. In addition, the sympathetic nervous system regulates renin release by β adrenergic stimulatory and α adrenergic inhibitory mechanisms. Furthermore, the secretion of renin is under the control of a negative feedback loop, in which plasma angiotensin II feeds back to inhibit renin release by a direct action on the juxtaglomerular cells. Aldosterone also feeds back to inhibit renin release. Finally, prostaglandins are potent stimulators of renin release. Renin secretion at any given time is apparently due to the combined effects of these various regulatory mechanisms.

Angiotensinogen
(renin substrate)
← Renin (active ⇌ inactive)
Angiotensin I   Asp - Arg - Val - Tyr - Ile - His - Pro - Phe - His - Leu
← Converting enzyme
Angiotensin II   Asp - Arg - Val - Tyr - Ile - His - Pro - Phe
← Angiotensinases
Peptide fragments
Angiotensin III   Arg - Val - Tyr - Ile - His - Pro - Phe

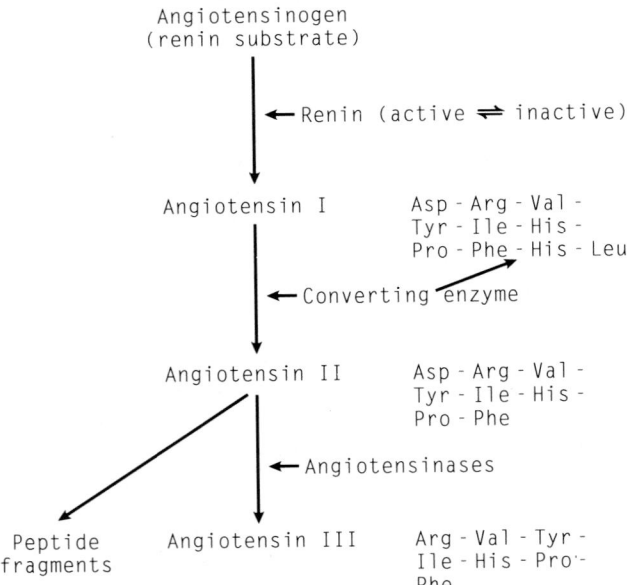

FIGURE 12–8. Production and amino acid sequence of the angiotensins.

Ontogeny of the Renin-Angiotensin System

The human kidney produces renin very early in gestation. At 5 to 6 weeks, renin-containing cells are detectable in the wall of the arterioles of the mesonephros.[78] By 8 weeks, it appears in the metanephros, and at this stage, renin granules are seen by transmission electron microscopy in the juxtaglomerular epithelial cells.[79] Thus, the granular cells of the kidney are one of the earliest endocrine cells detectable during human ontogenesis. In human fetuses from 12.5 to 25 weeks, total renal content of renin increases with gestation, but the specific activity of renin decreases during this period.[80] In spite of this decrease, renin specific activity in the fetal kidney is about 20 times greater than that in normal adult kidney. This high activity suggests that the fetal renin-angiotensin system is chronically stimulated, and may play an important role in the control of blood pressure and extracellular fluid volume during the fetal period. Indeed, studies in chronically catheterized fetal sheep have demonstrated that the renin-angiotensin system in the fetus is hyperactive and is responsive to stimuli such as hemorrhage or reductions in blood volume, hypotension, and renal arterial vasoconstriction.

Fetal Renin. Renin has a molecular weight of 43,000 and can exist in the activated or inactivated state; the latter is the precursor to the active hormone. Active renin reacts with its substrate at a physiological pH, while inactive renin is active only at acidic pH. Both active and inactive renin have been found in the fetal kidney. After trypsin treatment, which converts the precursor to the active form, renin activity in the fetal kidney increases by about 18% to 38%, suggesting that the amount of inactive renin present is limited.[80] Human fetal blood is also known to contain inactive renin in addition to the active hormone. Studies in chronically catheterized bilaterally nephrectomized fetal sheep show that renin does not cross the ovine placenta and that fetal renin activity is independent of maternal levels.

Plasma renin activity in the human fetus is highest in the first trimester and falls by the third trimester. These levels are greater than the normal levels found in nonpregnant adults. There are extrarenal sources of renin. These include the fetal male and female genital tracts, umbilical cord vessels, and the fetal lung. These tissues contain significant quantities of active or inactive renin. The production and release of renin from these sites may contribute to the high renin concentrations found in the fetal circulation. However, the absence of renin in the anephric fetus suggests that the kidneys are the primary source of plasma renin in the fetus. Renin release in the fetus appears to be activated by factors similar to those in the adult. In the fetal sheep, a reduction in fetal blood volume of as little as 3% to 5% can increase plasma renin activity. Hypotension, hypoxia, aortic constriction, and low maternal sodium intake can induce renin release from the fetal kidney. At birth, plasma renin activity in the fetal circulation is higher after vaginal delivery with normal labor than after cesarean section (Table 12-2).[81] This results from the combined increase in plasma renin concentration and plasma renin substrate levels. These increases are observed in both umbilical arterial and venous plasma. At vaginal delivery, plasma renin concentrations in the umbilical vein are higher than those in the umbilical artery, suggesting placental release of renin.[82] In newborns whose umbilical blood pH and oxygen tension are decreased, plasma renin concentrations are elevated (Figs. 12-9 and 12-10).[83] Growth-retarded fetuses and nonimmune hydropic fetuses also have elevated plasma renin activity.[61] Early studies have indicated that, in newborns of hypertensive patients, umbilical arterial and venous levels of plasma renin activity are higher than those in newborns of normotensive mothers.[84] Recent studies have found that newborns of hypertensive mothers have either an increased[85] or unchanged[86] umbilical renin activity.

TABLE 12–2. PLASMA RENIN ACTIVITY LEVELS DURING BIRTH IN THE HUMAN NEWBORN

TYPE OF DELIVERY	N	PLASMA RENIN ACTIVITY* ng/mL/hr
Cesarean section without labor	14	15.2 ± 2.3†‡
Cesarean section with labor	16	44.1 ± 8.9‡
Vaginal delivery	32	34.7 ± 4.3†

* Umbilical cord blood.

† Cesarean section without labor vs vaginal delivery ($P < 0.05$).

‡ Cesarean section without labor vs cesarean section with labor ($P < 0.02$), mean and SEM.

From Hadeed A, Sizgal SR. Plasma renin activity after birth and in the early newborn period. Am J Perinatal 1984;1:285.

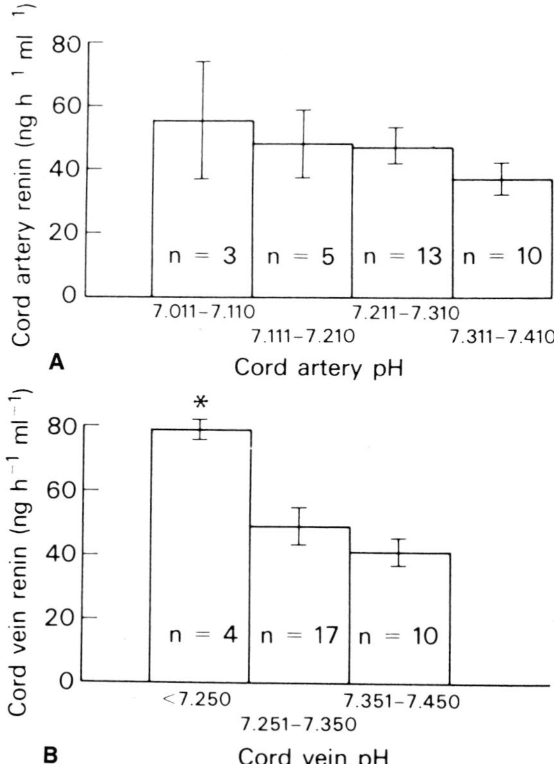

FIGURE 12–9. The effect of blood pH on renin concentration in umbilical artery (**A**) and vein (**B**) of newborns delivered vaginally. Each bar represents mean ± SEM. *$P < 0.001$. (From Tetlow HJ, Broughton Pipkin F. The effect of changes in blood gas tension upon the renin-angiotensin system of the newborn infant. Br J Obstet Gynecol 1983;90:898.)

Amniotic Fluid Renin. The amniotic fluid contains appreciable amounts of renin in both active and inactive forms. Other components of the renin-angiotensin system present in the amniotic fluid are angiotensin I, angiotensin-converting enzyme, and renin substrate. The most likely source of amniotic renin is the chorion, although contributions from the fetus cannot be ruled out. The presence of these components in the amniotic fluid allows the production of angiotensin II, which may act locally in the control of placental blood flow. In the amniotic fluid, a large molecular weight form of renin—"big renin"—has been reported, but its presence has not been confirmed.

Fetal Angiotensin II. In the fetus, circulating angiotensin II concentrations are similar to those in maternal circulation, and are higher than those in non-pregnant adults. Angiotensin II is important in the maintenance

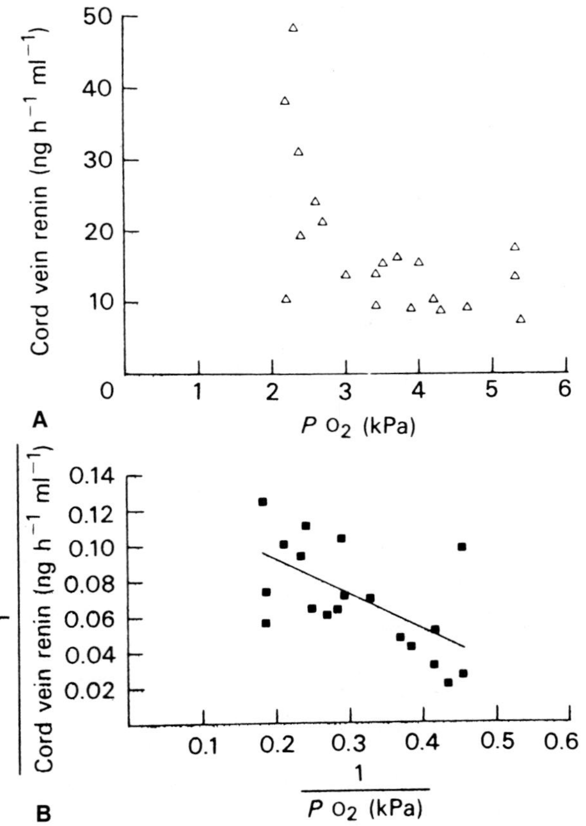

FIGURE 12–10. Correlation between umbilical vein renin concentration and oxygen tension in newborns at elective cesarean section. (**A**) Standard plot; (**B**) reciprocal plot. Solid line is the calculated linear regression line ($r = -0.60$, $P < 0.01$, $n = 19$). (From Tetlow HJ, Broughton Pipkin F. The effect of changes in blood gas tension upon the renin-angiotensin system of the newborn infant. Br J Obstet Gynaecol 1983;90:898).

of normal fetal blood pressure, and plays a major role in blood pressure regulation under stress conditions. These conclusions are supported by studies performed in the fetal sheep showing that intravenous infusion of the angiotensin II antagonist saralasin lowers fetal arterial pressure to levels below normal. In human newborns, umbilical arterial and venous angiotensin II concentrations are both significantly higher than maternal levels following vaginal delivery, but are not elevated if delivery is by cesarean section without labor.[87] Following normal labor, angiotensin II levels in umbilical venous blood exceed those in umbilical artery. This suggests that the placenta may be a site of angiotensin I to angiotensin II conversion, or that angiotensin II may be produced in the placenta and released into the fetal circulation. Transfer of angiotensin II across the human placenta is negligible, and maternal angiotensin II has little effect on the fetus. Angiotensin II infusion into pregnant women during the third trimester has little effect on fetal heart rate and fetal movement.[88] In the perifused human placenta, cotyledonary vessels on the fetal side can respond to angiotensin II by vasoconstriction.[89] In this preparation, angiotensin I is equally active, suggesting that the placenta may act as a site of conversion of angiotensin I to angiotensin II, which then acts locally to control blood flow.[90] The effect of the angiotensins is attenuated by prostacyclin.[91] Thus, the pressor effect of angiotensin II on the placental circulation can be counteracted by the prostacyclin. Angiotensin II receptors have been identified in human placenta.[92]

Renin-Angiotensin System in the Newborn

In newborn infants, plasma renin activity is elevated above that in the fetus. This is primarily due to an increase in renin release from the kidney rather than an increase in renin substrate level. The activity of the renin-angiotensin system in the newborn continues to increase for several hours after delivery, and rise further during the first few days of life. Plasma renin activity remains elevated throughout infancy, and adult levels are not achieved until 6 to 9 years of age.[93]

Fetal Production and Secretion of Aldosterone

The adrenal steroid aldosterone is the primary mineralocorticoid secreted in physiologically significant amounts by the zona glomerulosa of the adrenal cortex. The circulatory half-life of aldosterone is about 20 minutes, and in circulation it is bound to plasma proteins, but only to a small extent. Aldosterone promotes the reabsorption of sodium in the kidney by an action on the epithelium of the distal tubule and collecting duct. This action is mediated by an increase in active transport of sodium from the tubular lumen to the interstitium and then to the blood in exchange for potassium, resulting in kaliuresis.

The outer zone of the human fetal adrenal cortex is the definitive or adult zone, and comprises only 15% to 20% of the fetal adrenal cortex. This zone is relatively quiescent until the third trimester of pregnancy, when it secretes both aldosterone and cortisol. Aldosterone is present in low concentrations in the fetal adrenals at 12.5 weeks gestation. Thereafter, total tissue aldosterone content correlates positively with gestational age. Human fetal adrenocortical cells in culture use low-density lipoprotein-cholesterol as precursor for steroidogenesis, and secrete aldosterone in response to ACTH stimulation.[94] The fetal adrenal probably acquires the ability to synthesize aldosterone from precursor steroids in the second trimester. This may explain the low levels found prior to this period and the gradual increase in content from the second trimester on. The physiological role of aldosterone in the human fetus has not been investigated. In the sheep fetus, aldosterone infusion decreases urinary sodium excretion, suggesting that the fetal kidneys are responsive to physiological increases in aldosterone concentration. Plasma renin activity in these fetuses is suppressed, illustrating that a negative feedback inhibition of aldosterone on renin release is operative during the fetal period.[95]

Aldosterone crosses the human placenta. At term, fetal secretion of aldosterone is increased, resulting in transplacental passage of the steroid into the maternal circulation.[96] Similarly, in pregnant women in the third trimester, postural change from left lateral position to supine recumbency causes a reduction in uteroplacental blood flow, which activates the fetal renin-angiotensin-aldosterone system. Aldosterone secretion in these fetuses is stimulated, leading to passage into the maternal circulation.[97]

POSTERIOR PITUITARY HORMONES

In the human fetus, the posterior pituitary hormones AVP and oxytocin are present early in gestation. In addition, a third hormone, arginine vasotocin (AVT), is present in the posterior pituitary during the fetal period. These three nonapeptides are very similar in their amino acid sequence. Each consists of a six amino acid ring connected by a disulfide bridge and a three amino acid carboxyl terminal side chain. AVT is phylogenetically the ancestral peptide, with structural and functional similarities to both AVP and oxytocin (Fig. 12-11).

Development of the Posterior Pituitary Hormones

During embryonic development, an evagination of the floor of the third cerebral ventricle comes into contact with the posterior aspect of the primitive anterior pituitary. By the fifth gestational week, this downgrowth from the floor of the diencephalon forms the posterior pituitary and receives nerve fiber tracts from the hypothalamic nuclei paraventricular and supraoptic. The posterior pituitary hormones are produced in these hypothalamic nuclei and transported to the posterior pituitary for storage and release.

Each of the posterior pituitary hormones is synthesized by enzymatic conversion of a precursor molecule to the nine amino acid peptide hormone, together with a specific carrier protein neurophysin. AVP and oxytocin with their associated neurophysin are packaged into granules in the cell bodies of the supraoptic and paraventricular nuclei, and transported along the axons of the hypothalmo-hypophyseal tract to the terminals in the posterior pituitary for storage. Upon stimulation, the hormone along with its neurophysin is released into the circulation. AVP and oxytocin are synthesized by both hypothalamic nuclei with a preponderance of AVP in the supraoptic and oxytocin in the paraventricular nucleus. During the fetal period, the two hormones are also expressed in other hypothalamic nuclei, one of which is the suprachiasmatic nucleus.

Studies in the human fetus have shown that AVT is detectable in the fetal pituitary at 8 to 9 weeks gestation, while AVP is demonstrable at 12 weeks. At this age, the posterior pituitary contains a preponderance of AVT relative to AVP. Between 12 and 19 weeks, the ratio of AVT to AVP decreases, and at term the pituitary content of AVT is low.[98,99] Oxytocin appears in the pituitary 3 to 4 weeks later than AVP, and the AVP to oxytocin ratio is initially very high. The levels of these two hormones increase significantly over the next 20 weeks. During this time, the high AVP to oxytocin ratio gradually decreases, but does not reach unity until the neonatal period.[100] In the adult pituitary, the ratio of AVP to oxytocin is 1, while AVT is no longer present.

In the hypothalamus, the occurrence of AVP and oxytocin parallels that in the posterior pituitary. The AVP- and oxytocin-associated neurophysins appear at about 11 to 12 weeks. However, at this time AVP is detectable, while oxytocin is not detectable until 3 weeks later.[101] These observations indicate that the development and biosynthesis of the two hormone precursors proceed at a similar rate, and that the low content of oxytocin in the initial period is due to the lack of fully processed oxytocin, rather than to an excess of AVP. Experimental evidence in the rat reveals that the posttranslational processing of these two peptides is differentially regulated during development.[102]

Arginine Vasotocin

Cys - Tyr - Ile - Gln - Asn - Cys - Pro - Arg - Gly

Arginine vasopressin

Cys - Tyr - Phe - Gln - Asn - Cys - Pro - Arg - Gly

Oxytocin

Cys - Tyr - Ile - Gln - Asn - Cys - Pro - Leu - Gly

FIGURE 12–11. Amino acid sequence of the posterior pituitary hormones.

Posterior Pituitary Hormones in the Fetus

The AVP and oxytocin present in the fetal circulation originate from the fetal pituitary, because there is little evidence to suggest that either AVP or oxytocin crosses the human placenta during gestation. Both AVP and oxytocin are rapidly cleared from the circulation, with a half-life of 3 to 6 minutes. Clearance occurs in the kidney and, to a lesser extent, in the liver. Additionally, vasopressinases and oxytocinases produced by the cytotrophoblasts of the human placenta are found in cord blood, maternal plasma, and amniotic fluid. In the amniotic fluid, the activity of these enzymes increases with gestational age, and they probably play a role in the metabolism and degradation of AVP, AVT, and oxytocin.[103]

Oxytocin. Oxytocin is measurable by radioimmunoassay in the fetal pituitary at 14 to 17 weeks gestation. From 20 to 26 weeks, there is a three-fold increase in content; at 32 weeks, the levels are two to five times greater than those at 14 to 17 weeks. This increase in oxytocin content with gestational age is due to an increase in oxytocin concentration, rather than to an increase in the weight of the pituitary gland.[104] In human parturition, oxytocin levels in fetal blood rise. This increase may reflect limited transfer of oxytocin across the placenta when oxytocin concentrations in the maternal circulation reach high levels at this time. Because an umbilical arterial and venous difference exists in cord blood following labor in human newborn, fetal secretion of oxytocin must also be augmented during labor.

Arginine Vasotocin. In addition to its presence in the fetal pituitary, AVT is also found in the fetal pineal gland from 8 to 17 weeks gestation.[105] In vitro synthesis of AVT in human fetal pineal tissue can be demonstrated between 13 and 17 weeks of gestation. In the adult, the pineal gland and cerebrospinal fluid both contain AVT. The physiological role of AVT in the fetus is obscure. Studies in isolated fetal membranes have shown an osmoregulatory role for AVT. Hydrostatic and osmotic water movement from fetal to maternal side of the guinea pig amniotic membrane is slowed or reversed by AVT.[106] Similar effects of AVT have been subsequently reported in pregnant sheep, where AVT inhibits fetal to maternal water transfer.[107] Of interest is the finding in humans that fetal pituitary AVT levels decrease after midtrimester in conjunction with the increase in fetal urine production.

Arginine Vasopressin. During the fetal period, AVP is an important vasoactive hormone in the maintenance of cardiovascular function under stress conditions. Extensive research has been conducted in the chronically catheterized sheep fetus to elucidate the role of AVP in the fetus. It is well established that infusion of AVP into the fetal circulation elevates arterial pressure, decreases heart rate, and redistributes cardiac output to the vital organs. At high doses, AVP elevates venous pressure and decreases blood volume.[108] Fetal hypoxia or hemorrhage are potent stimuli for the release of AVP. In the sheep fetus, hypoxia not only elevates plasma AVP concentrations, but increases AVP levels in the cerebrospinal fluid as well.[109] The physiological implications of the rise in cerebrospinal fluid AVP is unclear at present. It is not unreasonable to speculate that, under these circumstances, AVP may influence brain water permeability and cerebrospinal fluid clearance, in addition to modifying central regulation of heart rate and arterial pressure.

In experimental animals, fetal plasma AVP concentration is positively correlated with urine osmolality, and high urine osmolality is associated with low urine output.[110] During the last third of gestation, the fetal kidney is functionally responsive to AVP, as demonstrated by increases in renal reabsorption of free water and urine osmolality in response to AVP administration. The responses are lesser in magnitude than those in the adult.[111] Administration of an AVP renal antagonist into the sheep fetus has little effect on basal urine flow, suggesting a lack of involvement of AVP in the maintenance of basal renal function. These findings support the view that the fetal kidney is immature and that renal AVP receptors are either present in reduced numbers or are not fully functional. In humans, the maturation and appearance of functional AVP receptors in the fetal kidney have not been investigated. In newborn infants, urinary osmolality does not correlate with urinary AVP levels.[112] This refractoriness of the neonatal kidney to AVP may suggest the presence of an AVP antagonist at the level of the renal collecting ducts, such as prostaglandin E_2.

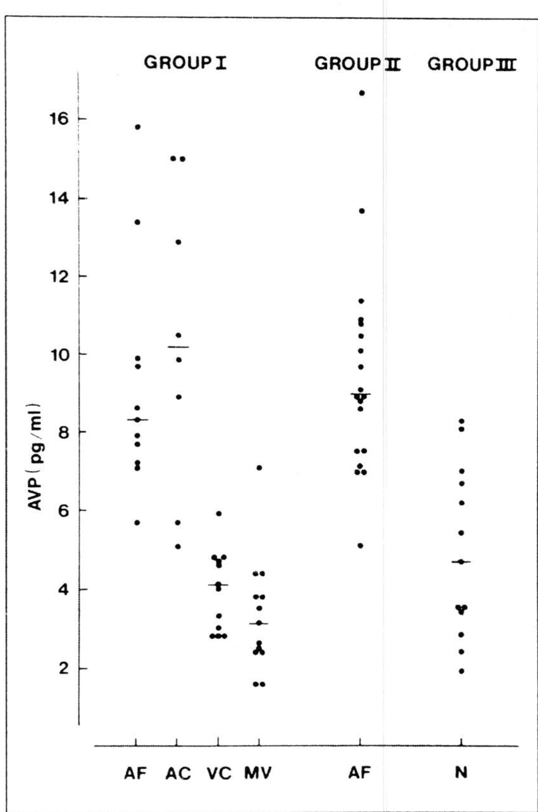

FIGURE 12–12. Arginine vasopressin (AVP) concentrations in amniotic fluid (AF), umbilical arterial (AC), umbilical venous (VC), maternal venous (MV) and nonpregnant venous (N) plasma. In Group I, the fetuses were delivered by elective cesarean section at 38 to 40 weeks. In Group II, amniocentesis was performed at 15 to 17 weeks of gestation in normal pregnancies. Group III consisted of healthy nonpregnant control subjects. (From Johannesen P, et al. Arginine vasopressin in amniotic fluid, arterial and venous cord plasma and maternal venous plasma. Gynecol Obstet Invest 1985;19:192.)

Amniotic Fluid Posterior Pituitary Hormones. All three posterior pituitary hormones, AVP, AVT, and oxytocin, have been measured in amniotic fluid from 16 weeks gestation to term.[113] The source of these hormones is presumably the fetus, because the fetus clears its circulating AVP partly by urinary excretion into the amniotic fluid. Amniotic fluid AVP concentrations at 15 to 17 weeks and at 38 to 40 weeks gestation are similar at around 9 pg/mL, and there is no significant correlation between amniotic fluid AVP levels and gestational age (Fig. 12-12). At term, umbilical arterial AVP concentration is 10 pg/mL. This is significantly higher than the levels of 4 pg/mL in umbilical venous blood.[114]

AVP and Fetal Stress

In the fetus in utero, stress is a potent stimulus for the release of AVP. Fetal hypoxia or hemorrhage elevates circulating AVP concentrations. This leads to increases in urinary excretion of AVP and high levels of AVP in the amniotic fluid. Thus, amniotic AVP concentration has been generally recognized as a marker for fetal stress. Patients affected with rhesus erythroblastosis have elevated levels of amniotic AVP.[115] In human neonates at birth, the umbilical plasma arteriovenous difference in AVP is maintained regardless of the mode of delivery or fetal stress. High concentrations of AVP in umbilical cord blood are associated with fetal conditions such as intrauterine growth retardation, multiple gestation, and fetal bradycardia. Passage of meconium into the amniotic fluid is usually accompanied by high concentrations of AVP in umbilical cord blood (Fig. 12-13).[116] In addition, the stress of vaginal delivery greatly elevates fetal secretion of AVP at birth by as much as 60-fold.[117] The physiological consequences of the high AVP concentrations in the stressed fetus are an increase in fetal blood pressure, a decrease in fetal heart rate, and a peripheral vasoconstriction resulting in reduced skin temperature.[118] Some investigators have attributed this enhanced release to the stress and hypoxia associated with delivery, but studies in human neonates at birth have found no correlation between AVP levels and fetal umbilical cord blood oxygen tension, pH, or Apgar score.

Other Fetal Sources of Posterior Pituitary Hormones

In addition to their presence in the posterior pituitary, AVP and oxytocin have been identified in the adrenal gland of the human fetus. AVP is localized in the definitive zone of the adrenal cortex, and oxytocin in the fetal zone. In anencephalic newborns, oxytocin can be measured in amniotic fluid, and oxytocin and AVP are also detectable in umbilical artery and vein. The source of the plasma and amniotic AVP and oxytocin in these

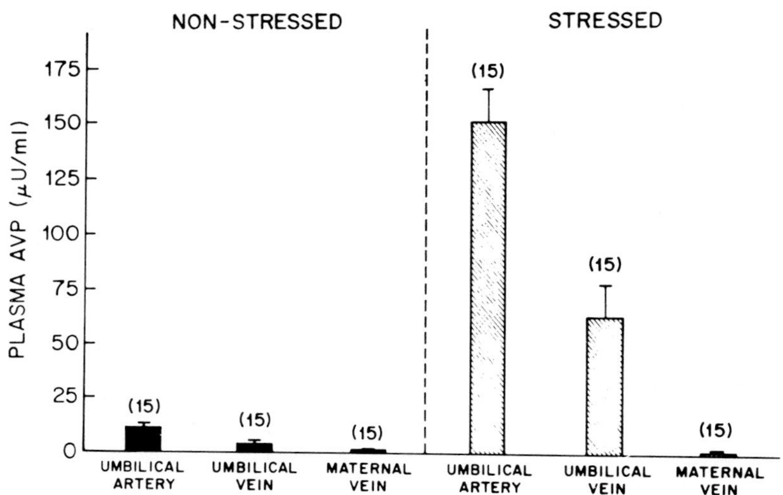

FIGURE 12–13. Arginine vasopressin (AVP) concentrations in umbilical arterial and venous plasma of term newborns, and maternal venous plasma at the time of labor and vaginal delivery. The status of the newborns at the time of delivery was either normal (nonstressed) or stressed, as judged by the presence of meconium in the amniotic fluid and by bradycardia and other abnormal cardiac rhythms. Each bar represents mean ± SEM and the number of observations in each group is given in the parentheses. Maternal plasma AVP concentrations were less than that in umbilical venous plasma of both groups of newborns ($P < 0.01$). Umbilical arterial and venous plasma AVP concentrations of the stressed newborns were greater than those in nonstressed newborns ($P < 0.01$). (From DeVane GW, Porter JC. An apparent stress-induced release of arginine vasopressin by human neonates. J Clin Endocrinol Metab 1980;51:1412.)

infants is probably the fetal adrenal cortex.[119] AVT, AVP, and oxytocin have been measured in cerebrospinal fluid of human neonates.[113]

CONCLUSION

The fetal endocrine system is unique in that it is autonomous from the maternal endocrine system and functions with minimal maternal influence. In the human fetus, the endocrine system develops very early in embryonic life. By midgestation, most of the endocrine functions are operative. Maturation of the endocrine system progresses as gestation advances. In the term fetus, the endocrine system plays an important role in the maintenance of homeostasis and in preparation for birth and extrauterine life.

REFERENCES

1. Gluckman PD, Grumbach MM, Kaplan SL. The neuroendocrine regulation and function of growth hormone and prolactin in the mammalian fetus. Endocr Rev 1981;2:363.
2. Winter JSD. Hypothalamic-pituitary function in the fetus and infant. Clin Endocrinol Metab 1982;11:41.
3. Fisher DA. The unique endocrine milieu of the fetus. J Clin Invest 1986;78:603.
4. Mulchahey JJ, DiBlasio AM, Martin MC, Blumenfeld Z, Jaffe RB. Hormone production and peptide regulation of the human fetal pituitary gland. Endocr Rev 1987;8:406.
5. Jaffe RB. Fetal neuroendocrinology. Contrib Gynecol Obstet 1989;17:104.
6. Pearse AGE, Takor Takor T. Neuroendocrine embryology and the APUD concept. Clin Endocrinol (Suppl) 1976;5:229.
7. Falin LI. The development of human hypophysis and differentiation of cells of its anterior lobe during embryonic life. Acta Anat 1961;44:188.
8. Mulchahey JJ, Jaffe RB. Detection of a potential progenitor cell in the human fetal pituitary that secretes both growth hormone and prolactin. J Clin Endocrinol Metab 1987;66:24.
9. Levina SE. Endocrine features in development of human hypothalamus, hyphophysis and placenta. Gen Comp Endocrinol 1968;11:151.
10. Siler-Khodr TM, Khodr GS. Studies in human fetal endocrinology. II: LH and FSH content and concentration in the pituitary. Obstet Gynecol 1980;56:176.
11. Siler-Khodr TM, Morgenstern LL, Greenwood FC. Hormone synthesis and release from human fetal adenohypophysis in vitro. J Clin Endocrinol Metab 1974;39:891.
12. Styne DM, Kaplan SL, Grumbach MM. Plasma glycoprotein hormone α-subunit in the neonate and in prepubertal and pubertal children: effects of luteinizing hormone-releasing hormone. J Clin Endocrinol Metab 1980;50:450.
13. Goodyer CG, Hall CSG, Guyda H, Robert F, Giroud JP. Human fetal pituitary in culture: hormone secretion and response to somatostatin, luteinizing hormone releasing factor, thyrotropin releasing factor and dibutyryl cyclic AMP. J Clin Endocrinol Metab 1977;45:73.
14. Dumesic DA, Goldsmith PC, Jaffe RB. Estradiol sensitization of cultured human fetal pituitary cells to gonadotropin-releasing hormone. J Clin Endocrinol Metab 1987;65:1147.
15. Huhtaniemi IT, Korenbrot CC, Jaffe RB. Content of chorionic gonadotropin in human fetal tissues. J Clin Endocrinol Metab 1978;46:994.
16. McGregor WG, Kuhn RW, Jaffe RB. Biologically active chorionic gonadotropin: synthesis by the human fetus. Science 1983;220:306.
17. Fukuchi M, Inove J, Abe H, Kumahaza Y. Thyrotropin in human fetal pituitaries. J Clin Endocrinol Metab 1970;31:565.
18. Fisher DA, Odel WD, Hobel CJ, Garza R. Thyroid function in the term fetus. Pediatrics 1969;44:526.
19. Fisher DA, Klein AH. Thyroid development and disorders of thyroid function in the newborn. N Engl J Med 1981;304:702.
20. Roti E, Gnudi A, Braverman LE, et al. Human cord blood concentrations of thyrotropin, thyroglobulin, and iodothyronines after maternal administration of thyrotropin-releasing hormone. J Clin Endocrinol Metab 1981;53:813.
21. Grasso S, Filetti S, Mazzone D, Pezzino V, Vigo R, Vigneri R. Thyroid-pituitary function in eight anencephalic infants. Acta Endocrinol 1980;93:396.
22. Klein AH, Oddie TH, Parslow M, Foley TP Jr, Fisher DA. Developmental changes in pituitary-thyroid function in the human fetus and newborn. Early Hum Dev 1982;6:321.
23. Fisher DA, Dussault JH, Sack J, Chopra IJ. Ontogenesis of hypothalamic-pituitary-thyroid function and metabolism in man, sheep and rat. Rec Prog Horm Res 1977;33:59.
24. Roti E. Regulation of thyroid-stimulating hormone (TSH) secretion in the fetus and neonate. J Endocrinol Invest 1988;11:145.
25. Kaplan SL, Grumbach MM, Aubert ML. The ontogenesis of pituitary hormones and hypothalamic factors in the human fetus: maturation of central nervous system regulation of anterior pituitary function. Rec Prog Horm Res 1976;32:161.
26. Suganuma N, Seo H, Yamamoto N, et al. Ontogenesis of pituitary prolactin in the human fetus. J Clin Endocrinol Metab 1986;63:156.
27. Aubert ML, Grumbach MM, Kaplan SL. The ontogenesis of human fetal hormones. J Clin Invest 1975;56:155.
28. Winters AJ, Colston C, MacDonald PC, Porter JC. Fetal plasma prolactin levels. J Clin Endocrinol Metab 1975;41:626.
29. Clements JA, Reyes FI, Winter JSD, Faiman C. Studies on human sexual development. IV: fetal pituitary and serum, and amniotic fluid concentrations of prolactin. J Clin Endocrinol Metab 1977;44:408.
30. Gluckman PD, Marti-Henneberg C, Thomsett MJ, Kaplan SL, Rudolph AM, Grumbach MM. Hormone ontogeny in the ovine fetus. VI: dopaminergic regulation of prolactin secretion. Endocrinology 1979;105:1173.
31. Riddick DH, Kusnik WF. Decidua: a possible source of amniotic fluid PRL. Am J Obstet Gynecol 1977;127:187.
32. Golander A, Hurley T, Barrett J, Hizi A, Handwerger S. Prolactin synthesis by human-chorion-decidual tissue: a possible source of prolactin in the amniotic fluid. Science 1978;202:311.
33. Suganuma N, Seo H, Yamamoto N, et al. The ontogeny of growth hormone in the human fetal pituitary. Am J Obstet Gynecol 1989;160:729.
34. Bugnon C, Fellman D, Bloch B. Immunocytochemical study of ontogenesis of the hypothalamic somatostatin-containing neurons in the human fetus. Metabolism 1978;27(Suppl 1):1161.
35. Bresson JL, Clavequin M-C, Fellman D, Bugnon C. Ontogeny of the neuroglandular system revealed with HPGRF44 antibodies in human hypothalamus. Neuroendocrinology 1984;39:68.
36. Roti E, Robuschi G, Alboni A, et al. Inhibition of foetal growth hormone (GH) and thyrotrophin (TSH) secretion after maternal administration of somatostatin. Acta Endocrinol 1984;106:393.
37. Gyevai A. Fine structure of, and ACTH production by, human fetal pituitaries taken at different periods of gestation. An in vitro study. Acta Biol Acad Sci Hung 1980;31:107.
38. Allen JP, Cook DM, Kendall JW, McGilvra R. Maternal-fetal ACTH relationships in man. J Clin Endocrinol Metab 1973;37:230.

39. Blumenfeld Z, Jaffe RB. Hypophysiotropic and neuromodulatory regulation of ACTH secretion in the human fetal pituitary. J Clin Invest 1986;78:288.
40. Johannison E. The foetal adrenal cortex in the human. Acta Endocrinol 1968;58(Suppl 130):7.
41. Séron-Ferré M, Lawrence CC, Siiteri PK, Jaffe RB. Steroid production by definitive and fetal zones of the human fetal adrenal gland. J Clin Endocrinol Metab 1978;47:603.
42. DiBlasio AM, Jaffe RB. Adrenocorticotropic hormone does not induce desensitization in human adrenal cells during fetal life. Biol Reprod 1988;39:617.
43. Fujieda K, Faiman C, Reyes FI, Winter JSD. The control of steroidogenesis by human fetal adrenal cells in tissue culture. III: the effects of various hormonal peptides. J Clin Endocrinol Metab 1981;53:690.
44. Simonian MH, Gill GN. Regulation of the fetal human adrenal cortex: effects of adrenocorticotropin on growth and function of monolayer cultures of fetal and definitive zone cells. Endocrinology 1981;108:1769.
45. Brace RA, Miner LK, Cheung CY. How ANF works during gestation. Contemporary OB/GYN 1988;31:69.
46. de Bold AJ, Borenstein HB, Veress AT, Sonnenberg H. A rapid and potent natriuretic response to intravenous injection of atrial myocardial extract in rats. Life Sci 1981;28:89.
47. Cantin M, Genest J. The heart and the atrial natriuretic factor. Endocr Rev 1985;6:107.
48. Kikuchi K, Nakao K, Hayashi K, et al. Ontogeny of atrial natriuretic polypeptide in the human heart. Acta Endocrinol (Copenh) 1987;115:211.
49. Sugawara A, Nakao K, Morri N, et al. α-human atrial natriuretic polypeptide is released from the heart and circulates in the body. Biochem Biophys Res Commun 1985;129:439.
50. Mercadier J-J, Zongazo M-A, Wisnewsky C, et al. Atrial natriuretic factor messenger ribonucleic acid and peptide in the human heart during ontogenic development. Biochem Biophys Res Commun 1989;159:777.
51. Gardner DG, Hedges BK, Wu J, LaPointe MC, Deschepper CF. Expression of the atrial natriuretic peptide gene in human fetal heart. J Clin Endocrinol Metab 1989;69:729.
52. Sirois P, Gutkowska J. Atrial natriuretic factor immunoreactivity in human fetal lung tissue and perfusates. Hypertension (Suppl 1) 1988;11:1.
53. Miyamoto S, Shimokawa H, Sumioki H, Touno A, Nakano H. Circadian rhythm of plasma atrial natriuretic peptide, aldosterone, and blood pressure during the third trimester in normal and preeclamptic pregnancies. Am J Obstet Gynecol 1988; 158:393.
54. Otsuki Y, Okamoto E, Iwata I, et al. Changes in concentration of human atrial natriuretic peptide in normal pregnancy and toxaemia. J Endocrinol 1987;114:325.
55. Hirai N, Yanaihara T, Nakayama T, Ishibashi M, Yamaji T. Plasma levels of atrial natriuretic peptide during normal pregnancy and in pregnancy complicated by hypertension. Am J Obstet Gynecol 1988;159:27.
56. Hatjis CG, Greelish JP, Kofinas AD, Stroud A, Hashimoto K, Rose JC. Atrial natriuretic factor maternal and fetal concentrations in severe preeclampsia. Am J Obstet Gynecol 1989; 161:1015.
57. Tulassay T, Rascher W, Hajdu J, Lang RE, Toth M, Seri I. Influence of dopamine on atrial natriuretic peptide level in premature infants. Acta Paediatr Scand 1987;76:42.
58. Castro LC, Arora CP, Roll KE, Sassoon DA, Hobel CJ. Perinatal factors influencing atrial natriuretic peptide levels in umbilical arterial plasma at the time of delivery. Am J Obstet Gynecol 1989;161:623.
59. Kikuchi K, Shiomi M, Horie K, et al. Plasma atrial natriuretic polypeptide concentration in healthy children from birth to adolescence. Acta Paediatr Scand 1988;77:380.
60. Yamaji T, Hirai N, Ishibashi M, Takaku F, Yanaihara T, Nakayama T. Atrial natriuretic peptide in umbilical cord blood: evidence for a circulating hormone in human fetus. J Clin Endocrinol Metab 1986;63:1414.
61. Weiner CP, Robillard JE. Atrial natriuretic factor, digoxin-like immunoreactive substance, norepinephrine, epinephrine, and plasma renin activity in human fetuses and their alteration by fetal disease. Am J Obstet Gynecol 1988;159:1353.
62. Panos MZ, Nicolaides KH, Anderson JV, Economides DL, Rees L, Williams R. Plasma atrial natriuretic peptide in human fetus: response to intravascular blood transfusion. Am J Obstet Gynecol 1989;161:357.
63. Kingdom JCP, Jardine AG, Doyle J, Connell JMC, Gilmore DH, Whittle MJ. Atrial natriuretic peptide in the fetus. Br Med J 1989;298:1221.
64. Cheung CY, Gibbs DM, Brace RA. Atrial natriuretic factor in maternal and fetal sheep. Am J Physiol (Endocrinology and Metabolism 15) 1987;252:E279.
65. Brace RA, Cheung CY. Cardiovascular and fluid responses to atrial natriuretic factor in sheep fetus. Am J Physiol (Regulatory Integrative and Comparative Physiology 22) 1987;253:R561.
66. Ervin MG, Ross MG, Castro R, et al. Ovine fetal and adult atrial natriuretic factor metabolism. Am J Physiol (Regulatory Integrative and Comparative Physiology 23) 1988;254:R40.
67. Brace RA, Bayer LA, Cheung CY. Fetal cardiovascular, endocrine, and fluid responses to atrial natriuretic factor infusion. Am J Physiol (Regulatory Integrative and Comparative Physiology 26) 1989;257:R580.
68. Varille VA, Nakamura KT, McWeeny OJ, Matherne GP, Smith FG, Robillard JE. Renal hemodynamic response to atrial natriuretic factor in fetal and newborn sheep. Pediatr Res 1989;25:291.
69. Nimrod C, Keane P, Harder J, et al. Atrial natriuretic peptide production in association with nonimmune fetal hydrops. Am J Obstet Gynecol 1988;159:625.
70. Robillard JE, Weiner C. Atrial natriuretic factor in the human fetus: effect of volume expansion. J Pediatr 1988;113:552.
71. Andersson S, Hallman M, Tikkanen I, Fyhrquist F. Birth stress increases fetal atrial natriuretic factor. Am J Obstet Gynecol 1990;162:872.
72. Ekblad H, Kero P, Arjamaa O, Erkkola R. Cord blood atrial natriuretic peptide (ANP) concentrations—lack of influence of labour stress. Acta Paediatr Scand 1988;77:312.
73. Ito Y, Matsumoto T, Ohbu K, et al. Concentrations of human atrial natriuretic peptide in the cord blood and the plasma of the newborn. Acta Paediatr Scand 1988;77:76.
74. Tulassay T, Seri I, Rascher W. Atrial natriuretic peptide and extracellular volume contraction after birth. Acta Paediatr Scand 1987;76:444.
75. Andersson S, Tikkanen I, Pesonen E, Meretoja O, Hynynen M, Fyhrquist F. Atrial natriuretic peptide in patent ductus arteriosus. Pediatr Res 1987;21:396.
76. Pesonen E, Merritt A, Heldt G, et al. Correlation of patent ductus arteriosus shunting with plasma atrial natriuretic factor concentration in preterm infants with respiratory distress syndrome. Pediatr Res 1990;27:137.
77. Shaffer S, Geer P, Goetz K. Elevated atrial natriuretic factor in neonates with respiratory distress syndrome. J Pediatr 1986;109:1028.
78. Phat VN, Camilleri JP, Bariety J, et al. Immunohistochemical characterization of renin-containing cells in the human juxtaglomerular apparatus during embryonal and fetal development. Lab Invest 1981;45:387.
79. Celio MR, Groscurth P, Inagami T. Ontogeny of renin immuno-

reactive cells in the human kidney. Anat Embryol 1985; 173:149.
80. Taylor GM, Peart WS, Porter KA, Zondek LH, Zondek T. Concentration and molecular forms of active and inactive renin in human fetal kidney, amniotic fluid and adrenal gland: evidence for renin-angiotensin system hyperactivity in 2nd trimester of pregnancy. J Hypertens 1986;4:121.
81. Hadeed A, Siegal SR. Plasma renin activity after birth and in the early newborn period. Am J Perinatol 1984;1:285.
82. Tetlow HJ, Broughton Pipkin F. Studies on the effect of mode of delivery on the renin-angiotensin system in mother and fetus at term. Br J Obstet Gynaecol 1983;90:220.
83. Tetlow HJ, Broughton Pipkin F. The effect of changes in blood gas tension upon the renin-angiotensin system of the newborn infant. Br J Obstet Gynaecol 1983;90:898.
84. Annat G, Raudrant D, Chappe J, et al. Maternal and fetal plasma renin and dopamine-β-hydroxylase activities in toxemic pregnancy. Obstet Gynecol 1978;52:219.
85. Brar H, Kjos S, Dougherty W, Do Y, Tam H, Hsueh W. Increased fetoplacental active renin production in pregnancy-induced hypertension. Am J Obstet Gynecol 1987;157:363.
86. Symonds E, Lamming G, Craven D. The fetal renin-angiotensin system in pregnancy-induced hypertension. Br J Obstet Gynaecol 1984;91:3.
87. Broughton Pipkin F, Symonds E. Factors affecting angiotensin II concentrations in the human infant at birth. Clin Sci Molec Med 1977;52:449.
88. Oney T, Kaulhausen H. Effect of angiotensin infusion during pregnancy on fetal heart rate and on fetal activity. Eur J Obstet Gynecol Reprod Biol 1982;13:133.
89. Abramovich D, Page K, Wright F. Effect of angiotensin II and 5-hydroxytryptamine on the vessels of the human foetal cotyledon. Br J Pharmacol 1983;79:53.
90. Glance D, Elder M, Bloxam D, Myatt L. The effects of the components of the renin-angiotensin system on the isolated perfused human placental cotyledon. Am J Obstet Gynecol 1984;149:450.
91. DeMoura RS. Effect of prostacyclin on the perfusion pressure and on the vasoconstrictor response of angiotensin II in the human isolated foetal placental circulation. Br J Clin Pharmacol 1987;23:765.
92. Cooke SF, Craven DJ, Symonds EM. A study of angiotensin II binding sites in human placenta, chorion, and amnion. Am J Obstet Gynecol 1981;140:689.
93. Pelayo JC, Eisner GM, Jose PA. The ontogeny of the renin-angiotensin system. Clin Perinatol 1981;8:347.
94. Higashijima M, Nawata H, Kato K-I, Ibayashi H. Studies on lipoprotein and adrenal steroidogenesis. I: roles of low density lipoprotein and high density lipoprotein-cholesterol in steroid production in cultured human adrenocortical cells. Endocrinol Jpn 1987;34:635.
95. Robillard JE, Nakamura KT, Lawton WJ. Effects of aldosterone on urinary kallikrein and sodium excretion during fetal life. Pediatr Res 1985;19:1048.
96. Bayard F, Ances IG, Tapper AJ, Weldon UV, Kowarski A, Migeon CJ. Transplacental passage and fetal secretion of aldosterone. J Clin Invest 1970;49:1389.
97. Oney T, Beer A, Kaulhausen H. Effect of postural change on plasma renin and aldoserone concentrations in third-trimester pregnancy. Obstet Gynecol 1981;58:31.
98. Skowsky WR, Fisher DA. Fetal neurohypophyseal arginine vasopressin and arginine vasotocin in man and sheep. Pediatr Res 1977;11:627.
99. Smith A, McIntosh N. Neurohypophysial peptides in the human fetus: presence in pituitary extracts of immuno reactive arginine-vasotocin. J Endocrinol 1983;99:441.
100. Schubert F, George JM, Rao MB. Vasopressin and oxytocin content of human fetal brain at different stages of gestation. Brain Res 1981;213:111.
101. Burford G, Robinson C. Oxytocin, vasopressin and neurophysins in the hypothalamo-neurohypophysial system of the human fetus. J Endocrinol 1982;95:403.
102. Gainer H, Altstein M, Whitnall M, Wray S. The biosynthesis and secretion of oxytocin and vasopressin. In: Knobil E, Neill J, eds. The physiology of reproduction. New York, Raven Press, 1988:2265.
103. Rosenbloom AA, Sack J, Fisher DA. The circulating vasopressinase of pregnancy: species comparison with radioimmunoassay. Am J Obstet Gynecol 1975;121:316.
104. Khan-Dawood FS, Dawood MY. Oxytocin content of human fetal pituitary glands. Am J Obstet Gynecol 1984;148:420.
105. Legros JJ, Louis F, Demoulin A, et al. Immunorective neurophysins and vasotocin in human foetal pineal glands. J Endocrinol 1976;69:289.
106. Vizsolyi E, Perks AM. The effects of arginine vasotocin on the isolated amniotic membrane of the guinea pig. Canadian Journal of Zoology 1974;52:371.
107. Leake RD, Palmer SM, Oakes GK, Artman HG, Morris AM, Fisher DA. Arginine vasotocin inhibits ovine fetal/maternal water transfer. Pediatr Res 1981;15:483.
108. Tomita H, Brace RA, Cheung CY, Longo LD. Vasopressin dose-response effects on fetal vascular pressures, heart rate, and blood volume. Am J Physiol (Heart and Circulatory Physiology 18) 1985;249:H974.
109. Stark RI, Daniel SS, Husain MK, Tropper PJ, James LS. Cerebrospinal fluid and plasma vasopressin in the fetal lamb: basal concentration and the effect of hypoxia. Endocrinology 1985;116:65.
110. Daniel SS, Stark RI, Husain MK, Baxi LV, James LS. Role of vasopressin in fetal homeostasis. Am J Physiol (Renal Fluid and Electrolyte Physiology 11) 1982;242:F740.
111. Robillard JE, Weitzman RE. Developmental aspects of the fetal renal response to exogenous arginine vasopressin. Am J Physiol (Renal Fluid and Electrolyte Physiology 7) 1980;238:F407.
112. Wiriyathian S, Rosenfeld CR, Arant BS Jr, Porter JC, Faucher DJ, Engle WD. Urinary arginine vasopressin: pattern of excretion in the neonatal period. Pediatr Res 1986;20:103.
113. Artman HG, Leake RD, Weitzman RE, Sawyer WH, Fisher DA. Radioimmunoassay of vasotocin, vasopressin, and oxytocin in human neonatal cerebrospinal and amniotic fluid. Dev Pharmacol Ther 1984;7:39.
114. Johannesen P, Pedersen EB, Rasmussen AB. Arginine vasopressin in amniotic fluid, arterial and venous cord plasma and maternal venous plasma. Gynecol Obstet Invest 1985;19:192.
115. Stegner H, Fischer K, Pahnke VG, Kitschke HJ, Commentz JC. There is evidence that amniotic fluid arginine vasopressin is a marker for foetal stress in rhesus erythroblastosis. Acta Endocrinol 1986;112:267.
116. DeVane GW, Porter JC. An apparent stress-induced release of arginine vasopressin by human neonates. J Clin Endocrinol Metab 1980;51:1412.
117. Pohjavuori M, Raivio KO. The effects of acute and chronic perinatal stress on plasma vasopressin concentration and renin activity at birth. Biol Neonate 1985;47:259.
118. Pohjavuori M, Fyhrquist F. Vasopressin, ACTH and neonatal haemodynamics. Acta Paediatr Scand 1983;305:79.
119. Oosterbaan HP, Swaab DF. Circulating neurohypophyseal hormones in anencephalic infants. Am J Obstet Gynecol 1987;157:117.

13

CHAPTER

FETAL HEMATOLOGY

F. Daffos and F. Forestier

FETAL HEMATOPOIESIS

Details of hematopoiesis in the newborn are well known, but because of the difficulties encountered in sampling, such is not the case with the fetus.

All blood cells are of mesenchymal origin. The mesenchyme, which stems from the cytotrophoblast surrounding the egg, forms the inner layers of the chorion and surrounds the unit created by the amniotic cavity, the embryonic button, and the yolk sac. The reunion of these two mesenchymal blades forms an embryonic film. When the first vascular elements appear, the conceptus is wholly embedded in the inner mucosa (Fig. 13-1).

FIRST STAGE: MESOBLASTIC HEMATOPOIESIS OF THE YOLK SAC

On the 19th day of pregnancy, the first blood cells outside the embryo become apparent in the many vascular islets that appear in the mesenchymal wall of the yolk sac. These islets appear as dark lumps of cells. Two systems—the vascular and the hematopoietic—originate from them; the peripheral cells of these lumps constitute the original endothelium of the developing vascular system. Some central cells of these islets leave the vascular walls, become free in the lumen, and form the primitive blood cells or hematocytoblasts. These cells will remain nucleated throughout their functional lives. The primitive erythroblasts or pronormoblasts stem directly from the hematocytoblasts. The separate islets will gradually become connected to each other to form an irregular network enveloping the yolk sac, which will give rise to the vitelline vessels.

Toward the 22nd day of pregnancy, similar vascular islets begin to appear in the mesenchyme of the chorion and all along the allantoic pedicle. These vascular islets create a further extraembryonic network—the chorioallantoic network—that constitutes the future umbilical vessels. In the both cases, hematopoiesis is intravascular; the two vascular networks connect to the vessels formed in the embryo at a later stage. Between the sixth and eighth weeks of pregnancy the vascular islets begin to regress, as does the intravascular hematopoiesis, with its large, nucleated "megaloblasts." The first-generation erythropoietic cells disappear completely from the embryo–placental circulation between the 12th and the 15th weeks.

The role of the yolk sac seems to be primary. Although the chorion's mesenchyme proves to be quantitatively greater—which means, in theory, a greater participation in hematopoiesis—the cells of the vascular islets in the wall of the yolk sac remain undifferentiated until the fourth week, whereas everywhere else the primitive vessels already contain erythroblasts.

SECOND STAGE: VISCERAL HEMATOPOIESIS

Visceral hematopoiesis begins in the liver around the fifth to sixth weeks of pregnancy and appears to reach an adequate development around the ninth week. Nests of hematopoiesis appear in the liver sinusoids and increase rapidly. Hematopoiesis becomes extravascular. Clear morphologic differences exist between the cells formed in the liver and the earlier lineages of the yolk sac. The former are smaller, and their nuclear structure is nearer the normoblast lineage of erythrocytic precursors. These are few in number when they appear in the blood around the fifth week, becoming predominant between the eighth and the ninth weeks of pregnancy (Fig. 13-2).

Although granulocytes and platelets are found in the circulation, the fetal liver seems to be the seat of an almost pure hematopoiesis, and from the third to the

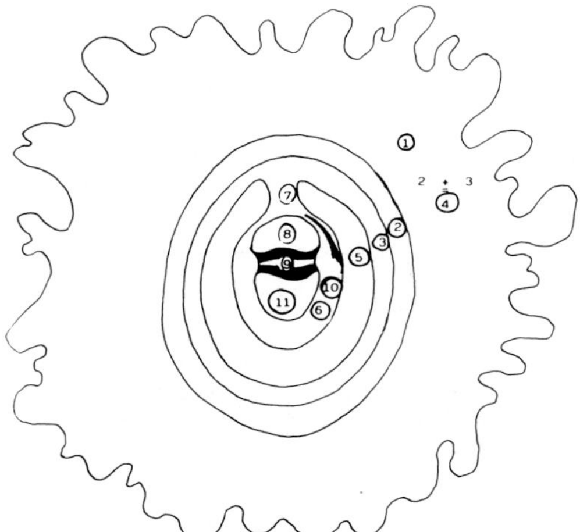

FIGURE 13–1. Schematic picture of the structures of the egg. (1) Undivided mass of the syncytiotrophoblast; (2) cytotrophoblast; (3) mesenchyme; (4) chorion; (5) extraembryonic coelom; (6) mesenchyme of the wall of the yolk sac; (7) mesenchyme of the embryonic pedicle; (8) amniotic cavity; (9) tridermal embryonic button: ectoblast, mésoblast, endoblast, (10) allantoic pedicle generated by the endoblast; (11) yolk sac.

fifth months of pregnancy, the erythrocytic precursors represent about 50% of the nucleated cells of this organ.

From the ninth to the 12th weeks some hematopoietic activity also can be observed in the thymus, the lymph nodes, and the kidneys. Nucleated red corpuscles are also observed in the spleen. Their presence has been interpreted in different ways: some consider that this corresponds to local production as well as sequestration and destruction; others, that it is nothing but sequestration at different stages of degeneration. In any case its role is only accessory in the human fetus. As for the yolk sac, it appears entirely fibrous at 11 weeks of pregnancy.

We have not been able to detect any erythrocytic activity elsewhere. Visceral, mainly hepatic, hematopoiesis reaches its highest level of production around the fifth and sixth months; then it gradually regresses until delivery. It can still be observed during the first week of postnatal life in the liver and occasionally even in the spleen.

Although it disappears almost entirely under normal conditions, extramedullary hematopoiesis is apt to increase noticeably in a large variety of diseases and infections in the fetus as well as in the newborn.

THIRD STAGE: MEDULLARY HEMATOPOIESIS

Medullary hematopoiesis begins about the fourth month. Medullary spaces develop in cartilaginous portions of the long bones by a resorptive process. Toward the fifth month, medullary cellularity is still poor and predominantly leukopoietic. The erythropoietic tissues multiply rapidly, and the marrow reaches its maximal cellularity toward the 30th week of pregnancy, each lineage being adequately represented. However, the volume of marrow occupied by the hematopoietic tissue continues to rise until full term. During the last 3 months, the marrow is the privileged seat of formation of the blood cells, the whole expanding medullary space being occupied by active hematopoietic tissues. However, its relative volume in the fetus and the newborn is smaller than that in the grown child or the adult, due to the fact that a large part of the fetal skeleton is cartilaginous and the bones are comparatively small.

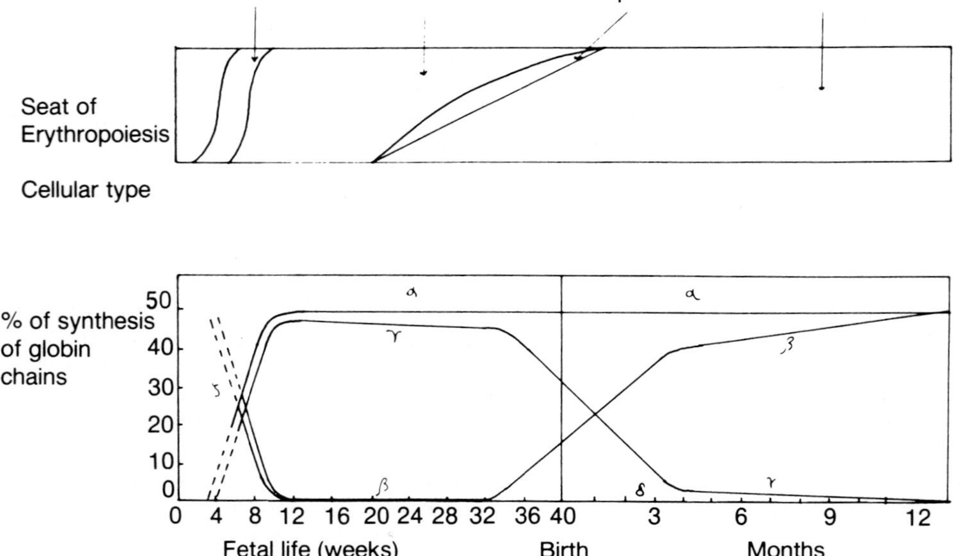

FIGURE 13–2. Ontogenesis of the chains of hemoglobins and erythropoiesis. (MCV = mean corpuscular volume.)

Nonerythroid Lineage

Leukocytes first develop in the wall of the yolk sac, then in the embryo. Very few circulating granulocytes are found during the first weeks of fetal life. At the eighth week of pregnancy, some myelocytes are observed, but mature polymorphonuclear leukocytes do not appear until around the 12th week. The circulating rate remains under 1000 elements/μL during the whole of the earlier part of pregnancy and does not increase significantly until the myeloid stage of hematopoiesis; it then increases rapidly until the 28th week. Lymphopoiesis begins in the lymphoid plexuses toward the eighth week and spreads first to the thymus, in the ninth week, and then to the lymph nodes from the third month on. After they have begun to appear, the circulating lymphocytes increase rapidly, reaching a peak of 10,000 elements/μL at the 20th week. The level then decreases gradually to 3000 elements/μL at birth. The megakaryocytes can be found in the wall of the yolk sac between the fifth and the sixth weeks, then in the liver after the visceral stage of hematopoiesis has begun. They persist there until the end of pregnancy and can be found in significant quantities in the marrow after the third month. Platelets are found in the blood from the 11th week of gestation and exist in numbers equal to those found in adult blood from the 18th week of gestation.

Origin and Differentiation of the Hematopoietic Cells

After years of controversy between the supporters of a unitary thesis and those of a pluricellular origin of the different hematopoietic lineages, the current opinion—based on experiments in animals, on clinical data in human pathology, and, more recently, on the cultures of hematopoietic cells from healthy subjects—is that there exists a pluripotent stem cell, the colony-forming unit (CFU), from which the various lineages stem. This pluripotent stem cell, which cannot be morphologically identified by maturation criteria, is capable of differentiation and self-renewal. It is the precursor of the erythroid, myeloid, and lymphoid lineages, and its existence was confirmed through the technique of splenic lineages described by Till and McCullough. We now distinguish a second generation of stem cells with a restricted differentiation potential in either the lymphoid lineages described by Iscove, Till, and McCullough.[1] We now distinguish a second generation of stem cells with a restricted differentiation potential in either the lymphoid lineage or the myeloid lineage, but their capacity for self-renewal persists. The stem cells are present in the marrow and the blood.

Kelemen, Calvo, and Fliedner, in their "Atlas of human haemopoietic development," suggest the following pattern: everything stems from a pool of stem cells appearing on the mesenchymal wall of the yolk sac.[2] It is the function of these first-generation intravascular stem cells, after the vascular intra- and extraembryonic networks have been connected together, to migrate into the embryo and multiply there. The necessity of this first migration has been demonstrated by the studies of Moore and Metcalf: there is no hematopoiesis in an embryo that has been prematurely separated from its yolk sac.[3] The seeding of the liver gives birth to a stem cell, called a second-generation stem cell, which is smaller than the first and nearer to the normoblastic lineage. These pluripotent cells proliferate in the liver, reaching a level of 50% of that of the liver's nucleated cells. Then they migrate toward and seed other areas of the embryo (marrow, spleen, lymph nodes, and thymus) as well as the extraembryonic areas. Some vascular islets of the yolk sac especially are colonized by second-generation stem cells (the first-generation cells are short-lived, with a half-life of about 8 to 12 weeks). A third generation of pluripotent cells corresponding to this medullary seeding will give birth to all the blood cells during pre- and postnatal life. Given what we know at present, it is difficult to speak of well-defined stages, and the modification in the population of stem cells is not proved, particularly as concerns the passage from primitive to fetal erythropoiesis. The current theory is that the passage from fetal to adult erythropoiesis represents a gradual modification of the stem cells rather than a change of population.

PURITY OF FETAL BLOOD SAMPLES

Fetal blood sampling under ultrasound guidance is a safe procedure that has enabled us to study fetal biology and to obtain prenatal diagnoses of an increasing variety of disorders.[4] The first step in establishing reference values and ensuring the accuracy of diagnosis is to be sure that the fetal blood sample is not contaminated.[5]

In our samples of fetal blood, contamination can be caused by maternal blood, amniotic fluid, or sodium citrate solution. The overall incidence of contamination in our study was small (1.8%) but must be viewed in relation to both the disorder under investigation and the type of contamination.

Each type of contamination has differing consequences, depending on the disorder under investigation. When diagnosing fetal infection in the presence of maternal infection, contamination with maternal blood will cause a false-positive result. The presence of amniotic fluid, which is also often collected for culture, will not affect the results, but the hematologic parameters and specific IgM must be evaluated with caution. Similarly, the presence of maternal blood cells in a specimen for investigation of fetal karyotype makes the specimen useless, but amniotic fluid or sodium citrate has negligible effects.

Investigation of disorders of hemostasis (platelets or coagulation factors) is severely affected by amniotic fluid contamination because amniotic fluid activates some coagulation factors and can cause platelet aggregation.

We evaluated the sensitivity of each method and

measured dilutions of maternal blood, amniotic fluid, and sodium citrate. We feel that each test must be done in all cases because of differing results under various conditions.

Depending on the gestational age and the indication for fetal blood sampling, between 2 mL and 3 mL of blood are collected. This is divided into 500 μL anticoagulated in lyophilized ethylenediamine tetraacetic acid K_2 (Sarstedt reference 32332), 400 μL collected in 0.129 mol/L sodium citrate solution (ratio 9:1), and 500 μL drawn into a lithium heparin dry mixture if karyotype is required. The remaining blood is not anticoagulated.

Hematologic indexes are determined with a Coulter Counter S Plus II. Leukocytes, erythrocytes, platelets, hemoglobin, hematocrit, and mean corpuscular volume are measured immediately after sampling. The distributions of the volumes of leukocytes, erythrocytes, and platelets are shown in Figures 13-3 and 13-4.

Smears are obtained after leukoconcentration and stained with the May-Grunwald Giemsa stain for the differential count. The Kleihauer-Betke test to differentiate fetal from adult red cells is performed with the Boehring kit.

Anti-I and anti-i cold agglutinins (against erythrocyte antigens), which are active at room temperature, are used in appropriate dilution.

The beta-subunit of human chorionic gonadotropic hormone (β-hCG) levels in maternal and fetal serum is determined with the enzyme-linked immunosorbent assay method using an anti-βhCG monoclonal antibody (Tandem Biotrol).

Coagulation factors IX and VIIIC are measured by a single-stage method, as described by Mibashan and colleagues, adapted for automated coagulation testing (KC 10 from DADE AHS).[6] Factor VIII activity is tested against the World Health Organization reference plasma 80/511. Factors II and V are measured by one-stage assay by means of thromboplastin, calcium, and substrate-deficient plasma. References are shown in Table 13-1.

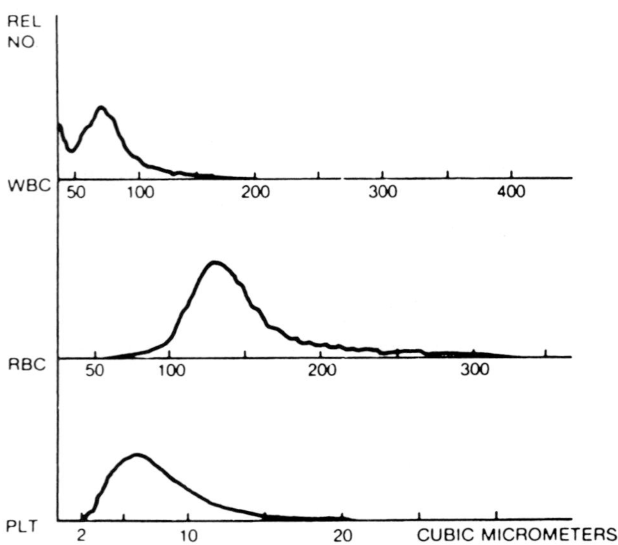

FIGURE 13–3. Graph that displays histograms of white blood cell, red blood cell, and platelet distribution curves of a fetus.

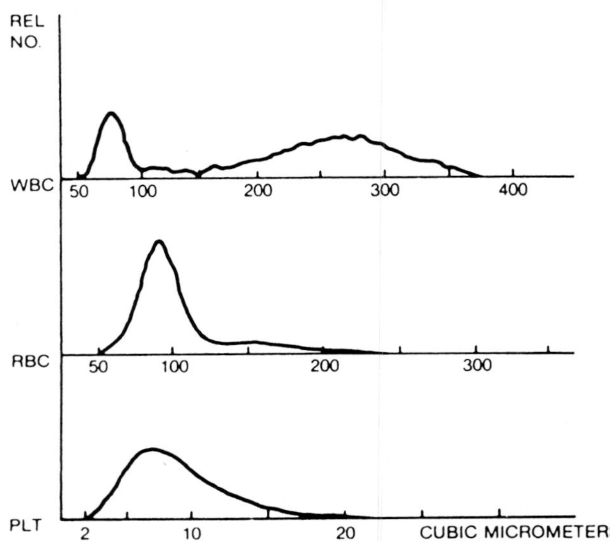

FIGURE 13–4. Graph that displays histograms of white blood cell, red blood, and platelet distribution curves of a mother.

The percentage of contamination detectable by each method is determined with fetal blood specimens by means of measured amounts of maternal blood, amniotic fluid, and sodium citrate until minimum detectable contamination is determined.

Each test is performed on all samples. Hematologic indexes are done immediately as an initial screening test before the patient leaves the hospital. It is possible, depending on the clinical circumstances, to repeat the fetal blood sampling if necessary. No individual test is infallible under all circumstances, and the reliability of each depends on the clinical situation and the type of contamination. The percentages of contamination detectable by each method are summarized in Table 13-2.

TABLE 13–1. FETAL HEMOSTASIS EXPRESSED AS PERCENTAGE (MEAN ± SD) OF NORMAL ADULT VALUE

COAGULATION	%	INHIBITORS	%
VIIIC	40 ± 12	Fibronectin	40 ± 10
VIIIRAg	60 ± 13	Protein C	11 ± 3
VII	28 ± 5	α_2-Macroglobulin	18 ± 4
IX	9 ± 3	α_1-Antitrypsin	40 ± 4
V	47 ± 10	AT III	30 ± 3
II	12 ± 3	α_2-Antiplasmin	61 ± 6
XII	22 ± 3		
Prekallikrein	19 ± 2		
Fibrin-stabilizing factor	30 ± 5		
Fibrinogen	40 ± 15		
Plasminogen	24 ± 15		

Data from fetuses of 19–27 weeks gestation.

TABLE 13-2. PERCENTAGE OF CONTAMINATION DETECTABLE BY EACH METHOD

METHOD	AMNIOTIC FLUID (%)	MATERNAL BLOOD (%)	SODIUM CITRATE (%)
Hematologic indexes	20	>5	20
Smear (Giemsa)	10	10	NC
Erythrocyte antigens	NC	5	NC
β-HCG	1	0.2	NC
Coagulation factors V or VII, IX or II	>0.1	30	10–50
Kleihauer-Betke test	NC	5*	NC

NC, Noncontributory.
* Depending on the gestational age.

Typical cell size distribution curves for hematologic indexes of a mother and fetus are shown in Figures 13-3 and 13-4. Three major differences distinguish maternal from fetal blood: there is only one peak of leukocytes in the fetus (corresponding to lymphocytes and nucleated erythrocytes); the average erythrocyte volume is much higher in the fetus; and red cell distribution width is broader in the fetus.

In cases of maternal blood contamination, a second peak of leukocytes is usually seen with a larger volume; this peak is the granulocyte peak. Using this approach, we are aware of contaminations of maternal blood in excess of 5%. The gestational age at the time of sampling must be taken into account because of the change in granulocytes toward term. Contamination of 10% or more by either amniotic fluid or sodium citrate causes a decrease in relation to the normal range of erythrocytes, leukocytes, and platelets in the same ratio.

The Kleihauer-Betke test relies on detecting differences in hemoglobins present in adult and fetal red cells. In theory this test should be able to detect a maternal blood contamination of as little as 0.5%. In practice, although the test is rapid and simple to perform, it is not possible to obtain absolutely accurate results because of the gradual appearance of hemoglobin A in fetal erythrocytes. After staining, erythrocytes containing only hemoglobin A appear as empty "cell ghosts." Those containing mainly or exclusively hemoglobin F stain darkly, and those with both hemoglobin A and F have an intermediate level of staining. This causes difficulties and technical errors in the differentiation of immature fetal cells from maternal erythrocytes. We have never demonstrated maternal blood contamination by this method after 30 weeks.

Blood smears stained for differential count will clearly show amniotic fluid squames if contamination with amniotic fluid has occurred. The presence of the squames depends on both the gestational age at the time of sampling and the percentage of contamination.

Erythrocyte antigen expression is different in the fetus compared with the adult. I antigen is present only on adult erythrocytes; i antigen is present only on fetal erythrocytes. Monoclonal antibody agglutination (anti-I and anti-i) is simple to perform and will detect a maternal blood contamination of 5%.

The β-hCG is of maternal origin, has a steep gradient across the placenta, and is found in only minute quantities in fetal blood, although higher levels are found in amniotic fluid. The ratio is approximately 1:100:400 (fetal blood:amniotic fluid:maternal blood). It is probably the most sensitive method to determine if the sample is contaminated and allows us to detect as little as 0.2% maternal blood or 1% amniotic fluid contamination. In practice, if we detect β-hCG in fetal serum, the specimen is regarded as contaminated. A markedly elevated level is suggestive of contamination by maternal blood rather than amniotic fluid, but β-hCG levels do not allow us to differentiate between the types of contamination, so other tests must be used for clarification.

Coagulation factors V and VIII detect both amniotic fluid and sodium citrate contamination but must be interpreted with caution. Less than 1% contamination with amniotic fluid activates coagulation and falsely increases the activities of factors V and VIII when tested against adult reference plasma. These values need to be compared with vitamin K–dependent factors, such as IX or II, which are not activated by amniotic fluid. In contrast, a large amniotic fluid contamination (greater than 10% and detectable on blood smears) will, by dilution, cause lower levels.

TABLE 13-3. EVOLUTION OF HEMATOLOGICAL VALUES OF 2860 NORMAL FETUSES DURING PREGNANCY (MEAN ± SD)

WK OF GESTATION	WBC ($\times 10^3/\mu L$)	Platelets ($\times 10^3/\mu L$)	RBC ($\times 10^6/\mu L$)	Hb (g/100 mL)	HT (%)	MCV (fL)
18–21 (n = 760)	4.68 ± 2.96	234 ± 57	2.85 ± 0.36	11.69 ± 1.27	37.3 ± 4.32	131.11 ± 10.97
22–25 (n = 1200)	4.72 ± 2.82	247 ± 59	3.09 ± 0.34	12.2 ± 1.6	38.59 ± 3.94	125.1 ± 7.84
26–29 (n = 460)	5.16 ± 2.53	242 ± 69	3.46 ± 0.41	12.91 ± 1.38	40.88 ± 4.4	118.5 ± 7.96
>30 (n = 440)	7.71 ± 4.99	232 ± 87	3.82 ± 0.64	13.64 ± 2.21	43.55 ± 7.2	114.38 ± 9.34

WBC, white blood cell count; RBC, red blood cell count; Hb, hemoglobin concentration; Ht, hematocrit; MCV, mean corpuscular volume.

TABLE 13–4. FETAL DIFFERENTIAL COUNT OF 732 NORMAL FETUSES ACCORDING TO THE STAGE OF GESTATION

WEEK OF GESTATION	LYMPHOCYTES (%)	NEUTROPHILS (%)	EOSINOPHILS (%)	BASOPHILS (%)	MONOCYTES (%)	NORMOBLASTS (% WHITE BLOOD CELLS)
18–21 (n = 186)	88 ± 7	6 ± 4	2 ± 3	0.5 ± 1	3.5 ± 2	45 ± 86
22–25 (n = 230)	87 ± 6	6.5 ± 3.5	3 ± 3	0.5 ± 1	3 ± 2.5	21 ± 23
26–29 (n = 144)	84 ± 6	8.5 ± 4	4 ± 3	0.5 ± 1	3 ± 2.5	21 ± 67
>30 (n = 172)	68.5 ± 15	23 ± 15	5 ± 3	0.5 ± 1	3 ± 2	17 ± 40

FETAL HEMATOLOGY

Starting from ultrasonically guided fetal blood samplings carried out between the 18th and the 29th weeks of pregnancy for various prenatal diagnoses (usually toxoplasmosis), we have been able to determine the reference values of some hematologic parameters in 2860 fetuses, for which prenatal diagnosis tests were normal and which were confirmed to be healthy at birth.[7]

Fetal blood was sampled into EDTA tubes, and we worked with a Coulter Counter S Plus II on prediluted samples.

Table 13-3 shows the main hematologic results obtained from 2860 normal fetuses between 18 and 36 weeks of pregnancy. There is no significant increase of the number of platelets (which stays around $250 \times 10^3/\mu L$). On the contrary, the red blood cell count gradually increases from 2.85 to $3.82 \times 10^6/\mu L$, and the white blood cell count increases from 4.7 to $7.7 \times 10^3/\mu L$. The concentration of hemoglobin also increases significantly during the second trimester of pregnancy. Conversely, one notices a significant decrease of the mean corpuscular volume, from 131.5 to 114 fL.

FETAL CYTOLOGY

The evolution of the fetal leukocyte differential according to the stage of pregnancy is shown in Table 13-4 and shows the distribution of polymorphonuclear leukocytes (neutrophils, eosinophils), monocytes, lymphocytes, and erythroblasts. Two reasons lead us to include the erythroblasts in the leukocyte differential, even though they belong to the red cell lineage and not to the white cells. Erythroblasts are a normal component of fetal blood, and the nuclei of these erythroblasts are counted as white blood cells by the Coulter Counter.

The first observation is that we found few or no basophils in the fetus. The second is that a very high lymphocytosis was present from the 18th week, along with erythroblastosis. The percentage of lymphocytes decreases from 88% at the 18th week to 68.5% by the 30th, and the erythroblast percentage gradually decreases from 45% at 18 weeks to 17% at the 30th. This reduction of the number of erythroblasts is made up for by a gradual increase of neutrophils as fetal life advances, from 6% at 18 weeks to 23% at 30 weeks.

The importance of this evolution of the fetal differential is threefold. First, we have been able retrospectively to establish reference values related to different stages of pregnancy. Second, the blood differential is an extremely useful tool to check the purity of fetal blood. For instance, blood that contains no erythroblasts at 18 weeks, or 40% neutrophils at 20 weeks, could have been contaminated by maternal blood or by blood of placental origin. Third, we have noticed that the fetal differential varies greatly in cases of parasitic (toxoplasmosis) or viral (rubella) infections.

FETAL RED BLOOD CELL ANTIGENS

We compared 72 samples of fetal blood ranging from 20 to 25 weeks of pregnancy with samples of full-term neonates (cord blood) and adults. We tested 37 red blood cell antigens, using specific antibodies:

TABLE 13–5. PERCENTAGE OF REACTIVITY OF SOME RED BLOOD CELL ANTIGENS IN ADULT, NEONATE (CORD), AND FETUS

	ANTIGENS (%)											
	A	A_1	B	H	Le^a	Le^b	Lu^a	Lu^b	P_1	P	I	i
Adult	45	35	9	100	20	70	7	100	75	100	100	0
Birth	45	37	12	90	0	4	3	100	38	100	12	100
Fetus	36	0	11	64	0	2	1	99	17	88	0	100

TABLE 13-6. PLATELET ANTIGENS IN FETUS (20 WEEKS) AND ADULT EXPRESSED AS MEAN FLUORESCENCE VALUES (±SEM)

PLATELETS	IMMUNOFLUORESCENCE INTENSITY (AUF) FETUS (Mean ± SD)	ADULTS (Mean ± SD)
Antigens		
PLA_1	433.0 ± 30.0	427 ± 13.5
Lek^a	441.5 ± 25.0	459 ± 15.0
Glycoproteins		
GPIIb IIIa, IgG	427.0 ± 23.0	420.0 ± 30.0
GPIIb IIIa, AP-2	459.5 ± 8.5	498.0 ± 11.0
GPIIIa, AP-3	536.0 ± 14.0	515.0 ± 13.0
GPIb, AN-51	491.5 ± 14.0	426.5 ± 9.0
GPIb, 6D1	479.0 ± 15.0	443.0 ± 8.7

- Polymorphic antigens: A, A_1, B, D, C, C^W, c, E, e, K, k, Kp^a, Fy^a, Fy^b, JK^a, JK^b, M, N, S, s, Lu^a, Lu^b, Le^a, Le^b, P_1, Xg^a.
- Monomorphic antigens: H, Rh17, Kp^b, Js^b, Fy^3, Jk^3, P, I, i, Ve^a, Ge^a, Emma.

Among these 37 antigens identical reactions were observed in fetus, newborn, and adult, except for A, A_1, B, H, Le^a, Le^b, Lu^a, Lu^b, P^1, P, I, and i.

Table 13-5 shows that some antigens are not expressed or have hardly developed in fetuses. Test results on newborns show an intermediate expression between the fetal and adult periods.

FETAL PLATELET ANTIGENS

From the 18th to the 29th weeks, the number of platelets remains stable at around $250 \times 10^3/\mu L$. On stained blood smears (with May-Grunwald Giemsa), fetal platelets present no particular cytologic differences as compared to adult platelets.

The study of the glycoproteins of platelet membranes has made it possible to identify glycoproteins Ib, IIb, IIIa, and IIIb. The PLA_1 antigen is present, which explains the risk of fetal anti-PLA_1 alloimmunization as early as the first trimester of pregnancy.

Working in cooperation with Y. Gruel we have been able to quantify PLA_1 and LeK^a antigens, as well as the membrane glycoproteins (Table 13-6).[8]

LYMPHOCYTE SUBPOPULATION

Lymphocyte Count

Leukocytes are numbered while monitoring the purity of fetal blood on the Coulter S Plus II. The absolute number of lymphocytes is observed from the leukocyte differential performed on a blood smear stained by May-Grunwald Giemsa.

Separation of the Mononucleated Cells

Separation of the mononucleated cells is carried out by differential centrifugation in a density gradient.

Lymphocyte phenotype

The development of hybridization techniques now permits the production of commercialized monoclonal antibodies and provides the means of investigating lymphocyte subpopulations.

The main markers of lymphocyte differentiation, as currently defined, have been characterized by using Coulter monoclonal antibodies labeled with fluorescein isothiocyanate. Detection was carried out by direct or indirect immunofluorescence. It proved necessary to implement a micromethod, considering the reduced volume of fetal blood.

The following monoclonal antibodies were used:

- Coulter Clone T_{11}—specific for the receptor of T-lymphocytes for the sheep erythrocytes and associated with an antigen 50,000 Da in molecular mass.
- Coulter Clone T_3—specific for an antigen T3, 30,000 Da in molecular mass. This antigen is present in the mature T-lymphocytes of peripheral blood and on 20% to 30% of thymocytes.
- Coulter Clone T_4—specific for an antigen 64,000 Da in molecular mass, present on 80% of thymocytes, 60% of circulating T-lymphocytes. It is associated with T-lymphocytes whose target is an antigen belonging to the major system of class II

TABLE 13-7. EVOLUTION OF T-LYMPHOCYTE SUBPOPULATIONS IN FETAL BLOOD, CORD BLOOD AT BIRTH, AND ADULT, EXPRESSED AS PERCENTAGE OF THE ABSOLUTE NUMBER OF LYMPHOCYTES (MEAN ± SD)

	T_{11}	T_3	T_4	T_8	T_4/T_8
Fetus 19–23 wks	44 ± 14	54.7 ± 9.6	39.9 ± 6.7	12.7 ± 3.7	3.5 ± 0.5
24–28 wks	—	61.9 ± 10.5	43.1 ± 9.3	14.4 ± 4.5	3.3 ± 1.4
29–32 wks	—	67.7 ± 7	45.5 ± 8.3	16.8 ± 6.1	3.1 ± 1.5
Neonate	71.4 ± 3.9	—	52.2 ± 10	—	—
Adult	78.3 ± 12.1	74.2 ± 6.9	46.2 ± 13.3	15.6 ± 4.1	3.1 ± 1.1

TABLE 13–8. B-LYMPHOCYTE MARKERS IN FETUS AND ADULT AS PERCENTAGE OF ABSOLUTE NUMBER OF LYMPHOCYTES

	B_1	B_4	E_{135}
Fetus (20–26 weeks)	4.4 ± 1.7	5 ± 3.8	28.6 ± 8.5
Adult	2.7 ± 2.3	3.2 ± 1.3	12.3 ± 1.5

histocompatibility. This antigen is stable and is not lost during the activation of the T-cells.

- Coulter Clone T_8—specific for an antigen present in the suppressive and cytotoxic T-subpopulations, 33,000 Da in molecular mass in its reduced state, 76,000 Da in its nonreduced state. This antigen can be found on 80% of human thymocytes and on about 35% of the T-lymphocytes of peripheral blood.
- Coulter Clone B_1—specific for an antigen of human B-lymphocytes, 35,000 Da in molecular mass. This antigen is found in the B-cells of peripheral blood, of the lymphoid organs, and of bone marrow.
- Coulter Clone B_4—specific for an antigen that is bimolecular in structure, 40,000 and 80,000 Da in molecular mass. It is expressed by the normal B-lymphocytes and is present in all isolated B-cells. Antigen B4 seems to be the first antigen associated with B-cells that can be detected in fetal tissues.
- E 135—monomorphic anti-DR, graciously provided by Professor Charron (Pitie–Salpetrière).
- Leu_7, Leu_{11} (Becton)—antibodies that recognize the "natural killer" (NK) cytotoxic cells of peripheral blood and some granulocytes.
  Antibody NKH_1A recognizes all the cells with NK activity; anti-NKH_2 determines a population of large-grained lymphocytes with poor cytotoxic activity.
- Coulter Clone My_4—recognizes macrophages and some granulocytes.

Results

The following outlines the results:

1. Lymphocyte count
   a. Fetal blood (20th–26th weeks of amenorrhea): $3.8 \pm 0.9 \times 10^3/\mu L$
   b. Cord blood at birth: $7.1 \pm 2.3 \times 10^3/\mu L$
   c. Adult blood: $2.5 \pm 0.95 \times 10^3/\mu L$
2. Phenotyping of lymphocyte subpopulations
   a. T-lymphocyte phenotyping is presented in Table 13-7; B-lymphocyte phenotyping is presented in Table 13-8.

The percentages of circulating mononucleated cells recognized by the Leu_{11}, NKH_1A, NKH_2 antibodies are, respectively, 21% ± 7%; 5.8% ± 2.3%; 2.5% ± 1.5% in the fetus between 20 and 26 weeks of gestation and 13% ± 5%; 12% ± 3%; 5% ± 1.5% in the adult. Of fetal circulating mononucleated cells, 10% ± 3% react with Coulter Clone My_4.

REFERENCES

1. Iscove NN, Till JE, McCulloch EA. The proliferative states of mouse granulopoietic progenitor cells. Proc Exp Biol Med 1970;134:33.
2. Kelemen E, Calvo W, Fliedner TM. Atlas of human haemopoietic development. Berlin:Springer-Verlag, 1979:1.
3. Moore MAS, Metcalf D. Ontogeny of the hematopoietic system. Yolk sac origin of in vivo and in vitro colony forming cells in the developing mouse embryo. Br J Haematol 1970;18:279.
4. Daffos F, Forestier F. Biologie du sang foetal. In: Medecine et Biologie du foetus humain. Paris: Maloine, 1988:100.
5. Forestier F, Cox W, Daffos F, Rainaut M. The assessment of fetal blood samples. Am J Obstet Gynecol 1988;158:1184.
6. Mibashan RS, Peake IR, Rodeck CH et al. Dual diagnosis of prenatal hemophilia A by measurement of fetal factor VIIIC and VIIIC antigen (VIIICAg). Lancet 1980;ii:994.
7. Forestier F, Daffos F, Catherine N, Renard M, Andreux JP. Developmental hematopoiesis in normal human fetal blood. Blood 1991;77:2360.
8. Gruel Y, Boizard B, Daffos F, Forestier F, Caen J, Wautier JL. Determination of platelet antigens and glycoproteins in the human fetus. Blood 1986;68:488.

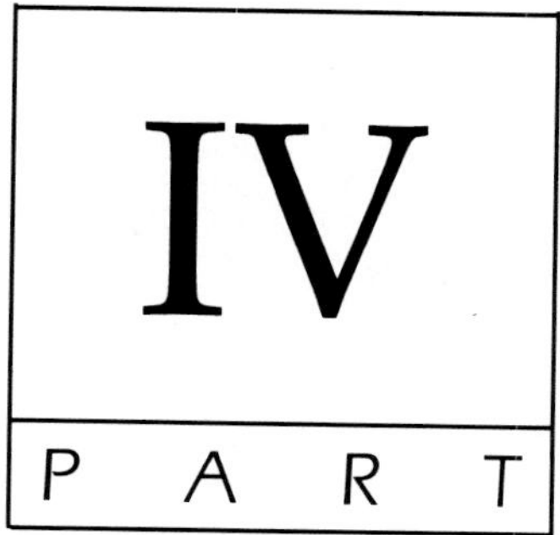

VARIATIONS IN EMBRYONAL AND FETAL GROWTH AND DEVELOPMENT

14

CHAPTER

ABNORMAL OVULATION AND IMPLANTATION

Ervin E. Jones

The efficiency of normal reproductive processes is very low when the number of gametes and conceptuses lost is compared to the number of viable offspring produced. Reproductive inefficiency is particularly marked among mammalian species, including the higher primates. Approximately 15% of all human pregnancies result in spontaneous abortion, with most occurring during the first trimester of gestation. To date, there is little information regarding the immediate peri-implantation period, particularly in humans, because of the difficulties in collecting such data. Clearly, if the means were available to assess the rate of utero death rates that occur soon after fertilization, the rate of reproductive waste would be considerably higher. Undoubtedly a large proportion of this wastage would be due to abnormalities of implantation. A number of abnormalities of physiology, endocrinology, and anatomy that contribute to a compromised reproductive performance add to what appears to be normal biological inefficiency of the reproductive process. In addition, there are genetic, environmental, and physical influences that infringe on reproductive outcome. Several facets of the biology of gametogenesis, ovulation, fertilization, and early implantation are well understood, and perturbations of these processes affect the success or failure of pregnancy. Although much of the available information pertaining to the peri-implantation period has been derived from studies involving laboratory or domestic animals, this information has contributed to our understanding of both normal and abnormal aspects of early implantation.

GENETIC ASPECTS OF IMPLANTATION FAILURE

A large part of embryonic mortality may be due to genetic causes that occur de novo during gametogenesis, and it may be that a considerable portion of this embryonic death should be regarded as nature's way of eliminating abnormal genotypes from a particular species.[1] Modern cytogenetics and molecular genetics has made it possible to investigate this subject in greater depth, and considerable attention has been directed toward understanding genetic aspects of early pregnancy and implantation failure.

ERRORS OF GAMETOGENESIS

Errors of gametogenesis are the most common cause of chromosomal abnormalities resulting in spontaneous abortion in humans, and such errors may account in part for our low fecundity. Certain errors of gametogenesis are independent and maternally derived, which may indicate that the oocyte undergoes detrimental changes during periods of arrest in the ovary over a period of several decades. Considerable information has been obtained from karyotypic studies pertaining to the etiology of early spontaneous abortion, and the findings are in general agreement. For example, in Bou'e and colleagues' study of 1500 spontaneous abortuses of less than 12 weeks gestation, 61.5% were found to have grossly abnormal karyotypes.[2] Almost all the chromosomal abnormalities identified were numerical and thus due to gross errors of chromosomal separation occurring at gametogenesis, at fertilization, or during early mitotic divisions of the fertilized egg. Abnormalities of male gametes are also involved in the production of genetically abnormal conceptuses. It has long been accepted that the haploid genotype of the spermatozoon is not expressed in its phenotype.[3] Thus, it seems unlikely that aneuploid spermatozoa would be selected out during ascent of the female reproductive tract unless, like diploid spermatozoa, they express their disability in terms of abnormal morphology, lifespan, or motility. In the absence of effective gamete selection, spontaneous abortion should be viewed as the inevitable price that a species has to pay for disorders of gametogenesis (Fig. 14-1).

DEFECTS OF FERTILIZATION

Abnormal fertilization accounts for a significant number of human abortions, apparently resulting from dispermy and the production of triploid embryos. This may be due to loss of the so-called block to polyspermy, a defective cortical granule reaction, or a defective zona pellucida. Lower animals only mate when the female is about to ovulate, but human sexual activity generally does not foster the close synchrony that normally exists between copulation and ovulation in lower species. In addition, as a result of aging, gametes may be more subject to polyspermy at the time of fertilization. Triploidy has been observed in pig blastocysts and can be reproduced by delayed matings that result in fertilization of eggs.[4] Interestingly, triploidy also can be induced by injecting progesterone, which apparently interferes with the normal block to polyspermy.

Molar pregnancy results from chromosomal errors occurring at fertilization, of which there are two types. Both complete and partial moles exhibit abnormal forms of implantation. The complete mole is associated with 46 chromosomes, all of paternal origin.[5] The partial mole, on the other hand, has 69 chromosomes because of an extra haploid complement of paternal origin.[6] Examination of a complete mole reveals marked hyperplasia of the trophoblasts, involving both cytotrophoblast and syncytial layers, edematous villi with cisterns, and early embryonic demise. The trophoblasts of the complete mole are highly "invasive" and often penetrate beyond the usual implantation site to involve the myometrium, occasionally eroding uterine veins. Approximately 2% of complete moles result in choriocarcinoma.[7] The partial mole is also characterized by a conceptus exhibiting a number of structural anomalies. The placenta reveals trophoblastic hyperplasia that is focally distributed but limited to the syncytial layer only, focal villous swelling, and the formation of cisterns. Trophoblastic inclusions are also observed, and the villous outline takes on a scalloped appearance.[8] Molar pregnancy represents an extreme form of abnormal implantation and reproductive failure (Fig. 14-2).

Prior to the relatively recent reports of studies involving embryos in vitro, no human studies were focused directly on the structural and genetic abnormalities of pre- and peri-implantation embryos. Hertig and colleagues found that of 34 early embryos found in reproductive organs and removed surgically, 10 were morphologically abnormal, including four of the eight preimplantation embryos.[9] Therefore, a minimum of approximately one third of these embryos was abnormal. This study provided powerful data suggesting that chromosomal anomalies play a major role in defects of implantation.

Evidence obtained from embryos studied in vitro also indicates that genetically defective preimplantation embryos are responsible for abnormalities of implantation in humans. Angell and colleagues described a method for analysis of the chromosomal status of early embryos fertilized and developed in vitro, and complete chromosomal analyses were performed on three oocytes, two of which were found to be chromosomally abnormal.[10] Data on the DNA content of the nuclei in another eight cases suggested that approximately 20% of embryos overall may be haploid. A more recent study published by the same group of investigators found evidence for chromosomal anomalies in human preimplantation embryos fertilized by donor sperm in vitro.[11] Despite the frequent occurrence of the XO karyotype in clinically recognized pregnancies, none were found among the 31 embryos studied. The most likely explanation for this finding has to do with the fact

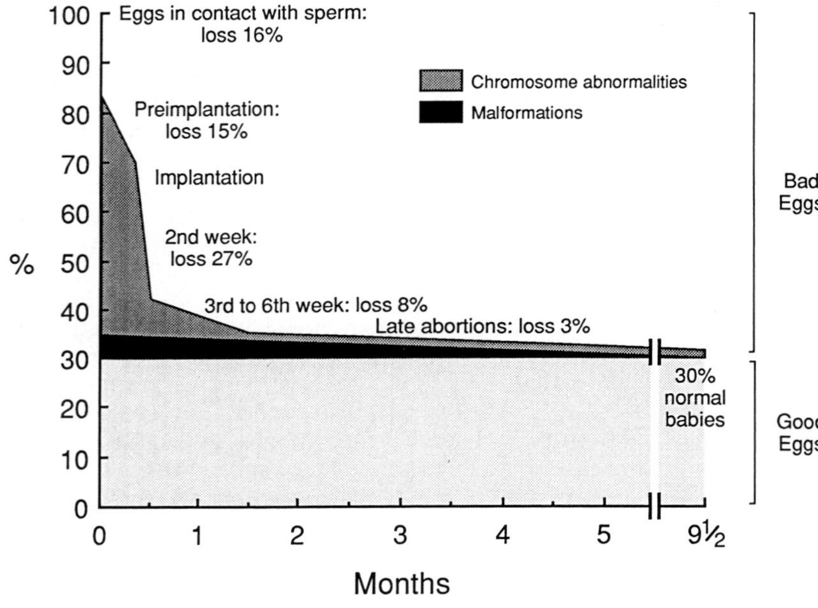

FIGURE 14–1. Bad eggs. Graph of the survival and development of eggs in humans following ovulation. It is assumed that under favorable conditions 30% of eggs develop to normal babies. Approximately 1% become live-born infants with cognitive defects. Therefore, 69% perish, are resorbed, or are aborted. (Witschi E. Teratogenic effects from overripeness of the egg. In: Fraser, FC, McKusick VA (eds). Congenital malformations. Amsterdam: Excerpta Medica, 1970: 157.)

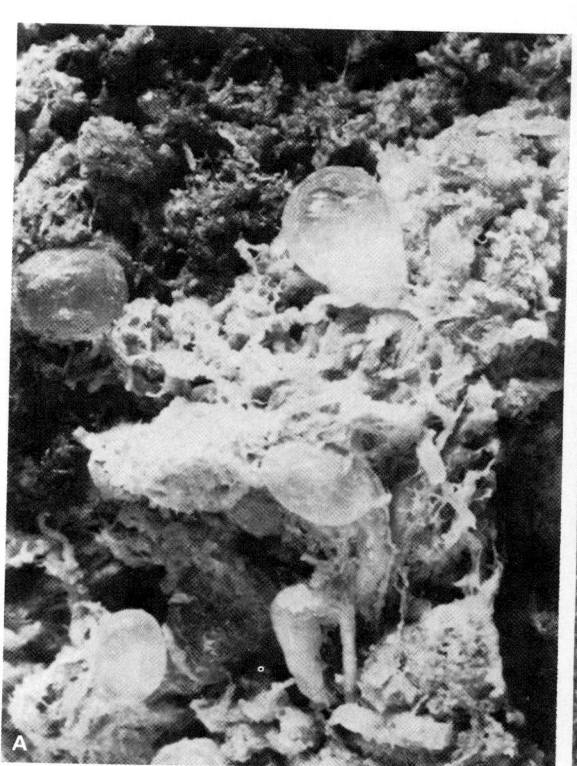

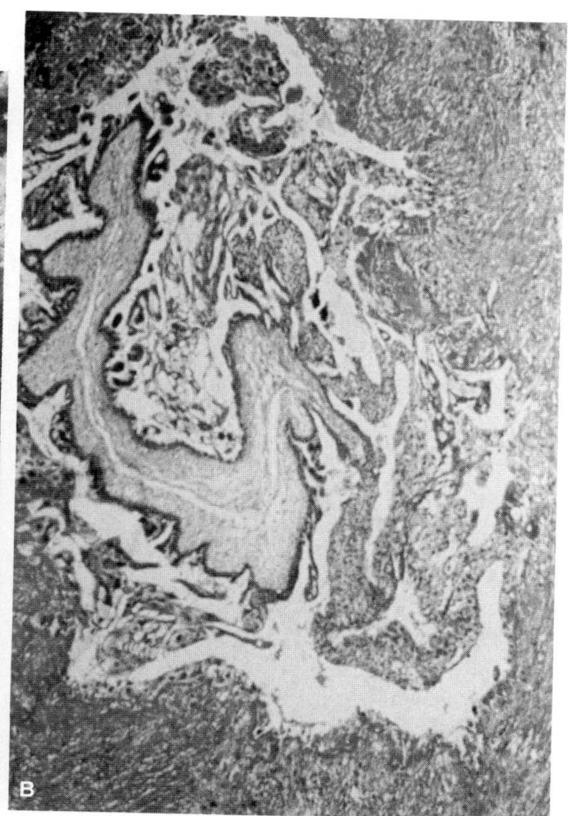

FIGURE 14–2. Gestational trophoblastic disease. (**A**) An incomplete hydatidiform mole. Large hydropic villi are seen among normal villi. (Reproduced with permission, from H Fox and CH Buckley, Pathology for gynecologists, University Park Press.) (**B**) Invasive mole; trophoblasts have invaded deep into the wall of the myometrium. (Courtesy of Dr E Kohorn, Yale Trophoblast Center.)

that the XO condition is associated with young maternal age, as described by Warburton and colleagues.[12] Evidence was also obtained for nondisjunction resulting in trisomy, monosomy, and nullisomy. Structural abnormalities, haploidy, and triploidy were also detected. Haploidy, like monosomy, is a condition that is not always lethal during the early cleavage stages of development but that is lethal once the embryo's coded genes begin expressing themselves. Haploidies appear to have a frequency of about 2% in oocytes fertilized in vitro.[13] Tripronuclear eggs are commonly identified after fertilization in vitro; different frequencies of tripronuclear eggs have been reported, ranging from 2% after clomiphene citrate stimulation to 12% after hMG.[14] Most tripronuclear embryos presumably arise through dispermy, although some could be due to the retention of the second polar body within the oocyte. The majority of such conceptuses can be identified in vitro during the pronuclear stage. These tripronuclear embryos could also arise due to abnormalities of follicular maturation rather than through the presence of too many spermatozoa around the oocyte. Although no hard data exist, it is not unreasonable to assume that once gene expression begins in the early chromosomally abnormal conceptus, implantation failure occurs (Fig. 14-3).

It has become apparent that lethal chromosomal anomalies contribute to the high failure rate of implantation, although the data were derived from preimplantation embryos studied in in vitro fertilization programs. Interestingly, when chromosomally abnormal preimplantation embryos are examined microscopically, there is no obvious evidence of abnormality, indicating that the apparent structural normality of embryos observed during in vitro fertilization contributes essentially no information about their chromosomes.[11] Lethal chromosomal abnormality, which does not allow development beyond the peri-implantation stage, is one possible reason for this high rate of implantation failure.

DISORDERS OF OVULATION–CONCEPTION CYCLE CHARACTERISTICS

Interactions between the embryo and the uterine endometrium that initiate establishment of the placenta, a hormonally regulated endometrial event, permit the in-

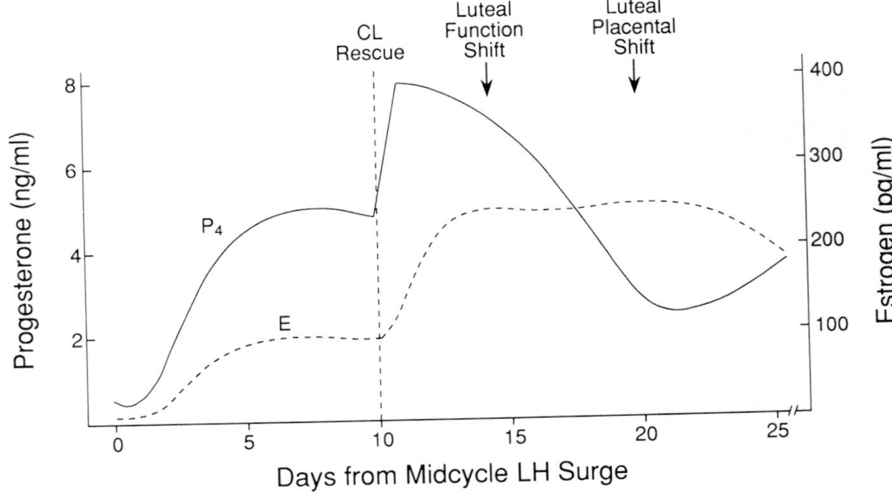

FIGURE 14–3. Luteal rescue. Changes in circulating levels of progesterone (P_4) and estrogen (E) during the luteal phase of the fertile menstrual cycle in rhesus monkeys. Note the timing of the luteal function shift and the luteal–placental shift. (Redrawn with permission from Stouffer et al.)

troduction of risk factors that may be detrimental to the process of implantation. When conception occurs in nonoptimum cycles, abnormalities such as poor endometrial maturation or the release of gametes of poor quality may result in improper implantation and problems of early pregnancy.

Endometrial maturation depends on appropriate quantities of estrogen and progesterone secreted by the ovary in the correct temporal order. Estrogen has a priming effect on the endometrium but is not obligatory for implantation, whereas progesterone is necessary for complete endometrial maturation. Furthermore, there is preferential retention of progestin receptors in decidual cells during the late luteal phase of the menstrual cycle, suggesting a shift in progestogenic actions from the epithelium to the stroma.[15] Progesterone production and secretion by the corpus luteum are essential for the maintenance of early pregnancy until the placenta takes over steroidogenesis and begins to synthesize adequate amounts of progesterone (ie, until the luteal–placental shift occurs).[16] Inadequate estrogen and progesterone secretion may cause inadequate endometrial maturation, a condition known as luteal phase insufficiency or luteal phase defect. Although it is not universally accepted, it is generally believed that inadequate endometrial maturation due to luteal phase insufficiency causes implantation failure in some women.

The importance of estrogen and progesterone production during the luteal phase has been studied in in vitro fertilization cycles. Forman and colleagues found a positive correlation between the follicular phase estradiol peak and the progesterone level on day 3 of the luteal phase of cycles stimulated for in vitro fertilization and embryo transfer.[17] Women who become pregnant had higher estradiol concentrations and lower progesterone–estradiol ratios than women who did not become pregnant. No correlation was found between the estradiol peak and the duration of the luteal phase or midluteal progesterone concentration. When comparing trials ending in failure to those resulting in clinical pregnancy for the same patients, pregnancies were obtained in cycles in which early luteal progesterone was higher and the early luteal estradiol–progesterone ratio was lower than that in failed cycles. In addition, there appeared to be a small but nonsignificant tendency for the pregnancy rate to decrease in association with increased luteal estradiol levels, suggesting that the progesterone–estradiol ratio is a better predictor of implantation than the absolute level of either hormone alone. Excessive estradiol levels resulting from ovulation induction with hCG had an apparent adverse effect on implantation. Gronow and colleagues suggested that some nonconception cycles may suffer early luteal regression based on studies of assessment of luteal function following in vitro fertilization and embryo transfer. They pointed out that women treated with hMG alone tend to have compressed cycles and that this group of patients should be given luteal phase support.[18] Estradiol levels also tended to decrease earlier in nonconception cycles than in conception cycles, although the differences were not statistically significant. Corroborating data showing that high progesterone levels influence the implantation process in human IVF were presented by Lejune and colleagues.[19] The importance of the ratio of estrogen to progesterone has also been shown by Gidley-Baird and colleagues, using a mouse model.[20] Thus, it has become clear that abnormal implantation following in vitro fertilization and embryo transfer may be associated with the methods of follicular stimulation utilized. Luteal phase abnormalities occur after 6 or 7 days and become extreme in many patients. Progesterone levels normally decrease in conception cycles before they rise again on days 10 to 12 in many patients, indicating that the secretion of hCG by the implanting conceptus must be capable of "rescuing" the corpus luteum.[21] Inadequate progesterone secretion during the luteal phase may also predispose to delayed implantation in many patients, since low levels of progesterone fail to maintain the full secretory status of the endometrium. Endometrium that is not synchronized with the developing conceptus may result in implantation failure (Fig. 14-4).

Clearly, the success of implantation depends on multiple factors, including pre- and postimplantation luteal function.[22] It appears that luteal phase insufficiency in some instances results from abnormal folliculogenesis; however, a recently reported study revealed that luteal phase defects exist after what appear to be completely normal follicular and periovular phases in some women, suggesting that follicular phase abnormalities do not contribute to luteal phase dysfunction in the human female.[23] In contrast, other investigators have found endocrine abnormalities during the follicular phases of cycles in which luteal insufficiency was identified. For example, one study revealed defects of follicular phase pulsatile luteinizing hormone (LH) secretion in women with luteal phase deficiency. Furthermore, during the luteal phase, the progestin pulse amplitude and mean serum progesterone levels were significantly lower in women with luteal phase insufficiency.[24] LH pulse frequencies were similar during the early and late follicular phases of women with luteal phase deficiency, whereas LH pulse frequency was highest during the late follicular phase in normal women, indicating that a too rapid LH pulse pattern in the early follicular phase may lead to inappropriate LH support of the corpus luteum, which becomes manifest as luteal phase deficiency. Decreased mean levels of serum inhibin during the early and mid-follicular phases of women with luteal phase insufficiency have also been reported.[25] Low levels of inhibin in the follicular phase of cycles with luteal phase insufficiency support the thesis that luteal phase insufficiency results from abnormal folliculogenesis.

UTERINE ABNORMALITIES AND IMPLANTATION FAILURE

Uterine leiomyomata, which are benign tumors of the myometrium, are usually characterized according to anatomical location as subserosal, intramural, or submucosal. Although the effects of leiomyomata on implantation and pregnancy maintenance have not been completely clarified, submucosal fibroids may decrease local blood flow to the endometrium and, as a result, interfere with implantation and the maintenance of early pregnancy. Local endometrial inflammation associated with submucosal leiomyomata may also interfere with the normal process of implantation. Although not conclusively demonstrated, it has been suggested that spatial uterine restrictions are teratogenic to human embryos.[26] Therefore, leiomyomata may create uterine spatial restrictions leading to teratogenesis and implantation failure. Matsunaga studied a total of 3614 well-preserved human embryos derived from *termination* of pregnancy to determine whether ectopic implantation or large myomas could enhance the prevalence of localized malformations in the embryos.[27] The frequency of malformed embryos was 11.6% among 43 recovered from ectopic pregnancies, 6.2% among 97 from uteri containing myomata, and 3.3% among those recovered from normally implanted pregnancies not complicated by myomata. Those women with myomata also had a

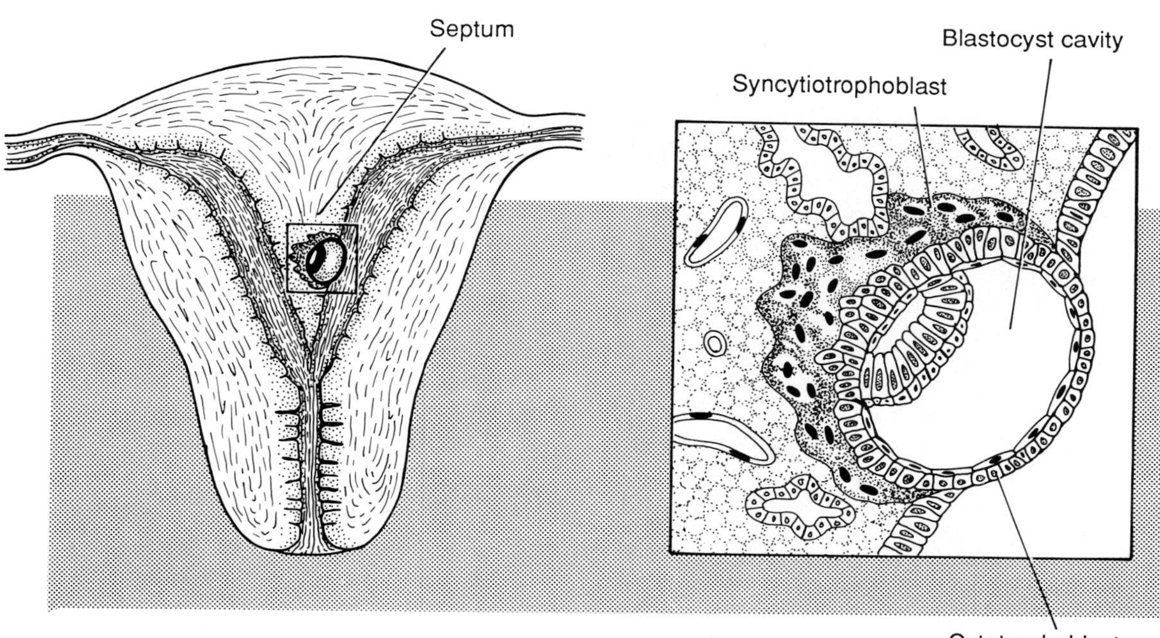

FIGURE 14–4. Implantation on a septum. This schema depicts the early conceptus implanting on a uterine septum. Since the blood supply to a uterine septum may be compromised, the risk of early implantation failure is increased.

higher frequency of previous pregnancy wastage, suggesting that uterine spatial anomalies such as myomata may cause implantation failure.

Scarification of the endometrial cavity may occur secondary to physical or infectious insults.[28] Irreversible damage to the endometrium occasionally occurs following intrauterine surgery such as curettage or following infection involving the uterine endometrium. The extent to which the uterine endometrium is damaged following such insults varies from intrauterine synechiae to complete destruction of the endometrial surface or obliteration of the uterine cavity. The blood supply to the affected areas of the uterus may be compromised. As a result, inadequate endometrial development would be insufficient to support implantation, and spontaneous abortion may occur. Congenital anomalies of the uterus are also associated with pregnancy wastage. Müllerian anomalies, which result from incomplete fusion of the müllerian ducts during embryologic development, such as the septate or bicornuate uterus, may be associated with implantation failure. Although no conclusive evidence exists, it may not be unreasonable to assume that a fibrous uterine septum develops, through which blood supply is limited and endometrial development is insufficient. When a blastocyst implants on or near a septum, implantation may be compromised, with the potential for early pregnancy loss (Fig. 14-5).

CONCEPTUS–ENDOMETRIAL ASYNCHRONY

Close synchronization between the developmental maturation of the embryo and the endometrium is necessary for successful implantation, and the width of the implantation window is probably not governed by endometrial maturation alone, but is determined instead by the coordinated development of the conceptus and the endometrium relative to one another. Thus, following fertilization, growth and development of the embryo must progress at a rate that is sufficient to ensure an appropriate stage of development prior to implantation.

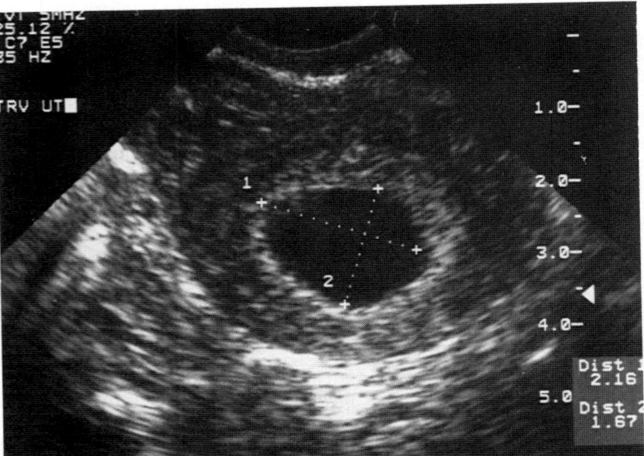

FIGURE 14–5. Blighted ovum. A so-called blighted ovum as seen on a vaginal ultrasound scan. This represents a gestation of approximately 8 weeks. Note that there is no fetal pole; only the empty gestational sac is visible (an embryonic gestation). (Courtesy Dr K Taylor, Department of Diagnostic Radiology, Yale University School of Medicine.)

PREIMPLANTATION EMBRYO CLEAVAGE

The cleavage potential of embryos in vitro is closely correlated with the progesterone production by granulosa cells of the cumulus–oocyte complex, and it has recently become apparent that the cleavage rate is directly related to the success of implantation.[29] Disparities between cleavage rates in vivo and in vitro were reported by Kreitman and colleagues using a monkey model.[30] Embryos developing in vitro kept pace with the expected time course for only about 24 hours, and extracorporeal conditions were inadequate to sustain normal cleavage rates. This suggests that asynchrony between cleavage rates and endometrial development contributes to prenidatory embryo wastage and subsequent implantation failure, even after successful in vitro fertilization. Buster and colleagues studied preimplantation human embryos obtained from the uterine cavity 93.5 to 130 hours following ovulation and observed that morphologic development varied from degenerating single-cell ova to mature blastocysts.[31] The relatively large variability in the state of development of intrauterine ova observed in the relatively fixed postovulatory interval of their study appears to be due to differences in viability and maturation, not to differences in age of the ovum. Thus, the maturational state of ova at the time of transfer appears to be a significant determinant of the likelihood of ensuing pregnancy. Claman and colleagues reported that embryo cleavage rate significantly influenced the pregnancy rate in their IVF-ET program.[32] Patients receiving at least one embryo that had reached the four-cell stage at 40 hours following insemination had a much higher pregnancy rate when compared with those receiving embryos cleaving at a slower rate. Additional culture time (24 hours) did not improve the pregnancy rate. This study further highlights the significance of embryo quality as a predictor of success in in vitro fertilization and embryo transfer.

ENDOMETRIAL RECEPTIVITY

Endometrial receptivity and pre-embryo quality as causal factors in normal implantation were investigated by Acosta and colleagues.[33] Eighty-one patients received a total of 325 embryos, resulting in multiple pregnancies with at least one reaching term. Total embryo loss reached 61% when the index embryo was excluded; thus, a mean of only 2.2 embryos were able to establish a normal pregnancy. Asynchrony of the pre-embryos had no apparent effect on the outcome, suggesting that with normal endometrial receptivity, the implantation potential of each pre-embryo is different. Additional evidence indicating that proper endometrial preparation is necessary to achieve the best pregnancy rate following in vitro fertilization, and embryo transfer was provided by Testart and colleagues, who studied 104 in vitro fertilization cycles in which 66 embryos were transferred fresh, while 151 embryos were frozen and transferred later.[34] Sixteen pregnancies (29.1%) originated from 55 embryo transfers or frozen–thawed embryos coming from IVF cycles in which pregnancy was not induced by fresh embryo transfer. Pregnancy rate after fresh embryo transfer (10.5%) was significantly lower than that obtained in the same group of patients receiving frozen–thawed embryos in later cycles (27.1%). Their findings indicate that a normal pregnancy rate may result if the embryos originating from unsuccessful cycles are transferred to a favorable uterus and that uterine inadequacy to embryo implantation in cycles stimulated for in vitro fertilization may be a determinant of pregnancy rate.

IMMUNOLOGIC FACTORS AND ABNORMAL IMPLANTATION

It is apparent that immunologic factors have major roles in implantation. The question of why the mother does not reject the fetal allograft persists. Several factors that are immune promoters or inhibitors during pregnancy have been identified. Some of these factors that are thought to be involved in implantation and the maintenance of pregnancy are produced by the conceptus; others are produced by the uterine endometrium or other maternal organs.

MATERNAL AND EMBRYO-DERIVED IMMUNE FACTORS

O'Neill and colleagues provided evidence showing that viable human embryos produce a platelet-activating factor in vitro that causes a reduction in the maternal platelet count after embryo transfer.[35] Their study revealed that the maternal platelet count is significantly reduced throughout the peri-implantation phase of pregnancy and returns to normal following embryo implantation. In some women there was no reduction in platelet count after transfer. Their embryos failed to produce a platelet-activating factor in vitro, and pregnancy was not established, which suggests that such platelet-derived factors are involved in the implantation process. Other evidence indicating the existence of immune factors that are toxic to the implanting blastocyst has been derived from studying the sera of women with histories of repeated pregnancy loss.[36] Incubation of peri-implantation mouse blastocysts in the presence of untreated human sera resulted in destruction of the blastocyst. Furthermore, heating the serum resulted in deactivation of the nonspecific toxic factor. Serum from men and from women with normal obstetric histories supported normal trophoblast attachment and outgrowth. Fractionation of the serum by affinity chromatography resulted in removal of the toxic factor with the IgG fraction, and absorption of the toxic serum on human trophoblast membranes resulted in serum that supported trophoblast outgrowth, indicating that the toxic factor was an antibody directed against trophoblast antigens. It has been suggested that factors produced in endometriotic lesions, such as macrophage-specific factors, are released and directly impair implantation.[37] Yovich has also suggested that there may be an implantation-inhibiting factor in women with severe endometriosis, as the pregnancy rate per embryo transfer and the number of gestational sacs identified per embryo transfer are significantly decreased in this group of patients.[38]

The uterine endometrium is different from other mucosal sites with respect to immune tolerance in that it tolerates sperm and the allogeneic fetus but resists microorganisms and other foreign antigens. Infection in the uterus causes local immune responses, as indicated by the secretion of IgA and IgG, and the secretion of these molecules is hormonally modulated. This proclivity of the endometrium to local immune function may be related to a sparse lymphatic supply to the endometrium and to local distribution of antigen-presenting cells. The development of the fetus, which is allogeneic, could stimulate production of maternal immune effectors, including macrophages, decidual cells, and T cells, which interact via soluble factors, causing local immune protection of the fetus. For example, it has been shown that progesterone-treated lymphocytes from pregnant women produce a 34-kDa protein (progesterone-induced blocking factor) that is capable of blocking lymphocyte function in vitro.[39] Lymphocytes from women with idiopathic-threatened preterm delivery failed to produce this factor. Furthermore, sera obtained at the time of delivery as well as those from women with preterm deliveries or spontaneous abortions contained significantly less progesterone-induced blocking factor than sera of healthy pregnant women. These data suggest that the production of soluble factors by lymphoid cells may be modulated by progesterone and that the determination of progesterone-induced blocking factor in pregnancy serum may contribute to the diagnosis of immunologically based preterm disruption of pregnancy. Progesterone also stimulates the production of uterine immunosuppressants as seen during pregnancy and prolongs the life of skin allografts placed in utero.[40] The supernatant of progesterone-treated pregnancy lymphocytes markedly suppressed natural cytotoxicity directed toward human embryonic fibroblast target cells as well as toward natural killer cell activity. Interestingly, the suppressive effect was not observed when progesterone was used in the presence of RU-486, a progesterone receptor-blocking agent. Suppression of natural cytotoxicity also was not observed with mixed lymphocyte reactions performed in the presence of supernatants from progesterone plus RU-486–treated peripheral blood lymphocytes. Therefore, in the presence of high local concentrations of progesterone, a suppressive pathway dependent on specific progesterone–lymphocyte interaction could be established, and this mechanism may play an important role in the maintenance of pregnancy.

First-trimester human decidua contains small lymphocytic suppressor cells that release 22- and 43-kDa soluble suppressor factors that block the action of interleukin-2.[41] Luteal phase endometrium, in contrast, contains large suppressor cells that do not release soluble immunosuppressive factors. If luteal phase endometrium from days 24 to 25 of the menstrual cycle is incubated with placental syncytial trophoblast membrane vesicles, suppressive factors having the same molecular weight as those found in late first-trimester pregnancy decidua are released into the supernatant. Based on these findings, fetal trophoblasts may activate two suppressor cell populations (large and small) in the endometrium via soluble long-range inducers and by contact with trophoblast membranes. Thus, trophoblast-dependent suppressor cells may have a role in inducing rejection of the conceptus, leading to occult or clinical abortion. T-cell suppressor factors (TsF) are present in maternal and fetal tissues of mice.

Blocking these factors with monoclonal antibody completely ablates pregnancy.[42] Monoclonal antibodies specific to TsF were also used to determine the time during gestation when TsF is most important to the maintenance of pregnancy. Significant decreases in the number of viable pregnancies were observed when monoclonal antibody was administered on days 3, 4, and 5, and increased levels of TsF in the uterus and the lymph nodes draining the uterus were observed when compared to the same tissues of non-pregnant animals. Thus, it appears that TsF is at least partially responsible for fetal specific immune suppression during pregnancy in allogeneic mice.

LUPUS ANTICOAGULANT

The antiphospholipid antibody, lupus anticoagulant (LAC), binds to certain phospholipids in cell membranes such as platelet factor III, a component of the platelet membrane.[43] The action of LAC is due to inhibition of binding of the phospholipid component of the platelet membrane and platelet factor III, which disturbs phospholipid-dependent coagulation via inhibition of thrombin formation.[44] Although LAC inhibits coagulation in vitro, its mechanism of action in vivo results in thrombosis of the microvasculature. This phenomenon may be explained on the basis of a reversal of the prostacyclin (PGI_2)–thromboxane (TxA_2) ratio. The net effect of PGI_2 is vasodilation and inhibition of platelet aggregation, whereas the primary effect of TxA_2 is vasoconstriction and increased platelet aggregation. Since LAC inhibits PGI_2 production, TxA_2 predominates, favoring constriction of the microvasculature and thrombosis. Although not all investigators agree, the available data support an association between recurrent spontaneous abortion and circulating LAC.[45,46] The pathophysiology of early recurrent abortion in women with LAC may involve thrombosis of the uterine microvasculature in and around the implantation site by compromising the supply of oxygen and nutrients to the developing conceptus, eventuating in early pregnancy loss.

ENVIRONMENTAL DETERMINANTS OF IMPLANTATION FAILURE

Two precepts have been introduced to explain teratogenesis during development. The first precept is that prior to implantation, the developing embryo is not susceptible to survival defects from chemical injury. The second is that developmental defects cannot be due to mutational events, since these rare occurrences seem unlikely to explain alterations in large populations of cells. These two fundamental precepts of developmental teratology were challenged in a study reported by Iannaccone.[47] Experimental evidence was presented that demonstrated that the effects of chemical exposure on blastocyst-stage embryos is manifested long after the insult and that subtle nonlethal mutations may have a role in poor fetal performance after early chemical exposure.

CHEMICAL INSULTS

The mother's occupational exposure to certain chemical agents may increase the risk of abortion.[48] Although alcohol consumption and smoking are both associated with increased risk of spontaneous abortion, whether smoking and drinking alcohol cause repeated abortion remains unclear. Sandor and colleagues found ethanol in oviductal and uterine luminal fluid in albino rats following chronic administration of ethanol in drinking water.[49] Although ethanol was found in both oviductal and uterine secretions at lower concentrations than those found in blood, their findings suggest possible direct noxious effects of ethanol on preimplantation development and that such effects may have adverse actions on the implantation potential of embryos. Maternal cigarette smoking increases the risk of spontaneous abortion.[50] Bou'e and colleagues studied a large number of spontaneous abortions and found a significant reduction in chromosomal aberrations in abortuses from women who inhaled cigarette smoke compared with noninhaling mothers.[2] The increase in abortuses with normal karyotypes in noninhaling mothers may be explained by an increase in the incidence of abortions in chromosomally normal embryos as a result of cigarette smoking. Mixed-function oxidase enzyme systems contained in human term placenta, such as aryl hydrocarbon hydroxylase, are induced by materials contained in cigarette smoke, such as polyaromatic hydrocarbons.[51–53] These enzyme systems convert polyaromatic hydrocarbons and other materials into water-soluble biotoxic radicals. Although it is not entirely clear if early human trophoblast metabolize these toxic radicals, recent evidence suggests that early human trophoblast also metabolize polyaromatic hydrocarbons.[54] Thus, it is possible that the generation of toxic radicals during the peri-implantation phase of pregnancy may be involved in disordered growth and differentiation resulting in implantation failure.

Disruption of embryonic and fetal development resulting from pre- and peri-implantation chemical insults may have a role in implantation failure. For example, Agarwal and colleagues reported results obtained when mice were exposed to di-2-ethyl-hexyl-phthalate.[55] An increased incidence of preimplantation losses and early fetal deaths was observed in treated animals when compared with controls, and their findings suggested a dominant lethal mutation effect based on the ratio of early fetal deaths to the number of pregnancies. Studies reported by Leonard and colleagues have shown that nickel is embryo-toxic, because of direct insults to the mammalian embryo as well as indirect effects through maternal damage.[56] Although no definite conclusions could be reached, these data suggest that the embryo and fetal toxicity of nickel may be related to its mutagenic properties and that nickel may induce changes in the mitotic apparatus, causing cellular death at critical phases of development, including the peri-implantation period.

EFFECTS OF RADIATION EXPOSURE ON IMPLANTATION

Fertile women may be exposed to ionizing radiation, and such exposures may result in radiation risk to the embryo or the fetus. Exposure to high doses of radiation probably increases the risk of chromosomal nondisjunction in the offspring of mothers who receive significant cumulative doses of radiation to the ovaries. For example, Michel reported an increase in spontaneous abortions as exposure to radiation increased, and the number of abortions with abnormal karyotypes also increased in proportion to the level of radiation exposure.[57] It remains unclear if early exposure of the conceptus to ionizing radiation during the peri-implantation period causes implantation failure. Because of known effects of radiation on growth and differentiation, it is likely that significant exposure has profound effects on the overall process of implantation and pregnancy maintenance. Fetter and colleagues presented evidence indicating risk to the embryo from radiation exposure prior to the period of organogenesis.[58] Russel reported that "irradiation during the (roughly) 9 day preimplantation period is virtually without risk of abnormality in a surviving child."[59] Much of what is known about the effects of radiation on perinatal development has been obtained from experiments performed on domestic animals and from the exposure of human embryos. It appears that doses between 10 and 100 rads relate to developmental anomalies and that other factors may modify the response.[57]

ABNORMAL GROWTH AND DIFFERENTIATION

Knowledge of abnormal implantation and embryonic growth in humans is difficult to obtain. Much of our knowledge of the process of implantation has been derived from analysis of the results of in vitro fertilization and embryo transfer. Most abnormalities of implantation probably involve defects of embryologic development or endocrine abnormalities. The information available about preimplantation development is restricted largely to morphology, and very little significant information is available pertaining to the biochemistry of the preimplantation embryo. Growth disorders in the preimplantation embryo and their relationship to defective implantation remain somewhat speculative. There may be extreme variation between embryos, because of nonsynchronous follicular maturation or because of the timing of fertilization. Embryos that implant late, relative to other embryos of the same cohort, could be due to slow embryonic growth in vitro. Implantation of these weak embryos could be facilitated by the stronger ones, and their eventual outcome may be what has been referred to as "vanishing fetuses" later in gestation. Another cause of slow or abnormal embryonic growth may be hardening of the zona pellucida in vitro, which could explain abnormal blastulation and hatching in vitro. Aberrant formation of the inner cell mass could result in a blastocyst with deficient numbers of embryonic cells that gives rise to a biochemical pregnancy, or, if damage to the embryonic disk is minimal and is expressed later in growth, the embryo could develop as a blighted ovum.[60]

There is very little knowledge about the growth of conceptuses in the oviducts and uterus in humans prior to implantation, although considerable information has been obtained pertaining to animal embryos in vitro and about those failing to progress beyond the period of implantation. Both direct observations of embryos and extensive use of hCG and other markers have indicated that many short-lived pregnancies abort at the time of menstruation or a day or so thereafter,[59,61] indicating that the early peri-implantation phase of development represents a critical period during embryonic development. It is apparent that many conceptuses die because of malformations of the inner cell mass and embryonic disk or because of the presence of chromosomal abnormalities, whereas other embryos die later because of abnormalities in the formation of the placenta or of failure of the embryonic disk to develop normally. Abnormalities of the trophoblast include hyperplasia, abnormal lamination of its layers, failure of formation of villi,[62] and the well-characterized "blighted ovum" or early embryonic demise. Immunologic conditions may also result in fetal death at this time; however, knowledge regarding this issue is scant. Other abnormal forms of implantation or placentation include the bilobed placenta, placenta previa, placenta accreta, and placental abruption. These occur later in gestation and may be due to abnormal implantation in some cases.[63]

TROPHOBLAST INSUFFICIENCY

To date, no specific markers allow assessment of pregnancy risk during the peri-implantation period. Peptide hormone markers that are expressed during this pivotal developmental process have been identified in in vitro laboratory models. Such trophoblastic signals are limited in their utility, particularly from the standpoint of extrapolation of these findings to human pregnancy. Such signals may serve to identify practical and sensitive markers to assess risk during early gestation in the future.[64] Extrapolation of experimental data has indicated that hCG may be used more effectively in the analysis of possible cause-and-effect relationships. Other peptide hormones that can serve to assess risk during the critical period of extraordinary sensitivity to toxic factors also may be useful.

The early trophoblast synthesizes and secretes many substances, a number of which appear to be necessary for normal implantation. Abnormal production or diminished secretion of certain materials produced by the trophoblast may be responsible for inadequate implantation. Hay and colleagues used monoclonal antibodies specific for dimer hCG (α,β), free beta subunit (β-hCG), free alpha subunit (α-hCG), and total β-hCG (dimer plus free β-hCG) to monitor discordant production of hCG during the early stages of embryo implantation.[65] The proportion of total measurable β-hCG due to free β-hCG subunits declined progressively from day 9 to less than 5% by day 22. Free α-hCG levels remained low, with rising levels first detected around day 18. A second group of patients had delayed or slowly rising levels of total β-hCG that were first detected at approximately 12.4 days, and this was associated mainly with biochemical pregnancies. In these patients, rising total β-hCG levels were due predominantly to free β-hCG production. Subsequent pregnancy losses may be due to poor luteal support, secondary to delayed increases in dimer hCG levels. In nonconception cycles, no significant rises were detected in dimer or free hCG subunits. Although the major form of hCG in circulation is the dimer, the origin of free β-hCG production in the early stages of implantation may be due to poorly differentiated trophoblastic tissue. Thus, falling levels of free β-hCG subunits associated with increasing dimer hCG production may reflect increasing α-hCG production by the proliferating layer of cytotrophoblastic cells.

DELAYED IMPLANTATION

The concept of delayed implantation was derived from observations of normal physiologic responses in certain groups of mammals, such as the marsupials, in which delayed implantation is a normal phenomenon. Delayed implantation may also be induced in other mammals by hormonal manipulation. Examples of delayed implantation following human embryo replacement have been reported based on delayed rises in the levels of luteal hCG, and the majority of these pregnancies developed to full term.[67] Whether delayed implantation or late opening of the implantation window causes abnormal implantation in humans remains to be determined. No clear evidence has been collected to explain why some implantations occur later than expected, and there have been no documented cases of delayed implantation caused by abnormalities of estradiol or progesterone secretion in humans. Thus, the term "delayed implantation" should be used with caution when referring to human pregnancies. It is not unreasonable to assume that abnormalities of the luteal phase may delay the opening of the implantation window in some women and that the embryos implant whenever the appropriate uterine conditions arise.

BLIGHTED OVUM SYNDROME

Hertig described a condition that he termed "blighted ovum".[62] This term is probably a misnomer, since the condition appears to arise following implantation because of the death or distortion of the embryonic disk after the trophoblast has differentiated. Blighted ova survive for longer periods of time than biochemical pregnancies, usually 30 days or longer, or even through the majority of the first trimester. On ultrasound, no fetal pole is visualized; at abortion no obvious fetal parts are found; and when examined microscopically, the tissue is entirely trophoblastic. It is possible that biochemical pregnancies and blighted ova are related, since both apparently occur because of the death of embryonic parts, an event that could occur earlier in biochemical pregnancies than in blighted ova. According to the work of Steptoe and colleagues, aborted fetuses resembling blighted ova secrete low amounts of hCG during pregnancy.[68] Some of the abortions arising after embryo replacement are due to blighted ova, and these generally can be characterized on ultrasound or by pathologic investigation (Fig. 14-6).

VANISHING FETUSES

It is not uncommon to observe a disappearing or "vanishing" twin or triplet that was detected earlier in the gestation by ultrasound. Thus, so-called blighted ova or other types of abortion can coexist with a normal living fetus. Steptoe and colleagues studied 17 vanishing gestations and reported the following: eight disappearances prior to 7 weeks, six between 7 and 10 weeks, and only three after 10 weeks. This suggests that the phenomenon usually occurs early during the first trimester.[68] Thus, vanishing fetuses arise at various times during pregnancy, and there is no information at this time to indicate whether the site or nature of implantation

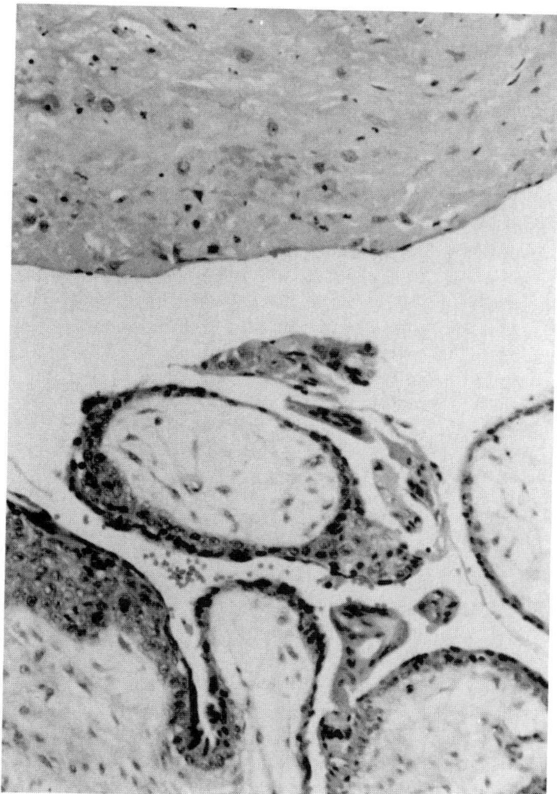

FIGURE 14–6. Photomicrograph depicting a tubal ectopic pregnancy. Note the presence of villi and trophoblastic invasion of the tubal epithelium. The tubal well is visible on the right. (Courtesy of Dr Maria Carcangiu, Department of Pathology, Yale University School of Medicine.)

influences the chances of embryonic death. The implantation efficiency of embryos resulting from singletons, twins, triplets, or quadruplets is difficult to determine. With the availability of modern ultrasonography, vanishing twins, triplets, and other multiple pregnancies can be visualized during early gestation, and it seems clear that the incidence of natural twinning has been underestimated because of the early unrecognized death of one fetus in twin pregnancies.[67]

ECTOPIC IMPLANTATION

The fallopian tube is highly functional, responds to the existing hormonal milieu, and is involved in the development of the preimplantation conceptus. The pathophysiology of ectopic implantation is not clearly understood but appears to be multifactorial and variable. The causes of ectopic gestation can be roughly divided between disease of the fallopian tube and defects of the conceptus or its investments, inasmuch as approximately 90% of all ectopic pregnancies occur in the fallopian tube. Tubal factors include infectious sequelae, endometriosis, tubal damage secondary to surgery, or a previous tubal pregnancy. The conceptus itself may also be a cause of ectopic implantation. For example, a greater number of abnormal karyotypes are found in ectopic pregnancies than in aborted intrauterine pregnancies.[69] It has also been postulated that abnormal hormone production by the cumulus oophorus, which *invests* the conceptus, results in aberrant tubal motility, and causes ectopic implantation (Fig. 14-7).[70]

EFFECTS OF MATERNAL AGE ON IMPLANTATION FAILURE

According to Leridon, the incidence of clinically recognizable spontaneous abortion in mothers over the age of 40 approximates 30%. Indications are that the majority of fetal deaths in this group are occult.[59] Experience with in vitro fertilization has shown that a substantially low proportion of embryos replaced will implant successfully in this age group when compared with younger patients, suggesting that conceptuses are lost at the peri-implantation stage as well as at later stages of gestation in older women.[67] Edwards and colleagues studied 1200 patients and were able to show that women under the age of 40 had favorable implantation, whereas beyond the age of 40 the rate of implantation decreased.[71] Conversely, another study done in humans reported by Ben-Rafael demonstrated no evidence of maternal age on implantation failure in cycles stimulated with clomiphene citrate for in vitro fertilization and embryo transfer.[72] Other studies performed using laboratory animals contributed useful information related to effects of aging on implantation failure. Page and colleagues published a study in which zygotes were transferred on the day of fertilization from young

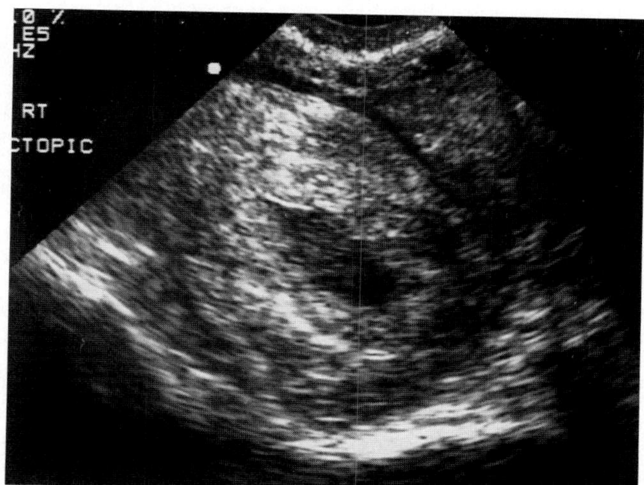

FIGURE 14–7. Tubal ectopic pregnancy as seen on high-resolution ultrasound scanning. Note the sonolucent region depicting the gestational sac surrounded by the edematous tubal well and what appear to be blood clots. (Courtesy of Dr K Taylor, Department of Diagnostic Radiology, Yale University School of Medicine.)

and old rats with 4- to 6-day estrus cycles to young recipients with 4-day cycles and vice versa.[73] Young rats with 4-day cycles served as controls for both donors and recipients. An increase in length of cycle or maternal age of donor caused an increase in the number of nonfertilized and/or abnormal eggs when examined at the pronuclear stage. Two factors contributed to the decline in implantation rate—the age of the donor and the age of the recipient. These findings provided compelling evidence that increasing maternal age has an adverse effect on implantation success. Changes in the biochemistry of the uterus also may be associated with declining implantation potential during aging. Thorpe and colleagues studied glycogen distribution in the uterus of young and old hamsters during implantation of the embryo.[74] Myometrial glycogen synthesis in the aged animal lagged behind that of the young animal throughout the period investigated. The role of delayed decidual cell response and the appearance of glycogen as possible causal factors in the decreased reproductive output observed in senescent animals may be significant.

Structural changes in the uterus may also contribute to early pregnancy loss in older women, since there are major changes in the noncellular components of uterine arterial walls resulting from aging and previous pregnancy. Sclerosis leads progressively to the obliteration of the lumina in both human and rodent uteri.[75–77] Human uterine smooth-muscle cells accumulate lipid particles during aging. These particles differ from lipid droplets seen in other cells in that they have a trilaminar membrane and a complex internal structure comprising several layers of differing electron density.[78] These are relatively large structures, measuring 1 to 3 μm in diameter, irrespective of age, and are not confined to toxemic patients, as has been suggested.[79] Implantation losses due to uterine aging may involve uterine fibrosis, abnormal surface architecture of the epithelium, and decreased capillary responses leading to attenuation or even absence of the decidual reaction. Growth retardation and death of implanted conceptuses with normal karyotypes may be due to ischemia of the uteroplacental circulation for which a considerable body of potential evidence exists.[80] Whatever the mechanism for uterine aging, it seems likely that a more hostile environment would encourage earlier and perhaps selective elimination of abnormal conceptuses. It remains unclear, however, whether this pregnancy wastage is due to a deteriorating uterine environment, deficient endocrine secretion during the cycle of conception, or chromosomally abnormal conceptuses.

REFERENCES

1. Bishop MWH. Paternal contribution to embryonic death. J Reprod Fertil 1964;7:383.
2. Bou'e J, Bou'e A, Lazar P. Retrospective and prospective epidemiological studies of 1500 karyotyped spontaneous abortions. Teratology 1975;12:11.
3. Beatty RA, Gluecksohn-Waelsch S. The genetics of the spermatozoon (Proceedings of an International Symposium), Edinburgh, 1972.
4. Hunter RHF. The effects of delayed insemination on fertilization and early cleavage in the pig. J Reprod Fertil 1967;13:133.
5. Kajii T, Ohama K. Androgenetic origin of hydatidiform mole. Nature 1977;268:633.
6. Jacobs PA, Szulman AE, Funkhouser J, Matsuura JS, Wilson CC. Human triploidy: relationship between parental origin of the additional haploid complement and development of partial hydatidiform mole. Ann Hum Genet 1982;46:223.
7. Szulman AE. Complete hydatidiform mole and partial hydatidiform mole. In: Szulman AE, Buchsbaum HJ, eds. Gestational trophoblastic disease. New York: Spring, 1987:27.
8. Sulzman AE. Syndromes of hydatidiform moles: partial versus complete. J Reprod Med 1984;29:788.
9. Hertig AT, Rock J, Adams EC, Menkin MC. Thirty-four fertilized human ova, good, bad, and indifferent, recovered from 210 women of known fertility. Pediatrics 1959;23:202.
10. Angell RR, Aitken RJ, van Look PF, Lumsden MA, Templeton AA. Chromosome abnormalities in human embryos after in vitro fertilization. Nature 1983;303:336.
11. Angell RR, Templeton AA, Aitken RJ. Chromosome studies in human in vitro fertilization. Hum Genet 1986;72:333.
12. Warburton D, Kline J, Stein Z, Susser M. Monosomy X: a chromosomal anomaly associated with young maternal age. Lancet 1980;i:167.
13. Angell RR, Aitken RJ, Van Look PFA, Lumsden MA, Templeton AA. Chromosome anomalies in human preimplantation embryos. J Embryol Exp Morphol (Suppl) 1984;82:193 (abstract).
14. Wentz AL, Repp JE, Maxon WS, Pittaway DE, Torbit CA. The problem of polysperm as in vitro fertilization. Fertil Steril 1982;40:748.
15. Benedetto MT, Tabanelli S, Gurpide E. Estrone sulfate sulfatase activity is increased during in vitro decidualization of stromal cells from human endometrium, J Clin Endocrinol Metab 1990;342:5.
16. Itskovitz J, Hodgen GD. Endocrine basis for the initiation, maintenance and termination of pregnancy in humans. Psychoneuroendocrinology 1988;13(1–2):155.
17. Forman R, Fries N, Testart J, Belaisch-Allart J, Hazout A, Frydman R. Evidence for an adverse effect of elevated serum estradiol concentrations on embryo implantation. Fertil Steril 1988;49:118.
18. Gronow MJ, Martin MJ, Hay D, Moro D, Brown JB. The luteal phase after hyperstimulation for in vitro fertilization. Ann NY Acad Sci 1985;442:391.
19. Lejeune B, Camus M, Deschacht J, Leroy F. Differences in the luteal phases after failed or successful in vitro fertilization and embryo replacement. J In Vitro Fert Embryo Transfer 1986;3(6):358.
20. Russel LB. Discussion: in biological risks of medical irradiation. In: Fullerton GD, Kopp DJ, Wiggins RG, Webster EW, eds. American Association of Physicists in Medicine, Monograph 5. New York: American Institute of Physics, YEAR:98.
21. Liu HC, Jones GS, Jones HW Jr, Rosenwaks Z. Mechanisms and factors of early pregnancy wastage in in vitro fertilization-embryo transfer patients. Fertil Steril 1988;(July)95:101.
22. Liu HC, Jones GS, Jones HW Jr, Rosenwaks Z. Mechanisms and factors of early pregnancy wastage in in vitro fertilization-embryo transfer patients. Fertil Steril 1988;50:95.
23. Grunfeld L, Sandler B, Fox J, Boyd C, Kaplan P, Navot D. Luteal phase deficiency after completely normal follicular and periovulatory phases. Fertil Steril 1989;(Dec)919:23.
24. Soules MR, Clifton DK, Cohen NL, Bremner WJ, Steiner RA. Luteal phase deficiency: abnormal gonadotropin and progesterone secretion patterns. J Clin Endocrinol Metab 1989;(Oct)813:20.

25. Soules MR, McLachlan RI, Ek M, Dahl KD, Cohen NL, Bremner WJ. Luteal phase deficiency: characterization of reproductive hormones over the menstrual cycle. J Clin Endocrinol Metab 1989;(Oct)804:12.
26. Duckering FA. The significance of myoma uteris in pregnancy. Am J Obstet Gynecol 1946;51:819.
27. Matsunaga E, Shiota K. Ectopic pregnancy and myoma uteri: teratogenic effects and maternal characteristics. Teratology 1980;21:61.
28. Schenker J, Margolioth E. Intrauterine adhesions: an updated appraisal. Fertil Steril 1982;37:593.
29. Wiswedel K. Granulosa cell metabolism and the assessment of oocyte quality in IVF. Hum Reprod 1987;(Oct)589:91.
30. Kreitmann O, Hodgen GD. Retarded cleavage rates of preimplantation monkey embryos in vitro. JAMA 1981;246:627.
31. Buster JE, Bustillo M, Rodi IA, Cohen SW, Hamilton M, Simon JA, et al. Biologic and morphologic development of donated human ova recovered by nonsurgical uterine lavage. Am J Obstet Gynecol 1985;153:211.
32. Claman P, Armant DR, Seibel MM, Wang TA, Oskowitz SP, Taymor ML. The impact of embryo quality and quantity on implantation and the establishment of viable pregnancies. J In Vitro Fert Embryo Transfer 1987;4(4):218.
33. Acosta AA, Moon SY, Oehninger S, Muasher SJ, Rosenwaks Z, Matta JF. Implantation potential of each pre-embryo in multiple pregnancies obtained by in vitro fertilization seems to be different. Fertil Steril 1988;50(6):906.
34. Testart J. Evidence of uterine inadequacy to egg implantation in stimulated in vitro fertilization cycles. Fertil Steril 1987;47:855.
35. ONeill C, Gidley-Baird AA, Pike IL, Porter RN, Sinosich MJ, Saunders DM. Maternal blood platelet physiology and luteal-phase endocrinology as a means of monitoring pre- and postimplantation embryo viability following in vitro fertilization. J In Vitro Fert Embryo Transfer 1985;2:87.
36. Chavez DJ, McIntyre JA. Sera from women with histories of repeated pregnancy losses cause abnormalities in mouse periimplantation blastocysts. J Reprod Immunol 1984;6:273.
37. Ory SJ. Pelvic endometriosis. Obstet Gynecol Clin North Am (Review) 1987;14:999.
38. Yovich JL, Matson PL, Richardson PA, Hilliard C. Hormonal profiles and embryo quality in women with severe endometriosis treated by in vitro fertilization and embryo transfer. Fertil Steril 1988;50:308.
39. Szekeres BJ, Varga P, Pejtsik B. ELISA test for the detection of an immunological blocking factor in human pregnancy serum. J Reprod Immunol 1989;(Sept)19:29.
40. Szekeres BJ, Autran B, Debre P, Andreu G, Denver L, Chaouat G. Immunoregulatory effects of a suppressor factor from healthy pregnant women's lymphocytes after progesterone induction. Dell-Immunol 1989;(Sept)281:294.
41. Daya S, Johnson PM, Clark DA. Trophoblast induction of suppressor-type cell activity in human endometrial tissue. Am J Reprod Immunol 1989;(Feb)65:72.
42. Ribbin SL, Hoversland RC, Beaman KD. T-cell suppressor factors play an integral role in preventing fetal rejection. J Reprod Immunol 1988;(Oct)83:95.
43. Bessman JD. Epitopes in medicine: the example of the lupus anticoagulant. JAMA 1988;259:573.
44. Lubbe WF, Liggins GC. Role of lupus anticoagulant and autoimmunity in recurrent pregnancy loss. Semin Reprod Endocrinol 1988;6:181.
45. Triplett DA. Antiphospholipid antibodies and recurrent pregnancy loss. Am J Reprod Immunol (Review) 1989;(June)52:67.
46. Petri M, Golbus M, Anderson R, Whiting-O'Keefe Q, Corash L, Hallmann D. Antinuclear antibody, lupus anticoagulant, and anticardiolipin antibody in women with idiopathic habitual abortions. A controlled, prospective study of forty-four women. Arthritis Rheum 1987;(June)601:6.
47. Iannaccone PM, Bossert NL, Connelly CS. Disruption of embryonic and fetal development due to preimplantation chemical insults: a critical review. Am J Obstet Gynecol 1987;157:476.
48. Pharoah POD, Alberman E, Doyle P, Chamberlain G. Outcome of pregnancy among women in anaesthetic practice. Lancet 1977;1:34.
49. Sandor S, Garban Z, Checiu M, Daradics L. The presence of ethanol in the oviductal and uterine luminal fluids of alcoholized rats. Morphol Embryol (Bucur) 1981;(Oct–Dec):303.
50. Kline J, Stein Z, Sussar M, Warburton D. Smoking: a risk factor for spontaneous abortion. N Engl J Med 1977;297:793.
51. Freinkel N, Cockroft DL, Lewis NJU, Gorman L, Akazawa S, Phillips LS, Shambaugh GE 3rd. The 1986 McCollum award lecture. Fuel-mediated teratogenesis during early organogenesis: the effects of increased concentrations of glucose, ketones, or somatomedin inhibitor during rat embryo culture. Am J Clin Nutr 1986;44:986.
52. Vaught JB, Gurtoo, HL, Parker NB, LeBoeuf R, Doctor G. Effects of smoking on benzo[a]pyrene metabolism by human placental microsomes. Cancer Res 1979;39:3177.
53. Fujino T, Gottlieb K, Manchester DK, Park SS, West D, Gurtoo HL, et al. Monoclonal antibody phenotyping of interindividual differences in cytochrome P-450-dependent reactions of single and twin human placenta. Cancer Res 1984;44:3916.
54. Sanyal MK, Biggers WJ, Satish J, Li YL, Barnea ER. Polynuclear aromatic hydrocarbon (PAH) metabolism potential of human placental tissues of the first trimester pregnancy (Personal Communication).
55. Agarwal DK, Lawrence WH, Autian J. Antifertility and mutagenic effects in mice from parenteral administration of di-2-ethylhexyl phthalate (DEHP). J Toxicol Environ Health 1985;71.
56. Leonard A, Jacquet P. Embryotoxicity and genotoxicity of nickel, IARC Sci Publ (Review) 1984;277.
57. Michel C. Radiation embryology. Experientia 1989;(Jan 15):69.
58. Vetter RJ. Radiation exposure of fertile women in medical research studies. Health Phys 1988;55:487.
59. Leridon, H. Human fertility: the basic components. Chicago: University of Chicago Press, 1977.
60. Landy HJ, Keith L, Keith B. The vanishing twin. Acta Genet Med Gemellol 1982;31:179.
61. Edmonds DK, Lindsay KS, Miller JF, Williamson E, Wood PJ. Embryonic mortality in women. Fertil Steril 1982;38:447.
62. Hertig, AT. Implantation of the human ovum: the histogenesis of some aspects of spontaneous abortion. In: Behrtman SJ, Kistner RW, eds. Progress in infertility. Boston: Little, Brown, 1975:411.
63. Torpin R. The human placenta, its shape, form, origin and development. Springfield, IL: Charles C Thomas, 1969.
64. Glasser SR, Julian J, Munir MI, Soares MJ. Biological markers during early pregnancy: trophoblastic signals of the periimplantation period. Environ Health Perspect 1987;74:129.
65. Hay DL. Discordant and variable production of human chorionic gonadotropin and its free alpha- and beta-subunits in early pregnancy. J Clin Endocrinol Metab 1985;61:1195.
66. Fishel SB, Edwards RG, Purdy JM. In vitro fertilization of human oocytes: factors associated with embryonic development in vitro, replacement of embryos and pregnancy. In: Seppala M, Edwards RG. Fertilization and embryo transfer, Helsinki, 1984. Ann NY Acad Sci. In press.
67. Edwards RGF, Steptoe PC Current status of in vitro fertilization and implantation of human embryos. Lancet 1983;ii:1265.
68. Steptoe PC et al. Am J Obstet Gynecol. In Press.
69. Elias S, LeBeau M, Simpson JL, et al. Chromosome analysis of ectopic human conceptuses. Am J Obstet Gynecol 1980;55:17.

70. Laufer N, DeCherney AH, Haseltine FP, et al. Steroid secretion by the human egg-corona-cumulus complex in culture. J Clin Endocrinol Metab, 1984;58:1153.

71. Edwards RG, Steptoe PC. Current status of in-vitro fertilization and implantation of human embryos. Lancet 1983;2:1265.

72. Ben-Rafael Z, Fateh M, Flickinger GL, Tureck R, Blasco L, Mastroianni L Jr. Incidence of abortion in pregnancies after in vitro fertilization and embryo transfer. Obstet Gynecol 1988;71:297.

73. Page RD, Kirkpatrick-Keller D, Butcher RL. Role of age and length of oestrous cycle in alteration of the oocyte and intrauterine environment in the rat. J Reprod Fertil 1983;69:23.

74. Thorpe LW, Connors TJ. The distribution of uterine glycogen during early pregnancy in the young and senescent golden hamster. J Gerontol 1975;30:149.

75. Lang WR, Aponte GE. Gross and microscopic anatomy of the aged female reproductive organs. Clin Obstet Gynecol 1967;10:454.

76. Naeye RL. Maternal age, obstetric complications, and the outcome of pregnancy. Obstet Gynecol 1983;61:210.

77. Wexler BC. Spontaneous artertiosclerosis in repeatedly bred Gosden RG, Gosden CA, Hawkins HK 1978. Autofluorescent particles of human uterine muscle cells. Am J Pathol 1964;91:155..

78. Gosden RG, Gosden CA, Hawkins HK. Autofluorescent particles of human uterine muscle cells. Am J Pathol 1978;91:155.

79. Haust MD, Hertas JL, Harding PG. Fat-containing uterine smooth muscle cells in "Toxaemia": possible relevance to arterioschlerosis. Science 1977;195:1353.

80. Ferguson-Smith MA, Yates JRW. Maternal age specific rates for chromosome aberrations and factors influencing them: report of a collaborative European study on 52965 amniocenteses. Prenat Diagn 1984;4:5.

15

CHAPTER

RECURRENT PREGNANCY LOSS

Charles J. Lockwood

Human reproduction is an inefficient process, with losses possibly following 70% to 80% of fertilizations.[1,2] A significant proportion (28%) of fertilized ova appear to be lost before implantation.[3] The cause of preimplantation losses remains obscure, although chromosomally abnormal animal zygotes are lost shortly after fertilization.[4] A number of investigators, using daily sensitive plasma and urine assays for human chorionic gonadotropin (hCG), have reported losses in 39% (217/560) of confirmed postimplantation pregnancies.[5–8] Two thirds of these postimplantation losses could not be detected clinically, consistent with the generally observed 10% to 15% clinical spontaneous abortion rate.[5–8]

Initial karyotype studies of abortus material suggested that 50% to 60% of spontaneous losses were chromosomally abnormal.[9–12] However, recent data derived from early gestational sonography and aggressive karyotype analysis have demonstrated a 77% chromosomal abnormality rate in very early losses.[13] Further study is needed, because not all investigators have confirmed this high correlation between early losses and chromosomal aberrations.[14] The high spontaneous loss rate observed in older women (>45% over age 40 years) supports the etiologic role of chromosomal abnormalities in early pregnancy loss, because these women are also at greater risk of meiotic nondisjunction.[15,16] However, it is uncertain whether aneuploidy alone is responsible for this maternal age-related increase in early pregnancy loss.[17]

Given the high rate of pregnancy wastage inherent in normal human reproduction, it would not be unusual for successive early losses to occur by chance. Earlier work by Malpas and Eastman[18,19] notwithstanding, the probability of a viable infant following three or more prior losses is 50% to 70% without intervention.[15,20,21] Indeed, the risk of a spontaneous abortion following one prior loss may not be appreciably different than the risk following four prior losses (23.7% versus 25.9%).[15] Therefore, any evaluation of possible causes for recurrent pregnancy loss or its treatment must take into account both the high background rate of pregnancy loss and the inherently high "spontaneous remission" rate.

Unfortunately, most studies of recurrent pregnancy loss inappropriately use patients' prior loss rates as statistical support for a given cause or as "controls" to document therapeutic efficacy. Ascertainment biases distort the relative frequencies of possible causes for recurrent pregnancy loss. For example, patients referred to genetic services are likely to have had infectious, uterine, and endocrine causes ruled out. An additional source of bias is the inherent tendency to identify a cause for which there is a treatment, particularly if the diagnostician is also the therapist. Finally, the preponderance of older patients in recurrent loss populations presents a particular challenge, because multiple causes are likely to be present in older patients, including an increased risk for aneuploidy, luteal phase dysfunction, myomas, and autoimmune disorders.

Despite the above reservations, this chapter assumes that recurrent pregnancy losses can occasionally occur other than by chance. Postulated causes for recurrent pregnancy loss are critically examined with discussion of their prevalence, pathogenic mechanisms, and clinical relevance. Appropriate diagnostic and therapeutic steps in the management of these patients are also outlined (Tables 16-1 through 16-7). Recurrent pregnancy loss is arbitrarily defined as two or more pregnancy losses occurring before 20 weeks gestation with or without prior live births, stillbirths, or fetal growth retardation. Early losses related to preterm labor are not included.

GENETIC ETIOLOGIES

As noted previously, chromosomal abnormalities may be associated with the majority of first trimester spontaneous abortions. Approximately 50% of these abnormalities are autosomal trisomies, most frequently trisomy 16.[22,23] Monosomy X and polyploidy each account for an additional 20% to 25% of cases.[22,23] Although cytogenetic abnormalities may account for most sporadic losses, chromosomal aberrations may also account for at least half of recurrent losses.[24] Single gene defects may also result in spontaneous abortions; however, our ability to characterize these defects or assess their clinical relevance is limited (Table 15-1).

CHROMOSOMAL CAUSES: RECURRENT ANEUPLOIDY

Logically, parental factors that increase the likelihood of a chromosomally abnormal conceptus should increase the likelihood of recurrent pregnancy losses. Purported factors include parental balanced translocations and chromosomal mosaicism, possible genetic predispositions to meiotic and mitotic nondisjunction, and paternal hyperspermia.

Parental Chromosomal Abnormalities

Larger studies and reviews of the literature suggest that 3% to 6% of couples experiencing two or more losses have identifiable chromosomal abnormalities.[25–27] This compares with a 0.2% prevalence in the general population.[28] Most (75% to 83%) abnormalities are balanced translocations, with two thirds reciprocal and one third Robertsonian.[25–27] An additional 12% to 16% are low-grade chromosomal mosaicisms, usually involving the X chromosome.[25,27] Some investigators have identified an even higher (36%) relative proportion of X-chromosomal mosaicism.[29] Couples with balanced translocations have spontaneous loss rates ranging from 50% for reciprocal translocations to 25% for Robertsonian translocations.[30] The greater the degree of resultant chromosomal imbalance, the more likely the pregnancy will be lost rather than result in an affected live born child. Nonalternate meiotic segregation patterns, adjacent 2 and 3:1, appear to produce the greatest imbalance and therefore the highest loss rates, while adjacent 1 segregation increases the risk of a malformed offspring.[25,30]

Minor chromosomal variants (1qh, 9qh, 16qh, Yqh, and satellites—p+) do not appear to be associated with increased rates of pregnancy loss.[31,32] Peri- and paracentric inversions are of uncertain significance, but could theoretically increase the risk of lethal chromosomal recombinants.[25,33,34]

In summary, a small but significant proportion of couples experiencing recurrent pregnancy loss will have abnormalities of chromosomal structure or number, which can be identified on parental karyotype analysis. Given these observations, it appears prudent to assess couples having two or more spontaneous losses with parental karyotype analysis before their next conception. Certainly, couples with either recurrent loss associated with an abnormal offspring or parental phenotypic abnormalities should be investigated with karyotype analysis. High-resolution banding techniques, if available, should be employed in these karyotypic assessments.[35] Obviously, couples with documented chromosomal abnormalities should be offered fetal karyotype analysis in subsequent ongoing pregnancies.

Confirmation of parental chromosomal abnormalities presents a therapeutic dilemma. The couple may wish to attempt repetitive conceptions, understanding that their success rate will be at least 50% per conception. Chromosomal analysis by amniocentesis should be offered to couples whose pregnancies progress past 8 weeks gestation. Alternatively, adoption, artificial insemination or, in the future, ova donations from in vitro fertilization programs may be opted for.

Parental Predispositions to Meiotic Nondisjunction

A number of investigators have demonstrated an increased incidence of hypermodal chromosomal spreads (mitotic nondisjunction) in lymphocyte cultures derived from recurrent aborters.[36–39] These involve both autosomes and the X chromosome.[36–39] Meiotic nondisjunctional events might also occur more frequently in these patients, accounting for their increased pregnancy loss rates. Potential mechanisms would include a genetic predisposition to nondisjunction (abnormal spindles, etc.), possible environmental factors, or exacerbation of age-related processes. The precise proportion of couples with recurrent loss who manifest a predisposition

TABLE 15-1. GENETIC ETIOLOGIES FOR RECURRENT PREGNANCY LOSS

ETIOLOGY	DIAGNOSIS	THERAPY
Recurrent Aneuploidy		
Parental chromosomal abnormalities	Parental karyotype	?Gamete donor
Predisposition to meiotic nondisjunction	Serial abortus karyotyping and serial sonography	?Gamete donor
Hyperspermia	Semen analysis	Sperm dilution
Lethal Genes or Gene Interactions		
X-linked disorders	Family history and serial sonography	None
Polygenic	Family history	None

to meiotic nondisjunction is unknown, and caution must be exercised because not all investigators have confirmed this phenomenon.[40]

Our ability to detect increased risks for meiotic nondisjunction in couples with normal parental karyotypes is limited. Therefore, it is essential to evaluate the karyotypes of each abortus in couples suffering recurrent pregnancy loss. High-resolution banding studies may be appropriate to rule out maternal contamination if a normal female karyotype is found. Detailed vaginal sonography early in pregnancy may also be of value in recurrent aborters. The presence of only a yolk sac-like structure within the gestational sac may be a marker for an abnormal karyotype.[41] Such a sonographic finding in a recurrent loss patient should prompt karyotype analysis of the products of conception or, possibly, chorionic villus sampling (CVS). Later in gestation, the finding of congenital heart defects,[42] gross fetal malformations,[43] and a number of relatively subtle sonographic findings may suggest aneuploidy.[44–47] In the setting of prior repetitive losses, these findings may also be an indication for karyotype evaluation.

Therapy in cases of recurrent aneuploidy of unknown cause is not possible beyond the use of donor gametes. Moreover, the couple's prognosis is difficult to predict because there is no a priori reason to believe that defects in germ cell chromosomal segregation will universally occur. However, persistent defects in meiosis II would produce a 50% aneuploidy rate, while persistent defects in meiosis I would indeed be universally associated with aneuploidy.[48] Karyotype assessment by amniocentesis may be indicated in pregnancies progressing past 8 weeks if recurrent aneuploid losses have been previously documented.

Hyperspermia

Higher sperm counts and superior sperm motility and morphology have been associated with recurrent pregnancy loss.[49,50] One proposed explanation for this phenomenon is polyspermia resulting in zygotic polyploidy.[49] However, these data have not been further evaluated, and the clinical utility of semen analysis in the partners of recurrent loss patients is unknown. If an elevated sperm count is incidentally identified, serial sonography in the next pregnancy may allow the early identification of a partial mole or triploid fetal phenotype. Such sonographic findings are certainly an indication for karyotype analysis.[47]

SINGLE GENE CAUSES AND LETHAL GENE INTERACTIONS

Mutations critical to cell function or tissue morphogenesis can lead to early embryonic loss.[51] Such mutations inherited in an autosomal recessive fashion are presumably quite rare and should only result in a 25% loss rate (eg, α-thalassemia) unless affected gametes are selected for. In contrast, a parental germ line lethal mutation would lead to a 50% loss rate or higher, if the mutation conferred a conceptive advantage. Certain disorders appear to be lethal in the hemizygous or heterozygous male, causing an increased spontaneous loss rate. Examples include focal dermal hypoplasia, incontinentia pigmenti, and oral-facial-digital syndrome (type I).[48,52] These disorders may have a X-linked recessive inheritance or be caused by an autosomal dominant mutation lethal in males. They should be suspected when the ratio of females to males in affected families is 2:1, where one half of female sibs are affected and if all male sibs are unaffected.[48,53] Lethal multiple pterygium syndrome (LMPS) appears to be an X-linked cause of recurrent midgestational loss without affected female heterozygotes.[54,55]

There appears to be an increased spontaneous loss rate in couples with a family history of either neural tube defects or cleft lip with or without cleft palate.[56,57] Because these polygenic anomalies may result in part from unfavorable gene interactions, the associated pregnancy losses may have an analogous cause. Interactions between HLA-linked and unlinked genes have been demonstrated to cause embryonic death in rats.[58] Weitkamp and Schacter have demonstrated an association between the human transferrin C3 allele and recurrent pregnancy loss.[59] They also noted an apparent distortion in paternal transferrin allele transmission rates and a possible association between neural tube defects, parental HLA-sharing, and transferrin genotypes.[59] These observations suggest that complex gene interactions between transferrin region gene products and other unlinked, perhaps HLA-associated, gene products may result in recurrent pregnancy loss or certain congenital malformations.

The potential for single gene disorders or complex gene interactions to cause recurrent euploid pregnancy loss is substantial. However, our ability to identify their frequencies or potential causes is rudimentary. This underscores the importance of a detailed genetic history in the assessment of affected couples. Serial high-resolution vaginal sonography may be of use in the detection of lethal single gene abnormalities (eg, LMPS), because postmortem evaluation of macerated tissue is often inadequate for phenotype ascertainment.[55]

MÜLLERIAN ANOMALIES AND OTHER UTERINE ABNORMALITIES

Abnormalities of müllerian duct fusion most commonly result in symmetric defects, including didelphic uterus, bicornuate uterus, and septate uterus, less commonly in unicornuate uterus with or without a rudimentary horn (Table 15-2).[60] Müllerian anomalies reportedly occur in 0.25% (0.1% to 0.5%) of patients; however, prevalence statistics are undoubtedly underestimated, because only in patients with pregnancy complications are these anomalies likely to be ascertained.[60–63] Conversely, in patients with recurrent pregnancy loss, the prevalence of müllerian anomalies is reportedly 15%.[21,64,65] This

TABLE 15–2. MÜLLERIAN AND OTHER UTERINE ABNORMALITIES

ETIOLOGY	DIAGNOSIS	THERAPY
Müllerian Anomalies		
Septate uterus	HSG/hysteroscopy with laparoscopy	Hysteroscopic resection
Didelphic and bicornuate uteri	HSG/hysteroscopy with laparoscopy	Strassman procedure
Unicornuate uterus	HSG/hysteroscopy with laparoscopy	None
Other Uterine Abnormalities		
Submucous myomas	HSG/hysteroscopy with laparoscopy	Myomectomy
Asherman's syndrome	HSG/hysteroscopy	Hysteroscopic resection or D & C
DES-Hypoplasia	HSG/hysteroscopy	? Cerclage

prevalence, however, is likely overestimated secondary to referral population selection biases. Müllerian anomalies appear to be associated with increases in abnormal fetal lie (20% to 30%), preterm delivery (13% to 23%), and spontaneous abortion (16% to 50%).[60–63,66] Again, however, ascertainment bias may overestimate the rate of pregnancy complications. Indeed, 80% of untreated patients with septate uteri will eventually deliver a liveborn infant.[60,67]

The mechanism whereby müllerian anomalies cause intermittent early loss is unclear. A commonly held view is that implantation onto a relatively avascular septum or uterine wall results in inadequate placentation.[60] Presumably, recurrent early losses that are purported to be caused by submucous myomas, uterine synechiae, and diethylstilbestrol (DES)-induced uterine hypoplasia have similar pathogeneses. The prognosis for successful pregnancies in patients with müllerian anomalies appears to be related to the type of malformation, with asymmetric fusion defects carrying the worst prognosis, followed by septate, bicornuate, and didelphis uterus, in that order.[60,62] Heinonen and coworkers, however, noted better fetal survival with septate (86%) compared to bicornuate (50%) uteri.[68] A dose-response curve has been suggested in patients with septate uterus, with larger septi resulting in more adverse outcomes.[69] Prior induced abortions are not associated with increased rates of spontaneous losses.[70]

The detection of müllerian anomalies, as well as acquired uterine structural abnormalities, relies on a proper index of suspicion. Patients with a history of spontaneous losses associated with preterm labor or abnormal fetal lie are appropriate candidates for diagnostic studies. A family history of uterine myomas, DES use, uterine or renal abnormalities, or a history of multiple prior uterine curettages are indicators of risk. Proper evaluation includes hysterosalpingography (HSG) or hysteroscopy with concomitant laparoscopy. All patients documented to have müllerian anomalies should undergo renal ultrasound and intravenous pyelography. The prevalence of concomitant urinary tract abnormalities in these patients is 20% to 60%[60,62]; conversely, up to 90% of women with unilateral renal anomalies may have concomitant genital tract abnormalities.[71]

The indication for therapy in patients with recurrent pregnancy loss accompanied by müllerian anomalies is open to question. Implantation in a vascular portion of the uterus would be expected to occur quite frequently, consistent with the observed high spontaneous remission rate.[60,67] Treatment does appear indicated for patients with müllerian and other uterine anomalies who demonstrate recurrent preterm deliveries early in gestation or recurrent spontaneous losses in the absence of other causes. Surgical success rates are, as expected, quite high (>80%).[60,65,72–77] Approaches to the septate uterus include hysteroscopic or resectoscopic resection of septi, in conjunction with laparoscopy[65,72–74] or the more traditional Tompkins-Jones metroplasty.[75–77] Results appear comparable.[60,65,72–77] The Strassman procedure has been employed for bicornuate uterus.[78] Patients with hypoplastic uteri secondary to in utero DES exposure are not surgical candidates. The unicornuate uterus is not amenable to repair, and pregnancies occurring in a rudimentary horn can result in rupture with extensive hemorrhage.[79] Myomectomy is employed for multiple large myomas. The treatment for uterine synechiae may employ a number of modalities including dilation and curettage (D & C) or hysteroscopic resection. Cerclage has been advocated as treatment for recurrent early loss; however, an appropriate control group was not employed.[80,81] Nonetheless, cerclage may be indicated in DES-exposed women with uterine or cervical abnormalities.[82]

INFECTIOUS ETIOLOGIES

A number of acute viral infections can result in the sporadic occurrence of spontaneous abortion, including herpes simplex,[83] mumps,[84] rubella,[85,86] and Epstein-Barr virus.[87] These organisms do not cause recurrent loss because the mother produces protective antibodies. The role of infectious agents in the genesis of recurrent pregnancy loss, if any, should therefore be limited to certain commensal organisms that provoke only a mod-

TABLE 15–3. INFECTIOUS ETIOLOGIES: MYCOPLASMA

ETIOLOGY	DIAGNOSIS	THERAPY
U. urealyticum	Cervical culture	Doxycycline
M. hominis	Cervical culture	Erythromycin ? Need

est host response or chronic infections by organisms of low virulence (Table 15-3). *Listeria monocytogenes*, a common commensal organism,[88] can cause intrauterine fetal demise but does not appear to be associated with recurrent early pregnancy losses.[64,89–91] Toxoplasmosis, a protozoan and obligate intracellular parasite, can cause congenital infection, hydrops, and fetal death. Although toxoplasmosis may form intrauterine tissue cysts,[92] it has not been clearly linked with either sporadic[93] or recurrent abortion.[92,94,95] Similarly, Chlamydia has not been consistently cultured from recurrent aborters, nor is there an increased mean antichlamydial antibody titer in recurrent loss patients.[96]

The link between recurrent loss and Mycoplasma species, self-replicating prokaryotes that lack a cell wall, has been intensively studied. The two primary genital mycoplasmas with pathogenic potential are *Mycoplasma hominis* and *Ureaplasma urealyticum*. Both are common commensal organisms with a population prevalence of 50% to 70% (greater for *U. urealyticum*).[97,98] The potential for *U. urealyticum* to induce spontaneous abortion is supported by the in vitro observation that it can induce chromosomal gaps, breaks, and polyploidy in human leukocyte and amnion cell cultures.[99–101] Furthermore, Quinn and colleagues postulate that mycoplasmas, and specifically *U. urealyticum*, may alter the maternal immune system to induce a nonspecific polyclonal B-cell activation.[96,102] Because recurrent loss patients appear to have elevated antibody titers to *U. urealyticum* when compared with controls,[103–105] it is possible that their pregnancy losses are in part a consequence of the production of autoantibodies (eg, antiphospholipid antibodies) injurious to the trophoblast.[96]

Unfortunately, the data linking mycoplasma with recurrent loss are far from convincing. Caspi and coworkers noted higher rates of both Mycoplasma-positive cervical cultures (43% versus 23%) and abortus cultures (34% versus 4%) in patients with spontaneous versus therapeutic abortions.[106] Similar findings were obtained by Sompolinsky and colleagues.[107] Quinn and associates noted a higher *M. hominis* and *U. urealyticum* culture rate among recurrent loss patients (84%) versus fertile controls (25%), and demonstrated an apparent salutary response to treatment compared with historical controls.[105,108] Higher antibody titers to *U. urealyticum*, particularly serotypes 4, 6, and 8, were also demonstrated in recurrent loss and pregnancy wastage patients, supporting a pathogenic role for *U. urealyticum*.[103–105] However, the high prevalence of these organisms in the general population and the high probability of a successful outcome in recurrent loss patients independent of therapy casts doubt on the clinical relevance of genital Mycoplasma colonization. Furthermore, the absence of a prospective, randomized, double-blind, placebo-controlled trial demonstrating that Mycoplasma eradication improves pregnancy outcomes prevents accurate assessment of the need for therapy.

Given the absence of definitive information, we recommend not treating all patients, but culturing patients with recurrent abortion for *M. hominis* and *U. urealyticum* and, if positive, treating both partners with doxycycline before attempting conception. Multiple courses may be required in some couples, particularly if colonized by both *U. urealyticum* and *M. hominis*.[105,108] Once pregnant, additional maternal erythromycin therapy may improve both Mycoplasma clearance and pregnancy success rates.[108]

ENDOCRINOLOGICAL AND METABOLIC ETIOLOGIES

Maternal endocrinological disorders have been implicated in the genesis of recurrent pregnancy loss, including luteal phase defects and poorly controlled diabetes mellitus (Table 15-4). There is no evidence that mild hyper- or hypothyroidism can cause recurrent pregnancy loss.[109,110] Untreated maternal metabolic disorders can also cause recurrent pregnancy loss, including homocystinuria[111,112] and Wilson's disease.[113,114] Fortunately, these latter disorders are sufficiently rare and, generally, although not always, obvious to the obstetrician so as not to pose a significant diagnostic concern.[114]

LUTEAL PHASE DEFECTS

Luteal phase defects (LPD) should be suspected in patients with short cycles, postovulatory intervals less than 14 days, or the association of secondary infertility with recurrent early losses. The reported prevalence of

TABLE 15–4. ENDOCRINOLOGICAL ETIOLOGIES

ETIOLOGY	DIAGNOSIS	THERAPY
Luteal phase defects	Endometrial biopsy Progesterone level	Clomid Progesterone suppositories
Poorly controlled diabetes mellitus	Serial blood glucose Hemoglobin A1-c	Insulin

LPD in recurrent aborters ranges from 20% to 60%,[109,115,116] although ascertainment biases undoubtedly inflate these numbers. Recurrent loss patients with LPD appear to have lower mean and peak progesterone concentrations in the luteal phase, as well as earlier peaks in their progesterone levels (day 21 versus day 22).[117] Potential causes for LPD include hyperprolactinemia, anorexia, rigorous exercise regimens, and congenital adrenal hyperplasia.

The pathogenesis of pregnancy loss in LPD is unclear. Postulated mechanisms include a dyssynchronous endometrium leading to inadequate placentation or poor coordination between the cessation of luteal progesterone production and increased placental progesterone secretion at 8 to 10 weeks gestation.[118] The diagnosis requires at least two luteal phase endometrial biopsies, preferably obtained within 4 days before the next anticipated menses, demonstrating more than 2 days histologic lag in endometrial development.[117] The biopsy should be obtained high on the anterior or posterior fundal wall, must contain adequate tissue, and should be read by an experienced interpreter.[117,119]

Treatment for LPD includes clomiphene citrate or vaginal progesterone suppositories. The latter therapy avoids potential clomiphene-induced embryotoxic effects.[119] Various regimens can be employed; one of these is 25 mg of micronized progesterone given intravaginally twice daily until 10 to 12 weeks.[120] Success rates of up to 90% compared with historical controls have been reported in recurrent aborters[109,117,121–123]; however, other investigators have noted no improvement in outcomes.[124–126] A large prospective, double-blind, placebo-controlled trial is necessary to establish the etiological validity of LPD.

INSULIN-DEPENDENT DIABETES MELLITUS

A number of studies have suggested that insulin-dependent diabetes mellitus is associated with an increased incidence of spontaneous abortion,[127–130] and that the increased loss rates are proportionate to the degree of maternal hyperglycemia.[128–131,133] Furthermore, rigorous preconceptional glucose control has been reported to decrease the risk of spontaneous loss in these patients.[134] However, a number of potential ascertainment biases are present in these studies.[135] In a meticulous evaluation of the incidence of spontaneous abortion among well-controlled, insulin-dependent diabetics and matched controls followed within 21 days of conception, no increased risk of miscarriage was observed (16.1% versus 16.2%).[135] Diabetics who spontaneously aborted had higher first trimester fasting and postprandial glucose concentrations than those whose pregnancies continued to term.[135] Thus, it appears that diabetic patients managed with contemporary insulin and glucose monitoring regimens that achieve good metabolic control have no higher risk of spontaneous abortion than nondiabetic women.

The mechanism for pregnancy loss in poorly controlled diabetes may be glucose-induced embryotoxicity.[136] Preliminary evidence suggests that a reduction in arachidonic acid may contribute to the embryopathic process.[137]

Poorly controlled diabetes is likely to account for only a fraction of recurrent loss patients. One should, however, not ascribe recurrent pregnancy loss in a diabetic to poor metabolic control unless all other potential causes have been ruled out, and fasting and postprandial glucoses are elevated along with glycosylated hemoglobin values. Therapy consists of optimizing the insulin regimen and aggressive home glucose monitoring. Subclinical glucose intolerance is not a cause for recurrent pregnancy loss and need not be searched for.[64]

HEMATOLOGICAL ETIOLOGIES

Hematological causes for recurrent pregnancy loss are rare, but unfortunately the presence or nature of the disorder may not be apparent to the obstetrician before pregnancy. Because these conditions may initially present as recurrent pregnancy loss, a working knowledge of their cause, pathogenesis, diagnosis, and treatment is necessary (Table 15-5).

DISORDERS OF FIBRIN METABOLISM

Physiologic placentation involves significant tissue and vascular architectural rearrangements. Fibrin deposition appears to play a critical role in these rearrangements. Fibrin deposition accompanies the transformation of placental bed spiral arteries[138] and may serve in the formation of villus anchoring sites. It is therefore not unexpected that disorders of fibrin metabolism, formation, and structure would be associated with recurrent pregnancy loss.

Factor XIII Deficiency

The mechanical strength of the fibrin clot is derived from monomer cross linking mediated by factor XIII (FXIII). In addition, FXIII also promotes the binding of α-2-antiplasmin to fibrin, rendering it less susceptible to plasmin digestion; FXIII facilitates the attachment of fibronectin to fibrin, anchoring the clot to damaged endothelial cells. A 320,000-dalton, tetrameric compound, FXIII is composed of two noncovalently bound α- and two noncovalently bound α-chains.[139] Factor XIII deficiency is a rare autosomal recessive disorder associated with both bleeding diathesis and poor wound healing.[139,140]

Recurrent abortion has also been described in affected females.[141] Kitchens and Newcomb described a large family in which none of the affected women successfully reproduced.[140] Fisher and colleagues reported 12 successive pregnancy losses associated with severe uterine bleeding in an affected patient.[142] Therapy in her next pregnancy with 300 mL of plasma every 10 days restored fibrin stability and allowed for an un-

TABLE 15-5. HEMATOLOGICAL CAUSES OF PREGNANCY WASTAGE

ETIOLOGY	DIAGNOSIS	THERAPY
Disorders of Fibrin Metabolism		
Factor XIII deficiency	Clot stability Quantitative RIA	Plasma therapy
Afibrinogenemia and hypofibrinogenemia	Fibrinogen level	Fibrinogen infusions
Dysfibrinogenemia	Chromatographic studies	Plasma therapy
Antithrombin III Deficiency	ATIII activity Quantitative RIA	Heparin
Thrombocythemia	Platelet count Aggregation studies	Aspirin Dipyridamole

eventful pregnancy productive of a 3000-gm healthy neonate.[142] The pathogenesis of pregnancy loss in FXIII deficiency may involve disruption of villus fibrin anchorage points. Alternatively, losses may follow hemorrhage and dissection into the tunica media of placental-bed spiral arteries secondary to unstable fibrin deposited during physiologic transformation.[138,143] Factor XIII deficiency is also associated a 25% incidence of maternal intracerebral hemorrhage in affected mothers and a greater than 90% incidence of spontaneous umbilical stump hemorrhage in affected mothers.[144]

Because patients generally develop bleeding diatheses only when FXIII concentrations are less than 1%,[140] the diagnosis of recurrent abortion secondary to FXIII deficiency can require a high index of suspicion. A family history of FXIII deficiency may be present; however, acquired deficiency is also possible.[140] Suggestive findings include several days' delay in soft tissue bleeding after trauma, chronic hemorrhagic cysts, and suboptimal wound healing. Pregnancy is normally accompanied by a decrease in FXIII activity, which can precipitate hemorrhagic episodes in susceptible patients.[140] The diagnosis of FXIII deficiency should be suspected with a history of recurrent abortion accompanied by exceptionally heavy uterine bleeding. Because routine coagulation indices will be within normal limits, confirmation of the diagnosis requires assessment of clot stability or a quantitative radioimmunoassay of FXIII concentrations.[140,146] Treatment goals include maintaining FXIII concentrations above 10% with one to two units of plasma every 3 weeks.[140] Given the risk of spontaneous umbilical stump hemorrhage, at-risk neonates should be tested and treated appropriately.

Afibrinogenemia and Hypofibrinogenemia

Fibrinogen is a complex glycoprotein, with a molecular weight of 340,000 daltons.[139] Hepatic fibrinogen synthesis increases dramatically in pregnancy, with mean concentrations of 432 mg/dL in the third trimester.[147] Afibrinogenemia is a rare autosomal recessive disorder associated with recurrent bleeding episodes after minor trauma. Untreated, afibrinogenemia results in recurrent abortion.[148–150] Hypofibrinogenemia, the heterozygous state, also results in recurrent abortion when fibrinogen levels fall below 60 mg/dL.[148,151] Both disorders are a consequence of inadequate hepatic synthesis of fibrinogen. The pathogenesis of pregnancy loss presumably involves inadequate fibrin generation with deficient fibrin trophoblast anchorage points or placental-bed spiral artery vascular disruption.

Detection is likely to depend on the severity of the fibrinogen deficiency. Although patients with afibrinogenemia or severe hypofibrinogenemia may manifest recurrent bleeding tendencies, mild hypofibrinogenemic patients may be asymptomatic. Also depending on the severity of the deficiency, routine coagulation indices may be prolonged or normal. The diagnosis can be strongly indicated by the quantitative findings of a low fibrinogen level.

Therapeutic regimens resulting in successful pregnancies have employed fibrinogen infusions of 2 to 4 gm/wk in cases of afibrinogenemia.[148] A reasonable therapeutic goal is the maintenance of fibrinogen concentrations > 75 mg/dL with either cryoprecipitate or fresh frozen plasma.[152] There is up to a 50% risk of a fetal bleeding dyscrasia in hypofibrinogenemic mothers, and consideration should be given to percutaneous umbilical cord sampling near term for the assessment of the fetal fibrinogen concentration. Low values may warrant in utero fibrinogen infusions or cesarean delivery.

Dysfibrinogenemia

Rare, qualitative abnormalities of fibrinogen structure can result from alterations in amino acid constituents. These dysfibrinogenemias are inherited in an autosomal dominant fashion. A single mutant allele will cause half of the fibrinogen monomers in a fibrin polymer to be abnormal, resulting in structural embarrassment. Recurrent abortion has been attributed to a number of abnormal fibrinogens. Pregnancy losses are frequently accompanied by either profuse uterine bleeding or paradoxical maternal thromboembolic phenomenon.[153–157] Aberrant placentation secondary to a deficient fibrin matrix or spiral artery vasculopathy may also be the mechanism for recurrent pregnancy loss in these disorders.

The diagnosis of a dysfibrinogenemia requires a very high index of suspicion, because most patients are asymptomatic.[158] Indeed, recurrent pregnancy loss may be the primary presentation. Bleeding dyscrasias tend to be mild, and routine coagulation studies can be normal or modestly prolonged. Definitive diagnoses require sophisticated chromatographic analysis.[157]

Treatment consists of cryoprecipitate infusions sufficient to restore fibrin integrity and stop hemorrhage.[157] There is a 50% risk of fetal dysfibrinogenemia, and consideration should be given to percutaneous umbilical cord sampling to assess fetal fibrinogen status and plan delivery.

ANTITHROMBIN III (ATIII) DEFICIENCY

The primary physiologic inhibitor of thrombin and factor Xa is antithrombin III (ATIII), accounting for 75% of the thrombin-inhibiting activity in plasma.[141] The 58,000-dalton ATIII molecule binds to and inactivates thrombin.[141] Heparin substantially accelerates (2000 X) ATIII binding.[141] Autosomal dominant ATIII deficiencies result in recurrent thromboembolic phenomenon when ATIII activity is less than 50%.[139] The prevalence of ATIII deficiency has been reported as 1/2000 to 1/5000.[159]

Pregnancy is not associated with a rise in ATIII concentrations,[160,161] and there is a 70% incidence of thromboembolic phenomenon in pregnant patients with ATIII deficiency.[162] Spontaneous abortions, stillbirth, and preeclampsia have been associated with ATIII deficiency.[162] Nelson and colleagues reported a 100% incidence of fetal growth retardation in five pregnancies occurring in two affected women.[163]

Pertinent clinical histories include recurrent thromboembolic events with or without adverse perinatal outcomes. Lupus anticoagulant, antiphospholipid antibodies, thrombocythemia, and protein C and S deficiencies should be ruled out. The diagnosis can be confirmed by either immunoassay or measurements of ATIII biological activity.[161]

Treatment for pregnant patients with ATIII deficiency should be implemented early in pregnancy with heparin at doses sufficient to prolong the activated partial thromboplastin time (PTT) by 5 to 10 seconds, or achieve plasma heparin levels of 0.1 to 0.2 IU/mL.[162] Therapeutic concentrations do not guarantee against thromboembolic events, and meticulous fetal and maternal surveillance is indicated. The fetal risk of ATIII deficiency is 50%, and because neonates normally have lower ATIII activity than adults, neonatal ATIII levels less than 30% of normal should be treated with fresh frozen plasma.[162]

ESSENTIAL THROMBOCYTHEMIA

Essential thrombocythemia is a myeloproliferative disorder. Fortunately, it is rarely found in the reproductive age group. Platelet counts exceed 800 × 10 mm, and the disorder may result in either hemorrhagic or thrombotic sequelae, depending on the functional capacity of platelets.[164] Although younger patients are frequently asymptomatic,[164] recurrent transient ischemic attacks can occur.

There have been multiple reports of recurrent pregnancy loss associated with maternal essential thrombocythemia. Snethlage and Ten Cate described a 26-year-old woman with three successive severely growth-retarded stillbirths at less than 28 weeks gestation.[165] Subsequent treatment with aspirin (250 mg twice daily) and dipyridamole (75 mg three times a day) from 17 weeks gestation resulted in a viable, although growth-retarded, term infant, despite a peak platelet count of 1,200 × 10 mm.[165] Earlier treatment with either aspirin and dipyridamole or heparin resulted in viable, non–growth-retarded infants in two subsequent pregnancies.[165] Murphy and associates reported fetal losses at 16 and 24 weeks in a 28-year-old woman who was presumably affected during these pregnancies and was subsequently diagnosed at the time of a superior sagittal sinus thrombosis.[166] Kaibara and colleagues described a patient whose first pregnancy ended in a 30-week stillbirth weighing 789 g; this was associated with multiple placental infarcts. She was subsequently diagnosed after an inferior myocardial infarction.[167] Her second pregnancy was managed with daily aspirin therapy (750 mg per day) and resulted in a viable 2790-g term infant. The pregnancy had been remarkable for a drop in her platelet count from 1219 × 10 mm at 7 weeks to 492 × 10 mm at 33 weeks, with a rise to 1570 × 10 mm 2 months postpartum.[167] Mercer and associates describe a similar decline in platelet count across gestation from 1370 × 10 mm at 9 weeks to 940 × 10 mm at 36 weeks in an untreated thrombocythemic patient whose pregnancy ended in a stillbirth with associated placental infarcts and a small abruption.[168] Falconer and colleagues describe six spontaneous abortions in two thrombocythemic patients.[169] Subsequent therapy with serial platelet phoresis in one patient was associated with a 34-week, growth-retarded fetus delivered abdominally for fetal distress.[169] The placenta demonstrated infarcts.[169]

Pregnancy wastage in patients with thrombocythemia may be a consequence of intervillous or spiral arterial thrombosis. Essential thrombocythemia should be suspected in patients with symptoms of transient ischemic events or peripheral arterial compromise. Patients with recurrent early or late pregnancy loss, particularly if associated with fetal growth retardation and placental infarction, should have a platelet count assessed. Splenomegaly is frequently present, and other myeloproliferative processes must be ruled out.

Treatment of pregnant patients with thrombocythemia appears to be indicated, although uneventful normal outcomes can apparently occur in untreated patients.[164] Regimens should be aimed at inhibiting pathologic platelet aggregation and include aspirin (325 or 80 mg per day) and or dipyridamole (75 mg three times a day). Maternal aspirin use in pregnancy has been associated with a slightly increased risk of congenital heart disease,[170] although exposure < 2 g per day does not appear to be associated with adverse ductal or pulmonary vascular sequelae in fetuses.[171–173] Even low dose (50 mg) aspirin therapy causes complete acetylation of fetal platelets,[174] which is of concern, given the reported increased incidence of hemorrhagic diatheses in neonates with in utero exposure to aspirin (300 to 1500 mg) during the last 10 days of pregnancy.[175] Given these concerns, therapy should be initiated only after consultation with a hematologist familiar with platelet disorders and after an assessment of platelet aggregatory potential. We prefer to treat thrombocythemic patients with evidence of platelet hyperaggregability and thrombotic risk using the lowest efficacious dose (80 to 325 mg every day) of aspirin, initiated after 8 weeks gestation and stopped at after 37 weeks gestation. Platelet phoresis is reserved for refractory cases. There are no reports on the safety and efficacy of anagrelide, an antiaggregant and thrombocytopenic agent[176] in pregnancy. Alkylating agents and 32P should be avoided in pregnancy unless the mother's condition is deteriorating. Fortunately, pregnancy itself appears to be associated with a diminution in platelet counts, perhaps secondary to the dilutional effects of plasma volume expansion[177] or increases in maternal estrogens and corticosteroids, both of which have been demonstrated to reduce platelet counts.[178,179] Meticulous fetal surveillance is necessary.

AUTOIMMUNE DISORDERS

The production of autoantibodies is far more common in women than men.[180] This gender difference has been theorized to result from unique human immunological requirements for successful reproduction (eg, the need for a response to semi-allogenic antigens).[181] Two distinct mechanisms have been proposed to account for the production of autoantibodies.[182] The first invokes a generalized impairment in immunoregulation, permitting previously suppressed B-cell clones to begin production of antibodies to various autoantigens. These autoantibodies are directed to the more ubiquitous "self" antigens such as DNA, ribonucleoproteins, IgG, and phospholipids. It is this mechanism of autoantibody production that appears to be responsible for adverse reproductive effects (Table 15-6).[181]

The second mechanism by which autoantibodies are generated appears to be a byproduct of normal humoral immunoregulation, namely, the production of anti-idiotypic antibodies.[182] Each antibody contains a unique protein-binding site (idiotype) that permits appropriate binding to newly exposed antigens. Because each idiotype represents a completely new polypeptide sequence (not even shared by monozygotic twins), the body generates an immune response against it, an anti-idiotype antibody. Multiple permutations on this theme are the basis for the network theory of humoral immunoregulation.[183] These anti-idiotypic antibodies may serendipitously react with self antigens, causing such autoimmune diseases as diabetes mellitus, Graves' disease, and myasthenia gravis.[182] The role of anti-idiotypic antibodies in recurrent pregnancy wastage is as yet unexplored.

LUPUS ANTICOAGULANT (ANTIPHOSPHOLIPID ANTIBODIES)

Laurell and Nilsson first described the association of a unique circulating anticoagulant and a false-positive Wasserman serology test with recurrent pregnancy wastage.[184] This phenomenon is now termed the lupus anticoagulant (LAC) because of its frequent occurrence in patients with systemic lupus erythematosus (SLE). The term is a misnomer, because its primary clinical effect is thrombosis. Lupus anticoagulants appear identical to or are very closely associated with IgG and IgM class antibodies whose epitopes are negatively charged phospholipids.[185,186] The genesis of these autoantibodies presumably reflects aberrant immunoregulation. Consistent with this theory is the evidence of concomitant polyclonal B-cell activation noted by some[187] but

TABLE 15–6. AUTOIMMUNOLOGICAL CAUSES

ETIOLOGY	DIAGNOSIS	THERAPY
Antiphospholipid Antibodies		
Lupus anticoagulant	aPTT KCT RVVT TTIT PNP	Aspirin and heparin ? Prednisone ? Plasmaphoresis
Other antiphospholipid antibodies, including: Anticardiolipin Antiphosphotidylserine Antiphosphatidic acid	ELISA or RIA	Same
Other Autoantibodies		
Antinuclear and DNA antibodies Antiribonucleoproteins	ANA, anti-DNA Abs SSA, SSB, Ro, La	? Need for prednisone

not all investigators.[188] Increasing attention has been given to the role of LAC and antiphospholipid antibodies in recurrent pregnancy loss[189,190]; however, their true clinical significance and optimal management remains unclear.

The prevalence of LAC among patients with SLE has been reported to be 5% to 15%,[189,191,194] whereas the prevalence of antiphospholipid antibodies in SLE patients is 25% to 61%.[191,193,194] Adverse pregnancy outcomes in SLE patients have been shown to correlate best with the presence of antiphospholipid antibodies by some[193,194] but not all investigators.[191] Among patients with recurrent abortion but without clinical connective tissue disease, the prevalence of antiphospholipid antibodies has been reported to be 11% to 44%.[192,195,196] Ascertainment biases may significantly inflate these figures. Further complicating an assessment of the pathogenicity of these antibodies are reports of normal pregnancy outcomes in the 2% to 3% of women in the general obstetric population incidentally found to have antiphospholipid antibodies.[196–198] There is also no clear correlation between adverse pregnancy outcomes or the response to therapy and antiphospholipid antibody levels.[198,199] The presence of LAC is far less common in the general obstetric population (0.2%), and may be more consistently linked to adverse pregnancy outcomes.[198]

Lupus anticoagulants are clearly associated with thromboembolic phenomena, including sundry neurological lesions (cerebral vascular accidents, spinal thrombosis, chorea, and Guillain-Barré syndrome),[189,200] pulmonary embolism,[201] Budd-Chiari syndrome,[202] renal vein thrombosis,[203] and verrucous endocardial lesions.[204,205] Approximately 50% of patients with LAC will eventually have a thrombotic event,[206] and the risk of thrombosis in patients with antiphospholipid antibodies may correlate with antibody concentrations.[193] Postulated mechanisms of thrombosis include antibody-induced platelet membrane instability and hyperaggregability[189] or an inhibition of endothelial prostacyclin synthetase activity,[207] both of which will promote arterial platelet deposition. Intravascular fibrin deposition may result from an inhibition of protein C or ATIII activity on endothelial cell phospholipids.[208,209] Fibrinolysis is also impeded by the antibody's interference with prekallikrein activity[210] and impairment of plasminogen activator release.[211]

Recurrent pregnancy loss is common in pregnant patients with LAC. Scott and colleagues reviewed the literature and described 242 untreated pregnancies in 65 women with lupus anticoagulant.[190] Spontaneous abortions or stillbirths occurred in 220 (91%), with approximately half of losses occurring before 20 weeks gestation.[190,189] Indeed, they report that only six untreated patients with LAC have had live births.[190] Additional obstetric complications include preeclampsia and hepatic-splenic rupture.[189] The association of adverse pregnancy outcomes in patients with antiphospholipid antibodies but without LAC appears less certain.[198] Pregnancy wastage, when present, may be mediated by uteroplacental thrombosis and vasoconstriction, although extensive placental infarction has been noted by some,[212] but not all[194] investigators. Spiral artery vasculopathy, termed "acute atherosis," may also contribute to adverse perinatal outcomes.[212] Additional mechanisms may include immune complex-mediated trophoblast damage[194] or trophoblast—reactive lymphocytotoxic antibody (see Alloimmune section).[213]

The diagnosis of recurrent pregnancy loss secondary to LAC/antiphospholipid antibody should be suspected in patients with recurrent abortion or intrauterine fetal growth retardation or demise. The combination of recurrent pregnancy wastage and maternal thromboembolic phenomenon is particularly suggestive. Patients with a history of false-positive syphilis serologies, prolonged PTT, or laboratory evidence of other autoantibody production should be evaluated. All patients with signs, symptoms, or a history of connective tissue disorders should be considered at high risk.

The LAC phenomenon can be detected by functional coagulation assays such as the activated partial thromboplastin time (aPTT). However, assays that employ low phospholipid concentrations appear to be more sensitive. These include the kaolin clotting time (KCT), Russell's viper venom time (RVVT), tissue thromboplastin inhibition test (TTIT), and the platelet neutralization procedure.[189,214–217] The paradoxical prolongation in coagulation identified by these assays is a consequence of antibody-mediated disruption of phospholipid micelles required as a substrate for the activation of prothrombin.[216] Definitive diagnosis requires mixing studies in which normal plasma is added to the patient's sample without correcting the prolonged coagulation time.[218] This essentially rules out a factor deficiency.

Alternatively, a direct assay for antiphospholipid antibodies can be carried out by either radioimmunoassay (RIA)[193] or enzyme-linked immunoassay (ELISA).[191,192] There is growing evidence that direct antibody identification by immunoassay is the more sensitive method of determining patients at risk.[191–193] It is not clear, however, whether the direct identification of antiphospholipid antibodies is as clinically relevant as their indirect detection via a functional coagulation assay because of the former's increased false positives.[196–198] If an antiphospholipid antibody ELISA or RIA is employed, it is important that each sample serum be assayed for specific and nonspecific binding to a given phospholipid, because generalized immunoglobulin elevations can cause spurious results. Also critical to the interpretation of results is the establishment of clinically rather than just statistically relevant cut-off values.[197,198]

Treatment for patients with antiphospholipid antibodies has had two aims: reducing the antibody burden with prednisone, azathioprine, or plasmaphoresis with or without immunoglobulin therapy; and reducing the antibody effect with low-dose aspirin (80 mg) or heparin. The literature suggests a 70% viable pregnancy rate for patients treated with some combination of the above modalities.[187,188,190,219–225] Such a success rate calls to mind the inherently high "spontaneous remission" rate present in recurrent aborters. Furthermore, there is a lack of double-blinded, randomized, placebo-controlled trials in the treatment of these patients.

Our success rate in treating patients with three previous losses who had LAC and high concentrations of antiphospholipid antibody is similar to that stated above. Treated with low-dose aspirin and high-dose prednisone or heparin, seven out of eleven patients had successful outcomes to their pregnancies. Successful perinatal outcomes are more common in my recurrent loss patients with modest or borderline antiphospholipid antibody levels and no LAC, with live births in ten out of eleven treated pregnancies. There is a recent report questioning the value of prednisone in the treatment of LAC/antiphospholipid antibody-mediated pregnancy wastage.[199]

Despite the above reservations, I recommend treatment for patients with a history of adverse pregnancy outcomes (or, if primigravid, prior thrombotic events) in whom LAC and high concentrations of antiphospholipid antibody are found. I currently employ combination therapy with aspirin 80 mg per day and heparin 10,000 U subcutaneously twice a day. Calcium supplementation is required because of the osteopenic effects of the heparin.

Additional maternal evaluations include initial echocardiography and serial assessment of renal and liver function. Fetal evaluations include serial sonography to evaluate fetal growth, and Doppler flow analysis, if available. Fetal heart rate testing and biophysical profiles should be initiated at 28 weeks gestation. Delivery is mandated by maternal indications, fetal distress, or the cessation of fetal growth.

The need to treat patients without LAC who have only modest elevations in antiphospholipid antibodies is unclear. Treatment in this group should be reserved for those patients with documented euploid recurrent pregnancy losses in whom all other causes have been ruled out. Pregnancy should be strongly discouraged in patients with refractory, life-threatening thrombotic disease secondary to LAC/antiphospholipid antibody syndrome.

OTHER AUTOIMMUNE-MEDIATED RECURRENT PREGNANCY LOSSES

Cowchock and associates reported a higher incidence of antinuclear antibodies (ANA) in patients with unexplained recurrent losses (29%) compared to patients with apparent explanations for their recurrent pregnancy losses (6%).[22] Petri and associates, however, failed to identify a higher incidence of elevated ANA titers in recurrent aborters (20%) when compared with controls (16%).[196] Antibodies to the ribonucleoprotein SS-A/Ro have been associated with fetal congenital heart block and neonatal lupus.[227–233] This mechanism could cause recurrent fetal demise. The etiologic significance of nonphospholipid autoantibodies in the genesis of recurrent pregnancy loss requires further evaluation.

ALLOIMMUNE MECHANISMS

Alloimmune refers to an immune response directed against a foreign or "non-self" antigen. Obstetrically pertinent alloimmune responses include rhesus and non-rhesus blood group fetal hemolytic disease and fetal alloimmune thrombocytopenia. Maternal antibodies to fetal P-blood group antigens produce a rare form of recurrent abortion that has been successfully treated with serial plasmaphoresis.[234] Recent insights into basic reproductive immunology have led to postulated alloimmune causes for recurrent early pregnancy loss (Table 15-7).

Theoretically, an exuberant maternal immune response, analogous to transplant rejection, could cause early pregnancy loss because the invading trophoblast presents a semi-allogeneic challenge to the mother's immune system. Yet growing evidence suggests that a rigorous maternal immune response to trophoblastic antigens is a prerequisite and not an impediment to vigorous placentation and a normal pregnancy. Prior concepts of passive maternal toleration of the trophoblast mediated by immunosuppressive hormones or limited trophoblast expression of HLA antigens have given way to a far more complex assessment of the maternal–fetal immune interaction.

Studies employing a murine model and human endometrial extracts indicate that decidual-associated suppressor cells can inhibit the proliferation of interleukin 2-dependent (IL-2) cells.[235–237] Thus, the ability of the mother to evoke a cytotoxic T-cell or natural killer cell response to the invading trophoblast is blunted.[238] Furthermore, the trophoblast itself may initiate the host suppressor cell response.[239] Because not all lymphokine and monokine production would be suppressed, potential trophoblast stimulatory factors may be preferentially produced by the maternal lymphocytes and macrophages that localize to the site of invasion.[240] A myriad of other maternal, fetal, or placental products

TABLE 15–7. ALLOIMMUNOLOGICAL CAUSES

ETIOLOGY	DIAGNOSIS	THERAPY
Maternal hyporesponse	Blocking factors Lymphocytotoxic Abs in a primary aborter	Paternal or 3rd party leukocyte transfusions
Maternal hyperresponse	Antipaternal lymphocytotoxins ? Autoantibodies	? Heparin

are also potentially immunoregulatory.[242] Examples include pregnancy-associated proteins A, B, and C, α-fetoprotein, Schwangerschaft's proteins 1, 2, and 3, β-1-glycoprotein, pregnancy-specific β-globulin, and placental proteins 1 through 6.[241]

Although cytotrophoblast cells contain Class I HLAG antigens, they do not appear to elicit a damaging maternal cytotoxic response.[242] Indeed, increased parental HLA antigen-sharing is paradoxically associated with reduced family size in Hutterite couples.[243] An increase in HLA-A, -B, -C, and D/DR loci sharing has been observed in recurrent aborter populations compared with controls by a number of groups.[244–247] Others, however, have found no such association.[249–250] An explanation for the negative findings may reside in inappropriate study populations or small sample sizes.[251]

An alternative explanation for these contradictory results may rest with the discovery of a distinct set of antigens found in both trophoblasts and lymphocytes, giving rise to the name trophoblast-lymphocyte cross-reactive (TLX) antigens. Antisera to TLX antigens do not recognize HLA or ABO blood group antigens.[253] However, the anti-TLX antibodies inhibit mixed lymphocyte cultures (MLC). Antisera to TLX TA-1 may bind near or on a portion of the transferring receptor protein (see genetic section) or interfere with the action of the NADH oxidase enzyme. In either case, anti-TA-1 antibodies could prevent cell proliferation by inhibition of the action of these critical enzymes.[252] Monoclonal antibodies to TLX antigens have been raised,[254] and couples with primary recurrent abortion (no live births) appear to share TLX antigens.[245] If the TLX loci were located near HLA loci (linkage disequilibrium) or if TLX gene expression were controlled by HLA-associated genes, the observed inconsistent association between HLA-sharing and recurrent abortion would be explained.

Maternal production of TLX antibodies and the subsequent generation of anti-TLX idiotype antibodies may regulate both the humoral and cellular arms of the maternal–fetal immune response.[252] Anti-idiotype antibodies may serve as local or circulating TLX antigen-equivalents that can block T-cell anti-TLX receptors or produce antigen–antibody complexes. Both arms of the immune response would then be prevented from damaging the trophoblast, but could exert stimulatory effects on trophoblast proliferation. Indeed, preimmunization with anti-idiotypic antibodies significantly reduced pregnancy wastage in a murine model for alloimmune pregnancy loss.[255]

ALLOIMMUNE-MEDIATED PREGNANCY LOSS (MATERNAL IMMUNE HYPORESPONSIVENESS)

A failure by the trophoblast to elicit decidual suppressor activity could result in pregnancy failure. Indeed, suppressor cell activity in the endometrium develops after ovulation and persists in the decidua of successful pregnancies, but not in cases of missed abortion.[235] Alternatively, a failure to establish the TLX or equivalent network for maternal–fetal immunoregulation could also result in recurrent pregnancy loss by generating a cytotoxic maternal immune response or paradoxically failing to stimulate trophoblast proliferation.[252] Three lines of evidence support this concept and have been employed as laboratory markers to identify couples at risk.

HLA Compatibility

As noted above, there is conflicting evidence that idiopathic recurrent aborters share a greater number of HLA antigens than do normally reproducing controls. Therefore, the assessment of HLA antigen-sharing cannot be recommended as a diagnostic test in the evaluation of couples with recurrent pregnancy loss.[256]

Blocking Factors

Normal pregnant sera contains a factor that reduces proliferative and cytotoxic responses to allogeneic cells in a one-way mixed lymphocyte culture.[257–261] This "blocking factor" appears to be an IgG that can inhibit the maternal cytotoxic response to inactivated paternal lymphocytes.[262,263] Blocking factors may also induce fetal suppressor cells.[247] Multiple investigations have demonstrated an absence of these blocking factors in the sera of women with recurrent early pregnancy losses.[262–268] Furthermore, it has been postulated that these blocking factors are anti-idiotype antibodies that mimic the lymphocyte antigens involved in the maternal versus paternal mixed lymphocyte reaction.[269] Alternatively, they could represent anti-TLX antibodies.[270] However, normal pregnancy outcomes can occur despite the absence of blocking factors and, conversely, pregnancy losses can occur despite their presence. Indeed, agammaglobulinemic women do not manifest recurrent losses.[271–273] It is therefore possible that these antibodies are merely a consequence and not a cause of normal pregnancy outcomes. In addition, there is great biological, assay, and interpretive variability present in the assessment of blocking activity laboratory results.[190] Despite these reservations, the absence of blocking factor in maternal sera has been cited as a reliable marker for alloimmune-mediated recurrent pregnancy loss.[190,247,256]

Lymphocytotoxic Antibodies

Pregnant women often produce antipaternal lymphocytotoxic antibodies, with levels increasing in the first trimester, falling at term, and transiently rising in the immediate postpartum period.[274] The prevalence of these antibodies is twice as common in multiparous (>40%) compared with primiparous (20%) women.[274–276] In contrast, primary recurrent aborters less often express antipaternal lymphocytotoxic antibodies (<20%).[246,277] Moreover, when patients are tested early in pregnancy, those undergoing spontaneous losses less often demonstrate cytotoxic antibodies when compared with those whose pregnancies are successful.[278] Maternal antibodies specifically directed to paternal Fc receptors may also be less common in patients with spontaneous abortions.[279] Although these antipaternal antibodies may represent an artifact of successful pregnancy, their absence has also been employed as a marker for alloimmune-mediated pregnancy loss.[247,280]

The diagnosis of alloimmune-mediated pregnancy loss should meet the following criteria:

1. An appropriate history: multiple early euploid pregnancy losses in a karyotypically normal couple without associated term births
2. An absence of all other causes for primary recurrent abortion or continued pregnancy loss despite treatment
3. Absent or low blocking factor activity
4. Absent maternal antipaternal lymphocytotoxic antibodies

Furthermore, these studies should be carried out at a center with an ongoing research interest in alloimmune-mediated pregnancy loss, where quality control is ensured by relatively high volumes.

Empiric therapy for presumed alloimmune-mediated pregnancy loss involves exposing the maternal immune system to the putative trophoblast antigens. This can be carried out by paternal[268,280] or third-party leukocyte injections or transfusions.[281–283] Other proposed therapeutic modalities include use of trophoblastic membrane antigens[270] and sperm antigens, which could be given in the form of vaginal suppositories.[284] Although the production of blocking factor has been documented following leukocyte transfusions and may have prognostic significance,[281,285] failure to induce blocking factors may be compatible with successful outcomes. To date, randomized placebo-controlled trials of leukocyte therapy in presumptive alloimmune recurrent abortion have produced inconclusive results.[285]

Potential risks of third-party donor therapy include HIV, hepatitis C, cytomegalovirus, and toxoplasmosis infections. Paternal leukocyte transfusions may increase the risk of blood group or platelet isoimmunization with untoward fetal sequelae. Additional fetal risks include an 11% incidence of severe intrauterine growth retardation.[286] A final caution must be raised on teleological grounds. Given an elaborate evolutionary mechanism to ensure genetic diversity, such as the proposed TLX system, one most question the wisdom and benefits of its circumvention, both for the resultant individual and the species as a whole.

Indeed, both the diagnosis and treatment of patients with presumptive alloimmune-mediated recurrent pregnancy loss remains controversial. Potential candidates should be referred to centers that are engaged in specific research in this area and are conducting well-designed clinical trials.[284]

ALLOIMMUNE-MEDIATED PREGNANCY LOSS (MATERNAL IMMUNE HYPERRESPONSIVENESS)

A couple who have had live births before, even when intermixed with multiple pregnancy losses, cannot have their losses attributed to a primary lack of maternal immune response to paternally derived trophoblastic antigens. Indeed, idiopathic "secondary" recurrent aborters may develop too vigorous a maternal immune response.[283,287] McIntyre and associates observed decreased HLA sharing, antipaternal lymphocytotoxins, and polyspecific lymphocytotoxins in secondary aborters.[283,287] It is theorized that these patients mount an inappropriate immune response to TLX antigens[287] that interferes with the anti-TLX, anti-TLX idiotype network regulation potentially required for successful reproduction. These patients may also produce embryotoxic autoantibodies[252] perhaps reflecting a generalized disturbance in immunoregulation. Interestingly, heparin therapy may alter this aberrant immune response, leading to successful gestations.[283] Further evaluation is needed to asses the validity of these theories and the actual existence of a maternal alloimmune cause for secondary recurrent abortion.

SUMMARY

As noted, the sporadic occurrence of early pregnancy loss is so common that recurrent pregnancy loss can be expected to occur frequently by chance. Sporadic losses appear to result most commonly from aneuploidy; however, lethal gene mutations or embryopathic gene interactions may be common. As anticipated, the prognosis for a viable pregnancy in a women with multiple prior losses is excellent without or despite "therapeutic" interventions. Although this information may provide solace for the perplexed clinician and hope for the anxious couple, it should not take the place of a thorough search for factors that may increase the risk for pregnancy loss. Moreover, because recurrent loss can persist despite a negative evaluation, affected couples should be presented with the limits of our knowledge and not with idle reassurances.

At least one half of recurrent pregnancy loss may be due to a recurrent aneuploidy. Uterine abnormalities, luteal phase defects, and Mycoplasma infections may contribute to losses, but it is unclear whether they represent primary causes. Immunologic causes are currently in vogue; however, their prevalence, clinical relevance, accurate diagnosis, and proper treatment are not yet well defined. Although scientific skepticism toward ill-defined causes and poorly tested therapies is required in our approach to recurrent loss patients, diagnostic and therapeutic nihilism is not. A methodical analysis of each of the potential etiological areas should be carried out as outlined in each section (see Tables 16-1 through 16-7). The treatment of one factor generally should not be undertaken until all others are ruled out.

The evaluation of these patients should not be limited to one or two sessions. Frequently, the most useful clinical data are accrued at the time of another loss, when an abortus karyotype or fetal morphological data can be obtained. We have noted patients with LAC and significant increases in antiphospholipid IgM levels present only at the time of their losses. Furthermore, long-term follow-up allows the clinician the opportunity to assess the psychological impact of recurrent loss on the couple and to intervene when appropriate. Long-term care itself may provide the necessary emotional support required to endure often difficult therapies or further losses if therapy fails. The clinician must also be prepared to discourage pregnancy attempts in patients with refractory, life-threatening thrombotic disease secondary to LAC/antiphospholipid antibodies. Perhaps our greatest challenge in caring for these anxious patients occurs when no therapy is indicated.

REFERENCES

1. Roberts CJ, Lowe CR. Where have all the conceptions gone? Lancet 1975;i:498.
2. Leridon H. Human fertility: the basic components. Chicago: University of Chicago Press, 1977.
3. Little AB. There's many a slip 'twixt implantation and the crib (Editorial). N Engl J Med 1988;319:241.
4. Sonta S, Fukui K, Yamamura H. Selective elimination of chromosomally unbalanced zygotes at the two-cell stage in the Chinese hamster. Cytogenet Cell Genet 1984;38:5.
5. Wilcox AJ, Weinberg CR, O'Connor JF, et al. Incidence of early loss of pregnancy. N Engl J Med 1988;319:189.
6. Edmonds DK, Lindsay KS, Miller JF, Williamson E, Wood PJ. Early embryonic mortality in women. Fertil Steril 1982;38:447.
7. Miller JF, Williamson E, Glue J, Gordon YB, Grudzinskas JG, Styles A. Fetal loss after implantation. A prospective study. Lancet 1980;ii:554.
8. Whittaker PG, Taylor A, Lind T. Unsuspected pregnancy loss in healthy women. Lancet 1983;i:1126.
9. Boue J, Boue A, Lazar P. Retrospective and prospective epidemiological studies of 1500 karyotyped spontaneous human abortions. Teratology 1975;12:11.
10. Kajii T, Dhama K, Niikawa N, Ferrier A, Avirachan S. Banding analysis of abnormal karyotypes in spontaneous abortion. Am J Hum Genet 1973;25:539.
11. Lauritsen JG, Jonasson J, Therkelsen AJ, Lass F, Lindsten J, Petersen GB. Studies on spontaneous abortions. Fluorescence analysis of abnormal karyotypes. Hereditas 1972;71:160.
12. Boue A, Boue J. Chromosome abnormalities and abortion. In: Hollaender A, ed. Basic life sciences. Physiology and genetics of reproduction, part B. New York: Plenum Press, 1974;317.
13. Guerneri S, Bettio D, Simoni G, Brambati B, Lanzani A. Prevalence and distribution of chromosome abnormalities in a sample of first trimester internal abortions. Hum Reprod 1987;2:735.
14. Hook EB, Porter IH, eds. Population cytogenetics: studies in humans. New York: Academic Press, 1977:64.
15. Warburton D, Fraser FC. Spontaneous abortion risks in man: data from reproductive histories collected in a medical genetics unit. Hum Genet 1964;16:1.
16. Harlap S, Shiono PH, Ramcharan S. A life table of spontaneous abortions and the effects of age, parity and other variables. In: Porter IH, Hook EB, eds. Human embryonic and fetal death. New York, Academic Press, 1980:145.
17. Stein ZA. A woman's age: childbearing and child rearing. Am J Epidemiol 1985;121:327.
18. Malpas P. A study of abortion sequences. J Obstet Gynaecol Br Empire 1938;45:932.
19. Eastman NJ. Habitual abortion. In: Meigs JV, Sturgis S, eds. Progress in gynecology, vol 1. New York: Grune and Stratton, 1946:262.
20. Poland BJ, Miller JR, Jones DC, Trimble BK. Reproductive counseling in patients who have had a spontaneous abortion. Am J Obstet Gynecol 1977;127:685.
21. Goldzieher JW, Benigno BB. The treatment of threatened and recurrent abortion: a critical review. Am J Obstet Gynecol 1958;75:1202.
22. Kajii T, Ferrier A, Niikawa N, Takahara H, Ohama K, Avirachan S. Anatomic and chromosomal anomalies in 639 spontaneous abortions. Hum Genet 1980;55:87.
23. Simpson JL, Golbus MS, Martin AO, Sarto GE. Genetics in obstetrics and gynecology. New York: Grune and Stratton, 1982:124.
24. Hassold TJ, Chi D, Yamane JA. Parental origin of autosomal trisomies. Ann Hum Genet 1984;48:129.
25. Campana M, Serra A, Neri G. Role of chromosome aberrations in recurrent abortion: a study of 269 balanced translocations. Am J Med Genet 1986;24:341.
26. Portnoi MF, Joye N, Van den Akker J, Morlier G, Taillemite JL. Karyotypes of 1142 couples with recurrent abortion. Obstet Gynecol 1988;72:31.
27. Avirachan TT, Tharapel SA, Bannerman RM. Recurrent pregnancy losses and parental chromosome abnormalities: a review. Br J Obstet Gynaecol 1985;92:899.
28. Jacobs PA. Epidemiology of chromosome abnormalities in man. Am J Epidemiol 1977;105:180.
29. Sachs ES, Jahoda MGJ, Van Hemel JO, Hoogeboom AJM, Sandkuyl LA. Chromosome studies of 500 couples with two or more abortions. Obstet Gynecol 1985;65:375.
30. Neri G, Serra A, Campana M, Tedeschi B. Reproductive risks for translocation carriers: cytogenetic study and analysis of pregnancy outcome in 58 families. Am J Med Genet 1983;16:535.
31. Blumberg BD, Shulkin JD, Rotter JI, et al. Minor chromosomal variants and major chromosomal anomalies in couples with recurrent abortion. Am J Hum Genet 1982;34:948.
32. Maes A, Staessen C, Hens L, et al. C heterochromatin variation in couples with recurrent early abortions. J Med Genet 1983;20:350.
33. Madan K, Seabright M, Lindenbaum RH, Bobrow M. Paracentric inversions in man. J Med Genet 1984;21:407.
34. Lyberatou-Moraitou E, Grigori-Kostaraki P, Retzepopoulou Z, Kosmaidou-Aravidou Z. Cytogenetics of recurrent abortions. Clin Genet 1983;23:294.
35. Mules EH, Stamberg J. Reproductive outcomes of paracentric inversion carriers: report of a liveborn dicentric recombinant and literature review. Hum Genet 1984;67:126.
36. Juberg RC, Knops J, Mowrey PN. Increased frequency of lymphocytic mitotic non-disjunction in recurrent spontaneous aborters. J Med Genet 1985;22:32.
37. Allen E, Rolland D, Ching E, Morse B. Frequency of sporadic chromosomally abnormal cells in patients referred for multiple spontaneous abortions. Am J Hum Genet 1982;34:116A.
38. Staessen C, Maes AM, Kirsch-Volders M, Susanne C. Is there a predisposition for meiotic non-disjunction that may be detected by mitotic hyperploidy? Clin Genet 1983;24:184.
39. Holzgreve W, Schonberg SA, Douglas RG, Golbus MS. X-chromosome hyperploidy in couples with multiple spontaneous abortions. Obstet Gynecol 1984;63:237.
40. Horsman DE, Dill FJ, McGillivray BC, Kalousek DK. X chromo-

some aneuploidy in lymphocyte cultures from women with recurrent spontaneous abortions. Am J Med Genet 1987;28:981.
41. Ferrazzi E, Brambati B, Lanzani A, et al. The yolk sac in early pregnancy failure. Am J Obstet Gynecol 1988;158:137.
42. Berg KA, Clark EB, Astemborski JA, Boughman JA. Prenatal detection of cardiovascular malformations by echocardiography: an indication for cytogenetic evaluation. Am J Obstet Gynecol 1988;159:477.
43. Platt LD, DeVore GR, Lopez E, Herbert W, Falk R, Alfi O. Role of amniocentesis in ultrasound-detected fetal malformations. Obstet Gynecol 1986;68:153.
44. Benacerraf BR, Miller WA, Frigoletto FD Jr. Sonographic detection of fetuses with trisomies 13 and 18: accuracy and limitations. Am J Obstet Gynecol 1988;158:404.
45. Benacerraf B, Frigoletto F. Soft tissue nuchal fold in the second-trimester fetus: standards for normal measurements compared with those in Down syndrome. Am J Obstet Gynecol 1987;157:1146.
46. Benacerraf B, Osathanondh R, Frigoletto F. Sonographic demonstration of hypoplasia of the middle phalanx of the fifth digit: a finding associated with Down syndrome. Am J Obstet Gynecol 1988;159:181.
47. Lockwood C, Scioscia A, Stiller R, Hobbins J. Sonographic features of the triploid fetus. Am J Obstet Gynecol 1987;157:285.
48. McDonough PG. Repeated first-trimester pregnancy loss: evaluation and management. Am J Obstet Gynecol 1985;153:1.
49. MacLeod J, Gold RZ. The male factor in fertility and infertility (IX): semen quality in relation to accidents of pregnancy. Fertil Steril 1957;8:36.
50. Joel CA. New etiologic aspects of habitual abortion and infertility with special reference to the male factor. Fertil Steril 1966;17:374.
51. Lohler J, Timpl R, Jaenisch R. Embryonic lethal mutation in mouse collagen I gene causes rupture of blood vessels and is associated with erythropoietic and mesenchymal cell death. Cell 1984;38:597.
52. Jones KL. Smith's recognizable patterns of human malformation. 4th ed. Philadelphia, WB Saunders, 1988:448.
53. Jones KL. Smith's recognizable patterns of human malformation. 4th ed. Philadelphia: WB Saunders, 1988:220.
54. Tolmie JL, Patrick A, Yates JRW. A lethal multiple pterygium syndrome with apparent x-linked recessive inheritance. Am J Med Genet 1987;27:913.
55. Lockwood C, Irons M, Troiani J, Kawada C, Chaudhury A, Cetrulo C. The prenatal diagnosis of lethal multiple pterygium syndrome: a heritable cause of recurrent abortion. Am J Obstet Gynecol 1988;159:474.
56. Dronamraju KR, Bixler D. Fetal mortality in oral cleft families (VII): birth intervals. Clin Genet 1984;25:318.
57. Alberman E, Creasy M, Polani PE. Spontaneous abortion and neural tube defects. Br Med J 1983;4:230.
58. Schaid DJ, Kunz HW, Gill TJ III. Genic interaction causing embryonic mortality in the rat: epistasis between the Tal and grc genes. Genetics 1982;100:615.
59. Weitkamp LR, Schacter BZ. Transferrin and HLA: spontaneous abortion, neural tube defects, and natural selection. N Engl J Med 1985;313:925.
60. Rock JA, Schlaff WD. The obstetric consequences of uterovaginal anomalies. Fertil Steril 1985;43:681.
61. Green LK, Harris RE. Uterine anomalies: frequency of diagnosis and associated obstetric complications. Obstet Gynecol 1976;47:427.
62. Semmens JP. Congenital anomalies of female genital tract: functional classification based on review of 56 personal cases and 500 reported cases. Obstet Gynecol 1962;19:328.
63. Jones WS. Obstetric significance of female genital anomalies. Obstet Gynecol 1957;10:113.
64. Stray-Pedersen B, Stray-Pedersen S. Etiologic factors and subsequent reproductive performance in 195 couples with a prior history of habitual abortion. Am J Obstet Gynecol 1984; 148:140.
65. DeCherney AH, Russell JB, Graebe RA, Polan ML. Resectoscopic management of mullerian fusion defects. Fertil Steril 1986;45:726.
66. Jewelewicz R, Husami N, Wallach EE. When uterine factors cause infertility. Contemp Obstet Gynecol 1980;16:95.
67. Thompson JP, Smith RA, Welch JS. Reproductive ability after metroplasty. Obstet Gynecol 1966;28:363.
68. Heinonen PK, Saarrikoski S, Pystynen P. Reproductive performance of women with uterine anomalies. Acta Obstet Gynecol Scand 1982;61:157.
69. Sorensen SS, Trauelsen AGH. Obstetric implications of minor mullerian anomalies in oligomenorrheic women. Am J Obstet Gynecol 1987;156:1112.
70. Harlap S, Shiono PH, Ramcharan S, Berendes H, Pellegrin F. A prospective study of spontaneous fetal losses after induced abortions. N Engl J Med 1979;301:678.
71. Collins DC. Congenital unilateral renal agensia. Ann Surg 1932;95:715.
72. Daly DC, Walters CA, Soto-Albors CE, Riddick DH. Hysteroscopic metroplasty: surgical technique and obstetric outcome. Fertil Steril 1983;39:623.
73. March CM, Israel R. Hysteroscopic management of recurrent abortion caused by septate uterus. Am J Obstet Gynecol 1987;156:834.
74. Fayez JA. Comparison between abdominal and hysteroscopic metroplasty. Obstet Gynecol 1986;68:399.
75. Muasher SJ, Acosta AA, Garcia JE, Rosenwaks Z, Jones HW. Wedge metroplasty for the septate uterus: an update. Fertil Steril 1984;42:515.
76. Rasmussen PE, Pedersen OD. Metroplasty and fetal survival. Acta Obstet Gynecol Scand 1987;66:117.
77. Thompson JP, Smith RA, Welch JS. Reproductive ability after metroplasty. Obstet Gynecol 1966;28:363.
78. Mattingly RF, Thomspon JD. Te Linde's operative gynecology. 6th ed. New York: JB Lippincott, 1985:365.
79. Muram D, McAlister MS, Winer-Muram HT, Smith WC. Asymptomatic rupture of a rudimentary uterine horn. Obstet Gynecol 1987;69:486.
80. Ayers JWT, Peterson EP, Ansbacher R. Early therapy for the incompetent cervix in patients with habitual abortion. Fertil Steril 1982;38:177.
81. Harger JH. Early cerclage in habitual abortion (letter). Fertil Steril 1983;39:244.
82. Ludmir J, Landon MB, Gabbe SG, Samuels P, Mennuti MT. Management of the diethylstilbestrol-exposed pregnant patient: a prospective study. Am J Obstet Gynecol 1987;157:665.
83. Brown ZA, Vontver LA, Benedetti J, et al. Effects on infants of a first episode of genital herpes during pregnancy. N Engl J Med 1987;317:1246.
84. Monif GRG. Maternal mumps infection during gestation: observations in the progeny. Am J Obstet Gynecol 1974;119:549.
85. Miller E, Cradock-Watson JE, Pollock TM. Consequences of confirmed maternal rubella at successive stages of pregnancy. Lancet 1982;i:781.
86. Peckham C. Congenital rubella in the United Kingdom before 1970: the prevaccine era. Rev Infect Dis 1985;7:11S.
87. Icart J, Didier J, Dalens M, et al. Prospective study of EBV infection during pregnancy. Biomedicine 1981;34:160.
88. Seeliger HPR, Finger H. Listeriosis. In: Remington JS, Klein JO,

eds. Infectious diseases of the fetus and newborn infant. Philadelphia: WB Saunders, 1976:333.
89. MacNaughton MC. Listeria Monocytogenes in abortion. Lancet 1962;ii:484.
90. Larsson S, Cronberg S, Winblad S. Listeriosis during pregnancy and neonatal period in Sweden 1958–1974. Acta Pediatr Scand 1979;68:485.
91. Kamplemacher EH, Huysinga L, Van Noorle Jansen L. The presence of Listeria monocytogenes in feces of pregnant women and neonates. Zentralbl Bakteriol Parist Infekt 1972;222:258.
92. Stray-Pedersen B, Lorentzen-Styr AM. Uterine toxoplasma infections and repeated abortions. Am J Obstet Gynecol 1977;128:716.
93. Ruoss CF, Bourne GL. Toxoplasmosis in pregnancy. Br J Obstet Gynaecol 1972;79:1115.
94. Dubey JP, Miller NL, Frenkel JK. Characterization of the new fecal form of Toxoplasma gondii. J Parasitol 1970;56:447.
95. Kimball AC, Kean BH, Fuchs F. The role of toxoplasmosis in abortion. Am J Obstet Gynecol 1971;111:219.
96. Quinn PA, Petric M, Barkin M, et al. Prevalence of antibody to Chlamydia trachomatis in spontaneous abortion and infertility. Am J Obstet Gynecol 1987;156:291.
97. Archer JF. "T" strain Mycoplasma in the female urogenital tract. Br J Vener Disease 1968;44:232.
98. McCormack WM, Rosner B, Lee YH. Colonization with genital mycoplasmas in women. Am J Epidemiol 1973;97:240.
99. Allison AC, Paton GR. Chromosomal abnormalities in human diploid cells infected with mycoplasma and their relevance to the etiology of Down's syndrome (Mongolism). Lancet 1966;ii:1229.
100. Kundsin RB, Ampola M, Streeter S, Neurath P. Chromosomal aberrations induced by T-strain mycoplasmas. J Med Genet 1971;8:181.
101. Fogh J, Fogh H. Chromosome changes in PPLO-infected FL human amnion cells. Proc Soc Exp Biol Med 1965;119:233.
102. Biberfeld G. Infection sequelae in autoimmune reactions in Mycoplasma pneumoniae infection. In: Razin S, Barile MF, eds. The mycoplasmas. IV. Mycoplasma pathogenicity. New York: Academic Press, 1985:293.
103. Quinn PA, Butany J, Chipman M, et al. A prospective study of microbial infection in still births and early neonatal death. Am J Obstet Gynecol 1985;151:238.
104. Quinn PA. Evidence of an immune response to Ureaplasma urealyticum in perinatal morbidity and mortality. Pediatr Infect Dis 1986;5:282S.
105. Quinn PA, Shewchuk AB, Shuber J, et al. Serologic evidence of Ureaplasma urealyticum infection in women with spontaneous pregnancy loss. Am J Obstet Gynecol 1983;145:245.
106. Caspi E, Solomon F, Sompolinsky D. Early abortion and Mycoplasma infection. Isr J Med Sci 1972;8:122.
107. Sompolinsky D, Solomon F, Weinraub Z, Bukovsky I, Caspi E. Infections with mycoplasma and bacteria in induced midtrimester abortion and fetal loss. Am J Obstet Gynecol 1975;121:610.
108. Quinn PA, Shewchuk AB, Shuber J, et al. Efficacy of antibiotic therapy in preventing spontaneous pregnancy loss among couples colonized with genital mycoplasmas. Am J Obstet Gynecol 1983;145:239.
109. Tho PT, Byrd JR, McDonough PG. Etiologies and subsequent reproductive performance of 100 couples with recurrent abortions. Fertil Steril 1979;32:289.
110. Harger JH, Archer DF, Marchese SG, Muracca-Clemens M, Garver KL. Etiology of recurrent pregnancy losses and outcome of subsequent pregnancies. Obstet Gynecol 1983;62:574.
111. Brenton DP, Cusworth DC, Biddle SA, Garrod PJ, Lasley L. Pregnancy and homocystinuria. Ann Clin Biochem 1977; 14:161.
112. Lamon JM, Lenke RR, Levy HL, Schulman JD, Shih VE. Selected metabolic diseases. In: Schulman JD, Simpson JL, eds. Genetic diseases in pregnancy: maternal effects and fetal outcome. New York: Academic Press, 1981:2.
113. Walshe JM. Pregnancy in Wilson's disease. Q J Med 1977;46:73.
114. Klee JG. Undiagnosed Wilson's disease as a cause of unexplained miscarriage. Lancet 1979;ii:423.
115. Wentz AC. Progesterone therapy of the inadequate luteal phase. Curr Probl Obstet Gynecol 1982;6:4.
116. Botella-Llusia J. The endometrium in repeated abortion. Int J Fertil 1962;7:147.
117. Daya S, Ward S, Burrows E. Progesterone profiles in luteal phase defect cycles and outcome of progesterone treatment in patients with recurrent spontaneous abortion. Am J Obstet Gynecol 1988;158:225.
118. DeCherney AH, Polan ML. Helping habitual aborters. Contemporary OB/GYN 1982;20:241.
119. Maxon WS. Hormonal causes of recurrent abortion. Clin Obstet Gynecol 1986;29:941.
120. Speroff L, Glass RH, Kase NG. Clinical gynecologic endocrinology and infertility. 4th ed. Baltimore: Williams & Wilkins, 1989:530.
121. Garcia J, Jones GS, Wentz AC. The use of clomiphene citrate. Fertil Steril 1977;28:707.
122. Wentz AC, Herbert CM, Maxon WS, Garner CH. Outcome of progesterone treatment of luteal phase inadequacy. Fertil Steril 1984;41:856.
123. Daly DC, Walters CA, Soto-Albors CE, Riddick DH. Endometrial biopsy during treatment of luteal phase defects is predictive of therapeutic outcome. Fertil Steril 1983;40:305.
124. Shearman RP, Garrett WJ. Double-blind study of effect of 17-hydroxyprogesterone caproate on abortion rate. Br Med J 1963;1:292.
125. Johansson EDB. Depression of progesterone levels in women treated with synthetic gestagens after ovulation. Acta Endocrinol 1971;68:779.
126. Klopper A, MacNaughton M. Hormones in recurrent abortion. J Obstet Gynaecol Br Commonwealth 1965;72:1022.
127. Sutherland HW, Pritchard CW. Increased incidence of spontaneous abortion in pregnancies complicated by maternal diabetes mellitus. Am J Obstet Gynecol 1986;155:135.
128. Miodovnik M, Lavin JP, Knowles HC, Holroyde J, Stys SJ. Spontaneous abortion among insulin-dependent diabetic women. Am J Obstet Gynecol 1984;150:372.
129. Miodovnik M, Mimouni F, Tsang RC, Ammar E, Kaplan L, Siddiqi TA. Glycemic control and spontaneous abortion in insulin-dependent diabetic women. Obstet Gynecol 1986;68:366.
130. Miodovnik M, Skillman C, Holroyde JC, Butler JB, Wendel JS, Siddiqi TA. Elevated maternal glycohemoglobin in early pregnancy and spontaneous abortion among insulin-dependent diabetic women. Am J Obstet Gynecol 1985;153:439.
131. Wright AD, Nicholson HO, Pollock A, Taylor KG, Betts S. Spontaneous abortion and diabetes mellitus. Postgrad Med 1983;59:295.
132. Goldman JA, Dicker D, Feldberg D, et al. Pregnancy outcome in patients with insulin-dependent diabetes mellitus with preconceptional diabetic control: a comparative study. Am J Obstet Gynecol 1986;155:293.
133. Sheridan-Pereira M, Drury M, Baumgart R, et al. Haemoglobin A1 in diabetic pregnancy: an evaluation. Ir J Med Sci 1983;152:261.
134. Dicker D, Feldberg D, Samuel N, Yeshaya A, Karp M, Goldman JA. Spontaneous abortion in patients with insulin-dependent diabetes mellitus: the effect of preconceptional diabetic control. Am J Obstet Gynecol 1988;158:1161.
135. Mills JL, Simpson JL, Driscoll SG, et al. Incidence of spontane-

ous abortion among normal women and insulin-dependent diabetic women whose pregnancies were identified within 21 days of conception. N Engl J Med 1988;319:1617.

136. Reece EA, Pinter E, Leranth CZ, et al. Ultrastructural analysis of malformations of the embryonic neural axis induced by hyperglycemic conceptus culture. Teratology 1985;32:363.
137. Pinter E, Reece EA, Leranth CZ, et al. Arachidonic acid prevents hyperglycemia-associated yolk sac damage and embryopathy. Am J Obstet Gynecol 1986;155:691.
138. De Wolf F, De Wolf-Peters C, Brosens I. Ultrastructure of the spiral arteries in the human placental bed at the end of normal pregnancy. Am J Obstet Gynecol 1973;117:833.
139. Lammle B, Griffin JH. Formation of the fibrin clot. The balance of procoagulant and inhibitory factors. Clin Haematol 1985;14:281.
140. Kitchens CS, Newcomb TF. Factor XIII. Medicine 1979;58:413.
141. Ikkala E, Myllyla G, Nevaliuna H. Transfusion therapy in factor III (FSF) deficiency. Scand J Haematol 1964;1:308.
142. Fisher S, Rikover M, Naor S. Factor 13 deficiency with severe hemorrhagic diathesis. Blood 1966;28:34.
143. Sheppard BL, Bonnar J. The ultrastructure of the arterial supply of the human placenta in early and late pregnancy. Br J Obstet Gynaecol 1974;81:497.
144. Duckert F. Documentation of the plasma factor XIII deficiency in man. Ann NY Acad Sci 1972;202:190.
145. Coopland A, Alkjaersig N, Fletcher A. Reduction in plasma factor XIII (fibrin stabilizing factor) concentration during pregnancy. J Lab Clin Med 1969;73:144.
146. Ikematsu S, McDonough R, Resiner H, et al. Immunochemical studies of human factor XIII. Radioimmunoassay for the carrier subunit of the zymogen. J Lab Clin Med 1981;97:662.
147. Kasper C, Hoag M, Aggeler P, et al. Blood clotting factors in pregnancy: factor VIII concentrations in normal and AHF deficient women. Obstet Gynecol 1964;24:242.
148. Inamoto Y, Terao T. First report of a case of congenital afibrinogenemia with successful delivery. Am J Obstet Gynecol 1985;153:803.
149. Matsuno K, Mori K, Amikawa H, et al. A case of congenital afibrinogenemia with abortion, intracranial hemorrhage and peritonitis. Jpn J Clin Hematol 1977;18:1438.
150. Dube B, Agarwal SP, Gupta MM, et al. Congenital deficiency of fibrinogen in two sisters. A clinical and haematological study. Acta Haematol 1970;43:120.
151. Hahn L, Lundberg PA. Congenital hypofibrinogenaemia and recurrent abortion. Br J Obstet Gynaecol 1978;85:790.
152. Mason DY, Ingram GIC. Management of the hereditary coagulation in disorders. Semin Hematol 1971;8:158.
153. Hasselback R, Marion RB, Thomas JW. Congenital hypofibrinogenemia in five members of a family. Can Med Assoc J 1963;88:19.
154. Bosch N, Araocha-Pinango C. An abnormal fibrinogen in a Venezuelan family [abstr]. Fifth Congress, International Society of Thrombosis and Haemostasis 1975;1:246.
155. Buraschi J, Sack E, Quiroga E, et al. A new fibrinogen anomaly: fibrinogen Buenos Aires [abstr]. Abstr Fifth Congr Int Soc Thomb Haemostasis 1975;1:244.
156. Fuchs G, Egbring R, Havemann K. Fibrinogen Marburg: a new genetic variant of fibrinogen. Blut 1977;34:107.
157. Grainick HR, Coller BS, Fratantoni JC, et al. Fibrinogen Bethesda III: a hypodysfibrinogenemia. Blood 1979;53:28.
158. Shapiro SS, Martinez J. Human prothrombin metabolism in normal man and in hypocoagulable subjects. J Clin Invest 1969;48;1292.
159. Thaler E, Lechner K. Antithrombin III deficiency and thromboembolism. Clin Haematol 1981;10:369.
160. Weiner CP, Brandt JT. Plasma antithrombin III activity in normal pregnancy. Obstet Gynecol 1980;56:601.
161. Weenink GH, Treffers PE, Kahle LH, et al. Antithrombin III in normal pregnancy. Thromb Res 1982;26:281.
162. Hellgren M, Tengborn L, Abildgaard U. Pregnancy in women with congenital antithrombin III deficiency: experience of treatment with heparin and antithrombin. Gynecol Obstet Invest 1982;14:127.
163. Nelson DM, Stempel LE, Brandt JT. Hereditary antithrombin III deficiency and pregnancy: report of two cases and review of the literature. Obstet Gynecol 1985;65:848.
164. Hoafland HC, Silverstein MN. Primary thrombocythemia in the young patient. Mayo Clin Proc 1978;53:578.
165. Snethlage W, Ten Cate JW. Thrombocythaemia and recurrent late abortions: normal outcome of pregnancies after antiaggregatory treatment. Case report. Br J Obstet Gynaecol 1986;93:386.
166. Murphy MF, Clarke CRA, Brearly RL. Superior sagittal sinus thrombosis and essential thrombocythaemia. Br Med J 1972;287:1244.
167. Kaibara M, Kobayashi T, Matsumoto S. Idiopathic thrombocythemia and pregnancy: report of a case. Obstet Gynecol 1985;65:18S.
168. Mercer B, Drouin J, Jolly E, d'Anjou G. Primary thrombocythemia in pregnancy: a report of two cases. Am J Obstet Gynecol 1988;159:127.
169. Falconer J, Pineo G, Blahey W, Bowen T, Docksteader B, Jadusingh I. Essential thrombocythemia associated with recurrent abortions and fetal growth retardation. Am J Hematol 1987;25:345.
170. Zierler S, Rothman KJ. Congenital heart disease in relation to maternal use of bendectin and other drugs in early pregnancy. N Engl J Med 1985;313:347.
171. Shapiro S, Monson RR, Kaufman DW, et al. Perinatal mortality and birth-weight in relation to aspirin taken during pregnancy. Lancet 1976;i:1375.
172. Beaufils M, Uzan S, Donsimoni R, et al. Prevention of preeclampsia by early antiplatelet therapy. Lancet 1985;i:840.
173. Wallenburg HCS, Dekker GA, Makovitz JW, et al. Low-dose aspirin prevents pregnancy-induced hypertension and preeclampsia in angiotensin-sensitive primigravidae. Lancet 1986;i:1.
174. Forestier F, Daffos F, Rainaut M. letter to the editor. Lancet 1985;i:1268.
175. Stuart MJ, Gross SJ, Elrad H, et al. Effects of acetylsalicylic-acid ingestion on maternal and neonatal hemostasis. N Engl J Med 1982;307:909.
176. Silverstein MN, Petitt RM, Solberg LA, Fleming JS, Knight RC, Schacter LP. Anagrelide: a new drug for treating thrombocytosis. N Engl J Med 1988;318:1292.
177. Pirani B, Campbell D, MacGillivray I. Plasma volume in normal first pregnancy. J Obstet Gynecol Br Commonwealth 1973;80:884.
178. Tyslowitz R, Dingemanse E. Effect of large doses of estrogens on the blood picture of dogs. Endocrinology 1941;29:817.
179. Cohen P, Gardner FH. Thrombocytopenic effect of sustained high dosage prednisone therapy in thrombocytopenic purpura. N Engl J Med 1961;265:611.
180. Talal N. Sex factors, steroid hormones and host response. Proceedings of the Kroc Foundation Conference. Arthritis Rheum 1979;22:1153.
181. Gleicher N, El-Roiy A. The reproductive autoimmune failure syndrome. Am J Obstet Gynecol 1988;159:223.
182. Shoenfeld Y, Schwartz RS. Immunologic and genetic factors in autoimmune diseases. N Engl J Med 1984;311:1019.

183. Geha RS. Regulation of the immune response by idiotypic-antiidiot interactions. N Engl J Med 1981;305:25.
184. Laurell A, Nilsson I. Hypergammaglobulinemia, circulating antiicoagulant and biologic false positive Wasserman reaction. J Lab Clin Med 1957;49:694.
185. Yin ET, Gaston LW. Purifications and kinetic studies on a circulating anticoagulant in a suspected case of lupus erythematous. Thromb Diath Haemorrh 1965;14:88.
186. Lechner K. A new type of coagulation inhibitor. Thromb Diath Haemorrh 1969;21:482.
187. Gleicher N, Friberg J. IgM Gammopathy and the lupus anticoagulant syndrome in habitual aborters. JAMA 1985;253:3278.
188. Branch DW, Scott JR, Kochenour NK, et al. Obstetric complications associated with the lupus anticoagulant. N Engl J Med 1985;313:1322.
189. Lubbe WF, Liggins GC. Lupus anticoagulant and pregnancy. Am J Obstet Gynecol 1985;153:322.
190. Scott JR, Rote NS, Branch DW. Immunologic aspects of recurrent abortion and fetal death. Obstet Gynecol 1987;70:645.
191. Petri M, Rheinschmidt M, Whiting-O'Keefe Q, et al. The frequency of lupus anticoagulant in systemic lupus erthematosus. Ann Intern Med 1987;106:524.
192. Cowchock S, Smith JB, Gocial B. Antibodies to phospholipids and nuclear antigens in patients with repeated abortions. Am J Obstet Gynecol 1986;155:1002.
193. Harris E, Gharvi A, Boey M, et al. Anticardiolipin antibodies: detection by radioimmunoassay and association with thrombosis in systemic erythematosus. Lancet 1983;ii:1211.
194. Lockshin MD, Druzin ML, Goei S, et al. Antibody to cardiolipin as a predictor of fetal distress or death in pregnant patients with systemic lupus erythematosus. N Engl J Med 1985;313:152.
195. Unander AM, Norberg R, Hahn L, Arfors L. Anticardiolipin antibodies and complement in ninety-nine women with habitual abortion. Am J Obstet Gynecol 1987;156:114.
196. Petri M, Golbus M, Anderson R, Whiting-O'Keefe Q, Corash L, Hellman D. Antinuclear antibody, lupus anticoagulant, and anticardiolipin antibody in women with idiopathic habitual abortion. Arthritis Rheum 1987;30:601.
197. El-Roeiy A, Gleicher N. Definition of normal autoantibody levels in an apparently healthy population. Obstet Gynecol 1988;72:596.
198. Lockwood CJ, Romero R, Feinberg RF, Clyne LP, Coster B, Hobbins JC. The prevalence and biological significance of lupus anticoagulant and anticardiolipin antibodies in a general obstetric population. Am J Obstet Gynecol 1989;161:369.
199. Lockshin MD, Druzin ML, Qamar T. Prednisone does not prevent recurrent fetal death in women with antiphospholipid antibody. Am J Obstet Gynecol 1989;160:439.
200. Englert H, Hughes GRV. Neurology and the lupus anticoagulant. Eur Neurol 1985;24:422.
201. Anderson NE, Ali MR. The lupus anticoagulant. Pulmonary thromboembolism, and fatal pulmonary hypertension. Ann Rheum Dis 1984;43:760.
202. Pomeroy C, Knodell RG, Swain WR, Arneson P, Mahowald ML. Budd-Chiari syndrome in a patient with lupus anticoagulant. Gastroenterology 1984;86:158.
203. Asherson RA, Lanham JG, Hull RG, Boey ML, Gharavi AE, Hughes GRV. Renal vein thrombosis in systemic lupus erythematosus: association with lupus anticoagulant. Clin Exp Rheum 1984;2:75.
204. Anderson D, Bell D, Lodge R, Grant E. Recurrent cerebral ischemia and mitral valve vegetation in a patient with antiphospholipid antibodies. J Rheumatol 1987;14:839.
205. Chartash EK, Paget SA, Lockshin MD. Lupus anticoagulant associated with aortic and mitral valve insufficiency. Arthritis Rheum 1986;13:416.
206. Boey ML, Colaco CB, Gharavi AE, Elkon KB, Loizou S, Hughes GRV. Thrombosis in systemic lupus erythematosus: striking association with the presence of circulating lupus anticoagulant. Br Med J 1983;287:1021.
207. Carreras LO, Defreyn G, Machin SJ, Vermylen J, Deman R, Spitz B, Van Assche A. Arterial thrombosis, intrauterine death and "lupus" anticoagulant: detection of immunoglobin interfering with prostacyclin formation. Lancet 1981;i:244.
208. Cariou R, Tobelem G, Soria C, et al. Inhibition of protein C activation by endothelial cells in the presence of lupus anticoagulant (letter). N Engl J Med 1986;314:1193.
209. Cosgriff TM, Martin BA. Low functional and high antigenic antithrombin III level in a patient with the lupus anticoagulant and recurrent thrombosis. Arthritis Rheum 1981;24:94.
210. San Felippo MJ, Drayna CJ. Prekallikrein inhibition associated with lupus anticoagulant. Am J Clin Pathol 1982;77:275.
211. Angeles-Cano E, Sultan Y, Chauvel JP. Predisposing factors to thrombosis in systemic lupus erythematosus: possible relation to endothelial cell damage. J Lab Clin Med 1979;94:313.
212. De Wolf F, Carrers LO, Moerman P, et al. Decidual vasculopathy and extensive placental infarction in a patient with repeated thromboembolic accidents, recurrent fetal loss, and a lupus anticoagulant. Am J Obstet Gynecol 1982;142:829.
213. Bresnihan B, Grigor RR, Oliver M, et al. Immunological mechanism for spontaneous abortion in systemic lupus erythematosus. Lancet 1977;ii:1205.
214. Exner T. Similar mechanism of various lupus anticoagulants. Thromb Haemost 1985;53:15.
215. Green D, Hougie C, Kazmier FJ, et al. Report of the working party on acquired inhibitors of coagulation: studies of the "lupus anticoagulant." Thromb Haemost 1983;49:144.
216. Shapiro S, Thiagarajan P. Lupus anticoagulant. Prog Hemost Thromb 1982;6:263.
217. Triplett DA, Brandt JT, Kaczor D, et al. Laboratory diagnosis of lupus inhibitors: a comparison of the tissue thromboplastin inhibition procedure with a new platelet neutralization procedure. Am J Clin Pathol 1983;79:678.
218. Clyne LP, Dainiak N, Hoffman R, Hardin J. In vitro correction of anticoagulant activity and specific clotting factor assays in SLE. Thromb Res 1980;18:643.
219. Junger P, Liote F, Dautzenberg F, et al. Lupus anticoagulant and thrombosis in systemic lupus erythamatosus. Lancet 1984;i:574.
220. Reece EA, Romero R, Clyne LP, Kriz NS, Hobbins JC. Lupus anticoagulant in pregnancy. Lancet 1984;ii:344.
221. Joffe AM, Hoskins CF, Ghitter-Mannes SC, Mant MJ. Anticoagulant therapy for prevention of spontaneous abortion in a patient with lupus anticoagulant. Am J Hematol 1988;29:56.
222. Kochenour NK, Branch DW, Hershgold EJ, et al. The lupus anticoagulant: a recently discovered and treatable cause of recurrent abortion and fetal death. Abstract 14, Society for Gynecological Investigation, 31st Annual Meeting, 1984.
223. Farquharson RG, Pearson JF, John L. Lupus anticoagulant and intrauterine death in the absence of systemic lupus. Lancet 1984;ii:228.
224. Garlund B. The lupus inhibitor in thromboembolic disease and intrauterine death in the absence of systemic lupus. Acta Med Scand 1984;215:293.
225. Lubbe WF, Pamer WF, Butler WS, et al. Fetal survival after prednisone suppression of maternal lupus anticoagulant. Lancet 1983;i:1361.
226. Cowchock S, Dehoratius RD, Wapner RJ, Jackson LG. Subclinical autoimmune disease and unexplained abortion. Am J Obstet Gynecol 1984;150:367.
227. Reed BR, Lee LA, Harmon C, et al. Autoantibodies to SS-A/Ro in infants with congenital heart block. J Pediatr 1983;103:889.
228. Lockshin MD, Gibofsky A, Peebles CL, et al. Neonatal lupus

erythematosus with heart block: family study of a patient with anti-SS-A and SS-B antibodies. Arthritis Rheum 1983;26:212.
229. Draznin TH, Esterly NB, Furey NL, et al. Neonatal lupus erythematosus. J Am Acad Dermatol 1979;1:437.
230. Miyagawa S, Katamura W, Yoshioka J, et al. Placental transfer of anticytoplasmic antibodies in annular erythema of newborns. Arch Dermatol 1981;117:569.
231. Franco HL, Weston WL, Peebles C, et al. Autoantibodies directed against sicca syndrome antigens in neonatal lupus syndrome. J Am Acad Dermatol 1981;1:437.
232. Weston WL, Harmon C, Peebles C, et al. A serological marker for neonatal lupus. Br J Dermatol 1982;107:377.
233. Kephart DC, Hood AF, Provost TT. Neonatal lupus erythematosus: new serologic findings. J Invest Dermatol 1981;77:331.
234. Rock JA, Shirey RS, Braine HG, Ness PM, Kickler TS, Niebyl JR. Plasmapheresis for the treatment of repeated early pregnancy wastage associated with anti-P. Obstet Gynecol 1985;66:57S.
235. Daya S, Clark DA, Devlin C, Jarrell J. Preliminary characterization of two types of suppressor cells in the human uterus. Fertil Steril 1985;44:778.
236. Hunt JS, Manning LS, Wood GW. Macrophages in murine uterus are immunosuppressive. Cell Immunol 1984;85:499.
237. Daya S, Rosenthal KL, Clark DA. Immunosuppressor factor(s) produced by decidual-associated suppressor cells: a proposed mechanism for fetal allograft survival. Am J Obstet Gynecol 1987;156:344.
238. Croy BA, Gambel P, Rossant J, Wegmann TG. Characterization of murine decidual natural killer (NK) cells and their relevance to the success of pregnancy. Cell Immunol 1985;93:315.
239. Daya S, Johnson PM, Clark DA. Mechanisms of activation of suppressor cells in the endometrium of the human uterus. J Reprod Immunol (Suppl) 1986;1:164.
240. Chaouat G, Clark DA, Wegmann TG. Genetic aspects of the CBA X DBA/2 and B10 X B10. A model of murine pregnancy failure and its prevention by lymphocyte immunisation. In: Beard RW, Sharp F, eds. Early pregnancy loss, mechanisms, and treatment. Ashton-under-Lyne: Peacock Press, 1988;89.
241. Gill TJ III. Immunity and pregnancy. CRC Crit Rev Immunol 1985;5:201.
242. Kovats S, Main EK, Librach C, et al. A-class I antigen, HLA-G expressed in human trophoblasts. Science 1990;248:220.
243. Ober C, Elias S, O'Brien E, Kostyu DD, Hauck WW, Bonmbard A. HLA sharing and fertility in Hutterite couples: evidence for prenatal selection against compatible fetuses. Am J Reprod Immunol Microbiol 1988;18:111.
244. Beer AE, Quebbeman JF, Ayers JWT, Haines RF. Major histocompatibility complex antigens, maternal and paternal immune responses, and chronic habitual abortions in humans. Am J Obstet Gynecol 1981;141:987.
245. McIntyre JA, Faulk WP. Recurrent spontaneous abortion in human pregnancy: results of immunogenetical, cellular, and humoral studies. Am J Reprod Immunol 1983;4:165.
246. Thomas ML, Harger JH, Wegener DK, Rabin BS, Gill TJ. HLA sharing and spontaneous abortion in humans. Am J Obstet Gynecol 1985;151:1053.
247. Unander M, Olding LB. Habitual abortion: parental sharing of HLA antigens, absence of maternal blocking antibody, and suppression of maternal lymphocytes. Am J Reprod Immunol 1983;4:171.
248. Cauchi MN, Koh SH, Tait B, Mraz G, Kloss M, Pepperell RJ. Immunogenetic studies in habitual abortion. Aust NZ J Obstet Gynaecol 1987;27:52.
249. Caudle MR, Rote NS, Scott JR, DeWitt C, Barney MF. Histocompatibility in couples with recurrent spontaneous abortion and normal fertility. Fertil Steril 1983;39:793.
250. Oksenberg JR, Persitz E, Amar A, Brautbar C. Maternal-paternal histocompatibility: lack of association with habitual abortions. Fertil Steril 1984;42:389.
251. Coulam CB, Moore SB, O'Fallon WM. Association between major histocompatibility antigen and reproductive performance. Am J Reprod Immunol Microbiol 1987;14:54.
252. McIntyre JA. In search of trophoblast-lymphocyte crossreactive (TLX) antigens. Am J Reprod Immunol Microbiol 1988;17:100.
253. McIntyre JA, Faulk WP. Allotypic trophoblast-lymphocyte crossreactive (TLX) cell surface antigens. Hum Immunol 1982;4:27.
254. Hsi BL, Yeh CJG, Fenichel P, Samson M, Grivaux C. Monoclonal antibody GB24 recognizes a trophoblast-lymphocyte crossreactive antigen. Am J Reprod Immunol Microbiol 1988;18:21.
255. Chaouat G, Lankar D. Vaccination against spontaneous abortion in mice by preimmunization with an anti-idiotypic antibody. Am J Perprod Immunol Microbiol 1988;16:146.
256. Stirrat GM. Recurrent miscarriage II: clinical associations, causes, and management. Lancet 1990;336:728.
257. Jones E, Curzen P, Gaugas JM. Suppressive activity of pregnancy plasma on the mixed lymphocyte reaction. J Obstet Gynaecol Br Commonwealth 1973;80:603.
258. Kasakura S. A factor in maternal plasma during pregnancy that suppresses the reactivity of mixed lymphocyte cultures. J Immunol 1971;107:1296.
259. Bissenden JG, Ling NR, Mackintosh P. Suppression of mixed lymphocyte reactions by pregnancy serum. Clin Exp Immunol 1980;39:195.
260. Barret DS, Rayfield LS, Brent L. Suppression of natural cell-mediated cytotoxicity in man by maternal and neonatal serum. Clin Exp Immunol 1982;47:742.
261. Fizet D, Bousquet J, Piquet Y, Cabantous F. Identification of a factor blocking a cellular cytotoxicity reaction in pregnant serum. Clin Exp Immunol 1983;52:648.
262. Rocklin RE, Kitzmiller JL, Carpenter CB, Garovoy MR, David JR. Maternal-fetal relation: absence of an immunologic blocking factor from the serum of women with chronic abortion. N Engl J Med 1976;295:1209.
263. Rocklin RE, Kitzmiller JL, Garvoy MR. Maternal-fetal relation (II): further characterization of an immunologuc blocking factor that develops during pregnancy. Clin Immunol Immunopathol 1982;22:305.
264. Anonymous. Maternal blocking antibodies, the fetal allograft, and recurrent abortion [editorial]. Lancet 1983;ii:1175.
265. Fizet D, Bousquet J. Absence of a factor blocking a cellular cytotoxicity reaction in the serum of women with recurrent abortion. Br J Obstet Gynaecol 1983;90:453.
266. Takeuchi S. Immunology of spontaneous abortion and hydatidiform mole. Am J Reprod Immunol 1980;1:23.
267. Stimson WH, Strachan AF, Sheperd A. Studies on the maternal immune response to placental antigens; absence of a blocking factor from the blood of abortion-prone women. Br J Obstet Gynecol 1979;86:41.
268. Takakuwa K, Kanazawa K, Takeuchi S. Production of blocking antibodies by vaccination with husband's lymphocytes in unexplained recurrent aborters: the role in successful pregnancy. Am J Reprod Immunol Microbiol 1986;10:1.
269. Suciu-Foca N, Reed E, Rohowsky C, et al. Anti-idiotypic antibodies to anti-HLA receptors induced by pregnancy. Proc Natl Acad Sci USA 1983;80:830.
270. McIntyre JA, Faulk WP. Trophoblast antigens in normal and abnormal human pregnancy. Clin Obstet Gynecol 1986;29:976.
271. Zak SJ, Good RA. Immunological studies of human serum gamma globulins. J Clin Invest 1959;38:579.
272. Holland NH, Holland P. Immunologic maturation in an infant of an agammaglobulinemic mother. Lancet 1966;ii:1152.
273. Kobayashi RH, Hymqan CJ, Steihm ER. Immunologic matura-

tion in an infant born to a mother with agammaglobulinemia. Am J Dis Child 1980;134:942.

274. Taylor PV, Hancock KW. Antigenicity of trophoblast and possible antigen masking effects during pregnancy. Immunology 1975;28:973.
275. Beard RW, Braude P, Mowbray JF, et al. Protective antibodies and spontaneous abortion. Lancet 1983;ii:1990.
276. Gill TJ III. Immunogenetics of spontaneous abortions in humans. Transplantation 1983;35:1.
277. Tongio MM, Berrebi A, Mayer S. A study of lymphocytotoxic antibodies in multiparous women having had at least four pregnancies. Tissue Antigens 1972;2:378.
278. Power DA, Mather AJ, MacLeod AM, Lind T, Catto GRD. Maternal antibodies to paternal B-lymphocytes in normal and abnormal pregnancy. Am J Reprod Immunol Microbiol 1986; 10:10.
279. Power DA, Catto GRD, Mason RJ, et al. The fetus as an allograft: evidence for protective antibodies to HLA-linked paternal antigens. Lancet 1983;ii:701.
280. Mowbray JF, Gibbings C, Liddell H, Reginald PW, Underwood JL, Beard RW. Controlled trial of treatment of recurrent spontaneous abortion by immunization with paternal cells. Lancet 1985;i:941.
281. Unander AM, Lindholm A, Olding LB. Blood transfusions generate/increase previously absent/weak blocking antibody in women with habitual abortion. Fertil Steril 1985;44:766.
282. McIntyre JA, Faulk WP, Nichols-Johnson VR, Taylor CG. Immunologic testing and immunotherapy in recurrent spontaneous abortion. Obstet Gynecol 1986;67:169.
283. Taylor CG, Faulk WP, McIntyre JA. Prevention of recurrent spontaneous abortions by leukocyte transfusions. J R Soc Med 1985;78:623.
284. Coulam CB. Treatment of recurrent spontaneous abortions [editorial]. Am J Reprod Immunol Microbiol 1988;17:149.
285. Beer AE, Semprini AE, Xiaoyu Z, et al. Pregnancy outcome in human couples with recurrent spontaneous abortions: HLA antigen profiles; HLA antigen sharing; female serum MLR blocking factors; and paternal leukocyte immunization. Exp Clin Immunogenetics 1985;2:137.

285a. Clark DA, Daya S. Trials and tribulations in the treatment of recurrent spontaneous abortion. Am J Reprod Immunol 1991;25:18.

286. Hill JA, Anderson DJ. Blood transfusions for recurrent abortion: Is the treatment worse than the disease [letter]? Fertil Steril 1986;46:152.
287. McIntyre JA, McConnachie, Taylor CG, Faulk WP. Clinical, immunologic, and genetic definitions of primary and secondary recurrent spontaneous abortions. Fertil Steril 1984;42:849.

16

CHAPTER

IMMUNOLOGIC ASPECTS OF PREGNANCY LOSS: ALLOIMMUNE AND AUTOIMMUNE CONSIDERATIONS

D. Ware Branch and James R. Scott

Although recurrent pregnancy loss is uncommon, it is a serious problem for the couple and the physician involved. This is particularly true in today's climate of high expectations for a favorable pregnancy outcome with each conception. However, in over half of cases of recurrent pregnancy loss, extensive evaluation fails to find a specific cause for the losses (Table 16-1). Recently, the concept that some unexplained pregnancy losses may be the result of the immunologic rejection of the conceptus, similar to that seen in transplant rejection, has gained popular acceptance. Because of the involvement of the alloimmune system, this type of pregnancy loss is referred to as alloimmune-mediated. In addition, autoimmunity has been recognized as a factor in recurrent pregnancy loss, even in women with no clinical autoimmune disease. This chapter focuses on these relatively new immunologic explanations for pregnancy loss.

ALLOIMMUNE CONCERNS

The term allogenicity refers to genetic dissimilarities between individuals of the same species. There are numerous readily recognized allogeneic traits in humans, including the ABO blood group system and the major histocompatibility (MHC) antigen system, also known as the human leukocyte antigen (HLA) system. The term alloimmune refers to the immune responses to these allogeneic antigens. Before the use of blood transfusions, alloimmune reactions in humans were limited to adverse fetal–maternal interactions such as Rh disease. But once modern medicine began to place the tissues of one human into another, the destructive nature of alloimmune rejection became apparent.

Nearly four decades of transplantation science have found that the usual mechanisms of immunologic rejection of an allograft (eg, a transplanted kidney) involve several important steps. The most important immunologic reactions appear to be cellular, and the allogeneic MHC antigens are particularly immunogenic. According to classic transplantation immunology, foreign donor MHC Class I antigens (as well as other cell surface antigens) are recognized by the recipient affector cells when presented in the context of the recipient's MHC Class II antigens. This step requires the participation of antigen-processing cells, such as macrophages, and takes place in local lymphatic tissues, where the primary affector cells are T-helper lymphocytes. Stimulated T-helper lymphocytes induce the proliferation of cytotoxic effector cells, including cytotoxic lymphocytes and macrophages. The cytotoxic lymphocytes recognize and kill the donor cells via the recognition of foreign MHC Class I molecules. Some T lymphocytes can recognize and kill donor cells via the foreign MHC Class I molecules, without the need for antigen-processing cells. It is now thought that this mechanism is particularly active in allograft rejection.

Antibodies also play a role in allograft rejection. T-helper lymphocytes, stimulated by their interaction with antigen-presenting cells, induce B lymphocytes to produce antibodies specific for graft cell-surface antigens. These antibodies may cause graft cell death through complement-mediated cell lysis or by coating the cells so that they may be attacked and lysed by effector cells, such as killer cells. The latter is known as antibody-dependent cellular cytotoxicity.

TABLE 16–1. ETIOLOGY OF RECURRENT PREGNANCY LOSS IN 209 WOMEN REFERRED TO THE UNIVERSITY OF UTAH DEPARTMENT OF OBSTETRICS AND GYNECOLOGY*

DIAGNOSIS	NUMBER OF PATIENTS	PERCENTAGE
Luteal phase deficiency	21	10
Uterine malformations	17	8
Antiphospholipid antibodies	8	4
Chromosome abnormalities	11	5
Unexplained	152	73

* All patients had three or more consecutive pregnancy losses and no more than one live birth.

The normal maternal response to pregnancy presents a fascinating interplay between maternal and paternal immunology. The maternal immune system functions perfectly well to guard the mother's body against infectious organisms, but allows the "semi-allograft" of the conceptus to lie in intimate contact with the maternal circulation and tissues for nearly 10 lunar months without apparent immunologic harm. From an immunological standpoint, there is substantial evidence that the mother recognizes the conceptus. Yet maternal immune rejection of the conceptus is subverted to allow the fetus to survive. To fully understand how this "selective immunotolerance" occurs would be to fully understand the science of immunology. As yet, only part of the story is revealed. Several factors play important roles in this unique process, and although each is discussed below as if it functioned independently, their complex interaction is crucial.

THE MATERNAL RESPONSE TO THE CONCEPTUS

Several investigators have established that syncytiotrophoblast lacks both Class I and II MHC antigens.[1–3] Thus, the vast majority of fetally-derived cells in contact with the maternal circulation are not immunogenic in the sense of classic transplantation recognition and rejection. Conversely, extravillous cytotrophoblastic cells express Class I MHC antigens, although they may be qualitatively different from those expressed by other fetal cells.[4,5] These cytotrophoblastic cells are in contact with the maternal tissues throughout pregnancy in trophoblast-anchoring columns, decidua, and the walls of the spiral arterioles. But again, classic transplantation immunologic recognition is limited by the failure of these cells to express Class II MHC antigens.[6,7]

It is now clear that trophoblast expresses antigens other than those of the MHC system. At least some of these antigens are immunogenic and may play an important role in maternal–fetal interaction. McIntyre and Faulk have described a trophoblast antigen system that induces antibodies that bind not only to the trophoblast but also to similar antigens on peripheral blood leukocytes.[8] Because of this cross reactivity, the antigen system was named the trophoblast-leukocyte cross-reactive (TLX) antigen system. TLX antigens are also found in seminal plasma and on platelets.[9] Other investigators have shown that human trophoblast can be used to generate murine monoclonal antibodies to non-MHC antigens.[10–12] Nearly 100 such antibodies have been produced, usually using preparations of trophoblast derived from villous trophoblast. However, it is generally conceded that only a handful of the monoclonal antibodies generated thus far are trophoblast specific. Several investigators presented work at the Fourth International Congress of Reproductive Immunology held in Kiel, Germany, in 1989 to show that three well-known, antitrophoblast, monoclonal antibodies may recognize a membrane co-factor, a surface glycoprotein involved in the regulation of complement activation. This surface glycoprotein is also found on peripheral blood lymphocytes and is a possible candidate for the TLX antigen.

Maternal humoral recognition of fetal–paternal antigens is well established. Antipaternal leukocytotoxic antibodies are found in 35% to 64% of multiparas and nearly a quarter of primiparas.[13–15] Many of these antibodies are directed against MHC antigens,[16] but a host of the less well-characterized trophoblast antigens may be involved. For example, Billington and colleagues have shown the presence of antitrophoblast antibodies devoid of MHC activity in the majority of primiparous and multiparous women, indicating the presence of an immunogenic non-MHC antigen(s).[17] At least some of the maternal antibodies against fetoplacental antigens would appear to be potentially destructive to the placenta. Not only can they agglutinate and kill paternal leukocytes, but they can also bind to trophoblastic cells in vitro.[18–20] Yet there is little evidence that the maternal antibodies to paternal antigens are damaging to the conceptus. To the contrary, some investigators consider their presence to be indicative of a normal immune response to pregnancy.[21]

But classic alloimmune recognition and rejection are cell-mediated, not humoral. Do mothers show evidence of such cell-mediated responses to fetal–paternal antigens? The data are conflicting. Circulating maternal leukocytes with weak cytotoxic activity against fetal cells have been found by some,[22,23] but not all, investigators.[7,24] Furthermore, at least two groups have found that maternal leukocytes are cytotoxic for trophoblast isolated from their own placentae.[25,26] But if cellular immunity to fetal–paternal antigens were part of pregnancy, one would expect a rapid, "secondary" maternal lymphocyte reaction to paternal cells in mixed lymphocyte culture (as well as in subsequent pregnancies). Indeed, several groups of investigators have reported such secondary maternal lymphocyte responses in mixed lymphocyte cultures of maternal and paternal cells.[27–29] But thorough investigation by Redman and colleagues found that neither primiparous nor multiparous women have a secondary proliferative or cytokine-release response to paternal antigens.[30,31]

In summary, maternal humoral alloreactivity to fetal–paternal antigens is common in normal pregnancy and indicates that the mother readily recognizes the fetus as foreign. In contrast, available methods have failed to demonstrate consistently maternal cell-mediated alloreactivity to the conceptus. In either event, there is little or no evidence that the conceptus is immunologically harmed during a normal pregnancy.

REGULATION OF MATERNAL–FETAL IMMUNOLOGY

The Placenta as an Immunologic Barrier

Not only are immunogenic fetal cells present on the trophoblast, but they are also commonly found in the maternal circulation.[32] In some circumstances these cells may induce a maternal immune response that is deleterious to the fetus, as in the case of maternal Rh immunization leading to fetal hemolytic disease. Why do other maternal responses to fetal–paternal antigens, such as anti-paternal MHC antibodies, not damage the fetus in the same fashion as anti-D antibody? Part of the answer to this perplexing question probably lies in the placenta as an anatomic barrier. In the case of MHC antigens, the extravillous trophoblast may serve a protective role for the fetus by acting as an "immunologic sponge," binding anti-[fetal]paternal MHC antibodies before they can gain access to the fetal tissues.[33] Neonates may have maternal antibodies to third-party MHC antigens, but not to paternal MHC antigens, in their circulation at birth,[34] suggesting that the trophoblast does exclude potentially damaging anti-paternal MHC antibodies from the fetus. But how does the trophoblast survive immunologic damage? As discussed below, many factors are probably involved, not the least of which is that trophoblastic cells, even those that express Class I MHC antigens, appear to be intrinsically resistant to attack and destruction by a variety of immunologically active cells, including antibody-dependent cellular cytotoxicity.[35,36]

Maternal Blocking Antibodies

One popular concept used to explain maternal immunotolerance of the fetus is that of maternal blocking factors, serum factors that inhibit cell-mediated immune function (as measured in vitro). Blocking factors were first described in the area of tumor immunology when it was observed that tumor cells were not destroyed in the presence of serum from the animal in which the tumor was grown.[37] In the late 1960s, the same group of investigators found that fetal cells were protected by blocking activity in the serum of pregnant animals.[38] The obvious conclusion was that the blocking factors played a role in the maternal immunotolerance of the conceptus. The blocking activity is in the immunoglobulin fraction of the maternal serum, suggesting that blocking factors are actually blocking antibodies. However, nonspecific serum factors, such as α-globulins, interleukin-2 (IL-2) inhibitors, and prostaglandins, may also be important.

Blocking factors may be demonstrated in several in vitro assays. The one-way mixed lymphocyte reaction (MLR) is commonly used in the field of recurrent pregnancy loss. In its simplest form, responder lymphocytes from the female (maternal) partner are cultured for several days with stimulator lymphocytes of the male (paternal) partner that have been irradiated to prevent replication. In unrelated control serum, the maternal lymphocytes proliferate in response to the antigenically foreign paternal lymphocytes. Responder-cell proliferation is primarily mediated by the response of T-helper lymphocytes to Class II MHC antigens on the irradiated stimulator cells. The degree of proliferation, and thus the degree of the response, is measured by adding radiolabeled thymidine to the culture. The proliferating cells incorporate the thymidine into their DNA, and the amount of incorporation can be measured using a radiocounter. In most maternal–paternal pairs, the presence of blocking factors is shown when the use of maternal serum in the assay modifies the MLR by suppressing the maternal proliferative response. Not only do blocking antibodies suppress the MLR to fetal–paternal cells, they often "nonspecifically" block the MLR to third-party unrelated cells.[39,40] Another kind of blocking activity may be measured in vitro using an assay of cell-mediated lympholysis (CML). This assay primarily measures the activity of stimulated maternal cytotoxic T lymphocytes against paternal lymphocytes bearing Class I MHC antigens. The maternal lymphocytes are first exposed to irradiated paternal cells so that they become alloactivated. The resultant lymphoblasts are then incubated with live paternal cells that have been labeled with ^{51}Cr. The release of the radiolabel into the culture media indicates target cell lysis. In the presence of serum-containing blocking factors, the cytotoxicity is suppressed or inhibited.

Blocking activity mediated by antibodies has received the most investigative attention. In pregnancy, these may be noncytotoxic antitrophoblast antibodies that bind to antigens on the trophoblast and thus simply "mask" recognition by maternal immune effectors. According to Faulk and McIntyre, a subset of the anti-TLX antibodies induced by TLX antigens, designated TA1, may cause this sort of blocking activity.[41] Alternatively, blocking antibodies may be anti-idiotypic antibodies specific for the maternal anti-(fetal)paternal idiotypes.[42] By binding to the recognition sites of the anti-paternal immunoglobulins, these antibodies would alter the function of the maternal immunoglobulins directed against the fetal–paternal antigens. Perhaps more importantly, anti-idiotypic antibodies could bind to recognition sites on maternal T lymphocytes to alter maternal cell-mediated immune responses.[43–45] They could also function to down-regulate the maternal immune response to fetal–paternal antigens according to the immunoregulatory role of anti-idiotypic antibodies proposed by Jerne.[46] Finally, blocking antibodies may be a unique kind of noncytotoxic antibody that binds to Fc receptors or to an Fc receptor-associated alloantigen present on paternal cells, thus inhibiting the ability of maternal effector cells to bind to antibody-coated trophoblastic cells.[47]

Several investigators have found blocking antibodies present in the sera of women with successful pregnancies and absent in the sera of women with spontaneous abortions.[48–51] These observations have led some to conclude that blocking antibodies are necessary for normal pregnancy. However, several observations run contrary to this hypothesis. Blocking antibodies are not detectable in maternal serum until the late first or early second trimester of the first pregnancy, yet the early part of the first pregnancy usually progresses normally.[49] Moreover, blocking antibodies are not present in the sera of all women with successful pregnancies.[52] Also, agammaglobulinemic women have been reported to have normal pregnancies.[53–55] Finally, mammals with hemochorial placentation that have been rendered incapable of producing immunoglobulins may have normal pregnancies.[56]

In our experience, blocking antibodies (as detected in MLR) develop in the vast majority of patients who progress into the second half of a pregnancy. However, they are categorically absent in the sera of nulliparous women and usually absent in the sera of women with first trimester pregnancy losses, even when the next pregnancy is successful. Thus, blocking antibodies do not seem to be an absolute requirement for normal pregnancy, suggesting that they are either epiphenomenal or expendable.

Decidual Immunosuppression

Recent studies suggest that most if not all of the maternal immunotolerance of the conceptus is mediated at the maternal interface with the placenta. Working primarily with rodent models, Clark and his colleagues have described two important uterine immunosuppressor cells. The first appears in the preimplantation uterine lining and is a relatively large cell known as the "large suppressor cell" or "phase A suppressor cell."[57] These cells act without MHC restriction to block the generation of cytotoxic T lymphocytes in the endometrium and draining lymph nodes. In the mouse, these cells have typical T-cell surface markers and lack macrophage markers.[58,59] Apparently analogous suppressor cells also appear in the luteal phase endometrium of the human, but they have not been as well characterized.[60] The induction of large suppressor cells in the uterus is dependent on gestational hormones present in the luteal phase[61]; trophoblast per se is not required.[57] Thus, local uterine immunosuppression is initiated at the time of conception, paving the way for immunologic tolerance of the implanting conceptus. Curiously, there appears to be a transient decrease in suppressive activity of the endometrium at the time of implantation,[58] a finding that is as yet unexplained.

Following implantation, a smaller, granulated lymphocytic immunosuppressive cell is found in the decidua under the site of placental implantation (decidua basalis). These cells are known as "small suppressor cells" or "phase B suppressor cells."[57] In mice, the small suppressor cells are induced by the presence of trophoblast,[62] probably via hormonal activity rather than immunologic activity.[63] Like large suppressor cells, the small suppressor cells inhibit the development of cytotoxic lymphocyte activity. Small suppressor cells similar to those found in the mouse have also been found in human decidua from first trimester elective pregnancy terminations.[58,60] One group of investigators has characterized the suppressive activity of early human decidua as being mediated by prostaglandin E_2 (PGE_2).[64] PGE_2 down-regulates IL-2 receptors on T lymphocytes, effectively blocking the usual proliferative response of T lymphocytes to this cytokine.[64,65] However, Clark and colleagues believe that the suppressive factor produced by the small suppressor cells is a unique member of the transforming growth factor-β family of molecules.[66] This factor can arrest ongoing IL-2 dependent cytotoxic lymphocyte responses, as well as the generation of IL-2 activated killer cells.

The decidua is also rich in macrophages[67,68]; in fact, these cells make up the majority of leukocytic-appearing cells in the decidua.[69] Macrophages can suppress lymphocyte proliferation by the production of PGE_2, and may be the source of suppressive PGE_2 in the decidua. Macrophages are present in limited numbers in early pregnancy, but increase to become a substantial population in the decidua basalis by midgestation.[70]

In areas of the decidua other than the decidua basalis, other cells of T-cell lineage are found.[71] These cells do not express surface markers typical of mature T cells and may be immature or inactivated lymphocytes.[72] The function of these cells is currently unknown.

Histocompatibility and the Immunotrophic Hypothesis

The mating of allogeneically different individuals is the rule in nature, and there is some evidence that maternal–fetal *histoincompatibility* provides a reproductive advantage. Because they can be easily manipulated immunogenetically, the best data come from studies of laboratory animals. In one investigation, histoincompatible mice were found to have larger litter sizes and larger placentas than histocompatible animals.[73] More recently, mating studies using an inbred strain of laboratory rat showed a strong preference for offspring heterozygous for genes at the histocompatibility locus.[74–76] These studies suggest an in utero selection for histoincompatible fetuses.

Numerous studies in humans have measured possible effects of MHC antigens on reproductive performance. Many investigators have reported a tendency for an increased sharing of HLA antigens between partners in couples with recurrent pregnancy loss.[77–79] In a detailed, prospective study of HLA in an isolated religious population that prohibits contraception, Ober and colleagues have found longer median intervals between births among couples who shared more than one HLA-A, -B, or -DR antigen.[80] On the average, couples who shared HLA-DR antigens had more spontaneous abortions and smaller completed family sizes than those not sharing HLA-DR antigens. However, many of these couples had fairly large completed family sizes.

Any complete hypothesis of maternal–fetal immunology must not only explain how the allogeneically different fetus survives immune rejection by the mother, but also how allogeneically disparate matings may have a reproductive advantage. One hypothesis, known as the immunotrophic hypothesis, holds that while immunoregulatory factors work to keep the mother's immune system from rejecting the fetus, other "immune" factors actually promote trophoblastic growth and thus fetal growth. As originally conceived, these immunotrophic factors are cytokines elaborated by maternal lymphoid cells recognizing fetal–paternal antigens. For example, activated maternal T cell may produce cytokines that stimulate trophoblast growth.[81] However, experimental support for immunotrophism is scant, and the original hypothesis has required modification. For a complete discussion of the relatively new concept of immunotrophism, the reader is referred to a recent review.[82]

ALLOIMMUNE-MEDIATED PREGNANCY LOSS

Numerous reproductive immunologists have used the data and ideas discussed above to formulate the hypothesis that some couples with unexplained recurrent pregnancy loss have an alloimmune-mediated problem. The particulars of the hypothesis vary from one authority to another, but the following is a reasonable synthesis. Some women with primary recurrent pregnancy loss share similar or identical alleles for trophoblast antigens (eg, MHC antigens or TLX antigens) with their male partners. In this situation, the pregnant woman fails to immunologically recognize the trophoblast as foreign, and the mechanisms that normally lead to maternal immunotolerance of the trophoblast (and possibly trophoblastic immunotrophism) are not triggered. The maternal alloimmune system "sees" the conceptus as foreign and rejects the pregnancy much in the same manner as an allograft is rejected. A woman with this supposed cause for her recurrent pregnancy losses would have a negative traditional evaluation for recurrent abortion and the following characteristics:

1. No pregnancy with the male partner involved in the abortions has progressed beyond the first or early second trimester.
2. The woman and her male partner often share more than the expected number of HLA antigens.[83]
3. The MLR between the woman's cells and those of her male partner in third-party serum is hyporeactive (because the couple is likely to share HLA antigens).[79]
4. Maternal blocking factor activity is absent.[84]

Although one group has found that anti-paternal leukocytotoxic antibodies are not present in this type of patient,[84] Beer suggests that they may be present because of immunization against fetal–paternal antigens other than those found on the trophoblast.[85] Work by Clark and colleagues suggests that the primary reason for pregnancy loss in this type of patient is the failure of uterine suppressor cells to appear.[58,86] Unfortunately, no convenient or practical test for these suppressor cells or their activity is currently available.

In the hypothesis proposed, women with secondary recurrent pregnancy loss caused by alloimmune factors do not have a failure of immune recognition of the trophoblast. Rather, these women are thought to have an inappropriate immunologic response to pregnancy wherein leukocytotoxic antibodies directed against trophoblast antigens have a pathologic effect. According to Faulk and McIntyre, the antibodies are damaging because regulating maternal anti-idiotypic antibodies against the leukocytotoxic antibodies are not produced. A woman with this cause for her recurrent pregnancy losses would have a negative traditional evaluation for recurrent abortion and the following characteristics:

1. One or more of the previous pregnancies with the male partner involved in the abortions resulted in a live born infant
2. The woman and her male partner do not share more than the expected number of HLA antigens.[83]
3. The MLR between the woman's cells and those of her male partner in third-party serum demonstrates a normal proliferative response.[87]
4. Maternal blocking factor activity is present.[84]

Although widely held, the direct evidence supporting this hypothesis in humans is scanty and circumstantial. In our experience, virtually all patients with unexplained primary recurrent pregnancy loss lack blocking factor activity. It is difficult for us to believe that *all* of these women have the same cause (ie, alloimmune-mediated) for their recurrent pregnancy loss. We believe that their lack of blocking activity may result from the fact that their previous pregnancies had never progressed to the point wherein blocking factors would normally develop. Nor have we found that the absence of blocking factors predicts another abortion in untreated pregnancies. In one of our ongoing studies, of eight women with unexplained pregnancy loss who lacked blocking factors by MLR assay, three had a successful next pregnancy without treatment.

ANIMAL MODELS OF IMMUNE-MEDIATED PREGNANCY LOSS

Animal models have played an important role in the development of the alloimmune-mediated pregnancy loss hypothesis. One interspecies murine model uses *Mus caroli* × *Mus caroli* embryos transferred to the uterus of suitably prepared *Mus musculus* recipients. Fetal resorption is the rule in this model,[88] and the losses appear to be due to an immune rejection phenomenon. The maternal decidua lacks suppressor cells,[89] and the resorbing fetuses are infiltrated with maternal lymphoid cells, including nonspecific killer cells.[90] If the *Mus caroli* embryos are enveloped in trophoblast (blastocyst) from *Mus musculus*, the fetuses are not rejected and live births result, suggesting that the induction of decidual immune suppression is dependent on species-specific aspects of the trophoblast.[82] The fetal losses in this model, however, are probably not exclusively due to an immune rejection mechanism because *Mus musculus* mothers rendered immunologically tolerant or immunodeficient remain incapable of bearing live *Mus caroli* offspring.[91]

In another model, developed by David Clark and colleagues, CBA/J (females) and DBA/2 (males) mice are used. This model is an allogeneic one, and thus more pertinent to the situation in humans. CBA/J × DBA/2 matings have a modestly high rate of fetal resorptions (from 13% to 50%), which investigators have linked to a lack of suppressor cells in the decidua. The resorbing fetuses appear to be undergoing immune rejection because they are infiltrated with natural killer and cytotoxic T lymphocytes.[92] Mating CBA/J females with males of similar MHC strains does not result in abnormally high resorption rates, suggesting that determinants other than those of the MHC are involved. Critics of this model have noted that the CBA/J × DBA/2 model is characterized by resorption of some but not a majority of fetuses. Clark has recently addressed this criticism[82] by pointing out that investigations in other murine strains show that the suppressor activity of the different implantation sites vary.[93,94] Those implantations associated with low suppressor activity were most susceptible to resorption.

The CBA/J × DBA/2 model has also provided evidence that immune rejection of the fetus is by nonclassical mechanisms. Treatment of the pregnant mice with anti-asialo-GM1, a surface marker for natural killer cells and precursors to cytokine-activated killer cells, reduces the resorption rate.[82,95] In contrast, treatment with antibodies that incapacitate T lymphocytes does not reduce the resorption rate. These findings suggest that non–antigen-specific, non–T-cell effectors, such as natural killer cells, are the most important component of immune rejection in this model.

TREATMENT OF ALLOIMMUNE-MEDIATED PREGNANCY LOSS

There are now many medical centers around the world that offer immunization with paternal or donor leukocytes, or other fractions containing MHC or trophoblast antigens, as a treatment for supposed alloimmune-mediated recurrent pregnancy loss. This treatment has come to be known as "immunotherapy." The rationale for immunotherapy is borrowed from transplantation medicine, wherein studies in animals and humans suggest that such immunizations may induce a beneficial immunosuppression in the graft recipient. Pretransplantation blood transfusions have been used for many years to decrease the risk of allograft rejection after renal transplantation,[96,97] and the beneficial effect has been localized to the leukocyte fraction.[98] The exact mechanism of immunosuppression is unknown, but various investigators have provided evidence for several possibilities. Leukocyte immunizations induce MLR-blocking antibodies,[99–101] which some have found to be anti-idiotypic in nature.[44,100] The immunizations may also generate peripheral suppressor T cells.[44,102]

The use of immunotherapy for the treatment of supposed alloimmmune-mediated pregnancy loss is backed by experiments in the CBA/J × DBA/2 murine model. Pre-pregnancy immunization of the CBA/J females with splenocytes from BALB/c mice and other strains that carry the same MHC determinants reduces resorption rates from about 30% to 7.4%.[103] Placental cells from the appropriate strains were also effective in reducing the resorption rate. The immunizations are correlated with the formation of anti-MHC antibodies,[104] the recruitment of decidual suppressor cells,[105,106] and the induction of MLR suppressor activity by decidual cell supernatants.[104] The protective effect of immunization can be adoptively transferred to virgin CBA/J females by administration of the serum or T cells from immunized mothers[104] The anti-MHC antibodies appear to be important, because absorption of the serum with MHC–antigen-bearing cells abrogates the protective effect.

Several immunization regimens have been used to induce a favorable immune response to pregnancy in women with supposed alloimmune-mediated recurrent pregnancy loss. Maternal immunization with paternal leukocytes was the first to be tried.[78] Other investigators have used unrelated, third-party leukocytes.[107–109] There is no consensus as to which patients are candidates for immunotherapy, but it is reasonable to exclude women who have a proven immune response to their male partner (eg, anti-paternal leukocytotoxic antibodies[21] or blocking factors to paternal stimulator cells in the MLR).[78,110] The group of investigators who described the TLX antigen system has suggested immunization with seminal plasma because they have found that it contains TLX antigens.[9] Along the same line of thinking, Johnson and colleagues are studying the effects of immunization with preparations of trophoblast membranes.[115]

Table 16-2 summarizes the reported studies to date.

TABLE 16–2. SUCCESSFUL PREGNANCIES AFTER IMMUNOTHERAPY IN PATIENTS WITH RECURRENT PREGNANCY LOSS

INVESTIGATOR	ANTIGEN SOURCE	ROUTE OF IMMUNIZATION	NUMBER OF PATIENTS	LIVE BIRTHS
Immunotherapy				
Beer[39]	Paternal leukocytes	Intradermal	37	26 (70%)
Mowbray[21]	Paternal leukocytes	Intradermal, subcutaneous, intravenous	22	17 (77%)
Takakuwa[110]	Paternal leukocytes	Intradermal	7	5 (71%)
McIntyre[108]	Unrelated donor	Intravenous	23	20 (87%)
Unander[109]	Unrelated donor	Intravenous	12	11 (92%)
Johnson[112]	Trophoblast	Intravenous	21	16 (76%)
Smith[113]	Paternal leukocytes	Intravenous, subcutaneous intradermal	58	29 (50%)
Ho[115a]	Paternal leukocytes or unrelated donor	Intradermal	38	18 (47%)
Cauchi[115b]	Paternal leukocytes	Intravenous, subcutaneous, intradermal	21	13 (62%)
Controls				
Mowbray[21]			27	10 (37%)
Bonara[114]			12	9 (75%)
Ho[115a]			37	14 (38%)
Cauchi[115b]			25	19 (76%)

Only three studies have appropriate control groups, and one could argue that the overall seemingly favorable results are no better than those achieved by supportive care.[115] The randomized, controlled study of Mowbray and coworkers[21] suggested that immunotherapy was indeed effective. The authors of that study immunized women who had unexplained recurrent pregnancy loss and no anti-paternal leukocytotoxic antibodies with paternal leukocytes. The control patients were immunized with their own leukocytes. The difference in pregnancy success between the two groups was statistically significant. However, two subsequent randomized controlled trials have failed to show a significant difference between immunized and control patients in terms of the next pregnancy outcome.[115a,115b] One of these attempted to repeat the work of Mowbray and coworkers in a paired sequential trial.[115b] Saline, rather than maternal leukocytes, was used in the control group. The proportion of successful pregnancies in the leukocyte-immunized patients and saline-injected controls was 62% and 76%, respectively.

The adverse effects of these immunization regimens are unknown, but it is encouraging that no one has reported transfusion reactions, anaphylaxis, or viral infection in the treated mothers. At the Third International Congress of Reproductive Immunology held in Toronto in 1986, investigators from around the world summarized the limited information available on the infants of immunized mothers. Adverse outcomes were rare: the list of those encountered included placental abruption, placenta accreta, oligohydramnios, preeclampsia, fetal growth retardation, preterm delivery, fetal death, cardiac anomalies, renal anomalies, trisomy 21 and 13, and an unusual case of an undefined neonatal immunodeficiency disease. Most authorities believe that the frequency of these abnormalities is no greater than expected; however, the undefined immunodeficiency disease is of particular concern because it could represent a form of graft-versus host-disease.

In spite of its use in several centers, immunotherapy remains controversial. Currently, the diagnosis of alloimmune-mediated recurrent pregnancy loss is one of exclusion; thus, there is no positive test or marker to distinguish these patients from all others who have unexplained recurrent pregnancy loss. There is also confusion as to what constitutes an appropriate response to the immunotherapy (apart from the obvious live birth). Several groups of investigators have reported that the therapy is successful if the patients develop blocking factors after the treatment.[39,110,116] Another investigator found that pregnancy success is correlated with the development of anti-paternal leukocytotoxic antibodies.[21] Finally, there is disagreement as to whether patients with secondary recurrent pregnancy loss should undergo immunotherapy, with some claiming that they should[21] and others saying no.[84] We believe that immunotherapy remains experimental at this time and that further randomized trials are needed to clarify the controversial issues in this new field. Documentation and confirmation of efficacy and safety are crucial before this treatment can be recommended.

AUTOIMMUNE CONCERNS

There is little question that women with certain frank autoimmune diseases, such as systemic lupus erythematosus, are at risk for pregnancy loss.[117] However, it is now apparent that some asymptomatic healthy women with previously unexplained pregnancy loss have evidence of autoimmunity, as demonstrated by the presence of autoantibodies. As a result, many physicians now measure one or several autoantibodies in their evaluation of the patient with the problem of pregnancy loss.

ANTINUCLEAR ANTIBODIES

Three retrospective studies link the presence of measurable antinuclear antibodies (ANAs) to unexplained pregnancy loss in asymptomatic women.[118–120] These studies found that 7.5% to 29% of patients have ANAs, while only 6.6% of the women with normal pregnancies[119] and 6% of the women with other known causes of pregnancy loss[120] had the antibodies. Such data suggest an association between unexplained pregnancy loss and subclinical autoimmunity, as reflected by the presence of ANAs. An additional, untested implication is that treatment—with immunosuppression, for example—could improve the next pregnancy outcome in these patients. Only one study considered this issue by showing that only four of seven untreated women with positive ANAs delivered a viable infant in the next pregnancy.[118]

At least two factors weigh against a cause-and-effect association between ANAs and pregnancy loss. In virtually all cases, the levels of ANAs found in the patients with recurrent pregnancy loss are low, suggesting that they may be clinically unimportant. Moreover, a substantial number of normal pregnant women can be found to have measurable ANAs, even though they eventually deliver healthy infants.[121] Neither of these points excludes the possibility that ANAs are important in some patients with pregnancy loss. But a larger prospective study is needed to compare ANAs in patients with unexplained and explained recurrent pregnancy loss and to determine their subsequent pregnancy outcomes without treatment.

ANTIPHOSPHOLIPID ANTIBODIES AND PREGNANCY LOSS

The association between antiphospholipid antibodies (aPLA) and pregnancy loss is well established; details may be found in recent reviews.[122,123] A substantial literature now indicates that some women have aPLA as their only "explanation" for pregnancy loss. Table 16-1 shows the cause of recurrent pregnancy loss in our series of 209 women with three or more consecutive losses with no more than one live birth. Nearly 4% had aPLA as the "cause" of their losses. In a separate population of women who had less than three consecutive losses or more than one previous live birth, nearly 7% had a diagnosis of aPLA.[124] A history of fetal death is particularly suspicious, because 30% to 40% of antiphospholipid antibody-associated pregnancy losses occur in the second or early third trimester.[122,123] A review of our experience shows that 33% of pregnancy losses attributable to aPLA are fetal deaths.[124] Moreover, over 90% of the patients with aPLA-associated losses had at least one fetal death.

The risk of pregnancy loss in women with aPLA is high. The only published prospective study included over 30 pregnancies in 25 women with moderate or high levels of aPLA.[125] The women were managed with either prednisone and aspirin, aspirin alone, or no therapy. The worst outcomes were among the women with previous fetal death and high levels of aPLA. In this group, 67% of the next pregnancies ended in fetal loss. Those women with high levels of aPLA but no history of previous pregnancy loss had a 33% rate of fetal death. For any level of aPLA, a history of previous pregnancy loss more than doubled the risk of fetal loss in the next pregnancy. The majority of the losses occurred during the second trimester.

Patients with antiphospholipid antibodies are also predisposed to thromboembolic disease.[122,123] The thrombotic episodes may be either venous or arterial and may be an important historical clue in a patient with pregnancy loss. In our series of patients, 22 of the 78 women (28%) ascertained because of pregnancy loss had a history of thrombotic episodes.[124] The majority were venous events, mostly occurring in the lower extremities. It is common for the thrombosis to have occurred in the setting of pregnancy or soon after the patient started oral contraceptives. We have recently described transient ischemic attacks as a feature of thromboembolic disease in pregnant patients with aPLA.[126]

Patients with antiphospholipid antibodies may have several other clinical problems, including thrombocytopenia. It has been recently suggested that the triad of fetal loss, thromboembolic disease, and thrombocytopenia form the clinical criteria for the "antiphospholipid syndrome."[127]

Diagnosis of Antiphospholipid Antibodies

It is generally accepted that there are three aPLA: the biologically false-positive serologic test for syphilis (STS), the lupus anticoagulant (LAC), and (3) anticardiolipin antibodies (ACA). Although false-positive STSs have been linked to pregnancy loss,[128] the latter two aPLA are most strongly associated.

The aPLA bind to negatively charged phospholipids,[129,130] and this feature of the antibodies is used for their detection in plasma or serum. LAC prolongs phospholipid-dependent coagulation tests, such as the partial thromboplastin time (PTT), by binding to the phospholipid portion of the prothrombin–prothrombinase complex.[131,132] In most hospital coagulation laboratories, LAC is the most common reason for an unexplained prolonged PTT,[133] but factor deficiencies must be excluded. To do so, the abnormal plasma is retested after mixing it with an equal volume of normal plasma. If the 1:1 mixture of LAC and normal plasma "corrects" to a normal clotting time, a factor deficiency is probably present. If the test remains abnormal (although it may "correct" somewhat), LAC is probably present. But this sequence of tests is not specific for LAC; for example, there are other immunoglobulin inhibitors of coagulation, such as antibodies to factor VIII. For this reason, authorities[134] have recently suggested that the suspicion of LAC be confirmed by demonstrating the phospholipid specificity of the anticoagulant using a phospholipid "bypass"[135] or "neutralizing"[136] procedure. The need for this third step in the diagnostic process will depend on the clinical situation and the prevalence of rare anticoagulants in the population being tested.

The numerous phospholipid-dependent coagulation tests that can be used for the detection of LAC vary in regard to sensitivity and specificity.[137–140] In general, phospholipid-poor or phospholipid-depleted assays are the most sensitive.[140–142] In the United States, a modified activated PTT (aPTT) is the most popular screening test.[134,141] The kaolin clotting time[134] and Russell's viper venom time[142] tests are also touted as being particularly sensitive and specific. Although several individual laboratories have done excellent work in the area of LAC detection testing, there are few interlaboratory comparisons of coagulation tests for the detection of LAC. In one international study of 20 coagulation laboratories with experience in the detection of LAC*, each laboratory was sent six plasma samples and asked to run their usual screening test(s) for LAC. Three of the samples contained varying amounts (10%, 20%, 50%) of well-characterized LAC plasma. One sample was normal plasma, another contained an anticoagulant enzyme, and the last contained 50% LAC with excess phospholipid. All but one of the laboratories detected both the 20% and 50% LAC samples, but several different coagulation assays were required in some cases, and the degree of positivity did not necessarily correspond to the amount of LAC in the sample. Two laboratories failed to find the 10% LAC positive, and three others found the specimen to be only equivocally positive. Thus, LAC results may vary remarkably from laboratory to laboratory, and weakly positive LAC plasmas may be missed. Even worse, six laboratories found the normal plasma to be a positive. Although international efforts at standardizing LAC assays are underway, the course is likely to be long and difficult. Currently, there is no single best test for detecting, quantifying, or specifying LAC, although the sensitivity of the kaolin clotting time[140] and specificity of the platelet neutralization procedure[136] may be slightly better than for other assays.

* T. Exner, personal communication, 1989

In contrast to LAC, ACA are detected in serum using immunoassay techniques. The most widely used technique is an enzyme-linked immunoabsorbent assay (ELISA), which employs a negatively charged phospholipid as the solid phase antigen. Many different laboratory methods for antiphospholipid ELISAs have been published,[130,143,144] but the well-characterized method of Loizou[145] using cardiolipin as the phospholipid antigen is now accepted as a standardized assay.[146] Standard positive ACA sera are now available that define a standard curve for IgG and IgM ACA activity (expressed in international units).[146] Although investigators may use different antiphospholipid assays for research purposes, this standardized ACA assay should be used for clinical testing. Results should be reported in international IgG or IgM units, and positive tests should be interpreted in a semiquantitative fashion, such as negative, low positive, medium positive, or high positive. The unpublished results of the Second International Anti-Cardiolipin Workshop show excellent agreement between laboratories using the standardized Loizou-type ACA assay in conjunction with the standard positive ACA sera (E. N. Harris, personal communication).

The correct interpretation of antiphospholipid antibody assays has been defined and tempered by experience. Like other autoimmune diagnoses, the diagnosis of antiphospholipid antibody syndrome rests on clinical and laboratory criteria (Table 16-3); it is not a diagnosis made by laboratory tests alone. Most patients with the syndrome have moderate or high levels of ACA.[127,147] Experienced investigators feel that low positive results are of questionable significance.[127,147]

TABLE 16–3. SUGGESTED CLINICAL AND SEROLOGIC CRITERIA FOR THE ANTIPHOSPHOLIPID ANTIBODY SYNDROME

CLINICAL FEATURES	LABORATORY FEATURES
Venous thrombosis Arterial thrombosis Recurrent fetal loss Thombocytopenia	IgG anticardiolipin antibody (>20 IU units) Positive lupus anticoagulant test* IgM anticardiolipin antibody (>20 IU units) and a positive lupus anticoagulant test

Note: Patients with the antiphospholipid antibody syndrome should have at least one clinical and one serologic feature at some time in their disease course. An antiphospholipid antibody test should be positive on at least two occasions more than 8 weeks apart.

* Lupus anticoagulant should be confirmed by demonstrating inhibition by phospholipids or by freeze-thawed platelets.

(Modified from Harris EN. Syndrome of the black swan. Br J Rheumatol 1987;26:324.)

Transient positive tests also occur (especially low positives) so that confirmation of a positive result is recommended. The relevant cut-off between low and medium positive or medium and high positive will probably always be debated. Currently, experienced laboratories consider a serum medium positive if it demonstrates over 15 to 20 international units of IgG or 10 to 20 units of IgM. In our experience, some isolated IgM positive results may result from nonspecific binding in the assay. Although some laboratories offer to test for IgA antiphospholipid antibody, the clinical meaning of IgA positive results is unclear.

There is a close relationship between LAC and ACA. One investigator found that the degree of coagulation prolongation correlates with the level of ACA antibody.[148] Another group showed that mouse and human monoclonal IgM antiphospholipid antibodies may have LAC and ACA activity.[149] These observations, coupled with the fact that the same clinical problems are associated with LAC and ACA, suggest that these two antibodies may be the same immunoglobulin measured by two different methods (coagulation versus immunoassay). Conversely, patients have been described with either LAC or ACA, but not both.[130,143,144,150] Also, our laboratory has not been able to confirm a linear correlation between the degree of prolongation of the coagulation time and the level of ACA.[130] Given the current uncertainty in this area, we recommend that patients with a suspicious history be assayed for *both* LAC and ACA by a reputable laboratory.

Prevalence of Antiphospholipid Antibodies

The highest prevalence of antiphospholipid antibodies is found among patients with autoimmune disease. Between 6% and 24% of patients with SLE have LAC[129,151,153]; about 40% have measurable levels of ACA.[152]

The frequency of antiphospholipid antibodies in the general population is unknown, but several small studies provide prevalence data for selected populations. One study found 10 patients with prolonged partial thromboplastin times in 813 patients having a coagulation screen;[139] 9 of the 10 were confirmed to have LAC, for a prevalence of 1.1%. None of the patients had SLE, but 2 had thrombocytopenia and 1 had thromboembolic disease. Another coagulation laboratory found that approximately 2% of patients screened using a PTT have LAC.[153] A recent study of 723 consecutive prenatal patients at a referral institution found two women who met coagulation criteria for LAC, for a prevalence of 0.3%.[154] Both patients suffered second trimester fetal losses.

If one includes low positives, the prevalence of ACA among normal non-pregnant controls is probably about 2% to 3%.[147,154] Thus, ACA is more frequently detected than LAC, probably because of the greater sensitivity of the ACA assays for low levels of antibody. Low levels of ACA are usually of little or no clinical importance[127,147]; however, higher levels may be associated with an increased risk of pregnancy loss. In one prospective study, a positive ACA at >5 standard deviations above the control mean predicted a pregnancy loss rate of about 20%.[154]

How frequently is LAC or ACA an explanation for recurrent pregnancy loss? Only a few studies have attempted to answer this important question. One group found that a surprisingly high percentage—48% of 29 women with unexplained recurrent pregnancy loss—had LAC.[156] Two other studies, more in line with our experience, found that about 10% of patients with unexplained recurrent pregnancy loss had LAC.[155,157] In regard to ACA, two published series have found a frequency of 11%[155] and 42%[158] among women with unexplained recurrent pregnancy loss. One large but unpublished observation holds that only 2.5% of more than 400 such women have ACA.† Our combined retrospective and prospective data show that about 5% of patients referred to a university clinic for recurrent pregnancy loss have significant levels of aPLA (LAC or ACA) (see Table 16-1). Another investigation of over 300 similarly chosen patients with recurrent pregnancy loss found a 6% prevalence of significantly positive aPLA.[159] In summary, the prevalence of aPLA is sufficient to warrant testing all patients with recurrent pregnancy loss, especially because the assays are relatively inexpensive and the condition may be treatable.

Pathophysiology of aPLA-Associated Pregnancy Loss

The pathology immediately responsible for pregnancy loss in patients with aPLA appears to be a necrotizing decidual vasculopathy at the maternal–placental interface. The vasculopathy is characterized predominantly by fibrinoid necrosis, but it also has several less consistent features, including infiltration of the vessel wall by cells with clear or foamy cytoplasm (so-called "atherosis") and a perivascular infiltrate composed of mononuclear and polymorphonuclear cells.[160] Other reports confirm the frequent finding of obvious infarction and decidual necrosis in the placentas of women with aPLA and fetal deaths.[143,161–163]

The evidence that a decidual vasculopathy is responsible for pregnancy loss in patients with aPLA is supported by recent investigations in our laboratory. We showed that IgG fractions from patients with antiphospholipid antibodies and fetal death can cause fetal loss in mice.[164] The immediate cause of the fetal loss appears to be deposition of IgG and fibrin in or around the decidual vasculature. But the typical decidual and vascular changes are not found in the placentas of all aPLA patients with unexplained fetal loss.[143,161,165] Also, in some cases, the extent of the placental pathology appears insufficient to explain the fetal death.[146] Finally, the abnormal histology found in the placentas of autoimmune patients is nonspecific, having been described in placentas from patients with preeclampsia[166,164] or unexplained fetal growth retardation.[164] Our

† J.F. Mowbray, personal communication, 1988

experience also shows that rather extensive macroscopic and microscopic placental pathology, indistinguishable from that found in some cases of fetal death, may be present in successful pregnancies.

The mechanism by which aPLA result in decidual vascular damage remains speculative. Investigators have focused on how aPLA might cause thrombosis, speculating that the same mechanism might result in the vasculopathy seen in the placenta. Our mouse experiments show the deposition of fibrin in the decidual circulation, strongly suggesting a role for intravascular thrombosis as an immediate cause of fetal loss.[164] But how does an IgG cause thrombosis? Several investigators have found that plasma or IgG fractions from patients with lupus anticoagulant inhibit vascular tissue or vascular endothelial prostacyclin production.[168–172] This may lead to vascular damage through a predisposition to marked vasoconstriction or thrombosis. It has been suggested, but not proved, that aPLA inhibit prostacyclin generation by vascular tissues because they bind to endothelial cell membranes. To date, however, no one has published evidence to show that antiphospholipid antibodies bind to normal, intact endothelial cells. Our attempts using live human umbilical vein endothelial monolayers have also been unsuccessful.[173] Moreover, we[173] and others[174] have been unable to confirm that aPLA inhibit endothelial cell prostacyclin generation, even when we perturbed the endothelial cells with trauma or peroxide.[173]

Several other possible mechanisms for antiphospholipid antibody-mediated vascular damage have been proposed.[175–178] One investigator proposed that antiphospholipid antibodies might bind to platelet membranes, thereby encouraging their aggregation, and lead to local thrombosis.[175] Circumstantial evidence supports this hypothesis. Antiphospholipid antibodies appear to bind to platelets when the latter are activated or damaged.[179,180] Nonactivated, intact platelets have little effect on lupus anticoagulant activity, suggesting that the appropriate membrane phospholipid epitope(s) may not be expressed unless the platelet membrane is dramatically altered. This may be due to the distribution of anionic phospholipids in the platelet membrane. The anionic phospholipids are available only when the platelets are activated or have the membrane fractured.[181] These observations suggest that activated or damaged platelets bind antiphospholipid antibodies. In turn, the antibody–platelet membrane complex could enhance further platelet aggregation and lead to local thrombosis.

Several recent investigations suggest that antiphospholipid antibodies may lead to thrombosis and vascular damage by interfering with the activation of protein C by thrombomodulin.[178,182,183] Protein C is an endogenous anticoagulant that circulates in an inactive form. It is activated by thrombin when the latter is bound to thrombomodulin, an endothelial cell membrane receptor. Once activated, protein C exerts an anticoagulant effect by degrading activated factor V and activated factor VIII. Limited data suggest that the antiphospholipid antibodies inhibit protein C activation by interfering with the function of anionic phospholipids in the thrombomodulin system.[182] The anionic phospholipids enhance the activity of thrombomodulin at least threefold.[184] The concept that the thrombotic tendency in patients with antiphospholipid antibodies is caused by inhibition of protein C activation is attractive. Like patients with antiphospholipid antibodies, patients with inherited protein C deficiency demonstrate recurrent thrombotic episodes. However, pregnancy loss is not an impressive feature of families with protein C deficiency.[185,186] To the authors' knowledge, only one report suggests a link between inherited protein C deficiency and recurrent pregnancy loss.[187] Unfortunately, antiphospholipid antibodies and other causes of fetal death were not specifically excluded. It is also of concern that one investigator found that IgG fractions from only two of seven patients with LAC inhibited protein C activation.[183]

Treatment of Autoimmune-Associated Pregnancy Loss

Aggressive treatment of patients with antiphospholipid antibodies and previous pregnancy loss may improve the chance of delivering a viable infant. The first report, published by Lubbe, showed that five of six women with LAC had successful pregnancy outcomes when treated with high doses of prednisone (at least 40 mg per day) combined with low doses of aspirin (75 mg per day).[188] The same investigator has now treated over 30 pregnancies and achieved live births in over 80% of cases.†† Using similar treatment regimens, successful pregnancy outcomes have been reported by groups throughout the world.[189–195] Our own experience is somewhat less optimistic than that of Lubbe. We have now treated 39 pregnancies in 32 women with aPLA with prednisone and low-dose aspirin. Fifty-nine percent of the pregnancies have resulted in the delivery of a viable infant, but two infants died of complications due to prematurity, leaving a corrected success rate of 54%. Fetal death occurred in 8 pregnancies, and spontaneous abortions occurred in 8 pregnancies. Moreover, many of the pregnancies were complicated and required preterm delivery, usually for severe preeclampsia.[124] Prednisone, especially in the high doses used, is a potentially dangerous drug with serious adverse effects. Reported adverse effects in treated pregnancies include oropharyngeal candidiasis, facial acne, facial abscess, postpartum adrenal insufficiency, pneumonia, mycobacterial infection, and osteoporosis leading to vertebral collapse.[189,196,197] It is quite clear that the use of high doses of prednisone does not guarantee a successful pregnancy.[124,196] Moreover, a recent investigation found that the use of prednisone may actually worsen fetal outcome in women with high levels of ACA.[125]

†† W.F. Lubbe, personal communication, 1988

The dangers of high-dose steroids, coupled with the notion that anticoagulation may be reasonable therapy in patients with antiphospholipid antibodies, led to the use of heparin therapy during pregnancy. The first published series was that of Rosove and coworkers.[198] Using a mean dose of 24,700 units of heparin daily started in the first trimester, 14 of 15 pregnancies (93%) were successful. In patients without LA, the heparin dose was adjusted to obtain a mid-interval PTT of 1.5 to 2.0 times normal. In patients with prolonged activated PTTs due to LA, the heparin dose was adjusted to achieve a thrombin time >100 seconds while not permitting the baseline PT to rise by more than 1.5 seconds. Cowchock and colleagues have recently completed a randomized trial comparing treatment with corticosteroids to heparin (both regimens included low-dose aspirin).[199] The mean dose of heparin used was 17,000 units daily. Although only 20 patients were randomized, the results suggest that the two treatments are of similar efficacy in achieving a successful pregnancy. Moreover, treatment with corticosteroids was associated with an increased neonatal morbidity (preterm delivery and low birth-weight) and maternal morbidity (gestational diabetes and pregnancy-induced hypertension). Our own experience using heparin and low-dose aspirin includes 17 patients. After checking to be sure that the patient's platelet count is normal, we use 7500 units of heparin by subcutaneous injection b.i.d. in the first trimester. Currently, we adjust the dose beginning in the second trimester to achieve anticoagulation. Fifteen of 18 pregnancies have resulted in live births, but in one case, neonatal death occurred due to prematurity. In our current management scheme, heparin is not started until the patient has had an ultrasound demonstrating a live embryo (usually at 5 to 7 weeks gestation); thus, early first trimester losses and anembryonic pregnancies are excluded. We continue to use low-dose aspirin in the treatment regimen since it may prevent or ameliorate preeclampsia in patients at risk.

A third, potentially useful treatment for antiphospholipid antibody-associated pregnancy loss is high-dose intravenous immunoglobulin. We recently successfully used this therapy in a patient with LAC and nine consecutive pregnancy losses, the last three occurring in spite of prednisone and low-dose aspirin therapy.[200] Three other investigators have also had favorable outcomes using intravenous immunoglobulin.§ However, we have recently been involved in two additional cases in which fetal death occurred in spite of the immunoglobulin. The lack of serious adverse effects makes this therapy attractive even though it is expensive.

The questions as to which treatment is best for women with aPLA and pregnancy loss remains unanswered. We believe that the differences between the treatment results of different investigators are due to the nature of the population selected and the "severity" of their aPLA syndrome. No published treatment series includes randomly selected, untreated controls, a problem that is likely to persist. Furthermore, our extended experience has generated a degree of concern and confusion. Which therapy is the most efficacious and safest for patients with aPLA and previous pregnancy loss must be addressed by multicenter cooperation in a carefully designed, randomized trial using strict standardization of aPLA testing.

§ W.F. Lubbe, A. Parke, L. Carreras, personal communications, 1988

REFERENCES

1. Faulk WP, Temple A. Distribution of B_2-microglobulin and HLA in chorionic villi of human placentae. Nature 1976; 262:799.
2. Goodfellow PN, Barnstable CJ, Bodmer WF, Snary D, Crumpton MJ. Expression of HLA system antigens on placenta. Transplantation 1976;22:595.
3. Sunderland CA, Naiem M, Mason Dy, Redman CWG, Stirrat GM. The expression of major histocompatibility antigens by human chorionic villi. J Reprod Immunol 1981;3:323.
4. Sunderland CA, Redman CWG, Stirrat GM. HLA, A, B, C antigens are expressed on nonvillous trophoblast of the early human placenta. J Immunol 1981;127:2614.
5. Redman CWG, McMichael AJ, Stirrat GM, Sunderland CA, Ting A. Class I major histocompatibility complex antigens on human extravillous trophoblast. Immunology 1984;52:457.
6. Galbraith RM, Kantor RRS, Ferrara GB, Ades EW, Galbraith GMP. Differential anatomical expression of transplantation antigens within the normal human placental chorionic villus. Am J Reprod Immunol 1981;1:331.
7. Redman CWG, Arenas J, Mason DY, Sargent IL, Sutton L. Maternal alloimmune recognition of the fetus in human pregnancy. In: Gill TS III, Wegmann TG, eds. Immunoregulation and fetal survival. New York: Oxford University Press, 1987:210.
8. McIntyre JA, Faulk WP, Verhulst ST. Human trophoblast lymphocyte cross reactive (TLX) antigens define a new alloantigen system. Science 1983;222:1135.
9. Faulk WP, McIntyre JA. Role of anti-TLX antibody in human pregnancy. In: Clark DA, Croys BA, eds. Reproductive immunology. Amsterdam, Elsevier Science Publishers, 1986:106.
10. Johnson PM, Cheng HM, Molloy CM, Stern CMM, Slade MB. Human trophoblast-specific surface antigens identified using monoclonal antibodies. Am J Reprod Immunol 1981;1:246.
11. Lipinski M, Parks DR, Rouse RV, Herzenberg LA. Human trophoblast cell-surface antigens defined by monoclonal antibodies. Proc Natl Acad Sci USA 1981;78:5147.
12. Bulmer JN, Billington WD, Johnson PM. Immunohistologic identification of trophoblast populations in early human pregnancy with the use of monoclonal antibodies. Am J Obstet Gynecol 1984;148:19.
13. Burke J, Johansen K. The formation of HLA antibodies in pregnancy. The antigenicity of aborted and term fetuses. J Obstet Gynaecol Br Commonwealth 1974;81:222.
14. Beard RW, Braude P, Mowbray JF, et al. Protective antibodies and spontaneous abortion. Lancet 1983;ii:1990.
15. Gill TJ III. Immunogenetics of spontaneous abortions in humans. Transplantation 1983;35:1.
16. Ahrons S. Leukocyte antibodies: occurrence in primigravidae. Tissue Antigens 1971;1:178.
17. Billington WD, Davies M. Maternal antibody to placental syncytiotrophoblast during pregnancy. In: Wegman TG, Gill TJ,

eds. Immunoregulation and fetal survival. New York: Oxford University Press, 1987:16.
18. van der Werf AJM. Are lymphocytotoxic iso-antibodies induced by the early human trophoblast? Lancet 1971;i:595.
19. Doughty RW, Gelsthorpe K. An initial investigation of lymphocyte antibody activity through pregnancy and in eluates prepared from placental material. Tissue Antigens 1974;4:291.
20. Gill TJ. Immunogenetic aspects of the maternal-fetal interactions. In: Wegmann TG, Gill TJ, eds. Immunobiology of reproduction. New York: Oxford University Press, 1983:55.
21. Mowbray SF, Gibbins C, Liddell H, et al. Controlled trial of treatment of recurrent spontaneous abortion by immunization with paternal cells. Lancet 1985;i:941.
22. Wattanasak K, Matangkasombut P. Specific human maternal lymphocyte cytotoxic effects on cord blood lymphocytes. In: Bratanov K, ed. Proceedings of Third International Symposium. Sofia, Bulgaria: Bulgarian Academy of Science, 1983:862.
23. Chardonnens X, Jeannet M. Lymphocyte mediated cytotoxicity and humoral antibodies in pregnancy. Int Arch Allergy Appl Immunol 1980;61:467.
24. Vanderbeeken Y, Vlieghe MP, Duchateau J, Delespesse G. Suppressor T lymphocytes in pregnancy. Am J Reprod Immunol 1984;5:20.
25. Taylor PV, Hancock KW. Antigenicity of trophoblast and possible antigen masking effects during pregnancy. Immunology 1975;28:973.
26. Timonen T, Saksela E. Cell-mediated anti-embryo cytotoxicity in human pregnancy. Clin Exp Immunol 1976;23:462.
27. Youtananukorn V, Matangkasombut P. Specific plasma factors blocking human maternal cell-mediated immune reactivity to placental antigens. Nature 1973;242:110.
28. Voisin GA. Immunological interventions of the placenta in maternal immunological tolerance to the fetus. In: Wegmann TG, Gill TJ, eds. Immunobiology of reproduction. New York: Oxford University Press, 1983:179.
29. Chaouat G, Voisin GA. Regulatory T cell subpopulations in pregnancy. I: evidence for suppressive activity of the early phase of MLR. J Immunol 1979;122:1383.
30. Sargent IL, Redman CWG, Stirrat GM. Maternal cell-mediated immunity in normal and pre-eclamptic pregnancy. Clin Exp Immunol 1982;50:601.
31. Moore MP, Sargent IL, Ting A, Redman CWG. Maternal cell-mediated immunity in pregnancy: lymphocyte responses of mothers and their non-pregnancy HLA-identical sisters to paternal HLA. Clin Exp Immunol 1983;54:91.
32. Herzenberg LA, Bianchi DW, Schroder J, Cann HM, Iverson GM. Fetal cells in the blood of pregnant women: detection and enrichment by fluorescence-activated cell sorting. Proc Natl Acad Sci USA 1979;76:1453.
33. Wegmann TG, Carlson GA. Allogeneic pregnancy as immunosorbent J Immunol 1977;119:1659.
34. Tongio MM, Mayer S. Transfer of HLA antibodies from mother to child. Transplantation 1975;20:163.
35. Zuckerman FA, Head JR. Possible mechanisms of nonrejection of the feto-placental allograft: trophoblast resistance to lysis by cellular immune effectors. Transplant Proc 1987;19:544.
36. Jenkinson EJ, Billington WD. Differential susceptibility of mouse trophoblast and embryonic tissue to immune cell lysis. Transplantation 1974;18:286.
37. Hellstrom KE, Hellstrom I. Lymphocyte-mediated cytotoxicity and blocking serum activity to tumor antigens. Adv Immunol 1974;18:209.
38. Hellstrom KE, Hellstrom I, Brawn J: Abrogation of cellular immunity to antigenically foreign mouse embryonic cells by a serum factor. Nature 1969;224:914.
39. Beer AE, Semprini AE, Xiaoyu Z, et al. Pregnancy outcome in human couples with recurrent spontaneous abortions: 1) HLA antigen profiles, 2) HLA antigen sharing; 3) female serum MLR blocking factors and 4) paternal leukocyte immunization. Exp Clin Immunogenet 1985;2:137.
40. Bissenden JG, Ling NR, Mackintosh P. Suppression of mixed lymphocyte reactions by pregnancy serum. Clin Exp Immunol 1980;39:195.
41. Faulk WP, Temple A, Lovins RE, Smith N. Antigens of human trophoblasts: a working hypothesis for their role in normal and abnormal pregnancies. Proc Natl Acad Sci USA 1978;75:1947.
42. Suciu-Foca N, Reed E, Rohowsky C, et al. Anti-idiotypic antibodies to anti-HLA receptors induced by pregnancy. Proc Natl Acad Sci USA 1983;80:830.
43. Burlingham WJ, Sparks EMF, Sondel PM, et al. Improved renal allograft survival following donor-specific transfusions. I: induction of antibodies that inhibit primary anti-donor MLC response. Transplantation 1985;39:12.
44. Takeuchi H, Sakagami K, Seki Y, et al. Anti-idiotypic antibodies and suppressor cells induced by DST in potential kidney transplant recipient. Transplant Proc 1985;17:1059.
45. Burlingham WJ, Sparks-Mackety EMF, Glass NR, et al. Induction of mixed lymphocyte culture-inhibitory antibodies by donor-specific transfusions plus azathioprine: heterogeneity of patient responses. Transplant Proc 1985;17:623.
46. Jerne NK. Towards a network theory of the immune system. Ann Inst Pasteur Immunol 1974;125C:373.
47. Power DA, Mason HJ, Stewart KN, et al. B-lymphocyte antibodies associated with successful pregnancy: evidence for MHC linkage. Transplant Proc 1983;15:890.
48. Rocklin RE, Kitzmiller JL, Carpenter CB, et al. Absence of an immunologic blocking factor from the serum of women with chronic abortion. N Engl J Med 1976;295:1209.
49. Rocklin RE, Kitzmiller JL, Garvoy MR. Further characterization of an immunologic blocking factor that develops during pregnancy. Clin Immunol Immunopathol 1982;22:305.
50. Stimson WH, Strachnan AF, Shepard A. Studies on the maternal immune response to placental antigens: absence of a blocking factor from the blood of abortion-prone women. Br J Obstet Gynaecol 1979;86:41.
51. Fizet D, Bousquet J. Absence of a factor blocking cellular cytotoxicity in the serum of women with recurrent abortion. Br J Obstet Gynaecol 1983;90:453.
52. Jonker M, van Leeuwen A, van Rood JJ. Inhibition of the mixed leukocyte reaction by alloantisera in man. II: incidence and characterization of MLC-inhibiting antisera from multiparous women. Tissue Antigens 1977;9:246.
53. Zak SJ, Good RA. Immunological studies of human serum gamma globulins. J Clin Invest 1959;38:579.
54. Holland NH, Holland P. Immunologic maturation in an infant of an agammaglobulinemic mother. Lancet 1966;ii:1152.
55, Kobayashi RH, Hyman CJ, Steihm ER. Immunologic maturation in an infant born to a mother with agammaglobulinemia. Am J Dis Child 1980;134:942.
56. Rodger JC. Lack of a requirement for a maternal humoral immune response to establish or maintain successful allogeneic pregnancy. Transplantation 1985;40:372.
57. Clark DA, Chapert A, Slapsys RM, et al. Suppressor cells in the uterus. In: Gill TJ III, Wegmann TG, eds. Immunoregulation and fetal survival. New York: Oxford University Press, 1987:63.
58. Clark DA. Host immunoregulatory mechanisms and the success of the conceptus fertilized in vivo and in vitro. In: Beard RW, Sharp F, eds. Early pregnancy loss. London: Springer-Verlag, 1988:215.
59. Brierley J, Clark DA. Characterization of hormone-dependent suppressor cells in the uteri of mated and pseudopregnant mice. J Reprod Immunol 1987;10:201.

60. Day S, Clark DA, Devlin MC, Jarrell J. Preliminary characterization of two types of suppressor cells in the human uterus. Fertil Steril 1985;44:778.
61. Brierley J, Clark DA. Identification of a trophoblast-independent hormone-regulated suppressor cell in the uterus of pregnant and pseudopregnant mice. Federation Proceedings 1985;44:1884.
62. Nagarkatti P, Clark DA. In vitro activity and in vivo correlates of alloantigen-specific murine suppressor T cells induced by allogeneic pregnancy. J Immunol 1983;131:638.
63. Slapsys RM, Beeson JH, Clark DA. The role of the trophoblast in the localization of decidua-associated suppressor cells. Am J Reprod Immunol 1984;6:66.
64. Lala PK, Kearns M, Parhar RS. Immunology of the decidual tissue. In: Gill TJ III, Wegmann TG, eds. Immunoregulation and fetal survival. New York: Oxford University Press, 1987:78.
65. Clark DA, Chaput A, Walker C, Rosenthal KL. Active suppression of host-versus-graft reaction in pregnant mice. VI: soluble suppressor activity obtained from decidua blocks the response to IL-2. J Immunol 1985;134:1659.
66. Clark DA, Falbo M, Rowley RB, Banwatt D, Stedronska-Clark J. Active suppression of host-versus-graft reaction in pregnant mice. IX: soluble suppressor activity obtained from allopregnant mouse decidua that blocks the response to interleukin 2 is related to TGF-beta. J Immunol 1988;141:3833.
67. Hunt JS, Manning LS, Mitchell D, et al. Localization and characterization of macrophages in murine uterus. J Leukoc Biol 1985;38:255.
68. Head JR, Gaede SD. Ia expression in the rat uterus. J Reprod Immunol 1986;9:137.
69. Bulmer JN, Johnson PM. Macrophage populations in the human placenta and amniochorion. Clin Exp Immunol 1984; 57:393.
70. Kearns M, Lala PK. Characterization of hematogenous cellular constituents of the murine decidua: a surface marker study. J Reprod Immunol 1985;8:213.
71. Bulmer JN, Sunderland CA. Immunohistological characterization of lymphoid cell populations in the early human placental bed. Immunology 1984;52:349.
72. Bulmer PN, Johnson PM, Bulmer D. Leukocyte populations in human decidua and endometrium. In: Gill TJ, Wegmann TG, eds. Immunoregulation and fetal survival. New York: Oxford University Press, 1987:111.
73. Beer AE, Scott JR, Billingham RE. Histoincompatibility and maternal immunologic status as determinants of fetoplacental weight and litter size in rodents. J Exp Med 1975;42:180.
74. Hings IM, Billingham RE. Maternal fetal immune interactions and the maintenance of major histocompatibility complex polymorphism in the rat. J Reprod Immunol 1985;7:337.
75. Michie D, Anderson NF. A strong selective effect associated with a histocompatibility gene in the rat. Ann NY Acad Sci 1966;192:88.
76. Hings IM, Billingham RE. Splenectomy and sensitization of Fischer female rats favors histoincompatibility of R2 backcross progeny. Transplant Proc 1981;13:1253.
77. Thomas ML, Harger JH, Wegener DK, et al. HLA sharing and spontaneous abortion. Am J Obstet Gynecol 1983;151:1053.
78. Beer AE, Quebbeman JF, Ayers JWT, Haines RF. Major histocompatibility complex antigens, maternal and paternal immune responses, and chronic habitual abortions in humans. Am J Obstet Gynecol 1981;141:987.
79. McIntyre JA, Faulk WP. Recurrent spontaneous abortion in human pregnancy: results of immunogenetical, cellular, and humoral studies. Am J Reprod Immunol 1983;4:165.
80. Ober CL, Hauck WW, Kostyu D, et al. Adverse effects of human leukocyte antigen-DR sharing on fertility: a cohort study in a human isolate. Fertil Steril 1985;44:227.
81. Athanassakis I, Bleackley RC, Paetkau V, Guilbert L, Barr PJ, Wegmann TG. The immunostimulatory effect of T cells and T cell lymphokines on murine fetally-derived placental cells. J Immunol 1987;18:37.
82. Clark DA, Chaouat G. What do we know about spontaneous abortion mechanisms? Am J Reprod Immunol Microbiol 1989;19:28.
83. Faulk WP, McIntyre JA. Immunological studies of human trophoblast: markers, subsets and functions. Immunol Rev 1983;75:139.
84. McIntyre JA, McConnachie PR, Taylor CG, Faulk WP. Clinical, immunologic and genetic definitions of primary and secondary recurrent spontaneous abortions. Fertil Steril 1984;42:849.
85. Beer AE. Immunologic aspects of normal pregnancy and recurrent spontaneous abortion. Seminars in Reproductive Endocrinology 1988;6:163.
86. Clark DA, Mowbray J, Underwood J, Lidell H. Histopathologic alterations in the decidua in human spontaneous abortion: loss of cells with large cytoplasmic granules. Am J Reprod Immunol 1987;13:19.
87. McIntyre JA, Faulk WP. Trophoblast antigens in normal and abnormal human pregnancy. Clin Obstet Gynecol 1986;29:976.
88. Frels WI, Rossant J, Chapman VM. Intrinsic and extrinsic factors affecting the development of hybrids between *Mus musculus* and *Mus caroli*. J Reprod Fertil 1980;59:387.
89. Clark DA, Slapsys RM, Croy BA, Rossant J. Suppressor cell activity in uterine decidua correlates with success or failure of murine pregnancy. J Immunol 1983;131:540.
90. Croy BA, Rossant J, Clark DA. Histological and immunological studies of post implantation death of *Mus caroli* embryos in the Mus musculus uterus. J Reprod Immunol 1982;4:277.
91. Rossant J, Croy BA. Properties of trophectoderm lineage in mouse development. In: Gill TJ III, Wegmann TG, eds. Immunoregulation and fetal survival. New York: Oxford University Press, 1987:156.
92. Clark DA, Chaput A, Tutton D. Active suppression of host-versus-graft reaction in pregnant mice. VII: spontaneous abortion of allogeneic CBA/J × DBA/2 fetuses in the uterus of CBA/J mice correlates with deficient non-T suppressor cell activity. J Immunol 1986;136:1668.
93. Clark DA, Head JR, Drake B, et al. Role of a factor related to transforming growth factor B_2 in successful pregnancy. In: Wegmann TG, Gill TJ, eds. Molecular biology of the fetomaternal interface. New York: Oxford University Press, 1989 (in press).
94. Clark DA, Damji N, Chaput A, Rosenthal KL, Brierley J. Decidua-associated suppressor cells and suppressor factors regulating interleukin 2: their role in the survival of the "fetal allograft." In: Cinader B, Miller RG, eds. Progress in immunology V. New York: Academic Press, 1986:1089.
95. de Fougerolles AR, Baines MG. Modulation of the natural killer cell activity in pregnant mice alters the spontaneous abortion rate. J Reprod Immunol 1987;11:147.
96. Opelz G, Terasaki PI. Dominant effect of transfusions on kidney graft survival. Transplantation 1980;29:153.
97. Sollinger HW, Burlinham WJ, Sparks EMF, et al. Donor-specific transfusions in unrelated and related HLA mismatched donor recipient combinations. Transplantation 1984;38:612.
98. Norman DJ, Barry JM, Fischer S. The beneficial effect of pretransplant third-party blood transfusions on allograft rejection in HLA identical sibling kidney transplants. Transplantation 1986;41:125.
99. Nagarkatti PS, Joseph S, Singal DP. Induction of antibodies by

blood transfusions capable of inhibiting responses in MLC. Transplantation 1983;37:695.

100. Singal DP, Fagnilli L, Joseph S. Blood transfusions induce anti-idiotypic antibodies in renal transplant patients. Transplant Proc 1983;15:1005.
101. MacLeod AM, Mason RJ, Stewart KN, et al. Fc-receptor blocking antibodies develop after blood transfusions and correlate with good graft outcome. Transplant Proc 1983;15:1019.
102. Leivestad T, Thorsby E. Effects of HLA-haploid identical blood transfusions on donor-specific immune responsiveness. Transplantation 1984;37:175.
103. Chaouat G, Clark DA, Wegmann TG. Genetic aspects of the CBA × DBA/2 and B10 × B10.A models of murine pregnancy failure and its prevention by lymphocyte immunization. In: Beard RW, Sharp F, eds. Early pregnancy loss. London: Springer-Verlag, 1988:89.
104. Chaouat G, Kolb JP, Riviere M, Chaffaux S. Local and systemic regulation of maternal antifetal cytotoxicity during murine pregnancy. In: Toder V, Beer AE, Karger S, eds. Gynaecology and obstetrics. Basel: S. Karger, 1985:55.
105. Clark DA. Local suppressor cells and the success or failure of the foetal allograft. Ann Inst Pasteur Immunol 1984;135:321.
106. Clark DA, Chaouat G, Guennet JL, Kiger N. Local active suppression and successful vaccination against spontaneous abortion in CBA/J mice. J Reprod Immunol 1987;10:79.
107. Taylor C, Faulk WP. Prevention of recurrent abortion with leukocyte transfusions. Lancet 1981;ii:68.
108. McIntyre JA, Faulk WP, Nichols-Johnson VR, et al. Immunologic testing and immunotherapy in recurrent spontaneous abortion. Obstet Gynecol 1986;67:169.
109. Unander AM, Linholm A. Transfusions of leukocyte-rich erythrocyte concentrates: a successful treatment in selected cases of habitual abortion. Am J Obstet Gynecol 1986;154:516.
110. Takakuwa K, Kanazawa K, Takeuchi S. Production of blocking antibodies by vaccination with husband's lymphocytes in unexplained recurrent aborters: the role in successful pregnancy. Am J Reprod Immunol Microbiol 1986;10:1.
111. Johnson PM, Chia KV, Risk JM. Immunological question marks in recurrent spontaneous abortion. In: Clark DA, Croy BA, eds. Reproductive immunology. New York: Elsevier, 1986:239.
112. Johnson PM, Chia KV, Hart CA, Griffith HB, Frances WJA. Trophoblast membrane infusion for unexplained recurrent miscarriage. Br J Obstet Gynaecol 1988;95:342.
113. Smith BJ, Cowchock FS. Immunological studies in recurrent spontaneous abortion: effects of immunization of women with paternal mononuclear cells on lymphocytotoxic and mixed lymphocyte reaction blocking antibodies and correlation with sharing of HLA and pregnancy outcome. J Reprod Immunol 1988;14:99.
114. Bonara P, Fabio G, Semprini M, et al. The autologous mixed lymphocyte reaction (MLR) in couples with recurrent abortions of unknown origin. Am J Reprod Immunol Microbiol 1985;7:136.
115. Stray-Pederson B, Stray-Pederson S. Etiologic factors and subsequent reproductive performance in 195 couples with a prior history of habitual abortion. Am J Obstet Gynecol 1984: 148:140.
115a. Ho HN, Gill TJ, Hsieh HJ, Jiang JJ, Lee TY, Hsieh CY. Immunotherapy for recurrent spontaneous abortions in a Chinese population. Am J Reprod Immunol 1991;25:10.
115b. Cauchi MN, Lim D, Young DE, Kloss M, Pepperell RJ. Treatment of recurrent aborters by immunization with paternal cells—controlled trial. Am J Reprod Immunol 1991;25:16.
116. Unander AM, Linholm A. Transfusions of leukocyte-rich erythrocytes concentrates: a successful treatment in selected cases of habitual abortion. Am J Obstet Gynecol 1986;154:516.
117. Branch DW, Ward K. Autoimmunity and pregnancy loss. Seminars in Reproductive Endocrinology 1989;7:168.
118. Harger JH, Archer DF, Marchese SG, et al. Etiology of recurrent pregnancy losses and outcome in subsequent pregnancies. Obstet Gynecol 1983;62:574.
119. Garcia-de la Torre I, Hernandez-Vazquez L, Angulo-Vazquez J, Romero-Ornelas A. Prevalence of antinuclear antibodies in patients with habitual abortion and in normal and toxemic patients. Rheumatol Int 1984;4:87.
120. Cowchock S, Dehoratius RD, Wapner RJ, Jackson LG. Subclinical autoimmune disease and unexplained abortion. Am J Obstet Gynecol 1984;150:367.
121. Rosenberg AM, Bingham MC, Fong K. Antinuclear antibodies during pregnancy. Obstet Gynecol 1986;68:560.
122. Branch DW. Immunologic disease and fetal death. Clin Obstet Gynecol 1987;30:295.
123. Scott JR, Rote NS, Branch DW. Immunologic aspects of recurrent abortion and fetal death. Obstet Gynecol 1987;70:645.
124. Branch DW. Clinical implications of antiphospholipid antibodies: the Utah experience. In: Harris EN, ed. Phospholipid binding antibodies. Boca Raton, FL: CRC Press, 1991:335.
125. Lockshin MD, Druzin ML, Qamar T. Prednisone does not prevent fetal death in women with antiphospholipid antibodies. Am J Obstet Gynecol 1989;160:439.
126. Digre KB, Durcan FJ, Branch DW, et al. Amaurosis fugax associated with antiphospholipid antibodies. Arch Neurol 1988; 25:228.
127. Harris EN. Syndrome of the black swan. Br J Rheumatol 1987;26:324.
128. Thornton JG, Foote GA, Page CE, et al. False positive results of tests for syphilis and outcome of pregnancy: a retrospective case-control study. Br J Med 1987;295:355.
129. Shapiro S, Thiagarajan P. Lupus anticoagulants. Prog Hemost Thromb 1982;6:263.
130. Branch DW, Rote NS, Dostal D, Scott JR. Association of lupus anticoagulant with antibody against phosphatidylserine. Clin Immunol Immunopathol 1987;42:63.
131. Thiagarajan P, Shapiro SS, DeMarco L. Monoclonal immunoglobulin M lambda coagulation inhibitor with phospholipid specificity: mechanism of a lupus anticoagulant. J Clin Invest 1980;66:397.
132. Pengo V, Thiagarajan P, Shapiro SS, Heine MJ. Immunological specificity and mechanism of action of IgG lupus anticoagulants. Blood 1987;70:69.
133. Kitchens CS. Prolonged activated partial thromboplastin time of unknown etiology: a prospective study of 100 consecutive cases referred for consultation. Am J Hematol 1988;27:38.
134. Triplett D, Exner T, Machin SJ, et al. Report of the lupus anticoagulant subcommittee. Presented at the Third International Symposium on Anti-phospholipid Antibodies. Kingston, Jamaica: January, 1988.
135. Rosove MH, Ismail M, Koziol BJ, et al. Lupus anticoagulant: improved diagnosis with kaolin clotting time using rabbit brain phospholipid in standard and high concentrations. Blood 1986;68:472.
136. Triplett DA, Brandt JT, Kaczor D, Schaeffer J. Laboratory diagnosis of lupus inhibitors: a comparison of the tissue thromboplastin inhibition procedure with a new platelet neutralization procedure. Am J Clin Pathol 1983;79:678.
137. Green D, Hougie FJ, Lechner K, et al. Report of the working party on acquired inhibitors of coagulation: studies of the "lupus" anticoagulant. Thromb Haemost 1983;49:144.
138. Brandt JT, Triplett DA, Musgrave K. The sensitivity of different

coagulation reagents to the presence of lupus anticoagulants. Arch Pathol Lab Med 1987;111:120.
139. Mannucci PM, Canciani MT, Mari D, Meucci P. The varied sensitivity of partial thromboplastin and prothrombin time reagents in the demonstration of the lupus-like anticoagulant. Scand J Haematol 1979;22:423.
140. Exner T. Richard KA, Kronenberg H. A sensitive test demonstrating lupus anticoagulant and its behavioral patterns. Br J Haematol 1978;40:143.
141. Alving BM, Baldwin PE, Richards RL, Jackson BJ. The dilute phospholipid APTT: a sensitive assay for verification of lupus anticoagulants. Thromb Haemost 1985;54:709.
142. Thiagarajan P, Pengo V, Shapiro SS. The use of the dilute Russell viper venom time for the diagnosis of lupus anticoagulants. Blood 1986;68:869.
143. Lockshin MD, Druzin ML, Goei S, et al. Antibody to cardiolipin as a predictor of fetal distress or death in pregnant patients with systemic lupus erythematosus. N Engl J Med 1985;313:152.
144. Triplett DA, Brandt JT, Musgrave KA, Orr CA. The relationship between lupus anticoagulants and antibodies to phospholipid. JAMA 1988;259:550.
145. Loizou S, McCrea JD, Rudge AC, et al. Measurement of anticardiolipin antibodies by an enzyme linked immunosorbent assay (ELISA): standardization and quantitation of results. Clin Exp Immunol 1985;62:738.
146. Harris EN, Gharavi AE, Patel SP, Hughes GRV. Evaluation of the anticardiolipin antibody test: report of a standardization workshop held April 4, 1986. Clin Exp Immunol 1987;68:215.
147. Branch DW, Rote NS, Li Y, Edwin S. Antiphospholipid antibodies: levels among women with the antiphospholipid antibody syndrome [abstract]. In: Proceedings of the 35th Annual Meeting, Society for Gynecologic Investigation, Atlanta, 1988:165.
148. Harris EN, Loizou S, Englert H, et al. Anticardiolipin antibodies and lupus anticoagulant. Lancet 1984;ii:1099.
149. Rauch J, Tannenbaum H, Senecal JL, et al. Polyfunctional properties of hybridoma lupus anticoagulant antibodies. J Rheumatol 1987;14:132.
150. Derue GJ, Englert HJ, Harris EN, et al. Fetal loss in systemic lupus in association with anti-cardiolipin antibodies. Obstet Gynecol 1985;5:207.
151. Feinstein DI, Rapaport SI. Acquired inhibitors of blood coagulation. In: Spaet TN, ed. Progress in hemostasis and thrombosis. New York: Grune and Stratton, 1972:75.
152. Harris EN, Gharavi AE, Hughes GRV. Anti-phospholipid antibodies. Clin Rheum Dis 1985;11:591.
153. Triplett DA, Brandt JT, Maas RL. The laboratory heterogeneity of lupus anticoagulants. Arch Pathol Lab Med 1985;109:946.
154. Lockwood C, Romero R, Costigan K, Hobbins J. The prevalence and significance of lupus anticoagulant and anticardiolipin antibodies in a general obstetric population [abstract]. In: Proceedings of the Eighth Annual Meeting, Society of Perinatal Obstetricians, Las Vegas, 1988:11.
155. Petri M, Golbus M, Anderson R, et al. Antinuclear antibody, lupus anticoagulant, and anticardiolipin antibody in women with idiopathic habitual abortion. A controlled, prospective study of 44 women. Arthritis Rheum 1987;30:601.
156. Howard MA, Firkin BG, Healy DL, Choong SCC. Lupus anticoagulant in women with multiple spontaneous miscarriage. Am J Hematol 1987;26:175.
157. Edelman P, Rouquette AM, Verdy E, et al. Autoimmunity, fetal losses, lupus anticoagulant: beginning of systemic lupus erythematosus or new autoimmune entity with gynaeco-obstetrical expression. Hum Reprod 1986;1:295.
158. Unander AM, Norberg R, Hahn L, Arfors L. Anticardiolipin antibodies and complement in 99 women with habitual abortion. Am J Obstet Gynecol 1985;156:114.
159. Wennerstrom H, Unander M, Norberg R, Haeger M. The occurrence of anti-cardiolipin antibodies among 337 women with habitual abortion and during normal pregnancy in 136 women [abstract]. In: Proceedings of the Fourth International Congress of Reproductive Immunology, Kiel, Germany, 1989:127.
160. DeWolf F, Carreras LO, Moerman P, et al. Decidual vasculopathy and extensive placental infarction in a patient with repeated thromboembolic accidents, recurrent fetal loss, and a lupus anticoagulant. Am J Obstet Gynecol 1982;142:829.
161. Nilsson IM, Astedt B, Hedner U, Berezin D. Intrauterine death and circulating anticoagulant, "antithromboplastin." Acta Med Scand 1975;197:153.
162. Garlund B. The lupus inhibitor in thromboembolic disease and intrauterine death in the absence of systemic lupus. Acta Med Scand 1984;215:293.
163. Lubbe WF, Butler WS, Palmer SJ, Liggins GC. Lupus anticoagulant in pregnancy. Br J Obstet Gynaecol 1984;91:357.
164. Branch DW, Dudley DJ, Mitchell MD, et al: IgG fractions from patients with antiphospholipid antibodies cause fetal death in Balb C mice: a model for autoimmune fetal loss. Am J Obstet Gynecol 1990;163:210.
165. Hanly JG, Gladman DD, Rose TH, et al. Lupus pregnancy. A prospective study of placental changes. Arthritis Rheum 1988;31:358.
166. Kitzmiller JL, Benirschke K. Immunofluorescent study of the placental bed vessels in pre-eclampsia of pregnancy. Am J Obstet Gynecol 1973;115:248.
167. Sheppard BL, Bonnar J. An ultrastructural study of the uteroplacental spiral arteries in hypertensive and normotensive pregnancy and fetal growth retardation. Br J Obstet Gynaecol 1981;88:695.
168. Carreras LO, Machin SJ, Defreyn G, et al. Arterial thrombosis, intrauterine death and "lupus" anticoagulant: detection of immunoglobulin interfering with prostacyclin formation. Lancet 1981;i:244.
169. Carreras LO, Vermylen J, Spitz B, Van Assche A. "Lupus" anticoagulant and inhibition of prostacyclin formation in patients with repeated abortion, intrauterine growth retardation and intrauterine death. Br J Obstet Gynaecol 1981;88:890.
170. Carreras LO, Vermylen JG. "Lupus" anticoagulant and thrombosis—possible role of inhibition of prostacyclin formation. Thromb Haemost 1982;48:38.
171. DeCastellarnau C, Vila L, Sancho MJ, et al. Lupus anticoagulant, recurrent abortion, and prostacyclin production by cultured smooth muscle cells. Lancet 1983;ii:1137.
172. Ros JO, Tarres MV, Baucells MV, et al. Prednisone and maternal lupus anticoagulant. Lancet 1983;ii:576.
173. Dudley DJ, Mitchell MD, Branch DW. Pathophysiology of antiphospholipid antibodies. Lack of effect on prostacyclin production on endothelial cells in culture. Presented at the Eighth Annual Meeting, American Gynecological and Obstetrical Society. Hot Springs, VA: September, 1989.
174. Marchesi D, Parbtani A, Frampton G, et al. Thrombotic tendency in systemic lupus erythematosus. Lancet 1981;i:719.
175. Harris EN, Asherson RA, Gharavi AE, et al. Thrombocytopenia in SLE and related disorders: association with anticardiolipin antibodies. Br J Haematol 1985;59:227.
176. Cosgriff TM, Martin BA. Low functional and high antigenic antithrombin III level in a patient with the lupus anticoagulant and recurrent thrombosis. Arthritis Rheum 1981;24:94.
177. Sanfelippo MJ, Drayna CJ. Prekallikrein inhibition associated with the lupus anticoagulant. A mechanism of thrombosis. Am J Clin Pathol 1982;77:275.
178. Cariou R, Tobelem G, Soria C, Caen J. Inhibition of protein C activation by endothelial cells in the presence of lupus anticoagulant. N Engl J Med 1986;314:1193.

179. Firkin BG, Hendrix L, Howard MA. Demonstration of a platelet bypass mechanism in the clotting system using an acquired anticoagulant. Am J Hematol 1978;5:81.
180. Howard MA, Firkin BG. Investigations of the lupus-like inhibitor bypassing activity of platelets. Thromb Haemost 1983; 50:775.
181. Zwaal RFA, Hemker HC. Blood cell membranes and haemostasis. Haemostasis 1982;11:12.
182. Freyssinet JM, Wiesel ML, Gauchy J, et al. An IgM lupus anticoagulant that neutralizes the enhancing effect of phospholipid on purified endothelial thrombomodulin activity—a mechanism for thrombosis. Thromb Haemost 1986;55:309.
183. Comp PC, DeBault LE, Esmon NL, Esmon CT. Human thrombomodulin is inhibited by IgG from two patients with nonspecific anticoagulants. Blood (Suppl) 1983;62:299a.
184. Freyssinet JM, Gauchy J, Cazemave JP. The effect of phospholipids on the activation of protein C by the human thrombin-thrombomodulin complex. Biochem J 1986;238:151.
185. Bertina RM, Broekmans AW, van der Linden IK, Mertens K. Protein C deficiency in a Dutch family with thrombotic disease. Thromb Haemost 1982;48:15.
186. Broekmans AW, Veltkamp JJ, Bertina RM. Congenital protein C deficiency and venous thromboembolism. A study of three Dutch families. N Engl J Med 1983;309:340.
187. Brenner B, Shapira A, Bahari C, et al. Hereditary protein C deficiency during pregnancy. Am J Obstet Gynecol 1987;157:1160.
188. Lubbe WF, Palmer SJ, Butler WS, et al. Fetal survival after prednisone suppression of maternal lupus anticoagulant. Lancet 1983;i:1361.
189. Branch DW, Kochenour NK, Scott JR, Hershgold E: Obstetric complications associated with lupus anticoagulant. N Engl J Med 1985;313:1322.
190. Faden D, Tincani A, Balestrieri G, et al. Pregnancy outcome and anti-phospholipid antibodies in systemic lupus [abstract]. Clin Exp Rheumatol 1988;6:202.
191. De Carolis S, Caruso A, Valesini A, et al. Anticardiolipin antibodies in pregnant women with systemic lupus erythematosus or lupus anticoagulant [abstract]. Clin Exp Rheumatol 1988; 6:201.
192. Lockwood CJ, Reece EA, Romero R, Hobbins JC. Antiphospholipid antibody and pregnancy wastage. Lancet 1986;ii:742.
193. Derksen RHWM, Brunise HW, Christiaens CCML, et al. A controlled clinical trial on the efficacy of medicamentous treatment of pregnancy patients with antiphospholipid antibodies — a preliminary report [abstract]. Clin Exp Rheumatol 1988;6:202.
194. Englert HJ, Derue GM, Loizou S, et al. Pregnancy and lupus: prognostic indicators and response to treatment. Q J Med 1988;66:125.
195. Hahn L, Norberg A, Stigendal L, et al. The anti-phospholipid antibody syndrome and pregnancy outcome — Swedish experiences [abstract]. Clin Exp Rheumatol 1988;6:204.
196. Quinn MJ, McHugh NJ, Barge A, et al. Persistent fetal loss (and venous thrombosis) in women with anticardiolipin antibodies receiving prednisone and aspirin [abstract]. Clin Exp Rheumatol 1988;6:211.
197. Lubbe WF, Liggins GC. Role of lupus anticoagulant and autoimmunity in recurrent pregnancy loss. Seminars in Reproductive Endocrinology 1988;6:181.
198. Rosove MH, Tabsh K, Wasserstrum N, et al. Heparin therapy for pregnant women with lupus anticoagulant or anticardiolipin antibodies. Obstet Gynecol 1990;75:630.
199. Cowchock FS, Reece EA, Balaban D, Branch DW, Plouffe L. Repeated fetal losses associated with antiphospholipid antibodies: a collaborative randomized trial comparing prednisone to low-dose heparin treatment. Am J Obstet Gynecol (in press).
200. Scott JR, Branch DW, Kochenour NK, Ward K: Intravenous globulin treatment of pregnant patients with recurrent pregnancy loss due to antiphospholipid antibodies and Rh immunization. Am J Obstet Gynecol 1988;159:1055.

17

CHAPTER

ECTOPIC AND HETEROTOPIC PREGNANCIES

Nicholas Kadar

Ectopic pregnancy (EP) has been the subject of intense clinical and epidemiological research in recent years, so much so that it is no longer possible to cover all aspects of these developments in the space of a single chapter. Therefore, we shall restrict our attention largely to the diagnosis and treatment of tubal pregnancies, because these are of most interest to clinicians.

Recent research into the epidemiology, etiology, and pathophysiology of EPs has raised larger issues. The incidence of this disease has increased two- to threefold throughout the industrialized world over the last 25 years.[1–6] Despite the fact that the risk of dying from an EP has fallen dramatically during the same period (from 35.2 to 5.3 per 10,000 cases during 1970–1983),[7] it has not fallen by as much as the risk of dying from other pregnancy-related causes. Consequently, the proportion of pregnancy-related deaths due to EP has doubled. EP is now the most common cause of maternal death among non-Caucasian women in the United States (accounting for almost 20% of the total). Regardless of race, it is the most common cause of death during the first 20 weeks of pregnancy. The risk of death from an EP is 10 times higher than that for childbirth and 50 times higher than that for induced abortion. About 50 women are estimated to die each year from EP in the United States, and two thirds of the deaths are still considered preventable. Overall, black women are three times more likely to die from EP than white women, and the relative risk is even higher for teenagers and women aged 35–44.[7]

ETIOLOGY

Because the rate of induced abortions and the number of women using intrauterine contraceptive devices (IUD) or undergoing sterilizations have all increased steadily during this same period, there has been some concern that the increase in the EP rate may be attributable, at least to some extent, to these factors. Fortunately, however, this concern has been shown to be largely unfounded.[8–11]

Past uncertainty about the risk of EP following induced abortions can be attributed to the effect of confounding variables, notably infection. In none of the controlled studies reported from the United States has a significant association been found between induced abortion and an increased risk of EP after confounding variables have been adjusted for.[11,12] Although many investigators still attribute a sizable portion of the rising incidence of EP to the use of IUDs[3] and, to a lesser extent, the minipill and sterilizations, none of the case-control studies published to date supports this suggestion.[8,9] Indeed, evidence that use of an IUD in fact protects women against EP has been available since 1970.[12]

If a woman who has been sterilized or who is a current user of the IUD or minipill becomes pregnant, her risk of having an EP is increased at least sevenfold,[3,12] but this occurs simply because these methods of contraception provide greater protection against intrauterine pregnancies than tubal pregnancies. The absolute risk of having an EP is in fact *lower* for women using one of these methods of contraception than it is for women who are not using any contraception.[8,9] Of all the interval methods of contraception studied,[8,9] the combined birth control pill (BCP) gave the highest protection against an EP (ninefold), and in the WHO study its protective effect was found to be equal to the protection afforded by sterilization.[9] Therefore, women who switch from a BCP to some other method of contraception would incur an increased risk of EP, and changing contraceptive practices could theoretically account for some of the recent rise in EP rates. There is, however, no evidence that this has happened. Although the number of married women using BCPs in the United States during 1973–1982 decreased by half, the number of sterilizations almost doubled, and the proportion of women using other methods of contraception remained constant.[7]

Although the minipill does not increase the absolute rate of EP, progesterone-bearing devices seem to do so, and there is further evidence to suggest that this is a dose-related effect. Devices that release progesterone at a rate of 25 or 65 μg/day, or levonorgestrel at 2 ug/day predispose to EP, whereas devices that release norgestrel at a rate of 20 μg/day do not.[13]

Pharmacologic doses of estrogens may also increase the risk of EP, because if postcoital contraception with diethylstilbestrol fails, 10% of the resulting pregnancies are ectopic.[14] A possible related finding is the apparent increase in the risk of EP among women who become pregnant after ovulation induction with Pergonal.[15,16] The risk of EP in this setting is related to hyperstimulation and high estrogen levels, but whether the critical factor is the high estrogen concentration in the plasma or the fact that multiple follicles were ovulated is a matter for speculation.

It is widely assumed that these pharmacologic effects of estrogen and progesterone are mediated through altered tubal transport. Direct evidence in humans is lacking, even though electrical activity along the human oviduct has recently been studied during different phases of the menstrual cycle and in cases of tubal pregnancy.[17,18] It is entirely possible that pharmacologic doses of estrogen or progesterone alter the implantation process by an effect on the zygote or the tubal epithelium or both. Whether nonpharmacologically induced hormonal imbalances can affect the oviduct or the process of implantation in a similar way, and so be a common cause of EP, is totally conjectural at this time.

Thus, although many theories have been advanced to explain the occurrence of tubal pregnancies, and several recent case-control studies have established an association between EP and a number of factors such as smoking,[19] douching,[20] and spontaneous abortions,[21] the only firmly established, noniatrogenic cause of EP is pelvic inflammatory disease (PID), and the consensus is that the rising incidence of PID probably accounts for much of the recent rise in the incidence of EP.[22] Cohort studies from Scandinavia have established conclusively that women who have laparoscopically proven PID are seven to 10 times more likely to have an EP than controls. EP rates for women who have had and who have never had PID have been estimated to be approximately 0.27 and 2.7 per 100 women years, respectively.[3] If one assumes that there are 500,000 first cases of PID annually in the United States (a conservative figure in the opinion of experts), then, based on the preceding figures, this cohort of women can be expected to contribute 13,500 cases of EP the first year they try to conceive, and a total of almost 27,000 EPs if on average they try to conceive twice, which is two thirds of the 1977 annual total of EPs in the United States.[22]

Although some epidemiological data show parallel increases in the rates of EP, PID, and sexually transmitted diseases,[4] the temporal relationship between the rising EP and PID rates is far from obvious.[22] In the United States, for example, no temporal correlation was found during the 1970s between hospitalization rates for PID and the incidence of EP in different segments of the population.[23] It is well established that gross pathologic or histologic evidence of PID cannot be found in at least 50% of EPs.[22] More recently, it has been shown that women with an EP are more likely than normal pregnant controls to be seropositive for antichlamydia IgG antibodies and to have higher mean titers, but at least a third of women with EPs are antibody negative.[24] The suggestion that many histologically normal tubes may still have sustained structural damage from previous infection remains unproven,[25] so the etiology of EP is clearly both multifactorial and uncertain in many cases. Some of the mechanisms that have been forwarded to explain the occurrence of tubal pregnancies in humans are listed in Figure 17-1, and a fuller discussion of these is available elsewhere.[26]

PATHOPHYSIOLOGY

Normal implantation is a process that lasts about a week. Very little is known about how this process operates at the cellular level or how it is regulated in humans. Whether the mechanisms of normal and extrauterine implantations are similar is not known, but Randall and coworkers found that the development of the placenta as seen in intrauterine pregnancies was replicated almost exactly in tubal gestations (see also Chapters 4 and 5).[27]

Budowick and colleagues were the first authors in recent years to describe in detail the behavior of the trophoblast in tubal pregnancies.[28] They stated that after implanting on the surface of the tubal mucosa, the trophoblast rapidly invades the lamina propria and tubal musculature. The pregnancy then grows in the potential space that exists between the outer wall of the fallopian tube and the overlying peritoneum. Growth of the conceptus at this extraperitoneal site occurs both in a direction parallel to the long axis of the tube and circumferentially. Tubal rupture actually entails rupture of the peritoneum overlying the tube. The authors pointed out that the peritoneum was more adherent at the isthmic portion of the tube than at the ampulla, which might explain the propensity of isthmic pregnancies to rupture.

Budowick and associates based their description on a retrospective review of 242 cases and dissection of 20 current cases of EP.[28] The authors described only one pattern of growth that, they implied, occurred in most tubal pregnancies. However, they neither gave quantitative information nor described the pattern of growth in those tubal pregnancies that had not developed in the previously mentioned way. Despite the discursive nature of their report, the authors deserve great credit

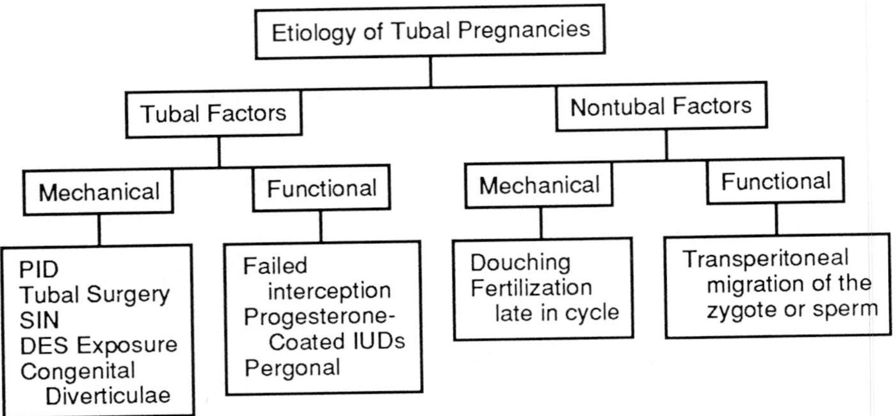

FIGURE 17–1. Etiology of tubal pregnancies.

for stimulating a new avenue of inquiry into the differences that might exist among pregnancies that implant in different portions of the oviduct and between those that rupture and those that do not.

In a planned, prospective study, Pauerstein and coworkers examined 25 consecutive fresh specimens under the dissecting microscope, and made scale drawings based on three-dimensional observations of their specimens.[29] Carefully marked step sections were also taken for histologic examination. They found that the pattern of growth described by Budowick and colleagues[28] (extraluminal) was present in only six cases. In 15 cases the growth of the pregnancy was predominantly intraluminal, and three cases manifested a mixed pattern of growth. There was an apparent association between the pattern of growth and the propensity to tubal rupture in that tubal rupture occurred in five out of six cases exhibiting extraluminal growth, but in only three out of 15 cases manifesting intraluminal growth.

In a more recent, but partly retrospective, study, Senterman and coworkers took these investigations a step further and attempted to determine whether there was a correlation between the pattern of trophoblastic growth and the site of the tubal pregnancy or the extent of tubal damage.[30] The authors examined 84 ampullary and seven isthmic pregnancies. Intraluminal growth was found to be uncommon in isthmic pregnancies (one out of seven) but to be the most common pattern in ampullary pregnancies (47 out of 84). Conversely, extraluminal growth was uncommon in ampullary pregnancies (six out of 84) but occurred in three out of seven isthmic pregnancies. A mixed trophoblastic growth pattern was present in roughly 40% of both ampullary (31 out of 84) and isthmic (three out of seven) pregnancies. Surprisingly, and contrary to the findings of Pauerstein and associates,[29] a purely extraluminal growth pattern was associated neither with tubal rupture nor with extensive tubal damage. In fact, tubal damage was least extensive when the trophoblast grew at an extraluminal site, and a mixed growth pattern produced the most extensive damage. In contrast to the observations of Budowick and coworkers,[28] these findings did not provide a compelling theoretical basis for treating isthmic pregnancies by segmental tubal resection rather than by linear salpingostomy, a matter that will be discussed more fully later in this chapter.

MANAGEMENT OF SUSPECTED ECTOPIC PREGNANCIES

The cardinal symptoms and signs associated with EP are well known and bear no repetition.[22] The clinical presentation of patients with EP falls into two more or less distinct categories. The minority (about 10%) present with a surgical abdomen and symptoms and signs of hypovolemia, if not frank shock. They present no diagnostic problem, require no special investigations, and need immediate laparoscopy or laparotomy. In most patients, however, the diagnosis is far less clearcut and immediate surgery is not mandatory. In some of these cases, the symptoms and signs will be, of course, much more suggestive of an EP than in others, but the gynecologist must accept that in the absence of shock or symptoms identical to that experienced in a previous pregnancy, EP cannot be reliably distinguished from other disorders on clinical grounds.[31] Past experience has repeatedly taught that unless all women of childbearing age who have lower abdominal pain or abnormal vaginal bleeding are suspected of having an ectopic pregnancy until proved otherwise, the diagnosis will often be missed initially and treatment will be delayed, often by more than a week. Furthermore, it is as imperative to exclude the diagnosis when the prior probability of an EP is felt on clinical grounds to be only, for example, 10%, as it is to exclude it when the probability of an EP is felt to be much higher. That is not to say that the history and physical examination are unimportant or that the identification of risk factors is merely an academic exercise. Women who have had a previous EP, tubal surgery, or sterilization, or who are current users of an IUD or the minipill, are at high risk of developing an EP if they become pregnant, and so they should be carefully investigated when they conceive, even if they are asymptomatic, to ensure that the pregnancy is intrauterine.

DIAGNOSTIC STUDIES

The literature pertaining to the diagnostic work-up of clinically stable women with suspected EP has become very large and to some extent conflicting and continues to grow as new methodologies become available. It is difficult, for a number of reasons, to interpret some of these data and to assess the relative utility of the various tests that have been proposed. Few of the diagnostic criteria or algorithms have been tested prospectively in centers other than those where they were originally defined, and some of the techniques (eg, serum or urinary progesterone measurements, endovaginal sonography) are so recent that there has been little opportunity yet to assess their utility prospectively. Another difficulty stems from the fact that many of the diagnostic criteria that have been suggested are not independent of each other. Consequently, it is impossible in many cases to determine precisely which criterion was central to reaching a diagnosis or whether the working diagnosis was changed by the addition of subsidiary criteria. It is not possible at this time for the clinician to establish an optimal algorithm for the work-up of women with suspected EPs. Nonetheless, it is possible to define the principles on which any diagnostic evaluation should be based and those that will serve as a logical framework for any future diagnostic algorithm, regardless of new developments.

LAPAROSCOPY AND CULDOCENTESIS

The first major advance in the diagnosis of EP was the introduction of laparoscopy, which enabled gynecologists to confidently exclude a diagnosis of EP without a laparotomy and which still represents the final decisive diagnostic test, short of laparotomy, today. Indispensable though it has been, laparoscopy is clearly not an ideal diagnostic technique, because besides requiring general anesthesia, it has potentially serious complications, even if they are uncommon. Also, to exclude an EP both tubes must be visible in their entirety. This may be impossible in women who have chronic PID, and a laparotomy will be required. Laparotomy is also required when laparoscopy is unsuccessful, and the laparoscopic appearances of the fallopian tube occasionally may mislead the gynecologist. For example, in a recent audit the author found that 67 out of 99 cases of suspected EP were subjected to a potentially avoidable laparoscopy because a sensitive pregnancy test had not been used. A laparotomy was required in 13 out of 67 cases either because laparoscopy was unsuccessful or because the pelvic organs could not be properly inspected, and in two cases part or all of a single remaining fallopian tube was removed because it was thought to contain, but did not in fact contain, an EP (Kadar, unpublished observations). Esposito has reported a similar experience.[32]

Two facts about women with a suspected EP largely govern how these patients should be investigated.[33–45] First, if a suitably high index of suspicion for the diagnosis is exercised, about 70% to 80% of patients investigated for a suspected EP will not have an EP. It follows immediately that a test that can reliably exclude a diagnosis of EP will be the most cost effective and should be administered first. Second, most women who are suspected of having, but who do not have, an EP are not pregnant at all. Consequently, a sensitive pregnancy test is the most cost effective and useful test in emergency gynecology, because by demonstrating that a pregnancy is not present, a diagnosis of EP can be excluded (in most cases) on the basis of a single test. At the present time, laparoscopy is the only available diagnostic test that enables one to exclude a diagnosis of EP reliably on the basis of a negative result. This is why culdocentesis, for example, is less useful in practice than some of the statistics cited about this procedure might suggest.

Culdocentesis has been found to be positive in about 80% of women with EP (although the figure is likely to fall as the diagnosis is made earlier).[46,47] In the remaining 20% of cases the result is nondiagnostic (dry tap). We have found that a hemoperitoneum was present in 75% of EPs associated with a nondiagnostic culdocentesis, and in 25% of these cases the fallopian tube had ruptured.[47] Therefore, clearly, a nondiagnostic finding cannot be used to reduce one's index of suspicion for the diagnosis. If one assumes that one third of the women with suspected EPs will have an EP (a relatively high figure), it follows from the preceding observations that if all women with suspected EPs are subjected to a culdocentesis, only about one fourth of the results will be positive. In most of the remaining 75% of cases of suspected EP, the result will be nondiagnostic, because negative results, though reliable, are uncommon.[46,47] Therefore, culdocentesis cannot be used to exclude a diagnosis of EP, and the test alters management only in that if the result is positive, further testing is not required. As only about one fourth of the women suspected of having an EP will have a positive culdocentesis and consequently have their management altered by the test, the place for this most unpleasant procedure is dwindling except where facilities for pregnancy testing and ultrasound are very limited.

PREGNANCY TESTS

Rapid and specific radioimmunoassays (RIA) for human chorionic gonadotropin (hCG) have been commercially available for about a decade. The need for a gamma counter and specially trained laboratory staff made the test relatively expensive for occasional use, and unavailable out of normal working hours. These last remaining obstacles to the routine use of sensitive pregnancy testing in all cases of suspected ectopic pregnancy have been removed by the development of enzyme-linked immunosorbent assays (ELISA).[37,38] In vitro, these assays are as sensitive as rapid RIAs, but no laboratory experience is required to perform them reliably.

The ELISA is based on the sandwich principle. Two monoclonal antibodies to hCG are used that recognize different epitopes on the molecule. One is bound to some solid phase such as filter paper, latex beads, or the side of a test tube; the other antibody is bound to an enzyme (Fig. 17-2). The specimen to be tested (urine or, in some cases, blood) is added to the solid phase and any hCG present is bound to the antibody. After washing, the second, enzyme-linked, antibody is added. This will only be bound to the solid phase if hCG is present. Finally, a suitable reagent is added that changes color when exposed to the enzyme. Thus, the color change is observed only if hCG has been bound by the first antibody (ie, if the woman is pregnant). The commercially available tests are qualitative, but quantitative ELISAs have been developed based on the spectrophotometric quantification of the color change.

A negative result of an RIA or ELISA is reliable, because if an EP is present, the tests will almost always be positive. Early reports on RIAs from Scandinavia cited false-negative rates (FNR) of 3% to 5%,[34,35,48] but the FNR has been far lower in almost all other series, ranging from 0 to less than 2%.[36] For example, recently we found that three out of 184 cases of EP were associated with hCG levels below the sensitivity of most ELISAs (<40 mIU/mL).[49] Also, most EPs that are associated with a negative hCG assay are destined for resorption, making serious hemorrhagic complications very unlikely.[35,50] Nonetheless, a few cases of ruptured tubal pregnancies have been reported in which an hCG assay was negative.[51] It appears that in some ectopic pregnancies there is a genuine defect in beta-hCG synthesis, and hCG simply is not produced.[52] Another theoretical concern about ELISAs is that only about 20% of hCG is in fact excreted in the urine, so that a serum hCG level of, for example, 80 mIU/mL, may be associated with urinary hCG levels below the sensitivity of the ELISA. The fact that urine is almost always more concentrated than blood compensates for this, and the available reports indicate that detection of hCG in urine is as good as measurement in serum.[53]

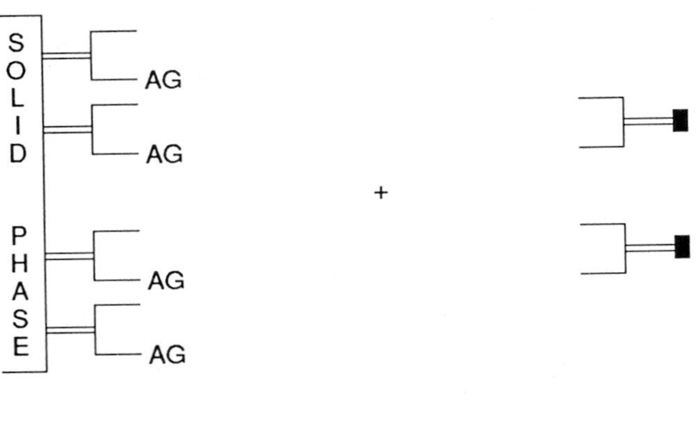

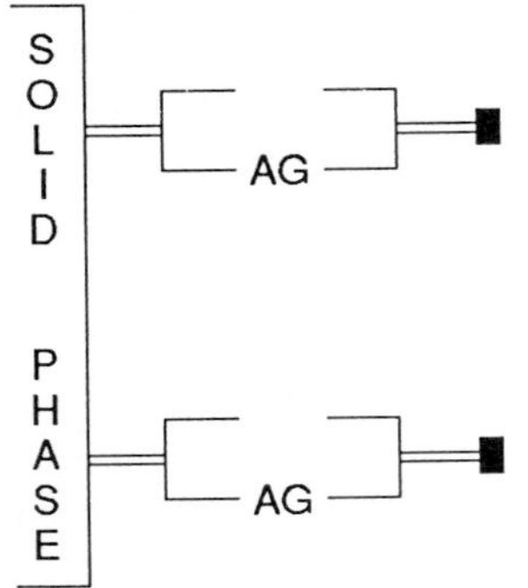

FIGURE 17–2. Two-site enzyme-linked immunosorbent assay (ELISA). AG, antigen; ■, enzyme.

ULTRASOUND

If a patient with a suspected ectopic pregnancy has a positive pregnancy test but does not have an EP, she will have an intrauterine pregnancy (IUP), or a threatened, missed, or complete abortion. In these patients ultrasound has its greatest value. In the absence of a positive pregnancy test, ultrasound is not helpful unless fetal heart activity (FHA) is detected inside or outside the uterus, which is uncommon.[37–45] Although the proportion of cases in which an ectopic fetus can be imaged has increased with the use of higher-resolution sonographic equipment such as the vaginal transducer, it is still not high enough to enable one to exclude an EP on the basis of a negative finding. For example, DeCrespigny reported a FNR of 19% and a FPR of 6.5% when endovaginal sonography alone was used to evaluate women with suspected EP, even though criteria much less specific for eccyesis than the imaging of an ectopic fetus or gestational sac were accepted in making a presumptive diagnosis of EP.[54] Therefore, ultrasound should be reserved for cases in which the pregnancy test is positive, and not used as a primary diagnostic test.[37–45,55–60]

INTRAUTERINE FINDINGS

The purpose of ultrasound in women with positive pregnancy tests is to try to localize the pregnancy, but usually the diagnosis of EP is still only presumptive, because in at least 80% of cases an ectopic fetus cannot be imaged even with transvaginal (TV) sonography.[44,54] Because simultaneous IUP and EP (heterotropic pregnancies) are uncommon, the presence of an IUP is taken to exclude an EP, and if an IUP cannot be detected, this is taken as presumptive evidence of an EP. Unfortunately, the situation is not so simple, for two reasons.

First, a pregnancy can be detected by a sensitive

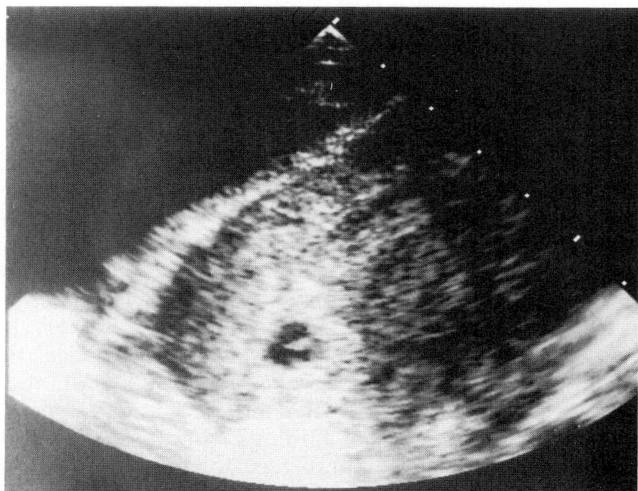

FIGURE 17–3. Gestational sac containing fetal parts.

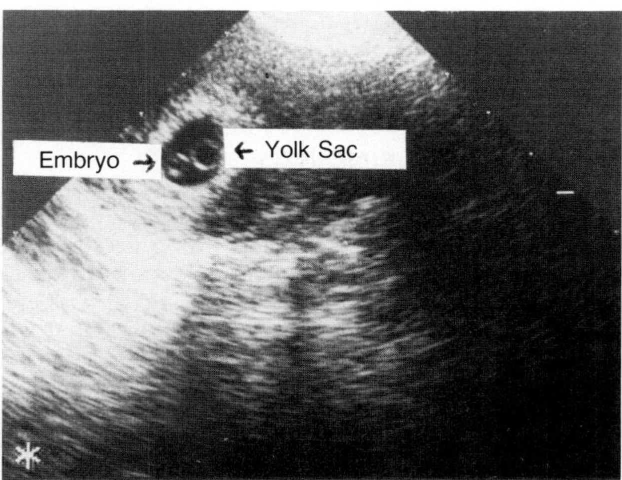

FIGURE 17–4. Gestational sac with a demonstrable yolk sac and embryo.

pregnancy test up to 2 weeks before it can be imaged by ultrasound. Therefore, failure to detect an IUP when an ultrasound test is positive does not necessarily mean that an early IUP is not present. A major advantage of endovaginal sonography is that IUPs can be detected much earlier, and the time period during which a pregnancy can be detected but cannot be localized has been greatly shortened.[55–58]

Second, sonographically detectable intrauterine "sacs" can be present in EPs (pseudogestational sac). (Blood in the endometrial cavity and a strong decidual reaction presumably give rise to this image.) One cannot automatically equate an intrauterine sac with an IUP. The demonstration of FHA or fetal products within the sac provides conclusive evidence that an IUP is present (Fig. 17-3). An equally reliable, but earlier, indicator of an IUP is the demonstration of the (secondary) yolk sac within an intrauterine sac (Fig. 17-4). In some cases, it is also possible to image the decidua capsularis and parietalis of an IUP, in which case the gestational sac has a double-walled appearance (Fig. 17-5). This so-called double ring sign can be detected in 30% of pseudogestational sacs[59] and is, therefore, not a reliable indicator of an IUP. With the use of TV sonography, a confident diagnosis of an IUP can be made. Hence EP can be excluded much earlier than by trans-

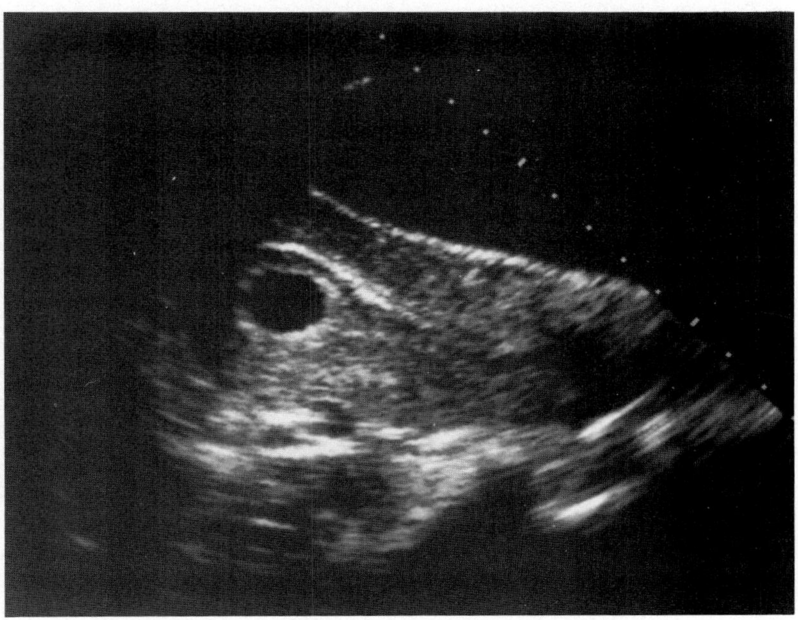

FIGURE 17–5. Gestational sac with double-ring image or sign.

abdominal (TA) ultrasound, because the yolk sac, fetus, or fetal cardiac activity can frequently be identified prior to their detection by TA ultrasound.

EXTRAUTERINE FINDINGS

The sonographic features of the adnexa or pouch of Douglas (POD) may also provide strong presumptive evidence for an EP, even if the findings are not specific for that condition.[60,61] One should look for a mass and fluid but must distinguish between masses that are purely cystic and those that have mixed echogenicity. In the presence of a positive hCG assay, a complex mass in the adnexa or POD is about 80% predictive of an EP, and the figure rises to about 95% if fluid is also present. Up to 50% of women with EP will have these findings, which are an indication for laparoscopy. A simple cyst or a small amount of fluid is no more predictive of an EP than a completely normal scan and should be regarded as nondiagnostic findings. When moderate to large amounts of fluid are present in isolation, as indicated by extension of the fluid collection in the POD to the adnexa or even the paracolic gutters,[60] the probability of an EP is increased. Theoretically, culdocentesis should be particularly useful in this situation,[61] but in practice large fluid collections are almost always associated with a mass.

It has become apparent in recent years that TV sonography is superior to TA ultrasound for the evaluation of women with suspected EPs and positive pregnancy tests. Most of the benefit accrues from the fact that normal and abnormal IUPs are detectable earlier when endovaginal sonography is used.[55–58] A positive diagnosis of EP can also be made more often (by imaging ectopic FHA or a fetus) by TV ultrasound, but this is still only possible in about 20% of cases. This should not be surprising, however, since it has been recognized for many years that a fetus is not identifiable pathologically in the majority of women with tubal pregnancies.[62] Among the other advantages of TV sonography are a much better image quality and the more frequent detection of adnexal masses, "sacs," and cul-de-sac fluid. As a result, the proportion of "nondiagnostic" studies in women with positive pregnancy tests, and hence the need for further testing, has been reduced. It should, however, be pointed out that the predictive values of the less specific adnexal findings, such as a complex mass with or without fluid, has not been specifically determined, and it is possible that the increased sensitivity of transvaginal sonography may prove to be a double-edged sword (Fig. 17-6*A* and *B*).

POSITIVE hCG ASSAYS AND NONDIAGNOSTIC SONAR FINDINGS

In approximately 20% of women with a suspected EP and positive pregnancy tests, ultrasound will be nondiagnostic; that is, an IUP cannot be demonstrated, and the extrauterine findings do not provide presumptive evidence of an EP. The management of these patients has reached a high level of sophistication in some centers and involves the use of a quantitative hCG as-

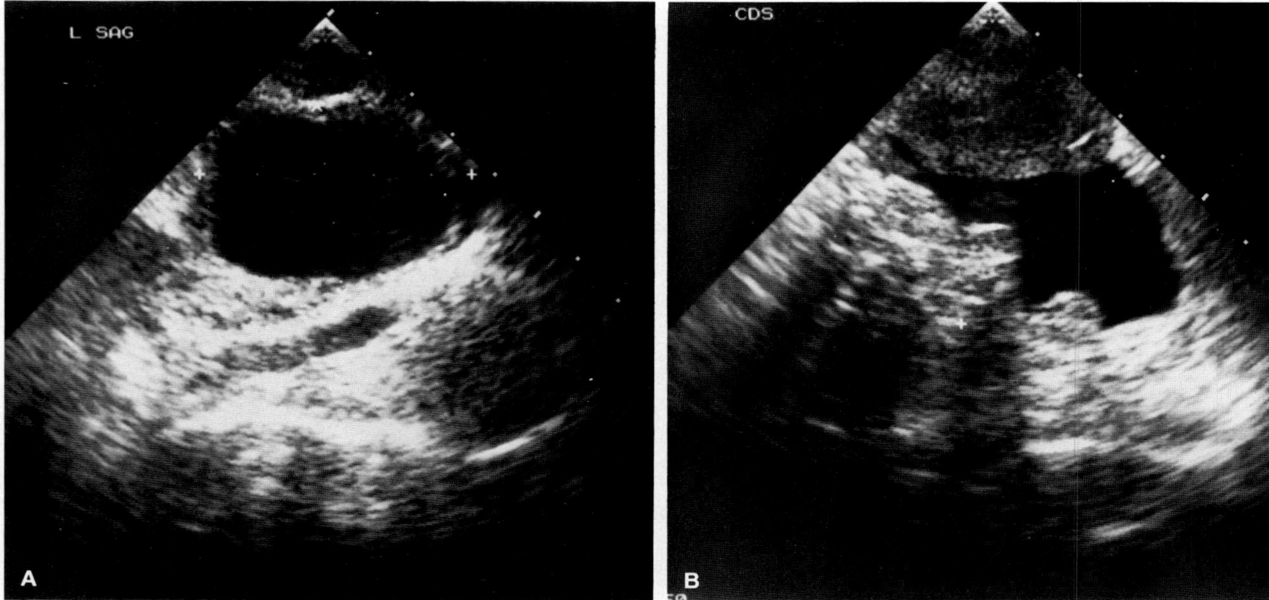

FIGURE 17–6. (A, B). Endovaginal sonograms showing an adnexal cyst with internal echoes and a large fluid collection in the cul-de-sac. The serum hCG was 571 mIU/mL (2nd-IS). Laparoscopy revealed no ectopic pregnancy, and the patient subsequently had a demonstrable intrauterine pregnancy.

say and serial hCG testing in some patients, as discussed later in this chapter.[63–66] However, this approach, which was first described by the author, may be either inappropriate to use or not cost effective in small centers with limited personnel in which only about 15–20 EPs are treated annually. The available alternative strategies are to laparoscope all women with positive hCG assays in which an intrauterine sac cannot be detected or to follow the women clinically and to repeat the scan in about a week.

In most of these patients the symptoms and signs present are not prominent and therefore do not help the gynecologist to choose between these two courses of action. If factors that place women at a high risk of having an EP can be identified (prior EP, tubal surgery, sterilization, or current use of IUD or minipill), then laparoscopy is probably the safest option. In the absence of high-risk factors the best strategy is to repeat the scan in about a week unless the symptoms change. If the repeat scan still reveals nothing specific, one will usually be dealing with a patient whose symptoms have abated (except perhaps for a slight amount of vaginal bleeding) and who has had a complete or missed abortion that will probably not require therapeutic curettage. The temptation to curette the uterus in this situation in the hope of securing a definite diagnosis usually should be resisted, as this strategy often confuses rather than clarifies the clinical picture, since villi may not be recovered if the pregnancy is already resorbing. The diagnostic approach based on an ELISA and ultrasound is summarized in Figure 17-7.

PROGESTERONE ASSAYS

An alternative method of evaluating women with nondiagnostic sonar findings (or indeed women with a positive pregnancy test prior to the performance of an ultrasound) may be to measure the serum progesterone with a rapid, direct RIA, or its urinary metabolite (pregnanediol-3-glucuronide) by an immunometric assay. Milwidsky and coworkers were the first to show that the EP is associated with a lower serum progesterone level than exists in IUP of the same gestational age.[67] However, the competitive binding assay used by these investigators was much too laborious to be of clinical use, and the results were unreliable for diagnostic purposes, as there was too much overlap in the serum hCG values between EPs and IUPs. Subsequently, Radwanska and colleagues, also using a competitive binding assay, found little overlap in the serum progesterone between normal IUPs and EPs or spontaneous abortions.[68] The authors suggested that a serum progesterone level of less than 10 ng/mL was a reliable indicator of a nonviable pregnancy. Since the serum progesterone in-

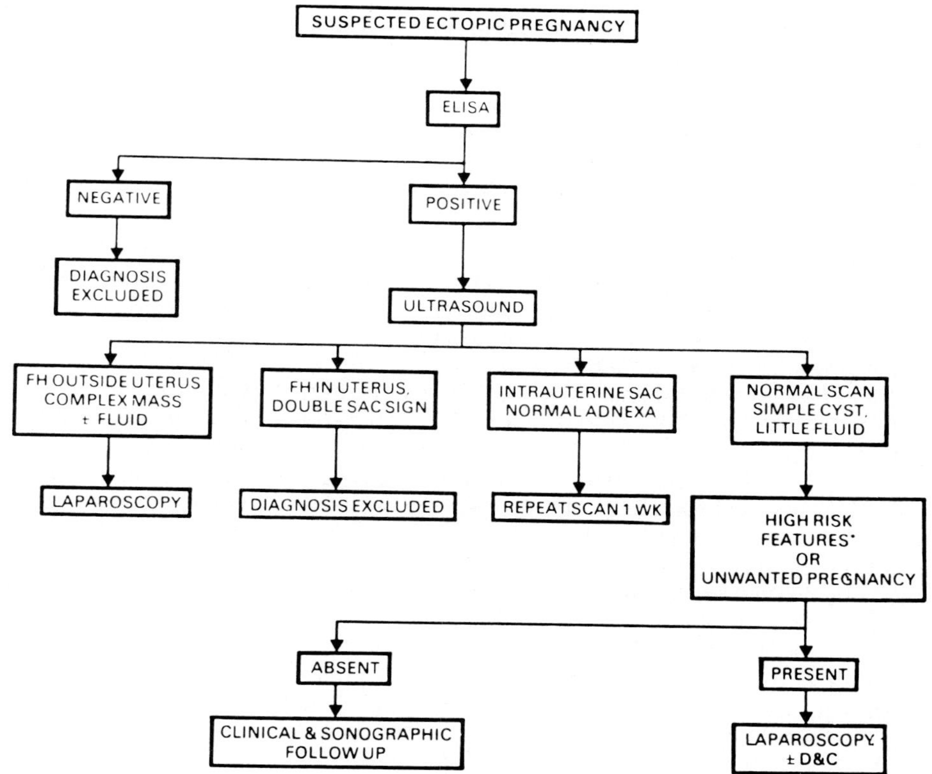

FIGURE 17–7. Algorithm for managing cases of suspected EP based on the availability of urinary ELISA and gray-scale sonography.

creased little during the first trimester of pregnancy, this same value was applicable in early pregnancy regardless of the precise gestational age.

The conventional approach to the RIA of progesterone required, among other things, extraction with an organic solvent to remove the progesterone that was bound to cortisol-binding globulin. Recently, cortisol or danazol has been used to displace progesterone from its binding site, and it has been shown neither one cross-reacts with the specific antiprogesterone antibody used in the assay. This technique has made it possible to assay progesterone in unextracted plasma or serum and has made the RIA suitable for clinical use, because the result is available in about 4 hours.[69,70]

Using direct RIA for progesterone, several authors have confirmed recently that there is little or no overlap in the serum progesterone levels between normal and abnormal (ectopic or abortions) pregnancies. However, ectopic pregnancies and abortions cannot be distinguished by serum progesterone measurements. Mathews and associates first demonstrated that there was no overlap between ectopic and normal pregnancies when a serum progesterone level of 15 ng/mL was taken as the critical value[71]; their findings were confirmed by Yeko and coworkers using a different direct RIA for progesterone.[72] In a much larger study, Buck and colleagues showed more recently that a serum progesterone level of 15 ng/mL (48 nM/L) corresponds approximately to the 5th percentile (50 nM/L) of the serum progesterone level associated with normal first-trimester pregnancy and that 77 out of 89 cases of EP had serum progesterone values below 50 nM/L. In other words, if 15 ng/mL is used as the critical value, the serum progesterone value has a sensitivity for EP of 87% and a false-positive rate of just under 5%.[73] At the lower level suggested by Radwanska and coworkers (10 ng/mL) serum progesterone measurements will be less sensitive but more specific for abnormal pregnancy.

More promising still is the use of an enzyme-multiplied immunoassay technique (EMIT) to measure pregnanediol glucuronide (PDG) in urine. This method has been used for evaluating spontaneous abortions. Recently, a commercially available kit for measuring PDG, which provides results in about 10 minutes, has been evaluated in ectopic pregnancies.[74] It was found that 75% of 60 EPs had PDG values below 9 μg/mL, and 90% had values below 15 μg/mL. By contrast, all 34 normal IUPs studied had PDG levels above 9 μg/mL, and 91% had values above 15 μg/mL. It must be stressed, however, that the technique has not been evaluated prospectively "in the field," and its usefulness is still to be evaluated. Nonetheless, the implications are clearly that with the use of two simple urine tests (ELISA for hCG and EMIT for PDG), the gynecologist may be able to discover most cases of EP within a matter of minutes in the office or emergency room. The next step would be to differentiate between an EP and an abortion. The obvious method that suggests itself is curettage, followed by frozen section examination of the curettings in cases of uncertainty.[75] A possible algorithm that merits further evaluation is shown in Figure 17-8.

The alternative approach to the evaluation of pregnant women with suspected EPs who have nondiagnostic sonar findings starts with a serum hCG determination (blood drawn at the time of the scan). If the serum hCG is found to be above a certain critical value (called the discriminatory zone [DZ]), and an IUP cannot be detected, one can safely assume that the patient has an EP. If the serum hCG is *not* above this critical value, then the patient may have an EP, a very early normal IUP, or an abortion. Serial hCG measurements are then obtained to try to distinguish between these possibilities.[63–66]

THE DISCRIMINATORY hCG ZONE

Kadar and coworkers first showed that if the serum hCG is more than 6500 mIU/mL (International Reference Preparation [IRP]; discussed later in this chapter) and an IUP cannot be detected sonographically, the probability is more than 95% that an EP is present.[63] The reason for this is twofold. First, if an IUP is present, the gestational sac can almost always be imaged when the serum hCG is above this critical level. Second, and equally important, it has been found empirically that if a pregnancy that has developed to the stage of sac formation is complicated by abortion, the serum hCG levels will fall before the sac disintegrates. Consequently, it is very uncommon to find an abortion when the serum hCG is more than 6500 mIU/mL (IRP) and the endometrial cavity does not contain a detectable gestational sac.[63,65]

It is vital for the reader to be aware that the DZ was originally described using an assay calibrated against the International Reference Preparation (IRP) and TA sonography.[78] Consequently, if a TV probe, or an assay calibrated against a different hCG standard, is being used, different hCG values must be used for the DZ. Many commercially available hCG assays are in fact still calibrated against the older Second International Standard (2nd-IS). This standard was developed by the WHO for use in bioassays and, unlike the IRP, is contaminated by free alpha and beta subunits. These subunits are inactive in bioassays but do react in immunoassays.[76] Hence, values obtained in an assay calibrated against the IRP are two to three times higher than the values obtained in assays calibrated against the 2nd-IS.[77] Some recent assay systems use monoclonal antibodies directed against epitopes (ie, antigenic sites) that are expressed only on the intact hCG molecule and not on its subunits. In such assay systems similar readings are obtained regardless of which standard is employed, as free subunits do not compete with hCG for antibody binding sites.

None of the published papers reported to date have used proper statistical methods (ie, probit or logit analysis) to arrive at a value for the DZ that corresponds to a defined fiducial limit.[55–58] It is probably safe for the

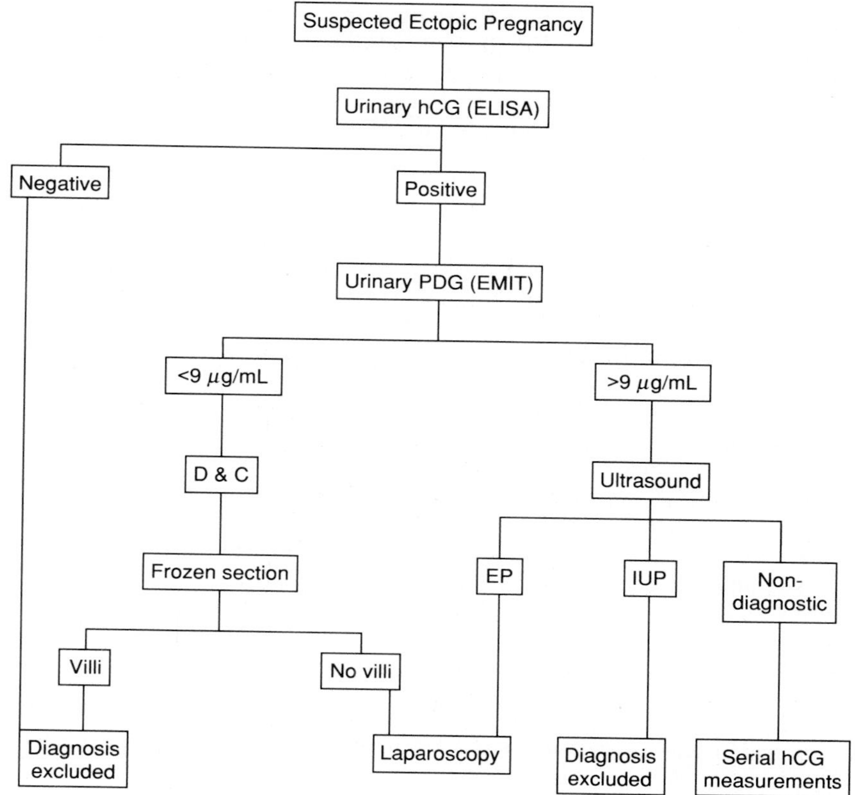

FIGURE 17–8. A possible algorithm for managing cases of EP based on a urinary ELISA for hC and a urinary EMIT for pregnanediol glucuronide (PDG).

reader to adopt the values shown in Figure 17-9 for the DZ, depending on which type of hCG assay the laboratory is running and which type of sonography is being performed. A fuller discussion of the principles underlying the use of the DZ, and of the correspondence between hCG values obtained in different hCG assays, is available elsewhere.[26]

SERIAL hCG TESTING

The serum hCG increases exponentially in normal pregnancies at hCG values that are below the original DZ (ie, the log hCG–time relationship is linear). The 15th percentile of the rate of hCG increase in normal pregnancies corresponds to a doubling time (DT) of 2.7 days, or to a slope of the log hCG–time regression line of 0.25 (or 0.11 if common logarithms [ie, base 10] are used).[79] In at least 87% of EPs the serum hCG increases at a slower rate, and the levels may in fact be falling.[63,65] The most suitable and practical way to determine the rate of hCG increase in serum among women with suspected EPs is to measure the hCG again in a blood sample drawn 48 hours (accurately timed) after the initial one. (Shorter sampling intervals cause potential problems, because the increase in hCG expected is less than twice the interassay variability of most assays.) The serum hCG should increase by 66% or more over this time period. Alternatively, one can compute the slope of the increase [log (hCG_2/hCG_1)-sampling interval], or the doubling time (DT) (log 2/slope). If the rate of increase is subnormal (ie, percentage of increase is less than 66%, DT is less than 2.7 days, or slope is less than 0.25), laparoscopy is indicated.

If the second hCG value is lower than the first one (ie, the levels are falling), one can be confident that the pregnancy is not viable, and in most cases it is appro-

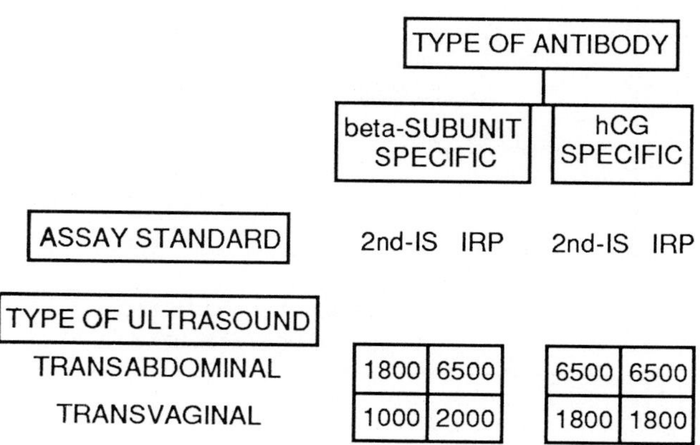

TYPE OF ANTIBODY	beta-SUBUNIT SPECIFIC		hCG SPECIFIC	
ASSAY STANDARD	2nd-IS	IRP	2nd-IS	IRP
TYPE OF ULTRASOUND				
TRANSABDOMINAL	1800	6500	6500	6500
TRANSVAGINAL	1000	2000	1800	1800

FIGURE 17–9. The hCG level (in mIU/mL) above which failure to detect a gestation should be taken as being indicative of an ectopic pregnancy is a function of both the type of ultrasound and the type of hCG assay being used.

priate to perform a D & C prior to laparoscopy to try to differentiate between an EP and an abortion. One should try to avoid having to give the patient a second anesthetic at a later date, so if there is uncertainty over the nature of the curettings obtained (in most EPs little or no tissue is obtained by gentle curettage) frozen section should be performed if possible.[75]

Kadar and Romero recently reported that when the serum hCG is below the DZ and the values are decreasing, the rate at which the serum hCG falls (half life [HL]) may also provide useful diagnostic information.[80] They found that if the HL was less than 1.4 days, the patient was very unlikely to have an EP, but villi could be recovered from only 10% of abortions. In other words, curettage is usually not helpful in these patients, and they are best managed expectantly, provided the clinical situation justifies this. By contrast, if the HL was more than 7 days, an EP was almost certainly present and was at risk of having already ruptured. Prompt laparoscopy is therefore indicated in this situation, and a D & C should only be performed if the curettings can be sent for frozen section. When the HL was between these values, the clearance rate of hCG could not be used to help separate EPs and abortions, and falling hCG levels should certainly *not* be used to sway the diagnosis in favor of an abortion. Failure to recover villi at curettage was more than 80% predictive of EP in these cases. An extension of the author's original algorithm incorporating these findings is shown in Figure 17-10.

Serial hCG monitoring was originally described for the evaluation of women with suspected EPs who had hCG values below the DZ. At higher hCG levels ultrasound always provides an extremely accurate (although not perfect) working diagnosis so serial hCG monitoring serves no useful diagnostic purpose. The DT of hCG also increases as the pregnancy advances, so the same cutoff above and below the DZ cannot be used to separate IUPs and EPs. In the attempt to explore other applications of serial hCG testing these points seem to have been forgotten. Our very simple yet effective approach to the evaluation of this subgroup of women with EPs has become embroiled in unnecessary complexity. These points will be commented on only briefly to highlight the salient points.

Batzer and coworkers used serial hCG monitoring to try to predict abortions among *asymptomatic* infertility patients.[81] Although 83% of the pregnancies that were destined to abort were identified on basis of "abnormal DTs," falling rather than subnormally increasing hCG values characterized many of these cases. By these authors' criteria, 18% of normal pregnancies had abnormal DTs, which is clearly unacceptably high, given the purpose of the test. Inasmuch as some asymptomatic

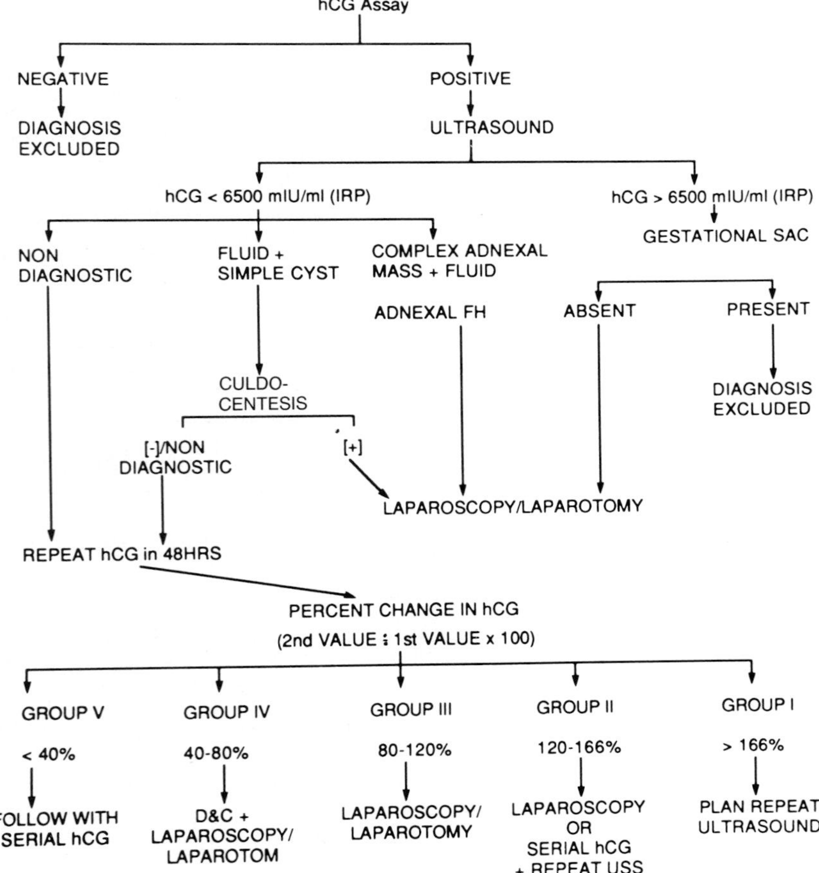

FIGURE 17–10. An extension of the original algorithm for managing patients with suspected EP based on transabdominal sonography and a quantitative hCG assay calibrated against the IRP.

women destined to abort their pregnancies had subnormally increasing hCG levels, it has been inferred from these findings that serial hCG monitoring in women with suspected EP would be less useful because of the inability to differentiate between EPs and abortions on the basis of serial hCG measurements. In fact, these theoretical concerns have not materialized, at least not in our experience, probably because most abortions are diagnosed clinically, and the vast majority of abortions that are not either clinically or ultrasonographically obvious are associated with falling hCG levels. Thus, in practice one simply does not encounter many cases of abortion associated with subnormally increasing hCG values below the DZ unless one looks for them specifically.

Another question that has taken on practical significance with the use of serial hCG testing focuses on the nature of the log hCG–time relationship in early pregnancy.[80,82,83] This issue cannot be explored fully here; the reader is referred to the original discussion.[84] Suffice it to say that Pittaway and colleagues suggested that this relationship was not linear but quadratic and that multiple "nomograms," rather than a single critical value, should be used to determine whether serum hCG levels were increasing normally or not in a particular patient.[82,83] They argued that the use of multiple nomograms would enhance the differentiation of IUPs and EPs, but as Kadar and Romero pointed out, the theory of ROC curve analysis would not predict this.[80] In fact, the multiple nomograms defined by Pittaway and associates did not improve the diagnosis of EP when they were applied to their data. The data to which Pittaway and colleagues fitted linear and quadratic curves included many observations above the DZ, and it is known that the hCG DT increases above this level. Despite the inclusion of these data points, a quadratic curve explained less than 4% more of the variability in the data than a linear one, and it was unclear from the presentation of the data whether a proper statistical test (the partial F-test) was ever carried out.[84] More recently, in a clearly presented analysis, Daya found that the log hCG–time relationship in normal pregnancy could be represented by a series of straight lines whose slope decreased progressively with advancing gestational age.[85] The log hCG–time relationship below the DZ was adequately described by a single straight line. Unfortunately, the message of the paper was that separate criteria are needed above the DZ, even though the value of serial hCG testing above the DZ has never been documented to the author's knowledge. One should also bear in mind that data obtained from a sample of asymptomatic pregnant women may not be applicable to women with symptomatic IUPs.[83]

THE TREATMENT OF TUBAL PREGNANCIES

The treatment of tubal pregnancies remains primarily surgical, even if no longer exclusively so. The primary goal of surgery is, of course, to remove the pregnancy and thereby arrest or prevent hemorrhage, which can be accomplished in many different ways. The first operation to be used successfully in this respect was salpingectomy, performed by Lawson Tait in Birmingham, England, in 1884.[86] (In fact, Tait had performed the operation the previous year but was unable to save the mother's life.) Following Lawson Tait's success, salpingectomy quickly became the standard method of treating tubal pregnancies and is probably still the most commonly used operation.

Many other operations have been used to treat tubal pregnancies.[87] Some of these operations were more radical than simple salpingectomy (ie, involved concurrent cornual resection and/or ipsilateral oophorectomy) and some were less radical (ie, involved preserving part or all of the affected fallopian tube). But the stimulus for considering both classes of operations was the same, namely, the endeavor to improve the woman's chance of giving birth to a living child and to reduce her risk of having another ectopic pregnancy (EP).

Although very firm views have been expressed in the literature, particularly about the merits of conservative operations, the extent to which the reproductive performance of women following an EP can be influenced by choosing different operations under different clinical circumstances remains very much undecided. The reason is that the available data are very hard to interpret, either because the treatment comparisons studied were confounded by other factors, because of other analytical inadequacies, or because of the heavy reliance that has been placed on nonsignificant results obtained in small retrospective studies.

FACTORS CONFOUNDING TREATMENT COMPARISONS

It is almost axiomatic that several factors besides the operative treatment used can affect both the live birth rate (LBR) and recurrent EP rate (REPR) following treatment of a tubal pregnancy. Should any "proof" be required of this, it is provided by the finding that vastly different results have been reported for identically treated women. For example, in two more or less equally sized studies, the LBR and REPR following abdominal salpingostomy on a sole remaining oviduct were, respectively, 100% and 0[88] and 50% and 17%.[89]

The best-established prognostic factor is a history of infertility or evidence of tubal disease at surgery. Pouly and coworkers found that prior infertility was associated with a significant reduction in the IUP rate (from 86% to 41%) and a significant increase in the recurrent EP rate (from 16% to 29%) following laparoscopic salpingostomy for tubal pregnancy.[90] Sherman and associates and Toumivara and Kaupilla also found that evidence of tubal disease at surgery impaired the subsequent LBR.[91,92] Some of the other factors that have been found to impair reproductive performance (nulliparity, prior PID, EP or tubal surgery, and increasing age) are probably also linked with infertility. Increasing size of the tubal pregnancy and the presence of tubal rupture may also influence reproductive performance adversely, whereas women with an EP who have an intrauterine device in place may have a more favorable reproductive outcome.

Despite the fact that a number of patient characteristics have a marked influence on reproductive outcome after an EP, in only three relatively recent studies have treatment comparisons been adjusted for these covariates.[91–93] The strength of the conclusions drawn from these studies must, therefore, be tempered accordingly. Indeed, in the only properly controlled study to date, the type of operation used did not affect reproductive performance.[93]

The preceding comments apply to retrospective comparisons between two or more operations performed in the same institution over roughly the same time period. Many tubal surgeons have, in addition, made comparisons between radical (ie, ablative) and conservative tubal operations on the basis of pooled data. Data from different institutions in different countries gathered over different time periods have been used for this purpose, and the pooling was carried out separately for the two types of procedures (ie, the radical and conservative operations were carried out in different sets of hospitals). Additional factors that confound these types of comparisons are the differential prevalence of various etiological factors between different countries, different regions within the same country, and different time periods, as well as other demographic and cultural differences. For example, there is some evidence that results may have improved slightly over time regardless of the operative treatment used.[94] Given the weight attached to these types of comparisons even today,[95] it is important to recognize that in reality they have very little scientific validity, and they will not be considered here.

ANALYTICAL INADEQUACIES

To determine the reproductive outcome after a particular operation for tubal pregnancy requires that only women who undergo the operation in question and who desire pregnancy be considered in the analysis. Although this may appear to be stating the obvious, it is commonplace to find different operations lumped together under an umbrella category such as "conservative surgery" for the purposes of analysis.[91–93,95] For example, in a recent paper, the procedures lumped together as "conservative" ranged from segmental resection of the tube to doing nothing to the tube as the pregnancy had already aborted, and the procedures were compared en masse with salpingectomy, even though there was a threefold variation in the REPR (10% to 30%) after these "conservative" procedures. In another report, the operations actually performed were not even stated, nor was any effort made to ascertain which patients were actually seeking pregnancy.[96] Although in many, but by no means all, reports the analysis was restricted to women seeking pregnancy, the method(s) used to identify which women were seeking pregnancy, or the way in which "nonresponse" was handled in the analysis, was rarely stated.

The merits of a particular operation are assessed from the number of subsequent pregnancies that reach viability and the number of subsequent recurrent EPs. However, all too frequently this information is not available, as pregnancies are often lumped together, regardless of type, to provide uninterpretable measures of outcome, such as the "conception rate." A more common, if less virulent, practice is to lump abortions and normal pregnancies together to arrive at the IUP rate. Presumably, this practice is designed to boost the apparent success of the operations in question, but inasmuch as the women seeking treatment are not interested in abortions, the figure is highly misleading.

Finally, women will have been followed up for different lengths of time after their operation, and the duration of follow-up will influence the statistics on conception. To take account of such differential follow-up, some form of survival analysis[97] (the simplest of which is the life table method) will be required to calculate the LBR and REPR. Unfortunately, the proper statistical methods of analysis have not been employed in a single report published to date.

THE MEANING OF NONSIGNIFICANT RESULTS

Many sweeping conclusions about the treatment of tubal pregnancies have been based on statistically nonsignificant results obtained in small retrospective studies. The much-quoted study of DeCherney and Kase provides an excellent example of many of the preceding points.[98] In some respects it is the best study to date in which the merits of conservative and ablative operations were compared, since only one type of tubal pregnancy was studied (unruptured ampullary) and only two operations were used, salpingectomy and salpingostomy (albeit with two methods of closing the tube). In addition, the patients were matched for age and parity. Nonetheless, any treatment effect was confounded with the effects of a number of other variables that were not controlled for, most notably the state of the contralateral tube and pelvis. The method of assessing the exposure or the desire of these women for pregnancy was not stated, and no mention was made of nonresponders, raising the suspicion that major assumptions were made when the relevant information was not available to the authors. Finally, full advantage was not taken of the case-control design, as methods of analysis appropriate to a matched pairs design (which one assumes the study was meant to be) were not used.

The results showed that the LBR and REPR after salpingostomy were 19 out of 48 (39.6%) and 9 out of 48 (18.75%), respectively; the LBR and REPR after salpingectomy were 21 out of 50 (42%) and 6 out of 50 (12%), respectively. In other words, the LBR was actually slightly higher and the REPR lower after salpingectomy than after salpingostomy, even though these differences did not reach statistical significance at the 5% level. One of the most astonishing facts about this study is that its findings have been consistently misquoted by DeCherney and his colleagues, as well as by other investigators, as having shown that the REPR after salpingostomy was variously 8%, 10%, or 12%.[98,130] Not surprisingly, therefore, despite the fact that the REPR after salpingostomy was 50% higher than that after salpingectomy, the results of this study have been cited repeatedly as evidence that tubal conservation does not increase the REPR.

Notwithstanding these errors, one might argue that the conclusions are still valid, since the difference between the REPR after the two operations does not reach statistical significance at the 5% level. Although this is undeniable, power calculations show that this study had only about a 15% chance of detecting a real difference of 6.75%. Even if the REPR after salpingostomy were to be twice as high as that after salpingectomy (ie, 24% and close to the highest overall REPR ever reported), the study had only a 35% chance of detecting this. What this study tells us, therefore, is that if the REPR after salpingectomy is 12%, then we can be 90% certain that the REPR after salpingostomy is not as high as 27%. This gives us a much better idea of just how sure we can be, from this evidence, that salpingostomy does not increase the REPR vis-à-vis salpingectomy. The answer is uncertain, because, given the very low power of the study, it might easily have failed to detect differences in the REPR of an important order of magnitude.

ABLATIVE OPERATIONS

Salpingectomy remains the standard operation whenever a tubal pregnancy is to be treated by removal of the affected tube. However, it is not the only ablative operation used, as two modifications to Lawson Tait's salpingectomy have been employed for a number of years: concurrent cornual resection and ipsilateral oophorectomy (sometimes called paradoxical oophorectomy).

CORNUAL RESECTION

The suggestion that the interstitial part of the fallopian tube should always be removed during salpingectomy originated at the turn of the century and was prompted by the occasional occurrence of an interstitial pregnancy after ipsilateral salpingectomy.[99] It was quickly realized, however, that cornual resection did not protect against a cornual recurrence unless excision of the intramural part of the tube was complete (ie, the incision was carried into the endometrial cavity). But this predisposed to rupture of the uterus in a subsequent pregnancy. Cornual resection appears to have been widely practiced in some centers[99,100] but has been condemned in recent years.[101] It can be shown by formal "cost–benefit" analysis that the risk associated with cornual resection in fact outweighs the benefits.[26] This is simply shown by estimating the probability of a homolateral interstitial recurrence (as the probability of a recurrent EP multiplied by the probability of an EP being interstitial) and the probability of a ruptured uterus following cornual resection.[26]

PARADOXICAL (IPSILATERAL) OOPHORECTOMY

The suggestion that ipsilateral oophorectomy should be performed at the time of salpingectomy in women who had normal contralateral adnexa and who wanted to conceive was first made by Jeffcoate.[102] However, his suggestion was based not on any data but entirely on theoretical arguments. He argued that removal of the ipsilateral ovary should facilitate ovum pick-up by ensuring that ovulation always occurred on the side of the remaining tube. This, in turn, could be expected to increase the number of fertilized ova made available for implantation, so that the live birth rate following an EP might be enhanced. In addition, by eliminating the possibility of transperitoneal migration of the fertilized ovum, the risk of a recurrent EP might also be reduced.

Salpingectomy (S) and salpingo-oophorectomy (SO) have been compared retrospectively in a number of studies, none of which corrected for extraneous variables, and in which both live births and abortions were classified as uterine pregnancies and both uterine and recurrent EPs were classified as "conceptions."[103–107] This has made for some absurdities. For example, Nagami and coworkers[107] cite the report by Schenker and associates[105] as having shown that the conception rate following SO was higher than that after S, a result that agreed with their own findings. Although factually accurate, the implication is most misleading, because in the study by Schenker and colleagues women who had SO fared better than women who had S, as regards both the REPR (which was lower) and the uterine pregnancy rate (which was slightly higher). This anomaly resulted from the fact that the uterine pregnancy rate was slightly higher after SO than S, and the REPR was markedly lower after SO than after S. When one combines the uterine pregnancies and recurrent EPs to obtain "conceptions," however, it turns out that there were fewer conceptions after SO than after S.

It is noteworthy that in every report, except for the one by Nagami and coworkers,[107] the uterine pregnancy rate after SO was higher than that after S, even if the difference did not reach statistical significance in any of the studies (Table 17-1). When such a situation occurs, it is possible to pool the data that show an association in the same direction and to examine the aggregate information for statistical significance, using the Mantel Haenszel statistic. When this is done, one finds that the difference in the IUP rate between the two operations reaches significance at the 5% level ($X^2 = 4.1$). By contrast, Nagami and colleagues found that the uterine pregnancy rate after salpingectomy (22

TABLE 17–1. UTERINE PREGNANCIES FOLLOWING TUBAL PREGNANCY TREATED BY SALPINGECTOMY OR SALPINGO-OOPHORECTOMY

AUTHOR(S)	SALPINGECTOMY	SALPINGO-OOPHORECTOMY
Bender, 1956[103]	67/187	25/51
Douglas, Shingleton, Crist, 1969[104]	33/78	15/28
Schenker, Eyal, Polishuk, 1972[105]	55/190	12/35
Franklin, Zeiderman, Laemmle, 1973[106]	26/67	95/251
Nagami, London, Amand, 1984[107]	22/37	15/34

out of 37) was higher than after salpingo-oophorectomy (15 out of 34).[107] The authors claimed statistical significance for this difference, which does not, however, occur.

The recurrent EP rates after the two operations are not amenable to such an analysis. Douglas and associates did not report the recurrent EP rates after SO and S.[104] Schenker and coworkers found a significantly lower recurrent EP rate after SO than after S.[105] Franklin and associates found that in fact the recurrent EP rate was significantly higher after SO than after S.[106] However, the authors found that in their study SO was used much more frequently than S in women who had PID, and they attributed the higher recurrent EP rate after SO not to the operation but to the characteristics of the patients in which the operation had been used preferentially. Nagami and colleagues found almost identical recurrent EP rates after SO (three out of 34) and salpingectomy (four out of 37).[107]

The effect of paradoxical oophorectomy on subsequent fertility has also been studied among infertile patients with unilateral tubal disease (ie, women who did not have a tubal pregnancy when treated). Scott and coworkers, in an uncontrolled study, reported a 67% conception rate following salpingo-oophorectomy in patients with unilateral tubal obstruction.[108] In a more recent comparative study, Trimbos-Kempers and associates offered unilateral salpingo-oophorectomy to 24 women with unilateral tubal disease who had failed to conceive after 1 year of follow-up.[109] The conception rate was significantly higher among women who had salpingo-oophorectomy (seven out of nine) than among women who refused to have the operation (four out of 15).

From these data it can be concluded that the chances of childbearing can be significantly enhanced by salpingo-oophorectomy among infertile women with unilateral tubal disease. It does not follow from the preceding observations that the fertility of all women with unilateral adnexal disease can be enhanced by this procedure, since only infertile women were selected for treatment. The preceding data justify treating women with a tubal pregnancy by salpingo-oophorectomy if the involved adnexum shows evidence of preexisting tubo-ovarian disease, the contralateral adnexum is normal and patent on intraoperative chromotubation, and the patient admits to a history of infertility of at least a year's duration. However, this set of circumstances will obtain in only a small minority of women with EP, perhaps 5%.

The preceding data do not justify *routine* salpingo-oophorectomy for women with normal contralateral adnexa. First, paradoxical oophorectomy carries the real risk, even if a very small one (less than 1%), of rendering the woman sterile if the contralateral ovary sustains irreparable damage from torsion of a benign cyst.[109] Second, in the pooled analysis carried out earlier, the advantage conferred by paradoxical oophorectomy was small, so the benefit as it applies to live births as opposed to IUPs is likely to be even smaller. Differences of this magnitude can easily be caused by the unequal distribution of confounding variables between the two treatment groups rather than by a real treatment effect. On the other hand, it is clearly misleading to claim that there is no evidence that paradoxical oophorectomy is beneficial. Further studies into this question are warranted to identify the subgroup(s) of women with EP who are most likely to benefit from the procedure. To recap, however, on the evidence presently available, women with a tubal pregnancy should be treated by salpingo-oophorectomy if the involved adnexum shows evidence of preexisting tubo-ovarian disease, the contralateral adnexum is normal and patent on intraoperative chromotubation, and the patient gives a history of antecedent infertility of at least a year's duration.

CONSERVATIVE OPERATIONS

The operations that are still used today to remove tubal pregnancies without sacrificing the gravid tube are salpingotomy, salpingostomy, segmental tubal resection, and manual expression (ME) of the pregnancy, also referred to as "milking" the tube or fimbrial expression. Of these, salpingotomy and salpingostomy are by far the most commonly performed procedures. For the sake of simplicity, the term *tubotomy* will be used to refer to either or both of these procedures in general terms. A tubotomy that is closed primarily will be referred to as a salpingotomy, and one that is left open to heal by secondary intention will be called a salpingostomy (although, strictly speaking, this is a misnomer, as it is not the surgeon's intention, when performing this operation, to fashion a "stoma").

SALPINGOTOMY/SALPINGOSTOMY

Salpingotomy was popularized and first described in the English literature by Stromme, although the procedure had apparently been practiced since about the turn of this century.[110] Irrefutable evidence that the operation can restore tubal function is provided by the results obtained when the procedure is performed to remove a pregnancy that is located in a woman's only remaining fallopian tube. The reproductive performance of women following tubotomy performed in this setting has been reported by a number of investigators.[88–90,95,96,110–113] Their findings are shown in Table 17-2.

In addition to the unevenness of reporting discussed previously, the series listed in Table 17-2 suffer from the fact that some authors included not only patients with a single tube but also those whose non-pregnant tube was blocked, and that the data are also heterogeneous with respect to the indications for which the missing tube was removed. The only exception is Tuladi's report, in which each patient's contralateral tube had been removed because of an antecedent tubal pregnancy.[114] In the remaining series, the indication for which the contralateral tube had been removed either was not specified[95,96,112,113] or, in 40% to 50% of cases, was a tubal pregnancy.[88,89]

Notwithstanding these limitations of the data, Table 17-2 shows that women who undergo a tubotomy for an ectopic pregnancy (EP) located in their only fallopian tube can expect to have an LBR of about 40% and a REPR of about 20%. Table 17-3 shows that, compared with women who have two fallopian tubes, patients with one oviduct who undergo tubotomy for an EP have a somewhat lower LBR and a somewhat higher REPR. The difference with respect to both outcomes reaches statistical significance when the pooled data are examined by the Mantel Haenszel statistic. Curiously enough, the figures reported by DeCherney and coworkers show an opposite trend, for reasons that are unclear.[89,98]

Although the preceding data show conclusively that the function of a fallopian tube containing a pregnancy can be restored by a tubotomy, they leave several questions about the procedure and the indications for it unanswered.

1. Should the tubal incision be closed primarily? Comparative data are not available to answer this question, but the findings shown in Figure 17-1 suggest that broadly similar results are obtained, regardless of whether the tube is closed primarily or left to heal by secondary intention. Preliminary data from animal research suggest that better results are obtained if the tubal incision is *not* closed primarily.[115] McComb and Gomel found that ovum transport in rabbits, subjected to bilateral tubotomy and primary closure of one of the incisions, was significantly delayed when the incision was closed compared to when it was left open to heal by secondary intention. The mucosal folds were also oriented transversely to the direction of

TABLE 17–2. REPRODUCTIVE PERFORMANCE FOLLOWING SALPINGOSTOMY PERFORMED FOR A TUBAL PREGNANCY LOCATED IN A WOMAN'S ONLY REMAINING FALLOPIAN TUBE

AUTHOR/YEAR	NO. SEEKING PREGNANCY	PREGNANCIES		
		IUP (%)	TERM (%)	TUBAL (%)
Salpingotomy				
Jarvinen, Nummi, Pietila, 1972[112]	10	? 7	?5 (50%)	3 (30%)
Stromme, 1973[110]	5	3 (60%)	1 (20%)	2 (40%)
Oelsen et al, 1986	17	7 (41%)	n/s	6 (35%)
Mostly Salpingotomy				
Langer, Bukovsky, Herman, Sherman, Sadovsky, Caspi, 1982[113]	8	5 (63%)	5 (63%)	2 (25%)
Salpingostomy				
Decherney, Maheaux, Naftolin, 1982[89]	12	–	6 (50%)	2 (17%)
Valle and Lifchez, 1983[88]	11	11 (100%)	11 (100%)	0
Tuladi, 1988[114]	16	8 (50%)	5 (31%)	3 (19%)
Laparoscopic Salpingostomy				
Pouly et al, 1987	24	11 (46%)	n/s	7 (29%)
Procedures Not Specified				
Hallatt, 1986[96]	n/s (26 treated)	10 (38%)	n/s	5 (19%)

TABLE 17–3. REPRODUCTIVE PERFORMANCE OF WOMEN SEEKING PREGNANCY AFTER SALPINGOSTOMY

AUTHOR/YEAR	NO. SEEKING PREGNANCY	PREGNANCIES		
		IUP (%)	TERM (%)	TUBAL (%)
Mostly Salpingotomy				
Langer, Burkovsky, Herman, Sherman, Sadovsky, Caspi, 1982[114]	Both tubes (N = 41)	34 (83%)	30 (73%)	4 (10%)
	Single tubes (N = 8)	5 (63%)	5 (63%)	2 (25%)
Oelsner, Morad, Carp, et al, 1987[95]	Both tubes (N = 25)	14 (56%)	n/s	3 (12%)
	Single tube (N = 26)	12 (46%)	n/s	10 (38%)
Salpingostomy				
DeCherney, et al, 1979[89] and 1982[98]	Both tubes (N = 42)	–	15 (36%)	9 (21%)
	Single tube (N = 12)	–	6 (50%)	2 (17%)
Laparoscopic Salpingostomy				
Pouly et al, 1987[90]	Both tubes (N = 94)	65 (69%)	n/s	19 (20%)
	Single tube (N = 24)	11 (46%)	n/s	7 (29%)
Procedures Not Specified	Both tubes (N = 174)	98 (57%)	n/s	24 (14%)
Hallatt, 1986	Single tube (N = 26)	10 (38%)	n/s	5 (19%)

tubal transport in the tubes subjected to primary closure.[115] These findings, coupled with the principle of surgical parsimony and simplicity, would commend salpingostomy rather than salpingotomy as the conservative operation of choice. Although tuboperitoneal fistulas can form when the tubes are left open,[116] in general healing seems to be both satisfactory and prompt.

2. Should salpingostomy ever be performed on a tube that has already been operated on either for a previous EP or blockage? Again, very little data are available to help answer these questions.

   Recurrent tubal pregnancies have been studied by a number of investigators, but few of the patients studied had two pregnancies in the same tube and salpingostomies performed at both operations. In Sandvei and colleagues' series of 74 cases this situation obtained in at most two patients, one of whom subsequently had a third tubal pregnancy.[117] In Hallatt's series of 123 repeat ectopic pregnancies, only six ipsilateral pregnancies occurred following a prior conservative operation (presumably a tubotomy), but it was unclear from the paper how these second tubal pregnancies were managed.[101] Shoen and Nowak describe 34 cases of repeat tubal pregnancies, in only two of which was the first pregnancy treated by a conservative operation; however, the authors did not specify how these patients' second tubal pregnancy was treated.[118] In Tuladi's report on 24 cases of repeat tubal pregnancy, the cases selected for study were specifically those in which the second tubal pregnancy was located on the side opposite the first one (which had been treated by a salpingectomy).[114] Finally, DeCherney and coworkers[119] describe three women who delivered live babies after two consecutive salpingostomies for pregnancies located in the same fallopian tube, and in one of these the tube in question was the woman's only remaining one. Although these cases demonstrate the possibility of normal childbearing after two salpingostomies have been performed on the same fallopian tube for an ectopic pregnancy, they give no indication of its probability, or of the probability of a third tubal pregnancy.

   Pouly and associates report on the reproductive performance of 17 women who had tubal pregnancies following a tuboplasty and who were treated by laparoscopic salpingostomy: four out of 17 (23%) had IUPs and seven out of 17 (41%) had recurrent tubal pregnancies. This IUP–EP ratio (0.6) is a third of that obtained from salpingostomy on a single fallopian tube (1.6).[90] In the author's opinion, a second salpingostomy should be considered only if the affected oviduct is the only one present and appears to be only minimally damaged.

3. When an oviduct is to be conserved, should a salpingostomy always be performed, or are there situations when manual expression (ME) or segmental resection and anastomosis produce better results? This question is discussed in the following sections.

MANUAL EXPRESSION

The present consensus among tubal surgeons is that ME should be abandoned, as it is associated with an inordinately high REPR, regardless of whether the procedure is performed at a laparotomy or through the laparoscope (Table 17-4).[95,120–123] Delayed hemorrhage from persistent trophoblastic activity also appears to be more common than after salpingostomy (see discussion later in this chapter). The histologic observations of Budowick and colleagues, which showed that tubal pregnancies penetrate the tubal wall at an early stage and in fact grow extraluminally rather than inside the tube, were quickly offered as an explanation for these findings.[28] However, as discussed earlier, these histologic findings were not entirely confirmed by more detailed, subsequent work, which showed that the type of growth exhibited by the developing trophoblast depended to a large extent on the location of the pregnancy within the tube and on whether the tube had ruptured.[29,30] Thus, the type of pregnancies that might be treated by ME (ie, unruptured ampullary–fimbrial ones) almost always exhibited intraluminal rather than extraluminal growth. In any case, the argument that pregnancies that penetrate the tubal wall and grow extraluminally cannot be expected to be removed by ME applies with equal force to salpingostomies, and so scarcely provides prima facie evidence for abandoning ME.

Recently, Sherman and coworkers reported that 23 out of 27 women attempting conception following fimbrial evacuation of a tubal pregnancy delivered one or more living children, and none had a repeat tubal pregnancy.[124] However, the number of cases in which the procedure was tried but was unsuccessful was not known, so the success rate of an *attempted* ME and the reproductive outcome following an unsuccessful ME remain unknown. Nonetheless, the impressive results obtained by Sherman and colleagues are difficult to reconcile with the data shown in Table 17-4. It is noteworthy that Sherman and coworkers have also reported the highest overall LBR and lowest REPR following conservative surgery for tubal pregnancies on record,[90] possibly because (1) a very low proportion of the author's patients gave a history of infertility (a factor that has been found to impair reproductive performance following treatment of a tubal pregnancy), and (2) a relatively high proportion of the author's patients were using an IUD when their EPs were diagnosed (a finding that has been linked with an improved prognosis for subsequent childbearing). In other words, the preceding results may be a reflection more of the patient population treated by these authors than of the operations they employed for the treatment of tubal pregnancies.

The data in Table 17-4 show a consistent trend toward a higher REPR following ME than after salpingostomy, which does not reach statistical significance when the data are subjected to pooled analysis using the Maentel Haenszel statistic. To some extent, therefore, Sherman and colleagues are perhaps justified in questioning the legitimacy of the notorious reputation that ME has gained in this regard.[124] However, one should not lose sight of the fact that there are no data to suggest that ME produces any better results than salpingostomy: the controversy is over whether ME does in fact increase the REPR, as first suggested by Timonen and Nieminen. Therefore, it is difficult to marshal a cogent argument for abandoning such a well-tried and simple procedure as salpingostomy for one that is at best no worse. If there is any place at all for ME, it is in fimbrial or infundibular pregnancies that have already almost completely aborted. Under these rather unusual conditions it is probably safe and appropriate to attempt the procedure.

SEGMENTAL TUBAL RESECTION

Segmental tubal resection is accepted as the procedure of choice whenever a gravid fallopian tube is to be conserved but the tubal wall is ruptured, or there is persistent or uncontrollable bleeding from the tube following

TABLE 17–4. REPRODUCTIVE OUTCOME FOLLOWING SALPINGOTOMY AND MANUAL EXPRESSION OF TUBAL PREGNANCIES

AUTHOR/YEAR	PROCEDURE	NO. SEEKING PREGNANCY	PREGNANCIES		
			IUP (%)	TERM (%)	TUBAL (%)
Timonen and Nieminen, 1967[121]	Salpingotomy	83	36 (43%)	25 (30%)	10 (12%)
	"Milking"	29	12 (41%)	6 (21%)	6 (21%)
Swolin and Fall, 1972[122]	Salpingotomy	24	4 (17%)	3 (13%)	4 (17%)
	"Milking"	16	4 (25%)	3 (19%)	3 (19%)
Bruhat, Mahnes, Mage, Pouly, 1980[123]	Salpingotomy	18	14 (78%)	n/s	1 (6%)
	"Milking"	7	3 (43%)	n/s	2 (14%)
Paavonen, Varjonen-Toivonen, Komulainen, Heinonen, 1985[124]	Salpingotomy	34	21 (62%)	18 (53%)	3 (8.8%)
	"Milking"	5	4 (80%)	4 (80%)	1 (20%)
Oelsner, Morad, Carp, et al, 1987[95]	Salpingotomy	38	19 (50%)	n/s	9 (24%)
	"Milking"	9	4 (44%)	n/s	3 (33%)

Mantel-Haenszel Chi Square = 3 for recurrent tubal pregnancies.

a salpingostomy. A few tubal surgeons have advocated that segmental resection with primary or delayed closure should be the primary treatment in all cases of tubal pregnancy.[125] They argue that salpingostomy conserves an abnormal implantation site, because the invading trophoblast is likely to have caused local damage to the tube in addition to any preexisting damage that might have caused the abnormal implantation in the first place. Although good results have been obtained from this procedure,[120–122] there is no evidence that better results are obtained than from salpingostomy (see Fig. 17-9). It is obviously a more complicated procedure, and the general consensus is that it is not the primary treatment of choice for most tubal pregnancies for which a conservative procedure is indicated (Table 17-5).

On the other hand, there appears to be a growing consensus that *unruptured* isthmic pregnancies should be treated by segmental tubal resection (and primary or delayed anastomosis) rather than by salpingostomy.[126,127] There is certainly some evidence that the reproductive performance of women following conservative surgery for an EP is less good if the pregnancy is located in the isthmic rather than in the ampullary portion of the oviduct. Hallatt stated, without giving figures, that the IUP–EP ratio after conservative surgery was about four times higher than that when the pregnancy was located in the ampulla as opposed to the isthmus.[96] Pouly and associates[90] found that the IUP rate following laparoscopic salpingostomy was 64 out of 96 (67%) for ampullary pregnancies and 12 out of 22 (55%) for isthmic pregnancies; the recurrent tubal pregnancy rates were 18 out of 96 (19%) and eight out of 22 (36%), respectively.

Whether the reproductive performance of women with isthmic pregnancies is any better following segmental tubal resection than after salpingostomy remains, however, far from clear. DeCherney and Boyers have argued strongly that it is, but their argument is based on meager evidence.[127] In a retrospective audit, they found that three of four women with unruptured isthmic pregnancies who were treated by salpingostomy had tubal occlusion on hysterosalpingography and none conceived, whereas three out of six women who were treated by segmental resection and delayed anastomosis delivered live infants and one out of six women so treated had a recurrent tubal pregnancy. However, these authors' dismal experience with salpingostomy in isthmic pregnancies was reflected neither in the results obtained by Pouly and coworkers[90] with laparoscopic salpingostomy nor in a subsequent, randomized prospective clinical study.[128]

Smith and colleagues randomly allocated the treatment of women with unruptured isthmic pregnancies to segmental resection and anastomosis (four cases) or to salpingostomy (nine cases).[128] (Some cases randomized to segmental resection in fact had a salpingostomy if a tubal surgeon was not available.) Cases of ruptured isthmic pregnancies were treated by segmental tubal resection alone (seven cases). All four tubes that were primarily anastomosed following segmental resection were patent on subsequent HSG, and one of the two women who were actively trying to conceive had an IUP. Four of the seven women who had segmental resection alone for a ruptured isthmic pregnancy were trying to conceive, and two had IUPs. Four of the nine women treated with salpingostomy subsequently had intrauterine pregnancies (two having delivered at the time of the report), whereas five were using contraception. Because the number of patients studied was so small, no meaning can be attached to the lack of statistical significance of the differences in outcome between the different treatment groups. Nonetheless, inasmuch as all women who tried to become pregnant after salpingostomy conceived IUPs, the results provide a striking contrast to those reported by DeCherney and Boyers.[127]

Therefore, the optimal treatment of isthmic pregnancies has yet to be determined. Although it is likely that the reproductive performance of women following an isthmic pregnancy really is less good than that after an ampullary one, the available data do not provide compelling evidence for treating women with isthmic and ampullary pregnancies differently. Certainly as far as the general gynecologist is concerned, salpingostomy should still be considered the operation of choice.

TABLE 17–5. COMPARISON OF SALPINGOTOMY WITH SEGMENTAL TUBAL RESECTION

AUTHOR/YEAR	PROCEDURE	NO. SEEKING PREGNANCY	PREGNANCIES		
			IUP (%)	TERM (%)	TUBAL (%)
Ploman and Wicksell, 1960[112]	Tubotomy	27	17 (63%)	16 (59%)	5 (19%)
	Seg. resec.	61	29 (48%)	25 (41%)	6 (10%)
Timonen and Nieminen, 1967[121]	Tubotomy	83	36 (43%)	25 (30%)	10 (12%)
	Seg. resec.	68	20 (29%)	12 (18%)	6 (9%)
Swolin and Fall, 1972[122]	Tubotomy	24	4 (17%)	3 (13%)	4 (17%)
	Seg. resec.	42	7 (17%)	4 (10%)	6 (14%)
Paavonen, Varjonen-Toivonen, Komulainen, Heinonen, 1985[124]	Tubotomy	34	21 (62%)	18 (53%)	3 (9%)
	Seg. resec.	18	13 (72%)	13 (72%)	3 (17%)

Mantel-Haenszel Chi Square = 1.3 for recurrent tubal pregnancies.

CONSERVATIVE VERSUS ABLATIVE TREATMENT OF TUBAL PREGNANCIES

The most common decision a gynecologist has to make in treating tubal pregnancies is whether to remove the oviduct. From the preceding discussion it is apparent that this decision almost always reduces to a choice between salpingectomy and salpingostomy. Furthermore, the question arises only in women who wish to have children, as tubal conservation serves no purpose in women who have completed their families, and it carries a higher complication rate than salpingectomy.

SALPINGOSTOMY VERSUS SALPINGECTOMY

Satisfactory comparisons between salpingostomy and salpingectomy are not available. As noted previously, the best available comparative data were reported by DeCherney and Kase,[98] which showed that the LBR was higher and the REPR lower after salpingectomy (42% and 12%, respectively) than after salpingostomy (39.6% and 18.75%), although the observed differences did not reach statistical significance. The available evidence is summarized in Tables 17-6 and 17-7.

It is apparent from Table 17-6 that with the possible exception of multiparas in the study by Timonen and Nieminen,[120] the LBR was almost identical, regardless of the operative treatment used, and there was certainly no consistent trend, however small, favoring one or another of these treatments. By contrast, Table 17-7 shows a consistent, and often quite marked, trend toward a higher REPR among patients treated by tubotomy, the only exception again being multiparas in Timonen and Nieminen's study, where the REPR was slightly higher after salpingectomy (9.8%) than after salpingotomy (8.2%). None of the preceding differences is statistically significant, even after examining the pooled data with the Mantel Haenszel statistic. However, to have a 90% chance of detecting a doubling of the REPR (from 10% to 20%) at the 5% significance level would require 263 patients in each of two equal-sized treatment groups (power is lost when the treatment groups are of unequal size).[129] Therefore, the consistent increase in the REPR after tubotomy cannot be ignored and in all probability reflects a real increase in the REPR after this procedure of at least 5%.

Data pertaining to the relative merits of radical and conservative operations are available in four other reports,[90,93,111] but they all suffer from some or all of the problems that were previously discussed, namely, that several different operations were lumped together under "conservative procedures," that the outcome of interest (term pregnancies and repeat tubal gestations) were not specified or analyzed by appropriate statistical methods, and that often the sample size was too small to detect differences in outcome of an important order of magnitude. Nonetheless, most ablative operations were salpingectomies, and most conservative operations were salpingostomies or salpingotomies. Therefore, a further comparison between conservative and ablative operations has been made using the two papers in which raw data were provided (Table 17-8).[91,111] It can be seen that the trend toward a higher REPR following tubal conservation persists. In these studies, however, there was also a trend toward a higher LBR following conservative surgery (Table 17-9).

THE INFLUENCE OF PATIENT CHARACTERISTICS ON SURGICAL RESULTS

In only three reports were the comparisons between the different operations used to treat EPs adjusted for some of the confounding variables that affect the outcome after surgery.[91–93] Studies by Sherman and coworkers and Toumivaara and Kauppila both found that when the contralateral tube was diseased, the subsequent IUP rate was higher after conservative than after ablative operations. Toumivaara and Kauppila found that the increase in the IUP rate was accompanied by an increase in the REPR.[91,92] Sherman and associates, however, found that the increase in the IUP rate was accompanied by a *decrease* in the REPR—a finding that, from first principles, is very difficult to accept without corroborating evidence.[91] In the only multivariate analysis reported to date, patient characteristics were also found to be a more important determinant of reproductive outcome than the operative treatment used.[93] The type of operation did not affect outcome even after accounting

TABLE 17–6. LIVE BIRTH RATES FOLLOWING SALPINGOSTOMY AND SALPINGECTOMY FOR TUBAL PREGNANCY

AUTHOR/YEAR	SALPINGOSTOMY	SALPINGECTOMY
Tiemonen and Nieminen, 1967[121]		
Nullipara	9/34 (29%)	46/160 (29%)
Multipara	16/49 (33%)	106/398 (27%)
Swolin and Fall, 1972[122]	4/44 (9.1%)	3/24 (12.5%)
Decherney and Kase, 1979[98]	19/48 (39.6%)	21/50 (42%)
Paavonen, Varjonen-Toivonen, Komulainen, Heinonen, 1985[124]	18/34 (53%)	20/39 (51%)

TABLE 17-7. RECURRENT TUBAL PREGNANCY RATES AFTER SALPINGOSTOMY AND SALPINGECTOMY

AUTHOR/YEAR	SALPINGOSTOMY	SALPINGECTOMY
Tiemonen and Nieminen 1967[121]		
Nullipara	6/34 (17.6%)	14/160 (8.8%)
Multipara	4/49 (8.2%)	39/398 (9.8%)
Swolin and Fall, 1972[122]	4/24 (16.7%)	7/44 (15.9%)
Decherney and Kase, 1979[98]	9/48 (18.75%)	6/50 (12%)
Paavonen, Varjonen-Toivonen, Komulainen, Heinonen, 1985[124]	3/34 (8.8%)	3/39 (7.3%)

for differences in patient characteristics, although the sample size was rather small and the number of operations considered quite numerous.

SITE OF RECURRENT TUBAL PREGNANCIES

It has been observed by a number of investigators that when both tubes are present, recurrent EPs after salpingostomy are located in the contralateral tube as often as in the conserved tube (see Table 17-8).[90,96,130,131] This finding has been uniformly interpreted as indicating that in general the conserved tube is at no greater risk of developing an EP than the contralateral one. Since the site of the recurrence has not been correlated with the state of the ipsilateral or contralateral tube, it is difficult to accept that this statement applies to all patients, not the least because the presence of contralateral tubal disease has been the major indication for tubal conservation in the past. Clearly, it is more than likely that patients who were subjected to a conservative operation were to some extent selected for having more extensive contralateral tubal disease, which would serve to minimize the disparity between the two oviducts' risk of an ectopic implantation.

Even in the absence of such selection biases, however, it does not follow from the preceding observation that the conserved tube necessarily delivers, as it were, the same IUP–EP ratio as the contralateral one. In fact, the available evidence suggests that it does not. For example, in the report by DeCherney and Kase, the IUP–EP ratios after salpingectomy and salpingostomy were 3.5 and 2.1, respectively, yet of nine recurrent EPs after salpingostomy five were in the contralateral tube.[98] In Table 17-7, the IUP–EP ratio following salpingostomy was consistently higher when both oviducts were present than when the contralateral one had been removed. In other words, these data seem to show that when a tubal pregnancy is treated by salpingostomy and both the conserved gravid tube and the contralateral oviduct are in place, the IUP–EP ratio is *lower* than when only the contralateral tube is present, but higher than when only the conserved tube is present. This finding strongly suggests (although, of course, by no means proves) that the conserved tube has a higher REPR for a given IUP rate. The IUP–EP ratio is an important measure of the relative efficacy of two procedures, because by focusing only on cases in which a conception occurred one not only corrects to some extent for other infertility factors but also avoids diluting the comparison by cases in which no conception occurred after either operation.

INDICATIONS FOR SALPINGOSTOMY

What, then, are the indications for salpingostomy? Clearly, salpingostomy is indicated whenever the woman wishes to have children and the pregnancy is located in her only remaining oviduct. The procedure is about three times more likely to result in a live birth than in vitro fertilization, and if conception occurs, a term pregnancy is at least twice as likely as an EP. The procedure is also indicated if the contralateral tube is blocked, but the results to be expected in this situation have been less clearly defined. Since unilateral tubal

TABLE 17-8. LIVE BIRTH AND RECURRENT TUBAL PREGNANCY RATES FOLLOWING CONSERVATIVE AND ABLATIVE OPERATIONS FOR TUBAL PREGNANCY

	PLOMAN AND WICKSALL[112]		SHERMAN, LANGER, SADOVSKY, ET AL[91]	
TYPE OF OPERATION	LIVE BIRTH RATE	RECURRENT EP RATE	LIVE BIRTH RATE	RECURRENT EP RATE
Conservative	16/27 (59%)	5/27 (18.5%)	39/47 (83%)	3/47 (6.4%)
Ablative	29/61 (48%)	5/61 (8.2%)	75/104 (72%)	5/105 (5.8%)

TABLE 17–9. SITES OF RECURRENT TUBAL IMPLANTATION FOLLOWING SALPINGOSTOMY IN WOMEN WITH TWO TUBES PRESENT

AUTHOR/YEAR	NO. RECURRENCES	IPSILATERAL	CONTRALATERAL
Abdominal Procedures			
Decherney, Sildker, Mezer, et al, 1985[120]	13	9	4
Hallatt, 1986	24	12	12
Laparoscopic Salpingostomy			
Pouly et al, 1986	18	7	11
Decherney and Diamond, 1987[99]	7	3	4
Reich, Johns, DeCaprio, McGlynn, Reich, 1988[131]	11	6	5

disease is uncommon, the ipsilateral tube is also likely to be damaged in this situation. Tubal conservation is inadvisable if the contralateral tube and ovary appear to be normal and patent on intraoperative chromotubation, but the gravid tube shows evidence of preexisting disease or has been operated on either for a previous EP or blockage. When both tubes show evidence of prior disease, the decision to conserve the gravid tube when it has been operated on previously, or when it appears to have been damaged much more than the opposite one, is not an easy one and has to be made on an individual basis, using as one's guide the extent to which the gravid tube has been damaged both in absolute terms (amount of scarring, mobility, and length) and relative to the other side.

If the contralateral adnexum appears to be completely normal and patent at intraoperative chromotubation, the case for tubal conservation is not compelling. Those who favor salpingostomy argue that if a salpingectomy is performed and an EP recurs, the opportunity to save what is then the only remaining tube may not present itself. This is the strongest argument justifying salpingostomy under these circumstances, but it is a weak one, because this eventuality is likely to occur in less than 5% of cases after salpingectomy (as judged from the average REPR and tubal rupture rate). It has also been argued that intraoperative chromotubation is unreliable and that a normal-appearing tube may nonetheless be diseased. However, the problem with chromotubation is that a patent tube may appear blocked (usually because blood or decidua occlude the cornua), and patency on intraoperative chromotubation is clearly a valid finding. The case against salpingostomy is that when the contralateral tube and ovary are normal, even the most favorable results obtained show no increase in the subsequent LBR. But tubal conservation probably does increase the recurrent tubal pregnancy rate even if only by about 5%, and the risk of early and late postoperative hemorrhage is also greater.

Based on the available information, therefore, one can legitimately adopt either a conservative or an ablative operation in the presence of a normal contralateral adnexa, but in the author's opinion the strength of one's adherence to a course of action should be commensurate with the strength of the supporting evidence. For example, if the pregnancy in the tube is small and unruptured and shells out easily at salpingostomy without bleeding, the tube should almost certainly be conserved. However, if there is a large ruptured tubal pregnancy present, or if after attempting a salpingostomy there is persistent bleeding from the tube, one should have a much lower "threshold" for removing the gravid tube, if the contralateral adnexa are normal, than if the affected tube is the patient's only oviduct or if the contralateral adnexa are severely diseased.

LAPAROSCOPIC SALPINGOSTOMY

Arguably the most important advance in the treatment of tubal pregnancies has been the introduction of laparoscopic surgery. Although Shapiro and coworkers[132] appear to have been the first to treat an EP endoscopically, the credit for pioneering the laparoscopic treatment of EPs must go in full measure to Professor Bruhat and his colleagues in France, who were the first to perform endoscopic salpingostomy and fimbrial expression.[7,20] During the 10-year period 1974–1984, this group treated 321 cases of tubal pregnancy endoscopically and currently treats 90% of tubal gestations in this way. Its early experience showed that what the authors called "tubal aspiration" (the endoscopic equivalent of manual expression of the pregnancy) was associated with a high incidence of incomplete evacuation (three out of 17 cases) compared with salpingostomy (0 out of 43 cases). Therefore, they now restrict the procedure to fimbrial pregnancies.[122]

During the past decade, laparoscopic salpingostomy as described by Bruhat and colleagues has been widely adopted in the United States and the indications for it have been extended.[130,131,133–136] Initially, the procedure was considered applicable only to a very select group of patients (unruptured ampullary pregnancies less than 3 cm in size, otherwise normal pelvis and contralateral tube).[130] However, Reich and coworkers, for example, who have reported the largest American series, have extended the indications for laparoscopic salpingostomy to patients with tubal rupture and nonampullary pregnancies.[131] Indeed, these authors consider that the laparoscopic treatment of tubal pregnancies, including salpingectomy, salpingo-oophorectomy, and segmental tubal resection when indicated, should be regarded as standard therapy in the future. Others have also shown that in practice most tubal pregnancies can be treated laparoscopically, the only absolute contraindications being shock or hemodynamic instability, a very large hemoperitoneum (more than 2 L), and very large pregnancies (>6 cm).[134] In practice, pregnancies that are larger than about 4 cm are difficult to remove because they tend to bleed more and are difficult to extract through the incision.[136]

The laparoscopic treatment of tubal pregnancies has proved to be surprisingly safe, even if not entirely complication-free. Secondary hemorrhage occurs in about 3% of patients,[130,131,133–137] and persistent EP, which is discussed in detail later, also occurs in a significant minority of cases (Table 17-10). Conservative laparoscopic procedures also seem to be as effective as their abdominally performed counterparts in terms of tubal patency and subsequent fertility.[90,130,136] The results of a recently published randomized clinical trial in which laparoscopic and abdominal salpingostomy were compared are shown in Table 17-11.[135] Interestingly, and for reasons that are unclear, the REPR seems to be higher after abdominal than after laparoscopic salpingostomy. A similar trend is apparent in the Yale data once one recognizes that the REPR after laparoscopic salpingostomy was 10% and not 16%, as the authors stated in their paper.[130] However, those data were retrospective and the results easily attributable, for example, to differences in the size of the tubal pregnancies treated by abdominal and laparoscopic salpingostomy. No such disparities were present in the data reported by Vermesh and associates.[136] Others have also found that the tubal incision heals, and tubal patency is restored, just as effectively after a laparoscopic salpingostomy as after an abdominal one, and the results obtained from the operation in women who had only one fallopian tube attest unequivocally to its efficacy (see Tables 17-2 and 17-12).

The advantages of laparoscopic surgery are decreased morbidity and lower cost of treatment. In a recent case-control study, Brumsted and coworkers found that patients treated laparoscopically had a significantly shorter hospital stay than patients undergoing laparotomy (1.34 + 0.8 versus 3.9 + 1.1 days), a shorter postoperative convalescence (8.7 + 7.8 versus 25.7 + 16.2 days), and a reduced requirement for analgesia after surgery.[134] Vermesh and colleagues[136] also found that the average length of hospitalization was 2 days shorter after laparoscopic salpingostomy, which would translate into a $50 million saving annually if half the annual number of tubal pregnancies in the United States were treated laparoscopically rather than abdominally.

PERSISTENT ECTOPIC PREGNANCY

In at least 40% of tubal pregnancies the trophoblast penetrates the tubal wall,[29,30] and some trophoblastic tissue is probably frequently left behind in the oviduct whenever the implantation site is not removed, as is the case with salpingotomy, salpingostomy, or fimbrial expression of the pregnancy. Usually, however, this tissue seems to degenerate, as late postoperative complications after these procedures are uncommon. Occasionally, however, instead of resorbing, the residual trophoblastic tissue persists and resumes growing, until the patient eventually develops symptoms again from intraperitoneal hemorrhage or a pelvic mass. The frequency of persistent ectopic pregnancy after conservative surgery depends on how this entity is defined (ie, whether seemingly abnormal hCG clearance patterns in asymptomatic women are counted as persistent pregnancies). Several case reports of delayed hemorrhage or pain referable to a pelvic mass have been reported after salpingotomy, salpingostomy, and fimbrial expression, but they give no indication of the frequency of the problem.

TABLE 17–10. IMMEDIATE AND DELAYED COMPLICATIONS OF LAPAROSCOPIC SURGERY FOR TUBAL PREGNANCY

			HEMORRHAGE		
AUTHOR/YEAR	NO.	FAILURES	IMMEDIATE	DELAYED	RISING hCG
Pouly et al, 1986[90]	321	n/s	n/s	0	15 (4.8%)
Cartwright, Herbert, Maxson, 1986[133]	27	0	1	0	2
DeCherney and Diamond, 1987[99]	79	n/s	2	0	0
Brumsted, Kessler, Gibson, Nakajima, Riddick, Gibson, 1988[134]	25	0	0	0	1
Reich, Johns, DeCaprio, McGlynn, Reich, 1988[131]	109	0	1	1	2
Silva, 1988[135]	22	0	0	0	1
Vermesh, Silva, Rosen, et al, 1989[136]	30	0	2	0	1

TABLE 17–11. TUBAL PATENCY AND FERTILITY FOLLOWING LAPAROSCOPIC AND ABDOMINAL SALPINGOSTOMY

	TUBAL PATENCY ON HSG	INTRAUTERINE PREGNANCY	TUBAL PREGNANCY
Laparoscopic salpingostomy (*N* = 30)	16/20 (80%)	9/18 (50%)	1/18 (6%)
Abdominal salpingostomy (*N* = 30)	17/19 (89%)	8/19 (42%)	3/19 (16%)

(Data from Vermesh M, Silva PD, Rosen GF, et al. Management of unruptured ectopic gestation by linear salpingostomy's prospective, randomized clinical trial of laparoscopy versus laparotomy. Obstet Gynecol 1989; 73:400.)

Since Kelly and associates first reported delayed hemorrhage following salpingotomy, it has become customary to obtain serial hCG measurements after any conservative operation (usually at weekly intervals) in the hope of forestalling this problem by identifying persistent trophoblastic activity at an asymptomatic stage.[138]

The disappearance rate of hCG following treatment of EPs has been studied by a number of investigators, but fiducial limits for the clearance rate of hCG have not been established, nor are they easy to establish, for reasons that are partly statistical and that will not be pursued here. Steier and coworkers studied 35 patients (one ovarian, 34 tubal pregnancies) treated in an unspecified manner.[139] Pretreatment hCG values ranged between 17 and 8680 mIU/mL (standard not specified), and the disappearance time ranged between 1 and 31 days (median 8.5 days).

Holtz obtained preoperative and at least one postoperative hCG value from 6 women undergoing salpingostomy, and constructed a nomogram that expressed the rate of fall of hCG as a percentage of the preoperative value.[140] His data suggest that 48 hours after surgery the serum hCG should be less than 20% of the preoperative value (based on the *slowest* clearance rate). This translates into an hCG half-life of 0.8 days or less, which seems inordinately rapid to me, even for such a short sampling interval.[79]

Kamrava and associates studied seven patients who underwent salpingectomy or segmental tubal resection, and nine patients who had undergone salpingostomy or fimbrial expression of the pregnancy.[141] The clearance patterns of hCG were broadly similar in these two groups of women. After excision of the implantation site, the serum hCG became "negative" by 14 days in six out of seven women, but required 24 days in the remaining patient. The serum hCG had become "negative" by the 12th postoperative day in eight out of nine conservatively treated patients. The remaining patient still had a positive hCG at 24 days, but she required no treatment.

In an ongoing study by the author, postoperative samples are being obtained from patients following operative treatment for a tubal pregnancy at 7 days. This value was chosen because of all cases of symptomatic sequelae following conservative procedures that had been reported at the commencement of the study, symptoms began at 10 days or later.[142–149] Also, it was felt that by 1 week between-patient variation in the first and fast component half-life of hCG clearance would not be reflected in the serum hCG values. Interestingly, the half-life of hCG as calculated from an intraoperative value and a single postoperative value was similar in patients undergoing salpingectomy and salpingostomy, and the mean value was almost identical to the hCG half-life associated with spontaneous resolution of missed abortions (1.4 days) in an entirely different

TABLE 17–12. TUBAL PATENCY AND PREGNANCY RATES FOLLOWING LAPAROSCOPIC SALPINGOSTOMY

AUTHOR/YEAR	TUBAL PATENCY	PREGNANCIES		
		UTERINE (%)	TUBAL (%)	BOTH
Pouly et al, 1986[90]	14/18 (78%)	76/118 (64%)	26/118 (22%)	5
Cartwright, Herbert, Maxson, 1986[133]	6/8 (75%)	3/8 (38%)	1/8 (13%)	1
Decherney and Diamond, 1987[129]	24/26 (92%)	36/69 (52%)	7/69 (10%)	?
Reich, Johns, DeCapria, McGlynn, Reich, 1988[131]	26/26 (100%)	19/38 (50%)	11/38 (29%)	?
Silva, 1988[135]	—	4/6 (66%)	0	0
Vermesh, Silva, Rosen, et al., 1989[136]	16/20 (80%)	9/18 (50%)	1/18 (6%)	0

study, conducted at another institution.[79] However, it is too early to say whether this approach will prove to be of practical use.

Recently, Vermesh and coworkers described the use of serial postoperative hCG and progesterone measurements following the conservative operative treatment of tubal pregnancies.[150] Serum samples were obtained at intervals of 3 days. Even in patients with persistent trophoblastic activity, hCG levels fell precipitously in the early postoperative period, reaching 13% to 25% of the baseline value by 3 days after surgery and 6% to 25% by 6 days. Thereafter, the serum hCG between the "persistent ectopic" and the "resolved ectopic" groups diverged, with no overlap at all between the groups by the 12th postoperative day. However, the definition of persistent trophoblastic activity was not made totally clear in the paper, inasmuch as two out of six patients with this diagnosis had continually decreasing hCG values and were managed by simple observation.

In summary, serial hCG monitoring after conservative operations for tubal pregnancy has been recommended by all clinical investigators, even though it is not certain how the results should be interpreted. Much more research is needed in this area to establish the various serial hCG patterns that may herald the development of clinical symptoms and the best way to manage these patients. In the interim it seems reasonable to suggest that in the absence of symptoms intervention should not be undertaken as long as the serum hCG continues to fall, however slowly. Rising values should be considered more ominous but do not inevitably presage continued trophoblastic growth. A reasonable compromise might be to intervene when the doubling time of hCG is in the normal range (less than 2.7 days) or to follow subnormally increasing titers for a few days before intervening to ensure that the pattern is persisting.

TREATMENT OF PERSISTENT PREGNANCY

The first few reported cases of persistent ectopic pregnancy presented with intraperitoneal hemorrhage or a pelvic mass and were managed by salpingectomy. Since the introduction of postoperative hCG monitoring, patients with rising hCG levels have been treated with chemotherapy on the assumption that rising hCG levels herald the development of the previously mentioned problems. It is clear from the cases reported to date that treatment with chemotherapy has been very effective (Table 17-13).[142–149] However, the uncertainties surrounding the significance of different serial hCG patterns as harbingers of overt clinical sequelae leave open the possibility that these cases might have resolved without any treatment. Nonetheless, the efficacy of chemotherapy in this setting is entirely in keeping with its effectiveness when used as primary treatment, since failure of primary therapy is generally confined to cases with detectable fetal heart rate activity (discussed later in this chapter). Whether chemotherapy will become the treatment of choice for the treatment of asymptomatic persistent ectopic pregnancies (as defined above or by future research) will depend on what the reproductive performance of women is following this form of therapy, which has not yet been established.

THE NONOPERATIVE TREATMENT OF TUBAL PREGNANCIES

For years, gynecologists have stressed the need to diagnose and treat EPs as early in their natural history as possible to reduce the mortality and morbidity associated with the disease. Therefore, one might be forgiven for regarding present-day attempts to treat tubal

TABLE 17–13. DELAYED HEMORRHAGE FOLLOWING CONSERVATIVE SURGERY FOR TUBAL PREGNANCY

AUTHOR/YEAR	PRIMARY OPERATION	POSTOPERATIVE PROBLEM	INTERVAL	hCG HALF-LIFE	TREATMENT
Kelly, Martin, Strickler, 1979[138]	Salpingotomy	Hemorrhage	18 days	N/K	Salpingectomy
Johnson, Sanborn, Wagner, Compton, 1980[142]	Expression	Pain/mass	10 days	N/K	Salpingectomy
	Expression	Hemorrhage	35 days	N/K	Salpingectomy
Richards, 1984[143]	Salpingostomy	Pain	14 days	7.4	Salpingectomy
Rivlin, 1985[144]	Salpingotomy	Mass	42 days	N/K	Salpingectomy
Higgins and Schwartz, 1986[145]	Salpingotomy	Rising hCG +	17 days	3.7	MTX
Cowan, McGehee, Bates, 1986[146]	Expression	Rising hCG	21 days	3.9	MTX
Bell, Awadalla, Mattox, 1987[147]	Salpingostomy	Mass	26 days	N/K	Salpingectomy
Kenigsberg, Porte, Hull, Spitz, 1987[147]	Salpingostomy	Rising hCG	14 days	2.4	RU 486/MTX
Patsner and Kenigsberg, 1988[149]	Salpingostomy	Rising hCG +	19 days	N/K	MTX
Vermesh, Silva, Sauer, et al, 1989[150]	Salpingostomy	Rising hCG	N/S	N/K	Salpingectomy

pregnancies nonoperatively as misguided and even as courting disaster.[151,152] However, it has been known for many years that some ectopic pregnancies resolve without sequelae.[153] Therefore, a number of investigators have managed selected patients with laparoscopically proven tubal pregnancies expectantly, in the hope of identifying those that may not require treatment.[154–157] The selection criteria used and the results obtained from expectant management by different investigators are summarized briefly in Table 17-14. In addition, following the successful use of chemotherapy in the treatment of some interstitial pregnancies,[158–160] three groups of investigators in the United States have studied the use of methotrexate for the treatment of unruptured tubal pregnancies.[158,161,162] More recently still, the technique of salpingocentesis has been described. This involves aspirating the pregnancy transvaginally using ultrasound guidance and injecting either potassium chloride or methotrexate.[163,164]

Much has been learned about the type of patient who may benefit from nonoperative treatment, even though this form of therapy is not yet ready for clinical application. The patients whose tubal pregnancies are likely to resolve without treatment are the ones who have low (1000 mIU/mL, 2nd-IS) and falling hCG levels, with no detectable FHA on ultrasound. Other prerequisites for expectant management are likely to be the absence of a pelvic mass or fluid on sonography and the rate of fall of hCG. When hCG levels are plateauing or rising, the pregnancy is unlikely to resolve without therapy. Resolution of the pregnancy can be achieved in these cases with chemotherapy, provided that FHA is not detectable by abdominal sonography, but the morbidity seems to be unacceptable vis-à-vis the morbidity from laparoscopic salpingostomy or salpingectomy. Salpingocentesis is likely to prove the only realistic competitor to laparoscopic surgery in these cases, but much more experience is required to determine whether this will prove to be a realistic method of treatment or simply an interesting, but passing, attempt at therapeutic innovation.

Until now, candidates for nonoperative treatment were identified by laparoscopy, and the patients have been monitored very closely in the hospital. Clearly, before this form of management can be accepted into routine clinical practice, further research will be needed to delineate the patients in whom it can be adopted safely without the need for preliminary laparoscopy or the intense surveillance that has been required up to now. If this proves to be impossible, the techniques will not be cost effective because the types of EPs that are amenable to nonsurgical therapy are precisely the ones that are easily treated with minimal morbidity via the laparoscope. If diagnostic laparoscopy continues to be necessary to identify the patients who are candidates for nonsurgical treatment, most of the advantages from this form of therapy will already have been lost. If in the interest of safety a more intensive surveillance program than that required after conservative surgical treatment also proves to be necessary, it is difficult to see what advantages could accrue from this form of treatment.

Besides maternal safety, the other major concern about the nonsurgical treatment of tubal pregnancies has been over the subsequent patency of the affected tube. From the evidence of isolated case reports, it appeared that unrecognized tubal pregnancies could sometimes result in tubal occlusion,[165–167] and delayed diagnosis of an ectopic pregnancy in some cases resulted in the formation of dense adhesions or an inflammatory mass[168] (the so-called chronic ectopic pregnancy). However, very little can be deduced from these data about the prognosis for tubal function following the nonsurgical treatment of tubal pregnancies. Indeed, preliminary evidence suggests that the tubal patency rate following nonsurgical management (approximately 80%) is about the same as that following salpingostomy (see Table 17-14).

HETEROTOPIC PREGNANCIES

Until now the discussion has centered on ectopically implanted singleton pregnancies, but one or more members of a multiple gestation may also implant out-

TABLE 17–14. THE EXPECTANT MANAGEMENT OF TUBAL PREGNANCIES

AUTHOR/YEAR	SELECTION CRITERIA	INITIAL hCG (MIU/ML)	SUBSEQUENT SURGERY	NORMAL PATIENT TUBE ON HSG	PREGNANCIES
Carp et al, 1986	hCG < 250 <2 × 2 CMS	14, 20, 100, 250, 20,000	1/5	1/1	1 Term 2 ABs 1 EP
Garcia, Aubert, Sama, Josimovich, 1987[155]	<4 CMS Falling hCG	All < 4000 10 < 1000 (Stand n/s)	1/13	7/10	3 Term 2 ABs
Fernandez, Rainhorn, Papianik, Bellet, Frydman, 1988[156]	Ampullary, <2 CMS, <50 mL Blood	All < 10,000 9 < 1000 (Stand n/s)	4/14	5/6	3 IUP
Sauer, Vermesh, Anderson et al., 1988[74]	<3 CMS Falling hCG	65–1010 (IRP)	0/5	3/4	n/s

side the endometrial cavity. Ectopic twins are curiosities whose clinical features do not differ from singleton EPs. However, when an EP is combined with an IUP, a potentially disastrous situation exists.

Coexistent intrauterine and extrauterine pregnancies are referred to as combined or heterotopic pregnancies. Based on a study of the Carnegie collection of embryos, Iffy[169] found that in these cases the ectopic pregnancy was always older than the intrauterine gestation (IUP), a finding that he cited in support of his menstrual reflux theory and that also supports superfetation (the occurrence of ovulation, fertilization, and implantation in a woman who is already pregnant) as the underlying cause of at least some combined pregnancies. However, inasmuch as the incidence of heterotopic pregnancies is increased among patients undergoing ovulation induction (see later), most heterotopic pregnancies probably arise from binovular twinning or possibly superfecundation (two synchronously released ova fertilized at different acts of coitus), but it is impossible to make this distinction in practice. The extrauterine pregnancy is almost always tubal, although ovarian,[170] interstitial,[171] abdominal,[172] and cervical pregnancies[173] have been described in association with IUPs.

INCIDENCE

Estimates of the incidence of heterotopic pregnancies are subject to the statistical uncertainties that bedevil the estimation of any uncommon events. (It is also debatable whether it is more meaningful to express the heterotopic pregnancy "rate" as a proportion of intrauterine, extrauterine, or multiple pregnancies, but this question will not be pursued further.) The important point is that in the case of heterotopic pregnancies, unlike other rare types of eccyesis, it is important to know what the current incidence rates are and how they vary in different patient populations, since the supposed rarity of heterotopic pregnancies has had an enormous influence on how the diagnosis of ectopic pregnancies is approached to this day.

For many years, the figure taken for the incidence of heterotopic pregnancies was 1 in 30,000 IUPs.[173] It is not widely recognized, however, that this figure was a theoretical one based on erroneous calculations. It was arrived at by using hypothetical figures for the rate of fraternal twinning and ectopic pregnancies and then making the assumption that the EP rate among singleton and multiple pregnancies was the same within a given population (ie, that the occurrences of EP and twins were independent events). DeVoe and Pratt took the fraternal twinning rate to be 0.8% and the EP rate to be 0.37%. On the assumption of independence, the joint occurrence of these events would then be approximately 1 in 15,000 IUPs $[(0.8/100) \times (0.37/100) \times 2]$, not 1 in 30,000, as DeVoe and Pratt calculated.[174] They omitted multiplying their figure by 2, which is required because in the case of fraternal twinning, each fertilized ovum is subjected to a 0.37% probability of ectopic implantation. It is noteworthy that the empirical heterotopic pregnancy rate among their clinical material was more than double this figure (two out of 13,527 IUPs),[174] suggesting that the figures used in the calculations were underestimates.

Regardless of whether the mathematically correct or incorrect figure is used, it is self-evident that the incidence of heterotopic pregnancies will increase if the incidence of either fraternal twinning or EP is increased. Since the ectopic pregnancy rate has increased quite markedly in recent years, one might expect the heterotopic pregnancy rate to have also increased during the same time period, which is precisely what has happened. The most recently available estimate of the EP rate across the United States as a whole showed this to be about 1.5% of reported pregnancies for the year 1983, and as high as 2.8% in some segments of the population (black women aged 35–44). This translates into a heterotopic pregnancy rate of about 1 out of 2000 to 1 out of 4000 reported pregnancies on the assumption that the rate of fraternal twinning is 0.8% of conceptions and that the EP rate among singleton and multiple pregnancies is the same. Interestingly, for the years 1981–1984, the heterotopic pregnancy rate at Mount Sinai Hospital in New York City was estimated (empirically, not theoretically) to be 1 in 3889 IUPs.[175] (The IUPs were estimated as 115% of the total deliveries plus the number of elective terminations that occurred at the hospital during this time period: a 15% increment was added to take account of spontaneous abortions.) For the years 1969–1977, the heterotopic pregnancy rate at the Sloane Hospital for Women in New York City was found by Reece and coworkers to be one in 7963 reported pregnancies.[176] The average EP rate nationwide during 1970–1977 was about 6.8 per 1000 reported pregnancies, which translates into a heterotopic pregnancy rate of about one in 9000 reported pregnancies. The fairly close correspondence between these empirical and theoretical figures suggests that the assumptions about the fraternal twinning rate in the general population and about the independence of twinning and ectopic implantations are probably valid.

There has been little fluctuation in the rate of fraternal twinning over the years. However, the rate is considerably higher than 0.8% of conceptions among some women. This is true of some racial groups, most notably Nigerians, but is especially the case among women who undergo induction of ovulation, particularly with gonadotropins, and among women undergoing in vitro fertilization–embryo transfer, since it has become standard practice to transfer up to four embryos.[177–181] A relatively high rate of heterotopic pregnancies can be expected among such women: indeed, at one center three out of 26 women who conceived after gonadotropin therapy developed heterotopic pregnancies. It is likely that other factors besides the increased number of fertilized ova made available for implantation influence the frequency of heterotopic pregnancies in this setting, such as the prevailing serum estrogen level at the time of implantation,[16,17] since women subjected to ovulation induction are generally a select group who have no evidence of tubal disease.

CLINICAL FEATURES AND DIAGNOSIS

Inasmuch as the diagnosis of EP has become largely nonsurgical, and in the course of a nonsurgical work-up the detection of an IUP is taken as presumptive evidence that an EP is not present, a heterotopic pregnancy can be expected a priori to pose formidable diagnostic problems and to represent a potentially disastrous situation whenever the IUP is diagnosed first. This will be the case if the IUP is aborted electively or spontaneously before the EP becomes symptomatic. However, even if the presenting symptoms are referable to the EP, it is more than likely that the IUP will be detected in the course of the work-up, and the possibility of an EP dismissed. The converse situation (ie, the EP is diagnosed but the IUP is unsuspected) can be equally disastrous, but for the fetus rather than for the mother.

The literature clearly shows that these concerns are amply borne out in practice. Generally speaking, a correct diagnosis is made in less than 10% of cases preoperatively, and even today many women with a heterotopic pregnancy end up hypovolemic, if not frankly shocked, from tubal rupture and a large hemoperitoneum. These women require transfusion. For example, a concatenation of one or more of these events was present in six out of nine cases described by Bello and coworkers in 1986,[175] and in three out of four cases reported even more recently by Laband and colleagues.[180]

The frequency with which heterotopic pregnancies are said to present with symptoms referable to the ecyesis has varied between 60% and 86%. The signs and symptoms are not markedly different from those associated with corresponding singleton ectopic pregnancies, except that vaginal spotting is said to be less common. However, this could not be corroborated by Reece and associates.[176] Numerous cases come to light after treatment for a supposed missed or incomplete abortion or after a termination of pregnancy. The presence of chorionic villi in the curettage specimen serves invariably to delay the diagnosis.

There are no specific features to help the clinician to diagnose heterotopic pregnancies at an earlier stage other than a general awareness of this possibility, particularly when symptoms and signs of abdominal pain and tenderness persist either after termination of pregnancy or evacuation of a spontaneous abortion, or in women who conceive after gonadotropin therapy, even if an IUP has been demonstrated. Determination of the hCG half-life may be helpful in the first situation if levels plateau (half-life or doubling time more than 7 days) or are rising, but early recourse to laparoscopy is likely to be required in the second group of patients. It is hoped that the earlier diagnosis of combined pregnancies will be a by-product of the widespread use of the vaginal probe in the sonographic evaluation of early pregnancy disorders.

TREATMENT

Treatment consists of removal of the ectopic pregnancy and avoidance of intrauterine instrumentation if the mother wishes to carry the intrauterine pregnancy. The prognosis for the intrauterine pregnancy is, in fact, excellent, provided that signs and symptoms of abortion are not present, as over 75% are carried to term. Indeed, the intrauterine pregnancy can be carried to term even after a cornual resection for a combined interstitial pregnancy.[172]

REFERENCES

1. Atrash H, Hughes JM, Hogue CJR. Ectopic pregnancy in the United States. 1970–1983. CDC Surveillance Summaries. MMWR 1986;35:29ss.
2. Robinson N, Beral V. Risk of ectopic pregnancy. Lancet 1979;2:1247.
3. Westrom L, Bengtsson LPH, Mardh P-A. Incidence, trends, and risks of ectopic pregnancy in a population of women. Br Med J 1981;282:15.
4. Hocking JC, Jessamine AG. Trends in ectopic pregnancy in Canada. Can Med Assoc 1984;131:737.
5. McIntosh MCM. Trends in ectopic pregnancy in New Zealand. Aust NZ J Obstet Gynecol 1986;26:145.
6. Makinen JI. Increase of ectopic pregnancy in Finland—combination of time and cohort effects. Obstet Gynecol 1989;73:21.
7. Atrash HK, Friede A, Hogue GR. Ectopic pregnancy mortality in the United States, 1970–1983. Obstet Gynecol 1987;70:817.
8. Ory HW. Ectopic pregnancy and intrauterine contraceptive devices: new perspectives. Obstet Gynecol 1981;57:137.
9. WHO Task Force. A multinational case-control study of ectopic pregnancy. Clin Reprod Fertil 1985;3:131.
10. Chung CS, Smith RG, Steinhoff PG, et al. Induced abortion and ectopic pregnancy in subsequent pregnancies. Am J Epidemiol 1982;115:879.
11. Levin AA, Schoenbaum SC, Stubblefield PG, et al. Ectopic pregnancy and prior induced abortion. Am J Public Health 1982;72:253.
12. Lehfeld H, Tietze C, Gorstein F. Ovarian pregnancy and the intrauterine device. Am J Obstet Gynecol 1970;108:1005.
13. Diczfaulsy E. New developments in oral, injectable and implantable contraceptives, vaginal rings and intrauterine devices: a review. Contraception 1986;33:7.
14. Morris JM, van Wagenen G. Interception: the use of postovulatory estrogens to prevent implantation. Am J Obstet Gynecol 1973;115:101.
15. McBain JC, Evans JH, Pepperell RJ, et al. An unexpectedly high rate of ectopic pregnancy following the induction of ovulation with human pituitary and chorionic gonadotrophin. Br J Obstet Gynaecol 1980;87:5.
16. Gemzell L, Guillome J, Wang FC. Ectopic pregnancy following treatment with human gonadotrophins. Am J Obstet Gynecol 1982;143:761.
17. Talo A, Pulkinen MO. Electrical activity in the human oviduct during the menstrual cycle. Am J Obstet Gynecol 1982;142:135.
18. Pulkinen MO, Talo A. Myoelectrical activity in the human oviduct with tubal pregnancy. Am J Obstet Gynecol 1984;148:151.
19. Chow WH, Daling JR, Weiss NS, et al. Maternal smoking and tubal pregnancy. Obstet Gynecol 1988;71:167.
20. Chow WH, Daling JR, Weiss NS, et al. Vaginal douching as a potential risk factor for ectopic pregnancy. Am J Obstet Gynecol 1985;153:727.

21. Fedele L, Acaia B, Parazzini F, et al. Ectopic pregnancy and recurrent spontaneous abortion: two associated reproductive failures. Obstet Gynecol 1989;73:206.
22. Kadar N. Ectopic pregnancy: a re-appraisal of aetiology diagnosis and treatment. Prog Obstet Gynaecol 1983;3:305.
23. Washington AE, Cates W, Zaidi AA. Hospitalizations for pelvic inflammatory disease. JAMA 1984;251:2529.
24. Walters MD, Eddy C, Gibb RS. Antibodies to chlamydia trachomatis and risk for tubal pregnancy. Am J Obstet Gynecol 1988;159:942.
25. Vasquez G, Winston RML, Brosens IA. Tubal mucosa and ectopic pregnancy. Br J Obstet Gynaecol 1983;90:468.
26. Kadar N. In: Extrauterine pregnancies. Chapter 4. New York: Raven Press, 1990.
27. Randall S, Buckley H, Fox H. Placentation in the fallopian tube. Int J Pathol 1987;6:132.
28. Budowick M, Johnson TRB, Genardy R, et al. The histopathology of the developing tubal ectopic pregnancy. Fertil Steril 1980;34:169.
29. Pauerstein CJ, Croxatto HB, Eddy CA, et al. Anatomy pathology of tubal pregnancy. Obstet Gynecol 1986;67:301.
30. Senterman M, Jibodh R, Tulandi T. Histopathologic study of ampullary and isthmic tubal ectopic pregnancies. Am J Obstet Gynecol 1988;159:939.
31. Halpin TJ. Ectopic pregnancy: the problem of diagnosis. Am J Obstet Gynecol 1970;106:227.
32. Esposito JM. Ectopic pregnancy: the laparoscope as a diagnostic aid. J Repr Med 1980;25:17.
33. Schwartz RO, DiPietro DL. B-hCG as a diagnostic aid for suspected ectopic pregnancy. Obstet Gynecol 1980;56:197.
34. Rutanen E-M, Tarjanne H, Huovinen J, et al. hCG-beta-subunit radioimmunoassay in gynaecologic emergencies. Lancet 1980;i:484.
35. Lindstedt G, Janson PO, Thorburn J. Sensitivity of serum chorionic gonadotropin assay for ectopic pregnancy. Lancet 1981;1:781.
36. Olson MC, Holt JA, Alenghat B, et al. Limitations of qualitative serum B-hCG assays in the diagnosis of ectopic pregnancy. J Reprod Med 1983;28:838.
37. Norman RL, Lowlings C, Chard T. Dipstick method for human chorionic gonadotrophin suitable for emergency use on whole blood and other fluids. Lancet 1985;i:19.
38. Burford GD, Naftalin AA, Shaw RM. The use of an enzyme linked immunosorbent assay for human chorionic gonadotrophin in gynaecological emergencies. Br J Obstet Gynaecol 1986;93:87.
39. Brown TL, Filly RA, Laing FC, et al. Analysis of ultrasonographic criteria in the evaluation for ectopic pregnancy. Am J Roentgenol 1978;131:967.
40. Lawson TL. Ectopic pregnancy: criteria and accuracy of ultrasonic diagnosis. Am J Roentgenol 1978;131:153.
41. Levi S, Leblieq P. The diagnostic value of ultrasonography in 342 suspected cases of ectopic pregnancy. Acta Obstet Gynecol Scand 1980;59:29.
42. Pedersen JF. Ultrasonic scanning in suspected ectopic pregnancy. Br J Radiol 1980;53:625.
43. Piiroinen O, Puonnonen R. The use of ultrasonography in the diagnosis of ectopic pregnancy. Clin Radiol 1981;32:331.
44. DeCrespigny LC. Demonstration of ectopic pregnancy by transvaginal ultrasound. Br J Obstet Gynecol 1988;95:1253.
45. Stabile I, Campbell S, Grudzinskas JG. Can ultrasound reliably diagnose ectopic pregnancy? Br J Obstet Gynecol 1988;95:1247.
46. Cartright PS, Vaughan B, Tuttle D. Culdocentesis and ectopic pregnancy. J Reprod Med 1984;29:88.
47. Romero R, Copel JA, Kadar N, et al. The value of culdocentesis in the diagnosis of ectopic pregnancy. Obstet Gynecol 1985;65:519.
48. Sandvei R, Stoa KF, Ulstein M. Radioimmunoassay of human chorionic gonadotropin B-subunit as an early diagnostic test in ectopic pregnancy. Acta Obstet Gynecol Scand 1981;60:389.
49. Romero R, Kadar N, Copel J, et al. The influence of the sensitivity of the hCG assay on pregnancy testing and screening for ectopic pregnancy. Am J Obstet Gynecol 1985;153:72.
50. Mashiah S, Carp HJA, Serr DM. Non-operative management of ectopic pregnancy: a preliminary report. J Reprod Med 1982;27:127.
51. Lonky NM, Sauer MV. Ectopic pregnancy with shock and undetectable beta-chorionic gonadotropin: a case report. J Reprod Med 1987;32:559.
52. Taylor RN, Padula C, Goldsmith PC. Pitfall in the diagnosis of ectopic pregnancy: immunocytochemical evaluation of a patient with false negative serum beta-hCG levels. Obstet Gynecol 1988;71:1035.
53. Norman RJ, Buck RH, Rom L, et al. Blood or urine measurement of human chorionic gonadotropin for detection of ectopic pregnancy? A comparative study of quantitative and qualitative methods in both fluids. Obstet Gynecol 1988;71:315.
54. Bernaschek G, Rudelstorfer R, Csaicsich P. Vaginal sonography versus serum human chorionic gonadotropin in early detection of pregnancy. Am J Obstet Gynecol 1988;158:608.
55. Dashefsky SM, Lyons EA, Levi CS, et al. Suspected ectopic pregnancy: endovaginal and transvesicle US. Radiology 1988;169:181.
56. Fossum GT, Davajan V, Kletzky OA. Early detection of pregnancy with transvaginal ultrasound. Fertil Steril 1988;49:788.
57. Goldstein SR, Snyder JR, Watson C, et al. Very early pregnancy detection with endovaginal ultrasound. Obstet Gynecol 1988;72:200.
58. Nyberg DA, Mack LA, Laing FC, et al. Early pregnancy complications: endovaginal sonographic findings correlated with human chorionic gonadotropin levels. Radiology 1988;167:619.
59. Nyberg DA, Mack LA, Harvey D, et al. Value of the yolk sac in evaluating early pregnancies. J Ultrasound Med 1988;7:129.
60. Mahoney BS, Filly RA, Nyberg DA, et al. Sonographic evaluation of ectopic pregnancy. J Ultrasound Med 1985;4:221.
61. Romero R, Kadar N, Castro D, et al. The value of adnexal sonographic findings in the diagnosis of ectopic pregnancy. Am J Obstet Gynecol 1988;158:52.
62. Poland BJ, Dill FJ, Styblo C. Embryonic development in ectopic human pregnancy. Teratology 1976;14:315.
63. Kadar N, DeVore G, Romero R. Discriminatory hCG zone: its use in the sonographic evaluation for ectopic pregnancy. Obstet Gynecol 1981;58:156.
64. Kadar N, Caldwell BV, Romero R. A method of screening for ectopic pregnancy and its indication. Obstet Gynecol 1981;58:162.
65. Romero R, Kadar N, Jeanty P, et al. Diagnosis of ectopic pregnancy: value of the discriminatory human chorionic gonadotropin zone. Obstet Gynecol 1985;66:357.
66. Romero R, Kadar N, Copel JA, et al. Serial hCG testing as a diagnostic tool in ectopic pregnancy. Am J Obstet Gynecol 1986;155:392.
67. Milwidsky A, Adoni A, Segal S, et al. Chorionic gonadotropin and progesterone levels in ectopic pregnancy. Obstet Gynecol 1977;50:145.
68. Radwanska E, Frankenberg J, Allen E. Plasma progesterone levels in normal and abnormal early human pregnancy. Fertil Steril 1978;30:398.
69. Haynes SP, Corcoran JM, Eastman CJ, et al. Radioimmunoassay of progesterone in unextracted serum. Clin Chem 1980;26:1607.
70. Ratcliffe WA, Corrie JE, Dalziel AH, et al. Direct ^{125}I-radioligand assay for serum progesterone compared with assays involving extraction of serum. Clin Chem 1982;28:1314.

71. Mathews CP, Coulson PB, Wild RA. Serum progesterone levels as an aid in the diagnosis of ectopic pregnancy. Obstet Gynecol 1986;68:390.
72. Yeko TR, Gorrill MJ, Hughes LH, et al. Timely diagnosis of early ectopic pregnancy using a single blood progesterone measurement. Fertil Steril 1987;48:1048.
73. Buck RH, Joubert SM, Norman RJ. Serum progesterone in the diagnosis of ectopic pregnancy: a valuable diagnostic test. Fertil Steril 1988;50:752.
74. Sauer MV, Vermesh M, Anderson RE, et al. Rapid measurement of urinary pregnanediol glucuronide to diagnose ectopic pregnancy. Am J Obstet Gynecol 1988;159:1531.
75. Legarth J, Nielsen PL. Freeze microscopy of the endometrium in ectopic pregnancy. Acta Obstet Gynecol Scand 1980;59:505.
76. Bangham DR, Storring PL. Standardization of human chorionic gonadotropin, hCG subunits, and pregnancy tests. Lancet 1982;i:390.
77. Rasor JL, Farber S, Braunstein GD. An evaluation of 10 kits for determination of human choriogonadotropin in serum. Clin Chem 1983;29:1828.
78. Kadar N, Romero R. hCG standardization. Fertil Steril 1987;47:742.
79. Kadar N, Romero R. Further observations on serial hCG patterns in ectopic pregnancy and abortions. Fertil Steril 1988;50:367.
80. Kadar N, Romero R. Observations on the log hCG-time relationship in early pregnancy and their practical implications. Am J Obstet Gynecol 1987;157:73.
81. Batzer FR, Weiner S, Corson SL, et al. Landmarks during the first forty-two days of gestation demonstrated by the B-subunit of human chorionic gonadotropin and ultrasound. Am J Obstet Gynecol 1983;146:973.
82. Pittaway DE, Reissh RL, Wentz AC. Doubling times of human chorionic gonadotropin increase in early viable intrauterine pregnancies. Am J Obstet Gynecol 1985;152:299.
83. Pittaway DE, Wentz AC. Evaluation of early pregnancy by serial chorionic gonadotropin determinations: a comparison of methods by receiver operating characteristic curve analysis. Fertil Steril 1985;43:529.
84. Kadar N. The log hCG-time relationship in early pregnancy (letter to the editor). Am J Obstet Gynecol 1986;154:692.
85. Daya S. Human chorionic gonadotropin increase in normal early pregnancy. Am J Obstet Gynecol 1987;156:286.
86. Tait RL. Five cases of extra-uterine pregnancy operated upon at the time of rupture. Br Med J 1884;1:1250.
87. Siegler AM, Wang CF, Westoff C. Management of unruptured tubal pregnancy. Fertil Steril 1981;36:599.
88. Valle JA, Lifchez AS. Reproductive outcome following conservative surgery for tubal pregnancy in women with a single fallopian tube. Fertil Steril 1983;39:316.
89. DeCherney AH, Maheaux R, Naftolin F. Salpingostomy for ectopic pregnancy in the sole patent oviduct. Fertil Steril 1982;37:619.
90. Pouly JL, Mahnes H, Canis M, et al. Conservative laparoscopic treatment of 321 ectopic pregnancies. Fertil Steril 1986;46:1093.
91. Sherman D, Langer R, Sadovsky G, et al. Improved fertility following ectopic pregnancy. Fertil Steril 1982;37:497.
92. Toumivara L, Kauppila A. Radical or conservative surgery for ectopic pregnancy? A follow-up study of fertility of 323 patients. Fertil Steril 1988;50:580.
93. Thorburn J, Philipson M, Lindblom B. Fertility after ectopic pregnancy in relation to background factors and surgical treatment. Fertil Steril 1988;49:595.
94. Fianu S, Ingleman-Sundberg A, Vaclavinkova V. The influence of an early diagnosis on the results of surgical treatment of ectopic pregnancy. Int J Gynecol Obstet 1983;21:247.
95. Oelsner G, Morad J, Carp H, et al. Reproductive performance following conservative microsurgical management of tubal surgery. Br J Obstet Gynaecol 1987;94:1078.
96. Hallatt JG. Tubal conservatism in ectopic pregnancy: a study of 200 cases. Am J Obstet Gynecol 1986;154:1216.
97. Kadar N, Cruddas M, Campbell S. Estimating the probability of spontaneous delivery conditional on time spent in the second stage. Br J Obstet Gynecol.
98. DeCherney AH, Kase N. The conservative surgical management of unruptured ectopic pregnancy Obstet Gynecol 1979;54:451.
99. Kalchman GG, Meltzer RM. Interstitial pregnancy following homolateral salpingectomy. Am J Obstet Gynecol 1966; 96:1139.
100. Bowbrow ML, Bell HG. Ectopic pregnancy: a 16-year survey of 905 cases. Obstet Gynecol 1962;20:500.
101. Hallatt JG. Repeat ectopic pregnancy: a study of 123 consecutive cases. Am J Obstet Gynecol 1975;122:520.
102. Jeffcoate TNA. Salpingectomy or salpingo-oophorectomy? J Obstet Gynecol Br Emp 1955;62:218.
103. Bender S. Fertility after tubal pregnancy. J Obstet Gynecol Br Emp 1956;63:400.
104. Douglas ES, Shingleton HM, Crist T. Surgical Management of tubal pregnancy: effect on subsequent fertility. South Med J 1969;62:954.
105. Schenker JG, Eyal F, Polishuk WZ. Fertility after tubal pregnancy. Surg Gynecol Obstet 1972;135:74.
106. Franklin EW, Zeiderman AM, Laemmle P. Tubal ectopic pregnancy. Etiology, obstetric and gynecologic sequelae. Am J Obstet Gynecol 1973;117:220.
107. Nagami M, London S, Amand PS. Factors influencing fertility after ectopic pregnancy. Am J Obstet Gynecol 1984;149:533.
108. Scott JS, Lynch EM, Anderson JA. Surgical treatment of female infertility: value of paradoxical oophorectomy. Br Med J 1976;1:631.
109. Trimbos-Kemper TCM, Trimbos JB, Van Hall EV. Management of infertile patients with unilateral tubal pathology by paradoxical oophorectomy. Fertil Steril 1982;37:623.
110. Stromme WB. Conservative surgery for ectopic pregnancy: a twenty year review. Obstet Gynecol 1973;41:215.
111. Ploman L, Wicksell F. Fertility after conservative surgery in tubal pregnancy. Acta Obstet Gynecol Scand 1960;39:143.
112. Jarvinen PA, Nummi S, Pietila K. Conservative operative treatment of tubal pregnancy with postoperative daily hydrotubations. Acta Obstet Gynecol Scand 1972;51:169.
113. Langer R, Bukovsky I, Herman I, Sherman D, Sadovsky G, Caspi E. Conservative surgery for tubal pregnancy. Fertil Steril 1982;38:427.
114. Tuladi T. Reproductive performance of women after two tubal ectopic pregnancies. Fertil Steril 1988;50:164.
115. Macomb P, Gomel V. Linear ampullary salpingostomy heals better by secondary versus primary closure (Abstr). Fertil Steril 1984;45S:41.
116. Cropp CS, Cowell PD, Rock JA. Failure of tubal closure following laser salpingostomy for ampullary tubal ectopic pregnancy. Fertil Steril 1987;48:887.
117. Sandvei R, Bergso P, Ulstein M, Steier JA. Repeat ectopic pregnancy. A twenty year hospital survey. Acta Obstet Gynecol Scand 1987;66:35.
118. Schoen JA, Nowak RJ. Repeat ectopic pregnancy: a 16-year clinical survey. Obstet Gynecol 1975;45:542.
119. DeCherney AH, Sildker JS, Mezer HC, et al. Reproductive outcome following 2 ectopic pregnancies. Fertil Steril 1985;43:82.
120. Timonen S, Nieminen U. Tubal pregnancy, choice of operative method of treatment. Acta Obstet Gynecol Scand 1967;46:327.
121. Swolin K, Fall M. Ectopic pregnancy. Acta Eur Fertil 1972;3:147.

122. Bruhat MA, Mahnes H, Mage G, Pouly JL. Treatment of ectopic pregnancy by means of laparoscopy. Fertil Steril 1980;33:411.
123. Paavonen J, Varjonen-Toivonen M, Komulainen M, Heinonen PK. Diagnosis and management of tubal pregnancy: effect on fertility outcome. Int J Gynaecol Obstet 1985;23:129.
124. Sherman D, Langer R, Herman A, Bukovsky I, Caspi E. Reproductive outcome after fimbrial evacuation of tubal pregnancy. Fertil Steril 1987;47:420.
125. Winston RML. Microsurgery of the fallopian tube: from fantasy to reality. Fertil Steril 1980;34:521.
126. Stangel J. Recent techniques for the conservative management of tubal pregnancy: surgery, laparoscopy and medicine. J Reprod Med 1986;31:99.
127. DeCherney AH, Boyers SP. Isthmic ectopic pregnancy: segmental resection as the treatment of choice. Fertil Steril 1985;44:307.
128. Smith HO, Toledo AA, Thompson JD. Conservative surgical management of isthmic cornual pregnancies. Am J Obstet Gynecol 1987;157:604.
129. Lachin JM. Introduction to sample size determination and power analysis for clinical trials. Controlled Clin Trials 1981;2:93.
130. DeCherney AH, Diamond MP. Laparoscopic salpingostomy for ectopic pregnancy. Obstet Gynecol 1987;70:948.
131. Reich H, Johns DA, DeCaprio J, McGlynn F, Reich E. Laparoscopic treatment of 109 consecutive ectopic pregnancies. J Reprod Med 1988;33:885.
132. Shapiro HI, Adler DH. Excision of an ectopic pregnancy through the laparoscope. Am J Obstet Gynecol 1973;117:290.
133. Cartwright P, Herbert CM, Maxson WS. Operative laparoscopy for the management of tubal pregnancy. J Reprod Med 1986;31:589.
134. Brumsted J, Kessler C, Gibson C, Nakajima S, Riddick DH, Gibson M. A comparison of laparoscopy and laparotomy for the treatment of ectopic pregnancy. Obstet Gynecol 1988;71:889.
135. Silva PD. A laparoscopic approach can be applied to most cases of ectopic pregnancy. Obstet Gynecol 1988;72:944.
136. Vermesh M, Silva PD, Rosen GF, et al. Management of unruptured ectopic gestation by linear salpingostomy: a prospective, randomized clinical trial of laparoscopy versus laparotomy. Obstet Gynecol 1989;73:400.
137. Mettler L, Semm K. Management of ectopic pregnancy: a shift from laparotomy to pelviscopy. Int J Fertil 1988;33:389.
138. Kelly RW, Martin SA, Strickler RC. Delayed hemorrhage in conservative surgery for ectopic pregnancy. Am J Obstet Gynecol 1979;133:225.
139. Steier JA, Bergso P, Myking OL. Human chorionic gonadotropin in maternal plasma after induced abortion, spontaneous abortion, and removed ectopic pregnancy. Obstet Gynecol 1984;64:391.
140. Holtz G. hCG regression following conservative surgical management of tubal pregnancy. Am J Obstet Gynecol 1983;147:347.
141. Kamrava MM, Taymor ML, Berger MJ, et al. Disappearance of hCG following removal of ectopic pregnancy. Obstet Gynecol 1983;62:486.
142. Johnson TRB, Sanborn JR, Wagner KS, Compton AA. Gonadotropin surveillance following conservative surgery for ectopic pregnancy. 1980;33:207.
143. Richards BC. Persistent trophoblast following conservative operation for ectopic pregnancy.
144. Rivlin ME. Persistent ectopic pregnancy: complication of conservative surgery. Int J Fertil 1985;30:10.
145. Higgins KA, Schwatrz MB. Treatment of persistent trophoblastic tissue after salpingostomy with methotrexate. Fertil Steril 1986;45:427.
146. Cowan BD, McGehee RP, Bates GW. Treatment of persistent ectopic pregnancy with methotrexate and leukovorum rescue: a case report. Obstet Gynecol 1986;67:505.
147. Bell OR, Awadalla SG, Mattox JH. Persistent ectopic syndrome: a case report and literature review. Obstet Gynecol 1987;69:521.
148. Kenigsberg D, Porte J, Hull M, Spitz IM. Medical treatment of residual ectopic pregnancy: RU 486 and methotrexate. Fertil Steril 1987;47:702.
149. Patsner B, Kenigsberg D. Successful treatment of persistent ectopic pregnancy with oral methotrexate therapy. Fertil Steril 1988;50:982.
150. Vermesh M, Silva PD, Sauer MV, et al. Persistent tubal ectopic gestation: patterns of circulating beta-human chorionic gonadotropin and progesterone, and managements options. Fertil Steril 1988;50:584.
151. Martin DC. Letter to the editor. Fertil Steril 1987;48:344.
152. Corsan GH, Carr BR. Letter to the editor. Fertil Steril 1988;50:380.
153. Lund JJ. Early ectopic pregnancy. J Obstet Gynaecol Br Emp 1955;62:70.
154. Maschiach S, Carp HJA, Serr DM. Nonoperative management of ectopic pregnancy. A preliminary report. J Reprod Med 1982;27:127.
155. Garcia AJ, Aubert JM, Sama J, Josimovich JB. Expectant management of presumed ectopic pregnancy. Fertil Steril 1987;48:395.
156. Fernandez H, Rainhorn JD, Papiernik E, Bellet D, Frydman R. Spontaneous resolution of ectopic pregnancy. Obstet Gynecol 1988;71:171.
157. Sauer MV, Gorrill MJ, Rodi IA, et al. Nonsurgical management of unruptured ectopic pregnancy: an extended clinical trial. Fertil Steril 1987;48:752.
158. Tanaka T, Hyashi H, Kutsuzawa T. Treatment of interstitial pregnancy with methotrexate. Report of a successful case. Fertil Steril 1982;37:851.
159. Brandes MC, Youngs DD, Goldstein DP, Parmley TH. Treatment of cornual pregnancy with methotrexate: case report. Am J Obstet Gynecol 1986;155:655.
160. Altaras M, Cohen I, Cordoba M, Ben-Nun I, Ben-Aderet N. Treatment of an interstitial pregnancy with actinomycin D. Case report. Br J Obstet Gynecol 1988;95:1321.
161. Ory SJ, Villanueva AL, Sand PK, Tamura R. Conservative treatment of ectopic pregnancy with methotrexate. Am J Obstet Gynecol 1986;154:1299.
162. Stovall TG, Ling FU, Buster JE. Outpatient chemotherapy of unruptured ectopic pregnancy. Fertil Steril 1989;51:435.
163. Feichtinger W, Kemeter P. Conservative treatment of ectopic pregnancy by transvaginal aspiration under ultrasonographic control and methotrexate injection. Lancet 1987;1:381.
164. Timor-Tritsch H, Baxi L, Peisner DB. Transvaginal salpingocentesis: a new technique for treating ectopic pregnancy. Am J Obstet Gynecol 1989;160:459.
165. Haney AF. Bilateral tubal occlusion secondary to asymptomatic ectopic pregnancy. Obstet Gynecol 1986;67:52s.
166. Gomel V, Filmar S. Arrested tubal pregnancy. Fertil Steril 1987;48:1043.
167. Tulandi T, Ferenczy A, Berger E. Tubal occlusion as a result of retained ectopic pregnancy: a case report. Am J Obstet Gynecol 1988;158:1116.
168. Cole T, Corlett RC. Chronic ectopic pregnancy. Obstet Gynecol 1982;59:63.
169. Iffy L. Embryological studies of time of conception in ectopic pregnancy and first trimester abortion. Obstet Gynecol 1965;76:490–498.
170. Phillips WDP. Clomiphene citrate-induced concurrent ovarian and intrauterine pregnancy. Obstet Gynecol 1979;53:37S.
171. Beckman CRB, Tomasi AM, Thomason JL. Combined intersti-

tial and intrauterine pregnancy: cornual resection in early pregnancy and caesarian delivery at term. Am J Obstet Gynecol 1984;149:83.

172. Felbo H, Fenger HJ. Combined extra- and intrauterine pregnancy carried to term. Acta Obstet Gynecol Scand 1966;45:140.
173. Phillips WDP. Twin pregnancy (intrauterine and cervical) after hemimysterectomy: case reports. Am J Obstet Gynecol 1978;130:603.
174. DeVoe RW, Pratt JH. Simultaneous intrauterine and extrauterine pregnancy. Am J Obstet Gynecol 1948;56:1119.
175. Bello GV, Schonholz D, Moshirpur J, Jeng D-Y, Berkowitz RL. Combined pregnancy: the Mount Sinai experience. Obstet Gynecol Surv 1986;41:603.
176. Reece EA, Petrie RH, Sirmans MF, Finster M, Todd WD. Combined intrauterine and extrauterine gestations: a review. Am J Obstet Gynecol 1983;146:323.
177. Berger MJ, Taymor ML. Simultaneous intrauterine and tubal pregnancies following ovulation induction. Am J Obstet Gynecol 1972;113:812.
178. Koroly MV, Belsky DH. Heterotopic pregnancy as a result of induced ovulation. A report of two cases. J Reprod Med 1982;27:476.
179. Yovich JL, Stanger JD, Tuvic A, Hahnel R. Combined pregnancy after gonadotropin therapy. Obstet Gynecol 1984; 63:855.
180. Laband SJ, Cherny WB, Finberg HJ. Heterotopic pregnancy: report of four cases. Am J Obstet Gynecol 1988;158:437.
181. Sondheimer SJ, Tureck RW, Blasco L, Strauss J, Arger P, Mennuti M. Simultaneous ectopic pregnancy with intrauterine twin gestations after in vitro fertilization and embryo transfer. Fertil Steril 1985;43:313.

18

CHAPTER

MULTIFETAL PREGNANCIES: EPIDEMIOLOGY, CLINICAL CHARACTERISTICS, AND MANAGEMENT

Diana M. Adams and Frank A. Chervenak

BACKGROUND

INCIDENCE AND PERINATAL SIGNIFICANCE

The incidence of multiple gestations is generally underestimated, because incidence rates reflect successful multiple gestations at advanced gestational ages rather than conception rates. The overall incidence of twins worldwide is about 1 in 80 pregnancies (1.13%).[1,2] The frequency of monozygotic (MZ) twins is relatively constant throughout the world, regardless of maternal age, parity, or race. The incidence is between 3.5 and 4 per 1000 births.[3] In contrast, the incidence of dizygotic (DZ) twins varies and is affected by a number of factors. In general, Asians have the lowest rate of DZ twinning, whites have an intermediate rate, and blacks have the highest incidence.[4] The lowest incidence, 4.3 per 1000, has been reported from Japan. Twelve of 1000 have been reported from the United States and 45 of 1000 have been reported from Nigeria.[5,6] Advancing maternal age and parity have independent positive effects on the incidence of DZ twins.[4] Taller, heavier women have a twinning rate 25% to 30% higher than short, nutritionally deprived women.[7] Greater coital frequency seems to increase the number of twin pregnancies.[8] Patients treated with clomiphene citrate have a twinning rate between 6.8% and 17%.[9] Treatment with gonadotropins may result in a rate between 18% and 53.5%.[9] The incidence of twins following in vitro fertilization using presently accepted methods is roughly equal to the rate following ovulation induction with human menopausal gonadotropins.[10] Interestingly enough, the rate of zygotic splitting and, therefore, monozygotic twins appears to be higher following ovulation induction therapy and in the setting of IVF.[11,12]

Higher-order gestations are rare except in cases in which fertility medications or IVF have been used. Most agree that the frequencies of triplets and other higher-order multiple gestations that occur naturally can be estimated using Hellin's hypothesis.[1] This calculation states that, if the incidence of twins in a given population is n, the incidence of triplets will be the square of n, the incidence of quadruplets will be the cube of n, and so on. In the United States, where $n = 85$, the incidence of triplets naturally occurring would be approximately 1 in 7000, quadruplets would be approximately 1 in 600,000, and so on. Again, with increasing use of ovulation induction and IVF, these rates are increasing.

Despite their relative rarity, multiple gestations contribute significantly to perinatal mortality. In a recent epidemiologic survey, twins accounted for 12.6% of the perinatal mortality, although they accounted for only 2.5% of the population.[13] Overall perinatal mortality for twins in developed countries ranges between 65 and 120 of 1000 births.[2] This corresponds to approximately a ninefold increase in incidence of perinatal death for the first twin and an 11-fold increase for the second twin when compared to singletons. With higher-order gestations, the greater prematurity and birth order are the most identifiable factors in relation to mortality. For example, with triplets the mortality rate for the infant born last is double that for the one born first and is intermediate for the one born second.[14] The perinatal mortality rate for triplets is 148 to 312 of 1000 births.[15,16]

Prematurity and intrauterine growth retardation (IUGR) leading to the high incidence of low–birth-weight infants in multiple gestations are the main causes of this significantly increased mortality. They also lead to most of the increased perinatal morbidity of multiple gestations. Studies reveal that more than 50% of twins weigh less than 2500 g.[17] Approximately 10%

of preterm deliveries are twin gestations.[18] Fifty percent of twins are delivered before 37 weeks,[18] a 12-fold increase in incidence compared to singletons.[19] The average length of gestation decreases inversely with the number of fetuses present (Table 18-1).[19] IUGR contributes to a higher incidence of stillborn babies,[17] and it is estimated that two thirds of twins show some signs of growth retardation at delivery.[21]

In addition to premature delivery and IUGR, congenital anomalies, placental abnormalities, cord accidents, preeclampsia, and malpresentations all have an increased incidence with twins and contribute to the overall morbidity and mortality.

DIAGNOSIS OF MULTIPLE GESTATION

Currently, more than 90% of twins are diagnosed before delivery,[22] a vast improvement over the frequently quoted figure of 50% from just 15 years ago.[23] This improvement is in large part due to the widespread availability of diagnostic ultrasound and maternal serum α-fetoprotein screening.

Clinical Indications

Clues that are suggestive of the diagnosis of multiple gestations include past or family history of twins, report of increased weight gain, and increased fetal activity. The most useful clinical screening tool is the finding of a fundal height greater than dates. Prior to the advent of obstetric ultrasound, antenatal diagnosis of twins was established by the auscultation of two fetal hearts differing by more than 10 beats per minute heard simultaneously by two examiners.[24] Complications indicative of a multiple gestation are unexplained anemias, hydramnios, or early onset of pregnancy-induced hypertension (PIH).

Maternal Serum α-Fetoprotein

No biochemical parameter will make the definitive diagnosis of more than one fetus. However, maternal serum α-fetoprotein elevation (>2.5 MOM) occurs in 20% to 30% of patients with twins. If the elevation is greater than 4 MOM and twins are seen, further evaluation is indicated.[25] If the extreme elevation remains unexplained after follow-up ultrasonography and amniocentesis, the pair still needs to be watched closely, as an associated poor perinatal outcome has been found for this group of twins.[25]

TABLE 18–1. AVERAGE LENGTH OF PREGNANCY RELATIVE TO THE NUMBER OF FETUSES (IN PREGNANCIES BEYOND 20 WEEKS GESTATION WITH ACCURATE DATES)

NO. OF FETUSES	NO. OF PREGNANCIES	DAYS GESTATION COMPLETED
One	82	271
Two	21	246
Three	5	234
Four	3	205

From Caspi E, Ronen J, Schreyer P, et al. The outcome of pregnancy after gonadotrophin therapy. Br J Obstet Gynaecol 1976;83:967.

Ultrasound

Given all the preceding clinical and biochemical clues, a differential diagnosis could still include poor dates, hydramnios, molar pregnancy, myomas, or neural tube defects. Ultrasound is clearly the diagnostic method of choice, as it will confirm both the diagnosis and the number of multiple fetuses.[26] In the first trimester, multiple sacs can be seen with transabdominal ultrasound at 6 weeks. Embryos within the sacs will be seen at 7 weeks, and fetal hearts can be identified between 7 and 8 weeks.[27] All these landmarks are seen approximately 1 to 2 weeks earlier with the transvaginal approach.[28] It is prudent to reserve the diagnosis of twins until two fetal poles with two fetal hearts are seen, because of the high frequency of twin "disappearance" in patients scanned in early pregnancy.[29]

Currently, the exact prevalence of this phenomenon of the "vanishing twin" has not been determined. It has been reported to range between 13% and 78% of patients scanned before 14 weeks of gestational age, with higher rates in those twins studied before 10 weeks.[29] From another perspective, it is estimated that 5% of patients presenting with first-trimester bleeding carry a diagnosis of a vanishing twin.[30] This disappearance phenomenon also occurs in multiple gestations of higher order. It is possible either that one twin was resorbed or that one twin was an anembryonic pregnancy (blighted ovum) from conception.[31] Two points need to be considered. First, a definitive diagnosis of twins on an early first-trimester sonogram should not be made simply on the basis of visualization of two cavities, as a blood clot or transducer pressure can mimic a twin gestation, or a "disappearing" twin might be present. Second, a therapeutic dilatation and curettage in the setting of an "inevitable abortion" should be done only after a sonogram is performed to rule out a potentially viable twin. Even with cramps, heavy bleeding, and a soft and dilated cervix, the remaining singleton usually carries to term without further complications, especially when the twin dies early in pregnancy.[31]

ZYGOSITY AND CHORIONICITY

There are two basic types of twin gestations, monozygous and dizygous. In describing them, one should avoid the terms *identical* and *fraternal*, which refer only to phenotypic likeness, although in general *identical* implies monozygosity and *fraternal* is meant to describe dizygosity. Overall, approximately 30% of multiple gestations are monozygous and 70% are dizygous.[32] Monozygous refers to progeny resulting from the fertilization of one ovum by one sperm. Then, after a variable number of divisions, the single zygote divides into two or more embryonic primordia, which explains their genotypic likeness. Dizygotic gestations result from the fertilization of two separate ova by two separate sperm, allowing for genotypic dissimilarity. Multiple gestations of higher order can be comprised of any combinations of monozygotic, dizygotic, or multizygotic gestations.

The cause of monozygous gestation is not known. It might be considered to be a teratogenic event occurring early in development of what would have become a singleton gestation. This concept of a twinning impetus, such as oxygen deprivation or other adverse environmental condition, has been supported by animal data.[33] The increased incidence of congenital anomalies associated with monozygotic twins also agrees with this hypothesis. It is generally assumed that dizygotic and multizygotic gestations are the result of multiple ovulation and that this in turn is secondary to elevated serum gonadotropins.[9,34–36] That two separate sperm are involved in dizygotic twins is supported by the rare but well-documented cases of superfecundation.[37] Theories other than multiple ovulation include the existence of two ova in one follicle, and the occurrence of irregular ovulation events such as polar body fertilization.[38]

Embryology

There are essentially three types of twin placentas—monoamnionic–monochorionic, diamnionic–mono chorionic, and diamnionic–dichorionic. All dizygous twins have dichorionic (diamnionic) placentas. Monozygous gestations, however, can result in any of the three possible configurations.[39] If the "twinning impetus" acts in the first 2 days after fertilization, a diamnionic dichorionic placenta will result (Fig. 18-1). About 30% of monozygous twins have this type of placenta.[39] It is felt that if the blastomeres separate within the first 10 days—at the two-cell stage while they still have full potential to form a morula, a blastula, and an embryo—each will have its own membranes and chorion. Amnion–chorion and chorion–amnion are the four layers of dividing membranes that show on histologic examination. Blood vessels and ghost villi might also be seen in the septum. Most diamnionic dichorionic placentas are the result of dizygous twinning. To identify the subset that are monozygous one must look at other parameters.

If twins arise between the third and the eighth days, the resulting placenta will be diamnionic monochorionic. About 70% of monozygous twins are of this type.[39] It is felt that the inner cell mass duplicates at the morula or blastula stage, that the trophoblast has already differentiated into the future chorion, but that the amnion has yet to form. Pathologic review of this placenta reveals a delicate, thin, translucent septum. This is in contrast to the thicker, opaque septum seen with dichorionic placentation. Separation of the membranes is easy. Microscopic examination reveals two layers of amnionic membranes in opposition with a central cleavage space and without chorion.

Finally, twins share the same sac if they arise after the amnion has formed, which occurs roughly about days 9 to 12. Monoamnionic monochorionic twins are the least common variety of monozygous gestations. They occur

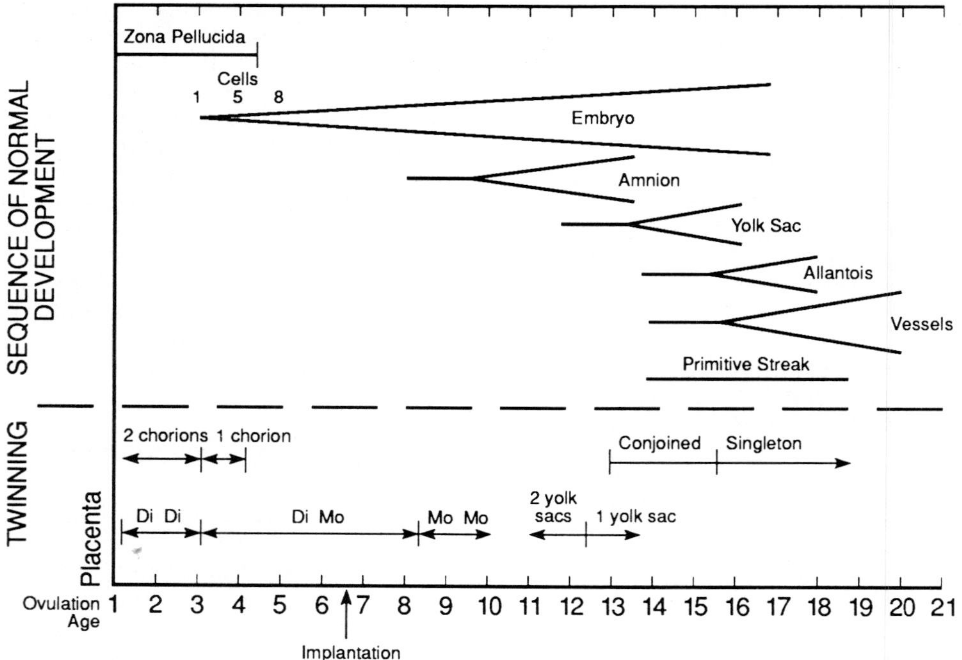

FIGURE 18–1. The embryology of twinning. (From Benirschke K. Twin gestation: incidence, etiology and inheritance. In: Creasy RK, Resnik R, eds. Maternal-fetal medicine: principles and practice. 2nd ed. Philadelphia: WB Saunders, 1989: 567.)

in about 1% of twin births.[39] This placenta will not have separating membranes, and pathologic confirmation is straightforward.

If the twinning process occurs even later, and duplication of the embryonic rudiment is thereby incomplete, conjoined twins can result. The phenomenon of "fetus in fetu" (an included twin) may be an even later form of incomplete twinning. Beyond the 17th day a singleton gestation will develop.

Placentas of higher orders of multiple gestations follow these same general developmental principles. Therefore, any combination of monochorionic and dichorionic, monoamnionic and diamnionic placentation can exist.

Examination of the placenta after birth aids in determination of zygosity. In approximately 35% of patients, differing sex establishes twins as dizygous. In an additional 20%, careful study of the placenta, as outlined previously, leads to the proper diagnosis. In the remaining 45% of like-sex dichorionic twins, most are dizygotic. In Cameron's study 37% were dizygotic and 8% were monozygotic.[40] Other methods to determine zygosity after birth in these cases are blood-grouping and DNA-mapping techniques. Antenatal determination of zygosity has now been worked out as well using molecular genetic techniques.[41] Determination is important in light of the immunobiology of tissue transplantation. Monozygous twins have the advantage of being able to accept tissue from one another as an isograft.

ABNORMALITIES OF MULTIPLE GESTATION

Fetal Anomalies

An overview of the abnormalities encountered in multifetal pregnancies appropriately begins with a discussion of fetal anomalies. The incidence is one and a half to three times higher than that of singleton gestations.[2,6,42] This increase is due to the higher percentage of structural defects found in monozygotic twin gestation.[6] Higher-order multiple gestations have an even greater chance of having an anomaly of one fetus.[42] When anomalies are detected, both twins are affected in only 14.8% of patients, and in none of them have all three triplets been affected by an anomaly.[43] Schinzel describes three helpful categories to organize the anomalies encountered in multifetal pregnancies.[44]

The first category of anomalies to be reviewed are those felt to be a consequence of the "teratogenic" event of twinning itself. Examples are sirenomelia, holoprosencephaly, exstrophy of the cloaca, anencephaly, and midline neural tube defects.[45] Nance proposes that this group of defects involving midline structures must be in some way linked to the twinning process.[46]

A more obvious result of twinning is the anomaly of conjoined twins, which deserves special mention as it is specific to multiple gestations. The incidence ranges from one in 50,000 to one in 100,000 births, or roughly one in 600 twin births.[47,48] The cause is felt to be incomplete division of the monozygotic embryo (13 to 16 days after ovulation). These twins are classified by site of union. Most commonly they are fused at the chest (thoracopagus).[48]

Fetus in fetu means "included twin," a vertebrate embryonic mass that develops inside of its companion embryo.[49,50] First clarified by Lord, this phenomenon is extremely rare, with fewer than 43 cases reported.[49] It is distinguishable from a teratoma by radiographic or sectional demonstrations of part or all of the vertebral column. The diagnosis is reinforced when the other bones or organs that are present are appropriately formed.[51]

The second category of anomalies to consider is made up of those resulting from the vascular interchange that is a potential complication of any monozygotic gestation. An acardiac twin is believed to arise when arterial–arterial and venous–venous anastomoses exist without any arterial–venous connections (Fig. 18-2.)[52] This provides for uncompensated reverse flow, which is then linked to absence of the heart. Whether the heart atrophied in this setting of a reversed circulation or did not properly develop is not known. This anomaly is rare and specific to multiple gestations, affecting approxi-

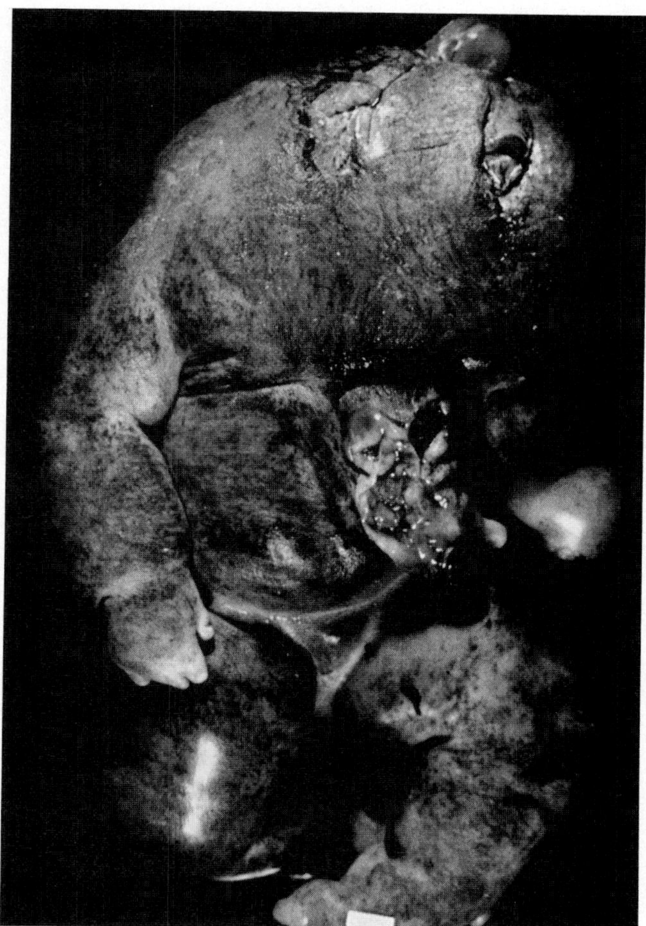

FIGURE 18–2. Postmortem photograph of an acardiac twin. (From Chervenak FA, Isaacson F, Lorber J. Anomalies of the fetal head, neck, and spine. Philadelphia: WB Saunders, 1988: 153.)

mately one in 30,000 infants or one in 100 monozygotic twin births.[47] Usually the heart is absent, but at times a misshapen one is found. Usually no head is present. These acardiac twins can be distinguished from teratomas because of the presence of a cord that is short and contains only one artery and one vein.[52]

Another type of vascular interchange that can lead to abnormalities is the embolization of necrotic material or development of disseminated intravascular coagulation (DIC) that can happen when one fetus is dead and vascular connections are present.[53] In this setting, the live twin can develop microcephaly, hydranencephaly, intestinal atresia, aplasia cutis, or limb amputation.[44,54]

The last type of anomaly related to multiple fetuses is that group of problems resulting from intrauterine crowding. Examples are minor foot deformities and skull asymmetry.[47] There also may be an increased frequency of congenital dislocation of the hip.[44,47]

Placental Anomalies

Anomalies of the placenta are also much more common among twins. These anomalies have an even higher incidence among higher-order multiple gestations. A bivascular (monoarterial) cord, found in only 1% of pregnancies, is found in closer to 4% of twins.[55] Prolapse of the umbilical cord occurs more frequently.[1] A velamentous cord complicates 1% of singleton pregnancies and 7% of twins.[1] The portion of cord that is unprotected is susceptible to thrombosis, compression, or rupture. The dreaded complication of rupture of a vasa previa must be anticipated. A circummarginate or circumvallate placenta is more frequently seen with twins.[56]

The Twin–Twin Transfusion Syndrome

The abnormality of vascular connections between placentas has been reported to complicate as many as 85% of monochorial placentas studied.[39] When arterial–venous connections are uncompensated and unidirectional flow results, the abnormality of the "twin–twin transfusion syndrome" can occur (Fig. 18-3).[1] The diagnosis as originally described by Corney consists of the three findings of hydramnios, a hemoglobin difference of at least 30% (4.4 g/100 mL), and morbid changes of the twins.[55] As many as 30% of monochorial twins have this syndrome to some degree. It is important to remember that there is a spectrum of involvement from the vascular abnormality, from very slightly affected to the full syndrome. In its most severe form, the donor fetus is growth retarded, or possibly hydropic due to high-output failure, with anemia and hypotension. The recipient of the transfusion will be more active, will have increased fluid due to increased urination, and will have congestive heart failure due to circulatory overload. This recipient twin will have hypovolemia, hypertension, plethora, and thromboses or peripheral vessels. The placenta will reveal pathologic changes in the respective areas.[57,58] The donor area should be boggy, pale, and edematous, and the receiving area should be red and congested. The vascular connections should be demonstrable. The degree of morbidity from the syndrome will depend not only on the quality and caliber of the vessels involved, but also on the gestational age of the pregnancy and the presence or absence of any compensatory connections (arterial–arterial or venous–venous). Perinatal mortality in the extreme cases may be as high as 70%.[39] Less affected twins have a much better prognosis. If the smaller twin dies, it is possible for the surviving twin to reach term as the hydramnios resolves.

PHYSIOLOGY

Compared to the singleton pregnancy, there is a greater maternal weight gain in multiple gestations. This increase begins as early as the first trimester, indicating that factors other than simply the size of the conceptus

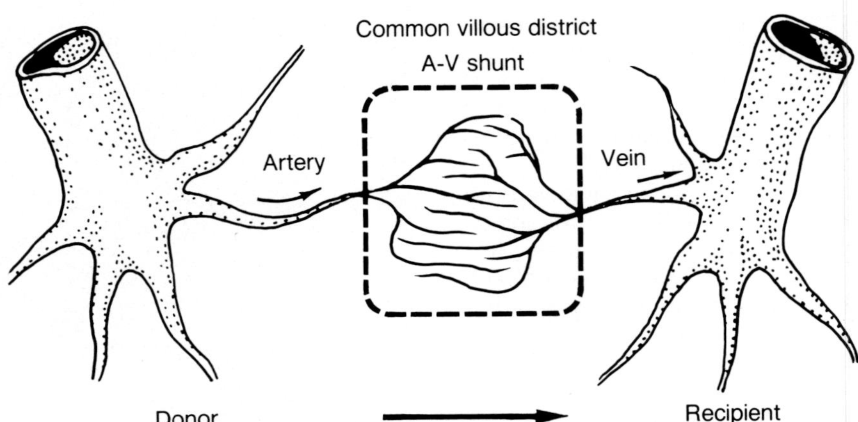

FIGURE 18–3. The pathologic arteriovenous connection in the twin transfusion syndrome. (Redrawn from Benirschke K. Twin gestation: incidence, etiology and inheritance. In: Creasy RK, Resnik R, eds. Maternal-fetal medicine: principles and practice. Philadelphia: WB Saunders, 1989.)

are involved.[59] Uterine growth is increased so that by 25 weeks gestation the total intrauterine volume with twins already equals that of a term singleton.[60] Hematologic changes are remarkable for the even greater hemodilution that takes place, as there is on average a hemodilution of 500 mL additional increase in plasma volume.[61] Recommended are 60 to 80 mg of iron and 1 mg of folate daily, in addition to a varied high-protein diet to meet these increased demands and avoid significant anemia.[61] Fibrinogen is increased even further.[62] The cardiovascular system is also affected in an exaggerated manner when compared with a singleton pregnancy.[63] There is an even greater drop in diastolic blood pressure in the second trimester, followed by a greater rise before delivery.[64] The incidence of pregnancy-induced hypertension is increased.[64] The respiratory system is notable for an even greater increase in tidal volume.[62] Carbohydrate metabolism may be affected; some data indicate that there is a higher incidence of gestational diabetes with multiple gestations.[62] Glomerular filtration rates are enhanced further.[62] Ureteral changes, such as dilatation from hormonal changes or compression at the pelvic brim, are exaggerated, which may lead to an increased stasis and more urinary tract infections.[65] The incidence of frank pyelonephritis may or may not be increased among multiple gestations.[65,66] One author has found a higher incidence of hyperemesis gravidarum among patients with twins.[61] Another author could not substantiate this observation from a review of the literature.[65]

Total concentration of serum protein and electrolytes is reduced because of the increased plasma volume. Total intravascular protein mass, however, is unchanged, as are serum sodium, potassium, chloride, and osmolality.[62] Maternal serum human chorionic gonadotropin levels are approximately two and a half times higher in twins than in singletons.[67] Human placental lactogen is also increased in maternal serum,[68] with levels from a dizygotic pregnancy on average higher than levels from a monozygotic pregnancy.[69] Because of increased DHEAS production by four fetal adrenals and increased 16-hydroxylation by two fetal livers, estriol levels are higher in twin pregnancies.[70] Serum estradiol and progesterone levels are also increased in the setting of a multiple gestation.[62,70]

ANTEPARTUM DIAGNOSIS AND MANAGEMENT

PREVENTION OF PREMATURITY

A review of the antepartum management of multifetal pregnancies appropriately begins with a discussion of premature delivery, which is the leading cause of morbidity and mortality in this group. The incidence of preterm birth among twins is between 20% and 50%,[71,72] and even higher for triplets (75%) and higher-order multiple gestations.[73] The average number of completed weeks of gestation at delivery is inversely related to the number of fetuses (Table 18-1).[19] Multiple gestations comprise 25% of the perinatal deaths related to prematurity.[71] Most of this mortality (50% to 80%) occurs before 32 weeks.[22,74] The critical period of gestation appears to be between 26 and 29 weeks,[22] and between 600 g and 900 g.[61] Preterm deliveries are the result of premature labor, premature rupture of the membranes, and third-trimester bleeding. Theories on the underlying causes for these complications include increased uterine tone from distention, increased intra-amniotic pressure, increased readiness of the myometrium, and uteroplacental insufficiency.[75] Because of their potentially significant impact on morbidity and mortality, many methods of preventing premature birth have been explored, with varying levels of success. But, overall, little progress has been made in this particular area of management of multiple fetuses. It becomes clear as we review these methods of combating prematurity that further clinical investigation in this area is needed.

DIAGNOSIS

Patient education, early referral to a specialist, and antepartum care in a special clinic are all measures aimed at earlier identification of the problem of premature labor.[5,76,77] Knowledgeable risk assessment, combined with serial cervical examinations, may also help identify patients at highest risk for premature birth (Table 18-2). Several authors have shown that subtle cervical changes warrant the use of additional measures to combat premature labor and delivery before they become inevitable.[5,77,78]

Home monitoring is a noninvasive modality that can lead to earlier identification and, therefore, treatment of premature uterine activity. One study has shown that baseline uterine activity is increased in twin pregnancies.[79] Other studies have shown that there is a characteristic increase in frequency of contractions as early as several weeks before development of preterm labor in those patients destined to have this complication.[80,81] Furthermore, a significant rise in contraction frequency is characteristic in the 24 hours immediately preceding the episode of preterm labor. (This apparently holds true for both singletons and twins, but not for triplets.)[81] The study by Katz and colleagues, which was controlled but not randomized, concluded that the home

TABLE 18–2. RISK FACTORS IN MULTIPLE GESTATIONS

Higher-order multiple gestations
Monozygosity
Single fetal death
Polyhydramnios
Anomaly
Growth discordancy
MSAFP > 4 MOM
Premature rupture of the membranes
Antepartum bleeding
Pregnancy-induced hypertension
Premature labor

monitoring device was helpful in making an earlier diagnosis of preterm labor, in that monitored patients had less cervical change when they presented.[82] In addition, the monitored patients had a lower incidence of failed tocolysis, gained more time in utero, and were more likely to deliver at term.[82] An appreciable reduction in incidence of prematurity with use of the home monitor would be difficult to prove, as often the patients using it have other risk factors for premature delivery. For the individual patient, however, it is our bias that outpatient uterine monitoring may be of value. The monitor should help identify the subset of twins that are in need of the initiation of the more invasive methods of combating prematurity.

MANAGEMENT

Tocolysis

Tocolysis has been looked at both as a prophylactic and as a therapeutic means of managing prematurity. The use of prophylactic beta-sympathomimetics was found by one researcher both to prolong gestation and to increase birth weight.[5] However, most studies to date have not shown a benefit, and the present consensus does not support the routine use of prophylactic tocolytics.[83–85] The use of ritodrine in the treatment of premature labor, on the other hand, has been shown to be beneficial.[86] The efficacy seen is similar to the benefit of ritodrine therapy for premature labor complicating a singleton pregnancy. Because of the increased maternal blood volume and cardiac output of a multiple pregnancy, the margin of safety with use of tocolytics is narrow.[87] Careful fluid management and monitoring of cardiovascular status are critical in the prevention of pulmonary edema and other maternal complications.

Bedrest

The value of bedrest in prevention of prematurity is controversial. Much of the confusion in the literature results from a lack of unanimity among protocols and a predominance of retrospective data. The nature of bedrest (inpatient vs. outpatient) and the gestational age at which bedrest was initiated vary from one study to the next. Saunders and colleagues, in a prospective randomized study, failed to show benefit from bedrest in the hospital starting at 32 weeks.[88] A large, prospective, controlled study, one that concentrates on the critical period, is needed. It has been found that up to 81% of perinatal mortality in twins occurs before the 29th week of gestation.[22] Therapeutic bedrest to prevent premature birth would be needed before this period. The authors feel that hospitalized bedrest is disruptive and costly. For these reasons alone it should not be routinely recommended until it has been proved to be beneficial. Of course certain complications, such as premature cervical dilatation, recurrent contractions, and suspected IUGR, may warrant prolonged hospitalization for rest and closer observation.

Cerclage

The placement of a cerclage to reinforce the cervix under the strain of a multiple gestation has been advocated by some.[89] Others have found no benefit from this procedure.[5,90–92] Because the procedure for twins does not yet have a proven benefit, and it is not without significant risks, the authors' view is that a cerclage should be placed only when suspected cervical incompetence is present in a twin pregnancy. The value of a cerclage for triplets, quadruplets, and greater multiple gestations is unproven at this time.

Steroid Administration

The use of steroids for treating known or suspected pulmonary immaturity has been shown to be efficacious in certain patients carrying singleton pregnancies.[93] Their use in multifetal pregnancies, however, has remained controversial. A collaborative study did not demonstrate a benefit from dexamethasone for twins or triplets, and they postulated that the dynamics and concentrations of the steroid might be altered when multiple fetuses are present.[93] A recent study using ambraxol found an effectiveness in reducing the incidence of respiratory distress syndrome for twins.[94] It should be kept in mind that when steroids are administered in multifetal pregnancies, especially when other tocolytic drugs are in use, the risk of maternal pulmonary edema may be greater.

Selective Reduction

Higher-order multiple fetuses are frequently delivered prematurely.[16,95] Antepartum management of these pregnancies should employ all available noninvasive measures to prolong gestation.[15,16] Bedrest and tocolytics should also be used liberally.[15,16] An invasive modality with potential benefit specific to this group of higher-order multiple gestations is that of embryo reduction. Selective termination of one or more embryos in the first trimester of a multiple gestation may be of value in reducing the complication of severe prematurity for this group.[96]

FETAL ASSESSMENT

A primary aim of antepartum management in multiple pregnancies should be serial fetal assessment to reduce the risks of IUGR, discordance, acute hypoxic stress in utero, and fetal death. The tools available to assess the fetus as a patient have been the focal point of the recent growth in obstetrics. Clearly, these modalities have a special role in the management of the fetus in a multiple pregnancy.

Diagnosis With Ultrasound Imaging

Fetal Growth. The use of ultrasound imaging is central to the diagnosis of the problems that twins face in utero. There is some controversy concerning the difference between normal fetal growth in twins and that in singletons. Most agree that progress is similar until at least the third trimester[97–99]; others believe the use of singleton nomograms is valid even beyond this point.[100,101] Studies indicate that femur length measurements between singletons and twins are similar throughout gestation,[100,101] although abdominal circumference growth is less after 32 weeks.[102,103] This is consistent with neonatal data showing that measurements such as body length and head circumference are not significantly reduced when compared to those for singletons.[102] It is technically possible to measure multiple parameters with ultrasound. These parameters are helpful in assessing fetal growth. Estimated fetal weight is especially useful in this regard.[104,105] In addition, because growth is a dynamic process, serial scanning is necessary.

Intrauterine Growth Retardation. To minimize the risks of intrauterine growth retardation (IUGR), fetal assessment by ultrasound is currently recommended every 3 to 4 weeks, beginning at 26 weeks, and as frequently as every 2 weeks if the diagnosis is suspected. The relative uteroplacental insufficiency that underlies IUGR in twin gestations is believed to become significant at about the onset of the third trimester. Multiple gestations of higher order may be at risk even sooner. Biparietal diameter (BPD) differences between twins will correlate with a higher incidence of IUGR, especially when those differences are greater than 4 to 6 mm,[106–108] but a discrepancy does not make the diagnosis. For instance, there will be no difference if both fetuses are growth retarded. IUGR can be predicted using an estimated fetal weight that is calculated using multiple parameters.[109] Of the individual parameters, abdominal circumference is the most accurate measurement.[110] IUGR in multiple gestations is not rare. It occurs in only 5% to 7% of singleton pregnancies, and it may complicate as many as 47% of multiple gestations.[103,105] Indeed, objective evidence of IUGR after delivery (neonatal body water turnover) has been found in up to 70% of twin neonates.[21,111] Therefore, a high index of suspicion for the problem, and careful, thorough examinations on a serial basis, are the best ways to ensure proper diagnosis of this complication.

Growth Discordance. As with IUGR, measurement of abdominal circumference is the most sensitive marker for significant growth discordance.[109,110] An intrapair difference of 20 mm should be followed with careful estimation of fetal weights based on abdominal circumferences, femur lengths, and BPDs. A difference in fetal weights of greater than 20% will then provide the best predictive value. Twin–twin transfusion syndrome, IUGR of one twin, and hydrops or macrosomia of one fetus are three underlying causes of weight discordance.

The diagnosis of the twin–twin transfusion syndrome has been made antenatally using ultrasound.[112] The sonographic findings are as follows. Midtrimester hydramnios is seen in the sac of a larger twin that may already have developed hydrops. The smaller twin classically is growth retarded with diminished fluid volume or frank oligohydramnios. This combination of findings is to be differentiated from a situation in which one twin has simple IUGR and the other twin is growing normally and is, therefore, larger. In this case the larger twin should be surrounded by a normal amount of amniotic fluid and should not be hydropic. With any growth-retarded fetus, the possibility of an underlying fetal anomaly should be considered. A less likely possibility is a patient with a normal fetus that is smaller relative to a twin that is hydropic or macrosomic. In this final instance the "smaller" twin should have a normal fluid volume and no other evidence of IUGR.

Amniotic Fluid Volume Assessment. Assessment of amniotic fluid volume with ultrasound is a mainstay of fetal surveillance for high-risk singleton pregnancies. Likewise, ultrasound evaluation of amniotic fluid is important when evaluating twins. Increased or decreased fluid may be the first sign of a new problem, such as IUGR, discordance from a transfusion syndrome, or hydrops. Abnormal fluid volume may lead to the discovery of an anomaly that had not previously manifested itself. And, certainly, altered fluid volume signals the need for closer surveillance with the other modes of fetal surveillance. The combination of polyhydramnios and oligohydramnios in twin gestations carries a very high perinatal mortality rate, especially if the finding is present before 26 weeks gestation.[113] The four-quadrant method of amniotic fluid assessment, which is widely used in singleton pregnancies, has not been established for use in twin pregnancies.[114]

Fetal Membranes. Ultrasound is instrumental in making the important diagnosis of a monoamniotic gestation. A monoamniotic sac is one without a visible separating membrane. This finding should be repeated on multiple examinations before a definitive diagnosis is made. Monoamniotic twins are rare, occurring in only 1% of twin gestations.[39] Antenatal diagnosis is important because of a mortality rate of 50% to 60% associated with monoamniotic twins. This mortality is predominantly the result of cord entanglement, which occasionally can be seen even by ultrasound.[115] In one reported case monoamniotic twins were seen by ultrasound. When variable decelerations were then seen on nonstress testing, delivery was accomplished, and entanglement of the twin cords was documented at cesarean section.[116]

After excluding a monoamniotic pregnancy, a systematic approach to diagnose chorionicity may be helpful.[117] This will begin with determination of sex. Discordant sex indicates that the pregnancy is dizygotic and, therefore, the placenta is dichorionic. Likewise, if two separate placental discs are seen, the gestation is dichorionic.

Dichorionic twins carry the lowest perinatal mortality rate, about 9%.[39] This type of placentation does not carry the potential for vascular communications and their associated complications of embolization and transfusion. In addition, most dichorionic placentas are associated with dizygotic twins, which do not have the greatly increased incidence of anomalies found among monozygotic twins. Difficulty at this step in determining chorionicity can arise if fetal position prevents sex determination or if an accessory lobe of placenta exists.

If evaluation of sex and number of placentas identifies twins of like sex and a shared placenta, attention is turned to the dividing membrane. Two methods of determining chorionicity have been described. The first method determines membrane thickness; this method correctly identifies chorionicity in 80% to 90% of patients.[118–121] A monochorionic membrane should be thin and hairlike. A dichorionic membrane is thick and more easily visualized. The second method involves actual counting of the layers in a dividing membrane. When this is possible, the correct diagnosis can be made in almost all cases.[122] Monochorionic dividing membranes should have only two layers; dichorionic membranes should consist of three or four visible layers. Evaluating the dividing membrane to determine chorionicity is optimally performed early in pregnancy. Factors that make the diagnosis more difficult are thinning of the membrane and intrauterine crowding, both of which become more of a problem as the pregnancy advances. A third situation that makes visualization of the membrane difficult is oligohydramnios of one twin. In this case the membrane may be completely apposed to the body of the fetus, which no longer has any fluid around it. If this is so, however, this fetus is trapped against the uterine wall. Therefore, even if the mother moves or a significant amount of time has elapsed, this "stuck twin" will not have moved. This sign aids in differentiating this situation from a monoamniotic pregnancy.[117]

Fetal Death in Utero. The diagnosis of single fetal death, which complicates 0.5% to 6.8% of multiple gestations, can be facilitated by ultrasound.[123,124] As previously discussed, early in pregnancy a vanishing twin may be a common event that usually does not lead to further problems. However, death of one fetus later in a multiple gestation can be associated with significant morbidity and mortality. The risk of major morbidity or death for the surviving twin has been reported to be as high as 46%.[125] Prognosis will depend on the cause of the initial demise, as well as the type of placentation—and therefore the degree of shared circulation—and the estimated gestational age or time of delivery. Potential fetal complications include DIC, thromboembolic phenomena from release of necrotic material into a shared circulation, and anemia from relaxation of the dead twin's vascular bed.[39,54,124,126,127] With a dead fetus in utero, the mother is also at risk for development of DIC from release of thromboplastic material.[128–130]

Antepartum Fetal Heart Rate Monitoring and the Biophysical Profile.

Ultrasound is used to monitor growth, monitor amniotic fluid volume, describe placentation, and diagnose fetal death, all of which are relatively long-term markers of fetal status in utero. Multiple gestations also should be monitored for acute changes in status, such as hypoxic stress in utero. Antepartum fetal heart rate monitoring and the biophysical profile (BPP) provide this immediate indication of fetal status.

Nonstress Test. At The New York Hospital–Cornell Medical Center, as at many centers, the nonstress test (NST) is the screening method of choice for fetal surveillance.[131] This method does not have contraindications and is less time-consuming because it is feasible to test multiple fetuses simultaneously.[132] The NST is reliable and has high predictive value when the results are normal.[133] When the results are abnormal the predictive value is lower, and vibroacoustic stimulation or another test of fetal well-being should be used to differentiate the sleeping fetus from the asphyxiated one.

Contraction Stress Test. Although a contraction stress test (CST) may be performed safely in some cases of multiple gestation, this form of fetal surveillance is rarely used. Often multiple pregnancies are complicated by conditions for which the CST is contraindicated, such as premature labor, abnormal placentation, or abnormal bleeding. If a spontaneous CST arises during a period of antepartum fetal heart rate testing, its interpretation may be of value.

Biophysical Profile. The fetal BPP is a reliable method of fetal surveillance and can be used as a means of follow-up of a nonreactive NST.[134] Of course it will be more time-consuming for a multiple gestation, but there are no contraindications to this procedure. Its sensitivity and specificity have been found to be as high for twins as for singletons.[134]

The time to initiate routine screening with these tests of fetal well-being is currently debated. Because they are noninvasive and potentially life-saving, many would begin testing at least weekly at the onset of fetal viability (26 weeks). Certainly they are indicated if a multiple gestation is complicated by other factors that place the fetus at even higher risk for acute hypoxic stresses in utero. These would be complications such as IUGR, premature labor, growth discordance, monozygosity, PIH, or any of the other complications listed earlier (see Table 18-2). In a case of dichorionic twins, the value of these tests as an adjunct to ultrasound is less certain.

Doppler Ultrasound. Doppler velocimetry is an accepted method of evaluating placental impedance in singleton pregnancies, during which it has been shown to predict in utero acid–base status and neonatal morbidity.[135,136] The role of Doppler in assessment of twins has been outlined by Pardi and Ferrazi.[137] Their technique uses continuous- and pulsed-wave Doppler coupled in a mechanical sector scanner to ensure proper localization of each twin. They found that for concordant sex pairs without anomalies a significant intrapair pulsatility index (PI) gradient was observed prior to 28 weeks in all pairs that subsequently had birth weight differences of more than 15%. They contend that this finding with Doppler preceded other evidence of growth difference by 4 to 8 weeks. Their recommendation is that Doppler assessment of twin fetuses should be initiated at 20 to 22 weeks to help identify pairs at risk for abnormal growth and in need of closer follow-up with the other methods of fetal assessment. In addition, other authors have found an abnormally high systolic/diastolic (S/D) ratio, combined with ultrasound findings, to be helpful in the diagnosis of both IUGR and the twin–twin transfusion syndrome.[138,139] Chapter 45 is devoted to the subject of Doppler velocimetry.

Percutaneous Umbilical Blood Sampling. Percutaneous umbilical blood sampling (PUBS) can be performed in a twin gestation for appropriate indications (see Chapter 51). A recent report described its use in determining fetal platelet counts.[140] Without cordocentesis the scalp of only the presenting twin can be sampled, and then only if the membranes are ruptured and the cervix is sufficiently dilated. Diagnosis of trisomy 18 has been confirmed in monozygous twins using PUBS.[141] And the technique has been described in the documentation of the twin–twin transfusion syndrome prior to selective feticide.[142] The exact risks of the procedure, however, are not well defined in multiple gestations.

MANAGEMENT

Intrauterine Growth Retardation

When IUGR afflicts one or more fetuses, management is similar to that of IUGR in a singleton. The risks of prematurity must be weighed against the risks of continued stress in utero. In addition, in multiple gestations the gestational age of the normal fetus(es) must be considered. If a decision is made to continue the pregnancy, close fetal surveillance should ensue, with biweekly ultrasound examination to assess fetal growth, frequent heart rate monitoring and BPPs, and possibly Doppler velocimetry. Ideally, delivery of the growth-retarded fetus should await fetal lung maturity of all the fetuses. If further evidence of fetal asphyxia becomes evident on the additional testing, delivery may become mandatory prior to documented maturity of all fetuses.

Growth Discordance

After careful ultrasound diagnosis of a twin–twin transfusion syndrome, management consists primarily of tocolysis for the premature labor that results from the progressive polyhydramnios. As with IUGR, bedrest and expectant management with close fetal surveillance are indicated. If fetal maturity is reached, delivery should be carried out. In contrast, for severely premature fetuses, allowing one fetus to die in utero in order to avoid severe prematurity for both is recommended. If the smaller twin dies, the hydramnios may resolve. The larger twin may reach a gestation at which survival is much more likely. Between the extremes of fetal lung maturity and severe prematurity, management of cases should be individualized. With the development of fetoscopy, occlusion of the pathologic arterial–venous connections might become possible.[39]

Acute and Chronic Polyhydramnios

"Acute" polyhydramnios is a phenomenon that complicates 5% to 8% of multiple gestations; it comprised 15% of all cases of hydramnios in one series.[61] It is usually associated with monozygotic twins.[143] A large amount of fluid accumulates rapidly, usually in the second trimester. This is to differentiate it from "chronic" polyhydramnios, which is more likely to be associated with an anomaly of the fetus.[144] This acute increase in fluid carries with it an extremely high rate of fetal mortality from severe prematurity. Weir recommends frequent amniocentesis to reduce fluid volume and delay delivery.[143] Others believe that the risks of this procedure, which include abruption, infection, and premature labor from the tap itself, outweigh the benefits.[75] The authors believe amniocentesis should be performed to relieve maternal respiratory embarrassment and in some manifestations of intractable premature labor.

Monoamniotic and Monochorionic Gestations

Diagnosis of amnionicity and chorionicity aids in perinatal management. Monoamnionic pregnancies need intensive fetal surveillance and early delivery to reduce their extremely high mortality rates. Monochorionic diamnionic gestations also deserve close monitoring. Monochorionic gestations have an increased perinatal mortality rate when compared to dichorionic gestations. Because they are monozygotic, they are at greater risk for anomalies, and they can have shared circulation, with its associated problems. With closer monitoring, an acute indication for earlier delivery may arise, as this group is at higher risk for hypoxic stress in utero. Dichorionic pregnancies progress with the fewest complications. Ultrasound is still indicated to follow fetal growth.

Single Fetal Death in Utero

After 34 weeks, delivery for all multiple gestations complicated by death of one fetus in utero is recommended after documentation of fetal lung maturity.[145] Before 34 weeks, expectant management with close surveillance seems prudent.[124] Both serial ultrasound and the other tests of fetal well-being and weekly determinations of maternal coagulation parameters are recommended. Delivery may become necessary prior to 34 weeks or documentation of fetal lung maturity if stress in utero of the surviving fetus(es) becomes apparent. The maternal coagulopathy that can occur develops slowly[128] and, if detected, can be successfully treated with heparin in cases remote from term.[129,130] Mode of delivery is usually determined by other obstetric indications but may be affected by the position of the dead twin.

Maternal Complications

Pregnancy-Induced Hypertension. Antepartum management of multiple fetuses includes the treatment of the many maternal complications of these pregnancies. Pregnancy-induced hypertension (PIH) is seen in as many as 37% of multiple gestations.[146] Not only is the incidence of PIH higher than that in singleton pregnancies, but the onset is often earlier and the severity greater. The risks of this disease to both mother and fetus, as well as the diagnosis and management of PIH, are similar in singleton and twin gestations (see Chapter 59). PIH is seen even more commonly with multiple gestations with more than two fetuses.[61]

Hemorrhage. Maternal hemorrhage is a major concern antepartum, intrapartum, and especially postpartum.[61,145] Placenta previa and abruptio placentae are both slightly more common with multiple fetuses.[147–149] There is an increased need for surgical intervention during the intrapartum period and, therefore, an increased risk of blood loss during this period.[150] Overdistention of the uterus, leading to uterine atony, can lead to a significant postpartum hemorrhage.[147]

Diagnosis

Ultrasound. Many anomalies are identifiable with ultrasound imaging. Conjoined twins are first suspected when ultrasound evaluation fails to reveal a dividing membrane.[151] Not only are the twins in the same sac but, on repeated examinations, their position relative to one another does not change.[152] Hydramnios is present in more than half the cases.[39] Longitudinal scanning of the heads, thoraces, and abdomens will then reveal any sharing of a major organ that is present.[152] A careful search must be made in all cases for other major congenital anomalies, as these often further complicate conjoined twins.[39]

For craniopagus pairs, junctions in the parietal and frontal areas are most favorable for separation and subsequent survival.[153] However, 40% of craniopagus twins have an intercerebral bridge, the location of which is critical in their prognosis.[152] One type of incomplete twinning results in one cephalic pole but two facial complexes, monocephalus–diprosopus (Fig. 18-4).[154] These twins usually also have major cardiac and neural tube abnormalities, which are important to consider in counseling.[155] Thoracopagus twins may have cardiac sharing or other major cardiovascular anomalies unsuitable for separation or correction.[152,156] The examination should be targeted to visualize two separate, four-chamber hearts, with normal inflow and outflow tracts. Echocardiography should be used to help determine if extrauterine life is possible and to document independent fetal heart rates if present. Any

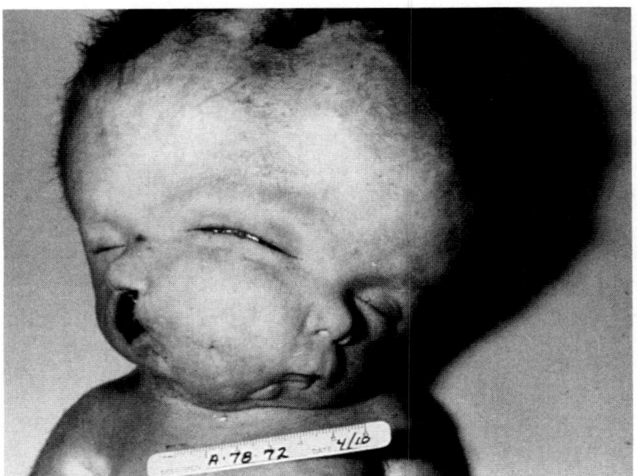

FIGURE 18–4. Postmortem photograph of infant with craniofacial duplication. (From Chervenak FA, Pinto MM, Heller CI, Norooz H. Obstetric significance of craniofacial duplication. J Reprod Med 1985;30:74.)

blood flow through communication sites should be studied with Doppler.[156] Omphalopagus twins should be ruled out by ultrasound of the umbilical cord insertion areas.[152] Separate umbilical vein Doppler flow should be documented. Joining at the level of the lower spines or below should be ruled out by visualizing free fetal movement at that level and uninhibited lower limb activity. Number and size of fetal urinary bladders should be documented, and potential cloacal anomalies should be explored.[152]

Fetus in fetu has been diagnosed antenatally using ultrasonography.[157] A complex mass with strong internal echoes was observed. Prenatal diagnosis led to prompt diagnosis and management in the neonatal period.

Some anomalies of multiple gestations are felt to be secondary to vascular interchange. The most striking example of this is reversed arterial perfusion, resulting in acardia. Hydramnios and a suspected dead smaller twin are clues to the diagnosis.[152] Signs of congestive heart failure and resultant death may be seen in the otherwise normal twin. Heart development in the perfused twin will vary from a rudimentary tube to complete absence of the heart. A series of complex echoes and repeated absence of heart motion will be seen in the "dead" twin, but unusual limb motion and evidence of growth may be detected.[152]

Chorionic Villous Sampling and Amniocentesis. Karyotype abnormalities are identifiable with chorionic villous sampling (CVS) and amniocentesis. There are special considerations to be aware of when proceeding with these diagnostic procedures in multiple gestations. If twins are newly diagnosed at the time of a scheduled procedure, the patient should be removed from the examination table and given time to reconsider.

CVS is feasible when twins have separate placentas.

The transcervical route and transabdominal route, or a combination of approaches, have been used. As with amniocentesis, the risk of fetal loss for twins, with CVS, is believed to be approximately equal to the risk for singletons.[158]

Amniocentesis for analysis of karyotype and AFP analysis requires sampling from both sacs. Tapping the cavities individually should begin with careful sonographic mapping.[159] If there is any uncertainty that separate sacs are being sampled, then the first sac should be identified with contrast. Indigo carmine or Evan's blue dye can be used. Methylene blue should be avoided because it is a chemical reducing agent with the ability to cause fetal hemolysis.[160] Red dyes cannot be used as they might be confused with blood.[161] Ultrasound guidance throughout the procedure is important. The fluid of the second sac should be free of contrast. Amniocentesis for twins in the second trimester, as with singletons, has been found to be a reliable and safe method for prenatal diagnostic testing.[162]

At times, documentation of fetal lung maturity by amniocentesis will aid in clinical management. It is felt that amniocentesis to document fetal lung maturity in most cases can be done by tapping only one sac.[161] Most studies indicate a close correlation between L/S ratios with twins. A ratio above 2.5 is felt to provide a margin of safety even in the setting of intersac variation.[61] Several situations, however, can lead to substantial differences between twins in L/S ratios. In fetuses in which the maturity indices may be altered significantly, the sac of the twin expected to be less mature should be sampled. For example, in the setting of premature rupture of membranes the twin in the unruptured sac should be tapped.[163] After onset of labor, the twin presenting second should be sampled.[161] If a significant discrepancy is present, the larger twin should have the amniocentesis.[161] One author continues to advocate amniocentesis of both sacs to assure fetal pulmonary maturity.[164]

MANAGEMENT

Conjoined twins are stillborn in 40% of births[152] and, in many instances, the remaining newborns are severely premature. If the fetuses are dead or have little chance of surviving and are small enough to be delivered vaginally, this route would be preferable. If conjoined twins have a possibility of survival, delivery should be by cesarean section, with appropriate neonatal support. For some patients, even when their fetuses are dead, abdominal delivery is necessary to avoid maternal trauma. Postnatal prognosis will depend on the site and degree of union, the presence or absence of any other major anomalies, and the degree of prematurity.

In cases of acardia, a method of obliterating a well-visualized vascular communication would be therapeutic, in that it would alleviate high output failure in the normal twin.[55] Steroids to enhance pulmonary maturity and early delivery might also have a role in limiting the damage to the normal twin. Mode of delivery may be affected by the position of the anomalous twin.

Management of any of the many other anomalies that can be seen with increasing frequency among twins, and management of any karyotype abnormality that is found, will depend on the severity of the anomaly, as well as on the gestational age at which it is diagnosed. The patient herself will have to make the final decision about management. One option is selective termination of one fetus.

INTRAPARTUM MANAGEMENT OF MULTIPLE FETUSES

LABOR

As with singletons, the average length of labor for primiparas with twins is longer than the average length of labor for multiparas.[165] In addition, primiparas with twins have a greater incidence of prolonged labor than multiparas with twins.[165] The patient with a multiple gestation is known to have a greater level of prelabor uterine activity.[79] Therefore, for both multiparas and primiparas the latent phase of labor is shorter,[166] because the patient usually presents with more advanced cervical changes. But the overall duration of labor is not significantly different when compared with singletons, because the active phase is often longer.[167,168] This frequent prolongation of the active phase may be due in part to the greater use of anesthetics and analgesics in women carrying twins, or the much higher incidence of prematurity. However, the main reason the active phase is longer with twins is that there is a greater incidence of dysfunctional labor. This in turn is believed to be due to uterine overdistention and the higher incidence of malpresentations.[166,169]

The patient with twins does not always have the advantage of awaiting spontaneous labor. Often one of the many potential complications facing a multiple pregnancy also necessitates induction of labor. Because an overdistended uterus is at higher risk for rupture, it is optimal to use an intrauterine pressure catheter to guide the infusion of oxytocin.

MONITORING AND THE INTERDELIVERY INTERVAL

In the past, the interval between delivery of twins was held to either 15 or 30 minutes because of the fear of premature separation of the placenta, prolapse of the cord, uterine inertia, and retraction of the cervix. With the availability of intrapartum ultrasound and continuous fetal heart rate monitoring, the time interval is no longer a critical factor in obtaining a successful outcome.[170,171]

Fetal status can be monitored throughout labor and delivery. It should be emphasized that antepartum care of twins should be carried out by those familiar with

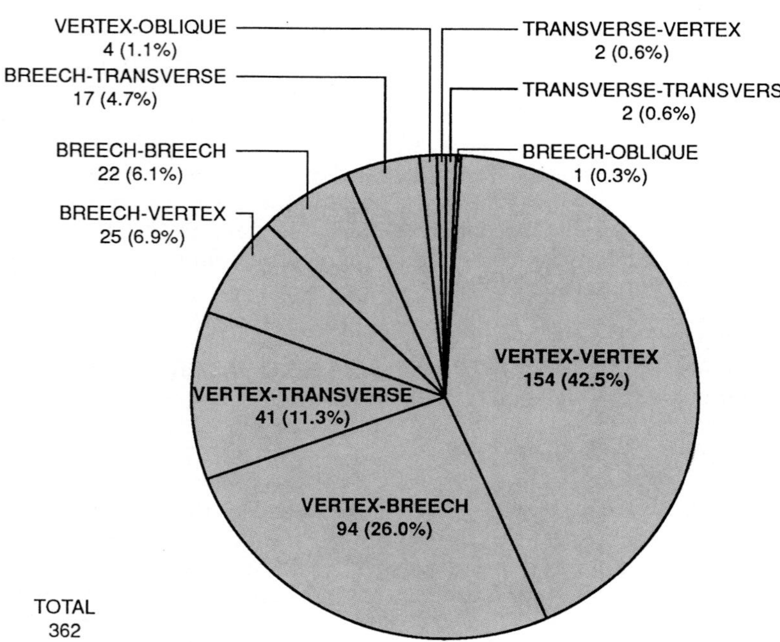

FIGURE 18–5. The relative occurrence rates of the possible combinations of twin presentations. (From Chervenak FA, Johnson RE, Youch S, et al. Intrapartum management of twin gestation. Obstet Gynecol 1985;65:119.)

their special needs. Likewise, twins should be delivered only in centers with capabilities for real-time ultrasound, electronic fetal heart rate monitoring, and immediate cesarean delivery when necessary. Monitoring of labor with twins usually involves a scalp electrode for twin A and an external fetal monitor for twin B. After delivery of twin A, electronic or sonographic monitoring of the fetal heart rate of twin B is carried out until its delivery.

MODE OF DELIVERY

Any meaningful discussion of the intrapartum management of twins should consider the relative presentations of twin A and twin B (Fig. 18-5). The possible combinations are varied, but three broad categories provide a working classification: vertex–vertex, vertex–nonvertex, and nonvertex twin A (Fig. 18-6). The authors' management plan is illustrated in Figure 18-7.

Twin A Vertex, Twin B Vertex

There is widespread agreement that vaginal delivery of vertex–vertex twins is appropriate.[22,170–172] After delivery of twin A, the status of twin B is assessed with ultrasound and fetal heart rate monitoring. Further labor should bring the vertex of twin B into the pelvis, whereupon amniotomy is performed and vaginal delivery is accomplished under continued monitoring. Oxytocin augmentation of uterine activity is used when indicated. If at any point close monitoring reveals fetal heart rate deterioration, the additional insult of an internal podalic version or difficult forceps delivery is not recommended. Instead, immediate cesarean delivery should be accomplished. In addition, cesarean section may become indicated for failure of descent.

One area of controversy involves the very low–birth-weight group, including those <1500 g.[173] (See Chapter 91 for a discussion of the topic of delivery of the very-low-birth-weight singleton.) The authors believe that vaginal delivery is appropriate for this group in the absence of convincing clinical data that cesarean section is beneficial.[171,172]

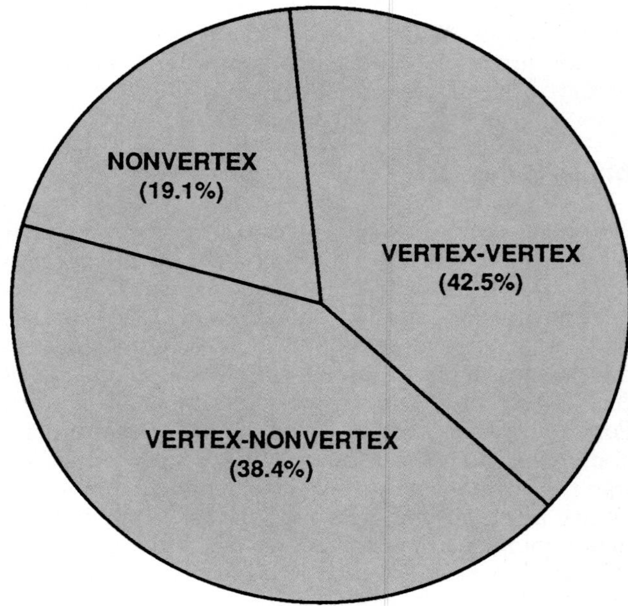

FIGURE 18–6. The relative occurrence rates of the three broad categories of twin presentations—vertex–vertex, vertex–nonvertex, and twin A nonvertex.

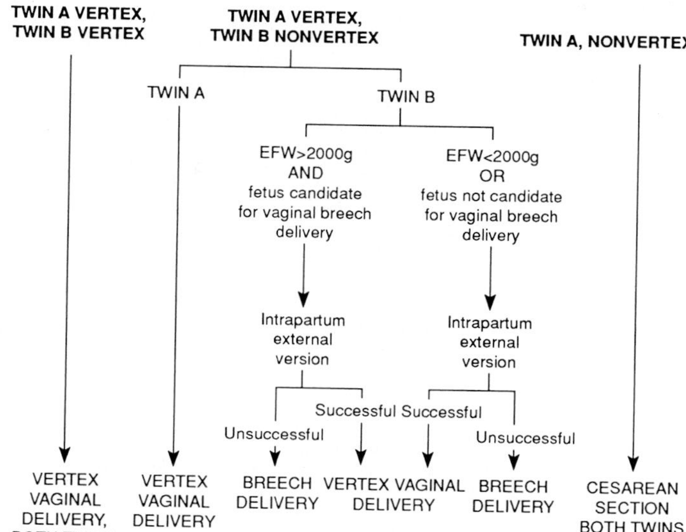

FIGURE 18–7. Outline of proposed intrapartum management of twin gestation. (Chervenak FA, Johnson RE, Youcha S, et al. Intrapartum management of twin gestation. Obstet Gynecol 1985;65:119.)

Twin A Vertex, Twin B Nonvertex

There is no definitive conclusion at this time regarding the optimum management of the vertex–nonvertex twin gestation. Cesarean delivery of all vertex–breech and vertex–transverse twin presentations is an option that is currently accepted.[172] This approach is recommended by some authors because of the possibility of birth trauma and birth asphyxia to the vaginally delivered nonvertex twin.[172,174] Two other options exist, however, to avoid routine cesarean section in this setting.

External cephalic version of the singleton is widely accepted both for its safety and for its efficacy.[175] Successful version of the second twin has been also reported by several investigators.[171,176] Sonographic assessment of the size of both fetuses should be carried out. If twin B is much larger (ie, >500 g difference), then version and attempted vaginal delivery are best avoided. If version is chosen, epidural anesthesia to provide abdominal wall relaxation is optimal. Ultrasound guidance facilitates the procedure, and continuous heart rate surveillance is performed. Under these guidelines, version has been found to be a safe and effective procedure to accomplish vaginal vertex delivery. In one series of 25 patients, external version was successful in 71% of transverse presentations and 73% of breech presentations. Neither neonatal nor maternal ill effect was seen.[177]

The specific maneuver is shown in Figure 18-8. Gentle pressure, either with the transducer or with one's hands, is used to guide the vertex toward the pelvis. The shortest arc between the vertex and the pelvic inlet should be followed initially. The version can be accomplished as either a forward or a backward roll, but in all patients undue force must be avoided. When the vertex is brought to the pelvic inlet, the membranes are rup-

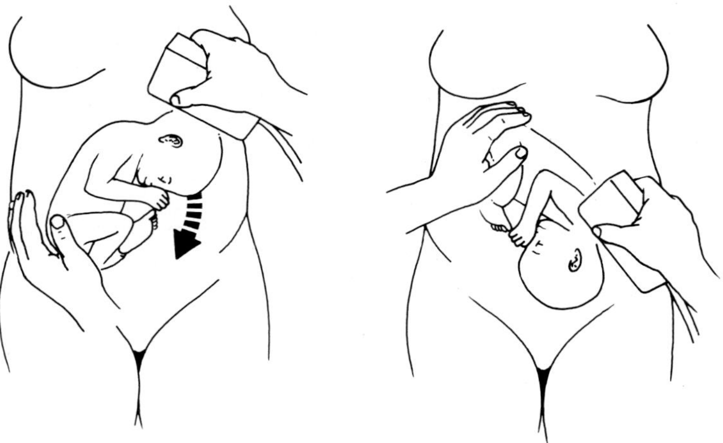

FIGURE 18–8. The maneuver of external version. (from Chervenak FA, Johnson RE, Berkowitz RL, et al. Intrapartum external version of the second twin. Obstet Gynecol 1983;62:160.)

tured and delivery is accomplished, with oxytocin augmentation as needed. If the version is unsuccessful, vaginal breech delivery or cesarean section is performed. If the fetal heart rate deteriorates, immediate cesarean section is carried out.

Vaginal breech delivery of the second twin is a second option to avoid routine abdominal delivery of vertex–nonvertex twins.[171,178–180] This approach will depend on estimated fetal weights. For twins estimated to be above 2000 g on ultrasound, several studies have not found an excessive risk of asphyxia or birth trauma when these second twins are delivered vaginally as a breech.[171,178–180] Neonatal mortality continues to result primarily from delivery of premature breeches. For breech delivery to be considered, the standard criteria for singleton pregnancy should be met: an adequate maternal pelvis, a flexed fetal head, and an estimated fetal weight of 2000 to 3500 g.[181]

For twins estimated to be below 2000 g and, therefore, potentially in the very low–birth-weight group, there is a lack of data demonstrating the safety of vaginal breech delivery.[171,182] At this time the authors are in agreement with others that these infants—whether singleton or breech—should be delivered through an adequate uterine incision.[171,182]

Twin A Nonvertex

There is no series documenting the safety of vaginal delivery of twins when twin A is nonvertex. For this reason the authors recommend cesarean section for this subgroup. Further clinical evaluation may establish that vaginal delivery is appropriate in this setting. If vaginal delivery is contemplated, the rare but potentially disastrous complication of interlocking of fetal heads must be considered.[183] It has been suggested that this complication can be successfully determined before delivery, and an attempt at vaginal delivery thereby would be avoided.[184]

There are several exceptions to the forgoing management plans. For some patients elective cesarean delivery should follow documentation of fetal lung maturity. For example, monoamniotic twins are optimally delivered by cesarean section at 36 weeks. This is done to minimize their already extremely high perinatal mortality rate and the risks of cord entanglement and fetal interlocking.[185] In most instances of conjoined twins abdominal delivery is indicated as described earlier.[186] Many of the other congenital anomalies seen more frequently among twins can also necessitate abdominal delivery. If one or both of a pair have severe IUGR, the stress of labor and vaginal delivery may be contraindicated. Triplets and multiple gestations of higher order warrant cesarean delivery to avoid birth trauma. However, some authors advocate vaginal delivery by an experienced operator, even when there may be three or more fetuses, because a clear improvement in outcome resulting from abdominal delivery has not been proven.[15,95]

REFERENCES

1. Benirschke K, Kim CK. Multiple pregnancy (first of two parts). N Engl J Med 1973;288:1276.
2. Kohl SG, Casey G. Twin gestation. Mt Sinai J Med 1975;42:523.
3. Bulmer MG. The familial incidence of twinning. Ann Hum Genet 1960;24:1.
4. Hrubec Z, Robinette CD. The study of human twins in medical research. N Engl J Med 1984;310:435.
5. Marivate M, Norman RJ. Twins. Clin Obstet Gynecol 1982;9:723.
6. MacGillivray I. Epidemiology of twin pregnancy. Semin Perinatol 1986;10:4.
7. Nylander PPS. Biosocial aspects of multiple births. J Biosoc Sci 1971;3:29S.
8. James WH. Dizygotic twinning, marital stage and status, and coital rates. Ann Hum Biol 1981;8:371.
9. Schenker JG, Yarkoni S, Granat M. Multiple pregnancies following induction of ovulation. Fertil Steril 1981;35:105.
10. Feldberg D, Laufer N, Dicker D, Goldman JA, DeCherney A. Quadruplet pregnancy in IVF. Eur J Obstet Gynecol Reprod Biol 1986;23:101.
11. Derom C, Derom R, Vlietinck R, Van Den Berghe H, Thiery M. Increased monozygotic twinning rate after ovulation induction. Lancet 1987;(May 30):1236.
12. Edwards RG, Mettler L, Walters DE. Identical twins in IVF. J IVF ET 1986;3:114.
13. Ghai V, Vidyasagar D. Morbidity and mortality factors in twins. An epidemiologic approach. In: Gall SA, ed. Twin pregnancy. Clin Perinatol 1988;15:123.
14. MacGillivray I. Twin pregnancies. In: Wynn RM, ed. Obstetrics and Gynaecology Annual. New York: Appleton-Century-Crofts, 1978.
15. Loucopoulos A, Jewelewicz R. Management of multifetal pregnancies: 16 years experience at the Sloane Hospital for women. Am J Obstet Gynecol 1982;143:902.
16. Holcberg G, Biale Y, Lewenthal H, Insler V. Outcome of pregnancy in 31 triplet gestations. Obstet Gynecol 1982;59:472.
17. Keith L, Ellis R, Berger GS, et al. The Northwestern University multihospital twin study. Am J Obstet Gynecol 1980;138:781.
18. Rush RW, Kierse MJNC, Howat P, et al. Contribution of preterm delivery to perinatal mortality. Br Med J 1976;2:965.
19. Caspi E, Ronen J, Schreyer P, Goldberg MD. The outcome of pregnancy after gonadotrophin therapy. Br J Obstet Gynaecol 1976;83:967.
20. Jeffrey RL, Bowes WA, DeLaney JJ. Role of bedrest in twin gestation. Obstet Gynecol 1974;43,822.
21. Miller HC, Merritt TA. Fetal growth in humans. Chicago: Year Book Medical Publishers, 1979.
22. Chervenak FA, Youcha S, Johnson RE, et al. Antenatal diagnosis and perinatal outcome in a series of 385 consecutive twin pregnancies. J Reprod Med 1984;29:727.
23. Farooqui MO. Grossman JH, Shannon RS. A review of twin pregnancy and perinatal mortality. Obstet Gynecol Surv 1973;28:144.
24. Keith L, Hughey MJ. Twin gestation. In: Gerbie AB, Sciarra JJ, eds. Gynecology and obstetrics. 2nd ed. New York: Harper & Row, 1986:1.
25. Redford DHA, Whitfield CR. Maternal serum alpha fetoprotein in twin pregnancies uncomplicated by neural tube defect. Am J Obstet Gynecol 1985;152:550.
26. Cetrulo CL, Ingardia CJ, Sbarra AJ. Management of multiple gestations. Clin Obstet Gynecol 1980;23:533.
27. Socol ML. In: Sabbagha R, ed. Diagnostic ultrasound applied to

obstetrics and gynecology. 2nd ed. Philadelphia: JB Lippincott, 1987:175.

28. Blumenfeld Z, Rottem S, Elgali S, et al. Transvaginal sonographic assessment of early embryological development. In: Obstetrical ultrasound. New York: McGraw-Hill, 1984.
29. Landy HJ, Keith L, Keith D. The vanishing twin. Acta Genet Med Gemellol 1982;31:179.
30. Jauniaux E, Elkazen N, Leroy F, et al. Clinical and morphological aspects of the vanishing twin phenomenon. Obstet Gynecol 1988;72:577.
31. Saidi MH. First trimester bleeding and the vanishing twin. A report of three cases. J Reprod Med 1988;33:831.
32. Benirschke K. Accurate recording of twin placentation. A plea to the obstetrician. Obstet Gynecol 1961;18:334.
33. Kaufman MH, O'Shea KS. Induction of monozygotic twinning in the mouse. Nature 1978;276:707.
34. Meyer WR, Meyer WW. Report on a very young dizygotic human twin pregnancy. Arch Gynecol 1981;231:51.
35. Nylander PPS. The factors that influence twinning rates. Acta Genet Med Gemellol 1981;30:189.
36. Soma H, Takayama M, Yokawa T, Akaedi T. Serum gonadotropin levels in Japanese women. Obstet Gynecol 1975;46:311.
37. Harris DW. Letter to the editor. J Reprod Med 1982;27:39.
38. Bieber FR. Nance WE, Morton CC, et al. Genetic studies of an acardiac monster: evidence of polar body twinning in man. Science 1981;213:775.
39. Benirschke K. Multiple gestation. Incidence, etiology, and inheritance. In: Creasy RK, Resnik R, eds. Maternal-fetal medicine: principles and practice. 2nd ed. Philadelphia: WB Saunders, 1989:565.
40. Cameron AH. The Birmingham twin survey. Proc Soc Med 1968;61:229.
41. Kovacs B, Shabahrami B, Platt LD. Molecular genetic prenatal determination of twin zygosity. Obstet Gynecol 1988;72:954.
42. Hendricks CH. Twinning in relation to birth weight, mortality, and congenital anomalies. Obstet Gynecol 1966;27:47.
43. Onyskowova A, Dolezal A, Jedlicka V. The frequency and the character of malformations in multiple births. Acta Univ Carol 1970;16:333.
44. Schinzel AA, Smith DW, Miller JR. Monozygotic twins and structural defects. J Pediatr 1979;95:921.
45. Windham GC, Bjerkedal T, Sever LE. The association of twinning and neural tube defects: studies in Los Angeles, California and Norway. Acta Genet Med Gemellol 1982;31:165.
46. Nance WE. Malformations unique to the twinning process. Prog Clin Biol Res 1981;69:123.
47. Little J, Bryan E. Congenital anomalies in twins. Semin Perinatol 1986;10:50.
48. Vaughn TC, Powell LC. The obstetrical management of conjoined twins. Obstet Gynecol (Suppl) 1979;53:67.
49. Lord JM. Intraabdominal foetus in foetu. J Pathol Bacteriol 1956;72:627.
50. Gross RE, Clatworthy Jr, HW. Twin fetuses in fetu. J Pediatr 1951;38:502.
51. Lewis RH. Foetus in foetu and the retroperitoneal teratoma. Arch Dis Child 1961;36:220.
52. Benirschke K, Harper VDR. The acardiac anomaly. Teratology 1977;15:311.
53. Romero R, Duffy TP, Berkowitz RL, et al. Prolongation of a preterm pregnancy complicated by death of a single twin in utero and disseminated intravascular coagulopathy. N Engl J Med 1984;310:772.
54. Hoyme HE, Higginbottom MC, Jones KL. Vascular etiology of disruptive structural defects in monozygotic twins. Pediatrics 1981;67:288.
55. Strong SJ, Corney G. The placenta in twin pregnancy. Elmsford, NY: Pergamon Press, 1967.
56. Benirschke K. Examination of the placenta. Obstet Gynecol 1961;18:309.
57. Aherne W, Strong SJ, Corney G. The structure of the placenta in the twin transfusion syndrome. Biol Neonat 1968;12:121.
58. Corney G, Aherne W. The placental transfusion syndrome in monozygotic twins. Arch Dis Child 1965;40:264.
59. MacGillivray I, Campbell DM. The physical characteristics and adaptation of women with twin pregnancy. In: Nance WE, ed. Twin research. Clinical studies. New York: Alan R Liss, 1978:81.
60. Redford DHA. Uterine growth in twin pregnancy by measurements of total intrauterine volume. Acta Genet Med Gemellol 1982;31:145.
61. Maclennan AH. Twin gestation. Clinical characteristics and management. In: Creasy RK, Resnick R, eds. Maternal-fetal medicine: principles and practice. 2nd ed. Philadelphia: WB Saunders, 1989:580.
62. MacGillivray I. Physiologic changes in twin pregnancy. In: MacGillivray I, Nylander PPS, Corney G, eds. Human multiple reproduction. Philadelphia: WB Saunders, 1975:107.
63. Rovinsky JJ, Jaffin H. Cardiac output and left ventricular work in multiple pregnancy. Am J Obstet Gynecol 1966;95:781.
64. Campbell DM, Campbell AJ. Arterial blood pressure—the pattern of change in twin pregnancies. Acta Genet Med Gemellol 1985;34:217.
65. Parsons M. Effects of twins: maternal, fetal, and labor. In: Gall SA, ed. Twin pregnancy. Clin Perinatol 1988;15:41.
66. Guttmacher AF. An analysis of 573 cases of twin pregnancy. Am J Obstet Gynecol 1939;38:277.
67. Campbell DM, Campbell AJ, MacGillivray I. Maternal characteristics of women having twin pregnancies. J Biol Sci 1975;6:463.
68. Spellacy WN, Buhi WC, Birk SA. Human placental lactogen levels in multiple pregnancies. Obstet Gynecol 1978;52:210.
69. Scheider L, Rigaud M, Taboste JL. Human placental lactogen level measurements: relationships with maternal weight gain in twin pregnancy. In: Nance WE, ed. Twin research: clinical studies. New York: Alan R Liss, 1978:123.
70. Tamby Raja RL, Ratnam SS. Plasma steroid changes in twin pregnancies. In: Gedda L, Parisi P, Nance WE, eds. Twin research: twin biology and multiple pregnancy. New York: Alan R Liss, 1981:189.
71. Mederis AL, Jonas HS, Stockbauer JW, Domke HR. Perinatal death in twins. Am J Obstet Gynecol 1979;134:413.
72. Watson P, Campbell DM. Preterm deliveries in twin pregnancies in Oxford. Acta Genet Med Gemellol 1986;35:193.
73. Syrop CH, Varner MW. Triplet gestation: maternal and neonatal implications. Acta Genet Med Gemellol 1985;34:81.
74. Hays PM, Smeltzer JS. Multiple gestation. Clin Obstet Gynecol 1986;29:264.
75. Newton ER. Antepartum care in multiple gestation. Semin Perinatol 1986;10:19.
76. O'Connor MC, Arias E, Royston JP, Dalrymple IJ. The merits of special antenatal care for twin pregnancies. Br J Obstet Gynaecol 1981;88:222.
77. Herron MA, Katz M, Creasy RK. Evaluation of a preterm birth prevention program: preliminary report. Obstet Gynecol 1982;59:452.
78. Houlton MCC, Marivate M, Philpott RH. Factors associated with preterm labour and changes in the cervix before labour in twin pregnancy. Br J Obstet Gynaecol 1982;89:190.
79. Newman RB, Gill PJ, Katz M. Uterine activity during pregnancy

in ambulatory patients: comparison of singleton and twin gestations. Am J Obstet Gynecol 1986;154:530.
80. Nageotte MP, Dorchester W, Porto M, et al. Quantitation of uterine activity preceding preterm, term, and postterm labor. Am J Obstet Gynecol 1988;158:1254.
81. Newman RB, Gill PJ, Campion S, et al. The influence of fetal number on antepartum uterine activity. Obstet Gynecol 1989;73:695.
82. Katz M, Gill PJ, Newman RB. Detection of preterm labor by ambulatory monitoring of uterine activity. A preliminary report. Obstet Gynecol 1986;68:773.
83. Skjaerris J, Aberg A. Prevention of prematurity in twin pregnancy by orally administered terbutaline. Acta Obstet Gynecol Scand (Suppl) 1982;108:39.
84. Cetrulo CL, Freeman RK. Ritodrine for the prevention of premature labor in twin pregnancies. Acta Genet Med Gemellol 1976;25:321.
85. O'Connor MC, Murphy H, Dalrymple IJ. Double blind trial of ritodrine and placebo in twin pregnancy. Br J Obstet Gynaecol 1979;86:706.
86. Rayburn W, Piehl E, Schork MA. Intravenous ritodrine therapy: a comparison between twin and singleton gestations. Obstet Gynecol 1986;67:243.
87. Katz M, Robertson PA, Creasy RK. Cardiovascular complications associated with terbutaline treatment for premature labor. Am J Obstet Gynecol 1981;139:605.
88. Saunders MC, Dick JS, McLBrown I, et al. The effects of hospital admission for bedrest on the duration of twin pregnancy: a randomized trial. Lancet 1985;2:793.
89. Zakut H, Insler V, Serr DM. Elective cervical suture in preventing premature delivery in multiple pregnancies. Isr J Med Sci 1977;13:488.
90. Weekes ARL, Menzies DN, DoBoer CH. Relative efficacy of bedrest, cervical suture, and no treatment in the management of twin pregnancy. Br J Obstet Gynaecol 1977;86:161.
91. Dor J, Shalev J, Mashiach S, et al. Elective cervical suture of twin pregnancies diagnosed ultrasonically in the first trimester following induced ovulation. Gynecol Obstet Invest 1982;13:55.
92. McGowan GW. Cervical incompetence in multiple pregnancy. Obstet Gynecol 1970;35:589.
93. Collaborative Group on Antenatal Steroid Therapy. Effects of antenatal dexamethasone administration on the prevention of respiratory distress syndrome. Am J Obstet Gynecol 1981;141:276.
94. Luerti M, Lazzarin A, Corbella E, et al. An alternative to steroids for prevention of respiratory distress syndrome (RDS): multicenter controlled study to compare ambraxol and betamethasone. J Perinat Med 1987;15:227.
95. Ron-El R, Caspi E, Schreyer P, et al. Triplet and quadruplet pregnancies and management. Obstet Gynecol 1981;57:458.
96. Berkowitz RL, Lynch L, Chitkara U, et al. Selective reduction of multifetal pregnancies in the first trimester. N Engl J Med 1988;318:1043.
97. McKeown T, Record RG. Observations on fetal growth in multiple pregnancy in man. J Endocrinol 1952;8:386.
98. Daw E, Walker J. Growth differences in twin pregnancy. Br J Clin Pract 1975;29:150.
99. Fenner A, Malm T, Kusserow U. Intrauterine growth of twins. Eur J Pediatr 1980;133:119.
101. Crane JP, Tomich PG, Kopta M. Ultrasonic growth patterns in normal and discordant twins. Obstet Gynecol 1980;55:678.
102. Socol ML, Tamura RK, Sabbagha RE, et al. Diminished biparietal diameter and abdominal circumference growth in twins. Obstet Gynecol 1984;64:235.
103. Grumback K, Coleman BG, Arger PH, et al. Twin and singleton growth patterns compared using ultrasound. Radiology 1986;158:237.
104. D'Alton ME, Dudley DKL. Ultrasound in the antepartum management of twin gestation. Semin Perinatol 1986;10:30.
105. Chitkara U, Berkowitz GS, Levine R, et al. Twin pregnancy: routine use of ultrasound examinations in the prenatal diagnosis of intrauterine growth retardation and discordant growth. Am J Perinatol 1985;2:49.
106. Haney AF, Crenshaw MC Jr, Dempsey PJ. Significance of biparietal differences between twins. Obstet Gynecol 1978;51:609.
107. Houlton MC. Divergent biparietal diameter growth rates in twin pregnancies. Obstet Gynecol 1977;49:542.
108. Leveno KJ, Santos-Ramos R, Duenhoelter JH, et al. Sonar cephalometry in twins: a table of biparietal diameters for normal twin fetuses and a comparison with singleton. Am J Obstet Gynecol 1979;135:727.
109. Estorlazzi AM, Vintzileos, Campbell WA, Nochimson DJ, Weinbaum PJ. Ultrasonic diagnosis of discordant fetal growth in twin gestations. Obstet Gynecol 1987;69:363.
110. Brown CEL, Guzick DS, Leveno KJ, Santos-Ramos R, Whalley PJ. Prediction of discordant twins using ultrasound measurement of biparietal diameter and abdominal perimeter. Obstet Gynecol 1987;70:677.
111. MacLennan AH, Millington G, Grieve A, et al. Neonatal body water turnover: a putative index of perinatal morbidity. Am J Obstet Gynecol 1981;139:948.
112. Wittman BK, Baldwin VJ, Nichol B. Antenatal diagnosis of twin transfusion syndrome by ultrasound. Obstet Gynecol 1981;58:123.
113. Chescheir NC, Seeds JW. Polyhydramnios and oligohydramnios in twin gestations. Obstet Gynecol 1988;71:882.
114. Rutherford SE, Phelan JP, Smith CV, et al. The four quadrant assessment of amniotic fluid volume: an adjunct to antepartum fetal heart rate testing. Obstet Gynecol 1987;70:353.
115. Nyberg DA, Filly RA, Golbus MS, et al. Entangled umbilical cords: a sign of monoamniotic twins. J Ultrasound Med 1984;3:29.
116. Lyndrup J, Schouenborg L. Cord entanglement in monoamniotic twin pregnancies. Eur J Obstet Gynecol Reprod Biol 1987;26:275.
117. Chitkara U, Berkowitz RL. Assessment of multiple gestations. In: Chervenak FA, Isaacson G, Campbell S, eds. Textbook of obstetric and gynecologic ultrasound. Boston: Little, Brown (in press).
118. Barss VA, Benacerraf BR, Frigoletto FD. Ultrasonographic determination of chorion type in twin gestation. Obstet Gynecol 1985;66:779.
119. Mahoney BS, Filly RA, Callen PW. Amnionicity and chorionicity in twin pregnancies: prediction using ultrasound. Radiology 1985;155:205.
120. Hertzberg BS, Kurtz AB, Choi HY, et al. Significance of membrane thickness in the sonographic evaluation of twin gestations. Am J Radiol 1987;148:151.
121. Townsend RR, Simpson GF, Filly RA. Membrane thickness in the ultrasound prediction of chorionicity of twin gestations. J Ultrasound Med 1985;7:327.
122. D'Alton ME, Dudley DKL. The ultrasonographic prediction of chorionicity in twin gestation. Abstract, 32nd Annual Convention of AIUM. New Orleans, LA, 1987;29.
123. Dudley DK, D'Alton ME. Single fetal death in twin gestations. Semin Perinatol 1986;10:65.
124. Hanna JH, Hill JM. Single intrauterine fetal demise in multiple gestation. Obstet Gynecol 1984;63:126.
125. Embom JA. Twin pregnancy with death of one twin. Am J Obstet Gynecol 1985;152:424.

126. Moore CM, McAdams AJ, Sutherland J. Intrauterine disseminated intravascular coagulation. A syndrome of multiple pregnancy with a dead twin fetus. J Pediatr 1969;74:523.
127. Yashioka H, Kadamoto Y, Mino M, et al. Multicystic encephalomalacia in a live-born twin with a stillborn macerated co-twin. J Pediatr 1979;95:798.
128. Pritchard JA, Ratnoff OD. Studies of fibrinogen and other hemostatic factors in women with intrauterine death and delayed delivery. Surg Obstet Gynecol 1955;101:467.
129. Skelly H, Marivate M, Norman R, Kenoyer G, Martin R. Consumptive coagulopathy following fetal death in a triplet pregnancy. Am J Obstet Gynecol 1982;142:595.
130. Romero R, Duffy TP, Berkowitz RL, et al. Prolongation of a preterm pregnancy complicated by death of a single twin in utero and disseminated intravascular coagulation: effects of treatment with heparin. N Engl J Med 1984;310:772.
131. Blake GD, Knuppel RA, Ingardia CJ, et al. Evaluation of nonstress fetal heart rate testing in multiple pregnancy. Obstet Gynecol 1984;63:528.
132. Devoe LD, Azor H. Simultaneous nonstress fetal heart rate testing in twin pregnancy. Obstet Gynecol 1981;58:450.
133. Lenstrup C. Predictive value of antepartum nonstress testing in multiple pregnancies. Acta Obstet Gynecol Scand 1984;63:597.
134. Lodeiro JG, Vintzileos AM, Feinstein SJ, et al. Fetal biophysical profile in twin gestations. Obstet Gynecol 1986;67:824.
135. Trudinger BJ, Giles WB, Cook CM, et al. Fetal umbilical artery flow velocity waveforms and placental resistance: clinical significance. Br J Obstet Gynaecol 1985;92:23.
136. Fleischer A, Schulman H, Farmakides G, et al. Umbilical artery velocity waveforms and intrauterine growth retardation. Am J Obstet Gynecol 1985;151:502.
137. Ferrazzi L, Pardi G. Doppler assessment of multiple gestation. In: Chervenak FA, Isaacson G, Campbell S, eds. Textbook of obstetric and gynecologic ultrasound. Boston: Little, Brown (in press).
138. Giles WB, Trudinger BJ, Cook CM. Fetal umbilical artery flow velocity-time waveforms in twin pregnancies. Br J Obstet Gynaecol 1985;92:490.
139. Pretorius DH, Manchester D, Barkin S, et al. Doppler ultrasound of twin transfusion syndrome. J Ultrasound Med 1988;7:117.
140. Moise KJ, Cotton DB. Discordant fetal platelet counts in a twin gestation complicated by idiopathic thrombocytopenic purpura. Am J Obstet Gynecol 1987;156:1141.
141. Shah DM, Jeanty P, Dev VG, Ulm JE, Phillips J. Diagnosis of trisomy 18 in monozygotic twins by cordocentesis. Am J Obstet Gynecol 1989;160:214.
142. Weiner CP. Diagnosis and treatment of twin to twin transfusion syndrome in the mid-second trimester of pregnancy. Fetal Ther 1987;2:71.
143. Weir PE, Ratten GJ, Beischer NA. Acute polyhydramnios—a complication of monozygotic twin pregnancy. Br J Obstet Gynaecol 1979;86:849.
144. Jones KL. Dysmorphology: an approach to a child with structural defects. Curr Prob Pediatr 1978;8:3.
145. Carlson NJ, Towers CV. Multiple gestation complicated by the death of one fetus. Obstet Gynecol 1989;73:685.
146. McMullen PF, Norman RJ, Marivate M. Pregnancy induced hypertension in twin pregnancy. Br J Obstet Gynaecol 1984; 91:240.
147. Brenner WE, Edelman DA, Hendricks CH. Characteristics of patients with placenta previa and results of "expectant management." Am J Obstet Gynecol 1978;132:180.
148. Karegard M, Gennser G. Incidence and recurrence rate of abruptio placenta in Sweden. Obstet Gynecol 1986;67:523.
149. Yla-outinen A, Palander M, Heinonen PK. Abruptio placentae —risk factors and outcome of the newborn. Eur J Obstet Gynecol Reprod Biol 1987;(May 25):23.
150. Wenstrom KD, Gall SA. Incidence, morbidity and mortality, and diagnosis of twin gestations. Clin Perinatol 1988;15:1.
151. Edmonds LD, Layde PM. Conjoined twins in the United States, 1970–77. Teratology 1982;25:301.
152. Mariona FG. Anomalies specific to multiple gestations. In: Chervenak FA, Isaacson G, Campbell S. Textbook of obstetric and gynecologic ultrasound. Boston: Little, Brown (in press).
153. Bucholz RD, et al. Temporo-parietal craniopagus. Case report and review of the literature. J Neurosurg 1987;66:72.
154. Chervenak FA, Pinto MM, Heller CI, Norooz H. Obstetric significance of fetal craniofacial duplication. A case report. J Reprod Med 1985;30:74.
155. Okazaki J, et al. Diprosopus: diagnosis in utero. Am J Radiol 1987;149:147.
156. Razavi, et al. Cardiovascular abnormalities in thoracopagus twins—embryological interpretation and review. Early Hum Dev 1987;15:33.
157. Nicolini U, Alberto DA, Ferrazzi E, et al. Ultrasonic prenatal diagnosis of fetus in fetu. J Clin Ultrasound 1983;11:321.
158. Wopner R. Personal communication. June 20, 1989.
159. Elias S, Gerbie AB, Simpson JL, et al. Genetic amniocentesis in twin gestations. Am J Obstet Gynecol 1980;138:169.
160. McEnerney JK, McEnerney LN. Unfavorable neonatal outcome after intraamniotic injection of methylene blue. Obstet Gynecol (Suppl) 1983;61:35.
161. Berkowitz RL. Multiple gestations. In: Gabbe S, Niebyl JR, Simpson JL, eds. Obstetrics: normal and problem pregnancies. New York: Churchill Livingston, 1986:739.
162. Pijpers L, Jahoda MG, Vosters RP. Genetic amniocentesis in twin pregnancies. Br J Obstet Gynaecol 1988;95:323.
163. Wender DF, Kandall C, Leppert PC, Berkowitz RL. Hyaline membrane disease in twin B following prolonged rupture of membranes for twin A. Conn Med 1981;45:83.
164. Obladen M, Gluck L. Respiratory distress syndrome and tracheal phospholipid composition in twins: independent of gestational age. J Pediatr 1977;90:799.
165. Ross CK, Philpott NW. Five year survey of multiple pregnancies. Can Med Assoc J 1953;69:247.
166. Friedman EA, Sachtleben MR. The effect of uterine overdistension on labor. I. Multiple pregnancy. Obstet Gynecol 1964;23:164.
167. Bender S. Twin pregnancy: a review of 472 cases. J Obstet Gynecol Br Emp 1952;59:510.
168. Garrett WJ, Phil D. Uterine over distension and the duration of labour. Med J Aust 1960;47:376.
169. MacGillivray I. Labour in multiple pregnancies. In: MacGillivray I, Nylander PPS, Corney G, eds. Human multiple reproduction. Philadelphia: WB Saunders, 1975:147.
170. Rayburn WF, Lavin JP, Miodovnik M, Varner MW. Multiple gestations: time interval between delivery of the first and second twins. Obstet Gynecol 1984;63:502.
171. Chervenak FA, Johnson RE, Youcha S, et al. Intrapartum management of twin gestation. Obstet Gynecol 1985;65:119.
172. Cetrulo C. The controversy of mode of delivery in twins: the intrapartum management of twin gestation. Semin Perinatol 1986;10:39.
173. Barrett JM, Staggs SM, Van Hooydonk JE, et al. The effect of type of delivery upon neonatal outcome in premature twins. Am J Obstet Gynecol 1982;143:360.
174. Kelsick F, Minkoff H. Management of the breech second twin. Am J Obstet Gynecol 1982;144:783.

175. Stine LE, Phelan JP, Wallace R, et al. Update on external cephalic version performed at term. Obstet Gynecol 1985;65:642.
176. Ranney B. The gentle art of external cephalic version. Am J Obstet Gynecol 1973;116:239.
177. Chervenak FA, Johnson RE, Berkowitz RL, et al. Intrapartum external version of the second twin. Obstet Gynecol 1983;62:160.
178. Acker D, Leiberman M, Holbrook H, et al. Delivery of the second twin. Obstet Gynecol 1982 59:710.
179. Chervenak FA, Johnson RE, Berkowitz RL, et al. Is routine cesarean section necessary for vertex-breech vertex-transverse twin gestation? Am J Obstet Gynecol 1984;148:1.
180. Collea JV, Chein C, Quilligan EJ. The randomized management of term frank breech presentation: a study of 208 cases. Am J Obstet Gynecol 1980;137:235.
181. Collea JV, Rabin SC, Weghorst GR, Quilligan EJ. The randomized management of term frank breech presentation: vaginal delivery versus cesarean section. Am J Obstet Gynecol 1978;131:186.
182. Kauppila O, Groncoos M, Aro P, et al. Management of low birth weight breech delivery: should cesarean section be routine? Obstet Gynecol 1981;57:289.
183. Nissen ED. Twins: collision, impaction, compaction, and interlocking. Obstet Gynecol ;11:514.
184. Hays PM, Smeltzer JS. Multiple gestation. Clin Obstet Gynecol 1986;29:264.
185. Sutter J, Arab H, Manning FA. Monoamniotic twins: antenatal diagnosis and management. Am J Obstet Gynecol 1986; 155:836.
186. Filler RM. Conjoined twins and their separation. Semin Perinatol 1986;10:82.

19

CHAPTER

THE BIOLOGY OF NORMAL AND DEVIANT FETAL GROWTH

Carl A. Nimrod

Fetal growth is a dynamic process that commences with a fertilized ovum and terminates with a newborn weighing approximately 3.2 kg. It involves orderly cell replication, differentiation, organogenesis, cell hypertrophy, and, eventually, functional maturity. The steps from the fertilized ovum to delivery at term involve approximately 44 cell divisions.[1] The numerous biological processes that dictate the sequencing of these events and the mechanisms involved in normal and deviant growth are discussed in this chapter.

Fetal growth is characterized by increase in cell number and cell size. Increase in cell number (mitotic activity) is assessed by evaluating the total DNA content in the organ. In the human fetus this equates to 6.0 picograms of DNA per cell nucleus.[2] Cell size is evaluated by expressing the weight or protein content of an organ per unit of DNA.[3] In normal human cell growth, the total DNA content (ie, cell number) increases in a linear fashion initially, then decelerates and reaches its maximum before organ size peaks. Three distinct phases of cell growth were identified by Winick[4]: hyperplasia, hyperplasia and associated hypertrophy, and hypertrophy only. Experimentally induced undernutrition during the period of hyperplasia results in a decrease in the number of cells. If this is prolonged, a permanent reduction in cell number results.[5] Fetal undernutrition during the period of hypertrophy results in a decrease in cell size that is reversible with improved nutrition. These fundamental differences correlate well with the two types of fetal growth restriction seen clinically. In the latter, preservation of normal fetal length occurs, but there is a deficiency in subcutaneous fat and possibly in skeletal muscle. This form of growth restriction occurs late in gestation and is referred to as headsparing growth restriction. The former situation generally occurs very early in pregnancy and gives rise to a symmetrically small fetus that is not necessarily underweight for height. Combinations of the two types of growth restriction can also occur. In addition, disturbances of overgrowth are possible. The two types of overgrowth described demonstrate the following characteristics: in some cases the fetus is normal in length but obese; in others, there are large body dimensions for gestational age but the fetus is not obese.

The ponderal index is one way of quantifying the degree of obesity or thinness of an infant. The index is expressed by the following equation:

$$\frac{\text{Birth weight in grams}}{(\text{Crown heel length})^3} \times 100$$

Its value is that it adjusts for gender, birth rank, race, and other variables and that it is more closely related to perinatal mortality than to birth weight percentile.[6] Infants are considered extremely obese if their ponderal index is above 2.93 and extremely malnourished if it is below 2.26.

CHANGES WITH ADVANCING GESTATION

As gestation advances, fetal nutritional needs are met by a wide variety of sources. The yolk sac of the human fetus appears to be a major provider before the development of the placenta. It plays an important role in the early establishment of fetal nutrition, organ differentiation, and growth. A portion of it becomes the primitive gut that lines the esophagus, trachea, and bronchial tracts. The endodermal portion of the yolk sac becomes the epithelia of the gallbladder, liver, bile ducts, pancreatic ducts, duodenum, and intestine. The cytoplasm in these endodermal cells contains glycogen as well as endoplasmic reticulum. Mitochondria and Golgi apparatus are also present, and in humans active protein synthetic function occurs in the yolk sac before the establishment of the liver. The placenta implants in a manner that has implications for fetal nutrition as gestation advances. Its role will be discussed later in this chapter.

Changes in skeletal muscle are responsible for 25% to 50% of birth weight increase during the second half of gestation,[7] so it can be used as a model for growth evaluation because of the two aspects of growth that occur in it: increase in muscle mass and changes in the functional differentiation of muscle that occur in the second half of pregnancy. There is an eightfold increase in the number of muscle cells present, whereas cell size increases by a factor of 2.6.[8] In the first half of gestation there is no differentiation within skeletal muscle; however, between 20 and 26 weeks of gestation, type I and type II muscle fibers appear in equal amounts.[9]

DETERMINANTS OF FETAL GROWTH

Genetic factors predominate in the first half of gestation. Although the genes of both parents are important in fetal growth, the maternal genes have the major influence on birth weight. Horse–pony breeding experiments have demonstrated that the offspring of maternal horse and paternal pony are significantly larger than those of maternal pony and paternal horse. Human studies also confirm these observations. The four major factors controlling growth in the second half of pregnancy are placental, metabolic, hormonal, and environmental. Overall the variance in human fetal weight at term can be explained by the relative contribution of the factors listed in Table 19-1.

Placental Factors

The placenta contributes, at several levels, to growth in the fetus. Its own growth as gestation advances and, consequently, the growth of villous surface area and its role in the provision of substrates for fetal metabolism, are of paramount importance. It must be remembered, however, that the maternal vascular supply to the placenta, placental hormone production, and mechanisms by which substrates are transported across the placenta (Table 19-2) all play a role in the growth of the fetus.

TABLE 19–1. FACTORS CONTRIBUTING TO VARIANCE IN HUMAN FETAL WEIGHT

FACTOR	PERCENTAGE
Maternal genotype	20%
Fetal genotype	15%
Y chromosome	2%
Maternal environment	31%
Intrauterine environment	31%

TABLE 19–2. PLACENTAL FACTORS IN FETAL GROWTH

MECHANISM OF PLACENTAL TRANSPORT	SUBSTANCE
Passive diffusion	Oxygen Carbon dioxide Fatty acids Ketones Fat-soluble vitamins
Facilitated diffusion	Sugars
Active transport	Amino acids
Pinocytosis	Proteins

The adequacy of maternal vascular supply to the placenta in part determines the rate at which nutrients are delivered to the fetus. Experimental interruption by vascular embolization can result in intrauterine growth restriction.[10,11] Placentas from women with pregnancy-induced hypertension who gave birth to small-for-date babies have been observed to have a lower total placental volume, a lower volume of parenchymal tissue, and smaller villous surface area.[12]

The margin of safety or placental reserve for oxygen and nutrient supply is obtained by calculating the ratio of delivery of the substrate (umbilical vein content × umbilical blood flow) to consumption (umbilical arteriovenous concentration difference × umbilical blood flow). Even though the placenta works more efficiently when its weight or fetal growth is decreased, the margin of safety at this time falls. This margin of safety is improved if 50% oxygen is given to the mother, as this does not result in an increase in oxygen consumption.

Abnormal Doppler flow velocity waveform patterns have been identified in the umbilical arteries of growth-retarded fetuses and have been shown to be associated with obliteration of the small arteries of the tertiary stem villi of the placenta.[13]

Significant placental reserve related to fetal need is present up to the end of the second trimester of gestation. Increasing fetal demands occur during the period of accelerated growth in early third trimester, and in the face of any form of placental compromise (eg, placental abruption), growth restriction can occur and placental insufficiency may arise. The physiologic mechanism accounting for this is the reduction of the villous surface area in the placenta across which nutrient transport occurs.

The human placenta is hemochorial in nature, with direct membrane contact of maternal blood with placental villi. In chronic fetal infection, edema of these villi decreases the efficiency of nutrient transport by increasing the distance between the maternal and fetal circulations.

Little is known about factors that limit placental growth, except that under normal circumstances, growth increases linearly until 36 weeks of gestation. Good correlation between fetal birth weight and placental weight has been demonstrated, and acceleration of fetal weight occurs during the last trimester.[14] This is manifested by an 11-fold increase in fat, 3.6-fold increases in protein, and an overall 2.5-fold increase in weight. The relative contribution of fat and proteins in the term fetus approximate to 525 g and 446 g, respectively.[15]

Metabolic Factors

Protein Metabolism. In the latter part of gestation the fetal liver serves as a major site for protein synthesis. Synthesis is regulated by substrate availability and modulation of synthetic apparatus by endocrine and other factors.

Substrate Availability. Protein synthesis and breakdown actively occur during gestation as the continuous remodeling of amino acid is maintained. Intracellular and extracellular amino acids comprise the essential building blocks and contribute to the pool utilized in protein synthesis.

Increased synthesis predominates during the last third of human gestation; however, this pattern is quite variable in other species. It is known to decrease in the second half of gestation in lambs.[16]

ATP and GTP provide the energy necessary for protein synthesis. Four molecules of ATP are necessary for the formation of each molecule of the peptide bond. This represents an energy cost of 0.86 kcal/g and consumes 17% of the fetal metabolic expenditure at this stage of gestation.[17] Growing fetuses at equivalent phases of development across several species use similar amounts of energy resources.

Modulation of Synthetic Apparatus. Ribosomes constitute the apparatus for protein biosynthesis in the fetus. The absolute number of ribosomes per cell increases as gestation advances and continues to increase in postnatal life. It is their absolute number and function that are important in synthesis.[18] In addition, the efficiency of the ribosomes at translating messenger RNA may improve during gestation. The mechanism of protein synthesis is no different in fetal life.

Situations in which excessive growth occurs suggest that this excessive growth can be due to decreases in protein turnover (eg, in skeletal tissue). This may result from insulin action in reducing protein breakdown and thus allowing its accumulation.

Induced hypoxia, created by decreased oxygen availability in fetal lambs, is associated with marked decreases in protein synthesis.[19] This response probably reflects the ability of fetuses to conserve energy and oxygen consumption during this period. In clinical practice, many of the conditions known to be associated with growth failure act via a decrease in oxygen transport to the fetus. These include high altitude, maternal cyanotic heart disease, maternal anemia, cigarette smoking, altered placental blood flow secondary to chronic maternal disease, umbilical cord occlusion, fetal anemia, and fetal heart disease.

During fetal life, glucose is the major metabolic fuel providing energy to maintain oxidative metabolism and tissue growth. It is unclear if the lack of availability of oxidized metabolic substrates (eg, glucose and lactate) affects protein synthesis directly.

These active metabolic processes contribute to the three- to fourfold increase in fetal protein seen in the last trimester of pregnancy.

Fetal Lipid Metabolism and Its Effect on Growth. Fetal fat stores increase from 1% to 15% of the fetal body weight during the last trimester of pregnancy. This develops because of the active placental lipid transport of at least 50% of the daily fatty acid requirement and all the essential fatty acids and the involvement of the fetal liver in the synthesis of fatty acids.

Placental Lipid Transport. Placental lipid transport depends on the nutritional status of the mother and the composition of her diet.[20] Two biochemical observations demonstrate this principle:

1. During maternal fasting, the fetus increases its storage of triacylglycerol in the liver and adipose tissue.
2. In uncontrolled diabetic mothers several metabolic changes occur, including increased fatty acid transport and placental storage of triacylglycerol. Fatty acid transport contributes significantly to the growth of the fetus in the third trimester.

Fatty Acid Metabolism in the Fetus. The fetus promotes the increase in lipid stores at the end of gestation to ensure that postnatal fuel stores are adequate for survival.[21] In addition, thermal insulation to protect the newborn from cold chill is desirable.

Several factors regulate fetal lipogenesis:

1. There is a transplacental fatty acid gradient.[22]
2. The availability of substrates, including glucose and lactate, facilitates the de novo synthesis of fat.[21]
3. Insulin affects lipogenesis by its action on fetal hepatocytes. In addition, the high insulin–glucagon ratio present in late gestation favors fatty acid synthesis.
4. Fetal albumin concentration facilitates the placental transfer of palmitic acid.
5. Medium-chain fatty acids are easier to transport across the placenta than long-chain fatty acids.[23]

Hormonal Factors

Peptide Regulatory Factors in Embryonic Development. Insulinlike growth factors (IGF-I and IGF-II) are bioactive mitogenic peptides that are homologous to proinsulin because of similarities in the amino acid sequence.[24] Previously described as somatomedins, they can act by endocrine, paracrine, and autocrine mechanisms[25] to influence growth and differentiation in a number of organs by the following:

1. Stimulation of glucose metabolism
2. DNA synthesis
3. Cell proliferation.

IGFs are present in the fetal circulation from 13 weeks gestation. Both maternal and fetal IGF-I levels rise during pregnancy and correlate with birth weight.[26] However, no relationship exists between fetal IGF-II levels and birth weight,[27] and amniotic fluid IGFs are unaltered during gestation.

At the cellular level, two types of IGF receptors have been identified.[28] Type I receptors are similar but not identical to the insulin receptor, whereas type II receptors bind only IGFs. IGF-binding proteins of two sizes are present in the blood. However, the precise mechanism by which the binding protein interacts at the level of the receptor with IGF-I is unknown.

It is postulated that IGF-binding protein modulates the mitogenic actions of IGF and promotes differentiation of the musculoskeletal system.

Insulin. Glucose is a major substrate used by the growing fetus. It is transported across the placenta by facilitated mechanisms. It is stored in the fetal liver as glycogen, and the stores there increase dramatically after 36 weeks. The reason for this is the need for an enhanced glycolytic capacity for the fetus during the periods of stress in the intrapartum and early newborn period. These stresses are generally associated with transient hypoxia, reduction of the umbilical blood flow, or neonatal cold stress.

Maternal and fetal glucose levels are closely related, and in situations with poor maternal glucose control there is increased fetal hyperglycemia and, consequently, fetal hyperinsulinemia. This hyperinsulinemia facilitates the uptake and storage of glucose as glycogen, lipogenesis, and the uptake and utilization of amino acids. Experiments of the effects of hyperinsulinemia on fetal growth in rhesus monkeys demonstrate organomegaly with a doubling of fetal weight, increase in placental weight, and increase in crown–heel length.[29] The storage of glucose as glycogen in the liver is facilitated by insulin but cannot by itself explain the changes that occur in liver size. In clinical practice, the macrosomic syndromes that include Beckwith-Wiedemann syndrome, B cell hyperplasia, or adenomatosis are all associated with fetal hyperinsulinism. When poor control of diabetes mellitus occurs, the fetal weight in the last 6 weeks of gestation exceeds that of age-matched controls by 500–600 g.

Other Hormones. In the normal fetus, the effect of growth hormone is minimal, as can be seen in anencephalics, in whom growth failure is rare. In addition, the liver is the only fetal tissue with receptors for growth hormone. Absence of thyroid hormone due to thyroid obliteration has a deleterious effect on growth, as evidenced by reduced size in kidney, heart, liver, muscle, and spleen. In some situations, however, the fetal weight can be above average.

Environmental Factors

Considerable deficiency of oxygen occurs at high altitude. The effect on fetal growth of the oxygen deficiency at 10,000 ft is noted to be three times greater than the effect of starvation.

The following lifestyle and physically related factors in the maternal environment contribute to altered growth.

Smoking. Impaired fetal growth secondary to smoking occurs as a result of several separate mechanisms. Nicotine produces vasoconstriction and results in compromise of the uteroplacental blood flow. In addition, carbon monoxide–induced hypoxia occurs by the displacement of oxygen from the hemoglobin in arterial blood and gives rise to a decrease in the oxygen-carrying capacity. Reduction in protein synthesis and lipid accumulation in cells is a by-product of the hypoxia.

Alcohol. Fetal and maternal alcohol concentrations are similar in exposed humans. Alcohol is easily distributed in body tissues in proportion to the water content of the tissue. As we age, our body water content decreases, and this results in higher peak levels of alcohol in older adults than in younger adults when they are exposed to equivalent quantities. This becomes more significant in the older gravida.

Clearance of alcohol from the fetus is slow and occurs by passive diffusion back through the placenta. This allows for greater exposure of the fetus to the alcohol and its metabolic by-products, which may not be effectively eliminated by the placenta.

Relatively small amounts of alcohol, on a consistent basis, affect fetal growth. The estimated impact is a decrease in birth weight of 160 g per ounce of alcohol per day consumed in late pregnancy. The greatest impact on birth weight is seen with third-trimester ingestion. The babies of alcoholics who have decreased or eliminated drinking before the third trimester do not experience as much growth retardation as those of mothers who have not eliminated this type of alcohol consumption.[30]

Cocaine Abuse. Drug abuse is associated with poor prepregnant weight and low maternal weight gain, both of which are implicated in growth failure. Cocaine also inhibits the presynaptic uptake of norepinephrine and causes a transient rise in the circulating catecholamine levels, thus leading to vasoconstriction, increases in maternal arterial blood pressure, and significant reduction in uterine blood flow.[31] Placental abruption is a common end result. Fetal oxygenation is impaired, and fetal cardiovascular vasoconstriction also occurs with the simple diffusion of cocaine across the placenta.

Congenital Infections. Congenital infections limit fetal growth rate. The herpes simplex virus in human embryonic cell culture causes destruction of cells, whereas the rubella virus in a similar medium shows no destructive effect other than a marked diminution of the ability of the cell to undergo mitosis. Infants with congenital rubella syndrome therefore have a decrease in the number of cells present per organ because of fewer mitoses; in a few of their organs (liver and spleen), however, a relative hyperplasia exists.

Physical Factors. It is conceivable that the space available to conduct growth limits the amount of actual growth that occurs. This is best exemplified in fetal lung growth, where the impact of chronic oligohydramnios is very apparent. It has been demonstrated that chronic amniotic fluid leak before 26 weeks gestation severely hinders fetal lung growth.[33]

Toward the end of gestation, fetal lung grows at a rate that is proportional to growth in the remainder of the fetus. This is usually due to an increase in cell number as the DNA concentration per gram of lung tissue remains constant. There is good clinical and experimental evidence to support the theory that the physical factors influencing growth are:

1. Adequate intrathoracic space
2. Adequate intrauterine space
3. Fetal breathing movements
4. The balance between lung liquid volume and pressure within the trachea and potential area spaces.

Investigators producing a chronic amniotic fluid leakage in the rhesus monkey[34] and sheep[35] have shown a reduction in the number and size of alveoli, though maturation was unaffected. In the sheep model Moessinger was able to demonstrate significant decreases in lung weight, lung volume, saccules, and elastic tissue length as compared to controls in which there was no chronic amniotic fluid leakage.[35] The maternal environment (patient size and uterine shape) may represent unsurmountable barriers to growth. These factors require comprehensive evaluation to determine their role.

CONCLUSION

Fetal growth is the complex development of a fertilized egg weighing less than a nanogram by an average daily increment of 10–15 g/day in humans. The anabolic and catabolic processes that must constantly occur result in the net gain of fat, protein, and carbohydrate at enormous rates. At the end of human gestation the increase in total body fat is about 5000-fold and that of protein is 400-fold. The human newborn at birth has more fat (16%) than any other newborn (eg, rat, 11%; cat, 2%; guinea pig, 9.5%). Fat accumulation to this degree in nature has only been seen in hibernating animals or migratory birds, usually for heat conservation and nutrition in the early newborn period.

Cordocentesis data, from fetuses with intrauterine growth restriction in which genetic causes and congenital infection have been excluded, indicate that stimulation of erythropoiesis and fetal biochemical liver injury are common. Elevations in lactic dehydrogenase and gamma glutamyl transferase that are seen reflect long-term stress.[32]

The early fertilized ovum brings to the uterine environment all its genetic endowment and proposes that growth follow a prescribed path. The realities of substrate availability, in utero–placental blood flow, interactions between substrates, and placental transfer mechanisms deliver the building blocks necessary for growth. The fetus acting in concert with these placental factors then ensures that growth proceeds in a manner that allows for appropriate organ differentiation and adequate insulation from the stresses of early newborn life.

REFERENCES

1. Milner RDG, Hill DJ. Fetal growth control: the role of insulin and related peptides. Clin Endocrinol 1984;21:415.
2. Musky AE, Ris H. Variable and constant components of chromosomes. Nature 1949;163:666.
3. Enesco M, LeBlond CP. Increase in cell number as a factor in the growth of the organs and tissues of the young male rat. J Embryol Exp Morphol 1962;10:530.
4. Winick M. Cellular changes during placental and fetal growth. Am J Obstet Gynecol 1971;109:166.
5. Winick M, Noble A. Cellular response in rats during malnutrition at various ages. J Nutr 1966;89:300.
6. Walther F, Namaekers LHJ. The Ponderal Index as a measure of the nutritional status at birth and its relation to some aspects of neonatal morbidity. J Perinatol Med 1982;10:42.
7. Cheek D, Hill D. Muscle and liver cell growth: role of hormones and nutritional factors. Med Proc 1970;29:1503.
8. Widdowson EM, Crabb D, Milner R. Cellular development of some human organs before birth. Arch Dis Child 1972;47:652.
9. Dubowitz V. Enzyme histochemistry of skeletal muscle. J Neurol Psychiatr 1965;28:516.
10. Creasy RK, Barrett CT, De Sweet M, et al. Experimental intrauterine growth retardation in the sheep. Am J Obstet Gynecol 1972;112:566.
11. Clapp JF, Szeot H, Larrow R, et al. Fetal metabolic response to experimental placental vascular damage. Am J Obstet Gynecol 1981;140:446.
12. Boyd PA, Scott A. Quantitative structural studies on human placentas associated with pre-eclampsia, essential hypertension and intrauterine growth retardation. Br J Obstet Gynecol 1985;92:714.
13. Giles WB, Trudinger B, Band PJ. Fetal umbilical artery flow velocity waveforms and placental resistance: pathological correlation. Br J Obstet Gynecol 1985;92:31.
14. Thompson AM. The weight of the placenta in relation to birth weight. J Obstet Gynecol Br Commonw 1967;76:865.
15. Widdowson EM. The demands of the fetal and maternal tissues for nutrients and the bearing of these on the needs of the mother to "eat for two." In: Dobbing J, ed. Maternal nutrition in pregnancy—eating for two? London: Academic Press, 1981:1.
16. Kennaugh JM, Bell AW, Teng C, et al. Ontogenetic changes in the rates of protein synthesis and leucine oxidation during fetal life. Pediatrics 1987;22:688.
17. Milley JR. Fetal protein metabolism. Semin Perinatol 1989; 13:192.
18. Goldspink DF, Rilly FJ. Protein turnover and growth in the whole

body, liver and kidney of the rat from the foetus to senility. Biochem J 1984;217:507.

19. Richardson B. Fetal adaptive responses to asphyxia. Clin Perinatol 1989;16:595.
20. Hill D, Stammers JP. Lipid metabolism during pregnancy and lactation. Biochem Soc Trans 1985;13:821.
21. Kiniuna RE. Fatty and metabolism in the fetus. Semin Perinatol 1989;13:202.
22. Hendriekse W, Stammers JP, Hill D. The transfer of free fatty acids across the human placenta. Br J Obstet 1985;92:945.
23. Dances J, Jansen V, Kayden JH, et al. Transfer across perfused human placenta III. Effect of chain length on transfer of free fatty acids. Pediatrics 1974;8:796.
24. Daughaday WH, Heath E. Physiological and possible clinical significance of epidermal and nerve growth factors. J Clin Endocrinol Metab 1984;13:207.
25. D'Ercole AJ, Stiles AD, Underwood LE. Tissue concentrations of somatomedin C: further evidence of multiple sites of synthesis and paracrine/autocrine mechanisms of action. Proc Natl Acad Sci USA 1984;81:935.
26. Gluckman PD, Barrett-Johnson JJ, Butler JH, et al. Studies of insulin like growth factor I and II by specific radioligand assays in umbilical cord blood. Clin Endocrinol 1983;19:405.
27. Ashton IK, Zapf J, Einschenk I, et al. Insulin-like growth factors (IGF) I and II in human foetal plasma and relationship to gestational age and fetal size during mid pregnancy. Acta Endocrinol 1985;10:558.
28. Shigematsu K, Niwa M, Kurihara M, et al. Receptor autoradiographic localization of insulin-like growth factor (IGF-I) binding sites in human fetal and adult adrenal glands. Life Sci 1985;45:383.
29. Susa JB, Schwartz R. Effects of hyperinsulinemia in the primate fetus. Diabetes 1985;34:36.
30. Rosett HL, Weiner L, Zuckerman B, et al. Reduction of alcohol consumption during pregnancy with benefits to the newborn. Alcoholism Clin Exp Res 1980;4:178.
31. Woods JR, Plessing MA, Clark KE. Effects of cocaine in uterine blood flow and fetal oxygenation. JAMA 1987;257:957.
32. Cox WL, Daffos F, Forestier F, et al. Physiology and management of intrauterine growth retardation: a biologic approach with fetal blood sampling. Am J Obstet Gynecol 1988;159:36.
33. Nimrod C, Varela-Gittings F, Machin G, Campbell D, Wesenberg R. The effect of very prolonged membrane rupture on fetal development. Am J Obstet Gynecol 1984;148(5):540.
34. Hislop A, Fairweather DVA, Blackwell RJ, et al. The effect of amniocentesis and drainage of amniotic fluid on lung development in Macaca fascicularis. Br J Obstet Gynecol 1984;91:835.
35. Moesseinger A, Fewell J, Stark R, et al. Lung hypoplasia and breathing movements following oligohydramnios in fetal lambs. In: The physiological development of the fetus and newborn. London: Academic Press, 1985:293.

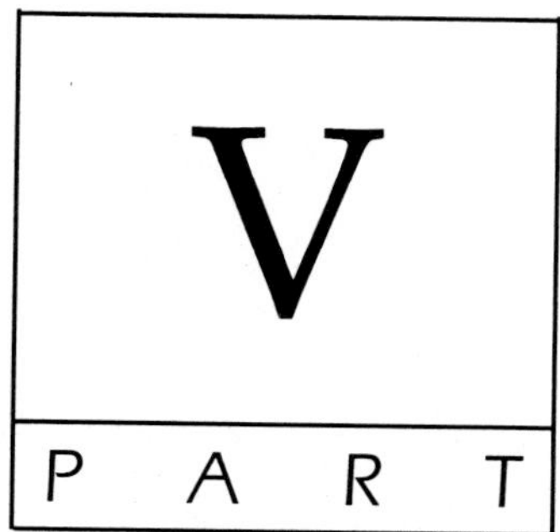

TERATOGENS AND TERATOGENESIS

20

CHAPTER

BASIC PRINCIPLES OF TERATOLOGY

David A. Beckman and Robert L. Brent

The etiology of abnormal embryonic development includes abnormalities of the genome (point mutations or chromosome abnormalities) and abnormalities of development related to environmental influences. We will not be concerned with the influence of genetic abnormalities on embryonic development in this presentation except to point out that variations in the genome within the normal range may alter the response of an embryo to an environmental reproductive toxin.

If we concentrate our attention on environmental influences or agents that interfere with embryonic development we must discuss those scientific or embryologic principles that have an important impact on the effect of various environmental agents on the developing embryo. These include the impact of embryonic stage, dose or magnitude of the exposure, threshold dose, pharmacokinetics and metabolism of the agent, placental transport, and species differences.

PRINCIPLES OF ENVIRONMENTALLY INDUCED MALFORMATIONS

A basic tenet of environmentally produced malformations is that the effects of the teratogens or the teratogenic milieu have certain characteristics in common and follow certain basic principles. These principles determine the quantitative and qualitative aspects of environmentally produced malformations.

EMBRYONIC STAGE

The induction of malformations by environmental agents usually results in a spectrum of malformations that varies somewhat because of variations in stage of exposure and dose. The developmental period at which an exposure occurs will determine which structures are most susceptible to the deleterious effects of the drug or chemical and to what extent the embryo can repair the damage. Furthermore, whether the period of sensitivity is narrow or broad depends on the environmental agent and the malformation in question. Limb defects produced by thalidomide have a very short period of susceptibility (Table 20-1), whereas microcephaly produced by radiation has a long period of susceptibility.

During the first period of embryonic development, from fertilization through the early postimplantation period, the embryo is most sensitive to the toxic effects of drugs and chemicals resulting in embryo lethality. Surviving embryos have malformation rates similar to the controls, not because malformations cannot be produced at this stage but because significant cell loss or chromosome abnormalities at these stages have a high likelihood of killing the embryo. Because of the omnipotentiality of early embryonic cells, surviving embryos have a much greater ability to have normal developmental potential than those affected later in their development. Wilson and Brent used ionizing x-irradiation as the experimental teratogen to demonstrate that the "all-or-none phenomenon" or marked resistance to teratogens disappears over a period of a few hours in the rat during early organogenesis.[1] The term *all-or-none phenomenon* has been misinterpreted by some investigators to indicate that malformations cannot be produced at this stage. On the contrary, it is likely that certain drugs, chemicals, or other insults during this stage of development can result in an increase in surviving malformed embryos.[2,3] However, the nature of embryonic development at this stage will still reflect the basic characteristic of the all-or-none phenomenon—a propensity for embryo lethality rather than for surviving malformed embryos.

The period of organogenesis (from day 18 through about day 60 of gestation in the human) is the period of greatest sensitivity to teratogenic insults and the period

TABLE 20–1. DEVELOPMENTAL STAGE SENSITIVITY OF THE HUMAN TO LIMB REDUCTION DEFECTS CAUSED BY THALIDOMIDE

DEVELOPMENTAL STAGE (DAYS)	LIMB REDUCTION DEFECT
24–29	Amelia, upper limbs
21–26	Thumb aplasia
24–33	Phocomelia, upper limbs
23–34	Hip dislocation
27–31	Amelia, lower limb
25–31	Preaxial aplasia, upper limb
28–33	Preaxial aplasia, lower limb
28–33	Phocomelia, lower limb
	Femoral hypoplasia
	Girdle hypoplasia

Adapted from Brent RL, Holmes LB. Clinical and basic science lessons from the thalidomide tragedy: what have we learned about the causes of limb defects? Teratology 1988;38:241.

when most gross anatomic malformations can be induced. Most major malformations are produced before the 36th day of gestation in the human. The exceptions are malformations of the genitourinary system, the palate, and the brain or those resulting from problems of constraint, disruption, or destruction. Severe growth retardation in the whole embryo or fetus may also result in permanent deleterious effects in many organs or tissues.

The fetal period is characterized by histogenesis involving cell growth, differentiation, and migration. Teratogenic agents may decrease the cell population by producing cell death or by inhibiting cell division or cell differentiation. There is, of course, some overlap, in that permanent cell depletion may be produced earlier than the 60th day. Effects such as cell depletion or functional abnormalities, not readily apparent at birth, may give rise to changes in behavior or fertility that may be apparent only later in life.

The last gestational day on which each of several malformations may be induced in the human is presented in Table 20-2.

DOSE OR MAGNITUDE OF THE EXPOSURE

The quantitative correlation of the magnitude of embryopathic effects to the dose of a drug, chemical, or other agent is referred to as the dose–response relationship. This is extremely important when comparing effects among different species because mg/kg doses are, at best, rough approximations. Dose equivalence among species can be accomplished only by performing pharmacokinetic studies, metabolic studies, and dose–response investigations in the human and the other species being studied.

Several considerations affect the interpretation of dose–response relationships:

1. The concentration of active metabolites may be more pertinent than the dosage of the original chemical (eg, the metabolites phosphoamide mustard and acrolein may produce maldevelopment resulting from exposure to cyclophosphamide).[4]
2. A chronic exposure at a low dose can contribute to an increased teratogenic risk (eg, anticonvulsant therapy).
3. Pregnancy alters the distribution and metabolism of drugs.[5]
4. It may be difficult to determine whether a maternal condition contributes to the etiology of malformations associated with the treatment for that condition during pregnancy (eg, etiologic factors that cause epilepsy may also contribute to the maldevelopment associated with exposure to diphenylhydantoin).[6,7]
5. Fat-soluble substances, such as polychlorinated biphenyls[8] and etretinate,[9] can produce fetal maldevelopment for an extended period after the last ingestion or drug exposure in a woman because they have an unusually long half-life.

Furthermore, the response should be interpreted in a biologically sound manner. One example is that a substance given in large enough amounts to cause maternal toxicity is likely also to have deleterious effects on the embryo, such as death, growth retardation, or retarded development. Another example is that because the steroid receptors that are necessary for naturally occurring and synthetic progestin action are absent from nonreproductive fetal mouse and monkey tissues, the evidence is against the involvement of progesterone or its synthetic analogs in nongenital teratogenesis.[10–13]

The interaction of two or more drugs or chemicals may potentiate their developmental effects. Although this hypothesis is extremely difficult to test in the human, it is an especially important consideration because multichemical or multitherapeutic exposures are common. Furthermore, Fraser warns that the actual existence of a threshold phenomenon when nonteratogenic doses of two teratogens are combined could easily be misinterpreted as potentiation or synergism.[14]

THRESHOLD DOSE

The threshold dose is the dosage below which the incidence of death, malformation, growth retardation, or functional deficit is statistically no greater than that of controls. The threshold level of exposure usually ranges from less than one to three orders of magnitude below the teratogenic or embryopathic dose for drugs and chemicals that kill or malform half the embryos. An exogenous teratogenic agent therefore has a no-effect dose, as compared to mutagens or carcinogens, which have a stochastic dose–response curve. Threshold phenomena are compared to stochastic phenomena in Table 20-3. The severity and incidence of malformations produced by every exogenous teratogenic agent that has been appropriately tested have exhibited threshold phenomena during organogenesis.[10]

TABLE 20–2. ESTIMATED OUTCOME OF 100 PREGNANCIES VERSUS TIME FROM CONCEPTION

TIME FROM CONCEPTION	SURVIVAL TO TERM* (PERCENTAGE)	DEATH DURING INTERVAL* (PERCENTAGE)	LAST TIME FOR INDUCTION OF SELECTED MALFORMATIONS†	
Preimplantation				
0–6 days	25	54.55		
Postimplantation				
7–13 days	55	24.66		
14–20 days	73	8.18		
3–5 weeks	79.5	7.56	Day 23:	Cyclopia; sirenomelia
			Day 26:	Anencephaly
			Day 28:	Meningomyelocele
			Day 34:	Transposition of great vessels
6–9 weeks	96	6.52	Day 36:	Cleft lip, limb reduction defects
			Week 6:	Diaphragmatic hernia, rectal atresia, ventricular septal defect, syndactyly
10–13 weeks	92	4.42	Week 9:	Cleft palate
			Week 10:	Omphalocele
			Week 12:	Hypospadias
14–17 weeks	96.26	1.33		
18–21 weeks	97.56	0.85		
22–25 weeks	98.39	0.31		
26–29 weeks	98.69	0.30		
30–33 weeks	98.98	0.30		
34–37 weeks	99.26	0.34		
38+ weeks	99.32	0.68	38+ weeks:	CNS cell depletion

An estimated 50% to 70% of all human conceptions are lost in the first 30 weeks of gestation (Hertig AT. The overall problem in man. In: Benirschke K, ed. Comparative aspects of reproductive failure. Berlin: Springer-Verlag, 1967:11), and 78% are lost before term (Robert CJ, Lowe CR. Where have all the conceptions gone? Lancet 1975;1:498).

* Data from Kline J, Stein Z. Very early pregnancy. In: Dixon RL, ed. Target organ toxicology series: Reproductive toxicology. New York: Raven Press, 1985:251.

† Modified from Schardein JL. Chemically induced birth defects. New York: Marcel Dekker, 1985.

PHARMACOKINETICS AND METABOLISM OF THE AGENT

The physiologic alterations of pregnancy and the bioconversion of compounds can significantly influence the teratogenic effects of drugs and chemicals by affecting absorption, body distribution, active form(s), and excretion of the compound.

Physiologic alterations in the mother during pregnancy that affect the pharmacokinetics of drugs include the following:

1. Gastrointestinal motility decreases and intestinal transit time increases, resulting in delayed absorption of drugs in the small intestine due to increased stomach retention and enhanced absorption of slowly absorbed drugs.
2. Decreased plasma albumin concentration alters the kinetics of compounds normally bound to albumin.
3. The increased plasma and extracellular fluid volumes affect concentration-dependent transfer of compounds.
4. Renal elimination is generally increased but is influenced by body position during late pregnancy.
5. Hepatic blood flow varies little during pregnancy; however, metabolic inactivation is inhibited during late pregnancy.
6. Although uterine blood flow varies during pregnancy, little is known about how this affects transfer across the placenta.[5,15,16]

The fetus also undergoes physiologic alterations that affect the pharmacokinetics of drugs:

1. Amount and distribution of fat varies with development and affects the distribution of lipid-soluble drugs.
2. The fetal circulation contains a higher concentration of free drug, largely because plasma fetal proteins are lower in concentration than the adult and may also be less able to bind drugs than in the adult or the newborn.
3. The functional development of pharmacologic receptors is likely to proceed at different rates in the various tissues.

TABLE 20-3. RELATIONSHIP BETWEEN DISEASES PRODUCED BY ENVIRONMENTAL AGENTS AND THE RISK OF OCCURRENCE

RELATIONSHIP	PATHOLOGY	SITE	DISEASES	RISK	DEFINITION
Stochastic phenomena	Damage to a single cell may result in disease	DNA	Cancer, mutation	Some risk exists at all dosages; at low exposures the risk is below the spontaneous risk.	The incidence of disease increases, but the severity and nature of the disease remain the same.
Threshold phenomena	Multicellular injury	Great variation in etiology, affecting many cell and organ processes	Malformation, growth retardation, chemical toxicity, etc.	Completely disappears below threshold dose	Both the severity and incidence of disease increase with dose

From Brent RL. Editorial comments on comments on teratogen update: bendectin. Teratology 31:429.

4. The excretion of drugs and metabolites by the fetus is a complex process involving the placenta and the possible recirculation of metabolites from the maternal circulation.[16]

The role the placenta plays in drug pharmacokinetics (reviewed by Juchau and Rettie[17] and Miller[18]) involves transport (discussed in detail later); the presence of receptor sites for a number of endogenous and xenobiotic compounds (β-adrenergic, glucocorticoid, epidermal growth factor, IgG-F_c, insulin, low-density lipoproteins, opiates, somatomedin, testosterone, transcobalamin II, transferrin, folate, retinoid)[18]; and the bioconversion of xenobiotics. Bioconversion of xenobiotics has been shown to be important in the teratogenic activity of several xenobiotics. There is strong evidence that reactive metabolites of cyclophosphamide, 2-acetylaminofluorene, and nitroheterocycles (niridazole) are the proximal teratogens.[19] There also is experimental evidence that suggests that other chemicals undergo conversion to intermediates that have deleterious effects on embryonic development.[19–22] These include phenytoin, procarbazine, rifampicin, diethylstilbestrol, some benzhydrylpiperazine antihistamines, adriamycin, testosterone, benzo(a)pyrene, methoxyethanol, caffeine, and paraquat.

The major site of bioconversion of chemicals in vivo is likely to be the maternal liver. Placental P450-dependent mono-oxygenation of xenobiotics will occur at low rates unless induced by such compounds as those found in tobacco smoke.[17] However, the rodent embryo and yolk sac have been shown to possess functional P450 oxidative isozymes capable of converting proteratogens to active metabolites during early organogenesis.[23] In addition, P450-independent bioactivation has been suggested. For example, there is strong evidence that the rat embryo can reductively convert niridazole to an embryotoxic metabolite.[24]

The embryo also possesses two general types of biochemical mechanisms for inactivating toxic intermediates. These mechanisms include thiol-dependent inactivation mediated primarily by reduced glutathione; and thiol-independent inactivation mediated by endogenous antioxidants and radical scavenging compounds such as tocopherols, ascorbate, β-carotene, and uric acid.[25]

Several experimental criteria defined by Juchau suggest that a suspected metabolite is responsible for the in vivo teratogenic effects of a chemical or drug[19]:

1. The chemical must be convertible to the intermediate.
2. The intermediate must be found in or have access to the tissue(s) affected.
3. The embryotoxic effect should increase with the concentration of the metabolite.
4. Inhibiting the conversion should reduce the embryotoxic effect of the agent.
5. Promoting the conversion should increase the embryotoxicity of the agent.
6. Inhibiting or promoting the conversion should not alter the target tissues.
7. Inhibition of biochemical inactivation should increase the embryotoxicity of the agent.

It is readily apparent why there may be marked qualitative and quantitative differences in the species responses to a teratogenic agent.

PLACENTAL TRANSPORT

The exchange between the embryo and the mother is controlled by the placenta, which includes the chorioplacenta, the yolk sac placenta, and the paraplacental chorion. The placenta varies in structure and function among species and for each stage of gestation. As an example, the rodent yolk sac placenta continues to function as an organ of transport for a much greater percentage of gestation than in the human. Thus, differences in placental function and structure may affect our ability to apply teratogenic data developed in one species directly to other species.[26] Yet as pharmacokinetic techniques and the actual measurement of metabolic products in the embryo become more sophisticated, the appropriateness of utilizing animal data to project human effects may improve.

Although it has been alleged that the placental barrier was protective, and therefore harmful substances did not reach the embryo, it is now clear that there is no "placental barrier" per se. Yet the package inserts on many drugs state that "this drug crosses the placental barrier."[27] The uninitiated may infer from this statement that this characteristic of a drug is both unusual and hazardous. The fact is that most drugs and chemicals cross the placenta. It is a rare substance that crosses the placental barrier in one species and cannot reach the fetus in another. This happens only with selected proteins whose actions are species-specific.

Even before there were chemical techniques to demonstrate the presence of drugs or chemicals in the embryo there was clear evidence that they had reached the fetus because of clinical manifestations of the drugs:

1. Anticoagulants such as warfarin can affect the clotting of fetal blood.
2. Many drugs can affect the fetal cardiac rate.
3. Changes in the fetal EEG can be demonstrated because of the many drugs that affect the central nervous system.
4. Newborns have exhibited withdrawal symptoms from drugs that their mothers have taken, either medications or substances of abuse, such as alcohol or opiates.

These observations demonstrate clinically significant placental transport of drugs only in the latter portion of gestation and may not be a means of evaluating embryonic exposure during early organogenesis.

Those factors that determine the ability of a drug or chemical to cross the placenta and reach the embryo include molecular weight, lipid affinity or solubility, polarity or degree of ionization, protein binding, and receptor mediation.

Those compounds with low molecular weight, lipid affinity, nonpolarity, and no protein-binding properties will cross the placenta with ease and rapidity. For example, ethyl alcohol is a chemical that reaches the embryo rapidly and in concentrations equal to or greater than the level in the mother. Thus, a low-molecular-weight, lypophilic, nonionized, nonprotein-bound molecule probably will readily reach the embryo.

High-molecular-weight compounds like heparin (molecular weight of 20,000) do not cross the placenta; therefore, heparin is used to replace warfarinlike compounds during pregnancy for the treatment of hypercoagulation conditions. Rose Bengal, a compound specifically concentrated in the liver, does not cross the placenta at all. Compounds with molecular weights of 1000 or greater do not readily cross the placenta, whereas 600-dalton compounds usually do; most drugs are 250–400 daltons and do cross the placenta.[28]

In addition to the particular properties of the drug or chemical, there are three other conditions that affect the quantitative aspect of placental transport: placental blood flow, the pH gradient between the maternal and fetal serum and tissues, and placental metabolism of the chemical or drug. The biotransformation properties of the placental or maternal organism are important because a number of chemicals or drugs are not teratogenic in their original form. Only certain metabolic products derived from these substances may be teratogenic.

Finally, the mechanism of transport can involve simple diffusion, facilitated diffusion, active transport, ultrafiltration, pinocytosis, or coupled transport.

The most important concept with regard to placental transport of teratogens must be reemphasized. An agent is teratogenic because it affects the embryo, either directly or indirectly, by its ability to produce an effect in the embryo or extraembryonic membranes at exposures that are attained in the human being, not because it crosses the placenta per se.

SPECIES DIFFERENCES

The genetic constitution of an organism is an important factor in the susceptibility of a species to a drug or chemical. More than 30 disorders of increased sensitivity to drug toxicity or effects due to an inherited trait have been reported in the human.[29] The effect of a drug or chemical depends on both the maternal and fetal genotypes and may result in differences in cell sensitivity, placental transport, absorption, metabolism (activation, inactivation, active metabolites), receptor binding, and distribution of an agent, and it accounts for some variations in teratogenic effects among species and in individual subjects.

TERATOGENIC INFECTIOUS AGENTS

There are viral, bacterial, and parasitic agents known to cause maldevelopment in humans: rubella, cytomegalovirus, herpes simplex, parvovirus B19, syphilis, toxoplasmosis, varicella zoster, and Venezuelan equine encephalitis.[30] The lethal or developmental effects of infectious agents are the result of mitotic inhibition, direct cytotoxicity, or necrosis. Repair processes may result in metaplasia, scarring, or calcification, which causes further damage by interfering with histogenesis. Infectious agents appear to be exceptions to some of the principles of teratogenesis because dose and time of exposure cannot be demonstrated as readily for replicating teratogenic agents. However, transplacental transmission of an infectious agent does not necessarily result in congenital malformations, growth retardation, or lethality.

IDENTIFICATION OF A HUMAN TERATOGEN

Without evidence of human teratogenicity it is difficult to provide estimates of the hazard that exposures to specific agents present to the human fetus. Uncritical evaluation of single reports suggesting causal associations between suspected agents and human malformations can be misleading,[31] such as the erroneous association of Bendectin with congenital defects.[32–35]

TABLE 20–4. PROOF OF TERATOGENESIS IN THE HUMAN

1. Controlled epidemiologic studies consistently demonstrate an increased incidence of a particular congenital malformation in exposed human population.
2. Secular trends demonstrate a relationship between the incidence of a particular malformation and exposures in human populations.
3. An animal model mimics the human malformation at clinically comparable exposures:
   a. Without evidence of maternal toxicity
   b. Without reduction in food and water ingestion
   c. With careful interpretation of malformations that occur in isolation, such as anophthalmia in the rat, cleft palate in the mouse, vertebral and rib malformations in the rabbit, and omphalocele in the ferret.
4. The teratogenic effects increase with dose.
5. The mechanisms of teratogenesis are understood or the results are biologically plausible.

After Brent RL. Evaluating the alleged teratogenicity of environmental agents. Clin Perinatol 13:609.

It should be noted that most human teratogens have been identified by alert physicians or scientists. Epidemiologic studies have been most helpful in understanding the frequency, trends, and incidence of congenital malformations. Although animal studies have been most useful in understanding the mechanism of action of known human teratogens, they also lend support to epidemiologic studies by the development of animal models.[36,37] Even with complete pharmacokinetic studies in the human and animal species, an animal model cannot be extrapolated with certainty to the human condition if one has no information on the teratogenicity in the human.[36,38–41]

Several criteria are required to establish that a drug or chemical exposure causes maldevelopment in the human (Table 20-4):

1. Epidemiologic studies should repeatedly report that exposure to a drug or chemical is associated with an increased incidence of a specific malformation or group of malformations.
2. For common exposures, secular trend data should support the allegation.
3. An animal model should be developed using exposures comparable to therapeutic doses in humans.
4. The teratogenic effects should increase in relation to the dose.
5. The alleged teratogenic response should be biologically plausible and should not contradict proven scientific principles.[42]

SUMMARY

Environmental influences that produce abnormal development have certain characteristics in common and follow certain basic principles. These principles determine quantitative and qualitative aspects of teratogenesis and include embryonic stage, the dose or magnitude of the exposure (threshold concept), pharmacokinetics and metabolism of the agent, placental transport, and species differences. Studies of environmentally induced malformations are important because these exposures are preventable; moreover, they may enable us to understand the mechanisms of teratogenesis from all etiologies.

ACKNOWLEDGMENTS

This work was supported in part by funds from NIH HD07075, NIH HD18167, the Foerderer Foundation, and Harry Bock Charities.

REFERENCES

1. Wilson JG, Brent RL, Jordan HC. Differentiation as a determinant of the reaction of rat embryos to x-irradiation. Proc Soc Exp Biol Med 1953;82:67.
2. Generoso WM, Rutledge JC, Cain KT, Hughes LA, Downing DJ. Mutagen-induced fetal anomalies and death following treatment of females within hours after mating. Mutat Res 1988;199:175.
3. Pampfer S, Streffer C. Prenatal death and malformations after irradiation of mouse zygotes with neutrons or x-rays. Teratology 1988;37:599.
4. Mirkes PE. Cyclophosphamide teratogenesis: a review. Teratogenesis Carcinog Mutagen 1985;5:75.
5. Mattison DR. Physiologic variations in pharmacokinetics during pregnancy. In: Fabro S, Scialli AR, eds. Drug and chemical action in pregnancy: pharmacologic and toxicologic principles. New York: Marcel Dekker, 1986:37.
6. Shapiro S, Slone D, Hartz SC, Rosenberg L, Siskind V, Monson RR, et al. Anticonvulsants and parental epilepsy in the development of birth defects. Lancet 1976;1:272.
7. Hanson JW. Teratogen update: fetal hydantoin effects. Teratology 1986;33:349.
8. Miller RW. Congenital PCB poisoning: a reevaluation. Environ Health Perspect 1985;60:211.
9. Lammer EJ. A phenocopy of the retinoic acid embryopathy following maternal use of etretinate that ended one year before conception. Teratology 1988;5:472.
10. Wilson JG. Environment and birth defects. New York: Academic Press, 1973.
11. Briggs MH, Briggs M. Sex hormone exposure during pregnancy and malformations. In: Briggs MH, Corbin A, eds. Advances in steroid biochemistry and pharmacology. Vol 7. London: Academic Press, 1979:51.
12. Wilson JG, Brent RL. Are female sex hormones teratogenic? Am J Obstet Gynecol 1981;114:567.
13. Hochner-Celnikier D, Marandici A, Iohan F, Monder C. Estrogen and progesterone receptors in the organs of prenatal Cynomolgus monkey and laboratory mouse. Biol Reprod 1986;35:633.
14. Fraser FC. Interactions and multiple causes. In: Wilson JG, Fraser FC, eds. Handbook of teratology. New York: Plenum Press, 1977:445.
15. Jackson MJ. Drug absorption. In: Fabro S, Scialli AR, eds. Drug and chemical action in pregnancy: pharmacologic and toxicologic principles. New York: Marcel Dekker, 1986:15.
16. Sonawane BR, Yaffe SJ. Physiologic disposition of drugs in the fetus and newborn. In: Fabro S, Scialli AR, eds. Drug and chemical action in pregnancy: pharmacologic and toxicologic principles. New York: Marcel Dekker, 1986:103.

17. Juchau MR, Rettie AE. The metabolic role of the placenta. In: Fabro S, Scialli AR, eds. Drug and chemical action in pregnancy: pharmacologic and toxicologic principles. New York: Marcel Dekker, 1986:153.
18. Miller RK. Placental transfer and function: the interface for drugs and chemicals in the conceptus. In: Fabro S, Scialli AR, eds. Drug and chemical action in pregnancy: pharmacologic and toxicologic principles. New York: Marcel Dekker, 1986:123.
19. Juchau MR. Bioactivation in chemical teratogenesis. Ann Rev Pharmacol Toxicol 1989;29:165.
20. Brown LP, Flint OP, Orton TC, Gibson CG. Chemical teratogenesis: testing methods and the role of metabolism. Drug Metab Rev 1986;17:221.
21. Juchau MR, Harris C, Beyer BK, Fantel AG. Reactive intermediates in chemical teratogenesis. In: Welsch, F, ed. Approaches to elucidate mechanisms in teratogenesis hemisphere. New York: 1987:167.
22. Slikker W Jr. The role of metabolism in the testing of developmental toxicants. Regul Toxicol Pharmacol 1987;7:390.
23. Yang HYL, Namkung MJ, Juchau MR. Cytochrome P450-dependent biotransformation of a series of phenoxazone ethers in the rat conceptus during early organogenesis: evidence for multiple P450 isozymes. Mol Pharmacol 1988;34:67.
24. Fantel AG, Person RE, Juchau MR. Niridazole metabolism by rat embryos in vitro. Teratology 1988;37:213.
25. Reed DJ. Cellular defense mechanisms against reactive metabolites. In: Anders MW, ed. Bioactivation of foreign compounds. Orlando: Academic Press, 1985:71.
26. Brent RL. Environmental factors: miscellaneous. In: Brent RL, Harris MI, eds. Prevention of embryonic, fetal and perinatal disease. DHEW Pub No NIH 76, Bethesda, MD, 1976:211.
27. Brent RL. Drugs and pregnancy: are the insert warnings too dire? Contemp OB-Gyn 1982;20:42.
28. Mirkin BL. Maternal and fetal distribution of drugs in pregnancy. Clin Pharmacol Ther 1973;14:643.
29. McKusick VA. Mendelian inheritance in man. 5th ed. Baltimore: The Johns Hopkins University Press, 1983.
30. Sever JL. Infections in pregnancy: highlights from the collaborative perinatal project. Teratology 1982;25:227.
31. Wilson JG. Misinformation about risks of congenital anomalies. In: Maurois M, ed. Prevention of physical and mental congenital defects. Part C: Basic and medical science, education, and future strategies. New York: Alan R Liss, 1985:165.
32. Brent RL. Editorial comments on comments on teratogen update: Bendectin. Teratology 1985;31:429.
33. Brent RL. Editorial: Bendectin and interventricular septal defects. Teratology 1985;32:317.
34. Holmes LB. Response to comments on teratogen update: Bendectin. Teratology 1985;31:432.
35. Shiono PH, Klebanoff MA. Bendectin and human congenital malformations. Teratology 1989;40:151.
36. Brent RL. Methods for evaluating the alleged teratogenicity of environmental agents. In: Marois M, ed. Prevention of physical and mental congenital defects. Part C: Basic and medical science, education, and future strategies. New York: Alan R Liss, 1985:191.
37. Brent RL, Beckman DA, Jensh RP. The relationship of animal experiments in predicting the effects of intrauterine effects in the human. In: Kriegel H, Schmahl W, Gerber GB, Stieve FE, eds. Radiation risks to the developing nervous system. New York: Gustav Fisher, 1986:367.
38. Brent RL. The indirect effect of irradiation on embryonic development. II. Irradiation of the placenta. Am J Dis Child 1960;100:103.
39. Brent RL. Drug testing in animals for teratogenic effects: thalidomide in the pregnant rat. J Pediatr 1964;64:762.
40. Brent RL. The prediction of human diseases from laboratory and animal tests for teratogenicity, carcinogenicity and mutagenicity. In: Lasagna L, ed. Controversies in therapeutics. Philadelphia: WB Saunders, 1981:134.
41. Fraser FC. Relationship of animal studies to man. In: Wilson JG, Fraser FC, eds. Handbook of teratology. New York: Plenum Press, 1977:75.
42. Brent RL. Evaluating the alleged teratogenicity of environmental agents. Clin Perinatol 1986;13:609.

21

CHAPTER

PRESCRIBED DRUGS, THERAPEUTIC AGENTS, AND FETAL TERATOGENESIS

Robert L. Brent and David A. Beckman

ETIOLOGIES OF CONGENITAL MALFORMATIONS

There have been dramatic advances in understanding of the causes of human birth defects. In earlier times, superstition, ignorance, and prejudice predominated in these explanations. The stigma associated with birth defects has primitive beginnings and persists today. In the minds of many, even the most sophisticated, a birth defect is felt to be some form of punishment. At the beginning of this century the predominant cause was believed to be genetic; the rest of the causes consisted of totally unsolvable clinical problems. At this point in the history of birth defect research, the etiology of congenital malformations can be divided into three categories: unknown, genetic, and environmental factors (Table 21-1). The etiology of the majority of human malformations, approximately 65% to 75%, is still unknown.[1-3] However, a significant proportion of congenital malformations of unknown etiology is likely to be polygenic (ie, due to two or more genetic loci[4,5]) or at least to have an important genetic component. Malformations with an increased recurrent risk, such as cleft lip and palate, anencephaly, spina bifida, certain congenital heart diseases, pyloric stenosis, hypospadias, inguinal hernia, talipes equinovarus, and congenital dislocation of the hip, can fit the category of multifactorial disease, as well as the category of polygenic inherited disease.[4,6] The multifactorial threshold hypothesis involves the modulation of a continuum of genetic characteristics by intrinsic and extrinsic (environmental) factors.[6] Although the modulating factors are not known, they probably include placental blood flow, placental transport, site of implantation, maternal disease states, infections, drugs, chemicals, and spontaneous errors of development.

Spontaneous errors of development may account for some of the malformations that occur without apparent abnormalities of the genome or environmental influence. We postulate that there is some probability for error during embryonic development based on the fact that embryonic development is a complicated process, similar to the concept of spontaneous mutations.[7,2] It has been estimated that up to 50% of all fertilized ova in the human are lost within the first 3 weeks of development.[8] The World Health Organization estimated that 15% of all clinically recognizable pregnancies end in a spontaneous abortion, with 50% to 60% of the spontaneously aborted fetuses having chromosomal abnormalities.[9-11] As a conservative estimate, 1173 clinically recognized pregnancies will result in approximately 173 miscarriages and 30 to 60 of the infants in the remaining 1000 live births will have congenital anomalies. The true incidence of pregnancy loss is much higher, but undocumented pregnancies are not included in this risk estimate. The 3% to 6% incidence of malformed offspring represents the background risk for human maldevelopment. Although we know little about the mechanisms that result in the in utero death of defective embryos, it is more important to understand the circumstances that permit abnormal embryos to survive to term.[12]

Understanding the pathogenesis for the large group of malformations with unknown etiology will depend on identifying the genes involved in polygenic or pleurogenic processes, the interacting genetic and environmental determinants of multifactorial traits, and the statistical risks for error during embryonic development.

The known etiologies of teratogenesis include genetic and environmental factors that affect the embryo during development (eg, drugs, chemicals, radiation, hyperthermia, infections, abnormal maternal metabolic states, or mechanical factors). Environmental and genetic causes of malformations have different pathologic processes that result in abnormal development. Congenital malformations due to genetic etiology have a spectrum of pathologic processes that are the result of a gene deficiency, a gene abnormality, chromosome deletion, or chromosome excess. The pathologic nature of this process is determined before conception, or at least before differentiation, because of inherited or newly acquired genetic abnormalities present in all or most of the cells of the embryo. Although environmental factors may modify the development of the genetically abnormal embryo, the genetic abnormality is usually the predominant contributor to the pathologic process.

The remainder of this review will focus on prescription drugs and therapeutic agents that cause congenital malformations in the human. Although these agents account for less than 1% of all malformations, they are important because these exposures are preventable.

TABLE 21-1. ETIOLOGY OF HUMAN MALFORMATIONS OBSERVED DURING THE FIRST YEAR OF LIFE

SUSPECTED CAUSE	PERCENT OF TOTAL
Unknown	65–75
Polygenic	
Multifactorial (gene–environment interactions)	
Spontaneous errors of development	
Synergistic interactions of teratogens	
Genetic	10–25
Autosomal and sex-linked genetic disease	
New mutations	
Cytogenetic (chromosomal abnormalities)	
Environmental	10
Maternal conditions: Alcoholism, diabetes, endocrinopathies, phenylketonuria, smoking and nicotine, starvation	4
Infectious agents: Rubella, toxoplasmosis, syphilis, herpes, cytomegalic inclusion disease, varicella, Venezuelan equine encephalitis, parvovirus	3
Mechanical problems (deformations): Amniotic band constrictions, umbilical cord constraint, disparity in uterine size and uterine contents	1–2
Chemicals, drugs, radiation, hyperthermia	<1

Adapted from: Brent RL. Environmental factors: miscellaneous. In: Brent RL, Harris MI, eds. Prevention of embryonic, fetal, and perinatal disease. DHEW Pub (NIH) 76-853. Bethesda, MD, 1976:211.

Brent RL. The magnitude of the problem of congenital malformations. In: Marois M, ed. Prevention of physical and mental congenital defects, part A: The scope of the problem. New York: Alan R Liss, 1985:55.

Brent RL, Holmes LB. Clinical and basic science lessions from the thalidomide tragedy: what have we learned about the causes of limb defects? Teratology 1988;38:241.

OVERALL TERATOGENIC RISK

To appreciate the difficulty in predicting the effect that an exposure to a drug or therapeutic agent will have on the developing embryo, we shall briefly discuss factors that influence this prediction.

The baseline risk of human reproduction is based on epidemiologic studies that have determined the incidence of fetal death and maldevelopment. Approximately 75% of all conceptions are lost before term, and 50% of those are lost within the first 3 weeks.[8,13] Of the liveborn infants, 3% to 6% will be recognized as congenitally malformed.

ENVIRONMENTAL RISK PARAMETERS OR (MODIFIERS)

The susceptibility of an embryo or fetus to teratogenic influences is related to the stage of development at which the exposure occurs. The explanation for this phenomenon is that the fetus is constantly changing during its development with respect to tissue receptors, metabolism, drug distribution, cell proliferation, and so on. Thus, tissue response to an exposure and the ability of the fetus to recuperate from the insult vary during gestation. Although detrimental effects can be induced at any time during pregnancy, most major malformations result from exposures during days 18–40 of gestation in the human. However, the palate, central nervous system, and genital structures can be affected at later stages of development. Our knowledge of the time of resistance or susceptibility of the embryo to various environmental influences has expanded over the past 30 years. This information is vital in evaluating the significance of individual exposures or epidemiologic studies.

Every teratogenic agent that has been validly tested has exhibited a dose–response relationship and a threshold dose response—that is, a dose below which there is no difference between the exposed and nonexposed in the incidence of malformations. The dose to which the fetus is exposed is determined by maternal pharmacokinetics, placental exchange, fetal and placental metabolism of the substance (and the teratogenic activity of the metabolites), the fetal distribution of the substance, and the presence of tissue-specific receptors. Factors that influence the response include maternal toxicity and drug–drug interactions. Additionally, more than 30 drug-related disorders are related to genotype.[13] Although genetic variations have not been proved to alter drug teratogenicity in human beings, such proof exists for experimental animals.[15,16]

Finally, maternal disease states may produce deleterious effects on the fetus that are difficult to separate from a possible teratogenic effect of a therapeutic agent. This is an especially relevant consideration for long-standing conditions such as diabetes.

When counseling patients, especially in our litigious climate, three confounding influences are at work:

1. Because of the anxiety created by unfounded reports and misinformation, reported associations of drugs and their effect on the fetus must be evaluated critically.[17]
2. Pregnancy is not without risk, and congenital malformations occur in the absence of drug or chemical exposures.
3. Teratogenic agents do exist and new ones could be introduced.

MECHANISMS OF TERATOGENESIS

Based on his review of the literature, Wilson provided a format of theoretical teratogenic mechanisms: mutation; chromosomal aberrations; mitotic interference; altered nucleic acid synthesis and function; lack of precursors, substrates, or coenzymes for biosynthesis; altered energy sources; enzyme inhibition; osmolar imbalance, alterations in fluid pressures, viscosities, and osmotic pressures; and altered membrane characteristics.[1] Even though an agent can produce one or more of these pathologic processes, exposure to such an agent does not guarantee that maldevelopment will occur. Furthermore, it is likely that a drug, chemical, or other agent can have more than one effect on the pregnant women and the developing conceptus, and therefore the nature of the drug or its biochemical or pharmacologic effects will not in themselves predict a human teratogenic effect. In fact, the discovery of human teratogens has come primarily from human epidemiologic studies. Animal studies and in vitro studies can be very helpful in determining the mechanism of teratogenesis and the pharmacokinetics related to teratogenesis.[18] We have proposed a list of mechanisms (Table 21-2) that we shall use in our discussion of the known teratogenic drugs and therapeutic agents in man. However, even if one understands the pathologic effects of an agent, one cannot predict the teratogenic risk of an exposure without taking into consideration the developmental stage, the magnitude of the exposure, and the reparability of the embryo.

What is known concerning the mechanism of action of drugs and therapeutic agents that have been shown to cause congenital malformations in man is summarized in Table 21-3.

TABLE 21-2. PROPOSED MECHANISMS OF TERATOGENESIS

Cell death beyond recuperative capacity of the embryo–fetus
Mitotic delay: increase in the length of the cell cycle
Retarded differentiation: slowing or cessation in the process of differentiation
Physical constraint and vascular insufficiency
Interference with histogenesis by processes such as cell depletion, necrosis, calcification, or scarring
Inhibited cell migration and cell communication

From Beckman DA, Brent RL. Mechanism of known environmental teratogens: drugs and chemicals. Clin Perinatol 1986;13:649.

TERATOGENIC THERAPEUTIC AGENTS AND DRUGS

AMINOPTERIN AND METHOTREXATE

Aminopterin-induced therapeutic abortions have been shown to result in malformations (hydrocephalus, cleft palate, meningomyelocele) in some of the abortuses.[19,20] Three case reports of children exposed to aminopterin in utero included observations of growth retardation, abnormal cranial ossification, high-arched palate, and reduction in derivatives of the first branchial arch.[21–23]

Aminopterin and methotrexate (methylaminopterin) are folic acid antagonists that inhibit dihydrofolate reductase, resulting in cell death during the S phase of the cell cycle.[24] The clinical literature has been reviewed by Warkany.[12]

Dyban and coworkers have reported abnormalities of cell proliferation and cytotoxicity employing rat blastomere cultures exposed to different doses of aminopterin.[25] Skalko and Gold demonstrated a threshold effect and a dose-dependent increase in malformations in mice exposed to methotrexate in utero.[26]

ANDROGENS

Masculinization of the external genitalia of the female has been reported following in utero exposure to large doses of testosterone, methyltestosterone, and testosterone enanthate.[27–29] The masculinization is characterized by clitoromegaly with or without fusion of the labia minora and no indication of nongenital malformations.

Many animal models show the masculinizing effects of androgens. Well-known studies were performed by Greene and coworkers in the rat, Raynaud in the mouse, Bruner and Witschi in the hamster, Jost in the rabbit, and Wells and Van Wagenen in the monkey.[30–34] These studies demonstrated the masculinization of the urogenital sinus, its derivatives, and the external genitalia, although there was little effect on the müllerian ducts, and ovarian inversion did not occur. Based on experimental animal studies, any effects of prenatal exposure to androgens on behavioral masculinization will be rare because the androgen must be aromatizable to an estrogen to affect sexual differentiation of the brain, and estrogen receptors in the brain have not been identified before birth in the mouse or rat.[35]

ANTICONVULSANTS

Although individual anticonvulsant drugs will be discussed in detail later, important aspects of anticonvulsants as a group should be discussed now.

Anticonvulsant drugs, with the exception of the succinimides (ethosuximide, methsuximide, phensuximide), have been associated with an increased teratogenic risk: barbiturates (phenobarbital, primaclone), hydantoins (phenytoin), oxazolidinediones (trimethadione, paramethadione) and a miscellaneous group (valproic acid, carbamazepine).[36] The increased teratogenic risk estimates for the anticonvulsants are 6% for barbiturate–hydantoin exposure, 80% for oxazolidinedione exposure, and about 1% for valproic acid. The mechanism of teratogenic action for the anticonvulsants has been difficult to define for several reasons: many are given in combination therapeutically, dose–response relationships are difficult to prove, and the exposure is chronic. Since the increased teratogenic risk is small relative to the risk in nontreated pregnancies, it is likely that the *chronic* nature of anticonvulsant therapy is an important contributor to the increased teratogenic risk.

CARBAMAZEPINE

Carbamazepine has been considered a relatively safe drug for pregnant women requiring anticonvulsant therapy. Reports in the literature suggested that carbamazepine presented no increased risk of major malformations.[37,38] However, other investigators reported an association between carbamazepine exposure and fingernail and toenail hypoplasia[39] or reduced birth weight, length, and head circumference.[40,41] Jones and coworkers[42] have recently documented a pattern of defects resulting from prenatal exposure to carbamazepine involving minor craniofacial defects, fingernail hypoplasia, and developmental delay. Based on the similarity between phenytoin and carbamazepine with respect to the defects seen after fetal exposure and to the metabolism of both drugs through the arene oxide pathway, Jones and coworkers[42] postulate that the epoxide intermediate is the teratogenic agent rather than the drug itself, but this is an unlikely explanation. Although the data were insufficient for a definitive estimation, carbamazepine does appear to present a significant risk to the fetus.

COUMARIN DERIVATIVES

Nasal hypoplasia following exposure to several drugs, including warfarin, during pregnancy was reported by DiSaia.[43] Kerber and colleagues[44] were the first to suggest warfarin as the teratogenic agent. Coumarin anticoagulants have since been associated with nasal hypoplasia, calcific stippling of the secondary epiphysis, and central nervous system (CNS) abnormalities.[44–47] Barr and Burdi[48] described warfarin embryopathy, and Warkany,[49,50] besides summarizing the clinical data, provides an excellent overview of the difficulties in relating a congenital malformation to an environmental cause. There is an estimated 10% to 25% risk for affected infants following exposure during the period from the eighth through the 14th week of pregnancy, although this risk has been reported to be much lower in some series, and other factors besides dose and gestational stage seem to play a role.

Coumarin has been shown to inhibit the formation of carboxyglutamyl residues from glutamyl residues, decreasing the ability of proteins to bind calcium.[51] The inhibition of calcium binding by proteins during embryonic–fetal development, especially during a critical period of ossification, could explain the nasal hypoplasia, stippled calcification, and skeletal abnormalities of warfarin embryopathy.[47] Microscopic bleeding does not seem to be responsible for these problems early in development.[48]

One case report was unique in that the time of exposure to warfarin was between 8 and 12 weeks of gestation, and the infant presented with Dandy-Walker malformation, eye defects, and agenesis of the corpus callosum.[52] Although this case report represents the clearest evidence for a direct effect of warfarin on the developing CNS rather than an effect mediated by hemorrhage, it is the only report with the exposure so well defined and occurring before the appearance of vitamin K–dependent clotting factors.

CYCLOPHOSPHAMIDE

Cyclophosphamide is a widely used antineoplastic agent with an apparent risk of malformation in the human of approximately 1:6.[36] The defects include growth retardation, ectrodactyly, syndactyly, cardiovascular anomalies, and other minor anomalies.[53,54] Six out of seven pregnancy outcomes have been reported to be normal after cyclophosphamide exposure.[55]

Experimental animal studies in the rat,[56,57] mouse,[58] and rabbit[59] have shown distinct developmental-stage specificity, dose–effect relationships, and a high sensitivity of nervous system and mesenchymal tissues.[60]

The current knowledge of the mechanism of cyclophosphamide teratogenesis has recently been reviewed: cytochrome P-450 monooxygenases convert cyclophosphamide to 4-hydroxycyclophosphamide, which in turn breaks down to phosphoramide mustard and acrolein.[60] Phosphoramide mustard may produce teratogenic effects by interacting with cellular DNA in an as yet undefined manner whereas acrolein appears to act differently, possibly by affecting sulfhydryl linkages in proteins.[61] Tissue sensitivity to phosphoramide mustard and acrolein is thought to be related to such processes as detoxification and cellular repair.

DIETHYLSTILBESTROL

The first abnormality reported following exposure to diethylstilbestrol (DES) during the first trimester was clitoromegaly in female newborns.[62] Much later, Herbst and coworkers[63,64] and Greenwald and associates[65] reported an association of vaginal adenocarcinoma in female offspring following first-trimester exposures. Fur-

Continued on page 306

TABLE 21–3. TERATOGENIC THERAPEUTIC AGENTS AND DRUGS*

ENVIRONMENTAL INFLUENCE	REPORTED EFFECTS OR ASSOCIATIONS	COMMENTS
Aminopterin, methotrexate	Microcephalus, hydrocephalus, cleft palate, meningomyelocele, IUGR, abnormal cranial ossification, reduction in derivatives of first branchial arch, mental retardation, postnatal growth retardation	Anticancer, antimetabolic agents; folic acid antagonists that inhibit dihydrofolate reductase, resulting in cell death
Androgens	Masculinization of female embryo: clitoromegaly with or without fusion of labia minora. Nongenital malformations are not a reported risk.	Effects are dose dependent; stimulates growth and differentiation of sex steroid receptor-containing tissue.
Angiotensin converting enzyme inhibitors (refer to text)	Exposures may cause fetal and neonatal death, oligohydramnios, pulmonary hypoplasia, neonatal anuria, IUGR, and skull hypoplasia.	Antihypertensive agents; adverse fetal effects are related to severe fetal hypotension over a long period of time during the second or third trimester. Risk appears to be low. Can be used in a woman of reproductive age because therapy can be changed without an increase in the risk of teratogenesis during the first trimester if the woman becomes pregnant, since this group of drugs does not interfere with organogenesis.
Carbamazepine	Minor craniofacial defects (upslanting palpebral fissures, epicanthal folds, short nose with long philtrum), fingernail hypoplasia, and developmental delay	Anticonvulsant; little is known concerning mechanism. Risk is not known but likely to be significant for minor defects.
Coumarin	Nasal hypoplasia; stippling of secondary epiphysis; IUGR; anomalies of eyes, hands, neck; variable CNS anatomical defects, such as absent corpus callosum, hydrocephalus, or asymmetrical brain hypoplasia.	Anticoagulant; bleeding is an unlikely explanation for effects produced in the first trimester. Risk from exposure 10% to 25% during 8th to 14th week of gestation. CNS anatomical defects may occur any time during second and third trimester and may be related to bleeding.
Cyclophosphamide	Growth retardation, ectrodactyly, syndactyly, cardiovascular anomalies, and other minor anomalies.	Anticancer, alkylating agent; requires cytochrome P450 mono-oxydase activation; interacts with DNA, resulting in cell death. Magnitude of risk unknown.
Diethylstilbestrol	Clear cell adenocarcinoma of the vagina occurs in between 1:1000 and 1:10,000 girls who were exposed in utero. Vaginal adenosis occurs much more frequently. Anomalies of the uterus and cervix may play a role in decreased fertility and an increased incidence of prematurity, although the majority of DES babies can conceive and deliver normal babies. Surprisingly, there are case reports of masculinization of the female fetus after high doses. The dose that increases risk of genitourinary abnormalities in the male is controversial.	Synthetic estrogen; stimulates estrogen receptor-containing tissue, may cause misplaced genital tissue, which has a greater propensity to develop cancer. Vaginal adenosis from exposures before 9th week of pregnancy, 75% risk; risk of adenocarcinoma is low (1 in 10,000).
Diphenylhydantoin	Hydantoin syndrome: microcephaly, mental retardation, cleft lip/palate, hypoplastic nails and distal phalanges; characteristic, but not diagnostic, facial features	Anticonvulsant; direct effect on cell membranes, folate, and vitamin K metabolism. Metabolic intermediate (epoxide) has been suggested as the teratogenic agent. Wide variation in reported risk. Associations documented only with chronic exposure.
Lithium carbonate	Although animal studies have demonstrated a clear teratogenic risk, the effect in humans is uncertain. Early reports indicated an increased incidence of Epstein's anomaly and other heart and great vessel defects, but as more studies are reported this association has diminished.	Antidepressant; mechanism has not been defined. Risk is low.
Oxazolidine-2,4-diones (trimethadione, paramethadione)	Fetal trimethadione syndrome: V-shaped eyebrows, low-set ears with anteriorly folded helix, high-arched palate, irregular teeth, CNS anomalies, severe developmental delay.	Anticonvulsants; affects cell membrane permeability. Actual mechanism of action has not been determined. Wide variation in reported risk. Characteristic facial features are associations documented only with chronic exposure.
Penicillamine	Cutis laxa, hyperflexibility of joints.	Copper chelating agent; produces copper deficiency, inhibiting collagen synthesis and maturation. Condition appears to be reversible and the risk is low.

(continued)

TABLE 21–3. (continued)

ENVIRONMENTAL INFLUENCE	REPORTED EFFECTS OR ASSOCIATIONS	COMMENTS
Progestins	Masculinization of female embryo exposed to *high* doses of some testosterone-derived progestins. The dose of progestins present in modern oral contraceptives presents no masculinization or feminization risks. All progestins present no risk for nongenital malformations.	Stimulates or interferes with sex steroid receptor-containing tissue.
Radioactive isotopes	Tissue- and organ-specific damage dependent on radioisotope element and distribution, eg, ^{131}I administered to pregnant mother can cause fetal thyroid hypoplasia after the 8th week of development.	Higher doses of radioisotopes can produce cell death and mitotic delay. Effect is dependent on dose, distribution, metabolism, and specificity of localization.
Radiation (external irradiation)	Microcephaly, mental retardation, eye anomalies, IUGR, and visceral malformations depend on dose and stage of exposure.	Diagnostic and therapeutic agents; produce cell death and mitotic delay. No measurable risk with exposures for 5 rad (0.05 Gy) or less of x-rays at any stage of pregnancy.
Retinoids (etretinate, isotretinoin)	Increased risk of central nervous system, cardioaortic, ear, and clefting defects. Microtia, anotia, thymic aplasia, and other branchial arch and aortic arch abnormalities.	Used in treatment of chronic dermatoses; retinoids can cause direct cytotoxicity and alter programmed cell death; affect many cell types, but neural crest cells are particularly sensitive.
Sonography (ultrasound)	No confirmed detrimental effects resulting from medical sonography.	The levels and types of medical sonography that have been used in the past have no measurable risks. It appears that if the embryonic temperature never exceeds 39°C, there is no measurable risk.
Tetracycline	Bone staining and tooth staining can occur with therapeutic doses. Persistent high doses can cause hypoplastic tooth enamel. No other congenital malformations are associated.	Antibiotic; effects seen only if exposure is late in the first or during second or third trimester, since tetracyclines have to interact with calcified tissue.
Thalidomide	Limb reduction defects (preaxial preferential effects, phocomelia); facial hemangioma; esophageal or duodenal atresia; anomalies of external ears, kidneys, and heart. The thalidomide syndrome, while characteristic and recognizable, can be mimicked by some genetic diseases.	Sedative-hypnotic agent; multiple theories have been proposed. Although it is likely that one or more of the theories have elements of the truth, the etiology of thalidomide teratogenesis has not been definitively determined.
Thyroid: Iodine deficiency, iodides, radioiodine, antithyroid drugs (propylthiouracil)	Hypothyroidism or goiter; neurologic and aural damage is variable.	Fetopathic effect of endemic iodine occurs early in development. Fetopathic effect of iodides, antithyroid drugs, and radioiodine involves metabolic block, decreased thyroid hormone synthesis, and gland development. Maternal intake of 12 mg or more of iodide per day increases the risk of fetal goiter.
Valproic acid	Malformations are primarily facial dysmorphology and neural tube defects. Although there are some facial characteristics associated with this drug, they are not diagnostic. Small head size and developmental delay have been reported with high doses.	Anticonvulsant; little is known about the teratogenic action of valproic acid. The risk for spina bifida is about 1%, but the risk for facial dysmorphology may be greater.
Vitamin A	The same malformations that have been reported with the retinoids have been reported with very high doses of vitamin A. Exposures below 10,000 IU present no risk to the fetus.	Retinoic acid is cytotoxic; it may interact with DNA to delay differentiation and/or inhibit protein synthesis.
Vitamin D	Large doses given in vitamin D prophylaxis are possibly involved in the etiology of supravalvular aortic stenosis, elfin faces, and mental retardation.	Mechanism is likely to involve a disruption of cell calcium regulation. Genetic susceptibility and excessive doses are probably responsible.
Streptomycin	Hearing deficiency	Although only rarely reported, streptomycin and a group of ototoxic drugs can interfere with hearing. It is a relatively low risk phenomenon and would be associated with long-duration maternal therapy during pregnancy.
Bendectin (doxylamine succinate pyridoxine)	Not teratogenic as used in doses to treat nausea and vomiting of pregnancy.	This drug is mentioned because it was involved in so much litigation as an alleged teratogen. It is a drug with no measurable risk.

Updated from Beckman DA, Brent RL. Mechanism of known environmental teratogens: drugs and chemicals. Clin Perinatol 1986;13:649.
* Does not include non-therapeutic drugs, chemicals, and environmental agents.

ther studies revealed that almost all the cancers occurred after 14 years of age and only in those exposed before the 18th week of gestation.[66–68] There is a 75% risk for vaginal adenosis for exposures occurring before the ninth week of pregnancy; however, the risk of developing adenocarcinoma is extremely low (1 in 10,000).[69]

Although there does not appear to be an adverse effect on the rate of conception,[70] it is not clear whether the anatomical abnormalities of the uterus and cervix induced by intrauterine exposure to DES increase the probability of reproductive problems such as spontaneous abortions.[71,72]

There have been reports that males exposed to DES in utero exhibited genital lesions and abnormal spermatozoa, but no malignancies were observed.[73] A more recent epidemiologic study by Leary and coworkers reported no increase in the risk for the male for genitourinary abnormalities, infertility, or testicular cancer.[74] The controversial nature of the effects of DES exposure on the male may be attributable to study design or, more likely, to the fact that dose levels have varied greatly according to different regimens.

DES is a potent nonsteroidal estrogen and, as in the case of steroidal estrogens, must interact with the receptor proteins present only in estrogen-responsive tissues before exerting its effects by stimulating RNA, protein, and DNA synthesis. The carcinogenic effect of DES is most likely indirect: DES exposure results in the presence of columnar epithelium in the vagina, and this "misplaced tissue" may have a greater susceptibility to developing the adenocarcinoma—much as teratomas and other misplaced tissues are more susceptible to malignant degeneration.

Teratogenic and transplacental carcinogenic effects following in utero exposure to DES have been demonstrated in the rat,[75] mouse,[5,76] and hamster.[65] A major difficulty in studies of the mechanism of action of DES is the extensive biotransformation that occurs in the adult mammal, reviewed by Metzler.[77] These transformations recently have been demonstrated in the hamster fetus.[78]

DIPHENYLHYDANTOIN

Chronic exposure to diphenylhydantoin has been suggested to present a maximum of 10% risk for the full syndrome and a maximum of 30% risk for some anomalies.[79–82] Although cleft lip and palate, congenital heart disease, and microcephaly have been reported, hypoplasias of the nails and distal phalanges may be more specific malformations in the exposed fetuses.[45,83] Hanson and associates noted that, although the hydantoin syndrome is observed in 11% of the subjects in their study, three times that number exhibit mental deficits.[84,85] Prospective studies demonstrate a much lower frequency of effects, and some do not demonstrate any effect; thus, the overall prospective risk may be much lower for the classically reported effects.

Factors associated with epilepsy may contribute to the etiology of these malformations: based on the United States Collaborative Perinatal Project and a large Finnish registry, the incidence of malformations was 10.5% when the mother was epileptic, 8.3% when the father was epileptic, and 6.4% when neither parent was affected.[23]

Cleft lip and palate, as well as limb defects, have been produced in rabbits[86] and in mice,[87,88] and the malformation rate was dose-dependent.[89]

The teratogenic action of diphenylhydantoin has been postulated to involve the cytochrome P-450 metabolism of phenytoin to produce a reactive epoxide metabolite. The arene oxide would covalently bind to macromolecules and interfere with their function.[90–93]

LITHIUM CARBONATE

Lithium carbonate, widely used for treatment of manic–depressive disorders, was first associated with human congenital malformations in 1970.[94,95] The malformations described include heart and large-vessel anomalies, Epstein's anomaly, neural tube defects, talipes, microtia, and thyroid abnormalities.[96,36,97] Although lithium does cross the placenta,[98] its mechanism of teratogenic action is not understood. Lithium carbonate appears to be a human teratogen at therapeutic dosages but it presents a very small risk. Because of the value of lithium carbonate for treating manic–depressive psychosis, the risk associated with psychiatric relapse on removing the drug may be greater than the teratogenic risk.

Although lithium can induce abnormal development in several laboratory animals, its mechanism of teratogenic action is unknown. The neurotropic activity of lithium suggests that central nervous system malformations may result from cell membrane disturbances that affect neural tube closure.[99]

OXAZOLIDINE-2,4-DIONES

Trimethadione and paramethadione are antiepileptic oxazolidine-2,4-diones that distribute uniformly throughout body tissues and exert their effects by means of the action of their metabolism. These drugs affect cell membrane permeability and vitamin K–dependent clotting factors, but their primary mode of action is unknown.

Zackai and colleagues described the fetal trimethadione syndrome characterized by development delay, V-shaped eyebrows, low-set ears with anteriorly folded helix, high-arched palate, and irregular teeth.[100] German and coworkers reported similar findings plus cardiac anomalies.[101] Feldman and associates and Goldman and Yaffe have reviewed the clinical findings in the literature and from their own observations.[102,103] There are wide variations in reported risk, with estimates as high as 80% for major or minor defects. Because the number of exposures is small, the actual risk could vary considerably from these figures. It is unlikely that we will ever be able to ascertain the risk accurately, because the drug should not be used in pregnant women.

Mice exposed to high doses of trimethadione on days 8 to 10 or 11 to 13 of gestation had a high incidence of fetal growth retardation and abnormalities of the viscera and skeleton; aortic arch and vertebral defects were especially common.[104]

PENICILLAMINE

Human exposure to D-penicillamine can induce a connective tissue defect, including generalized cutix laxa, hyperflexibility of the joints, varicosities, and impaired wound healing.[105] The exposure must be long enough to induce a copper deficiency sufficient to inhibit collagen synthesis and maturation. However, the condition appears to be reversible, and the risk is low,[106] approximately 4% to 5%.[36]

D-penicillamine is a copper chelator shown to induce cleft palate and skeletal defects in the rat.[107,108] Copper deficiency appears to be the mechanism for teratogenicity.[109]

PROGESTINS (FEMALE SEX HORMONES)

For the purpose of discussion, expediency justifies grouping together many compounds by generically using the term "sex hormones." Similarly, there are common references to "progestogens" or "progestational agents." This expediency is unfortunate when it occurs in epidemiologic studies, which do not list the composition of sex hormone exposures.[110–112] It also is often overlooked that, although various progestogens act by means of similar receptors, their potential androgenic effects can differ markedly. This point is critical to the appreciation of the virilizing effects of these compounds in the human. It has been shown, for example, that the pharmacokinetic parameters that estimate steroid bioavailability and metabolism show great variability among subjects and between steroids conveniently grouped together, such as "progestins."[113] One must assume that these differences in bioavailability and metabolism reflect differences in the biologic activity of these steroids in humans.

In contrast to progesterone and 17-alpha-hydroxyprogesterone caproate, high doses of some of the synthetic progestins have been reported to cause virilizing effects in humans. Exposure during the first trimester to large doses of 17-alpha-ethinyltestosterone has been associated with masculinization of the external genitalia of female fetuses.[114,115] Similar associations result from exposure to large doses of 17-alpha-ethinyl-19-nortestosterone (norethandrolone)[115] and 17-alpha-ethinyl-17-OH-5(10)estren-3-one (Enovid-R).[116] The synthetic progestins, like progesterone, can influence only those tissues with the appropriate steroid receptor proteins. The preparations with androgenic properties may cause abnormalities in the genital development of females only if present in sufficient amounts during critical periods of development.[114,115,117] In 1959, Grumbach and coworkers pointed out that labioscrotal fusion could be produced with large doses if the fetuses were exposed before the 13th week of pregnancy, whereas clitoromegaly could be produced after this period, illustrating that a specific form of maldevelopment can be induced only when the susceptible embryonic tissues are in a restricted stage of development.[116]

The World Health Organization reported that there is a suspicion that combined oral contraceptives or progestogens may be weakly teratogenic but that the magnitude of the relative risk is small.[118] In a large retrospective study, Heinonen and associates reported a positive association between cardiovascular defects and in utero exposure to female sex hormones.[110] A revaluation of some of the base data by Wiseman and Dodds-Smith, however, did not support the reported association.[119] Another retrospective study, conducted by Ferencz and colleagues, did not find a positive association between female sex hormone therapy and congenital heart defects.[120] Although neither study disproved the positive association reported by Heinonen and coworkers, their findings made the association less likely.[110]

Epidemiologic studies have reported an association between exposures to female sex hormones, hormone pregnancy tests, oral contraceptives or progestogens, and congenital neural tube defects[121,122] and limb defects.[111,112] Further studies and revaluations have not supported either of these associations.[123–126] Several reviews have discussed the evidence against the involvement of female sex hormones in nongenital teratogenesis.[1,127,128]

Further support for the absence of a nongenital effect of progestins comes from a negative correlation between sex hormone usage during pregnancy and malformations,[129] no increased incidence in malformations following progesterone therapy to maintain pregnancy,[130] and no increased incidence in malformations following first-trimester exposure to progestogens (mostly medroxyprogesterone) administered to pregnant women who had signs of bleeding.[131,132] The Food and Drug Administration has recently recognized that the evidence does not support an increased risk of limb reduction defects, congenital heart disease, or neural tube defects following exposure to oral contraceptives or progestins.[133]

As has been stated, it is generally accepted that the actions of steroid hormones are mediated by specific steroid receptors,[134,135] and therefore only those tissues with the specific receptors can be affected by steroid hormones. It has been shown that 17-alpha-hydroxyprogesterone caproate (Delalutin) does not cause developmental abnormalities in nonreproductive organs of mice.[136]

RADIOACTIVE ISOTOPES

All forms of irradiation are not identical. The effects of external irradiation (discussed later) with x-rays or gamma rays differ from those of radioisotopes. Medically administered radioactive isotopes (or the compound containing the isotope) have a predictable distribution in the embryo determined by several factors that include placental exchange, tissue affinity, and nature of the radiation(s) emitted (alpha particle, beta particle, gamma ray).

In addition to the administered isotope, background radiation contributes to the total exposure. Background radiation has been estimated to contribute less than 100 mrad over the course of pregnancy to the dose absorbed by soft tissue, which presents no increased risk of deleterious effects for the embryo.[137] This is an important concept because many of the exposures from nuclear medicine procedures are within the same order of magnitude as background radiation.

Estimating the absorbed dose and hazard to the fetus is complex because the radioisotope may locate on specific target organs, it may or may not cross the placenta, the distribution of irradiation may not be random, metabolism of the element or compound may be affected by disease or genotype, and the radiation dose rate increases exponentially with time.

Radioactive iodine in the form of ^{131}I is used primarily for uptake studies and radioactive scanning. It may be in the form of the inorganic ion or it may be bound to protein. ^{125}I is used to label hormones for in vivo and in vitro studies. Radioactive iodine is a potential risk to the fetal thyroid, especially once the fetal thyroid begins to concentrate iodide at 10 to 12 weeks of gestation. Inorganic iodides readily cross the placenta, and in time, a substantial amount of bound iodide will be released and become available to the fetus.[138] In all likelihood, there is no compound containing radioisotope of iodide that does not expose the fetus to some radioactivity.

Fetal thyroid avidity for iodides is greater than maternal thyroid avidity.[139] Reported fetal effects from therapeutic (ablative) doses of ^{131}I administered to pregnant women include total fetal thyroid destruction. In a retrospective study of fetuses accidentally exposed to ^{131}I during the first or first and second trimesters, six neonates out of 178 live births had hypothyroidism, although other anomalies were statistically increased above the general population.[140] Although there are few case reports in the literature, there is a definite risk of thyroid dysfunction in the offspring.

The use of radioactive iodine should be avoided during pregnancy unless it is essential for the medical care of the mother and there is no substitute.

Inorganic radioactive potassium, sodium, phosphorus, cesium, thallium, selenium, chromium, iron, and strontium cross the placenta readily. Experiments in animals with radioactive phosphorus and strontium indicate that if the dose is large enough, embryonic abnormality and death can result.[141] These isotopes are used in less than 1% of procedures; only radioactive phosphorus or gold may be used therapeutically (eg, in the treatment of polycythemia or management of malignancies involving peritoneal surfaces). Most new isotopic agents are bound to some complex macromolecule or macroaggregate, cross the placenta in minuscule amounts, and therefore deliver extremely low doses to the embryo.

When radioisotopes are to be used in a woman of childbearing age, the following procedure is recommended:

1. Record the date of the last menstrual period and determine whether the woman could be pregnant.
2. If pregnancy is a possibility, determine the stage of gestation and the estimated dose to the fetus or fetal target organs.
3. Communicate this information to the patient or a responsible member of the family. Record this information, the time and place of the communication, and an informed consent in the patient's record.

For each procedure, the dose to the embryo must be calculated individually and is dependent on the form of the isotope, the site of administration, and the nature of the disease. Estimates of approximate fetal and maternal exposure for standard doses and procedures have been published.[137] In the vast majority of instances a careful analysis will reveal that the exposure is too low to present a significant risk to the embryo.

EXTERNAL IRRADIATION

The classic effects of radiation are cell death or mitotic delay. These effects are due to direct damage to the cell chromatin and are expressed in the offspring as gross malformations, intrauterine growth retardation, or embryonic death, each having a dose–response relationship and a threshold exposure below which no difference between an exposed and a nonexposed control population can be demonstrated.[142] Offspring born to patients receiving radiation therapy for various conditions exhibited growth retardation, eye malformations, and CNS defects.[143–145] Microcephaly is probably the most common manifestation observed following in utero exposure to high levels of radiation in the human.[146] Fetal exposure to radiation at Hiroshima and Nagasaki resulted in microcephaly, growth retardation, and mental retardation.[147–149] In a recent review of radiation teratogenesis, Brent pointed out that no malformation of the limb, viscera, or other tissue has been observed unless the child also exhibits intrauterine growth retardation, microcephaly, or eye malformations.[142] The risk of major anatomical malformations is not increased by in utero exposure of 5 rads or less.[142]

Experimental animal models have shown that radiation-induced effects on the developing organism are the result of the direct action of ionizing radiation on the embryo and are not due to a maternal effect.[142] Prior to implantation, the mammalian embryo is minimally sensitive to the teratogenic and growth-retarding effects of radiation and very sensitive to the lethal effects.[150–152] Organogenesis is a stage sensitive to the teratogenic, growth-retarding, and lethal effects, but the embryo has some recuperative capacity.[150,153–155] Sensitivity to the teratogenic effects of radiation decreased during the fetal stage, but the fetus may still sustain permanent cell depletion, since the recuperative capacity is less.[142] Permanent growth retardation is thus more severe following midgestation radiation.[156,157] Because of its extended periods of organogenesis and histogenesis, the CNS retains the greatest sensitivity of all organ systems to the detrimental effects of radiation through the later fetal stages. The documented effects of prenatal exposure to ionizing radiation, which leads to histopathologic abnormalities of the brain in experimental animals, are cell death and inhibition of cell migration.[158]

RETINOIDS

There are few case reports of congenital defects in humans associated with massive vitamin A ingestion during pregnancy: two have cited urogenital anomalies,[159,160] and one described Goldenhar's syndrome.[161] Historically, vitamin A has played an important role in experimental and clinical teratology. Vitamin A deficiency in swine was the first experimental model of teratogenesis in a mammal.[162–165] Vitamin A congeners—including retinol, retinal, all-*trans*-retinoic acid (tretinoin) and 13-*cis*-retinoic acid (isotretinoin)—are all teratogenic in numerous species (reviewed by Schardein[36]).

Both isotretinoin (Accutane), marketed for treating severe acne, and etretinate (Tegison), marketed for treating psoriasis, contained warnings by the manufacturers against exposure during pregnancy. Unfortunately, exposures occurred. Analyses of the resulting malformations have been reviewed.[166,167] Human malformations include malformations of the central nervous system, cardioaortic malformations, microtia, and clefting defects. Similar defects may result from vitamin A supplements (as retinol–retinyl esters) at high dosage. "Recommendations for Vitamin A Use During Pregnancy" is a position paper published by the Teratology Society reviewing the literature concerning retinoids and birth defects.[168] Supplementation of 8000 IU vitamin A per day should be the maximum during pregnancy, and high dosages (25,000 IU or more) are not recommended.

Experimental evidence[169] suggests that endogenous retinoic acid may act as a natural morphogen. Cellular binding protein–retinoic acid complexes enter the nucleus to affect gene activity, and the resulting regulation of gene transcription influences digit formation. Exogenous retinoids appear to act either directly, to result in cytotoxicity, or via receptor-mediated pathways, to interact with DNA and alter programmed cell death.[170–174]

We are beginning to understand how retinoid metabolism and placental transfer affect the teratogenic potency of various retinoids. In mice, the metabolites of isotretinoin, 4-oxo-isotretinoin and tretinoin, are more efficiently transferred across the placenta than isotretinoin and are more potent teratogens.[182,183] It is likely that different specificities of retinoid-binding proteins[184] account for the variations in placental transfer. Although retinoids can influence many types of cells, Lammer has recently emphasized that neuroectodermally derived cells of the rhomboencephalon are particularly sensitive and that the resulting neural crest cell abnormality differs from that resulting in oculoauriculo-vertebral dysplasia or Goldenhar syndrome.[174] It has been postulated that the susceptibility of specific cell types to the effects of the retinoids is determined by the intracellular concentration of cellular retinoic binding protein.[174]

TETRACYCLINE

The antimicrobial tetracyclines inhibit bacterial protein synthesis by preventing access of aminoacyl transfer RNA (tRNA) to the messenger RNA (mRNA)–ribosome complex.[185]

Tetracycline crosses the placenta but is not concentrated by the fetus. It has been shown to discolor teeth,[186] and very high doses may depress skeletal bone growth and result in hypoplasia of tooth enamel.[187] No congenital malformations of any other organ system have been associated with antenatal tetracycline exposures. Several case reports of limb reduction defects in human embryos exposed to tetracycline are not supported by epidemiologic studies or animal studies. Tetracyclines complex with calcium and the organic matrix of newly forming bone without altering the crystalline structure of hydroxyapatite.[180]

Although stunting has been produced in rats,[181] other experimental animal studies have found either no teratogenic effect[182] or ambiguous effects.[183]

THALIDOMIDE

Lenz and Knapp were the first to describe the thalidomide-induced limb reduction defects and other features of the thalidomide syndrome.[184–186] Limb defects resulted from exposure limited to a 2-week period from the 22nd to the 36th days of gestation: exposures from the 27th to the 30th days most often affected only the arm, whereas exposures from the 30th to the 33rd days resulted in abnormalities of both leg and arm.[185–187] Although there was no association of mental retardation, brain malformations, or cleft palate, other abnormalities included facial hemangioma, microtia, esophageal or duodenal atresia, deafness, and anomalies of the kidneys, heart, and external ears.[184,187,188] A high proportion of the fetuses exposed during the critical period were affected.

McCredie proposed that the segmental pattern of limb reduction defects was determined by the peripheral nerves derived from the neural crest.[189] Stephens and McNulty confirmed that limb development exhibits a segmental pattern.[190] However, recent studies by Strecker and Stephens have refuted the proposed role of peripheral nerve damage in thalidomide-induced embryopathy.[191] A foil barrier was placed lateral to the chick neural tube to block the innervation of the wing field by the brachial plexus. A reduced source of innervation from spinal nerves anterior or posterior to the brachial plexus resulted in muscular atrophy but not in reductions or malformations of the skeleton of the wing. Therefore, the two proposals—that the segmental pattern of the limb is determined by level-specific nerves and that diminished levels of innervation will result in skeletal malformations—are controversial.

Lash and Saxen have postulated that thalidomide indirectly exerts its effects on limb chondrogenesis by acting on the kidney primordia.[192] Based on an association between nephric tissue and limb development[193,194] Lash and Saxen have in vitro evidence suggesting that thalidomide inhibits an interaction between metanephric tissue and associated mesenchymal tissue necessary for normal limb development.[192]

Although the mechanism of teratogenic action for thalidomide is not yet defined, the subject has been critically reviewed by Stephens.[195]

THYROID: IODINE DEFICIENCY, IODIDES, ANTITHYROID DRUGS

Iodine deficiency, reviewed by Warkany,[196] is the primary cause of endemic cretinism. The damage to the embryo is due to iodine deficiency, occurs early in gestation, and results in irreversible neurologic and aural damage with variable severity. Goiter in a female of reproductive age due to endemic iodine deficiency is an indicator for iodine supplementation prior to conception to prevent harmful teratogenic effects.

Several drugs used to treat maternal hyperthyroidism (^{131}I and antithyroid drugs) and nonthyroid conditions (especially iodide-containing compounds for bronchitis and asthma) affect thyroid function. In utero exposure to these drugs may result in congenitally hypothyroid infants who will not reach their potential for physical or mental development unless treated very early after birth with thyroid hormone.

There are several case reports of congenital goiter due to in utero exposures to iodide-containing drugs.[197,198] Maternal intake as low as 12 mg per day may result in fetal goiter.[198] Iodinated diagnostic x-ray contrast agents used for amniofetography have been reported to affect fetal thyroid function adversely.[199]

Propylthiouracil and methimazole, used to treat thyrotoxicosis, readily cross the placenta.[200] Methimazole has been associated with aplasia cutis.[201,202] Propylthiouracil is safer because the incidence of fetal goiter is low,[200,203] and there have been no observed detrimental effects on mental development.[204,205]

VALPROIC ACID

Valproic acid (dipropylacetic acid) is approved for the treatment of absence seizure disorders in the United States, and is used in other countries for the treatment of various types of epilepsy. Valproic acid had been identified as a teratogen in animal studies,[206–210] but Dalens and coworkers were the first to report the association of valproic acid and congenital malformations in the human.[211] Although other reports followed, Robert and colleagues described the associated malformations, consisting primarily of neural tube defects, and their incidence in detail.[212–214] Therapeutic dosages during pregnancy present a teratogenic risk for spina bifida of about 1%,[36] but the risk for facial dysmorphology may be greater.

Valproic acid crosses the human placenta,[215,216] but the fetal serum concentrations are not known. In the rhesus monkey, the fetus is exposed to approximately one half of the free valproic acid concentration present in the maternal plasma.[217] Little is known of its mechanism of action or of the effects of various dosages of valproic acid on human development. A recent review by Lammer and colleagues underscores the importance of birth defect surveillance and the alert physician in identifying human teratogens.[218]

VITAMIN D

Because the vitamins as a group are essential for normal metabolism, it seems unlikely that a severe deficiency would be compatible with reproduction and therefore would result in reproductive loss. There is some evidence, however, for an association between folic acid deficiency and increased frequency of neural tube defects.[124,219] Excess of vitamin D has been associated with increased incidence of congenital malformations. Huge doses of vitamin D administered for rickets prophylaxis resulted in a markedly increased incidence of a syndrome consisting of supravalvular aortic stenosis, elfin facies, and mental retardation in the human.[220,221]

OTHER HUMAN TERATOGENIC AGENTS: ALCOHOL

Table 21-4 lists other human teratogenic agents. Alcohol will be discussed here because of its relatively large social impact. Jones and associates described the fetal alcohol syndrome (FAS) in children with intrauterine growth retardation, microcephaly, mental retardation,

TABLE 21-4. HUMAN ENVIRONMENTAL TERATOGENIC AGENTS

Alcohol	Maternal conditions
Cocaine	Diabetes
Infectious agents	Phenylketonuria
Rubella	Endocrinopathies
Cytomegalovirus	Nutritional deprivation
Herpes simplex	Mechanical problems
Parvovirus B19	Methylmercury
Syphilis	Polychlorinated biphenyls
Toxoplasmosis	Smoking and nicotine
Varicella zoster	
Venezuelan equine encephalitis	

maxillary hypoplasia, flat philtrum, thin upper lip, and reduction in the width of palpebral fissures (cardiac abnormalities also were seen).[222] Many children of alcoholic mothers had FAS, and all the affected children evidenced developmental delay.[223-225]

A period of greatest susceptibility and a dose–response relationship have not yet been established. Although we are reluctant to claim that malformations are due to single exposures to alcohol in the human, binge drinking early in pregnancy has been suggested to be associated with neural tube defects.[226] Actually, the neural tube defects, if real, are a minor risk when compared to the risk of decreased brain growth and differentiation that results from high alcohol consumption during the second and third trimester. Chronic consumption of 6 ounces of alcohol per day constitutes a high risk, whereas FAS is not likely when the mother drinks fewer than two drinks (equivalent to 2 ounces of alcohol) per day.[227] Reduction of alcohol consumption at any time in pregnancy reduces the severity of FAS but may not significantly reduce the risk of some degree of physical or behavioral impairment. The human syndrome is likely to involve the direct effects of ethanol and the indirect effects of genetic susceptibility and poor nutrition. Although alcoholic mothers frequently smoke and consume other drugs, there is little doubt that alcohol ingestion alone can have a disastrous effect on the developing embryo or fetus. It is estimated that at least several hundred children each year are born with the full FAS and probably several thousand children are born with fetal alcohol effects.

SUMMARY

Environmental causes of human malformations account for approximately 10% of malformations, and fewer than 1% of all human malformations are related to prescription drug exposure, chemicals, or radiation. However, malformations caused by drugs and other therapeutic agents are important because these exposures are preventable. As we better understand the mechanisms of teratogenesis from all etiologies we may learn how best to predict and test for teratogenicity.

ACKNOWLEDGMENTS

We thank Mrs. Yvonne G. Edney and Mrs. Margaret D. Rauner for their assistance in the preparation of this manuscript. This work was supported in part by funds from NIH HD07075, NIH HD18167, the Foerderer Foundation, and Harry Bock Charities.

REFERENCES

1. Wilson JG. Environment and birth defects. New York: Academic Press, 1973.
2. Brent RL. Environmental factors: miscellaneous. In: Brent RL, Harris MI, eds. Prevention of embryonic, fetal, and perinatal disease. DHEW Pub (NIH) 76-853. Bethesda, MD, 1976:211.
3. Heinonen OP, Sloane D, Shapiro S. Birth defects and drugs in pregnancy. Littleton, MA: Publishing Sciences Group, 1977.
4. Carter CO. Genetics of common single malformations. Br Med Bull 1976;32:21.
5. McLaughlin JA. Prenatal exposure to diethylstilbestrol in mice: toxicological studies. J Toxicol Environ Health 1977;2:527.
6. Fraser FC. The multifactorial/threshold concept-uses and misuses. Teratology 1976;14:267.
7. Brent RL. Drug testing in animals for teratogenic effects: thalidomide in the pregnant rat. J Pediatr 1964;64:762.
8. Hertig AT. The overall problem in man. In: Benirschke K, ed. Comparative aspects of reproductive failure. Berlin: Springer-Verlag, 1967:11.
9. Boue J, Boue A, Lazar P. Retrospective and prospective epidemiological studies of 1,500 karyotyped spontaneous abortions. Teratology 1975;12:11.
10. World Health Organization. Spontaneous and induced abortion. World Health Organization Technical Report Series, Number 461, Geneva World Health Organization, 1970.
11. Simpson JL. Genes chromosomes and reproductive failure. Fertil Steril 1980;33:107.
12. Warkany J. Aminopterin and methotrexate: folic acid deficiency. Teratology 1978;17:353.
13. Robert CJ, Lowe CR. Where have all the conceptions gone? Lancet 1975;1:498.
14. McKusick VA. Mendelian inheritance in man: catalogs of autosomal dominant, autosomal recessive, and x-linked phenotypes. 8th ed. Baltimore: Johns Hopkins University Press, 1988.
15. Biddle FG, Fraser FC. Genetics of cortisone-induced cleft palate in the mouse-embryonic and maternal effects. Genetics 1976;84:743.
16. Biddle FG. Use of dose-response relationships to discriminate between the mechanisms of cleft-palate induction by different teratogens: an argument for discussion. Teratology 1978;18:247.
17. Wilson JG. Misinformation about risks of congenital anomalies. In: Maurois M, ed. Prevention of physical and mental congenital defects. Part C: Basic and medical science, education, and future strategies New York: Alan R Liss, 1985:165.
18. Brent RL. Predicting teratogenic and reproductive risks in humans from exposure to various environmental agents using in vitro techniques and in vivo animal studies. Cong Anom (Suppl) 1988;28:S41.
19. Thiersch JB. Therapeutic abortions with a folic acid (4-amino PGA). Am J Obstet Gynecol 1952;63:1298.

20. Goetsch C. An evaluation of aminopterin as an abortifacient. Am J Obstet Gynecol 1962;83:1474.
21. Meltzer HJ. Congenital anomalies due to attempted abortion with 4-aminopteroglutamic acid. JAMA 1956;161:1253.
22. Warkany J, Beautry PH, Horstein S. Attempted abortion with aminopterin (4-aminopteroylglutamic acid). Am J Dis Child 1959;97:274.
23. Shapiro S, Slone D, Hartz SC, Rosenberg L, Siskind V, Monson RR, et al. Anticonvulsants and parental epilepsy in the development of birth defects. Lancet 1976;1:272.
24. Skipper HT, Schabel FM Jr. Quantitative and cytokinetic studies in experimental tumor models. In: Holland JF, Frei E III, eds. Cancer medicine. Philadelphia: Lea & Febiger, 1973:629.
25. Dyban AP, Sekirina GG, Golinsky GF. The effect of aminopterin on the preimplantation rat embryo cultivated in vitro. Ontogenez 1977;82:121.
26. Skalko RG, Gold MP. Teratogenicity of methotrexate in mice. Teratology 1974;9:159.
27. Grumbach MM, Conte FA. Disorders of sex differentiation. In: Williams RH, ed. Textbook of endocrinology. Philadelphia: WB Saunders, 1981:422.
28. Moncrieff A. Nonadrenal female pseudohermaphroditism associated with hormone administration in pregnancy. Lancet 1958;2:267.
29. Hoffman F, Overzier C, Uhde G. Zur frage der hormonalen erzengung fotaler zwittenbildugen beim menschen. Geburtshife Frauerheikd 1955;15:1061.
30. Greene RR, Burrill MW, Ivy AC. Experimental intersexuality: the effect of antenatal androgens on sexual development of female rats. Am J Anat 1939;65:415.
31. Raynaud A. Observations sur le développement normal des ébauches de la glande mammaire des foetus mâles et femelles de souris. Ann Endocrinol 1947;8:349.
32. Bruner JA, Witschi E. Testosterone-induced modifications of sexual development in female hamsters. Am J Anat 1946;79:293.
33. Jost A. Problems of fetal endocrinology: the gonadal and hypophyseal hormones. Rec Prog Horm Res 1953;8:379.
34. Wells LJ, Van Wagenen G. Androgen-induced female pseudo hermaphroditism in the monkey (Macaca mulatta) anatomy of the reproductive organs. Carnegie Institute Contrib Embryol 1954;35:93.
35. Dohler KD, Hancke JL, Srivastava SS, Hofman C, Shryne JE, Gorski RR. Participation of estrogens in female sexual differentiation of the brain: neuroanatomical, neuroendocrine and behavioral evidence. Prog Brain Res 1984;61:99.
36. Schardein JL. Chemically induced birth defects. New York: Marcel Dekker, 1985.
37. Niebyl JR, Blake DA, Freeman JM, Luff RD. Carbamazepine levels in pregnancy and lactation. Obstet Gynecol 1979;53:139.
38. Nakane Y, Okuma T, Takahashi R, Sato Y, Wada T, Sato T, et al. Multi-institutional study on the teratogenicity and fetal toxicity of antiepileptic drugs: a report of a collaborative study group in Japan. Epilepsia 1980;21:663.
39. Nielsen M, Froscher W. Finger- and toenail hypoplasia after carbamazepine monotherapy in late pregnancy. Neuropediatrics 1985;16:167.
40. Hiilesmaa VK, Teramo K, Granstrom ML, Bardy AH. Fetal head growth retardation associated with maternal antiepileptic drugs. Lancet 1981;2:165.
41. Bertollini R, Kallen B, Mastroiacovo P, Robert E. Anticonvulsant drugs in monotherapy: effect on the fetus. Eur J Epidemiol 1987;3:164.
42. Jones KL, Lacro RV, Johnson KA, Adams J. Pattern of malformations in the children of women treated with carbamazepine during pregnancy. New Engl J Med 1989;320:1661.
43. DiSaia PJ. Pregnancy and delivery of a patient with a Starr-Edwards mitral valve prosthesis: report of a case. Obstet Gynecol 1966;29:469.
44. Kerber IJ, Warr OS, Richardson C. Pregnancy in a patient with prosthetic mitral valve. JAMA 1968;203:223.
45. Barr M, Pozanski AK, Schmickel RD. Digital hypoplasia and anticonvulsants during gestation, a teratogenic syndrome. J Pediatr 1974;4:254.
46. Pettiflor JM, Benson R. Congenital malformations associated with the administration of oral anticoagulants during pregnancy. J Pediatr 1975;86:459.
47. Hall JG, Pauli RM, Wilson RM. Maternal and fetal sequelae of anticoagulation during pregnancy. Am J Med 1980;68:122.
48. Barr M, Burdi AR. Warfarin-associated embryopathy in a 17-week abortus. Teratology 1976;14:129.
49. Warkany J. A warfarin embryopathy? Am J Dis Child 1975;129:287.
50. Warkany J. Warfarin embryopathy. Teratology 1976;14:205.
51. Stenflo J, Suttie JW. Vitamin K-dependent formation of gamma-carboxyglutamic acid. Ann Rev Biochem 1977;46:157.
52. Kaplan LC. Congenital Dandy Walker malformation associated with first trimester warfarin: a case report and literature review. Teratology 1985;32:333.
53. Greenberg LH, Tanaka KR. Congenital anomalies probably induced by cyclophosphamide. JAMA 1964;188:423.
54. Toledo TM, Harper RC, Moser RH. Fetal effects during cyclophosphamide and irradiation therapy. Ann Intern Med 1971;74:87.
55. Blatt J, Mulvihill JJ, Ziegler JL, Young RC, Poplack DG. Pregnancy outcome following cancer chemotherapy. Am J Med 1980;69:828.
56. Chaube S, Kury G, Murphy ML. Teratogenic effects of cyclophosphamide (NSC-26271) in the rat. Cancer Chemother Rep 1967;51:363.
57. Singh S. The teratogenicity of cyclophosphamide (Endoran-Asta) in rats. Indian J Med Res 1971;59:1128.
58. Gibson JE, Becker BA. The teratogenicity of cyclophosphamide in mice. Cancer Res 1968;28:475.
59. Fritz H, Hess R. Effects of cyclophosphamide on embryonic development in the rabbit. Agents Actions 1971;2:83.
60. Mirkes PE. Cyclophosphamide teratogenesis: a review. Teratogen Carcinog Mutagen 1985;5:75.
61. Hales BF. Effects of phosphoramide mustard and acrolein, cytotoxic metabolites of cyclophosphamide, on mouse limb development in vitro. Teratology 1989;40:11.
62. Bongiovanni AM, DiGeorge AM, Grumbach MM. Masculinization of the female infant associated with estrogenic therapy alone during gestation: four cases. J Clin Endocrinol Metab 1959;19:1004.
63. Herbst AL, Ulfelder H, Poskanzer DC. Adenocarcinoma of the vagina: association of maternal stilbestrol therapy with tumor appearance in young women. N Engl J Med 1971;284:878.
64. Herbst AL, Kurman RJ, Scully RE, Poskanzer DC. Clear-cell adenocarcinoma of the genital tract in young females. N Engl J Med 1972;287:1259.
65. Greenwald P, Barlow JJ, Nasca PC, Burnett WS. Vaginal cancer after maternal treatment with synthetic estrogens. N Engl J Med 1971;285:390.
66. Herbst AL, Poskanzer DC, Robboy SJ, Friedlander L, Scully RE. Prenatal exposure to stilbestrol: a prospective comparison of exposed female offspring with unexposed controls. N Engl J Med 1975;292:334.
67. Herbst AL, Scully RE, Robboy SJ. Effects of maternal DES ingestion on the female genital tract. Hosp Pract 1975;10:51.

68. Ulfelder H. DES-transplacental teratogen and possibly also carcinogen. Teratology 1976;13:101.
69. O'Brien PC, Noller KL, Robboy SJ, Barnes AB, Kaufman RH, Tilley BC, Townsend DE. Vaginal epithelial changes in young women enrolled in the National Cooperation Diethylstilbestrol Adenosis (DESAD) Project. Obstet Gynecol 1979;53:300.
70. Barnes AB, Colton T, Gundersen J, Noller KL, Tilley BC, Strama T, et al. Fertility and outcome of pregnancy in women exposed in utero to diethylstilbestrol. N Engl J Med 1980;302:609.
71. Berger MJ, Goldstein DP. Impaired reproductive performance in DES-exposed women. Obstet Gynecol 1980;55:25.
72. Veridiano NP, Delk I, Rogers J, Tancer ML. Reproductive performance of DES-exposed female progeny. Obstet Gynecol 1981;58:58.
73. Gill WB, Schumacher GFB, Bibbo M. Structural and functional abnormalities in the sex organs of male offspring of mothers treated with diethylstilbestrol (DES). J Reprod Med 1976;16:147.
74. Leary FJ, Resseguie LJ, Kurland LT, O'Brien PC, Emslander RF, Noller KL. Males exposed to diethylstilbestrol. JAMA 1984;252:2984.
75. Miller RK, Heckmann ME, McKenzie RC. Diethylstilbestrol: placental transfer, metabolism, covalent binding, and fetal distribution in the Wistar rat. J Pharmacol Exp Ther 1982;220:358.
76. Newbold RR, Bullock BC, McLachlan JA. Exposure of diethylstilbestrol during pregnancy permanently alters the ovary and oviduct. Biol Reprod 1983;28:735.
77. Metzler M. The metabolism of diethylstilbestrol. CRC Crit Rev Biochem 1981;10:171.
78. Madl R, Metzler M. Oxidative metabolites of diethylstilbestrol in the fetal Syrian golden hamster. Teratology 1984;30:351.
79. Speidel BD, Meadow SR. Maternal epilepsy and abnormalities of the fetus and newborn. Lancet 1972;2:839.
80. Federick J. Epilepsy and pregnancy: a report from Oxford record linkage study. Br Med J 1973;2:442.
81. Monson RR, Rosenberg L, Hartz SC, Shapiro S, Heinonen OP, Sloane D. Diphenylhydantoin and selected malformations. N Engl J Med 1973;289:1049.
82. Albengres E, Tillement JP. Phenytoin in pregnancy: a review of the reported risks. Biol Res Pregnancy Perinatol 1983;4:71.
83. Hill RM, Veriand WM, Horning MG, McCulley LB, Morgan NF. Infants exposed in utero to antiepileptic drugs. Am J Dis Child 1974;127:645.
84. Hanson JW, Myrianthopoulos NC, Harvey MAS, Smith DW. Risks to the offspring of women treated with hydantoin anticonvulsants, with emphasis on the fetal hydantoin syndrome. J Pediatr 1976;89:662.
85. Hanson JW. Teratogen Update: fetal hydantoin effects. Teratology 1986;33:349.
86. McClain RM, Langhoff L. Teratogenicity of diphenylhydantoin in the New Zealand white rabbit. Teratology 1980;21:371.
87. Elshave J. Cleft palate in the offspring of female mice treated with phenytoin. Lancet 1969;2:1074.
88. Harbinson RD, Becker BA. Relation of dosage and time of administration of diphenylhydantoin to its teratogenic effect in mice. Teratology 1969;2:305.
89. Finnell RH. Phenytoin-induced teratogenesis: a mouse model. Science 1981;211:483.
90. Blake DA, Fallinger C. Embryopathic interaction of phenytoin and trichloropropene oxide in mice. Teratology 1976;13:17A.
91. Martz F, Failinger C, Blake DA. Phenytoin teratogenesis: correlation between embryopathic effect and covalent binding of putative arene oxide metabolite in gestational tissue. J Pharmacol Exp Ther 1977;203:231.
92. Harbinson RD. Proposed mechanism for phenylhydantoin-induced teratogenesis. Pharmacologist 1977;19:179.
93. Spielberg SP, Gordon GB, Blake DA, Mellits ED, Bross DS. Anticonvulsant toxicity in vitro: possible role of arene oxides. J Pharmacol Exp Therap 1981;217:386.
94. Lewis WH, Suris OR. Treatment with lithium carbonate: results in 35 cases. Tex Med 1970;66:58.
95. Vacaflor L, Lehmann HE, Ban TA. Side effects and teratogenicity of lithium carbonate treatment. J Clin Pharmacol 1970;10:387.
96. Frankenberg RR, Lipinski JF. Congenital malformations. N Engl J Med 1983;309:311.
97. Warkany J. Teratogen update: lithium. Teratology 1988;38:593.
98. Rane A, Tomson G, Bjarke B. Effects of maternal lithium therapy in a newborn infant. J Pediatr 1974;93:296.
99. Jurand A. Teratogenic activity of lithium carbonate: an experimental update. Teratology 1988;38:101.
100. Zackai EH, Melman WJ, Neiderer B, Hanson JW. The fetal trimethadione syndrome J Pediatr 1975;87:280.
101. German J, Kowal A, Ehlers KH. Trimethadione and human teratogenesis. Teratology 1970;3:349.
102. Feldman GL, Weaver DD, Lovrien EW. The fetal trimethadione syndrome. Am J Dis Child 1977;131:1389.
103. Goldman AS, Yaffe SJ. Fetal trimethadione syndrome. Teratology 1978;17:103.
104. Brown NA, Schull G, Fabro S. Assessment of the teratogenic potential of trimethadione in the CD-1 mouse. Toxicol Appl Pharmacol 1979;51:59.
105. Mjolnerod OK, Rasmussen K, Dommerud SA, Gjeruldsen ST. Congenital connective-tissue defect probably due to penicillamine treatment in pregnancy. Lancet 1971;1:673.
106. Endres W. D-penicillamine in pregnancy—to ban or not to ban. Klin Wochenschr 1981;59:535.
107. Steffek AJ, Verrusio AC, Watkins CA. Cleft palate in rodents after maternal treatment with various lathrogenic agents. Teratology 1972;5:33.
108. Mark-Savage P, Keen CL, Lonnerdal B, Hurley LS. Teratogenicity of D-penicillamine in rats. Teratology 1981;23:50A.
109. Keen CL, Mark-Savage P, Lonnerdal B, Hurley LS. Teratogenesic and low copper status resulting from D-penicillamine in rats. Teratology 1982;26:163.
110. Heinonen OP, Sloane D, Monson RR, Hook EB, Shapiro S. Cardiovascular birth defects and antenatal exposure to female sex hormones. N Engl J Med 1977;296:67.
111. Janerich DT, Piper JM, Glebatis DM. Oral contraceptives and congenital limb-reduction defects. N Engl J Med 1974;291:697.
112. Janerich DT, Dugan JM, Standfast SJ, Strite L. Congenital heart disease and prenatal exposure to exogenous sex hormones. Br Med J 1977;1:1058.
113. Fotherby K. A new look at progestins. Clin Obstet Gynecol 1984;11:701.
114. Wilkins L, Jones HW, Holman GH, Stempfel RS. Masculinization of the female fetus associated with administration of oral and intramuscular progestins during gestation: nonadrenal female pseudohermaphroditism. J Clin Endocrinol Metab 1958;18:559.
115. Wilkins L. Masculinization due to orally given progestins. JAMA 1960;172:1028.
116. Grumbach MM, Ducharine JR, Moloshok RE. On the fetal masculinizing action of certain oral progestins. J Clin Endocrinol Metab 1959;19:1369.
117. Van Wyk J, Grumbach MM. Disorders of sex differentiation. In: Williams RH, ed. Textbook of endocrinology. Philadelphia: WB Saunders, 1968:537.
118. World Health Organization. The effect of female sex hormones

on fetal development and infant health World Health Organization, Technical Report Series, Number 657, Geneva World Health Organization, 1981:2.
119. Wiseman RA, Dodds-Smith IC. Cardiovascular birth defects and antenatal exposure to female sex hormones: a reevaluation of some base data. Teratology 1984;30:359.
120. Ferencz C, Matanoski GM, Wilson PD, Rubin JD, Neill CA, Gutberlet R. Maternal hormone therapy and congenital heart disease. Teratology 1980;21:225.
121. Gal I, Kirman B, Stern J. Hormonal pregnancy tests and congenital malformation. Nature 1967;216:83.
122. Gal I. Risks and benefits of the use of hormonal pregnancy test tablets. Nature 1972;240:241.
123. Laurence M, Miller M, Vowles M, Evans K, Carter C. Hormonal pregnancy tests and neural tube malformations. Nature 1971;233:495.
124. Laurence KM, James N, Miller MH, Tennant GB, Campbell H. Double-blind randomized controlled trial of folate treatment before conception to prevent recurrence of neural tube defects. Br Med J 1981;282:1509.
125. Laurence KM. Reply to Gal. Nature 1972;240:242.
126. Sever LE. Hormonal pregnancy tests and spina bifida. Nature 1973;242:410.
127. Briggs MH, Briggs M. Sex hormone exposure during pregnancy and malformations. In: Briggs MH, Corbin A, eds. Advances in steroid biochemistry and pharmacology. Vol 7. London: Academic Press, 1979:51.
128. Wilson JG, Brent RL. Are female sex hormones teratogenic? Am J Obstet Gynecol 1981;114:567.
129. Wiseman RA. Negative correlation between sex hormone usage and malformations. In: Maurois M, ed. Prevention of physical and mental congenital defects. Part C: Basic and medical science, education, and future strategies. New York: Alan R Liss, 1985:171.
130. Rock JA, Wentz AC, Cole KA, Kimball AW Jr, Zacur HA, Early SA, Jones GS. Fetal malformations following progesterone therapy during pregnancy: a preliminary report. Fertil Steril 1985;44:17.
131. Katz K, Lancet M, Skornick J, Chemke J, Mogilner BM, Klingberg M. Teratogenicity of progestogens given during the first trimester of pregnancy. Obstet Gynecol 1985;65:775.
132. Yovich JL, Turner SR, Draper R. Medroxyprogesterone acetate therapy in early pregnancy has no apparent fetal effects. Teratology 1988;38:135.
133. Brent RL. Editorial comment: Kudos to the Food and Drug Administration: reversal of the package insert warning for birth defects for oral contraceptives. Teratology 1989;39:93.
134. King RJB, Mainwaring WIP. Steroid-cell interactions. Baltimore: University Park Press, 1974:1.
135. O'Malley BW, Schrader DT. The receptors of steroid hormones. Sci Am 1976;234:32.
136. Seegmiller RE, Nelson BW, Johnson CK. Evaluation of the teratogenic potential of Delautin (17a-hydroxyprogesterone caproate) in mice. Teratology 1983;28:201.
137. Brent RL, Beckman DA, Jensh RP. The relationship of animal experiments in predicting the effects of intrauterine effects in the human. In: Kriegel H, Schmahl W, Gerber GB, Stieve FE, eds. Radiation risks to the developing nervous system. New York: Gustav Fisher, 1986:367.
138. Speert H, Quimby EH, Werner SC. Radioiodine uptake by the fetal mouse thyroid and resultant effects in later life. Surg Gynecol Obstet 1951;93:230.
139. Book S, Goldman M. Thyroidal adioiodine exposure of the fetus. Health Phys 1975;29:874.
140. Stoffer SS, Hamber JI. Inadvertent 131I therapy for hyperthyroidism in the first trimester of pregnancy. J Nucl Med 1976;17:146.
141. Sikov MR, Noonan TR. Anomalous development induced in embryonic rat by the maternal administration of radiophosphorus. Am J Anat 1958;103:137.
142. Brent RL. Radiation teratogenesis. Teratology 1980;21:281.
143. Goldstein L, Murphy DP. Microcephalic idiocy following radium therapy for uterine cancer during pregnancy. Am J Obstet Gynecol 1929;18:189.
144. Murphy DP, Goldstein L. Micromelia in a child irradiated in utero. Surg Gynecol Obstet 1930;50:79.
145. Dekaban AS. Abnormalities in children exposed to x-radiation during various stages of gestation: tentative timetable of radiation injury to the human fetus. J Nucl Med 1968;9:471.
146. Miller RW, Mulvihill JJ. Small head size after atomic irradiation. Teratology 1976;14:355.
147. Miller RW. Delayed radiation effects in atomic bomb survivors. Science 1969;166:569.
148. Wood JW, Johnson KG, Omori Y. In utero exposure to the Hiroshima atomic bomb. An evaluation of head size and mental retardation: twenty years later Pediatrics 1967;39:385.
149. Wood JW, Johnson KG, Omori Y, Kawamoto S, Keehn RJ. Mental retardation in children exposed in utero to the atomic bombs in Hiroshima and Nagasaki. Am J Public Health 1967;57:1381.
150. Russell LB. X-ray-induced developmental abnormalities in the mouse and their use in the analysis of embryological patterns. I. External and gross visceral changes. J Exp Zool 1950;114:545.
151. Russell LB, Russell WL. The effects of radiation on the preimplantation stages of the mouse embryo. Anat Res 1950;108:521.
152. Brent RL, Bolden BT. The indirect effect of irradiation on embryonic development. IV. The lethal effects of maternal irradiation on the first day of gestation in the rat. Proc Soc Exp Biol Med 1967;125:709.
153. Russell LB. X-ray-induced developmental abnormalities in the mouse and their use in the analysis of embryological patterns. II. Abnormalities of the vertebral column and thorax. J Exp Zool 1956;131:329.
154. Russell LB, Russell WL. An analysis of the changing radiation response of the developing mouse embryo. J Cell Comp Physiol 1954;43:103.
155. Brent RL, Bolden BT. The indirect effect of irradiation on embryonic development. III. The contribution of ovarian irradiation, uterine irradiation, oviduct irradiation, and zygote irradiation of fetal mortality and growth retardation in the rat. Radiat Res 1967;30:759.
156. Jensh RP, Brent RL. Effects of prenatal X-irradiation on the 14th–18th days of gestation on postnatal growth and development in the rat. Teratology 1988;38:431.
157. Jensh RP, Brent RL. Effects of prenatal X-irradiation on postnatal testicular development and function in the Wistar Rat: development/teratology/behavior/radiation. Teratology 1988; 38:443.
158. Ferrer I, Xumetra A, Santamaria J. Cerebral malformation induced by prenatal x-irradiation: an autoradiographic and Golgi study. J Anat 1984;138:81.
159. Bernhardt IB, Dorsey DJ. Hypervitaminosis A and congenital renal anomalies in a human infant. Obstet Gynecol 1974;43:750.
160. Fantel AG, Shepard TH, Newell-Morris LL, Moffett BC. Teratogenic effects of retinoic acid in pigtail monkeys (Macaca nemistrinal). Teratology 1977;15:65.
161. Mounoud RL, Klein D, Weber F. A propos d'un cas de syndrome de Goldenhar intoxication aigue à la vitamine A chez la mère pendant la grossesse. J Genet Hum 1975;23:135.
162. Zilva SS, Golding J, Drummond JC, Coward KH. The relation of

the fat-soluble factor to rickets and growth in pigs. Biochem J 1921;15:427.

163. Hale F. Pigs born without eyeballs. J Hered 1933;24:105.

164. Hale F. Relation of vitamin A to anophthalmos in pigs. Am J Ophthalmol 1935;18:1087.

165. Hale F. Relation of maternal vitamin A deficiency to microphthalmia in pigs. Tex State J Med 1937;33:228.

166. Rosa FW, Wilk AL, Kelsey FO. Teratogen update: vitamin A congeners. Teratology 1986;33:355.

167. Lammer EJ. Developmental toxicity of synthetic retinoids in humans. Prog Clin Biol Res 1988;281:193.

168. Teratology Society. Teratology Society position paper: recommendations for vitamin A use during pregnancy. Teratology 1987;35:269.

169. Thaller C, Eichele G. Identification and spatial distribution of retinoids in the developing chick limb bud Nature 1987;327:625.

170. Kay ED. Craniofacial dysmorphogenesis following hypervitaminosis A in mice. Teratology 1987;35:105.

171. Sulik KK, Johnson MC, Dehart DB. Potentiation of programmed cell death by 13-cis retinoic acid: a common mechanism for early craniofacial and limb malformations? Teratology 1987;35:32A.

172. Yasuda Y, Konishi H, Kihara T, Tanimura T. Developmental anomalies induced by all-trans-retinoic acid in fetal mice. II. Induction of abnormal neuroepithelium. Teratology 1987; 35:355.

173. Sulik KK, Dehart DB. Retinoic-acid-induced limb malformations resulting from apical ectodermal ridge cell death. Teratology 1988;37:527.

174. Alles AJ, Sulik KK. Retinoic-acid-induced limb-reduction defects: perturbation of zones of programmed cell death as a pathogenetic mechanism. Teratology 1989;40:163.

175. Creech-Kraft J, Kochhar DM, Scott WJ, Nau H. Low teratogenicity of 13-cis-retinoic acid (isotretinoin) in the mouse corresponds to low embryonic concentrations during embryogenesis: comparisons to the all-trans isomer. Toxicol Appl Pharmacol 1987;87:474.

176. Kochhar DM, Penner JD. Developmental effects of isotretinoin and 4-oxo-isotretinoin: the role of metabolism in teratogenicity. Teratology 1987;36:67.

177. Ong DE, Chytil F. Changes in levels of cellular retinol- and retinoic-acid-binding proteins of liver and lung during perinatal development of rat. Proc Natl Acad Sci USA 1976;73:3976.

178. Weisblum B, Davies J. Antibiotic inhibitors of the bacterial ribosome. Bacteriol Rev 1968;32:493.

179. Baden E. Environmental pathology of the teeth. In: Gorlin RJ, Goldman HM, eds. Thomas' oral pathology. 6th ed. St Louis: CV Mosby, 1970:189.

180. Cohlan SQ, Bevelander G, Tiamsic T. Growth inhibition of prematures receiving tetracycline: clinical and laboratory investigation. Am J Dis Child 1963;105:453.

181. Bevelander G, Cohlan SW. The effect of the rat fetus of transplacentally acquired tetracycline. Biol Neonate 1962;4:365.

182. Hurley LS, Tuchmann-Duplessis H. Influence de la tétracycline sur le développement pré- et post-natal du rat. CR Acad Sci (Paris) 1963;257:302.

183. Fillippi B. Antibiotics and congenital malformations: evaluation of the teratogenicity of antibiotics. In: Woollam DHM, ed. Advances in teratology. Vol 2. New York: Academic Press, 1967:237.

184. Lenz W, Knapp K. Thalidomide embryopathy. Arch Environ Health 1962;5:100.

185. Lenz W. Thalidomide embryopathy in Germany 1959. In: Maurois M, ed. Prevention of physical and mental congenital defects. Part C: Basic and medical science, education, and future strategies. New York: Alan R Liss, 1985:77.

186. Lenz W. A short history of thalidomide embryopathy. Teratology 1988;38:203.

187. Brent RL, Holmes LB. Clinical and basic science lessons from the thalidomide tragedy: what have we learned about the causes of limb defects? Teratology 1988;38:241.

188. Knapp K, Lenz W, Nowack E. Multiple congenital abnormalities. Lancet 1962;2:725.

189. McCredie J. Sclerotome subtraction: a radiologic interpretation of reduction deformities of the limbs. In: Bergsman D, Lowry RB, eds. Birth defects: original article series. Vol 13. No 3D. New York: Alan R Liss, 1977:65.

190. Stephens TD, McNulty TR. Evidence for a metameric pattern in the development of the chick humerus. J Embryol Exp Morphol 1981;61:191.

191. Strecker TR, Stephens TD. Peripheral nerves do not play a trophic role in limb skeletal morphogenesis. Teratology 1983;27:159.

192. Lash JW, Saxen L. Human teratogenesis: in vitro studies on thalidomide-inhibited chondrogenesis. Dev Biol 1972;28:61.

193. Lash JW. Studies on the ability of embryonic mesonephros explants to form cartilage. Develop Biol 1963;6:219.

194. Lash JW. Normal embryology and teratogenesis. Am J Obstet Gynecol 1964;90:1193.

195. Stephens TD. Proposed mechanisms of action in thalidomide embryopathy. Teratology 1988;38:229-239.

196. Warkany J. Teratogen update: iodine deficiency. Teratology 1985;31:309.

197. Martin MM, Rento RD. Iodide goiter with hypothyroidism in 2 newborn infants. J Pediatr 1962;61:94.

198. Carswell F, Kerr MM, Hutchison JH. Congenital goiter and hypothyroidism produced by maternal ingestion of iodides. Lancet 1970;1:1241.

199. Rodesch F, Camus M, Ermans AM, Dodion J, Delange F. Adverse effect of amniofetography on fetal thyroid function. Am J Obstet Gynecol 1976;126:723.

200. Cheron RG, Kaplan MM, Lasen PR, Selenkow HA, Crigler JF Jr. Neonatal thyroid function after propylthiouracil therapy for maternal Graves' disease. N Engl J Med 1981;304:525.

201. Milham S Jr, Elledge W. Maternal methimazole and congenital defects in children. Teratology 1972;5:125.

202. Mujtaba Q, Burrow GM. Treatment of hyperthyrodism in pregnancy with propylthiouracil and methimazole. Obstet Gynecol 1975;46:282.

203. Burrow GN. Neonatal goiter after maternal propylthiouracil therapy. J Clin Endocrinol 1965;25:403.

204. McCarroll AM, McCarroll AM, Hutchinson M, McAuley R, Montgomery DAD. Long-term assessment of children exposed in utero to carbimazole. Arch Dis Child 1976;51:532.

205. Burrow GN, Klatski EH, Genel M. Intellectual development in children whose mothers received propylthiouracil during pregnancy. Yale J Biol Med 1978;41:151.

206. Whittle BA. Pre-clinical teratological studies on sodium valproate (Epilim) and other anticonvulsants. In: Legg NJ, ed. Clinical and pharmacological aspects of sodium valproate (Epilim) in the treatment of epilepsy. Tunbridge Wells, England: MCS Consultants, 1976:105.

207. Kao J, Brown NA, Schmid B, Goulding WH, Fabro S. Teratogenicity of valproic acid: in vivo and in vitro investigations. Teratogen Carcinogen Mutagen 1981;1:367.

208. Bruckner A, Lee YJ, O'Shea KS, Henneberry RC. Teratogenic effects of valproic acid and diphenylhydantoin on mouse embryos in culture. Teratology 1983;27:29.

209. Nau H, Spielmann H. Embryotoxicity testing of valproic acid. Lancet 1983;1:763.
210. Loscher W ,Nau H, Marescaux C, Vergnes M. Comparative evaluation of anticonvulsant and toxic potencies of valproic acid and 2-envalproic acid in different animal models of epilepsy. Eur J Pharmacol 1984;99:211.
211. Dalens B, Raynaud E-J, Gaulme J. Teratogenicity of valproic acid. J Pediatr 1980;97:332.
212. Robert E. Valproic acid and spina bifida: a preliminary report—France. MMWR 1982;31:515.
213. Robert E, Guibaud P. Maternal valproic acid and congenital neural tube defects. Lancet 1982;2:1142.
214. Robert E, Rosa F. Valproate and birth defects. Lancet 1983;2:1142.
215. Dickinson RG, Hapland RC, Lynn RK, Smith WB, Gerber N. Transmission of valproic acid across the placenta: half-lives of the drug in mother and baby. J Pediatr 1979;94:832.
216. Nau H, Zierer R, Spielmann H, Neubert D, Gansau C. A new model for embryotoxicity testing: teratogenicity and pharmacokinetics of valproic acid following constant-rate administration in the mouse using human therapeutic drug and metabolite concentrations. Life Sci 1981;29:2803.
217. Hendrickx AG, Nau H, Binkerd P, Rowland JM, Rowland JR, Cukierski MJ, Cukierski MA. Valproic acid developmental toxicity and pharmacokinetics in the Rhesus monkey: an interspecies comparison. Teratology 1988;38:329.
218. Lammer EJ, Sever LE, Oakley GP Jr. Valproic acid. Teratology 1987;35:465.
219. Smithells RW. Neural tube defects: prevention by vitamin supplements. Pediatrics 1982;69:498.
220. Garcia RE, Friedman WF, Kaback MM, Rowe RD. Idiopathic hypercalcemia and supravalvular stenosis: documentation of a new syndrome. N Engl J Med 1964;271:117.
221. Friedman WF. Vitamin D and the supravalvular aortic stenosis syndrome. In: Woollam DHM, ed. Advances in teratology. Vol 3. New York: Academic Press, 1968:83.
222. Jones KL, Smith DW, Ulleland CN, Streissguth AP. Pattern of malformation in offspring of chronic alcoholic mothers. Lancet 1973;1:1267.
223. Jones KL, Smith DW. Recognition of the fetal alcohol syndrome in early infancy. Lancet 1973;2:99.
224. Jones KL, Smith DW. The fetal alcohol syndrome. Teratology 1975;12:1.
225. Jones KL, Smith DW, Streissguth AP, Myrianthopoulous NC. Outcome in offspring of chronic alcoholic women. Lancet 1974;1:1076.
226. Graham JM Jr. The effects of alcohol consumption during pregnancy. In: Marois M, ed. Prevention of physical and mental congenital defects. Part C: Basic and medical science, education, and future strategies. New York: Alan R Liss, 1985:335.
227. Streissguth AP, Landesman-Dwyer C, Martin JC, Smith DW. Teratogenic effects of alcohol in humans and laboratory animals. Science 1980;209:353.

22
CHAPTER

NONPRESCRIPTION DRUGS AND ALCOHOL: ABUSE AND EFFECTS IN PREGNANCY

Donald R. Coustan

In modern American society the use of "recreational" drugs and alcohol has reached epidemic proportions, reaching pervasively into every socioeconomic class and becoming so important that presidential campaigns have seized on the drug problem as a major political issue. It is not the intent of the author of this chapter to describe the vast societal, legal, economic, and moral consequences of the use of illicit drugs. Rather, this chapter will be limited to a discussion of the effect of such chemicals on the mother and her fetus.

ALCOHOL

Ethyl alcohol, or ethanol, is a social drug that apparently offers no benefit to the pregnant woman or her fetus. The Old Testament carries the admonition "Behold, thou shalt conceive, and bear a son; and now drink no wine or strong drink. . ."(Judges 13:7).[1]

FETAL ALCOHOL SYNDROME

Effects of maternally ingested alcohol on the unborn fetus may have been recognized by the middle of the 18th century, when the artist William Hogarth created "Gin Lane," an engraving that depicted a British street scene during the "gin mania," when gin was available at very low prices, and untaxed, in order to create a market for overproduced grains. A central figure in this engraving is a small child with short palpebral fissures; this may have been an observation of the prenatal effects of alcohol on the child.[2] It was in 1973 that the term *fetal alcohol syndrome* (FAS) was coined by Jones and coworkers, who observed 11 children of alcoholic mothers with characteristic features (Table 22-1).[3,4] In 1980, specific criteria for FAS were proposed by the Fetal Alcohol Study Group of the Research Society on Alcoholism, requiring that at least one feature from each of three categories be present for the diagnosis to be made[5]:

1. Growth retardation before or after birth.
2. A pattern of abnormal features of the face and head (including small head circumference and small eyes) or evidence of retarded formation of the midfacial area (including a flattened bridge and short length of the nose, and flattening of the vertical groove between the nose and mouth—that is, the philtrum).
3. Evidence of central nervous system abnormality (eg, abnormal neonatal behavior, mental retardation, or other evidence of abnormal neurobehavioral development).

In general, it should be possible to diagnose FAS without any knowledge of the mother's drinking history, since the facial abnormalities are so characteristic. The intrauterine growth retardation may also be expressed as failure to thrive during childhood. The original FAS children were followed for 10 years, and their growth deficiency and mental handicaps persisted. Females were found to be obese at the time of menarche, whereas males were thin at the time of puberty.[6]

ALCOHOL-RELATED BIRTH DEFECTS

Other abnormalities associated with alcohol exposure in utero have subsequently been described, including ophthalmologic anomalies, otic anomalies, cardiac sep-

TABLE 22-1. ALCOHOL AND THE FETUS

Fetal alcohol syndrome: At least one from each of the following categories:
Growth retardation
Craniofacial abnormalities
Central nervous system abnormalities
Alcohol-related birth effects: Any of the preceding problems in the offspring of an alcoholic individual

tal defects, hemangiomas, undescended testes, hernias, unusual fingerprint patterns, and palmar creases. The presence of any of these abnormalities in the offspring of an alcohol-using mother raises the question of a causal relationship. Because these abnormalities also occur in children who were not exposed to alcohol in utero, they can only be ascribed to maternal drinking when seen with the characteristic features of FAS. Another category of problems, "alcohol-related birth effects" (ARBE), consists of pregnancy complications and adverse outcomes that can be attributed to maternal alcohol use in the epidemiologic sense when potentially confounding variables have been controlled for.[7] The birth of a small-for-dates baby to an alcoholic mother is an example of such an ARBE.

PREVALENCE

Researchers have had considerable difficulty in estimating the prevalence of FAS, and particularly in constructing a dose–response curve for levels of alcohol exposure necessary to produce this problem, primarily because it is virtually impossible to quantitate alcohol intake in alcoholic persons. The amount of alcohol used is invariably underestimated. In addition, specific features of the FAS may be brought about by exposure to alcohol at different times of gestation. For example, craniofacial anomalies may occur during embryogenesis, whereas disorders of central nervous system function may be brought about later in gestation, and growth disturbances may reflect alcohol exposure over a broad range of gestational ages. Given these limitations, a general picture has emerged.

The amount of alcohol consumed is expressed in terms of absolute alcohol, since different alcoholic beverages contain different percentages. Beer contains approximately 5% alcohol; wine, 12%; fortified wines (sherry, port, muscatel), 20%; and "hard liquor," 40% to 50%. The alcohol concentration of hard liquor is doubled to arrive at the "proof"; thus, 80 proof vodka is 40% alcohol.[8] Conveniently, the usual unit of alcohol consumption contains approximately the same amount of absolute alcohol, no matter what the type of drink. Thus, a 12-ounce can of beer, a 4-ounce glass of table wine, and a shot of 100 proof whiskey each contain 15 mL, or approximately 0.5 ounce, of absolute alcohol.

The prevalence of FAS among the offspring of "heavy drinkers" (variously defined) ranges from 2.5% to 10% in prospective studies.[9] Although it is difficult to obtain more specific data, it is clear that all cases of full-blown FAS have been reported in chronic alcoholic mothers who drank "heavily" throughout pregnancy. Ernhart and colleagues performed a prospective observational study of 359 pregnancies, in which they demonstrated the existence of a dose–response curve for craniofacial abnormalities as a function of alcohol intake during the embryonic period, with a very clear excess of anomalies among the offspring of those mothers who were believed to have ingested more than 3 ounces of absolute alcohol (six drinks) per day.[10] Drinking behavior during the embryonic period was estimated rather than observed.

The effect of the chronic ingestion of less than 3 ounces of absolute alcohol per day has also been investigated. Rosett and coworkers noted a 32% incidence of intrauterine growth retardation (IUGR) (<10th percentile) among the offspring of "heavy" drinkers (average 154 mL, or 5 ounces, absolute alcohol per day), compared with 3% in "rare" drinkers.[11] There was no apparent excess of IUGR among "moderate" drinkers, or "heavy" drinkers who reduced their intake before the third trimester. Little found that the ingestion of an average of 1 ounce of absolute alcohol per day in late pregnancy was associated with an average decrease in birth weight of 160 g.[12] In a large prospective study of 31,604 pregnancies, Mills and associates demonstrated a dose–response curve, with the proportion of newborns under 2500 g being 4% in nondrinkers and those who drank less than one drink per day, doubling among those drinking one or two drinks per day, reaching 11% at three to five drinks per day, and 13.5% in those drinking six or more drinks per day.[13] This difference persisted even when corrections were made for potential confounding variables, such as smoking, maternal age, hypertension, and so on.

Spontaneous abortion has also been reported to occur with increased frequency among mothers who drink alcohol. In a case-control study of 616 spontaneous abortions and 632 deliveries at or beyond 28 weeks, Kline and colleagues found that women who experienced an abortion were twice as likely to report drinking two or more times per week.[14] Neurobehavioral abnormalities in infancy have also been associated with exposure to alcohol in utero, even in children without fetal alcohol syndrome.[7]

Before the advent of other tocolytic agents, intravenous alcohol was the drug of choice for stopping preterm labor. There have been only a few studies in which the offspring exposed to brief but high doses of ethanol in utero have been followed up. Although no significant adverse physical or neurobehavioral outcomes were reported,[15] one study noted that the subset of infants who were born within 15 hours of discontinuance of ethanol infusion had worse developmental test scores than controls at 4–7 years of age.[16] However, since only seven children were in this group, it is not possible to draw firm conclusions.

PATHOPHYSIOLOGY

The pathophysiologic mechanism for the adverse effects of alcohol on the developing fetus is poorly understood. Ethanol levels in maternal and fetal blood are identical in the sheep, and studies in sheep have shown that there is a time lag before the appearance of this substance in the amniotic fluid.[17] A similar time lag has been found in the appearance of ethanol in amniotic fluid in human pregnancies.[18] It has been suggested that amniotic fluid may function as a reservoir, exposing the fetus to ethanol long after the mother has cleared it from her system. Acetaldehyde, which is a potentially toxic metabolic product of ethanol, behaves similarly with respect to the amniotic fluid. Either alcohol itself, acetaldehyde, or both bear responsibility for the disruption of fetal growth and development. Alcohol is metabolized via a number of different systems, including alcohol dehydrogenase in the cytosol fraction of the liver, the hepatic microsomal ethanol-oxidizing system, and the peroxisomal–catalase system. There are genetic differences in some of these enzymes, and different individuals may induce such enzymes at different rates when exposed to the same concentrations of ethanol. Differential enzyme induction may lead to differential susceptibility to cell injury or disruption by other agents.[19] Alternatively, ethanol or acetaldehyde may interfere with placental transport of vital nutrients such as amino acids, leading to a form of "fetal malnutrition."[20]

The ingestion of alcohol by the mother has been shown to decrease fetal breathing movements, while not changing gross body movements or the fetal heart rate.[21] Alcohol withdrawal effects have been described, even in infants without the stigmata of fetal alcohol syndrome.[22] The fetal effects of alcohol, although poorly characterized, appear to be multifactorial.

MANAGEMENT

There is no treatment or "cure" for fetal alcohol syndrome or alcohol-related birth effects. Therefore, the only possible strategy at the present time is prevention. The first component of prevention is education, so that women of childbearing age are aware of the risks of drinking during pregnancy. Education campaigns have been carried out in this country at the federal, state, and local levels, as well as by private charitable institutions. In an epidemiologic study in Seattle the proportion of gravidas reporting any alcohol use in early pregnancy fell from 81% in 1974–1975 to 42% in 1980–1981.[23] Although the prevalence of "heavy" drinking (defined in this study as 1 ounce or more of absolute alcohol per day) prior to the discovery of pregnancy was unchanged at 6% to 7% during each time period, such use after pregnancy was discovered fell from 2.3% to 0.8% of women. In a population-based study in Finland during 1983–1985, 55% of women drank at least 2 ounces of absolute alcohol during the week in which conception occurred, and only 16% were totally abstinent during the first trimester.[24] By 32 weeks, 50% were totally abstinent, and by term, 80% took no alcohol at all. The remaining 20% continued some alcohol intake throughout gestation.

To prevent fetal alcohol syndrome, it is first necessary to identify mothers at risk (ie, those who are alcoholic). It is clear that we tend to "gloss over" alcohol intake when we take a history, perhaps out of a subconscious desire not to insult our patients or make them uncomfortable. A number of approaches have been developed to taking an alcohol history, including the "Ten Question Drinking History" (TQDH) and the Michigan Alcohol Screening Test (MAST), which are standardized lists of questions to be asked.[25,26] Perhaps the simplest and easiest to use is the CAGE approach, in which four basic questions are asked[27]:

Have you ever
- Felt the need to *C*ut down drinking?
- Felt *A*nnoyed by criticism of your drinking?
- Had *G*uilty feelings about drinking?
- Taken a morning *E*ye-opener?

Depending on the study cited, either two or three positive answers (out of four) are highly suggestive of alcoholism. It is appropriate to administer the CAGE questions, or some other instrument for diagnosing alcoholism, to every patient at the time of obtaining a history.

Currently, investigations focusing on detection of alcoholism and possible risk for FAS, using biochemical markers such as gamma-glutamyl transferase and mean red cell volume measurements, are being carried out in some centers. Results to date have been mixed.[28,29]

Having identified the individual with a problem of alcohol intake, who is at increased risk for having a child with FAS, attention should next be turned to intervention. Rosett and coworkers found that 67% of 49 pregnant problem drinkers reduced their alcohol intake when enrolled in a counseling program.[30] They have demonstrated that cessation of heavy alcohol intake before the third trimester can benefit the fetus.[11] Similar results have been reported by Halmesmaki in Finland.[31]

The use of disulfiram to increase the motivation of alcoholics to avoid consumption of alcohol is generally considered contraindicated in pregnancy.[32] A suspected but not proven teratogen, disulfiram, when taken in combination with alcohol, leads to very high circulating acetaldehyde concentrations.

Because alcohol has no known therapeutic value for either mother or fetus and because no threshold for adverse effects has been convincingly demonstrated, pregnant women should be advised to avoid alcohol altogether. However, this advice certainly should not be construed as suggesting interruption of pregnancy when a history of alcohol consumption has been elicited; the risks of low-level alcohol consumption, or even occasional binges of marked consumption, have not been demonstrated to date.

COCAINE

PHARMACOLOGY

Until recently cocaine was perceived by many as a benign, nonaddictive agent whose recreational use was harmless. This belief was, in all likelihood, based on a lack of data. In the years between 1985 and 1990 cocaine use increased to the point where some experts believe that it represents our most significant societal problem. Along with this skyrocketing use of cocaine has come a plethora of data documenting major morbidity and mortality associated with its use.

Cocaine is an alkaloid originating in the leaves of the *Erythroxylon coca* plant that has a molecular weight of 339.81.[33] It can be administered intranasally ("snorting"), orally, vaginally, sublingually, rectally, and by intravenous, subcutaneous, or intramuscular injection. Although at one time the most popular form of administration was intranasal, the emergence of a very inexpensive, pure, and portable form of cocaine ("crack cocaine") that when smoked gives a very immediate effect as it is absorbed by the pulmonary circulation has superseded the more traditional snorting. Cocaine is detoxified by cholinesterases, and cocaine and its metabolites are excreted in the urine, where they may be present for up to 3 days. Cocaine blocks the presynaptic reuptake of norepinephrine and dopamine, with the resultant accumulation of these neurotransmitters at receptor sites. Vasoconstriction, hypertension, myocardial irritability, and seizures may result. Euphoria may result from the accumulation of dopamine, a mechanism that may also be responsible for addiction. In the pregnant ewe cocaine has been shown to induce vasoconstriction, decreased uterine blood flow, maternal and fetal hypertension, and fetal hypoxemia due to impaired oxygen transfer.[34,35]

ADVERSE EFFECTS ON THE MOTHER

Medical complications reported with cocaine include acute myocardial infarction, cardiac arrhythmias, aortic rupture, subarachnoid hemorrhage, strokes, ischemic bowel damage, and various other problems.[33] It would be expected that these same complications could occur in pregnant women, and a recent report of intracerebral hemorrhage during the postpartum period confirms that expectation (Table 22-2).[36]

TABLE 22–2. REPORTED EFFECTS OF COCAINE ON THE FETUS AND PREGNANCY

Abruptio placentae
Intrauterine growth retardation
Preterm labor
Premature rupture of membranes
Meconium
Spontaneous abortion
Intrauterine cerebral infarctions
?Urinary tract abnormalities
Neurobehavioral disorders

ADVERSE EFFECTS ON THE PREGNANCY

In 1983 Acker and associates reported two cases of abruptio placentae occurring 30 minutes to "a few hours" after intravenous or intranasal administration of cocaine.[37] Two years later, Chasnoff and colleagues reported four more such cases, and in 1987 Bingol and coworkers reported abruptio placentae with fetal death in 4 of 50 pregnancies among cocaine users.[38,39] Although not all studies have been confirmatory, it is highly likely that cocaine use can acutely trigger abruptio placentae by causing vasoconstriction in the uterine circulation, as evidenced by hypertension, with diminished placental perfusion. However, a more recent study found that women who used cocaine only in the first trimester demonstrated a high rate of abruption (9%), as did women who used the drug throughout gestation (15%).[40] The authors suggested that cocaine may alter the placental or uterine vasculature early in pregnancy, with adverse effects showing up nearer to term. A number of other reports of increased perinatal morbidity in cocaine users have appeared. Types of morbidity include intrauterine growth retardation,[41,42] preterm labor and delivery,[41,44] premature rupture of membranes,[41] meconium passage,[43,44] and spontaneous abortion.[38] Cerebral infarcts occurring in utero have been reported in offspring of cocaine-using mothers.[45] The possible teratogenicity of cocaine has proven difficult to evaluate, since many cocaine users take other potentially toxic substances as well, and patterns of cocaine use during the time of organogenesis are difficult to document. In one study there was an excess of infants with cardiac malformations born to cocaine users compared to infants who had not been exposed to cocaine.[44] Another study reported a major malformation rate of 10% among 50 cocaine users, compared to 2% of 340 drug-free pregnancies ($p < 0.01$).[39]

ADVERSE EFFECTS ON THE NEONATE

A further problem may be "behavioral teratogenesis," a condition in which cocaine-exposed newborns have been described as demonstrating poor organizational responses to their environment.[39,43] Signs of possible withdrawal have been reported in cocaine-exposed neonates,[40,41,46] as have long-lasting abnormalities of the electroencephalogram[46] and abnormal visual evoked potentials.[47] Cocaine babies have been described as "difficult to comfort," perhaps because they do not respond normally to their environments. This inability to interact with the environment in an appropriate way may interfere with parent–infant bonding. Whether child abuse will be more common among these children remains to be discovered.

Cocaine use by pregnant women is widespread. In one public hospital approximately 10% of mothers reported using cocaine.[48] It is becoming clear that cocaine exposure has potentially devastating effects on the fetus as well as the mother. Currently, the only available approach for preventing these problems appears to be education of pregnant and potentially pregnant women, in the hope that they will avoid cocaine use during pregnancy. Stopping cocaine after the first trimester appears to decrease some (low birth weight, preterm delivery) but not all of the risk.[40]

HEROIN

PHARMACOLOGY

Heroin (diacetylmorphine) is not used medically in the United States. Its effects are similar to those of morphine, except that it appears to cross the blood–brain barrier more effectively than does morphine. Heroin is hydrolyzed to monoacetylmorphine and morphine and is excreted in the urine. Its effects are similar to those of other opioids, and physical dependence leading to abstinence-related withdrawal symptoms is induced with chronic use. Gynecologic problems such as galactorrhea–amenorrhea have been reported in female heroin addicts.[49] Heroin is highly addictive, and this addiction is a major medical, economic, social, and legal problem in our society. Although the "cocaine epidemic" has tended to shift attention away from perinatal heroin addiction, this problem remains a challenge for obstetricians and other caregivers (Table 22-3).

FETAL EFFECTS

One study suggests that multiple gestations may be more common among heroin-addicted mothers.[50] Heroin crosses the placenta, and addiction is common among fetuses of heroin-addicted mothers. Fetal withdrawal with intrauterine convulsions has been postulated.[51,52] Heroin-addicted mothers are likely to deliver premature infants of low birth weight,[53] although respiratory distress syndrome may actually occur with less frequency in such children.[54] Teratogenicity has not been conclusively demonstrated. However, "behavioral teratogenicity" is highly likely, with neonates of heroin addicts demonstrating impairment of interactive abilities and motor changes.[55] It has long been recognized that sudden infant death syndrome (SIDS) occurs with greater frequency among offspring of heroin-addicted mothers, but the mechanism has not been elucidated.[56,57] Chasnoff has suggested that this high rate of SIDS may be associated with sleep apnea in such infants and has used theophylline treatment to prevent it.[55] One series has provided evidence of a remarkably high incidence of strabismus at age 3 among infants of heroin addicts.[58]

TABLE 22–3. REPORTED EFFECTS OF HEROIN ON PREGNANCY

Fetal addiction
Intrauterine withdrawal
Neonatal abstinence syndrome
Low birth weight
Behavioral teratogenesis
Sudden infant death syndrome

NEONATAL ABSTINENCE SYNDROME

The most striking finding with perinatal heroin addiction is neonatal withdrawal, or abstinence syndrome. It occurs in infants both of mothers addicted to heroin and of mothers treated with methadone. This syndrome, thoroughly described by Finnegan,[59] includes tremors, restlessness, hyperreflexia, high-pitched cry, sneezing, sleeplessness, tachypnea, yawning, sweating, fever, and, in severe cases, seizures. The onset of symptoms occurs from birth to as long as 2 weeks of age and may persist for up to 4–6 months.[60] Treatment has ranged from supportive measures to the use of medications such as diazepam, barbiturates, and opioids such as paregoric and methadone.[55] There is some evidence that withdrawal is less severe in infants whose mothers' methadone dose was down to 20 mg/day or less prior to delivery.[61]

TREATMENT IN PREGNANCY

The heroin-addicted mother is usually treated with methadone maintenance. There is no clear-cut advantage to methadone over heroin from the fetal point of view, and, in fact, methadone may be associated with worse withdrawal symptoms. However, heroin is not available for treatment in this country. Thus, the only way an addict can procure heroin is to do so illegally. Street heroin varies in its purity, and its availability depends on the ability of the addict to pay for it. Thus, the heroin addict is subject to periodic withdrawal symptoms that may put the fetus at risk. Therefore, most methadone maintenance programs give priority to pregnant addicts in order to offer some protection to the fetus. Specific programs for management of drug dependency during pregnancy have met with some success in lowering the various morbidities encountered in such extremely high-risk pregnancies.[62]

AIDS

The most significant problem facing intravenous drug users and their offspring now is the danger of acquired immunodeficiency syndrome (AIDS). Intravenous drug use accounts for the majority of HIV positivity among women, with some areas reporting a 50% seropositivity rate among IV drug users.[63] Any patient acknowledging a history of IV drug use should be offered HIV testing early enough in gestation to allow an informed decision about whether to continue pregnancy.

HALLUCINOGENS

In the 1960s and 1970s hallucinogenic drugs such as lysergic acid (LSD) were commonly taken recreationally. A great deal of interest was generated, but few credible studies were performed regarding the effects of such chemicals on the pregnant woman and her fetus. Because these substances were illegal, controlled trials were virtually impossible. Even retrospective studies were confounded by variables such as polydrug use, life-style differences, and reporting bias. Although there have been studies reporting chromosome damage from in vitro exposure of leukocytes to LSD, and increased prevalence of chromosome breaks in vivo in those exposed to this agent,[64] no definitive conclusions have been drawn as to possible human teratogenicity for LSD. In one observational study, eight of 83 liveborn offspring of mothers who admitted LSD use by themselves or their sexual partners prior to or during pregnancy had major anomalies.[64] Although this malformation rate (10%) is considerably higher than that reported in the general population, it was impossible to control for confounding variables, such as the fact that all patients also smoked marijuana and that the LSD was obtained on the street with no way to ascertain its true composition. Because LSD use seems to have declined in recent years, little recent data are available.

Phencyclidine (PCP, or "angel dust") was also a drug of the 1960s and 1970s, but it has apparently continued to be used as a hallucinogen to a greater extent than LSD. This drug was originally developed as an anesthetic agent but was not approved for human use because of its severe side effects. Patients recovering from phencyclidine anesthesia often manifested hallucinations, disorientation, agitation, and delirium. It is easy to produce PCP, and the drug is inexpensive on the street, so that it has become a popular hallucinogen because of the very side effects that limited its use as an anesthetic agent.[65] Animal studies demonstrated that phencyclidine readily crosses the placenta and appears in murine breast milk in concentrations 10 times those in maternal plasma.[66] The drug has been shown to appear in umbilical cord plasma and amniotic fluid from human pregnancies,[67] and the human placenta has been shown to be an active site for conversion of PCP to its metabolic products in vitro.[68] In one case in which both maternal and umbilical cord levels were measured, the concentration of PCP in the fetus was double that in the mother.[69] Animal studies have demonstrated reduced birth weight and embryotoxicity.[70] In one prospective epidemiologic study of 2327 pregnant women who were assessed by questionnaire and urinary assays, 12 (0.5%) admitted PCP use during the index pregnancy and an additional 7 (0.3%) tested positive for this drug in their urine.[71] Abnormal neonatal behavior in infants chronically exposed in utero to PCP has been described in case reports, but no epidemiologic studies have quantitated the risk.[65,72,73] The possibility of structural or behavioral teratogenesis remains unproven.

Newer "designer drug" hallucinogens have appeared in recent years, but there are virtually no data concerning the risk or lack thereof to the developing fetus.

TOBACCO

Cigarette smoke contains nicotine, carbon monoxide, and a countless number of other potentially toxic substances. There is a diverse literature relating chronic in utero exposure to maternal smoking to a variety of adverse perinatal outcomes. There appears to be little disagreement that maternal smoking is associated with a significant reduction in birth weight of the offspring.[74] This effect may,[75,76] or may not,[77] be associated with decreased food intake and decreased weight gain by the mother. There also appears to be an increased likelihood of preterm birth,[78] antepartum hemorrhage,[79] and perinatal mortality of low-birth-weight infants.[80] Maternal smoking has been associated with reduced placental blood flow in humans.[81] Clinical studies have demonstrated variable effects on fetal breathing,[82] and increased fetal heart rate with decreased beat-to-beat variability,[83] during acute maternal exposure to cigarette smoke. However, no effect was demonstrated on the reactivity of non-stress tests.[84] Chronic cigarette exposure was associated with lower Apgar scores in some,[85] but not other[86] studies. Vascular injury to the intimal lining of umbilical arteries of newborns from smoking mothers has been demonstrated,[87] as have placental changes.[88,89] Maternal smoking has been associated with both low[90,91] and high[92] human placental lactogen levels, and with a failure in expansion of total body water and mean plasma volume during pregnancy.[93] Changes in hemostatic function[94] and platelet function[95] have also been associated with maternal smoking. It is difficult to determine whether these changes are due to the effects of nicotine, carbon monoxide, or some other substance(s). Nicotine administered to the mother has been associated with decreased uterine blood flow in the rhesus monkey,[96] but in the human fetus it has been associated with increased umbilical blood flow.[97] Its administration to the pregnant ewe is associated with a rapid fall in fetal pO_2 and a decline in the frequency of fetal breathing movements.[98] Its oral administration to pregnant rats has been associated with damage to the fetal brain stem.[99] On the other hand, both standard cigarette smoke and smoke from nicotine-free cigarettes were associated with a drop in fetal pO_2 when inhaled by pregnant rhesus monkeys.[100] This effect has been attributed to carbon monoxide, since carboxyhemoglobin is preferentially trapped on the fetal side of the placenta.[101] The relative hypoxia induced by increased carboxyhemoglobin levels in the fetus could be responsible for a wide variety of adverse effects.

Maternal cigarette smoking has been implicated in the genesis of congenital malformations such as cleft lip and palate,[102] but this association has not been universally present.[103] A recent epidemiologic study suggests that only isolated oral clefts, unassociated with other birth defects, are increased in the offspring of cigarette smokers.[104]

Maternal smoking during pregnancy has been associated with a decreased risk of respiratory distress syndrome in the prematurely delivered offspring, an effect that has generally been attributed to enhanced pulmonic maturation secondary to intrauterine hypoxic stress.[105,106] Effects on cord blood immunoglobulin levels have also been demonstrated.[107] One epidemiologic study was unable to demonstrate any effect of maternal smoking on the prevalence of childhood cancer in the offspring.[108] On the other hand, maternal smoking during pregnancy has been associated with apparently adverse behavioral and developmental outcomes in the offspring.[109,110]

It is difficult to assess the relative contributions of in utero exposure to smoking versus passive smoking by the child who is raised in a smoking household. Such passive smoking has been associated with slower development of lung function in children and adolescents.[111] Although it is possible to detect the effects of household smoking exposure on infants,[112] one study found it impossible to demonstrate maternal–fetal transmission of thiocyanate acquired passively by the mother exposed to a smoking environment but not herself a smoker.[113] However, another study was able to show such an effect,[114] and a recent report demonstrated a significant reduction in birth weight among the offspring of mothers exposed passively to cigarette smoke, as evidence by raised maternal cotinine levels during the second trimester.[115]

Nieburg and colleagues[116] have suggested the term *fetal tobacco syndrome* to describe infants meeting the following four conditions:

1. A mother who smoked five or more cigarettes a day throughout the pregnancy.
2. No evidence of hypertension during the pregnancy.
3. Symmetrical growth retardation at term.
4. No other obvious cause of growth retardation.

They postulated that this label would increase the awareness of the medical and lay communities to the adverse effects of maternal smoking and would lead to greater efforts to help pregnant women discontinue this habit. Over 10 years ago, the Commissioner of Public Health in Massachusetts suggested that physicians consider obtaining a carboxyhemoglobin level or expired carbon monoxide level on each patient at her first prenatal visit. Patients with elevated levels would be so informed, and the dangers should be described.[117] In 1979 the American College of Obstetricians and Gynecologists published a Technical Bulletin on this subject that recommended that pregnant women be encouraged to stop smoking.[118] Identification of the smoker at the first prenatal visit should be coupled with intensive education about the risks of smoking during pregnancy. Again the use of carboxyhemoglobin measurements to help motivate patients was encouraged. Prohibition of smoking within the office, clinic, and hospital settings was strongly urged. Community-based smoking cessation programs were encouraged.

Although there have been great strides in American society in prohibiting smoking in public areas and in decreasing the number of cigarette-smoking citizens, smoking during pregnancy continues to be a problem. In a recent epidemiologic study, 28% of women smoked before pregnancy, and 23% continued to smoke during pregnancy.[119] A study of 26 states demonstrated that 21% of pregnant women currently smoke, as compared to 30% of nonpregnant women.[120] Clearly, intervention is necessary to help women stop smoking. Encouraging developments have included a randomized intervention study, in which pregnant smoking women treated with a cessation program demonstrated a significant increase in birth weight and length of their offspring when compared to untreated smoking controls.[121] It is clear that the major responsibility rests with caregivers for pregnant women. We must find out if our patients are smoking, educate them about the risks, and refer them to smoking cessation programs in our communities. Recent preoccupation among patients and caregivers about the details and environment of "the birthing experience" seems less compelling if that "childbirth environment" is smoke-filled.

CAFFEINE

Caffeine, a dioxypurine, is 1,3,7-trimethylxanthine. It is chemically related to the xanthines theophylline and theobromine. The xanthines exert most of their systemic effects by increasing intracellular cyclic AMP, altering ionized calcium levels, and potentiating the action of catecholamines. These systemic effects include central nervous system excitation, smooth muscle relaxation, increased heart rate, and increased cardiac output. There is also an increase in gastric acid secretion and diuresis.[122] Caffeine is contained in coffee and tea (100–150 mg per average cup, but with wide variations), nondietetic cola drinks (35–55 mg per 12-ounce serving), and cocoa (200 mg theobromine per average cup).[122] Pregnant women near term have been shown to eliminate caffeine considerably more slowly than nonpregnant controls.[123,124] Caffeine is fat soluble and has been demonstrated to cross the placenta in sheep and humans.[125,126]

The administration of caffeine to pregnant sheep has been shown to result in a mild fall in uterine blood flow, but to have no effect on oxygenation or acid–base status.[125,127] In human pregnancies near term, the maternal ingestion of two cups of coffee was associated with a small but significant fall in intervillous blood flow.[128] Chronic coffee drinkers were found to have increased fetal breathing activity, but acute ingestion of 200 mg of caffeine had no significant effect on fetal breathing.[129]

High-dose bolus studies in rodents have demonstrated teratogenicity with caffeine, but only at maternal blood levels higher than is likely to be achieved in human pregnancies. In one study, in which rats were gavage fed caffeine in a single dose of 100 mg/kg each day, limb abnormalities were produced. The publication of this abstract received a lot of media attention in 1982–1983, but the bolus nature and high circulating levels, coupled with the differences in xanthine metabolism between rats and humans, make it difficult to apply these data to human pregnancies.[130] A report of three pregnancies in which high maternal caffeine intake was associated with ectrodactyly in the offspring created a great deal of interest in the possibility; each mother was estimated to have consumed between 1100 and 1777 mg of caffeine on an average day during her pregnancy.[131] However, at least three large epidemiologic studies in humans have failed to detect any increase in congenital anomalies related to caffeine intake among pregnant women.[132–134] A single study has suggested an increase in the rate of spontaneous late first- and second-trimester abortions among moderate to heavy caffeine users.[135] Although animal studies have suggested an effect of increasing doses of caffeine in lowering birth weight, human studies have been less convincing.[136]

In summary, there is no convincing evidence supporting a teratogenic or other adverse role on pregnancy for caffeine when taken in amounts equivalent to less than 10 cups of coffee per day. Pregnant women should be advised to use moderation in their caffeine intake, but it need not be avoided altogether.

REFERENCES

1. Clarren SK, Smith DW. The fetal alcohol syndrome. N Engl J Med 1978;298:1063.
2. Rodin AE. Infants and gin mania in 18th-century London. JAMA 1981;245:1237.
3. Jones KL, Smith DW. Recognition of the fetal alcohol syndrome in early infancy. Lancet 1973;1:999.
4. Jones KL, Smith DW, Uelland CN, Streissguth AP. Pattern of malformation in offspring of chronic alcoholic mothers. Lancet 1973;1:1267.
5. Rosett HL. Editorial: a clinical perspective on the fetal alcohol syndrome. Alcoholism: Clin Exp Res 1980;2:119.
6. Streissguth AP, Clarren SK, Jones KL. A natural history of the fetal alcohol syndrome: a 10-year followup of 11 patients. Alcohol Health Res World 1985;101:13.
7. National Institute on Alcohol Abuse and Alcoholism. Program Strategies for Preventing Fetal Alcohol Syndrome and Alcohol-Related Birth Defects. Washington, DC: US Department of Health and Human Services, 1987 [DHS Public No. (ADM) 87-1482].
8. Rosett HL, Weiner L. Alcohol and the adult. In: Alcohol and the fetus: a clinical perspective. New York: Oxford University Press, 1984:13.
9. Rosett HL, Weiner L. Fetal alcohol syndrome. In: Alcohol and the fetus: a clinical perspective. New York: Oxford University Press, 1984:3.
10. Ernhart CB, Sokol RJ, Martier S, Moron P, Nadler D, Ager JW, Wolf A. Alcohol teratogenicity in the human: a detailed assessment of specificity, critical period, and threshold. Am J Obstet Gynecol 1987;156:33.
11. Rosett HL, Weiner L, Lee A, Zuckerman B, Dooling E, Oppenheimer E. Patterns of alcohol consumption and fetal development. Obstet Gynecol 1983;61:539.
12. Little RE. Moderate alcohol use during pregnancy and decreased infant birth weight. Am J Public Health 1977;67:1154.
13. Mills JL, Graubard BI, Harley EE, Rhoads GG, Berendes H. Maternal alcohol consumption and birth weight: how much drinking during pregnancy is safe? JAMA 1984;252:1875.
14. Kline J, Stein Z, Shrout P, Susser M, Warburton D. Drinking during pregnancy and spontaneous abortion. Lancet 1980;2:176.
15. Halmesmaki E, Ylikorkala O. A retrospective study on the safety of prenatal ethanol treatment. Obstet Gynecol 1988; 72:545.
16. Sisenwein FE, Tejani NA, Boxer HS, DiGiuseppe R. Effects of maternal ethanol infusion during pregnancy on the growth and development of children at four to seven years of age. Am J Obstet Gynecol 1983;147:52.
17. Brien JF, Clarke DW, Richardson B, Patrick J. Disposition of ethanol in maternal blood, fetal blood, and amniotic fluid in third-trimester pregnant ewes. Am J Obstet Gynecol 1985;152:583.
18. Brien JF, Loomis CW, Tranmer J, McGrath M. Disposition of ethanol in human maternal venous blood and amniotic fluid. Am J Obstet Gynecol 1983;146:181.
19. Lieber C. Biochemical and molecular basis of alcohol-induced injury to liver and other tissues. New Engl J Med 1988;319:1639.
20. Fisher SE. Selective fetal malnutrition: the fetal alcohol syndrome. J Am Coll Nutr 1988;7:101.
21. McLeod W, Brien J, Loomis C, Carmichael L, Probert C, Patrick J. Effect of maternal ethanol ingestion on fetal breathing movements, gross body movements, and heart rate at 37 to 40 weeks' gestational age. Am J Obstet Gynecol 1983;145:251.
22. Coles CD, Smith IE, Fernhoff PM, Falek A. Neonatal ethanol withdrawal: characteristics in clinically normal, nondysmorphic neonates. J Pediatr 1984;105:445.
23. Streissguth AP, Darby BL, Barr HM, Smith JR, Martin DC. Comparison of drinking and smoking patterns during pregnancy over a six-year period. Am J Obstet Gynecol 1983;145:716.
24. Halmesmaki E, Raivio KO, Ylikorkala O. Patterns of alcohol consumption during pregnancy. Obstet Gynecol 1987;69:594.
25. Rosett HL, Weiner L, Edelin KC. Strategies for prevention of fetal alcohol effects. Obstet Gynecol 1981;57:1.
26. Selzer ML. The Michigan Alcoholism Screening Test: the quest for a new diagnostic instrument. Am J Psychiatry 1971;127:1653.
27. Ewing JA. Detecting alcoholism: the CAGE questionnaire. JAMA 1984;252:1905.
28. Larsson G, Ottenblad C, Hagenfeldt L, Larsson A, Forsgren M. Evaluation of gamma-glutamyl transferase as a screening method for excessive alcohol consumption during pregnancy. Am J Obstet Gynecol 1983;147:654.
29. Ylikorkala O, Stenman U, Halmesmaki E. Gamma-glutamyl transferase and mean cell volume reveal maternal alcohol abuse and fetal alcohol effects. Am J Obstet Gynecol 1987;157:344.

30. Rosett HL, Weiner L, Edeline KC. Treatment experience with pregnant problem drinkers. JAMA 1983;249:2029.
31. Halmesmaki E. Alcohol counselling of 85 pregnant problem drinkers: effect on drinking and fetal outcome. Br J Obstet Gynaecol 1988;95:243.
32. Berkowitz RL, Coustan DR, Mochizuki TK. Handbook for prescribing medications during pregnancy. 2nd ed. Boston: Little, Brown, 1986:112.
33. Creigler LL, Mark H. Special report: medical complications of cocaine abuse. N Engl J Med 1986;315:1495.
34. Moore TR, Sorg J, Miller L, Key T, Resnik R. Hemodynamic effects of intravenous cocaine on the pregnant ewe and fetus. Am J Obstet Gynecol 1986;155:883.
35. Woods JR Jr, Plessinger MA, Clark KE. Effect of cocaine on uterine blood flow and fetal oxygenation. JAMA 1987;157:957.
36. Mercado A, Johnson G Jr, Calver D, Sokol RJ. Cocaine, pregnancy, and postpartum intracerebral hemorrhage. Obstet Gynecol 1989;73:467.
37. Acker D, Sachs BP, Tracey KJ, Wise WE. Abruptio placentae associated with cocaine use. Am J Obstet Gynecol 1983;146:220.
38. Chasnoff IJ, Burns WJ, Schnoll SH, Burns KA. Cocaine use in pregnancy. N Engl J Med 1985;313:666.
39. Bingol N, Fuchs M, Diaz V, Stone RK, Gromisch DS. Teratogenicity of cocaine in humans. J Pediatr 1987;110:93.
40. Chasnoff IJ, Griffith DR, MacGregor S, Dirkes K, Burns KA. Temporal patterns of cocaine use in pregnancy: perinatal outcome. JAMA 1989;261:1741.
41. Cherukuri R, Minkoff H, Feldman J, Parekh A, Glass L. A cohort study of alkaloidal cocaine ("crack") in pregnancy. Obstet Gynecol 1988;72:147.
42. Chouteau M, Namerow PB, Leppert P. The effect of cocaine abuse on birth weight and gestational age. Obstet Gynecol 1988;72:351.
43. Chasnoff IJ, Burns KA, Burns WJ. Cocaine use in pregnancy: perinatal morbidity and mortality. Neurotoxicol Teratol 1987;9:291.
44. Little BB, Snell LM, Klein VR, Gilstrap LC III. Cocaine abuse during pregnancy: maternal and fetal implications. Obstet Gynecol 1989;73;:157.
45. Chasnoff IJ, Bussey ME, Savich R, Stack CM. Perinatal cerebral infarction and maternal cocaine use. J Pediatr 1986;108:456.
46. Doberczak TM, Shanzer S, Senie RT, Kandall SR. Neonatal neurologic and electroencephalographic effects of intrauterine cocaine exposure. J Pediatr 1988;113:354.
47. Dixon SD, Coen R, Crutchfield S. Visual dysfunction in cocaine-exposed infants. Pediatr Res 1987;21:359A.
48. Little BB, Snell LM, Palmore MK, Gilstrap LC III. Cocaine use in pregnant women in a large public hospital. Am J Perinatol 1988;5:206.
49. Pelosi MA, Sama JC, Caterini H, Kaminetzky HA. Galactorrhea–amenorrhea syndrome associated with heroin addiction. Am J Obstet Gynecol 1974;118:966.
50. Rementeria JL, Janakammal S, Hollander M. Multiple births in drug-addicted women. Am J Obstet Gynecol 1975;122:958.
51. Rementeria JL, Nunag NN. Narcotic withdrawal in pregnancy: stillbirth incidence with a case report. Am J Obstet Gynecol 1973;116:1152.
52. Zuspan FP, Gumpel JA, Mejia-Zelaya A, Madden J, Davis R. Fetal stress from methadone withdrawal. Am J Obstet Gynecol 1975;122:43.
53. Stone ML, Salerno LJ, Green M, Zelson C. Narcotic addiction in pregnancy. Am J Obstet Gynecol 1971:109:716.
54. Glass L, Rajegowda BK, Evans HE. Absence of respiratory distress syndrome in premature infants of heroin-addicted mothers. Lancet 1971;2:685.
55. Chasnoff IJ. Perinatal addiction: consequences of intrauterine exposure to opiate and nonopiate drugs. In: Chasnoff IJ, ed. Drug use in pregnancy: mother and child. Boston: MTP Press, 1986:52.
56. Pierson PS, Howard P, Klaber HD. Sudden deaths in infants born to methadone-maintained addicts. JAMA 1972;220:1733.
57. Chavez CJ, Ostrea EM Jr, Stryker JC, Smialek Z. Sudden infant death syndrome among infants of drug-dependent mothers. J Pediatr 1979;95:407.
58. Nelson LB, Ehrlich S, Calhoun JH, Matteucci T, Finnegan LP. Occurrence of strabismus in infants born to drug-dependent women. Am J Dis Child 1987;141:175.
59. Finnegan LP, Connoughton JF, Kron RE, Emich JP. Neonatal abstinence syndrome: assessment and management. In: Harbison RD, ed. Perinatal addiction. New York: Spectrum, 1975:141.
60. Chasnoff IJ, Hatcher R, Burns WJ. Early growth patterns of methadone-addicted infants. Am J Dis Child 1980;134:1049.
61. Madden JD, Chappel JN, Zuspan F, Gumpel J, Mejia A, Davis R. Observation and treatment of neonatal narcotic withdrawal. Am J Obstet Gynecol 1977;127:199.
62. Rosner MA, Keith L, Chasnoff I. The Northwestern University Drug Dependence Program: the impact of intensive prenatal care on labor and delivery outcomes. Am J Obstet Gynecol 1982;144:23.
63. Weinberg DS, Murray HW. Coping with AIDS: the special problems of New York City. M Engl J Med 1987;317:1469.
64. Jacobson CB, Berlin CM. Possible reproductive detriment in LSD users. JAMA 1972;222:1367.
65. Golden NL, Sokol RJ, Rubin IL. Angel dust: possible effects on the fetus. Pediatrics 1980;65:18.
66. Nicholas JM, Lipshitz J, Schreiber EC. Phencyclidine: its transfer across the placenta as well as into breast milk. Am J Obstet Gynecol 1982;143:143.
67. Kaufman KR, Petrucha RA, Pitts FN Jr, Kaufman ER. Phencyclidine in umbilical cord blood: preliminary data. Am J Psychol 1983;140:450.
68. Rayburn WF, Holsztynska EF, Domino EF. Phencyclidine: biotransformation by the human placenta. Am J Obstet Gynecol 1984;148:111.
69. Petrucha RA, Kaufman KR, Pitts FN. Phencyclidine in pregnancy: a case report. J Reprod Med 1982;27:301.
70. Fico TA, Vanderwende C. Phencyclidine during pregnancy: behavioral and neurochemical effects in the offspring. Ann NY Acad Sci 1989;562:319.
71. Golden NL, Kuhnert BR, Sokol RJ, Martier S, Bagby BS. Phencyclidine use during pregnancy. Am J Obstet Gynecol 1984;148:254.
72. Strauss AA, Modanlou HD, Bosu SK. Neonatal manifestations of maternal phencyclidine (PCP) abuse. Pediatrics 1981;68:550.
73. Chasnoff IJ, Burns KA, Burns WJ, Schnoll SH. Prenatal drug exposure: effects on neonatal and infant growth and development. Neurotoxicol Teratol 1986;8:357.
74. US Dept of Health and Human Services. The health consequences of smoking for women: a report of the surgeon general 1983. Washington, DC: US Government Printing Office, Publication 410–889/1284:808.
75. Davies DP, Gray OP, Ellwood PC, Abernethy M. Cigarette smoking in pregnancy: associations with maternal weight gain and fetal growth. Lancet 1976;1:385.
76. Papoz L, Eschwege E, Pequignot G, Barrat J, Schwartz D. Maternal smoking and birth weight in relation to dietary habits. Am J Obstet Gynecol 1982;142:870.
77. Haworth JC, Ellestad-Sayed JJ, King J, Dilling LA. Fetal growth retardation in cigarette-smoking mothers is not due to de-

creased maternal food intake. Am J Obstet Gynecol 1980;137:719.
78. Shiono PH, Klebanoff MA, Rhoads GG. Smoking and drinking during pregnancy. JAMA 1986;255:82.
79. Meyer MB, Tonascia JA. Maternal smoking, pregnancy complications, and perinatal mortality. Am J Obstet Gynecol 1977;128:494.
80. Terrin M, Meyer MB. Birth weight-specific rates as a bias in the effects of smoking and other perinatal hazards. Obstet Gynecol 1981;58:636.
81. Andersen KV, Hermann N. Placenta flow reduction in pregnant smokers. Acta Obstet Gynecol Scand 1984;63:707.
82. Thaler I, Goodman JDS, Dawes GS. Effects of maternal cigarette smoking on fetal breathing and fetal movements. Am J Obstet Gynecol 1980;138:282.
83. Kariniemi V, Lehtovirta P, Rauramo I, Forss M. Effects of smoking on fetal heart rate variability during gestational weeks 27 to 32. Am J Obstet Gynecol 1984;149:575.
84. Barrett JM, Vanhooydonk JE, Boehm FH. Acute effect of cigarette smoking on the fetal heart rate nonstress test. Obstet Gynecol 1981;57:422.
85. Garn SM, Johnston M, Ridella SA, Petzold AS. Effect of maternal cigarette smoking on Apgar scores. Am J Dis Child 1981;135:503.
86. Hingson R, Gould JB, Morelock S, Kayne H, Heeren T, Alpert JJ, et al. Maternal cigarette smoking, psychoactive substance use, and infant Apgar scores. Am J Obstet Gynecol 1982;144:959.
87. Asmussen I, Kjeldsen K. Intimal ultrastructure of human umbilical arteries: observations on arteries from newborn children of smoking and nonsmoking mothers. Circ Res 1975;36:579.
88. Rush D, Kristal A, Blanc W, Navarro C, Chauhan P, Brown MC, et al. The effects of maternal cigarette smoking on placental morphology, histomorphometry, and biochemistry. Am J Perinatol 1986;3:263.
89. Brown HL, Miller JM Jr, Khawli O, Gabert HA. Premature placental calcification in maternal cigarette smokers. Obstet Gynecol 1988;71:914.
90. Mochizuki M, Maruo T, Masuko K, Ohtsu T. Effects of smoking on fetoplacental-maternal system during pregnancy. Am J Obstet Gynecol 1984;149:413.
91. Moser RJ, Hollingsworth DR, Carlson JW, Lamotte L. Human chorionic somatomammotropin in normal adolescent primiparous pregnancy. I. Effect of smoking. Am J Obstet Gynecol 1974;120:1080.
92. Spellacy WN, Buhi WC, Birk SA. The effect of smoking on serum human placental lactogen levels. Am J Obstet Gynecol 1977;127:232.
93. Pirani BBK, MacGillivray I. Smoking during pregnancy: its effect on maternal metabolism and fetoplacental function. Obstet Gynecol 1978;52:257.
94. Condie RG, Pirani BBK. The influence of smoking on the haemostatic mechanism in pregnancy. Acta Obstet Gynecol Scand 1977;56:5.
95. Leuschen MP, Davis RB, Boyd D, Goodlin RC. Comparative evaluation of antepartum and postpartum platelet function in smokers and nonsmokers. Am J Obstet Gynecol 1986;155:1276.
96. Suzuki K, Minei LJ, Johnson EE. Effect of nicotine upon uterine blood flow in the pregnant rhesus monkey. Am J Obstet Gynecol 1980;136:1009.
97. Lindblad A, Marsal K, Anderson KE. Effect of nicotine on human fetal blood flow. Obstet Gynecol 1988;72:371.
98. Manning F, Walker D, Feyerabend C. The effect of nicotine on fetal breathing movements in conscious pregnant ewes. Obstet Gynecol 1978;52:563.
99. Krous HF, Campbell GA, Fowler MW, Catron AC, Farber JP. Maternal nicotine administration and fetal brain stem damage: a rat model with implications for sudden infant death syndrome. Am J Obstet Gynecol 1981;140:743.
100. Socol ML, Manning FA, Murata Y, Druzin ML. Maternal smoking causes fetal hypoxia: experimental evidence. Am J Obstet Gynecol 1982;142:214.
101. Longo LD. The biological effects of carbon monoxide on the pregnant woman, fetus, and newborn infant. Am J Obstet Gynecol 1977;129:69.
102. Ericson A, Kallen B, Westerholm P. Cigarette smoking as an etiologic factor in cleft lip and palate. Am J Obstet Gynecol 1979;135:348.
103. Hemminki K, Mutanen P, Saloniemi I. Smoking, the occurrence of congenital malformations and spontaneous abortions: multivariate analysis. Am J Obstet Gynecol 1983;145:61.
104. Khoury MJ, Gomez-Farias M, Mulinare J. Does maternal cigarette smoking during pregnancy cause cleft lip and palate in offspring? Am J Dis Child 1989;143:333.
105. Curet LB, Rao AV, Zachman RD, Morrison J, Burkett G, Poole WK, and The Collaborative Group on Antenatal Steroid Therapy. Maternal smoking and respiratory distress syndrome. Am J Obstet Gynecol 1983;147:446.
106. White E, Shy KK, Daling JR, Guthrie RD. Maternal smoking and infant respiratory distress syndrome. Obstet Gynecol 1986;67:365.
107. Cederqvist LL, Eddey G, Abdel-latif N, Litwin SD. The effect of smoking during pregnancy on cord blood and maternal serum immunoglobulin levels. Am J Obstet Gynecol 1984;148:1123.
108. Neutel CI, Buck C. Effect of smoking during pregnancy on the risk of cancer in children. J Natl Cancer Inst 1971;47:59.
109. Naeye RL, Peters EC. Mental development of children whose mothers smoked during pregnancy. Obstet Gynecol 1984;64:601.
110. Fried PA, Watkinson B, Dillon RF. Neonatal neurological status in a low-risk population after prenatal exposure to cigarettes, marijuana, and alcohol. Develop Behav Pediatr 1987;8:318.
111. Tager IB, Weiss ST, Munoz A, Rosner B, Speizer FE. Longitudinal study of the effects of maternal smoking on pulmonary function in children. N Engl J Med 1983;309:699.
112. Greenberg RA, Haley NJ, Etzel RA, Loda FA. Measuring the exposure of infants to tobacco smoke. N Engl J Med 1984;310:1075.
113. Hauth JC, Hauth J, Brawbaugh RB, Gilstrap LC III, Pierson WP. Passive smoking and thiocyanate concentrations in pregnant women and newborns. Obstet Gynecol 1984;63:519.
114. Bottoms SF, Kuhnert BR, Kuhnert PM, Reese AL. Maternal passive smoking and fetal serum thiocyanate levels. Am J Obstet Gynecol 1982;144:787.
115. Haddow JE, Knight GJ, Palomaki GE, McCarthy JE. Second-trimester serum cotinine levels in nonsmokers in relation to birth weight. Am J Obstet Gynecol 1988;159:481.
116. Nieburg P, Marks JS, McLaren NM, Remington PL. The fetal tobacco syndrome. JAMA 1985;253:2998.
117. Fielding JE. Smoking and pregnancy. N Engl J Med 1978;298:337.
118. American College of Obstetricians and Gynecologists. Cigarette smoking and pregnancy. 1979;ACOG Technical Bulletin 53, 1.
119. Kruse J, LeFevre M, Zweig S. Changes in smoking and alcohol consumption during pregnancy: a population-based study in a rural area. Obstet Gynecol 1986;67:627.
120. Williamson DF, Serdula MK, Kendrick JS, Binkin NJ. Comparing the prevalence of smoking in pregnant and nonpregnant women, 1985 to 1986. JAMA 1989;261:70.
121. Sexton M, Hebel JR. A clinical trial of change in maternal smoking and its effect on birth weight. JAMA 1984;251:911.
122. Berkowitz RL, Coustan DR, Mochizuki TK. Xanthines. Hand-

book for prescribing medications during pregnancy. 2nd ed. Boston: Little, Brown, 1986:303.

123. Knutti R, Rothweiler H, Schlatter C. Effect of pregnancy on the pharmoacokinetics of caffeine. Eur J Clin Pharmacol 1981;21:121.
124. Parsons WD, Pelletier JG. Delayed elimination of caffeine by women in the last 2 weeks of pregnancy. Can Med Assoc J 1982;127:377.
125. Wilson SJ, Ayromlooi J, Errick JK. Pharmacokinetic and hemodynamic effects of caffeine in the pregnant sheep. Obstet Gynecol 1983;61:486.
126. Abdul-Karim, RW. Methylxanthines. Drugs during pregnancy: clinical perspectives. Philadelphia: Stickley, 1981:74.
127. Conover WB, Key TC, Resnik R. Maternal cardiovascular response to caffeine infusion in the pregnant ewe. Am J Obstet Gynecol 1983;145:534.
128. Kirkinen P, Jouppila P, Koivula A, Vuori J, Puukka M. The effect of caffeine on placental and fetal blood flow in human pregnancy. Am J Obstet Gynecol 1983;147:939.
129. McGowan J, Devoe LD, Searle N, Altman R. The effects of long- and short-term maternal caffeine ingestion on human fetal breathing and body movements in term gestations. Am J Obstet Gynecol 1987;157:726.
130. Smith SE, McElhatton PR, Sullivan FM. How can two "identical" caffeine teratology studies produce different results? Teratology 1982;26:21A.
131. Jacobson MF, Goldman AS, Syme RH. Coffee and birth defects. Lancet 1981;1:1415.
132. Linn S, Schoenbaum SC, Monson RR, Rosner B, Stubblefield PG, Ryan KJ. No association between coffee consumption and adverse outcomes of pregnancy. N Engl J Med 1982;306:141.
133. Rosenberg L, Mitchell AA, Shapiro S, Slone D. Selected birth defects in relation to caffeine-containing beverages. JAMA 1982;247:1429.
134. Furuhashi N, Sato S, Suzuki M, Hiruta M, Tanaka M, Takahashi T. Effects of caffeine ingestion during pregnancy. Gynecol Obstet Invest 1985;19:187.
135. Srisuphan W, Bracken MB. Caffeine consumption during pregnancy and association with late spontaneous abortion. Am J Obstet Gynecol 1986;154:14.
136. Update on caffeine. Reproductive toxicology: a medical letter. 1987;6:13.

23

CHAPTER

RISK ASSESSMENT FOR DEVELOPMENTAL TOXICITY: EFFECTS OF DRUGS AND CHEMICALS ON THE FETUS

Donald R. Mattison and Frederick R. Jelovsek

Structural or functional developmental defects complicate a significant number of pregnancies. Between 3% and 5% of all infants are born with a congenital malformation, and 1% to 2% have a severe malformation. As the child grows and develops, more congenital defects are identified.[1] The causes of these congenital defects fall into three general areas:

1. The action of a mutated gene or chromosome anomaly (eg, achondroplasia or maternal phenylketonuria[2])
2. The action of an environmental agent (eg, congenital rubella, ionizing radiation, or aminopterin[3,4])
3. A combination of genetic and environmental factors (eg, fetal phenytoin syndrome[5,6]).

Among all congenital defects, 20% to 25% are associated with a chromosomal or genetic (spontaneous or Mendelian inheritance) anomaly, 7% to 10% are due to infection or maternal disease, and drugs and environmental chemicals account for approximately 2%. Approximately two thirds of all developmental defects have no identifiable cause. It has been estimated that 7% to 10% of developmental defects are potentially preventable.[7] Identification of the etiology of congenital defects and prevention of those caused by environmental factors represent a significant challenge for modern maternal–fetal medicine.

The challenge to define the impact of drug or chemical exposure on pregnancy is becoming more common and much more difficult for the practicing obstetrician.[3,8] For example, imagine that you are called upon to assess the following scenarios:

A nurse phones about a patient who has been taking lithium carbonate, 300 mg four times a day, for the last year for severe manic depression. The psychiatrist put her on this after several years of trying many different medications, none of which worked as well as lithium. The patient has just found out that she is pregnant, 8 weeks from her last menstrual period. Is she at any increased risk for having a baby with a birth defect? If so what are the defects and what proportion of the women receiving this medication have a malformed child? Should she reduce or discontinue her dose, or can she continue taking the medication since it is working well and she really needs it? If she continues the medication, do alterations in pharmacokinetics during pregnancy mandate alterations in dose or treatment interval to maintain blood levels in the therapeutic range?

A lawyer phones and says he has a client with a child with multiple defects, including structural and functional CNS defects. His client thinks that some chemical exposures at work (she is a laboratory technician in a hospital) may be responsible for this malformation. Geneticists consulted about the defects think that if there is any relationship to an exposure, it must have occurred before the 10th week of pregnancy. During the fifth through the eighth week of pregnancy the mother was exposed to a volatile solvent containing toluene and xylene. Is there a causal relationship?

These and other scenarios are not unusual questions asked of today's health professional. Patients individually and collectively are very concerned about the environment and exposures to drugs or chemicals that can affect their fertility or their offspring.[8-10] It is important for obstetricians to understand how to define exposures that represent potential risks to the fetus. Similarly, it is important to identify exposures correctly that do not represent a risk to the fetus. In either situation the obstetrician must provide accurate and appropriate guidance concerning the extent of fetal risk. It is inappropriate to suggest termination of pregnancy when there is little or no excess risk to the fetus. Similarly, it is important to suggest exposure modifications in situations when reproduction or development may be impaired.

The need for accurate, responsible counsel about reproductive and developmental hazards is growing. For example, in 1986 California voters adopted a law (Proposition 65) to protect themselves against, and to be informed about, chemicals that cause cancer, birth defects, or other reproductive harm.[8,10] Under Proposition 65 the state has an obligation to protect the public from chemicals that cause birth defects or reproductive harm, or at least warn the public about such hazards.

Proposition 65 requires the state to list those substances it identifies as hazardous to reproduction or development. Listing automatically prohibits discharge of the chemical into sources of drinking water. If the substance is present in a product at a level that exceeds 0.001 of the no-observed-adverse-effect level (the highest dose associated with no measurable toxicity in experimental animal studies), Proposition 65 requires that consumers be warned that the product contains a chemical or chemicals known to the state of California to cause reproductive or developmental toxicity. The listing process contained in Proposition 65 will substantially increase the number of questions about fetal and reproductive risk addressed to obstetricians. These patients will expect their physicians to provide estimates of the magnitude of risk resulting from their exposure, which may be extremely difficult. In addition, most obstetricians have not had formal training in the evaluation of reproductive or developmental risks from occupational or environmental exposures, the communication of the magnitude of those risks to the patient and her family, or the development of strategies for risk management.[8-11]

Although Proposition 65 obligates the governor of California to provide information on possible reproductive and developmental hazards, it fails to provide a means of management of the concerns engendered by "informing" the public. Managing patient concern after exposure to a chemical identified as a reproductive or developmental toxicant under Proposition 65 is especially critical, since a pregnant woman learning after the fact that exposure to a "known" developmental toxicant has occurred may have various options (amniocentesis, ultrasound, magnetic resonance imaging, counseling, terminating the pregnancy, etc.).

Warning of the possibility of reproductive or developmental hazard from exposure may lead individuals to decide whether or not to limit or avoid exposure based on an individual assessment of personal risks and benefits of the exposure. To allow individual discretion in decision making, access to the data and to appropriately trained, knowledgeable health-care practitioners is essential. The goal of this chapter is to address the steps that are used in risk assessment for developmental toxicity, whether on a public health or an individual basis, and to provide some guidance for the physician in communicating that risk (if any) to the patient and assisting the patient in the management of that risk.

PROBLEMS FACING OBSTETRICIANS

In defining the magnitude of the problems faced by obstetricians who want to provide accurate advice to patients concerning developmental toxicity, several issues should be explored: existing data on the developmental toxicity of drugs and chemicals in animals and humans, potential for occupational and environmental exposure, and potential for drug exposure.

AVAILABLE DATA ON THE DEVELOPMENTAL TOXICITY OF CHEMICALS

It is estimated that there are approximately 90,000 chemicals in commerce in the United States.[12] About 3000 of those chemicals have been tested for developmental toxicity in experimental animals and reported in the scientific literature.[6,13,14] This means that many compounds of interest to the patient and her physician may have no published data from which any advice about the potential for developmental toxicity can be derived. For some chemicals for which published data are unavailable, the manufacturer may have collected and submitted data to a federal regulatory agency. However, obtaining and interpreting these data can be very problematic indeed for the busy obstetrician.

Of the approximately 3000 chemicals for which published data are available on developmental toxicity, between 500 and 1000 are teratogenic in animals.[4,6,15] If the ratio of hazardous to safe compounds (between 1:6 and 1:3) among tested chemicals remains the same among chemicals not tested, it suggests that 15,000 to 30,000 of the chemicals in commerce have the potential to be developmental toxicants in experimental animals. Of interest with respect to prediction of human risk for developmental toxicity, approximately 30 chemicals are thought to be developmental toxicants in humans.[4,6,15-18]

If that ratio of risk for developmental hazard persists over all chemicals, then approximately 1000 of the chemicals in use would be expected to be human developmental toxicants. If this is correct there are two interpretations: (1) the vast majority of chemicals in commerce may have little potential for human developmental toxicity, and (2) there are chemicals in use that have not been identified as developmental toxicants that may represent hazards for human fetal development.

WOMEN IN THE WORKFORCE

It is estimated that approximately 44% of the workforce (more than 45 million) are women.[12] Of these, about 75% are between 16 and 44 years old and considered to be of reproductive age. Unfortunately, because of substantial gaps in the identification of reproductive or developmental hazards, it is difficult, if not impossible, to estimate the number of women exposed to chemical, physical, or biological hazards to reproduction or development. In addition, because men are considered fertile at all ages beyond puberty, all men in the workforce have the potential to be exposed to reproductive or developmental toxicants.

DRUG USE DURING PREGNANCY

Several surveys of drug use during pregnancy have been undertaken over the past 25 years.[11,19,20] The common significant finding of these studies is that a large number of drugs are ingested during pregnancy. On average, 60% to 75% of pregnant women use from 3 to 10 medications during pregnancy. Excluded from these reviews were illicit and recreational drugs. Recent surveys have suggested that between 20% and 30% of pregnant women abuse some chemical substance during pregnancy.[21]

Uniformly, the drugs most frequently used during pregnancy fall into broad categories of analgesics and antipyretics, followed by antimicrobials and antiemetics. Many exposures involve common substances such as vitamins, caffeine, acetaminophen, alcohol, and nicotine. However, of women calling a teratogen information service, many are concerned about exposures to x-rays (14%), benzodiazepines (9%), codeine (8%), hydrocarbons/solvents (8%), pesticides (7%), amphetamines/diet pills (6%), and paint/inks/stains (6%).[22]

Given the large number of women in the workforce, the concern about environmental exposures in the home and neighboring environment and the number of women who consume licit and illicit drugs during pregnancy, it would be an unusual obstetrical practice that did not generate one or two questions about the effect of these exposures on pregnancy each week. To answer these questions obstetricians need training and ready access to animal and human data concerning the effects of chemical, biological, and physical agents on reproduction and development. At the present time both of these areas represent substantial training and information gaps.

DEVELOPMENTAL TOXICANTS

A developmental toxicant is a drug, chemical, virus, bacteria, physical agent, or deficiency state that if present before conception, during the embryonic or fetal period, or during neonatal development alters the morphology or subsequent development or function of the newly formed individual.[6,8,15,23,24] Developmental toxicology is the science that deals with the causes, mechanisms, manifestation, and prevention of developmental deviations of a structural or functional nature produced by developmental toxicants.

Many teratologists think that any chemical given in large enough amounts may affect embryonic or fetal development,[25] especially if maternal toxicity is produced. When chemicals produce toxic effects deleterious to maternal health, they also have the potential to produce fetal toxicity, which may be expressed as embryonic or fetal death, fetal growth retardation, or retardation of osseous development. Note that existing data[6,15,16,18] suggest that not all chemicals are developmental toxicants in experimental animals. As discussed previously, these data suggest that between one sixth and one third of the chemicals tested are developmental toxicants in experimental animals. The difference between the existing data on developmental toxicity and the hypothesis of Karnofsky may reflect inadequate testing, inadequate protocols, or simply the fact that not every chemical is a developmental toxicant.

Of special interest are data suggesting that reproductive and development end points are not always the most sensitive end points for toxicity. Koeter reviewed toxicity data from 37 chemicals tested for both systemic and reproductive toxicity.[26] For one third of the chemicals, reproduction was the most sensitive end point. For another one third the systemic end points of toxicity were equally sensitive. Among the compounds tested, 46% produced alterations in reproduction or development at the minimal effect level, and 54% had no effect on reproduction or development at the minimal effect level. Therefore, although reproduction and development are critical end points for toxicologic evaluation—and clearly of concern for obstetricians—these data suggest that not all chemicals will adversely effect reproduction or development. Clearly, then, each chemical needs to be evaluated for toxicity to reproduction and development as well as systemic toxicity. Regulatory approaches to protect human health should be directed to the most sensitive toxic end point. Physicians must recognize the spectrum of toxicity and not assume that reproduction and development are the most sensitive or even vulnerable.

PATTERNS OF DEVELOPMENTAL ABNORMALITY

As illustrated by the two scenarios in the introduction, when obstetricians are asked for advice on the relationship between environmental exposure and adverse developmental outcome, the questions typically represent one of two different concerns: "What is the effect of this exposure on my fetus?" or "My baby has a malformation. Was it caused by any exposures during my pregnancy?" To help understand approaches to both questions it is important to understand the types of malformations observed and the proposed etiologies of those malformations. Spranger and colleagues as well as several other investigators proposed a practical classification for developmental abnormalities.[2,27,28,32] This system separates developmental defects into several categories: malformations, disruptions, and deformations.

MALFORMATION

"A malformation is a defect that results from an intrinsically abnormal developmental process."[2,27,28] This implies that the developmental potential of the structure was abnormal from the beginning, at conception or very early in embryogenesis. Many malformations are considered to be defects of a developmental region. The whole developmental region responds as a coordinated unit during embryonic development. Therefore, abnormal development of the developmental region can result in complex or multiple malformations. For example, defects associated with Down syndrome can include abnormalities of the central nervous system, face, skeleton, cardiovascular system, skin, hair, and reproductive systems. The impact of this intrinsically abnormal developmental process is manifest in multiple developmental regions.

DISRUPTION

"A disruption is a developmental defect that results from an extrinsic or intrinsic factor producing the breakdown of, or interference with, an originally normal developmental process."[27,32] In the absence of the extrinsic or intrinsic factor (a deficiency state or chemical, biological, or physical exposure), development would have been normal. Therefore, developmental alterations following exposure to developmental toxicants should be considered disruptions. A disruption cannot be inherited. However, the genetic composition of the maternal or fetal organism may predispose to and influence the development of a disruption. For example, in some cases development of fetal phenytoin syndrome has been demonstrated to depend on fetal genotype.[5,6] Similarly, experiments using genetically defined experimental animals have demonstrated clearly the interaction of extrinsic factors with genotype in the production of developmental defects, including orofacial clefts or neural tube defects.[29,30]

DEFORMATION

"A deformation is an abnormal form, shape, or position of a part of the body that is caused by mechanical forces acting on that part of the body during development."[31] For example, in pregnancies complicated by oligohydramnios, intrauterine compression can produce alterations in the shape of the legs and feet. Another example of a deformation is the hypoplastic lung associated with herniation of the gut into the thorax during fetal development.

MULTIPLE DEVELOPMENTAL DEFECTS

Investigation of the child with multiple anomalies requires detailed consideration of the developmental processes to determine which represents the earliest malformation and temporal sequence of subsequent malformations. Once the developmentally earliest malformation is identified, consideration of the subsequent developmental processes altered may indicate that all the malformations resulted from the first. For example, if fetal kidneys do not form—a malformation—amniotic fluid volume will be lower than normal. In the absence of amniotic fluid, multiple deformations of the fetus will occur. These multiple anomalies are all secondary to the renal malformation and so would form a malformation sequence known as the oligohydramnios sequence or Potter syndrome.[2]

Identification of the initial event in abnormal development assists in understanding the etiology and classification of the abnormalities. Terms that have evolved to express pathogenesis in the child with multiple birth defects include the following.[2,27,31,32]

Polytopic field defect—multiple anomalies that result from disturbance of a single developmental field
Sequence—multiple anomalies that result from a single known or presumed malformation, deformation, or disruption
Syndrome—multiple anomalies thought to be related developmentally to a single malformation and not a polytopic field defect or sequence
Association—the occurrence of multiple anomalies thought to be associated with a malformation (although it may not be identified) in two or more individuals.

RISK ASSESSMENT FOR DEVELOPMENTAL TOXICITY

The process of risk assessment for human developmental toxicity encompasses four interrelated activities.[15,33,34] The first is hazard identification: Can this agent produce adverse developmental effects in humans or experimental animals at any exposure short of a maternally toxic or lethal dose? If so, what type of effect is produced and what is the developmental window of susceptibility for the effect(s)? The second step is hazard characterization, which, at a minimum, requires dose–response data. Note that dose–response relationships in developmental toxicity can be complicated by multiple competing end points, such as reduced fetal weight, disruption of fetal development, and fetal death. Because of this, dose–response relationships may not have the familiar sigmoidal shape.[35,36] In addition, because the use of the toxicity data in risk assessment implies extrapolation of animal data to humans, it is important to get as much information as possible on the site of toxicity and mechanism of action of the toxicant. The third step is exposure assessment: What is the likely amount of agent that the person was actually exposed to, and how much of the agent was absorbed and distributed to the fetus or placenta? The final step is risk characterization: How likely is the given exposure to result in an adverse developmental outcome, and what degree of uncertainty is inherent in that estimation?[8,10,13,16,24,37–40]

HAZARD IDENTIFICATION

In considering developmental end points of concern, two different perspectives are required: effects in humans and effects in animals. The goal of developmental toxicology is to identify exposures to chemical, physical, or biological agents that alter or impair development, before humans are exposed and suffer developmental toxicity. This means that chemical, physical, or biological agents are initially evaluated in experimental animals and data from those experiments are translated into exposure levels that are thought to protect human populations from developmental toxicity. However, as the past has demonstrated, it is not always possible to identify all developmental toxicants in animal models. Therefore, epidemiologic studies are also conducted to define the human effects of the exposure(s) of interest or concern.[36,41] This means that it is necessary to consider both animal and human end points of concern for developmental toxicity and define methods for relating these end points across species.[8,10,13,16,18,24,37,38,40,42,43]

Developmental End Points in Humans

Human outcomes of interest as measures of developmental toxicity include alterations of growth, structure, and function, in addition to death (Table 23-1). It is important, however, to recognize that many of these end points may not be independent events. For many developmental toxicants there is a spectrum of adverse developmental outcomes that may vary in frequency, severity, and type.[2,35,36] In addition, some investigators believe there is a spectrum of severity of effect. For example, at low doses a toxicant may produce growth retardation. At higher doses a specific malformation, malformation syndrome, malformation sequence, or polytopic field effect may occur. At even higher doses, fetal death may occur. It is uncommon among an exposed population to find individuals who display all the structural and functional consequences attributable to that exposure. For additional complexity, some investigators have suggested that exposures associated with neural tube defects act by preventing spontaneous abortion of the malformed fetus,[44] although more recent data do not support this view.[45] In other words, variability of both outcome and severity of effect is the rule. The sources of this variability include differences in dose, timing of exposure, host susceptibility (both maternal and fetal), and interactions with other environmental factors.

TABLE 23–1. EXAMPLES OF HUMAN END POINTS OF DEVELOPMENTAL TOXICITY

Fetal death (early and late)
Stillbirth
Perinatal death
Placental, cord, and fetal membrane abnormalities
Intrauterine growth retardation
Postnatal growth retardation
Proportionate, disproportionate
Symmetrical, asymmetrical
System limited, generalized
Change in gestational age at delivery (premature, postmature)
Altered sex ratio
Birth defects
Major, minor, mild
Malformations, deformations, disruptions
Single defects, syndromes, sequences, patterns
Mutations, chromosomal defects, monogenic disorders
Infancy and childhood morbidity and mortality
Abnormal maturation
Abnormal sexual development or function
Mental retardation/ learning disability
Specific organ system dysfunction
Developmental disabilities
Visual impairment
Hearing impairment
Cerebral palsy and other motor handicaps
Other sensory disturbances
Behavioral disorders
Transplacental carcinogenesis and mutagenesis (genotoxicity)

From Mattison DR, Hanson J, Kochhar DM, Rao KS. Criteria for identifying and listing substances known to cause developmental toxicity under California's Proposition 65. Reproductive Toxicol 1989;3:3.

It is also important to note that structural defects as an outcome of hazardous environmental exposures occur in characteristic patterns, not as random aggregates of defects.[2,4,6,15,18] Furthermore, individual defect categories (especially when classified by organ system or body region) are both etiologically and pathogenetically heterogeneous. In addition, many of the adverse outcomes (see Table 23-1) are measured and classified in different ways (and in some cases in greater detail) in humans than in animal experiments. This is especially true for birth defects, growth disturbances, and abnormalities of function, such as learning and behavior.

The classification of human structural abnormalities is different from that for animal abnormalities. Human structural abnormalities include malformations, disruptions, and deformations as previously described.[2,27] These types of abnormalities may have different pathogenic and etiologic implications from those for animals. Furthermore, some structural defects in humans may be considered to be normal variations with no clinical significance while nonetheless being important clues to mechanisms of abnormal development.[2] From the standpoint of developmental anatomy and pathology, congenital malformations may be classified as shown in Table 23-2.[32]

TABLE 23–2. CLASSIFICATION SCHEME FOR DEVELOPMENTAL ABNORMALITIES

DEVELOPMENTAL ABNORMALITY	EXAMPLES
Agenesis—developmental failure	Renal agenesis, anophthalmia
Hypoplasia—developmental arrest	Infantile uterus, cleft palate
Hyperplasia—developmental excess	Polydactyly, diabetic macrosomia
Abnormal development of skeleton	Phocomelia
Persistence of vestigial structures Failure of involution	Patent ductus arteriosus, imperforate anus
Failure to divide or canalize	Syndactyly, esophageal atresia
Dysraphia—failure to fuse	Spina bifida, cleft lip or palate
Atypical differentiation	Renal teratoma, neuroblastoma
Accessory (several centers or organogenesis) or ectopic (abnormal site of) development	Supernumerary nipples and ectopic ureters

Adapted from Persaud TVN, Chudley AE, Skalko RG. Basic concepts in teratology. New York: Alan R Liss, 1985.

Thus, there are many different types of end points or outcomes in humans that are identified as developmental effects. These end points are measured differently and may be interpreted differently from those observed in animal studies. Skilled laboratory scientists and clinicians should be involved in the interpretation of human studies, especially those in which postnatal functional abnormalities (eg, learning and behavior) are end points of concern.

Developmental End Points in Animals

Developmental toxicity in animals is defined as the adverse effect of a chemical on the conceptus associated with exposure during pregnancy or during postnatal development. These effects may be manifest during the embryonic or fetal periods or postnatally. Developmental toxicity can include growth retardation, death of the conceptus, structural malformation, and functional deficits (Table 23-3).[37]

The end points of developmental toxicity encountered in experimental animals do not and should not necessarily be expected to mimic those observed in humans exposed to the same toxicant. This is an important concept to grasp so as not to discard the results from animal studies when they have different outcomes from those observed or suspected in humans. Similarly, specific substance-related end points in humans are not always reproduced in experimental animals. The absence of absolute uniformity of response is not surprising, however, when the differences that exist between the conditions of human and experimental animal exposure are considered. For example, differences in dosage, placentation, metabolism, pharmacokinetics, critical periods of development, durations of gestation, and so on, can be expected to influence expression of developmental toxicity.

In general, mammalian developmental toxicity experiments should include a dose that is toxic to the mother. This may or may not result in toxic effects in the conceptus (death, morphologic alteration, delayed development, or functional impairment). As previously discussed, one criterion for identifying a development toxicant is determination of the relative toxicity of the

TABLE 23–3. EXAMPLES OF DEVELOPMENTAL ALTERATIONS OBSERVED IN LABORATORY ANIMALS

MAJOR EFFECTS	VARIATIONS
Cleft lip/palate	Delayed ossification of bones
Aphakia	Lumbar ribs
Anophthalmia	Wavy ribs
Renal agenesis	Unfused centers of ossification
Malformed heart valves, vessels	Extra center of sternebral ossification
Gastroschisis	Increased renal pelvic cavitation
Missing ribs, vertebrae	Hemorrhages at some sites
Exencephaly	Displaced testes
Spina bifida	Some types of hydroureter
Missing or malformed limbs	
Fetal death	
Increased number of resorptions	

From Wang GM, Schwetz BA. An evaluation system of ranking chemicals with teratogenic potential. Teratogenesis Carcinog Mutagen 1987;7:133.

substance to the adult mother and the developing conceptus.[46] In humans there appear to be exposures that produce developmental toxicity in the absence of maternal toxicity (eg, thalidomide, diethylstilbestrol, ionizing radiation) and exposures that produce developmental toxicity at exposure levels that are used therapeutically or that result in maternal physiologic or toxicologic changes (eg, tobacco, steroidal hormones, alcohol, methylmercury, 13-*cis*-retinoic acid, phenytoin, and valproic acid).

Timing of Exposure

One definition of developmental toxicity used by some regulatory agencies is "adverse effects on the developing organism that may result from exposure prior to conception to either parent, during prenatal development or if a result of prenatal exposure, postnatal to the time of sexual maturity."[47] Most developmental toxicants, however, produce their effects during specific critical developmental periods, which vary across both compounds and species. A fundamental concept of developmental toxicology is that some stages of embryonic development are more vulnerable than others. The time of exposure to a developmental toxicant determines not only severity of damage, but the type of defect (Table 23-4).

For some animal developmental toxicants, critical periods have not been reliably established because exposure to the conceptus continues throughout pregnancy. For some compounds, however, detailed studies have been conducted at different doses and times during pregnancy.[6,15] For these chemicals clear definition of critical period and sensitive developmental processes can be defined. These studies indicate that the susceptible period is generally the time of maximal tissue proliferation and differentiation in a particular organ. Time specificity has also been found in nearly all cases where developmental toxicity of the human has been proven and studied in detail.

The period of development during which the conceptus is exposed to an agent largely determines its sensitivity to developmental toxicity. It is generally thought that exposure during the preimplantation or presomite periods (0–14 days after fertilization) produces little altered morphogenesis because the ovum either dies or regenerates completely. Recent data from Generoso, however, suggest that this hypothesis may be incorrect.[48–50] During organogenesis (up to 60 days) the embryo is highly sensitive to developmental toxicity, and exposure can produce major morphologic changes. After this period the fetus is less sensitive to morphologic alterations, but functional changes can occur in selected organs throughout pregnancy and even during postnatal development (eg, effects of lead on the central nervous system).

By the third trimester much of the structure of the fetus has been defined. During this period, however, many of the functional characteristics of the fetus are being developed. For example, cellular communication (eg, neuronal contacts) is being developed, as is the cell number in many organ systems. In addition, the fetus remains vulnerable to cytotoxic or disruptive processes during the third trimester. Finally, during the third trimester, issues of fetal toxicity from environmental exposure remain a substantial concern.

TABLE 23–4. CRITICAL PERIODS FOR DEVELOPMENTAL TOXICITY IN THE HUMAN

DAYS FROM LMP	DAYS FROM CONCEPTION*	BIOLOGICAL EVENT
14	0	Ovulation
15–16	1	Conception
19–21	5–7	Implantation/Blastula
38–39	24–25	Anterior neuropore closes
40–41	26–27	Posterior neuropore closes
41–42	27–28	Upper limb bud develops
43–44	29–30	Lower limb bud develops
51	37	Crown–rump 10 mm
60–61	46–47	Heart septation
70–72	56–58	Palate closed
98	84	Second trimester begins

* Based on 28-day menstrual cycle.

HAZARD IDENTIFICATION WITH INCOMPLETE DATA

Although regulatory agencies may have the luxury of silence in the face of uncertainty or missing data, physicians are still expected to provide rational guidance to their patients. The general principles outlined later suggest some approaches that may assist the process of providing advice.[43] Equally important, patients must understand the quality and quantity of data from which advice is derived.

If no animal or human evidence is available that addresses the developmental hazard posed by a chemical, it is difficult to assign a risk at any exposure dose. The most that can be said is that the risk is unknown. The one caveat to this is if exposure is at a level that produces maternal toxicity, then an indirect effect is always possible.[25] If, however, any human reports or animal studies suggest a possible hazard or if there are physical or chemical properties of the compound that would make it more or less likely to be a hazard, then, depending upon the weight of the evidence, it is important to proceed further in calculating effect and exposure doses.[43]

It would be important to know if the physical structure is similar to a known developmental toxicant (eg, methyltestosterone and testosterone). Does the compound belong to a class of compounds known to be developmental toxicants (eg, antimetabolites or antithyroid compounds)? Does the drug or compound have a mechanism of action similar to a known developmental toxicant (eg, bind with an estrogen receptor)? Is the compound a mutagen or cytotoxic agent (eg, cyclophosphamide)? Any of these characteristics heighten suspicion, suggesting the potential for developmental toxicity even if no animal or human data are available.

If there are human studies that look for developmental toxicity from the substance, it is important to define the outcome pattern for each study and the timing of exposure that would produce that outcome. Often, however, human data are not available or are so sketchy that interpretation is almost impossible.

If there are any animal studies that look for developmental toxicity from the substance, it is important to characterize the pattern of toxicity in each animal species, as well as the highest no-observed-abnormal effect level for each study. Are there any weaknesses of the study design that would lower confidence in the study?

Implicit in this first step in risk assessment is the assumption that reproductive or developmental hazards identified in animals are predictive of reproductive or developmental hazard in humans. Note that the converse, failure to demonstrate reproductive or developmental hazard, is also generally assumed to reflect safety following human exposure. It is important to review critically the accuracy of this assumption.[6,15,18,42,43]

Frankos has reviewed the concordance of animal and human data for 38 drugs reported to be developmental toxicants in humans and 165 reported not to produce developmental toxicity.[16] Of the 38 drugs identified as human teratogens, 37 were positive in at least one species of experimental animal and 29 were positive in more than one test species. Among the 165 compounds identified as nonteratogenic in humans, only 47 were negative in all species tested.

Recently, we have also conducted a detailed analysis of the predictive power of developmental toxicity testing in experimental animals using statistical techniques.[18,42] These studies suggest that combining animal data using statistical models, although generally useful for predicting human developmental toxicants, may be inadequate for regulation, causation, or clinical guidance.[18] Thus, positive or negative animal studies do not always mean hazard or safety for humans. However, that evidence should be evaluated for hazard identification. A more detailed assessment of the rules used by developmental toxicologists to assign hazard for developmental toxicity has been assembled and may assist the process of hazard identification.[43]

HAZARD CHARACTERIZATION

At a minimum, hazard characterization requires demonstration of the dose–response relationship for the developmental toxicant. Given the species differences in development as well as the tendency for animal studies to have a high false-positive rate,[16,18,42] it would be much better to have information on the site and mechanism of action of the developmental toxicant in the animal species studied. Like hazard identification, hazard characterization suffers from the lack of published peer-reviewed data.[3,14] As a result, even the minimal requirement for dose–response information is often not available to health professionals charged with risk assessment.

For any chemical that has been identified as a developmental toxicant in either a human or animal study, it is important to know if the offending agent is the parent compound or a metabolite. This is especially true when animal studies are positive, because the metabolic pathway may be different in humans, so that the metabolite that produced an animal malformation may not be produced in the human. What is the compound's absorption by different likely routes of exposure and what is the likely fetal exposure at different maternal doses (extent of placental transport)? In addition, it is important to extract from the studies the different levels of effect (eg, lowest-observed-abnormal-effect level, the no-observed-abnormal-effect level, the maternal toxic effect level) and for drugs the maternal therapeutic effect level. All these levels will play a role in assessing the likelihood that a given exposure is above or below the threshold for developmental toxicity.[51]

EXPOSURE ASSESSMENT

During exposure assessment, it is important to determine if there was exposure to a dose that could cause an indirect or direct developmental effect. If the exposure was at or near maternally toxic levels, or if the exposed individual manifests toxic side effects, then there is always the possibility of an indirect effect whether or not the compound is known or suspected to be a hazard. If the compound is a known or suspected hazard, the toxic side effects are evidence that the chemical(s) did get into the maternal bloodstream and thus the fetus is presumably at greater risk. The route of exposure and the absorption via that route considering gestational age bring into play our knowledge of the physiology of pregnancy and its likely effects on the pharmacokinetics of the compound.[52,53] All this information is used to estimate the dose to which the fetus was exposed and its likely range.

Because of unique windows of vulnerability for developmental toxicants, exposure assessment requires accurate determination of the dose, the duration of exposure, and the relationship of exposure to windows of developmental vulnerability. If, for example, the exposure occurred prior to conception and clearance of the parent compound and any metabolites also occurred prior to conception, it is unlikely that any excess fetal risk would result. Although the physician or health care professional may have some knowledge of dose, duration of exposure, and relationship of exposure to stages of fetal development for prescription drugs, information on environmental or occupational exposures is likely to be scanty.

RISK CHARACTERIZATION

The final step of risk assessment, risk characterization, requires a methodology for translating the developmental toxicity data in animals and humans and estimates of

Continued on page 338

TABLE 23-5. IMPACT OF DRUGS ON THE FETUS

CLASS AND COMPOUND	RISK	COMMENT
Analgesics and Antipyretics		
Aspirin	S	Large doses may be toxic to mother and fetus
Acetaminophen	S	Fetal renal and maternal and fetal hepatic toxicity in large doses
Narcotic Analgesics		
Codeine	C	Respiratory malformations, withdrawal
Pentazocine	S	Withdrawal with chronic use
Meperidine	S	Withdrawal with chronic use
Antibiotics		
Penicillins	S	Routine use for infections during pregnancy
Cephalosporins	C	Probably safe, few epidemiologic studies
Tetracyclines	N	Incorporation in teeth and bones, maternal hepatic toxicity and acute fatty metamorphosis
Streptomycin	C	Ototoxicity at high doses, interaction with $MgSO_4$
Gentamicin	C	Ototoxicity not reported, interaction with $MgSO_4$
Tobramycin	C	Ototoxicity not reported, interaction with $MgSO_4$
Amikacin	C	Ototoxicity not reported
Chloramphenicol	C	Cardiovascular collapse (gray syndrome)
Sulfonamides	S	Displace bilirubin from albumin hemolysis, anemia and hyperbilirubinemia in G6PD deficiency
Nitrofurantoin	S	
Metronidazole	C	Avoid during first trimester
Trimethoprim–sulfamethoxazole	C	Folic acid antagonist
Antituberculosis		
Isoniazid	S	Drug of choice for tuberculosis treatment during pregnancy
Rifampin	S	Drug of choice for tuberculosis treatment during pregnancy
Ethambutol	C	
Para-aminosalicylic acid	C	
Immunizing Agents		
Live-virus vaccines	N	
Attenuated vaccines	N	
Killed-virus vaccines	S	
Tetanus toxoid	C	
Diphtheria toxoid	C	
Antinauseant		
Cyclizine	S	
Buclizine	S	
Meclizine	S	
Prochlorperazine	S	
Trimethobenzamide	S	
Antihistamines		
Diphenhydramine	C	Gentiourinary malformations
Chlorpheniramine	S	
Brompheniramine	S	
Sedatives		
Barbiturates	C	Conflicting data on malformations, dependence with prolonged use
Ethanol	N	Fetal alcohol syndrome, craniofacial and limb abnormalities, microcephaly
Tranquilizers		
Chlordiazepoxide	C	Conflicting data on malformations, dependence with prolonged use
Meprobamate	C	Conflicting data on malformations, dependence with prolonged use
Diazepam	C	Oral clefts
Antidepressants		
Lithium carbonate	N	Cardiovascular anomaly
Imipramine	C	Neonatal withdrawal
Amitriptyline	C	Neonatal withdrawal
Doxepin	C	
Anesthetics		
Inhalational	C	Spontaneous abortion

(continued)

TABLE 23–5. (continued)

CLASS AND COMPOUND	RISK	COMMENT
Anticonvulsants		
Phenytoin	C	Fetal hydantoin syndrome, define benefit:risk ratio
Carbamazepine	C	Conflicting data on malformations
Ethosuximide	C	Conflicting data on malformations, drug of choice for petit mal in pregnancy
Primidone	C	Conflicting data on malformations
Valproic acid	N	CNS, neural tube defects
Trimethadione	N	Congenital malformations, abortion
Paramethadione	N	Congenital malformations, abortion
Aminophyllines		
Theophylline	S	Bronchodilator of choice in pregnancy
Diuretics	C	Initiation of use during pregnancy discouraged
Reserpine and Rauwolfia		
Alkaloids		
Reserpine	C	
Methyldopa	C	
Vasodilators		
Hydralizine	C	Drug of choice in preeclampsia, eclampsia
Sodium nitroprusside	C	Produces increased cyanide levels in fetus
Digitalis	S	
Hypoglycemic		
Tolbutamide	N	Not indicated during pregnancy
Antithyroid and Iodine		
Propylthiouracil	N	Mild fetal hypothyroidism and goiter, drug of choice for hyperthyroidism in pregnancy
Potassium iodide	N	Fetal hypothyroidism and goiter
Povidone iodide	N	Fetal hypothyroidism and goiter
Steroids		
Cortisone	C	
Betamethasone	C	Prevention of respiration distress
Diethylstilbestrol	N	Uterine and vaginal malformations (adenosis), epididymal cysts, hypotrophic testes, infertility
Estradiol	N	Congenital defects
Medroxyprogesterone	C	Possible congenital defects
Methyltestosterone	N	Masculinization
Anticoagulants		
Heparin	S	Anticoagulant of choice, prolonged use associated with maternal osteopenia
Coumarins	N	Nasal hypoplasia, shortened extremities, abortion
Antimalarials		
Chloroquine	C	Drug of choice for malaria, small increased risk for malformations
Quinine	C	Abortion, conflicting data on malformations
Pyimethamine	C	Folic acid antagonist
Cancer Chemotherapeutic		
Aminopterin	N	Malformations, spontaneous abortions
Busulfan	N	Multiple visceral malformations, abortion
Chlorambucil	N	Renal agenesis
Cyclophosphamide	N	Conflicting data on malformations, ovarian and testicular toxicity
Cytarabine	N	Malformations and chromosome abnormalities
Fluorouracil	N	Multiple anomalies
Mechlorethamine	N	
Methotrexate	N	Malformations similar to aminopterin, folic acid antagonist
Procarbazine	N	Malformations, decreased spermatogenesis
Antiacne		
Retinoids	N	Spontaneous abortion, hydrocephalus, microcephalus, ear and eye abnormalities, cardiovascular malformations
Miscellaneous		
Penicillamine	N	Skin lesion (cutis laxa)
Disulfiram	N	Multiple anomalies

S, Safe in normal exposure doses.
C, Caution, therapeutic indication should outweigh possible small risk.
N, Human developmental toxicant; use during pregnancy requires careful risk benefit analysis.

time and duration of exposure into a qualitative or quantitative estimate of excess risk. On a population level there are methods for estimating human risk for developmental toxicity from animal studies.[38,43] However, there is still considerable disagreement on the validity of these methods, because they do not consider species differences in reproduction or development, nor do they consider species differences in site or mechanism of action of the reproductive or developmental toxicants.

If the window of exposure is inconsistent with a known or suspected effect and the compound is a known teratogen, how much reassurance will the patient get from our calculations? It is at this point that the risk assessment procedure becomes somewhat subjective and we must admit the lack of hard-and-fast rules for assigning the final risk. Having completed the data-gathering process of risk assessment, whatever conclusions are drawn are more likely to represent the actual risk of developmental toxicity than if one merely guesses ("In my professional opinion. . .") or counsels, "Don't worry," or, "When in doubt, terminate the pregnancy." Again, it is important that our patients understand that not all pregnancies end with the birth of a normal child. Finally, we must clearly communicate the quality and quantity of data from which our estimates of reproductive and developmental risk are derived.

IMPACT OF DRUGS AND CHEMICALS ON THE FETUS

Using the approach outlined earlier, we have formulated a listing of drugs (Table 23-5) and chemicals (Table 23-6) and attempted to characterize their risk to the fetus, if any. The data on these two tables reflect a qualitative attempt at hazard identification. It is important to reemphasize that existing data suggest that many more chemicals are developmental toxicants in experimental animals than have been identified as developmental toxicants in humans. This may reflect several factors, including differences in species sensitivity, level of exposure, or epidemiologic insensitivity (see Hemminki and Vineis,[17] for a discussion of this issue). The listing of drugs and chemicals in Tables 23-5 and 23-6 indicates an estimate of their hazard for human development and comments on the effects observed. This listing utilizes review material and interpretation of several other authors.[6,15,18] We may not agree with all the classifications, but we present them for consideration by the reader.

ANALGESICS AND ANTIPYRETIC DRUGS

High doses of aspirin can be toxic during pregnancy, prolonging gestation and increasing the risk of maternal and fetal hemorrhage. Acetaminophen is suspect for producing both maternal and fetal renal toxicity with chronic use of high doses.

NARCOTIC ANALGESICS

Among the narcotic analgesics, codeine has been associated with respiratory malformations, and heroin has been associated with a high incidence of chromosome variations. In these studies, however, it is important to try to distinguish life-style factors such as nutrition and infection from fetal and maternal toxicity associated directly with substance abuse. That unfortunately has not been clearly defined. Medical use, however, appears to carry little, if any, fetal risk.

ANTIBIOTICS

Among the antibiotics, penicillin and cephalosporins are believed to be safe for use in pregnancy. Tetracyclines are associated with discoloration of teeth due to enamel hypoplasia and are incorporated into bone. Streptomycin, gentamycin, tobramycin, and amikacin all carry the potential for damage of the eighth cranial nerve in both mother and fetus. Among women treated near term, chloramphenicol has the potential for neonatal cardiovascular collapse because of its slow clearance. In addition, treatment near term with sulfonamides, drugs demonstrated to compete with bilirubin for binding sites on albumin, may increase bilirubin levels in the newborn and increase risk for kernicterus. Nitrofurantoin use during pregnancy may be associated with hemolysis, anemia, and hyperbilirubinemia, especially in glucose-6-phosphate dehydrogenase-deficient infants, if this drug is used near term. Although there are no data that suggest that the use of metronidazole during pregnancy carries with it any increased risk, it is best to avoid the use of this drug during the first trimester. Among the drugs used to treat tuberculosis, available evidence suggests that use during pregnancy with vitamin B_6 supplementation carries no increased risk to the fetus.

IMMUNIZATIONS

Immunizing agents or vaccines that contain live viruses should not be used during pregnancy. However, killed virus vaccines in general are safe.

ANTIHISTAMINES

Among the antihistamines, diphenhydramine has been associated with genitourinary malformation. However, these data are not strong.

SEDATIVES

Among the sedatives, alcohol has certainly been associated with fetal structural and functional malforma-

TABLE 23–6. IMPACT OF CHEMICALS IN INDUSTRY AND THE ENVIRONMENT ON THE FETUS

CLASS AND COMPOUND	RISK	COMMENT
Methyl mercury	N	Microcephaly, mental retardation, cerebral palsy
Acetone	C	Sacral abnormalities, campomelic syndrome
Benzene	C	Spontaneous abortions, premature births
Boric acid	C	Conflicting data on malformation rate
Carbon disulfide	C	Spontaneous abortions, sperm abnormalities, abnormal menses
Carbon monoxide	C	Stillbirth with maternal toxicity
Chloroprene	C	Possible mental defects, chromosomal abnormalities
1,2-dibromo-3-chloropropane	C	Testicular toxicity, spontaneous abortion
Dichloromethane	C	Spontaneous abortion
Dinitrodipropylsulfanilamide	C	Miscarriage, heart defects
Ethylene dibromide	C	Decreased fertility
Formaldehyde	C	Spontaneous abortion
Hexachlorobenzene	C	Stillbirth
Lead	N	Increased abortion rate, stillbirth, central nervous system toxicity
Mercuric chloride	C	Spontaneous abortion
Methylethyl ketone	C	Spontaneous abortion
Methylparathion	C	Malformations
Polychlorinated biphenyls	N	Brown skin in newborns, growth retardation, exophthalmos
Sodium selenite	C	Spontaneous abortions, limb defects
Styrene	C	Spontaneous abortion
Toluene	C	Growth retardation, malformations
Trichloroethylene	C	Malformations, sacral agenesis
Vinyl chloride	C	Spontaneous abortions
Xylene	C	Sacral agenesis

C = Caution; may pose risk of developmental toxicity during pregnancy.
N = Known human developmental toxicant.

tions. Among the tranquilizers, chlordiazepoxide, meprobamate, and diazepam in general are felt to be safe to use during pregnancy.

ANTIDEPRESSANTS

Lithium carbonate is associated with cardiovascular anomalies, and so careful attention to risk versus benefit for use during pregnancy is important. Among the monoamine oxidase inhibitors limited data are available. In general, their use should be balanced by consideration of benefit.

ANTICONVULSANTS

As seizure disorders will require treatment during pregnancy it is important to balance risk versus benefit. This class of patients, along with any patients on chronic medication, should be evaluated carefully and counseled prior to conception. Among the anticonvulsant drugs considered to be relatively safe to use during pregnancy, the barbiturates, ethosuximide, and primidone appear to be safest.

INDUSTRIAL AND ENVIRONMENTAL EXPOSURES

Among the occupational and environmental exposures listed, only three are identified as known human developmental toxicants: methyl mercury, lead, and polychlorinated biphenyls. Caution is indicated for all the others. Does that mean that these chemicals actually pose risks to human reproduction and development? The data for each chemical are quite variable, and careful assessment of potential for reproductive or developmental hazard is necessary. Even if the chemical of concern is determined to represent a reproductive or developmental hazard, additional information is needed to define the actual risk to the reproductive or developmental process. These steps, outlined earlier, include hazard characterization, exposure assessment, and the final step of qualitative or quantitative risk assessment. Only when all these steps have been completed can the assessment of risk be defined.

SUMMARY

As suggested by the scenarios at the beginning of this chapter, by legislative changes like California's Proposition 65, and by general patient concern, the need for obstetricians to become familiar with risk assessment in reproductive and developmental toxicity is becoming more acute. This will require training in risk assessment methodology, including hazard identification, hazard characterization, exposure characterization, and quantitative risk characterization. In addition to the need for training, there are substantial data gaps in developmental toxicity that will need to be addressed as a national priority in toxicology and public health.

An important consideration in all risk assessment methodology is the utility of animal studies in predicting human toxicity. Existing data suggest that despite shortcomings, developmental toxicity assessment in experimental animals is useful for regulatory policy development and human health protection. Limitation in animal developmental toxicity data will be corrected by increasing the number of compounds tested and improving our understanding of the toxicokinetics, site, and mechanism of action of developmental toxicants.

One of the constants in medicine is the need to make recommendations, provide guidance, and make decisions based on inadequate data. This is especially true in developmental toxicology. It is important for physicians providing counsel about the risk for developmental toxicity to define clearly the quality and quantity of information used in providing that advice.

The challenges facing developmental toxicology are substantial. Quantitative risk assessment methodology needs to be improved. Enormous data gaps exist, frustrating health care professionals charged with providing guidance. The number of health care professionals trained in risk assessment for reproductive and developmental toxicology is much too small. Our ability to address and meet these challenges will clearly reflect our commitment to the future.

ACKNOWLEDGMENT

This chapter draws upon the previous writing and research of both authors individually and collectively. In the preparation of this chapter we have drawn from previous publications,[8,10,18,42,43] the proceedings of two expert committee reports on the criteria for identifying reproductive[10] and developmental toxicants,[8] and a chapter entitled Environmental and Occupational Exposures scheduled for publication in Reproductive Risks and Prenatal Diagnosis edited by M. Evans and to be published by Appleton.

REFERENCES

1. Myrianthopoulos, NC. Malformations in children from one to seven years: a report from the perinatal project. New York: Alan R Liss, 1985.
2. Jones KL. Smith's recognizable patterns of human malformation. 4th ed. Philadelphia: WB Saunders, 1988.
3. Barlow SM, Sullivan FM. Reproductive hazards of industrial chemicals: an evaluation of animal and human data. New York: Academic Press, 1982.
4. Sever JL, Brent RL Teratogen update: environmentally induced birth defect risks. New York: Alan R Liss, 1986.
5. Hanson JW. Fetal hydantoin effects. In: Sever JL, Brent RL (eds). Teratogen update: environmentally induced birth defect risks. New York: Alan R Liss, 1986:29.
6. Shepard TH. Catalog of teratologic agents. 5th ed. Baltimore: Johns Hopkins University Press, 1986.
7. Brent RL. The complexities of solving the problem of human malformations. In: Sever JL, Brent RL (eds). Teratogen update: environmentally induced birth defect risks. New York: Alan R Liss, 1986:189.
8. Mattison DR, Hanson J, Kochhar DM, Rao KS. Criteria for identifying and listing substances known to cause developmental toxicity under California's Proposition 65. Reproductive Toxicol 1989;3:3.
9. Koren G, Bologa M, Long D, Feldman Y, Shear NH. Perception of teratogenic risk by pregnant women exposed to drugs and chemicals during the first trimester. Am J Obstet Gynecol 1989;160:1190.
10. Mattison DR, Working PK, Blazak WF, Hughes CL Jr, Killinger JM, Olive DL, Rao, KS. Criteria for identifying and listing substances known to cause reproductive toxicity under California's Proposition 65. Reproductive Toxicol 1990;4:163.
11. Koren G. Maternal-fetal toxicology: a clinicians guide. New York: Marcel Dekker, 1990.
12. Reproductive health hazards in the workplace. Office of Technology Assessment. Washington, DC: Congress of the United States; 1985. US Government Printing Office OTA-BA-266.
13. Schardein JL. Teratogenic risk assessment: past, present, and future. In: Kalter H, ed. Issues and reviews in teratology. Vol 1. New York: Plenum Press, 1983:181.
14. National Research Council Toxicity Testing. Strategies to determine needs and priorities. Steering Committee on Identification of Toxic and Potentially Toxic Chemicals for Consideration by the National Toxicology Program. Board on Toxicology and Environmental Health Hazards. Commission on Life Sciences. Washington, DC: National Academy Press, 1984.
15. Schardein JL. Chemically induced birth defects. New York: Marcel Dekker, 1985.
16. Frankos VH. FDA perspectives on the use of teratology data for human risk assessment. Fundam Appl Toxicol 1985;5:615.
17. Hemminki K, Vineis P. Extrapolation of the evidence on teratogenicity of chemicals between humans and experimental animals: chemicals other than drugs. Teratogenesis Carcinog Mutagen 1985;5:251.
18. Jelovsek FR, Mattison DR, Chen J. Prediction of risk for human development toxicity: how important are animal studies? Obstet Gynecol 1989;74(4):624.
19. Quirk JG. Use and misuse of drugs in pregnancy. In: Fabro S, Scialli A, eds. Drug and chemical action in pregnancy: pharmacologic and toxicologic principles. New York: Marcel Dekker, 1986:477.
20. Heinonen OP, Slone D, Shapiro S. Birth defects and drugs in pregnancy. Littleton, MA: John Wright PSG Inc, 1983.
21. Chasnoff IJ, Landress HJ, Barrett ME. The prevalence of illicit-drug or alcohol use during pregnancy and discrepancies in mandatory reporting in Pinellas County, Florida. N Engl J Med 1990;322(17):1202.
22. Vogt BL. Teratogen information programs. In: Koren G, ed. Maternal-fetal toxicology: a clinicians guide. New York: Marcel Dekker, 1990:329.
23. Stein Z, Kline J, Kharrazi M. What is a teratogen? In: Kalter H, ed. Epidemiologic criteria issues and reviews in teratology. Vol 2. New York: Plenum Press, 1984:23.
24. Fabro S. On predicting environmentally-induced human reproductive hazards: an overview and historical perspective. Fundam Appl Toxicol 1985;5:609.

25. Karnofsky DA. Drugs as teratogens in animals and man. Ann Rev Pharmacol 1965;5:447.
26. Koeter HBWM. Relevance of parameters related to fertility and reproduction in toxicity testing. In: Mattison DR, ed. Reproductive toxicology. New York: Alan R Liss 1983:81.
27. Spranger J, Bernischke K, Hall JG, Lenz W, Lowry RB, Opitz JM, et al. Errors of morphogenesis: concepts and terms. J Pediatr 1982;100:160.
28. Persaud TVN, Chudley AE, Skalko RG. Basic concepts in teratology. New York: Alan R Liss, 1985.
29. Seller MJ. Neural-tube defects: cause and prevention. In: Matteo A, Benson P, Giannelli F, Seller M, eds. Pediatric research: a genetic approach. Spastics International Medical Publication. Lavenham, Suffolk: The Lavenham Press, 1982.
30. Pratt RM. Hormones, growth factors, and their receptors in normal and abnormal prenatal development. In: Kalter H, ed. Issues and reviews in teratology. Vol 2. New York: Plenum Press, 1984:189.
31. Graham JM Jr. Smith's recognizable patterns of human deformation. 2nd ed. Philadelphia: WB Saunders, 1988.
32. Persaud TVN. Classification and epidemiology of developmental defects. In: Persaud TVN, Chudley AE, Skalko, RG, eds. Basic concepts in teratology. New York: Alan R Liss, 1985:13.
33. National Research Council. Committee on the Institutional Means for the Assessment of Risks to Public Health. Risk assessment in the Federal government; managing the process. Commission on Life Sciences, National Research Council. Washington, DC: National Academy Press, 1983.
34. Sheehan DM, Young JF, Slikker W Jr, Gaylor DW, Mattison, DR. Workshop on risk assessment in reproductive and developmental toxicology: addressing the assumptions and identifying the research needs. Regul Toxicol Pharmacol 1989;10:110.
35. Selevan SG, Lemasters GK. The dose-response fallacy in human reproductive studies of toxic exposures. J Occup Med 1987;29(5):451.
36. Kline J, Stein Z, Susser M. Conception to birth: epidemiology of prenatal development. New York: Oxford University Press, 1989.
37. Wang GM, Schwetz BA. An evaluation system of ranking chemicals with teratogenic potential. Teratogenesis Carcinog Mutagen 1987:7:133.
38. Hart WL, Reynolds RC, Krasavage WJ, Ely TS, Bell RH, Raleigh RL. Evaluation of developmental toxicity data: a discussion of some pertinent factors and a proposal. Risk Analysis 1988;8:59.
39. Kimmel CA, Wellington DG, Farland W, Ross P, et al. Overview of a workshop on quantitative models for developmental toxicity risk assessment. Environ Health Perspect 1989;79:209.
40. Schardein JL, Schwetz BA, Kenel MF. Species sensitivities and prediction of teratogenic potential. Environ Health Perspect 1985;61:55.
41. Bracken MB. Perinatal epidemiology. New York: Oxford University Press, 1984.
42. Mattison DR, Jelovsek FR. Pharmacokinetics and expert systems as aids for risk assessment in reproductive toxicology. Environ Health Perspect 1987;76:107.
43. Jelovsek FR, Mattison DR, Young JF. Eliciting principles of hazard identification from experts. Teratology. 42;521:1990.
44. Roberts CJ, Lloyd S. Area differences in spontaneous abortion rates in South Wales in their relation to neural tube defect incidence. Br Med J 1973;4:20.
45. Byrne J, Warburton D. Neural tube defects in spontaneous abortion. Am J Med Genet 1986;25:327.
46. Fabro S, Schull G, Brown NA. The relative teratogenic index and teratogenic potency: proposed components of developmental toxicity risk assessment. Teratogenesis Carcinog Mutagen 1982;2:61.
47. US Environmental Protection Agency. Guidelines for the health assessment of suspect developmental toxicants. Federal Register 1986;51:340280.
48. Rutledge JC, Generoso WM. Fetal pathology produced by ethylene oxide treatment of the murine zygote. Teratology 1989;39(6):563.
49. Katoh M, Cacheiro NL, Cornett CV, Cain KT, et al. Fetal anomalies produced subsequent to treatment of zygotes with ethylene oxide or ethyl methanesulfonate are not likely due to the usual genetic causes. Mutat Res 1989;210(2):337.
50. Generoso WM, Katoh M, Cain KT, Hughes LA, et al. Chromosome malsegregation and embryonic lethality induced by treatment of normally ovulated mouse oocytes with nocodazole. Mutat Res 1989;210(2):313.
51. Gaylor DW, Sheehan DM, Young JF, Mattison DR. The threshold dose question in teratogenesis. Teratology 1988;8:389.
52. Mattison DR. Physiological variations in pharmacokinetics during pregnancy. In: Fabro S, Scialli AR, eds. Drug and chemical action in pregnancy. New York: Marcel Dekker, 1986:37.
53. Mattison DR, Malek A, Cistola C. Physiological adaptations to pregnancy: impact on pharmacokinetics. In: SJ Yaffe, J Aranda, eds. Pediatric pharmacology: therapeutic principles in practice. 2nd ed. In press.

24

CHAPTER

VIRAL-INDUCED TERATOGENESIS

John L. Sever

Five viruses are known to be teratogenic to humans: cytomegalovirus, rubella, herpes simplex, Venezuelan equine encephalitis, and varicella viruses. Other viruses that can infect and produce disease or death of the fetus are influenza, rubeola, Western equine encephalitis, variola, vaccinia, hepatitis B, echoviruses, poliovirus, parvovirus B-19, and human immunodeficiency virus (HIV). The teratogenic effects of infections with these five viruses during pregnancy are reviewed in this chapter.

Epidemiologic studies using clinical data, virus isolation, and serology have provided estimates for the frequencies of these five viral infections in pregnant women and their children (Table 24-1). Factors that influence the data for the frequency of these infections include the population sampled, the occurrence of epidemics, the method of diagnosis used, the use of vaccines for rubella, delivery by cesarean section when maternal herpes infection is present, changing social behavior, and the use of therapeutic abortions.

CYTOMEGALOVIRUS

Maternal infections with cytomegalovirus are frequent. In most studies, 3% to 5% of women shed this virus at term.[1] Almost all of these women are asymptomatic. About one third of the children of infected women are also infected at birth, and many more acquire this infection in the first months of life. Severe damage due to congenital cytomegalovirus infection occurs at a rate of about 1 in 5,000 to 1 in 20,000 births. Studies of asymptomatic infected newborns, however, suggest that as many as 10% to 15% of these children have some damage due to this infection. The most frequent problems are low intelligence and some degree of deafness.

The most common cause of congenital infection is cytomegalovirus (CMV) (Table 24-2). Several serologic surveys in the United States have shown that approximately one half of adult women have antibody to this virus.[2] In addition, CMV can be isolated from the cervix or urine of 3% to 5% of pregnant women.[1] The great majority of infected women are asymptomatic. Occasionally, cervicitis and illness resembling infectious mononucleosis are caused by infection with these viruses. Infection can be documented by isolation of the virus from the urine or cervical area, or by the production of antibody. The fluorescent and ELISA tests appear to be the most practical and reliable methods for detecting antibody and seroconversions.[3]

Congenital infection with CMV occurs in 0.5% to 1.5% of births.[4] Present information indicates that as many as 10% to 15% of these children exhibit permanent damage in the form of mental or motor retardation or deafness. Children with normal neurologic findings at 2 years of age generally have a good prognosis. The severe form of cytomegalic inclusion disease occurs in 1 in 5,000 to 1 in 20,000 live births. Congenital infection can be documented by isolation of the virus from the nasopharynx or urine. Specific IgM cytomegalovirus antibody is also present in many of the infected newborns.

Fetal infection apparently results from hematogenous spread from the mother. The infection is usually widely disseminated, and the virus can be isolated from many tissues. Damage to the brain includes direct tissue destruction with the formation of calcified areas. Similarly, chorioretinitis is associated with direct infection by the virus. Infected children shed the virus for many months, and spread of infection from the baby to other members of the family has been well documented. Vaccines are not yet available in the United States, but they are being tested in special populations.

A number of studies have shown that about 1% to 4% of pregnant women have a primary infection (seroconversion) with CMV.[5] The reported annual rates are

TABLE 24–1. FREQUENCY OF TERATOGENIC VIRAL INFECTIONS IN PREGNANT WOMEN AND THEIR CHILDREN

	MOTHER/10,000	CHILD/10,000
Cytomegalovirus	300–500	50–150
Rubella virus		20–40
Epidemic	200–400	20–40
Nonepidemic	10–20	1–2
Current United States	<1	<0.1
HSV-1 and HSV-2	50–150	0.5–5
Venezuelan equine encephalitis virus	With epidemics	
Varicella virus	1–2	<0.01–1

higher for low-income women (6.8%) and day care workers with young children in their care (11%).[5,6]

RUBELLA VIRUS

Rubella has almost disappeared in the United States, and no major epidemics have occurred since 1964. The great majority of children are immunized. At present, however, approximately 10% of women of childbearing age in the United States are at risk for this infection.

We are fortunate that this high proportion of women who are currently at risk are rarely or very infrequently exposed to rubella. As a result, there are now less than 25 reported cases of congenital rubella each year. When "mini" epidemics occur or if susceptible women travel to other countries, the opportunity for risk of infection is great. For this reason, immunization programs must continue to emphasize the use of rubella vaccines for women at risk.

The defects due to congenital rubella are associated primarily with infection during the first 5 months of pregnancy (Table 24-3). The frequency of abnormal children following maternal infection is highest with rubella in the first month of gestation (50%), decreasing to 22% in the second month, 10% in the third month, and 6% in the fourth and fifth months. In the United States, approximately 10% of the women of childbearing age are at risk for rubella infection. With infections, clinical manifestations occur in approximately two thirds of women of this age group. The most useful laboratory test is the ELISA method for antibody determination. With this method, susceptible individuals can be identified on the basis of absence of antibody, and seroconversions can be documented. IgM rubella-specific antibody is also detectable for a number of weeks following infection, so this determination can be used to document recent infection.

The usual manifestations of congenital rubella include malformations of the heart and great vessels, deafness, cataracts, microcephaly, and mental retardation. The newborns may also exhibit hepatosplenomegaly, hepatitis, pneumonitis, and encephalitis. Most infected newborns have rubella-specific IgM antibody, which persists for a number of months. Rubella virus can be isolated from throat swabs and urine of congenitally infected children for a period of several months. The children are infectious, and contact with pregnant women should be avoided.

Rubella virus is spread hematogenously from the mother through the placenta to the fetus. Maternal infection in the first months of pregnancy almost always results in placental infection. Only about one third of the fetuses, however, show evidence of the virus. The virus in the fetus may be localized to one or a few organs, or it may be widely disseminated. Chronic infection of the fetus and child persists, even in the presence of high titers of specific antibody. The shedding of virus, however, ceases in almost all infants between approximately 6 months and 1 year of age, suggesting that some change in the immune status of the child has taken place. The nature of the immune deficiency in congenital infections is not known, but it may be related to absence of specific cellular immune responses. In

TABLE 24–2. CONGENITAL CYTOMEGALOVIRUS INFECTION

Birth defects	Microcephaly, chorioretinitis, deafness, mental retardation, hepatosplenomegaly, epilepsy, hydrocephalus, cerebral palsy, death
Detection	
Mother	No clinical symptoms (rarely, infectious mononucleosis-like symptoms), virus isolation from urine and cervix, seroconversion (fluorescence, ELISA)
Child	Wide spectrum of clinical findings (listed above), only severely affected are usually recognized; lab tests—CMV-specific IgM, virus isolation from nasopharynx and urine
Prevention	Avoid contact, chemotherapy (?), vaccines (?)

TABLE 24–3. CONGENITAL RUBELLA

Defects	Malformations of heart and great vessels, microcephaly, deafness, cataracts, mental retardation, newborn bleeding, hepatosplenomegaly, pneumonitis, hepatitis, encephalitis, death
Detection	
Mother	Exposure, rash, nodes; lab tests—antibody response ELISA IgM specific antibody, virus isolation from nasopharynx
Child	Congenital rubella syndrome; lab tests—rubella-specific IgM, persisting rubella IgG antibody after 6 months of age, virus isolation from nasopharynx or cerebrospinal fluid
Prevention	Rubella vaccine, abortion

rare cases, in the second decade of life, the persisting virus spreads slowly throughout the brain, causing progressive rubella panencephalitis, which is fatal.

Rubella vaccines are now used routinely in the United States. These vaccines produce a low incidence of side reactions, primarily arthritis and arthralgia, most marked in women of childbearing age. Immunity produced by the vaccines appears to be permanent. There is no satisfactory animal model for the teratogenic effects of congenital rubella.

HERPES SIMPLEX VIRUS

Herpes infections continue at a high frequency. It is estimated that there are over 300,000 new cases each year in the United States, and because of recurrences, over 5 million people experience genital herpes each year. In addition to the pain and discomfort associated with the infection, virus present in the vagina at term can be transmitted to the child during the birth process. In over 50% of cases, this leads to severe, often fatal, disease in the newborn. The use of cesarean section for delivery significantly reduces the frequency of infections in the newborn.

Congenital herpes simplex virus (HSV) infections usually are acquired at birth (Table 24-4). Maternal infection is transmitted as a venereal disease, and 90% of such infections are due to HSV-2. HSV-1, conversely, usually affects the mouth, face, or upper part of the trunk. The congenital infections studied in detail in the Collaborative Perinatal Project Study were all related to primary HSV-2 infection occurring late in gestation. Other studies, however, have shown that HSV-1 can also result in severe fetal damage. Prior maternal infection with either strain does not completely protect the child; however, the severity of lesions is often reduced.[7] Most women with vaginal HSV infection do not exhibit lesions; thus, infection is underreported. The diagnosis can be made by recognition of the typical inclusions in the cells of Papanicolaou smear, fluorescent staining, or by direct virus isolation.

The child with congenital infection usually appears normal at birth, but signs and symptoms of the disease develop during the first 1 to 3 weeks of life. The disease is manifested in three general forms:

1. Vesicular lesions of the skin or throat with or without conjunctivitis (15% of cases)
2. Central nervous system involvement, characterized by spinal fluid pleocytosis, elevated pressure, increased protein content, and convulsions (15% of cases)

TABLE 24–4. PERINATAL HERPES SIMPLEX INFECTION

Defects	Three groups Limited—vesicular lesions on skin, throat, and sometimes conjunctivitis Central nervous system—convulsions Systemic—hepatitis, jaundice, hepatomegaly, thrombocytopenia, petechiae, hemolytic anemia, pulmonary disease
Detection	
Mother	Many asymptomatic and no herpetic lesions, virus isolation most sensitive, vaginal–cervical infection, some ulcerative lesions, husband may also have infection; lab tests—Papanicolaou smear often shows cells with inclusions, fluorescent tests often positive, antigen ELISA, virus isolation from cervix
Child	Often difficult to recognize initially, skin lesions present in about 50% of cases, most later develop severe brain or systemic disease (listed above); lab tests—isolation of virus from skin lesions, throat, eyes, or tissues; specific herpes IgM antibody
Prevention	Delivery by cesarean section, chemotherapy, particularly for limited infections; vaccines (?)

3. Systemic disease, manifested by hepatitis, jaundice, pulmonary disease, hemolytic anemia, petechiae, hepatomegaly, and thrombocytopenia (70% of cases).

The prognosis in children with localized vesicular lesions (and conjunctivitis) is good, although about 50% of them progress to more extensive disseminated infection. Systemic infection is fatal in over 90% of cases. Laboratory tests useful in the diagnosis of HSV infection are the isolation of virus from lesions, the pharynx, or the conjunctiva, or the presence of specific HSV IgM antibody.

Chemotherapy for congenital infection using acyclovir has been helpful. This drug reduces the frequency of morbidity and mortality. If there is only limited infection, the drug is particularly effective in reducing the number of permanent neurologic sequelae. Vaccines are not presently available, but are being investigated. Delivery by cesarean section is recommended in order to avoid contact between the child and the infected vaginal lesions, if these are found to be present near term.

The prevalence of HSV infections appears to be increasing. The infection is transmitted as a venereal disease. Primary infection of the mother at term is of greatest importance in the production of congenital disease. Only rarely is there evidence of intrauterine infection.

VENEZUELAN EQUINE ENCEPHALITIS VIRUS

Venezuelan equine encephalitis can be transmitted to humans during epidemics. This in turn can result in spread of the virus to the baby, where severe infection of the brain and eyes can occur. Affected children may have hydrocephaly, porencephalic cysts, and cataracts.[8] Most of the epidemics occur in the Caribbean or Central and South America.

Epidemics of Venezuelan equine encephalitis occur in South America, Central America, Mexico, Texas, and Florida. The infection can be transmitted by mosquitoes of many different species, and is both endemic and epidemic. There are many hosts among wild animals, including monkeys, rats, mice, opossums, jackrabbits, foxes, and bats. Domestic animals other than horses that have been infected include cattle, pigs, goats, and sheep. In humans, infection results in a mild febrile illness, usually without neurologic complications. There is no age or sex predominance. The incubation period is approximately 2 to 5 days. The primary symptoms are headache, fever, malaise, and myalgia. Occasionally patients have seizures, mental confusion, coma, tremors, and encephalitis (Table 24-5). The symptoms usually last 3 to 8 days, and the virus can be isolated from the serum or spinal fluid.

An epidemic in Venezuela in 1962 resulted in over 6000 officially registered cases, 389 of which were severe, and 43 individuals died. Frequent abortions were noted among pregnant women who suffered encephalitis in the first 3 months of pregnancy. In addition, women who contracted encephalitis between the 13th and 36th week of pregnancy were found to have children with severe central nervous system damage. In three cases in which encephalitis occurred at 13 to 20 weeks gestation, the newborns had microphthalmia and no cerebellum, and the cranial cavities were filled with fluid. Only small nests of nervous tissue were found. In four cases of maternal encephalitis at about the eighth month of pregnancy, the infant's central nervous system showed massive necrosis, softening, and hemorrhage in the cerebrum and, to a lesser degree, in the cerebellum. Experimental studies have been reported in which pregnant rhesus monkeys of approximately 100 days gestation were inoculated with live Venezuelan equine encephalitis virus vaccine by the direct intracerebral route. The offspring of these pregnancies also had congenital microcephaly, hydrocephalus cataracts, and porencephaly.[9]

TABLE 24–5. CONGENITAL VENEZUELAN EQUINE ENCEPHALITIS INFECTION

Defects	Abortion, microphthalmia, absent cerebrum, massive CNS necrosis, hydrocephalus
Detection	
Mother	Exposure (epidemic in area), febrile illness, myalgia, encephalitis, specific antibody
Child	Microphthalmia, hydrocephalus, severe brain damage, specific antibody
Prevention	Vaccines to animals, possible danger of vaccines in pregnant women

Venezuelan equine encephalitis can be controlled by immunization of animals and quarantine. Vaccines for this virus have also been used in human beings. When administered directly to the rhesus fetuses, however, the vaccines produced severe damage to the brain and eyes. This should be considered, because the vaccine virus is being advocated for administration to women of childbearing age.

VARICELLA VIRUS

Varicella (chickenpox) is recognized as a teratogen.[10] Infection of the mother in the first half of pregnancy can lead to severe skeletal and brain damage of the child in approximately 1% to 5% of cases. In addition, varicella at term can be transmitted intravenously to the child. This direct infection in the last few days of gestation may result in generalized varicella, which is fatal for approximately one third of the infected children.

Varicella (chickenpox) and herpes zoster (shingles) are caused by the same virus. In the United States, approximately 15% of women of childbearing age are susceptible to varicella infection, and some of those infected during pregnancy have produced children with congenital defects (Table 24-6). In the tabulation of defects in 11 cases from the literature, cataracts, mi-

TABLE 24–6. CONGENITAL VARICELLA

Defects	Cataracts, microphthalmus, Horner's syndrome, anisocoria, optic atrophy, nystagmus, chorioretinitis, mental retardation, skin scarring, hypoplasia of limbs
Detection	
Mother	Rash, antibody response (fluorescence, ELISA)
Child	Defects (listed above); specific IgM antibody to varicella (some positive)
Prevention	Avoid exposure, vaccines (?), abortion (?)

crophthalmia, Horner's syndrome, anisocoria, optic atrophy, nystagmus, and chorioretinitis were reported in nine infants; brain damage was seen in seven, and skin scars and hypoplasia of specific parts could have been due to the degeneration of the nerve supply to that particular area.[10]

Varicella very late in pregnancy is often manifested at birth or in the newborn by the presence of the characteristic chickenpox skin lesion or severe pneumonia with other complications. Maternal infection 5 to 10 days before delivery may produce disease in the infant, and symptoms usually develop within 4 days of delivery. These infants usually escape severe effects of infection, presumably because maternal antibody confers some protection. However, maternal infection 0 to 5 days before delivery or 0 to 2 days after delivery may result in infection of the infant, and approximately 30% of infected children die of disseminated disease. The use of high-titered varicella zoster immune globulin (VZIG) shortly after birth prevents the disseminated disease.

SUMMARY

There are five viruses that are recognized to be causes of fetal infections and malformation: cytomegalovirus, rubella virus, herpesvirus, Venezuelan equine encephalitis virus, and varicella virus. Fortunately, rubella can now be prevented through the use of safe and effective vaccines. Clinical approaches to the prevention and treatment of congenital herpesvirus infections are already being used in many parts of the world. These include the use of cesarean section delivery to avoid exposure of the child to the virus, and treatment with chemotherapy. The use of immune globulin at the time of birth prevents disseminated varicella in the newborn. New methods for the detection of several other virus teratogens now provide opportunities for the study of the frequency and pathogenesis of these diseases. It is hoped that this will aid in the control of these infections. Intensive use of vaccines and other methods of prevention are needed for the control of congenital infections. New studies are also needed to develop methods to prevent congenital cytomegalovirus, Venezuelan equine encephalitis, and congenital varicella infections, and to detect new, unrecognized agents of importance in humans.

REFERENCES

1. Hildebrandt RJ, Sever J, Margileth AM. Cytomegalovirus in the normal pregnant female. Am J Obstet Gynecol 1967;98:1125.
2. Adler, SP. Cytomegalovirus transmission among children in day care, their mothers and caretakers. Pediatr Dis J 1988;7:279.
3. Castellano GA, Hazzard GT, Madden DL, Sever JL. Comparison of the enzyme linked immunosorben assay and the indirect hemagglutination test for detection of antibody to cytomegalovirus. J Infect Dis 1977;136:337.
4. Birnbaum G, Lynch JI, Margileth AM, Lonergan WM, Sever JL. Cytomegalovirus infections in newborn infants. J Pediatr 1969;75:789.
5. Adler SP. Cytomegalovirus and child day care, evidence for an increased infection rate among day care workers. N Engl J Med 1989;321:1290.
6. Stagno S, Pass RF, Cloud G, et al. Primary cytomegalovirus infection in pregnancy: incidence, transmission to fetus, and clinical outcome. JAMA 1986;256:1904.
7. Yeager AS, Arvin AM, Urbani JL, Kempf JA. Relationship of antibody to outcome in neonatal herpes simplex virus infections. Infect Immun 1980;29:532.
8. Wenger F. Massive cerebral necrosis of the fetus in cases of Venezuelan equine encephalitis. Investigations Clinica (Maracaibo) 1967;21:13.
9. London WT, Levitt NH, Kent SG, Wang VG, Sever JL. Congenital cerebral and ocular malformations induced in rhesus monkeys by Venezuelan equine encephalitis virus. Teratology 1977;16:285.
10. Williamson A. The varicella-zoster virus in the etiology of severe congenital defects. Clin Pediatr 1975;14:553.

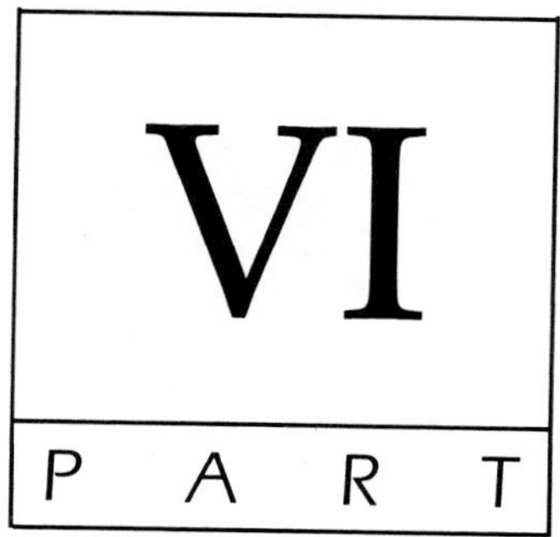

FETAL INFECTIONS OF MATERNAL ORIGIN AND TREATMENT

25 CHAPTER

TORCH VIRUS–INDUCED FETAL DISEASE

Barbara M. Nies, Jean M. Lien, and John H. Grossman III

The acronym TORCH was coined by Nahmias to describe a group of perinatal infections with similar clinical features (Table 25-1).[1] This group initially included *Toxoplasma gondii,* rubella virus, cytomegalovirus, and herpes simplex virus. Gregg's report of maternal rubella associated with congenital cataracts was the first description of malformations caused by in utero viral infection.[2] Since that time, other pathogens have been accepted as causes of congenital infection. Epstein-Barr virus, a member of the herpesviridae family, will be discussed in this chapter. Other viruses, such as Parvovirus and varicella zoster virus, will be discussed in the chapter on nonbacterial infections of the fetus.

TOXOPLASMOSIS

EPIDEMIOLOGY

The incidence of toxoplasmosis varies throughout the world. For example, in Paris, France, more than 80% of reproductive-age women are seropositive for toxoplasmosis,[3] whereas in Birmingham, Alabama, the corresponding rate is only approximately 30%.[4] Acute infection during pregnancy occurs in 10 in 1000 in France[3] but only 1.1 in 1000 in the United States.[5] Because of the higher prevalence of the disease, there has been a greater emphasis on screening, prenatal diagnosis, and treatment programs in France than in the United States.

TRANSMISSION

Fetal infection only occurs with acute maternal toxoplasmosis. The likelihood of transmission and the severity of the risk to the fetus varies with gestational age. Congenital toxoplasmosis is more frequent but usually less apparent when maternal infection occurs in later gestations. Desmonts and Couvreur found that 17% of first-trimester pregnancies with acute maternal toxoplasmosis, 24% of the second-trimester pregnancies, and 62% of the third-trimester pregnancies resulted in infected infants.[1] More than 90% of the infections acquired in the third trimester are asymptomatic.

MICROBIOLOGY/IMMUNOLOGY

The organism responsible for toxoplasmosis infection is *Toxoplasma gondii,* a protozoan parasite with a complex life cycle. It exists in three forms: trophozoite (or tachyzoite), cyst, and oocyst. Trophozoites are the proliferative and invasive forms, whereas cysts are the latent forms, persisting in tissue for the lifetime of the host. Oocysts are found in cats that have ingested rodents infected with cysts. Humans become infected if they eat uncooked, or undercooked, fresh (never frozen) meat from infected animals. Human infection may also occur with hand-to-mouth contact with oocysts excreted in cat feces. Inhalation of aerosolized oocysts is another possible mechanism for infection. Parasitemia in a pregnant woman with acute toxoplasmosis may result in transplacental migration of the parasites, with subsequent fetal infection. An infected fetus can produce IgM antibodies to *Toxoplasma,* but this response may be suppressed by maternal IgG antibodies acquired transplacentally.[6]

CLINICAL MANIFESTATIONS: MATERNAL

An immunocompetent adult with acute toxoplasmosis is often only minimally symptomatic. When the disease is clinically apparent, symptoms similar to infectious mononucleosis, including malaise, myalgias, sore throat, and fever, may be present. Painful but nonsup-

TABLE 25–1. TORCH-VIRUS INFECTIONS

	TOXOPLASMOSIS	RUBELLA
Laboratory Diagnosis		
Maternal	IgG seroconversion, T-IgM	IgG seroconversion, R-IgM virus isolation (throat)
Fetal/Neonatal	Cord IgM, placental histology, abnormal CSF	Cord IgM, IgG + >6 months
Fetal Signs	IUGR, NIH, microcephaly, anencephaly, hydranencephaly, cerebral calcifications	Microcephaly, IUGR, VSD
Neonatal Signs	Chorioretinitis, fever, hydrocephaly, hepatosplenomegaly, thrombocytopenia, seizures	Deafness, cataracts, mental retardation, hepatosplenomegaly, rash, thrombocytopenia
Treatment	Pyrimethamine, sulfa antibiotics, spiramycin	No antiviral therapy
Prevention	Avoid raw meat, cat feces	Preconception testing and vaccine for susceptibles
Laboratory Diagnosis	**CMV**	**Herpes**
Maternal	Virus isolation, IgG seroconversion, C-IgM	Virus isolation (lesion, cervix) Tzanck smear, Pap smear
Fetal/Neonatal serology	Serology, virus isolation (urine, possibly fetal blood)	Virus isolation (lesion, eye, CSF) Tzanck smear, H-IgM at <6 months
Fetal Signs	IUGR, NIH, microcephaly, hydrocephaly, cerebral calcifications, hepatosplenomegaly, SVT, heart block	Microcephaly, SAb, IUGR, cerebral calcifications
Neonatal Signs	Hepatosplenomegaly, chorioretinitis, jaundice, purpura	Chorioretinitis, vesicles, jaundice, bleeding, CNS abnormalities
Treatment	Symptomatic for mother, no antiviral therapy	Acyclovir, vidarabine
Prevention	Hygienic measures vaccines being studied	Cesarean section if virus present at parturition

C-IgM, CMV-specific IgM; CNS, central nervous system; CSF, cerebrospinal fluid; H-IgM, HSV IgM; IUGR, intrauterine growth retardation; NIH, nonimmune hydrops; R-IgM, rubella-specific IgM; SAb, spontaneous abortion; SVT, supraventricular tachycardia; T-IgM, toxoplasmosis-specific IgM; VSD, ventricular septal defect.

purative lymph node enlargement, most commonly involving the posterior cervical nodes, is a frequent finding in acute toxoplasmosis. Other associated findings include maculopapular rash, hepatosplenomegaly, and lymphocytosis. Ocular symptoms such as blurred vision, photophobia, and eye pain may be present with chronic disease. In the immunocompromised patient, severe disease with pulmonary and central nervous system involvement can be seen.

CLINICAL MANIFESTATIONS: FETAL

Some investigators have reported an increased incidence of spontaneous abortion and preterm delivery in acute primary toxoplasmosis.[7,8] Clinical manifestations that may prompt suspicion of infection include intrauterine growth retardation, nonimmune hydrops, hydrocephaly, microcephaly, anencephaly, and hydranencephaly.[9–13] A case of fetal toxoplasmosis presenting with fetal ascites and hepatosplenomegaly without other hydropic manifestations on ultrasound has been described.[14] Toxoplasmosis has also been reported in multiple gestations.[15,16]

CLINICAL MANIFESTATIONS: NEONATAL

Most infants with congenital toxoplasmosis are asymptomatic in the newborn period. In a symptomatic infant, chorioretinitis is the most common finding. There are no pathognomonic findings; the classic triad of periventricular calcifications, chorioretinitis, and hydrocephaly is actually uncommon. Severe congenital toxoplasmosis, which complicates one in 4000–8000 pregnancies,[3,17] may also be associated with fever, microcephaly, abnormal cerebrospinal fluid, jaundice, anemia, hepatosplenomegaly, thrombocytopenia, convulsions, lymphadenopathy, cataracts, microphthalmia, maculopapular rash, pneumonia, vomiting, and diarrhea. Serious long-term complications include mental retardation, severe visual deficits, and seizures. Adverse sequelae have been detected in long-term follow-up of infants with subclinical infection at birth.[10,18]

DIAGNOSIS

Serologic techniques are the usual methods for diagnosis. However, serologic tests for toxoplasmosis are some of the most error-prone assays performed by clinical labs.[19] Traditionally, Sabin-Feldman dye test, indirect fluorescent assays (IFA), indirect hemagglutination assays (IHA), and complement fixation (CF) tests have been used. More recently, enzyme-linked immunosorbent assay (ELISA) tests have been used. Most labs no longer perform the Sabin-Feldman dye test. The assays that are used most commonly measure IgG, IgM, or both. IgM can appear as early as 1 week after an acute infection and persist for several weeks or months. IgG usually does not appear until several weeks after the IgM rise, but low titers usually persist for years.

Optimally, IgG antibody to toxoplasmosis should be measured before conception; the presence of *Toxoplasma*-specific IgG would indicate protection from further infection. In pregnant women of unknown serologic status, the presence of a high *Toxoplasma* IgG titer should prompt testing for *Toxoplasma*-specific IgM. The presence of IgM is suggestive of a recent infection, especially if the titer is high, but it must be remembered that IgM may be present for up to 4 months when a fluorescent antibody test is used and for up to 8 months with an ELISA test.[20] Prenatal diagnosis of congenital toxoplasmosis is possible using cordocentesis and amniocentesis with serologic tests for IgM and IgG on fetal blood and with isolation of the organism by inoculation into mice.[21,22] However, IgM-specific antibodies may not be detected even in culture-proven cases because antibody synthesis may be delayed in the fetus and neonate; in Desmonts' study these antibodies were present in only four of nine cases.[23] Isolation of parasites may also be unsuccessful because parasitemia may be intermittent and the samples of fetal blood or amniotic fluid may be limited in quantity.[23] After delivery, a placental specimen, fixed in formalin (not refrigerated or frozen, since this may result in false-negative tests due to lysis of the organisms), should be examined for *Toxoplasma* cysts (Fig. 25-1).

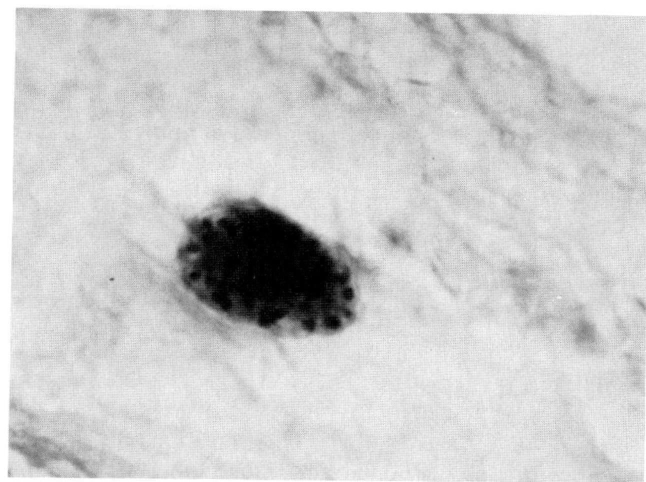

FIGURE 25–1. Toxoplasma cyst in placenta (hematoxylin-eosin, original magnification 500×). (Courtesy of Dr. M. Renate Dische, Department of Pathology, Mount Sinai School of Medicine.)

TREATMENT/PREVENTION

Usually, therapy is not necessary for toxoplasmosis in the mother and isolation is not required. Several medications are used to diminish the consequences of fetal infection, but the estimated efficacy of these is only approximately 50%. If acute toxoplasmosis is diagnosed early in pregnancy, the option of termination should be discussed. The combination of pyrimethamine (a folic acid antagonist) and sulfa drugs (sulfadiazine or triple sulfonamides) is the only effective medication generally available in the United States. Folinic acid should be used with pyrimethamine to minimize its potential side effects of bone marrow depression and pancytopenia. Sulfa drugs displace bilirubin, and if given near term may result in neonatal hyperbilirubinemia and kernicterus. The combination of pyrimethamine and sulfonamides has been shown to be teratogenic in animals and therefore should be avoided in the first trimester. Spiramycin, a macrolide antibiotic, used extensively in Europe but not approved for use in the United States, has been used frequently in the first trimester without adverse effects. Spiramycin crosses the placental barrier minimally; therefore, its effectiveness in the treatment of intrauterine infection is unclear.

The primary method of prevention of congenital toxoplasmosis is the application of certain hygienic measures.[13] The pregnant woman should be advised to wash her hands thoroughly after contact with raw meat, cats, and materials potentially contaminated by cat feces. She should also eat meat only when it has been cooked to ≥66°C. The brown color of well-done meat is due to myoglobin turning to metmyoglobin at this temperature, which is also the temperature at which the cysts are rendered noninfectious. It is too early to tell if a primary prevention program will significantly reduce the incidence of acquired toxoplasmosis. A prospectively evaluated prevention program reduced the rate of seroconversion by 34%, but this was not statistically significant.[24]

Mandatory serologic screening for toxoplasmosis during pregnancy is required by law in France and Austria and has been advocated by some as a means of improving treatment and prenatal diagnosis in the United States.[25] Because of the low prevalence of the disease in the United States, the high cost of a systematic screening program, and concern about the reliability of serologic testing, it has been suggested that toxoplasmosis testing be reserved for use as a preconceptional screen or for patients with clinical symptoms or exposure to infection.

RUBELLA

EPIDEMIOLOGY

The epidemiology of rubella infection was altered by the introduction of the vaccine in 1969. Before this, immunity to rubella through primary infection was acquired by 85% of the population by adolescence. The highest incidence was in the age group of 5–9 years, accounting for 38.5% of cases in 1966–1968. Although the incidence of rubella has declined by 99% between 1966 and 1986, 32% of all cases now occur in the 15–29-year age group.[26] Despite immunization, 10% to 20% of the US population is susceptible to rubella.[27] After the initial decrease in the incidence of CRS, the incidence has plateaued at approximately 0.05 per 100,000 live births (Fig. 25-2) for the past 10 years because of continued rubella infection in women of child-bearing age. If all these women had been vaccinated (in the ideal case) the incidence of CRS would have decreased to zero.

Before the implementation of large-scale vaccination policies in the United States, epidemics of rubella occurred every 6–9 years. The last epidemic before introduction of the vaccine was in 1964. It is estimated that over 20,000 cases of CRS and 11,000 pregnancy losses occurred due to this epidemic.[28] The vaccine was originally targeted at young children, but this had little impact on attack rates in the over-15-year age group. Now efforts are also made to vaccinate susceptible adults,[27] but opportunities to do so are missed, including the postpartum period. According to data from CRS surveillance, almost one half of mothers of CRS infants have had a previous live birth. All these cases of CRS could presumably have been prevented by postpartum vaccination after the birth of the first child.[27]

Rubella outbreaks occur in colleges, camps, the Armed Forces, and the workplace. In a 1983 outbreak in a Manhattan bank, the attack rate for women was significantly higher than that for men (2.1% versus 0.8%) and was significantly higher in women under 45 years of age.[29]

The goal of immunization should be the eradication of congenital rubella infection (CRI). The number of reported cases of CRS has declined by 99% since 1969, but increased numbers of cases are seen after outbreaks such as the one in New York City. Until the 10% to 20%

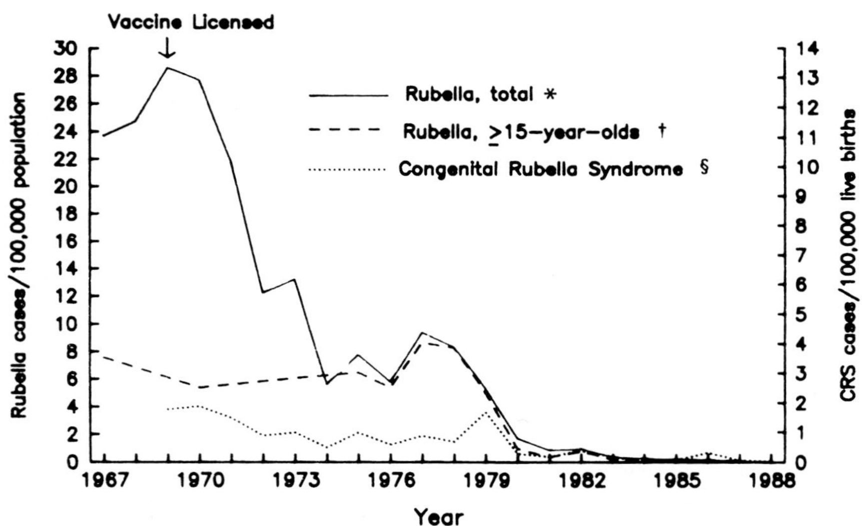

*1988 provisional data.

†Includes proration of patients ≥15 years old for whom age was unreported. Average annual U.S. estimate based on data from Illinois, Massachusetts, and New York City for the 3-year periods 1966–1968, 1969–1971, and 1972–1974.

§Confirmed and compatible cases, by year of birth. Provisional data due to delayed diagnosis and reporting.

FIGURE 25–2. Incidence rates of reported rubella and congenital rubella syndrome (CRS) cases—United States, 1967–1988. (From Centers for Disease Control. Rubella and congenital rubella syndrome—United States, 1985–1988. MMWR 1989;38:173.)

incidence of susceptible adults is eliminated, CRS cannot be eradicated.

TRANSMISSION

Rubella virus is spread by respiratory droplets. This requires prolonged, close exposure. The virus is present in the nasopharynx and spreads via the lymphatics and then blood. It is less communicable than varicella, with an 80% attack rate. Fetal infection requires maternal viremia and placental transmission. Viremia has been thought to occur only with primary infection. Rare cases of reinfection leading to CRS have been reported.[30] Serologic evidence of fetal exposure to rubella has been documented after inadvertent vaccination in pregnancy. To date, no cases of congenital defects of CRS have been reported due to vaccine.[31,32] Nevertheless, vaccine administration is contraindicated in pregnancy because the theoretical risk of CRS following vaccination, although low, may not be zero.[33] Virus is shed in breast milk as well. Neonatal exposure to rubella during breast feeding has not been associated with morbidity.[34] Prolonged viral shedding from the CRS infant may be a source of infection. Virus has been isolated in the urine, the CSF, and even the lens of CRS patients.[35,36]

The variable risk of CRS at different gestational ages has long been recognized. Rubella infection before implantation has been implicated in spontaneous abortion, stillbirth, neonatal death, and CRS.[28] Enders and coworkers reported that rubella occurring from 12 days to 12 weeks after the last menstrual period (LMP) resulted in an 81% to 90% fetal infection rate. No infection was noted if the rash appeared before the LMP or up to 11 days after the LMP.[37] Cradock-Watson and colleagues reviewed rates of rubella infection after the first trimester.[38] The overall rate of CRI (seropositivity, with or without clinical disease) was 29% based on rubella-specific IgM and 49% based on persistence of rubella-specific IgG after 8 months of age. Gestational-age-specific rates of CRI ranged from 12% when infection occurred at 24–28 weeks to 58% at 36–40 weeks. This study focused on the immunologic aspects of rubella and did not comment on clinical results of these pregnancies.

The type of malformation is gestational age specific. Cataracts and cardiac lesions were present when infection occurred before 8 weeks. Deafness occurs with infection before 16 weeks; retinopathy, before 130 days. It must be remembered that timing of fetal exposure is, at best, estimated due to difficulties in dating gestational age and lack of information regarding the incubation period of fetal rubella infection.[28]

Contrary to the prior perception that second- and third-trimester rubella infections were without clinical consequence in the fetus, Hardy and coworkers found abnormalities in 15 out of 24 infants exposed to rubella between 14 and 31 weeks' gestation. Developmental delay, hearing loss, growth retardation, pulmonic stenosis, and thrombocytopenia were some of the abnormalities seen.[39]

Most studies of placental rubella infection have analyzed first-trimester placentas. A study of 18 second- and third-trimester placentas showed a sparsity of villous trunci and terminal villi, and presence of intracytoplasmic and intranuclear inclusion bodies. One hundred percent of third-trimester placentas had necrotic, proliferative villitis and viral inclusions. None of the fetuses had gross anomalies, although visceral evidence of fetal infection was present.[40]

MICROBIOLOGY/IMMUNOLOGY

Rubella is an RNA virus of the Togavirus family, measuring 40–50 nm. Infection causes cytolysis and decreased mitotic activity.[41] Primary infection leads to production of rubella-specific IgM within 14 days. Viremia is characteristic in primary infection but may occur rarely with reinfection, as suggested by reports of CRS in those cases.[42] Rubella-specific IgM persists for 3 months. IgG response is slower and usually persists indefinitely. Reinfection or vaccination of a previously infected individual leads to a booster response of IgG only. This occurs even in patients who no longer have detectable antibody.[43] It is felt that these individuals are functionally immune to rubella, since a booster response is evident with revaccination. The booster response is also seen in children who were exposed to vaccine virus during breast-feeding.[34]

Seroconversion after vaccination occurs in 96% of patients. If antibody is measured by hemagglutination inhibition (HAI), 36% of patients may become seronegative with time. Detection of antibody by ELISA is more sensitive and therefore more predictive of immune status.

Congenital rubella leads to chronic, persistent infection; the immune response may lead to ongoing damage. Temporary and permanent immune defects were found in CRI when studied.[44] The virus may persist in spite of an active immune response. Defective cell-mediated immunity may underlie the pathogenesis of some late effects of CRI. The cell-mediated immunity response is lowest in children infected in the first 4 months of gestation and is less in all CRI children than for immune controls. Fucillo demonstrated absence of cell-mediated cytotoxicity in CRS.[45]

CLINICAL MANIFESTATIONS: MATERNAL

Postnatally acquired rubella is a mild infection that is asymptomatic in 30% of adults. The incubation period is 14 to 21 days, with viral shedding beginning 1 week before onset of rash. The rash is macular and lasts 3 days, hence the name *3-day measles.* Malaise, fever, and postauricular and suboccipital adenopathy are also common. Arthralgias are common in adult women; arthritis, neuritis, encephalitis, and thrombocytopenia are rare in postnatal infection. Symptoms are nonspecific. Therefore, diagnosis should be made on serologic rather than clinical grounds.[46]

CLINICAL MANIFESTATIONS: FETAL/NEONATAL

First-trimester rubella infection is believed to cause abortion. This was difficult to confirm during the 1964 epidemic because of the small numbers of women who were both exposed in the first trimester and registered in the study early in the pregnancy.[28] Current surveillance practices do not provide information on the incidence of pregnancy loss.[27] The Centers for Disease Control (CDC) classification of CRS is shown in Table 25-2. Congenital infection may be divided into three categories based on its manifestations: CRS, extended CRS, and delayed CRS. Newborn rubella, or CRS, and extended CRS are apparent at birth. Delayed manifestations of congenital infection may not be apparent for years or decades.

The pathogenesis of congenital defects includes defects in organogenesis due to decreased mitosis and damage due to scarring and persistent infection.[47] Abnormalities due to impaired organogenesis result when maternal infection occurs in the first trimester. Other abnormalities, such as progressive hearing loss and pulmonic or aortic stenosis, are due to ongoing damage due to persistent infection and immune response. Deafness may be a result of either mechanism.

Four major defects in CRS, in order of frequency, are deafness, mental retardation, heart lesions, and ophthalmologic abnormalities. Sever and associates, in the Collaborative Perinatal Research Study (CPRS) of 1964, reported that deafness was the most common single defect and is present in 100% of infants with multiple defects resulting from first-trimester infection.[28] Conversely, eye defects were present only with other abnormalities; cataracts and glaucoma were most frequent. Cardiac lesions include ventricular septal defect, patent ductus arteriosus, and peripheral pulmonic stenosis. Thrombocytopenic purpura (blueberry muffin rash; Fig. 25-3), hepatosplenomegaly, osseous lesions, meningoencephalitis, and rubelliform rash may also be present in CRS.

The spectrum of extended CRS includes cerebral palsy, mental retardation, developmental and language delay, seizures, cirrhosis, growth retardation, and immunologic disorders (eg, hypogammaglobulinemia).[48]

Delayed manifestations of CRI include endocrinopathies, late-onset deafness and ocular damage, renovascular hypertension, and encephalitis. Long-term follow-up of CRS patients revealed a 20% incidence of

TABLE 25–2. CLASSIFICATION OF CONGENITAL RUBELLA SYNDROME (NATIONAL CONGENITAL RUBELLA SYNDROME REGISTER)

1. CRS confirmed. Defects and one or more of the following present in the infant:
   - Rubella virus isolated
   - Rubella-specific IgM present
   - Persistent rubella-specific IgG (ie, does not decrease at rate of one twofold dilution per month)
2. CRS compatible. Defects present but insufficient laboratory confirmation. Two defects from item a or one each from items a and b are necessary:
   a. Cataracts and/or congenital glaucoma, congenital heart disease, hearing loss, pigmentary retinopathy
   b. Purpura, splenomegaly, jaundice, microcephaly, mental retardation, meningoencephalitis, radiolucent bone disease
3. CRS possible. Clinical defects that do not fulfill criteria for CRS compatible
4. Congenital rubella infection only (CRI). Serologic evidence of infection without defects
5. Stillbirths: Stillbirths attributed to maternal rubella
6. Not CRS. The following laboratory findings are inconsistent with CRS in the absence of an immunodeficiency disease:
   - Absent rubella antibody in child younger than 24 months of age
   - Absent rubella antibody in the mother
   - Rate of decline of rubella antibody consistent with decline of passively acquired antibody (one twofold dilution per month)

Adapted from CDC. Rubella and congenital rubella—United States, 1984–1986. MMWR 1987;36:664.

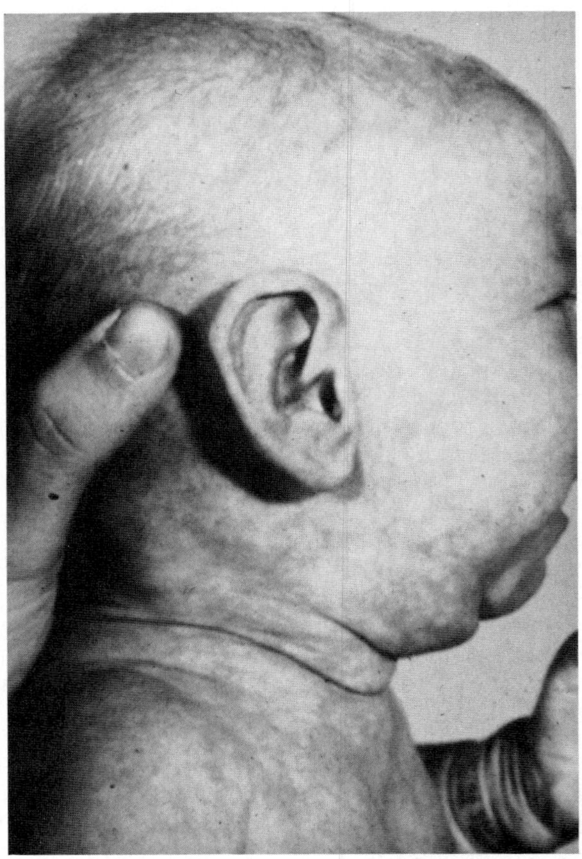

FIGURE 25–3. Blueberry muffin rash of congenital rubella syndrome.

diabetes mellitus by the age of 35.[47] Other endocrinopathies include thyroid dysfunction and growth hormone deficiency. Deafness and ocular and vascular damage may be due to ongoing infection with scarring and inflammation. Delayed manifestations of CRS are thought to be due to circulating immune complexes.[49,50]

Delayed manifestations occur in more than 20% of those with initially symptomatic CRS.[47] The incidence of delayed defects in those with asymptomatic CRI and their gestational-age-related risk are not clear. Data from the CPRS showed delayed effects in almost two thirds of those infected in the third trimester.[51] Although major malformations due to infection in the first trimester may be devastating, the adverse effects from later infection are clearly not minor.

Progressive rubella panencephalitis (PRP) has been likened to subacute sclerosing panencephalitis (SSPE) due to rubeola infection and is a different entity than the encephalitis present at birth. By 1984, 12 cases of PRP had been reported.[52] It is progressively fatal, with onset in the second decade of life. Like SSPE, PRP is associated with presence of defective viral particles. Their role in the pathogenesis of PRP has not been fully elucidated.

Hypogammaglobulinemia may be a delayed result of CRI; altered cell-mediated immunity is necessary for continued latent viral infection.[45] Because of altered cell-mediated immunity, the rubella virus persists in the congenitally infected person for up to a year and perhaps longer.[46]

DIAGNOSIS

Clinical diagnosis of postnatal infection is unreliable and must be confirmed by serology. Before the availability of serologic tests of rubella infection and immunity, virus isolation was attempted. The rubella virus is difficult to isolate. Serologic evidence of maternal primary infection includes presence of rubella-specific IgM, or presence of a fourfold rise in HAI titer on acute and convalescent sera.

Prenatal diagnosis of congenital rubella infection is possible. The presence of rubella-specific IgM in fetal blood confirms infection. Fetal immunocompetence is attained in the mid–second trimester; therefore, fetal blood sampling must be delayed until that time, to avoid a false negative result.[53,54] First-trimester confirmation of fetal infection was described by Terry and colleagues by detecting virus specific antigen and RNA in a chorionic villus sample.[55] This method is superior to virus isolation in products of conception.[56] Though experience with detection of rubella infection in utero is limited, these reports demonstrate the potential for early diagnosis. There are no abnormalities specific to rubella that are visible on prenatal ultrasound. The presence of nonspecific findings, such as VSD or microcephaly, in an at-risk pregnancy may aid in counseling the patient.

PREVENTION/TREATMENT

Prevention of in utero rubella infection requires the acquisition of immunity by all persons before the childbearing years. Programs to ensure vaccination of all schoolchildren, susceptible college students and military personnel help, but they cannot eradicate CRI. Missed opportunities for vaccination of adults still occur and contribute to the continued existence of CRS.[26] Congenitally infected neonates are also a source of virus.

There is no specific antiviral therapy for rubella infection. If in utero exposure to rubella virus is documented, the woman should be counseled as to the risks and consequences of CRI. Prenatal diagnosis, even in the first trimester, is possible. With the potentially devastating effects of first-trimester infection, a patient may choose to terminate the affected pregnancy if the diagnosis is made in a timely manner.

CYTOMEGALOVIRUS

EPIDEMIOLOGY

Cytomegalovirus (CMV) is considered to be the most common viral cause of congenital infection. An estimated 0.2% to 2.2% of all neonates are infected in utero, with 5% to 10% of these infants symptomatic at birth.[57] Over 30,000 infants are born with congenital CMV infection in the United States every year.[58] Primary CMV occurs in 1% to 2% of pregnant women.[59] Approximately 50% of reproductive-age women are susceptible to CMV infection. The rate of seroreactivity, the risk of congenital infection, and the incidence of recurrent infection is greater in lower socioeconomic groups. CMV infection is spread through infected secretions or body fluids such as endocervical mucus, semen, blood, urine, saliva, breast milk, and tears. "High-risk" environments for exposure to CMV include child-care centers, newborn nurseries, renal dialysis units, and areas of hospitals providing care for immunocompromised individuals.

TRANSMISSION

Fetal infection can occur with both primary and recurrent maternal infection; however, the likelihood and severity of congenital disease appears to be greater with a primary infection.[60] Transmission to the fetus occurs in approximately 40% of pregnancies with primary CMV.[61] Congenital infection can rarely occur in a mother with a prior infected infant. Transmission can occur at any time during pregnancy, but there is evidence that CMV infection acquired earlier in gestation results in a more severely affected infant.[62]

MICROBIOLOGY/IMMUNOLOGY

Cytomegalovirus is an enveloped, double-stranded DNA virus of the herpesvirus family. The virus, which is very species-specific, infects by adsorbing to host cells. IgG and IgM antibodies may be detectable several weeks after infection. Many different strains of cytomegalovirus have been identified by restriction endonuclease analysis. Studies indicate that recurrent infections and transmission to the fetus in immune women are more frequently due to reactivation than to reinfection.[63]

CLINICAL MANIFESTATIONS: MATERNAL

CMV infection in the immunocompetent mother is generally asymptomatic. In some patients a heterophile-negative mononucleosis-like syndrome may be present. Fever, malaise, myalgias, mild pharyngitis, minimal lymphadenopathy, lymphocytosis, and abnormal liver function tests may be present in such cases.[64]

CLINICAL MANIFESTATIONS: FETAL

Characteristics of fetal infection that may aid in prenatal diagnosis include intrauterine growth retardation, microcephaly, hydrocephaly, periventricular calcifications, and hepatosplenomegaly. CMV has been reported to be the cause of nonimmune hydrops in 1.6% to 5% of cases.[65,66] In such cases, the proposed pathophysiologic process appears to be CMV hepatitis, causing low serum protein and portal hypertension. Intrauterine resolution of hydropic features but with subsequent neonatal CMV manifestations has been reported.[67] In another case, autopsy of a 30-week fetus after preterm delivery revealed massive ascites and pulmonary hypoplasia as the only clinical evidence of CMV.[68] CMV has also been implicated in myocarditis; there have been reports of fetal heart block and of fetal supraventricular tachycardia.[69–71] There is also some evidence that CMV infection may result in second-trimester elevation of maternal serum alphafetoprotein.[72] Ultrasound visualization of periventricular calcifications due to CMV has been reported, even in the second trimester (Fig. 25-4).[73]

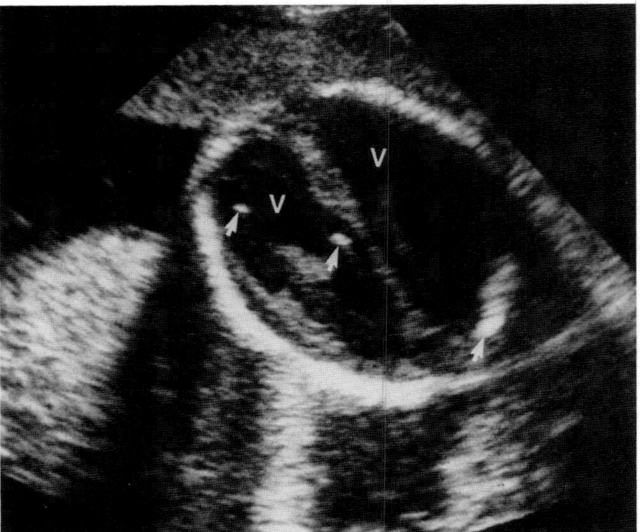

FIGURE 25–4. Cytomegalovirus-induced intracranial calcifications. (Arrow indicates periventricular hyperechoic deposits.) (From Ghidini A, Sirtori M, Vergani P, et al. Fetal intracranial calcifications. Am J Obstet Gynecol 1989; 160:86.)

CLINICAL MANIFESTATIONS: NEONATAL

Only approximately 10% of infants with congenital infection are symptomatic at birth. Common clinical findings associated with cytomegalic inclusion disease (CID) include hepatosplenomegaly, growth retardation, microcephaly, hydrocephaly, cerebral calcifications, chorioretinitis, sensorineural hearing deficits, microphthalmia, jaundice, thrombocytopenia, purpura, mental retardation, and dental abnormalities. The mortality rate for the infants with clinical evidence of disease at birth is about 20%.[57] Approximately 5% to 15% of the initially asymptomatic infants develop evidence of disease by 2 years of age, with sensorineural hearing deficits (5% to 10% of cases) and subsequent learning disabilities being the most important long-term sequelae.[58]

DIAGNOSIS

The most definitive method for diagnosis of CMV infection is by isolation of the virus from blood, urine, or cervix, but the cytopathic effects of the virus may not be seen for 2 to 6 weeks. A number of serologic studies are available for the detection of antibody to CMV, including indirect hemagglutination assay (IHA), enzyme-linked immunosorbent assay (ELISA), immunofluorescent assay (IFA), neutralization tests, and complement fixation (CF). CF assays are often inaccurate because of a high false-positive rate due to cross reactivity with other herpesviruses. CMV-specific IgM antibody tests are helpful but of limited value because 30% of women with primary infections are initially seronegative and the test is positive in 10% of women with recurrent infection.[59] Acute and convalescent paired specimens demonstrating a significant rise in titer are suggestive of a primary infection. IgG crosses the placenta; therefore, it is not very helpful in the detection of neonatal infection acquired in utero. The presence of cord blood CMV-specific IgM, which is detectable in 60% of infants with congenital infection, establishes the diagnosis.[60] Other methods of diagnosis under investigation include simultaneous measurement of CMV-specific IgM and IgE antibody by ELISA,[74] immunofluorescent staining of cells after 24 hours of culture, electron microscopy, and DNA hybridization.[75] Cytomegalovirus has been isolated from amniotic fluid.[76–78] However, in utero infection may occur even with negative amniotic fluid cultures. Another possible method of diagnosis is cordocentesis to obtain fetal blood for detection of CMV-specific IgM or isolation of the virus. There is insufficient clinical experience with these approaches to establish their sensitivity for detecting congenital infection.

TREATMENT/PREVENTION

No treatment other than symptomatic therapy is necessary for the immunocompetent adult with CMV infection. A variety of therapeutic agents—adenosine arabinoside (ara-A), acyclovir, idoxuridine, cytosine arabinoside (ara-C), 5-fluoro-2′-deoxyuridine, leukocyte interferon, and transfer factor—have been administered for the treatment of congenital CMV infection, but none have been found to be satisfactory, because of toxicity or recurrence of infection after drug administration is terminated. Vaccines have been investigated.[79,80] However, there have been concerns that the vaccine virus itself could be reactivated, causing infection in subsequent pregnancies. The clinical evidence that even women with prior congenitally infected infants and presence of CMV antibody can deliver subsequent CMV-infected infants makes it unclear whether immunization with currently configured vaccines could prevent congenital CMV. Even if a vaccine were efficacious against a specific CMV serotype, it is unclear whether it would prevent reinfection by a different strain of CMV.

Routine antepartum serologic screening for CMV is not recommended at this time. The detection of maternal CMV antibody before conception indicates prior infection, but the degree of protection that this immunity provides against congenital infection in subsequent pregnancies is unclear. Also, the implications of a single antibody titer obtained during pregnancy are difficult to interpret. Even in a "high-risk" environment, the extent of risk by exposure for a seronegative pregnant woman is uncertain. On the other hand, there is some evidence to suggest that the risk of CMV infection, even in "high-risk" settings, may be minimized by good hand washing and other hygienic measures.[81]

HERPES SIMPLEX VIRUS

EPIDEMIOLOGY

Herpes simplex virus (HSV) infection is ubiquitous. Seropositivity to type 1 of HSV (HSV-1) is acquired by a majority of persons by age 7. The incidence of seropositivity to HSV-2 varies with age, sexual habits, and economic status.[82] HSV-1 is the serotype found in most oral lesions; HSV-2 causes most lesions below the waist.[83] Eighty-five percent of genital HSV in adults is due to HSV-2.

Genital HSV infection was first described in 1736.[84] By the end of the 19th century, vesicular eruptions due to the pox virus and herpes virus were known to have characteristic cytopathic effects.[84] The virus was discovered in 1924, but the concept of two distinct serotypes was not accepted until the 1960s.

The actual incidence of genital HSV is unknown in the United States, as it is not a reportable disease. Population-based studies show a 15-fold increase in office consultations for genital HSV from 1966 to 1984.[85] The largest number of visits were by adults 20–29 years old. Although some of the increase in care seeking may be due to increased awareness of the disease by the public, the true incidence has probably increased dramatically.

Neonatal HSV has also increased in occurrence in some areas. In King County, Washington, neonatal infection rose from 2.6 per 100,000 live births in 1966–1969 to 11.9 per 100,000 live births in 1978–1981.[86] These figures are necessarily based on small numbers of cases, and their statistical validity may be questioned.

Excretion of HSV from the genital tract accompanies 0.1% to 0.4% of deliveries. The incidence of neonatal disease is 10 times lower, 0.01% to 0.04% of deliveries.[87]

TRANSMISSION

Transmission of genital HSV requires intimate contact of infectious secretions with susceptible mucous membranes or skin. Mechanical friction is necessary for efficient transfer.[88] Transmission by fomites or nonvenereal means appears to be less frequent. There is a high rate of unsuspected genital transmission; 57% of partners of pregnant women had serologic evidence of HSV infection, yet only 6% had a history of HSV. Thus, the clinical history may not provide reliable information regarding the likelihood of sexual transmission.[85]

Analysis of survival characteristics of HSV in water and on plastic surfaces supports the possibility of fomite spread.[88] There was no documented transmission of virus from these sources, however. Most cases of genital herpes are probably sexually transmitted, and genital HSV-1 is usually due to oral–genital contact.[89]

Nonvenereal transmission may occur by autoinoculation or may represent reactivation of infection initially acquired by a nongenital route. Cases of genital HSV-1 in children support this theory.[90]

Neonatal transmission occurs intrapartum in the vast majority of cases—virus is encountered in the infected maternal genital tract. Postnatal acquisition has been documented, especially in cases of HSV-1 neonatal infection. Since 1% of the population has HSV-1 infection at any given time, the risk of transmission must be low, as HSV-1 remains a rare source of neonatal disease. Although there may be considerable reporting bias, a review of the literature revealed a 66% mortality rate in postnatally acquired HSV infection.[91] Sources include mothers, fathers, and health care workers with lesions on the mouth or fingers.

Transplacental infection with HSV has been reported but is not well understood.[92,93] Evidence for teratogenic potential of HSV is circumstantial. The concept of transplacentally spread HSV is consistent with in utero infection due to cytomegalovirus (CMV), varicella zoster virus (VZV), and Epstein-Barr virus (EBV), which are also Herpesviridae. Reported cases of congenital HSV are rare, and serologic and virologic confirmation is incomplete.[94] Factors affecting rates of transmission are not well understood. Cervical shedding of virus is more frequent in primary episodes: 87% versus 4% of recurrences.[95] Duration of shedding and virus inoculum are also less in recurrent disease. These facts plus the transplacental passage of neutralizing antibody in recurrent infection may account for the lower risk of neonatal infection in recurrent episodes.[95] Infection has been estimated to occur in over 50% of exposures during a primary infection versus less than 5% with recurrences.[96]

MICROBIOLOGY/IMMUNOLOGY

Herpes simplex virus is a double-stranded DNA virus of the same family as VZV, CMV, and EBV. HSV enters the host via skin or mucosa; after initial infection antibody is produced and the virus becomes latent in the ganglia of sensory neurons.[91] Reactivation occurs in response to stimuli such as fever, ultraviolet light, menses, or emotional upset.[89] The subtypes 1 and 2 contain many different strains distinguishable by DNA fingerprinting.[97] Serotypes 1 and 2 are biochemically and morphologically distinct, and specific serologic assays are available to distinguish them.

HSV-2 appears to have a predilection for genital mucosa. Most primary infections of external genitalia are symptomatic, but infection of the cervix may be subclinical.[98] Reactivation may result in asymptomatic viral shedding. Antibody to HSV-1, present in most adults, may modify the course of primary genital infection by HSV-2. This may account for asymptomatic cases of primary genital infection. Hormonal modification of HSV effects has also been investigated.[104] Anecdotal reports of disseminated disease in pregnancy raise the question of a predisposition to more severe disease in pregnant women.[105] Recent work, however, does not support this contention.[89]

Presence of antibody alters the course of disease in adults; transplacental antibody may also modify neonatal infection. This is supported by animal studies[95] and the documented lower risk of neonatal herpes with recurrent as opposed to primary maternal infection.[96]

Wilson and, recently, Kohl outlined the immune mechanisms necessary for containment of HSV, and characterized the greater susceptibility of neonates.[100,101] Disseminated disease is rare in immunocompetent adults when compared to the neonate, especially the preterm infant.

The initial containment phase depends on macrophages, natural killer cells (NK), interferon, and transplacentally acquired antibody. Lymphocyte- and monocyte-mediated lysis of HSV-infected cells is deficient in neonates, as is NK cytotoxicity. Interferon production is normal, but NK cell response to interferon and other lymphokines is absent in 25% of neonates' cells.[101] The late "curative" phase of immune response produces two main types of anti-HSV antibodies, neutralizing antibody and antibody-dependent cell cytotoxicity antibody. Antibody production in neonates is variable. An adequate titer of neutralizing antibody may attenuate the severity of HSV infection. High titers of actively or passively acquired antibodies can protect against a small viral inoculum.[101]

Integration of antibody-mediated effector cells, humoral antibody, and interferon or acyclovir results in optimal control of infection. It may become possible to direct immune therapy toward these deficient neonatal systems (eg, by administration of immunoglobulin or interferon).[102,103]

The immunocompetence of preterm infants is less than that of term infants; altered skin integrity may also be a factor in the higher infection rates and mortality of preterm neonates.

CLINICAL MANIFESTATIONS: MATERNAL

Corey and coworkers reviewed clinical manifestations of genital HSV. Sixty percent of first episodes were serologically primary, 90% were HSV-2.[98] Systemic symptoms such as fever, malaise, myalgia, and headache were present in 68% of women with primary infection and in 16% of recurrences. Local symptoms include pain, discharge, adenopathy, and dysuria. Urinary retention due to nerve involvement or local pain is common. Lesions follow primary exposure in 2–10 days and are painful vesicles. These ulcerate and then heal without scarring. Lesions were present for a mean of 11 days in primary cases and 7 days in recurrences. Viral shedding persists until the lesions heal. Cervical shedding is present with primary infection in over 80% of patients and in up to 30% of recurrences.[106] Asymptomatic shedding occurs in less than 1% of pregnancies.[107]

CLINICAL MANIFESTATIONS: FETAL

Infection of the conceptus by transplacental spread of HSV has been linked with spontaneous abortion, preterm labor, and congenital malformations.[108] The spectrum of anomalies is similar to congenital CMV infection. Microcephaly, periventricular calcifications, chorioretinitis, intrauterine growth retardation, and vesicular eruptions have been described.[109] Some of these nonspecific abnormalities may be apparent on ultrasound. In most reports, virus isolation and serologic confirmation are incomplete. Granat and associates recommended the following investigations in cases of suspected congenital HSV: viral cultures of mother, placenta, and fetus; HSV-specific IgM of maternal and cord blood; and histologic examination of the placenta.[94] Complete prospective data are needed to define more clearly the congenital syndrome. Prenatal diagnosis of transplacental HSV is theoretically possible by demonstration of HSV IgM in fetal blood. Presently, the low risk of transmission may not justify invasive methods of prenatal diagnosis. Termination of pregnancy is not required in cases of first-trimester primary HSV infection, because of the apparent low risk of fetal infection in those pregnancies that continue.

CLINICAL MANIFESTATIONS: NEONATAL

Infection acquired intrapartum has an average incubation period of 6–12 days.[110] Infection may be *localized* to the skin, eye, or oral mucosa; may be *disseminated*; or may involve the *central nervous system* (CNS). Neonatal HSV is rarely asymptomatic. Almost 50% of infections are in premature neonates.

Local infection occurs in 15% of cases. Signs include mucocutaneous vesicles, keratoconjunctivitis, and chorioretinitis. Mortality is lower than that for CNS or disseminated disease. Chorioretinitis or keratoconjunctivitis may result in blindness; 30% of infants with local disease develop major neurologic sequelae such as spastic quadriplegia or microcephaly. Seventy-five percent of localized infection will disseminate unless early therapy is instituted.

Neonatal HSV confined to the CNS occurs in 15% to 30% of cases. Onset is at 3 weeks of age; 65% have skin vesicles. Seizures, poor feeding, irritability, and other nonspecific signs are present. Mortality is greater than 50% and devastating neurologic sequelae are the rule in survivors.

Disseminated infection occurs in 70% of neonates. Forty-five percent of affected neonates are premature. Onset is at 9–11 days of life; 90% have the characteristic vesicular rash. Involvement of liver and adrenal glands in 70% accounts for signs of jaundice, hemorrhage, and shock. CNS involvement occurs in 75%; pneumonitis is present in half of these infants. Mortality is over 50% and is usually due to disseminated intravascular coagulopathy or pneumonitis.[110]

DIAGNOSIS

A rapid assay for HSV with a high specificity and positive predictive value is needed to prevent neonatal transmission and infection. Virus identification by presence of cytopathic effect in tissue culture is the gold standard but necessarily takes time. The majority of cultures with clinically significant virus will be positive 48 hours after inoculation.[111] Methods for amplification of virus by immunofluorescent antibody or ELISA techniques still require more than 24 hours.[112] A rapid ELISA test for detection of HSV was reported to have 97.5% sensitivity and 98% to 100% specificity.[113] The clinical relevance of the presence of HSV antigen has not yet been determined.

A potential benefit of rapid detection of HSV antigen in the maternal genital tract is the early identification of exposed neonates. Some investigators feel that early or prophylactic antiviral therapy may benefit these infants.[114] Identification of virus in the maternal genital tract at the onset of labor or rupture of membranes should be the diagnostic goal. In 1979, Amstey and colleagues recommended weekly cervical and labial cultures to screen high-risk patients for the presence of virus at delivery. This allowed for the presumed safe vaginal delivery of women with negative antepartum cultures and would ideally decrease the rate of cesarean sections in this group.[115] Further study has shown that antepartum HSV cultures do not predict either presence or absence of virus at the time of parturition.[116] Virus is shed in 1.4% of parturients regardless of their antepartum culture status.[99] Additionally, 50% of HSV-infected neonates are born to mothers with no history of genital herpes,[117] thus discounting the value of screening only the high-risk patient.

The diagnosis of neonatal herpes is complicated by its nonspecific presentation and clinical resemblance to bacterial sepsis.[117] Diagnosis may be unsuspected until after the failure of antibiotic therapy. Only half of infected neonates have skin lesions, and in the case of focal HSV encephalitis, virus may only be recoverable by brain biopsy.[117]

Direct immunologic identification of viral antigens without intermediate tissue culturing sacrifices sensitivity for speed. Direct immunologic detection has a sensitivity of 70%, equivalent to exfoliative cytology.[112] Genetic diversity of HSV complicates the use of antigen probes.

Serologic identification of antibody to HSV indicates exposure at some earlier time. Viral typing or subtyping by restriction endonuclease may be useful for epidemiologic studies, but their clinical utility is limited.[97]

PREVENTION

A rational approach to the prevention of neonatal HSV infection requires understanding of the natural history of transmission. Screening of all parturients is not currently feasible, screening of patients at risk is not adequate, and cesarean section does not prevent all cases of neonatal infection.[118] The greater risk of infection of preterm infants must be considered also.

Binkin and coworkers estimated that weekly antepartum cultures would predict only 25% of asymptomatic shedding at delivery.[116] Culture results would lead to approximately three additional maternal deaths related to cesarean section. The protocol would cost $1.8 million per case of neonatal herpes averted. Clearly, a cost-effective, targeted approach to the detection of HSV at parturition is needed.

A 1988 editorial by the Infectious Disease Society for Obstetrics and Gynecology proposed an alternate approach to the once standard practice of weekly HSV cultures after 32 weeks in patients with recurrent genital herpes.[119] Their recommendations include the following: abandon weekly prenatal cultures; culture patients only when they are symptomatic. Obtain cultures of the mother or neonate at the time of delivery in all patients with a history of genital herpes or a partner with HSV, to identify potentially exposed neonates.

Harger and colleagues documented duration of viral presence by culturing patients with active lesions every 2–3 days.[118] This strategy, although likely to be more clinically useful than antepartum cultures, still does not solve the problem of the preterm neonate or the woman with no history of HSV. Another problem is the lack of 100% correlation of maternal cultures and neonatal cultures. Transplacental infection is one possible explanation for neonatal herpes simplex infection in infants born to mothers with negative HSV cultures at delivery. Failure to recover maternal virus may also occur.

Cesarean section of all patients with a history of herpes would not prevent neonatal HSV, not even the cases due to recurrent infection. At least 19 cases of neonatal infection have occurred after abdominal delivery before rupture of membranes. Until a rapid, reliable method for detection of HSV is available, the approach outlined by the Infectious Disease Society for Obstetrics and Gynecology may prevent most neonatal HSV, while minimizing unnecessary cesarean sections.

TREATMENT

Acyclovir and vidarabine are specific antiviral therapies against HSV. Acyclovir has selective activity against herpes viruses, with little effect on uninfected cells.[120] Its selectivity is due to activation by HSV-specific thymidine kinase. The activated form inhibits HSV DNA polymerase. Acyclovir is excreted primarily by the kidneys and has a wide margin of safety. Adverse reactions are rare with oral or topical forms.[120]

When used for primary infection, acyclovir decreases duration of shedding, pain, new lesion formation, and time to complete healing.[98] Duration of shedding may be decreased by 80%. Oral acyclovir is effective in suppressing recurrences with long-term use.[121]

Routine indications for antiviral therapy in pregnancy have not been established.[122] Potential uses include treatment of cases of disseminated herpes, severe primary infection, uncomplicated primary infection, and possibly as prophylaxis against recurrence at term. Acyclovir is considered by many to be appropriate for treatment of disseminated HSV in pregnancy. Primary HSV infection in pregnancy increases the risk of adverse perinatal outcome (eg, preterm delivery, intrauterine growth retardation, and congenital anomalies). Although acyclovir may be beneficial in uncomplicated primary HSV or may decrease the risk of intrapartum exposure when given at term, favorable risk–benefit analyses for these uses have not been clearly established.

Both acyclovir and vidarabine have been used for neonatal HSV. Vidarabine was available before acyclovir. Unlike acyclovir, a large fluid volume is needed for parenteral administration of vidarabine. Acyclovir has been associated with decreased production of humoral antibody in adults and neonates. This has been implicated in late relapses of neonatal HSV, and for this reason some investigators are reluctant to use acyclovir in asymptomatic infants.[114]

EPSTEIN-BARR VIRUS

EPIDEMIOLOGY

Epstein-Barr virus (EBV) is considered by some to be the most common herpes virus.[123] At least 95% of pregnant women demonstrate seroreactivity to EBV antigens.[124] In general, prior infection and serologic conversion confers immunity and prevents reinfection. In three large prospective studies conducted in Pennsylvania, Alabama, and California on approximately 14,000 pregnant women, only three seroconversions were detected in serosusceptible women.[125–127] None of their infants had documented congenital EBV infection.

MICROBIOLOGY/IMMUNOLOGY

Epstein-Barr virus, a lymphotropic herpesvirus, is the etiologic agent of infectious mononucleosis. After a primary infection, viral excretion may continue for weeks or months. Antibodies to EBV viral capsid antigen (VCA) and early antigen (EA) develop early, whereas antibodies to EBV nuclear antigen (EBNA) may take weeks or months to develop.[128] Reactivation of latent, persistent EBV infection has been found to occur more frequently in pregnancy, often occurring very early in gestation.[129]

TRANSMISSION

Transplacental transmission of EBV can occur but is very rare. Congenital defects were first associated with EBV infection in 1949 among three children of mothers who had had infectious mononucleosis in the first trimester.[130] Placental studies by Ornoy in women with infectious mononucleosis in the first 2 months of pregnancy revealed necrotizing deciduitis, villitis, and chorioamnionitis.[131] Reactivation of latent, persistent EBV infection has not been associated with adverse perinatal outcome.[129]

CLINICAL MANIFESTATIONS: MATERNAL

More than half of all patients with primary EBV infections are asymptomatic.[124] The most common clinical manifestations are the sore throat, fever, malaise, and lymph node enlargement characteristic of infectious mononucleosis. Rare complications of EBV infection include splenic rupture, meningitis, airway obstruction, Guillain-Barré syndrome, and death.

CLINICAL MANIFESTATIONS: FETAL/NEONATAL

There have thus far been no reported cases of antenatal diagnosis of EBV congenital infection. As noted earlier, EBV has been implicated as the possible cause of congenital malformations (cardiovascular defects and cataracts) in several infants of mothers who developed infectious mononucleosis during the first trimester.[130] EBV has been more strongly implicated as a cause of in utero infection by two case reports in which there was serologic confirmation. Joncas and coworkers described a term infant with microcephaly, cerebral calcifications, hepatosplenomegaly, seizures, petechiae, and limb spasticity.[132] This child had pathologic, immunologic, and biochemical evidence of simultaneous infection with CMV and EBV. It was presumed that the EBV in this case was acquired late in pregnancy. Another case reported by Goldberg and associates described a male infant with micrognathia, cryptorchidism, cataracts, hypotonia, thrombocytopenia, monocytosis, proteinuria, and metaphyseal lucencies.[133] The most likely period of acute maternal EBV infection in this case was in the fifth to sixth week. No other associated infections were documented in this case.

DIAGNOSIS

Laboratory diagnosis of EBV infection depends primarily on serology. The detection of heterophil antibodies in a patient with clinical symptoms of infectious mononucleosis is usually diagnostic for an acute EBV infection. In patients with a negative heterophil antibody, EBV-specific serology can be used. Antibodies to VCA are present in all individuals by the third week of infection. IgM–VCA declines over the next 3 months, whereas IgG–VCA persists for life.[134] IgG–EA appears after the VCA antibodies and declines over the next 6 months.[134] IgG–EBNA can sometimes be detected by the third to fourth week of infection and may persist indefinitely.[134] IgM antibody to VCA is diagnostic for a primary EBV infection, but if there is no IgM–VCA, the presence of IgG antibody to VCA and EA, along with an absence of IgG to EBNA, is suggestive of primary or postacute infection.[124] Acute or recent infection can also be diagnosed by an antibody titer to VCA of 1:160 or higher, even if anti-EBNA is absent.[135] Congenital infection can be identified by testing umbilical cord blood lymphocytes for spontaneous transformation or by testing oropharyngeal secretions for EBV.[127]

TREATMENT/PREVENTION

There are no specific treatment or preventative measures for EBV. Treatment of infectious mononucleosis is primarily supportive. In the rare patients with severe complications, corticosteroids and acyclovir have been used. Pregnant women should avoid contact with infectious mononucleosis patients to diminish their risks for infection, but it has been demonstrated that even with intimate contact with EBV excreters, serosusceptible women may not necessarily acquire an infection.[136] Women who develop EBV infections during pregnancy should be informed about the rare cases of congenital malformations that have been reported. In view of the limited number of such cases, it is presently impossible to render an exact estimate of malformation risk to the fetus following documented EBV infection in pregnancy.

REFERENCES

1. Nahmias AJ, Walls KW, Stewart JA, Herrmann KL, Flynt WJ. The TORCH complex—perinatal infections associated with toxoplasma and rubella, cytomegol-[sic] and herpes simplex viruses. Pediatr Res 1971;5:405.
2. Gregg NM. Congenital cataract following German measles in the mother. Trans Ophthalmol Soc Aust 1941;3:35.
3. Desmonts G, Couvreur J. Congenital toxoplasmosis. A prospective study of 378 pregnancies. N Engl J Med 1974;290:1110.
4. Hunter K, Stagno S, Capps E, Smith RJ. Prenatal screening of pregnant women for infections caused by cytomegalovirus, Epstein-Barr virus, herpesvirus, rubella, and Toxoplasma gondii. Am J Obstet Gynecol 1983;145:269.
5. Sever JL, Ellenberg JH, Ley AC, et al. Toxoplasmosis: maternal and pediatric findings in 23,000 pregnancies. Pediatrics 1988;82:181.
6. Naot Y, Desmonts G, Remington JS. IgM enzyme-linked immunosorbent assay test for the diagnosis of congenital Toxoplasma infection. J Pediatr 1981;98:32.
7. Alford CA, Stagno S, Reynolds DW. Congenital toxoplasmosis: clinical, laboratory, and therapeutic considerations, with special reference to subclinical disease. Bull NY Acad Med 1974;50:160.
8. Stray-Pederson B, Lorentzen-Styr AM. Uterine toxoplasma infections and repeated abortions. Am J Obstet Gynecol 1977;128:716.
9. Stagno S, Reynolds D, Amos C. Auditory and visual defects resulting from symptomatic and subclinical congenital cytomegalovirus and Toxoplasma infections. Pediatrics 1977;59:699.
10. Wilson CB, Remington JS, Stagno S, Reynolds DW. Development of adverse sequelae in children born with subclinical congenital Toxoplasma infection. Pediatrics 1980;66:767.
11. Zornes SL, Anderson PG, Lott RL. Congenital toxoplasmosis in an infant with hydrops fetalis. South Med J 1988;81:391.
12. Bambirra EA, Pittella JE, Rezende M. Toxoplasmosis and hydranencephaly. N Engl J Med 1982;306:1112.
13. Frenkel JK. Congenital toxoplasmosis: prevention or palliation? Am J Obstet Gynecol 1981;141:359.

14. Blaakaer J. Ultrasonic diagnosis of fetal ascites and toxoplasmosis. Acta Obstet Gynecol Scand 1986;135:618.
15. Couvreur J, Desmonts G, Girre JY. Congenital toxoplasmosis in twins. J Pediatr 1976;89:235.
16. Wiswell TE, Fajardo JE, Bass JW, Brien JH, Forstein SH. Congenital toxoplasmosis in triplets. J Pediatr 1984;105:59.
17. Sever JL. Perinatal infections affecting the developing fetus and newborn. The prevention of mental retardation through the control of infectious diseases. Public Health Service Publication No. 1692. Washington, DC: NIH, 1968:37.
18. Koppe JG, Loewer-Sieger DH, De Roever-Bonnet H. Results of 20-year follow-up of congenital toxoplasmosis. Lancet 1986;1:254.
19. Fucillo D, Madden D, Tzan N, et al. Problems associated with the diagnosis of acquired toxoplasmosis with an indirect enzyme-linked immunosorbent assay and fluorescent-antibody immunoassay for immunoglobulin M antibodies. American Society for Microbiology. Eighty-Fifth Annual Meeting. Session 31, C24, Las Vegas, 1985.
20. Sever JL. TORCH tests and what they mean. Am J Obstet Gynecol 1985;152:495.
21. Daffos F, Forestier F, Capella-Pavlovsky M, et al. Prenatal management of 746 pregnancies at risk for congenital toxoplasmosis. N Engl J Med 1988;318:271.
22. Teutsch SM, Sulzer AJ, Ramsey JE, Murray WA, Juranek DD. Toxoplasma gondii isolated from amniotic fluid. Obstet Gynecol 1980;55:2S.
23. Desmonts G, Forestier F, Thulliez P, et al. Prenatal diagnosis of congenital toxoplasmosis. Lancet 1985;1:500.
24. Foulon W, Naessens A, Lauwers S, De Meuter F, Amy J. Impact of primary prevention on the incidence of toxoplasmosis during pregnancy. Obstet Gynecol 1988;72:363.
25. McCabe R, Remington JS. Toxoplasmosis: the time has come. N Engl J Med 1988;318:313.
26. Centers for Disease Control. Rubella and congenital rubella syndrome—United States, 1985–1988. MMWR 1989;38:173.
27. Centers for Disease Control. Rubella and congenital rubella—United States, 1984–1986. MMWR 1987;36:664.
28. Sever JL, Nelson KB, Gilkeson MR. Rubella epidemic, 1964: effect on 6,000 Pregnancies. Am J Dis Child 1965;110:395.
29. Centers for Disease Control. Rubella outbreak among office workers—New York City. MMWR 1983;32:349.
30. Saule H, Enders G, Bernsau U. Congenital rubella infection after previous immunity of the mother. Eur J Pediatr 1988;147:195.
31. Levine JB, Berkowitz CD, St Geme JW. Rubella virus reinfection during pregnancy leading to late-onset congenital rubella syndrome. J Pediatr 1982;100:589.
32. Preblud SR, Williams NM. Fetal risk associated with rubella vaccine: implications for vaccination of susceptible women. Obstet Gynecol 1985;66:121.
33. Bart SW, Stetler HC, Preblud SR, et al. Fetal risk associated with rubella vaccine: an update. Rev Infect Dis 1985;7:S95.
34. Losonsky GA, Fishaut JM, Strussenberg J, Ogra PL. Effect of immunization against rubella on lactation products. II. Maternal-neonatal interactions. J Infect Dis 1982;145:661.
35. Dudgeon JA. Congenital rubella. J Pediatr 1975;87:1078.
36. Menser MA, Forrest JM, Slinn RF, Nowak MJ, Dorman DC. Rubella viruria in a 29-year-old woman with congenital rubella. Lancet 1971;2:797.
37. Enders G, Nickerl-Pacher U, Miller E, Cradock-Watson JE. Outcome of confirmed periconceptional maternal rubella. Lancet 1988;1:1445.
38. Cradock-Watson JE, Ridehalgh MKS. Fetal infection resulting from maternal rubella after the first trimester of pregnancy. The Journal of Hygiene [Cambridge] 1980;85:381.
39. Hardy JB, McCracken GH, Jr, Gilkeson MR, Sever JL. Adverse fetal outcome following maternal rubella *after* the first trimester of pregnancy. JAMA 1969;207:2414.
40. Garcia AGP, Marques RLS, Lobato YY, Fonesca MEF, Wigg MD. Placental pathology in congenital rubella. Placenta 1985;6:281.
41. Zeichner SL, Plotkin SA. Mechanisms and pathways of congenital infections. Clin Perinatol 1988;15:163.
42. Eilard T, Strannegard O. Rubella reinfection in pregnancy followed by transmission to the fetus. J Inf Dis 1974;129:594.
43. Schiff GM, Young BC, Stefanovic GM, et al. Challenge with rubella virus after loss of detectable vaccine-induced antibody. Rev Infect Dis 1985;7:S157.
44. Buimovici-Klein E, Cooper LZ. Cell-mediated immune response in rubella infections. Rev Infect Dis 1985;7:S123.
45. Fuccillo DA, Steele RW, Hensen SA, Vincent MM, Hardy JB, Bellanti JA. Impaired cellular immunity to rubella virus in congenital rubella. Infect Immun 1974;9:81.
46. Freij BJ, South MA, Sever JL. Maternal rubella and the congenital rubella syndrome. Clin Perinatol 1988;15:247.
47. Sever JL, South MA, Shaver KA. Delayed manifestations of congenital rubella. Rev Infect Dis 1985;7:S164.
48. Hancock MP, Huntley CC, Sever JL. Congenital rubella syndrome with immunoglobulin disorder. J Pediatr 1968;72:636.
49. Verder H, Dickmeiss E, Haahr S, et al. Late-onset rubella syndrome: coexistence of immune complex disease and defective cytotoxic effector cell function. Clin Exp Immunol 1986;63:367.
50. Tardieu M, Grospierre B, Durandy A, Griscelli C. Circulating immune complexes containing rubella antigens in late-onset rubella syndrome. J Pediatr 1980;97:370.
51. South MA, Sever JL. The congenital rubella syndrome. Teratology 1985;31:297.
52. Johnson RT. Progressive rubella encephalitis. N Engl J Med 1975;292:1023.
53. Daffos F, Forestier F, Grangeot-Keros, et al. Prenatal diagnosis of congenital rubella. Lancet 1984;2:1.
54. Enders G, Jonathan W. Prenatal diagnosis of intrauterine rubella. Infection 1987;15:12.
55. Terry GM, Ho-Terry L, Warren RC, Rodeck CH, Cohen A, Rees KR. First trimester prenatal diagnosis of congenital rubella: a laboratory investigation. Br Med J 1986;292:930.
56. Cradock-Watson JE, Miller E, Ridehalgh MKS, Terry GM, Ho-Terry L. Detection of rubella in fetal and placental tissues and in the throats of neonates after serologically confirmed rubella in pregnancy. Prenatal Diag 1989;9:91.
57. Stagno S, Pass RF, Dworsky ME, Alford CA. Maternal cytomegalovirus infection and perinatal transmission. Clin Obstet Gynecol 1982;25:563.
58. Stagno S, Whitley RJ. Herpesvirus infections of pregnancy. Part I: cytomegalovirus and Epstein-Barr virus infections. N Engl J Med 1985;313:1270.
59. Sever JL, Larsen JW, Grossman JH. Handbook of perinatal infections. 2nd edition. Boston: Little, Brown, 1989:38.
60. Stagno S, Pass RF, Dworsky ME, et al. Congenital cytomegalovirus infection: the relative importance of primary and recurrent maternal infection. N Engl J Med 1982;306:945.
61. Stagno S, Pass RF, Cloud G, et al. Primary cytomegalovirus infection in pregnancy. JAMA 1986;256:1904.
62. Monif GR, Egan EA, Held B, et al. The correlation of maternal cytomegalovirus infection during varying stages in gestation with neonatal involvement. J Pediatr 1972;80:17.
63. Huang E, Alford CA, Reynolds DW, Stagno S, Pass RF. Molecular epidemiology of cytomegalovirus infections in women and their infants. N Engl J Med 1980;303:958.
64. Weller TH. The cytomegaloviruses: ubiquitous agents with protean clinical manifestations. (Parts 1 and 2.) N Engl J Med 1971;285:203.

65. Perlin BM, Pomerance JJ, Schifrin BS. Nonimmunologic hydrops fetalis. Obstet Gynecol 1981;57:584.
66. Hutchinson AA, Drew JH, Yu VY, Williams ML, Fortune DW, Beischer NA. Nonimmunologic hydrops fetalis: a review of 61 cases. Obstet Gynecol 1982;59:347.
67. Fadel HE, Ruedrich DA. Intrauterine resolution of nonimmune hydrops associated with cytomegalovirus infections. Obstet Gynecol 1988;71:1003.
68. Stocker T. Congenital cytomegalovirus infection presenting as massive ascites with secondary pulmonary hypoplasia. Hum Pathol 1985;16:1173.
69. Lewis PE, Cefalo RC, Zaritsky AL. Fetal heart block caused by cytomegalovirus. Am J Obstet Gynecol 1980;136:967.
70. Karn K, Julian TM, Ogburn PL. Fetal heart block associated with congenital cytomegalovirus infection. J Reprod Med 1984;29:278.
71. Filloux F, Kelsey DK, Bose CL, Veasy LG, Gooch WM. Hydrops fetalis with supraventricular tachycardia and cytomegalovirus infection. Clin Pediatr 1985;24:534.
72. Katz VL, Cefalo RC, McCune BK, Moos M. Elevated second trimester maternal serum alpha-fetoprotein and cytomegalovirus infection. Obstet Gynecol 1986;68:580.
73. Ghidini A, Sirtori M, Vergani P, Mariani S, Tucci E, Scola GC. Fetal intracranial calcifications. Am J Obstet Gynecol 1989; 160:86.
74. Nielsen SL, Ronholm E, Sorensen I, Jaeger P, Andersen HK. Improvement of serological diagnosis of neonatal cytomegalovirus infection by simultaneously testing for specific immunoglobulins E and M by antibody-capture enzyme-linked immunosorbent assay. J Clin Microbiol 1987;25:1406.
75. Freij BJ, Sever JL. Herpesvirus infections in pregnancy: risks to embryo, fetus, and neonate. Clin Perinatol 1988;15:203.
76. Davis LE, Tweed GV, Chin TD, Miller GL. Intrauterine diagnosis of cytomegalovirus infection: viral recovery from amniocentesis fluid. Am J Obstet Gynecol 1971;109:1217.
77. Yambao TJ, Clark D, Weiner L, Aubrey RH. Isolation of cytomegalovirus from the amniotic fluid during the third trimester. Am J Obstet Gynecol 1988;158:1189.
78. Huikeshoven FJ, Wallenburg HC, Jahoda MG. Diagnosis of severe fetal cytomegalovirus infection from amniotic fluid in the third trimester of pregnancy. Am J Obstet Gynecol 1982;142:1053.
79. Elek SD, Stern H. Development of a vaccine against mental retardation caused by cytomegalovirus infection in utero. Lancet 1974;1:1.
80. Osburn JE. Cytomegalovirus: pathogenicity, immunology, and vaccine initiatives. J Infect Dis 1981;143:618.
81. Balfour CL, Balfour HH. Cytomegalovirus is not an occupational risk for nurses in renal transplant and neonatal units. JAMA 1986;256:1909.
82. Nahmias AJ, Josey WE, Naib ZM, Luce CF, Duffey A. Antibodies to *Herpesvirus hominis* types 1 and 2 in humans. I. Patients with genital herpetic infections. Am J Epidemiol 1970;91:539.
83. Josey WE, Nahmias AJ, Naib ZM. The epidemiology of type 2 (genital) herpes simplex virus infection. Obstet Gynecol Surv 1972;27:295.
84. Nahmias AJ, Keyserling HL, Kerrick GM. Herpes simplex. In: Remington SJ, Klein JO, eds. Infections of the fetus and newborn infant. Philadelphia: WB Saunders, 1983:636.
85. Becker TM, Stone KM, Cates W, Jr. Epidemiology of genital herpes in the United States. The current situation. J Reprod Med 1986;31:359.
86. Sullivan-Bolyai J, Hull HF, Corey L. Neonatal herpes simplex virus infection in King County, Washington. Increasing incidence and epidemiologic correlates. JAMA 1983;250:3059.
87. Brown ZA, Berry S, Vontver LA. Genital herpes simplex virus infections complicating pregnancy. Natural history and peripartum management. J Reprod Med 1986;31:420.
88. Nerurkar LS, West F, May M, Madden DL, Sever JL. Survival of herpes simplex virus in water specimens collected from hot tubs in spa facilities and on plastic surfaces. JAMA 1983;250:3081.
89. Harger JH, Pazin GJ, Breinig MC. Current understanding of the natural history of genital herpes simplex infections. J Reprod Med 1986;31:365.
90. Nahmias AJ, Dowdle WR, Naib ZM, Josey WE, Luce CF. Genital infection with *Herpesvirus hominis* types 1 and 2 in children. Pediatrics 1968;42:659.
91. Light IJ. Postnatal acquisition of herpes simplex virus by the newborn infant: a review of the literature. Pediatrics 1979;63:480.
92. South MA, Tompkins WAF, Morris R, Rawls WE. Congenital malformation of the central nervous system associated with genital type (type 2) herpesvirus. J Pediatr 1969;75:13.
93. Hutto C, Arvin A, Jacobs R, et al. Intrauterine herpes simplex virus infections. J Pediatr 1987;110:97.
94. Granat M, Morag A, Margalioth EJ, Leviner E, Ornoy A. Fetal outcome following primary herpetic gingivostomatitis in early pregnancy. Morphologic study and updated appraisal. Isr J Med Sci 1986;22:455.
95. Yeager AS, Arvin AM, Urbani LJ, Kemp JA, III. Relationship of antibody to outcome in neonatal herpes simplex virus infections. Infect Immun 1980;29:532.
96. Prober CG, Sullender WM, Yasukawa LL, Au DS, Yeager AS, Arvin AM. Low risk of herpes simplex virus infections in neonates exposed to the virus at the time of vaginal delivery to mothers with recurrent genital herpes simplex virus infections. N Engl J Med 1987;316:240.
97. Buchman TG, Roizman B, Adams G, Hewitt Stover B. Restriction endonuclease fingerprinting of herpes simplex virus DNA: a novel epidemiological tool applied to a nosocomial outbreak. J Infect Dis 1978;138:488.
98. Corey L, Adams HG, Brown ZA, Holmes KK. Genital herpes simplex virus infections: clinical manifestations, course, and complications. Ann Intern Med 1983;98:958.
99. Arvin AM, Hensleigh PA, Prober CG, et al. Failure of antepartum maternal cultures to predict the infant's risk of exposure to herpes simplex at delivery. N Engl J Med 1986;315:796.
100. Wilson CB. Immunologic basis for increased susceptibility of the neonate to infection. J Pediatr 1986;108:1.
101. Kohl S. The neonatal human's immune response to herpes simplex virus infection: a critical review. Pediatr Infect Dis J 1989;8:67.
102. Stanberry LR, Burke RL, Myers MG. Herpes simplex virus glycoprotein treatment of recurrent genital herpes. J Infect Dis 1988;157:156.
103. Pazin GJ, Harger JH, Armstrong JA, et al. Leukocyte interferon for treating first episodes of genital herpes in women. J Infect Dis 1987;156:891.
104. Amstey MS. Effect of pregnancy hormones on herpesvirus and other deoxyribonucleic acid viruses. Am J Obstet Gynecol 1977;129:159.
105. Young EJ, Killam AP, Greene JF. Disseminated herpes virus infection in association with primary genital herpes in pregnancy. JAMA 1976;235:2731.
106. Guinan ME, MacCalman J, Kern ER, et al. The course of untreated recurrent genital herpes simplex infection in 27 women. N Engl J Med 1981;304:759.
107. Bolognese RJ, Corson SL, Fuccillo DA, Traub R, Moder F, Sever JL. Herpesvirus hominis type II infections in asymptomatic pregnant women. Obstet Gynecol 1976;48:507.
108. Nahmias AJ, Josey WE, Naib ZM, Freeman MG, Fernandez RJ, Wheeler JH. Perinatal risk associated with maternal genital

herpes simplex virus infection. Am J Obstet Gynecol 1971;110:825.

109. Honig PJ, Holzwanger J, Leyden JJ. Congenital herpes simplex virus infections. Report of three cases and review of the literature. Arch Dermatol 1979;115:1329.

110. Whitley RJ. Neonatal herpes simplex virus infections. Presentation and management. J Reprod Med 1986;31:426.

111. Sever JL. New tissue culture-fluorescent method speeds detection of herpes simplex virus. JAMA 1983;250:3045.

112. Grossman JH. Diagnostic techniques for evaluating herpes simplex virus infections. Laboratory considerations. J Reprod Med 1986;31:384.

113. Baker DA, Gonik B, Milch PO, Berkowitz, Lipson S, Verma U. Clinical evaluation of a new herpes simplex virus ELISA: a rapid diagnostic test for herpes simplex virus. Obstet Gynecol 1989;73:322.

114. Overall JC, Whitley RJ, Yeager AS, McCracken GH, Nelson JD. Prophylactic or anticipatory antiviral therapy for newborns exposed to herpes simplex virus infection. Pediatr Infect Dis 1984;3:193.

115. Amstey MS, Monif GRG, Nahmias AJ, Josey WE. Cesarean section and genital herpesvirus infection. Obstet Gynecol 1979;53:641.

116. Binkin NJ, Koplan JP, Cates W. Preventing neonatal herpes. The value of weekly viral cultures in pregnant women with recurrent genital herpes. JAMA 1984;251:2816.

117. Arvin AM, Yaeger AS, Bruhn FW, Grossman M. Neonatal herpes simplex infection in the absence of mucocutaneous lesions. J Pediatr 1982;100:715.

118. Harger JH, Amortegui AJ, Meyer MP, Pazin GJ. Characteristics of recurrent genital herpes simplex infection in pregnant women. Obstet Gynecol 1989;73:367.

119. Gibbs RS, Amstey MS, Sweet RL, Mead PB, Sever JL. Management of genital herpes infection in pregnancy. Obstet Gynecol 1988;71:779.

120. Baker DA, Milch PO. Acyclovir for genital herpes simplex virus infections. A review. J Reprod Med 1986;31:433.

121. Baker DA, Blythe JG, Kaufman R, Hale R, Portnoy J. One-year suppression of frequent recurrences of genital herpes with oral acyclovir. Obstet Gynecol 1989;73:84.

122. Brown ZA, Baker DA. Acyclovir therapy during pregnancy. Obstet Gynecol 1989;73:526.

123. Stagno S, Whitley RJ. Herpesvirus infections of pregnancy. Part I: Cytomegalovirus and Epstein-Barr virus infections. N Engl J Med 1985: 313:1270.

124. Freij BJ, Sever JL. Herpesvirus infections in pregnancy: risks to embryo, fetus, and neonate. Clin Perinatol 1988;15:203.

125. Fleisher G, Bolognese R. Epstein-Barr virus infections in pregnancy: a prospective study. J Pediatr 1984;104:374.

126. Hunter K, Stagno S, Capps E, Smith RJ. Prenatal screening of pregnant women for infections caused by cytomegalovirus, Epstein-Barr virus, herpesvirus, rubella, and *Toxoplasma gondii*. Am J Obstet Gynecol 1983;145:269.

127. Le CT, Chang RS, Lipson MH. Epstein-Barr virus infections during pregnancy. A prospective study and review of the literature. Am J Dis Child 1983;137:466.

128. Sumaya CV. Epstein-Barr virus serologic testing: Diagnostic indications and interpretations. Pediatr Infect Dis 1986;5:337.

129. Fleisher G, Bolognese R. Persistent Epstein-Barr virus infection and pregnancy. J Infect Dis 1983;147:982.

130. Miller HC, Clifford SH, Smith CA, et al. Study of the relation of congenital malformation to maternal rubella and other infections: preliminary report. Pediatrics 1949;3:259.

131. Ornoy A, Dudai M, Sadovsky E. Placental and fetal pathology in infectious mononucleosis: a possible indicator for Epstein-Barr virus teratogenicity. Diagn Gynecol Obstet 1982;4:11.

132. Joncas JH, Alfieri C, Leyritz-Wills M, et al. Simultaneous congenital infection with Epstein-Barr virus and cytomegalovirus. N Engl J Med 1981;304:1399.

133. Goldberg GN, Fulginiti VA, Ray CG, et al. In utero Epstein-Barr virus (infectious mononucleosis) infection. JAMA 1981; 246:1579.

134. Radetsky M. A diagnostic approach to Epstein-Barr virus infections. Pediatr Infect Dis 1982;1:425.

135. Andiman WA. The Epstein-Barr virus and EB virus infections in childhood. J Pediatr 1979;95:171.

136. Chang RS, Le CT. Failure to acquire Epstein-Barr virus infection after intimate exposure to the virus. Am J Epidemiol 1984;119:392.

26

CHAPTER

FETAL INFECTIONS FROM NON-TORCH VIRUSES

Ronald S. Gibbs

HUMAN PAPILLOMA VIRUS

Human papilloma virus (HPV) is a common genital tract virus that causes anogenital warts. These viruses are of great interest not only because of a dramatic increase in frequency, but because of their potential roles in genital tract malignancy and juvenile respiratory papilloma virus. Although HPV has not yet been cultured, it is known to be a DNA virus. Presently, there are over 20 subtypes recognized, with the most common types being numbers 6, 11, and 16.[1]

EPIDEMIOLOGY

Within the last 15 years there has been a fully fourfold increase in genital warts (condylomata acuminata). If one considers the recently described cervical "flat warts," it is estimated that approximately 2% of reproductive-age females carry HPV. It is most likely that HPV infections are spread by direct skin-to-skin contact, with sexual activity being the most common mode of spread. Contagion is thought to be relatively high, and condylomata acuminata have been reported on infants at birth. Respiratory papillomatosis results in warts of the larynx and trachea and is thought to result from contact with an infected maternal genital tract at delivery. In about 60% of juveniles with respiratory papillomatosis, genital condyloma has been present in the mother at delivery. Although the incubation period is variable, it is estimated to be relatively long—generally from about 3 to 8 months. Women who have genital warts may also be infected with other sexually transmitted diseases. Most women who have genital warts fall in the age range of 16–25.

DIAGNOSIS

Classically, the genital wart appears as a soft verrucous lesion, several millimeters in diameter. These warts may occur either singly or in clusters and occasionally appear as giant condylomata up to 3 cm or more in diameter. These warts, which often have a pebble surface, are soft and round. They have a predilection for moist areas and are commonly found in the vaginal introitus, the vagina, and the vaginal vestibule. With more common use of colposcopy, minute flat warts are now recognized commonly on the cervix. The diagnosis of condyloma acuminata is usually made on the basis of these classic clinical findings. However, condyloma of secondary syphilis should be ruled out by determining a serologic test for syphilis (ie, VDRL). When the lesion appears atypical or if the diagnosis is suspect, a biopsy may be performed to confirm the diagnosis.

JUVENILE RESPIRATORY PAPILLOMATOSIS

Respiratory papillomatosis has been recognized in both young children and adults, with approximately one third of cases evident by age 5. The most frequent symptom is hoarseness due to involvement of the vocal cords. On occasion, papillomas may be so extensive as to produce respiratory obstruction. In view of the similarity in histology between respiratory papillomas and genital warts, HPV has been suspected as an etiology in both. Recent studies have determined that warts on these two locations are indistinguishable from a virologic viewpoint. In both locations, over 90% of the HPV types are either 6 or 11.[2]

Over 30 years ago it was recognized that HPV might

be transmitted perinatally, as the prevalence of HPV in mothers delivering children afflicted with laryngeal papillomas is much greater than in the general population. In the former group of women, over 50% are afflicted with genital warts, whereas in the general population, the prevalence is approximately 1% to 2%. It has also been speculated that perinatal transmission may occur by ascent of the virus into the uterus or by direct contact at birth. The rate of transmission during vaginal delivery has not been established. However, Shah and colleagues recently estimated this risk with indirect information. They examined the frequency of cesarean delivery in 109 cases of respiratory papillomas with onset before age 14.[2] It was presumed by these investigators that cesarean delivery before rupture of the membranes would prevent intrapartum transmission but would not prevent other modes of spread. Because of the rarity of respiratory papillomatosis, cases were collected from three sources. In all cases, the diagnosis of respiratory papillomas was proved by culture. In only 1 of the 109 cases was there a history of cesarean birth. The authors reasoned that on the basis of the national cesarean section rate in the relevant years, there would have been 10 cesarean births in these 109 patients. Thus, the authors concluded that in juvenile onset respiratory papillomatosis, mother-to-infant transmission occurs most often during vaginal delivery but that in utero infection is also possible, as the child who developed respiratory papillomatosis was born by cesarean section before membrane rupture. Further, in view of the frequency of genital warts and the rarity of juvenile respiratory papillomatosis, it was estimated that the risk of developing disease for a child born vaginally to an infected mother would be low, probably in the range of one in 80 to one in 1500. Based on this estimate, some might suggest that mothers with genital warts be delivered by cesarean section to prevent respiratory papillomatosis. There is little general support for this position, for three reasons:

1. The risk of transmission of the disease is very small.
2. Cesarean delivery does not offer a complete protection.
3. The risk of cesarean section for all women with any genital warts probably would outweigh the potential benefit.[2]

TREATMENT OF CONDYLOMATA ACUMINATA IN PREGNANCY

In general, predisposing features, including vaginitis, should be treated and the areas involved should be kept clean and dry. In addition to the problem of transmission of HPV to the neonate, warts in pregnancy may lead to bleeding during delivery and to tears. We believe that genital warts in pregnancy should be treated when recognized. It has been noted that condyloma acuminata exacerbate in pregnancy, perhaps due to a degree of maternal immunosuppression. Specific treatment recommendations for the non-pregnant woman must be modified in pregnancy. Podophyllin should be avoided, as it may be absorbed if applied to large areas and may be toxic to the fetus. For an isolated large condyloma, surgical incision would be the most appropriate treatment. For smaller lesions, treatment may be performed with carbon dioxide laser, with electrocoagulation with curettage, or with cryotherapy.

HEPATITIS

Viral hepatitis is a common infection that affects predominantly the liver. Of all hospitalized cases of hepatitis in pregnancy, approximately 80% are caused by hepatitis B. Hepatitis A is responsible for approximately 7%, and non-A, non-B hepatitis is responsible for the remainder. Laboratory diagnosis can confirm the presence of hepatitis A or B infection, whereas non-A, non-B is established only by exclusion. Hepatitis A is also referred to as "infectious" hepatitis or "short-incubation" hepatitis, and hepatitis B has been referred to as "serum" hepatitis, "long-incubation" hepatitis, and hepatitis B "surface antigen positive" hepatitis. Other infections that may cause a secondary hepatitis include Epstein-Barr virus infection, Coxsackie B infection, cytomegalovirus infection, and others. In this chapter the main emphasis will be on perinatal consequences of hepatitis B infection in pregnancy.

EPIDEMIOLOGY

Hepatitis B is a worldwide problem with an estimated 5% prevalence. Thus, over 200 million carriers are estimated throughout the world. In the United States, which is a low-prevalence area, it is estimated that the prevalence is from 0.01% to 0.5% of the population (an estimated 1 million HBV carriers).[3] Women in the United States most at risk for hepatitis B surface antigenemia (HBsAg) are as follows:

Asian Pacific Basin or Native Alaskan women, whether immigrants or US-born, 15%
Haitian, Sub-Saharan African, Eastern European, Middle Eastern, Caribbean, Central or South American women, 15%
Women with occupational exposure (ie, medical or dental), 0.5% to 1%
Women working or residing in custodial institutions, 3%
Women with acute or chronic liver disease, illicit drug users, or women with multiple blood transfusions, 7% to 10%
Women living in a household with an HBV-infected person, 6% to 13%.

The impact of HBV infection is immense. Its consequences include chronic hepatitis, cirrhosis, and primary hepatocellular carcinoma. Of an estimated

300,000 new cases yearly in the United States, 75,000 of these will become clinically ill, including 15,000 requiring hospitalization. A small number, estimated at 375, will die of fulminant disease. Six percent to 10% will become chronic carriers, and as many as 25% of these HBV carriers eventually will die of cirrhosis or hepatocellular carcinoma. Despite the availability of an effective vaccine, the incidence of HBV reported to the Centers for Disease Control (CDC) has continued to increase. In 1981, the incidence was 9.2 per 100,000, and in 1985 it was 11.5 per 100,000. The incidence of hepatitis B infection in pregnant women is the same as that in the general population, and the course of the disease in pregnancy is probably not altered.

HBV infection is spread by sexual transmission, blood transfusion, IV drug abuse, and intrauterine or perinatal transmission from the mother to the fetus/newborn (Table 26-1). The major concern in pregnancy is transmission to the infant. In the Far East, approximately 40% of HBV cases in mothers result in vertical transmission to the fetus or newborn.[4] In the United States, the reported overall risk of perinatal HBV transmission from HBV surface antigen-positive mothers ranges from 20% to 50%, with the rate of transmission depending on population characteristics. These influencing characteristics include ethnic background, life-style, and persistence of the HBe antigen. Nonfulminant hepatitis probably does not increase fetal wastage but may be associated with an increased risk of prematurity. Finally, there is no apparent increase in congenital anomalies associated with maternal hepatitis B infection in pregnancy.

VIROLOGY AND SEROLOGY OF HBV INFECTION

Hepatitis B virus is a DNA virus 42 nm in diameter. The outer protein coat is the so-called surface, the HBsAg. This antigen is produced in excess by the virus and appears in the serum of individuals with active infection. The central core contains DNA, a DNA polymerase, and the core antigen, HBcAg. The core antigen is found only in infected liver cells, not in the serum. The third antigen, HBeAg, is found in the serum and is a marker of high rates of perinatal transmission.

TABLE 26-1. HEPATITIS TRANSMISSION RATES FROM THE MOTHER TO THE FETUS/NEONATE

MOTHER'S CLINICAL AND SEROLOGIC STATUS	INFECTION RATE IN INFANT (%)
Acute HBV in third trimester or within 1 month of delivery	80–90
Asymptomatic, HBeAg pos	90
Asymptomatic, HBeAg neg	10–30
Asymptomatic, anti-HBe pos	0–10

Each of these three HBV antigens has a corresponding antibody, called anti-HBs, anti-HBc, and anti-HBe. The serologic pattern that is followed in 90% of cases of HBV infection is that within 6 months of infection, all antigens are cleared from the serum. This individual becomes noninfectious. The antibodies to HBs and to HBc are life-long markers of prior infection.

In the remaining 10% of individuals with HBV infection, there is persistence of HBsAg beyond 6 months. Approximately 60% of these women with persistence of infection will develop chronic persistent hepatitis. About 10% will have asymptomatic HBsAg antigenemia, and approximately 30% will have chronic active hepatitis. All these groups are potentially infective of others, including, in pregnant women, transmission to the offspring. This is a group that is the target for prenatal screening. Transmission rates from the mother to the fetus–neonate are shown in Table 26-1.[5,6]

CLINICAL MANIFESTATIONS

After an incubation period of 45–160 days, hepatitis B may become clinically evident. Initial symptoms often include fever, headache, and abdominal pain, followed in several days by spontaneous resolution. At this point, the urine may become dark and jaundice may be evident. The liver is usually somewhat enlarged and tender. As the jaundice resolves, the patient spontaneously feels better and usually recovers rapidly. As noted, in approximately 10% of patients with hepatitis B, a form of chronic disease continues. Rarely, hepatitis B may present as an acute fulminated form that may become fatal, although this is quite rare in well-nourished Western populations. Fulminant hepatitis is heralded by a rapidly shrinking liver, rapidly rising bilirubin, and abnormalities in prothrombin time with development of encephalopathy and ascites. The mortality rate in such cases of fulminant hepatitis is greater than 80%.

In the neonate, the most frequent presentation of hepatitis infection is an asymptomatic child with chronic infection. Clinical illness is relatively infrequent with congenital hepatitis, but about 10% of neonates with asymptomatic disease become jaundiced within the first 3–4 months of life.

TREATMENT

Most women with hepatitis B infection during pregnancy can be managed on an outpatient basis. There is no specific treatment, but supportive measures include increased bedrest and a high-protein, low-fat diet. Specific indications for hospitalization of women with viral hepatitis include severe anemia, diabetes, protracted nausea and vomiting, abnormalities in prothrombin time, a rapidly falling or low serum albumin level, and high serum bilirubin greater than approximately 15 mg/dL.

PREVENTION

Women with a definite exposure to hepatitis B virus should be given hepatitis B immune globulin (HBIG) as soon as possible within a 7-day period of exposure, with a second dose 30 days after the first. Such passive immunization would be indicated for hospital exposures and inoculation with contaminated needles. Until June 1988, the Centers for Disease Control had recommended screening of pregnant women for asymptomatic hepatitis B infection on a selective basis.

However, in mid-1988, the Centers for Disease Control[7] overhauled recommendations based on several recent studies that demonstrated that selective screening identified only 50% of women who were HBsAg positive.[7–10] The study populations were medically indigent women located in Cleveland, New Orleans, and Miami, for example. In middle-class populations, the sensitivity of selective screening has not been well studied. Yet a cost analysis study carried out at the CDC concluded that even in extremely low-prevalence populations (with a prevalence of less than 0.1%), the universal screening program would be cost effective.[11]

The purpose of universal screening is to allow treatment of newborns of HBsAg-positive women with hepatitis B immune globulin (HBIG) and hepatitis B vaccine —a regimen that is 90% effective in preventing the development of HBV chronic carrier state in the newborn. The specifics of the recommendation are that women should be tested for HBsAg during an early prenatal visit. Testing for additional markers is considered unnecessary. Even though women who have HBeAg are at a much higher risk for perinatal transmission, there is still a risk of about 10% to 15% in perinatal transmission in women who do not have the e antigen but who have HBsAg. If a woman is identified as being HBsAg positive, she should be evaluated for active liver disease. Infants born to HBsAg-positive women should receive HBIG (0.5 mL) IM once they are stable, preferably within 12 hours of birth. In addition, these infants should receive the recombinant HBV vaccine (5 μg per dose), or they may receive the plasma-derived vaccine (10 μg per dose). Either of these vaccines should be given intramuscularly in the following sequence of three doses: the first at birth, and the second and third at 1 and 6 months of age, respectively. It is estimated that the direct cost to prevent one newborn from becoming a chronic HBV carrier would be approximately $12,700 if the prevalence of HBsAg in a given population is approximately five in 1000.[12]

Household members and sexual partners of women identified as being HBsAg positive should be tested to determine susceptibility to HBV infection. Susceptible individuals should receive the HBV vaccine.[12]

Since few women in low-risk populations for HBV infection will have a change in the HBsAg antigen status during subsequent pregnancies, it may be argued that routine testing in each pregnancy is unnecessary. However, because of the expected benefits of routine testing and the possibility of omission if done selectively, the CDC currently recommends testing during each pregnancy. On the other hand, routine follow-up testing later in pregnancy is not necessary. Women who deliver without prenatal care should be tested as early as possible on delivery admission so that infants at risk can begin to receive their prophylaxis within 48 hours after birth. It is further recommended that hospitals that cannot rapidly test for HBsAg either develop this capability or test at another laboratory.[12]

As a further preventive measure it is recommended that during delivery of HBsAg-positive women, gloves, masks, and glasses or goggles be worn by delivery room personnel to keep infectious fluids away from mouth, nose, eyes, and breaks in the skin. All these precautions are equally important in guarding against HBV infection and in preventing transmission of the AIDS virus. Thus, to prevent both of these serious infections, universal blood and body fluid precautions are the best measures of preventing nosocomial transmission.[12]

VARICELLA

A member of the herpesvirus group, varicella zoster (VZ) virus is a DNA virus that exhibits a viral latency. Primary infection usually occurs in childhood, clinically presenting as chickenpox. As a highly contagious disorder, varicella zoster infection is acquired by most children in the United States prior to reproductive age and is generally a self-limited disease characterized by typical skin lesions.[13] It is recognized that when adults contract the disease both constitutional and pulmonary symptoms may be more severe. Reactivation of latent zoster infection clinically presents as shingles, generally occurring in the older population or in immunocompromised individuals. Zoster presents as painful crops of vesicular lesions occurring along the distribution of a segmental dermatome.

The remainder of this discussion will be limited to the effects of VZ infection in pregnancy. There are two major concerns for the perinatologist. The first is the risk the infection imposes for the mother; the second is the risk of either teratogenesis or perinatal acquisition to the fetus or neonate.

EPIDEMIOLOGY

Over 150,000 cases of chickenpox occur annually in the United States.[14] Yet, because of widespread underreporting, it is estimated that the actual number of cases is 2–3 million.[15,16] Over 90% of the population has been infected during childhood. The incidence of varicella zoster infection in pregnancy is estimated at approximately five in 10,000 pregnancies.

CLINICAL PRESENTATION

After an incubation period of from 10 to 20 days (usually 13–17 days), fever and rash commonly occur simultaneously in children. In adults, fever and generalized malaise usually precede the rash by several days. The rash usually begins on the face and scalp and then spreads to the trunk. There is usually minimal involvement of the extremities. The skin lesion begins as a macule and proceeds to a vesicular and then pustular stage. Healing is heralded by the presentation of crusts and scabs. The prominent feature of the disease is itching. Over a period of 2–5 days, new crops of lesions occur, and lesions in various stages of progression usually are present at the same time.

Bacterial infection of the skin is the common secondary complication of chickenpox.[13] Encephalitis, meningitis, myocarditis, glomerulonephritis, and arthritis are all rare complications in childhood. The most serious complication of varicella infection is pneumonia. It occurs more commonly in adults, but the pneumonia does not appear to have an increased prevalence in pregnant women as opposed to other adults.[15–17] Currently, it is estimated that approximately 5% to 10% of adults with chickenpox develop pneumonia. In a review of the literature on varicella pneumonia in pregnancy, Young and Gershon noted in 1983 that of 77 cases of chickenpox in pregnancy, 29% developed pneumonia. Because of selectivity, we estimate that this incidence of varicella pneumonia in pregnancy is high. Ten deaths occurred —all in women who had pneumonia. The mortality of varicella pneumonia in this series was 45%. There were no severe complications in women who did not develop pneumonia.[13] Accordingly, it appears that uncomplicated chickenpox poses no major threat to the pregnant woman, especially in view of current critical care abilities to manage severe respiratory distress and failure. We believe that mortality now would be improved.

For the clinician, the main objective is to maintain a high index of suspicion for pneumonia in women who have varicella infection in pregnancy. Pulmonary symptoms usually begin on the second to sixth day after appearance of the rash and usually present with a mild nonproductive cough. If the disease is more severe, there may be additional symptoms, including hemoptysis, dyspnea, pleuritic chest pain, or progression to frank cyanosis. Physical examination in women who develop pneumonia would include fever, rales, and wheezes. The chest x-ray characteristically shows a miliary pattern or a diffuse nodular pattern. On the chest x-ray, the perihilar regions are more likely to be involved. Women who have varicella infection without complications in pregnancy do not need to be hospitalized. However, women with this infection must be warned to contact their physician immediately in the event of any pulmonary symptoms, including a mild cough. At this point, hospitalization with full respiratory support, if necessary, should be indicated.

In a recent series of 43 pregnancies complicated by maternal varicella, Paryani and Arvin noted that nine women had developed associated morbidity.[18] Varicella pneumonia developed in four of these women (9%), one of whom died. Premature labor developed in four out of 42 (10%), with premature delivery occurring in two (5%). Another woman developed herpes zoster infection.

If a pregnant woman is exposed to varicella infection, it is very likely that she is immune, but if she is not immune, it is most probable that she will become infected. McGregor and colleagues recently pointed out that most pregnant women have detectable antibody even if they have a negative history of chickenpox.[19] In their series, 12 out of 17 (71%) of such women were already antibody-positive. Of those women with indeterminate histories, approximately 90% were immune. On the basis of these data, it appears appropriate and cost effective to test for maternal antibody by any of the following antibody tests: fluorescent antibody to membrane antigen (FAMA), enzyme-linked immunosorbent assay (ELISA), enhanced neutralization test, and immune adherence hemagglutination.

If it is found that a woman has been exposed and is susceptible, varicella zoster immune globulin (VZIG) may be given. When administered intramuscularly within 3 days of exposure, it is likely that VZIG ameliorates the course of the maternal disease as it does in children.[20] However, it is not at all certain that passive immunization with VZIG prevents fetal infection. Currently, there is no reason to believe that VZIG in pregnancy is harmful. Thus, the only disadvantage of providing VZIG to nonimmune pregnant women with exposure to varicella is the cost, currently a few hundred dollars.

VARICELLA IN THE NEWBORN

Acquisition by the fetus of maternal antibody usually is protective. However, in an infant born after maternal viremia but before maternal development of antibodies, the infant is at high risk for potentially life-threatening neonatal varicella infection. Infants at risk are those whose mothers develop clinical varicella within 5 days of birth or within the first 5 days after delivery. Congenital varicella infection has been reported in approximately 20% of term infants born to mothers with varicella within this time frame, and the case fatality has been reported at approximately 30%. Infants born 5 or more days after maternal development of clinical illness develop either a mild varicella infection or none whatsoever. Both zoster immunoglobulin (ZIG) and varicella zoster immunoglobulin (VZIG) have been shown to modify or prevent varicella in normal children, leading Brunell to recommend their use in preventing severe neonatal infections.

Accordingly, infants at risk, as outlined earlier, should receive ZIG or VZIG as passive immunization at a dose of 1.25 mL. Weibel and colleagues have recently reported excellent results using a live attenuated varicella vaccine.[21] The seroconversion rate was 94% and the vaccine was 100% effective in preventing varicella. In a placebo-controlled group, approximately 10% of children developed varicella.

EFFECT OF ZOSTER VARICELLA INFECTION IN EARLY PREGNANCY

Congenital birth defects due to varicella in early pregnancy were not recognized until about 40 years ago.[22] The syndrome of congenital varicella infection consists of limb hypoplasia, cicatricial skin lesions, atrophic digits, psychomotor retardation, growth retardation, and even bilateral cortical atrophy.[22] We now recognize that maternal varicella infection in the first trimester of pregnancy may be responsible for such a syndrome, but the risk of the fetus developing these anomalies with first-trimester chickenpox has only recently been recognized. Of 11 infants of women with first-trimester varicella, one (9%) developed findings consistent with congenital varicella syndrome.[18]

EFFECT OF ZOSTER IN PREGNANCY

Herpes zoster infection, as noted, is caused by the same virus that causes clinical chickenpox. Zoster occurs very rarely in pregnancy, and because it is a reactivation, maternal antibodies are already present. In healthy women, zoster poses no special threat to the fetus or newborn.

MEASLES (RUBEOLA)

Measles is a common acute illness, most likely occurring in childhood. Among the most communicable of childhood exanthems, rubeola is characterized by fever, coryza, cough, maculopapular rash, and conjunctivitis. Rubeola virus is an RNA virus belonging to the paramyxovirus group.

EPIDEMIOLOGY

With an incubation time between 10 and 14 days, measles is spread chiefly by droplets expectorated by infected persons. The virus gains access to susceptible individuals via the nose, oropharynx, and conjunctiva. It is most communicable during the prodromal as well as catarrhal stages of infection. Three fourths of exposed susceptible individuals develop the infection. Prior to the availability of live measles vaccines, epidemics occurred in the United States at 2- to 3- year intervals.[24,25] Since 1963, the introduction of the attenuated measles vaccine has had a major impact in decreasing measles in the United States.

Occurring less frequency than either chickenpox or mumps in pregnancy, measles has a rate of approximately of 0.4–0.6 per 10,000 pregnancies.

CLINICAL MANIFESTATIONS

The clinical prodrome that consists of fever and malaise usually begins 10–11 days after exposure. The coryza, sneezing, conjunctivitis, and cough usually begin approximately 24 hours later. This catarrhal phase worsens over the next few days, often leading to marked conjunctivitis and photophobia. The so-called Koplik's spots, pathognomonic of measles, appear at the end of the prodrome. These characteristic lesions are tiny granular, slightly raised, white lesions surrounded by erythema and located on the lateral buccal mucosa. The characteristic rash begins 12–14 days after exposure and begins on the head and neck, especially in the posterior auricular region. The rash, maculopapular in character, spreads to the trunk, upper extremities, and finally the lower extremities.

Pulmonary complications are the most frequent complications of measles, with otitis media and croup also occurring frequently. Bacterial pneumonia is the complication with most frequent association with mortality. Encephalitis is a less common serious complication, occurring in an estimated one case of measles out of 1000. Rare complications of measles include thrombocytopenic purpura, myocarditis, and subacute sclerosing panencephalitis.

EFFECTS OF MEASLES ON THE MOTHER

It is unclear whether pregnant women with measles are at greater risk for serious complications or death than nonpregnant adults. Recent studies have noted that measles in pregnant women is very rarely associated with major complications such as pneumonia.[26]

EFFECT OF MEASLES ON THE FETUS

Recent reviews of the literature note that there is an increased rate of prematurity in pregnancies complicated by measles, especially when the disease occurs in the third trimester. However, measles does not appear associated with an increased risk for spontaneous abortion. No fetal syndrome of abnormalities has been found among the sporadic instances of congenital defects occurring in women who reported maternal measles.[27] Thus, if there is any increased risk of congenital malformations from measles occurring in pregnancy, the risk appears to be very small. When measles becomes clinically apparent in the first 10 days of life, it is considered to be congenital, that is, transplacental in origin. Cases becoming clinically evident at 14 days or after are considered to be acquired postnatally. Postnatally acquired measles is usually a very mild disorder, whereas the spectrum of congenital measles varies from a mild illness to a rapidly fatal disease. We note that the presence of maternal measles immediately prior to delivery does not involve the fetus and neonate commonly. In cases of congenital measles, a mortality rate of 32% has been reported (seven out of 22). Premature infants with congenital measles have a significantly higher death rate (56%) than do term infected infants (20%). We do not know whether transplacentally acquired antibodies to measles virus diminish the case fatality rate in congenital measles if the mother's rash occurs more than 48 hours before delivery. It is important to note that the reported cases of mortality due to congenital measles all occurred in the preantibiotic era. Accordingly, with antimicrobial therapy effective against secondary bacterial pneumonia and modern support, we anticipate that fatal outcomes of rubeola infection are much less likely.

DIAGNOSIS

Diagnosis of measles relies on the clinical history and typical clinical presentation. Elements in the differential diagnosis include rubella, scarlet fever, meningococcemia, roseola, Rocky Mountain spotted fever, infectious mononucleosis, other enterovirus infections, toxoplasmosis, and drug eruptions.

TREATMENT

Uncomplicated measles is treated symptomatically. If secondary otitis media or pneumonia occur, then an appropriate antibiotic should be instituted.

PREVENTION

Susceptible exposed pregnant women, neonates, and their contacts should receive passive immunization. Immune serum globulin (ISG) in a dose of 0.25 mg/kg as soon as possible after an exposure may prevent or at least modify the infection.

Children born to women who have measles in the last week of pregnancy or first week postpartum should also be given the immune serum globulin as soon as possible in the same dose.[28]

MUMPS

Mumps is an acute generalized infection in childhood that has a predilection for the parotid and salivary glands. There is no characteristic rash. The mumps virus is also an RNA virus and a member of the paramyxovirus family.

EPIDEMIOLOGY

The virus is spread by saliva and droplet contamination. It has been recovered from salivary and respiratory secretions from approximately 7 days before the onset of clinical parotitis until 9 days afterward. The usual incubation period runs approximately 2–2.5 weeks. Only approximately 10% of cases occur after the age of 15, because most adults are immune as a consequence of childhood illness. Approximately one third of cases are subclinical. Mumps is less contagious than measles or chickenpox, and the attack rate, even among exposed, susceptible household members, is low. Mumps occurs more frequently in pregnant women than measles or chickenpox, with an estimated incidence of approximately 0.8–10 cases per 10,000 pregnancies.[29]

CLINICAL MANIFESTATIONS

Mumps begins with a prodrome of fever, malaise, myalgia, and anorexia and then develops into parotitis within approximately 24 hours. This stage is characterized by tender, painful, swollen parotid glands. On physical examination, the orifice of Stenson's duct is red and swollen. Most commonly, parotitis is bilateral. The submaxillary glands are less involved and never become involved without parotid gland involvement. It is unusual for sublingual glands to be affected. Mumps is usually self-limited, and complications are rare.[30]

In approximately 20% of postpubertal males, orchitis occurs. This is the most common manifestation other than parotitis in this group. Oophoritis is much less common and presents with adnexal pain. Aseptic meningitis is a rare but recognized neurologic complication of mumps. Mumps meningitis is almost always benign and self-limited. Rare complications of mumps include pancreatitis, mastitis, thyroiditis, myocarditis, arthritis, and nephritis.

EFFECT ON MOTHER AND FETUS

In pregnancy, mumps is generally benign and not more involved than in nonpregnant patients. Similarly, asymptomatic meningitis in pregnant patients is neither more frequent nor severe. Mortality is extremely rare in both pregnant and nonpregnant adults.

In retrospective studies, mumps occurring in the first trimester of pregnancy has been associated with a twofold increase in the rate of spontaneous abortion.[31] Mumps, however, has not been associated with prematurity, growth retardation, or excess perinatal mortality. It is uncertain whether mumps leads to any congenital disease. Definite evidence of teratogenic potential for mumps virus in humans has not been presented. In a controlled prospective study, Siegal noted that congenital malformations were no more common in neonates whose mothers had mumps during pregnancy than in controls.[32] In both groups, the rates of congenital anomalies were approximately 2%.

Of concern in the past decade and a half has been the purported association between maternal mumps infection and development of the congenital cardiac defect endocardial fibroelastosis.[33,34] Data are currently conflicting and the low incidence of mumps in pregnancy makes it unlikely that prospective and controlled data will be gathered in the near future.

DIAGNOSIS

As with measles, the diagnosis of mumps is usually made on clinical grounds. The diagnosis is straightforward with the typical presentation of acute bilateral parotitis and the history of recent exposure. In more difficult cases, the diagnosis may depend on virus isolation or on demonstration of a rising antibody of the complement fixation, hemagglutination inhibition, or neutralizing antibody type.

TREATMENT

Again, the treatment of mumps is symptomatic in both pregnant and non-pregnant individuals. Supportive treatment includes bedrest, application of cold or heat to the parotids, and analgesics. Maternal mumps is not an indication for termination of pregnancy.

Live attenuated mumps vaccine has been effective in preventing primary mumps, because 95% of susceptible individuals develop antibodies. Clinical adverse reactions have been infrequent and mild. Immunization of mumps with live-virus vaccine in pregnancy is contraindicated on the theoretical grounds that the developing fetus might be harmed. Although the risk to the fetus seems negligible, the innocuous nature of mumps in pregnancy suggests that any risk from vaccination should be avoided.

INFLUENZA

Influenza viruses belong to the myxovirus group and cause the clinical entity of influenza that occurs in epidemics. Type A influenza is responsible for most epidemics and is associated with more severe disease, whereas types B and C occur less frequently.[35]

EPIDEMIOLOGY

The frequency and severity of influenza outbreaks have been related to changes in the viral antigens.[35] The major antigenic changes occur at 10- to 30-year intervals and are associated with severe infection because of the absence of protective antibodies.

Two major pandemics occurred in 1918 and in 1957–1958. More than 20 million deaths occurred worldwide during the pandemic of 1918.[36]

CLINICAL PRESENTATION

With a short incubation period of 1–4 days, influenza presents with abrupt onset of an upper respiratory infection, fever, malaise, myalgia, and headache. With wide clinical variability, the major portion of the disease lasts approximately 3 days in most cases.

Definitive diagnosis can be made by isolation of virus from throat washings during acute illness or by serologic confirmation of a fourfold rise in antibody. Although these antibodies are of either the complement fixation or hemagglutination inhibition types, they are rarely indicated clinically.

MATERNAL EFFECTS OF INFLUENZA

For the obstetrician, the major concern of influenza infection in pregnancy is the increased likelihood for potentially life-threatening pneumonia. From reports of epidemics in both 1918 and 1957, it appears that pregnant women were disproportionately represented in individuals dying of influenza. In addition, reported estimates of maternal mortality rate are approximately 27%, with a mortality rate of almost 50% in cases complicated by pneumonia. It is not certain, however, whether pregnant women are more likely to develop influenza or whether they are more likely to develop influenza pneumonia. Yet if influenza pneumonia develops in pregnancy, then it is more severe. Deaths among pregnant women with influenza may result from secondary bacterial infection and from primary influenza pneumonia without secondary superinfection.

EFFECTS OF INFLUENZA ON THE FETUS

Contradictory data address the issues of the effect of influenza on abortion, prematurity, and congenital anomalies.[37] These studies may be summarized as noting that the vast majority of women who have influenza in pregnancy have normal outcomes and that there seems to be little influence on congenital abnormalities, intrauterine growth, prematurity, or stillbirth.

TREATMENT

As in other adults, management of uncomplicated pregnant women with influenza is symptomatic, consisting of bedrest, analgesics, liberal fluid intake, and antipyretics (acetaminophen). If signs of pneumonia occur in pregnant women with influenza, prompt evaluation and hospitalization are indicated. Broad-spectrum antibiotic coverage for presumed bacterial superinfection is required.

In nonpregnant individuals, use of amantadine, a blocker of the replication of influenza A virus, has been efficacious in preventing symptoms, shortening the clinical disease, and improving pulmonary function. Since this drug has been associated with teratogenic effects in animals, it is not recommended for use in pregnant women.[38]

PREVENTION

In years of epidemics, it is generally considered advisable to vaccinate pregnant women. However, during the 1977 swine flu vaccination program, pregnancy (in and of itself) was not considered among the high-risk conditions. Influenza vaccines are as immunogenic in pregnant women as in other adults, and no specific complications have been encountered in pregnant women. Because the vaccines are killed virus preparations, they are safe for use during pregnancy.

HUMAN PARVOVIRUS INFECTION IN PREGNANCY

Human parvovirus (B19) infection, recently recognized as a cause of fetal death, has caused great concern in physicians, public health officials, and pregnant women. Information has been developing rapidly, and this chapter will attempt to summarize the current state of knowledge.

B19, first discovered in England in 1975, is now recognized as the causative agent of erythema infectiosum, a worldwide illness most common in children.[39] B19 is also the primary etiologic agent of transient aplastic crisis in patients with chronic hemolytic anemias. As noted, B19 has been associated with both spontaneous abortions and stillbirths and may be involved in acute arthralgia and arthritis as well as chronic anemia in immunodeficient patients. The virus is a member of the Parvoviridae family.

CLINICAL FEATURES OF B19 INFECTION

Erythema infectiosum is characterized by a facial rash commonly referred to as "slapped cheek" appearance.[39] There is also a lacelike rash on the trunk and extremities. The rash may also reappear several weeks later, following exposure to temperature, sunlight, and emotional stress. Otherwise, the patient is well at the onset of the rash but may give a history of mild systemic symptoms a few days before the rash's onset. Pruritus may be a common feature in some outbreaks. Erythema infectiosum is more common in the winter and spring and usually lasts approximately 5–9 days in children. Headache, fever, anorexia, sore throat, and gastrointestinal symptoms occur in a minority of children. Complications such as lymphadenopathy, arthralgia, or arthropathy rarely occur in children. As with other viral infections (eg, rubella), erythema infectiosum (also known as "fifth disease") tends to be more severe in adults. Here fatigue, fever, adenopathy, and arthritis are common. There have also been reports of more serious complications, such as encephalitis, pneumonia, and hemolytic anemia.

In investigations of outbreaks, asymptomatic infection has been reported in up to 20% of adults and children. B19 infection is also associated with a condition known as transient aplastic crisis with asymmetrical peripheral polyarthropathy and with severe chronic anemia in patients who are immunodeficient.

The major concern for the obstetrician, however, is infection with B19 in pregnant women.[40–50] In most of the reported B19 infections during pregnancy, there has been no adverse outcome. However, in some cases fetal death, usually involving hydrops fetalis, has occurred. Preliminary results are now being gathered to estimate the risk of fetal death after maternal B19 exposure.[39]

Studies in both the United States and the United Kingdom have suggested that the risk of fetal death in a woman with documented B19 infection is less than 10%. In data cited by the CDC, a British study reported on 174 pregnant women with IgM antibody to B19, followed prospectively toward delivery.[39] Fetal loss occurred in 17%, but not all fetal deaths resulted directly from B19 infection. An estimate of the number of fetal deaths linked to B19 infection was made by determining whether fetal tissues contained B19 DNA. Tests for B19 DNA were available on a subset of infants who died. By extrapolating these results to all fetal deaths, it was estimated that less than 10% of the 174 B19-infected women might have had a B19-associated fetal loss.

In the United States, studies are also ongoing to determine the rate of fetal death.[39] At this time, with 95 pregnant women with IgM antibody to B19 being followed, fetal deaths have so far occurred in 4% of 49 women followed to term, but it is not known whether these fetal deaths were caused by B19 infection. In one instance, the fetus was hydropic. Since antibody status of women may not be commonly available, it is important to estimate the risk of fetal death after exposure. These estimates must take into account the rate of susceptibility in the general population and the risk of infection after exposure. The CDC estimates that by taking these factors into account, the risk of fetal death would be less than 2.5% after exposure of a pregnant woman to a household member with a documented infection. The upper limit of the risk of fetal death would be less than 1.5% in a pregnant woman who has prolonged exposure to B19 infection in the workplace. Further, it is estimated that the upper limit of risk of fetal death occurring in pregnant women with other types of exposure (eg, limited exposure to students with erythema infectiosum) would be substantially less.

Current data suggest that B19 is not responsible for a substantial proportion of fetal deaths in the general population. As noted by Kinney and colleagues, the rate of serologically confirmed B19 infection was the same in a group of 96 stillbirths and in controls (1% each group).[40] Further, in a survey of 50 fetuses with nonimmune hydrops fetalis, four (8%) had positive tests for B19 DNA.

There is currently no evidence that the rate of congenital anomalies exceeds background rates following B19 infection.

Tissues that are positive for B19 DNA have been identified in 20 fetal deaths and in 17 cases with associated pathologic findings; nonimmune hydrops fetalis was present in all.[39] The mechanism of fetal death is undetermined, but it is likely that severe anemia may precipitate congestive heart failure and hydrops. The fetus appears to be especially vulnerable to B19 infection because fetuses have short red blood cell survival time and the fetal red cell volume expands rapidly.

DNA specific for B19 has been identified in respiratory secretions of viremic patients, suggesting this as a major mode of spread. At the time that erythema infectiosum develops, however, patients are probably past the point of greatest infectiousness. After close contact exposure, the virus appears to be transmitted effectively; during school outbreaks, 10% to 60% of students develop erythema infectiosum. In the settings of outbreaks it is not clear whether the major mode of transmission involves direct contact of person-to-person, large-particle droplets; small-particle droplets; or fomites. It is also known that the virus can be transmitted parenterally through transfusion and vertically from mother to fetus.

DIAGNOSIS

Diagnostic testing is available in only a few sites—primarily research laboratories—and through the Centers for Disease Control. At the time of writing, however, the CDC is accepting specimens from only selected patients, including pregnant women exposed to B19 or with symptoms suggestive of B19 and from cases of nonimmune hydrops fetalis probably related to B19 infection.[39] The CDC is not accepting specimens for routine antibody testing. B19 antibody assays are available, with the most sensitive test to detect recent infection being the IgM antibody assay. This can be performed by a captured antibody radioimmunoassay or by enzyme immunoassay. There is also an IgG, B19 antibody assay that is usually positive by the seventh day of illness. IgG persists for years. The IgM antibody, on the other hand, begins to decline after 30–60 days. The most sensitive test for detecting the virus is the B19 DNA nucleic acid hybridization.

TREATMENT AND PREVENTION

Currently, no treatment is available in individuals with presumed B19 infection. They are treated with supportive measures. In otherwise healthy individuals, B19 infection usually produces a mild self-limited infection.

Further, there is no vaccine to prevent B19 infection and no studies have been conducted to assess the value of commercially available immunoglobulin. At this point, the CDC does not recommend routine prophylaxis with immunoglobulin. In health care settings where exposures to B19 may be possible through contact with patients with B19 infection (such as transient aplastic crisis), the CDC has recommended infection control measures such as admission of patients with transient aplastic crisis due to chronic B19 infection to private rooms. It is noteworthy that most patients with erythema infectiosum are past their period of infectiousness by the time clinical symptoms develop, and these individuals do not present a risk for further transmission. Thus, isolation precautions are not necessary.[39]

Hospital personnel who may be pregnant or who might wish to become pregnant should know about the potential risks to their fetus from exposure to B19 infection. In homes, school, and the workplace, the greatest risk of transmitting B19 occurs before the symptoms of erythema infectiosum develop. Therefore, transmission cannot truly be prevented by excluding contact with persons who have erythema infectiosum. The only measure that is currently recommended is handwashing.

MANAGEMENT OF THE PREGNANT WOMAN WITH DOCUMENTED INFECTION

For women with documented infection, diagnostic ultrasound examinations and maternal serum α-fetoprotein levels have been employed in an attempt to identify the adversely affected fetus. It is uncertain whether these tests have high sensitivity and specificity. Intrauterine blood transfusion to the fetus has been attempted for the fetus with B19-induced severe anemia, but the benefits of this approach are not yet evaluated. In view of the recentness of the association between B19 infection and adverse pregnancy outcome, there is great concern in the community. Because of great and intensive interest, it is likely that new information will develop promptly.

REFERENCES

1. Lynch PJ. Condylomata acuminata (anogenital warts). Clin Obstet Gynecol 1985;28:142.
2. Shah K, Kashima H, Polk BF, et al. Rarity of cesarean delivery in cases of juvenile-onset respiratory papillomatosis. Obstet Gynecol 1986;68:795.
3. Sever JL, Larsen JW Jr, Grossman JH III. Handbook of perinatal infections. Boston: Little, Brown, 1979:37.
4. Derso A, Boxall EH, Tarlow MJ, Flewett TH. Transmission of HBsAg from mother to infant in four ethnic groups. Br Med J 1978;1:949.
5. Stevens CE, Neurath RA, Beasley RP, Szmuness W. HBeAg and anti-HBe detection by radioimmunoassay: correlation with vertical transmission of hepatitis B virus in Taiwan. J Med Virol 1979;3:237.

6. Lee AKY, Ip HMH, Wong VCW. Mechanisms of maternal-fetal transmission of hepatitis B virus. J Infect Dis 1978;138:668.
7. Jonas MM, Schiff ER, O'Sullivan MJ, et al. Failure of Centers for Disease to identify hepatitis B infection in large municipal obstetrical populations. Ann Intern Med 1987;107:335.
8. Summers PR, Biswas MK, Pastorek JG, et al. The pregnant hepatitis B carrier: evidence favoring comprehensive antepartum screening. Obstet Gynecol 1987;69:701.
9. Kumar ML, Dawson NV, McCullough AJ, et al. Should all pregnant women be screened for hepatitis B? Ann Intern Med 1987;107:273.
10. Wetzel AM, Kirz DS. Routine hepatitis screening in adolescent pregnancies: is it cost effective? Am J Obstet Gynecol 1987;156:166.
11. Arevalo JA, Washington AE. Cost-effectiveness of prenatal screening and immunization for hepatitis B virus. JAMA 1988;259:365.
12. Prevention of perinatal transmission of hepatitis B virus: prenatal screening of all pregnant women for hepatitis B surface antigen. MMWR 1988;37:341.
13. Young NA, Gershon AA. Chicken pox, measles, and mumps. In: Remington JS, Klein JO, eds. Infectious diseases of the fetus and newborn. Philadelphia: WB Saunders, 1983:375.
14. Centers for Disease Control. Annual summary 1982. Reported morbidity and mortality in the United States. MMWR 1983;31:21.
15. Hermann KL. Congenital and perinatal varicella. Clin Obstet Gynecol 1982;25:605.
16. Preblud SR, D'Angelo LJ. Chickenpox in the United States 1972–1977. J Infect Dis 1979;140:257.
17. Brunell PA. Varicella-zoster infections in pregnancy. JAMA 1967;199:315.
18. Paryani SG, Arvin AM. Intrauterine infection with varicella zoster virus after maternal varicella. N Engl J Med 1986;314:1542.
19. McGregor JA, Mark S, Crawford GP, et al. Varicella zoster antibody testing in the care of pregnant women exposed to varicella. Am J Obstet Gynecol 1987;157:281.
20. Brunell PA. Fetal and neonatal varicella-zoster infections. Semin Perinatol 1983;7:47.
21. Weibel RE, Neff BJ, Kuter BJ, et al. Live attenuated varicella virus vaccine. Efficacy trial in healthy children. N Engl J Med 1984;310:1409.
22. LaForet E, Lynch CL. Multiple congenital defects following maternal varicella. N Engl J Med 1947;236:534.
23. Meyers JD. Congenital varicella in term infants: risk considered. J Infect Dis 1974;129:215.
24. Siegal M, Fuerst H. Low birth weight and maternal virus diseases. A prospective study of rubella, measles, mumps, chicken pox, and hepatitis. JAMA 1966;197:88.
25. Young NA, Gershon AA. Chicken pox, measles and mumps. In: Remington JS, Klein JO, eds. Infectious diseases of the fetus and newborn infant. Philadelphia: WB Saunders, 1983:375.
26. Sever JL, Larsen JW Jr, Grossman JH III. Handbook of perinatal infections. Boston: Little, Brown, 1979:63.
27. Siegal M. Congenital malformations following chicken pox, measles, mumps, and hepatitis. Results of a cohort study. JAMA 1973;226:1521.
28. American Academy of Pediatrics. Report of the Committee on Infectious Diseases. 17th ed. Evanston, IL, 1974:74.
29. Siegal M, Fuerst HT. Low birth weight and maternal virus diseases. A prospective study of rubella, measles, mumps, chicken pox, and hepatitis. JAMA 1966;19:197.
30. Bowers D. Mumps during pregnancy. West J Surg Obstet Gynecol 1953;61:72.
31. Siegal M, Fuerst HT, Peress NS. Comparative fetal mortality in maternal virus disease. A prospective study on rubella, measles, mumps, chicken pox, and hepatitis. N Engl J Med 1966;274:768.
32. Siegal M. Congenital malformations following chicken pox, measles, mumps, and hepatitis. Results of a cohort study. JAMA 1973;226:1521.
33. St Geme JW Jr, Noren GR, Adams P. Proposed embryopathic relation between mumps virus and primary endocardial fibroelastosis. N Engl J Med 1966;275:339.
34. St Geme JW Jr, Peralta H, Farias E, et al. Experimental gestational mumps virus infection and anocardial fibroelastosis. Pediatrics 1971;48:82.
35. Sever JL, Larsen JW Jr, Grossman JH II. Handbook of perinatal infections. Boston: Little, Brown, 1980:45.
36. Finland M. Influenza complicating pregnancy. In: Charles D, Finland M, eds. Obstetrics and perinatal infections. Philadelphia: Lea & Febiger, 1973:355.
37. Griffiths PD, Ronalds CJ, Heath RB. A prospective study of influenza infections during pregnancy. J Epidemiol Commun Health 1980;34:1224.
38. Larsen JW Jr. Influenza and pregnancy. Clin Obstet Gynecol 1982;25:599.
39. Centers for Disease Control. Risks associated with human parvovirus B19 infection. MWMR 1989;38(6):81.
40. Kinney JS, Anderson LJ, Farrar J, et al. Risk of adverse outcomes of pregnancy human parvovirus B19 infection. J Infect Dis 1968;157:663.
41. Anand A, Gray ES, Brown T, et al. Human parvovirus infection in pregnancy and hydrops fetalis. N Engl J Med 1987;316:183.
42. Woernle CH, Anderson LJ, Tatersall, et al. Human parvovirus B19 infection during pregnancy. J Infect Dis 1987;156:17.
43. Anderson LJ, Hurwitz ES. Human parvovirus B19 and pregnancy. Clin Perinatol 1989;15:273.
44. Porter HJ, Khong TY, Evans MF, Chan VT-W, Fleming KA. Parvovirus as a cause of hydrops fetalis: detection by in situ DNA hybridisation. J Clin Pathol 1988;41:381.
45. Anderson MJ, Khousam MN, Maxwell DJ, Gould SJ, Happerfield LC, Smith WJ. Human parvovirus B19 and hydrops fetalis (letter). Lancet 1988;1:535.
46. Weiland HT, Vermey-Keers C, Salimans MM, Flueren GJ, Verway RA, Anderson MJ. Parvovirus B19 associated with fetal abnormality (letter). Lancet 1987;1:682.
47. Carrington D, Gilmore DH, Whittle MJ, et al. Maternal serum α-fetoprotein—a marker of fetal aplastic crisis during intrauterine human parvovirus infection. Lancet 1987;1:433.
48. Brond PR, Caul EO, Usher J, Cohen BJ, Clewley JP, Field AM. Intrauterine infection with human parvovirus (letter). Lancet 1986;1:448.
49. Maeda H, Shimokawa H, Satoh S, Nakano H, Nunoue T. Nonimmunologic hydrops fetalis resulting from intrauterine human parvovirus B-19 infection: report of two cases. Obstet Gynecol 1988;72:482.
50. Schwarz TF, Roggendorf M, Hottentrager B, et al. Human parvovirus B19 infection in pregnancy (letter). Lancet 1988;2:566.

27

CHAPTER

BACTERIAL, PARASITIC, AND MICROBIAL INFECTIONS IN THE FETUS

Philip B. Mead

For practical purposes, there are only two important routes of fetal infection: the ascending, or transcervical route; and the transplacental route. The ascending route, by far the more common, results in intra-amniotic infection and transorificial fetal infections. It is characterized histologically by a polymorphonuclear leukocytic infiltration of the chorion and amnion—"chorioamnionitis," often associated with acute umbilical angiitis. The etiologic agents are usually bacteria.

Transplacentally acquired fetal infections are nearly always secondary to maternal bloodstream infections but may rarely result from spread from the decidua to the fetus, either from a focus of dormant endometritis or by the ascending decidual pathway.[1] Parenchymal placental lesions, chiefly villous inflammation, are the hallmark of transplacental fetal infections.[2] The great majority of transplacental infections are caused by viruses, but bacteria, fungi, protozoa, and helminths have been implicated as well (Table 27-1).

This chapter reviews nonviral fetal infections that are acquired transplacentally and that are not covered in other chapters (viral infections are covered in Chapters 24 and 25; toxoplasmosis in Chapter 24; syphilis, chlamydia and HIV in Chapter 72). The nonviral transplacental fetal infections discussed in this chapter are rare and often exotic, occur throughout pregnancy, may have devastating effects on the pregnancy, but have not been proven to be a cause of congenital anomalies.

TRANSPLACENTALLY ACQUIRED BACTERIAL INFECTIONS

LISTERIOSIS

Listeria monocytogenes is a small, aerobic, non–spore-forming, gram-positive rod that is beta-hemolytic on blood agar. Major serotypes causing infection are Ia, Ib, IVa, and IVb. *L. monocytogenes* is widely distributed in the environment and in animals, but the source of human infections is poorly understood. Food-borne outbreaks have been traced to soft cheeses, milk, raw vegetables, and shellfish. Asymptomatic fecal and vaginal carriage occurs in humans and may account for sporadic cases. *L. monocytogenes* has been recognized as a cause of human disease since 1929 and primarily affects pregnant women, neonates, individuals with immune system dysfunction, and the elderly. Neonatal disease was first described in 1936; maternal and fetal infections currently account for 50% of reported cases. Although most maternal infections are mild, *Listeria* infection in pregnancy may result in abortion, preterm labor, and fetal infection, with reported rates of neonatal mortality ranging from 7% to more than 50%.

Reiss and coworkers have described the pathogenesis of fetal *Listeria* infection.[3] Maternal hematogenous infection leads to placental infection, which results in fetal septicemia and multiorgan involvement. Amniotic fluid becomes infected by excretion of the organism in fetal urine. Aspiration and swallowing of infected amniotic fluid result in respiratory tract involvement. Variend and Blumenthal report two cases that lend support to this proposed transplacental route of infection: early-onset neonatal listeriosis following elective cesarean section at term, and vaginal birth of twins, where twin A was uninfected and twin B had blood cultures positive for *Listeria*.[4] Alternatively, an ascending route of infection from cervicovaginal colonization with *L. monocytogenes* may account for some fetal infections.

Maternal infection with *Listeria* is often asymptomatic, but patients may present with a flulike syndrome characterized by chills, fever, and back pain, occasionally mimicking a pyelonephritis. Although diarrhea is commonly believed to be a symptom of listeriosis, it was not reported by any pregnant patients in a recent

TABLE 27-1. NONVIRAL TRANSPLACENTAL FETAL INFECTIONS

Bacteria
Listeria monocytogenes
Mycobacterium tuberculosis
Mycobacterium leprae
Campylobacter fetus and *C. jejuni*
Salmonella typhi
Francisella tularensis
Treponema pallidum
Borrelia burgdorferi
Borrelia hermsii
Leptospira
Brucella abortus and *B. melitensis*
Yersinia pestis
Bacillus anthracis
Staphylococcus aureus
Coxiella burnetii
Protozoa
Toxoplasma gondii
Plasmodia
Trypanosomes
Leishmania donovani
Babesia microti
Helminths
Ascaris lumbricoides
Ancylostoma duodenale and *Necator americanus*
Trichinella spiralis
Schistosomes
Fungi
Cryptococcus neoformans
Coccidioides immitis

outbreak.[5] Most infected gravidas present with fever, active preterm labor, and brown-stained amniotic fluid that is frequently mistaken for meconium.[6] Intrapartum fetal monitoring commonly shows nonspecific abnormalities consistent with intrauterine infection (eg, fetal tachycardia, decreased variability, and absence of accelerations).

Both early- and late-onset forms of neonatal listeriosis occur, similar to group B streptococcal infection. The early type presents within 2 days of birth with signs of septicemia and is felt to be due to transplacental infection. Early-onset disease is most commonly associated with serotypes Ia and IVb. The late form of the disease appears after the fifth day of life and usually presents as meningitis. Late-onset neonatal listeriosis is associated with serotype IVb and is felt to result from infection acquired during delivery.[7]

In a recent report of listeriosis identified at perinatal autopsy, gross pathologic lesions were encountered in only one of seven cases and consisted of a skin rash and small hepatic abscesses. Microscopic lesions in six cases consisted of rare, localized microabscesses and granulomalike lesions. One case had no gross or microscopic findings. Placental lesions, consisting of chorioamnionitis and villitis, were found in all cases, whereas three of five examined cords showed acute funisitis.[8]

Infants with early-onset disease characteristically are preterm, are of appropriate weight for gestational age, and have respiratory distress at birth and evidence of congenital pneumonia.

Maternal listeriosis should be suspected in a pregnant woman with a flulike syndrome, especially if she has back pain and premature labor. Blood cultures, which are often positive, and vaginal cultures and gram stains should be performed as part of the evaluation of such a patient. Antimicrobial therapy (ampicillin plus gentamicin) of infection diagnosed during pregnancy is essential, since it may prevent fetal infection and its consequences.[9]

Congenital listeriosis should be considered in the differential diagnosis of a depressed preterm infant after a labor complicated by fetal distress and meconium or brown-stained amniotic fluid. A gram stain should be performed of amniotic fluid, the newborn's throat and skin, or eye lesions. Gram stain of a fecal smear from an infected newborn may show the organism in profusion. The findings of gram-positive rods or coccobacillary forms should prompt a presumptive diagnosis of listeriosis. One must inform the microbiologist that *Listeria* is a concern, since *L. monocytogenes* can easily be mistaken for diphtheroids and ignored.

Presumptive diagnosis of *Listeria* by gram stain demands immediate institution of therapy; awaiting confirmation by culture may result in fatal delay. The optimal therapeutic regimen for the infected newborn is unknown, but initial therapy with ampicillin plus gentamicin is recommended, because this combination is highly effective in animal models of *Listeria* infection.

TUBERCULOSIS

Congenital tuberculosis is a rare but well-defined entity that has been reported in over 150 newborns.[10] Tuberculosis can be acquired by the fetus by one of two routes: transplacental spread via the umbilical vein from a mother with primary hematogenous tuberculosis; or aspiration in utero of amniotic fluid infected through direct extension of a focus of tuberculous endometritis.[11] This second pathway is extremely rare, because most women with tuberculous endometritis are sterile because of concomitant tubal involvement. Congenital tuberculosis most commonly follows maternal miliary disease; women who have only pulmonary tuberculosis are not likely to infect their fetus until after delivery. Three prerequisites must be met to establish the diagnosis of congenital tuberculosis:

1. The primary tuberculous complex must be present in the liver.
2. Extrauterine acquisition of infection must be definitely excluded.
3. The tuberculous lesions must be present at birth.

Monif advises that the diagnosis of congenital tuberculosis be actively sought in neonates born to women with active cavitary, pelvic, or military tuberculosis who are not receiving therapy.[12] Diagnosis of perinatal tuberculosis is frequently delayed, because disease in the mother is often undiagnosed. Findings in the newborn include loss of appetite, failure to gain weight, progressive bilateral interstitial pneumonia (without abnormal chest auscultation), and ascites. If infection occurred via a placental source, the liver will be extensively involved early. Lymphadenopathy, splenomegaly, and biliary obstruction are common. Infants infected through aspiration of infected amniotic fluid following erosion of tuberculous endometritis usually succumb quickly to tuberculous bronchopneumonia.

Acid-fast stains of the placenta have been touted as effective in the rapid diagnosis of congenital tuberculosis. However, sampling errors can produce false negatives, and false positives are also common, since placental involvement occurs far more frequently than infection of the fetus.

If the infant is suspected of having congenital tuberculosis, 5 tuberculin units of purified protein derivative (TU PPD) skin testing and chest x-rays should be obtained promptly. Cutaneous tuberculin reactivity is unlikely before 4–6 weeks of life and can be delayed for many months. Regardless of the skin test results, treatment of the infant should be initiated promptly with isoniazid and rifampin.[13]

It is commonly stated that maternal tuberculosis does not increase the incidence of congenital malformations or spontaneous abortion. Congenital tuberculosis, however, frequently results in spontaneous abortion or stillbirth, in part because hypersensitivity to the tubercle bacillus that might help to control the infection cannot be transferred significantly from mother to fetus.[14]

LEPROSY

Placental transmission of *Mycobacterium leprae* remains a subject of conjecture, but there is growing evidence for an influence of leprosy on fetal development and for intrauterine infection of the fetus. Cerruti and Bechelli[15] and Inaba[16] found placental involvement to be uncommon and to occur only with advanced lepromatous disease. King and Marks[17] found no placental involvement in treated patients. Transplacental transmission of disease is suspect in mice[18] but still not proved in humans.[19] However, IgA and IgM antibodies for *M. leprae* are found in the cord blood of 30% to 50% of babies from mothers with lepromatous leprosy.[20] This is strong evidence for fetal antibody synthesis to *M. leprae* or associated antigens.

Estrogen excretion levels at 32–40 weeks gestation are reduced in leprosy patients, suggesting fetoplacental dysfunction.[21]

CAMPYLOBACTER INFECTIONS

Campylobacters are motile, non–spore-forming, comma-shaped gram-negative rods. Six species are recognized. The major pathogen of humans, *Campylobacter jejuni*, causes acute enteritis; a case of midtrimester abortion caused by *C. jejuni* has also been reported.[22]

Campylobacter fetus more commonly causes a prolonged relapsing illness characterized by fevers, chills, myalgias, bacteremia, meningitis, and vascular infections. Infections during pregnancy typically present with upper respiratory symptoms, pneumonitis, fever, and bacteremia. Fever and pneumonitis may be prolonged, lasting several weeks, and unless appropriately treated, symptoms usually resolve only after spontaneous abortion or premature delivery. Gribble has reviewed the reported cases of *Campylobacter* infection in pregnancy and concludes that abortion, stillbirth, and early neonatal meningitis are due to transplacental spread.[23]

Campylobacter enteric infections are treated with fluid and electrolyte replacement and erythromycin. The need for treating septic or bacteremic episodes with agents other than erythromycin has not been established. For patients who appear very toxic, and those with endovascular infections, gentamicin is probably the agent of choice.[24]

SALMONELLOSIS

Nearly all cases of neonatal salmonellosis are acquired during the perinatal period via the ascending route. Transplacental infection is extremely rare, but it has been reported and is almost exclusively due to *Salmonella typhi*. Pregnancy does not alter the maternal prognosis in typhoid fever, but the disease can have a major effect on perinatal morbidity. During the early 1900s, typhoid fever was a common complication of pregnancy, with the frequent outcome of either spontaneous abortion or premature labor.[25] The early termination of pregnancy was probably caused by high fever, anoxia, circulating toxins, or metabolic derangements in the mother, not by in utero infection. The effectiveness of the placental barrier is evident from the observation that, when fetal exposure to maternal disease has been less than 2 or 3 weeks, the typhoid bacillus has not been isolated at autopsy from the spleen, bone marrow, or liver of fetuses that have aborted.[25–27]

Later in the course of disease, transplacental fetal infection may occur.[25,27–29] Both Diddle[25] and Wing[28] have reported on women convalescing from typhoid fever who gave birth to infants with evidence of intrauterine dissemination. In Wing's report the cord blood gave a positive Widal reaction. Since this reaction is dependent on IgM antibody, which does not cross the placenta, the presence of such agglutinins in cord blood is strong evidence for intrauterine exposure.

Finally, noninvolvement of the fetus despite clear evidence of placental infection has also been described in a mother who harbored *S. choleraesuis* in her blood for at least 6 days prior to delivery,[30] and in a mother who was an *S. typhi* carrier throughout pregnancy.[31]

In uncomplicated gastroenteritis caused by nontyphi *Salmonella* species, antimicrobials do not shorten the duration of disease. In invasive *Salmonella* disease, such as typhoid fever, non–*S. typhi* bacteremia, or *S. choleraesuis* infections, chloramphenicol, ampicillin, or amoxicillin is indicated, depending on susceptibility studies. Chloramphenicol should be avoided near delivery because of "gray syndrome."

Typhoid vaccine is a killed bacterial vaccine that offers some protection for those working or traveling in endemic areas. However, its use is commonly associated with systemic febrile reactions. Since febrile illness has been linked with spontaneous pregnancy loss, typhoid vaccine is not routinely recommended during pregnancy. Emphasis should be placed on water purification techniques and a safe supply of drinking water rather than on typhoid immunization.[32]

TULAREMIA

Francisella tularensis, the causative agent of tularemia, is a small gram-negative coccobacillus. Sources of the organism include wild mammals and blood-sucking arthropods. In the United States rabbits are the most important reservoir. Transmission is by indirect contact via insect bites; direct contact with infected animals; ingestion of contaminated, inadequately cooked meat or water; or inhalation of contaminated particles by laboratory technicians working with this highly infectious organism.

Tularemia is usually characterized by high fever and severe, flulike symptoms; however, clinically mild disease is being recognized with increasing frequency. Five tularemic syndromes are described: ulceroglandular, occuloglandular, oropharyngeal, glandular, and typhoidal.

Several cases of tularemia during pregnancy, with maternal recovery and subsequent delivery of a normal infant, have been reported. A review of the literature, however, identified only a single case of transplacentally acquired congenital tularemia. Maternal ulceroglandular disease occurred in the eighth month of pregnancy. A rise in the patient's temperature and development of leukocytosis in the fourth week of illness suggested maternal reinfection by the fetus. Shortly thereafter, fetal heart tones were lost and the patient spontaneously delivered a macerated fetus, after which her temperature fell to normal. Subsequently, she developed jaundice and hepatosplenomegaly that began on the third day and cleared rapidly. At autopsy necrotic granulomas, similar to those seen in adults, were found in various fetal organs and in the placenta, predominantly in the intervillous spaces. Gram-negative coccobacilli consistent morphologically with *F. tularensis* were demonstrated in chorionic villi.[33]

RELAPSING FEVER

Relapsing fever is a vector-borne bacterial infection characterized by recurring febrile attacks separated by periods of relative well-being. Spirochetes of the genus *Borrelia* cause the disease. Most cases in the United States are caused by *B. hermsii*, transmitted by infective ticks in forested western mountain areas.

Acute infection with relapsing fever during pregnancy often results in spontaneous abortion; in one study 92% of women aborted.[34] Although most early losses are probably secondary to the maternal response to systemic illness, some are probably due to direct involvement of the products of conception. The diagnosis of congenital infection requires both the onset of disease prior to the third day of life (the incubation prior of relapsing fever is 3–10 days), and the demonstration of spirochetes in peripheral blood smears or placental tissue. Three reports clearly demonstrate that transplacental transmission of *Borrelia* occurs. Fuchs and Oyama,[35] Correa (cited by Fuchs), and Steenbarger[36] have each presented cases fulfilling the criteria for transplacental infection. In Fuchs' case, *Borrelia* spirochetes were documented in the blood of the mother and infant and in the CSF of the infant. Autopsy of the baby, who died 39 hours after birth, showed meningitis and typical splenic lesions with numerous spirochetes. In Steenbarger's case, microscopic sections revealed *Borrelia* spirochetes in placental villi, in other areas of the placenta, and in the umbilical cord. This was the first demonstration of *Borrelia* spirochetes in placental tissue. Steenbarger recommends examining stained placental sections in suspected cases of congenital relapsing fever as a rapid and sensitive method for accurate diagnosis of this disease. Warthin-Starry silver stains and a standard acridine orange stain are both effective.

LYME DISEASE

Lyme disease is a tick-borne illness caused by a newly identified spirochete, *Borrelia burgdorferi*. In the United States there are three distinct foci of Lyme disease: the northeastern states from Massachusetts to Maryland, the upper midwestern states of Minnesota and Wisconsin, and four western states, including parts of California, Oregon, Nevada, and Utah. There are scattered reports of cases elsewhere, such as Texas.[37] Lyme disease has received unusual media attention, and obstetricians both within and outside of endemic areas can expect to be asked questions about the effect of the illness on the fetus.

Lyme disease usually begins with a characteristic skin lesion, erythema chronicum migrans, accompanied by a flulike syndrome and neurologic abnormalities, including headache, photophobia, dysesthesias, and stiff neck. Some patients later develop cardiac abnormalities, such as atrioventricular heart block or myopericarditis, neurologic complications, or intermittent attacks of arthritis.

Spirochetes, including the agents of syphilis, relapsing fever and leptospirosis, are known to cause transplacental infections, and maternal infections are associated with an increased risk of fetal loss. Because Lyme disease is also caused by a spirochete there has been understandable concern about the effect of maternal Lyme disease on the fetus and the risk of transplacental transmission of infection. Preliminary epidemiologic data have begun to emerge.

Twenty-two cases of Lyme disease in pregnancy have been reported to date. Schlesinger and colleagues described the first case of transplacental transmission of *Borrelia burgdorferi* in a young pregnant woman who acquired Lyme disease while camping in Wisconsin. Her infant died 39 hours after birth of complications related to a complex congenital cardiac malformation (tubular hypoplasia of the ascending aorta and aortic arch, marked endocardial fibroelastosis, and a persistent left superior vena cava draining into the coronary sinus). Although spirochetes were not found in the myocardium, rare spirochetes were seen in fetal kidney, spleen, and bone marrow. No attempt was made to culture spirochetes from autopsy tissues. Maternal serum was reactive against *B. burgdorferi* by IFA and ELISA methods.[38]

The following year the Centers for Disease Control reported 19 cases of Lyme disease during pregnancy that were identified between 1976 and 1984. Eight of the women were affected during the first trimester, seven during the second trimester, and two during the third trimester; in two the trimester of onset was unknown. Thirteen received appropriate antibiotic therapy for Lyme disease. Of the 19 pregnancies, five had adverse outcomes, including syndactyly, cortical blindness, intrauterine fetal death, prematurity, and rash in the newborn. Three of 13 patients who received antimicrobial therapy had an abnormal outcome (two serious), as did two of the six who did not receive antimicrobials (none serious). Adverse outcomes occurred in cases with infection during each of the trimesters. In the one death the fetus had no congenital anomalies. Microscopic evaluation revealed autolysis of fetal tissues and an immature placenta. There were no inflammatory infiltrates. Culture and IFA of the placenta and fetal tissues were negative for *B. burgdorferi*.

Umbilical cord blood was obtained from five normal infants in this study. Four were tested for IgM to *B. burgdorferi*, and none had an elevated titer. One infant, tested by IFA, had an antibody titer of 1:512 at birth but had no detectable antibody at 7 months of age. No umbilical cord blood was obtained from any of the infants with abnormalities.[39]

No infant in this study had a congenital heart defect. However, since heart defects due to teratogens result from exposure in the first trimester and only eight women had onset of disease during the first trimester, the power of the study to detect a congenital heart defect was limited. Although five (26%) of the pregnancies in this study had an adverse outcome, several were minor, no two adverse outcomes were the same, and none was documented to be due to Lyme disease. For no abnormality, however, was another etiology implicated.

MacDonald and colleagues reported a case of stillbirth at term in a patient who retrospectively remembered a suggestive skin lesion during the pregnancy. The only fetal malformation found at autopsy was an atrioventricular canal ventricular septal defect. Spirochetes were identified in the placenta, fetal myocardium, adrenal gland, liver, and brain. Lyme serologic studies on postpartum maternal blood were positive by IFA and ELISA methods.[40]

Mikkelsen and Palle have reported the case of a woman who developed Lyme disease during pregnancy that was recognized and treated with penicillin, with the subsequent birth at term of a normal infant. *Borrelia* antibody titer in the cord blood was not elevated and the placenta was said to be normal.[41]

Although these 22 cases undoubtedly represent an incomplete picture of the impact of Lyme disease on pregnancy, several observations seem appropriate:

1. The frequency of adverse outcomes in reported cases, 7 of 22, or 32%, warrants close surveillance and epidemiologic and laboratory studies of pregnant women with Lyme disease.
2. Although no specific congenital anomaly has been associated with Lyme disease, cardiac abnormality would appear the most likely candidate. Two cases of *Borrelia burgdorferi* infection have been associated with fetal death and cardiac malformation. Different anomalies were found in each case; therefore, a cause-and-effect relationship cannot be concluded. However, fetal cardiac malformations should be sought in pregnancies where Lyme disease occurs in the first trimester. Additionally, unexplained congenital cardiac anomalies should prompt the retrospective search for a history or serologic evidence of maternal Lyme disease, or a search for spirochetes in the tissues of stillborn infants with such cardiac abnormalities.
3. Although antibiotic treatment of gravidas with Lyme disease is strongly endorsed, such treatment apparently will not always assure a normal outcome.
4. Even classical symptoms or signs of Lyme disease may be overlooked by the patient and her physician unless they are informed about disease manifestations and the potential implications in pregnancy.
5. Because results of serologic tests for Lyme disease are often negative during the first several weeks of infection, the diagnosis of Lyme disease should be made on the basis of clinical criteria,[42] and treatment should be begun immediately. Many obstetricians now regularly prescribe prophylactic treatment for deer tick bites during pregnancy. The usual regimen is 3 weeks of either amoxicillin 500 mg tid, or penicillin V 500 mg qid. Erythromycin 250–500 mg q.i.d. can be prescribed for women allergic to penicillin. Antibiotic therapy for clinical disease is often chosen according to the stage of disease. Oral antibiotics are administered for the rash and flulike symptoms of early Lyme disease; intravenous antibiotics are used if the disease is recognized later, when the patient is suffering from arthritic or neurologic complications.

However, other physicians feel it is best to administer intravenous treatment immediately to a pregnant woman with Lyme disease at any stage. The most common oral regimen is amoxicillin 500 mg tid or penicillin V 500 mg qid, given for 3 or more weeks. Intravenous therapy can be either 20 million units of penicillin G given in divided doses every 4 hours for 2–3 weeks, or ceftriaxone 2 g once daily for 14–21 days.[43]

It would seem prudent for pregnant women to avoid tick exposure assiduously in endemic areas.

At the time of delivery of women who have acquired Lyme disease during pregnancy, the placenta should be examined microscopically for spirochetes.

LEPTOSPIROSIS

Leptospirosis—together with syphilis, Lyme disease, and relapsing fever—is the fourth illness caused by a spirochete that has been associated with transplacental transmission of infection. *Leptospira* produce a group of syndromes with protean manifestations, including fever, headache, chills, severe malaise, vomiting, myalgia, and conjunctivitis. Intrauterine infection of the human fetus has been demonstrated. Chung isolated leptospires from the liver and kidney of a 5-month-old abortus of a patient suffering from leptospirosis caused by serotype Kasman.[44] Lindsay and Luke reported a fatal case of leptospirosis occurring within hours of parturition, presumably because of intrauterine infection. Histologic study revealed hepatocellular necrosis with relative sparing of the periportal areas. Sections of the kidneys demonstrated extensive tubular epithelial cell degeneration involving particularly the proximal and distal convoluted tubules. *L. icterohemorrhagica* was demonstrated in both organs. It should be noted that the maternal illness was subclinical.[45] Involvement of the fetal liver has also been documented with intrauterine infection due to *L. pomona*[46] and *L. canicola*.[47] Although these case reports clearly document the occasional occurrence of transplacental infection, it is likely that the majority of fetal wastage observed is secondary to maternal disease rather than to direct fetal involvement.

BRUCELLOSIS

Porreco and Haverkamp have summarized the literature concerning Brucellosis in pregnancy, concluding that documentation exists for transplacental infection with *Brucella abortus* and *Brucella melitensis*.[48] The rarity of human fetal wastage resulting from maternal *Brucella* infection, as compared with the common problem in domestic animals, may be explained by the lack of the carbohydrate erythritol in the human placenta. This substance is the preferred nutrient for growth of the brucellae species and is present in the placentas of animal hosts who commonly abort as a major manifestation of the illness.

PLAGUE

Plague, like other severe systemic illnesses acquired during pregnancy, may cause spontaneous abortion. The fetal wastage resulting from maternal infection with plague probably results from the systemic effects of illness rather than from direct placental or fetal infection. However, true intrauterine infection with *Yersinia pestis,* the plague bacillus, has been described.[49]

ANTHRAX

In 1923, Regan reported a case of probable transplacental *Bacillus anthracis* infection with the following documentation: positive maternal cultures at necropsy, positive cultures from fetal heart blood and liver, and typical long gram-positive bacilli in the microscopic sections of fetal liver.[50] In a review of anthrax meningitis, Haight[51] refers to a case report from 1887 describing a newborn infant who died of hemorrhagic anthrax meningitis that was presumed to have been acquired from the bloodstream of the mother, who was infected with the anthrax bacillus.

COMMON AEROBIC BACTERIA

Although aerobic bacteria such as group B streptococci and *Escherichia coli* are by far the commonest causes of ascending fetal infection, they are virtually unmentioned in the etiology of transplacental infection. A single report, published in 1951, describes a case of intrauterine meningitis and hydrocephalus caused by *Staphylococcus aureus.* The mother had undergone a tooth extraction during the third month of pregnancy and had multiple upper-respiratory infections until delivery. At no time was there a significant temperature elevation, however. She underwent elective cesarean section at 38 weeks because of hydrocephalus diagnosed by x-ray. The course of the infant in the hospital showed no evidence of acute infection. The infant underwent craniotomy at 2 months of age, revealing a chronic bacterial leptomeningitis that was estimated to have been present since the sixth month of pregnancy. The authors postulated a transient bacteremia in the mother, with subsequent transplacental transmission.[52]

Whether the common aerobic bacteria are truly rare causes of transplacental fetal infection or transplacental infection caused by them is mistakenly interpreted as resulting from ascending infection is not addressed in the literature. The only other reference to transplacental infection by common aerobic bacteria is the report of Patrick, who was able to isolate *E. coli* from the amniotic fluid, fetal circulation, placentas, and umbilical cords of infants of bacilluric mothers.[53] The following observations support this experience. Certain bacteria, including *E. coli*, are known to stimulate blood group antibodies (isohemagglutinins). Several studies have shown increased titers of isohemagglutinins in infants of mothers with *E. coli* bacilluria. Other studies have shown that lymphocytes of infants born to mothers with *E. coli* bacilluria demonstrate blast transformation when cultured in the presence of an extract of *E. coli* antigen. These reports suggest previous intrauterine exposure of the fetus to *E. coli* or one of its products. If such is the case, it would appear that significant maternal bacilluria, even without symptoms, might result in the dissemination of organisms into the maternal circulation, intervillous space, and ultimately the fetus.[54] It is important to recognize, however, that Patrick's work in this area has not been confirmed by other investigators.

An increased frequency of abortions or stillbirths in pregnant women with bacteriuria has been reported by several investigators, whereas others have found no such increase. Similarly, some authors report a significant decrease in the incidence of abortions and stillbirths when bacteriuria is eradicated with antimicrobial therapy, whereas others find no difference in the rates between treated and untreated women with bacteriuria.[55] An association between maternal bacteriuria and congenital anomalies has also been proposed by Patrick,[53] Savage and coworkers,[56] and Kincaid-Smith and Bullen.[57] Establishment of a causal relationship awaits further investigation.

Finally, a recent report describes a putative case of transplacentally acquired gonococcal infection.[58] The authors concluded that this was not a case of ascending infection because the membranes were intact; however, several observations cast doubt on this conclusion. Ruptured membranes are not a prerequisite for ascending infection, because bacteria are capable of crossing intact membranes, especially in the setting of labor that was present in this case. Moreover, the pathologic lesion described was chorioamnionitis, not villus inflammation, and therefore is more consistent with an ascending route of infection.

Q FEVER

Q fever is a zoonosis caused by the rickettsia *Coxiella burnetii*. In humans the illness is characterized by fever to 40°C (104°F), chills, malaise, myalgia, chest pain, and occasionally pneumonia and hepatitis. Humans are usually infected by inhaling infectious aerosols.[59]

C. burnetii has been isolated from placentas and breast milk of mothers who acquired Q fever from 3 years to 2 months before delivery.[60–62] These reports suggest that the fetus may become infected in utero with *C. burnetii*. The most compelling evidence for transplacental infection in humans was presented by Fiset and coworkers.[63] In this report the cord serum of four infants had high levels of IgM antibodies specific for *C. burnetii*. The children were normal at birth. A recent report describes a 19-year-old woman with a history of spontaneous abortions and delivery of abnormal children. At 29 weeks gestation she gave birth to an infant who died at 6 days of age. An elevated titer of antibody to phase-II antigen was demonstrated in the serum obtained from the infant's blood. Serum from the mother had positive titers of both phase-I and phase-II antigens. The same report describes a 9-month-old girl who died of sudden infant death syndrome with diagnostic levels of Q fever antibodies.[64]

Although Q fever was formerly considered an occupational hazard only for persons working with animals or in bacteriology laboratories, a recent outbreak among adults exposed to a parturient house cat raises concern that Q fever risk may be widespread.[65]

TRANSPLACENTALLY ACQUIRED PROTOZOAL AND HELMINTHIC INFECTIONS

MALARIA

Human malaria is caused by four species of *Plasmodium: P. falciparum, P. vivax, P. malariae*, and *P. ovale*. It is transmitted from person to person by female *Anopheles* mosquitoes. Malaria is indigenous in 102 countries, with 56% of the world's population living in areas where malaria is present. The resettling of refugees from Southeast Asia has created the need for US physicians to have greater awareness and knowledge of plasmodial infection.

Malaria has well-documented and complex effects on pregnancy. Both prevalence and density of parasitemia are increased in pregnant women as compared with nonpregnant controls from similar geographic areas. A theoretic basis for this observation exists: maturation of Plasmodial schizonts occurs in "deep sinuses" within the bloodstream (eg, the spleen). The placenta, which does not contain a macrophage system, appears to provide an additional and immunologically privileged site for parasitic reproduction.[66] Interestingly, the greatest degree of placental infestation is observed in highly immune patients, suggesting evasion of the immune system.

Galbraith reported histologic and ultrastructural findings in placentas heavily infested with *P. falciparum*. Intervillous spaces contained large numbers of parasitized red blood cells and monocytes with ingested pigment associated with focal syncytial microvilli and proliferation of cytotrophoblastic cells. Basement membrane thickening and immunopathologic lesions were present even in treated malarial infection.[67] It has been suggested that these latter changes may decrease nutrient and oxygen exchange between mother and fetus, causing intrauterine growth retardation. Placental parasitemia is associated with lower maternal plasma estradiol concentration, and some authors have questioned an increased risk of abruption.[66]

Malaria causes an increased rate of abortions and is the most important cause of low birth weight in the tropics. Premature labor may begin during a malarial attack or shortly thereafter, probably as a response to maternal fever and systemic illness. Intrauterine growth retardation has been referred to earlier. Using the Dubowitz method for calculating gestational age, Reinhardt found that most low-birth-weight infants born to women with malaria were premature rather than small for gestational age.[68] Low-birth-weight infants occur more frequently in primigravidas with malaria, not only because birth weight increases with parity, but because parasitemia and placental infection are more common in primiparous women. Density of placental infection correlates inconsistently with birth weight.[66]

Evidence that malaria causes stillbirths is sparse. Fetal distress is said to be common in mothers with acute malaria and may be caused by high fever or hypoglycemia.

Congenital malaria has been reported for all four species of *Plasmodia* and is more common among infants of women who have clinical attacks of malaria during pregnancy than in those with chronic subclinical infections. It is more common in infants of women who have immigrated to areas in which malaria is endemic than in women who have been raised to maturity in such areas, because levels of immunity in the former group are lower than those of the native population. Conversely, congenital malaria is also more common among women who immigrate from areas where malaria is endemic to areas free of malaria, since lack of frequent exposure leads to loss of immunity.

MacLeod has summarized studies of congenital malaria in Africa reported since 1950.[69] In six studies from low-frequency areas the incidence was zero to 0.2%. In six other studies from high-frequency areas the incidence ranged between 4% and 44%. There were no consistent differences between the low- and high-frequency groups, and these marked variations in incidence of congenital disease remain unexplained. It is probable that IgG antibody transmitted from mother to baby is an important factor in determining whether or not parasites that reach the fetal circulation establish an infection. Additionally, placental infection is much more common than congenital infection, indicating that the placenta serves as a relatively effective barrier to fetal infection.

For most North American women, travel represents the only real threat of acquiring malaria. In areas where chloroquine-sensitive *P. falciparum* is present, prophylactic regimens that are safe in pregnancy have been developed. Pregnant women must realize, however, that no prophylactic regimen can ensure complete protection against malaria, that the most severe complications of malaria are more common in pregnant women, and that these drug regimens occasionally produce unwanted side effects.

In areas where chloroquine-resistant *P. falciparum* is present there is no safe regimen for pregnant women and travel should be avoided unless the need is imperative. Barry has recently reviewed malarial prophylaxis in pregnancy.[32] Detailed recommendations for the prevention of malaria may be obtained 24 hours a day by calling the CDC Malaria Hotline at (404) 332-4555.

AFRICAN SLEEPING SICKNESS

African trypanosomiasis (African sleeping sickness) is caused by *Trypanosoma brucei gambiense* or *Trypanosoma brucei rhodesiense*.[70] Congenital transmission of African trypanosomiasis has infrequently been reported, with most cases caused by *T. gambiense* infection. Vertical transmission of the parasite is proved if the infant of an infected mother has never been in an endemic area or if the parasite is found in the newborn within 5 days of birth. Debroise reviewed 18 cases of trypanosomiasis in children, seven of which were probably transplacental in origin. The clinical picture in these infants included low birth weight, somnolence, fever hepatomegaly, and neurologic symptoms of hypertonicity, trembling, and abnormal movements.[71] Early passage of parasites into the central nervous system (CNS) is said to be a characteristic feature of congenital infections.

Reinhardt has suggested that the apparent rarity of congenital disease is likely due to the lack of study in endemic areas. Also, endocrine abnormalities in severely ill mothers may result in amenorrhea and infertility, and intrauterine infection may lead to early fetal wastage.[72]

The diagnosis of congenital infection can be made if parasites are found in the infant's peripheral blood or cerebrospinal fluid (CSF). High IgM levels in serum and CSF are also noted, although newborns may have normal CSF IgM levels in spite of the presence of parasites in the CSF.

Reinhardt has recently reviewed treatment options.[72]

CHAGAS' DISEASE

Chagas' disease (American trypanosomiasis) is caused by the flagellate *Trypanosoma cruzi*. It occurs from the southern portion of the United States to Argentina and is a major public health problem in South and Central America. *T. cruzi* is transmitted to humans by insect vectors, by blood transfusion, and transplacentally. Congenital transmission occurs when trypomastigotes, present in the intervillous space, penetrate the villus through the trophoblastic epithelium. Necrosis of the trophoblast follows, and maternal mononuclear cells collect around the necrotic area. The trypomastigotes transform into amastigotes in Hofbauer cells within the stroma of the villus, where they multiply until they are liberated as trypomastigotes. These forms gain access to the fetus through the villus fetal vessels.[73]

Chagas documented congenital transmission of *T. cruzi* infection in 1911, 2 years after he described the first case of the disease that now bears his name. Bittencourt has recently summarized the 200 cases of congenital Chagas' disease reported in the literature from South America.[74] Congenital transmission may occur during any stage of maternal disease. Maternal parasitemia is greatest in the acute phase of the infection, but this period of intense parasitemia is brief. Thus, most congenital infections occur in infants born to women who may be asymptomatic but have the chronic form of the disease.

Congenital Chagas' disease may cause abortion, prematurity, intrauterine growth retardation, and intrauterine and neonatal death. Congenital infections occur in 1% to 4% of women with serologic evidence of having had Chagas' disease and are very rare among infants with a birth weight of greater than 2500 g. Congenitally infected low-birth-weight infants can be either premature or small for gestational age. Symptoms may be present from birth or develop days, weeks, or even months later. Early-onset jaundice, anemia, and petechiae are common. Hepatosplenomegaly, cardiomegaly with congestive heart failure, esophageal involvement with regurgitation, myxedematous edema, and encephalitis with convulsions have been described in congenitally infected infants.

The diagnosis of congenital Chagas' disease in the newborn is based on the demonstration of trypomastigotes in the circulating blood. When available, cord blood should be centrifuged and examined directly. Otherwise the leukocyte layer obtained from a microhematocrit tube should be examined.[75] In stillbirths and neonatal deaths, the diagnosis is based upon histologic examination of the placenta and fetal tissues. Placentas, which have a gross appearance similar to that seen in erythroblastosis fetalis, should be examined microscopically for the amastigote of *T. cruzi.*

No satisfactory chemotherapy for Chagas' disease is currently available; nifurtimox is being evaluated. Information regarding treatment can be obtained from the Parasitic Disease Division, Centers for Disease Control, Atlanta, Georgia.

VISCERAL LEISHMANIASIS (KALA-AZAR)

Leishmaniasis is the general name given to infection caused by any member of the protozoan genus *Leishmania* and includes visceral, cutaneous, and mucocutaneous syndromes. *L. donovani* is the etiologic agent responsible for visceral leishmaniasis (kala-azar, Dumdum fever, Assam fever, or infantile splenomegaly), which is characterized by a subacute or chronic course with fever, hepatosplenomegaly, anemia, leukopenia, hyperglobulinemia, and progressive emaciation.

Visceral leishmaniasis occurs in widely scattered areas throughout the world, including Central and South America, the Mediterranean region, China, East Africa, Central Asia, and India. Various animals serve as the reservoir of disease, and an intermediate insect vector is involved in nearly all cases. Transmission in India is by a *Phlebotomus* species that is anthropophilic (thereby promoting indirect person-to person spread), whereas in other regions it is by sandflies that feed on the appropriate animal host as well as humans.

Two probable cases of transplacentally acquired visceral leishmaniasis have been reported.[76,77] The most convincing of the two was unique in that a pregnant woman suffering from kala-azar moved from India to England in the seventh month of pregnancy and subsequently delivered a child infected with *L. donovani.* However, since one adult case of direct person-to-person transmission has been reported, even this case may be suspect.

AMEBIASIS

Amebiasis is caused by a protozoan, *Entamoeba histolytica,* that is found in all areas of the world. There are no reported cases of congenital amebiasis and no well-documented data on direct fetal morbidity due to maternal amebiasis.[78] Amebiasis affects the fetus indirectly, causing premature labor and possibly stillbirth, when severe electrolyte imbalances or shock occur in the mother. No placental changes secondary to amebiasis have been reported. The same mechanism that prevents pregnant women from developing amebic liver abscesses (possibly hormonally mediated) may prevent the occurrence of placental and fetal infection as well.[79]

BABESIOSIS

Babesiosis is a protozoan tick-borne disease of domestic and wild animals that is occasionally transmitted to humans. Most case reports in the United States have come from Long Island, Nantucket, and Martha's Vineyard. A single case of transplacentally acquired babesiosis has recently been reported.[80] The infant was delivered by cesarean section 1 week after the mother was bitten by a tick. Although the mother remained asymptomatic, the infant became ill 1 month after birth, developing fever, hepatosplenomegaly, anemia, and thrombocytopenia. *Babesia microti* organisms were found in the infant's erythrocytes, although the mother's peripheral blood smears at the time of delivery and 1 month later revealed no parasites. Serologic studies in both mother and infant showed evidence of babesiosis. The infant responded to therapy with quinine plus clindamycin.

ASCARIASIS

Ascaris lumbricoides, the giant roundworm of humans, is distributed worldwide. A single case of congenital ascariasis was reported by Chu and colleagues in 1972.[81] During preparations for a cesarean section occasioned by prolonged premature labor and fetal distress, one worm passed from the vagina and another was found in the vagina. When the placenta was removed, 10 worms were found on the maternal surface. The infant passed two female worms, 28 and 30 cm long, on the second and sixth days of life. Fertilized ova of *A. lumbricoides* were found in the amniotic fluid and in the infant's feces. Chu discussed three possible mechanisms of infection in this case. Direct invasion of *A. lumbricoides* worms from the mother's intestine to the placenta and amniotic cavity seemed unlikely, because bleeding and severe placental injury, which would have been caused by the worms' penetration, were not observed. Could fertilized eggs have been laid by female worms in the placenta, where, by an intracorporeal hatching process, they became infective and reached the amniotic cavity, after which they were swallowed by the fetus and developed into mature worms in the small intestine? This appears untenable, because the eggs require oxygen for maturation, and bile and gastric secretions are needed for hatching. Thus, the most plausible explanation seems to be transplacental transmission—migration of the larvae from the mother's intestine to the maternal lymphatics and bloodstream, to the placenta and into the fetal circulation, then to the fetus's small intestine, where they developed into adult worms.

OTHER INTESTINAL NEMATODES

Neither whipworm infection (*Trichuris trichiura*) nor pinworm infestation (*Enterobius vermicularis*) is associated with transplacental transmission, since systemic migration of larvae does not occur.

Congenital hookworm infection (*Ancylostoma duodenale, Necator americanus*) was first reported in 1917.[82] In addition, several cases of severe hemorrhage due to hookworm infestation have been reported in infants less than 4 months old. In at least some of these cases it is possible that transplacental passage of larvae resulted in infection.[83]

TRICHINOSIS

Trichinosis is a well-known zoonotic parasitic infection caused by the tissue nematode *Trichinella spiralis.* Infection results from the consumption of undercooked meat of animals infected with *T. spiralis* cysts. *T. spiralis* has been identified in the placenta,[84] and sporadic reports of intrauterine infection by *Trichinella* have been published. Kuitunen-Ekbaum found four encapsulated *T. spiralis* larvae in the diaphragm of a 7-month fetus.[85] Bourns found 22 larvae in the diaphragm of an immature infant who died at 6 weeks.[86] Hood and Olson found *T. spiralis* in pressed muscle preparations from four of 48 infants zero to 12 months of age.[87]

SCHISTOSOMIASIS

Several trematodes (blood flukes) of the genus *Schistosoma* can infect human beings. The most frequently encountered species are *S. haematobium, S. japonicum,* and *S. mansoni. Schistosoma* infection of the placenta has been sporadically reported. Although the frequency of placental infection is as high as 25% in endemic areas, the infestations are light and cause little histologic reaction. A cause-and-effect relationship between schistosomiasis and abortion, prematurity, and intrauterine growth retardation has yet to be clearly demonstrated.[88,89]

In 1916, Narabayashi reported congenital *S. japonicum* infection in three out of 22 newborns examined for infection.[90] No subsequent cases of congenitally acquired schistosomiasis have been documented, although experimental congenital infection in laboratory animals has been induced. Finally, sensitization to *S. mansoni* antigen in uninfected children born to infected mothers has been demonstrated by intradermal skin tests.[91]

OTHER TREMATODE INFECTIONS

Trematode infections other than schistosomiasis (ie, fasciolopsiasis, heterophyiasis, metagonimiasis, clonorchiasis, opisthorchiasis, fascioliasis, and paragonimiasis) produce no known adverse effects on the fetus. Goldsmith and Mankell have recently published treatment regimens for pregnant women infected with these parasites.[92]

CANDIDIASIS

Despite the frequency with which *Candida* species colonize the pregnant vagina, reports of fetal *Candida* infections are rare. Only 50 cases have been reported[93–95] since Benirschke and Raphael described the first definite case in 1958.[96] The method of transmission is not entirely clear, but ascending infection through either ruptured or even intact membranes seems most likely. Although candidemia has been reported during pregnancy,[97] hematogenous transmission from mother to fetus has never been described. Thus, fetal *Candida* infections are *not* transplacentally acquired; they are included in this chapter because they represent a unique fetal infection, unlike most bacterial infections acquired by the ascending route.

The hallmark of fetal *Candida* infection is the presence of discrete rounded yellow plaques, varying in size from 0.5 to 2 mm, on the surface of the umbilical cord and membranes. The fungal nature of these lesions can be confirmed by a frozen section if necessary, but Whyte has emphasized the importance of obstetricians identifying them with the naked eye and recognizing their importance, since they are virtually pathognomonic for this seldom-encountered fetal infection.[94]

The pattern of fetal organ involvement suggests slowly spreading infection affecting the skin and contiguous mucosal surfaces, with spread due to aspiration and swallowing of contaminated material. Histologic sections of chorionic villi fail to reveal evidence of inflammatory changes, supporting an ascending rather than a transplacental mode of transmission.

One additional feature of congenital fetal *Candida* infection is worthy of note. The majority of such gestations are complicated by the presence of an intrauterine foreign body, either a retained intrauterine contraceptive device or, less commonly, a cervical suture. Smith and colleagues reported the interesting case of an asymptomatic pregnant patient with a retained intrauterine contraceptive device. Intrauterine infection with *Candida albicans* was discovered serendipitously at the time of genetic amniocentesis when the cell cultures were overgrown with *Candida* species.[95]

Although congenital *Candida* infection is rare, it can be anticipated by its association with foreign bodies in the genital tract in pregnancy and diagnosed by careful inspection of the cord and membranes in the delivery room. Appreciation of these facts will allow early recognition and treatment of this disease.

TRANSPLACENTALLY ACQUIRED FUNGAL INFECTIONS

CRYPTOCOCCOSIS

Infection with *Cryptococcus neoformans* follows inhalation of the fungus; the respiratory tract is the primary focus of infection. Hematogenous dissemination may then occur to any organ in the body, the central nervous system being the most common site of infection following dissemination. The fact that bloodstream dissemination occurs suggests the potential for transplacental spread in pregnancy. Data regarding congenital cryptococcosis are extremely scanty, but six infants who developed this infection in the first month of life have been reported.[98–101] All these neonates died, and in each, organisms with the morphologic appearance of *Cryptococcus* were identified by microscopic examination of tissue obtained at autopsy or by culture. Miller has reviewed these cases.[102] The mother of one of these infants had *Cryptococcus* isolated from her cervix, suggesting this may have been a case of ascending fetal infection.[99]

COCCIDIOIDOMYCOSIS

Coccidioidomycosis is a dust-borne disease common in certain arid regions of the western hemisphere, including parts of southern California, Nevada, Arizona, and the western part of Texas. It is caused by *Coccidioides immitis*, a dimorphic fungus.

Primary infection may be entirely asymptomatic or may resemble an acute influenzal illness with fever, chills, cough, and pleural pain. Disseminated coccidioidomycosis is a progressive, frequently fatal granulomatous disease characterized by lesions and abscesses throughout the body, especially in subcutaneous tissues, skin, bone, peritoneum, thyroid, and the CNS. An estimated one in every 1000 cases of symptomatic coccidioidomycosis becomes disseminated. Dissemination is more common in blacks, in Filipinos, and during pregnancy. In pregnancy both the incidence of dissemination (10%) and its resultant mortality (90%) rise markedly.

Placental coccidioidomycosis is well documented. Harris reported seven cases of placental involvement with coccidioidomycosis.[103] Smale and Waechter identified three additional cases in which placental involvement occurred during systemic dissemination.[104]

Although coccidioidal dissemination occurs frequently during pregnancy, with occasional invasion of the placenta, infants are nearly always born free of infection. A few cases of transplacental fetal coccidioidomycosis have been reported, however. Smale and Waechter reported a case of probable fetal intrauterine infection in a preterm infant dying of coccidioidomycosis at 29 days of age.[104] Shafai reported twins born to a woman who died of disseminated coccidioidomycosis 24 hours after she delivered. Both infants died with widespread disease thought to have been acquired in utero.[105] Cohen described an infant, born of a mother with active disease, who developed pulmonary disease at 1 week of age, suggesting that the infection was acquired in utero.[106] With these few exceptions, fetuses have been spared in pregnancies complicated by dissemination. Monif has speculated that the infrequency of congenital infection is a reflection of limitation of infection to the placenta because of either the size of the coccidioidal spherules, resulting in their physical exclusion from the fetal circulation, or the severity of the host reaction, resulting in thrombosis of the adjacent vascular spaces and generation of an acute inflammatory response.[107]

REFERENCES

1. Blanc WA. Pathology of the placenta, membranes, and umbilical cord in bacterial, fungal and viral infections in man. In: Naeye RA, Kissane JM, Kaufman N, eds. Perinatal diseases. Baltimore: Williams & Wilkins, 1981:67.
2. Driscoll SG. Pathology of the developing fetus. Pediatr Clin N Am 1965;12:493.
3. Reiss HJ, Potal J, Krebs A. Granulomatosis infanti septica. Klin Wochenschr 1951;29:29.
4. Variend S, Blumenthal I. Neonatal listeriosis. Postgrad Med J 1975;55:99.
5. Linnan MJ, Mascola L, Lou XD, et al. Epidemic listeriosis associated with Mexican-style cheese. N Engl J Med 1988;319:823.
6. Teberg AJ, Yonekura ML, Salminen C, Pavlova Z. Clinical manifestations of epidemic neonatal listeriosis. Pediatr Infect Dis J 1987;6:817.
7. Khong TY, Frappell JM, Steel HM, Stewart CM, Burke M. Perinatal listeriosis: a report of six cases. Br J Obstet Gynaecol 1986;93:1083.
8. Klatt EC, Pavlova Z, Teberg AJ, Yonekura ML. Epidemic perinatal listeriosis at autopsy. Hum Pathol 1986;17:1278.
9. Cruikshank DP, Warenski JC. First-trimester maternal *Listeria monocytogenes* sepsis and chorioamnionitis with normal neonatal outcome. Obstet Gynecol 1989;73:469.

10. Pai PM, Parikh PR. Congenital miliary tuberculosis. Clin Pediatr 1976;15:376.
11. Smith MHD, Marquis JR. Tuberculosis and other mycobacterial infections. In: Feign RD, Cherry JD, eds. Textbook of pediatric infectious diseases. 2nd ed. Philadelphia: WB Saunders, 1987:1366.
12. Monif GRG. Infectious diseases in obstetrics and gynecology. 2nd ed. Philadelphia: Harper & Row, 1982:310.
13. Peter G, Giebink GS, Hall CB, Plotkin SA, eds. Report of the committee on infectious diseases. 20th ed. Elk Grove Village, IL: American Academy of Pediatrics, 1986:387.
14. Huber GL. Tuberculosis. In: Remington JS, Klein JO, eds. Infectious diseases of the fetus and newborn infant. 2nd ed. Philadelphia: WB Saunders, 1983:577.
15. Cerruti H, Bechelli LM. Congenital infection and lepra reaction in pregnancy. Int J Lepr 1938;6:583.
16. Inaba T. A histologic and bacteriologic examination of the placenta. Int J Lepr 1940;8:394.
17. King JA, Marks RA. Pregnancy and leprosy. Am J Obstet Gynecol 1958;76:438.
18. Sushida I, Hirano N. Placental infection in fetuses of pregnant murine leprous mice. Yokohama Med Bull 1970;21:21.
19. Maurus JN. Hansen's disease in pregnancy. Obstet Gynecol 1978;52:22.
20. Melsom R, Harboe M, Duncan ME, et al. IgA and IgM antibodies against *Mycobacterium leprae* in cord sera and in patients with leprosy: an indication of intrauterine infection in leprosy, Scand J Immunol 1981;14:343.
21. Duncan ME, Oakey RE. Estrogen excretion in pregnant women with leprosy: evidence of diminished fetoplacental function. Obstet Gynecol 1982;60:82.
22. Gilbert GL, Davoren RA, Cole ME, et al. Midtrimester abortion associated with septicaemia caused by *Campylobacter jejuni.* Med J Aust 1981;1:585.
23. Gribble MJ, Salit IE, Isaac-Renton J, et al. *Campylobacter* infections in pregnancy. Am J Obstet Gynecol 1981;140:423.
24. Blaser MJ. *Campylobacter* species. In: Mandell GL, Douglas RG, Bennett JE, eds. Principles and practice of infectious diseases. 2nd ed. New York: John Wiley & Sons, 1985:1221.
25. Diddle AW, Stephens RL. Typhoid fever in pregnancy. Probable intrauterine transmission of disease. Am J Obstet Gynecol 1939;38:300.
26. Riggall F, Salkind G, Spellacy W. Typhoid fever complicating pregnancy. Obstet Gynecol 1974;44:117.
27. Hicks HT, French H. Typhoid fever and pregnancy with special reference to fetal infection. Lancet 1905;1:1491.
28. Wing ES, Troppoli DV. The intrauterine transmission of typhoid. JAMA 1930;95:405.
29. Griffith JPC, Ostheimer M. Typhoid fever in children of two and a half years and under. Am J Med Sci 1902;124:868.
30. Neter E. Observations on the transmission of salmonellosis in man. Am J Pub Health 1950;40:929.
31. Kramer J. Salmonellen-Ubertragung von der mutter auf das neugerborene. Dtsch Med Wochenschr 1977;102:84.
32. Barry M, Bia F. Pregnancy and travel. JAMA 1989;261:728.
33. Lide TN. Congenital tularemia. Arch Pathol 1947;43:165.
34. Omar ME. Rare complication of louse borne relapsing fever. J Egypt Public Health Assoc 1946;2:195.
35. Fuchs PC, Oyama AA. Neonatal relapsing fever due to transplacental transmission of *Borrelia*. JAMA 1969;208:690.
36. Steenbarger JR. Congenital tick-borne relapsing fever: report of a case with first documentation of transplacental transmission. Birth Defects 1982;18:39.
37. Duffy J. Lyme disease. Infect Dis Clin N Am 1987;1:511.
38. Schlesinger PA, Duray PH, Burke BA, Steere AC, Stillman MT. Maternal-fetal transmission of the Lyme disease spirochete, *Borrelia burgdorferi*. Ann Int Med 1985;103:67.
39. Markowitz LE, Steere AC, Benach JL, Slade JD, Broome CV. Lyme disease during pregnancy. JAMA 1986;255:3394.
40. MacDonald AB, Benach JL, Burgdorfer W. Stillbirth following maternal Lyme disease. New York State J Med 1987;87:615.
41. Mikkelsen AL, Palle C. Lyme disease during pregnancy. Acta Obstet Gynecol Scand 1987;66:477.
42. Shrestha M, Grodzichi RL, Steere AC. Diagnosing early Lyme disease. Am J Med 1985;78:235.
43. Williams CL, Strobino BA. Lyme disease transmission during pregnancy. Contemp Ob/Gyn 1990;35:48.
44. Chung H, Ts'ao W, Mo P, et al. Transplacental or congenital infection of leptospirosis. Clinical and experimental observations. Chin Med J 1963;82:777.
45. Lindsay S, Luke IW. Fetal leptospirosis in a newborn infant. J Pediatr 1949;34:90.
46. Gsell HO, Olafsson A, Sonnabend W, et al. Intrauterine *Leptospirosis pomona*. Dtsch Med Wochenschr 1971;96:1263.
47. Cramer HHW. Abortus bein *Leptospirosis canicola*. Arch Gynecol 1950;177:167.
48. Porreco RP, Haverkamp AD. Brucellosis in pregnancy. Obstet Gynecol 1974;44:597.
49. Pollitzer R, cited by: Mann JM, Moskowitz R. Plague and pregnancy. JAMA 1977;237:1854.
50. Regan PC, Litvak A, Regan C. Intrauterine transmission of anthrax. JAMA 1923;80:1769.
51. Haight TH. Anthrax meningitis: review of literature and report of two cases with autopsies. Am J Med Sci 1952;224:57.
52. Crosby RMN, Mosberg WH, Smith GW. Intrauterine meningitis as a cause of hydrocephalus. J Pediatr 1951;39:94.
53. Patrick MJ. Influence of maternal renal infection on the foetus and infant. Arch Dis Child 1967;42:208.
54. Mead PB. Asymptomatic bacteriuria in pregnancy. In: de Alvarez RR, ed. The kidney in pregnancy. New York: John Wiley & Sons, 1976:63.
55. Sweet RL, Gibbs RS, eds. Infectious diseases of the female genital tract. Baltimore: Williams & Wilkins, 1985:302.
56. Savage WE, Hajj SN, Kass EH. Demographic and prognostic characteristics of bacteriuria in pregnancy. Medicine 1967;46:385.
57. Kincaid-Smith P, Bullen M. Bacteriuria in pregnancy. Lancet 1965;1:395.
58. Smith LG, Summers PR, Miles RW, et al. Gonococcal chorioamnionitis associated with sepsis: a case report. Am J Obstet Gynecol 1989;160:573.
59. Sawyer LA, Fishbein DB, McDade JE. Q fever: current concepts. Rev Infect Dis 1987;9:935.
60. Babudieri B. Q fever: a zoonosis. Adv Vet Sci 1959;5:81.
61. Syrucek L, Sobeslavsky O, Gutvirth I. Isolation of *Coxiella burnetii* from human placentas. J Hyg Epidemiol Microbiol Immunol 1958;2:29.
62. Wagstaff DJ, Janney JH, Crawford KL, et al. Q fever studies in Maryland. Public Health Rep 1965;80:1095.
63. Fiset P, Wisseman CL, El Batawi Y. Immunologic evidence of human fetal infection with *Coxiella burnetii.* Am J Epidemiol 1975;101:65.
64. Ellis ME, Smith CC, Moffat MAJ. Chronic or fatal Q fever infection: a review of 16 patients seen in northeast Scotland (1967–1980). Q J Med 1983;52:54.
65. Langley JM, Marrie TJ, Covert A, et al. Poker players' pneumonia. An urban outbreak of Q fever following exposure to a parturient cat. N Engl J Med 1988;319:354.
66. McGregor IA, Wilson ME, Billewicz WZ: Malaria infection of the placenta in Gambia, West Africa. Trans R Soc Trop Med Hyg 1983;77:232.

67. Galbraith RM, Fox H, Hsi B, et al. The human materno-foetal relationship in malaria. II. Histological, ultrastructural and immunopathological studies of the placenta. Trans R Soc Trop Med Hyg 1980;74:61.
68. Reinhardt MC, Ambroise-Thomas P, Cavallo-Serra R, et al. Malaria at delivery in Abidjan. Helv Paediatr Acta 33 (Suppl) 1978;41:65.
69. MacLeod C. Malaria. In: MacLeod C, ed. Parasitic infections in pregnancy and the newborn. New York: Oxford University Press, 1988:8.
70. Eyckmans L. *Trypanosoma* species. In: Mandell GL, Douglas RG, Bennett JE, eds. Principles and practice of infectious diseases. 2nd ed. New York: John Wiley & Sons, 1985:235.
71. Debroise A, Debroise-Ballereau C, Satge P, et al. La trypanosomiase africaine du jeune enfant. Arch Fr Pediatr 1968;25:703.
72. Reinhardt MC, MacLeod C. African trypanosomiasis. In: MacLeod C, ed. Parasitic infections in pregnancy and the newborn. New York: Oxford University Press, 1988:43.
73. Delgado MA, Santos Buch CA. Transplacental transmission and fetal parasitosis of *Trypanosoma cruzi* in outbred white Swiss mice. Am J Trop Med Hyg 1978;27:1108.
74. Bittencourt AL. Congenital Chagas disease in Bahia. Rev Baiana Saude Publ 1984;11:159.
75. Bittencourt AL, Mota E, Ribeiro FR, et al. Incidence of congenital Chagas disease in Bahia, Brazil. J Trop Pediatr 1985;31:242.
76. Banerji D. Possible congenital infection of kala-azar. J Indian Med Assoc 1955;24:433.
77. Low GC, Cooke WE. A congenital case of kala-azar. Lancet 1926;2:1209.
78. Czeizel E, Hancsok M, Palkovich I, et al. Possible relation between fetal death and *E. histolytica* infection of the mother. Am J Obstet Gynecol 1966;96:264.
79. Wagner VP, Smale LE, Lischke JH. Amebic abscess of the liver and spleen in pregnancy and the puerperium. Obstet Gynecol 1975;45:562.
80. Esernio-Jenssen D, Scimeca PG, Benach JI, Tenenbaum MJ. Transplacental/perinatal babesiosis. J Pediatr 1987;110:570.
81. Chu WG, Chen PM, Huang CC, et al. Neonatal ascariasis. J Pediatr 1972;81:783.
82. Howard HH. Prenatal hookworm infection. South Med J 1917;10:793.
83. MacLeod C. Intestinal nematode infections. In: MacLeod C, ed. Parasitic infections in pregnancy and the newborn. New York: Oxford University Press, 1988:192.
84. Salzer BF. A study of an epidemic of 14 cases of trichinosis with cures by serum therapy. JAMA 1916;67:579.
85. Kuitunen-Ekbaum E. The incidence of trichinosis in humans in Toronto. Findings in 420 autopsies. Can Public Health J 1941;32:569.
86. Bourns TKR. The discovery of trichina cysts in the diaphragm of a six-week-old child. J Parasitol 1952;38:367.
87. Hood M, Olson SW. Trichinosis in the Chicago area. Am J Hyg 1939;29:51.
88. Renaud R, Brettes P, Costanier C, et al. Placental bilharziasis. Int J Gynecol Obstet 1972;10:25.
89. Bittencourt AL, de Almeida MAC, Ivres MAF, et al. Placental involvement in Schistosomiasis mansoni. Am J Trop Med Hyg 1980;29:571.
90. Narabayashi H, cited by Cort WW. Prenatal infestation with parasitic worms. JAMA 1921;76:170.
91. Camus D, Carlier Y, Bina JC, et al. Sensitization to *Schistosoma mansoni* antigen in uninfected children born to infected mothers. J Infect Dis 1976;134:405.
92. Goldsmith R, Mankell EK. Other trematode infections. In: MacLeod C, ed. Parasitic infections in pregnancy and the newborn. New York: Oxford University Press, 1988:252.
93. Mead PB. *Candida albicans*. In: Monif GRG, ed. Infectious diseases in obstetrics and gynecology. 2nd ed. Philadelphia: Harper & Row, 1982:323.
94. Whyte RK, Hussain Z, De Sa D. Antenatal infections with *Candida* species. Arch Dis Child 1982;57:528.
95. Smith CV, Horenstein J, Platt LD. Intraamniotic infection with *Candida albicans* associated with a retained intrauterine contraceptive device. Am J Obstet Gynecol 1988;159:123.
96. Benirschke K, Raphael SI. *Candida albicans* infection of the amniotic sac. Am J Obstet Gynecol 1958;75:200.
97. Schonebeck J, Segerbrand E. *Candida albicans* septicemia during first half of pregnancy successfully treated with 5-fluorocytosine. Br Med J 1973;4:337.
98. Oliverio Campos J. Congenital meningoencephalitis due to torulosis neoformans. Preliminary report. Bol Clin Hopit Civis (Lisbon) 1954;18:609.
99. Neuhauser EBD, Tucker A. The roentgen changes produced by diffuse torulosis in the newborn. Am J Roentgenol 1948;59:805.
100. Nassau E, Weinberg-Heiruti C. Torulosis of the newborn. Harefuah (Tel Aviv) 1948;35:50.
101. Heath P. Massive separation of retina in full-term infants and juveniles. JAMA 1950;144:1148.
102. Miller MJ. Fungal infections. In: Remington JS, Klein JO, eds. Infectious diseases of the fetus and newborn infant. 2nd ed. Philadelphia: WB Saunders, 1983;464.
103. Harris RE. Coccidioidomycosis complicating pregnancy. Obstet Gynecol 1966;28:401.
104. Smale LE, Waechter KG. Dissemination of coccidioidomycosis in pregnancy. Am J Obstet Gynecol 1970;170:356.
105. Shafai T. Neonatal coccidioidomycosis in premature twins. Am J Dis Child 1978;132:634.
106. Cohen R. Coccidioidomycosis: case studies in children. Arch Pediatr 1949;66:241.
107. Monif GRG. *Coccidioides immitis*. In: Monif GRG, ed. Infectious diseases in obstetrics and gynecology. 2nd ed. Philadelphia: Harper & Row, 1982:345.

28

CHAPTER

ANTIBIOTICS AND OTHER ANTIMICROBIAL AGENTS IN PREGNANCY AND DURING LACTATION

Jennifer R. Niebyl

Antibiotics are widely used during pregnancy. Because of the potential for maternal and fetal side effects, they should be used only when the indication is clear and the risk : benefit ratio justifies their use. Pregnant patients should be warned that they are particularly susceptible to yeast infections and may need therapy later with antifungal agents should such symptoms occur.

PENICILLINS

The penicillins are probably the class of antibiotics most widely used in pregnancy. They have a wide margin of safety and lack toxicity for both the pregnant woman and the fetus.[1] Penicillin is the antibiotic of choice in the treatment of numerous serious bacterial infections, including gonorrhea and syphilis. Ampicillin, on the other hand, is one of the most frequently used drugs in the treatment of respiratory and urinary tract infections during pregnancy. Adverse effects, however, may include nausea, epigastric distress, diarrhea, and candidal vaginitis.

Before therapy it is important to ascertain that the patient is not allergic to penicillin. The severity of reactions ranges from a mild rash to anaphylaxis. One patient had a stillborn infant attributed to an anaphylactic reaction to penicillin.[2]

There is no evidence that penicillin or its derivatives are teratogenic. In the Collaborative Perinatal Project, 3546 mothers took penicillin derivatives in the first trimester of pregnancy, with no increased risk of anomalies.[1] In another controlled study of 110 patients,[3] penicillin G was given for a total of 107 weeks in the first trimester, and the incidence of birth defects was no different from that in the nontreated controls. There is little experience in pregnancy with the new penicillins such as piperacillin, mezlocillin, and azlocillin. These drugs, therefore, should be used in pregnancy only when another, better-studied antibiotic is not effective.

PHARMACOLOGY

The pharmacokinetics of the penicillin group of antibiotics have been relatively well studied. Several studies have revealed that the serum levels of these drugs are lower and their renal clearance is higher throughout pregnancy when compared to the non-pregnant state.[4–6] The increase in maternal renal function, because of an increase in both renal blood flow and glomerular filtration rate, results in a higher renal excretion of drugs excreted in the urine, which is the case with the penicillins. The expansion of the maternal intravascular volume during the late stages of pregnancy is another factor that affects antibiotic therapy. If the same dose of penicillin or ampicillin is given to both non-pregnant and pregnant women, lower serum levels are attained during pregnancy, because of the distribution of the drug in a larger intravascular volume.

The transplacental passage of penicillin is by simple diffusion. The free circulating portion of the antibiotic crosses the placenta, resulting in a lower maternal serum level of the unbound portion of the drug. The data indicate that the maternal administration of penicillins with high protein binding (eg, oxacillin, cloxacillin, dicloxacillin, and nafcillin) results in lower fetal tissue and amniotic fluid levels than the administration of poorly bound penicillins (eg, penicillin G, ampicillin, and methicillin).[7,8]

The antibiotic is ultimately excreted in the fetal urine and thus into the amniotic fluid. The delay in appearance of different types of penicillins in the amniotic fluid depends primarily on the rate of transplacental diffusion, the amount of protein binding in fetal serum, and the adequacy of fetal enzymatic and renal function. A time delay may occur before effective levels of the antibiotic appear in the amniotic fluid.

At term maternal serum and amniotic fluid concentrations of penicillin G are equal at 60–90 minutes after intravenous administration,[9] representing rapid passage into the fetal circulation and amniotic fluid. Continuous intravenous infusions caused equal concentrations of penicillin G at 20 hours in maternal serum, cord serum, and amniotic fluid.[9] Ampicillin rapidly crosses the placenta and fetal serum levels can be detected within 30 minutes, and equilibrate in an hour.

Amoxicillin is similar to ampicillin in its spectrum of activity but is stable in the presence of gastric acid and may be given without regard to meals. It has been used effectively as a 3-g single dose to treat bacteriuria in pregnancy.[10]

Methicillin crosses rapidly into the fetal circulation and amniotic fluid. Following a 500-mg intravenous dose over 10–15 minutes, equilibration occurred within 1 hour in fetal tissues.[11]

Carbenicillin crosses the placenta and distributes to fetal tissues. Following a 4-g intramuscular dose, mean peak concentrations in cord and maternal serum occurred at 2 hours and were similar.[12] Ticarcillin rapidly crosses the placenta into the fetal circulation and amniotic fluid.[13]

Oxacillin and dicloxacillin cross the placenta only in low concentrations because of the high degree of maternal protein binding. Cord serum and amniotic fluid levels of oxacillin were less than 0.3 μg/mL in 15 of 18 patients given 500 mg orally 0.5–4 hours prior to cesarean section.[14] Following a 500-mg intravenous dose of dicloxacillin, the peak fetal serum level was only 8% of the maternal peak level.[11]

Most penicillins are primarily excreted unchanged in the urine with only small amounts being inactivated in the liver. This is of significance in patients with impaired renal function, which requires reduction in dosage.

BREAST-FEEDING

Penicillin G is excreted into breast milk in low concentrations. Milk : plasma ratios vary between 0.2 and 0.13.[15] Although no adverse effects are clearly attributable to penicillin in breast milk, there are three problems that theoretically might be seen in the nursing infant:

1. Modification of bowel flora (possible diarrhea, candidiasis)
2. Allergic response
3. Interference with the interpretation of culture results.

The benefits of continued breast-feeding usually outweigh these potential risks. When these drugs are used to treat mastitis or other infections in nursing mothers, continued nursing is usually allowed. Ampicillin is excreted into breast milk in low concentrations. Milk : plasma ratios up to 0.2 have been reported.[16] Amoxicillin is excreted into breast milk in low concentrations, with a maximum milk : plasma ratio of 0.04.[17]

Oxacillin and dicloxacillin are highly protein bound and are excreted into breast milk in only very small amounts. Ticarcillin is excreted in low concentrations also. After a 1-g intravenous dose was given to five patients, only trace amounts of the drug were measured at intervals up to 6 hours.[13]

CEPHALOSPORINS

The use of cephalosporins in obstetrics has been extensive. They are used as prophylactic agents in cesarean section and in the treatment of septic abortion, pyelonephritis, and amnionitis.

There is no evidence of teratogenicity of these agents. However, they are sufficiently new that they were not included in the Collaborative Perinatal Project, and so studies in very large numbers of patients have not been performed. The third-generation agents have had limited use during pregnancy.

PHARMACOLOGY

Maternal serum levels attained with these drugs during pregnancy are lower than those in non-pregnant patients receiving equivalent dosages, due to a shorter half-life in pregnancy and an increased volume of distribution. This is true not only for well-established cephalosporin drugs (eg, cephalothin,[18] cephalexin, and cephazolin), but also for the newer cephalosporins (eg, cephoxitin, cephradine, and cefuroxime).[19–21]

These drugs readily cross the placenta to the fetal bloodstream and ultimately the amniotic fluid. While the blood level in the mother is decreasing after an intramuscular injection, the concentration in the cord blood rises and then decreases, and the amniotic fluid level rises.[22]

Transplacental transfer of these drugs is fairly rapid, and adequate bactericidal concentrations are attained in both fetal soft tissues and the amniotic fluid.[19–21,23–25] Repeated high-bolus doses of cephalosporins have been shown to result in higher levels in fetal serum and amniotic fluid than continuous intravenous infusions of the same amount of drug.[26]

The average fetal cord blood level achieved ranges from 10% to 40% of the maternal serum levels, depending on the timing and the particular drug used. Studies reporting cord levels only a few hours after a drug dose may not reveal the full picture. For example, when ceftizoxime was administrated in a 2-g intravenous dose, the mean fetal : maternal ratio was 0.28. However, after reaching steady state after three doses of 2 g every 8 hours, ceftizoxime was concentrated on the fetal side of the placenta, achieving a fetal serum level of two times that in the maternal serum and, in the amniotic fluid, a level of four times that of the maternal serum.[27]

BREAST-FEEDING

The cephalosporins are excreted into breast milk in sufficiently low concentrations that the infant receives an insignificant dose. Although the same theoretical concerns exist as with penicillins, the advantages of continued breast-feeding during treatment usually outweigh these risks.

SULFONAMIDES

The sulfonamides are often used for treatment of urinary tract infections in pregnancy. Among 1455 human infants exposed to sulfonamides during the first trimester, no teratogenic effects were noted.[1]

The administration of sulfonamides should be avoided in glucose-6-phosphate dehydrogenase-deficient women. A dose-related toxic reaction may occur in these individuals, resulting in red cell hemolysis. This is also a theoretical risk to the fetus if the drug is used near the time of delivery, because fetal red cells are always relatively deficient in glutathione, but this has not been reported.

Sulfonamides cause no known damage to the fetus in utero because the fetus can clear free bilirubin through the placenta. These drugs might theoretically have deleterious effects if present in the blood of the neonate after birth, however. The sulfonamides compete with bilirubin for binding sites on albumin, thus raising the levels of free bilirubin in the serum and increasing the risk of hyperbilirubinemia or kernicterus in the neonate.[28,29] For that reason it is recommended that an alternate antibiotic be used in the third trimester, if possible. However, kernicterus in the neonate following in utero exposure has not been reported.

PHARMACOLOGY

The sulfonamides are easily absorbed orally, and they readily cross the placenta, achieving fetal plasma levels 50% to 90% of those attained in the maternal plasma.[30] Ylikorkala and colleagues studied the pharmacokinetics of trimethoprim-sulfamethoxazole in 10 pregnant women in the first trimester and found the maternal serum levels of the drug to be comparable to nonpregnant individuals.[31] The elimination half-life of this combination drug was shorter, however, in the pregnant women, and trimethoprim was cleared faster from the maternal serum than sulfamethoxazole.[31]

USE WITH TRIMETHOPRIM

Sulfa is often given with trimethoprim in treatment of urinary tract infections. Controlled trials have failed to show any increased risk of birth defects after first-trimester exposure.[32,33] Although trimethoprim antagonizes folic acid in bacteria, it does not affect the human enzyme system with similar potency.

SULFASALAZINE

Sulfasalazine is used for treatment of ulcerative colitis and Crohn's disease because of its relatively poor oral absorption. However, it does cross the placenta to the fetal circulation, with fetal concentrations approximately the same as maternal concentrations, although both are low. Neither kernicterus nor severe neonatal jaundice has been reported following maternal use of sulfasalazine, even when the drug was given up to the time of delivery.[34,35]

BREAST-FEEDING

Sulfonamides are excreted into breast milk in low concentrations. The milk : plasma ratio is approximately 0.5.[36] The amount of sulfonamide ingested by an infant would be sufficiently low not to have any toxicity (less than 1% of the maternal dose) and so breast-feeding is usually continued during administration of these drugs. When sulfasalazine was taken by breast-feeding mothers, the drug was undetectable in all milk samples. However, during the first 5 days of life or with premature infants when hyperbilirubinemia may be a problem, sulfa drugs are best avoided.[37]

NITROFURANTOIN

Nitrofurantoin is an antimicrobial agent used in the treatment of acute uncomplicated lower urinary tract infections as well as for long-term suppression in patients with chronic bacteriuria. Nitrofurantoin is capable of inducing hemolytic anemia in patients deficient in G6PD and in patients whose red blood cells are deficient in glutathione.[38] Since the red blood cells of newborns are deficient in glutathione, the use of this drug might be a problem for the fetus at delivery. However, hemolytic anemia in the newborn as a result of in utero exposure to nitrofurantoin has not been reported to date, despite this theoretical concern.

No reports linking the use of nitrofurantoin with congenital defects have been located. In the Collaborative Perinatal Project,[1] 590 infants were exposed, 83 in the first trimester, with no significantly increased risk of anomalies or other adverse effects. In a retrospective analysis of another 91 pregnancies, there was no evidence of fetal toxicity.[39] Other studies also suggested no fetal toxicity from nitrofurantoin exposure.[40]

PHARMACOLOGY

Nitrofurantoin absorption from the gastrointestinal tract varies with the form administered. The macrocrystalline form is absorbed more slowly than the crystalline and is associated with less gastrointestinal intolerance. Because of rapid elimination, the serum half-life is 20–60 minutes. Therapeutic serum levels are not achieved; therefore, this drug is not indicated when there is a possibility of bacteremia. Approximately one third of an oral dose appears in the active form in the urine.

BREAST-FEEDING

Nitrofurantoin is excreted into breast milk in very low concentrations. In one study the drug could not be detected in 20 samples from mothers receiving 100 mg four times a day.[41] Although these amounts are negligible, an infant with G6PD deficiency might be susceptible to hemolytic anemia from this exposure.[42]

TETRACYCLINES

The tetracyclines readily cross the placenta and are firmly bound by chelating to calcium in developing bone and tooth structures. This produces brown discoloration of the teeth, hypoplasia of the enamel, inhibition of bone growth,[44] and other skeletal abnormalities. The yellowish brown staining of the teeth usually occurs in the second or third trimesters of pregnancy after 24 weeks, whereas bone incorporation can occur earlier. Depression of skeletal growth was particularly common among premature infants treated with tetracycline. A 40% inhibition of fibular growth in the second trimester was demonstrated in patients who subsequently underwent termination of pregnancy, but the effect was reversible when the drug was stopped. Alternate antibiotics are currently recommended during pregnancy.

Hepatotoxicity has been reported in pregnant women treated with large doses of tetracyclines, usually for pyelonephritis with intravenous administration. This has been presumed to be an overdose effect and has not been reported with brief courses of therapy at lower doses. Tetracycline-induced hepatotoxicity differs from acute fatty liver of pregnancy in that it is not unique to pregnant women and reversal of the disease does not occur with pregnancy termination.

First-trimester exposure to tetracycline has not been found to have any teratogenic risk in 341 women in the Collaborative Perinatal Project[1] or in 174 women in another study.[45]

BREAST-FEEDING

Tetracycline is excreted into breast milk in low plasma concentrations, with milk : plasma ratios varying between 0.2 and 1.5. Tetracycline was not detectable in the serum of breast-feeding infants, and delayed bone growth from tetracycline has not been reported after the drug was taken by breast-feeding mothers. This may be due to the high binding of the drug to calcium and protein, limiting absorption from the milk.

AMINOGLYCOSIDES

Aminoglycosides are commonly used with penicillin or clindamycin in the treatment of postpartum endometritis, septic abortion, or endometritis. They should be given during pregnancy only when serious gram-negative infections are suspected. Gentamicin is preferred over tobramycin and amikacin, as it has been more extensively studied.

Streptomycin and kanamycin have been associated with congenital deafness in the offspring of mothers who took these drugs during pregnancy. Ototoxicity was reported with doses as low as 1 g of streptomycin biweekly for 8 weeks during the first trimester, and it is recommended to limit dosages to a total of 20 g during the last half of pregnancy.[46] Eighth cranial nerve damage has been reported following in utero exposure to kanamycin. Of 391 mothers who had received 50 mg/kg for prolonged periods during pregnancy, nine children were found to have hearing loss (2.3%).[47] Although ototoxicity in the fetus has not been reported with use of aminoglycosides other than kanamycin and streptomycin, it may occur with the others. Ototoxicity may be increased with simultaneous use of ethacrynic acid.[48]

Nephrotoxicity may be increased when the drug is given in combination with cephalosporins, and this should be avoided. Neuromuscular blockade may be potentiated by the combined use of these drugs and curariform drugs; therefore, the dosages should be reduced appropriately. Potentiation of magnesium sulfate–induced neuromuscular weakness has also been reported in a neonate exposed to magnesium sulfate and gentamicin.[49]

No known teratogenic effect is associated with the use of these drugs in the first trimester other than ototoxicity. In 135 infants exposed to streptomycin in the Collaborative Perinatal Project[1] no teratogenic effects were observed. In a group of 1619 newborns whose mothers were treated for tuberculosis during pregnancy with multiple drugs, including streptomycin, the incidence of congenital defects was the same as that of the healthy control group.[50]

PHARMACOLOGY

The aminoglycosides are poorly absorbed after oral administration and are rapidly excreted by the normal kidney. Because the rate of clearance is related to the glomerular filtration rate, dosage must be reduced in the face of abnormal renal function.

The serum aminoglycoside levels are usually lower in pregnant than in non-pregnant patients receiving equivalent doses due to more rapid elimination. Thus, it is important to monitor levels to prevent subtherapeutic dosing.[51,52] Wide interpatient variation in gentamicin levels has been observed in obstetric patients, varying with the volume of distribution of the drug.[52] The concentrations in fetal blood are lower than those in maternal blood at full term.[53] Following 40–80-mg intramuscular doses given to patients in labor, peak cord serum levels averaging 30% to 40% of maternal levels were obtained at 1–2 hours.[52,53] At term, cord serum levels of amikacin are one half to one third of maternal serum levels, and measurable amniotic fluid levels appear at about 5 hours postinjection.[54]

BREAST-FEEDING

Limited information is available about excretion of gentamicin into breast milk. Other aminoglycosides (eg, amikacin, kanamycin,[55] streptomycin, and tobramycin) are known to be excreted in low levels into breast milk. Since oral absorption of these drugs by the infant is poor, ototoxicity or other side effects would not be expected.

ERYTHROMYCIN

Erythromycin is the alternate drug of choice to penicillin for many diseases in pregnancy, including gonorrhea or syphilis, and is used for primary treatment for other diseases, such as mycoplasma and chlamydia. It is also an adequate substitute in the treatment of urinary tract infection, provided the urine can be adequately alkalized.[56]

Erythromycin estolate has been associated with subclinical reversible hepatotoxicity during pregnancy.[57] Thus, other forms that are felt to be relatively nontoxic are usually recommended.

No teratogenic risk of erythromycin has been reported. In 79 patients in the Collaborative Perinatal Project[1] and 260 in another study,[45] no increased risk of birth defects was noted.

PHARMACOLOGY

Erythromycin and its salts are not consistently absorbed from the gastrointestinal tract of pregnant women, and their transplacental passage is unpredictable. Both maternal and fetal serum levels achieved after the administration of the drug in pregnancy are low and vary considerably.[58,59] Thus, some authors have recommended that penicillin be administered to every newborn whose mother received erythromycin for the treatment of syphilis.[60] Fetal tissue levels increase after multiple doses.[59] Fetal plasma concentrations are 5% to 20% of those in maternal plasma. The usual oral dose is 250–500 mg every 6 hours, but the higher dose may not be well tolerated in pregnant women who are susceptible to nausea and gastrointestinal symptoms.

BREAST-FEEDING

Erythromycin is excreted into breast milk in small amounts with milk : plasma ratios at about 0.5. No reports of adverse effects of infants exposed to erythromycin in breast milk have been noted.

CLINDAMYCIN

Clindamycin should be used in pregnancy only when anaerobic infections are suspected that are not sensitive to other antibiotics. Most authorities would agree that this drug should not be used for prophylaxis prior to cesarean section, reserving its use for therapeutic indications.

If diarrhea develops during the administration of this drug, the patient should be evaluated for the possibility of pseudomembranous colitis, which has been reported in up to 10% of patients.

No reports linking the use of clindamycin with congenital defects have been noted, although this drug is sufficiently new that it was not included in the Collaborative Perinatal Project.[1]

PHARMACOLOGY

Clindamycin crosses the placenta, achieving maximum cord serum levels of about 50% of the maternal serum.[59] It is 90% bound to serum protein, and fetal tissue levels increase following multiple dosing.[59] Maternal serum levels after dosing at various stages of pregnancy are similar to those of non-pregnant patients.[51]

Clindamycin is nearly completely absorbed after oral administration, and a small percentage is absorbed after topical application. Most of the drug is metabolized in the liver to products excreted in the urine and bile, and only 10% of the drug is excreted unchanged in the urine.

BREAST-FEEDING

Clindamycin is excreted into breast milk in low levels, and nursing is usually continued during administration of this drug. Two bloody stools were observed in one nursing infant whose mother was receiving clindamycin and gentamicin[61]; this symptom cleared when the breast-feeding was stopped. Except for this one case, no other adverse effects in nursing infants have been reported.

METRONIDAZOLE

Metronidazole possesses trichomonacidal and amebicidal activity as well as effectiveness against certain bacteria, especially anaerobes.

Controversy regarding the use of metronidazole during pregnancy was initiated when the drug was shown to be positive in the Ames test, which correlates with carcinogenicity in animals. However, doses used were much higher than the doses used clinically, and carcinogenicity in humans has not been confirmed.[62] As some have advised against the use of this drug in pregnancy,[63] it should only be used for clear-cut indications.

Several studies have failed to show any increase in the incidence of congenital defects or other adverse pregnancy outcomes among newborn infants of mothers treated with metronidazole during pregnancy. In one study, four out of 55 infants treated in early pregnancy had a variety of minor defects.[64] In the Collaborative Perinatal Project, two out of 31 infants were abnormal, both close to the expected incidence.[1] In an additional study of 880 infants exposed in the three trimesters of pregnancy, no difference in any adverse outcome was noted compared to controls.[65]

Metronidazole remains the most effective drug for trichomoniasis. Because of the controversy surrounding this drug, deferring therapy until after the first trimester is probably wise.

PHARMACOLOGY

Metronidazole crosses the placenta to the fetus throughout gestation with a cord : maternal plasma ratio at term of approximately 1.0.[66]

BREAST-FEEDING

Metronidazole is excreted into breast milk in small amounts with milk : plasma ratios about 1.0. One infant had diarrhea while the mother was receiving metronidazole; otherwise, no adverse effects in metronidazole-exposed nursing infants have been reported. The American Academy of Pediatrics recommends interrupting breast-feeding after a single 2-g oral dose for 12–24 hours to allow clearance of the drug.[37]

LINDANE (QUELL)

Lindane has been administered to pregnant women for the treatment of scabies and lice. Treatment should be such that only a minimal amount of the drug is absorbed percutaneously, as high doses applied in this way have produced convulsions.

Toxicity in humans after topical use of 1% lindane has been observed almost exclusively after overexposure to the agent. However, about 10% of the dose is recovered in the urine after application to the skin. As this drug is a potent neurotoxin, its use during pregnancy should be limited. The manufacturer recommends no more than two treatments during pregnancy. Although no specific reproductive damage attributable to lindane has been reported, pregnant women should be advised to wear gloves when shampooing their children's hair, as absorption could easily occur across the skin of the hands of the mother. Alternate drugs are usually recommended, specifically pyrethrins with piperonyl butoxide (RID).

PHARMACOLOGY

Lindane is absorbed through the skin after local application, and more is absorbed in patients with excoriated skin.

BREAST-FEEDING

No reports describing the use of lindane in lactating women have been noted. However, the amount of lindane ingested in breast milk would be less than the amount absorbed from direct topical application to the infant.

PYRETHRINS WITH PIPERONYL BUTOXIDE (RID)

Pyrethrins with piperonyl butoxide constitute a combination product used topically for the treatment of lice. This product is considered the drug of choice for lice in pregnancy, as topical absorption is poor, so potential toxicity should be less than that with lindane.

ANTIFUNGAL AGENTS

Nystatin, miconazole, and clotrimazole are commonly used during pregnancy for monilial infections. Nystatin is poorly absorbed from intact skin and mucous membranes; consequently, topical use would not be expected to be associated with teratogenesis. In the Collaborative Perinatal Project,[1] however, of 142 exposures there were 14 malformations, which was a statistically increased risk. This was attributed to adjunctive use with other drugs, particularly tetracycline therapy. Another study of 176 infants has not confirmed any risk with use in pregnancy.[45]

Clotrimazole has not been implicated as a teratogen. Only small amounts are absorbed from the skin and vaginal mucosa.[67] Only 0.15% of the dose was recovered in the urine after it had been applied to inflamed skin and serum levels of only 0.05 μg/mL were achieved after administration of a 100-mg vaginal tablet.[68]

Miconazole is also absorbed in small amounts from the vagina. Use in pregnancy is not known to be associated with congenital malformations. However, in one study a slightly increased risk of first-trimester abortion was noted after use of this drug, although many associations were examined. These findings were considered not to be definitive evidence of risk.[69] However, use of these drugs should be postponed until after the first trimester, if possible, for theoretical reasons.

BREAST-FEEDING

Since nystatin is poorly absorbed orally, it is unlikely to be found in serum and breast milk.

No data are available with miconazole or clotrimazole in breast milk, but as only small amounts are absorbed vaginally, this would not be expected to be a problem.

CONCLUSIONS

Most antibiotics are safe to use during pregnancy, but as there is potential for fetal effects that are still unrecognized, they should be used only when clearly indicated.

REFERENCES

1. Heinonen PO, Slone D, Shapiro S. Birth defects and drugs in pregnancy. Littleton, MA: Publishing Sciences Group, 1977.
2. Kosim H. Intrauterine fetal death as a result of anaphylactic reaction to penicillin in a pregnant woman. Dapim Refuiim 1959;18:136.
3. Ravid R, Toaff R. On the possible teratogenicity of antibiotic drugs administered during pregnancy: a prospective study. In: Klingberg M, Abramovici A, Chemki J, eds. Drugs and fetal development. New York: Plenum Press, 1972:505.
4. Philipson A. Pharmacokinetics of antibiotics in pregnancy and labour. Clin Pharmacokinetics 1979;4:297.
5. Bastert G, Muller WG, Wallhauser KH, et al. Pharmacokinetische Untersuchungen zum Ubertritt von Antibiotika in das Fruchtwasser am Ende der Schwagerschaft. 3. Tiel: Oxacillin. Zietschrift fur Geburtshilfe und Perinatologie 1975;179:346.
6. Philipson A. Pharmacokinetics of ampicillin during pregnancy. J Infect Dis 1977;136:370.
7. Kunin CM. Clinical pharmacology of the new penicillins. I. The importance of serum protein binding in determining antimicrobial activity and concentration in serum. Clin Pharmacol Ther 1966;7:166.
8. Macaulay MA, Berg SA, Charles D. Placental transfer of dicloxacillin at term. Am J Obstet Gynecol 1968;102:1162.
9. Woltz J, Zintel H. The transmission of penicillin to amniotic fluid and fetal blood in the human. Am J Obstet Gynecol 1945;50:338.
10. Masterson RG, Evans DC, Strike PW. Single-dose amoxicillin in the treatment of bacteriuria in pregnancy and the puerperium: a controlled clinical trial. Br J Obstet Gynaecol 1985;92:498.
11. Depp R, Kind A, Kirby W, Johnson W. Transplacental passage of methicillin and dicloxacillin into the fetus and amniotic fluid. Am J Obstet Gynecol 1970;107:1054.
12. Elek E, Ivan E, Arr M. Passage of penicillins from mother to foetus in humans. Int J Clin Pharmacol Ther Toxicol 1972;6:223.
13. Cho N, Nakayama T, Vehara K, Kunii K. Laboratory and clinical evaluation of ticarcillin in the field of obstetrics and gynecology. Chemotherapy (Tokyo) 1977;25:2911.
14. Prigot A, Froix C, Rubin E. Absorption, diffusion, and excretion of new penicillin, oxacillin. Antimicrob Agents Chemother 1962;402.
15. Greene H, Burkhart B, Hobby G. Excretion of penicillin in human milk following parturition. Am J Obstet Gynecol 1946;51:732.
16. Wilson J, Brown R, Cherek D, et al. Drug excretion in human breast milk: principles, pharmacokinetics and projected consequences. Clin Pharmacol Ther 1980;5:1.
17. Kafetzis D, Siafas C, Georgakopoulos P, Papadatos C. Passage of cephalosporins and amoxicillin into the breast milk. Acta Paediatr Scand 1981;70:285.
18. Morrow S, Palmisano P, Cassady G. The placental transfer of cephalothin. J Pediatr 1968;73:262.
19. Dubois M, Delapierre D, Deresse A, et al. Transplacental transfer of cefuroxime. 11th International Congress of Chemotherapy and 19th Interscience Conference on Antimicrobial Agents and Chemotherapy. Boston, 1979.
20. Dubois M, Delapierre D, Demonty J, et al. Transplacental and mammary transfer of cephoxitin. 11th International Congress of Chemotherapy and 19th Interscience Conference on Antimicrobial Agents and Chemotherapy. Boston, 1979.
21. Philipson A, Stiernsted TG. Pharmacokinetics of cephradine in pregnancy. 11th International Congress of Chemotherapy and 19th Interscience Conference on Antimicrobial Agents and Chemotherapy. Boston, 1979.
22. Sheng KT, Huang NN, Promadhattavedi V. Serum concentrations of cephalothin in infants and children and placental transmission of the antibiotic. Antimicrob Agents Chemother 1964:200.
23. Dubois M, Delapierre D, Demonty J, et al. Transplacental and mammary transfer of cephoxitin. 11th International Congress of Chemotherapy and 19th Interscience Conference on Antimicrobial Agents and Chemotherapy. Boston, 1979.
24. Craft I, Mullinger BM, Kennedy MRK. Placental transfer of cefuroxine. 11th International Congress of Chemotherapy and 19th Interscience Conference on Antimicrobial Agents and Chemotherapy. Boston, 1979.
25. Macaulay MA, Charles D. Placental transfer of cephalothin. Am J Obstet Gynecol 1968;100:940.
26. Hirsch HA, Herbst S, Lang R, et al. Transfer of a new cephalosporin antibiotic to the foetus and the amniotic fluid during a continuous infusion (steady state) and single repeated intravenous injections to the mother. Arkh fur Gynakologie 1974;216:1.
27. Fortunato SJ, Bawdon RE, Welt SI, et al. Steady-state cord and amniotic fluid ceftizoxime levels continuously surpass maternal levels. Am J Obstet Gynecol 1988;159:570.
28. Harris RC, Lucey JF, MacLean JR. Kernicterus in premature infants associated with low concentration of bilirubin in the plasma. Pediatrics 1950;23:878.

29. Nyhan WL. Toxicity of drugs in the neonatal period. J Pediatr 1961;59:1.
30. Monif GFG. Infectious diseases in obstetrics and gynecology. New York: Harper & Row, 1974:26.
31. Ylikorkala O, Sjostedt E, Jarvinen PA, et al. Trimethoprim-sulfonamide combination administered orally and intravaginally in the first trimester of pregnancy: its absorption into serum and transfer to amniotic fluid. Acta Obstet Gynecol Scand 1973;52:229.
32. Ochoa AG. Trimethoprim and sulfamethoxazole in pregnancy. JAMA 1971;217:1244.
33. Brumfitt W, Pursell R. Double-blind trial to compare ampicillin, cephalexin, co-trimoxazole, and trimethoprim in treatment of urinary infection. Br Med J 1972;2:673.
34. Jarnerot G, Into-Malmberg MB, Esbjorner E. Placental transfer of sulphasalazine and sulphapyridine and some of its metabolites. Scand J Gastroenterol 1981;16:693.
35. Modadam M. Sulfasalazine IBD, Pregnancy: reply. Gastroenterology 1981;81:194.
36. Foster FP. Sulfanilamide excretion in breast milk: report of a case. Proc Staff Meet Mayo Clin 1939;14:153.
37. Committee on Drugs. American Academy of Pediatrics. Transfer of drugs and other chemicals into human breast milk. Pediatrics 1989;84:924.
38. Briggs GG, Freeman RK, Yaffe SJ. Drugs in pregnancy and lactation. Baltimore: Williams & Wilkins, 1986:311.
39. Hailey FJ, Fort H, Williams JR, et al. Foetal safety of nitrofurantoin, macrocrystals therapy during pregnancy: a retrospective analysis. J Int Med Res 1983;11:364.
40. Lenke RR, VanDorsten JP, Schifrin BS. Pyelonephritis in pregnancy: a prospective randomized trial to prevent recurrent disease evaluating suppressive therapy with nitrofurantoin and close surveillance. Am J Obstet Gynecol 1983;146:953.
41. Hosbach RE, Foster RB. Absence of nitrofurantoin from human milk. JAMA 1967;202:1057.
42. Varsano I, Fischl J, Shochet SB. The excretion of orally ingested nitrofurantoin in human milk. J Pediatr 1973;82:886.
43. Kline AH, Blattner RJ, Lunin M. Transplacental effects of tetracycline on teeth. JAMA 1964;118:178.
44. Cohlan SQ, Bevelander G, Tiamsic T. Growth inhibition of prematures receiving tetracycline. Am J Dis Child 1963;105:453.
45. Aselton P, Jick H, Milunsky A, et al. First-trimester drug use and congenital disorders. Obstet Gynecol 1985;65:451.
46. Robinson GC, Cambon KG. Hearing loss in infants of tuberculous mothers treated with streptomycin during pregnancy. N Engl J Med 1964;271:949.
47. Nishimura H, Tanimura T. Clinical aspects of the teratogenicity of drugs. Amsterdam: Excerpta Medica, 1976:131.
48. Jones HC. Intrauterine ototoxicity: a case report and review of literature. J Natl Med Assoc 1973;65:201.
49. L'Hommedieu CS, Nicholas D, Armes DA, et al. Potentiation of magnesium sulfate-induced neuromuscular weakness by gentamicin, tobramycin, and amikacin. J Pediatr 1983;102:629.
50. Marynowski A, Sianozecka E. Comparison of the incidence of congenital malformations in neonates from healthy mothers and from patients treated because of tuberculosis. Ginekol Pol 1972;43:713.
51. Weinstein AJ, Gibbs RS, Gallagher M. Placental transfer of clindamycin and gentamicin in term pregnancy. Am J Obstet Gynecol 1976;124:688.
52. Zaske DE, Cipolle RJ, Strate RG, Malo JW, Koszalka MF. Rapid gentamicin elimination in obstetric patients. Obstet Gynecol 1980;56:559.
53. Yoshioka H, Monma T, Matsuda S. Placental transfer of gentamicin. J Pediatr 1972;80:121.
54. Matsuda C, Mori C, Maruno M, Shiwakura T. A study of amikacin in the obstetrics field. Jpn J Antibiot 1974;27:633.
55. Wilson JT. Milk/plasma ratios and contraindicated drugs. In: Wilson JT, ed. Drugs in breast milk. Balgowlah, Australia: ADIS Press, 1981:79.
56. Sabath LD, Gerstein DA, Loder PB, et al. Excretion of erythromycin and its enhanced activity in urine against gram negative bacilli with alkalinization. J Lab Clin Med 1968;72:916.
57. McCormack WM, George H, Donner A, et al. Hepatotoxicity of erythromycin estolate during pregnancy. Antimicrob Agents Chemother 1977;12:630.
58. Philipson A, Sabath LD, Charles D. Erythromycin and clindamycin absorption and elimination in pregnant women. Clin Pharmacol Ther 1976;19:68.
59. Philipson A, Sabath LD, Charles D. Transplacental passage of erythromycin and clindamycin. N Engl J Med 1973;288:1219.
60. South MA, Short DH, Knox JM. Failure of erythromycin estolate therapy in in utero syphilis. JAMA 1964;190:70.
61. Mann CF. Clindamycin and breast-feeding. Pediatrics 1980; 66:1030.
62. Beard CM, Noller KL, O'Fallon WM, et al. Lack of evidence for cancer due to use of metronidazole. N Engl J Med 1979;301:519.
63. Finegold SM. Metronidazole. Ann Intern Med 1980;93:585.
64. Peterson WF, Stauch JE, Ryder CD. Metronidazole in pregnancy. Am J Obstet Gynecol 1966;94:343.
65. Morgan FK. Metronidazole treatment in pregnancy. International Congress and Symposium Series. Roy Soc Med 1979;18:245.
66. Karhunen M. Placental transfer of metronidazole and tinidazole in early human pregnancy after a single infusion. Br J Clin Pharmacol 1984;18:254.
67. Tan CG, Good CS, Milne LJR, Loudon JDO. A comparative trial of six day therapy with clotrimazole and nystatin in pregnant patients with vaginal candidiasis. Postgrad Med 1974;50:102.
68. Lindeque BG, Niekirk WA. Treatment of vaginal candidiasis in pregnancy with a single clotrimazole 500 mg vaginal pessary. S Afr Med J 1984;65:123.
69. Rosa FW, Baum C, Shaw M. Pregnancy outcomes after first-trimester vaginitis drug therapy. Obstet Gynecol 1987;69:751.

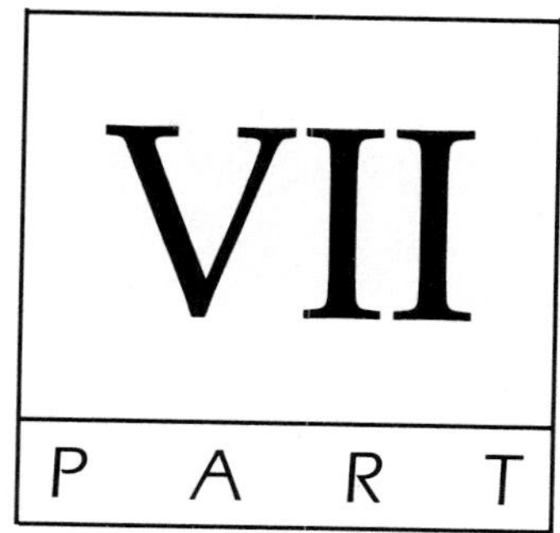

FETAL DISEASES

A. Genetic Disorders

29 CHAPTER

PRINCIPLES OF HUMAN GENETICS

Joe Leigh Simpson

Genetic disorders can result from any of several mechanisms: numerical or structural alterations in chromosomal constitution, mutation involving a single genetic locus (mendelian), or the cumulative effect of several genes (polygenic) possibly interacting with environmental factors (multifactorial). In this chapter we shall review major principles underlying these genetic mechanisms, perturbations of which are responsible for most of the disorders whose diagnosis will be considered elsewhere in this section.

CHROMOSOME ABNORMALITIES

CHROMOSOMAL IDENTIFICATION

A characteristic number of chromosomes exists in each species. In humans there are 46 chromosomes in all nuclei except germ cells: 22 pairs of autosomes (nos. 1–22) and one pair of sex chromosomes (XX in females, XY in males) (Figs. 29-1, 29-2). Chromosomes are numbered according to size and centromere position. The centromere divides a chromosome into a short arm (p) and a long arm (q). The relative centromere position permits chromosomes to be classified as *metacentric* (p and q equal in length), *submetacentric* (q slightly greater than p), *acrocentric* (q much greater than p, the centromere nearly terminal), or *telocentric* (the centromere terminal) (Fig. 29-3).

A variety of the banding techniques (Table 29-1) allow identification of specific chromosomes, a result of characteristic horizontal stripes, as illustrated in Figures 29-1 and 29-2. The first banding technique involved staining chromosomes with quinacrine, followed by fluorescent microscopy (Q-banding). Later, other methods became available, with G-banding techniques (see Figs. 29-1, 29-2) perhaps most widely used at present (see Table 29-1).

CYTOGENETIC NOMENCLATURE

An official chromosomal nomenclature is accepted.[1] Normal or abnormal, the chromosomal complement is designated by the following:

1. The total number of chromosomes
2. A comma
3. The sex chromosomal complement (XY in normal males; XX in normal females)
4. The specific abnormality, if any.

Thus, the normal male chromosomal complement is designated 46,XY (Table 29-2). A complement containing an abnormal number of chromosomes is designated by listing the total number of chromosomes and the appropriate sex chromosomal complement. For example, 45,X is the complement most commonly associated with Turner syndrome. A complement containing additional or missing autosomes is signified by + or − followed by the specific chromosome responsible. Thus, a male with trisomy 21 (Down syndrome) is designated 47,XY,+21; a female with monosomy 21 would be designated 45,XX,−21. When + or − signs are placed after a symbol, it indicates an increase in the length of chromosome (eg, 46,XX,+8q+). Complements containing structurally abnormal chromosomes require the symbol for the aberration present, as well as the number of the aberrant chromosome(s).

Table 29-3 lists symbols used to designate parts of chromosomes and certain rearrangements. Chromosome bands are designated as shown in Figure 29-3. A band is designated by listing first the chromosome, the arm (p or q), the region, and finally the specific band. Bands are numbered consecutively from the centromere distally. Standardized methods to designate translocations and other rearrangements are reviewed elsewhere in much greater detail.[1]

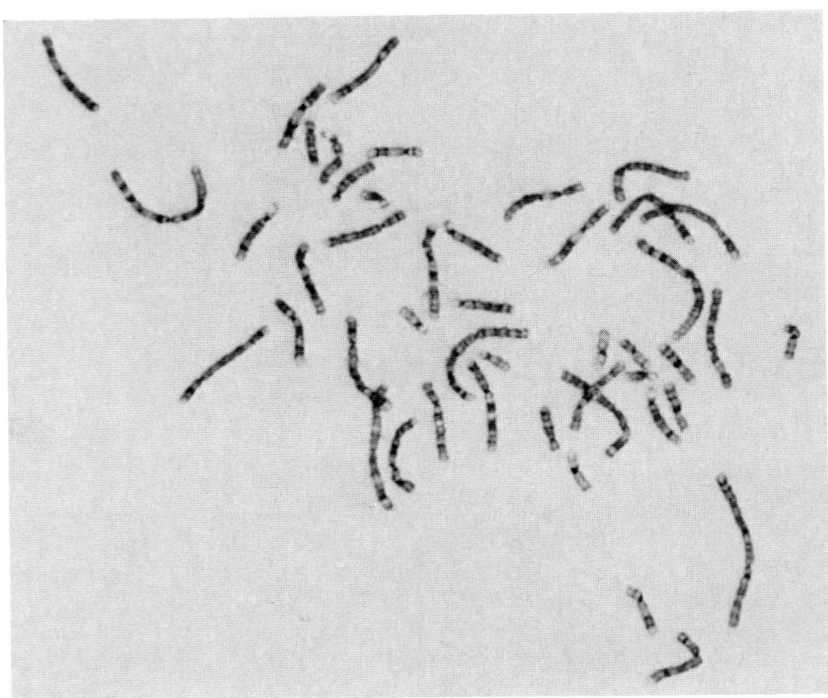

FIGURE 29–1. Metaphase derived from a normal female (46,XX, G-banding technique). (From Simpson JL, Tharapel AT. Principles of cytogenetics. In: Philipp E, Barnes J, eds. Scientific foundations of obstetrics and gynaecology. 4th ed. London: Heinemann, in press.)

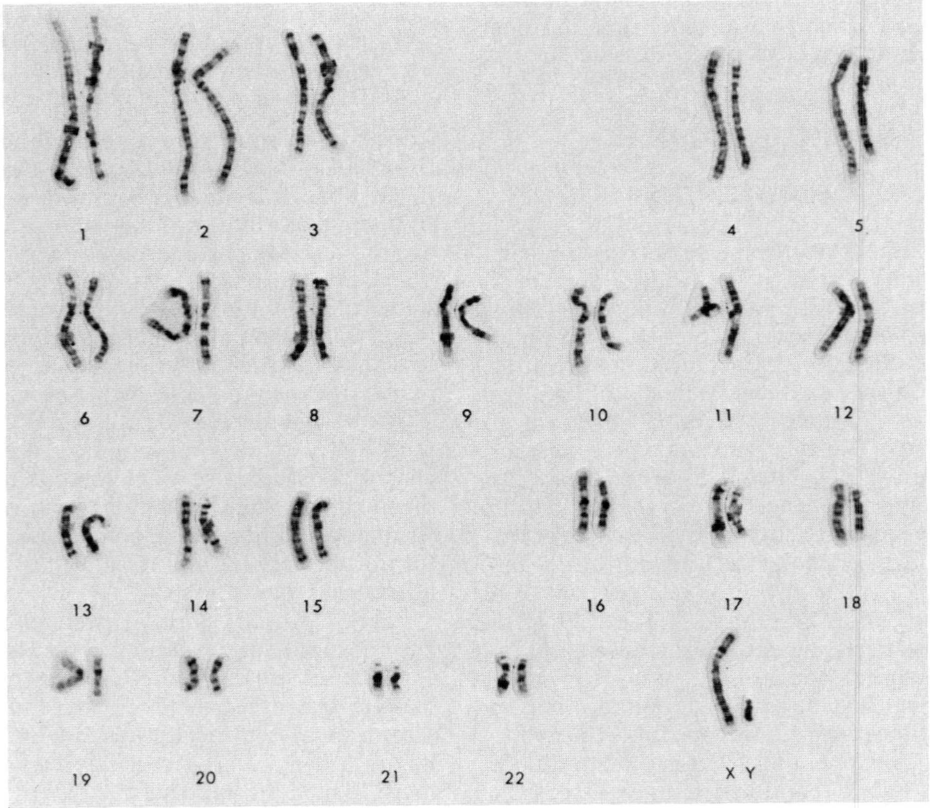

FIGURE 29–2. Karyotype of a normal male (46,XY) G-bands. (From Simpson JL, Tharapel AT. Principles of cytogenetics. In: Philipp E, Barnes J, eds. Scientific foundations of obstetrics and gynaecology. 4th ed. London: Heinemann, in press.)

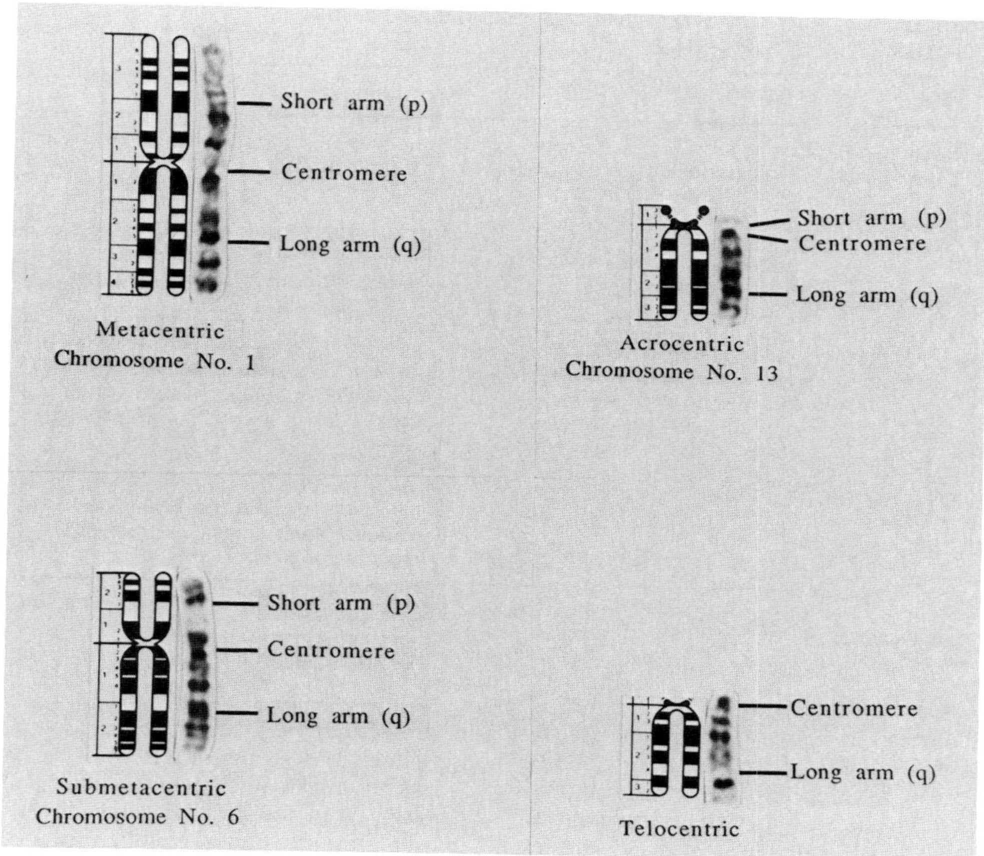

FIGURE 29–3. Parts of chromosome, illustrated in actual and schematic chromosomes. The short arm is abbreviated p and the long arm is abbreviated q. (From Simpson JL, Tharapel AT. Principles of cytogenetics. In: Philipp E, Barnes J, eds. Scientific foundations of obstetrics and gynaecology. 4th ed. London: Heinemann, in press.)

CHROMOSOMAL ANALYSIS

Chromosomal analyses are usually performed on peripheral blood (lymphocytes) or fibroblasts cultured from skin, gonads, chorionic villi (mesenchyme), or amniotic fluid cells. Very rapidly dividing cells (eg, bone marrow, chorionic villi, trophoblasts, fetal cord blood, newborn cord blood, or cancer cells) may sometimes be analyzed without culturing. Of relevance here is a rapid technique our group has developed, suitable for use in cord blood or percutaneous umbilical cord blood.[2]

If cultures are necessary, cells are grown in nutrient media to which fetal calf serum and perhaps antibiotics and other growth factors are added. A specified period of growth is required for a given tissue: overnight for bone marrow, cord blood, and chorionic villi trophoblasts; 48–72 hours for peripheral blood; 7–14 days for chorionic villi mesenchyme, or amniotic fluid cells. Preparation of cells for chromosomal analysis requires the sequential addition of (1) colchicine or desoxymethylcolchicine, (2) a hypotonic solution that causes cells to swell, (3) an acetic acid–methanol fixative, and (4) a dye to enhance chromosome visibility. Metaphases are photographed, photographic prints are developed, and individual chromosomes are cut out and realigned. Published karyotypes usually portray realigned chromosomes, not the original metaphase. Analysis generally requires counting 20–25 cells and karyotyping perhaps two to five. Not all cells will be intact. Some will have been damaged ("broken") in preparation and will have hypodiploid counts. This technical point is clinically relevant, for approximately 2% of chorionic villi or amniotic fluid specimens contain one or more spurious cells.

Sometimes two or more cell lines exist in a single individual, a phenomenon called mosaicism. Since mosaicism arises during embryogenesis, not all tissues show the same complements. Of additional relevance to the obstetrician is that the complements in chorionic villus trophoblasts may differ from those not only of cultured chorionic villus mesenchyme but also of the embryo. The frequency and management of this phenomenon is discussed by Ledbetter and colleagues.[3]

Routine cytogenetic analysis usually reveals about 450–500 bands per haploid set of chromosomes. Using high-resolution chromosome analysis, it is often possi-

TABLE 29–1. BANDING TECHNIQUES COMMONLY USED IN HUMAN CYTOGENETICS

NAME	TECHNIQUE	PATTERN
Q-banding	Staining with fluorescent dyes (eg, quinacrine dihydrocholoride); analysis by fluorescent microscopy	Positive bands fluorescent; negative bands nonfluorescent
G-banding	Pretreatment by buffers and salt solutions of specific pH at high temperature (eg, 60°C) proteolytic enzymes or other method	Positive bands darkly staining; negative bands lightly staining; pattern corresponds closely to that of Q-bands
R-banding	Pretreatment by high temperature and controlled pH; staining with Giemsa. Fluorescent methods may also produce R-bands	Positive bands darkly staining; negative bands lightly staining; pattern usually the reverse of that seen with Q- and G-bands
C-banding	Pretreatment by bases, acids, or other method; followed by staining with Giemsa	Positive bands darkly staining; negative bands lightly staining. Positive bands usually present only at centrometric regions and Yq.

Modified from Simpson JL, Golbus MS. Genetics. In: Obstetrics and gynecology. 2nd ed. Philadelphia: WB Saunders, in press.

ble to obtain resolution of about 1000 bands. At this level each band will consist of approximately 3000–4000 kilobases (kb) of DNA, capable of translating 30–40 genes. Predictably, small deletions, duplications, and other rearrangements can pass undetected even with high-resolution chromosome analysis. Application of various molecular techniques to cytogenetics is necessary to detect yet more minute abnormalities.

Identifying small cytogenetic abnormalities can be facilitated by in situ hybridization. In this molecular approach, an appropriate genetic probe is hybridized directly on a chromosome preparation under controlled conditions. A probe is a DNA fragment, usually labeled (eg, biotin). The single-stranded DNA fragment will hybridize with its complementary DNA sequence, the biotin label enabling one to verify the hybridization. The region of the chromosome to which a DNA probe hybridizes indicates the location of a specific gene on that chromosome. For example, immunoglobulin genes

TABLE 29–2. REPRESENTATIVE CHROMOSOMAL COMPLEMENTS WRITTEN ACCORDING TO THE RECOMMENDATIONS OF THE PARIS CONFERENCE (1971) AND SUPPLEMENT (1975)*

OFFICIAL DESIGNATION	DESCRIPTION
46,XY	Normal male karyotype
46,XX	Normal female karyotype
45,X	Monosomy X
47,XXX	Polysomy X
47,XY,+21	Trisomy 21
46,XX,lq+	Increase in length of the long arm of No. 1
46,X,del(X)(p21) or 46,X,del(X)(qter→p21:)	Terminal deletion of the short arm of X distal to band 21
46,X,i(Xq) or 46,X,i(X)(qter→qter)	Isochromosome of the long arm of X
46,X,r(Y)	Ring Y chromosome
46,X,t(X;3)(q21;q31)	Balanced translocation between band 21 of the long arm of X and band 31 of the long arm of No. 3
45,X/46,XX or mos 45,X/46,XX	45,X/46,XX mosaicism

* The shortened system is illustrated for each complement; the detailed system is also illustrated for deletions and isochromosomes. Simpson JL, Martin AO. Cytogenetic nomenclature. Am J Obstet Gynecol 1977;128:167.

TABLE 29–3. SOME SYMBOLS RECOMMENDED BY THE PARIS CONFERENCE (1971) AND SUPPLEMENT (1975)

Centromeres	cen
Short arm	p
Long arm	q
Isochromosome	i
Deletion	del
Translocation	t
Reciprocal translocation	rcp
Mosaicism	mos
Chimerism	chi
Ring	r
Dicentric	dic
Duplication	dup
Inversion	inv
Break without reunion (eg, terminal deletion)	:
Break and join	::
From. . . to. . .	→

Simpson JL, Martin AO. Cytogenetic nomenclature. Am J Obstet Gynecol 1977;128:167.

are known to be clustered on chromosome 14 (band 14q32.3→qter). In situ hybridization using DNA probes for immunoglobulin genes could be performed. If hybridization occurs to a chromosome other than No. 14, existence of a translocation from 14q would be identified. This technique is applicable not only to metaphases but also to interphase nuclei, where the presence and number of a given chromosome can be determined (Fig. 29-4).

NUMERICAL CHROMOSOMAL ABNORMALITIES

Definitions and Cytologic Origin

If a haploid gamete or diploid cell lacks the expected number of chromosomes (n or $2n$), *aneuploidy* exists. If an additional chromosome is present ($2n + 1$), *trisomy* exists. The term *polysomy* is sometimes applied if the additional chromosome is a sex chromosome (eg, 47,XXY).

Trisomy may arise from several mechanisms, but in humans it usually arises de novo following meiotic or mitotic nondisjunction. Nondisjunction may originate following failure of homologous chromosomes to disjoin in meiosis I or failure of sister chromatids to disjoin in either meiosis II or mitosis. In humans maternal meiosis I is most common.[4] Nondisjunction during meiosis produces aneuploid gametes, with the resulting zygote having the identical chromosomal constitution in all cells. By contrast, nondisjunction during mitosis produces two or more cell lines (mosaicism). A rare mechanism for trisomy involves normal meiotic segregation in a trisomic parent (secondary trisomy).

Monosomy ($2n - 1$) arises by mechanisms similar to those that result in trisomy. Indeed, meiotic nondisjunction leading to a disomic gamete also produces a complementary gamete lacking that chromosome. In addition, monosomy may result from a chromosome merely lagging behind and failing to pass to daughter cells (*anaphase lag*).

In *polyploidy* more than two haploid sets of chromosomes exist. Polyploidy is detected frequently among human abortuses but rarely among neonates. The most common form of polyploidy is triploidy ($3n = 69$), which may be characterized by either two maternal or two paternal haploid complements. In humans, dispermy is the most common mechanism for polyploidy. Triploidy accounts for 25% of chromosomally abnormal abortuses, or about 10% to 15% of all first-trimester abortuses.

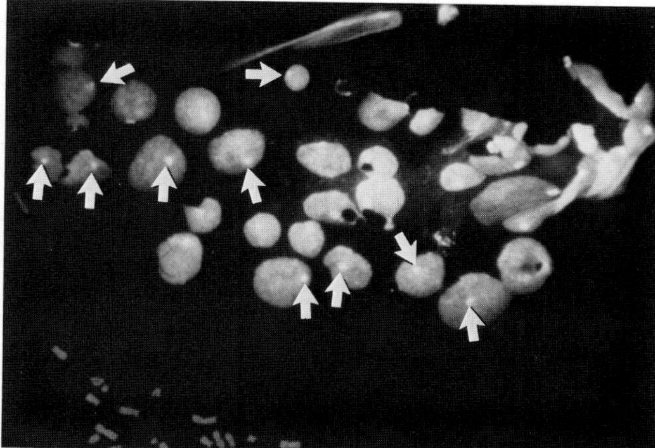

FIGURE 29–4. In situ hybridization. A Y-specific probe hybridizes to male cells.

Causes

Although trisomies are presumed to result from nondisjunction, the actual cause of nondisjunction is unknown. It is well known that various trisomies increase with increasing maternal age (Table 29-4). However, the biological basis of this epidemiologic observation is unknown. The leading possibility is that the phenomenon merely reflects intrinsic ovarian aging. Indeed,

TABLE 29–4. CHROMOSOME ABNORMALITIES IN LIVEBORNS

MATERNAL AGE	RISK OF DOWN SYNDROME	TOTAL RISK FOR CHROMOSOME ABNORMALITIES*
20	1/1667	1/526*
21	1/1667	1/526*
22	1/1429	1/500*
23	1/1429	1/500*
24	1/1250	1/476*
25	1/1250	1/476*
26	1/1176	1/476*
27	1/1111	1/455*
28	1/1053	1/435*
29	1/1000	1/384*
30	1/952	1/385*
31	1/909	1/322*
32	1/769	1/317*
33	1/625	1/260
34	1/500	1/204
35	1/385	1/164
36	1/294	1/130
37	1/227	1/103
38	1/175	1/82
39	1/137	1/65
40	1/106	1/51
41	1/82	1/40
42	1/64	1/32
43	1/50	1/25
44	1/38	1/20
45	1/30	1/15
46	1/23	1/12
47	1/18	1/10
48	1/14	1/7
49	1/11	

Data from Hook EB. Rates of chromosome abnormalities at different maternal ages. Obstet Gynecol 1981;58:282. Because sample size for some intervals is relatively small, confidence limits are sometimes relatively large. Nonetheless, these figures are suitable for genetic counseling.

* 47,XXX excluded for ages 20–32 (data not available).

older mice show fewer ovarian chiasmata than younger mice, and decreased chiasmata predispose to nondisjunction.[5] It is also possible that ova initially selected for ovulation are more likely to be normal than those remaining in older women (production-line hypothesis). On the other hand, increased risk for aneuploidy with age could merely reflect accumulation of exogenous factors. One possibility that seems unlikely is that the mother is unable to reject trisomic fetuses (relaxed selection).[6]

It is relevant to the clinician that few specific factors are known to increase the risk for aneuploidy to such an extent that prenatal diagnosis would be offered to a woman who otherwise would not be a candidate.

A genetic predisposition toward aneuploidy probably exists, although the mechanism of gene(s) action is unknown. After one liveborn aneuploid child, the likelihood of a second trisomic offspring is increased. The same chromosome is not necessarily involved in successive pregnancies (ie, trisomy 21 might occur in one pregnancy and trisomy 13 in the next). Data involving repetitive abortuses support the existence of a genetic predisposition. If the first abortus is trisomic, the second is also likely (70%) to be trisomic.[7,8] If the first is chromosomally normal, the second is likewise (80%). Whether a trisomic abortus confers an increased risk for having a liveborn trisomic child is actually unknown, and there is indeed controversy on the topic of recurrent aneuploidy.[8] Nonetheless, it would seem prudent to offer antenatal cytogenetic studies to couples having either trisomic abortuses or liveborns, regardless of age.

Advanced *paternal* age does not predispose to aneuploidy.[9]

Transmission of Chromosomal Abnormalities

Trisomies. Autosomal trisomy usually leads either to lethality or to such severe anomalies that trisomic women are rarely pregnant. In fact, 47,XXY Klinefelter syndrome is associated with sterility. However, 47,XXX and 47,XYY individuals are usually fertile, and 47,XX,+21 women may become pregnant. Moreover, gonadal mosaicism may exist in phenotypically normal individuals whose germ cells are trisomic. In fact, parental germinal mosaicism is frequently offered as an explanation for recurrent aneuploid offspring.

Although direct human or even mammalian data are limited, one principle derived from plant studies is worth summarizing. Fewer than expected (50%) $2n + 1$ progeny are recovered, especially among liveborns from $2n + 1$ parents. Small chromosomes (eg, No. 21) are especially likely to be eliminated, presumably because their short length minimizes the opportunity for chiasmata formation.

Only about one third of the liveborn offspring of women with trisomy 21 had trisomy 21, and other chromosomal abnormalities are rare.[10] Likewise, it is uncommon for 47,XYY men and 47,XXX women to produce aneuploid offspring. Despite these reassuring facts, antenatal cytogenetic studies should at least be discussed with such couples.

Monosomy. Transmission of monosomies is not of great clinical relevance. (See the chapter by Simpson and Tharapel[11] for theoretical considerations.)

STRUCTURAL CHROMOSOMAL ABNORMALITIES

Definitions and Cytologic Origin

Minor structural variation (*polymorphism*) exists among human chromosomes without apparent phenotypic consequences. Examples include prominent satellites on acrocentric chromosomes and variation in length of the Y long arm. Such "variants" are transmitted in dominant fashion.

On the other hand, major structural alterations clearly cause phenotypic abnormalities. One can assume that many genes are duplicated or deficient. Phenotypic abnormalities might also result if the position of a gene with respect to its neighbors is altered (*position effect*). Several different types of chromosomal abnormalities are of clinical relevance.

First, chromosomal deletion involves loss of one portion of one chromosome, either terminal or interstitial. Deficiencies usually result from breakage and loss of an acentric fragment. Deficiencies may also arise following crossing over within a pericentric inversion loop, as will be discussed later. Autosomal deficiency usually leads to embryonic death or malformation, but deficiency in a sex chromosome is not necessarily as damaging.

If, following chromosome breakage, material is exchanged between two or more chromosomes, a *translocation* is said to have occurred (Fig. 29-5). Rearrangement of genes need not necessarily be deleterious, provided genes are neither lost nor gained. If the individual is phenotypically normal, it is assumed that no genetic material is lost. Such a translocation is said to be balanced. If a translocation has led to deficiency or excess of genetic material, the rearrangement is said to be unbalanced. Even if it is not evident on banding analysis, this can be assumed if the individual is phenotypically abnormal. If offspring show the same translocation as a normal parent, it can be assumed that the translocation is balanced. However, deductive reasoning is hazardous when a de novo balanced translocation is detected in villi or amniotic fluid cells, even if ostensibly balanced. A subtle rearrangement may be unappreciated, accounting for the concomitant 10% to 15% risks of phenotypic abnormalities.

Translocations may be either reciprocal or Robertsonian. In *reciprocal* translocations, breaks and rearrangement occur in two or more chromosomes but do not involve centromeres (see Fig. 29-5). Heterozygotes thus have 46 chromosomes, albeit one or more pair will differ in morphology and composition from one another. In *Robertsonian* translocations, acrocentric chromosomes (Nos. 13, 14, 15, 21, 22) fuse at their centromere. Since no single acrocentric short arm is essential, heterozygotes are phenotypically normal. They have, of course, 45 chromosomes (centromeres).

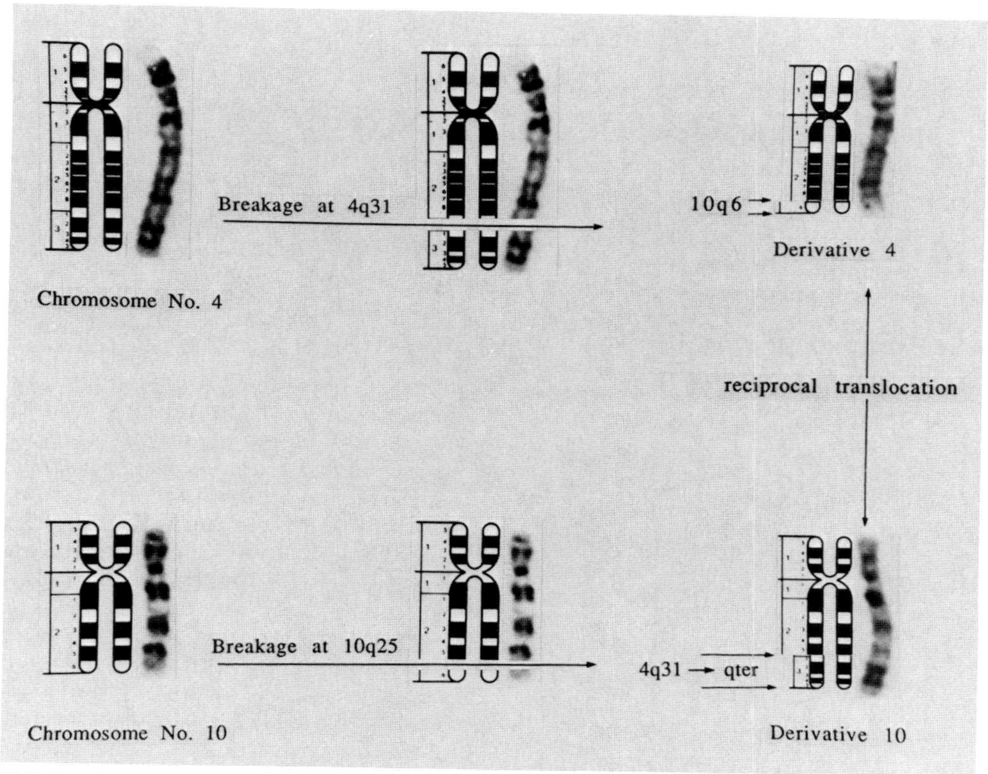

FIGURE 29–5. A reciprocal translocation between chromosomes 4 and 10. Origin of derivative chromosomes is shown. (From Simpson JL, Tharapel AT. Principles of cytogenetics. In: Philipp E, Barnes J, eds. Scientific foundations of obstetrics and gynaecology. 4th ed. London: Heinemann, in press.)

An *inversion* (Fig. 29-6) is an intrachromosomal rearrangement in which the sequence of genes in the inverted segment is reversed. Such a rearrangement is usually caused by two chromosomal breaks, followed by reversal and reinsertion of the chromosomal segment produced by the breaks. There are two types of inversions, those in which the region includes the centromere (*pericentric*) and those in which it does not (*paracentric*). Heterozygotes for either type may be normal if genes are neither lost, gained, nor altered as a result of the breaks leading to the inversion.

Isochromosomes are chromosomes with identical arms. They arise if the centromere divides in horizontal rather than longitudinal fashion (Fig. 29-7). One product is acentric and thus is lost at the next cell division. The other product is telocentric, capable of replicating itself at the next S period to form a metacentric chromosome. The isochromosome thus formed consists of complete duplication of one arm and complete deficiency of the other arm. Isochromosome for the X long arm [i(Xq)] is the most common structural abnormality associated with gonadal dysgenesis.[12]

A *dicentric* chromosome has two centromeres. Its formation most often begins with an isochromatid break in G2 (Fig. 29-8). Regardless of how a dicentric chromosome arises, the presence of two centromeres (dicentric) confers mitotic instability because the centromeres may migrate to opposite poles during telophase. The dicentric stretches until breaking, followed by either loss of chromosomal material or secondary rearrangements (breakage–fusion–bridge cycle).

A *ring chromosome* arises following a break in both the long arm and the short arms (Fig. 29-9). Chromosomal regions contiguous with the centromeres fuse; telomeric regions of each arm are acentric, lost, and thus deficient. Like decentrics, ring chromosomes are inherently unstable.

Duplications may originate by several mechanisms. Often duplications for certain loci are accompanied by deficiencies for other loci. This is the usual situation when duplication arises following meiotic segregation in a parent having a chromosomal translocation. However, duplications not associated with concomitant deficiencies exist.

Causes

Structural chromosomal abnormalities usually originate following chromosomal breakage. Breakage is caused by irradiation, chemicals, or viruses, or it may arise spontaneously.

Agents that break chromosomes are termed *clastogens*. In vitro studies have identified many agents as clastogens. Whether in vivo exposure to agents that are

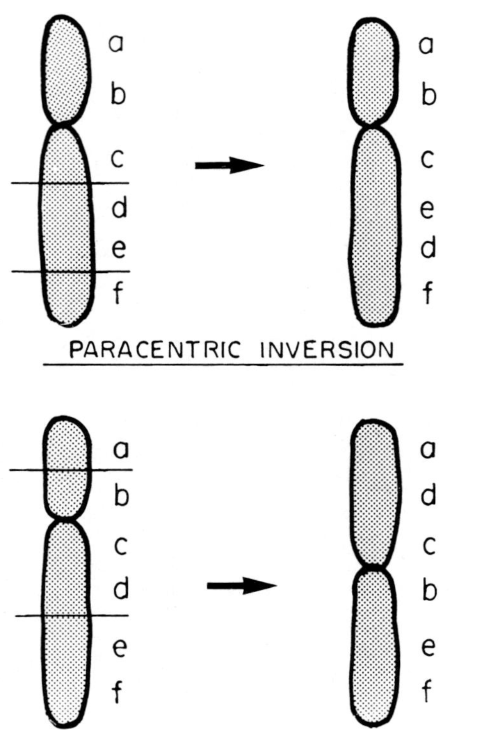

FIGURE 29–6. Origin of paracentric (top) and pericentric (bottom) inversions. (From Simpson JL. Disorders of sexual differentiation: Etiology and clinical delineation. New York: Academic Press, 1976:250.)

clastogens in vitro confers increased risks for abnormal liveborn or even abortuses is unknown. In fact, couples can usually be reassured concerning the consequences of exposure to clastogens.

Transmission of Structural Abnormalities

Chromosomal Variants. Chromosomal variants segregate in autosomal dominant fashion, recoverable in approximately 50% of offspring of individuals having a given variant.

Deletions and Duplications. Deletions or duplications affecting large chromosomal regions produce such severe phenotypic abnormalities that affected individuals rarely reproduce. Reproduction by individuals with isolated deletions or duplications should theoretically yield 50% gametes with the parental abnormality. Analogous to other chromosomal abnormalities, however, the empiric likelihood of transmission should be far less.

Dicentric and Ring Chromosomes. Dicentric and ring chromosomes are mitotically unstable, as already noted. Although in theory offspring of parents with dicentric or ring chromosomes may inherit the same dicentric or ring as their parent, it is more likely that they will inherit a secondarily rearranged chromosome or show no derivative chromosome (being monosomic because the chromosome became broken and was lost). No empiric data are available.

Robertsonian Translocations. Robertsonian translocations involve members of group D (Nos. 13–15) and group G (Nos. 21–22). The most important single translocations involve chromosomes Nos. 14 and 21 (Fig. 29-10). Of individuals with Down syndrome, 2% to 3% are affected as a result of this translocation. In theory, one third of viable offspring of translocation heterozygotes should have Down syndrome. However, empiric data show that only 10% to 14% of viable offspring of female heterozygotes and only 2% to 4% of viable offspring of male heterozygotes have Down syndrome.[13,14] Liveborn normal offspring have equal likelihood of showing either translocation heterozygosity ($2n = 45$) like their parents, or normal chromosomal complements ($2n = 46$).

If a Robertsonian translocation involves homologous chromosomes, the prognosis is bleak. Translocations involving both Nos. 13[t(13;13)] or both Nos. 21[t(21;21)] yield only abnormal liveborns or abortions (trisomy 13

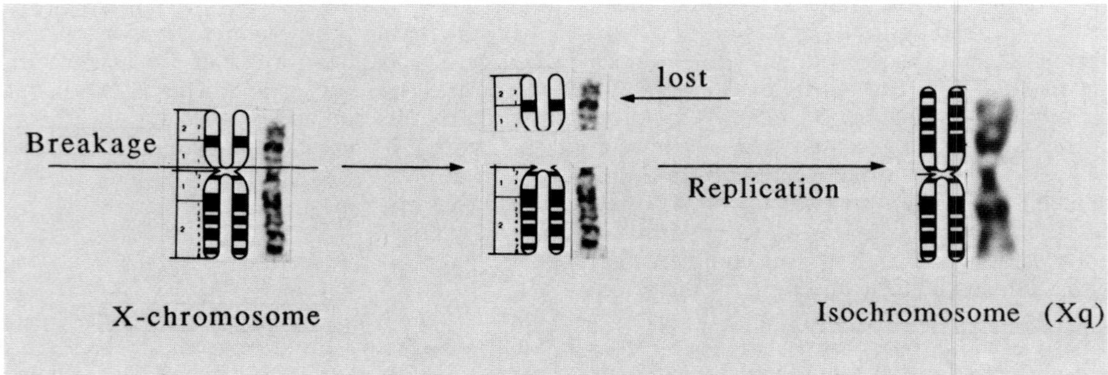

FIGURE 29–7. Origin of an isochromosome from Xq. (From Simpson JL, Tharapel AT. Principles of cytogenetics. In: Philipp E, Barnes J, eds. Scientific foundations of obstetrics and gynaecology. 4th ed. London: Heinemann, in press.)

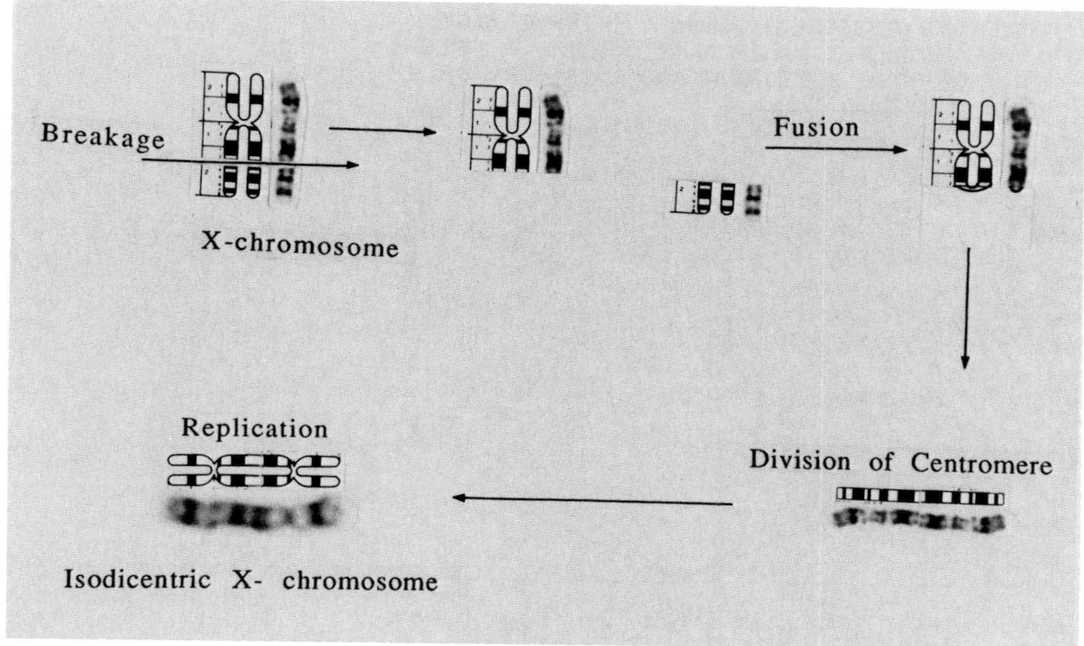

FIGURE 29–8. Origin of a dicentric chromosome. A dicentric can also arise following crossing-over within a paracentric loop. (From Simpson JL, Tharapel AT. Principles of cytogenetics. In: Philipp E, Barnes J, eds. Scientific foundations of obstetrics and gynaecology. 4th ed. London: Heinemann, in press.

or trisomy 21); all other conceptions would terminate in spontaneous abortions. Homologous translocations for Nos. 14, 15, and 22 virtually all result in abortions, liveborns with these trisomies being very rare. Females with homologous translocations should be informed about sterilization or embryo transfer techniques. Artificial insemination can be offered for male heterozygotes.

In t(21;22), female and male heterozygotes appear on the basis of antenatal cytogenetic surveillance to be at relatively high (10% to 15%) risk for Down syndrome offspring.[13,14] Abnormal liveborn infants are uncommon in most other Robertsonian translocations. In t(13;14), less than 1% of offspring have trisomy 13. These empiric findings are not surprising because trisomies 14 and 15 are lethal, rarely resulting in liveborns. Nonetheless, individuals with any Robertsonian translocation should be counseled concerning antenatal chromosomal studies.

Reciprocal Translocations. Many different reciprocal translocations exist. Ideally, for each translocation empiric data should be available; however, at present only data for general categories exist. In addition, counseling requires attention to the mode of ascertainment.

A reciprocal translocation may be ascertained through a balanced (normal) proband—incidentally during the course of a survey, or through a couple with repeated abortions, or through term unbalanced progeny. The risk of having a liveborn child with chromosomal duplication or deficiency is higher in the latter situation than in the former two.[14,15] The lower risk in the former probably reflects selection against unbalanced segregants. Overall, antenatal amniocentesis surveillance involving couples in

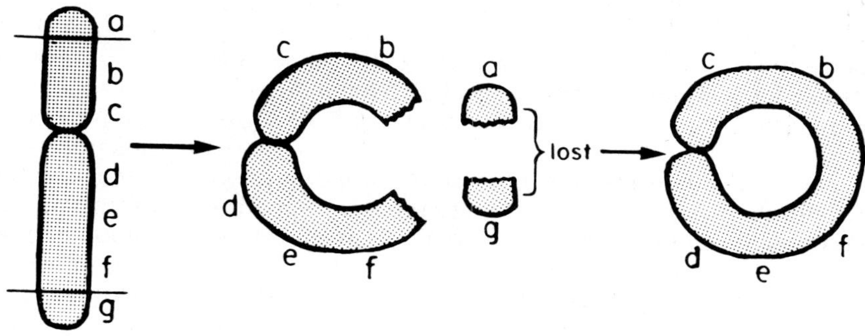

FIGURE 29–9. Origin of a ring chromosome. (From Simpson JL. Disorders of sexual differentiation: Etiology and clinical delineation. New York: Academic Press, 1976:22.)

RESULTS OF SEGREGATION IN A HETEROZYGOTE FOR A ROBERTSONIAN TRANSLOCATION BETWEEN CHROMOSOME NUMBERS 14 AND 21 (A FORM OF D/G TRANSLOCATION)

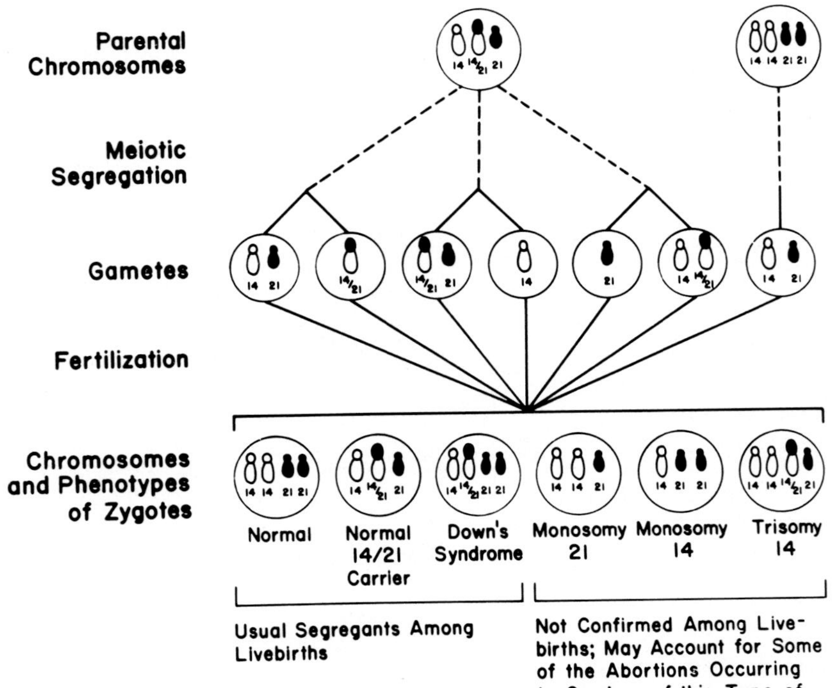

FIGURE 29–10. Diagram of possible gametes and progeny of a phenotypically normal individual heterozygous for a translocation between chromosomes 14 and 21. Three of the six possible gametes are incompatible with life. The likelihood that an individual with such a translocation would have a child with Down syndrome is thus 33%. However, the empirical risk is considerably less. (Simpson JL, Gerbie AT. Antenatal detection of genetic disorders. Postgrad Med 1976;59:133.)

which either male or female showed a reciprocal translocation suggests that their risk of unbalanced fetuses is about 10%.[13,14] These risks are substantial, but they are still less than the theoretical risks, which, assuming random segregation and no crossing over, could be as high as 50% to 60% (proportion of unbalanced gametes). If ascertained through a full-term unbalanced neonate, Daniel and colleagues calculate risks in unbalanced amniotic fluid specimens to be 19.3% and 23.8% for female and male carriers.[14] If ascertained through a couple with repetitive abortions, risks are 3.5% and 1.5%. If ascertained incidentally, risks are 5.1% and 3.8%. Liveborn offspring who are phenotypically normal are equally likely to inherit either normal chromosomes (46,XY or 46,XX) or the same two balanced translocation chromosomes as present in the carrier parent. Although most reciprocal translocations carry an empiric risk of only about 10%, the risk is higher for complex rearrangements involving more than two chromosomes[14] and for situations in which 3:1 segregation occurs.

An unresolved question of obstetric importance is whether a translocation ascertained through repetitive abortions confers a risk for abnormal liveborns as high as that conferred by ascertainment through an abnormal liveborn. Risks appear lower.[14] The question will arise frequently because about 2% to 3% of couples experiencing repetitive abortions will show a translocation.[16]

Pericentric Inversions. Abnormal reproductive outcome among offspring of individuals with either pericentric or paracentric inversions is actually the result of normal meiotic phenomena. Recall that genes seek to pair with their alleles on homologous chromosomes, not only to exchange genetic information but also to facilitate orderly disjunction. Whenever pairing occurs, genetic exchanges (crossing over) may also occur. For inversions to achieve pairing, a loop is commonly formed (Fig. 29-11). Crossing over may or may not occur within an inversion loop, but it is likely to do so if the loop encompasses a large portion of the chromosome. A single crossover anywhere within a pericentric loop leads to four types of gametes. Two of the four have the parental sequences: one normal, one inverted; the other two gametes are characterized by combinations of genes not present in either parent (recombinants; see Fig. 29-11). The crossover results in the ends of the chromatids being duplicated for those genes distal to one breakpoint.

It is the chromosomal region *outside* the inverted segment that is duplicated or deficient in unbalanced gametes. As result, the *smaller* the inversion, the *greater*

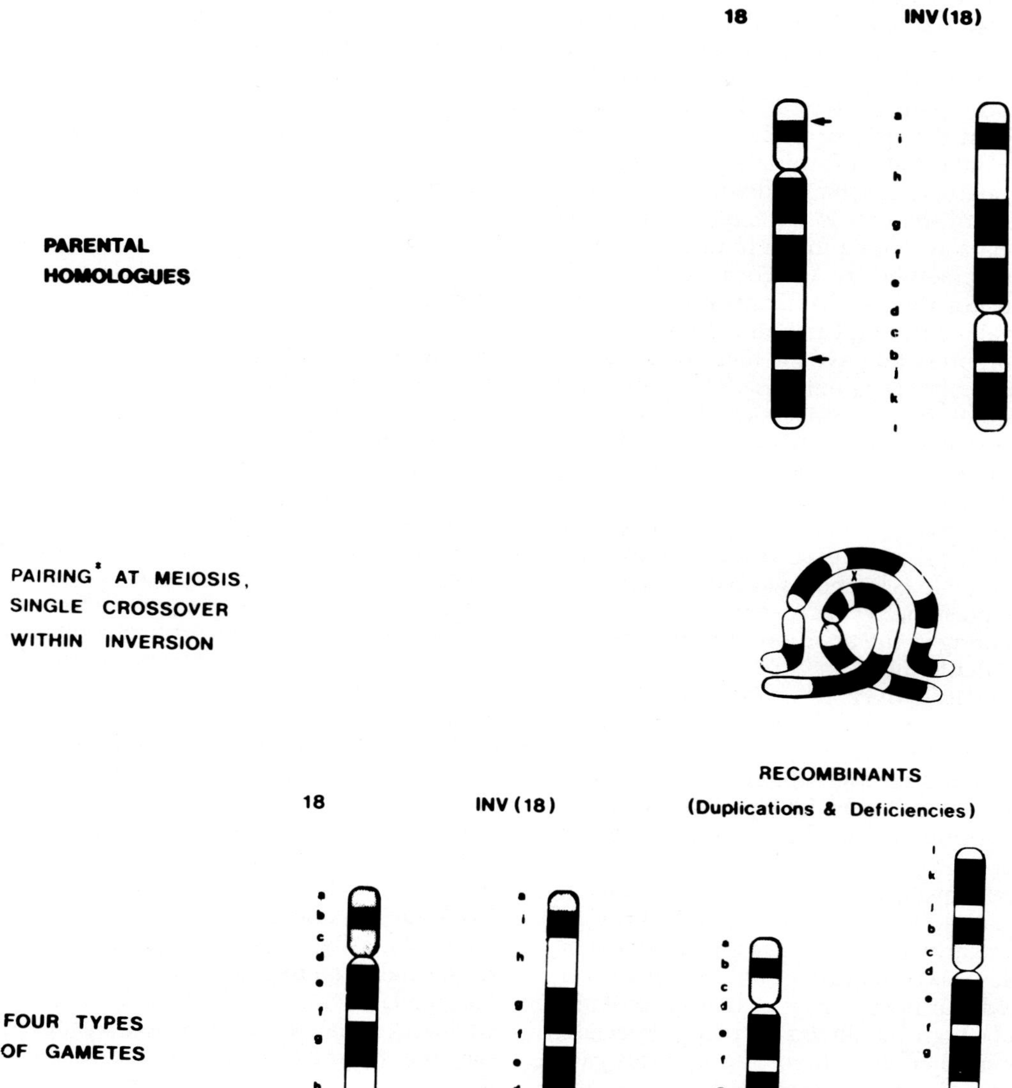

FIGURE 29-11. The effects of a single crossover within a pericentric inversion loop. Other mechanisms of crossing over need not involve formation of a loop. (Martin AO, Simpson JL, Deddish R, et al. Clinical implications of chromosomal inversions: a pericentric inversion in No. 18 segregating in a family ascertained through an abnormal proband. Am J Perinatal 1983;1:84.)

the genetic imbalance in recombinant gametes and the more severe the expected phenotype effect. That is, crossing over in inversions encompassing only a small portion of the total chromosomal length leads to large duplications and deficiencies. In fact, such imbalances are usually so great that lethality results. Inversions of intermediate length, namely, those involving 30% to 60% of total chromosomal length, most often lead to duplications and deficiencies compatible with survival.

Counseling about the risks of pericentric inversions requires empiric data, but unfortunately only limited data exist.[17,18] Nonetheless, some guidelines may be derived on the basis of theoretical principles and on the basis of clinical data accumulating in humans. As with translocations, the method by which an inversion is ascertained indicates the risk to offspring. Pericentric inversions ascertained through an anomalous (presumably recombinant) proband have the highest likelihood of recurrence of an abnormal outcome.[14,15] Pooled empiric data indicate that an inversion heterozygote usually carries approximately 8% to 15% risk for an abnormal liveborn,[14] probably higher if the female is the carrier.[17] Antenatal cytogenetic studies clearly should be offered. Inversions ascertained among couples having repetitive spontaneous abortions may carry lower risks for anomalous liveborns or second-trimester fetuses.[14] This is presumably because recombinants are often lethal, resulting in the abortions that brought the patient to medical attention.

Similarly, pericentric inversions ascertained through phenotypically normal probands (eg, surveys) also appear much less likely to lead to abnormal liveborns[15,18] than those ascertained through abnormal clinical consequences. Risks may not even be increased, although counseling concerning antenatal cytogenetic studies is still appropriate.

Analogous to translocations, de novo inversions ascertained in amniotic fluid pose special problems. Chromosomal integrity cannot be assumed, despite ostensible normalcy. Data indicating that de novo inversions ascertained during prenatal diagnosis probably carry a relatively high likelihood of being associated with an abnormal phenotype (two of nine cases gathered by Warburton[19]) are consistent with the existence of subtle rearrangements.

Paracentric Inversions. A single crossover within a *paracentric* inversion results in both dicentric and acentric chromatids. Both chromatids are characterized by duplications and deficiencies, albeit for different regions. Acentric fragments cannot persist in subsequent cell divisions because a centromere is required for orderly chromosomal disjunction. The fate of dicentric chromosomes varies, as we have already observed. However, production of acentric and dicentric gametes clearly can lead to reproductive problems. Very few liveborns with abnormalities occur, presumably again because recombinants are usually lethal. Nonetheless, it is not unreasonable to offer prenatal diagnosis for couples in which one parent has a paracentric inversion.

SINGLE-GENE ABNORMALITIES (MENDELIAN INHERITANCE)

In mendelian inheritance, a gene mutation usually involves only a single genetic locus. A chromosome carrying a single mutant gene but no other abnormality appears structurally normal because the change involves only a minute deletion or a change in a single nucleotide sequence. Analysis of a mutant gene is therefore not ordinarily facilitated by cytogenetic studies. Instead, one studies pedigrees, measures a gene product or its metabolite, or examines the DNA coding for the gene.

DEFINITIONS

Chromosomes exist in pairs, one maternally derived and one paternally derived. Chromosomes contain genes; thus, genes exist in pairs. More properly, it is alleles—different states of a single gene—that exist in pairs. Alleles occupy identical places on homologous chromosomes and can become interchanged during meiotic recombination.

If alleles are identical, *homozygosity* exists. If alleles are dissimilar, *heterozygosity* exists. An allele capable of expression in its heterozygous state is dominant, whereas an allele capable of expression only in homozygous form is recessive. The preceding definitions apply cleanly to autosomal loci. However, different circumstances exist for X-linked loci. A recessive trait whose allele is located on the X chromosome is expressed by all males (46,XY) carrying the recessive allele. Affected males are said to be *hemizygous.*

A related phenomenon particularly relevant to autosomal recessive inheritance is *compound heterozygosity.* In compound heterozygosity, two alleles are dissimilar, but both are abnormal. Compound heterozygosity is often clinically indistinguishable from homozygosity for a single mutant allele. Use of molecular techniques has made it clear that compound heterozygosity is a frequent explanation for genetic disorders. For example, many cystic fibrosis cases are compound heterozygotes. In addition to affected individuals homozygous for deletion of three nucleotides at position (ΔF508), other cystic fibrosis patients have one such mutant allele and one other dysfunctional allele at the same locus.[20,21]

TRANSMISSION OF MUTANT GENES IN FAMILIES

The familial patterns followed by mendelian traits depend not only on whether the mutant gene is dominant or recessive, but also on whether the gene is located on an autosome or a sex chromosome. There are five potential patterns of transmission: autosomal dominant, autosomal recessive, X-linked dominant, X-linked recessive, and Y-linked.

Autosomal Dominant Inheritance

An autosomal dominant allele is recognized by its ability to be expressed in more than one generation (Fig. 29-12). In autosomal dominant traits, equal numbers of males and females are usually affected. The likelihood is 50% that an individual carrying a mutant autosomal dominant gene (allele) will transmit that allele to any given offspring, male or female. If penetrance (see later for definition) is complete, no unaffected individual will have an affected offspring.

Autosomal dominant patterns are not always associated with the idealized characteristics defined earlier. Some individuals may be more severely affected than others, a phenomenon known as variable expression. Variable expression occurs not only among families but also among different affected members of a single family (intrafamilial variability). A single mutant gene may also be responsible for several ostensibly distinct phenotypic effects (*pleiotropy*). An autosomal dominant allele may exert its effect only on individuals of one sex (*sex limitation*). Another characteristic of autosomal dominant inheritance is that some individuals may be phenotypically normal yet carry a mutant autosomal dominant allele. Such a mutant allele is said to show lack of penetrance in the phenotypically normal individual. Actually, lack of penetrance probably reflects only our inability to study gene products or DNA directly. If molecular analysis were possible in all disorders, "nonpenetrant" individuals surely would show an abnormality in their DNA.

In the absence of ability to measure DNA or its gene products, an autosomal dominant allele in humans must be recognized clinically. Usually one of the following clinical characteristics must exist for dominant inheritance to be recognized:

1. Lack of interference with reproductive ability (eg, polydactyly)
2. Manifestation only after reproduction is completed (eg, Huntington's chorea)
3. Characterization by lack of penetrance or variable expressivity (ie, a minimally affected parent might have severely affected progeny).

The more severe the trait, the more likely it is that an affected individual has a new mutation. Relatively few cases of polydactyly represent new mutations, but 90% of achondroplasia does. All individuals with a dominant trait conferring sterility must represent a new mutation.

Autosomal Recessive Inheritance

An autosomal recessive trait is expressed only when an individual is homozygous for the mutant allele. At a given genetic locus both alleles show an identical mutation. As noted, different but equally dysfunctional alleles could also exist (compound heterozygosity). An individual with a recessive trait is usually the product of a mating between parents who are both heterozygous (carriers) for the same mutation (Table 29-5). If two heterozygotes mate, the likelihood is 25% that a given offspring will be affected (see Fig. 29-12). If multiple affected siblings of both sexes exist, autosomal recessive inheritance definitely should be considered. Consanguineous parents are more likely to carry an identical allele (mutant or normal) than nonconsanguineous parents. Thus, an individual with a recessive trait is relatively more likely to arise from a consanguineous than from a nonconsanguineous union. The rarer a trait, the higher the proportion of affected individuals who arise from consanguineous unions. For common

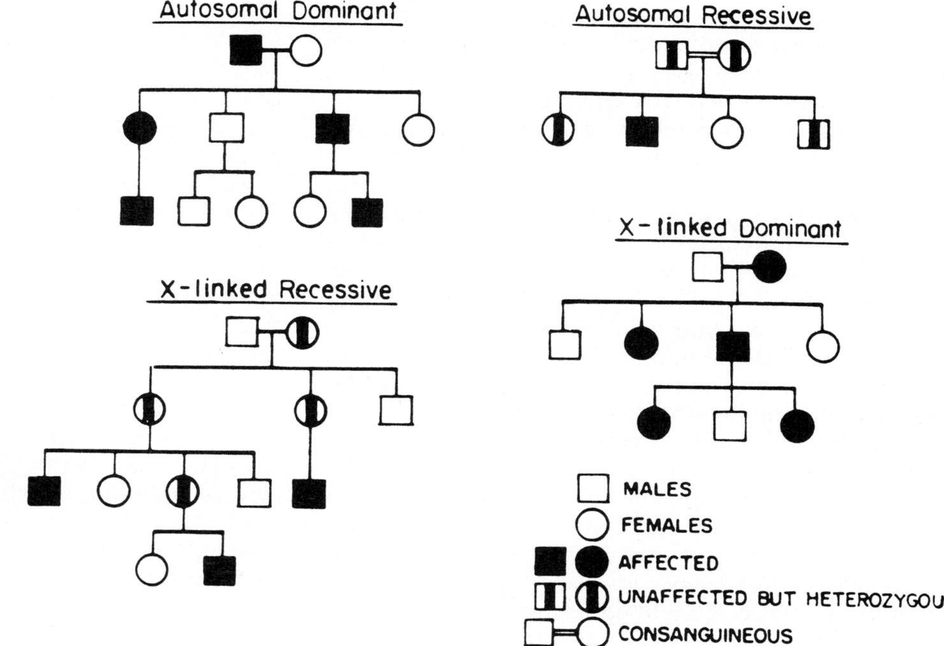

FIGURE 29–12. Idealized pedigree of common modes of Mendelian inheritance. (Simpson JL. Disorders of sexual differentiation: Etiology and clinical delineation. New York: Academic Press, 1976:34.)

TABLE 29-5. AUTOSOMAL RECESSIVE INHERITANCE GAMETES

PARENTAL	D	d
D	DD	Dd
d	dD	dd

Progeny expected of a mating between two individuals heterozygous for the same mutant recessive allele (d). D represents the normal allele. The probability is 0.25 that a given offspring will inherit both mutant alleles (dd) and be affected. The probability is 0.50 that a given offspring will be heterozygous (Dd). If geneotype dd can be excluded, the likelihood of heterozygosity can be calculated as 0.67.

traits (cystic fibrosis, sickle cell anemia), parents of affected offspring will usually not be consanguineous.

Autosomal recessive inheritance also occurs if a homozygous individual mates with a heterozygous individual. Half (50%) the offspring would be affected (pseudoautosomal dominant inheritance). This phenomenon is becoming more frequent for serious traits, as survival to reproduction is becoming less unusual for serious autosomal recessive traits (eg, cystic fibrosis, sickle cell anemia).

The relationship between the frequencies of homozygotes and heterozygotes is clinically important. This relationship is expressed by the Hardy-Weinberg equilibrium. Suppose the normal allele is A and the mutant allele is a. The normal allele A is said to have the frequency p, and the mutant allele is said to have the frequency q. Since the frequencies of alleles at a given locus add up to 1, $p + q = 1$. After squaring both sides of the equation, $p^2 + 2pq + q^2 = 1$. In this binomial expansion, p^2 becomes the frequency of individuals homozygous for allele $A(AA)$; q^2 is the frequency of individuals homozygous for allele $a(aa)$; $2pq$ is the frequency of the heterozygote (Aa). The frequency of a mutant allele (q) is usually much less than the frequency of a normal allele (p). If q is much less than 0.5, q^2 is very much less than $2pq$ because p is nearly equal to 1.

Consideration of the relative magnitudes of $2pq$ and q^2 makes it obvious that the "load" for deleterious recessive traits is carried mostly by heterozygotes; relatively few homozygotes exist. To illustrate, suppose the incidence of a trait (q^2) is 1/10,000. Thus, $q = 1/100$; $p = 99/100$, or almost 1; $2pq = 2 \times 1 \times 1/100 = 1/50$, much more frequent than 1/10,000 (q^2). This mathematical exercise becomes clinically relevant when addressing proposals for eliminating mutant alleles from the population by selecting against homozygous fetuses. Eliminating heterozygous individuals might also be theoretically unwise, because heterozygotes may possess an advantage over homozygously normal individuals that was responsible for maintaining the mutant allele in the population. In fact, "normal" individuals may be heterozygous for at least five to six deleterious recessive genes.

Clinically unaffected individuals who have a sibling with an autosomal recessive disorder often inquire about risks of their own offspring having that disorder. Assuming that they and their mate are not related, the risk of having affected offspring can be shown to be very low if the recessive disorder is rare. If heterozygote detection tests are not available, the a priori likelihood that the unaffected individual is a heterozygote can still be calculated. The unaffected individual who inquires about his or her offspring is known clinically not to be homozygously abnormal (affected). Of course, one hopes that a test to detect heterozygosity is available, as is increasingly the case with molecular techniques. If not, one is left with three equally likely genotypes: two connote heterozygosity and one connotes homozygosity for the normal allele (see Table 29-5). The likelihood of heterozygosity is thus 2/3. The likelihood of the individual's mate being heterozygous for the same mutant gene will reflect gene frequency in the general population, as discussed earlier (Hardy-Weinberg equilibrium). For example, a trait whose incidence is 1/8100 births shows a heterozygote frequency of only 1/45 ($q^2 = 1/8100$; $q = 1/90$; $2pq = 1/45$). The likelihood that any given offspring will be affected is thus $2/3 \times 1/45 \times 1/4 = 2/540 = 1/270$. Rarer traits naturally confer correspondingly lower likelihoods. Risks for other family members can be calculated on the basis of assuming that a heterozygous individual has equal likelihood of either transmitting or not transmitting a mutant gene. Thus, a normal individual whose uncle was affected would have a likelihood of only 1/3 of being heterozygous (ie, $2/3 \times 1/2 = 2/6 = 1/3$).

X-Linked Recessive Inheritance

A mutant recessive gene located on the X chromosome is expressed by all males (46,XY) who carry it. Such individuals are said to be hemizygous. X-linked recessive alleles are usually transmitted through phenotypically normal yet actually heterozygous females (see Fig. 29-12). In a family in which an X-linked recessive mutant is segregating, affected individuals might include male siblings, maternal uncles, maternal nephews, maternal male first cousins, and certain other maternal male relatives.

The probability is 0.5 that a heterozygous female will transmit an X-linked recessive allele to any given offspring. Males inheriting the allele will be affected, whereas females inheriting the allele will be heterozygous like their mother. An affected male transmits the allele to all his daughters but to none of his sons. Male-to-male transmission thus excludes X-linked inheritance. All offspring of an affected male will be phenotypically normal, unless his wife is heterozygous for the same mutant. In such a case, four genotypes are possible, and females may be affected. This is unlikely for severe traits (eg, Duchenne muscular dystrophy) but quite possible for mild traits (color blindness) or successfully treatable traits (hemophilia).

Phenotypic females can occasionally be affected with X-linked recessive traits; 46,XX individuals can be affected if homozygous, a circumstance that could result if their mother were heterozygous and their father hemizygous. Occasionally, vicissitudes of X inactivation (preferential inactivation of normal X) can be so extreme that phenotypic effects approximating those present in hemizygous males exist. Alternatively, females with only one X chromosome (45,X) may manifest X-linked recessive traits.

The pedigree relationships portrayed earlier have not taken into account the possibility of new mutations. Actually, one cannot necessarily assume that the mother of a child with an X-linked recessive mutation is heterozygous. The child may represent a new mutation arising in the ovum. If the trait is lethal with respect to fertility and if no other relatives are affected, the likelihood of a new mutation can be shown to be 1/3.

In counseling individuals at risk for X-linked recessive traits, it is frequently helpful to utilize Bayesian calculations. Conceptually simple, but sometimes complex in application, Bayesian calculations take into account all available data, rather than merely restricting one to a priori calculations. For example, common sense dictates that a woman at theoretical risk for offspring having an X-linked recessive trait is actually less likely to be heterozygous if four consecutive sons prove unaffected.

As an example, suppose that a prospective mother (proband) relates that her two brothers have an X-linked disorder for which neither metabolic nor DNA analysis is possible. We can counsel that her mother is an obligate heterozygote; thus, the prospective mother has a 50% likelihood of being heterozygous. This is the proband's a priori risk or prior probability. Suppose now that the same mother relates that she has had three unaffected males. She might still be heterozygous and fortunate enough to have had no affected sons (probability 1/8 of a heterozygote having three consecutive unaffected sons). On the other hand, the greater likelihood is that the woman is in fact not heterozygous. Table 29-6 illustrates how the occurrence of three unaffected males can be taken into account. The newly calculated likelihood of being heterozygous is only 1/9, considerably lower than if one had continued to use only a priori expectations.

Bayesian calculations are also useful in estimating likelihood of heterozygosity for a trait lacking a completely reliable assay and in estimating risk for a trait with varying ages of onset. Clinical geneticists are quite familiar with their use, but obstetricians and gynecologists ordinarily need to be aware only of the existence of bayesian calculation.

X-Linked Dominant Inheritance

In X-linked dominant traits the incidence of affected females is twice that of affected males. However, females are usually less severely affected. In fact, some X-linked dominant traits are lethal in males. A male carrying an X-linked dominant allele transmits the mutant to all his daughters but to none of his sons (Table 29-7). The probability that a female with an X-linked

TABLE 29-6. BAYESIAN ANALYSIS

	PROBAND HETEROZYGOUS	PROBAND NOT HETEROZYGOUS
Prior probability	$\frac{1}{2}$	$\frac{1}{2}$
Conditional probability	$\left(\frac{1}{2}\right)^3 = \frac{1}{8}$	1
Joint probability (prior and conditional)	$\frac{1}{16}$	$\frac{1}{2}$
Posterior probability (joint and prior)	$\dfrac{\frac{1}{16} \text{ or } \frac{8}{16}}{\frac{1}{16}+\frac{1}{2}\left(\text{or } \frac{8}{16}\right)} = \dfrac{\frac{1}{16}}{\frac{9}{16}} = \frac{1}{9}$	$\dfrac{\frac{1}{2} \text{ or } \frac{8}{16}}{\frac{1}{16}+\frac{1}{2}} = \dfrac{\frac{8}{16}}{\frac{9}{16}} = \frac{8}{9}$

This analysis calculates the likelihood of heterozygosity for a woman whose two brothers have Duchenne muscular dystrophy, an X-linked recessive disorder. The a priori risk (prior probability) of heterozygosity is 1/2, inasmuch as the woman's mother is an obligate heterozygote. Suppose the woman has three unaffected sons. What is the likelihood that she is nevertheless heterozygous? Multiplying prior by conditional probability yields joint probability. The newly derived heterozygosity risk, taking into account the three unaffected sons, is the posterior probability calculated as shown: 1/9.

TABLE 29–7. X-LINKED DOMINANT INHERITANCE

	AFFECTED MALE			NORMAL MALE	
	X	Y		X	Y
Normal Female			Affected Female		
x	xX	xY	x	xx	xY
x	xX	xY	X	Xx	XY

X-linked dominant inheritance. **X** carries an X-linked dominant allele; x does not carry the allele. For offspring of affected males, all females are affected, but no males. For offspring of affected females, 50% of females and 50% of males are affected.

dominant allele will pass that allele to any offspring, male or female, is 0.5. Only a few X-linked dominant traits are known, the best example being vitamin D–resistant rickets.

Y-Linked Inheritance

A male would pass a Y-linked gene to each of his sons but to none of his daughters. Y-linked inheritance for monogenic traits remains unproved in humans; however, several features are controlled by factors on the Y, notably testicular determination.

CAUSES OF GENE MUTATION

Gene mutations are individually rare, but overall 1% of all infants have a disorder resulting from a single mutant gene. Sometimes affected individuals inherit a mutant gene, but at other times they are the first in their family to have the disorder. Spontaneous mutation rates average 10^{-5} to 10^{-6} per locus per gamete per generation. Overall, each gamete is estimated to contain 20–30 mutations. Most mutations are neutral or lethal. Otherwise, many more than 2% to 3% of liveborns would be abnormal.

Mutation rates increase with increasing paternal age. Fathers in their fifth and sixth decade have increased likelihood of certain gene mutations arising in their germ cells. This applies to some but not to all X-linked recessive and autosomal dominant disorders. This increase is believed to reflect germ cell replication (spermatogenesis) continuing throughout a male's fertile lifetime, although the manner by which repeated replications lead to mutation remains obscure. Unlike the situation for chromosomal abnormalities, advanced maternal age is not associated with increased gene mutations.

Among recognized causes, ionizing irradiation is a well-established mutagen. X-rays are the major source of ionizing irradiation, although ultraviolet light also causes mutations. Ultrasound and microwave are not ionizing and probably not mutagenic. Likewise, exposure to a video display terminal is probably not mutagenic. Even x-ray exposures of 50–100 rads only double mutation rates. Thus, the absolute risk following all except massive exposure is relatively low.

Numerous chemicals cause mutations in animals and in vitro testing systems. Well-known examples include alkylating agents, DNA base analogs (eg, 5-bromouracil), antimetabolites, nitrous acid, and acridine dyes. Even inorganic salts, caffeine, nitrites, and other ubiquitous agents are mutagenic under certain circumstances. It is difficult to determine the likelihood of these compounds being mutagenic in humans, especially in specific circumstances. Retrospective clinical data are rarely satisfactory. Fortunately, even substantive exposure to alkylating agents or antimetabolites leads to little if any increase in abnormal liveborns. Individuals treated prior to pregnancy with chemotherapeutic agents show no increased abnormalities in subsequent progeny. This suggests that most induced mutations are lethal.

Both DNA and RNA viruses can be mutagenic. Again, viruses induce gene mutations frequently, but only a few survive.

LINKAGE

Genes are located on chromosomes at given locations and in definite linear relationship to one another. Genes on the same chromosome are said to be linked or to exhibit linkage. Specifically, genes show linkage if during meiosis, with its opportunity for recombination, they are more likely to remain on the same chromosome in parental combination than to behave as if they were on different chromosomes.

If the frequency of recombination between two linked genes is 1%, those genes are defined to be 1 map unit or 1 centimorgan apart (percentage recombination = centimorgans). Genes 50 centimorgans apart on the same chromosome fail, by definition, to show linkage, because such genes segregate indistinguishably from genes on nonhomologous chromosomes. Linkage analysis is increasingly useful in antenatal diagnosis as a more complete map of the human genome becomes available. Linkage analysis in prenatal diagnosis usually relies on some polymorphic locus. (Polymorphism exists when two or more alleles are present at a given locus, such that the less frequent allele is still present in 1% of the population.)

Let us illustrate linkage analysis. A decade ago hemophilia could not be detected directly. Still diagnosis was possible if a mother were heterozygous both for the polymorphic enzyme G6PD and for hemophilia A. Loci for G6PD and hemophilia A are on the X chromosome. An individual can be heterozygous for either locus. Individuals may or may not carry the hemophilia mutant. Independently, they may or may not differ in G6PD electrophoretic characteristics. In females, genotypes AA, AB, and BB are possible. In males, only types A and B are possible. If a female is heterozygous at both G6PD (ie, type AB) and hemophilia, there are two possible relationships between the various G6PD and hemophilia alleles. If the G6PD-A allele and hemophilia A allele are located on the same X chromosome, G6PD-B and the normal allele at the hemophilia A locus can be deduced to exist on the homologous X chromosome. Conversely, if the G6PD-A allele and the normal allele at the hemophilia locus are located on the same X chromosome, G6PD-B and the hemophilia allele must exist on the homologous X chromosome. In the family illustrated in Figure 29-13, G6PD-A and hemophilia are located on the same chromosome because the male child with hemophilia is G6PD-A. If amniotic fluid fibroblasts in the next pregnancy are both 46,XY and G6PD-A, the likelihood is 95% (5% chance for recombination) that the fetus will have hemophilia. On the other hand, if 46,XY amniotic fluid fibroblasts are G6PD-B, the likelihood that the fetus will be affected is low, although greater than zero because of the possibility of recombination. Antenatal diagnosis of hemophilia can now be accomplished directly through DNA analysis. For many other disorders linkage analysis remains the only method to achieve prenatal diagnosis. Usually the polymorphic locus near the mutant gene is a polymorphism with respect to nucleotide sequences identified by whether a given restriction endonuclease does or does not cut the DNA.

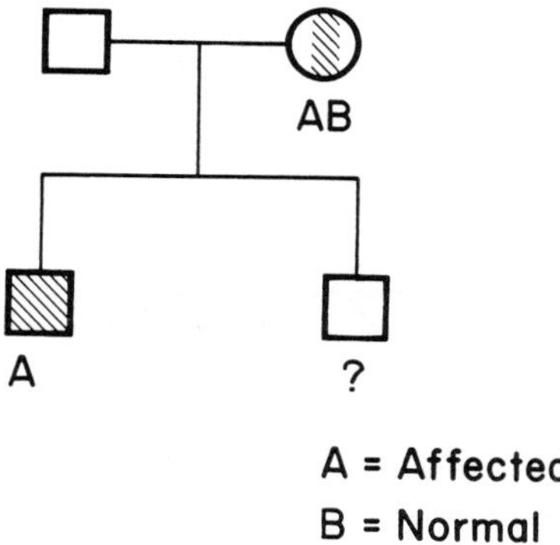

FIGURE 29–13. Principles of linkage analysis. Pedigree of family in which G6PD typing could be used for prenatal diagnosis of hemophilia. G6PD and hemophilia are closely linked on the X chromosome. Hemophilia can now be diagnosed directly. (Simpson JL. Antenatal diagnosis of genetic disorders. In: Sciarra JJ, ed. Gynecology and obstetrics, vol 3, Chap 104. Philadelphia: JB Lippincott, 1979:14.)

MOLECULAR BASIS OF THE GENE

DNA exists in the form of a double helix, which may be envisioned as a twisted ladder (Fig. 29-14*A*). Each vertical column consists of alternating phosphate and deoxyribose carbohydrate residues. Carbohydrate and phosphate residues of opposite sides are connected by various nitrogenous bases called nucleotides. The DNA nucleotides consist of the purines adenine (A) or guanine (G) and the pyrimidines thymine (T) or cytosine (C). One purine is always connected to one pyrimidine, joined by hydrogen bonds (base pairing) (Fig. 29-14*B*). Adenine is bound to thymine by two hydrogen bonds; cytosine is bound to guanine by three hydrogen bonds. As a result, the two DNA strands are complementary. If the sequence of bases on the one strand is ATTGC (adenine–thymine–thymine–guanine–cytosine), the sequence on the opposite strand must be TAACG. The ratio of adenine to thymine is always 1:1, as is the ratio of guanine to cytosine. However, the ratio of adenine–thymine (AT) pairs to guanine–cytosine (GC) pairs varies in different portions of even a single chromosome, as well as among different chromosomes. This variation is one basis for chromosomal banding.

Genetic information, specifically amino acid sequence, is determined by the sequence of nucleotides on one of the two DNA strands. A sequence of three bases forms a codon. A codon signifies one and only one of the 20 amino acids, but some codons connote other signals (eg, "stop" or cessation of transcription).

Structural Organization of the Gene

Genes interspersed along chromosomes that are capable of coding for protein are termed *unique* sequences of DNA. By contrast, *repetitive* sequences of DNA are not capable of coding for protein. There also are sequences essential for DNA transcription and RNA translation, and other types of DNA less immediately relevant to our discussion (eg, *pseudogenes,* which code for only part of a protein). Unique-sequence DNAs are generally interspersed within repetitive DNAs (Fig. 29-15).

Let us consider further the structure of a gene that will code for a protein. Figure 29-16 shows the sequence of events by which DNA is first transcribed into messenger RNA (mRNA) and then translated into protein. The hereditary information is read in the 5′ to 3′ direction. Prior to (5′ to, or "upstream" from) the nucleotide sequence actually coding for amino acids, there lie base sequences assumed to be involved in transcription regulation. Little is known about regulation in humans, but there are some intriguing observations. The nucleotide sequence TATA ("TATA box") is consistently found 30 base pairs (bp) before (5′ to) the site at

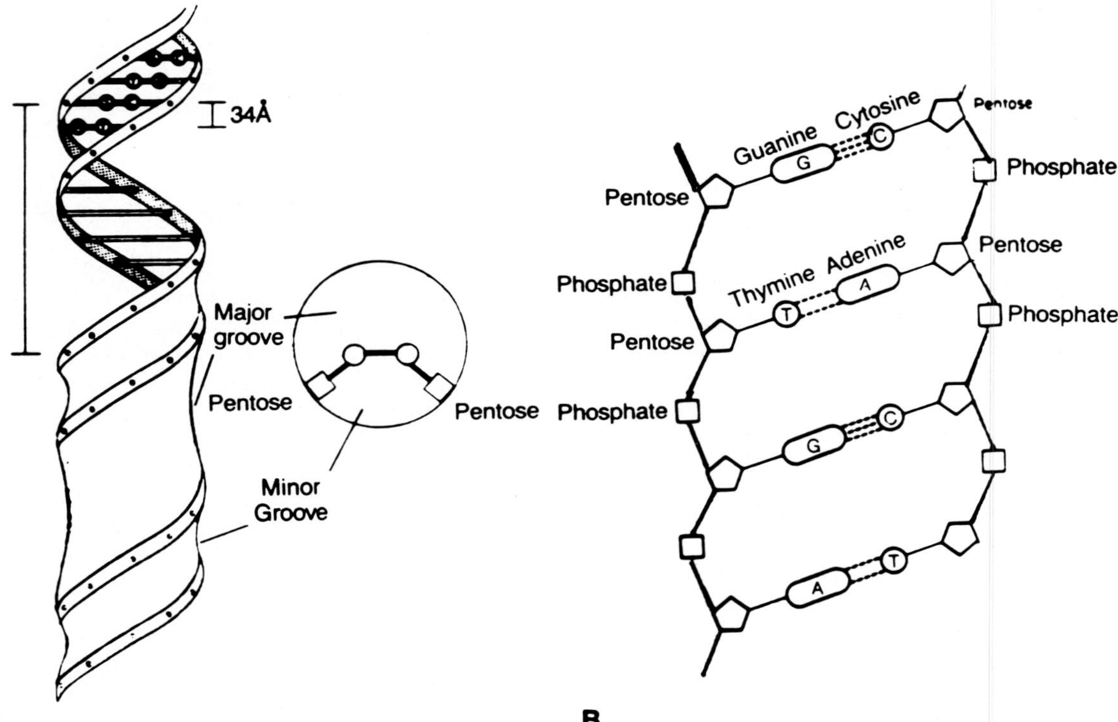

FIGURE 29–14. The double helix configuration of DNA, illustrating helix (A) and base pairing (B). Each vertical column consists of alternating deoxyribose sugar (pentrose) and phosphate. The pentose residues of opposite sides are connected transversely by nitrogenous bases: the purine adenine (A) or guanine (G) and pyrimidine thymine (T) or cytosine (C). Each transverse connection consists of one purine and one pyrimidine (AT or CG), held together by hydrogen bonds (dotted lines). (Ford EHR. Human chromosomes. New York: Academic Press, 1973:95, 97.)

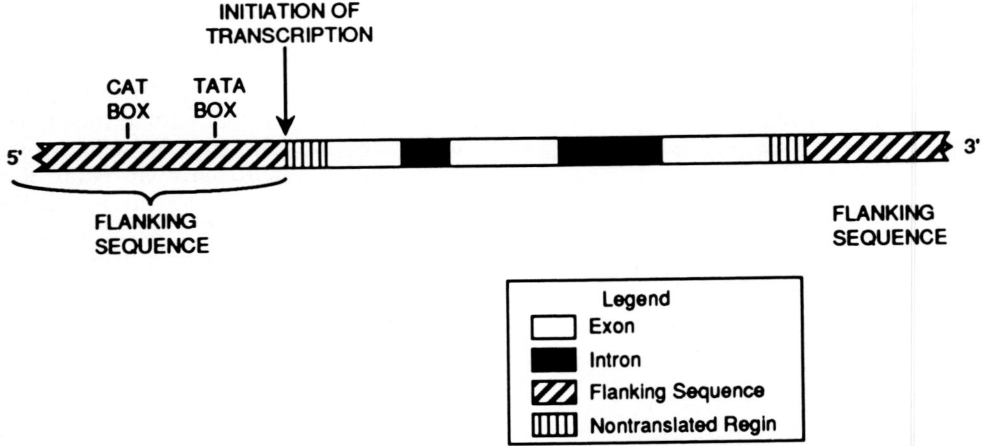

FIGURE 29–15. Organization of a human gene, specifically β-globin. The gene consists of three coding regions (exons) interspersed with three intervening sequences (introns). Upstream (5′) of the coding region lie sequences necessary for regulation.

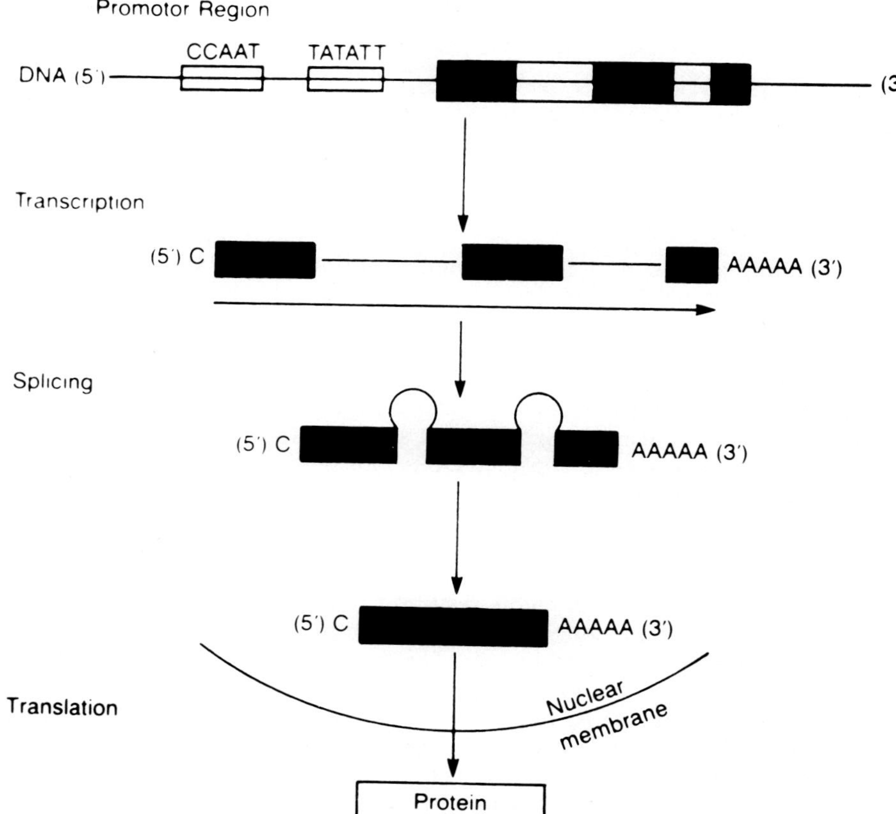

FIGURE 29–16. Transcription and translation. Intervening sequences (introns) must be excised, leaving exons to be translated to proteins. (Simpson JL. Antenatal diagnosis of genetic disorders. In: Sciarra JJ, ed. Gynecology and obstetrics. Vol. III. Philadelphia: JB Lippincott, 1979: 54.)

which transcription begins. The TATA box therefore may be involved in positioning RNA polymerase II, the enzyme essential for transcribing mRNA from DNA. Another pivotal sequence is CAAT, located 50–75 bp upstream from the transcription site. The "CAAT box" may be that site at which RNA polymerase II actually binds. Nevertheless, transcription proceeds in the 5′ to 3′ direction, extending beyond the region of unique-sequence DNA. The signal terminating transcription is also unknown, but the sequence AATAAA is consistently observed 15–30 bases 5′ to that site at which the polyadenylated [poly(A)] tail will be added.

Posttranscriptional Events

The entire sequence (5′ region, unique-sequence region with its intervening repetitive sequences, 3′ region) has now been transcribed into mRNA. Several posttranscriptional processes are necessary before the protein can be synthesized (translated).

A precise splicing mechanism also exists, apparently involving nucleotides GT on the 5′ side of the intervening sequence to be removed (intron) and nucleotides AG on the 3′ side (see Fig. 29-16).

Translation

The transcribed mRNA can now direct polypeptide synthesis (translation), a process that takes place in the cytoplasm. The first step in translation is that mRNA moves into the cytoplasm to associate with ribosomes, structures consisting of both protein and a special high-molecular-weight RNA (ribosomal RNA or rRNA). Adenosine triphosphate next reacts with the carboxyl end of specific amino acids to form an amino acid–specific transfer tRNA that lines up on the ribosome complex at that point signified by its appropriate codon. The amino acids that make up the polypeptide chain are thus brought into correct sequence.

Transporting Proteins to Their Proper Cellular Location

After being synthesized on ribosomes, proteins must find their way to the appropriate location either inside the cell (eg, lysosome) or outside the cell (extracellular fluid). Specific pathways must exist by which proteins reach their destinations. Perhaps certain amino acids bind to a receptor on the endoplasmic reticulum (ER), allowing the still-growing polypeptide sequence to be transferred across the ER. Additional signals must later direct the polypeptide to more distant locations.

MOLECULAR ANALYSIS OF THE GENE AND ITS CLINICAL APPLICABILITY

Analytical Techniques

Understanding the use of molecular genetics for prenatal diagnosis requires brief review of several analytic techniques.

Restriction Endonucleases and Restriction Fragment Length Polymorphisms. *Restriction endonucleases* are bacterial enzymes that recognize and cut specific nucleotide sequences in double-stranded DNA molecules. The sites at which DNA is cut are called *restriction sites.* Approximately 200 different restriction enzymes are known, each recognizing a unique sequence of bases. Figure 29-17 illustrates the recognition sequence of one particular enzyme. DNA fragments resulting from restriction enzymes differ in length in direct proportion to the distance between recognition sites. The greater the distance between recognition sites, the longer the length of intervening DNA. *Restriction fragments* are specified according to numbers of bases (eg, 8000 bases = 8 kilobases, or 8 kb). Usually there is more than one restriction site per gene, but occasionally the sites are situated in such a way that the entire gene lies between two sites. If a gene contains more than one restriction site, its DNA would ordinarily be subdivided into fragments of different lengths.

DNA from ostensibly normal individuals will not always show the same spectrum of DNA fragments after exposure to a given restriction enzyme. The reason is that differences in DNA sequences exist among the population. These differences confer no advantage or disadvantage. Thus, polymorphism exists with respect to the presence or absence of restriction sites. The term *restriction fragment length polymorphism* (RLFP) connotes this phenomenon. These differences among individuals are in contrast to differences in DNA sequence that cause disorders (eg, sickle cell anemia). Many RFLPs have been identified in the human genome, providing innumerable markers for linkage analysis (see the discussion of linkage in the section Single-Gene Abnormalities). If a given RFLP is closely linked to a locus conferring a disease, following linkage analysis to detect the presence or absence of a disorder may be possible. Since RFLPs exist every few centimorgans, linkage analysis will eventually permit prenatal diagnosis for almost all loci. At present, RFLP linkage analysis forms the basis for prenatal diagnosis of many cases of cystic fibrosis, Duchenne muscular dystrophy, hemophilia, and other common disorders when the exact mutation is not known in a family.

Southern Blotting. Distinguishing DNA fragments of differing size requires a technique called Southern blotting. DNA digested by restriction endonucleases yields fragments of various lengths. If allowed to migrate through an agarose gel, heavier DNA fragments prove less mobile and remain near the origin of the gel. Lighter fragments migrate further (Fig. 29-18). The gel can be laid on a piece of nitrocellulose paper, and the buffer can be allowed to flow through the gel into the nitrocellulose filter. DNA fragments concomitantly migrate out of the gel and bind to the filter, creating a replica of the DNA fragment pattern. If the nitrocellulose replicate is exposed to a specific gene probe (see the next paragraph), the probe will hybridize only to that portion of the filter containing complementary DNA. The probe will thus locate its complementary DNA sequence, and only that sequence. To identify such a fragment and its length, the probe is made radioactive or more commonly biotinylated. Thus, a gene (or more specifically a DNA sequence that is part of a gene) can

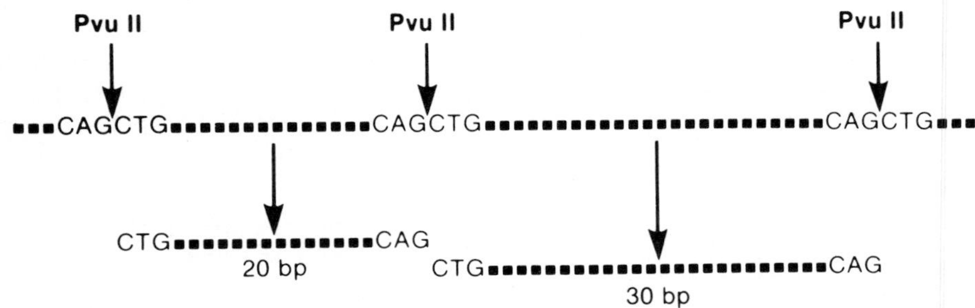

FIGURE 29–17. Simplification of the manner in which a restriction endonuclease cuts DNA at a specific nucleotide sequence. DNA nucleotide sequence is shown as single-stranded. Pvu II recognizes the sequence CAGCTG and only that sequence. DNA can be separated into fragments of different lengths on the basis of distances between restriction enzyme recognition sites. The greater the distance between sites, the longer the length of intervening DNA. (From Gabbe S, Niebyl J, Simpson JL. Obstetrics: Normal and problem pregnancies. New York: Churchill-Livingstone, 1986:238.)

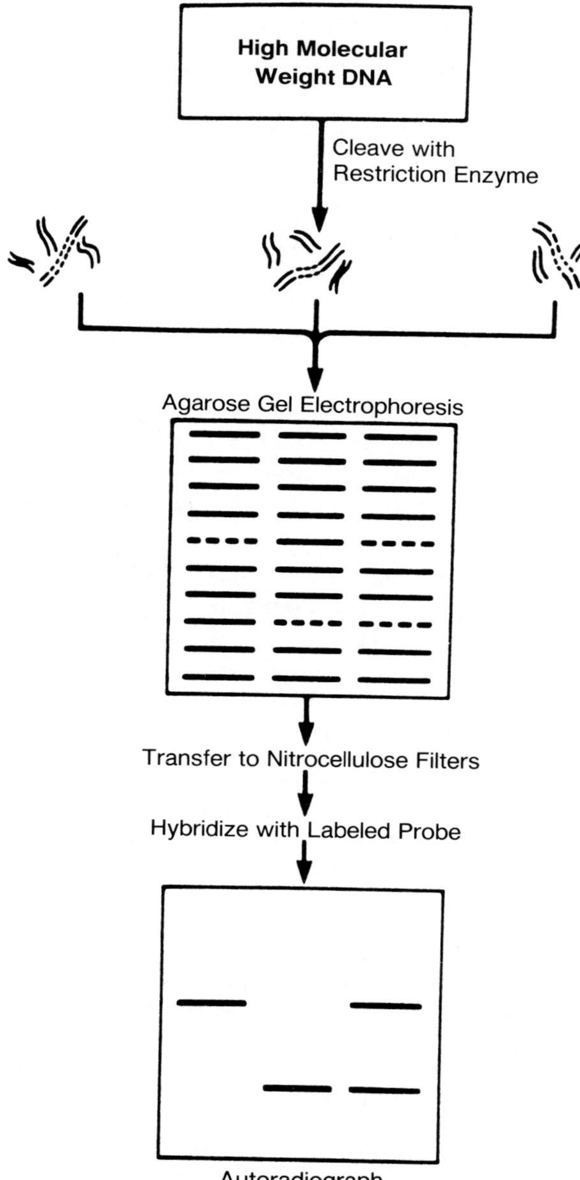

FIGURE 29–18. Southern blotting. DNA is cleaved with restriction enzymes, and the cleaved DNA is separated by size, using agarose gel electrophoresis. The gel is then laid on a piece of nitrocellulose and buffer is allowed to flow through the gel onto the nitrocellulose. DNA fragments migrate out of the gel and bind to the filter. A replica of the DNA fragment pattern of the gel is thus created on the filter. The filter can then be hybridized to a suitably labeled probe, with DNA fragments that hybridize to the probe signaled by autoradiography. (From Gabbe S, Niebyl J, Simpson JL. Obstetrics: Normal and problem pregnancies. New York: Churchill-Livingstone, 1986:240.)

be identified among thousands of fragments, categorized according to length.

Gene Probes. For a specific gene—or more precisely, a specific DNA sequence—to be located from among thousands of DNA fragments DNA probes must be available. These in turn are made from cloned DNA. If purified mRNA is available, single-stranded DNA probes can be made readily by use of an enzyme called *reverse transcriptase*. This enzyme, present in viruses whose hereditary information is not DNA but RNA, directs the synthesis of DNA from RNA (the reverse of the situation in humans). Exposing human mRNA to viral reverse transcriptase produces *complementary* single-stranded human DNA called cDNA. Probes are made by injecting DNA into a vector (eg, a plasmid). Plasmids have the property of replicating their DNA separately from that of their bacterial host. Bacteriophage or synthetic systems (cosmids) can also be used as vectors. A vector will synthesize many copies, both of itself and of inserted DNA (eg, cDNA). If these copies are labeled, a "probe" will have been constructed (Fig. 29-19). The DNA inserted can either be of known DNA sequence or of unknown sequence.

Oligonucleotide Probes. A natural extension of the techniques described earlier is the development of oligonucleotide or allele-specific probes. One can construct DNA probes for sequences of any desired number of nucleotides, usually 15–20. These sensitive probes will hybridize only to sequences complementary for every single nucleotide. If only a single nucleotide is absent (or altered), the oligonucleotide probe will fail to hybridize. Usually this technique is used in conjunction with the polymerase chain reaction (PCR), described later.

Polymerase Chain Reaction (PCR). All laboratory techniques require a minimum amount of material for testing, whether it is serum, nuclei, or other structures. A highly useful procedure is the *polymerase chain reaction* (PCR). In PCR a target sequence of up to 1 kb can be amplified 10^5 to 10^6 times (Figs. 29-20, 29-21). The prerequisite for this amplification is the identification of unique DNA primers that flank and are specific for the DNA region in question. The region in question may consist of a portion of a gene (eg, that containing a mutation), a polymorphic DNA sequence closely linked to a given locus, or a repetitive DNA sequence characteristic of regions of a given chromosome (the Y long arm). A heat-stable DNA polymerase extracted from Thermas aquaticus is then used (thus, the term *Taq polymerase*). A tube containing the DNA in question, the unique primers, and *Taq polymerase* is then placed together, resulting in amplification. When the temperature is raised, denaturation into single-stranded DNA occurs. On cooling, another amplification cycle occurs. Amplification increases the DNA between primes in logarithmic fashion, allowing with automation some 30 cycles in perhaps 3–4 hours.

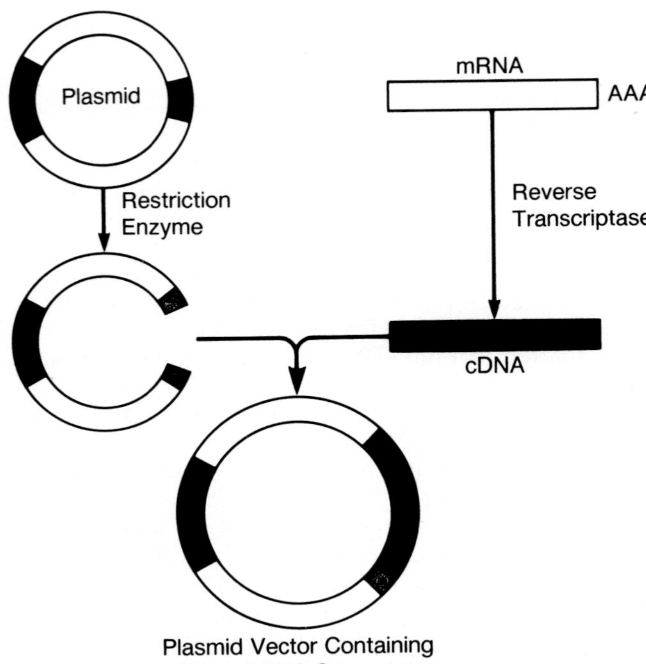

FIGURE 29–19. Cloned DNA. A DNA fragment is inserted in a plasmid vector, which synthesizes many copies of not only itself but also the inserted fragment. The clone can be labeled radioactively to constitute a gene probe. (From Gabbe S, Niebyl J, Simpson JL. Obstetrics: Normal and problem pregnancies. New York: Churchill-Livingstone, 1986:239.)

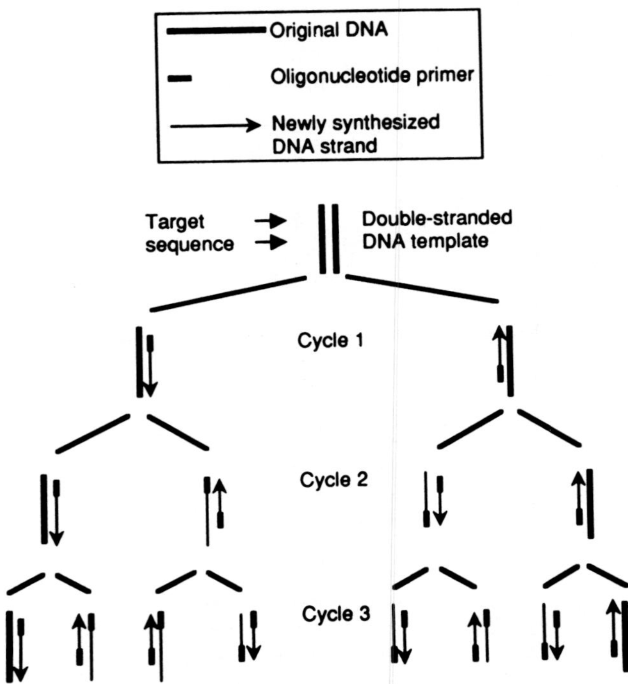

FIGURE 29–21. Polymerase chain reaction (PCR). Placing the DNA in question, unique primers, and Taq polymerase together results in amplification (cycle 1). When the temperature is raised, denaturation into single-stranded DNA occurs. Upon cooling, a second amplification cycle occurs. Continued amplification increases the DNA between primers in logarithmic fashion.

This technique is so successful that DNA diagnoses can be made literally from a single cell. In fact, this was illustrated by Handyside and colleagues,[22] who used this technique in an embryonic blastomere biopsy from a preimplantation embryo and by Lo and coworkers.[23] In that example PCR was specific for a repetitive sequence on the Y long arm that contained many copies of DNA.

In theory, one can use PCR to test for a sequence not ordinarily present in the mother. This technique could be used to confirm the existence of fetal cells in maternal blood and could be used diagnostically (eg, in a homozygous pregnant SS mother, presence of DNA connoting hemoglobin A would indicate a heterozygous fetus). PCR works quite well on a single cell. However, the technique has limitations if the single cell is not analyzed in isolation but rather is to be analyzed in the presence of a variety of other cells. Under these circumstances results are less satisfactory or totally unreliable when the concentration of the cell in question falls below perhaps 0.001. Another major limitation is that of contamination. The extraordinary sensitivity of PCR dictates extraordinary precautions to exclude contamination. For example, contamination from ambient cells is a genuine concern of technicians responsible for setting up equipment or transporting laboratory specimens.

Diagnostic Application by Molecular Genetics

Detailed discussion of prenatal diagnosis is not the goal of this chapter. However, it will be useful to illustrate

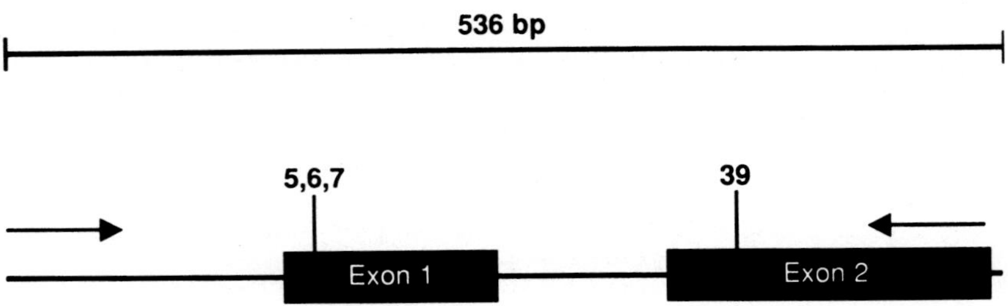

FIGURE 29–20. Region of the β-globin gene that contains mutation for sickle cell anemia (codon 6) and one for β-thalassemia (codon 39). Amplification of this region by PCR would allow one to arrive at prenatal diagnosis, after challenge by specific oligonucleotide probes (allele-specific).

β^a	**Codon**	**5**	**6**	**7**
	Amino Acid	**Pro**	**Glu**	**Glu**
	Nucleotide	**CCT**	**GAG**	**GAG**
β^s	**Codon**	**5**	**6**	**7**
	Amino Acid	**Pro**	**Val**	**Glu**
	Nucleotide	**CCT**	**GTG**	**GAG**

Mst II Recognition Sequence, CCTNAGG, Absent in β^s

FIGURE 29–22. Loss of Mst II restriction recognition site in β^s (sickle cell anemia). Mutation of adenine to thymine results in a new nucleotide sequence, no longer recognized by Mst II. N = any nucleotide. (From Gabbe S, Niebyl J, Simpson JL. Obstetrics: Normal and problem pregnancies. New York: Churchill-Livingstone, 1986:240.)

how the molecular techniques described earlier can be applied to specific clinical circumstances.

Known Molecular Basis of a Disorder. Let us first consider mutation resulting from a known alteration in DNA. Diagnosis may be caused by complete absence of DNA (deletions) or by presence of a single abnormal nucleotide (point mutation). An obvious way to detect a disorder characterized by absence of DNA would be to determine whether or not a DNA probe for the normal gene hybridizes to DNA of an unknown individual. If the latter's DNA does not hybridize, he or she must lack the DNA sequence and thus must be affected. DNA from the fetus in question could originate from any available nucleated cell (eg, chorionic villi or amniotic fluid cells).

A second general approach becomes applicable whenever the nucleotide sequence producing a mutation is known. Knowing the altered nucleotide sequence potentially allows one to select a restriction enzyme that acts at the altered site. If a useful restriction enzyme exists, prenatal diagnosis becomes possible. An example is sickle cell anemia, a disorder in which codon 6 (the triplet signifying the sixth amino acid) has undergone a mutation from adenine to thymine. Restriction enzymes exist capable of recognizing the normal nucleotide sequence, but not capable of recognizing the mutant sequence (Fig. 29-22). The enzyme MstII requires the normal nucleotide sequence at codon 6. Use of a β-globin DNA probe can differentiate DNA containing the mutant gene from DNA containing the normal gene. The probe highlights a longer fragment in the former as a result of the missing restriction site (Fig. 29-23).

An alternative approach, applicable when either a deletion or altered nucleotide sequence exists, is to use an oligonucleotide probe, as illustrated in Figure 29-24. The probe will hybridize only to DNA containing each of a specified sequence of nucleotides (mutation or normal).

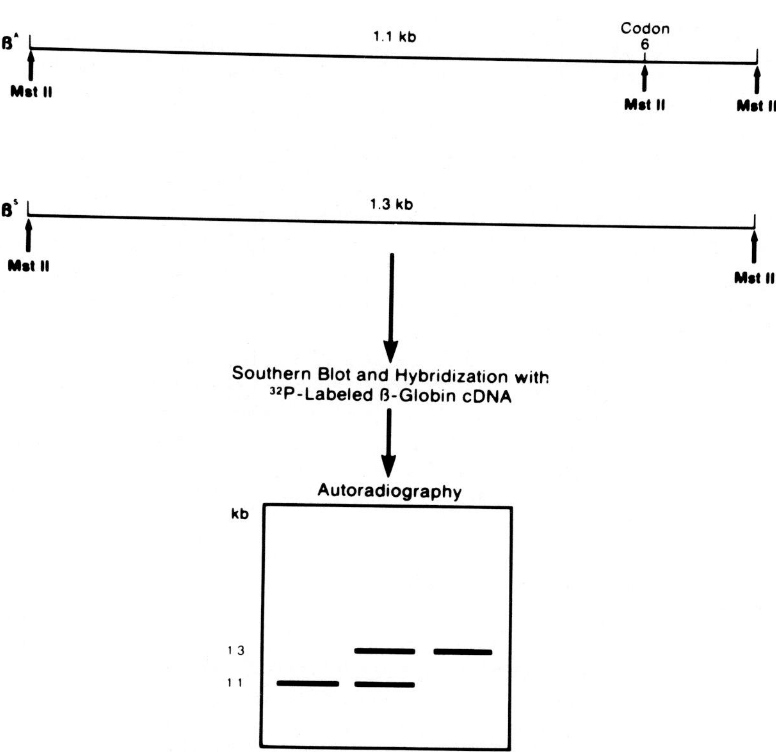

FIGURE 29–23. Use of radioactively labeled gene probe for β-globin to diagnose sickle cell anemia. (From Gabbe S, Niebyl J, Simpson JL. Obstetrics: Normal and problem pregnancies. New York: Churchill-Livingstone, 1986:241.)

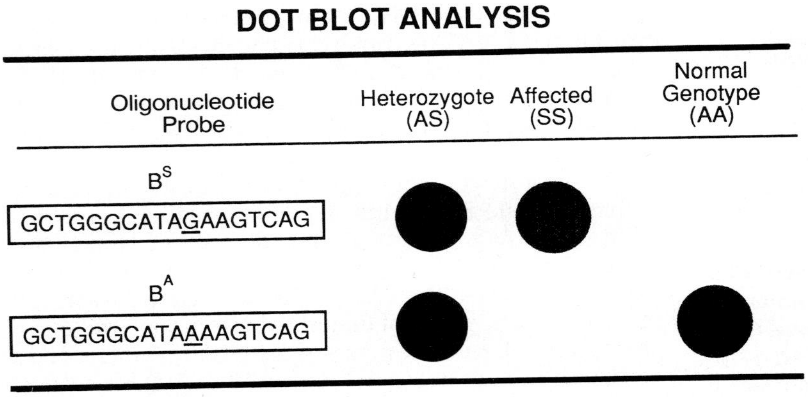

DOT BLOT ANALYSIS

Oligonucleotide Probe	Heterozygote (AS)	Affected (SS)	Normal Genotype (AA)
B^S GCTGGGCATA<u>G</u>AAGTCAG	●	●	
B^A GCTGGGCATA<u>A</u>AAGTCAG	●		●

FIGURE 29-24. Oligonucleotide and dot blot analysis.

Unknown Molecular Basis (RFLP Linkage Analysis)

If the nucleotide sequence responsible for a given disorder is not known, one can still use molecular techniques if the mutant gene has been localized to a chromosome and if an RFLP is nearby. These RFLPs serve as markers, permitting linkage analysis by following segregation of mutant genes in a given family.

The difficulty lies in finding a RFLP closely linked to the mutant gene under study. If a probe is available, one must determine whether an informative situation even exists in a given family. Suppose, for example, that a probe sometimes highlights a fragment of DNA 5700 bp long. Still other individuals might show 2400-bp and 3300-bp bands as well. The basis of this polymorphism is presence or absence of restriction site B (Figure 29-25). Sites A and C are relatively constant. Suppose further that this RFLP has already been proved to be closely linked to the locus corresponding to a given mutant. Figure 29-25 illustrates RFLP analysis. In the family, the normal allele is signified by the 5700-bp fragment, the mutant by the presence of the 3300-bp fragment. Recall that the RFLP pattern that will connote an affected fetus in this family may connote just the opposite in another family. The RFLP merely serves as a marker; its presence or absence is functionally independent from the disease.

The attraction of RFLP linkage analysis is that diagnosis can be accomplished without knowledge of the molecular basis of a disorder. Moreover, a limitless number of RFLPs exist throughout the human genome, eventually assuring prenatal diagnosis for any disorder whose chromosomal localization is known.

POLYGENIC–MULTIFACTORIAL INHERITANCE

Genetic tendencies, rather than merely shared environmental factors, very often are responsible for physiologic and anatomical variation, as well as for common anomalies affecting a single organ system (eg, cleft palate). Most of the latter show recurrence risks of 1.5% for first-degree relatives (siblings, offspring, parents). This can also be deduced from twin studies. Monozygotic twins are much more likely to be concordant for any given anomaly than are dizygotic twins. Since either monozygotic or dizygotic twins are exposed to the same intrauterine environment, genetic factors must be invoked to explain the differences.

Basis of Polygenic Inheritance

The logical explanation for either anatomical and physiologic variation for a trait whose recurrence risk is 1% to 5% is involvement of several genes. To illustrate the logic, let us consider the progressively increasing number of genotypes whenever more than one gene influences a single characteristic. Suppose only one gene controls a trait and that this gene has two alleles. If the frequency of allele *A* equals the frequency of allele *a*, 25% of the population is *AA* ($p = q = 0.5$; $p^2 = q^2 = 0.25$), 25% is *aa*, and 50% is *Aa* ($2pq = 0.50$). Now suppose that not one but two genes influence the trait. At the second locus, alleles *B* and *b* exist. Nine genotypes are now possible: *AABB, AABb, AAbb, AaBB, AaBb, Aabb, aaBB, aaBb, aabb*. The population will contain nine distinct classes of individuals if *A, B, a,* and *b* all exert dissimilar influences (Table 29-8). As the number of genes controlling a trait increases, the number of genotypic classes increases rapidly. If one gene has two alleles, there are three classes. If two genes exist, each with two alleles, there will be nine classes and thus nine histographic bars. If one continues to represent histographically the proportion of individuals in each genotypic class, normal distribution will be approximated as more and more genotypes became possible (Fig. 29-26). Thus, continuous variation will be approximated in the population.

A trait controlled by more than one gene is said to be inherited in polygenic fashion. Although the term *polygenic inheritance* is often used synonymously with continuous variation, the latter may also result from other mechanisms—namely, a single multiple-allele locus influenced by environmental factors. If environmental as well as ge-

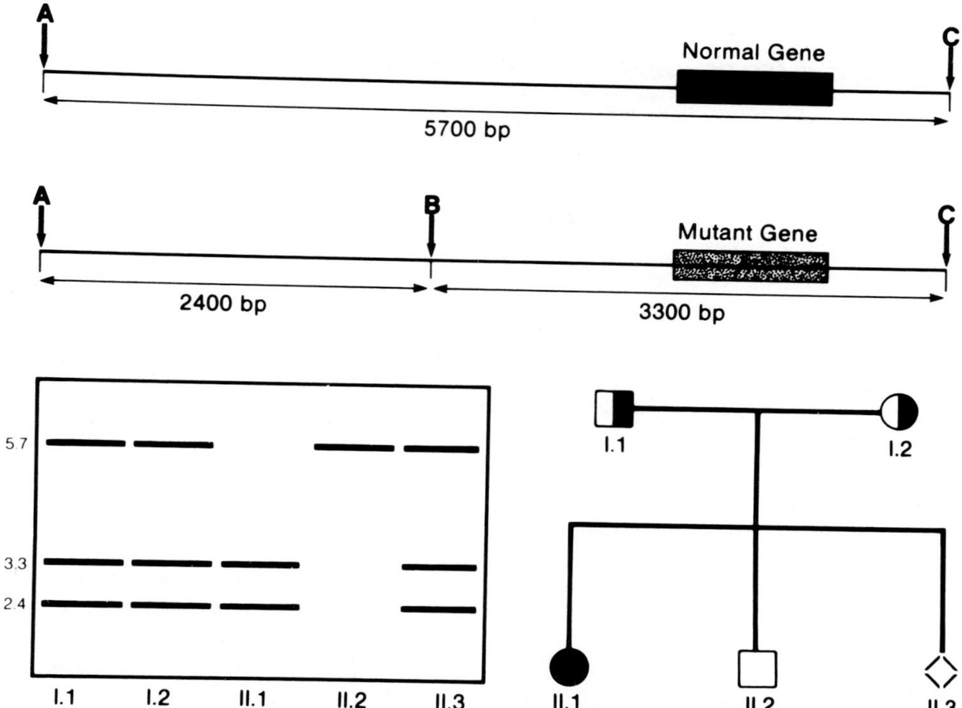

FIGURE 29–25. Prenatal diagnosis achieved by use of restriction fragment length polymorphism linked to the locus causing a disease. Suppose a restriction site (B) is closely linked to a gene. This restriction site is present in some individuals but not in others (polymorphism). A probe that hybridizes to DNA containing the polymorphic site will identify 2400-bp and 3300-bp fragments in individuals with the restriction site, but only a single 5700-bp fragment in those without the restriction site. On agarose gel electrophoresis, individuals homozygous for the restriction site will display two bands (II.1). Homozygous individuals lacking the restriction site will display only one band (II.2). In this family, parents (I.1, I.2) are doubly heterozygous. They are each heterozygous both for the restriction site and for an autosomal recessive mutant (pedigrees). DNA analysis of the affected child (II.1) shows only two bands (3.3 and 2.4 kb). We can conclude that in both parents the mutant gene is located on the chromosome characterized by the presence of restriction site B. DNA analysis reveals that their unaffected son (II.2) is not heterozygous but homozygous normal. DNA analysis from amniotic fluid cells or chorionic villi reveals that the fetus (II.3) is normal but heterozygous. (From Gabbe S, Niebyl J, Simpson JL. Obstetrics: Normal and problem pregnancies. New York: Churchill-Livingstone, 1986:242.)

netic factors influence a trait, the term *multifactorial* is more appropriate. Polygenic and multifactorial inheritance usually cannot be distinguished in humans, although comparisons between monozygotic and dizygotic twins theoretically permit such a distinction.

Polygenic–multifactorial inheritance is invoked to explain the inheritance of normal anatomical and physiologic variables that display *continuous variation*—height, skin color, hair color, blood pressure, age of menarche, ability to metabolize a given drug or toxin. However, polygenic inheritance ostensibly cannot explain discontinuous variation. In discontinuous variation the population consists of two discrete groups, one affected (eg, cleft palate) and one unaffected. Either one has a cleft palate or one does not. There is no continuum in the population. To explain such dichotomy (discontinuity) on a polygenic basis, one must postulate a threshold beyond which the accrued genetic liability for developing a specific trait becomes so great that a malformation is manifested (Fig. 29-27). Phenotypically normal parents delivered of a child with a polygenic–multifactorial trait (anomaly) are assumed to have genetic liabilities nearer the threshold than most other individuals in the general population. This model is biologically reasonable if "liability" reflects rate of embryonic growth. Growth occurring too slowly could preclude a key embryonic step being accomplished by a certain crucial time, thus leading to anomalous development. For example, if the paired palatine shelves reach the midline before a certain day of development, they fuse to form a secondary palate. After that day the shelves are too widely separated ever to fuse, thus re-

TABLE 29-8. RELATIONSHIP BETWEEN NUMBERS OF GENES CONTROLLING A TRAIT AND NUMBERS OF CLASSES OF INDIVIDUALS IN A POPULATION

NUMBERS OF GENES	CLASSES OF INDIVIDUALS	NUMBER OF CLASSES
1 (A, a)	AA, Aa, aa	3
2 (A, a; B, b)	AABB, AABb, AAbb AaBB, AaBb, Aabb aaBB, AABb, aabb	9
n		3^n

A and a represent alleles at one locus, B and b at another. If one gene controls the presence or absence of a given trait, the population consists of three genotypes; if two genes control a trait, the population consists of nine genotypes. If there are more than two alleles at a given locus, the number of genotypes would increase. (Data from Simpson JL. Disorders of sexual differentiation: etiology and clinical delineation. New York: Academic Press, 1976.)

sulting in cleft palate. Inherited factors influencing presence or absence of this anomaly might indicate velocity of growth, size of mandible and tongue, and rapidity of palatine migration.

Characteristics of Polygenic–Multifactorial Inheritance

In humans, several empirical characteristics are indicative of polygenic–multifactorial inheritance:

1. The trait usually involves a single organ system or embryologically related organ system. Table 29-9 lists some traits considered inherited in this fashion.
2. Unlike mendelian inheritance, the recurrence risk increases after two affected progeny. However, the risk never approaches the 25% expected for recessive traits or the 50% expected for dominant traits.
3. If the trait occurs more frequently among members of a single sex, the risk for relatives is higher if the proband (index case) is of the less frequently affected sex. Pyloric stenosis occurs more frequently in males; thus, the recurrence risk is higher if the proband is female. The converse is true for congenital hip dislocation.
4. The more serious the defect, the higher the recurrence risk. Bilateral cleft palate carries a higher recurrence risk than unilateral cleft palate. Long-segment aganglionosis (Hirshsprung disease) carries a higher recurrence risk than short-segment aganglionosis.
5. The frequency of similarly affected co-twins (concordance) is higher among monozygotic than dizygotic twins. However, dissimilarly affected

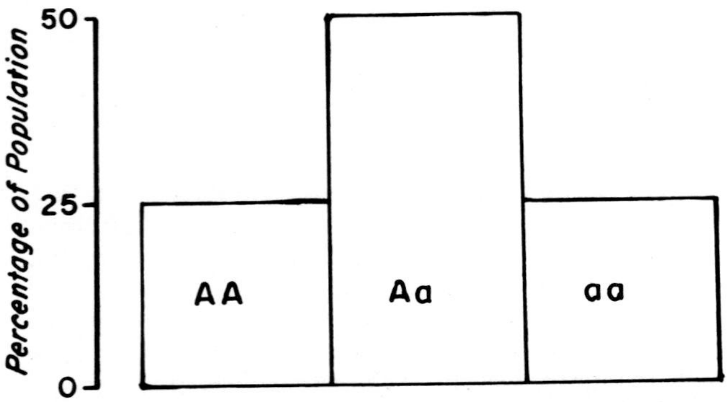

FIGURE 29–26. Histogram showing the relative proportions of individuals with various genotypes (AA, Aa, aa) if a trait is influenced by a single gene that can exist in two allelic forms (A or a). If A = a = 0.5, $p^2 = q^2 = 0.25$ and $2pq = 0.50$ (Hardy-Weinberg equilibrium). Thus, 25% of the population is AA, 25% is aa, and 50% is Aa. If A = 0.9, 81% are AA, 18% are Aa, and 1% are aa. (From Simpson JL. Disorders of sexual differentiation: Etiology and clinical delineation. New York: Academic Press, 1976:42.)

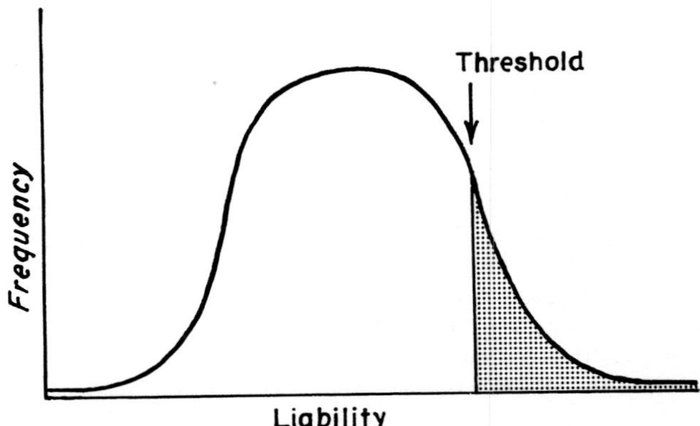

FIGURE 29–27. Schematic presentation of one model for polygenic or multifactorial inheritance, assuming a threshold beyond which liability is so great that an abnormality is manifested. Parents of affected individuals presumably have a greater liability (ie, are closer to the threshold) than most other individuals in the population. (From Simpson JL. Disorders of sexual differentiation: Etiology and clinical delineation. New York: Academic Press, 1976:43.)

TABLE 29–9. COMMON POLYGENIC/ MULTIFACTORIAL TRAITS

Neural tube defects (most cases)
Hydrocephaly (most cases)
Cleft lip, with or without cleft palate
Cleft lip (alone)
Cardiac defects (most types)
Diaphragmatic hernia
Omphalocele and gastroschisis
Renal agenesis
Ureteral anomalies
Hypospadias
Posterior urethral values
Uterine (müllerian fusion) defects (probable)
Hip dislocation
Limb reduction defects
Talipes equinovarus (clubfoot)

co-twins (discordance) still are seen among monozygotic twins, in contrast to identity for mendelian traits.

6. As the degree of the relationship decreases, the recurrence risk to relatives decreases more rapidly than that for autosomal dominant traits.

In humans it is nearly impossible to differentiate between polygenic and multifactorial causes. Geneticists are, moreover, often guilty of loosely terming as polygenic any trait whose inheritance is complex. Nonetheless, it is appropriate to invoke the concept of polygenic inheritance or multifactorial inheritance for traits carrying recurrence risks of 1% to 5% for first-degree relatives.

REFERENCES

1. ISCN: An international system for human cytogenetic nomenclature. Basel: S Karger, 1985.
2. Tipton RE, Tharapel AT, Chang HT, et al. Rapid chromosome analysis with the use of spontaneously dividing cells derived from umbilical cord blood (fetal and neonatal). Am J Obstet Gynecol 1986;161:1546.
3. Ledbetter DH, Gilbert F, Jackson L, et al. Cytogenetic results of chorionic villus sampling: high success rate and diagnostic accuracy in the United States Collaborative Study. Am J Obstet Gynecol, in press.
4. Hassold TJ, Jacobs PA. Trisomy in man. Adv Hum Genet 1984;18:69.
5. Henderson SA, Edwards RG. Chiasma frequency and maternal age in mammals. Nature 1968;218:22.
6. Hook EB. Rates of chromosome abnormalities at different maternal ages. Obstet Gynecol 1981;58:282.
7. Hassold TJ. A cytogenetic study of repeated abortions. Am J Hum Genet 1980;32:723.
8. Warburton D, Kline S, Stein Z, et al. Does the karyotype of a spontaneous abortion predict the karyotype of a subsequent abortion? Am J Hum Genet 1987;41:465.
9. Stene J, Fischer G, Stene E, et al. Paternal age effect in Down's syndrome. Ann Hum Genet 1977;40:299.
10. Rani AS, Jyothi PP, Reddy OS. Reproduction in Down's syndrome. Int J Gynecol Obstet 1990;31:81.
11. Simpson JL, Tharapel AT. Principles of cytogenetics. In: Philipp E, Barnes J, eds. Scientific foundations of obstetrics and gynaecology. 4th ed. London: Heinemann Medical Books, in press.
12. Simpson JL. Disorders of sexual differentiation: etiology and clinical delineation. New York: Academic Press, 1976.
13. Boué A, Gallano B. A collaborative study of inherited chromosome structural rearrangements in 13,356 prenatal diagnoses. Prenat Diagn 1984;4:45.
14. Daniel A, Hook EB, Wulf G. Risk of unbalanced progeny at amniocentesis to carriers of chromosome rearrangements: data from the United States and Canadian Laboratories. Am J Med Genet 1989;33:14.
15. Jacobs PA, Frachiezicz A, Law P, et al. The effect of structural aberrations of the chromosomes on reproductive fitness in man II. Results. Clin Genet 1975;8:169.
16. Simpson JL, Meyers CM, Martin AO, et al. Translocations are infrequent among couples having repeated spontaneous abortions but no other abnormal pregnancies. Fertil Steril 1989;51:811.
17. Sutherland GR, Gardiner AJ, Carter RF. Familial pericentric inversion of chromosome 19, inv(19)(p13q13) with a note on genetic counseling of pericentric inversion carriers. Clin Genet 1976;10:54.
18. Martin AO, Simpson JL, Deddish R, et al. Clinical implications of chromosomal inversions: a pericentric inversion in No. 18 segregating in a family ascertained through an abnormal proband. Am J Perinatal 1983;1:81.
19. Warburton D. Outcome of cases of de novo structural rearrangements diagnosed at amniocentesis. Prenatal Diagn 1984;4:69.
20. Riordan JR, Rommens JM, Kerem BS, et al: Identification of the cystic fibrosis gene: cloning and characterization of complementary DNA. Science 1989;245:1066.
21. Lemma WK, Feldman GL, Kerem BS, et al. Mutation analysis for heterozygote detection and the prenatal diagnosis of cystic fibrosis. N Engl J Med 1990;322:219.
22. Handyside AH, Penketh RJA, Winston RML, et al: Biopsy of preimplantation embryos and sexing by DNA amplification. Lancet 1989;1:347.
23. Lo TMD, Patel P, Wainscoat JS, et al: Prenatal sex determination by DNA amplification from maternal peripheral blood. Lancet 1989;2:1363.

30

CHAPTER

CHROMOSOMAL DISORDERS

Lillian Y. F. Hsu

At the beginning of the third decade of prenatal cytogenetic diagnosis, it is probable that more than 1 million mid-trimester genetic amniocenteses have been performed throughout the world. Although we have accumulated extensive experience and data from cytogenetic diagnosis through amniocentesis and have made significant progress in terms of success rate, turnaround time (TAT), and quality of preparation, we still sometimes face problems and pitfalls in diagnosis and counseling.

The development in the early 1980s of chorionic villi sampling (CVS) for first-trimester diagnosis is one further step forward in prenatal diagnosis. Today over 80,000 CVS have been carried out worldwide. However, experience here also has shown considerable diagnostic problems, such as maternal cell contamination and discrepancies between CVS and amniocytes and/or fetal cells.

In this chapter discussion will focus primarily on the problems related to prenatal diagnosis of chromosome abnormalities. Armed with all available data from amniocentesis and CVS, physicians or geneticists may be better equipped to deal with the complexities of prenatal cytogenetic diagnosis.

INDICATIONS FOR PRENATAL CYTOGENETIC DIAGNOSES

Today genetic laboratories (including commercial ones) are readily available, so that any pregnant woman should be able to choose to have a genetic amniocentesis if there is no financial barrier. Nevertheless, prenatal cytogenetic diagnosis is still offered primarily to pregnant women with an increased risk of having a child affected with a chromosome abnormality. On the other hand, more and more institutions have become less stringent in their definition of indications and tend to accept more cases under the category of maternal anxiety.

ADVANCED MATERNAL AGE

The risk of carrying a fetus with a trisomy clearly increases with the age of the mother. Specific maternal-age–related frequencies for trisomy 21 and for all chromosome abnormalities from both live-born statistics and mid-trimester amniocentesis data are listed in Table 30-1. Although the CVS data are preliminary, the rate of abnormal chromosomes detected in CVS is, as expected, considerably higher than the rate at amniocentesis.

The advanced maternal age group (ie, 35 years and over at the time of confinement) currently represents the major target population for prenatal cytogenetic diagnosis. However, the decision to use age 35 as a dividing line is arbitrary, since the risks increase gradually along with the age. It is probably not wise to deny prenatal cytogenetic diagnosis to any pregnant woman. One option is to offer young women maternal serum α-fetoprotein screening (MSAFP) to detect patients with increased risk for bearing a fetus with trisomy 21. However, it must be realized that this is not a highly sensitive screening test (see the section Low Maternal Serum α-Fetoprotein).

Advanced paternal age is generally not considered a valid indication for prenatal cytogenetic diagnosis, as several recent studies have found no evidence for a positive paternal age effect.[1]

CARRIER OF A BALANCED STRUCTURAL REARRANGEMENT

The risk that a carrier parent with a balanced structural rearrangement will have a child with an unbalanced chromosome complement is significantly higher than that for the advanced maternal age group. The risk for such a carrier varies, depending on the type of rearrangement, the method of ascertainment, whether

TABLE 30–1. CRUDE MATERNAL AGE-SPECIFIC RATES (%) FOR CHROMOSOME ABNORMALITIES

MATERNAL AGE (YEARS)	LIVE-BORN STATISTICS*		AT AMNIOCENTESIS†		AT CVS‡
	47, +21	ALL CHROMOSOME ABNORMALITIES	47, +21	ALL CHROMOSOME ABNORMALITIES	ALL CHROMOSOME ABNORMALITIES
33	0.16	0.29	0.24	0.48	—
34	0.20	0.36	0.30	0.66	—
35	0.26	0.49	0.40	0.76	0.78
36	0.33	0.60	0.52	0.95	0.80
37	0.44	0.77	0.67	1.20	2.58
38	0.57	0.97	0.87	1.54	3.82
39	0.73	1.23	1.12	1.89	2.67
40	0.94	1.59	1.45	2.50	3.40
41	1.23	2.00	1.89	3.23	6.11
42	1.56	2.56	2.44	4.00	8.05
43	2.00	3.33	3.23	5.26	5.15
44	2.63	4.17	4.00	6.67	10.00
45	3.33	5.26	5.26	8.33	7.14

* Estimated live-born statistics. (Schreinemacher DM, Cross PK, Hook EB. Rates of trisomies 21, 18, 13 and other chromosome abnormalities in about 20,000 prenatal studies compared with estimated rate in live births. Hum Genet 1982;61:318.)

† Data compiled from 20,000 genetic amniocenteses. (Schreinemacher DM, Cross PK, Hook EB. Rates of trisomies 21, 18, 13 and other chromosome abnormalities in about 20,000 prenatal studies compared with estimated rate in live births. Hum Genet 1982;61:318.)

‡ Data derived from 4122 CVS; corrected from unconfirmed aberrations, especially mosaicism. (Mikkelsen M, Ayme A. Chromosomal findings in chorionic villi. A collaborative study. In: Vogel F, Sperling K, eds. Proceedings of the 7th International Congress of Human Genetics. Berlin: Springer-Verlag, 1987:598.)

the father or the mother is the carrier, and the specific chromosome involved.[2,3]

Reciprocal Translocation

Reciprocal translocation is a result of chromosome breaks of two nonhomologous chromosomes and subsequent exchange of chromosome segments. When a germ cell with a reciprocal translocation undergoes meiosis, the two translocation chromosomes and their homologues will form a quadrivalent configuration (Fig. 30-1). Theoretically, a gamete can receive any combination of the two chromosomes, any three chromosomes, all four, any one, or none. However, there are three major ways of segregation—alternate segregation, adjacent I (adjacent nonhomologous), and adjacent 2 (adjacent homologous). Fertilization of gametes from alternate segregation would result in fetuses with either a normal chromosome constitution or a balanced reciprocal translocation like that of the parent. Fertilization of gametes from adjacent 1 or adjacent 2 segregation will lead to unbalanced rearrangements with chromosome duplication and deficiency, which would cause either fetal loss or a live-born with abnormalities.

An earlier report,[2] as well as a revised and updated analysis,[3,4] showed an overall risk of 11% to 13% for producing a child with an unbalanced chromosome constitution. Mother carriers do not carry a higher risk than father carriers, in contrast to what was once believed.[5] However, there is an obvious difference in the frequency of detection of fetuses with an unbalanced chromosome constitution when different methods of ascertainment are used (Table 30-2). The proportion of chromosomally unbalanced progeny is rather high (18% to 28%) when ascertained through live births with an unbalanced karyotype in comparison to the frequency of unbalanced progeny ascertained through recurrent miscarriage or other means (3% to 5%). According to the most recent data, the risk is highest (approximately 50%) for carriers of complex chromosome rearrangements, insertions, and reciprocal transloca-

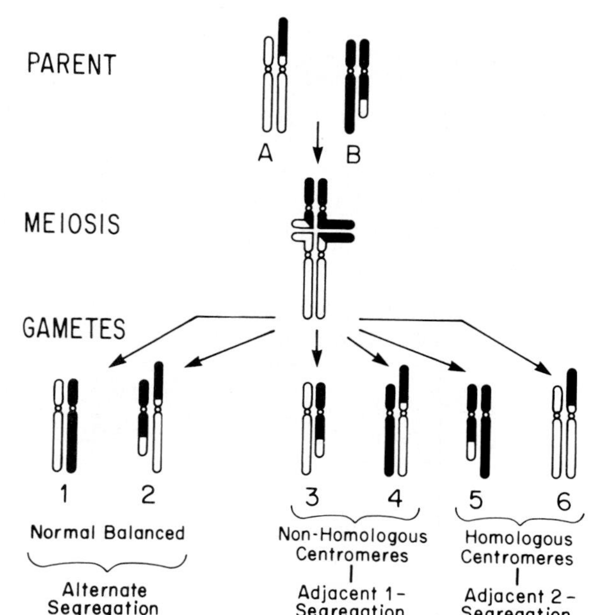

FIGURE 30–1. Meiotic segregation in a balanced reciprocal translocation involving two nonhomologous chromosomes (A and B) illustrating how the six major types of gametes may be produced. (Courtesy of Dr. Dagmar Kalousek, 1988.)

TABLE 30–2. OUTCOME OF PRENATAL DIAGNOSIS FOR PREGNANCIES OR RECIPROCAL TRANSLOCATION CARRIERS (N = 596) FREQUENCIES (%) OF NORMAL AND BALANCED VERSUS UNBALANCED FETAL CHROMOSOMES IN RELATION TO METHODS OF ASCERTAINMENT*

METHOD OF ASCERTAINMENT	FATHER CARRIER (N = 243)		MOTHER CARRIER (N = 353)		TOTAL NO. OF CASES
	BALANCED AND NORMAL (%)	UNBALANCED (%)	BALANCED AND NORMAL (%)	UNBALANCED (%)	
By unbalanced progeny	71.4	28.6	81.9	18.1	235
By recurrent miscarriages	97.3	2.7	95.3	4.7	180
By other means	93.7	6.3	92.2	7.8	181
Overall	86.4	13.6	88.9	11.1	596

* (Daniel A, Boué A, Gallano P. Prospective risk in reciprocal translocation in heterozygotes at amniocentesis as determined by potential chromosome inbalance sizes. Data of the European collaborative prenatal diagnosis centres. Prenat Diagn 1986;6:315.)

tions ascertained through an unbalanced proband with "small" unbalanced segments.[3]

In a European collaborative CVS study of 75 parents who are carriers of a reciprocal translocation, 17 (22.7%) of the analyses showed unbalanced progeny; 24 (32%), normal chromosomes; and 34 (45.3%), balanced carriers.[6] There was no difference in the frequencies of unbalanced fetuses when mother carriers and father carriers were compared.

Robertsonian Translocation

Robertsonian translocation is also referred to as centric-fusion type translocation. It is a fusion of the entire long arms of two acrocentric chromosomes after breakage at the centromeres. In humans, an individual with a "balanced" Robertsonian translocation shows only 45 chromosomes, with the translocation chromosome containing the two complete long arms of the two acrocentric chromosomes involved. The short arms of the two chromosomes are absent. It is known that individuals with a "balanced" Robertsonian translocation usually have a normal phenotype. Apparently, the short arms of acrocentric chromosomes do not carry important genetic material. However, when a germ cell with a Robertsonian translocation undergoes meiosis, the translocation chromosome and its homologues will form a trivalent. Fertilization of gametes resulting from alternate segregation would result in a fetus with either a normal chromosome constitution or a "balanced" Robertsonian translocation like the parent's. Since it is not possible to identify the origin of the centromere of this translocation chromosome, one cannot distinguish adjacent 1 from adjacent 2 segregation in Robertsonian translocations.

In a collaborative study, a total of 517 prenatal diagnoses were provided to couples in which one member was a carrier for a Robertsonian translocation.[2] All 216 D/D translocation carriers produced offspring with either a normal karyotype or a "balanced" translocation like the parent's. No fetus was found to have an unbalanced D/D translocation (Table 30-3). It made no difference whether the mother or the father was the carrier. Therefore, couples with a D/D translocation appear to carry a low risk for producing offspring with an unbalanced translocation. This probably indicates that D/D unbalanced fetuses tend to be aborted early in pregnancy (before mid-trimester). On the other hand, the European collaborative study,[2] as well as data from United States and Canadian laboratories,[3] showed that

TABLE 30–3. SEGREGATION OF ROBERTSONIAN TRANSLOCATION NOT INVOLVING CHROMOSOME 21 (DATA FROM AMNIOCENTESIS ONLY)

TYPE OF TRANSLOCATION	NUMBER OF DIAGNOSES	OFFSPRING		
		NORMAL	BALANCED	UNBALANCED
13q14q	230	96	134	—
13q15q	15	4	11	—
14q15q	6	4	2	—
13q22q	3	—	2	1*
14q22q	3	—	3	—
15q22q	5	2	3	—

(Data from Boué A, Gallano P. A collaborative study of the segregation of inherited chromosome structural rearrangements in 1356 prenatal diagnoses. Prenat Diagn (Special Issue), 1984;4:45.)
* Mother is carrier.

TABLE 30–4. FREQUENCIES OF UNBALANCED FETAL CHROMOSOMES IN PREGNANCIES OF CARRIERS WITH A ROBERTSONIAN TRANSLOCATION INVOLVING CHROMOSOME 21

	AMINOCENTESIS*				CHORIONIC VILLI SAMPLE (CVS)†			
	MOTHER CARRIER		FATHER CARRIER		MOTHER CARRIER		FATHER CARRIER	
	TOTAL NUMBER	UNBALANCED (%)	TOTAL NUMBER	UNBALANCED (%)	TOTAL NUMBER	UNBALANCED (%)	TOTAL NUMBER	UNBALANCED (%)
13q21q	20	2 (10.0)	11	0	3	1 (33.3)††	—	—
14q21q	137	21 (15.3)	51	0	33	4 (12.1)††	7	0
15q21q	9	1 (11.1)	5	0	2	1 (50.0)††	2	0
21q22q	19	3 (15.8)	3	0	4	0	—	—

*Data from Boué A, Gallano P. A collaborative study of the segregation of inherited chromosome structural rearrangements in 1356 prenatal diagnoses. Prenat Diagn (Special Issue), 1984;4:45.

† Mikkelsen M, Ayme A. Chromosomal findings in chorionic villi. A collaborative study. In: Vogel F, Sperling K, eds. Proceedings of the 7th International Congress of Human Genetics. Berlin: Springer-Verlag, 1987:598.

†† Insufficient data for accurate assessment.

a female carrier of a Robertsonian translocation involving chromosome 21 has a high risk (10% to 15%) (Table 30-4) of carrying a fetus with an unbalanced chromosome constitution. The preliminary CVS data are compatible with amniocentesis data but are still too few to be meaningful (Table 30-4).

Inversion

An inversion results when there has been a double break in one chromosome, reversal of a segment, and repair in the inverted sequence. If the inversion includes the centromere, a pericentric inversion results. If it is confined to a single arm of the chromosome, it is called paracentric. Prenatal diagnosis should be recommended to couples when one is a carrier of a pericentric inversion. When a germ cell with a pericentric inversion undergoes meiosis, the inverted chromosome forms a loop in order to line up all homologous segments for proper pairing. A crossover within the loop of the inversion may result in a gamete with an unbalanced chromosome constitution. The risk of having an abnormal child from carriers with a paracentric inversion is low, because a crossover within the loop would result in unstable gametes with acentric fragments or dicentric chromosomes.

The risk of a pericentric inversion carrier parent's producing a fetus with an unbalanced karyotype is reported as 5.9% (Table 30-5). However, recent data from Daniel and colleagues suggest that carriers of pericentric inversions of small distal segments have a higher risk (10% to 15%).[3]

Inv(9)qh, a common chromosome polymorphism, is a pericentric inversion of chromosome 9 involving only the heterochromatic secondary constriction region. This type of inversion is not considered a justified indication for prenatal diagnosis.

PREVIOUS CHILD WITH CHROMOSOME ABNORMALITIES

When a pregnant woman has had a child or fetus with a noninherited chromosome aberration, the risk for a chromosomally abnormal fetus is significantly increased, especially when the woman is under the age of 30 years.[1] Of 2890 prenatal diagnoses through amniocentesis, performed because of a previous child with a noninherited chromosome aberration, the overall risk for a chromosomally abnormal fetus was 1.42%. The risk ranged from 1.0% to 1.9% in five different maternal age groups (20 to 24, 25 to 29, 30 to 34, 35 to 39, and over 40), with no significant differences.[7] Of 2353 amniocenteses performed because of an index case with trisomy-21, 35 fetuses (1.49%) were found to have abnormal karyotypes, including 19 cases of trisomy 21

TABLE 30–5. SEGREGATIONS OF INVERSIONS

CARRIER	TOTAL NUMBER OF DIAGNOSES	OFFSPRING NORMAL	BALANCED	UNBALANCED (%)
Father	51	14	35	2 (3.9)
Mother	67	32	30	5 (7.5)
Total	118	46	65	7 (5.9)

Data from Boué A, Gallano P. A collaborative study of the segregation of inherited chromosome structural rearrangements in 1356 prenatal diagnoses. Prenat Diagn (Special Issue), 1984;4:45.

(0.80%) and 16 cases of other abnormalities (0.69%) (Table 30-6).

Of 556 CVS cases studied because of a previous child or fetus with a noninherited chromosome aberration, 12 cases (2.15%) were found to have chromosome aberrations.[6]

The CVS data for recurrence of viable autosomal trisomies are comparable to those from amniocentesis: roughly 1% for younger mothers. Of 369 pregnancies in women aged 34 years or younger, four (1.08%) resulted in a trisomic fetus, and of 185 pregnancies in women aged 35 years or older, two (1.05%) carried a trisomic fetus.

LOW MATERNAL SERUM α-FETOPROTEIN

An association between low maternal serum α-fetoprotein (MSAFP) and fetal chromosome aneuploidy was first suggested by Merkatz and colleagues.[8] The correlation more specifically with trisomy 21 (Down syndrome) was subsequently confirmed.[9] By combining the maternal serum AFP concentration with the gestational age of the fetus and the mother's weight and age, the risk for Down syndrome can be estimated. Several groups have generated risk figures for use by genetic counselors in advising prospective mothers.[10–16] Since there are variations among all these published studies, Hook suggests that caution be used before quoting the published risk figures during genetic counseling, especially to older women where the data are insufficient. An established risk table from one laboratory may not be completely applicable for another laboratory.[17] Because the MSAFP level varies with gestation, it is essential to verify the gestational age by ultrasound before quoting a risk. If the risk figure for Down syndrome is greater than or equal to 1 in 270 (the risk of a 35-year-old woman having a live-born with Down syndrome), it is considered an increased risk and an indication for amniocentesis.

It must be kept in mind, however, that a normal (or high) MSAFP level does not preclude the possibility of a Down syndrome fetus. By using low MSAFP levels to screen pregnant women under 35 years of age, only 20% to 30% of all Down syndrome pregnancies can be expected to be detected.[14,18] When patients are offered MSAFP screening, careful counseling may help to prevent the intense anxiety exhibited by some patients when told they have a low MSAFP. They should be informed beforehand that although a low MSAFP may lead to a diagnosis of Down syndrome, by itself it is merely an indication for amniocentesis. Normal chromosome finding is still by far the most likely outcome of amniocentesis. Thus, it should be clear that MSAFP screening is not a substitute for amniocentesis.

Because of the low detection rate and high false-positive rate of MSAFP for fetal Down syndrome, investigators have tried other biochemical assays, such as maternal serum unconjugated estriol (uE_3) and serum human chorionic gonadotrophin (hCG).[19–22] Correlations were demonstrated between fetal Down syndrome and low serum unconjugated estriol, as well as high serum hCG concentration. A combination of MSAFP, estriol, and hCG (ie, a triple testing) would probably increase the detection rate and reduce the false-positive rate from MSAFP alone.

TABLE 30–6. OBSERVED RISK FOR CHROMOSOME ABNORMALITIES IN CONCEPTIONS AFTER A PREVIOUS CHILD/FETUS WITH A NONINHERITED CHROMOSOME ABERRATION (AMNIOCENTESIS DATA)

INDEX CASE	TOTAL PRENATAL DIAGNOSES	ABNORMAL FETAL CHROMOSOME (%)
Trisomy 21	2353	35 (1.5)
Trisomy 18	171	2 (1.2)
Trisomy 13	99	0
Sex chromosome aberration	91	1 (1.1)
De novo translocation	58	0
Deletion	40	1 (2.5)
Mosaic	24	1 (4.2)
Triploidy	10	1 (10.0)

Data from Stene J, Steine E, Mikkelsen M. Risk for chromosome abnormality at amniocentesis following a child with a non-inherited chromosome aberration. Prenat Diagn (Special Issue), 1984;4:81.

OTHER INDICATIONS

History of Unexplained Fetal Wastage, Subfertility, or Unexplained Perinatal Death

Each case with such history should be evaluated individually to determine the priority of prenatal cytogenetic diagnosis. It is known that approximately 40% of first-trimester spontaneous abortions are associated with a major chromosome abnormality.[1] In studies of couples experiencing multiple spontaneous abortions, a mean of 5.1% (with a range from 2.2% to 7.4%) had chromosome abnormalities in one of the partners (such as a balanced reciprocal translocation).[1] There is apparently a positive relationship between the number of spontaneous abortions and the frequency of parental chromosome aberrations. Couples with a history of a stillborn or malformed infant have a greater frequency of chromosomal abnormalities (16.7%) than couples with no such history (5.4%). Therefore, if parental chromosome studies cannot be done first, couples with repeated spontaneous abortions and a history of stillbirths or a malformed infant should receive higher priority in obtaining prenatal diagnosis than couples with repeated fetal loss but no such history.

Subfertility may be associated with chromosome abnormalities.[1] Over 5% of oligozoospermic or azoospermic men had constitutional chromosome abnormalities. Subfertility or repeated spontaneous abortions have been reported in females with 45,X or 47,XXX mosaicism.

Abnormal Parental Karyotype (Other Than a Balanced Structural Rearrangement)

If a parent has a sex chromosome aneuploidy not affecting his or her reproductive ability, such as XYY or XXX, the risk of producing offspring with a sex chromosome abnormality is increased. Individuals may also be mosaic for an autosome trisomy or a sex chromosome abnormality. These individuals must be considered to have an increased risk. Trisomy-21 mosaicism has been found in both mothers and fathers of Down syndrome patients.[1] Several of these reported mosaic parents had two affected children with trisomy 21. Prenatal cytogenetic diagnosis should be offered. But since the vast majority of XYY males and XXX females remain unidentified because of a grossly normal phenotype, prenatal diagnosis for this indication is infrequent.

Previous Affected Child With Fragile-X Syndrome or Mother Known to Be a Carrier for Fragile X

Fragile X syndrome, one common form of X-linked mental retardation, is an inherited abnormality of the X chromosome that causes disabilities ranging from varying degrees of learning problems to mental retardation.[22a] The fragile X chromosome has a narrowing of chromosomal material or a break at the distal end of the long arm at q27.3. Features most commonly associated with the syndrome are severe language delays, behavior problems, autism or autistic-like behaviors, delayed motor development, macroorchidism, large or prominent ears, and prominent jaw.[22a]

The fragile X was first recognized by Lubs in 1969.[22b] It was not until 1977 that Sutherland[23] demonstrated that the expression of the fragile site was dependent on the cell culture conditions. Folic acid and thymidine inhibit expression of the fragile X, whereas folate antagonists induce expression. Folate antagonists have been especially useful in detection of the fragile X in fibroblasts, lymphoblasts, and cultured amniotic fluid cells. Even under optimal conditions, the fragile X is usually observed in less than half of metaphases from affected males and not at all in cells from certain carrier females. The structural nature of the fragile X and the relationship of the fragile site to mental retardation are not known. It is estimated that one to two of every 2000 to 3000 males carries a fragile X gene, yet a significant proportion of these males (transmitting males) might not show fragile X or such a syndrome. Currently, with cytogenetic methods, fragile X is prenatally diagnosable through amniocentesis, chorionic villous sampling, and PUBS.[23a,23b] In experienced laboratories, a positive result can be considered reliable; a negative result is only 90% to 95% reliable. By and large, amniocytes have been used for diagnosis. Use of CVS is still considered experimental.[23b] Negative results from CVS should be confirmed by molecular methods or by a cytogenetic method using another tissue.[23b]

Recently, a gene containing a CGG repeat (designated FMR-1) was identified as the candidate gene for fragile X syndrome.[24] With newer molecular methods using specific DNA probes such as Ox 1.9[24a] and St B 12.3,[24b] the reliability of prenatal diagnosis of fragile X can be further enhanced.

Previous Affected Child With a Chromosome Breakage Syndrome

Fanconi anemia, Bloom syndrome, ataxia telangiectasia, xeroderma pigmentosum, and Werner syndrome are the five major autosomal recessive diseases associated with an increased incidence of chromosome breakage and rearrangement. Prenatal diagnosis of Fanconi anemia is reported to be reliable in both cultured amniotic fluid cells and CVS when baseline chromosome breakage and breakage induced by diepoxybutane (DEB) are studied.[25,26] Ataxia telangiectasia is also prenatally diagnosable by a combined scoring of spontaneous breakage rate and the clastogenic potential of at-risk amniocytes.[27] Since sister chromatid exchange (SCE) can be scored in both cultured amniotic fluid cells and CVS, prenatal diagnosis of diseases characterized by changes in the SCE rate is potentially feasible.

Previous Affected Child With Robert Syndrome (SC Phocomelia Syndrome)

Robert syndrome is inherited in an autosomal recessive fashion. Cytogenetically, it is characterized by premature centromere separation, readily noticeable in cultured metaphase cells if the examiner is alerted to its significance.

Prenatal Sex Determination for X-Linked Disorders Not Prenatally Diagnosable

The category of X-linked disorders that are not diagnosable prenatally is rapidly shrinking and will become obsolete once all X-linked disorders are prenatally diagnosable. Prenatal fetal sex determination is acceptable only for an X-linked disorder that is not prenatally diagnosable; it is not acceptable solely for social reasons.

Miscellaneous Considerations

Maternal anxiety is often given as an indication for prenatal diagnosis when the reason for the amniocentesis is not within the generally accepted medical guidelines. Couples who desire amniocentesis even though there are no specific medical indications for such testing must be fully counseled regarding the risks and limitations of prenatal cytogenetic diagnosis.

For a short time there was serious concern about a possible association between carriers of a double NOR variant and increased risk for having children with Down syndrome. The association was suggested by Jackson-Cook and colleagues.[28] Recent studies provide evidence to reject this speculation, however.[29,30]

Questions still remain. For example, does maternal radiation exposure or exposure to chemotherapy or to a mutagen increase the frequency of aneuploid progeny? If such exposures are accepted as indications, they should be regarded as low priority or maternal anxiety.

TECHNICAL CONSIDERATIONS FOR PRENATAL CYTOGENETIC DIAGNOSIS

AMNIOTIC FLUID CELL CULTURES

The 1979 International Workshop on Prenatal Diagnosis made the following recommendations[31]:

1. Prenatal cytogenetic diagnosis should be a team effort combining expertise in obstetrics, ultrasonography, genetic counseling, cytogenetics, clinical genetics, and biochemical genetics.
2. One cytogeneticist at the doctoral level should supervise every four or five technical staff members.
3. The annual case load per technologist should not exceed 150 fluid specimens for fetal karyotype.
4. A minimum of 100 amniotic fluid specimens per year should be required to maintain the technical competency of a cytogenetics laboratory providing prenatal cytogenetic diagnoses.
5. A new cytogenetic laboratory should achieve successful diagnoses in 20 to 30 "split specimens" (split with established laboratories). The minimum success rate should be 95%, and case completion should be within 21 days for 20 consecutive specimens.
6. Final diagnosis should be reported no later than 21 days.
7. Regardless of the cell culture method employed (eg, trypsinized cells or in situ clones), cytogenetic analysis should be derived from a minimum of two separate primary cultures.
8. Chromosome banding techniques should be used in all laboratories providing prenatal diagnosis.

Today most of these earlier recommendations are adopted as minimal requirements. In general, it is now believed that a trained technician can be responsible for four or five cases a week and an experienced technologist can handle six cases per week, with an annual case load of over 250 cases. The average turn-around time (TAT) has also been significantly improved. Although a completion time of 20 days is still considered acceptable, many laboratories have reduced TAT to less than 15 days. Some report a TAT of 10 days or less.

It is advisable to have a minimum of three containers set up as primary cultures and grown in a minimum of two incubators, preferably using two different types of medium. It is recommended that a minimum of 20 metaphases or 10 to 15 colonies (for in situ techniques) from two containers be counted and a minimum of three metaphases be analyzed under the microscope. A minimum of two additional cells should be karyotyped by photography or using an automated system. All karyotypes should be banded with either G-, Q-, or R-banding. A minimum of approximately 400 bands per haploid set is required.

CHORIONIC VILLI PREPARATION AND CULTURE

Although no guidelines for cytogenetic diagnosis using CVS have been published, it is generally understood that any cytogenetic laboratory that wishes to accept a diagnostic chorionic villi specimen must first complete a set number of experimental CVS studies from noncontinuing pregnancies so as to develop and establish its competency in achieving a diagnosis. Such a laboratory must have adequate procedures for dissecting villi from maternal decidual tissues. Both direct preparation (to study cytotrophoblasts) and long-term culture (to assay mesenchymal-core cells) are to be set up and used for final cytogenetic diagnosis. Although direct CVS preparation can minimize the risk of maternal cell contamination, long-term villi culture can provide better-quality metaphase cells for cytogenetic analysis. Whenever there is suspicion of maternal cell contamination, a comparison of chromosome polymorphisms of the 46,XX cells with those of the mother's should be made.

Other requirements, such as the number of cells to be counted in each type of these two preparations, the number of cells to be karyotyped, and the quality of banding, are yet to be determined. Currently, it appears that counting 15 to 20 cells, analysis of four, and karyotyping of two cells from each of the two methods (direct and culture) is considered more than adequate.[32,33] Whenever the diagnosis is uncertain, especially in findings of unusual aneuploidies or possible mosaicism, it is highly advisable to use amniocentesis as a backup study to determine the significance of the findings in question.

BACKUP LABORATORY

A cytogenetic laboratory providing prenatal diagnosis should have a backup agreement with a second cytogenetic laboratory to prevent interruption of services caused by a potential laboratory catastrophe, such as equipment failure, massive laboratory microbial contamination, and so on.

LIMITATIONS OF A ROUTINE PRENATAL CYTOGENETIC DIAGNOSIS

The limitations of a routine prenatal cytogenetic diagnosis must be carefully explained to the prospective parents during the genetic counseling session before amniocentesis or CVS. Most important, all patients must be advised that a normal karyotype does not necessarily imply a normal phenotype. Many varieties of birth defects cannot be detected by chromosome analysis. Although other methods of prenatal diagnosis are available for the detection of a number of nonchromosomal birth defects and genetic disorders, they are generally performed only when a specific indication is present.

A routine prenatal cytogenetic diagnosis is designed primarily to detect numerical abnormalities and major structural aberrations. With a generally accepted standard protocol, neither high-resolution banding nor fragile-X studies are carried out unless there is an indication for such studies. Therefore, a subtle structural abnormality may easily go undetected and a fragile-X chromosome cannot be diagnosed. Low-level chromosome mosaicism could also be missed. A minute or subtle structural abnormality may require molecular confirmation in addition to high-resolution banding. For example, even in postnatal cytogenetic study two children with Wolf-Hirschhorn syndrome were found to have normal-appearing chromosomes; yet on the molecular level they were proved to have a very small deletion of 4p.[34,35]

In addition, one must realize that maternal cell contamination is not a rare event. Occasionally, maternal cells may outgrow fetal cells, leading to a misdiagnosis. Patients should also be informed that both parents may be called for studies to confirm maternal cell contamination or to identify the origin and the nature of chromosome polymorphism or a structural abnormality.

Patients undergoing CVS diagnosis should be informed that if there is an uncertain diagnosis, they may be advised to have amniocentesis for further evaluation. It would be wise to cover all these crucial points in the informed consent. Every effort should be made to have patients read and understand the contents of the consent form.

PROBLEMS AND PITFALLS IN PRENATAL CYTOGENETIC DIAGNOSIS

Although the major problems and pitfalls are quite similar for both genetic amniocentesis and CVS, much of the data and experience that have been accumulated come from studies of amniocytes rather than of chorionic villi.

GENETIC AMNIOCENTESIS

Chromosome Mosaicism

The findings of cells with both normal and abnormal karyotypes in the same amniotic fluid specimen lead to the diagnostic dilemma of distinguishing true chromosome mosaicism (an in vivo abnormality) from pseudomosaicism (an in vitro finding). It is now well accepted that a diagnosis of true mosaicism should be accepted only when two cell populations with different karyotypes are found in multiple independent culture vessels. If one uses in situ harvesting and analyzes cells from colonies, the findings of an identical aneuploidy from a minimum of two different culture vessels should still be a major criterion for diagnosing true chromosome mosaicism. The findings of identical aneuploidy cells from two or more clones restricted to one culture vessel do not meet this criterion because cell migration occurs from one colony to another, and colonies may be formed by aggregates of cells of independent origin.

It must be realized that chromosome mosaicism can never be completely ruled out. According to a statistical analysis, a routine analysis of 15 to 20 cells or clones can detect only mosaicism with 14% to 19% of aneuploid cells at 95% confidence level.[36] This means that a low-level mosaicism (containing less than 14% of aneuploid cells) may go undetected. Benn and colleagues estimated that even when up to three separate cultures are extensively analyzed with an average of 24 cells per culture examined, a minimum of 4.5% of cases of true mosaicism could be undiagnosed and 7% could be diagnosed as pseudomosaicism.[37]

With in situ harvesting there are three different types of chromosome pseudomosaicism, namely, one region (in a colony) with an abnormal karyotype, an entire single colony with the same aberrant karyotype, and multiple colonies within the same culture vessel showing an identical abnormal karyotype.[38] With trypsinized amniocytes there are two types of pseudomosaicism (ie, multiple cells showing an identical abnormality and a single cell showing an aberrant karyotype). In the latter system, one cannot distinguish whether the multiple cells are derived from one initial clone or multiple clones.

According to three large surveys, the frequency of true chromosome mosaicism in cultured amniocytes ranged from 0.1% to 0.3% (Table 30-7). The frequency of pseudomosaicism with multiple cells showing an identical abnormality but restricted to one culture vessel ranged from 0.64% to 1.1% (see Table 30-7). The frequency of finding a single cell or a single clone with an aberrant karyotype is not at all rare, ranging from 2.47% to 7.1%. All three surveys showed that the most frequent in vitro finding in cultured amniocytes is trisomy 2. In addition, there are indications that five other chromosomes are more frequently involved in pseudomosaicism for trisomies than the remaining chromosomes. They are chromosomes 7, X, 17, 20, and 9.[1] The vast majority of these cases diagnosed as pseudomosaicism appeared grossly normal at birth, were not rekaryotyped, and consequently had no follow-up. The risk for an apparent pseudomosaicism to be true mosaicism is not known, but it should not be confused with the risk of showing phenotypic abnormalities, which is far lower than that for true mosaicism.

Autosome Mosaicism. Various chromosome mosaicisms involving numerical and structural abnormalities have been diagnosed prenatally. The six most common types of autosome mosaicism are 46/47,+20,

TABLE 30–7. FREQUENCY OF MOSAICISM AND PSEUDOMOSAICISM IN AMNIOTIC FLUID STUDIES

ORIGIN OF DATA	MOSAICISM		PSEUDOMOSAICISM			
			MULTIPLE CELLS OR CLONES*		SINGLE CELL OR CLONE*	
	TOTAL CASES STUDIED	PERCENT SHOWING MOSAICISM	Cases Studied	% Showing Pseudomosaicism	Cases Studied	% Showing Pseudomosaicism
United States Survey†	62,279	0.25	48,442	0.70	30,754	2.47
European Survey‡	44,170	0.10	44,170	0.64	44,170	2.84
Canadian Survey§	12,386	0.30	12,386	1.10	12,386	7.10

* Restricted to one culture vessel.

† United States Survey. (Hsu LYF, Perlis T. United States survey on chromosome mosaicism and pseudomosaicism in prenatal diagnosis. Prenat Diagn [Special Issue], 1984;4:97.)

‡ European Survey. (Bui TH, Iselius L, Lindsten J. European collaborative study on prenatal diagnosis: mosaicism, pseudomosaicism and single abnormal cell in amniotic fluid cell cultures. Prenat Diagn [Special Issue] 1984;4:145.)

§ Canadian Survey. (Worton RG, Stern R. A Canadian collaborative study of mosaicism in amniotic fluid cell cultures. Prenat Diagn (Special Issue), 1984;4:131.)

46/47,+21, 46/47,+9, 46/47,+8, 46/47,+13, and 46/47,+18.

Trisomy-20 mosaicism is the most common autosome mosaicism diagnosed from genetic amniocentesis.[39,40] It remains a dilemma in diagnosis and counseling. A review of 103 such cases (Table 30-8) gave the following conclusions:

1. Approximately 90% of cases were associated with grossly normal phenotype.
2. There is a strong likelihood that in the majority of cases, the cells with trisomy 20 were extraembryonic in origin (or confined to the placenta) and thus were not representative of the fetus. This possibility is supported by the following facts:
   a. In one case, trisomy 20 was identified in 100% of cells cultured from the amnion, but not in fetal tissues.[41] In five other cases, some cells with trisomy 20 were detected in placental tissues and membranes.[39,40] Confinement of chromosome mosaicism (not necessarily trisomy 20) to the placenta was demonstrated by Kalousek and Dill in 1983.[42]
   b. Although trisomy-20 mosaicism is the most frequently seen autosome mosaicism, it is the one least likely to be associated with major birth defects.
3. Of the 11 cases with phenotypic abnormalities the description of facial dysmorphism in six abortuses was vague and uninformative, and it is doubtful that trisomy-20 mosaicism was the underlying cause of the unilateral cleft lip in one live-born and William syndrome in another. The major concern should still be the urinary tract abnormalities found in three abortuses and the congenital heart defects in two. Detailed ultrasound scan of the fetus with special emphasis on the renal and cardiovascular systems could help the prospective parents in their decision making.
4. In those cases where cells with trisomy 20 were recovered, it is only in certain specific fetal tissues —such as kidney (six cases), lung (two cases), esophagus (one case), and rectum (one case)—that it appears that trisomy 20 could be tissue specific or that such a trisomy is more likely to be confined to specific tissues.
5. Trisomy 20 has thus far not been recovered from blood cultures. Therefore, fetal blood sampling is unhelpful for further evaluation of trisomy-20 mosaicism.
6. For cytogenetic confirmation in live-borns—in addition to studies of placenta, skin, and blood cells—urine sediment cell culture is strongly recommended. In fact, one recent case was confirmed by this method.[43] We know that if the mosaicism is real, kidney cells would be a good source for finding trisomy-20 cells.
7. Only 18 cases had follow-up of 1 year or more. Longer follow-up and careful developmental evaluation of all pregnancies continued to term are needed.

Trisomy-21 mosaicism is the second most frequent autosomal mosaicism diagnosed prenatally. Of 53 cases with 46/47,+21 mosaicism (Table 30-9),[1,44] termination was elected in 47 (88.7%). Phenotypic information was available in only 24 cases. Of these, 17 were described as abnormal and compatible with Down syndrome; seven appeared to be phenotypically normal. Of 36 cases with successful follow-up cytogenetic studies, mosaicism was confirmed in 28 and straight trisomy 21 was confirmed in three.

The next most frequent prenatally diagnosed group of autosome trisomy mosaicisms includes mosaicism for trisomy 9, trisomy 18, trisomy 13, and trisomy 8 (Table 30-10).

Of 18 cases with 46/47,+9, 16 patients elected to terminate their pregnancies. Of 15 cases with available

TABLE 30–8. 46/47,+20 MOSAICISM*

PHENOTYPE	NUMBER OF CASES		
Grossly normal (90)	73 live-borns†; 17 abortuses		
Grossly abnormal (11)	3 live-borns; 8 abortuses		
	Abnormal live-borns		
	1—Unilateral cleft lip		
	1—Williams syndrome		
	1—MCA, including facial asymmetry, microcephaly, low-set abnormal ears, etc.		
	Abnormal abortuses		
	1—Facial dysmorphism and microcephaly		
	1—Renal anomalies (megapelvis and kinky ureters)		
	1—Slight facial dysmorphism and microretrognathia		
	1—Facial dysmorphism		
	1—Facial dysmorphism, congenital heart disease (transposition of great arteries, pulmonary stenosis, hypoplasia of right ventricle, and hypoplasia of tricuspid and bicuspid valves), anal fistula, camptodactyly		
	1—Micrognathia, abnormal ears, renal anomalies (pelvic horseshow kidneys), and congenital heart disease (stenosis of ductus Botalli, hypoplasia of right ventricle, and hypertrophy of ventricle walls)		
	1—Slight facial dysmorphism, epicanthal folds, microretrognathia, abnormal ears, and meandering of left ureter		
	1—Occipital and cervical meningocele		
Turner syndrome	1 (abortus with monosomy X)		
Hydrops	1 (abortus with Rh incompatibility)		
CYTOGENETIC CONFIRMATORY STUDIES	**NUMBER OF CASES**		
46/47,+20	19 cases‡		
	Cells with 47,+20 were recovered from kidney (6 cases); skin/muscle/fascia (5 cases); lung (2 cases); esophagus (1 case); rectum 1 case; urine sediment (1 case); placental tissues/membrane/amnion (6 cases).		
Normal Chromosomes	68 cases		
Blood only	43	Skin only	2
Blood and skin	6	Placenta only	2
Blood and placenta	5	Skin and other tissue	2
Blood, skin and placenta	4	Placenta and other tissue	2
		Abortion fluid only	2
No Study or Unsuccessful Study	16 cases		

Total number of cases:	103	(from 102 pregnancies including one pair of twins)
Pregnancy Continued	75	(one carried twins)
Pregnancy Terminated	26	
Spontaneous abortion	1	(hydrops—Rh incompatibility)

* Data from Reference 39 (67 cases); reference 40 (36 cases).

† Eighteen cases with follow up ≥1 year, one was noted to have borderline psychomotor delay; all others were reported to be normal.

‡ Four cases showed cells with 47,+20 from more than one source.

information, eight abortuses were described as grossly abnormal, and one live-born had intrauterine growth retardation. Five abortuses had multiple congenital malformations (four had congenital heart disease), and three were without a specific description of the abnormality. Six abortuses were recorded as grossly normal with no noticeable abnormalities. No information was available on the remaining two abortuses. One live-born, whose trisomy-9 mosaicism was confirmed in blood culture, was small for gestation at birth and was reported to have delayed psychomotor development. One live-born was reported to have a normal karyotype; there was no phenotypic description. Overall, trisomy-9 mosaicism was confirmed in seven of 14 cases with successful cytogenetic studies.

At least 15 cases of trisomy-18 mosaicism have been diagnosed prenatally. Six of seven abortuses with available information were described as phenotypically abnormal. The mosaicism was confirmed in all successful cytogenetic follow-up studies.

Of 11 cases with 46/47,+13, four of 10 with available information showed phenotypic abnormalities. Three of seven successful cytogenetic follow-up studies confirmed 46/47,+13.

TABLE 30–9. 46/47,+21 MOSAICISM

Total Number of Cases	53
Outcome of Pregnancy	
Continued	6
Terminated	47
Phenotype	
Abnormal, compatible with Down syndrome	17 (15 abortuses, 2 live-borns)
Grossly normal	7 (6 abortuses, 1 live-born)
No information	29
Cytogenetic Confirmatory Studies	
46/47,+21	28 (19 fetal tissues; 7 abortion fluids; 2 live-born blood)
Normal karyotype	5 (2 fetal tissues; 1 liveborn blood; 2 abortion fluids;
All trisomy 21	3 (All fetal tissues)
No study or unsuccessful study	17 cases

Data from references 1 (37 cases) and 44 (16 cases).

Interestingly, of 10 cases with 46/47,+8, only one abortus was reported to be phenotypically abnormal (with no detailed description), yet cytogenetic confirmation of 46/47,+8 was achieved in 75% (six of eight) of cases with successful follow-up studies. It is known that clinical diagnosis of trisomy 8 or trisomy-8 mosaicism in a live-born is difficult. Therefore, it is conceivable that recognition of subtle phenotypic abnormalities in an abortus could be even more difficult. It is important to remember the minimum criterion for diagnosis of chromosome mosaicism, namely, detection of two cell populations in at least two independent culture vessels. One case clearly demonstrated the value of this criterion.[49] In this case, only two cells of 47,+8 were found in the amniotic fluid culture (one of 20 cells in each of two flasks). However, 16 of 20 skin fibroblasts from the abortus showed 47,+8. Camurri and colleagues reported a case with an initial diagnosis of pseudomosaicism that resulted in a grossly normal liveborn but proved to be a true 46/47,+8 mosaic.[48]

As to the rare autosome trisomy mosaicisms, 33 cases of various types have been diagnosed prenatally (Table 30-11). Of 28 cases with phenotypic information, 11 were reported to be abnormal (two with 46/47,+2; one each with 46/47,+4, 46/47,+5, 46/47,+12, 46/47,+14, 46/47,+15, 46/47,+17; and three with 46/47,+22). Except for one case each with 46/47,+2, 46/47,+14, 46/47,+17, and 46/47,+22, these cases were cytogenetically confirmed in follow-up studies. Therefore, if such rare trisomies are found in two or more culture vessels, they should not be disregarded. Serial detailed ultrasound examinations of the fetus and fetal blood sampling may help the parents to decide about the pregnancy. Confined placental mosaicism may still be one of the contributing factors for some of these rare mosaicisms. Some trisomic cells may also be confined to certain specific tissues. If parents choose to continue the pregnancy, a urine sediment culture for cytogenetic confirmation should be pursued in addition to postnatal studies of blood or skin fibroblasts, placental tissues, or membranes. One case of 46/47,+12 was confirmed cytogenetically in a urine sediment study, even though the infant was described as phenotypically normal.[55] If parents elect termination, it is advisable to study kidney tissue, placenta, or a membrane in addition to other fetal tissues to detect cells with trisomy.

Thirteen cases with possible monosomy mosaicism have been diagnosed prenatally (eight cases by Hsu,[1] four cases by Hsu,[44] and one case by Wilson and colleagues[57]). These include five cases of 46/45,−21; three cases of 46/45,−22; two cases of 46/45,−17; and one case each of 46/45,−9, 46/45,−19 and 46/45,−20. Of seven cases with phenotypic information and four cases with successful cytogenetic follow-up studies, only one case with 46/45,−22 was associated with multiple congenital abnormalities, congenital heart disease, and mosaicism confirmed in blood culture. One case with 46/45,−21 was confirmed cytogenetically but was reported to be phenotypically normal.

There have been at least 53 cases of mosaicism involving autosome structural aberrations (Hsu, 27 cases[1]; Hsu, 25 cases[44]; and Wilson and colleagues, one case[57]). Thirty-eight cases contained at least one cell line with an unbalanced aberration. In this category, 52.9%

TABLE 30–10. TRISOMY MOSAICISM INVOLVING CHROMOSOMES 9, 18, 13, AND 8

KARYOTYPE	NO. OF CASES	OUTCOME OF PREGNANCY: CONTINUED	OUTCOME OF PREGNANCY: TERMINATED	PHENOTYPE: NO. WITH ABNORMAL PHENOTYPE / TOTAL W/INFO. (%)	FOLLOW-UP CYTOGENETIC CONFIRMATION: NO. WITH CONFIRMATION OF MOSAICISM / TOTAL SUCCESSFUL STUDIES (%)
46/47,+9	18*	2	16	9/15 (60.0)	7/14 (50.0)
46/47 +18	15†	1	14	6/7 (85.7)	8/8 (100)
46/47,+13	11†	—	10	4/10 (40.0)	3/7 (42.9)
46/47,+8	10††	2	8	1/9 (11.1)	6/8 (75.0)

* Data from references 1, 44–47.
† Data from references 1 and 44.
†† Data from references 1 and 44; one case was diagnosed as pseudomosaicism due to the findings of one affected clone in one of 8 cultures, yet 46/47,+8 was confirmed in the live-born's blood. The infant was phenotypically normal.

TABLE 30–11. RARE AUTOSOMAL TRISOMY MOSAICISM

KARYOTYPE	NUMBER OF CASES	OUTCOME OF PREGNANCY: CONTINUED	OUTCOME OF PREGNANCY: TERMINATED	PHENOTYPE: NO. W/ABNORMALITIES / TOTAL W/INFORMATION (%)	FOLLOW-UP CYTOGENETIC CONFIRMATION: NO. W/CONFIRMATION OF MOSAICISM / TOTAL SUCCESSFUL STUDIES (%)	REFERENCES
46/47,+2	2	—	2	2/2* (100)	1/1 (100)	Bui et al (1984)[50]
46/47,+4	1	1	0	1/1† (100)	1/1 (100)	Priest, J. (personal communication)[51]
46/47,+5	3	3	0	1/3 (33.0)	1/3 (33.3)	Cassmassima et al (1989)[52]; Richkind et al (1987)[53]; Penchaszadeh et al (1988)[54]
46/47,+6	2	2	0	0/2	0/1	Hsu (1986)[1]
46/47,+7	2	1	1	0/1	1/2 (50.0)	Hsu (1986)[44]; Hsu (unpublished data)
46,47,+11	1	0	1	0/1	0/1	Hsu (1986)[1]
46/47,+12	4	2	2	1/2‡ (50.0)	2/3§ (66.7)	Hsu (1986)[1]; Hsu (unpublished data)[44]; Leschot et al (1988)[55]; Von Koskull et al, (1989)[56]
46/47,+14	2	1	1	1/2 (50.0)	0/1	Hsu (1986)[1]; Hsu (unpublished data)[44]
46/47,+15	3	1	2	1/3 (33.3)	1/2 (50.0)	Hsu (1986)
46/47,+16	2	2	0	0/2	1/1‖ (100)	Hsu (1986)[1]; Hsu (unpublished data)[44]
46/47,+17	4#	2	1	1/3 (33.3)	0/3	Hsu (1986)[1]; Hsu (unpublished data)[44]; Wilson et al (1989)—1 case[57]
46/47,+22	7	3	4	3/6** (50.0)	3/6 (50.0)	Hsu (1986)—2 cases[1]; Hsu (unpublished data)—4 cases[44]; Stioui et al, 1989—1 case[58]

* One abortus had transversal hemimelia and the other had ambiguous external genitalia.
† Features of 4p trisomy.
‡ One live-born had seizure disorder and hypoglycemia with otherwise unremarkable phenotype.
§ Cells with 47,+12 were detected in urine sediment in one (reference 55).
‖ Cells with 47,+16 were confined to the placenta.
\# Outcome of one case in unknown.
** One live-born had intrauterine growth retardation and confined placental chromosome mosaicism.

(18/34) were reported to be phenotypically abnormal and 64.2% (18/28) were cytogenetically confirmed. Ten of these 18 confirmed cases were also phenotypically abnormal.

Eleven cases contained a cell line with a balanced translocation, either reciprocal or Robertsonian. Here no abnormal phenotypes were observed, although mosaicism was confirmed in two of five cases with successful studies.

Four cases of inversion mosaicism resulted in three phenotypically normal offspring and one spontaneous abortion.[1,44] Among three cases with successful cytogenetic follow-up studies, only normal karyotypes were detected.

The overall data indicate that mosaicism for a structural aberration, although rare, does occur. When there is an unbalanced cell line, the risk for an abnormal phenotype should not be underestimated.

Sex Chromosome Mosaicism. Mosaicism involving sex chromosomes has been observed with almost as high a frequency as that observed for all the autosomes together. By and large, the percentage of noticeable phenotypic abnormalities in prenatally diagnosed sex chromosome mosaicism is far less than the frequency observed in autosome mosaicism (other than 46/47,+20 and mosaicism with a balanced structural rearrangement). The three more commonly seen sex chromosome mosaicisms are 45,X/46,XX; 45,X/46,XY; and 46,XY/47,XXY.

Because of the drastic difference in phenotypic outcome between postnatal and prenatal diagnosis of 45,X/46,XY, this mosaicism deserves our special attention. As reviewed by Hsu[59] in 1989, 100% of all postnatally diagnosed cases with 45,X/46,XY mosaicism were phenotypically abnormal, with the majority of patients having mixed gonadal dysgenesis and a female phenotype with Turner syndrome. However, this reflects biased ascertainment, since phenotypically normal cases are not likely to come to medical attention postnatally. In contrast, among 61 prenatally diagnosed cases of 45,X/46,XY (Table 30-12), only three of 53 with information on phenotype resulted in phenotypically abnormal fetuses with mixed gonadal dysgenesis. The vast majority (48 cases, or 92.3%) resulted in normal male offspring. The two other cases were classified as borderline abnormal. Another recent survey also indicated that a normal phenotypic male can be expected in 90% of cases diagnosed prenatally as 45,X/46,XY mosaic.[61]

Ultrasound visualization of the external genitalia of the fetus could be helpful to the parents in their decision making. Identification of male external genitalia would probably be more reassuring than a risk figure for an abnormal outcome of 10%.

The most common sex chromosome mosaicism is 45,X/46,XX. At least 103 cases with X/XX mosaicism have been diagnosed prenatally (Table 30-13). Of 70 cases with some information about the phenotypic outcome, five were reported to have some features of Turner syndrome, three had other anomalies, and two resulted in stillbirths. However, one must realize that even in patients with 45,X without mosaicism, the typical features of Turner syndrome, such as short stature and sexual infantilism, are not manifested perinatally.

TABLE 30–12. 45,X/46,XY MOSAICISM

Total Number of Cases	61
Pregnancy continued	30
Pregnancy terminated	25
Fetal demise	1
Stillbirth (cord compressed)	1
Unknown outcome	4
Phenotype	
Grossly normal male	48 (30 live born* 16 abortuses; 1 stillbirth; 1 fetal demise)
Mixed gonadal dysgenesis	3 (all abortuses)†
Phenotypic male with penile chordae and hypoplastic scrotum	1 (abortus)
Phenotypic female	1 (abortus)
No information	8
Cytogenetic Confirmatory Studies	
45,X/46,XY	35
46,XY	9
No study or unsuccessful study	17

Data from references 44, 57, 59, 60.
* Nine had follow-up at 3 months to 4 years.
† External phenotype: one female, one male, one abnormal.

The third most common prenatally diagnosed sex chromosome mosaicism is 46,XY/47,XXY. (The second most common is 45,X/46,XY, discussed earlier.) Of 40 cases collected (see Table 30-13), 26 cases had outcome information. Twenty-five were associated with a normal male phenotype and one live-born with intrauterine growth retardation. Again, as with Turner syndrome, the typical features for nonmosaic 47,XXY, such as hypogonadism and infertility, cannot be diagnosed perinatally.

Other common sex chromosome mosaicisms are 45,X/47,XXX; 46,XX/47,XXX; and 46,XY/47,XYY (see Table 30-13). Two cases with 45,X/47,XXX were reported to be abnormal; one live-born was small for gestation and one abortus had some minor abnormalities. One live-born with 46,XY/47,XYY had short neck and left hydronephrosis. The vast majority of cases were associated with a grossly normal phenotype, although over 90% of successful follow-up studies confirmed the mosaicism.

As to mosaicism involving a structurally abnormal sex chromosome, all six cases mosaic for a structurally abnormal X chromosome and a normal 46,XX cell line resulted in phenotypically normal female fetuses or live-borns. Of five successful follow-up studies, mosaicism was confirmed in three and normal chromosomes were found in two. Twelve other cases were mosaic for a structurally abnormal X and another abnormal cell line (without a Y chromosome). Of nine informative cases, four had some features of Turner syndrome and five were reported to be normal. Mosaicism was confirmed in eight cases with successful cytogenetic studies (including three phenotypically abnormal cases).[44]

There were two cases involving a structurally abnormal Y chromosome. Both had a normal 46,XY cell line and were associated with a normal male phenotype.

Triploidy Mosaicism. At least three cases with triploidy mosaicism have been diagnosed prenatally. One resulted in a grossly abnormal stillborn and another was spontaneously aborted with multiple congenital abnormalities. One abortus, however, appeared to be normal. Cytogenetic confirmation was achieved in the first two but failed in the third.[1,44]

Summary of Chromosome Mosaicism. Of 601 cases diagnosed through amniocentesis as chromosome mosaicism, phenotypic information was available in 461 (Table 30-14). The frequency of noticeable phenotypic abnormalities, as described in the pathologic examination of abortuses or in the physical examination of live-borns, was 31.5% for autosome mosaicism. This frequency increased to 45.3% when cases with 46/47,+20

TABLE 30–13. MAJOR SEX CHROMOSOME MOSAICISM (EXCLUDING 45,X/46,XY)

KARYOTYPE	NUMBER OF CASES	OUTCOME OF PREGNANCY: CONTINUED	TERMINATED	UNKNOWN	PHENOTYPE: NO. WITH ABNORMALITY / TOTAL W/INFORMATION (%)	FOLLOW-UP CYTOGENETIC CONFIRMATION: NO. WITH CONFIRMATION OF MOSAICISM / TOTAL SUCCESSFUL STUDIES (%)
45,X/46,XX[1,44,57,62]	103	53*	38	12	8/70 (11.4)†	49/56 (87.5)
46,XY/47,XXY[1,44]	40	21	16	3	1/26 (3.8)††	22/22 (100)
45,X/47,XXX[1,44]	20	6	9	5	2/8 (25.0)§	8/8 (100)
46,XX/47,XXX[1,44]	19	16	3	0	0/18	13/13 (100)
46,XY/47,XYY[1,44]	18	12	5	1	1/12 (8.3)‖	8/9 (88.9)
45,X/46,XX/47,XXX[44]	4	1	3	0	0/1	3/3 (100)
45,X/46,XY/47,XYY[1,44,57]	4	2	2	0	0/2	2/3 (66.6%)
45,X/47,XYY[60]	1	0	1	—	0/1	1/1 (Chorion)

* Two of the X/XX pregnancies resulted in stillbirths.
† Of these 8, 5 had Turner syndrome and 3 had other anomalies.
†† One live-born with XY/XXY had intrauterine growth retardation.
§ One live-born was small for gestational age; one abortus had clinodactyly, widespread nipples, and hypertelorism.
‖ One live-born with XY/XYY had right undescended testis, short neck, and right hydronephrosis.

were excluded. In the majority of cases of 46/47,+20, the cells with trisomy 20 were probably extraembryonic in origin and not representative of the fetus. As to sex chromosome mosaicism, the overall frequency of noticeable abnormalities was 10.1%. We also know that 90% of cases with 45,X/46,XY were associated with a normal male phenotype.

It must be realized that the frequency of noticeable abnormalities is likely to be underestimated because it is difficult to recognize minor dysmorphic features in mid-trimester fetuses; for live-borns a physical evaluation at birth would not reveal mental retardation or other subtle abnormalities. The overall cytogenetic confirmation of mosaicism was over 50%.

At the genetic counseling regarding a prenatal diagnosis of chromosome mosaicism, it is important to include the following points:

1. It must be explained to the parents that the respective proportions of each cell line in an amniotic fluid culture do not necessarily reflect cell proportions in various somatic tissues of the fetus and that in some cases the abnormal cell line might be derived from extraembryonic tissues and may not be found in any fetal tissue.
2. It should be pointed out that it is impossible to predict the phenotype of the fetus. The spectrum of possible phenotypes should be presented.

TABLE 30–14. SUMMARY OF PRENATAL DIAGNOSIS MOSAICISM DIAGNOSED THROUGH AMNIOCENTESIS

TYPE OF MOSAICISM	NUMBER OF CASES	NO. W/ABNORMAL PHENOTYPE / TOTAL W/INFORMATION (%)
All autosome mosaicism	309	79/251 (31.5)
Autosome mosaicism (excluding 46/47,+20)	206	68/150 (45.3)
46/47,+20 only	103	11/101 (10.9)
Sex chromosome mosaicism	289	21/207 (10.1)
Triploid mosaicism	3	2/3 (66.7)
Total	601	102/461 (22.1)

3. The counseling should be as nondirective as possible and the decision about continuation of the pregnancy or termination must be left to the parents.

Fetal blood sampling for chromosome analysis and serial detailed ultrasound examinations of the fetus may be helpful to parents in their decision making. However, fetal blood is only one tissue type and sonography has its limitations. Thus, one must be very careful not to provide a false sense of security when fetal blood does not show any aneuploid cells and the ultrasound examination is negative. Fetal blood sampling should not be recommended for further evaluation of 46/47,+20, since cells with trisomy 20 have never been detected in blood studies.

All attempts should be made to obtain cytogenetic confirmation or to perform a careful examination of the live-born or abortus. If it is feasible, one should try to study placental tissue, especially the amnion, to determine whether certain chromosome abnormalities are more frequently confined to those tissues. In addition to studying blood cells, skin fibroblasts and urine sediments from a live-born can be used for culture. Information on long-term follow-up of all mosaic live-borns is urgently needed for geneticists and obstetricians providing prenatal diagnosis.

Maternal Cell Contamination

Maternal cell contamination (MCC) in cultured amniotic fluid cells is a source of potential error in prenatal diagnosis (MCC in CVS will be discussed later). The vast majority of cases of MCC were detected through an admixture of XY and XX cells. A few were ascertained when an unexpected pregnancy outcome revealed a discrepancy—where the prenatal diagnosis had been 46,XX but the live-born was either 46,XY or had a major chromosome abnormality. At least four cases of trisomy 21 are known to have been misdiagnosed as 46,XX because of MCC.[1] According to data from three large surveys (Table 30-15), the overall frequency of diagnosed MCC is 0.157%, or 1 in 637. Since MCC cannot be recognized when the fetal sex is female, the true incidence of MCC is probably twice the observed frequency. Considerable variability exists between laboratories in the frequency of MCC.[63] A high incidence of MCC has been observed at the centralized Prenatal Diagnosis Laboratory of New York City (PDL), where awareness of this possibility is stressed.[44,64] It was 0.5% in the first 3000 cases and has remained unchanged in the last 10 years. In the first 22,000 cases analyzed by PDL (Table 30-16), there were 114 cases of MCC; 113 cases were diagnosed through an admixture of XY and XX cells. One case was diagnosed prenatally as 46,XX, but a normal boy with 46,XY chromosomes was born. The 46,XX cells from the amniotic fluid showed the same chromosome polymorphisms as the mother's chromosomes. Among the cases with MCC detected through admixture of XY and XX, 25.4% showed a single 46,XX cell, 60.5% showed multiple 46,XX cells from one flask, and 13.2% showed multiple 46,XX cells from two or more flasks. According to a United States survey on MCC, the frequencies of detected MCC are comparable for in situ preparations and the trypsinized flask method.[63]

The data from this survey bring out several major points:

1. The incidence of MCC is two and a half times lower when the first few milliliters of amniotic fluid are not used for culture.
2. MCC seems to be more frequent when wider-gauge needles are used for the amniocentesis. A needle of gauge 20 or less was associated with MCC incidence of 0.15%, whereas incidence of 0.11% was observed when a smaller needle of gauge 21 or higher was used. The difference, however, is statistically insignificant.
3. The incidence of MCC is more common in cultures established from bloody fluids. Approximately 35% of all cases with MCC in the US survey were associated with bloody samples.

TABLE 30–15. FREQUENCY OF MATERNAL CELL CONTAMINATION (MCC)

SURVEY	MCC RATIOS NO. OF CASES W/MCC / TOTAL NO. OF SAMPLES	PERCENTAGE
U.S. Survey*	134/91,131	0.15
European Study†	79/45,806	0.17
Canadian Study‡	22/12,386	0.18
Overall MCC Frequency	235/149,323	0.157

* Benn PA, Hsu LYF. Maternal cell contamination of amniotic fluid cell cultures: Results of a U.S. nationwide survey. Am J Med Genet 1983;15:297.

† Bui TH, Iselius L, Lindsten J. European collaborative study on prenatal diagnosis: mosaicism, pseudomosaicism and single abnormal cell in amniotic fluid cell cultures. Prenat Diagn (Special Issue) 1984;4:145.

‡ Worton RG, Stern R. A Canadian collaborative study of mosaicism in amniotic fluid cell cultures. Prenat Diagn (Special Issue), 1984;4:131.

TABLE 30–16. FREQUENCY OF MATERNAL CELL CONTAMINATION AT PDL

Total Cases Studied	22,000
Cases with admixture of 46,XY and 46,XX	113 (100%)
Cases showing a single cell with 46,XX	29 (25.7%)
Cases showing multiple cells with 46,XX (restricted to one flask)	69 (61.0%)
Cases showing multiple cells with 46,XX (from 2 or more flasks)	15 (13.3%)
Cases with only 46,XX cells	1
Overall MCC frequency	114/22,000 (0.518%)

4. Cultures with MCC showed no unusual growth patterns. The harvesting time did not differ for cultures with or without MCC.
5. MCC was detected in more than one culture in 41% of the MCC cases.
6. In the majority of cases where MCC was not detected and a misdiagnosis was made, only one culture and/or less than 20 cells had been examined.
7. A comparison of chromosome polymorphisms in the amniotic fluid cells and in parents' cells, especially the mother's, is generally helpful in diagnosing MCC.

It appears that fragments of maternal tissue removed by the needle are the main source of MCC. This possibility is supported by (1) the increased incidence of MCC when the first few milliliters of amniotic fluid are used for analysis, with fragments of maternal tissue probably having been introduced into the amniotic fluid sample; and (2) the repeat observations of MCC in amniotic fluids from two consecutive pregnancies complicated by fibroids where the shedding of cells or fibroid fragments into the amniocentesis needle has led to the MCC.[64a]

To reduce the frequency of MCC, recommendations for the amniocentesis procedure should include carefully monitoring with ultrasound, using a smaller-gauge needle with stylet in place, and discarding the first 1 or 2 milliliters of amniotic fluid sample.

Recommendations for the laboratory procedure include performing chromosome analysis of a minimum of 20 metaphases from two independent cultures or 10 to 15 clones from two culture dishes and, when an admixture of XY and XX cells is found, attempting to compare Q-banding chromosome polymorphism of the amniotic fluid (or CVS) cells with the mother's.

Although nearly all cases with an admixture of XY and XX turn out to be MCC in XY fetuses, the remote possibility of XX/XY chimerism still exists. In fact, three such cases from prenatal diagnosis are known—two reported by Hsu[1] and one by Freiberg and colleagues.[65]

When a diagnosis of MCC is entertained, it is advisable for the clinical geneticist or the referring physician to recommend a careful ultrasound examination of the fetal external genitalia. Visualization of male genitalia may provide reassurance to the parents.

Supernumerary Marker Chromosomes

A marker chromosome simply means an unidentifiable, structurally altered chromosome. The finding of such a supernumerary marker chromosome in amniotic fluid cell culture (or CVS preparation) poses problems in diagnosis and counseling. The overall incidence of supernumerary marker chromosome from amniocentesis ranges from 0.6 to 0.86 per 1000. These figures are much higher than the incidence of marker chromosomes detected in newborn series (Table 30-17). However, one must consider the methodological differences between amniocentesis data and newborn surveys. The real frequency of marker chromosomes in newborn surveys could be higher simply because marker mosaicism or minute markers were undetected. In the amniocentesis data there were more de novo cases than inherited ones. In addition, these data show a strong positive maternal age effect for de novo marker chromosomes.[66] Evidence for elevated maternal age in de novo marker chromosomes has also been reported in postnatal cases.[67,68] The relatively high incidence of marker chromosomes in amniocentesis compared to that in newborn series can also be attributed to the fact that advanced maternal age is the indication for the vast majority of patients referred for amniocentesis.

Whenever a supernumerary marker chromosome is detected prenatally, both parents should be studied immediately, regardless of the cytogenetic characteristics of the marker chromosomes. Since it is possible that one parent is mosaic for the marker, a careful search for an identical marker in a minimum of 50 cells must be pursued. It is extremely important to determine whether the marker chromosome is de novo or inherited. Available data indicate that all familial cases resulted in phenotypically normal offspring. Only de novo cases carry an increased risk for offspring with congenital abnormalities.

A satellited de novo marker may carry a better prognosis than a non-satellited de novo marker.[69] Recent data indicate a 10.9% risk for satellited de novo marker chromosomes and a 15.6% risk for non-satellited de novo marker chromosomes[69a] (Table 30–18).

Apparently, the prognosis does not differ between mosaic and nonmosaic groups,[69] because there may be a tendency for a supernumerary marker chromosome to be lost either by anaphase lag or by mitotic nondisjunction, resulting in cell lines with no marker or two markers.[70] Familial markers may be perpetuated for many generations, and the de novo appearance of a marker chromosome may be relatively frequent.

Cytogenetic studies such as C-banding, DA-DAPI (distamycin A and 4′, 6-diamidino-2-phenylindole) staining, NOR-silver staining and R-banding may help to characterize the cytogenetic nature of the marker chromosome and thereby provide some clues for as-

TABLE 30–17. INCIDENCE OF SUPERNUMERARY MARKER CHROMOSOMES

SOURCE OF DATA	NUMBER STUDIED	INCIDENCE (per thousand)		
		OVERALL	DE NOVO	INHERITED
Amniocentesis	75,000*	0.64	0.32 to 0.40	0.23 to 0.32
Amniocentesis	52,965†	0.60	—	—
Amniocentesis	98,745‡	—	0.22	—
Amniocentesis	22,000§	0.86	0.59	0.27
Newborns	59,452#	0.18	0.05	0.10

* Hook EB, Cross PK. Extra structurally abnormal chromosomes (ESAC) detected at amniocentesis: frequency in approximately 75,000 prenatal cytogenetic diagnoses and association with maternal and paternal age. Am J Hum Genet 1987;40:83.

† Ferguson-Smith MA, Yates JRW. Maternal age specific rates for chromosome aberrations and factors influencing them: Report of a collaborative European study on 52,965 amniocenteses. Prenatal Diagnosis (Special Issue) 1984;4:5.

‡ Warburton D. Outcome of cases of de novo structural rearrangements diagnosed at amniocentesis. Prenat Diagn 1984;4:69 and personal communication of unpublished data.

§ Hsu (unpublished data).

Jacobs PA. Mutation rates of structural chromosome rearrangements in man. Am J Hum Genet 1981;33:44.

sessing the prognosis. Several markers were identified as inversion duplication of chromosome 15 (inv dup [15]).[71,72] It was suggested that a de novo DA-DAPI positive marker, such as an inv dup(15), presents a low risk for fetal anomalies,[72] because it was believed that only regions on the short arm of chromosome 15 fluoresced brightly with DA-DAPI. However, recent reports indicating a lack of specificity in DA-DAPI staining for 15p make identification of 15p inconclusive.[73,74]

Steinbach and colleagues suggested that a de novo bisatellited marker chromosome with a single C-band or a bipartite C-band carries less risk than a marker chromosome with a discrete G-band or R-band between two distinct C-bands or near a single C-band.[75] Very recently, the use of the fluorescence in situ hybridization techniques (FISH) and panels of biotinylated pericentric repeat probes have made it possible to identify the chromosomal origin of a marker chromosome.[75a]

From our own first 22,000 cases, 19 cases of marker chromosomes were diagnosed. Six were inherited and 13 (including two new cases) were de novo in origin.[76] Of the 13 de novo cases, only two resulted in fetuses with an abnormal phenotype; both of these cases had a bisatellited marker chromosome (NOR positive). We believe that the extent of euchromatin material in a de novo marker chromosome is the crucial factor in determining the risk for fetal anomalies. It appears that a minute marker or a fragmentlike marker that is made almost entirely of C-positive material carries a low risk for fetal abnormalities.

One or more detailed ultrasound examinations should be recommended to the prospective parents to help them in their decision making. In fact, in both of our de novo cases with an abnormal phenotype, the parents chose to terminate their pregnancies because fetal anomalies were demonstrated by ultrasound examination.

Chromosome Polymorphisms

Chromosome polymorphisms or heteromorphisms are structural variants of chromosomes that are widespread in human populations and that have no effect on the phenotype. These variants are most often found at certain chromosome segments, including the highly variable centromeric regions of chromosomes 1, 9, 16; the distal two thirds of the long arm of the Y chromosome; and the short arms and satellites of the acrocentric chromosomes. In inexperienced hands a rare chromosome polymorphism may be misdiagnosed as a structural aberration. By and large, such misdiagnoses can be avoided by studies of the parents' chromosomes and by further characterization of the chromosome in question with additional banding techniques.

TABLE 30–18. OUTCOME OF CASES WITH DE NOVO MARKER CHROMOSOMES

TYPE	NO. OF CASES WITH KNOWN OUTCOME	PHENOTYPE	
		NORMAL	ABNORMAL
Satellited	55	49	6 (10.9%)
Nonsatellited	64	54	10 (15.6%)
Total	119	103	16 (13.4%)

Warburton D. De novo balanced chromosome rearrangements and extra marker chromosomes identified at prenatal diagnosis: clinical significance and distribution of break points. Am J Hum Genet 1991;49:995.

Morphologic variations of the heterochromatic secondary constriction regions (qh) of chromosomes 1, 9, 16, and the Y chromosome primarily include pericentric inversion involving the constitutive heterochromatin secondary constriction region and enlarged heterochromatic region (qh+). Among unusual Y chromosomes are a large Y (larger than chromosome 18), a small Y (smaller than chromosome 21), and those with pericentric inversion.

The incidence of specific chromosome polymorphisms varies in different racial groups.[77] Although the general incidence of complete pericentric inversion of 9qh [inv(9) (p11q13)] is 1% to 2%, the incidence is highest in the black population (3.5%), moderate among Hispanics (2.4%), and relatively low among whites (0.73%) and Asians (0.26%) (Table 30-19). The Y chromosome appears to be more polymorphic among Asians, with a higher frequency of large Y chromosome. The overall incidence of inv(Y) was found to be 1 per 1000 males and apparently is more prevalent in the Asian and Hispanic population (see Table 30-19). In this series 9qh+ is more frequently seen than 1qh+ or 16qh+, with no indication of any racial prevalence.

The size of satellites, stalks, and short arms of acrocentric chromosomes varies a great deal. Occasionally, the entire short arm can be absent with no visible satellites. In our first 23,000 genetic amniocenteses, 21ps− and 13ps− were the most frequently seen variants, with frequencies of 0.7 and 0.3 per 1000, respectively; 15ps−, 22ps−, and 14ps− occurred less often, with frequencies of 0.17, 0.13, and 0.09 per 1000. Apparently, an absence of the short arm in an acrocentric chromosome is without any deleterious effect.

Among the acrocentric chromosomes, the short arm of chromosome 15 is the most polymorphic one. It differs from the other short arms of acrocentric chromosomes in that it possesses a large amount of 5-methylcytosine and stains positively with DA-DAPI.[78] A large short arm (not a large satellite) of chromosome 15 (15p+) can be a diagnostic concern. If such a chromosome is observed to be involved in satellite association with another acrocentric chromosome, one would know that at least it functions like a short arm of an acrocentric chromosome and most likely represents a benign polymorphism. A prominent or enlarged short arm in chromosomes 13, 14, 21, and 22 has also been observed as chromosome polymorphism. Again, searching for satellite association involving the short arm of the chromosome in question probably should be the first step. Additional cytogenetic studies and studies of the parents' chromosomes will further help to identify the origin and nature of the polymorphism.

Polymorphisms of constitutive heterochromatin have been found at the centromeric regions of many autosomes other than 1, 9, and 16. A large heterochromatic region has been reported for chromosome 3,[79] chromosome 4,[80,81] and chromosome 5.[82,83] An additional G-band positive and C-band negative segment have been found in the proximal region of the short arm of chromosome 16 (16 pt) in four cases; three were familial and one unknown.[84] Chromosome variants have also been reported for 17p and 18p, such as, 17ph+,[85] 18ph+,[86] and 20ph+.[87] Variable staining of chromosome 19, including pericentric inversion, is also known.[88,89]

De Novo Structural Rearrangement

When a structural chromosome rearrangement is detected in every cultured cell from either amniocentesis or CVS, the chromosomes of both parents should be studied immediately, regardless of whether the rearrangement appears to be balanced or unbalanced. If both parents are found to have normal karyotypes, the diagnosis of a de novo rearrangement is established. A comparison of chromosome polymorphisms of the fetal cells and the parents' cells could help to rule out questionable paternity.

De novo structural chromosome rearrangements fall into three categories:

1. Apparently balanced rearrangements, which include translocations (reciprocal, Robertsonian, and insertional) and inversions (paracentric and pericentric)
2. Apparently unbalanced rearrangements
3. Small supernumerary marker chromosomes (discussed earlier under Supernumerary Marker Chromosomes).

TABLE 30–19. INCIDENCE OF INV(9), LARGE Y, SMALL Y, AND INV(Y) IN FOUR RACIAL GROUPS

RACIAL GROUP	CASES STUDIED	PERCENT WITH INV(9)	CASES STUDIED	PERCENT WITH Yq+	PERCENT WITH Yq−	PERCENT WITH INV(Y)
White	2,334	0.73	1,139	0.53	0.53	N.D.
Black	1,795	3.57	909	0.66	0.11	N.D.
Hispanic	1,737	2.42	877	0.57	1.00	0.23
Asian	384	0.26	208	1.92	0.96	0.48
Total	6,250	1.98	3,133	0.67	0.57	0.10

N.D.—Not Detected.

From Hsu LYF, Benn PA, Tannenbaum HL, et al. Chromosomal polymorphisms of 1, 9, 16, and Y in 4 major ethnic groups: a large prenatal study. Am J Med Genet 1987;26:95.

The finding of a de novo unbalanced autosome rearrangement is generally indicative of an unfavorable phenotypic outcome; the risk of being associated with an abnormal phenotype is 60% or higher.[69] Additional cytogenetic studies, including the use of molecular probes (when a specific duplication or deletion is suspected), may help to identify the origin and nature of the abnormality.

De novo balanced rearrangements, however, fall into the "gray" zone of prognosis. The incidence of balanced de novo rearrangements was increased eightfold among mentally retarded individuals as compared with the incidence in newborn surveys.[90] It is possible that an increased risk for mental retardation or congenital anomalies is caused by one or more of the following factors: minute submicroscopic chromosome deletion or duplication, mutation of the translocation or the rearranged site, and position effect of the rearranged genetic material.

According to the North American survey by Warburton,[69a] 13 (5.75%) of 226 cases with a prenatal diagnosis of a de novo balanced rearrangement had an abnormal phenotype (Table 30-20). De novo reciprocal translocations and inversions carry a risk of 5% to 10% of a phenotypically abnormal offspring. De novo balanced Robertsonian translocations are more likely to be associated with normal phenotypes (>95%). Unfortunately, there is a lack of long-term follow-up data on cases diagnosed prenatally and continued to term, but some information is available. One recent report presented outcome data on eight cases of de novo balanced reciprocal translocations.[91] Except for one that was terminated at 18 weeks after diagnosis of anencephaly, all these cases went to term. All seven children were reported to be normal at follow-up examination, their ages ranging from 16 months to 10 years. Three children of school age were reported to be performing satisfactorily in a class appropriate to their age.

There have been two conflicting reports in terms of mental development of children detected to have de novo balanced translocations at birth. One report indicated normal physical and mental development in five children with de novo balanced translocations (three reciprocal and two Robertsonian) in comparison to children with familial translocations.[92] The other reported a significantly lower IQ in 10 children with de novo balanced translocations (seven reciprocal and three Robertsonian) compared to 20 children with familial translocations ($p < 0.01$).[93] It should be noted that all children in the study attended regular school.

A worldwide collaborative effort to follow up all children with prenatal diagnosis of a de novo balanced rearrangement would be most useful for clinical geneticists who provide counseling and for parents who have to decide whether to continue or terminate the pregnancy.

Other Problems in Cell Culture and Diagnosis

Mycoplasma Contamination. The seriousness of mycoplasma contamination is largely due to its insidious damaging effect. The contaminated cells may at first show no noticeable difference in terms of cell growth or cell morphology, but mycoplasma infection should be suspected if there is an abrupt cessation of cell growth or if there is a significant increase of chromosome breaks and rearrangements. A rapid in situ staining method using DNA A-T-specific fluorochromes can diagnose mycoplasma infection readily. Contaminated cultures, when fixed and stained with Hoechst 33258[94] or DAPI[95] reveal small, brightly fluorescent particles surrounding cell nuclei. For practical purposes, once mycoplasma contamination is diagnosed, immediate disposal of the contaminated culture is probably the method of choice. When all cultures from a given case are infected, it is better to request a repeat amniocentesis immediately than to attempt to salvage the cultures with antibiotics. Meanwhile, all likely sources of the infection should be removed and incubators emptied and cleaned.

Toxic Syringes or Tubes. Amniotic fluid cell culture failure has been associated with various brands of syringes or tubes. In the United States the following constitute a partial list: Jelco syringes, Monoject syringes, Venoject tubes, and Vacutainers from Becton-Dickinson.[1] The Gillette "Sabre" syringe in the United King-

TABLE 30–20. PHENOTYPIC OUTCOME OF DE NOVO BALANCED REARRANGEMENTS DIAGNOSED AT AMNIOCENTESIS

	TOTAL NUMBER	PERCENTAGE W/ABNORMAL OUTCOME	LIVEBIRTH		ELECTIVE ABORTION		FETAL DEATH	
			NORMAL	ABNORMAL	NORMAL	ABNORMAL	NORMAL	ABNORMAL
Reciprocal translocation	144	5.5	118	6	15	2	3	0
Robertsonian translocation	51	3.9	48	2	1	0	0	0
Inversion	31	9.7	27	1	1	1	0	1
Total	226	5.75	193	9	17	3	3	1

Warburton D. De novo balanced chromosome rearrangements and extra marker chromosomes identified at prenatal diagnosis: clinical significance and distribution of break points. Am J Hum Genet 1991;49:995.

dom and Omnifix syringes in Israel were also reported to cause culture failure.[1] Although some of these situations may have been corrected, there may be other toxic syringes or tubes that have not been identified. The possibility of a toxic syringe, tube, or container must be considered when there is repeated culture failure from the same referring source.

Tetraploidy. Tetraploidy is a frequent observation in cultured amniotic fluid cells. In one study two thirds of all cases showed more than 10% of the cultured cells to be tetraploid.[96] Occasionally, the frequency of tetraploid cells reached over 80%, even approaching 100%. Although today tetraploidy in cultured amniotic fluid cells is not considered clinically significant by the vast majority of cytogeneticists, several published cases of live-borns with tetraploidy mosaicism have once again aroused cytogenetic concern.[97,98] Since it is impossible to distinguish between tetraploidy of in vitro origin and that of in vivo origin and since the risk of its being in vivo is remote, it is probably more practical not to be too concerned about tetraploidy. On the other hand, if the frequency of tetraploidy in multiple-culture vessels is consistently high, options of repeat amniocentesis and fetal blood sampling may be considered.

Twin Pregnancy. Occasionally, only one specimen can be obtained from a dichorionic twin pregnancy. Thus, the prenatal diagnosis will apply to only one of the twins. In this situation the limitations of the diagnosis should be explained to the patient. When two fluids are obtained and one twin is found to be normal and the other abnormal, the dilemma in counseling and management is obvious. Each such case requires extensive medical and legal counseling and management needs to be individualized. Selective abortion of the abnormal fetus has been attempted over 30 times. In a series of 22 selective terminations of the abnormal twin, 18 resulted in the delivery of a normal infant, although six of those were prematurely delivered.[99]

Error Rates in Diagnosis From Amniocentesis. The overall error rate for prenatal cytogenetic diagnosis from genetic amniocentesis ranges from 0.1% to 0.6%.[1] The vast majority of cases involved wrong sex assignment due to either maternal cell contamination (MCC) or laboratory error. At least four cases of trisomy 21 misdiagnosed as 46,XX represent the most serious consequence of MCC. These error rates do not include undetected subtle structural aberrations or chromosome mosaicism and fragile X.

CHORIONIC VILLI SAMPLING

First-trimester diagnosis through chorionic villi sampling (CVS) no doubt has a number of significant medical, social, and psychological advantages. However, as more data and experience are being accumulated, more diagnostic problems are becoming obvious. The following discussions cover two special major problems.

Maternal Cell Contamination in CVS

Maternal cell contamination (MCC) has been one of the major concerns in CVS prenatal diagnosis. With careful dissection of visible maternal decidual tissue, the risk of MCC could be significantly reduced, but it would still remain much greater than that in amniocentesis. Direct preparation of CVS is generally considered to carry a very small risk of MCC compared to that of cultured CVS preparations. Nevertheless, MCC has been detected in direct preparations as well (Table 30-21). The vast majority of cases of MCC were found in long-term CVS culture (see Table 30-21). As many as 10% to 13% of cases have been reported to have MCC.[104,105] It appears that MCC tends to occur more often in CVS cultures as cultivation time increases.[101,104] On the other hand, a different report did not find any significant difference in the cultivation time between those cultures showing MCC and those without MCC.[106] It has also

TABLE 30–21. FREQUENCIES OF MATERNAL CELL CONTAMINATION IN CVS PREPARATION

SOURCE	TOTAL NO. OF CASES STUDIED	CVS: DIRECT PREP	CVS: LONG-TERM CULTURE	PERCENT
Karkut et al, 1985[100]	60	0	5	8.3
Cooke et al, 1986[101]	82	1	5	7.3
Olson et al, 1986[102]	50	1	3	8.0
Simoni et al, 1986[103]	477	2	—	0.4
Williams III et al, 1987[104]	45	0	6	13.3
Cheung et al, 1987[105]	(A) 36	0	9	25.0
	(B) 107	0	12	11.2
Roberts et al, 1988[106]	140	1	11	8.5

Prep = Preparation.
(A) = Noncontinuing pregnancies.
(B) = Continuing pregnancies.

been observed that either decidual maternal cells or villi cells can outgrow the other in a mixed culture.[103,107] Roberts and colleagues recommended that Chang's medium (Hana Biologics, Inc) be used in CVS culture because their observations suggested a possible correlation between low frequency of MCC and use of this medium.[106] However, without further investigation this recommendation cannot be considered seriously.

Today, based on all published information, the following procedures are recommended to minimize MCC in CVS:

1. Careful dissection and washing of villi tissue to remove all decidual tissue, preferably under a dissecting microscope
2. Requirement of both direct CVS preparation and long-term villi culture (preferably using two or more culture vessels) for final cytogenetic analysis
3. Comparison of chromosome heteromorphisms of the 46,XX CVS cells and the mother's lymphocytes when MCC is suspected.

Discordance Between CVS and Amniocytes and/or Fetus

With worldwide CVS data exceeding 80,000 cases, the problem of potential discordance between the CVS karyotype and fetal karyotype has become a major concern for physicians or geneticists providing prenatal diagnosis based on CVS. The frequencies of such discrepancies have been reported to be from 0.7 to 3.6% (Table 30-22). In the pooled data of 13,774 cases from 11 reports the overall frequency of discrepancy was 1.2% (see Table 30-22). The recent European collaborative study showed an overall discordance rate of 2.1% (247/11,855) (see Table 30-22).[118] This included non-mosaic discordance in 0.9% of cases (106/11,855) and mosaicism in 1.2% of cases (141/11,855). This relatively high discordance rate in comparison to amniocentesis data can be attributed primarily to the facts that chorionic villi biopsy samples only extraembryonic tissues[119] and chromosome mosaicism may be confined to placental or chorionic tissues, a condition called "confined placental mosaicism."[42]

According to Kalousek's hypothesis, the direct CVS preparation or short-term culture basically studies the karyotype of the cytotrophoblasts; the fibroblasts of the long-term CVS cultures represent primarily the mesenchymal villus core.[120] Theoretically, there could be three types of chromosome mosaicism (Fig. 30-2): mosaicism type 1—generalized chromosome mosaicism present in both the placenta and the fetus; mosaicism type 2a—mosaicism confined to the placenta; and mosaicism type 2b—mosaicism confined to the fetus.

Kalousek has further classified confined placental mosaicism (CPM) into three categories (Table 30-23).

CPM type I shows aneuploid or mosaic-aneuploid cells in direct preparation (cytotrophoblast preparation) but normal diploidy in cultured CVS (placental stroma) and the fetus. This is apparently the most common type. Of over 100 cases showing discrepancies (Table 30-24), approximately half could be considered as CPM type I, although only 10% could be definitely classified as such, with a clear indication of aneuploidy in direct preparation and normal diploidy in both long-term culture and the fetus.

The available data (see Table 30-24) also signal a more frequent, possibly nonrandom involvement of certain chromosomes in forming mosaic trisomies.

TABLE 30–22. DISCREPANCIES BETWEEN CHROMOSOME COMPLEMENTS OF CVS PREPARATIONS, AMNIOCYTES, AND/OR FETAL TISSUES (EXCLUDING MATERNAL CELL CONTAMINATION)

SOURCE	TOTAL NUMBER OF CVS	NUMBER OF CASES WITH DISCREPANCY	%
Heim et al, 1985[108]	100	2	2.0
Wapner et al, 1985[109]	857	9	1.1
Martin et al, 1986[110]	103	3	2.9
Simoni et al, 1986[111]	912	8	0.9
Hogge et al, 1986[112]	1,000	17	1.7
Leschot et al, 1987[113]	412	15	3.6
Mikkelsen and Ayme, 1987[6]	6,125	42	0.7
Callen et al, 1988[114]	1,312	22	1.7
Green et al, 1988[115]	940	12	1.3
Breed et al, 1990[116]	1,447	21	1.5
Schwinger et al, 1989[117]	568	14	2.5
Total of studies cited above	13,774	165	1.2
European (1989) Collaborative Study: Verjerslev and Mikkelsen[118]	11,855	247	2.1

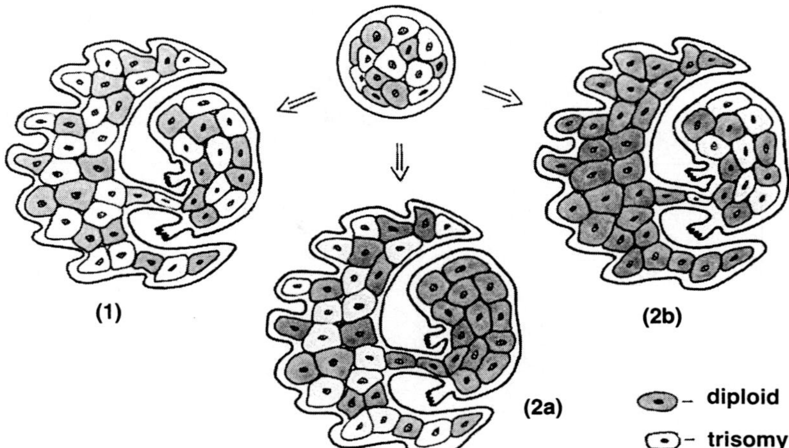

FIGURE 30–2. Diagrammatic representation of three types of constitutional chromosomal mosaicism: (1) generalized, (2a) confined to the placenta, and (2b) confined to the embryo. (Courtesy of Dr. Dagmar Kalousek, 1988.)

Among them are chromosome 18 (16 cases), chromosome 16 (12 cases), chromosome 3 (nine cases), chromosome 13 (six cases), and chromosome 7 (five cases). Monosomy X for either 46,XY/45,X or 46,XX/45,X was frequently seen.

CPM type II is less common. Perhaps approximately 25% of the cases listed in Table 30-24 could be assigned to this category, having aneuploidy or mosaic aneuploidy in cultured CVS and normal diploidy in fetus. However, many of these cases did not have a direct preparation or data on a direct preparation to show whether there was concordance or discordance with the cultured CVS or the fetus.

CPM type III is defined as the finding of mosaic or (straight) diploidy in direct preparation and nonmosaic (straight) aneuploidy in both cultured CVS and the fetus. Here a diagnosis of normal karyotype could be derived from direct CVS preparation (if a long-term CVS culture is not carried out) while the fetus may have a nonmosaic aneuploidy. Such false-negative diagnoses from direct preparation have been reported at least eight times.[110,113,114,135,138,140,141,141b] In six of these cases, mosaic or nonmosaic aneuploidy was demonstrated in the long-term CVS culture. CPM type III fortunately is the least common type. Yet the consequence could be serious. A normal diploid cell line (from 12% to 100%) with or without a trisomic cell line in the direct preparation was found in all 14 placentas from 14 pregnancies (either live-borns or abortuses with trisomy 13 or 18).[141b] They speculate that the presence of a normal diploid cell line in the placenta may have some protective effect for the nonmosaic aneuploid or trisomic fetus. A CVS direct preparation of these trisomic cases would have resulted in a false-negative diagnosis.

Thus far there have been no well-defined guidelines for the diagnosis of true chromosome mosaicism in CVS. The European collaborative study reported 1.2% chromosome mosaicism (141 cases out of 11,855 CVS diagnostic samples), but of these, 99 cases (70%) turned out to be associated with a nonmosaic fetus, and in 87% (86/99) the initial diagnosis of mosaicism had been based on the direct preparation alone. Seventy-seven of 141 mosaic cases were followed up with amniocentesis, and the initial diagnosis was confirmed in only four cases; a nonmosaic aneuploidy was found in four other cases. This collaborative study indicated that long-term villus culture is a clinically more reliable procedure than direct CVS preparation for diagnosing true chromosome mosaicism and for reducing discrepancies.

In conclusion, although considerable concern has been raised about the predictive value or accuracy of CVS due to its relatively high rate of false positives and false negatives compared to amniocentesis,[142,143] we

Continued on page 450

TABLE 30–23. THE TYPES OF CONFINED PLACENTAL MOSAICISM: DISCREPANCIES BETWEEN THE CYTOGENETIC FINDINGS IN CYTOTROPHOBLASTS, VILLOUS STROMA, AND FETAL TISSUES

TISSUES	CPM TYPE I	CPM TYPE II	CPM TYPE III
Cytotrophoblasts (direct preparation)	Mosaic or nonmosaic aneuploidy	Normal diploidy	Mosaic or nonmosaic diploidy
Placental stroma (CVS culture)	Normal diploidy	Mosaic	Nonmosaic aneuploidy
Fetus	Normal diploidy	Normal diploidy	Nonmosaic aneuploidy

TABLE 30–24. DISCREPANCIES BETWEEN VARIOUS CELL PREPARATIONS CLASSIFIED BY ANEUPLOIDIES*

	CVS					
REFERENCES	DIRECT PREPARATION	LONG-TERM CULTURE	PLACENTA	AMNIO	FETUS	LIVE-BORN
Brambati et al, 1985[121]	46/47,+3	—	—	—	46	—
Mikkelsen, 1985[122]	—	46/47,+3	47,+3	—	46	—
Simoni et al, 1985[123]	46/47,+3	46	—	—	46	—
Schulze et al, 1987[124]	46/47,+3	46	—	—	46	—
Callen et al, 1988[114]	46/47,+3	—	—	—	—	—
Callen et al, 1988[114]	46/47,+3	—	—	46	—	—
Green et al, 1988[115]	46/47,+3	—	—	46	—	—
Schwinger et al, 1989[117]	46/47,+3	—	—	46	—	†
Schwinger et al, 1989[117]	46/47,+3	—	—	—	—	†
Verjaal et al, 1987[125]	46/47,+5	—	—	46	—	—
Schwinger et al, 1989[117]	46/47,+5	—	46/47,+5	46	—	†
Schwinger et al, 1989[117]	47,+6	—	46/47,+6	—	—	—
Bartels et al, 1986[126]	46/47,+7	46/47,+7	—	—	46	—
Leschot et al, 1987[113]	46/47,+7	—	—	46	—	†
Callen et al, 1988[114]	46/47,+7	—	—	—	46	—
Callen et al, 1988[114]	46/47,+7	—	—	46	—	—
Delozier-Blanchett et al, 1988[127]	47,+7	—	Central—46 Peripheral —46/47,+20 t(2;21)	46	46	—
Wapner et al, 1985[109]	47,+8	46	—	46	—	—
Hogge et al, 1986[112]	—	46/47,+8	—	46	—	—
Green et al, 1988[115]	46/47,+8	—	—	46	—	—
Leschot et al, 1987[113]	47,+11	—	—	46	—	†
Callen et al, 1988[114]	46/47,+11	—	—	—	46	—
Green et al, 1988[115]	46/47,+11	—	—	46	—	—
Kalousek et al, 1987[128]	46/47,+12	46	—	—	46	—
Verjaal et al, 1987[125]	46/47,+12	—	—	46	—	46
Wapner et al, 1985[109]	46/47,+13	46	—	46	—	—
Wapner et al, 1985[109]	46/47,+13	46	—	—	46	—
Cheung et al, 1987[105]	46/47,+13	46	—	—	—	46
Kalousek et al, 1987[128]	46/47,+13	46	—	46	—	46
Callen et al, 1988[114]	46/47,+13	—	46/47,+13	—	46	—
Callen et al, 1988[114]	46/47,+13	46	46/47,+13	—	46	—
Kalousek et al, 1987[128]	—	46/47,+14	—	46/47,+14	46	—
Wegner et al, 1988[129]	46/47,+14	(11 week 47,+14; 12 week 46)	—	—	46/47,+14	—
Hogge et al, 1988[112]	—	46/47,+15	—	46	—	—
Martin et al, 1986b[130]	46/47,+15	—	—	46	—	—
Schulze et al, 1987[124]	46/47,+15	46/47,+15	—	—	46	—
Callen et al, 1988[114]	46/47,+15	46/47,+15	—	46	—	†
Breed et al, 1990[116]	47, +15	—	—	—	46	—
Brambati et al, 1985[121]	46/47,+16	—	—	—	46	—
Mikkelsen, 1985[122]	—	47,+16	47,+16	—	46	—
Simoni et al, 1985[123]	47,+16	—	—	—	46	—
Simoni et al, 1985[123]	47,+16	46/47,+16	—	—	—	—
Hogge et al, 1986[112]	—	47,+16	—	—	46	—
Leschot et al, 1987[113]	46/47,+16	—	46	—	Spontaneous abortion	—
Callen et al, 1988[114]	46/47,+16	—	Amnion 46/47,+16	46	—	†
Callen et al, 1988[114]	47,+16	—	47,+16	—	46	—
Tharapel et al, 1989[137]	47,+16	47,+16	Amnion 46/47,+16 Placenta-46 Pla. Nodule 46/47,+16	46	—	46

(continued)

TABLE 30–24. (continued)

REFERENCES	CVS		PLACENTA	AMNIO	FETUS	LIVE-BORN
	DIRECT PREPARATION	LONG-TERM CULTURE				
Schwinger et al, 1989[117]	46/47,+16	—	—	—	—	†
Verp et al, 1989[132]	46/47,+16	47,+16	47,+16	46	—	46†
Williams et al, 1989[133]	47,+16	47,+16	46/47,+16	46	—	46 (VSD)
Kalousek et al, 1987[128]	—	46/47,+17	46/47,+17 Amnion-46	—	—	46
Heim et al, 1985[108]	47,+18	—	46	—	—	—
Mikkelsen, 1985[122]	—	47,+18	47,+18	—	46	—
Simoni et al, 1985[123]	47,+18	—	—	—	46	—
Simoni et al, 1985[123]	46/47,+18	46/47,+18	—	—	46	—
Hogge et al, 1986[112]	—	46/47,+18	—	46	—	—
Martin et al, 1986a[110]	46	47,+18	—	47,+18	47,+18	—
Schulze and Miller et al, 1986[134]	—	46/47,+18	—	46	—	—
Callen et al, 1988[114]	46/47,+18	—	—	—	46	—
Callen et al, 1988[114]	47,+18	—	—	—	46/47,+18	—
Callen et al, 1988[114]	46/47,+18	—	—	46	—	—
Green et al, 1988[115]	46/47,+18	—	—	46	—	—
Green et al, 1988[115]	46/47,+18	—	—	46	—	—
Leschot et al, 1988[55]	46	—	Site A—46 Site B—47,+18	47,+18	—	Stillborn 47,+18
Wirtz et al, 1988[135]	46	—	—	47,+18	47,+18	—
Breed et al, 1990[116]	47, +18	—	—	—	46	—
Schwinger et al, 1989[117]	46/47,+18	—	46/47,+18	—	47,+18	—
Leschot et al, 1987[113]	46/47,+19	—	—	46	—	—
Green et al, 1988[115]	46/47,+19	—	—	46	—	—
Mikkelsen, 1985[122]	—	47,+20	47,+20	—	46	—
Mikkelsen, 1985[122]	—	46/47,+20	47,+20	—	46	—
Wapner et al, 1985[109]	47,+20	47,+20	—	46/47,+20	—	—
Schwinger et al, 1989[117]	46/47,+20	46	—	46	—	†
Callen et al, 1988[114]	46/47,+21	46/47,+21	—	46	—	—
Callen et al, 1988[114]	46	46/47,+21	46	46/47,+21	—	—
Crane and Cheung, 1988[136]	46/47,+21	47,+21	—	—	47,+21	—
Nisani et al, 1989[137]	46	47,+21 (1st CVS 46/47,+21 2nd CVS)	—	46/47,+21	46	46/47,+21
Mikkelsen, 1985[122]	—	46,XY/45,X	—	46,XY	—	—
Mikkelsen, 1985[122]	—	46,XY/45,X	46,XY/45,X	—	46,XY	—
Mikkelsen, 1985[122]	—	46,XY/45,X	—	46,XY	—	—
Simoni et al, 1985[123]	46,XY/45,X	46,XY	—	—	46,XY	—
Hogge et al, 1986[112]	—	45,X	—	—	46,XY	—
Hogge et al, 1986[112]	—	46,XY/45,X	—	46,XY	—	46,XY
Hogge et al, 1986[112]	—	46,XY/45,X	—	46,XY	—	—
Hogge et al, 1986[112]	—	46,XY/45,X	—	46,XY	—	—
Smidt-Jensen and Lind, 1987[138]	46,XY	46,XY/45,X	—	—	46,XY/45,X	—
Mulcahy et al, 1989[139]	45,X	46,XY	—	—	Term'd NA	
Schwinger et al, 1989[117]	46,XY/45,X	—	46,XY/45,X	46,XY	—	46,XY†
Eichenbaum et al, 1986[140]	46,XY	46,XY/47,XXY	—	—	46,XY/47,XXY	—
Linton & Lilford, 1986[141]	46,XY	47,XXY	—	46,XY/47,XXY	46,XY/47,XXY	—
Cheung et al, 1987[105]	46,XY/47,XXY	46,XY	—	46,XY	—	— 46,XY
Hogge et al, 1986[112]	—	46,XX/45,X	—	46,XX	—	—
Martin et al, 1986b[130]	46,XX/45,X	46,XX/45,X	—	—	46,XX	—
Schulze & Miller, 1986[134]	—	46,XX/45,X	—	46,XX	—	—
Cheung et al, 1987[105]	46,XX/45,X	46,XX	—	—	—	46,XX

(continued)

TABLE 30–24. (continued)

REFERENCES	CVS DIRECT PREPARATION	CVS LONG-TERM CULTURE	PLACENTA	AMNIO	FETUS	LIVE-BORN
Leschot et al, 1987[113]	46,XX/45,X	—	—	46,XX	—	—
Green et al, 1988[115]	46,XX/45,X	—	—	46,XX	—	—
Green et al, 1988[115]	46,XX/45,X	—	—	46,XX	—	—
Green et al, 1988[115]	46,XX/45,X	—	—	46,XX	—	—
Breed et al, 1990[116]	45,X	—	—	—	46,XX	—
Mikkelsen, 1985[122]	—	46,XX/47,XXX	—	46,XX	—	—
Wapner et al, 1985[109]	46,XX/47,XXX	46,XX	—	46,XX	—	—
Schulze et al, 1986[124]	46,XX	46,XX/47,XXX	—	46,XX	—	—
Cheung et al, 1987[105]	46,XX	46,XX/47,XXX	—	—	—	46,XX
Verjaal et al, 1987[125]	—	—	46,XX	46,XX/47,XXX	—	46,XX/47,XXX
Karkut et al, 1985[100]	46	46/47,+mar	—	—	—	—
Cheung et al, 1987[105]	46/47,+mar	46	—	46	—	46
Kalousek et al, 1987[128]	47,+mar	46	Amnion—46 Chorion—46	—	—	46
Leschot et al, 1987[113]	47,+mar	—	47,+mar	—	46	—
Leschot et al, 1987[113]	46/47,+mar	—	—	46	—	†
Green et al, 1988[115]	46/47,+mar	—	—	46	—	—
Ammala et al, 1989[116]	46/47,+mar	46	—	—	—	46
Heim et al, 1985[108]	—	92,XXY	—	46,XY	—	—
Wapner et al, 1985[109]	92,XXYY	46,XY	—	—	—	—
Wapner et al, 1985[109]	92,XXXX	46,XX	—	—	—	—
Leschot et al, 1987[113]	92,XXYY	—	—	46,XY	—	†
Leschot et al, 1987[113]	46,XY/92,XXYY	—	—	46,XY	—	†
Schwinger et al, 1988[117]	46,XY/92,XXYY	—	46/92	—	Spontaneous abortion	—

* Aneuploidies involving more than one chromosome or more than two cell lines or structural rearrangements are not listed here.
† Normal Liveborn.
NA = Not Available.

also know now that these risks can be significantly reduced if both direct CVS preparation and long-term villus culture are mandated for chromosome analysis. More important, whenever there is a doubtful diagnosis, such as chromosome mosaicism or an unusual aneuploidy, amniocentesis must be recommended as a backup study.

CONCLUSION

The increased public awareness of genetic amniocentesis, the trend among career women to plan a family late in their 30s, and the growing use of maternal serum AFP screening (for both high and low values) have all resulted in a greater demand for genetic prenatal diagnosis. Limitations of resources and trained technical personnel are hurdles yet to be overcome, but the expansion of these services is likely to continue. Since commercial facilities can provide services only to affluent consumers, a significantly large proportion of patients still needs to be financially subsidized for these important services.

Although chorionic villi sampling has demonstrated the great advantage of providing a diagnosis in the first trimester, the relatively high fetal loss rate from the procedure, as well as its high cytogenetic discrepancy rate, must be addressed and the results improved. Meanwhile, for at least several years, genetic amniocentesis will remain the more popular method for the vast majority of patients requesting prenatal cytogenetic diagnosis, and the only method for patients with low MSAFP.

Although the advent of molecular genetic technology will not eliminate the basic cytogenetic technologies, it has become more and more necessary for a cytogenetics laboratory either to have molecular components or to affiliate with a molecular cytogenetics facility for the capability to diagnose subtle abnormalities not detectable with regular banding methods.

Recent development using biotinylated chromosome-specific probes for the identification of specific human chromosomes ("chromosome painting") appears to be a practical addition for cytogenetic laboratories. The biotinylated probes are nonradioactive. Thus, with a fluorescent microscope one can readily examine fluorescence in situ hybridization.[144–147]

Less invasive methods for early prenatal testing, such as sorting out fetal cells from the maternal circulation, are currently being investigated.

ACKNOWLEDGMENT

This work was supported by New York City Health Department, Maternal and Child Health Block Grant.

I thank Eva Kahn for her helpful suggestions, Carmen Vazquez and Janet Rivera for the preparation of the manuscript, and Theresa Perlis and Alena Leff for the proofreading of the manuscript.

REFERENCES

1. Hsu LYF. Prenatal diagnosis of chromosome abnormalities. In: Milunsky A, ed. Genetic disorders and the fetus. New York: Plenum Press, 1986:115.
2. Boué A, Gallano P. A collaborative study of the segregation of inherited chromosome structural rearrangements in 1356 prenatal diagnoses. Prenatal diagnosis (Special Issue) 1984;4:45.
3. Daniel A, Hook EB, Wulf G. Risks of unbalanced progeny at amniocentesis to carriers of chromosome rearrangements: data from United States and Canadian Laboratories. Am J Med Genet 1989;33:14.
4. Daniel A, Boué A, Gallano P. Prospective risk in reciprocal translocation in heterozygotes at amniocentesis as determined by potential chromosome inbalance sizes. Data of the European collaborative prenatal diagnosis centres. Prenat Diagn 1986;6:315.
5. Hamerton JL. Chromosome mutation II:IV Reciprocal translocation in man. In: Human cytogenetics. Vol I. New York: Academic Press, 1971:254.
6. Mikkelsen M, Ayme A. Chromosomal findings in chorionic villi. A collaborative study. In: Vogel F, Sperling K, eds. Proceedings of the 7th International Congress of Human Genetics. Berlin: Springer-Verlag, 1987:598.
7. Stene J, Steine E, Mikkelsen M. Risk for chromosome abnormality at amniocentesis following a child with a non-inherited chromosome aberration. Prenat Diagn (Special Issue) 1984; 4:81.
8. Merkatz JR, Nitowsky HM, Macri JN, Johnson WE. An association between low maternal serum alpha-fetoprotein and fetal chromosomal abnormalities. Am J Obstet Gynecol 1984; 148:886.
9. Cuckle HS, Wald NJ, Lindenbaum RH. Maternal serum alpha-fetoprotein measurement: a screening test for Down syndrome. Lancet 1984;I:926.
10. Hershey DW, Crandall BF, Perdue S. Combining maternal age and serum alpha-fetoprotein to predict the risk of Down syndrome. Obstet Gynecol 1986;68:177.
11. Martin AO, Liu K. Implications of "low" maternal serum alpha-fetoprotein levels: are maternal age risk criteria obsolete? Prenat Diagn 1986;6:243.
12. Ashwood ER, Cheng E, Luthy DA. Maternal serum alpha-fetoprotein and fetal trisomy 21 in women 35 years and older. Implications for alpha-fetoprotein screening programs. Am J Med Genet 1987;26:531.
13. Cuckle HS, Wald NJ, Thompson SG. Estimating a woman's risk of having a pregnancy associated with Down's syndrome using her age and serum alpha-fetoprotein level. Br J Obstet Gynecol 1987;94:387.
14. DiMaio MS, Baumgarten A, Greenstein RM, Saal HM, Mahoney MJ. Screening for fetal Down's syndrome in pregnancy by measuring maternal serum alpha-fetoprotein levels. N Engl J Med 1987;317:342.
15. Palomaki GE, Haddow JE. Maternal serum alpha-fetoprotein, age and Down syndrome risk. Am J Obstet Gynecol 1987;156:460.
16. Tabor A, Larsen SO, Neilsen J, et al. Screening for Down's syndrome using an iso-risk curve based on maternal age and serum alpha-fetoprotein level. Br J Obstet Gynecol 1987;94:636.
17. Hook EB. Variability in predicted roles of Down syndrome associated with elevated maternal serum alpha-fetoprotein levels in older women. Am J Hum Genet 1988;43:160.
18. New England Regional Genetics Group. Prenatal Collaborative Study of Down Syndrome Screening. Combining maternal serum alpha-fetoprotein measurements and age to screen for Down syndrome in pregnant women under 35. Am J Obstet Gynecol 1989;160:575.
19. Canick JA, Knight GJ, Palomaki GE, Haddow JE, Cuckle HS, Wald NJ. Low second trimester maternal serum unconjugated estriol in pregnancies with Down syndrome. Br J Obstet Gynecol 1988;95:330.
20. Ruta DA, Leece JG. Screening policy for Down syndrome. Lancet 1988;II:752.
21. Wald NJ, Cuckle HS, Densem JW, et al. Maternal serum screening for Down's syndrome in early pregnancy. Br Med J 1988;297:883.
22. Osathanondh R, Canick JA, Abell KB, et al. Second trimester screening for trisomy 21. Lancet 1989;II:52.
22a. Nussbaum RL, Ledbetter DH. The fragile X syndrome. In Scriver C, et al, eds. The metabolic basis of inherited diseases. 6th ed. New York: McGraw Hill, 1989:327.
22b. Lubs HA. A marker X chromosome. Am J Hum Genet 1969;21:231.
23. Sutherland GR. Fragile sites on human chromosome: Demonstration of their dependence on the type of tissue culture medium. Science 1977;197:265.
23a. Jenkins EC, Michael S, Krawczun, et al. Improved prenatal detection of fra(X) (q27.3): Methods for prevention of false negatives in chorionic villus and amniotic fluid cell cultures. Am J Med Genet 1991;38:447.
23b. Shapiro LR, Wilmot PL, Murphy PD. Prenatal diagnosis of the fragile X syndrome: Possible end of the experimental phase for amniotic fluid. Am J Med Genet 1991;38:453.
24. Verkerk AJMH, Pieretti M, Sutcliffe JS, et al. Identification of a gene (FMR-1) containing a CGG repeat coincident with a break point cluster region exhibiting length variation in fragile X syndrome. Cell 1991;65:905.
24a. Hirst M, Knight S, Davis K, et al. Prenatal diagnosis of fragile X syndrome. Lancet 1991;338:956.
24b. Dobkin CS, Ding XH, Jenkins EC, et al. Prenatal diagnosis of fragile X syndrome. Lancet 1991;338:957.
25. Auerbach AD, Sagi M, Adler B. Fanconi anemia: prenatal diagnosis in 30 fetuses at risk. Pediatrics 1985;76:794.
26. Auerbach AD, Min Z, Ghosh R, et al. Clastogen-induced chromosomal breakage as a marker for first trimester prenatal diagnosis of Fanconi anemia. Hum Genet 1986;73:86
27. Schwartz S, Flannery DB, Cohen MM. Tests appropriate for the prenatal diagnosis of ataxia telangiectasia. Prenat Diagn 1985;5:9.
28. Jackson-Cook CK, Flannery DB, Corey LA, Nance WE, Brown JA. Nucleolar organizer regions variants as a risk factor for Down syndrome. Am J Hum Genet 1985;37:1049.
29. Schwartz S, Roulston D, Cohen MM. Invited editorial: dNORs and meiotic nondisjunction. Am J Hum Genet 1989;44:627.
30. Green JE, Rosenbaum KN, Rapoport SI, Schapiro MB, White

BJ. Variant nucleolus organizing regions and the risk of Down syndrome. Clin Genet 1989;35:243.
31. Hamerton JL, Boué A, Cohen MM, de la Chapelle A, Hsu LYF, Lindsten J, et al. Section 2: chromosome disease. Prenatal diagnosis (Special Issue). Prenatal diagnosis—past, present and future (report of an international workshop), 1980:11.
32. Canadian Collaborative CVS-Amniocentesis Clinical Group. Multiple center randomized clinical trial of chorion villus sampling and amniocentesis. First report. Lancet 1989;I:1.
33. Chromosome analysis guidelines preliminary report. Karyogram 1989;15(6):131.
34. Driscoll DA, Zackai EH, Minnuti MT, McDonald DM, Budarf M, Emanuel BS. Molecular detection of a submicroscopic 4p deletion in Wolf-Hirschhorn syndrome (WHS). Pediatr Res (Abstract 826) 1989;25:140A.
35. Greenberg F, Elder FFB, Ledbetter DH, Altherr M, Wasmuth JJ. Molecular confirmation of Wolf-Hirschhorn syndrome with apparently normal chromosomes. Pediatr Res (Abstract 443) 1989;25:76A.
36. Hook EB. Exclusion of chromosome mosaicism: tables of 90%, 95% and 99% confidence limits and comments on use. Am J Hum Genet 1977;29:94.
37. Benn PA, Hsu LYF, Perlis T, Schonhaut AG. Prenatal diagnosis of chromosome mosaicism. Prenat Diagn 1984a;4:1.
38. Boué J, Nicholas H, Barichard F, Boué A. Leclonage des cellules du liquide amniotique, aide dans l'interpretation des mosaiques chromosomiques en diagnostic prenatal. Annales de Genetique 1979;22:3.
39. Hsu LYF, Kaffe S, Perlis TE. Trisomy 20 mosaicism in prenatal diagnosis—a review and update. Prenat Diagn 1987b;7:581.
40. Hsu LYF, Kaffee S, Perlis TE. A revisit of trisomy 20 mosaicism in prenatal diagnosis—an overview of 103 cases. Prenat Diagn 1991;11:7.
41. Baldinger S, Millard C, Schmeling D, Bendel RP. Prenatal diagnosis of trisomy 20 mosaicism indicating an extra embryonic origin. Prenat Diagn 1987;7:273.
42. Kalousek DK, Dill FJ. Chromosomal mosaicism confined to the placenta in human conceptions. Science 1983;221:665.
43. Miny P, Karabacak Z, Hammer P, Schulte-Vallentin M, Holzgreve W. Chromosome analysis from urinary sediment: postnatal confirmation of a prenatally diagnosed trisomy 20 mosaicism. N Engl J Med 1989;320:809.
44. Hsu, unpublished data.
45. Purvis-Smith AG, Saville T, Osborn RA. Prenatal diagnosis of trisomy 9 mosaicism. Pathology 1983;15:109.
46. Zadeh TM, Peters J, Sandlin C. Prenatal diagnosis of mosaic trisomy 9.Prenat Diagn 1987;7:67.116.
47. Schwartz S, Roulston D, Cohen MM. dNORs and meiotic nondisjunction. Am J Hum Genet 1989a;44:627.
48. Camurri L, Caselli L, Manent E. True mosaicism and pseudomosaicism in second trimester fetal karyotyping. A case of mosaic trisomy 8. Prenat Diagn 1988;8:168.
49. Kaffe S, Benn PA, Hsu LYF. Fetal blood sampling in investigation of chromosome mosaicism in amniotic fluid cell culture. Lancet 1988;II:284.
50. Bui TH, Iselius L, Lindsten J. European collaborative study on prenatal diagnosis: mosaicism, pseudomosaicism and single abnormal cell in amniotic fluid cell cultures. Prenat Diagn (Special Issue) 1984;4:145.
51. Priest J. Personal communication.
52. Casamassima AC, Wilmot PL, Mahoney MJ, Scott RV, Shapiro LR. Trisomy 5 mosaicism in amniotic fluid with normal outcome. Clin Genet 1989;35:282.
53. Richkind KE, Apostol RA, Puck SM. Prenatal detection of trisomy 5 mosaicism with normal outcome. Prenat Diagn 1987;7:143.
54. Penchaszadeh VB, Morejon DP, Gervis J, Schwartz M, Mahoney MJ, Babu A. Prenatally detected trisomy 5 mosaicism in amniotic fluid confirmed in the newborn. Am J Hum Genet (Abstract 256) 1988;43:A64.
55. Leschot NJ, Wilmsen-Linders EJ, VanGeijn HP, Samson JF, Smit LM. Karyotyping urine sediment cells confirms trisomy 12 mosaicism detected at amniocenteses. Clin Genet 1988;34:145.
56. Von Koskull H, Ritvanen A, Ammala P, Gahmberg N, Salonen R. Trisomy 12 mosaicism in amniocytes and dysmorphic child despite normal chromosomes in fetal blood sample. Prenat Diagn 1989;9:433.
57. Wilson MG, Lin MS, Fujimoto A, Herbert W, Kaplan FM. Chromosome mosaicism in 6,000 amniocenteses. Am J Med Genet 1989;32:506.
58. Stioui S, Silvestris M De, Molinari A, Stripparo L, Ghisoni L, Simoni G. Trisomy 22 placenta in a case of severe intrauterine growth retardation. Prenat Diagn 1989;9:673.
59. Hsu LYF. Prenatal diagnosis of 45,X/46,XY mosaicism—a review and update. Prenat Diagn 1989;9:31.
60. McFadden DE, Kalousek DK. Confirmation of prenatal diagnosis of sex chromosome mosaicism. Am J Med Genet 1989; 32:495.
61. Chang HJ, Clark RD, Bachman H. Prenatally diagnosed 45,X/46,XY and normal phenotype. Lancet 1989;I:961.
62. Kulkarni R, Hawkins J, Bradford WP. Prenatal diagnosis of 45,X/46,XX mosaicism in the fetus. Should the pregnancy be terminated? Prenat Diagn 1989;9:439.
63. Benn PA, Hsu LYF. Maternal cell contamination of amniotic fluid cell cultures: results of a U.S. nationwide survey. Am J Med Genet 1983;15:297.
64. Benn PA, Schonhaut AG, Hsu LYF. A high incidence of maternal cell contamination of amniotic fluid cell cultures. Am J Med Genet 1983;14:361.
64a. Benn PA, Gilbert F, Hsu LYF. Maternal cell contamination of amniotic fluid cultures from two consecutive pregnancies complicated by fibroids. Prenat Diagn 1984;4:151.
65. Freiberg AS, Blumberg B, Lawce H, Mann J. XX/XY chimerism encountered during prenatal diagnosis. Prenat Diagn 1988;8:423.
66. Hook EB, Cross PK. Extra structurally abnormal chromosomes (ESAC) detected at amniocentesis: frequency in approximately 75,000 prenatal cytogenetic diagnoses and association with maternal and paternal age. Am J Hum Genet 1987;40:83.
67. Wisniewski L, Hassold T, Heffelfinger J, Higgins JV. Cytogenetic and clinical studies in five cases of inv dup(15). Hum Genet 1979;50:259.
68. Buckton KE, Spowart G, Newton MS, Evans HJ. Forty-four probands with an additional "marker" chromosome. Hum Genet 1985;69:353.
69. Warburton D. Outcome of cases of de novo structural rearrangements diagnosed at amniocentesis. Prenat Diagn 1984;4:69.
69a. Warburton D. De novo balanced chromosome rearrangements and extra marker chromosomes identified at prenatal diagnosis: clinical significance and distribution of break points. Am J Hum Genet 1991;49:995.
70. Benn PA, Hsu LYF. Incidence and significance of supernumerary marker chromosomes in prenatal diagnosis. Am J Hum Genet 1984;36:1092.
71. Stetten G, Sroka-Zaczek B, Corson VL. Prenatal detection of an accessory chromosome identified as an inversion duplication (15). Hum Genet 1981;57:357.
72. Sachs ES, Van Hemel JO, Den Hollander JC, Jahoda GJ. Marker chromosomes in a series of 10,000 prenatal diagnoses. Cytogenetic and follow-up studies. Prenat Diagn 1987;7:81.

73. Buhler EM, Malik NJ. DA/DAPI heteromorphisms in acrocentric chromosomes other than 15. Cytogenet Cell Genet 1988;47:104.
74. Lin MS, Zhang A, Wilson MG, Fujimoto A. DA/DAPI-fluorescent heteromorphism of human Y chromosome. Hum Genet 1988;79:36.
75. Steinbach P, Djalali M, Hamsmann I, et al. The genetic significance of accessory bisatellited marker chromosomes. Hum Genet 1983;65:155.
75a. Callen DF, Eyre HJ, Baker E, et al. Molecular characterization of marker chromosomes in man. Am J Hum Genet 1990;43:A27 (Abstract #0099).
76. Kaffe S, Hsu LYF. Supernumerary marker chromosomes in a series of 19,000 prenatal diagnoses: pregnancy outcome of satellited vs. nonsatellited de novo markers. Am J Hum Genet (Abstract 944) 1988;43:A237.
77. Hsu LYF, Benn PA, Tannenbaum HL, et al. Chromosomal polymorphisms of 1, 9, 16, and Y in 4 major ethnic groups: a large prenatal study. Am J Med Genet 1987;26:95.
78. Werner W, Herman FH. Analysis of a familial 15p+polymorphism: exclusion of Y/15 translocation. Clin Genet 1984;26:204.
79. Petrovic V. A new variant of chromosome 3 with unusual staining properties. J Med Genet 1988;25:781.
80. Bardhan S, Singh DN, Davis K. Polymorphism in chromosome 4. Clin Genet 1981;20:44.
81. Dogherty Z, Bowser-Riley SM. A rare heterochromatic variant of chromosome 4. J Med Genet 1984;21:470.
82. Seabright M, Gregson NM, Johnson M. A familiar polymorphic variant of chromosome 5. J Med Genet 1980;17:444.
83. Fineman RM, Issa B, Weinblatt V. Prenatal diagnosis of a large heteromorphic region in a chromosome 5: implications for genetic counseling. Am J Med Genet 1989;32:498.
84. Thompson PW, Roberts SH. A new variant of chromosome 16. Hum Genet 1987;76:100.
85. Kubien E, Kleczkowska A. Familial occurrence of chromosome variant 17ph+. Clin Genet 1977;12:39.
86. Hoo JJ, Robertson A. 18ph+ is a normal chromosomal variant. Clin Genet 1987;32:79.
87. Fryns JP, Kleczkowska A, Smeets E, VanDenBergh H. A new centromeric heteromorphism in the short arm of chromosome 20. J Med Genet 1988;25:636.
88. Crossen PE. Variation in the centromeric banding of chromosome 19. Clin Genet 1975;8:218.
89. Alessandro ED, DeMatteis Vaccarella C, LoRe ML, et al. Pericentric inversion of chromosome 19 in three families. Hum Genet 1988;80:203.
90. Jacobs PA. Correlation between euploid structural chromosome rearrangements and mental subnormality in humans. Nature 1974;249:164.
91. Macgregor DJ, Imrie S, Tolmie JL. Outcome of de novo balanced translocations ascertained prenatally. J Med Genet 1989;26:590.
92. Nielsen J, Krag-Olsen B. Follow-up of 32 children with autosomal translocations found among 11,148 consecutively newborn children from 1964–1974. Clin Genet 1981;20:48.
93. Tierney I, Axworthy D, Smith L, Ratcliffe SG. Balanced rearrangements of the autosomes: results of a longitudinal study of a newborn survey population. J Med Genet 1984;21:45.
94. Chen TR. In situ detection of mycoplasma contamination in cell cultures by fluorescent Hoechst 33258 stain. Exp Cell Res 1977;104:255.
95. Russell WC, Newman C, Williamson DH. A simple cytochemical technique for demonstration of DNA in cells infected with mycoplasmas and viruses. Nature 1975;253:461.
96. Milunsky A. The prenatal diagnosis of chromosomal disorders. In: Milunsky A, ed. Genetic disorders and the fetus. New York: Plenum Press, 1979:93.
97. Scarbrough PR, Hersh J, Kukolich MK, et al. Tetraploidy: a report of three live-born infants. Am J Med Genet 1984;19:29.
98. Quiroz E, Orozco A, Salamanca F. Diploid-tetraploid mosaicism in a malformed boy. Clin Genet 1985;27:183.
99. Golbus MS, Cunningham N, Goldberg JD, Anderson R, Filly R, Callen P. Selective termination of multiple gestations. Am J Med Genet 1988;31:339.
100. Karkut I, Zakrzewski S, Sperling K. Mixed karyotypes obtained by chorionic villi analysis: mosaicism and maternal contamination. In: Fraccaro M, Simoni G, Brambati B, eds. First trimester fetal diagnosis. Berlin: Springer-Verlag, 1985:144.
101. Cooke HMG, Penketh RJA, Delhanty JDA. An evaluation of maternal cell contamination in cultures of chorionic villi for the prenatal diagnosis of chromosome abnormalities. Clin Genet 1986;30:458.
102. Olson S, Buckmaster J, Bissonnette J, Magenis E. Comparison of maternal and fetal chromosome heteromorphisms to monitor maternal cell contamination in chorionic villus samples. Prenat Diagn 1986;7:413.
103. Simoni G, Rossella F, Lalatta F, Fraccaro M. Maternal metaphases on direct preparation from chorionic villi and in cultures of villi cells. Hum Genet 1986a;72:104.
104. Williams J III, Medearis AL, Chu WH, Kovacs GD, Kaback MM. Maternal cell contamination in cultured chorionic villi: comparison of chromosome Q-polymorphisms derived from villi, fetal skin and maternal lymphocytes. Prenat Diagn 1987;7:315.
105. Cheung SW, Crane JP, Beaver HA, Burgess AC. Chromosome mosaicism and maternal cell contamination in chorionic villi. Prenat Diagn 1987;7:535.
106. Roberts E, Duckett DP, Lang GD. Maternal cell contamination in chorionic villus samples assessed by direct preparations and three different culture methods. Prenat Diagn 1988;8:635.
107. Blakemore K, Mahoney MJ. Chorionic villus sampling. In: Milunsky A, ed. Genetic disorders and the fetus. New York: Plenum Press, 1986:625.
108. Heim S, Kristoffersson U, Mandahl N, et al. Chromosome analysis in 100 cases of first trimester trophoblast sampling. Clin Genet 1985;27:451.
109. Wapner R, Jackson L, Davis G, Barr M, Hux C. Cytogenetic discrepancies found at chorionic villus sampling (CVS). Am J Hum Genet (Abstract 358) 1985;37:A122.
110. Martin AO, Elias S, Rosinsky B, Bombard AT, Simpson JL. False negative finding on chorionic villus sampling. Lancet 1986a;II:391.
111. Simoni G, Gimelli G, Cuoco C, et al. First trimester fetal karyotyping: one thousand diagnoses. Hum Genet 1986b;72:203.
112. Hogge WA, Schonberg SA, Golbus MS. Chorionic villus sampling: experience of the first 1000 cases. Am J Obstet Gynecol 1986;154:1249.
113. Leschot N, Wolf H, Verjaal M, et al. Chorionic villi sampling: cytogenetic and clinical findings in 500 pregnancies. Br Med J 1987;295:407.
114. Callen DF, Korban G, Dawson G, et al. Extraembryonic/fetal karyotypic discordance during diagnostic chorionic villus sampling. Prenat Diagn 1988;8:453.
115. Green JE, Dorfmann A, Jones SL, Bender S, Patton L, Schulman JD. Chorionic villus sampling: experience with an initial 940 cases. Obstet Gynecol 1988;71:208.
116. Breed ASPM, Martingh A, Beekhuis JR, et al. The predictive value of cytogenetic diagnosis after CVS: 1500 cases. Prenat Diagn 1990;10:101.
117. Schwinger E, Seidl E, Klink F, Rehder H. Chromosome mosa-

icism of the placenta. A cause of developmental failure of the fetus. Prenat Diagn 1989;9:639.
118. Vejerslev LO, Mikkelsen M. The European collaborative study on mosaicism in chorionic villus sampling: data from 1986 and 1987. Prenat Diagn 1989;9:575.
119. Koulischer L, Hustin J, Gillerot Y. Histologic study of tritiated thymidine incorporation by trophoplastic villi in first trimester. In: Fraccaro M, Simoni G, Brambati B, eds. First trimester fetal diagnosis. Berlin: Springer-Verlag, 1985:161.
120. Kalousek DK. The role of confined chromosomal mosaicism in placental function and human development. Growth, Genetics and Hormones 1988;4:1.
121. Brambati B, Simoni G, Danesino C, et al. First trimester fetal diagnosis of genetic disorders. Clinical evaluation of 250 cases. J Med Genet 1985;22:92.
122. Mikkelsen M. Cytogenetic findings in first trimester chorionic villi biopsies: a collaborative study. In: Fraccaro M, Simoni G, Brambati B, eds. First trimester fetal diagnosis. Berlin: Springer-Verlag, 1985:109.
123. Simoni G, Gimelli G, Cuoco C, et al. Discordance between prenatal cytogenetic diagnosis after chorionic villi sampling and chromosomal constitution of the fetus. In: Fraccaro M, Simoni G, Brambati B, eds. First trimester fetal diagnosis. Berlin: Springer-Verlag, 1985:137.
124. Schulze B, Schlesinger CH, Miller K. Chromosomal mosaicism confined to chorionic tissue. Prenat Diagn 1987;7:451.
125. Verjaal M, Leschot NJ, Wolf H, Treffer PE. Karyotypic differences between cells from placenta and other fetal tissues. Prenat Diagn 1987;7:343.
126. Bartels I, Rauskolb R, Hansmann I. Chromosomal mosaicism of trisomy 7 restricted to chorionic villi. Am J Med Genet 1986;25:161.
127. Delozier-Blanchet CD, Engel E, Extermann P, Pastori B. Trisomy 7 in chorionic villi: follow-up studies of pregnancy, normal child, and placental clonal anomalies. Prenat Diagn 1988;8:281.
128. Kalousek DK, Dill FJ, Pantzar T, McGillivray BC, Yong SL, Wilson RD. Confined chorionic mosaicism in prenatal diagnosis. Hum Genet 1987;77:163.
129. Wegner RD, Hohle R, Karkut G, Sperling K. Trisomy 14 mosaicism leading to cytogenetic discrepancies in chorionic villi sampled at different times. Prenat Diagn 1988;8:239.
130. Martin AO, Simpson JL, Rosinsky BS, Elias S. Chorionic villus sampling in continuing pregnancies. II. Cytogenetic reliability. Am J Obstet Gynecol 1986b;154:1353.
131. Tharapel AT, Elias S, Shulman LP, Seely L, Emerson DS, Simpson JL. Resorbed co-twin as an explanation for discrepant chorionic villus results: non-mosaic 47,XX,+16 in villi (direct and culture) with normal (46,XX) amniotic fluid and neonatal blood. Prenat Diagn 1989;9:467.
132. Verp MS, Rosinsky B, Sheikh Z, Amarose AP. Non-mosaic trisomy 16 confined to villi. Lancet 1989;2:915.
133. Williams J, Wang B, Rubin C, Clark R, Mohandas T. Apparent non-mosaic trisomy 16 in chorionic villi: diagnostic dilemma or clinically significant finding? Am J Hum Genet (Abstract 1077) 1989;45:A273.
134. Schulze B, Miller K. Chromosomal mosaicism and maternal cell contamination in chorionic villi cultures. Clin Genet 1986; 30:239.
135. Wirtz A, Seidel H, Brusis E, Murkey J. Another false-negative finding on placental sampling. Prenat Diagn 1988;8:321.
136. Crane JP, Cheung SW. An embryogenic model to explain cytogenetic inconsistencies observed in chorionic villus versus fetal tissue. Prenat Diagn 1988;8:119.
137. Nisani R, Chemke J, Voss R, et al. The dilemma of chromosomal mosaicism in chorionic villus sampling: direct versus long-term cultures. Prenat Diagn 1989;9:223.
138. Smidt-Jensen S, Lind AM. A case of first trimester chromosomal mosaicism confined to the cultivation of the gestational products. Clin Genet 1987;32:133.
139. Mulcahy MT, Murch AR, Rose A, Chabros V. Another case of completely discordant findings at CVS. Prenat Diagn 1989;9:221.
140. Eichenbaum SZ, Krumins EJ, Fortune DW, Duke J. False-negative finding on chorionic villus sampling. Lancet 1986;II:391.
141. Linton G, Lilford RJ. False-negative finding on chorionic villus sampling. Lancet 1986;II:630.
141a. Miny P, Basaran S, Holgreve W, Horst J, Pawlowitzki IH, Kim Nhan Ngo T. False negative cytogenetic result in direct preparations after CVS. Prenat Diagn 1988;8:633.
141b. Kalousek D, Barrett IJ, McGillivray BC. Placental mosaicism and intrauterine survival of trisomies 13 and 18. Am J Hum Genet 1989;44:338.
142. Hunter A. False-positive and false-negative findings on chorionic villus sampling. Prenat Diagn 1988;8:475.
143. Tomkins DJ, Vekemans MJJ. False positive and false negative cytogenetic findings on chorionic villus sampling. Prenat Diagn 1989;9:139.
144. Lau YF. Detection of Y-specific repeat sequences in normal and variant human chromosomes using in situ hybridization with biotinylated probes. Cytogenet Cell Genet 1985;39:184.
145. Julien C, Bazin A, Guyot B, Forestier F, Daffos F. Rapid prenatal diagnosis of Down's syndrome with in-situ hybridization of fluorescent DNA probes. Lancet 1986;II:863.
146. Pinkel D, Straume T, Gray JW. Cytogenetic analysis using quantitative, high-sensitivity, fluorescence hybridization. Proc Natl Acad Sci USA 1986;83:2934.
147. Guyot B, Bazin A, Sole Y, Julien C, Daffos F, Forestier F. Prenatal diagnosis with biotinylated chromosome specific probes. Prenat Diagn 1988;8:485.

31

CHAPTER

SINGLE GENE DISORDERS

Maurice J. Mahoney

Genetic disorders are commonly classified into three large categories:

- Disorders due to single gene mutations, often termed Mendelian disorders.
- Disorders due to chromosomal abnormalities
- Disorders due to an interaction of several genetic and environmental factors, termed multifactorial or polygenic disorders

Although this classification represents some oversimplification, especially in light of such phenomena as small chromosome deletions and differential expression of genes in different environments, it provides a useful focus for understanding current approaches to prenatal diagnosis.

Single gene disorders represent a very large group of individually infrequent, often rare, conditions numbering in the hundreds. Diagnoses depend mostly on gene analysis or analysis of a gene's product, and occasionally on effects secondary to deficient gene function. This chapter will address prenatal diagnosis of these single gene disorders.

Chromosomal abnormalities such as Down syndrome or trisomy 18 are by far the most frequent disorders addressed by current diagnostic activities that use invasive techniques. At most prenatal diagnosis centers 90% or more of amniocenteses or chorionic villus samplings for genetic diagnosis will have determination of the fetal karyotype as their primary goal. This area is discussed in detail in Chapter 30.

Multifactorial disorders have complex etiologies, often depicted as combining small effects of several hypothetical factors. Neural tube defects, facial clefts, and dysplastic kidneys are examples of disorders in this category. At present, if prenatal diagnosis of a multifactorial disorder is successful, it is usually accomplished by sonographic imaging of altered anatomy. It may be that eventually a small number of genetic or nongenetic factors, perhaps as few as one or two, may be recognized as having the major causative role in generating the anomaly; then that factor or factors could become the target for diagnostic efforts. Progress in this direction may change prenatal diagnosis of multifactorial disorders to resemble the laboratory-based diagnosis of chromosomal and single gene disorders.

The continuing rapid progress in molecular and biochemical genetics makes futile any attempt to compile a complete list of possible diagnoses and the appropriate methodology to accomplish a specific diagnosis. When an obstetrician or genetic counselor is faced with questions in this area, consultation with specialists or referral to prenatal diagnosis centers is necessary. This chapter will consider first, the major methods by which diagnoses are sought, with examples of specific diagnoses that use each method, and second, groups of disorders that are diagnosable today, again with examples of specific diagnoses within each group. The reader is referred for further details to textbooks devoted to prenatal diagnosis[1,2] and to a catalog that lists diagnosed conditions.[3]

METHODS OF DIAGNOSIS

The primary abnormality in a single gene disorder is presumed to lie at the level of the gene, usually in the structure of the gene at fault, or, less often, in a controlling element of that gene. The most elementary and proximate method of diagnosis would be analysis of the gene. Recently this has become possible for more than two dozen genes, and the pace of gene discovery from current efforts to clone genes and to sequence the human genome ensures that there will be a rapid increase in that number. For many disorders, however, the gene either is not yet known or has not yet been isolated and studied, so other diagnostic strategies are necessary. These parallel the methods of postnatal genetic diagnosis that have been established for many decades. Even when a gene has been isolated and studied, diagnosis of a disease state may be made more efficiently through analysis of the gene product or some other effect secondary to the primary gene defect. This is true, for example, when a disease state arises from a large number of different mutations in a specific gene (allelic variation or allelic heterogeneity) or when the disease state arises from mutations in more than one gene, each affecting a final common pathway that leads to disease expression (genetic heterogeneity). Thus, a number of strategies that are one or more steps away from the primary gene defect have been used.

At present most prenatal diagnoses of single gene disorders require tissue or cells that contain the fetal genome and fetal gene products, usually cells external to the fetus itself but within the womb. These are recovered by amniocentesis or chorionic villus sampling. Occasionally cells obtained directly from the fetus via fetal blood sampling (cordocentesis) or fetal organ biopsy (from skin, liver, or muscle) are required. Use of the least dangerous approach that will achieve accurate information is axiomatic to the discipline of prenatal diagnosis. Thus, fetal organ biopsy is rarely used, being reserved for situations where a disease is expressed in that organ but not in amniotic fluid cells or chorionic villi. Diagnostic techniques that avoid invasion of the womb altogether would be preferable, and this should become possible as progress is made in the isolation of fetal cells that cross into the maternal circulation and can be recovered from a small sample of the pregnant woman's blood.[4,5]

In addition to analysis of genes and gene products, several other approaches have been successful in the prenatal diagnosis of single gene disorders. These approaches generally depend on expression of the disease phenotype in one way or another. Sometimes they are not applicable at early stages of pregnancy but must await expression of the disease as the fetus develops. Sonographic imaging, fetoscopic imaging, measurement of metabolite concentrations, histology of biopsies, and chromosomal analysis have been among the successful approaches.

SONOGRAPHIC IMAGING

Pedigree analysis has established single gene mutations as the presumed or probable etiology of a large number of malformations and birth defect syndromes,[6,7] but progress in understanding the underlying gene defect or the cellular pathology leading to the malformations has been very slow. The pathologic events most often take place during early embryogenesis. Some processes may be ongoing and still amenable to detection during the fetal stage, but many will already have been completed, leaving the malformations as the evidence of earlier cell malfunction. When altered anatomy can be visualized sonographically, imaging can be used to reach a diagnosis. X-linked aqueductal stenosis, for example, often produces ventriculomegaly in the second trimester. This example also points out significant limitations of this approach to diagnosis. Early diagnosis, in the first trimester, has not yet been possible because demonstration of ventriculomegaly is currently achieved only in the second trimester or later. The pathologic process may not even progress to ventriculomegaly in the early weeks. In some cases demonstrable ventriculomegaly will not occur until late in pregnancy or even until hydrocephalus is evident after birth. For these late manifesting cases, pregnancy interruption would probably not be a consideration because the surgical placement of an intracranial shunt after delivery would likely prove successful. Diagnostic accuracy for the condition itself, however, is limited by these variations in expression.

Other genetic malformation syndromes always or almost always manifest an anatomic abnormality. The severe skeletal dysplasia achondrogenesis, a recessive disorder, always shows extremely short ribs and limb bones; type II osteogenesis imperfecta, most often a dominant disorder, will show compacted, deformed limb bones in virtually all cases by the second trimester.

In some syndromes one manifestation will be much less constant than another. Chondroectodermal dysplasia (Ellis-van Creveld syndrome), a recessive disorder, has six fingers as a cardinal feature but a heart defect in only about half of cases. Meckel-Gruber syndrome, also a recessive disorder, usually shows the triad of encephalocele, polydactyly, and cystic kidneys, but any one of the three may be absent or rudimentary in a specific case. The variability in disease expression and the time during gestation at which altered anatomy occurs and can be visualized become crucial factors in sonographic diagnosis. Thorough knowledge of the disease and its expression are important. In many circumstances positive findings can be accepted as establishing a diagnosis, but negative findings will not exclude a diagnosis. When family history shows a high risk for an inherited malformation syndrome, that specific diagnosis can be inferred from an anatomic finding. Without the family history that same finding can generate several considerations in a differential diagnosis.

FETOSCOPIC IMAGING

Fetoscopy for direct optical visualization of the fetus in the second trimester was introduced in the 1970s.[8] Its main use was to obtain samples of fetal blood or skin during procedures, but it also had the capacity to visualize the surface of the fetus and allow diagnoses based on anatomic findings. The remarkable improvements in sonographic imaging since that time and the risk of miscarriage associated with fetoscopy have rendered the technique essentially obsolete either for fetal visualization or as an aid during biopsies or other intrauterine procedures.

The advantage of the fetoscope over sonographic

imaging was the viewing of small areas of anatomy, such as the tips of the digits, details of the genitalia, or features of facial anatomy. Syndactyly, hypospadias, or preauricular sinuses could be visualized and enable a diagnosis of a malformation syndrome beyond the capability of ultrasound. Occasionally, fetoscopic imaging might still be of use in these types of circumstances, but indications are few today and very few perinatologists have developed or maintained the skills necessary to make the procedure as safe as it can be. Visualization of the embryo with an embryoscope in the first trimester is now being investigated.[9] How useful the technique will be for prenatal diagnosis and how well sonographic imaging will compete for first trimester visualization are questions that will be answered in the next few years.

METABOLITE ANALYSIS

Inborn errors of metabolism, in which there typically is a block in a metabolic pathway, can usually be characterized by an accumulation or deficiency of one or more metabolites. The concentrations of these metabolites in various body fluids or tissues then become useful for diagnosis. If the metabolite in excess is present in fetal blood, it will probably be transferred to the maternal blood stream and further metabolized or excreted. Unfortunately, prenatal diagnosis by measurement of the metabolite in the mother's blood or urine has not proved useful as yet, for several reasons. The metabolite would rarely be unique to the fetus but would also be present in the mother, such that the mother's large volume of fluids and tissues, compared to that of the fetus, would provide rapid and large scale dilution. The mother presumably would have substantial metabolic capacity and well developed excretory mechanisms. Occasionally the concentration of the metabolite in the mother might be altered because of her own metabolism, reflecting a heterozygous carrier state of the homozygous disease state present in the fetus. More investigations are necessary if analyses of maternal metabolite concentrations are to contribute very much to prenatal diagnosis. If metabolites are unique to the fetus, however, there is reason to be encouraged about eventual success.

Fluids or tissues from the fetal compartment offer a much better opportunity for diagnosis via metabolite analysis. Here there is access to the metabolite before it has been acted on by maternal dilution or metabolism. A few disorders have been accurately diagnosed through measurements of metabolites in amniotic fluid. Amniotic fluid has some of the characteristics of a fetal plasma transudate, especially in the first trimester, and some of the characteristics of fetal urine, in the second and third trimesters. Of course, many metabolites from the maternal plasma also find their way into amniotic fluid, thereby making the composition of amniotic fluid complex.

Analysis of amniotic fluid is akin to analyzing fetal urine. In methylmalonic acidemias, for example, a greatly increased concentration of methylmalonate is found in amniotic fluid, both early and late in gestation, when the fetus has disease.[10] The same is true of methylcitrate in propionic acidemia[11] and of 17-OH progesterone in adrenogenital syndrome due to 21-hydroxylase deficiency.[12] Many other inborn errors are probably diagnosable in this way as well, but extensive efforts are required to establish the chemical methods for diagnosis, and the number of pregnancies at risk for most inborn errors of metabolism is very small. One group of inborn errors for which the results from amniotic fluid analyses have been disappointing is the disorders of amino acid metabolism characterized by high concentrations of one or more amino acids in blood or urine (eg, phenylketonuria). This may reflect the efficient dialysis and transport that occur within the placenta for amino acids, thereby preventing a large build-up in fetal blood of these common molecules.

HISTOLOGIC EXAMINATION

Tissue biopsies have played a limited role in prenatal diagnosis. The two tissues that are usually available with low risk to the fetus are cells from the amniotic fluid and chorionic villi (placenta), neither of which is part of the fetus per se. Fetal blood sampling and skin, liver, and muscle biopsy increase the risks of miscarriage and fetal demise. Unfortunately, uncultured amniotic fluid cells are a variable mixture of many cell types dominated in the second trimester by desquamated epithelial cells in varying stages of disintegration. Chorionic villi, on the other hand, are healthy tissue when biopsied; they consist of only a few cell types, essentially trophoblasts and a few types of mesenchymal cells. Thus far most of the success from histology has come from examination of skin biopsies for diagnosis of inherited skin diseases including ichthyoses, epidermolysis bullosa syndromes, and ectodermal dysplasias.[13] Pathologic changes diagnostic of the disease are sought. One major drawback is that diagnosis must be delayed until the skin has developed to a stage that can demonstrate disease and the pathologic process has indeed caused histologic abnormalities.

CHROMOSOME ANALYSIS

A few single gene disorders show abnormalities of chromosome structure when cells are examined by cytogenetic techniques. In many of these cases the conditions of laboratory analysis will have to be altered and tightly controlled in comparison to usual conditions for chromosome analysis. In general, the abnormality is demonstrable in any cell type as long as the cells are dividing and can be arrested in prophase or metaphase for examination. Many children with Roberts-SC phocomelia syndrome have shown premature separation at centromeres of chromosomes, and this phenomenon has been described in amniotic fluid cells.[14] Chromosome breakage syndromes, in which the affected individual's chromosomes have an increased number of breaks and perhaps rearrangements, have had prenatal diagnoses attempted. Examination for breaks and rearrangements has been very successful in the diagnosis of Fanconi pancytopenia syndrome.[15]

The fragile X syndrome, which is due to an abnormal gene on the X-chromosome and is one of the most common mental deficiency syndromes, has posed difficult prenatal diagnosis problems. One of the characteristics of the syndrome has been a fragile site on the distal part of the long arm of the X-chromosome (Xq27). Reliable demonstration of the fragile site in amniotic fluid cells, chorionic villi cells, or even fetal lymphocytes has been difficult. The recent isolation of the gene whose mutations putatively cause the syndrome should alter the situation dramatically and allow a much easier approach to prenatal diagnosis of fragile X by DNA analysis.[16,17]

GENE PRODUCTS

Single gene disorders are most often defined by a deficiency, alteration, or excess of a gene product. Even in this age of gene analysis and description of specific gene mutations, definition of a disorder is likely to remain tied to a gene product as long as pathophysiology and the basis for therapeutic intervention are most easily understood by reference to the gene product. Certainly, analysis of gene products for diagnosis continues to be very important both postnatally and prenatally and, as mentioned earlier, may have a major advantage when a disease shows important allelic or genetic heterogeneity.

Today, most, if not all, gene products that are associated with a disease process are proteins or peptides. (Abnormal RNAs that do not code for peptides will presumably be discovered, but they are not yet important to genetic diagnosis.) Most protein analyses in single gene disorders are measurements of enzyme activities, whereas a few analyses depend on physical attributes of the protein such as electrophoretic mobility or recognition of the protein by antibodies. The protein must be present, of course, in the cells or tissue used for diagnosis, ie, the gene must be expressed in that tissue. The large majority of prenatal diagnoses based on protein gene products have been able to use amniotic fluid cells and chorionic villi. For example, iduronidase activity is measured for the diagnosis of Hurler syndrome,[18] and collagens are analyzed for diagnosis of osteogenesis imperfecta syndromes.[19] Occasionally, another specialized tissue, such as liver or blood cells has been required, because of limited expression of the gene. For instance, ornithine transcarbamylase (OTC) is present in liver but not in measurable amounts in chorionic villi or amniotic fluid cells[20]; similarly, globins are present only in red blood cells.[21]

Healthy, living tissue is usually necessary for accurate protein analyses. Amniotic fluid cells, obtained by amniocentesis, are almost always cultured to provide this healthy tissue. Biopsies of chorionic villi or blood cell aspirates, on the other hand, consist almost entirely of healthy cells and thus can be used without being cultured as well as being used as a source of cultured cells. Because the culture process takes many days, analyses on uncultured biopsies have the advantage of providing a more rapid diagnosis.

GENE ANALYSIS

Understanding a genetic disease at the molecular level means isolating the gene responsible for the disease and demonstrating molecular abnormalities in that gene. The pace of discovery and study of these genes is accelerating, with the result that diagnoses for several diseases can now be accomplished by DNA or gene analyses. Cystic fibrosis,[22] Duchenne/Becker muscular dystrophy,[23] and most hemoglobinopathies[24] are some common single gene disorders that can be diagnosed in this way.

The sequence of gene discovery usually begins with an initial phase of gene mapping, in which the gene's approximate location on a chromosome or its relation to neighboring genetic material will be found, followed by eventual isolation of the gene and documentation of its mutations. During the first phase, DNA diagnosis will depend on linkage relationships to neighboring markers that can be followed from the parents to the fetus. These markers, known as restriction fragment length polymorphisms (RFLPs), arise because of naturally occurring polymorphic sites in human DNA. Because linked markers rather than the disease gene itself are being followed, the relationship of those markers to the mutant and normal alleles of the disease gene must be established individually for each family that requests prenatal diagnosis. These studies should be carried out, if at all possible, before a pregnancy has commenced. Major limitations of a DNA diagnosis that depends on linkage analysis are the possibility that RFLPs are unavailable in the family to distinguish mutant and normal alleles (ie, the polymorphism is not informative in that family), a family member who is crucial to establishing linkage relationships is not available, and the possibility of crossover events between the linked marker and the gene of interest during meiosis. The last of these limitations is minimized when informative markers are on both sides and thus flank the gene of interest.

When the gene and its structure are known and mutations have been discovered, possibilities of direct DNA diagnoses are generated based on the mutations present in the family. There may be large deletions in the gene or only single nucleotide substitutions as mutations. Sometimes the gene can be sequenced in a family to detect previously unrecognized mutations. Again, family studies should be started well before prenatal diagnosis is necessary, although direct gene analysis can sometimes be accomplished during a pregnancy for disorders in which there has been intensive study of the gene and its mutations. Fetal DNA, the diagnostic material required for gene analysis, is present in any fetal or extraembryonic tissue derived from the conceptus. Chorionic villi and amniotic fluid cells are the two sources used at present; fetal cells recovered from the maternal circulation may become an alternative in the future. Sometimes uncultured amniotic fluid cells will not provide sufficient DNA of requisite quality, and diagnosis must await a period of cell culture. This delay is usually not necessary when chorionic villi are used. The polymerase chain reaction (PCR) provides a method of amplifying tiny amounts of DNA and can help to minimize the time to diagnosis. To use PCR, however, considerable knowledge of the sequence of the gene is necessary.

PRENATAL DIAGNOSIS OF SPECIFIC DISORDERS

The following sections list specific disorders that can be diagnosed prenatally. The lists are not complete, and new information is constantly appearing in journals. It is especially important to consult with specialists in prenatal diagnosis when dealing with single gene disorders, because there are hundreds of these disorders and there are sometimes several possible methods by which a diagnosis might be approached. Specialty texts are also available.[1,2,3] As more and more genes are isolated and previously unknown gene products are discovered, disorders become diagnosable for the first time. In addition, a different and better method may become available to improve the accuracy, safety, or timing of a diagnosis. For example, diagnosis of hemoglobinopathies and hemophilias at one time required umbilical blood sampling midway through pregnancy, whereas diagnosis is now possible in most cases using DNA obtained in the first trimester.

Another caveat to the diagnosis of single gene disorders is the absolute requirement of accurate diagnosis in a proband or gene carrier in the family in order to use many of the diagnostic tests. For example, if an enzyme assay or a mutation analysis is to be used, it must already be known from prior studies in the family that the proposed test is the appropriate one. Correct information about paternity is also required, sometimes for several matings in the family, if a DNA linkage method is being used.

MALFORMATION SYNDROMES

Sonographic imaging and, to a lesser extent, x-ray or magnetic resonance imaging can detect malformations of many organ systems. When a specific diagnosis is being sought because of a previously affected child, a specific malformation can be essentially diagnostic. Absence of a demonstrable malformation is often much less reassuring about absence of the disorder, however, Examples of malformation syndromes are presented in Table 31-1.

In autosomal dominant adult polycystic kidney disease, which is only rarely manifested in fetal life as cystic kidneys, diagnosis can also be approached by DNA linkage methods. Unfortunately, not all families demonstrate the linkage of the putative gene to chromosome 16 markers indicating some genetic heterogeneity in the disorder.

TABLE 31–1. MALFORMATION SYNDROMES

SYNDROME	INHERITANCE PATTERN*
Aqueductal stenosis[31]	XL (and others)
Walker-Warburg syndrome[32]	AR
Holoprosencephaly[33]	AR (and others)
Achondrogenesis[34]	AR
Ellis-van Creveld syndrome[34]	AR
Asphyxiating thoracic dystrophy[35]	AR
Thanatophoric dysplasia[36]	?AD, AR
Short rib–polydactyly syndromes[37,38]	AR
Thrombocytopenia–absent radius syndrome[39]	AR
Adult polycystic kidney disease[40,41]	AD
Infantile polycystic kidney disease[42]	AR
Arthrogryposis syndromes[43,44]	AR, AD
Multiple pterygium syndrome[45,46]	AR, XL
Meckel-Gruber syndrome[47]	AR
Noonan syndrome[48]	AD
Roberts syndrome[14]	AR

* Some malformation syndromes occur sufficiently often in families to warrant designation of an inheritance pattern; they may occur sporadically as well, raising possibilities of AD inheritance, if reproduction is sharply limited, or multifactorial etiologies.

AD, autosomal dominant; AR, autosomal recessive; XL, X-linked.

TABLE 31–2. SKIN DISORDERS

DISORDER	INHERITANCE PATTERN
Epidermolysis bullosa syndromes[49]	AR, AD
Ichthyosis syndromes[50]	AR
Anhidrotic ectodermal dysplasia[51]	XL, AR
Sjögren-Larsson syndrome[52]	AR
Oculocutaneous albinism[53]	AR

AD, autosomal dominant; AR, autosomal recessive; XL, X-linked.

SKIN DISORDERS

Severe skin disorders have been diagnosed using skin biopsies (Table 31-2). Specific proteins and the genes associated with the diseases are not well understood as yet; progress should allow alternative methods of diagnosis in the future.

CHROMOSOME BREAKAGE SYNDROMES, DNA REPAIR DEFECTS, AND FRAGILE X SYNDROME

Fanconi pancytopenia syndrome has been successfully diagnosed many times.[15] Experience with Bloom syndrome[25] and ataxia telangiectasia,[26] which also show increased chromosome breakage, has been limited. Xeroderma pigmentosum syndromes show faulty repair of induced DNA damage; prenatal diagnosis based on this phenomenon has had some success.[27]

Cytogenetic demonstration of the fragile X phenomenon has had considerable use in prenatal diagnosis, but results have been inconsistent.[28] Linkage analysis to markers on the X chromosome has improved attempts at diagnosis. Now new information about the gene and its abnormalities should greatly change prenatal diagnosis of the fragile X syndrome through the use of DNA analysis.[16,17]

HEMATOLOGIC DISORDERS

Several different types of hematologic disorders have been diagnosed prenatally (Table 31-3). These include globin abnormalities (especially the thalassemias and sickle cell disorders), hemophilias, and immune deficiency syndromes. Increasingly, DNA methods have become available for this group of disorders.

CYSTIC FIBROSIS

The gene and gene product for cystic fibrosis were discovered simultaneously with a common mutation in the cystic fibrosis gene that is present in 30% to 70% of persons from different ethnic populations who carry cystic fibrosis mutations.[29,30] This common mutation is a deletion of the three nucleotides coding for a phenylalanine at position 508 of the cystic fibrosis protein. The mutation can be easily diagnosed with DNA, but unidentified mutations, all individually uncommon, pose difficulties. If DNA diagnosis cannot be accomplished, analysis of intestinal microvillar enzyme activities in amniotic fluid at 17 to 18 menstrual weeks offers reasonably good diagnostic results for couples at high risk of having a baby with the disease.[30] These enzymes enter amniotic fluid from the intestinal tract less well when the fetus has cystic fibrosis. Both false positive and false negative diagnoses exist.

INBORN ERRORS OF METABOLISM

Measurements of enzyme activities define most inborn errors of metabolism that are diagnosable prenatally. A few disorders are diagnosed by other types of protein analysis or by measurement of secondary effects of the metabolic block. Tables 31-4, 31-5, 31-6, and 31-7 list many of the inborn errors that have been diagnosed.

TABLE 31–3. HEMATOLOGIC DISORDERS

DISORDER	INHERITANCE PATTERN
Beta thalassemias[21,24]	AR
Alpha thalassemias[24]	AR
Sickle cell disorders[21,24]	AR
Hemophilia A[54,55]	XL
Hemophilia B[54]	XL
von Willebrand's disease[54]	AD
Wiskott-Aldrich syndrome[56]	XL
Chronic granulomatous disease[57]	XL, AR
Severe combined immunodeficiency diseases[58,59]	AR, XL
Hereditary elliptocytosis[60]	AR

AD, autosomal dominant; AR, autosomal recessive; XL, X-linked.

TABLE 31–4. INBORN ERRORS OF LIPID METABOLISM

DISORDER	INHERITANCE PATTERN
Fabry disease[61]	XL
Gaucher disease[62]	AR
Tay-Sachs disease[63]	AR
Sandhoff disease[64]	AR
Metachromatic leukodystrophy[65]	AR
Adrenoleukodystrophy[66]	XL, AR
Zellweger syndrome[67]	AR
Krabbe disease[68]	AR
Mucolipidoses[69,70]	AR

AD, autosomal dominant; AR, autosomal recessive; XL, X-linked.

TABLE 31–5. INBORN ERRORS OF AMINO ACID AND FATTY ACID METABOLISM

DISORDER	INHERITANCE PATTERN
Ornithine transcarbamylase (OTC) deficiency[20,71]	XL
Citrullinemia[72]	AR
Argininosuccinic acidemia[73]	AR
Propionic acidemias[11,74]	AR
Methylmalonic acidemias[10,75]	AR
Isovaleric acidemia[76]	AR
Glutaric acidemias[77,78]	AR
Phenylketonuria[79]	AR
Maple syrup urine disease[80]	AR
Biotinidase deficiency[81]	AR
Tyrosinemia[82]	AR
Nonketotic hyperglycinemia[83]	AR
Cystinosis[84]	AR
Homocystinuria[85]	AR
Medium chain acyl-CoA dehydrogenase (MCAD) deficiency[86]	AR
Canavan disease[87]	AR

AD, autosomal dominant; AR, autosomal recessive; XL, X-linked.

TABLE 31–6. INBORN ERRORS OF CARBOHYDRATE METABOLISM AND RELATED DISORDERS

DISORDER	INHERITANCE PATTERN
Galactosemia[88]	AR
Glycogen storage diseases[89,90]	AR
Sialidoses[91,92]	AR
Mucopolysaccharidoses[18,93,94]	AR, XL
Mucolipidoses[69,70]	AR
Pyruvate carboxylase deficiency[95]	AR
Mannosidosis[96]	AR
Fucosidosis[97]	AR

AD, autosomal dominant; AR, autosomal recessive; XL, X-linked.

TABLE 31–7. MISCELLANEOUS INBORN ERRORS

DISORDER	INHERITANCE PATTERN
Lesch-Nyhan disease[98]	XL
Menkes disease[99]	XL
Osteogenesis imperfecta[19]	AD, AR
Porphyrias[100,101]	AD, AR
Adrenogenital syndrome due to 21-hydroxylase deficiency[12,102]	AR
Hypophosphatasia[103]	AR

AD, autosomal dominant; AR, autosomal recessive; XL, X-linked.

MUSCLE AND NERVE DISORDERS

Mapping and then cloning of genes have made possible prenatal diagnosis of a few muscle and nerve disorders for which little basic information had previously been known (Table 31-8). Most of the diagnostic activity has been with Duchenne/Becker muscular dystrophy, and the gene product, dystrophin, has proved useful in clarifying presence or absence of disease in muscle obtained by biopsy or autopsy.

There appear to be at least two gene loci that can cause spinal muscular atrophy (Werdnig-Hoffman disease), so ambiguities will exist for many families. Only one locus has been identified for myotonic dystrophy and for type I neurofibromatosis.

SUMMARY

Single gene disorders represent an extremely heterogeneous category of inherited problems. Many of the features that define a disorder in postnatal life can be sought in prenatal diagnosis, but extreme care must be taken to examine variability of expression and onset of the disorder, possible genetic heterogeneity underlying the phenotype, and accuracy of diagnosis within the family that is requesting a prenatal diagnosis.

TABLE 31–8. MUSCLE AND NERVE DISORDERS

DISORDER*	INHERITANCE PATTERN
Duchenne/Becker muscular dystrophy[23]	XL
Werdnig-Hoffman disease[104]	AR
Myotonic dystrophy[105]	AD
Neurofibromatosis, type I[106]	AD

* Many disorders that affect muscle and/or the nervous system are classified as inborn errors of metabolism or malformation syndromes. Prenatal diagnosis of those listed here has depended on recent discoveries about the genes causing the disorders.

AD, autosomal dominant; AR, autosomal recessive; XL, X-linked.

REFERENCES

1. Milunsky A, ed. Genetic disorders and the fetus: Diagnosis, prevention, and treatment. 2nd ed. New York: Plenum Press, 1986.
2. Filkins K, Russo JF, eds. Human prenatal diagnosis. 2nd ed. New York: Marcel Dekker, 1990.
3. Weaver DD. Catalog of prenatally diagnosed conditions. Baltimore: Johns Hopkins University Press, 1989.
4. Herzenberg LA, Bianchi DW, Schroder J, Cann HM, Iverson GM. Fetal cells in the blood of pregnant women: Detection and enrichment by fluorescence-activated cell sorting. Proc Natl Acad Sci USA 1989;76:1453.
5. Bianchi DW, Flint AF, Pizzimenti MF, Knoll JHM, Latt SA. Isolation of fetal DNA from nucleated erythrocytes in maternal blood. Proc Natl Acad Sci USA 1990;87:3279.
6. Jones KL. Smith's recognizable patterns of human malformation. 4th ed. Philadelphia: WB Saunders, 1988.
7. Buyse ML, ed. Birth defects encyclopedia. Cambridge, MA: Blackwell, 1990.
8. Romero R, Hobbins JC, Mahoney MJ. Fetal blood sampling and fetoscopy. In Milunsky A, ed. Genetic disorders and the fetus: Diagnosis, prevention, and treatment. 2nd ed. New York: Plenum Press, 1986:571.
9. Cullen MT, Reece EA, Whetham J, Hobbins JC. Embryoscopy: description and utility of a new technique. Am J Obstet Gynecol 1990;162:82.
10. Zinn AB, Hine DG, Mahoney MJ, Tanaka K. The stable isotope dilution method for measurement of methylmalonic acid: a highly accurate approach to the prenatal diagnosis of methylmalonic acidemia, Pediatr Res 1982;16:740.
11. Sweetman L. Prenatal diagnosis of the organic acidurias. Journal of Inherited Metabolic Diseases 1984;7(Suppl 1):18.
12. Hughes IA, Lawrence KM. Antenatal diagnosis of congenital adrenal hyperplasia. Lancet 1979;ii:7.
13. Holbrook KA, ed. Prenatal diagnosis of genetic skin disease. Seminars in Dermatology 1984;3:155.
14. Willner JP, Radu M, Hobbins JC, Kereny T, Strauss L, Desnick RJ. Roberts syndrome: prenatal diagnosis by cytogenetic and ultrasonic studies. Pediatr Res 1979;13:428.
15. Auerbach AD, Sagi M, Adler BA. Fanconi anemia: prenatal diagnosis in 30 fetuses at risk. Pediatrics 1985;76:794.
16. Hirst M, Knight S, Davies K, et al. Prenatal diagnosis of fragile X syndrome. Lancet 1991;338:956.
17. Dobkin CS, Ding X, Jenkins EC, et al. Prenatal diagnosis of fragile X syndrome. Lancet 1991;338:957.
18. Kleijer WJ, Thompson EJ, Niermeijer MF. Prenatal diagnosis of the Hurler syndrome: report on 40 pregnancies at risk. Prenat Diagn 1983;3:179.

19. Shapiro JE, Phillips JA III, Byers PH, et al. Prenatal diagnosis of lethal perinatal osteogenesis imperfecta (OI Type II). J Pediatr 1982;100:127.
20. Rodeck CH, Patrick AD, Pembrey ME, Tzannatos C, Whitfield AE. Fetal liver biopsy for prenatal diagnosis of ornithine carbamyl transferase deficiency. Lancet 1982;2:297.
21. Alter BP, Modell CB, Fairweather D, et al. Prenatal diagnosis of hemoglobinopathies: a review of 15 cases. N Engl J Med 1976;295:1437.
22. Kerem B, Rommens JM, Buchanan JA, et al. Identification of the cystic fibrosis gene: genetic analysis. Science 1989;245:1073.
23. Darras BT, Koenig M, Kunkel LM, Francke U. Direct method for prenatal diagnosis and carrier detection in Duchenne/Becker muscular dystrophy using the entire dystrophin cDNA. Am J Med Genet 1988;29:713.
24. Boehm C, Kazazian HH. Prenatal diagnosis of the hemoglobinopathies by DNA analysis. CRC Crit Rev Oncol Hematol 1984;4:155.
25. German J, Bloom D, Passarge E. Bloom's syndrome. VII. Progress report for 1978. Clin Genet 1979;15:361.
26. Shaham M, Voss R, Becker Y, Yarkoni S, Ornoy A, Kohn G. Prenatal diagnosis of ataxia telangiectasia. J Pediatr 1982;100:134.
27. Halley DJJ, Keijzer W, Jaspers NGJ, et al. Prenatal diagnosis of xeroderma pigmentosum (group C) using assay of unscheduled DNA synthesis and postreplication repair. Clin Genet 1979; 16:137.
28. Sutherland GR, Baker E, Purvis-Smith S, Hockey A, Krumins E, Eichenbaum SZ. Prenatal diagnosis of the fragile X using thymidine induction. Prenat Diagn 1987;7:197.
29. Lemna WK, Feldman GL, Kerem B, et al. Mutation analysis for heterozygote detection and the prenatal diagnosis of cystic fibrosis. N Engl J Med 1990;322:291.
30. Buffone GJ, Spence JE, Fernbach SD, Curry MR, O'Brien WE, Beaudet AL. Prenatal diagnosis of cystic fibrosis: microvillar enzymes and DNA analysis compared. Clin Chem 1988;34:933.
31. Pilu G, Rizzo N, Orsini LF, Bovicelli L. Antenatal recognition of cerebral anomalies. Ultrasound Med Biol 1986;12:319.
32. Crowe C, Jassani M, Dickerman L. The prenatal diagnosis of the Walker-Warburg syndrome. Prenat Diagn 1986;6:177.
33. Chervenak FA, Isaacson G, Hobbins JC, Chitkara U, Tortora M, Berkowitz RL. Diagnosis and management of fetal holoprosencephaly. Obstet Gynecol 1985;66:322.
34. Filly RA, Golbus MS. Ultrasonography of the normal and pathologic fetal skeleton. Radiol Clin North Am 1982;20:311.
35. Lipson M, Waskey J, Rice J, et al. Prenatal diagnosis of asphyxiating thoracic dysplasia. Am J Med Genet 1984;18:273.
36. Chervenak FA, Blakemore KJ, Isaacson G, Mayden K, Hobbins JC. Antenatal sonographic findings of thanatophoric dysplasia with cloverleaf skull. Am J Obstet Gynecol 1983;146:984.
37. Gembruch U, Hansmann M, Fodisch HJ. Early prenatal diagnosis of short rib-polydactyly (SRP) syndrome type I (Majewski) by ultrasound in a case at risk. Prenat Diagn 1985;5:357.
38. Johnson VP, Petersen LP, Holzwarth DR, Messner FD. Midtrimester prenatal diagnosis of short-limb dwarfism (Saldino-Noonan syndrome). Birth Defects 1982;18(3A):133.
39. Filkins K, Russo J. Prenatal diagnosis of thrombocytopenia absent radius syndrome using ultrasound and fetoscopy. Prenat Diagn 1984;4:139.
40. Zerres K, Weiss H, Bulla M, Roth B. Prenatal diagnosis of an early manifestation of autosomal dominant adult-type polycystic kidney disease. Lancet 1982;ii:988.
41. Novelli G, Frontali M, Baldini D, et al. Prenatal diagnosis of adult polycystic kidney disease with DNA markers on chromosome 16 and the genetic heterogeneity problem. Prenat Diagn 1989;9:759.
42. Luthy DA, Hirsch JH. Infantile polycystic kidney disease: Observations from attempts at prenatal diagnosis. Am J Med Genet 1985;20:505.
43. Goldberg JD, Chervenak FA, Lipman RA, Berkowitz RL. Antenatal sonographic diagnosis of arthrogryposis multiplex congenita. Prenat Diagn 1986;6:45.
44. Socol ML, Sabbagha RE, Elias S, et al. Prenatal diagnosis of congenital muscular dystrophy producing arthrogryposis. N Engl J Med 1985;313:1230.
45. Hogge WA, Golabi M, Filly RA, Douglas R, Golbus MS. The lethal multiple pterygium syndrome: Is prenatal detection possible? Am J Med Genet 1985;20:441.
46. Tolmie JL, Patrick A, Yates JRW. A lethal multiple pterygium syndrome with apparent X-linked recessive inheritance. Am J Med Genet 1987;27:913.
47. Wapner RJ, Kurtz AB, Ross RD, Jackson LG. Ultrasonographic parameters in the prenatal diagnosis of Meckel syndrome. Obstet Gynecol 1981;57:388.
48. Witt D, Hall J, Lau A, McGillivray B, Manchester D. Prenatal diagnosis and fetal edema in Noonan syndrome. Am J Hum Genet 1984;36:82S.
49. Anton-Lamprecht I. Prenatal diagnosis of epidermolysis bullosa hereditaria: a review. Seminars in Dermatology 1984;3:229.
50. Blanchet-Bardon C, Dumez Y. Prenatal diagnosis of a harlequin fetus. Seminars in Dermatology 1984;3:225.
51. Arnold ML, Anton-Lamprecht I, Rauskolb R. Prenatal diagnosis of ectodermal dysplasias. Seminars in Dermatology 1984;3:247.
52. Trepeta R, Stenn KS, Mahoney MJ. Prenatal diagnosis of Sjogren-Larsson syndrome. Seminars in Dermatology 1984;3:221.
53. Robin AJ, Eady MB. Prenatal diagnosis of oculocutaneous albinism: implications for other hereditary disorders of pigmentation. Seminars in Dermatology 1984;3:241.
54. Mibashan RS, Millar DS. Fetal haemophilia and allied bleeding disorders. Br Med Bull 1983;39:392.
55. Malcolm S, Robertson E, Harper K, et al. Prenatal assessment of haemophilia A using DNA probes. J Med Genet 1986;23:470.
56. Schwartz M, Mibashan RS, Nicolaides KH, et al. First-trimester diagnosis of Wiskott-Aldrich syndrome by DNA markers. Lancet 1989;ii:1405.
57. Huu TP, Dumez Y, Marquetty C, Durandy A, Boue J, Hakim J. Prenatal diagnosis of chronic granulomatous disease (CGD) in four high risk male fetuses. Prenat Diagn 1987;7:253.
58. Durandy A, Griscelli C, Dumez Y, et al. Antenatal diagnosis of severe combined immunodeficiency from fetal cord blood. Lancet 1982;1:852.
59. Hirschhorn R, Beratis N, Rosen RS, Parkman R, Stern R, Polmar S. Adenosine-deaminase deficiency in a child diagnosed prenatally. Lancet 1975;i:73.
60. Dhermy D, Feo C, Garbarz M, et al. Prenatal diagnosis of hereditary elliptocytosis with molecular defect of spectrin. Prenat Diagn 1987;7:471.
61. Kleijer WJ, Hussaarts-Odijk LM, Sachs ES, Jahoda MGJ, Niermeijer MF. Prenatal diagnosis of Fabry's disease by direct analysis of chorionic villi. Prenat Diagn 1987;7:283.
62. Schneider EL, Ellis WG, Brady RO, McCulloch JR, Epstein CJ. Infantile (type II) Gaucher's disease: In utero diagnosis and fetal pathology. J Pediatr 1972;81:1134.
63. Grabowski GA, Kruse JR, Goldberg JD, et al. First-trimester prenatal diagnosis of Tay-Sachs disease. Am J Hum Genet 1984;36:1369.
64. Warner TG, Turner MW, Toone JR, Applegarth D. Prenatal diagnosis of infantile GM_2 gangliosidosis type II (Sandhoff disease) by detection of N-acetylglucosaminyl-oligosaccharides in

amniotic fluid with high-performance liquid chromatography. Prenat Diagn 1986;6:393.
65. Wiesmann UN, Meier C, Spycher MA, et al. Prenatal metachromatic leukodystrophy. Helv Paediatr Acta 1975;30:31.
66. Moser HW, Moser AB, Powers JM, et al. The prenatal diagnosis of adrenoleukodystrophy: Demonstration of increased hexacosanoic acid levels in cultured amniocytes and fetal adrenal gland. Pediatr Res 1982;16:172.
67. Schutgens RBH, Schrakamp G, Wanders RJA, et al. The cerebro-hepato-renal (Zellweger) syndrome. Prenat Diagn 1985; 5:337.
68. Kleijer WJ, Mancini GMS, Jahoda MGJ, et al. First-trimester diagnosis of Krabbe's disease by direct enzyme analysis of chorionic villi. N Engl J Med 1984;311:1257.
69. Hug G, Bove KE, Soukup S, et al. Increased serum hexosaminidase in a woman pregnant with a fetus affected by mucolipidosis II (I-cell disease). N Engl J Med 1984;311:988.
70. Ornoy A, Arnon J, Grebner EE, Jackson LG, Bach G. Early prenatal diagnosis of mucolipidosis IV. Am J Med Genet 1987;27:983.
71. Fox J, Hack AM, Fenton WA, et al. Prenatal diagnosis of ornithine transcarbamylase deficiency with use of DNA polymorphisms. N Engl J Med 1986;315:1205.
72. Fleisher LD, Harris CJ, Mitchell DA, Nadler HL. Citrullinemia: Prenatal diagnosis of an affected fetus. Am J Hum Genet 1983;35:85.
73. Goodman SI, Mace JW, Turner B, Garrett WJ. Antenatal diagnosis of argininosuccinic aciduria. Clin Genet 1973;4:236.
74. Sweetman L, Weyler W, Shafai T, Young PE, Nyhan WL. Prenatal diagnosis of propionic acidemia. JAMA 1979;242:1048.
75. Ampola MG, Mahoney MJ, Nakamura E, Tanaka K. Prenatal therapy of a patient with vitamin-B_{12}-responsive methylmalonic acidemia. N Engl J Med 1975;293:313.
76. Hine DG, Hack AM, Goodman SI, Tanaka K. Stable isotope dilution analysis of isovalerylglycine in amniotic fluid and urine and its application for the prenatal diagnosis of isovaleric acidemia. Pediatr Res 1986;20:222.
77. Goodman SI, Gallegos DA, Pullin CJ, et al. Antenatal diagnosis of glutaric acidemia. Am J Hum Genet 1980;32:695.
78. Jakobs C, Sweetman L, Wadman SK, Duran M, Saudubray JM, Nyhan WL. Prenatal diagnosis of glutaric aciduria type II by direct chemical analysis of dicarboxylic acids in amniotic fluid. Eur J Pediatr 1984;141:153.
79. Lidsky AS, Guttler F, Woo SLC. Prenatal diagnosis of classic phenylketonuria by DNA analysis. Lancet 1985;1:549.
80. Cox RP, Hutzler J, Dancis J. Antenatal diagnosis of maple-syrup urine disease. Lancet 1978;ii:212.
81. Wolf B, Grier RE, Parker WK Jr, Goodman SI, Allen RJ. Deficient biotinidase activity in late-onset multiple carboxylase deficiency. N Engl J Med 1983;308:161.
82. Jakobs C, Kvittingen EA, Berger R, Haagen A, Kleijer W, Niermeijer M. Prenatal diagnosis of tyrosinaemia type I by use of stable isotope dilution mass spectrometry. Eur J Pediatr 1985;144:209.
83. Applegarth DA, Levy HL, Shih VE, et al. Prenatal diagnosis of non-ketotic hyperglycinemia. Prenat Diagn 1986;6:257.
84. Patrick AD, Young EP, Mossman J. First trimester diagnosis of cystinosis using intact chorionic villi. Prenat Diagn 1987;7:71.
85. Fowler B, Borresen AL, Boman N. Prenatal diagnosis of homocystinuria. Lancet 1982;ii:875.
86. Bennett MJ, Allison F, Lowther GW, et al. Prenatal diagnosis of medium-chain acyl-coenzyme A dehydrogenase deficiency. Prenat Diag 1987;7:135.
87. Matalon R, Michals K, Sebesta D, Deanching P, Gashkoff P, Casanova J. Aspartoacylase deficiency and N-acetylaspartic aciduria in patients with Canavan disease. Am J Med Genet 1988;29:463.
88. Kleijer WJ, Janse HC, van Diggelen OP, et al. First-trimester diagnosis of galactosaemia. Lancet 1986;i:748.
89. Niermeijer MF, Koster JF, Jahoda M, Fernandes J, Heukel-Dully MJ, Galjaard H. Prenatal diagnosis of type II glycogenosis (Pompe's disease) using microchemical analyses. Pediatr Res 1975;9:498.
90. Besley GT, Cohen PT, Faed MJ, Wolstenholme J. Amylo-1,6-glucosidase activity in cultured cells: a deficiency in type III glycogenosis with prenatal studies. Prenat Diagn 1983;3:13.
91. Mueller TO, Wenger DA. Mucolipidosis I: Studies of sialidase activity and a prenatal diagnosis. Clin Chim Acta 1981;109:313.
92. Renlund M, Aula P. Prenatal detection of Salla disease based upon increased free sialic acid in amniocytes. Am J Med Genet 1987;28:377.
93. Kleijer WJ, Van Diggelen OP, Janse HC, Galjaard H, Dumez Y, Boue J. First trimester diagnosis of Hunter syndrome on chorionic villi. Lancet 1984;ii:472.
94. Kleijer WJ, Janse HC, Vosters RPL, Niermeijer MF, van de Kamp JJP. First-trimester diagnosis of mucopolysaccharidosis IIIA (Sanfilippo A disease). N Engl J Med 1986;314:185.
95. Robinson BH, Toone JR, Benedict RP, Dimmick JE, Oei J, Applegarth DA. Prenatal diagnosis of pyruvate carboxylase deficiency. Prenat Diagn 1985;5:67.
96. Poenaru L, Girard S, Thepot F, et al. Antenatal diagnosis of three pregnancies at risk for mannosidosis. Clin Genet 1979;16:428.
97. Robinson D, Thorpe R. Fluorescent assay of α-L-fucosidase. Clin Chim Acta 1974;55:65.
98. Stout JT, Jackson LG, Caskey CT. First trimester diagnosis of Lesch-Nyhan syndrome: Application to other disorders of purine metabolism. Prenat Diagn 1985;5:183.
99. Horn N. Menkes X-linked disease: Prenatal diagnosis of hemizygous males and heterozygous females. Prenat Diagn 1981;1:107.
100. Sassa S, Solish G, Levere RD, Kappas A. Studies in porphyria: IV. Expression of the gene defect of acute intermittent porphyria in cultured skin fibroblasts and amniotic cells: Prenatal diagnosis of the porphyric trait. J Exp Med 1975;142:722.
101. Kaiser, IH. Brown amniotic fluid in congenital erythropoietic porphyria. Obstet Gynecol 1980;56:383.
102. Mornet E, Boue J, Raux-Demay M, et al. First trimester prenatal diagnosis of 21-hydroxylase deficiency by linkage analysis to HLA-DNA probes and by 17-hydroxyprogesterone determination. Hum Genet 1986;73:358.
103. Mulivor RA, Mennuti M, Zackai EH, Harris H. Prenatal diagnosis of hypophosphatasia: Genetic, biochemical, and clinical studies. Am J Hum Genet 1978;30:271.
104. Gilliam TC, Brzustowicz LM, Castilla LH, et al. Genetic homogeneity between acute and chronic forms of spinal muscular atrophy. Nature 1990;345:823.
105. Norman AM, Floyd JL, Meredith AL, Harper PS. Presymptomatic detection and prenatal diagnosis for myotonic dystrophy by means of linked DNA markers. J Med Genet 1989;26:750.
106. Wallace MR, Marchuk DA, Andersen LB, et al. Type 1 neurofibromatosis gene: Identification of a large transcript disrupted in three NF1 patients. Science 1990;249:181.

32

CHAPTER

DISORDERS OF FETAL HEMOGLOBIN AND BLOOD CELLS

Mitchell S. Golbus and James D. Goldberg

BLOOD AND BLOOD-FORMING TISSUES

PRODUCTION

Sites

Embryonic red blood cell production starts by 2 weeks after conception. The original site of production is the yolk sac, but at 7 to 9 fetal weeks (9 to 11 menstrual weeks) production switches to the fetal liver, and production of white blood cells and platelets begins. At mid-gestation, hematopoiesis begins in the bone marrow and rapidly increases to fill the marrow; concurrently, hematopoiesis in the liver decreases. The site changes are thought to occur by progressive seeding of totipotential stem cells, first from the yolk sac to the liver and then from the liver to the bone marrow (Fig. 32-1). The shifts occur when the microenvironment of the recipient tissue is prepared to support hematopoiesis.

Production Rates

Fetal hematocrit increases from a mean of 30% at 12 weeks to 40% at 22 weeks and 50% at term. The red blood cell count increases more, from $1.5 \times 10^6/mm^3$ at 12 weeks to $4.7 \times 10^6/mm^3$ at term. Hematocrit rises less rapidly because the cells progressively decrease in size during gestation. The mean red cell volume decreases from 180 femtoliters (fL) at 12 weeks to 108 fL at term. The fact that fetal red blood cells are larger than maternal cells allows us to determine whether blood obtained by percutaneous umbilical blood sampling is truly fetal. Examining samples with a Coulter counter and channalyzer distinguishes between fetal and maternal blood (Fig. 32-2).

Another difference between fetal and postnatal blood is that fetal blood has a greater proportion of reticulocytes and nucleated red blood cells, reflecting active erythropoiesis. The proportion of nucleated red blood cells is high enough to require correction of white blood cell counts.

HEMOGLOBIN

The peripheral red blood cell is one of the most specialized cells in the body: 95% of its protein is hemoglobin. Hemoglobin has four subunits, each containing one iron atom attached to a porphyrin ring to form heme, which is attached to a globin chain. Each hemoglobin molecule's four globins consist of two pairs of identical chains.

The globins are divided into the alpha-like globins, with genes located on chromosome 16, and the beta-like globins, with genes located on chromosome 11. The alpha-like family includes an embryonic form (zeta) and an adult form (alpha). The beta-like family includes an embryonic form (epsilon), a fetal form (gamma), a major adult form (beta), and a minor adult form (delta). Through development there is a progression from embryonic hemoglobins, Gower I ($\zeta_2\epsilon_2$), Portland $(\zeta_2\gamma)_2$, and Gower II ($\alpha_2\epsilon_2$), to fetal hemoglobin ($\alpha_2\gamma_2$), to adult hemoglobins ($\alpha_2\beta_2$ and $\alpha_2\delta_2$). The human globin genes share a common general structure, suggesting a common origin as a single ancestral globin gene.

COAGULATION

Blood proteins that are related to coagulation are of special interest to obstetricians. The prenatal diagnosis of congenital bleeding disorders has been an important and highly successful field of endeavor.

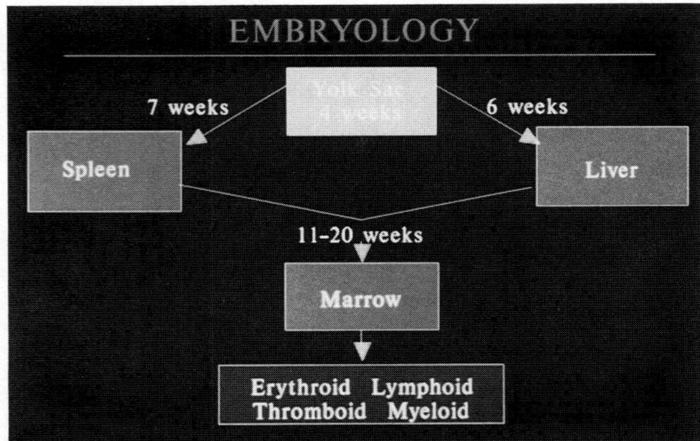

FIGURE 32–1. Embryology of hematopoiesis.

Hemophilia A (Factor VIII Deficiency)

Hemophilia A is the most common example of a coagulation-factor deficiency that produces severe clinical manifestations. Its estimated incidence is 1:10,000 Caucasian male births. It is transmitted as an X-linked deficiency of factor VIII. Males with 0% to 1% of normal activity have severe disease, those with 1% to 5% activity have moderate hemophilia, and those with more than 5% activity generally have only mild manifestations.

Despite greatly improved replacement therapy, hemophilia A continues to exact a heavy medical and socioeconomic cost. This has produced an increased demand for prenatal diagnosis. Some parents seek such information for the purpose of not delivering affected sons, others so they can begin specialized intrapartum care. As always, prenatal diagnosis includes verifying the diagnosis in the proband, carrier testing, risk calculation, and appropriate nondirectional counseling.

Originally, prenatal diagnosis of hemophilia A was done by fetal blood sampling and determining factor VIII activity by coagulant and antigen determinants.[1–3] More than 200 male fetuses at risk were tested using this method. However, since the isolation of the factor VIII gene, almost all prenatal diagnoses of hemophilia A have been made using recombinant DNA techniques.[4] At present, three intragenic and two extragenic probes allow a DNA diagnosis in more than 95% of women carrying an at-risk fetus.[5] Thus, couples can obtain information at 10 to 12 menstrual weeks by chorionic villus sampling instead of at 18 to 20 weeks by fetal blood sampling.

Hemophilia B (Factor IX Deficiency)

About 15% of patients with hemophilia have hemophilia B. Its clinical manifestations are similar to those of hemophilia A, and the disease is also inherited as an X-linked trait. Replacement therapy is available, but as

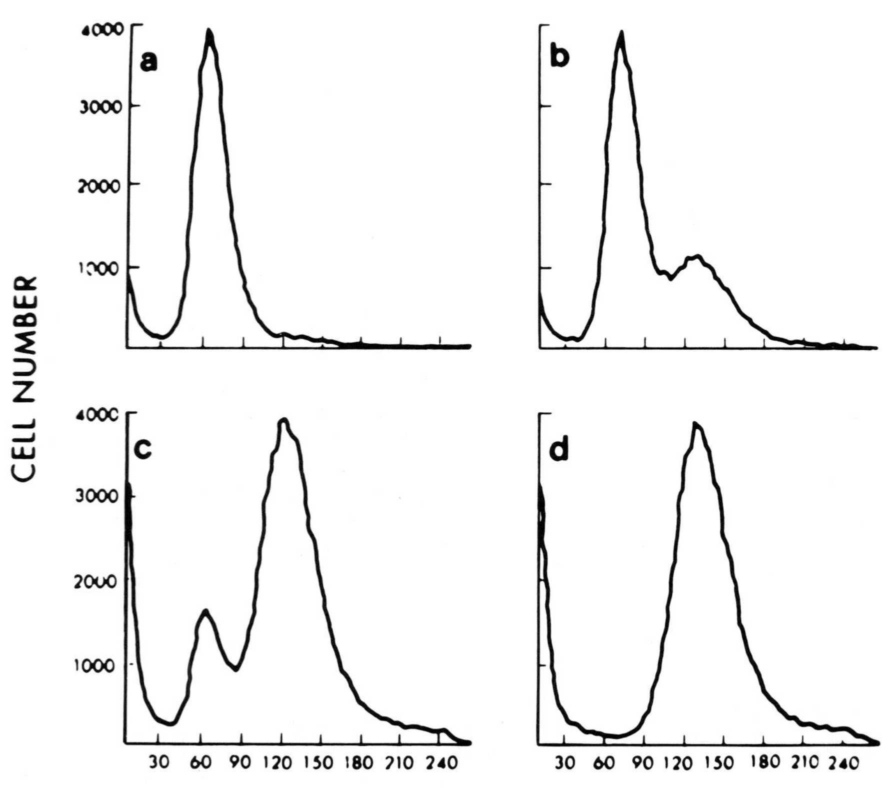

FIGURE 32–2. Coulter Channelyzer analysis of fetal and maternal red blood cells. (**A**) 100% maternal; (**B**) 30% fetal, 70% maternal; (**C**) 80% fetal, 20% maternal; and (**D**) 100% fetal.

in hemophilia A prenatal diagnosis has been popular. Prenatal diagnosis using fetal blood samples has been difficult for the following reasons:

- Levels of fetal factor IX are normally low.
- Factor IX is present in amniotic fluid, which means that the fetal blood sample must be pure.
- Positive cross-reactive material in the proband is prevalent, ruling out the use of immunologic methods.

These difficulties notwithstanding, dozens of at-risk fetuses have been tested using immunologic and coagulant tests.[2,6] The gene for factor IX has been cloned and intragenic probes used for recombinant DNA prenatal diagnoses.[7,8] More recently, gene amplification by the polymerase chain reaction, followed by DNA sequencing to identify the mutation in specific families, has been applied to carrier testing and prenatal diagnosis.[9]

Von Willebrand's Disease

Von Willebrand's disease, a relatively common and usually mild autosomal dominant trait, is characterized by a prolonged bleeding time and abnormalities of the factor VIII complex. Rarely, homozygosity for the von Willebrand's gene or a severe form of the disease leads to a request for prenatal diagnosis. Fetal blood samples have been used successfully to identify both unaffected and affected fetuses, using coagulant activity and immunologic measurements.[2,10]

Other Factor Deficiencies

Deficiencies of nearly all the clotting factors have been reported. The only one recognized prenatally (although retrospectively) was a fetus diagnosed as having asymmetric ventricular dilation at 28 menstrual weeks on the basis of intraventricular hemorrhage. The neonate suffered additional intraventricular bleeding and was found to have only 2% of normal factor V activity.[11]

Theoretically, any of these factor deficiencies should be recognizable prenatally using a pure fetal blood sample. This assumes that the factor is normally expressed during fetal life, and that would have to be demonstrated using samples from fetuses having blood sampling for other indications.

RED BLOOD CELLS

HEMOGLOBINOPATHIES

Alpha Thalassemia

The thalassemias are hereditary microcytic anemias caused by defects in the rate of hemoglobin synthesis.[12] Each thalassemia is named for the globin chain that is insufficiently produced. The diseases are inherited as autosomal recessive traits; thalassemia minor is the carrier state, thalassemia major the affected homozygote. There are normally four alpha globin genes per diploid genome, and alpha thalassemia is usually due to the deletion of all four genes. If three alpha globin genes are deleted or nonfunctional, too much hemoglobin H (β_4) is produced; this is called hemoglobin H disease. Deletion of two alpha globin genes produces the carrier state. Deletion of one alpha globin gene produces a "silent carrier" with no clinical or laboratory manifestations. Less commonly, non-deletion alpha thalassemia is due to a point mutation.

Alpha thalassemia major is a lethal fetal disorder; only a few liveborns have been reported. The hydrops fetalis and markedly enlarged edematous placenta associated with the fetal disorder produces a 50% incidence of preeclampsia in the mother. This has been a significant factor in the drive to provide prenatal diagnosis for women with at-risk pregnancies. In fact, prenatal diagnosis of the hemoglobinopathies was the driving force behind the development of fetal blood sampling. Originally, prenatal diagnosis was done by analyzing fetal blood samples for globin chain synthesis and composition by carboxymethyl cellulose columns, electrophoresis, or high-performance liquid chromatography. However, the advent of recombinant DNA techniques has caused a drop in the number of diagnoses made by fetal blood sampling and an increase in prenatal diagnoses for alpha thalassemia. New techniques have made the diagnosis even more straightforward.[13]

Beta Thalassemia

In beta thalassemia, the normal production of beta globin chains is reduced. Dozens of mutations have been identified that cause this decrease and lead to the common clinical presentation.[12] These mutations are inherited in a codominant fashion that produces the disease state in an autosomal recessive mode of inheritance. The fetus with beta thalassemia major does well in utero because gamma globin is the predominant beta-like globin produced, but the switch to beta globin production after birth causes a corresponding decrease in hemoglobin level. The infant rapidly becomes dependent on transfusions.

The severity of this disorder has led to prenatal diagnosis of more than 10,000 at-risk fetuses.[14] Prenatal diagnosis methods are essentially the same as for alpha thalassemia and have progressed from globin chain synthesis in fetal blood samples to recombinant DNA techniques. Currently, the combination of polymerase chain reaction amplification of the beta globin gene and allele-specific oligonucleotide hybridization offers rapid results and is applicable to any source of fetal DNA.

Structurally Abnormal Hemoglobins

Humans can produce a structurally abnormal globin chain with altered biochemical and biological properties. Although there are a large number of such abnormal globins, the most significant clinically is sickle-cell disease. This includes homozygotes for hemoglobin S and also the mixed heterozygotes for hemoglobin S and either another beta globin structural variant or one of the beta thalassemias. The symptomatology varies markedly among these various combinations and even among patients with the same mutation.[15] This great variability in clinical status is one reason why there is less demand for prenatal diagnosis of at-risk fetuses.

The methodology for prenatal diagnosis has undergone the same changes as described for the thalassemias. The safer, earlier diagnoses made possible by recombinant DNA technology have caused some increase in the use of prenatal diagnosis.[14] Interestingly, the uncertainty about the desirability of prenatal diagnosis has been reflected in the increased proportion of parents who, when told that the fetus has sickle-cell disease, elect to continue the pregnancy. When prenatal diagnosis of sickle-cell disease required fetal blood sampling, 9% of affected fetuses were carried (as opposed to 1% for beta thalassemia). Since DNA techniques have been available, 51% of affected fetuses have been carried.[14]

Methemoglobinemia

Congenital methemoglobinemia is due to homozygous deficiency of red blood cell NADH-diaphorase (methemoglobin reductase), which normally reduces methemoglobin.[16] The disease has two presentations. Type I, which is due to an enzyme deficiency only in red blood cells, is a benign treatable condition. Type II, which is due to an enzyme deficiency in all cells, is associated with a progressive neurologic disorder that is lethal. Because the status of the fetus at risk for type II methemoglobinemia is reflected in amniocytes, prenatal diagnosis is possible.[16] Presumably, this could be done using chorionic villi, but this has not yet been reported.

MEMBRANE ABNORMALITIES

Spherocytosis

Hereditary spherocytosis is the most common congenital hemolytic anemia in people of northern European origin. In the United States the incidence is about 1:4500. Spherocytosis is most likely due to a structural or functional abnormality in spectrin. Because spherocytes are more rigid than normal red blood cells, they are less likely to traverse the spleen and more likely to be hemolyzed. The hemolytic anemia is successfully treated by splenectomy. The trait is inherited in an autosomal dominant fashion. Due to the mildness of the condition, there has been no demand for prenatal diagnosis, but such diagnosis should be possible by spectrin analysis or by osmotic fragility testing of fetal red blood cells.

Elliptocytosis

Hereditary elliptocytosis is a clinically and molecularly heterogenous group of disorders. A common finding is defective dimer–dimer spectrin association, producing an increased proportion of spectrin dimers, cell membrane fragility, and in severe cases hemolysis. These disorders are inherited in an autosomal dominant mode and are generally clinically mild. However, one couple who each had elliptocytosis had an affected child who was transfusion-dependent. In a subsequent pregnancy they had prenatal diagnosis, and fortunately the spectrin analysis demonstrated a heterozygous fetus, which was confirmed after birth.[17]

Type II Hereditary Pyropoikilocytosis

This disorder, reported in only a few families, may represent a compound heterozygous state for elliptocytosis and is reflected in spectrin abnormalities. Therefore, the condition appears to be inherited in an autosomal recessive mode. It causes a transfusion-dependent hemolytic anemia. Prenatal diagnosis of an at-risk fetus has diagnosed one unaffected pregnancy.[18]

METABOLIC ABNORMALITIES

Hexose Monophosphate Shunt

Enzyme deficiencies of the hexose monophosphate shunt can cause hemolysis due to oxidative damage to red blood cells. The most common enzyme deficiency of this group is X-linked glucose-6-phosphate dehydrogenase deficiency. Probably because of the usually mild nature of this disorder and the ability to prevent hemolysis by avoiding certain drugs, there has been no demand for prenatal diagnosis.

Glycolysis Disorders

There are eight enzymes in the Embden-Meyerhof glycolysis pathway whose deficiencies produce variable hemolysis. All are inherited as autosomal recessive traits (except phosphoglycerate kinase, which is X-linked). Glucose phosphate isomerase deficiency in some families has produced sufficient hemolysis to cause hydrops fetalis or transfusion-dependent anemia. Prenatal diagnoses in two such families showed one affected fetus (using amniocytes) and one heterozygous fetus (using chorionic villus cells).[19,20] Triose phosphate isomerase deficiency may also produce a severely affected child. Clark and Szobolotzky have reported diagnosis of a heterozygote by amniocentesis.[21] Heterozygotes also have been diagnosed by fetal blood sampling and by chorionic villus sampling.[22–24] Both triose phosphate isomerase activity and thermal stability of the enzyme should be measured, because an overlap in affected and heterozygote enzyme values has been reported.[21,25]

OTHER DISORDERS

Fanconi Anemia

Fanconi anemia is an autosomal recessive disorder characterized clinically by progressive pancytopenia, variable physical abnormalities, and a predisposition to the development of malignancies. Although the molecular defect in Fanconi anemia is unknown, the cells of affected patients show a marked susceptibility to chromosome breakage, and this characteristic has been used for prenatal diagnosis. Prenatal diagnoses have been done on dozens of at-risk fetuses by examining amniocytes or chorionic villus cells for spontaneous and diepoxybutane-induced chromosome breakage.[26]

Blackfan-Diamond Syndrome

Blackfan-Diamond syndrome is an autosomal recessive disorder characterized by pure red blood cell anemia due to a congenital deficiency of erythroid precursors. One affected fetus of a couple known to be at risk demonstrated an altered blood flow velocity pattern by echocardiography at 28 menstrual weeks.[27] Prenatal diagnosis should be possible by measuring the fetal hematocrit and red blood cell count.

LYMPHOCYTES

STRUCTURAL AND NUMERICAL DISORDERS

Bare Lymphocyte Syndrome

The bare lymphocyte syndrome, characterized by an absence of lymphocyte surface antigens, has been diagnosed by membrane immunofluorescence using monoclonal antibodies for HLA class I and II molecules.[28]

Agammaglobulinemia

X-linked agammaglobulinemia has been excluded by examining B lymphocytes with a monoclonal antibody in fetal blood.[29] There is some concern about this approach because of the variable numbers of B cells in fetal blood.[30] Malcolm and colleagues recently demonstrated close linkage of this disorder to the X-chromosome markers DXS94 and DXS17.[31] Lau and coworkers have excluded the diagnosis in one fetus at risk by linkage analysis, but they found non-allelic linkage heterogeneity in 10% of cases.[32]

FUNCTIONAL DISORDER

Severe Combined Immunodeficiency

The diagnosis of severe combined immunodeficiency (SCID) has been reported by fetal blood analysis.[29,33] This diagnosis is performed by enumeration of T and B lymphocytes using specific monoclonal antibodies and functional evaluation of phytohemagglutinin-induced T-cell proliferation in fetal blood obtained at 18 to 20 menstrual weeks. Because of the heterogenous nature of this disorder, the specific defect must be well characterized in a specific family. In about 25% of cases of the autosomal recessive form of SCID, there is a deficiency of adenosine deaminase, which may be measured in chorionic villi or amniocytes.[34–36] Because there have been reports of residual activity in affected patients, fetal blood sampling with multiple functional tests would be more reliable in these cases.[36] Purine nucleoside phosphorylase deficiency, another enzyme deficiency cause of SCID, has been diagnosed in amniocytes and chorionic villi and excluded in fetal blood.[35,37] The X-linked form of SCID has recently been shown to be tightly linked to the DXS159 probe on the X chromosome.[38] In addition, abnormal patterns of X-chromosome inactivation in T cells of carriers of X-linked SCID have been demonstrated.[39,40] The above approaches have been used to identify the mother as a female carrier in a family with an isolated affected male and to perform prenatal diagnosis in a subsequent pregnancy by linkage analysis.[41]

GRANULOCYTES

FUNCTIONAL DISORDERS

Chronic Granulomatous Disease

Chronic granulomatous disease causes recurrent pyogenic infections with catalase-positive organisms due to impaired activation of neutrophil oxygen metabolism. Death occurs by age 7 in one third of affected patients. Type I, the most common form (66% of cases), is inherited as an X-linked recessive trait. This disorder has been diagnosed using fetal granulocytes' presence or absence of nitroblue tetrazolium reduction, which measures superoxide production.[29,42] This gene has recently been cloned, but no informative polymorphisms are useful for prenatal diagnosis (except for the 10% of cases that show deletions).[43]

Chédiak-Higashi Disease

Chédiak-Higashi syndrome, a generalized disorder of cellular dysfunction, is characterized by large neutrophil cytoplasmic granules and an increased susceptibility to pyogenic infections. This autosomal recessive disorder has been excluded in three at-risk fetuses.[29]

PLATELETS

STRUCTURAL AND NUMERICAL DISORDERS

The congenital inherited platelet disorders are most easily grouped into quantitative or qualitative disorders. The quantitative disorders may be further subdivided into disorders of decreased platelet production or enhanced platelet destruction.

Several disorders of decreased platelet production have been diagnosed prenatally. Fanconi anemia, a genetic aplastic anemia that includes thrombocytopenia, has been discussed above.

The most common cause of enhanced platelet destruction in pregnancy is immune-mediated, resulting in autoimmune or alloimmune thrombocytopenia. These disorders are discussed in other chapters.

Thrombocytopenia Absent Radius Syndrome

Thrombocytopenia absent radius syndrome is an autosomal recessive disorder that may also include bilateral aplasia of the radii, renal and cardiac malformations, and an allergy to cow's milk. Symptoms generally improve with age, but serious hemorrhage can occur in infancy, usually associated with stress. There is a marked deficiency of megakaryocytes in the bone marrow. In all cases, the radii are absent, and almost all patients have thrombocytopenia at birth.[44] This disorder has been prenatally diagnosed by demonstration of absent radii at 16 to 20 menstrual weeks. This has been done by radiographs, ultrasound, and visualization of an abnormally positioned hand by fetoscopy in a case of oligohydramnios.[45–47]

Amegakaryocytic Thrombocytopenia

Amegakaryocytic thrombocytopenia is a rare, predominantly X-linked disorder that presents at birth with thrombocytopenia that gradually develops into pancytopenia. Millar and colleagues have reported prenatal diagnoses in three at-risk cases; one affected fetus had an in utero platelet count of 9×10^9/L (9000/μL).[48]

Wiskott-Aldrich Syndrome

Wiskott-Aldrich syndrome is an X-linked disorder that presents in the first year of life with thrombocytopenia, eczema, and recurrent infections. Fatal hemorrhage, infection, or a malignant reticuloendothelioma is common. Although it is unclear whether affected fetuses have a reduced platelet count in utero, it is thought that they do demonstrate the reduced platelet volume characteristic of this disorder. Several cases have been excluded when fetal blood sampling analysis showed a normal platelet volume.[48,49] No affected cases have been diagnosed by this approach. Recently, the gene for Wiskott-Aldrich has been mapped to a 20-centimorgan region on the X chromosome.[50] Schwartz and coworkers have reported first-trimester prenatal diagnoses of the syndrome by using flanking markers (DXS7 and DXS14) with more than 98% accuracy.[51] This approach will be useful for couples who are fully informative for both flanking markers. Parkman and colleagues have also reported the absence of a specific glycoprotein in platelets and lymphocytes of patients with the syndrome; this may prove useful in the future for prenatal diagnosis.[52]

FUNCTIONAL DISORDERS

Glanzmann Thrombasthenia

Glanzmann thrombasthenia, a rare autosomal recessive disorder, is characterized by a normal platelet count but a lack of ADP-induced platelet aggregation, causing severe bleeding. An abnormality of the platelet membrane glycoprotein IIb/IIIa complex has been identified in most cases of this disorder.[53] This abnormality has been analyzed by fetal blood sampling for prenatal diagnosis.[48,54] Champeix and associates have reported prenatal diagnosis of a variant form of Glanzmann thrombasthenia with normal glycoprotein IIb/IIIa values using functional assessment of ADP-induced platelet aggregation.[55] Of note, fetal exsanguination after blood sampling has been reported.[48,54]

Bernard-Soulier Syndrome

Bernard-Soulier syndrome, an autosomal recessive disorder of platelet adhesion, is characterized by a prolonged bleeding time and very large platelets. A defect in platelet glycoprotein Ib has been described and could potentially be used for prenatal diagnosis.[53]

Grey Platelet Syndrome

The Grey platelet syndrome, a rare defect of platelet alpha granules, has been prenatally excluded by measuring platelet beta thromboglobulin, which is reduced in this disorder.[56]

REFERENCES

1. Firshein SI, Hoyer LW, Lazarchick MD, et al. Prenatal diagnosis of classic hemophilia. New Engl J Med 1979;300:937.
2. Mibashan RS, Millar DS. Fetal hemophilia and allied bleeding disorders. Br Med Bull 1983;39:392.
3. Hoyer LW, Carta CA, Golbus MS, et al. Prenatal diagnosis of hemophilia (hemophilia A) by immunoradiometric assays during a 6-year period. Blood 1985;65:1312.
4. Gitscher J, Wood WI, Goralka TM, et al. Characterization of the human factor VIII gene. Nature 1984;312:326.
5. Antonarakis SE, Waber PG, Kittur SD, et al. Detection of molecular defects and of carriers by DNA analysis. N Engl J Med 1985;313:842.
6. Holmberg L, Gustavii B, Cordesius E, et al. Prenatal diagnosis of hemophilia B by an immunoradiometric assay of factor IX. Blood 1980;56:397.
7. Choo KH, Gould KG, Rees DJG, et al. Molecular cloning of the gene for human anti-hemophilic factor IX. Nature 1982;299:178.
8. Giannelli F, Anson DS, Choo KH, et al. Characterization and use of an intragenic polymorphic marker for detection of carriers of haemophilia B (factor IX deficiency). Lancet 1984;1:239.
9. Bottema CDK, Koeberl DD, Sommer SS. Direct carrier testing in 14 families with haemophilia B. Lancet 1989;2:526.
10. Hoyer LW, Lindsten J, Blomback M, et al. Prenatal evaluation of fetus at risk for severe von Willebrand's disease. Lancet 1979;2:191.
11. Whitelaw A, Haines ME, Bolsover W, et al. Factor V deficiency and antenatal intraventricular haemorrhage. Arch Dis Child 1984;59:997.
12. Spritz RA, Forget BG. The thalassemias; molecular mechanisms of human genetic disease. Am J Hum Genet 1983;35:333.
13. Lebo RV, Saiki RK, Swanson K, et al. Prenatal diagnosis of α-thalassemia by PCR and dual restriction enzyme analysis. Hum Genet 1990;in press.
14. Alter BP. Prenatal diagnosis: general introduction, methodology, and review. Hemoglobin 1988;12:763.

15. Harkness DR. Hematological and clinical features of sickle-cell diseases: a review. Hemoglobin 1980;4:313.
16. Junien C, Leroux A, Lostanlen D, et al. Prenatal diagnosis of congenital enzymopenic methaemoglobinaemia with mental retardation due to generalized cytochrome b_5 reductase deficiency: first report of two cases. Prenat Diagn 1981;1:17.
17. Dhermy D, Feo C, Garbaz M, et al. Prenatal diagnosis of hereditary elliptocytosis with molecular defect of spectrin. Prenat Diagn 1987;7:471.
18. Morris SA., Ohanian V, Lewis ML, et al. Prenatal diagnosis of hereditary red cell membrane defect. Br J Haematol 1986;62:763.
19. Whitelaw AGL, Rogers PA, Hopkinson DA, et al. Congenital haemolytic anaemia resulting from glucose phosphate isomerase deficiency: genetics, clinical picture, and prenatal diagnosis. J Med Genet 1979;16:189.
20. Dallapiccola B, Novelli G, Ferranti G, et al. First-trimester monitoring of a pregnancy at risk for glucose phosphate isomerase deficiency. Prenat Diagn 1986;6:101.
21. Clark ACL, Szobolotsky MA. Triose phosphate isomerase deficiency: prenatal diagnosis. J Pediatr 1985;106:417.
22. Rosa R, Prehu MO, Calvin MC, et al. Possibility of prenatal diagnosis of hereditary triose phosphate isomerase deficiency. Prenat Diagn 1986;6:231.
23. Bellingham AJ, Lestas AN, Williams LHP, et al. Prenatal diagnosis of a red-cell enzymopathy: triose phosphate isomerase deficiency. Lancet 2:419.
24. Dallapiccola B, Novelli G, Cuoco C, et al. First-trimester studies of a fetus at risk for triose phosphate isomerase deficiency. Prenat Diagn 1987;7:289.
25. Dallapiccola B, Novelli G. Prenatal diagnosis of triose phosphate isomerase deficiency. Lancet 1989;2:871.
26. Auerbach AD, Sagi M, Adler B. Fanconi anemia: prenatal diagnosis in 30 fetuses at risk. Pediatrics 1985;76:794.
27. Visser GHA, Desmed MCH, Meijboom EJ. Altered fetal cardiac flow patterns in pure red cell anaemia (the Blackfan-Diamond syndrome). Prenat Diagn 1988;8:525.
28. Durandy A, Cerf-Bensussan N, Dumez Y, et al. Prenatal diagnosis of severe combined immunodeficiency with defective synthesis of HLA molecules. Prenat Diagn 1987;7:27.
29. Durandy A, Dumez Y, Griscelli C. Prenatal diagnosis of severe inherited immunodeficiencies: a 5-year experience. In: Progress in immunodeficiency research and therapy II. Amsterdam: Elsevier, 1986.
30. Lau YL, Levinsky RJ. Prenatal diagnosis and carrier detection in primary immunodeficiency disorders. Arch Dis Child 1988; 63:758.
31. Malcolm S, de Saint Basile G, Arveiler B, et al. Close linkage of random DNA fragments from Xq21.3–22 to X-linked agammaglobulinemia (XLA). Hum Genet 1987;77:172.
32. Lau YL, Levinsky RJ, Malcolm S, et al. Genetic prediction in X-linked agammaglobulinemia. Am J Med Genet 1988;31:437.
33. Gelfand EW, Dosch H. Diagnosis and classification of severe combined immune deficiency disease. In: Primary immunodeficiency diseases. New York: Alan R. Liss, 1983.
34. Dooley T, Fairbanks LD, Simmonds HA, et al. First-trimester diagnosis of adenosine deaminase deficiency. Prenat Diagn 1987;7:561.
35. Linch DC, Levinsky RJ, Rodeck CH, et al. Prenatal diagnosis of three cases of severe combined immunodeficiency: severe T cell deficiency during the first half of gestation in fetuses with adenosine deaminase deficiency. Clin Exp Immunol 1984;56:223.
36. Pérignon JL, Durandy A, Peter MO, et al. Early prenatal diagnosis of inherited severe immunodeficiencies linked to enzyme deficiencies. J Pediatr 1987;111:595.
37. Kleijer WJ, Hussaarts-Odijk LM, Los FJ, et al. Prenatal diagnosis of purine nucleoside phosphorylase deficiency in the first and second trimesters of pregnancy. Prenat Diagn 1989;9:401.
38. de Saint Basile G, Arveiler B, Oberlé I, et al. Close linkage of the locus for X chromosome-linked severe combined immunodeficiency to polymorphic DNA markers in Xq11–q13. Proc Natl Acad Sci USA 1987;84:7576.
39. Puck JM, Nussbaum RL, Conley ME. Carrier detection in X-linked severe combined immunodeficiency based on patterns of X chromosome inactivation. J Clin Invest 1987;79:1395.
40. Conley ME, Lavoie A, Briggs C, et al. Nonrandom X chromosome inactivation in B cells from carriers of X chromosome-linked severe combined immunodeficiency. Proc Natl Acad Sci USA 1988;85:3090.
41. Puck JM, Krauss CM, Puck SM, et al. Prenatal test for X-linked severe combined immunodeficiency by analysis of maternal X-chromosome inactivation and linkage analysis. N Engl J Med 1990;322:1063.
42. Newburger PE, Cohen HJ, Rothchild SB, et al. Prenatal diagnosis of chronic granulomatous disease. N Engl J Med 1979;300:178.
43. Royer-Pokera B, Kunkel LM, Monaco AP, et al. Cloning the gene for an inherited human disorder—chronic granulomatous disease—on the basis of its chromosomal location. Nature 1986;322:32.
44. Hall JG. Thrombocytopenia and absent radius (TAR) syndrome. J Med Genet 1987;24:79.
45. Luthy DA, Hall JG, Graham CB. Prenatal diagnosis of thrombocytopenia with absent radii. Clin Genet 1979;15:495.
46. Luthy DA, Hack L, Hirsch J, et al. Prenatal ultrasound diagnosis of thrombocytopenia with absent radii. Am J Obstet Gynecol 1981;141:350.
47. Filkins K, Russo J. Prenatal diagnosis of thrombocytopenia absent radius syndrome using ultrasound and fetoscopy. Prenat Diagn 1984;4:139.
48. Millar DS, Mibashan RS, Pagliuca A, et al. Prenatal diagnosis of severe inherited platelet disorders by early second-trimester analysis of pure fetal blood (abstract). Br J Haematol 1988;69:109.
49. Holmberg L, Gustavii B, Jönsson A. A prenatal study of fetal platelet count and size with application to fetus at risk for Wiskott-Aldrich syndrome. J Pediatr 1983;102:773.
50. Kwan S, Sandkuyl LA, Blaese M, et al. Genetic mapping of the Wiskott-Aldrich syndrome with two highly linked polymorphic DNA markers. Genomics 1988;3:39.
51. Schwartz M, Mibashan RS, Nicolaides KH, et al. First-trimester diagnosis of Wiskott-Aldrich syndrome by DNA markers. Lancet 2:1405.
52. Parkman R, Kenney DM, Remold-O'Donnell E, et al. Surface protein abnormalities in lymphocytes and platelets from patients with Wiskott-Aldrich syndrome. Lancet 2:1387.
53. Montgomery RR, Kunicki TJ, Taves C. Diagnosis of Bernard-Soulier syndrome and Glanzmann's thrombasthenia with a monoclonal assay on whole blood. J Clin Invest 1983;71:385.
54. Seligsohn U, Mibashan RS, Rodeck CH, et al. Prevention program of Type I Glanzmann thrombasthenia in Israel: prenatal diagnosis. Curr Stud Hematol Blood Transfus 1988;55:174.
55. Champeix P, Forestier F, Daffos F, et al. Prenatal diagnosis of a molecular variant of Glanzmann's thrombasthenia. Curr Stud Hematol Blood Transfus 1988;55:180.
56. Wautier JL, Gruel Y. Prenatal diagnosis of platelet disorders. Ballière's Clin Haematol 1989;2:569.

33

CHAPTER

GENETIC COUNSELING IN PRENATAL AND PERINATAL MEDICINE

Aubrey Milunsky

It is important to keep genetics in mind in every patient encounter. Genetics has a role in virtually every illness, in either causation, predisposition and susceptibility, immune response, modulation, or reaction to medical treatment. Current estimates are that each of us carries about 20 harmful genes. About one in 13 conceptions results in a conceptus with a chromosome abnormality. About 50% of first-trimester spontaneous abortions are associated with chromosome anomalies.[1] Live-born infants have a 0.4% rate of chromosome defects and an additional 0.2% rate of balanced chromosomal rearrangements.[2] Some 3% to 4% of all births are associated with a major congenital malformation, mental retardation, or genetic disorder, a rate that doubles by 7–8 years of age, given later-appearing and/or later-diagnosed genetic disorders.[3] The burden of genetic disease is sufficiently significant in childhood to account for between 28% and 40% of hospital admissions in North America, Canada, and England.[4,5] Catalogued single-gene traits or disorders now exceed 4000.[6] The extent and importance of the role of genetics in disease causation becomes apparent immediately when one includes later-onset disease, such as heart disease, hypertension, diabetes, and the polygenic disorders in general. If chromosomal, monogenic, and polygenic disorders are combined, about 60% of all sick individuals have genetically influenced diseases.[7] It is appropriate and important that parents be fully informed about the risks they normally undertake in having a child[8] and about any significant additional risks of 0.5% to 1.0% or more.

PRECONCEPTION CARE AND COUNSELING

Major and continuing efforts must be made to educate the public at large about the importance of pregnancy planning and, in particular, of preconception care and counseling. Our knowledge of embryonic and fetal development and the sophisticated developments of the "new genetics" make the matter more compelling than ever. Physicians need to inculcate the wisdom not only of planning pregnancy but of initiating care in the preconception period. Many issues that influence fetal development and maternal welfare need to be addressed at the preconception visit.

Careful attention is necessary in eliciting the *medical history and examination*. Medical disorders may be detected that have a bearing on pregnancy, fetal development, delivery, and the newborn. For example, the significance of excessive joint laxity may be recognized for the first time at the preconception visit and point to diagnoses such as the Ehlers-Danlos syndrome, with its associated complications of premature delivery and tissue fragility.[9,10] Excess bruisability may reflect a disorder of coagulation. A history of panic attacks may alert the physician to the associated possible presence of mitral valve prolapse, requiring antibiotic prophylaxis.[11] These few examples exemplify opportunities for the early detection of potential later complications and facilitates anticipatory obstetric and perinatal management.

The preconception visit is also the time to secure *control and treatment of specific disorders* that may affect an otherwise successful pregnancy. Prospective mothers with insulin-dependent diabetes need help and advice to achieve tight control of their hyperglycemia. They need to understand that the poorer the control of their diabetes, the higher the frequency of congenital malformations and the more severe they may be, and vice versa.[12,13] Women with epilepsy, in particular, require review by their own neurologists concerning anticonvulsant medication. Where appropriate, anticonvulsants could be changed to those that might pose lesser risks of fetal anomalies without risking maternal health. Women with sickle cell disease[14,15] or cystic fibrosis[16,17] who face serious personal and fetal risks need special attention and treatment to secure the best chance for successful pregnancy and survival if that is their wish. Recognition of systemic lupus erythematosus allows appropriate careful medical surveillance and later monitoring of the fetal and neonatal heart for early detection and treatment of congenital heart block, which occurs much more frequently in this condition.[18]

The *obstetric and gynecologic* history, taken at the preconception visit, provides important opportunities again for intervention. Patients with prolonged infertility of unknown cause or current spontaneous abortion, who may face a 3% to 10% risk of a parental chromosome abnormality,[19,20] require chromosome analysis, as do their spouses. Failure to detect a parental chromosome translocation or other rearrangement may later be followed by the conception and birth of a child with an unbalanced karyotype. Such a patient would not have been offered prenatal genetic studies and, hence, could become a victim of an unmitigated catastrophe.

History of a previous stillbirth should raise questions about the need for parental chromosome analysis. Between 6% and 11% of stillbirths have a chromosome abnormality,[21] and a small portion of such cases indeed may have a transmitting parent with a chromosome rearrangement or disorder. The preconception visit, in addition, facilitates determination of whether the prospective mother is susceptible to rubella, cytomegalovirus, or toxoplasmosis, or has herpes or AIDS. Timely vaccination for rubella, where indicated, should be taken care of before conception.

Nutritional considerations that bear on fetal development have become more important. Our recent data indicate that multivitamins containing folic acid taken during the preconception period and continuing at least through the first 6 weeks of pregnancy reduce the frequency of neural tube defects by between 50% and 70%.[22] The preponderance of the evidence points in the same direction,[23–25] except for one flawed study.[26] Therefore, even though it is not entirely certain that folic acid is the key ingredient or essential nutrient that facilitates such protection, it seems prudent for patients to be advised of this potential benefit that is achievable through normal dosage. The minimum dose of folic acid required to achieve this level of protection against neural tube defects is not yet established. Thus far, 400 μg to 1 mg daily of folic acid seems to have been sufficient to reduce the frequency of neural tube defects significantly.

The *clinical genetic history* focuses first on analysis of the family pedigree. An obvious pattern of inheritance may emerge without a known named disorder. For example, a *maternal* history of nephews, brothers, or uncles with mental retardation may point to sex-linked mental retardation that may require further study. A previous living child with a specified genetic defect might require additional specific diagnostic studies, parental examination, or other appropriate investigations. Carrier detection tests using DNA analysis for conditions such as Duchenne or Becker muscular dystrophy, chronic granulomatous disease, and ornithine transcarbamylase deficiency are among the many disorders now approachable through molecular analysis.

Attention to the patient's *ethnicity* may be the only warning to the obstetrician of potential genetic risks. Virtually all ethnic groups carry some "genetic burden."[8] For example, whites have a risk of about 1 in 20 of carrying the gene for cystic fibrosis. About 68% of such carriers share the same common mutation—a simple 3–base pair (bp) deletion of phenylalanine.[27] Less common mutations in the cystic fibrosis gene continue to be elucidated. At least for the common mutation, it is already feasible to extract DNA from peripheral blood leukocytes and, using the polymerase chain reaction, to determine the presence of the common mutation in 1 day. Prenatal diagnosis using this same technique is also possible—also in 1 day. Individuals of Mediterranean extraction have a risk of about 1 in 12 of carrying the gene for β-thalassemia. Once again, a simple blood examination for mean cell volume and for hemoglobins A_2 and F will assist in carrier detection. Ashkenazi Jews, who have a risk that about a 1 in 30 will carry the gene for Tay-Sachs disease, also should be routinely offered the necessary carrier detection test (hexosaminidase A assay in serum or leukocytes) for this degenerative neurologic disorder. For all the autosomal recessive disorders just mentioned, only if both parents are carriers would there be a 25% risk of bearing an affected child. In all these instances, prenatal diagnosis would be available.[28] This information becomes important for individuals who might select prenatal diagnosis as an option or for couples who prefer to avoid the possibilities of abortion and prefer artificial insemination from a donor known not to carry that specific gene.

Dramatic and continuing advances in molecular genetics increasingly enable *predictive tests* for disorders not previously detectable by any method.[29] Hence, even asymptomatic individuals may be able to determine whether they have a particular dominant gene for which there is a risk of 50% for transmission in each pregnancy, or whether they carry autosomal or X-linked genes, with their associated risks. Selected examples of such disorders for which presymptomatic and prenatal diagnosis and carrier detection are feasible are listed in Table 33-1. Hence, for example, once a parent is shown to carry the gene for myotonic muscular dystrophy, preconception studies of the family could assist in determining whether prenatal diagnosis, using DNA analysis, can be accomplished and with what degree of certainty. These tests further allow detection of maternal myotonic dystrophy, facilitating prenatal diagnosis, anticipation,[30] optimal surveillance, and possible early intervention or prevention of the frequently serious intrapregnancy, labor, delivery, postpartum, and neonatal complications (Table 33-2).

Advances in human genetics are expected to escalate rapidly during the last decade of this century with the planned mapping of the entire human genome. Obstetricians and all physicians who care for patients in their childbearing years should remain alert to these advances. In the future, preimplantation diagnosis may require discussion during the preconception visit. It is

TABLE 33–1. EXAMPLES OF MONOGENIC DISORDERS FOR WHICH DNA DIAGNOSTIC TESTS NOW FACILITATE PRESYMPTOMATIC AND PRENATAL DIAGNOSIS AS WELL AS CARRIER DETECTION

	GENE LOCATION
Autosomal Dominant Disorder	
Huntington's disease	4p
Myotonic muscular dystrophy	19q
Retinoblastoma	13q
Familial hypercholesterolemia	19p
Von Willebrand's disease	12p
Familial amyloidotic polyneuropathy	18q
Neurofibromatosis	17p
Autosomal Recessive Disorder	
Cystic fibrosis	7q
Sickle cell anemia	11p
Phenylketonuria	12q
Friedreich's ataxia	9q
β-Thalassemia	11p
α-Thalassemia	16p
Wilson's disease	13q
Sex-Linked Disorders	
Duchenne/Becker muscular dystrophy	Xp
Hemophilia A	Xq
Chronic granulomatous disease	Xp
Lymphoproliferative disease	Xq
Lesch-Nyhan syndrome	Xq
Ornithine transcarbamylase deficiency	Xp
Charcot-Marie-Tooth disease	Xq
Adrenoleukodystrophy	Xq

likely that in some cases, and for some individuals, this eventually may be an expensive, but possible, option. Finally, among the more important aspects of the preconception visit is the provision of *genetic counseling,* the details of which now follow.

GENETIC COUNSELING

Genetic counseling is a communication process concerning the occurrence and the risks of recurrence of genetic disorders within a family. The aim of such counseling is to provide the patient with a clear and comprehensive understanding of all the important implications of the disorder in question, as well as the possible options. The purpose is also to help families through their problems, necessary decision making, and emotional adjustments and adaptations, where indicated. Although the physician may wish to prevent or minimize the suffering of both patient and family and to decrease the incidence of serious genetic disease, the primary strategy must be to achieve clear understanding by prospective parents, facilitating rational decision making.[31,28,8] All prospective parents have a right to know if they have an increased risk of having children with a genetic disorder, or other defect, and what their options are. The physician's duty is to communicate this information clearly and in simple language (with a translator if required), to offer specific tests (serially, if necessary), or to refer couples for second expert opinion.

The primary reasons couples seek genetic counseling in the context of risks and prenatal diagnosis are circumscribed:

1. Advanced maternal age. An arbitrary age of 35 years has long functioned as the standard of expected care, at which age maternal age-related risks of chromosome defects should be discussed and prenatal genetic studies recommended.[28] Increasingly, geneticists consider it appropriate to inform parents of their gradually escalating risks related to maternal age, and many recommend amniocentesis by 34 years of age. Indeed, the decision to have an amniocentesis or not should reflect the balance of risks between fetal loss and fetal defects. Although decisions made for or against such studies should be primarily parental, based on appropriate consultation with their physician, third-party payors continue to influence many of these decisions through cost considerations.
2. High or low maternal serum α-fetoprotein (AFP) values. Neural tube defects or other leaking structural abnormalities reflect the need for discussing high values, whereas low values of AFP initiate discussions on the risks of chromosome defects, with a view to both ultrasound and amniocentesis.[32,28]
3. A previous fetus or child with a chromosome, monogenic, or polygenic disorder.
4. A family history of a specific family disorder.
5. One prospective parent with a suspected or known chromosomal, monogenic, or polygenic disorder.
6. A maternal disorder with or without specific drug treatment, associated with an increased risk of congenital defects.
7. A known or suspected carrier state for a certain genetic disorder on the basis of previous or required tests or ethnicity.
8. Exposure during, or prior to, pregnancy, to po-

TABLE 33–2. MYOTONIC MUSCULAR DYSTROPHY: POTENTIAL PREGNANCY, NEONATAL, AND OTHER COMPLICATIONS

1. Potential abortion
2. Fetal death
3. Polyhydramnios
4. Prolonged labor
5. Fetal distress
6. Uterine atony
7. Postpartum hemorrhage
8. Cardiac arrhythmias
9. Increased sensitivity to anesthetic and relaxant agents
10. Postoperative respiratory depression
11. Neonatal death
12. Arthrogryposis
13. Mental retardation

Data from references 42, 46, and 47.

tentially hazardous medications, infectious organisms, x-rays, toxins, or occupational hazards.
9. Known or suspected consanguinity.
10. The random risk of congenital defects and genetic disorders.

In general, genetic counseling is best provided by a clinical geneticist. In both the United States and Canada, board-certified specialists in clinical genetics and medical genetics are available for referral. If an obstetrician is well informed, he or she should be able to provide the necessary counseling for advanced maternal age and, increasingly, for high and low maternal serum AFP values. Caution should guide the physician in avoiding areas outside expected expertise. Quotation of risk figures through intuitive judgments are strictly contraindicated. Clinical geneticists who provide counseling are expected to provide a letter to the referring physician, with a copy to the patient (or two separate letters, if preferred). Either way, documentation of the key elements transmitted during counseling would be regarded as mandatory, regardless of who provides such services.

THE GENETIC BASIS FOR COUNSELING

Genetic disorders that affect fetal development may be either chromosomal, monogenic or multifactorial in origin. Acquired disorders, which complicate fetal development (eg, infectious diseases, medications, toxins), will not be discussed here, even though their actions may be mediated through individual genetic susceptibility. Chromosomal disorders arise as a consequence of chromosome number (too many or too few) or from structural rearrangements of one or more chromosomes. Single-gene disorders may be inherited or arise de novo as a consequence of mutation. The modes of inheritance for single-gene disorders are classified as autosomal dominant, autosomal recessive, or X-linked. Multifactorial disorders result from an interaction between multiple genes and one or more environmental factors. The arbitrary distinction between chromosomal and single-gene inheritance should be understood, since many examples exist in which structural alteration of a chromosome results in deletion or interruption of one or more genes. Notwithstanding such arbitrary classifications, it is simpler, when trying to determine the origin of a specific phenotype, to think in terms of the preceding categorical classification.

Chromosomal Disorders

Each of our somatic cells contains 46 chromosomes, with 23 derived from each parent. There are 44 non–sex chromosomes (called autosomes) and two sex chromosomes. Females have two X chromosomes (XX) and males have one X chromosome and one Y chromosome (XY). The chromosomes can be distinguished from each other on the basis of size; location of the centromere, which divides a chromosome into long or short arms; and the unique banding pattern. Not only can subtle details of chromosome structure now be delineated (eg, deletions), but the origin of an extra or abnormal chromosome can be determined frequently and precisely. For example, the extra chromosome 18 in trisomy 18 derives from a maternal source in 95% of cases, whereas the structurally abnormal chromosome (with a deletion) in the Prader-Willi syndrome appears to be uniformly of paternal origin (Table 33-3). High-resolution chromosome analysis of prophase chromosomes, rather than metaphase, allows easier recognition of structural defects (Fig. 33-1).

Chromosomal disorders can be classified into either numerical or structural rearrangement groups. Numerical disorders are characterized by extra, or absent, chromosomes. For example, the most common numerical chromosome disorder in newborns is characterized by an entire extra No. 21 chromosome, resulting in trisomy 21. Among first-trimester abortuses, an absent sex chromosome, resulting in a 45,X fetus, is the most common numerical chromosome disorder. A single cell division, soon after fertilization, may go awry, resulting in a numerical chromosome abnormality in the daughter cells of that division and, consequently, in chromosomally abnormal cells from that original stem cell. These abnormal cells continue to divide and multiply alongside the subjacent chromosomally normal cells and eventually result in an individual who has two or more different cell lines—a chromosomal mosaic. Chromosomal mosaicism is found most frequently among the sex chromosome disorders. Extra segments, due to duplication of either an entire region (resulting in par-

TABLE 33–3. EXAMPLES OF PARENTAL ORIGIN OF SPECIFIC CHROMOSOMES IN ANEUPLOIDY OR WITH CERTAIN STRUCTURAL ARRANGEMENTS

CHROMOSOMAL DISORDER	PARENTAL ORIGIN OF "INVOLVED" CHROMOSOME
Trisomy 21 (Down's syndrome)	95% extra No. 21 maternal
Trisomy 18 (Edward's syndrome)	95% extra No. 18 maternal
Prader-Willi syndrome	Paternal No. 15
Angelman "Happy Puppet" syndrome	Maternal No. 15
Wilms' tumor	Nonrandom loss of No. 11 maternal
Turner's syndrome (45,X)	Paternal X absent ± 76%

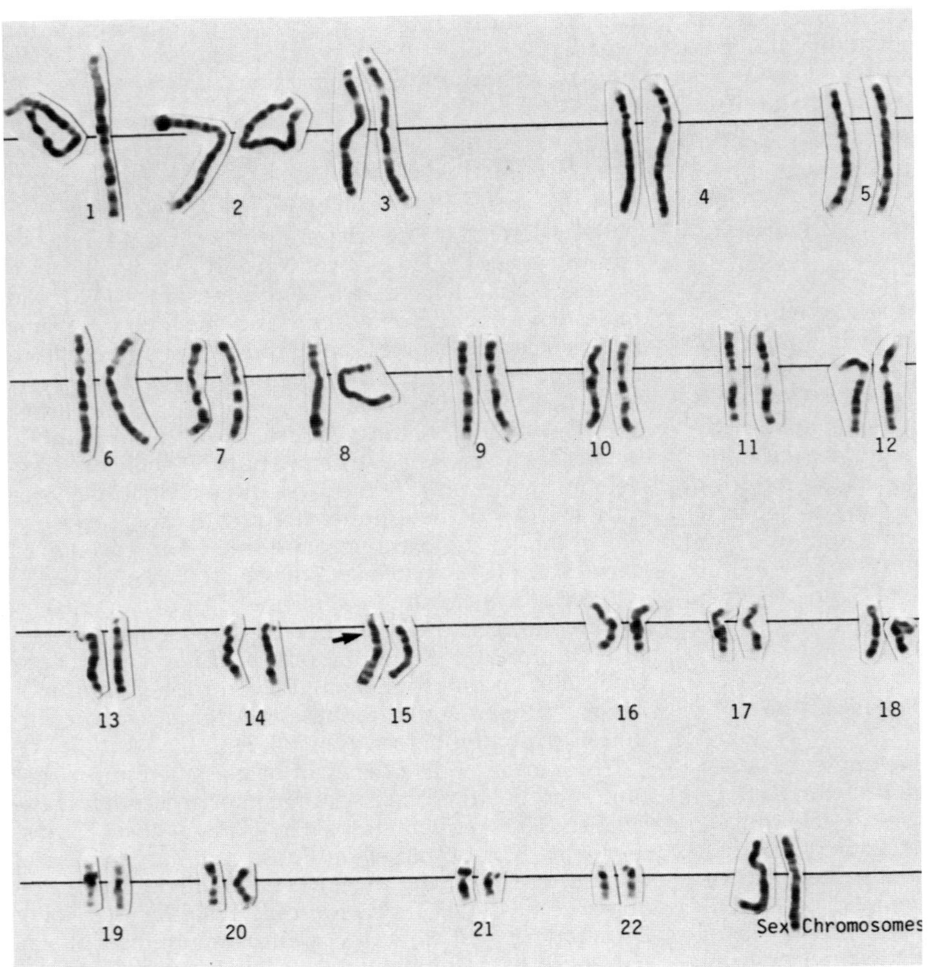

FIGURE 33–1. Karyotype of a patient with Angelman "happy puppet" syndrome showing a deletion of a band at 15q12. Arrow points to band 15q12 in the normal homologue. This band is deleted in the other homologue.

tial trisomy of the long or short arm of a specific chromosome) or a tiny segment of a chromosome arm, may all result in catastrophic malformations, with or without mental retardation.

Structural chromosome defects may result from the breakage and loss of a variable-sized piece of a long or short arm (deletion) or the breakage of two chromosomes and transfer with fusion of parts of the broken fragments onto the residual chromosomes (translocation). About one in 500 live-borns has a balanced chromosomal translocation, whereas an unbalanced translocation occurs in one in 2000 live-born infants.

Translocations involving the acrocentric chromosomes in one parent are associated with risks of an unbalanced translocation, ranging mostly from 4% to 20%, with higher risks for maternal carriers (Table 33-4).[13–15,21,22] Reciprocal translocations between autosomes are associated, almost invariably, with much lower risks for unbalanced karyotypes, mostly below 3% and frequently around 1%. One remarkable exception is shown in Figure 33-2. Abnormal splitting of a centromere during meiosis occurs infrequently but may cause the loss of an entire chromosome arm and duplication of the remaining arm, resulting in a single symmetric chromosome with two genetically identical arms (called an isochromosome).

Chromosome inversions, which occur following breakage at two sites along a chromosome length, followed by inversion and reattachment, are not uncommon. Such inversions, which involve the centromere (called pericentric inversions)[33] or occur away from the centromere (called paracentric inversions),[34] are generally thought to be associated with a risk of up to 5% of congenital defects, with or without mental retardation, when they occur de novo (see Table 33-4). The exception is the pericentric inversion involving the long arm of chromosome 9, which appears to have no clinical significance.

Subtle chromosome deletions pose serious diagnostic difficulties when they occur de novo. Virtually all microdeletion syndromes are associated with serious or fatal genetic disease (Table 33-5). The finding of a microdeletion in an infant should lead automatically to chromosome analysis (of both parents) that seeks a translocation or other chromosomal rearrangement. For many years, many of these microdeletion syndromes were considered to be mendelian monogenic conditions. Only after high-resolution chromosome analysis

TABLE 33–4. THE RISKS OF RECURRENCE AND THE RISKS OF HAVING UNBALANCED PROGENY FOR THE MORE COMMON CHROMOSOME DISORDERS ENCOUNTERED IN CLINICAL PRACTICE

CHROMOSOME DISORDERS	RISK OF RECURRENCE (%)	NOTES
Numerical Abnormalities		
A previous child with trisomy 21	1–1.5	Includes risks for all aneuploidy and applies to all women age ≤ 30 years. Those >30 have maternal age–associated risks of aneuploidy
A previous child with trisomy 18	<1	
A previous child with trisomy 13	<1	
A previous child with Turner syndrome (45X)	Population risk	As long as mother is not a Turner syndrome mosaic, risks of recurrence will approximate population risk (±1 in 4000 females)
A previous child with XXX syndrome	Population risk	As long as neither parent has sex chromosome mosaicism and mother is <35 years, risk of recurrence will approximate population risk (one in 1000 females)
A previous child with Klinefelter's syndrome (47,XXY)	Population risk	As long as neither parent has sex chromosome mosaicism and mother is <35 years, risk of recurrence will approximate population risk (one in 1000 males)
A previous child with 47,XYY	Population risk	Population risk approximates one in 1000 males
CHROMOSOME DISORDERS	**RISK OF UNBALANCED PROGENY (%)**	**NOTES**
Structural Rearrangements		
Robertsonian translocations		
t(13;14)	Rare	
t(14;21) maternal	11–15	
t(14;21) paternal	1–2	
t(13;21) maternal	11–15	
t(13;21) paternal	1–2	
t(15;21) maternal	11–15	
t(15;21) paternal	1–2	
Reciprocal translocations		
In general maternal	5–20	Risks depend on how original case was ascertained If through recurrent miscarriage lower figure applies
In general paternal	3–30	Risks depend on how original case was ascertained If through recurrent miscarriage lower figure applies
t(11;22) maternal	6	
t(11;22) paternal	5	
Inversions (autosomal)		
Pericentric	5–10	If original case ascertained through a previous child with a structural rearrangement
Pericentric	1–3	If original case ascertained fortuitously and without phenotypic abnormality
Paracentric	<1	

Data from references 33–36.

was introduced did it become increasingly possible to detect these disorders with the light microscope. Submicroscopic deletions for each of these conditions undoubtedly exist or have already been recognized, using molecular DNA probes, and result in the same or similar abnormal phenotypes.

Indications for chromosome analysis in the context of reproduction and perinatal medicine can be considered in the following groups:

1. For *both* prospective parents with prolonged infertility or three or more spontaneous abortions, or two or more stillbirths
2. When one parent has a chromosome abnormality (most commonly a sex chromosome defect) or is a known carrier of a chromosomal translocation or other structural rearrangement
3. For all the offspring of one parent who carries a structural chromosome rearrangement

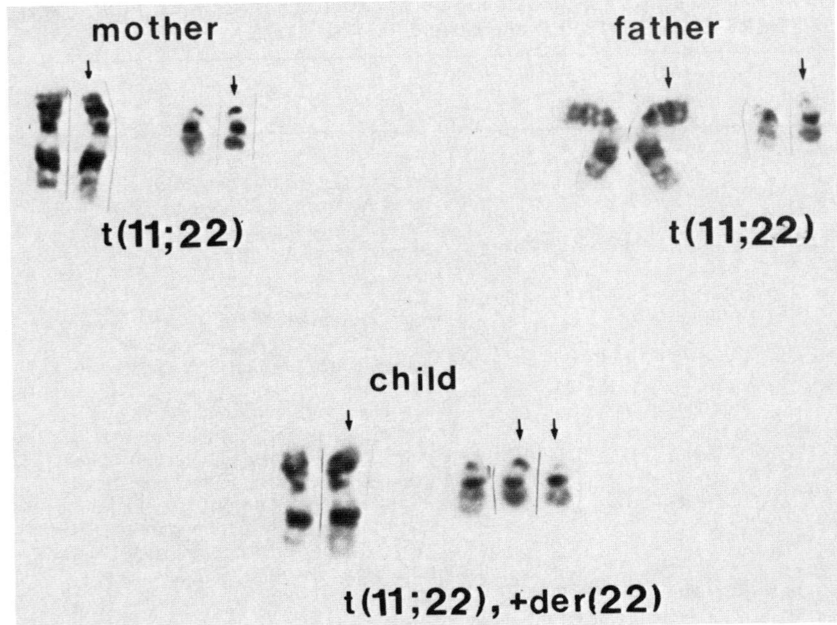

FIGURE 33–2. An unusual translocation family in which the mother and father both carry identical balanced reciprocal translocations between chromosomes 22 and 11. Their child has trisomy for proximal 22 and the distal band of 11q (small arrows point to translocation chromosomes). The child has two copies of the derivative 22 [ie, der(22)], but these copies are not identical. Variation in the size and staining intensity of satellite regions of the der(22)'s of the two parents indicated recombination in the satellite region that apparently occurred in a common ancestor. Hence, a der(22) was contributed by each parent to the child's karyotype. The most likely mechanism is that the maternal contribution resulted from a 3:1 segregation at meiosis and that the paternal contribution resulted from either an alternate or an adjacent I segregation. (Courtesy of Dr. Herman Wyandt.)

4. For the prospective parent who has genital malformations or abnormalities of sexual development
5. On all stillborns (with or without dysmorphic features or malformation) or babies following neonatal death without a specific diagnosis
6. In newborns with dysmorphic features, or those who exhibit serious growth retardation, with or without a single major congenital malformation
7. In infants or children with developmental delay, with or without dysmorphic features or associated malformations.

Despite remarkable advances in human genetics, there is still a lack of knowledge about those factors that cause chromosomal disorders. Because of the frequency of chromosomal anomalies (Table 33-6), careful consideration should be given to such possibilities in all cases of aberrant fetal development, including those detected in the third trimester. Advancing maternal age is associated with an increasing frequency of numerical chromosome disorders resulting from nondisjunction and include not only trisomy 21, but also trisomies 13 and 18, triple-X, and the 47,XXY male (Klinefelter's) syndrome. The risks of recurrence, following the birth of babies with different trisomies, are shown in Table 33-4. Certainly, one numerical chromosome abnormality, caused by nondisjunction, may be followed by a different one caused by the same basic mechanism. Hence, following conception of an offspring with trisomy 21, recurrence of a numerical abnormality has been different in some 50% of subsequent chromosomally abnormal offspring.[28] Available data suggest no increased risk of chromosome abnormality in future pregnancies after spontaneous abortions of lethal trisomies or recurrent abortion with normal parental karyotypes.[37]

Monogenic Disorders

Single-gene disorders occur in approximately 10 per 1000 live births, with about 7 in 1000 being due to autosomal dominant genes, about 2.5 in 1000 being due to recessive genes, and 0.4 per 1000 being due to X-linked genes. Thus far, over 300 genetic disorders with biochemical defects have been recognized.[38] Their single mutant genes have involved mainly abnormalities in enzymes and, increasingly, of specific proteins. A reduced lifespan is associated with over half of all monogenic disorders, whereas reproductive capacity is reduced in about 69% of such disorders.[38]

Clinically, dominant disorders are viewed as those in which symptomatic individuals are heterozygotes, whereas those with autosomal recessive disorders are symptomatic and are considered homozygotes. The distinction between dominant and recessive disorders is largely arbitrary, but useful clinically. It is known, for example, that for the autosomal recessive sickle cell disease, heterozygotes have subtle physiologic abnormalities, affecting renal concentrating ability as well as demonstrating a selective advantage for resistance to malaria. Heterozygotes for ataxia telangiectasia are known to be at an increased risk for developing malignancy. Hence, carriers of recessive genes may manifest disorders, just as do those individuals with dominant genes. Concerning the concept of dominant and recessive genes, other subtleties are recognized. For example, retinoblastoma is typically transmitted as an autosomal dominant disorder with virtually full penetrance. It is now established that the deletion, or point mutation on

TABLE 33–5. EXAMPLES OF CHROMOSOME MICRODELETION SYNDROMES

SYNDROME	MAIN FEATURES	CHROMOSOME DELETION SITE
Cri du chat	Mental retardation, mewing cry, mild dysmorphic facies	5p
Langer-Giedion (Trichorhinophalangeal syndrome type 2)	Mental retardation, sparse hair, typical facial features, exostoses	8q24
Aniridia-Wilms' tumor	Nephroblastoma, absent irises, genitourinary tract abnormalities, growth retardation, and variable mental retardation	11p13
Retinoblastoma	Intraocular malignancy, typical facies, possible mental retardation	13q14
Prader-Willi	Variable intellectual deficits, hypotonia, obesity, typical facies and body habitus, hypogonadism	15q11
DiGeorge	Absent/hypoplastic thymus and parathyroid, congenital heart defects, mental retardation, dysmorphic facies	22q11
Duchenne/Becker muscular dystrophy	Ascending muscle weakness, cardiomyopathy, possible mental retardation	Xp21
Steroid sulfatase deficiency	Frequent stillbirths, ichthyosis, low maternal estriol in urine and plasma	Xp22
Congenital adrenal hypoplasia	Early death (without treatment), features of Addison's disease	Xp21
Chronic granulomatous disease	Recurrent bacterial or fungal infections due to defective microbicidal capacity of phagocytes	Xp21
Lymphoproliferative disease	Fatal Epstein-Barr virus infection, malignant lymphomas, hypogammaglobulinemia	Xq26

one of the No. 13 chromosomes, has to be associated with another mutation in the homologous allele on the other No. 13 chromosome for retinoblastoma to develop. In other words, "two hits" are necessary, as though for this classical, dominant disorder, a recessive gene mechanism is effective. Notwithstanding continued progress in understanding complex mechanisms resulting in genetic disorders due to dominant or recessive genes, it still remains useful to consider them clinically in their well-established categories.

Autosomal Dominant Disorders

Since the genes for autosomal dominant disorders exist on one of the 22 autosomes, both males and females may be affected. An individual who is affected has a 50% risk of transmitting the gene to each of his or her offspring. The phenomenon of pleiotropy is especially important in this category of disorders. A single gene that has several different effects is regarded as pleiotropic (eg, the single gene causing tuberous sclerosis may result in retardation, achromic spots, and subungual fibromas). In contrast, genetic heterogeneity means that several genes have the same effect. A good example is deafness, which results from a variety of different single-gene disorders. Mutations commonly cause autosomal dominant disorders. For example, about seven of eight offspring with achondroplasia are due to a dominant gene mutation. Moreover, the frequency of such mutations rises with advancing paternal age. Variability in clinical expression (called expressivity) is also especially important in dominantly inherited disorders. One excellent example is the multiple endocrine neoplasia syndrome, in which individual affected family members may have either hyperplasia or malignancy or both, in various endocrine organs. Also typical of autosomal dominant disorders is the variation seen in the age of onset, even for the same condition. Hence, Huntington's disease may manifest in childhood or not until old age, even though the mutant gene has been present from the time of conception. Molecular analysis allows determination of the presence of the mutant gene, but does not provide any ability to predict onset time. Some guidance on this point is likely to emerge from a study of disease onset ages within specific families.

Autosomal Recessive Disorders

The mutant genes that cause this group of disorders are located on one of the 22 autosomes, and therefore both males and females may be affected. Clinically obvious autosomal recessive disorders exist only in the homozygous state (each parent contributing one of the mutant genes). Hence, when both parents are carriers, they have a 25% risk of having affected offspring in each pregnancy. In recent years, proof has emerged that an autosomal recessive disorder can result in an offspring inheriting the same harmful gene from each parent,

TABLE 33–6. FREQUENCY OF CHROMOSOME ABNORMALITIES IN LIVE-BORN INFANTS

CHROMOSOME ABNORMALITY	APPROXIMATE FREQUENCY
Numerical Disorders	
Autosomal trisomies	
47,+21	1:800
47,+18	1:7500
47,+13	1:22,700
Other	1:34,000
Sex chromosome abnormalities	
47,XYY	1:1000 males
47,XXY	1:1000 males
Other (males)	1:1300 males
45,X	1:4000 females
47,XXX	1:1000 females
Other (females)	1:2700 females
Structural Rearrangements	
Structural balanced	
Robertsonian translocation Reciprocal and insertional translocation Inversion	1:500
Structural unbalanced	
Robertsonian Reciprocal and insertional Inversion Deletion Supernumerary Other	1:1600

Data from references 2, 28.

even though the site of the mutation within the gene may be different. These so-called compound heterozygotes still develop the disease, but the nature of its clinical manifestations and time of onset may be altered. Important examples include cystic fibrosis, Tay-Sachs disease, and metachromatic leukodystrophy.

Typically, the rarer the mutant recessive gene, the greater the likelihood that those affected will result from consanguineous unions, or those where the couple have ethnicity in common. Although new mutations that result in recessive disorders may occur, they have not been easy to distinguish clinically. With increasing use of DNA analysis, the frequency and nature of recessive mutations are likely to be better understood. Meanwhile, for the more common autosomal recessive disorders, the physician needs to recognize the patient's ethnicity and provide the straightforward carrier detection tests for that specific group. Hence, couples who share Mediterranean, Ashkenazi Jewish, black, or Oriental extraction should be routinely offered preconception carrier detection tests for β-thalassemia, Tay-Sachs disease, sickle cell disease, and α-thalassemia, respectively.

X-Linked Disorders

The mutant genes that result in X-linked disorders are located on the X chromosome. Given that the male has only one X chromosome and the female has two, both the risk and severity of X-linked disease will vary between the sexes. Males will usually manifest the fullest expression of the disorder, whereas random X inactivation will largely influence expression in females. In contrast to females who carry autosomal recessive genes, those heterozygous for X-linked genes frequently manifest some sign(s) of the disease in question (Table 33-7).

Characteristically, male-to-male transmission does not occur in X-linked disease. This is because, normally, a male never contributes his X chromosome to a son. An affected male, by contributing his only X chromosome to all his daughters, will render them all carriers of the trait in question. In examining the pedigree of a family with possible X-linked disease, attention is usually given to whether the disease has occurred in maternal nephews, uncles, or first cousins and through the female line. Female heterozygotes have a 50% risk of having male offspring.

X-linked dominant traits are characterized by an affected male transmitting the condition to all his daughters and none of his sons and by an affected female, with a 50% likelihood of transmitting the disorder to her sons *or* daughters. X-linked dominant disorders occur about twice as often in females as males and may be less severe in affected females. Rarely, an X-linked dominant trait may be lethal in affected males, resulting in a disorder that appears to occur, clinically, only in females and in which an affected female has a 50% likelihood of transmitting the trait to her daughters. These affected women have an increased frequency of miscarriage, representing affected male fetuses. Incontinentia pigmenti is a good example.

TABLE 33–7. SIGNS IN X-LINKED RECESSIVE DISEASE CARRIERS

Fragile-X syndrome	Mild–moderate mental retardation
Fabry disease	Corneal dystrophy
Duchenne muscular dystrophy	Pseudohypertrophy and weakness
Alport's syndrome	Hematuria and hearing impairment
Ectodermal dysplasia (hypohidrotic)	Sparse hair: decreased sweating
Choroideremia	Chorioretinal dystrophy

Mutations of X-linked genes are not uncommon and are most often associated with the occurrence of a sporadic affected male within a family. Because of advances in molecular genetics, we now know that even in some of these families, despite the presence of a normal gene in the mother of such an affected male, germline mosaicism may account for recurrence in a future pregnancy. Hence, genetic counseling following sporadic occurrence of a male with X-linked Duchenne muscular dystrophy, should provide, notwithstanding negative DNA carrier testing of the mother, prenatal genetic studies in all subsequent pregnancies.

Fragile-X Syndrome. Special attention must be given to the X-linked disorder known as fragile-X syndrome, which represents the most common single cause of inherited mental retardation in males. Typical features include mental retardation of varying severity; macroorchidism; typical facial features, including a large head, prominent ears, forehead, and jaw; signs suggestive of a connective tissue disorder, including hyperextensibility, pectus excavatum, flat feet, possible mitral valve prolapse, and dilatation of the aortic root; and behavioral disorders, seizures, stereotypies, speech disorders, some autistic signs, and other neurologic features. The fragile-X syndrome occurs in one or two of every 2600 males, and about one in 866 females carry the gene.[39] About one third of female heterozygotes may be variably mentally retarded. This disorder is named for the appearance of the chromosomal fragile site, located on the distal long arm of the X chromosome and demonstrated by using folic acid–depleted culture medium for blood chromosome study. About 20% of males carrying the mutant gene are thought to be physically and cytogenetically normal; nevertheless, they transmit the gene to all their daughters and none of their sons. Families with one or more males with mental retardation of otherwise unknown etiology, should always have such sons checked for fragile-X syndrome. Some families also have more mildly affected females, which should not prevent diagnostic consideration of this extremely important X-linked disorder.

Multifactorial Genetic Disorders

Many disorders result from the interaction of multiple genes with one or more environmental factors. Typical birth defects in this category include cleft lip and palate, congenital heart disease, and neural tube defects. Generally, risks of recurrence tend mostly to range between 3% and 5%; important exceptions (such as pyloric stenosis) are well known. Recurrence risks typically vary from family to family and are particularly influenced by the number of affected family members and the severity of the condition in the index case. In general, if there are more affected relatives with more severe disease, the risk to their other relatives will be higher.

Consideration of phenocopies is particularly important in determining the etiology of what might be considered a multifactorial disorder. For example, cleft lip and palate may also occur as a consequence of a monogenic disorder, a chromosome abnormality, or a specific medication.

EVALUATING THE CAUSE OF STILLBIRTH OR PERINATAL DEATH

The full spectrum of grief can be expected to attend all stillbirths and perinatal deaths. Therefore, the physician can, and should, anticipate feelings of denial, expressions of guilt, experience of depression, and expressed or contained anger from the parents. Although the intensity and duration of such *normal* responses by parents may vary, active steps to evaluate the cause(s) of their loss serves to assist in turning anguish into action and to possibly providing important information that would help alleviate the grieving process. A summary protocol for such evaluation is suggested in Table 33-8.

Following stillbirth or perinatal death, careful review of the family (genetic) history and of the medical and obstetric history is recommended. Assessment of consanguinity should include determination of possible common ancestral origins of the parents, as well as consideration of last names of grandparents or great-grandparents. Autopsy should automatically be recommended in all such cases, unless an absolute and definitive diagnosis is already known. During the overwhelming grief at such times, one or both parents frequently are not inclined to allow an autopsy. Experience has taught that many such parents later regret having lost the opportunity to determine specific answers to very definite questions. If the ward, medical, and nursing staffs have been unable to obtain permission for autopsy, judicious action would include requesting the senior attending physician to meet with the parents immediately, lending experience and authority to the recommendation, urging that information gained at autopsy may benefit their other or future chil-

TABLE 33–8. PROTOCOL FOR EVALUATING THE CAUSE OF STILLBIRTH OR PERINATAL DEATH

1. Review genetic, medical, and obstetric history.
2. Determine possible consanguinity.
3. Gently and persistently recommend that parents permit a complete autopsy.
4. Obtain photographs, including full face and profile, whole body, and, where applicable, detailed pictures of any specific abnormality (eg, of digits).
5. Obtain full-body skeletal radiographs.
6. Carefully document any dysmorphic features.
7. Obtain heparinized cord or fetal blood sample for chromosomal or DNA analysis.
8. Obtain fetal serum for infectious disease studies (eg, parvovirus, cytomegalovirus, toxoplasmosis).
9. Obtain fetal tissue sample (sterile fascia best) for cell culture aimed at chromosome analysis, biochemical, or DNA studies.
10. Obtain parental bloods for chromosome analysis, where indicated.
11. Communicate final autopsy results and conclusions of special analyses.
12. Provide follow-up counseling, including a summary letter.

dren. Keeping the deceased child on the ward for a few hours pending this decision will sometimes prove helpful.

Photographs of the face, including profile views, and whole-body pictures, including detailed photographs of any specific abnormality (eg, of digits) would be helpful to a dysmorphologist later. Full-body skeletal x-rays may prove similarly important later. Any dysmorphic features should be carefully documented. Heparinized cord or fetal blood samples should be obtained for chromosome analysis in all cases. Between 6% and 11% of all such offspring will have a chromosome abnormality, whether or not an abnormal physical phenotype is present. A fetal serum sample should also be obtained for infectious disease studies, which might include, for example, parvovirus, cytomegalovirus, and toxoplasmosis.

Fetal tissue samples (a few millimeters of internal fascia of the thigh is a good choice) should be obtained for cell culture, either to determine the chromosome complement; to determine the biochemical phenotype, where applicable; or to analyze DNA subsequently, where indicated. The obstetrician is expected to ensure that sterile culture medium is kept available for these often unexpected circumstances, thereby avoiding submission to the laboratory of pieces of fetal tissue in dry gauze or in a container, without any culture medium whatsoever. Parental blood samples for chromosome analysis may be useful if fetal karyotyping fails or if a specific chromosomal anomaly is detected (eg, translocation). Results of the autopsy, as well as those of any special tests performed, should be communicated directly to the parents. Many weeks may elapse before such communication can occur. Nevertheless, face-to-face consultation with *both* parents is recommended to reiterate any previous counseling, especially since anxiety block to the reception of information may have lessened somewhat by that time. This communication and counseling should be followed by a summary letter explaining their future risks and options and emphasizing any necessary recommendations.

GUIDELINES TO GENETIC COUNSELING

The principles guiding the delivery of genetic counseling have been discussed extensively elsewhere.[31,28,40] The quintessential points will be summarized briefly here.

Accurate Diagnosis

Current expectations demand that a careful and sharp focus be kept on fetal development throughout pregnancy. Discrepancy between gestational age and fetal growth, disparity in specific measurements (eg, femur length, size of lateral ventricles), or questions of organ presence or normality (eg, large or absent kidneys) will alert the perinatologist to the need for further study, including serial examinations, in order to seek accurate diagnosis. Reliable genetic counseling cannot begin if an accurate diagnosis has not been established. This same exhortation applies to the history obtained at the first obstetric visit (ideally, the preconception visit), when pregnancy planning has been initiated. At this visit, expectations include careful review of the family pedigree and formal confirmation of specific congenital defects or genetic disorders that bear on the risk of the proband in the current or future pregnancies. Examination of previous autopsy reports, x-rays, and photographs—including those of previous stillborns—is often necessary for confirmation or for help in establishing a diagnosis not made earlier. Now more than ever, the advent of molecular genetic diagnosis makes it incumbent on the physician to determine precisely whether a history of "muscular dystrophy" was, in fact, Duchenne, myotonic, or some other type. Failure to check a history of "encephalocele" in a previous deceased newborn could result in counseling with an approximate 3% risk estimate. The autopsy record, however, may have revealed polydactyly and polycystic kidneys, which, in combination with the encephalocele, constitute Meckel syndrome, an autosomal recessive disorder with a 25% risk of recurrence.

Nondirective Counseling

Most therapeutic medicine involves paternalistic management, with directions to the patient to take a specific medication that will restore them to good health. The consensus among medical geneticists in the Western world is to provide nondirective genetic counseling, where the physician is expected to dispense the most complete information available while remaining impartial and objective. In contrast, a directive approach invites, consciously or subconsciously, the opportunity for the physician to insinuate his or her own religious, racial, eugenic, or other beliefs or dictates of conscience into the counseling process. Hence, whether they have antiabortion views or personal judgments of the estimated burden of a specific disease on a family, physicians are strongly encouraged to avoid directing patients' decisions. Efficacy in genetic counseling means helping the clients to rational decision making, which may not necessarily result in a reduction in the frequency of a genetic disease.

Concern for the Individual

A physician's paramount concern is for the individual patient. The physician is *not* an advocate for society when in the midst of patient care and counseling. Hence, if a patient does not wish to terminate a pregnancy in the face of a serious fetal genetic disease, it is inappropriate for the physician to try to influence that decision, either on behalf of other family members or because of the "cost to society." This principle does not, however, preclude the requirement to inform the patient fully about all aspects, both advantageous and disadvantageous, of the decision they are making. An informative discussion, therefore, should range over issues that the patient may not be cognizant of to include future interrelationships of the couple, the effect on their other children, the suffering of the affected child, anticipated reactions by relatives and the public at large, and the many economic and other societal implications.

Truth in Counseling

There are relatively few instances in genetic counseling where the abiding principle of telling the truth is threatened. Detection of unexpected nonpaternity perhaps ranks first in frequency and is likely to retain its favored status with increasing use of DNA diagnostic studies. Detection of nonpaternity during routine prenatal chromosome studies is not at all uncommon. Such discoveries are usually predicated on recognition or suspicion of a potential fetal chromosome abnormality, necessitating blood samples from both "parents." Determination of what might appear to be a de novo translocation, rather than an inherited one, brings the issue into sharp relief. Because risk counseling for fetal normality will be decidedly different for the de novo versus inherited translocation and because the other male is invariably unaware of his possible translocation, every effort needs to be made to arrange a face-to-face consultation with the pregnant patient herself. These not infrequent encounters raise tricky ethical and legal questions and require considerable finesse in management.

Discovery of nonpaternity during DNA diagnostic studies in members of the family distant to the proband (her own father, an uncle, a first cousin) represents the same thematic challenge. Once again, considerable judgment and insight is required by the physician in determining whether to transmit such information; ethical and legal issues exist and cannot be ignored. Nevertheless, where sufficient information (eg, to set "phase" for genotype evaluation through DNA studies) is available, communication concerning nonpaternity might best be avoided. Only in situations in which life-threatening circumstances are clear is there an absolute need for communication and disclosure. Even then great sensitivity and finesse are required.

Confidentiality and Trust

The traditional and expected confidentiality and trust relationship between physician and patient is no different in the genetics arena. This principle may be challenged, for example, when the need arises to inform the sisters of a proven X-linked disease carrier about their own risks and need for testing. Difficulty arises if the patient insists on not communicating with her family and specifically instructs the physician also to desist. Although statutes of conditional immunity cover physicians communicating private information concerning highly infectious diseases (eg, meningococcemia), such immunity may not safeguard the physician transmitting genetic risk information. Notwithstanding this difference in informing about germs and genes, the advent of AIDS and the associated privacy issues further add to the dilemma in managing these kinds of genetic cases.

Information transmitted to the physician's or institution's employees about patients' serious genetic neurologic genetic disorders (eg, Huntington's disease) add a further dimension in which confidentiality and trust may be questioned. The physician's first and clearest duty is to the patient, and great caution must be exercised to safeguard this critical relationship.

Timing of Genetic Counseling

The need for preconception counseling has been emphasized. Notwithstanding this frequently repeated recommendation, huge numbers of couples emerge for genetic counseling *during* pregnancy. Professional and public education is needed to reverse this practice if couples are to benefit from available options (not to have children, adoption, in vitro fertilization, artificial insemination by donor, embryo transfer, vasectomy, tubal ligation, carrier detection tests, prenatal diagnosis, treatment, and selection or avoidance of abortion).

The timing of genetic counseling, following the birth

of a child with a serious congenital defect, is also important. Although communication and support are critical during these first unhappy days, formal genetic counseling should not be attempted. Anxiety block effectively prevents anguished parents from assimilating or comprehending the important information being communicated. Essential diagnostic information must be communicated, but not in a corridor, not to the patient alone without her mate, and not to the patient who is still under the effects of anesthesia. Sadly, examples of all these practices are well known. Although a formal appointment should be scheduled with such a couple within 6 weeks of the birth, access by telephone should also be made available for response to urgent questions and concerns.

Parental Counseling

Contribution of half the genome by the father is not the only reason the physician should insist on the father accompanying his mate for genetic counseling. Not only may outright diagnostic information be obtained from such a face-to-face visit, but a more reliable paternal family history may be obtainable. Moreover, issues to be discussed are frequently complex and invariably involve questions of guilt, family prejudices, religious obstacles, fear, and serious differences of opinion between mates. Physicians should systematically insist, at the time appointments are made, that a couple attend together for counseling. Even though a letter summarizing the essential points made during counseling should be routinely sent to the referring doctor and counselees, the male partner must be urged to attend.

Knowledge, Jargon, and Empathy

Enormous advances in human genetics over the past three decades have led to a huge and exponentially increasing body of specialized knowledge. As a consequence of these developments, a board-certified specialty in medical genetics was initiated in 1982 in the United States and, shortly thereafter, in Canada. Physicians who are not medical geneticists need to be especially careful about venturing into areas in which they lack expertise. Communication concerning risks, based on DNA studies for a rapidly increasing number of prenatally detectable disorders, serves as one example where caution and referral would be appropriate. Understanding the full expression of a disease not only in the fetus or newborn, but also in the child and adult, and its wider consequences for the family, requires special knowledge and experience.

Communications concerning genetic disorders are frequently based on complex information. An important principle is to avoid technical jargon in communication and to make no assumptions about a patient's basic knowledge or understanding. Some patients, especially professionals, are embarrassed to reveal their ignorance or lack of understanding even after an explanation has been provided. Great sensitivity is always necessary, and sufficient insight in these circumstances may encourage repetition of the communication then and there or at a subsequent, planned appointment.

The birth of a child with a fatal or serious genetic defect is invariably associated with complex responses and reactions from both parents. After the anticipated shock, self-incrimination or guilt, anger, and (one hopes) final adaptation will come the associated dashed expectations and dreams, fear of recurrence, anxiety about disability and/or death, economic woes, concern about social stigmatization, and stress between partners (often for not planning). The physician should be able to dispense empathy and sensitivity and to project warmth, understanding, and support. Together with knowledge, these essential prerequisites take time—the final ingredient for effective counseling. Genetic counseling cannot be brief and hurried.

Do No Harm

The classical exhortation *primum non nocere* ("do no harm") is no less pertinent to clinical genetics than to medicine generally. In this context, however, a primary new dimension to be considered is whether the perinatologist will be willing (the ability now exists) to predict fatal genetic diseases from first-trimester prenatal diagnostic studies, using DNA analysis, of conditions that will manifest decades after birth. The prime example is Huntington's disease, although an increasing number of molecular prenatal diagnoses have already been achieved in this category (eg, myotonic muscular dystrophy,[41,42] Friedreich's ataxia,[43] familial amyloidotic polyneuropathy[44]). Valuable experience in the presymptomatic testing for Huntington's disease has been reported.[45] The inherent danger in such presymptomatic testing (as opposed to immediate predictive testing, prenatally) is the depression and possible demoralization a patient might experience. For a disorder without curative, let alone meaningful palliative, treatment, the wisdom of providing presymptomatic diagnoses must be seriously considered. Although 50% of individuals at risk will receive good news, relieving them of a burdensome yoke of anxiety, the other 50% face an effective death sentence. Given the high suicide rate in individuals at risk for Huntington's disease, it may reasonably be questioned whether one does more harm than good by providing this 50% with a death sentence years before manifestations appear. Given the pace of advances in human genetics, it might well be possible in the foreseeable future to develop a system that enhances the mechanism already in place and to delay the manifestations of Huntington's disease for decades after birth. It would be sad to find a life ruined by severe depression or suicide, only to be followed shortly thereafter by discoveries that delay the manifestations of Huntington's disease by decades or permanently. Difficult as these decisions may be for individual patients at risk, such undertakings can only be regarded as acceptable if performed with the extreme care, concern, and professionalism displayed by the Johns Hopkins

Group.[45] Although patients retain the right to make the choice for presymptomatic testing, there is reason to remain concerned about the wisdom of such choices for those who find themselves affected.

Duty

The physician has a duty to inform the patient, impartially, fully, and in a nondirective way, providing a clear delineation of available risks and options. Where facts are uncertain or new advances possible, there is a clear duty for the physician to refer the patient to or consult with a medical geneticist. All communications with the patient must be documented and, preferably, summarized in a letter to the patient. Physicians have a duty to support patients and to remain nonjudgmental about their decisions. No confusion should arise about the paradox of wishing to diminish the frequency of genetic disease (and, hence, suffering) while not directing the decisions of patients. Finally, the physician has a duty to remain aware of new advances and progress in human genetics so that patients may benefit from them in a timely manner.

REFERENCES

1. Boue J, Boue A, Lazar P. Retrospective and prospective epidemiological studies of 1500 karyotyped spontaneous human abortions. Teratology 1975;12:11.
2. Hook EB, Hamerton JL. The frequency of chromosome abnormalities detected in consecutive newborn studies—differences between studies—results by sex and by severity of phenotypic involvement. In: Hook FB, Porter IH, eds. Population cytogenetics: studies in humans. New York: Academic Press, 1977.
3. Myrianthopoulos NC. Malformations in children from one to seven years. New York: Alan R Liss, 1985.
4. Galjaard H. Genetic metabolic diseases: early diagnosis and prenatal analysis. Amsterdam: Elsevier North-Holland, 1980.
5. Scriver CR, Neal JL, Saginur R, et al. The frequency of genetic disease and congenital malformation among patients in a pediatric hospital. Can Med Assoc J 1973;108:1111.
6. McKusick VA. Mendelian inheritance in man. 8th ed. Baltimore: Johns Hopkins University Press, 1988.
7. Baird PA, Anderson TW, Newcombe HB, et al. Genetic disorders in children and young adults: a population study. Am J Hum Genet 1988;42:677.
8. Milunsky A. Choices, not chances: an essential guide to your heredity and health. Boston: Little, Brown, 1989.
9. Beighton P. Obstetrical aspects of the Ehlers-Danlos syndrome. J Obstet Gynaecol Br Commonw 1969;76:97.
10. Taylor DJ, Wilcox I, Russell JK. Ehlers-Danlos syndrome during pregnancy: a case report and review of the literature. Obstet Gynecol Semin 1981;36:277.
11. Devereux RB, Perloff JK, Reiche N, et al. Mitral valve prolapse. Circulation 1976;54:3.
12. Miller E, Hare JW, Cloherty JP, et al. Elevated maternal hemoglobin A1C in early pregnancy and major congenital anomalies in infants of diabetic mothers. N Engl J Med 1981;304:1331.
13. Ylinen K, Aula P, Stenman U-H, et al. Risk of minor and major fetal malformations in diabetics with high haemoglobin A1C values in early pregnancy. Br Med J 1984;289:345.
14. Horger, EO. Sickle cell and sickle cell-hemoglobin C disease during pregnancy. Obstet Gynecol 1972;39:873.
15. Serjeant, GR. Sickle haemoglobin and pregnancy. Br Med J 1983;287:628.
16. Cohen LF, di Sant'Agnese PA, Friedlander J. Cystic fibrosis and pregnancy. Lancet 1980;2:842.
17. Palmer J, et al. Pregnancy in patients with cystic fibrosis. Ann Intern Med 1983;99:596.
18. Chameides L, Truex RC, Vetter V, et al. Association of maternal systemic lupus erythematosus with congenital complete heart block. N Engl J Med 1977;297:1204.
19. Tharapel AT, Tharapel SA, Bannerman RM. Recurrent pregnancy losses and parental chromosome abnormalities: a review. Br J Obstet Gynaecol 1985;92:899.
20. Sachs ES, Jahoda MG, Van Hemel JD, et al. Chromosome studies of 500 couples with two or more abortions. Obstet Gynecol 1985;65:375.
21. Alberman ED, Creasy MR. Frequency of chromosomal abnormalities in miscarriages and perinatal deaths. J Med Genet 1977;14:313.
22. Milunsky A, Jick H, Jick SS, et al. Multivitamin/folic acid supplementation in early pregnancy reduces the prevalence of neural tube defects. JAMA 1989;262:2847.
23. Mulinare J, Cordero JF, Erickson JD, et al. Periconceptional use of multivitamins and the occurrence of neural tube defects. JAMA 1988;260:3141.
24. Smithells RW, Sheppard S, Wild J, et al. Prevention of neural tube defect recurrences in Yorkshire: final report. Lancet 1989;2:498.
25. Nevin NC, Seller MJ. Prevention of neural tube defect recurrences. Lancet 1990;1:178.
26. Mills JL, Rhoads GG, Simpson JL, et al. The absence of a relation between the periconceptional use of vitamins and neural-tube defects. N Engl J Med 1989;321:430.
27. Kerem B, Rommens JM, Buchanan JA, et al. Identification of the cystic fibrosis gene: genetic analysis. Science 1989;245:1073.
28. Milunsky A, ed. Genetic disorders and the fetus: diagnosis, prevention and treatment. New York: Plenum Press, 1986.
29. Cooper DN, Schmidtke J. Diagnosis of genetic disease using recombinant DNA. 2nd ed. Hum Genet 1989;83:307.
30. Milunsky JM, Skare JS, Milunsky A. Presymptomatic and prenatal diagnosis of myotonic muscular dystrophy with linked DNA probes. Am J Med Sci 1991;301:231.
31. Milunsky A, ed. The prevention of genetic disease and mental retardation. Philadelphia: WB Saunders, 1975.
32. Milunsky A, Jick SS, Bruell C, et al. Predictive values, relative risks and overall benefits of high and low maternal serum alpha-fetoprotein screening in singleton pregnancies: new epidemiologic data. Am J Obstet Gynecol 1989;161:291.
33. Groupe de cytogénéticiens français. Paracentric inversions in man. A French collaborative study. Ann Genet 1986;29:169.
34. Groupe de cytogénéticiens français. Pericentric inversions in man. A French collaborative study. Ann Genet 1986;29:129.
35. Daniel A, ed. The cytogenetics of mammalian autosomal rearrangements. New York: Alan R Liss, 1988.
36. Gardner RJM, Sutherland GR. Chromosome abnormalities and genetic counseling. New York: Oxford University Press, 1989.
37. Warburton D, Kline J, Stein Z, et al. Does the karyotype of a spontaneous abortion predict the karyotype of a subsequent abortion?—evidence from 273 women with two karyotyped spontaneous abortions. Am J Hum Genet 1987;41:465.
38. Scriver CR, Beaudet AL, Sly WS, Valle D, eds. The metabolic basis of inherited disease. 6th ed. New York: McGraw-Hill, 1989.
39. Nussbaum RL, Ledbetter DH. The fragile X syndrome. In: Scriver CR, Beaudet AL, Sly WS, Valle D, eds. The metabolic basis of inherited disease. 6th ed. New York: McGraw-Hill, 1989:327.

40. Hsia YE, Hirschhorn K, Silverberg RL, Godmilow L, eds. Counseling in genetics. New York: Alan R Liss, 1979.
41. Norman AM, Floyd JL, Meredith AL, et al. Presymptomatic detection and prenatal diagnosis for myotonic dystrophy by means of linked DNA markers. J Med Genet 1989;26:750.
42. Milunsky A, Skare JC, Milunsky JM, et al. Diagnosis of myotonic muscular dystrophy with linked deoxyribonucleic acid probes. Am J Obstet Gynecol 1991;164:751.
43. Wallis J, Shaw J, Wilkes D, et al. Prenatal diagnosis of Friedreich ataxia. Am J Med Genet 1989;34:458.
44. Nichols WC, Padilla LM, Benson MD. Prenatal detection of a gene for hereditary amyloidosis. Am J Med Genet 1989;34:520.
45. Brandt J, Quaid KA, Folstein SE, et al. Presymptomatic diagnosis of delayed-onset disease with linked DNA markers: the experience in Huntington's disease. JAMA 1989;261:3108.
46. Sarnat HB, O'Connor T, Byrne PA. Clinical effects of myotonic dystrophy on pregnancy and the neonate. Arch Neurol 1976;33:459.
47. Webb D, Muir I, Faulkner J, Johnson G. Myotonia dystrophica: obstetric complications. Am J Obstet Gynecol 1978;132:265.

B. Prenatal Diagnosis of Congenital Anomalies

34

CHAPTER

BASIC PRINCIPLES OF ULTRASONOGRAPHY

E. Albert Reece and Joshua Copel

Ultrasonic examination during pregnancy has become an important obstetric tool for assessing a variety of factors during pregnancy. There are two types of examination: the routine basic exam and the targeted examination of a fetus suspected of anatomical or functional defects. The latter examination is covered extensively in Chapters 34 through 43 of this text. Other applications of ultrasound, such as the assessment of fetal well-being or adjunctive use when performing invasive techniques, are also covered separately. In this chapter we review the fundamentals of ultrasonography: physical basis, approach to examination, and safety.

BASIC PHYSICS

Sound consists of waves, and these waves have properties common to all waves, including frequency, wavelength, amplitude, intensity, and propagation speed.

For ultrasound, the frequency is higher than that audible to the human ear. Frequency, amplitude, and intensity are determined by the source of the sound. Frequency is described in units called Hertz (Hz), defined as 1 cycle per second. Audible sounds may be between 20 and 20,000 Hz, whereas diagnostic ultrasound for fetal imaging usually operates at 3 to 7.5 million cycles per second (megahertz, or MHz). Because frequency is defined as the number of waves per second and is determined by the length of each wave, the wavelength and frequency are inversely related.

The generation of the ultrasound signals used for fetal imaging depends on the piezoelectric phenomenon of certain materials, such as resins, crystals, or ceramics. Electrical stimulation induces mechanical deformation, which stimulates the generation of waves at ultrasonic frequencies. The phenomenon also operates in reverse: the echoed mechanical waves generate electrical signals. Thus, we can stimulate the ultrasound carrier frequency electrically and then generate an electrical signal from the returning echoes.

All ultrasound transducers rely on similar principles. A sound is generated as a pulse; then the same crystal that transmitted the sound listens for the returning echoes. The propagation speed of sound in tissue is known (1540 m/s), allowing the distance to the source of the returning echoes to be calculated. The intensity of the echo determines the brightness of the dot at that point on the screen.

Accumulation of the returning information allows the signal processor to paint an image and update it at very brief intervals. To create the illusion of a moving image, the frame rate (ie, the rate at which the image is updated) must be greater than the flicker-fusion rate of the eye, which is about 15 cycles per second—the speed at which rapidly updated pictures appear to be moving rather than flickering.[1]

ULTRASOUND TRANSDUCERS

Although the operating principles or the physics of ultrasound transducers may be similar, the path to that end, as evidenced in the mechanical designs, may vary. There are several basic designs. The type used most often for obstetric sonography is the linear-array transducer, so-called because its numerous crystals are arranged along a straight, flat surface and are fired electronically in a predetermined order. The image thereby generated is rectangular. Currently available linear arrays typically have 64 or 128 elements (Fig. 34-1).

Mechanical-sector transducers use either moving crystals or rocking mirrors to create the image. In the former design, the crystal(s) rotate on a wheel or rock back and forth. In the latter design—less frequently used at present—the crystal remains stationary and a mirror rocks and reflects the sound. Both types create a

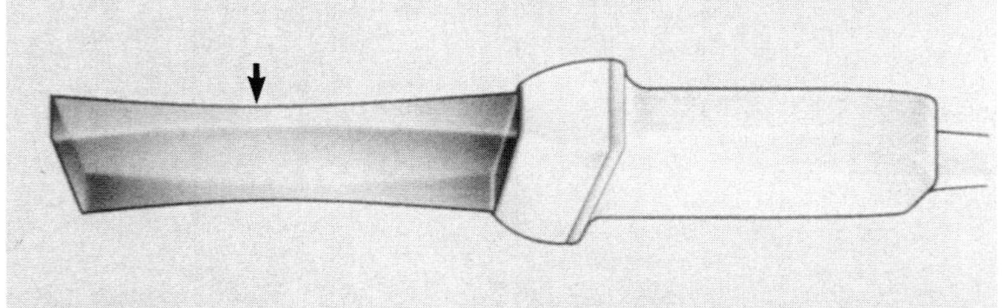

FIGURE 34–1. Linear-array transducer, depicting the relatively parallel discharge of sound waves. (Courtesy of Advanced Technology Laboratories.)

sector image, which looks like a wedge whose apex is at the tip of the transducer (Fig. 34-2).

A third type of transducer is the phased-array sector. This uses electronic steering to generate a wedge-shaped image, which also features a small "footprint," from a lightweight source without moving parts (see Fig. 34-2). The most recent variation in transducer technology has been the introduction of curvilinear transducers, which combine the advantages of both linear and sector designs (Fig. 34-3).

Linear-array transducers are the easiest to master and are often favored by obstetric sonologists. Sector transducers, although they offer more flexibility in terms of the number of different angles from which a desired structure can be visualized, are somewhat harder to learn to use. Sector technology also offers the advantage of a wide field of view below the skin's surface and is very useful for first-trimester abdominal imaging and gynecologic sonography. It also offers a sufficiently expanded "far field" to see third-trimester fetal heads and abdomens in their entirety.

It has become evident that for certain obstetric applications, placement of the transducer close to the target is desirable. This is especially true for first-trimester vaginal imaging, when high-frequency transducers can provide optimal resolution of small structures. Unfortunately, image quality is lost when the transducer is applied abdominally. Vaginal probes have been introduced with 5- or even 7.5-MHz transducers, which may be either mechanical or phased array in design (Fig. 34-4). In the first trimester, patients having vaginal sonography need not have full bladders—a definite advantage from the patients' point of view. In fact, a full bladder may unacceptably displace the uterus out of the focal plane of the transducer. In late pregnancies, vaginal probes can also be useful for examining the fetal head in the vertex presentation or the spine of breech presentation fetuses with suspected anomalies.

RESOLUTION

All transducers produce an ultrasound beam focused through some type of lens. As the beam leaves the transducer, the signal is not infinitely thin but has a thickness known as its azimuthal resolution. Any echo sources within the beam reflect back to the transducer and end up superimposed on the screen image. Thus, two adjacent objects within this plane may appear superimposed. The lens portion of the transducer serves to focus the beam at a depth that may be controlled by the operator, providing optimal resolution (ie, the thinnest slice) at a desired portion of the image. However, the further the beam travels, the more it diverges, causing deterioration in the image quality. In mechanical sector transducers, the thickness of the ultrasound beam is the same as the lateral resolution and generally has a fixed optimal depth. In linear, curved, and annular-array transducers, this thickness is determined by a lens and can be manipulated by the operator.

The ultrasound image is characterized by two other types of resolution, known as "axial" and "lateral." These can be thought of as the ability of the scan to distinguish between two separate objects; the closest juxtaposition at which they can be differentiated defines the resolution. Axial resolution (parallel to the direction of the sound waves leaving the transducer) is related to the length of the ultrasound pulse according to the following formula:

$$\text{axial resolution (mm)} = \frac{\text{pulse length}}{2}$$

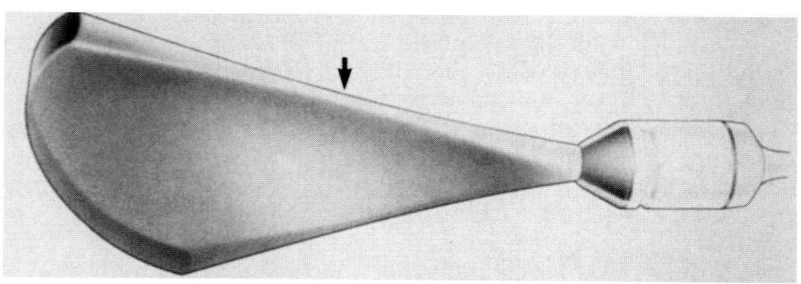

FIGURE 34–2. Sector transducer, illustrating the pie-shaped discharge of sound waves. (Courtesy of Advanced Technology Laboratories.)

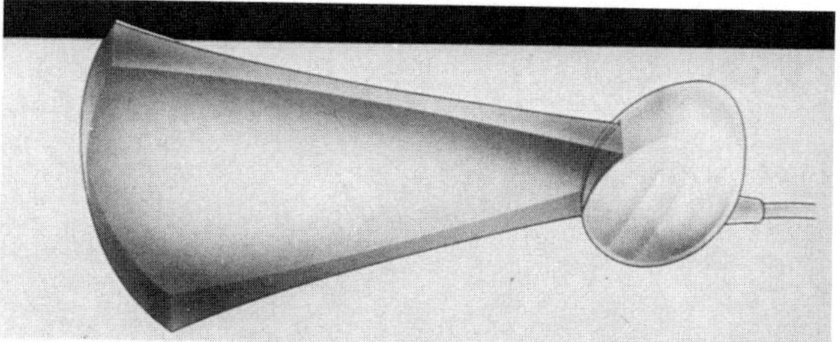

FIGURE 34–3. Curvilinear transducer, which is essentially a cross between the linear and the sector. The waves are less divergent than the sector but more divergent than the linear. (Courtesy of Advanced Technology Laboratories.)

In soft tissue this can also be expressed as follows:

$$\frac{0.77 \times \text{number of cycles in the pulse}}{\text{frequency of the transducer (MHz)}}$$

Therefore, higher-frequency transducers generally provide better axial resolution.

Lateral resolution (perpendicular to the axial) is inevitably poorer than axial resolution. For mechanical-sector transducers, this resolution is equal to the beam diameter in millimeters, increasing with depth, and is equivalent in millimeters to the azimuthal resolution.

The optimal lateral resolution in linear, annular, phased, and convex-array transducers is determined by the operator, based on the focal requirements of the scan. The optimal depth of focus can be found and several depths may be obtained with electronically steered transducers. Although selecting "multiple depths" will provide better resolution at those levels in the scan and can be useful for obtaining selected still images, it also slows the frame rate significantly, resulting in a very choppy image (similar to watching movement under a strobe light). This can detract from the quality of the fetal image and outweigh the advantages of multiple focal depths.

BASIC "KNOBOLOGY"

Optimal resolution is generally obtained by using the highest possible transducer frequency. For prenatal diagnosis by abdominal sonography, this is best accomplished with 5-MHz crystals. The improved resolution of higher-frequency transducers comes at the cost of decreased tissue penetration, and they have generally proved inadequate for abdominal sonography. With term pregnancies or obese patients in the second trimester it may be necessary to use even lower-frequency (3- or 3.5-MHz) transducers, which enhance tissue penetration but decrease resolution.

The depth of "minimal beam diameter" is the area of optimal resolution. On many systems, the operator can select this by setting the focal depth. When desired, several bands of depth can even be selected, but this comes at the expense of a significant slowing of the frame rate. In obstetric sonography, one or at most two focal points are usually sufficient.

The intensity (the gain) of the transmitted sound can be varied on most ultrasound machines, as can the amplification of the returning echoes. Most currently available machines also allow selective manipulation of the gain at desired depths. Since the machine translates time into distance, this type of control is known as time-gain compensation (TGC) or depth-gain compensation (DGC). Increasing the gain equally amplifies all information (ie, both true signal and random noise), so it in fact does not increase clarity.

A final control common to most obstetric ultrasound systems is "dynamic range," which defines the way the returning echoes are assigned shades of gray on the screen. A wide dynamic range produces a gray image; a narrow range results in a high-contrast image. Operator preference is important in setting this control.

THE BASIC ULTRASOUND EXAMINATION

The technical bulletin for the American College of Obstetricians and Gynecologists indicates that, in general, a basic ultrasound examination should include evaluation and documentation of the following[2]:

1. Fetal number
2. Fetal presentation (in second and third trimesters)
3. Fetal lie
4. Placental location
5. Amniotic fluid volume
6. Gestational dating (preferably by multiple parameters)
7. Detection and evaluation of maternal pelvic masses (best done in the first trimester)
8. Survey of fetal anatomy for gross examinations (in second and third trimesters).

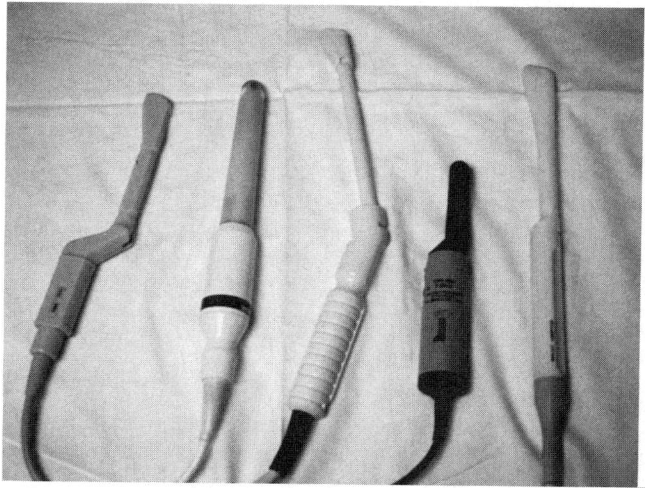

FIGURE 34–4. Multiple vaginal transducers with varying frequencies. The sizes and lengths of these transducers are very similar, although there may be some variation in shape.

No single method can detect all fetal abnormalities, but a systematic approach such as the preceding will minimize the likelihood of errors. Most obstetric ultrasound examinations are performed to document gestational age when clinical dating is equivocal, or when there is a discrepancy between the uterine size and the gestational age as based on the last menstrual period.

The optimal date for the ultrasound exam is determined by its purpose; furthermore, the date affects its accuracy in achieving different goals. An ultrasound exam for gestational dating is best done as early as possible in the pregnancy, because that is when fetal biometry is most accurate. A targeted ultrasound to exclude congenital anomalies should wait until midgestation, when organogenesis is complete and the structures of interest are large enough to permit accurate evaluation. Assessment of fetal well-being should be done in the third trimester, after extrauterine fetal viability is reached.

EXAMINATION DURING EARLY GESTATION

The first trimester is a time of rapid embryonic–fetal development. Highly accurate first-trimester dating can be obtained by measuring the crown–rump length of the fetus. Because of the concurrent anatomical development of the fetus and the improving ability of ultrasound to see structures throughout their longitudinal growth, the sonologist should have some familiarity with embryology to avoid potential pitfalls. For example, the physiologic bowel herniation into the proximal umbilical cord at 9 weeks can be mistaken for an omphalocele.

Ultrasound is most commonly used in the estimation of gestational age, thus circumventing the use of indirect means such as fundal height measurement, fetal heart tone auscultation, or the recording of fetal movement. Ultrasound permits the measurement of embryonic–fetal structure in a noninvasive manner.[3]

A number of studies have demonstrated that fetal crown–rump length is the most accurate measurement for estimating gestational age (Fig. 34-5). Chervenak and colleagues have suggested that ultrasound measurement of crown–rump length can be more accurate in estimating gestational age in the first trimester than measurement of human chorionic gonadotropin.[4] The crown–rump length is also a useful biometric parameter because it has a high reproducibility and can be measured reliably until about 12 weeks gestation.

Reece and associates have introduced trunk circumference as another way to estimate gestational age in the first trimester. This measurement involves obtaining a circumference of the trunk, perpendicular to the long axis at the point below the cardiac pulsation. This measurement is highly accurate in estimating gestational age, with an error rate of ±3 days.[5]

The biparietal diameter (BPD) can also be obtained late in the first trimester (Fig. 34-6). This versatile measurement is commonly used in both early and late pregnancy, although its accuracy decreases with advancing gestation and increased BPD size. In early pregnancy, the accuracy of the BPD measurement is ±6 days. When the BPD and crown–rump length are combined, there is 20% less variability in predicting gestational age than when either parameter is used independently.[6] As early as the late first trimester separate fetal body structures can be examined.

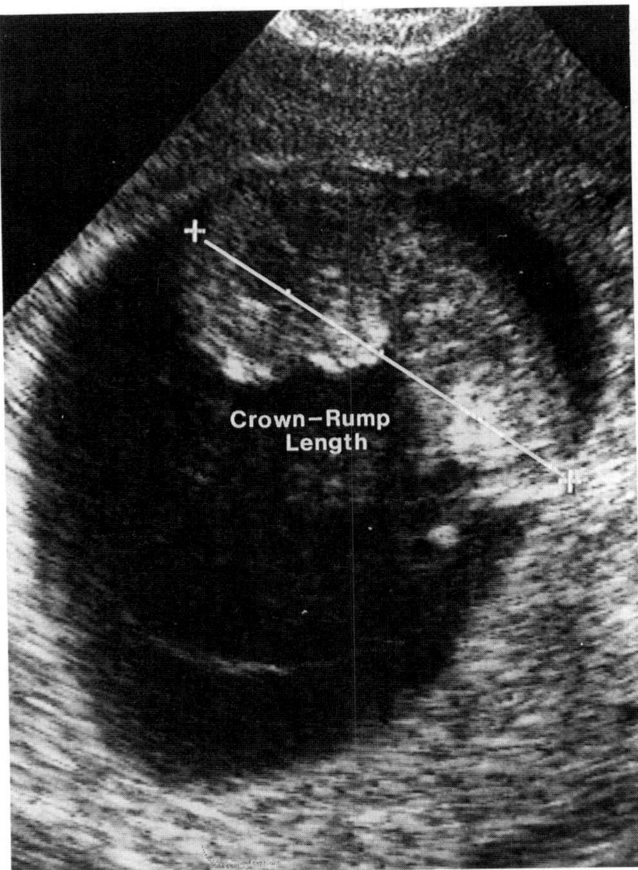

FIGURE 34–5. Embryo of about 9 weeks gestation depicting the crown–rump length measurement.

Head

The oval outline of the fetal head should be sought in all examinations. On rare occasions, a fetal head may present deep in the pelvis and a cursory examination may suggest that the head measurement is unobtainable, when in fact the fetus is anencephalic. Also, the intracranial anatomy ought to be examined to ascertain that midline structures are present (Fig. 34-7). Besides the BPD, other frontal head measurements include the orbital distances (Fig. 34-8); the occipital frontal distance (OFD); and the cephalic index, which is the ratio of BPD to OFD (normal being 75% to 85%). Major intracranial anatomic abnormalities such as overt hydrocephalus should be excluded.

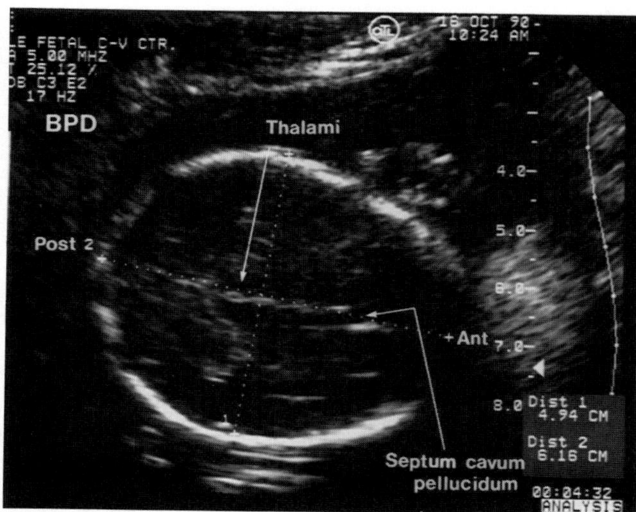

FIGURE 34–6. Ultrasound picture at the level of BPD showing landmarks such as the septum cavum pellucidum, anteriorly, and the thalami in the center. The dotted line goes from anterior to posterior (occipitofrontal diameter) and from side to side (BPD).

Fetal Spine

The fetal spine ossifies as early as 10 weeks and is seen as parallel sets of echoes representing the articulating facets. These facets can be seen from the cervical region through the sacral spine, where the converging facets come to a point. In targeted examinations for neural tube defects, the spine should be examined in both longitudinal (coronal) and transverse planes (Fig. 34-9).

Heart

A four-chamber image of the fetal heart should be part of all examinations after 18 to 20 weeks of gestation. Major structural anomalies of the heart, which can distort the normal four-chamber view, may be excluded by demonstrating ventricles and atria of equal and appropriate size on either side of a normal-looking ventricular septum. Although some significant lesions that result in critical neonatal illness may not be detected with this approach (eg, transposition of the great vessels), it is a rapid and easy-to-perform screen for congenital heart disease (Fig. 34-10).

Abdomen

The fetal abdomen and stomach can be visualized as early as 14 weeks gestation, and the kidneys can often be observed at that time as well. Ventral wall defects can be excluded by the demonstration of an intact abdomen in the area of the umbilical cord insertion. Other normal structures that should be sought are the single cystic area representing the stomach, on the left side of the abdomen, and the umbilical vein, which hooks toward the right in the liver. Occasionally, the gallbladder

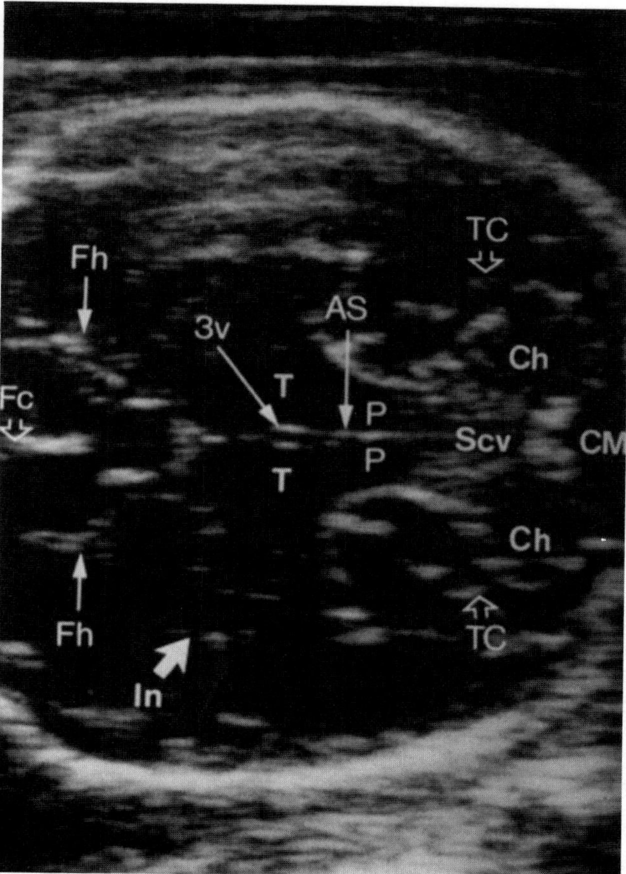

FIGURE 34–7. Ultrasound picture of the fetal head imaged obliquely and depicting major identifiable structures. FC, falx cerebri; FH, frontal horn; 3V, ventricle; t, thalami; P, peduncles of cerebellum; AS, aqueduct of Sylvius; CV, cerebellar vermis; Ch, cerebellar hemisphere; cm, cystemia magna.

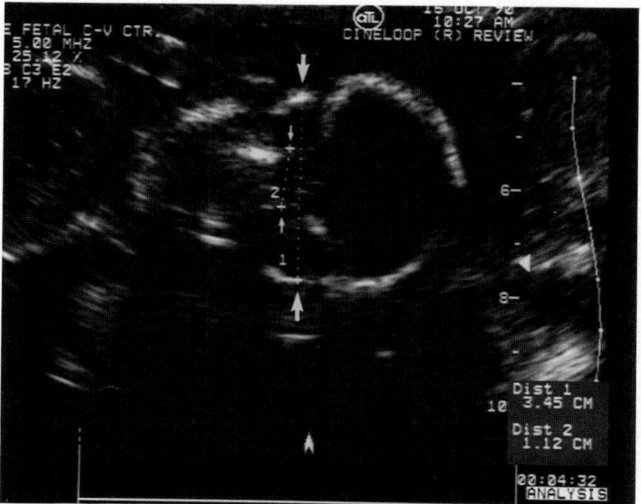

FIGURE 34–8. Ultrasound picture of fetal face depicting the orbits and measurements taken from the outer orbital distances (*thick arrows*) and inner orbital distances (*thin arrows*).

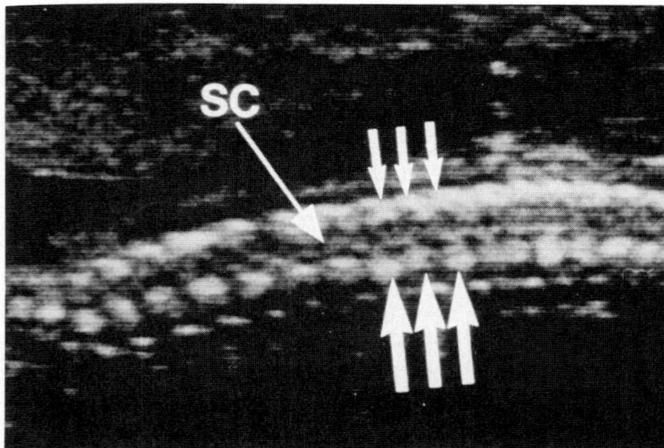

FIGURE 34–9. Fetal spine (*arrows*) with spinal cord (SC) on the inside of the bony spine.

may be seen, inferior to the liver on the right. During the course of a routine examination, the fetal bladder is usually visible as a fluid-filled structure in the midline, low in the pelvis. In fact, the bladder may visibly fill and empty over the course of an examination (Fig. 34-11).

Extremities

The four fetal limbs should be identified routinely during any second- or third-trimester examination. Standard growth curves are available for the proximal and distal segments of the bones in the upper and lower extremities. Although it is not necessary to measure all six tubular bones in every fetus, the sonologist should measure at least one or two segments and ascertain that there is no noticeable shortening of any segment. Both bones of the normal distal segments should be present (eg, tibia and fibula, radius and ulna) (Fig. 34-12).

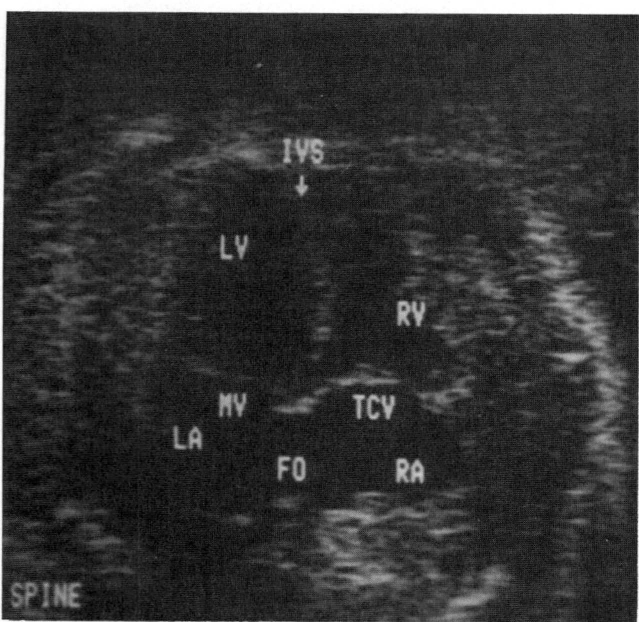

FIGURE 34–10. Ultrasound picture of a four-chamber view of the fetal heart. RV, right ventricle; RA, right atrium; LV, left ventricle; LA, left atrium; IVS, interventricular septum; FO, foramen ovale; TCV, tricuspid valve; MV, mitral valve.

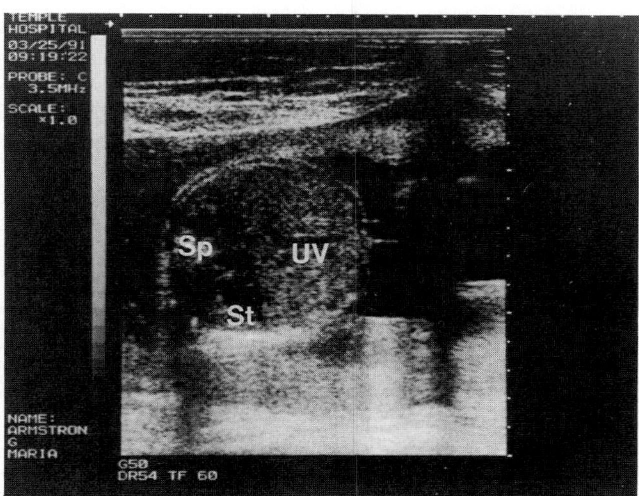

FIGURE 34–11. Ultrasound picture of fetal abdominal circumference. Sp, spine; UV, umbilical vein; St, stomach.

EXAMINATION DURING MIDGESTATION

By midpregnancy the fetal anatomy can be visualized in greater detail, thereby permitting prenatal diagnosis of many structural congenital anomalies. In the midtrimester, the biparietal diameter (BPD) remains the "gold

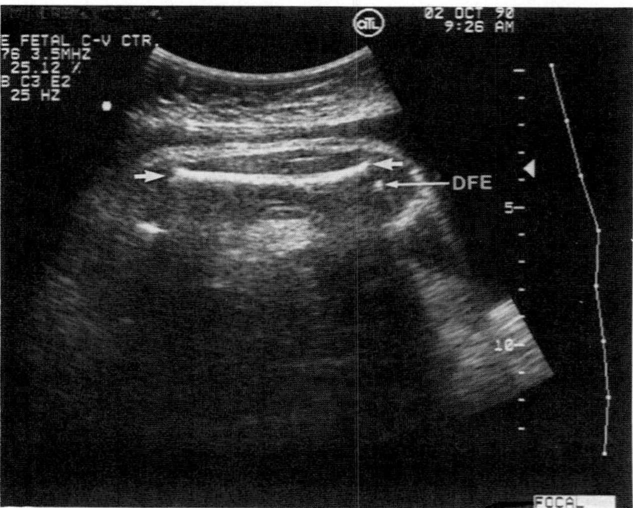

FIGURE 34–12. Ultrasound picture showing long bone imaged (between thick arrows) with the distal femoral epiphyses (DFE) shown.

standard" for gestational-age determination, because it is easily identifiable and highly reproducible. Unfortunately, the BPD cannot always be measured, even in early gestation, because of certain fetal positions, such as direct occiput anterior or posterior, fetal compression, fetal crowding, multiple gestation, or even fetuses that are deep in the pelvis. In other situations, such as anomalous fetuses, the BPD may be distorted as part of the structural anomaly.

To circumvent these problems, another intracranial landmark, the transcerebellar diameter (TCD), has been used.[7,8] The TCD can be obtained from the latter part of the first trimester onward (Fig. 34-13). The corresponding gestational age is easy to remember, because up to 24 weeks the gestational age is the same as the TCD in millimeters. However, later in pregnancy this close relationship no longer holds. Measuring the TCD allows gestational dating independent of the shape of the fetal head, making it extremely useful when the fetal head is compressed. The TCD is also useful in the evaluation of intrauterine growth retardation because it remains constant, even when the growth of other fetal parameters has been compromised.

Other parameters that may prove useful during this period are the clavicular length and the foot length.[9–11] Foot length measurement may be useful in select circumstances, such as in fetuses with hydrocephaly or limb dysplasia (Fig. 34-14).[12,13]

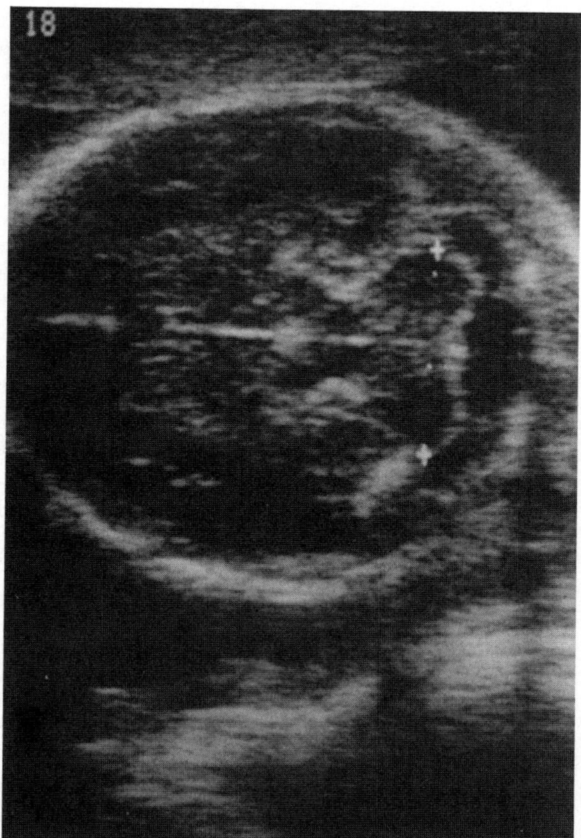

FIGURE 34–13. Ultrasound image of the posterior fossa depicting the cerebellum and the transverse cerebellar distance (*dotted lines*). The cerebellum can be seen easily as a butterfly-shaped object in the posterior fossa.

EXAMINATION DURING LATE GESTATION

In the third trimester, fetal gestational-age assignment from biometry becomes more difficult because of the normal biological variation, which is most prominent in later gestation. On the other hand, the size of the fetus can be evaluated accurately by estimates of fetal weight derived from various combinations of abdominal circumference and BPD, femur length, and/or head circumference (see Chapter 44). Gestational age in the third trimester may also be estimated by nonbiometric parameters, which can be tied to fetal maturation.

A high degree of correlation between gestational age and fetal intestinal appearance has been reported.14,15 Goldstein and colleagues demonstrated that colonic echogenicity and colonic diameter correlated with gestational age and, in some instances, may even be superior to BPD or femur length measurement.

Correlations have also been observed between fetal lung maturation and the ultrasonic detection of epiphyseal ossification centers in the fetal long bones.[16,17] Goldstein and colleagues reported that sonographic detection of lower limb epiphyseal ossification centers was an accurate indicator of gestational age during the third trimester (see Fig. 34-12). A significant correlation was observed between the distal femoral epiphyses, the proximal tibial epiphyses, and the lecithin–sphingomyelin (LS) ratio in nondiabetics. For example, a distal femoral epiphysis greater than 3 mm and the presence

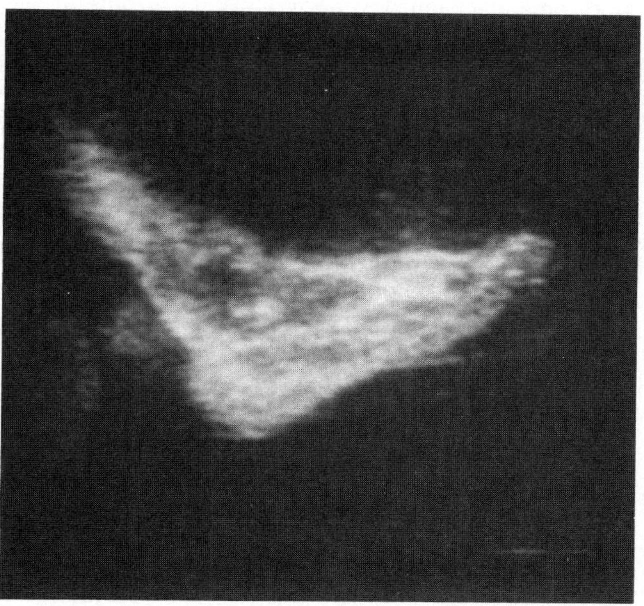

FIGURE 34–14. Ultrasound image of the fetal foot.

of a proximal tibial epiphysis of any size was seen with LS ratios indicative of fetal lung maturity in almost all cases. This combination of findings may substitute acceptably for amniocentesis in selected cases when pulmonic maturity should be assessed but amniocentesis is contraindicated.

In another study, Goldstein and colleagues demonstrated that a highly accurate estimation of term gestation could be obtained by combining the colonic grade with the detection of proximal humeral epiphyses.[18] For example, a fetus with a proximal humeral epiphysis equal to or greater than 3 mm and a mature colonic pattern (grade 3) had almost a 95% probability of being full term.

ULTRASOUND SAFETY

Diagnostic ultrasound has been available for over 25 years and has now become a widely accepted clinical tool in almost all branches of medicine.[19] It has been estimated that more than half of all pregnant women in the United States are examined with ultrasound.[20] This widespread acceptance is due to its clinical utility, convenience, and noninvasiveness. In addition to being used in fetal biometry and in the detection of fetal anomalies, newer techniques in ultrasound make it useful in such areas as fetal echocardiography and uterine and fetal–placental blood flow evaluations through Doppler waveform analysis.

Our examinations deal with human fetuses, and therefore the topic of safety is of fundamental importance.[21] Initial concerns regarding ultrasound safety were raised by MacIntosh and Davey, who suggested that chromosomal aberrations could be induced by an ultrasonic fetal pulse detector.[22] Subsequently, Liebeskind and colleagues reported sister chromatid exchanges in human lymphocytes after exposure to diagnostic ultrasound.[23] Neither of these findings, however, has been replicated by other investigators.[24]

A recent review of studies on the effects of ultrasound concluded that many experiments have used inconsistent methodology, resulting in unpredictable outcomes and uninterpretable conclusions.[25] These experiments have caused confusion by using not only small mammals, but insects, plants, and cell suspensions. It is almost impossible to extrapolate from the inconsistent positive findings of such experiments to humans.[21]

In animal experiments and therapeutic applications involving sufficiently high exposure levels of ultrasound, modification of biological structures and functions does occur.[20] However, no confirmed ultrasonically induced adverse effects in humans have yet been reported when diagnostic levels of ultrasound are used.[21,26] The acoustic outputs, carrier frequencies, and pulse lengths of diagnostic ultrasound are all significantly less than those used for the reviewed experiments.

BIOLOGICAL EFFECTS OF ULTRASOUND

Ultrasound in higher intensities than those used for diagnostic purposes can produce biological effects, mainly via thermal changes and the induction of microcavitation.[27]

Thermal Changes

As ultrasound propagates through tissues, its energy is absorbed and converted into heat. This heat is dissipated by adjacent tissues and by blood flowing through the insonated area. During a normal diagnostic scan, tissue temperature rises less than 1°C.[20] Such aberrations occur normally during the human diurnal cycle, and temperature increases of 3° to 4°C occur in febrile states. It therefore seems unlikely that tissue damage would be caused by such minor increases in temperature.[20,21] Moreover, during diagnostic ultrasonography, there is no significant tissue heating because of the very low average intensity to which the tissue is exposed—less than 20 milliwatts per square centimeter (20 mW/cm^2). Computer modeling suggests that such exposures do not cause temperature rises greater than 1°C. In the same way, the continuous-wave Doppler devices used externally to monitor the fetal heart rate operate at these same intensities and therefore seem equally unlikely to produce hazardous increases in temperature.

At this time there are no studies of adverse effects to living mammals from increases in body temperatures of 1°C or less.[20,21] A recent report by Miller and Ziskin uncovered no effects to animals at temperatures below 39°C.[28] They also showed that the generation of heat-shock protein may be protective against tissue injury at certain elevated temperatures. Soothill and colleagues, using a thermocouple probe during ultrasound exams in humans, revealed that the mean fetal muscle temperature is 36.9°C and the mean amniotic fluid temperature is 36.6°C.[29]

From the information available thus far, a few conclusions can be drawn regarding fetal temperature elevation in utero and its relationship to fetal anomalies:

1. An association seems to exist between elevated temperatures and fetal anomalies in animal models.
2. This elevated temperature must be several degrees above normal and depends on the duration of exposure; the higher the temperature, the shorter the exposure time required to induce adverse effects.
3. This relationship (between elevated temperature and adverse effects) is stronger in animal models and is reproducible in them.
4. A relationship between elevated temperature and adverse effects has not been demonstrated clearly in humans, as is evident by the lack of adverse effects during febrile states.
5. Current ultrasound equipment is almost incapable of inducing significant thermal effects in the human fetus.

Microcavitation

The term *cavitational mechanism* refers to the interaction of sound with the microscopic gas bubbles that preexist in tissues, causing the bubbles to increase and decrease rapidly in size. Plant and insect tissues contain these gas bubbles, and there is evidence that diagnostic ultrasound can produce adverse effects in these lower organisms. Mammalian tissues also contain such gaseous nuclei, but little is known about conditions under which they occur or could produce biological effects.[30] In humans, there is no direct evidence to suggest that, under clinical conditions, ultrasound-induced microcavitation produces biological effects.[30] Diagnostic ultrasound involves short pulses with long intervals between adjacent pulses.[31] Andrews and colleagues found that the median exposure time was 105 seconds.[32] They also found that the median maternal exposure time was 131 microseconds and that the exposure to the fetus was even less. The combination of low intensity and minimum exposure time suggests that any adverse effects on the human fetus would be unlikely.

EXPERIMENTAL EVIDENCE OF ULTRASOUND-ASSOCIATED TISSUE INJURY

Many investigators have tested the potentially deleterious effects of ultrasound on sensitive cell functions. They have paid particular attention to experiments relating to sister chromatid exchange (SCE).[23,33–35] This phenomenon involves the exchange of portions of two chromatids in the same chromosome. SCE can occur spontaneously; however, an increase in SCE frequency may indicate a risk of other types of chromosomal cross-over, as well as abnormal exchanges. Agents that have strong mutagenic effects—such as ionizing radiation, certain chemicals, and alcohol—can cause small increases in SCE frequency. By comparison, even weak carcinogens produce marked increases in SCE rates.[33,34]

Liebeskind and colleagues described a small but statistically significant increase in the SCE rate in human lymphocytes after exposure to diagnostic levels of ultrasound.[23] However, these results have not been subsequently corroborated. In a recent review, Gross examined 14 papers dealing with ultrasound and SCE; 11 of them concluded that diagnostic ultrasound did not cause an increase in SCE rates.[35]

Recently, Barnett and colleagues exposed lymphocytes from healthy women to pulsed Doppler ultrasound for prolonged periods in order to involve the full mitotic cell cycle.[36] Even after extended exposure, no changes in SCEs were observed.[21]

The cell nucleus has also been investigated for possible bioeffects following exposure to ultrasound. MacIntosh and Davey in 1970[22] observed an increase in chromosomal aberrations in human lymphocytes exposed to ultrasound; however, those data also remain unconfirmed.

The effects of diagnostic ultrasound on the bone marrow and its products have been variable. Sanada and colleagues did observe pseudopod formation in platelets (an early sign of activation) after in vivo exposure to pulsed Doppler.[38] Several other authors, however, reported no damage to blood cells in vivo after exposure to therapeutic intensities of continuous wave ultrasound.[18–21]

EVIDENCE IN HUMANS FOR ULTRASOUND-ASSOCIATED TISSUE INJURY

Human epidemiologic data have been used to evaluate potentially adverse effects of ultrasound. Table 30-1[39–48] summarizes a number of studies examining possible effects of ultrasound exposure in utero. The majority of the reports fail to identify specific adverse outcomes related to ultrasound exposure.

Scheidt and colleagues did, however, find neurologic abnormalities in those exposed to diagnostic ultrasound.[43] In this study, data from the Amniocentesis Registry of the National Institute of Child Health and Human Development were analyzed for possible effects of diagnostic ultrasound exposure in the second trimester of pregnancy. The first group, 297 newborns of mothers who had undergone both amniocentesis and diagnostic ultrasound, was compared with 661 newborns of mothers who had amniocentesis only and with 949 newborns whose mothers had undergone neither ultrasound nor amniocentesis. The investigators initially studied the neonatal outcome for weight, length, head circumference, and detailed neurologic examination. They found a significantly higher rate of abnormal grasp and tonic neck reflexes among neonates exposed to ultrasound. However, a year later they reevaluated the data for infections, abnormal hearing, convulsions, and neurologic development and found no difference between the three groups. The authors therefore suggested that the initial findings in the ultrasound group could have been coincidental.

The potential relationship of ultrasound exposure to childhood malignancies has been investigated by Kinnier-Wilson and Waterhouse.[44] The mothers of 1731 children who died of cancer in the United Kingdom between 1972 and 1981 and the mothers of 1731 matched control children were asked about exposure to diagnostic ultrasound during pregnancy. There was no difference in ultrasound exposure between the sick and control children. Although a difference between cases and controls exposed during the earlier years of ultrasound use was found, it was felt to be the result of the selective application of ultrasound to abnormal pregnancies.

Cartwright and colleagues examined whether a relationship exists between exposure to ultrasound in utero and cancer in childhood.[45] In an epidemiologic study, they analyzed information obtained by interviewing the parents of 555 children with malignancies diagnosed between 1980 and 1983. The parents of 1110 healthy children were used as a control group. They

TABLE 34–1. STUDIES IN HUMANS OF ULTRASOUND EXPOSURE IN UTERO

AUTHOR	TYPE OF STUDY	NO. OF SUBJECTS	FINDINGS
Bernstine[39]	Retrospective	720 newborns exposed to Doppler in utero	No significant abnormality rate
Hellman et al[40]	Retrospective	1114 fetuses ultrasound exposed	2.7% incidence fetal anomalies
Serr et al[41]	Retrospective	150 newborns	No difference in abnormality rates
Falus et al[42]	Retrospective	171 newborns exposed to ultrasound in utero	No significant developmental disorders at ages 6 months to 3 years
Scheidt et al[43]	Retrospective Follow-up	297 ultrasound and amniocentesis; 661 amniocentesis; 949 neither	Abnormal grasp and tonic neck reflexes; no difference for 122 other outcomes
Kinnier-Wilson et al[44]	Retrospective	1731 mothers whose children died of cancer; 1731 matched controls	No difference in ultrasound exposure duration between sick and control subjects
Cartwright et al[45]	Retrospective	555 children with malignancy; 1110 control children	No significant association between exposure to ultrasound in utero and cancer risk
Bakketeig et al[46]	Retrospective	510 ultrasound; 499 controls	No adverse short-term biological effects
Stark et al[47]	Retrospective Follow-up	425 ultrasound exposed 381 not exposed	Increased risk of dyslexia; no difference for any other neurologic outcomes
Lyons et al[48]	Retrospective Follow-up	149 sibling pairs of the same sex; one exposed and one not	No growth difference between siblings at birth and at 6 years of age

Reece EA, Assimakopoulos E, Zheng X, Hobbins JC. The safety of obstetric ultrasonography: concern for the fetus. Obstet Gynecol 1990;76:139.

found no significant association between exposure to ultrasound in utero and risk for childhood cancer.

Bakketeig and colleagues studied the benefits of ultrasound examination during pregnancy.[46] In 510 ultrasound cases and 499 controls, they reported that for screened women, twins were diagnosed earlier, post-term inductions were fewer (2.8% versus 4.0%), and low birth weights were fewer (2.2% versus 3.6%). However, none of these differences were statistically significant. In relation to ultrasound, they reported that their study revealed no adverse short-term bioeffects.

A well-designed, long-term epidemiologic study by Stark and associates examined outcomes such as growth, immunologic and neurologic maturation, and childhood behavior after exposure in utero to diagnostic ultrasound.[47] Gestational age, Apgar scores, birth weight, length, head circumference, congenital anomalies, and congenital and neonatal infections were also scrutinized. The children were later examined between 7 and 12 years of age, when they were tested for hearing performance, visual acuity and color vision, cognitive function, behavior, and neurologic status. No significant biological differences between the two groups were found, although there was a higher incidence of dyslexia in the exposed group. Many of these children had low birth weights. In many cases, this was probably the reason for the ultrasound examination itself, thus making it difficult to interpret the results.[20]

A more recent epidemiologic study analyzed 149 sibling pairs of the same sex with one child exposed to diagnostic ultrasound in utero and one not exposed.[48] It found no statistically significant difference in head circumference, height, weight at birth, or weight at 6 years of age. Furthermore, there was no difference in the pattern of growth between the two groups over the 6-year postnatal evaluation period.

CONCLUSION

Despite the relatively large number of studies on the bioeffects of ultrasound, unequivocal conclusions cannot be drawn. A review of the available information reveals that although ultrasound at high intensities is associated with biological effects, similar bioeffects are not reproducible at diagnostic levels. This is in concert with the position statement by the American Institute of Ultrasound in Medicine in which it was concluded that there are "no confirmed biological effects on patients or instrument operators caused by exposure at intensities typical of present diagnostic ultrasound instruments."[20] Although the possibility exists that such biological effects may be identified in the future, current data indicate that the benefits to patients exposed to prudent levels of diagnostic ultrasound outweigh the risks, if any, that might be present.

REFERENCES

1. Kremkau FW. Diagnostic ultrasound: principles, instruments, and exercises. 3rd ed. Philadelphia: WB Saunders, 1989.
2. ACOG Technical Bulletin. American College of Obstetrics and Gynecology Technical Bulletin No. 116, May 1988, pp 1–3.

3. Reece EA, Gabrielli S, DeGennaro N, Hobbins JC. Dating through pregnancy: a measure of growing up. Obstet Gynecol Surv 1989;44:544.
4. Chervenak FL, Brightman RC, Thornton J, Berkowitz GS. An analysis of sonographically determined fetal crown rump length and human chorionic gonadotropin as predictive of gestational age. ABST, Proceedings of the 33rd Annual Meeting of the Society of Gynecologic Investigation, Toronto, Ontario, Canada. March 26–29, 1986.
5. Reece EA, Scioscia AL, Green J, O'Connor TZ, Hobbins JC. Embryonic trunk circumference in the estimation of gestational age. Am J Obstet Gynecol 1987;156:713.
6. Bovicilli L, Orsini LF, Rizzo ON, et al. Estimation of gestational age during the first trimester. Real-time measurement of fetal crown rump length and biparietal diameter. J Clin Ultrasound 1981;9:71.
7. Goldstein I, Reece EA, Pilu G, et al. Cerebellum measurements with ultrasonography in the evaluation of fetal growth and development. Am J Obstet Gynecol 1987;156:1065.
8. Reece EA, Goldstein I, Pilu G, Hobbins JC. Fetal cerebellum growth unaffected by intrauterine growth retardation: a new parameter for prenatal diagnosis. Am J Obstet Gynecol 1987;157:632.
9. Yarkoni S, Schmidt W, Jeanty P, et al. Clinical measurements: a new biometric parameter for fetal evaluation. J Ultrasound Med 1985;4:467.
10. Jeanty P, Dramaix-Willmet M, Van Kem J, et al. Ultrasound echovalues and fetal limb growth. Part II. Radiology 1982;143:751.
11. Hadlock FP, Harris RB, Dieter RL, Park SK. Fetal length as a predictor of menstrual age: sonographically measured. Am J Obstet Gynecol 1982;138:875.
12. Mercer BM, Sklar S, Shariatmader A, et al. Fetal foot length as a predictor of gestational age. Am J Obstet Gynecol 1987;156:350.
13. Goldstein I, Reece EA, Hobbins JC. The sonographic appearance of the fetal heel, ossification centers and foot length measurements provide independent marks for gestational age estimation. Am J Obstet Gynecol 1988;159:923.
14. Zilanti M, Fernandez S. Correlation of ultrasonic images of fetal intestine and gestational age in fetal maturity. Obstet Gynecol 1983;62:569.
15. Goldstein I, Lockwood CJ, Hobbins JC. Ultrasound assessment of fetal intestinal development in the evaluation of gestational age. Obstet Gynecol 1987;70:682.
16. Tabsh KMA. Correlation of ultrasonic epiphyseal center and lecithin:sphingomyelin ratio. Obstet Gynecol 1984;64:92.
17. Goldstein I, Lockwood C, Belanger K, et al. Ultrasonic assessment of gestational age with the distal, femoral and proximal tibial ossification centers in the third trimester. Am J Obstet Gynecol 1988;158:127.
18. Goldstein I, Reece EA, Hobbins JC. Estimating gestational age in the term pregnancy using a model based on multiple indices of fetal maturity. Am J Obstet Gynecol 1989;161:1235.
19. Kossoff G. President's address, Ultrasound '85: challenges and opportunities. Ultrasound Med Biol 1986;12:3.
20. AIUM. Bioeffects consideration for the safety of diagnostic ultrasound. J Ultrasound Med 1988;7:51.
21. Reece EA, Assimakopoulos E, Zheng X, Hobbins JC. The safety of obstetrical ultrasound: concern for the fetus. Obstet Gynecol 1990;162:82.
22. MacIntosh IJC, Davey DA. Chromosome aberrations induced by ultrasonic fetal pulse detector. Br Med J 1970;4:92.
23. Liebeskind D, Bases R, Mendez F, Elequin F, Koeningsberg M. Sister chromatid exchanges in human lymphocytes after exposure to diagnostic ultrasound. Science 1979;205:1273.
24. Meire HB. The safety of diagnostic ultrasound. Br J Obstet Gynaecol 1987;94:1121.
25. Wells PNT. The safety of diagnostic ultrasound. Report of a British Institute of Radiology Working Group. Br J Radiol 1987;(20S):1.
26. Thompson HE. Introduction. First Symposium on Safety and Standardization of Ultrasound in Obstetrics. Ultrasound Med Biol 1986;12:679.
27. Williams AR. Ultrasound: biological effects and potential hazards. London: Academic Press, 1983.
28. Miller MW, Ziskin, MC. Biological Consequences of Hypothermia. Ultrasound Med Biol 1989;15;8:707.
29. Soothill PW, Nicolaides KH, Rodeck CH, Campbell S. Amniotic fluid and fetal tissues are not heated by obstetric ultrasound scanning. Br J Obstet Gynaecol 1987;94:675.
30. Carstensen EL. Acoustic cavitation and the safety of diagnostic ultrasound. Ultrasound Med Biol 1987;13:597.
31. Taylor JWK, Dyson M. Experimental insonation of animal tissues and fetuses. In: Sanders CR, James AE, eds. The principles and practice of ultrasonography in obstetrics and gynecology. New York: Appleton-Century-Crofts, 1980:15.
32. Andrews M, Webster M, Fleming JEE, McNay MB. Ultrasound exposure time in routine obstetric scanning. Br J Obstet Gynaecol 1987;94:843.
33. Gebhart E. Sister chromatid exchange (SCE) and structural chromosome aberration in mutagenicity testing (review article). Hum Genet 1981;58:235.
34. Wolff S. Sister chromatid exchange. Annu Rev Genet 1977;11:183.
35. Gross AS. Sister chromatid exchange and ultrasound. J Ultrasound Med 1984;3:463.
36. Barnett SB, Barnstable SM, Kossoff G. Sister chromatid exchange, frequency in human lymphocytes after long duration exposure to pulsed ultrasound. J Ultrasound Med 1987;6:637.
37. MacIntosh IJC, Brown RC, Brown RC, Coakley WT. Ultrasound and in vitro chromosome aberrations. Br J Radiol 1975;48:230.
38. Sanada M, Hattori A, Watanabe T, et al. The in vivo effect of ultrasound upon human blood platelets. Nippon Choompa Igakukai. Koen-Rombunshu 1977;37:149.
39. Bernstine RL. Safety studies with ultrasonic Doppler technic: a clinical follow-up of patients and tissue culture-study. Obstet Gynecol 1969;34:707.
40. Hellman LM, Duffus GM, Donald I, Sunden B. Safety of diagnostic ultrasound in obstetrics. Lancet 1970;i:1133.
41. Serr DM, Padeh B, Zakut H, et al. Studies on the effects of ultrasonic waves on the fetus. In: Huntingford PJ, ed. Proceedings 2nd European Congress on Perinatal Medicine. Basel: Karger, 1971:302.
42. Falus M, Koranyi G, Sobel M, et al. Follow-up studies on infants examined by ultrasound during fetal age. Orv Hetil 1972;113:2119.
43. Scheidt PD, Stanley F, Bryla DA. One year follow-up of infants exposed to ultrasound in utero. Am J Obstet Gynecol 1978;121:742.
44. Kinnier-Wilson LM, Waterhouse JAH. Obstetric ultrasound and childhood malignancies. Lancet 1984;ii:997.
45. Cartwright RA, McKinney PA, Hopton PA, et al. Ultrasound examinations in pregnancy and childhood. Lancet 1984;ii:999.
46. Bakketeig L, Eik-Nes SH, Jacobsen G, et al. Randomized controlled trial of ultrasonographic screening in pregnancy. Lancet 1984;ii:207.
47. Stark CR, Orleans M, Haverkamp AD, Murphy J. Short and long-term risks after exposure to diagnostic ultrasound in utero. Obstet Gynecol 1984;63:194.
48. Lyons EA, Dyke C, Toms M, Cheang N. In utero exposure to diagnostic ultrasound; a 6-year follow-up. Radiology 1988;166:687.

35

CHAPTER

PRENATAL DIAGNOSIS OF ANOMALIES OF THE HEAD AND NECK AND CENTRAL NERVOUS SYSTEM

Sandro Gabrielli and Gianluigi Pilu

Because of the frequency and severity of congenital anomalies arising from or involving the central nervous system, the investigation of this area of fetal anatomy has always been a major concern for obstetric sonographers. In the early 1970s prenatal diagnosis was possible for only a small group of catastrophic lesions, namely, anencephaly[1] and gross hydrocephalus.[2]

In more recent years rapid advances in ultrasound technology have resulted in the introduction of gray scale imaging and high resolution real time ultrasound, providing equipment able to identify very subtle details of fetal anatomy. Nevertheless, the prominent developmental changes that occur in the cerebrum well beyond the end of embryogenesis and throughout the entire gestation have proved to be a significant source of confusion for sonographers. It took years before the different fetal intracranial structures could be accurately mapped.

Johnson, Fiske and Filly, and Hidalgo must all be given credit for providing considerable insight into the sonographic interpretation of ventricular and vascular anatomy of the brain prior to birth.[3–5] Nomograms of the normal size of the head,[6] ventricular system,[7,8] and parts of the cerebrum, including the frontal lobe[9] and cerebellum,[10] have been developed to assist the early recognition of intracranial anomalies.

The purpose of this chapter is to review the principles of embryogenesis and gestational development of the brain and to provide guidelines for both sonographic identification and management of fetal abnormalities.

EMBRYOGENESIS AND DEVELOPMENTAL ANATOMY OF THE CENTRAL NERVOUS SYSTEM

The differentiation and development of the neural axis have been extensively reviewed.[11–14] In this section, we shall not try to give a comprehensive overview of this exceedingly complex topic. Rather, we shall focus mainly on those aspects of embryogenesis that are relevant for the understanding of congenital abnormalities amenable to prenatal diagnosis. We shall also consider the morphologic modifications that normally occur during the first half of pregnancy and can be recognized with ultrasound.

The nervous system originally derives from the neural plate, a dorsal thickening of the ectoderm that can be recognized as early as the 14th day of development. The essential steps leading to the formation and early differentiation of the cerebrum are summarized in Figure 35-1. The faster growth rate of the lateral portions of the plate results in the formation of two longitudinal folds demarcating an internal groove. The folds fuse with each other in the midline, starting the transformation of the groove into a tube at about the midportion of the embryonic disk. Closure then proceeds cephalad and caudad. From 20 to 24 days the neural tube is almost entirely closed, with the only exception being two openings at the extremities—the anterior and posterior neuropore. The anterior neuropore undergoes obliteration first, followed by the posterior neuropore at

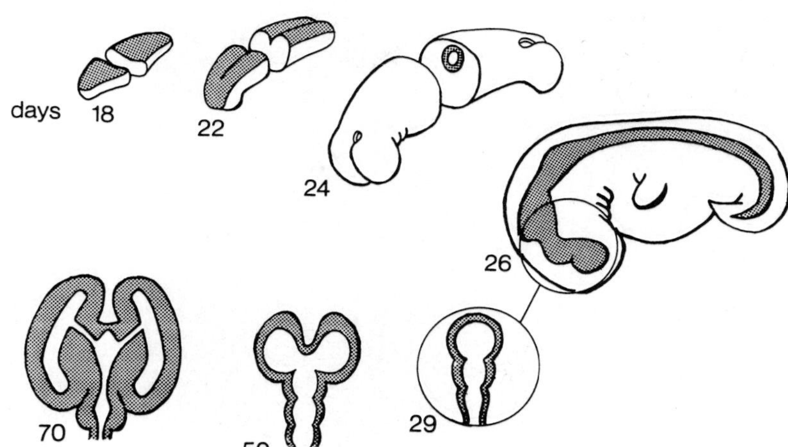

FIGURE 35–1. Schematic representation of human central nervous system development. Two main stages can be recognized. The first one, commonly referred to as dorsal induction, leads to the closure of the neural tube. The second stage, ventral induction, leads to the sagittal sepimentation and differentiation of the nervous axis.

about 24 to 26 days. This first stage of nervous development is often referred to as *dorsal induction.*

At 26 days, the rostral portion of the neural tube is cleaved along the horizontal planes, giving rise to the three primary vesicles of the brain: the prosencephalon, mesencephalon, and rhombencephalon. Two further cleavages occur in the following weeks, leading to the subdivision of the prosencephalon into telencephalon and diencephalon, and of rhombencephalon into metencephalon and myelencephalon.

The cerebral hemispheres originate from two paired diverticula ballooning out of the telencephalon. At the same time, the diencephalon—the primordium of the optic thalami—gives rise to two anterior paired diverticula, the optic bulbs, and two unpaired buds on the median plane, the anterior neurohypophysis and the posterior pineal body. The mesencephalon will form the cerebral peduncles and quadrigeminal plate. The metencephalon will develop into the pons, cerebellum, and rostrad portion of the fourth ventricle, and the myelencephalon will be the origin of the medulla oblongata and caudad portion of the fourth ventricle.

Cleavage of the primitive cerebrum along four horizontal planes leading to the formation of the five primary cerebral vesicles results in constriction and secondary enlargements of the cavity of the neural tube that in time will originate the ventricular system. The cavity contained within the telencephalon (telocoele) undergoes paired symmetrical division and diverticularization along the sagittal plane with formation of two distinct cavities that will give rise to the lateral ventricles. This process of paired diverticularization is commonly referred to as *ventral induction,* and it is closely related to the development of the median facial structures.

Cavities are now formed within the cerebrum. The ones contained within the diencephalon (diocoele), mesencephalon (mesocoele), and metencephalon–myelencephalon (metacoele, myocoele) will form the third ventricle, aqueduct of Sylvius, and fourth ventricle, respectively. The remaining portion of the neural tube cavity will develop into the ependymal canal, which runs within the spinal cord.

The rapidly growing hemispheres rotate inwardly, enfolding the thin membranous roof of the telocoele (the thela choroidea) deep into the brain. The hemispheres are now separated by a thin mesenchymal layer that is the primordium of the falx cerebri. The cerebral cortex is thin at this point in gestation, most of the hemispheres being occupied by the primitive ventricular cavities. At about the sixth week of gestation, the medial wall of the lateral ventricles is seen bulging within the cavity, thus forming a fold that is rapidly covered by pseudostratified epithelium and molded by the proliferation of the underlying blood vessels into a villous structure—the choroid plexus. Both anatomic studies on animal models[15] and sonographic investigation of the human fetus in utero[16] have outlined the generous size of the choroid plexus, which fills almost entirely the lateral ventricles from about 8 to 16 weeks. The peculiar echogenicity of this structure in vivo (Fig. 35-2) has been attributed to a high glycogenic content, which is thought to represent a major energetic supply for the rapidly growing cerebrum.

Whereas the choroid plexuses decrease in size relative to both brain mass and ventricular volume, the lateral ventricles are stretched and molded by the many developing processes occurring within the forebrain (growth of cerebral lobes, basal ganglia and thalami, formation and deepening of the cerebral sulci). Assessment of the developmental anatomy of the ventricular system in the fetus has depended mainly on complex dissection procedures and barium casting techniques.[13]

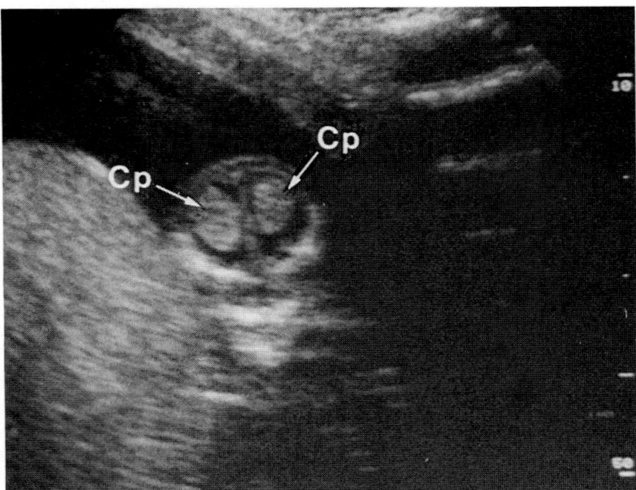

FIGURE 35-2. Coronal scan of the head in a normal 11-week-old fetus. Most of the intracranial cavity is occupied by the large echogenic choroid plexuses (CP). The thin cerebral cortex is seen as hypoechoic crescent interposed between the prominent choroid plexuses and the calvarium.

More recently, real-time ultrasound equipment has allowed us to document in a large number of living fetuses the observations originally made on abortion specimens (Fig. 35-3). By the fourth month of gestation the lateral ventricles are large when compared to the cortex and intracranial cavity. At this time, the bodies and the frontal horns are short, the atrium being by far the most prominent portion. Both ontogenetically and phylogenetically, the last modification in the shape of the lateral ventricle to occur is the formation of the occipital horns, as only higher mammals and mature fetuses have an occipital lobe large enough to allow a well-defined internal cavity. The lateral ventricles are fully developed at about the 30th week of gestation. As the fetus usually lies on one side inside the amniotic cavity, ultrasound examination of the intracranial contents relies mainly on axial scans. The obstetric sonographer should be familiar with the tomographic anatomy of the brain. Figure 35-4 displays three views that can be easily obtained in the vast majority of fetuses and that enable a proper assessment of the relevant cerebral anatomy. The most rostrad section plane is especially useful for assessing the integrity of the lateral ventricles (Fig. 35-5). By using this scanning plane, nomograms of frontal horns and atria have been established (Fig. 35-6). Moving the transducer slightly caudad, it is possible to image the plane that is commonly used for measuring the biparietal diameter and head circumference. Eventually, a posterior angulation of the transducer allows the demonstration of the posterior fossa structures (Fig. 35-7).

A few other anatomic structures will be considered in this section. The cavum septi pellucidi is a fluid-filled cavity comprised between the leaves of the septum pellucidum. The cavum is largely patent in the fetus, and it decreases progressively in size during gestation, being sonographically recognizable in 40%[17] to 60%[18] of normal newborn infants. A caudad prolongation of the cavum septi pellucidum, the cavum vergae, can be seen at times (Fig. 35-8).

The development of cerebral fissure and sulci has been extensively reviewed by Doroviv-Zis and Dolman.[14] The distinct feature of the human brain prior to

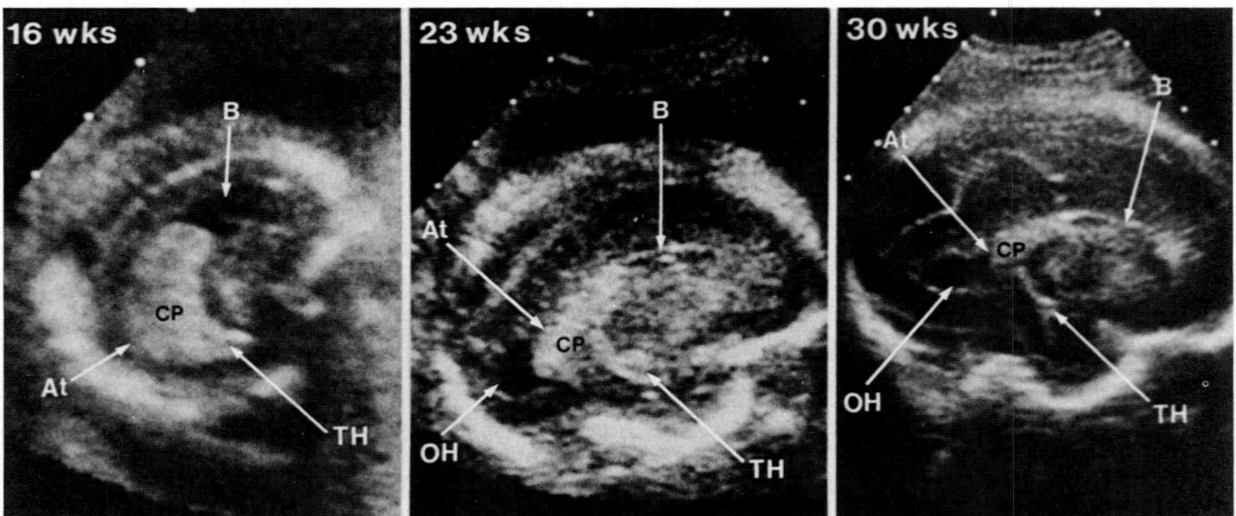

FIGURE 35-3. Parasagittal scans of the fetal head at 16, 23, and 30 weeks. Note the modifications in the size and shape of the body (B), atrium (At), and temporal horns (TH) of lateral ventricles. At 16 weeks the atrium is prominent and ends blindly posteriorly, with the occipital horn (OH) appearing only at about midgestation. At any gestational interval, the choroid plexus (CP) is seen filling the atrium entirely.

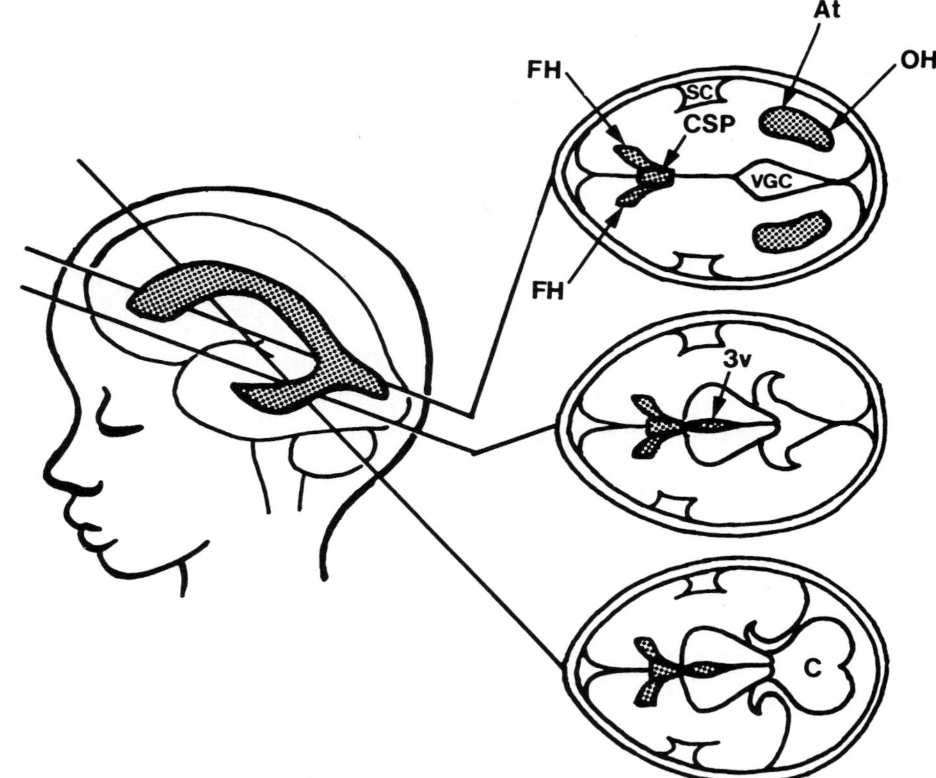

FIGURE 35–4. A schematic representation of three scanning planes that can be obtained rapidly with ultrasound in most fetuses after the midtrimester and that allow identification of the relevant details of intracranial anatomy. (FH, frontal horns; At, atria; OH, occipital horns; 3v, third ventricle; SC, Sylvian cistern; VGC, cistern of the vein of Galen; C, cerebellum.)

the 22nd week of gestation is a peculiar smoothness. Only the calcarine and parieto-occipital fissures are discernible. In the following 8 weeks the rapid growth of the cerebral cortex leads to the formation of the Rolandic fissure and of the cingulate, frontal, and parietal sulci. The formation of cortical convolutions proceeds steadily up to the 40th week, when tertiary sulci can be finally seen. Evaluation of the convolutional pattern is a well-established method to assess maturity in both pathologic[14] and neonatal ultrasound studies.[19] Cerebral sulci can be appreciated sonographically in utero as well (Fig. 35-9). However, adequate visualization requires the use of transfontanellar coronal and sagittal scans. As these views can be obtained only in a minority of cases, such otherwise promising approaches to the intrauterine estimation of fetal maturity have important limitations.

Development of the brain results in a conspicuous modification of the subarachnoid cisterns. This issue has been the subject of both anatomical[20] and sonographic studies.[21] Knowledge of the normal sonographic anatomy of the subarachnoid space is useful both in avoiding misinterpretation of normal sonograms and in diagnosing congenital anomalies differentially. The main features of the cisterns that are particularly relevant for the obstetric sonographer will be briefly considered. The interested reader is referred to specific works on the subject.[21,22]

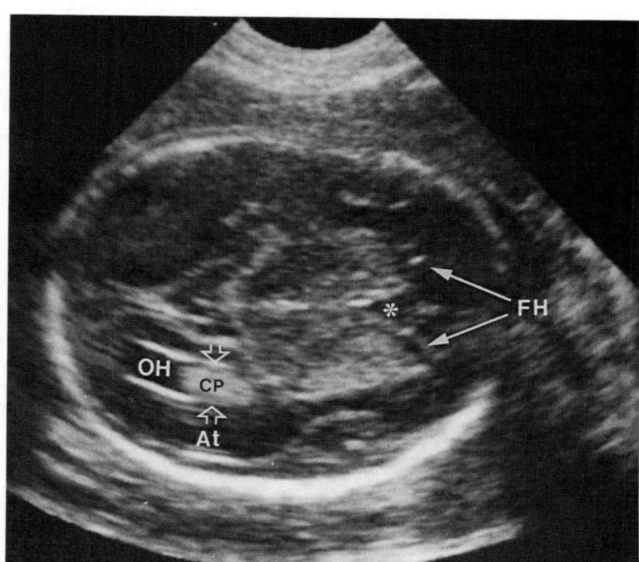

FIGURE 35–5. Axial scan of the fetal head at the level of frontal horns (FH), atria (At), and occipital horns (OH) of lateral ventricles. The choroid plexus (CP) fills the atrium entirely, being closely apposed to both the medial and lateral wall (*open arrows*). (*, cavum septi pellucidum.)

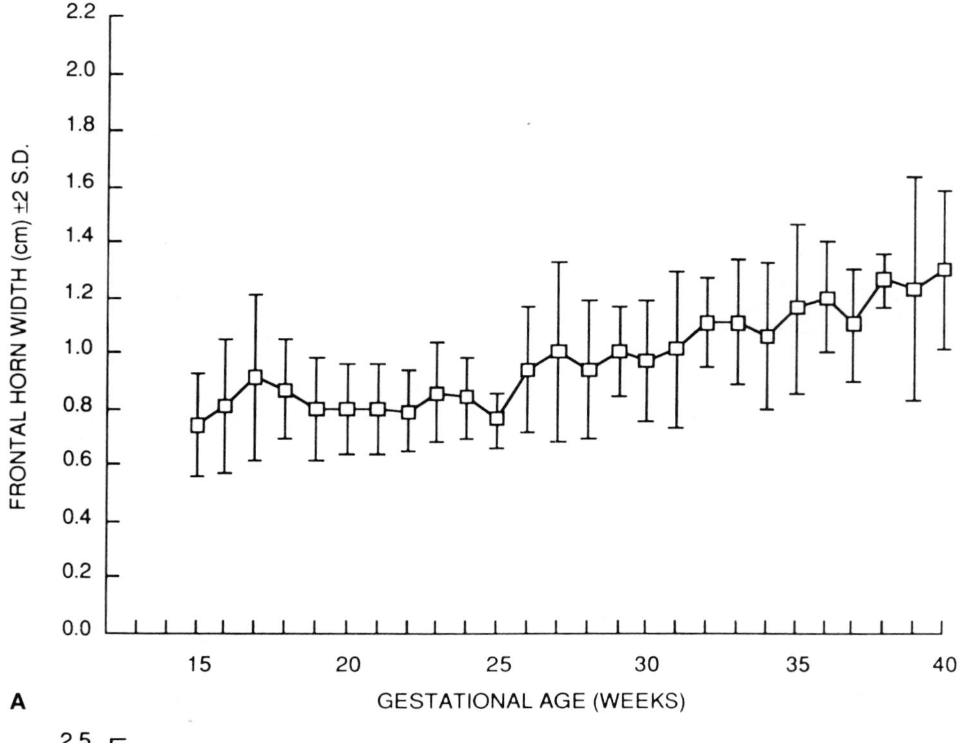

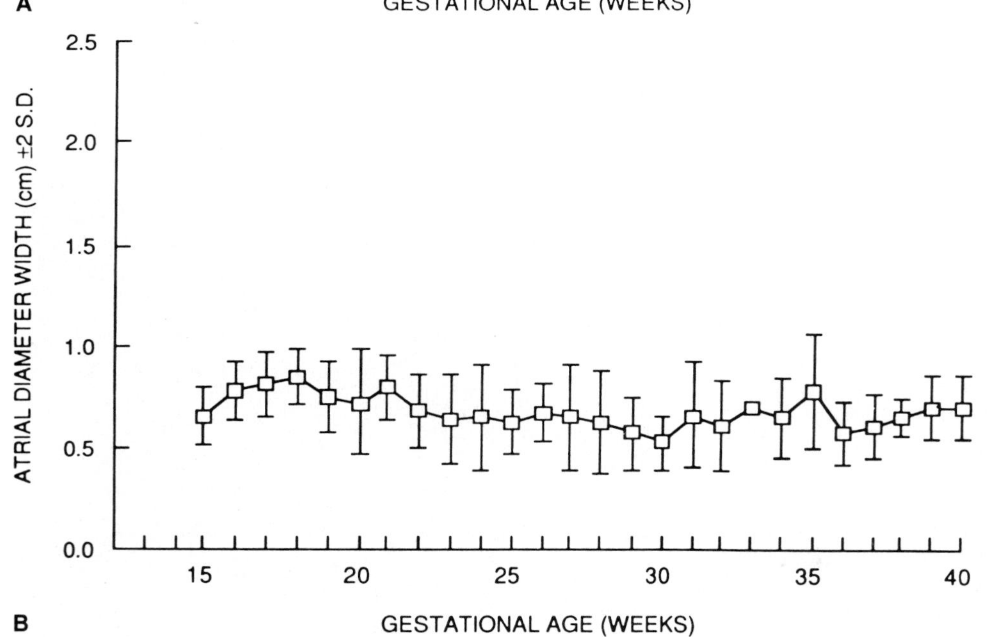

FIGURE 35-6. (**A**) Normal values of the frontal horn width (mean and two standard deviations) from 15 weeks to term. (**B**) Normal values of the internal diameter of the atria of lateral ventricles from 15 weeks to term (mean and two standard deviations). (**A** from Goldstein I, Reece EA, Pilu G, et al. Sonographic evaluation of the normal developmental anatomy of the fetal cerebral ventricles. I. The frontal horn. Obstet Gynecol 1988;72:588, **B** from Pilu G, Reece EA, Goldstein I, et al. Sonographic evaluation of the normal developmental anatomy of the fetal cerebral ventricles. II. The atria. Obstet Gynecol 1989;73:250.)

The extracortical space overlying the cerebral convexities is very prominent early in gestation and decreases steadily, starting from about the fifth month, until it becomes of minimal dimensions in the adult (Fig. 35-10). Prior to the sixth month of gestation, the frontal and temporal lobes adjacent to the insula—the opercula—are separated by an ample space, the base of which is the insula. The opercula get progressively closer, until they meet to form the Sylvian fissure. The beginning of Sylvian fissure demarcation is already visible at 22 weeks of gestation. However, it is not until 32 to 34 weeks of gestation that the opercularization is complete. The cistern of the vein of Galen (or quadrigeminal cistern), which lies in the angle between the superior surfaces of the cerebellum and mesencephalon, can be seen on sonographic scans as early as the 15th week (Fig. 35-11). The cisterna magna, which is situated between the inferior surface of the cerebellum

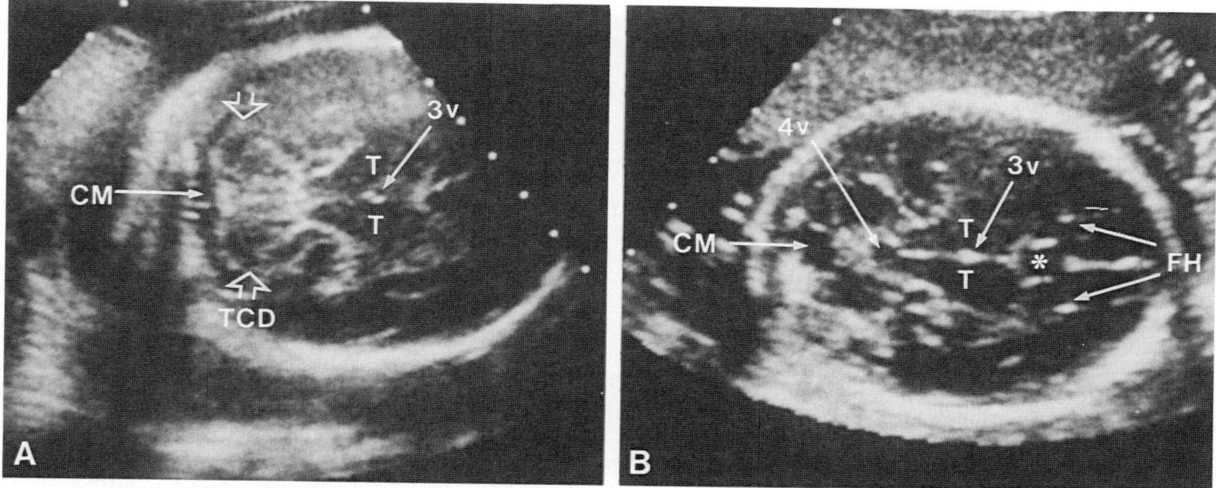

FIGURE 35–7. Axial scans of the fetal head demonstrating the posterior fossa. The normally generous cisterna magna (CM) outlines the cerebellum. In **A** measurement of transverse cerebellar diameter (TCD) is demonstrated. In **B** a slight posterior movement of the transducer allows visualization of the fourth ventricle (4v). (T, thalami; 3v, third ventricle; FH, frontal horns; *, cavum septi pellucidum.)

and the posterior aspect of the medulla oblongata, can be consistently visualized with ultrasound, and it is large up to the third trimester.[21,22]

HYDROCEPHALUS

INCIDENCE AND CLASSIFICATION

The incidence of congenital hydrocephalus ranges between 0.3 and 1.5 in 1000 births in different series.[23] Hydrocephalus can result from pathologic entities that differ both in etiology and clinical course. In a series of 205 infants with congenital isolated hydrocephalus, aqueductal stenosis was found in 43%, communicating hydrocephalus was found in 38%, and Dandy-Walker malformation occurred in 13%.[24] However, pediatric data may not apply to cases recognized prior to birth. In our experience, fetal ventriculomegaly usually enters one of three main entities: triventricular hydrocephalus (which may result from both aqueductal stenosis or communicating hydrocephalus), Dandy-Walker malformation, and hydrocephalus associated with other ce-

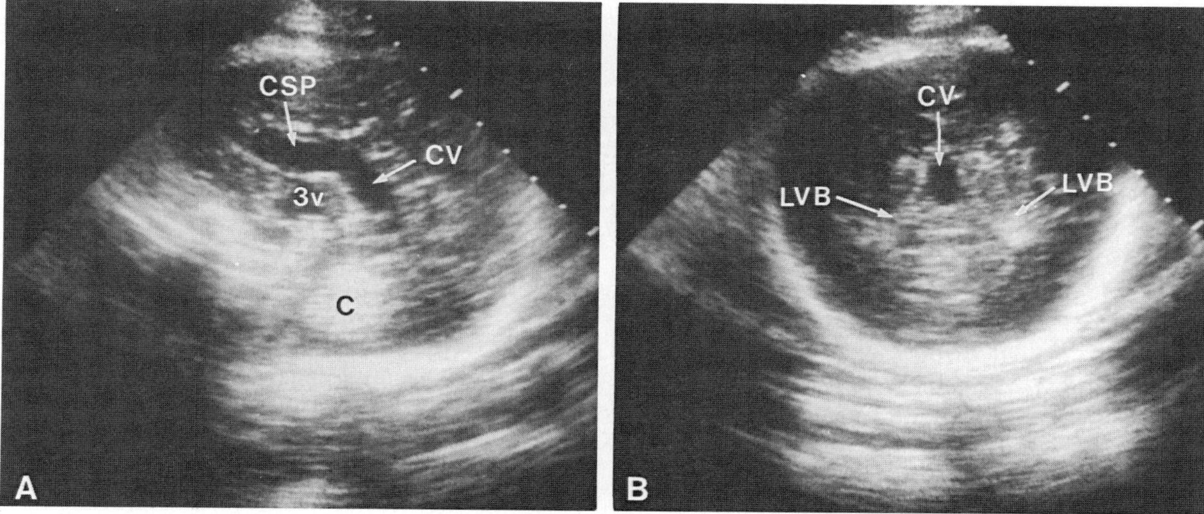

FIGURE 35–8. In this third-trimester fetus, axial (**A**) and coronal (**B**) scans of the head reveal a normally generous cavum septi pellucidum (CSP) posteriorly connected to a patent cavum vergae (CV). (3v, third ventricle; C, cerebellum; LVB, bodies of lateral ventricles.)

rebral anomalies (most frequently, disorders of dorsal induction, disorders of ventral induction, and disruptive lesions).

ETIOLOGY AND RECURRENCE RISK

Congenital infections and genetic factors are both involved in the pathogenesis of aqueductal stenosis. Infectious agents include toxoplasmosis, syphilis, cytomegalovirus, mumps, and influenza virus.[25] Many familial cases indicate an X-linked pattern of transmission that is thought to account for 25% of lesions occurring in males.[24] Multifactorial etiology has also been suggested.[24] Infections result in gliotic stenosis of the aqueduct. True malformations include narrowing and forking (multicanalization); less frequently, a transverse septum obstructs the lumen. In an autopsy series, 50% of cases of aqueductal stenosis were due to gliosis, 46% to forking, and 4% to simple narrowing.[26] Congenital tumors such as gliomas, pinealomas, and meningiomas cause aqueductal stenosis by external compression.

Communicating hydrocephalus usually results from failure of reabsorption of cerebrospinal fluid. It has been found in access of agenesis[27] or blockage or arachnoid granulation due to subarachnoid hemorrhage,[28] venous occlusion of the superior sagittal sinus, torcular herophili or lateral sinuses,[29] and overproduction of cerebrospinal fluid by a choroid plexus papilloma.[30] A multifactorial etiology with a recurrence risk of 1% to 2% has been suggested.[24] Communicating hydrocephalus in its most typical manifestation is characterized by a variable degree of enlargement of the entire ventricular system associated with dilatation of the subarachnoid spaces. However, a radiologic study has outlined the natural history of this lesion, demonstrating that in the earliest stage enlargement is confined to the subarachnoid channels overlying the cerebral hemispheres.[31] In a further stage, a simultaneous dilatation of both the subarachnoid spaces and the ventricular system is seen. Eventually, only ventriculomegaly can be demonstrated.

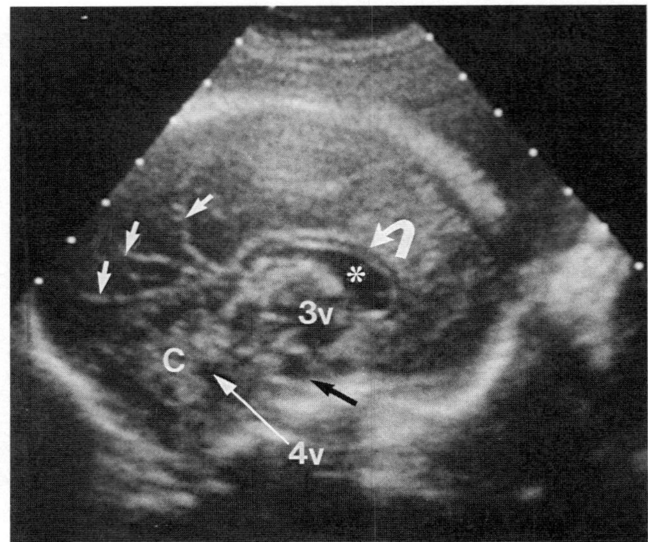

FIGURE 35–9. Midsagittal scan of the fetal head at 29 weeks. The corpus callosum is seen as a thin, sonolucent crescent interposed between the echogenic pericallosal cistern (*curved arrow*) and the patent cavum septi pellucidum (*). Anteriorly to the third ventricle (3v) the chiasmatic cistern is seen (*black arrow*). The cerebellar vermis (C) is anteriorly indented by the fourth ventricle (4v). Well-developed cerebral sulci (parieto-occipital, calcarine, and collateral) are seen on the medial surface of the hemisphere (*straight arrowheads*).

It should be stressed that the traditional view that

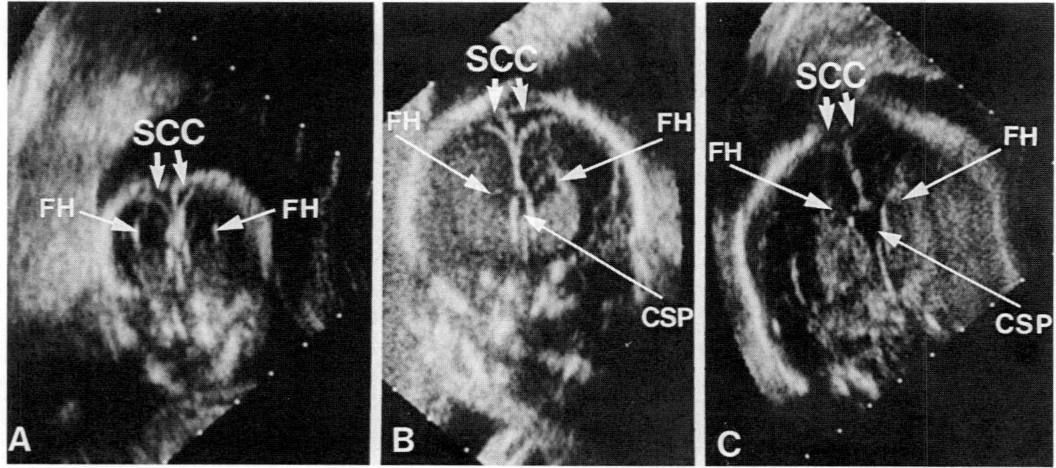

FIGURE 35–10. Coronal scans of the fetal head at 16 (**A**), 24 (**B**), and 30 (**C**) weeks, demonstrating the progressive reduction in size of the subarachnoid space overlying the cerebral convexities (*arrows*). A patent cavum septi pellucidum (CSP) separating the frontal horns of lateral ventricles (FH) is seen in **B** and **C**.

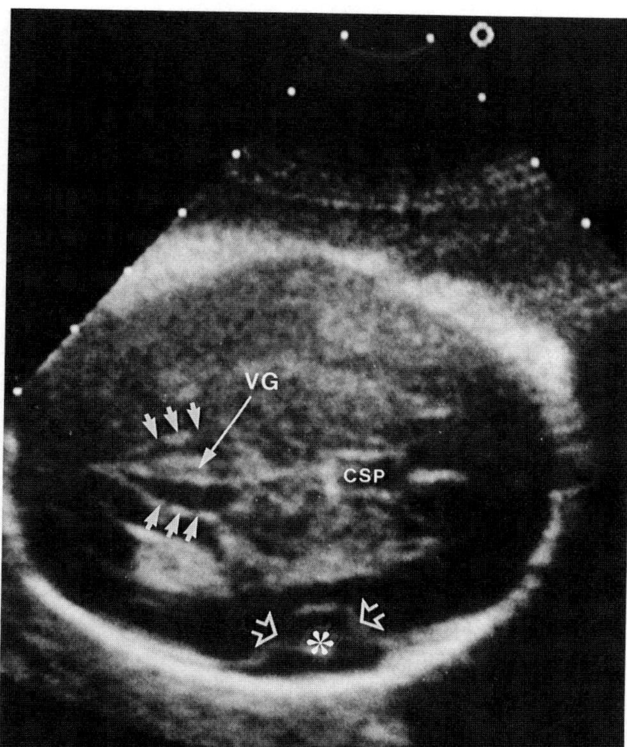

FIGURE 35–11. Axial scan of the fetal head at 25 weeks passing through frontal horns and atria of lateral ventricles (unlabeled). The vein of Galen cistern is seen as a triangular sonolucent space demarcated on both sides by the medial surface of the occipital lobes (*arrowheads*). Within this cistern the great cerebral vein of Galen (VG) is clearly seen. The frontal and temporal opercula (*open arrowheads*) are widely separated, and the sylvian cistern (*) appears as an ample, square-shaped area extending from the base of the insula to the inner calvarium (CSP, cavum septi pellucidum).

considers stenosis of the aqueduct and communicating hydrocephalus as two separate entities has been challenged by the hypothesis that ventriculomegaly may be the cause instead of the consequence of aqueductal stenosis.[32]

The etiology of Dandy-Walker malformation is still unclear. Genetic factors probably play a major role. Familial cases have been reported by many authors and reviewed by Brown and by Hirsch and coworkers.[33,34] They seem to indicate that an autosomal recessive transmission is implicated in at least some instances. More recently, this view has been challenged, and a multifactorial etiology with an empiric recurrence risk of 1% to 5% has been advocated.[35] Dandy-Walker malformation is frequently associated with other nervous system abnormalities, such as agenesis of corpus callosum, heterotopia, polymicrogyria, agyria and macrogyria, systemic anomalies such as congenital heart disease (mainly ventricular septal defects), polydactyly–syndactyly, cleft palate, and polycystic kidneys.[33–35] It may also be related to a number of genetic and nongenetic syndromes that have been extensively reviewed.[35]

PATHOLOGY

In aqueductal stenosis, outlet obstruction of the third ventricle results in severe enlargement of the lateral and third ventricles (triventricular hydrocephalus). In communicating hydrocephalus, at least in early stages, distention of the lateral, third, and fourth ventricles (tetraventricular hydrocephalus) is seen in association with enlarged subarachnoid cisterns. In advanced stages, however, the fourth ventricle and subarachnoid cisterns may appear normal or even small, probably as a consequence of the compression operated by the large lateral ventricles.

Dandy-Walker malformation is featured by the association of three distinct anomalies: hydrocephalus, a retrocerebellar cyst, and a defect in the cerebellar vermis through which the posterior fossa cyst communicates with the fourth ventricle. The embryology of this lesion is still unclear. The original view of Dandy and Taggart and of Walker considered the condition to be secondary to primary atresia of the exit foramina of the fourth ventricle, progressively leading to disruption of the cerebellar vermis.[36,37] Both Benda and Hart suggested that the primary disorder was a defective formation of the cerebellar vermis resulting in secondary maldevelopment and atresia of the foramina of the fourth ventricle.[38,39] Gardner and co-workers have suggested that Dandy-Walker malformation results from embryonic ventriculomegaly, which would lead to an abnormal expansion of the primordia of the roof of the fourth ventricle.[40]

Despite the classical definition of Dandy-Walker malformation, it has been demonstrated that in 80% of cases hydrocephalus is absent at birth and develops only after several months or years.[34] This observation is relevant for the obstetric sonographer, as it indicates that the Dandy-Walker malformation cannot be excluded on the pure basis of the absence of ventriculomegaly.

PRENATAL DIAGNOSIS

Many investigators have addressed the issue of prenatal diagnosis of hydrocephalus by sonography. As macrocrania usually does not develop until late in gestation, head measurements are unreliable, and the identification of hydrocephalus should depend on the direct demonstration of the enlargement of the ventricular system. Nomograms of the normal size of frontal horns,[7] atria,[8,41] and occipital horns[42] of the lateral ventricles throughout gestation are now available. Measurement of the lateral ventricular ratio[3] has been probably the most used approach to the evaluation of the integrity of the ventricular system in the last 10 years. However, it has been recently demonstrated that the echogenic lines that were originally interpreted as the lateral wall of the midbody of the lateral ventricle originate from the white matter and are therefore unreliable for predicting mild to moderate hydrocephalus.[43]

Several authors have demonstrated that a qualitative evaluation of the intracranial structures is most useful in cases of early hydrocephalus. Chinn and co-workers have observed that the large fetal choroid plexus entirely fills the cavity of the lateral ventricle at the level of the atria, being closely apposed to both the medial and the lateral wall.[44] In early hydrocephalus, the choroid plexus cyst is shrunken and anteriorly displaced, thus being clearly detached from the medial wall (Fig. 35-14). This simple approach is very effective in screening for fetal hydrocephalus. However, we found that in a finite number of normal fetuses there is some disproportion between the choroid plexus and the atrial lumen.[8] Under these circumstances, a quantitative evaluation of ventricular dimensions is required. We favor the measurement of the internal diameter of the atria of lateral ventricles.[8] Our experience is in agreement with other reports in indicating that this diameter does not vary in the second half of gestation.[41] We have found that from 16 weeks to term a measurement of 1 cm or less is indicative of normalcy (see Fig. 35-6). However, because an evolutive course is a distinctive feature of fetal hydrocephalus, caution is necessary and dubious cases may require serial examinations performed by an experienced sonologist.

Once hydrocephalus has been recognized, the site of the obstruction may be inferred by identifying the enlarged portion of the ventricular system. Marked dilatation of the lateral and third ventricles suggests aqueductal stenosis (Fig. 35-12). Tetraventricular enlargement in the presence of a normal cerebellar vermis associated with distention of the subarachnoid cisterns suggests communicating hydrocephalus[21,45] (Fig. 35-13). A defect in the cerebellar vermis through which the fourth ventricle communicates with a posterior fossa cyst indicates Dandy-Walker malformation (Fig. 35-17).[46] An attempt to differentiate the anatomical type of hydrocephalus should always be made, as each form carries a different prognosis.[47,48] In most cases, however, distinction between aqueductal stenosis and communicating hydrocephalus is not possible, as has been demonstrated by noncontrast computed tomographic studies in infants.[49,50] In our prenatal series, in only 22% of cases of communicating hydrocephalus could the enlarged subarachnoid spaces be demonstrated clearly.[45]

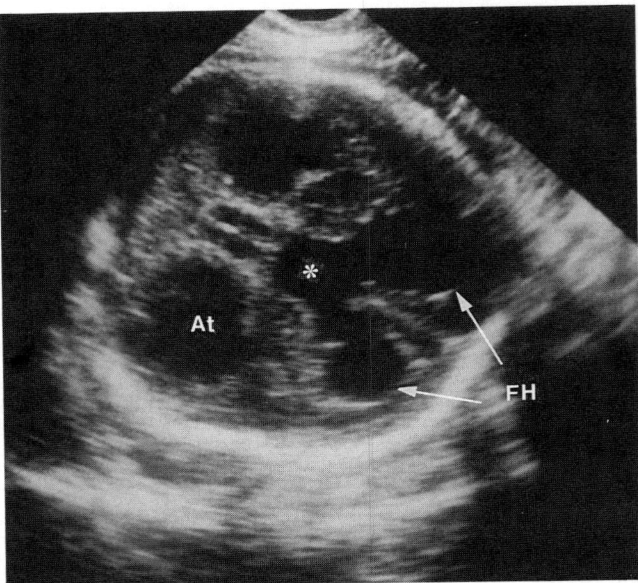

FIGURE 35–12. Fetal triventricular hydrocephalus. Gross enlargement of the lateral ventricles and particularly of the third ventricle (*). The fourth ventricle appeared small. The infant was found at birth to have aqueductal stenosis (FH, frontal horns; At, atria of lateral ventricles.)

PROGNOSIS

Neurosurgical studies of infants with aqueductal stenosis indicate a mortality rate ranging between 10% and 30%.[47,48] In one study only 50% of infants developed normal intelligence following surgical correction.[47] In a more recent study, the mean IQ of treated infants was 71.[48]

According to recent experience, isolated communicating hydrocephalus carries a good prognosis. In a series of 13 treated infants no deaths occurred and the intelligence was normal in all cases.[48]

Infants with Dandy-Walker malformation have an overall mortality rate ranging between 12% and 26% and an IQ above 80 in 30% to 40% of cases.[34,51]

Much work has been done trying to correlate the outcome of ventriculomegalic infants with the extent of ventricular enlargement. Such measurements as the frontal cerebral mantle thickness[52] and the brain mass, calculated on the basis of the frontal cerebral mantle thickness and the occipitofrontal diameter,[48,53] were used. All these studies uniformly indicate that the prognosis is unpredictable on the basis of a quantitative evaluation of the spared cerebral cortex. Many reports indicate that even infants with a cerebral mantle thickness of a few millimeters have sometimes developed a normal or superior intelligence following treatment. At present, the outcome of affected infants seems to depend more on the nature of the underlying lesion than on the degree of ventriculomegaly.

OBSTETRICAL MANAGEMENT

Difficulties in establishing a reliable prognosis in utero are reflected in uncertainties in electing the proper obstetrical management. When the diagnosis of hydrocephalus is made prior to viability, many parents would probably request termination of pregnancy. When this option is not accepted, and in those cases recognized

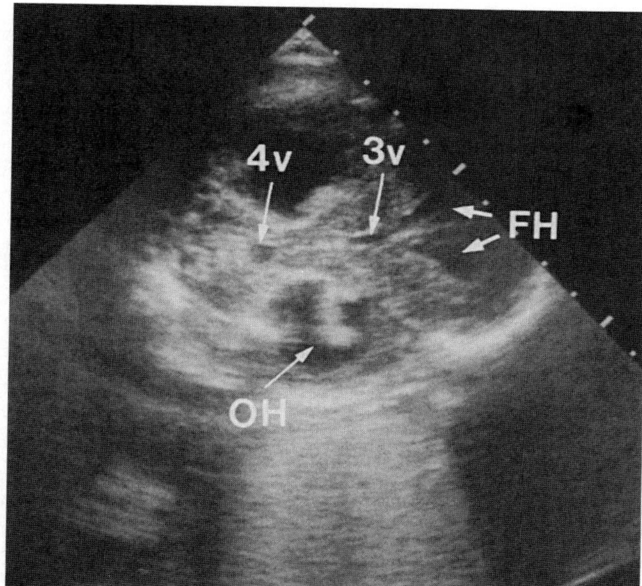

FIGURE 35–13. Fetal tetraventricular hydrocephalus. Enlargement of the frontal and occipital horns of lateral ventricles (FH, OH) and of the third ventricle (3v) is attested to by this scan. There is also questionable enlargement of the fourth ventricle (4v). This infant was found at birth to have communicating hydrocephalus.

later on in pregnancy, a thorough discussion with the couple of the possible choices is recommended. Many authors feel that delivery as soon as fetal maturity is achieved and prompt neurologic treatment will maximize the chances of survival and normal development for the affected infants.[54–56] A cesarean section is recommended in those cases with associated macrocrania. As a chance of normal intellectual development appears possible, cephalocentesis to allow vaginal delivery in cases of fetopelvic disproportion is strongly contraindicated, in view of the significant risk associated with such procedure.[56]

It should be stressed that one of the factors that has an important influence on the outcome of hydrocephalic fetuses is the possible association with other important life-threatening anomalies. In our experience, the incidence of severe associated anomalies, including chromosomal aberrations and extranervous malformations, was almost 30%.[45] In view of these figures, an effort to identify associated anomalies should always be made before considering aggressive obstetrical management. Detailed examination of the entire fetal anatomy by high-resolution ultrasound, echocardiography, and karyotyping is strongly recommended. If severe anomalies are found, suggesting that postnatal survival is unlikely, a conservative management can be offered to the parents.

Intrauterine treatment of congenital obstructive hydrocephalus by ventriculoamniotic shunting has recently been suggested. Experimental studies on animal models hold promise.[57] The preliminary experience on human fetuses is less encouraging. The Registry of the International Society of Fetal Medicine and Surgery indicates that out of a total of 44 fetuses who underwent shunting between 1982 and 1985, the procedure-related death rate was 10%, and of survivors, 53% had a severe handicap, 12% had a mild handicap, and only 35% were developing normally at the time of follow-up.[58]

DISORDERS OF DORSAL INDUCTION

INCIDENCE

The incidence of neural tube defects varies considerably according to geographic and ethnic factors. A figure of one in 1000 to 2000 births is commonly quoted for the general population. In South Wales, the frequency rises to about seven in 1000 births.[59,60]

ETIOLOGY AND PATHOGENESIS

The etiology is multifactorial, with a recurrence risk after the birth of one affected child of 1% to 3%. The interested reader is referred to the review compiled by Brocklehurst.[59]

Two pathogenetic hypotheses have been suggested. Failure of closure of the anterior (anencephaly) or posterior (spina bifida) neuropore have been advocated by the vast majority of authors. Gardner postulated a secondary opening of the already formed neural tube following embryonic hydrocephalus.[61]

PATHOLOGY

In anencephaly the cranial vault is absent, as well as the telencephalic and diencephalic structures. Necrotic remnants of the brain stem and rhombencephalic structures are covered by a vascular membrane. Associated malformations are common and include spina bifida, cleft lip and palate, clubfoot, and omphalocele. Polyhydramnios is frequently found.

Spina bifida is subdivided into occulta and aperta. Spina bifida occulta is characterized by vertebral schisis covered by normal soft tissues. Large defects are usually associated with pigmented and dimpled lesions overlying skin and subcutaneous lipomas. Spina bifida aperta is characterized by a defect of the skin, underlying soft tissues, and vertebral arches exposing the neural canal. The defect may be covered by a thin meningeal membrane (meningocele). In the presence of neural tissue inside the sac the lesion is defined as a *myelomeningocele,* a term often used to indicate all cases of spina bifida aperta. The defect may vary considerably in size. The lumbar, thoracolumbar, or sacrolumbar areas are most frequently affected. Spina bifida aperta is almost always associated with a typical intracranial malformation (Arnold-Chiari type II) consisting of displacement of the cerebellar vermis, fourth ventricle, and medulla oblongata through the foramen magnum inside the upper cervical canal.[59] Hydrocephalus of variable degree is present in virtually all cases of spina bifida aperta.[62] Hydrocephalus is thought to arise from the low position of the exit foramina of the fourth ventricle, which either can be obstructed by the surrounding bony structures or can be open inside the spinal canal. In the latter case, the cerebellum impacted within the posterior fossa would prevent return of cerebrospinal fluid to the intracranial subarachnoid spaces and reabsorption sites.[63] Deformities and obstruction of the aqueduct are found in almost all cases[64] and are thought to derive from the external compression operated by the enlargement of the lateral ventricles.[32] Infants with spina bifida aperta often have associated anomalies, such as kyphoscoliosis and clubfoot.

The term *cephalocele* indicates a protrusion of intracranial contents through a bony defect of the skull.[65] Cephaloceles may occur either as isolated defects or as a part of genetic and nongenetic syndromes, which have been extensively reviewed.[66] Classical examples include Meckel syndrome (autosomal recessive transmission, also featured by microcephaly, polydactyly, polycystic kidneys, and multiple visceral anomalies)[67] and the amniotic band syndrome (sporadic, featured by asymmetrical or multiple cephaloceles, gastroschisis, facial clefts, amputation, and ring constrictions of the limbs).[68] In most cases, the lesion arises from the midline, in the occipital area; less frequently it arises from the parietal or frontal bones. Encephaloceles are characterized by the presence of brain tissue inside the lesion. When only meninges protrude, the term *cranial meningocele* should be used. Cephaloceles often cause impaired cerebrospinal fluid circulation and hydrocephalus. Massive encephaloceles may be associated with microcephaly.

PRENATAL DIAGNOSIS

The association between fetal neural tube defects and elevated amniotic[69] and maternal serum α-fetoprotein[70] and amniotic acetylcholinesterase[71] is well established. The combined use of α-fetoprotein determination and ultrasound as a screening tool for the prenatal diagnosis of these lesion has been advocated and is presently routinely used in several countries, including Great Britain and the United States. In this chapter we consider only the role of sonography. The interested reader is referred to works on this subject.[70–77]

Anencephaly was the first congenital anomaly recognized in utero by ultrasound.[1] The diagnosis is easy and relies on the demonstration of the absence of the cranial vault. Because the fetal head can be positively identified by modern ultrasound equipment as early as the first trimester, anencephaly is recognizable at that time.

We are not aware of cases of spina bifida occulta diagnosed in utero by ultrasound. It seems unlikely that such lesions can be detected even by the most experienced operators. Open defects can be recognized by demonstrating the defect of the neural arches and overlying soft tissues (Fig. 35-14). The accuracy of ultrasound in predicting fetal spinal lesions is a critical issue. It is clear that the predictive value of the technique largely depends on the quality of the equipment, the experience of the operator, and the amount of time dedicated to any single patient. No data are available with regard to level 1 or basic untargeted examinations. However, there is little doubt that the sensitivity of these examinations is quite low.

Level 2 examinations on patients at risk because of either familial history or elevated α-fetoprotein are much more accurate. The use of sonography for antenatal detection of spina bifida was first suggested by Campbell and colleagues.[78] In the original report, ultrasound was successful in identifying one affected fetus and ruling out lesions in one normal fetus, but failed to recognize a lumbosacral defect in a third fetus. Ten years later, the same group reported a sensitivity and specificity of level 2 ultrasound very close to 100%. A similar trend was reported by Roberts and colleagues, who described the results of a large multicentric study performed in South Wales.[73] The sensitivity of the technique was 30% in the first 3 years and rose to 80% over the following 3 years. The false-positive rate decreased from 57% to 9% in the second period of the study. Both the increased experience of the operators and the introduction of high-resolution real-time ultrasound equip-

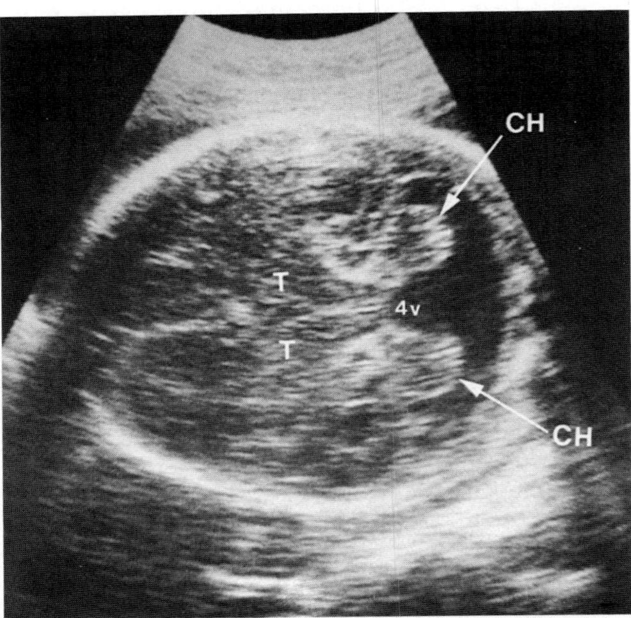

FIGURE 35–14. Fetal Dandy-Walker malformation. A wide defect is seen at the level of the cerebellar vermis. Through this defect the cystic cisterna magna amply communicates with the area of the fourth ventricle (4v). The cerebellar hemispheres (CH) are widely separated. (T, thalami.)

ment were probably responsible for this dramatic diagnostic improvement.

Sonologists have focused recently on the evaluation of intracranial anatomy in fetuses with spina bifida. Several reports indicate that typical cranial signs are consistently found. These findings include frontal bossing (the "lemon sign"), hypoplasia of the posterior fossa structures, attested by an abnormal configuration of the cerebellum (the "banana sign"),[79] an abnormally reduced transverse cerebellar diameter, failure to recognize the cerebellum, and obliteration of the cisterna magna.[80] These signs can be demonstrated easily even by less experienced sonographers and are therefore potentially useful for sonographic mass screening of spina bifida (Fig. 35-15).

Fetal cephaloceles should be suspected when a paracranial mass is seen on sonography. The diagnosis of encephaloceles is easy, as the presence of brain tissue inside the sac is striking on ultrasound (Fig. 35-16). Differentiation of a cranial meningocele (Fig. 35-17) from soft-tissue edema or a cystic hygroma of the neck may be difficult.[81] Demonstration of the bony defect in the skull would allow a proper diagnosis, but cranial meningoceles are often associated with extremely small (a few millimeters) defects that are not amenable to antenatal sonographic recognition. Certain clues can assist a correct diagnosis. Cranial cephaloceles are very often associated with ventriculomegaly. Cystic hygromas arise from the region of the neck, have multiple internal septations and a thick wall, and are often associated with generalized soft-tissue edema and hydrops. Some cephaloceles protrude through the base of skull inside the pharynx. These lesions are obviously inaccessible to prenatal ultrasound identification unless derangement of intracranial morphology is present. As cephaloceles are often associated with other anomalies, a careful investigation of the entire fetal anatomy is recommended.

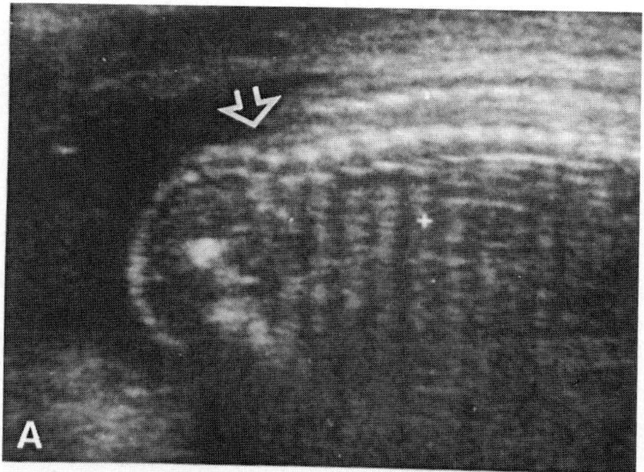

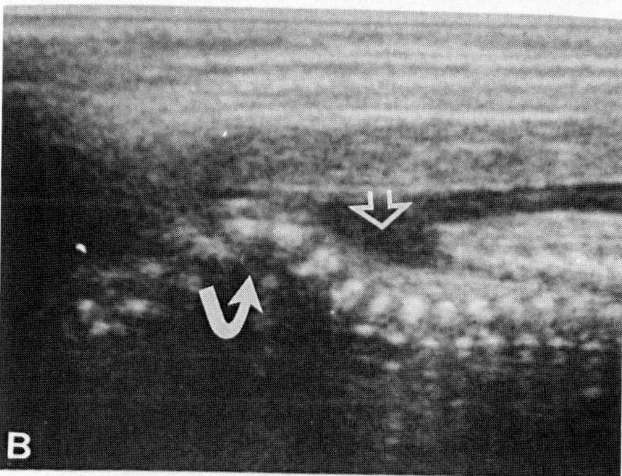

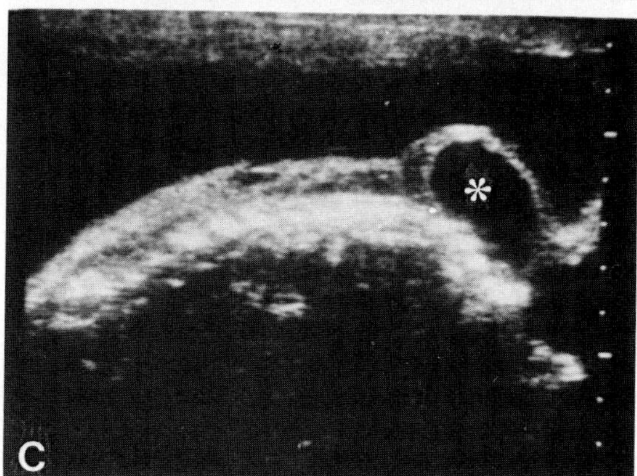

FIGURE 35–15. Spectrum of spina bifida recognizable in utero with sonography. Longitudinal scans of the fetal spine allows us to identify the site and extension of the lesion. In **A** a small sacral defect is demonstrated (*open arrow*). In **B** a large thoracolumbar defect with severe associated kyphoscoliosis (*curved arrow*) is seen. In **C** a cervical meningocele (*) with complete rachischisis is seen.

PROGNOSIS

Anencephaly is invariably fatal. The outcome for infants with spina bifida is dictated by the site and extension of the lesion. The mortality is high, with the 7-year survival rate being only 40% despite early treatment.[82] Many of the survivors will suffer from significant disabilities, such as lower limb paralysis or dysfunction and incontinence. The association of spina bifida and severe hydrocephalus was traditionally considered a poor prognostic factor for intellectual development.[82] More recent studies indicate that in many cases control of intracranial hypertension by shunting results in a normal and even superior intelligence.[48,83]

The outcome of infants with cephalocele is primarily related to the presence or absence of brain tissue inside the lesion. Encephaloceles carry a neonatal mortality rate of about 40% and an incidence of intellectual impairment and neurologic sequelae of 80%. Infants with cranial meningoceles develop a normal intelligence in 60% of cases.[84]

OBSTETRIC MANAGEMENT

As anencephaly is an invariably fatal lesion, termination of pregnancy can be offered at any time in pregnancy.[85] When the diagnosis of spina bifida is

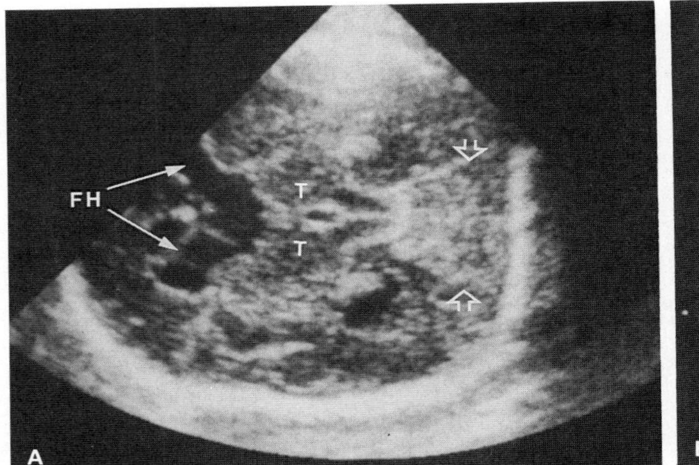

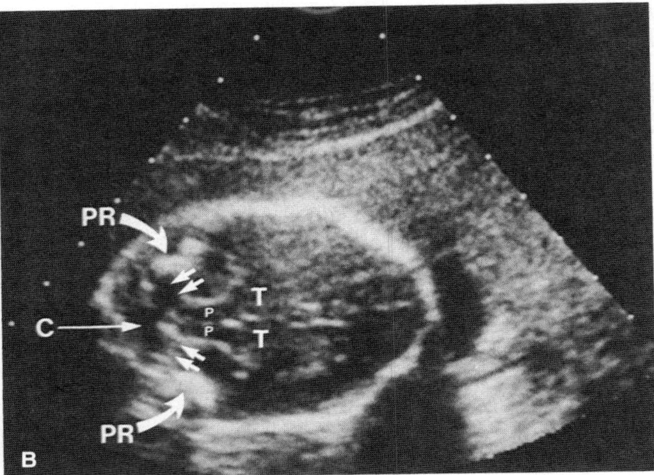

FIGURE 35–16. (**A**) Typical intracranial anatomy in a fetus with spina bifida. Obliteration of the cisterna magna, reduced transverse cerebellar diameter (*open arrows*), enlarged third ventricle, and frontal horns of lateral ventricles (FH) are demonstrated. (**B**) In this second-trimester fetus, the small cerebellum (C) has a very low position and is obscured by the acoustic shadowing arising from the petrous ridges of the skull base (PR). Failure to visualize the cerebellum is frequent in fetuses with open neural tube defects. Note the typical elongation of cerebral peduncles (P) and frontal bossing (the "lemon sign"). (T, thalami.)

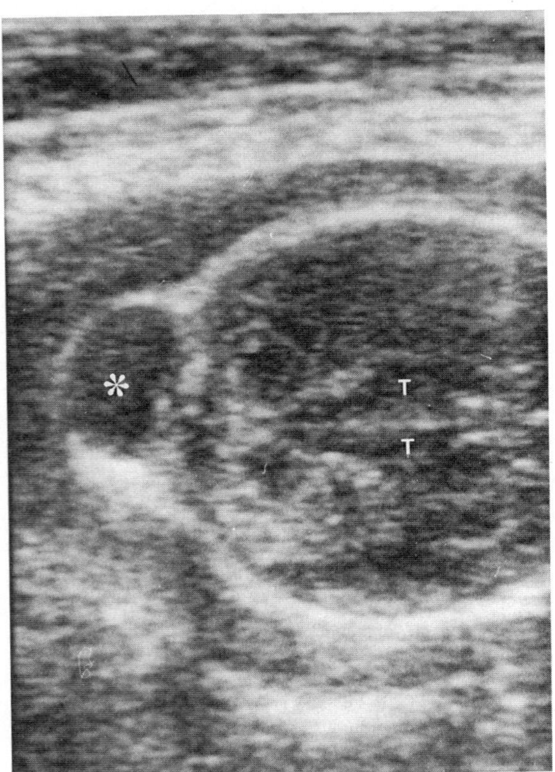

FIGURE 35–17. Occipital meningocele (*). (T, thalami.)

made prior to viability, termination of pregnancy can be offered to the parents. When this is refused, and in those cases recognized later or in gestation, an attempt to identify the site and the extent of the lesion should be made to give a tentative prognosis. Options should be discussed with the couples. Several reports indicate that birth injury is frequent in fetuses with spina bifida and represents a major prognostic shortcoming.[86–88] Therefore, cesarean delivery is recommended.[10]

When a prenatal diagnosis of cephalocele is made, termination of pregnancy can be offered prior to viability. In continuing pregnancies, a cesarean section should be considered to avoid birth trauma. However, as infants with massive encephaloceles and microcephaly have a dismal prognosis, conservative management can be offered in these cases.

DISORDERS OF VENTRAL INDUCTION

The term *ventral induction* refers to the interrelated developmental events that occur in the embryonic forebrain starting from the fifth week of gestation and that lead to the separation of the cerebral hemispheres and to the formation of the midline structures. The differentiation of these nervous structures is closely related to the development of the midface. Disorders of ventral induction include a group of midline cerebral defects that encompass a wide spectrum of severity and are typically associated with craniofacial malformations.[89]

HOLOPROSENCEPHALY

INCIDENCE

The incidence of holoprosencephaly is unknown as milder forms are probably unrecognized. Two subtypes of this anomaly, cyclopia and cebocephaly, have been reported to occur in one in 40,000 and one in 16,000 births, respectively.[90] An incidence of four in 1000 abortions has also been reported,[91] suggesting a high intrauterine fatality rate from this defect.

ETIOLOGY AND PATHOGENESIS

The etiology of holoprosenchephaly is heterogeneous.[92] In most cases, the anomaly is isolated and sporadic. In some cases, however, chromosomal abnormalities have been found as well as other congenital anatomical deformities, such as anencephaly, encephalocele, DiGeorge syndrome, and Meckel's syndrome.[92] Several familial cases suggest genetic inheritance with autosomal dominant transmission.[93] The overall recurrence risk is 6%.[92]

Holoprosencephaly is the consequence of a failed diverticularization of the embryonic prosencephalon into its components, the cerebral hemispheres and the diencephalic structures. The primary disorder seems to reside in the precordal mesenchyma, which is thought to induce both cleavage of the primitive forebrain and development of the median facial structures (orbits, nose, median upper lip, and palate). This concept provides an explanation of the typical association of brain anomalies and facial dysmorphism seen in this malformation sequence.[90]

PATHOLOGY

Failure of the forebrain to undergo paired symmetrical division along the sagittal plane and diverticularization results in varying degrees of fusion of the cerebral structures. In the alobar variety, the most severe one, this interhemispheric fissure and the falx cerebri are totally absent, there is a single primitive ventricle (holoventricle), the thalami are fused on the midline, and the third ventricle, neurohypophysis, olfactory bulbs, and tracts are absent. In semilobar holoprosencephaly, the two cerebral hemispheres are partially separated posteriorly, but there is still a single ventricular cavity. In both the alobar and semilobar forms, the roof of the ventricular cavity, the thela choroidea, normally enfolded within the brain, may balloon out between the cerebral convexity and the skull to form a cyst of variable size—the dorsal sac. Alobar and semilobar holoprosencephaly are often associated with microcephaly. They are associated less frequently with macrocephaly, which is invariably due to internal obstructive hydrocephalus. In the lobar variety, the interhemispheric fissure is well developed posteriorly and anteriorly, but there is still a variable degree of fusion of the cingulate gyrus and of the lateral ventricles, and the septum pellucidum is absent. The facial anomalies are pleomorphic. According to the classification suggested by DeMyer and co-workers, five categories can be recognized: cyclopia, which is featured by a single eye or partially divided eyes in a single orbit; arhinia; median cleft palate and/or lip; face with median philtrum–premaxilla anlage; and flat nose.[94] Cyclopia and etmocephaly are invariably associated with alobar holoprosencephaly. Cebocephaly and median cleft lip face may be found in either the alobar or semilobar variety. The face with median philtrum–premaxilla anlage is indicative of either semilobar or lobar varieties. It should be stressed that infants with any kind of holoprosencephaly may have a normal face.[90]

PRENATAL DIAGNOSIS

Several cases of sonographic antenatal diagnosis of holoprosencephaly have been reported in the literature. A variety of findings has been described: microcephaly and absence of the midline[95]; absence of the midline and intracranial cyst[96]; absence of the midline and cyclopia[97]; absence of the midline and enlarged holoventricle[5]; microcephaly, intracranial fluid collection, and proboscis[98]; holoventricle and hypotelorism[99]; cyclopia and unspecified intracranial anomalies[100]; and holoventricle, fused thalami, dorsal sac, and cyclopia.[101] In our experience, the most valuable finding was the demonstration of the single primitive ventricle, which was possible in all cases (see Fig. 35-17). We were also able to recognize the dorsal sac, when present (Fig. 35-18), and to predict facial anomalies such as cyclopia, hypotelorism, anophthalmia, arhinia, and proboscis and median cleft lip (Figs. 35-19, 35-20).[102,103] Demonstration of facial anomalies strengthens the diagnosis of holoprosencephaly based on central nervous system findings. Conversely, should any of the aforementioned facial features be serendipitously encountered, a careful examination of the intracranial contents is recommended.

Only one case of antenatal diagnosis of semilobar holoprosencephaly has been reported thus far.[104] The ultrasonic findings were very similar to the ones described in cases of alobar holoprosencephaly. In newborns, semilobar holoprosencephaly can be confirmed by visualizing well-developed occipital horns.[105,106]

The lobar variety of holoprosencephaly can be identified by demonstrating fusion and squaring of the roof of the frontal horns (Fig. 35-21).[107]

PROGNOSIS

The invariably poor prognosis for infants affected by alobar and semilobar holoprosencephaly is well estab-

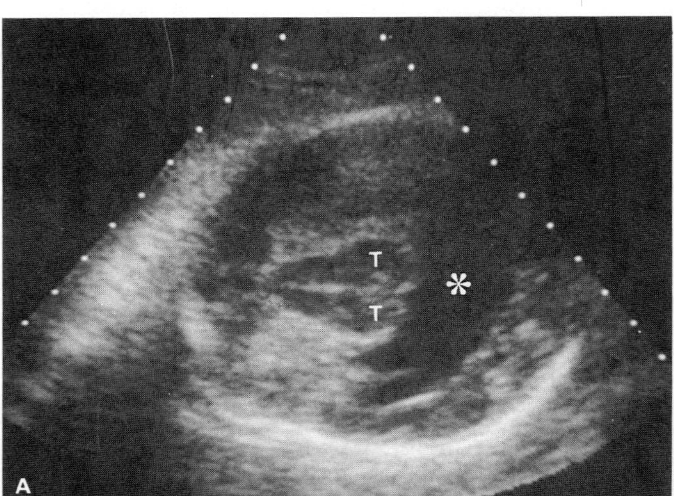

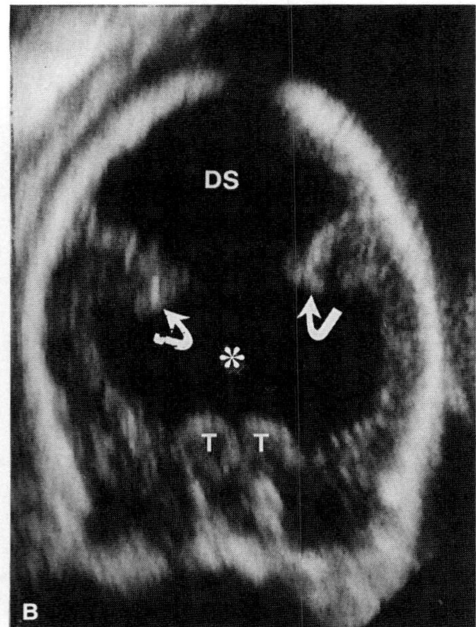

FIGURE 35–18. Alobar holoprosencephaly. (**A**) Axial scan of the head, demonstrating the single central ventricle (*) and bulblike undivided thalami. (**B**) Coronal scan in a different fetus, demonstrating the relationship between single ventricle (*), the uncompletely formed brain mantle (*curved arrows*), and the dorsal sac (DS).

lished.[90,108] Although precise prognostic figures are not available, infants with the lobar variety may have both a normal lifespan and a normal intelligence.[90,108]

OBSTETRICAL MANAGEMENT

When either alobar or semilobar holoprosencephaly is identified in utero, termination of pregnancy can be offered prior to viability. A conservative management is strongly recommended in continuing pregnancies. The prognosis of lobar holoprosencephaly is unclear, and this is reflected in uncertainties about obstetric management.

AGENESIS OF THE CORPUS CALLOSUM

INCIDENCE

The incidence of agenesis of the corpus callosum is highly controversial and depends mainly on the techniques used to ascertain it. Figures ranging from one in 100 to one in 19,000 have been reported.[109]

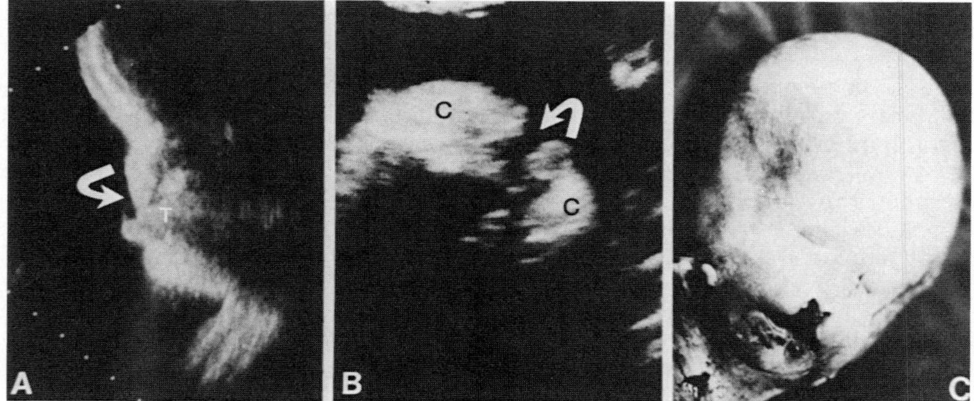

FIGURE 35–19. Alobar holoprosencephaly with median cleft lip and palate. In **A** a view of the profile of the fetal face reveals absence of the nose (*curved arrow*). In **B** an axial scan of the palate reveals a large central cleft (*arrow*). In **C** an image of the stillborn fetus is provided for comparison. Extreme hypotelorism can be noted. C, cheeks.

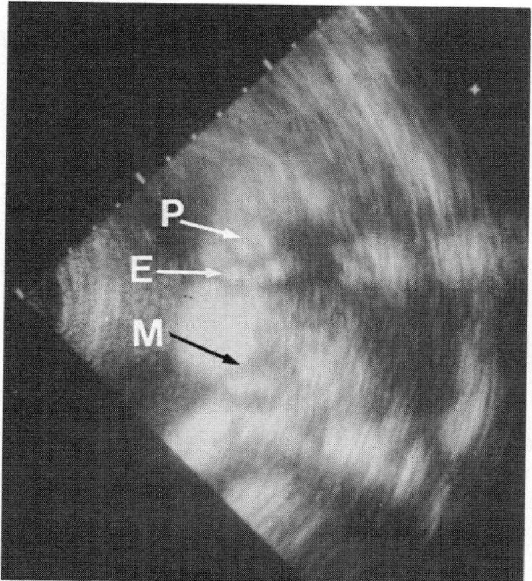

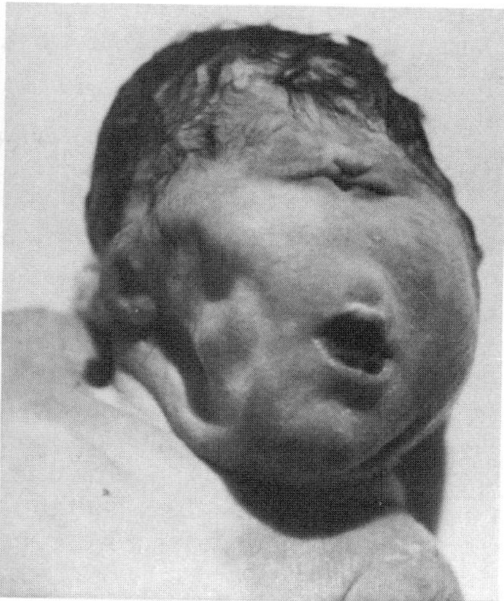

FIGURE 35–20. Alobar holoprosencephaly with cyclopia. (P, proboscis; E, median eyelid; M, mouth.)

ETIOLOGY

The etiology is unknown. Agenesis of the corpus callosum can be found in association with chromosomal aberrations (trisomy 13 and 18), mostly as part of the holoprosencephalic malformative sequence. Various teratogens can produce agenesis of the corpus callosum in animal models[110]. The familial cases reported in the literature have been recently reviewed by Young and co-workers.[111] A marked genetic heterogeneity was found, with evidence supporting autosomal dominant, autosomal recessive, and X-linked inheritance. Agenesis of the corpus callosum may be a part of genetic syndromes, such as Aicardi syndrome (seizures, chorioretinal lacunae, mental retardation, microcephaly, and vertebral anomalies; sex-linked dominant inheritance)[112]; Andermann syndrome (mental retardation and progressive motor neuropathy, autosomal recessive transmission)[113]; acrocallosal syndrome (mental retardation, macrocephaly, polydactyly, autosomal recessive transmission)[114]; and FG syndrome (mental retardation, macrocephaly, hypotonia).[115] The high frequency of associated malformations suggests that agenesis of the corpus callosum may be part of a widespread developmental disturbance.

PATHOLOGY

The corpus callosum is a white matter structure connecting the two cerebral hemispheres. Embryologically it derives from the massa commissuralis, which is formed by fusion of the lateral margins of the groove that separates the two primitive telencephalic ventricles. The anterior portion of the corpus callosum is the first one to be formed. Growth proceeds then caudally, with the definitive configuration of the corpus callosum being assumed only by the 20th week.[116] Agenesis may be complete or partial. In the latter case aplasia affects the posterior portion, which is ontogenetically the last one to be formed. In a review of the literature, associated central nervous system anomalies, including microcephaly, abnormal convolutional patterns, neural tube defects, Dandy-Walker malformation, and aplasia or hypoplasia of the pyramidal tracts were found in 85% of the cases.[117] Systemic anomalies, including a

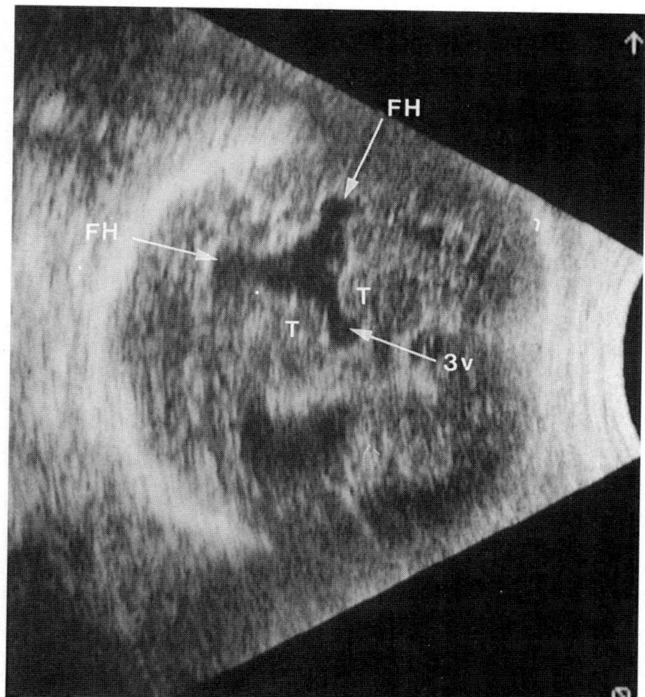

FIGURE 35–21. In this fetus, lobar holoprosencephaly is inferred by the wide central fusion of the frontal horns (FH) with the inferior third ventricle (3v). The flattened roof of the frontal horns and the bulblike thalami (T) can also be noted.

variety of musculoskeletal, cardiovascular, genitourinary, and gastrointestinal malformations were found in 62% of cases.

PRENATAL DIAGNOSIS

The criteria for the postnatal diagnosis of agenesis of the corpus callosum by diagnostic imaging techniques, such as ventriculography,[118] computed tomography,[119] and ultrasound,[120,121] are well established. They depend mainly on the demonstration of the typical alterations of the cerebral architecture that are found in this condition. The bodies of the lateral ventricles are invariably widely separated, and the atria and occipital horns are enlarged (colpocephaly). The third ventricle is frequently enlarged and dorsally extended, being found at the same level as or higher than the bodies of lateral ventricles. Two cases of prenatal sonographic diagnosis of agenesis of the corpus callosum have been reported by Comstock and colleagues.[122] In both cases, colpocephaly and upward displacement of the third ventricle were observed. In our own series the most valuable sonographic finding was the demonstration of colpocephaly.[123] The wide separation of the bodies of lateral ventricles and the enlargement of the atria resulted in a very typical image (Fig. 35-22). Dorsal extension of the third ventricle appears to be an inconsistent finding, as it was present in only 45% of our cases (Fig. 35-23). A very valuable, although inconstant finding, is the demonstration of a widening of the interhemispheric fissure, which results in triplication of the midline echo (Fig. 35-24). Meticulous scanning may also sometimes allow the direct demonstration of the absence of the corpus callosum (Fig. 35-25).

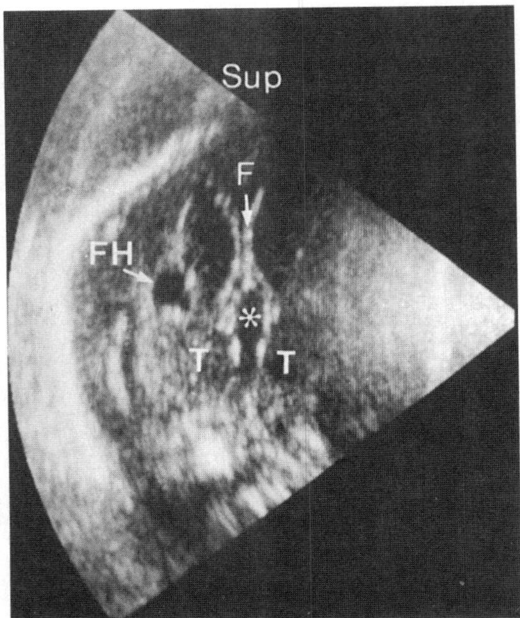

FIGURE 35–23. Coronal scan in the same case of the previous figure. Upward displacement of the third ventricle (*) that can be seen at the same level of frontal horns (FH) is demonstrated. The close proximity between the third ventricle and the superior falx cerebelli (F) excludes the presence of the corpus callosum. The interhemispheric fissure is typically enlarged.

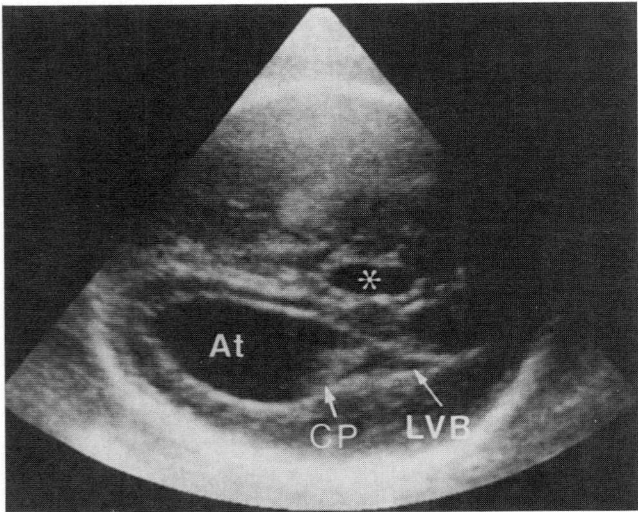

FIGURE 35–22. Colpocephaly demonstrated by an axial scan of the head in a fetus with agenesis of the corpus callosum. The atria of lateral ventricles (At) are considerably enlarged; the bodies of lateral ventricles (LVB) are normal in size but widely separated. The third ventricle is enlarged and displaced upward, thus resulting in a median cystic structure (*) that can be seen at the same level as the bodies of the lateral ventricles. (CP, choroid plexus.)

PROGNOSIS

Establishing a reliable prognosis for agenesis of the corpus callosum is extremely difficult. Many patients suffer from mental retardation, neurologic abnormalities —including increased muscle tone and seizures—and are psychologically abnormal.[109] However, in some cases the condition is totally asymptomatic. It is likely that disabilities depend more on the amount and extent of associated anomalies than on agenesis of the corpus callosum. No specific figures are available at present.

Difficulties in assessing the prognosis are reflected in uncertainties as to parental counselling and obstetrical management. A careful search for associated anomalies, including echocardiography and karyotyping, is mandatory. However, it should be stressed that the ability of prenatal ultrasound to identify several of the anomalies classically associated with agenesis of the corpus callosum, such as abnormal convolutional patterns, has not been tested yet. Abnormalities of the pyramidal tracts, which may cause significant disability, are obviously unpredictable. Termination of pregnancy

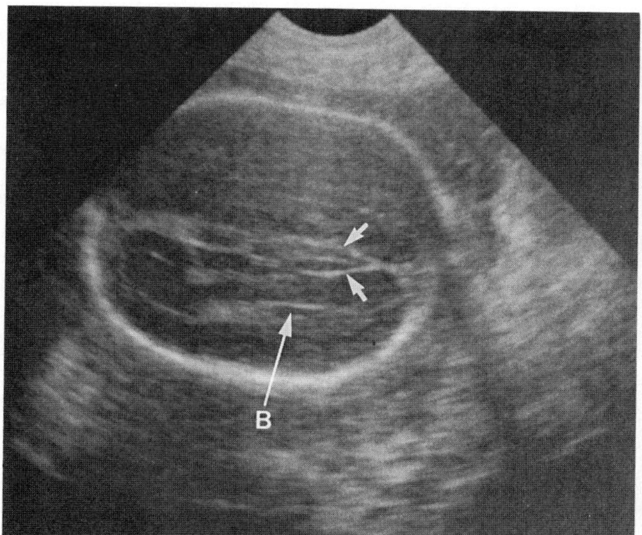

FIGURE 35–24. Second-trimester fetus with complete agenesis of the corpus callosum. Enlargement of the interhemispheric fissure results in a triplication of the midline echo (*arrowheads*). The bodies of lateral ventricles (B) are separated, but there is not significant enlargement of the atria.

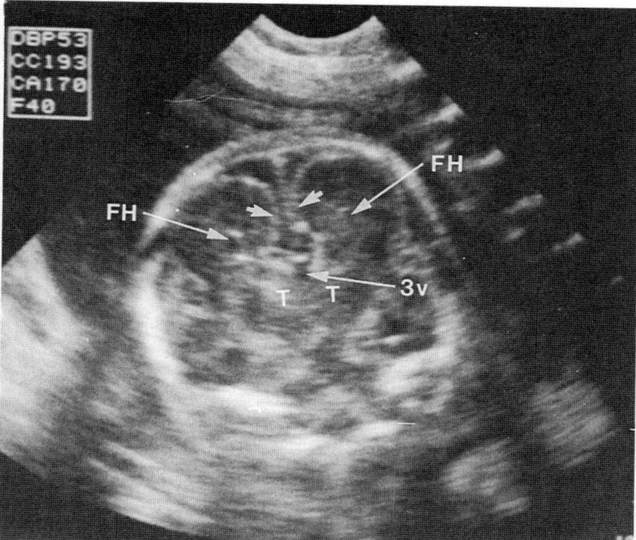

FIGURE 35–25. Same case as the previous figure. Coronal scans are mostly informative in cases of agenesis of the corpus callosum. The wide separation between the medial surfaces of the cerebral hemispheres (*arrowheads*) allows us to infer the absence of the corpus callosum. The frontal horns (FH) are widely separated. The third ventricle (3v) is not displaced upward.

can be offered prior to viability, but the parents should be informed that there is a chance of entirely normal intellectual and neurologic development. In continuing pregnancies, no specific obstetric management is required. Agenesis of the corpus callosum may be associated with macrocephaly. In these cases, a cesarean delivery is definitely indicated.

DESTRUCTIVE CEREBRAL LESIONS

PORENCEPHALY

Incidence and Etiology

The incidence of porencephaly is rare. The etiology is unknown. The acquired form may be the consequence of thrombosis of cerebral vessels resulting from embolization or infection.

Pathology

The term *porencephaly* refers to a condition in which cystic cavities are found within the brain matter. It may be either the consequence of a morphogenetic disorder (true porencephaly or schizencephaly) or the result of an intrauterine or postnatal destructive process (pseudoporencephaly or encephaloclastic porencephaly).[124,125] The cavities usually communicate with either the ventricular system, the subarachnoid space, or both. The development form is often bilateral and symmetrical. In pseudoporencephaly a unilateral lesion is usually found; in both cases, there is a wide variability in the size of the lesion. Hydrocephalus is frequently associated.

Prenatal Diagnosis

Prenatal sonographic identification of intracerebral cystic cavities is easy[45] (Fig. 35-26), but the differential diagnosis with intracranial cysts of different nature, such as arachnoid cysts and congenital tumors,[126] may be impossible.

Prognosis

Both true porencephaly and congenital pseudoporencephaly are severe anomalies with a dismal prognosis. The vast majority of patients are affected by severe mental retardation and important neurologic sequelae such as blindness and tetraplegia.[127]

Obstetric Management

When a confident diagnosis of porencephaly is made prior to viability, termination of pregnancy should be offered to the parents. In continuing pregnancies, conservative obstetric management is recommended.

HYDRANENCEPHALY

Incidence

Hydranencephaly is very rare.

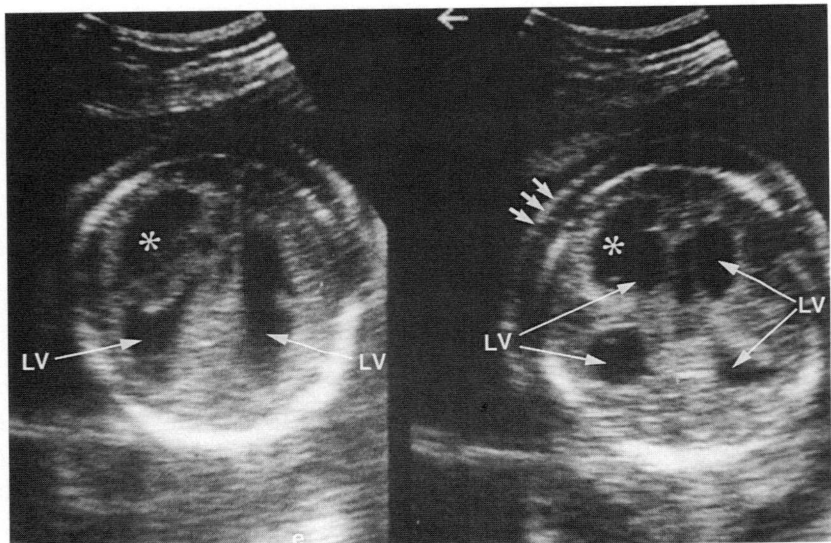

FIGURE 35–26. Porencephaly in a second-trimester fetus with multiple anomalies and nonimmune hydrops. The lateral ventricles are enlarged (LV) and loss of cerebral tissue in the parietal region can be appreciated (*). Significant scalp edema is present (*arrowhead*).

Etiology and Pathogenesis

Hydranencephaly is thought to result from an intrauterine destructive process and may be considered as an extreme form of pseudoporencephaly. The etiology is heterogeneous. Congenital infections, including toxoplasmosis and cytomegalovirus, and intrauterine strangulation or atresia of the internal carotid arteries have been reported.[128–131]

Pathology

Most of the cerebral hemispheres are absent and the intracranial cavity is filled with fluid. Remnants of the temporal and occipital lobes can be found. The brain stem and rhombencephalic structures are usually spared. The head may be either small, of normal size, or extremely enlarged.[132]

Prenatal Diagnosis

Even if replacement of intracranial structures with fluid is easily detected by antenatal sonography, certain identification of hydranencephaly may be difficult. The differential diagnosis includes severe hydrocephalus and holoprosencephaly. However, even in the most devastating forms of ventriculomegaly, it is possible to demonstrate the falx cerebri and some spared cortex. In alobar holoprosencephaly, the falx is absent, but a crescent-shaped frontal cortex can usually be seen. In hydranencephaly, the falx is absent or incomplete in the vast majority of cases. In our experience, the most valuable finding for a specific diagnosis is the demonstration of the bulblike brain stem, which, in the absence of the surrounding cortex, bulges inside the fluid-filled intracranial cavity (Fig. 35-27).[45] The sonographic appearance is somewhat similar to that of the hypoplastic thalami that can be seen in cases of alobar or semilobar holoprosencephaly. Obviously, confusion between holoprosencephaly and hydranencephaly is without serious consequences, as both conditions share a dismal prognosis and the obstetrical management does not differ.

Prognosis and Obstetric Management

Prognosis is severe. Long survival has been reported.[133] However, these infants are obviously incapable of any intellectual achievement. When a confident diagnosis of hydranencephaly is made in a fetus, conservative management is suggested.

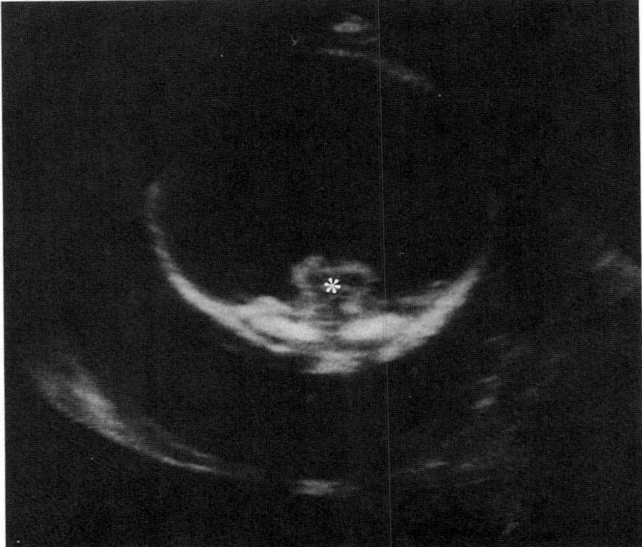

FIGURE 35–27. Hydranencephaly. The cerebral hemispheres are entirely replaced by fluid. The brain stem (*) is relatively spared.

MICROCEPHALY

DEFINITION AND INCIDENCE

The definition of microcephaly is highly controversial. Some authors suggest that we use as a diagnostic criterion a head circumference two standard deviations below the mean.[134] Others believe that a threshold of three standard deviations below the mean should be used.[135] Differences in diagnostic modalities probably account for the wide variability of the incidence of this condition reported in different studies. Figures ranging from 1.6 in 1000 births[23] to one in 25,000 to 50,000[135] can be found in the literature.

ETIOLOGY

The etiology is extremely heterogeneous. Microcephaly should be considered not as a separate entity but as a symptom of many etiologic disturbances. Genetic and environmental causative factors are both well accepted, and the reader is referred to the extensive reviews on the subject.[136,137] The widely accepted classification suggested by Book and co-workers includes two main categories: microcephaly resulting from nongenetic insults such as infections, anoxia, radiations, and so on, and genetic microcephaly, which includes all those cases in which microcephaly is a part of inherited syndromes.[135]

PATHOLOGY

Microcephalic individuals share in common a typical disproportion size between the splanchnocranium and neurocranium. The forehead is sloping. The correlation between a small head circumference and reduced brain mass and total cell number is well established.[138] The cerebral hemispheres are affected more than the diencephalic and rhombencephalic structures. Abnormal convolutional patterns (macrogyria, microgyria, agyria) are frequently found. The ventricles may be enlarged. Microcephaly is frequently found in cases of porencephaly, lissencephaly, and holoprosencephaly.

PRENATAL DIAGNOSIS

Many difficulties arise in attempting to identify fetal microcephaly. The utility of head measurements alone is limited, as these can be markedly biased by factors such as incorrect dating or intrauterine growth retardation. Furthermore, the natural history of fetal microcephaly is largely unknown. Campbell and co-workers have described a progressive intrauterine development of the lesion that would render early prenatal diagnosis impossible in some cases.[139] This observation is in agreement with our own experience. Nevertheless, recognition before viability is of paramount importance, as microcephaly has genetic implications, and many couples with a positive familial history demand prenatal diagnosis. A comparison of biometric parameters, such as the ratio of head circumference to abdominal circumference[95,139] and the ratio of femur length to biparietal diameter,[140] has been suggested. In this regard, Chervenak and associates have provided nomograms that are extremely useful for diagnostic practice.[141] Nevertheless, both false-positive and false-negative diagnoses have been reported.[141] It is clear that the predictive value of ultrasound biometry has several limitations at present.[142] A qualitative evaluation of the intracranial structures is a very useful adjunct to biometry, as cerebral malformations are found in a significant proportion of infants with microcephaly.[143] Measurement of the fetal frontal lobe may assist the diagnosis (Fig. 35-28).[9]

PROGNOSIS

Establishing a reliable prognosis for infants affected by microcephaly is difficult. Associated anomalies obviously have a major influence on the outcome. Controversial clinical data exist with regard to isolated microcephaly. In one series of 134 infants with head circumference two standard deviations below the mean, only one had normal intelligence.[134] More recent studies are in disagreement with these observations. Avery and co-workers reported a group of 28 infants with head circumference two standard deviations below the mean and found either a normal intellectual development or only mild retardation in 50%.[144] Martin

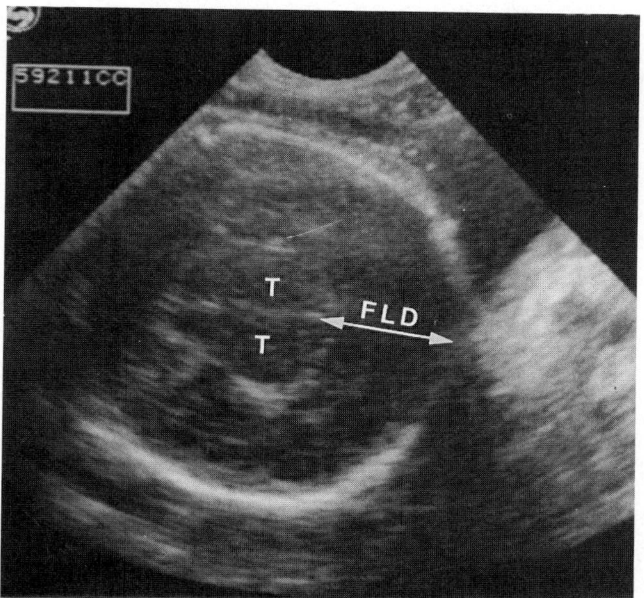

FIGURE 35–28. Reduction of the frontal lobe distance (FLD) in a fetus with severe microcephaly. (T, thalami.)

found a normal intellectual development in 82% and 28% of infants with a head circumference between two and three standard deviations below the mean, respectively.[145] Even if it is hard to derive precise prognostic figures from these studies, there is evidence to indicate that a small head size does not necessarily imply mental retardation.

OBSTETRIC MANAGEMENT

When a confident prenatal diagnosis of microcephaly is made in a pregnancy at risk, the couple will most likely request termination of pregnancy. A conservative management is certainly indicated also in cases of fetal microcephaly with associated cerebral or extracerebral anomalies. A confident diagnosis of isolated microcephaly in a pregnant patient who has no risk factors occurs quite rarely in our experience. The infrequency of these observations is responsible for an uncertainty in obstetrical management. In any case, it is necessary to remember that infants with a small head may have a normal intelligence and that at present there is no established correlation between head measurement and intellectual development.

CHOROID PLEXUS CYSTS

INCIDENCE

Prenatal sonographic identification of choroid plexus cysts has been reported with increasing frequency (Fig. 35-29).[146,147] Although other authors have reported a very low incidence of fetal choroid plexus cysts,[147] we have documented this finding in almost 3% of routine second-trimester sonograms.[148]

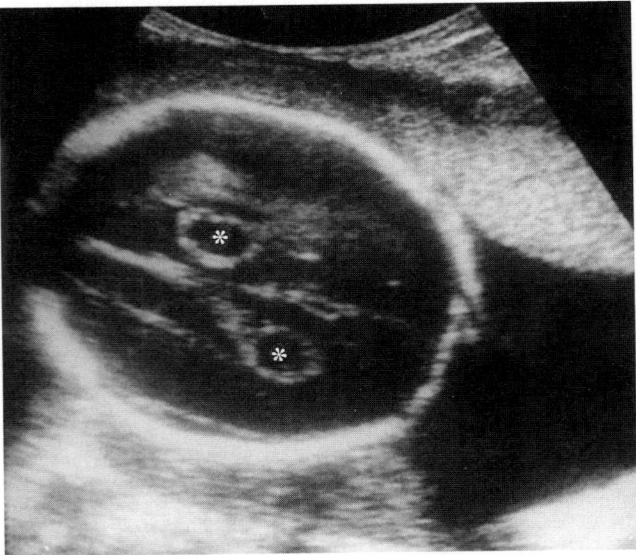

FIGURE 35–29. Bilateral choroid plexus cysts in a second-trimester fetus.

ETIOLOGY

The etiology is unknown.

PATHOLOGY

Although choroid plexus cysts are a frequent finding in antenatal sonography, there are no pathologic studies in the literature. It is commonly assumed that fetal choroid plexus cysts demonstrated with sonography are probably the same entity as the "neuroepithelial" cysts that have been described in autopsy studies of adults (ie, simple fluid-filled cysts lined by normal choroid plexus tissue).[149,150]

PRENATAL DIAGNOSIS

Choroid plexus cysts can be easily demonstrated with sonography (see Fig. 35-29). In most cases, the cyst is single and unilateral. However, bilateral cysts are very frequently seen. Rarely, bizarre clusters of multiple cysts can be found.

PROGNOSIS

Although the pediatric literature indicates that small choroid plexus cysts have no clinical significance, their detection in utero may increase the risk of chromosomal aberrations, and specifically of trisomy 18. However, only limited series are available at present. We have recently reported our preliminary experience with 82 cases.[148] Fetal karyotype was available in 65 and trisomy 18 was found in four (6.2%). The prognosis for infants with isolated choroid plexus cysts is excellent. In our experience, as well as in that of others, most of the cysts detected in the second trimester disappear within the third trimester. Neurologic examination at birth has always been unremarkable. It is of note, however, that a few cases of very large choroid plexus cysts have been reported to be associated with intracranial hypertension and required neurosurgery.[151] Furthermore, choroid plexus cysts are frequently encountered in infants with Sturge-Weber angiomatosis.[152]

OBSTETRIC MANAGEMENT

In our early experience, all cases with choroid plexus cysts and trisomy 18 had associated malformations that were easily detected with ultrasound (congenital heart disease and skeletal abnormalities were the most frequent findings).[148] More recently, we have encountered two fetuses with choroid plexus cysts and trisomy 18 in which ultrasound performed at 16 and 20 weeks' gestation failed to demonstrate abnormalities clearly. We have also seen choroid plexus cysts in one fetus with trisomy 21 and in one fetus with trisomy 20 in mosaic. We were not able to document any difference in the sonographic appearance of the cyst in normal and trisomic fetuses. Disappearance of the cyst documented at serial scans is not reassuring, as this occurred in two cases in our series.

Identification of a choroid plexus cyst is an indication for a careful survey of fetal anatomy. At present, it is controversial whether karyotype determination should be offered to the parents in those cases in which no associated anomalies can be detected. No risk figures can be established at present. However, it is expected that anatomical abnormalities will not be sonographically recognized in all fetuses with trisomy 18. The experience of the sonologist and the gestational age probably will have a major influence with this regard. Furthermore, our experience seems to suggest that a choroid plexus cyst can be found with other chromosomal abnormalities that are inconsistently associated with ultrasound-detectable malformations.

Current experience indicates that in the presence of a normal karyotype the prognosis is excellent. However, serial sonographic examinations are suggested, as a disproportionate increase of the cyst with symptoms of intracranial pressure has been described in rare cases.[150]

CONCLUSIONS

Modern ultrasound equipment has a unique potential for the evaluation of the normal and abnormal fetal central nervous system since very early in pregnancy. A large number of congenital anomalies can be consistently recognized. Criteria for identification of nervous malformations are well established. However, it should be stressed that many uncertainties exist as to parental counseling and obstetrical management. At present, the prognostic figures derived by pediatric studies are used in most instances. It is important to realize that these figures may not apply to the fetus. The natural history of many congenital anomalies is still unknown. Establishing reliable prognostic figures to be applied to affected fetuses and drawing precise guidelines for obstetrical management are one of the priorities for the next decade.

REFERENCES

1. Campbell S, Johnstone FD, Holt EM, et al. Anencephaly: early ultrasonic diagnosis and active management. Lancet 1972;2:1226.
2. Freeman RK, McQuown DS, Secrist LJ, et al. The diagnosis of fetal hydrocephalus before viability. Obstet Gynecol 1977;49:109.
3. Johnson ML, Dunne MG, Mack LA, et al. Evaluation of fetal intracranial anatomy by static and real-time ultrasound. Journal of Clinical Ultrasound 1980;8:311.
4. Fiske CE, Filly RA. Ultrasound evaluation of the normal and abnormal fetal neural axis. Radiol Clin North Am 1982;20:285.
5. Hidalgo H, Bowie J, Rosenberg ER, et al. In utero sonographic diagnosis of fetal cerebral anomalies. Am J Roentgenol 1982;139:143.
6. Jeanty P, Cousaert E, Hobbins JC, et al. A longitudinal study of fetal head biometry. Am J Perinatol 1984;1:118.
7. Goldstein I, Reece EA, Pilu G, et al. Sonographic evaluation of the normal developmental anatomy of the fetal cerebral ventricles. I. The frontal horn. Obstet Gynecol 1988;72:588.
8. Pilu G, Reece EA, Goldstein I, et al. Sonographic evaluation of the normal developmental anatomy of the fetal cerebral ventricles. II. The atria. Obstet Gynecol 1989;73:250.
9. Goldstein I, Reece EA, Pilu G, et al. Sonographic assessment of the fetal frontal lobe: a potential tool for the diagnosis of microcephaly. Am J Obstet Gynecol 1988;158:1057.
10. Goldstein I, Reece EA, Pilu G, et al. Cerebellar measurement using sonography in the evaluation of fetal growth and development. Am J Obstet 1987;156:1065.
11. O'Rahilly R, Gardner E. The developmental anatomy and histology of the human central nervous system. In: Vinken PJ, Bruyn GW, eds. Handbook of clinical neurology. Vol 30. Amsterdam: Elsevier, 1977:15.
12. Crelin ES. Development of the nervous system. A logical approach to neuroanatomy. Clin Symp 1974;26:1.
13. Kier EL. The cerebral ventricles: a phylogenetic and ontogenetic study. In: Newton TH, Potts DG, eds. Radiology of the skull and brain: anatomy and pathology. St Louis: CV Mosby, 1977:2787.
14. Dorovini-Zis K, Dolman CL. Gestational development of brain. Arch Pathol Lab Med 1977;101:192.
15. Tennyson VM, Pappas GD. The fine structure of the developing telencephalic and myelencephalic choroid plexus in the rabbit. J Comp Neurol 1964;123:379.
16. Crade M, Patel J, McQuown D. Sonographic imaging of the glycogen stage of the fetal choroid plexus. Am J Neuroradiol 1981;2:345.
17. Farruggia S. Babcock DS. The cavum septi pellucidi: its appearance and incidence with cranial ultrasonography in infancy. Radiology 1981;139:147.
18. Cerisoli M, Sandri F, Pilu G, et al. Ultrasound recognition of the cavum septi pellucidi and the cavum Vergae in the newborn. J Nucl Med Allied Sci 1984;28:163.
19. Worthen NJ, Gilbertson V, Lau C. Cortical sulcal development seen on sonography: relationship to gestational parameters. J Ultrasound Med 1984;5:163.
20. Lanman JT, Partanen Y, Ullberg S, et al. Extracortical cerebrospinal fluid in normal human fetuses. Pediatrics 1958;21:403.
21. Pilu G, DePalma L, Romero R, et al. The fetal subarachnoid cisterns: an ultrasound study with report of a case of congenital communicating hydrocephalus. J Ultrasound Med 1986;5:365.
22. Mahony BS, Callen PW, Filly RA, et al. The fetal cisterna magna. Radiology 1984;153:773.
23. Myrianthopoulos NC. Epidemiology of central nervous system malformations. In: Vinken PJ, Bruyn GW, eds. Handbook of clinical neurology. Amsterdam: Elsevier, 1977:139.
24. Burton BK. Recurrence risks for congenital hydrocephalus. Clin Genet 1979;16:47.
25. Salam MZ. Stenosis of the aqueduct of Sylvius. In: Vinken PJ, Bruyn GW, eds. Handbook of clinical neurology. Vol 30. Amsterdam: Elsevier, 1977:609.
26. Milhorat TH. Hydrocephalus and the cerebrospinal fluid. Baltimore: Williams & Wilkins, 1972
27. Gutierrez Y, Friede RL, Kaliney AJ. Agenesis of arachnoid granulations and its relationship to communicating hydrocephalus. J Neurosurg 1975;43:553.

28. Ellington G, Margolis G. Block of arachnoid villus by subarachnoid hemorrhage. J Neurosurg 1969;30:651.
29. Kalbag RM, Woolf AL. Cerebral venous thrombosis. London: Oxford University Press, 1967.
30. Gradin WC, Taylor C, Fruin AH. Choroid plexus papilloma: case report and review of the literature. Neurosurgery 1983;12:217.
31. Robertson WC, Gomez MR. External hydrocephalus: early finding in congenital communicating hydrocephalus. Arch Neurol 1978;35:541.
32. Williams B. Is aqueduct stenosis a result of hydrocephalus? Brain 1973;96:399.
33. Brown JR. The Dandy-Walker syndrome. In: Vinken PJ, Bruyn GW, eds. Handbook of clinical neurology. Vol 30. Amsterdam: Elsevier, 1977:623.
34. Hirsch JF, Pierre Kahn A, Reiner D, et al. The Dandy-Walker malformation: a review of 40 cases. J Neurosurg 1984;61:515.
35. Murray JC, Johnson JA, Bird TD. Dandy-Walker malformation: etiologic heterogeneity and empiric recurrence risks. Clin Genet 1985;28:272.
36. Dandy WE. The diagnosis and treatment of hydrocephalus due to occlusion of the foramina of Magendie and Luschka. Surg Gynecol Obstet 1921;32:112.
37. Taggart JK, Walker AE. Congenital atresia of the foramen of Luschka and Magendie. Arch Neurol Psychiatry 1942;48:583.
38. Benda CE. The Dandy-Walker syndrome or the so-called atresia of the foramen Magendie. J Neuropathol Exp Neurol 1954;13:14.
39. Hart MN, Malamud N, Ellis WG. The Dandy-Walker syndrome: a clinico-pathological study based on 28 cases. Neurology 1972;22:771.
40. Gardner WJ, Smith JL, Padget DH. The relationship of Arnold-Chiari and Dandy-Walker malformations. J Neurosurg 1972;36:481.
41. Siedler DE, Filly RA. Relative growth of the higher fetal brain structures. J Ultrasound Med 1987;6:573.
42. Goldstein I, Reece EA, Pilu G, et al. Sonographic evaluation of the normal developmental anatomy of the fetal cerebral ventricles: IV. The posterior horn. Am J Perinatol 1990;7:79
43. Hertzberg BS, Bowie JD, Burger PC, et al. The three lines: origin of sonographic landmarks in the fetal head. American Journal of Roentgenology 1987;149:1009.
44. Chinn DH, Callen PW, Filly RA. The lateral cerebral ventricle in early second trimester. Radiology 1983;148:529.
45. Pilu G, Rizzo N, Orsini LF, et al. Antenatal recognition of cerebral anomalies. Ultrasound Med Biol 1986;12:319.
46. Pilu G, Romero R, De Palma L, et al. Antenatal diagnosis and obstetrical management of Dandy-Walker syndrome. J Reprod Med 1986;31:1017.
47. Guthkelch AN, Riley NA. Influence of aetiology on prognosis in surgically treated infantile hydrocephalus. Arch Dis Child 1969;44:29.
48. McCullough DC, Balzer-Martin LA. Current prognosis in overt neonatal hydrocephalus. J Neurosurg 1982;57:378.
49. Raybaud C, Bamberger-Bozo C, Laffont J, et al. Investigations of nontumoral hydrocephalus in children. Neuroradiology 1978;16:24.
50. Naidich TP, Schott LH, Baron RL. Computed tomography in evaluation of hydrocephalus. Radiol Clin North Am 1982;20:143.
51. Sawaja R, McLaurin RL. Dandy-Walker syndrome: clinical analysis of 23 cases. J Neurosurg 1981;55:89.
52. Yashon D, Jane JA, Sugar O. The course of severe untreated infantile hydrocephalus: prognostic significance of the cerebral mantle. J Neurosurg 1965;23:509.
53. Shurtleff DB, Foltz EL, Loeser JD. Hydrocephalus: a definition of its progression and relationship to intellectual function, diagnosis and complication. Am J Dis Child 1973;125:688.
54. Cochrane DD, Myles ST. Management of intrauterine hydrocephalus. J Neurosurg 1982;57:590.
55. Vintzileos AM, Ingardia CJ, Nochimson DJ. Congenital hydrocephalus: a review and protocol for perinatal management. Obstet Gynecol 1983;62:539.
56. Chervenak FA, Romero R. Is there a role for fetal cephalocentesis in modern obstetrics? Am J Perinatol 1984;1:170.
57. Michejda M, Hodgen GD. In utero diagnosis and treatment of nonhuman primate fetal skeletal anomalies. I. Hydrocephalus. JAMA 1981;246:1093.
58. Manning FA, Harrison MR, Rodeck E, et al. Catheter shunts for fetal hydronephrosis and hydrocephalus. Reports of the International Fetal Surgery Registry. N Engl J Med 1986;315:336.
59. Brocklehurst G. Spina bifida. In: Vinken PJ, Bruyn GW, eds. Handbook of clinical neurology. Vol 30. Amsterdam: Elsevier, 1978:519.
60. Laurence KM, Carter CO, David PA. Major central nervous system malformations in South Wales. I. Incidence, local variations and geographical factors. Br J Prev Soc Med 1968;22:146.
61. Gardner WJ. Myelocele: rupture of the neural tube? Clin Neurosurg 1968;15:57.
62. Lorber J. Systematic ventriculographic studies in infants born with meningomyelocele and encephalocele. The incidence and development of hydrocephalus. Arch Dis Child 1961;36:381.
63. Russell DS, Donald C. The mechanism of internal hydrocephalus in spina bifida. Brain 1935;58:203.
64. Emery JL. Deformity of the aqueduct of Sylvius in children with hydrocefalus and myelomeningocele. Dev Med Child Neurol (Suppl) 1974;32:40.
65. Schulman K. Encephalocele. In: Bergsma D, ed. Birth defect compendium. 2nd ed. New York: Alan R Liss, 1979:390.
66. Cohen MM, Lemire RJ. Syndromes with cephaloceles. Teratology 1982;25:161.
67. Mecke S, Passarge E. Encephalocele, polycystic kidneys and polydactyly as an autosomal recessive trait simulating certain other disorders. The Meckel syndrome. Ann Genet 1971;14:97.
68. Seeds JW, Cefalo RC, Herbert WP. Amniotic band syndrome. Am J Obstet Gynecol 1982;144:243.
69. Brock DJH, Sutcliffe RG. Alphafetoprotein in the antenatal diagnosis of anencephaly and spina bifida. Lancet 1972;2:197.
70. Clarke PC, Gordon YB, Kitau MJ, et al. Screening for fetal neural tube defects by maternal plasma alpha-fetoprotein determination. Br J Obstet Gynaecol 1977;84:568.
71. Haddow JE, Morin ME, Holman MS, et al. Acetylcholinesterase and fetal malformations: modified qualitative technique for diagnosis of neural tube defects. Clin Chem 1981;27:61.
72. United Kingdom Collaborative Study on Alphafetoprotein in Relation to Neural Tube Defects. Maternal serum alpha-fetoprotein measurements in antenatal screening for anencephaly and spina bifida in early pregnancy. Lancet 1977;1:1323.
73. Roberts CJ, Evans KT, Hibbard BM, et al. Diagnostic effectiveness of ultrasound in detection of neural tube defects: the South Wales experience of 2509 scans (1977–1982) in high-risk mothers. Lancet 1983;2:1068.
74. Macri JN, Haddow JE, Weiss RR. Screening for neural tube defects in the United States. A summary of the Scarborough Conference. Am J Obstet Gynecol 1979;133:119.
75. Hobbins JC, Venus I, Tortora M, et al. Stage II ultrasound examination for the diagnosis of fetal abnormalities with an elevated amniotic fluid alpha-fetoprotein concentration. Am J Obstet Gynecol 1982;142:1026.
76. Allen LC, Doran TA, Miskin M, et al. Ultrasound and amniotic fluid alpha-fetoprotein in the prenatal diagnosis of spina bifida. Obstet Gynecol 1982;60:169.

77. Hashimoto BE, Mahony BS, Filly RA, et al. Sonography, a complementary examination to alpha-fetoprotein testing for fetal neural tube defects. J Ultrasound Med 1985;4:307.
78. Cambell S, Pryse-Davies J, Coltart TM, et al. Ultrasound in the diagnosis of spina bifida. Lancet 1975;1:1065.
79. Nicolaides KH, Campbell S, Gabbe SG, et al. Ultrasound screening for spina bifida: cranial and cerebellar signs. Lancet 1986;2:72.
80. Pilu G, Romero R, Reece EA, et al. Subnormal cerebellum in fetuses with spina bifida. Am J Obstet Gynecol 1986;158:1052.
81. Nicolini U, Ferrazzi E, Minonzio M, et al. Prenatal diagnosis of cranial masses by ultrasound: report of five cases. Journal of Clinical Ultrasound 1983;11:170.
82. Lorber J. Results of treatment of myelomeningocele. Dev Med Child Neurol 1971;13:279.
83. Mapstone TB, Rekate HL, Nulsen FE, et al. Relationship of CSF shunting and IQ in children with myelomeningocele: a retrospective analysis. Childs Brain 1984;11:112.
84. Lorber J. The prognosis of occipital encephalocele. Dev Med Child Neurol 1971;13:279.
85. Chervenak FA, Farley MA, Walters L, et al. When is termination of pregnancy during the third trimester morally justifiable? N Engl J Med 1984;310:501.
86. Stark G, Drummond M. Spina bifida as an obstetric problem. Dev Med Child Neurol (Suppl 12) 1970;22:157.
87. Ralis Z, Ralis HM. Morphology of peripheral nerves in children with spina bifida. Dev Med Child Neurol (Suppl 14) 1972;27:109.
88. Ralis ZA. Traumatizing effect of breech delivery on infants with spina bifida. J Pediatr 1975;87:613.
89. Leech RW, Shuman RM. Holoprosencephaly and related midline cerebral anomalies. J Child Neurol 1986;1:3.
90. DeMyer W. Holoprosencephaly. In: Vinken PJ, Bruyn GW, eds. Handbook of clinical neurology. Vol 30. Amsterdam: Elsevier, 1977:431.
91. Matsunaga E, Shiota Y. Holoprosencephaly in human embryos: epidemiological studies of 150 cases. Teratology 1977;16:261.
92. Cohen MM. An update on the holoprosencephalic disorders. J Pediatr 1982;101:865.
93. Roach E, DeMyer W, Palmer K, et al. Holoprosencephaly: birth data, genetic and demographic analysis of 30 families. Birth Defects 1975;11:294.
94. DeMyer W, Zeman W, Palmer CG. The face predicts the brain. Diagnostic significance of median facial anomalies for holoprosencephaly (arhinencephaly). Pediatrics 1964;34:259.
95. Kurtz AB, Wapner RJ, Rubin CS, et al. Ultrasound criteria for in utero diagnosis of microcephaly. Journal of Clinical Ultrasound 1980;8:11.
96. Hill LM, Breckle R, Bonebrake CR. Ultrasonic findings with holoprosencephaly. J Reprod Med 1982;27:172.
97. Blackwell DE, Spinnato JA, Horsch G, et al. Prenatal diagnosis of cyclopia. Am J Obstet Gynecol 1982;143:848.
98. Lev-Gur M, Maklad NF, Patel S. Ultrasonic findings in fetal cyclopia. A case report. J Reprod Med 1983;28:554.
99. Chervenak FA, Isaacson G, Mahoney MJ, et al. The obstetric significance of holoprosencephaly. Obstet Gynecol 1984;63:114.
100. Benacerraf BR, Frigoletto FD, Bieber FR. The fetal face. Ultrasound examination. Radiology 1984;153:495.
101. Filly RA, Chinn DH, Callen PW. Alobar holoprosencephaly. Ultrasonographic prenatal diagnosis. Radiology 1984;151:455.
102. Pilu G, Romero R, Rizzo N, et al. Criteria for the antenatal diagnosis of holoprosencephaly. Am J Perinatol 1987;4:41.
103. Pilu G, Reece EA, Romero R, et al. Prenatal diagnosis of craniofacial malformations by sonography. Am J Obstet Gynecol 1986;155:45.
104. Cayea PD, Balcar I, Alberti O, et al. Prenatal diagnosis of semilobar holoprosencephaly. Am J Roentgenol 1984;142:455.
105. Fitz CR. Holoprosencephaly and related entities. Neuroradiology 1983;25:255.
106. Altman NR, Altman DH, Sheldon JJ, et al. Holoprosencephaly classified by computed tomography. Am J Neuroradiol 1984;5:433.
107. Hoffman-Tretin JC, Horoupian DS, Koenigsberg M, et al. Lobar holoprosencephaly with hydrocephalus: antenatal demonstration and differential diagnosis. J Ultrasound Med 1986;5:691.
108. DeMyer W, Zeman W. Alobar holoprosencephaly (arhinencephaly) with median cleft lip and palate: clinical electroencephalographic and nosologic considerations. Confin Neurol 1963;23:1.
109. Ettlinger G. Agenesis of the corpus callosum. In: Vinken PJ, Bruyn GW, eds. Handbook of clinical Neurology. Vol 30. Amsterdam: Elsevier, 1977:285.
110. Warkany J. Congenital malformations. Notes and comments. Chicago: Year Book Medical Publishers, 1971.
111. Young ID, Trunce JQ, Levene MI, et al. Agenesis of the corpus callosum and macrocephaly in siblings. Clin Genet 1985;28:225.
112. Aicardi J, Lefebvre J, Lerique-Koechlin A. A new syndrome: spasms in flexion, callosal agenesis, ocular abnormalities. Electroencephalogr Clin Neurophysiol 1965;19:609.
113. Andermann F, Andermann E, Joubert M, et al. Familial agenesis of the corpus callosum with anterior horn cell disease. A syndrome of mental retardation, areflexia and paraplegia. Trans Am Neurol Assoc 1972;97:242.
114. Schinzel A. Four patients including two sisters with the acrocallosal syndrome (agenesis of the corpus callosum in combination with preaxial hexadactyly). Hum Genet 1982;62:382.
115. Opitz JM, Kaveggia EG. The FG syndrome. An X-linked recessive syndrome of multiple congenital anomalies and mental retardation. Z Kinderheilk 1974;117:1.
116. Loeser JD, Alvord EC. Agenesis of the corpus callosum. Brain 1968;91:553.
117. Parrsh M, Roessman U, Levinsohn M. Agenesis of the corpus callosum: a study of the frequency of associated malformations. Ann Neurol 1979;6:349.
118. Davidoff LM, Duke CG. Agenesis of the corpus callosum. Its diagnosis by encephalography. Report of 3 cases. American Journal of Roentgenology 1934;32:1.
119. Byrd SE, Harwood-Nash DC, Fitz CR. Absence of the corpus callosum: computed tomographic evaluation in infants and children. J Can Assoc Radiol 1978;29:108.
120. Gebarski SS, Gebarski KS, Bowerman RA, et al. Agenesis of the corpus callosum: sonographic features. Radiology 1984;151:443.
121. Babcock DS. The normal, absent and abnormal corpus callosum: sonographic findings. Radiology 1984;151:449.
122. Comstock CH, Culp D, Gonzalez J, et al. Agenesis of the corpus callosum in the fetus: its evolution and significance. J Ultrasound Med 1985;4:613.
123. Sandri F, Pilu G, Cerisoli M, et al. Sonographic diagnosis of agenesis of the corpus callosum in the fetus and newborn infant. American Journal of Perinatology 1988;5:226.
124. Yakovlev PI, Wadsworth RC. Schizencephalies; a study of the congenital clefts in the cerebral mantle. I. Clefts with fused lips. J Neuropathol Exp Neurol 1946;5:116.
125. Yakovlev PI, Wadsworth RC. Schizencephalies; a study of the congenital clefts in the cerebral mantle. II. Clefts with hydrocephalus and lips separated. J Neuropathol Exp Neurol 1946;5:169.
126. Sauerbrei EE, Cooperberg PL. Cystic tumors of the fetal and

neonatal cerebrum: ultrasound and computed tomographic evaluation. Radiology 1983;147:689.

127. Gross H, Simanyi M. Porencephaly. In: Vinken PJ, Bruyn GW, eds. Handbook of clinical neurology. Vol 30. Amsterdam: Elsevier, 1977:681.
128. Lange-Cossack R. Die Hydranencephalie (Blasehirn) als sanderform der Grobhirnlosigkeit. Arch Psychiatr Nervenkr 1944; 1:117.
129. Johnson EE, Warner M, Simonds JP. Total absence of the cerebral hemispheres. J Pediatr 1951;38:69.
130. Norman RM. Malformation of the nervous system, birth injury and diseases in early life. In: Greenfield JG, eds. Neuropathology. London: Arnold, 1958:23.
131. Aicardi J, Goutieres F, Deverbois AH. Multicystic encephalomalacia of infants and its relation to abnormal gestation and hydranencephaly. J Neurol Sci 1972;15:357.
132. Alsey JH, Allen N, Chamberlin HR. Hydranencephaly. In: Vinken PJ, Bruyn JW, eds. Handbook of clinical neurology. Vol 30. Amsterdam: Elsevier, 1977:661.
133. Halsey JH, Allen N, Chamberlin HR. The chronic decerebrate state of infancy. Arch Neurol 1968;19:339.
134. O'Connell EJ, Feldt RH, Stickler GB. Head circumference, mental retardation and growth failure. Pediatrics 1965;36:62.
135. Book JA, Schut JW, Reed SC. A clinical and genetical study of microcephaly. Am J Ment Defic 1953;57:637.
136. Wimsmuller HF, Koch G. Microzephalie. Erlangen, Germany: Palm and Enke, 1975.
137. Ross JH, Frias JL. Microcephaly. In: Vinken PJ, Bruyn JW, eds. Handbook of clinical neurology. Vol 30. Amsterdam: Elsevier, 1977:507.
138. Winick M, Rosso P. Head circumference and cellular growth of the brain in normal and marasmic children. J Pediatr 1969;74:774.
139. Campbell S, Allan L, Griffin D, et al. The early diagnosis of fetal structural abnormalities. In: Lerski A, Morley P, eds. Ultrasound '82. Oxford, England: Pergamon Press, 1983:547.
140. Hohler CW, Quetal TA. Comparison of ultrasound femur length and biparietal diameter in late pregnancy. Am J Obstet Gynecol 1981;141:759.
141. Chervenak FA, Jeanty P, Cantraine F, et al. The diagnosis of fetal microcephaly. Am J Obstet Gynecol 1984;149:512.
142. Chervenak FA, Rosenberg J, Brightman RC, et al. A prospective study of the accuracy of ultrasound in predicting fetal microcephaly. Obstet Gynecol 1987;69:908.
143. Jaworski M, Hersh JH, Donat J, et al. Computed tomography of the head in the evaluation of microcephaly. Pediatrics 1986;78:1064.
144. Avery GB, Meneses L, Lodge A. The clinical significance of measurement microcephaly. Am J Dis Child 1972;123:214.
145. Martin HP. Microcephaly and mental retardation. Am J Dis Child 1970;119:128.
146. Chudleigh P, Pearce MJ, Campbell S. The prenatal diagnosis of transient cysts of the fetal choroid plexus. Prenat Diagn 1984;4:135.
147. Ricketts NEM, Lowe EM, Patel NB. Prenatal diagnosis of choroid plexus cyst. Lancet 1987;1:213.
148. Gabrielli S, Reece EA, Pilu G, et al. The clinical significance of prenatally diagnosed choroid plexus cysts. Am J Obstet Gynecol 1989;160:1207.
149. Fakhry J, Schechter A, Tenner MS, et al. Cysts of the choroid plexus in neonates. Documentation and review of the literature. J Ultrasound Med 1985;4:561.
150. Shuangshoti S, Netsky MG. Neuroepithelial (colloidal) cysts of the nervous system: further observations on pathogenesis, location, incidence and histochemistry. Neurology (NY) 1966; 16:887.
151. Neblett CR, Robertson JW. Symptomatic cysts of the telencephalic choroid plexus. J Neurol Neurosurg Psychiatr 1971;34:324.
152. Flodmark O. Computed tomography and magnetic resonance imaging of the neonatal central nervous system. In: Levene Mi, Bennett MJ, Punt J, eds. Fetal and neonatal neurology and neurosurgery. London: Churchill Livingstone, 1988:122.

36

CHAPTER

FETAL THORACIC MALFORMATIONS

E. Albert Reece

Fetal thoracic malformations represent a relatively rare group of potentially lethal congenital anomalies. Traditionally, these conditions have received relatively little attention, possibly because they are rare or because sonographic visualization of these structures is complicated by acoustic shadowing of the fetal limbs, making prenatal diagnosis difficult. However, in recent years improvement in real-time ultrasonography has permitted the prenatal diagnosis of a variety of congenital malformations, including thoracic anomalies, and this has led to the increasing interest in this group of developmental abnormalities.

Respiratory tract development begins around the 26th postconceptual day, resulting in formation of the laryngotracheal groove. After the tracheoesophageal folds fuse, the laryngotracheal bud is separated from the foregut. This series of distal branchings from the initial bud results in the formation of the bronchial tree. Although the epithelium of the bronchial system is derived from the endoderm, its connective tissue, muscle, cartilage, and terminal sacs are derived from splanchnic mesenchymal or mesodermal differentiation. The lungs are supplied by two distinct sets of arteries: the pulmonary arteries arising from the right ventricle, and the bronchial arteries derived directly or indirectly from the thoracic aorta. Lymphatic drainage includes both pleural and parenchymal systems, which eventually drain into the thoracic duct system.[1] Aberrant development in the aforementioned sequence of events will result in a variety of malformations, as outlined in Table 36-1.

BRONCHOGENIC CYSTS

ETIOPATHOLOGY

Bronchogenic cysts arise from abnormal budding of the laryngotracheal tube. They often remain attached to the tracheobronchial tree and are found in the area of the trachea, mediastinum, or pulmonary lung tissue.[2] When aberrant budding occurs in early bronchial development, these cysts assume a periesophageal or mediastinal location, as is present in about 30% of cases. If development occurs later, intraparenchymal lesions are observed in about 70% of the cases.[3] These cysts may be single or multiple, contain a mucoid fluid, and are lined by pseudostratified columnar epithelium. The lower lobes are more often involved than the upper lobes; however, right and left lung fields and male and female fetuses are equally affected.[3]

PRENATAL DIAGNOSIS

Sonographic diagnosis of intraparenchymal lesions requires identification of thin-walled sonolucent cysts without associated diaphragmatic defect or echodense septae (Fig. 36-1).[4,5] When these lesions are suspected, other potential defects should be excluded, such as diaphragmatic hernia or macrocystic adenomatoid malformations. If the lesion is mediastinal, a greater challenge may be experienced, because midline lesions such as goiters, teratomas, and vascular malformations must be excluded.[6]

MEDICAL MANAGEMENT AND OUTCOME

Prenatal diagnosis of intrathoracic cysts should not evoke a need for any special medical management. Ultrasound examinations throughout pregnancy are advised in order to look for evidence of hydrops or polyhydramnios. It is most important that these infants be immediately evaluated postnatally so that, if necessary, respiratory assistance can be initiated immediately and medical or surgical management promptly instituted.

Bronchogenic cysts may be well tolerated, especially if they appear as isolated lesions. They can, however, cause postnatal obstruction of bronchioles, leading to

TABLE 36–1. INTRINSIC INTRATHORACIC MALFORMATIONS

Bronchogenic cysts
Isolated
Coexisting cardiac and thoracic anomalies
Congenital cystic adenomatoid malformations
Macrocystic
Microcystic
Bronchopulmonary sequestration
Intralobar
Extralobar
Primary pulmonary hypoplasia (scimitar syndrome)
Congenital pleural effusion (chylothorax/hydrothorax)
Idiopathic
Inheritable (possibly X-linked)

Modified from Reece EA, Lockwood CJ, Rizzo N, Pilu G, Boviccelli L, Hobbins JC. Intrinsic intrathoracic malformations of the fetus: sonographic detection and clinical presentation. Obstet Gynecol 1987;70:627, with permission.

recurrent respiratory tract infection or airway compression.[7] Following surgical excision of these lesions, infants often do very well.[8,9]

CYSTIC ADENOMATOID MALFORMATION

ETIOPATHOLOGY

This is a unilateral hamartoma that usually presents during the first day of life, often as a serious respiratory emergency. These patients present clinically in three ways: stillborn, or neonatal or perinatal death; progressive respiratory distress in the newborn; and acute or chronic pulmonary infection in the older infant and child.[10–12] Associated fetal anasarca and maternal polyhydramnios have been emphasized in the literature as characteristically associated antepartum features of this lesion.[13–18]

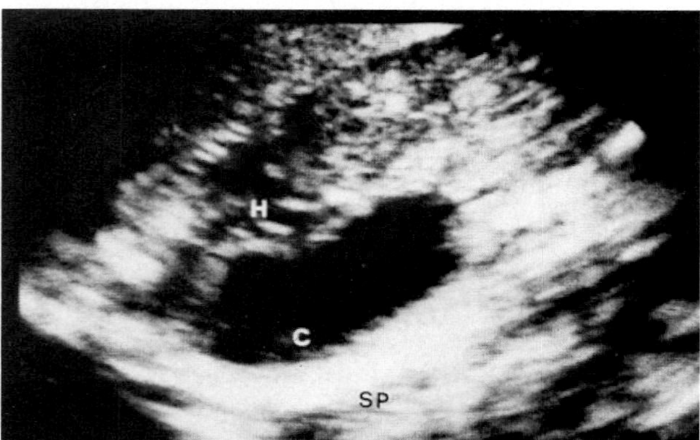

FIGURE 36–1. Bronchogenic cyst. Longitudinal section of the fetal chest demonstrating a large unilocular cyst (C) posterior to the heart (H). Spine (SP) is located posterior to the cyst. (From Reece EA, Lockwood CJ, Rizzo N, Pilu G, Bovicelli L, Hobbins JC. Intrinsic intrathoracic malformations of the fetus: sonographic detection and clinical presentation. Obstet Gynecol 1987; 70: 628.)

Cystic adenomatoid malformations result from abnormal induction of surrounding mesenchymal differentiation by the ramifying bronchial buds, leading to the overgrowth of bronchioles with adjacent but noncommunicating alveolar ducts and sacs. There are two subtypes based on variations in size: the macrocystic variety, which contains single or multiple cysts of 5 mm or greater in diameter, and the microcystic type, which is predominantly solid cysts, generally smaller than 5 mm in diameter.[21] Males show a slight predominance, but no significant racial predilection is seen. This lesion also occurs equally in term and preterm births, and with equal frequency in the right and left lung. Both single- and multiple-lobe involvement have been described.[19,20]

Typical morphologic and pathologic features of cystic adenomatoid malformations have been described.[21,22] This lesion has been categorized into three subtypes. Type I typically has one large cystic cavity with trabeculations of the wall, with smaller cavities adjacent to normal lung parenchyma. In Type II, there are multiple small cysts of up to 1 cm in diameter. Type III is predominantly solid. All three types share common histologic features: an adenomatoid increase in terminal bronchiolar structures; a polypoid configuration of the cuboidal/columnar epithelium lining the cystic structures; an increase in elastic tissue in areas lined by cuboidal/columnar epithelium, often associated with polypoid projections; and absence of inflammation.

There is aberrant lymphatic drainage with this lesion, resulting in pleural effusion and hydrops.[16,20,23] Progressive worsening of this disorder with increased fluid accumulation would enhance the likelihood of pulmonary hypoplasia.[24]

Polyhydramnios is a commonly associated feature of cystic adenomatoid malformations resulting from either esophageal obstruction or excessive lung fluid production. There has also been an association between maternal hydramnios and fetal anasarca.[13,15–17] The reported incidence of maternal hydramnios occurring in association with cystic adenomatoid malformation varies from 30%[21] to as much as 80%.[25] Miller reported a 15% incidence of cases with both hydrops and hydramnios, of which nearly 50% were stillborn.[21] This increased amniotic fluid may be secondary to either excess secretion by the abnormal lung or decreased absorption by the malformed or hypoplastic adjacent lung. Alternately, obstruction of the esophagus by the expanding chest mass could interfere with fetal absorption of amniotic fluid.[25] Fetal hydrops could also be caused by lymphatic obstruction of the mass or by direct compression of the heart by the expanding lesion, resulting in a decrease in the cardiac output. It has been reported, however, that as much as 65% of patients with cystic adenomatoid malformations remain asymptomatic during the perinatal period.[26] Unfortunately, such a determination cannot be made prospectively.

PRENATAL DIAGNOSIS

Prenatal diagnosis of macrocystic tumors requires identifying small peripheral cysts (Fig. 36-2). The microcystic variety poses more of a challenge and appears as an echodense mass replacing the lung (Fig. 36-3). Both types may result in a significant shift of the mediastinum with cardiac displacement.[6,18,27]

Type III cystic adenomatoid malformations have been described previously. In one report, a fetus presented at 32 weeks gestation with polyhydramnios and an abnormally thick hydropic placenta. The lung was described as voluminous, with the heart displaced to the right. The echogenicity was consistent with that of a solid organ. Autopsy and histologic examination confirmed Type III congenital cystic adenomatoid malformation.[28] In another report, Garrett and colleagues described the sonographic appearance of the Type III lesion to be very echogenic.[29] Despite these two cases with seemingly characteristic sonographic features, such lesions could be mistaken for a solid tumor or even other lung lesions, such as extralobar pulmonary sequestration. The finding of a solid, space-occupying lung lesion with gross mediastinal shift and often associated with maternal polyhydramnios and fetal hydrops but without other detectable associated anomalies should raise the possibility of congenital cystic adenomatoid malformation.

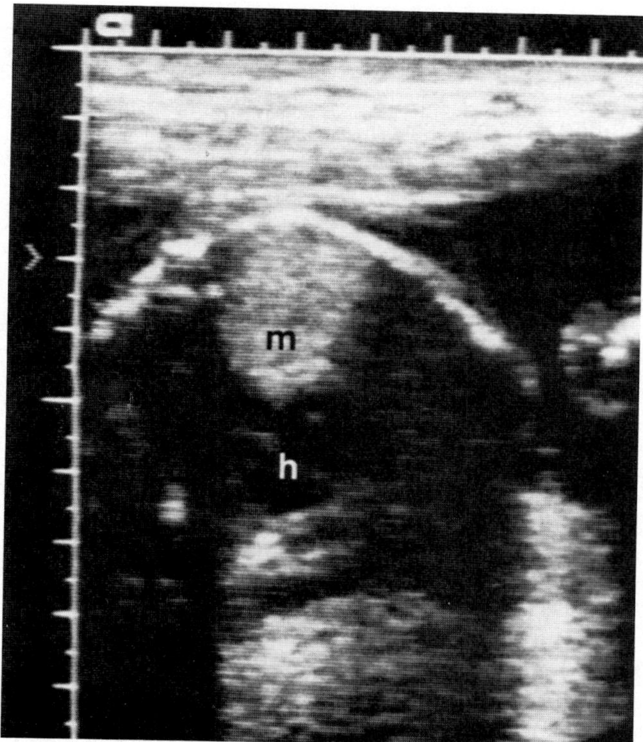

FIGURE 36–3. Microcystic adenomatoid malformation. Transverse section of the fetus demonstrating an echodense mass (m) filling the right hemithorax. The mediastinum and heart (h) are deviated to the left. (From Reece EA, Lockwood CJ, Rizzo N, Pilu G, Bovicelli L, Hobbins JC. Intrinsic intrathoracic malformations of the fetus: sonographic detection and clinical presentation. Obstet Gynecol 1987; 70: 631.)

MEDICAL MANAGEMENT AND OUTCOME

Respiratory distress and cyanosis are the common initial signs in the vast majority of children born with cystic adenomatoid malformation.[30] The respiratory distress is believed to be due to compression and displacement of the normal pulmonary tissue, and the pressure caused by the cyst is associated with pulmonary hypoplasia.[10,31,32]

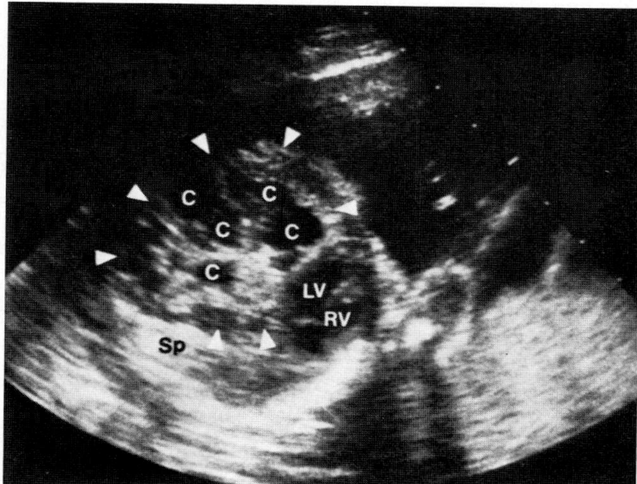

FIGURE 36–2. Macrocystic adenomatoid malformation. Transverse section through the fetal thorax demonstrating dextrorotation of the fetal heart (LV, left ventricle; RV, right ventricle) caused by a large, multilocular cystic mass (C) (outlined by arrowheads). Spine (SP) is located posteriorly. (Romero R, Chervenak FA, Kotzen J, et al. Antenatal sonographic findings of extralobar pulmonary sequestrations. J Ultrasound Med 1982; 1: 131.)

Management will depend on the time of diagnosis and the presence or absence of hydrops or polyhydramnios. For example, in the absence of hydrops or polyhydramnios, the outcome is quite good. In these cases, repeated thoracentesis has been shown to improve the chance of survival.[20] The fetus, however, that is anomalous and has hydrops or associated polyhydramnios has an extremely poor prognosis.[13,25,33] Therefore, if the diagnosis is made prior to 24 weeks, in light of the poor performance of these fetuses termination of the pregnancy may be advised. Conversely, for diagnoses made after 24 weeks with hydrops or polyhydramnios, a nonaggressive neonatal approach may be recommended.

Because associated anomalies are rare and the malformations are almost always unilateral, the afflicted infant without hydrops or other anomalies presents the surgeon with an opportunity to cure a congenital lesion which, if neglected, results either in death or protracted infirmity due to infection.[33]

The prognosis is better for patients with the macrocystic variety, who have an overall survival rate as high as 70% compared to 20% with the microcystic lesion.[20] Fetuses without associated anomalies, hydrops, or pulmonary hypoplasia tend to have a better outcome.[13,33] The survival rate for the Type I lesion is 69%, whereas the mortality rate for Type III has been almost 100%. The mortality rate for the latter appears to be related to the extreme mediastinal shift associated with circulatory and respiratory embarrassment.[34]

Almost all infants with congenital adenomatoid malformation have respiratory distress. It has been reported by Madewell and associates that about two thirds of affected infants have onset of respiratory distress on the first day of life, but about one quarter may remain asymptomatic for a week or longer.[35] Respiratory functions compromised by pulmonary hypoplasia or by compression of the thoracic viscera can result in heart failure.[36]

There is a tendency for this cystic mass to expand progressively after birth, leading to air trapping.[12,33] Immediate surgical decompression, the treatment of choice, has been shown to be well tolerated by infants.[27] Survival depends on both the extent of the hypoplasia and the state of lung maturation.[14]

Ueda and colleagues reported a case of asymptomatic congenital cystic adenomatoid lung malformation discovered at 18 months.[37] Subsequently, a small embryonal rhabdomyosarcoma was diagnosed in this lesion. This case represents one of the few cases of a malignant tumor arising within a congenital malformation.

BRONCHOPULMONARY SEQUESTRATION

ETIOPATHOLOGY

Bronchopulmonary sequestration is a rare congenital thoracic defect in which a systemic artery supplies an accessory or dysplastic segment of lung that may be anatomically distinct from the remainder of the lobe (extralobar) or may be included in the substance of the lung, in which case it may or may not have bronchial communication with the rest of the bronchial tree.[38–40]

The sequestration of pulmonary tissue has been defined by Potter as masses of pulmonary tissue that have no communication with the bronchial tree. Within the subgroups there are three types:

1. Intralobar, that is, part of the lobe of a lung
2. Extralobar, that is, a separate lobe still attached to the main pulmonary mass
3. Complete sequestration, that is, entirely independent of the lungs.[38,41]

Intralobar bronchopulmonary sequestrations are confined within the visceral pleura with adjacent normal lung tissue and venous drainage, which goes into the left atrium.[1] This form is generally located basally and vertebrally. Either side of the lung is involved with similar frequency. The lower lobes are affected in about 98% of cases. The arterial supply is generally from the thoracic aorta, whereas the pulmonary veins almost always drain this lesion.[39,42] The extralobar type are enclosed within their own pleura and drain into the right atrium.[43] The latter is the most common variety observed in newborns. Approximately 90% of extralobar lesions reside in the posterior left costaphrenic sulcus.[2] The arterial supply and venous drainage are primarily from the systemic vessels.[44,46] In contrast to the intralobar variety, which may be either cystic or solid in appearance, the extralobar type tends to resemble normal lung tissue.[2,46] Rarely do sequestrations of both types coexist involving an entire lung or occurring bilaterally.[47,48]

Although the pathogenesis of these lesions remains obscure, a spectrum of anatomical variables may be associated with this lesion:

1. A sequestered mass of pulmonary parenchyma may exist within or outside the visceral pleura of the ipsilateral normal lung.
2. The arterial supply may be from a systemic or a pulmonary artery or both.
3. The venous drainage may be to a systemic or a pulmonary vein or both.
4. Communication with the gastrointestinal tract may or may not be present.
5. The diaphragm may or may not be defective.[38,45,49]

Some investigators call attention to the aberrant systemic artery and the developing bronchial bud that sequesters this from the rest of the respiratory tract.[1,45,49,50] There appears also to be a slight male preponderance, and the left lung field is more commonly involved.[38,43,44,51]

PRENATAL DIAGNOSIS

Sonographic prenatal diagnosis of either form (intralobar or extralobar), although possible, may be difficult and requires a certain degree of sophistication.[52] The extralobar lesion may present as a discrete, echodense lesion in the left costaphrenic sulcus (Fig. 36-4). Prenatal diagnosis of the intralobar variety does not seem feasible at this time.[1]

MEDICAL MANAGEMENT AND OUTCOME

As we have described in previous sections, lung masses of significant size associated with or without pleural effusion and diagnosed prior to 24 weeks tend to have a poor outcome. Therefore, pregnancy termination may be offered in such circumstances. Of course, adequate diagnosis and workup will be necessary in order to provide appropriate counseling. If this diagnosis is made after 24 weeks, the prognosis would be related to

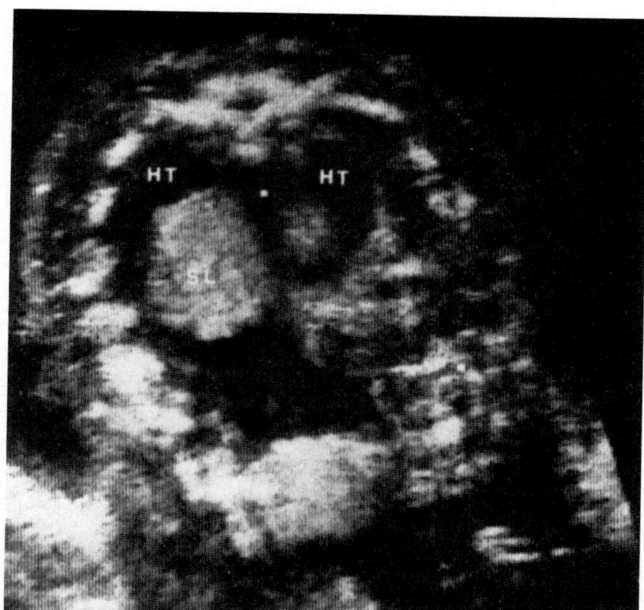

FIGURE 36–4. Bronchopulmonary sequestration. Transverse section through the fetal thorax demonstrating sequestered extralobar lung segment (SL) and hydrothorax (HT). (Romero R, Chervenak FA, Kotzen J, et al. Antenatal sonographic findings of extralobar pulmonary sequestrations. J Ultrasound Med 1982; 1: 131.)

whether or not there is polyhydramnios, pleural effusion, fetal hydrops, or mediastinal shift.

Fetal outcome in the presence of the above complications is uniformly poor, with mortality rates as high as 100%.[53]

PRIMARY PULMONARY HYPOPLASIA (THE SCIMITAR SYNDROME)

ETIOPATHOLOGY

Primary pulmonary hypoplasia is a very rare thoracic anomaly characterized by total anomalous pulmonary venous drainage with connection to the left innominate vein by a vertical or scimitar vein.[1]

This pulmonary malformation is frequently associated with hypoplasia of the right lung with bronchial anomalies, dextroposition or dextrorotation of the heart, hypoplasia of the right pulmonary artery, and anomalous systemic arterial supply to the lower lobe of the right lung directly from the aorta or its main branches. Neill and associates coined the term "scimitar syndrome" to describe this complex of defects.[54]

Associated findings include hypoplasia of the right lung, vertical scimitar vein, bronchial anomalies, hypoplasia of the right pulmonary artery, and anomalous subdiaphragmatic systemic arterial supply to the lower lobe of the right lung.[55,56]

PRENATAL DIAGNOSIS

Sonographic diagnosis may be suspected with the identification of severe dextrocardia, mediastinal shift, or intrinsic cardiac defects.

MEDICAL MANAGEMENT AND OUTCOME

If such a diagnosis is suspected and there are other congenital anomalies, the option of pregnancy termination may be advised. For example, cardiac defects, most commonly ventricular septal defects, frequently coexist and may significantly influence the prognosis. In general, the prognosis is poor.[1,55]

CONGENITAL CHYLOTHORAX

ETIOPATHOLOGY

Although pleural effusions are unusual during fetal or even early neonatal life, chylothorax is the most common form of thoracic effusion encountered in the prenatal period.[2,57,58] This disorder occurs at an incidence of 1 in 10,000, with males affected twice as commonly as females.[2] About 60% of effusions appear on the right, but occasionally bilateral collection of fluid occurs.[2,57,59–61] Chylothorax represents accumulation within the pleural cavity of a fluid called chyle, which is clear, with abundant lymphocytes of about 60% (Table 36-2).[2,62,63]

The cause of chylothorax is unknown. Some investigators have indicated that this disorder may result from rupture or failed fusion of the thoracic lymphatic channels.[7,10,64] Chylothorax has also been reported in the presence of monosomy X or trisomy 21, or occurring in each male offspring within families, indicating a possible X-linked inheritance.[10,62,65,66]

TABLE 36–2. CONGENITAL CHYLOTHORAX

Characteristics of chyle
Milky appearance
Separated into two distinct layers on standing
Clear when fat is extracted by alkali and ether
Most of the fat present is neutral fat
Odorless
Sterile
Bacteria static
Alkaline reaction
Fat content 0.4 to 4 grams per 100 mL
Specific gravity greater than 1.012
Protein content generally between 1.0 and 6 grams per 100 mL

From Diwan RV, Brennan JN, Philipson EH, Jain S, Bellon EM. Ultrasonic prenatal diagnosis of type III congenital cystic adenomatoid malformation of lung. J Clin Ultrasound 1983;11:218, with permission.

PRENATAL DIAGNOSIS

Sonographic findings include unilateral or rarely bilateral effusion, with or without collapsed lungs (Fig. 36-5).[60] It should be pointed out, however, that these sonographic findings are indistinguishable from nonchylothorax effusion. Thoracentesis has been used to demonstrate a marked lymphocytosis, with the fluid remaining clear before birth but becoming cloudy neonatally following feeding.[2] The precise prenatal diagnosis using these hematologic indices remains unsettled.[61,63,66–68]

Tachypnea, retractions, and cyanosis occur with many pulmonary disorders in the newborn. When these symptoms occur in association with maternal polyhydramnios, the diagnosis of spontaneous chylothorax should be considered.[65]

MEDICAL MANAGEMENT AND OUTCOME

In Brodman's analysis of 34 cases, 64% were symptomatic within 24 hours of birth, and there was a predominance of males. Only three effusions were bilateral, and no correlations could be found among the type of labor or mode of delivery, birth weight, onset of symptoms, site of infusion, or onset of respiratory distress.[69,70]

Management depends on the severity of the disorder and the gestational age at which it is identified. As indicated previously, chylothorax may be associated with chromosomal abnormalities. Therefore, if this lesion is identified prior to 24 weeks, karyotypic analysis ought to be conducted and appropriate counseling given based on the laboratory results. The accumulation of fluid before 24 weeks might adversely affect lung development and, therefore, might lead to pulmonary hypoplasia and neonatal death, even in the otherwise normal fetus. If the diagnosis is made at or beyond 24 weeks, such fetuses should be managed expectantly.[35] Thoracentesis should be performed as fluid accumulation increases.[58,64,65,71,72] In our experience, such procedures might prevent the development of pulmonic hypoplasia.

Spontaneous resolution of these effusions is rare, so the prognosis for these fetuses, especially when this condition occurs early in pregnancy, is poor. Mortality statistics range from 15% to 50%.[66,69,73] Fetuses, however, that survive the initial neonatal period might expect to have resolution of chylothorax with surgical ligation of the thoracic duct.[58,65]

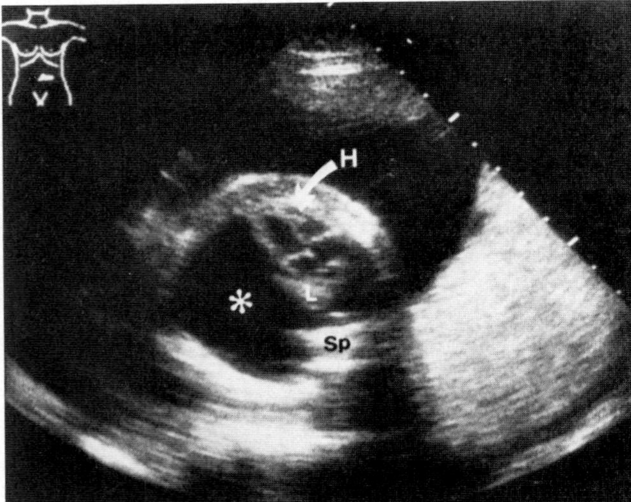

FIGURE 36–5. Chylothorax/hydrothorax. Transverse section of the fetal thorax demonstrating the fetal heart (H), lung (L), and spine (Sp). Fluid surrounding the heart (*) represents idiopathic hydrothorax or chylothorax. (Romero R, Pilu G, Ghidini A, et al. Prenatal diagnosis of congenital anomalies. Norwalk, CT: Appleton & Lange, 1987: 196.)

REFERENCES

1. Reece EA, Lockwood CJ, Rizzo N, Pilu G, Boviccelli L, Hobbins JC. Intrinsic intrathoracic malformations of the fetus: sonographic detection and clinical presentation. Obstet Gynecol 1987;70:627.
2. Ryckman FC, Rosenkrants JG. Thoracic surgical problems in infancy and childhood. Surg Clin North Am 1955;65:1423.
3. Rogers LF, Osmer JC. Bronchogenic cyst. A review of 46 cases. AJR 1964;91:273.
4. Lebrun D, Avni EF, Goolaaerts JP, et al. Prenatal diagnosis of a pulmonary cyst by ultrasonography. Eur J Pediatr 1985;144:399.
5. Mayden KL, Tortora M, Chervenak FA, et al. The antenatal sonographic detection of lung masses. Am J Obstet Gynecol 1984;148:349.
6. Newnham JP, Crues JV, Vinstein AL, et al. Sonographic diagnosis of thoracic gastroenteric cyst in utero. Prenat Diagn 1984;4:467.
7. Eraklis AJ, Griscom NT, McGovern JB. Bronchogenic cysts of the mediastinum in infancy. N Engl J Med 1969;281:1150.
8. Ramenofsky ML, Leape LL, McCauley RGK. Bronchogenic cyst. J Pediatr Surg 1979;14:219.
9. Bower RJ, Kiesewetter WB. Mediastinal masses in infants and children. Arch Surg 1977;112:1003.
10. Randolph JG, Gross RE. Congenital chylothorax. Arch Surg 1957;74:405.
11. Frenckner B, Freyschuss U. Pulmonary function after lobectomy for congenital lobar emphysema and congenital cystic adenomatoid malformation: a follow-up study. Scand J Thorac Cardiovasc Surg 1982;16:293.
12. Moncrieff MW, Cameron AH, Astley R, et al. Congenital cystic adenomatoid malformation of the lung. Thorax 1969;24:476.
13. Kohler HG, Rymer BA. Congenital cystic malformation of the lung and its relation to hydramnios. J Obstet Gynaecol Br Commonwealth 1973;80:130.
14. Aslam PA, Korones SB, Richardson RL, et al. Congenital cystic adenomatoid malformation with anasarca. JAMA 1970;212:622.
15. Glaves J, Baker JL. Spontaneous resolution of maternal hydramnios in congenital cystic adenomatoid malformation of the lung. Antenatal ultrasound features. Case report. Br J Obstet Gynaecol 1983;90:1065.

16. Johnson JA, Rumack CM, Johnson ML, et al. Cystic adenomatoid malformation: Antenatal demonstration. AJR 1984;142:483.
17. Harvey JG, Houlsby W, Sherman K, et al. Congenital chylothorax: report of unique case associated with "H"-type tracheoesophageal fistula. J Surg 1979;66:485.
18. Haller JA, Golladay ES, Pickard LR, et al. Surgical management of lung bud anomalies: lobar emphysema, bronchogenic cyst, cystic adenomatoid malformation, and intralobar pulmonary sequestration. Ann Thorac Surg 1979;28:33.
19. Fisher JE, Nelson ST, Allen JE, Holzman RS. Congenital cystic adenomatoid malformation of the lung. A unique variant. Am J Dis Child 1982;136:1071.
20. Adzick NS, Harrison MR, Glick PL, et al. Fetal cystic adenomatoid malformation: prenatal diagnosis and natural history. J Pediatr Surg 1985;20:483.
21. Miller RK, Sieber WK, Unis EJ. Congenital adenomatoid malformation of the lung. Pathol Annu 15 [Part 1] 1980;387.
22. Stocker JT, Madewell JE, Drake RM. Congenital cystic adenomatoid malformation of the lung. Classification and morphologic spectrum. Hum Pathol 1977;8:155.
23. Graham D, Winn K, Dex W, et al. Prenatal diagnosis of cystic adenomatoid malformation of the lung. J Ultrasound Med 1982;1:9.
24. Knochel JQ, Lee TG, Melendez MG, et al. Fetal anomalies involving the thorax and abdomen. Radiol Clin North Am 1982;20:297.
25. Oestoer AG, Fortune DW. Congenital cystic adenomatoid malformation of the lung. Am J Clin Pathol 1978;70:595.
26. Wolfe SA, Hertzler JH, Philippart AO. Cystic adenomatoid display of the lung. J Pediatr Surg 1980;15:925.
27. Stauffer UG, Salvoldelli G, Mieth D. Antenatal ultrasound diagnosis in cystic adenomatoid malformation of the lung: case report. J Pediatr Surg 1984;19:141.
28. Cave APD, Adam AE. Cystic adenomatoid malformation of the lung (Stocker Type III) found on antenatal ultrasound examination. Br J Radiol 1984;57:176.
29. Garrett WJ, Kossoff G, Lawrence R. Gray scale echography in the diagnosis of hydrops due to fetal lung tumor. J Clin Ultrasound 1975;3:45.
30. Sawyer DR, Mosadomi A. A case of congenital cystic adenomatoid malformation of the lung with associated anomalies. Afr J Med 1980;26:220.
31. Cachia R, Sobonya RE. Congenital cystic adenomatoid malformation of the lung with bronchial atresia. Hum Pathol 1981;12:947.
32. Birdsell DC, Wentworth P, Reilly BJ, et al. Congenital cystic adenomatoid malformation of the lung: a report of eight cases. Can J Surg 1966;9:350.
33. Halloran LG, Silverberg SG, Salzberg AM. Congenital cystic adenomatoid malformation of the lung. Arch Surg 1972;104:715.
34. Diwan RV, Brennan JN, Philipson EH, Jain S, Bellon EM. Ultrasonic prenatal diagnosis of type III congenital cystic adenomatoid malformation of lung. J Clin Ultrasound 1983;11:218.
35. Madewell JE, Stocker JT, Korsower JM. Cystic adenomatoid malformation of the lung. AJR 1975;124:436.
36. Donn SM, Martin JN Jr, White SJ. Antenatal ultrasound findings in cystic adenomatoid malformation. Pediatr Radiol 1981; 10:180.
37. Ueda K, Gruppo R, Unger F, et al. Rhabdomyosarcoma of lung arising in congenital cystic adenomatoid malformation. Cancer 1977;40:383.
38. Khalil KG, Kilman JW. Pulmonary sequestration. J Thorac Cardiovasc Surg 1975;70:928.
39. Sade RM, Clouse M, Ellis FH Jr. The spectrum of pulmonary sequestration. Ann Thorac Surg 1974;18:644.
40. Choplin RH, Siegel MJ. Pulmonary sequestration: six unusual presentations. AJR 1980;134:695.
41. Horowitz RN. Extralobar sequestration of lung in newborn infant. Am J Dis Child 1965;110:195.
42. Savic B, Birtell FJ, Tholen W, et al. Lung sequestration: report of seven cases and review of 540 published cases. Thorax 1979;34:96.
43. Kilman JW, Battersby JS, Taybi H, et al. Pulmonary sequestration. Arch Surg 1965;90:648.
44. Carter R. Pulmonary sequestration. Ann Thorac Surg 1969;7:68.
45. Demos NJ, Teresi A. Congenital lung malformations. A unified concept and a case report. J Thorac Cardiovasc Surg 1975;70:260.
46. Buntain WL, Woolley MM, Mahour GH, et al. Pulmonary sequestration in children: a twenty-five year experience. Surgery 1977;81:413.
47. Jona JZ, Raffensperger JG. Total sequestration of the right lung. J Thorac Cardiovasc Surg 1975;69:361.
48. Wimbish KJ, Agha FP, Brady TM. Bilateral pulmonary sequestration: computed tomographic appearance. AJR 1983;140:689.
49. Iwai K, Shindo G, Hajikano H, et al. Intralobar pulmonary sequestration, with special reference to developmental pathology. Am Rev Respir Dis 1973;107:911.
50. Pryce D. Lower accessory pulmonary artery with intralobar sequestration of lung: a report of seven cases. J Pathol 1946;58:457.
51. Stocker JT, Kagan-Hallet K. Extralobar pulmonary sequestration. Analysis of 15 cases. Am J Clin Pathol 1979;72:917.
52. Romero R, Chervenak, Kotzen J, et al. Findings of extralobar pulmonary sequestrian. J Clin Ultrasound 1986;5:283.
53. Weiner C, Varner M, Pringle K, et al. Antenatal diagnosis and palliative treatment of nonimmune hydrops fetalis secondary to pulmonary extralobar sequestration. Obstet Gynecol 1986; 68:275.
54. Neill CA, et al. The familial occurrence of hypoplastic right lung with systemic arterial supply and venous drainage: scimitar syndrome. The Bulletin of Johns Hopkins Hospital 1960;107:1.
55. Jue KL, Amplatz K, Adams P, et al. Anomalies of great vessels associated with lung hypoplasia. Am J Dis Child 1966;11:35.
56. Mathey J, Galey JJ, Logeais Y, et al. Anomalous pulmonary venous return into inferior vena cava and associated bronchovascular anomalies (the scimitar syndrome). Report of three cases and review of the literature. Thorax 1968;23:398.
57. Doolittle WM, Ohmart D, Egan EA. Congenital bilateral pleural effusions. A cause for respiratory failure in the newborn. Am J Dis Child 1973;125:435.
58. Andersen EA, Hertel J, Pedersen SA, et al. Congenital chylothorax: management by ligature of the thoracic duct. Scand J Thorac Cardiovasc Surg 1984;18:193.
59. Yancy WS, Spock A. Spontaneous neonatal plural effusion. J Pediatr Surg 1967;2:313.
60. Defoort P, Thiery M. Antenatal diagnosis of congenital chylothorax by gray scale sonography. J Clin Ultrasound 1978;6:47.
61. Petres RE, Redwine FO, Cruikshank DP. Congenital bilateral chylothorax. Antepartum diagnosis and successful intrauterine surgical management. JAMA 1982;248:1360.
62. Yoss BS, Lipsitz PJ. Chylothorax in two mongoloid infants. Genet 1977;12:357.
63. Lange IR, Manning FA. Antenatal diagnosis of congenital pleural effusions. Am J Obstet Gynecol 1981;140:839.
64. Perry RE, Hodgman J, Cass AB. Pleural effusion in the neonatal period. J Pediatr 1963;62:838.
65. Van Aerde J, Campbell AN, Smyth JA, et al. Spontaneous chylothorax in newborns. Am J Dis Child 1984;138:961.
66. Chernick V, Reed MH. Pneumothorax and chylothorax in the neonatal period. J Pediatr 1970;76:624.

67. Jaffa AJ, Barak S, Kaysar N, et al. Case report. Antenatal diagnosis of bilateral congenital chylothorax with pericardial effusion. Acta Obstet Gynecol Scand 1985;64:455.

68. Thomas DB, Anderson JC. Antenatal detection of fetal pleural effusions and neonatal management. Med J Aust 1979;2:435.

69. Brodman RF. Congenital chylothorax. Recommendations for treatment. NY J Med 1975;553.

70. Koffler H, Papile LA, Burstein RL. Congenital chylothorax: two cases associated with maternal polyhydramnios. Am J Dis Child 1978;132:638.

71. Benacerraf BR, Frigoletto FD. Mid-trimester fetal thoracentesis. J Clin Ultrasound 1985;13:202.

72. Benacerraf BR, Frigoletto FD, Wilson M. Successful midtrimester thoracentesis with analysis of the lymphocyte population in the pleural effusion. Am J Obstet Gynecol 1986;155:398.

73. Jouppila P, Kirkinen P, Herva R, et al. Prenatal diagnosis of pleural effusions by ultrasound. J Clin Ultrasound 1983;11:516.

37

CHAPTER

PRENATAL DIAGNOSIS OF CARDIOVASCULAR ANOMALIES

Gianluigi Pilu

INCIDENCE AND ETIOLOGY OF CONGENITAL HEART DISEASE

Congenital heart defects (CHD) are among the most frequent malformations encountered at birth. They are currently estimated to occur in 8% to 9% of live births,[1,2] and an even higher frequency has been documented in spontaneous abortions.[3] Spontaneous selection of fetuses with severe CHD, chromosomal aberrations, or multiple anomalies most likely accounts for the discrepancy between prenatal and postnatal series.

Congenital heart disease probably results from a wide variety of causes. Chromosomal aberrations are found in 4% to 5%. Mendelian transmission and environmental factors have been documented, but they probably account for only a minority of cases. An unusually high frequency of cardiac anomalies has been reported recently in children of mothers with CHD. These observations have prompted the hypothesis that cytoplasmic inheritance or teratogens may play a major role in the etiology of CHD. Table 37-1 reports the recurrence risks of CHD that are suggested by Nora and Nora. The interested reader is referred to the many publications on this complex subject.[4,5]

This chapter reviews prenatal diagnosis of CHD. The categorization and nomenclature of cardiac anomalies that we have adopted follows the approach suggested by Becker and Anderson.[6] Tentative guidelines for obstetric management, based on the experience of the author and on the current literature, have been suggested. However, at the time of writing, prenatal diagnosis of CHD has been formulated in only a limited number of cases. Increasing experience may modify some of these views in the near future.

THE TECHNIQUE OF FETAL ECHOCARDIOGRAPHY

Sonography has been used for the investigation of the fetal heart since the early 1970s,[7–9] although detailed and reproducible examinations of the fetal heart were not possible until the late 1970s, when high-resolution real-time ultrasound apparatuses were introduced into clinical practice. At present, fetal echocardiography is a well-established technique for the prenatal diagnosis of CHD.[10–13] However, the use of this technique is not yet widespread, as it requires both a very experienced operator and meticulous scanning. Therefore, fetal echocardiography is necessarily used only in a selected number of pregnancies carrying a higher than normal risk of fetal cardiac anomalies. A tentative list of indications is reported in Table 37-2. However, although at present detailed cardiac scanning is not recommended in all pregnancies, the use of some views of the heart during routine sonographic evaluation of fetal anatomy has been advocated. The use of such views—the four-chamber view being the most representative example[12]—is a reasonable compromise between screening the entire obstetric population and entirely ignoring the fetal heart during obstetric ultrasound examination.

By using a high-frequency transducer (5 to 7 MHz), the main cardiac connections can be consistently imaged starting from 14 weeks of gestation. From a technical point of the view, however, the optimal time for fetal echocardiography is between 20 and 26 weeks. In later gestation, increasing calcification of the fetal ribs and relative decrease in amniotic fluid volume hinder the examination, and it is rare that this can be satisfyingly accomplished at term.

TABLE 37–1. RECURRENCE RISKS OF CONGENITAL HEART DISEASE

DEFECT	RECURRENCE RISKS (PERCENTAGE) ONE SIBLING AFFECTED*	FATHER AFFECTED†	MOTHER AFFECTED†
Aortic stenosis	2	3	13–18
Atrial septal defect	2.5	1.5	4–4.5
Atrioventricular canal	2	1	14
Coarctation	2	2	4
Patent ductus arteriosus	3	2.5	3.5–4
Pulmonary stenosis	2	2	4–6.5
Tetralogy of Fallot	2.5	1.5	2.5
Ventricular septal defect	3	2	6–10

*Data derived from Nora JJ, Nora AH. Genetics and counseling in cardiovascular disease. Springfield, IL: Charles C Thomas, 1978.

† Data derived from Nora JJ, Nora AH: Maternal transmission of congenital heart disease: new recurrence risk figures and the questions of cytoplasmic inheritance and vulnerability to teratogens. Am J Cardiol 1987;59:459.

The sequential approach to the evaluation of cardiac anatomy, originally suggested for pathologic and angiographic studies,[6] is very suitable for fetal echocardiography. The left and right sides of the fetus are assessed by determining the position of the head and spine. The visceral situs is then assessed by demonstrating the relative position of the stomach, hepatic vessels, abdominal aorta, and inferior vena cava (Fig. 37-1). A transverse cross section of the fetal chest provides a four-chamber view (Fig. 37-2). This view is easily obtained even by sonographers who do not have specific training in fetal echocardiography, and it permits the identification of many cardiac anomalies.[12] The elements that are relevant in the analysis of the four-chamber view are as follows: position of the heart inside the thorax (the heart is normally positioned in the left side of the chest, with the apex pointing to the left); integrity of the ventricular and atrial septum; and equal size of the left and right ventricles and atria. The patency of the atrioventricular valves can be demonstrated by real-time imaging of the movements of the leaflets. Additional elements that can be visualized in the four-chamber view include the more apical insertion of the tricuspid valve with regard to the mitral valve and the presence of the moderator band of the trabeculae septomarginalis at the apex of the right ventricle. These elements are both of value in distinguishing the morphologic left ventricle from the morphologic right ventricle.

TABLE 37–2. INDICATIONS FOR FETAL ECHOCARDIOGRAPHY

Maternal and Familial Indications
Familial history of congenital heart disease
Maternal diabetes
Maternal drug exposure during pregnancy*
Maternal infections during pregnancy*
Maternal alcoholism*
Maternal connective tissue disease
Maternal phenylketonuria
Fetal Indications
Polyhydramnios
Nonimmune hydrops
Dysrhythmias
Extracardiac anomalies*
Chromosomal aberrations*
Symmetrical intrauterine growth retardation

* The interested reader is referred to Copel JA, Pilu G, Kleinman CS. Congenital heart disease and extracardiac malformations. Associations and indications for fetal echocardiography. Am J Obstet Gynecol 1986;154:1121.

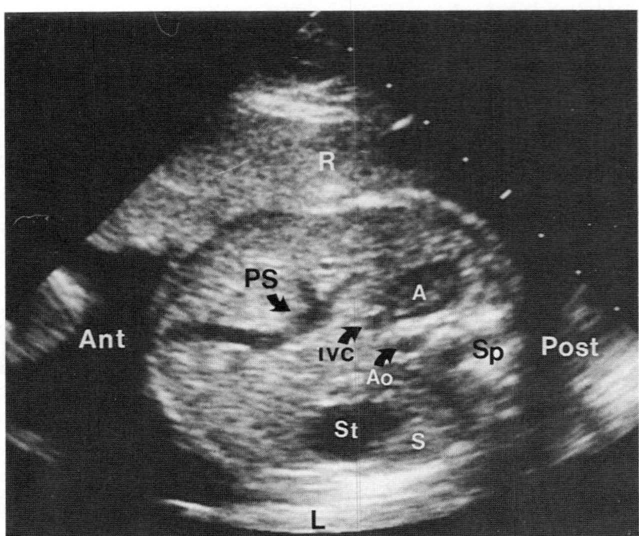

FIGURE 37–1. Transverse cross section of the upper abdomen in a second-trimester fetus, demonstrating visceral situs. The portal situs (PS), the anatomical landmark of the hilus of the liver, can be clearly recognized. The stomach (St), spleen (S), inferior vena cava (IVC), and abdominal aorta (Ao) are demonstrated. (Ant, anterior; Post, posterior; R, right; L, left; A, right adrenal gland.)

Tilting the transducer cephalad, the left and right ventriculoarterial connection can be identified, and further angulation allows the visualization of the right outflow tract and main pulmonary artery, ductus arteriosus, and aortic arch. M-mode ultrasound evaluation of the fetal heart is easily performed by using the currently available real-time directed M-mode apparatuses.[14,15] Movements of the cardiac valves and walls can be studied with this technique (Fig. 37-3). The tracings are remarkably similar to those that have been described after birth. M-mode has also been used to derive nomograms of the normal size of the ventricular chambers and great vessels.[14,16,17] Measurement of ventricular chambers and determination of contractility have been suggested as a way of assessing cardiac function,[16] although the clinical value of such an evaluation

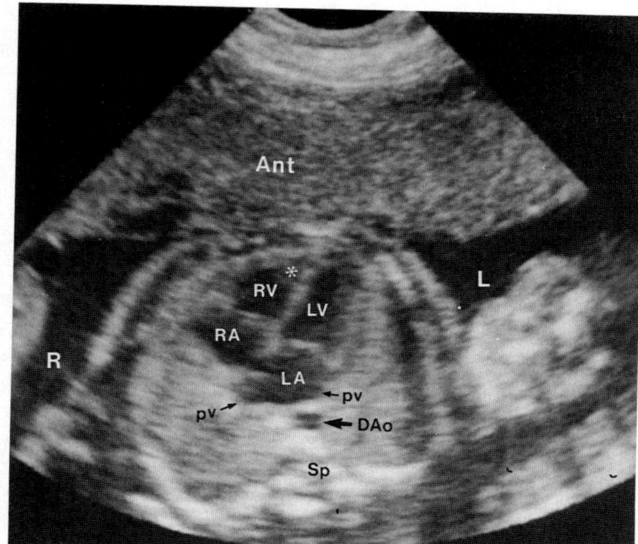

FIGURE 37–2. Four-chamber view of the heart in a second-trimester fetus. (RV, right ventricle; LV, left ventricle; RA, right atrium; La, left atrium; PV, pulmonary veins; DAo, descending aorta; Sp, spine; *, the moderator band of the trabecula septomarginalis. Other abbreviations are as in previous figure.)

is still undetermined. At present, M-mode ultrasound is particularly valuable in the identification and differential diagnosis of fetal dysrhythmias.[18–21]

Pulsed Doppler ultrasound evaluation has recently been applied to the study of the heart function in the live human fetus.[22–30] Adequate recordings of velocity waveforms of the blood flow through the atrioventricular valves, great vessels, and inferior vena cava can be obtained in almost all cases after 18 to 20 weeks gestation (Fig. 37-4). Several authors have pointed out remarkable differences between in utero and postnatal Doppler studies. The higher velocity in the flow at the ventricular inlet that is dependent on atrial contraction when compared to passive venous filling has been interpreted as a sign of the physiologic "stiffness" of the fetal myocardium.[24] Pulsed Doppler ultrasound, in combination with two-dimensional and M-mode sonography, has proved useful in the evaluation of both fetal dysrhythmias and structural anomalies. In this regard, Doppler is of value for documenting atrioventricular valve insufficiency (Fig. 37-5). It has been demonstrated recently that the association of structural heart disease, hydrops, and atrioventricular valve insufficiency carries a very poor prognosis.[23] It has also been found that in normal fetuses, the peak velocity in both ascending aorta and pulmonary artery is less than 1 m/s.[26] This observation is relevant for the prenatal diagnosis of pulmonic and aortic stenosis, which are associated with poststenotic turbulence. However, the use of Doppler in the fetus is still an area of ongoing research. Sophisticated analyses of cardiac function are appearing with increasing frequency.

The accuracy of fetal echocardiography in the prenatal identification of CHD seems to be high. However, some defects are easily identified and others are extremely difficult to recognize. Intracardiac anomalies, such as those involving the ventricular septum and those associated with hypoplasia or enlargement of the cardiac chambers, probably can be rapidly identified even by sonographers who lack specific training in fetal cardiac evaluation. Abnormal connections between the ventricles and the great arteries require meticulous scanning and sometimes are a challenge for even the experienced sonologist.

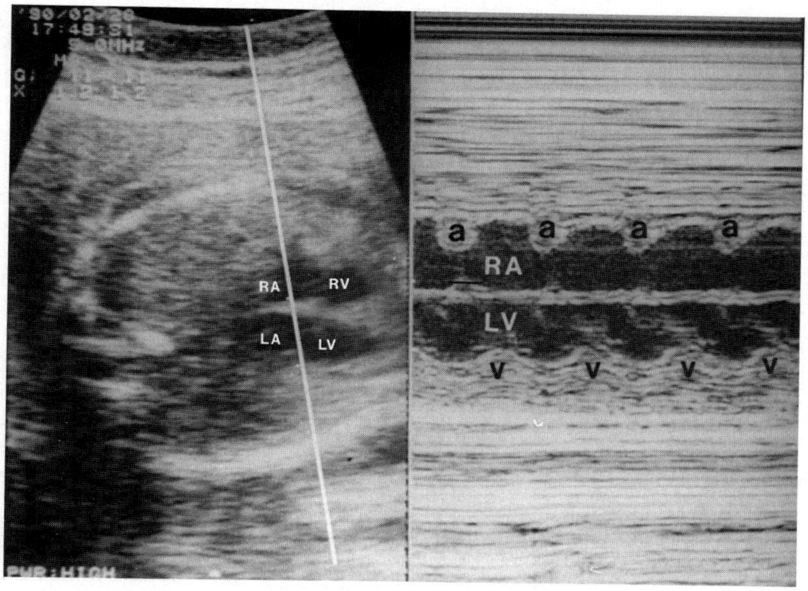

FIGURE 37–3. TM-mode evaluation of cardiac chambers. The M line is directed across the right atrium (RA) and left ventricle (LV). Undulations of the walls of the cardiac chambers indicate atrial (a) and ventricular (v) contractions. This sonogram allows precise calculation of atrial and ventricular frequency. The atrioventricular sequence of excitation can be inferred as well.

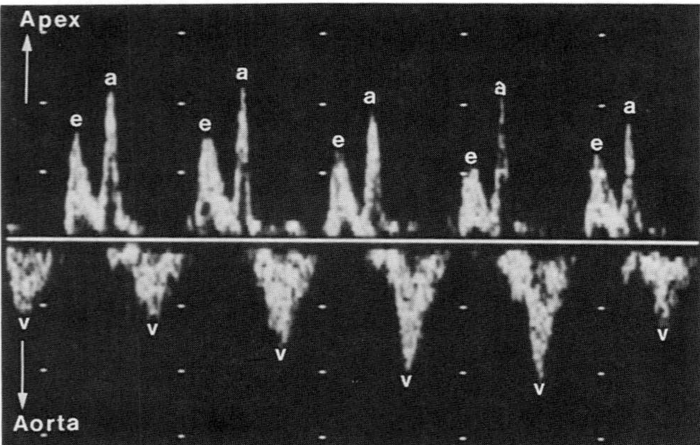

FIGURE 37–4. Doppler sonogram of the left ventricle in a 20-week-old fetus obtained by positioning a 4-mm large sampling gate below the mitral valve. Blood flow coursing along both inflow and outflow tract is registered. During dyastole, blood moves away from the atrioventricular valve toward the cardiac apex. Two distinct velocity peaks can be recognized: the e peak, corresponding to passive venous filling, and the a peak, corresponding to atrial systole. During ventricular systole, blood flows in the opposite direction (v), moving toward the aortic valves. This sonogram allows us to infer the atrioventricular sequence of excitation.

ATRIAL AND VENTRICULAR SEPTAL DEFECTS

Atrial septal defects (ASD) are commonly divided into *primum* and *secundum* types. Primum ASD is the simplest form of the atrioventricular septal defects, which cover a wide spectrum of severity, the most severe of which is the complete atrioventricular defect. Atrioventricular septal defects (according to a different terminology, *atrioventricular canals*) are found in more than 50% of infants with trisomy 21.[31] Secundum ASD may be a part of the Holt-Oram syndrome, with autosomal dominant transmission.

Because of the patency of the foramen ovalis, it is usually difficult to assess properly the integrity of the septum secundum in the fetus, and it is questionable whether isolated, small defects in this area can be recognized in utero. Conversely, primum ASDs are easily seen. Septum primum ASD, or partial atrioventricular septal defects, lack the lower portion of the atrial septum, usually associated with atrioventricular valves that insert at the same level (Fig. 37-6). Complete atrioventricular septal defects have an ASD with a ventricular septal defect and a common atrioventricular valve (Fig. 37-7). ASDs are not a cause of impairment of cardiac function in utero, as a large right-to-left shunt at the level of the atria is a physiologic condition in the fetus. Most affected infants are asymptomatic even in the neonatal period. In complete atrioventricular septal defects the common atrioventricular valve may be incompetent, and systolic blood regurgitation from the ventricles to the atria may give rise to congestive heart failure.[32] Pulsed Doppler ultrasound is valuable in assessing these defects, as it allows the identification of the regurgitant jet.[23]

Atrioventricular septal defects are among the most frequent types of CHD found in cardiosplenic syndromes (asplenia and polysplenia, also defined as right and left isomerism, respectively). Diagnosis of these conditions is possible by evaluation of the visceral situs (Fig. 37-8).

Ventricular septal defects (VSD) are probably the most common form of CHD. The echocardiographic diagnosis depends on the demonstration of a dropout of echoes in the ventricular septum (Fig. 37-9). However, VSDs smaller than 1 to 2 mm will fall beyond the resolution power of current ultrasound equipment and

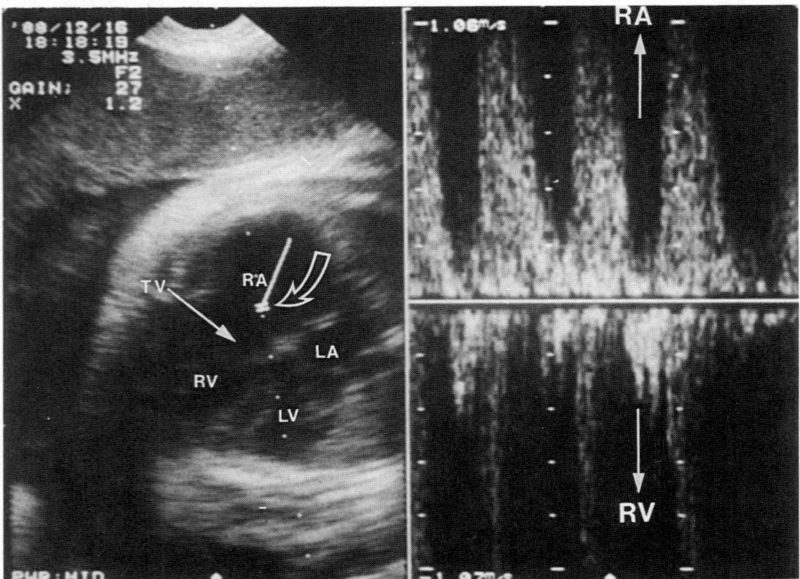

FIGURE 37–5. Pulsed Doppler demonstration of tricuspid insufficiency in a third-trimester fetus that was referred for fetal echocardiography due to obvious enlargement of the right atrium and ventricle (RA, RV). The sampling gate (*curved arrow*) is positioned within the right atrium just above the tricuspid valve. A high-velocity (more than 1 m/s) regurgitant jet in systole is clearly demonstrated.

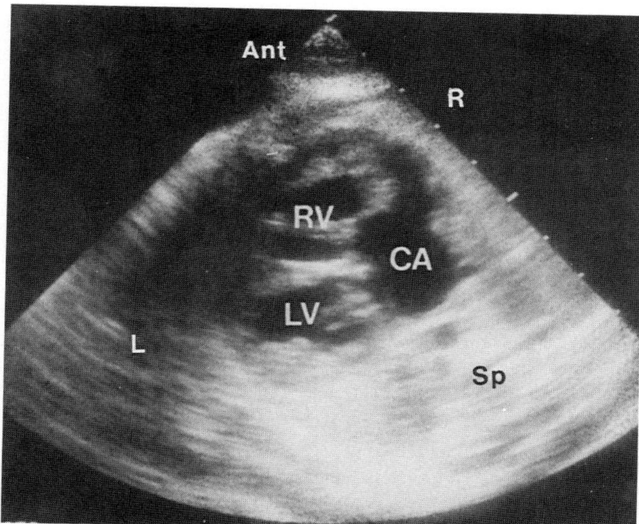

FIGURE 37–6. Partial atrioventricular septal defect in a third-trimester fetus with complex congenital heart disease. A common atrium (CA) is demonstrated. The two atrioventricular valves insert at the same level on the ventricular septum (other abbreviations as in the previous figures).

escape detection. There is no evidence that VSDs are responsible for hemodynamic compromise in utero. Even considerable interventricular communication probably gives rise only to small, bidirectional shunts in the fetus, as during intrauterine life the right and left ventricular pressures are believed to be equal.[33] The vast majority of infants are not symptomatic in the neonatal period.[34]

PULMONARY AND AORTIC STENOSIS

There are different anatomic types of pulmonic and aortic stenosis, and probably only a minority of these lesions are amenable to prenatal diagnosis. Pulmonic stenosis increases both the work of the right ventricle and the pressure, leading to myocardial hypertrophy. In the most severe cases, right ventricular overload may cause insufficiency of the tricuspid valve and congestive heart failure. Aortic stenosis includes three different lesions: subaortic stenosis, valvar stenosis, and supravalvular stenosis. Subaortic stenosis includes a fixed type, which is the consequence of a fibrous or fibromuscular obstruction, and a dynamic type, which is due to a thickened ventricular septum obstructing the outflow tract of the left ventricle. The latter is also known as asymmetric septal hypertrophy (ASH) or idiopathic hypertrophic subaortic stenosis. Hypertrophy of the ventricular septum and free walls of the left ventricle, giving rise to subaortic stenosis, is also commonly found in infants of diabetic mothers. In the most severe cases of aortic stenosis, the association of left ventricular pressure overload and decreased coronary perfusion may result in early intrauterine impairment of cardiac function.[35] Insufficiency of the mitral valve and systolic regurgitation may ensue. Intrauterine hemodynamic perturbation following aortic stenosis is indirectly suggested by the very high incidence of intrauterine growth retardation in infants affected by this anomaly.[36] Neither supravalvular nor subaortic stenosis is usually clinically manifest in newborns.

Postnatal ultrasound diagnosis of pulmonary or aortic stenosis depends on demonstration of doming of the cusps with real-time and poststenotic turbulence detected by Doppler ultrasound.[37] Prenatal diagnosis is probably difficult, as only a few, very severe cases have been described thus far, mainly in association with enlargement of the ventricles or poststenotic enlargement or hypoplasia of the great vessels.[36,38] Pulsed Doppler ultrasound is valuable in assessing the presence of atrioventricular valve insufficiency.[23]

Asymmetric septal hypertrophy has been identified in a fetus.[39] The only reported case, however, is likely to be an exception, as there is evidence indicating that this anomaly usually evolves over time, and it is not apparent in the neonatal period.[40] We are not aware of any case of supravalvular aortic stenosis detected in utero.

TETRALOGY OF FALLOT

Tetralogy of Fallot is defined by the association of a ventricular septal defect (usually in the perimembranous area), infundibular pulmonic stenosis, aortic valve overriding the ventricular septum, and hypertrophy of the right ventricle. However, both pathologic studies in infants and echocardiographic studies in live fetuses

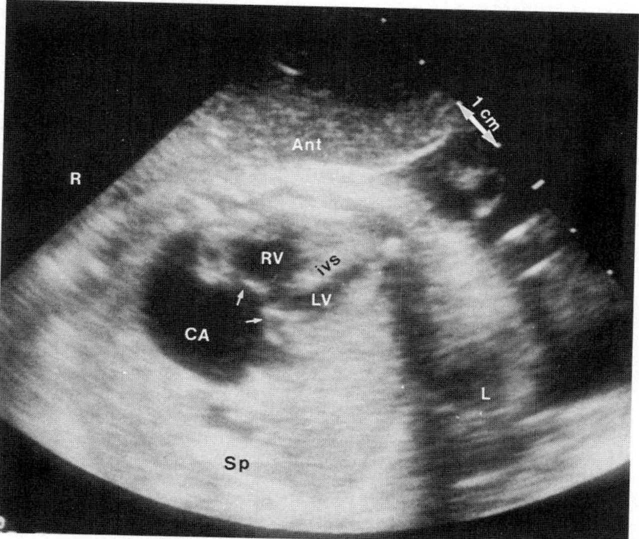

FIGURE 37–7. Complete atrioventricular septal defect. A common atrium (CA) is demonstrated in association with a common atrioventricular valve with central opening (*arrows*) and a large ventricular septal defect. (Other abbreviations as in the previous figures.)

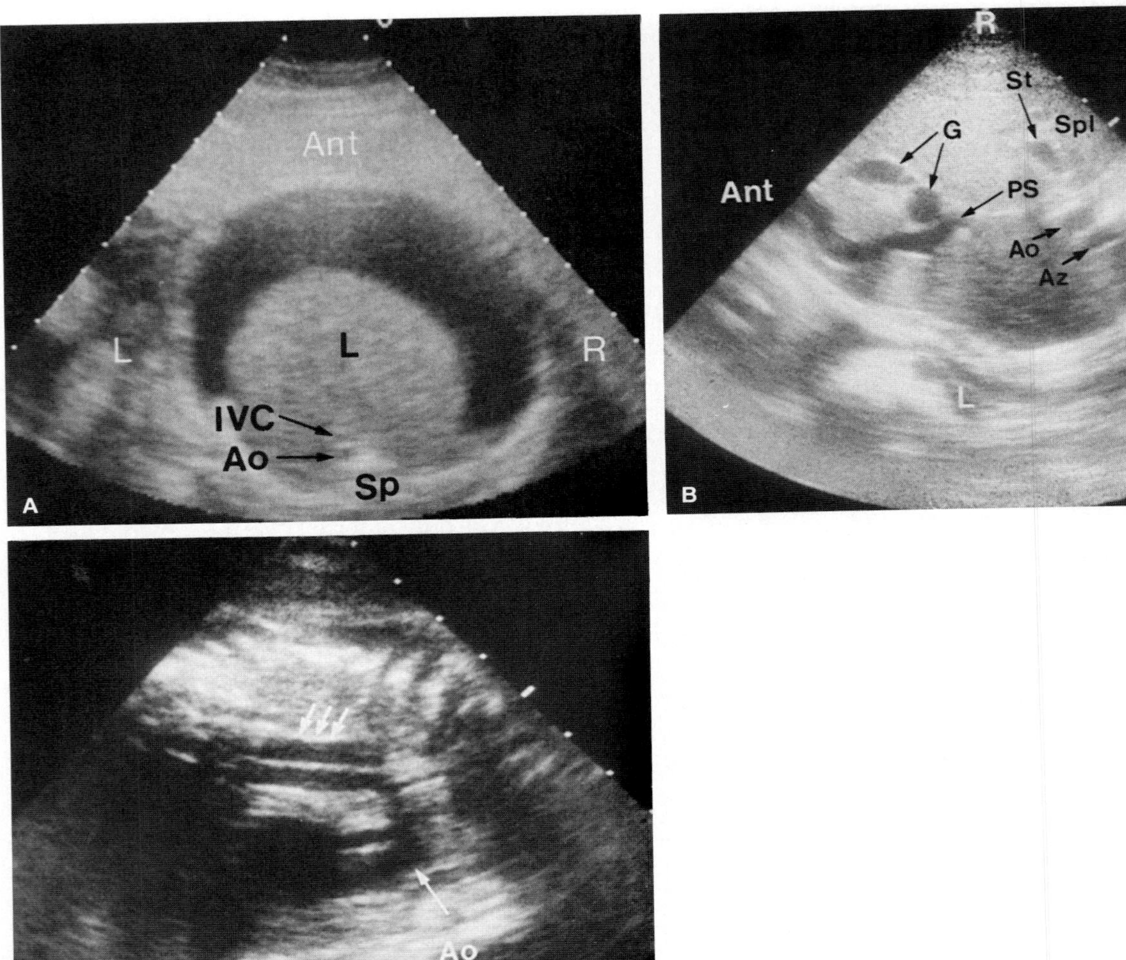

FIGURE 37–8. (**A**) Asplenia syndrome in a fetus with complex heart disease and nonimmune hydrops. A large layer of ascites delineates a symmetric liver, and both the inferior vena cava (IVC) and descending aorta (Ao) are demonstrated on the same side of the spine (Sp). (Other abbreviations as in previous figures.) (**B**) Polysplenia syndrome. Same case as Figure 37-6. A transverse section of the upper abdomen reveals a considerable alteration in the topographic disposition of abdominal organs. The stomach (St) was seen on the right side, as well as a splenic mass (Spl). The umbilical vein, left portal vein, and portal sinus (PS) are tortuous. The main abdominal vessels are seen on the same side of the spine. Careful sonographic examination along different planes revealed the most anterior vessel to be the descending aorta (Ao). The posterior vessel was eventually identified as an enlarged anomalous azygos vein (Az). Absence of the inferior vena cava with an azygous vein draining the lower portion off the body is pathognomonic of left isomerism, or polysplenia syndrome. (**C**) Same case as Figure 37-8*B*. Longitudinal section of the fetal chest. A large vessel (*arrows*) in which pulsed Doppler sonography revealed venous blood flow is seen coursing within the thorax posterior to the descending aorta (Ao). This venous vessel can be positively identified with an anomalous azygous vein draining the lower portion of the body. Such a finding is pathognomonic of absence of the inferior vena cava and left isomerism.

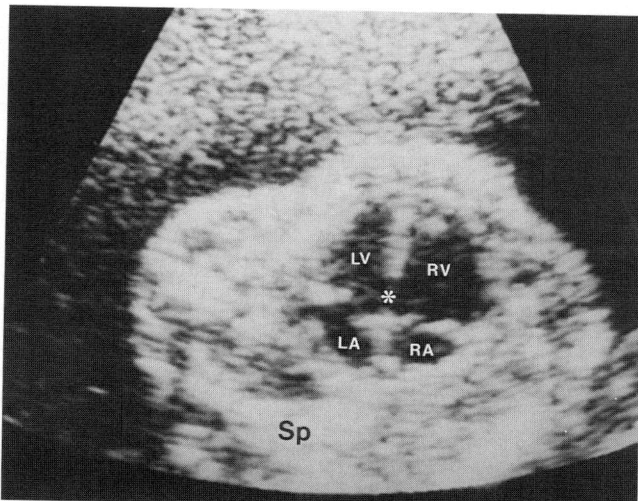

FIGURE 37–9. Four-chamber view in a second-trimester fetus with a large perimembranous ventricular septal defect (*). There is evidence indicating that ventricular septal defects are well tolerated during intrauterine life. However, in our experience large defects are often associated with some degree of enlargement of the right ventricle. Color Doppler has revealed that in these cases, a left-to-right shunt is a frequent finding even prior to birth. (Abbreviations are as in previous figures.)

suggest that right ventricular hypertrophy does not occur until late in the neonatal period.[11,41]

Associated defects, including atrial septal defects and bicuspid or absent pulmonary valve, are frequently seen. The main factor affecting hemodynamics is the degree of hypoplasia of the right ventricular outflow tract, as this causes both a decrease in pulmonary blood flow and a right-to-left shunt at the level of the ascending aorta, with decreased oxygen saturation. However, tetralogy of Fallot does not seem to cause hemodynamic compromise in utero. Even in the case of very tight infundibular stenosis or pulmonary atresia, the combined output of both ventricles will be directed toward the aorta, and the pulmonary vascular bed will be supplied by reverse flow through the ductus arteriosus. This concept is supported by the observation of normal intrauterine fetal growth in affected fetuses.[37] Congestive heart failure is very rarely seen in neonates, and it usually occurs only in those with an absent pulmonary valve.

Echocardiographic diagnosis can be made by demonstrating the aorta overriding the ventricular septum (Fig. 37-10).[11,32] Caution is recommended, as artifacts are frequently seen. In our experience, all fetuses with tetralogy of Fallot have an enlargement of the ascending aorta that is striking on real-time examination and that should increase the index of suspicion. Study of the right ventricular outflow tract and pulmonary artery provides important clinical information by allowing us

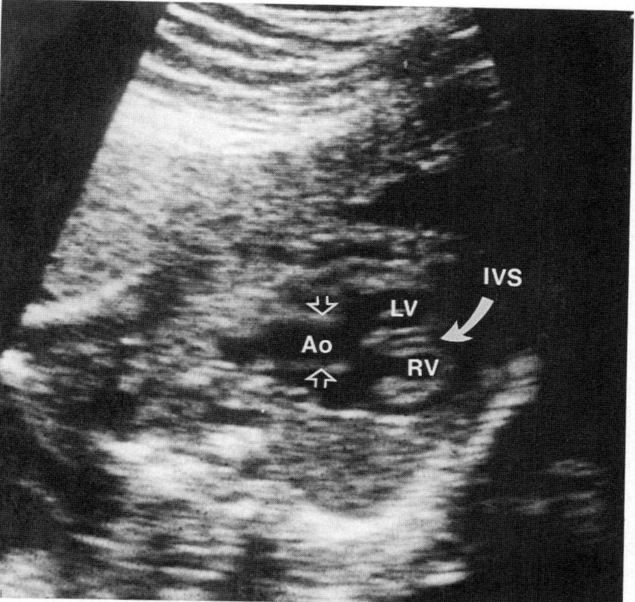

FIGURE 37–10. Tetralogy of Fallot. A large aortic root (Ao) is clearly seen overriding by almost 50% the ventricular septum (IVS). (Other abbreviations as in previous figures.)

to assess the degree of infundibular stenosis (Fig. 37-11). Doppler ultrasound is valuable in assessing the presence of blood flow in the pulmonary artery. Enlargement of the right ventricle, main pulmonary trunk, and pulmonary artery suggests absence of the pulmonary valve.[32]

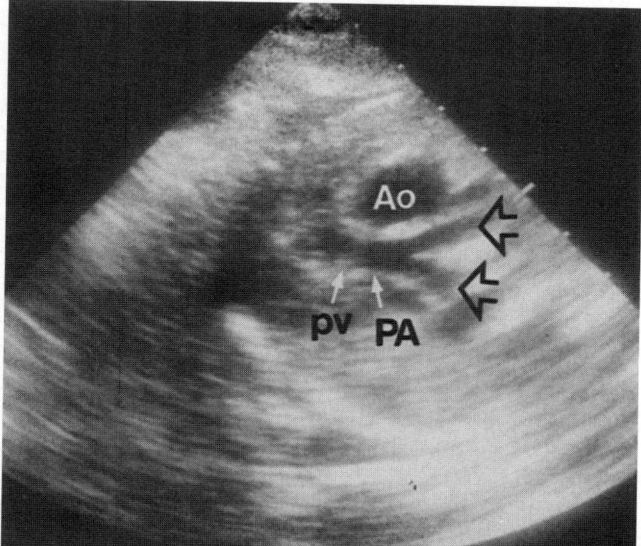

FIGURE 37–11. Pulmonic stenosis is a constant finding in tetralogy of Fallot. In this third-trimester fetus, a typically small pulmonary artery is seen (PA). The aortic root is quite large. (pv, pulmonary valve; arrows indicate the right and left pulmonary artery.)

TRANSPOSITION OF THE GREAT ARTERIES

Transposition of the great arteries (TGA) includes two anatomical forms: complete TGA and corrected TGA. In complete TGA, the aorta arises from the morphologic right ventricle and the pulmonary artery arises from the left ventricle in the presence of a normal atrioventricular connection. Associated cardiac anomalies are frequently found. According to Becker and Anderson, three main varieties can be distinguished: transposition with intact ventricular septum, with or without pulmonic stenosis; transposition with ventricular septal defect; and transposition with ventricular septal defect and pulmonic stenosis.[6] Other anomalies commonly found include abnormalities of the atrioventricular valves, underdevelopment of either the right ventricle or the left ventricle, and coarctation of the aorta.

Corrected transposition of the great arteries is marked by the association of an atrioventricular and a ventriculoarterial discordance. The right atrium is connected to the left ventricle, which is connected to the pulmonic aorta; the left atrium is connected to the right ventricle, which is connected to the ascending aorta.

Fetal echocardiography allows us to identify abnormalities of the ventriculoarterial connection, but meticulous scanning is required. In both complete and corrected transposition, the two great vessels arise parallel from the base of the heart. By careful scanning, the aorta and pulmonic artery can be identified and their relationship with each ventricle can be assessed (Fig. 37-12). Differential diagnosis between complete and corrected transposition depends on identification of the morphologic right and left ventricles by visualization of the moderator band, papillary muscles, and insertion of atrioventricular valves. The atrioventricular connection can be further recognized by the demonstration of the systemic and pulmonary venous return.

Fetuses with uncomplicated complete transposition should not undergo hemodynamic compromise in utero. Survival after birth depends on the persistence of fetal circulation. In corrected transposition, discordance between atrioventricular and ventriculoarterial connection cancel each other, and ideally there should not be any hemodynamic imbalance. Corrected transposition may indeed be an occasional finding at autopsy. However, important associated cardiac anomalies are found in the vast majority of cases (ventricular septal defects, pulmonic stenosis, abnormalities of the atrioventricular valves, atrioventricular block).

DOUBLE OUTLET RIGHT VENTRICLE

Double outlet right ventricle (DORV) is commonly defined as a cardiac lesion in which most of the aorta and the pulmonary artery arise from the right ventricle. The relative position of the two great vessels is variable. A defect of the ventricular septum is almost always associated, as are other anomalies, such as atrial septal defects, pulmonary stenosis, abnormalities of the atrioventricular valves. By definition, the term *DORV* includes those cases of tetralogy of Fallot in which the aorta arises predominantly from the right ventricle. Prenatal

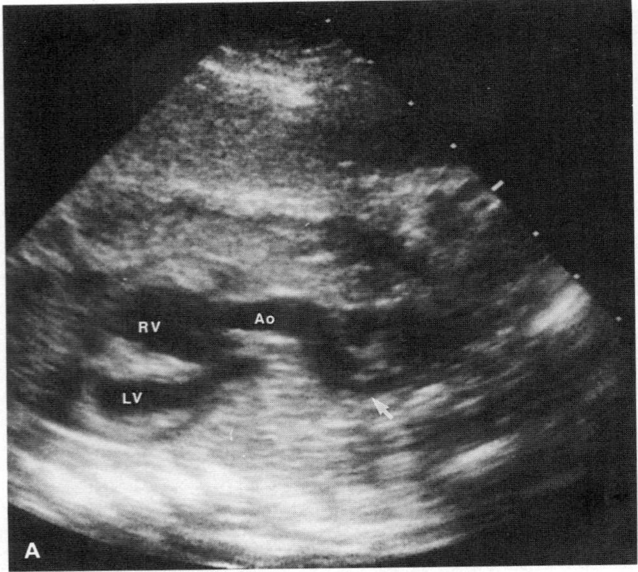

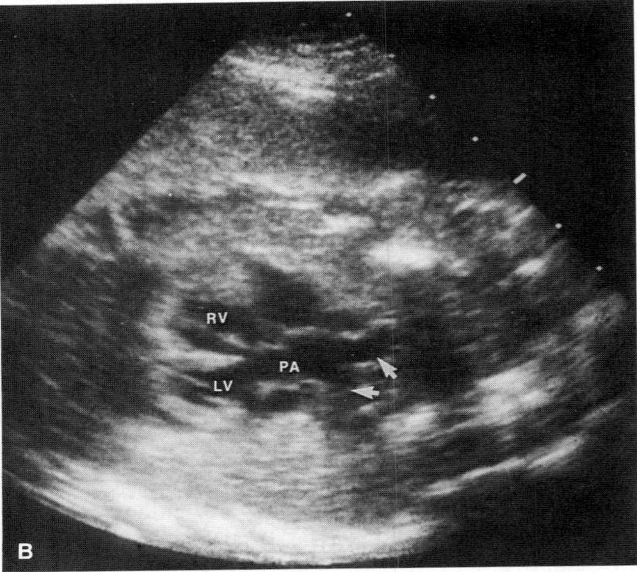

FIGURE 37–12. Evaluation of ventriculoarterial connections in a fetus with complete transposition of the great arteries. (**A**) The vessel that is connected to the right ventricle (RV) has a long upward course and gives rise to the brachiocephalic vessels (*arrow*). This finding allows us to identify this vessel with the aorta (Ao). (**B**) The vessel that arises from the left ventricle (LV) bifurcates (*arrows*). This indicates that this vessel is the pulmonary artery (PA).

diagnosis of DORV has been reported.[42] However, differentiation from other conotruncal anomalies, such as transposition of the great vessels and tetralogy of Fallot, is notoriously difficult.[43] An example of fetal DORV is shown in Figure 37-13.

HYPOPLASTIC LEFT HEART SYNDROME

Hypoplastic left heart syndrome (HLHS) is characterized by a very small left ventricle, with mitral and/or aortic atresia. Blood flow to the head and neck vessels and coronary artery is supplied in a retrograde manner via the ductus arteriosus. HLHS is frequently associated with intrauterine heart failure. The prognosis has classically been regarded as extremely poor. Untreated infants usually die in the very first days of life. However, palliative procedures have been proposed and long-term survivors have been reported. Recently, cardiac transplantation in the neonatal period has also been attempted. The success of these procedures may be enhanced in the near future by prenatal diagnosis, as this will allow prompt treatment of the infants, thus preventing the severe hemodynamic, respiratory, and metabolic complications that always occur in the early neonatal period.

Ultrasound recognition of HLHS in the fetus depends on the demonstration of a small left ventricle (Fig. 37-14).[44,45] The ascending aorta is severely hypoplastic. The right ventricle, right atrium, and pulmonary artery are usually enlarged. By the use of pulsed Doppler ultrasound it may be possible to demonstrate retrograde blood flow in the ascending aorta and a systolic regurgitant jet within the right atrium in those cases with tricuspid insufficiency. However, the small size of the aorta renders it difficult to obtain satisfying Doppler waveforms in a moving fetus. In most cases, the two-dimensional ultrasound appearance is striking, and the diagnosis is easy.

PULMONARY ATRESIA WITH INTACT VENTRICULAR SEPTUM

Pulmonary atresia with intact ventricular septum (PA:IVS) in infants is usually associated with an hypoplastic right ventricle. In fetuses, cases with enlarged right ventricle and atrium have been described with unusual frequency (Fig. 37-15).[46] Although prenatal series are small, the discrepancy with the pediatric literature may be due to the very high proportion of perinatal losses in "dilated" cases. Enlargement of the ventricle and atrium is probably the consequence of tricuspid insufficiency. Prenatal diagnosis of PA:IVS relies on the demonstration of a small pulmonary artery with an atretic pulmonary valve. We have recently been able to confirm real-time two-dimensional diagnosis of pulmonary atresia by demonstrating with Doppler ultrasound the absence of forward blood flow within the main pulmonary trunk and the presence of reverse flow through the ductus arteriosus.

UNIVENTRICULAR HEART

According to Becker and Anderson, the term *univentricular heart* defines a group of anomalies unified by the presence of an atrioventricular junction that is entirely connected to only one chamber in the ventricular mass.[6] By adhering to this approach, which we find very suitable for fetal echocardiographic studies, the univentricular heart includes both those cases in which two atrial chambers are connected, by either two distinct atrioventricular valves or a common one, to a main ventricular chamber (classic "double-inlet" single ventricle) and those cases in which, because of the absence of one atrioventricular connection (tricuspid or mitral atresia), one of the ventricular chambers is either rudimentary or absent. The main ventricular chamber may be either of left or right type, and in some cases may be

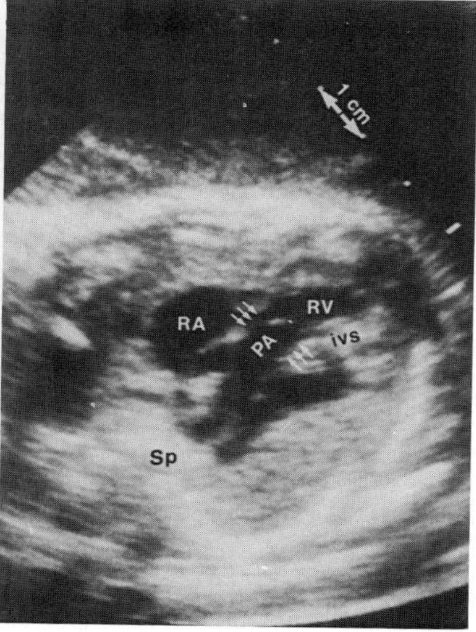

FIGURE 37–13. Double-outlet right ventricle. The aorta (Ao) overrides the interventricular septum (IVS), being predominantly connected to the right ventricle (RV). The pulmonary artery (PA) is connected as well with the right ventricle. (Other abbreviations are as in previous figures.)

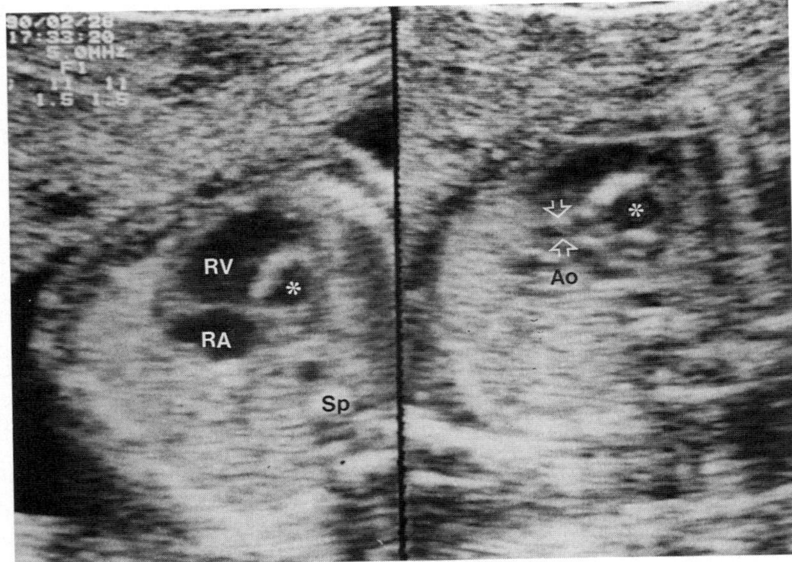

FIGURE 37–14. In this second-trimester fetus, the demonstration of a diminutive left ventricle (*), connected with a very small ascending aorta (Ao) within which Doppler ultrasound did not reveal any blood flow, prompted the diagnosis of hypoplastic left heart syndrome. (Other abbreviations are as in previous figures.)

of indeterminate type. A rudimentary ventricular chamber lacking atrioventricular connection is a frequent but not constant finding. Antenatal echocardiographic diagnosis is usually easy (Fig. 37-16). The hemodynamics may vary greatly from case to case, depending on the type of ventriculoarterial connection and the sum of the associated cardiac anomalies, which are very frequently seen.

CARDIOMYOPATHIES

Congenital cardiomyopathies include a heterogeneous group of myocardial disorders, commonly subdivided into nonobstructive and obstructive forms. The etiology of the former type includes inborn errors of metabolism, muscular dystrophies, and infections. Obstructive forms include hypertrophic cardiomyopathy of infants of diabetic mothers and asymmetric septal hypertrophy, which has been previously considered. Hypertrophic cardiomyopathy is found in 30% to 50% of infants of diabetic mothers, even though it is clinically manifest in a much smaller proportion.[47] The etiology of this condition is controversial, but it is commonly accepted that it represents the final consequence of fetal hyperglycemia and hyperinsulinemia.

Cardiomyopathies of both obstructive and nonobstructive types share in common, either as a conse-

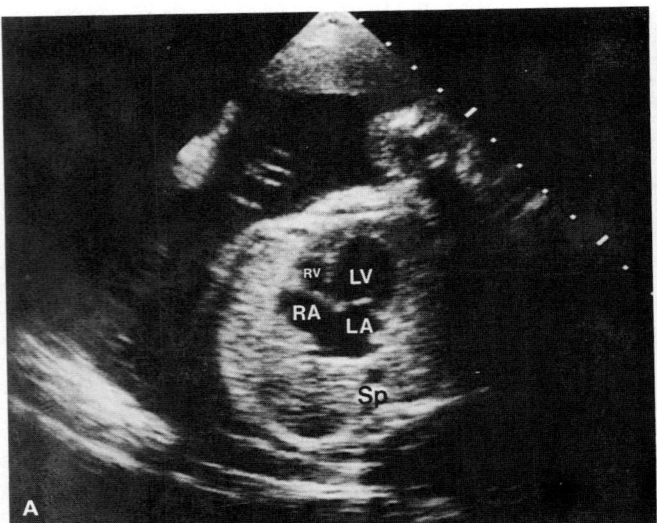

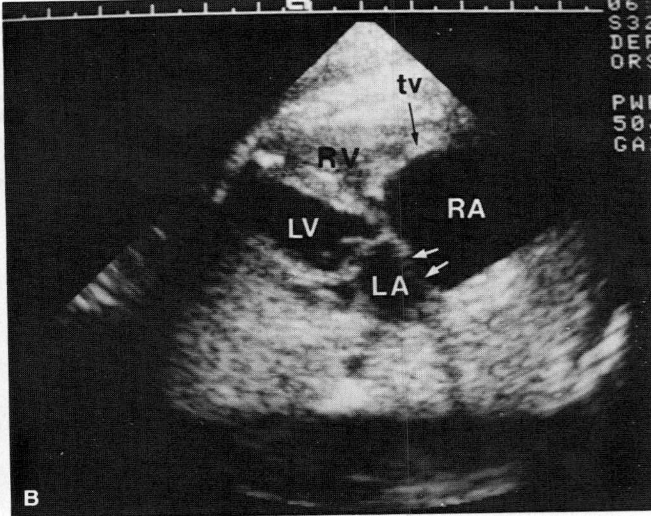

FIGURE 37–15. Spectrum of presentation of pulmonary atresia with intact ventricular septum in the fetus. (**A**) Hypoplastic right ventricle (RV). (**B**) Grossly enlarged right ventricle (RV) and right atrium (RA). In the latter case, pulsed Doppler sonography revealed massive tricuspid regurgitation. (Other abbreviations are as in previous figures.)

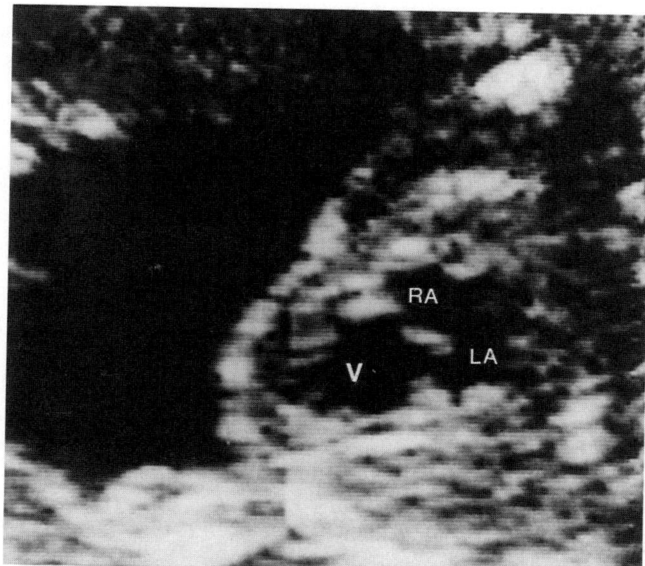

FIGURE 37–16. Double-inlet single ventricle in a second-trimester fetus. Two distinct atrioventricular valves are seen emptying into a single ventricular cavity (V). (Other abbreviations are as in previous figures.)

quence of pump failure or valvular regurgitation or as a consequence of obstruction of ventricular outflow, a more or less marked tendency to congestive heart failure. The onset and extent of symptoms are extremely variable from case to case. Although most newborns are asymptomatic, cases associated with intrauterine heart failure have been described.[11,48]

Echocardiographic diagnosis of nonobstructive forms relies on demonstration of cardiomegaly and poor contractility of ventricular chambers.[48] In obstructive forms, thickening of the interventricular septum and free walls of the ventricles has been reported (Fig. 37-17).[39,49]

COARCTATION OF THE AORTA

The pathogenesis of coarctation of the aorta is controversial. Three hypotheses were suggested. According to these different views, coarctation may be a true malformation, arising from an embryogenetic abnormality; the consequences of aberrant ductal tissue in the aortic wall, resulting in narrowing of the isthmus at the time of closure of the ductus (the so-called Skodaic theory); or the anatomical result of an intrauterine hemodynamic perturbation, caused by an intracardiac anomaly diverting blood flow from the aorta into the pulmonary artery and the ductus arteriosus. There is clinical as well as pathologic evidence to support at least the last two hypotheses.

A discrete shelf between the isthmus and the descending aorta is the most common finding at anatomical dissection. Tubular hypoplasia of a segment of the aortic arch is seen less frequently. Coarctation may be a postnatal event, and this limits prenatal diagnosis in many cases. However, this anomaly has been described in the fetus, although only in late pregnancy.[50] In one case seen in our laboratory, echocardiography was negative at 20 weeks. At 30 weeks, enlargement of the right ventricle was found and the aortic isthmus appeared severely narrowed (Fig. 37-18). As the blood flow through the isthmus is minimal during intrauterine life, with the descending aorta being supplied mainly via the ductus arteriosus, isolated coarctation is not expected to alter hemodynamics significantly. However, cases with tubular hypoplasia of the aortic arch may

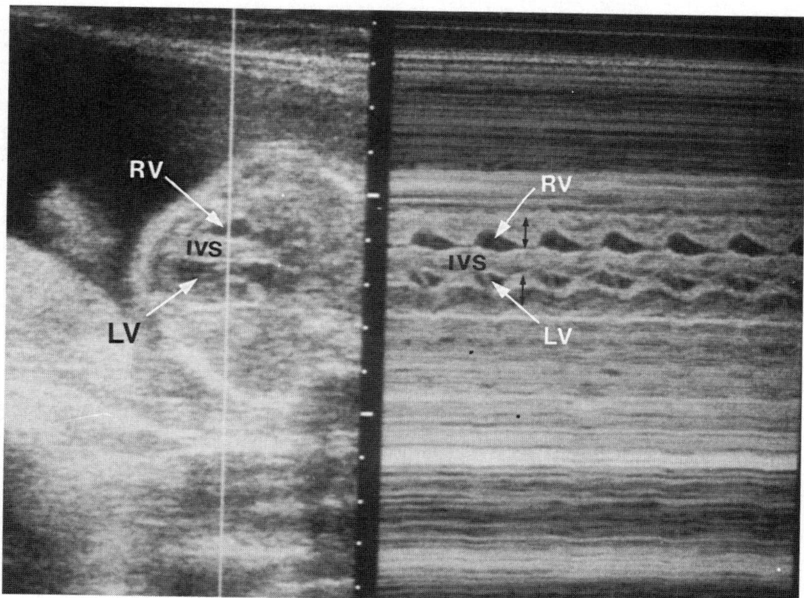

FIGURE 37–17. Hypertrophic cardiomyopathy in a second-trimester fetus. Thickened free walls of the ventricles and ventricular septum (IVS) are clearly demonstrated in both real-time and TM-mode sonograms. The ventricular cavities (RV, LV) are significantly reduced in size.

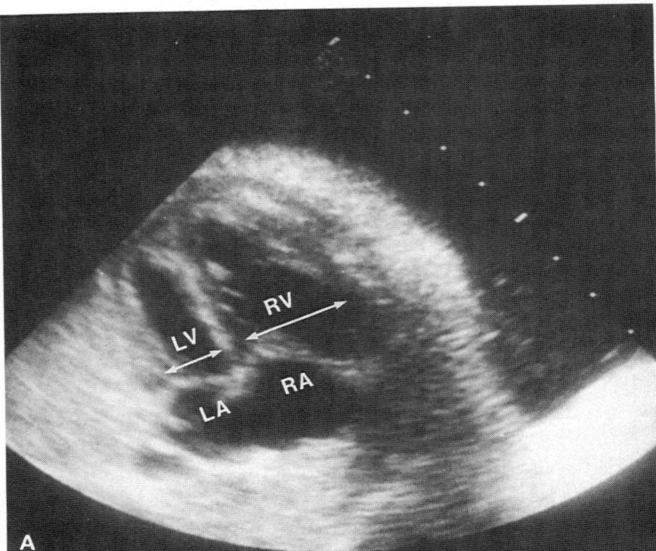

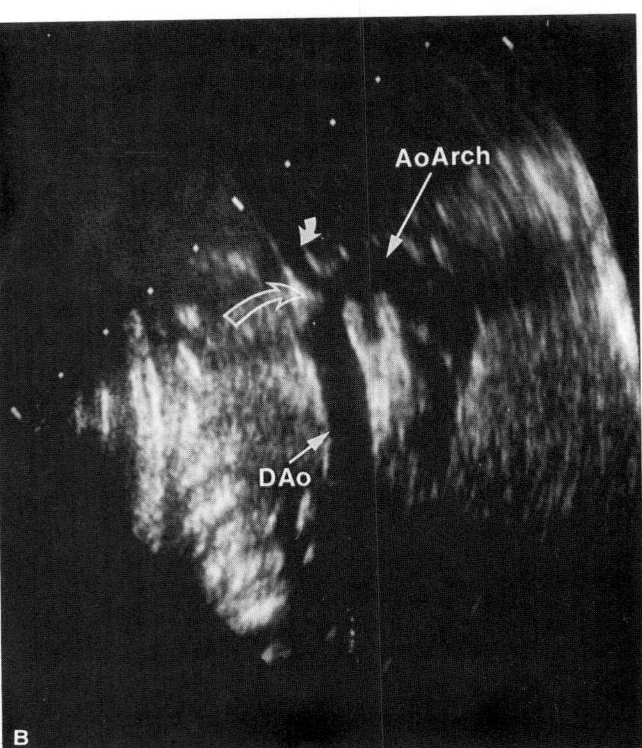

FIGURE 37–18. Coarctation of the aorta in a third-trimester fetus. This case was initially referred for fetal echocardiography at 20 weeks because of a positive familial history. At that time the examination was negative. At 30 weeks a disproportion in the size of the ventricles was noted. Enlargement of the right ventricle (RV) associated with a possible reduction in size of the left ventricle (LV) was observed (A). A longitudinal view of the aortic arch (B) suggested constriction of the aortic isthmus (*long curved arrow*). Severe preductal coarctation was confirmed after birth.

result in a greater hemodynamic burden, and this could explain the dilatation of the right heart that has been documented with echocardiography prior to birth.

FETAL DYSRHYTHMIAS

Irregular patterns of fetal heart rhythms are a frequent finding. Brief periods of tachycardia, bradycardia, and ectopic beats are very commonly seen and in the vast majority of cases have no clinical significance. The electric instability of the fetal heart has not yet been explained satisfactorily. It has been suggested that catecholamine release or accessory pathways may play a role. Even realizing that a clear differentiation between physiologic variations and pathologic alterations is not possible in many cases, a distinction must be attempted for practical clinical purpose. According to the pragmatic approach suggested by Allan and colleagues, a sustained bradycardia of less than 100 beats per minute, a sustained tachycardia of more than 200 beats per minute, and irregular beats occurring more than one in 10 must be considered abnormal and require further investigation.[18]

The fetal electrocardiogram is of little value in the prenatal diagnosis of dysrhythmias, as a satisfactory transabdominal recording can be obtained in a minority of cases. At present, M-mode and pulsed Doppler ultrasound are the most suitable techniques for the assessment of irregular fetal heart rhythm.

The study of the mechanical events of the sequence of contraction may be accomplished in different ways.[18–20] Simultaneous visualization of atrioventricular valves and ventricular wall motion, visualization of aortic valve opening and atrial wall movement with M-mode, and sampling of the ventricular inlet or inferior vena cava with M-mode can be used from time to time. The sequence of excitation can be reasonably inferred by the sequence of contraction.

PREMATURE ATRIAL AND VENTRICULAR CONTRACTIONS

Premature atrial and ventricular contractions are the most frequent fetal dysrhythmias.[19] Repeated premature contractions can give rise to complex rhythm patterns. Premature atrial contractions may be either conducted to the ventricles or blocked, depending on the time of the cardiac cycle in which they occur, thus resulting in either an increased or a decreased ventricular rate. Blocked premature atrial contractions must be differentiated from atrioventricular block. Premature atrial and ventricular contractions are considered a benign condition.[19] They probably do not induce any hemodynamic perturbation, do not appear to be associated with an increased risk of structural abnormalities, and usually disappear in utero or soon after birth. However, as there is at least a theoretical possibility that in a few cases an ectopic beat could trigger a reentrant tachyarrhythmia, serial monitoring of the fetal heart during pregnancy is suggested.[19] Prenatal diagnosis of fetal extrasystoles is easy by using TM-mode (Fig. 37-19). Pulsed Doppler ultrasound evaluation of blood flow in fetuses with premature beats suggests that the fetal heart is capable of postextrasystolic potentiation (Fig. 37-20) and that the Frank-Starling mechanism is operative beginning in the early stages of fetal development.[27]

SUPRAVENTRICULAR TACHYARRHYTHMIAS

Supraventricular tachyarrhythmias include supraventricular paroxysmal tachycardia (SVT), atrial flutter, and atrial fibrillation. SVT is characterized by an atrial frequency between 200 and 300 beats per minute (bpm) and a 1:1 atrioventricular conduction rate (Fig. 37-21). It can occur by one of two mechanisms: automatically or on reentry. In the former case an irritable ectopic focus discharges at high frequency. In the latter case an electrical impulse reenters the atria, giving rise to repeated electrical activity. Reentry may occur at the level of the sinoatrial node, the atrium, the atrioventricular node, and the His-Purkinje system. Reentry may also occur along an anomalous atrioventricular connection such as the Kent bundle in the Wolff-Parkinson-White (WPW) syndrome. In atrial flutter the atrial rate ranges from 300 to 460 bpm. Because of variable degrees of atrioventricular block, the ventricular rate ranges between 60 and 200 bpm (Fig. 37-22). In atrial fibrillation the atrial rate is more than 400 bpm and the ventricular rate ranges between 120 and 200 bpm. Atrial flutter and fibrillation often alternate and are thought to arise from similar mechanisms, which include circus movement of the electrical impulse, ectopic formation, multiple reentry, and multifocal impulse formation. SVT is by far the most common tachyarrhythmia in children. The most frequent form is the one caused by atrioventricular nodal reentry.

Diagnosis of fetal tachyarrhythmia can be accomplished easily by direct auscultation or continuous Doppler examination. M-mode and/or pulsed Doppler ultrasound allow us to identify the precise heart rate and to recognize the atrioventricular sequence of contraction.

The association between fetal tachyarrhythmia and nonimmune hydrops is well established.[32,51] It has been postulated that a fast ventricular rate results in suboptimal filling of the ventricle. This would lead to decreased cardiac output, right atrial overload, and congestive heart failure.[51] Pulsed Doppler analysis of ventricular filling in tachyarrhythmic fetuses would seem to support such a view (Fig. 37-23).[51] For unknown reasons, the frequency of nonimmune hydrops is variable. We have seen fetuses with SVT that did well in utero and

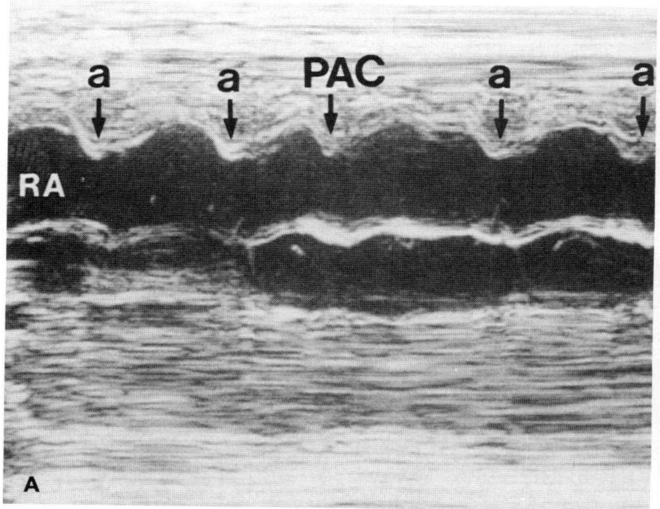

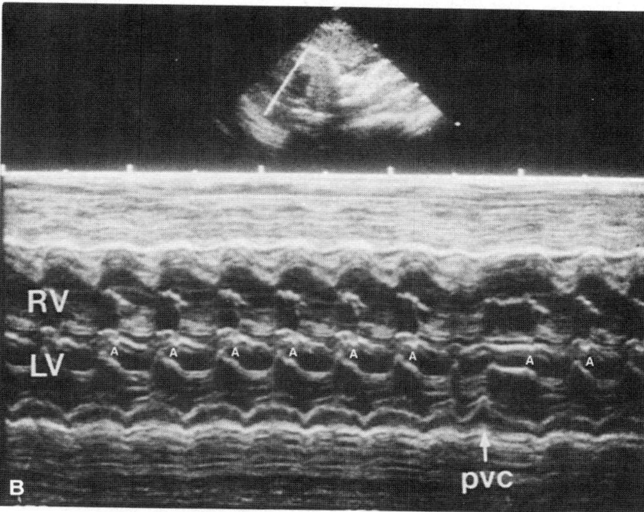

FIGURE 37–19. (**A**) TM-mode evaluation of the movement of the wall of the right atrium in a fetus with supraventricular extrasystoles. Regular atrial rhythm (a) is interrupted by a premature atrial contraction (PAC). (**B**) In this fetus, TM-mode reveals a premature ventricular contraction that is not preceded by atrial systole (absence of the a wave on the mitral valve). This indicates ventricular extrasystoles.

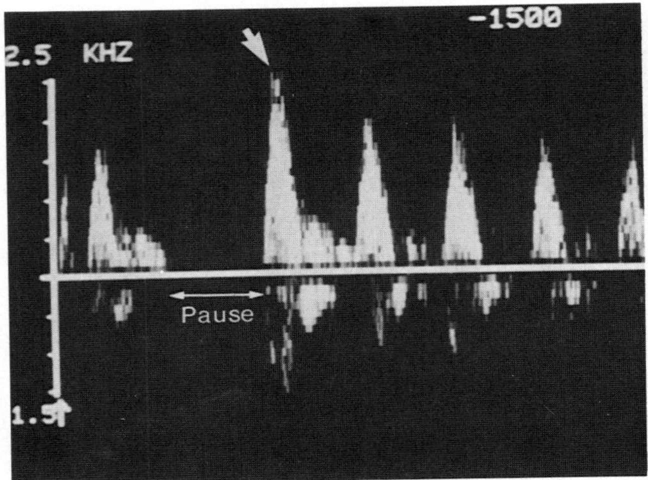

FIGURE 37–20. Blocked atrial extrasystoles in a second-trimester fetus. Doppler ultrasound evaluation of the ascending aorta reveals increased peak velocity (*arrow*) following a ventricular pause. This observation suggests the presence of the Frank-Starling mechanism.

that were successfully treated after birth. It can be postulated that in those cases in which a reentry mechanism is involved, the fetus alternates phases of tachycardia and phases of normal rhythm.

Intrauterine pharmacologic cardioversion of fetal tachyarrhythmia by maternal administration of drugs has been attempted with success in many cases. The optimal approach to the treatment of these conditions is still uncertain. Digoxin, verapamil, propranolol, quinidine, procainamide, and amiodarone have all been used from time to time. The interested reader is referred to specific works on this subject.[51]

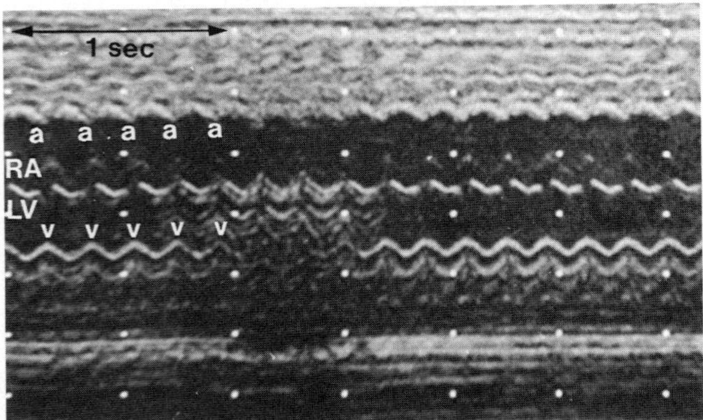

FIGURE 37–21. Supraventricular tachycardia in a third-trimester fetus. The TM-mode sonogram indicates an atrial rhythm of about 220 bpm and a one-to-one ventricular response (v). Return to a normal sinus rhythm was noted following maternal administration of a daily dose of 240 mg of verapamil. Digoxin and procainamide had been previously administered without any beneficial effect.

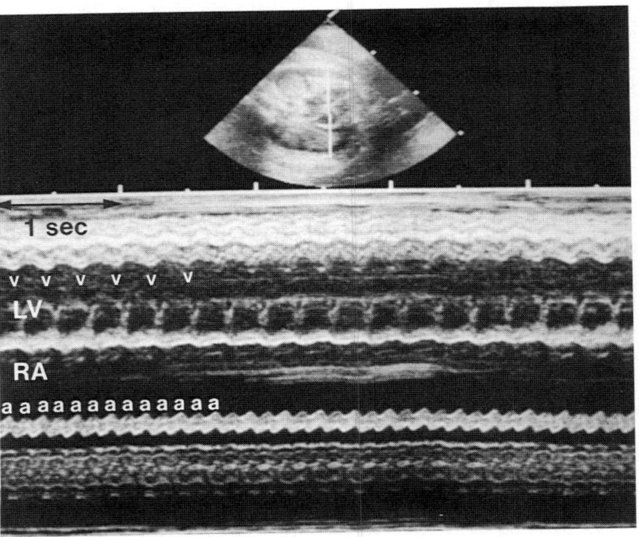

FIGURE 37–22. Atrial flutter. The TM-mode sonogram reveals an atrial rate (a) of about 440 bpm, and a two-to-one ventricular response. This 36-week-old infant converted spontaneously to a normal sinus rhythm a few hours after this sonogram was obtained. Wolff-Parkinson-White syndrome was diagnosed after vaginal delivery at term.

ATRIOVENTRICULAR BLOCK

Atrioventricular (AV) block can result from immaturity of the conduction system, absence of connection to the AV node, or abnormal anatomical position of the AV node. AV block is commonly classified into three types: first-, second-, and third-degree AV block. First-degree AV block corresponds to a simple conduction delay, which is associated with a prolongation of the PR interval on the electrocardiogram. Second-degree AV block is subdivided into Mobitz types I and II. Mobitz type I consists of a progressive prolongation of the PR interval that finally leads to the block of one atrial impulse (Luciani-Wenckebach phenomenon). In Mobitz type II the ventricular rate is a submultiple of the atrial rate (eg, 2:1, 3:1). Third-degree, or complete, AV block involves complete dissociation of atria and ventricles, usually with independent and slow activation of the ventricles (Fig. 37-24). Third-degree AV block is widely reported to be associated in over half of the cases with cardiac structural anomalies,[52] including corrected transposition, univentricular heart, cardiac tumors, and cardiomyopathies. Although in the cases without structural cardiac disease the etiology is unknown, growing evidence suggests an association with the presence of maternal antibodies against SSA and SSB antigens. Transplacental passage of these antibodies would lead to inflammation and damage of the conduction system. Anti-SSA antibodies have been reported in over 80% of mothers that delivered infants with AV block, although only 30% had clinical evidence of connective tissue disease (mostly lupus erythematosus).[53–55]

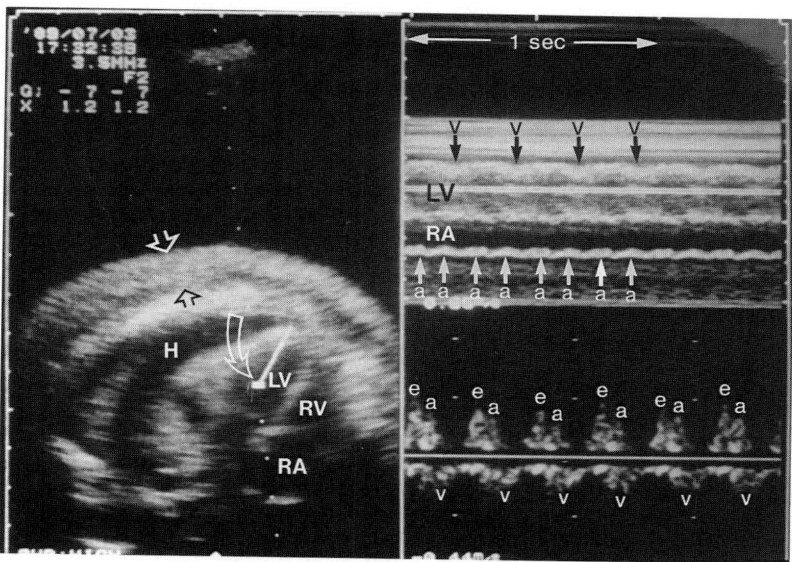

FIGURE 37–23. Simultaneous real-time, TM-mode, and duplex sonography in a third-trimester fetus with atrial flutter. The TM-mode sonogram reveals an atrial rate of 480 bpm and a ventricular rate of 240 bpm. Doppler ultrasound reveals an inversion between the size of the e and a peak (compare with normal sonogram displayed in Fig. 38-4) that is thought to represent failure of diastolic filling. Real-time sonography demonstrates polyhydramnios, pleural effusion (H), and subcutaneous edema (*arrowheads*). Although sinus rhythm could never be obtained, a significant reduction of the frequency with amelioration of hydropic manifestation was observed following maternal administration of amiodarone. Digoxin, procainamide, and verapamil were all ineffective. The infant was delivered by cesarean section at 34 weeks and survived.

First- and second-degree AV block are not usually associated with any significant hemodynamic perturbation. Third-degree AV block may lead to important bradycardia, with decreased cardiac output and congestive heart failure in utero.[19,32]

Intrauterine ventricular pacing has been attempted in one case. A lead was inserted through the maternal abdominal and uterine wall and the fetal thorax and placed inside the right ventricle.[56]

OBSTETRIC MANAGEMENT OF PREGNANCIES WITH FETAL STRUCTURAL CHD

Currently, most series of prenatally diagnosed CHD include mainly cases that were referred because of either associated extracardiac anomalies or very severe cardiac alterations resulting in gross cardiomegaly or intrauterine heart failure. It is not surprising that the outcome of these cases has generally proved to be dismal. Nevertheless, the experience thus far seems to indicate that fetal echocardiography has great potential in accurately identifying correctable cardiac defects whose prognosis could be ameliorated by prompt neonatal assistance. Although these cases are a minority at present, there is reason to believe that their number will grow in the near future.

The development of many types of CHD can be reliably predicted from the early stages of pregnancy. The "parallel" model of cardiac circulation during intrauterine life renders most cardiac defects asymptomatic until birth. Ventricular and atrial septal defects, tetralogy of Fallot, and transpositions are not causes of significant hemodynamic compromise during fetal life. Because these forms of CHD are well tolerated prior to birth, there does not seem to be any contraindication to a vaginal delivery at term. Cardiosurgery is available for many of these conditions, and it yields excellent results. Prenatal diagnosis could be highly beneficial under these circumstances, by allowing the mother to be referred for delivery in a tertiary care center where imme-

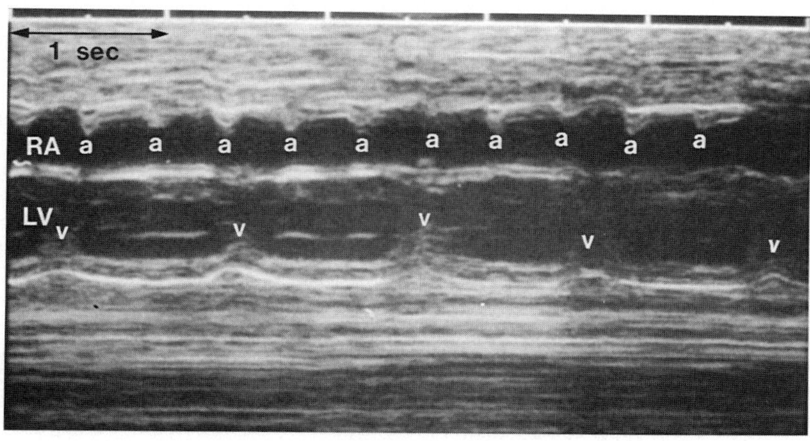

FIGURE 37–24. Complete atrioventricular block. The TM-mode sonogram reveals a regular atrial activity (a) with a frequency of about 120 bpm and a slow, independent ventricular activity (v) with a frequency of about 60 bpm. This infant was delivered at term by cesarean section. A pacemaker had to be installed on the third day of life.

diate neonatal assistance by a skilled pediatric team is available.

On the other hand, cardiac lesions associated with either pump failure, high cardiac output, or atrioventricular valve insufficiency may be associated with intrauterine heart failure. Because of the presence of an ample communication at the level of the atria, fetal cardiac failure is usually of the right type, and it is manifest with polyhydramnios, hepatosplenomegaly, and hydrops. It is uncertain if prenatal diagnosis can ameliorate the prognosis for this group of fetuses, although it is theoretically possible that in some cases, early atraumatic delivery and immediate postnatal treatment could be beneficial. The association of fetal CHD and overt hydrops is, however, to be considered at present a lethal condition and should be managed conservatively.

CONCLUSIONS

Fetal echocardiography is an established technique for the prenatal diagnosis of structural cardiac lesions and dysrhythmias. Although the time and expertise involved in fetal cardiac scanning limits its application to selected pregnancies, the inclusion of some views of cardiac anatomy in routine ultrasound examination may increase the antenatal detection rate of congenital heart disease. Criteria for the recognition of the most frequent types of cardiac anomalies have been described. It is expected that antenatal recognition of certain types of cardiac lesions and a rational perinatal management can ameliorate the prognosis for the affected infants.

REFERENCES

1. Mitchell SC, Korones SB, Berendes HW. Congenital heart disease in 56,109 births. Incidence and natural history. Circulation 1971;43:323.
2. Hoffman JI, Christianson R. Congenital heart disease in a cohort of 19,502 births with long-term follow-up. Am J Cardiol 1978;42:641.
3. Gerlis LM. Cardiac malformations in spontaneous abortions. Int J Cardiol 1985;7:29.
4. Nora JJ, Nora AH. Genetics and counselling in cardiovascular disease. Springfield, IL: Charles C Thomas, 1978.
5. Nora JJ, Nora AH. Maternal transmission of congenital heart disease: new recurrence risk figures and the questions of cytoplasmic inheritance and vulnerability to teratogens. Am J Cardiol 1987;59:459.
6. Becker AE, Anderson RH. Pathology of congenital heart disease. London: Butterworths, 1981.
7. Winsberg F. Echocardiography of the fetal and newborn heart. Invest Radiol 1972;7:152.
8. Ianniruberto A, Iaccarino M, De Luca I, et al. Analisi delle strutture cardiache fetali mediante ecografia. Nota tecnica. Proceedings of the 3rd National Congress of the SISUM. Terlizzi, September 24–25, 1977:285.
9. De Luca I, Ianniruberto A, Colonna L. Aspetti ecografici del cuore fetale. G Ital Cardiol 1978;8:776.
10. Kleinman CS, Hobbins JC, Jaffe CC, et al. Echocardiographic studies of the human fetus: prenatal diagnosis of congenital heart disease and cardiac dysrhythmias. Pediatrics 1980;65:1059.
11. Allan LD, Crawford DC, Anderson RH, et al. Echocardiographic and anatomical correlates in fetal congenital heart disease. Br Heart J 1984;52:542.
12. Copel JA, Pilu G, Greene J, et al. Fetal echocardiographic screening for congenital heart disease: the importance of the four-chamber view. Am J Obstet Gynecol 1987;157:648.
13. Pilu G, Baccarani G. Prenatal diagnosis of cardiac structural abnormalities. Fetal Ther 1986;1:73.
14. Allan LD, Joseph MC, Boyd EGCA, et al. M-mode echocardiography in the developing human fetus. Br Heart J 1982;47:573.
15. DeVore GR, Donnerstein RL, Kleinman CS, et al. Fetal echocardiography. I. Normal anatomy as determined by real-time directed M-mode ultrasound. Am J Obstet Gynecol 1982;144:249.
16. DeVore GR, Siassi B, Platt LD. Fetal echocardiography. IV. M-mode assessment of ventricular size and contractility during the second and third trimester of pregnancy in the normal fetus. Am J Obstet Gynecol 1984;150:981.
17. St John Sutton MG, Gewitz MH, Shah B, et al. Quantitative assessment of growth and function of the cardiac chambers in the normal human fetus. A prospective longitudinal echocardiographic study. Circulation 1984;69:645.
18. Allan LD, Anderson RH, Sullivan ID, et al. Evaluation of fetal arrhythmias by echocardiography. Br Heart J 1983;50:240.
19. Kleinman CS, Donnerstein RL, Jaffe CC, et al. Fetal echocardiography. A tool for evaluation of in utero cardiac arrhythmias and monitoring of in utero therapy: analysis of 71 patients. Am J Cardiol 1983;51.237.
20. De Vore GR, Siassi B, Platt LD. Fetal echocardiography. III. The diagnosis of cardiac arrhythmias using real-time directed M-mode ultrasound. Am J Obstet Gynecol 1983;146:792.
21. Stewart PA, Tonge HM, Wladimiroff JW. Arrhythmias and structural abnormalities of the fetal heart. Br Heart J 1983;50:550.
22. Huhta JC, Strasburger JF, Carpenter RJ, et al. Pulsed Doppler fetal echocardiography. J Clin Ultrasound 1985;13:247.
23. Silverman NH, Kleinman CS, Rudolph AM, et al. Fetal atrioventricular valve insufficiency associated with nonimmune hydrops. A two-dimensional echocardiographic and pulsed Doppler ultrasound study. Circulation 1985;72:825.
24. Reed KL, Sahn DJ, Scagnelli S, et al. Doppler echocardiographic studies of diastolic function in the human fetal heart. Changes during gestation. J Am Coll Cardiol 1986;8:391.
25. Kenny JF, Plappert T, Doubilet P, et al. Changes in intracardiac blood flow velocities and right and left ventricular stroke volumes with gestational age in the normal human fetus: a prospective Doppler echocardiographic study. Circulation 1986; 74:1208.
26. Reed KL, Meijboom EJ, Sahn DJ, et al. Cardiac Doppler flow velocities in human fetus. Circulation 1986;73:41.
27. Lingman G, Marsal K. Circulatory effects of fetal cardiac arrhythmias. Pediatr Cardiol 1986;7:67.
28. Kenny JF, Plappert T, Doubilet P, et al. Effects of heart rate on ventricular size, stroke volume, and output in the normal human fetus: a prospective Doppler echocardiographic study. Circulation 1987;76:52.
29. Machado MVL, Chita SC, Allan LD. Acceleration time in the aorta and pulmonary artery measured by Doppler echocardiography in the midtrimester normal human fetus. Br Heart J 1987;58:15.
30. De Smedt M, Visser GHA, Meijboom EJ. Fetal cardiac output estimated by Doppler echocardiography during mid- and late gestation. Am J Cardiol 1987;60:337.
31. Rowe RD, Uchida IA. Cardiac malformation in mongolism. A prospective study of 184 mongoloid children. Am J Med 1961;31:726.
32. Kleinman CS, Donnerstein RL, DeVore GR, et al. Fetal echocardi-

ography for evaluation of in utero congestive heart failure: a technique for study of nonimmune fetal hydrops. N Engl J Med 1982;306:568.

33. Rudolph AM. Congenital disease of the heart. Chicago: Year Book Medical Publishers, 1974.
34. Hoffman JIE, Rudolph AM. The natural history of ventricular septal defects in infancy. Am J Cardiol 1965;16:634.
35. Allan LD, Little D, Campbell S, et al. Fetal ascites associated with congenital heart disease. Care report. Br J Obstet Gynaecol 1981;88:453.
36. Reynolds JL. Intrauterine growth retardation in children with congenital heart disease. Its relation to aortic stenosis. Birth Defects Original Articles Series 1972;8:143.
37. Feigenbaum H. Echocardiography. 3rd ed. Philadelphia: Lea & Febiger, 1981.
38. Huhta JC, Carpenter RJ, Moise KJ, et al. Prenatal diagnosis and postnatal management of critical aortic stenosis. Circulation 1987;75:573.
39. Stewart PA, Buis-Liem T, Verwey RA, et al. Prenatal ultrasonic diagnosis of familial asymmetric septal hypertrophy. Prenat Diagn 1986;6:249.
40. Wright GB, Keane JF, Nadas AS, et al. Fixed subaortic stenosis in the young. Medical and surgical course in 83 patients. Am J Cardiol 1983;52:830.
41. Lev M, Rimoldi HJA, Rowlatt UF. The quantitative anatomy of cyanotic tetralogy of Fallot. Circulation 1964;30:531.
42. Stewart PA, Wladimiroff JW, Becker AE. Early prenatal detection of double outlet right ventricle by echocardiography. Br Heart J 1985;54:340.
43. Sanders SP, Bierman FZ, Williams RG. Conotruncal malformations. Diagnosis in infancy using subxyphoid 2-dimensional echocardiography. Am J Cardiol 1982;50:1361.
44. Sahn DJ, Shenker L, Reed KL, et al. Prenatal ultrasound diagnosis of hypoplastic left heart syndrome in utero associated with hydrops fetalis. Am Heart J 1982;104:1368.
45. Silverman NH, Enderlein MA, Golbus MS. Ultrasonic recognition of aortic valve atresia in utero. Am J Cardiol 1984;53:391.
46. Allan LD, Crawford DC, Tynan MJ. Pulmonary atresia in prenatal life. J Am Coll Cardiol 1986;8:1131.
47. Walther FJ, Siassi B, King J, et al. Cardiac output in infants of insulin-dependent diabetic mothers. J Pediatr 1985;107:109.
48. Bovicelli L, Picchio FM, Pilu G, et al. Prenatal diagnosis of endocardial fibroelastosis. Prenat Diagn 1984;4:67.
49. Romero R, Pilu G, Jeanty P, et al. Cardiomyopathies. In: Prenatal diagnosis of congenital anomalies. Norwalk, CT: Appleton & Lange, 1987:178.
50. Allan LD, Crawford DC, Tynan MJ. Evolution of coarctation of the aorta in intrauterine life. Br Heart J 1984;52:471.
51. Kleinman CS, Copel JA, Weinstein EM, et al. In utero diagnosis and treatment of fetal supraventricular tachycardia. Sem Perinatol 1985;9:113.
52. Griffiths SP. Congenital complete heart block. Circulation 1971;43:615.
53. Chameides L, Truex RC, Vetter V, et al. Association of maternal systemic lupus erythematosus with congenital complete heart block. N Engl J Med 1977;297:1204.
54. Scott JS, Maddison PJ, Taylor PV, et al. Connective tissue disease, antibodies to ribonucleoprotein and congenital heart block. N Engl J Med 1983;309:209.
55. Singsen BH, Akther JE, Weinstein MM, et al. Congenital complete heart block and SSA antibodies. Obstetric implications. Am J Obstet Gynecol 1985;152:655.
56. Carpenter RJ, Strasburger JF, Garson A, et al. Fetal ventricular pacing for hydrops secondary to complete atrioventricular block. J Am Coll Cardiol 1986;8:1434.

38

CHAPTER

GASTROINTESTINAL AND GENITOURINARY ANOMALIES

Sandro Gabrielli and E. Albert Reece

EMBRYOLOGICAL NOTES

During the fourth week of gestation, significant changes in size and shape of the embryo result from the process of folding the flat embryonic disk into a cylindrical structure.[1] Folding of the embryo in a transverse plane produces right and left lateral folds. Each lateral body wall folds toward the midline ventrally, forming a roughly cylindrical structure. During this process, the flat endodermal roof of the yolk sac that lies below the embryonic disk is incorporated into the embryo as a tubular structure (the primitive gut). The cranial end of the roof of the yolk sac will become the foregut, and the caudal end develops into the hindgut. In the body of the embryo, the section of the roof of the yolk sac between the cranial and the caudal end will become the midgut, which was originally connected to the extraembryonic portion of the yolk sac. This connection is progressively reduced to a narrow yolk stalk or vitelline duct. As the midgut separates from the yolk sac, it connects to the dorsal abdominal wall by a thin dorsal mesentery.

The foregut gives origin to the following structures: pharynx and lower respiratory system, esophagus, stomach, duodenum (cranial to the common bile duct), liver, pancreas, and biliary apparatus. The midgut gives rise to the duodenum (distal to the common bile duct), jejunum, ileum, cecum, appendix, ascending colon, and right proximal one half to two thirds of the transverse colon.

The left or distal one half to one third of the transverse colon, the descending and sigmoid colon, the rectum, and the upper portion of the anal canal derive from the hindgut. The remaining portion of the anal canal develops from the anal pit or proctodeum.

The urinary tract originates from the intermediate mesoderm and cloaca. The kidneys and ureters begin to develop during the fifth week of gestation as a structure called metanephron, which is derived in turn from two different components: the ureteral bud and the metanephric blastema of mesoderm. The ureteral bud enlarges cranially, surrounded by the metanephric blastema, which forms a cap around it. The ureteral bud gives origin to the ureter in its distal portion, and to the renal pelvis in its caudal end. A process of induction leads to the formation of calices and collector ducts, which branch several times. At the blind extremity of the collector ductus, groups of mesenchymal cells constitute the metanephric ducts. The distal convolute tubule eventually fuses itself with a collector ductus. Therefore, each urinary tubule consists of two portions: a nephron, derived from metanephric blastema, and a collector ductus, derived from the ureteral bud. The urinary bladder derives from the division of endodermal cloaca through the rectourinary septum into a dorsal portion (rectum) and a ventral portion (urogenital sinus). The cranial part of the urogenital sinus is the vesicourethral canal. The epithelium of the bladder takes origin from the vesicourethral canal, while surrounding mesenchyma provides the lamina propria, muscular layers, and peritoneal cover. As the bladder enlarges, the mesonephric ducts are incorporated into the dorsal wall of the bladder, and ureters open separately into the bladder itself. The allantois involutes and becomes a tubule, which is called the urachus. In postnatal life, the urachus is transformed into a fibrous string, extending from the apex of the bladder to the umbilicus.

NORMAL ULTRASOUND ANATOMY

The outline of the fetal abdomen can be demonstrated by ultrasound by early midtrimester. Abdominal circumference is measured on an axial section at the level of the confluence of the umbilical vein into the portal sinus (Fig. 38-1).[2] Additional cross sections parallel to the latter can be performed to detect any possible defects. Normal insertion of the umbilical cord on the abdominal wall can be visualized as an interruption of the abdominal outline connected to a cylindrical structure formed by two or more echogenic parallel lines. Normal insertion is also visible on a longitudinal scan, allowing the detection of the direction of the umbilical vein inside the abdomen (Fig. 38-2).

The liver occupies most of the upper abdomen, showing a homogeneous, echogenic ultrasound pattern. Measurement of the right lobe from the diaphragm to the tip plotted against biparietal diameter (BPD) has been used in the diagnosis of fetal hepatomegaly (in case of erythroblastosis fetalis, for example) (Fig. 38-3). The gallbladder is often distended in utero, appearing as a pear-shaped, fluid-filled structure arising from the hilum, and angles from the anteroposterior axis of the abdomen at 45 degrees. The stomach is almost constantly distended, and in a transverse scan appears as a semilunar, fluid-filled, and neatly outlined area. Stomach dimensions can vary significantly at each gestational age, due to the filling and emptying state. The stomach volume has been calculated in normal pregnancies from 14 to 24 weeks gestation.[3] The fetal bowel is usually uniformly echogenic, and it may be difficult to distinguish bowel from liver, particularly in second and early third trimester. Late in pregnancy, loops distended by the accumulating meconium are easily visualized (Fig. 38-4). Changes occurring in bowel ultrasound pattern have been correlated with increasing fetal maturation.[4] The variety of bowel ultrasound pattern has been recently suggested as an aid in dating the pregnancy during third trimester.[5]

All components of the urinary system, except ureters,

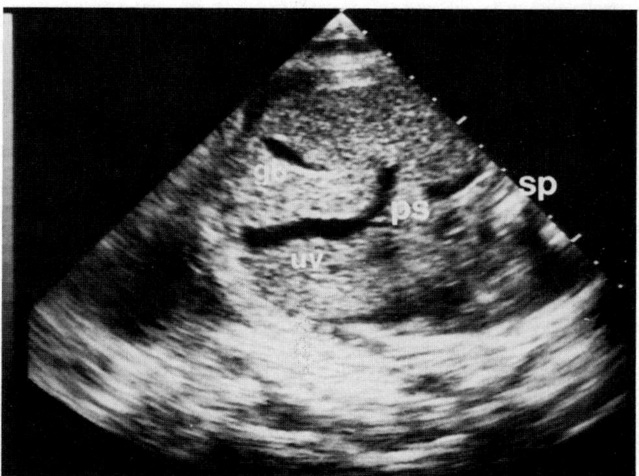

FIGURE 38–1. Cross section of the abdomen at the level of cord insertion and slightly angled cranially, showing the umbilical vein bending sharply at the portal sinus (uv, umbilical vein; ps, portal sinus; sp, spine; gb, gallbladder).

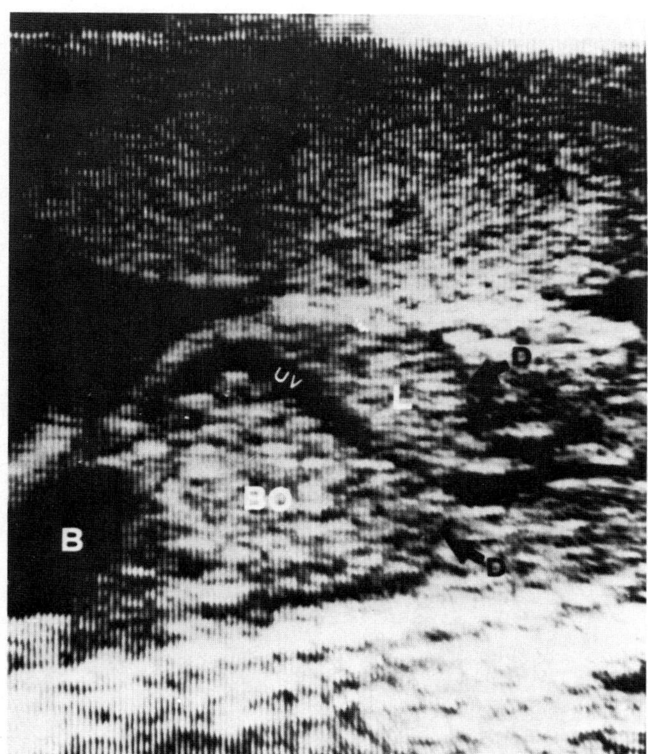

FIGURE 38–2. Longitudinal scan of the trunk in a fetus of 28 weeks gestation, showing a replete urinary bladder (B), loops of bowel (BO), the normal direction of umbilical vein (UV). L, liver; D, diaphragm.

can be visualized in utero from the beginning of the early second trimester. Using a cross section of the abdomen, as early as 14 weeks and up to 20 weeks gestation, kidneys appear circular and slightly hypoechoic, compared to the liver and bowel loops, at both sides of vertebral bodies.[6]

At 20 weeks, the kidneys show a hyperechoic capsule, the parenchyma is less hyperechoic, and calices sometimes surround a minimally physiologically dilated pelvis. This dilated pelvis has nothing to do with hydronephrosis, and is probably due to a more efficient diuresis than in later gestation. At this gestational age, the cortical area is slightly more echogenic than the medulla.[7]

With progressing gestation, fat tissue accumulates around the kidneys, enhancing the borders of the kidneys in contrast with the other splanchnic organs. Around 26 to 27 weeks gestation, renal pyramids can be detected, and the arcuate arteries can be seen pulsating in their proximity in real-time ultrasonography.

During midtrimester, kidneys should be differentiated from adrenals, which can be easily confused with them. Differential diagnosis is made by looking for the renal pelvis.

Longitudinal and transverse sections of the abdomen can be used to study the kidneys. In a longitudinal scan, kidneys appear as elliptical areas, while on transverse scan they appear as roundish structures at both sides of

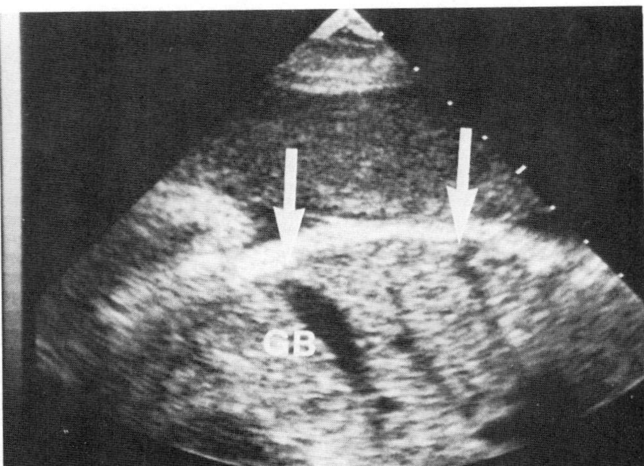

FIGURE 38–3. Longitudinal section of the upper abdomen, demonstrating the mode of measuring the length of the right hepatic lobe, from the diaphragm to the tip (arrows). GB, gallbladder.

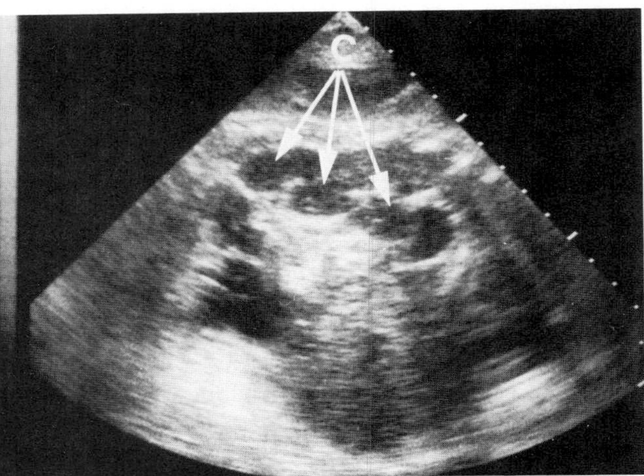

FIGURE 38–4. Meconium accumulating in the colon (C) in the third trimester of pregnancy.

the spine (Figs. 38-5, 38-6). Using a cross section of the abdomen, it is possible to estimate the size of the kidneys. Generally, they cover less than one third of the surface of the entire abdomen. Biometry of the kidneys has been suggested by various authors to diagnose congenital anomalies.[8–10]

The fetal bladder can be detected as a fluid-filled area in the anterior lower abdomen from early midtrimester, when urine formation begins. The contribution of the kidneys to the amniotic fluid dynamics is little before 16 weeks, but it steadily increases throughout gestation, so that in the second half of gestation amniotic fluid is formed mostly by urine.[11]

Changing of shape and volume depends on alternate emptying and filling. It has been demonstrated that micturition occurs approximately every 110 minutes.[12] The fetal bladder, however, should be always visualized, due to the incomplete emptying. A simple diagnostic test has been proposed when the bladder has not been seen: Lasix is administered to the mother, and if the bladder is not seen in 1 hour, there is a strong suspicion of urinary tract anomaly.[13] However, absence of urine in the fetal bladder after furosemide administration does not necessarily imply a diagnosis of bilateral renal agenesis. Severe intrauterine growth retardation (IUGR), for instance, is almost invariably associated with oligohydramnios, despite normal renal function.[14,15]

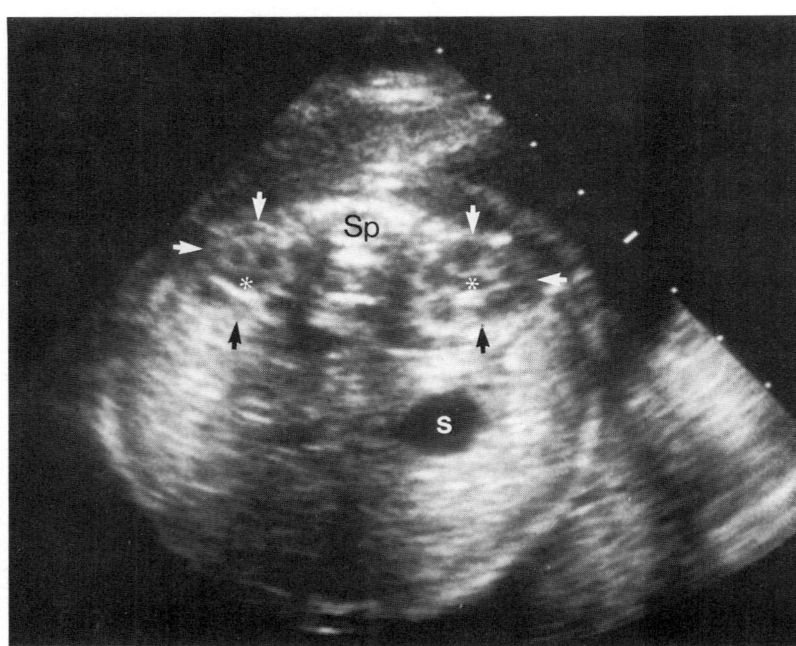

FIGURE 38–5. Transverse section of the abdomen in a 35-week fetus, demonstrating normal kidneys (arrows) at both sides of the spine (Sp). *, renal pelvis; S, stomach.

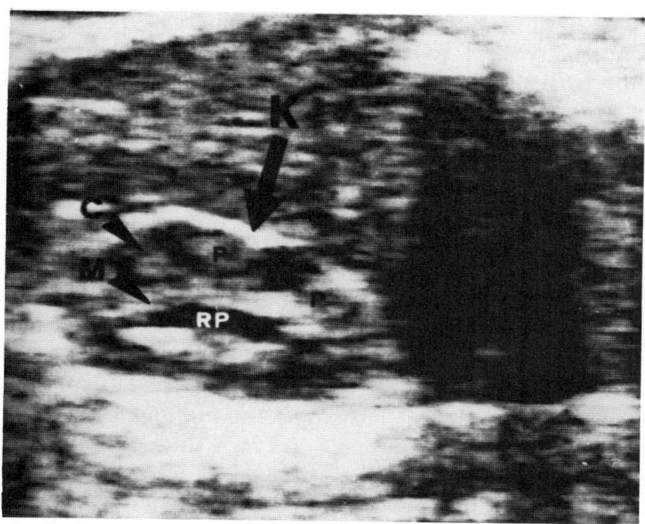

FIGURE 38-6. Longitudinal scan of the fetal trunk at 36 weeks gestation, demonstrating the kidney (K) as an elliptical mass. RP, renal pelvis; C, cortex; M, medulla; P, pyramids.

GASTROINTESTINAL ANOMALIES

Structural anomalies of the gastrointestinal (GI) tract are relatively common. Fetuses with GI anomalies, which often allow a good quality of life after postnatal surgical correction, largely benefit from prenatal diagnosis.[16] Anomalies can be subdivided into two groups: intestinal obstructions and ventral wall defects.

OBSTRUCTIONS

The echo-free areas resulting from fluid collection and progressive dilation of the bowel cranial to the obstruction site are easily detected by ultrasound. Furthermore, a GI obstruction is often associated with hydramnios, allowing a better visualization.[17] A proximal obstruction can be expected approximately in 1 in 15 pregnancies with polyhydramnios.[18] GI obstructions can involve the esophagus, duodenum, and small bowel; they can be intrinsic or extrinsic (eg, intrathoracic cyst or annular pancreas). Conversely, distal obstructions are not usually associated with hydramnios, and their detection is rather more difficult.

ESOPHAGEAL ATRESIA

PATHOGENESIS

Esophageal atresia is a relatively frequent anomaly, occurring in 1 in 3000 to 3500 live births. It is caused by an impairment in the process of recanalization of the primitive esophagus. An abnormal connection between trachea and esophagus is usually derived from an imperfect development of the respiratory diverticulum (Fig. 38-7). In the most common type of fistula (90% to 95%), the upper portion of the esophagus ends blindly (esophageal atresia), and the lower portion develops from the trachea near the bifurcation. The two portions of the esophagus may be connected by a solid cord. Less common are (1) the upper portion ending in the trachea, the lower portion being of variable length; (2) double fistula, where upper and lower portions end in the trachea; (3) tracheo-esophageal fistula without esophageal atresia; (4) esophageal atresia without tracheo-esophageal fistula; and (5) tracheal aplasia (lethal).

ASSOCIATED ANOMALIES

Severe structural anomalies are associated in nearly 50% of the cases, including heart, GI, and genitourinary (GU) tract anomalies; skeletal deformities; cleft defects of the face; and central nervous system (CNS) lesions such as meningoceles or hydrocephalus. Chromosomal anomalies, particularly trisomy 21, are also commonly present.

PRENATAL DIAGNOSIS

Prenatal diagnosis is based on indirect findings. Rarely, an elongated upper mediastinal and retrocardiac anechoic structure, interpreted as the dilated proximal esophageal pouch, can be observed (Fig. 38-8).[19] Ultrasound criteria for diagnosis are polyhydramnios and failed visualization of the stomach (Fig. 38-9).[20] The bowel appears uniformly echogenic, even in late pregnancy, due to the absence of amniotic fluid. In the majority of the cases, a fistula between the respiratory

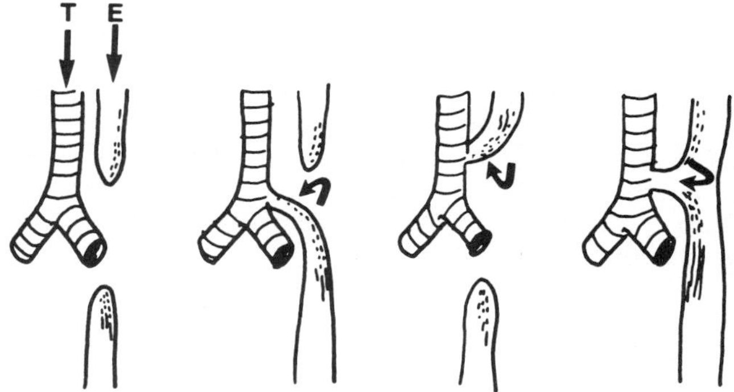

FIGURE 38-7. Different types of esophageal atresia with and without tracheoesophageal fistula. Esophageal atresia without fistula, atresia of the upper esophagus with a fistula connecting the lower portion of the esophagus and the trachea (more common), atresia of the lower esophagus with a fistula connecting the upper portion of the esophagus and the trachea, and double fistula (upper and lower portions of the esophagus) ending in the trachea.

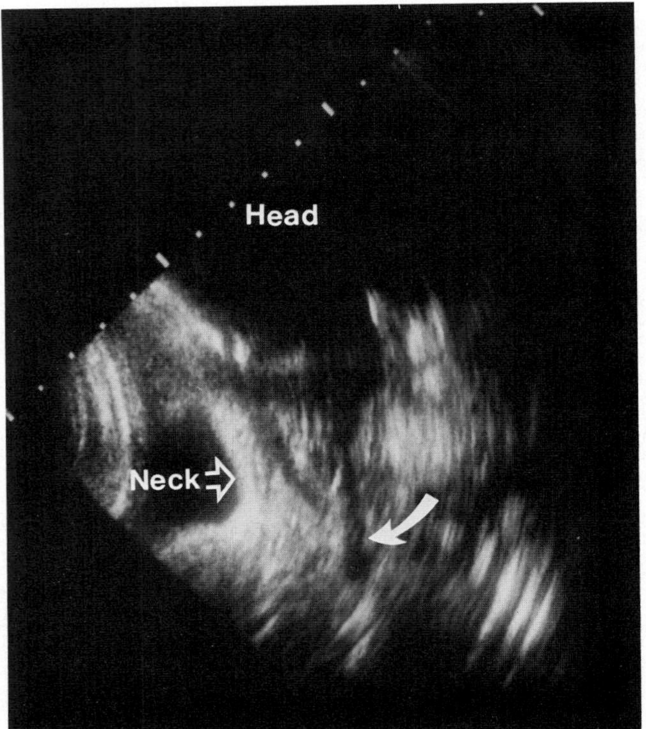

FIGURE 38–8. Coronal section of the neck in a fetus with esophageal atresia, showing the blind end of the esophagus (*arrow*). (From Romero et al. Prenatal diagnosis of congenital anomalies. Norwalk, CT: Appleton and Lange, 1988: 235.)

and the GI tract distal to the obstruction allows ingestion of amniotic fluid. Conversely, absence of amniotic fluid in the GI tract does not mean absence of tracheoesophageal fistula, because a small quantity of fluid cannot be seen with ultrasound or a fistula may be obstructed in utero.[19] Increased amniotic fluid α-fetoprotein (AFP) concentration has a limited diagnostic value, because amniotic fluid levels of the protein can be within normal range, due to the dilutional effect caused by polyhydramnios.[21] As an additional diagnostic test, Holzgreve and coworkers suggested determination of amniotic acetylcholinesterase secretory isoenzyme, which can be high even when amniotic fluid AFP levels are normal.[22]

PROGNOSIS AND MANAGEMENT

We are not aware of any case of esophageal atresia that was diagnosed or even suspected earlier than during the early third trimester of pregnancy. Because the prognosis of the affected newborn is worse if severe congenital anomalies are associated with it, an accurate ultrasound examination of the entire fetal anatomy should be performed. Time and mode of delivery are not influenced by prenatal diagnosis. Delay in postnatal recognition, however, results in increased neonatal morbidity and mortality.[23] Prenatal diagnosis alerts the pediatrician, facilitates prompt neonatal diagnostic confirmation, and enables prevention of possible complications, such as aspiration pneumonia, which can be lethal.

DUODENAL OBSTRUCTION

PATHOGENESIS

Duodenal obstruction occurs in approximately 1 in 7500 to 10,000 live births. The anomaly can be either intrinsic or extrinsic. Extrinsic lesions are mainly the consequence of a compression of the duodenum by the surrounding annular pancreas or by peritoneal fibrous bands. With intrinsic obstructions in duodenal atresia or stenosis, either defect derives from an incomplete developmental process during the second and third month of fetal life.[24] As the intestine turns from a solid structure into an empty tubular one, persistence of one or more septa, resulting in a diaphragm, is defined as stenosis. Complete atresia develops from the separation of solid intestine into two or more blind portions, which can be either totally isolated from each other or connected by fibrous bands.

ASSOCIATED ANOMALIES

Duodenal atresia is very often associated with other malformations. Nearly 30% of the fetuses have trisomy 21. Other common anomalies include structural cardiac anomalies (20%), malrotation of the colon (22%) and, less frequently, tracheo-esophageal fistula and renal malformations.

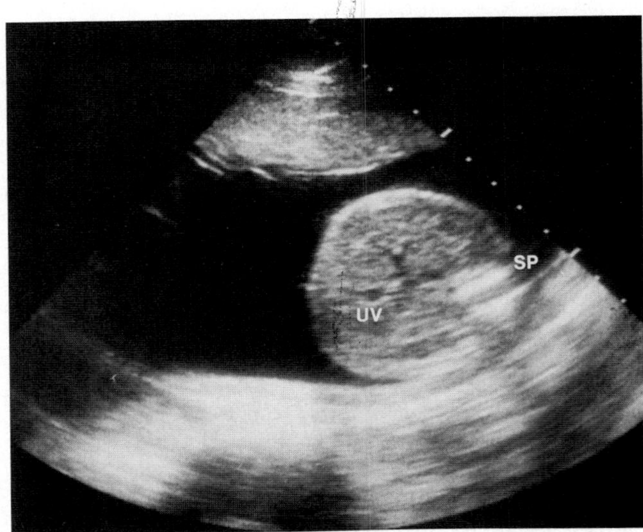

FIGURE 38–9. Transverse scan of the fetal abdomen in a fetus with esophageal atresia. The stomach is not visualized.

PRENATAL DIAGNOSIS

Since Loveday reported the first intrauterine ultrasound diagnosis of duodenal atresia in 1975,[25] many other cases have been described in the literature. Detection of two echo-free areas inside the abdomen ("double-bubble" sign), representing the dilated stomach and first portion of the duodenum, is crucial for prenatal diagnosis (Fig. 38-10). Polyhydramnios is a constant associated finding. An appropriate oblique scan of the fetal abdomen may demonstrate a single anechoic mass showing a connection between the fluid-filled stomach and duodenum.[26] Furthermore, a double-bubble image can also be produced by a curved stomach or by gastric peristaltic activity (Fig. 38-11). Bovicelli and associates[27] in 1983 reported a prenatal ultrasound diagnosis at 26 weeks gestation; previous ultrasound examinations had revealed normal fetal anatomy until 23 weeks. It would be interesting to determine whether that gestational age represents a threshold for ultrasound in utero detection of duodenal atresia. The majority of the cases diagnosed in utero have had previous ultrasound examinations performed during pregnancy, which were negative for anomalies. In summary, prenatal diagnosis of duodenal atresia on the basis of the double-bubble sign mostly depends on sonographer's expertise. Fetal vomiting has been observed by ultrasound[28] and related to upper GI tract obstruction.[29,30] Amniotic fluid levels of AFP may be elevated in cases of duodenal atresia.[31]

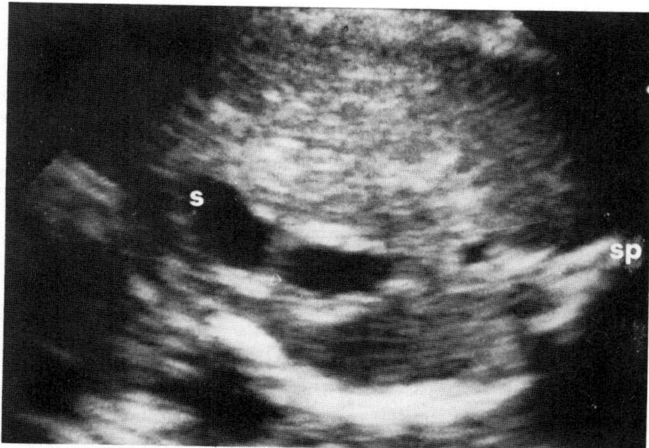

FIGURE 38–11. Double-bubble sign produced by gastric peristaltic activity. s, stomach; sp, spine.

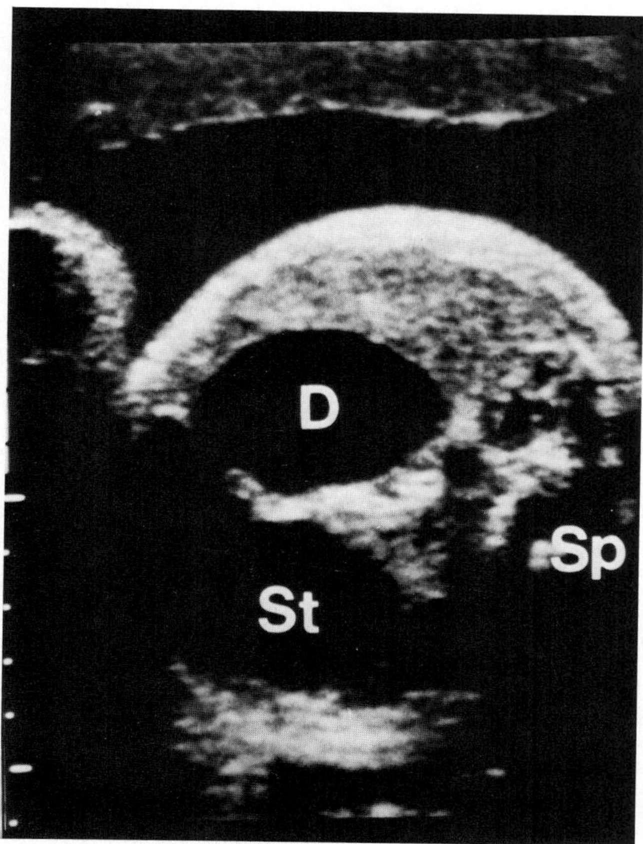

FIGURE 38–10. Transverse scan of the upper fetal abdomen in case of duodenal atresia. The double-bubble sign is evident. St, stomach; D, dilated duodenal bulb; Sp, spine.

PROGNOSIS AND MANAGEMENT

Postnatal prognosis of duodenal atresia depends mainly on the following: associated anomalies, birth weight, and prompt confirmation of prenatal diagnosis.

A thorough survey of the entire fetal anatomy and fetal karyotyping are of paramount importance. Isolated anomaly is compatible with a good quality of life after postnatal surgical correction. Obstetrical management is not influenced by prenatal diagnosis of duodenal atresia; however, spontaneous premature labor is a frequent complication due to polyhydramnios. Prenatal detection of the anomaly allows prevention of neonatal vomiting or aspiration pneumonia through early aspiration of gastric contents.

INTESTINAL OBSTRUCTIONS (BELOW THE LEVEL OF THE DUODENUM)

PATHOGENESIS

Intestinal obstructions are a quite common congenital anomaly, occurring in 1 in 300 to 1500 live births. Obstructions can be intrinsic or extrinsic. Intrinsic lesions result from absent (atresia) or partial (stenosis) recanalization of the intestine. In atresia, the two segments of the gut may be either completely separated or connected by a fibrous cord. In stenosis, the lumen of the gut is narrowed or the two intestinal segments are separated by a septum with a central diaphragm. Extrinsic obstructions are caused by malrotation of colon with volvulus, peritoneal bands, meconium ileus, and agangliosis (Hirschsprung's disease).

ASSOCIATED ANOMALIES

Intestinal atresias or stenosis are infrequently associated with other anomalies. However, GI anomalies can be slightly more frequent than in the general population.

PRENATAL DIAGNOSIS

With GI obstructions below the level of the duodenum, multiple echo-free areas within distended fetal abdomen are usually seen (Fig. 38-12).[20,32] The more distal the site of the obstruction, the greater is the number of anechoic structures.

Although polyhydramnios is almost invariably present in cases of duodenal atresia, it is only an occasional finding in cases of lower small bowel obstructions. The severity of the polyhydramnios depends on the level of the obstruction: "high" obstructions are often associated with a certain degree of polyhydramnios, whereas obstructions of the colon are generally not accompanied with increased volume of amniotic fluid.[33] Atresia and stenosis produce comparable ultrasound findings.

Once prenatal diagnosis of obstruction is made, attention should be paid to the possible complications of the anomaly. Perforation as a consequence of impaired blood supply to the distended bowel can be suspected by ultrasound demonstrating ascites that was previously absent (Fig. 38-13).

Because meconium begins to accumulate in fetal bowel at 4 months, any perforation occurring after that time could bring the outflow of meconium into the peritoneal cavity. As a result, an intense reaction occurs, leading to extensive adhesions. If it is localized at the site of perforation, a calcified mass develops. At ultrasound, this appears as a highly echogenic mass, often visible near the liver (Fig. 38-14). Ascites may be also present (Fig. 38-15).[34,35]

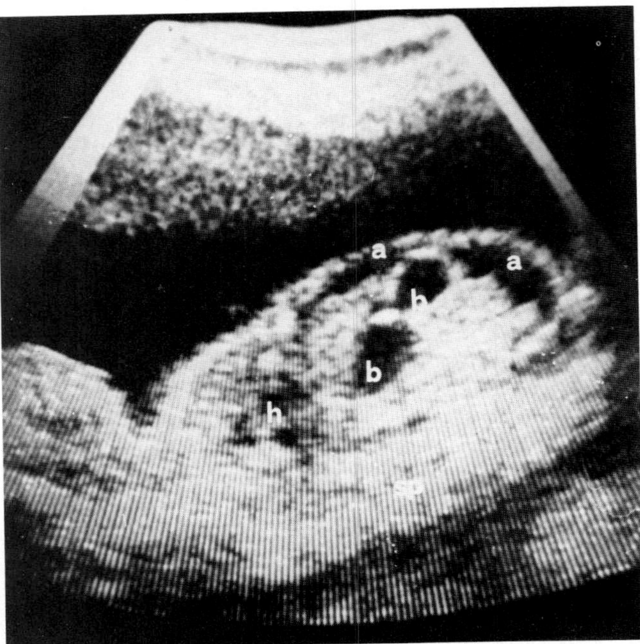

FIGURE 38–13. Longitudinal scan of the fetal abdomen showing perforation of the distended bowel occurring in a case of bowel obstruction (a, ascites; b, distended bowel; h, heart).

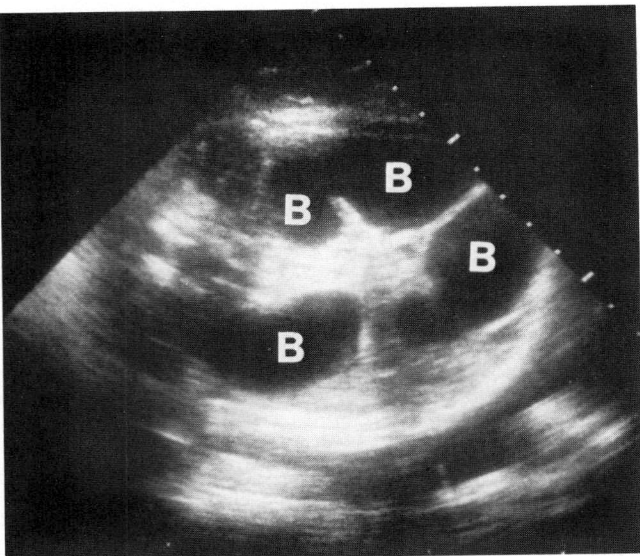

FIGURE 38–12. Transverse scan of the abdomen in a fetus with small bowel atresia. Multiple distended loops of bowel are visible. In real time, increased peristalsis was noted. B, distended loops of bowel.

PROGNOSIS AND MANAGEMENT

The mortality rate of babies affected by intestinal obstructions greatly depends on the postnatal complications due to delayed recognition: severe bronchopneumonia, gangrene of intestinal segments, postnatal perforation, and bacterial peritonitis.[36] When prenatal diagnosis is made, delivery should be planned in a center where prompt postnatal correction can be performed, thus improving the infant's prognosis.

The survival rate of surgically treated infants depends on prematurity and associated anomalies. Associated anomalies are far less common than in case of duodenal atresia. Chromosomal anomalies are rare, too. In case of meconium ileus, cystic fibrosis is a possibility.

Fetuses with uncomplicated intestinal obstruction can be delivered vaginally at term. Induction of preterm delivery should be considered when perforation occurs and ascites are seen. In these cases, Baxi and coworkers[37] suggested fetal paracentesis in order to decrease abdominal pressure on the diaphragm, thus allowing expansion of the lung. Decompression of fetal abdomen could permit normal vaginal delivery. If perforation and bleeding into the abdominal cavity occur,

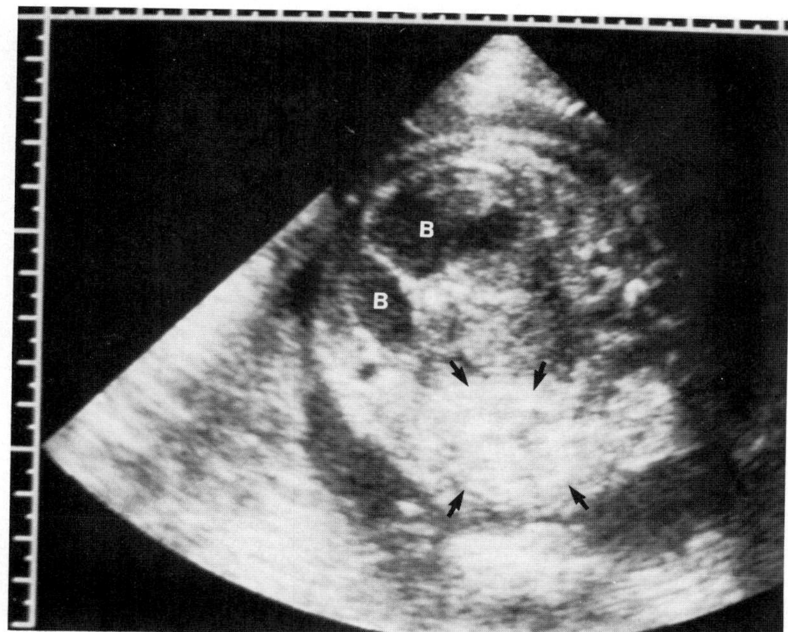

FIGURE 38–14. Transverse scan of the fetal abdomen showing a highly hyperechogenic mass (*arrows*) in a fetus with meconium peritonitis. Note the distended loops of bowel (*). Sp, spine.

delay in delivery may cause hydrops fetalis, owing to severe anemia, decreased oncotic pressure, and loss of plasma volume.[38]

ABDOMINAL WALL DEFECTS

Congenital abdominal wall defects are always associated with external herniation of viscera. Depending on the site and extent of the lesion, two separate pathologic entities are described—omphalocele, or exomphalos, and gastroschisis. Omphalocele is an herniation of the bowel through the umbilical ring. Gastroschisis is a lateral abdominal wall defect with eviscerated bowel and intact umbilicus. Congenital abdominal wall defects can be successfully corrected after birth.[39,40] Intrauterine diagnosis allows appropriate management of the affected fetus.

OMPHALOCELE

Pathogenesis

Omphalocele is a sporadic anomaly with a risk of occurrence of 1 in 6000 live births. It results from an alteration of the vital mechanism of closing of the body of the embryo. Impaired embryonic folding at the level of the lateral folds causes a herniation of intra-abdominal contents through the open umbilical ring into the base of the umbilical cord. Protrusion is covered by a translucent, avascular membrane, consisting of peritoneum inside and amniotic membrane outside, separated by Wharton's jelly.[41] When omphalocele is small, the umbilical cord is inserted into its apex; in cases of large defects, the cord is attached inferiorly and the umbilical vein and arteries are splayed out in the wall of the sac.[42] If the sac ruptures in utero, its remnants with the umbilical vessels are still visible on the border of the lesion. The defect varies greatly in size, from a small opening through which only one or two loops of the small intestine or a Meckel's diverticulum protrude, to an enormous defect containing all abdominal contents.

ASSOCIATED ANOMALIES

Omphalocele is often associated with other abnormalities, as a result of general interference with embryonic development during early gestation. Malrotation of the gut and duodenal obstruction are frequent. GU anomalies, including exstrophy of the bladder, penile anoma-

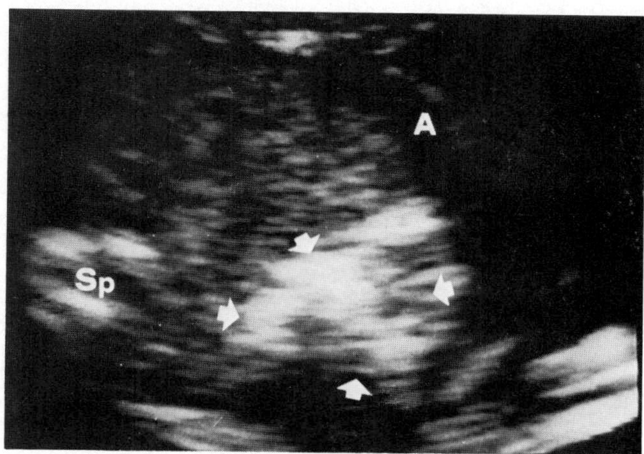

FIGURE 38–15. Transverse section of fetal abdomen, showing a disomogeneous mass (arrows) in a fetus with perforation complicating a meconium peritonitis. Sp, spine; A, ascites.

lies, and undescended testes, are also very common. Congenital heart diseases are frequent and represent the most important cause of death for the affected child. Craniofacial anomalies are quite rare. Chromosomal anomalies occasionally occur, particularly trisomies 13, 18, and 21. If macrosomia is present, one should suspect Beckwith-Wiedemann syndrome (EMG syndrome). This syndrome includes multiple malformations, such as omphalocele, macroglossia occasionally requiring partial glossectomy to prevent mandibular prognathism, and macrosomia with hyperplastic fetal visceromegaly; a severe resistant neonatal hypoglycemia may be expected in 50% of the cases. Omphalocele is also present in pentalogy of Cantrell, which includes a large upper abdominal omphalocele, an anterior diaphragmatic hernia, a sternal cleft, ectopia cordis, and various cardiac anomalies such as ventricular septal defect or tetralogy of Fallot. A low omphalocele is frequently associated with bladder or cloacal exstrophy, and other anomalies, including anal atresia or myelomeningocele and lower limb anomalies.[43,44]

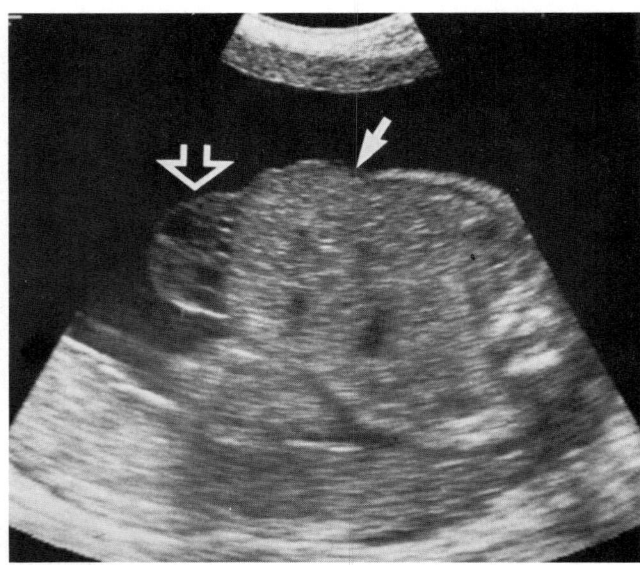

FIGURE 38–17. Transverse section of a 30-week fetus with large omphalocele. The solid arrow is pointing at the defect in the abdominal wall; the open arrow indicates the amnioperitoneal membrane surrounding the herniated viscera.

PRENATAL DIAGNOSIS

Omphalocele is relatively easy to detect with ultrasound from early midtrimester.[45–48] As normal migration of the midgut back into the abdomen occurs between the ninth and 12th gestational weeks, the diagnosis of ventral wall defects should not be made before 14 weeks.[49,50] A dense, echogenic mass outside the abdomen, covered by amnioperitoneal membrane, can be seen (Fig. 38-16). Protrusion generally consists of bowel alone, but in severe cases, liver and stomach can also be herniated (Figs. 38-17, 38-18). Exceptionally, heart and bladder are contained in the herniated sac.[51] In small defects, umbilical cord insertion is on top of the mass, whereas in large lesions, the cord is attached to its lower border. A cystic structure associated with the umbilical cord, representing an allantoic cyst often associated with omphalocele, can be interpreted as protrusion of abdominal contents through a defect of the abdominal wall.[52] Polyhydramnios is of-

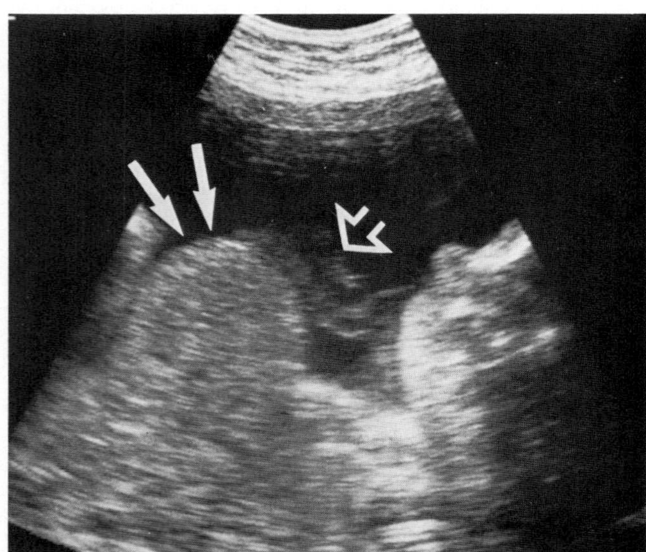

FIGURE 38–16. Longitudinal view of a fetus with omphalocele. The amnioperitoneal membrane (*arrows*) covering a dense, echogenic mass protruding through the defect and the umbilical cord (*open arrow*) originating from the apex of the defect are clearly visible.

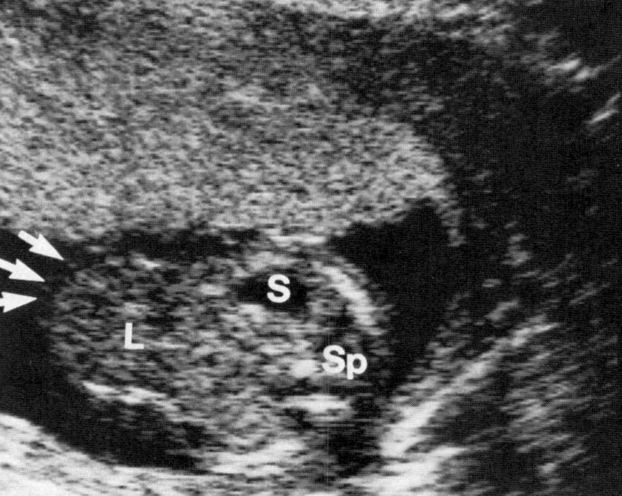

FIGURE 38–18. Transverse section of a 21-week fetus with large omphalocele. The liver (L) is protruded from the abdominal wall defect. S, stomach; Sp, spine; arrows, amnioperitoneal membrane.

ten present, and levels of amniotic fluid AFP are significantly raised,[53] due to diffusion through peritoneal membrane.[54]

PROGNOSIS AND MANAGEMENT

Omphalocele, unlike gastroschisis, is often associated with additional congenital anomalies (45% versus 5%); the mortality rate is therefore higher (34% versus 12.7%).[55] Cardiovascular malformations are present in 40% of the cases. They are more common in cases of trisomy 13, whereas the association of holoprosencephaly with omphalocele suggests the diagnosis of trisomy 18. Thus, in cases of omphalocele, a thorough sonographic evaluation of the fetus and fetal karyotype should be performed. In particular, abdominal wall defects can be a part of amniotic band syndrome, which is characterized by protrusion of abdominal contents, often attached to the placenta (see Fig. 38-18), and severe CNS, facial, and limb deformities. EMG syndrome or Beckwith-Wiedemann syndrome has a poor prognosis, because it is associated with resistant neonatal hypoglycemia and mental retardation in 50% of the surviving infants. The volume of the protruded viscera is also critical for determining fetal prognosis: giant defects are frequently associated with liver evisceration and ectopia cordis, having a much worse prognosis than small defects, in which only bowel loops are extruded.

When prenatal diagnosis is of giant omphalocele, or when multiple malformations are found, termination of pregnancy may be considered. If pregnancy is continued, the obstetrician should be able to select the most appropriate time and mode of delivery and plan adequate therapy for the newborn and subsequent surgical correction. In cases of small defects or isolated anomaly, if omphalocele is intact, there appears to be no need to anticipate early delivery.[56] In cases of ruptured omphalocele, Harrison and associates suggest a preterm cesarean section to avoid the pathologic alterations of the bowel being exposed to the amniotic fluid, which can compromise the outcome of postnatal surgical correction.[57] However, risks of prematurity should be taken into account. There is no agreement in the literature regarding the route of delivery. Large or ruptured omphalocele probably should be delivered by cesarean section, in strictly sterile conditions, to avoid trauma and infection of the herniated viscera and to decrease the risk of dystocia. However, it has yet to be demonstrated whether this kind of management improves the fetal outcome. Kirk and Wah in 1983, in a large retrospective study of 112 cases of abdominal wall defects, found no adverse effects related to vaginal delivery or to the success of surgical postnatal correction.[58] However, because the mortality rate of newborns affected by abdominal wall defects largely depends on the clinical condition of the malformed baby at the time of admission,[59] maternal transport to a specialized center and an accurately planned cesarean delivery probably avoid the risks of a sudden, unexpected delivery leading to a delay in surgical care.

GASTROSCHISIS

PATHOGENESIS

Gastroschisis represents the herniation of some of the intra-abdominal content through a paraumbilical defect of the abdominal wall. The umbilical cord is normally inserted and no sac is visible. At 5 to 6 weeks, as the intestine elongates to enter the umbilical cord, it ruptures at the base of the cord as a consequence of a failure of umbilical coelom to form. Rupture occurs on the right of the abdomen, where the right umbilical vein has been absorbed, causing a locus minoris resistentiae.[60] Other pathogenetic theories suggest that gastroschisis results from an intrauterine rupture of an incarcerated hernia into the cord,[61] or from a vascular accident involving the omphalomesenteric artery, leading to disruption of the umbilical ring and herniation of abdominal contents.[62] Occasionally, only a short tract of the intestine is herniated; in most cases, however, all of the small and large intestines protrude. Stomach, gallbladder, urinary bladder, testes or uterus, and adnexae are also prolapsed. Chemical peritonitis is an ominous complication due to amniotic fluid exposure of eviscerated abdominal contents. In such cases, the intestine shows marked dilation of the lumen and increased thickness of the walls, which appear edematous, of leathery consistency, and matted together and encased in a net of fibrinous material. In many cases, the intestine reveals an abnormal shortening. Single or multiple atretic sites of the protruded gut can be detected.

ASSOCIATED ANOMALIES

Associated anomalies are uncommon in gastroschisis compared to omphalocele, and usually involve the intestinal tract (malrotation). Occasionally, intestinal obstruction due to angulation of gut, adhesions, or atresia secondary to vascular impairment of the wall can be seen as ancillary complications.

PRENATAL DIAGNOSIS

Multiple rounded, thick-walled, echo-free structures within the amniotic cavity along the anterior surface of fetal abdomen, representing freely floating herniated loops of bowel, suggest a diagnosis of gastroschisis (Fig. 38-19).[63] Hypoechogenic areas can sometimes be identified within the bubble-like structures, suggesting the presence of meconium. The extruded structures are not covered by amnioperitoneal membrane, and normal umbilical cord insertion is present (Fig. 38-20). Polyhydramnios is a common feature, as well as increased amniotic fluid AFP levels. An impairment of fetal growth is

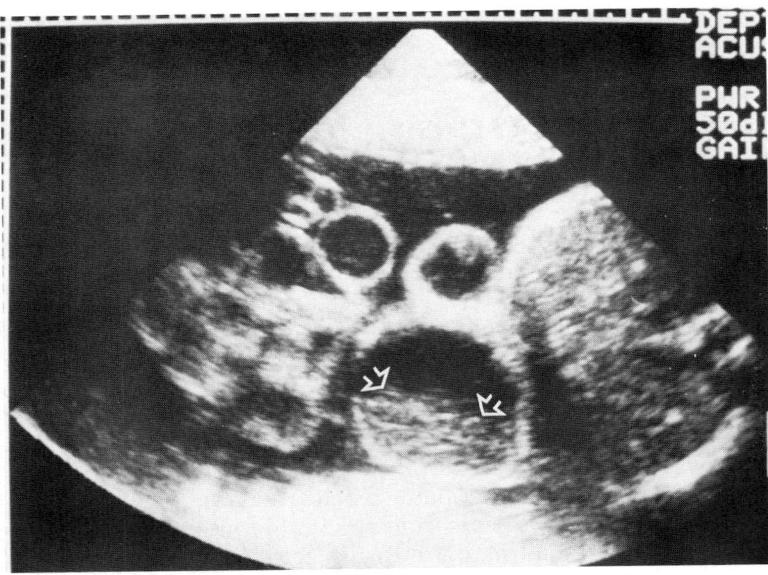

FIGURE 38–19. Free-floating loops of bowel in a fetus with gastroschisis. Levels are seen into the lumen of the loops (*arrow*).

often associated with gastroschisis.[64] On this occasion, the volume of amniotic fluid can be reduced and visualization is suboptimal.

PROGNOSIS AND MANAGEMENT

Prognosis for a fetus affected by gastroschisis has improved dramatically during the last three decades.[65–68] Perinatal mortality decreased from 82% in 1960 to less than 10% in 1984. This is likely to be attributable to improved surgical technique and the use of parenteral nutrition. Gastroschisis is less frequently associated with other congenital anomalies than omphalocele. As with omphalocele, it can be a part of amniotic band syndrome. Unlike omphalocele, gastroschisis is often associated with IUGR and oligohydramnios, which occasionally renders the diagnosis rather difficult. In light of the association with IUGR, risks connected to prematurity should be balanced with benefits of decreasing the time of exposure to the action of amniotic fluid. As with omphalocele, a fetus affected by gastroschisis should preferably be delivered by cesarean section in a center where the neonate can receive intensive care and where neonatal surgical correction is promptly available. Delay in pediatric care, in fact, increases the risk of sepsis and may be the cause of severe dehydration and rapid heat loss, which may compromise the outcome of surgical correction. Long-term follow-up of survivors is excellent: children show normal growth and development in follow-up to 5 years of age.[69]

FIGURE 38–20. Loops of bowel protruding through a lateral defect of the abdominal wall. Note the intact insertion of the cord (*arrow*). B, bowel; uv, umbilical vein.

URINARY TRACT ANOMALIES

Antenatal ultrasonography permits accurate identification of the fetal urinary tract. Therefore, ultrasound can reliably detect most urinary tract lesions, which previously were undetected until later in postnatal life. Fetal GU lesions are the major cause of neonatal abdominal masses. The antenatal sonographic detection of such anomalies is dramatically important for choosing the appropriate prenatal and postnatal management, and has improved the prognosis of children affected by these anomalies.[70] The sonographer has to be particularly careful in the evaluation of the volume of the amniotic fluid. Significant diminution of amniotic fluid volume heralds the presence of many GU anomalies, and when detected after the second trimester is an ominous prognostic factor, because of the association with pulmonary hypoplasia.[71]

Congenital malformations of the GU tract are relatively frequent anomalies, probably due to the complexity of embryologic development. The most important anomalies, which will be the subject of this section, are the following:

1. Bilateral renal agenesis
2. Cystic dysplasias of the kidneys, which have been classified by Potter as Types I, II, and III[13]
3. Obstructive uropathies
4. Ovarian cysts.

BILATERAL RENAL AGENESIS

Bilateral renal agenesis is a relatively rare condition, occurring in 1% to 3% of liveborn infants.

Pathogenesis

The anomaly can be isolated, or it can be a feature of a genetic syndrome. When isolated, it can be transmitted as a multifactorial character, with a risk of recurrence of 2.5%. Sporadic X-linked and autosomal recessive cases also have been described.[72]

Renal agenesis derives from failure of development of ureteric bud or nephrogenic blastema, because both components concur at the formation of normal kidneys.

Associated Anomalies

Renal agenesis can be part of Potter's syndrome, which includes pulmonary hypoplasia, skeletal deformities, and typical facies, characterized by low-set ears. Oligohydramnios is considered responsible for pulmonary hypoplasia and skeletal deformities, which are also present in some cases of prolonged rupture of membranes or IUGR.[73] Conversely, when oligohydramnios is not severe, characteristic features of Potter's syndrome are uncommon.[74] Other structural anomalies, such as cardiac and GI tract anomalies, are associated with variable incidence.

Prenatal Diagnosis

Failed visualization of kidneys and bladder, associated with oligohydramnios and IUGR, prompts the diagnosis of bilateral renal agenesis (Fig. 38-21). Prenatal diagnosis can be rather difficult due to the lack of amniotic fluid and to the posture of the fetus, which impairs detection of the kidneys. Additionally, adrenals are usually hypertrophic in cases of bilateral renal agenesis and can be confused with normal kidneys (Fig. 38-22). Identification of the renal capsule and renal pelvis enables the two structures to be distinguished.[75,76]

When a bilateral renal agenesis is suspected, the presence or absence of fetal bladder has to be confirmed by ultrasound or with a furosemide test. The latter, however, although somewhat controversial, may not discriminate between bilateral renal agenesis and other causes of compromised renal function.[77] In 1984, Goldenberg[78] reported a case in which a fetus with severe oligohydramnios did not respond to the furosemide test and required dialysis at birth. Therefore, a positive test seems to be useful to exclude bilateral renal agenesis, but a negative test cannot confirm such an anomaly. Currently, saline solution, when instilled in the amniotic cavity, permits a better view of splanchnic viscera.

Differential diagnosis between bilateral renal agenesis and other conditions associated with oligohydramnios, such as premature rupture of the membranes (PROM) and polycystic kidney, is rather difficult, particularly at early gestation.

Ultrasound and the additional tests mentioned above are routinely used to ruled out pathologic conditions.

Prognosis and Management

Prognosis is poor, because bilateral renal agenesis is not compatible with life; affected fetuses die either in utero or soon after birth due to pulmonary hypoplasia.

Termination of pregnancy can be offered to the couple when diagnosis is made during the second trimes-

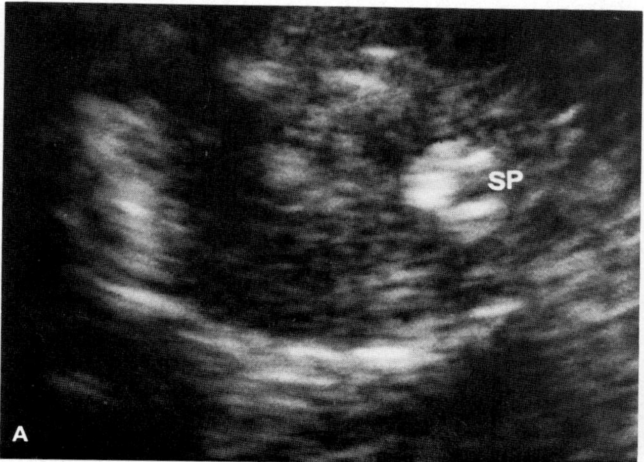

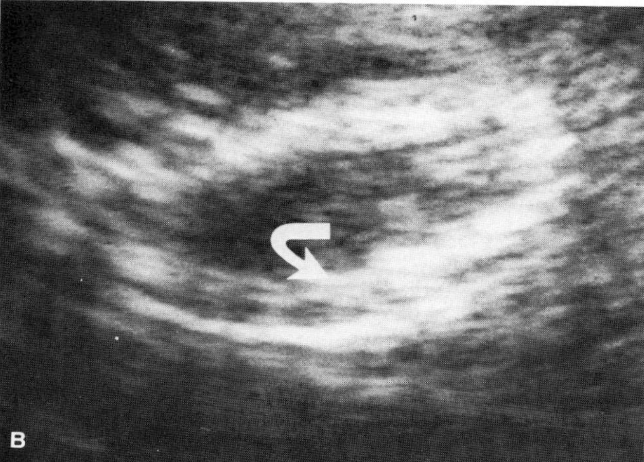

FIGURE 38–21. Transverse (top) and longitudinal (bottom) section of the abdomen of a fetus with bilateral renal agenesis. Note the empty renal fossa. Sp, spine.

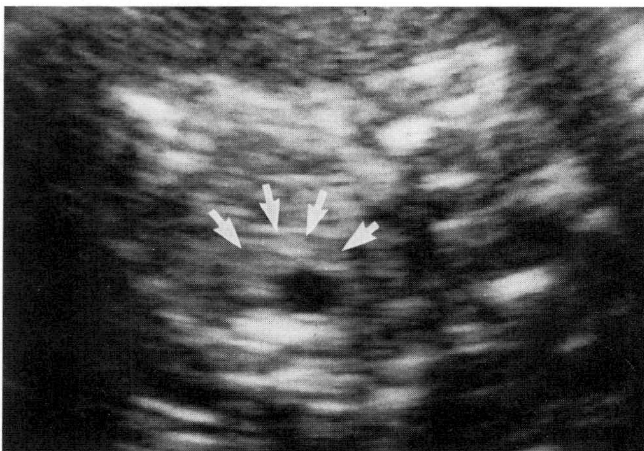

FIGURE 38–22. Fetus with bilateral renal agenesis. The renal fossa is empty and a hyperplastic adrenal gland is seen (*arrows*).

ter, whereas conservative management is the treatment of choice in the infrequent cases of third trimester diagnosis, particularly when the diagnosis is uncertain.

INFANTILE POLYCYSTIC KIDNEY DISEASE

Infantile polycystic kidney (IPKD), or Potter's Type I dysplasia, invariably involves both kidneys, which appear symmetrically enlarged and containing multiple minute cysts. Periportal fibrosis of the liver and biliary ductal ectasia are often associated with the kidney anomaly.

Pathogenesis

IPKD is an autosomal recessive disease, with a recurrence risk of 25% in a subsequent pregnancy after an affected child. A defect of the collecting system seems to be responsible for the anomaly. Kidneys are symmetrically enlarged, and the parenchyma is totally occupied by numerous cysts of minute dimensions. At section, the cysts present a cubic epithelium. According to the patient's age at the time of clinical presentation, the disease has been classified into four types: perinatal, neonatal, infantile, and juvenile.[79] The most common variety is the perinatal one.[80]

Associated Anomalies

In severe cases, compromised renal function leads to a marked oligohydramnios, which in turn is responsible for the pulmonary hypoplasia and skeletal deformities typical of Potter's syndrome.

Prenatal Diagnosis

On ultrasound, both kidneys usually appear extremely enlarged and hyperechogenic (Fig. 38-23).[81] The hyperechogenicity seems to be due to multiple minute cysts, which fall below the resolution power of the ultrasound equipment, thus increasing the acoustic transmission. In severe cases, the bladder is absent and oligohydramnios is extreme. Despite suboptimal visualization, however, alteration of the anatomy of the kidneys is often striking. Prenatal ultrasound diagnosis is possible at varying gestational ages, depending on the severity of the anomaly. In two cases, diagnoses have been performed in the third trimester, after a number of normal examination results.[82] At the moment, therefore, prenatal diagnosis of IPKD is restricted to severe cases, and it is not always possible to diagnose during midtrimester. Differential diagnosis has to be made with bilateral renal agenesis, Potter's Type II, and Potter's Type III renal dysplasia. The main criterion for distinction is morphology of the cysts: for example, in cases of Potter's Type II cystic dysplasia, cysts appear of variable size, mainly located in the periphery. In most cases, kidneys are enlarged (Fig. 38-24), but occasionally both are small. Distinction between Potter's Type I and Potter's Type III cystic dysplasia is almost impossible in utero, but an enlarged kidney is extremely rare in case of Potter's Type III.[83] Severe oligohydramnios renders the differential diagnosis between bilateral renal agenesis and Potter's Type I cystic dysplasia extremely difficult.

Prognosis and Management

Prognosis of IPKD (Potter's Type I cystic dysplasia) is poor, depending on the severity of the disease. The perinatal variety is usually the most severe, leading to stillbirth or neonatal death due to pulmonary hypopla-

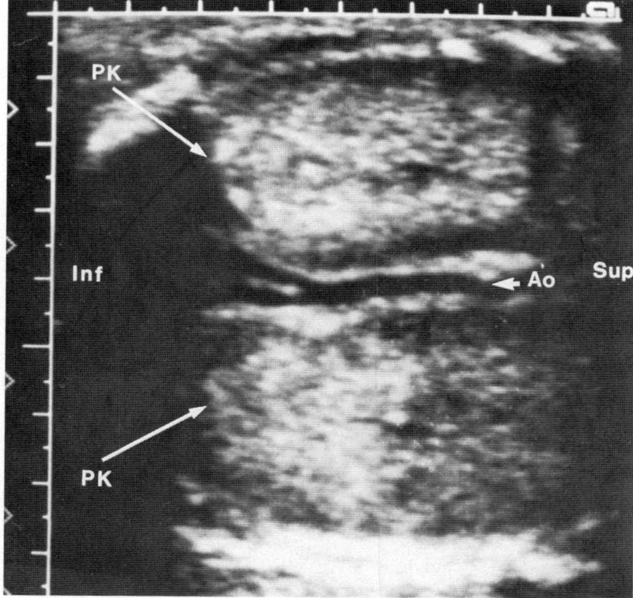

FIGURE 38–23. Coronal section of a fetus with infantile polycystic kidney disease (IPKD). Kidneys appear enlarged and hyperechogenic at both sides of the fetal aorta (Ao). PK, polycystic kidney; Inf, inferior; Sup, superior.

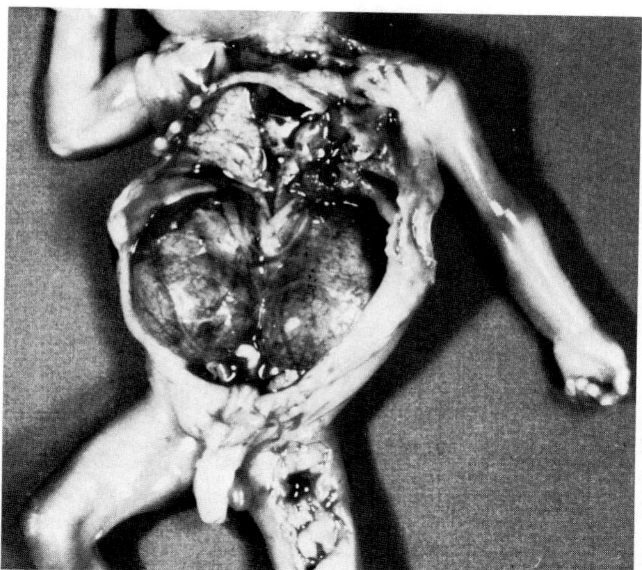

FIGURE 38–24. Dissection of a fetus with polycystic kidneys. Note the extremely enlarged kidneys occupying most of the fetal abdomen.

sia.[84,85] If diagnosis is made within the second trimester, termination of pregnancy is an option that can be offered to the parents. If diagnosis is made in the third trimester, conservative management is advisable. Occasionally, when the fetal abdomen is excessively distended, a cesarean section should be performed to avoid the risk of soft tissue dystocia.

MULTICYSTIC DYSPLASTIC KIDNEY DISEASE

Multicystic dysplastic kidney disease (MDKD) or Potter's Type IIA renal dysplasia are synonymous terms describing one of the most common congenital renal anomalies. Renal parenchyma is replaced by a number of cysts of variable size. One kidney is affected in the vast majority of cases, although bilateral renal involvement has been reported.[86] The dysplastic process is usually limited to the medulla, but can involve the cortex as well. The prevalence of unilateral MDKD is unknown; bilateral involvement is estimated to occur in 1 out of 1000 live births.[87]

Pathogenesis

MDKD is a sporadic disease. However, few examples of familial cases have been described.[88,89] MDKD also can be a feature of genetic syndromes, usually as a secondary event. Pathogenesis of the anomaly is controversial; however, there is almost general agreement on the theory that the anomaly is secondary to atresia of either the ureter or the pelvis or both during the metanephric stage of development.[90,91]

Associated Anomalies

MDKD is often associated with other congenital anomalies. Zerres and Fodisch reported an incidence of 50%; we recently reported an incidence of 37%.[92] Associated anomalies include CNS, GI, and congenital heart diseases, and chromosomal aberrations. MDKD may be frequently associated with contralateral renal anomalies, including contralateral renal agenesis and hydronephrosis. In cases of agenesis, such a diagnosis is prompted by failure of visualization of kidney and bladder, together with the detection of severe oligohydramnios. Misdiagnosis can occur when contralateral kidney is ectopic. In 10% of cases, MDKD is associated with contralateral hydronephrosis, usually from obstruction at the ureteropelvic junction (UPJ). Because the obstructed kidney is the only functioning one, serial examination should be planned to control dilation of the pelvis and the amount of amniotic fluid.

Prenatal Diagnosis

The criteria for prenatal ultrasound diagnosis are multiple cysts of various sizes, separated by thin layers of hyperechoic tissue (Fig. 38-25).[93-98] Affected kidneys

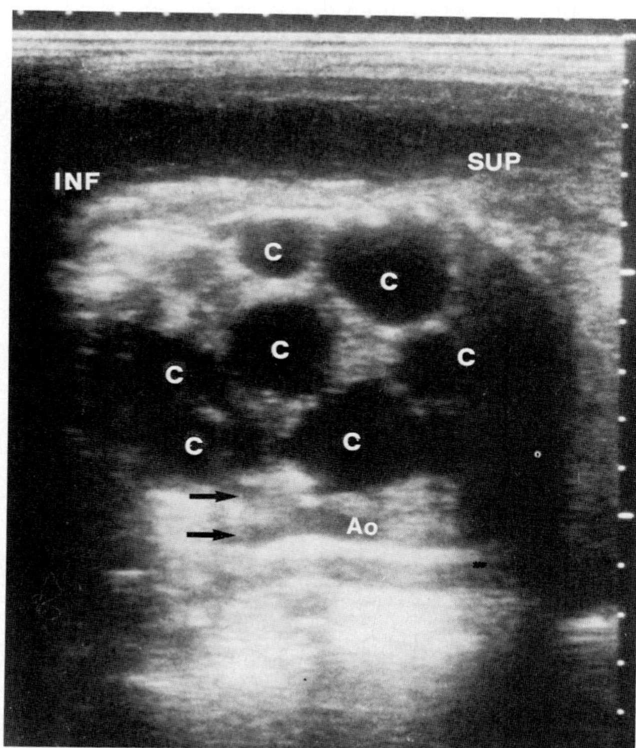

FIGURE 38–25. Coronal scan of the trunk of a fetus of a 35-week fetus with unilateral MDKD. The cysts (C) are clearly separated by echoic tissue. The bifurcation of the abdominal aorta (Ao) in the common iliac arteries (*black arrows*) is demonstrated in this scanning plane. Sup, superior; Inf, inferior. (From Rizzo N, et al. Prenatal diagnosis and obstetrical management of multicystic dysplastic kidney disease. Prenat Diagn 1987; 7:112.)

are usually extremely enlarged (Fig. 38-26). The hypoplastic or atretic collecting system is undetectable by ultrasound. In the unilateral variant, contralateral kidney and bladder are normal, as is the amount of amniotic fluid. Occasionally, the contralateral renal pelvis appears slightly enlarged due to compensatory urine flow. When both kidneys are affected, the bladder is not detected and amniotic fluid is decreased.

Differential diagnosis between MDKD and adult polycystic kidney (APKD) will be discussed in the next section. Distinction between MDKD and obstructions at the UPJ in prenatal sonograms can be extremely difficult.[99] Coronal scans seem to be most specific, because in UPJ obstructions they clearly demonstrate the connection between renal pelvis and the dilated calyceal system (Fig. 38-27). Conversely, in MDKD the cysts are separated. Such a distinction is much easier when ultrasound examination is performed in early pregnancy, with the progression of obstructive uropathy resulting in a sonographic appearance similar to that of MDKD. Although, using coronal scans, we were able to distinguish between these two conditions even in close to term pregnancies, the distinction between severe UPJ obstruction and MDKD with a large central cyst surrounded by smaller cysts would seem impossible with currently available ultrasound equipment (Fig. 38-28). Similarly, differential diagnosis between UVJ and MDKD is rather difficult, frequently leading to misinterpretations of the ultrasound picture (Fig. 38-29).

Prognosis and Management

In case of unilateral MDKD, with no sign of failure of renal function and no associated anomalies, prognosis is good and the fetus can be safely delivered vaginally at term. The need for postnatal nephrectomy is currently under discussion: it is required when the size of the kidney is inconvenient to the patient,[100] and it has to be considered in all cases, because complications, including GI infections, hypertension, and malignant mixed tumors, may originate from a retained affected kidney.[101,102]

Bilateral MDKD has an invariably poor prognosis, and termination of pregnancy can be offered to the couple when diagnosis is made prior to viability.

When other anomalies are associated, prognosis and management vary according to the type and severity of the diseases. In these cases, we recommend a detailed survey to exclude associated anomalies, and perform fetal karyotype.

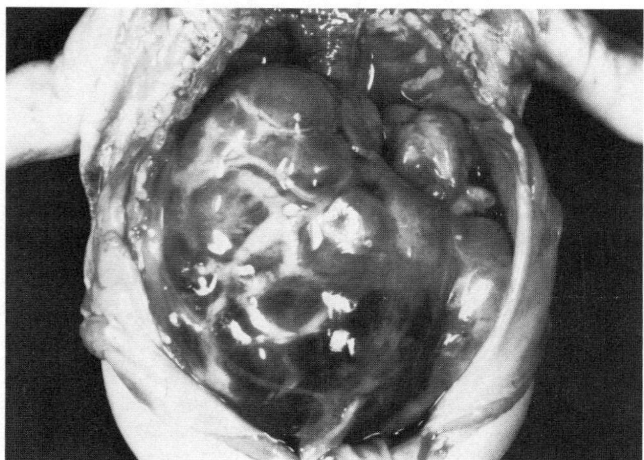

FIGURE 38–26. Dissection of the affected kidney (Potter II renal dysplasia). Note the extremely enlarged kidney, with multiple cysts of various sizes.

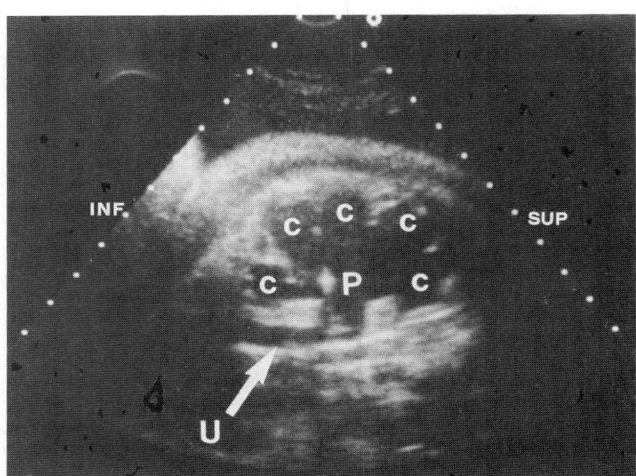

FIGURE 38–27. A coronal scan of the fetal trunk demonstrating renal cysts (C) radially distributed and communicating with an enlarged renal pelvis (P). The proximal portion of the dilated ureter (U) is also visualized in this scanning plane. The contralateral kidney appeared normal on ultrasound. A diagnosis of unilateral ureterovesical junction obstruction was made at this point and confirmed after birth. Inf, inferior, Sup, superior. (From Rizzo N, et al. Prenatal diagnosis and management of multicystic dysplastic kidney disease. Prenat Diagn 1987;7:115.)

ADULT POLYCYSTIC KIDNEY DISEASE

Adult polycystic kidney disease (APKD), or Potter's Type III renal dysplasia, almost invariably affects both kidneys, although often asymmetrically.[103,104] Although the malformation process begins in utero, in most cases the disease is clinically manifested in adulthood, or more rarely in early infancy.

Pathogenesis

APKD may be inherited as an autosomal dominant trait, and it may be a feature of genetic and nongenetic syndromes. Sporadic diseases have also been reported in the literature.[103]

Prenatal Diagnosis

APKD has been detected in the third trimester.[103,105] We were able to make a diagnosis during the second trimester. Ultrasound revealed a grossly enlarged left kid-

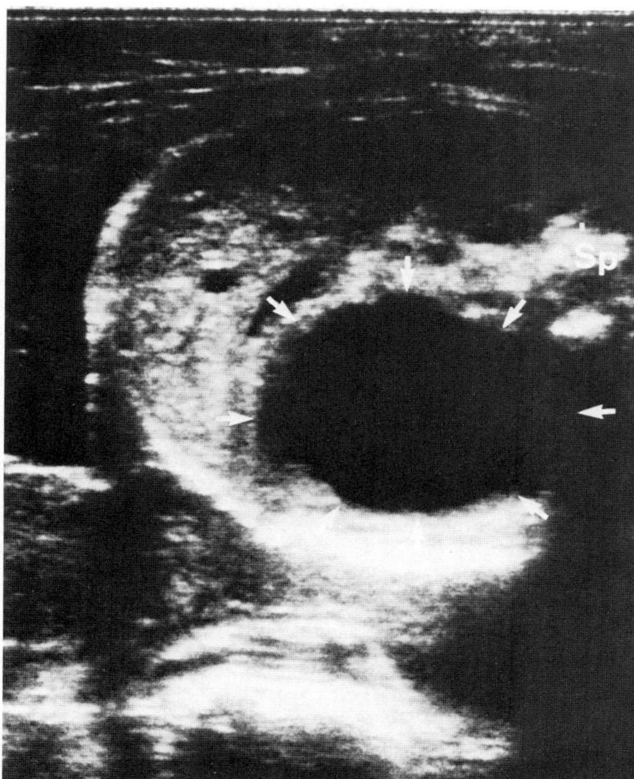

FIGURE 38–28. Transverse section of a fetus with a cystic mass in the lower abdomen (*arrows*), prompting a diagnosis of ureteropelvic junction. Postnatal evaluation made a diagnosis of multicystic kidney with a large central cyst surrounded by smaller cysts, which fell below the resolution power of the ultrasound equipment.

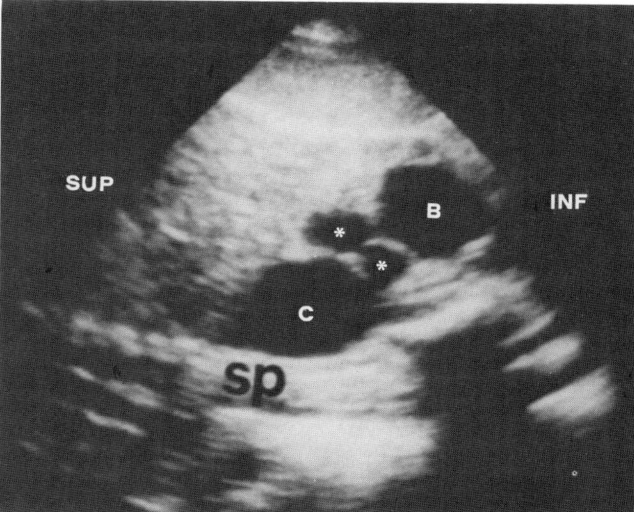

FIGURE 38–29. Oblique sagittal scan of the lower abdomen of a 32-week fetus. The largest sonolucent area (C) was erroneously thought to be a massively enlarged renal pelvis, while the two smaller cysts (*) were interpreted as cross sections of a dilated and tortuous ureter, thus prompting the diagnosis of ureterovesical junction obstruction. The newborn infant was subsequently found to have unilateral multicystic dysplastic kidney disease (MDKD). B, bladder; Sup, superior; Inf, inferior. (From Rizzo N, et al. Prenatal diagnosis and management of multicystic dysplastic kidney disease. Prenat Diagn 1987;7:114.)

ney, which contained multiple cysts of variable size intermixed with well-represented, hyperechogenic solid tissue (Fig. 38-30). The contralateral kidney and the bladder were normal (Fig. 38-31). The amniotic fluid was within normal range. Careful survey of fetal anatomy did not reveal other abnormalities. The couple was informed of the likelihood of APKD, and opted to terminate the pregnancy. A male, 450-gram fetus was aborted one day after intra-amniotic administration of prostaglandin E_2 (PGE_2). Cytogenetic analysis performed on amniotic fluid cells sampled at the time of prostaglandin administration revealed normal karyotype. Pathologic examination revealed gross enlargement of the left kidney. The largest diameter was 4 cm. Dissection showed the presence of multiple cysts of variable size filled with fluid within both the medulla and cortex (Fig. 38-32). Histology demonstrated the presence of normal renal parenchyma. Nephrons and collecting tubules were poorly defined, as were papillae and calices. The cysts were lined by cuboidal cells (Fig. 38-33). The contralateral kidney and the liver were normal. Both parents and the sibling underwent subsequent ultrasound examinations, which failed to demonstrate any morphological derangement of renal structures.

In other cases, bilateral involvement can occur. Differential diagnosis between MDKD and APKD is possible, because in APKD renal parenchyma interposed between the cysts is well preserved in most cases. When APKD has been found in a newborn or in a fetus, both parents should be carefully examined.

Using a highly polymorphic DNA probe genetically

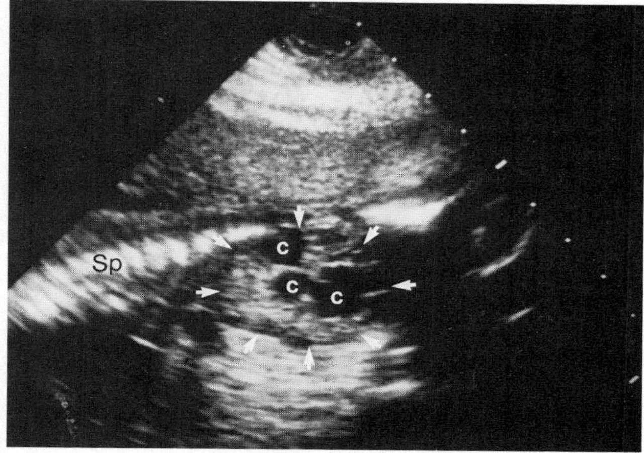

FIGURE 38–30. Longitudinal scan of the fetal trunk demonstrating a grossly enlarged kidney with multiple cysts (C) intermixed with abundant parenchyma. Sp, spine.

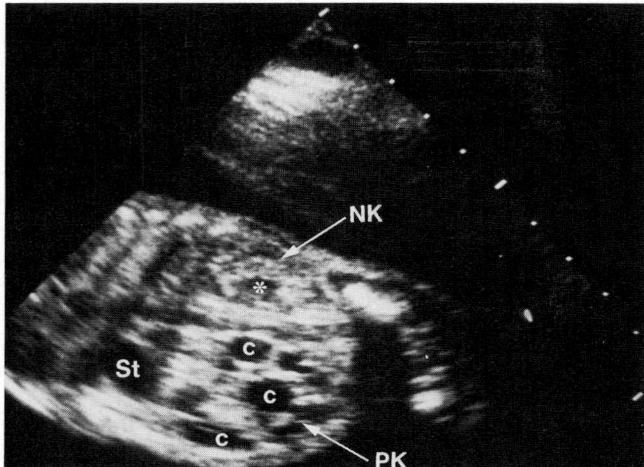

FIGURE 38–31. Coronal view of the fetal trunk demonstrating the polycystic kidney (PK) and the normal contralateral kidney (NK) with a normal pelvis (*). St, stomach; C, renal cysts.

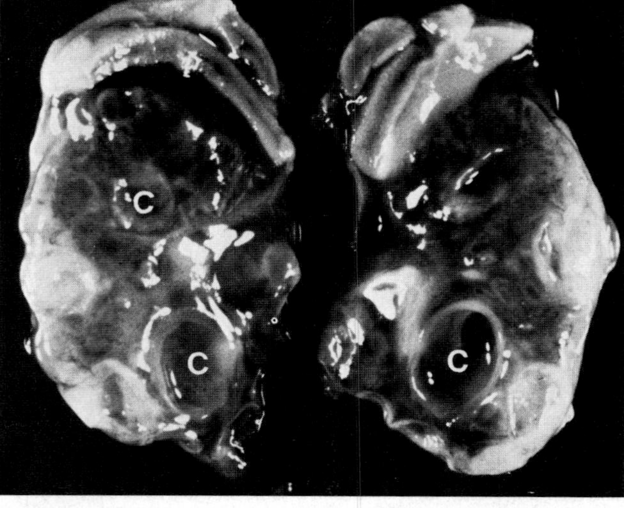

FIGURE 38–32. Dissection of the affected kidney, revealing multiple cysts (C) located in both the renal cortex and medulla.

linked to the mutant gene, prenatal diagnosis is possible.[107]

Associated Anomalies

APKD is often part of malformation complexes, which have been extensively reviewed.[45] Detection of Potter's Type III cystic dysplasia associated with occipital encephalocele enables the diagnosis of Meckel-Gruber syndrome, which is a lethal anomaly, recurring in an autosomal recessive manner (25% recurrence risk for subsequent pregnancies). Therefore, careful survey of the entire fetal anatomy is mandatory (Fig. 38-34).

Prognosis and Management

Because experience with prenatal diagnosis is limited, no data regarding the natural history of the disease are available. In the largest series reported in the literature,[107] four out of seven infants had normal renal function, one had hypertension, one fetus was terminated in the second trimester, and one neonate died soon after birth. Based on postnatal course, APKD is a chronic disease that can be asymptomatic and detected at autopsy only. It can manifest itself at any age, from the newborn period to adulthood.

Parents at risk should be informed of the possibility

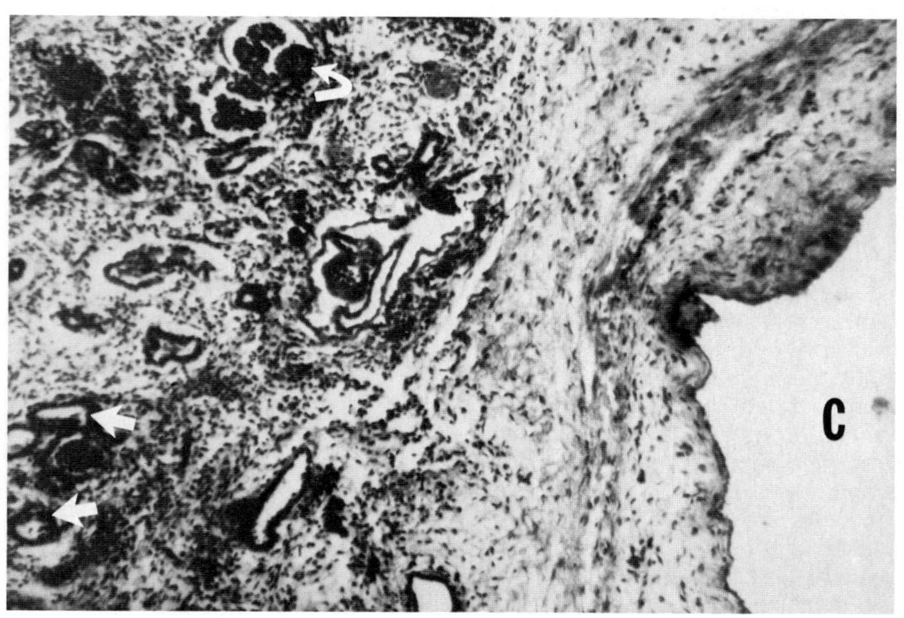

FIGURE 38–33. Histologic specimen of the polycystic kidney revealing the cuboidal lining of the cyst (C) and the presence of well-developed glomeruli (curved arrow) and tubules (T) (hematoxylin and eosin, ×240).

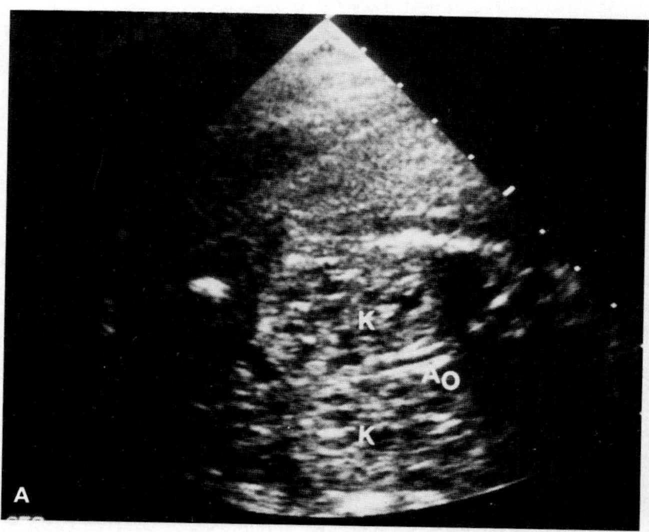

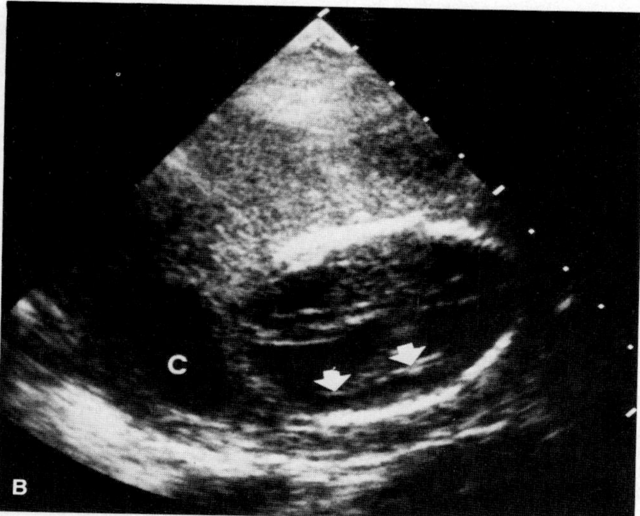

FIGURE 38–34. Polycystic kidneys (Potter III cystic dysplasia) associated with an encephalocele prompt the diagnosis of Meckel-Gruber syndrome. K, kidneys; Ao, aorta; C, encephalocele; arrows, dilated lateral cerebral ventricles.

of first trimester prenatal diagnosis. When diagnosis is made before viability, the option to terminate the pregnancy can be offered to the couple. Conservative management should be the rule when diagnosis is made after viability.

OBSTRUCTIVE UROPATHIES

GU tract obstructions are among the most common congenital anomalies. The prevalence of obstructive uropathies is unknown, although it has been estimated in 1 out of 6000 live births[108]; however, because severe cases often end in intrauterine or neonatal death, whereas mild cases are usually diagnosed later in postnatal life, the number of affected fetuses is probably larger. These anomalies are usually sporadic, but a few familiar cases also have been described. Prenatal ultrasound diagnosis is based on the recognition of dilated GU tract. Prognosis and management vary considerably according to the type and severity of the obstruction, and also in relation to associated anomalies. According to the level of the obstruction, it is possible to distinguish high (at the level of ureteropelvic junction), median (at the level of ureterovesical junction), and low (at the level of the urethra) obstructions. High and median obstructions can be either bilateral or unilateral.

URETEROPELVIC JUNCTION OBSTRUCTION

The prevalence of the disease is unknown. Male neonates seem to be more frequently affected (male to female ratio, 5:1).[109]

Pathogenesis

In most cases sporadic, familial occurrence[110] or autosomal dominant cases[111] have been reported. The etiology seems to be referred to anatomical or functional causes: spiral muscular layers are replaced by longitudinal muscular or fibrous tissue, determining a defective peristaltic wave.

Associated Anomalies

Urinary anomalies, such as vesicoureteral reflux, kidney duplication, contralateral renal agenesis, and meatal stenosis, are commonly associated. GI and cardiac anomalies and neural tube defects are variably present in association.

PRENATAL DIAGNOSIS

Prenatal ultrasound diagnosis is based on the finding of a dilated renal pelvis (Fig. 38-35). Particularly at advanced gestational age, a slightly enlarged pelvis is fairly common. Quantitative criteria for diagnosis have been suggested: anteroposterior diameter >1 cm, and the ratio between maximal transverse diameter of the pelvis and renal diameter measured at the same level (>0.5).[112] The severity of the anomaly varies from mild dilation to enormous cystic masses, without any chance of recognizing the calyces. If unilateral, the contralateral kidney is normal, the bladder is visible, and the amniotic fluid is preserved. Bilateral diseases, when severe, may determine compromised renal function (Fig. 38-36). Occasionally, mild hydronephrosis detected by ultrasound in utero has not been confirmed on postna-

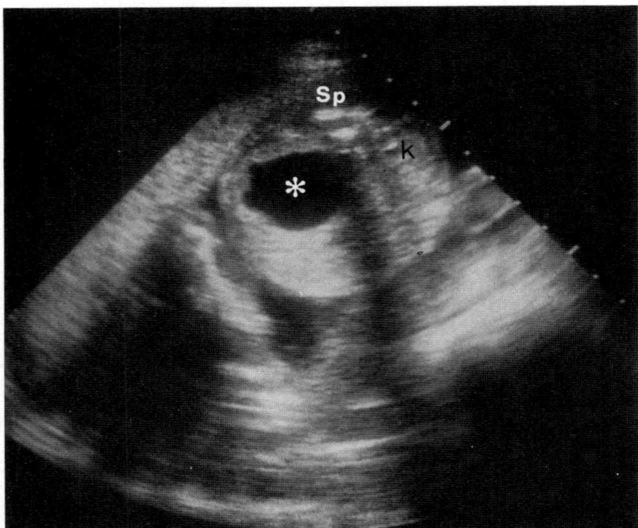

FIGURE 38–35. Transverse section of the fetal abdomen showing an enlarged renal pelvis (*) and a contralateral normal renal parenchyma (k). Sp, spine.

tal examination; therefore, spontaneous resolution can occur. Differential diagnosis has to be established with multicystic kidney (see the earlier section on MDKD). In late gestation, it is sometimes impossible to distinguish the two conditions; however, neither of them requires alteration of standard obstetric management. Duplication of the kidney is commonly associated with dilation of one or both renal pelves (Fig. 38-37).

Prognosis and Management

Prognosis is good, unless associated anomalies are present. In most cases, obstruction is not particularly tight and probably develops late in gestation. Rarely, and particularly in cases of bilateral involvement, the process progresses to compromised renal function. There is generally no need to alter standard obstetric management; affected fetuses should be vaginally delivered at term.

URETEROVESICAL JUNCTION OBSTRUCTION

Pathogenesis

Ureterovesical junction (UVJ) obstruction is a sporadic disease in most cases; however, familial inheritance has been described. It can be unilateral and bilateral. The anomaly is caused by a deficiency of muscular fibers at the distal end of the ureter, limiting peristalsis, or by the presence of fibrous tissue instead of muscular fibers in the ureter wall. Urine, therefore, cannot enter the bladder, accumulating in the proximal portion of the ureter, and eventually causing dilation of the renal pelvis.

Associated Anomalies

Various urinary anomalies can be associated with UVJ obstruction, such as contralateral renal agenesis, ectopic kidney, renal cystic dysplasia, and horseshoe kidney. Cardiac and GI anomalies can occasionally occur.

Prenatal Diagnosis

In cases of UVJ obstruction, the ureter is dilated and tortuous, and on ultrasound appears as a collection of cysts of variable size, localized between the renal pelvis, which is variably dilated, and the bladder, which is of normal morphology and dimensions (Fig. 38-38).[113,114] Sometimes, it is clearly visible as a ureterocele, which is represented by a thin-walled and fluid-filled small circular area inside the bladder (Fig. 38-39). Amniotic fluid is present in normal amounts. Differential diagnosis must be made with multicystic kidney and particularly with ureterovesical reflux, where an enlarged bladder is a distinctive element (Fig. 38-40). Duplication of the kidneys is sometimes associated with bilateral hydroureteronephrosis (Fig. 38-41). Distinction between urinary and GI tract obstruction is possible on the basis of increased peristalsis and detection of feces in the lumen.

Prognosis and Management

Prognosis is good, unless in cases of bilateral involvement renal function deteriorates. In most cases, obstetrical management remains unchanged. When the pathological process worsens along with gestation, preterm induction of labor can be attempted so that postnatal surgical correction can be performed soon after birth.

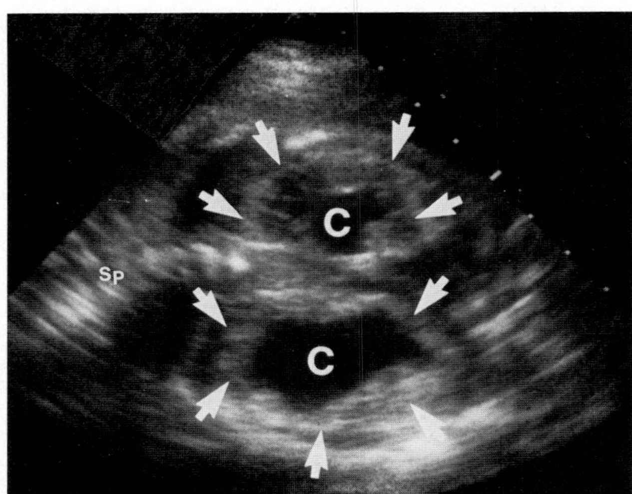

FIGURE 38–36. Coronal view of the lower abdomen in a fetus with bilateral ureteropelvic junction obstruction. Both renal pelves (C) appear dilated. Sp, spine.

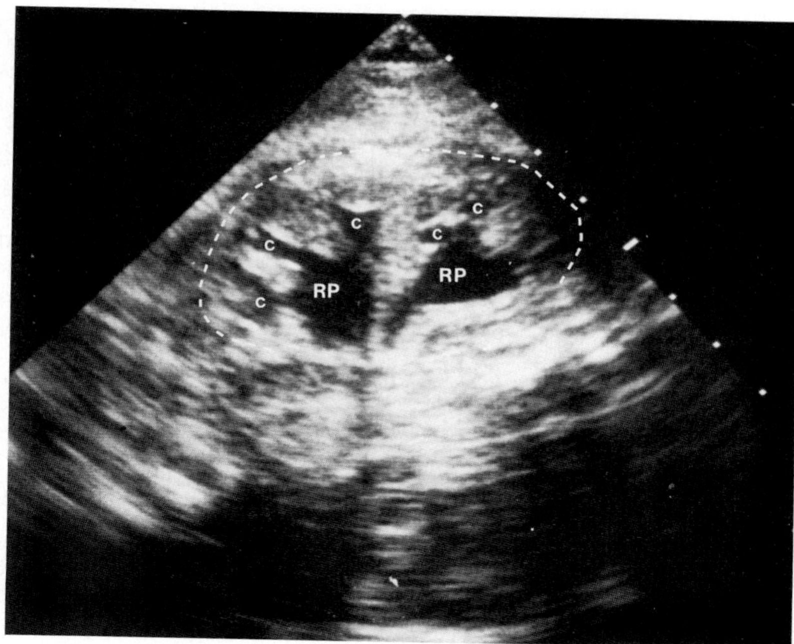

FIGURE 38–37. Longitudinal scan of the abdomen of a fetus with duplication of the kidneys. Note that the two renal pelves (RP) and calyces (c) appear moderately dilated.

URETHRAL LEVEL OBSTRUCTION

Pathogenesis

The anomaly is generally sporadic; however, in some cases it has a genetic basis.[115] In the majority of the cases, obstruction is caused by two semicircular membranous plicae at the level of verumontanum.[72] Those plicae, as urine flows from the bladder, adhere and close the upper portion of the urethra. Upper urinary tract anatomy (bladder, ureters, and renal pelvis) is dilated. Increased upstream pressure with time is responsible for kidney dysplasia. An early obstruction is more likely to determine compromised renal function, compared to cases that are diagnosed only in late pregnancy.[116]

Prenatal Diagnosis

Urethral valves cannot be detected by ultrasound. Diagnosis has been suggested by dilation of the entire GU tract in a male fetus (Fig. 38-42).[117] The urinary bladder is overdistended, often reaching the transverse

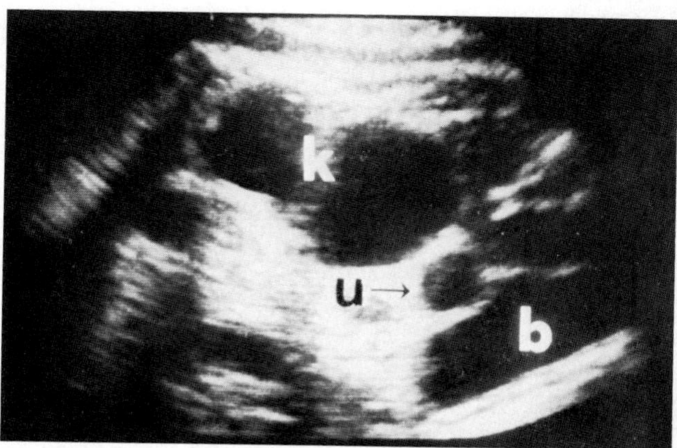

FIGURE 38–38. Paramedian longitudinal scan of the lower abdomen in a fetus with unilateral ureterovesical junction obstruction. Between the dilated renal pelvis (k) and the normal-size bladder multiple cystic areas are seen, representing hydroureter (u). B, bladder.

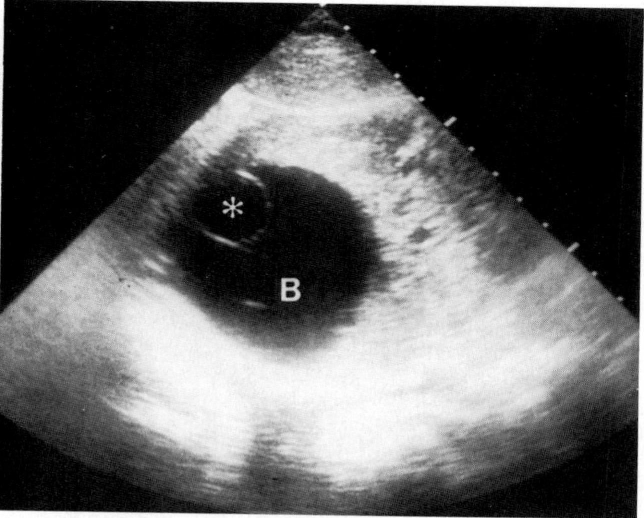

FIGURE 38–39. Thin-walled, fluid-filled small circular area (*) inside the bladder (B) representing a ureterocele in a fetus with ureterovesical junction obstruction.

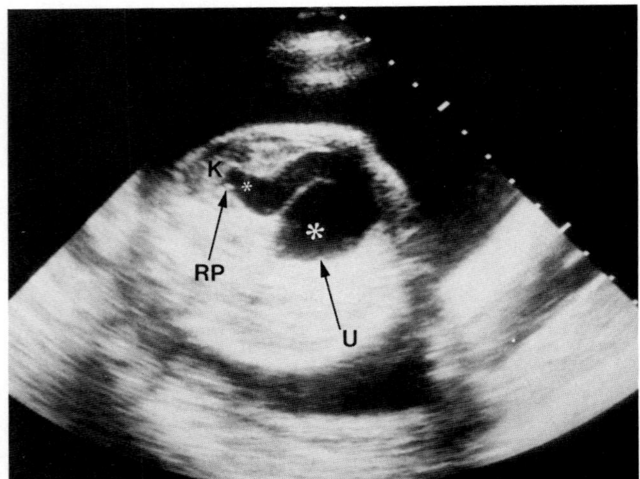

FIGURE 38–40. Vesicoureteral reflux simulating a ureterovesical junction obstruction. Note the enlarged distal portion of the ureter close to the bladder (U). RP, renal pelvis; K, kidney.

umbilical line. The initial portion of the urethra is often visible, giving a peculiar "keyhole" image (Fig. 38-43). The increased intravesical pressure sometimes leads to a dilation of the urachus, which presents as a cystic mass anterior to the bladder (Fig. 38-44). Ureters are usually moderately dilated and tortuous. The renal pelvis can be only minimally dilated, particularly in cases of compromised renal function. The increased pressure in the urinary system may lead to a severe kidney dysplasia, which is characterized by hyperechogenicity of the kidneys and the presence of cortical cysts (Fig. 38-45). More or less severe oligohydramnios is present. Occasionally, the increased pressure in the urinary tract causes fluid transudation, leading to urinary ascites and abdominal distension. The association of low obstructive uropathy and ascites is typical of the so-called prune-belly syndrome, which is also characterized by distended abdomen and abdominal wall hypoplasia.

In our experience, 40 cases of fetal megacystis have been diagnosed with ultrasound. Of those, 26 (65%) were posterior urethral valves, 4 (10%) were caused by urethral atresia, in 3 cases bilateral vesicoureteral reflux was found at postnatal examination, in 3 cases there was a common cloaca (Fig. 38-46), in 3 cases megacystis was unexplained, and in 1 case diagnosis of megacystis–microcolon syndrome was made. Therefore, although posterior urethral valves are the most common anomaly underlying a fetal megacystis, one should not forget other, less frequent defects.

Associated Anomalies

Associated anomalies are present in a minority of cases of low obstructive uropathies. In our experience, for instance, 80% (32/40) of the cases were isolated megacystis; in the rest of the cases, 7 were skeletal, 1 was cardiac, 3 had intestinal anomalies, and 1 had trisomy 21.

Prognosis and Management

Among fetal kidneys with obstructive uropathies, sonographic demonstration of renal dysplasia indicates irreversible renal damage that is probably consequent to elevated pressures within the developing nephron system.[88] The presence of cortical cysts is suggestive of dysplasia. However, absence of the cysts does not exclude renal dysplasia, because not all dysplastic kidneys have cysts, or the cysts may be smaller than the ultrasound resolution power. An increased renal echogen-

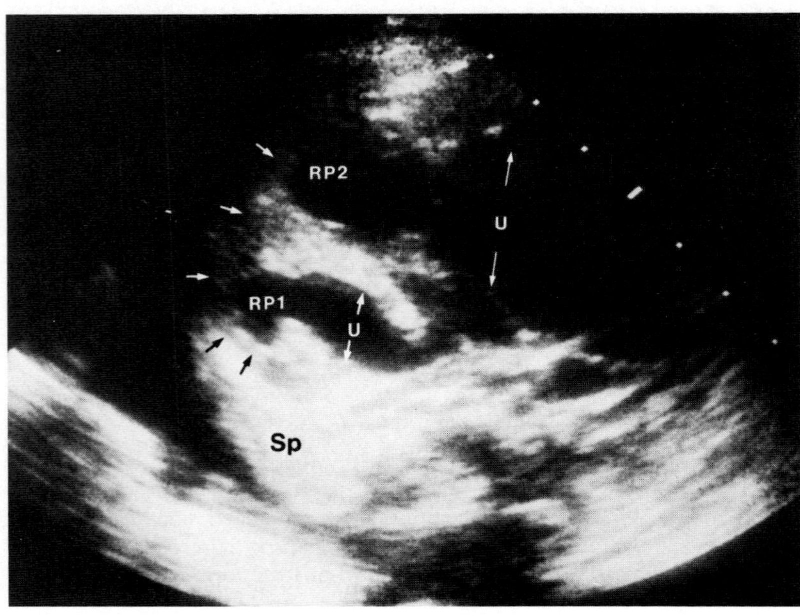

FIGURE 38–41. Cross section of a fetus with duplication of the kidneys. Both the renal pelves (RP) are dilated, as well as the two ureters (U), although the renal pelvis identified as RP2 and its corresponding ureter are comparably more dilated.

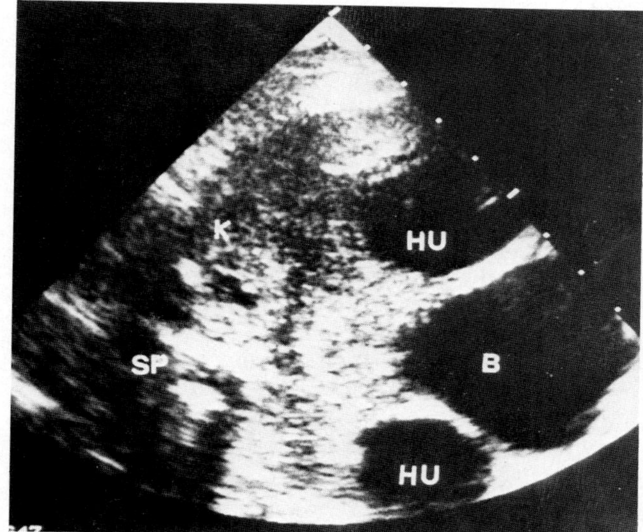

FIGURE 38–42. Cross section of a fetus with severe Potter IV cystic dysplasia. The bladder (B) is markedly distended, as are both ureters (HU). The kidneys (K) appear small and hyperechoic. SP, spine.

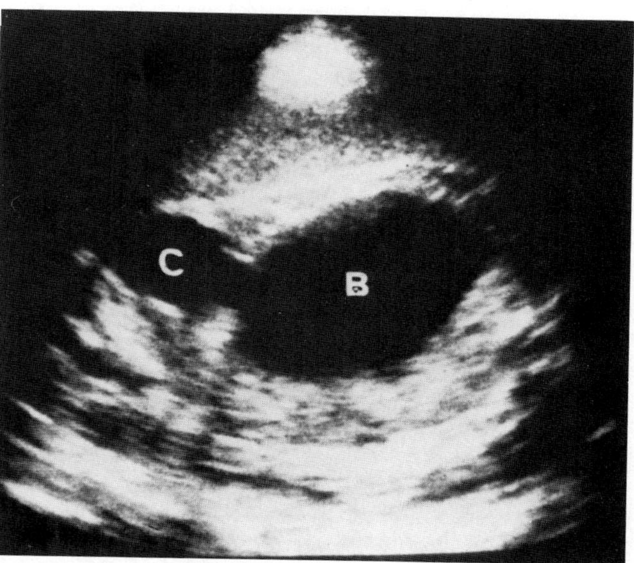

FIGURE 38–44. Oblique transverse section of the abdomen of a fetus affected by lower obstructive uropathy (urethral valves). The bladder (B) is communicating anteriorly with a cystic mass (C), representing the dilated urachus.

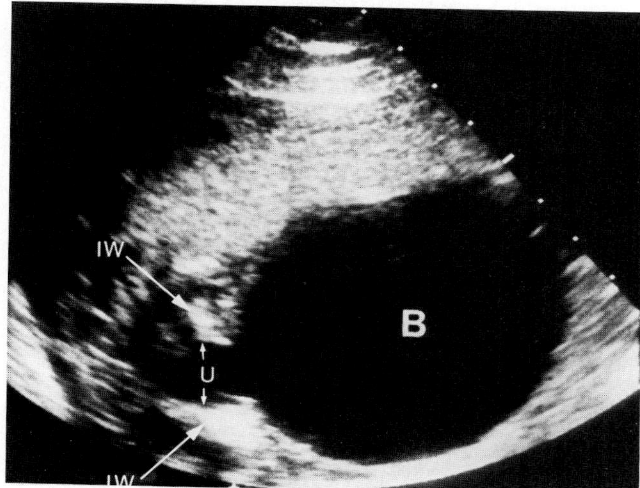

FIGURE 38–43. Longitudinal scan of the lower abdomen in a fetus with lower obstructive uropathy (Potter IV). The dilatation of the proximal tract of the ureter (U) is evident. B, enlarged bladder; IW, iliac wings.

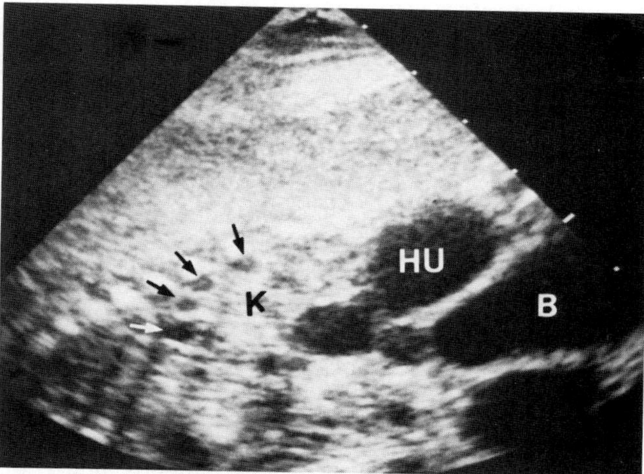

FIGURE 38–45. Oblique transverse section of the abdomen of a fetus affected by posterior urethral valves. The dilated pelvis has a disomogeneous structure, suggesting the presence of a cystic dysplasia (*arrows*). K, kidney; HU, hydroureter; B, bladder.

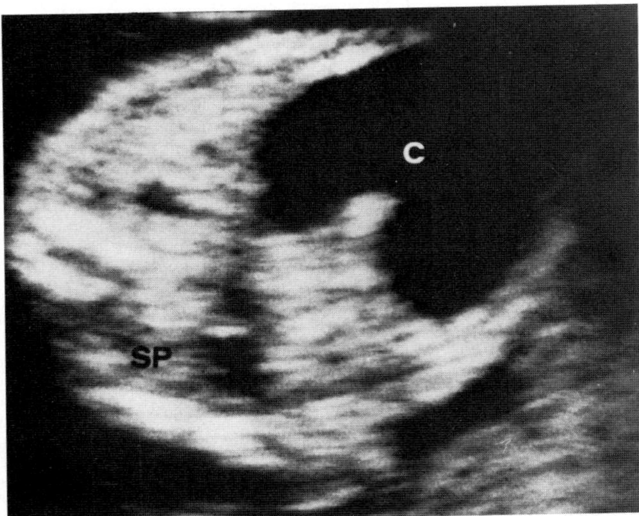

FIGURE 38–46. Transverse section of the lower abdomen of a 25-week fetus showing a large cyst (C), which was interpreted as megacystis consequent to a low obstructive uropathy. After the termination of pregnancy, autopsy revealed a common cloaca.

icity is occasionally found in cases of renal dysplasia, due to the presence of abundant fibrous tissue. Not all the dysplastic kidneys are hyperechogenic and, conversely, 20% of hyperechogenic kidneys are not dysplastic.[118] Therefore, increased renal echogenicity cannot predict renal dysplasia with certainty. Because ultrasound has a limited accuracy, evaluation of renal function is enhanced by analysis of the urine sampled by intrauterine cystocentesis. Poor prognostic factor is a decreased output (<2 mL/hr) of isotonic urine (osmolarity, >210 mOsm; sodium, >100 mEq/mL; chloride, >90 mEq/mL). Conversely, normal glomerular and tubular function is implied by hypotonic fetal urine. When in utero diagnosis of low obstructive uropathies is made, prognosis is relatively poor. Affected neonates carry a high risk for death (32% to 50%), as a consequence of pulmonary hypoplasia, associated congenital anomalies, renal failure, and surgical complications after decompressive surgery.[119] Most patients show an improvement in renal function after surgery, although progressive renal failure may occur despite correction.

Obstetrical management depends on associated congenital anomalies, gestational age at diagnosis, and status of renal function. Careful survey of the anatomy is mandatory, although it is hampered by oligohydramnios. Infusion of saline may be useful. Fetal karyotype by amniocentesis or, when this is not feasible, by cordocentesis, should be undertaken, because various prevalences of associated chromosomal anomalies (up to 23% of the cases) are reported in the literature. When an anatomical or chromosomal defect that is incompatible with life is diagnosed, the option of terminating the pregnancy can be offered to the couple. Next, renal function needs to be studied. Poor prognostic factors are oligohydramnios, the presence of cortical cysts, and the urine parameters reported above. With poor prognostic criteria, termination of pregnancy or conservative management are the available options. If prognosis is good, further management depends on gestational age at diagnosis. If diagnosis is made during the third trimester and fetal lung maturity is proved by an L\S ratio, the fetus should be delivered vaginally, if not clinically contraindicated, where pediatric surgery is available. If the diagnosis is made after viability but before lung maturity, preventive in utero decompression may be attempted, or, in cases of decreasing amniotic fluid, conservative management and intervention only may be chosen. The outcome of infants who have undergone vesicoamniotic shunt is reported in the Registry of the International Fetal Medicine and Surgery

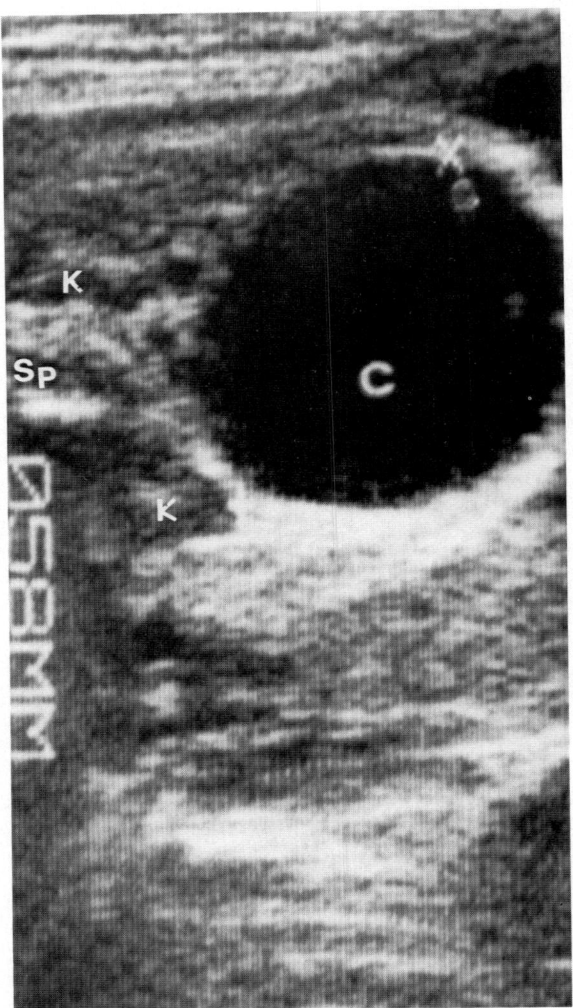

FIGURE 38–47. Cross section of the abdomen of a 31-week fetus with a large ovarian cyst (C). Sp, spine; K, kidney. (From Rizzo N, et al. Prenatal diagnosis and management of fetal ovarian cysts. Prenat Diagn 1989; 9: 98.)

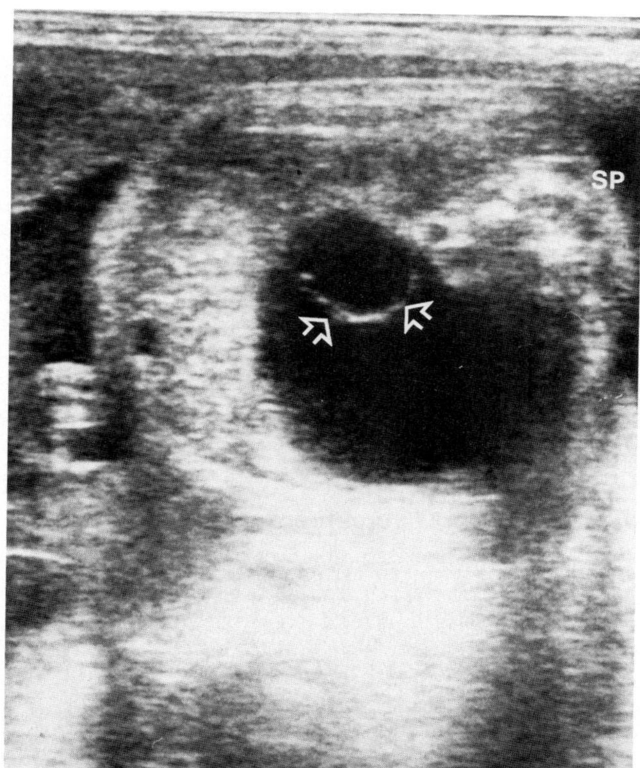

FIGURE 38–48. Cross section of the abdomen of a fetus showing a cystic mass with a subtle septum (*arrows*). SP, spine.

Society.[120] Forty percent (35/87) of the fetuses with obstructive uropathies who underwent in utero surgery survived. Thirteen (14.9%) were electively terminated after shunt placement because of abnormal karyotype (7/13) or because of compromised renal function (6/13). Of the remaining 74, 35 fetuses (47.3%) survived. Fetuses with posterior urethral valves had a higher survival rate (68%). Only 3 of 35 survivors (8.6%) developed significant complications after birth. One of the three is affected by posterior urethral valves and has developed chronic renal failure, requiring hemodialysis. One child has mild renal insufficiency, and a third child has required extensive and ongoing surgical correction for persistent cloacal syndrome. Vesicoamniotic shunt has a death rate of 4.7% (4 of 85). The survival rate in our experience of 16 cases of low obstructive uropathies is 30% (5 of 16). Three of five were vesicoureteral refluxes; in one case, the dilated bladder appeared small on a subsequent scan, suggesting a spontaneous in utero decompression. We attempted to perform two vesicoamniotic shunts; in both cases, the fetus died soon after birth from pulmonary hypoplasia. Because the vesicoamniotic shunt cannot be the ideal long-term treatment for obstructive uropathies, Harrison and coworkers, with a small group of five patients, have used a technique for open fetal urinary tract decompression.[121] All fetuses were delivered by cesarean section at 32 to 35 weeks. Three fetuses showed normal pulmonary function at birth. Two fetuses died soon after birth of pulmonary hypoplasia. Of the three surviving infants, two had normal renal function, but one required renal transplantation for worsening of renal function. Open fetal surgery is therefore feasible, and may prevent pulmonary hypoplasia at birth; however, the effect of decompression on the development of renal dysplasia and ultimate renal function is still unknown.

FETAL OVARIAN CYSTS

Ovarian cysts are one of the most common causes of abdominal mass in the female neonate.[122,123] They are the most significant genital anomaly presenting in the prenatal period.

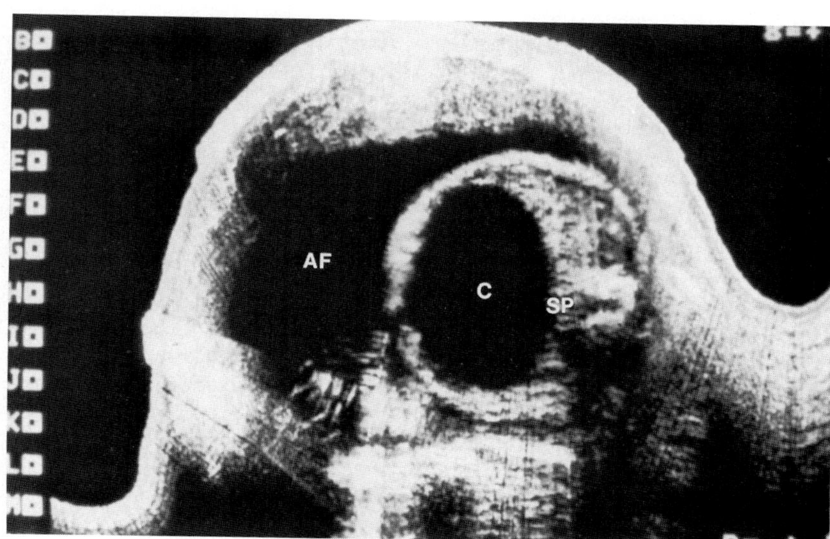

FIGURE 38–49. Cross section of the abdomen of a 34-week fetus with a large ovarian cyst (C). Polyhydramnios is present. AF, amniotic fluid; SP, spine; K, kidneys. (From Rizzo N, et al. Prenatal diagnosis and management of fetal ovarian cysts. Prenat Diagn 1989;9:100.)

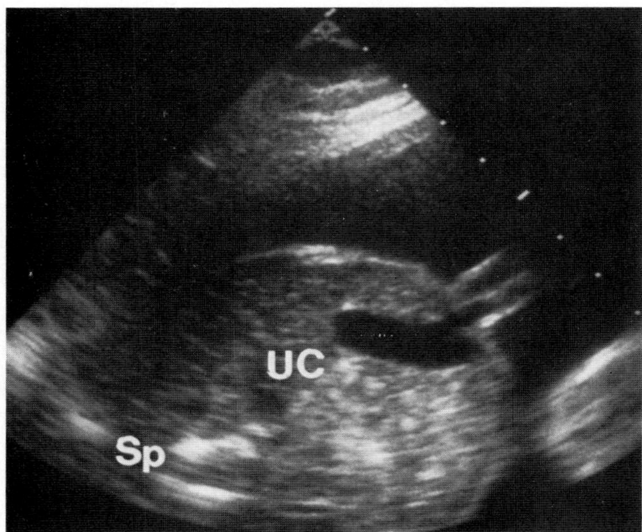

FIGURE 38–50. Longitudinal scan of the trunk of a fetus with a urachal cyst (UC). Sp, spine.

Pathogenesis

Although classically related to hormonal stimulation, the cause of the anomaly is still uncertain. Interestingly, congenital ovarian cysts occurred in association with hypothyroidism.[124]

Prenatal Diagnosis

Prenatal ultrasound diagnosis is possible from the second trimester of pregnancy.[125–127] Cystic mass in the fetal lower abdomen, integrity of GI and GU tracts, and female sex are the main ultrasound criteria for diagnosis of fetal ovarian cyst. In the majority of cases, the cyst is completely fluid (Fig. 38-47); sometimes it is septated (Fig. 38-48).[128] Polyhydramnios is often present (Fig. 38-49). However, diagnosis is always presumptive, because rare conditions including mesenteric and urachal cysts (Fig. 38-50), enteric duplication anomalies, cystic teratoma, and low intestinal obstructions cannot be ruled out with certainty in utero. Serial examinations of the anomaly allow the detection of structural changes of the cyst, which prompt the diagnosis of a complication of the cyst (Fig. 38-51).[129]

Associated Anomalies

Associated anomalies are uncommon, although an increased amniotic fluid is often present, probably secondary to partial GI obstruction.[130] In our experience, large cysts are commonly associated with more or less massive polyhydramnios.

Prognosis and Management

Prognosis and management of fetal ovarian cysts depends largely on the natural history of the mass.[131] The cyst may increase in size, decrease, or even disappear, or lead to complications such as torsion, infarction, and rupture. In this light, once prenatal ultrasound diagnosis has been made, serial examinations should be performed throughout gestation to detect any structural change in the mass. Enlargement of the mass, causing distension of fetal abdomen, is an indication for cesarean section to avoid the risk of soft tissue dystocia. Ultrasound-guided fine-needle aspiration of large fetal ovarian cysts may eliminate the need for a cesarean section and theoretically may diminish the risk of intrauterine torsion. However, the benefit of such an invasive procedure is unclear, and it may possibly cause intraperitoneal bleeding. Sudden development of intense hyperechogenicity within the mass, followed by a complex, heterogeneous appearance, should be considered to result from an intrauterine torsion of the cyst with infarction. When this occurs, immediate delivery

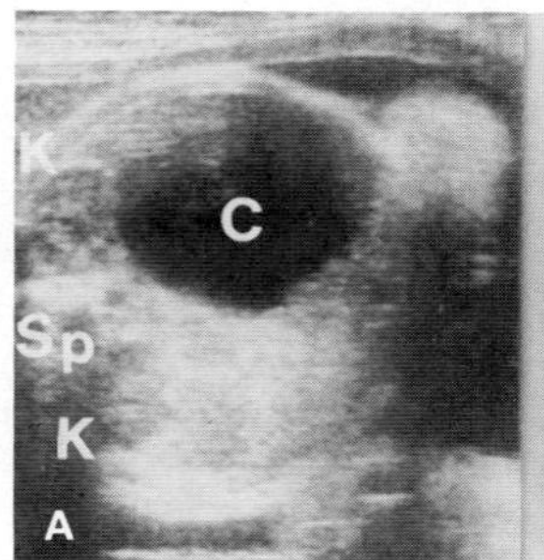

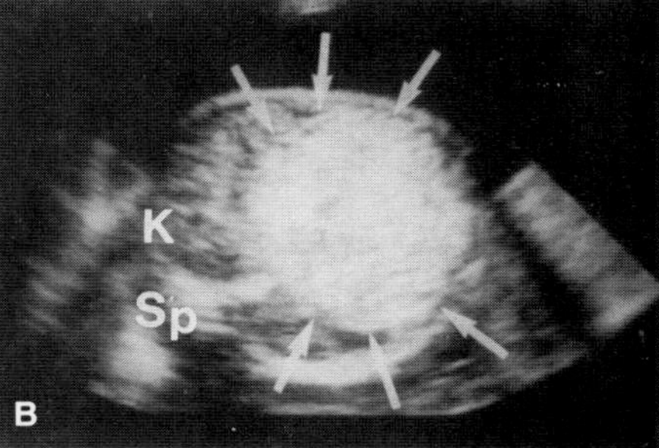

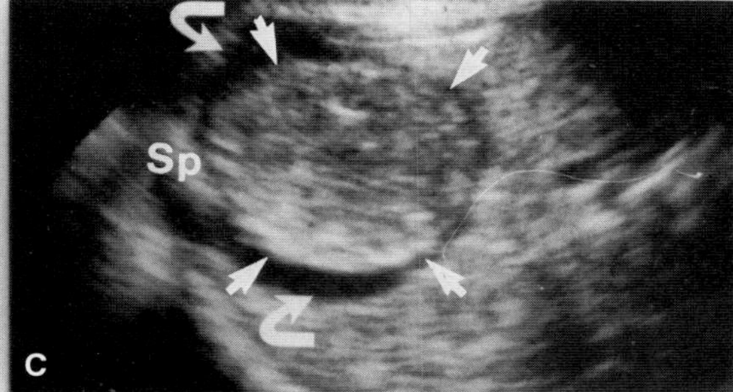

FIGURE 38–51. (**A**) Cross section of the abdomen of a 28-week fetus with an ovarian cyst (C). Sp, spine; K, kidney. (**B**) Cross section of the abdomen of the same fetus at 30 weeks. Note the highly hyperechoic mass (*arrows*), which was considered to represent an intrauterine torsion of the cyst and subsequent infarction. Sp, spine; K, kidney. (**C**) Cross section of the abdomen of the same fetus at 32 weeks. A heterogeneous mass, considered to be the evolution of the infarction, was found (*arrows*). Ascites (*curved arrows*) were present. K, kidney; Sp, spine. (From Rizzo N, et al. Prenatal diagnosis and management of fetal ovarian cysts. Prenat Diagn 1989;9:100.)

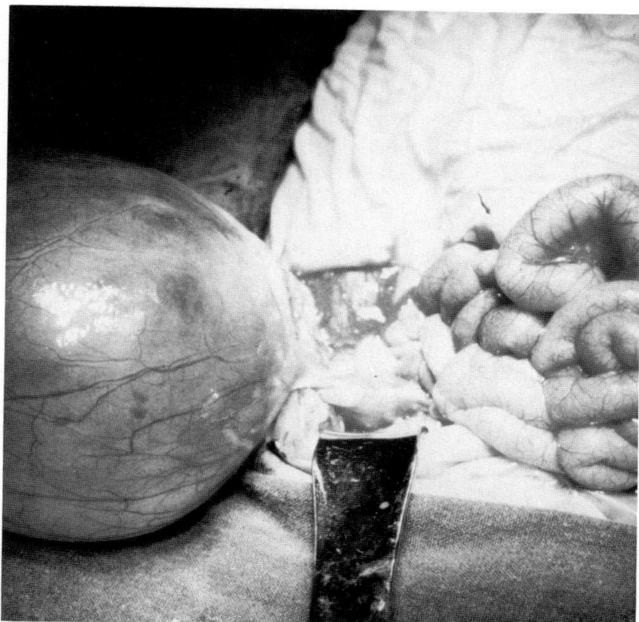

FIGURE 38–52. A large ovarian cyst at laparotomy. (From Rizzo N, et al. Prenatal diagnosis and management of fetal ovarian cysts. Prenat Diagn 1989;9:101.)

should be considered. Conversely, small cysts detected in utero can subsequently disappear and may not be present on a postnatal ultrasound evaluation.

In summary, prenatal diagnosis of fetal ovarian cysts per se does not modify standard obstetrical management, whereas complications occurring during gestation, such as torsion and rupture, may require active obstetric intervention.

Fetuses with confirmed diagnosis often require postnatal ovariectomy soon after birth (Fig. 38-52).

REFERENCES

1. Moore KL. The digestive system. In: The developing human: clinically oriented embryology. 4th ed. Philadelphia: WB Saunders, 1988.
2. Campbell S, Wilkin D. Ultrasonic measurement of fetal abdominal circumference in estimation of fetal weight. Br J Obstet Gynaecol 1975;82:689.
3. Rizzo N, Orsini LF, Calderoni P, et al: Lo studio anatomobiometrico dello stomaco fetale. In: Proceedings of the 6th National Congress of SISUM—Florence, October 29–31, 1981. Rome: Ed Novappia 1981:79.
4. Picker RH. A scoring system for the morphological ultrasonic assessment of foetal well-being and maturation. In: Lerski RA, Morley P, eds. Ultrasound '82. Pergamon Press, 1982:597.
5. Goldstein I, Lockwood C, Hobbins JC. Ultrasound assessment of fetal intestinal development in the evaluation of gestational age. Obstet Gynecol 1987;70:682.
6. Lawson TL, Foley WD, Berland LL, et al. Ultrasonic evaluation of fetal kidneys: analysis of normal size and frequency of visualization as related to stage of pregnancy. Radiology 1981; 138:153.
7. Bowie JD, Rosemberg ER, Andreotti MD, et al. The changing sonographic appearance of fetal kidneys during pregnancy. J Ultrasound Med 1983;2:505.
8. Bertagnoli L, Lalatta F, Gallicchio MD, et al. Quantitative characterization of the growth of the fetal kidney. J Clin Ultrasound 1983;11:349.
9. Jeanty P, Dramaix-Wilmet M, Elkhazen N. Measurement of fetal kidney growth on ultrasound. Radiology 1982;144:159.
10. Grannum P, Bracken M, Silverman R, et al. Assessment of fetal kidney size in normal gestation by comparison of ratio of kidney circumference. Am J Obstet Gynecol 1980;136:249.
11. Abramovich DR. The volume of amniotic fluid and its regulating factors. In: Fairweather DVI, Eskes TKA, eds. Amniotic fluid research and clinical application. 2nd Ed. Amsterdam: Excerpta Medica, 1978:31.
12. Campbell S, Wladimiroff JW, Dewhurst CJ. The antenatal measurement of fetal urine production. J Obstet Gynaecol Br Commonwealth 1973;80:680.
13. Wladimiroff JW. Effect of furosemide on fetal urine production. Br J Obstet Gynaecol 1985;82:221.
14. Rosenberg ER, Bowie JD. Failure of furosemide to induce diuresis in a growth-retarded fetus. AJR 1984;142:485.
15. Harmon CR. Maternal furosemide may not provoke urine production in the compromised fetus. Am J Obstet Gynecol 1984;150:322.
16. Touloukian RJ, Hobbins JC. Maternal ultrasonography on the antenatal diagnosis of surgically correctable fetal abnormalities. J Pediatr Surg 1980;15:373.
17. Queenan JT, Gadow ED. Amniography for detection of congenital malformations. Obstet Gynecol 1970;35:648.
18. Duenholter JH, Santos-Ramos R, Rosenfeld CR, et al. Prenatal diagnosis of gastrointestinal tract obstruction. Obstet Gynecol 1976;47:976.
19. Eyheremendy E, Pfister M. Antenatal real-time diagnosis of esophageal atresia. J Clin Ultrasound 1983;11:395.
20. Hobbins JC, Venus I. Congenital anomalies. In: Hobbins JC, ed. Diagnostic ultrasound in obstetrics. New York: Churchill Livingstone, 1979:95.
21. Seppala M. Increased α-fetoprotein in amniotic fluid associated with a congenital esophageal atresia of the fetus. Obstet Gynecol 1973;42:613.
22. Holzgreve W, Beller FK, Pawlowitzki IH. Amniotic fluid acetylcholinesterase as a marker in prenatal diagnosis of esophageal atresia. Am J Obstet Gynecol 1983;145:641.
23. Andrassy RJ, Mahour GH. Gastrointestinal anomalies associated with oesophageal atresia or tracheoesophageal fistula. Arch Surg 1979;114:1125.
24. Gross RE. The surgery of infancy and childhood. Philadelphia: WB Saunders, 1953.
25. Loveday BJ, Barr JA, Aitken J. The intrauterine demonstration of duodenal atresia by ultrasound. Br J Radiol 1975;48:1031.
26. Farrant P, Dewbury KC, Meire HB. Antenatal diagnosis of duodenal atresia. Br J Radiol 1981;54:633.
27. Bovicelli L, Rizzo N, Orsini LF, Pilu G. Prenatal diagnosis and management of fetal gastrointestinal anomalies. Semin Perinatol 1983;7:109.
28. Bowie JD, Clair MR. Fetal swallowing and regurgitation: observation of normal and abnormal activity. Radiology 1982;144:877.
29. Dunne ME, Johnson ML. The ultrasonic demonstration of fetal abnormalities in utero. J Reprod Med 1979;23:195.
30. Deleze G, Sideropoulos D, Paumgartner G. Determination of the acid concentration in human amniotic fluid for prenatal diagnosis of intestinal obstruction. Pediatrics 1977;59:657.
31. Weinberg AG, Milunski A, Harrod HJ. Elevated amniotic fluid α-fetoprotein and duodenal atresia. Lancet 1975;2:496.

32. Wrobleski D, Wesselhoef C. Ultrasonic diagnosis of prenatal intestinal obstruction. J Pediatr Surg 1979;14:598.
33. Nikapota VLB, Loman C. Gray-scale sonographic demonstration of fetal small bowel atresia. J Clin Ultrasound 1979;7:307.
34. Blumenthal DH, Rushovich AM, Williams RK, et al. Prenatal sonographic findings of meconium peritonitis with pathological correlations. J Clin Ultrasound 1982;10:350.
35. Garb M, Riseborough J. Meconium peritonitis presenting as fetal ascites on ultrasound. Br J Radiol 1980;53:602.
36. Lister J, Rickham PP. Intestinal atresia and stenosis, excluding the duodenum. In: Rickham PP, Lister J, Irving IM, eds. Neonatal surgery. 2nd ed. London: Butterworths, 1978:353.
37. Baxi LV, Yeh MN, Blanc WA, et al. Antepartum diagnosis and management of in utero intestinal volvulus with perforation. N Engl J Med 1983;308:1519.
38. Seward JF, Zusman J. Hydrops fetalis associated with small bowel volvulus. Lancet 1978;52.
39. Martin LW, Torres AM. Omphalocele and gastroschisis. Surg Clin North Am 1985;65:1235.
40. King DR, Savrin R, Boles ET, et al. Gastroschisis update. J Pediatr Surg 1980;15:553.
41. Morison JE. Fetal and neonatal pathology. 2nd ed. London: Butterworths, 1963.
42. Moore TC, Stokes GE. Gastroschisis. Surgery 1953;33:112.
43. Meizner I, Bar-Ziv J. In utero prenatal ultrasound diagnosis of a rare case of cloacal exstrophy. J Clin Ultrasound 1985;13:500.
44. Mirk P, Calisti A, Fileni A. Prenatal sonographic diagnosis of bladder exstrophy. J Ultrasound Med 1986;5:291.
45. Cameron GM, McQuown DS, Modanlou HD, et al. Intrauterine diagnosis of an omphalocele by diagnostic ultrasonography. Am J Obstet Gynecol 1978;131:821.
46. Brown BSJ. The prenatal ultrasonographic features of omphalocele: a study of 10 patients. J Can Assoc Radiol 1985;36:312.
47. Redford DH, McNay MB, Whittle MJ. Gastroschisis and exomphalos: recise diagnosis by midpregnancy ultrasound. Br J Obstet Gynaecol 1985;92:54.
48. Bair JH, Russ PD, Pretorius DH, et al. Fetal omphalocele and gastroschisis: a review of 24 cases. AJR 1986;147:1047.
49. Cyr DR, Mack LA, Schoenecker SA, et al. Bowel migration in the normal fetus: US detection. Radiology 1986;161:119.
50. Schmidt W, Jarkoni S, Crelin ES, et al. Sonographic visualization of physiologic anterior abdominal wall hernia in the first trimester. Obstet Gynecol 1987;69:911.
51. Harrison MR, Filly RA, Stauger P, et al. Prenatal diagnosis and management of omphalocele and ectopia cordis. J Pediatr Surg 1982;17:64.
52. Fink IJ, Filly RA. Omphalocele associated with umbilical cord allantoic cyst: sonographic evaluation in utero. Obstet Gynecol 1983;149:473.
53. Clarke PC, Gordon YB, Kitan MJ, et al. Alphafetoprotein levels in pregnancies complicated by gastrointestinal abnormalities of the fetus. Br J Obstet Gynaecol 1977;84:285.
54. King CR, Prescott GH: Amniotic fluid alpha-fetoprotein elevation with fetal omphalocele and a possible mechanism for its occurrence. Am J Obstet Gynecol 1978;130:279.
55. Mayer T, Black R, Matlak M, et al. Gastroschisis and omphalocele. An eight year review. Ann Surg 1980;192:783.
56. Nakajama DK. Management of the fetus with an abdominal wall defect. In: Harrison MR, Golbus MS, Filly RA, eds. The unborn patient: prenatal diagnosis and treatment. Orlando, FL: Grune & Stratton, 1984:217.
57. Harrison MR, Golbus MS, Filly RA. The management of the fetus with a correctable congenital defect. JAMA 1981;246:744.
58. Kirk EP, Wah RM. Obstetrics management of a fetus with omphalocele or gastroschisis. Am J Obstet Gynecol 1983;146:512.
59. Klein MD, Kosloske AM, Hertzier JH. Congenital defects of abdominal wall. A review of the experience in New Mexico. JAMA 1981;245:1643.
60. Shaw A. The myth of gastroschisis. J Pediatr Surg 1975;10:235.
61. Thomas DFM, Atwell JD. The embryology and surgical management of gastroschisis. Br J Surg 1976;63:893.
62. Hoyme EH, Higginbotton CM, Jones LK. The vascular pathogenesis of gastroschisis: intrauterine interruption of the omphalomesenteric artery. J Pediatr 1981:98:228.
63. Giulian BB, Alvear DT. Prenatal ultrasonographic diagnosis of fetal gastroschisis. Radiology 1978;129:473.
64. Colombani PM, Cunningham MD. Perinatal aspects of omphalocele and gastroschisis. Am J Dis Child 1977;131:1386.
65. Mabogunje OOA, Mahour GH. Omphalocele and gastroschisis: trends in survival across two decades. Am J Surg 1984;148:679.
66. Luck SR, Sherman J, Raffensperger JG, Goldstein IR. Gastroschisis in 106 consecutive newborn infants. Surgery 1985;98:677.
67. Schwaitzenberg SD, Pokorny WJ, McGill CW, et al. Gastroschisis and omphalocele. Am J Surg 1982;144:650.
68. Stringel G, Filler RM. Prognostic factors in omphalocele and gastroschisis. J Pediatr Surg 1979;14:515.
69. Swartz KR, Harrison MW, Campbell JR, Campbell TJ. Long-term follow-up of patients with gastroschisis. Am J Surg 1986;151:546.
70. Schwoebel MG, Sacher P, Bucher HU, et al. Prenatal diagnosis improves the prognosis in children with obstructive uropathy. J Pediatr Surg 1984;19:187.
71. Barss VA, Benacerraf BR, Frigoletto FD. Second trimester oligohydramnios, a predictor of poor fetal outcome. Obstet Gynecol 1984;64:608.
72. Osathanondh V, Potter EL. Pathogenesis of polycystic kidneys. Arch Pathol 1964;77:459.
73. Pashayan H, Dowd T, Nigro AV. Bilateral absence of the kidneys and ureters. Three cases reported in one family. J Med Genet 1977;14:205.
74. Perlman M, Levin M. Fetal pulmonary hypoplasia, anuria and oligohydramnios: clinico-pathologic observations and review of the literature. Am J Obstet Gynecol 1974;118:1119.
75. Thomas IT, Smith DW. Oligohydramnios: cause of the non-renal features of Potter's syndrome, including pulmonary hypoplasia. J Pediatr 1974;84:811.
76. Dubbins PA, Kurtz AB, Wapner RJ, et al. Renal agenesis: spectrum of in utero findings. J Clin Ultrasound 1981;9:189.
77. Romero R, Cullen M, Grannum P, et al. Antenatal diagnosis of renal anomalies with ultrasound. III: bilateral renal agenesis. Am J Obstet Gynecol 1985;151:38.
78. Goldemberg RL, Davis RO, Brumfield CG. Transient fetal anuria of unknown etiology: a case report. Am J Obstet Gynecol 1984;149:87.
79. Blyth H, Ockenden BG. Polycystic disease of kidneys and liver presenting in childhood. J Med Genet 1971;8:257.
80. Bosniak MA, Ambos MA. Polycystic kidney disease. Semin Roentgenol 1975;10:133.
81. Romero R, Cullen M, Jeanty P, et al. The diagnosis of congenital renal anomalies with ultrasound. II: infantile polycystic renal disease. Am J Obstet Gynecol 1984;150:259.
82. Simpson JL, Sabbagha RE, Elias S, et al. Failure to detect polycystic kidneys in utero by second trimester ultrasonography. Hum Genet 1982;60:295.
83. Sumner TE, Volberg FM, Martin JF. Real-time ultrasonography of congenital cystic kidney disease. Urology 1982;20:97.
84. Madewell JE, Hartman DS, Lichtenstein JE. Radiologic-pathologic correlations in cystic disease of the kidney. Radiol Clin North Am 1979;133:580.
85. Spence HM, Singleton R. Cysts and cystic disorders of the kidneys: types, diagnosis and treatment. Urol Surv 1972;22:131.

86. Johannessen JV, Haneberg B, Moe PJ. Bilateral multicystic dysplasia of the kidneys. Beitr Pathol Bd 1973;148:290.
87. Sanders RC, Hartman DS. The sonographic distinction between neonatal multicystic kidney and hydronephrosis. Radiology 1984;151:621.
88. Bernstein J. Heritable cystic disorders of the kidney: the mythology of polycystic disease. Pediatr Clin North Am 1971;18:435.
89. Bernstein J, Kissane JM. Hereditary disorders of the kidney. Perspect Pediatr Pathol 1973;1:117.
90. Pathak IG, Williams DI. Multicystic and cystic dysplastic kidneys. Br J Urol 1964;36:318.
91. Potter EL, Craig JM. The pathology of the fetus and infant. 3rd ed. Chicago: Yearbook Medical Publishers, 1975.
92. Rizzo N, Gabrielli S, Pilu G, et al. Prenatal diagnosis and obstetrical management of multicystic dysplastic kidney disease. Prenat Diagn 1987;7:109.
93. Bartley JA, Golbus MS, Filly RA, et al. Prenatal diagnosis of dysplastic kidney disease. Clin Genet 1977;11:375.
94. Dunne MG, Johnson ML. The ultrasonic demonstration of fetal abnormalities in utero. J Reprod Med 1979;23:195.
95. Friedberg JE, Mitnick JS, David DA. Antepartum ultrasonic detection of multicystic kidney. Radiology 1979;131:198.
96. Henderson SC, van Holken RJ, Rahatzad M. Multicystic kidney with hydramnios. J Clin Ultrasound 1980;8:249.
97. Older RA, Hinman CG, Craine LM, et al. In utero diagnosis of multicystic kidney by grey scale ultrasonography. AJR 1979;133:130.
98. Santos-Ramos R, Duenholter JH. Diagnosis of congenital fetal abnormalities by sonography. Obstet Gynecol 1975;45:279.
99. Beretsky I, Laukin DH, Rusoff JH, Phelan L. Sonographic differentiation between the multicystic dysplastic kidney and the uretero-pelvic junction obstruction in utero using high-resolution real-time scanners employing digital detection. J Clin Ultrasound 1984;12:429.
100. Kelalis PP, King LR. Clinical pediatric urology. Philadelphia: WB Saunders, 1976.
101. King LR. Editorial comment. In: Yearbook of urology. Chicago: Yearbook Medical Publishers, 1974:61.
102. Gütter W, Hermanek P. Maligner tumor der Nierengegend unter dem Bilde der Knolleniere. Urol Int 1957;4:164.
103. Zerres K, Weiss H, Bulla M. Prenatal diagnosis of an early manifestation of autosomal dominant adult-type polycystic kidney disease. Lancet 1982;2:988.
104. Zerres K, Volpel MC, Weiss H. Cystic kidneys. Genetics, pathologic anatomy, clinical picture, and prenatal diagnosis. Hum Genet 1984;68:104.
105. Main D, Mennuti MT, Cornfeld D, et al. Prenatal diagnosis of adult polycystic kidney disease. Lancet 1983;2:337.
106. Reeders ST, Zerres K, Ga IA, et al. Prenatal diagnosis of autosomal dominant polycystic kidney disease with a DNA probe. Lancet 1986;2:6.
107. Pretorius DH, Lee ME, Manco-Johnson ML, et al. Diagnosis of autosomal dominant polycystic kidney disease in utero and in the young infant. J Ultrasound Med 1987;6:249.
108. Hobbins JC, Romero R, Grannum P, et al. Antenatal diagnosis of renal anomalies with ultrasound. I: obstructive uropathy. Am J Obstet Gynecol 1984;148:868.
109. Ahmed S, Savage JP. Surgery of pelviureteric obstruction in the first year of life. Aust N Z J Surg 1985;55:253.
110. Atwell JD. Familial pelviureteric junction hydronephrosis and its association with a duplex pelvicaliceal system and vesicoureteric reflux. A family study. Br J Urol 1985;57:365.
111. Buscemi M, Shanske A, Mallet E, et al. Dominantly inherited ureteropelvic junction obstruction. Urology 1985;26:568.
112. Arger PH, Coleman BG, Mintz MC, et al. Routine fetal genitourinary tract screening. Radiology 1985;156:485.
113. Jeffrey RB, Laing FC, Wing VW, et al. Sonography of the fetal duplex kidney. Radiology 1984;153:123.
114. Montana MA, Cyr DR, Lenke RR, et al. Sonographic detection of fetal ureteral obstruction. AJR 1985;145:595.
115. Levine PM, Delaune J, Gonzales ET Jr. Genetic etiology of posterior urethral valves. J Urol 1983;130:781.
116. Beck AD. The effect of intrauterine urinary obstruction upon the development of fetal kidney. J Urol 1971;105:784.
117. Mahony BS, Callen PW, Filly RA. Fetal urethral obstruction: US evaluation. Radiology 1985;157:221.
118. Harrison MR, Golbus MS, Filly RA. Congenital hydronephrosis. In: The unborn patient. Orlando, Grune & Stratton, 1984:277.
119. Krueger RP, Hardy BE, Churchill BM. Growth in boys with posterior urethral valves. Primary valve resection vs. upper tract diversion. Urol Clin North Am 1980;7:265.
120. Evans M. Newsletter, International Fetal Medicine and Surgery Society, 1989.
121. Crombleholme TM, Harrison MR, Langer JC, et al. Early experience with open fetal surgery for congenital hydronephrosis. J Pediatr Surg 1988;23:1114.
122. Ahmed S. Neonatal and childhood ovarian cyst. J Pediatr Surg 1971;6:702.
123. Carlson DH, Griscom NT. Ovarian cysts in the newborn. J Roentgenol Radium Ther Nucl Med 1972;116:664.
124. Jafri SZ, Bree RL, Silver TM, et al. Fetal ovarian cysts: sonographic detection and association with hypothyroidism. Radiology 1984;150:809.
125. Valenti C, Kassner EG, Yermankov V, et al. Antenatal diagnosis of a fetal ovarian cyst. Am J Obstet Gynecol 1975;123:216.
126. Lee TG, Blake S. Prenatal fetal abdominal ultrasonography and diagnosis. Radiology 1977;124:475.
127. Kirkinen PJP, Tuononen S. Ultrasonic detection of bilateral ovarian cyst in the fetus. Eur J Obstet Gynecol Reprod Biol 1982;131:87.
128. Sandler MA, Smith SJ, Pope SG, et al. Prenatal diagnosis of septated ovarian cysts. J Clin Ultrasound 1985;13:55.
129. Rizzo N, Gabrielli S, Perolo A, et al. Prenatal diagnosis and management of fetal ovarian cysts. Prenat Diagn 1989;9:97.
130. Tabsh KMA. Antenatal sonographic appearance of a fetal ovarian cyst. J Clin Ultrasound 1982;1:329.
131. Preziosi P, Pariello G, Maiorana A, et al. Antenatal sonographic diagnosis of complicated ovarian cysts. J Clin Ultrasound 1986;14:196.

39

CHAPTER

FETAL SKELETAL ANOMALIES

Roberto Romero and Jose Nores

Skeletal dysplasias are a heterogeneous group of disorders that affect the development of chondro-osseous tissues and result in abnormalities in the size and shape of different segments of the skeleton. Little is known about their etiology, but genetic factors are clearly important, because a Mendelian pattern of inheritance has been described in many of these conditions. Sporadic cases suggest the appearance of new spontaneous mutations or environmental factors. Exposure to drugs (eg, thalidomide, warfarin), ionic radiation, hyperthermia, hyperglycemia (diabetes mellitus), mechanical factors, and vascular disruption with hypoperfusion of specific areas in the embryo have been implicated in the etiology of some skeletal dysplasias.

The prenatal diagnosis of these disorders is particularly challenging. This chapter reviews the birth prevalence and classification of skeletal dysplasias and provides an approach to the diagnosis of conditions identifiable at birth.

BIRTH PREVALENCE AND CONTRIBUTION TO PERINATAL MORTALITY

The birth prevalence of skeletal dysplasias, excluding limb amputations, recognizable in the neonatal period has been estimated to be 2.4 of 10,000 births.[1] In a large series, 23% of affected infants were stillborn, and 32% died during the first week of life. The overall frequency of skeletal dysplasias among perinatal deaths was 9.1 out of 1000. The birth prevalence of the different skeletal dysplasias and their relative frequency among perinatal deaths in this study are shown in Table 39-1. The four most common skeletal dysplasias found were thanatophoric dysplasia, achondroplasia, osteogenesis imperfecta, and achondrogenesis. Thanatophoric dysplasia and achondrogenesis accounted for 62% of all lethal skeletal dysplasias.[1] The most common nonlethal skeletal dysplasia was achondroplasia.

In another large series, reporting the prevalence and classification of lethal neonatal skeletal dysplasias in west Scotland, the prevalence was 1.1 in 10,000 births, and the most frequently diagnosed conditions were thanatophoric dysplasia (1/42,000), osteogenesis imperfecta (1/56,000), chondrodysplasia punctata (1/84,000), campomelic syndrome (1/112,000), and achondrogenesis (1/112,000).[2]

CLASSIFICATION OF SKELETAL DYSPLASIAS

The existing nomenclature for skeletal dysplasias is complicated, and definition criteria are not uniform. For example, disorders may be referred to by eponyms (eg, Ellis-van Creveld syndrome, Larsen dysplasia), by Greek terms describing a salient feature of the disease (eg, diastrophic [twisted], metatropic [angeable]), or by terms related to the presumed pathogenesis of the disease (eg, osteogenesis imperfecta, achondrogenesis). The fundamental problem with any classification of skeletal dysplasias is that the pathogenesis of these diseases is largely unknown. Therefore, the current system relies on purely descriptive findings of either clinical or radiologic nature.

In an attempt to develop a uniform terminology (Fig. 39-1), a group of experts met in Paris in 1977 and proposed an International Nomenclature for Skeletal Dysplasias that has recently been revised (Table 39-2).[3,4] The system subdivides the diseases into five different groups:

1. Osteochondrodysplasias—abnormalities of cartilage and/or bone growth and development

TABLE 39–1. BIRTH PREVALENCE (PER 10,000 TOTAL BIRTHS) OF SKELETAL DYSPLASIAS

	BIRTH PREVALENCE (PER 10,000)	FREQUENCY AMONG PERINATAL DEATHS
Thanatophoric dysplasia	0.69	1:246
Achondroplasia	0.37	—
Achondrogenesis	0.23	1:639
Osteogenesis imperfecta type II	0.18	1:799
Osteogenesis imperfecta (other types)	0.18	—
Asphyxiating thoracic dysplasia	0.14	1:3196
Chondrodysplasia punctata	0.09	—
Camptomelic dysplasia	0.05	1:3196
Chondroectodermal dysplasia	0.05	1:3196
Larsen syndrome	0.05	—
Mesomelic dysplasia (Langer's type)	0.05	—
Others	0.46	1:800
Total skeletal dysplasias	2.44	1:110

Camera G, Mastroiacovo P. Birth prevalence of skeletal dysplasias in the Italian multicentric monitoring system for birth defects. In: Papadatos CJ, Bartsocas CS, eds. Skeletal dysplasias. New York: Alan R Liss, 1982:441.

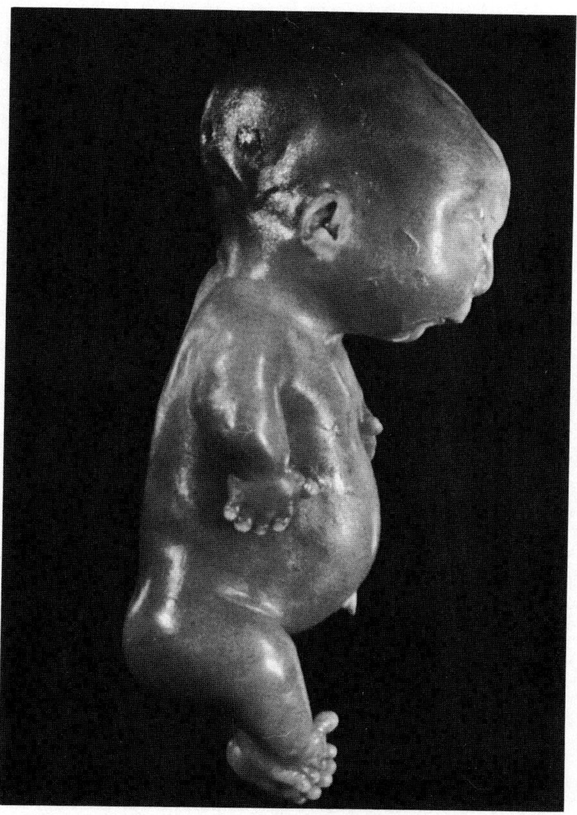

FIGURE 39–1. Micromelic fetus affected by a lethal skeletal dysplasia. Discrepancies among authorities have led to the classification of this entity as atelosteogenesis type II, diastrophiclike dysplasia, de la Chapelle dysplasia, and McAlister dysplasia.

2. Dysostoses—malformations of individual bones singly or in combination
3. Idiopathic osteolysis—disorders associated with multifocal resorption of bone
4. Skeletal disorders associated with chromosomal aberrations
5. Primary metabolic disorders.

Recently, Spranger and Maroteaux have classified lethal osteochondrodysplasias in 11 groups based on the radioanatomical manifestations (Table 39-3). The purpose of this classification is to facilitate differential diagnosis, and the groups do not necessarily constitute pathogenetic "families."[5]

A comprehensive description of these diseases is beyond the scope of this chapter; the interested reader is referred to genetics textbooks for a full discussion of the subject. This chapter focuses primarily on the osteochondrodysplasias that are recognizable at birth. Although more than 200 skeletal dysplasias have been described, and more will probably be identified as distinct entities, the number that can be recognized with the use of sonography in the antepartum period is considerably smaller. Most of these disorders result in short stature; the term "dwarfism" has been used to refer to this clinical condition. However, because this term carries a negative connotation, we use the term "dysplasia" instead.

TERMINOLOGY FREQUENTLY USED IN THE DESCRIPTION OF BONE DYSPLASIAS

Shortening of the extremities can involve the entire limb (micromelia), the proximal segment (rhizomelia), the intermediate segment (mesomelia), or the distal segment (acromelia). The diagnosis of rhizomelia or

Continued on page 585

TABLE 39–2. INTERNATIONAL CLASSIFICATION FOR DYSPLASIAS

Osteochondrodysplasias							
Abnormalities of cartilage and/or bone growth and development							
A. Defects of growth of tubular bones and/or spine							
a. Identifiable at birth							
(a.) Usually lethal before or shortly after birth							
1. Achondrogenesis type I (Parenti-Fraccaro)				AR	**		
2. Achondrogenesis type II (Langer-Saldino)					**		
3. Hypochondrogenesis		*					
4. Fibronchondrogenesis	AR	*					
5. Thanatophoric dysplasia			***				
6. Thanatophoric dysplasia with cloverleaf skull					**		
7. Atelosteogenesis			*				
8. Short-rib syndrome (with or without polydactyly)							
a. Type I (Saldino-Noonan)		AR	**				
b. Type II (Majewski)	AR	*					
c. Type III (lethal thoracic dysplasia)			AR	*			
(b.) Usually nonlethal dysplasia							
9. Chondrodysplasia punctata							
a. Rhizomelic form autosomal recessive			AR	**			
b. Dominant X-linked form (lethal in male)				XLD	**		
c. Common mild form (Sheffield)							
Exclude: symptomatic stippling (warfarin, chromosomal aberration)							**
10. Camptomelic dysplasia				AR	*		
11. Kyphomelic dysplasia				AD	****		
12. Achondroplasia				AR		***	
13. Diastrophic dysplasia				AR, AD		**	
14. Metatropic dysplasia (several forms)							
15. Chondroectodermal dysplasia (Ellis-van Creveld)				AR		***	
16. Asphyxiating thoracic dysplasia (Jeune)				AR		**	
17. Spondyloepiphyseal dysplasia congenita							
a. Autosomal dominant form				AD		**	
b. Autosomal recessive form				AR		**	
18. Kniest dysplasia				AR		**	
19. Dyssegmental dysplasia				AR		*	
20. Mesomelic dysplasia							
a. Type Nievegelt				AD		*	
b. Type Langer (probable homozygous dyschondrosteosis)				AR		*	
						*	
c. Type Robinow				AD		*	
d. Type Rheinardt						***	
e. Others							
21. Acromesomelic dysplasia				AR		**	
22. Cleidocranial dysplasia				AD		****	
23. Otopalatodigital syndrome							
a. Type I (Langer)				XLSD		**	
b. Type II (Andre)				XLR		**	
24. Larsen syndrome				AR, AD		**	
25. Other multiple dislocation syndromes (Desbuquois)				AR			
b. Identifiable late in life							
1. Hypochondroplasia				AD	***		
2. Dyschondrosteosis				AD	***		
3. Metaphyseal chondrodysplasia type Jansen				AD	*		
4. Metaphyseal chondrodysplasia type Schmid				AD	**		
5. Metaphyseal chondrodysplasia type McKusick				AR	**		

(continued)

TABLE 39-2. (continued)

6. Metaphyseal chondrodysplasia with exocrine pancreatic insufficiency and cyclic neutropenia	AR	**	
7. Spondylometaphyseal dysplasia			
a. Type Kozlowski	AD	**	
b. Other forms		***	
8. Multiple epiphyseal dysplasia			
a. Type Fairbank	AD	****	
b. Other forms			***
9. Multiple epiphyseal dysplasia with early diabetes (Wolcott-Rallisson)	AR	**	
10. Arthro-ophthalmopathy (Stickler)	AR	***	
11. Pseudoachondroplasia			
a. Dominant	AD	***	
b. Recessive	AR	**	
12. Spondyloepiphyseal dysplasia tarda (X-linked recessive)	XLR	**	
13. Progressive pseudorheumatoid chondrodysplasia	AR	**	
14. Spondyloepiphyseal dysplasia, other forms			***
15. Brachyolmia			
a. Autosomal recessive	AR	*	
b. Autosomal dominant	AD	*	
16. Dyggve-Melchior-Clausen dysplasia	AR	**	
17. Spondyloepimetaphyseal dysplasia (several forms)			***
18. Spondyloepimetaphyseal dysplasia with joint laxity	AR	**	
19. Otospondylomegaepiphyseal dysplasia (OSMED)	AR	*	
20. Myotonic chondrodysplasia (Catel-Schwartz-Jampel)	AR	**	
21. Parastremmatic dysplasia	A	*	
22. Trichorhinophalangeal dysplasia	AD	**	
23. Acrodysplasia with retinitis pigmentosa and nephropathy (Saldino-Mainzer)	AR	**	
B. Disorganized development of cartilage and fibrous components of skeleton			
1. Dysplasia epiphyseal hemimelica			**
2. Multiple cartilaginous exostoses	AD	***	
3. Acrodysplasia with exostoses (Giedion-Langer)			**
4. Enchondromatosis (Ollier)			***
5. Enchondromatosis with hemangioma (Maffucci)			**
6. Metachondromatosis	AD	**	
7. Spondyloenchondroplasia	AR	*	
8. Osteoglophonic dysplasia			*
9. Fibrous dysplasia (Jaffe-Lichtenstein)			***
10. Fibrous dysplasia with skin pigmentation and precocious puberty (McMune-Albright)			***
11. Cherubism (familial fibrous dysplasia of the jaws)	AD	**	
C. Abnormalities of density of cortical diaphyseal structure and/or metaphyseal modeling			
1. Osteogenesis imperfecta (several forms)	AD, AR		****
2. Juvenile idiopathic osteoporosis			**
3. Osteoporosis with pseudoglioma	AR	*	
4. Osteopetrosis			
a. Autosomal recessive lethal	AR	**	
b. Intermediate recessive	AR	**	
c. Autosomal dominant	AD	***	
d. Recessive with tubular acidosis	AR	**	
5. Pycnodysostosis	AR	***	

(continued)

TABLE 39-2. (continued)

6. Dominant osteosclerosis type Stanescu	AD	**		
7. Osteomesopycnosis	AD	**		
8. Osteopoikilosis	AD	***		
9. Osteopathia striata	AD	***		
10. Osteopathia striata with cranial sclerosis	AD	**		
11. Melorheostosis			***	
12. Diaphyseal dysplasia (Camurati-Engelmann)		AD	***	
13. Craniodiaphyseal dysplasia	AR	**		
14. Endosteal hyperostosis				
a. Autosomal dominant (Worth)	AD	**		
b. Autosomal recessive (Van Buchem)	AR	**		
c. Autosomal recessive (sclerosteosis)	AR	**		
15. Tubular stenosis (Kenny-Caffey)	AD	*		
16. Pachydermoperiostosis	AD	**		
17. Osteodysplasty (Melnick-Needles)	AD	**		
18. Frontometaphyseal dysplasia	XLR	**		
19. Craniometaphyseal dysplasia (several forms)	AD	***		
20. Metaphyseal dysplasia (Pyle)	AR or AD		**	
21. Dysosteosclerosis	AR or XLR		**	
22. Osteoectasia with hyperphosphatasia	AR	**		
23. Oculo-dento-osseous dysplasia				
a. Mild type	AD	***		
b. Severe type	AR	*		
24. Infantile cortical hyperostosis (Caffey disease, familial type)	AD	**		
Dysostoses				
Malformation of individual bones, singly or in combination				
A. Dysostoses with cranial and facial involvement				
1. Craniosynostosis (several forms)			***	
2. Craniofacial dysostosis (Crouzon)				***
3. Acrocephalosyndactyly				
a. Type Apert	AD		***	
b. Type Chotzen	AD		**	
c. Type Pfeiffer	AD	**		
d. Other types			***	
4. Acrocephalopolysyndactyly (Carpenter and others)	AR		**	
5. Cephalopolysyndactyly (Greig)	AD	*		
6. First and second branchial arch syndromes				
a. Mandibulofacial dysostosis (Treacher-Collins, Franceschetti)	AD	***		
b. Acrofacial dysostosis (Nager)			**	
c. Oculo-auriculo-vertebral dysostosis (Goldenhar)	AR	***		
d. Hemifacial microsomia			***	
e. Others			***	
(Probably parts of a large spectrum)				
7. Oculomandibulofacial syndrome (Hallermann-Streiff-François)				
B. Dysostoses with predominant axial involvement				
1. Vertebral segmentation defects (including Kippel-Feil)			**	
2. Cervico-oculo-acoustic syndrome (Wildervanck)			***	
3. Sprengel anomaly				***
4. Spondylocostal dysostosis				
a. Dominant form	AD		**	
b. Recessive form	AR		**	
5. Oculovertebral syndrome (Weyers)				*

(continued)

TABLE 39-2. (continued)

6. Osteo-onychodysostosis	AD	***		
7. Cerebrocostomandibular syndrome	AR	**		
C. Dysostoses with predominant involvement of extremities				
1. Acheiria				**
2. Apodia				**
3. Tetraphocomelia syndrome (Roberts) (SC pseudothalidomide syndrome)	AR		**	
4. Ectrodactyly				
a. Isolated			***	
b. Ectrodactyly-ectodermal dysplasia, cleft palate-syndrome	AD	**		
c. Ectrodactyly with scalp defects	AD		**	
5. Oro-acral syndrome (aglossia syndrome, Hanhart syndrome)				*
6. Familial radioulnar synostosis				**
7. Brachydactyly, types A, B, C, D, E (Bell's classification)	AD		****	
8. Symphalangism	AD	***		
9. Polydactyly (several forms)				****
10. Syndactyly (several forms)				****
11. Polysyndactyly (several forms)				***
12. Camptodactyly				****
13. Manzke syndrome				*
14. Poland syndrome				***
15. Rubinstein-Taybi syndrome				**
16. Coffin-Siris syndrome				**
17. Pancytopenia-dysmelia syndrome (Franconi)	AR	***		
18. Blackfan-Diamond anemia with thumb anomalies (Aase syndrome)	AR	**		
19. Thrombocytopenia–radial-aplasia syndrome	AR	**		
20. Orodigitofacial syndrome				
a. Type Papillon-Leage (lethal in males)	XLD		**	
b. Type Mohr	AR	**		
21. Cardimelic syndromes (Holt-Oram and others)	AD	***		
22. Femoral focal deficiency (with or without facial anomalies)				**
23. Multiple synostoses (includes some forms of symphalangism)	AD	***		
24. Scapuloiliac dysostosis (Kosenow-Sinios)	AD	**		
25. Hand–foot–genital syndrome	AD		**	
26. Focal dermal hypoplasia (Goltz) (lethal in males)	XLD		**	
Idiopathic osteolyses				
1. Phalangeal (several forms)				**
2. Tarsocarpal				
a. Including François form and others	AR		**	
b. With nephropathy	AD	**		
3. Multicentric				
a. Hajdu-Cheney form	AD	**		
b. Winchester form	AR	*		
c. Torg form	AR	*		
d. Other forms			**	
Miscellaneous disorders with osseous involvement				
1. Early acceleration of skeletal maturation				
a. Marshall-Smith syndrome			*	
b. Weaver syndrome			*	
c. Other types			*	
2. Marfan syndrome	AD	****		
3. Congenital contractural arachnodactyly	AD	**		

(continued)

TABLE 39-2. (continued)

4. Cerebrohepatorenal syndrome (Zellweger)					**
5. Coffin-Lowry syndrome		SLR	**		
6. Cockayne syndrome		AR	**		
7. Fibrodysplasia ossificans congenita		AD	***		
8. Epidermal nervus syndrome (Solomon)					**
9. Nevoid basal cell carcinoma syndrome					**
10. Multiple hereditary fibromatosis					**
11. Neurofibromatosis		AD	****		
Chromosomal aberrations					
Primary metabolic abnormalities					
A. Calcium and/or phosphorus					
1. Hypophosphatemic rickets		XLD		****	
2. Vitamin D dependency or pseudodeficiency rickets					
a. Type I with probable deficiency in 25-hydroxy vitamin D 1-alpha-hydroxylase	AR	***			
b. Type II with target-organ resistance		AR	**		
3. Late rickets (McCance)					**
4 Idiopathic hypercalciuria					***
5. Hypophosphatasia (several forms)		AR	***		
6. Pseudohypoparathyroidism (normo- and hypocalcemic forms, including acrodysostosis)		AD	***		
B. Complex carbohydrates					
1. Mucopolysaccharidosis, type I (alpha-L-iduronidase deficiency)					
a. Hurler form		AR	***		
b. Scheie form		AR	**		
c. Other forms		AR		**	
2. Mucopolysaccharodosis, type II (Hunter) (sulfoiduronate sulfatase deficiency)		XLR	***		
3. Mucopolysaccharidosis, type III (Sanfilippo)					***
a. Type III A (heparin sulfamidase deficiency)		AR			
b. Type III B (*N*-acetyl-alpha-glucosaminidase)		AR			
c. Type III C (alpha-glucosaminide-*N*-acetyl transferase deficiency)		AR			
d. Type III D (*N*-acetyl-glucosamine-6 sulfate sulfatase deficiency)		AR			
4. Mucopolysaccharidosis, type IV					**
a. Type IV A—Morquio (*N*-acetyl-galactosamine-6 sulfate sulfatase deficiency)		AR			
b. Type IV B (Beta-galactosidase deficiency)		AR			
5. Mucopolysaccharidosis, type VI-(Maroteaux-Lany) (arylsulfatase B deficiency)		AR			
6. Mucopolysaccharidosis, type VII (beta-glucuronidase deficiency)		AR		**	
7. Aspartyl glucosaminuria (aspartylglucosaminidase deficiency)		AR		**	
8. Mannosidosis (alpha-mannosidase deficiency)	AR	**			
9. Fucosidosis (alpha-fucosidase deficiency)		AR	**		
10. GMI-gangliosidosis (beta-galactosidase deficiency) (several forms)		AR	**		
11. Multiple sulfatase deficiency (Austin-Thieffry)		AR	**		

(continued)

TABLE 39-2. (continued)

12. Isolated neuroaminidase deficiency —several forms, including						**
a. Mucolipidosis I				AR		
b. Nephrosialidosis				AR		
c. Cherry red spot myoclonia syndrome				AR		
13. Phosphotransferase deficiency—several forms, including						**
a. Mucolipidosis II (I cell disease)				AR		
b. Mucolipidosis III (pseudopolydystrophy)				AR		
14. Combined neuroaminidase beta-galactosidase deficiency				AR	*	
15. Salla disease			AR	*		
C. Lipids						
1. Niemann-Pick disease (sphingomyelinase deficiency) (several forms)		AR	***			
2. Gaucher disease (beta-glucosidase deficiency) (several types)				AR	****	
3. Farber disease lipogranulomatosis (cereaminidase deficiency)	AR	**				
D. Nucleic acids						
1. Adenosine-deaminase deficiency and others				AR	**	
E. Amino acids						
1. Homocystinuria and others				AR	**	
F. Metals						
1. Menkes syndrome (kinky hair syndrome and others)				AR	***	

Kozlowski K, Beighton P. Gamut Index of Skeletal Dysplasias (an aid to radiodiagnosis). Berlin: Springer-Verlag, 1986.

a, Mode of transmission; b, Frequency; AR, autosomal recessive; XLD, X-linked dominant; AD, autosomal dominant; XLR, X-linked recessive; SLR, sex-linked recessive.

**** 1000+ cases
*** 100–1000 cases
** 20–100 cases
* Fewer than 20 cases
(Estimates of the relative frequency of these conditions are based on the compilers' experience and a review of the literature.)

mesomelia requires the comparison of the dimensions of the bones of the legs and forearm with those of the thigh and arm. Figures 39-2 and 39-3 display the relationship between the humerus and ulna, and the femur and tibia, and can be used in the assessment of rhizomelia and acromesomelia. Table 39-4 presents skeletal dysplasias characterized by rhizomelia, mesomelia, acromelia, and micromelia.

Several skeletal dysplasias feature alterations of the hands and feet. The term "polydactyly" refers to the presence of more than five digits. It is classified as postaxial if the extra digits are on the ulnar or fibular side, and preaxial if they are located on the radial or tibial side. Syndactyly refers to soft-tissue or bony fusion of adjacent digits. Clinodactyly consists of deviation of a finger (or fingers). The most common spinal abnormality seen in skeletal dysplasias is platyspondylia, which consists of flattening of the vertebrae (Fig. 39-4). Kyphosis and scoliosis can also be identified in utero (Fig. 39-5). Prenatal diagnosis of hemivertebra[6] (Fig. 39-6) and coronal clefting of vertebral bodies (Fig. 39-7) has been made.

BIOMETRY OF THE FETAL SKELETON IN THE DIAGNOSIS OF BONE DYSPLASIAS

Long-bone biometry has been used extensively in the prediction of gestational age. Nomograms available for this purpose use the long bone as the independent variable and the estimated fetal age as the dependent variable. However, the type of nomogram required to assess the normality of bone dimensions uses gestational age as the independent variable and the long bone as the dependent variable. For the proper use of these nomograms, the clinician must accurately know the gestational age of the fetus. Therefore, patients at risk for skeletal dysplasias should be advised to seek prenatal care at an early gestational age to assess all clinical estimators of gestational age. Tables 39-5 and 39-6 present nomograms for the assessment of limb biometry for the upper and lower extremities, respectively. For those patients presenting with uncertain gestational age, comparisons between limb dimensions and the head perimeter can be used (Figs. 39-8 and 39-9). Other authors have employed the biparietal diameter for this purpose.

TABLE 39-3. NOSOLOGY OF LETHAL OSTEOCHONDRODYSPLASIAS

1. Hypophosphatasia and morphologically similar disorders
1.01 Hypophosphatasia
1.02 Probable hypophosphatasia
1.03 Lethal metaphyseal dysplasia
2. Chondrodysplasia punctata and similar disorders
2.01 Rhizomelic chondrodysplasia punctata
2.02 Lethal chondrodysplasia punctata, X-linked dominant
2.03 Greenberg dysplasia
2.04 Dappled diaphysis dysplasia
3. Achondrogenesis and similar disorders
3.01 Achondrogenesis I-A (Houston-Harris)
3.02 Achondrogenesis I-B (Fraccaro)
3.03 New lethal osteochondrodysplasia
3.04 Achondrogenesis II (Langer-Saldino)
3.05 Hypochondrogenesis
4. Thanatophoric dysplasia, and similar disorders
4.01 Thanatophoric dysplasia, type 1
4.02 Thanatophoric dysplasia, type 2
4.03 Homozygous achondroplasia
4.04 Lethal achondroplasia
4.05 Glasgow variant
5. Platyspondylic lethal chondrodysplasias
5.01 Platyspondylic chondrodysplasia, Torrance type
5.02 Platyspondylic chondrodysplasia, San Diego type
5.03 Platyspondylic chondrodysplasia, Luton type
5.04 Platyspondylic chondrodysplasia, Shiraz type
5.05 Opsismodysplasia
5.06 Sixth form of platyspondylic chondrodysplasia
5.07 Seventh form of platyspondylic chondrodysplasia
6. Short-rib–polydactyly syndromes
6.01 Short-rib–polydactyly syndrome, type I (Saldino-Noonan)
6.02 Short-rib–polydactyly syndrome, type II (Verma–Naumoff)
6.03 Short-rib–polydactyly syndrome, type III (Le Marec)
6.04 Short-rib–polydactyly syndrome, type IV (Yang)
6.05 Asphyxiating thoracic dysplasia (Jeune)
6.06 Short-rib–polydactyly syndrome, type VI (Majewski)
6.07 Short-rib–polydactyly syndrome, type VII (Beemer)
7. Lethal metatropic dysplasia and similar disorders
7.01 Lethal metatropic dysplasia (hyperchondrogenesis)
7.02 Isolated case
7.03 Isolated case
7.04 Fibrochondrogenesis
7.05 Schneckenbecken dysplasia
7.06 Isolated case
7.07 Isolated case
7.08 Isolated case
8. Kniest-like disorders
8.01 Dyssegmental dysplasia, Silverman type
8.02 Dyssegmental dysplasia, Rolland-Desbuquois type
8.03 Lethal Kniest disease
8.04 Chondrodysplasia resembling Kniest dysplasia
8.05 Isolated case
8.06 Blomstrand chondrodysplasia
9. Lethal osteochondrodysplasias with pronounced diaphyseal abnormalities
9.01 Campomelic syndrome
9.02 Stuve-Wiedemann syndrome
9.03 Boomerang dysplasia
9.04 Atelosteogenesis
9.05 Disorder resembling atelosteogenesis
9.06 De la Chapelle dysplasia
9.07 McAlister dysplasia
9.08 Pseudodiastrophic dysplasia
10. Osteogenesis imperfecta and similar disorders
10.01 Osteogenesis imperfecta II-A
10.02 Osteogenesis imperfecta II-B
10.03 Osteogenesis imperfecta II-C
10.04 Isolated case
10.05 Astley-Kendall dysplasia
11. Lethal disorders with gracile bones
11.01 Fetal hypokinesia phenotype
11.02 Lethal osteochondrodysplasia with gracile bones
11.03 Lethal osteochondrodysplasia with intrauterine overtubulation

Spranger J, Maroteaux P. The lethal osteochondrodysplasias. Adv Hum Genet 1989;19:3.

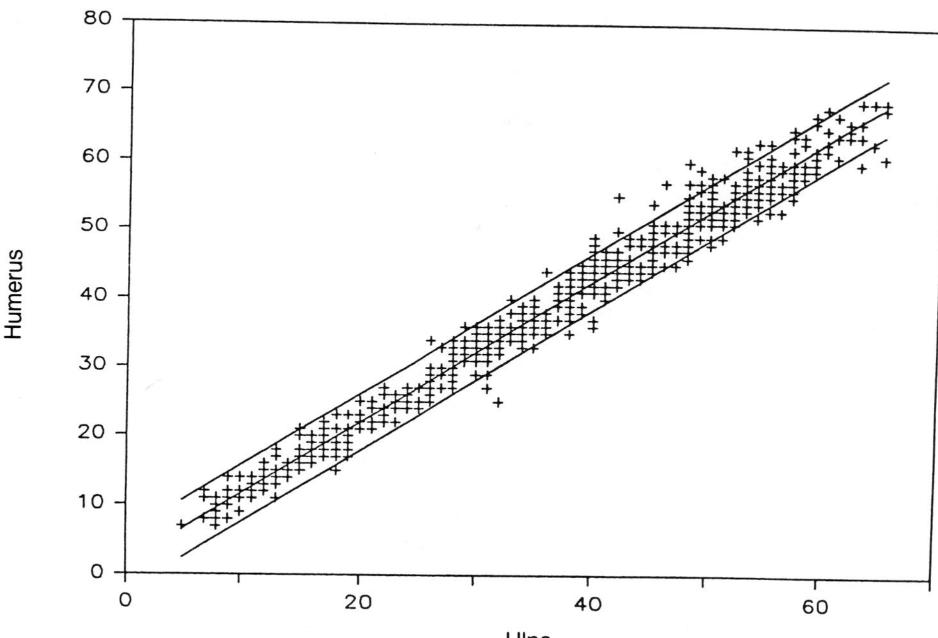

FIGURE 39–2. Relationship between the ulna and the humerus.

The head perimeter has the advantage of being shape independent. A limitation of this approach is that it assumes that the cranium is not involved in the dysplastic process, and this may not be the case in some skeletal dysplasias.

The nomograms and figures in this chapter provide the mean, 5th, and 95th percentiles of limb biometric parameters. The reader should be aware that 5% of the general population will fall outside these boundaries. Ideally, a more stringent criterion—such as the 1st percentile of limb growth for gestational age—should be used for diagnosis. Unfortunately, none of the currently available nomograms have been based on enough patients to provide an accurate discrimination between the 5th and the 1st percentiles. However, most skeletal dysplasias diagnosed in utero or at birth are associated with dramatic long-bone shortening, and under these circumstances, the precise boundary used (1st or 5th percentile) is not critical. An exception to this is achondroplasia, in which limb biometry is mildly affected until the third trimester, when abnormal growth can be detected by examining the slope of growth of femur length.[7]

Continued on page 590

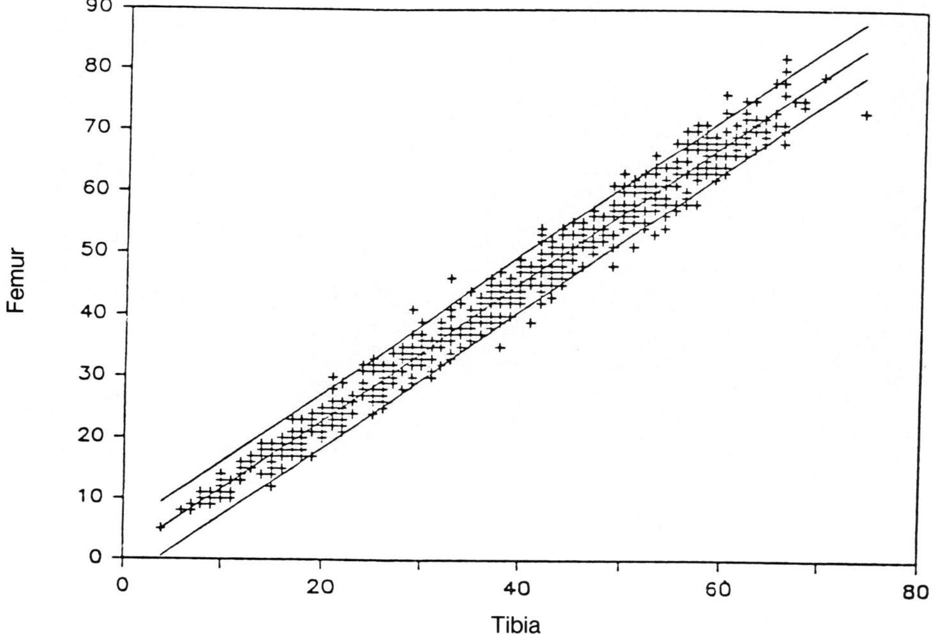

FIGURE 39–3. Relationship between the tibia and the femur.

TABLE 39–4. CLASSIFICATION OF SKELETAL DYSPLASIAS BY RHIZOMELIA, MESOMELIA, ACROMELIA, AND MICROMELIA

Rhizomelia
Thanatophoric dysplasia
Atelosteogenesis
Chondrodysplasia punctata (rhizomelic type)
Diastrophic dysplasia
Congenital short femur
Achondroplasia
Mesomelia
Mesomelic dysplasia (Langer, Reinhardt, and Robinow types)
COVESDEM association
Acromelia
Ellis-van Creveld syndrome (Chondroectodermal dysplasia)
Micromelia
Achondrogenesis
Atelosteogenesis
Short-rib–polydactyly syndrome (type I and type II)
Diastrophic dysplasia
Fibrochondrogenesis
Osteogenesis imperfecta (type III)
Kniest dysplasia
Dyssegmental dysplasia
Roberts syndrome

Reproduced with permission from Romero R, Athanassiadis AP, Sirtori M, Inati M. Fetal skeletal anomalies. In: Fleischer AC, Romero R, Manning FA, Jeanty P, James AE Jr, eds. The principles and practice of ultrasonography in obstetrics and gynecology, 4th ed. Norwalk, CT: Appleton & Lange, 1991:286.

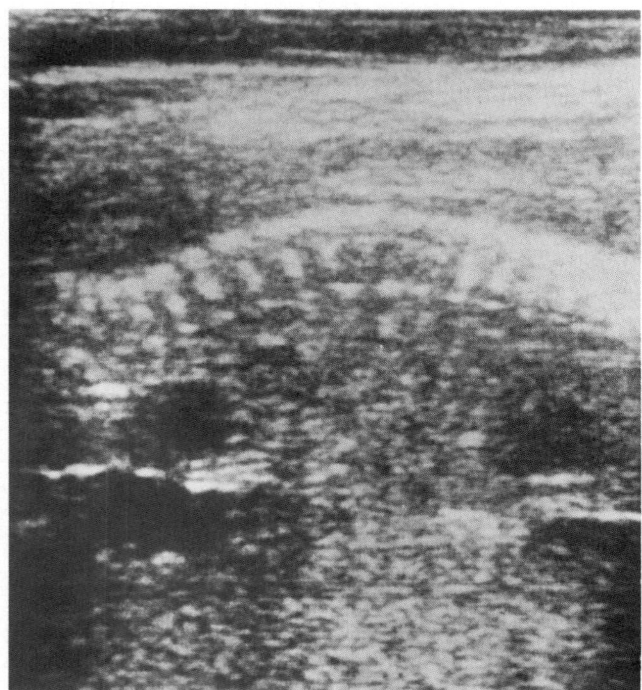

FIGURE 39–4. Sagittal scan of a fetus with platyspondyly.

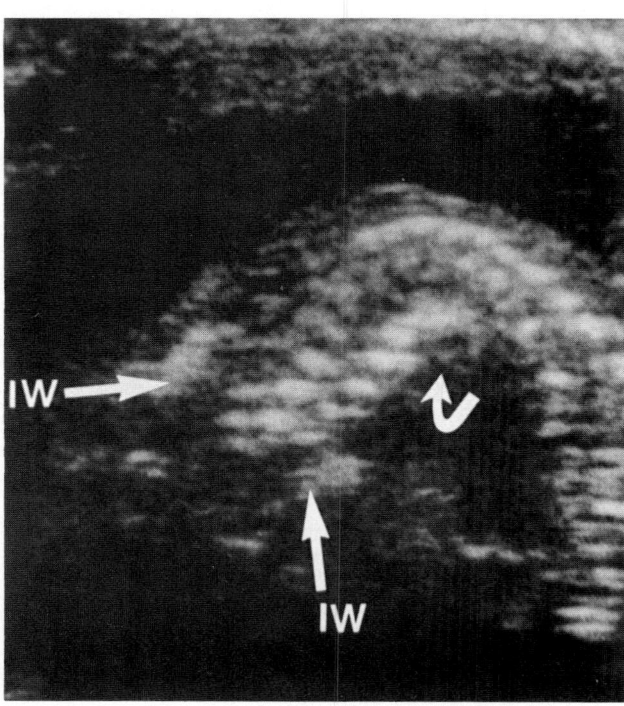

FIGURE 39–5. Coronal scan demonstrating severe scoliosis (curved arrow). (IW = iliac wings.)

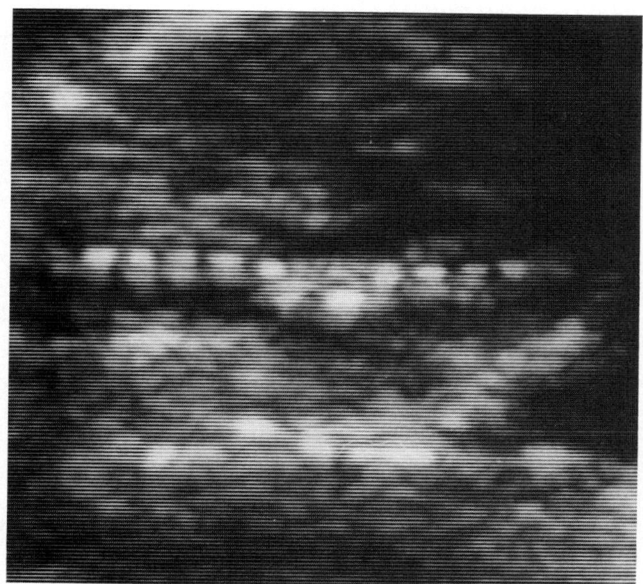

FIGURE 39–6. Hemivertebra longitudinal scan of the thoracolumbar spine showing abnormal ossification of the vertebral body.

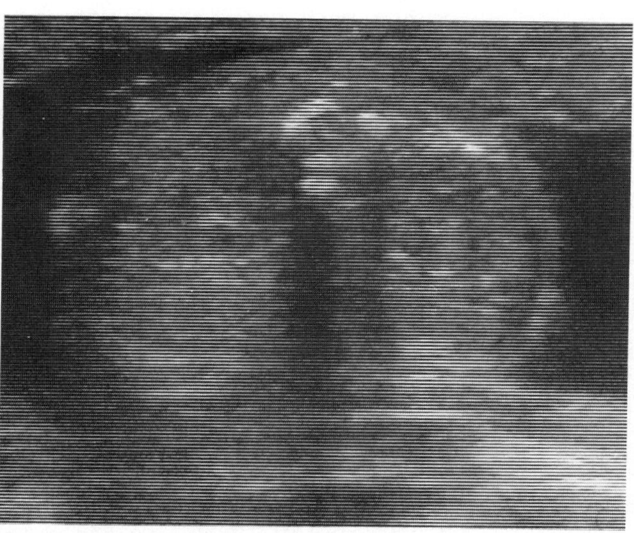

FIGURE 39–7. Transverse scan at the level of L-2 demonstrating a coronal cleft in the vertebral body.

TABLE 39–5. NORMAL VALUES FOR THE ARM (mm)

	HUMERUS			ULNA			RADIUS		
	PERCENTILE			PERCENTILE			PERCENTILE		
WEEK	5th	50th	95th	5th	50th	95th	5th	50th	95th
12	—	9	—	—	7	—	—	7	—
13	6	11	16	5	10	15	6	10	14
14	9	14	19	8	13	18	8	13	17
15	12	17	22	11	16	21	11	15	20
16	15	20	25	13	18	23	13	18	22
17	18	22	27	16	21	26	14	20	26
18	20	25	30	19	24	29	15	22	29
19	23	28	33	21	26	31	20	24	29
20	25	30	35	24	29	34	22	27	32
21	28	33	38	26	31	36	24	29	33
22	30	35	40	28	33	38	27	31	34
23	33	38	42	31	36	41	26	32	39
24	35	40	45	33	38	43	26	34	42
25	37	42	47	35	40	45	31	36	41
26	39	44	49	37	42	47	32	37	43
27	41	46	51	39	44	49	33	39	45
28	43	48	53	41	46	51	33	40	48
29	45	50	55	43	48	53	36	42	47
30	47	51	56	44	49	54	36	43	49
31	48	53	58	46	51	56	38	44	50
32	50	55	60	48	53	58	37	45	53
33	51	56	61	49	54	59	41	46	51
34	53	58	63	51	56	61	40	47	53
35	54	59	64	52	57	62	41	48	54
36	56	61	65	53	58	63	39	48	57
37	57	62	67	55	60	65	45	49	53
38	59	63	68	56	61	66	45	49	54
39	60	65	70	57	62	67	45	50	54
40	61	66	71	58	63	68	46	50	55
	mm	mm	mm	mm	mm	mm	mm	mm	mm

Romero R, Athanassiadis AP, Sirtori M, Inati M. Fetal skeletal anomalies. In: Fleischer AC, Romero R, Manning FA, Jeanty P, James AE Jr, eds. The principles and practice of ultrasonography in obstetrics and gynecology, 4th ed. Norwalk, CT: Appleton & Lange, 1991:283.

TABLE 39–6. NORMAL VALUES FOR THE LEG (mm)

	TIBIA			FIBULA			FEMUR		
	PERCENTILE			PERCENTILE			PERCENTILE		
WEEK	5th	50th	95th	5th	50th	95th	5th	50th	95th
12	—	7	—	—	6	—	4	8	13
13	—	10	—	—	9	—	6	11	16
14	7	12	17	6	12	19	9	14	18
15	9	15	20	9	15	21	12	17	21
16	12	17	22	13	18	23	15	20	24
17	15	20	25	13	21	28	18	23	27
18	17	22	27	15	23	31	21	25	30
19	20	25	30	19	26	33	24	28	33
20	22	27	33	21	28	36	26	31	36
21	25	30	35	24	31	37	29	34	38
22	27	32	38	27	33	39	32	36	41
23	30	35	40	28	35	42	35	39	44
24	32	37	42	29	37	45	37	42	46
25	34	40	45	34	40	45	40	44	49
26	37	42	47	36	42	47	42	47	51
27	39	44	49	37	44	50	45	49	54
28	41	46	51	38	45	53	47	52	56
29	43	48	53	41	47	54	50	54	59
30	45	50	55	43	49	56	52	56	61
31	47	52	57	42	51	59	54	59	63
32	48	54	59	42	52	63	56	61	65
33	50	55	60	46	54	62	58	63	67
34	52	57	62	46	55	65	60	65	69
35	53	58	64	51	57	62	62	67	71
36	55	60	65	54	58	63	64	68	73
37	56	61	67	54	59	65	65	70	74
38	58	63	68	56	61	65	67	71	76
39	59	64	69	56	62	67	68	73	77
40	61	66	71	59	63	67	70	74	79
	mm	mm	mm	mm	mm	mm	mm	mm	mm

Romero R, Athanassiadis AP, Sirtori M, Inati M. Fetal skeletal anomalies. In: Fleischer AC, Romero R, Manning FA, Jeanty P, James AE Jr, eds. The principles and practice of ultrasonography in obstetrics and gynecology, 4th ed. Norwalk, CT: Appleton & Lange, 1991:284.

CLINICAL PRESENTATION

The challenge of the antenatal diagnosis of skeletal dysplasias generally presents itself in one of two ways: (1) a patient who has delivered an infant with a skeletal dysplasia and desires antenatal assessment of a subsequent pregnancy; or (2) the incidental finding of a shortened, bowed, or anomalous extremity during a routine sonographic examination. The task is easier when a particular phenotype is looked for in a patient at risk. The inability to obtain reliable information about skeletal mineralization and the involvement of other systems

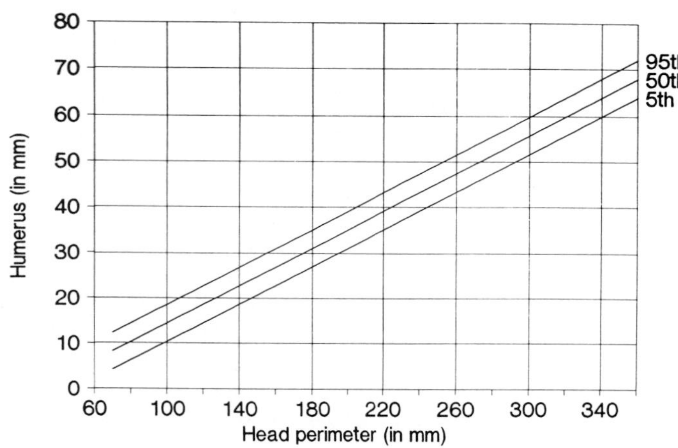

FIGURE 39–8. Relationship between the head perimeter and the humerus.

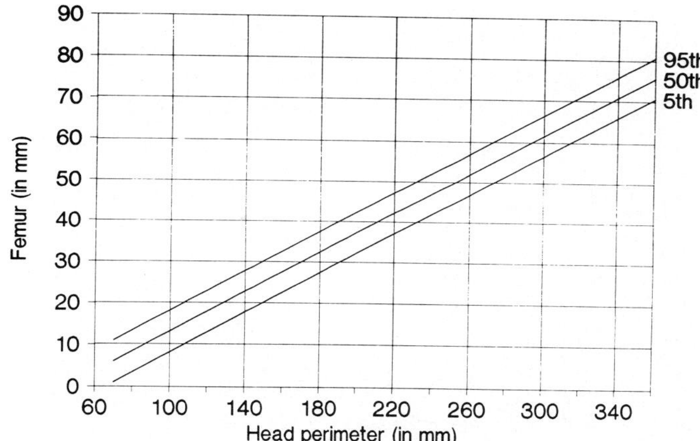

FIGURE 39–9. Relationship between the head perimeter and the femur.

(eg, skin) with sonography is a limiting factor in the establishment of an accurate diagnosis after the identification of an incidental finding. Another limitation is the paucity of information about the in utero natural history of these disorders.

Despite these difficulties and limitations, there are good medical reasons for attempting an accurate prenatal diagnosis of skeletal dysplasias. A number of these disorders are uniformly lethal, and a confident antenatal diagnosis would present the patient with options for the termination of the pregnancy. Table 39-7 lists such disorders. Other skeletal dysplasias are associated with mental retardation,[8] and this information is important in prenatal counseling. There is a group of disorders associated with thrombocytopenia. Vaginal delivery may expose these infants to the risk of intracranial hemorrhage.

APPROACH TO THE DIAGNOSIS OF SKELETAL DYSPLASIAS

Our approach to the diagnosis of skeletal dysplasias follows an organized plan of examination of the fetus, which is performed in the following manner:

1. *Evaluation of long bones.* All long bones should be measured in all extremities. Comparisons with other segments should be performed to establish whether the limb shortening is predominantly rhizomelic, mesomelic, or acromelic, or whether it involves all segments (Fig. 39-10). A detailed examination of each bone is necessary to exclude the absence or hypoplasia of individual bones (fibula, tibia, scapula, radius), which are frequently absent in certain conditions.[9–12]

   An attempt should be made to characterize the degree of mineralization. This can be assessed by examining the acoustic shadow behind the bone

TABLE 39–7. LETHAL SKELETAL DYSPLASIAS

Achondrogenesis
Thanatophoric dysplasia
Short-rib–polydactyly syndromes (types I, II, and III)
Fibrochondrogenesis
Atelosteogenesis
Homozygous achondroplasia
Osteogenesis imperfecta, perinatal type
Hypophosphatasia

Romero R, Athanassiadis AP, Sirtori M, Inati M. Fetal skeletal anomalies. In: Fleischer AC, Romero R, Manning FA, Jeanty P, James AE Jr, eds. The principles and practice of ultrasonography in obstetrics and gynecology. 4th ed. Norwalk, CT: Appleton & Lange, 1991:287.

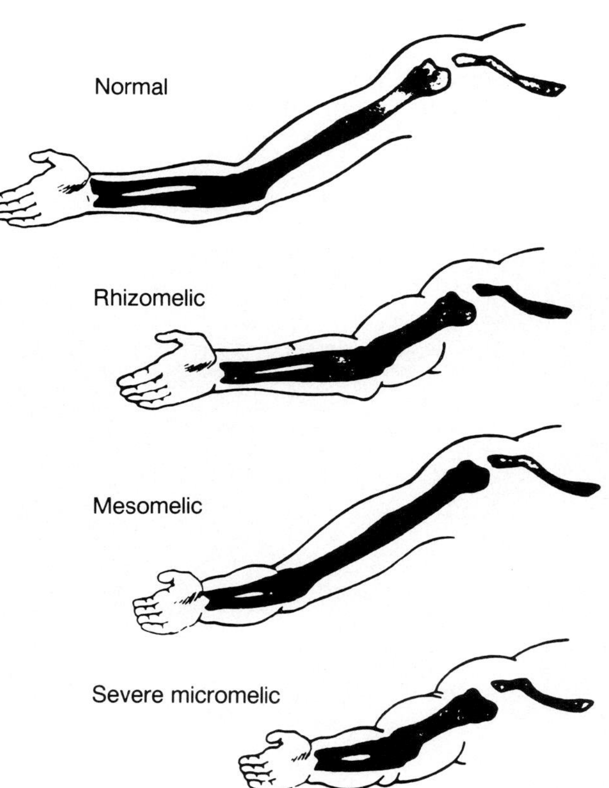

FIGURE 39–10. Varieties of short limb dysplasia according to the segment involved.

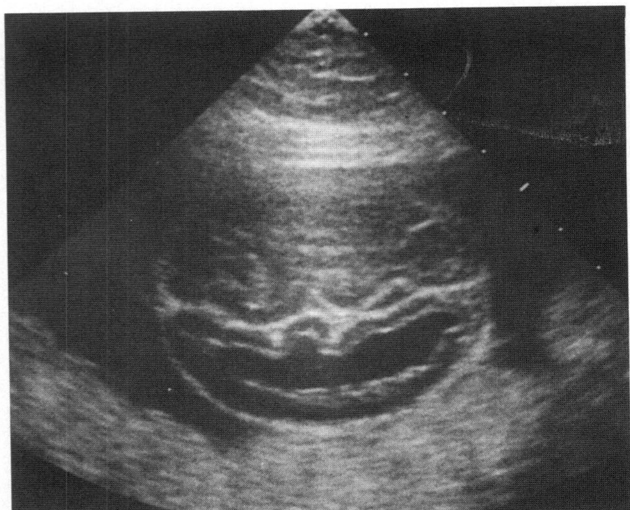

FIGURE 39–11. Demineralization of the skull in a case of congenital hypophosphatasia.

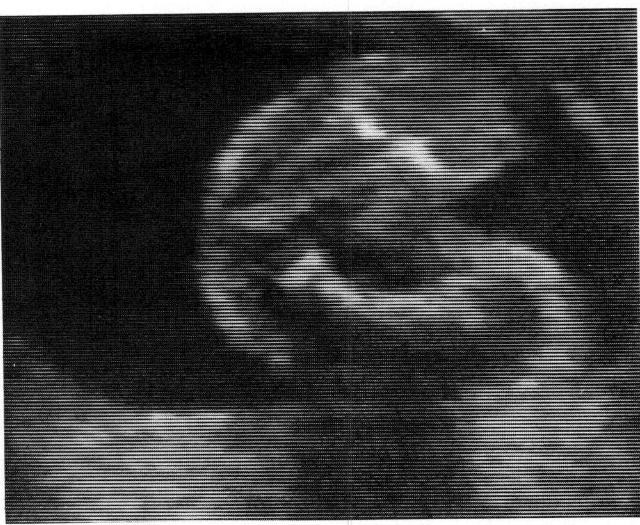

FIGURE 39–13. Shortening and bowing of the humerus with short but straight ulna and radius in a fetus with micromelia.

and the echogenicity of the bone itself. Signs of demineralization are the visualization of an unusually prominent falx and the absent or decreased echogenicity of the spine. It should be stressed that there are limitations in the sonographic evaluation of mineralization of long bones and that other structures, such as the skull, may be better suited for this assessment (Figs. 39-11 and 39-12). The degree of long-bone curvature should be examined. At present, there is no objective means of assessing this sign, and experience is the only means by which the operator can discern the boundary between normality and abnormality (Fig. 39-13). Campomelia (excessive bowing) is characteristic of certain disorders (eg, campomelic dysplasia). Finally, the possibility of fractures should also be considered, as they can be detected in some conditions (eg, osteogenesis imperfecta) (Fig. 39-14). The fractures may be extremely subtle or may lead to angulation and separation of the segments of the affected bone (Fig. 39-15).

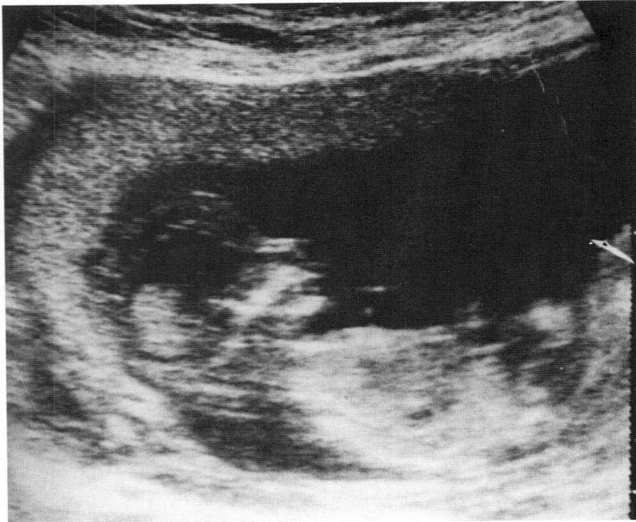

FIGURE 39–12. Sagittal scan of a fetus with severe demineralization of the calvarium.

2. *Evaluation of thoracic dimensions.* Several skeletal dysplasias are associated with a hypoplastic thorax. Such a finding is extremely important because chest restriction leads to pulmonary hypoplasia, a frequent cause of death in these conditions. The appropriateness of thoracic dimensions can be assessed by measuring the thoracic circumference at the level of the four-chamber view of the heart. The thoracic circumference can be measured or calculated using the following formula: thoracic circumference = (anteroposterior diameter + transverse diameter) × 1.57. The thoracic length is measured from the boundary between the neck and the chest to the diaphragm. Tables 39-8 and 39-9 illustrate nomograms used to evaluate the thoracic dimensions in fetuses with known gestational age. When gestational age is uncertain, age-independent ratios can be used. The thoracic-to-abdominal circumference ratio (normal value: 0.77–1.01) and the thoracic-to-head circumference ratio (normal value: 0.56–1.04) permit evaluation of the transverse thoracic dimensions.[13]

Evaluation of thoracic dimensions is a critical part of the work-up because the cause of death in most lethal skeletal dysplasias is pulmonary hypoplasia secondary to an underdeveloped rib cage (Fig. 39-16). Table 39-10 displays skeletal dys-

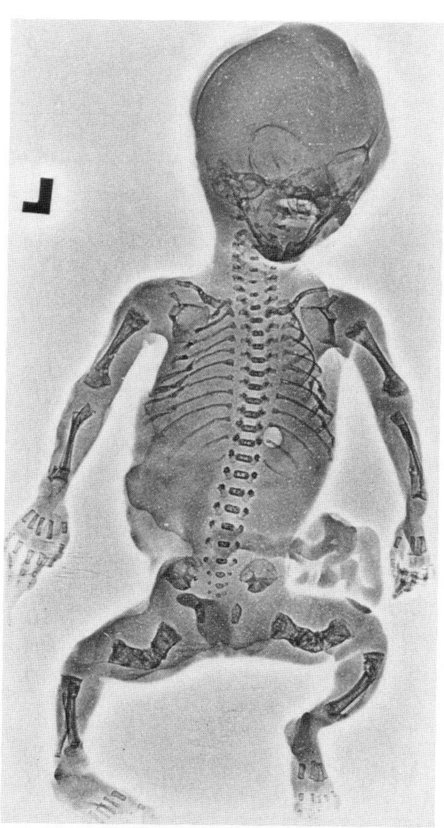

FIGURE 39–14. Osteogenesis imperfecta type II. Multiple fractures in long bones and ribs are present. Note the severe bowing and shortening of both femurs.

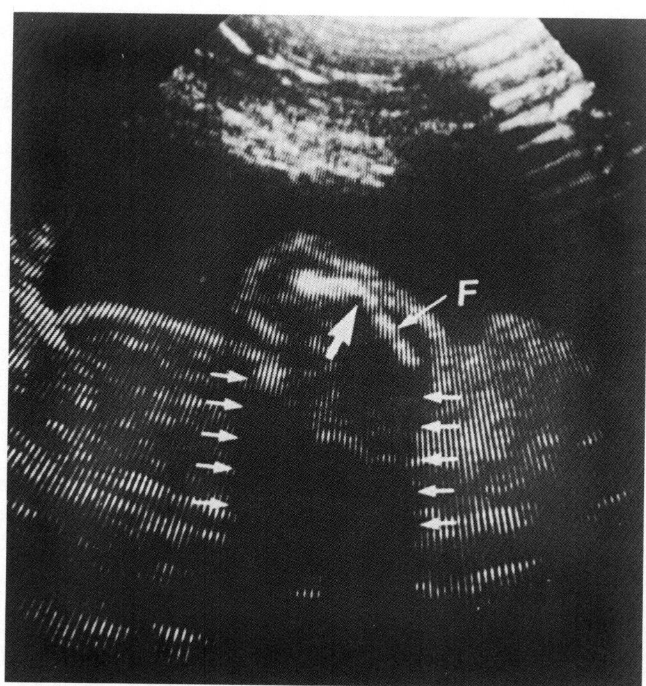

FIGURE 39–15. In utero fracture in a case of osteogenesis imperfecta. The large arrow corresponds to the fracture site. The small arrows outline the decreased shadowing cast by the bone. (F, femur.)

TABLE 39–8. FETAL THORACIC CIRCUMFERENCE MEASUREMENTS (in cm)

GESTATIONAL AGE (WK)	NO.	PREDICTIVE PERCENTILES								
		2.5	5	10	25	50	75	90	95	97.5
16	6	5.9	6.4	7.0	8.0	9.1	10.3	11.3	11.9	12.4
17	22	6.8	7.3	7.9	8.9	10.0	11.2	12.2	12.8	13.3
18	31	7.7	8.2	8.8	9.8	11.0	12.1	13.1	13.7	14.2
19	21	8.6	9.1	9.7	10.7	11.9	13.0	14.0	14.6	15.1
20	20	9.5	10.0	10.6	11.7	12.8	13.9	15.0	15.5	16.0
21	30	10.4	11.0	11.6	12.6	13.7	14.8	15.8	16.4	16.9
22	18	11.3	11.9	12.5	13.5	14.6	15.7	16.7	17.3	17.8
23	21	12.2	12.8	13.4	14.4	15.5	16.6	17.6	18.2	18.8
24	27	13.2	13.7	14.3	15.3	16.4	17.5	18.5	19.1	19.7
25	20	14.1	14.6	15.2	16.2	17.3	18.4	19.4	20.0	20.6
26	25	15.0	15.5	16.1	17.1	18.2	19.3	20.3	21.0	21.5
27	24	15.9	16.4	17.0	18.0	19.1	20.2	21.3	21.9	22.4
28	24	16.8	17.3	17.9	18.9	20.0	21.2	22.2	22.8	23.3
29	24	17.7	18.2	18.8	19.8	21.0	22.1	23.1	23.7	24.2
30	27	18.6	19.1	19.7	20.7	21.9	23.0	24.0	24.6	25.1
31	24	19.5	20.0	20.6	21.6	22.8	23.9	24.9	25.5	26.0
32	28	20.4	20.9	21.5	22.6	23.7	24.8	25.8	26.4	26.9
33	27	21.3	21.8	22.5	23.5	24.6	25.7	26.7	27.3	27.8
34	25	22.2	22.8	23.4	24.4	25.5	26.6	27.6	28.2	28.7
35	20	23.1	23.7	24.3	25.3	26.4	27.5	28.5	29.1	29.6
36	23	24.0	24.6	25.2	26.2	27.3	28.4	29.4	30.0	30.6
37	22	24.9	25.5	26.1	27.1	28.2	29.3	30.3	30.9	31.5
38	21	25.9	26.4	27.0	28.0	29.1	30.2	31.2	31.9	32.4
39	7	26.8	27.3	27.9	28.9	30.0	31.1	32.2	32.8	33.3
40	6	27.7	28.2	28.8	29.8	20.9	32.1	33.1	33.7	34.2

Chitkara U, Rosenberg J, Chervenak FA, et al. Prenatal sonographic assessment of the fetal thorax: normal values. Am J Obstet Gynecol 1987;156:1069.

TABLE 39–9. FETAL THORACIC LENGTH MEASUREMENTS (in cm)

GESTATIONAL AGE (WK)	NO.	PREDICTIVE PERCENTILES								
		2.5	5	10	25	50	75	90	95	97.5
16	6	0.9	1.1	1.3	1.6	2.0	2.4	2.8	3.0	3.2
17	22	1.1	1.3	1.5	1.8	2.2	2.6	3.0	3.2	3.4
18	31	1.3	1.4	1.7	2.0	2.4	2.8	3.2	3.4	3.6
19	21	1.4	1.6	1.8	2.2	2.7	3.0	3.4	3.6	3.8
20	20	1.6	1.8	2.0	2.4	2.8	3.2	3.6	3.8	4.0
21	30	1.8	2.0	2.2	2.6	3.0	3.4	3.7	4.0	4.1
22	18	2.0	2.2	2.4	2.8	3.2	3.6	3.9	4.1	4.3
23	21	2.2	2.4	2.6	3.0	3.4	3.8	4.1	4.3	4.5
24	27	2.4	2.6	2.8	3.1	3.5	3.9	4.3	4.5	4.7
25	20	2.6	2.8	3.0	3.3	3.7	4.1	4.5	4.7	4.9
26	25	2.8	2.9	3.2	3.5	3.9	4.3	4.7	4.9	5.1
27	24	2.9	3.1	3.3	3.7	4.1	4.5	4.9	5.1	5.3
28	24	3.1	3.3	3.5	3.9	4.3	4.7	5.0	5.4	5.4
29	24	3.3	3.5	3.7	4.1	4.5	4.9	5.2	5.5	5.6
30	27	3.5	3.7	3.9	4.3	4.7	5.1	5.4	5.6	5.8
31	24	3.7	3.9	4.1	4.5	4.9	5.3	5.6	5.8	6.0
32	28	3.9	4.1	4.3	4.6	5.0	5.4	5.8	6.0	6.2
33	27	4.1	4.3	4.5	4.8	5.2	5.6	6.0	6.2	6.4
34	25	4.2	4.4	4.7	5.0	5.4	5.8	6.2	6.4	6.6
35	20	4.4	4.6	4.8	5.2	5.6	6.0	6.4	6.6	6.8
36	23	4.6	4.8	5.0	5.4	5.8	6.2	6.5	6.8	7.0
37	22	4.8	5.0	5.2	5.6	6.0	6.4	6.7	7.0	7.1
38	21	5.0	5.2	5.4	5.8	6.2	6.6	6.9	7.1	7.3
39	7	5.2	5.4	5.6	6.0	6.4	6.8	7.1	7.3	7.5
40	6	5.4	5.6	5.8	6.1	6.5	6.9	7.3	7.5	7.7

Chitkara U, Rosenberg J, Chervenak FA, et al. Prenatal sonographic assessment of the fetal thorax: normal values. Am J Obstet Gynecol 1987;156:1069.

plasias associated with alteration of thoracic dimensions.

3. *Evaluation of hands and feet.* Hands and feet should be examined to exclude polydactyly, brachydactyly (Figs. 39-17 and 39-18), and extreme postural deformities such as those seen in diastrophic dysplasia. Table 39-11 shows a nomogram of the fetal foot size throughout gestation. Table 39-12 displays disorders associated with hand and foot deformities. Disproportion between hands and feet and the other parts of the extremity may also be a sign of a skeletal dysplasia. Figure 39-19 illustrates the relationship between femur length and foot length. The femur length–foot length ratio is nearly constant from the 14th to the 40th week. The mean is 0.99 (SD = 0.06). A ratio below 0.87 should be considered abnormal.[14] Although fetuses with skeletal dysplasias have been reported to have abnormally low ratios, more experience is required to test the diagnostic value of this method.[15] It is expected that a small proportion of normal fetuses may have an abnormal ratio. As in the case of other limb biometric parameters, large deviations from the lower limit of normal are likely to be significant.

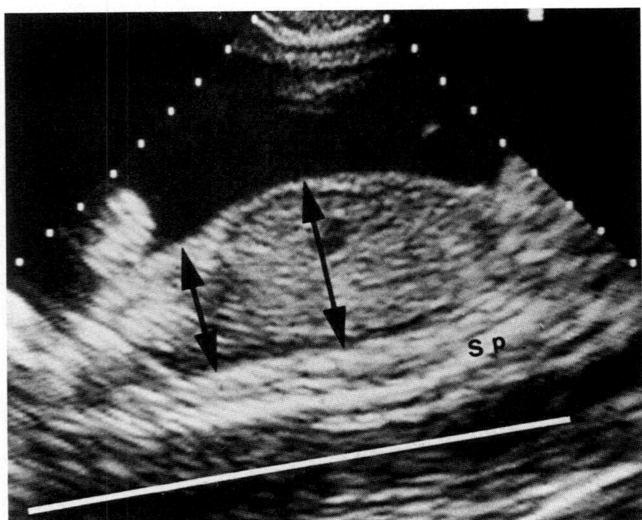

FIGURE 39–16. Longitudinal section of a fetus affected with thanatophoric dysplasia. Note the significant disproportion between the chest and the abdomen. (Sp, spine.) (Reproduced with permission from P Jeanty and R. Romero. Obstetrical ultrasound. New York: McGraw-Hill, 1983.)

4. *Evaluation of the fetal cranium.* Several skeletal dysplasias are associated with defects of membranous ossification and, therefore, affect skull bones. Orbits should be measured to exclude hypertelorism.[16,17] Other findings that should be searched for are micrognathia,[18] short upper lip, abnormally shaped ear,[19] frontal bossing (Fig. 39-20), and cloverleaf skull deformity (Fig. 39-21). Table 39-13 presents abnormalities of the skull and face in the different skeletal dysplasias.

TABLE 39–10. SKELETAL DYSPLASIAS ASSOCIATED WITH ALTERED THORACIC DIMENSIONS

Long, Narrow Thorax
Asphyxiating thoracic dysplasia (Jeune)
Chondroectodermal dysplasia (Ellis–van Creveld)
Metatropic dysplasia
Fibrochondrogenesis
Atelosteogenesis
Campomelic dysplasia
Jarcho-Levin syndrome
Achondrogenesis
Osteogenesis imperfecta congenita
Hypophosphatasia
Dyssegmental dysplasia
Cleidocranial dysplasia
Short Thorax
Osteogenesis imperfecta (type II)
Kniest dysplasia (metatropic dysplasia type II)
Pena-Shokeir syndrome
Hypoplastic Thorax
Short-rib–polydactyly syndrome (type I, type II)
Thanatophoric dysplasia
Cerebro-costo-mandibular syndrome
Cleidocranial dysostosis syndrome
Homozygous achondroplasia
Melnick-Needles syndrome (osteodysplasty)
Fibrochondrogenesis
Otopalatodigital syndrome type II

Romero R, Athanassiadis AP, Sirtori M, Inati M. Fetal skeletal anomalies. In: Fleischer AC, Romero R, Manning FA, Jeanty P, James AE Jr, eds. The principles and practice of ultrasonography in obstetrics and gynecology. 4th ed. Norwalk, CT: Appleton & Lange, 1991:292.

5. *Evaluation of the internal organs.* A detailed examination of the cardiovascular, genitourinary, gastrointestinal, and central nervous system organs should be performed in all fetuses with skeletal anomalies. Some syndromes present with specific abnormalities of the internal organs, thus helping in the differential diagnoses of these entities. For example, congenital heart disease is a prominent feature of Ellis-van Creveld syndrome and Holt-Oram syndrome.

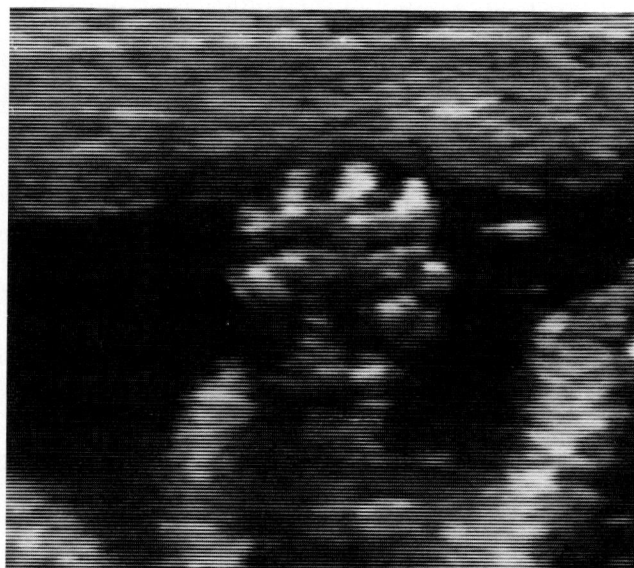

FIGURE 39–17. Brachydactyly in a fetus with severe micromelia.

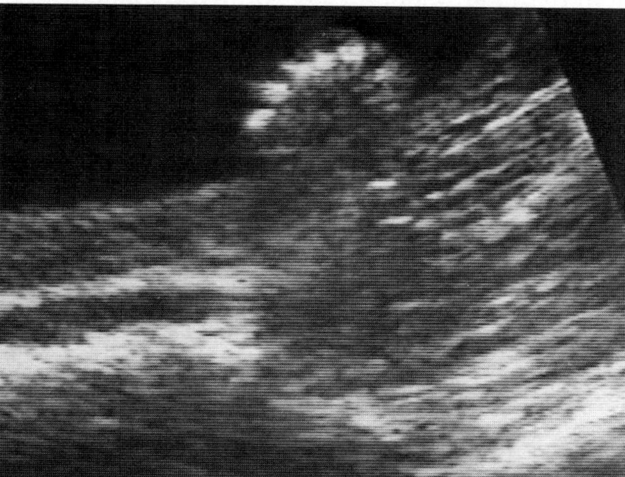

FIGURE 39–18. Transverse scan of a fetus with chondroectodermal dysplasia showing postaxial polydactyly. Six digits are easily identified.

TABLE 39–11. NOMOGRAM OF FETAL FOOT SIZE THROUGHOUT GESTATION (mm)

GESTATIONAL AGE WEEK	PERCENTILE 10th	50th	90th
14	16	18	21
15	16	19	22
16	18	22	28
17	19	22	22
18	19	27	30
19	25	30	39
20	33	33	33
21	24	24	24
22	25	36	40
23	41	41	40
24	46	46	46
25	40	47	53
26	40	47	54
27	45	50	56
28	51	53	55
29	49	54	58
30	61	61	61
31	51	56	52
32	54	57	62
33	59	59	59
34	60	65	71
35	71	71	71

Romero R, Athanassiadis AP, Sirtori M, Inati M. Fetal skeletal anomalies. In: Fleischer AC, Romero R, Manning FA, Jeanty P, James AE Jr, eds. The principles and practice of ultrasonography in obstetrics and gynecology. 4th ed. Norwalk, CT: Appleton & Lange, 1991:294.

Despite all efforts to establish an accurate prenatal diagnosis, a careful study of the newborn will be required in all instances. The evaluation should include a detailed physical examination performed by a geneticist or an individual with experience in the field of skeletal dysplasias and radiograms of the skeleton. The latter should include anterior, posterior, lateral, and Towne views of the skull and anteroposterior views of the spine and extremities, with separate films of hands and feet. Examination of the skeletal radiographs will permit precise diagnoses in the overwhelming majority of cases, since the classification of skeletal dysplasias is largely based on radiographic findings. In lethal skeletal dysplasias, histologic examination of the chondro-osseous tissue should be performed, as this information may help reach a specific diagnosis. Chromosomal studies should be included, as there is a specific group of constitutional bone disorders associated with cytogenetic abnormalities. Biochemical studies are helpful in rare instances (eg, hypophosphatasia). DNA restrictions and enzymatic activity assays should be considered in those cases in which the phenotype suggests a metabolic disorder such as a mucopolysaccharidosis. Although a full discussion of such disorders is beyond the scope of this text, they are well-known causes of constitutional bone diseases.

OSTEOCHONDRODYSPLASIAS

A growing number of skeletal dysplasias have been recognized in utero. A complete account of each disorder is beyond the scope of this chapter, and we refer the reader to texts on the subject for further details.[20] The following discussion presents only a few of the most common disorders relevant to prenatal diagnosis.

THANATOPHORIC DYSPLASIA, FIBROCHONDROGENESIS, ATELOSTEOGENESIS

Thanatophoric dysplasia is the most common lethal skeletal dysplasia in fetuses and neonates. It is characterized by extreme rhizomelia, a normal trunk length with a narrow thorax, and a large head with a prominent forehead. It occurs in 0.24 to 0.69 of 10,000 births.[1,2] Two subtypes have been identified: type 1, with typical bowed "telephone receiver" femurs (Fig. 39-22) and without cloverleaf skull; and type 2, with cloverleaf skull (see Fig. 39-21) and short, straight long bones.[21] However, mild cloverleaf skull has been described in type 1.[22] The differential diagnosis between the two depends on the radiographic findings and histology. There is no agreement about the pattern of inheritance of this condition. The majority of cases of thanatophoric dysplasia (all type 1 and most cases of type 2) are sporadic.[23] Some familial cases of type 2 have been reported.[24]

The prenatal sonographic findings depend on the specific variety. The association of cloverleaf skull and micromelia is specific for thanatophoric dysplasia. The other skeletal dysplasia associated with cloverleaf skull is campomelic syndrome. However, micromelia is not a feature of this condition. Cloverleaf skull may result from premature closure of the coronal and lambdoid sutures, defective development of the cranial base with secondary synostosis, or a primary developmental disorder of the brain with secondary deformation of the skull. Hydrocephaly and polyhydramnios are frequently seen. There is a relatively large calvarium with a prominent forehead (see Fig. 39-20), a saddle nose, and hypertelorism. Additional findings are short ribs, platyspondylia (see Fig. 39-4), and short and broad tubular bones in hands and feet. The differential diagnoses include short-rib–polydactyly syndrome, homozygous achondroplasia (both parents are affected), and asphyxiating thoracic dysplasia (slight shortening of long bones and normal vertebrae). On review of the radiologic findings of several cases of thanatophoric dysplasia, Horton and colleagues were able to discern a group of distinct entities characterized by severe platyspondylia.[25] These disorders include the Torrance, San Diego, Lutton, and Shiraz types of platyspondylic lethal osteochondrodysplasias. Differential diagnosis among these entities is based on histologic and radiologic characteristics.[5] Thanatophoric dysplasia is a uniformly

TABLE 39–12. SKELETAL DYSPLASIAS ASSOCIATED WITH POLYDACTYLY AND SYNDACTYLY

Postaxial Polydactyly
Chondroectodermal dysplasia
Short-rib–polydactyly syndrome (type I, type II)
Asphyxiating thoracic dysplasia
Otopalatodigital syndrome
Mesomelic dysplasia, Werner type (associated with absence of thumbs)
Preaxial Polydactyly
Chondroectodermal dysplasia
Short-rib–polydactyly syndrome, type II
Carpenter syndrome
Syndactyly
Poland syndrome
Acrocephalosyndactylies (Carpenter syndrome, Apert syndrome)
Otopalatodigital syndrome, type II
Mesomelic dysplasia, Werner type
TAR syndrome
Jarcho-Levin syndrome
Roberts syndrome
Brachydactyly
Mesomelic dysplasia, Robinow type
Otopalatodigital syndrome
Hitchhiker Thumbs
Diastrophic dysplasia
Clubfoot Deformity
Diastrophic dysplasia
Osteogenesis imperfecta
Kniest dysplasia
Spondyloepiphyseal congenita
Metatropic dysplasia
Mesomelic dysplasia Nievergelt type
Chondrodysplasia punctata
Larsen syndrome
Roberts syndrome
TAR syndrome
Pena-Shokeir syndrome

Romero R, Athanassiadis AP, Sirtori M, Inati M. Fetal skeletal anomalies. In: Fleischer AC, Romero R, Manning FA, Jeanty P, James AE Jr, eds. The principles and practice of ultrasonography in obstetrics and gynecology. 4th ed. Norwalk, CT: Appleton & Lange, 1991:294.

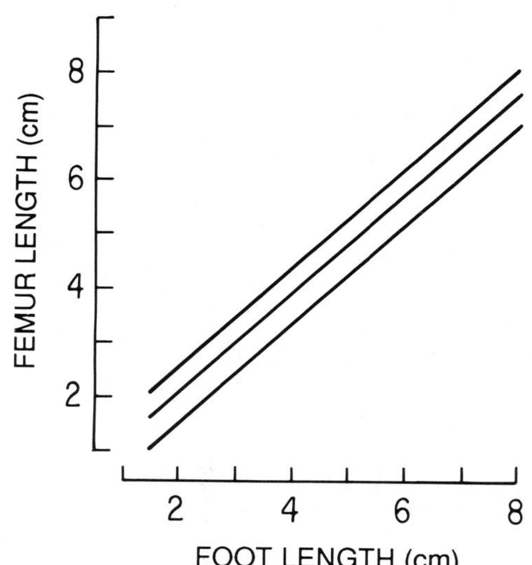

FIGURE 39–19. Relationship between the femur length and the foot length.

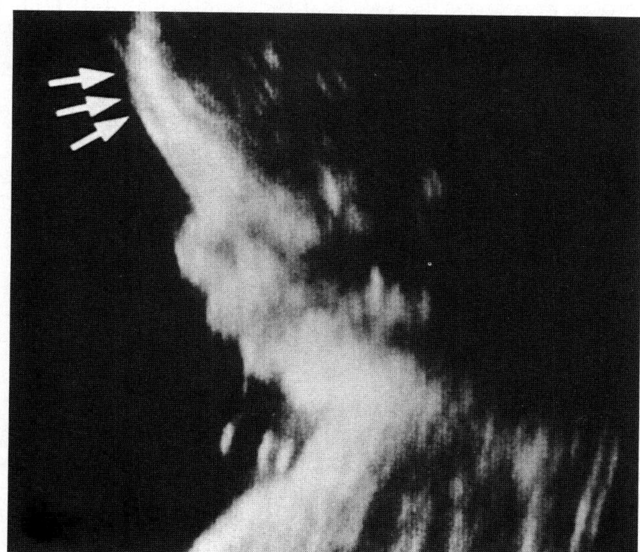

FIGURE 39–20. Frontal bossing in a sagittal scan. The arrows point to the prominent frontal bone.

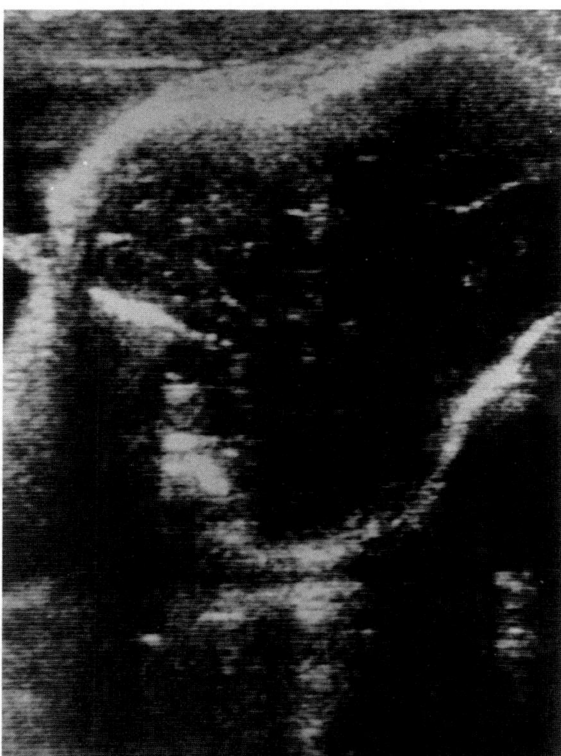

FIGURE 39–21. Coronal scan of the head of a fetus with thanatophoric dysplasia and cloverleaf skull.

lethal disorder, although survival of several months has been reported in some isolated cases.[26,27] Prenatal diagnosis has been documented on several occasions.[28–35]

Fibrochondrogenesis and atelosteogenesis have a clinical presentation similar to that of thanatophoric dysplasia. A differential diagnosis between these disorders in utero is extremely difficult. Fibrochondrogenesis is a lethal chondrodysplasia inherited with an autosomal recessive pattern and characterized by micromelia with significant metaphyseal flaring, normal head size, undermineralized skull, platyspondylia, clefting of the vertebral bodies, and narrow and bell-shaped thorax.[36,37] Metaphyseal flaring is not a feature of thanatophoric dysplasia.[38] Other conditions to be considered in the differential diagnosis include metatropic dysplasia and Kniest dysplasia.

Atelosteogenesis is also a lethal chondrodysplasia characterized by severe micromelia (with hypoplasia of the distal segments of the humerus and femur), bowing of long bones, narrow chest with short ribs, coronal (see Fig. 39-7) and sagittal vertebral clefts, and dislocation at the level of the elbow and knee. Clubfoot deformities may also be present.[39] Three subtypes of atelosteogenesis have been described based on radiologic and pathologic findings.[40–46] Atelosteogenesis types I and III are sporadic; type II is inherited with an autosomal recessive pattern (see Fig. 39-1). Differential diagnosis includes diastrophic dysplasia and de la Chapelle dysplasia.[47,48] Three cases of a lethal dysplasia termed boomerang syndrome ("boomerang-like tibia") may actually represent the same disorder as atelosteogenesis type I.[49] Fibrochondrogenesis and atelosteogenesis are extremely rare, and only a few cases of each have been reported.

TABLE 39–13. SKELETAL DYSPLASIAS ASSOCIATED WITH SKULL AND FACE DEFORMITIES

Large Head
Achondroplasia
Achondrogenesis
Thanatophoric dysplasia
Osteogenesis imperfecta
Cleidocranial dysplasia
Hypophosphatasia
Campomelic dysplasia
Short-rib–polydactyly syndrome, type III
Robinow mesomelic dysplasia
Otopalatodigital syndrome
Cloverleaf Skull
Thanatophoric dysplasia (rare variant)
Campomelic syndrome
Other Craniostenosis
Apert syndrome
Carpenter syndrome
Hypophosphatasia
Congenital Cataracts
Chondrodysplasia punctata
Cleft Palate
Asphyxiating thoracic dysplasia
Kniest dysplasia
Diastrophic dysplasia
Spondyloepiphyseal dysplasia
Campomelic syndrome
Jarcho-Levin syndrome
Ellis-van Creveld syndrome
Short-rib–polydactyly syndrome, type II
Metatropic dysplasia
Dyssegmental dysplasia
Otopalatodigital syndrome, type II
Roberts syndrome
Short Upper Lip
Chondroectodermal dysplasia
Micrognathia
Camptomelic dysplasia
Diastrophic dysplasia
Weissenbacher-Zweymuller syndrome
Oto-palato-digital syndrome
Pena-Shokeir syndrome
TAR syndrome
Langer syndrome

Romero R, Athanassiadis AP, Sirtori M, Inati M. Fetal skeletal anomalies. In: Fleischer AC, Romero R, Manning FA, Jeanty P, James AE Jr, eds. The principles and practice of ultrasonography in obstetrics and gynecology. 4th ed. Norwalk, CT: Appleton & Lange, 1991:296.

ACHONDROGENESIS

Achondrogenesis, or anosteogenesis, is a lethal chondrodystrophy characterized by extreme micromelia, short trunk, and macrocrania. The birth prevalence is

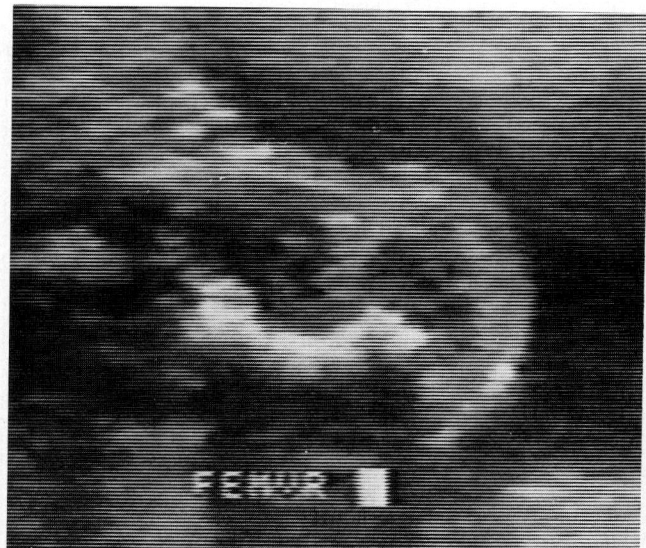

FIGURE 39–22. Bowed and short femur with the typical "telephone receiver" appearance.

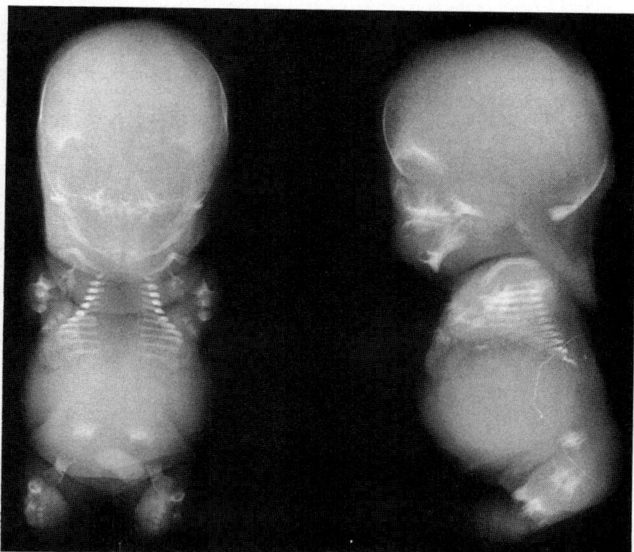

FIGURE 39–23. Frontal and lateral views in a case of achondrogenesis type II. There is no mineralization of the spine and ischial bones. The thorax is bell shaped, with short and straight ribs and no fractures. Long bones are short, with metaphyseal flaring and cupping.

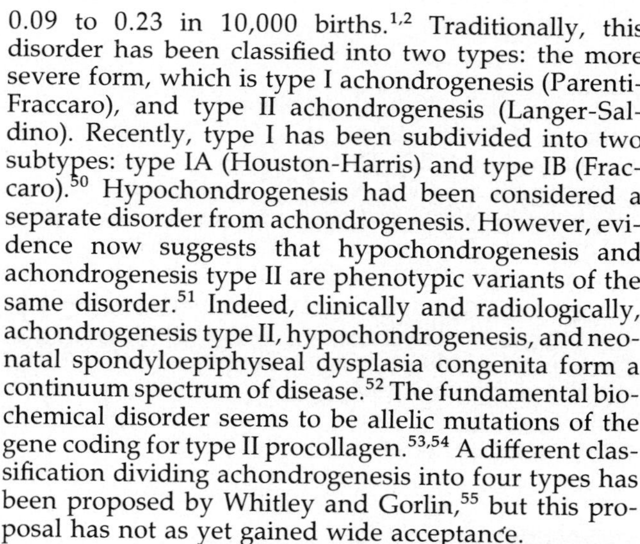

0.09 to 0.23 in 10,000 births.[1,2] Traditionally, this disorder has been classified into two types: the more severe form, which is type I achondrogenesis (Parenti-Fraccaro), and type II achondrogenesis (Langer-Saldino). Recently, type I has been subdivided into two subtypes: type IA (Houston-Harris) and type IB (Fraccaro).[50] Hypochondrogenesis had been considered a separate disorder from achondrogenesis. However, evidence now suggests that hypochondrogenesis and achondrogenesis type II are phenotypic variants of the same disorder.[51] Indeed, clinically and radiologically, achondrogenesis type II, hypochondrogenesis, and neonatal spondyloepiphyseal dysplasia congenita form a continuum spectrum of disease.[52] The fundamental biochemical disorder seems to be allelic mutations of the gene coding for type II procollagen.[53,54] A different classification dividing achondrogenesis into four types has been proposed by Whitley and Gorlin,[55] but this proposal has not as yet gained wide acceptance.

Type IA achondrogenesis (Houston-Harris) is characterized by micromelia, lack of ossification of vertebral bodies but ossification of the pedicles in the cervical and upper thoracic region, and short ribs with multiple fractures. The calvarium is demineralized. Type IB (Fraccaro) is similar to type IA, but the calvarium is ossified, and fractured ribs are not seen. Although the vertebral bodies are minimally ossified or not at all ossified, the pedicles show some ossification. Type II achondrogenesis is characterized by micromelia, lack of mineralization of all or many vertebral bodies, sacrum and ischion, enlarged calvarium with normal ossification, variable shortening of the ribs, and absence of fractures (Fig. 39-23).[56] Table 39-14 illustrates the characteristics of the different types of achondrogenesis. An association between cytic hygromas and achondrogenesis has been reported in a fetus with normal chromosomal constitution.[57]

Prenatal diagnosis should be suspected on the basis of micromelia, lack of vertebral ossification, and a large head with various degrees of ossification of calvarium.[58–64] Polyhydramnios and hydrops have been associated with achondrogenesis. However, sonographic examinations of affected fetuses do not demonstrate fluid accumulation in body cavities. The hydropic appearance of these fetuses and neonates is probably attributable to redundancy of soft-tissue mass over a limited skeletal frame. Achondrogenesis type IA and type IB is inherited with an autosomal recessive pattern, whereas most cases of achondrogenesis type II and hypochondrogenesis have been sporadic (new autosomal dominant mutations). Some severe cases of type II achondrogenesis follow an autosomal recessive pattern.[56]

ACHONDROPLASIA

The most common nonlethal skeletal dysplasia is achondroplasia. It is characterized by rhizomelic shortening, limb bowing, lordotic spine, and enlarged head. It is inherited with an autosomal dominant pattern, and its prevalence is one out of 66,000.[1] This is probably an overestimation of the real incidence because of incorrect overdiagnosis of this entity in the past. Advanced paternal age is a risk factor for achondroplasia. This disease is the result of anomalous growth of cartilage,

TABLE 39–14. RADIOLOGIC DIFFERENCES BETWEEN ACHONDROGENESIS, TYPE I (A–B), TYPE II, AND HYPOCHONDROGENESIS

	TYPE IA (HOUSTON-HARRIS)	TYPE IB (FRACCARO)	TYPE II (LANGER-SALDINO)	HYPOCHONDROGENESIS
Skull	Membranous calvarium	All parts of ossified skull well seen	Normal ossification	Normal ossification
Long Bones	Extremely shortened with metaphyseal cupping and spurs. "Rectangular bones"	Arms and legs shorter than type IA with minimal ossification; abundant metaphyseal spiking or spurring in lower leg bones. "Square or stellate bones"	Short and bowed with metaphyseal flaring and cupping. "Mushroom stem bones"	Less bowed and shortened with irregular or smooth metaphyses
Spine	Vertebral bodies unossified, with partly ossified pedicles	Vertebral bodies minimally or not ossified, pedicles ossified	Variable pattern of ossified or unossified vertebral bodies and pedicles	Thoracic and upper lumbar vertebral bodies ossified but still platyspondylic. Cervical and lower lumbar bodies unossified
Pelvis	Poorly formed and ossified, with crenated iliac bones. Ischial bones poorly ossified, pubic bones unossified	Iliac bones same aspect as in type IA. Ischial and pubic bones unossified	Halberdlike iliac bones with unossified ischial and pubic bones	Near normally developed iliac bones with partial ossification of ischial bones and unossified pubic bones
Thorax	Short and barrel-shaped. Short ribs with cupped metaphyses and multiple fractures	Same as in type IA with unfractured ribs	Short and barrel- or bell-shaped with short unfractured ribs	Near normal but shallow cage with short unfractured ribs

Van der Harten HJ, Brons JTJ, Dijkstra PF, et al. Achondrogenesis-hypochondrogenesis: the spectrum of chondrogenesis imperfecta: a radiological, ultrasonographic, and histopathologic study of 23 cases. Pediatr Pathol 1988;8:571.

followed by abnormal endochondral ossification, which is responsible for the shortness of long bones. The bones of the hands and feet are short (brachydactyly). The head is large; a flattened nasal bridge, frontal bossing, and broad mandible are frequent features. The problems in the prenatal diagnosis of this condition have been discussed in detail by Kurtz and colleagues.[65] The major difficulty in the antenatal diagnosis is that the long-bone growth in this disease is not clearly appreciated in most cases until the third trimester of pregnancy. Therefore, it is usually not possible to detect this disorder in time to allow for pregnancy termination.[66,67] Heterozygous achondroplasia is compatible with a normal life and intellectual development. The disease is lethal in the homozygous state. A 37-month survivor has been reported.[68] The radiologic characteristics of homozygous achondroplasia lie between those of thanatophoric dysplasia and heterozygous achondroplasia.

Hypochondroplasia is a disorder that resembles achondroplasia.[69,70] The differential diagnosis between these two conditions is based on the sparing of the head and the lack of tibial bowing in hypochondroplasia. Although this condition is generally first detected during childhood, prenatal diagnosis in a patient at risk has been made at 22 weeks.[71] Hypochondroplasia and achondroplasia are probably allelic diseases.[72]

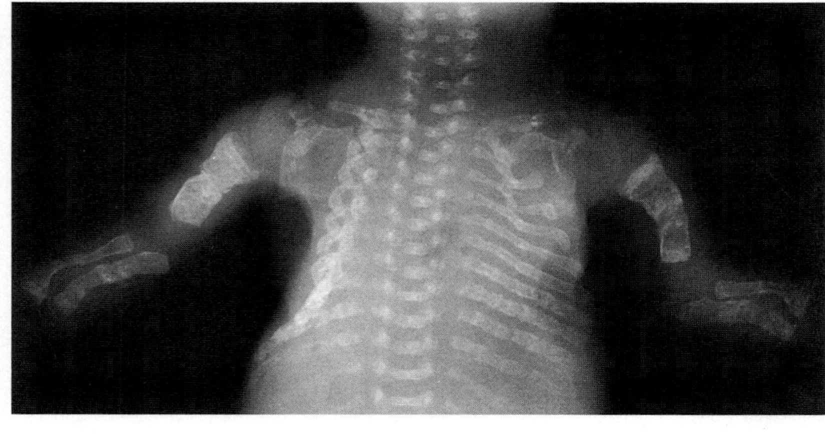

FIGURE 39–24. Osteogenesis imperfecta type IIA. Multiple skeletal fractures are present. Note the contiguous beading of the ribs and other long bones. The spine shows platyspondyly.

OSTEOGENESIS IMPERFECTA AND HYPOPHOSPHATASIA

Osteogenesis imperfecta and hypophosphatasia are discussed together because they are characterized by significant skeletal demineralization.

The term "osteogenesis imperfecta"(OI) was introduced over a century ago to describe a newborn with extremely brittle bones (Fig. 39-24). Currently, the term refers to a heterogeneous group of disorders caused in most cases by mutations in one or two structural genes for type I procollagen.[73] The prevalence of OI is 0.18 per 10,000 births.[1,2]

The most popular classification is that proposed by Sillence and colleagues.[74] In type I (autosomal dominant), patients have bone fragility, blue sclera (all ages), and hearing loss. There is osteoporosis and a normal calvarium; fractures range from none to multiple. Type II (new dominant mutations; less than 5% autosomal recessive) is also known as the perinatal variety and is uniformly lethal. There is almost no ossification of the skull; beaded ribs; shortened, crumpled long bones; and multiple fractures in utero (Fig. 39-25). The thorax is short but not narrow. Type II is subclassified into three subtypes—IIA, IIB, and IIC—according to radiologic criteria.[75] Type III (autosomal recessive, rare) is a nonlethal variety characterized by blue sclera and multiple fractures present at birth. The sclera becomes white with time. The membranous skull is severely deossified and the long bones are mildly shortened but with marked angulations. Type IIB and type III OI are difficult to distinguish and may represent different degrees of severity of the same disorder.[76,77] Type IV (autosomal dominant) is the mildest form. Long bones and sclera are normal. There is mild to moderate osseous fragility, and 25% of the newborns have fractures. There is significant heterogeneity in the expression of the disease even within the same family.

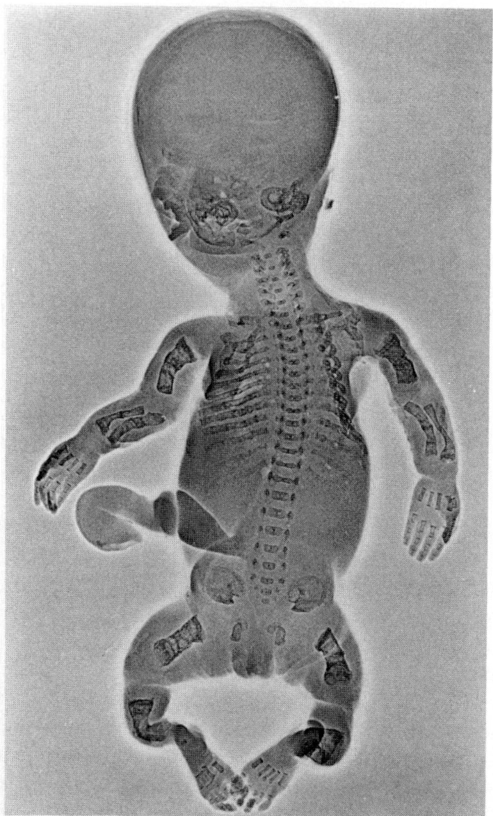

FIGURE 39–25. Xerogram of the fetus shown in Figure 39-23. There is extreme osteopenia of the cranial vault. Note the severe angulation of the bones in the lower leg.

The natural history of OI in utero is quite variable. In some cases fractures and limb shortening can be observed in the early second trimester; in other cases abnormalities are not detectable until the third trimester. Type IIA OI has been diagnosed as early as 15 weeks.[78] It seems that prenatal diagnosis of OI types IIB, IIC, and III may require a longer observation period because of the later onset of the disease.[79,80]

The prognosis for types I and IV is much better than that for types II and III. Antenatal diagnosis of OI type II has been reported several times.[81–84] Type I OI and type III OI diagnoses have also been reported.[78–80,85,86] Linkage analysis has been used effectively for prenatal diagnosis.[87]

Hypophosphatasia is a group of disorders characterized by demineralization of bones and low alkaline phosphatase in serum and other tissues. Alkaline phosphatase acts on pyrophosphate and other phosphate esters, leading to the accumulation of inorganic phosphates that are critical for the formation of bone crystals. Bone fragility is thought to be the result of deficient generation of bone crystals.

Hypophosphatasia is a condition that has been subdivided into three clinical types according to the age of onset: congenital-infantile, childhood, and adult. The congenital-infantile and childhood varieties have an autosomal recessive pattern of inheritance, whereas the adult form is autosomal dominant.[23] The congenital (neonatal) form is associated with early neonatal death or stillbirth.

Fetuses with congenital hypophosphatasia have generalized demineralization of the skeleton, with shortening and bowing of tubular bones. Multiple fractures are present. The marked demineralization of the cranial vault results in deformation of the skull after external compression (Fig. 39-26). This sonographic sign is also present in some cases of osteogenesis imperfecta type II and achondrogenesis type IA. Prenatal diagnosis of this condition has been reported with ultrasound[87,88] and by assaying alkaline phosphatase in tissue obtained by chorionic villous sampling[89] and alkaline phosphatase in amniotic fluid cell culture. Alkaline phosphatase measurement in amniotic fluid is not a reliable means of making a diagnosis of hypophosphatasia because most of the alkaline phosphatase in amniotic fluid is of intestinal origin.[90,91] The involved enzymes in hypophosphatasia are bone and liver alkaline phosphatases.

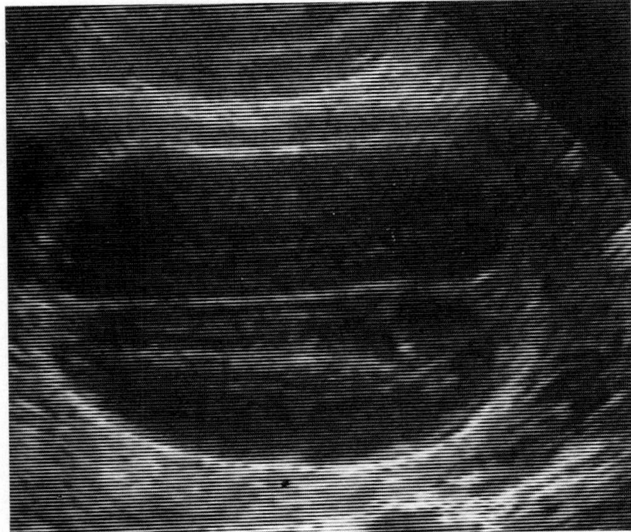

FIGURE 39–26. Deformation of the cranial vault after compression of the maternal abdomen with the transducer. No ossification of the calvarium was noted in postmortem radiographs.

These isoenzymes contribute only 16% of the total amniotic fluid enzymatic activity.[92]

SKELETAL DYSPLASIAS CHARACTERIZED BY A HYPOPLASTIC THORAX

The dysplastic process involves the ribs and other bones of the rib cages in many skeletal dysplasias. A reduction in thoracic dimensions leads to restriction of lung growth and, consequently, pulmonary hypoplasia. Lung hypoplasia is the main cause of death in lethal skeletal dysplasias. There is a specific group of dysplasias in which thoracic hypoplasia is a cardinal feature. These include asphyxiating thoracic dysplasia, Ellis-van Creveld syndrome, short-rib–polydactyly syndrome, and campomelic syndrome. Table 39-13 illustrates the criteria for the differential diagnoses of the first three of these conditions. Other disorders presenting with altered thoracic dimensions are thanatophoric dysplasia, atelosteogenesis, fibrochondrogenesis, achondrogenesis, and Jarcho-Levin syndrome (Fig. 39-27).[93]

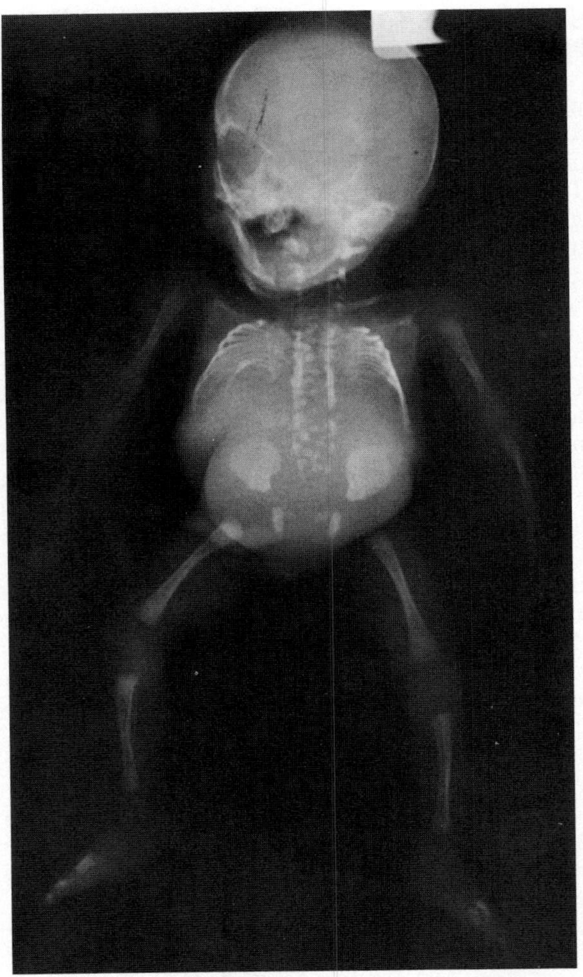

FIGURE 39–27. Jarcho-Levin syndrome. There is dramatic spinal shortening with disorganization of the vertebral bodies, a characteristic chest deformity ("crablike appearance" with posterior fusion and anterior flaring of the ribs), and unaffected long bones.

Asphyxiating Thoracic Dysplasia

Asphyxiating thoracic dysplasia, known as Jeune syndrome, is rare. Its prevalence is 0.14 in 10,000 births, and it is inherited in an autosomal recessive pattern.[1] It is characterized by a narrow and "bell-shaped" thorax, with short, horizontal ribs. Long bones are normal or mildly shortened. Polydactyly and cleft lip and/or palate can occur in association. The presence of a proximal femoral ossification center at birth is characteristic.[94] Asphyxiating thoracic dysplasia has a wide spectrum of clinical manifestations varying from lethal to mild forms; long-term survivors have been reported.[95,96] The clinical course of individuals surviving the neonatal period is complicated by respiratory distress of varying severity, nephropathy, and hepatic and pancreatic problems. Prenatal diagnosis has been reported.[97–100]

Short-Rib–Polydactyly Syndromes

Short-rib–polydactyly syndromes are a group of disorders characterized by micromelia, constricted thorax, and postaxial polydactyly (Fig. 39-28). Traditionally, three different types have been recognized (Saldino-Noonan, Majewski, and Naumoff). These conditions have been identified prenatally (Fig. 39-29).[101,102] Table 39-15 illustrates the differential diagnosis and features

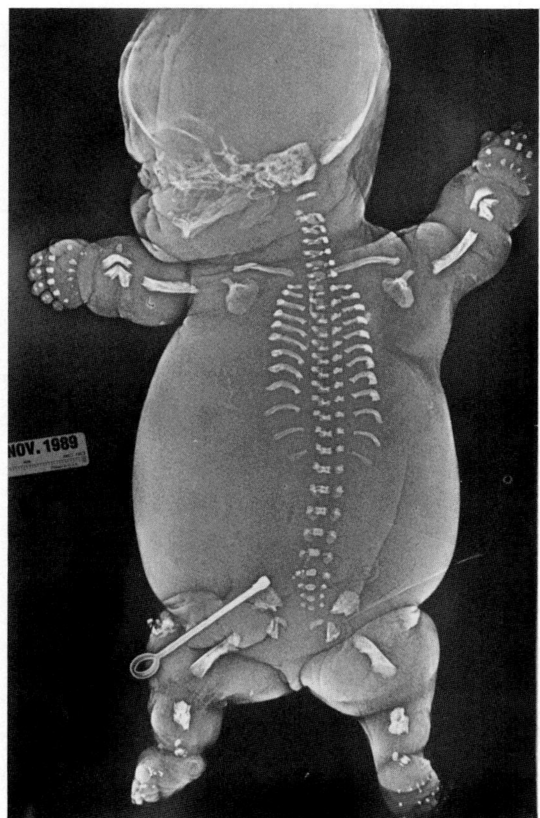

FIGURE 39–28. Short rib polydactyly syndrome. There is severe shortening of all long bones, very short and horizontal ribs, and postaxial polydactyly in all four extremities. Note the angulation of the bones in the forearm.

of these conditions. Recently, some authorities have expanded the definition of short-rib–polydactyly syndrome to encompass at least seven disorders, including the three previously mentioned entities plus the Yang, Le Marec, and Beemer varieties, and asphyxiating thoracic dysplasia.[5] Spranger and Maroteaux have indicated that the absence of polydactyly does not exclude the diagnosis of this entity.[5]

Chondroectodermal Dysplasia

Chondroectodermal dysplasia, also known as Ellis-van Creveld syndrome, is inherited with an autosomal recessive pattern. There is a high incidence in Amish communities.[103] It is characterized by acromesomelia with normal spine and skull, postaxial polydactyly (Figs. 39-30 and 39-31), long and narrow thorax with short ribs (Fig. 39-32), and congenital heart disease (60% of the cases). Polydactyly is a constant finding. The supernumerary digit usually has well-formed metacarpal and phalangeal bones. One third of affected individuals die in the postnatal period because of cardiopulmonary disease. Survivors who reach adulthood present with short stature but normal intelligence.[104] Prenatal diagnosis has been reported.[105–107]

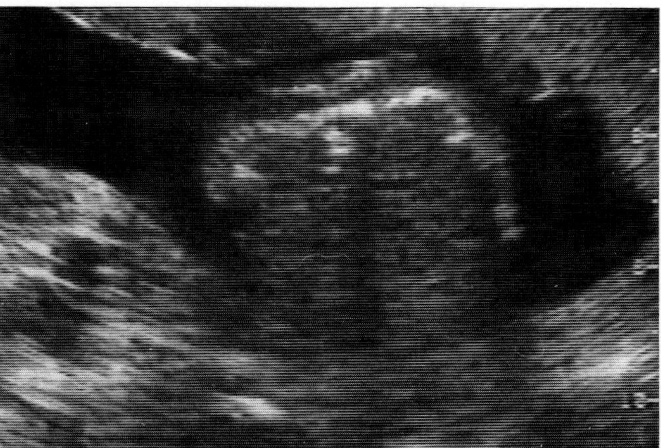

FIGURE 39–29. Transverse scan of the fetus shown in Figure 39–27. Note the severe shortening of the ribs.

Campomelic Dysplasia

Campomelic dysplasia is characterized by bowing of the long bones of the lower extremities, an enlarged and elongated skull with a peculiar small facies, hypoplastic scapulae, and several associated anomalies, such as cleft palate, micrognathia, hydrocephalus, hydronephrosis, and congenital heart defects. Campomelic syndrome has a prevalence of 0.05 in 10,000 births.[1] The most important feature is bowing of femur and tibia; other tubular bones are normal in length. The thorax is narrow and can be "bell-shaped." Cervical vertebrae are hypoplastic and poorly ossified.[108] Sporadic cases as well as some with an autosomal recessive pattern of inheritance have been described. There are two "short-bone varieties" of campomelic dysplasia representing distinct syndromes: the normocephalic form is known as kyphomelic dysplasia, and the craniostenotic type appears to be identical to the Antley-Bixler syndrome. Differential diagnoses include OI, thanatophoric dysplasia, and hypophosphatasia. Antenatal diagnosis of campomelic dysplasia has been reported in patients at risk.[109–112] The condition is frequently lethal in infancy, but some survivors have been reported.[113–114]

Diastrophic Dysplasia

Diastrophic dysplasia is characterized by micromelia, clubfoot, hand deformities, multiple joint flexion contractures, and scoliosis. This disorder is inherited as an autosomal recessive trait. Because of phenotypic variability, the diagnosis may be difficult at birth, and milder cases are diagnosed later.[115] The clinical features include rhizomelic-type micromelia, contractures, hand deformities with abducted position of the thumbs ("hitchhiker thumb"), and severe talipes equinovarus. The head is normal, but micrognathia and cleft palate may be associated. This dysplasia is a generalized disorder of cartilage with destruction of the cartilage matrix with formation of fibrous scar tissue and subse-

TABLE 39–15. DISORDERS WITH THORACIC DYSPLASIA AND POLYDACTYLY

	ASPHYXIATING THORACIC DYSPLASIA (JEUNE)	CHONDROECTODERMAL DYSPLASIA (ELLIS–VAN CREVELD)	SHORT-RIB–POLYDACTYLY SYNDROME, TYPE I (SALDINO-NOONAN)	SHORT-RIB–POLYDACTYLY SYNDROME, TYPE II (MAJEWSKI)	SHORT-RIB SYNDROME, TYPE III (DAVIDOFF)
Relative prevalence	Common	Uncommon	Common	Extremely rare	Rare
Clinical features					
Thoracic constriction	++	+	+++	+++	+++
Polydactyly	+	++	++	++	++
Limb shortening	+	+	+++	+	++
Congenital heart disease	–	++	++	++	–
Other abnormalities	Renal disease	Extodermal dysplasia	Genitourinary and gastrointestinal anomalies	Cleft lip and palate	Renal abnormality
Radiographic features					
Tubular bone shortening	+	+	+++	++	+++
Distinct features in femora	–	–	Pointed ends	–	Marginal spurs
Short, horizontal ribs	++	++	+++	+++	+++
Vertical shortening of ilia and flat acetabula	++	++	++	–	++
Defective ossification of vertebral bodies	–	–	++	–	+
Shortening of skull base	–	–	–	–	+

Cremin BJ, Beighton P. Bone dysplasias of infancy: a radiological atlas. Berlin: Spring-Verlag, 1978.
+, not common; ++, common; +++, most common; –, absent.

quent ossification. The latter process is responsible for the contractures.

The prenatal diagnosis of diastrophic dysplasia has been made in patients at risk,[116–119] based on severe shortening and bowing of all long bones. This disorder has a wide spectrum, and some cases may not be diagnosable in utero. This disease is not lethal, and intellectual development is unaffected. However, death in the neonatal period[120] and mental retardation have been reported in some patients. Differential diagnoses include arthrogryposis multiple congenita, atelosteogenesis type II, and pseudodiastrophic dysplasia. Pseudodiastrophic dysplasia has a similar presentation as diastrophic dysplasia[121] and is inherited with an autosomal recessive pattern.[23] Histologic examination is required for a differential diagnosis. The distinctive morphologic abnormalities of the growth plate noted in diastrophic dysplasia have not been observed in pseudodiastrophic dysplasia.[5]

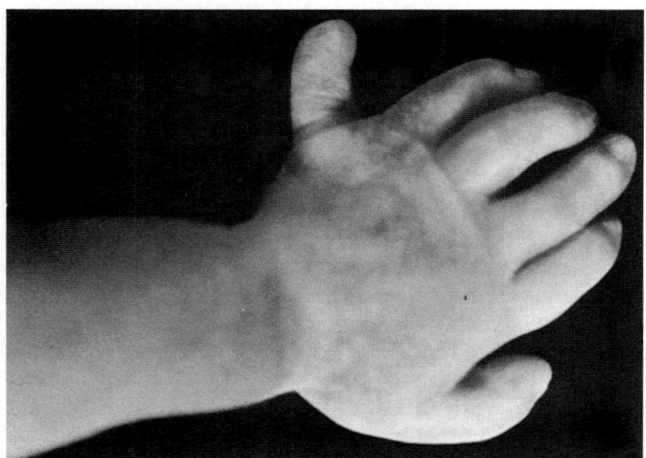

FIGURE 39–30. Postaxial polydactyly in a fetus with Ellis–van Creveld syndrome.

Kniest Syndrome

Kniest syndrome is an autosomal dominant disorder characterized by involvement of the spine (platyspondylia and coronal clefts) and the tubular bones (shortened and metaphyseal flaring), with a broad and short thorax.[122] There is a wide spectrum of disease.[123] Most commonly, the disorder is compatible with life. However, lethality in the neonatal period has been reported.[5,124] Abnormalities of type 2 collagen may be involved in the pathogenesis of the disease.[125] The term "Kniest-like disorders" is used to refer to a group of conditions that share histologic and radiologic characteristics with Kniest syndrome but differ in terms of clinical presentation and inheritance.[94]

Dyssegmental dysplasia is another entity related to Kniest dysplasia.[126] Two distinct types of dyssegmental dysplasia have been recognized: the mild, Rolland-Desbuquois form and the lethal Silverman-Handmaker.[128] The latter is characterized by anarchic ossifi-

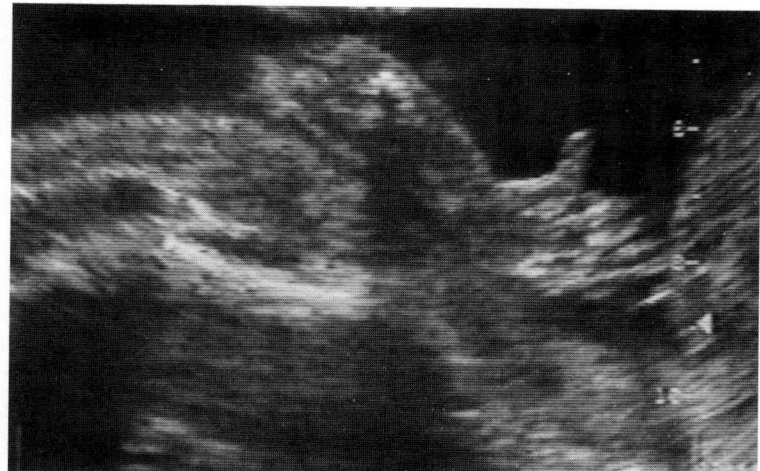

FIGURE 39–31. Sonographic image of the hand shown in Figure 39–29. Note the abnormal angulation of the extra digit in the ulnar side of the forearm.

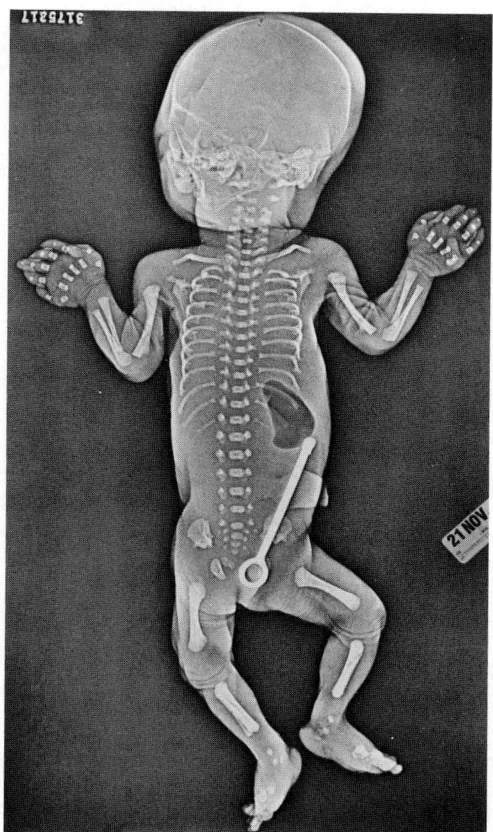

FIGURE 39–32. Xerogram of a fetus with chondroectodermal dysplasia. Note the disproportion between the limbs and the trunk. Long bones are moderately shortened. A sixth digit with its own metacarpal is present in the left hand.

cation of the vertebral bodies, metaphyseal flaring, and severe bowing of the long bones. The Rolland-Desbuquois type has essentially the same features, but the defects are much milder. Prenatal identification has been made in patients at risk.[129,130] Other conditions associated with vertebral disorganization are Jarcho-Levin syndrome and mesomelic dysplasia. A cephalocele is present in 50% of cases of Silverman-Handmaker type and has been attributed to defective segmentation at the level of the occiput. The disease is autosomal recessive.[23]

LIMB DEFICIENCY OR CONGENITAL AMPUTATIONS

On occasion, the only identifiable anomaly is the absence of an extremity (limb deficiency) or a segment of an extremity (congenital amputation) (Table 39-16). These constitute a group of disorders different from osteochondrodysplasias. The overall incidence of congenital limb reduction deformities is approximately 0.49 in 10,000 births (Table 39-17).[131] It has been estimated that 51% of these limb reduction defects are simple transverse reduction deficiencies of one forearm or hand without associated anomalies. The remainder consists of multiple reduction deficiencies, with an approximate 23% incidence of additional anomalies of the internal organs of craniofacial structures.[131]

Limb deficiencies can present alone or as part of a specific syndrome. An isolated limb deficiency of the upper extremity (eg, distal segment of an arm) is generally an isolated anomaly. In contrast, congenital amputation of the leg generally occurs within the context of a syndrome, as do bilateral amputations or reduction of all limbs.[132]

Isolated amputation of an extremity can be due to amniotic band syndrome, exposure to a teratogen, or a

TABLE 39–16. CONGENITAL AMPUTATIONS

Absent limb(s) only
  Single absent limb
  Multiple absent limbs
Absent limbs with rings
  Congenital ring constriction syndrome
Absent limbs and face anomaly
  Aglossia–adactylia syndrome
  Möbius syndrome
Absent limbs with other anomalies
  Ichthyosiform skin (CHILD syndrome)
  Fibula agenesis–complex brachydactyly (Dupan syndrome)
  Splenogonadal fusion
  Skull and scalp defects (Adams-Oliver syndrome)
Phocomelia
  Thalidomide
  Thrombocytopenia with absent radii (TAR) syndrome
  Roberts pseudothalidomide-SC syndrome
  Grebe syndrome
Proximal femoral focal deficiency
  Femoral hypoplasia–unusual facies syndrome
  Femur–fibula–ulna complex
  Femur–tibia–radius complex
Split-hand/split-foot (SH/SF) syndromes
  Only split hand/split foot
  SH/SF and absent long bones
  Ectrodactyly, ectodermal dysplasia, cleft lip/palate (EEC syndrome)
  Some others
    Split foot and triphalangeal thumb, autosomal dominant
    Split foot, or split hand and central polydactyly (see central polydactyly)
    SH/SF and congenital nystagmus (Karsch-Neugebauer syndrome)
    SH/SF and renal malformations (acrorenal syndrome)
    Split foot and mandibulofacial dysostosis (Fontaine syndrome), autosomal dominant

Goldberg MD. The dysmorphic child: an orthopedic perspective. New York: Raven Press, 1987.

vascular accident. In most cases, the anomaly is sporadic, and the risk of recurrence is negligible. However, recurrence of upper-limb deficiencies has been reported.[133,134]

The following section will review syndromes in which a limb amputation or deficiency is associated with other anomalies. We will follow the classification proposed by Goldberg.[132]

TABLE 39–17. INCIDENCE OF DIFFERENT TYPES OF LIMB REDUCTION MALFORMATIONS IN HUNGARY, 1975–1977

TYPE	TOTAL NO.	POPULATION INCIDENCE (PER 1000 BIRTHS)
Terminal transverse	79	0.14
Radial	13	0.09
Ulnar and fibular	41	0.11
Split hand and/or foot	20	0.04
Ring constriction	62	0.11
Total	274	0.49

Adapted from Bod M, Czeizel A, Lenz W. Hum Genet 1983;65:27.

SYNDROMES WITH ABSENT LIMBS AND FACIAL ANOMALIES

The aglossia–adactylia syndrome consists of transverse amputations of the limbs and malformations of the mouth, including micrognathia, vestigial tongue (hypoglossia), dental abnormalities, and ankylosis of the tongue to the hard palate, the floor of the mouth, or the lips (glossopalatine ankylosis). The spectrum of anomalies of the extremities is variable, ranging from absent digits to severe deficiencies of all four extremities. Intelligence is generally normal. The condition is sporadic and has been attributed to a vascular accident.[135] Although some authors have considered the Hanhart syndrome and the glossopalatine ankylosis syndrome as distinct entities,[136] differential diagnosis is extremely difficult.

The Möbius sequence consists of a number of facial anomalies attributed to paralysis of the sixth and seventh cranial nerves. Limited jaw mobility and micrognathia are present. Ptosis is also a common feature. The Möbius sequence is generally sporadic,[137] but autosomal dominant and recessive forms have been described.[138] The associated limb reduction anomalies (25% of cases) are generally present in the upper extremities and range from transverse deficiencies to absent digits. Mental retardation occurs in 10% of the cases.[94] The Möbius, Poland, and Klippel-Feil syndromes have been considered subclavian artery supply disruption sequences, based on the hypothesis that interruption of the early embryonic blood supply to the subclavian artery, vertebral artery, and/or their branches may lead to these conditions.

Limb Reduction Defects Associated With Other Anomalies

Congenital hemidysplasia with ichthyosiform erythroderma and limb defects (CHILD syndrome) is a defect characterized by strict demarcation of the skin lesions to one side of the midline. The presence of unilateral defects of long bones is an important feature of the syndrome.[139] Limb deficiencies may vary from hypoplasia of phalanges or metacarpals to complete absence of an extremity. The calvarium, scapulae, or ribs also may be involved. Zellweger syndrome, chondrodysplasia punctata, and warfarin embryopathy may present with similar findings. Visceral anomalies include congenital heart disease, unilateral hydronephrosis, hydroureter, and unilateral absence of the kidney, fallopian tube, ovaries, adrenal gland, and thyroid. The CHILD syndrome affects females predominantly (by a ratio of 19:1).[139]

Fibula aplasia–complex brachydactyly (Du Pan syndrome) is an extremely rare condition characterized by bilateral agenesis of the fibula with abnormalities of the metacarpals and proximal phalanges. Limb reduction defects can involve the lower extremities.[140] An autosomal recessive pattern of inheritance has been suggested.

The splenogonadal fusion syndrome is characterized by limb reduction defects and splenogonadal fusion.[141] Most reported cases have occurred in males. Typically, there is a mass in the scrotum, and an ectopic spleen is identified during surgery.[142] There is a continuous type in which the normally located spleen is connected to the gonad by bands or cords of splenic tissue.[143] A review of 14 reported cases indicates that there is some overlap between this syndrome and the aglossia–adactylia syndrome or Hanhart syndrome.

The Adams-Oliver syndrome is a group of disorders characterized by the association of limb reduction defects and scalp anomalies (aplasia cutis and deficiency of bony calvarium).[144] Sporadic and familial cases have been reported.

Phocomelia

In phocomelia the extremities resemble those of a seal. Typically, the hands and feet are present, but the intervening arms and legs are absent. Hands and feet may be normal or abnormal. Three syndromes must be considered in the differential diagnosis of phocomelia: Robert's syndrome, some varieties of the thrombocytopenia with absent radius (TAR) syndrome, and Grebe syndrome. Phocomelia also can be caused by exposure to thalidomide, but this is only of historical interest.[145]

Robert's syndrome is an autosomal recessive disorder characterized by the association of tetraphocomelia and facial dysmorphisms (hypertelorism, facial clefting defects, hypoplastic nasal alae).[146] The upper extremities are generally more severely affected than the lower extremities. The spine is not involved. Polyhydramnios has been noted, and other anomalies associated with the syndrome include horseshoe kidney, hydrocephaly, cephalocele, and spina bifida.[147]

Grebe syndrome is a condition described among inbred Indian tribes from Brazil. It is an autosomal recessive disorder characterized by marked hypomelia of upper and lower limbs increasing in severity from proximal to distal segments. In contrast to Robert's syndrome, the lower limbs are more affected than the upper extremities.[148] Many affected fetuses die in utero or during the first year of life. Survivors have normal intelligence and develop normal secondary sexual characteristics.

TAR syndrome is discussed in detail in the section on radial clubhand deformities.

Proximal Femoral Focal Deficiency, or Congenital Short Femur

Proximal femoral focal deficiency, or congenital short femur, refers to a group of disorders encompassing a wide range of congenital developmental anomalies of the femur. The disorder has been classified into five groups: type I, simple hypoplasia of the femur; type II, short femur with angulated shaft; type III, short femur with coxa vara (the most common); type IV, absent or defective proximal femur; and type V, absent or rudimentary femur.[149] One or both femurs can be affected. The right femur is more frequently involved. Anomalies of the upper limbs can also be present and do not exclude the diagnosis.[9] The proximal femoral focal deficiency syndrome may be associated with umbilical or inguinal hernias. If both femurs are affected, it is important to examine the face carefully. The disorder may be femoral hypoplasia and unusual face syndrome B,[150,151] which consists of bilateral femoral hypoplasia and facial defects, including short nose with broad tip, long philtrum, micrognathia, and cleft palate (Fig. 39-33). Long-bone abnormalities can extend to other segments of the lower extremity (absent fibula) and to the upper extremity. The syndrome is sporadic and has been associated with maternal diabetes mellitus. A familiar form has been described.[152] This diagnosis has been made in utero.

If the defect is unilateral, it may correspond to the femur–fibula–ulna or femur–tibia–radius complex. These two syndromes have different implications for genetic counseling: the former is nonfamilial, whereas the second has a strong genetic component.[153]

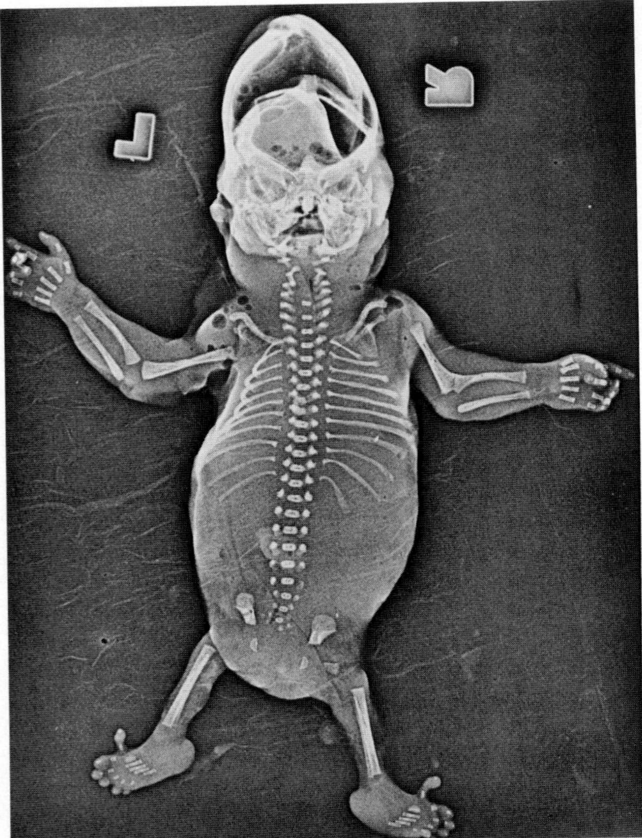

FIGURE 39–33. Unusual facies–femoral hypoplasia syndrome. Note the absence of the left femur and only a tiny portion of ossified bone in the right side. There is partial fusion of the tibia and fibula. Of interest is the presence of preaxial polydactyly in both feet.

Split Hand and Foot Deformities

The term "split-hand-and-foot syndrome" is used to refer to a group of disorders characterized by splitting of the hand and foot into two parts. Other terms include "lobster-claw deformity," "ectrodactyly," and "aborted fingers." The conditions are classified into typical and atypical varieties.[154] The typical form consists of absence of both the finger and the metacarpal bone, resulting in a deep V-shaped central defect that clearly divides the hand into an ulnar and a radial part. It occurs in one out of 90,000 live births and has a familial tendency (usually inherited with an autosomal dominant pattern).[155] The atypical variety is characterized by a much wider cleft formed by a defect of the metacarpals and the middle fingers. As a consequence, the cleft is U-shaped and wide, with only thumb and small finger remaining. It occurs in one in 150,000 live births.[155]

A complex system for the classification of these disorders, based on the distribution of remaining fingers, has been proposed.[156] However, this system is not helpful in differential diagnosis and syndrome classification.

Split-hand-and-foot deformities can occur as isolated anomalies or as part of a more complex syndrome. The syndromic types are the ones more frequently encountered.[132]

The split-hand-and-foot and absent-long-bones syndromes include two conditions in which there is split hand and aplasia of the tibia or split foot with aplasia of the ulna. However, skeletal anomalies are not limited to these bones; the clavicle, femur, and fibula can also be affected. The pattern of inheritance of these disorders has not been clearly determined. Autosomal dominant, recessive, and X-linked recessive patterns have been proposed.[157,158]

The ectrodactyly–ectodermal dysplasia–cleft lip/palate syndrome (EEC syndrome) generally involves the four extremities, with more severe deformities of the hands. The spectrum of ectodermal defects is wide, including hypopigmentation, dry skin, sparse hair, and dental defects.[159] Tear duct anomalies and decreased lacrimal secretions lead to chronic keratoconjunctivitis and severe loss of visual acuity. The cleft lip is generally bilateral. Obstructive uropathy often occurs in this condition.[160] The pattern of inheritance is autosomal dominant. Intelligence is generally normal.[161]

There is a different group of syndromes that involves associations of the split-hand-and-foot deformity with other anomalies. These entities include split foot and triphalangeal thumb, split foot and hand and central polydactyly, Karsch-Neugebauer syndrome (split hand and foot with congenital nystagmus), acrorenal syndrome, and mandibulofacial dysostosis (Fontaine syndrome).[162–165]

CLUBHANDS

Clubhand deformities are classified into two main categories: radial and ulnar. Radial clubhand includes a wide spectrum of disorders that encompass absent thumb, thumb hypoplasia, thin first metacarpal, and absent radius (Table 39-18). Ulnar clubhand is much less frequent than radial clubhand and ranges from mild deviations of the hand of the ulnar side of the forearm to complete absence of the ulna. Although radial clubhand is frequently syndromatic, ulnar clubhand is usually an isolated anomaly.[132] Table 39-19 displays conditions that present with ulnar ray defects.

Whenever a clubhand is identified, it is important to conduct a thorough examination of the fetus and newborn to delineate associated anomalies that may suggest a syndrome. Fetal blood-sampling procedures and fetal echocardiography are recommended. A complete blood cell count, including platelets, is important to establish the diagnosis of Fanconi's pancytopenia, TAR syndrome, and Aase syndrome. A fetal karyotype is indicated because several chromosomal abnormalities (eg,

TABLE 39–18. RADIAL RAY DEFECTS: A DIFFERENTIAL DIAGNOSIS OF CONGENITAL DEFICIENCY OF THE RADIUS AND RADIAL RAY

I. Isolated: nonsyndromatic
II. Syndromes with bood dyscrasias
  Fanconi's anemia
  Thrombocytopenia with absent radii (TAR) syndrome
  Aase syndrome: congenital anemia, nonopposable triphalangeal thumb, scaphoid and distal radius hypoplasia, radioulnar synostosis, short stature with narrow shoulders, autosomal recessive (see Diamond-Blackfan syndrome for a similar, perhaps identical, syndrome)
III. Syndromes with congenital heart disease
  Holt-Oram syndrome
  Lewis upper limb–cardiovascular syndrome: more extensive arm malformations and more complex heart anomalies than Holt-Oram, but probably not a separate syndrome, autosomal dominant
IV. Syndromes with craniofacial abnormalities
  Nager acrofacial dysostosis
  Radial clubhand and cleft lip or cleft palate: sporadic
  Juberg-Hayward syndrome: cleft lip and palate, hypoplastic thumbs, short radius, radial head subluxation, autosomal recessive
  Baller-Gerold syndrome: craniosynostosis, bilateral radial clubhand, absent/hypoplastic thumb, autosomal recessive
  Rothmund-Thomson syndrome: prematurely aged skin changes, juvenile cataract, sparse gray hair, absent thumbs, radial clubhands, occasional knee dysplasia (see progeria syndromes)
  Duane–radial dysplasia syndrome: abnormal ocular movements: inability to abduct and eyeball retraction with adduction, radius and radial ray hypoplasia, vertebral anomalies, renal malformation, autosomal dominant (see Klippel-Feil variants)
  The IVIC syndrome (Instituto Venezolano de Investigaciones Cientificas): radial ray deficiency, hypoplastic or absent thumbs and radial clubhands, impaired hearing, abnormal movements of extraocular muscles with strabismus, autosomal dominant
  LARD syndrome (lacrimo-auriculo-radial-dental; Levy-Hollister): absent lacrimal structures, protuberant ears, thumb and radial ray hypoplasia, abnormal teeth, autosomal dominant
  Radial defects with ear anomalies and cranial nerve 7 dysfunction
  Radial hypoplasia, triphalangeal thumb, hypospadias, diastema of maxillary central incisors, autosomal dominant
V. Syndromes with congenital scoliosis
  The VATER association
  Goldenhar syndrome (oculoauriculovertebral dysplasia
  Klippel-Feil syndrome
VI. Radial aplasia and chromosome aberrations
  Trisomy 18, may include all the features of VATER association
  Chromosome 13 (long arm deletion 13 q-)
  Chromosome 4 (ring formation 4r; short arm deletion 4p-)
  Trisomy 21 (Down syndrome, a very rare association)
VII. Syndromes with mental retardation
  Seckel syndrome (bird-headed dwarfism): microcephaly, beaklike protrusion of nose, mental retardation, absent/hypoplastic thumbs, bilateral dislocated hips.
VIII. Thalidomide embryopathy
  Of historical interest, but some 60% had radial clubhand.

Goldberg MD. The dysmorphic child: an orthopedic perspective. New York: Raven Press, 1987.

trisomy 18, trisomy 21, and other structural aberrations) have been reported in association with clubhand deformities. Congenital heart disease is an important feature of the Holt-Oram syndrome, of the Lewis upper limb–cardiovascular syndrome, and of some cases of TAR syndrome.

Radial Clubhand

The term "isolated radial clubhand" indicates that the clubhand is not part of a recognized syndrome. However, this does not exclude that other anomalies may be present (eg, scoliosis, congenital heart disease). Isolated nonsyndromic radial clubhand is generally a sporadic disorder.[166]

Radial clubhand may be part of the three syndromes characterized by hematologic abnormalities: Fanconi's pancytopenia, TAR syndrome, and Aase syndrome.

Fanconi's anemia (pancytopenia) is an autosomal recessive disease characterized by the association of bone marrow failure (anemia, leukopenia, and thrombocytopenia) and skeletal anomalies, including a radial clubhand with absent thumbs, radial hypoplasia, and a high frequency of chromosomal instability (demonstrated in

TABLE 39–19. ULNAR RAY DEFECTS: A DIFFERENTIAL DIAGNOSIS OF CONGENITAL DEFICIENCY OF THE ULNA AND ULNAR RAY

I. Isolated, nonsyndromatic absent ulna

II. Ulna hypoplasia and skeletal deficiency elsewhere
   Ulna aplasia with lobster-claw deformity of hand and/or foot, autosomal dominant
   Femur–fibula–ulna complex.

III. Syndromes with ulna deficiency
   Cornelia de Lange syndrome
   Miller syndrome (postaxial acrofacial dysostosis): absent ulna and ulnar rays and absent fourth and fifth toes: Treacher Collins mandibulofacial hypoplasia, autosomal recessive; distinguish from Nager preaxial acrofacial dysostosis
   Pallister ulnar–mammary syndrome. Hypoplasia of ulna and ulnar rays; hypoplasia of the breast and absence of apocrine sweat glands, autosomal dominant
   Pillay syndrome (ophthalmo-mandibulo-melic dysplasia): absent distal third of ulna, absent olecranon, hypoplastic trochlea and proximal radius, fusion of interphalangeal joints in ulnar fingers, knee dysplasia; corneal opacities, fusion of temporo-mandibular joint, autosomal dominant
   Weyers oligodactyly syndrome: deficiency of ulna and ulnar rays, antecubital webbing, short sternum, malformed kidney and spleen, cleft lip and palate, sporadic
   Schnizel syndrome: absent/hypoplastic fourth, fifth metacarpals and phalanges, hypogenitalism, anal atresia, autosomal dominant
   Mesomelic dwarfism, Reinhardt-Pfeiffer type (ulno-fibula dysplasia): a generalized bone dysplasia but with a disproportionate hypoplasia of the ulna and fibula, autosomal dominant
   Mesomelic dwarfism, Langr type: a generalized bone dysplasia, but with aplasia of the distal ulna and proximal fibula and hypoplasia of the mandible

Goldberg MD. The dysmorphic child: an orthopedic perspective. New York: Raven Press, 1987.

amniotic fluid cells or fetal lymphocytes as a high frequency of chromosomal breakage after incubation with diepoxy-butane).[167,168] Approximately 25% of affected individuals do not have limb reduction anomalies. Associated findings include microcephaly, congenital dislocation of the hip, scoliosis, and cardiac, pulmonary, and gastrointestinal anomalies. Intrauterine growth retardation is common. Prenatal diagnosis has been reported many times.[169] Up to 25% of the patients will show some degree of mental deficiency.

TAR syndrome is an autosomal recessive disorder characterized by thrombocytopenia (platelet count of less than 100,000/mm^3) and bilateral absence of the radius.[170] The thumb and metacarpals are always present. The ulna and humerus may be absent, and clubfoot deformities may be present. Congenital heart disease is present in 33% of the cases (tetralogy of Fallot and septal defects). Delivery by cesarean section is recommended, as these fetuses are at risk for intracranial hemorrhage.[11,12,171]

Aase syndrome is an autosomal recessive condition characterized by congenital hypoplastic anemia and a radial clubhand with bilateral triphalangeal thumb and a hypoplastic distal radius. Cardiac defects (ventricular septal defects, coarctation of the aorta) may be present.[172,173] Triphalangeal thumbs are a feature of several bone dysostoses and malformation syndromes. They may also occur in random association with other defects, and as isolated, often familial, anomalies. Other disorders with this condition are the Holt-Oram syndrome, Diamond-Blackfan syndrome, chromosomal abnormalities, and the fetal hydantoin syndrome.

The association of upper limb defects and congenital heart disease has been recognized for decades. The Holt-Oram syndrome is an autosomal dominant disorder characterized by congenital heart disease (mainly atrial septal defects, secundum type, and ventricular septal defects), aplasia or hypoplasia of the radius, and triphalangeal or absent thumbs. Limb defects are often asymmetric, with the left side being more affected than the right side. There is no correlation between the severity of the limb defects and the cardiac anomaly. Indeed, some individuals only have a skeletal anomaly. Other findings include hypertelorism, chest wall, and vertebral anomalies.[174] This condition has been diagnosed prenatally.[175,176] The upper limb–cardiovascular syndrome described by Lewis and colleagues is probably not a separate entity from the Holt-Oram syndrome.[177]

Radial clubhand is also associated with congenital scoliosis. The three syndromes that should be considered part of the differential diagnosis include VATER association, some cases of the Goldenhar syndrome, and the Klippel-Feil syndrome.[178,179]

The VATER association is the result of a defective mesodermal development during embryogenesis before the 35th day of gestation. The typical findings are vertebral segmentation (70%), anal atresia (80%), tracheo-esophageal fistula (70%), esophageal atresia, and radial and renal defects (65% and 53%, respectively).[180,181] Other anomalies include a single umbilical artery (35%) and congenital heart disease, occurring in nearly 50% of the patients. The VATER association occurs sporadically, although recurrence within a sibship has been reported.[182]

The Goldenhar syndrome is characterized by hemifacial microsomia, vertebral anomalies, and radial defects.[183] Alterations in the morphogenesis of the first and second brachial arches result in hypoplasia of the malar, maxillary, or mandibular region; microtia; and ocular and oropharyngeal anomalies.[184] Prenatal diagnosis has been reported.[185]

Radial clubhand has been reported in association with several chromosomal anomalies, including trisomies 18 and 21, deletion of the long arm of 13, and ring formation of chromosome 4.[186,187]

Finally, there is a different group of syndromes that present with craniofacial abnormalities and radial clubhand deformities. These syndromes are sporadic and have common features that make a prenatal differential diagnosis difficult. The most common craniofacial anomaly is cleft lip and palate. Uuspaa's study of 3225 cases with orofacial cleft showed a 2.8% association with upper-extremity deformities.[188]

Ulnar clubhand occurs as an isolated, nonsyndromic anomaly in most cases. It can also be associated with a variety of syndromes (eg, Poland complex) (see Table 39-17).[189]

POLYDACTYLY

Polydactyly is the presence of an additional digit (see Fig. 39-18). The extra digit may range from a fleshy nubbin to a complete digit with controlled flexion and extension (see Figs. 39-30 and 39-31). Polydactyly can be classified as postaxial (the most common form), preaxial, and central (see Table 39-11). Postaxial polydactyly occurs on the ulnar side of the hand and fibular side of the foot. Preaxial polydactyly is present on the radial side of the hand and the tibial side of the foot (see Fig. 39-33).

The majority are isolated conditions with an autosomal dominant mode of inheritance. Some of them are part of a syndrome, usually an autosomal recessive one. Preaxial polydactyly, especially triphalangeal thumb, is most likely to be part of multisystem syndrome. Central polydactyly consists of an extra digit that is usually hidden between the long and the ring finger. It is often bilateral and is inherited with an autosomal mode of inheritance. It can be associated with other hand and foot malformations.[190–193]

ARTHROGRYPOSIS

The term "arthrogryposis multiplex congenita" (AMC) refers to multiple joint contractures present at birth. Normal fetal movement is important for the development of the joints; limitation of the fetal joint motion leads to the development of contractures and AMC.[194] Therefore, AMC is a syndrome, not a specific disorder. Neurologic, muscular, connective tissue, skeletal abnormalities, or intrauterine crowding can lead to impaired fetal motion and AMC.[195] Table 39-20 illustrates motor systems that can lead to AMC. In a series of 74 children, Banker found that the most common cause of AMC was a neurogenic disorder followed by myopathic disorders.[196] The condition is present in 0.03% live births.[197] The pattern of inheritance depends on the specific cause of AMC. In a series of 350 cases, Hall found that 46% of cases corresponded to a syndrome with no recurrence risk, 23% corresponded to disorders inherited with a mendelian pattern (autosomal dominant, recessive, or X-linked), 20% were unknown conditions,

TABLE 39–20. DISORDERS OF THE DEVELOPING MOTOR SYSTEM ON ALL LEVELS, LEADING TO IMMOBILIZATION

Disorders of the Developing Neuromuscular System
Loss of anterior horn cells
Radicular disease with collagen proliferation
Peripheral neuropathy with neurofibromatosis
Congenital myasthenia
Neonatal myasthenia (maternal myasthenia gravis)
Amyoplasia congenita
Congenital muscular dystrophy
Central core disease
Congenital myotonic dystrophy
Glycogen accumulation myopathy
Disorders of Developing Connective Tissue or Connective Tissue Disease
Muscular and articular connective tissue dystrophy
Articular defects by mesenchymal dysplasia
Increased collagen synthesis
Disorders of Developing Medulla or Medullar Disease
Congenital spinal epidural hemorrhage
Congenital duplication of the spinal canal
Disorders of Brain Development (eg, Porencephaly or Brain Disease)
Congenital encephalopathy

Romero R, Athanassiadis AP, Sirtori M, Inati M. Fetal skeletal anomalies. In: Fleischer AC, Romero R, Manning FA, Jeanty P, James AE Jr, eds. The principles and practice of ultrasonography in obstetrics and gynecology. 4th ed. Norwalk, CT: Appleton & Lange, 1991:303.

6% were associated with environmental disorders, 3% were chromosomal, and 2% were multifactorial in origin.[198]

The deformities are usually symmetric. In most cases of AMC, all four limbs are involved (Fig. 39-34), followed by deformities of the lower extremities only, or bimelic involvement. The severity of the deformities increases distally in the involved limb, with the hands and feet typically being the most deformed.

Many congenital anomalies are associated with AMC. The most frequent are cleft palate, Klippel-Feil syndrome, meningomyelocele, and congenital heart disease. Ten percent of patients with AMC have associated anomalies of the central nervous system.[194]

The prenatal diagnosis of AMC with ultrasound has been reported only five times.[199–203] The cardinal findings are absent fetal movement on real-time examination and severe flexion deformities.[198]

The prognosis of AMC depends on the specific cause. Although some cases are uniformly lethal, others are associated with mild to moderate handicap.

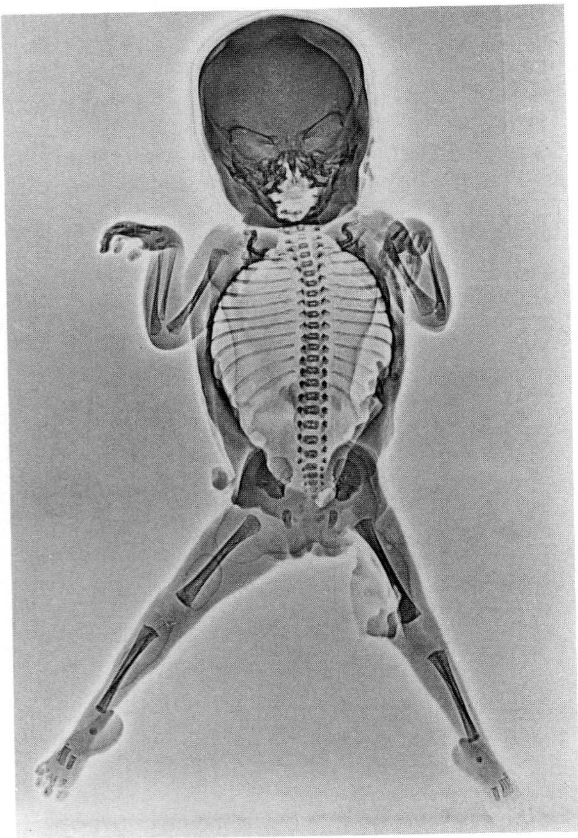

FIGURE 39–34. Arthrogryposis multiplex congenita. There is flexion of the upper limbs with hyperextension of the lower limbs.

REFERENCES

1. Camera G, Mastroiacovo P. Birth prevalence of skeletal dysplasias in the Italian multicentric monitoring system for birth defects. In: Papadatos CJ, Bartsocas CS, eds. Skeletal dysplasias. New York: Alan R Liss, 1982:441.
2. Connor JM, Connor RAC, Sweet EM, et al. Lethal neonatal chondrodysplasias in the West of Scotland 1970–1983 with a description of a thanatophoric, dysplasialike, autosomal recessive disorder, Glasgow variant. Am J Med Genet 1985;22:243.
3. International nomenclature of constitutional diseases of bone. J Pediatr 1978;93:614.
4. International nomenclature of constitutional diseases of bone. Ann Radiol 1984;27:275.
5. Spranger J, Maroteaux P. The lethal osteochondrodysplasias. Adv Hum Genet 1989;19:1.
6. Benaceraff BR, Greene MF, Barss VA. Prenatal sonographic diagnosis of congenital hemivertebra. J Ultrasound Med 1986;5:257.
7. Kurtz AB, Wapner RJ. Ultrasonographic diagnosis of second trimester skeletal dysplasias: a prospective analysis in a high-risk population. J Ultrasound Med 1983;2:99.
8. Coffin GS, Siris E, Wegienka LC. Mental retardation with osteocartilaginous anomalies. Am J Dis Child 1966;112:205.
9. Graham M. Congenital short femur: prenatal sonographic diagnosis. J Ultrasound Med 1985;4:361.
10. Pashayan H, Fraser FC, McIntyre JM, et al. Bilateral aplasia of the tibia, polydactyly and absent thumbs in father and daughter. J Bone Joint Surg 1971;53B:495.
11. Filkins K, Russo J, Bilinki I, et al. Prenatal diagnosis of thrombocytopenia absent radius syndrome using ultrasound and fetoscopy. Prenat Diagn 1984;4:139.
12. Luthy DA, Hall JG, Graham CB, et al. Prenatal diagnosis of thrombocytopenia with absent radii. Clin Genet 1979;15:495.
13. Chitkara U, Rosenberg J, Chervenak FA, et al. Prenatal sonographic assessment of the fetal thorax: normal values. Am J Obstet Gynecol 1987;156:1069.
14. Campbell J, Henderson A, Campbell S. The fetal femur/foot length ratio: a new parameter to assess dysplastic limb reduction. Obstet Gynecol 1989;72:181.
15. Hershey DW. The fetal femur/foot length ratio: a new parameter to assess dysplastic limb reduction. Obstet Gynecol 1989;73:682.
16. Galli G. Craniosynostosis. Boca Raton, FL: CRC Press, 1984.
17. Kozlowski K, Robertson F, Middleton R. Radiographic findings in Larsen's syndrome. Aust Radiol 1974;18:336.
18. Pilu G, Romero R, Reece EA, et al. The prenatal diagnosis of Robin anomalad. Am J Obstet Gynecol 1986;154:630.
19. Pilu G, Reece EA, Romero R, et al. Prenatal diagnosis of craniofacial malformations with ultrasonography. Am J Obstet Gynecol 1986;155:45.
20. Romero R, Pilu G, Jeanty P, et al. Prenatal diagnosis of congenital anomalies. Norwalk, CT: Appleton & Lange, 1988:311.
21. Iannaccone G, Gerlini G. The so-called "cloverleaf skull syndrome": a report of three cases with a discussion of its relationships with thanatophoric dwarfism and craniostenosis. Pediatr Radiol 1974;2:175.
22. Yang SS, Heidelberger KP, Brough AJ, et al. Lethal short-limbed chondrodysplasia in early infancy. In: Rosenberg HS, Boland RP, eds. Perspectives in pediatric pathology. Chicago: Year Book Medical Publishers, 1976;3:1.
23. McKusick VA, Francomano CA, Antonarakis SE. Mendelian inheritance in man: catalogs of autosomal dominant, autosomal recessive, and x-linked phenotypes. 9th ed. Baltimore: The Johns Hopkins University Press, 1990.

24. Partington MW, Gonzales-Grassi F, Khakee SG, Wallin DG. Cloverleaf skull and thanatophoric dwarfism, a report of four cases, two in the same sibship. Arch Dis Child 1971;46:656.
25. Horton WA, Rimoin DL, Hollister DW, Lachman RS. Further heterogeneity within lethal neonatal short-limbed dwarfism: the platyspondylic types. J Pediatr 1979;94:736.
26. Moir DH, Kozlowski K. Long survival in thanatophoric dwarfism. Pediatr Radiol 1976;5:123.
27. Stensvold K, Hovland AR. An infant with thanatophoric dwarfism surviving 169 days. Clin Genet 1986;29:157.
28. Fink IJ, Filly RA, Callen PW, et al. Sonographic diagnosis of thanatophoric dwarfism in utero. J Ultrasound Med 1982; 1:337.
29. Beetham FGT, Reeves JS. Early ultrasound diagnosis of thanatophoric dwarfism. J Clin Ultrasound 1984;12:43.
30. Burrows PE, Stannard MW, Pearrow J, et al. Early antenatal sonographic recognition of thanatophoric dysplasia with cloverleaf skull deformity. AJR 1984;143:841.
31. Mahony BS, Filly RA, Callen PW, et al. Thanatophoric dwarfism with the cloverleaf skull: a specific antenatal sonographic diagnosis. J Ultrasound Med 1985;4:151.
32. Elejald BR, de Elejalde MM. Thanatophoric dyplasia: fetal manifestations and prenatal diagnosis. Am J Med Genet 1985; 22:669.
33. Weiner CP, Williamson RA, Bonsib SM. Sonographic diagnosis of cloverleaf skull and thanatophoric dysplasia in the second trimester. J Clin Ultrasound 1986;14:463.
34. van der Harten JJ, Brons JTJ, Dijkstra PF, et al. Some variants of lethal neonatal short-limbed platyspondylic dysplasia: a radiologic, ultrasonographic, neuropathologic and histopathologic study of 22 cases. In: Brons JTJ, van der Harten JJ, eds. Skeletal dysplasias, pre- and postnatal identification: an ultrasonographic, radiologic and pathologic study. Amsterdam: Free University Hospital, 1988:111.
35. Chervenak FA, Blakemore KJ, Isaacson G, et al. Antenatal sonographic findings of thanatophoric dysplasia with cloverleaf skull. Am J Obstet Gynecol 1983;146:984.
36. Eteson DJ, Adomian GE, Ornoy A, et al. Fibrochondrogenesis: radiologic and histologic studies. Am J Med Genet 1984;19:277.
37. Lazzaroni-Fossati F, Stanescu F, Stanescu R, Serra G, Magliano P, Maroteaux P. La fibrochondrogenèse. Arch Fr Pediatr 1978;35:1096.
38. Whitley CB, Langer LO, Ophoven J, et al. Fibrochondrogenesis: lethal, autosomal recessive chondrodysplasia with distinctive cartilage histopathology. Am J Med Genet 1984;19:265.
39. Chevernak FA, Isaacson G, Rosenberg JC, et al. Antenatal diagnosis of frontal cephalocele in a fetus with atelosteogenesis. J Ultrasound Med 1986;5:111.
40. Maroteaux P, et al. Atelosteogenesis. Am J Med Genet 1982;13:15.
41. Sillence DO, et al. Spondylo-humero-femoral hypoplasia (giant cell chondroplasia). Am J Med Genet 1982;13:7.
42. Yang, et al. Two lethal chondrodysplasias with giant chondrocytes. Am J Med Genet 1983;15:615.
43. McAlister W, et al. A new neonatal short-limbed dwarfism. Skeletal Radiol 1985;13:271.
44. Sillence DO, et al. Atelosteogenesis: evidence for heterogeneity. Pediatr Radiol 1987;17:112.
45. Herzberg AJ, et al. Variant of atelosteogenesis? Report of a 20-week fetus. Am J Med Genet 1988;29:883.
46. Stern HJ, et al. Atelosteogenesis type 3: a distinct skeletal dysplasia with features overlapping atelosteogenesis and oto-palato-digital syndrome type 2. Am J Med Genet (in press).
47. De la Chapelle A, Maroteaux P, Havu N, Granroth G. Une rare dysplasie osseuse létale de transmission récessive autosomique. Arch Fr Pediatr 1972;29:759.
48. Whitley CB, Burke BA, Granroth G, Gorlin RJ. De la Chapelle dysplasia. Am J Med Genet 1986;25:29.
49. Kozlowski K, Sillence D, Cortis-Jones R, Osborn R. Boomerang dysplasia. Br J Radiol 1985;58:369.
50. Borochowitz J, Lachman R, Adomian E, Spear G, Jones K, Rimoin DL. Achondrogenesis type I: delineation of further heterogeneity and identification of two distinct subgroups. J Pediatr 1988;112:23.
51. Borochowitz Z, Ornoy A, Lachman R, et al. Achondrogenesis II–hypochondrogenesis: variability versus heterogeneity. Am J Med Genet 1986;24:273.
52. Spranger J. Pattern recognition in bone dysplasias. In: Papadatos CJ, Bartsocas CS, eds. Endocrine genetics and genetics of growth. New York: Alan R Liss, 1985:315.
53. Godfrey M, Keene DR, Blank E, et al. Type II achondrogenesis-hypochondrogenesis: morphologic and immunohistopathologic studies. Am J Hum Genet 1988;43:894.
54. Murray LW, Rimoin DL. Abnormal type II collagen in the spondylepiphyseal dysplasias. Pathol Immunopathol Res 1988; 17:99.
55. Whitley CB, Gorlin RJ. Achondrogenesis: new nosology with evidence of genetic heterogeneity. Radiology 1983;148:693.
56. Van der Harten HJ, Brons JTJ, Dijkstra PF, et al. Achondrogenesis, hypochondrogenesis, the spectrum of chondrogenesis imperfecta: a radiologic, ultrasonographic and histopathologic study of 23 cases. Pediatr Pathol 1988;8:571.
57. Wenstrom KD, Williamson RA, Hoover WW, Grant SS. Achondrogenesis type II (Langer-Saldino) is associated with jugular lymphatic obstruction sequence. Prenat Diagn 1989;9:527.
58. Golbus MS, Hall BD, Filly RA, Poskanzer LB. Prenatal diagnosis of achondrogenesis. J Pediatr 1977;91:464.
59. Johnson VP, Yiu-Chiu VS, Wierda DR, et al. Midtrimester prenatal diagnosis of achondrogenesis. J Ultrasound Med 1984;3:223.
60. Mahony BS, Filly RA, Cooperberg PL. Antenatal sonographic diagnosis of achondrogenesis. J Ultrasound Med 1984;3:333.
61. Glenn LW, Teng SSK. In utero sonographic diagnosis of achondrogenesis. J Clin Ultrasound 1985;13:195.
62. Chen H, Liu CT, Yang SS. Achondrogenesis: a review with special consideration of achondrogenesis type II (Langer-Saldino). Am J Med Genet 1981;10:379.
63. Benacerraf B, Osathanondh R, Bieber FR. Achondrogenesis type I: ultrasound diagnosis in utero. J Clin Ultrasound 1984;12:357.
64. Smith WL, Breitweiser TD, Dinno N. In utero diagnosis of achondrogenesis, type I. Clin Genet 1981;19:51.
65. Kurtz AB, Filly RA, Wapner RJ, et al. In utero analysis of heterozygous achondroplasia: variable time of onset as detected by femur length measurements. J Ultrasound Med 1986;5:137.
66. Elejalde BR, de Elejalde MM, Hamilton PR, et al. Prenatal diagnosis in two pregnancies of an achondroplastic woman. Am J Med Genet 1983;15:437.
67. Filly RA, Golbus MS, Carey JC, et al. Short-limbed dwarfism: ultrasonographic diagnosis by mensuration of fetal femoral length. Radiology 1981;138:653.
68. Pauli RM, Conroy MM, Langer LO, et al. Homozygous achondroplasia with survival beyond infancy. Am J Med Genet 1983;16:459.
69. Hall BD, et al. Hypochondroplasia: clinical and radiological aspects in 39 cases. Radiology 1979;133:95.
70. Scott CL. Achondroplastic and hypochondroplastic dwarfism. Clin Orthop 1976;114:18.
71. Stoll C, et al. Prenatal diagnosis of hypochondroplasia. Prenat Diagn 1985;5:423.

72. McKusick V, et al. Observations suggesting allelism of the achondroplasia and hypochondroplasia genes. J Med Genet 1973;10:11.
73. Prockop DJ, Baldwin CT, Constantinou CD. Mutations in type I procollagen genes that cause osteogenesis imperfecta. Adv Hum Genet 1989;19:105.
74. Sillence DO, Senn A, Danks DM. Genetic heterogeneity in osteogenesis imperfecta. J Med Genet 1979;16:101.
75. Sillence DO, Barlow KK, Garber AP, et al. Osteogenesis imperfecta type II: delineation of the phenotype with reference to genetic heterogeneity. Am J Med Genet 1984;17:407.
76. Sillence DO, Barlow KK, Cole WG, Dietrich S, Garber AP, Rimoin DL. Osteogenesis imperfecta type III. Delineation of the phenotype with reference to genetic heterogeneity. Am J Med Genet 1986;23:821.
77. Spranger J. Osteogenesis imperfecta: a pasture for splitters and lumpers. Am J Med Genet 1984;17:425.
78. Van der Harten JJ, Brons JTJ, Dijkstra PF. Perinatal lethal osteogenesis imperfecta: radiologic and pathologic evaluation of seven prenatally diagnosed cases. Pediatr Pathol 1988;8:233.
79. Aylsworth AS, Seeds JW, Bonner-Guilford W, et al. Prenatal diagnosis of a severe deforming type of osteogenesis imperfecta. Am J Med Genet 1984;19:707.
80. Robinson LP, Worthen NJ, Lachman RS, et al. Prenatal diagnosis of osteogenesis imperfecta type III. Prenat Diagn 1987;7:7.
81. Mertz E, Goldhofer W. Sonographic diagnosis of lethal osteogenesis imperfecta in the second trimester: case report and review. J Clin Ultrasound 1986;14:380.
82. Brons JTJ, van der Harten JJ, Wladimiroff JW. Prenatal ultrasonographic diagnosis of osteogenesis imperfecta. Am J Obstet Gynecol 1988;159:176.
83. Elejalde BR, de Elejalde MM. Prenatal diagnosis of perinatally lethal osteogenesis imperfecta. Am J Med Genet 1983;14:353.
84. Ghosh A, Woo JSK, Wan CW, et al. Simple ultrasonic diagnosis of osteogenesis imperfecta type II in early second trimester. Prenat Diagn 1984;4:235.
85. Hobbins JC, Bracken MB, Mahoney MJ. Diagnosis of fetal skeletal dysplasias with ultrasound. Am J Obstet Gynecol 1982;142:306.
86. Chervenak FA, Romero R, Berkowitz RL, et al. Antenatal sonographic findings of osteogenesis imperfecta. Am J Obstet Gynecol 1982;143:228.
87. Tsipouras P, Schwartz RC, Goldberg JD, Berkowitz RL, Ramirez F. Prenatal prediction of osteogenesis imperfecta (OI type IV): exclusion of inheritance using a collagen gene probe. J Med Genet 1987;24:406.
88. Wladimiroff JW, Niermeijen MF, van der Harten JJ, et al. Early prenatal diagnosis of congenital hypophosphatasia: case report. Prenat Diagn 1985;5:47.
89. Warren RC, McKenzie CF, Rodeck CH, et al. First trimester diagnosis of hypophosphatasia with a monoclonal antibody to the liver/bone/kidney isoenzyme of alkaline phosphatase. Lancet 1985;2:856.
90. Mulivor RA, Mennuti M, Zackai EH, et al. Prenatal diagnosis of hypophosphatasia: genetic, biochemical, and clinical studies. Am J Hum Genet 1978;30:271.
91. Rudd NL, Miskin M, Hoar DI, et al. Prenatal diagnosis of hypophosphatasia. N Engl J Med 1976;1:146.
92. Rattenbury JM, Blau K, Sandler M, et al. Prenatal diagnosis of hypophosphatasia. Lancet 1976;1:306.
93. Romero R, Ghidini A, Eswara MS, Seashore MR, Hobbins JC. Prenatal findings in a case of spondylocostal dysplasia type I (Jarcho-Levin syndrome). Obstet Gynecol 1988;71:988.
94. Hooshang T, Ralph SL. Radiology of syndromes, metabolic disorders, and skeletal dysplasias. 3rd ed. Chicago: Year Book Medical Publishers, 1983.
95. Kozlowski K, Masel J. Asphyxiating thoracic dystrophy without respiratory distress. Report of 2 cases of the latent form. Pediatr Radiol 1976;5:30.
96. Friedman JM, Kaplan HG, Hall JG. The Jeune syndrome (asphyxiating thoracic dystrophy) in an adult. Am J Med 1975;59:857.
97. Elejalde BR, de Elejalde MM, Pansch D. Prenatal diagnosis of Jeune syndrome. Am J Med Genet 1985;21:433.
98. Lipson M, Waskey J, Rice J, et al. Prenatal diagnosis of asphyxiating thoracic dysplasia. Am J Med Genet 1984;18:273.
99. Schinzel A, Savoldelli G, Briner J, et al. Prenatal sonographic diagnosis of Jeune Syndrome. Radiology 1985;154:777.
100. Skiptunas SM, Weiner S. Early prenatal diagnosis of asphyxiating thoracic dysplasia (Jeune's syndrome): value of fetal thoracic measurement. J Ultrasound Med 1987;6:41.
101. Wladimiroff JW, Niermeijer MF, Laar J, et al. Prenatal diagnosis of skeletal dysplasia by real-time ultrasound. Obstet Gynecol 1984;63:360.
102. Muller LM, Cremin BJ. Ultrasonic demonstration of fetal skeletal dysplasia. SAMJ 1985;67:222.
103. McKusick VA, Egeland JA, Eldridge R, Krusen DE. Dwarfism in the Amish. The Ellis-van Creveld syndrome. Bull Johns Hopkins Hosp 1964;115:306.
104. Smith DW. Recognizable patterns of human malformation: genetic, embryologic and clinical aspects. Philadelphia: WB Saunders, 1982:266.
105. Bui TH, Marsk L, Ekloef O. Prenatal diagnosis of chondroectodermal dysplasia with fetoscopy. Prenat Diagn 1984;4:155.
106. Mahoney MJ, Hobbins JC. Prenatal diagnosis of chondroectodermal dysplasia (Ellis-van Creveld syndrome) with fetoscopy and ultrasound. N Engl J Med 1977;297:258.
107. Zimmer EZ, Weinraub Z, Raijman A, et al. Antenatal diagnosis of a fetus with an extremely narrow thorax and short limb dwarfism. J Clin Ultrasound 1984;12:112.
108. Houston CS, Opitz JM, Spranger JW, et al. The campomelic syndrome. Am J Med Genet 1982;15:3.
109. Fryns JP, van der Berghe K, van Assche A, et al. Prenatal diagnosis of campomelic dwarfism. Clin Genet 1981;19:199.
110. Winter R, Rosenkranz W, Hofmann H, et al. Prenatal diagnosis of campomelic dysplasia by ultrasonography. Prenat Diagn 1985;5:1.
111. Slater CP, Ross J, Nelson MM, Coetzee EJ. The campomelic syndrome—prenatal ultrasound investigations: a case report. SAMT 67:863.
112. Balcar I, Bieber FR. Sonographic and radiologic findings in campomelic dysplasia. AJR 1983;141:481.
113. Opitz JM. Comment to: Genetical and clinical aspects of campomelic dysplasia. Beluffi G, Fraccaro M. Prog Clin Biol Res 1982;104:66.
114. Beluffi G, Fraccaro M. Genetical and clinical aspects of campomelic dysplasia. Prog Clin Bio Res 1982;104:53.
115. Horton WA, Rimoin DL, Lachman RS, et al. The phenotypic variability of diastrophic dysplasia. J Pediatr 1978;93:609.
116. Kaitila I, Ammala P, Karjalainen O, et al. Early prenatal detection of diastrophic dysplasia. Prenat Diagn 1983;3:237.
117. Mantagos S, Weiss RR, Mahoney M, et al. Prenatal diagnosis of diastrophic dwarfism. Am J Obstet Gynecol 1981;139:1111.
118. Gembruch U, Niesen M, Kehrberg H, Hansmann M. Diastrophic dysplasia: a specific prenatal diagnosis by ultrasound. Prenat Diagn 1988;8:539.
119. Gollop TR, Eigier A. Brief clinical report: prenatal ultrasound diagnosis of diastrophic dysplasia at 16 weeks. Am J Med Genet 1987;27:321.
120. Gustavson K-H, Holmgren G, Jagell S, Jorulf H. Lethal and non-lethal diastrophic dysplasia: a study of 14 Swedish cases. Clin Genet 1985;28:321.

121. Eteson DJ, et al. Pseudodiastrophic dysplasia: a distinct newborn skeletal dysplasia. J Pediatr 1986;109:635.
122. Siggers D, Rimoin D, Dorst J, et al. The Kniest syndrome. Birth Defects 1974;10(9):193.
123. Rimoin DL, Hughes GNF, Kaufman RL, et al. Metatropic dwarfism: morphological and biochemical evidence of heterogeneity. Clin Res 1969;17:317.
124. Chen H, Yang SS, Gonzales E. Kniest dysplasia: neonatal death with necropsy. Am J Med Genet 1980a;6:171.
125. Poole AR, Pidoux I, Reiner A, Rosenberg L, Hossiter D, Murray L, Rimoin DL. Kniest dysplasia is characterized by an apparent abnormal processing of the C-propeptide of type II cartilage collagen resulting in imperfect fibril assembly. J Clin Invest 1988;81:579.
126. Maisonneuve J, Armand JP, Louis JJ, Guibaud P. Nanisme dyssegmentaire. Pédiatrie 1984;39:273.
127. Fasanelli S, Kozlowski K, Reiter S, Sillence D. Dyssegmental dysplasia. Skeletal Radiol 1985;14:173.
128. Handmaker SD, Campbell IA, Robinson LD, et al. Dyssegmental dwarfism: a new syndrome of lethal dwarfism. Birth Defects 1977;13(3D):79.
129. Andersen PE Jr, Hauge M, Bang J. Dyssegmental dysplasia in siblings: prenatal ultrasonic diagnosis. Skeletal Radiol 1988;17:29.
130. Kim HJ, Costales F, Bouzouki M, Wallach RC. Prenatal diagnosis of dyssegmental dwarfism. Prenat Diagn 1986;6:143.
131. Bod M, Creizel A, Lenz W. Incidence at birth of different types of limb reduction abnormalities in Hungary, 1975–1977. Hum Genet 1983;65:27.
132. Goldberg MJ. The dysmorphic child: an orthopedic perspective. New York: Raven Press, 1987.
133. Pilarski RT, Pauli RM, Engber WD. Hand-reduction malformations: genetic and syndrome analysis. J Pediatr 1985;5:274.
134. Hecht JT, Scott CI Jr. Recurrent unilateral hand malformations in siblings. Clin Genet 1981;20:225.
135. Tunobileck E, Yalcin C, Atasu M. Aglossia-adactylia syndrome (special emphasis on the inheritance pattern). Clin Genet 1977;11:421.
136. Baraitser M. Genetics of Moebius syndrome. J Med Genet 1977;14:415.
137. Chicarilli ZN, et al. Oromandibular limb hypogenesis syndromes. Plast Reconstr Surg 1985;76:13.
138. Sugarman GI, Stark HH. Moebius syndrome with Poland's anomaly. J Med Genet 1973;10:192.
139. Happle R, Koch H, Lenz W. The CHILD syndrome: congenital hemidysplasia with ichthyosiform erythroderma and limb defects. Eur J Pediatr 1980;134:27.
140. Martin Du Pan CH. Absence congénitale du péroné sans déformation du tibia. Revue d'Orthopédie 1924;3:227.
141. Tank ES, Forsyth M. Splenic gonadal fusion. J Urol 1988;139:798.
142. Pauli RM, Greenlaw A. Limb deficiency and splenogonadal fusion. Am J Med Genet 1982;13:81.
143. Bearss RW. Splenic-gonadal fusion. Urology 1980;16:277.
144. Bonafede RP, Beighton P. Autosomal dominant inheritance of scalp defects with extrodactyly. Am J Med Genet 1979;3:35.
145. Claus GH, Newman CGH. The thalidomide syndrome: risks of exposure and spectrum of malformations. Teratology 1986;13:555.
146. Freeman MVR, Williams DW, Schimke N, et al. The Roberts syndrome. Clin Genet 1974;5:1.
147. Waldenmaier C, Aldenhoff P, Klemm T. The Roberts' syndrome. Hum Genet 1978;40:345.
148. Romeo G, Zonana J, Lachman RS, Opitz JM, Scott CI, Spranger JW, Rimoin DL. Grebe chondrodysplasia and similar forms of severe short-limbed dwarfism. Birth Defects 1977;13:109.
149. Hamanishi C. Congenital short femur. J Bone Joint Surg 1980;62:307.
150. Daentl DL, Smith DW, Scott C. Femoral hypoplasia—unusual facie syndrome. J Pediatric 1975;86:107.
151. Burn J, Winter RJ, Baraitser M, Hall CM, et al. The femoral hypoplasia—unusual facies syndrome. J Med Genet 1984;21:331.
152. Gupta DKS, Gupta SK. Familial bilateral femoral focal deficiency. J Bone Joint Surg 1984;66-A:1470.
153. Tentamy S, McKusick V. Birth defects. National Foundation—March of Dimes, XIV(3), March of Dimes. New York: Alan R Liss, 1978.
154. Miura T, Suzuki M. Clinical differences between typical and atypical cleft hand. J Hand Surg 1984;9:311.
155. Barsky AJ. Cleft hand: classification, incidence, and treatment. J Bone Joint Surg 1964;46:1707.
156. Tada K, Yonenobu K, Swanson AB. Congenital central ray deficiency in the hand—a survey of 59 cases and subclassification. J Hand Surg 1981;6:434.
157. Van den Berghe H, Dequeker J, Fryns JP, et al. Familial occurrence of severe ulnar aplasia and lobster claw feet: a new syndrome. Hum Genet 1978;42:109.
158. Verma IC, Joseph R, Bhargava S, Mehta S. Split-hand and split-foot deformity inherited as an autosomal recessive trait. Clin Genet 1976;9:8.
159. Rudiger RA, Haase W, Passarge E. Association of ectrodactyly, ectodermal dysplasia, and cleft lip-palate, Am J Dis Child 1970;120:160.
160. Leiter E, Lipson J. Genitourinary tract anomalies in lobster claw syndrome. J Urol 1976;115:339.
161. Penchaszadeh VB, De Negrotti TC. Ectrodactyly-ectodermal dysplasia-clefting (EEC) syndrome: dominant inheritance and variable expression. J Med Genet 1976;13:281.
162. Halal F, Homsy M, Perreault G. Acro-renal-ocular syndrome: autosomal dominant thumb hypoplasia, renal ectopia, and eye defect. Am J Med Genet 1984;17:753.
163. Chan KM, Lamb DW. Triphalangeal thumb and five-fingered hand. Hand 1983;15:329.
164. Wood VE. Congenital thumb deformities. Clin Orthop 1985;195:7.
165. Bujdoso G, Lenz W. Monodactylous splithand-splitfoot. Eur J Pediatr 1980;133:207.
166. Carroll RE, Louis DS. Anomalies associated with radial dysplasia. J Pediatr 1974;84:409.
167. Glanz A, Fraser FC. Spectrum of anomalies in Fanconi anaemia. J Med Genet 1982;19:412.
168. Nilsson LR. Chronic pancytopenia with multiple congenital abnormalities (Fanconi's anaemia). Acta Paediatrica 1960; 49:518.
169. Auerbach AD, Sagi M, Adler B. Fanconi anemia: prenatal diagnosis in 30 fetuses at risk. Pediatrics 1985;76:794.
170. Hedberg VA, Lipton JM. Thrombocytopenia with absent radii: a review of 100 cases. Am J Pediatr Hematol Oncol 1988; 10(1):51.
171. de Vries LS, Connell J, Bydder GM, et al. Recurrent intracranial haemorrhages in utero in an infant with alloimmune thrombocytopenia. Case report. Br J Obstet Gynaecol 1988;95:299.
172. Higginbottom MC, Jones KL, Kung FH. The Aase syndrome in a female infant. J Med Genet 1978;15:484.
173. Jones B, Thompson H. Triphalangeal thumbs associated with hypoplastic anemia. Pediatrics 1973;52:609.
174. Zhang KZ, Sun QB, Tsung OC. Holt-Oram syndrome in China: a collective review of 18 cases. Am Heart J 1986;111:573.
175. Muller LM, et al. The antenatal ultrasonographic detection of the Holt-Oram syndrome. S Afr Med J 1985;68:313.
176. Brons JTJ, van Geijn HP, Wladimiroff JW. Prenatal ultrasono-

graphic diagnosis of the Holt-Oram syndrome. Prenat Diagn 1988;8:175.
177. Lewis KB, Bruce RA, Baum D, et al. The upper limb-cardiovascular syndrome. JAMA 1965;193:1080.
178. Chemke J, Nisani R, Fischel RE. Absent ulna in the Klippel-Feil syndrome: an unusual associated malformation. Clin Genet 1980;17:167.
179. Tentamy SA, Miller JD. Extending the scope of the VATER association: definition of a VATER syndrome. J Pediatr 1974; 85:345.
180. Quan L, Smith DW. The VATER association: vertebral defects, anal atresia, tracheoesophageal fistula with esophageal atresia, radial dysplasia. Birth Defects 1972;8:75.
181. Fernbach SK, Glass RBJ. The expanded spectrum of limb anomalies in the VATER association. Pediatr Radiol 1988;18:215.
182. Auchterlonie IA, White MP. Recurrence of the VATER association within a sibship. Clin Genet 1982;21:122.
183. Rollnick BR, Kaye Cl, Nagatoshi K, Hauck W, Martin AO. Oculoauriculovertebral dysplasia and variants: phenotypic characteristics of 294 patients. Am J Med Genet 1987;26:361.
184. Setzer ES, Reiz-Castaneda N, Severn C, et al. Etiologic heterogeneity in the oculoauriculovertebral syndrome, J Pediatr 1981;98:88.
185. Tamas DE, Mahony BS, Bowie JD, Woodruff III WW, Kay HH. Prenatal sonographic diagnosis of hemifacial microsomia (Goldenhar-Gorlin syndrome). J Ultrasound Med 1986;5:461.
186. Swanson AB, Tada K, Yonenubo K. Ulnar ray deficiency: its various manifestations. J Hand Surg 1984;9A:658.
187. Gausewitz SH, Meals RA, Setocuchi Y. Severe limb deficiency in Poland's syndrome. Clin Orthop 1984;185:9.
188. Uuspaa V. Upper extremity deformities associated with the orofacial clefts. Scand J Plast Reconstr Surg 1978;12:157.
189. David TJ. Preaxial polydactyly and the Poland complex. Am J Med Genet 1982;13:333.
190. Lowry RB. Variability in the Smith-Lemli-Opitz syndrome: overlap with the Meckel syndrome. Am J Med Genet 1983;14:429.
191. Goodman RM, Sternberg M, Shem-Tob Y, et al. Acrocephalopolysyndactyly type IV: a new genetic syndrome in 3 sibs. Clin Genet 1979;15:209.
192. Khaldi F, Bennaceur B, Hammou A, et al. An autosomal recessive disorder with retardation of growth, mental deficiency, ptosis, pectus excavatum and camptodactyly. Pediatr Radiol 1988;18:432.
193. Christophorou MN, Nicolaidou P. Median cleft lip, polydactyly, syndactyly and toe anomalies in a non-Indian infant. Br J Plast Surg 1983;36:447.
194. Hageman G, Willemse J. Arthrogryposis multiplexa congenita. Review with comments. Neuropediatrics 1983;14:6.
195. Swinyard CA, Bleck EE. The etiology of arthrogryposis (multiple congenital contracture). Clin Orthop 1985;194:15.
196. Banker BQ. Neuropathologic aspects of arthrogryposis multiplex congenita. Clin Orthop 1985;194:30.
197. Thompson GH, Bilenker RM. Comprehensive management of arthrogryposis multiplex congenita. Clin Orthop 1985;194:6.
198. Hall JG. Genetic aspects of arthrogryposis. Clin Orthop 1985;194:44.
199. Gorczyca DP, McGahan JP, Kindfors KK, Ellis WG, Grix A. Arthrogryposis multiplex congenita: prenatal ultrasonographic diagnosis. J Clin Ultrasound 1989;17:40.
200. Kirkinen P, Herva R, Leisti J. Early prenatal diagnosis of a lethal syndrome of multiple congenital contractures. Prenat Diagn 1987;7:189.
201. Goldberg JD, Chervenak FA, Lipman RA, Berkowitz RL. Antenatal sonographic diagnosis of arthrogryposis multiplex congenita. Prenat Diagn 1986;6:45.
202. Miskin M, Rothberg R, Rudd N, Benxie R, Shine J. Arthrogryposis multiplex congenita—prenatal assessment with diagnostic ultrasound and fetoscopy. J Pediatr 1979;95:463.
203. Socol ML, Sabbagha RE, Elias S, Tamura RK, Simpson JL, Dooley SL, Depp R. Prenatal diagnosis of congenital muscular dystrophy producing arthrogryposis. N Engl J Med 1985; 313:1230.

40

CHAPTER

FETAL NEOPLASM

E. Albert Reece

Fetal neoplasms represent a rare and heterogeneous group of abnormalities. Some have suggested that fetal neoplasms may be caused by faulty histogenesis and organogenesis.[1] The precise mechanism by which these tumors arise is as poorly understood as the occurrence of neoplasms in adults. Neoplasms may be divided into five main categories: tumors of the head and neck, brain, heart, chest, and abdominal/pelvic areas (Table 40-1). Since tumors of the chest are described in detail in Chapter 36, they will not be discussed here.

TUMORS OF THE HEAD AND NECK

CYSTIC HYGROMA

Etiopathology

Cystic hygroma, the most frequent fetal tumor of the head and neck, is found in one in 200 spontaneous abortuses.[2] These lesions result from lymphatic system abnormalities, in which the jugular lymphatic sacs fail to drain into the internal jugular vein, resulting in dilated lymphatic channels and giving a cystic appearance sonographically. These cysts present as sacs with or without multiple septations (Fig. 40-1).[1]

The lymphatic system is a complex network of thin-walled vessels that return tissue fluid to the jugular lymphatic sac, which in turn empties into the jugular vein. This system is established as early as the sixth week of pregnancy, and obstruction of these channels alters the development of the vessel systems, causing dilation of the lymphatic channels with backup of tissue fluid.[1–3] When this obstructive process occurs at the level of the jugular lymphatics, it leads to dilation of these vessels and results in the characteristic cystic hygroma.[3] It is also believed that a more severe obstructive process with failure in communication can lead to progressive, severe lymphedema or nonimmune hydrops.[4] Chervenak and colleagues have suggested that resorption of this fluid, or possibly the use of alternate channels for fluid drainage, sometimes results in the resolution of cystic hygromas.[4] The persistence of redundant skin folds is seen at birth as webbing of the neck (pterygium coli), which is also observed in Turner's syndrome, Noonan syndrome, or familial pterygium coli.

Prenatal Diagnosis

Cystic hygromas have been diagnosed successfully prenatally and reported in the literature. Prenatal diagnosis of cystic hygromas is not very difficult and can be made as early as the first trimester of pregnancy (see Fig. 40-1).[5] These lesions are easily recognized by the distorted appearance of the fetal neck, characterized by pericervical cystic structures located in the posterolateral area, some with septations, others without; however, most are associated with fetal hydrops (see Fig. 40-1). The size of these lesions is also variable; some may be small and confined to the neck region, whereas others may extend down to the back, trunk, or even pelvic area.

Because cystic hygroma is associated with a number of other abnormalities, both structural and chromosomal, it is important to carry out a careful anatomical survey of the entire fetal anatomy. Renal abnormalities, cardiac anomalies, single umbilical artery, and adrenal masses should all be ruled out. Fetal karyotyping should also be performed, since this lesion is associated with Turner's syndrome in about half of the cases. Other chromosomal abnormalities—such as trisomy 13, 18, and 21—have also been reported (Table 40-2).[1,5]

The differential diagnosis includes other cervical abnormalities, such as cephalocele, cystic teratoma of the neck, or cephalomeningocele. Cystic hygromas can be distinguished from the previously mentioned structures by the fact that cystic hygroma presents as an echolucent, fluid-filled, posterolateral sac originating in the

TABLE 40–1. PRENATAL ULTRASOUND DIAGNOSIS OF FETAL TUMORS

Tumors
Head and Neck Tumors
Cystic hygroma
Epignathus
Goiter
Hemangioma
Neuroblastoma
Proboscis
Thyroid teratoma
Intracranial Tumors
Choroid plexus papilloma
Choroid plexus cyst
Craniopharyngioma
Glioblastoma
Teratoma
Cardiac Tumors
Fibroma
Rhabdomyoma
Chest Tumors
Bronchogenic cyst
Cystic adenomatoid malformation
Extralobar sequestration
Abdominal and Pelvic Tumors
Appendiceal abscess
Cavernous hemangioma
Choledochal cyst
Extrathoracic pulmonary sequestration
Meconium ileus
Mesoblastic nephroma
Neuroblastoma
Ovarian cyst and teratoma
Multicystic kidney disease
Polycystic kidney disease
Sacrococcygeal teratoma
Urachal cyst

Modified from Kurjak A, Zalud I, Jurkovic D, et al. Ultrasound diagnosis and evaluation of fetal tumors. J Perinat Med 1989; 17: 173.

pericervical area. Conversely, encephalocele, cystic teratoma, and cephalomeningocele all contain areas of echodensity consistent with herniation of brain tissue or neural elements. Additionally, a herniating lesion may indicate a smaller biparietal diameter or even the presence of ventriculomegaly.[6]

Medical Management and Outcome

Medical management depends largely on the karyotypic and sonographic findings. For example, if the diagnosis of cystic hygroma is made in the first trimester and karyotypic analysis reveals trisomy 18, then pregnancy termination may be offered to the patient. Similarly, if the diagnosis is made later, but before 24 weeks, and there are multiple congenital malformations or nonimmune hydrops, pregnancy termination may also be considered. When this diagnosis is made after 24 weeks and neither major congenital malformations nor nonimmune hydrops are present and the karyotype is normal (which occurs in 25% of cases), then such patients should be followed expectantly with serial ultrasound examinations. Cystic hygroma with the presence of hydrops occurs in 50% to 90% of cases and is associated with a mortality rate of almost 100%.[7,8]

Patient counseling should indicate that some cystic hygromas can resorb spontaneously, depending on the initial size of the lesion. If resorption occurs, a favorable neonatal outcome can be expected, although cosmetic surgery may be necessary postnatally.

EPIGNATHUS

Etiopathology

An epignathus is a large, disfiguring teratoma that arises out of the fetal mouth and may involve the sphenoid bone, pharynx, tongue, and/or jaw.

Prenatal Diagnosis

Epignathuses are rare lesions, and prenatal diagnosis has only been reported twice (Fig. 40-2).[9,10] Both cases were described as huge masses emanating from the mouth, containing solid and cystic components.

Medical Management and Outcome

Since these lesions can be of variable size and involve multiple structures, management depends on both size and location. For example, some lesions may alter the facial anatomy significantly or grow into the face or head. If such cases are diagnosed before 24 weeks gestation, termination may be offered; otherwise management should be expectant.

FETAL GOITER

Etiopathology

Fetal goiter is an enlargement of the thyroid gland, presenting as a solid neck mass with some echolucent areas when observed with ultrasound. The usual cause is maternal ingestion of iodine preparations.[11] Fetal goiter may also be caused by maternal diseases such as Graves' disease or the treatment of hyperthyroidism with iodine or, rarely, with propylthiouracil. In cases involving maternal Graves' disease, there is transplacental passage of a thyroid-stimulating substance, IgG immunoglobulin, which crosses the placenta and can cause hyperthyroidism of the fetus as well.

Goiters resulting from maternal hypothyroidism may be caused by treatment given to the mother, deficiency of iodine, or a congenital metabolic disorder of thyroid synthesis. Congenital hypothyroidism, however, is rare.[12] Carswell and colleagues have reported the association of congenital hypothyroidism with maternal ingestion of as little as 12 mg/day of iodine preparations.[13] It is often recommended that treatment should be tailored to the maternal symptoms rather than attempting to achieve the non-pregnant, normal levels for thyroid hormones. Another cause of hypothyroid-

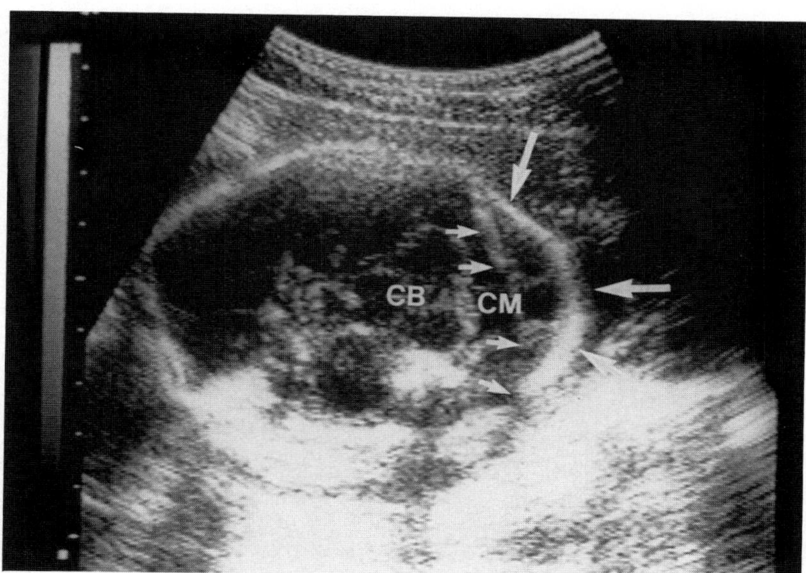

FIGURE 40-1. Fetal head scan at a level slightly inferior to the thalami, depicting the cerebellum (CB) and the cisterna magna (CM). Posterior to these structures is a septated echolucent sac representing a cystic hygroma.

ism includes thyroid hormone-enzyme deficiency, which can also result in goiter with varying effects, ranging from hypothyroidism to a euthyroid state.

Prenatal Diagnosis

The antenatal diagnosis of fetal goiter may be difficult but is based solely on the identification of a mass in the neck region of the fetus that causes hyperextension of the fetal head (Fig. 40-3). This mass may be solid but have a fairly homogenous and echolucent consistency.[11,14] When the mass compresses the fetal esophagus, polyhydramnios may result. Conversely, the mass may become so large that it actually precludes normal vaginal delivery, primarily because of the hyperextension of the fetal head.

Absolute prenatal diagnosis of a fetal goiter is difficult, since differential diagnosis of a neck mass in the fetus may include hemangiomas, cystic hygromas, teratomas, and bronchial cleft cysts. Clearly, the possibility of prenatal diagnosis is enhanced by the size of the lesion, the homogeneity of the mass, and the clinical setting. Few prenatal diagnoses of fetal goiter have been reported.[15–17]

Medical Management and Outcome

Medical management depends largely on the cause of the fetal goiter. For example, fetal goiter resulting from aggressive maternal propylthiouracil therapy would be best managed by a significant reduction in medication, and patients taking iodide would require discontinua-

TABLE 40-2. SUMMARY OF REPORTS OF PRENATAL DIAGNOSES OF CHOROID PLEXUS CYSTS BY ULTRASONOGRAPHY AND EVALUATED BY KARYOTYPE

REFERENCE	CASES	KARYOTYPE	FETAL OUTCOME
Furness et al	30	27 normal; 3 trisomy 18	Follow-up not reported
Chudleigh et al	5	All normal	Cysts disappeared in all cases by 20–23 weeks; all neonates were normal
Nicolaides et al	4	1 normal; 3 trisomy 18	3 TOP. Cyst disappeared in one case by 23 weeks; neonate was normal
Ricketts et al	4	3 normal; 1 trisomy 21	Cysts disappeared in two cases by 21 weeks and in one case by 36 weeks. Cyst was detected in trisomic case at 23 weeks. No follow-up reported
Benacerraf et al	2	2 normal	Cysts resolved by 22 and 28 weeks. Both neonates were normal
Ostlere et al	11	All normal	Cysts resolved in all cases by 21–34 weeks; all neonates were normal
Bundy et al	1	Trisomy 18	1 TOP. Postmortem examination was not available
Gabrielli et al	65	61 normal; 4 trisomy 18	5 TOP. All cysts disappeared by early third trimester except one; all neonates were normal

Reprinted with permission from Gabrielli S, Reece EA, et al. The clinical significance of prenatally diagnosed choroid plexus cysts. Am J Obstet Gynecol 1989;160:1207.

* TOP, Termination of pregnancy.

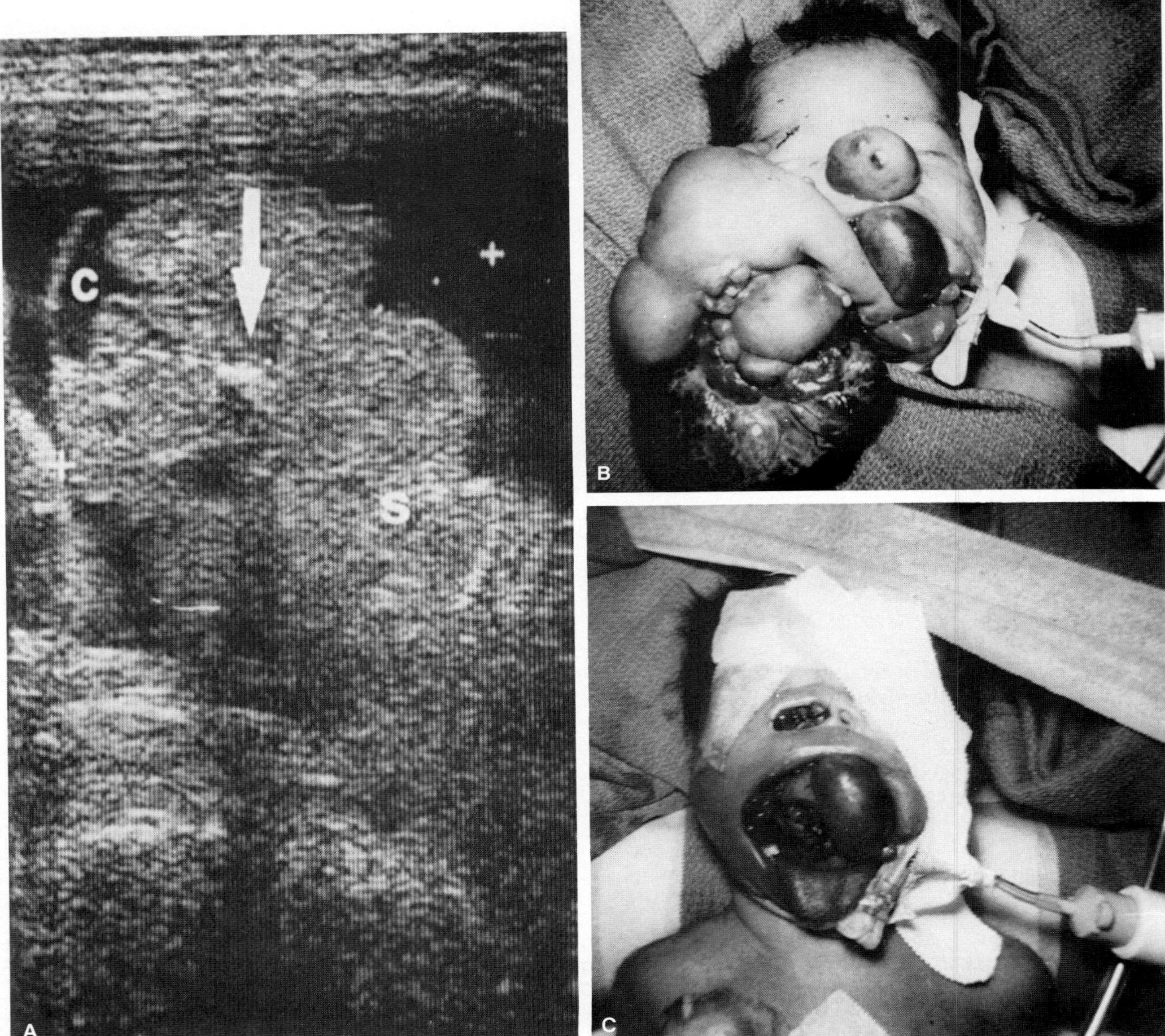

FIGURE 40–2. (**A**) Sonogram of a 32-week fetus, demonstrating a complex mass with solid (S) and cystic (C) components. The arrow points to areas of calcification with acoustic shadowing. (**B**) Mass arising from the palate, obstructing the mouth and nostrils of the neonate. (**C**) Appearance of mass after initial resection. (Reproduced with permission from Chervenak FA, Tortora M, Moya FR, et al. Antenatal sonographic diagnosis of epignathus. J Ultrasound Med 1984;3:235.)

tion of the drug. Similarly, the prognosis is relative to the cause of the fetal goiter. If hypothyroidism is diagnosed at birth, then aggressive supplemental treatment is necessary, since prolonged hypothyroidism may be associated with severe mental retardation.

Prenatal diagnosis of fetal goiter accompanied by a large lesion and hyperextension of the head may preclude vaginal delivery, making cesarean section the optimal mode of delivery. On the other hand, if the mass is small and the head is not hyperextended, vaginal delivery could be attempted.

OTHER NECK TUMORS

Other neck tumors include neuroblast of the neck with nodules within or on the surfaces of most of the abdominal organs and heart. Hemangiomas and teratomas of

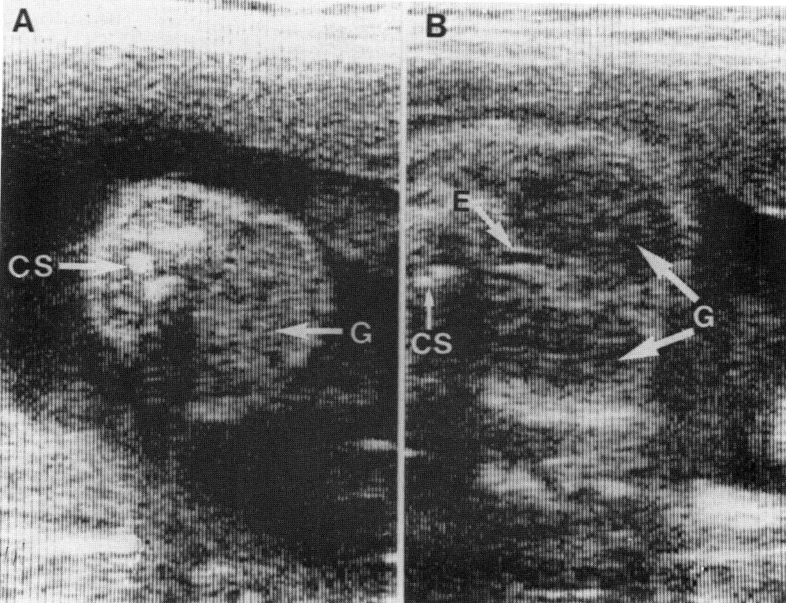

FIGURE 40-3. (**A**) Fetal goiter at 27 weeks. The back of the neck and cervical spine (CS) are on the left. Echolucent areas are evident within the substance of the goiter (G). (**B**) Fetal goiter at 36 weeks. The cervical spine is again on the left. Swallowed amniotic fluid is visible within the esophagus (E). The goiter is clearly bilobed in this view. (Kourides IA, Berkowitz RL, Pan S, et al. Antepartum diagnosis of goitrous hypothyroidism by fetal ultrasonography and amniotic fluid thyrotropin concentration. J Clin Endocrinol Metab 1984;59:1016.)

the neck can also appear as a mixture of solid and cystic components. Like fetal goiter, these neck masses may compress the esophagus and, when very large, can lead to polyhydramnios.

INTRACRANIAL TUMORS

CHOROID PLEXUS PAPILLOMA

Etiopathology

Papillomas are usually benign tumors of variable size attached to the normal choroid plexus, occurring in one or both of the cerebral ventricles. However, in the majority of cases, the lesion is unilateral and found in the atrial portion of the lateral ventricle.

Prenatal Diagnosis

Papillomas are often recognized following the diagnosis of hydrocephalus. A unilateral dilation of the lateral ventricle, associated with an echogenic mass in the ipsilateral atrium of the lateral ventricle, would be highly indicative of a choroid plexus papilloma (Fig. 40-4).

Medical Management and Outcome

If the diagnosis is made antenatally, obstetric management should be unaltered. Patients should be allowed to go full term, or if severe hydrocephalus and polyhydramnios exist, pregnancy should be continued until there is pulmonic maturity. Postnatal surgery is the preferred treatment.[18] A good prognosis depends on the successful surgical removal of the tumor.

CHOROID PLEXUS CYST

Etiopathology

Choroid plexus cysts are thought to result from the folding of the neuroepithelium, which becomes filled with fluid and cellular debris.[19] The pediatric literature reports that many choroid plexus cysts occur as asymptomatic findings in children; however, some are reportedly associated with chromosomal anomalies, particularly trisomy 18.[19] At autopsy, these cysts are usually found to be less than 1 cm in diameter.[20,21]

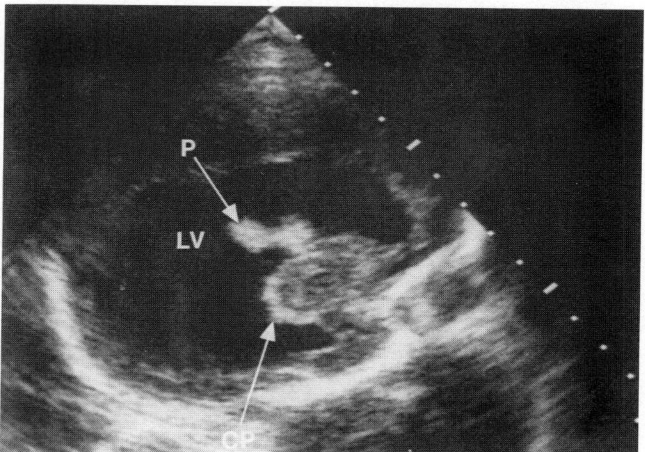

FIGURE 40-4. Parasagittal scan in a 30-week fetus with hydrocephalus secondary to a choroid plexus papilloma. The papilloma (P) is seen as an echogenic mass attached to the normal choroid plexus (CP) and protruding inside the dilated lateral ventricle (LV). (Pilu G, Rizzo N, Orsini LF, et al. Antenatal recognition of cerebral anomalies. Ultrasound Med Biol 1986;12:319.)

Prenatal Diagnosis

Choroid plexus cysts are usually located in the atrium of the lateral ventricle, in a location similar to where the choroid plexus papillomas are found (Fig. 40-5). Papillomas, however, are characterized by hyperechogenicity, in contrast to the characteristic echolucency of choroid plexus cysts.[20] On rare occasions, these cysts may be found at the level of the body of the lateral ventricle and, therefore, might be misdiagnosed as hydrocephaly.[19] Important diagnostic criteria for the choroid plexus cyst include the thick hyperechogenic wall of these lesions. Many of these cysts disappear in later gestation.

Medical Management and Outcome

Choroid plexus cysts are believed to be benign, and serial ultrasound examinations are recommended to exclude the development of hydrocephalus.[22] Otherwise, obstetric care should remain unaltered. It has been reported that these cysts are associated with aneuploidy.

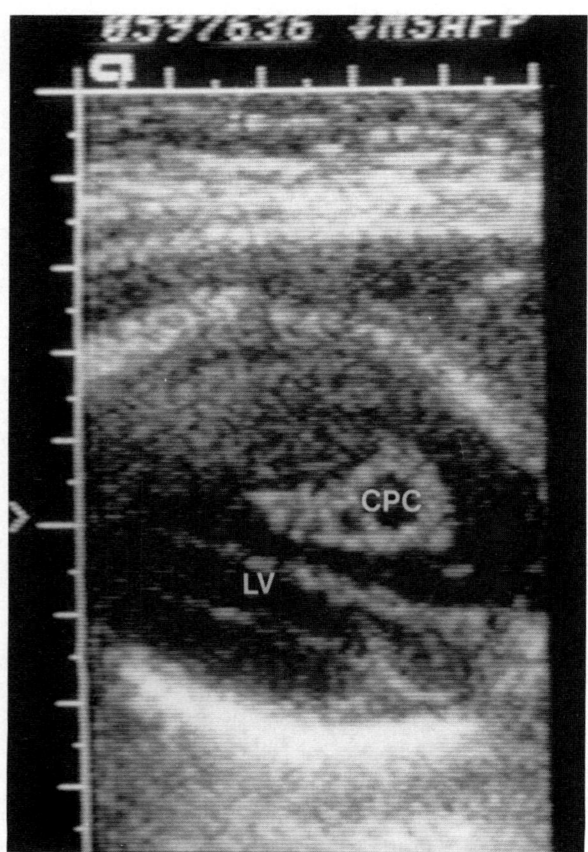

FIGURE 40–5. Scan of fetal head at the level of the lateral ventricles. In the near field is shown the choroid plexus containing a cystic area, choroid plexus cyst (CPC). In the far field, the lateral wall of the lateral ventricle can be seen delineating the borders of the lateral ventricle.

We have found the incidence of these lesions to be 6.1% in a select referral group of patients. This incidence was not significantly different from the 5.7% determined from a general-population screening program.[19] In this study, we noted that when a choroid plexus cyst was associated with an abnormal karyotype, other structural malformations were usually present and detectable by sonography. It remains to be determined whether the sonographic finding of an isolated choroid plexus cyst or the size of the cyst also carries an increased risk of a chromosomal anomaly. We believe that if such an increased risk exists, it is small when structural malformations are excluded. Some studies have suggested that many of these isolated choroid plexus cysts disappear spontaneously[23] and provided there is no evidence of associated malformations, and that these infants do well.[24–26] Persistently large cysts, however, have been noted to be associated with hydrocephalus.

TERATOMAS

Etiopathology

Teratomas are the most frequent intracranial tumors, accounting for 0.5% of all intracranial neoplasms.[26,27] Greenhouse and Neubauer reviewed 25 cases of intracranial teratomas and identified three groups of neonates with characteristic clinical and pathologic features.[26] Group 1 consisted of stillborn infants. In several of these newborns, the normal brain was completely replaced by teratomas. Others had large tumors with obstructive hydrocephalus. The newborns in group 2 were born alive but with enlarged heads. Tumors in group 3 were generally of intermediate size. Other teratomas diagnosed prenatally include the sacrococcygeal teratoma[29] which is discussed in the section Abdominal and Pelvic Tumors.

Prenatal Diagnosis

Fetuses with teratomas usually present with a sudden onset of large-for-dates size in otherwise normal pregnancies. The rapid growth in maternal abdominal girth usually results from the development of associated polyhydramnios. An enlarged mass with distortion of the anatomy is usually present in prenatally diagnosed cases. Multiple cystic spaces within a solid tumor were described in some of the reported cases. Calcification was noted by ultrasound in others; however, varying echodensities within the tumors were common features (Fig. 40-6; Table 40-3).

Medical Management and Outcome

In light of the poor prognosis associated with this lesion, termination of pregnancy should be offered to those patients who have not yet reached 24 weeks ges-

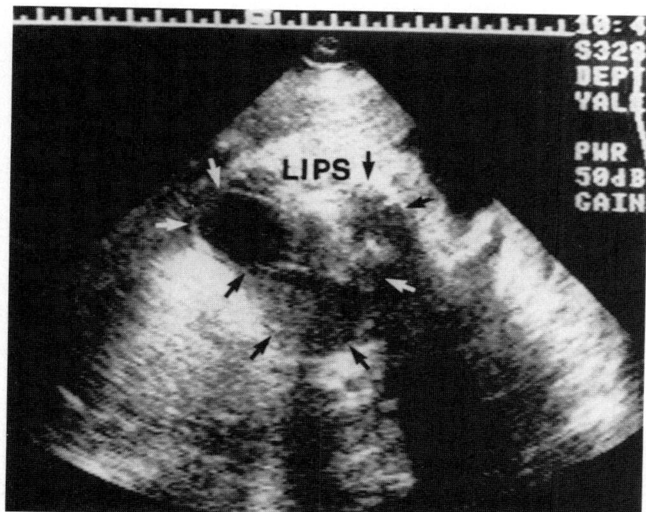

FIGURE 40–6. Frontal view depicting a semisolid mass below the fetal lips (see mass outlined with arrows).

tation. Beyond the latter gestational age, obstetric care should be otherwise unaltered. A pediatric surgeon should be consulted, because attempts should be made to resect the tumor postnatally.[28] There have been ten reported cases of surgically treated neonatal intracranial teratomas. The operative experience and outcome for neonates with this lesion have been reviewed by Whittle and Simpson and Ventureyra and Herder, who found that three deaths out of the ten reported cases occurred within 1 month of surgery.[28,29] Ventureyra and Herder reported a successful excision from a 6-day-old male with no evidence of recurrence at 4 months of age.[29] One of the patients of Whittle and Simpson, however, had a benign teratoma with a malignant recurrence 8 months postoperatively.[28] Takaku and colleagues reported one child whose tumor recurred at 2 years. Although long-term survival may be possible, the risk of neurologic impairment is high.[30] In two cases, treatment of unresectable lesions by shunting also resulted in early failure. In both cases, the high protein content of the cerebrospinal fluid resulted in repeated shunt obstruction, and death occurred within 3 months.[31,32]

CARDIAC TUMORS

Etiopathology

The most frequent cardiac tumor in the fetus or neonate is rhabdomyoma, which typically arises from the interventricular septum and interrupts electrical conduction within the heart.[33]

The overwhelming majority of primary cardiac tumors are benign and are usually incidental findings at autopsy. They include lipoma, fibroma, leiomyoma, hamartoma, myxoma, rhabdomyoma, and hemangioma. In the fetus, a cardiac mass may produce congestive heart failure and hydrops, which may lead to fetal demise.[34] Cardiac masses may be associated with arrhythmia, pericardial infusion, obliteration of the cardiac chamber, and embolic phenomena. Higher complication rates are expected with rapidly growing malignancies, such as rhabdomyosarcoma.[35]

Fibromas are seen less frequently than rhabdomyomas, but they present with similar symptoms. Both can be removed surgically after delivery, and both can appear as solid masses and must enter into the differential diagnosis when an echodense lesion is seen within the heart and a tumor is suspected.

Prenatal Diagnosis

Prenatal sonographic diagnosis of cardiac tumors has been reported. The usual findings include a solid echogenic mass in the right ventricle that abuts on the intraventricular septum (Fig. 40-7). In the case reported by Schaffer and colleagues, there was no evidence of fetal hydrops.[36] This fetus was delivered by cesarean section and did well immediately after birth. Postnatal echocardiographic examination confirmed the prenatal findings. The presumptive diagnosis of tuberous sclerosis was made based on the coexistence of café-au-lait spots, seizures, periventricular calcifications, and the cardiac mass. It should be pointed out that the diagnosis of rhabdomyoma cannot be made with confidence, since other solid tumors may present in a similar manner. Persistent tachyarrhythmia in the fetus may be associated with congestive heart failure, fetal hydrops, or death. The likelihood of poor outcome is increased when there is coexistent structural heart disease.[37]

Medical Management and Outcome

Cardiac neoplasm in the fetus may result in stillbirth or early neonatal death. These rare tumors are almost exclusively rhabdomyomas, although atrial hemangioma has been described.[38]

ABDOMINAL AND PELVIC TUMORS

Abdominal masses can represent neoplasms, as well as displaced or enlarged organs, such as the spleen, kidneys, or lungs.[1] Many of these lesions are part of systemic abnormalities (eg, multicystic kidney disease, the most common of all neonatal abdominal masses). This condition has been reported to represent 20% of all abdominal masses.[39] These lesions are covered in greater detail elsewhere in this book (see Chapter 38). Table 40-4 lists the masses of the fetal abdomen and pelvis that may present as solid, cystic, or mixed lesions. In this section the following lesions are discussed: ovarian cyst and teratoma, sacrococcygeal teratoma, and urachal cyst. Others, because of their rarity, are not covered.

TABLE 40–3. TERATOMAS DIAGNOSED BY ULTRASONOGRAPHY: REVIEW OF THE LITERATURE

AUTHOR	PRESENTING SYMPTOM	GESTATIONAL AGE AT DETECTION (WK)	HEAD SIZE, BPD (EXPECTED BPD FOR GA)
DeVore and Hobbins[67]	N/R	N/R	N/R (N/R)
Hoff and McKay[68]	Large for gestation date	28	Grossly enlarged
Crade[69]	Evaluate for placenta previa	Near term	10.5 (9.7)
Gadwood and Reynes[70]	Large for gestation date	31	Grossly enlarged
Vinters et al.[71]	Acute polyhydramnios	30	15.0 (7.4)
Kirkinen et al.[72]	Large for gestation date, sudden onset	32	14.8 (7.8)
Paes et al.[73]	Prior spontaneous abortions	32	Large
Lipman et al.[32] (case 1)	Large for gestation date	30	9.6 (7.4)
Lipman et al.[32] (case 2)	Breech presentation	36.5	10.0 (8.9)
Lipman et al.[32] (case 3)	Large for gestation date	20	12.3 (4.5)
Rostad et al.[65] (case 1)	Breech presentation	36	N/R
Rostad et al.[65] (case 2)	Persistent back pain	20	Massively enlarged N/A
Odell et al.[66]	N/R	22/28	14 cm (9.5)
Chervenak et al.[27]	N/R	N/R	N/R

AUTHOR	HYDROCEPHALUS	SONOGRAPHIC FEATURES	POLYHYDRAMNIOS	OUTCOME
DeVore and Hobbins[67]	N/R	Complex mass with multiple cysts	N/R	N/R
Hoff and MacKay[68]	No	Complex array of echoes of varying intensities replacing normal brain	Yes	Cesarean section; newborn survived a few seconds
Crade[69]	No	Cranial vault filled by bizarre cystic and echogenic regions	N/R	Cesarean section; newborn survived 2 hours
Gadwood and Reynes[70]	No	Solid and cystic areas with variable intensities	N/R	Cesarean section; newborn died shortly after delivery
Vinters et al.[71]	N/R	Solid mass with multiple cystic spaces	Yes	Cesarean section (prior cesarean section); stillborn
Kirkinen et al.[72]	N/R	Mass with high-level, irregularly arranged echoes	Yes	Vaginal delivery following cranial decompression; stillborn
Paes et al.[73]	N/R	Central echogenic mass with peripheral fluid-filled spaces	No	Vaginal delivery following cranial decompression; stillborn
Lipman et al.[32] (case 1)	N/R	Solid mass with multiple cysts; loss of normal brain architecture	No	Vaginal delivery following cranial decompression; stillborn
Lipman et al.[32] (case 2)	N/R	Solid mass with multiple low-level echoes and hyperechoic densities with shadowing	Yes	Cesarean section; newborn survived 3 minutes
Lipman et al.[32] (case 3)	N/R	Solid mass with multiple cysts	Yes	Cesarean section; newborn survived 5 minutes
Rostad et al.[65] (case 1)	Yes	Displacement of the right lateral ventricle by a large cystic mass		Cesarean section; newborn died within minutes of birth; spontaneous breathing
Rostad et al.[65] (case 2)	N/R	Massive tumor distorted extension of tumor into left side of face and neck	N/R	—
Odell et al.[66]	N/R	Dilation of left ventricles (22) with large mass (28)	Yes	Cesarean section survived 9.5 hours
Chervenak et al.[27]	Yes	Solid and cystic mass; hydrocephalus	N/R	Cesarean section survived 1 hour

N/R = not recorded.

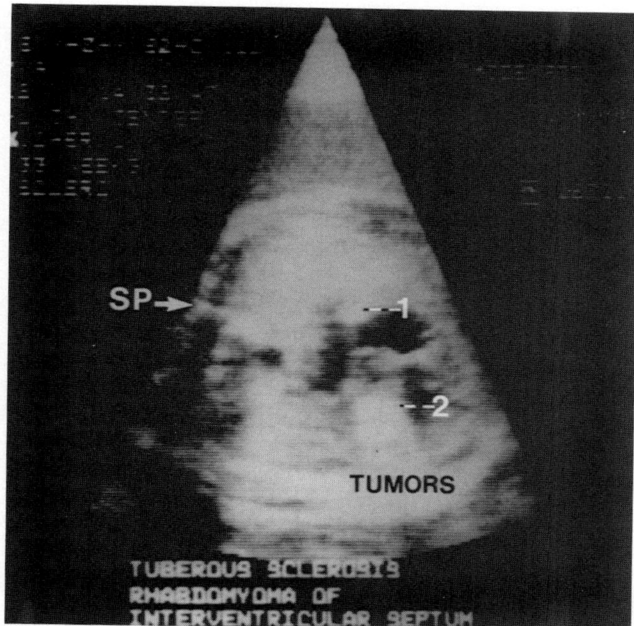

FIGURE 40–7. Transverse scan showing rhabdomyoma in a patient with tuberous sclerosis. sp, spine. (Courtesy of Dr. Joshua Copel, Yale University School of Medicine.)

OVARIAN CYST

Etiopathology

Ovarian cysts are one of the most common causes of abdominal–pelvic masses in female neonates. These cysts are unilateral and unilocular with a high variation in size. The cause of this disease is still uncertain; however, excessive ovarian stimulation by gonadotropins is considered to be a likely cause.[40–43] Usually derived from the germinal or graafian follicle, these cysts may initially develop as follicle cysts or corpus luteum cysts.

It has been demonstrated that these cysts appear earlier than the 30th week of pregnancy and may decrease in size during the remainder of the gestation. This decrease is thought to reflect the decline in gonadotropin near term and presumably results from the maturation of the hypothalamus in response to the negative feedback of estrogen.[40]

The association between ovarian cysts and juvenile hypothyroidism is well known. More recently, Jaffrey and colleagues reported two cases of congenital hypothyroidism associated with neonatal ovarian cyst.[43]

Prenatal Diagnosis

Ovarian cysts should be considered when a fetus presents with a unilateral, unilocular, echolucent structure in the abdominal–pelvic region, especially if the bladder and stomach can be seen separately (Fig. 40-8).[44] Prenatal diagnosis of large fetal ovarian cysts with ultrasonography has been reported on several occasions based on the following criteria: presence of a cystic structure that is symmetrical in shape, usually unilateral, and separate from the gastrointestinal and urinary tracts in a female fetus.[44,46–52] Rizzo and colleagues reported 14 pregnancies in which prenatal diagnosis of ovarian cysts was made and confirmed prenatally in 11 of the cases (78.5%).[51] In one case, the diagnosis was erroneously interpreted prior to birth as an ovarian cyst but was found neonatally to be a kidney duplication. In two cases, the cysts spontaneously disappeared prior to birth. In another case, an intra-abdominal cyst, presumably arising from the ovary, was detected at 34 weeks.

Polyhydramnios has been reported in 10% of cases of fetal ovarian cysts and probably results from intestinal obstruction.[51] Other lesions that ought to be excluded when one observes a unilateral echolucent cyst in the abdominal–pelvic region of a female fetus include urachal and mesenteric cysts. It may be very difficult to differentiate these cysts from one another. The urachal cysts usually present anteriorly, extending from

TABLE 40–4. MASSES OF THE FETAL ABDOMEN AND PELVIS

Solid
Ectopic spleen
Normal gastrointestinal system
Mesoblastic nephroma
Extrathoracic pulmonary sequestration
Wilms' tumor
Polycystic kidney
Chondroma
Chordoma
Sacrococcygeal teratoma
Cystic
Hydrometrocolpos
Choledochal cyst
Hemangioma of liver
Duplications of stomach
Cloacal dysgenesis
Cystic hygroma
Mesenteric, omental, or retroperitoneal cyst
Meconium pseudocyst
Urachal cyst
Renal cyst
Adrenal cyst
Sacrococcygeal teratoma
Myelomeningocele
Mesenchymal hamartoma of liver
Adrenal neuroblastoma
Mixed
Adrenal neuroblastoma
Multicystic kidney
Degenerating mesoblastoma
Normal small bowel
Meconium pseudocyst
Anterior myelomeningocele
Ovarian teratoma
Appendiceal abscess
Sacrococcygeal teratoma
Mesenchymal hamartoma
Cavernous hemangioma of liver

Kurjak A, Latin V. Fetal and placental abnormalities. In: Kurjak A, ed. Progress in medical ultrasound. II. Amsterdam: Excerpta Medica, 1981.

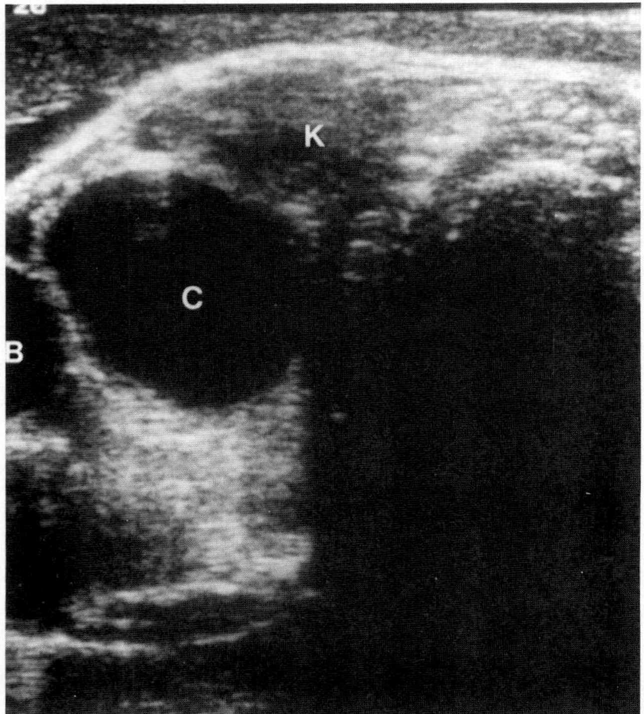

FIGURE 40–8. Oblique scan of the abdomen of a female fetus with an ovarian cyst. The cystic lesion (C) can be seen separately from the bladder (B) or the kidney (K). (From Romero et al., Prenatal diagnosis of congenital anomalies. Norwalk, CT: Appleton Lange, 1988:308).

the bladder to the umbilicus, whereas the ovarian cyst is midline, separate from and not contiguous with the bladder. The diagnosis of mesenteric cyst is usually made by exclusion. These subtle differences might be helpful in differentiating these very similar lesions.

Medical Management and Outcome

Management of a fetus with an ovarian cyst depends on the size and echopattern of the cyst. Serial ultrasound examinations, however, permit the evaluation of possible changes in size or structure. Many of these cysts undergo complete resolution before delivery or show changes suggesting complications such as endocystic bleeding.

Following the prenatal diagnosis of a probable ovarian cyst, serial ultrasound examinations can be used to detect any structural changes in the mass. An increase in size can cause distention of the fetal abdomen and, if persistent, may result in prune belly syndrome. If the mass is enlarged and the fetal abdomen is distended, it may be necessary to remove excess fluid by needle aspiration, thereby relieving the pressure on the abdominal wall and preventing the development of pulmonic hypoplasia. The latter condition can result from diaphragmatic elevation with compression of the lung parenchyma.

The mere presence of ovarian cysts should not lead to any alteration in standard obstetric care. Vaginal delivery at term is possible,[53] but evaluation prior to delivery should be carried out, since cystic growth occasionally leads to dystocia. Cesarean section was performed routinely for these conditions in the past; however, sonographically guided needle aspiration may be conducted so as to permit normal vaginal delivery.[51] Infrequent complications such as distention of the fetal abdomen and torsion of the cyst may require active obstetric intervention.[52] Surgery should be reserved for such complications as torsion.[41,52] Adherence to the preceding conservative recommendations usually ensures a good prognosis for the infant. Postnatal laparotomy may be necessary for cysts that are large and do not resolve spontaneously.

SACROCOCCYGEAL TERATOMA

Etiopathology

Sacrococcygeal teratoma is one of the most common tumors seen in the newborn; of affected infants, 80% are female.[54] It is observed in the perinatal period, with approximately 60% arising from the sacrococcygeal region. These tumors are true neoplasms, arising from the presacral area and composed of cells representative of more than one germ layer. They are thought to be derived embryologically from multipotential cells segregated from primitive Hensen's node.[55] A classification system developed by the surgical section of the American Academy of Pediatrics is as follows: type I lesion is external and has no identifiable pelvic extension; type II shows an intrapelvic component, but the majority of the mass is external; type III, the presacral component, predominates over the external portion; and type IV, teratomas, is entirely intrapelvic and not externally identifiable. The combination of cystic and solid areas within the mass is the most common presentation.[56] Scattered calcifications are frequently present in these tumors, which probably represent fragments of bone. Type I and type II account for more than 80% of the cases.[57]

Although in 5% to 25% of cases there are associated anomalies, no specific types have been identified. These anomalies include spina bifida, obstructive uropathy, and cleft palate.[58]

The reported incidence of sacrococcygeal teratoma is one in 35,000 live births. Most of these cases are asymptomatic during pregnancy and are frequently not diagnosed until birth.[59] Reviewing the literature, Flake and colleagues reported that the vast majority of cases present from 20 to 34 weeks gestation with the uterus large-for-dates or with symptoms of acute polyhydramnios.[60] Presentation after 30 weeks is a relatively good prognostic sign, with fetal survival in six of eight reported cases, compared with survival in one of 14 cases presenting prior to 30 weeks. The presence of placentomegaly and hydrops was associated with in utero fetal demise soon after diagnosis in seven of 40 cases. Although chromosomal abnormalities or associated life-threatening congenital anomalies are rare,[61] the mortality rate is very high, appearing to result from a secondary effect of the tumor. Preterm labor with premature delivery is also common and associated with polyhydramnios. Other complications connected with this lesion include massive hemorrhage into the tumor with secondary high-output cardiac failure or fetal exsanguination, occurring both in utero and intrapartum.

Prenatal Diagnosis

Prenatal diagnosis of types I, II, and III involves the identification of the external mass arising from the sacral area. This mass, as mentioned earlier, may be multicystic with solid components and areas of calcification (Fig. 40-9).[57] The presence of fetal hydrops is a very poor prognostic sign.[61,63,64]

Real-time ultrasound and Doppler studies in afflicted fetuses have revealed a dilation of both ventricles (two standard deviations above the mean), higher mean combined ventricular output, higher abdominal aortic flow, and dilated inferior vena cava.[61] Some cases have shown an enlargement of the middle sacral artery, as this artery usually provides the vast majority of blood supply to the tumor.[62] Embolization of the middle sacral artery has been suggested as a reasonable surgical approach to fetuses with early signs of congestive heart failure.

Amniotic fluid α-fetoprotein and acetylcholinesterase enzyme values have been reported to be either high-normal or elevated, making it difficult to distinguish between neural tube defects and sacrococcygeal teratoma. In cases of severe polyhydramnios, as the volume of amniotic fluid increases, the dilution effect of α-fetoprotein by the amniotic fluid worsens and can result in a false-normal finding.

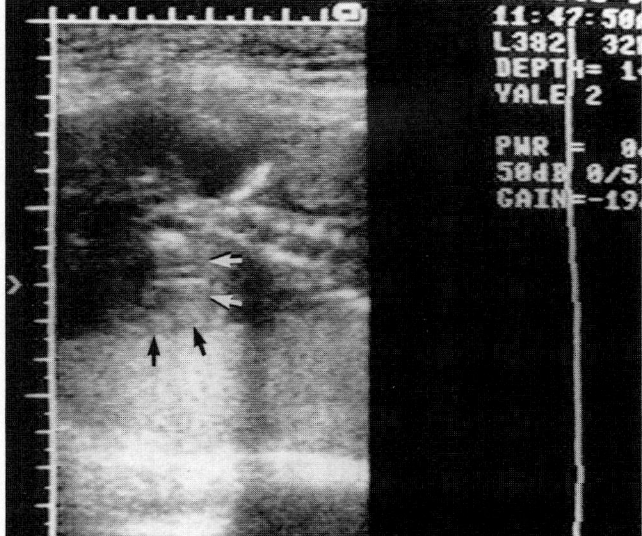

FIGURE 40–9. Sagittal scan of fetal spine depicting the lumbosacral area with a large semisolid mass attached to the posterior aspect of the spine (*arrows*).

Medical Management and Outcome

Appropriate treatment for fetal sacrococcygeal teratoma remains undefined. For cases diagnosed after 30 weeks, cesarean section is indicated following pulmonic maturity to avoid dystocia, uterine rupture, fetal hemorrhage of the tumor, or traumatic injury to the mother and fetus. When these lesions are diagnosed prior to 30 weeks, a high fetal death rate is observed and is often associated with the development of hydrops and placentomegaly. In both cases, serial ultrasound examinations should be done, provided neither hydrops nor placentomegaly has occurred, and attempts should be made to carry all pregnancies to pulmonic maturity.

There may be an evolving role for in utero surgical intervention. Flake and colleagues described their experience with six cases with sacrococcygeal teratoma associated with the development of hydrops and placentomegaly that resulted in fetal death.[60] In one case, open uterine fetal surgery was attempted and the tumor was excised. The procedure resulted in a reversal of the hydrops, a decrease in the cardiac output, and a reduction in the placentomegaly. This experience demonstrates that hydrops and fetal death may be caused by high-output cardiac failure resulting from arteriovenous shunting through the tumor, thus making a case for surgical intervention, particularly in subjects that present after 30 weeks.[63]

CONCLUSION

Fetal tumors constitute an eclectic group of neoplastic lesions that arise at varied times during fetal development. Fortunately, the majority are rare and can be diagnosed early in the prenatal period.

REFERENCES

1. Kurjak A, Zalud I, Jurkovic D, et al. Ultrasound diagnosis and evaluation of fetal tumors. J Perinat Med 1989;17:173.
2. Byrne J, Blancwa, Warburten O, et al. The significance of cystic hygroma in fetuses. Hum Pathol 1984;15:61.
3. Smith DW, Jones KL. Recognizable patterns of human malformation. Genetic embryologic and clinical aspects. 3rd ed. Philadelphia: WB Saunders, 1982:472.
4. Chervenak FA, Isaacson G, Blakemore KJ, et al. Fetal cystic hygroma: cause and natural history. N Engl J Med 1983;309:822.
5. Gustavii B, Edval H. First trimester diagnosis of cystic nuchal hygroma. Acta Obstet Gynecol Scand 1984;63:377.
6. Pearce JM, Griffin D, Campbell S. The differential diagnosis of cystic hygromata and cephalocele by ultrasound. J Clin Ultrasound 1985;13:317.
7. Pijpers L, Renss A, Stuart PA, et al. Fetal cystic hygroma: prenatal diagnosis and management. Obstet Gynecol 1988;72:233.
8. Chervenak FA, Isaacson G, Tortora M. A sonographic study of fetal cystic hygromas. J Clin Ultrasound 1985;13:317.

9. Chervenak FA, Tortora M, Moya FR, et al. Antenatal sonographic diagnosis of epignathus. J Ultrasound Med 1984;3:235.
10. Kang KW, Hissong SL, Langer A. Prenatal ultrasound diagnosis of epignathus. J Clin Ultrasound 1978;6:330.
11. Weiner S, Scarf JI, Bolognesi RJ, et al. Antenatal diagnosis and treatment of fetal goiter. J Reprod Med 1980;24:39.
12. Fisher DA, Dussault JH, Foley TP Jr, et al. Screening for congenital hypothyroidism. Results of screening one million North American infants. J Pediatr 1979;94:700.
13. Carswell F, Kurr MM, Hutchinson JH. Congenital goiter and hypothyroidism produced by maternal injection of iodides. Lancet 1970;1:1241.
14. Barone CM, Van Natta FC, Kourides IA, et al. Sonographic detection of fetal goiter and unusual causes of hydramnios. J Ultrasound Med 1985;4:625.
15. Kurjak A, Latin V. Fetal and placental abnormalities. In: Kurjak A, ed. Progress in medical ultrasound II. Amsterdam: Excerpta Medica, 1981.
16. Kourides IA, Heath CV, Ginsberg F. Measurement of thyroid simulating hormone in human amniotic fluid. J Clin Endocrinol Metal 1982;54:635.
17. Kourides IA, Berkowitz RL, Pan S, et al. Antepartum diagnosis of goitrous hypothyroidism by fetal ultrasonography and amniotic fluid thyrotropin concentration. J Clin Endocrinol Metab 1984;59:1016.
18. Matson DD, Crofton FDL. Papilloma of the choroid plexus in childhood. J Neurosurg 1960;17:1002.
19. Gabrielli S, Reece EA, Pilu G, et al. The clinical significance of prenatally diagnosed choroid plexus cysts. Am J Obstet Gynecol 1989;160:1207.
20. Shuangshoti S, Netsky MG. Neural epithelial (colloid) cysts of the nervous system: further observation on pathogenesis location in histochemistry. Neurology 1966;16:887.
21. Shuangshoti S, Netsky MG. Histogenesis of choroid plexus. Neurosci Res 1970;3:131.
22. Benacerraf BR, Laboda LA. Cyst of the fetal choroid plexus: a normal variant? Am J Obstet Gynecol 1989;160:319.
23. Lodeiro JG, Feinstein SJ, Lodeiro SB. Late disappearance of fetal choroid plexus cyst: case report and review of the literature. Am J Perinatol 1989;6:450.
24. Nicolaides KH, Rodeck CH, Gosden CM. Rapid karyotyping in nonlethal fetal malformations. Lancet 1986;1:283.
25. Ostlere SJ, Irving HC, Lilford RJ. A prospective study of the incidence and significance of fetal choroid plexus cyst. Prenat Diagn 1989;9:205.
26. Greenhouse AH, Neubauer KT. Intracranial teratoma of the newborn. Neurology 1960;3:126.
27. Chervenak FA, Isaacson G, Touloukian R, et al. Diagnosis and management of fetal teratomas. Obstet Gynecol 1985;66:666.
28. Whittle JR, Simpson DA. Surgical treatment of neonatal intracranial teratomas. Surg Neurol 1981;15:268.
29. Ventureyra ECG, Herder S. Neonatal intracranial teratomas. J Neurol Surg 1983;59:879.
30. Takaku A, Kodama N, O'Hara, H, et al. Brain tumor in newborn babies. Brain 1978;4:365.
31. Hirsh LF, Rorke LB, Schmidt HH. The usual cause of relapsing hydrocephalies congenital intracranial teratoma. Am Neurol 1977;34:505.
32. Lipman SP, Pretorius DH, Rumack CM, et al. Fetal intracranial teratoma: ultrasound diagnosis of three cases and a review of the literature. Radiology 1985;157:491.
33. Riggs T, Sholl JS, Ilbawi M, et al. Neonatal diagnosis of pericardial tumor with successful surgical repair. Pediatr Cardiol 1984;5:23.
34. Nadus AS, Ellison RC. Cardiac tumors in infancy. Am J Cardiol 1968;21:363.
35. Harrison MR, Goldbus MS, Phili RA. The unborn patient: prenatal diagnosis and treatment. Orlando, FL: Grune and Stratton, 1984.
36. Schaffer RM, Cabbad M, Minkoff H, et al. Sonographic diagnosis of fetal cardiac rhabdomyoma. J Ultrasound Med 1986;5:531.
37. Birnbaum SE, McGahan JP, Janos GG, et al. Fetal tachycardia and intramyocardial tumors. Am Coll Cardiol 1985;6:1358.
38. Gresser CD, Shime J, Rakowski H, et al. Fetal cardiac tumor: a prenatal echocardiographic marker for tuberous sclerosis. Am J Obstet Gynecol 1987;156:689.
39. Kurjak A, Latin V, Mandruzzat OG, et al. Ultrasound diagnosis and perinatal management of fetal genital urinary abnormalities. J Perinat Med 1984;12:291.
40. Ahmed S. Neonatal and childhood ovarian cyst. J Pediat Surg 1971;6:702.
41. Carlson DH, Griscom NT. Ovarian cyst in the newborn. American Journal of Roentgenology, Radium Therapy, & Nuclear Medicine 1972;116:664.
42. Morrison JE. Fetal and neonatal pathology. 3rd ed. London: Buttersworth. 1970:204.
43. Jaffrey SZ, Bree RL, Silver TM, et al. Fetal ovarian cyst: sonographic detection association with hypothyroidism. Radiology 1984;150:809.
44. Jaffe R, Ambramowicz J, Fejgin M, et al. Giant fetal abdominal cyst. Ultrasonic diagnosis and management. J Ultrasound Med 1987;6:45.
45. Valenti C, Kasner EG, Yerkamnov V, et al. Antenatal diagnosis of a fetal ovarian cyst. Am J Obstet Gynecol 1975;123:261.
46. Lee TJ, Blake S. Prenatal female abdominal ultrasonography and diagnosis. Radiology 1977;124:475.
47. Kraid M, Gilloly L, Taylor KJM. In utero demonstration of an ovarian cystic mass in ultrasound. J Clin Ultrasound 1980;8:251.
48. Touloukian RJ, Hobbins JC. Maternal ultrasonography and the antenatal diagnosis of surgical correctable fetal abnormalities. J Pediatr Surg 1980;15:373.
49. Mitsutake K, Abe T, Masumoto R, et al. Prenatal diagnosis of fetal dome masses by real-time ultrasound. Kurume Med J 1981;28:329.
50. Tabsh KM. Antenatal sonographic appearance of a fetal ovarian cyst. J Clin Ultrasound or J Ultrasound Med 1982;1:329.
51. Rizzo N, Gabrielli S, Perolo A, et al. Prenatal diagnosis and management of fetal ovarian cysts. Prenat Diagn 1989;9:97.
52. Lindeque BG, duToit JP, Muller LMM, et al. Ultrasonographic criteria for the conservative management of antenatally diagnosed fetal ovarian cysts. J Reprod Med 1988;33:196.
53. Breen JL, Bonamo JF, Maxson WS. Genital tract tumors in children. Pediatr Clin North Am 1981;28:355.
54. Donnellan WA, Swenson O. Benign and malignant sacrococcygeal teratomas. Surgery 1968;64:834.
55. Gross FE, Clatworthy W, Mekur IA. Sacrococcygeal teratomas in infants and children: a report of 40 cases. Surg Gynecol Obstet 1951;92:341.
56. Ein SH, Adeyemi SD, Marker K. Benign sacrococcygeal teratomas in infants and children. A 25 year review. Ann Surg 1980;191:382.
57. Gonzales-Crussi, Winkler RF, Mirkin DL. Sacrococcygeal teratomas in infants and children: relationship of histology and prognosis in 40 cases. Arch Pathol Lab Med 1978;102:420.
58. Pantojae, Lopez E. Sacrococcygeal teratomas in infants and childhood. NY State J Med 1978;78:813.
59. Gergely RZ, Eden R, Schriffin BS, et al. Antenatal diagnosis of congenital sacral teratoma. J Reprod Med 1980;24:229.
60. Flake AW, Harrison MR, Adzick NS, et al. Fetal sacrococcygeal teratoma. J Pediatr Med 1986;21:563.
61. Schmidtt KG, Silverman NA, Harrison MR, et al. High output of the cardiac failing fetus with large sacrococcygeal teratoma: diag-

nosis about echocardiography and Doppler ultrasound. J Pediatr 1989;114:1023.

62. Holzgreve W, Mahoney BS, Glick P, et al. Sonographic demonstration of fetal sacrococcygeal teratoma. Prenat Diagn 1985;5:245.
63. Alter DN, Reid KL, Marx GR, et al. Prenatal diagnosis of congestive heart failure in the fetus with sacrococcygeal teratoma. Obstet Gynecol 1988;71:978.
64. Pringel KC, Weiner CP, Sopper RT, et al. Sacrococcygeal teratoma. Fetal Therapy. 1987;2:80.
65. Rostad S, Kleinschmidt-DeMasters BK, Manchester DK. Two massive congenital intracranial immature teratomas with neck extension. Teratology. 1985;32(2):163.
66. Odell JM, Allen JK, Badura RJ, Weinberger E. Massive congenital intracranial teratoma: a report of two cases. Pediatr Pathol 1987;7(3):333.
67. Devore G, Hobbins J. Diagnosis of structural abnormalities in the fetus. Clin Perinatol 1979;6:293.
68. Hoff NR, Mackay IM. Prenatal ultrasound diagnosis of intracranial teratoma. J Clin Ultrasound 1980;8:247.
69. Crade M. Ultrasonic demonstration in utero of an intracranial teratoma. JAMA 1982;247:1173.
70. Gadwood KA, Reynes CJ. Intracranial teratoma. Illinois Med J 1983;164:196.
71. Vinters HV, Murphy J, Wittman B, Norman MG. Intracranial teratoma, antenatal diagnosis at 31 weeks' gestation by ultrasound. Acta Neuropathol 1982;58:233.
72. Kirkinen P, Suramo I, Jouppila P, Ilerva R. Combined use of ultrasound and computed tomography in the evaluation of fetal intracranial abnormality. J Perinatol Med 1982;10:257.
73. Paes BA, DeSa DJ, Hunter DJ, Pirani M. Benign intracranial teratoma—prenatal diagnosis influencing early delivery. Am J Obstet Gynecol 1982;143:600.

41

CHAPTER

FIRST-TRIMESTER PRENATAL DIAGNOSIS

John C. Hobbins and E. Albert Reece

The virtual explosion of technology in the last 10 years has given physicians special insight into fetal growth and development. This chapter is devoted to only one portion of the unfolding fetal story: early development.

Recently, prenatal diagnostic techniques have been directed toward early diagnosis, thus reducing the anxiety-laden waiting period and also permitting early termination of pregnancy. If that option is chosen by parents at an early gestational age, the overall risks are less. Opponents of prenatal diagnostic testing argue that its only function is to identify an anomalous fetus for "extinction." Although today's techniques do allow patients to know whether their fetus has a devastating problem, an affected fetus is not always aborted. For example, armed with the knowledge that a fetus has a major anomaly, optimal management can be achieved by arranging delivery in a tertiary-care center with experienced pediatricians and surgeons readily available. Further, patients can become psychologically prepared for the delivery of an anomalous child. When this information can be made available, it would be inexcusable not to allow patients at high risk for anomalies to have prenatal testing.

The major factor responsible for our enhanced ability to diagnose abnormal fetal development has been the exponential improvement in ultrasound imagery. In addition to providing a detailed view of embryonic/fetal anatomy even very early in pregnancy, sonography has enabled physicians to perform invasive procedures safely and obtain samples of amniotic fluid, chorionic villi, and fetal blood. With these techniques, we can conservatively estimate that at least half of all major fetal anomalies can be diagnosed before birth.

In this chapter, we will discuss the diagnostic possibilities now available in the United States. The material has been selected for its importance in today's diagnostic setting.

ULTRASOUND

Entire textbooks have been devoted to the diagnosis of fetal anomalies with ultrasound, so it is beyond the scope of this chapter to explore every diagnostic facet comprehensively. Rather, we will focus on the comprehensive first-trimester evaluation.

Even before the inception of real-time ultrasound, it was clear that the embryo could be visualized with static scanners. In fact, the first-trimester crown–rump length (CRL) initially described by Robinson remains one of the most precise measurements for predicting gestational age.[1]

Real-time ultrasound enables us to focus on an often mobile first-trimester target. Previously it was a triumph simply to identify the embryonic poles, but over the past 7 years significant improvements in gray-scale imagery have enabled us to scrutinize the embryo in detail. The newest technology uses a transvaginal approach to the ultrasound evaluation of the first-trimester conceptus. The transvaginal probe can be directed to within a few centimeters of the embryo, and since there is less dissipation of sound over a shorter pathway, very high frequency probes can be used. Coupled with the ability to use highly focused transducers, this technology dramatically improves both axial and lateral resolution. Remarkable detail can be obtained with transvaginal ultrasound examination of embryos magnified several times.

CROWN-RUMP LENGTH

Using transabdominal ultrasound, a gestational sac can be visualized as early as 5 menstrual weeks, and an embryo can be identified as early as 6.5 menstrual weeks. Using transvaginal probes, these structures can be visualized about a week earlier (Fig. 41-1). If an embryo can clearly be seen, an actively beating heart should also be visualized; failure to do so may indicate an early embryonic demise.

By 7 menstrual weeks, the investigator should be able to distinguish two fetal poles and to measure the CRL by both transabdominal and transvaginal techniques. CRL correlates closely with gestational age until about 12 weeks; after that, the measurement is less reliable.

Brambati and associates reported that embryos ultimately diagnosed as having aneuploidy tended to have smaller CRLs than normals.[2] Pedersen and Molsted-Pedersen found that embryos of diabetic patients had a mean CRL less than that of embryos of nondiabetic patients.[3] In both cases, the temptation was to conclude that both chromosomal abnormalities and diabetes result in early (primary) growth curtailment. On the other hand, we have been unable to confirm the association between aneuploidy and decreased CRL.[4] Others have also failed to reproduce an early growth delay in diabetic patients associated with anomalies.[5] Further investigation in this area is needed.

YOLK SAC

The primary and early secondary yolk sacs play an essential role in early embryonic development. The structure that can be identified in virtually all pregnancies between 7 and 11 weeks of gestation is a remnant of the secondary yolk sac and a vestige of its active forerunner (Fig. 41-2). The early secondary yolk sac produces the gonadocytes, blood vessels and red blood cells, and the epithelia for the digestive and respiratory tracts, and invaginates to generate portions of the mid-gut. The yolk sac is also the site of early protein synthesis; alpha-fetoprotein is the principal protein synthesized.

In experiments with rodents, we have demonstrated that diabetes-associated congenital malformations in the embryo are associated with cytoarchitectural changes in the yolk sac, observed with both light and electron microscopy. Further, these changes were not thought to be parallel to the embryopathy, as selective yolk sac injury in our laboratory and those of others have resulted in anomalous embryos (Fig. 41-3). We have therefore hypothesized that the yolk sac is the target site for insults resulting in diabetes-associated embryopathy (Fig. 41-4). We also believe that these findings are not unique to diabetes and may underlie other maldevelopmental events as well.

Unfortunately, the vestigial remnant of the secondary yolk sac seems to convey little information about early embryonic/fetal development. There are, however, data to suggest that failing to visualize a yolk sac or finding one either less than 2 mm in diameter or solid in appearance may be associated with a missed abortion or a fetal anomaly.[6] An association between a yolk sac greater than 5 mm in diameter and fetal abnormalities was also noted.[6]

ULTRASOUND DIAGNOSIS OF CONGENITAL ANOMALIES

Cranial Anomalies

In the first trimester the fetal cranium undergoes some developmental changes that can easily be chronicled with ultrasound.[6,7] Between 6 and 8 menstrual weeks, a large echospared area can normally be seen in the posterior cranium, reflecting the confluence of the third and

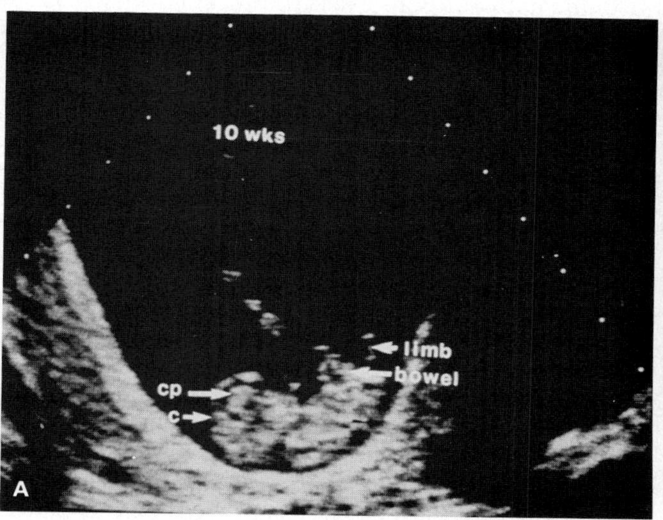

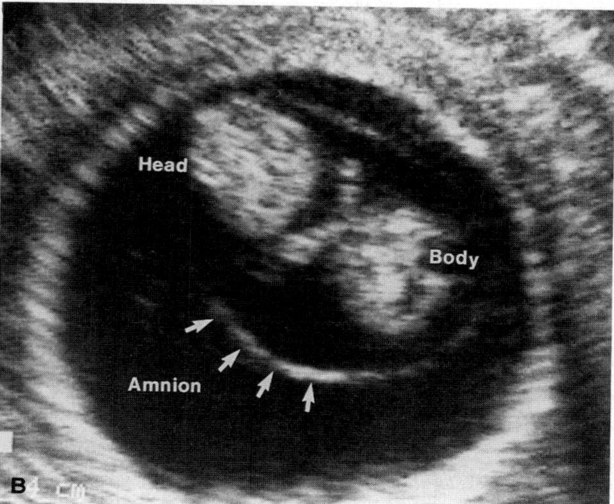

FIGURE 41-1. First trimester fetus. (**A**) Some structures are recognizable: choroid plexus (cp), calvarium (c), herniated bowel, cord (extending anteriorly), and the lower limbs. Crown–rump length is measured from the calvarium to the end of the rump. (**B**) The amnion is not yet in apposition with the chorion. Head, body, and upper limbs are easily recognized.

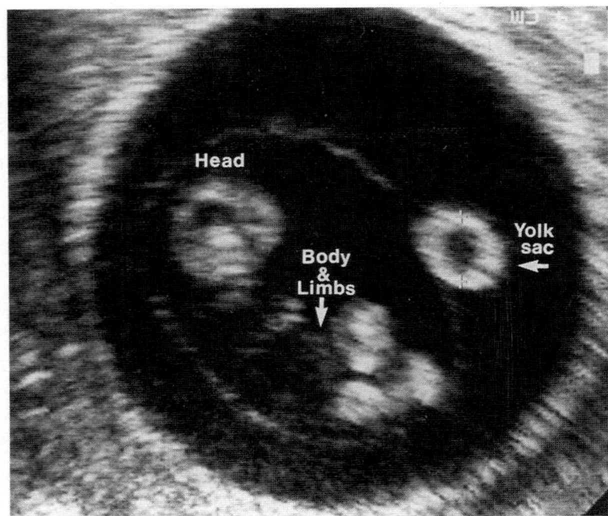

FIGURE 41–2. The yolk sac is seen outside the amnion as a clearly defined spherical structure with an echodense border and echolucency inside. The head, body, and limbs can also be seen.

fourth ventricles. This completely normal finding can be mistaken for a posterior fossa cyst. Throughout the first and early second trimesters, the lateral ventricles appear large, leading the inexperienced observer to suspect ventriculomegaly. In addition, the earliest we have noted the calvarium to be well demonstrated is at 10

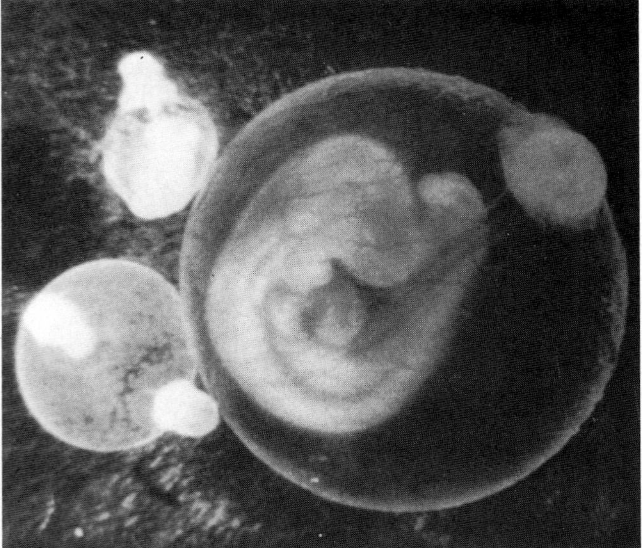

FIGURE 41–3. (Right) A normal-appearing 12-day-old rat embryo grown in normal male rat serum for 48 hours. Confluent and vitelline blood vessels course between the embryo and the ectoplacental cone. The embryo within the yolk sac appears normal, with primordial organs recognizable. (Left) Two rat conceptuses grown in male rat serum for 48 hours, but with added D-glucose. The entire conceptus is abnormal in each case: note the smaller size, absence of vascularization, and abnormal embryos.

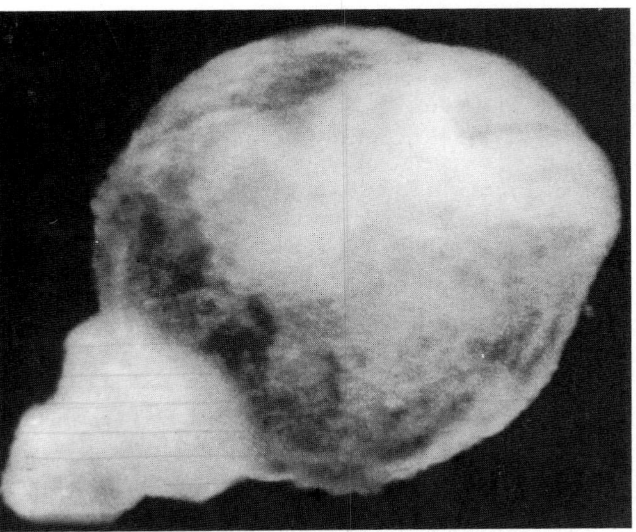

FIGURE 41–4. Magnified picture of the abnormal yolk sac and embryo shown in Figure 41-3. Note the lack of normal blood-vessel pattern throughout the surface of the yolk sac. The yolk sac membrane is opaque with the embryo with clearly malformed.

menstrual weeks, so anencephaly is a diagnosis best made beyond this gestational age. Despite the potential difficulties encountered in diagnosing cranial abnormalities in the first trimester, many cephalic anomalies can be identified, such as acrania, encephalocele, and anencephaly (Fig. 41-5).

It has become apparent that there are many variations on the cystic hygroma theme. When first using the vaginal probe, we occasionally began seeing a posterior nuchal membrane that extended from the fetal occiput to the upper dorsal surface of the fetus. Since then, we have observed lateral nuchal cysts, large septated echolucent cysts (classic cystic hygroma), and general body-wall edema (Fig. 41-6).

Because the fate of embryos displaying these "abnormalities" had not been clarified in the literature, we collected cases from Yale University and combined them with those identified by our colleagues at the University of Bologna, Italy.[8] Thus far, we have outcome data on 30 such embryos. Karyotypic information was available on 29: 15 had aneuploidy, while 14 had normal chromosomes. Six patients chose to terminate pregnancy and eight continued the pregnancy, delivering morphologically normal infants at term. In all eight cases, the nuchal findings disappeared by the middle of the second trimester, as did the generalized edema and pleural effusions previously noted.

It is noteworthy that no particular finding seemed to correlate with the presence or absence of aneuploidy. In other words, since there was an even mixture of modest and severe nuchal aberrations in the group with aneuploidy and the group with normal chromosomes, it was impossible to predict outcome based on the severity of ultrasound findings. As stated previously, this ob-

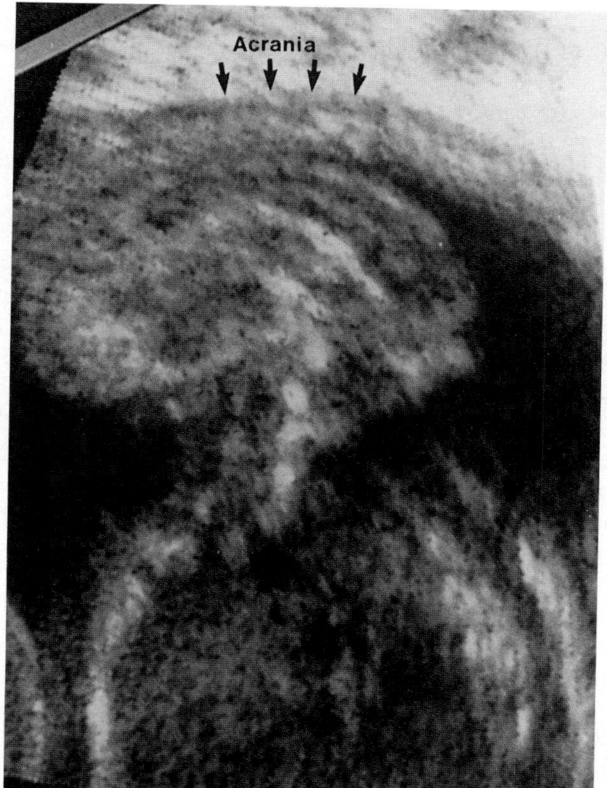

FIGURE 41–5. Ultrasound picture of a fetus with acrania. The calvarium calcifies at about 10 weeks; therefore, the absence of a calcified skull (black arrows) suggests a diagnosis of acrania.

servation resulted from our study of first-trimester development.

Cardiac Anomalies

Using the transvaginal transducer, the beating heart can be observed inside the embryo's chest cavity as early as 7 menstrual weeks. Using the same technique, a four-chamber view of the heart has been obtained as early as 12 menstrual weeks, allowing the diagnosis of major cardiac defects by the end of the first trimester in some cases.

Fetal cardiac malformation is one of the most common developmental abnormalities, occurring in as many as 8 per 1000 live births.[9] Our group has demonstrated the theoretical potential of identifying more than 90% of cardiac defects with an ultrasonically derived four-chamber view of the heart, accomplished in the second or third trimester.[10] With transvaginal scanning, gross cardiac anomalies such as large interventricular septal defects and hypoplastic chambers could well be identified before 14 weeks of gestation. Obviously, however, this theoretical possibility must be borne out by further investigation. Ventricular hypoplasia, which may represent a late change, cannot be excluded by a first-trimester examination.[11] Conversely, there is a suspicion that some interventricular septal defects may close in late gestation. Earlier examination is preferable in the identification of cardiac defects, especially those often associated with chromosomal anomalies, since over 90% of fetuses with trisomy 13 and 18 and 30% of fetuses with trisomy 21 have cardiac defects.[12,13] The ability to image the embryonic heart with transvaginal sonography now takes on added significance.

Abdominal Anomalies

Fetal kidneys can be visualized as early as 10 weeks (Fig. 41-7), and the fetal bladder can be seen by 12 weeks in most cases.[6] Renal agenesis may be easier to diagnose in the first trimester because at that time there is enough amniotic fluid to aid in imaging intra-abdominal structures. On two recent occasions megacystis has been identified at or before 13 menstrual weeks.[14] Although in utero shunting of obstructive uropathies has been controversial, there is no doubt that early identification of the condition is critical to the suc-

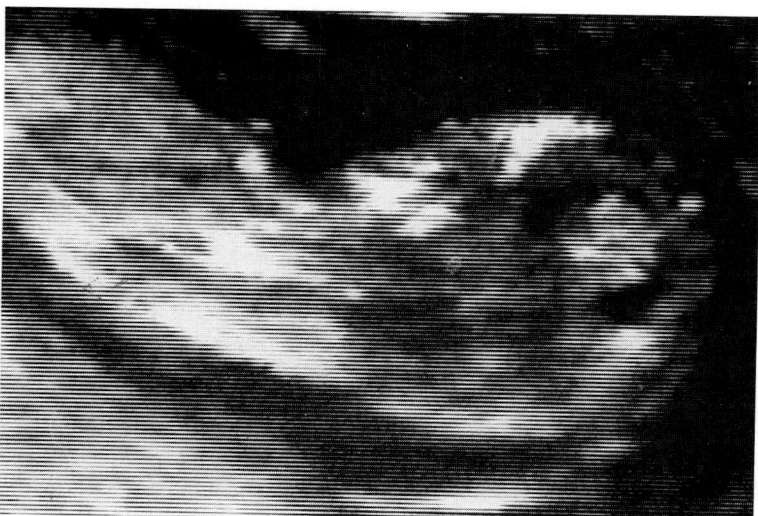

FIGURE 41–6. A large echolucent area envelops the back and sides of the fetal head and neck. These are typical features of a cystic hygroma.

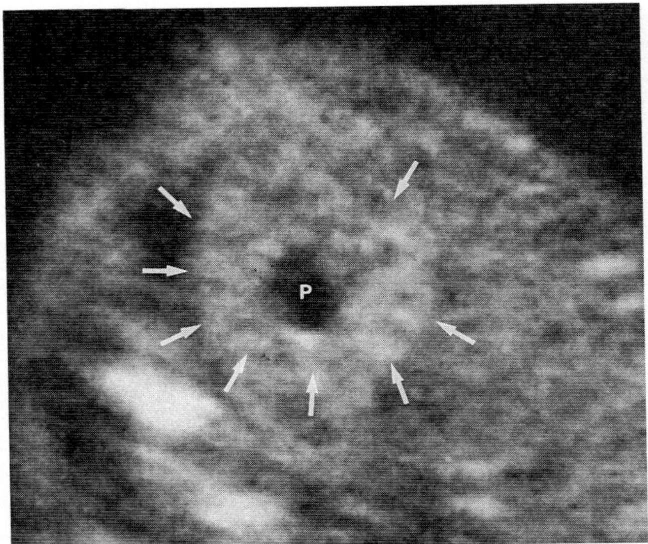

FIGURE 41–7. Kidney in an 11-week-old fetus with a dense echogenic rim (arrows) and a slightly dilated renal pelvis (P).

cess of intrauterine "surgery" in cases of fetal lower urinary tract obstruction. Demonstrating the presence of a normal urinary tract greatly allays the fears of a patient in the first trimester who has previously delivered a baby with a severe renal anomaly.

Occasionally, highly echogenic structures in the fetal abdomen can be demonstrated. In most cases, this represents an unusually echogenic small bowel. In the second trimester, this finding has been correlated with a variety of conditions, including cytomegalovirus infection, cystic fibrosis, Down syndrome, and early signs of necrotizing enterocolitis.[15] Thus far, it has been our experience that increased bowel echogenicity in the first trimester is of no significance and usually disappears by the second trimester.

Spinal/Skeletal Anomalies

Neural tube defects can be definitively diagnosed as early as the late first trimester.[6] Both lateral pedicles and the spinal body ossify by the 10th menstrual week, allowing the visualization of the spinal column and potential defects (Fig. 41-8). Our group has identified a low sacral defect at 11 weeks using transvaginal sonography.[4] Long bone lengths can consistently be measured by the 12th week of gestation. Although severe skeletal dysplasias (eg, phocomelia, amniotic band syndrome) could well be diagnosed at this time, little is known about the early development of many of the other short-limb dysplasias (eg, osteogenesis imperfecta, thanatophoric dysplasia, camptomelic dysplasia). Certainly in some forms of skeletal dysplasias, such as heterozygous achondroplasia, significantly shortened limbs are not noted until late in the second trimester.[16] With transvaginal sonography, fetal hands, feet, and even digits can be visualized by the 12th menstrual week (Fig. 41-9).

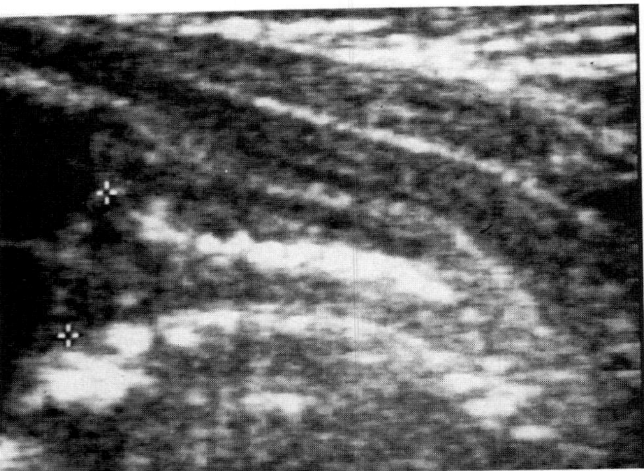

FIGURE 41–8. A 12-week-old fetus with spine depicted as parallel lines extending from the neck to the sacrum. At the posterior aspect of the head can be seen the cerebellum (asterisks).

Investigators have begun to explore the relationship of aneuploidy and ultrasound findings in the fetal hand. Benacerraf has found that some fetuses with Down syndrome have a hypoplastic or absent middle phalanx of the fifth digit.[17] The concept is limited somewhat by the facts that some normal fetuses have this fifth-finger abnormality and that in some cases the phalangeal hypoplasia was quite subtle. Given that the middle phalanx of the fifth digit of a 12-week-old fetus is normally minute, a "positive" finding would have to be the absence of the middle phalanx.

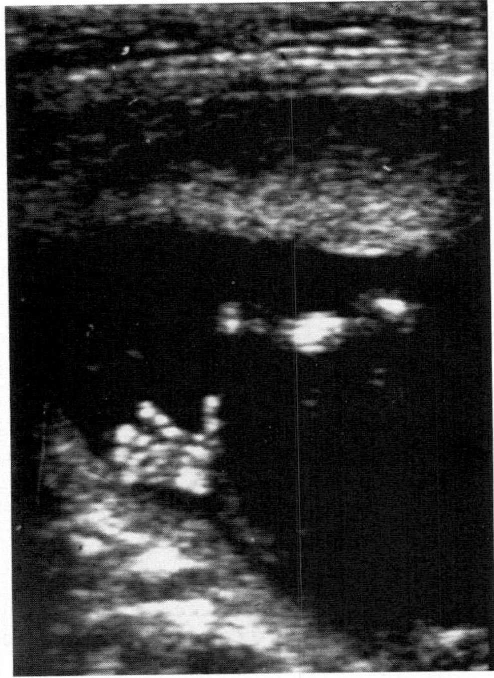

FIGURE 41–9. Hand of an 11-week-old fetus, with fingers and digits clearly delineated.

In some syndromes such as chondroectodermal dysplasia (Ellis-van Creveld syndrome), polydactyly (a diagnosis distinctly possible at 12 weeks with ultrasound) is uniformly associated with the condition, which has an autosomal recessive pattern of inheritance. In fact, polydactyly may be the first of many signs to be identified in this condition. A patient whose fetus is at risk for this devastating condition would derive significant psychological benefit from an early diagnosis.

A variety of conditions such as amniotic band syndrome, tibular radial aplasia syndrome, and body stalk anomalies can be diagnosed with ultrasound in the first trimester.[9]

BIOCHEMICAL SCREENING

Maternal serum alpha-fetoprotein (MSAFP) screening has become almost uniformly accepted as an efficacious way to identify patients at greater risk of having a fetus with a neural tube defect. High MSAFP levels have also been associated with fetal conditions such as ventral wall defects, renal agenesis, obstructive uropathies, and gastrointestinal obstructions, all of which can be potentially diagnosed with ultrasound.

In the early days of MSAFP screening, it was noted that mothers with fetuses eventually diagnosed with Down syndrome tended to have lower MSAFP levels than mothers with normal fetuses.[18,19] Subsequent investigation allowed the calculation of a "corrected" risk of Down syndrome for a given patient based on her age, weight, and MSAFP level.[20]

Since MSAFP can be quantified with very sensitive assays before 14 weeks, it was originally hoped that MSAFP screening could be pushed back into the first trimester, but initial results have been puzzling.[21–23] Thus far, the association between high MSAFP and neural tube defects has been inconsistent. However, one study has found an association between low MSAFP and aneuploidy in the first trimester. Since this may be highly assay-dependent, this finding must be confirmed by other investigators; if valid, extensive study will be needed to accurately assess the predictive value of this method. We have found that in second-trimester MSAFP screening, one aneuploidy is identified for every 120 patients having an amniocentesis (for low MSAFP).[23] Since invasive testing (chorionic villus sampling or early amniocentesis) ultimately is required for the diagnosis of aneuploidy, the benefits of early MSAFP screening must be carefully evaluated.

CHORIONIC VILLUS SAMPLING

Because the placental villi and the fetus are derived from the same tissue, villi sampling has become an attractive source of data for genetic studies on the fetus. Further, these cells are actively growing; they come from a single cell line, and tissue culture of these cells can be obtained more rapidly than that of amniotic fluid cells. The indications for CVS are similar to those for amniocentesis. The specimens obtained can be directly examined for karyotyping, or cultured for biochemical studies, gene mapping, or karyotypic analysis.

TRANSCERVICAL CVS

Although Hahnemann[24] first described an endoscopic technique to obtain trophoblast, Brambati[25] was the first to describe the technique used in most centers today. The procedure involves advancing a catheter under ultrasound direction to the thickest part of the placenta (Fig. 41-10). Trophoblast is then aspirated through the catheter into a syringe attached to the hub of the catheter. Generally, 5 mg or more is needed for direct chromosome analysis, but results can be obtained after cell culture with a sample of less than 5 mg. More sophisticated DNA studies using restriction fragment length polymorphisms or enzyme assays may require up to 40 mg of villus tissue.

TRANSABDOMINAL CVS

Hahnemann was also the first to describe this technique.[26] The major advantage is that the cervix, which may be responsible for infectious morbidity, is circumvented. The transabdominal CVS procedure is a modification of an amniocentesis technique. Either a needle-aspiration transducer or a freehand technique can be used. The operator simply places a needle tangentially through the placental substance under ultrasound guidance. While aspirating through a syringe attached to the

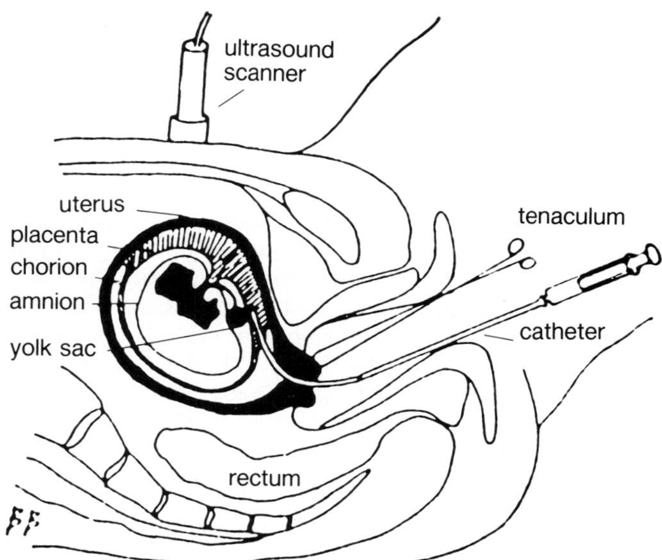

FIGURE 41–10. Schematic representation of transvaginal chorionic villus sampling, showing instruments and pertinent landmarks.

hub of the needle, the needle tip is moved up and down through the placenta until adequate tissue is obtained for analysis. Some investigators prefer to use a double-needle technique in which a smaller needle is advanced through an "introducer" needle.

ADVANTAGES AND DISADVANTAGES

The transcervical approach to CVS has been the most widely used. Although more than 80,000 procedures are estimated to have been performed by late 1991, the actual risks of the procedure have yet to be accurately measured. Patients undergoing CVS are at higher risk of pregnancy loss because of their indications for the procedure (ie, chromosomally abnormal fetuses have a higher spontaneous abortion rate than do normal fetuses). Any comparison of pregnancy loss must be made to patients of similar maternal age.

One source of information about CVS risks is a Philadelphia-based registry overseen by Laird Jackson. The registry has accumulated data on more than 57,000 pregnancies.

There have been two prospective clinical trials, one in the United States[27] and one in Canada.[28] The results from the six-center American trial indicate a 0.7% greater risk for transcervical CVS when compared with second-trimester amniocentesis. A Canadian randomized clinical trial yielded similar results. However, since some patients in the chromosomally normal CVS group chose to terminate their pregnancies, if the study subject denominator were adjusted accordingly, the increased risk of CVS could reach 1.7%.[29,30] From these data it appears that CVS carries a slightly higher risk of pregnancy loss than does second-trimester amniocentesis.

Initial studies evaluating the risks of transabdominal CVS indicate that it may well be safer than transcervical CVS, but the verdict must await the results of the randomized clinical trials in progress.

AMNIOCENTESIS

Bevis introduced the modern era of diagnostic amniocentesis with his report of the technique in 1952.[31] Liley was the first to demonstrate the ability to assess the severity of erythroblastosis fetalis by indirectly determining the amount of bilirubin in amniotic fluid in patients sensitized to the Rh factor.[32] In 1966, it became clear that fetal cells obtained from amniotic fluid could be cultured and later karyotyped.[33] This stimulated some institutions to offer second-trimester amniocentesis to women at significant risk for fetal chromosomal abnormalities.

Today, few women over age 35 are not offered amniocentesis, and millions of women to date have had the peace of mind of knowing that their fetuses had a normal chromosome complement. Stimulated by the demand to provide earlier information to couples at risk for fetal conditions that were generally diagnosed by second-trimester amniocentesis and frustrated by the governmental regulatory aspects of CVS investigation, some investigators began exploring the possibility of performing early amniocentesis before the 14th week of gestation.[34]

RISKS OF SECOND-TRIMESTER AMNIOCENTESIS

Since few studies deal with the risks of early amniocentesis, it is useful to review the results of second-trimester studies. Those who counsel patients weighing their diagnostic options may have the impression that the risks of second-trimester amniocentesis are small. But it has been difficult to quantify these risks precisely, primarily because there is little information on spontaneous fetal loss rates. Many studies deal with the risks of amniocentesis, but many of these suffer from insufficient numbers or inadequate control data; sometimes older techniques of amniocentesis were used.

Since 1979, 17 studies have emerged on the risk of second-trimester amniocentesis. Most offer no control data. The average total fetal loss rate was 3.3% (2.4% to 5.2%), and the spontaneous abortion rate was 1.3% (0.1% to 1.5%). The average loss rate to 28 weeks was 2.4% (0.3% to 2.9%); at about the same time, spontaneous abortion rates (15 to 17 weeks) in the United Kingdom were 1.3%, United States 2.6%, and Denmark 2.7%.[35]

The most comprehensively designed study undertaken has only recently been reported.[36] In this study 4606 Danish women under age 35 were randomized into two groups: women in Group I had an ultrasound and an amniocentesis, whereas women in Group II had an ultrasound examination alone. The amniocenteses were performed by a few skilled physicians under simultaneous real-time ultrasound guidance. There was a 1% difference in spontaneous abortion rates between the amniocentesis and controls (1.7% versus 0.7%). The stillbirth rate was identical (0.5%). These results correlate with the findings of a British study[38] and underscore the fact that amniocentesis is not a completely innocuous procedure and results in spontaneous abortion in up to 1% of cases.

A United Kingdom MRC study in 1978 showed that infants born after a second-trimester amniocentesis had a higher rate of respiratory difficulties than controls.[37] However, Crandall found no difference in respiratory distress syndrome rates.[38] The recent Danish study showed a statistically significant difference between amniocentesis patients and controls in the rate of respiratory distress syndrome (1.1% versus 0.5%) and infant pneumonia (0.7% versus 0.3%).[36] The most likely mechanism for respiratory difficulties would be the effect on the developing lung of a sudden decrease in amniotic fluid volume.

RISKS OF EARLY AMNIOCENTESIS

Although the gestational age of study populations varies, "early" amniocenteses have generally been performed between 10 and 14 weeks of gestation. Initial results have suggested fetal loss rates comparable to those of second-trimester amniocentesis.[39,40] However, the studies have problems that make the results difficult to evaluate. For example, the number of patients in these studies was small, and the study populations were heavily laden with 14-week pregnancies. It would be unfair to a patient about to have an 11-week amniocentesis to quote a loss rate derived from a study composed mostly of 14-week pregnancies.

Of theoretical concern is the fact that proportionally more amniotic fluid is taken from the amniotic cavity in early amniocentesis than at 16 weeks or later. We have recently evaluated the intra-amniotic fluid volumes in pregnancies between 9 and 14 weeks of gestation using a vaginal ultrasound probe.[40] This new technique allows the visualization of both the amnion and chorion. In many cases we have found a marked discrepancy between the intracavitary and the intra-amniotic volumes; in some 12- and 13-week pregnancies, the intra-amniotic fluid volume is as little as 30 mL. If 13 mL of fluid were aspirated from one of these patients, the embryo would be temporarily deprived of almost half its aquatic environment. It could well be that this would not pose a problem to the fetus, but given the results of second-trimester studies in which higher rates of respiratory distress syndrome and pneumonia were found among infants born after amniocenteses, more information must be accumulated to assess the long-term effects of early amniocentesis. Until then, we cannot confidently counsel patients who wish to have an early amniocentesis about the potential risk of the procedure.

EMBRYOSCOPY

Endoscopic techniques for direct visualization of the fetus allow detailed, direct observations of fetal anatomical structures and integument. Fetal visualization was used previously to diagnose structural anomalies and to guide sampling of fetal blood and skin.[41–43] Current approaches include fetoscopy in the second trimester and the recently developed embryoscopy in the first trimester. Visualization of the fetus by fetoscopy is limited to small segments, due to the limited field of view and the larger size of the second-trimester fetus. Hence, this technique has been superseded by ultrasound in the diagnosis of structural anomalies and by percutaneous umbilical blood sampling when fetal blood is needed for prenatal diagnosis.

Embryoscopy, however, is a relatively new and evolving procedure in which a rigid endoscope is inserted transcervically. The procedure was first used by Hahnemann to identify the placenta for CVS.[24] No attempt was made to visualize the fetus at that time, but Gallinat later suggested using the technique for fetal observation.[44] A contact hysteroscope (CO_2 insufflation, 6 mm outer diameter) was used to see the embryo through the intact chorion before elective termination of pregnancy. Cervical dilation and instillation of air were often needed. The results were disappointing; limited visualization and significant bleeding were often encountered. No reports of ongoing pregnancies were made with this technology.

Dumez and Oury were the first to use embryoscopy effectively in first-trimester prenatal diagnosis and have initiated a study in continuing pregnancies.[45] The procedures were performed to diagnose facial and limb abnormalities (personal communication, 1990). Our group has been using a modification of their original

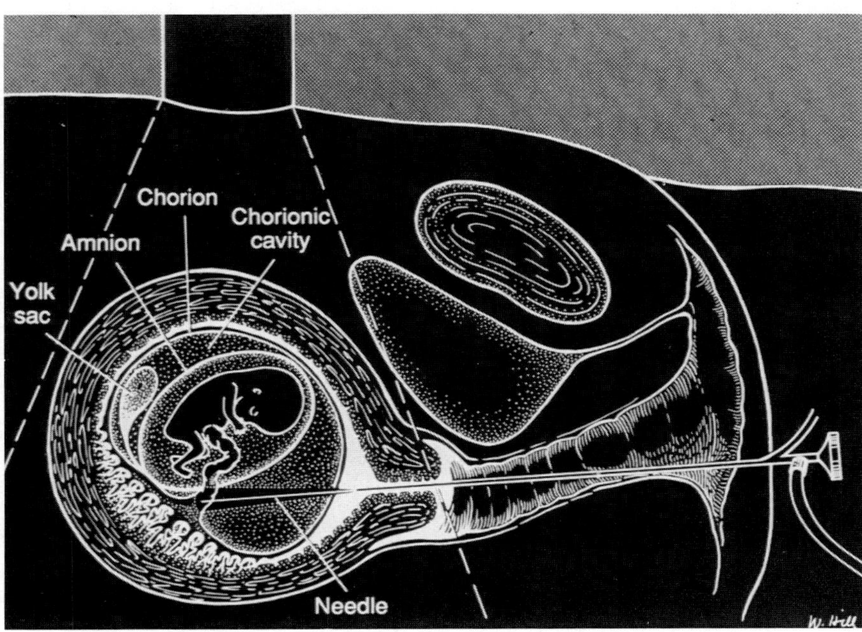

FIGURE 41–11. Schematic representation of embryoscopy, with the endoscope inserted transvaginally under ultrasound guidance. Pertinent anatomical landmarks are labelled.

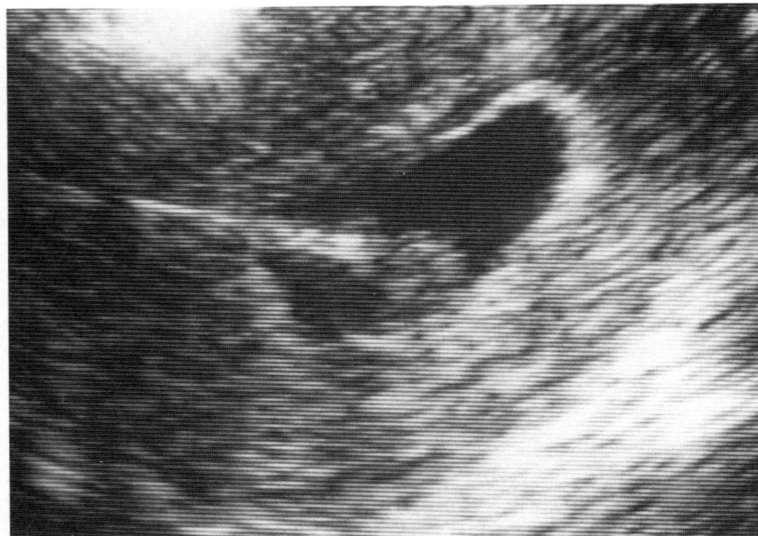

FIGURE 41–12. The endoscope is seen via sonography as it is inserted into the exovolemic space approaching the embryo. Entry and subsequent manipulations are under sonographic view.

technique. We use ultrasound to guide the rigid endoscope through the cervix and chorion into the extracoelomic cavity.[46] The chorion is ruptured with the tip of the endoscope, but the amnion remains intact. The yolk sac and placenta are directly visualized, while the embryo is seen through the amnion (Figs. 41-11 through 41-13). The endoscopes used have an outer diameter of 1.7 to 3.5 mm and have a visual field with no offset from the vector of the embryoscope. Wide-angle lenses are available that permit complete visualization of the conceptus. A bright halogen light source is used, but no heat is dissipated from the end of the fiber-optic part of the endoscope. The embryo can be seen directly through the endoscopic eyepiece or via a video camera and monitor (Figs. 41-14, 41-15).

In an initial feasibility study of 100 pregnancies before elective termination, the embryo was successfully visualized in 96, with structural anomalies suggested by ultrasound and later confirmed in 5.[47] Inadvertent amnion rupture did not occur in those pregnancies examined between 7 and 10 weeks but was a problem in two cases later in pregnancy.

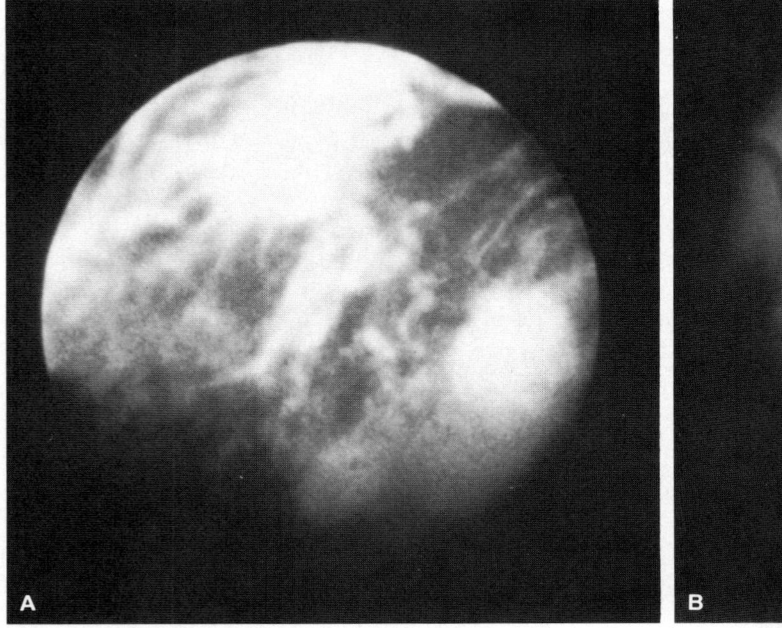

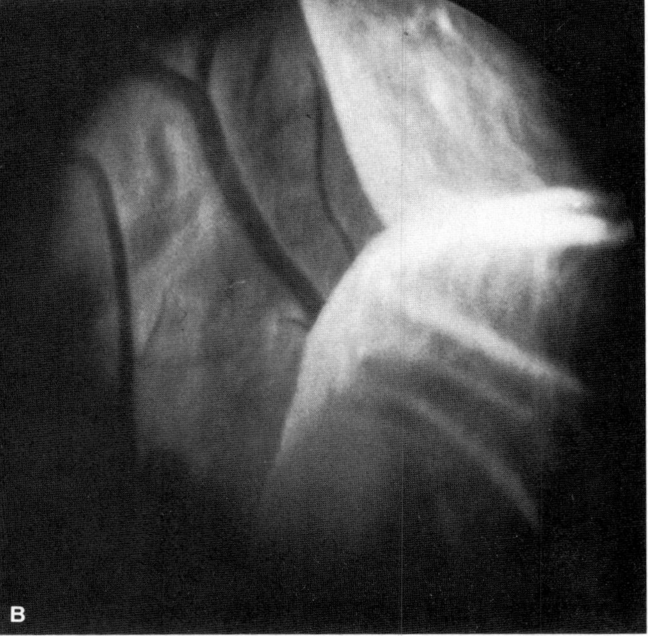

FIGURE 41–13. The view via the eyepiece of the video monitor as the endoscope is inserted through the cervical canal (**A**) or into the exocoelemic cavity (**B**). In the latter the filmy transparent amnion can be seen with the prominent placental vessel in focus.

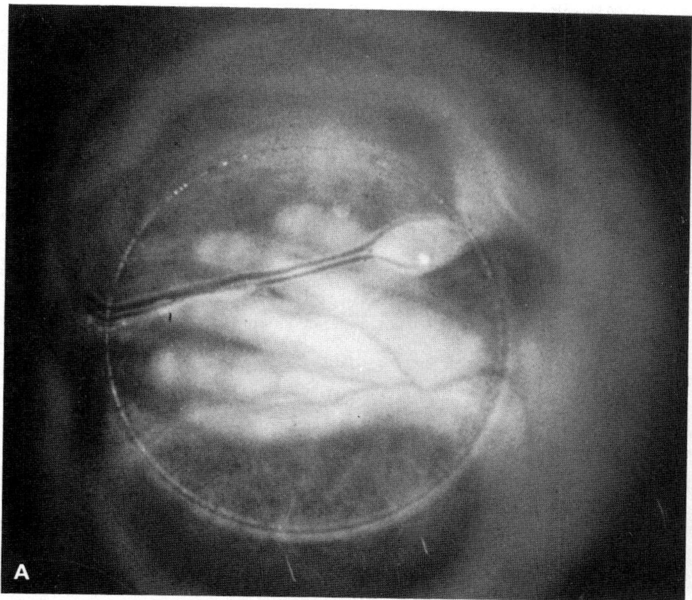

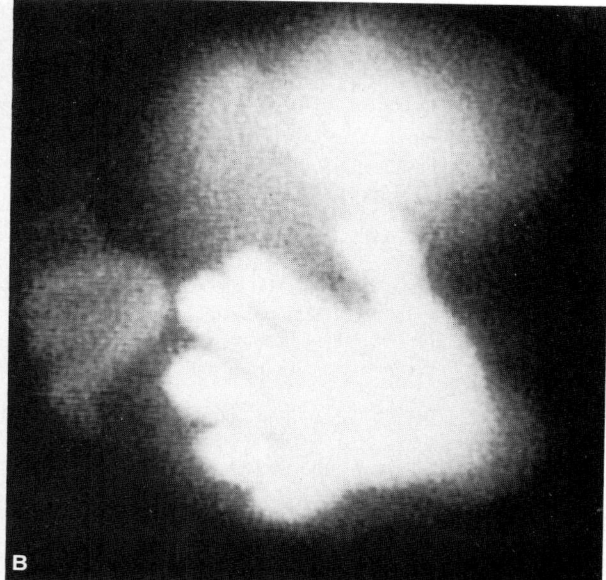

FIGURE 41–14. The fetal structures can easily be seen following endoscopic insertion into the exocoelemic space. (**A**) A normal hand of a 10-week-old fetus. (**B**) Polydactyly in an 11-week-old fetus.

Among the problems anticipated with this technique are bleeding, amnion rupture, infection, and damage to the developing eye from the bright light source. The risks of bleeding and infection should be similar to those of CVS performed with good technique, although careful documentation of experience with continuing pregnancies is needed to confirm this. The fetal neural optic axis does not completely develop until the second trimester, suggesting that the risk of eye damage should be minimal. Confirmation will also require extensive follow-up of any continuing pregnancies.

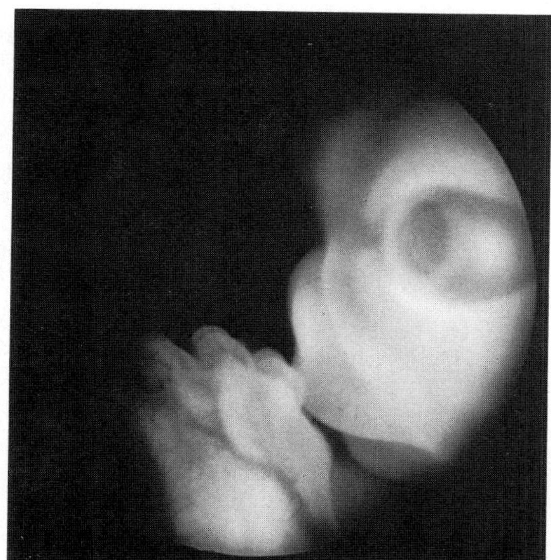

FIGURE 41–15. The face of a 10-week-old fetus visualized via embryoscopy.

While improvements in ultrasound resolution, especially as applied to transvaginal ultrasound, may eclipse embryoscopy for the practical diagnosis of first-trimester fetal abnormalities, we find the most important current application of embryoscopy to be in the confirmation of anomalies diagnosed by ultrasound before elective pregnancy termination. Because fetal tissues and external structures are disrupted by operative terminations, embryoscopic visualization in the operating room may be helpful in confirming the presence of externally visible fetal abnormalities. Additionally, with embryoscopy we can gain access into the embryonic circulation through the vitelline vessels that course through the extraembryonic coelom. This would enable injection of hemopoietic stem cells or cloned genes into embryos with hemoglobinopathies or single gene defects.

REFERENCES

1. Robinson HP, Fleming JEE. A critical evaluation of sonar "crown-rump length" measurements. Br J Obstet Gynecol 1975;82:702.
2. Brambati B, Tului L, Simoni G, Travi M. Prenatal diagnosis at six weeks. Lancet 1988;2(8607):397.
3. Pedersen JF, Molsted-Pedersen L. Early growth retardation in diabetic pregnancy. Br Med J 1979;1(6155):18.
4. Copel JA, Cullen M, Green JJ, Mahoney MJ, Hobbins JC, Kleinman CS. The frequency of aneuploidy in prenatally diagnosed congenital heart disease: an indication for fetal karyotyping. Am J Obstet Gynecol 1988;158:409.
5. Cousins L, Key TC, Schorzman L, Moore TR. Ultrasonographic assessment of early fetal growth in insulin-treated diabetic pregnancies. Am J Obstet Gynecol 1988;159:1186.

6. Green JJ, Hobbins JC. Abdominal ultrasound examination of the first-trimester fetus. Am J Obstet Gynecol 1988;159:165.
7. Timor-Tritsch IE, Farine D, Rosen MG. A close look at early embryonic development with the high-frequency transvaginal transducer. Am J Obstet Gynecol 1988;159:676.
8. Cullen MT, Green JJ, Whetham J, Salafia C, Gabrielli S, Hobbins JC. Transvaginal ultrasonographic detection of congenital anomalies in the first trimester. Am J Obstet Gynecol 1990;163:466.
9. Hoffman JI, Christianson R. Congenital heart disease in a cohort of 19,502 births with long-term follow-up. Am J Cardiol 1978;42:641.
10. Copel JA, Pike G, Green J, et al. The application of fetal echocardiography to prenatal care. Hospimedica 1987;5:29.
11. Hill LM, Thomas ML, Kislak S, Runco CJ. Sonographic assessment of the first-trimester fetus: a cautionary note. Am J Perinatol 1988;5:13.
12. Nora JJ, Nora AH. Genetics and counseling in cardiovascular diseases. Springfield: Charles C. Thomas, 1978.
13. Simpson AT, Golbus MS, Martin AO, et al. Genetics in obstetrics and gynecology. Orlando: Grune & Stratton, 1982.
14. Stiller RJ. Early ultrasonic appearance of fetal bladder outlet obstruction. Am J Obstet Gynecol 1989;160:584.
15. Nyberg DA, Hastrup W, Watts H, Mack LA. Dilated fetal bowel: a sonographic sign of cystic fibrosis. J Ultrasound Med 1987;6:257.
16. Filly RA, Golbus MS, Carey JC, Hal JG. Short-limbed dwarfism: ultrasonographic diagnosis by mensuration of fetal femoral length. Radiology 1981;138:653.
17. Benacerraf BR, Osathanondh R, Frigoletto FD. Sonographic demonstration of hypoplasia of the middle phalanx of the fifth digit: a finding associated with Down syndrome. Am J Obstet Gynecol 1988;159:181.
18. Merkatz IR, Nitowsky HM, Macri JN, Johnson WE. An association between low maternal serum alpha-fetoprotein and fetal chromosomal abnormalities. Am J Obstet Gynecol 1984;147:886.
19. Wald N, Cuckle H. Reporting the assessment of screening and diagnostic tests. Br J Obstet Gynecol 1989;96:389.
20. Stiller RJ, Lockwood CJ, Belanger K, Baumgarten A, Hobbins JC, Mahoney MJ. Amniotic fluid alpha-fetoprotein concentrations in twin gestations: dependence on placental membrane anatomy. Am J Obstet Gynecol 1988;158:1088.
21. Milunsky A, Wands J, Brambati B, Bonacchi I, Currie K. First-trimester material serum alpha-fetoprotein screening for chromosome defects. Am J Obstet Gynecol 1988;159:1209.
22. Stiller RJ, de Regt RH, Suntag S, Baumgarten A, Hobbins JC, Mahoney MJ. Elevated material serum alpha-fetoprotein concentration and fetal chromosomal abnormalities. Obstet Gynecol 1990;75:994.
23. DiMaio MS, Baumgarten A, Greenstein RM, Saal HM, Mahoney MJ. Screening for fetal Down's syndrome in pregnancy by measuring maternal serum alpha-fetoprotein levels. New Engl J Med 1987;317:342.
24. Hahnemann N, Mohr J. Antenatal fetal diagnosis in the embryo by means of biopsy from the extra-embryonic membranes. Bull Eur Soc Hum Genet 1968;2:33.
25. Brambati B, Oldrini A, Ferrazzi E, Lanzani A. Chorionic villus sampling: an analysis of the obstetric experience of 1,000 cases. Prenat Diagn 1987;7:157.
26. Smidt-Jensen S, Hahnemann N. Transabdominal fine-needle biopsy from chorionic villi in the first trimester. Prenat Diagn 1984;4:163.
27. Rhoads GG, Jackson LG, Schlesselman SE, et al. The safety and efficacy of chorionic villus sampling for early prenatal diagnosis of cytogenetic abnormalities. New Engl J Med 1989;320:609.
28. Canadian Collaborative CBS Amniocentesis Clinical Trial Group. Multicentre randomized clinical trial of chorion villus sampling and amniocentesis: first report. Lancet 1989;1(8628):1.
29. Chorionic villus sampling versus amniocentesis. Lancet 1989; 1(8639):678.
30. Chorionic villus sampling or amniocentesis. Lancet 1989; 1(8633):334.
31. Bevis DCA. The antenatal prediction of haemolytic disease of the newborn. Lancet 1952;1:395.
32. Liley AW. Liquor amnii analysis in the management of the pregnancy complicated by rhesus sensitization. Am J Obstet Gynecol 1961;82:1359.
33. Steele MW, Breg WR. Chromosome analysis of human amniotic fluid cells. Lancet 1966;1(7434):383.
34. Johnson A, Godmilow L. Genetic amniocentesis at 14 weeks or less. Clin Obstet Gynecol 1988;31:345.
35. Ager RP, Oliver RW. The risks of midtrimester amniocentesis. Salford, U.K.: , 1986.
36. Tabor A, Madsen M, Obel EB, Philip J, Bang J, Norgaard-Pedersen B. Randomized controlled trial of genetic amniocentesis in 4,606 low-risk women. Lancet 1986; :1287.
37. Medical Research Council. An assessment of the hazards of amniocentesis. Br J Obstet Gynecol 1978;85: suppl. 2.
38. Crandall B, Howard J, Legher TB, et al. Follow-up of 2,000 second-trimester amniocenteses. Obstet Gynecol 1980;56:625.
39. Hanson FW, Zorn EM, Tennany FR, Marianos S, Samuels S. Amniocentesis before 15 weeks' gestation: outcome, risks and technical problems. Am J Obstet Gynecol 1987;156:1524.
40. Hobbins J, Green J. Early amniocentesis (manuscript in preparation).
41. Hobbins JC, Mahoney MJ. Fetoscopy in continuing pregnancies. Am J Obstet Gynecol 1977;129:440.
42. Daffos F, Forestier F, Kaplan C, Cox W. Prenatal diagnosis and management of bleeding disorders with fetal blood sampling. Am J Obstet Gynecol 1988;158:939.
43. Eady RAJ, Gunner DB, Garner A, Rodeck CH. Prenatal diagnosis of oculocutaneous albinism by electron microscopy of fetal skin. J Invest Dermatol 1983;80:210.
44. Gallinat A, Lueken RP, Lindemann HJ. A preliminary report about transcervical embryoscopy. Endoscopy 1978;10:47.
45. Dumez Y. Embryoscopy and congenital malformations. Proceedings of the international conference on chorionic villus sampling and early prenatal diagnosis, May 1988, Athens, Greece.
46. Cullen MT, Reece EA, Whetham J, Hobbins JC. Embryoscopy: description and utility of a new technique. Am J Obstet Gynecol 1990;162:82.
47. Cullen MT, Green JJ, Reece EA, Hobbins JC. A comparison of transvaginal and abdominal sonography ultrasound in visualizing the first-trimester conceptus. J Ultrasound Med 1989;8:565.

42 CHAPTER

AMNIOCENTESIS, SKIN BIOPSY, AND UMBILICAL CORD BLOOD SAMPLING IN THE PRENATAL DIAGNOSIS OF GENETIC DISEASES

Lauren Lynch and Richard L. Berkowitz

AMNIOCENTESIS

The medical literature contains scattered reports of amniocentesis performed as early as the 19th century. During the early experience the procedure was utilized for various indications, such as polyhydramnios and instillation of hypertonic solutions to induce abortion. These reports remained sporadic until the 1950s, when analysis of amniotic fluid bilirubin was found to be useful in assessing fetal compromise secondary to isoimmunization.

Amniocentesis for genetic studies was first performed in the 1950s, when Serr and colleagues and Fuchs and Riis reported that antenatal sex determination could be made by examination of the X-chromatin body in human amniotic cells.[1,2] Subsequently, in 1966 Steele and Breg were able to culture amniotic cells and analyze their karyotypes.[3] Since then amniocentesis for prenatal diagnosis has been used not only for karyotype determination but also for the diagnosis of a variety of disorders by either enzymatic analysis of the fetal cells or analysis of the fetal DNA.

The indications for prenatal genetic testing are discussed elsewhere in this book. This chapter discusses the technique, risks, and complications of genetic amniocentesis.

TECHNIQUE

Genetic amniocentesis is most commonly performed at approximately 16 weeks of gestation. At this time the uterus has enlarged sufficiently so that amniotic fluid can easily be aspirated transabdominally. In addition, the ratio of viable to nonviable cells is greatest at this gestational age.[4] However, this procedure has been successfully performed as early as 9 weeks of menstrual age. The subject of early amniocentesis will be discussed later in this chapter.

Before performing an amniocentesis a thorough ultrasound examination should be performed for the following reasons:

1. To document fetal viability
2. To determine the number of fetuses
3. To detect major fetal structural abnormalities
4. To locate the placenta
5. To confirm gestational age
6. To confirm adequate amniotic fluid volume
7. To select an optimal pocket of fluid for sampling
8. To rule out significant uterine or adnexal pathology.

The evidence documenting improved safety when ultrasound is used as an adjunct to amniocentesis is scanty. Existing publications both support and deny this premise. These data have been reviewed in detail by Elias and Simpson.[5] A major problem with virtually all the studies, however, is that they were conducted at a time when ultrasound was much less sophisticated than it is today. Nevertheless, primarily because it makes excellent sense, preamniocentesis ultrasound evaluation has become the standard of care in the United States. Furthermore, most authorities now recommend that direct ultrasound guidance be used so that the needle can be visualized throughout the insertion process.

Amniocentesis is performed in a room where ultrasound scanning is performed. The patient is asked to empty her bladder prior to the procedure to avoid uterine displacement. After performing a thorough ultrasound examination the optimal site for needle placement is selected. Ideally, this site should be one where there is adequate amniotic fluid volume, no fetal parts are present, and the placenta does not have to be traversed to reach the fluid. Even when the placenta is anterior, it is almost always possible to find an area devoid of placental tissue or, at least, an area where it is thinned out. The area where the umbilical cord inserts into the placenta should always be avoided because of the possibility of perforating one of the large chorionic plate vessels that abound in this location.

Once the sampling site has been selected, the abdominal wall is thoroughly cleansed with iodine solution. The ultrasound transducer is then placed in a sterile plastic bag or glove. We sterilize bags that are commercially available for food storage, which fit the transducer very nicely. Either sector or linear-array transducers can be used, the difference being the placement of the transducer in relation to the needle. A sector transducer should be placed several centimeters away from the needle, whereas a linear-array transducer should be placed immediately adjacent to it. Sterile gel is placed on the abdomen, and again the appropriateness of the selected site is reassessed. Using the freehand technique while observing the ultrasound screen, a 20- to 22-gauge needle is introduced under direct visualization. Once satisfactory placement of the needle is obtained, the stylet is removed and in most instances free flow of amniotic fluid will follow. With the smaller needles this does not always occur and gentle suction must be applied to the needle in order to verify adequate placement of its tip. A 10- to 30-mL syringe is attached to the needle and 20 to 30 mL of fluid are removed. Occasionally, the fluid will be blood-tinged initially, in which case syringes should be changed and the bloody fluid discarded. If fluid cannot be aspirated, the needle can be rotated in place or the stylet replaced to reposition the tip. One cause of failure to obtain fluid is tenting of the membranes, which usually can be seen by ultrasound. Often this can be overcome by withdrawing the needle a few centimeters and then thrusting it forward in a quick, controlled motion to the desired depth. Care must be taken not to "overshoot" the targeted area when performing this maneuver. Inability to pierce the membranes despite attempting this approach should prompt the operator to remove the needle and select another insertion site. If the flow of fluid stops during the procedure, it is often because the negative pressure created by aspiration of the fluid causes obstruction of the tip with membranes, cord, or fetal skin. In this situation rotating the needle 90° to 180° often solves the problem. In some cases cessation of flow may be due to a uterine contraction at the insertion site. In these cases the stylet should be replaced and the needle repositioned. Once the fluid has been obtained, fetal cardiac activity within the normal range should be visualized and shown to the patient for her reassurance.

If an initial attempt is unsuccessful a second needle can be inserted in another location. However, no more than two needle insertions should be performed on any given occasion, and the procedure should not be reattempted until several days or a week later. The rationale for this is that the fetal loss rate has been shown to increase in proportion to the number of needle insertions, but not to the number of separate procedures performed (see Risks and Complications). If the patient is Rh negative she should be given Rh-immune globulin (300 μg) unless the father has also been documented to be Rh negative. After the procedure the patient can resume normal activities.

RISKS AND COMPLICATIONS

There are a large number of publications dealing with the safety of amniocentesis. A comprehensive review of that literature is beyond the scope of this chapter. Our discussion of this subject will be limited to five studies that have included a control group of patients for comparison.

United States Collaborative Study

The United States Collaborative Study was the first large prospective collaborative study designed to assess the safety and accuracy of amniocentesis.[6] It included 1040 subjects and 992 controls, most of whom were matched for race, gravity, income, age, and gestational age. Nine centers participated in the study between 1971 and 1973.

Ultrasound examination for placental localization was performed in only 29% of the procedures. The amniocentesis group had a total fetal loss rate (spontaneous abortions, stillbirths, and neonatal deaths) of 3.5%, compared with 3.2% in the controls, a difference that was not statistically significant. Factors correlating with a higher loss rate were increasing number of needle insertions per procedure and the use of needles that were 18-gauge or larger. Placental localization with ultrasound did not affect the loss rate, nor did the number of separate procedures performed to obtain fluid. Two percent of the subjects had immediate complications (vaginal bleeding or leakage of fluid). The incidence of bleeding correlated with the number of needle insertions but not with the size of the needle, gestational age, or use of ultrasound prior to the procedure. There was no difference in the incidence of late pregnancy complications except for a higher rate of cesarean sections in the study group. Newborn examination indicated no significant differences between the two groups in the incidence of congenital anomalies and no evidence of physical injury resulting from amniocentesis. In addition, the two groups of infants did not differ significantly in physical, neurologic, or developmental status at 1 year of age.

Canadian Collaborative Study

The Canadian collaborative study included 1020 pregnancies monitored by amniocentesis that were compared with two different control groups.[7] The number of stillbirths and neonatal deaths in the amniocentesis group were compared with those of women of the same age obtained from vital statistics records of two provinces. The incidence of spontaneous abortions after the procedure was compared with that of patients admitted to several hospitals with a pregnancy-related diagnosis. In addition, statistics of one of the prenatal clinics were used. Thirteen centers participated in the study from 1973 to 1976. Ultrasound was used in only some cases. The total pregnancy loss rate in the amniocentesis group was 5.2%, which was not significantly different from that of the controls. A higher loss rate correlated with more than two needle insertions per procedure and needles 19-gauge or larger, but not with the use of ultrasound or the number of amniocenteses performed in a given pregnancy. The incidence of immediate complications was 1.4% and correlated with a gestational age of 15 weeks or less and the use of 19-gauge or larger needles. The use of ultrasound did not affect the incidence of complications but decreased both the number of needle insertions and the number of procedures required. Neonatal morbidity was not studied, and there was no long-term follow-up.

British Collaborative Study

The British collaborative study included 2428 amniocentesis subjects, an equal number of matched controls, and another 506 unmatched subjects.[8] Nine centers participated in the study between 1973 and 1976. The use of ultrasound for placental localization was not uniform among the centers. In contrast to the previous two studies, this one concluded that there was a significant excess of 1% to 1.5% in fetal losses in the amniocentesis group. In addition, infants born to amniocentesis subjects had a higher incidence of unexplained respiratory difficulties lasting more than 24 hours and of orthopedic postural abnormalities than the controls. Although this study showed significantly higher rates of adverse outcomes in the amniocentesis group, the study design has been criticized for the following reasons:

- Matching criteria for controls and subjects were changed during the course of the study
- A significant proportion of women underwent amniocentesis because of elevated maternal serum α-fetoprotein, which in itself is associated with adverse pregnancy outcome.
- The incidence of pregnancy complications in the control group was unusually low.

University of California Center for the Health Sciences Study

In 1980 Crandall and colleagues reported on 2000 consecutive midtrimester amniocentesis subjects compared to two control groups of 2000 women each.[9] One group consisted of women followed from about 16 weeks gestation, when a maternal serum α-fetoprotein determination was obtained as part of a neural tube defect screening program, and the other group was composed of women delivered at this institution between 1975 and 1978 who were 28 years or older. As expected, the women in both control groups were significantly younger than those in the study group. One outstanding aspect of this study was that the infants underwent physical and developmental testing at 10, 24, and 48 months of age. All but 200 patients had ultrasound examinations before the amniocentesis. These authors found that the total fetal loss rate was 2.7%, compared with 2.2% in the control groups. They found no difference in the incidence of neonatal respiratory difficulties or orthopedic abnormalities. Subsequent developmental testing showed no significant difference between the groups.

Danish Collaborative Study

The Danish collaborative study published in 1986 is the only randomized trial to have been performed to date.[10] Five centers participated between 1980 and 1984. The study population consisted of 4606 low-risk women, ranging in age from 25 to 34 years, who were randomized to have either amniocentesis or no procedure. All amniocenteses were done under direct ultrasound guidance, and the majority (83.5%) of the controls underwent ultrasound examination at comparable gestational ages (16 to 17 weeks). The rate of spontaneous abortion was 1.7% in the study group compared to 0.7% in the control group, and this difference was statistically significant. The observed difference of 1% corresponded to a relative risk of 2.3 for the amniocentesis group. Factors associated with a higher risk of spontaneous pregnancy loss were a raised maternal serum α-fetoprotein before the amniocentesis, placental perforation, and the presence of discolored amniotic fluid. There was no correlation between the rate of spontaneous abortion and location of the placenta, number of needle insertions (but none of the patients had more than two at any given time), or experience of the operator. There was no significant difference in the perinatal mortality rates. The frequency of postural malformations was the same in both groups, but in the study group respiratory distress syndrome was diagnosed more often and more babies were treated for pneumonia. This study has been criticized because the initial publication stated that 18-gauge needles were used; however, the authors responded in a letter to the editor by saying that larger needles were used only for a few months at the beginning of the study, and after that only 20-gauge needles were used.

Conclusion

The older collaborative studies, with the exception of that performed in Britain, reported loss rates due to amniocentesis of approximately 0.3% to 0.5%. These studies, however, were conducted when amniocentesis was a relatively new procedure, ultrasound was not uniformly used, and none of them were randomized. The Danish study, which used ultrasound guidance and was randomized, found an excess fetal loss rate of 1%. Therefore, it seems reasonable to assume that even in highly skilled hands amniocentesis carries a risk that may approach this figure. Technical factors that may be associated with higher risk of spontaneous abortion are needle gauges larger than 20, placental perforation, and more than two needle insertions at any given time. Other factors include a raised α-fetoprotein before the procedure and the presence of discolored amniotic fluid.

SPECIFIC RISK FACTORS

Placental Localization

The collaborative studies in which ultrasonic placental localization was performed in only some of the patients showed no reduction in fetal loss rate when ultrasound was used. One problem with these studies is that the ultrasound examinations were sometimes performed hours or days before the procedure, thus substantially reducing their potential usefulness. Several authors have reported conflicting results regarding the benefits of localizing the placenta prior to the procedure.[11–15]

In 1980 Mennuti and colleagues determined pre- and postamniocentesis maternal serum α-fetoprotein values as an indicator of fetal–maternal transfusion.[16] All the placentas were localized before insertion of the needle. Those patients with post-AFP elevations were found to have higher spontaneous abortion rates and a higher frequency of anterior placentas. In 1982 Porreco and colleagues reviewed their experience with 2300 amniocenteses and found that anterior placentation was associated with a twofold increase in pregnancy losses when compared to posterior placentation.[17] This study does not mention whether attempts were made to avoid traversing the placenta, and 18-gauge needles were used in some cases. More recently, Crane and Kopta reported 998 amniocenteses performed with 22-gauge needles under ultrasound guidance.[18] The placenta was avoided whenever possible, or its thinnest portion was traversed when this was necessary. Using this approach, the authors found placental location did not affect the loss rates. The Danish collaborative study, which also used ultrasound guidance, found that placental puncture was associated with an increased risk of spontaneous abortion. In conclusion, the available data suggest that the placenta should be avoided whenever possible and that, when this is not possible, its thinnest portion should be traversed. To achieve this, ultrasound localization is necessary to select the optimal sampling site. Furthermore, the literature contains a number of reports of fetal trauma attributed to midtrimester amniocenteses performed without ultrasound guidance, making its use even more justified.[5]

Rhesus Isoimmunization

Disruption of the fetal–maternal circulation during amniocentesis can cause isoimmunization in Rh-negative women carrying Rh-positive fetuses. Quantifying the risk, however, has been difficult, since it is potentially related to such variables as ABO incompatibility, number of needle insertions, needle gauge, placental location, and amount of fetal blood introduced into the maternal circulation. Mennuti and colleagues found that 8.4% of the patients had a postprocedure AFP elevation representing transfer of fetal blood or amniotic fluid into the maternal circulation.[16] These authors used 18- or 20-gauge needles and ultrasonic placental localization but not ultrasound guidance during needle insertion. This paper did not address the issue of isoimmunization. Similarly, Lele and colleagues, using maternal serum AFP measurements, found a 7% incidence of fetal–maternal hemorrhage following amniocentesis.[19] All Rh-negative women in this study received Rh-immune globulin, and none became sensitized. Bowman and Pollock, using postamniocentesis Kleihauer-Betke tests, determined that women undergoing midtrimester procedures had a 2.6% higher incidence of fetal–maternal hemorrhage than controls.[20] The control group consisted of Rh-negative women at 28 weeks gestation just before antenatal administration of Rh immunoglobulin. Based on their findings, they recommend administration of 300 μg of Rh-immune globulin to Rh-negative women undergoing amniocentesis.

It is clear that a number of women will experience transplacental hemorrhage secondary to amniocentesis. The significance of this observation in regard to the actual development of isoimmunization, however, is less clear. The British collaborative study reported three cases (5.2%) of sensitization among 59 Rh-negative untreated subjects delivering Rh-positive infants, and no instances of sensitization among 58 similar patients given Rh-immune globulin following the amniocentesis.[8] In 1980 Hill and colleagues found a 5.4% incidence of isoimmunization compared with the 2.1% rate of spontaneous sensitization during pregnancy reported by Bowman.[21] Although this difference was not statistically significant, the authors recommended administering Rh immunoglobulin. Golbus and colleagues, on the other hand, reported an incidence of only 2.1% sensitization among 615 Rh-negative women at risk who did not receive Rh-immune globulin after midtrimester amniocentesis.[22] This number was not significantly different from the rate of spontaneous sensitization during the antepartum period. However, the majority of the sensitizations in the amniocentesis group occurred before 34 weeks, whereas most of the spontaneous sensitizations were noted later in pregnancy. This suggests a causal relationship with the procedure. By pooling their data with those of Hill and Golbus, Murray and colleagues estimated that amniocentesis increases the risk of Rh sensitization approximately 1% above the background risk.[23] Consistent with this estimate, the Danish collaborative study found that seven (1.9%) out of 370 amniocentesis patients became sensitized during pregnancy as compared to three (0.9%) of the 347 control patients. Antepartum Rh-immune globulin was not used in Denmark at the time of the study. In summary, it appears that approximately 1% of Rh-negative women at risk will become sensitized as a result of amniocentesis if Rh-immune globulin is not given. The American College of Obstetricians and Gynecologists recommends administration of 300 μg of Rh-immune globulin following second-trimester procedures.[24] If further amniocenteses are performed 6 or more weeks after the initial procedure, Bowman and Pollock recommend a second dose of 300 μg of Rh-immune globulin.[20]

Discolored Amniotic Fluid

Discolored amniotic fluid has been reported in 1% to 7% of midtrimester amniocenteses.[25–28] Brown or green discoloration has been found to be due to the presence of soluble blood breakdown products in the vast majority of cases, although meconium also has been detected in a small number.[25,26] A history of vaginal bleeding prior to the amniocentesis has been reported in 38% to 75%[25–27] of these cases. The significance of this finding has been the subject of much debate, with some authors reporting fetal demise in as many as 30% of pregnancies with discolored fluid and others finding little or no increase in adverse outcomes. Some of these series, however, have included procedures performed without prior ultrasound evaluation for fetal viability. In recent controlled studies where amniocentesis was preceded by ultrasound examination, fetal loss rates between 7% and 16% have been reported for women with discolored fluids.[10,25,27] These rates were significantly higher than those of the controls. Other authors have reported no difference in fetal losses among patients with this finding.[26,28] Thus, it appears that discolored amniotic fluid may imply a greater risk of fetal loss, and these pregnancies should be monitored accordingly. The reason for this association is not currently known, but whatever caused the initial episode of bleeding may compromise placental function or cause further bleeding in some cases.

MATERNAL RISKS

The risks of life-threatening maternal complications after amniocentesis are almost nonexistent. The incidence of amnionitis secondary to the procedure is approximately one per 1000 women.[29] Although this will lead to loss of the pregnancy, if recognized and treated promptly amnionitis generally does not seriously affect the mother.

OTHER PREGNANCY COMPLICATIONS

Complications occurring shortly after amniocentesis are not uncommon, but they are usually self-limited. Postprocedure amniotic fluid leakage occurs in 1% to 2% of patients.[6,7,10] Although in the majority of cases this is a transient occurrence, some patients experience persistent leakage throughout the pregnancy. Several cases have been reported in which the patients continued to leak amniotic fluid throughout the pregnancy and delivered normal neonates.[30] Unfortunately, these reports are sporadic, and in some cases ultrasound assessment of amniotic fluid volume was not done. Since leakage of fluid is transient in most cases, these patients should be managed expectantly. Ultrasound examinations should be performed periodically to evaluate amniotic fluid volume and appropriate fetal growth. Persistent leakage and severe oligohydramnios are probably associated with a much worse prognosis than when amniotic fluid volume is normal. In the former the risk of pulmonary hypoplasia and skeletal abnormalities may be significant and termination of the pregnancy should be considered. The risk of amnionitis in patients with transient leakage of fluid is low because in most cases the defect in the membranes is distant from the cervix. Women with frank rupture of membranes with oligohydramnios may be at higher risk of ascending infection and should be monitored accordingly if the pregnancy is not terminated.

Vaginal spotting and uterine contractions are also not uncommon, but they are almost always transient and of little consequence.

NEEDLE INJURIES

In the early amniocentesis studies, when ultrasound was not routinely used, several cases of cutaneous scarring were observed in the neonates. A small number of more serious needle injuries were also reported.[5] Since the advent of ultrasound guidance this has become an extremely rare occurrence.

AMNIOCENTESIS IN MULTIPLE GESTATIONS

The incidence of twins in the general population is approximately one in 80, whereas the incidence of twinning in women over the age of 35 is more frequent. Thus, genetic amniocenteses in twin pregnancies are relatively common. The counseling issues in twins are more complicated than those in singletons. If the multiple gestation is initially discovered at the time of a scheduled genetic amniocentesis, we feel that the amniocentesis should be postponed until all the relevant issues have been discussed and the couple has had time to consider them. The first point is that the risk of an abnormal result is doubled. Furthermore, the risk of losing the pregnancy may be increased because of the necessity of having a minimum of two needle insertions. A more complicated issue is the possibility of discordant results (ie, finding that one fetus is normal while the other is not). The couples should at least consider what they would do under these circumstances. At the present time three options are available: continuation of the pregnancy, termination of both fetuses, or selective termination of the affected twin.

As is true for singletons, the technique of amniocentesis in twins requires a careful ultrasound exam before the procedure. In addition to the usual parameters, one must identify the membrane separating the sacs and the lie of each fetus within its sac. The needle should be introduced into the first sac under ultrasound guidance; after aspiration of the amniotic fluid sample, a small amount of dye is injected before the needle is removed. Indigo carmine is the dye most commonly used. Methylene blue should be avoided because it can cause methemoglobinemia. The other sac is then entered with a different needle; aspiration of clear fluid indicates that the initial reservoir has not been resampled. Blue amniotic fluid, on the other hand, indicates that the same sac has been sampled twice, although a slight blue tinge may result from transmembranous diffusion of the dye in monochorionic pregnancies. If the same sac has been sampled twice, the needle should be removed, a different area identified, and another amniocentesis performed in an attempt to aspirate clear fluid. No more than four needle insertions should be attempted at any given time.

Several authors have reported their experience with amniocentesis performed in twin pregnancies. Those who routinely used ultrasound report success rates approaching 100% in sampling both fetuses. It is difficult to quantify the risks of amniocentesis in twin pregnancies because all of the studies report a small number of patients and none of them have a group of matched controls. The spontaneous abortion rates (less than 28 weeks), range from 2% to 17%,[31–36] but as mentioned, the significance of these figures is uncertain.

In cases in which only one fetus is abnormal, selective termination may be considered.[37,38] This procedure involves selective termination of the affected twin while allowing the unaffected one to continue to develop in utero. Several techniques have been used, but the most widely accepted is intracardiac injection of potassium chloride. It is obviously essential that the affected fetus be correctly identified if selective termination is to be performed. Identification is relatively easy if a structural abnormality is involved or the fetuses are of different sexes. Otherwise, accurate identification of each twin at the time the amniocentesis was done is critical. Thus, it is *essential* to note the location of each sac on a diagram at the time of amniocentesis and to label the amniotic fluid samples correctly.

EARLY AMNIOCENTESIS

Although genetic amniocentesis is usually performed at approximately 16 weeks gestation, it has been done as early as 9 weeks. The safety and success rate in obtaining a diagnosis in these early procedures are still unknown, as is the volume of fluid that can be removed safely from the uterus. With the advent of chorionic villus sampling (CVS), which is performed at 8 to 12 weeks, physicians are being asked to perform genetic testing earlier in pregnancy. Of particular concern in this regard are those patients who present at a gestational age too advanced for first-trimester CVS but too early for the more traditional amniocentesis.

Although several series of early amniocentesis have been presented at various scientific meetings, few have appeared in the literature. In 1987 Hanson and colleagues reported 541 amniocenteses performed between 11 and 14 weeks gestation, although follow-up was available in only 298 of these cases.[39] Volumes of amniotic fluid removed ranged from 15 mL to 35 mL, with an average of 25 mL. The procedures were performed with 20-gauge needles under ultrasound guidance. There were no amniotic fluid cell culture failures in this series. The total fetal loss rate was 4.7%, with 2.7% of the losses occurring before 28 weeks. This study, however, was not controlled; more importantly, the vast majority of the patients were in their 14th week. Therefore, the results cannot be extrapolated to earlier gestational ages.

FETAL BLOOD SAMPLING

Amniocentesis opened the door for invasive fetal diagnosis; however, there are still many disorders that cannot be diagnosed with amniotic fluid studies. In 1973 Valenti obtained fetal blood by introducing a modified pediatric cystoscope directly into the uterus before hysterotomy for second-trimester abortions.[40] In 1974 Kan and colleagues obtained fetal blood by blind aspiration of anterior placentas.[41] By this technique fetal cells were obtained in 58% of cases, but most of the specimens were contaminated with maternal blood. In 1974 Hobbins and Mahoney were the first to use the percutaneous fetoscopic approach for obtaining fetal blood.[42] These authors visualized fetal vessels beneath the chorionic plate through the fetoscope and aspirated blood, which in most cases was contaminated with amniotic fluid and/or maternal blood. This report, however, proved that fetal blood could be obtained in the majority of cases and without exposing the patient to general anesthesia and laparotomy. In 1979 Rodeck and Campbell reported drawing blood directly from the umbilical cord under fetoscopic visualization.[43] This approach yielded uncontaminated fetal blood in the majority of the cases. Fetal blood obtained by fetoscopy made possible the prenatal detection of several hematologic disorders that could not be diagnosed by amniocentesis. Fetoscopy, however, was a relatively cumbersome procedure that could be performed only during the early second trimester because visualization progressively deteriorated in later gestation. Furthermore, fetal loss rates of 2.5% to 6% were reported with this technique.[44,45] A major breakthrough came in 1983, when Daffos and colleagues reported percutaneous umbilical blood sampling (PUBS) by introducing a standard spinal needle into the umbilical cord vessels under ultrasound guidance.[46] This procedure was much easier to perform than fetoscopy, and the associated fetal loss rates proved to be lower. Since then numerous groups around the world have adopted this technique, not only for prenatal diagnostic purposes but for the administration of fetal therapy as well. (During the remainder of this section we will be referring to PUBS whenever fetal blood sampling is mentioned.)

INDICATIONS

With the development of DNA technology an expanding number of genetic diseases are now diagnosed on cells obtained from amniotic fluid or chorionic villi. The most common indications for fetal blood sampling in the 1970s were the detection of hemoglobinopathies and coagulation defects, which in most cases can now be diagnosed by DNA analysis. Nevertheless, there are still many situations in which fetal blood sampling is necessary for the prenatal diagnosis of genetic disorders. Furthermore, the list of nongenetic indications for PUBS is constantly growing.

FETAL KARYOTYPING

Karyotyping cultured amniocytes can take anywhere from 1 to 3 weeks. However, quicker results are sometimes necessary. Results from karyotypes performed on fetal white blood cells are usually available within 48 to 72 hours. Common indications for rapid fetal karyotyping are the detection of structural malformations or intrauterine growth retardation because management decisions may need to be made within days. If the need for karyotyping arises at a critical gestational age (ie, close to the time when a legal termination of pregnancy is no longer possible, or if delivery is imminent), analysis of fetal blood is also indicated.

Another indication for karyotyping fetal white blood cells is mosaicism in amniotic fluid or chorionic villus sampling. In 1988 Gosden and colleagues reported a series of 41 pregnancies in which mosaicism had been found on amniotic fluid culture and subsequent fetal blood sampling had been performed.[47] None of the autosomal trisomies or sex chromosome mosaicisms were confirmed in fetal blood. Five out of 11 chromosome rearrangements and four out of six supernumerary markers, however, were confirmed. Possible explanations for such discrepancies include maternal cell contamination, culture artifacts, and mosaicism of extraembryonic tissues. By studying fetal cells directly these factors can be ruled out and the pregnancy can be managed accordingly.

FETAL BLOOD DISORDERS

Although the majority of hemoglobinopathies and coagulopathies can be diagnosed by analyzing DNA obtained by amniocentesis or chorionic villus sampling, there are still situations in which fetal blood sampling is necessary. Examples are those families that are not informative for the DNA probes available, or cases in which the affected individuals are deceased. In these cases globin chain synthesis and coagulation factors can be measured directly in the fetal blood. Congenital thrombocytopenias can also be diagnosed by fetal platelet count determination.

FETAL INFECTION

Intrauterine fetal infection is discussed in previous chapters; however, in discussing fetal blood sampling, several basic concepts should be mentioned. Before this technique was available, patients exposed to teratogenic viruses or other microbes were counseled according to neonatal rates of infection. Many of these patients chose to terminate their pregnancies, but in the majority of cases their fetuses were not infected. It is now clear that fetal infection can be detected in utero by studying fetal blood. The first infectious disease studied was toxoplasmosis. In 1988 Daffos and colleagues investigated more than 700 pregnancies exposed to *Toxoplasma gondii* infection and accurately showed that the vast majority of fetuses were not infected.[48] As a consequence needless termination of pregnancy was avoided in these cases. Furthermore, by detecting those fetuses who were infected they were able to administer treatment in utero, which significantly reduced the incidence of sequelae of this disorder. Other infections—such as rubella, cytomegalovirus, and parvovirus—have been diagnosed subsequently in utero by fetal blood analysis.

Direct isolation of an organism in fetal blood or amniotic fluid is the most reliable evidence of fetal infection. This, however, is not always possible because culturing techniques may be either very difficult to perform or extremely lengthy. In these cases other evidence of infection may be helpful. Like the adult, fetal responses to infection may be either specific or nonspecific. The former response includes production of IgM antibodies that are directed specifically at the offending organism. The production of such antibodies, however, depends on the maturity of the fetal immune system, and consequently, gestational age. In most cases detection of this marker of infection has proved to be very reliable when present, but its absence does not rule out fetal exposure to the organism. Nonspecific evidence of infection has proved to be very useful in these cases. Some of these signs include thrombocytopenia, erythroblastosis, leukocytosis, eosinophilia, elevated γ-glutamyltransferase, and lactic dehydrogenase and elevated total IgM. These findings are not pathognomonic of fetal infection, and some of them can be seen in other fetal conditions, such as intrauterine growth retardation. Nevertheless, when fetal infection is a possibility, positive nonspecific findings may be very helpful in either expediting a positive isolation of the organism or informing the patient that the chances of infection are high.

TECHNIQUE

Fetal blood sampling is performed as an outpatient procedure. Fetal blood can be aspirated from the cord root, free-floating loops of cord, or the hepatic vein within the fetal liver. The placental insertion of the cord root is usually the preferred site. The type of transducer used varies from one operator to another, but linear-array, sector scanner, or curvilinear transducers can all be used. At the Mount Sinai Medical Center we use a linear-array transducer. After identification of the cord insertion site the maternal abdomen is cleaned with an antiseptic solution and the transducer is placed in a sterile plastic bag. A 20- to 22-gauge needle is introduced under direct ultrasound guidance through the maternal abdominal wall into the targeted vessel. Once the needle is in place a 1-mL disposable syringe that has been flushed with heparin is attached to the needle. Gentle aspiration will yield pure fetal blood if the needle is placed correctly. Once blood has been aspirated its fetal origin should be confirmed. This should be done in the sampling room, if possible, so that another sample can be drawn if the first proves to be maternal. The volume of blood withdrawn depends on the indication for sampling and the gestational age. In general, we do not exceed 4 mL during the second trimester and 6 mL during the third. Once an adequate sample is obtained, the needle is withdrawn and the duration of bleeding from the puncture site is determined. Fetal cardiac activity should be assessed during and after the procedure.

If the placenta is posterior, entry into the amniotic cavity becomes necessary. This poses several potential problems. First, the distance between the maternal abdominal wall and the cord insertion is greater than that with anterior placentas. This means that longer needles are necessary, and these may be somewhat difficult to manipulate. Second, the fetus may be lying directly on top of the cord, making it inaccessible. Several maneuvers, such as changing the maternal position, applying pressure to the maternal abdomen to displace the fetus, or simply waiting for the fetus to move, will allow sampling in most cases. Finally, when the placenta is posterior and the needle has to traverse the amniotic cavity, fetal movements may dislodge the needle, possibly tearing the cord vessel and causing significant fetal bleeding. Some authors have advocated paralyzing the fetus with a neuromuscular blocking agent immediately after entry into the vessel to avoid this complication. Fetal paralysis can also be achieved by administering the drug intramuscularly into the fetal thigh or buttock before the cord is punctured. Several neuromuscular blocking agents have been used, including d-tubocurarine (1.5 to 3 mg/kg),[49] pancuronium (0.3 mg/kg),[50] and atracurium besylate (0.4 mg/kg).[51] Although paralyzing the fetus appears to be safe, it is usually unnecessary for fetal blood sampling because the sampling time is usually short. However, during longer procedures, such as intravascular transfusions, fetal paralysis is often very helpful.

ASSESSMENT OF FETAL BLOOD SAMPLES

It is critical to confirm that the sample of blood obtained is fetal in origin and to be aware of any contamination with either amniotic fluid or maternal blood. Depending on the disorder under investigation, each type of contamination has differing consequences. When attempting to diagnose fetal infection, contamination with maternal blood may cause a false-positive result. Contamination with amniotic fluid will not have this effect, but it may alter the hematologic parameters. The presence of maternal blood cells in a specimen obtained for fetal karyotyping renders the sample almost useless, especially if the fetus is female, but amniotic fluid contamination has no effect in this case. On the other hand, investigation of hemostasis (platelet counts or coagulation factors) is very severely affected by amniotic fluid contamination because it activates some coagulation factors and causes platelet aggregation. In their series of 1553 samples, Forestier and colleagues found an overall incidence of contamination of 1.8%.[52] The most frequent sources of contamination were amniotic fluid, or citrate solution that was used to flush the collection syringes. Since no single test is reliable in all situations, these authors recommend performing a series of tests on each sample of blood to guarantee its purity. The tests include hematologic indexes determined with a Coulter counter (eg, hemoglobin, hematocrit, mean corpuscular volume, and leukocyte, erythrocyte, and platelet counts). These parameters should always be assessed, if possible, in the procedure suite to determine if the blood is of fetal origin. The mean corpuscular volume of fetal red cells is much larger than that of the adult, so by comparing the red cell size distribution of the aspirated sample to that of the mother this distinction can be made. These parameters are not very sensitive in detecting small degrees of sample contamination, since they are only reliable with more than 5% maternal blood and 20% amniotic fluid contamination. When greater assurance is necessary Forestier and colleagues recommend a blood smear with Giemsa stain; human chorionic gonadotropin B-subunit (B-hCG) analysis; coagulation factors II, V, VII, and IX assays; and red cell (I/i) antigen determination to detect very small degrees of contamination.

When assessing fetal hematologic parameters it is essential that they be compared with reference values for that specific gestational age.

RISKS AND COMPLICATIONS

The population of patients undergoing fetal blood sampling is unique because, in general, there is no alternative diagnostic procedure to offer them. Thus, the risks of the procedure cannot be compared to those of any other, and controlled studies are not possible. In addition, some of these patients have very sick or anomalous fetuses that are already at a greater risk of death in utero, so that determining which poor outcomes are due to the procedure itself may be difficult.

Despite these drawbacks the fetal loss rate related to fetal blood sampling appears to be relatively low. In 1985 Daffos and colleagues reported their experience with 606 procedures performed in 562 patients.[53] In this series there was a total fetal loss rate of 1.9%, but only two of seven losses appeared to be related to the procedure. In 1989 the same group reported 1770 cases with a total fetal loss rate of 2.3%, and a procedure-related loss rate of 0.4%. The rate of premature delivery was 4.2%.[54] A national fetal blood sampling registry for North America is being kept by the group at Pennsylvania Hospital.[55] As of October 1989, 3002 procedures in 2501 pregnancies had been reported from 16 centers in the United States and Canada. In this group 1.4% of the patients lost the pregnancy because of the sampling (1.2% loss rate per procedure).

The populations studied in France and the United States are somewhat different because the main indication for sampling in the former was exposure to toxoplasmosis. Since most of the fetuses in the French series were normal, a relatively small background loss rate would be expected. In theory this lower loss rate more accurately represents that related to the procedure itself. On the other hand, the most common indication for sampling in the North American series was rapid karyotyping (Table 42-1), and presumably a higher proportion of these fetuses had anomalies or severe growth retardation. Both of these conditions are associated with higher background loss rates. In summary, the exact risk of fetal blood sampling cannot be assessed at this time; however, it appears to be between 1% and 2%, which is not very much higher than that with amniocentesis.

The most common complication of fetal blood sampling is transient fetal bradycardia. Daffos reported that this occurred in 9% of his cases but the vast majority were of short duration.[54] Only four patients in that series had bradycardias lasting more than a total of 5 minutes. The etiology of the bradycardia is unclear. In some cases cord hematomas have been identified, but in the majority no obvious cause has been found. Some postulate that when an umbilical artery is punctured instead of the vein, arterial vasospasm may occur. In any case, since prolonged bradycardia is a potentially serious complications, PUBS should be performed in an area where immediate operative delivery is possible whenever the fetus is of a viable gestational age.

Fetal bleeding from the puncture site can be observed in a number of cases when the needle is removed, but this also is usually very short-lived. Daffos and colleagues reported that the duration of bleeding was 5 to 60 seconds in 32% of their cases, 1 to 2 minutes in 6%, and more than 2 minutes in 2%.[53] This bleeding seemed to be of very little clinical significance, because those fetuses that had repeated sampling were found to have normal hemoglobin concentrations. Many fetuses with severe coagulation defects have been sampled without complications. It appears that some hemostatic property of Wharton's jelly or amniotic fluid may have an important role in preventing significant fetal hemorrhage.

Severe chorioamnionitis secondary to fetal blood sampling has been reported.[56] This, in fact, was the most common cause of fetal loss in the cases reported to the North American registry (Table 42-2). Daffos and colleagues encountered only one case in their expanded series. This may be related to the fact that in the latter series only one needle insertion was required in 97% of the cases. Some centers have advocated the use of prophylactic antibiotics, but their benefit has not been substantiated. It may be possible to avoid amnionitis more efficiently by limiting the number of needle insertions and the duration of the procedure.

TABLE 42–1. INDICATIONS FOR FETAL BLOOD SAMPLING IN THE UNITED STATES AND CANADA

INDICATION	PERCENTAGE OF CASES
Karyotype	37.0
Red cell isoimmunization	34.0
Non-immune hydrops fetalis	6.5
Fetal infections	5.5
Idiopathic thrombocytopenic purpura	5.3
Alloimmune thrombocytopenia	2.1
Hemoglobinopathies	2.0
Other	7.6

Data from Ludomirski A. National PUBS Registry. Fourth International Conference, Philadelphia, 1989.

TABLE 42–2. ETIOLOGY OF FETAL LOSSES AFTER FETAL BLOOD SAMPLING

CAUSE	PERCENTAGE OF LOSSES
Chorioamnionitis	47
Rupture of membranes	17
Bleeding from puncture site	14
Fetal bradycardia	8
Thrombosis	3
Unexplained	11

Data from Ludomirski A. National PUBS Registry. Fourth International Conference, Philadelphia, 1989.

FETAL SKIN BIOPSY

Some skin disorders or systemic diseases with cutaneous manifestations may now be diagnosed by such techniques as chorionic villus sampling, amniocentesis, or fetal blood sampling.[57] Ataxia telangiectasia, Bloom syndrome, and xeroderma pigmentosa, for example, can be diagnosed by cytogenetic analysis because they exhibit specific chromosomal aberrations. DNA analysis can be used in the prenatal diagnosis of neurofibromatosis, tuberous sclerosis, hypohidrotic ectodermal dysplasia, and dyskeratosis congenita. A specific enzymatic defect has been identified in some disorders, such as Ehlers-Danlos types VI and VII, and biochemical studies can be used for prenatal diagnosis in these cases. Other diseases with hematologic manifestations, such as Wiskott-Aldrich syndrome (abnormal platelets) and the Chediak-Higashi syndrome (abnormal neutrophils), can be studied by fetal blood sampling. Elevated amniotic fluid α-fetoprotein and the presence of acetylcholinesterase have been reported in association with aplasia cutis congenita and epidermolysis bullosa dystrophica.[58]

Despite these advances, most primary skin disorders must be diagnosed by directly studying the fetal skin. Originally, fetal skin biopsies were performed "blindly" or by fetoscopic guidance. Recently, percutaneous insertion of the biopsy forceps under ultrasound guidance has replaced the earlier methods. At Mount Sinai Medical Center we use the percutaneous approach. Before starting the procedure, an ultrasound examination is performed to identify the best site of entry into the amniotic cavity. Because of the relatively large-bore instrument utilized, the placenta should never be punctured. In addition, the pocket selected should not contain loops of umbilical cord or fetal parts. The optimum site for fetal skin biopsy is the fetal back, buttocks, or thighs. However, for disorders of pigmentation, areas with abundant hair follicles (scalp) are preferred. Once the insertion site is selected and has been prepared aseptically, local anesthesia is injected into the maternal skin, subcutaneous tissue, and fascia. A 3- to 4-mm incision is then made with a scalpel in the skin down to the fascia, and under ultrasonic guidance a 14-gauge trocar with stylet is inserted into the amniotic cavity. The stylet is then removed and a flexible fetal skin biopsy forceps with a diameter of 1 mm is introduced through the sleeve.

Several samples of fetal skin can be taken from the same general area or from different locales. Care must be taken always to visualize the area being sampled with ultrasound because inadvertent biopsy of the amniotic sac may cause rupture of the membranes. Once adequate samples have been obtained, the instruments are removed and the skin incision is closed with a single suture. Fetal heart activity should be monitored during and after the procedure.

The loss rate due to fetal skin biopsy is not known. The main reason is that the number of fetuses requiring the procedure is extremely small. It seems reasonable to assume, however, that the risk is no greater than that of fetoscopy (2.5% to 6%),[44,45] and it may be even lower, since the instruments currently being used are smaller.

Several congenital skin diseases have been diagnosed in utero by fetal tissue biopsy. In the normal fetus keratinization does not occur until 24 to 26 weeks gestation.[59] However, prenatal diagnosis of keratinization disorders has been possible at 20 to 22 weeks by a combination of both light and electron microscopy examination. Within the group of keratinizing disorders the following have been diagnosed: lamellar ichthyosis (nonbullous congenital ichthyosiform erythroderma),[60] epidermolytic hyperkeratosis (bullous ichthyosiform erythroderma),[61] and harlequin syndrome.[62] Several forms of blistering disorders have also been diagnosed in utero, such as epidermolysis bullosa letalis[63] and some of the recessive and dominant types of epidermolysis bullosa dystrophica.[64] Prenatal diagnosis of disorders of pigmentation, such as oculocutaneous albinism, has been possible by observing a lack of melanin synthesis in hair bulb melanocytes.[65] This diagnosis can be made as early as 16 weeks gestation because in normal fetuses at least 50% of the melanosomes are fully pigmented at this age.[66] More complete reviews of this subject have been published.[67,68]

CONCLUSION

During the last two decades we have witnessed a revolution in prenatal diagnosis. Significant advances in ultrasound technology have allowed us not only to assess fetal morphology but also to develop techniques for safely sampling a variety of fetal tissues. This capability, coupled with spectacular developments in the field of genetics, has made possible the detection in utero of a growing list of pathologic entities. This chapter has reviewed some of the techniques currently being used to obtain fetal tissue.

Because invasive testing carries an inherent, albeit small, risk to the fetus, this diagnostic approach has been limited primarily to patients at significant risk for specific problems. At this time, however, noninvasive modalities, such as isolation of fetal cells in the maternal circulation, are being investigated as a way of screening low-risk populations. Furthermore, since we are now able to diagnose a large number of genetic disorders reliably, in utero therapy of some of these conditions will become the focus of intense research in the near future. In summary, the fetus has truly become an approachable patient in its own right.

REFERENCES

1. Serr DM, Sachs L, Danon M. Diagnosis of sex before birth using cells from the amniotic fluid. Bull Res Council Isr 1955;58:137.
2. Fuchs F, Riis R. Antenatal sex determination. Nature 1956;177:330.
3. Steele MW, Breg WR. Chromosome analysis of human amniotic cells. Lancet 1966;i:383.
4. Emery AEH. Antenatal diagnosis of genetic disease. Mod Trends Hum Genet 1970;1:267.
5. Elias S, Simpson JL. Amniocentesis. In: Milunsky A, ed. Genetic disorders and the fetus. New York: Plenum Press, 1986:31.
6. NICHD National Registry for Amniocentesis Study Group. Midtrimester amniocentesis for prenatal diagnosis: safety and accuracy. JAMA 1976;236:1471.
7. Simpson NE, Dallaire L, Miller JR, Siminovich L, Hemerton JL, Miller J, McKeen C. Prenatal diagnosis of genetic disease in Canada: report of a collaborative study. Can Med Assoc J 1976;15:739.

8. Working Party on Amniocentesis. An assessment of the hazards of amniocentesis. Br J Obstet Gynaecol (Suppl 2) 1978;85:1.
9. Crandall BF, Howard J, Lebherz TB, Rubinstein L, Sample WF, Sarti D. Follow-up of 2000 second trimester amniocenteses. Obstet Gynecol 1980;56:625.
10. Tabor A, Phillip J, Madsen M, Bang J, Obel EB, Nϕrgaard-Pedersen B. Randomized controlled trial of genetic amniocentesis in 4606 low-risk women. Lancet 1986;i:1287.
11. Kerenyi TD, Walker B. The preventability of "bloody taps" in second trimester amniocentesis by ultrasound scanning. Obstet Gynecol 1977;50:61.
12. Karp LE, Rothwell R, Conrad SH, Hoen HW, Hickok DE. Ultrasonic placental localization and bloody taps in midtrimester amniocentesis for prenatal genetic diagnosis. Obstet Gynecol 1977;50:589.
13. Levine SC, Filly RA, Golbus MS. Ultrasonography for guidance of amniocentesis in genetic counseling. Clin Genet 1978;14:133.
14. Harrison R, Campbell S, Craft I. Risks of fetomaternal hemorrhage resulting from amniocentesis with and without placental localization. Obstet Gynecol 1975;46:389.
15. Gerbie AB, Shlolnik AA. Ultrasound prior to amniocentesis for genetic counseling. Obstet Gynecol 1975;46:716.
16. Mennuti MT, Brummond W, Crombleholme WR, Schwarz RH, Arvan DA. Fetal-maternal bleeding associated with genetic amniocentesis. Obstet Gynecol 1980;55:48.
17. Porreco RP, Young PE, Resnick R, Cousins L, Jones OW, Richards T, et al. Reproductive outcome following amniocentesis for genetic indications. Am J Obstet Gynecol 1982;143:653.
18. Crane JP, Kopta MM. Genetic amniocentesis: impact of placental position upon the risk of pregnancy loss. Am J Obstet Gynecol 1984;150:813.
19. Lele AS, Carmody PJ, Hurd ME, O'Leary JA. Fetomaternal bleeding following diagnostic amniocentesis. Obstet Gynecol 1982;60:60.
20. Bowman JM, Pollock JM. Transplacental fetal hemorrhage after amniocentesis. Obstet Gynecol 1985;66:749.
21. Hill LM, Platt LD, Kellogg B. Rh sensitization after genetic amniocentesis. Obstet Gynecol 1980;56:459.
22. Golbus MS, Stephens JD, Cann HM, Mann J, Hensleigh PA. Rh isoimmunization following genetic amniocentesis. Prenat Diagn 1982;2:149.
23. Murray JC, Karp LE, Williamson RA, Cheng EY, Luthy DA. Rh isoimmunization related to amniocentesis. Am J Med Genet 1983;16:527.
24. American College of Obstetricians and Gynecologists. Management of isoimmunization in pregnancy (ACOG Technical Bulletin 90). Washington, DC: ACOG, 1986.
25. Zorn EM, Hanson FW, Greve C, Phelps-Sandall B, Tennant FR. Analysis of the significance of discolored amniotic fluid detected at midtrimester amniocentesis. Am J Obstet Gynecol 1986;154:1234.
26. Hankins GD, Rowe J, Quirk JG, Trubey R, Strickland DM. Significance of brown and/or green amniotic fluid at the time of second trimester genetic amniocentesis. Obstet Gynecol 1984;64:353.
27. Hess LW, Anderson RL, Golbus MS. Significance of opaque discolored amniotic fluid at second trimester amniocentesis. Obstet Gynecol 1986;67:44.
28. Allen R. The significance of meconium in midtrimester genetic amniocentesis. Am J Obstet Gynecol 1985;152:413.
29. Murken JA, Stengel-Rutkowski S, Schwinger E. In: Prenatal diagnosis. Proceedings, 3rd European Conference on Prenatal Diagnosis of Genetic Disorders. Stuttgart: Ferdinand Enke, 1979:132.
30. Crane JP, Rohland BM. Clinical significance of persistent amniotic fluid leakage after genetic amniocentesis. Prenat Diagn 1986;6:25.
31. Palle C, Andersen JW, Tabor A, Lauritsen JG, Bang J, Phillip J. Increased risk of abortion after genetic amniocentesis in twin pregnancies. Prenat Diagn 1983;3:83.
32. Goldstein AI, Stills SM. Midtrimester amniocentesis in twin pregnancies. Obstet Gynecol 1983;62:6559.
33. Librach CL, Doran TA, Benzie RJ, Jones JM. Genetic amniocentesis in seventy twin pregnancies. Am J Obstet Gynecol 1984;148:585.
34. Filkins K, Russo J. Genetic amniocentesis in multiple gestation. Prenat Diagn 1984;4:223.
35. Tabsh KMA, Crandall B, Lebherz TB, Howard J. Genetic amniocentesis in twin pregnancy. Obstet Gynecol 1985;65:843.
36. Pijpers L, Jahoda MGJ, Vosters RPL, Niermeijer MF, Sachs ES. Genetic amniocentesis in twin pregnancies. Br J Obstet Gynaecol 1988;95:323.
37. Chitkara U, Berkowitz RL, Wilkins IA, Lynch L, Mehalek KE, Alvarez M. Selective second trimester termination of the anomalous fetus in twin pregnancies. Obstet Gynecol 1989;73:690.
38. Golbus MS, Cunningham N, Goldberg JD, Anderson R, Filly R, Callen P. Selective termination of multiple gestation. Am J Med Genet 1988;31:339.
39. Hanson FW, Zorn EM, Tennant FR, Marianos S, Samuels S. Amniocentesis before 15 weeks gestation: outcome, risks, and technical problems. Am J Obstet Gynecol 1987;156:1524.
40. Valenti C. Antenatal detection of haemoglobinopathies. Am J Obstet Gynecol 1973;115:851.
41. Kan YW, Valenti C, Carnazza V, Guidotti R, Rieder RF. Fetal blood sampling in utero. Lancet 1974;1:79.
42. Hobbins JC, Mahoney MJ. In utero diagnosis of hemoglobinopathies. N Engl J Med 1974;290:1065.
43. Rodeck CH, Campbell S. Umbilical cord insertion as source of pure fetal blood for prenatal diagnosis. Lancet 1979;1:1244.
44. Rodeck CH, Nicolaides KH. Fetoscopy and fetal tissue sampling. Br Med Bull 1983;39:332.
45. International Fetoscopy Group. The status of fetoscopy and fetal tissue sampling. Prenatal Diagn 1984;4:79.
46. Daffos F, Capella-Parlovsky M, Forestier F. A new procedure for fetal blood sampling in utero: preliminary results of fifty-three cases. Am J Obstet Gynecol 1983;146:985.
47. Gosden C, Nicolaides KH, Rodeck CH. Fetal blood sampling in investigations of chromosome mosaicism in amniotic fluid cell culture. Lancet 1988;i:613.
48. Daffos F, Forestier F, Capella-Parlovsky M, Thulliez P, Aufrant C, Valenti D, Cox WL. Prenatal management of 746 pregnancies at risk for congenital toxoplasmosis. N Engl J Med 1988;318:271.
49. Moise KJ, Carpenter RJ, Deter RL, Kirshon B, Diaz SF. The use of fetal neuromuscular blockade during intrauterine procedures. Am J Obstet Gynecol 1987;157:874.
50. Copel JA, Grannum PA, Harrison D, Hobbins JC. The use of intravenous pancuronium bromide to produce fetal paralysis during intravascular transfusions. Am J Obstet Gynecol 1988;158:170.
51. Bernstein HH, Chitkara U, Plosker H, Gettes M, Berkowitz RL. Use of atracurium besylate to arrest fetal activity during intravascular transfusions. Obstet Gynecol 1988;72:813.
52. Forestier F, Cox WL, Daffos F, Rainaut M. The assessment of fetal blood samples. Am J Obstet Gynecol 1988;158:1184.
53. Daffos F, Capella-Parlovsky M, Forestier F. Fetal blood sampling during pregnancy with use of a needle guided by ultrasound: a study of 606 consecutive cases. Am J Obstet Gynecol 1985;153:655.
54. Daffos F. Fetal blood sampling. Presented at the 27th Annual Meeting of the American College of Obstetrics and Gynecology. Atlanta, Georgia, May 1989.
55. Ludomirski A. National PUBS Registry. Fourth International Conference, Philadelphia, 1989.

56. Wilkins I, Mezrow G, Lynch L, Bottone EJ, Berkowitz RL. Amnionitis and life-threatening respiratory distress after percutaneous umbilical blood sampling. Am Obstet Gynecol 1989; 160:427.
57. Soothil PW. Prenatal diagnosis of skin diseases. Arch Dis Child 1988;63:1175.
58. Bick DP, Balkite MS, Baumgarten A, Hobbins JC, Mahoney MJ. The association of congenital skin disorders with acetylcholinesterase in amniotic fluid. Prenat Diagn 1987;7:543.
59. Arnold ML, Anton-Lamprecht I. Problems in prenatal diagnosis of the ichthyosis congenita group. Hum Genet 1985;71:301.
60. Perry TB, Hollbrook KA, Hoff MS, Hamilton EF, Senikas V, Fisher C. Prenatal diagnosis of congenital non-bullous ichthyosiform erythroderma (lamellar ichthyosis). Prenat Diagn 1987; 7:145.
61. Golbus MS, Sagebiel RW, Filly RA, Gindhart TD, Hull JD. Prenatal diagnosis of congenital bullous ichyosiform erythroderma (epidermolytic hyperkeratosis) by fetal skin biopsy. N Engl J Med 1980;302:93.
62. Elias S, Mazur M, Sabbagha R, Esterly NB, Sympson JL. Prenatal diagnosis of Harlequin ichthyosis. Clin Genet 1980;17:275.
63. Rodeck CH, Eady RAJ, Gosden CM. Prenatal diagnosis of epidermolysis bullosa letalis. Lancet 1980;i:949.
64. Bauer EA, Ludmen MD, Goldberg JD, Berkowitz RL, Hollbrook KA. Antenatal diagnosis of recessive dystrophic epidermolysis bullosa: collagenase expression in cultured fibroblasts as a biochemical marker. J Invest Dermatol 1986;87:597.
65. Eady RA, Gunner DB, Garner A, Rodeck CH. Prenatal diagnosis of oculocutaneous albinism by electron microscopy of fetal skin. J Invest Dermatol 1983;80:210.
66. Haynes ME, Robertson E. Can oculocutaneous albinism be diagnosed prenatally? Prenat Diagn 1981;1:85.
67. Holbrook KA, ed. Prenatal diagnosis of genetic skin disease. Seminars in dermatology. Vol 3, part 3. New York: Thieme-Stratton, 1984:155.
68. Gedde-Dahl T, Wuepper KD, eds. Prenatal diagnosis of heritable skin diseases. Current problems in dermatology. Vol 16. Basel: Karger, 1987:129.

43

CHAPTER

MATERNAL PROTEIN ENZYME ANALYSES

James E. Haddow and Glenn E. Palomaki

α-FETOPROTEIN

In 1956 Bergstrand and Czar described a band of protein in fetal serum, located in the α_1 region on electrophoresis, that was not present in adult serum.[1] This band, subsequently labeled α_1-fetoprotein, was found to have both a molecular weight similar to that of albumin (about 69,000 d) and considerable structural homology.[2] α-Fetoprotein (AFP) is the major serum protein in fetal blood early on, peaking in concentration at about 12 weeks gestation and then falling slowly for the remainder of the pregnancy. For practical purposes it can be considered fetospecific, being present in minute concentrations in non-pregnant adult serum (<0.5 to 2.0 ng/mL).

MEASURING α-FETOPROTEIN IN AMNIOTIC FLUID TO DETECT OPEN FETAL NEURAL TUBE DEFECTS

The present era of biochemical testing for fetal disorders dates from the discovery that AFP levels in amniotic fluid are elevated in the presence of open fetal neural tube defects.[3] The investigation that led to that discovery was prompted by a high birth prevalence of the two major neural tube defects, anencephaly and spina bifida (three to seven births out of every 1000), in certain areas of the United Kingdom and by the accompanying psychological and physical burdens. Following confirmation that AFP measurements could be used reliably for diagnostic purposes, many laboratories in Europe and the United States began to offer such testing to pregnant women who were known to be at high risk for having an affected fetus, usually by virtue of family history. Although helpful to these women, the overall diagnostic effectiveness of amniotic fluid AFP testing to the general pregnancy population was severely restricted; only 3% to 5% of the annual births affected by open neural tube defects occur in families known to be at high risk. Realizing this to be the case, a number of investigators turned their attention to measuring AFP in maternal serum, to learn whether open neural tube defects might be associated with higher AFP levels in that compartment as well.

BROADENING THE APPLICATION OF AFP MEASUREMENT TO INCLUDE MATERNAL SERUM

The excitement accompanying confirmation that this was, in fact, the case[4,5] was tempered by an appreciation that both sensitivity and specificity of AFP elevations were reduced in maternal serum for detecting open neural tube defects, requiring that maternal serum α-fetoprotein (MSAFP) measurements be applied to the general pregnancy population for screening purposes only. Pregnancies identified by the MSAFP screening process as being at high risk would then become candidates for amniocentesis, in similar fashion to pregnancies identified as being at high risk because of a positive family history.

DEVELOPING ACETYLCHOLINESTERASE TESTING IN AMNIOTIC FLUID AS A SECOND DIAGNOSTIC TEST

Although analysis of AFP in amniotic fluid proved highly sensitive, false-positive results did occur occasionally, and the search therefore continued for additional biochemical products that might both serve as markers for open neural tube defects and be more specific. Acetylcholinesterase (AChE) was found to be such a marker,[6] and its introduction as a second diagnostic test, along with AFP, has significantly improved the laboratory's ability to distinguish affected from unaffected pregnancies (Fig. 43-1). AChE cannot be measured, however,in maternal serum.

THE DISCOVERY THAT LOWER MSAFP LEVELS ARE ASSOCIATED WITH FETAL TRISOMY 21

AFP screening and diagnostic protocols for detecting open neural tube defects were well established by 1984, when a new and unexpected association was discovered between lower MSAFP levels and certain autosomal trisomies (trisomy 21, trisomy 18).[7] This discovery, prompted by a query from a patient whose MSAFP value was low and who subsequently gave birth to an infant with trisomy 18, was rapidly confirmed,[8] and over the succeeding years, interpretation of low MSAFP values became incorporated into the routine of most MSAFP screening programs in the United States.

MSAFP AS A SCREENING TEST FOR FETAL TRISOMY 21 IN PREGNANT WOMEN UNDER AGE 35

Applying MSAFP screening to trisomy 21 detection was initially restricted to pregnant women under age 35, because of the already well-established practice of offering amniocentesis to all pregnant women aged 35 and older, because of their age-related increased risk for having a fetus affected with trisomy 21. Prior to MSAFP screening, no method existed of identifying a high-risk group for trisomy 21 among younger women (other than the unusual circumstance of a known balanced translocation). MSAFP measurement, although relatively low in sensitivity for detecting trisomy 21, was still capable of identifying approximately 25% of the cases among younger women, thereby doubling the total number of the cases potentially identifiable by using age alone as a screening test.

OTHER FETOPLACENTAL BIOCHEMICAL PRODUCTS THAT ARE ALTERED WITH TRISOMY 21

The relatively low sensitivity of MSAFP as a screening test for trisomy 21 stimulated a search for other possible biochemical markers in maternal blood, and human chorionic gonadotropin (hCG)[9] and unconjugated estriol (uE3)[10] were subsequently found to occur in different concentrations from unaffected pregnancies, when trisomy 21 was present in the fetus. A subsequent study analyzed the extent of interdependence of these new markers with AFP, concluding that there was a high degree of independence and that the three markers together could identify 60% of all pregnancies affected by trisomy 21 at a screening cut-off that selected 5% of the screened population for amniocentesis.[11]

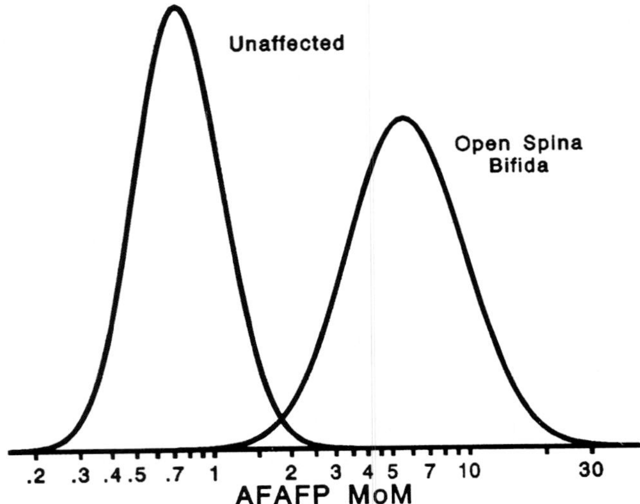

FIGURE 43–1. Amniotic fluid α-fetoprotein (AFAFP) distributions in singleton, unaffected pregnancies and in pregnancies affected by open spina bifida, during the second trimester. AFAFP measurements are expressed as multiples of the unaffected population median (MoM) on a logarithmic scale. Distributions of AFAFP values are log Gaussian for both of the populations, and a small degree of overlap is present, forming the basis for defining detection and false-positive rates at various AFAFP cut-offs. The odds of being affected, given a positive AFAFP measurement, can also be estimated using these distributions and the individual's prior risk.

PROJECTED APPLICATIONS FOR THESE NEWER SCREENING MARKERS

The application of AFP and the other screening and diagnostic biochemical markers described earlier continues to evolve and expand rapidly, and it is likely that hCG and uE3 will be added to the prenatal screening armamentarium within the next few years. It is also likely that other biochemical markers will be discovered whose use will further refine and extend our collective ability to detect fetal disorders. The remainder of this chapter is devoted to providing more detailed and comprehensive information about AFP and other biochemical products as screening or diagnostic tests for a variety of fetal disorders.

AFP IN AMNIOTIC FLUID AS A DIAGNOSTIC MARKER FOR FETAL OPEN NEURAL TUBE DEFECTS AND OTHER FETAL DISORDERS

WHY AFP IS UNIQUELY SUITED TO SERVE AS A MARKER FOR OPEN FETAL DEFECTS

Brock and Sutcliffe selected AFP as a likely candidate to indicate the presence of an open fetal defect, because AFP was produced almost solely by the fetus.[3] They reasoned that AFP might transudate into amniotic fluid from the open fetal lesion and that it might prove to be a more sensitive marker than a protein shared by both fetus and mother. The bulk of amniotic fluid protein is now known to be maternally derived,[12,13] and no other major serum protein has been found helpful in identifying open fetal defects. For their initial analyses Brock and Sutcliffe relied heavily on banked amniotic fluid samples from the third trimester whose outcomes were known. In that study AFP proved relatively insensitive for detecting open spina bifida, but subsequent studies demonstrated AFP to be highly sensitive in the second trimester, at a time when prenatal diagnostic studies are ordinarily performed.

ELECTROPHORESIS AS A TECHNIQUE FOR MEASURING AFP IN AMNIOTIC FLUID

"Rocket" electrophoresis was the most commonly used technique for measuring AFP in amniotic fluid during the early introduction for routine testing. This method, described by Laurell in 1966,[14] combined traditional electrophoresis with a specific antiserum mixed into the gel, in this case antiserum against AFP. When AFP moved into the gel during electrophoresis, it reacted with the antibody and formed a precipitate, shaped like a rocket. The height of the rocket was directly proportional to the concentration of AFP, and this technique's level of sensitivity was well suited for measuring accurately the amounts of AFP normally found in amniotic fluid during the second trimester (1 to 15 μg/mL).

THE ORIGIN OF NORMAL BACKGROUND LEVELS OF AFP IN AMNIOTIC FLUID

AFP is normally present in amniotic fluid during the second trimester, as a result of leakage through the fetal kidney into fetal urine. For this reason it became necessary to define normal ranges for each gestational week during the second trimester, during which time AFP normally decreases steadily in concentration in a similar pattern to the AFP concentration in fetal serum.

SENSITIVITY AND SPECIFICITY OF AFP MEASUREMENT IN AMNIOTIC FLUID TO DETECT OPEN NEURAL TUBE DEFECTS

A collaborative study was carried out in the United Kingdom to gain a better understanding of the sensitivity and specificity of amniotic fluid AFP measurements to detect open neural tube defects during the second trimester.[15] The 20 collaborating laboratories each had their own AFP standards; therefore, it became necessary for the study organizers to convert each contributing center's AFP measurements into multiples of its own unaffected population's median (MoM) as a first step toward a combined analysis. Using this approach, it became possible to define distributions of AFP concentrations in both unaffected and affected pregnancies. Figure 43-1 illustrates the relationship between amniotic fluid AFP values in unaffected pregnancies and pregnancies affected with open spina bifida, demonstrating a small degree of overlap. A stepwise cut-off was then defined, based on gestational age, that allowed 99.5% of anencephaly cases and 98% of open spina bifida cases to be identified at a false-positive rate of approximately seven out of 1000 amniotic fluid samples analyzed. With this information it became possible to estimate the likelihood of an amniotic fluid AFP elevation being a true positive, and it became clear that the likelihood depended heavily on the woman's prior risk of having an affected pregnancy. For example, if the woman's prior risk for having a fetus affected with an open neural tube defect were that of the general population (two per 1000 in the United States), then an AFP elevation would provide her with a 2:7 odds of having an affected pregnancy. However, if her prior risk were defined by a previous affected pregnancy (20 per 1000 in the United States), the odds of having an affected pregnancy would be 20:7.

REASONS FOR FALSELY ELEVATED AFP MEASUREMENTS IN AMNIOTIC FLUID

Most false-positive AFP elevations in amniotic fluid could be traced to fetal blood contamination related to the procedure. If the amniotic fluid sample were visibly bloodstained and if the blood could be documented as fetal in origin (either by Kleihauer-Betke analysis or by counterelectrophoresis to detect hemoglobin F), then any accompanying AFP elevation would need to be viewed as a false-positive until proved otherwise. Sometimes the presence of fetal blood can only be determined retrospectively, since samples may be centrifuged and the red cells removed prior to being sent to the AFP laboratory. In such cases, hemoglobin F can often be detected in the supernatant, leading to heightened suspicion of a false positive. Once fetal blood contamination has been excluded by all available means, the likelihood of a false positive is considerably reduced but is not eliminated. Unexplained AFP elevations do occasionally occur in amniotic fluid, even in the absence of blood contamination. Appreciation of the less-than-absolute ability of AFP measurements to diagnose open fetal defects had led prenatal diagnostic laboratories to emphasize interpreting positive test results to patients in relative terms.

OTHER FETAL DISORDERS ASSOCIATED WITH AFP ELEVATIONS IN AMNIOTIC FLUID

A variety of other fetal disorders are now known to be associated with AFP elevations in amniotic fluid, among them open ventral wall defects (omphalocele and gastroschisis), congenital nephrosis, and a severely distressed or recently dead fetus.[16] These can be factored into the interpretation of an elevated AFP measurement, depending on their local prevalence. Congenital nephrosis, an autosomal recessive disorder, is rare in most of the world but occurs frequently in Finland, where it figures prominently among the fetal disorders diagnosed prenatally.[17] In the United States open ventral wall defects are the second most common major open fetal malformation identified by AFP elevations in amniotic fluid, occurring at an approximate rate of three per 10,000 second-trimester pregnancies.[18] Many cases of omphalocele and gastroschisis are now identified prior to amniocentesis, in which case amniotic fluid AFP measurements either may be ordered to confirm the diagnosis or may be unnecessary. When the amniotic fluid AFP elevation is the first indication of this group of disorders, ultrasound studies provide a highly reliable next diagnostic step to identify the specific condition (ie, omphalocele versus gastroschisis) and to document the extent and severity of the lesion.

ACETYLCHOLINESTERASE (AChE) IN AMNIOTIC FLUID AS A DIAGNOSTIC MARKER FOR FETAL OPEN NEURAL TUBE DEFECTS AND OTHER FETAL DISORDERS

EARLY, UNSUCCESSFUL ATTEMPTS TO APPLY QUANTITATIVE MEASUREMENTS TO DETECT OPEN NEURAL TUBE DEFECTS

During the 1970s several investigators examined the relationship between fetal open neural tube defects and concentrations of AChE in amniotic fluid samples from the affected pregnancies. Such an association seemed reasonable, given the known high concentrations of AChE in neural tissues and cerebrospinal fluid. Were it possible to differentiate between affected and unaffected pregnancies using this type of analysis, the problem of false-positive AFP results might be reduced or avoided altogether. The early studies were carried out with quantitative assays that measured AChE enzyme activity, using a relatively nonspecific substrate. Results of the studies were not encouraging, probably because of the high background enzyme activity from other cholinesterases.

QUALITATIVE AChE ANALYSIS BY GEL ELECTROPHORESIS FOR DETECTING OPEN NEURAL TUBE DEFECTS

In 1979 Smith and colleagues reported a different and successful approach to measuring AChE activity in amniotic fluid.[6] The assay relied on first separating AChE from other cholinesterases in amniotic fluid and then developing the gel with a substrate that allowed the AChE enzyme band to be magnified for easy visibility. This qualitative assay provided a clear definition between affected and unaffected pregnancies, in that a discrete band was visible in amniotic fluid in the presence of open neural tube defects, whereas no band could be seen in unaffected pregnancies. This analytic system not only proved highly sensitive for detecting open neural tube defects (99% of anencephaly cases, 98% of open spina bifida cases with positive AFP results), but also was found negative in nine out of 10 cases where the amniotic fluid AFP measurement was falsely elevated. AChE activity is not visible by gel electrophoresis in human adult serum but is visible in fetal blood during the second trimester. This characteristic of AChE helps to explain why most, but not all, of the false-positive measurements can be reclassified correctly. In the presence of a larger fetal hemorrhage into amniotic fluid, both AFP and AChE are likely to be detectable in higher concentrations.

SENSITIVITY AND SPECIFICITY OF GEL AChE ANALYSIS TO DETECT OPEN NEURAL TUBE DEFECTS

A collaborative study was carried out in the United Kingdom to test the extent to which gel AChE analysis might add power to AFP as a diagnostic test for open neural tube defects in amniotic fluid.[19] Results of that study demonstrated that AChE analysis, by correctly identifying most false-positive and nearly all true-positive AFP results, strengthened the diagnostic process by a substantial margin.

GEL AChE ANALYSIS TO DETECT OPEN VENTRAL WALL DEFECTS

The presence of an AChE band has also been documented in approximately 75% of amniotic fluid samples associated with open ventral wall defects. It is likely that the origin of this AChE is the fetal circulation, rather than the central nervous system; other nonneural cholinesterases are increased in these cases as well. Further, visible amniotic fluid AChE bands are seen about 95% of the time when gastroschisis is present but are seen much less frequently in association with omphalocele. The most likely explanation for this difference is that omphalocele is membrane covered, whereas gastroschisis is not.

THE AChE/PChE RATIO TO DIFFERENTIATE BETWEEN NEURAL TUBE AND VENTRAL WALL DEFECTS

It has also been discovered that the ratio between the densities of the pseudocholinesterase (PChE) and acetylcholinesterase bands in amniotic fluid gel analyses is a reliable means of differentiating between open neural tube and open ventral wall defects.[20] Open ventral wall defects are associated with PChE bands that are relatively more dense in relation to AChE bands than open neural tube defects. This distinction can be helpful in guiding follow-up sonographic studies in cases where a lesion is difficult to visualize. Calculating AChE/PChE ratios is not helpful in detecting false positives.

Congenital nephrosis, a frequently diagnosed disorder in certain areas of the world (eg, Finland and Puerto Rico), is nearly always associated with AFP elevations in amniotic fluid. AChE bands are not visible in the presence of this lesion, however. The fetal kidney in congenital nephrosis allows AFP to filter into fetal urine and, via that route, into amniotic fluid in markedly increased concentrations, but the large molecular size of AChE appears to prevent it from following a similar path.

GEL AChE STUDIES AND FETAL DEATH

Fetal death is associated frequently with both AFP elevations and the presence of AChE bands in amniotic fluid.[21] The gel AChE electrophoresis in such cases often shows a characteristic smeared pattern. When the identification of fetal death has not been made at amniocentesis, recognizing this smeared pattern can help resolve the case. This type of situation occurs increasingly less often as ultrasound diagnosis becomes more refined.

FETAL CALF SERUM CONTAMINATION AS A SOURCE OF FALSELY POSITIVE GEL AChE STUDIES

One source of false-positive AChE gel studies in amniotic fluid has been found to result from contamination with fetal calf serum.[21] Fetal calf serum is rich in acetylcholinesterase and is used in culturing amniotic fluid cells for chromosome analysis. Small amounts of fetal calf serum, when accidentally introduced into an amniotic fluid sample prior to analysis, can produce a visible AChE band. When this is suspected, testing for bovine serum albumin via counter immunoelectrophoresis can identify the cause of the false-positive result.

AFP LEVELS IN MATERNAL SERUM IN RELATION TO FETAL OPEN NEURAL TUBE DEFECTS AND OTHER FETAL DISORDERS

DEFINING REFERENCE RANGES FOR MSAFP DURING THE SECOND TRIMESTER

The discovery that maternal serum α-fetoprotein (MSAFP) levels were higher in association with fetal open neural tube defects than with unaffected singleton pregnancies in the second trimester led to a multicenter study in the United Kingdom, aimed at testing the feasibility of using this biochemical marker for screening or diagnostic purposes.[22] MSAFP concentrations rise steadily throughout the second trimester in unaffected singleton pregnancies (by approximately 15% per week), and so it was necessary for each participating center to establish normative data against which MSAFP measurements from affected pregnancies could be compared. Figure 43-2 displays data recently analyzed from a single center, demonstrating a typical pattern of increasing MSAFP concentration between 14 and 21 weeks gestation. Because of this relationship between MSAFP concentration and gestational age, it is important to ensure accuracy of dating. Any laboratory carrying out MSAFP screening needs to be capable of demonstrating a rise in MSAFP values similar to that displayed in the figure. The higher AFP levels in maternal blood found in association with pregnancy are contributed from the fetus. There is no evidence that maternal production of AFP is altered.

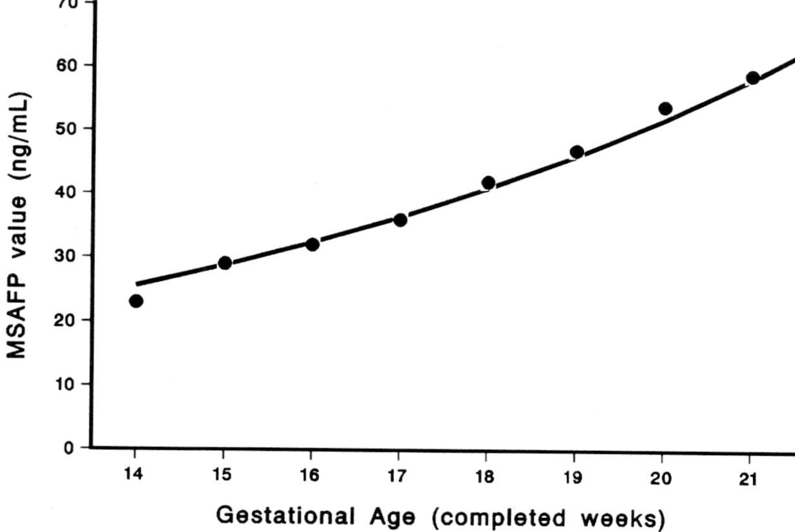

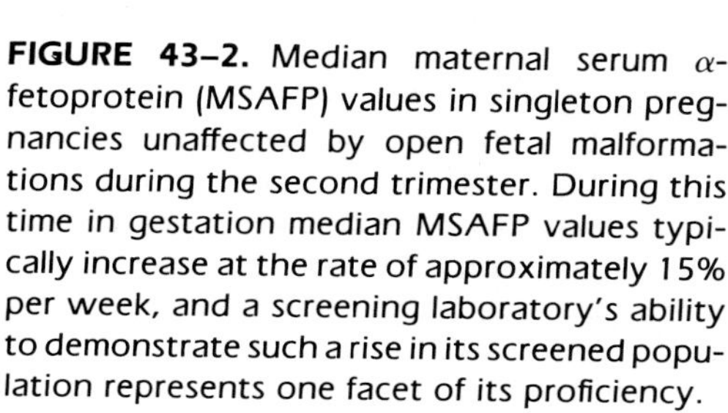
FIGURE 43-2. Median maternal serum α-fetoprotein (MSAFP) values in singleton pregnancies unaffected by open fetal malformations during the second trimester. During this time in gestation median MSAFP values typically increase at the rate of approximately 15% per week, and a screening laboratory's ability to demonstrate such a rise in its screened population represents one facet of its proficiency.

TYPES OF ASSAYS EMPLOYED TO MEASURE AFP IN MATERNAL SERUM

Radioimmunoassay (RIA) was the type of assay employed by nearly all centers for measuring MSAFP levels, because of the relatively low concentrations (about one 150th of the concentration in amniotic fluid). Rocket electrophoresis lacked sufficient sensitivity to detect such low levels. RIA continues to be used for measuring MSAFP levels, but assays that rely on enzyme or other labels instead of radioactivity are now the dominant method. These assays, when properly designed and used, can measure AFP accurately and precisely in maternal serum over the required range, and several of these assays are now commercially available in the United States.

CONDITIONS OTHER THAN OPEN FETAL DEFECTS ASSOCIATED WITH MSAFP ELEVATIONS

During the multicenter trial it became apparent that a variety of conditions in pregnancy could result in higher MSAFP levels, among them multiple gestations (twin pregnancies had MSAFP levels twice as high, on average, as singletons; triplets, three times as high; and so on) and fetal death, which often are associated with very increased MSAFP levels. Higher MSAFP levels were also found to be associated with increased risk for preterm delivery and intrauterine growth retardation, once multiple gestation, fetal death, and open fetal malformations had been ruled out. This all indicated that an elevated MSAFP measurement was relatively nonspecific in relation to open fetal defects and might be suitable as a screening, but not as a diagnostic, test.

THE USE OF MULTIPLES OF THE MEDIAN TO NORMALIZE MSAFP MEASUREMENT

In analyzing the multicenter study, Wald and Cuckle began by converting data from all the centers into multiples of the unaffected populations' median (MoM).[22] At the time of the study, large differences in assay standards existed between the contributing centers, meaning that an MSAFP level of 40 ng/mL as measured in one center might be measured as 75 ng/mL in a second center. Although both of these measurements would be found correct, when analyzed according to the normative data for their respective laboratories, it would be impossible to compare them without using a conversion factor. Wald and Cuckle chose the median as a reference point for each laboratory's unaffected population data, because it was the most stable and reliable measure of the midpoint, being less subject to the influence of occasional outlying measurements than the mean. This conversion also allowed the midpoint value for each gestational week to be designated as 1.0 MoM, thereby avoiding confusion that might arise from having to consider different within-laboratory differences in mass unit values for each gestational week. Unifying the midreference point for each laboratory meant that it was now possible to establish the median for twin pregnancies (2.0 multiples of the singleton unaffected population median), for pregnancies affected with open spina bifida (3.8 MoM), for pregnancies associated with anencephaly (7.7 MoM), and for a number of other well-defined disorders whose MSAFP values differed in distribution from the singleton, unaffected pregnancies. Figure 43-3 demonstrates the distributions of MSAFP values in unaffected singleton pregnancies and in pregnancies affected by open spina bifida. Being able to define the distributions of MSAFP values in MoM as well as the midpoints meant that the extent of overlap between unaffected and affected populations could also be analyzed, meaning that both collective and individual odds could be estimated for a pregnancy with a given fetal disorder.

ESTIMATING INDIVIDUAL AND COLLECTIVE ODDS FOR OPEN SPINA BIFIDA, BASED ON THE MSAFP MEASUREMENT

The ability to estimate individual and collective odds for a lesion such as open spina bifida provided a rational basis for decision making that allowed the background population risk to be combined with MSAFP measurements as a means of deciding a reasonable cutoff for high-risk classification. For example, the first

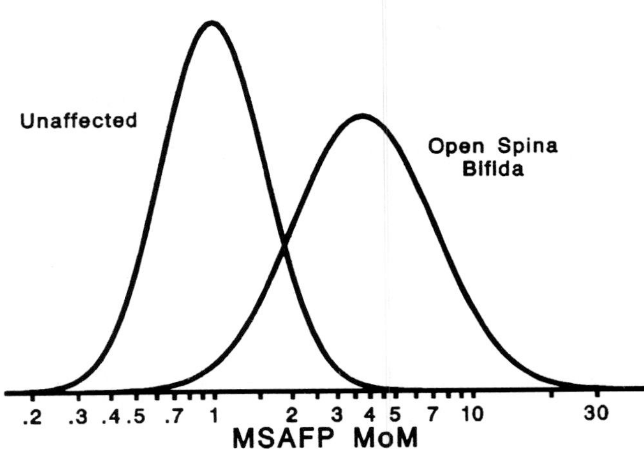

FIGURE 43–3. Maternal serum α-fetoprotein (MSAFP) distributions in singleton, unaffected pregnancies and in pregnancies affected by open spina bifida, during the second trimester. MSAFP measurements are expressed as multiples of the unaffected population median (MoM) on a logarithmic scale. Distributions of MSAFP values are log Gaussian for both of the populations, and a moderate degree of overlap is present. These distributions form the basis for estimating both collective and individual odds for being affected with open spina bifida, once the MSAFP value and prior risk of the individual or population are known.

U.K. collaborative study demonstrated that 3.4% of screened pregnancies from the general population and 85% of open spina bifida pregnancies were associated with MSAFP values at, or above, 2.5 MoM. The birth prevalence of open spina bifida at that time was approximately two in 1000. Given this information, it was possible to estimate that for every 10,000 pregnancies screened, 340 would initially be classified as at high risk and 17 of those (one in 19) actually would be affected with open spina bifida. In the United States, where the birth prevalence of open spina bifida was one per 1000, one in 38 of the pregnancies initially classified as at high risk would be affected by open spina bifida. It also became possible to assign individual risk estimates for open spina bifida, based on the woman's initial MSAFP value. To accomplish this, a line was first drawn vertically from the point on the baseline where the woman's MSAFP value was located to intersect the two curves (one curve representing the distribution of the unaffected population, and the other representing that of the open spina bifida population). Measurements were then made of the distance from baseline to unaffected curve intersection and from baseline to open spina bifida curve intersection (Fig. 43-4). These two measurements were expressed as a ratio of affected to unaffected, called the likelihood ratio. If the height of the affected were four times that of the unaffected, the likelihood ratio would be 4. This ratio could then be multiplied by the rate in the general population to determine the woman's new risk, based on her MSAFP value. If the background risk were one in 1000, this would be multiplied by 4, to produce a new risk of four in 1000.

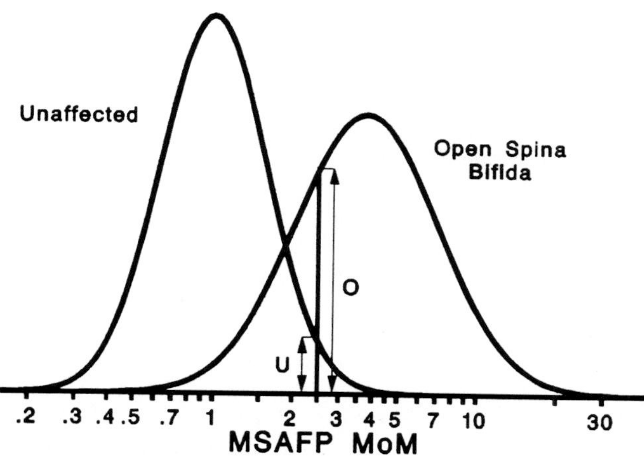

FIGURE 43–4. Estimating a pregnant woman's individual odds during the second trimester for carrying a fetus affected by open spina bifida, once her maternal serum α-fetoprotein (MSAFP) value has been determined. The distributions of MSAFP values for unaffected and affected populations, expressed as multiples of the median (MoM), are the same as those in Fig. 43-3. In this example, the woman's MSAFP level is 2.5 MoM, and the measurements from that point on the baseline to intersection with the unaffected and affected curves are 1.0 and 4.0 units, respectively, producing a likelihood ratio of 4:1. Based on her MSAFP level, the woman's individual odds for a pregnancy affected by open spina bifida are now four times as great as those in the general population.

These odds estimates do not take into account the impact of follow-up steps, such as repeating the MSAFP measurement, reinterpreting the MSAFP value after misdating errors have been corrected, and identifying multiple gestations. Approximately half of the pregnancies initially classified as being at high risk are removed from that category by these follow-up steps, and nearly all the pregnancies associated with open spina bifida remain in the high-risk group. The net effect is to increase both the collective and individual risks of those women who remain at high risk, by a factor of approximately 2.

A further factor influencing collective and individual odds estimates has evolved in recent years, as a result of improved MSAFP assay performance. It is now common for a laboratory to have coefficients of variability below 5%, in contrast to the mid-1970s, when figures ranging from 8% to 25% were common. This improvement in assay performance has little impact on median MSAFP values but substantially changes the proportion of values found in the tails of both the unaffected and affected population distributions. The proportion of pregnancies with MSAFP values above 2.5 MoM was 3.4% in the U.K. collaborative study; most individual laboratories now find rates of 1% to 2%. A similar reduction in positives has occurred at a lower 2.0 MoM cut-off—7.7% in the U.K. collaborative study as opposed to 3% to 5% in individual laboratories currently. This assay improvement has essentially no impact on the sensitivity of the screening process, but it has a significant impact on specificity, again leading to an increase in both collective and individual risk at any given MSAFP value above the cut-off. A precise method for taking these improved performance characteristics into account when estimating risk has not yet been developed.

REPEATING THE MSAFP MEASUREMENT AFTER AN INITIALLY ELEVATED RESULT: THE CONCEPT OF REGRESSION TO THE MEAN

Considerable debate has taken place as to the merit of analyzing a second maternal serum sample for AFP once a positive result has been discovered. During the first several years after MSAFP screening was introduced in the United States, only elevated MSAFP test results were considered positive, because screening was restricted to open neural tube defects. Many centers called for a second serum sample to be analyzed for AFP during that time, reasoning that the risk of open neural tube defects would be reduced, if the second measurement was lower and fell within the normal range. This assumption was correct, but much of the time the centers did not fully appreciate the mathematical principle that provided the basis for this phenomenon: regression to the mean.[23] This principle states that when a measurement is located away from the center of its population, the tendency will be for it to move toward the center when the measurement is repeated, and the further away that the initial measurement is from its population's center, the greater will be that tendency.

The midpoints of the unaffected singleton population and the open spina bifida population are widely separated (1.0 MoM for unaffected, 3.8 MoM for open spina bifida), and MSAFP measurements above the cut-offs used by most centers (2.0 to 2.5 MoM) often are located between the central points of the two populations. A repeat MSAFP measurement, in such cases, is highly likely to move in one direction for unaffected pregnancies (lower) and in another if the pregnancy is affected with open spina bifida (higher) (Fig. 43-5). Other major open fetal malformations associated with MSAFP elevations also have MSAFP MoM midpoints widely separated from the unaffected population (eg, anencephaly, open ventral wall defects), and the principle of regression to the mean applies in those cases as well.

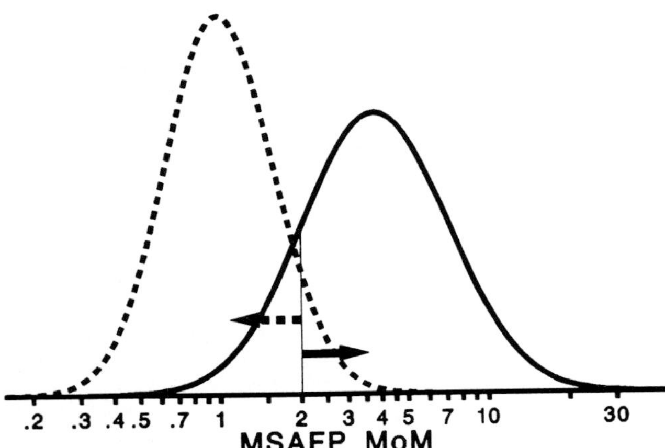

FIGURE 43–5. The effect of repeating the maternal serum α-fetoprotein (MSAFP) measurement when the initial value falls above the screening cut-off for detecting open spina bifida and other open fetal malformations. In this example, the woman's initial MSAFP value falls at 2.0 multiples of median (MoM), a commonly used screening cut-off. This value falls between the center points of the unaffected (MSAFP = 1.0 MoM) population distribution and the population distribution for open spina bifida (MSAFP = 3.8 MoM). The line drawn vertically from 2.0 MoM indicates that the woman's individual odds for having an affected pregnancy are equivalent to those of the general population (the heights of the curves are approximately equal, making the likelihood ratio 1). When a second serum sample is obtained and measured for AFP, there will be a tendency for the value to be lower when the pregnancy is unaffected and to be higher, if open spina bifida is present. This is an example of regression to the mean.

Repeating MSAFP measurements following an initial elevation has proved helpful to many screening programs as a way to sort out falsely positive screening results.[24] A repeat MSAFP measurement that falls within the normal range does not, however, exclude the possibility of an open fetal malformation; it only reduces its likelihood, and this is a particularly important aspect of the screening process to explain to the patient.

WHY REPEATING THE MSAFP MEASUREMENT AFTER AN INITIAL LOW VALUE IS CONTRAINDICATED

When screening for Down syndrome using MSAFP measurements was first introduced, it seemed natural to call for repeat testing after an initial positive test result. Unfortunately, the MSAFP distributions of the unaffected singleton and Down syndrome populations overlap considerably, and the midpoints are close together. For that reason nearly all the MSAFP measurements labeled as positive fall away from the two medians in the same direction. The tendency to regress, therefore, is in the same direction, whether or not the pregnancy is associated with Down syndrome (Fig. 43-6). The net effect of repeating is to decrease the sensitivity of the screening test, and a number of cases of Down syndrome are known to have been missed using this type of approach. It is now generally recommended that repeat MSAFP testing not be done when screening for Down syndrome.[25]

LIMITATIONS OF SENSITIVITY OF MSAFP SCREENING TO DETECT OPEN FETAL DEFECTS

Among the major open fetal malformations detected by MSAFP screening, anencephaly is the most readily detected, being associated with MSAFP values above the screening cut-off in more than 90% of cases. Gastroschisis is also readily detected, and MSAFP screening sensitivity for that condition approaches that for anencephaly.[26] Open spina bifida is associated with MSAFP values that more often overlap with the unaffected population, and screening sensitivity for detecting that condition is approximately 75%.[22] A smaller proportion of omphalocele cases is detected than of open spina bifida (about 60%).[26] The reasons for not identifying a greater proportion of cases through screening are not always correctly perceived. For example, some believe that faulty MSAFP assay performance is largely responsible for diminished detection of the open lesions and that improvement in the assay will lead to better detection. This perception is incorrect, except in extreme cases, such as where an assay might be measuring a substance other than AFP or where technical performance is so poor that samples are constantly mixed up. Commercially available assays now perform very satisfactorily,[27] and nearly all laboratories carry out their duties

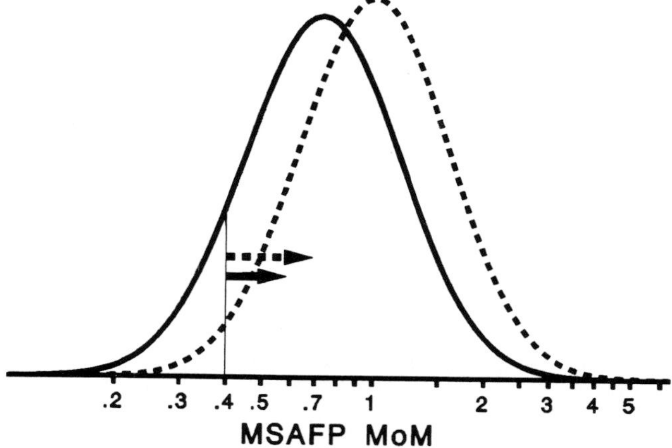

FIGURE 43–6. The effect of repeating the maternal serum α-fetoprotein (MSAFP) measurement, when the initial value falls below the screening cut-off for detecting Down syndrome. In this example, the woman's initial MSAFP value falls at 0.4 multiples of the median (MoM). At age 28 or greater, this places her in a high-risk category for having a fetus affected with Down syndrome. The MSAFP value falls considerably below the center points of both the unaffected (MSAFP = 1.0 MoM) population distribution and the population distribution for Down syndrome (MSAFP = 0.75 MoM). The line drawn vertically from 0.4 MoM indicates that the woman's individual odds for having an affected pregnancy are about three times that of unscreened pregnancies of the same age. When a second serum sample is obtained and measured for AFP, there will be a tendency for the value to be higher, regardless of whether the pregnancy is affected with Down syndrome. The net effect of using repeat measurements will be to reduce both Down syndrome detection and false positives equally. This is also an example of regression to the mean.

responsibly. The actual reason that detection is limited for the various open fetal lesions is that their MSAFP distributions do overlap to varying degrees with the unaffected population, making certain proportions impossible to detect. This characteristic of the MSAFP screening process also needs to be understood by physicians, their office personnel, and their patients, so that expectations do not exceed the capacity of the screening test.

IMPROVED GESTATIONAL DATING AND BIPARIETAL DIAMETER MEASUREMENTS AS WAYS TO IMPROVE SCREENING SENSITIVITY

With this limitation clearly in mind, certain steps can be undertaken by both physician and laboratory that will lead to some improvement in both sensitivity and specificity of the screening process. The first of these has to do with gestational dating. Most pregnancies are still dated from the first day of the last menstrual period (LMP) at the time in gestation when MSAFP testing is performed, and the original estimates for both sensitivity and specificity were made, using LMP dates. Even when LMP dates are carefully obtained, they are incorrect by more than 2 weeks about 20% of the time.[28] Furthermore, there is a tendency to think a pregnancy is further advanced than it really is. This diminishes screening sensitivity, on the one hand, and yields false-positive screening results, on the other, because MSAFP measurements normally rise by about 15% per week during the second trimester, and normative data are based on this rise.

In 1980 the biparietal diameters (BPD) of fetuses with spina bifida were found to be smaller, on average, at a given gestational week in the second trimester, than their unaffected counterparts.[29] Other measurements did not differ. The net effect of dating pregnancies via BPD measurements is to date fetuses with spina bifida incorrectly as being less far advanced than they really are. If BPD measurements were to be used routinely in dating for MSAFP screening, the MSAFP measurements would appear higher for the pregnancies with open spina bifida because of this artifact, and sensitivity for detecting the lesion would be increased, possibly to above 90%. Furthermore, a brief ultrasound study would correct the dates of pregnancies further advanced than predicted by LMP and would also identify twins, thereby reducing false-positive screening results. Cases of anencephaly would also be identified at that point. Systematically using BPD measurements would reduce screening program costs and avoid unnecessary anxiety for many of the women.

THE RELATIONSHIP BETWEEN A WOMAN'S WEIGHT AND HER MSAFP CONCENTRATION

A second refinement in interpreting MSAFP screening results came in 1981, when it was reported that the AFP concentration in the mother's blood was partly dependent on her weight: the larger the woman, the lower the average MSAFP concentration, presumably because of a dilution effect from the larger vascular compartment (Fig. 43-7).[30,31] This source of variability could be corrected for mathematically, and most screening centers now take this into account in their test interpretations. Concern has been expressed that correcting for maternal weight might diminish sensitivity for detecting open spina bifida. Such would be the case if women with affected fetuses were smaller as a group than their unaffected counterparts. One analysis from England reports a slightly lower average weight among women with affected pregnancies,[31] whereas a second, from the United States, reports a slightly higher average weight.[32] Neither of these reported differences is significant. A third 16-center collaborative study from the United States finds no difference.[33] On the assumption that no weight differences exist, adjusting for the woman's weight might be expected to result in slightly increased detection of open spina bifida, because of the very heavy women in the upper tail of the weight dis-

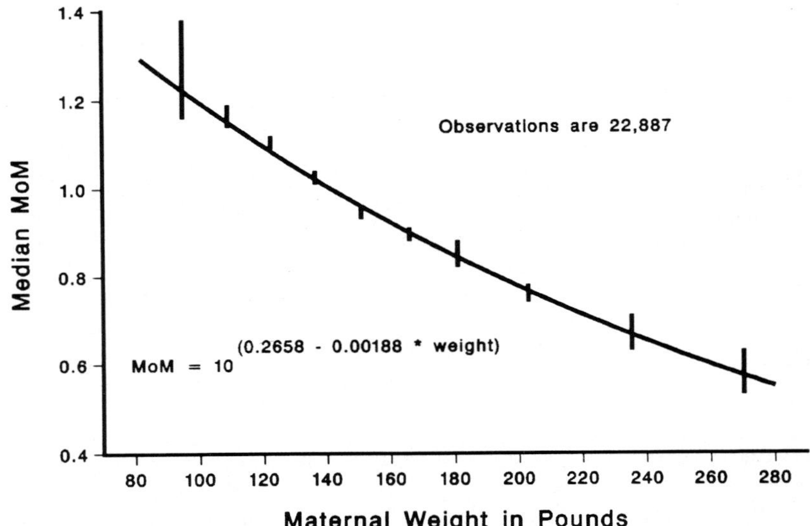

FIGURE 43–7. The relationship between a woman's weight and her maternal serum α-fetoprotein (MSAFP) level during the second trimester. During the second trimester a nearly twofold difference exists in average MSAFP concentrations between very light-weight and very heavy women, and a steady downward progression in MSAFP concentration occurs as weight increases. This relationship exists for both unaffected pregnancies and pregnancies affected with open fetal malformations. It is possible to take the woman's weight into account when interpreting her MSAFP measurement by using the formula shown in the figure.

tribution. This has been found to be the case in the U.S. collaborative study mentioned earlier. A greater advantage from correcting MSAFP values for maternal weight results from reducing false-positive test results associated with the lighter-weight women by about 10%, translating into fewer amniocenteses and fewer women being made anxious. The relationship between weight and MSAFP concentration appears to be independent of both the woman's age and her geographic location.

A WOMAN'S RACE IN RELATION TO HER MSAFP CONCENTRATION

Sometimes a woman's race independently influences her MSAFP level.[34] Black women have, on average, MSAFP screening measurements that are 15% higher than those of white women.[35] In mixed population screening, where this is not taken into account, an inappropriately high proportion of black pregnant women will be identified as having positive screening results and will be sent on for further diagnostic procedures. The inappropriateness of this action is compounded by a lower risk among black women for having pregnancies affected by neural tube defects. Until recently, it was not known whether the higher average MSAFP value in the black population was restricted to the unaffected pregnancies or whether pregnancies with open spina bifida also were associated with higher values. The 16-center U.S. collaborative study documented a higher average MSAFP level in the pregnancies affected with open spina bifida and thereby documented the feasibility of adjusting the MSAFP values to reflect a more appropriate proportion of women with positive screening results.[36]

INSULIN-DEPENDENT DIABETES AND MSAFP CONCENTRATION

A more occasional variable that influences MSAFP measurements is maternal insulin-dependent diabetes, which is associated with 20% lower MSAFP values, on average, than the unaffected singleton population.[37,38] Women with insulin-dependent diabetes also are at greater risk for having pregnancies affected by open neural tube defects. No MSAFP differences have been observed for gestational diabetes. It is not presently known whether insulin-dependent diabetic women with pregnancies associated with open spina bifida also have lower average MSAFP values, but this is not a critical point, since correcting MSAFP values in diabetic pregnancies will always increase screening sensitivity. Adjusting MSAFP measurements in diabetic women is now carried out routinely in most screening centers. Currently, a scientific discussion is in progress as to whether the level of diabetic control, as measured by the hemoglobin $A1_C$, influences the MSAFP concentration.[39,40] The issue is not yet completely resolved.

THE BIOLOGY OF AFP AS IT RELATES TO SCREENING AND DIAGNOSTIC TESTING

AFP PRODUCTION AND CIRCULATION IN FETAL AND MATERNAL COMPARTMENTS

α-Fetoprotein is the major circulating fetal protein early in pregnancy, reaching a peak concentration of approximately 3000 mg/L at 12 weeks gestation and then slowly falling in concentration. AFP is thought to be the fetal albumin equivalent, and its molecular structure is similar to that of albumin, even though antibodies raised against AFP have virtually no cross-reactivity with albumin. This latter characteristic is critical in allowing a variety of antibody-based assays to be developed for measuring AFP in amniotic fluid, maternal serum, and other body fluids as well (all of which also contain very high concentrations of albumin). For practical purposes, AFP can be thought of as feto-specific (the circulating level in non-pregnant adults is up to 2 μg/L). This property of AFP separates it from all the other major circulating proteins and makes it uniquely suitable to serve as a marker for certain of the major fetal disorders. The major source of AFP production in the fetus is the liver, and production continues constant into the third trimester, with actual circulating concentrations falling, because the fetal circulatory compartment is enlarging steadily.

NORMAL TRANSPORT OF AFP INTO AMNIOTIC FLUID AND MATERNAL SERUM

Normally, AFP levels are relatively high in amniotic fluid during the second trimester, because of sieving through the fetal kidney (about 20 mg/L at 14 weeks gestation, and falling at a constant rate thereafter). The steady fall in concentration coincides with the increasing amniotic fluid volume, and it is necessary to establish a reference range for amniotic fluid AFP that takes gestational age into account. Fetal AFP normally appears in the maternal circulation via two routes: transplacental and transamniotic.[41] About 70% of the fetal contribution of AFP to the maternal circulation has been estimated to be transplacental; the rest is estimated to be transamniotic, under normal conditions.

NORMAL PATTERNS OF AFP CONCENTRATIONS IN AMNIOTIC FLUID AND MATERNAL SERUM

Normally, median levels of MSAFP rise steadily at the rate of about 15% per week during the second trimester, at a time when both amniotic fluid and fetal serum levels are falling. This paradox has not been explained experimentally, but one possible explanation is that the placenta is growing rapidly during this time and provides a larger surface area for both transplacental and transamniotic diffusion.

TRANSPORT OF AFP INTO AMNIOTIC FLUID AND MATERNAL SERUM IN THE PRESENCE OF FETAL MALFORMATIONS

Understanding this transfer process helps us to appreciate why maternal serum AFP measurements are less sensitive and specific for detecting open fetal malformations. When open spina bifida is present in the fetus, AFP leaks directly from the exposed surface into the amniotic fluid, leading to levels raised sufficiently that the lesion can be detected 97% of the time. The same mechanism operates with anencephaly, where the lesion is usually larger and leaks even higher amounts of AFP (leading to 99% detection).

The increased concentrations of AFP in amniotic fluid are reflected in maternal serum, because of diffusion across the amnion. But the amnion is a barrier with some variability in sieving characteristics.[41] Furthermore, the transplacental contribution is not likely to be increased in the presence of fetal lesions and stands as a constant background source of AFP that may interfere with the signal being provided by the transamniotic AFP. The higher the amniotic fluid AFP concentration, the more AFP, on average, appears in the maternal circulation, explaining why MSAFP levels are higher with anencephaly than with open spina bifida.

ABNORMAL TRANSPORT OF AFP WITH IMPENDING OR PREEXISTING FETAL DEATH

When a fetus has died just prior to MSAFP screening, the amniotic fluid contains higher than normal concentrations of AFP, and MSAFP levels are also elevated. It is likely that these higher AFP levels result from a general breakdown in the normal fetal tissue barriers to diffusion and filtration. MSAFP levels are also elevated in some instances when the fetus is viable at the time of MSAFP screening but dies subsequently, in some cases several weeks later. In those instances, the amniotic fluid AFP level is normal at the time of screening, and the mechanism to explain the higher MSAFP level is unclear. It is possible, however, that placental hemorrhage has occurred as a premorbid event or that "fetal distress" led to a compromise in the integrity of the placental interface. Recognizing that elevated MSAFP measurements indicate a high risk for subsequent fetal death after other conditions have been ruled out, many clinicians have increased surveillance of such pregnancies, but no strategy has yet been found successful in preventing those deaths. Risk of fetal death is approximately 6 times higher with MSAFP elevation than when the MSAFP measurement is not elevated.

ABNORMAL TRANSPORT OF AFP IN CASES OF FALSE POSITIVES

Fetal blood is often a problem when either amniotic fluid or maternal serum AFP levels are being measured. If, during amniocentesis, the fetal circulation is inadvertently breached, the fetal blood in the amniotic fluid sample will carry high concentrations of AFP with it and can produce false-positive test results.[15] This can be especially difficult to identify if the sample has been centrifuged prior to being sent for AFP analysis. Under such conditions an analysis for hemoglobin F in the supernatant usually provides the clue. Visibly bloody amniotic fluid of fetal origin is sufficient to produce false positives. Fetal blood in the maternal circulation is a second and frequent source of false-positive test results, this time for the MSAFP screening test. Fetal blood can enter the maternal circulation through a placental hemorrhage (the usual source)[42] or may enter in conjunction with a procedure, such as amniocentesis.

ABNORMAL TRANSPORT OF AFP INTO MATERNAL SERUM AND RISK FOR LOW BIRTH WEIGHT

Elevated MSAFP values in conjunction with normal amniotic fluid AFP values also signal a high risk for low-birth-weight outcomes, some due to prematurity and others to intrauterine growth retardation.[43] This is a further example of the nonspecificity of MSAFP as a screening test but also demonstrates that even false-positive screening results (in relation to open fetal malformations) are providing additional information about high-risk pregnancies. Just as with fetal deaths, no management protocol has been discovered that reduces risk of low birth weight. This risk is increased between three and four times over the risk in pregnancies with normal MSAFP measurements.

VAGINAL BLEEDING AND ABNORMAL TRANSPORT OF AFP INTO MATERNAL SERUM

Vaginal bleeding during pregnancy is associated with higher risk for fetal morbidity and mortality and is associated with placental hemorrhage.[44] When the presence or absence of vaginal bleeding is considered in relation to MSAFP measurements, it is found to be an independent risk factor for both low birth weight and fetal death. It is therefore helpful to know if a woman with an elevated MSAFP measurement also has vaginal bleeding; when both risk factors are present, the risk for fetal death is considerably higher.

AN UNEXPLAINED ASSOCIATION BETWEEN MSAFP ELEVATIONS AND OLIGOHYDRAMNIOS

Oligohydramnios is another condition found occasionally in association with elevated MSAFP measurements.[45] In some instances the reason for oligohydramnios becomes apparent with the ultrasound study, including conditions such as urinary tract anomalies and extrauterine pregnancies. Whether or not an explanation is found, the prognosis for viability of the pregnancy is poor, with the survival rate being estimated at less than 20%.[46]

TRANSPORT OF AFP INTO MATERNAL SERUM IN ASSOCIATION WITH TWINS

Twin pregnancies are associated with MSAFP values that are, on average, twice as high as those of singleton pregnancies, and if a cut-off for MSAFP screening is set at 2.0 MoM, half of the twin pregnancies will fall above that cut-off.[22] Unsuspected twin pregnancies are therefore a frequent source for false-positive screening results. There has been much discussion as to what should be an appropriate cut-off for twin pregnancies when screening for open neural tube defects. Most centers simply double their singleton cut-off, a policy that is both reasonable and easy to remember. Screening sensitivity for open fetal malformations in twins is reduced at any given cut-off, however, because in most instances only one of the twins is affected when an open fetal lesion is present in the pregnancy. Other risk factors, such as fetal death and low birth weight, can also be roughly estimated, using the two times higher cut-off.

MSAFP LEVELS IN ASSOCIATION WITH FETAL DOWN SYNDROME AND OTHER CONDITIONS

VERY LOW MSAFP LEVELS IN RELATION TO FETAL DEATH AND MISDATED PREGNANCY

Prior to 1984, low MSAFP values were of limited interest to screening centers. Values of less than 10 μg/L were found to be associated with several conditions, the most frequent of which was gross misdating of the pregnancy.[47] When the screened pregnancies were dated by LMP, between 50% and 75% of the very low MSAFP values could subsequently be explained by correcting the dates via ultrasound. This was, and continues to be, of some importance. Because screening for open fetal defects is not reliable until 15 weeks gestation, nearly all the grossly misdated pregnancies would be candidates for rescreening at the appropriate gestational age. Also found in association with very low MSAFP measurements were fetal deaths that had occurred a long time prior to the blood sample being obtained. In such cases the AFP had simply undergone autolysis. Miscellaneous other conditions were also discovered when very low MSAFP values were followed up, including molar pregnancy and non-pregnancy. It did appear worthwhile to perform ultrasound studies when the MSAFP values were under 10 μg/L, and if no obvious explanation was found, the pregnancy could then be considered at low risk for subsequent fetal death and other pregnancy complications.

COMBINING LOW MSAFP MEASUREMENTS WITH WOMEN'S AGE TO SCREEN FOR TRISOMY 21

The potential significance of low MSAFP values changed in 1984, when Merkatz and colleagues reported that MSAFP values were lower in pregnancies where the chromosomal constitution of the fetus was trisomy 21 (Down syndrome) or trisomy 18 (Edwards syndrome).[7] Cuckle and colleagues subsequently confirmed the observation and proposed that MSAFP screening might be extended to include Down syndrome by combining a woman's prior, age-related risk with the risk as defined by her MSAFP level to derive a composite risk.[8] Until this time the screening test for determining whether a woman's risk was sufficient to warrant amniocentesis was a question: asking her age. Pregnant women aged 35 and older were judged to be at high risk, and women younger than that age were not offered amniocentesis because their risk was relatively low. The additional information provided by the MSAFP measurement now offered the potential to identify a group of younger pregnant women whose individual risk for having a pregnancy affected by Down syndrome was comparable to that of women aged 35 and older. Just over 5% of all pregnancies annually occur in women aged 35 and older, and approximately 20% of the cases of Down syndrome are born to those women. The remaining 80% of the births of Down syndrome babies are to women younger than age 35, and it was estimated that 20% of the cases of Down syndrome could be identified in that younger population by using a combination of MSAFP and age-related risk. Although this represents a relatively insensitive screening process when judged against screening for open fetal defects, it is comparably sensitive to the traditional screening by a woman's age, and it provides the opportunity to nearly double the number of cases of Down syndrome detected within a given population. Figures 43-4 and 43-5 can be compared to appreciate the extent of overlap between the unaffected population and populations affected by either open spina bifida or Down syndrome.

Many prenatal screening centers subsequently analyzed and reported their MSAFP measurements in relation to Down syndrome, and all but one confirmed the two original observations. The median MSAFP value for pregnancies with Down syndrome fetuses was identified as being 0.75 multiples of the unaffected singleton population median, with a log Gaussian distribution. Similarly, amniotic fluid AFP measurements were found to be lower in the presence of a fetus with Down syndrome.[48] Cord blood levels of AFP were also lower, on average, when the baby suffered from Down syndrome.[49] This all suggested that fetal liver AFP production or disposition was altered with Down syndrome. A recent analysis of second-trimester fetal blood AFP levels failed to identify lower concentrations when Down syndrome was present.[50] Further work needs to be done to understand better the mechanism leading to the lower MSAFP levels in the presence of fetal Down syndrome.

A MULTICENTER FIELD TRIAL TO DETERMINE THE EFFICACY OF MSAFP SCREENING FOR FETAL TRISOMY 21

An eight-center collaborative field trial was initiated in New England in 1985, sponsored by the New England Regional Genetics Group, to determine the efficacy of applying MSAFP screening routinely to the pregnancy population.[51] All the centers used a screening cut-off based on individual risk, set to the second-trimester risk of a 35-year-old woman for carrying a fetus with Down syndrome (1:270). The centers all limited MSAFP interpretation for Down syndrome to women under the age of 35, to avoid conflict with accepted medical practice, and all recommended that a second MSAFP determination not be done after an initially positive result, to avoid reducing sensitivity (as discussed earlier in this chapter). During the 14-month enrollment period 77,273 pregnancies were screened with MSAFP measurements by the eight centers. Out of that number, 4.7% were initially classified as being at high risk for Down syndrome, and 2.7% of the pregnancies remained at high risk after gestational dates had been confirmed. Seventy-six percent of these high-risk women elected to have amniocentesis, and 18 fetuses with Down syndrome and four fetuses with trisomy 18 were identified in this group. One fetus with Down syndrome was identified per 89 amniocenteses performed (approximately one per 150 amniocenteses performed in women aged 35 and older is associated with Down syndrome), and an additional three Down syndrome births were identified from among the women who refused amniocentesis. It was estimated that approximately 25% of the fetal Down syndrome cases could be identified in younger pregnant women, and the study concluded that this type of screening was feasible. A recent survey of MSAFP screening centers in the United States indicates that more than 1 million pregnancies were being provided with screening for Down syndrome in 1988.

ADDITIONAL BIOCHEMICAL MARKERS OF POTENTIAL VALUE IN SCREENING FOR TRISOMY 21

More recently, two additional biochemical products in a pregnant woman's blood, human chorionic gonadotropin (hCG) and unconjugated estriol (uE3), have been identified as potential screening markers for Down syndrome during the second trimester. Unconjugated estriol is synthesized in three steps: production of dehydroepiandrosterone (DHEAs) in the fetal adrenal, conversion of DHEAs to 16αOH-DHEAs in the fetal liver, and conversion of 16αOH-DHEAs to uE3 in the placenta. Unconjugated estriol is then released into the maternal serum circulation and excreted. Canick and colleagues have reported that maternal uE3 levels are lower, on average, in the presence of fetal Down syndrome.[52] Wald and colleagues have found that uE3 levels are largely independent of AFP levels, making uE3 a suitable candidate for an additional screening test.[53] Bogart and colleagues have studied hCG and found that its levels in maternal serum during the second trimester are, on average, considerably higher in the presence of fetal Down syndrome.[9] Wald and colleagues have confirmed this finding and have discovered that hCG levels also are largely independent of both uE3 and AFP.[11] They have estimated that, using a combination of these three tests, it may be possible to raise the sensitivity for detecting fetal Down syndrome to approximately 60%, while keeping the false-positive rate similar to that for AFP alone. Field trials are now underway to evaluate the feasibility of this new, and more demanding, process.

REFERENCES

1. Bergstrand CG, Czar B. Demonstration of a new protein fraction in serum from the human fetus. Scand J Clin Lab Invest 1956;174:8.
2. Ruoslahti E. Isolation and biochemical properties of alpha-fetoprotein. In: Crandall BR, Brazier MAB, eds. Prevention of neural tube defects: the role of alpha-fetoprotein. New York: Academic Press, 1978:9.
3. Brock DJH, Sutcliffe RG. Alpha-fetoprotein in the antenatal diagnosis of anencephaly and spina bifida. Lancet 1972;ii:197.
4. Wald NJ, Brock DJH, Bonnar J. Prenatal diagnosis of spina bifida and anencephaly through maternal serum alpha-fetoprotein. Lancet 1974;i:765.
5. Brock DJH, Bolton AE, and Scrimgeour JB. Prenatal diagnosis of spina bifida and anencephaly through maternal plasma alpha-fetoprotein measurement. Lancet 1974;i:767.
6. Smith AD, Wald NJ, Cuckle HS, Stirrat GM, Bobrow M, Lagercrantz H. Amniotic fluid acetylcholinesterase as a possible diagnostic test for neural tube defects in early pregnancy. Lancet 1979;i:685.
7. Merkatz IR, Nitowsky HM, Macri JN, Johnson WE. An association between low maternal serum α-fetoprotein and fetal chromosomal abnormalities. Am J Obstet Gynecol 1984;148:886.
8. Cuckle HS, Wald NJ, Lindenbaum RH. Maternal serum alpha-fetoprotein measurement: a screening test for Down syndrome. Lancet 1984;i:926.
9. Bogart MH, Pandian MR, Jones OW. Abnormal maternal serum chorionic gonadotropin levels in pregnancies with fetal chromosome abnormalities. Prenat Diagn 1987;7:623.
10. Canick JA, Knight GJ, Palomaki GE, Haddow JE, Cuckle HS, Wald NJ. Low second trimester maternal serum unconjugated oestriol in pregnancies with Down's syndrome. Br J Obstet Gynaecol 1988;95:330.
11. Wald NJ, Cuckle HS, Densem JW, et al. Maternal serum screening for Down's syndrome in early pregnancy. Br Med J 1988;297:883.
12. Johnson AM, Umansky I, Alper CA, Everett C, Greenspan G. Amniotic fluid proteins: maternal and fetal contributions. J Pediatr 1974;84:588.
13. Haddow JE, Cowchock FS, Macri JN, Munson M, Baldwin P, Aldrich N. Second trimester amniotic fluid protein values from normal, neural tube defect, and fetal demise pregnancies after exclusion of maternal blood contamination by testing for pregnancy-associated macroglobulin. Pediatr Res 1978;12:243.
14. Laurell C-B. Quantitative estimation of proteins by electrophoresis in agarose gel containing antibodies. Anal Biochem 1966;15:45
15. Amniotic-fluid alpha-fetoprotein measurement in antenatal diagnosis of anencephaly and open spina bifida in early pregnancy. Second report of the U.K. Collaborative Study on alpha-fetoprotein in relation to neural tube defects. Lancet 1979;ii:651.
16. Wald NJ, Cuckle HS. Open neural tube defects. In: Wald NJ, ed. Antenatal and neonatal screening. Oxford: Oxford University Press, 1984:53.
17. Seppala M, Aula P, Rapola J, Karjalainen O, Hottunen NP, Ruoslahti E. Congenital nephrotic syndrome: prenatal diagnosis and genetic counseling by estimation of amniotic fluid and maternal serum alpha-fetoprotein. Lancet 1976;ii:123.
18. Goldfine C, Haddow JE, Knight GJ, Palomaki GE. Amniotic fluid acetylcholinesterase measurements in pregnancies associated with gastroschisis. Prenat Diagn 1989;9:697.
19. Amniotic fluid acetylcholinesterase electrophoresis as a secondary test in the diagnosis of anencephaly and open spina bifida in early pregnancy. Collaborative acetylcholinesterase study. Lancet 1981;ii:321.
20. Goldfine C, Miller WA, Haddow JE. Amniotic fluid gel cholinesterase density ratios in fetal open defects of the neural tube and ventral wall. Br J Obstet Gynaecol 1983;90:238.
21. Haddow JE, Goldfine C. The evolving role of amniotic fluid acetylcholinesterase analysis for identifying open fetal defects during the second trimester. In: Mizejewski GJ, Porter IH, eds. Alpha-fetoprotein and congenital disorders. San Diego: Academic Press, 1985:215.
22. Maternal serum alpha-fetoprotein measurement in antenatal screening for anencephaly and spina bifida in early pregnancy. Report of the UK collaborative study on alpha-fetoprotein in relation to neural tube defects. Lancet 1977;i:1323.
23. James KE. Regression toward the mean in uncontrolled clinical studies. Biometrics 1973;29:121.
24. Haddow JE, Kloza EM, Smith DE, Knight GJ. Data from an alpha-fetoprotein screening program in Maine. Obstet Gynecol 1983;62:556.
25. Haddow JE, Palomaki GE, Wald NJ, Cuckle HS. Maternal serum alpha-fetoprotein screening for Down syndrome and repeat testing. Lancet 1986;ii:1460.
26. Palomaki GE, Hill LE, Knight GJ, Haddow JE, Carpenter M. Second trimester maternal serum alpha-fetoprotein levels in pregnancies associated with gastroschisis and omphalocele. Obstet Gynecol 1988;71:906.
27. Knight GJ, Palomaki GE, Haddow JE. Assessing reliability of AFP test kits. Contemp Obstet Gynecol 1987;October:1.
28. Wald NJ, Cuckle HS, Boreham J. Effect of estimating gestational age by ultrasound cephalometry on the specificity of α-fetoprotein screening for open neural tube defects. Br J Obstet Gynaecol 1982;89:1050.
29. Wald NJ, Cuckle HS, Boreham J, Stirrat G. Small biparietal diameter of fetuses with spina bifida: implications for antenatal screening. Br J Obstet Gynaecol 1980;87:219.
30. Haddow JE, Knight GJ, Kloza EM, Smith DE. Relation between maternal weight and serum alpha-fetoprotein concentration during the second trimester. Clin Chem 1981;27:133.
31. Wald NJ, Cuckle HS, Boreham J, Terzian E, Redman C. The effect of maternal weight on maternal serum alpha-fetoprotein levels. Br J Obstet Gynaecol 1981;88:1094.
32. Haddow JE, Smith DE, Sever J. Effect of maternal weight on

maternal serum alpha-fetoprotein. Br J Obstet Gynaecol 1982;89:93.

33. Johnson AM, Palomaki GE, Haddow JE. The effect of adjusting maternal serum alpha-fetoprotein levels for maternal weight in pregnancies with fetal open spina bifida: a United States collaborative study. Am J Obstet Gynecol 1990;163:9.
34. Johnson AM. Racial differences in maternal serum alpha-fetoprotein screening. In: Mizejewski GJ, Porter IH, eds. Alpha-fetoprotein and congenital disorders. New York: Academic Press, 1985:183.
35. Baumgarten A. Racial differences and biological significance of maternal serum alpha-fetoprotein. Lancet 1986;ii:573.
36. Johnson AM, Palomaki GE, Haddow JE. Maternal serum alpha-fetoprotein levels in black and Caucasian pregnancies with fetal open spina bifida: a United States collaborative study. Am J Obstet Gynecol 1990;162:328.
37. Wald NJ, Cuckle HS, Boreham J, Stirrat GM, Turnbull AC. Maternal serum alpha-fetoprotein and diabetes mellitus. Br J Obstet Gynaecol 1979;86:101.
38. Milunsky A, Alpert E, Kitzmiller JL, Younger MD, Neff RK. Prenatal diagnosis of neural tube defects VIII. The importance of serum alpha-fetoprotein screening in diabetic pregnant women. Am J Obstet Gynecol 1982;142:1030.
39. Baumgarten A, Robinson S. Prospective study of an inverse relationship between maternal glycosylated hemoglobin and serum α-fetoprotein concentrations in pregnant women with diabetes. Am J Obstet Gynecol 1988;159:77.
40. Greene MF, Haddow JE, Palomaki GE, Knight GJ. Maternal serum alpha-fetoprotein levels in diabetic pregnancies. Lancet 1988;ii:345.
41. Haddow JE, Macri JN, Munson M. The amnion regulates movement of fetally derived alpha-fetoprotein into maternal blood. J Lab Clin Med 1979;94:343.
42. Los FJ, deWolf BTHM, Huisjes JH. Raised maternal serum alpha-fetoprotein levels and spontaneous fetomaternal transfusion. Lancet 1979;ii:210.
43. Brock DJH, Barron L, Labb GM. The potential of mid-trimester maternal plasma alpha-fetoprotein measurement in predicting infants of low birthweight. Br J Obstet Gynaecol 1980;87:582.
44. Haddow JE, Knight GJ, Kloza EM, Palomaki GE. Alpha-fetoprotein, vaginal bleeding and pregnancy risk. Br J Obstet Gynaecol 1986;93:589.
45. Stirrat GM, Gough JD, Bullock S, Wald NJ, Cuckle HS. Raised maternal serum AFP, oligohydramnios and poor fetal outcome. Br J Obstet Gynaecol 1981;88:231.
46. Richards DS, Seeds JW, Katz VL, Lingley LH, Albright SG, Cefalo RC. Elevated maternal serum alpha-fetoprotein with oligohydramnios: ultrasound evaluation and outcome. Obstet Gynecol 1988;72:337.
47. Haddow JE, Hill LE, Palomaki GE, Knight GJ. Very low versus undetectable maternal serum alpha-fetoprotein values and fetal death. Prenat Diagn 1987;7:401.
48. Cuckle HS, Wald NJ. Amniotic fluid alpha-fetoprotein levels in Down's syndrome. Lancet 1986;ii:290.
49. Cuckle HS, Wald NJ. Cord serum alpha-fetoprotein and Down's syndrome. Br J Obstet Gynaecol 1986;93:408.
50. Scioscia A, Blakemore K, Inati M, et al. Midtrimester fetal serum AFP levels in normal and Down syndrome fetuses. Am J Hum Genet 1988;43:A250.
51. Combining maternal serum alpha-fetoprotein measurements and age to screen for Down syndrome in pregnant women under age 35. An eight center prospective collaborative study. Am J Obstet Gynecol 1989;160:575.
52. Canick JA, Knight GJ, Palomaki GE, Haddow JE, Cuckle HS, Wald NJ. Low second trimester maternal serum unconjugated oestriol in Down syndrome pregnancy. Br J Obstet Gynaecol 1988;95:330.
53. Wald NJ, Cuckle HS, Densem JW, et al. Maternal serum unconjugated oestriol as an antenatal screening test for Down syndrome. Br J Obstet Gynaecol 1988;95:334.

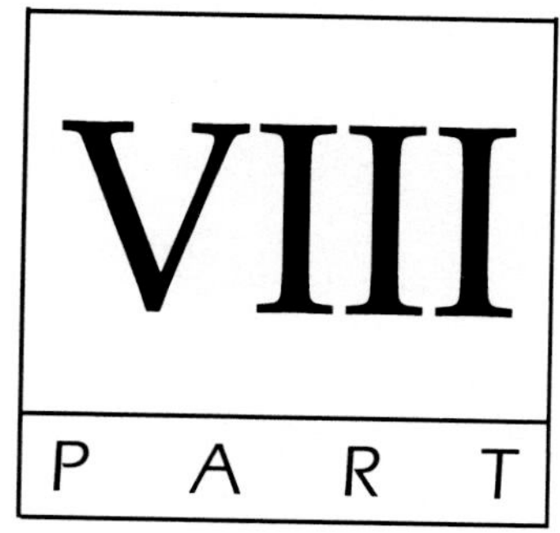

METHODS OF EVALUATION OF FETAL DEVELOPMENT AND WELL-BEING

44

CHAPTER

PRENATAL DIAGNOSIS OF DEVIANT FETAL GROWTH

E. Albert Reece and Zion Hagay

Fetal growth is a fundamental characteristic of the continuity of life and fetal well-being. Cell divisions, cell hyperplasia, and cell hypertrophy are the cornerstones of fetal growth. Winick has suggested that early in pregnancy, growth of fetal organs takes place first by cell hyperplasia or cell division, then by cell hypertrophy, and finally by the cessation of hyperplasia, after which growth continues by cellular hypertrophy alone.[1] Despite this apparent orderly sequence of events, fetuses grow at different rates, become different sizes, and have different shapes. It has been observed in sheep that up until 130 days gestation growth seems to be very similar between fetuses, but after this point varying patterns of growth may be recognized.

In this chapter we will discuss the two extreme types of deviant fetal growth–accelerated (macrosomia) and diminished (intrauterine growth retardation). In addition, prenatal diagnosis of these conditions will be discussed.

INTRAUTERINE GROWTH RETARDATION

ETIOLOGY AND DEFINITION

Intrauterine growth retardation (IUGR) is an abnormality of fetal growth and development that affects 3% to 7% of all deliveries, depending on the diagnostic criteria used.[2–4] The growth-retarded fetus is at greater risk for mortality and morbidity. It is estimated that perinatal mortality is 5 to 10 times higher in the growth-retarded neonate than in the neonate who is sized appropriately for gestational age.[5] Several associated morbid conditions of serious concern following different periods of growth failure in utero include birth asphyxia, neonatal hypoglycemia, hypocalcemia, polycythemia, meconium aspiration, and persistent fetal circulation. Investigators have reported poorer neurodevelopmental outcome in small-for-gestational-age infants, particularly when there is also associated prematurity.[6–8] The incidence of major neurologic handicaps in preterm small-for-gestational-age infants may affect 35% of neonates.[9]

There are several causes of IUGR. These may be conceptually divided into three main categories: maternal, fetal, and uteroplacental (Table 44-1). It should be stressed, however, that in almost one half of the cases of IUGR, the etiology is unknown. Furthermore, it has been found that the single most important maternal clinical risk factor is a previous history of IUGR.[10] Therefore, suspicion of IUGR should not be based only on the existence of clinical risk factors during the index pregnancy.

One point of confusion and disagreement is the criteria that are used to define IUGR. Intrauterine growth retardation has been defined variously as an infant whose birth weight is below the 3rd,[11] 5th,[12] and 10th[13] percentile for gestational age or whose birth weight is more than 2 standard deviations below the mean for gestational age.[15] The ponderal index is determined in the neonate by the following formula:

$$\text{ponderal index} = \text{birth weight} \times 100/(\text{crown-heel length}).$$

The ponderal index may identify a neonate who has a small amount of soft tissue clinically evident by loss of subcutaneous tissue and muscle mass, even though the birth weight is normal for gestational age. Neonates with a ponderal index below the 10th percentile for gestational age are probably suffering from malnutrition in utero. For example, a fetus of 2900 g born at 38

TABLE 44–1. RISK FACTORS OF INTRAUTERINE GROWTH RETARDATION

Maternal Risk Factors
Alcohol
Smoking
Drugs
Steroids
Propranolol
Dilantin
Coumadin
Heroin
Anemia
Malnutrition
Prepregnancy weight < 50 kg
Cyanotic heart disease
Chronic hypertension
Pregnancy-induced hypertension
Diabetes mellitus (with vasculopathy)
Connective tissue disease
Fetal Risk Factors
Genetic disorders (eg, dwarf syndromes)
Chromosomal abnormalities (eg, trisomies 13, 18, 21)
Congenital anomalies (eg, gastroschisis)
Fetal infection (eg, viral, protozoan)
Uterine and Placental Risk Factors
Müllerian anomalies (eg, septate uterus)
Placental insufficiency due to:
Infarctions
Infection
Chorioangioma
Multifetal pregnancy
Circumvallate placenta
Previa
Focal abruption
Marginal insertion of the cord

weeks gestation would have been larger (ie, 3500 g) under normal nutritional conditions. Such an infant may be identified as IUGR only when using the ponderal index definition for this condition.

In an interesting study by Weiner and Robinson, results of sonographic diagnoses of IUGR were compared to the postnatal ponderal indices.[16] The study showed that 40% of small-for-gestational-age infants identified by birth-weight percentiles were not growth retarded by their ponderal index. In contrast, 53% of the neonates diagnosed as IUGR by postnatal ponderal index were average for gestational age by birth weight percentile. Since the importance of antenatal diagnosis of IUGR is to identify those infants at high risk for the intrapartum and neonatal complications, the ponderal index is more closely related to perinatal morbidity and mortality than is the birth-weight percentile.[17] Therefore, it would be important to be able to employ the ponderal index in attempting to diagnose IUGR in utero. Unfortunately, there is presently no practical method to evaluate ponderal index in utero. Hence, the most commonly used definition of IUGR is a fetal weight below the 10th percentile for gestational age.

Another index, the crown–heel length, has been used to evaluate neonatal size. However, prediction from femur length measurement (FL) has been found to be too imprecise to be useful.[18]

One unresolved problem concerns which growth curve should be used. Goldenberg and colleagues have shown that the 10th percentile birth weights at each gestational age differ substantially among published charts, occasionally by more than 500 g.[19] One of the most widely used birth-weight curves is that of Battaglia and Lubchenco, which was derived from 5635 liveborn Caucasians and Hispanics living at approximately 8000 feet above sea level in Denver, Colorado.[2] Obviously, this growth curve cannot be applied to a different ethnic and geographic population.

It has been suggested that much of the confusion that presently surrounds IUGR would be eliminated, at least in the United States, if we used a clearly defined American population to derive the percentiles for defining IUGR.[19] In fact, discrepancies between different birth-weight charts from different geographic areas underscore the need for generating birth-weight curves from the population to which they will be applied.

CLASSIFICATION OF IUGR

Clinically, three categories of IUGR may be recognized. Each of them reflects the time of onset of the pathologic process (Fig. 44-1).[21–23]

Type 1 or Symmetrical IUGR

Type 1 IUGR refers to the infant with decreased growth potential. This type of IUGR begins early in gestation, and the entire fetus is proportionally small for gestational age. Head and abdominal circumferences, length, and weight are all below the 10th percentile for gestational age. However, those infants have a normal ponderal index.

Type 1 IUGR is a result of growth inhibition early in gestation. This early stage of embryonic-fetal development is characterized by active mitosis from 4 to 20 weeks gestation and is called the hyperplastic stage.[24–26] Any pathologic process during this stage may lead to a reduced number of cells in the fetus.

Symmetric IUGR accounts for 20% to 30% of growth retarded fetuses.[22,27] This condition may result from the inhibition of mitosis, as is seen in intrauterine infection (eg, herpes simplex, rubella, cytomegalovirus, toxoplasmosis), chromosomal disorders, and congenital malformations. It should be remembered, however, that symmetrically small fetuses may be constitutionally small and suffer from no abnormality at all.[20]

In general, type 1 IUGR is associated with a poor prognosis; this is in direct relation to the pathologic condition that causes it. Weiner and Williamson showed that in the absence of an identifiable maternal factor and sonographically detected abnormality, approximately 25% of fetuses evaluated for severe, early-onset growth retardation have aneuploidy.[28] Therefore, the performance of percutaneous umbilical blood sampling is strongly recommended to search for karyotypic abnormality.

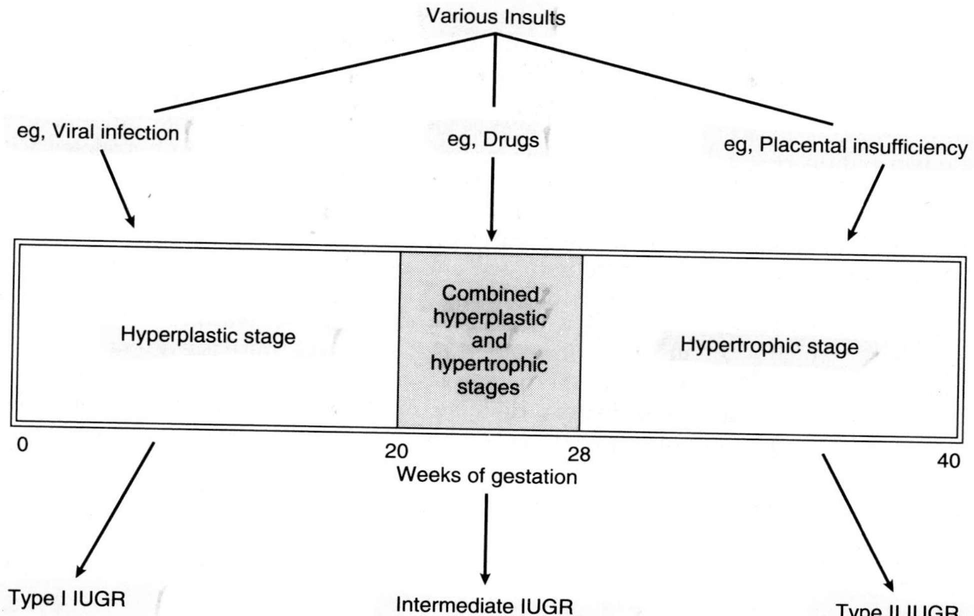

FIGURE 44-1. A schematic illustration of possible insults during the three stages of embryonic-fetal development and the corresponding IUGR that may develop

Type 2 or Asymmetrical IUGR

This term refers to the neonate with restricted growth, and is most frequently due to utero-placental insufficiency.[21] Type 2 IUGR is a result of a later growth insult than type 1 and usually occurs after 28 weeks gestation. As has been shown by Vorherr and colleagues, in the late second trimester normal fetal growth is characterized by a process of hypertrophy.[26] In this hypertrophic stage, there is a rapid increase in cell size and formation of fat, muscle, bone and other tissues. In this phase, the process of hyperplasia is decreased (Fig. 44-2).

The symmetrically growth-retarded fetuses have a near normal total number of cells, but these cells are decreased in size. Asymmetrical IUGR fetuses have low ponderal indices with below-average infant weight but normal head circumference (HC) and fetal length. In these cases of asymmetrical IUGR, fetal growth is nor-

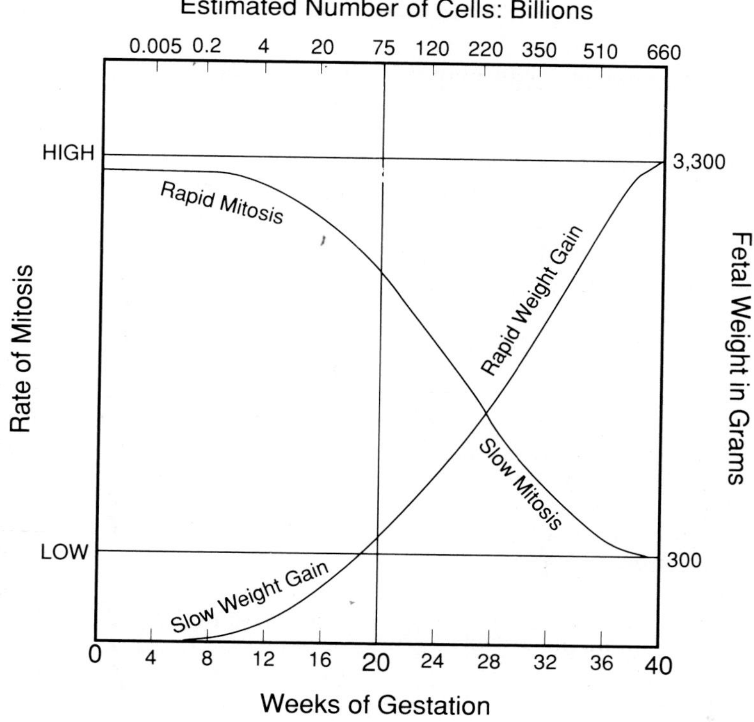

FIGURE 44–2. Cell number and rate of mitosis in relation to embryonic-fetal growth. Embryonic weight gain is slow (small initial cell number) even though the rate of mitosis is very high. Around weeks 16 to 20 of gestation, a substantial fetal cell mass is reached. Thereafter, however, mitosis is slowed (organ differentiation and function). Even though slowed, division of a large number of fetal cells produces a rapid fetal weight gain. (Redrawn from Vorherr H. Factors influencing fetal growth. Am J Obstet Gynecol 1982;142:579.)

mal until late in the second trimester or early in the third, when head growth remains normal while abdominal growth slows (brain-sparing effect). This asymmetry is a result of a fetal compensatory mechanism that responds to a state of poor placental perfusion. Redistribution of fetal cardiac output occurs with increased flow to the brain, heart, and adrenals, and decreased glycogen storage and liver mass.[30] However, if placental insufficiency is aggravated during late pregnancy, the head growth may be flattened and its size may drop below the normal growth curve.

It is estimated that 70% to 80% of growth-retarded fetuses are type 2 IUGR.[31] This form of IUGR is frequently associated with maternal diseases such as chronic hypertension, renal disease, diabetes mellitus with vasculopathy, and others (see Table 44-1).

Intermediate IUGR

Indeterminate IUGR refers to growth retardation that is a combination of types 1 and 2 IUGR. The insult to fetal growth in intermediate IUGR most probably occurs during the middle phase of fetal growth–that of hyperplasia and hypertrophy (see Figs. 44-1 and 44-2)–which corresponds to 20 to 28 weeks gestation. At this stage, there is a decrease in mitotic rate and a progressive overall increase in cell size.

This form of IUGR is less common than types 1 and 2; it is estimated at being responsible for 5% to 10% of all growth-retarded fetuses. Chronic hypertension, lupus nephritis, or other maternal vascular diseases that are severe in nature and begin early in the second trimester may result in an intermediate IUGR with symmetrical growth and no significant brain-pairing effect.

ULTRASONIC MEASUREMENTS USED IN THE DIAGNOSIS OF IUGR

The intrauterine detection of retarded fetal growth by clinical means is possible in approximately 30% of affected pregnancies.[32] Ultrasonography offers an objective, reliable, and effective means of identifying retarded intrauterine fetal growth. However, in order to make a proper diagnosis and appropriately manage the growth-retarded fetus, it is crucial to determine the gestational age as accurately as possible.

Pregnancy dating has traditionally been based on historical and clinical clues. The certain date of a patient's last menstrual period had been regarded as the most reliable method of estimating a fetus' gestational age.[33] However, it has been reported that 20% to 40% of pregnant women fail to recall the exact date of their last menstrual period.[34]

Therefore, ultrasonography may be of help in dating a pregnancy. In the first trimester, crown-rump length measurement allows for an estimation of gestational age with a range of 4.7 days at the 95% confidence level. Between 12 to 24 weeks gestation, the biparietal diameter (BPD) measurement provides reliable estimates comparable to that of the crown-rump measurement performed in the first trimester of pregnancy. Beyond 28 to 30 weeks gestation, there is a progressive increase in BPD variations, and the establishment of accurate gestational age is less satisfactory.

The FL correlates with gestational age, particularly during 14 to 22 weeks gestation, with a range of 6.7 days at the 95% confidence level.[35]

Accurate antenatal diagnosis of IUGR may prevent the high perinatal morbidity and mortality associated with this condition and permits appropriate management and obstetrical intervention when fetal compromise is evident. Most authorities believe that whenever IUGR is diagnosed after 37 weeks gestation, delivery is indicated in order to decrease the risk of fetal death.[36]

There are several sonographic parameters that may be used in the diagnosis of IUGR. In the following section these parameters are critically reviewed.

BIPARIETAL DIAMETER

Nomograms of BPD or HC are available to provide calculated estimates of weekly increments for the size of the fetal head (Tables 44-2 through 44-4).[37] Hence, when comparing the observed increase in BPD with the expected rate of growth, the physician should be able to identify growth-retarded fetuses when the head is affected in the growth curtailment. In fact, the BPD was the first ultrasonic parameter used for detection of IUGR.[23,38] The detection rates of IUGR with single and serial BPD measurements alone have been reported to be of poor value by most authors.[39,40–42] Reported accuracy rates have ranged from 43% to 82%.[40,44–47] Rosendahl and Kivinen studied the efficiency of a single BPD measurement at 34 weeks gestation to identify infants with birth weights below the 10th percentile.[48] Single BPD measurements at 34 weeks gestation detect only 26.9% of the small-for-gestational-age infants with a positive predictive value of 30.9%, which means that 69% of the fetuses with retarded BPD actually proved to be normally grown. The study of Warsof and colleagues indicates that a single BPD measurement in the third trimester is a poor predictor of IUGR.[49]

Other studies used serial BPD determinations in the hope of improving accuracy; however, their results were equally disappointing. Kurjak and colleagues have shown that only 48% of fetuses with small BPD (below the 10th percentile) had birth weights below the 10th percentile and actually resulted in delivery of small-for-gestational-age infants.[43]

From the previously mentioned data it is clear that BPD alone cannot be used as a good predictor of IUGR. This is not surprising, because almost two thirds of IUGR cases are of the asymmetric or late-flattening type, which have normal growth of the head until late in pregnancy as a consequence of the brain-sparing process. Therefore, BPD in asymmetric IUGR may be normal until late in gestation. Another reason for the low sensitivity of BPD measurements in detecting IUGR is the distortion of the fetal head shape that may occur as

TABLE 44–2. GESTATIONAL AGE FROM THE BPD

	PERCENTILE				PERCENTILE		
BPD (mm)	5TH	50TH	95TH	BPD (mm)	5TH	50TH	95TH
10	7	10 + 1	13 + 1	39	14	17 + 1	20 + 1
11	7 + 2	10 + 2	13 + 3	40	14 + 2	17 + 3	20 + 3
12	7 + 3	10 + 4	13 + 4	41	14 + 4	17 + 5	20 + 5
13	7 + 5	10 + 5	13 + 5	42	14 + 6	18	21
14	7 + 6	10 + 6	14	43	15 + 1	18 + 2	21 + 2
15	8 + 1	11 + 1	14 + 1	44	15 + 3	18 + 4	21 + 4
16	8 + 2	11 + 2	14 + 3	45	15 + 6	18 + 6	21 + 6
17	8 + 4	11 + 4	14 + 4	46	16 + 1	19 + 1	22 + 1
18	8 + 5	11 + 5	14 + 6	47	16 + 3	19 + 3	22 + 4
19	9	12	15	48	16 + 5	19 + 5	22 + 6
20	9 + 1	12 + 2	15 + 2	49	17	20 + 1	23 + 1
21	9 + 3	12 + 3	15 + 3	50	17 + 3	20 + 3	23 + 3
22	9 + 4	12 + 5	15 + 5	51	17 + 5	20 + 5	23 + 6
23	9 + 6	12 + 6	16	52	18	21	24 + 1
24	10 + 1	13 + 1	16 + 1	53	18 + 2	21 + 3	24 + 3
25	10 + 2	13 + 3	16 + 3	54	18 + 5	21 + 5	24 + 5
26	10 + 4	13 + 4	16 + 5	55	19	22	25 + 1
27	10 + 6	13 + 6	17	56	19 + 2	22 + 3	25 + 3
28	11	14 + 1	17 + 1	57	19 + 5	22 + 5	25 + 6
29	11 + 2	14 + 3	17 + 3	58	20	23 + 1	26 + 1
30	11 + 4	14 + 4	17 + 5	59	20 + 3	23 + 3	26 + 3
31	11 + 6	14 + 6	18	60	20 + 5	23 + 6	26 + 6
32	12 + 1	15 + 1	18 + 1	61	21 + 1	24 + 1	27 + 1
33	12 + 3	15 + 3	18 + 3	62	21 + 3	24 + 4	27 + 4
34	12 + 4	15 + 5	18 + 5	63	21 + 6	24 + 6	27 + 6
35	12 + 6	16	19	64	22 + 1	25 + 2	28 + 2
36	13 + 1	16 + 2	19 + 2	65	22 + 4	25 + 4	28 + 5
37	13 + 3	16 + 4	19 + 4	66	22 + 6	26	29
38	13 + 5	16 + 6	19 + 6	67	23 + 2	26 + 2	29 + 3

(Reproduced with permission from Jeanty P, Romero R. *Obstetrical Ultrasound*, New York McGraw-Hill, 1984.)

in dolichocephaly, or may be seen in cases of breech presentation when the BPD may be falsely small.

BPD determinations, when utilized singly, fail to identify about 20% to 50% of IUGR infants and therefore cannot be used as the only parameter in screening for IUGR.[39]

TRANSVERSE CEREBELLAR DIAMETER

The cerebellum can be easily visualized as early as the first trimester as a butterfly-shaped figure in the posterior fossa of the fetal head, behind the thalami and in front of the echolucent area (cisterna magna) (Fig. 44-

TABLE 44–3. ESTIMATED VARIABILITY ASSOCIATED WITH DETERMINING MENSTRUAL AGE FROM BPD VALUES

GROUP (MENSTRUAL AGE)	HADLOCK ET AL.*	DAYS	KURTZ ET AL.†	DAYS
1 (12–18 weeks)	±0.85 weeks (r^2 = 90.4%)	5.9	±0.80 weeks	5.6
2 (18–24 weeks)	±1.29 weeks (r^2 = 87.6%)	9.03	±1.70 weeks	11.9
3 (24–30 weeks)	±1.40 weeks (r^2 = 89.1%)	9.8	±1.34 weeks	9.38
4 (30–36 weeks)	±1.96 weeks (r^2 = 76.5%)	13.7	±1.42 weeks	9.94
5 (36–42 weeks)	±2.06 weeks (r^2 = 25.6%)	14.42	±1.23 weeks	8.61

* 95% confidence interval.

† 90% confidence interval (of mean values).

(Modified from Hadlock FP, Deter R, Harrist R, et al: Fetal biparietal diameter: A critical re-evaluation of the relation to menstrual age by means of real-time ultrasound. *J. Ultrasound Med* 1982;1:91 and Kurtz AB, Wapher RJ et al. Analysis of biparietal diameter as an accurate indicator of gestational age. JCU 1986;8:319.)

TABLE 44–4. GESTATIONAL AGE FROM THE HEAD CIRCUMFERENCE

	PERCENTILE				PERCENTILE		
HC (mm)	5TH	50TH	95TH	HC (mm)	5TH	50TH	95TH
60	8 + 6	10 + 5	12 + 3	205	19 + 5	21 + 4	23 + 2
65	9 + 1	11	12 + 5	210	20 + 2	22	23 + 5
70	9 + 3	11 + 2	13	215	20 + 5	22 + 3	24 + 1
75	9 + 6	11 + 4	13 + 2	220	21 + 1	22 + 6	24 + 5
80	10 + 1	11 + 6	13 + 4	225	21 + 4	23 + 3	25 + 1
85	10 + 3	12 + 1	14	230	22 + 1	23 + 6	25 + 4
90	10 + 5	12 + 4	14 + 2	235	22 + 4	24 + 3	26 + 1
95	11 + 1	12 + 6	14 + 4	240	23 + 1	24 + 6	26 + 4
100	11 + 3	13 + 1	14 + 6	245	23 + 4	25 + 3	27 + 1
105	11 + 5	13 + 4	15 + 2	250	24 + 1	25 + 6	27 + 4
110	12 + 1	13 + 6	15 + 4	255	24 + 4	26 + 3	28 + 1
115	12 + 3	14 + 1	16	260	25 + 1	26 + 6	28 + 5
120	12 + 6	14 + 4	16 + 2	265	25 + 5	27 + 3	29 + 1
125	13 + 1	14 + 6	16 + 5	270	26 + 1	28	29 + 5
130	13 + 4	15 + 2	17	275	26 + 5	28 + 4	30 + 2
135	13 + 6	15 + 5	17 + 3	280	27 + 2	29	30 + 6
140	14 + 2	16	17 + 6	285	27 + 6	29 + 4	31 + 2
145	14 + 5	16 + 3	18 + 1	290	28 + 3	30 + 1	31 + 6
150	15	16 + 6	18 + 4	295	29	30 + 5	32 + 3
155	15 + 3	17 + 2	19	300	29 + 4	31 + 2	33
160	15 + 6	17 + 4	19 + 3	305	30 + 1	31 + 6	33 + 4
165	16 + 2	18	19 + 6	310	30 + 5	32 + 3	34 + 1
170	16 + 5	18 + 3	20 + 1	315	31 + 2	33	34 + 5
175	17 + 1	18 + 6	20 + 4	320	31 + 6	33 + 4	35 + 2
180	17 + 4	19 + 2	21	325	32 + 3	34 + 1	36
185	18	19 + 5	21 + 3	330	33	34 + 6	36 + 4
190	18 + 3	20 + 1	21 + 6	335	33 + 5	35 + 4	37 + 1
195	18 + 6	20 + 4	22 + 3	340	34 + 2	36	37 + 5
200	19 + 2	21	22 + 6				

(Reproduced with permission from Jeanty P, Romero R, *Obsterical Ultrasound,* New York: McGraw-Hill, 1984.)

3). The transverse cerebellar diameter (TCD) in millimeters has been shown to correlate with gestational age in weeks up to 24 week. Above 24 weeks gestation, the growth curves turn upward, and this uniform correlation no longer exists. Goldstein and colleagues have constructed a nomogram of the TCD throughout pregnancy (Table 44-5).[50]

Reece and colleagues subsequently evaluated the TCD measurement in IUGR fetuses.[51] They reported that TCD measurement was not significantly affected by retarded fetal growth, and therefore the TCD could be used as a reliable predictor of gestational age even in cases of IUGR. This parameter is particularly useful because it is a standard against which other parameters can be compared. Duchatel and colleagues have corroborated these findings in their report of 12 cases of IUGR below the 3rd percentile in which the TCD remained unaltered.[52] Other investigators have provided additional support for the usefulness of the TCD by constructing a nomogram of the ratio between TCD and abdominal circumference (AC) ratio.[53] In a small series, these investigators have shown that this ratio permits the identification of IUGR by demonstrating the fairly consistent growth of the TCD relative to the decrease in AC in cases of IUGR. In yet another study by Hill and colleagues, the TCD was found to be within 2 standard

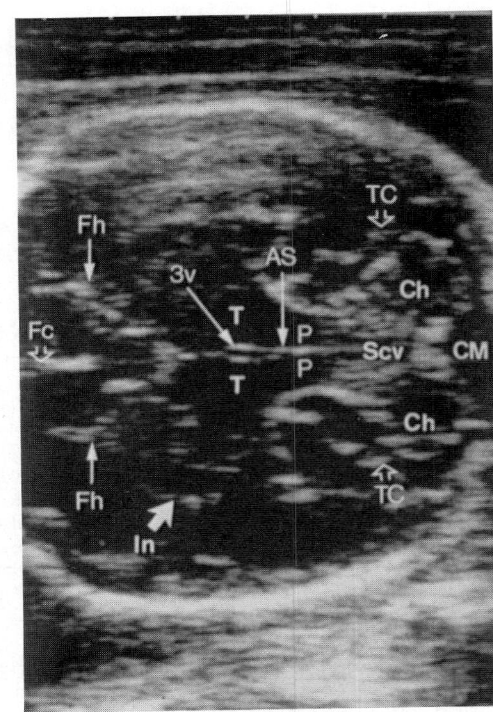

FIGURE 44–3. Intracranial anatomy of fetal head.

TABLE 44–5. A NOMOGRAM OF THE TRANSVERSE CEREBELLAR DIAMETER, BIPARIETAL DIAMETER, AN HEAD CIRCUMFERENCE ACCORDING TO PERCENTILE DISTRIBUTION

GESTATIONAL AGE (WK)	CEREBELLUM (mm)					BIPARIETAL DIAMETER (mm)					HEAD CIRCUMFERENCE (mm)				
	10	25	50	75	90	10	25	50	75	90	10	25	50	75	90
15	10	12	14	15	16	30	31	33	34	35	12	12	126	128	128
16	14	16	16	16	17	34	34	35	36	38	123	125	130	136	141
17	16	17	17	18	18	36	37	38	40	43	134	136	138	149	160
18	17	18	18	19	19	38	40	42	43	44	142	147	154	158	160
19	18	18	19	19	22	42	43	45	46	48	147	154	159	170	178
20	18	19	20	20	22	45	46	47	48	53	146	164	173	190	190
21	19	20	22	23	24	48	49	50	52	57	185	185	191	208	211
22	21	23	23	24	24	50	51	53	54	55	193	193	193	200	203
23	22	23	24	25	26	53	54	56	58	60	203	203	206	222	222
24	22	24	25	27	28	56	59	60	61	64	219	220	224	228	230
25	23	21.5	28	28	29	61	61	63	66	68	219	224	234	248	251
26	25	28	29	30	32	63	64	65	66	67	235	237	241	246	246
27	26	28.5	30	31	32	64	67	68	69	70	237	237	243	246	246
28	27	30	31	32	34	68	69	70	71	72	246	247	253	261	264
29	29	32	34	36	38	71	72	74	76	79	254	264	274	288	301
30	31	32	35	37	40	72	74	75	75	79	253	261	277	288	298
31	32	35	38	39	43	75	78	76	81	84	274	277	291	301	303
32	33	36	38	40	42	75	78	80	81	83	275	280	288	307	308
33	32	36	40	43	44	80	80	81	82	87	292	292	297	316	322
34	33	38	40	41	44	81	82	84	86	91	326	326	326	327	327
35	31	37	40.5	43	47	78	83	87	89	93	300	300	301	303	303
36	36	29	43	52	55	84	85	88	89	91	309	309	313	318	318
37	37	37	45	52	55	87	87	89	92	92	303	303	313	324	324
38	40	40	48.5	52	55	87	87	90	93	94					
39	52	52	52	55	55	92	92	92	92	92					

deviations in only 40% of IUGR cases, and in 60% of cases, the TCD was greater than 2 standard deviations below the mean.[54] The results of this paper is at variance with the three reports discussed earlier. Nevertheless, the majority of data available would suggest that the use of the TCD when gestational age is unknown or IUGR is suspected is extremely valuable. The accuracy of the TCD can be enhanced by using biometric ratios, especially FL:AC, as well as amniotic fluid volume and the presence or absence of fetal ossification centers.

ABDOMINAL CIRCUMFERENCE

The abdominal circumference (AC) has been reported to be the best fetal biometric parameter that correlates with fetal weight and is the most sensitive parameter for detecting IUGR.[55] Warsof and colleagues studied the effectiveness of three ultrasonic growth parameters —BPD, HC, and AC—to detect IUGR in a large group of obstetric populations.[49] They demonstrated that AC measurements are more predictive of IUGR than BPD or HC, singly or in combination. In this study, it was shown that screening at 34 weeks gestation for IUGR results in a sensitivity of approximately 70% and a positive predictive value of 50%. However, the authors used the 25th rather than 10th percentile measurement to determine a positive result to maximize sensitivity of the screening test.

It is noteworthy that the sensitivity and true positive rates are influenced by the incidence of IUGR in the population studied. This is demonstrated in the study by Geirsson and colleagues, who have shown that the measurement of the abdominal area at 36 weeks gestation to detect fetuses below the 10th percentile for weight results in a sensitivity of 72% in a high risk group, but only 56% when the entire obstetric population was screened.[56,57] The positive predictive values were 68% in the high risk group and 50% in the unselected group.

Others have found results that further demonstrate that AC is the single best predictor of IUGR, with accuracy that may reach 96% of cases.[43,58] In fact, in contrast to the BPD measurement, AC is smaller in both symmetric and asymmetric types of IUGR, and therefore its measurement has higher sensitivity. Animal studies have shown that the liver is the most affected organ in IUGR. Since the liver is the largest intra-abdominal organ, assessment of the AC at the level of the liver is actually an indirect indication of the nutritional status of the fetus.

Unfortunately, AC has more intra-observer and inter-observer variation than either BPD or FL.[36] Furthermore, AC variability may result from fetal breathing movements, compression, or position of the fetus. To obtain the proper AC, the section should be round and at the level of the fetal stomach and the portal umbilical vein (or the bifurcation of the main portal vein into the right and left branches). Normal values of AC are presented in Table 44-6.[59]

TABLE 44-6. NORMAL VALUES FOR THE ABDOMINAL CIRCUMFERENCE

WEEK NUMBER	JEANTY 5TH	JEANTY 50TH PERCENTILE	JEANTY 95TH	DETER 50TH PERCENTILE
12	35	57	80	63
13	45	67	90	74
14	55	77	100	84
15	65	88	110	95
16	76	98	120	106
17	86	109	131	117
18	97	119	142	128
19	108	130	152	139
20	119	141	163	150
21	129	152	174	161
22	140	163	185	172
23	151	173	196	183
24	162	184	206	194
25	172	195	217	205
26	183	205	227	216
27	193	215	238	227
28	206	225	248	238
29	213	235	257	249
30	222	244	267	260
31	231	254	276	271
32	240	262	285	282
33	248	271	293	293
34	256	279	301	304
35	264	286	309	315
36	271	293	316	326
37	278	300	322	337
38	283	306	328	348
39	289	311	333	359
40	294	316	338	370

Geirrson RT, Patel NB, Christie AD. Efficiency of intrauterine volume, fetal abdominal area and biparietal diameter measurements with ultrasound in screening for small-for-dates babies. Br J Obstet Gynaecol 1985;92:929.

LONG BONES

The FL is another important parameter in evaluating fetal growth (Table 44-7). Long bones other than the femur can be equally useful in the assessment of gestational age (Tables 44-8 and 44-9). It has been demonstrated by several authors that there is a linear relationship between FL specifically and long bones in general and crown-heel length of a newborn.[60,18] These long bones are generally decreased in symmetrically growth-retarded fetuses, but may be of normal length in asymmetric IUGR. In fact, the fetal head and long-bone length in asymmetric IUGR tend to be affected late in gestation.[60] Since the measurement of most long bones is relatively simple, they become a useful means of estimating gestational age on a routine basis. Like most other biometric parameters, the standard deviation tends to expand with increasing gestational age. Hence, accuracy is greatest in early gestation.

TOTAL INTRAUTERINE VOLUME

The rationale for measuring total intrauterine volume derives from the fact that in IUGR intrauterine content is reduced (fetal, placental mass, and the amount of amniotic fluid). Gohari and colleagues calculated total intrauterine volume using the formula of an ellipsoid volume.[61] Although these results were encouraging because 75% of IUGR were correctly diagnosed, this method has been abandoned by most centers because of the widespread use of real-time ultrasonography and the fact that a static scanner is needed to measure total intrauterine volume.

AMNIOTIC FLUID VOLUME ASSESSMENT

In the growth-retarded fetus, decreased amounts of amniotic fluids may be observed. This is a direct result of decreased renal perfusion and reduced urine production. Manning and colleagues have shown that oligohydramnios, determined by ultrasound as the absence of a pocket of amniotic fluid greater than 1 cm in its largest diameter, may predict that the fetus is growth retarded with high accuracy.[62] Their study group included patients at high risk for IUGR. In this group, oligohydramnios was found to be highly sensitive (84%) and (97%), with a predictive value approaching 90%. Unfortunately, progressive growth curtailment usually occurs without evidence of significant amniotic fluid reduction. Hence, this parameter is not very sensitive to detect evolving IUGR. As shown above, its utility is greatest in diagnosing frank IUGR.

When amniotic fluid volume evaluation was tested as a screening method in the detection of IUGR in the general obstetric population, the results were quite disappointing. Philipson and colleagues studied 2453 pregnant patients and found the oligohydramnios test to be poorly sensitive (16%); in other words, in 84% of IUGR infants, there was no evidence of oligohydramnios and therefore the problem would have been missed by this test.[63] In summary, it seems that this ultrasonic method to detect fetal growth retardation is unsatisfactory because of low accuracy.

PLACENTAL GROWTH

Grannum and colleagues were the first to present an ultrasonic classification of placental maturity.[64] This classification grades placentae from 0 to 3 according to specific ultrasonic findings at the basal and chronic plates, as well as within substances of the organ itself (Table 44-10). It is noteworthy that placentas do not all necessarily go through the full maturational process during pregnancy. This is demonstrated by the fact that in normal pregnancies at term, only 20% of placentas are classified as grade 3.[65] Furthermore, ultrasound examination of placental maturation, or examination after 42 weeks gestation, shows that 45% of placentas are of grade 3 and all of the others are grade 2.[66] Therefore, it has been assumed that the appearance of a grade 3 placenta prior to 35 weeks gestation should alert the physician to the possibility of the presence or subsequent development of IUGR. However, there are still

TABLE 44-7. GESTATIONAL AGE ESTIMATED FROM THE FEMUR LENGTH

FEMUR LENGTH (mm)	PERCENTILE 5TH	50TH	95TH	FEMUR LENGTH (mm)	PERCENTILE 5TH	50TH	95TH
10	10 + 3	12 + 4	14 + 6	46	23 + 1	25 + 3	27 + 4
11	10 + 5	12 + 6	15 + 1	47	23 + 4	25 + 6	28
12	11 + 1	13 + 2	15 + 4	48	24	26 + 1	28 + 3
13	11 + 3	13 + 4	15 + 6	49	24 + 3	26 + 4	28 + 6
14	11 + 5	13 + 6	16 + 1	50	24 + 6	27	29 + 1
15	12	14 + 1	16 + 3	51	25 + 1	27 + 3	29 + 4
16	12 + 3	14 + 4	16 + 6	52	25 + 4	27 + 6	30
17	12 + 5	14 + 6	17 + 1	53	26	28 + 1	30 + 3
18	13	15 + 1	17 + 3	54	26 + 3	28 + 4	30 + 6
19	13 + 3	15 + 4	17 + 6	55	26 + 6	29 + 1	31 + 2
20	13 + 5	15 + 6	18 + 1	56	27 + 2	29 + 4	31 + 5
21	14 + 1	16 + 2	18 + 4	57	27 + 5	29 + 6	32 + 1
22	14 + 3	16 + 4	18 + 6	58	28 + 1	30 + 2	32 + 4
23	14 + 5	16 + 6	19 + 1	59	28 + 4	30 + 5	32 + 6
24	15 + 1	17 + 2	19 + 4	60	28 + 6	31 + 1	33 + 2
25	15 + 3	17 + 4	19 + 6	61	29 + 3	31 + 4	33 + 6
26	15 + 6	18	20 + 1	62	29 + 6	32	34 + 1
27	16 + 1	18 + 2	20 + 4	63	30 + 1	32 + 3	34 + 4
28	16 + 4	18 + 5	20 + 6	64	30 + 5	32 + 6	35 + 1
29	16 + 6	19	21 + 1	65	31 + 1	33 + 2	35 + 4
30	17 + 1	19 + 3	21 + 4	66	31 + 4	33 + 5	35 + 6
31	17 + 4	19 + 6	22	67	32	34 + 1	36 + 3
32	17 + 6	20 + 1	22 + 2	68	32 + 3	34 + 4	36 + 6
33	18 + 2	20 + 4	22 + 5	69	32 + 6	35	37 + 1
34	18 + 5	20 + 6	23 + 1	70	33 + 2	35 + 4	37 + 5
35	19	21 + 1	23 + 3	71	33 + 5	35 + 6	38 + 1
36	19 + 3	21 + 4	23 + 6	72	34 + 1	36 + 3	38 + 4
37	19 + 6	22	24 + 1	73	34 + 3	36 + 6	39
38	20 + 1	22 + 3	24 + 4	74	35 + 1	37 + 2	39 + 4
39	20 + 4	22 + 5	24 + 6	75	35 + 4	37 + 5	39 + 6
40	20 + 6	23 + 1	25 + 2	76	36	38 + 1	40 + 3
41	21 + 2	23 + 4	25 + 5	77	36 + 3	38 + 4	40 + 6
42	21 + 5	23 + 6	26 + 1	78	36 + 6	39 + 1	41 + 2
43	22 + 1	24 + 2	26 + 4	79	37 + 2	39 + 4	41 + 5
44	22 + 4	24 + 5	26 + 6	80	37 + 6	40	42 + 1
45	22 + 6	25	27 + 1				

(Reproduced with permission from Jeanty P, Romero R: *Obstetrical Ultrasound*, New York: McGraw-Hill, 1984.)

no substantial data to support this assumption. Kazzi and colleagues studied the value of placental grading in the diagnosis of IUGR in a high-risk group of patients.[67] They have shown that grade 3 placentas accurately diagnose IUGR in 62% of cases with a positive predictive value of 59%. Therefore, the prenatal diagnosis of IUGR using placental grading is rather limited. In fact, the utility of placental grading in general has been supplanted by more sensitive tests, and, therefore, this grading system is infrequently used in clinical practice today.

BODY PROPORTIONALITY

Investigators examined the possibility that the use of fetal body proportionality may improve ultrasonic accuracy in the diagnosis of IUGR. Indices of body proportionality that have been studied and found clinically useful include the HC:AC ratio (Table 44-11) and the FL:AC ratio.

Head Circumference:Abdominal Circumference Ratio

The use of the ratio of HC to AC in determining IUGR was proposed by Campbell and Thoms in 1977.[37] The rationale for this was based on the observation that type 2 IUGR may have a disturbed HC:AC ratio as a result of the brain-sparing effect. Although this method has been shown to have a sensitivity of approximately 70% in detecting asymmetric IUGR, its use is limited by its high false-positive rate in screening a general population.[37,68]

Further limitations of this technique are its inability to detect asymmetric growth retardation and the need for accurate knowledge of gestational age in order to make the diagnosis of IUGR. It is therefore believed that the value of the HC:AC ratio lies in the assessment of proportionality, and thus it may assist the clinician to classify IUGR as symmetrical or asymmetrical. Obviously, an elevated ratio suggests symmetrical IUGR (see Table 44-11).

TABLE 44–8. GESTATIONAL AGE IN WEEKS AND DAYS AS OBTAINED FROM THE LONG BONES

BONE LENGTH (mm)	HUMERUS PERCENTILE			ULNA PERCENTILE			TIBIA PERCENTILE		
	5TH	50TH	95TH	5TH	50TH	95TH	5TH	50TH	95TH
10	9 + 6	12 + 4	15 + 2	10 + 1	13 + 1	16 + 1	10 + 4	13 + 3	16 + 2
11	10 + 1	12 + 6	15 + 4	10 + 4	13 + 4	16 + 4	10 + 6	13 + 5	16 + 4
12	10 + 3	13 + 1	15 + 6	10 + 6	13 + 6	16 + 6	11 + 1	14 + 1	17
13	10 + 6	13 + 4	16 + 1	11 + 1	14 + 1	17 + 2	11 + 4	14 + 3	17 + 2
14	11 + 1	13 + 6	16 + 4	11 + 4	14 + 4	17 + 5	11 + 6	14 + 6	17 + 5
15	11 + 3	14 + 1	16 + 6	11 + 6	15	18	12 + 1	15 + 1	18
16	11 + 6	14 + 4	17 + 2	12 + 2	15 + 3	18 + 3	12 + 4	15 + 4	18 + 3
17	12 + 1	14 + 6	17 + 4	12 + 5	15 + 5	18 + 6	13	15 + 6	18 + 6
18	12 + 4	15 + 1	18	13 + 1	16 + 1	19 + 1	13 + 2	16 + 1	19 + 1
19	12 + 6	15 + 4	18 + 2	13 + 4	16 + 4	19 + 4	13 + 5	16 + 4	19 + 4
20	13 + 1	15 + 6	18 + 5	13 + 6	16 + 6	20	14 + 1	17	19 + 6
21	13 + 4	16 + 2	19 + 1	14 + 2	17 + 2	20 + 3	14 + 4	17 + 3	20 + 2
22	13 + 6	16 + 5	19 + 3	14 + 5	17 + 5	20 + 6	14 + 6	17 + 6	20 + 5
23	14 + 2	17 + 1	19 + 6	15 + 1	18 + 1	21 + 1	15 + 1	18 + 1	21 + 1
24	14 + 5	17 + 3	20 + 1	15 + 4	18 + 4	21 + 4	15 + 4	18 + 4	21 + 3
25	15 + 1	17 + 6	20 + 4	16	19	22 + 1	16	18 + 6	21 + 6
26	15 + 4	18 + 1	21	16 + 3	19 + 3	22 + 4	16 + 3	19 + 2	22 + 1
27	15 + 6	18 + 4	21 + 3	16 + 6	19 + 6	22 + 6	16 + 6	19 + 5	22 + 4
28	16 + 2	19	21 + 6	17 + 2	20 + 2	23 + 3	17 + 1	20 + 1	23
29	16 + 5	19 + 3	22 + 1	17 + 5	20 + 6	23 + 6	17 + 4	20 + 4	23 + 4
30	17 + 1	19 + 6	22 + 4	18 + 1	21 + 1	24 + 2	18 + 1	21	23 + 6
31	17 + 4	20 + 2	23	18 + 4	21 + 5	24 + 6	18 + 4	21 + 3	24 + 2
32	18	20 + 5	23 + 4	19 + 1	22 + 1	25 + 1	18 + 6	21 + 6	24 + 5
33	18 + 3	21 + 1	23 + 6	19 + 4	22 + 5	25 + 5	19 + 2	22 + 1	25 + 1
34	18 + 6	21 + 4	24 + 2	20 + 1	23 + 1	26 + 1	19 + 5	22 + 4	25 + 4
35	19 + 2	22	24 + 6	20 + 4	24 + 4	26 + 5	20 + 1	23 + 1	26
36	19 + 5	22 + 4	25 + 1	21 + 1	24 + 1	27 + 1	20 + 4	23 + 4	26 + 3
37	20 + 1	22 + 6	25 + 5	21 + 4	24 + 4	27 + 5	21	23 + 6	26 + 6
38	20 + 4	23 + 3	26 + 1	22 + 1	25 + 1	28 + 1	21 + 4	24 + 3	27 + 2
39	21 + 1	23 + 6	26 + 4	22 + 4	25 + 4	28 + 5	21 + 6	24 + 6	27 + 5
40	21 + 4	24 + 2	27 + 1	23 + 1	26 + 1	29 + 1	22 + 3	25 + 2	28 + 1
41	22	24 + 6	27 + 4	23 + 4	26 + 5	29 + 5	22 + 6	25 + 5	28 + 4
42	22 + 4	25 + 2	28	24 + 1	27 + 1	30 + 2	23 + 2	26 + 1	29 + 1
43	23	25 + 5	28 + 4	24 + 5	27 + 5	30 + 6	23 + 5	26 + 4	29 + 4
44	23 + 4	26 + 1	29	25 + 1	28 + 2	31 + 2	24 + 1	27 + 1	30
45	24	26 + 5	29 + 4	25 + 6	28 + 6	31 + 6	24 + 4	27 + 4	30 + 4
46	24 + 4	27 + 1	30	26 + 2	29 + 3	32 + 3	25 + 1	28	30 + 6
47	25	27 + 5	30 + 4	26 + 9	29 + 6	33	25 + 4	28 + 4	31 + 3
48	25 + 4	28 + 1	31	27 + 3	30 + 4	33 + 4	26 + 1	29	31 + 6
49	26	28 + 6	31 + 4	28	31 + 1	34 + 1	26 + 4	29 + 3	32 + 2
50	26 + 4	29 + 2	32	28 + 4	31 + 4	34 + 5	27	29 + 6	32 + 6
51	27 + 1	29 + 6	32 + 4	29 + 1	32 + 1	35 + 2	27 + 4	30 + 3	33 + 2
52	27 + 4	30 + 2	33 + 1	29 + 5	32 + 6	35 + 6	28	30 + 6	33 + 6
53	28 + 1	30 + 6	33 + 4	30 + 2	33 + 3	36 + 3	28 + 4	31 + 3	34 + 2
54	28 + 5	31 + 3	34 + 1	30 + 6	34	37	29	31 + 6	34 + 6
55	29 + 1	32	34 + 5	31 + 4	34 + 4	37 + 5	29 + 4	32 + 3	35 + 2
56	29 + 6	32 + 4	35 + 2	32 + 1	35 + 1	38 + 2	30	32 + 6	35 + 6
57	30 + 2	33 + 1	35 + 6	32 + 6	35 + 6	38 + 6	30 + 4	33 + 3	36 + 2
58	30 + 6	33 + 4	36 + 3	33 + 3	36 + 3	39 + 4	31	33 + 6	36 + 6
59	31 + 1	34 + 1	36 + 6	34	37 + 1	40 + 1	31 + 4	34 + 3	37 + 2
60	32	34 + 6	37 + 4	34 + 4	37 + 5	40 + 6	32	34 + 6	37 + 6
61	32 + 4	35 + 2	38 + 1	35 + 2	38 + 2	41 + 3	32 + 4	35 + 4	38 + 2
62	33 + 1	35 + 6	38 + 5	35 + 6	39	42	33	35 + 6	38 + 6
63	33 + 6	36 + 4	39 + 2	36 + 4	39 + 4	42 + 5	33 + 4	36 + 4	39 + 3
64	34 + 3	37 + 1	39 + 6	37 + 1	40 + 2	43 + 2	34 + 1	37	39 + 6
65	35	37 + 5	40 + 4				34 + 4	37 + 4	40 + 3
66	35 + 4	38 + 2	41 + 1				35 + 1	38	41
67	36 + 1	38 + 6	41 + 5				35 + 5	38 + 4	41 + 4
68	36 + 6	39 + 4	42 + 4				36 + 1	39 + 1	42
69	37 + 3	40 + 1	42 + 6				36 + 6	39 + 5	42 + 4

(Reproduced with permission from Jeanty P, Rodesch F, Delbeke D, et al: Estimation of gestational age from measurements of fetal long bones. *J. Ultrasound Med* 1984;3:75.)

TABLE 44–9. GESTATIONAL AGE AS OBTAINED FROM CLAVICLE LENGTH

CLAVICLE LENGTH (mm)	GESTATIONAL AGE (WEEKS AND DAYS) PERCENTILE		
	5TH	50TH	95TH
11	8 + 3	13 + 6	17 + 2
12	9 + 1	14 + 4	18 + 1
13	10	14 + 3	19 + 6
14	11 + 6	15 + 2	20 + 5
15	12 + 5	16 + 1	21 + 4
16	12 + 3	18	21 + 3
17	13 + 2	18 + 5	22 + 2
18	14 + 1	19 + 4	23
19	16	19 + 3	24 + 6
20	16 + 6	10 + 2	25 + 5
21	17 + 4	21 + 1	26 + 4
22	17 + 3	22 + 6	26 + 2
23	18 + 2	23 + 5	27 + 1
24	19 + 1	24 + 4	28
25	21	24 + 3	29 + 6
26	21 + 5	25 + 1	30 + 5
27	22 + 4	26	30 + 3
28	22 + 3	27 + 5	31 + 2
29	23 + 2	28 + 5	32 + 1
30	24	29 + 4	34
31	25 + 6	29 + 2	34 + 6
32	26 + 5	30 + 1	35 + 4
33	27 + 4	31	35 + 3
34	27 + 3	32 + 6	36 + 2
35	28 + 1	33 + 5	37 + 1
36	29	33 + 3	39
37	30 + 6	34 + 2	39 + 5
38	31 + 5	35 + 1	40 + 4
39	32 + 4	37	40 + 3
40	32 + 2	37 + 6	41 + 2
41	33 + 1	38 + 4	41
42	35	38 + 3	43 + 6
43	35 + 6	39 + 2	44 + 5
44	36 + 5	40 + 1	45 + 4
45	36 + 3	41 + 6	45 + 3

(Reproduced with permission from Yarkoni S, Schmidt W, Reece EA, Jeanty P: Clavicular measurement: A new biometric parameter for fetal evaluation. *J Ultrasound Med* 1985;4:467.)

Femur Length:Abdominal Circumference Ratio

The ratio of FL:AC is the equivalent of the postnatal ponderal index and has been proposed as a useful method in detecting asymmetrical IUGR.[69] This ratio has the advantage of being age-independent and thus may help in the diagnosis of IUGR when gestational age is unknown. In fact, FL:AC ratios have a constant value of 22% ± 2% after 21 weeks gestation. Hadlock and colleagues evaluated this method in the diagnosis of IUGR and reported that 63% of growth-retarded fetuses were accurately diagnosed when a ratio above 23.5% was considered abnormal.[69] However, these authors and others have indicated the poor predictive value of a positive test that is less than 25%.[70] In spite of this, the FL:AC ratio still has its merits, since it is the only ultrasonic technique that enables the physician to identify IUGR when gestational age is unknown.

ESTIMATED FETAL WEIGHT

Several formulas that use multiple ultrasonic parameters are used to estimate fetal weight.[71–73] The most widely used formula is that of Shepard and colleagues, in which estimated fetal weight (EFw) is derived from the BPD and AC.[74] This equation predicts fetal weight with an accuracy of 15% to 20%.75 Hadlock and colleagues[76] and Warsof and colleagues[77] also have introduced equations to estimate fetal weight using combinations of BPD, AC, and FL.

Ott and Doyle reported accurate predictions of IUGR in 90% of cases in a high-risk population when EFw was determined by BPD and AC.[78] The use of this formula may introduce errors that are related to the variations in BPD which usually occur as a result of changes in head shape in the last weeks of pregnancy, in malpresentation, and in pregnancies complicated by spontaneous rupture of membranes.[79,80] Biparietal diameter may be inaccurate if there is dolichocephaly or brachy-

TABLE 44–10. SUMMARY OF PLACENTAL GRADING

	GRADE 0	GRADE I	GRADE II	GRADE III
Chorionic plate	Straight and well-defined	Subtle undulations	Indentations extending to but not into the basal layer	Indentations communicating with the basal layer
Placental substance	Homogeneous	Few scattered echogenic areas	Linear echogenic densities (comma-like densities)	Circular densities with echo-spared areas in center, large irregular densities which cast acoustic shadowing
Basal layer	No densities	No densities	Linear arrangement of small echogenic areas (basal stipling)	Large and somewhat confluent basal echogenic areas can create acoustic shadows

Grannum PA, Hobbins J. The placenta. Radiology Clin North Am 1982;20:353.

TABLE 44–11. HEAD CIRCUMFERENCE/ABDOMINAL CIRCUMFERENCE RATIO COMPARED WITH GESTATIONAL AGE

GESTATIONAL AGE (WEEKS)	HEAD CIRCUMFERENCE		
	−2SD	MEAN	+2SD
14	1.085	1.230	1.375
15	1.080	1.225	1.365
16	1.075	1.215	1.350
17	1.070	1.205	1.340
18	1.065	1.195	1.330
19	1.060	1.185	1.320
20	1.055	1.178	1.305
21	1.050	1.177	1.295
22	1.045	1.165	1.285
23	1.040	1.155	1.275
24	1.030	1.145	1.265
25	1.025	1.135	1.255
26	1.050	1.125	1.245
27	1.010	1.120	1.235
28	1.000	1.110	1.225
29	0.999	1.095	1.215
30	0.975	1.085	1.200
31	0.965	1.075	1.190
32	0.945	1.060	1.175
33	0.935	1.045	1.163
34	0.925	1.030	1.150
35	0.915	1.020	1.135
36	0.910	1.005	1.120
37	0.905	0.995	1.100
38	0.900	0.980	1.085
39	0.896	0.970	1.065
40	0.895	0.965	1.046
41	0.894	0.960	10.25

From Campbell S, Metreweli C (eds). Practical abdominal ultrasound. Chicago; Year Book Medical Publishers, 1978.

cephaly. We therefore strongly recommend that the physician calculate the cephalic index in each case. If the cephalic index is abnormal (<75% or >80%), one should not rely on estimated weight formulas that include the BPD.

Weiner and colleagues have proposed the use of another formula for prediction of fetal birth weight that incorporates HC and FL in order to avoid errors related to changes in head shape.[81] The authors suggest that the prediction of IUGR fetuses may be more accurate using this formula.

In an effort to further increase the accuracy of ultrasonic estimation of fetal weight, Hadlock and colleagues advocate the use of HC, AC, and FL measurements in combination.[76] They have shown that the prediction of fetal weight has a standard deviation of ±15% (2 standard deviations). However, the accuracy in predicting fetal weight decreases in small-sized fetuses (<1500 g), and the error may approach ±20%.

Various ultrasound methods are used to estimate fetal weight with essentially equal accuracy when low-risk obstetrical populations are studied. It is thought that as many as 80% of IUGR fetuses can be detected; however, there is still a relatively low positive predictive value that only approaches 40%. Therefore, 60% of fetuses suspected of IUGR because of low EFw will actually be normally grown.

DOPPLER ULTRASOUND

The introduction of Doppler ultrasonography to obstetrics has made possible a non-invasive method of evaluation of the fetal–placental circulation.[82,83] Investigators have suggested that abnormal Doppler waveforms, from either the uterine or the umbilical artery, may be identified several weeks before the development of IUGR.[84,85] The King's College group has shown that abnormal uterine waveforms detected in early pregnancy may predict the development of IUGR and pregnancy-induced hypertension with a sensitivity of 68% and a positive predictive value of 42%.[86] Thus, more than one half of the pregnant patients with abnormal waveforms from the uterine artery had normal outcomes, which indicates a high false-positive test.

Fleischer and colleagues studied umbilical artery flow velocity waveforms of 189 pregnant patients between 31 and 39 weeks gestation and have shown that 78% of IUGR fetuses were accurately identified by this test.[85] However, there was still only a 49% positive predictive value for IUGR.

Sijmons and colleagues, in a prospective blind study, evaluated the efficacy of Doppler examination of the umbilical arteries in an unselected obstetrical population as a screening procedure for predicting IUGR.[87] In contrast to the study by Fleischer and colleagues, Doppler examinations were performed at fixed gestational ages (28 to 34 weeks) and not serially.[85] The authors found that a single umbilical artery Doppler examination (pulsatility index) at 28 or 34 weeks gestation is a poor predictor of fetal growth retardation. Their screening results at 28 and 34 weeks gestation show a sensitivity of 16.9% and 22%, respectively, in predicting IUGR. The reason for these poor results could be explained by the fact that the authors studied Doppler waveforms only at 28 or 34 weeks gestation. Screening at these gestational ages might have been too early, since placental insufficiency could occur in later gestation. Another possible reason for the failure of Doppler velocity waveforms to detect a large number of IUGR fetuses may be related to the fact that certain cases of IUGR are not due to placental lesions, and therefore no change in the umbilical arterial waveforms would be expected.

Investigators who have studied the ability of Doppler velocimetry to predict IUGR have shown conflicting results. More prospective blind studies are needed in order to clarify the role of this technique in predicting fetal growth retardation.

MACROSOMIA

The etiology of fetal macrosomia is believed to be multifactorial. Although this condition is often associated with diabetes mellitus in pregnancy, especially in women without vasculopathy, macrosomia may also occur in non-diabetics. Fetal macrosomia is defined either as an EFw >4000 g at term or EFw >90th percentile for gestational age.

Macrosomic infants and their mothers are at increased risk for intrapartum injury, and perinatal mortality is more common among these fetuses. The principal causes of injury include shoulder dystocia, fractures, and neurologic damage.[88–91]

Accurate prenatal diagnosis of fetal macrosomia would permit fetuses to be delivered by cesarean section, thus obviating these complications. On the other hand, liberal cesarean section may expose the mother to unnecessary operative risks.

Prenatal diagnosis of macrosomic fetuses is often difficult because <40% of such infants are born to mothers with identifiable risk factors for macrosomia.[92]

A number of sonographic parameters have been used in an attempt to diagnose altered fetal growth, including the BPC, HC, HC:AC or HC:thoracic circumference ratio, the macrosomic index, and the EFw. Miller and colleagues conducted a study of 382 patients with singleton pregnancies whose infants were born within one week of the ultrasound examination.[93] Of the 382 pregnancies, 58 delivered macrosomic infants (>4500 g). Ultrasonically determined BPD, FL, AC, and EFw were analyzed for their ability to predict the macrosomic newborn. EFw was found to be superior to BPD or FL in the prenatal diagnosis of fetal macrosomia. Elliott and colleagues calculated a macrosomic index for 70 diabetic pregnancies by subtracting the BPD from the chest diameter.[94] Thirty-three macrosomic infants (>4500 g) were delivered. In this study 20/23 (87%) of infants weighing greater than 4500 g had a chest BPD >0.4 cm. In this study, the authors reported four cases of shoulder dystocia among 15 infants with macrosomic indices of >0.4 cm. They recommended cesarean section for all fetuses with a chest BPD of >0.4 cm because this approach would decrease the incidence of traumatic morbidity from 27% to 9%.

In yet another study, Tamura and colleagues[95] showed that the EFw determined by Shepard and colleagues,[96] when greater than the 90th percentile, correctly predicted macrosomia at birth in 74% of cases. When both the AC and the EFw exceeded the 90th percentiles, macrosomia was correctly diagnosed in 88.8% of pregnant women with diabetes mellitus. The BPD and HC percentiles were significantly less predictive of macrosomia.

Although the etiology of IUGR is variable, prenatal diagnosis is possible using a variety of biometric parameters. When the gestational age is certain, IUGR is diagnosed if sonographic predictors of gestational age reflect an age significantly reduced from the expected, or an EFw less than the 10th percentile. Adjunctive indices which can enhance the prenatal diagnosis include reduced amniotic fluid volume, early third trimester grade 3 placenta, abnormal Doppler waveform analysis, and abnormal biometric ratios.

When the gestational age is unknown or uncertain, it is necessary to differentiate between the IUGR fetus and the normally grown fetus identified at an inaccurate gestational age. The transverse cerebellum is a useful parameter for estimating gestational age even in IUGR fetuses and can be a parameter against which other biometric indices are compared. Biometric ratios, especially FL:AC, may also be useful adjuncts in the prenatal diagnosis of IUGR.

The prenatal diagnosis of macrosomia is best accomplished by the use of EFw. However, a certain amount of caution should be exercised in light of the fact that a margin of error exists with this method of weight estimation. EFw is reported to be accurate within 10% of the actual birth weight 85% of the time. In the remaining 15%, EFw is less accurate, and the error can range from 15% to 20% of the actual birth weight.

REFERENCES

1. Winick M. Fetal malnutrition. Clin Obstet Gynecol 1970;13:3.
2. Battaglia FC, Lubchenco LO. A practical classification of newborn infants by weight and gestational age. J Pediatr 1967;71:159.
3. Berkowitz RL, Hobbins JC. Ultrasonography in the antepartum patient. In Bolognese RJ, Schwartz R, eds. Perinatal medicine: management of the high risk fetus and neonate. Baltimore: Williams & Wilkins, 1977:85.
4. Galbraith RS, Karchmar EJ, Pievey WN, et al. The clinical predication of intrauterine growth retardation. Am J Obstet Gynecol 1979;133:281.
5. Ounsted M, Moar V, Scott WA. Perinatal morbidity and mortality in small-for-dates babies: the relative importance of some maternal factors. Early Hum Dev 1981;5:367.
6. Commey JOO, Fitzhardinge PM. Handicap in the preterm small-for-gestational age infant. J Pediatr 1979;94:779.
7. Pena IC, Teberg AJ, Finello K. Neurodevelopmental outcome of the small for gestational age preterm infant during the first year of life. Pediatr Res [Abstract] 1986;20:165.
8. Pena IC, Teberg AJ, Finello K. Effect of intrauterine growth retardation on premature infants of similar gestational age. Pediatr Res [Abstract] 1987;21:183.
9. Fitzhardinge PM, Kalman E, Ashby S, et al. Present status of the infant of very low birth weight treated in a referral neonatal intensive care unit in 1974. In Elliott K, O'Connor M, eds. Major mental handicap: methods and cost of prevention. Ciba Foundation Symposium 59. Amsterdam: Elsevier, 1978:139.
10. Scott A, Moar V, Ounsted M. The relative contributions of different maternal factors in small-for-gestational age pregnancies. Eur J Obstet Gynecol Reprod Biol 1981;12:157.
11. Fitzhardinge PM, Steven EM. The small-for-date infant. II. Neurological and intellectual sequelae. Pediatrics 1972;50:50.
12. Michaeleis R, Schulte F, Nolte R. Motor behavior of small for gestational age newborn infants. J Pediatr 1970;76:208.
13. Lubchenco LO, Hansman C, Dressler, et al. Intrauterine growth as estimated from liveborn birth-weight data at 24 to 42 weeks of gestation. Pediatrics 1963;32:793.
14. Gruenwald P. Growth of the human fetus. Am J Obstet Gynecol 1966;94:1112.
15. Daikoku NH, Tyson JE, Graf C, et al. The relative significance of human placental lactogen in the diagnosis of retarded fetal growth. Am J Obstet Gynecol 1979;135:516.

16. Weiner CP, Robinson D. The sonographic diagnosis of intrauterine growth retardation using the postnatal ponderal index and the crown-heel length as standards of diagnosis. Am J Perinatol 1989;6:375.
17. Walther FJ, Ramaekers LHJ. The ponderal index as a measure of the nutritional status at birth and its relation to some aspects of neonatal morbidity. J Perinat Med 1982;10:42.
18. Hadlock FP, Deter RL, Roecker E, et al. Relation of fetal femu length to neonatal crown-heel length. J Ultrasound Med 1984;3:1.
19. Goldenberg RL, Cutter GR, Hoffman HJ, et al. Intrauterine growth retardation: standards for diagnosis. Am J Obstet Gynecol 1989;161:271.
20. Seeds JW. Impaired fetal growth: definition and clinical diagnosis. Obstet Gynecol 1984;64:303.
21. Johnson MP, Evans MI. Intrauterine growth retardation pathophysiology and possibilities for intrauterine treatment. Fetal Therapy 1987;2:109.
22. Mintz M, Landon M. Sonographic diagnosis of fetal growth disorders. Clin Obstet Gynecol 1988;31:44.
23. Lockwood CJ, Weiner S. Assessment of fetal growth. Clin Perinatol 1986;13:3.
24. Enesca M, LeBlond CP. Increase in cell number as a factor in the growth of the organs and tissues of the young male rat. J Embryol Exp Morphol 1962;10:530.
25. Winick M, Noble A. Cellular response in rats during malnutrition at various ages. J Nutr 1966;89:300.
26. Vorherr H. Factors influencing fetal growth. Am J Obstet Gynecol 1982;142:577.
27. Little D, Campbell S. Ultrasound evaluation of intrauterine growth retardation. Radiol Clin North Am 1982;20:335.
28. Weiner CP, Williamson RA. Evaluation of severe retardation using cordocentesis–hematologic and metabolic alterations by etiology. Obstet Gynecol 1989;73:225.
29. Meschia G. Supply of oxygen to the fetus. J Reprod Med 1979;23:160.
30. Evans MI, Mukherjee AB, Schulman JD. Animal models of intrauterine growth retardation. Obstet Gynecol Surv 1983;38:183.
31. Harbander S, Rutherford SE. Classification of intrauterine growth retardation. Semin Perinat 1988;12:2.
32. Shabbagha RE. Intrauterine growth retardation. In Sabbagha RE, ed: Diagnostic ultrasound. Hagerstown, MD: Harper & Row, 1980:112.
33. Anderson HF, Johnson TRB, Flora JD, Barclay ML. Gestational age assessment. II. Prediction from combined clinical observations. Am J Obstet Gynecol 1981;140:770.
34. Callen PW. Ultrasonography in obstetrics and gynecology. Philadelphia: WB Saunders, 1983:21.
35. Hobbins JC, Winsberg F, Berkowitz RL. Ultrasonography in obstetrics and gynecology. 3rd ed. Baltimore: Williams & Wilkins, 1983:203.
36. Romero R, Jeanty P. The detection of fetal growth disorders. Seminars in Ultrasound 1984;5:130.
37. Campbell S, Thoms A. Ultrasound measurement of the fetal head to abdomen circumference ratio in the assessment of growth retardation. Br J Obstet Gynaecol 1977;84:165.
38. Geirsson RT, Persson PH. Diagnosis of intrauterine growth retardation using ultrasound. Clin Obstet Gynaecol 1982;11:457.
39. Seeds JW. Impaired fetal growth: ultrasonic evaluation and clinical management. Obstet Gynecol 1984;63:577.
40. Arias F. The diagnosis and management of intrauterine growth retardation. Obstet Gynecol 1977;49:293.
41. Sabbagha RE. Intrauterine growth retardation—antenatal diagnosis by ultrasound. Obstet Gynecol 1978;52:252.
42. Queenan JT, Kubarych SF, Cook LN, et al. Diagnostic ultrasound for detection of intrauterine growth retardation. Am J Obstet Gynecol 1976;124:865.
43. Kurjak A, Kirkinen P, Latin V. Biometric and dynamic ultrasound assessment of small-for-dates infants: report of 260 cases. Obstet Gynecol 1980;56:281.
44. Campbell S, Dewhurst C. Diagnosis of the small-for-date fetus by serial ultrasound cephalometry. Lancet 1971;ii:1002.
45. Deter RL, Harrist RB, Hadlock FP, et al. The use of ultrasound in the detection of intrauterine growth retardation. A review. J Clin Ultrasound 1982;10:9.
46. Shool JS, Woo D, Rubin JM, et al. Intrauterine growth retardation risk detection for fetuses of unknown gestational age. Am J Obstet Gynecol 1982;144:709.
47. Fescina RH, Martell M, Martinez G, et al. Small for dates: evaluation of different diagnostic methods. Acta Obstet Gynecol Scand 1987;66:221.
48. Rosendahl H, Kivinen S. Routine ultrasound screening for early detection of small for gestational age fetuses. Obstet Gynecol 1988;71:518.
49. Warsof SL, Cooper DJ, Little D, et al. Routine ultrasound screening for antenatal detection of intrauterine growth retardation. Obstet Gynecol 1986;67:33.
50. Goldstein I, Reece EA, Pilu G, Bovicelli L, Hobbins JC. Cerebellar measurements with ultrasonography in the evaluation of fetal growth and development. Am J Obstet Gynecol 1987;156:1065.
51. Reece EA, Goldstein I, Pilu G, Hobbins JC. Fetal cerebellar growth unaffected by intrauterine growth retardation: a new parameter for prenatal diagnosis. Am J Obstet Gynecol 1987;157:632.
52. Duchatel F, Mennesson B, Berseneff H, Oury JF. Antenatal echographic measurement of the fetal cerebellum. Significance in the evaluation of fetal development. J De Gynecologi, Obstetrique Et Biologie De La Reproduction 1989;18:879.
53. Campbell WA, Narci D, Vintzileos AM, Rodis JF, Turner GW, Egan JF. Transverse cerebellar diameter/abdominal circumference ratio throughout pregnancy: a gestational age-independent method to assess fetal growth. Obstet Gynecol 1991;77:893.
54. Hill LM, Guzick D, Rivello D, Hixson J, Peterson C. The transverse cerebellar diameter cannot be used to assess gestational age in the small for gestational age fetus. Obstet Gynecol 1990;75:329.
55. Campbell S, Wilkin D. Ultrasonic measurement of fetal abdomen circumference in the estimation of fetal weight. Br J Obstet Gynaecol 1975;82:689.
56. Geirsson RT, Patel NB, Christie AD. Efficiency of intrauterine volume, fetal abdominal area and biparietal diameter measurements with ultrasound in screening for small-for-dates babies. Br J Obstet Gynaecol 1985;92:929.
57. Geirsson RT, Patel NB, Christie AD. Intrauterine volume, fetal abdominal area and biparietal diameter measurements with ultrasound in the prediction of small-for-dates babies in a high risk obstetric population. Br J Obstet Gynaecol 1985;92:936.
58. Wittman BK, Robinson HP, Aitchison T, et al. The value of diagnostic ultrasound as a screening test for intrauterine growth retardation: comparison of nine parameters. Am J Obstet Gynecol 1979;134:30.
59. Jeanty P, Coussaert E, Contraine F. Normal growth of the abdominal perimeter. Am J Perinatol 1984;1:129.
60. O'Brien GD, Queenan JR. Ultrasound fetal femur length in relation to intrauterine growth retardation. Am J Obstet Gynecol 1982;144:34.
61. Gohari P, Berkowitz RL, Hobbins JC. Prediction of intrauterine growth retardation by determination of total intrauterine volume. Am J Obstet Gynecol 1977;127:255.
62. Manning FA, Hill LM, Platt LD. Qualitative amniotic fluid vol-

ume determination by ultrasonic antepartum detection of intrauterine growth retardation. Am J Obstet Gynecol 1981;139:254.
63. Philipson EH, Sokol RJ, Williams T. Oligohydramnios: clinical associations and predictive value for intrauterine growth retardation. Am J Obstet Gynecol 1983;146:271.
64. Grannum PA, Berkowitz RL, Hobbins JC. The ultrasonic changes in the maturing placenta and their relationship to fetal pulmonic maturity. Am J Obstet Gynecol 1979;133:915.
65. Petrucha R, Platt LD. Relationship of placenta grade to gestational age. Am J Obstet Gynecol 1982;144:733.
66. Grannum PA, Hobbins JC. The placenta. Radiol Clin North Am 1982;20(2):353.
67. Kazzi GM, Gross TL, Sokil RJ, et al. Detection of intrauterine growth retardation—a new use for sonographic placental grading. Am J Obstet Gynecol 1983;145:733.
68. Deter RL, Hadlock FP, Harrist RB. Evaluation of normal fetal growth and the detection of intrauterine growth retardation. In Callen PW, ed: Ultrasonography in obstetrics and gynecology. Philadelphia: WB Saunders, 1983:113.
69. Hadlock FP, Deter RL, Harrist RB, et al. A date-independent predictor of intrauterine growth retardation: femur length/abdominal circumference ratio. Am J Roentgenol 1983;141:979.
70. Benson, CB, Doubilet PM, Saltzman DH, et al. FL/AC ratio: poor predictor of intrauterine growth retardation. Invest Radiol 1985;20:727.
71. Stocker J, Maward R, Deleon A, et al. Ultrasonic cephalometry. Its use in estimating fetal weight. Obstet Gynecol 1975;45:278.
72. Sampson MB, Thomason JL, Kelly SL, et al. Prediction of intrauterine fetal weight using real-time ultrasound. Am J Obstet Gynecol 1982;142:554.
73. Eik-Nes SH, Grottum P. Estimation of fetal weight by ultrasound measurement. I. Development of a new formula. Acta Obstet Gynecol Scand 1982;61:299.
74. Shepard MJ, Richards VA, Verkowitz RL, et al. An evaluation of two equations for predicting fetal weight by ultrasound. Am J Obstet Gynecol 1982;142:47.
75. Deter RL, Harrist RB, Hadlock FP, et al. Evaluation of three methods of obtaining fetal weight estimates using dynamic image ultrasound. J Clin Ultrasound 1981;9:421.
76. Hadlock FP, Harrist RB, Sharman RS, et al. Estimation of fetal weight with the use of head, body and femur measurements—a prospective study. Am J Obstet Gynecol 1985;151:333.
77. Warsof SL, Gohar P, Berkowitz RL, et al. The estimation of fetal weight by computer-assisted analysis. Am J Obstet Gynecol 1977;128:881.
78. Ott WJ, Doyle S. Ultrasonic diagnosis of altered fetal growth by use of a normal ultrasonic fetal weight curve. Obstet Gynecol 1984;63:201.
79. Hadlock FP, Deter RL, Carpenter RJ, et al. Estimating fetal age: effect of head shape on BPD. Am J Roentgeol 1981;137:83.
80. Divon MY, Chamberlain PF, Sipos L, Platt LD. Underestimation of fetal weight in premature rupture of membranes. J Ultrasound Med 1984;3:529.
81. Weiner CP, Sabbagha RE, Vaisrub N, Socol ML. Ultrasonic fetal weight prediction: the role of head circumference and femur length. Obstet Gynecol 1985;65:812.
82. Tudinger BJ, Giles WB, Cook CM. Uteroplacental blood flow velocity-time waveforms in normal and complicated pregnancy. Br J Obstet Gynaecol 1985;92:39.
83. Reuwer PJHM, Sijmons EA, Rietman GW, et al. Intrauterine growth retardation: prediction of perinatal distress by Doppler ultrasound. Lancet 1987;ii:415.
84. Reuwer PJHM, Bruinse HW, Stoutenbeek PH, Haspels AA. Doppler assessment of the fetoplacental circulation in normal and growth retarded fetuses. Eur J Obstet Gynecol Reprod Biol 1984;18:199.
85. Fleischer A, Schulman H, Farmakides G, et al. Umbilical artery velocity waveforms and intrauterine growth retardation. Am J Obstet Gynecol 1985;151:502.
86. Campbell S, Pearce JM, Hackett G, et al. Qualitative assessment of uteroplacental blood flow: early screening test for high risk pregnancies. Obstet Gynecol 1986;68:649.
87. Sijmons EA, Reuwer PJHM, Van Beek E, Bruinse HW. The validity of screening for small-for-gestational age and low-weight-for-length infants by Doppler ultrasound. Brit J Obstet Gynecol 1989;96:557.
88. Sack RA. The large infant: a study of maternal, obstetric, fetal and newborn characteristics, including a long-term pediatric follow-up. Am J Obstet Gynecol 1969;104:195.
89. Nelson JH, Rovner IW, Barter RH. The large baby. South Med J 1958;51:23.
90. Posner AC, Friedman S, Posner LB. The large fetus: a study of 547 cases. Obstet Gynecol 1955;5:268.
91. Parks DG, Ziel HK. Macrosomia: a proposed indication for primary cesarean section. Obstet Gynecol 1978;52:407.
92. Boyd ME, Usher RH, McLean FH. Fetal macrosomia: prediction, risks, proposed management. Obstet Gynecol 1983;61:715.
93. Miller JM, Brown HL, Khawli OF, Pastorek JG, Gabert HA. Ultrasonographic identification of the macrosomic fetus. Am J Obstet Gynecol 1988;159:1110.
94. Elliott JP, Garite TJ, Freeman RK, McQuown DS, Patel JM. Ultrasonic prediction of fetal macrosomia in diabetic patients. Obstet Gynecol 1982;60:159.
95. Tamura RK, Sabbagha RE, Depp R, Dooley SL, Socol ML. Diabetic macrosomia: accuracy of third trimester ultrasound. Obstet Gynecol 1986;67:828.
96. Shepard MJ, Richards VA, Berkowitz RL et al. An evaluation of two equations for predicting fetal weight by ultrasound. Am J Obstet Gynecol 1982;47:142.

45

CHAPTER

MAGNETIC RESONANCE IMAGING IN OBSTETRICS

Richard R. Viscarello and Ruben Kier

During the past century various diagnostic imaging modalities have been developed that permit the perinatologist to view the internal contents of the pregnant uterus, to evaluate maternal anatomy and pathology, and to assess fetal growth and development. Conventional roentgenography, fluoroscopy, and computed tomography can serve in this capacity, but all necessarily expose the fetus to ionizing radiation and are limited in visualization of soft tissue.[1] Both transabdominal and endovaginal ultrasonography offer high-resolution, noninvasive imaging without the use of ionizing radiation or other side effects to mother or fetus, but ultrasonography clearly has its limitations in some diagnostic situations.[2,3]

Over the past decade a new diagnostic tool, magnetic resonance imaging (MRI), which relies on radio-frequency radiation, has become available. MRI can produce images of unsurpassed contrast and tissue resolution, as well as biochemical information, providing access to a new frontier in medical diagnosis and clinical management of pregnancy.[4] Since its first reported use in pregnancy by Smith[5] in 1983, numerous investigators have verified its utility in the diagnosis of a variety of maternal and fetal pathologies. The purpose of this chapter is to present the basic principles of MRI, its potential utility, and its present limitations in perinatal medicine.

PRINCIPLES OF MRI

MRI is a noninvasive technique employing nonionizing radio-frequency radiation to produce high-resolution, direct, multiplanar images containing biochemical information of great diagnostic potential.[6] The images are derived from the nuclear magnetic moments present in the nuclei of hydrogen atoms from the tissue. Although quantum physics can provide precise explanations of the complicated phenomena of nuclear magnetic moments, such a discussion is beyond the limits of this chapter. To comprehend the basic technique of MRI and to appreciate sufficiently its applications and potential in obstetrics and diagnostic medicine a few basic concepts will be presented.

MRI is based upon the phenomenon of nuclear magnetic resonance (NMR) and was reported first in 1946 by two groups working at Stanford and Harvard. Bloch and Purcell were awarded the 1952 Nobel Prize for their recognition of small magnetic moments in the nuclei of certain atoms.[4] NMR refers to the resonant absorption and remission of radio waves exhibited by these nuclei.[7] For some time after its discovery, NMR remained relegated to physical investigation of the behavioral properties of nuclear magnetic moments such as quantifying the magnetogyric ratio and spin of various nuclei. Subsequently, the recognition of the chemical and biochemical applications of NMR has been appreciated.[8] This information about molecular structure and the interactions of molecules opened up the world of nuclear magnetic moments and launched widespread applications in physics, chemistry, biology, and medicine.[2–4,6,7] As a result of this discovery the imaging technology now known as MRI evolved in 1973.

NMR and MRI depend on the physical properties of nuclear magnetism possessed by some atomic nuclei (eg, ^{1}hydrogen, ^{31}phosphorous, ^{23}sodium, and ^{13}carbon) and the behavioral parameters of these nuclei in an external magnetic field.[9] The hydrogen nucleus is most widely used in MRI because of its abundance in biological tissue. The charged hydrogen nucleus has an inherent spin or rotation about its axis that results in a nuclear magnetic moment. Generally, only nuclei with an odd number of nuclear particles possess nuclear magnetic moments, since pairs of neutrons or protons align in a way that effectively cancels each other's spin. The spinning hydrogen proton behaves as a small bar magnet with a north and south pole.[10]

In the absence of an external magnetic field, the magnetic moments generated by these nuclei are oriented randomly. If the nuclei (eg, hydrogen protons in tissue) are placed into an external magnetic field, their magnetic moments will orient themselves either parallel and aligned with or antiparallel and opposed to the external magnetic field. The antiparallel situation is a high-energy, or "excited," state; the parallel orientation is a low-energy, or "ground," state. Since the majority of magnetic moments will be in the ground state at equilibrium, the net magnetization vector (M) will be aligned parallel to the external magnetic field.

In NMR and MRI, radio-frequency energy expressed in the form of a pulse is used to move nuclear magnetic moments from a "ground state" to an "excited state." Measuring this transition in energy levels in the nuclear magnetic moments is how biochemical information is determined by NMR and MRI. The radio frequency or *resonant frequency* needed to produce the transition in energy levels is proportional to the strength of the magnetic field, as determined by a constant termed the magnetogyric ratio. This resonant or Larmor frequency is equal to the strength of the field measured in tesla (T) multiplied by the magnetogyric ratio.[9,10]

As noted, each species of nuclei has a specific magnetogyric ratio. By selecting the appropriate frequencies, specific nuclei can be isolated, and observations of their behavior in a magnetic field can be studied. Most medical applications of MRI obtain images using resonances from hydrogen nuclei (protons) because of their abundance in human tissue and its inherent sensitivity to MRI, which results from its unique atomic configuration. For the hydrogen atom, with a magnetogyric ratio of 42.7 MHz/T, the frequency at which transitions in energy levels take place in a 1-T field is 42.7 MHz. This has practical implications for design, as the radio-frequency transmitter as well as the receiver coils used in the MRI scanner must be maximally sensitive at 42.7 MHz for best imaging quality.

The extent to which the radio-frequency pulses move the nuclear magnetic moments depends on the strength and duration of the pulse, termed a pulse sequence. The pulses are classified by the angle through which they move magnetic moments. A pulse of 90° will rotate a nuclear magnetic moment through an angle of 90° and then stop. If the magnetic moment was originally along a Z axis, a 90° pulse will move it into a magnetic vector aligned with the XY plane. Similarly, a longer pulse of 180° will rotate the spinning and precessing magnetic moment through 180°, simply inverting the starting position (Fig. 45-1).[4]

Currently, the spin-echo (SE) pulse sequences are used predominantly to view maternal and fetal anatomy. The SE method employs first a 90° "excitation" pulse to rotate the macromagnetic moments into the XY plane; they next begin to dephase. After a specified interval, a "rephasing" pulse of 180° induces partial rephasing of the magnetization, producing an echo signal. This rephasing neutralizes the dephasing that occurs as a product of the inhomogeneities in the field. If the 90° pulse is followed by a 180° pulse 20 milliseconds (msec) later, the peak of the echo will occur 20 msec after the 180° pulse, since the time to rephase equals the time required to dephase. The time to echo (TE) is the time from the beginning of the 90° excitation pulse to the peak of the echo. For routine image acquisition, the data from multiple sequential excitation–rephasing cycles must be collected to allow spatial encoding. The time between the sequential excitation pulses is termed the repetition time (TR). Diagnostic information in the MR image depends on contrast between tissues that can be manipulated by varying the TR or TE of the pulse sequence.[6,10]

The MRI signal intensity or brightness of a structure depends on the density of protons that can give rise to signals, the relaxation rate of the protons after an excitation pulse, and flow effects. Although air appears black because of low proton density, most soft tissues

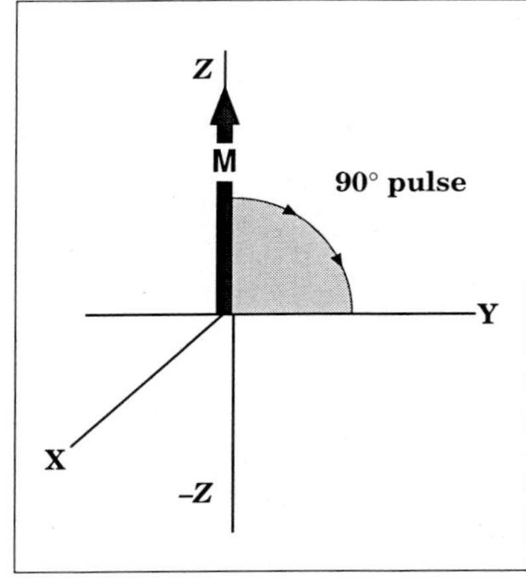

A

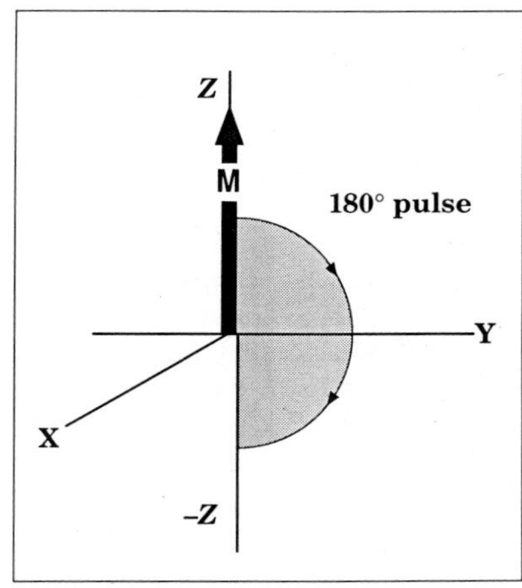

B

FIGURE 45–1. When placed in an external magnetic field oriented in the Z axis, the net magnetization vector (M) of the spinning protons aligns parallel to the external magnetic field. (**A**) When a radiofrequency pulse of the proper duration is applied, the net magnetic moment can be tipped 90° into the XY plane. (2) A pulse that is twice the amplitude or duration of a 90° pulse will rotate the net magnetic moment 180°, essentially inverting the net magnetic vector of the spinning protons.

have a similar proton density, so that other factors are needed to provide tissue contrast. The major contribution to contrast reflects measurement of the relaxation time, during which the protons lose the pulsed-energy and return to a state of equilibrium. This process involves two distinct, quantifiable times for relaxation. The spin-lattice relaxation time (T1) represents the time required for a magnetic moment to return to its original orientation with the external magnetic field. The spin-spin relaxation time (T2) is the time required for the nuclear motion to dephase and transfer energy to other protons (Fig. 45-2). By definition, T1 is always longer than T2. Different tissues generally have inherently different T1 and T2 relaxation times, which vary with magnetic field strength. This enables MRI to demonstrate various soft-tissue characteristics by differentiation of the level of intensity or brightness.[4–6,10,11]

MR images can be T1- or T2-weighted to exploit the spin-spin or spin-lattice relaxation times inherent in tissue and to enhance the intensity and contrast of tissues. Whether or not an image is T1- or T2-weighted depends on the length of TE and TR. T1-weighted images usually have a TR between 300 and 600 msec and a TE between 11 and 30 msec. These images will show fluid-containing structures as low-intensity signal (dark gray), soft-tissue structures as intermediate-intensity signal (medium gray), and fat as high-intensity signal (white). T2-weighted images usually have a TR between 1500 and 2500 msec and a TE between 70 and 100 msec. These images usually increase contrast between different soft tissues, especially the uterus and ovaries (Fig. 45-3). No single-pulse sequence will maximize contrast and intensity for all tissue types.

In whole-body MRI the patient is placed in a supine position in a static magnetic field. A viewing plane is selected: axial, coronal, or sagittal; and the desired region of imaging is stimulated with an oscillating magnetic field in the form of radio-frequency energy. The effects of this stimulation on the nuclear magnetic moments in the selected region are measured in multiple

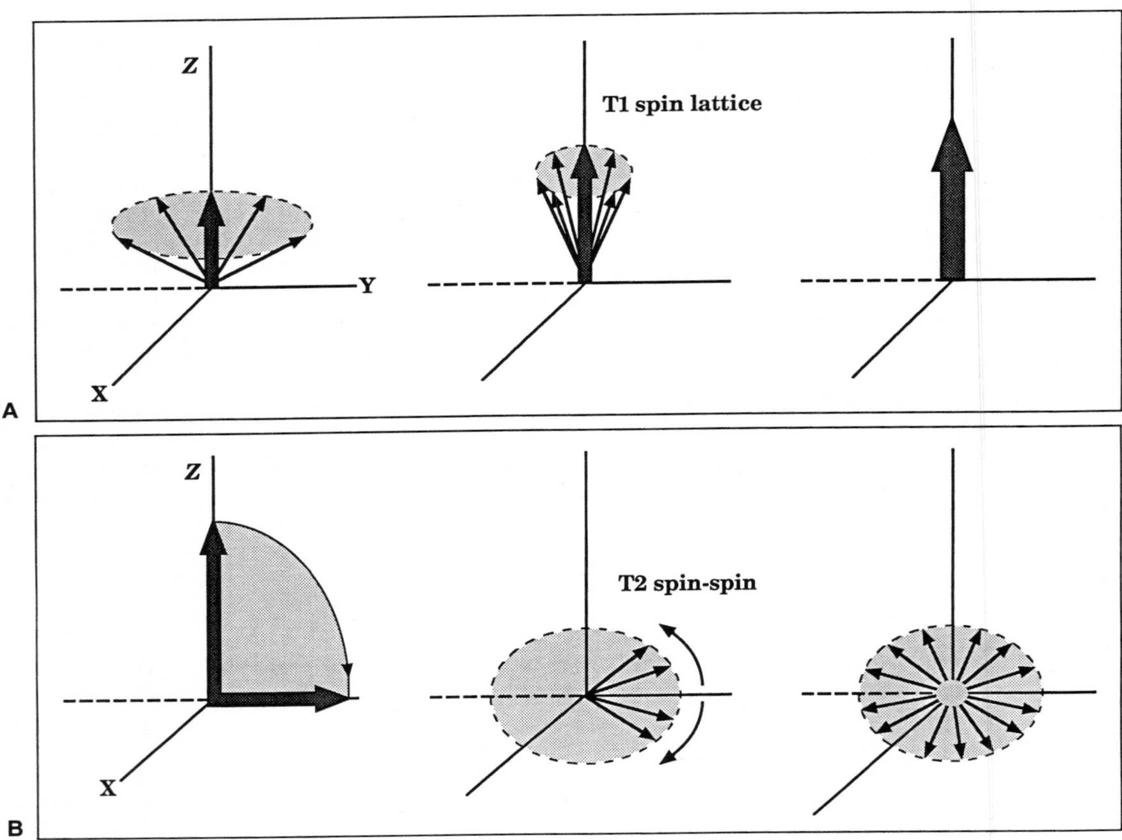

FIGURE 45–2. Following radiofrequency excitation, the net magnetic vector returns to its original orientation at a rate determined by two discrete time constants. (**A**) The T1 relaxation time represents the time constant for the recovery of longitudinal magnetization along the Z axis. (**B**) The T2 relaxation time reflects the time constant for decay of the magnetic vector along the XY axis. Initially, the protons tipped into the XY plane are in phase, generating a net vector that is rotating through the XY plane. With T2 decay, the protons lose coherence by dephasing.

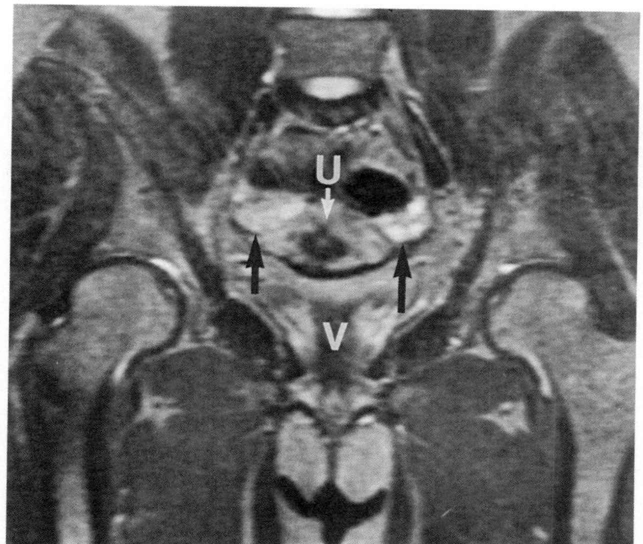

FIGURE 45–3. Normal ovaries (arrows) on coronal T2-weighted image, containing several small follicles that appear high signal. (U, uterus; V, vagina.)

directions using a receiving coil. A cross-sectional image or slice is generated and is reconstructed via computer. Information for the image can be limited to specific areas, allowing variations in thickness of slice and region without repositioning the patient. Information from several planes may be obtained simultaneously.

LIMITATIONS IN THE USE OF MRI

The utility of MRI for fetal diagnosis during the first and second trimesters of pregnancy may be hindered by fetal motion and resulting artifact. At the present time, the only real-time capability available with MRI, the echo planar technique, offers poor resolution and requires special equipment.[12] The relatively long imaging time of 2 to 10 minutes with conventional spin-echo techniques makes image degradation by fetal motion almost unavoidable before 26 weeks of gestation,[13] possibly earlier with oligohydramnios (Fig. 45-4). Fetal motion is random; therefore, gating techniques are of no use.[13–15] A new "fast spin-echo" pulse sequence, representing a hybrid between echo-planar and spin-echo methods, has reduced imaging times to under 1 minute with suppression of motion.

Success at reducing fetal motion by inducing transient fetal paralysis by selective fetal neuromuscular blockade has been recorded with pancuronium bromide[16] and with direct, fetal intravascular infusion of vercuronium bromide.[17] No objective measurement of decreased fetal motion resulted from maternal intravenous sedation with diazepam.[12] Motion artifact resulting from maternal aortic pulsation may be precluded by left lateral tilt and will improve maternal comfort during a long examination.[16]

Another limiting factor may be the lack of expertise in the area of prenatal diagnosis using MRI, because experience with the technique is small at present. As investigative and clinical use of MRI increases, appro-

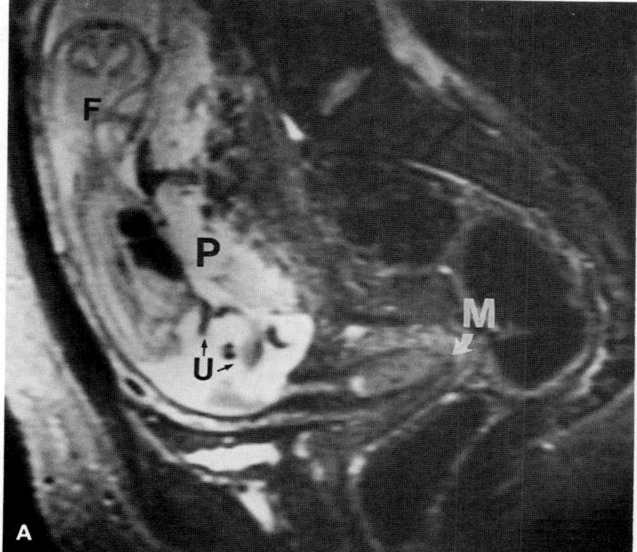

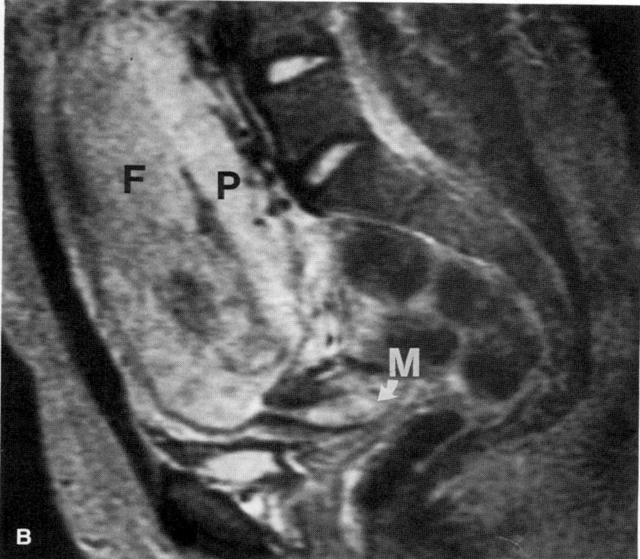

FIGURE 45–4. A 15-week fetus in a patient with cervical carcinoma. (**A**) Routine T2-weighted spin echo sequence demonstrates a posterior placenta (P) and an abnormal mass (M) within the cervical canal. The fetus (F) is poorly visualized because of the extensive fetal motion during the long imaging time (8 minutes). (**B**) A "fast spin echo" pulse sequence obtained T2-weighted images in less than 1 minute in the same patient. The fetus (F) and umbilical cord (U) are defined more clearly. The placenta (P) and cervical mass (M) are also well defined.

priate technical parameters to facilitate the diagnosis of specific congenital anomalies are sure to evolve, just as parameters were developed using ultrasonography.

There are other, more general limitations to consider. Women undergoing MRI must not have pacemakers or be wearing metal objects. The cost of an MRI facility is considerable. A single imaging unit may cost several millions of dollars to build, not including additional protective shielding for the surrounding environment.[18] This is reflected in the high cost of an individual examination, requiring highly trained personnel to maintain a safe, successful operation.[19]

SAFETY AND EFFICACY OF MRI

Since the use of MRI in obstetrics is still in its infancy, much clinical investigation is still needed to assess the safety to the mother and fetus. It is crucial to remember that during an MRI examination the patients are exposed to magnetic fields from 2500 to 20,000 times more intense than the earth's magnetic field, with examination times as long as several hours. The length of the examinations may vary, depending on the purpose of the examination, and will shorten as the level of expertise and knowledge in assessing maternal, fetal, and uterine anatomy increases.

Although caution is indicated, there are no reported biological hazards or deleterious effects to the mother, fetus, or placenta. The fetus seems to incur no known risk from MRI. There is no empirical evidence of mutagenicity or adverse fetal effects.[4] Although there is no evidence to suggest that MRI is hazardous to the embryo at the magnetic field strength and radio frequency used for clinical MRI,[20] the first trimester represents the critical period of organogenesis, which poses at least a theoretical risk. Thus, both the British National Radiological Protection Board and scientists at the National Institutes of Health Consensus Development Conference on MRI agree that "it might be prudent to exclude pregnant women during the first trimester" and that MRI "should be used during the first trimester only when there are clear medical indications and it offers a definite advantage over other available tests."[21,22] A recently published study evaluated the umbilical blood flow and fetal cardiotocography before and after MRI and found no changes in fetal well-being.[23]

CLINICAL USES FOR MRI

Some of the earliest imaging studies using MRI were done on cells and secretions from the female reproductive tract. The physical parameters that form the basis of MRI (ie, proton density, T1- and T2- relaxation times, pulse sequence, and imaging time) can be exploited not only to provide optimum differentiation of specific tissues and anatomical structures, but also to visualize perfusion without the use of intravenous contrast materials. Unlike ultrasound, MRI does not require the presence of urine in the bladder, or of amniotic fluid in the uterus. It can be used to view the uterus, cervix, ovaries, fetus, and placenta.[14,15,24,25] The physiologic changes in structure and relationship that occur during pregnancy can be measured due to the biological sensitivity of T1 and T2 to the tissue distribution of water and concentration of lipids.[14,15] Additionally, since slow flow of blood may produce a large MRI signal, venous congestion and venous stasis can be monitored.[2,24]

CERVIX

Maternal anatomy can be well defined using MRI and can be very useful for early diagnosis of cervical incompetence during pregnancy. Spin-echo, T2-weighted pulse sequences provide good definition of the cervix.[3] The cervix is best viewed in the sagittal plane (Fig. 45-5). MRI offers a distinct advantage over ultrasound in its ability to portray maternal anatomy accurately, because it does not require a distended bladder.[4,14,26] The spurious elongated appearance of a truly shortened, incompetent cervix caused by compression from bladder distention can occur with ultrasound.[4] In addition, a full bladder can express the membranes and amniotic fluid normally invaginated into the cervical canal, concealing this sign of cervical incompetence.[24]

It has also been suggested that it may be possible to diagnose cervical incompetence using MRI in nonpregnant women by observing the change in the size, shape, structure, and appearance of the cervical stroma.[6,26] The pregnant cervix has a characteristic trilaminar appearance when uneffaced.[27] There is an outer zone of intermediate intensity surrounding a low-intensity band believed to be stromal tissue high in collagen.[14] The cervical mucous plug and epithelial glands comprise the high-intensity central zone.[24]

It has been shown that ripening of the cervix can be assessed more accurately with MRI than by clinical evaluation with a metal dilator or digital examination. With softening and effacement, the central lumen containing the glandular tissue appears widened superiorly and loses the previous distinction seen between the two contrasting layers prior to the process of effacement (Fig. 45-6).[24] The positions of the external and internal ostia are clearly demonstrated, as is their relationship to the presenting part and to the vagina.[24]

PLACENTA

The exact location and size of the placenta can be visualized with MRI, thus making this technique very helpful in the diagnosis of placental abnormalities. The use of a T2-weighted spin-echo sequence with long excitation (TE) and relaxation times (TR) produces a high-intensity signal from the placenta and clearly contrasts with the surrounding amniotic fluid (Fig. 45-7).[27] Since the cervical os is also very apparent, a diagnosis of placenta previa can be made with confidence (Fig. 45-8).

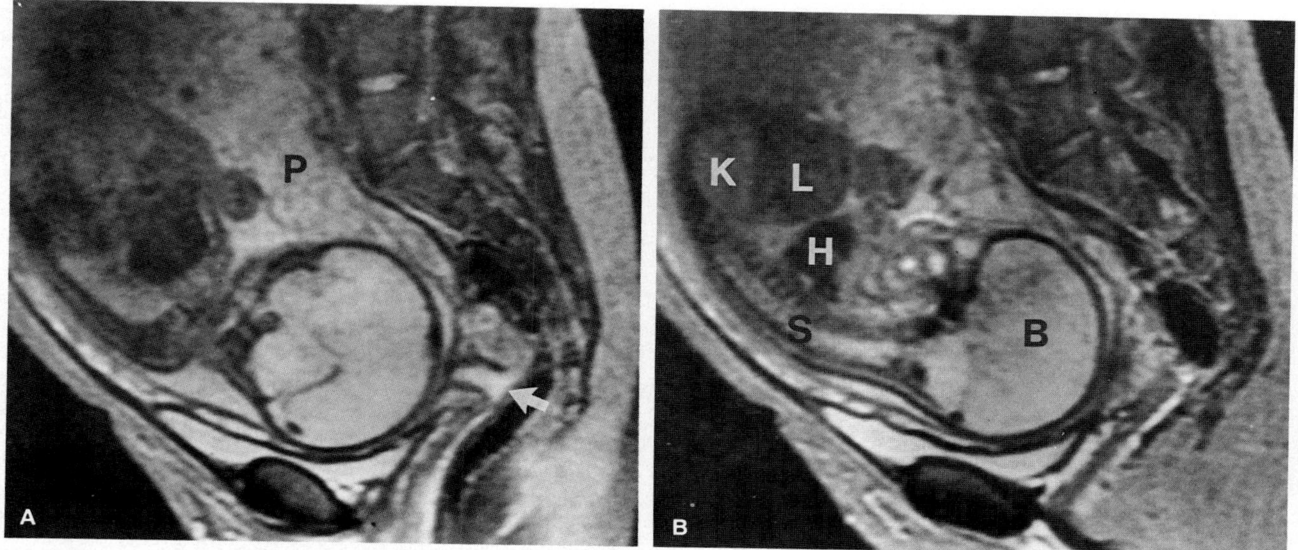

FIGURE 45–5. Normal third-trimester pregnancy on sagittal T2-weighted images. (**A**) The cervix (arrowheads) contains a central, high-signal mucus plug (arrow). The posterior placenta (P) is well seen, without evidence of previa. (**B**) On an adjacent image, the fetal anatomy is better demonstrated: brain (B), spine (S), heart (H), kidney (K), liver (L).

This is especially relevant in posterior implantations, a situation where ultrasound is limited with respect to assessing the degree of previa, whether marginal, low-lying, or total posterior previa. MRI can delineate the exact relationship of the placental edge to the internal cervical os, thereby directly affecting clinical management and possibly avoiding an extended hospitalization and eliminating unnecessary surgery.[27]

Other conditions that are difficult to visualize with ultrasonography, such as placental infarction, retroplacental clots, and impaired placental perfusion, can be delineated better with MRI.[14] An additional advantage to the patient and technician performing the examination is that MRI does not require a full bladder, which may distort the uterus and create a false impression of a previa.

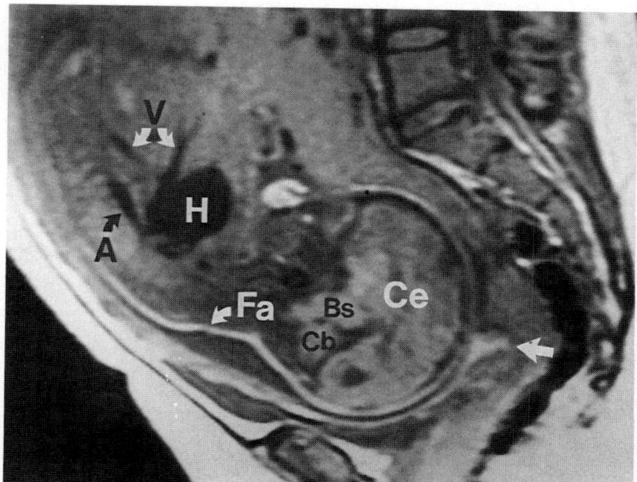

FIGURE 45–6. Pregnancy near term on a sagittal proton density-weighted image. The central lumen of the cervix (arrow) is beginning to widen superiorly. Internal anatomy of the fetus can be identified: cerebrum (Ce), cerebellum (Cm), brain stem (Bs), heart (H), aorta (A), hepatic veins (V). Note the normal thin layer of subcutaneous fat (F).

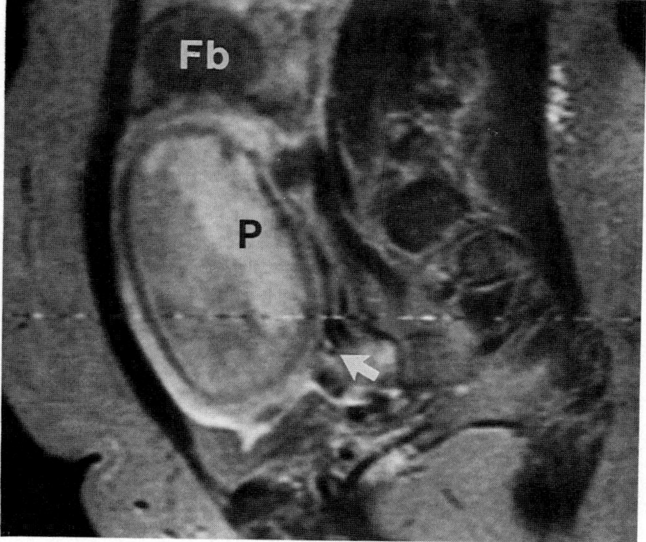

FIGURE 45–7. First-trimester pregnancy with marginal placenta previa (P) seen on a sagittal T2-weighted image. The internal cervical os (arrow) can be identified. With progression of pregnancy, this previa may resolve. A subserosal uterine fibroid (Fb) is noted at the fundus.

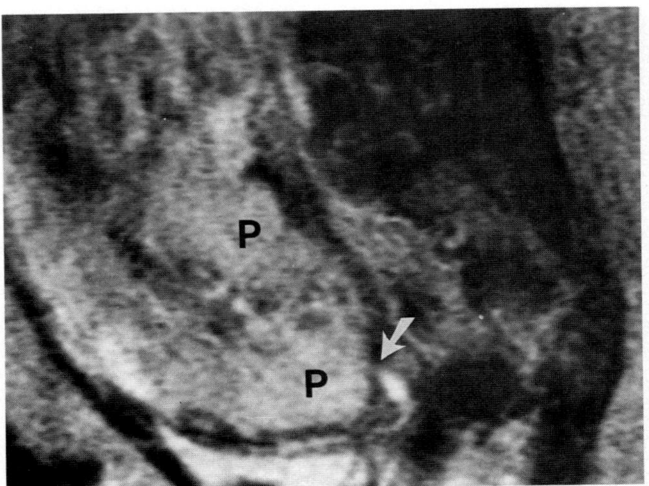

FIGURE 45–8. Complete placenta previa on a sagittal T2-weighted image. Despite image degradation by motion artifact, the predominantly posterior placenta (P) completely covers the region of the internal cervical os (arrow).

AMNIOTIC FLUID

Oligohydramnios often precludes ultrasonic visualization of fetal anatomy and, therefore, sonographic detection of fetal anomalies. Reduced volume of amniotic fluid actually enhances the quality of MRI by restricting fetal motion and resulting artifact.[4,27] Amniotic fluid has a long T1; with the appropriate pulse sequence this property can be exploited to provide contrast with adjacent tissue, such as subcutaneous fat, with its short T1 and long T2. A T1-weighted spin-echo sequence with short relaxation time (500 msec) best highlights this contrast (Fig. 45-9).[28]

One cause of oligohydramnios is poor renal function in the fetus. MRI has been used in the diagnosis of a fetus with Potter's syndrome that could not be visualized utilizing ultrasound.[23] MRI has also been shown to be useful in the identification of fetal hydronephrosis.[29,30]

The T1 relaxation time of amniotic fluid can be altered by the passage of meconium in utero.[23] The shorter T1 and T2 of meconium-stained amniotic fluid decreases the image intensity. This may serve as a useful, noninvasive marker of fetal distress.[6]

FETAL LUNG MATURITY

The possibility of assessing fetal lung maturity by MRI is currently being explored. Lung maturation commences around 24 weeks and develops with an increasing water content and a rise in the phospholipid concentration resulting from the production of surfactant.[15] This physiologic change is reflected in a shortening of both the T1 and T2 relaxation times of the lung tissue. Currently, no noninvasive method of determining lung maturity exists; rather, an amniocentesis is required to obtain a sample to perform a lecithin–sphingomyelin ratio. This procedure is not without some risk (estimated at 0.5%) and may be impossible in cases of severe oligohydramnios. Lung maturity assessment using parameters of T1 and T2 could be of tremendous clinical utility if confirmed.

FETAL ANATOMY

The significant expense, the lack of widespread availability, and current technical limitations restrict the role and use of MRI for the purpose of routine viewing of the fetus. Although ultrasound remains the primary modality for the screening and diagnosis of fetal anomalies, the improved tissue characterization and contrast provided by MRI can provide additional needed information. In situations where sonography is limited, suboptimal, or equivocal, MRI can be used to demonstrate fetal anatomy in great detail (Fig. 45-10).[30]

The use of tissue characteristics other than sound impedance may actually enhance depiction of fetal anatomy and pathology.[23] There have been reports describing the advantage of MRI over ultrasound in depicting details of fetal dysmorphology.[25,29] In view of the wide range of therapeutic alternatives available, the value of a more precise diagnosis cannot be overlooked.

The anatomy of the fetus is best visualized with MRI during the third trimester, when fetal motion is more restricted, because of fetal size (see Figs. 45-5, 45-6, and 45-9). Although current MRI technology allows images to be obtained in any maternal body plane or section, sagittal images appear to be most helpful in prenatal diagnosis of fetal anomalies. This plane provides a coronal or parasagittal view of the fetus. Usually, structures

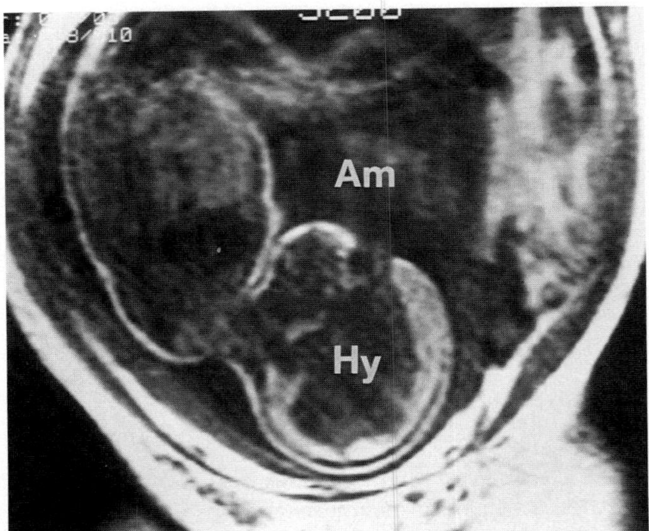

FIGURE 45–9. Thirty-three-week fetus with hydrocephalus (Hy), and borderline increase amnionic fluid volume (Am). These fluid-containing structures appear low in signal intensity on this T1-weighted coronal image.

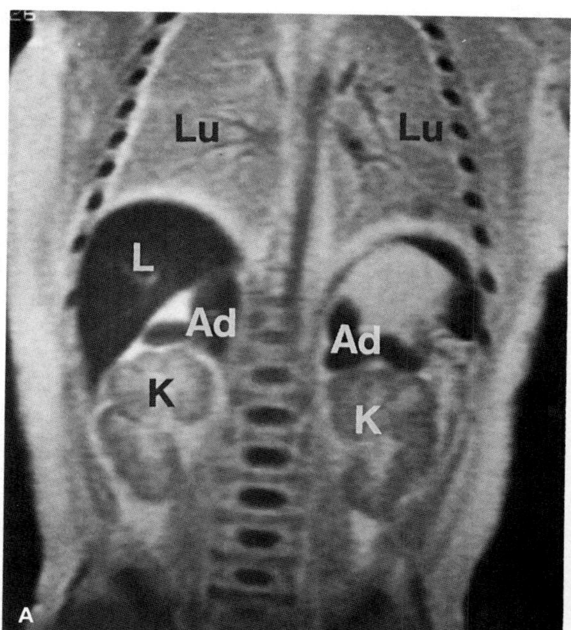

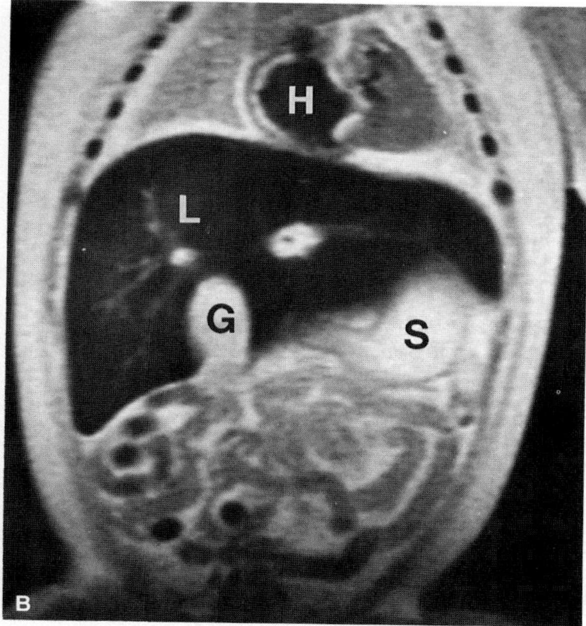

FIGURE 45–10. Fetal anatomy demonstrated in a 22-week abortus, imaged in vitro with T2-weighted coronal images. These images demonstrate the potential of MRI of the fetus if motion artifacts can be suppressed completely. (**A**) Lobulations in the fetal kidneys (K) are demonstrated. The lungs (Lu) appear relatively high in signal intensity because of their water content in the fetus. The adrenal glands (Ad) are also well seen. (**B**) More anteriorly, the liver (L), gallbladder (G), stomach (S), and heart (H) are clearly demonstrated.

are imaged most clearly using a T1-weighted, spin-echo pulse sequence, since the short TR and TE reduce fetal motion artifact. Muscle, cortical bone, marrow-containing bone, and subcutaneous fat of limbs are visible but may not be well delineated because of fetal motion.[25]

The fetal brain and central nervous system can be well demonstrated during the third trimester of pregnancy by MRI (see Fig. 45-6). This is the only imaging modality that can display in utero the process of physiologic myelination and, therefore, any delays or deficits in its development.[15] Because of the greater water and lower protein content of the fetal brain, the T2-weighted, spin-echo pulse sequence highlights the T2 contrast between brain tissue and optimizes detailed imaging of the premyelinated brain with its long T2 relaxation time.[25] Late in the pregnancy, the decrease in the water content of the CNS and brain is reflected in a decreased T1 as myelinization begins to occur.[13]

The posterior fossa is well demonstrated by MRI, presenting an area of potential use, since abnormalities of this region can be difficult to assess using sonography.[2] The tentorium cerebelli and falx cerebri separate the cerebellum and the cerebral hemispheres with low-intensity stripes indicative of a lack of mobile protons, similar to other fibrous tissues.[25] A T1-weighted, spin-echo sequence provides the best delineation of cerebrospinal fluid (low signal) from spinal cord (intermediate signal), although imaging of the spinal cord itself is difficult. Fetal cerebrospinal fluid increases in intensity with greater T2 weighting.[25] MRI may define intrinsic brain anatomy better than existing imaging modalities. This may enhance outcome of fetal surgery, such as intrauterine shunting procedures for hydrocephalus, by eliminating concurrent undiagnosed brain abnormalities.

The fetal liver is the most readily visualized organ in the fetal abdomen because of its size and its contrast with the fetal lungs and abdominal fat on T2-weighted images.[25] It is seen as a homogeneous structure of moderate intensity (see Fig. 45-5). Early in gestation, the liver has a different relaxation time and signal, because of its erythropoietic function (see Fig. 45-10). The portal and hepatic veins also are visible in the third trimester of pregnancy (see Fig. 45-6).[25]

Normal fetal kidneys are not readily imaged because of their small size and the lack of contrast that results from scarcity of retroperitoneal fat.[15] When visualized, they appear light gray to white because of the strong signal from blood and urine in T1 images (see Figs. 45-5 and 45-10). Pelviectasis, cysts, hydronephrosis, and renal dysplasia can be seen with MRI.[25] NMR is being studied in the evaluation of fetal kidney function by the analysis of fetal urine.[16]

Although abnormal conditions such as bowel distention may be seen by MRI, normal fetal bowels are generally not visible. Loops of bowel have been imaged prenatally in a fetus with a diaphragmatic hernia.[16]

Fluid-filled sacs with long T1 values, such as the stomach, gall bladder, and urinary bladder, are easily identified, especially in contrast to abdominal fat.[13]

From the second trimester, the fetal heart is seen as a low-intensity structure (see Figs. 45-5 and 45-6). By the third trimester, it may be seen as having four distinct chambers, as the interventricular septum is usually visualized.[13,15] The major vessels of the fetus are visible as low-intensity structures on T2-weighted sequences. The low signal is dependent on the rate of flow, the degree of turbulence, and the image slice chosen.[13,15] Sonography provides an excellent depiction of the heart from early in gestation, and the diagnosis of most cardiac anomalies is possible with ultrasound alone.[15] In assessing the fetal cardiovascular system, MRI is able to provide unique information and measurements on the flow of blood through the placenta and umbilical vessels.

FETAL GROWTH

MRI has demonstrated the ability to assess disorders of fetal growth. MRI may prove superior to ultrasound in the diagnosis of such conditions as intrauterine growth retardation or macrosomia, since ultrasound-derived fetal growth parameters do not always correlate with the soft-tissue wasting present at birth in the former, or the abundance of subcutaneous fat in the latter, as in the fetus of the diabetic mother (Fig. 45-11).[15] MRI provides excellent resolution of fetal fat stores and exhibits high contrast with both amniotic fluid and skeletal muscle.[28]

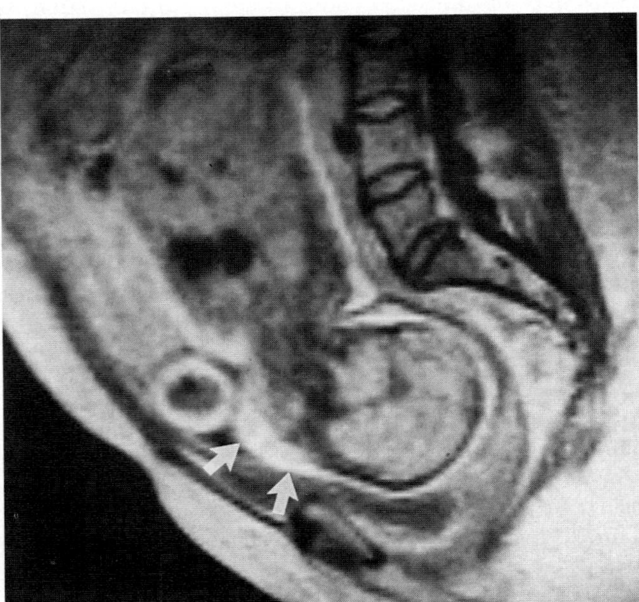

FIGURE 45–11. Abnormally increased thickness of subcutaneous fat (arrows) in the fetus of a diabetic mother. (Compare to Figure 45–6.)

In one study, 11 pregnancies determined to be at high risk between 32 and 37 weeks were examined utilizing T1-weighted, spin-echo pulse sequences.[28] This technique provided the best discrimination between subcutaneous adipose tissue and adjacent muscle, as well as between amniotic fluid and skin. The findings indicate a correlation between decreased subcutaneous tissue mass as estimated by MRI and malnourishment of the fetus independent of fetal size. MRI has also been used to demonstrate significant intra-twin birth weight discordance, associated with poor perinatal outcome, and intrauterine growth retardation for one or both of the twins.[31]

MOLAR PREGNANCIES

Recently, MRI has been used to detect molar pregnancies.[32] On T2-weighted MR images, molar pregnancies appear as a diffuse area of mixed high-intensity signal comparable to placenta filling the entire uterus (Fig. 45-12).[6] T1-weighting images can differentiate the heterogeneous elements of the signal into a high-intensity signal representing blood and a low-intensity signal from trophoblastic tissue.[14] As MRI is highly specific for trophoblastic disease, it may be used to detect the extent of invasion into the myometrium, the position and extent of the spread of malignancy, response to therapy, and recurrent trophoblastic disease when indicated by a rising human chorionic gonadotrophin titer.[33]

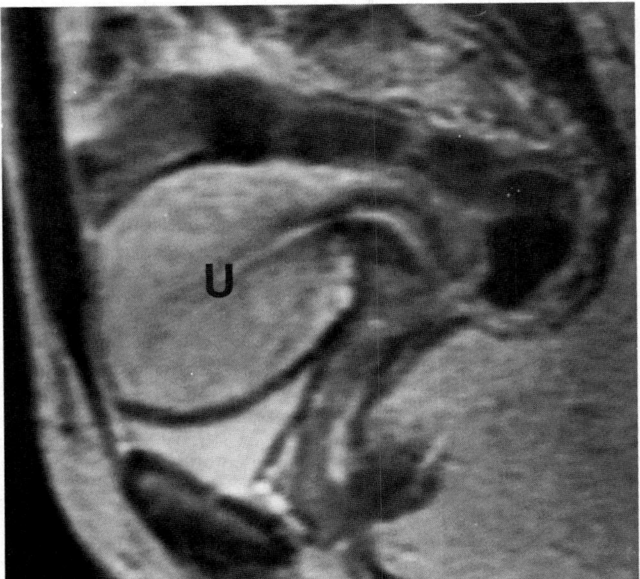

FIGURE 45–12. Gestational trophoblastic disease diffusely involving the uterus (U), seen on a sagittal T2-weighted image. Unlike the normal intermediate signal of the myometrium and low signal intensity of the junctional zone of the myometrium, diffuse trophoblastic disease leads to abnormal high signal throughout the uterus.

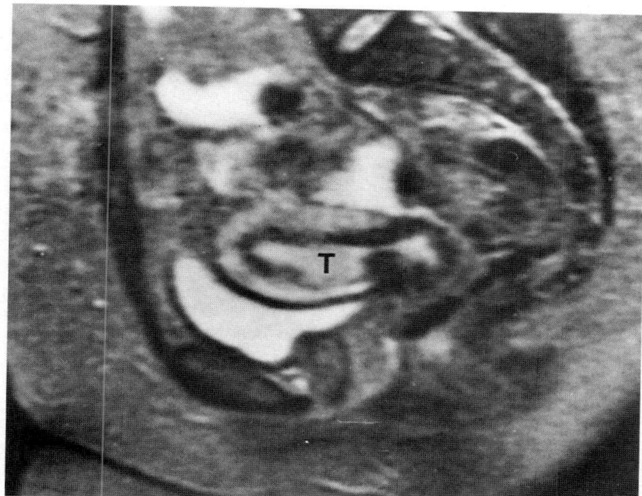

FIGURE 45–13. Endometrial carcinoma seen on sagittal T2-weighted image. The tumor (T) is slightly lower in signal intensity than the endometrial stripe but disrupts the normal low-signal-intensity "junctional zone" in the anterior wall of the uterus, indicating myometrial invasion. The junctional zone along the posterior wall of the uterus remains intact.

ABDOMINAL PREGNANCIES

There have been recent reports of successful diagnosis and management of a viable abdominal pregnancy that have been attributed to MRI.[34–36] This technique was able to confirm location of the fetus, amniotic fluid, uterus, and placenta prior to surgery and to follow placental involution after delivery. Sonographic diagnosis of an abdominal pregnancy may be hindered by bowel gas, adjacent soft tissue, or lack of an acoustic window secondary to oligohydramnios. MRI can clearly define the area of placental implantation and its proximity to the pelvic organs and their vascular supply. The inadvertent dislodgment of the placenta and consequent hemorrhaging would be less likely with the precise information provided by the MRI to aid in locating the incision for laparotomy.[37]

EVALUATION OF MALIGNANCY

Primary malignancy in the female pelvis has been shown to increase signal intensity in the MR image,[3,37,38] although the cystic and hemorrhagic nature of ovarian neoplasm results in high signal intensity as well.[39] It has been suggested that MRI may be helpful in staging certain malignancies in pregnant patients. MRI is unique among imaging modalities in its ability to depict the layers of the myometrium, stratum basale, endometrium, fibrous stroma, and parametrium.[40] MRI produces images of superior detail, revealing information about the myometrium and endometrium that may result in recognition and management of pathologic conditions during pregnancy.

Although MRI may be useful in the diagnosis of stage I or early stage II endometrial carcinoma,[33,38,40] histologic diagnosis remains necessary. Although MRI cannot discriminate between adenomatous hyperplasia or blood clot, with long T2 weighting, endometrial adenocarcinoma has inherently high signal intensity; the myometrium has an intermediate signal. Thus, any myometrial invasion of the tumor can be assessed.[33,38] Attenuation or disruption of the low-intensity band or "junctional zone" between the myometrium and endometrium generally indicates myometrial invasion. The absence of the low-intensity band has a high correlation with histologic diagnosis of deep myometrial invasion (Fig. 45-13).[38] Metastatic endometrial carcinoma also has inherently high-intensity signal with long T2 weighting. This facilitates evaluation of the spread of

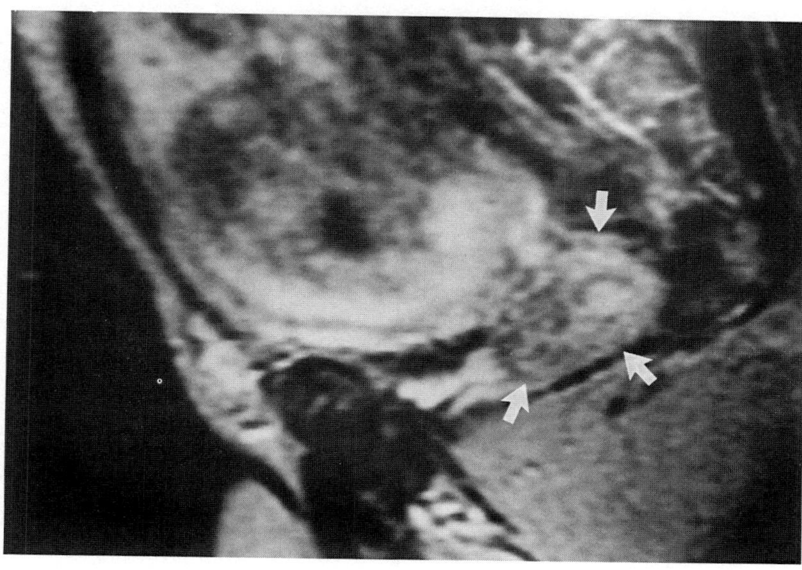

FIGURE 45–14. Cervical carcinoma imaged in the 14th week of pregnancy on a sagittal T2-weighted image. This stage 2A lesion (arrows) demonstrates disruption of the normal architecture of the cervix, with extension to the upper portion of the vagina.

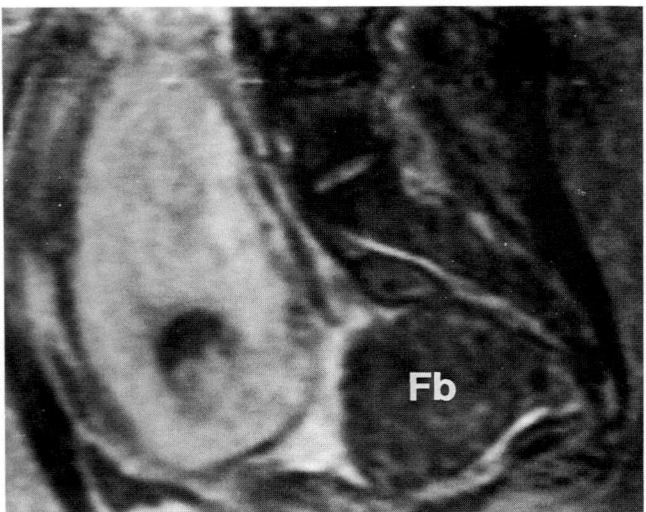

FIGURE 45–15. Subserosal fibroid (Fb) in the lower uterine segment, appearing as a well-circumscribed low-signal-intensity mass lesion on this T2-weighted sagittal image.

tumor outside the uterus and subsequently may aid in the detection of recurrence.[33] MRI also demonstrates lymph node involvement.[38,40]

MRI is useful in the diagnosis and identification of stage I or early stage II cervical carcinoma, especially since cervical carcinoma exhibits distortion of the characteristic trilaminar appearance and interruption of the low-intensity band (Fig. 45-14). SE long T2-weighted sequences will show cervical neoplasm to have a medium increase in signal intensity contrasted with nonpathologic tissue.[33] An uncharacteristic asymmetrical appearance of the parametrium or tumor signal intensity expanding into the parametrium indicates parametrial extension. Involvement of the cervical stroma and vagina also can be depicted with MRI.[38] Clearly presented pelvic relations allow assessment of cervix, parametrium, pelvic sidewalls, rectum, and lymph nodes in spite of the gravid uterus.

Although MRI can discern simple fluid and other types of lesion, it cannot differentiate between benign and malignant ovarian neoplasm, although depiction of lymphadenopathy in MR images may aid in the detection of malignancy. Ovarian cystadenoma may be indistinguishable from cystadenocarcinoma with MRI.[39] Sarcomatous change in degenerative leiomyoma cannot be differentiated from myxomatous degeneration.[41] Heavy T2-weighted SE pulse sequences will allow differentiation of late posttreatment fibrosis from recurrent pelvic neoplasm.[40] The recurrent tumor is visualized as a region of increased signal intensity with long TR and TE.

Benign and malignant ovarian masses may display manifestation of bleeding on MR images; however, the absence of a solid component accompanying a homogeneous hemorrhagic appearance would indicate diagnosis of endometrioma rather than hemorrhagic cyst.[42]

PELVIC MASSES IN PREGNANCY

Pelvic masses are especially problematic when suspected during pregnancy. Localizing a mass by physical examination is difficult after the first trimester. Sonography may be limited in its capacity to locate and characterize pelvic masses by the gravid uterus itself, uterine retroversion, or maternal obesity, or by the size and location of the mass.[43] Pelvic masses associated with pregnancy can be diagnosed and located more accurately using MRI.[23,42]

It is suggested that MRI be used after the first trimester for several reasons. The most common lesion presenting during early pregnancy is the corpus luteum

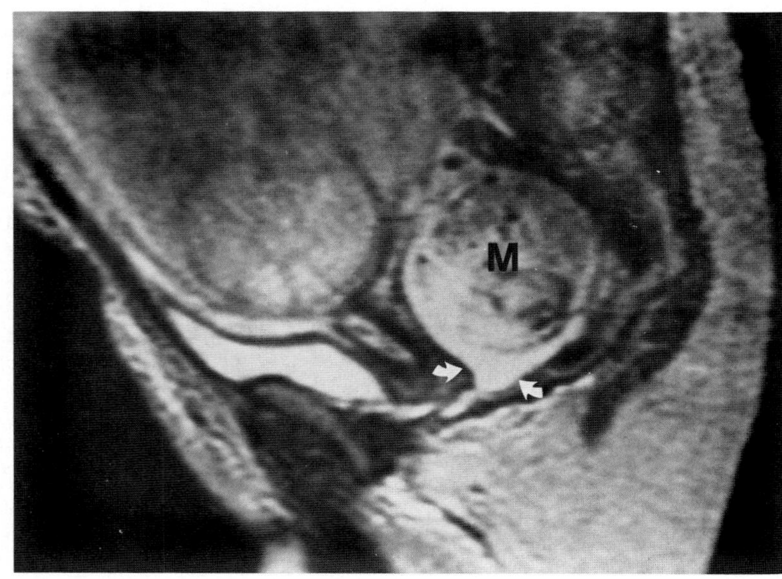

FIGURE 45–16. Fibrothecoma of the ovary appearing as a well-circumscribed heterogeneous mass (M) on this sagittal T2-weighted image. A small amount of free fluid is identified in the cul de sac (arrows).

cyst, whose regression usually can be demonstrated using ultrasonography by the end of the first trimester.[24,38] Surgical intervention is usually delayed until the second trimester, when the chances of fetal loss from spontaneous abortion are reduced. Waiting until the second trimester minimizes the chances of postoperative fetal death from anesthesia-related causes and avoids the period of fetal organogenesis and possible teratogenesis.[42]

Uterine leiomyomas during pregnancy may cause spontaneous abortion, premature rupture of membranes, postpartum hemorrhage, disseminated intravascular coagulation, and hemoperitoneum. MRI has demonstrated a superior ability for preoperative location of uterine leiomyomas in non-pregnant patients.[41,44] In a study of 16 pregnant patients MRI detected leiomyomas more often than transabdominal ultrasound. Successful myomectomy may lessen complications of pregnancy and delivery. T2 weighting produces the best contrast between intramural and submucosal leiomyomas, and myometrium[44]; it also defines the tumor margin from myometrium in the case of endometrial cancer.[45] MRI imaging may help differentiate the leiomyoma from adenomyosis by distinguishing the sharp margin of leiomyoma from the indistinct border of adenomyosis in the myometrium. Leiomyomas without degeneration exhibit a homogeneous low-intensity signal, whereas areas of hyaline fatty and myomatous degeneration have a higher signal intensity (Fig. 45-15).[41]

MRI's demonstrated ability to locate and characterize adnexal masses may positively influence clinical management of pregnancy and delivery of the patient with a pelvic mass.[42] Localizing tumor may help determine the optimum route of delivery. Ovarian neoplasms can cause dystocia and other obstetric complications.

The ovaries are best viewed in coronal or transverse planes with no gap between slices.[40] T2-weighted pulse sequences identify normal ovaries as well-circumscribed, oval structures containing small follicles of high signal intensity (see Fig. 45-3). Most ovarian masses are seen as either homogeneous or heterogeneous areas of high-intensity signal on T2-weighted images and low-intensity signal on T1-weighted images (Figs. 45-16 to 45-

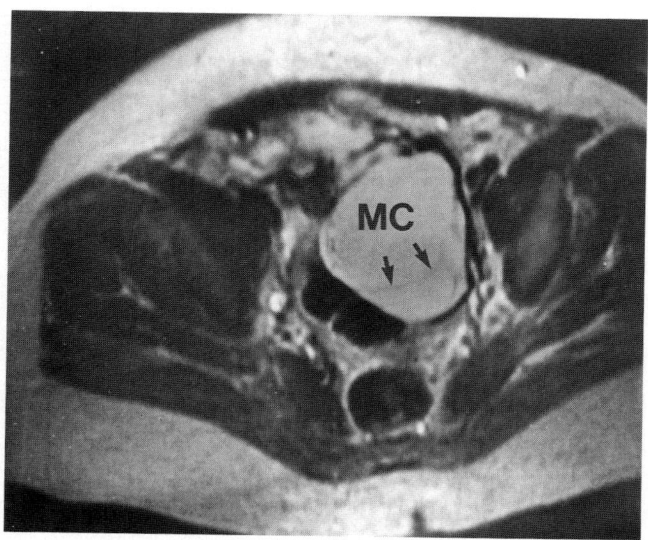

FIGURE 45–18. Mucinous cystadenoma (MC) appearing as a multiseptated but otherwise homogeneous high-signal mass on this T2-weighted axial image. The presence of septations (small arrows) is the only feature that may help distinguish this lesion from a simple corpus luteal cyst in this pregnant patient.

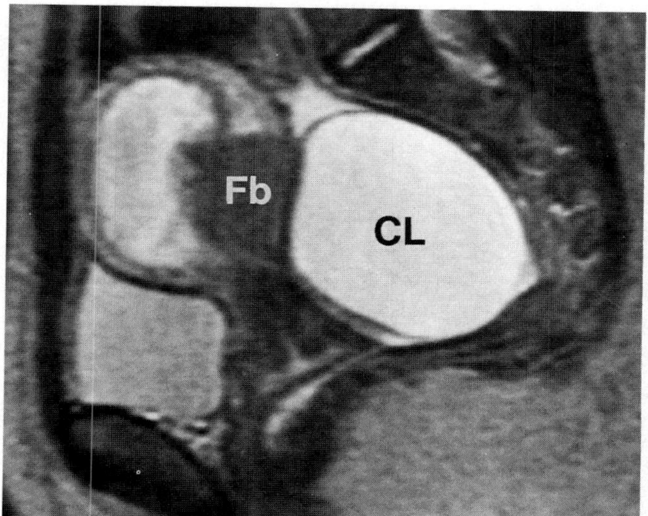

FIGURE 45–17. Corpus luteal cyst (CL) of pregnancy appearing as a homogeneous high-signal, well-circumscribed mass on this sagittal T2-weighted image. An intramural fibroid (Fb) is also noted in this pregnant patient.

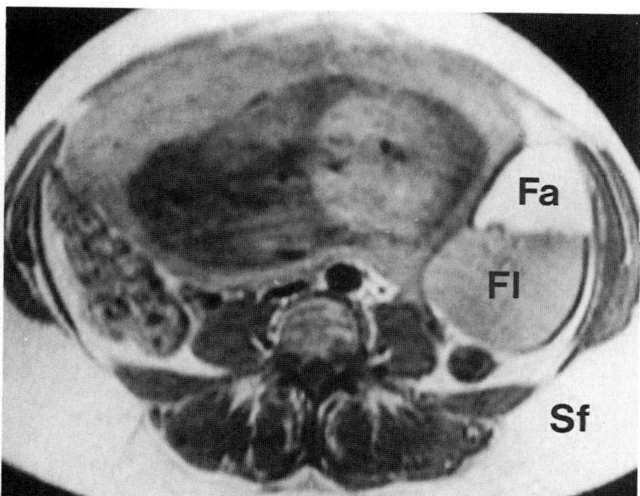

FIGURE 45–19. Mature cystic teratoma occurring in a pregnant patient, identified on this axial T1-weighted image. The fatty component of the tumor (Fa) floats above the fluid component (Fl) of the tumor. On this pulse sequence, fat in the tumor has the same high signal intensity as subcutaneous fat (Sf) in the patient's body.

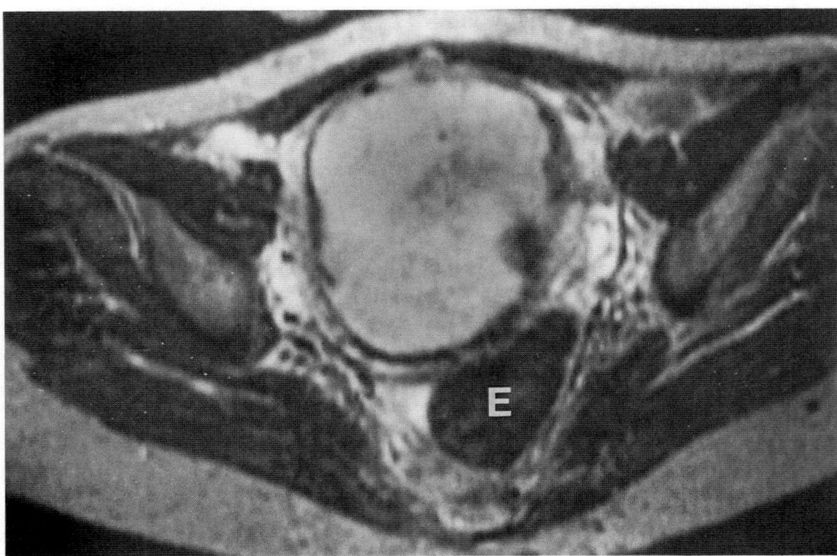

FIGURE 45–20. An endometrioma (E) is identified as a low-signal-intensity structure on this axial T2-weighted image of a second-trimester pregnancy.

18).[39,46] In cases of suspected pelvic mass, T1-weighted sequences should be performed for improved tissue characterization of blood or fat. Although MRI is unable to detect calcium in adnexal masses such as teratomas,[23] the high signal intensity of fat on T1-weighted images may allow confident diagnosis of mature cystic teratoma, the most common benign ovarian neoplasm among younger women (Fig. 45-19).

Endometriomas have a varied appearance on MRI. Those with recent hemorrhage may have an MRI signal of high intensity on T1-weighted images with high, intermediate, or low signal intensity on T2-weighted images (Fig. 45-20). This variability in the signal intensity of blood is due to the differing paramagnetic effects of the degradation products of hemoglobin.[2]

ECTOPIC PREGNANCY

MRI can also display the morphologic changes that frequently accompany an ectopic pregnancy (Fig. 45-21).[47] An enlarged uterus and hyperplasia of the supporting vasculature may be shown along with an empty uterine cavity. The adnexal mass may also be located with signal intensity consistent with hemorrhagic contents. MRI has been used during gestation to assess ovarian torsion and chorioangiomas.[23]

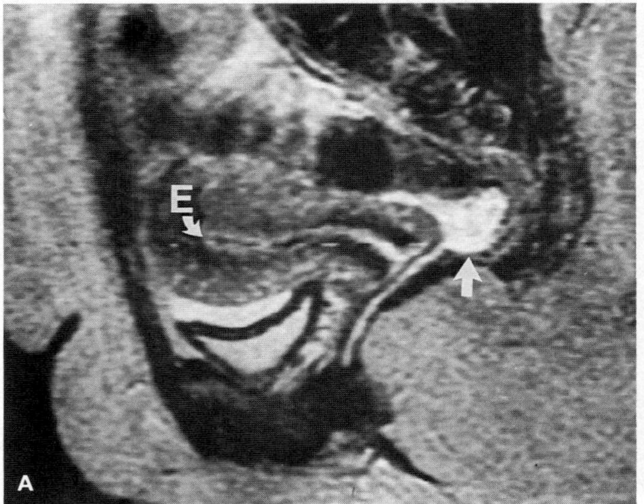

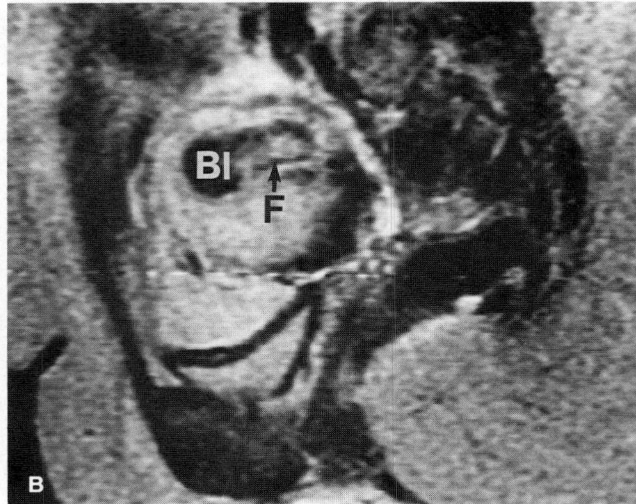

FIGURE 45–21. Ectopic pregnancy seen on sagittal T2-weighted images. (**A**) At the midline the uterus demonstrates no evidence for intrauterine pregnancy, with a thin endometrial stripe (E). A small amount of free fluid is noted in the cul de sac (arrow). (**B**) In the adnexa, a complex mass is identified with a small fetus (F) inside a gestational sac filled with low-signal blood (B1).

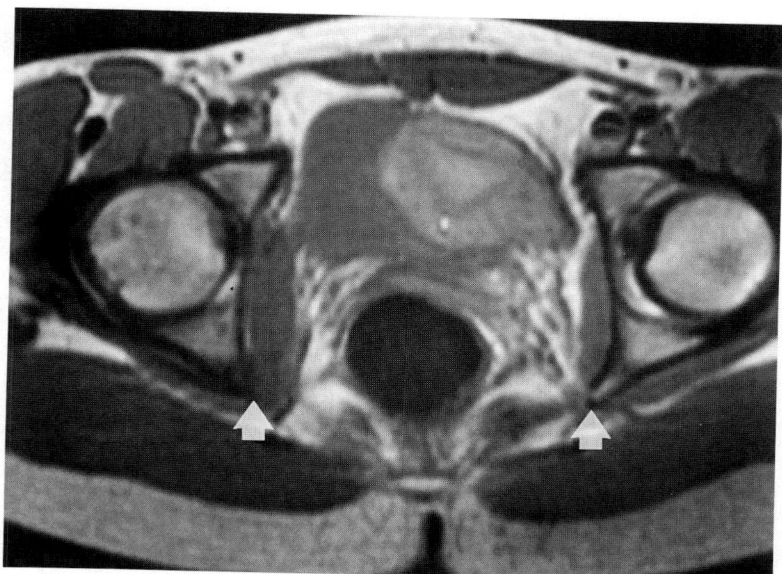

FIGURE 45-22. MR pelvimetry. With its multiplanar capability, MRI can identify the pertinent anatomical relationships for pelvimetry. In this axial proton-density-weighted image, the ischial spines (arrows) are well seen, permitting accurate determination of interspinous distance.

PELVIMETRY

MRI has been used successfully to assess maternal pelvic structure in anticipation of a vaginal delivery. Soft-tissue dystocia appears to be a more frequent cause of fetopelvic disproportion than bony dystocia.[10] The direct advantage of MRI over conventional x-ray pelvimetry is the ability to define soft-tissue structures better, to measure pelvic dimensions, and to assess the exact position of the fetal head. The anteroposterior diameter, the transverse pelvic diameter, and posterior interspinous distances can be obtained from sagittal and axial images, with total imaging time of as little as 8 minutes (Fig. 45-22).[24] Since MRI pelvimetry does not require the use of ionizing radiation, it would eliminate a major source of radiation for as many as 6% of all pregnancies in the United States.

CONCLUSION

The capacity to alter and enhance image intensity and contrast by varying the nuclear, tissue-specific, or imaging-specific factors is what makes MRI such a dynamic and promising technique in the field of maternal–fetal medicine. Spatial information is derived from the use of a gradient placed across the magnetic field. The gradient produces a known variation in the magnetic field across the patient. The variation in magnetic field produces a variation in resonance frequencies across the patient; as a result, each position is encoded by a known frequency. Since position now corresponds to frequency, signals received from the patient are spatially encoded. A phase-encoding gradient may also be applied for additional spatial information.

The quality of the MR image depends on factors specific to the tissues, such as the proton density, T1, T2, flow, paramagnetic concentrations, chemical shift, and motion. It also depends on the technical parameters of the imaging apparatus, such as the magnetic field strength, pulse sequence chosen, and time parameters of TR and TE. The nuclear parameters of spin magnetogyric ratio and relative sensitivity also contribute to the contrast and intensity of the image.

Although no harmful side effects have been associated with MRI, its utility at present may lie in confirmation of conditions and abnormalities where sonograms are inconclusive or equivocal. MRI also may play a useful role in characterizing and staging pelvic masses, in establishing cervical incompetence and placenta previa, and in monitoring molar and abdominal pregnancies and venous stasis during late pregnancy. Additionally, MRI may provide crucial information about fetal anomalies, growth, and development, and it may provide such information when ultrasound is compromised by maternal obesity, bowel gas, oligohydramnios, or acoustic shadowing. In the future, the increased information MRI affords about soft-tissue structures may eliminate the need to employ ionizing examinations during pregnancy.

Acknowledgments

We would like to acknowledge the significant contribution made by Sandra Kalison Peccerillo in the overall preparation of this manuscript. In addition, we would like to thank Nancy J. DeGennaro, RN, BSN, and Kim Huber for their help and support throughout the project.

REFERENCES

1. Filly RA. Alternative imaging techniques: computed tomography and magnetic resonance imaging. In: Harrison MR, Golbus MS, Filly RA, eds. The unborn patient: prenatal diagnosis and treatment. Philadelphia: WB Saunders, 1991:131.

2. McCarthy S. Magnetic resonance imaging in obstetrics and gynecology. Magn Reson Imaging 1986;4(1):59.
3. Hricak H. MRI of the female pelvis: a review. AJR 1986; 146:1115.
4. Mattison D, Angtuaco T, Long C. Magnetic resonance imaging in obstetrics and gynecology. Contemp Ob/Gyn 1987;27:48.
5. Smith FW, Adam AH, Phillips WDP. NMR-imaging in pregnancy. Lancet 1983;1:61.
6. Mattison DR, Angtuaco T. Magnetic resonance imaging in prenatal diagnosis. Clin Obstet Gynecol 1988;31(2):353.
7. Shulman R. NMR spectroscopy of living cells. Sci Am 1985;5:86.
8. Margulis A, Shea W Jr. Advances in imaging technology and their impact on medicine. Br J Radiol 1986;59(700):309.
9. Partain CL, Price RR, Patton JA, et al. Nuclear magnetic resonance imaging. Radiograph 1984;4:5.
10. Mattison D, Kay H, Miller R, Angtuaco T. Magnetic resonance imaging: a noninvasive tool for fetal and placental physiology. Biol Reprod 1988;38:39.
11. Kneeland JB, Whalen JP. Magnetic resonance imaging and female health care. Female Patient 1984;9:63.
12. Lowe T, Weinreb J, Santos-Ramos R, Cunningham F. Magnetic resonance imaging in human pregnancy. Obstet Gynecol 1985;66(5):629.
13. Smith F. The potential use of nuclear magnetic resonance imaging in pregnancy. J Perinat Med 1985;13:265.
14. Powell M, Worthington B, Buckley J, Symonds E. Magnetic resonance imaging (MRI) in obstetrics. I. Maternal anatomy. Br J Obstet Gynaecol 1988;95:31.
15. Powell M, Worthington B, Buckley J, Symonds E. Magnetic resonance imaging (MRI) in obstetrics. II. Fetal anatomy. Br J Obstet Gynaecol 1988;95:38.
16. Williamson R, Weiner C, Yuh W, Abu-Yousef M. Magnetic resonance imaging of anomalous fetuses. Obstet Gynecol 1989;73:952.
17. Daffos F, Forestier F, Aleese J, et al. Fetal curarization for prenatal magnetic resonance imaging. Prenat Diagn 1988;8:311.
18. Mun SK. Operating magnetic field strength for nuclear magnetic resonance imaging. Radiograph 1984;4:44.
19. Barman M. Sites, magnets, action: obtaining an MRI unit. Contemp Ob/Gyn 1987;4:84.
20. Budinger TF, Cullander C. Health hazards in nuclear magnetic resonance in vivo studies. Radiograph 1984;4:74.
21. Radiological Protection Board N. Revised guidance on acceptable limits of exposure during magnetic resonance clinical imaging. Br J Radiol 1983;56:974.
22. Abrahms HL, Berne AS, Dodd GD, et al. Magnetic resonance imaging. National Institutes of Health Consensus Development Conference. Bethesda, Md: National Institutes of Health, 1987.
23. Weinreb J, Lowe T, Santos-Ramos R, Cunningham F, Parkey R. Magnetic resonance imaging in obstetric diagnosis. Radiology 1985;154:157.
24. McCarthy S, Stark D, Filly R, Callen P, Hricak H, Higgins C. Obstetrical magnetic resonance imaging: maternal anatomy. Radiology 1985;154:421.
25. McCarthy S, Filly R, Stark D, et al. Obstetrical magnetic resonance imaging: fetal anatomy. Radiology 1985;154:427.
26. Klimek R. Nuclear magnetic resonance in obstetrics and gynecology. Int J Gynaecol Obstet 1990;32:199.
27. Powell M, Buckley J, Price H, Worthington B, Symonds E. Magnetic resonance imaging and placenta previa. Am J Obstet Gynecol 1985;154(3):565.
28. Stark D, McCarthy S, Filly R, Callen P, Hricak H, Parer J. Intrauterine growth retardation: evaluation by magnetic resonance. Radiology 1985;155:425.
29. McCarthy S, Filly R, Stark D, Callen P, Golbus M, Hricak H. Magnetic resonance imaging of fetal anomalies in utero: early experience. AJR 1985;145:677.
30. Benson RC, Colleti PM, Platt LD, Ralls PW. MR imaging of fetal anomalies. AJR 1991;156:1205.
31. Brown C, Weinreb J. Magnetic resonance imaging appearance of growth retardation in a twin pregnancy. Obstet Gynecol 1988;71(6):987.
32. Hricak H, Demas BE, Braga CA, Fisher MR, Winkler ML. Gestational trophoblastic neoplasm of the uterus: MR assessment. Radiol 1986;161:11.
33. Powell M, Symonds E, Worthington B. The application of magnetic resonance imaging to gynaecology. Br J Hosp Med 1986;5:393.
34. Spanta R, Roffman L, Grissom T, Newland J, McManus B. Abdominal pregnancy: magnetic resonance identification with ultrasonographic follow-up of placental involution. Am J Obstet Gynecol 1987;157(4):887.
35. Cohen JM, Weinreb JC, Lowe TW, Brown C. MR imaging of a viable full-term abdominal pregnancy. AJR 1985;145:407.
36. Murphy WD, Feiglin DH, Cisar CC, Al-Malt AM, Bellon EM. Magnetic resonance imaging of a third trimester abdominal pregnancy. Magn Reson Imaging 1990;8:657.
37. Harris M, Angtuaco T, Frazier C, Mattison D. Diagnosis of a viable abdominal pregnancy by magnetic resonance imaging. Am J Obstet Gynecol 1988;159(1):150.
38. Hricak H, Stern J, Fisher M, Shapero L, Winkler M, Lacey C. Endometrial carcinoma staging by MR imaging. Radiology 1987;162:297.
39. Mitchell D, Mintz M, Spritzer C, et al. Adnexal masses: MR imaging observations at 1.5 T, with US and CT correlation. Radiology 1987;162:319.
40. Hricak H, Lacey C, Schriock E, et al. Gynecologic masses: value of magnetic resonance imaging. Am J Obstet Gynecol 1985;153(1):31.
41. Hricak H, Tscholakoff D, Heinrichs L, et al. Uterine leiomyomas: correlation of MR histopathologic findings, and symptoms. Radiology 1986;158:385.
42. Kier R, McCarthy S, Scoutt L, Viscarello R, Schwartz P. Pelvic masses in pregnancy: MR imaging. Radiology 1990;176:709.
43. Bezjian A. Pelvic masses in pregnancy. Clin Obstet Gynecol 1984;27(2):402.
44. Dudiak C, Turner D, Patel S, Archie J, Silver B, Norusis M. Uterine leiomyomas in the infertile patient: preoperative localization with MR imaging versus US and hysterosalpingography. Radiology 1988;167:627.
45. Togashi K, Nishimura K, Itoh K, et al. Adenomyosis: diagnosis with MR imaging. Radiology 1988;166:111.
46. Mitchell D, Gefter W, Spritzer C, et al. Polycystic ovaries: MR imaging. Radiology 1986;160:425.
47. Roth G, Kleinstein J, Kuhnert A, Kunzel W. Nuclear magnetic resonance imaging of a patient with an ectopic pregnancy. Gynecol Obstet Invest 1987;23:135.

46

CHAPTER

DOPPLER ULTRASONOGRAPHY AND FETAL WELL-BEING

Brian J. Trudinger

Obstetricians have long desired to be able to measure blood flow, particularly to the placenta. Diagnoses such as "placental insufficiency" were created to express a hypothetical reduction in blood flow almost without any actual basis. Doppler ultrasound has provided the noninvasive clinical tool to assess blood flow in pregnancy in the circulations that are precluded from direct study because of risk to the fetus caused by such procedures. The information obtained from such studies has expanded our knowledge of the physiology of pregnancy and the pathophysiology of a variety of disorders, and provided a diagnostic tool for evaluation of the welfare of the fetus.

DOPPLER INSTRUMENTATION

When an ultrasound beam strikes a blood vessel, the moving column of red blood cells scatters and reflects the ultrasound beam with a new frequency. The change in frequency or Doppler frequency shift (incident frequency − reflected frequency) is proportional to the velocity of the red blood cell scatterers. This change in frequency may be displayed and used to calculate blood flow. Various devices have been designed for this purpose (Fig. 46-1).

The transducer of the Doppler flowmeter or velocimeter can act as both the emitting source of the ultrasound beam and the receiver of the reflected signal. In continuous wave systems, there are separate crystals, usually mounted side by side for each role, whereas in a pulsed system, the single crystal emits an ultrasound pulse and then functions as a receiver. Activation of the crystal causes the conversion of electrical energy to an ultrasound beam during emission, and the returning ultrasound signal reverses this process. The weak returning signals are amplified and fed to the Doppler shift detector, which filters out unwanted frequencies (including the original ultrasound frequency) so that the Doppler frequency shift remains. This information is nondirectional. To separate the Doppler signals produced by flow toward and away from the transducer (forward and reverse flow), phase domain processing is commonly used. This requires two detectors with their reference inputs differing in phase by 90°; the filtered output signals are referred to as quadrature Doppler shift signals. Two types of Doppler systems are in use—continuous wave and pulsed. They differ in a number of ways. Continuous wave systems are continuously emitting from one crystal and receiving through another. They are relatively simple, cheap, and portable. The reflected echoes from any moving structure within the ultrasound beam are detected, so that there is no spatial resolution. Positioning the transducer and line of sight of the ultrasound beam is more readily done. In the pulsed system, a short burst of the ultrasound wave is transmitted, and the crystal then acts as a receiver. A range gate circuit allows recording only at a specified time after the pulse emission, so the Doppler shift detected originates from a fixed depth. This type of processing may be referred to as setting the sample volume to a known depth. These Doppler velocimeters may exist as stand-alone items, but are also built into ultrasound imaging systems. Integration with an imaging facility provides the ability to steer the ultrasound beam and, for pulsed Doppler systems, to locate the sample volume precisely over the vessel to be studied. In addition, the dimensions of the vessel under study may be measured.

The chosen frequency of the ultrasound beam is a compromise among a number of considerations.[1] The depth of penetration (tissue attenuation) is inversely

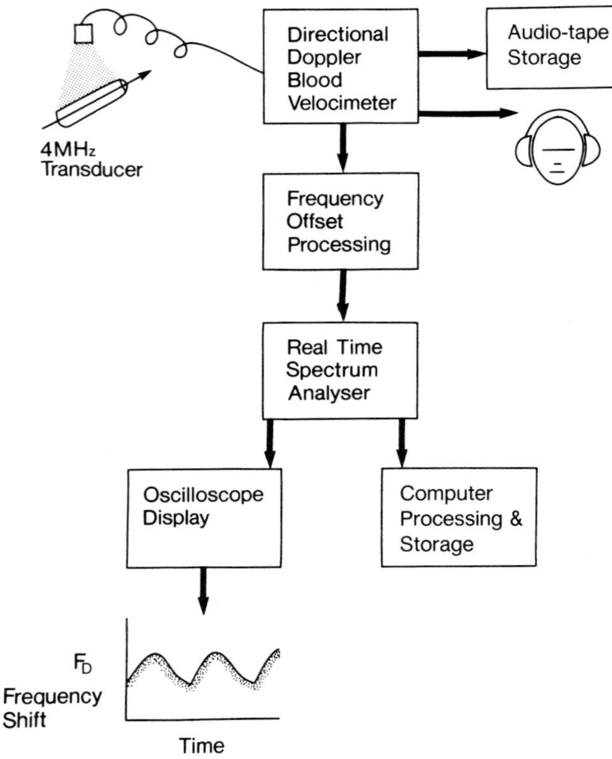

FIGURE 46–1. A block diagram of the components of a typical system used for recording and displaying the blood flow velocity.

proportional to the square of the frequency. The degree of scattering is proportional to the fourth power of the frequency. The higher the transmitting frequency, the greater the Doppler frequency shift. With pulsed Doppler systems, there must be sufficient time to characterize the Doppler shift frequency before the next pulse is emitted. The laws of signal processing state that any Doppler signal with frequency greater than the "Nyquist limit" (equal to half the pulse repetition rate) will be grossly distorted, suffering "frequency aliasing" and so appearing with quite different frequencies. In general, the highest frequency producing a reliable signal is used.

With medical equipment and vascular studies, the Doppler shift frequency usually falls in the audible range; therefore, the simplest display of the Doppler frequency shift is an audio signal. The method of choice is spectral analysis. If the vessel is totally insonated, the frequency spectrum represents all the different velocities across its lumen. The process of spectral analysis is carried out by a spectrum analyzer and is therefore also subject to the possibility of frequency aliasing if too fast a sampling rate is required. Equipment usually carries out the spectral analysis sufficiently quickly (less than 10 msec per spectrum) so that it is available in real time. A recent development is to display the frequency and direction of blood flow by color coding superimposed on the real-time ultrasound two-dimensional image ("color flow mapping").

Because blood flow velocity is directly proportional to Doppler frequency shift, the information made available to the clinician by the Doppler instrumentation is a blood flow velocity waveform (FVW). The envelope of this wave is the maximum flow velocity. Beneath this is a frequency distribution, representing the various velocities of blood flow in the vessel under study. Both instantaneous and temporal mean flow velocities can be determined from this. If the angle between the ultrasound beam and vessel is known, then velocity can be calculated absolutely. This requires the use of pulsed Doppler systems. Volume blood flow may be determined as the product of mean velocity and vessel area.

THE BLOOD FLOW VELOCITY WAVEFORM

Blood flow is pulsatile. With each contraction of the heart, a pressure pulse or wave propagates down the aorta and its branches with an initial wave speed of 5 m/sec. This creates a time-varying pressure gradient between neighboring points along the arterial tree. Blood flows ahead of this pressure gradient from high to low pressure. The blood flow is also pulsatile—the flow velocity waveform. Doppler ultrasound systems record this flow velocity waveform. Early in systole the pressure and flow waveforms are in phase, but this breaks down later in systole because of the arrival of waves reflected from points of branching along the arterial tree and the periphery. The flow velocity wave travels more slowly than the pressure wave, and its amplitude decreases as it moves away from the heart. In the ascending aorta following the opening of the aortic valve, blood flow velocity increases to a peak and then falls. After closure of the aortic valve, the blood is close to stationary for the remainder of the cardiac cycle.

The pressure and flow waveforms are influenced by the cardiac contraction, physical properties of the arterial walls and the blood within, and outflow impedance from the arterial tree. Traditionally, blood flow is described in terms of pressure and flow. Resistance has been defined as the ratio of mean pressure difference (or pressure head) across a vascular bed to mean flow through it. Resistance may also be conceptualized as how difficult it is to force blood through the circulation or the energy dissipation required for blood flow.[2] It is an artificial concept insofar as blood flow is not steady but pulsatile. Changes in resistance in clinical physiology are more often than not due to changes in the caliber of small blood vessels, but resistance is not necessarily an index of arteriolar caliber. It also depends on the distensibility of the arterial walls (and transmural pressure) and blood viscosity.[3] Impedance takes into consideration the pulsatile nature of blood flow, being the ratio of pulsatile pressure to pulsatile flow.[4] A consequence of pulsatile blood flow in comparison to steady flow is the requirement for more energy to move a given volume of blood, and much of this extra energy is used to distend the large arteries. The mean term resistance depends much more on arteriolar caliber than large artery distension. Various indices derived from the FVW pattern have been defined to assess "resistance." They would appear to depend most on the size of the peripheral vascular bed.

When a blood vessel is interrogated with an ultrasound beam, not one but a spectrum of Doppler frequencies is found. This corresponds to all the different velocities across the flowing stream of blood. Each point across the vessel may be represented by a velocity vector, and a line through the tips of these vectors creates the velocity profile (Fig. 46-2). The variations in velocity result from the nonviscous and inhomogeneous nature of blood. The velocity profile also varies through the cardiac cycle, and in some circumstances flow may not always be forward or in the same direction (Fig. 46-3).

If the lumen of the blood vessel has been totally insonated, all this information is available in the Doppler FVW. In order to recreate the exact velocity profile, it would be necessary to use a pulsed Doppler system and sample from each point across the vessel. If the vessel is uniformly insonated, the mean Doppler frequency shift is proportional to the mean velocity, and this fact is used in the calculation of volume flow.[5] In a blood vessel with an established flow, the "boundary layer" is the region of flow in which velocity is increasing with distance from the wall. Here viscosity is important, because there is shear between adjacent flow lamina. In the central stream, the movement is "en masse" and inertia is more important. If the disturbances of local geometry are ignored, then in large arterial vessels inertial forces dominate blood flow, whereas in small vessels viscous forces are more important. Reynold's number expresses the relative importance of these two forces.[3]

The Doppler FVW has been analyzed in a variety of different ways. In clinical applications, inferences about the cardiovascular system are made using empirical indices. The connection between an empirical index and a physiological variable may be based on a statistical association or experimental models. In many situations, only the maximum velocity waveform (or the waveform envelope) is used. This is the easiest waveform to locate and is relatively error free. It does ignore all the information about the velocity profile contained within the frequency spectrum. The problems of analysis of the maximum mean and first moment of the velocity waveform in the fetal circulation have been reviewed.[6,7] The shape of the waveform envelope can be considered a characteristic of the vascular site. Waveforms recorded from arteries supplying low-impedance vascular beds (eg, internal carotid, umbilical, and uterine artery in pregnancy) exhibit relatively high forward velocities throughout diastole. A triphasic waveform shape, where there is a period of reverse flow in diastole, is characteristic of sites with high distal impedance. The peripheral impedance, vessel wall elasticity, the degree and geometry of any proximal stenoses, and the condition of the upstream pump all affect the waveform. All of these factors are important, all can be affected in the disease state being investigated, and none can be independently eliminated or controlled in clinical practice. Even in normal, presumably healthy subjects, blood flow patterns at a site with complicated geometry such as the carotid bifurcation are very complex.

The fetal circulation is uniquely suited to Doppler waveform analysis by simple empirical indices. This is because of the absence of degenerative arterial disease. The indices used in the fetal circulation have been directed toward assessing downstream resistance. Three are in common usage (Fig. 46-4). All of these are highly correlated. Coefficients in excess of 0.9 have been demonstrated when the indices are compared.[6,8] This means that the indices are all providing the same information about the same physiological variables. Choice of index then is a matter of convenience relative to the investiga-

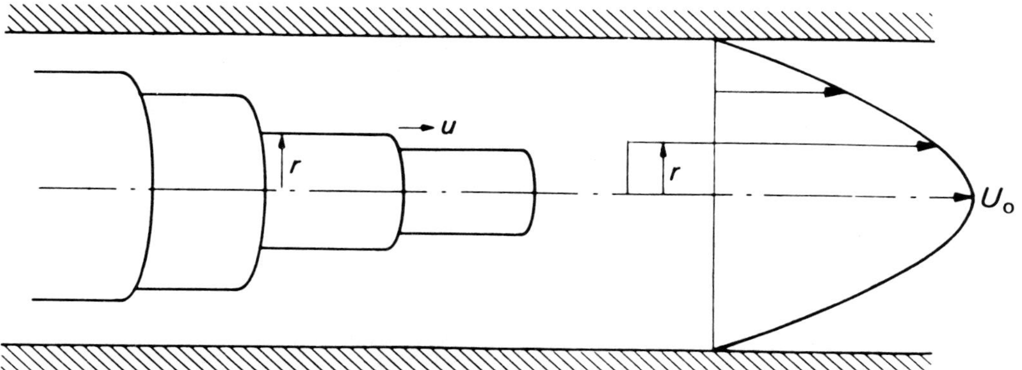

FIGURE 46–2. The blood flow velocity profile across a vessel. U_0, center line velocity; u, velocity at radial position *r*. (Modified from Caro CG, Pedley TJ, Schroter CW, Seed WA. The mechanics of circulation. Oxford: Oxford University Press, 1978:47.)

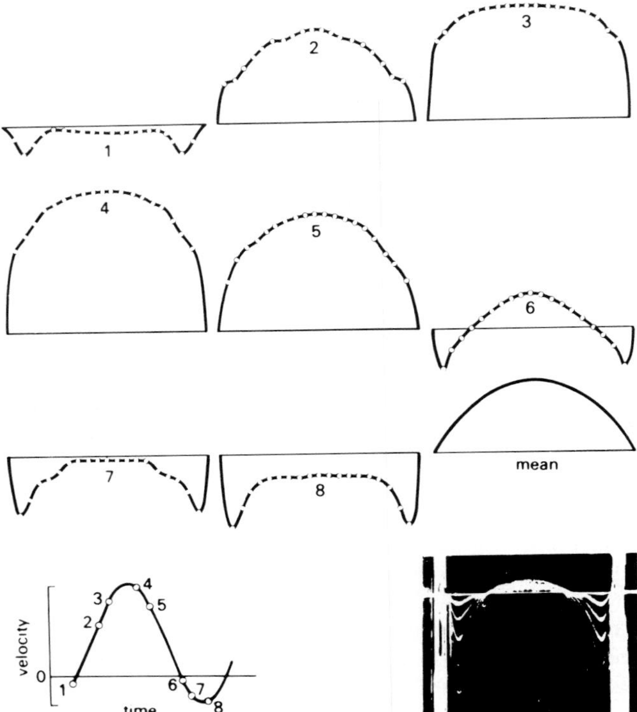

FIGURE 46–3. Instantaneous velocity profiles across a rigid pipe at eight different times during a cycle produced by an oscillating pump. The time of each profile on the mean flow velocity waveform is shown at bottom left. Measurements were made by serial photographs of flow lines of tiny hydrogen bubbles (bottom right). (From Caro CG, Pedley TJ, Schroter CW, Seed WA. The mechanics of the circulation. Oxford: Oxford University Press, 1978:320.)

tional task. The systolic:diastolic ratio is easiest to calculate. Abnormally high values when there is little or no diastolic value tend to infinity and become meaningless. The pulsatility index has a precise mathematical definition. It requires determination of the mean velocity, and this is usually an inaccurate estimate. The resistance index is the only one normally distributed and has the advantage that the maximum value attainable is one. It has an extra arithmetic step in comparison to the systolic:diastolic ratio. All these indices, when used to interpret the maximum velocity waveform, should be seen as simple descriptors of the waveform pattern. They are not precisely estimatable quantities. There is an inherent systematic error of 10% to 20% in their calculation.[8]

THE UMBILICAL CIRCULATION

The umbilical cord, linking the fetus and placenta, is long and suspended in amniotic fluid, and so is ideal for Doppler studies. The two umbilical arteries travel along this without branching or changes in lumen diameter. The radius of curvature of the loops of cord is large in comparison to the diameter of the umbilical arteries, and so is unlikely to significantly influence flow patterns.

However, this spiralling course means that it is not possible to image a length of artery or vein sufficient to permit determination of the angle between the ultrasound beam and vessel, and so it is not possible to make Doppler volume flow measurements. Studies of the umbilical artery flow velocity waveform using the indices of resistance have been carried out to assess the downstream vascular bed—the fetal placenta.

NORMAL PREGNANCY

Blood flow through the umbilical circulation increases throughout pregnancy and represents some 40% of combined ventricular output of the fetus.[9] The actual flow in the fetal lamb has been measured at 180 to 200 mL/kg fetus/min;[10] in human pregnancy it is less, 100 to 110 mL/kg fetus/min.[11,12] The umbilical placental vascular bed is not innervated, and indeed is refractory to such circulating vasoconstrictors as epinephrine and norepinephrine.[10] Blood flow to the placenta appears to be the result of the balance between resistance to other fetal vascular beds and the placenta.[9] Almost certainly there are local controls of placental blood flow that regulate the perfusion to keep a balance between the fetal and maternal placental flows.[13] It has been pointed out that the fetus does not need to regulate umbilical blood flow finely, because it has the capacity to vary tissue oxygen extraction ratios and, consequently, oxygen uptake.[14] The fetus requires from the placenta oxygenated blood for distribution to the fetal tissues, where uptake and delivery may be regulated.

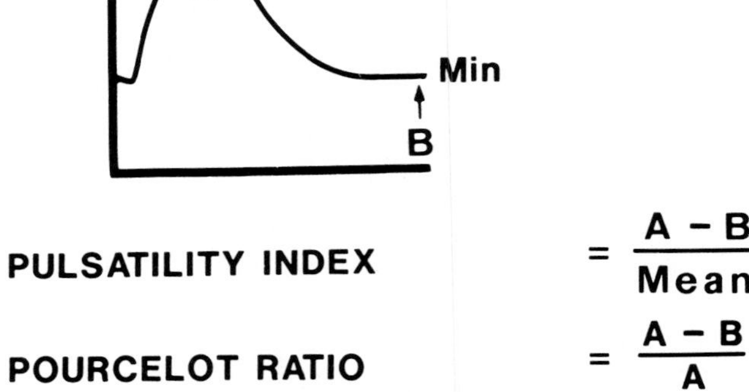

PULSATILITY INDEX $= \dfrac{A - B}{Mean}$

POURCELOT RATIO $= \dfrac{A - B}{A}$

SYSTOLIC/DIASTOLIC RATIO $= A/B$

FIGURE 46–4. The three indices of downstream resistance in common clinical use for the analysis of arterial flow velocity waveforms.

The umbilical circulation is a low-resistance vascular bed, which is reflected in the pattern of the umbilical artery FVW (Fig. 46-5). Throughout pregnancy, the increase in umbilical blood flow is achieved by a decrease in resistance rather than an increase in driving pressure, although this also occurs in the last part of pregnancy.[10]

Gestational age is an important influence in determining the normality of the umbilical FVW (Fig. 46-5). In early pregnancy, diastolic flow velocities may be absent. The range of variation in waveform pattern is much greater in early pregnancy. This is clearly apparent in the normal ranges of the various indices of resistance used to describe the umbilical waveform pattern (Fig. 46-6).

There has been debate about the influence of fetal heart rate (FHR) on the umbilical FVW. Two careful studies observed a weak relationship between FHR and waveform index over the physiological range of heart rates.[6,15] Others have reported strong associations, but included values outside the normal range, especially below 100/minute. Over the normal range of FHR, the correction suggested is less than the systematic error present in calculation of the various indices and very small in comparison to the difference between normal and abnormal waveform patterns. The suggestion that a correction factor is necessary is based in part on the assumption that the decay in the diastolic component of the maximum velocity is passive. This is unfounded.

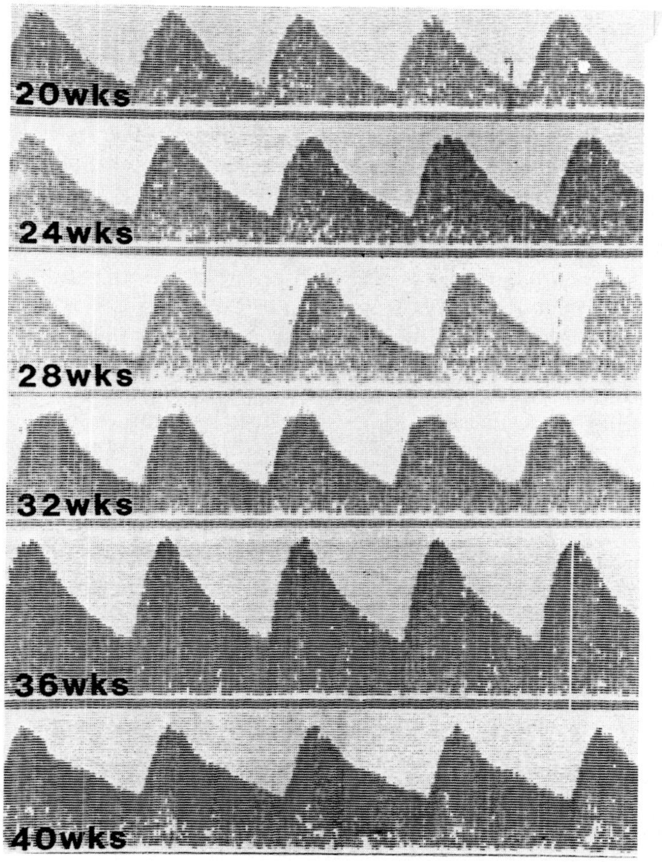

20wks

24wks

28wks

32wks

36wks

40wks

FIGURE 46–5. The changing form of the umbilical artery flow velocity waveform recorded from one patient at varying periods of gestation.

Fetal breathing movements do alter the flow velocity waveform. During "inspiration," both peak systolic and least diastolic values are decreased, so that the systolic:diastolic ratio is increased (Fig. 46-7). It is interesting to speculate on the reason for this change. During inspiration, more of the right ventricular output has been directed through the pulmonary circulation and less bypasses this through the ductus arteriosus to the aorta and umbilical circulation. This implies that fetal breathing is associated with opening of the fetal pulmonary circulation.

Behavioral states do not influence the FVW pattern or indices of resistance in the umbilical circulation. This is in contrast to the aortic waveform.[16] Such an observation is not unexpected, because the aortic waveform is influenced by flow to various fetal organs under autonomic control, whereas the placenta is not so regulated.

There has been debate about variations in the umbilical FVW along the length of the cord. Close to the fetus, a higher value may be obtained for the systolic:diastolic ratio.[17] There is a transition from the typical aortic to umbilical waveform. At the placental end, the resistance indices have been reported lower than the values recorded from free-floating loops of cord. This difference is very small in comparison to differences between normal and abnormal pregnancy.

In recording the umbilical FVW, it is necessary to review a sequence of 10 to 20 cycles to confirm that variations due to fetal activity are absent. Ideally, at least five waveforms should be measured and averaged. To minimize errors, the measured waveforms should be those displaying the maximum obtainable peak systolic and least diastolic flow velocities. This requires that the angle between the ultrasound beam and vessel is small and can be sought by small movements of the transducer. Simultaneous display of flow in the umbilical artery and vein allows confirmation of the origin of the signal from the umbilical cord by the characteristic pattern, and eliminates the possibility of superimposition of signals from the vein and artery, giving a false value for the diastolic velocity.

MODELS AND EXPERIMENTAL STUDIES OF THE UMBILICAL CIRCULATION TO AID FVW INTERPRETATION

Two quite different approaches have been taken to establish models of the umbilical placental circulation for the study and understanding of the blood FVW. The placental vasculature has been modelled as a lumped electrical circuit equivalent, and animal preparations have been used in experimental studies.

Two groups have suggested that a lumped electrical circuit equivalent could be used to model the umbilical placental circulation.[18,19] This approach has been used extensively in modeling blood flow in other circula-

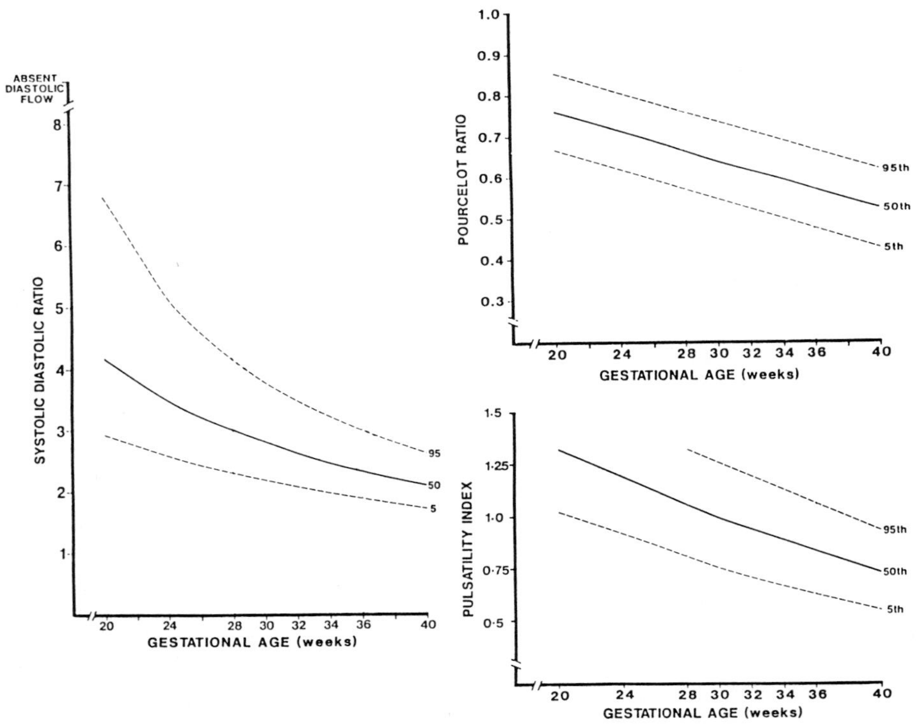

FIGURE 46–6. The normal range of values for the umbilical artery downstream resistance indices. (From Thompson RS, Trudinger BJ, Cook CM, Giles WB. Umbilical artery velocity waveforms: normal reference values for AB ratio and Pourcelot ratio. Br J Obstet Gynecol 1988;95:590.)

tions. Thompson and Stevens[18] developed a computer-based model that was used to study pulsatile blood flow (Fig. 46-8). In that study, detailed attention was given to recreating the branching structure of the villus tree. Each arterial vessel was represented by a resistor and a capacitor in parallel. A schematic diagram of the circuit is shown.

This approach is simple and attractive. The only assumption is that each artery can indeed be represented by a resistor and capacitor. The validity of this approach was confirmed by substituting physiologically realistic values for vessel size, resistance, capacitance, and pressure, and demonstrating that calculated and clinically measured umbilical flow were similar. This model was used to examine the influence of obliteration of a fraction of the terminal arterial branches of the umbilical placental vascular tree on the FVW pulsatility index.[20] It was also used to examine the influence of physiological variables such as pressure, heart rate, and volume flow on the FVW. Using this model, it can be shown that the pulsatility index (PI) of the FVW is proportional to the pulsatility of the pressure waveform and the resistance of the umbilical placental villus vascular tree.

$$PI = (P^1/P^0)(1 + R_2/R_1)$$

where

P^1 = peak systolic pressure

P^0 = mean pressure

R^2 = resistance of umbilical placental vascular bed

R^1 = resistance of main umbilical artery

Assuming a diffuse vascular pathology, it can be shown that the FVW index of resistance increases as the fraction (q) of terminal arterial vessels obliterated increases. This increase is not linear (Fig. 46-9).

It is not until some 50% to 60% of the vessels have been obliterated that the PI is increased beyond the "normal range." Thereafter it rises rapidly. This relationship is the result of obliteration of a vascular bed arranged as the placenta. It highlights the presence of extensive disease before Doppler detection is possible, and emphasizes the reserve capacity of the placenta.

The electrical circuit equivalent placental model also demonstrated that variations in blood pressure will alter the pulsatility index, but this variation is small.[20] Over the physiological range of blood pressures, the

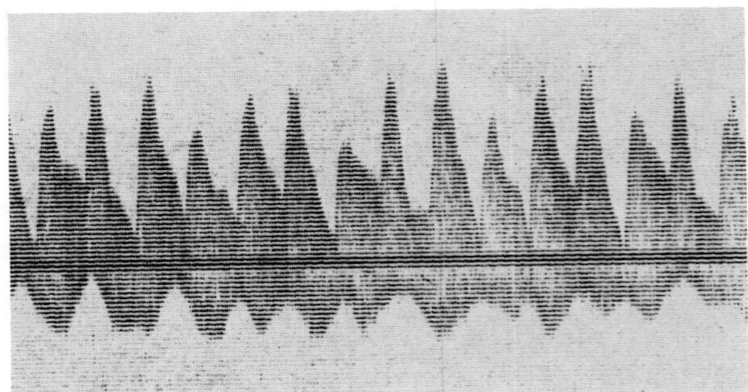

FIGURE 46–7. The influence of fetal breathing movements on the flow velocity waveform of the umbilical artery (upper trace) and umbilical vein (lower trace).

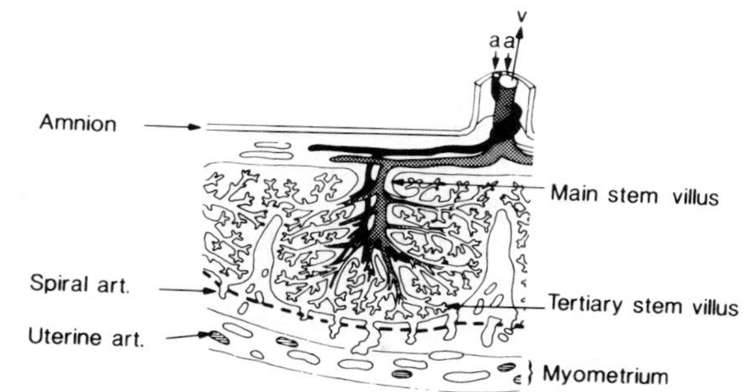

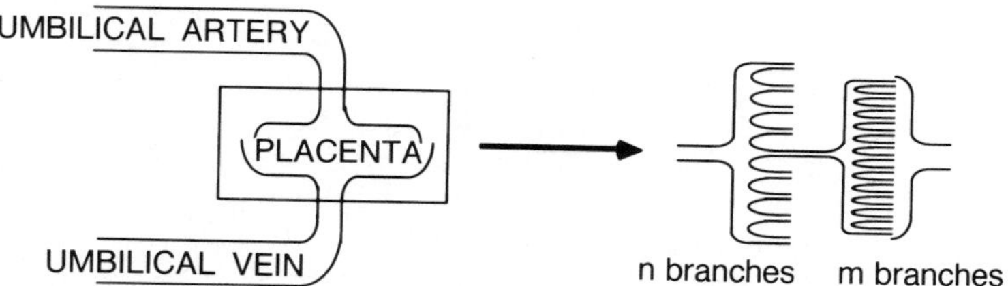

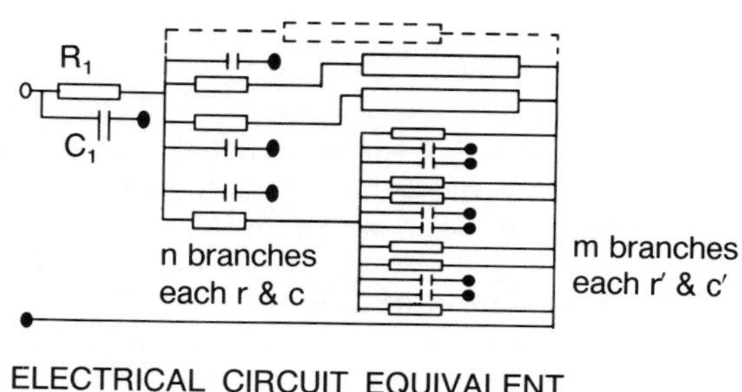

FIGURE 46–8. The vascular branching pattern of the umbilical placental circulation and the electrical circuit equivalent model created by detailed matching of this pattern. (Thompson RS, Trudinger BJ. Doppler waveform pulsatility index and resistance pressure and flow in the umbilical circulation: an investigation using a mathematical model. Ultrasound Med Biol 1990;16:451.)

FIGURE 46–9. Using a mathematical model of the umbilical placental circulation, the change in the umbilical artery pulsatility index was calculated in the presence of an increasing obliteration of an increasing fraction (q) of the umbilical placental vascular bed. (From Thompson RS, Trudinger BJ. Doppler waveform pulsatility index and resistance, pressure and flow in the umbilical placental circulation: an investigation using a mathematical model. Ultrasound Med Biol 1990;16:454, with permission.)

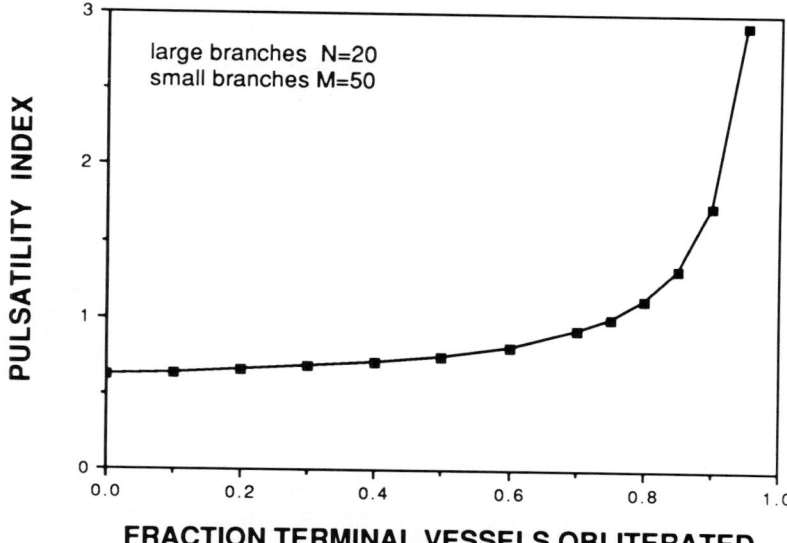

very high values of PI seen in fetal compromise could not be obtained. The PI was demonstrated independent of heart rate over the range 100 to 180 beats/minute. The effect of a fetal response (by increase in blood pressure) following placental vascular bed obliteration was examined using this mathematical model. If terminal vessels in the placenta were obliterated, the placental resistance increased, as did the PI, while umbilical volume flow decreased. However, a small, physiologically realistic increase in systolic pressure was sufficient to maintain umbilical flow until approximately 80% of the terminal arterial vessels were obliterated. Beyond this point, the pressure increase required was unrealistic (outside the physiological range).

This model of the placental circulation was used to examine the influence of growth (more vascular channels) of the placenta on PI. With advancing gestation, the decrease in PI as the placenta grows was predicted by the model. A major difference was shown between the response of a large and a small vascular bed to superimposed vascular obliteration. The same fraction obliteration (q) produced a much greater increase in PI when the placenta was small. It follows from this prediction that a large, late third trimester placental vascular bed can accommodate a considerably greater obliteration with minimal change in resistance index in comparison to a smaller, second trimester placenta. This parallels recent clinical reports that indicate Doppler studies have a low sensitivity in predicting fetal compromise in post-date pregnancies.[21,22] Doppler umbilical studies are a far more sensitive test for the detection of placental vascular pathology earlier in pregnancy.

The umbilical circulation in the fetal lamb has been studied with Doppler ultrasound. In ovine pregnancy, it is possible to demonstrate the same decrease in the FVW indices of resistance seen in human pregnancy.[23] The Doppler indices have been demonstrated to be a measure of resistance in the umbilical circulation in the fetal lamb. Embolization of the umbilical cotyledon circulation with 15-μm microspheres was carried out to increase the resistance of the peripheral vascular bed.[24] This caused a rise in the umbilical systolic:diastolic ratio and a rise in calculated vascular resistance (Fig. 46-10). The large reserve of the ovine umbilical cotyledon vascular bed was shown by the fact that these increases in systolic:diastolic ratio and calculated resistance were quite small, despite embolization with large numbers ($>20\times10^6$) of microspheres. This work has been repeated with larger microspheres and a greater dose, producing a greater increase in the systolic:diastolic ratio.[25]

The animal model has also been used to investigate the relationship between the abnormal umbilical artery Doppler waveform and the uterine circulation. Fetal constraint and growth failure in placental insufficiency has been thought to follow a reduction in uteroplacental blood flow. In the ewe, pre-pregnancy carunculectomy has been performed to induce fetal growth retardation. It has been suggested that this caused a reduction in the uterine vascular bed. However, Doppler recordings of the umbilical waveform from growth-retarded fetal lambs where the ewe had undergone pre-pregnancy carunculectomy were normal and did not show the high resistance indices seen in human disease.[23] This evidence supports a primary vascular pathology in the fetal umbilical circulation in placental insufficiency, identified by the abnormal umbilical Doppler study.

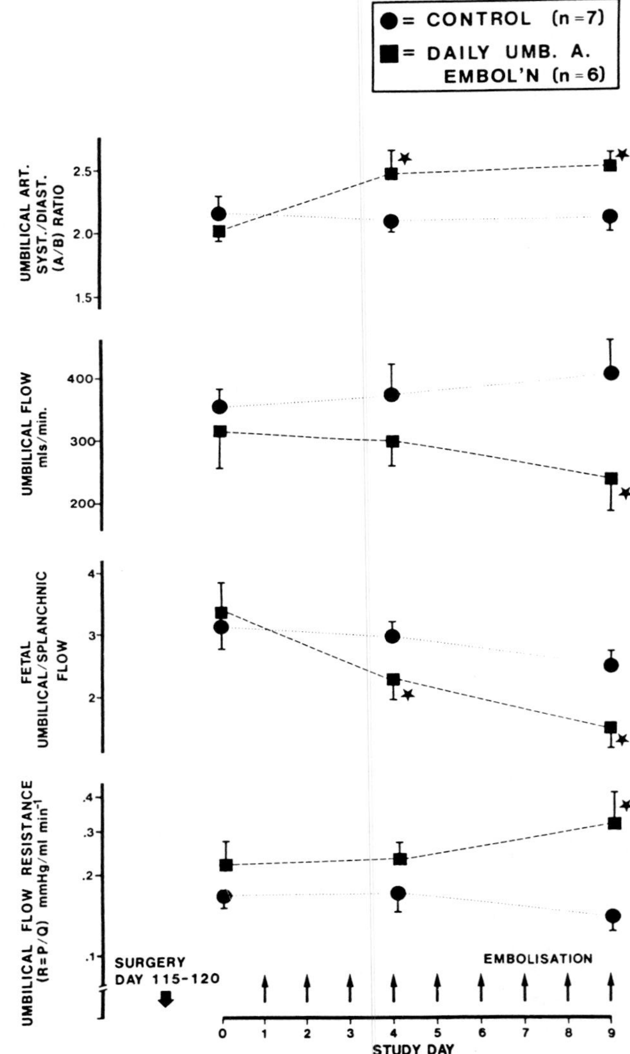

FIGURE 46–10. Progressive embolization of the umbilical circulation was carried out in fetal lambs at 120 days gestation. There was an increase in calculated vascular resistance and umbilical artery S/D, whereas umbilical flow (relative to splanchnic flow) decreased. (From Trudinger BJ, Stevens D, Connelly A, et al. Umbilical artery flow velocity waveforms and placental resistance: the effects of embolization on the umbilical circulation. Am J Obstet Gynecol 1987;157:1445.)

To investigate the pathophysiology of abnormal Doppler waveforms, pharmacological studies have been carried out in fetal lambs. Alterations in prostacyclin to thromboxane production ratios by placental tissue have been reported in pregnancy hypertension.[26] Infusion of the stable thromboxane analogue U46619 caused a decrease in the umbilical diastolic flow velocity and also an increase in the systolic:diastolic ratio[27] matching in vitro reports of an increase in vascular resistance in isolated perfused placenta.[28,29] This observation is consistent with local thromboxane release in the placenta, producing the waveform changes seen in human pregnancy. This effect of thromboxane was in marked contrast to infusions of catecholamines, which had no demonstrable effect (unpublished observation).

PATHOPHYSIOLOGY OF ABNORMAL UMBILICAL DOPPLER FVW

In normal pregnancy, placental growth continues throughout, as demonstrated by the progressive increase in the weight of the placenta. The overall increase in placental size is associated with an increase in the number of tertiary stem villi and, therefore, total small arterial channels. The continuing expansion of the umbilical placental vascular tree matches the decreasing vascular resistance directly measured in fetal lambs.[10] The normal decrease in the umbilical artery FVW indices of resistance is consistent with this. The abnormal umbilical Doppler FVW waveform is characterized by a change in the opposite direction, with decreasing diastolic flow velocities relative to the systolic peak and, in extreme cases, by absent or even reversal of blood flow in diastole. This is a high resistance pattern and contrasts with the normal FVW discussed and illustrated above.

A histological study to correlate the umbilical artery FVW pattern with the "resistance" vessels in the umbilical placental vascular tree has been carried out.[30] Because the major drop in arterial pressure across the umbilical placental vascular bed occurs in the small arteries and arterioles of the tertiary villi, these are the "resistance vessels." When these placental vessels were examined after delivery in pregnancies classified according to whether the antenatal umbilical Doppler studies were normal or abnormal, significant differences were found. The modal tertiary villus small arterial vessel count was significantly less in the group with the abnormal umbilical artery FVW (1 to 2 arteries/high-power field) in comparison to the normal one (7 to 8 arteries/field) (Fig. 46-11).

There was a small increase in the small arterial vessel count in the tertiary stem villi of the placenta with increasing gestational age, but the magnitude of this was much less than the difference between normal and abnormal pregnancy. This work has recently been confirmed by others.[31,32] This placental lesion of vascular sclerosis, with obliteration of the small muscular arteries of the tertiary stem villi, could be expected to cause an increase in flow resistance in the umbilical placenta. This lesion in the fetal placenta could best be described as "umbilical placental insufficiency." There has been

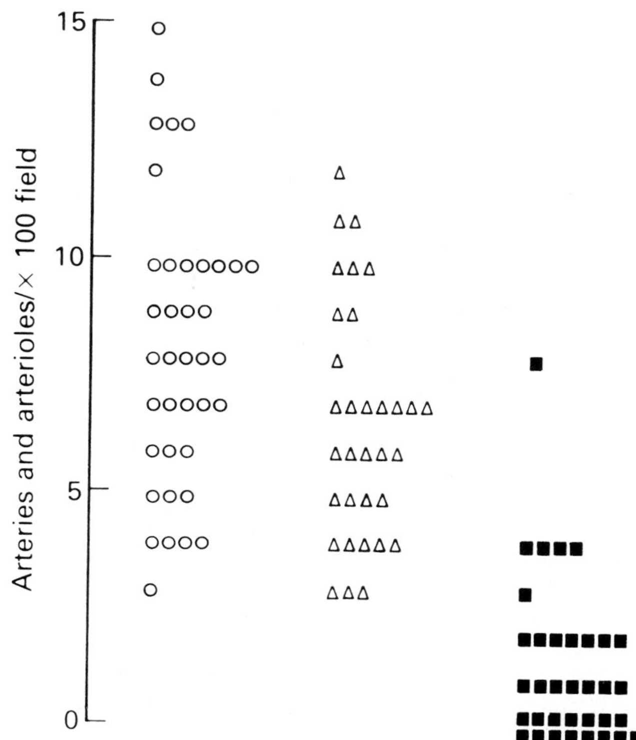

FIGURE 46–11. The modal count (per ×100 field) of small vascular arteries (<90 μm diameter) in tertiary villi from placentae from normal, complicated pregnancies with normal umbilical flow velocity waveforms (FVW) (control) and complicated pregnancies with abnormal umbilical FVW. (From Giles WB, Trudinger BJ, Baird P. Fetal umbilical artery flow velocity waveforms and placental resistance: pathological correlation. Br J Obstet Gynaecol 1985;92:34.)

discussion as to whether this vascular lesion is a disappearance of vessels or whether these channels were never present in the villus tree. An increase in the systolic:diastolic ratio may be seen on serial studies of pregnancies with fetal compromise, suggesting vessel obliteration. A recent report of change in the walls of these resistance vessels may be an earlier feature in the development of this vascular lesion.[33]

In the past, a variety of histological findings have been defined by investigators as possible indicators of placental insufficiency. These include the syncytial knot count, placental infarction, cytotrophoblast hypertrophy, deficiency of vasculo-endothelial membranes, fibrinoid necrosis of villi, basement membrane thickening, stromal fibrosis, stromal edema, apparent placental hypovascularity, and villus maturation.[34] These findings are extremely variable and are not consistently found in complicated pregnancies or those associated with fetal compromise. Fox has stated that a pathological basis for placental insufficiency cannot be defined.[34] The author suggests that failure to recognize this specific lesion in the past has been a consequence of patients being classified by maternal disease or fetal effect, rather than by the disturbance in the arterial flow pattern. This is not to imply that the umbilical placental lesion is necessarily primary; it may be determined by factors of fetal or uterine origin.

The finding of a reduction in the number of terminal arterial resistance vessels in the placenta of fetuses in whom the Doppler waveform index of resistance is elevated matches the predictions of the physical model of the placenta concerning the genesis of the abnormal Doppler pattern by vessel obliteration. The origin of the umbilical placental vascular obliteration remains to be determined. It is attractive to implicate the vasoactive prostaglandins, prostacyclin and thromboxane (for which animal experimental evidence has been provided). Thromboxane is believed to be released predominantly on platelet activation, whereas prostacyclin is a product of endothelial cells. These two prostanoids have opposite actions. Thromboxane-mediated vasoconstriction and, ultimately, vessel obliteration could well account for the increase in Doppler resistance index.[27] Further support for a role for thromboxane has been provided by the demonstration that fetuses in whom the umbilical Doppler study is abnormal have a significantly lower platelet count than controls.[35] This finding in the fetal circulation was independent of the maternal platelet count and whether or not pregnancy hypertension was present.

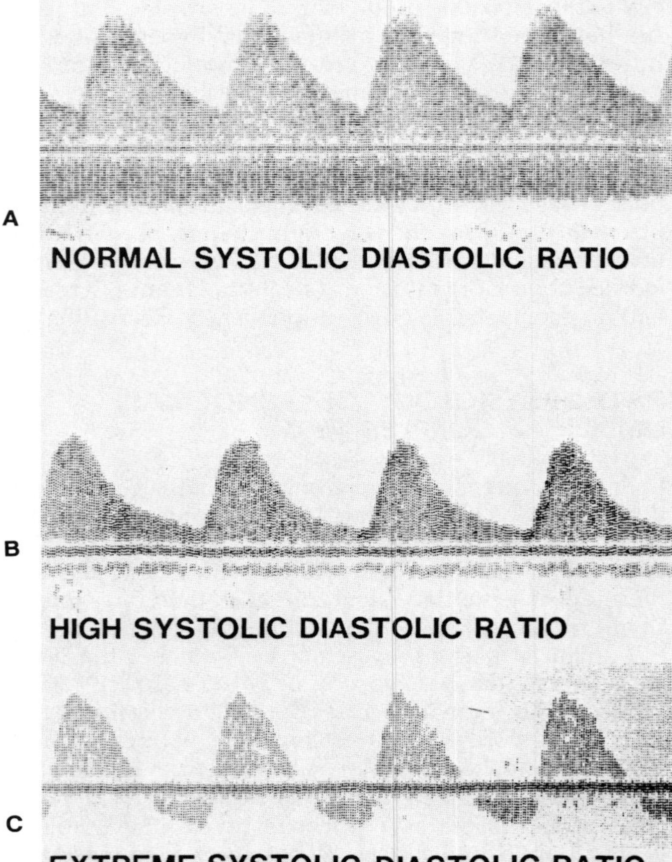

FIGURE 46–12. Examples of (**A**) a normal umbilical artery waveform, (**B**) a waveform in which the systolic diastolic ratio is high, and (**C**) an extremely abnormal waveform, in which the diastolic flow velocities are reversed.

CLINICAL CORRELATES OF ABNORMAL UMBILICAL DOPPLER FVW IN HIGH-RISK PREGNANCY

The abnormal umbilical artery Doppler FVW is characterized by a pattern of reduced, absent, or even reversed diastolic flow velocities relative to the systolic peak velocity (Fig. 46-12). In this situation, the indices of resistance are increased. Review of the normal ranges for these measures (see Fig. 46-6) illustrates the importance of knowledge of gestational age before an index is called abnormal. Before 24 weeks, absent diastolic flow may be seen in normal pregnancies. Particularly in early pregnancy, serial studies are necessary to determine if the normal growth of the placental vascular tree is occurring, because the normal range is wide.

Before considering the clinical correlates of the abnormal umbilical FVW, it is worth restating that analyzing the umbilical artery FVW with the various indices of resistance does not indicate a fetal condition, but rather the presence of a vascular lesion in the placenta—umbilical placental insufficiency. It is believed that this Doppler-defined umbilical placental insufficiency precedes the fetal deprivation. The fetal effects consequent upon this vascular lesion are the clinical correlates. Poor fetal outcome, particularly in terms of birth of an infant small for gestational age (SGA), is the major clinical association reported. This has been the consistent finding in many reports of the results of Doppler studies in high-risk pregnancy.[36–40] However, the point has been made on many occasions that what matters most to the obstetrician is not the recognition of the small fetus, but rather the fetus at risk of death in utero, distress in labor, and neonatal morbidity. To enable the association between Doppler test result and fetal outcome to be further assessed, I have reviewed the clinical outcome of all studies (2178 patients) from my laboratory over a 6-year period (Table 46-1).[41]

The most abnormal studies (highest systolic:diastolic ratio group) had the greatest incidence of fetal growth failure as indexed by the centile birth weight. Both fetal and neonatal deaths were highest in this group. The requirement for neonatal Level 3 nursery care and the duration of stay provide indices of neonatal morbidity that also correlated with the antenatal Doppler result. These differences remained when the data were corrected for gestation at delivery.

Comparison of fetal outcome in the group with an elevated (95th to 99th centile), high (>99th centile), or extreme (absent diastolic flow) study suggests the possibility of grading fetal risk by the degree of waveform abnormality. Neonatal problems were far more likely if the waveform was high or extreme (see Table 46-1).

TABLE 46–1. OUTCOME CHARACTERISTICS OF A HIGH RISK PREGNANCY POPULATION STUDIED BY DOPPLER UMBILICAL VELOCIMETRY

	LAST STUDY UMBILICAL ARTERY FVW RESULT				
	WHOLE GROUP	<95	95–99	>99	ABSENT DIASTOLIC FLOW
No. Patients	2178	1650 (76%)	193 (9%)	239 (11%)	96 (4%)
Delivery					
Gestational age	37.7	38.3	37.6‡	35.8§	31.1§
Labor planned					
Spontaneous	790	691 (42%)	56 (29%)‡	35 (15%)§	8 (8%)§
Induced	818	642 (39%)	86 (45%)	85 (36%)	5 (5%)§
Elective CS	570	317 (19%)	51 (26%)	119 (50%)§	83 (86%)§
Labor outcome					
Vaginal	1371	1145	122	95	9
Emergency CS	237	188	20	25	4
Neonate					
Birth weight (g)	2875	3097	2713§	2148§	1198§
Length in cm (mean)	47.8	48.8	47§	44.2§	37.6§
Ponderal index	26.0	26.4	25.9	24.6§	21.8§
Centile weight (mean)	36.2	41.9	27.0§	15.1§	9.0§
SGA Infants					
<10th	588 (27%)	293 (18%)	73 (38%)§	144 (60%)§	78 (81%)§
<5th	389 (18%)	165 (10%)	44 (23%)§	111 (46%)§	69 (72%)§
Apgars					
1 min ≤6	531 (24%)	335 (20%)	53 (27%)*	78 (33%)§	65 (68%)§
5 min ≤6	131 (6%)	62 (4%)	16 (8%)*	27 (11%)§	26 (27%)§
Admission NICU	548	303	45	113§	87§
NICU stay (mean days)	18.5	10.0	18.9	25.0§	43.7§
Perinatal deaths					
Fetal deaths (no.)	21	8	4†	3	6§
Neonatal deaths (no.)					
Day 0–7	38	16	4	9‡	9§
Day 8–28	10	2	0	0	8
PNM rate/1000	31.7	15.8	41.5‡	50.2§	239.6§
Corrected PNM	18.2	7.9	21.2*	13.0	206.5§
Major fetal anomaly					
Total	61	27	9†	16§	9§
Survived 1st 28 days	31	14	5*	7‡	5§
Not surviving (includes SBs)	30	13	4	9§	4‡

Results are shown as number (percent of grouping) unless otherwise stated. Differences significant in comparison to the normal (<95th centile) grouping are shown: *, $p < 0.05$; †, $p < 0.01$; ‡, $p < 0.001$; §, $p < 0.0001$.

PNM rate/1000 total births corrected for fetal anomaly.

(Data from Trudinger BJ, Cook CM, Giles WB, Ng S, Fong E, Connelly A, Wilcox W. Fetal umbilical artery velocity waveforms and subsequent neonatal outcome. Br J Obstet Gynaecol, 1991;98:378.)

Despite this, I am unhappy with this approach, because the umbilical waveform detects a placental vascular lesion. An effect on fetal condition in this truly "at risk" group should be sought using the other fetal tests before delivery. Some fetuses in the high and extreme groups have a good outcome. There has been considerable discussion about the group of patients that shows an umbilical FVW pattern of absent diastolic flow. Statements about the poor pregnancy outcome of this group and the need for delivery appear in the literature. It has been suggested that it constitutes a watershed for fetal risk.[42,43] The outcome of patients with this finding after 26 weeks may be seen in my series (see Table 46-1).[41] The outcome of high and extreme groups was similar, between 28 and 32 weeks. Although morbidity and mortality are high in this group, there is almost always the opportunity to seek other evidence of fetal compromise before clinical intervention. Absent diastolic flow is then a part of the spectrum of FVW change from normal to extremely abnormal. It is not a level at which fetal morbidity starts to appear. It has been noted above that absent diastolic flow may be a feature of normal pregnancy before 24 weeks. This finding varies with gestational age and may occasionally result from error of technique. There would seem to be no reason to fix on a single abnormal waveform type for clinical intervention. The greater incidence of hypoxemia in this group of fetuses is not surprising, but a number have normal gas tensions.[44]

Among a group of fetuses born small for gestational age, an abnormal Doppler umbilical study predicted those more likely to require early delivery and neonatal intensive care and those with the highest mortality (Table 46-2).[45] Those cases with an abnormal result were delivered earlier, required more Level 3 nursery care, and exhibited a higher mortality. Others have reported similar findings.[46]

The trend of umbilical Doppler results proved a very useful measure of neonatal morbidity in those patients with serial studies.[41] This was analyzed among 794 high-risk pregnancies with three or more umbilical Doppler studies available.[41] A decreasing systolic:diastolic ratio was associated with a good outcome, even if the values were outside the normal range (Table 46-3). Such a result suggests continuing placental growth. Such a trend in serial studies is also important in identifying the false-positive results. Serial studies will also be helpful in determining the response to therapy.

TABLE 46–2. RESULTS OF THE LAST STUDY PRIOR TO DELIVERY IN THE GROUP OF 53 SMALL-FOR-GESTATIONAL AGE FETUSES

	UMBILICAL ARTERY WAVEFORMS	
	NORMAL	ABNORMAL
No. of fetuses	19	34
Mean gestational age at delivery	37.6	34.6
Admission to neonatal intensive care	3	23
Neonatal deaths	0	7

(Data from Trudinger BJ, Cook CM, Giles WB, Ng S, Fong E, Connelly A, Wilcox W. Fetal umbilical artery velocity waveforms and subsequent neonatal outcome. Br J Obstet Gynaecol 1991;98:378.)

UMBILICAL DOPPLER FVW AND SPECIFIC PREGNANCY COMPLICATIONS

Hypertensive Disease of Pregnancy

Hypertensive disease of pregnancy may be associated with abnormal umbilical FVWs. In one report, it was suggested that the incidence of abnormal umbilical Doppler studies was related to the degree of severity of hypertension.[47] However, the hypertensive patients in that report were quite a mixed group. The suggestion from these studies was that those pregnancies with an abnormal Doppler study were most likely to be associated with fetal compromise. It was further suggested that this was consequent to the hypertension. In contrast, in a large and more homogeneous series of pregnancies with severe proteinuric hypertension, an abnormally elevated systolic:diastolic ratio was present in two-thirds of cases (Fig. 46-13).[48] In this study there was no relationship between the duration of hypertension and the umbilical flow result. Fetal morbidity and mortality were significantly associated with the abnormal systolic:diastolic ratio, not the period of hypertension. Furthermore, in serial studies I have noted a number of patients in whom the abnormal umbilical study preceded the hypertension. I believe that the placental lesion, detected by the abnormal Doppler study, is present before the clinical features of preeclampsia in the mother. It is suggested that those mothers with normal umbilical Doppler studies and severe preeclampsia have a vascular pathology in the placenta that has not yet reached the extent of vessel obliteration at which the Doppler study becomes abnormal. Further studies are necessary to establish this.

TABLE 46–3. PREGNANCY OUTCOME IN RELATION TO TREND IN SERIAL UMBILICAL ARTERY FLOW STUDIES

	PATTERN OF SERIAL DOPPLER STUDIES		
OUTCOME PARAMETER	NORMAL	ABNORMAL/ IMPROVING	ABNORMAL/ DETERIORATING
Total cases	567	117	110
Gestational age at delivery	38.5	37.5*	34.5†
Birth weight (mean g)	3164	2708†	1906†
Centile birth weight (mean)	43.8	26.5†	12.4†
Small for gestational age (<10th C) no. (%)	97 (17%)	47 (40%)†	78 (71%)†
Admission to NICU (no.)	101 (18%)	27 (23%)	65 (59%)†
Duration of stay in NICU (mean days)	6.1	11.1	34†
Perinatal mortality			
Number	7	2	7
Rate per 1,000	12.3	17.1	63.6†

Results shown are the number of patients in each grouping unless otherwise stated. The level of significance of results different from the normal Doppler study group is shown: *, $p < 0.001$; †, $p < 0.0001$.

(Data from Trudinger BJ, Cook CM, Giles WB, Ng S, Fong E, Connelly A, Wilcox W. Fetal umbilical artery velocity waveforms and subsequent neonatal outcome. Br J Obstet Gynaecol 1991;98:378.)

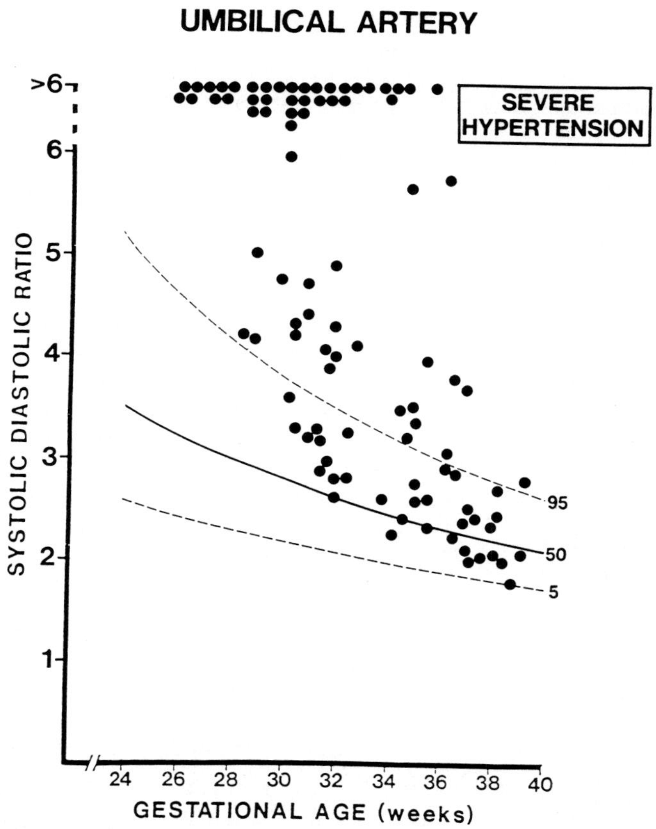

UMBILICAL ARTERY

SEVERE HYPERTENSION

SYSTOLIC DIASTOLIC RATIO

>6
6
5
4
3
2
1

95
50
5

24 26 28 30 32 34 36 38 40

GESTATIONAL AGE (weeks)

FIGURE 46–13. The last study before delivery of umbilical artery systolic/diastolic ratio in a group of 94 patients with severe pregnancy hypertension. (From Trudinger BJ, Cook CM. Doppler umbilical and uterine flow waveforms in severe pregnancy hypertension. Br J Obstet Gynaecol 1990;97:144.)

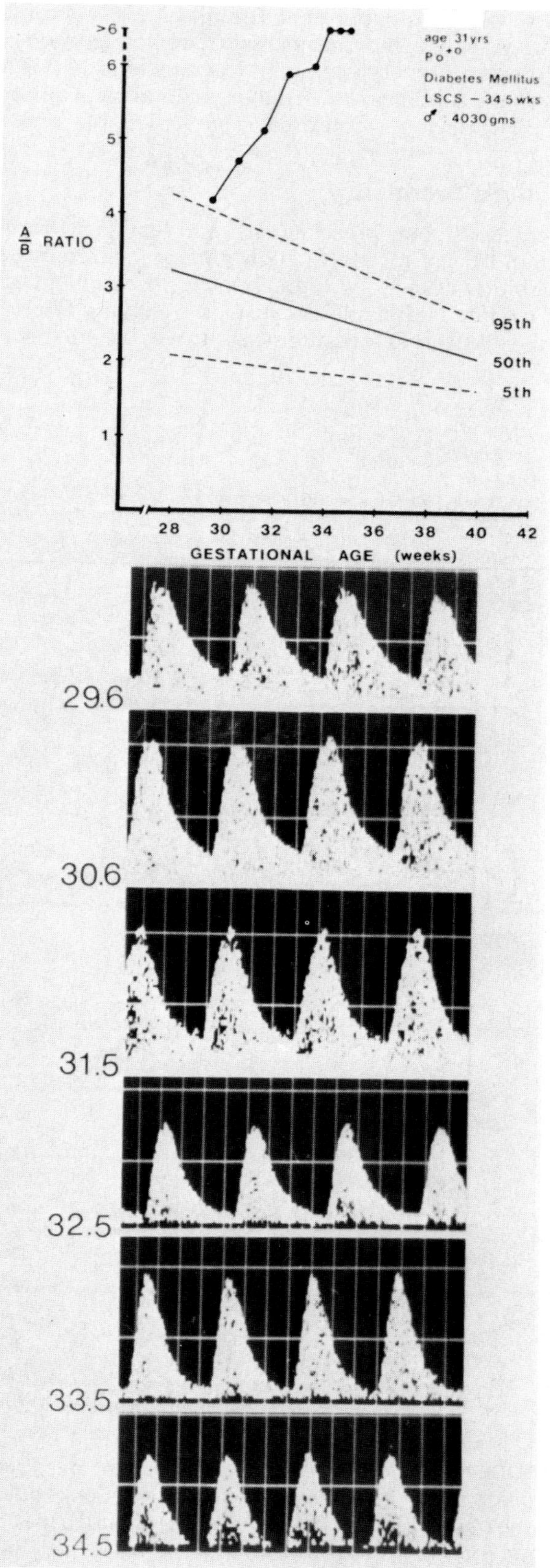

Diabetes Mellitus

Umbilical artery FVWs have also been used in the management of diabetic pregnancies.[49] My experience suggests that normal studies are recorded from the macrosomic fetus continuing to grow, but that cessation of growth, even if the fetus is macrosomic (ie, earlier in pregnancy the growth stimulus had been excessive), is associated with the development of a high resistance pattern in the umbilical artery waveform (Fig. 46-14).

Mothers with long-standing diabetes and vascular disease affecting the small vessels of the uterus may have a fetus that is small, and here growth cessation is

FIGURE 46–14. Sequential studies of the umbilical artery flow velocity waveforms in one patient with poorly controlled diabetes mellitus. Although the fetus was large, there was evidence of ultrasound fetal growth failure at the end of the pregnancy. (From Trudinger BJ, Giles WB, Cook CM, Bombardieri J, Collins L. Fetal umbilical artery flow velocity waveforms and placental resistance: clinical significance. Br J Obstet Gynaecol 1985;92:29.)

associated with abnormal umbilical FVW studies. I have also observed mothers with previously good control become hyperglycemic and ketoacidotic. In this situation, the umbilical FVW may remain normal although the FHR tracing is abnormal (Fig. 46-15).

Multiple Pregnancy

Premature labor, preeclampsia, and fetal growth retardation all contribute to high perinatal mortality and morbidity rates in twin pregnancies. Assessment of fetal welfare is difficult, because an overlying fetus may make ultrasound measurements unreliable and because

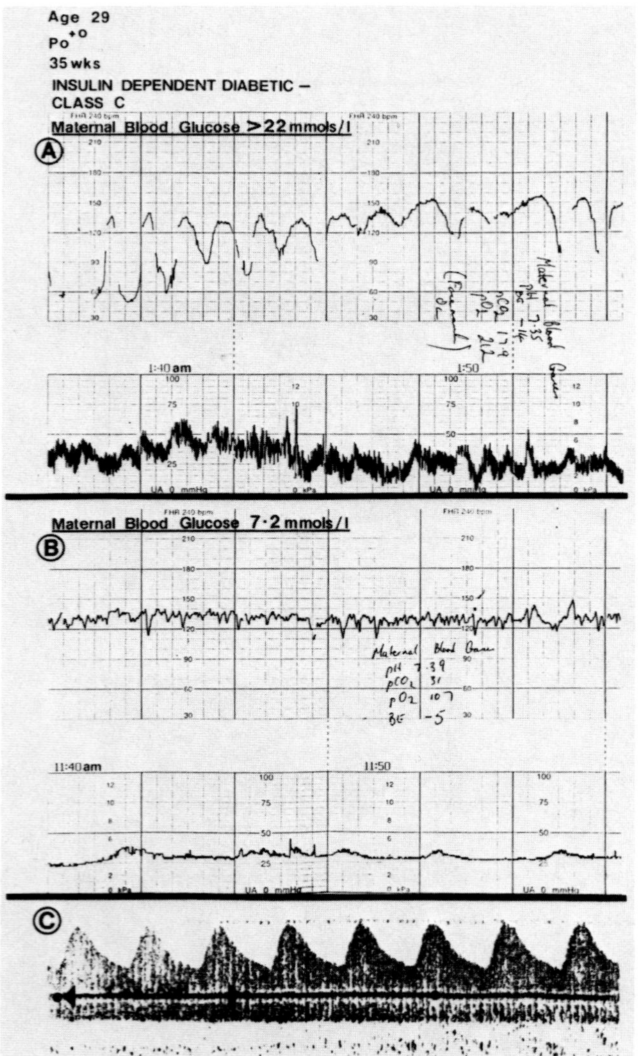

FIGURE 46–15. In one diabetic mother, with an episode of hyperglycemia and acidosis, the fetal heart rate (FHR) monitoring trace was abnormal (upper panel), although the umbilical artery Doppler flow velocity waveform appeared normal. After correction for the metabolic problem, the FHR monitoring was normal (middle panel).

fetal heart rate monitoring presents problems of identification. Doppler umbilical studies are especially useful. The umbilical recordings must be matched against real-time observation of the fetal heart to ensure the identity of the fetus being studied.[50]

The great value of Doppler studies in twin pregnancy management lies in the early recognition of the fetus at risk. An evaluation of the benefits of Doppler studies in the management of twin pairs has been carried out.[51] A comparison was made between two groups of 100 twin pairs studied before and after the Doppler study results were made clinically available. The Doppler studies were done at 28 weeks. It was shown that perinatal mortality and, in particular, fetal deaths could be significantly reduced. The perinatal mortality was reduced from 58 per 1000 to 18 per 1000 ($P < 0.05$). It was suggested that the abnormal Doppler study identified patients who could be followed by a program of intensive fetal surveillance and that the improved outcome was the consequence of this.

Although a consistent Doppler picture in the case of twin transfusion syndrome has been disputed,[50,52–55] I believe it is possible to suspect this diagnosis. Discordance in ultrasound measures of fetal size, cord diameter, and amniotic fluid volume between the members of the twin pair exists, yet similar umbilical waveforms for the two fetuses are recorded. It is suggested that the absence of obliterative vascular disease in the placenta explains the normal study in the smaller fetus.[55] It is now possible to check for hemoglobin discrepancy by percutaneous umbilical blood sampling of the members of the twin pair. Doppler studies have also been reported useful in fetal assessment of triplet pregnancy.[56]

Isoimmunization and Fetal Anemia

The systolic:diastolic ratio has been reported low in association with fetal anemia. Fetal transfusion in utero has been observed to increase toward normal the low systolic:diastolic ratio index of resistance in the umbilical placental circulation.[57] An inverse correlation has been reported between the hematocrit of fetal blood and the resistance index, but this is weak and not of clinical value.[58] In fetuses at risk of sickle hemoglobinopathy by virtue of its presence in the mother, it has been found that fetal growth retardation is predicted by an increase in the umbilical systolic:diastolic ratio.[59]

Lupus Obstetric Syndrome

A high incidence of both early and late pregnancy fetal wastage and maternal hypertension is associated with the presence in maternal blood of the "lupus anticoagulant." Such mothers may have systemic lupus erythematosus (SLE) or other autoimmune phenomena, but the obstetric manifestations may be the only clinical feature.[60] Fetal deterioration is predicted by the development of an abnormal umbilical artery waveform, and these studies have aided the management of such pregnancies. Frequent studies, at least weekly in the third trimester, are recommended because fetal demise may occur over a short time.[61]

Major Fetal Anomaly

Major fetal anomaly is not consistently associated with an abnormal umbilical artery waveform, although such a finding is more common in this group.[62] The systolic:diastolic ratio has been reported high in association with fetuses with trisomy 13, 18, and 21.[62,63] Care should be taken before extrapolating these findings to a total population, because the reported cases studied by Doppler had come to the attention of the clinician before the Doppler study, and the reported findings may be the result of this selection bias. An incidence of abnormal karyotype of 16% has been reported in a series of profoundly growth-retarded fetuses confirmed by ultrasound scan (abdominal circumference < 3rd centile). Most of these fetuses had an abnormal Doppler study.[64]

Postdate Pregnancy

It appears that the Doppler studies of the umbilical artery FVW do not predict fetal compromise in postdate pregnancy.[21,22] This may be due to the fact that the mechanism of fetal demise in this group differs from that operating before term. However, on the basis of mathematical modelling of the placental vascular tree, we have shown that the larger the placental size, the greater the fraction of the vascular tree that needs to be obliterated to cause a detectable increase in the systolic:diastolic ratio.[20] This, combined with a greater susceptibility of the mature fetus to the effects of hypoxemia, could account for the poor Doppler predictive value. Doppler umbilical surveillance is not recommended for postdate pregnancies.

UMBILICAL VEIN VOLUME FLOW STUDIES

Doppler ultrasound measurement of volume flow in the umbilical circulation is possible by recording from the umbilical vein as it traverses the fetal liver.[5] The dimensions of the vessel need to be measured at the same time, and flow calculated as the product of average velocity and of vessel lumen. In normal pregnancy, flow in the umbilical vein increases with gestation. Flow per unit of fetal weight is relatively constant at 110 $mL/min^{-1}/kg\ fetus^{-1}$.[12]

Studies in high-risk pregnancy suggest that a reduced umbilical vein flow is associated with growth retardation, but only 40% of low flow studies were associated with birth weight below the tenth centile.[65] The relationship between umbilical artery FVW and umbilical vein volume flow measurements has been examined.[66] The FVW was more sensitive and recognized more SGA fetuses. It had a higher predictive value and similar specificity. The ratio of umbilical vein flow to aortic flow was also measured in this series. In the normal fetuses, this was 39%; in those fetuses with an abnormal umbilical artery FVW systolic:diastolic ratio, it was 25%. This result suggests that the fetus is able to maintain umbilical placental circulation at least initially by an increase in cardiac output. The same observation has been made in experimental growth retardation in fetal lambs.[67] Thus, there is experimental and clinical evidence to suggest that the umbilical artery FVW will detect the compromised fetus earlier than volume flow measurements. A high umbilical vein volume flow has been seen in association with fetal hydrops caused by rhesus isoimmunization[68] and Bart's hemoglobin.[64] The high umbilical vein volume flow has been reduced in rhesus isoimmunization by fetal transfusion.

The application of measures of umbilical vein volume flow to obstetric practice has been limited by the need for a detailed technique, measurement errors, and complex equipment.

THE RELATIONSHIP OF UMBILICAL DOPPLER TO FETAL WELFARE TESTS

Tests of fetal welfare exist to identify the potentially compromised fetus (sometimes termed the "at risk" fetus) and to quantitate fetal condition. The recognition of imminent fetal demise (ie, the fetus in a terminal state) may be too late to prevent damage or loss of potential. It has been stated above that the umbilical Doppler study recognizes a vascular pathology in the fetal placenta that may lead to a fetal effect. Evaluative studies against other fetal tests support this.

Antenatal nonstressed FHR monitoring is widely used in fetal surveillance protocols for high-risk pregnancy. Several comparative studies have demonstrated a greater sensitivity (the proportion of abnormal outcomes identified by the test) for umbilical Doppler in comparison to nonstressed FHR monitoring in recognizing the SGA fetus.[69,70] Because antenatal FHR monitoring is not a test to recognize the SGA fetus, this may not be the correct endpoint. It is important to identify the small fetus before birth, but it is even more important to identify those fetuses at risk of further morbidity. Although the predictive value of an abnormal Doppler was similar to that of an abnormal FHR tracing in relation to such measures of prenatal asphyxia as operative delivery for fetal distress, low 5-minute Apgar score, and admission to neonatal Level 3 care, the Doppler study did have a greater sensitivity.[69] It appears that the association of an abnormal nonstressed FHR test with an abnormal Doppler study selects a group with a very high risk of morbidity.[70] The above observations suggest that the abnormal FHR monitoring occurs later in fetal compromise than the abnormal umbilical Doppler study.

The relationship between umbilical Doppler and ultrasonic estimation of fetal size has been examined.[71,72] Although sonographic biometry was a more sensitive technique for identifying the small fetus, the umbilical artery systolic:diastolic ratio was noted to be abnormal at a significantly earlier gestation when serial studies were available.[71] The biophysical profile has not been widely compared to umbilical Doppler studies.

Because fetal compromise is not confined to the SGA fetus, larger fetuses in whom growth has stopped may also be identified by umbilical Doppler, although the ultrasonic measurements are not small. Serial ultrasound measurements could be expected to reveal the growth failure in these fetuses, but this requires at least 2 weeks. In contrast, the genetically small infant whose only problem is a birth weight below the tenth percentile for gestational age would not be expected to present with any abnormal measure of fetal welfare, apart from the small size and reduced ultrasonic estimates of fetal weight. However, serial studies should demonstrate growth. Good fetal outcome has been reported in the ultrasonically small fetus with a normal umbilical Doppler study.[71] Serial umbilical Doppler studies in such cases should reveal the normal decrease in systolic:diastolic ratio as the placenta grows. It has also been demonstrated that, among a group of fetuses clinically suspected of being SGA, Doppler umbilical studies identified the fetus at risk of adverse perinatal outcome in comparison to ultrasonic abdominal circumference, which better identified the small size only.[72] A Swedish study of all small fetuses identified from a total obstetric population, screened for ultrasound weight estimation at 32 weeks, reported operative delivery for fetal distress more likely in the group also exhibiting an abnormal Doppler study.[73,74]

CLINICAL STRATEGIES

The approach of the obstetrician to fetal compromise progresses through a sequence of steps, which can be summarized as:

1. Recognition of high-risk pregnancy on the basis of clinical history and examination, supported by the ancillary aids of maternal–fetal movement counting and fundal height measurement (Is it a high-risk pregnancy?)
2. Confirmation of fetal risk by identifying the placental vascular lesion with Doppler ultrasound studies of the umbilical artery FVW (Is there a placental pathology threatening the fetus?)
3. Determination of the extent to which the fetus is affected using the direct fetal assessments of biophysical profile, ultrasound growth, and FHR monitoring (How sick is the fetus?)
4. Therapy aimed at improving the intrauterine environment by treating mother or fetus, and delivery if the risk to the fetus of intrauterine death or damage exceed that of delivery.

Included in this approach is the use of Doppler umbilical studies interposed between the clinical identification of the high-risk pregnancy and a full fetal surveillance testing to quantitate the degree to which the fetus is affected. This assumes that the placental vascular lesion identified by umbilical Doppler underlies all fetal compromise. Although this is common in the "chronic" situation, it is not always the case. Acute fetal deterioration (eg, abruption) is not recognized. Fetal anemia, whether due to isoimmunization or other causes such as fetal–maternal hemorrhage, is also not identified. However, chronic "placental insufficiency" is operating in the majority of cases, and these are identified. The one fourth to one third of infants born SGA with normal umbilical Doppler studies have a good outcome (see Table 46-1) and include the cases of low growth potential where the growth velocity of the small fetus is normal and there is no placental constraint.[41] The concept of identification of umbilical placental insufficiency by umbilical Doppler studies also implies that the various clinical situations in which this is present operate through a final, common pathological pathway. This is recognized by the abnormal umbilical FVW.

The above scheme involves the use of the Doppler umbilical waveform study as a discriminator or doorway test to determine which fetuses are truly at risk and in need of intensive fetal surveillance. The relationship of the various direct fetal assessments to the umbilical FVW has been described above.

It cannot be too frequently stated that the Doppler umbilical artery waveform provides a guide to the presence of a placental pathology important in terms of the equation:

$$\text{placental lesion} \rightarrow \text{fetal effect.}$$

It is not a direct fetal test and should not in itself be used as a measure of fetal condition, but rather as the need for detailed assessment of fetal welfare.

Doppler umbilical studies have also been used to guide specific therapies aimed at reversing the placental lesion. The demonstrated placental vascular obliteration[30] and fetal platelet consumption[35] suggested a role for thromboxane activity in the fetal placenta. This is quite consistent with reports of alterations in the thromboxane prostacyclin balance toward thromboxane activity in the fetal placenta.[26] It was the rationale for the evaluation of low-dose aspirin as a therapy.[75] In a randomized clinical trial, soluble aspirin 150 mg/day was administered to mothers with pregnancies identified by an umbilical artery waveform systolic:diastolic ratio above the 95th centile. The treated pregnancies yielded infants with a 25% greater birth weight. There was an increase in head circumference. The placentas from the treated pregnancies showed the same proportional increase in size. This improvement was not seen in pregnancies in which the umbilical Doppler study was extremely abnormal, with absent diastolic flow velocities. It is quite likely that lower doses of aspirin will exert the same benefit. Low-dose aspirin provides a means of treatment of placental insufficiency if the Doppler diagnosis can be made early and before marked fetal effect. There is currently much interest in developing specific thromboxane antagonists as an alternative to aspirin.

SCREENING OF ALL PREGNANCIES BY UMBILICAL DOPPLER STUDIES

The possible use of umbilical Doppler studies to screen all pregnancies or low-risk pregnancy has been investigated by several groups. The largest patient group examined was 2097, and these patients were seen at 28, 34, and 38 weeks.[76] There was a significant association between abnormal Doppler result and low centile birth weight, but the authors suggested from receiver operating curves that this lacked sufficient sensitivity for clinical usage. The most important result was the presence of an abnormal waveform in all three of the unexplained stillbirths and one of two fetal deaths associated with placental abruption. This was emphasized in correspondence subsequent to the original report.[77] Other studies of smaller numbers from unselected low-risk pregnancy groups reported poor prediction of the small-for-date infants and adverse perinatal outcomes.[78] The statistical power of these reports was low, because adverse outcome is infrequent in an unselected pregnancy population. In contrast, another group of investigators has suggested that a screening umbilical Doppler study at 26 weeks was associated with clinically useful identification of adverse perinatal outcome.[79] The issue remains unresolved, although it is the writer's opinion that identification of potentially high-risk pregnancies will always require the input of a clinician.

OTHER FETAL DOPPLER STUDIES

Within the fetal body, the aortic and cerebral circulations are the two most studied vascular trees, although reports of FVW in the renal and external iliac arteries have been made.[80]

FETAL AORTA

A pulsed Doppler system integrated with a real-time B-mode image is necessary to record from the fetal aorta.[81] This permits location of the sample volume over the desired part of the aorta, because the waveform varies along its length. It also excludes interfering signals from the heart or other vessels within the beam path. Insonation angles of the aorta should not exceed 60 degrees. The most common site used for recording is the midthoracic part of the descending aorta (above the diaphragm) (Fig. 46-16). The fetal aortic blood FVW has been analyzed using the same indices of downstream resistance described in the assessment of umbilical artery FVW. Volume blood flow in the aorta may be calculated from the mean blood flow velocity and the mean diameter, and is usually expressed in relation to the estimated fetal weight. Measuring aortic dimensions from a "frozen" screen image is not satisfactory because of the changing diameter with pulsatile flow, and it has been estimated that this adds an error of 6% to the volume flow measurement. Because of the vulnerability to the various errors inherent in volume blood flow measurement, most clinical studies of the fetal aortic circulation now use the analysis of the blood flow velocity waveform and the blood flow velocity itself.

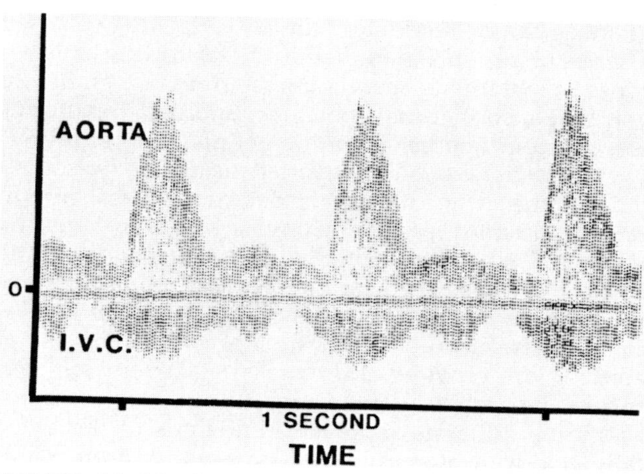

FIGURE 46–16. The normal flow velocity waveform recorded from the thoracic aorta in the third trimester. I.V.C., inferior vena cava.

Normal Pregnancy

The pulsatility index of the maximum velocity waveform in the thoracic aorta (1.68 ± 0.28) does not change with gestation.[82] This index is significantly affected by changes in FHR. Within the normal FHR range, there is a negative correlation with thoracic descending aorta pulsatility index ($r = 0.43$). This index is also affected by behavioral state.[16] These observations are not surprising, because 60% of aortic blood is distributed to nonplacental fetal vascular beds in which the vasomotor tone will be regulated according to fetal behavioral and metabolic states. In clinical studies, the use of a high cut-off value for pulsatility index (mean + 2 standard deviations) to distinguish normal and abnormal eliminates the effect of FHR over the normal range.[83] The same effects on pulsatility index of FHR and behavioral state have been reported in the growth-retarded fetus.[84] Fetal breathing movements affect the aortic flow waveform, and studies should be carried out during fetal apnea to ensure reproducible results.

Volume blood flow measurement in the fetal descending thoracic aorta increases with gestation to 36 to 37 weeks, when a plateau is attained, whereas flow per unit fetal weight decreases during the third trimester.[85]

High-Risk Pregnancy

Studies of aortic FVW have been evaluated as predictors of fetal growth retardation and fetal distress (diagnosed on the basis of cardiotocographic changes). A grading score has been developed to classify changes in the aortic waveform.[81] The degree of abnormality is quantified into "blood flow classes" (Fig. 46-17). When a series of patients identified in the third trimester because of small fetal size on ultrasound were graded, it was demonstrated that the most abnormal waveforms were seen in fetuses exhibiting perinatal morbidity.[86]

The predictive ability reported using the pulsatility index of the aortic FVW for the detection of fetal growth retardation and perinatal asphyxia has been noted by others.[87–90] The likely explanation for the change in the aortic FVW seen in these pregnancy complications is the increase in downstream flow resistance in the placenta. There is no evidence to suggest that the use of aortic FVWs provides additional predictive value over that of the umbilical artery waveform.

A quite different approach to analysis of the aortic flow velocity waveform has been reported from Kings College Hospital in London. This group has determined the peak mean velocity of the aortic waveform and demonstrated its correlation with hypoxemia, hypercarbia, hyperlactemia, and acidemia as determined from fetal blood obtained at cordocentesis.[91] These end points were used to compare the various methods of analysis of flow velocity waveforms from aortic, cerebral, and umbilical fetal circulations. Again, the peak mean velocity of the aortic waveform was the most sensitive.[92] Many growth-retarded infants do not show these changes in blood gas analysis. They are present when the fetus is in extremis. The use of such end points is not valid for the evaluation of Doppler techniques for the prediction of fetal compromise, but rather for the assessment of severity of compromise.

Assessment of volume blood flow in the fetal aorta has not proved helpful in the assessment of fetal growth retardation. In the assessment of fetal cardiac arrhythmias, measures of aortic volume flow and the FVW have provided valuable information and allowed determination of the adequacy of ventricular output. In fetal tachycardia, the high heart rate (eg, supraventricular tachycardia) may mean insufficient time for filling. The upper limit of the FHR above which failure is imminent seems to be about 240 beats/minute. In bradycardia (eg, heart block) the slow rate may be associated with insufficient output. Measure of aortic volume flow and the FVW may also provide useful information as to the effect of antenatal treatment, such as transplacental digoxin therapy. Studies of ventricular output (aortic flow) in relation to heart rate confirm that the Frank-Starling mechanism operates in fetal life and contradicts the former belief that the fetus could only increase cardiac output by an increase in rate.

BFC 0 PI < + 2 SD and continuous forward diastolic flow (normal)

BFC 1 PI ≥ + 2 SD and continuous forward diastolic flow

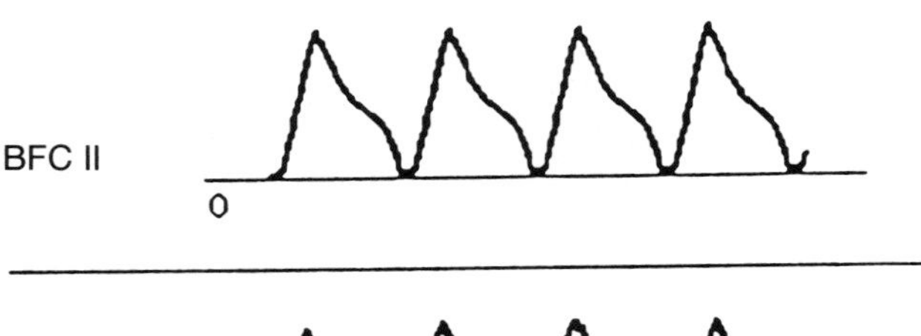

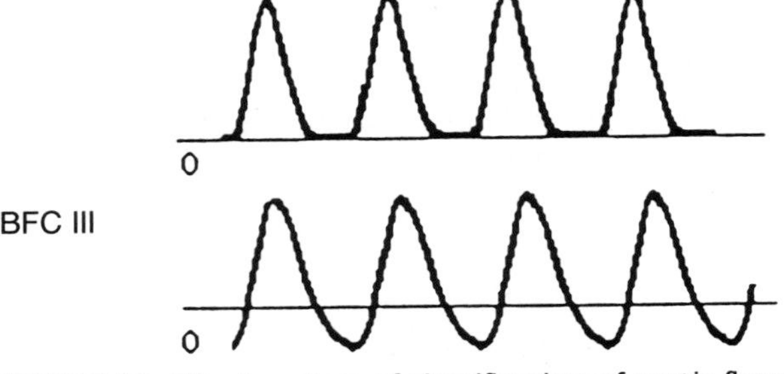

FIGURE 46–17. A system of classification of aortic flow velocity waveforms into classes by degree of abnormality. (Laurin J, Lingman G, Marsal K, Persson RH. Fetal blood flow in pregnancies complicated by intrauterine growth retardation. Obstet Gynecol 1987;69:895.)

FETAL CEREBRAL CIRCULATION

The combined use of duplex B-mode imaging and pulsed Doppler ultrasound system has enabled the recording of FVWs from the fetal internal carotid artery and, more recently, the individual arteries of the human fetal cerebral circulation. The internal carotid artery is best located at the level of its bifurcation into the middle and anterior cerebral artery.[93] This particular point can be readily identified on a transverse cross section of the fetal cerebrum. The standard plane for measuring the biparietal diameter, which includes the thalamus and the cavum of the septum pellucidum, is visualized. The middle cerebral artery can be seen pulsating at the level of the insula. If the transducer is now moved in a parallel fashion toward the base of the skull, a plane is reached that demonstrates a heart-shaped cross section of the brain stem with the anterior lobes representing the cerebral peduncles. Anterior to this heart-shaped structure, on either side of the midline, is an oblique cross section of the internal carotid artery as it divides into its middle and anterior cerebral branches. Transducers with carrier frequencies of 3.5 and 5 MHz have been used for this. The sample volume size of the pulsed Doppler system should not exceed 3 to 4 mm. This allows clear flow velocity signals from the internal carotid artery and reduces the likelihood of interference from other nearby vessels, such as the basilar artery.

Normal Pregnancy

The waveform of the fetal internal carotid artery is a typical low-resistance pattern. With advancing gestation through the third trimester, this waveform reveals a small decrease in resistance. A normal range for the pulsatility index of the fetal internal carotid artery FVW has been reported.[94] A value below 1.1 in the third trimester is regarded as low—less than 5th centile value. These measurements are affected by fetal breathing movements and behavioral state.[15] For clinical studies, the fetus should be inactive and apneic.

High-Risk Pregnancy

Intrauterine fetal growth retardation may be associated with a fetal internal carotid FVW pulsatility index lower than normal.[95–97] In one series of 35 infants with a birth weight below the fifth centile, 19 were observed with an internal carotid pulsatility index below the normal range.[98] This result was compared to umbilical FVWs in the same fetuses. A lesser number exhibited an abnormal cerebral artery study in comparison to the number with a high umbilical artery pulsatility index. The presence of a normal fetal carotid FVW and a high-resistance umbilical FVW was suggested to indicate the maintenance of normal cerebral flow. Later, with a deteriorating fetal condition, cerebral vasodilation occurs and the cerebral FVW shows a lower pulsatility index. Whether this effect is adaptive to maintain cerebral oxygen supply or consequent on the occurrence of fetal hypoxia and hypercarbia is not know at present. The possibility of monitoring the anterior cerebral artery FVW waveform during labor has also been studied.[99]

MATERNAL UTERINE CIRCULATION

Both pulsed[100] and continuous wave[101] ultrasound have been used to record flow velocity waveforms from the uterine circulation. The fundamental problem with the study of uteroplacental circulation is in reproducibility, because a number of different vessels may be studied. It is hoped that the introduction of color Doppler will allow precise localization of the uterine and arcuate vessels and therefore remove the problem of vessel identification.[102] Pulsed Doppler systems allow simultaneous imaging and recording from the main internal iliac artery, as well as from branches of the uterine artery in the myometrium.[103] Color Doppler systems enable the main uterine artery to be imaged. It has been stated that the pattern of the waveform in normal pregnancy allows this same distinction about recording site to be made using continuous wave systems.[104] This claim cannot be extended to complicated pregnancy. The signal recorded from the site of placental implantation is a lower resistance pattern in comparison to the nonplacental site.[105] Problems of vessel identification limit studies with continuous wave ultrasound systems to the myometrial segments of the uterine artery, either within the placental bed or away from it.

The same indices of downstream resistance as described in the assessment of umbilical artery FVWs are used to assess flow velocity waveforms of uteroplacental arteries. Attention has also been focused on the presence of an early diastolic "notch," which has been suggested to be due to increased downstream resistance.[47]

NORMAL PREGNANCY

The process of trophoblast invasion of the spiral arteries of the decidual and inner third of the myometrium occurs during the first 20 weeks of gestation. The spiral artery is stripped of its musculoelastic coat. It is widely believed that this lowers the resistance to blood flow in the uterine artery branches opening into the intervillous

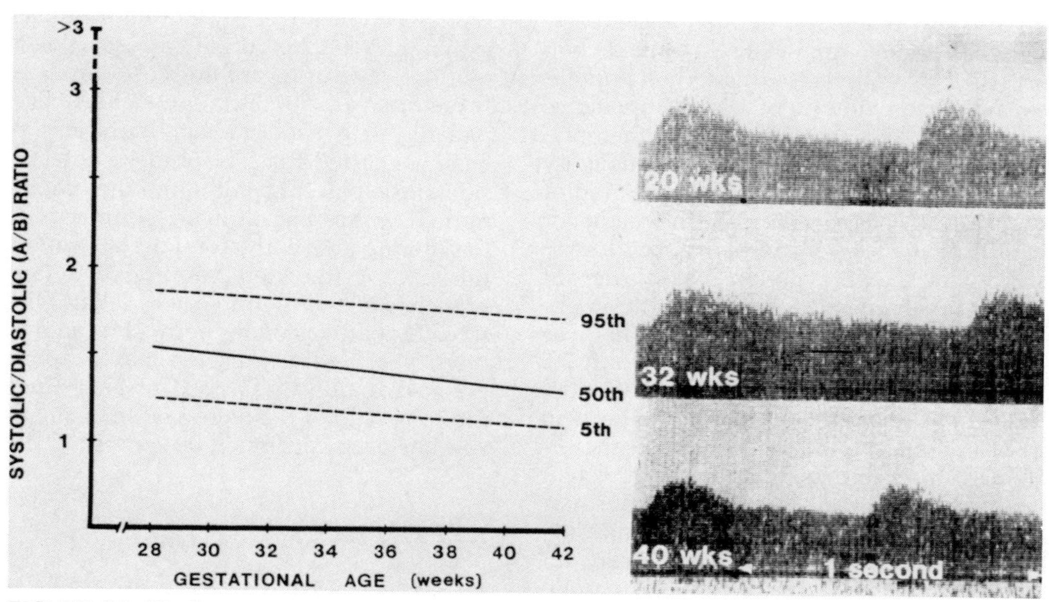

FIGURE 46–18. Sequential studies of arterial flow velocity waveforms recorded from the uteroplacental bed during normal pregnancy, along with a normal range for the systolic/diastolic ratio from such vessels.

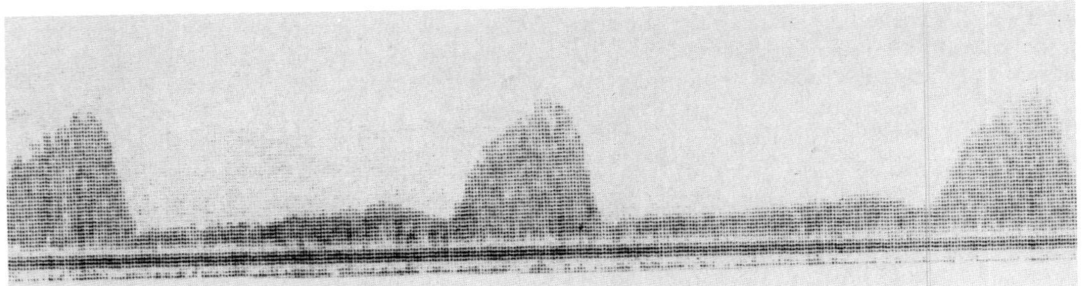

FIGURE 46–19. An abnormal pregnancy with a high resistance pattern, uteroplacental bed, arterial flow velocity waveform.

space. A decrease in resistance in uterine artery branches causes higher end diastolic flow velocities, and this can be detected in early pregnancy. After 20 weeks of gestation, there is little change in the waveform of the uteroplacental arteries throughout the remainder of the pregnancy. A pattern of low pulsatility and high end diastolic velocity relative to peak systolic velocity is seen (Fig. 46-18).[101] It is, however, relevant to realize that there is no direct evidence linking the trophoblast invasion of the spiral arteries with uterine blood flow or flow velocity waveform changes.

The early diastolic "notch" of uteroplacental FVW has been reported in normal pregnancy until approximately 26 weeks gestation. However, on the side of the uterus of the placental bed, it has been reported to be rarely found after 20 weeks gestation.[103]

HIGH-RISK PREGNANCY

Both severe growth retardation and maternal hypertension may be associated with uteroplacental waveforms demonstrating a high systolic:diastolic ratio (Fig. 46-19).[101] A study of 31 patients with pregnancies complicated by hypertension or IUGR identified two groups: those with FVWs similar to the normal population and those who had evidence of a high impedance to flow.[100] In this second group, there was a higher incidence of proteinuric hypertension, the time of delivery was significantly shorter, and the birth weight ratio of the infants (actual birth weight/mean birth weight for gestational age corrected for sex and parity) was lower. In a group of 72 women with hypertensive disorders of pregnancy of varying degrees, 28 patients with an abnormal uterine waveform were identified.[47] This was defined by a systolic:diastolic ratio of greater than 2.6 and persistence of the notch after 26 weeks of gestation. There was a significantly higher maternal uric acid level, shorter gestational period, higher cesarean section rate for fetal distress, and lower infant birth weight than the 43 patients with normal waveforms. Furthermore, in the pathologic group, there was a significantly higher incidence of SGA babies and a significant increase in stillbirths. Whether the reduction of uteroplacental circulation is the cause or effect of pregnancy hypertension remains an open question. Others have not been able to demonstrate consistently abnormal studies in hypertension of pregnancy.[106,107]

Based on the hypothesis that trophoblast invasion of the spiral arteries causes the change in the uterine waveforms during the first half of pregnancy, and that this invasion is less developed in pregnancy hypertension, these studies have also been evaluated for screening in early pregnancy. In a study of 126 consecutive pregnancies screened between 16 and 18 weeks gestation, an abnormal waveform predicted these complications with a sensitivity and specificity of 69%.[108] Others have made similar claims.[109] These preliminary results have been disputed by other groups, and it has been pointed out that many normal pregnancy outcomes occur in the large group with "abnormal" uterine waveforms.[107]

RELATIONSHIP OF UMBILICAL AND UTERINE FVW STUDIES

Study of umbilical and uterine waveforms allows classification into four groups, depending on whether these waveforms are normal or abnormal.[45] The two subgroups characterized by normal umbilical waveforms exhibit little fetal morbidity, irrespective of whether the uterine waveforms are normal or not. If the umbilical waveforms are abnormal, fetal morbidity is present. In patients with a normal uterine artery pattern, it has been suggested that the primary defect is on the fetal side of the placenta. Although the uterine waveform is normal, indicating normal resistance in that branch of the uterine artery, the total uterine flow may be low if the size of the uteroplacental bed (and number of branches of the uterine artery feeding it) is not extensive. In patients with both abnormal umbilical and uterine waveforms, disease may exist in the maternal uteroplacental vascular bed, and it is this that produces the constraint of the fetal–placental circulation. This result has been confirmed by others.[110,111]

REFERENCES

1. Gill RW. Doppler ultrasound—physical aspects. Semin Perinatol 1987;11:292.
2. Milnor WR. Pulsatile blood flow. N Engl J Med 1972;187:27.

3. Caro CG, Pedley TJ, Schroter CW, Seed WA. The mechanics of the circulation. London: Oxford University Press, 1978.
4. O'Rourke MF. Vascular impedance in studies of arterial and cardiac function. Physiol Rev 1982;62:571.
5. Gill RW. Pulsed Doppler with B-mode imaging for quantitative blood flow measurement. Ultrasound Med Biol 1979;5:223.
6. Thompson RS, Trudinger BJ, Cook CM. A comparison of Doppler ultrasound waveform indices in the umbilical artery. I: indices derived from the maximum velocity waveform. Ultrasound Med Biol 1986;12:835.
7. Thompson RS, Trudinger BJ, Cook CM. A comparison of Doppler ultrasound waveform indices in the umbilical artery. II: indices derived from the mean velocity and first moment waveforms. Ultrasound Med Biol 1986;12:845.
8. Thompson RS, Trudinger BJ, Cook CM. Doppler ultrasound waveform indices. AB ratio pulsatility index and Pourcelot ratio. Br J Obstet Gynaecol 1988;95:581.
9. Rudolph AM, Heymann MA. Circulatory changes during growth in the fetal lamb. Circ Res 1970;26:289.
10. Dawes GS. The umbilical circulation. In: Fetal neonatal physiology. Chicago: Year Book Medical Publishers, 1968:66.
11. Eik-Nes SH, Brubakk AO, Ulstein MK. Measurement of human fetal blood flow. Br Med J 1980;280:283.
12. Gill RW, Trudinger BJ, Garrett WJ, Kossoff G, Warren PS. Fetal umbilical venous flow measured in utero by pulsed Doppler and B-mode ultrasound. I: Normal pregnancy. Am J Obstet Gynecol 1981;139:720.
13. Rankin JHG, McLaughlin MK. The regulation of placental blood flows. J Dev Physiol 1979;1:3.
14. Itskovitz J, LaGamma EF, Rudolph AM. The effect of reducing umbilical blood flow on fetal oxygenation. Am J Obstet Gynecol 1983;145:813.
15. van Eyck J, Wladimiroff JW, Winjngaard JAGW, et al. The blood flow velocity waveform in the fetal internal carotid and umbilical artery: its relationship to fetal behavioural states in normal pregnancy at 37–38 weeks of gestation. Br J Obstet Gynaecol 1987;94:736.
16. van Eyck J, Wladimiroff JW, Noordam MJ, Tonge HM, Prechtle HRF. The blood flow velocity waveform in the fetal descending aorta: its relationship to fetal behavioural state in normal pregnancy at 37–38 weeks. Early Hum Dev 1985;12:137.
17. Mehalex KE, Rosenberg J, Berkowtiz GS, Chitkara U, Berkowitz RL. Umbilical and uterine artery flow velocity waveforms effect of the sampling site on Doppler ratios. J Ultrasound Med 1989;8:171.
18. Reuwer PJ, Nuyen WC, Beijer HJM, et al. Characteristics of flow velocities in the umbilical arteries, assessed by Doppler ultrasound. Eur J Obstet Gynaecol Reprod Biol 1984;17:397.
19. Thompson RS, Stevens RJ. A mathematical mode for interpretation of Doppler velocity waveform indices. Med Biol Eng Comput 1989;27:269.
20. Thompson RS, Trudinger BJ. Doppler waveform pulsatility index and resistance, pressure and flow in the umbilical placental circulation: an investigation using a mathematical model. Ultrasound Med Biol 1990;16:449.
21. Guidetti DA, Diven MY, Cavalieri RL, et al. Fetal umbilical artery flow velocimetry in postdate pregnancies. Am J Obstet Gynecol 1987;1157:1521.
22. Farmakides G, Schulman H, Winter D, et al. Prenatal surveillance using non-stress testing and Doppler velocimetry. Obstet Gynecol 1988;71:184.
23. Giles WB, Trudinger BJ, Stevens D, et al. Umbilical artery flow velocity waveform analysis in normal ovine pregnancy and after caruncelectomy. J Dev Physiol 1989;11:135.
24. Trudinger BJ, Stevens D, Connelly A, et al. Umbilical artery flow velocity waveforms and placental resistance: the effects of embolization on the umbilical circulation. Am J Obstet Gynecol 1987;157:1443.
25. Morrow RJ, Adamson SL, Bull SB, Ritchie JWK. Effect of placental embolization on the umbilical arterial velocity waveform in fetal sheep. Am J Obstet Gynecol 1989;161:1056.
26. Walsh SW. Preeclampsia: an imbalance in placental prostacyclin and thromboxane production. Am J Obstet Gynecol 1985;152:335.
27. Trudinger BJ, Connelly AJ, Giles WB, Hales JR, Wilcox GR. The effects of prostacyclin and thromboxane analogue (U46619) on the fetal circulation and umbilical flow velocity waveforms. J Dev Physiol 1989;11:179.
28. Mak KKW, Gude NM, Walters WAW, Boura ALA. Effects of vasoactive autocoids on the human umbilical-fetal placental vasculature. Br J Obstet Gynaecol 1984;91:99.
29. Glance DG, Elder MG, Mytatt L. The actions of prostaglandins and their interactions with angiotensin II in the isolated perfused human placental cotyledon. Br J Obstet Gynaecol 1986;93:488.
30. Giles WB, Trudinger BJ, Baird P. Fetal umbilical artery flow velocity waveforms and placental resistance: Pathological correlation. Br J Obstet Gynaecol 1985;92:31.
31. McCowan LM, Mullen BM, Ritchie K. Umbilical artery flow velocity waveforms and the placental vascular bed. Am J Obstet Gynecol 1987;157:900.
32. Bracero LA, Beneck D, Kirshenbaum N, Pfeiffer M, Stalter P. Doppler velocimetry and placental disease. Am J Obstet Gynecol 1989;161:388.
33. Fok R, Parlova Z, Benirschke K, Paul R. The correlation of arterial lesions with umbilical artery Doppler velocimetry in the placentas of small for date pregnancies. Obstet Gynecol 1990;75:578.
34. Fox H. Pathology of the placenta. In: Bennington JL, ed. Major problems in pathology. Vol 3. Philadelphia: WB Saunders, 1978:169, 238.
35. Wilcox GR, Trudinger BJ, Cook CM, Wilcox WR, Connelly AJ. Reduced fetal platelet counts in pregnancies with abnormal Doppler umbilical flow waveforms. Obstet Gynecol 1989;75:639.
36. Trudinger BJ, Giles WB, Cook CM, Bombardieri J, Collins L. Fetal umbilical artery flow velocity waveforms and placental resistance: clinical significance. Br J Obstet Gynaecol 1985;92:23.
37. Schulman H, Fleischer A, Stern W, Farmakides G, Jagani N, Blottner P. Umbilical velocity wave ratios in human pregnancy. Am J Obstet Gynecol 1984;148:986.
38. Reuwer PJHM, Bruinse HW, Stoutenbeek P, Haspels AA. Doppler assessment of the feto-placental circulation in normal and growth retarded fetuses. Eur J Obstet Gynaecol Reprod Biol 1984;18:199.
39. Erskine RLA, Ritchie JWK. Umbilical artery blood flow characteristics in normal growth retarded fetuses. Br J Obstet Gynaecol 1985;92:605.
40. Gudmundsson S, Marsal K. Umbilical and uteroplacental blood flow velocity waveforms in pregnancies with fetal growth retardation. Eur J Obstet Gynecol Reprod Biol 1988;27:187.
41. Trudinger BJ, Cook CM, Giles WB, et al. Fetal umbilical artery velocity waveforms and subsequent neonatal outcome. Br J Obstet Gynaecol 1991;98:378.
42. Woo JS, Liang ST, Lo RLS. Significance of an absent or reversed end diastolic flow in Doppler umbilical artery waveforms J Ultrasound Med 1987;6:291.
43. Rochelson B, Schulman H, Farmakides G, et al. The significance of absent end-diastolic velocity in umbilical artery velocity waveforms. Am J Obstet Gynecol 1987;156:1213.
44. Nicholaides KH, Bilardo CM, Soothill PW, Campbell S. Ab-

sence of end diastolic frequencies in umbilical artery: a sign of fetal hypoxia and acidosis. Br Med J 1988;297:1026.
45. Trudinger BJ, Giles WB, Cook CM. Flow velocity waveforms in the maternal uteroplacental and fetal umbilical placental circulation. Am J Obstet Gynecol 1985;92:155.
46. Rochelson BC, Schulman H, Fleischer A, et al. The clinical significance of Doppler umbilical artery velocimetry in the small for gestational age fetus. Am J Obstet Gynecol 1987;156:1223.
47. Fleischer A, Schulman H, Farmakides G, et al. Uterine artery Doppler velocimetry in pregnant women with hypertension. Am J Obstet Gynecol 1986;154:807.
48. Trudinger BJ, Cook CM. Doppler umbilical and uterine flow waveforms in severe pregnancy hypertension. Br J Obstet Gynaecol 1990;97:142.
49. Landon MB, Gabbe SG, Bruner JP, Ludmir J. Doppler umbilical artery velocimetry in pregnancy complicated by insulin-dependent diabetes mellitus. Obstet Gynecol 1989;73:961.
50. Giles WB, Trudinger BJ, Cook CM. Fetal umbilical artery flow velocity time waveforms in twin pregnancies. Br J Obstet Gynaecol 1985;92:490.
51. Giles WB, Trudinger BJ, Cook CM, Connelly A. Umbilical artery flow velocity waveforms and twin pregnancy outcome. Obstet Gynecol 1988;72:894.
52. Farmakides G, Schulman H, Saldana LR, et al. Surveillance of twin pregnancy with umbilical arterial velocimetry. Am J Obstet Gynecol 1985;153:789.
53. Pretorius DH, Manchester D, Barkin S, Parker S, Nelson TR. Doppler ultrasound of twin transfusion syndrome. J Ultrasound Med 1988;7:117.
54. Giles WB, Trudinger BJ, Cook CM. Letter. J Ultrasound Med 1989;8:531.
55. Giles WB, Trudinger BJ, Cook CM, Connelly AJ. Doppler umbilical artery studies in the twin-twin transfusion syndrome. Obstet Gynecol 1990;76:1097.
56. Giles WB, Trudinger BJ, Cook CM, Connelly AJ. Umbilical artery waveforms in triplet pregnancy. Obstet Gynecol 1990; 75:813.
57. Copel JA, Grannum PA, Belanger K, Green J, Hobbins JC. Pulsed Doppler flow velocity waveforms before and after intrauterine intravascular transfusions for severe erythroblastosis fetalis. Am J Obstet Gynecol 1988;158:768
58. Rightmmire DA, Nicolaides KH, Rodeck C, Campbell S. Fetal blood velocities in rhesus isoimmunisation: relationship to gestational age and to fetal haematocrit. Obstet Gynecol 1986;68:233.
59. Anyaegbunam A, Langer O, Brustman L, Damus K, Halpert R, Merkatz IR. The application of uterine and umbilical artery velocimetry to the antenatal supervision of pregnancies complicated by maternal sickle hemoglobinopathies. Am J Obstet Gynecol 1988;159: 544.
60. Dombroski RA. Autoimmune disease in pregnancy. Med Clin North Am 1989;73:650.
61. Trudinger BJ, Stewart G, Cook CM, Connelly A, Exner T. Monitoring lupus anticoagulant positive pregnancies with umbilical artery flow velocity waveforms. Obset Gynecol 1988;72:215.
62. Trudinger BJ, Cook CM. Umbilical and uterine artery flow velocity waveforms in pregnancy associated with major fetal abnormality. Br J Obstet Gynaecol 1985;92:666.
63. Rochelson B, Kaplan C, Guzman E, Arato M, Hansen K, Trunca C. A quantitative analysis of placental vasculature in the third-trimester fetus with autosomal trisomy. Obstet Gynecol 1990;75:59.
64. Campbell S. In: Sharp F, Fraser RB, Milner RDG, eds. Fetal growth. London: Springer-Verlag, 1989:255.
65. Gill RW, Kossoff G, Warren PS, Garrett WJ. Umbilical venous-flow in normal and complicated pregnancies. Ultrasound Med Biol 1984;10:349.
66. Giles WB, Trudinger BJ, Cook CM. Fetal volume blood flow and umbilical artery flow velocity waveform analysis. A comparison. Br J Obstet Gynaecol 1986;93:461.
67. Block BSB, Llanos AJ, Creasy RK. Response of the growth retarded fetus to acute hypoxemia. Am J Obstet Gynecol 1984;148:879.
68. Warren PS, Gill RW, Fisher CC. Doppler flow studies in rhesus isoimmunization. Semin Perinatol 1987;11:375.
69. Trudinger BJ, Cook CM, Jones L, Giles WB. A comparison of fetal heart rate monitoring and umbilical artery waveforms in the recognition of fetal compromise. Br J Obstet Gynaecol 1986;93:171.
70. Farmakides G, Schulman H, Winter D, et al. Prenatal surveillance using non-stress testing and Doppler velocimetry. Obstet Gynecol 1988;71:184.
71. Berkowitz GS, Chitkara U, Rosenberg J, et al. Sonographic estimation of fetal weight and Doppler analysis of umbilical artery velocimetry in the prediction of intrauterine growth retardation: a prospective study. Am J Obstet Gynecol 1988;158:1149.
72. Chambers SE, Hoskins PR, Haddad NG, Johnstone FD, McDicken WN, Muir BB. A comparison of fetal abdominal circumference measurements and Doppler ultrasound in the prediction of small-for-dates babies and fetal compromise. Br J Obstet Gynaecol 1989;96:803.
73. Laurin J, Marsal K, Persson P-H, et al. Ultrasound measurement of fetal blood flow in predicting fetal outcome. Br J Obstet Gynaecol 1987;94:940.
74. Marsal K, Persson P. Ultrasonic measurement of fetal blood velocity waveform as a secondary diagnostic test in screening for intrauterine growth retardation. J Clin Ultrasound 1988;16:239.
75. Trudinger BJ, Cook CM, Thompson RS, Giles WB, Connelly A. Low dose aspirin therapy improves fetal weight in umbilical placental insufficiency. Am J Obstet Gynecol 1988;159:681.
76. Beattie RB, Dornan JC. Antenatal screening for intrauterine growth retardation with umbilical artery Doppler ultrasonography. Br Med J 1989;298:631.
77. Martin DH, Antenatal screening with umbilical artery Doppler ultrasonography. Br Med J 1989;298:1097.
78. Hanretty KP, Primrose MH, Neilson JP, Whittle MJ. Pregnancy screening by Doppler uteroplacental and umbilical artery waveforms. Br J Obstet Gynaecol 1989;96:1163.
79. Schulman H, Winter D, Farmakides G, et al. Pregnancy surveillance with Doppler velocimetry of uterine and umbilical arteries. Am J Obstet Gynecol 1989;160:192.
80. Vyas S, Nicolaides KH, Campbell S. Renal artery flow velocity waveforms in normal and hypoxemic fetuses. Am J Obstet Gynecol 1989;161:168.
81. Marsal K, Laurin J, Lindblad A, Lingman G. Blood flow in the fetal descending aorta. Semin Perinatol 1987;11:322.
82. Marsal K, Eik-Nes SH, Lindblad A, Lingman G. Blood flow in the fetal descending aorta, intrinsic factors affecting fetal blood flow in fetal breathing movements and cardiac arrhythmia. Ultrasound Med Biol 1984;10:339.
83. Lingman G, Marsal K. Fetal central blood circulation in the third trimester of normal pregnancy. A longitudinal study. II: aortic blood velocity waveform. Early Hum Dev 1986;13:151.
84. van Eyck J, Wladimiroff JW, Noordam MJ, Tonge HM, Prechtle HFR. The blood flow velocity waveform in the fetal descending aorta: its relationship to behavioural state in the growth retarded fetus at 37–38 weeks of gesation. Early Hum Dev 1986;14:99.
85. Lingman G, Marsal K. Fetal central blood circulation in the third trimester of normal pregnancy. A longitudinal study. I: aortic and umbilical blood flow. Early Hum Dev 1986;13:137.
86. Laurin J, Lingman G, Marsal K, Persson RH. Fetal blood flow in

pregnancies complicated by intrauterine growth retardation. Obstet Gynecol 1987;69:895.

87. Griffin D, Bilardo K, Masini L, et al. Doppler blood flow waveforms in the descending thoracic aorta of the human fetus. Br J Obstet Gynaecol 1984;91:997.
88. Jouppila P, Kirkinen P. Increased vascular resistance in the descending aorta of the human fetus in hypoxia. Br J Obstet Gynaecol 1984;91:853.
89. Tonge HM, Wladimiroff JW, Noordam MH, van Kooten C. Blood flow velocity waveforms in the descending fetal aorta: comparison between normal and growth retarded pregnancies. Obset Gynecol 1986;17:851.
90. van Lierde M, Oberweiss D, Thomas K. Ultrasonic measurement of aortic and umbilical blood flow in the human fetus. Obstet Gynecol 1984;63:801.
91. Soothill PW, Nicolaides KH, Bilardo CM, Campbell S. Relation of fetal hypoxia in growth retardation to mean blood velocity in the fetal aorta. Lancet 1986;2:1118.
92. Bilardo CM, Nicolaides KH, Campbell S. Doppler measurements of fetal and uteroplacental circulations: relationship with umbilical venous blood gases measured at cordocentesis. Am J Obstet Gynecol 1990;162:115.
93. Wladimiroff JW, van Bel F. Fetal and neonatal cerebral blood flow. Semin Perinatol 1987;11:335.
94. van den Winjngaard JAGW, Groenenberg IAL, Wladimiroff JW, Hop WCJ. Cerebral Doppler ultrasound of the human fetus. Br J Obstet Gynaecol 1989;96:845.
95. Woo JSK, Liang ST, Lo RLS, Chan FY. Middle cerebral artery Doppler flow velocity waveforms. Obstet Gynecol 1987; 70:613.
96. Kirkener P, Muller R, Huch R, Huch A. Blood flow velocity waveforms in human fetal intracranial arteries. Obstet Gynecol 1987;70:617.
97. Arbeille Ph, Roncin A, Berson M, Patat F, Pourcelot L. Exploration of the fetal cerebral blood flow by duplex Doppler-linear array system in normal and pathological pregnancies. Ultrasound Med Biol 1987;13:329.
98. Waldimiroff JW, Tonge HM, Stewart PA. Doppler ultrasound assessment of cerebral blood flow in the human fetus. Br J Obstet Gynaecol 1986;93:471.
99. Mirro R, Gonzalez A. Perinatal anterior cerebral artery Doppler flow indexes: methods and preliminary results. Am J Obstet Gynecol 1987;156:1227.
100. Campbell S, Diaz-Recasens J, Griffin DR, Pearce J, et al. New Doppler technique for assessing uteroplacental blood flow. Lancet 1983;1:675.
101. Trudinger BJ, Giles WB, Cook CM. Uteroplacental blood flow velocity time waveforms in normal and complicated pregnancy. Br J Obstet Gynaecol 1985;92:39.
102. Campbell S, Vyas S, Beweley S. Doppler uteroplacental waveforms. Lancet 1988;1:1287.
103. Cohen-Overbeek T, Pearce JM, Campbell S. The anteantal assessment of utero-placental and feto-placental blood flow using Doppler ultrasound. Ultrasound Med Biol 1985;11:329.
104. Schulman H, Fleischer A, Farmakides G, et al. Development of uterine artery compliance in pregnancy detected by Doppler ultrasound. Am J Obstet Gynecol 1986;155:1031.
105. Chambers SE, Johnstone FD, Muir BB, Hoskins P, Haddad NG, McDicken WN. The effects of placental site on the arcuate artery flow velocity waveform. J Ultrasound Med 1988;7:671.
106. Hanretty KP, Whittle M, Rubin PC. Doppler uteroplacental waveforms in pregnancy induced hypertension: a reappraisal. Lancet 1988;1:850.
107. Jacobson S-L, Imhof R, Manning N, et al. The value of Doppler assessment of the uteroplacental circulation in predicting preeclampsia or intrauterine growth retardation. Am J Obstet Gynecol 1989;162:110.
108. Campbell S, Pearce KMF, Hackett G, Cohen-Overbeek T, Hernandex C. Qualitative assessment of uteroplacental blood flow: early screening test for high risk pregnancies. Obstet Gynecol 1986;69:649.
109. Steele SA, Pearce JKM, Chamberlain GVP. Doppler ultrasound of the uteroplacental circulation as a screening test for severe preeclampsia with intra-uterine growth retardation. Eur J Obstet Gynecol Reprod Biol 1988;28:279.
110. Schulman H. The clinical implications of Doppler ultrasound examination of the uterine and umbilical arteries. Am J Obstet Gynecol 1987;136:889
111. Gudmundsson S, Marsal K. Ultrasound Doppler evaluation of uteroplacental and fetoplacental circulation in pre-eclampsia. Arch Gynecol Obstet 1988;243:199.

47

CHAPTER

FETAL BIOPHYSICAL PROFILE SCORING: APPLICATIONS IN HIGH-RISK OBSTETRICS

Frank A. Manning

In medicine in general, accurate methods for diagnosis of disease states and for prospective monitoring of the pathologic processes form the cornerstone for innovation and for implementation of strategies for therapeutic intervention. In perinatal medicine in particular, prenatal recognition of fetal disease states and intrauterine events, which may ultimately lead to fetal compromise, has been hampered by the relative inability to examine the intrauterine patient. Traditional methods of fetal risk assessment were limited until recently to relatively nonspecific clinical methods or to monitoring of a single fetal biophysical variable, the fetal heart rate. Since fetal disease encompasses a spectrum of conditions—including acute and chronic asphyxia of diverse etiologies, as well as functional and/or structural developmental anomalies—it is not surprising that clinical examination of the gravid uterus and heart rate monitoring alone may not provide a completely accurate prediction of impending fetal trouble. The advent of high-resolution dynamic ultrasound methods has created wide new vistas for fetal imaging and, in so doing, has incontrovertibly altered both the practical and the psychological basis of the practice of perinatal medicine. Instead of having only limited access to fetal biophysical events, the obstetrician is now presented with a wide array of fetal biophysical variables and responses that may be monitored accurately. As the knowledge base expands through application of this new tool, it is becoming increasingly evident that the limitations to fetal biophysical variable monitorings are due not to inaccessibility of monitoring methods, but to the practical clinical time restraints of monitoring all available data. In more graphic terms, the issue facing prenatal diagnosticians is which of the many variables to select for construction of a risk-assessment analysis. Because the etiology of fetal compromise is so diverse, biophysical markers of both acute fetal asphyxia and more long-standing chronic fetal asphyxial states must be included. These data must then be interpreted within the informational context of fetal structural integrity and the presence or absence of other hostile environmental factors that may involve fetal support structures, such as the placenta and umbilical cord. This new information source is beginning to create important changes in the practical and philosophical basis of the practice of perinatal medicine. Foremost among these changes are the following:

1. *The presence of fetal disease is determined more accurately.* Whereas the clinical significance of such improvement for the affected fetus is obvious, the corollary of the statement may be of even greater clinical importance. Improved discrimination of the fetus who is *not* at immediate risk even in the presence of risk factors in the mother permits selective conservative management, thereby avoiding potential maternal and perinatal iatrogenic complications.
2. *The progressive pathophysiology of fetal disease is defined with greater accuracy.* Balancing fetal and neonatal risks remains an integral part of perinatal management decisions. A rational decision about the need for and the timing of perinatal intervention can be reached by knowing the rate at which a perinatal disease process is progressing in a given fetus. Consider, for example, the severely growth-retarded but immature fetus exhibiting functional biophysical signs of impending fetal death. In our center we have intervened for such fetuses with birth weights of less than 600 g, which has resulted in intact perinatal survival. Alternately, the corollary is again as important clinically. In the

immature growth-retarded fetus without any functional biophysical signs of immediate compromise, conservative management based on close fetal surveillance may permit continued maturation in utero, thereby reducing the risk of neonatal immaturity-related complications.

3. *In some fetal disease states fetal prognosis may be assigned with certainty.* The risks of perinatal management decision must always be contrasted with maternal risks. For some fetal pathologic conditions, usually those involving developmental anomalies, a hopeless prognosis may be assigned with certainty. Consider, for example, the fetus with renal agenesis (Potter's syndrome). Classically, these fetuses present with early-onset severe intrauterine growth retardation and exhibit a very high frequency of intrapartum fetal distress. In the absence of accurate forewarning, operative intervention, with its attendant maternal risks, may lack any benefit for the fetus. The high incidence of fetal distress in labor in this and other anomalous fetal conditions is well described.[1] Further forewarning of fetal disease and expected prognosis can help to decide where and when delivery should take place. In the fetus with a developmental anomaly for which either in utero or neonatal therapy is an option, referral to a center capable of providing the needed care may be life-saving.
4. *Disease-specific testing schemes are becoming a practical reality.* Until recently, the method selected for antepartum fetal surveillance and the frequency of testing have been determined using arbitrary criteria. Fitting such an arbitrary model to the spectrum of fetal disease and fetal disease progression has never been satisfactory. Thus, for example, it is unclear why some centers advocate once-weekly testing for the fetus whose mother is hypertensive, since the effect of this disease state on both mother and fetus is widely variable. A more rational approach would involve initial testing to determine fetal condition and then tailoring subsequent testing in accordance with the change, if any, in maternal and fetal condition. Similarly, the application of one testing modality (eg, antepartum fetal cardiotocography) to all fetal diseases is not easily understood, since in some conditions, such as the postdates fetus, assessment of other biophysical markers of impending fetal trouble may yield superior information.[2,3] The concept of disease-specific testing, applicable with all forms of antepartum testing but best achieved with dynamic fetal ultrasound evaluation, implies consideration of both pathophysiologic characteristics and progression in selecting the method and frequency of antepartum testing. Consider again, for example, the postdates fetus (>42 completed weeks) in whom induction is difficult because of an unfavorable cervix. Frequent evaluation of amniotic fluid volume done at least twice weekly may be the preferable method of management. The fetus severely affected by the alloisoimmunization syndrome also exemplifies this principle. In the isoimmunized fetus, except in extreme circumstances, antepartum fetal heart rate monitoring offers little insight into fetal condition and prognosis. In contrast, daily assessment by a dynamic ultrasound method allows for determination of rate of change of physical signs (eg, ascites) of the disease process long before the fetal heart rate may be affected. Fetal biophysical profile scoring is a method of fetal risk surveillance based on a composite assessment of both acute and chronic markers of fetal disease. Since the method uses dynamic ultrasound monitoring, it also yields fetal morphologic and morphometric fetal data as well as information concerning the contiguous fetal structures (placenta and umbilical cord). This envelope of fetal information is then interpreted within the clinical context to arrive at a management decision. The method may be viewed as doing a physical examination of the fetus, including determination of vital signs. Specific details of the criteria for performing the test, for interpretation of results, and the impact of this method on reducing perinatal mortality and morbidity in the at-risk population are described in this chapter.

The spectrum of perinatal compromise ranges from the extremes of death and debilitating major handicap to minor, nearly imperceptible functional or structural defects. Adverse perinatal outcome, although rare, still remains a major life tragedy for the expectant couple. The goal of any prenatal fetal surveillance method is to detect disease state and to initiate therapeutic intervention when possible at an early enough stage to avoid major sequelae. By convention the perinatal death rate has been used as the end point to measure efficacy of antepartum fetal surveillance schemes, since this end point is clearly defined and not subject to observer bias or error and since it is assumed that a measurable change in this "hard" end point is associated with a concomitant change in less easily categorized "soft" measures of perinatal morbidity. In our unscreened, untested population perinatal death occurred at a rate of 12.5 per 1000 live births; this rate is disproportionately increased to 65 per 1000 in patients with recognizable maternal high-risk factors.[4] Fetal asphyxia of varying chronicity is the major contributing factor to perinatal death in about 60% of the recorded cases, with major developmental anomalies accounting for about 10% to 20% of the remaining cases. Theoretically, an effective prenatal fetal surveillance method should be expected to reduce overall perinatal mortality by recognition and intervention for those fetuses suffering from intrauterine asphyxia and those fetuses with structural or functional development anomalies for whom in utero or neonatal corrective measures are possible. Therefore, besides producing an absolute reduction in the number of deaths, an effective program should produce proportional deaths due to developmental anomalies for which no effective therapy exists. As discussed subsequently, fetal assessment by dynamic ultrasound fetal biophysical profile scoring appears to approximate these theoretical constraints.

It is important to emphasize, however, that recognition of fetal anomaly, an important contributor to perinatal disease, remains a basic advantage of fetal assessment by dynamic ultrasound methods. In our ongoing experience in some 60,000 pregnant patients, the detection rate of major life-threatening anomalies exceeds 85%.[5]

An understanding of the fetal biophysical response to hypoxemia and acidemia (asphyxia) is essential to interpret the fetal biophysical profile score (BPS). In the animal models fetal hypoxemia, usually induced by maternal isocapnic hypoxemia, results in a profound alteration in CNS-regulated fetal biophysical activities. Thus, the fetus, like its extrauterine counterpart, responds to central hypoxemia by an alteration in its movement, tone, breathing, and heart rate patterns. Specifically, hypoxemia in the fetal lamb or monkey model causes profound reduction or even cessation of breathing movements[6,7]; in the fetal lamb model it causes a significant and sustained reduction in fetal limb movements.[8] Direct experimental confirmation of a response similar to hypoxemia in the human fetus obviously falls outside accepted ethics, but indirect evidence from observation of fetuses whose mothers are hypoxemic from disease or of fetuses whose mothers smoke suggests the human fetus may react similarly.[9–11] The mechanism by which fetal hypoxemia causes a change in biophysical activities is not known but is presumed to be the result of hypoxemia-induced central nervous system cellular dysfunction. The corollary of this hypothesis is of major importance: in the presence of normal fetal biophysical activities, CNS tissue is functional and is therefore not hypoxemic. Fetal aortic body chemoreceptor responses to arterial hypoxemia create a second and important set of recognizable fetal adaptations. In the fetal lamb aortic body chemoreceptor hypoxemic stimulation induced by direct intra-arterial injection of minute amounts of cyanide or by inducing isocapnic hypoxemia in the ewe produces a profound redistribution in cardiac output such that blood flow to the brain, heart, adrenals, and placenta increases, whereas blood flow to the remaining fetal organ decreases.[12,13] In particular, aortic body chemoreceptor stimulation results in a reduction in pulmonary and renal perfusion.[13] In the last half of pregnancy the fetal kidneys and lungs are the major source of amniotic fluid production.[14] Diminished perfusion of these organs is postulated to cause reduced fluid production, leading to oligohydramnios. The relationship between oligohydramnios, as measured by an objective ultrasound method and adverse perinatal outcome in fetuses with functional renal tissue, is well described in a recent large clinical study by Chamberlain and colleagues.[15] This asphyxia-induced reflex redistribution of fetal cardiac output, when sustained or repetitive, will cause a net fall in trunk and limb and selective organ perfusion, and this phenomenon may ultimately explain the pathophysiologic process of intrauterine growth retardation in the human fetus. Furthermore, many of the asphyxia-related neonatal complications—including the occurrence of respiratory distress syndrome in the mature perinate, the increased severity of pulmonary disease in the immature perinate, necrotizing enterocolitis, and neonatal oliguria–renal failure—may be explained by this reflex response.

Fetal biophysical responses to asphyxia may then be divided into two general categories (Fig. 47-1). These are (1) acute or immediate responses (ie, a change in or a loss of CNS-regulated activities) and (2) chronic responses (ie, a reduction in amniotic fluid production [oligohydramnios], impaired fetal growth, and an increased probability of neonatal complication). In a given fetus the mix of these acute and chronic biophysical markers of asphyxial disease will vary with the se-

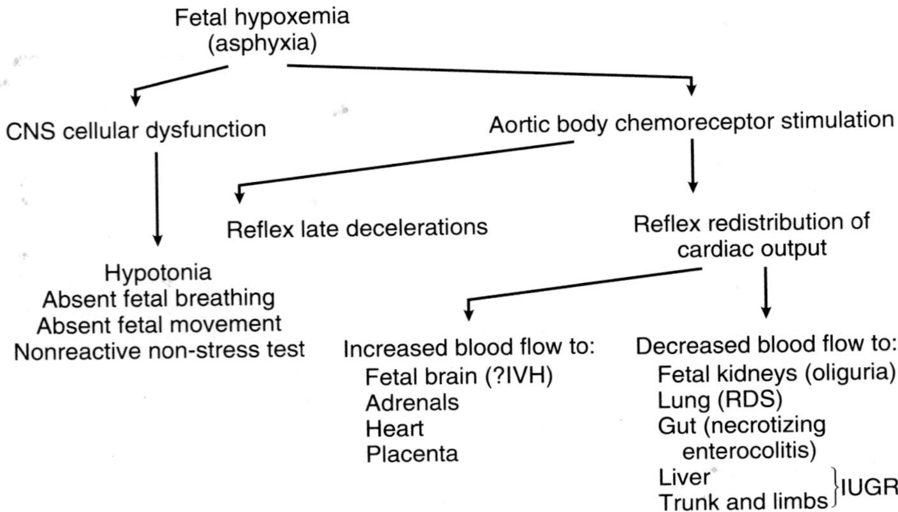

FIGURE 47–1. Schematic of the fetal biophysical effects of hypoxemia on the fetus. The conditions in parentheses refer to neonatal sequelae of fetal asphyxia. (CNS, central nervous system; IUGR, intrauterine growth retardation; IVH, intraventricular hemorrhage; RDS, respiratory distress syndrome.)

verity, the repetitive frequency, and the chronicity of the asphyxial process. From practical clinical experience it is well recognized that human fetal asphyxial insults present as a wide spectrum, ranging from acute catastrophic asphyxia (as seen with massive sudden placental abruption) to progressive indolent asphyxia (as seen in the growth-retarded fetus in the hypertensive mother). It is further recognized that in the human the superimposed effect of uterine contraction on the failing uteroplacental unit is an obvious and major compounding factor. Experimental animal models to study fetal asphyxia commonly use maternal hypoxemia as the initiating event, but in the pregnant woman maternal hypoxemia is a rare cause of fetal disease. In the compromised human fetus the nature of the asphyxial insult is most certainly different from the experimental animal model. In the human fetus the degree of fetal asphyxia varies with both the severity and progression of uteroplacental failure and with the frequency, intensity, and duration of urine contraction. Further, the CNS and reflex responses of the fetus will vary with the extent of hypoxemia. Thus, in human pregnancy a wide range of fetal biophysical response may be expected. With mild to moderate chronic uteroplacental failure fetal hypoxemia may occur only during uterine contraction with normal fetal oxygen tension between contractions. If the contractions are widely spaced in time or vary widely in intensity, then the only cumulative fetal effect may be the aortic arch chemoreceptor redistribution reflex, leading to oligohydramnios. The postmature human fetus presenting with oligohydramnios but normal CNS-regulated biophysical variables is the most common clinical example of this phenomenon. With mild to moderate uteroplacental failure and frequent and intense uterine contractions or, in severe uteroplacental failure, with or without uterine contraction, fetal hypoxemia may be severe and prolonged and result in both CNS depression (loss of acute biophysical variable) and intense aortic body chemoreceptor stimulation (oligohydramnios). In clinical practice the dysmature IUGR fetus most closely approximates this model. Acute onset of severe uteroplacental failure produces yet another clinical picture. Serial studies of the rate of decrease of amniotic fluid volume in fetuses destined to develop oligohydramnios indicate the time for progression from normal fluid to marginal fluid (largest pocket < 2 cm) to be on average 9 days, and that to decreased fluid (largest pocket < 1 cm) to be 11 days (Fig. 47-2). Therefore, with acute onset of fetal asphyxia the CNS-regulated variables may be absent while amniotic fluid volume may still be normal. Left untreated, many of these fetuses will die before there is sufficient time to develop a measurable change in amniotic fluid volume. Finally, in some clinical conditions a pathologic increase in amniotic fluid volume may occur coincidentally with an exaggerated risk of fetal asphyxia. These fetuses may also present with a loss of CNS-regulated biophysical variables alone. (The diabetic and alloisoimmunized pregnancies are good examples.)

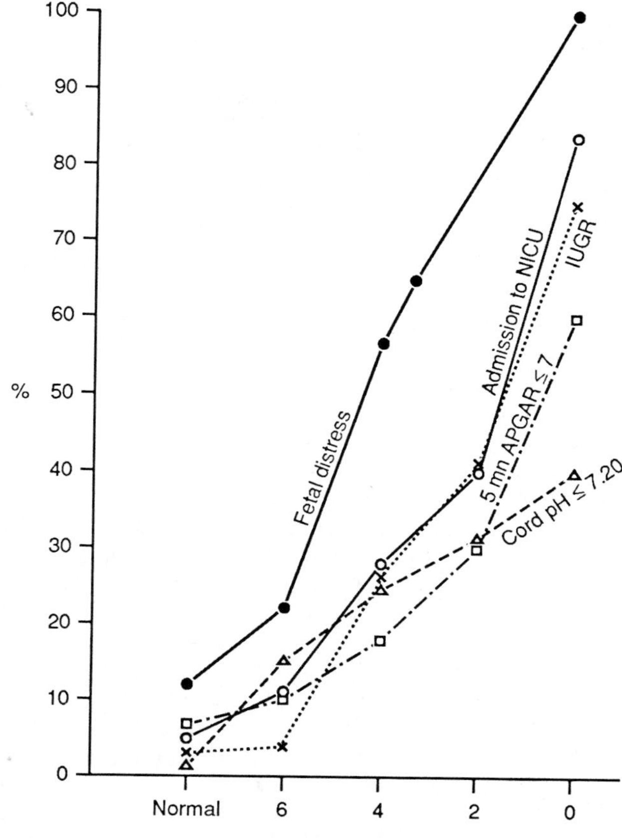

FIGURE 47–2. The relationship between any perinatal morbidity and the presence of fetal distress, admission to NICU, IUGR, 5-minute Apgar < 7, and umbilical vein pH < 7.20, either alone or in any combination. A highly significant inverse linear correlation is observed. In contrast, no relationship was observed between meconium staining of amniotic fluid and the presence of a major anomaly.

FETAL BIOPHYSICAL PROFILE SCORING: THE METHOD

At Women's Hospital of the University of Manitoba, fetal biophysical profile scoring is used only in referred patients with recognized high-risk factors; indications for testing among the first 12,620 referred high-risk patients have been reported.[16] The gestational age at which testing is begun has been arbitrarily set at the minimal gestational age at which intervention would be considered should an abnormal result be encountered. Over the years since the inception of the program, the lower limit of fetal age for testing has fallen. At present, initial testing is begun as early as 26 weeks. At each testing, in addition to the fetal BPS, fetal morphometric data are obtained (biparietal diameter, femur length, abdominal circumference), an anatomical screen for structural or functional anomaly is done, and the placenta and umbilical cord are assessed. The fetal BPS is obtained by components. The uterine cavity is scanned to identify the largest pocket of amniotic fluid and the largest vertical or near vertical axis of the fluid pocket is measured and recorded. In patients with normal amniotic fluid the presence of loops of umbilical cord with the fluid pocket do not influence the measurement. However, when oligohydramnios is present, some additional care is exercised in selecting a cord-free fluid pocket, since approximation of the umbilical vein due to looping of the cord can give a false impression of the actual size of the fluid pocket. The fetus is then scanned in a longitudinal plane such that the fetal face, forelimbs, and particularly hand(s) and thorax are visualized. On achieving the proper scan plane the time is noted and observation is continued until either normal activity is seen or 30 consecutive minutes of scanning have elapsed. Attention is paid to the presence or absence of three discrete biophysical variables:

1. Fetal breathing movements are defined by initial inward movement of the thorax with descent of the diaphragm and abdominal contents, followed by a return to the original position. Recognition of both the thoracic and abdominal component of fetal breathing is important so that extrinsic chest wall movement, which may occur with fetal movements, is not misinterpreted as representing fetal breathing. Fetal "hiccups" are interpreted as a variant of normal fetal breathing. At present the rate and pattern of the breathing movements are not considered clinically significant except in extreme cases.[17] Fetal breathing movements are said to be normal when at least 30 seconds of breathing activity have been observed.
2. Fetal movements are defined as single or clusters of activity involving the limbs or the fetal body. In our method isolated hand and arm movements are considered to represent normal movements. Fetal movements are considered as normal if at least three episodes are observed in the study period. At present other movements (eg, facial grimace, thumb sucking, tongue extension, swallowing, and eye movement), although easily seen, are not included in our criteria for normal movement.
3. The definition of fetal tone has changed as the imaging quality of ultrasound equipment has improved. In our initial reports we described tone as normal when at least one fetal movement characterized by limb or trunk extension with return to flexion was observed. With the more sophisticated ultrasound equipment we have refined the definition of fetal tone. At present, normal fetal tone is defined as at least one episode of opening of the hand with finger and thumb extension with a return to closed fist formation. In the absence of any hand movement fetal tone is still recorded as normal if the hand remains in fist formation for the entire 30-minute observation period. Abnormal fetal tone is defined by the fetal hand remaining in an open position with fingers and thumb extended despite the presence or absence of fetal movements.

Each of the four variables of the BPS is coded as normal or abnormal according to fixed criteria and is then assigned an arbitrary score of 2 if normal and 0 if abnormal (Table 47-1). In the original and early prospective clinical studies of the method, nonstress test results were also included, yielding a maximal score of 10 (five variables). Subsequently, we modified the method by selective use of the nonstress test; at the time of writing, it is our policy to perform a nonstress test only when one or more of the ultrasound-monitored variables are abnormal. The modification has caused no change in our negative predictive accuracy and has limited the use of nonstress test to less than 5% of tests.[18]

TABLE 47–1. BIOPHYSICAL PROFILE SCORING: TECHNIQUE AND INTERPRETATION

BIOPHYSICAL VARIABLE	NORMAL (SCORE = 2)	ABNORMAL (SCORE = 0)
Fetal breathing movements	≥1 episode of ≥30 sec in 30 min	Absent or no episode of ≥30 sec in 30 min
Gross body movements	≥3 discrete body–limb movements in 30 min (episodes of active continuous movement considered)	≤2 episodes of body/limb movements in 30 min as single movement
Fetal tone	≥1 episode of active extension with return to flexion of fetal limb(s) or trunk. Opening and closing of hand considered normal tone	Either slow extension with return to partial flexion movement of limb in full extension or absent fetal movement
Reactive fetal heart rate	≥2 episodes of acceleration of ≥15 bpm and of >15 sec associated with fetal movement in 20 min	>2 episodes of acceleration fetal heart rate or acceleration of <15 bpm in 20 min
Qualitative amniotic fluid volume	≥1 pocket of fluid measuring 2 cm in vertical axis	Either no pockets or largest pocket <2 cm in vertical axis

Contraction stress testing is done very infrequently (approximately three CSTs per 10,000 tests per year) and estriols are not done at all.

Clinical management is based on the test score result as interpreted against obstetrical factors (eg, favorability of the cervix for induction), the extent and progression of maternal disease, and other fetal factors—including the presence or absence of anomalies and, in selected cases, confirmation of pulmonary maturity by amniotic fluid phospholipid profile (Table 47-2).

The fetal BPS provides an accurate estimate of the risk of fetal death in the immediate future. When this risk is low, as with a normal score, intervention is indicated only for obstetrical or maternal factors. Thus, in the postdates pregnancy with a favorable cervix (obstetrical factor), we would induce labor regardless of the test score. In contrast, in the postdates fetus with an unfavorable cervix and a normal score, we would delay induction and rely on serial fetal assessment. When an abnormal score or oligohydramnios is encountered, we would induce labor regardless of the cervical state. With serious maternal disease (eg, preeclampsia), we would intervene despite a normal fetal biophysical score if the maternal condition was deteriorating. However, in the same patient with severe but stable disease, we would use a normal test score result to delay intervention until the fetal maturity was certain and the cervix was favorable for induction. Oligohydramnios in the presence of a normal fetus, with functioning renal tissue (as evidenced by fetal bladder emptying and filling) and with intact membranes, is always considered an indication for induction, despite the presence of normal movement, breathing, tone, and heart rate reactivity. This approach is based on an extensive review of the relationship of ultrasound-defined oligohydramnios to perinatal mortality,[15] and the subsequent prospective study indicating that intervention for oligohydramnios can improve perinatal outcome.[19] In the mature fetus with an equivocal test but normal fluid (score 6 of 10) we advocate delivery; when the cervix is not favorable for induction, repeat testing is undertaken within 24 hours. If subsequent testing is normal, as it will be in 75% of all cases, no intervention for fetal indication is contemplated. If the repeat test remains equivocal, or becomes abnormal, intervention for fetal indications is indicated. In the fetus with an abnormal score (<4 of 10), we would always advocate immediate intervention unless there are recognized, and remedial, compounding factors. Such factors might include a history of fetal trauma, an intrauterine condition for which treatment

TABLE 47–2. RECOMMENDED CLINICAL MANAGEMENT BY FETAL BIOPHYSICAL PROFILE SCORE

TEST SCORE	INTERPRETATION	RECOMMENDED MANAGEMENT
10/10 8/10 (NST-not done)* 8/10 (N-AFV)†	No evidence of acute or chronic asphyxia	Conservative management. No active intervention for fetal indication. Serial testing as per protocol.
8/10 (ABN-AFV)†	No evidence of acute asphyxia; chronic asphyxia likely	Deliver if gestational age > 36 weeks. If <36 weeks serial testing. Deliver if BPS < 6.
6/10 (N-AFV)	Acute asphyxia possible	If gestational age > 34 weeks, deliver. If <34 weeks repeat test within 24 hours; delivery for repeat score <6.
6/10 (ABN-AFV)	Acute asphyxia possible; chronic asphyxia likely	Deliver if gestational age > 26 weeks.
4/10 (N-AFV)	Acute asphyxia likely	If gestational age > 32 weeks, deliver. If <32 weeks repeat test same day; repeat test < 6 deliver.
4/10 (ABN-AFV)	Acute asphyxia likely; chronic asphyxia likely	Deliver if gestational age > 26 weeks.
2/10	Acute (± chronic asphyxia) very likely	Extend test in time to 60 minutes. Deliver if score remains <6 and gestational age > 26 weeks.
0/10	Acute/chronic asphyxia nearly certain	Deliver if gestational age > 26 weeks.

* Socol ML, Manning FA, Murata Y, et al. Maternal smoking causes fetal hypoxemia: experimental evidence. Am J. Obstet. Gynecol. 1982; 142: 214.

† Normal (N) and abnormal (ABN) amniotic fluid volume (AFV), from Manning FA, Wyn-Puch E, Boddy K. Effect of cigarette smoking on fetal breathing movements in normal pregnancies. Br Med J 1975; 1: 552.

is possible (eg, rhesus isoimmunization), maternal drug effects on the fetus (eg, recent narcotic or sedative administration), or a gestational age (<26 weeks) that renders extreme fetal immaturity certain.

FETAL BIOPHYSICAL PROFILE SCORING: CLINICAL RESULTS

PERINATAL OUTCOME: BLINDED STUDY

The concept of fetal biophysical profile scoring was first tested in a prospective blind study of 216 referred high-risk patients.[20] In these patients, a fetal BPS was obtained within 1 week of delivery and, in more instances (52%), it was obtained within 2 days of delivery. The mean gestational age at the time of delivery was 38.7 weeks ±0.2 SEM (range of 30 to 44 weeks). Fetal biophysical profile scores were not revealed before delivery and therefore did not influence perinatal outcome. A relationship was noted between the last fetal biophysical score and perinatal outcome, as measured by the 5-minute Apgar score, fetal distress in labor, and perinatal mortality. The incidence of low 5-minute Apgar score (<7) varied inversely with the profile score of 0. A similar increased relationship between the last fetal BPS and the incidence of fetal distress in labor was noted. Perinatal mortality increased progressively as the score decreased; the perinatal mortality with a score of 10 was 1, and increased to 600 per 1000 when the score before delivery was 0.

PERINATAL MORTALITY: CLINICAL STUDY

Recently Baskett reviewed the relationship between the fetal BPS and perinatal mortality.[21] The results of seven published series are given in Table 47-3.[16,21–26] The two largest series, which came from Canadian hospitals, were performed in an identical manner and comprise 95% of the reported experience of fetal biophysical profile scoring and perinatal mortality.[16,21] The corrected perinatal mortality rate for these two series, involving 16,804 high-risk referred patients, was 2.2 per 1000. In one of these studies Manning and colleagues contrasted perinatal mortality among 12,620 high-risk tested patients with 65,979 nontested historical controls.[16] The control population, the majority of whom were low risk, yielded a gross perinatal mortality rate of 14.3 per 1000 as compared to a rate of 7.37 per 1000 in the tested population, a decrease in mortality of 48.5%. In this study the corrected stillbirth rate among tested patients was 1.18 per 1000 as compared to a rate of 6.35 per 1000 among historical controls, a decrease of 81%. These collective data strongly suggest the application of fetal biophysical profile scoring to the high-risk pregnant population results in a dramatic improvement in perinatal mortality rates.

The false-negative rate of the testing method, defined by fetal death within a week of a last normal test result, is of considerable clinical importance, since it may permit conservative management of the high-risk pregnancy, thereby reducing the risk of perinatal immaturity and the maternal risks attendant upon expedited delivery. The false-negative rate is reported to range from 0.645 to 7 per 1000. In the two large Canadian studies involving some 24,105 high-risk fetuses there are 17 reported false-negative deaths (rate 0.7 per 1000).[21,27]

PERINATAL MORBIDITY: CLINICAL STUDY

Although perinatal mortality is an unequivocal end point against which to measure test performance, it is clearly not the ideal clinical end point, since a method of fetal assessment in which abnormal test results correlate with a high perinatal mortality rate is too late to be of clinical value. Early intervention for the abnormal score has been shown to reduce mortality, but what is the relationship test score and perinatal morbidity? This measure of test performance is more difficult to mea-

TABLE 47–3. THE RELATIONSHIP OF BIOPHYSICAL PROFILE SCORING TO PERINATAL DEATH

AUTHOR	NO. OF PATIENTS	NO. OF TESTS	PERINATAL MORTALITY (PER 1000) TOTAL	CORRECTED*	FALSE-NEGATIVE RATE (PER 1000)	FALSE-POSITIVE RATE (%)
Manning et al (1985)[16]	12620	26257	93 (7.4)	24 (1.9)	8 (0.6)	—
Baskett et al (1987)[21]	4184	9624	45 (8.6)	13 (3.1)	4 (1.0)	71.8
Platt et al (1983)[22]	286	1112	4 (14.0)	2 (7.0)	2 (7.0)	71.4
Shime et al (1984)[23]	274	274	0	0	0	100.0
Schifrin et al (1981)[24]	158	240	7 (44.3)	2 (12.7)	1 (6.3)	42.6
Vintzileos et al (1983)[25]	150	342	5 (33.3)	4 (26.6)	0	60.0
Golde et al (1984)[26]	107	459	2 (18.7)	0	0	75.0
Total	23780	54337	206 (8)	59 (2.27)	18 (0.77)	42.6–100

* Lethal anomalies excluded.

sure, because morbidity end points are "softer" (ie, more subject to intercurrent events and to observer bias). Despite these limitations the two largest studies, again both emanating from Canadian universities, have shown a strong relationship between last test score and perinatal morbidity variables.[21,28]

In our most recent study, the relationship between last test score and individual perinatal outcome variables fell into three general categories. First, a highly significant *inverse linear* correlation was observed for five variables. These were fetal distress, admission to a neonatal intensive care unit, intrauterine growth retardation, 5-minute Apgar score of ≤7, and cord pH of ≤7.20 (see Fig. 47-2). Combinations of these variables also exhibited the same highly significant inverse linear correlation with test score. The second relationship was observed between last test score and perinatal mortality both in total and by components; this relationship was *inverse and exponential* and demonstrated a highly significant correlation (Fig. 47-3). The third relationship (or *lack thereof*) was that between last test score and the incidence of meconium staining of amniotic fluid and the incidence of major anomaly (Fig. 47-4). The incidence of meconium staining rose significantly between the last normal score and the equivocal score but then remained essentially unchanged for deteriorating test scores (see Fig. 47-4). In contrast, the incidence of major anomaly was similar for all last test scores except for the very abnormal score (BPS = 0), where a significant increase is recorded (see Fig. 47-4). The explanation for these observed relationships is intriguing and may offer considerable insight into the nature of fetal compromise and the characteristics of fetal adaptive responses.

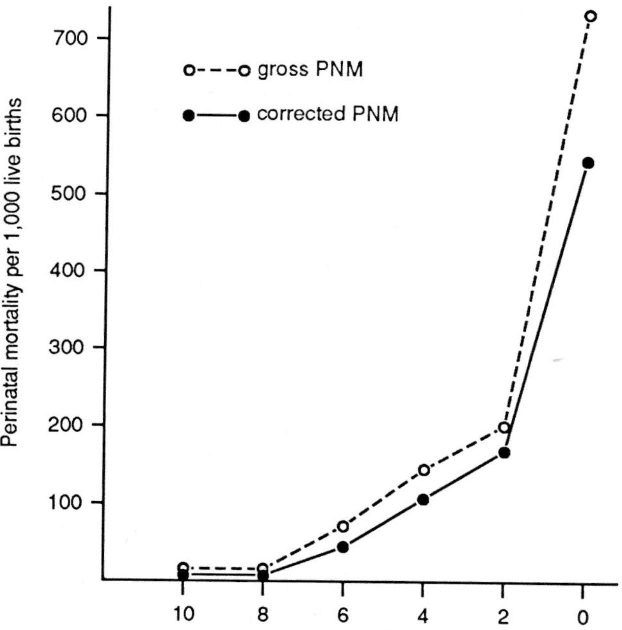

FIGURE 47–3. The relationship between perinatal mortality, either total or corrected for major anomaly, and the last BPS result. This relationship is exponential, yielding a highly significant inverse correlation using log 10 conversion.

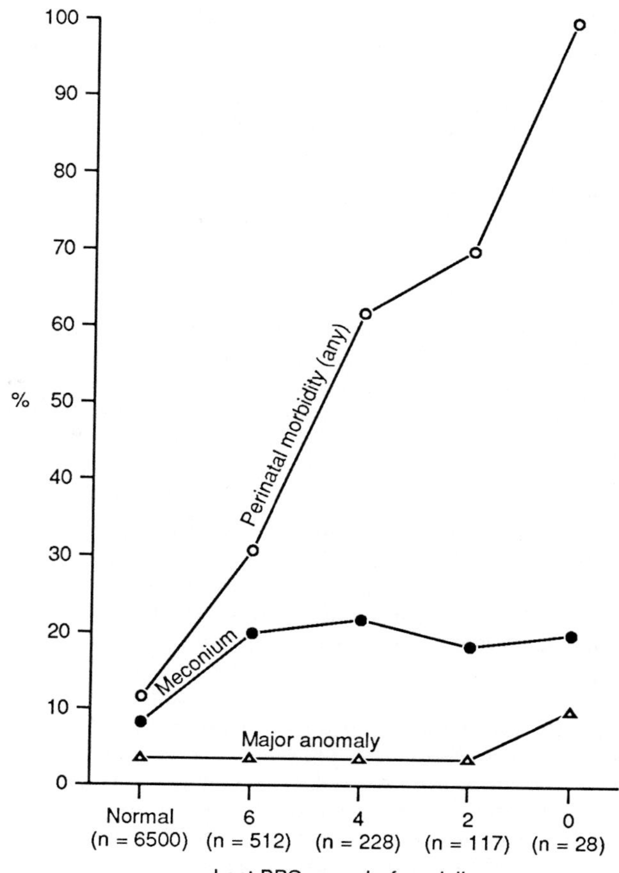

FIGURE 47–4. The relationship between the last test score and the incidence of meconium staining of amniotic fluid and the incidence of major anomaly.

The effect of hypoxemia on the human fetus may be expected to vary according to the characteristics of the hypoxemia and the fetal response. From both serendipitous observation in the human fetus and experimental observation of the animal fetus it is known that hypoxemia abolishes CNS-generated acute biophysical activities[6,9] and that the duration of abolition of activities exceeds the duration of hypoxemia, often by a considerable margin.[6–8] Variation in sensitivity of discrete CNS signal sources to graded hypoxemia is suspected but as of yet incompletely characterized. Oligohydramnios is also a consequence of hypoxemia, but it evolves more slowly and is due to different mechanisms. In the human, fetal hypoxemia, at least in the evolving stages, is unlikely to be sustained; rather, it is likely to be intermittent, the modulation of episodes that result from superimposed reduction of perfusion of the failing uteroplacental unit induced by spontaneous uterine contraction. According to this hypothesis, changes in measured fetal biophysical variables and the net effect, a change in the fetal BPS, indicate the cumulative effect of episodes of hypoxemia.

The observations reported in this study are well described by this hypothesis. The sequential loss of biophysical variables yielding the range of equivocal to abnormal score results reflects the magnitude and the repetitive frequency of antepartum episodes of fetal hypoxemia and therefore serves as a marker of the degree of placental dysfunction. As would be predicted by this theory, all markers of adverse perinatal outcome should increase as the last test score falls. The results of this study confirm these relationships. The variation in slope (defined as the incremental increase as the score falls) between select end points is also predicted by this theory. The steepest slope would be expected for fetal distress, since this end point is a nearly direct reflection of the degree of placental dysfunction as unmasked by uterine contraction. In this study the steepest slope was observed for the incidence of fetal distress reaching unity (100%) with a BPS of 0. The need for admission to a neonatal intensive care unit most likely reflects the cumulative effects of hypoxemia (both acute and chronic) and as such is a more obtuse marker. A rise in the frequency or severity of hypoxemic episodes would be predicted to increase the need for intensive postnatal care. A highly significant but slightly less steep inverse linear correlation with the last test score was observed for this variable. Depression of the 5-minute Apgar scores is interpreted as reflective of more severe central effects of fetal hypoxemia and may be predicted to occur less commonly than the reflex heart rate manifestations of hypoxemia. Similarly, umbilical vein acidosis would reflect the cumulative effects of more severe fetal hypoxemia and may be expected to occur less frequently than fetal distress. In this study the slope of the inverse linear correlation for both the low 5-minute Apgar score and umbilical vein acidosis were considerably less steep than that observed for fetal distress. The slope of the inverse linear correlation for the incidence of intrauterine growth retardation requires an additional explanation. Intrauterine growth retardation is a reflection of more chronic uteroplacental dysfunction of sufficient severity to produce a net reduction in metabolite and energy-constituent transfer, including respiratory gases.

The inverse exponential relationship observed between last test score and perinatal mortality is complex. At least two factors probably explain this curve. First, the degree and nature of fetal adaptive responses are not well studied but are likely to be substantial. Accordingly, the sharp rise in perinatal mortality with the abnormal and very abnormal scores may suggest a terminal failure of adaptive responses to chronic fetal hypoxemia. In addition, in accordance with the concept presented, it is likely that the very abnormal scores reflect the most severe degree of hypoxemia. Since death is the most severe manifestation of severe hypoxemia, it would follow that this occurrence should be restricted primarily to those fetuses who have the most severe forms of placental dysfunction. We would speculate that both explanations are involved in this exponential relationship. Thus, it appear that this spectrum of response in end points ranging from fetal distress through perinatal death is representative of the degree of compromise of placental function and that this compromise is being accurately reflected by last fetal BPS. In this context, the profile scoring method probably offers the unique method for determining not only the presence of placental dysfunction but its degree and progressive nature.

Clinical application of these data requires consideration of other obstetrical and maternal factors in addition to the test of fetal well-being. The object is not to treat the test score but to interpret test score data within the overall clinical context. In our experience it is in this context that the test scoring method has been most valuable. We would consider, for example, a score of 6 of 10 to be indicative of compromise and an indication for delivery in the mature fetus. In contrast, in the very immature fetus (<28 weeks gestation) repeat testing may be in order before intervention is recommended. Although the correlation between adverse perinatal outcome and mortality is well defined in this study, it is equally apparent that the converse of positive predictive accuracy (ie, the false-positive rate) is directly related to test scoring. We note that almost 40% of fetuses with the last score of 6 exhibited none of the markers of fetal compromise, whereas no fetuses with a score of 0 demonstrated absence of perinatal disease. Furthermore, whereas fetal hypoxemia appears to be one cause of suppression of fetal biophysical variables, it cannot be the only cause. Rhythmic variation in the frequency of biophysical activities is known to occur in the fetus. Since the study was interventional in design, it offers only incomplete information regarding the natural progression of the abnormal or equivocal score. Nonetheless, we are aware of several cases in which a score of 6 reverted to a score of normal on repeat testing and was not associated with adverse outcome. This occurrence was less frequent with a score of 4 or 2 and has not occurred with a score of 0.

The object of any method of antepartum fetal surveillance is to identify that point in the natural progression of a perinatal disease process at which the risks attendant with a continued fetal existence exceed those of delivery and neonatal life. These data confirm there is a progressive rise in the risk of adverse outcome, as measured by several end points as the fetal BPS deteriorates. On reflection, however, it is also evident that the relationships between test scores and perinatal outcome must be complex. The overt dynamics of the natural rhythm in biophysical activities, of advancing gestation age, of the rate of progression of placental dysfunction, of the recruitment of adaptive and compensatory responses of both mother and fetus to disease states, and of the superimposition of the uterine activity of labor must all influence the relationship between test score and outcome. The very complexities of these interacting factors argue for the need for gathering as many bits of data as possible to arrive at an accurate estimate of fetal risk. This principle, which forms the very basis of fetal biophysical profile scoring, is underscored by the data in this study. We speculate that the addition of the newer modalities of fetal assessment, such as arterial velocimetry and antepartum fetal blood gas determination, to the existing method of fetal biophysical profile scoring will further help to define the critical point of intervention. In contrast, reliance on any single variable to define fetal risk may no longer be acceptable.

DISEASE-SPECIFIC TESTING: BPS

THE DIABETIC PREGNANCY

The application of dynamic ultrasound monitoring, including fetal biophysical profile scoring, has yielded encouraging results in the pregnancy complicated by chemical- and insulin-dependent diabetes. Johnson and colleagues have recently reviewed an experience in 238 referred diabetic pregnancies managed by these methods.[29] There were no perinatal deaths in structurally normal infants, and the neonatal morbidity was principally that of prematurity. Morbidity in term fetuses was low, requiring only limited use of resuscitative and intensive care resources. Management predicated on the BPS achieved these results while allowing conservative management, with a low induction rate (32% overall) and a high proportion (57.4%) who labored spontaneously. Forty-five percent of the entire diabetic population had spontaneous labor and vaginal delivery at term. Considering the general risk of this population, and the high incidence of large babies (26% over 4000 g), the cesarean section rate of 23.9% overall (11.7% elective, 12.1% in labor) seems reasonable.

This management is in contrast to most conventional protocols, which rely on a policy of active intervention in the presence of fetal lung maturity and which are associated with higher rates of cesarean section, induction of labor, and neonatal morbidity. It is notable that although amniocentesis was used only 14% of the time, hyaline membrane disease was confined to five of the 33 unavoidable preterm deliveries. This may be seen as a direct consequence of safe prolongation of pregnancy beyond 37 weeks in the large majority of patients studied.

The overall incidence of infants weighing over 4000 g was high (26%), compared to the general non-diabetic population (14%). Although this might reflect less than ideal metabolic control, the incidence of true macrosomia (abdominal circumference > 90th percentile, excess fetal fat, and hydramnios on ultrasound) was much less frequent (<10%), corroborated by the low rate of reactive neonatal hypoglycemia (6.3%).

When neonatal morbidity in the 206 term fetuses is used as the end point, the accuracy of biophysical profile scoring in predicting fetal well-being (negative predictive value) was 96.5%. Seven of 200 term fetuses experienced morbidity not predicted by their normal BPS (a false-negative rate of 3.5%), but there were no significant long-term sequelae in any of these. Thus, a normal BPS conveys a low risk of neonatal morbidity, as well as a low risk of stillbirth.

Of the infants with an abnormal score (eight fetuses, 3.3%), 37.5% experienced significant morbidity. This relatively low positive predictive value (63.5% of infants with an abnormal BPS had no morbidity) may well be related to a high frequency of intervention. For example, although a normal BPS carries a stillbirth rate of only 0.65 per 1000, scores of 6 and 4 have stillbirth rates of 33 per 1000 and 56 per 1000, respectively, justifying the intervention in these cases.[16]

In addition to the reliable evaluation of fetal status by the BPS, composite ultrasound fetal assessment offers other advantages. Accurate assessment of fetal growth parameters and amniotic fluid volume on a serial basis is used to detect fetal macrosomia, indirectly reflecting the adequacy of maternal metabolic control. Ultrasound evidence of fetal macrosomia, in the presence of a normal maternal blood glucose profile, may be associated with the intrapartum complications of macrosomia and with metabolic instability in the newborn. In the Johnson study, such patients were managed with increased dietary restriction, on occasion with insulin, and elective delivery, even with normal BPS. This may have contributed to the low rate of neonatal complications and the absence of abrupt fetal death.

As expected, the incidence of congenital anomalies was increased in these diabetics (3.3%), compared to the general population (1.5%). Major anomalies were almost all confined to group I diabetics, who accounted for all deaths in this study. As mortality in diabetic pregnancies from other causes declines, congenital anomalies will become the most important cause of perinatal mortality and morbidity. This demonstrates the significance of both early pregnancy ultrasound anomaly screening and strict periconceptional diabetic control.

In summary, these data suggest that ultrasound-based fetal assessment using the BPS is well suited for fetal surveillance in the diabetic pregnancy. It is notable that no deaths among structurally normal fetuses occurred within the prescribed testing intervals. This is consistent with previous observations that a normal BPS conveys a low risk of stillbirth. The reported rate is 0.65 per 1000 among 19,221 high-risk patients.[27] Recently, we have observed a fetal death in a well-controlled insulin-dependent diabetic within 7 days of a last normal BPS. It may well be that such nonasphyxial ("acute metabolic") fetal deaths will escape detection by BPS, owing to their rapid progression. Despite this recent setback, it is clear that accurate intervention in the few who required it and a confident conservative approach in the majority led to significant clinical advantages to both mother and infant.

THE POSTDATES PREGNANCY: THE ROLE OF ULTRASOUND

The appropriate management of the obstetric patient whose gestation has exceeded 42 completed weeks (postmaturity or postdates syndrome) remains one of the most difficult problems in modern perinatal medicine. The perinatal risks of the postdates syndrome are well established; perinatal mortality doubles for each additional week after the 42nd week.[30] One simple solution to this problem would be to deliver all patients by the end of the 42nd week. However, such a nonselective approach, although done to prevent perinatal morbidity and mortality, may create iatrogenic morbidity for the mother. This nonselective approach to timing of delivery yields in our center a cesarean section rate of 42%, more than 2.5 times the rate for the general population to our institution (16.5%).

A more logical approach may be to consider both fetal and maternal prognostic factors in selecting the most appropriate management strategy. Fetal biophysical profile scoring, as measured in a study population of 12,620 high-risk patients, has proved to be a very accurate method of determination of fetal well-being and risk.[16]

Johnson and colleagues have applied this method, using a standard protocol, to 307 postdates pregnancies (Fig. 47-5).[3] In those fetuses with normal biophysical activities and normal amniotic fluid volume (n = 211) who were managed according to protocol, there were no perinatal deaths or fetal distress, low Apgar scores were infrequent (3.31% and 1.89%, respectively), and subsequent neonatal morbidity was unusual (1.9%). In contrast, in those fetuses exhibiting an abnormal BPS or oligohydramnios (n = 32), fetal distress (22%), low Apgar scores (12.5%), and neonatal morbidity (19%) were all substantially and significantly increased. When considered collectively, neonatal morbidity ranged from 3.7% when the fetal BPS was normal to 18.7% when the score was abnormal. These data indicate that fetal biophysical profile scoring facilitates differentiation of the normal noncompromised fetus from the compromised fetus within a population of postdates pregnancies. Accurate recognition of fetal risk, in turn, combined with maternal obstetric assessment (including cervical findings), allows for a rational and selective approach to patient care. The potential beneficial impact of such a selective approach in reducing maternal morbidity is clear. In the Johnson study some of this benefit was realized. The cesarean section rates for patients with a normal fetus managed conservatively and those with a normal fetus delivered because of favorable cervical findings were similar (15% and 13%, respectively) and were not increased as compared to the population at large (16.5%). In contrast, both were sharply and significantly lower than the cesarean section rate observed in patients induced in a nonselective manner on the basis of gestational age alone (42%). Perinatal mortality was absent, morbidity was low, and intervention rates were reduced, at least as compared with those observed among patients with nonselective intervention based on gestational age alone. Based on these findings, it may no longer be reasonable to elect routine delivery of all patients at or beyond 42 completed weeks of gestation. In view of the proved reliability of fetal assessment methods and the potential risk of nondiscriminative intervention, selective patient care appears to be the method of choice.

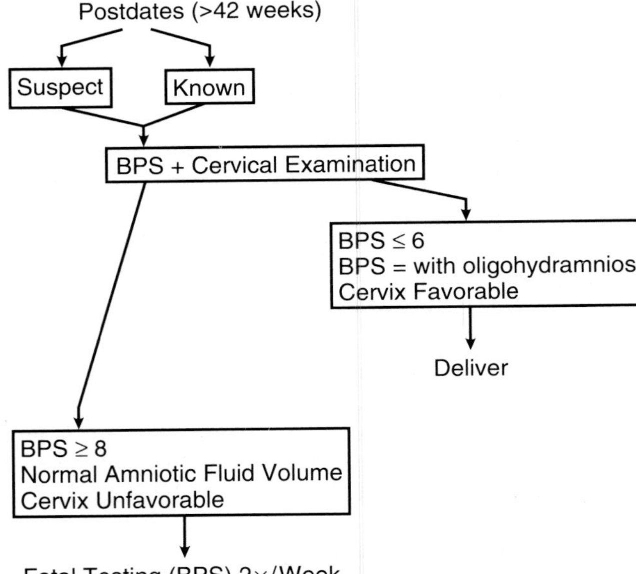

FIGURE 47–5. A management protocol for postdates pregnancy (>42 weeks) based on clinical assessment of the cervix and fetal assessment by the fetal biophysical profile scoring method. The experience with this protocol in 243 postdates pregnancies has been reported recently. (Data from Johnson JM, Harman CR, Lange IR, et al., Biophysical profile scoring in the management of the post term pregnancy: An analysis of 307 patients. Am J Obstet Gynecol 1986;154:269).

MANAGEMENT OF IUGR: INTEGRATION OF ULTRASOUND DATA

In view of the now extensive diverse information that may be accumulated by ultrasound assessment, it has become possible to recognize, categorize, and ultimately treat integration of ultrasound data (IUGR) with ever-increasing clinical precision. Application of these principles can result in a significant and sustained reduction in the mortality and morbidity of the condition. From the outset it is necessary to recognize that for the most part delivery remains the only effective therapy for the condition, although intriguing therapy of the affected fetus in utero is under study.[31] It then follows that after recognition of the condition the remaining role of ultrasound evaluation is to provide the input to balancing the equation of fetal and neonatal risks. In this context ultrasound data have moved beyond the recognition component directly into the management component, and this shift no doubt accounts for the dramatic reduction in morbidity and mortality now being reported. The algorithm for diagnosis and management of IUGR is complex and subject to variation by preference and experience. The algorithm used in our center is presented in graphic and descriptive terms (Fig. 47-6). The patient enters the diagnostic point from a variety of routes, most notably by either clinical suspicion of IUGR or recognition of suggestive signs in the course of ultrasound examination for other purposes. At initial assessment both morphometric and functional data are considered. The determination of IUGR at the outset is almost always based on the fetal morphometric data. Nonderived morphometric indices (eg, abdominal circumference) are recommended over derived indices (eg, fetal weight estimate) since the risk of compounding error is eliminated. Morphometric index ratios such as the head to abdomen ratio against gestational age are not of any real clinical value.

Normal morphometrics and normal functional signs virtually exclude the diagnosis of IUGR in the fetuses of known gestational age. Repeat assessment would be indicated only if the maternal condition were to change or the clinical impression of IUGR were to persist or exacerbate. In the patient with unknown menstrual dates, repeat assessment at an interval sufficient to measure fetal growth (or absence thereof), usually 2 weeks, is indicated. If at repeat assessment the functional signs remain normal and normal growth parameters are demonstrated, the patient may be safely assumed to have mistaken data and can be discharged from the algorithm with the previously cited provisos. If at first visit in a patient with known dates or at repeat visits in a patient with unknown dates the selected growth variable is below the lower limit ascribed (5th percentile), a diagnosis of IUGR is established and efforts are directed toward determining etiology, severity, and prognosis. In such fetuses ultrasound assessment should be done at a frequent interval (at least weekly) and conservative management should be continued, provided fetal growth is demonstrated and functional signs remain normal. Intervention in such fetuses may take place when fetal maturity is affirmed and delivery may be instituted with minimal difficulty. In the fetus with proved major anomaly a decision toward total conservative management with a view to absolute minimization of maternal risk is the usual role. In our center either a confirmed abnormal BPS (<4) or the isolated observation of oligohydramnios by defined criteria (<2 cm largest vertical pocket), or both, in an IUGR fetus of at least 25 weeks gestation are considered an indication for prompt delivery regardless of gestational age. In our center umbilical artery velocimetry and intrafetal proportion are used not to precipitate intervention but to guide the frequency of fetal surveillance. In the presence of a distinctly abnormal pulsatility index or absent diastolic flow, fetal well-being surveillance should be intensified. The use of reverse diastolic flow to prompt delivery in the IUGR fetus remains undefined at present, but it seems likely that with further experience this

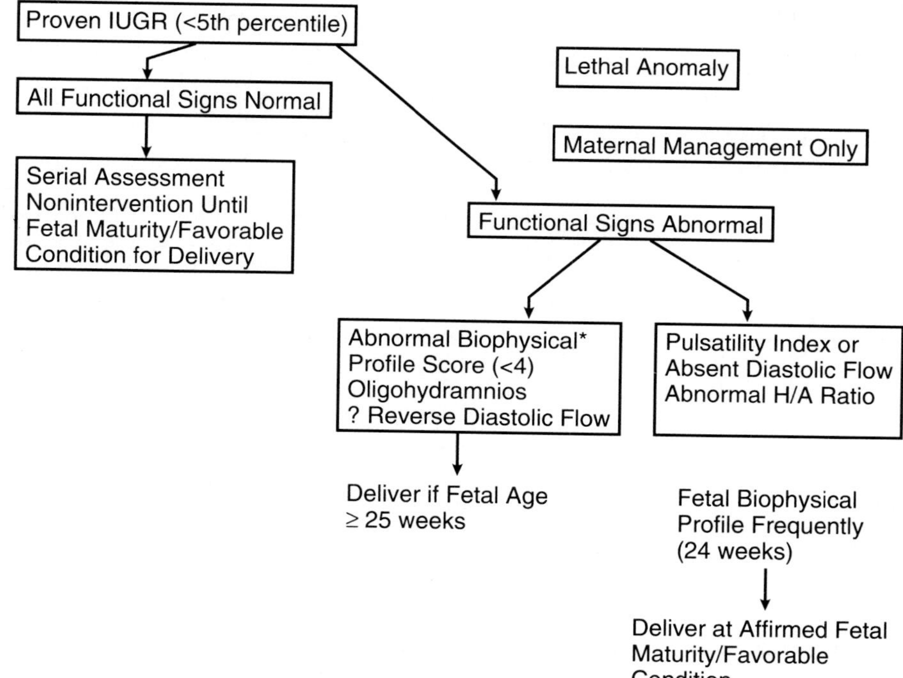

FIGURE 47–6. Proposed management of the fetus with proven IUGR as defined by morphometric indices at or below the 5th percentile for gestational age. Provided functional signs are normal, conservative management (observation) may be safely continued until low-risk delivery may be accomplished. In contrast, if functional signs are abnormal, intervention is recommended at any gestational age beyond which neonatal survival is possible.

finding will also be used to precipitate immediate delivery. In the dysmature IUGR fetus, as well as other types, it has been our policy to continue conservative management only until fetal maturity is confirmed and delivery can be accomplished with minimal maternal risk. This method of management has been applied now to more than 1200 proved IUGR fetuses, yielding a corrected perinatal mortality (anomaly exclusion) of 12.5 per 1000, a very significant reduction from the expected rate among IUGR fetuses (60 to 80 deaths per 1000). It remains our consistent policy that the observation of oligohydramnios in a fetus known to have a functional genitourinary tract and with intact membranes is always considered an indication for delivery, provided extrauterine survival is possible. This policy is derived from extensive clinical observation with or without an interventional protocol.[15,19]

OTHER CONSIDERATIONS

COMPARISON WITH OTHER METHODS

Until recently, antepartum fetal heart rate testing based on either the presence or the absence of heart rate acceleration with fetal movement (nonstress test, or NST) or the presence of fetal heart rate deceleration with induced or spontaneous uterine contraction (contraction stress test, or CST) was the primary method for antepartum fetal risk assessment.

The comparative accuracy and clinical applicability of fetal biophysical profile scoring and the nonstress test has been an area of investigation. Lavery has reviewed the perinatal mortality among patients in whom nonstress testing was the primary method of fetal assessment.[32] In nine separate studies involving 7759 patients, he noted a gross perinatal mortality rate of 12.5 per 1000 and a death rate within a week of a reactive (normal) test of 6.41 per 10,000. As noted previously, the gross perinatal mortality rate in our experience of 10,000 patients is less than seven in 1000, and the death rate within 1 week of a normal test result is less than 1 per 1000. These comparative data suggest that fetal biophysical profile scoring may be a more accurate method for identification of the fetus at risk for asphyxia. Also the observation of fetal movements and breathing (or their absence) is unequivocal and there are no interobserver discrepancies in interpretation, which exists with electronic monitoring tracings.

LIMITATIONS OF THE METHOD

Despite the advantages, fetal biophysical profile scoring remains an incomplete method for fetal risk assessment, and several important questions have yet to be answered. The exact relationship between the duration and degree of insult and the sequence of loss of activities is speculative. The interval of testing frequency (1 to 2 per week) is arbitrary, and more frequent testing is recommended when the maternal or fetal conditions are judged to be unstable. This decision is often a matter of individual judgment based on a pragmatic assessment of the situation rather than on scientific fact. In the future it may be possible to determine the need for more frequent testing by the use of additional tests in preselected high-risk situations or as more is learned about fetal pathophysiology. This is particularly true since the occurrence of fetal death within a short time after a normal score, although infrequent, indicates that the loss of biophysical variable can occur fairly rapidly sometimes.

In this connection it is important to appreciate that the interpretation of the test has always included clinical obstetric factors. For example, as already alluded to, delivery can be recommended in the face of a normal biophysical profile examination in cases of preeclampsia or postmaturity if the cervical findings are favorable. Conversely, the interpretation of absent biophysical variables must recognize the inherent periodicity of these activities or the other factors that influence fetal behavior.

The ease with which these observations can be made and their unequivocal nature can lead to a false sense of simplicity if these limitations to interpretation are not appreciated. For example, a normal BPS of 10 has been observed to change to an abnormal score over a period of hours in the presence of an initially minor but progressive marginal separation of the placenta. Obstetric training and experience are a prerequisite and greatly enhance the interpretation and use of this method.

The test is designed for particular application in cases where there is an increased risk of death or morbidity because of hypoxemia and placental dysfunction. The limitations, if any, in other situations where fetal jeopardy has a different cause have not yet been elucidated. For instance, the cause of fetal death in the diabetic mother may not necessarily be asphyxial. The heterogeneity of the underlying pregnancy complication must be a consideration in the interpretation of the test, particularly with normal results.

The subjective or semiqualitative nature of some of the measurements (eg, tone, qualitative amniotic fluid volume) is a potential source of difficulty, although in practice this is more theoretical than real. The observation of fetal tone rarely is a cause for disagreement among experienced observers. Decreased amniotic fluid is more liable to observer interpretation, but the limitations here apply more to the inexperienced observer. Measurement of an amniotic fluid pocket of 2.1 cm, for example, is not incompatible with the diagnosis of oligohydramnios by two experienced observers. Overreliance on marginal measurements of fluid in providing reassurance suggests a degree of scientific precision that is impossible to justify by the very nature of the imaging process.

It is obvious that changes and modification will occur to the system as attempts continue to substitute more objective measurements for some of the qualitative aspects of the examination. Undoubtedly, the method will evolve as more information on fetal physiology and pathology becomes available.

FUTURE MODIFICATIONS

Some changes to the current system have been reported already. The use of the NST in association with measurement of amniotic fluid volume has been reported.

Since the ultimate long-term outcome of the infant with abnormal biophysical variables has not yet been determined, modifications may be required as results become available. These modifications would be in the direction of earlier intervention, perhaps for a particular combination of variables.

The role of the contraction stress test or oxytocin challenge test in conjunction with the biophysical profile system, if any, has yet to be explored fully. Doppler waveforms or umbilical artery blood flow measurements undoubtedly will have a role in the future but as yet their precise place in clinical management is not clear. Modifications in the future will be important because with the trend to delivery at ever-earlier gestations, it becomes essential to increase the predictive accuracy to ensure that only the fetus at greatest risk will be delivered prematurely. The development of probability curves in association with other methods of assessment such as Doppler studies may refine the decision of the timing of the delivery for the clinician.

The pathophysiology of biophysical behavior during labor needs to be studied, since this information may complement fetal heart rate monitoring and its interpretation. As further work progresses in all these areas it will certainly afford the clinician even more information on which to make a considered decision.

THE FUTURE ROLE OF FETAL BIOPHYSICAL PROFILE SCORING IN OBSTETRICS

As yet there is no unanimity about which of the various methods of fetal assessment should be employed routinely. Some centers continue to use the NST almost exclusively; some combine electronic fetal monitoring testing with selected scanning for amniotic fluid; and others have moved to a greater reliance on the biophysical profile examination. Another question is the selection of patients for ancillary testing. Clinical examination is well known to be an imprecise method for the diagnosis of intrauterine growth retardation or congenital anomalies. Maternal high-risk factors do not necessarily or invariably lead to a compromised fetus. An alternative solution is to screen the general obstetric population. To date, however, legitimate concerns have been expressed in relation to cost benefit, the availability of adequately trained personnel, and the production of undue patient anxiety. These concerns need to be addressed because the obstetric benefits of ultrasound screening continue to accumulate.[33]

The question of who should be responsible for obstetric fetal assessment has not yet been resolved in this country. In many centers organized obstetric ultrasound services are the exclusive province of radiologists and obstetricians separately explore and expand various future applications of fetal assessment. Genetic amniocentesis, chorionic villus sampling, fetal surgery, and interpretation of biophysical variables in the context of the complete obstetric situation are all obstetrically oriented. "Obstetric" and "radiological" uses for ultrasound in pregnancy can be complementary, but the current situation remains confused and needs to be resolved.

Standards of training have not yet been defined clearly and are not universal throughout the country. Observation of fetal biophysical variables is simple and unequivocal, yet it is well acknowledged that detection of fetal congenital anomalies requires considerable experience. There has been no general agreement about whether different levels of skills need to be defined and whether the capability of assessing fetal condition in utero should also require the ability to carry out a complete fetal examination.

Finally, both professional and public expectations about the advantages and limitations of fetal assessment and biophysical profile scoring are sometimes unrealistic, often because of an inadequate understanding of the methods employed. Because this can be a source of misinterpretation that affects the patient's management and expectations of outcomes, the issue of education for both professional and lay persons is important and needs to be addressed. These and other questions related to the future of the biophysical examination and other forms of fetal assessment need to be considered now and answered soon.

CONCLUSION

It seems reasonable to assume that application of the traditional extrauterine methods of assessment of health and disease will continue to be of value. However, the availability of highly accurate dynamic ultrasound now permits a more detailed examination of the fetus. Biophysical responses appear to be useful in the discrimination of the fetus at risk. The issue of who is best qualified to evaluate, interpret, and act on these results is part of the evolutionary process of this method of assessment. Historic precedent and logic imply an increasingly active role for the obstetrician and perinatologist in this new frontier.

REFERENCES

1. Powell-Phillips WP, Towel M. Abnormal fetal heart rate associated with congenital anomalies. Br J Obstet Gynecol 1980;87:270.
2. Phelan JP, Platt LD, Sze-Ya Y, et al. The role of ultrasound assessment of amniotic fluid volume in the management of the post-dates pregnancy. Am J Obstet Gynecol 1985;151:304.

3. Johnson JM, Harman CR, Lange IR, et al. Biophysical profile scoring in the management of the post term pregnancy: an analysis of 307 patients. Am J Obstet Gynecol 1986;154:269.
4. Perinatal and Maternal Welfare Committee. Annual report—1985, College of Physicians and Surgeons of Manitoba. Winnipeg, Manitoba, Canada.
5. Lange IR. Congenital anomalies: detection and strategies for management. Semin Perinatol 1985;9:151.
6. Boddy K, Dawes GS, Fisher R, et al. Fetal respiratory movement, electrocortical and cardiovascular responses to hypoxemia and hypercapnia. J Physiol 1974;243:599.
7. Martin DB Jr, Murato Y, Petrie RH, Parer TT. Respiratory movements in fetal rhesus monkeys. Am J Obstet Gynecol 1974;119.
8. Natale R, Clewlow F, Dawes GS. Measurement of fetal limb movements in the lamb in utero. Am J Obstet Gynecol 1981;140:545.
9. Manning FA, Platt LD. Maternal hypoxemia and human fetal breathing movements. Obstet Gynecol 1979;53:758.
10. Manning FA, Wyn-Puch E, Boddy K. Effect of cigarette smoking on fetal breathing movements in normal pregnancies. Br Med J 1975;1:552.
11. Socol ML, Manning FA, Murata Y, et al. Maternal smoking causes fetal hypoxemia: experimental evidence. Am J Obstet Gynecol 1982;142:214.
12. Dawes GS, Duncan SLB, Lewis BV, et al. Cyanide stimulation of the systemic arterial chemoreceptors in fetal lambs. J Physiol (Lond) 1969;201:117.
13. Cohn HE, Sacks GT, Heyman M, et al. Cardiovascular responses to hypoxemia and acidemia in fetal lambs. Am J Obstet Gynecol 1974;120:817.
14. Seeds AE. Current concepts of amniotic fluid dynamics. Am J Obstet Gynecol 1980;138:575.
15. Chamberlain PF, Manning FA, Morrison I, et al. Ultrasound evaluation of amniotic fluid volume. I. The relationship of marginal and decreased amniotic fluid volumes to perinatal outcome. Am J Obstet Gynecol 1984;150:245.
16. Manning FA, Morrison I, Lange I, et al. Fetal assessment based upon fetal biophysical profile scoring: experience in 12,620 referred high risk pregnancies. I. Perinatal mortality by frequency and etiology. Am J Obstet Gynecol 1985;151:343.
17. Manning FA, Heaman M, Boyce D, et al. Intrauterine fetal tachypnea. Obstet Gynecol 1981;58:398.
18. Manning FA, Harman CR, Lange IR, et al. Modified fetal biophysical profile scoring by selective use of the non-stress test. Am J Obstet Gynecol 1987;156:709.
19. Bastide A, Manning FA, Harman CR, et al. Ultrasound evaluation of amniotic fluid: outcome of pregnancies with severe oligohydramnios. Am J Obstet Gynecol 1986;154:895.
20. Manning FA, Platt LD, Sipos L. Antepartum fetal evaluation: development of a fetal biophysical profile score. Am J Obstet Gynecol 1980;136:787.
21. Baskett TF, Allen AC, Gray JH, et al. Fetal biophysical profile and perinatal death. Obstet Gynecol 1987;70:357.
22. Platt LD, Eglinton GS, Sipos L, Broussard PM, Paul RH. Further experience with the fetal biophysical profile. Obstet Gynecol 1983;61:480.
23. Shime J, Gare JD, Andrews J, Bertrand M, Salgado J, Whillans G. Prolonged pregnancy: surveillance of the fetus and the neonate and the course of labour and delivery. Am J Obstet Gynecol 1984;148:547.
24. Schifrin BS, Guntes V, Gergley RC, et al. The role of real-time scanning in antenatal surveillance. Am J Obstet Gynecol 1981;140:525.
25. Vintzileos AM, Campbell WA, Ingardia CJ, Nochimson DJ. The fetal biophysical profile and its predictive value. Obstet Gynecol 1983;62:271.
26. Golde SH, Montero M, Anderson BG, et al. The role of nonstress tests, fetal biophysical profile and contraction stress tests in the outpatient management of insulin requiring diabetic pregnancies. Am J Obstet Gynecol 1984;148:269.
27. Manning FA, Morrison I, Harman CR, et al. Fetal assessment based on fetal biophysical profile scoring: experience in 19,221 referred high risk pregnancies. II. An analysis of false negative fetal deaths. Am J Obstet Gynecol 1987;157:880.
28. Manning FA, Harman CR, Morrison I, et al. Fetal assessment based on fetal biophysical profile scoring. IV. An analysis of perinatal morbidity and mortality. Am J Obstet Gynecol 1990; 162:703.
29. Johnson JM, Lange IR, Harman CR, et al. Biophysical profile scoring in the management of the diabetic pregnancy. Obstet Gynecol 1988;72:841.
30. Beischer NA, Brown JB, Smith MA, Townsend L. Studies in prolonged pregnancy. I. The incidence of prolonged pregnancy. Am J Obstet Gynecol 1969;103:476.
31. Nicolaides K, Bradley RJ, Soothill P, et al. Maternal oxygen therapy for intrauterine growth retardation. Lancet 1987;1:942.
32. Lavery JP. Non-stress fetal heart rate testing. Clin Obstet Gynecol 1982;25:689.
33. Waldenstrom U, Nilsson S, Fall O, et al. Effects of routine one-stage ultrasound screening in pregnancy: a randomized controlled trial. Lancet 1988;2:585.

48

CHAPTER

ANTEPARTUM FETAL HEART RATE MONITORING

Jaye M. Shyken and Roy H. Petrie

Since its first use, electronic fetal heart rate monitoring has become an important part of antepartum and intrapartum surveillance. Initial fetal monitoring efforts used intravaginal and abdominal leads to obtain fetal electrocardiograms (ECG). However, the fetal ECG waveform proved insensitive to the occurrence and characterization of fetal distress. In 1958, Edward Hon published one of the first preliminary investigations of the use of electronic monitoring to record instantaneous fetal heart rate.[1] It was with this technology that the association between intrapartum fetal heart rate and fetal distress came to be elucidated. By 1978, electronic fetal monitoring (EFM) in labor was widely used.[2] Despite controversy regarding its value, EFM has largely supplanted intermittent intrapartum auscultation of the fetal heart rate in the United States.[3–5]

The increased use of intrapartum EFM in the 1970s was inversely proportional to the perinatal mortality rate over that period of time. Yeh and coworkers demonstrated that the majority of the decrease in perinatal mortality was due to a decrease in neonatal and intrapartum death rates.[5] The reduction in the intrapartum death rate associated with EFM was highly significant.[5,6] The amelioration in neonatal outcome statistics reflects antepartum, intrapartum, and postpartum events and improvements in obstetric, anesthetic, and neonatal intensive care over that period of time.

With the decrease in intrapartum fetal and neonatal losses, antepartum fetal loss becomes a greater determinant of perinatal mortality. Focus on prevention of these in utero fetal deaths leads to the development of antepartum testing schemes directed at the fetus at risk for perinatal demise. One of the initial applications of antepartum fetal heart rate testing was in the form of stress testing, first in the form of graded maternal exercise, and later with uterine contractions.[7] Uterine contractions increase myometrial pressure, which results in occlusion of spiral arteries and increased intra-amniotic pressure. The net result is a stress characterized by diminution of circulation in the intervillous space.[8] The rationale behind antepartum monitoring is to identify the fetus in a suboptimal intrauterine environment before the onset of irreversible damage. Fetuses with uteroplacental insufficiency who perform normally in the basal state would thereby be identified by compromise with the addition of the hypoxic stress from uterine activity. The oxytocin challenge test (OCT) was first reported in the United States in 1972 by Ray and associates.[9] The presence of late decelerations was thought to represent impairment of fetal respiratory reserves. Freeman and others have continued to be proponents of the OCT as primary antepartum surveillance.[7]

In the late 1960s, European investigators used unstressed antepartum fetal heart rate tracings to assess fetal well-being. Hammacher[10] and Kubli[11] observed that antepartum fetal heart rate accelerations predicted a healthy newborn. In 1975, Lee and colleagues classified intrapartum fetal heart rate accelerations and characterized them as the "responses of the healthy fetus to various stimuli and stresses."[12] Furthermore, observation of baseline fetal activity and heart rate accelerations was proposed to replace the OCT in cases in which the latter was contraindicated. Trierweiler and coworkers retrospectively studied baseline fetal heart rate characteristics and found no positive OCTs in the presence of fetal heart rate accelerations prior to the infusion of oxytocin.[13] Lee and associates[14] proposed the "fetal acceleration test" as an alternative for the OCT for primary surveillance, and others confirmed its worthiness in the 1970s.[15–17] The fetal acceleration test has come to be known as the nonstress test (NST).

The controversy regarding which mode of antepartum testing is most prognostic continues.[18–20] Regardless of this, antepartum testing for the at-risk fetus has become the standard of care in the United States.[21] Recent technological advances in fetal monitoring and ultrasound have made the fetus more accessible for examination. Newer techniques, are therefore being used more extensively to replace or augment the traditional NST and contraction stress test (CST). The current clinical armamentarium of antepartum surveillance techniques includes fetal movement counts, nonstress testing, contraction stress testing, fetal "stimulation" studies that augment nonstress testing, the biophysical profile, ultrasound-determined amniotic fluid volume status, Doppler ultrasound, and fetal acid–base status via funicentesis.

DEMOGRAPHIC IDENTIFICATION OF INFANTS AT RISK

Currently, fetal death after 20 weeks gestation occurs in about 1% of all pregnancies. In 50% of cases, antepartum risk factors are present; of these, 25% to 70% are amenable to prenatal modification.[22] The purpose of identifying epidemiologic risk factors for fetal death is to begin antepartum evaluation and risk-appropriate interventions in view of reducing perinatal morbidity and mortality. Ideally, preconceptional identification of risk factors is accomplished and education is begun. Failing an opportunity at preconception counseling, a history for possible antepartum perils is sought. A high-risk pregnancy is defined as one in which the relative risk of perinatal mortality over normal is 1.5. Other, more vague definitions, such as "a pregnancy with an increased risk of poor outcome,"[23] or a pregnancy with increased probability of fetal metabolic acidosis in labor, also prevail.[24] Various risk scoring systems have been devised to predict the fetus in danger of antepartum and intrapartum compromise.[25,26] Table 48-1 reflects a compilation of the major indications for antepartum testing.

The concept of uteroplacental insufficiency underlies the basis for selection of individuals who are candidates for improvement in obstetric performance by the application of antepartum surveillance techniques. Uteroplacental insufficiency implies inadequate nutritive and respiratory exchange due to decreased uterine blood flow or decreased placental surface area. Various maternal and fetal conditions predispose to uteroplacental compromise. Fetuses at risk should be observed in utero until it is believed that maximum benefit from the intrauterine environment has been achieved and that extrauterine life is superior to continued gestation.

One of the newer indications for the application of antepartum surveillance techniques is elevation of maternal serum α-fetoprotein (MSAFP). Data suggest that elevations of midtrimester MSAFP in the absence of a malformed fetus are associated with low birth weight and increased perinatal loss due to prematurity and intrauterine growth retardation,[27,28] even when amniotic

TABLE 48–1. INDICATIONS FOR ANTEPARTUM SURVEILLANCE

Hypertensive disorders
Chronic hypertension
Mild preeclampsia
Insulin-dependent diabetes mellitus
Chronic renal disease
Collagen vascular disorders
Maternal cyanotic heart disease
Hemoglobinopathies (SS, SC, S-Thal)
Decreased maternal perception of fetal movements
Elevated maternal serum AFP with normal amniotic fluid AFP
Certain medications/drugs (indomethacin, methadone)
Third trimester bleeding
Placenta previa
Preterm rupture of membranes
Suspected oligohydramnios
Intrauterine growth retardation
Post dates pregnancy (>42 weeks)
Isoimmunization
Multiple gestation
Previous unexplained fetal demise
Selected fetal anomalies
Other medical complications
Other obstetric complications

fluid α-fetoprotein (AFP) determination is normal.[29] These associations appear to be stronger when MSAFP is elevated on two occasions[27,30] and when the magnitude of MSAFP elevation is high.[31] The pathophysiologic explanation of this phenomenon may be due to midtrimester placental abnormalities in the form of chronic villitis, placental infarction, or intervillous thrombosis.[32] Elevations of MSAFP on two occasions has emerged as an indication for early third trimester ultrasound to rule out intrauterine growth retardation, with subsequent antepartum testing as needed.

Advanced maternal age (over 35 years) is epidemiologically associated with an increased risk of fetal mortality of 13.6/1000 for maternal age 35 to 39 years and 22.8/1000 for maternal age ≥ 40 years.[33] When corrected for confounding medical conditions such as diabetes, chronic hypertension, and congenital anomalies, some authors have found no increased perinatal mortality.[34–36] It appears that maternal age is not an independent risk factor for increased perinatal mortality, but is due to increases in chromosomal abnormalities,[37] in concurrent medical complications,[36] and in dizygotic multiple gestation.[38] The authors do not perform antepartum fetal heart rate testing for the indication of advanced maternal age over 35 years alone; rather, all risk factors are taken into consideration.

A number of authors feel that all pregnant patients, high-risk and low-risk alike, should undergo antepartum surveillance.[23,39] Indeed, it is unusual for a fetus under antepartum surveillance to die in utero. Wilson and Schifrin reported in 1980 that "low-risk" pregnancies contributed to half of all perinatal mortality in their review of the literature.[23] Because a reduction in perinatal mortality over the last two decades is partially due to high-risk interventions, they postulate that further reductions are possible. A universal program of antepartum fetal heart rate surveillance would prevent the problem of inaccurate risk classification or demise occurring in a patient without previously identified risk. Of course, diagnostic accuracy as measured by positive predictive value declines when the prevalence of fetal distress occurs rarely in a given population. The rare occurrence of perinatal mortality, in general, poses such a statistical problem. For each new fetus identified to be in antepartum jeopardy, a far greater number will have false-positive tests with which to contend. Ambrose stated the problem nicely: "Each obstetrician must determine the number of normal pregnancies he is willing to accept with a false positive label, considering possible iatrogenic morbidity from early delivery, in order to save the truly compromised fetus."[40] This question can only be resolved through prospective randomized trials and detailed cost analysis.

TECHNIQUES OF SURVEILLANCE

The major forms of antepartum fetal surveillance available to the clinician are fetal movement counts, the nonstress test, the contraction stress test, fetal stimulation tests (in association with fetal heart rate monitoring), the biophysical profile, amniotic fluid volume assessment, Doppler ultrasound, and funicentesis for determination of fetal acid–base status. The focus of this chapter is primarily antepartum heart rate testing. Other methods of biophysical monitoring are mentioned for completeness, but are discussed in detail elsewhere in this text.

Discussion of the relative merits of one form of testing over another is predicated on an understanding of the terms: sensitivity, specificity, positive predictive value, and negative predictive value. These terms are displayed in Table 48-2. The term "false-positive test" refers to a positive diagnostic test that occurs for a fetus with an ultimate normal perinatal outcome. A false-negative test refers to a negative result on a diagnostic test that occurs for a fetus with an abnormal perinatal outcome. The interpretation of a test result as a false positive or false negative is dependent on the outcome parameter that is measured.

TABLE 48–2. DIAGNOSTIC TESTS AND PERINATAL OUTCOMES

	ABNORMAL PERINATAL OUTCOME	NORMAL PERINATAL OUTCOME	TOTAL
Abnormal Test	a	c	a + c
Normal Test	b	d	b + d
Total	a + b	c + d	a + b + c + d

$$\text{Sensitivity} = \frac{a}{a+b}$$

$$\text{False positive rate} = \frac{c}{a+c}$$

$$\text{Negative predictive value} = \frac{d}{b+d}$$

$$\text{False negative rate} = \frac{b}{b+d}$$

$$\text{Specificity} = \frac{d}{c+d}$$

$$\text{Prevalence} = a + b + c + d$$

$$\text{Positive predictive value} = \frac{a}{a+c}$$

FETAL MOVEMENT COUNTS

Systematic assessment of fetal movements has been advocated as a method of antepartum surveillance because it is inexpensive, noninvasive, carries no contraindications, and is a reliable mode of fetal surveillance.[41,42] The observation of fetal activity in utero gives indirect evidence of an intact central nervous system.

Spontaneous fetal movements are discernible on ultrasound as early as 7.5 weeks gestation and represent one of the earliest expressions of neural activity. Maturation and integration of fetal motor expression become apparent throughout the first and early second trimester. By the age of 15 weeks, all types of newborn movements are present.[43] At 16 to 18 weeks, most women become aware of fetal activity. Timor-Tritsch,[44] among others,[43] has exhaustively classified types of fetal movements. The work of Edwards and Edwards indicates that the number of fetal movements per day increases rapidly until about midgestation, then increases steadily and is maintained at 12 to 60 movements per hour until term.[45] However, Rayburn[46] and Pearson and coworkers[47] describe perceived fetal activity to be maximal at 28 to 32 weeks gestation and to decrease gradually until delivery (Fig. 48-1). There is not, as is commonly believed, a sharp diminution in fetal activity in the days preceding delivery.

Diurnal and shorter periodic variations in fetal activity have been described by several authors who have monitored fetal activity for prolonged periods of time.[48–50] Fetuses demonstrate alternating periods of ac-

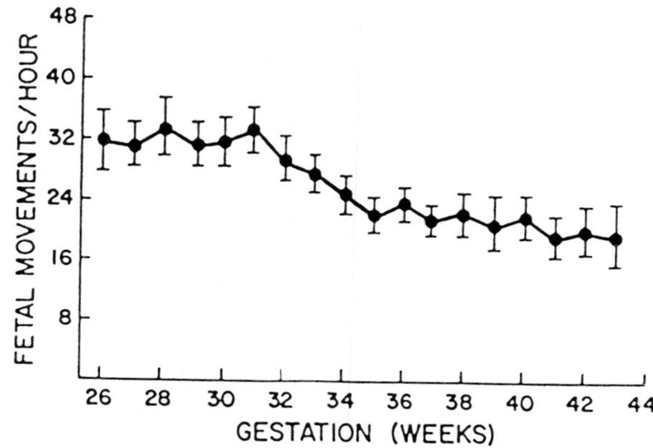

FIGURE 48–1. Comparison between perceived fetal movements per hour (mean ± 1 SD) and week of gestation. (Rayburn WF. Clinical implications from monitoring fetal activity. Am J Obstet Gynecol 1982;144:967.)

tivity with periods of inactivity that tend to be characteristic for that gestation. The longest period of lack of gross body movements in a group of fetuses in good health with normal obstetric outcome was 75 minutes.[48]

Besides gestational age and time of day, other factors that affect perceived fetal movements are preterm rupture of the membranes, tobacco, and certain medications. Tobacco[51] and certain depressant medications[52] may acutely diminish fetal motor activity. Fetal movements were increased with rupture of the membranes, as determined by Rayburn in 1980.[53] Ohel and associates, however, found no difference in the perception of fetal movements in women with premature rupture of the chorioamniotic membrane compared to uncomplicated pregnancies at any gestational age.[54] There appears to be no relationship between maternal meals[48,49] or activity[45] and the pattern of fetal activity.

Fetal movements can be quantitated by tocodynamometry, direct ultrasound techniques, or maternal assessment and tabulation. Maternal perception of fetal movements correlates well with real-time observations of fetal activity. It has been demonstrated that maternally perceived movements are visible ultrasonically, and 55% to 88% of major ultrasonically visualized movements are perceived by the mother.[53,55–57] Sadovsky and coworkers used an electromagnetic recording device and demonstrated that women perceived 87% of the observed movements.[58] When Doppler recordings were used, mothers felt 88% of fetal movements.[59] Certain variability in women's sensitivity to fetal movements is to be expected. Small fetus movements may be below the threshold for maternal perception, but can be detected with real-time and Doppler ultrasound. Most authors agree that women feel fewer than 100% of fetal movements, which makes fetal "kick counting" prone to false-positive results.[53,55–59]

The technique of fetal kick counting by the gravida is not complicated. Women at 26 or greater weeks gestation are asked to count fetal movements for an hour, 2 hours after a meal, while positioned in the left lateral recumbent position. The minimum number of fetal movements thought to be reassuring varies among investigators from ten per 2 hours to four per 12 hours.[41,42,60] Another frequently used method to assess fetal activity is to count the time necessary to achieve ten fetal movements. Fetal kick counting allows the gravida to participate in monitoring for fetal well-being and ensures at least 1 hour per day of optimal uterine perfusion in the left lateral decubitus position. Women are instructed to contact their physician if ten movements are not experienced in 2 hours.

The significance of decreased fetal activity has been addressed by several authors. Experimentally, fetal sheep demonstrate decreased movements in the face of hypoxia.[61] It appears that the fetus with inadequate reserve first seeks to conserve oxygen consumption by decreasing body movements. Sadovsky and associates observed that a marked decreased in fetal movement preceded an abnormal fetal heart rate by at least 24 hours.[62] Rayburn demonstrated that an active fetus predicted a favorable perinatal outcome as well as a reassuring antepartum fetal heart rate testing. The presence of an inactive fetal movement pattern (fewer than four fetal movements in 1 hour on 2 successive days) was less sensitive than abnormal antepartum fetal heart rate evaluation in the prediction of fetal distress or adverse perinatal outcome. Both fetal inactivity and poor antepartum heart rate testing together were highly predictive of poor obstetric outcome.[42]

Although fetal movement counting is not generally disputed among high-risk populations, should routine kick counting be introduced into general obstetric practice for low-risk women? Several investigators recommend routine fetal movement surveys in order to reduce unexpected perinatal mortality.[42,63] Neldam first demonstrated a decrease in the number of intrauterine fetal demises in women performing fetal movement counts in a prospective, randomized, clinical trial.[41] A recent, large prospective study by Moore and colleagues revealed a significant reduction in perinatal mortality from 8.7% to 2.1%, associated with the implementation of a program of routine fetal movement assessment using the count-to-ten method.[63] However, this study involved recent historical controls. In a prospective, randomized, multicenter trial by Grant and coworkers involving over 68,000 women, the application of routine fetal movement counting did not prevent fetal demise in utero in late gestation.[64] The definition of reduced fetal movements in the latter two studies varied significantly. Moore set the fetal movement alarm at fewer than ten movements in 2 hours, and Grant set the fetal movement alarm at fewer than ten movements in 10 hours on 2 successive days, or no movements in 24 hours. In addition, the former study counted movements in the evening and the latter in the morning. It is difficult, therefore, to compare protocols or to discuss the relative merit of routine screening of all pregnancies in this light. Despite the fact that the latter study was both prospective and randomized, the fetal alarm signal was set such that the false-negative rate was intentionally low and, as such, sacrificed some sensitivity.

Maternal assessment of fetal movements appears to be an effective screening test when the minimum number of fetal movements that triggers the "alarm" is not set too low. A scheme of daily kick counting also augments other forms of antepartum testing by providing day-to-day assessment of fetal condition. As with other forms of antepartum surveillance, a reassuring test has better predictive value than an abnormal one. Therefore, with our present level of understanding, abnormal kick counts should be followed with other antepartum assessment techniques.

THE NONSTRESS TEST

The nonstress test (NST) is predicated on the normal neurologic development and central control of the fetal heart. Specifically, fine-tuning of baseline heart rate and expression of accelerative patterns is dependent on the normal integration of central nervous system activity and maturing sensitivity to endogenous neurotransmitters. Baseline fetal heart rate is the product of sympathetic and parasympathetic influences. Stimulation of sympathetic nerves located in the heart releases norepinephrine, causing increased cardiac rate and contractility. Parasympathetic stimulation via the vagus nerve causes reflex slowing of conduction at the sinoatrial and atrioventricular nodes, thus decelerating fetal heart rate. *Variability* of fetal heart rate is likely more dependent on parasympathetic rather than sympathetic input. Fetal heart rate decreases with advancing gestation, indicating progressive maturation of tonic, parasympathetic expression.[65]

An expression of maturation of the normal central nervous system is the coordinated association of fetal activity and acceleration of the fetal heart rate.[66] Fetal heart rate accelerations arise with fetal movements and in response to uterine contractions or external stimuli. An acceleration occurs almost simultaneously with the onset of a fetal movement, or with a mean delay of only 1.3 seconds. Delgado demonstrated in dogs that stimulation or destruction of specific hypothalmic centers could induce or repress exertion-related acceleration of the heart rate.[67] These data indicate that these events are under coordinated control by higher brain centers.[68] Nonperiodic fetal heart rate accelerations appear to be mediated by a transient decrease in parasympathetic tone or a transient increase in sympathetic tone.[69] Regardless, movement associated acceleration of the fetal heart rate requires an intact brain stem and normal responsiveness of the myocardium.

Numerous studies have validated the association between movement-related fetal heart rate accelerations and successful perinatal outcome.[12,13,16,70–72] All accelerations do not necessarily follow maternally perceived fetal movements, but are associated with virtually all ultrasonographically visualized ones.[73] For this reason, it does not appear that accelerations in the absence of maternally identified fetal movements are any less prognostic. Some of these accelerations are likely associated with fetal movements small enough to escape maternal detection.

In the pathological condition, lack of fetal heart rate accelerations can be a manifestation of fetal hypoxia. During hypoxemia, the fetus redistributes blood flow preferentially toward the brain stem, cerebral cortex, coronary arteries, and adrenals.[74] Sheep demonstrate a decrease in forelimb movements in the presence of hypoxia.[61] Murata and coworkers demonstrated in chronically instrumented animals that loss of heart rate accelerations occurs when fetal arterial pH drops significantly from baseline levels.[75] Although late decelerations develop in the pre-acidotic fetus, lack of accelerations represents loss of central nervous system function in the hypoxic, acidotic fetus. Accelerations of the fetal heart rate in labor are uniformly associated with reassuring scalp blood pH of 7.29 ± 0.05[76] and mean fetal tissue pH of 7.27.[77] Indeed, fetal heart rate accelerations do not occur in the face of significant acid–base disturbances.[76] Decrease in fetal movements and blunted acceleratory responses both serve to cause the nonstress test to be nonreactive in hypoxic fetuses.

Gestational age has considerable influence on the result of the nonstressed cardiotocogram. Accelerations of the fetal heart rate become apparent by 25 weeks gestation and become more frequent thereafter. The ratio of fetal heart rate accelerations with fetal movements to fetal movements increases linearly after 25 weeks, from 20%, to 65% at 40 weeks.[78] Therefore, with advancing gestational age, a greater number of reactive NSTs are encountered. This relationship is depicted in Table 48-3. After 32 weeks, the vast majority (90% to 99%) of NSTs in normal fetuses should be reactive.[79,80] In addition, the amplitude of accelerations appears to increase with increasing duration of pregnancy, and appears to relate to the falling fetal heart rate baseline.[81,82] These findings have caused some investigators to question the current criteria for reactivity at gestational ages prior to 30 to 32 weeks.[81,83] Gagnon and colleagues, in a study of the effect of gestational age on fetal heart rate accelerations, found several maturational changes that occurred between 28 and 30

TABLE 48–3. THE INFLUENCE OF GESTATIONAL AGE ON FETAL HEART RATE REACTIVITY

GESTATION (WK)	TOTAL NO. OF NONSTRESS TESTS	REACTIVE NONSTRESS TESTS		NONREACTIVE NONSTRESS TESTS	
		n	%	n	%
23–27	36	6	16.7	30	83.3
28–32	32	21	65.6	11	34.4
33–37	42	38	90.5	4	9.5
38–42	18	17	94.4	1	5.6

(From Smith CV, Phelan JP, Paul RH: A prospective analysis of the influence of gestational age on the baseline fetal heart rate and reactivity in a low-risk population. Am J Obstet Gynecol 1985;153:780.)

weeks.[82] These changes are (1) a decrease in basal fetal heart rate by five beats per minute, (2) an increase in the amplitude of fetal heart rate accelerations by four beats per minute, (3) an increase in the long-term variability, and (4) the appearances of "a significant negative correlation between the mean amplitude of fetal heart rate accelerations and the mean basal fetal heart rate." Interestingly, no additional significant changes occurred between 30 and 40 weeks.[82] The consensus appears to be that a considerable number of NSTs will be expected to be nonreactive at early gestational ages due to relative immaturity of the fetal central nervous system.[79–82]

Certainly, fetal state is an important determinant of fetal heart rate variability and accelerations. Nihuis and associates demonstrated a coordinated clustering of the biophysical variables, rapid eye movements, fetal heart rate pattern, fetal breathing, and fetal movements, in utero.[66] These emerged as well-organized constellations at 36 weeks gestation and are analogous to newborn behavioral states. Timor-Tritsch and coworkers also described comparable epochs of quiet sleep, active sleep, and transitional periods clustered into longer time periods representing behavioral states.[84] In quiet states, fetal movements and fetal heart rate accelerations are largely absent and have a mean duration of 22.8 minutes. In studies of fetuses during the last 10 weeks of gestation, there is evidence that fetal movements, breathing, heart rate, and heart rate variability are governed by nonrandom repeat patterns. One must be certain that errors in the assessment of a fetus's overall pattern are not incurred by ignoring inherent periodicities. One could easily observe a fetus for less than an hour, during a sleep cycle, and make inaccurate inferences as to the overall behavioral activity of that fetus. The time between two fetal heart rate accelerations of ten beats per minute for 6 seconds in healthy term fetuses may be as long as 37 minutes.[85] Thus, current arbitrary cutoffs of 20 or 40 minutes for NST durations ignore inherent fetal biorhythms.

Besides hypoxia, fetal state, and gestational age, other factors impact on the presence or absence of antepartum fetal heart rate accelerations. Moderate maternal exercise appears to increase fetal heart rate baseline, but dose not decrease NST reactivity.[86] Smoking, conversely, is associated with decreased NST reactivity.[87] Phenobarbital, previously used frequently in the treatment of preeclampsia, has been demonstrated to result in a greater number of nonreactive nonstress tests.[88] Propranolol has also been implicated in the genesis of a nonreactive NST.[89] Lack of accelerations may therefore be a reflection of normal fetal sleep–wake cyclicity, external influences, or hypoxia.

The NST is accomplished in a noninvasive manner and carries no specific contraindications; it is performed with the woman in left lateral tilt position with her head elevated 15 to 20 degrees. Blood pressure is assessed before the NST and at every 15 minutes of testing. All attempts are made to avoid supine hypotension. In general, fetal heart rate tracings are recorded using phonocardiographic or Doppler-derived techniques. Fetal ECG derived from the maternal abdomen is also reliable for interpretation.[90] Uterine activity is recorded using a strain gauge secured to the maternal abdomen by means of an elastic strap. The mother is asked to record fetal movements via a hand-held "event marker," and the results are then displayed on the tocodynamometric channel of the fetal monitor. Fetal movements can thus be related to fetal heart rate accelerations.

Technical difficulties in obtaining adequate fetal heart rate tracings may be encountered in the presence of morbid maternal obesity, excessive fetal activity, polyhydramnios, or fetal hiccoughs. Maternal hypotension or discomfort may also hamper attempts at fetal monitoring. These same obstacles also pertain to the adequate achievement and assessment of the CST.

The NST is interpreted as reactive or nonreactive. Throughout the brief history of the NST in the United States, a variety of interpretive schemes have been devised to realize the best predictive value. Anywhere from one[15] to five[91] accelerations per 20-minute window have been used for the criteria for reactivity. The standard of practice adopted by the American College of Obstetricians and Gynecologists as of 1987 is to define a reactive test by the occurrence of two accelerations of at least 15 beats per minute sustained for at least 15 seconds, within a 20-minute period. Failure to meet reactive criteria within a 40-minute period constitutes a nonreactive or abnormal test.[21] It should be noted that comparison studies of nonstress testing, contraction stress testing, and other tests of fetal well-being are plagued with the problems of lack of standardization of the NST, and make relative evaluation difficult. The problem of lack of uniformity in the criteria for interpretation of the nonstress test has been addressed by Devoe[92] and others.[18]

The predictive value of a negative test is uniformly high in reviews of the literature, with a range of 72% to 100%. Overall, a reactive NST predicts a good perinatal outcome (absence of intrapartum fetal distress, mortality, neonatal depression, or complications) in 95% of cases.[93]

False-positive NST results continue to be a source of diagnostic error in the interpretation of this form of surveillance. The predictive value of a positive test remains low at 11.5% to 86%, but is below 40% in most studies.[93] In a large review, Thacker found the false-positive rate with respect to perinatal mortality to be 57% to 100%, and 44% to 92% with respect to perinatal morbidity.[18] Although excellent specificity is achieved with a reactive NST, the nonreactive NST would result in a large number of unnecessary interventions if used as the only measure of fetal well-being. Interestingly, Devoe and colleagues found the greatest test sensitivity in populations with a high percentage of Rh-sensitized and diabetic gravidas, and the lowest in populations that were largely post-dates.[93] Given our present level of understanding, a nonreactive NST must be confirmed with other tests of fetal well-being, such as the CST or biophysical profile. Several acceptable options for follow-up of the nonreactive NST exist: CST, biophysical profile, or stimulation of the monitored fetus.

False-negative nonstress test results fortunately occur infrequently. They are reported to be 0% to 2% for perinatal mortality and 1% to 15% for the occurrence of fetal distress in labor.[18] In a review by Phelan and coworkers, of 1564 women who delivered within 7 days of a reactive NST, there were four fetal deaths, for a rate of 0.26%.[94] These deaths were due to cord accidents and abruptio placenta. Twice-weekly testing would have prevented, at most, one of these deaths. Among post-date patients, however, the majority of fetal deaths occur within 3 to 5 days of testing.[95] Investigators have therefore questioned the reliability of once-weekly nonstress testing in the post-date population,[95,96] in favor of increased frequency of testing and assessment of amniotic fluid volume.[97] It is not always possible to anticipate acute, cord-related events unless variable decelerations are noted at the time of NST. When variable decelerations are noted during the NST in a post-date patient, delivery should be accomplished.

Boehm and colleagues demonstrated a significant reduction in perinatal mortality when nonstress tests were performed twice weekly in a high-risk population.[98] His study was retrospective in nature, using a historical comparison group. However, the stillbirth rate following a reactive NST fell from 6.1/1000 to 1.9/1000 after institution of twice-weekly NSTs. Schneider and associates noted that the stillbirth rate at Columbia University was lower within 4 days of a normal antepartum fetal heart rate test (0.027%), compared with a test interval of 5 to 7 days (0.11%).[99] These studies question the current concept of once-weekly, instead of twice-weekly, nonstress testing. We have also adopted the twice-weekly surveillance regimen with the understanding that the problem of false-positive NSTs are compounded.

When interpreting NST monitor strips, attention should also be directed toward other unusual fetal heart rate features. At times, variable decelerations or bradycardia may be noted. The incidence of variable decelerations or bradycardia ranges from 1.3% to 5.5% in reported series.[100–102] The presence of these decelerative patterns has been demonstrated to be associated with fetal death,[102] intrauterine growth retardation,[102] and neonatal mortality.[100] Furthermore, there is a higher incidence of fetal distress in labor, low Apgar scores, neonatal intensive care unit admissions, and nuchal cord location.[101] The presence of fetal heart rate accelerations concomitant with variable decelerations is more likely to indicate a favorable perinatal outcome.[99,101] Fetal bradycardia in the antepartum period may be due to supine hypotension or spontaneous uterine hyperstimulation. In the absence of explanatory conditions and fetal heart rate reactivity, the presence of repetitive variable decelerations should give cause to deliver the term fetus. The preterm fetus under similar conditions should have management individualized with regard to the risk of prematurity versus the risk of continued gestation. Whenever variable decelerations (whether moderate or prolonged) are found on NST, search should ensue for nuchal cord or oligohydramnios.

Modifications of the Nonstress Test

Due to the relative lack of predictive value for a nonreactive NST, several investigators have tried to modify the NST in favor of greater selectivity. Devoe described the distribution of movement-associated FHR accelerations in fetuses with normal outcomes using diagnostic windows of different sizes.[92] When short windows were chosen—10 minutes to 40 minutes—significant numbers of false-positive scores resulted. Extending the diagnostic window for the occurrence of one acceleration of 15 beats per minute for 15 seconds decreased the false-positive rate from 19.5% to 5%. Therefore, the nonreactive nonstress test rate, in the face of a normal outcome, could be improved but could not be eliminated. Mendenhall and coworkers reported success in predicting stillbirth with a nonreactive test and normal outcome with a reactive test when the criterion of one acceleration of ten beats per minute during a 30-minute observation was used.[103] Even so, 68% of women with nonreactive NSTs in the week prior to delivery had normal labor and delivery outcomes. Greater positive predictive value is possible by increasing the length of the NST to 90 minutes[104] or 120 minutes.[105] When 120 minutes was allowed to elapse in order to achieve five accelerations in 20 minutes, the predictive value of a nonreactive test was increased to 85.7% and the negative predictive value for a reactive NST was 98.5%.[105] Given that fetal activity is episodic, it is reasonable to expect that extension of the testing time would eliminate some false-positive results due to quiet sleep states of the normoxemic fetus.

Another modification of the NST proposed to decrease the number of false-positive readings and improve positive predictive value involves relaxing the criteria for reactivity in the fetus under 30 weeks gestational age. Using an acceleration amplitude of ten beats per minute for a 15-second duration, Gagnon decreased the false-positive rate from 65% by current standard criteria to 4%.[82] Using the modified criteria, Nicolaides found reactive patterns in 19 of 25 (76%) fetuses between 20 and 26 weeks demonstrated to be normoxemic via funicentesis.[106] Unfortunately, application of age-dependent criteria at different gestational ages would serve to increase the prevailing confusion, especially if the gestational age of the fetus is uncertain.

Several scoring systems have been devised using multiple parameters for NST interpretation.[107–109] Krebs and Petres achieved relatively high sensitivity (55%), specificity (99%), and positive predictive value (86%) by the use of a multiple parameter scoring system that included the evaluation of baseline fetal heart rate, fetal heart rate oscillatory frequency and oscillatory amplitude, accelerations, decelerations, and fetal movements.[109] The false-positive rate was 14%, much less than that achieved by the nonscored test (47%). All proponents of multiparameter scoring state that these systems more accurately distinguish prepathologic from pathologic situations and obviate unnecessary interventions. However, interobserver variability using multiple criteria tabulation is high, leading to low reproducibility.[110] Another potential problem with this method is that each parameter is weighted equally, assuming equal prognostic ability of each variable. Furthermore, many question the ability to read beat-to-beat variability on external tracings. Scoring systems for the nonstress test have not enjoyed widespread popularity in the United States. Rather, NSTs have been augmented with other procedures.

FETAL STIMULATION TESTS

Several investigators have aspired to decrease the incidence of false-positive tests by attempting to stimulate the fetus toward a reactive pattern. The intent of such fetal stimulation devices is to awaken a sleeping, healthy fetus and thereby distinguish it from the fetus in jeopardy. Such stimuli include ringing a bell,[15] deep palpation of the maternal abdomen,[111] administration of glucose,[112] and vibroacoustic stimulation.[113–116]

The basal frequency of spontaneous fetal movements under ordinary circumstances is very high,[43] and evaluation of stimuli intended to provoke increases in fetal activity should take this fact into consideration. Fetuses characteristically spend proportions of their time in "sleeping" and "active" states that have periodicity independent of stimulation. It may be at times difficult to prove that a putative stimulus actually invoked the desired activity response. Carefully designed studies take this information into consideration.

Manual manipulation of the fetus does not appear to improve the incidence of nonreactive results.[111,117] Maternal administration of neither orange juice[118] nor glucose[112] results in a decreased incidence of nonreactive tests or a reduction in testing time. Despite experimental evidence of futility, both dispensing orange juice and pushing the mother's abdomen continue to be performed.

The use of vibroacoustic stimulation, or fetal acoustic stimulation (FAS), generally in the form of an artificial larynx or other sound source, has been demonstrated effective in fetal arousal. When visualized with ultrasound, fetuses "startle" in response to sound stimulus applied to the maternal abdomen, beginning at about 26 weeks gestation. At 31 weeks and older, 96% of fetuses respond with increased motor activity.[113] Fetuses also respond with an increase in heart rate, which may exceed 160 beats per minute and persist for more than 15 minutes. Also, a significant shift to "awake" fetal heart rate patterns is noted.[115] In a prospective, randomized trial of NST versus NST augmented by FAS, a reduction in the length of testing and the number of nonreactive tests was demonstrated.[114]

Bradycardia or fetal heart rate decelerations have been demonstrated in association with the FAS. In these situations, the abnormal fetal heart rate response likely resulted from cord compression in association with growth retardation and oligohydramnios,[119] or a tight nuchal cord.[120] One should exercise caution in the application of FAS in the presence of oligohydramnios.

Romero and associates reviewed the available literature on FAS. Despite the number of studies performed, there was disparity of sources of stimuli, intensity and duration of stimuli, primary and secondary outcome measures, and interpretation of results. It appears that evaluation of FASs bears the same difficulties as evaluation of other tests of antepartum condition; that is, lack of standardization. They caution not to adopt wholesale this form of fetal assessment until critical assessment of efficacy and safety has been established.[121]

NEWER DEVELOPMENTS

Reliability of NST readings are dependent on the experience of the reviewer, the quality of the fetal heart rate tracing, and number of persons reviewing monitor strips. Interobserver variability can be sizable when using visual techniques.[122] Recently, computer-assisted analysis of fetal heart rate tracings has been developed that uses standard microcomputer technology.[123] Accurate determination of mean fetal heart rate and quantitation of accelerations and decelerations are then possible. Potentially, computerized techniques could improve reliability and aid the clinician in archiving and comparing an individual's NSTs over time. Clearly, such methods will not replace physician judgment.

It is now possible for the gravida to monitor fetal heart rate at home using a portable monitoring device, and then transmit the fetal heart rate recording to the hospital or clinic by telephone.[124] Home monitoring could obviate the necessity for long drives to the hospital and excessive activity, especially when bed rest is prescribed. Again, clinical trials to scrutinize this technology adequately are appropriate before wholesale acceptance of domiciliary fetal heart rate monitoring.

CONTRACTION STRESS TEST

The CST is a test of fetal well-being that involves evaluation of the fetal heart rate response to uterine contractions. In effect, fetal respiratory or oxygen reserve is assessed. When a fetus with adequate reserve is subjected to the stress of relative circulatory stasis in the intervillous space caused by uterine contractions, no ominous heart rate pattern will develop. That is, late decelerations will not be seen. Conversely, if fetal respiratory reserves are inadequate, as in the case of uteroplacental insufficiency, uterine contractions may cause fetal oxygen levels to drop to a critical level. Hypoxia stimulates fetal carotid chemoreceptors with resultant α-adrenergic response. The peripheral vasoconstriction and sudden hypertension produced via this reflex stimulate baroreceptors, which results in vagal-mediated bradycardia, manifested as late decelerations. This mechanism of late decelerations produced through the reflex arc occurs even in the absence of fetal acidemia.[125] If left unchecked, chronic hypoxic stress will lead to fetal reliance on anaerobic metabolism and acidosis. The second mechanism of late decelerations occurs in the already acidotic fetus who suffers direct myocardial depression.[126]

In general, exogenous oxytocin is used to evoke uterine contractions and is known as the oxytocin challenge test (OCT). The CST rationale and technique is explained to the patient at or prior to the first testing session. Blood pressure is measured prior to initiation of the study and every 15 minutes throughout. In semi-Fowler position, on a bed or in a recliner, the gravida has tocodynamometer and Doppler transducers applied, as in the procedure for the NST. A baseline 20-minute recording of fetal heart rate and uterine activity is accomplished. If three spontaneous contractions occur in 10 minutes, oxytocin is withheld and the procedure is considered completed. Failing a spontaneous CST, oxytocin is administered through a free-flowing intravenous line at a keep-open rate, beginning with an infusion rate of 0.5 mIU/hour. The rate is doubled every 20 minutes until three contractions in 10 minutes are achieved. When criteria for adequate uterine frequency are reached, the oxytocin is discontinued. The patient is instructed to record fetal movements by depressing a button, which represents an "event" on the uterine activity channel. At our institutions, the OCT is performed on labor and delivery, because this study follows one or more nonreassuring fetal surveillance examinations.

Nipple stimulation, rather than oxytocin, may be used to induce uterine activity. The technique of Huddelston is described.[127] The gravida is instructed to gently stroke one nipple, through her clothes, with the palmar surface of her fingers for 2 minutes. After a rest period of 5 minutes, stimulation for 2 minutes is resumed. The stimulation–rest cycle is repeated until adequate contractions are achieved. Mothers are instructed to cease breast stimulation at the onset of uterine activity until the frequency of contractions can be assessed. The use of this methodology resulted in a 2% hyperstimulation rate, with no failed tests in 345 trials.[127] Regardless of the method employed to evoke uterine contractions, the patient is monitored until uterine contractions diminish to pretest frequency and any late decelerations resolve.

Interpretation of the CST according to Freeman's criteria is outlined in Table 48-4.[7] Each tracing is evaluated for the presence or absence of late decelerations associated with contractions and the presence or absence of fetal heart rate accelerations. Initial reports of the CST employed response of the fetal heart rate to uterine contractions as the sole criterion for interpretation.[9,128] Later, criteria of the NST and heart rate accelerations were added to the interpretation of the CST to decrease the false-positive rate.[129] As in the interpretation of the NST, reactivity of the fetal heart rate indicates fetal well-being. A reactive fetal heart rate pattern in the context of the CST is defined as any acceleration of at least 15 beats per minute and of at least 15 seconds duration at any time during the testing procedure. The acceleration(s) may precede or follow the period of uterine contractions. A nonreactive tracing is defined as the absence of accelerations that qualify for a reactive reading. A positive CST is defined by the presence of consistent and persistent late decelerations associated with uterine contractions. Although several authors have used other criteria to further delineate a positive result,[9,130] it appears that late decelerations associated with 50% of uterine contractions would satisfy most authorities. A CST is said to be suspicious if late decelerations occur in association with uterine contractions but are neither consistent nor persistent. Therefore, a suspicious CST is defined by late decelerations occurring with fewer than 50% of contractions. An unsatisfactory CST occurs in the presence of insufficient tracing of fetal heart rate or inability to achieve the critical uterine contractile pattern of three contractions in 10 minutes. If late decelerations persistently accompany contractions, it is not necessary to achieve three contractions in 10 minutes to assign a positive test result.

TABLE 48–4. INTERPRETATION OF THE CONTRACTION STRESS TEST

INTERPRETATION	CRITERIA
Nonreactive	No acceleration of at least 15 bpm in amplitude or of 15-second duration during test
Reactive	Any acceleration ≥15 bpm for ≥15 seconds during test
Negative	No late deceleration with a contraction frequency of at least 3 per 10 min
Positive	Consistent, persistent late decelerations, regardless of contraction frequency, in the absence of uterine hyperstimulation
Equivocal	
Suspicious	Nonpersistent late decelerations
Hyperstimulation	Fetal heart rate deceleration in the presence of uterine activity exceeding 5 per 10 minutes or duration >90 seconds

A negative, reactive contraction stress test is thought to signify adequate placental respiratory reserve. The incidence of antepartum fetal deaths within 1 week of study per negative CST is 0.2% to 0.7%.[131] Proponents of the CST recommend subsequent examinations weekly in the presence of a stable maternal condition when the OCT is reactive and negative. The exception is insulin-dependent diabetes, in which some type of testing should occur twice weekly.

A positive, nonreactive CST is suggestive of uteroplacental insufficiency. Animal studies of intrapartum fetal demise demonstrate that late decelerations precede the loss of heart rate accelerations. Late decelerations occur with small degrees of hypoxia prior to the onset of acidemia, and loss of accelerations with late decelerations occur in the phase prior to intrauterine death.[75] Absence of fetal heart rate accelerations in the presence of repetitive late decelerations predicts persistent late decelerations in labor or in utero fetal demise in 70% of cases.[132] In 1977, Braly and Freeman reported that, in 12 patients with a positive, nonreactive CST, all had late decelerations in labor, and concluded that a trial of labor in these individuals should be avoided.[133] It should be remembered that older studies did not extensively use fetal scalp blood analysis for pH for the diagnosis of intrapartum acidosis and, in many cases, true positivity was assigned to test results based on the presence of late decelerations in labor. Based on this criterion alone, it is unclear how many of the "true positives" were premorbid infants. The position of automatic cesarean section for positive, nonreactive CSTs is somewhat extreme in view of the fact that fetal acid–base status can be monitored in labor if the fetal scalp is accessible. In the absence of other indicators of fetal well-being and inability to monitor fetal pH and base excess, cesarean section is warranted.

The positive, reactive CST may pose some clinical dilemmas for the obstetrician. Bissonette and coworkers demonstrated that 70% of their patients with fetal heart rate accelerations in the presence of a positive CST tolerated labor without distress.[132] Braly and Freeman reported that although 53% developed late decelerations in labor, all had good fetal outcomes in the absence of traumatic delivery or extreme prematurity.[133] Compared to a group of women with positive, nonreactive CSTs, women with positive, reactive CSTs have significantly lower rates of perinatal mortality, intrapartum fetal distress, low 5-minute Apgar scores, neonatal morbidity, and primary cesarean sections.[134] These data indicate that a trial of labor is warranted when there is evidence of fetal heart rate reactivity. In the preterm fetus, delivery is not indicated when the heart rate tracing is reactive. A positive, reactive CST likely represents the fetus who suffers some degree of relative hypoxia with uterine activity, but who has an intact central nervous system. Under basal conditions in the absence of uterine contractions, this fetus is well oxygenated. In cases of prematurity with a stable maternal condition, fetuses can be observed, but with heightened vigilance.

Negative, nonreactive contraction stress tests are somewhat controversial. Druzin and colleagues reported a significantly higher rate of fetal death within 7 days of a negative, nonreactive CST than of a reactive NST.[135] Grundy and associates did not substantiate their findings and found a 12% rate of congenital malformations in fetuses with negative, nonreactive results.[136] Freeman found no difference in neonatal outcome in fetuses with reactive-negative and nonreactive-negative CSTs.[137] Others have not demonstrated poor perinatal outcome with a nonreactive nonstress test followed by a negative CST.[138] Lack of reactivity of the fetal heart rate may be due to fetal sleep cycle in the short term,[68] maternal depressant medications,[88] or congenital malformations.[99] One should search for congenital malformations rather than fetal distress in the fetus with a persistently nonreactive, negative CST tracing.

The suspicious CST has been evaluated by several investigators. Bruce and coworkers found 16% of studies to be suspicious. Of 107 patients with suspicious CST results, there were no antepartum losses. Of the 67 retested, 7% converted to positive, 54% to negative, and 39% remained suspicious. All of those fetuses who converted to a positive test lacked heart rate reactivity. The lack of reactivity also strongly correlated with a persistently suspicious test.[139] Staisch found no association between suspicious CST results and neonatal morbidity or mortality.[140] Conversely, Garite described 26% of patients with a suspicious result to proceed to a positive result or perinatal demise.[141] The suspicious CST should be repeated in 24 hours or followed up with other forms of antepartum assessment. Alternatively, the patient may be delivered if there is evidence of pulmonic maturity or there are other indications for termination of pregnancy.

Equivocal tests occur as a result of uterine hyperstimulation or inability to obtain satisfactory fetal heart rate information. These always deserve a follow-up study within 24 hours. Repetition of equivocal CSTs with late decelerations due to hyperstimulation generally results in satisfactory, reactive-negative tests that predict fetal health.[142] Unsatisfactory contraction stress tests may be caused by excessive fetal activity, polyhydramnios, or maternal activity. Variable decelerations on antepartum heart rate testing in the presence of other reassuring parameters represent cord compressions. One should be suspicious for the presence of oligohydramnios which, without apparent cause, may be a result of chronic uteroplacental insufficiency.

Certain other antepartum fetal heart rate patterns deserve special attention. The loss of apparent short-term variability (which cannot reliably be recorded with indirect, external techniques) in the presence of deep, repetitive, variable decelerations on CST has been reported to signify chronic fetal asphyxic changes.[143] However, the post-term fetus with variable decelerations, even in the presence of fetal heart rate reactivity, is at risk of fetal compromise.[144] Antepartum demonstration of significant bradycardia, a reduction in heart rate of more than 40 beats per minute below baseline for 50 seconds or longer, or a heart rate of 90 beats per minute or below for 50 seconds or longer correlates with oligohydramnios, fetal distress in labor,[145,146] and stillbirth.[145] Spontaneous bradycardia during antepartum heart rate testing appears to be due to vagal reflex response to cord compromise. Some recommend increased fetal surveillance and consideration of delivery in the presence of oligohydramnios and bradycardia.[145] When these conditions coexist in the fetus with pulmonic maturity or at term, delivery is indicated. If continued gestation is chosen for the very preterm fetus, a low threshold for intervention should be considered.

The object of the CST, as with other forms of antepartum testing, is to prevent perinatal mortality. It is effective in this regard,[137] but it is not a perfect test. Staisch and coworkers performed 435 OCTs on 217 high-risk patients and blinded the attending physicians to the results. Pregnancies were terminated spontaneously or as a result of clinical indications. The worst test, rather than the last test, was used for stratification. Fetuses who had a positive CST had a statistically significant higher incidence of late decelerations in labor, low Apgar scores, and low neonatal performance scores. The perinatal mortality rate was 114/1000, compared to 31/1000 in the negative group. The negative CST group experienced a substantially lower incidence of low Apgar scores and neonatal morbidity. Moreover, 67% of the positive tests were falsely positive and 17% of the negative tests were falsely negative with respect to the occurrence of late decelerations in labor.[140] Specificity of the CST is reportedly variable, but is over 90% in half of the studies reviewed by Thacker.[18]

The incidence of false-negative CSTs is variably reported to be 3% to 21% when fetal distress in labor is considered.[18,140,147,148] It is 0% to 8% with respect to perinatal mortality in a recent large review.[18] Of course, perinatal mortality due to congenital malformations, cord accidents, abruptio placenta, or changing maternal condition may not be uniformly preventable. Another issue of import is the accuracy with which the CST is read. Freeman reported potentially preventable perinatal mortality as a result of misread antepartum heart rate tests.[137]

False-positive results are particularly problematic in the overall assessment of the efficacy and reliability of contraction stress testing. The false-positive rate is reported as high as 57%,[141] but is somewhat dependent on the outcome criteria used. Review of the literature reveals the incidence of false-positive results to be greater than 50% in 19 of 30 studies.[18] Unfortunately, intervention based on a false-negative test result could result in unnecessary morbidity due to prematurity. Therefore, unless several surveillance techniques (generally NST or CST and biophysical profile) reveal fetal compromise, attempts should be made to ascertain fetal maturity.

As an alternative to the use of oxytocin, the CST can be performed via nipple stimulation to invoke uterine contractions.[127,149–151] Nipple stimulation results in release of endogenous oxytocin, which is measurably increased at the conclusion of both successful and unsuccessful tests.[152] Failure to achieve uterine activity meeting the criteria for an adequate CST occurs in 0% to 31% of reported series requiring follow-up with the classic OCT.[149–151,153] Nipple-stimulation CST has been reported to result in uterine hyperstimulation with resultant fetal bradycardia.[154] Although Capeless and Mann[151] found no increase in uterine hyperstimulation associated with breast stimulation, when oxytocin was administered following breast stimulation, a significant increase in prolonged contractions occurred. Several investigators report predictability to be similar to the classic OCT[149–151] or to spontaneously occurring CSTs,[155] but with considerable savings in time.[149–151] Rosenzweig and associates, in a prospective, randomized trial, found the nipple-stimulation CST not to save time overall when the time necessary to perform OCT following a failed test was taken into account.[153]

Contraindications to the contraction stress test are described in Table 48-5. Essentially, any clinical situation that may predispose to preterm labor or that carries a contraindication to labor contractions would make performance of the CST imprudent. In a nonrandomized study by Braly and coworkers, the incidence of preterm labor following OCT in patients without contraindications was not increased.[156]

Disadvantages of the oxytocin challenge CST include the following:

1. The procedure is invasive, requiring peripheral access, unless spontaneous contractions or a nipple-stimulation CST is performed.
2. The time taken to achieve the desired contraction pattern may be considerable—90 to 120 minutes.
3. The occurrence of equivocal results may further add to the time necessary to achieve a prognostic test.
4. The cost is greater than that of other testing techniques that do not require intravenous access and constant attendance of personnel capable of administering an OCT.

These reasons, and the rise in popularity of ultrasonic methods of biophysical assessment, have kept the CST as a secondary method of antepartum surveillance in many institutions. When the advantages and disadvantages of the NST and CST are compared, it appears that the NST is more suitable for large-scale screening.

ANTEPARTUM TESTING TECHNIQUE COMPARISONS

It should be considered that the primary goal of both methods of antepartum heart rate testing is the timely termination of pregnancy in order to prevent perinatal mortality. In fact, to this end, both the CST and the NST have low rates of false-negative results.[94,141]

As previously outlined, the NST measures fetal well-being by assessment of functional and neurologic integration of the parasympathetic and sympathetic ner-

TABLE 48-5. CONTRAINDICATIONS TO THE CONTRACTION STRESS TEST

Classical cesarean section scar (or previous myomectomy)
Placenta previa
Premature rupture of membranes
Preterm labor in current gestation
Multiple gestation
Incompetent cervix

vous system as predicted by fetal heart rate. The CST evaluates functional respiratory reserve of the fetus by classification of fetal heart rate response to reduced intervillous space blood flow caused by uterine contractions. In general, these two tests of antepartum surveillance are considered to be interchangeable. In fact, each test evaluates different, yet overlapping, aspects of fetal condition. The presence of fetal heart rate accelerations on the CST may represent a somewhat different physiologic phenomenon than accelerations associated with fetal movements. Heart rate accelerations in the NST occur in association with movements, and accelerations during the CST occur in association with fetal movements or, at times, with uterine contractions. A uterine contraction may cause partial cord occlusion, resulting in a fall in fetal blood pressure, which stimulates fetal heart rate acceleration via carotid baroreceptor reflexes.[12] Both types of accelerations reflect autonomic integrity.

In 1982, in a multicenter trial involving over 9000 patients, Freeman reported that fetal death was significantly higher with a reactive NST than with a negative CST. He recommended the CST be used as primary surveillance.[20] This study included several centers that did not apply the criteria for performance and interpretation of the NST uniformly and did not use a single set of criteria for the performance of one test or another. Although data collection was prospective, randomization did not occur. Possibly, women who had contraindications to the CST were at higher risk for perinatal morbidity. Due to lack of randomization, population characteristics were not balanced among the NST and CST groups.

There have been only a few randomized trials that assess the efficacy of the NST, and none for the CST.[157–159] The total number of patients in these studies do not contain enough subjects to achieve the statistical power to make meaningful negative conclusions. A prospective study comparing the extended NST and nipple-stimulation tests for primary surveillance was performed using uniform protocols, criteria for interpretation, and follow-up of abnormal results. Similar results were obtained with either test, and no false-negative tests occurred.[160] Devoe reviewed the literature regarding the nonstress test as a diagnostic tool. In 26 studies, the CST was used as a back-up for a persistently nonreactive NST and in seven the CST was not used. No difference in the incidence of abnormal outcomes was seen.[93] The nonstress test and the contraction stress test have been found to be of similar predictive value in the identification of an unhealthy fetus.[18,99]

Correlation between a reactive NST and a negative CST is excellent (99.4%), but between a nonreactive NST and a positive CST is poor (24.9%).[138] Although this suggests that the CST is a better indicator of morbidity, this is only true in the presence of a nonreactive NST. Prevailing data support the continued use of the NST as a primary method of surveillance, with other testing techniques, including the CST and biophysical profile, as adjuncts for the nonreactive result.

The limitations of antepartum heart rate testing must also be recognized. The brain stem rather than the cerebral cortex controls fetal heart rate modulation. A fetus with cortical damage is capable of normal antepartum heart rate testing, yet will not have normal neurological development. An infant who has suffered in utero compromise but has an intact brain stem may not show alterations in antepartum testing. It is then possible for an anencephalic fetus to have a reassuring fetal heart rate tracing.[7]

CONGENITAL ANOMALIES

A proportion of fetuses with congenital malformations display aberrations in antepartum heart rate testing and abnormal fetal activity profiles.[161,162] As many as 51% demonstrate abnormal fetal heart rate tracings in the antepartum period or during labor.[163] An abnormal NST or CST is associated with a lethal anomaly in 2.54% of cases, whereas the general population incidence of anomalies is about 1%.[99] Loss of long-term variability and periodic abrupt decelerations as well as overt distress in labor have been described. Peculiarities of fetal movement patterns in congenitally malformed fetuses have also been described. Sadovsky warns that every attempt should be made to exclude fetal malformations when decreased fetal activity is identified in the antepartum period.[60] Indeed, fetuses identified as having persistently abnormal NSTs should undergo ultrasonic anatomic survey, most conveniently performed at the time of biophysical profile.

AMNIOTIC FLUID VOLUME

The biophysical profile, discussed elsewhere in this text, was developed to decrease false-positive results and improve diagnostic accuracy of antepartum heart rate testing methods. The concept of biophysical testing involves the detection of both acute and chronic indicators of adverse pregnancy conditions. During hypoxemia, as the fetus redistributes blood flow to essential organs, renal perfusion decreases.[74] As a result, it is hypothesized that, over time, oligohydramnios follows.

The association of oligohydramnios and poor pregnancy outcome is well documented. Factors responsible for the genesis of decreased amniotic fluid may manifest as uteroplacental insufficiency. However, variable decelerations on antepartum heart rate evaluations, often associated with oligohydramnios, may signal poor perinatal outcome, even in the absence of overt uteroplacental insufficiency.[164] Post-date pregnancies, in the presence of decreased amniotic fluid volume, are at particular risk of cord compromise.[97]

Nonstress testing at our institution is augmented by amniotic fluid volume assessment using the four-quadrant technique described by Phelan and associates.[165,166] The maternal abdomen is divided into four quadrants, with the linea nigra and umbilicus serving as landmarks. The ultrasound transducer is held perpendicular to the floor and along the longitudinal axis of the mother. The largest vertical pocket of amniotic fluid (exclusive of those filled with umbilical cord) in each quadrant is measured. The sum of the four vertical pockets of fluid constitutes the amniotic fluid index (AFI). Pregnancies complicated by suspected intrauterine growth retardation, post-dates, chronic hypertension, preeclampsia, preterm rupture of membranes, indomethacin tocolysis, diabetes, and multiple fetuses have an amniotic fluid index measured at the time of surveillance. In any case of biophysical profile performed for a nonreactive nonstress test, a four-quadrant AFI is also performed. Recently, standards for amniotic fluid volumes using this technique have been developed by Moore and coworkers.[167] An AFI of 5 cm or less is abnormal at any time in gestation, and a value of 5 to 8 cm is considered decreased. Poor perinatal outcome has been documented with AFIs of $\leq$5 cm.[165]

Clark and colleagues report no unexpected fetal demises among 5973 examinations using an antepartum testing protocol of increased intensity.[168] Nonstress testing with sound stimulation, performed twice weekly in diabetics, post-date patients, and those with intrauterine growth retardation, and weekly in all others, was used in conjunction with assessment of amniotic fluid volume employing the four-quadrant AFI.

FUNICENTESIS

The most recent addition to the clinical armamentarium for the antepartum assessment of fetal well-being is percutaneous umbilical cord blood sampling, or funicentesis. In limited clinical situations, assessment of fetal acid–base status may be used as an adjunct to other assessment techniques in order to decrease the false-positive rate and avoid unnecessary preterm delivery. In situations of extreme prematurity or in the term fetus prior to the capability of fetal scalp blood sampling, funicentesis has been performed.[169] Normal curves have been developed for fetal acid–base parameters in utero as a result of blood analyzed in fetuses studied via funicentesis for genetic indications.[170,171]

There are several situations in which knowledge of antepartum fetal acid–base status may be beneficial. A fetus who does not move in utero as a result of a neuromuscular disorder may not necessarily demonstrate normal biophysical testing. In this situation, normal acid–base status will modify the interpretation of abnormal antepartum testing results. In another situation the route of delivery, cesarean section versus a trial of labor, in a fetus with poor antepartum heart rate testing, may be decided with determination of the presence or absence of fetal respiratory reserve. Delivery of the very premature fetus on the basis of false-positive antepartum testing techniques has potentially disastrous implications. Thus, intrauterine assessment of fetal status can avoid unnecessary iatrogenic prematurity. Furthermore, Nicolaides and associates suggest that maternal hyperoxygenation by mask may be used to improve oxygenation of even hypoxemic, immature, growth-retarded fetuses in order to prolong gestation.[172]

Funicentesis for rapid fetal karyotyping may be indicated in the third trimester fetus with newly diagnosed congenital malformations and a persistently nonreactive nonstress test. The association between fetal malformations and abnormal antepartum cardiotocography is well known.[39,162,163] Likewise, fetuses with major malformations are at particular risk for fetal distress in labor.[162] When there is enough time to wait for results of peripheral blood karyotype, cesarean section for the fetus with lethal abnormalities can be avoided, should fetal distress in labor occur.

Unfortunately, blood chemistry and acid–base values give only short-term information regarding fetal well-being. Practically, repeated use of percutaneous umbilical blood sampling is impractical and potentiates the possibility of procedure-related morbidity. At present, this procedure has definite, but limited, clinical utility.

THE WASHINGTON UNIVERSITY–BARNES HOSPITAL PROTOCOL FOR ANTEPARTUM TESTING

Antepartum testing should begin at 28 weeks for most fetuses at risk for uteroplacental insufficiency. In those not previously identified as belonging to a high-risk group, testing is begun at the time of diagnosis. Some fetuses also deserve monitoring at 26 weeks, a point in gestation at which intervention by cesarean section might be performed for fetal compromise. Monitoring is begun at 26 weeks for those fetuses with severe or labile maternal diseases such as collagen vascular disease, diabetes with vascular involvement, or severe hypertensive disease. From 26 to 31 weeks, the NST is repeated weekly, and twice weekly at 32 weeks and thereafter. In cases of deteriorating fetal condition or potentially unstable maternal status, testing frequency may be performed more frequently and is individualized.

The NST is reactive if two accelerations of at least 15 beats per minute and of at least 15 seconds duration occur in any 20-minute interval. If the NST is nonreactive after 42 minutes (the duration of two typical sleep cycles), vibroacoustic stimulation is performed with a Model 5C electronic artificial larynx (AT&T, New York,

NY).[84] Monitoring is continued for another 42 minutes, or until a reactive pattern is identified. If the NST is still nonreactive, or if variable decelerations are recognized, a biophysical profile is performed. In addition, pregnancies complicated by preterm prolonged rupture of membranes, oligohydramnios, intrauterine growth retardation, indomethacin tocolysis, or postdates have amniotic fluid measurements using the four-quadrant technique. Doppler ultrasound is also employed for fetuses at risk for intrauterine growth retardation or other selected perinatal complications. Contraction stress tests are performed rarely, in the situation of a persistently nonreactive NST or a biophysical profile score of 6 or less.

SUMMARY

Current forms of antepartum heart rate testing are conspicuously more successful in correctly identifying the fetus who is normal than in identifying the fetus in jeopardy. There is no consensus regarding the best antepartum routine to evaluate fetal well-being. The biophysical tests outlined have different end points that must be considered, and measure somewhat different aspects of uteroplacental function. It is inappropriately believed by some clinicians that a reassuring antepartum heart rate test is a 1-week life insurance policy for the fetus. It should be remembered that the obstetric and metabolic stability of the mother is tantamount to a successful outcome, even in the face of a normal test. It is unrealistic to ignore the complex relationship among maternal, placental, and fetal function in favor of prognostication on the basis of a single examination.

REFERENCES

1. Hon EH. The electronic evaluation of the fetal heart rate. Am J Obstet Gynecol 1958;75:1215.
2. Williams RL, Hawes WE. Cesarean section, fetal monitoring and perinatal mortality in California. Am J Public Health 1979;69:864.
3. Low JA, Cox MJ, Karchmar EJ, McGrath MJ, Pancham SR, Piercy WN. The prediction of intrapartum fetal metabolic acidosis by fetal heart rate monitoring. Am J Obstet Gynecol 1981;139:299.
4. Shy KK, Luthy DA, Bennett FC, et al. Effects of electronic fetal-heart-rate monitoring, as compared with periodic auscultation, on the neurologic development of premature infants. N Engl J Med 1990;322:588.
5. Yeh S-Y, Diaz F, Paul RH. Ten-year experience of intrapartum fetal monitoring in Los Angeles County/University of Southern California Medical Center. Am J Obstet Gynecol 1982;143:496.
6. Shamsi HH, Petrie RH, Steer CM. Changing obstetrical practices and amelioration of perinatal outcome in a university hospital. Am J Obstet Gynecol 1979;133:855.
7. Freeman RK, Lagrew DC. The contraction stress test. In: Eden RD, Boehm FH, eds. Assessment and care of the fetus: physiological, clinical and medicolegal principles. Norwalk, CT: Appleton and Lange, 1990:351.
8. Hendricks CH. Amniotic fluid pressure recordings. Clin Obstet Gynecol 1966;9:535.
9. Ray M, Freeman RK, Pine S, Hesselgesser R. Clinical experience with the oxytocin challenge test. Am J Obstet Gynecol 1972;114:1.
10. Hammacher K. The clinical significance of cardiotocography. In: Huntingford P, Hunter M, Saling E, eds. Perinatal medicine. New York: Academic Press, 1970:80.
11. Kubli F, Boss R, Ruttgers H, et al. Antepartum fetal heart rate monitoring. In: Bear R, Campbell S, eds. The current status of FHR monitoring and ultrasound in obstetrics. London: Royal College of Obstetrics and Gynecology, 1977:28.
12. Lee CY, di Loreto PC, O'Lane JM. A study of fetal heart rate acceleration patterns. Obstet Gynecol 1975;45:142.
13. Trierweiler MW, Freeman RK, James J. Baseline fetal heart rate characteristics as an indicator of fetal status during the antepartum period. Am J Obstet Gynecol 1976;125:618.
14. Lee CY, DiLoreto PC, Logrand B. Fetal activity acceleration determination for the evaluation of fetal reserve. Obstet Gynecol 1976;48:19.
15. Rayburn WF, Duhring JL, Donaldson M. A study of fetal acceleration tests. Am J Obstet Gynecol 1978;132:33.
16. Rochard F, Schifrin BS, Goupil F, Legrand H, Blottiere J, Sureau C. Nonstressed fetal heart rate monitoring in the antepartum period. Am J Obstet Gynecol 1976;126:699.
17. Nochimson DJ, Turbeville JS, Terry JE, Petrie RH, Lundy LE: The nonstressed test. Obstet Gynecol 1978;51:419.
18. Thacker SB, Berkelman RL. Assessing the diagnostic accuracy and efficacy of selected antepartum fetal surveillance techniques. Obstet Gynecol Surv 1986;41:121.
19. Lee CY, Drukker B. The nonstress test for the antepartum assessment of fetal reserve. Am J Obstet Gynecol 1979;134:460.
20. Freeman RK, Anderson G, Dorchester W. A prospective multi-institutional study of antepartum fetal heart rate monitoring. II: contraction stress test versus nonstress test for primary surveillance. Am J Obstet Gynecol 1982;143:778.
21. Antepartum fetal surveillance. ACOG technical bulletin #107. Washington, D.C.: American College of Obstetricians and Gynecologists, 1987:1.
22. Pitkin RM. Fetal death: diagnosis and management. Am J Obstet Gynecol 1987;157:583.
23. Wilson RW, Schifrin BS. Is any pregnancy low risk? Obstet Gynecol 1980;55:653.
24. Low JA, Karchmar J, Broekhoven L, et al. The probability of fetal metabolic acidosis during labor in a population at risk as determined by clinical factors. Am J Obstet Gynecol 1981;141:941.
25. Hobel CJ, Hyvaninen MA, Okada DM, Oh W. Prenatal and intrapartum high risk screening. I: prediction of the high risk neonate. Am J Obstet Gynecol 1973;117:1.
26. Halliday HL, Jones PK, Jones SL. Method of screening obstetric patients to prevent reproductive wastage. Obstet Gynecol 1980;55:656.
27. Hamilton MPR, Abdalla HI, Whitfield CR. Significance of raised maternal serum alpha-fetoprotein in singleton pregnancies with normally formed fetuses. Obstet Gynecol 1985;65:465.
28. Wald N, Cuckle H, Stirrat GM, Bennet JM, Turnbull AC. Maternal serum alpha-fetoprotein and low birth-weight. Lancet 1977;ii:268.
29. Brumfield CG, Cloud GA, Finley SC, Cosper P, Davis RO, Huddleston JF. Amniotic fluid alpha-fetoprotein levels and pregnancy outcome. Am J Obstet Gynecol 1987;157:822.
30. Brock DJH, Barron L, Duncan P, Scrimgeour JB, Watt M. Significance of elevated midtrimester maternal plasma alpha-fetoprotein values. Lancet 1979;i:1281.

31. Wald NJ, Cuckle HS, Boreham J, Turnbull AC. Maternal serum alpha-fetoprotein and birth weight. Br J Obstet Gynaecol 1980;87:860.
32. Salafia CM, Silberman L, Herrera NE, Mahoney MJ. Placental pathology at term associated with elevated midtrimester maternal serum alpha-fetoprotein concentration. Am J Obstet Gynecol 1988;158:1064.
33. Pettiti DB. The epidemiology of fetal death. Clin Obstet Gynecol 1987;30:253.
34. Berkowitz GS, Skovron ML, Lapinski RH, Berkowitz RL. Delayed childbearing and the outcome of pregnancy. N Engl J Med 1990;322:659.
35. Grimes DA, Gross GK. Pregnancy outcomes in black women aged 35 and older. Obstet Gynecol 1981;58:614.
36. Kirz DS, Dorchester W, Freeman RK. Advanced maternal age: the mature gravida. Am J Obstet Gynecol 1985;152:7.
37. Hook EB. Rates of chromosome abnormalities at different maternal ages. Obstet Gynecol 1981;58:282.
38. Bulmer MG. The effect of parental age, parity and duration of marriage on the twinning rate. Ann Hum Genet 1959;23:454.
39. Schifrin BS, Foye G, Amato JC, Kates R, MacKenna J. Routine fetal heart rate monitoring in the antepartum period. Obstet Gynecol 1979;54:21.
40. Ambrose SE, Petrie RH. Antenatal detection of fetal compromise. Fetal Medicine Review 1989;1:27.
41. Neldam S. Fetal movements as an indicator of fetal well-being. Lancet 1980;i:1222.
42. Rayburn W, Zuspan F, Motley ME, Donaldson M. An alternative to antepartum fetal heart rate testing. Am J Obstet Gynecol 1980;138:223.
43. de Vries JIP, Visser GHA, Prechtl HFR. The emergence of fetal behaviour. I: qualitative aspects. Early Hum Dev 1982;7:301.
44. Timor-Tritsch I, Zador I, Hertz RH, Rosen MG. Classification of human fetal movement. Am J Obstet Gynecol 1976;126:70.
45. Edwards DD, Edwards JStal movement: development and time course. Science 1970;169;95.
46. Rayburn WF. Clinical implications from monitoring fetal activity. Am J Obstet Gynecol 1982;144:967.
47. Pearson JF, Weaver JB. Fetal activity and fetal wellbeing: an evaluation. Br Med J 1976;1:1305.
48. Patrick J, Campbell K, Carmichael L, Natale R, Richardson B. Patterns of gross fetal body movements over 24-hour observation intervals during the last 10 weeks of pregnancy. Am J Obstet Gynecol 1982;142:363.
49. Birkenfeld A, Laufer N, Sadovsky E. Diurnal variation of fetal activity. Obstet Gynecol 1980;55:417.
50. Campbell K. Ultradian rhythms in the human fetus during the last ten weeks of gestation: a review. Semin Perinatol 1980;4:301.
51. Goodman JDS, Visser FGA, Dawes GS. Effects of maternal cigarette smoking on fetal trunk movements, fetal breathing movements and the fetal heart rate. Br J Obstet Gynaecol 1984;91:657.
52. Rayburn WF. Antepartum fetal assessment: monitoring fetal activity. Clin Perinatol 1982;9:231.
53. Rayburn WF. Clinical significance of perceptible fetal motion. Am J Obstet Gynecol 1980;138:210.
54. Ohel G, Sadovsky E, Aboulafia Y, Simon A, Zajicek G. Fetal activity in premature rupture of membranes. Am J Perinatol 1986;3:337.
55. Hertogs K, Roberts AB, Cooper D, Griffin DR, Campbell S. Maternal perception of fetal motor activity. Br Med J 1979;2:1183.
56. Gettinger A, Roberts AB, Campbell S. Comparison between subjective and ultrasound assessments of fetal movement. Br Med J 1978;2:88.
57. Neldam S, Jessen P. Fetal movements registered by the pregnant woman correlated to retrospective estimations of fetal movements from cardiotocographic tracing. Am J Obstet Gynecol 1980;136:1051.
58. Sadovsky E, Mahler Y, Poleshuk WZ, Malkin A. Correlation between electromagnetic recording and maternal assessment of fetal movement. Lancet 1973;i:1141.
59. Johnson TRB, Jordan ET, Paine LL. Doppler recordings of fetal movements. II: comparison with maternal perception. Obstet Gynecol 1990;76:42.
60. Sadovsky E, Ohel G, Simon A, Aboulafia Y. Decreased fetal activity in complications of pregnancy. Int J Gynaecol Obstet 1986;24:443.
61. Natale R, Clelow F, Dawes GS. Measurement of fetal forelimb movements in lambs in utero. Am J Obstet Gynecol 1981;140:545.
62. Sadovsky E, Weinstein D, Even Y. Antepartum fetal evaluation by assessment of fetal heart rate and fetal movements. Int J Obstet Gynecol 1981;19:21.
63. Moore TR, Piacquadio K. A prospective evaluation of fetal movement screening to reduce the incidence of antepartum fetal death. Am J Obstet Gynecol 1989;160:1075.
64. Grant A, Elbourne D, Valentin L, Alexander S. Routine formal fetal movement counting and risk of antepartum late death in normally formed singletons. Lancet 1989;i:345.
65. Parer JT. Fetal heart rate. In: Creasy RK, Resnik R, eds. Maternal-fetal medicine: principles and practice. Philadelphia: WB Saunders, 1989:314.
66. Nijhuis JG, Prechtl HFR, Martin CB, Bots RSGM. Are there behavioural states in the human fetus? Early Hum Dev 1982;6:177.
67. Delgado FMR. Circulatory effects of cortical stimulation. Physiol Rev 1960;40:146
68. Timor-Tritsch IE, Dierker LJ, Zador I, Hertz RH, Rosen MG. Fetal movements associated with fetal heart rate accelerations and decelerations. Am J Obstet Gynecol 1978;131:276.
69. Weingold AB, Yonekura ML, O'Kieffe J. Nonstress testing. Am J Obstet Gynecol 1980;138:195.
70. Flynn AM, Kelly J. Evaluation of fetal well-being by antepartum fetal heart monitoring. Br Med J 1977;1:936.
71. Visser GHA, Huisjes JH. Diagnostic value of the unstressed antepartum cardiotocogram. Br J Obstet Gynecol 1977;84:321.
72. Phelan JP. The nonstress test: a review of 3,000 tests. Am J Obstet Gynecol 1981;139:7.
73. Rabinowitz R, Persitz E, Sadovsky E. The relation between fetal heart rate accelerations and fetal movements. Obstet Gynecol 1983;61:16.
74. Sheldon RE, Peeters LLH, Jones MD, Makowski EL, Meschia G. Redistribution of cardiac output and oxygen delivery in the hypoxemic fetal lamb. Am J Obstet Gynecol 1979;135:1071.
75. Murata Y, Martin CB, Ikenoue T, et al. Fetal heart rate accelerations and late decelerations during the course of intrauterine death in chronically catheterized rhesus monkeys. Am J Obstet Gynecol 1982;144:218.
76. Polzin GB, Blakemore KJ, Petrie RH, Amon E. Fetal vibro-acoustic stimulation: magnitude and duration of fetal heart rate accelerations as a marker of fetal health. Obstet Gynecol 1988;72:621.
77. Young BK, Katz M, Klein SA. The relationship of heart rate patterns and tissue pH in the human fetus. Am J Obstet Gynecol 1979;134:685.
78. Navot D, Yaffe H, Sadovsky E. The ratio of fetal heart rate accelerations to fetal movements according to gestational age. Am J Obstet Gynecol 1984;149:92.
79. Smith CV, Phelan JP, Paul RH. A prospective analysis of the influence of gestational age on the baseline fetal heart rate and

reactivity in a low-risk population. Am J Obstet Gynecol 1985;153:780.
80. Druzin ML, Fox A, Kogut E, Carlson C. The relationship of the nonstress test to gestational age. Am J Obstet Gynecol 1985;153:386.
81. Natale R, Nasello C, Turliuk R. The relationship between movements and accelerations in fetal heart rate at twenty-four to thirty-two weeks' gestation. Am J Obstet Gynecol 1984; 148:591.
82. Gagnon R, Campbell K, Hunse C, Patrick J. Patterns of human fetal heart rate accelerations from 26 weeks to term. Am J Obstet Gynecol 1987;157:743.
83. Sorokin Y, Dierker LJ, Pillay SK, Zador IE, Schreiner ML, Rosen MG. The association between fetal heart rate patterns and fetal movements in pregnancies between 20 and 30 weeks' gestation. Am J Obstet Gynecol 1982;143:243.
84. Timor-Tritsch IE, Dierker LJ, Hertz RH, Deagan NC, Rosen MG. Studies of antepartum behavioral state in the human fetus at term. Am J Obstet Gynecol 1978;132:524.
85. Patrick J, Carmichael L, Chess L, Staples C. Accelerations of the human fetal heart rate at 38 to 40 weeks' gestational age. Am J Obstet Gynecol 1984;148:35.
86. Hauth JC, Gilstrap LC, Widmer K. Fetal heart rate reactivity before and after maternal jogging during the third trimester. Am J Obstet Gynecol 1982;142:545.
87. Phelan JP. Diminished fetal reactivity with smoking. Am J Obstet Gynecol 1980;136:230.
88. Keegan KA, Paul RH, Borussard PM, McCart D, Smith MA. Antepartum fetal heart rate testing. III: the effect of phenobarbital on the nonstress test. Am J Obstet Gynecol 1979;133:579.
89. Margulis E, Binder D, Cohen AW. The effect of propranolol on the nonstress test. Am J Obstet Gynecol 1984;148:340.
90. Petrie RH. Antepartum surveillance of fetal well-being. In: Rathi M, ed. Clinical aspects of perinatal medicine. Vol 2. New York: Macmillan, 1986:46.
91. Evertson LR, Paul RH. Antepartum fetal heart rate testing: the nonstress test. Am J Obstet Gynecol 1978;132:895.
92. Devoe LD, McKenzie J, Searle N, Sherline DM. Nonstress test: dimensions of normal reactivity. Obstet Gynecol 1985;66:617.
93. Devoe LD, Castillo RA, Sherline DM. The nonstress test as a diagnostic test: a critical reappraisal. Am J Obstet Gynecol 1985;152:1047.
94. Phelan JP, Cromartie AD, Smith CV. The nonstress test: the false negative test. Am J Obstet Gynecol 1982;142:293.
95. Barss VA, Frigoletto FD, Diamond F. Stillbirth after nonstress testing. Obstet Gynecol 1985;65:541.
96. Miyazaki FS, Miyazaki BA. False reactive nonstress tests in postterm pregnancies. Am J Obstet Gynecol 1981;140:269.
97. Eden RD, Gergely RZ, Schifrin BS, Wade ME. Comparison of antepartum testing schemes for the management of the postdate pregnancy. Am J Obstet Gynecol 1982;144:683.
98. Boehm FH, Salyer S, Shah DM, Vaughn WK. Improved outcome of twice weekly nonstress testing. Obstet Gynecol 1986;67:566.
99. Schneider EP, Hutson JM, Petrie RH. An assessment of the first decade's experience with antepartum fetal heart rate testing. Am J Perinatol 1988;5:134.
100. Pazos R, Vuolo K, Aladjem S, Lueck J, Anderson C. Association of spontaneous fetal heart rate decelerations during antepartum nonstress testing and intrauterine growth retardation. Am J Obstet Gynecol 1982;144:574.
101. Anyaegbunam A, Brustman L, Divon M, Langer O. The significance of antepartum variable decelerations. Am J Obstet Gynecol 1986;155:707.
102. Bourgeois FJ, Thiagarajah S, Harbert GM. The significance of fetal heart rate decelerations during nonstress testing. Am J Obstet Gynecol 1984;150:213.
103. Mendenhall HW, O'Leary JA, Phillips KO. The nonstress test: the value of a single acceleration in evaluation the fetus at risk. Am J Obstet Gynecol 1980;136:87.
104. Devoe LD, McKenzie J, Searle N, Sherline DM. Clinical sequelae of the extended nonstress test. Am J Obstet Gynecol 1985;151:1074.
105. Brown R, Patrick J. The nonstress test: how long is enough? Am J Obstet Gynecol 1981;141:646.
106. Nicolaides KH, Sadovsky G, Visser GHA. Heart rate patterns in normoxemic, hypoxemic, and anemic second-trimester fetuses. Am J Obstet Gynecol 1989;160:1034.
107. Pearson JF, Weaver JB. A six-point scoring system for antenatal cardiotocographs. Br J Obstet Gynaecol 1978;85:321.
108. Lyons ER, Bylsma-Howell M, Shamsi S, Towell ME. A scoring system for nonstressed antepartum fetal heart rate monitoring. Am J Obstet Gynecol 1979;133:242.
109. Krebs H-B, Petres RE. Clinical application of a scoring system for evaluation of antepartum fetal heart rate monitoring. Am J Obstet Gynecol 1978;130:765.
110. Lotgering FK, Wallenburg HCS, Schouten HJA. Interobserver and intraobserver variation in the assessment of antepartum cardiotocograms. Am J Obstet Gynecol 1982;144:701.
111. Druzin ML, Gratacos J, Paul RH, Broussard P, McCart D, Smith M. Antepartum fetal heart rate testing. XII: the effect of manual manipulation of the fetus on the nonstress test. Am J Obstet Gynecol 1985;151:61.
112. Druzin ML, Foodim J. Effect of maternal glucose ingestion compared with maternal water ingestion on the nonstress test. Obstet Gynecol 1986;67:425.
113. Crade M, Lovett S. Fetal response to sound stimulation: preliminary report exploring use of sound stimulation in routine obstetrical ultrasound examinations. J Ultrasound Med 1988;7:499.
114. Smith CV, Phelan JP, Platt LD, Broussard P, Paul RH. Fetal coustic stimulation testing. II: a randomized clinical comparison with the nonstress test. Am J Obstet Gynecol 1986;155:131.
115. Thomas RL, Johnson TRB, Besinger RE, Rafkin D, Treanor C, Strobino D. Preterm and term fetal cardiac and movement responses to vibratory acoustic stimulation. Am J Obstet Gynecol 1989;161:141.
116. Ohel G, Birkenfeld A, Rabinowitz R, Sadovsky E. Fetal response to vibratory acoustic stimulation in periods of low heart rate reactivity and low activity. Am J Obstet Gynecol 1986;154:619.
117. Visser GHA, Zeelenberg HJ, de Vries JIP, Dawes GS. External physical stimulation of the human fetus during episodes of low heart rate variation. Am J Obstet Gynecol 1983; 145:579.
118. Eglinton GS, Paul RH, Broussard PM, Walla CA, Platt LD. Antepartum fetal heart rate testing. XI: stimulation with orange juice Am J Obstet Gynecol 1984;150:97.
119. Gagnon R, Hunse C, Fellows F, Carmichael L, Patrick J. Fetal heart rate and activity patterns in growth-retarded fetuses: changes after vibratory acoustic stimulation. Am J Obstet Gynecol 1988;158:265.
120. Sherer DM, Menashe M, Sadovsky E. Severe fetal bradycardia caused by external vibratory acoustic stimulation. Am J Obstet Gynecol 1988;159:334.
121. Romero R, Mazor M, Hobbins JC. A critical appraisal of fetal acoustic stimulation as an antenatal test for fetal well-being. 1988;71:781.
122. Hage ML. Interpretation of nonstress tests. Am J Obstet Gynecol 1985;153:490.
123. Searle JR, Devoe LD, Phillips MC, Searle NS. Computerized analysis of resting fetal heart rate tracings. Obstet Gynecol 1988;71:407.

124. James D, Peralta B, Porte S, et al. Fetal heart rate monitoring by telephone. II: clinical experience in four centers with a commercially produced system. Br J Obstet Gynaecol 1988;95:1024.
125. Myers RE, Mdueller-Heubach E, Adamsons K. Predictability of the state of fetal oxygenation from a quantitative analysis of the components of late deceleration. Am J Obstet Gynecol 1973;115:1083.
126. Martin CB, De Haan J, Wilot BVD, et al. Mechanisms of late deceleration in the fetal heart rate. A study with autonomic blocking agents in fetal lambs. Eur J Obstet Gynecol Reprod Biol 1979;9:361.
127. Huddleston JF, Sutliff G, Robinson D. Contraction stress test by intermittent nipple stimulation. Obstet Gynecol 1984;63:669.
128. Freeman RK. The use of the oxytocin challenge test for antepartum clinical evaluation of uteroplacental respiratory function. Am J Obstet Gynecol 1975:121:481.
129. Fox HE, Steinbrecher M, Ripton B. Antepartum fetal heart rate and uterine activity studies. I: preliminary report of accelerations and the oxytocin challenge test. Am J Obstet Gynecol 1976;126:61.
130. Farahani G, Vasudeva K, Petrie R, Fenton AN. Oxytocin challenge test in high-risk pregnancy. Obstet Gynecol 1976;47:159.
131. Evertson LR, Gauthier RJ, Collea JV. Fetal demise following negative contraction stress tests. Obstet Gynecol 1978;51:671.
132. Bissonnette JM, Johnson K, Toomey C. The role of a trial of labor with a positive contraction stress test. Am J Obstet Gynecol 1979;135:292.
133. Braly P, Freeman RK. The significance of fetal heart rate reactivity with a positive oxytocin challenge test. Obstet Gynecol 1977;50:689.
134. Devoe LD. Clinical features of the reactive positive contraction stress test. Obstet Gynecol 1984;63:523.
135. Druzin ML, Gratacos J, Paul RH. Antepartum fetal heart rate testing. VI: predictive reliability of "normal" tests in the prevention of antepartum death. Am J Obstet Gynecol 1980;137:746.
136. Grundy H, Freeman RK, Lederman S, Dorchester W. Nonreactive contraction stress test: clinical significance. Obstet Gynecol 1984;64:337.
137. Freeman RK, Anderson G, Dorchester W. A prospective multi-institutional study of antepartum fetal heart rate monitoring. I: risk of perinatal mortality and morbidity according to antepartum fetal heart rate test results. Am J Obstet Gynecol 1982;143:771.
138. Keane MWD, Horger EO, Vice L. Comparative study of stress and nonstress antepartum fetal heart rate testing. Obstet Gynecol 1980;57:320.
139. Bruce SL, Petrie RH, Yeh S-Y. The suspicious contraction stress test. Obstet Gynecol 1978;4:415.
140. Staisch KJ, Westlake JR, Bashore RA. Blind oxytocin challenge test and perinatal outcome. Am J Obstet Gynecol 1980;138:399.
141. Garite TJ, Freeman RK, Hochleutner I, Linzey EM. Oxytocin challenge test: achieving the desired goals. Obstet Gynecol 1978;51:614.
142. Elliott JP, Barry MK. Contraction stress test after hyperstimulation patterns during antepartum fetal heart rate monitoring. J Reprod Med 1988;33:761.
143. Freeman RK, James J. Clinical experience with the oxytocin challenge test. II: an ominous atypical pattern. Obstet Gynecol 1975;46:255.
144. Small ML, Phelan JP, Smith CV, et al. The impact of an active management approach to the postdate fetus with a reactive nonstress test and FHR decelerations. Obstet Gynecol 1987;70:636.
145. Dashow EE, Read JA. Significant fetal bradycardia during antepartum heart rate testing. Am J Obstet Gynecol 1984;148:187.
146. Druzin ML, Gatacos J, Keegan KA, Paul RH. Antepartum fetal heart rate testing. VII: the significance of fetal bradycardia. Am J Obstet Gynecol 1981;139:194.
147. Freeman RK, Goebelsmann U, Nochimson D, Cetrulo C. An evaluation of the significance of a positive oxytocin challenge test. Obstet Gynecol 1976;47:8.
148. Schifrin BS, Lapidus M, Doctor GE, Leviton A. Contraction stress test for antepartum fetal evaluation. Obstet Gynecol 1975;45:433.
149. Lenke RR, Nemes JM. Use of nipple stimulation to obtain contraction stress test. Obstet Gynecol 1984;63:345.
150. Palmer SM, Martin JN, Moreland ML, Ewing J, Bucovaz ET, Morrison JC: Contraction stress test by nipple stimulation: efficacy and safety. South Med J 1986;79:1102.
151. Capeless EL, Mann LI. Use of breast stimulation for antepartum stress testing. Obstet Gynecol 1984;64:641.
152. Finley BE, Amico J, Castillo M, Seitchik J. Oxytocin and prolactin responses associated with nipple stimulation contraction stress tests. Obstet Gynecol 1986;67:836.
153. Rosenzweig BA, levy JS, Schipiour P, Blementhal PD. Comparison of the nipple stimulation and exogenous oxytocin contraction stress tests. J Reprod Med 1989;34:950.
154. Schellpfeffer MA, Hoyle D, Johnson JWC. Antepartal uterine hypercontractility secondary to nipple stimulation. Obstet Gynecol 1985;65:588.
155. Owen J, Hauth JC, Williams G, Davis RO, Goldenberg RL, Brumfield CG. A comparison of perinatal outcome in patients undergoing contraction stress testing performed by nipple stimulation versus spontaneously occurring contractions. Am J Obstet Gynecol 1989;160:1081.
156. Braly PS, Freeman RK, Garite TJ, Anderson GG, Dorchester W. Incidence of premature delivery following the oxytocin challenge test. Am J Obstet Gynecol 1981;141:5.
157. Lumley J, Lester A, Anderson I, Renou P, Wood C. A randomized trial of weekly cardiotocography in high-risk obstetric patients. Br J Obstet Gynecol 1983;90:1018.
158. Flynn AM, Kelly J, Mansfield H, Needham P, O'Conor M, Viegas O. A randomized controlled trial of non-stress antepartum cardiotocography. Br J Obstet Gynaecol 1982;89:427.
159. Brown VA, Sawers S, Parsons RJ, Duncan SLB, Cooke ID. The value of antenatal cardiotocography in the management of high-risk pregnancy: a randomized controlled trial. Br J Obstet Gynaecol 1982;89:716.
160. Devoe LD, Morrison J, Martin J, et al. A prospective comparative study of the extended nonstress test and the nipple stimulation contraction stress test. Am J Obstet Gynecol 1987;157:531.
161. Rayburn WF, Barr M. Activity patterns in malformed fetuses. Am J Obstet Gynecol 1982;142:1045.
162. Garite TJ, Linzey EM, Freeman RK, Dorchester W. Fetal heart rate patterns and fetal distress in fetuses with congenital anomalies. Obstet Gynecol 1979;53:716.
163. Phillips WDP, Towell ME. Abnormal fetal heart rate associated with congenital abnormalities. Br J Obstet Gynaecol 1980;87:270.
164. Phelan JP, Lewis PE. Fetal heart rate decelerations during a nonstress test. Obstet Gynecol 1981;57:228.
165. Rutherford SE, Phelan JP, Smith CV, Jacobs N. The four-quadrant assessment of amniotic fluid volume: an adjunct to antepartum fetal heart rate testing. Obstet Gynecol 1987;70:353.
166. Phelan JP, Smith CV, Broussard P, Small M. Amniotic fluid volume assessment with the four-quadrant technique at 36–42 weeks' gestation. J Reprod Med 1987;32:540.
167. Moore TR, Cayle JE. The amniotic fluid index in normal human pregnancy. Am J Obstet Gynecol 1990;162:1168.
168. Clark SL, Sabey P, Jolley K. Nonstress testing with acoustic

stimulation and amniotic fluid volume assessment: 5973 tests without unexpected fetal death. Am J Obstet Gynecol 1989:160:694.

169. Pardi G, Buscaglia M, Ferrazzi E, et al. Cord sampling for the evaluation of oxygenation and acid-base balance in growth-retarded human fetuses. Am J Obstet Gynecol 1987;157:1221.
170. Soothill PW, Nicolaides KH, Rodeck CH, et al. The effect of gestational age on blood gas and acid-base values in human pregnancy. Fetal Therapy 1986;1:168.
171. Soothill PW, Nicolaides KH, Rodeck CH, Gamsu H. Blood gases and acid-base status of the human second-trimester fetus. Obstet Gynecol 1986;68:173.
172. Nicolaides KH, Campbell S, Bradley RJ, et al. Maternal oxygen therapy for intrauterine growth retardation. Lancet 1987;i:942.

49

CHAPTER

INTRAPARTUM SURVEILLANCE FOR FETAL OXYGEN DEPRIVATION

Roy H. Petrie

Before the mid-1940s, the fetus was free for the most part from significant intrusion into the mother's uterus and questions regarding the health of the fetus. Since that time, investigators have steadily learned more about the fetus during both the ante- and intrapartum intervals.[1–9]

From the mid-1940s to the mid-1960s, intermittent stethoscopic fetal heart rate monitoring was evaluated, and it was found that a fetal heart rate that remained within the normal range generally correlated with a healthy newborn.[10] When the fetal heart rate fell outside the range generally accepted as normal, particularly when this was associated with the presence of meconium, the presence of a depressed or damaged fetus was more likely, but the diagnostic precision was disappointing. Normal fetal heart rate data allow the obstetrician to leave the fetus in utero with the expectation of a good outcome.

Intermittent fetal capillary blood acid–base surveillance was introduced in the early 1960s. This extended the period of time during which the fetus could safely be left in utero with the expectation of a healthy newborn, as long as the acid–base data were within what was accepted to be a normal range.[1,11–13] Initially, the acid–base value relied on was pH. Later, base excess or base deficit was added to further extend the period of time that the fetus could safely be left in utero in the presence of repetitive stress with the potential for a rapidly deteriorating acid–base status.

In the early 1970s, continuous electronic fetal heart rate/uterine activity (cardiotocography) was introduced in order to further refine and define normal fetal heart rate and acid–base values that would allow the obstetrician to leave the fetus in utero with the expectation of a healthy newborn.[14–18] Fetal cardiotocography had many advantages. As a robot, it could continuously and accurately calculate and record heart rate at the same time it continuously recorded uterine activity.[19] It could work 24 hours a day in a continuous fashion in a much more economical manner than one-on-one nursing. Moreover, aspects of continuous fetal heart rate monitoring could detect quite early the stress potential of uterine contractions and diminution of blood flow to the fetus from the placenta, as well as blood flow to the uterus from the mother.[15] Nevertheless, once again the ability of data that were outside the accepted ranges of normal to predict an abnormal or depressed newborn was disappointing. During this period, many clinical scientists believed that a significant amount of neurological damage secondary to fetal oxygen deprivation during labor could be avoided by the use of intrapartum cardiotocography. This has been shown to be possible in a number of centers around the world; however, statistics from the overall global experience during the past decade has not demonstrated that the average obstetrician has been able to use this technique with any improvement in outcome. Rather, the increased use of intrapartum fetal cardiotocography has been associated with an increased use of cesarean section to attempt to avoid these problems.[14,20–32] Furthermore, it has now been demonstrated that far less neurological damage secondary to fetal oxygen deprivation exists in the intrapartum interval than had been thought previously. Accordingly, because no objective improvement in neurological outcome could be demonstrated with the use of electronic cardiotocography, some investigators propose a return to the simpler intermittent form of fetal heart rate surveillance. Other clinical investigators propose the use of cardiotocography without complementary acid–base commentary from fetal capillary blood sampling because of its complexity, relying on fetal stimulation and, by inference, perhaps a slightly higher cesarean section rate, to avoid the failure to identify the few fetuses truly at risk for fetal oxygen deprivation. It is unlikely that obstetrics will revert to intermittent stethoscopic/Doppler fetal heart rate monitoring on a large scale simply because of the economics involved, the overwhelming reliability that normal continuous fetal heart rate data provide, and the fact that cardiotocography does indeed provide markers of potential problems that can be used in an altered management scheme to both correct and manage potential problems with fetal oxygenation.

Because the technology of acid–base evaluation[1,2,33–35] and fetal electronic cardiotocography[14–17,36] are recent introductions into the arena of intrapartum fetal surveillance, it has become obvious that the "normal" ranges of data that correlate with a healthy newborn may have been drawn too strictly. Recent work in this area suggests that the upper and lower ranges of fetal heart rate as well as the lower ranges of fetal acidosis and the expectations of fetal/neonatal outcome require reconsideration and, probably, clinical alterations.[37,38]

This chapter will be aimed at what I consider to be mainline, classical as well as practical, intrapartum fetal surveillance. Recent surveillance and management innovations that both expand and simplify the process will be discussed.

THE REASON FOR INTRAPARTUM FETAL SURVEILLANCE

The principal reason to monitor the fetus during labor is to evaluate the fetal oxygenation status. A number of causes for fetal/newborn morbidity and mortality may be evident at birth. These include developmental, immunologic, genetic, infectious, traumatic, metabolic, and other problems that have been recognized for some time. The only cause for fetal/newborn morbidity and mortality that has a potentially remediable origin during the labor process is fetal oxygen deprivation. As a result of the labor process, there may be sufficient fetal oxygen deprivation to bring about various organ system damage and even death. It is damage to the neurological system that is of the greatest concern to the obstetrician inasmuch as damage in this system is permanent, irreversible, and may limit to varying degrees the future well-being, lifestyle, and long-term performance of the newborn. If fetal oxygen deprivation can be identified sufficiently early, before neurological damage has occurred, the fetus may be appropriately managed in utero or removed from the uterus prior to the occurrence of permanent neurological loss.

Historically, it is well known that such conditions as prolapse of the umbilical cord and hemorrhage secondary to a placenta previa fall into the category of remediable oxygen deprivation. To this end, it is well understood that if operative intervention can be carried out sufficiently early, the fetus/newborn may be spared problems with oxygen deprivation. If operative intervention is delayed beyond a critical point, fetal oxygen deprivation may lead to permanent neurological damage or even death. For these reasons, intrapartum fetal surveillance for potential fetal oxygen deprivation has been carried out in some form for as long as the obstetrician has had the ability to safely and rapidly intervene in a delivery process by an early, instrument-assisted delivery or a cesarean section. Recent studies have demonstrated that remediable fetal oxygen deprivation-induced neurological damage occurring during labor is considerably less common than prior expectations had calculated.

All living things, including the human fetus, require energy to carry out the various life functions and processes. The energy form under consideration here is adenosine triphosphate (ATP). The fetus requires ATP to function and carry out appropriate metabolic functions. Normally, ATP is produced by Kreb's cycle, where ATP, water, and carbon dioxide are produced. To function optimally, an adequate supply of oxygen is required in Kreb's cycle. When fetal oxygen deprivation occurs and Kreb's cycle does not produce sufficient ATP, then a nonoxidative process is employed to produce ATP. The Embden-Meyerhof pathway produces smaller amounts of ATP, and the byproducts are pyruvic and lactic acid. Pyruvic acid is rapidly converted into lactic acid. Lactic acid in sufficiently great concentration will cause brain cell damage. The brain cell wall becomes permeable to water, causing the cytoplasm to swell to a point at which cell wall integrity can no longer be maintained, and the brain cell undergoes lysis. Obviously, with sufficient concentrations of lactic acid and the corresponding loss of sufficient numbers of brain cells, fetal neurological damage or even death may ensue.

As it is currently understood, fetal oxygen deprivation is a function of an inadequate supply of oxygen delivered to the fetus as a result of blood flow from the maternal circulation to the placenta and the intervillous space. This form of fetal oxygen deprivation, uteroplacental insufficiency, may have its clinical cause in problems such as maternal hypotension, maternal hypertension, uterine hyperactivity, severe forms of anemia, etc. In the placental intervillous space, oxygen from the maternal red cell is exchanged for carbon dioxide coming from the fetal circulation as the fetal red cell then takes up oxygen from the mother. Oxygen is then transported to the fetus via the fetal–placental circulation through the funis or umbilical cord. Because the umbilical cord has no rigid protective support, it is possible to interrupt blood flow and the delivery of oxygen to the fetus by umbilical cord compression. Varying degrees of umbilical cord compression, ranging from minor repetitive compression with contractions to the somewhat devastating potential of an umbilical cord prolapse through the cervix with major or total compression, are noted in the majority of all labor processes. Usually, these are minor and do not require major interventions; however, on occasion cord compression may produce sufficient oxygen deprivation to necessitate an early delivery by the use of early, instrument-assisted delivery or by cesarean section.

Alteration in blood flow resulting in oxygen deprivation to the fetus may vary in the degree of reduction and duration. It is now understood that certain hypertensive disorders, such as pregnancy-induced hypertension, may actually initiate some flow reduction at a time quite early in gestation, with continuation through the time of delivery. This is known as chronic oxygen deprivation, and although it is poorly understood, it appears that the fetus tolerates varying degrees of reduced oxygen supply over the long period much better than it tolerates acute oxygen deprivation. Although a fetus may be exposed to reduced oxygenation that is sufficient to cause intrauterine growth retardation over many months, it may cause minimal or no obvious effect on or damage to brain cells. The obstetrician may recognize that chronic fetal oxygen deprivation can be expected in certain disorders, such as the hypertensive diseases in pregnancy, intrauterine growth retardation, diabetes, and prolonged gestation, and that there are few techniques available to detect the degree or severity of chronic fetal oxygen deprivation. In some instances, there may be sufficient oxygen deprivation prior to the onset of labor to cause brain damage. Blood flow and fetal oxygen supply may subsequently be ameliorated, with normal surveillance parameters of fetal oxygenation during labor, and a resultantly impaired neonate may be noted some time following delivery.

The form of intrapartum fetal oxygen deprivation which the obstetrician is currently equipped to recognize and manage is acute fetal oxygen deprivation due to alterations in uteroplacental or fetal–placental blood flow delivery of oxygen to the fetus. Although it is well recognized that severe forms of anemia, abnormal hemoglobin structure, and various anatomical abnormalities may result in fetal oxygen deprivation, by far the most common causes are uteroplacental insufficiency and fetal–placental insufficiency. It is recognized that labor itself provides the potential for primary fetal oxygen deprivation, as well as an additive amount of deprivation that may cause a prelabor borderline supply of oxygen to the fetus to become an overt fetal oxygen deprivation sufficient to cause morbidity or mortality. The manner in which this occurs is relatively simple. The intramyometrial pressure rises during a uterine contraction, as a function of that contraction. If this elevation in pressure becomes greater than the pressure responsible for providing blood flow to the placenta, then a decrease in flow occurs. Normally, the fetus is able to tolerate this; however, if uterine activity is too great in either duration or intensity, there may be sufficient oxygen deprivation to cause a problem. Likewise, fetal–placental blood flow may be interrupted, causing fetal oxygen deprivation by umbilical cord compression, as previously described.

An infant that is markedly depressed at birth, as evidenced by very low Apgar scores, marked fetal metabolic acidosis, seizure activity shortly after birth, and evidence of other neonatal organ system insult or damage, can point to intrapartum fetal oxygen deprivation of the acute type, which is sufficiently severe to bring about permanent neurological impairment.[37]

GESTATIONAL STATUS

For centuries it has been recognized that certain women and certain disease states are more likely than others to present problems with human reproduction. Erythroblastosis fetalis and diabetes mellitus are prime examples. During the 1950s blood banking, antibiotics, and improved operative and anesthetic techniques made the cesarean section a safe and viable option to labor and delivery. A pure preparation of oxytocin enabled the obstetrician to initiate labor safely prior to the onset of spontaneous labor. As a result of these advances, it became prudent to attempt to evaluate those conditions and states that were more likely to result in an adverse outcome for either the mother or the fetus. Furthermore, it became important to determine which of these maternal or fetal conditions were potentially remediable during the intrapartum interval, secondary to fetal oxygen deprivation.

In the 1950s, epidemiologic and demographic data were evaluated that yielded a relative risk status for mother and fetus during a pregnancy and during labor. By convention, risk for an adverse outcome to either mother or fetus at the level of one and a half times normal was chosen as a marker to establish risk. Accordingly, gestations with a one and a half times normal or greater likelihood of an adverse outcome have been designated as "high-risk" gestations. When the likelihood of an adverse outcome did not reach the level of one and a half times normal, the pregnancy was considered to be a "low-risk" gestation. High-risk gestations are not all subject to special risk during labor, but may be at risk at another point in pregnancy or for another reason, such as the high-risk gestation of advanced maternal age. This gravida is at risk at the time of conception for a genetically abnormal fetus. Once the fetus has been found to be normal, then the likelihood of potential problems during labor may be only slightly higher than that of a completely normal pregnancy. The woman with insulin-dependent diabetes mellitus may be at risk at the time of conception, during the period of embryogenesis for a developmental abnormality, and again during the fetal growth period as well as during the intrapartum interval for the potential of intrapartum fetal oxygen deprivation or delivery trauma. The prolonged gestation achieves a risk level of one and one half times normal for an adverse outcome at 42 weeks, and the gestation may be at risk for an adverse outcome if the principal clinical markers of affected prolonged gestation are noted, including the large fetus, an abnormal labor partogram, oligohydramnios, or abnormal fetal physiologic functions such as heart rate.

Fetuses known to have the potential for acute oxygen deprivation during labor may be selected, if the appropriate markers are present, for more intense surveillance during the intrapartum interval. The intensity of fetal surveillance for low-risk versus high-risk patients at present remains somewhat vague, arbitrary, and indistinct. The ability to identify and evaluate chronic fetal oxygen deprivation as opposed to acute fetal oxygen deprivation is somewhat theoretical and philosophical. Nevertheless, when the potential for chronic fetal oxygen deprivation exists, it is logical, reasonable, and prudent to increase the intensity of fetal surveillance for the potential addition of acute fetal oxygen deprivation during labor.

METHODS OF SURVEILLANCE FOR FETAL OXYGEN DEPRIVATION

Inasmuch as it is fetal oxygen deprivation that is the rate-limiting step that yields production of lactic acid, which ultimately causes brain damage or death, it is reasonable to expect that one should be able to measure fetal oxygen levels and determine which fetuses have sufficient oxygen deprivation to cause morbidity or mortality. Recently, the use of pulse oximetry electrodes has improved our ability to determine oxygenation in the adult. The use of these electrodes and other oxygen electrodes for the fetus has not been fruitful for the detection of fetal oxygenation deprivation. There are a number of reasons for the deficiency; however, the chief problem revolves around the wide fluctuations of fetal oxygen levels, particularly from the fetal scalp or presenting part. Historically, a drift in an oxygen electrode's reading has made fetal oxygen evaluation somewhat less than reliable. At the same time, pH and pCO_2 electrodes have been considerably more reliable for the collection of data and more specific for the determination of significant levels of acidosis, which in turn can be related to the overall fetal oxygenation state. In the early 1960s, intermittent intrapartum fetal surveillance by the collection of fetal capillary blood for determination of pH was introduced. Subsequently, with the use of fetal pH and pCO_2 levels, bicarbonate and base excess have been available to evaluate fetal oxygenation. This advance occurred at a time when intermittent stethoscopic evaluation of fetal heart rate was the only reliable method of intrapartum fetal surveillance. Normal intermittent intrapartum fetal heart rate data were very reliable indicators to allow the labor to continue without worry of fetal oxygen deprivation. A number of fetuses demonstrated abnormal fetal heart rate data during labor, which caused the obstetrician to think about methods that would enhance the diagnosis of significant fetal oxygen deprivation. The use of intermittent pH determinations from fetal scalp capillary blood collection in instances of normal values enabled the obstetrician to extend the time that a fetus could be comfortably left in utero when abnormal fetal heart rate data were obtained. With abnormal pH values, there is an increased probability of fetal oxygen deprivation when both fetal heart rate and acid–base surveillance indicate that the fetus may be experiencing fetal oxygen deprivation. The principal problems with intermittent intrapartum fetal surveillance with acid–base determinations are that it is intermittent, somewhat difficult to obtain, and uncomfortable for some patients. Accordingly, it has remained a secondary form of surveillance. Although continuous acid–base data relating to pH, pCO_2, and base excess is possible with the use of electrodes attached to the fetal presenting part, this form of surveillance has not yet moved from the laboratory to the clinical labor and delivery setting.

A number of investigators have demonstrated that detection of fetal movement, including fetal breathing, is highly significant when correlated with fetal well-being. For the most part, this is evaluated in the antepartum interval prior to the onset of labor. This technique may be used in early labor as a gross screening technique to evaluate the fetal well-being. Its utility in the intrapartum period beyond latent labor has not been evaluated fully because of the difficulty in detecting fetal motion as opposed to uterine contractions.

For almost two centuries, fetal heart rate has been used as a way to determine whether the fetus was alive or dead. More recently, when it became important to evaluate fetal oxygenation, a number of investigators have found that normal intrapartum fetal heart rate data are highly predictive of a healthy fetus. Abnormal fetal heart rate data are considerably less predictive of a fetus with significant oxygen deprivation. Accordingly, the principal value of fetal heart rate surveillance is that normal data, being the most predictive value for a healthy fetus, allow the labor to continue toward its completion without significant concern for fetal damage or death secondary to oxygen deprivation.

Surveillance of the amniotic fluid as a potential marker for fetal oxygen deprivation involves an evaluation for volume as well as for the presence of meconium in the amniotic fluid. The presence of a normal amount of amniotic fluid without the presence of meconium is more significantly associated with a normal fetal oxygenation state than the presence of oligohydramnios or polyhydramnios is associated with fetal oxygen deprivation. Nevertheless, the presence of oligohydramnios, particularly in conditions such as prolonged gestation, may be associated with an increased likelihood for problems during the intrapartum period, including the potential for fetal oxygen deprivation. Developmental abnormalities, including abnormal karyotypic states, and various metabolic and infectious problems, may be associated with abnormal amniotic fluid volumes.

Although most investigators do not consider the presence of meconium in the amniotic fluid a distinct marker of potential fetal oxygen deprivation, there is no argument that fetal oxygen deprivation is encountered more frequently when meconium is noted in the amniotic fluid. Even with the presence of meconium in prolonged gestation and normal fetal heart rate data, the fetal acid–base markers of potential fetal oxygenation remain in a low normal range. The presence of meconium with abnormal fetal heart rate data appears to enhance the probability of potential fetal oxygen deprivation. Most investigators consider that in a normal gestation, the presence of meconium alone is not considered to be a marker of fetal oxygen deprivation; however, in the presence of another marker for potential fetal oxygen deprivation, meconium becomes a valid second marker.

SURVEILLANCE TECHNIQUES FOR FETAL OXYGEN DEPRIVATION

The principal screening surveillance technique for the intrapartum evaluation of the fetal oxygenation state is *fetal heart rate monitoring*.[39] The presence of normal fetal heart rate data during the intrapartum period usually indicates that there is no fetal oxygen deprivation. With normal fetal heart rate data, most investigators consider that it is safe to allow labor to continue toward completion and delivery. Fetal heart rate monitoring is accomplished by two methods: intermittent determinations of the fetal heart rate and continuous electronic calculation and recording of the fetal heart rate.

Intermittent fetal heart rate monitoring is currently performed by three different methods. The first is the use of a Doppler/ultrasound device that is hand-held with a transducer placed over the gravid abdomen. The fetal heart tones are detected and manual counting is carried out. Each time that the fetal heart rate is determined, it should be recorded in the patient's chart. In a similar technique, a stethoscope is placed over the gravid abdomen and the actual heart tones are obtained, counted, and manually recorded in the patient's chart. The third technique involves the intermittent use of continuous electronic fetal heart rate monitor (either external or internal) to detect, instantaneously calculate, and automatically record the fetal heart rate on graphic tracing.

Intermittent fetal heart rate monitoring is generally performed according to guidelines provided by the American College of Obstetricians and Gynecologists[39] as well as the Nurses Association of the American College of Obstetricians and Gynecologists (NAACOG).[40] The technique for the evaluation of fetal oxygenation can be used in almost all low-risk labors, as well as most appropriately selected high-risk pregnancy labors. A stethoscope (fetoscope) or a hand-held Doppler device is used to listen to the fetal heart tones for evaluation. The interval used for counting fetal heart rate varies from several brief intervals (5 to 15 seconds) to longer intervals (30 to 60 seconds). Occasionally, listening for several minutes continuously in order to ensure a rate is recommended. The recommended procedure for intermittent fetal heart rate monitoring as outlined by NAACOG is given below:[40]

Palpate the maternal abdomen to identify the fetal presentation and position (Leopold's maneuvers).

Place the bell of the fetoscope or Doppler device over the area of maximum intensity of the fetal heart sounds (usually over the fetal back).

Place a finger over the maternal radial pulse to differentiate maternal–fetal heart rate.

Palpate for uterine contractions using the period of fetal heart rate auscultation to clarify relationship between fetal heart rate and uterine contractions.

Count fetal heart rate during a uterine contraction and for 30 seconds thereafter to identify fetal response.

Count fetal heart rate between uterine contractions for at least 30 to 60 seconds to identify average baseline rate.

If distinct differences are made between counts, recounts for longer periods are appropriate to clarify the presence of possible periodic fetal heart rate changes such as abrupt versus gradual changes.

To clarify accelerations, recounts for multiple brief periods of 5 to 10 seconds may be particularly helpful.

The frequency of fetal heart rate determinations vary depending on the probability of fetal oxygen deprivation (high risk versus low risk). It is recommended that for low-risk patients the fetal heart rate should be determined at least every hour in the latent phase of labor, every 30 minutes in the active phase of labor, and every 15 minutes during the second stage of labor. When monitoring high-risk patients, it is recommended that the fetal heart rate be determined every 30 minutes during the first stage of labor and in latent labor, every 15 minutes in active phase labor, and every 5 minutes during the second stage of labor. It is critically important that, when intermittent fetal heart rate surveillance is used, the frequency of fetal heart rate determination not only be adhered to by patient risk category, but the rate must be also recorded in the patient's chart on each and every occasion that the fetal heart rate is determined. In addition to these intervals, it is further recommended that the fetal heart rate be taken during labor in the following situations: initiation of labor-enhancing procedures (eg, artificial amniotomy); periods of ambulation; administration of medication and administration or initiation of anesthesia/analgesia, including recognition of abnormal uterine activity patterns such as increased basal tones or tachysystole; evaluation of oxytocin (maintenance, increase, or decrease of doses); administration of medicine (at a time of peak action); expulsion of an enema; urinary catheterization; vaginal examination; and evaluation of anesthesia or analgesia (maintenance, increase, or decrease of doses).

When using intermittent Doppler/stethoscopic fetal heart rate monitoring, traditionally reassuring rates have varied from 110 to 120 beats per minute at the lower range and 150 to 160 beats per minute at the upper range. It is normal to note the presence of fetal heart rate accelerations in the absence of decelerations following contractions. The fetal rate of 100 to 119 beats per minute in the absence of other nonreassuring fetal heart rate data is generally not associated with fetal compromise. Nonreassuring fetal heart rate data include baseline fetal heart rate of less than 100 beats per minute (it should be noted that a moderate bradycardia of 80 to 100 beats per minute may be associated with fetal head compression and not necessarily associated with nonreassuring patterns), a fetal heart rate of less than 100 beats per minute 30 seconds after a contraction, an unexplained fetal baseline tachycardia greater than 160 beats per minute, especially if the patient is at risk and that tachycardia persist through three or more contractions in spite of corrective measures.

Using the intermittent stethoscopic/Doppler form of fetal heart rate monitoring during labor, when it is ascertained that an abnormality may exist, the use of additional methods of evaluation for potential fetal oxygenation are employed and include external continuous fetal cardiotocography, internal continuous fetal cardiotocography, fetal scalp blood sampling for acid–base determinations, or fetal stimulatory data that correlates fetal heart rate accelerations to acid–base data to gain commentary regarding fetal acid–base status. This often includes umbilical cord arterial and venous respiratory blood gas determinations at delivery.

Continuous electronic fetal heart rate monitoring is performed by two methods.[15,16] External continuous fetal heart rate monitoring is carried out extra-amniotically from transducers that are placed on the gravid abdomen overlying the fetal heart. Currently, the most commonly used technique is that of an Doppler/ultrasound device that detects one of four cardiac events (aortic opening, aortic closing, mitral opening, or mitral closing); with each beat of the fetal heart, the cardiotachometer instantaneously calculates and causes the rate to be recorded on a graph. Other signals used for external or extra-amniotic fetal heart rate monitoring include use of an abdominal microphone to detect the "lub dub" of the fetal heart and instantaneously calculate and record rate. This can also be accomplished by the use of multiple electrocardiographic electrodes placed on the maternal abdomen to obtain the fetal electrocardiogram (ECG) and thus calculate rate from the "R" wave of the fetal ECG. Phonocardiographic and electrocardiographic techniques, while they can be used for some patients during labor, are not generally applicable for technical reasons, and the most commonly used external technique for continuous fetal heart rate monitoring is that of Doppler ultrasound. A tocodynamometer is positioned over the gravid uterus to detect uterine activity from the changing uterus curvature during a contraction.

Once the cervix dilates to 1 to 2 cm and the chorioamnion is or has been ruptured, one may apply an electrode to the fetal presenting part for the collection of fetal electrocardiographic signal as well as the placement of intrauterine pressure catheter for the collection of uterine activity data in the form of intra-amniotic pressures. The transducers from the intra-amniotic or internal fetal heart rate monitoring are attached to an electronic monitor, where continuous instantaneously calculated and recorded fetal heart rate is displayed on a continuous graphic tracing. The value of internal continuous electronic monitoring over external continuous fetal heart rate monitoring and intermittent fetal heart rate monitoring is that, with an electrode attached to the fetal presenting part and with an intrauterine pressure catheter positioned, precise information regarding fetal heart rate and uterine activity is available on a continuous basis. With external monitoring, some degree of variation in rate may occur due to nonpredictability in the selection of one of the four cardiac events (aortic opening, aortic closing, mitral opening, and mitral closing). At the same time, when a tocodynamometer is used to detect uterine activity, precision relating to quantitation of uterine activity in terms of frequency, duration, and amplitude of a contraction is lost, whereas the use of intrauterine pressure to represent uterine contractions is a continuous and quantitatively precise database for evaluation.

Some critics of continuous fetal heart rate monitoring believe that monitoring requires the patient to stay in bed once monitoring begins, not allowing her to be up walking and moving about. Both internal and external monitoring by radio telemetry is now possible. Telemetry will allow the entire labor to be accomplished away from a labor bed while still providing continuous information regarding fetal heart rate and uterine activity.

Using internal monitoring, the "R" wave from the fetal ECG is obtained and the temporal interval between each "R-R" interval is measured in milliseconds. A calculation for rate is made based on the assumption that the "R-R" interval would be uniform for a whole minute. Each "R-R" interval's rate is individually recorded. For a rate of 120 beats per minute, the "R-R" interval is 500 milliseconds. Instantaneously calculated fetal heart rate and intrauterine pressure are recorded on graph paper that moves uniformly at a given speed. Usually the graph paper speed is 3 cm/min, although 1 cm/min may be used to save paper. Vertical scaling is from 30 to 240 beats per minute and covers a 7-cm vertical distance and from 0 to 100 mm Hg over a 4-cm vertical distance. Generally, wider vertical lines occur once every minute (Fig. 49-1). Although graph paper or tracing can be used to write notes upon and record vital signs and time markers for the labor, some manufacturers provide spontaneous documentation of time and the ability to record other clinical information that may be important. After delivery, the fetal heart rate tracing is generally microfilmed or electronically stored and becomes available as a permanent part of the patient's medical record.

When using continuous fetal heart rate monitoring, the *baseline rate* is that rate in between contractions and represents persistent periods for an interval of 10 minutes or greater of heart rate at a given level. Fetal heart rate above 160 beats per minute is classified as a baseline tachycardia, while rates below 120 beats per minute are classified as fetal bradycardia. It is generally thought that rates between 120 and 160 beats per minute are in the normal range; however, rates of 90 to 180 beats per minute are not uncommon or necessarily abnormal in the absence of other abnormal fetal heart rate markers. Persistent fetal bradycardia or tachycardia,

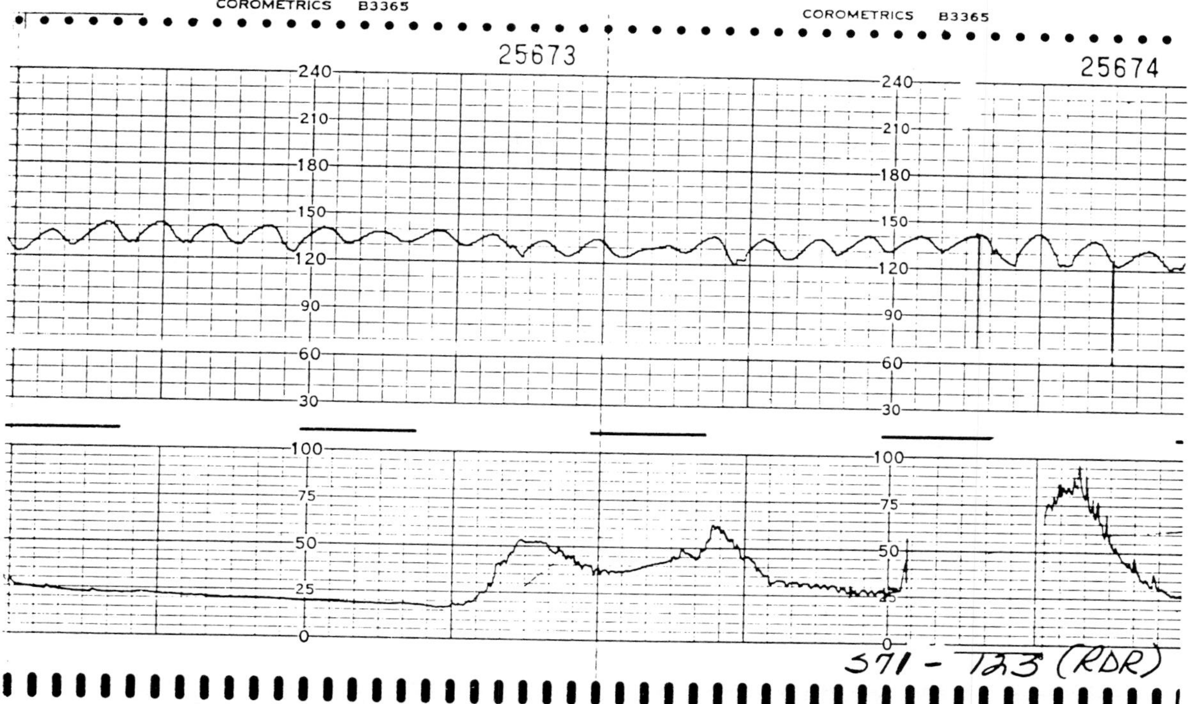

FIGURE 49–1. Monitoring graph or trace demonstrating vertical and horizontal scaling. A sinusoidal fetal heart rate tracing. (Modified from Paul RH, Petrie RH. Fetal intensive care. Vol. I. North Haven, William Mack, 1979: 19.)

without other markers, while representing a relatively low potential fetal oxygen deprivation or acidosis, is slightly more likely to be associated with some degree of fetal oxygen deprivation than a normal rate. Other conditions may cause a fetal tachycardia or a fetal bradycardia. These include maternal fever, fetal infection, maternal thyrotoxicosis, fetal anemia, and fetal tachyrhythmias that cause fetal tachycardia. A fetal bradycardia may be observed in patients managed with pharmacologic agents such as beta-blockers (eg, propranolol), in the fetus with cephalic presentation in a posterior position, and in the fetus with a congenital heart block. In instances in which the mother receives certain drugs such as beta-sympathomimetic tocolytic agents or vagolytic agents such as scopolamine or atropine, a fetal tachycardia may be observed. In instances where the mother has systemic lupus erythematosus, an antibody may be produced that crosses the placenta and damages the fetal heart's conduction system, causing a congenital heart block.

A *sinusoidal fetal heart rate* occurs infrequently, but may be of considerable clinical importance. This baseline rate is usually within the normal range of 120 to 160 beats per minute. There usually is an absence of short-term variability. The rate is relatively smooth and has a somewhat undulating pattern of uniform, long-term variability with an aptitude of 5 to 20 beats per minute that resembles a sine wave (see Fig. 49-1). A sinusoidal fetal heart rate is often noted with fetal anemia, particularly with Rh isoimmunization. Physiologic mechanisms for this rate are unknown. A number of investigators believe that this may represent an abnormal neurologic control of the heart rate, which may result from varying degrees of fetal oxygen deprivation. The sinusoidal-like heart rate can be seen following the administration of narcotic analgesic and related agents. The presence of a persistent nonpharmacologically induced fetal sinusoidal heart rate is generally thought to represent potential fetal oxygen deprivation. To allow labor to continue, it is necessary to obtain information regarding fetal anemia and fetal acid–base status. This may be obtained either by direct capillary blood collection for acid–base status and hematocrit or by stimulation of the fetus to evoke a fetal heart rate acceleration.

Fetal heart rate variability in the form of normal beat-to-beat heart rate variability is perhaps the most reliable indicator of fetal well-being that is available to the obstetrician. Short-term fetal heart rate variability or irregularity can be appreciated only when the heart rate is continuously and instantaneously calculated and recorded on a beat-to-beat basis using the fetal electrocardiographic "R" wave signal to trigger the cardiotachometer (Fig. 49-2). Long-term variability can be appreciated using an external ultrasonographic Doppler system for the detection of fetal heart rate activity. Fetal heart rate variability represents an interplay between the cardio-accelerator and cardio-inhibitor centers in the fetal brain stem. Physiologically under normal ner-

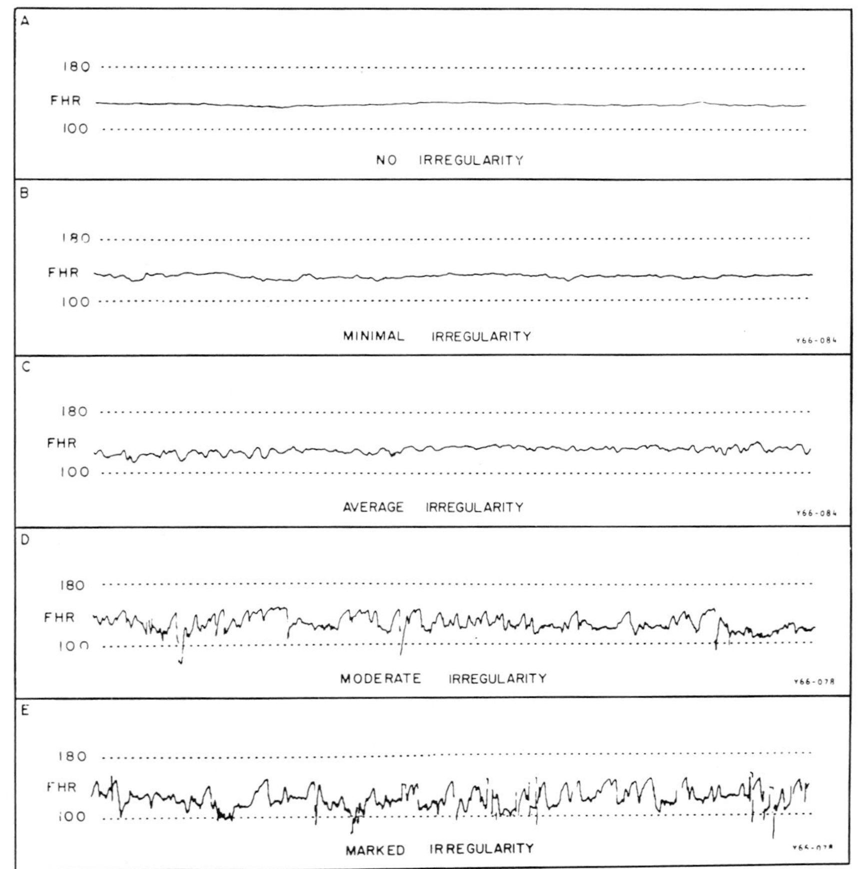

FIGURE 49–2. Classification of fetal heart rate variability or irregularity. (Modified from Hon EH. An atlas of fetal heart rate patterns. New Haven, Harty Press, 1968: 69.)

vous system control, it is unusual for the fetal heart rate to be steady at one constant number. There is considerable variation or short-term variability on a beat-to-beat basis, which usually varies between three to eight beats per minute around an imaginary average heart rate. Fluctuation in long-term variability occurs as well, generally representing a cyclicity of three to five cycles per minute.[41] Normal fetal heart rate variability recorded on a graph represents one of the best indicators of intact integration between the nervous system of the fetus and the fetal cardiovascular system. Although the loss of fetal heart rate variability potentially may suggest fetal hypoxia, other factors may be responsible, including fetal sleep state, pharmacologic agents that depress the central nervous system, a fetal tachycardia greater than 180 beats per minute, and anomalies of the heart and central nervous system. It is possible for a fetus of a gestational age of 28 or more weeks to demonstrate normal fetal heart rate variability.

Exaggerated or increased fetal heart rate variability ($\geq$25 beats per minute) may indicate a shift in the pO_2–pCO_2 relationship, which the barochemoreceptors mediate without the presence of significant or repetitive fetal heart rate decelerations. There generally is no significant clinical alteration in fetal oxygenation. The presence of increased fetal heart rate variability that is followed by loss of beat-to-beat variability may indicate potential fetal oxygen deprivation. Without other significant markers of potential fetal oxygen deprivation, a reduction or loss of fetal heart rate variability represents a potential of less than 2% for a significant degree of fetal oxygen deprivation.[42]

Fetal arrhythmias are suspected with certain regular and irregular irregularities of the fetal heart rate. When these occur, a continuous tracing of the electrocardiographic signals that the fetal monitor is using may be traced via an electrocardiographic monitor. In this manner, the obstetrician may evaluate the presence of P, QRS, and T waves of the fetal cardiac signals. Although most fetal cardiac arrhythmias are transient and of little clinical significance, some have been associated with potential fetal compromise. Fetal supraventricular tachycardia may evoke heart failure and hydrops. A persistent rate of 50 to 70 beats per minute may represent a complete heart block. Approximately 40% of fetuses with a rate between 50 and 70 beats per minute will have congenital heart disease; ventricular septal defects especially are noted. Fetal heart failure and hydrops have been associated with congenital heart block. A persistent fetal rate between 40 and 80 beats per minute can be evaluated by fetal capillary blood sampling or stimulatory test for accelerations to gain commentary regarding acid–base status. A number of fetuses with a persistent bradycardia secondary to an arteriovenous block in this range will have a normal acid–base status and can tolerate labor well.

Periodic heart rate or *fetal heart rate patterns* are transient alterations in the fetal heart rate associated with uterine contractions. These may be transient increases or transient decreases in heart rate, which are referred to as accelerations or decelerations. Generally, these transient changes are temporally related to the onset of a contraction and return to baseline heart rate prior to the onset of the next contraction. An *acceleration* in the fetal heart rate may occur at any time, but is frequently associated with a contraction and may be seen with a breech presentation (Fig. 49-3). Generally, the acceleration is thought to represent early or mild cord compression and is a sympathetic nervous system response. The fetal heart rate acceleration is perhaps the single best indicator of adequate fetal oxygenation and generally is thought to represent a healthy fetus.

There are four forms of fetal heart decelerations that may be noted during the course of labor. *Early deceleration* is generally thought to be secondary to fetal head compression as the head moves through the dilating cervix and the bony pelvis. Early deceleration is termed such inasmuch as deceleration begins as the contraction begins, and it represents an inverted mirror image of the uterine contraction, reaching its greatest point of deceleration as the acme of the contraction is reached and returning to baseline as the contraction is terminated (Fig. 49-4). Early deceleration is mediated by the vagus nerve with the release of acetylcholine at the sinoatrial node. It does not fall below 110 to 100 beats per minute. Classical early deceleration has been demonstrated by a number of studies to be completely innocuous and does not represent any degree of fetal oxygen deprivation or acidosis (see Tables 49-2 and 49-3).

Variable deceleration may begin before, at the onset of, or following the onset of a uterine contraction. On occasion, it may be seen independent of an uterine contraction. Variable deceleration usually drops many beats per minute in absolute rate within a few fetal heartbeats. It is occasionally referred to as the V or W shape deceleration because of this sudden drop and often a sudden return to baseline (see Fig. 49-4). It is somewhat jagged, irregular, or sawtoothed in nature and may last from just a few seconds to a minute or more. The criteria for grading the severity of variable deceleration are given in Table 49-1. Mild variable deceleration is usually innocuous. Repetitive and severe variable deceleration, particularly if it is prolonged, when associated with rising baseline heart rate, loss of beat-to-beat variability, and loss of acceleration prior to the deceleration, may herald the onset of significant fetal oxygen deprivation. This pattern is thought to be mediated by the vagus nerve through the barochemoreceptors when the umbilical cord is compressed, causing fetal peripheral vascular resistance with a fall in fetal pO_2 and a rise in pCO_2. To be significant, the fetal heart rate usually falls below 90 beats per minute. Variable deceleration is the most common periodic pattern noted during the course of labor. As the umbilical cord is compressed, via the vagus nerve, acetylcholine is released at the sinoatrial node, causing a parasympathetic response or fall in fetal heart rate commensurate with the degree of cord compression, as long as the fetal heart rate does not fall below 80 beats per minute or the duration of the deceleration is not too long. It is uncommon for cord compression, even when repetitive, to be of major clinical significance; however, with moderate and severe variable decelerations, significant reduction in umbilical blood flow may occur with the accumulation of significant amounts of carbon dioxide in the fetal compartment, thus causing a respiratory acidosis (Tables 49-2 through 49-4). When the decelerations become severe, repetitive, or prolonged in duration, fetal oxygen

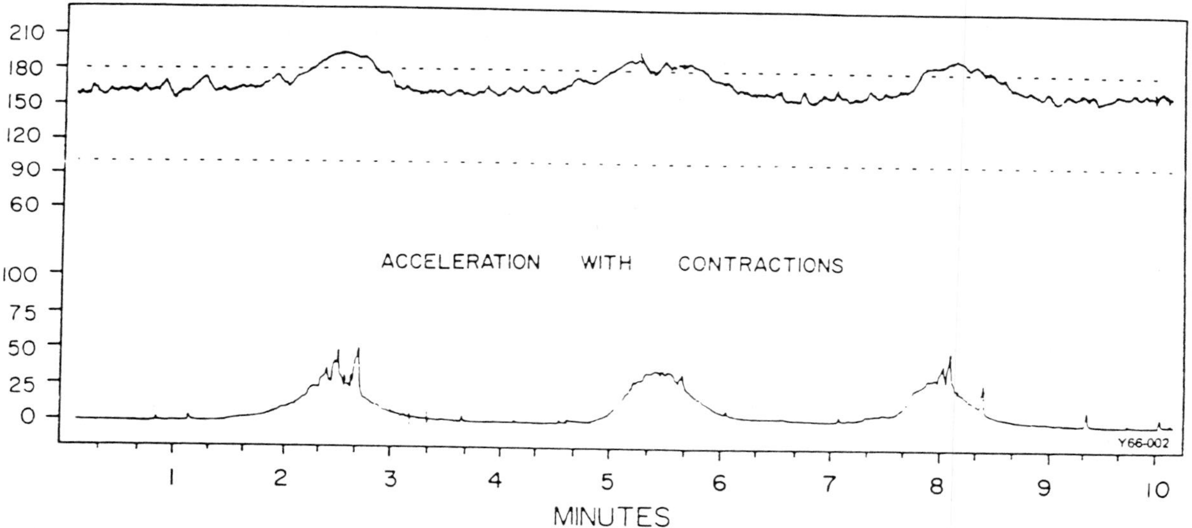

FIGURE 49–3. Fetal heart rate accelerations. (Modified from Hon EH. An atlas of fetal heart rate patterns. New Haven, Harty Press, 1968: 77.)

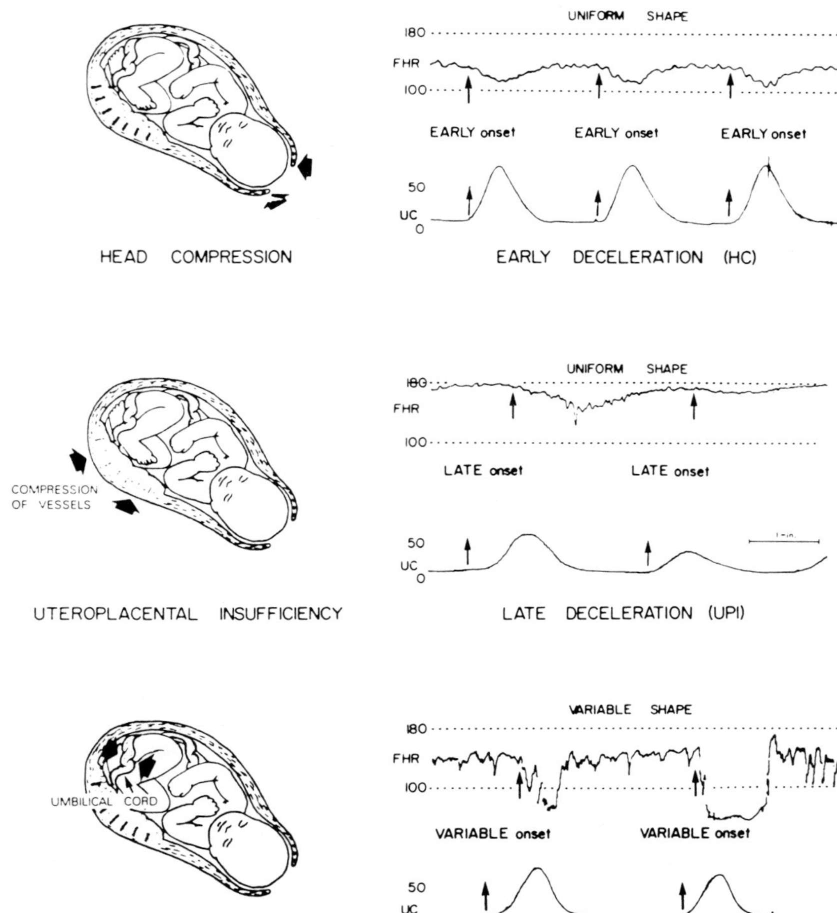

FIGURE 49–4. Examples of early, late, and variable fetal heart rate decelerations. (Modified from Hon EH. An atlas of fetal heart rate patterns. New Haven, Harty Press, 1968: 49.)

deprivation, resulting in a metabolic acidosis, may occur. When this occurs and there is potential for significant fetal oxygen deprivation, a delay in recovery of the fetal heart rate to the baseline level may be noticed. When this is seen, steps should be taken to correct this pattern by alternation of maternal position, amnioinfusion, or use of a tocolytic agent to remove the stress of uterine activity.

Below 60 beats per minute, nodal control of the fetal heart may be lost. At the depth of a severe variable deceleration, a transient "cardiac arrest" for a few seconds may be noted. This is uncommon and, although it may be tempting to treat the finding with a vagolytic pharmacologic agent such as atropine, this should not be done because it only clouds the marker and does not improve fetal oxygenation. Management should follow the standard management for severe variable deceleration. This brief "cardiac arrest," even if repetitive, does not require an early instrument-assisted delivery or cesarean section. Fetal death or damage is almost never encountered.

Late decelerations are transient slowings of the fetal heart rate that are noted to occur after the onset of the contraction or late in the contraction phase of uterine activity. The deceleration reaches its lowest point following the acme of the contraction, and it returns to baseline well after the contraction is over (see Fig. 49-4). In many instances, the late deceleration will appear very much as an early deceleration that is delayed in onset. For this pattern to become clinically significant, it must be repetitive in nature. Most investigators believe that there is no such entity as a single late deceleration and that this pattern must be seen following three or more contractions to be called a late deceleration pattern. When the late deceleration is first noted, the deceleration may represent a reflex vagally mediated response, which is associated with normal heart rate variability. It has been noted that late decelerations develop from fetal myocardial hypoxia, trigger a chemoreceptor response, and cause transient fetal hypotension, thereby stimulating fetal baroreceptors. The degree of potential fetal oxygenation deprivation for a deceleration pattern is related to the duration and depth of the deceleration, as well as the interval from the onset of the contraction to the onset of the deceleration. The shorter the interval from onset of contractions to onset

TABLE 49–1. PRINCIPLES OF GRADING VARIABLE AND LATE DECELERATIONS

CRITERIA OF GRADING	MILD	MODERATE	SEVERE
Variable deceleration; level to which FHR drops and duration of deceleration	<30 sec duration, regardless of level >80 bpm, regardless of duration 70–80 bpm, <60 sec	<70 bpm, >30–<60 sec 70–80 bpm, >60 sec	<70 bpm, >60 sec
Late deceleration; amplitude of drop in FHR	<15 bpm	15–45 bpm	>45 bpm

bpm, beats per minute; FHR, fetal heart rate.
(From Kubli FW, Hon EH, Khazin AF, et al. Observations on heart rate and pH in the human fetus during labor. Am J Obstet Gynecol 1969;104:1190.)

of the deceleration, the greater is the likelihood of a greater degree of oxygenation deprivation. The same is true for the deceleration's duration and depth. The longer a deceleration pattern persists, the greater the likelihood is of significant fetal oxygenation deprivation.[43]

Late decelerations may indicate that uteroplacental insufficiency with decreased intervillous exchange between the mother and the fetus may exist, with persistent or intermittent fetal oxygen deprivation. The criteria for grading the severity of late deceleration are given in Table 49-1. Fetal oxygenation may be impaired as the uterine contraction peaks, thus limiting intervillous space blood flow. Poorly oxygenated blood ultimately reaches the fetus—thus the late timing of the fetal heart rate deceleration (see Tables 49-2 through 49-4). Late decelerations are noted with placental abruption, excessive uterine activity of either a spontaneous or oxytocin-induced nature, maternal hypotension, anemia, or ketoacidosis. Mild, repetitive late decelerations of only five to ten beats per minute may indicate a significant potential for fetal oxygen deprivation such that metabolic acidosis and neurologic damage may result. When the clinician notes the pattern of recurrent repetitive late deceleration, the pattern must be corrected by the usual common steps, inasmuch as up to 35% to 40% of these fetuses may have significant fetal oxygen deprivation. The temporal interval between the onset of fetal heart rate data that may indicate the potential for significant fetal oxygen deprivation and actual damage is unknown, but the interval probably ranges from approximately 0.5 to 2.0 hours.[43] The customary correction plan consists of improvement of maternal hypotension, appropriate repositioning of the patient, administration of maternal oxygen, or reduction of the intensity and duration of uterine contractions with a tocolytic agent. For labor to continue with the presence of repetitive late decelerations, normal acid–base values must be obtained at a regular interval of every 15 to 20 minutes or commentary from fetal stimulation for evaluation of fetal well-being with the presence of fetal accelerations. The continuation of labor in the presence of repetitive late deceleration and reassuring acid–base or fetal stimulatory test is most commonly carried out in the active phase of labor, when a delivery process is not too distant. This situation is most often applicable to a multipara whose delivery is expected quite shortly. It has been demonstrated that the cesarean section rate in

TABLE 49–2. RELATIONSHIP BETWEEN QUALITATIVE PERIODIC FETAL HEART RATE CHANGES AND MEAN FETAL pH

PATTERN	KUBLI (1969)*	BEARD (1971)†	TEJANI (1975)‡
Normal	7.30 ± 0.04	7.34 ± 0.06	7.33 ± 0.01
Accelerations		7.34 ± 0.03	7.34 ± 0.01
Early decelerations	7.30 ± 0.04	7.33 ± 0.05	7.33 ± 0.01
Variable decelerations (all)		7.31 ± 0.05	7.30 ± 0.01
Moderate	7.26 ± 0.04		
Severe	7.15 ± 0.07		
Late decelerations (all)		7.28	7.29 ± 0.01
Moderate	7.21 ± 0.05		
Severe	7.12 ± 0.07		

* From Kubli FW, Hon EH, Khazin AF, et al. Observations on heart rate and pH in the human fetus during labor. Am J Obstet Gynecol 1969;104:1190.
† From Beard RW, Filshie GM, Knight CA, et al. The significance of the changes in the continuous fetal heart rate in the first stage of labor. Br J Obstet Gynaecol 1971;78:865.
‡ From Tejani N, et al. Obstet Gynecol 1975;46:392 and Obstet Gynecol 1976;48:460.

TABLE 49–3. RELATIONSHIP OF FETAL HEART RATE PATTERN, FETAL ACID–BASE, 5-MINUTE APGAR SCORE, AND UMBILICAL ACID–BASE

PATTERN	5-MINUTE FETAL SCALP BLOOD pH	APGAR SCORES ≥ 7 (%)	UMBILICAL pH ≥ 7.25 (%)
Normal tracing	7.33 ± 0.01	92	91
Accelerations	7.34 ± 0.01	91	97
Early decelerations	7.33 ± 0.01	92	93
Variable decelerations	7.30 ± 0.01	78	77
Late decelerations	7.29 ± 0.01	63	66

Correlation of fetal heart rate–uterine contraction patterns with fetal scalp blood pH (1975). (Data from Tejani N, et al. Obstet Gynecol 1975;46:392, and Correlation of fetal heart rate patterns and fetal pH with neonatal outcome. Obstet Gynecol 1976;48:460.)

this situation can be significantly lowered with the use of dual fetal surveillance with fetal heart rate and commentary regarding acid–base status.

Prolonged deceleration occurs infrequently and unexpectedly. Usually, the fetal heart rate will fall below 80 beats per minute and the deceleration can last for several minutes, in the manner of a prolonged variable or reflex deceleration. These sudden, prolonged decelerations can be related to uterine activity, fetal manipulation, conduction anesthesia with hypotension, supine hypotension, and a maternal respiratory arrest secondary to intravenous narcotic use. Although the mechanism for the deceleration is usually a reflex mechanism, as with a variable deceleration pattern, if there is no demonstrable, readily apparent, and correctable cause for the sudden prolonged deceleration, the fetal heart rate following recovery should be observed carefully. When a second or third sudden prolonged deceleration occurs, the patient may be moved to an operating room for corrective measures such as would be performed with a severe variable deceleration pattern, including maternal evaluation of blood pressure, repositioning, oxygenation, and so forth.[44] The possibility of a prolapsed cord should be investigated. Intravenous fluid may be increased and oxygen may be given to the mother. If delivery is not too far distant, substantiation of a satisfactory fetal acid–base commentary may allow the labor to continue. If this pattern repeats with evidence of fetal oxygen deprivation by acid–base determinations, particularly when associated with the rising fetal base excess and a falling pH, an early vaginal delivery or an operative delivery may be prudent.

On occasion, fetal heart rate decelerations will be noted that appear to be a combination or mixture of two or more decelerations in point of timing, cause, or a visual nature of the pattern. This is referred to as *combination* or *mixed deceleration*. Often this is a combination of late and variable decelerations, but on occasion there may be combinations of early and late or early and variable decelerations. In some instances, there may be combinations of accelerations and decelerations. When this mixed pattern deceleration is noted to be repetitive in nature, the labor should be managed according to the most ominous aspect of the mixed or combined pattern of deceleration. Frequently, this will occur in the active phase of labor or in the second stage of labor. If there is any doubt regarding the potential for fetal oxygen deprivation, additional fetal surveillance or commentary regarding the fetal acid–base status will enable the obstetrician to make a logical decision regarding the continuation of labor or the potential need for an early, instrument-assisted delivery or an operative delivery by cesarean section.

Fetal acid–base evaluation by fetal scalp capillary

TABLE 49–4. FETAL SCALP CAPILLARY BLOOD BASE DEFICIT CORRELATION (COLLECTED WITHIN 30 MINUTES PRIOR TO DELIVERY) WITH FETAL HEART RATE PATTERNS

FETAL HEART RATE PATTERN	MEAN (mEq/L) ± SE	RANGE (mEq/L)
Normal	6.98 ± 0.16	0.3–15.5
Early decelerations	6.97 ± 0.44	1.0–13.4
Mild variable decelerations	7.84 ± 0.19	2.0–13.4
Moderate variable decelerations	8.98 ± 0.44	2.5–21
Severe variable decelerations	10.44 ± 0.93	2.5–15.7
Mild late decelerations	9.29 ± 0.49	2.0–15.5
Moderate late decelerations	10.79 ± 0.43	4.8–16.8
Severe late decelerations	12.88 ± 0.77	10.1–18.8

Adapted from Hon EH, Khazin A. Observation of fetal heart rate and fetal biochemistry I. Base deficit. Am J Obstet Gynecol 1969;105:721, with permission.

blood sampling for fetal acidosis was used to monitor the well-being of the known high-risk fetus before continuous fetal cardiotocography was introduced in the late 1960s and early 1970s.[42,45] Fetal acid–base monitoring represents an intermittent commentary regarding the acid–base status or well-being of the fetus.[46] Generally, to collect fetal capillary blood from the presenting part, the cervix will need to be dilated approximately 2 cm with the presenting part at least at a −3 station. The chorioamnion will have to be ruptured, and the patient will need to cooperate. The technique involves positioning the patient in the lateral Sims' or dorsolithotomy position or with hips elevated on an object such as an inverted bed pan so that an elongated cone can be placed into the vagina to rest against the fetal presenting part. The mucus, blood, and fluid is cleared from the scalp or buttocks, and a 2-mm scalpel is used to make a single "stab-like" incision into the scalp or skin. Free-flowing fetal capillary blood is collected by gravity into a long (355 μL volume), preheparinized capillary tube. Approximately 40 μL of blood (about 2 inches in the capillary tube) is needed to obtain a complete set of respiratory blood gases, including pH, pO_2, pCO_2, bicarbonate, and base excess. Following the collection, the incisional site is inspected and pressure from a forceps-held swab is applied through three contractions. The site is subsequently inspected through a contraction, and if there is no bleeding, the cone is removed. Ideally, the equipment for analysis of p^H and respiratory blood gases will be by the patient's bedside or in the labor and delivery suite. Using modern equipment and with minimal training, labor suite personnel can perform these analyses.

When the technique was first introduced, fetal scalp capillary blood samples were used for pH determination; later pCO2, pO2, bicarbonate, and base excess (base deficit) were added. At first Doppler/stethoscopic-determined alterations in fetal heart rate would be followed up by the collection of fetal blood for pH determinations. When there was no alteration in the intermittent form of fetal heart rate monitoring, fetal capillary blood samples would be collected randomly during high-risk labors as a dual intermittent surveillance system, especially when chronic fetal oxygen deprivation could be present. This included labors of prolonged gestation, pregnancy-induced hypertension, intrauterine growth retardation, or otherwise unexplained thick meconium. Because most obstetricians are comfortable with the diagnostic accuracy of normal fetal heart rate data, intermittent acid–base determinations are used only when fetal heart rate monitoring is unclear or confusing. Currently, determinations of the fetal acid–base status represent the most precise information that the obstetrician has available for the diagnosis of the loss of fetal health or significant likelihood of clinically pertinent fetal oxygen deprivation. The intrapartum use of fetal capillary respiratory blood gas values with the presence of a maternal temperature greater than 103° to 104°F should not be relied on as the sole indicator to continue labor, especially if a long labor is anticipated. False values may result from alterations in fetal metabolism with a temperature of this level. Fetal temperatures usually exceed the maternal level by 0.5°C. After the introduction of fetal capillary blood for the determination of respiratory gases, its use became an integral aspect of intrauterine surveillance in many institutions (see Tables 49-5 and 49-6). Its use in the United States has been limited until very recently, when there appeared to be a resurgence of interest regarding acid–base commentary. A number of investigators have demonstrated that fetal stimulation and an evoked heart rate acceleration may be correlated to a known fetal acid–base status.

Both human and animal work regarding fetal capillary blood sampling during labor for the determination of acid–base status has revealed that there is a correlation between the fetal heart rate pattern, the severity of that pattern, and the fetal/newborn outcome (see Tables 49-2 through 49-4).[17,36] During labor, fetal acidosis may result from fetal oxygen deprivation secondary to impaired maternal–fetal exchange in the intervillous space. A transient fall in fetal pH may be secondary to acute umbilical cord compression, leading to the accumulation of carbon dioxide with a resultant fetal respiratory acidosis. Of greater importance is fetal oxygen deprivation, which is due to impaired fetal oxygen–carbon dioxide exchange in the intervillous space. When there is fetal oxygen deprivation sufficient to cause use of the anaerobic (Embden-Meyerhof) pathway for energy production, lactic acid will be accumulated and the fetal pH level will fall. If sufficient fetal oxygen deprivation and acidosis develop, neurological damage or death may result. There is a close relationship between fetal capillary blood gas values that are collected just prior to birth and umbilical cord arterial values collected at birth.[1,34]

Data collection regarding fetal blood pH and respiratory gas evaluation performed at the appropriate time may enable the obstetrician to recognize potential fetal oxygen deprivation prior to damage and allow fetal oxygen deprivation correction from the underlying problem or even a delivery by a route considered to be the safest for both mother and fetus. a number of investigators have considered pH values of 7.25 or greater to be

TABLE 49–5. ONE-MINUTE APGAR SCORE (355 PATIENTS)

	APGAR SCORE	
FETAL pH	1–6	7–10
≥7.20	10.4% (false normal)	64.4%
≤7.19	17.6%	7.6% (false abnormal)

From Hutson JM, Bowe ET, Petrie RH: The reliability of fetal acid-base determinations for prediction of normal Apgar scores: a reappraisal using the 5-minute score. Society of Perinatal Obstetricians Abstracts 1982:99, with permission.

TABLE 49–6. FIVE-MINUTE APGAR SCORE (355 PATIENTS)

	APGAR SCORE	
FETAL pH	1–6	7–10
≥7.20	1.7% (false normal)	—
≤7.19	—	—

From Hutson JM, Bowe ET, Petrie RH: The reliability of fetal acid-base determinations for prediction of normal Apgar scores: a reappraisal using the 5-minute score. Society of Perinatal Obstetricians Abstracts 1982:99, with permission.

normal. They consider that a pH range of 7.20 to 7.24 is pre-acidotic. A fetal capillary pH value of 7.19 or less has been believed to represent potential fetal acidosis and, if sustained on two collections 5 to 10 minutes apart, may represent sufficient acidosis to warrant termination of labor. Recent studies have demonstrated that it is uncommon to find significant fetal neurological damage until a pH range of less than 7.10 is noted,[38] and it is possible that the value may be as low as 7.00.[37] Normal umbilical cord blood and fetal capillary pH and respiratory gas values are given in Tables 49-2 through 49-8. Fetal capillary scalp pH values will normally fall in early labor, from approximately 7.35 to 7.25 at delivery. In clinical practice, it has been determined that serial pH determinations correlate best with the clinical setting and are probably of greater significance than an absolute value of one or two determinations of pH. Fetal heart rate variability provides important commentary on the severity of periodic patterns that may herald potential fetal oxygen deprivation.

A maternal acidosis can cause an apparent fetal acidosis secondary to the equilibration of H^+ ions across the placenta. The presence of a maternal and fetal acidotic state may indicate one of two things. Both the mother and fetus may be producing H+ ions, or the fetus may be a recipient of H+ ions but not truly have fetal oxygen deprivation. Maternal and fetal base excess can be compared to distinguish between the fetus with true fetal oxygen deprivation and the fetus who receives H+ ions from the mother. Maternal venous blood that is freely flowing without the use of a tourniquet can be collected for determinations of maternal respiratory blood gas values. The fetal pH is usually about 0.1 pH units below the maternal value. When a maternal acidosis is found, efforts should be made to determine the cause, such as ketoacidosis, sepsis, or dehydration. Appropriate corrective therapy then may be initiated. When there is maternal respiratory alkalosis associated with hyperventilation, falsely elevated fetal pH values have been reported.

A *base excess* (deficit) value is an indicator of fetal buffer reserves that are present to neutralize H+ ions or fixed acids. The base excess/deficit value can be clinically useful as an indicator of impending loss of fetal well-being when fetal pH values are satisfactory but the fetal heart rate pattern is the cause for concern (Tables 49-4 and 49-9). The longer the fetus is exposed to recurrent stress, the more likely it is that its acid–base status will suddenly deteriorate. With recurrent stress, evidenced by fetal heart rate deceleration, stable pH values, and a rising base excess/deficit status, the temporal interval before deterioration of the fetal status becomes progressively shorter. As with intermittent and continuous fetal heart rate and pH surveillance, base excess also has an indistinct border between normal and abnormal. Oxygen deprivation-induced fetal/newborn neurologic damage is not observed below a base excess of −12 to −14 mEq/L; nevertheless, even at a base excess level of −25 mEq/L or greater, only approximately 40% of newborns will have neurologic damage. When fetal base excess/deficit values are compared with fetal pH determinations and fetal heart rate patterns, there is a more reliable association of base excess/deficit with the severity of fetal heart rate patterns than with pH alone. Thus, judicious clinical use of base excess/deficit as an indicator of fetal well-being, especially when there are confusing fetal heart rate patterns, is of significant potential benefit. Now that instrumentation is available that can determine pH and base excess/deficit fetal capillary blood samples as small as 25 to 40 μL, this is especially important. On some occasions, before the cervix is sufficiently dilated to collect fetal capillary blood, it may be important to obtain commentary regarding acid-base status or other laboratory information. It is now possible with the use of ultrasound to guide an amniocentesis needle early in labor, prior to cervical dilatation sufficient to allow transcervical fetal scalp blood sampling, to do a funicentesis (funipuncture, cordocentesis, percutaneous umbilical blood sampling) to collect fetal blood. The use of funicentesis for this purpose is limited, but it is of real potential value in situations in which blood flow problems are likely, such as prolonged gestation, intrauterine growth retardation, pregnancy-induced hypertension, and perhaps diabetes mellitus.

TABLE 49–7. FETAL CAPILLARY BLOOD RESPIRATORY GAS VALUES

NORMAL	RESPIRATORY ACIDOSIS	METABOLIC ACIDOSIS
pH 7.25–7.40	Decreased	Decreased
pO_2	Usually stable	Decreased
PCO_2	Increased	Usually stable
Base deficit 0–12	Usually stable	Increased

TABLE 49-8. NORMAL UMBILICAL CORD ACID-BASE VALUES

	pH	pO_2	PCO_2	BASE EXCESS
Umbilical Arterial	7.242 (7.10–7.37)	16.6 (6.8–33.4)	49.9 (37.2–59.5)	−6.8 (−3.2−−13.6)
Umbilical Venous	7.312 (7.20–7.42)	28.9 (16.5–42.0)	39.1 (33–49.8)	−5.5 (2.7−−8.6)

Adapted from Wible JL, Petrie RH, Koons A, et al. The clinical use of umbilical cord acid-base determinations in perinatal surveillance and management. Cl in Perinatology 1982;9:387, with permission.

Fetal capillary blood collection for the determination of pH and respiratory blood gases has been considered by many to be too difficult for routine clinical use. Accordingly, these individuals relied on fetal heart rate information alone as a single surveillance technique during labor. Recently, fetal stimulation for evoking a fetal heart rate acceleration or comparison to pH/buffer evaluation has become somewhat widely used as commentary regarding fetal acid–base status. This allows use of fetal acid–base status without the actual collection of fetal blood for determinations of pH and respiratory gases by a machine. A number of stimuli, including injections of cold sterile water through an intrauterine pressure catheter, pain from the pinching of the fetal scalp, physical movement of the fetus, or a noise as in a vibroacoustic stimulation of the fetal auditory system, have gained popularity in recent years.

Fetal stimulation in some form has been used on a limited basis for three to four decades; recent investigators have studied the use of an evoked fetal heart rate acceleration during fetal scalp sampling as a stimulation at the time of the collection of fetal capillary blood. It was observed that, during the fetal capillary blood collecting process, when the scalp was stimulated an acceleration of 15 beats per minute with an excursion away from baseline for 15 seconds or greater was almost always indicative of a pH value of 7.22 or greater.[45] Conversely, the absence of a fetal heart acceleration when the fetus was stimulated is not absolutely predictive of a fetus who is acidotic; although some of the fetuses will be acidotic, the remainder will have a normal acid–base status. An acceleration in response to fetal scalp stimulation generally is accepted as a sufficient acid–base commentary to allow labor to continue. As long as an abnormal fetal heart rate is noted, normal acid–base commentary or acid–base determinations performed at intervals of every 15 to 20 minutes have been reliable to safely continue labor (see Tables 49-5 and 49-6).[47] When this intermittent form of acid–base commentary is to be used over a prolonged period of time, it is probably prudent to collect a sample of fetal capillary blood, as well as a sample of free-flowing maternal venous blood, occasionally to substantiate a satisfactory acid–base status inasmuch as fetal stimulation and correlation to accelerations for acid–base commentary is a relatively recent innovation.

Some investigators have used vibroacoustic stimulation during labor to bring about a fetal heart rate acceleration.[48] An artificial larynx (AT&T, Parsippany, NJ 07054) that generates 81 decibels of mixed noise and vibration can be placed on the maternal abdomen, approximately one third the distance from the symphysis pubis to the xiphoid process, to stimulate the fetus. Stimulation intervals of from 2 to 5 seconds are commonly used. Such a stimulation may evoke a fetal heart rate acceleration. With such fetal heart rate accelerations, generally, the fetus is in good condition from the physiologic and acid–base status. When using the internal form of fetal heart rate monitoring, a 5-second vibroacoustic stimulation to the fetus that results in either a ten beats per minute acceleration with a 10-second excursion away from baseline or a 15 beats per minute acceleration with a 15-second excursion away from baseline as correlated with a mean pH of 7.29 ± 0.07.[49] Again, some healthy fetuses as well as some fetuses with loss of fetal health will not respond with an acceleration. Accordingly, if an acceleration is not achieved through a vibroacoustic stimulation, then it is prudent to collect fetal capillary blood for pH and base excess determination to clarify the picture.

Umbilical cord pH and respiratory blood gas values are frequently used at birth to compare intrapartum fetal heart rate data with acid–base status and newborn condition (see Table 49-8).[50] These values frequently help identify the degree of fetal/newborn oxygenation at delivery. Following the delivery, 10 to 30 cm of a doubly clamped segment of the umbilical cord is obtained, and using two preheparinized small syringes, samples of umbilical cord blood from the artery and vein are collected separately. The blood samples are

TABLE 49-9. BASE DEFICIT (EXCESS)* IN FETAL CAPILLARY BLOOD

0 to 9 mEq/liter	Normal
9 to 11	Borderline
>12	Potential metabolic acidosis

* Base deficit and base excess have the same numerical value; however, a positive value is used for base deficit and negative value for base excess, ie, a base deficit of 6 is the same as a base excess of −6.

analyzed for pH and respiratory gases and correlated to both newborn conditions and fetal heart rate data during labor. By placing the umbilical cord segment or the blood samples on ice, one may delay the actual determination by a half hour or more but still obtain reliable determinations. Many obstetricians now include umbilical artery and vein, pH and respiratory gases as an integral part of the delivery process.

For almost 20 years, the potential of continuous fetal pH and respiratory gases from the fetal presenting part has been the aspiration of many obstetricians. A number of electrodes have been evaluated, and continuous pH, pCO_2, pO_2, and base excess/deficit has been available in a few laboratories. In Europe, continuous fetal pCO_2 is becoming more common. Unfortunately, continuous pH and respiratory gases are still under investigation, and it does not appear that they will be available for several years.

The evaluation of amniotic fluid as a surveillance technique for potential fetal oxygen deprivation represents a small role of primary consideration but a very valuable complementary role of fetal surveillance. The contribution of evaluation of amniotic fluid lies in two aspects: evaluation of volume and evaluation for the presence of meconium. *Amniotic fluid volume* can be carried out by manual palpation, observation of the amount of fluid lost when the chorioamnion has ruptured, or by ultrasonographic techniques to estimate either quantitatively or semiquantitatively the volume of amniotic fluid. It has been known for some time that less than the normal amount of fluid (oligohydramnios) or greater than normal volume of amniotic fluid (hydramnios or polyhydramnios) may indicate potential problems, either in terms of physiology or developmental, congenital, metabolic, or infectious processes. When excessive or diminished amounts of amniotic fluid are present, the obstetrician must be alert for potential problems and should be ready to evaluate the fetus in depth and perhaps with dual surveillance systems.

At present, perhaps the most reliable technique for evaluating amniotic fluid is ultrasonography; although used mostly in the antepartum period, intrapartum evaluation may also be valuable, particularly when conditions such as intrauterine growth retardation, pregnancy-induced hypertension, prolonged gestation, and diabetes mellitus are concerned. Amniotic fluid volume can be evaluated by many techniques. One of the most common is the amniotic fluid index.[51] The abdomen is divided into four quadrants and, with the transducer perpendicular to the plane of the table, the greatest depth of amniotic fluid found in each quadrant is obtained. The quadrants are summed and represent the relative amniotic fluid volume. Values of less than 8 to 10 cm and especially less than 5 cm will cause the obstetrician to be on the lookout for such problems as those involving cord compression.

Meconium evaluation is a reasonably soft marker for potential fetal oxygen deprivation. Two groups of investigators have evaluated the significance of meconium in the amniotic fluid and its relationship to fetal heart rate. Fenton and Steer correlated meconium, fetal heart rate, and newborn outcome using intermittent fetal heart rate monitoring prior to fetal cardiotocography.[10] Miller and coworkers[52] and Miller and Read[53] have looked at the significance of meconium, fetal heart rate, and newborn outcome using continuous fetal heart rate monitoring. In both instances, the conclusions have been similar. Generally, it is thought that meconium alone, in an otherwise normal fetus, is not a significant marker for the potential of fetal oxygen deprivation. When meconium is present with other markers of potential fetal oxygen deprivation, meconium then becomes an additional marker. The presence of meconium early in a labor, particularly when placental function may be suspect, such as in prolonged gestation, fetal growth retardation, maternal hypertension, maternal diabetes, etc, may cause a number of clinicians to be concerned about the overall acid–base status of the fetus. The evaluation of acid–base by either direct capillary blood sampling or fetal stimulation may be performed quite early in the labor to establish acid–base status and to identify those fetuses already exposed to chronic fetal oxygen deprivation. It is easy to evaluate meconium from amniotic fluid when the membranes are ruptured. Prior to rupture of the membranes, the use of an amniocentesis or transcervical amnioscopy to evaluate the presence of meconium have been used.

Both the evaluation of fetal breathing[54,55] and the evaluation of fetal movement or fetal kicking have been established by investigators such as Sadovsky[30] and Rayburn[56] to have significant potential for the detection of possible fetal oxygen deprivation during the antepartum interval. Although the evaluation of both fetal breathing and fetal movement or kicking during labor can be carried out to a limited degree, their use is usually limited to the early latent period of labor and becomes more difficult as uterine contractions become more frequent, because the fetus tends to move less and it is more difficult to differentiate fetal movement from uterine activity.

Uterine activity evaluation is an exceedingly important part of intrapartum fetal surveillance. Many clinicians believe that manual palpation of the uterus for contractions or tocodynametric or external uterine monitoring is sufficient to carry out a successful intrapartum fetal surveillance protocol. Often, this is the case; nevertheless, a careful evaluation of uterine activity that can be quantitated and evaluated may be critical in the high-resolution protocol. The early detection of dysfunctional labor secondary to inadequate uterine activity, while not totally dependent on internal quantitated monitoring of uterine activity, certainly is benefited by it. The early detection of a placental abruption can be very rewarding in some instances, and the evaluation of uterine activity for the establishment of the effects of drugs on labor and uterine activity, or progress in labor is equally rewarding. It is the use of uterine activity data for the proper identification of periodic patterns that is critically important. In many instances, the fetal heart rate data may be good and clear, but uterine activity surveillance, using an external form of fetal monitoring, is of such poor quality that the true identity of fetal heart rate changes cannot be easily appreciated. For this reason, the use of an intrauterine pressure catheter to evaluate uterine activity is recommended. Although many people believe that the presence of a foreign body such as an intrauterine pressure catheter is a cause of infection, the data do not support this.[57–59] In fact, the presence of an intrauterine pressure catheter frequently decreases the number of cervical examinations that are required during labor, and a reduction in the number of vaginal examinations may lead to reduced incidence of post-partum endomyometritis. Quantitation of uterine activity for the identification of dysfunctional labor requiring oxytocin or the presence of uterine activity related fetal heart rate abnormalities can best be evaluated with the use of an internal pressure catheter. Rising baseline tone, frequent, strong contractions developing into a tachysystole or tetanic contraction may be seen with spontaneous excessive uterine activity, and in drug-induced excessive uterine activity in the presence of certain pathophysiologic states such as abruptio placentae. Oxygenation of the fetus is obviously proportionate in some of these disorders to the amount of uterine activity. Thus, it may be prudent when evaluating fetal heart rate and acid–base data for interpretation of the fetal oxygenation status to always be mindful of the potential stress that the fetus is encountering in the form of uterine activity.

FETAL INTRAPARTUM MANAGEMENT

Management options used to avoid the potential of significant fetal oxygen deprivation include control of maternal hypotension, control of uterine activity–hyperactivity, control or alleviation of umbilical cord compression, and appropriate intravenous fluid administration.

Fetal surveillance during labor is principally surveillance with fetal heart rate monitoring. As long as fetal heart rate monitoring data are normal, the low-risk patient needs no additional monitoring. High-risk patients with the potential for intrapartum fetal oxygen deprivation may benefit from a baseline acid–base commentary; however, usually as long as the fetal heart rate data remain normal, no additional surveillance techniques are required. When heart rate changes are noted, such as significant tachycardia, bradycardia, late, variable, or prolonged decelerations, or significant loss of fetal heart rate variability, particularly when it had been present previously or following significant fetal stress such as significant uterine hyperactivity, the patient usually responds to correction of maternal supine hypotension, position change, administration of maternal oxygen, or reduction in oxytocin administration. When simple measures such as these and the use of intravenous fluids do not correct the problem, and long-term (> than 30 minutes) or repetitive late or variable decelerations are present, one may look for accelerations as a marker of well-being. One may also consider stimulation of the fetus to provoke accelerations or the actual collection for capillary blood acid–base determinations. It should be kept in mind that with increasing temporal duration, repetitive fetal heart rate decelerations are more likely to result in significant fetal oxygen deprivation, although the acid–base status at the time may be satisfactory.[43] Accordingly, dual surveillance that allows the continuation of labor in the presence of questionable or abnormal fetal heart rate data should be carried out only when the delivery process can be expected within 1 to 2 hours and intermittent acid–base commentary can be obtained at an interval of every 15 to 20 minutes. On occasion, when uterine activity is excessive, causing an immediate fetal heart rate abnormality, such as with significant variable decelerations, the temporary use of a tocolytic agent such as intravenous magnesium sulfate by an intravenous injection of 4 to 6 g over a 15- to 20-minute interval or 0.25 to 0.5 mg of terbutaline subcutaneously may reduce uterine activity sufficiently to allow the fetus to recover and then return to a productive labor.[60] When such a technique is used, careful attention to fetal well-being must be utmost in the clinician's mind.

In conditions where reduced amniotic fluid is a potential, such as labor with a premature fetus, intrauterine growth retardation, prolonged gestation, pregnancy-induced hypertension, and even diabetes mellitus, the use of an *amnioinfusion* to buffer the umbilical cord can be of considerable help, especially with significant cord compression in a premature fetus.[61–63] The use of amnioinfusion in gestations complicated by meconium has been demonstrated to be of benefit. Sadovsky and coworkers have found that amnioinfusion for the elimination of meconium was safe, simple, and effective.[64] Amnioinfusion has been demonstrated to significantly reduce the thickness of meconium, the incidence of neonatal acidemia, and the incidence of significant meconium below the vocal cords at delivery. A number of protocols are used for amnioinfusion. Miyazaki[61] and Nageotte[62,63] have advocated the use of amnioinfusion for cord compression, and they use 0.5 to 1 L of normal saline infused at 150 to 200 mL/hour as long as the decelerative pattern persists. Once the pattern has been ameliorated, a maintenance infusion of 10 to 20 mL/hour is used. Until recently, amnioinfusion required warming of the saline solution to body temperature prior to infusion; recently, however, it has been reported that saline at room temperature has been found to be as effective as fluid warmed to body temperature.

POTENTIAL PROBLEMS OF FETAL SURVEILLANCE

The critics of continuous fetal heart rate monitoring point out that this technique has caused the cesarean section rate to soar for obstetrically unwarranted reasons. There is no doubt that increased surveillance of the fetus has caused the cesarean section rate to rise to some degree; however, the impact of the increased attention paid to intrapartum fetal surveillance by the legal/justice system is impossible to evaluate. There is no doubt that in programs where dual surveillance systems are used, the incidence of cesarean sections for fetal distress has actually declined.[23]

Regarding acid–base monitoring, the problems of infection and bleeding following the collection of fetal scalp blood are real but small. When the scalp puncture site is viewed through three contractions following the collection of capillary blood, significant bleeding thereafter is quite uncommon. In fact, significant bleeding is quite uncommon outside of a pharmacologically induced coagulopathy.[24] The most common of these is with the use of phenobarbital and diphenylhydantoin.[65] Once continued fetal bleeding is identified, usually a small clip placed across the incision site to add pressure to the scalp will take care of the problem. Occasionally, an early instrument-assisted vaginal delivery or a cesarean section may be required. A small pustule or local infection may be noted at the incision site. Bowe gives the incidence of this as approximately 1 in 1000 cases.[33] In most instances, simple drainage will take care of the problem; however, on occasion, antibiotics may be needed for more serious infections. Bleeding and infection may be noted at the site of a scalp electrode attachment. Bleeding is almost unheard of, and infections occur at about the same rate as they do for fetal capillary blood sampling.

The use of fetal stimulation to obtain a fetal heart rate acceleration as a marker of fetal acid–base status without collecting fetal capillary blood is being used with increasing frequency. This form of fetal surveillance would appear to be without problem, except for the possibility of not being able to identify the fetus with good acid–base status who does not respond with an acceleration. Nevertheless, some investigators have questions regarding potential problems, which may be as grave as damage to the fetal auditory system.[66] Considerable investigation in this area is presently underway to substantiate its safety.

On occasion, a uterine perforation will occur when the uterine pressure catheter is inserted. Almost uniformly, this occurs when the stiff catheter guide is inserted beyond the operator's fingertip. Case reports indicate that complications may occur from time to time, including problems with attachment of the fetal scalp electrode; however, these complications are exceedingly rare.

Intrauterine infection following the use of internal fetal heart rate monitoring is a fear of a number of obstetricians; however, the infection rate as evidenced by incidence of endomyometritis is not outside the normal range.[58,59] Gassner and Ledger confirmed these findings, but included the fact that in cases in which internal fetal heart rate monitoring was used for several hours and the patient underwent cesarean section, there was an increased incidence of intrauterine infections.[57] A cause and effect relationship has not been established.

Some obstetricians are somewhat uncomfortable following a patient with repetitive heart rate indicators of potential fetal oxygen deprivation in the presence of normal fetal acid–base evaluation. In an obstetrical unit that routinely uses acid–base determinations as a secondary surveillance system, especially when base excess is used, dual fetal surveillance is rarely found to be a problem. The 1- and 5-minute Apgar score data by Bowe and Hutson and coworkers demonstrate that this is a reasonably safe protocol.[34,47] From the work of Fleischer and associates, it is known that, with repetitive stress, a normal acid–base status can deteriorate over a period of time; thus, it is important that as long as the fetal heart rate pattern is suggestive of potential fetal oxygen deprivation, commentary regarding acid–base status is necessary every 15 to 20 minutes.[43] In this particular instance, the use of fetal capillary blood pH and base excess will be more reassuring than pH alone. Base excess will enable the obstetrician to determine when the fetal buffer reserves are being exhausted, to be shortly followed by a deterioration in the pH values.

Some patients believe that both continuous electronic fetal heart rate and acid–base surveillance is too technical and too restrictive, and they think these techniques interfere with the natural birth process. The patients believe that they are not in control, and that monitoring in any form is unwarranted.[67–71] Generally, when the patient expresses this form of doubt, a careful and complete explanation of the means and benefits of this form of monitoring will make her more comfortable. In spite of appropriate antepartum screening, some patients arrive on a delivery service refusing any form of fetal surveillance. When this happens, a careful explanation of the procedure and what is expected of her should be given to the patient, and if the patient continues to refuse appropriate fetal surveillance, in the presence of witnesses, it should be verified in the chart that the patient was offered fetal monitoring and the reasons for needing fetal monitoring were explained to her. Fetal heart rate data should then be collected when maternal vital signs are collected. Fortunately, the incidence of intrapartum fetal oxygen deprivation is quite small, and it is hoped that neither the patient nor her fetus will adversely be affected by her decision not to use intrapartum fetal surveillance on the frequent basis that current protocols suggest are important.

On occasion, the obstetrician will be required to monitor a multiple gestation in labor. Many commercial monitors now have the ability to monitor two fetuses on one unit. It is possible, by using two monitors, to evaluate up to three fetuses concomitantly. If internal monitoring is being used for the first fetus, a sterile tubing can be run from the dome of the strain gauge of the first monitor to the dome of the strain gauge on the second monitor. With appropriate filling of the tube connecting the two domes, intrauterine pressure can be available on both monitors for the proper evaluation of heart rate data in relation to uterine contractions. In the high-risk multiple gestation, some maternal–fetal medicine specialists believe that if one is unable to adequately monitor a fetus during labor, a delivery by cesarean section may be in order.

REFERENCES

1. Adamsons K, Beard RW, Cosmi E, et al. The validity of capillary blood in the assessment of the acid-base state of the fetus. In: Adamsons K, ed. Diagnosis and treatment of fetal disorders. New York: Springer-Verlag, 1968:175.
2. Apgar V. A proposal for a new method of evaluation of the newborn infant. Anesth Analg 1953;32:260.
3. Barcroft J. Researches on pre-natal life. Springfield, IL: Charles C Thomas, 1947.
4. Barron DH. The exchange of the respiratory gases in the placenta. Neonatal Studies 1952;1:3.
5. Caldeyro-Barcia R, Magãna JM, Castillo JB, et al. A new approach to the treatment of acute intrapartum fetal distress. Perinatal factors affecting human development. Proceedings of the Special Session held during the Eight Meeting of the PAHO Advisory Committee on Medical Research, Washington, DC, June 1969.
6. Caldeyro-Barcia R, Casacuberta C, Busros R, et al. Correlation of intrapartum changes in fetal heart rate with fetal blood oxygen and acid-base balance. In: Adamsons K ed. Diagnosis and treatment of fetal disorders. New York: Springer-Verlag, 1968:205.
7. Dawes GS, Handler JJ, Mott JC. Some cardiovascular responses in fetal, newborn and adult rabbits. J Physiol 1957;139:123.
8. Freda V. Hemolytic disease. Clin Obstet Gynecol 1973;16:72.
9. James LS, Weisbrot IM, Prince CE, et al. The acid-base status of human infants in relation to birth asphyxia and the onset of respiration. J Pediatr 1958;52:379.
10. Fenton AN, Steer CM. Fetal distress. Am J Obstet Gynecol 1962;83:354.
11. Assali NS, Holm L, Parker H. Regional blood flow and vascular resistance in response to oxytocin in the pregnant sheep and dog. J Appl Physiol 1961;16:1087.
12. Saling E. Technik der endoskopischen microblutent-nahme am feten. Geburtshilfe Frauenheilkd 1964;24:464.
13. Saling E. Neues Vorgehen zur Untersuchung des Kindes unter der Gebrut. Archiv für Gynäkologie 1961;197:108.
14. Hammacher K, Huter KA, Bokelmann J, et al. Foetal heart frequency and perinatal condition of foetus and newborn. Gynaecologia (Basel) 1968;166:348.
15. Hon EH, Quilligan EJ. The classification of fetal heart rate. II: a revised working classification. Conn Med 1967;31:779.
16. Hon EH. The electronic evaluation of the fetal heart rate. Am J Obstet Gynecol 1958;75:1215.
17. Kubli FW, Hon EH, Khazin AF, et al. Observations on heart rate and pH in the human fetus during labor. Am J Obstet Gynecol 1969;104:1190.
18. Low JA, Cox MJ, Karchmar EJ, et al. The prediction of intrapartum fetal metabolic acidosis by fetal heart rate monitoring. Am J Obstet Gynecol 1981;139:299.
19. Miller FC, Pearse KE, Paul RH. Fetal heart rate pattern recognition by the method of auscultation. Obstet Gynecol 1984;64:332.
20. Boylan P, MacDonald D, Grant A, et al. The Dublin fetal monitoring trial [abstract]. Proceedings of the Society of Perinatal Obstetricians, Fourth Annual Meeting in San Antonio [Abstracts] 1984, page 18.
21. Kelso IM, Parsons RJ, Lawrence GF, et al. An assessment of continuous fetal heart rate monitoring in labor. A randomized trial. Am J Obstet Gynecol 1978;131:526.
22. Renou P, Chang A, Anderson I, et al. Controlled trial of fetal intensive care. Am J Obstet Gynecol 1972;113:573.
23. Shamsi HH, Petrie RH, Steer CM. Changing obstetrical practices and amelioration of perinatal outcome in a university hospital. Am J Obstet Gynecol 1979;133:855.
24. Wood C, Lumbley J, Renou P. A clinical assessment of foetal diagnostic methods. J Obstet Br Commonwealth 1967;74:832.
25. Banta HD, Thacker S. Assessing the costs and benefits of electronic fetal monitoring. Obstet Gynecol Surv 1979;34:627.
26. Brown NA, Scialli AR. Editorial: congenital "brain damage." Reproductive Toxicology 1987;6(1):1.
27. Jenkins HM. Thirty years of electronic intrapartum fetal heart rate monitoring: discussion paper. J R Soc Med 1989;82:210.
28. Newell SJ, Green SH. Diagnostic classification of the etiology of mental retardation in children. Br Med J 1987;294:163.
29. Prentice A, Lind T. Fetal heart rate monitoring during labour—too frequent intervention, too little benefit? Lancet 1987;2:1375.
30. Rosen MG. Consensus report by the Task Force on Cesarean Childbirth. Hyattsville, MD: U.S. Department of Health and Human Services, Public Health Service, National Institutes of Health publication #82–2067, 1981.
31. Sims ME, Turkel SB, Halterman G, Paul RH. Brain injury and intrauterine death. Am J Obstet Gynecol 1985;151:721.
32. Shy KK, Luthy DA, Bennett FC, et al. Effects of electronic fetal-heart-rate monitoring, as compared with periodic auscultation, on the neurologic development of premature infants. N Engl J Med 1990;322:588.
33. Beard RW. Fetal blood sampling. Br J Hosp Med 1970;3:523.
34. Bowe ET, Beard RT, Finster M, et al. Reliability of fetal blood sampling. Am J Obstet Gynecol 1970;107:279.
35. Bowe ET. Fetal blood sampling. Bulletin of the Sloane Hospital for Women 1967;13:11.
36. Hon EH, Khazin AF. Biochemical studies of the fetus. II: fetal pH and Apgar scores. Obstet Gynecol 1969;33:237.
37. Gilstrap LC, Leveno KJ, Burris J, Williams ML, Little BB. Diagnosis of birth asphyxia on the basis of fetal pH, Apgar score, and newborn cerebral dysfunction. Am J Obstet Gynecol 1989;161:825.
38. Wible JL, Petrie RH, Koons A, et al. The clinical use of umbilical cord acid-base determinations in perinatal surveillance and management. Clin Perinatol 1982;9:387.
39. Intrapartum fetal heart rate monitoring. ACOG Technical Bulletin number 132, September 1989.
40. Fetal heart rate auscultation. NAACOG Abstracts of Clinical Care Guidelines 1990;2:1.
41. Martin CB. Physiology and clinical use of fetal heart rate variability. Clin Perinatol 1982;9:339.
42. Zalar RW Jr, Quilligan EJ. The influence of scalp sampling on the cesarean section rate for fetal distress. Am J Obstet Gynecol 1975;123:206.
43. Fleischer A, Schulman H, Jagani N, et al. The development of fetal acidosis in the presence of an abnormal fetal heart rate tracing. Am J Obstet Gynecol 1982;144:55.
44. Hutson JM, Mueller-Heubach E. Diagnosis and management of intrapartum reflex fetal heart rate changes. Clin Perinatol 1982;9:325.
45. Clark SL, Gimovsky ML, Miller FC. Fetal heart rate response to scalp blood sampling. Am J Obstet Gynecol 1982;144:706.
46. Assessment of fetal and newborn acid-base status. ACOG Technical Bulletin number 127, April 1989.
47. Hutson JM, Bowe ET, Petrie RH. The reliability of fetal acid-base determinations for prediction of normal Apgar scores: a reappraisal using the 5 minute score [abstract]. Proceedings of the Society of Perinatal Obstetricians, Second Annual Meeting in San Antonio S.P.O. [abstracts], 1984, page 99.
48. Edersheim TG, Hutson JM, Druzin MD, et al. Fetal heart rate

response to vibratory acoustic stimulation predicts fetal pH in labor. Am J Obstet Gynecol 1987;157:1557.

49. Polzin GB, Blakemore KJ, Petrie RH, Amon E. Fetal vibroacoustic stimulation: magnitude and duration of fetal heart rate accelerations as a marker of fetal health. Obstet Gynecol 1988;72:621.
50. Thorp JA, Sampson JE, Parisi VM, Creasy RK. Routine umbilical cord blood gas determinations? Am J Obstet Gynecol 1989;161:600.
51. Moore TR, Cayle JE. The amniotic fluid index in normal human pregnancy. Am J Obstet Gynecol 1990;162:1168.
52. Miller FC, Sacks DA, Yeh S-Y. Significance of meconium during labor. Am J Obstet Gynecol 1978;130:473.
53. Miller FC, Read JA. Intrapartum assessment of the postdate fetus. Am J Obstet Gynecol 1981;141:516.
54. Patrick J, Challis J. Measurement of human fetal breathing movements in healthy pregnancies using a real-time scanner. Semin Perinatol 1980;4:275.
55. Patrick J, Campbell LK, Carmichael L, et al. Patterns of human fetal breathing during the last 10 weeks of pregnancy. Obstet Gynecol 1980;56:24.
56. Rayburn WF. Clinical significance of maternal perceptible fetal motion. Am J Obstet Gynecol 1980;138:210.
57. Gassner CB, Ledger WJ. The relationship of hospital-acquired maternal infection to invasive intrapartum monitoring techniques. Obstet Gynecol 1976;126:33.
58. Gibbs RS, Listwa HM, Read JA. The effect of internal fetal monitoring on maternal infection following cesarean section. Obstet Gynecol 1976;48:653.
59. Ledger WJ. Complications associated with invasive monitoring. Semin Perinatol 1978;2:187.
60. Reece EA, Chervenak AF, Romero R, Hobbins JC. Magnesium sulfate in the management of acute intrapartum fetal distress. Am J Obstet Gynecol 1984;148:104.
61. Miyazaki FS, Taylor NA. Saline amnioinfusion for relief of variable or prolonged decelerations. Am J Obstet Gynecol 1983;146:670.
62. Nageotte MP, Bertucci L, Towers CV, Lagrew DC, Mondanlou H. Prophylactic amnioinfusion in pregnancies complicated by oligohydramnios or thick meconium: a prospective study. Society of Perinatal Obstetricians, Tenth Annual Meeting, Houston [abstracts] 1990, page 78.
63. Nageotte MP, Freemen RK, Garite TJ, Dorchester W. Prophylactic intrapartum amnioinfusion in patients with preterm premature rupture of membranes. Am J Obstet Gynecol 1985;153:557.
64. Sadovsky Y, Amon E, Bade M, Petrie RH. Prophylactic amnioinfusion during labor complicated by meconium: a preliminary report. Am J Obstet Gynecol 1989;161:613.
65. Mountain KR, Hirsh J, Gallus AS. Neonatal coagulation defect due to anticonvulsant drug treatment in pregnancy. Lancet 1970;1:265.
66. Richards DS. The fetal virbroacoustic stimulation test: an up date. Semin Perinatol 1990;14:305.
67. Dulock HL, Herron M. Women's response to fetal monitoring. J Obstet Gynecol Neonatal Nurs 1976;5:68.
68. Jackson JE, Vaughan M, Black P, et al. Psychological aspects of fetal monitoring: maternal reaction to the position of the monitor and staff behavior. Journal of Psychosocial Obstetrics and Gynecology 1983;2:97.
69. Molfese V, Sunshine P, Bennett A. Reactions of women to intrapartum fetal monitoring. Obstet Gynecol 1982;59:706.
70. Shields D. Maternal reactions to fetal monitoring. Am J Nurs 1978;3:2110.
71. Starkman M. Psychological responses to the use of the monitor during labor. Psychosom Med 1976;38:269.

50

CHAPTER

AMNIOTIC FLUID ASSESSMENT AND SIGNIFICANCE OF CONTAMINANTS

Jeffrey P. Phelan

The clinical significance of amniotic fluid has puzzled practitioners for centuries. In the past, it was believed that the fetus was nourished in part from the amniotic fluid.[1] These mysteries gradually abated as the concepts of amniotic fluid dynamics changed over time.[2–4] Recent evidence demonstrates that 4 liters of water accumulates in the uterus during pregnancy. In the third trimester, intrauterine water accumulates from 30 to 40 mL per day.[4] The accumulation of amniotic fluid is of vital importance to the fetus. For example, normal and above normal amniotic fluid volumes permit regular fetal movement. At the same time, a normal volume protects the fetus from cord compression during fetal activity, by permitting the cord to move away from the fetus. Finally, the amniotic fluid volume helps to maintain an even temperature for the fetus.

Because of the known clinical importance of amniotic fluid for the developing fetus, this chapter will focus on the physiologic aspects of amniotic fluid during pregnancy, newer techniques to assess the amniotic fluid volume, disorders in amniotic fluid volume, such as oligo- and polyhydramnios and, finally, the clinical applications of amniotic fluid volume assessment during pregnancy in antepartum fetal surveillance, the fetal admission test, premature rupture of the membranes, amnioinfusion, and polyhydramnios.

PHYSIOLOGIC ASPECTS OF AMNIOTIC FLUID

The amniotic sac is created approximately 12 days after fertilization, as follows: A cleft enclosed in the primitive amnion is found adjacent to the embryonic plate. It rapidly enlarges and fuses to the body stock. When it fuses with the chorion, the amniotic sac is created. Once formed, this sac fills with a colorless liquid, presumably from maternal plasma. This is the amniotic fluid.

With advancing gestation, the composition of the amniotic fluid changes. In the first half of pregnancy, the amniotic fluid is isotonic and similar to maternal plasma,[3] but the amniotic fluid contains less protein concentration than maternal plasma and is devoid of particulate matter. By 20 weeks gestation, the osmolality and concentration of sodium and urea are similar to maternal serum concentrations.[5] In the second half of pregnancy, the composition changes with increases in particulate matter.[2] In particular, desquamated fetal cells, lanugo and scalp hair, and vernix caseosa increase in the latter half of pregnancy. While this is occurring, the osmolality of the amniotic fluid decreases. In effect, the amniotic fluid becomes hypotonic.[6] In comparison with the first half of pregnancy, there is a 20 to 30 mOsm, or 10%, decrease with advancing gestation. Moreover, the osmolality of the amniotic fluid is approximately 92% of that of the maternal serum.[5]

In many respects, amniotic fluid represents extracellular fluid, with a composition similar to fetal urine. The kidney, with its importance in urine production, appears to be the major contributor to the changes in the amniotic fluid in the latter half of pregnancy. For instance, there are noticeable increases in urea, creatinine, and uric acid. By 24 weeks gestation,[7] the concentration of these urinary by-products is two to three times higher than fetal plasma; this change represents a 70% to 250% increase in the concentration of these compounds. Electrolyte changes similarly occur in the latter half of pregnancy. The amniotic fluid concentrations of sodium, potassium, and chloride are usually 20% to 33% less than the fetal and maternal plasma levels.[7] In fact, the amniotic fluid sodium level is 92% of that of maternal serum.[5]

In contrast, amniotic fluid protein increases progressively during the first 6 months of pregnancy. From 32 weeks to term, there is a progressive decline in the amniotic fluid protein concentration.[7]

With the changes in amniotic fluid content, the amniotic fluid volume changes dramatically during pregnancy (Fig. 50-1). For example, the amniotic fluid volume increases progressively to the early third trimester. From then until term, the amniotic fluid volume remains constant. During the period from 37 weeks to 41 weeks, amniotic fluid volume declines 10%. Once the patient becomes post dates, there is a 33% decline in amniotic fluid volume per week.[8–11]

These changes in amniotic fluid volume are frequently related to the mechanisms responsible for amniotic fluid production. For example, in the first half of pregnancy, the amniotic fluid volume is proportional to the increases in fetal weight. It is during this time that the fetal skin is highly permeable to water and sodium and can transport urea. By 25 weeks gestation, the skin becomes keratinized[5] and becomes impermeable to the fluid in the uterine cavity.

In the latter half of pregnancy, the turnover in amniotic fluid increases. Hutchinson has estimated that 3600 mL per hour per day are transported in the maternal and fetal compartment.[12] In fact, Vosburgh has demonstrated there is a complete turnover in the amniotic fluid every 2.9 hours.[13] Previous work by Pritchard, however, has demonstrated a turnover of approximately 500 mL per day.[14]

In contrast to the first half of pregnancy, amniotic fluid regulation involves the complex interaction between fetal swallowing, tracheal fluid production, and urination. For example, while the role of fetal swallowing in controlling amniotic fluid volume is undefined, fetal swallowing does play a dominant role when the amniotic fluid volume is normal. Using radioactively labeled red blood cells, Pritchard was able to determine the impact of fetal swallowing during pregnancy.[14] From 16 weeks until term, he showed that the fetus swallowed 7 to 20 mL/hr. This amounted to over 500 mL over a 24-hour period, equivalent to half the amniotic fluid volume in the term gestation. When the amount swallowed was correlated with the fetal weight, a three-fold increase in the amount swallowed was observed in a 24-hour period.[5] This amounted to a change from 50 to 150 mL/kg over a 24-hour period.

Fetal pulmonary or tracheal fluid increases with advancing gestation. Based on animal studies,[5] the amount of fetal pulmonary fluid increases 1.7 times during the last 4 weeks of pregnancy. It is estimated that at term, 50 to 80 mL of fluid per hour are generated.[15] The true origin of the fetal tracheal fluid is less clear as to whether it represents previously swallowed or "aspirated" amniotic fluid or the respiratory tree's contribution to the amniotic fluid volume. However, tracheal fluid does play an important role in amniotic fluid volume dynamics, and may be a critical factor in the evolution of polyhydramnios.

In the latter half of pregnancy, fetal urine production is estimated to be 500 mL per day, and constitutes the major source of amniotic fluid. According to Pritchard, urine flow (output) equals swallowing (input), or 500 mL per day.[14] This has also been confirmed in investigations by Chez and coworkers.[16] In that latter investigation, Chez was able to show that the fetus excreted approximately 500 mL/kg/hr. Subsequent investigations by Kurjak and associates demonstrated a twelvefold increase in the hourly urine production from 22 to 41 weeks gestation.[17] In fact, hourly urine production increased from 2.2 mL/hr to 26.3 mL/hr at term.

According to Kurjak, renal function was also maxi-

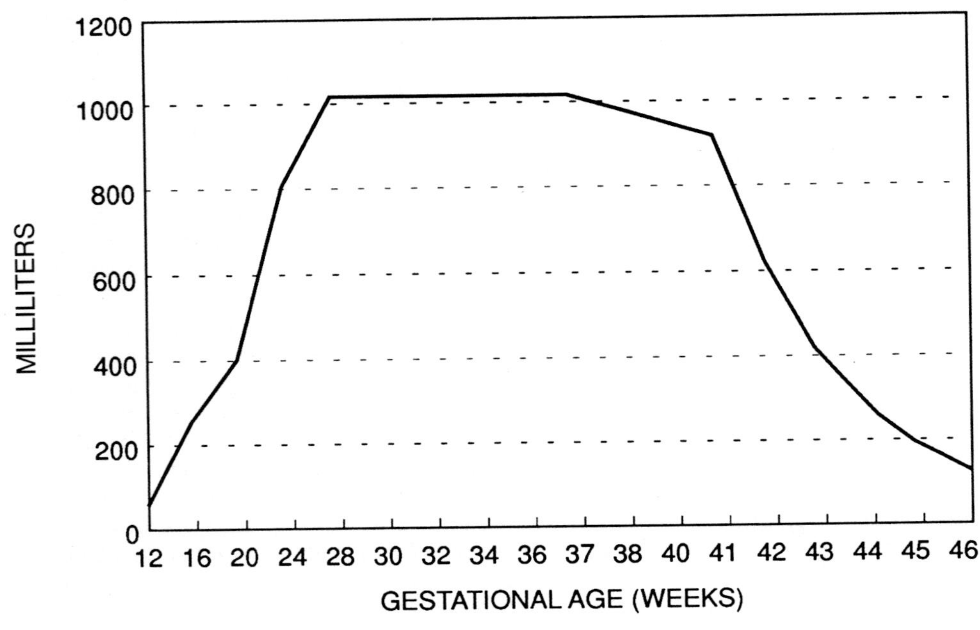

FIGURE 50–1. Mean amniotic fluid volume changes during pregnancy.

mal at term.[17] For example, the term fetus had demonstrated a glomerular filtration rate of 2.6 mL/min and a tubular water reabsorption rate of 78%. In the postdate period, fetal urine production declines and probably accounts for the reductions in amniotic fluid volume that are frequently observed.[8,9]

TECHNIQUES TO ASSESS AMNIOTIC FLUID VOLUME

A variety of techniques have been developed to assess amniotic fluid volume.[8,9,13,18–23] These methods have included invasive techniques, such as dye dilution techniques that require amniocentesis,[8,9,13,18] and noninvasive ones that employ ultrasonography.[19–23] To accurately assess the amniotic fluid volume with the dye dilution technique requires an amniocentesis with its attendant risks and potential complications. It is interesting to note that W. J. Dieckmann, in his address before the Chicago Gynecologic Society on June 17, 1932, commented favorably on this "invasive" technique. In his address, he stated, "We have been interested in finding a method to determine the amount of liquor amnii in utero without disturbing the fetus," and concluded that Congo red infusion after amniocentesis was a reliable method to quantify amniotic fluid volume without disturbing the fetus.[24]

With the introduction of ultrasonography, invasive techniques were no longer medically necessary. Instead, an array of ultrasound techniques were developed to estimate the amniotic fluid volume (Table 50-1). Initially, contact "B-scanners" were used to estimate the amniotic fluid volume.[19] With the use of these scanners, Gohari was able to visualize and measure the entire intrauterine cavity. By so doing, he was able to calculate the total intrauterine volume. He then correlated his findings with pregnancy outcome, and was able to quantify an abnormal amniotic fluid volume and reliably predict the likelihood of intrauterine growth retardation.

With real-time ultrasound, a total intrauterine image could not be readily accomplished in a single view. As a consequence, newer techniques to assess the amniotic fluid volume were sought.[20–23] These techniques focused on a single amniotic fluid pocket. Thus, to estimate the amniotic fluid volume, the vertical diameter of the largest amniotic fluid pocket was measured and correlated with subsequent fetal outcome.

TABLE 50–1. TECHNIQUES TO ASSESS AMNIOTIC FLUID VOLUME DURING PREGNANCY

	TECHNIQUE
Gohari[19]	Total intrauterine volume
Manning[20]	"One-centimeter rule"*
Chamberlain[21]	"Two-centimeter rule"*
Crowley[22]	"Three-centimeter rule"*
Phelan[23]	Amniotic fluid index

* Vertical diameter of the largest pocket.

First, the "one centimeter rule" was developed to identify a normal amniotic fluid volume.[20] This qualitative assessment of the amniotic fluid volume was used primarily to predict intrauterine growth retardation, but later served as an indicator of oligohydramnios. For example, the finding of a single amniotic fluid pocket of 1 cm or less was associated with a 90% chance of intrauterine growth retardation.[18]

Phelan[25] and Eden[26] demonstrated that the volume associated with a single pocket less than 1 cm represented severe oligohydramnios. Moreover, these investigators found a volume larger than 1 cm that was also associated with significantly greater risk of perinatal morbidity and mortality.

Subsequently, Chamberlain and coworkers developed what is known as the "two centimeter rule."[21] These investigators found that the 1-centimeter rule was too restrictive to properly identify those fetuses at the greatest risk of an adverse perinatal outcome. With the use of the 2-centimeter rule, Chamberlain found they could reliably predict those fetuses at risk for intrauterine growth retardation, oligohydramnios, and perinatal mortality. This risk was the greatest in patients whose largest amniotic fluid pocket was less than 2 cm. Those patients with pockets in excess of 2 cm were considered to have a normal amniotic fluid volume and were at low risk for these complications.

As an outgrowth of these two approaches, Crowley developed what has been described as a "three centimeter rule."[22] In her investigation, she once again showed a significant difference in outcome between patients above and below the 3 cm line.

In 1987, Phelan and associates described the amniotic fluid index.[23] This technique was an outgrowth of the external cephalic version protocol to assess amniotic fluid volume. During the course of external cephalic version, Phelan found it extremely difficult to successfully convert breech fetuses to a cephalic lie whenever the amniotic fluid volume appeared to be more than 1 cm, but at the same time subjectively decreased. Therefore, the four-quadrant technique, known as the amniotic fluid index, was developed to assess the amniotic fluid volume prior to an attempted version.

This technique for assessing amniotic fluid volume is illustrated in Figure 50-2. Using the umbilicus as one reference point, the uterus is divided into upper and lower halves. The linea nigra is then used to divide the uterus into right and left halves. The transducer is then placed on the maternal abdomen along the longitudinal axis of the mother, with the transducer perpendicular to the floor. The vertical diameter of the largest pocket in each quadrant is measured (Fig. 50-3). The numbers obtained from each quadrant are summed. This summation represents the amniotic fluid index in centimeters for that patient.

In low-risk pregnancies, the mean amniotic fluid index was 16.2 ± 5.3 cm (Fig. 50-4). As part of their investigation, these investigators established definitions for

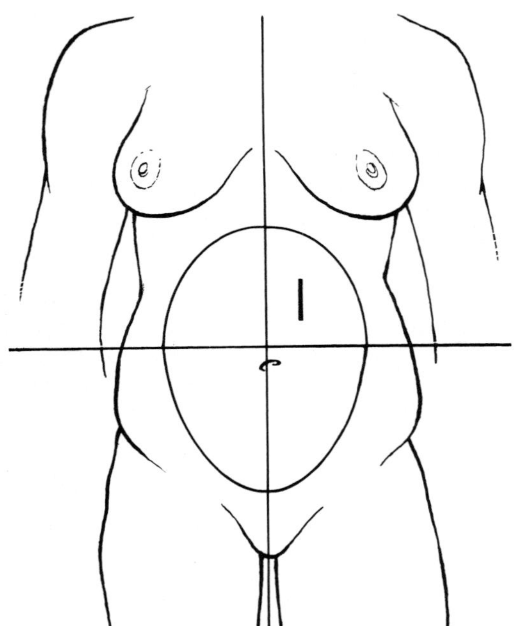

FIGURE 50–2. The uterus is divided into four quadrants. The linea nigra divides the uterus into right and left halves; the umbilicus divides the uterus into upper and lower halves. (From Phelan JP, Smith CV, Broussard P, et al. Amniotic fluid volume assessment using the four-quadrant technique in the pregnancy between 36 and 42 weeks. J Reprod Med 1987; 32: 540.)

oligo- and polyhydramnios. Oligohydramnios was defined as an amniotic fluid index ≤ 5.0 cm,[23] and polyhydramnios was considered whenever the amniotic fluid index was in excess of 25.0 cm.[27,28]

When the various techniques are compared, the amniotic fluid index appears superior to the currently available methods of amniotic fluid volume assessment. For example, Eden[26] and Phelan[24] first noted that Manning's[18] 1-cm rule was inadequate and that a larger volume was necessary to describe an abnormal volume. Chamberlain[21] and Crowley[22] attempted to address these concerns by expanding the volume to 2 cm and 3 cm, respectively. But Rutherford[29] was able to show comparable to superior results with the amniotic fluid index over these single-packet techniques[20–22] without substantial inter- and intraobserver differences.[30]

Subsequent work has demonstrated that the amniotic fluid index is simple, easy to perform, and reproducible, and provides a semiquantitative measurement of the amniotic fluid volume.[31,32] Recent evidence also suggests that 1 cm is approximately equal to 50 mL of amniotic fluid.[33] In comparison with the other techniques available to measure the amniotic fluid volume, the amniotic fluid index has the additional advantage that it can be correlated with changes in amniotic fluid volume during pregnancy.[27] These findings suggest that it may be clinically useful for following the amniotic fluid volume in patients with premature rupture of the membranes[34] or who are on amniotic fluid volume reduction therapy with indomethacin.[35]

AMNIOTIC FLUID VOLUME DISORDERS

POLYHYDRAMNIOS

Polyhydramnios is the pathologic accumulation of amniotic fluid. It is associated with a high maternal and perinatal morbidity and mortality.[28,36–44] Quantitatively, polyhydramnios is considered whenever the amniotic fluid volume is in excess of 2000 mL.[36] However, dye dilution techniques have given way to ultrasound methods of assessing this condition. Presently, polyhydramnios is considered whenever the amniotic fluid index is in excess of 25 cm.[27] Under these circumstances, the incidence of polyhydramnios in a general population ranges from 0.2% to 1.6%.[40–44] However, this incidence is considerably less when referral patients are excluded from these reports.[41]

With the dye dilution techniques of the past, the diagnosis of polyhydramnios was confirmed by actual volume measurements. Recently, ultrasound has facilitated the diagnosis of polyhydramnios. To determine a cause for the polyhydramnios depends to a large extent on its severity. For example, Hill and associates found the cause to be apparent in 17% of patients with mild polyhydramnios and in 91% of those with moderate or severe polyhydramnios.[41] When a basis for the polyhydramnios can be found, the diagnosis usually falls into the following categories[28]: fetal malformations and genetic disorders, diabetes mellitus, Rh sensitization, and congenital infections.[45] The incidence of these conditions is also directly proportional to the severity of the hydramnios.[41]

Thus, the management of patients with suspected polyhydramnios begins with the referral to a maternal–fetal medicine specialist skilled in the art of ultrasonography. There, the polyhydramnios will need to be confirmed. Once confirmed, a targeted ultrasound evaluation focusing on the more commonly identified fetal malformations is necessary (Table 50-2).

Commonly, polyhydramnios is associated with some impairment of the fetal swallowing mechanism. In the case of central nervous system abnormalities, the pathophysiologic mechanism may also be related to transudation of fluid across the fetal meninges or the lack of antidiuretic hormone and resultant polyuria.[46]

In contrast, gastrointestinal tract abnormalities are not associated with an inability of the fetus to swallow, but are frequently due to an obstructive process, such as duodenal atresia. Moreover, the closer the obstruction is to the oropharynx, the greater is the likelihood of a pathologic accumulation of amniotic fluid. In the case of an omphalocele or gastroschisis, the polyhydramnios is believed to be due to transudation of fluid. Impaired swallowing in chromosomal errors such as trisomies 13 and 18 might also contribute.

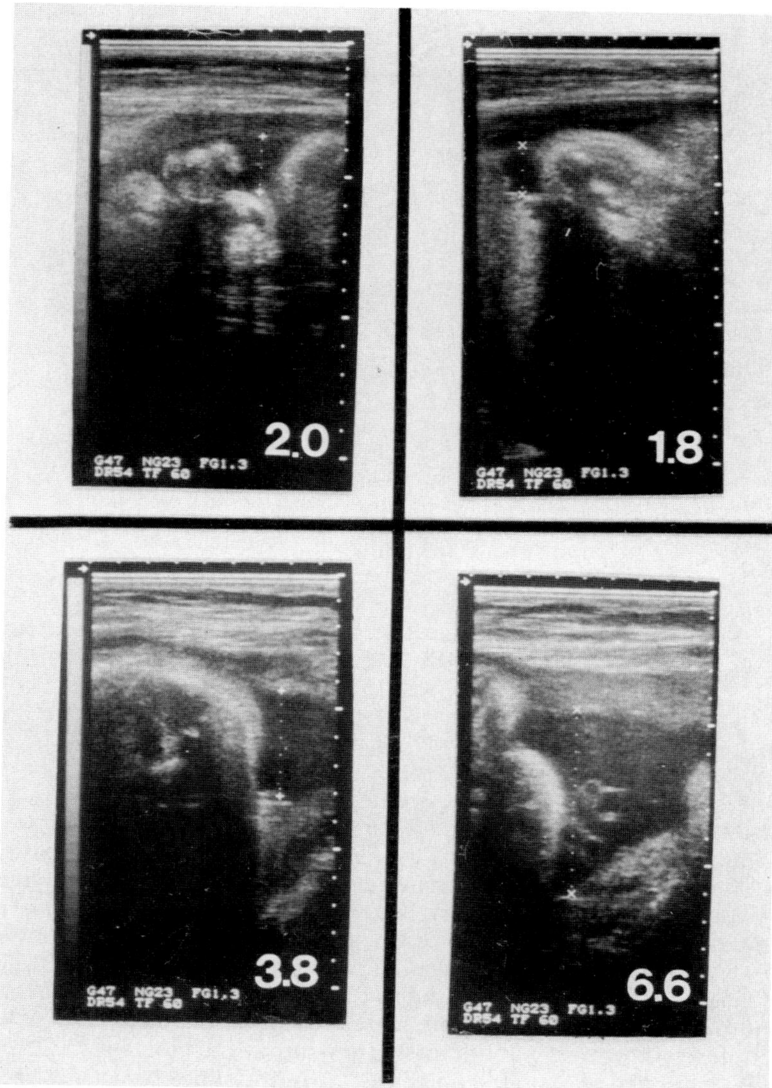

FIGURE 50–3. With the uterus divided into four quadrants, the vertical diameter of the largest pocket in each quadrant is measured. The summation of all four quadrants equals the amniotic fluid index. In the patient presented, the amniotic fluid index is 14.2 cm and is within normal limits.

Amniotic fluid also plays a direct role in pulmonary development and contributes in part to lung growth. In the fetal lungs, the flow of tracheal fluid is bidirectional. If there is an interruption of this exchange process across the surface area of the lungs, polyhydramnios can occur,[47] as in conditions such as pulmonary hypoplasia.

In addition to fetal structural malformations, chromosomal and genetic abnormalities are also increased in polyhydramnic patients. In fact, the incidence of chromosomal abnormalities may approach 35%.[48] The most common chromosomal abnormalities involve the trisomies 13, 18, and 21. Neuromuscular disorders may also be manifested clinically as polyhydramnios.

In the absence of a sonographic abnormality, the evaluation should also include screening tests for toxoplasmosis and cytomegalovirus, diabetes mellitus, and Rh sensitization. If these evaluations are negative, amniotic fluid volume reduction with prostaglandin synthetase inhibitors would seem reasonable.[35]

OLIGOHYDRAMNIOS

Oligohydramnios, little or scant amniotic fluid, is considered whenever the amniotic fluid volume is less than 400 mL[8,9,36] or when there is an amniotic fluid index ≤ 5.0 cm.[23,27,30–32] Multiple causes (Table 50-3) and consequences (Table 50-4) for this condition have been identified. Thus, the clinical focus will depend to a large extent on the trimester of pregnancy. For example, the finding of second trimester oligohydramnios should alert the clinician to the possibility of urinary tract malformations or preterm premature rupture of the membranes,[5] whereas third trimester oligohydramnios should alert the clinician to the possibility of intrauter-

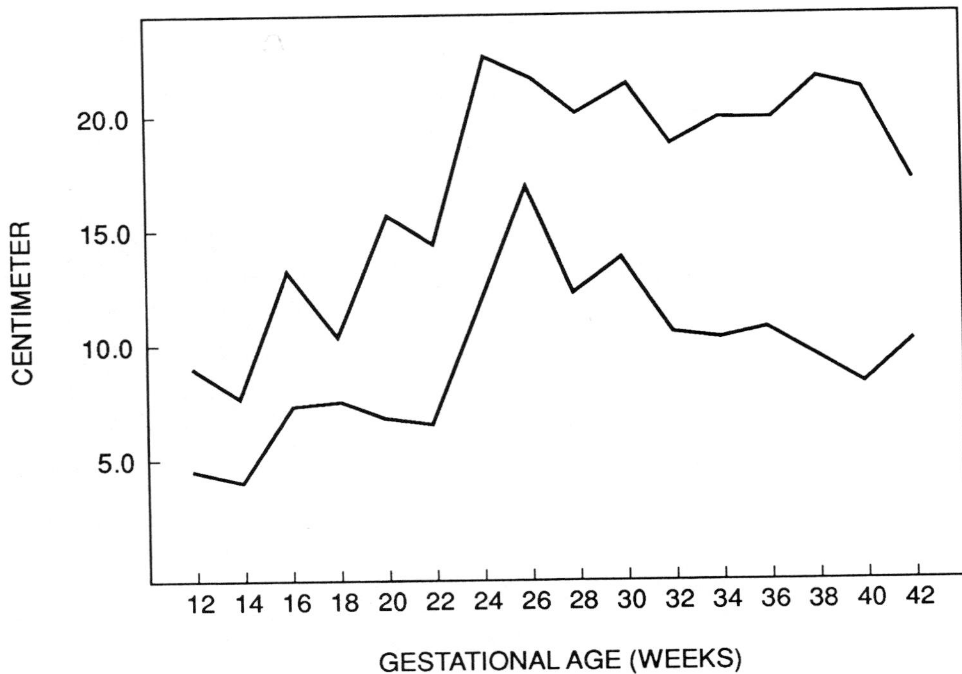

FIGURE 50–4. Amniotic fluid index changes during pregnancy. (Adapted from Phelan JP, Ahn MO, Smith CV, et al. Amniotic fluid index measurements during pregnancy. J Reprod Med 1987; 32: 627.)

ine growth retardation or postdate pregnancy. In the latter circumstance, the estimated incidence of oligohydramnios is 20%.[49]

Second trimester oligohydramnios is associated with a poor prognosis for the fetus. For example, of 34 pregnancies without premature rupture of the membranes, 9 (27%) fetuses had congenital malformations, 11 (32%) fetuses died in utero, and 6 (18%) had an entirely normal outcome.[50] In contrast, patients with premature rupture of the membranes remote from term were more likely to have a favorable outcome.[51,52] In the series by Garite, the probability of a favorable prognosis for both mother and fetus was 25%.[51] Thus, the finding of second trimester oligohydramnios should not be considered hopeless for the parents in either situation.

TABLE 50–2. FETAL MALFORMATIONS COMMONLY ASSOCIATED WITH POLYHYDRAMNIOS

Central nervous system
Anencephaly
Hydrocephaly
Encephalocele
Gastrointestinal
Gastroschisis
Omphalocele
Tracheo-esophageal fistula
Duodenal atresia
Respiratory tract
Pulmonary hypoplasia
Chylothorax

(From Phelan JP, Martin GI. Polyhydramnios: fetal and neonatal implications. Clin Perinatol 1989;16:987.)

The potential for long-term sequelae as a consequence of prolonged exposure to oligohydramnios should be considered. For example, prolonged exposure to oligohydramnios can lead to the deformation syndrome, such as cranial, facial, or skeletal abnormalities, or pulmonary hypoplasia. Of patients with oligohydramnios, 10% to 15%[53,54] will develop the deformation syndrome, and 17% are at risk for pulmonary hypoplasia.[55,56]

Of patients with oligohydramnios unrelated to premature rupture of the membranes, urinary tract malformations are the most common abnormality (Table 50-5). In addition to a targeted ultrasound evaluation, the Lasix test may be necessary to confirm a renal abnormality.[5] As part of the evaluation, if possible, amniocentesis to assess the fetal chromosomal complement is also helpful in the subsequent management of these pregnancies.

Third trimester oligohydramnios should alert the clinician to these aforementioned possibilities, but should also give rise to the clinical suspicion of intrauterine growth retardation or a postdate pregnancy. The finding of oligohydramnios in the third trimester is asso-

TABLE 50–3. CLINICAL CONDITIONS COMMONLY ASSOCIATED WITH OLIGOHYDRAMNIOS

Intrauterine growth retardation
Urinary tract malformations
Ruptured membranes
Postdate pregnancy

TABLE 50–4. POTENTIAL CONSEQUENCES OF OLIGOHYDRAMNIOS

Umbilical cord compression
Meconium-stained amniotic fluid
Fetal demise
Deformation syndrome
Pulmonary hypoplasia
Maternal/neonatal infection

ciated with increased incidence of cord compression, with variable fetal heart rate decelerations, meconium-stained amniotic fluid, nonreactivity, and adverse perinatal outcome. Unlike the patient with premature rupture of the membranes, this kind of oligohydramnios is probably related to fetal compromise[49] and associated with a less favorable outcome for the fetus. As shown by Rutherford and associates, there is an inverse relationship between amniotic fluid volume and pregnancy outcome.[57] The lower the amniotic fluid volume, the greater the percentage of fetal heart rate abnormalities, such as decelerations and nonreactivity, meconium-stained amniotic fluid, and perinatal morbidity and mortality. Thus, in the case of third trimester oligohydramnios, ultrasound evaluation will often need to be complemented by fetal heart rate monitoring to determine the extent of fetal compromise. Regardless of the nonstress test results, oligohydramnios in a third trimester pregnancy unrelated to a premature rupture of the membranes should alert the clinician to the potential for fetal compromise; these patients ought to be considered for delivery.

CLINICAL APPLICATIONS

ANTEPARTUM FETAL SURVEILLANCE

An outgrowth of amniotic fluid volume assessment is its implementation in the area of antepartum fetal surveillance (Table 50-6). Its present use is in combination with current fetal heart rate techniques, such as the nonstress test or contraction stress test.[58] Thus, each patient who presents for testing undergoes a nonstress test and amniotic fluid index measurement (Fig. 50-5). The underlying rationale for this approach stems from the work of Rutherford and associates.[57] In that article, she demonstrated not only an inverse relationship between pregnancy outcome and the amniotic fluid index, but also that this risk, although lessened by the presence of a reactive nonstress test, was significantly greater in the low amniotic fluid index group. Thus, patients undergoing testing for whatever indication will have an assessment of immediate (nonstress test) and previous (amniotic fluid index) fetal condition at each visit (see Fig. 50-5).

If the nonstress test (NST) is reactive and the amniotic fluid index is in excess of 5 cm, the patient is retested in 1 week or sooner, depending on the indication for testing. For example, patients with a history of diabetes mellitus, postdate pregnancy, and intrauterine growth retardation are tested twice weekly. All other patients are tested once a week, unless circumstances dictate earlier retesting. Those patients who manifest a nonreactive NST complete the remaining portions of the fetal biophysical profile (Table 50-7). If the fetal biophysical profile score is considered normal, the patient is retested at her usual testing interval. If the fetus has a score of 6, the test is considered suspicious and a repeat test is recommended within 12 to 24 hours. If,

TABLE 50–5. URINARY TRACT MALFORMATIONS ASSOCIATED WITH OLIGOHYDRAMNIOS

Renal agenesis
Dysplastic kidneys
Polycystic kidney
Uteropelvic obstruction
Posterior urethral valve

(From King JC. Oligohydramnios. In: Charles D, Glover DD, eds. Current therapy in obstetrics. Philadelphia: BC Decker, 1988:46.)

TABLE 50–6. CLINICAL APPLICATION OF AMNIOTIC FLUID VOLUME ASSESSMENT

Antepartum fetal surveillance
Fetal admission test
Premature rupture of the membranes
Amnioinfusion
Polyhydramnios

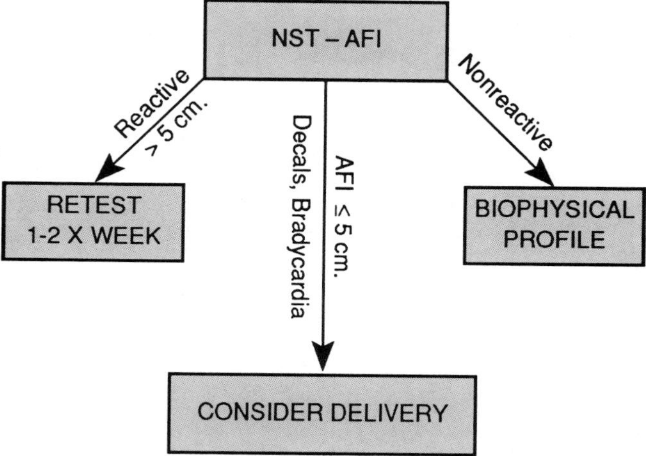

FIGURE 50–5. Management scheme for patients who undergo primary fetal surveillance with the nonstress test (NST) and amniotic fluid index (AFI). Decels, fetal heart rate decelerations. (Adapted from Phelan JP. Antepartum fetal assessment: newer techniques. Semin Perinatol 1988; 12: 57.)

TABLE 50–7. BIOPHYSICAL PROFILE SCORING SYSTEM AS MODIFIED BY THE USE OF THE AMNIOTIC FLUID INDEX FOR A 30-MINUTE OBSERVATION PERIOD

COMPONENT	POINTS
Nonstress—Reactive	2
Fetal breathing movements	2
Fetal movement	2
Fetal tone	2
Amniotic fluid index > 5 cm	2

however, the patient manifests a fetal biophysical profile score of 4 or less, she is considered for delivery. In the term and postterm fetus, the indications for intervention include the presence of oligohydramnios (amniotic fluid index ≤ 5 cm), a fetal heart rate bradycardia, or a fetal biophysical profile score of ≤4. With term fetuses who exhibit a fetal heart rate deceleration during the NST and have a normal amniotic fluid index (>5 cm), repeat testing within 3 to 4 days is recommended. If, at the time of repeat testing in the term fetus, the fetal heart rate deceleration pattern persists, consideration should be given for delivery by a trial of labor. In the postdate pregnancy, the fetus who exhibits a fetal heart rate deceleration is at significant risk for perinatal morbidity and mortality.[59,60] As a consequence, induction of labor with oxytocin and continuous fetal surveillance during labor should be considered in order to reduce the morbidity associated with this fetal heart rate pattern.[60] With this combination approach, perinatal morbidity and mortality can be significantly reduced.[60] For example, as demonstrated by Clark and associates, the combined use of the NST and amniotic fluid index was not associated with an unexpected fetal death in 5973 tests.[61]

FETAL ADMISSION TEST

The natural extension of the principles of antepartum fetal surveillance is the early detection of those patients at risk for intrapartum fetal distress.[62–64] As pointed out by Ingemarsson and associates, the "test can detect fetal distress already present at admission and unnecessary delay(s) can be avoided."[62,63] Moreover, third world countries have capitalized on this concept and used the fetal admission test to reallocate risk status in labor. For example, patients with normal fetal surveillance test results are allocated to auscultation rather than continuous fetal monitoring. However, those patients with an abnormal admission test (a nonreactive fetal heart rate pattern with or without decelerations) undergo continuous fetal surveillance because of the significantly higher rates of intrapartum fetal distress.[62–64]

Although fetal heart rate patterns have been the basis for the fetal admission test, amniotic fluid volume assessment also appears to be a reasonable consideration.[64] For example, a normal amniotic fluid volume in the nonlaboring patient is associated with a favorable fetal outcome.[25,57] Similar results are seen in patients with normal amniotic fluid volume on admission to labor and delivery.[64] Although these results suggest that amniotic volume assessment with the amniotic fluid index may be an effective screening tool in detecting intrapartum fetal distress, more research is needed to confirm these observations.

PRETERM PREMATURE RUPTURE OF THE MEMBRANES

Preterm premature rupture of the membranes affects 6% of all patients and is responsible for 30% of preterm deliveries. It is the leading cause of admission to neonatal intensive care units in the United States today.[65] In the clinical management of patients with preterm premature rupture of the membranes, ultrasound assessment of amniotic fluid volume appears to be helpful in predicting subsequent duration of pregnancy,[66] identifying patients at risk for intrauterine infection[67,68] and the potential selective use of amniocentesis,[69] and in the antepartum assessment of fetal well-being.[70,71]

Early ultrasound evaluation of the amniotic fluid volume in patients admitted with preterm premature rupture of the membranes is useful in counseling these patients as to the likelihood of early delivery. Although these observations are not absolute, patients with a normal amniotic fluid volume are four times more likely to be undelivered after 1 week.[66] In fact, Vintzileos has shown that a normal amniotic fluid volume is associated with a significantly lower rate of cesarean delivery, Apgar scores of less than 7 at 1 and 5 minutes, and perinatal mortality.[66]

Either on admission or subsequently, the assessment of amniotic fluid can serve as an indicator of potential underlying amnionitis.[67,68] As demonstrated by Vintzileos, a low amniotic fluid volume or nonreactive fetal heart rate pattern is associated with a 67% probability of intrauterine infection.[67,68] This is six to seven times higher than that encountered in patients with a normal test result. Thus, patients with abnormal fetal surveillance tests on or subsequent to admission would appear to be candidates for amniocentesis to determine the presence of fetal infection.[69]

With combined fetal surveillance testing with the NST and amniotic fluid index done on a daily[70,71] or less frequent basis,[72] one can clinically monitor the changes in fetal status. For example, changes such as variable decelerations or a declining amniotic fluid index may represent a sign of early fetal infection. Late manifestations of an underlying fetal infection appear to be a loss of fetal movement and tone. Thus, with heightened scrutiny of fetal condition, intrauterine infection or impending fetal distress can be detected earlier.

Fetal assessment in the patient with preterm premature rupture of the membranes is similar to the patient with intact membranes (see Fig. 50-5). The key difference is that in the patient with preterm premature rupture of the membranes, the goal is to avoid, when possible, preterm delivery. Here, testing provides a basis for which to resort to continuous fetal surveillance in labor and delivery. For instance, the management protocol outlined in Figure 50-5 is followed, except that testing is done more frequently.[70,71] Then, if fetal heart rate decelerations or oligohydramnios (amniotic fluid index ≤ 5 cm) are observed, the patient is referred to labor and delivery for continuous electronic fetal monitoring. There, the patient is monitored to determine the extent or frequency of an abnormal fetal heart rate pattern or evidence of infection. Criteria for delivery are not well delineated. There does not appear to be a bright line to dictate the appropriate time of delivery in these circumstances. Thus, clinical judgment remains the mainstay of subsequent management. In this circumstance, options could include continuous fetal surveillance, delivery, or less frequent fetal surveillance testing.

AMNIOINFUSION

Ultrasound assessment of the amniotic fluid volume may be used to determine candidates for amnioinfusion.[73–79] As previously demonstrated by Rutherford and associates, there is an inverse relationship between the amniotic fluid volume as measured by the amniotic fluid index and the incidence of fetal heart rate abnormalities and pregnancy outcome.[29] For example, the lower the amniotic fluid volume, the greater the likelihood of umbilical cord compression producing fetal heart rate decelerations.

Thus, many patients who present with repetitive variable decelerations during labor undergo cesarean delivery to remedy the fetal situation. However, restoration of the amniotic fluid volume with saline amnioinfusion has been shown to be effective in reducing the requirement for cesarean delivery for patients with this intrapartum fetal heart rate abnormality.[73–77] In those series published to date (Table 50-8), the overall cesarean delivery rate for fetal distress was reduced 87% in patients undergoing saline amnioinfusion.

In an effort to better identify those patients at risk for intrapartum fetal distress, Strong infused saline in a group of patients with sonographic evidence of oligohydramnios (amniotic fluid index ≤ 5 cm).[78] This approach was based on the previous work by Sarno and associates, who demonstrated a significantly higher rate of cesarean delivery for fetal distress and low Apgar scores whenever an amniotic fluid index value ≤ 5 cm was encountered in early labor.[79] In the Strong series, the group receiving amnioinfusion had significantly lower rates of meconium passage, severe variable decelerations, end-stage bradycardias, and operative deliveries for fetal distress. Moreover, as demonstrated by Nageotte[74] and Strong,[79] higher umbilical arterial blood pH values were also observed in the infusion group.

As pointed out by Strong and associates, saline amnioinfusion is useful for the correction of repetitive variable decelerations or prolonged fetal heart rate decelerations, but also for the restoration of an inadequate amniotic fluid volume.[79] If amnioinfusion is implemented to expand the fluid volume, repeated infusions may be necessary to maintain it during labor. Therefore, ultrasound assessment of the amniotic fluid volume during labor is essential in order to ensure that the patient has evidence of a normal amniotic fluid volume. As a rule, an amniotic fluid index of 1 cm is equivalent to approximately 50 mL of amniotic fluid. In the Strong series, the amniotic fluid index was kept in excess of 8 cm.[78] At this level, significantly lower risk of an adverse perinatal outcome was observed.

TABLE 50–8. EFFECTIVENESS OF SALINE AMNIOINFUSION IN REDUCING THE INCIDENCE OF CESAREAN DELIVERY FOR FETAL DISTRESS

	NUMBER	CESAREAN FETAL DISTRESS
Sadovsky[73]	19	0 (%)
Nageotte[74]	29	1 (3%)
Ogita[75]	84	8 (10%)
Miyazaki[76]	42	11 (26%)
Miyazaki[77]	49	9 (18%)

POLYHYDRAMNIOS—VOLUME REDUCTION

Ultrasound is helpful in confirming polyhydramnios and determining the cause for the extra-amniotic fluid. At the same time, ultrasound can be used to monitor attempts to reduce the amniotic fluid volume. For example, uncorrected polyhydramnios can be associated with a number of obstetrical complications (Table 50-9). Theoretically, these risks could be reduced with volume reduction.

Amniocentesis or prostaglandin inhibitors are the techniques commonly used for this purpose.[35,79,80] The use of repeated amniocentesis to reduce the amniotic fluid volume is fraught with tremendous difficulty. For example, the amniotic fluid volume appears to turn over every 2.9 hours.[13] As a consequence, any effort to reduce the amniotic fluid volume with amniocentesis would require placement of a catheter to permit amniotic fluid drainage or repeated amniocentesis. Either approach is associated with considerable discomfort for

TABLE 50–9. POTENTIAL COMPLICATIONS ASSOCIATED WITH POLYHYDRAMNIOS

Premature labor
Placental abruption
Puerperal hemorrhage
Perinatal mortality
Maternal respiratory difficulties

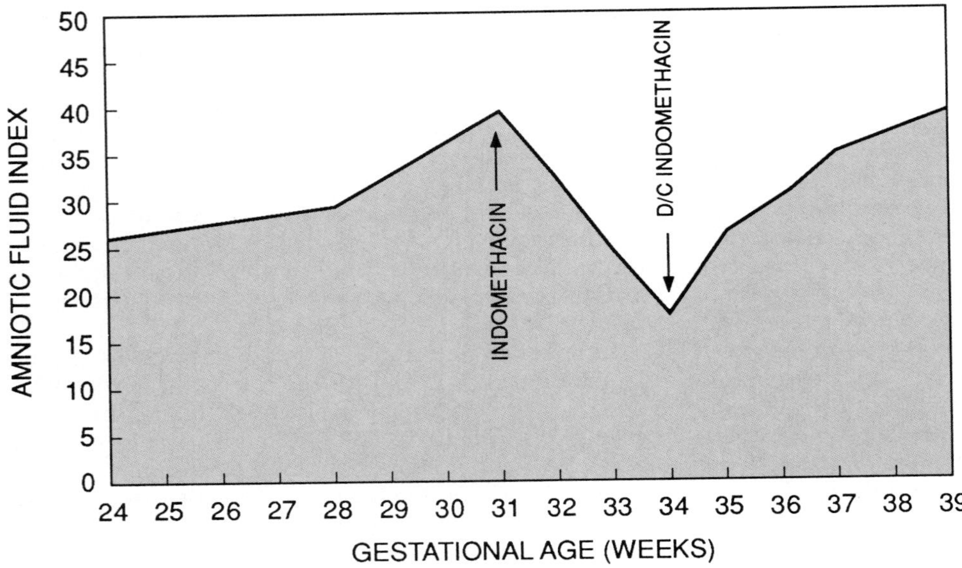

FIGURE 50–6. Amniotic fluid index measurements used to follow a patient with idiopathic polyhydramnios on indomethacin therapy.

the patient and exposes the patient to a greater risk of infection or decompression-related complications, such as abruption.

Therefore, prostaglandin synthetase inhibitors have been suggested as an alternative to reduce the amniotic fluid volume.[35,80,81] Indomethacin at a dose of 25 mg orally every 6 hours appears to operate by decreasing fetal urinary output or the amnion–chorion production of amniotic fluid. For example, studies done with the invasive para-amino hippuric acid dilution technique before and during indomethacin therapy confirmed a reduction in amniotic fluid volume with indomethacin therapy. In a similar study by Hickok, prostaglandin inhibitors rather than beta-mimetics or magnesium sulfate reduced the amniotic fluid volume.

While patients are on indomethacin therapy, the amniotic fluid volume should be monitored frequently. Rather than using invasive techniques, the amniotic fluid index appears to be ideally designed to assist in the clinical management of these patients. For example, Figure 50-6 represents the amniotic fluid index changes in a patient with idiopathic polyhydramnios on indomethacin therapy. At 31 weeks gestation, she had symptomatic polyhydramnios with an amniotic fluid index of 41 cm. After a negative clinical evaluation, she was placed on indomethacin, 25 mg every 6 hours. Her amniotic fluid index was measured weekly. At 34 weeks gestation, her amniotic fluid index measured 18 cm and she had improved symptomatically. The indomethacin therapy was then discontinued. As demonstrated by Figure 50-6, the amniotic fluid index rose progressively each week. By the 39th week of gestation, she had returned to pretreatment levels. Soon thereafter, she went into labor and delivered a healthy child. This case illustrates the importance of amniotic fluid volume assessment with the amniotic fluid index in patients who are on indomethacin therapy for amniotic fluid volume reduction or premature labor.

REFERENCES

1. Denman T. An Introduction to the Practice of Midwifery. London: Bliss and White, 1815.
2. Hellman LM, Pritchard JA. Williams Obstetrics. 14th ed. New York: Appleton-Century-Crofts, 1971:226.
3. Queenan JT. Amniotic fluid. In: Eden RD, Boehm RH, eds. Assessment and care of the fetus: physiological, clinical and medicolegal principles. Norwalk, CT: Appleton & Lange, 1990:179.
4. Seeds AE. Current concepts of amniotic fluid dynamics. Am J Obstet Gynecol 1980;138:575.
5. King JC. Oligohydramnios. In: Charles D, Glover DD, eds. Current therapy in obstetrics. Philadelphia: BC Decker, 1988:46.
6. Gillibrand PN. Changes in amniotic fluid volume with advancing pregnancy. J Obstet Gynaecol Br Commonwealth 1969;76:527.
7. Mandelbaum B, Evans TN. Life in the amniotic fluid. Am J Obstet Gynecol 1969;104:365.
8. Gadd RL. The volume of the liquor amnii in normal and abnormal pregnancies. J Obstet Gynaecol Br Commonwealth 1966;73:11.
9. Beischer NA, Brown JB, Townsend L. Studies in prolonged pregnancy. III: amniocentesis in prolonged pregnancy. Am J Obstet Gynecol 1969;193:496.
10. Queenan JT. Amniocentesis. In: Queenan JT, ed. Management of high risk pregnancy. Oradell, NJ: Medical Economics Books, 1985:201.
11. Queenan JT, Thompson W, Whitfield CR, et al. Amniotic fluid volumes in normal pregnancies. Am J Obstet Gynecol 1972;114:34.
12. Hutchinson DL, Gray MJ, Plentl AA. The role of the fetus in the water exchange of the amniotic fluid of normal and hydramniotic patients. J Clin Invest 1959;38:971.
13. Vosburgh GH, Flexner LB, Cowie DB, Hellman LM, Proctor NK, Wilde WS. The rate of renewal in woman of the water and sodium of the amniotic fluid as determined by tracer techniques. Am J Obstet Gynecol 1948;56:1156.
14. Pritchard JA. Deglutition by normal and anencephalic fetuses. Obstet Gynecol 1965;25:289.
15. Goodlin R, Lloyd D. Fetal tracheal excretion of bilirubin. Biol Neonate 1968;12:1.

16. Chez RA, Smith FG, Hutchinson DL. Renal function in the intrauterine primate fetus. Am J Obstet Gynecol 1964;90:128.
17. Kurjak A, Kirkinen P, Latin V, Ivankovic D. Ultrasonic assessment of fetal kidney function in normal and complicated pregnancies. Am J Obstet Gynecol 1981;141:266.
18. Dieckmann WJ, Davis ME. The volumetric determination of amniotic fluid with congo red: a preliminary report. Am J Obstet Gynecol 1933;25:623.
19. Gohari P, Berkowitz RL, Hobbins JC, et al. Prediction of IUGR by total intrauterine volume. Am J Obstet Gynecol 1977;127:255.
20. Manning FA, Hill LM, Platt LD. Qualitative amniotic fluid volume determination by ultrasound: antepartum detection of intrauterine growth retardation. Am J Obstet Gynecol 1981;139:254.
21. Chamberlain PF, Manning FA, Morrison I, et al. Ultrasound evaluation of amniotic fluid volume. I: the relationship of marginal and decreased amniotic fluid volumes to perinatal outcome. Am J Obstet Gynecol 1984;150:245.
22. Crowley P, O'Herlihy C, Boylan P. The value of ultrasound measurement of amniotic fluid volume on the management of prolonged pregnancies. Br J Obstet Gynaecol 1984;91:444.
23. Phelan JP, Smith CV, Broussard P, et al. Amniotic fluid volume assessment using the four quadrant technique in the pregnancy between 36 and 42 weeks. J Reprod Med 1987;32:540.
24. Dieckman WJ, Davis ME. The volumetric determination of amniotic fluid with congo red: a preliminary report. Am J Obstet Gynecol 1933;25:623.
25. Phelan JP, Platt LD, Yeh SY, et al. The role of ultrasound assessment of amniotic fluid volumes in the management of the post date pregnancy. Am J Obstet Gynecol 1985;151:304.
26. Eden RD, Gergely RZ, Schifrin BS, Wade M. Comparison of antepartum testing schemes for the management of the post date pregnancy. Am J Obstet Gynecol 1982;144:683.
27. Phelan JP, Ahn MO, Smith CV, et al. Amniotic fluid index measurements during pregnancy. J Reprod Med 1987;32:627.
28. Phelan JP, Martin GI. Polyhydramnios: fetal and neonatal implications. Clin Perinatol 1989;16:987.
29. Rutherford SE, Phelan JP, Smith CV, et al. The four quadrant assessment of amniotic fluid volume: an adjunct to antepartum fetal heart rate testing. Obstet Gynecol 1987;70:533.
30. Rutherford SE, Phelan JP, Smith CV, et al. The four quadrant assessment of amniotic fluid volume: interobserver and intraobserver variation. J Reprod Med 1987;32:597.
31. Moore TR, Cayle JE. The amniotic fluid index in normal human pregnancy. Am J Obstet Gynecol 1990;162:1168.
32. Jeng CJ, Jou TJ, Wang KG, Yang YC, Lee YN, Lan CC. Amniotic fluid index measurement with the four-quadrant technique during pregnancy. J Reprod Med 1990;35:674.
33. Strong T, Hetzler G, Paul RH. Amniotic fluid volume increase after amnioinfusion of a fixed volume. Am J Obstet Gynecol 1990;162:746.
34. Smith CV, Greenspoon J, Phelan JP, Platt LD. The clinical utility of the nonstress test in the conservative management of patients with preterm spontaneous premature rupture of the membranes. J Reprod Med 1987;32:1.
35. Cabrol D, Landesman R, Muller J, Uzan M, Sureau C, Sacena BB. Treatment of polyhydramnios with prostaglandin synthetase inhibitor (indomethacin). Am J Obstet Gynecol 1987;157:422.
36. Pritchard JA, MacDonald PC. Diseases and abnormalities of the placenta and fetal membranes. In: Williams' Obstetrics. 15th ed. New York: Appleton Century Crofts, 1976:476.
37. Phelan JP, Park YW, Ahn MO, Rutherford SE. Polyhydramnios and perinatal outcome. J Perinatol 1990;4:347.
38. Cardwell MS. Polyhydramnios: a review. Obstet Gynecol Surv 1987;42:612.
39. Quinlan RW, Amelia CC, Martin M. Hydramnios: ultrasound diagnosis and its impact on perinatal management and pregnancy outcome. Am J Obstet Gynecol 1983;145:306.
40. Alexander EX, Spintz HB, Clark RA. Sonography of polyhydramnios. AJR 1982;138:343.
41. Hill L, Breckle R, Thomas ML, Fries JK. Polyhydramnios: ultrasonically detected prevalence and neonatal outcome. Obstet Gynecol 1987;69:21.
42. Hobbins JC, Grannum PA, Berkowitz RL, et al. Ultrasound in the diagnosis of congenital anomalies. Am J Obstet Gynecol 1979;134:331.
43. Kramer E. Hydramnios, oligohydramnios and fetal malformations. Clin Obstet Gynecol 1966;9:508.
44. Barry AP. Hydramnios: a survey of 100 cases. Br J Med Sci 1953;61:257.
45. Ledger WF. Maternal infection with adverse fetal and newborn outcomes. In: Infection in the female. Philadelphia: Lea & Febiger, 1986:197.
46. Wallenburg HC, Wladimiroff JW. The amniotic fluid: polyhydramnios and oligohydramnios. J Perinat Med 1977;5:233.
47. Mendelsohn G, Hutchins GM. Primary pulmonary hypoplasia. Am J Dis Child 1977;131:1220.
48. Platt LD, Devore GR, Lopez E, et al. Role of amniocentesis in ultrasound-detected fetal malformations. Obstet Gynecol 1986;68:153.
49. Phelan JP. The postdate pregnancy an overview. Clin Obstet Gynecol 1989;32:221.
50. Mercer LJ, Brown LG. Fetal outcome with oligohydramnios in the second trimester. Obstet Gynecol 1986;67:840.
51. Garite TJ. Premature rupture of the membranes: the enigma of the obstetrician. Am J Obstet Gynecol 1985;151:1001.
52. Wilson JC, Levy DL, Wilds PL. Premature rupture of membranes prior to term: consequences of nonintervention. Obstet Gynecol 1982;60:601.
53. King JC, Mitzner W, Butterfield AB, Queenan JT. Effect of induced oligohydramnios on fetal lung development. Am J Obstet Gynecol 1986;154:823.
54. Nimrod C, Varela-Bittings F, Machin G, Campbell D, Wesenberg R. The effect of very prolonged membrane rupture on fetal development. Am J Obstet Gynecol 1984;148:540.
55. Perlman M, Williams J, Hirsch M. Neonatal pulmonary hypoplasia after prolonged leakage of amniotic fluid. Arch Dis Child 1976;51:349.
56. Nimrod C, Davies D, Iwanicki S, Harder J, Persaud D, Nicholson S. Ultrasound prediction of pulmonary hypoplasia. Obstet Gynecol 1986;68:495.
57. Rutherford SE, Phelan JP, Smith CV, Jocobs N. The four quadrant assessment of amniotic fluid volume: an adjunct to antepartum fetal heart rate testing. Obstet Gynecol 1987;70:353.
58. Phelan JP. Antepartum fetal assessment: newer techniques. Semin Perinatol 1988;12:57.
59. Phelan JP, Platt LD, Yeh SY, et al. Continuing role of the nonstress test in the management of the postdates pregnancy. Obstet Gynecol 1984;64:624.
60. Small ML, Phelan JP, Smith CV, et al. The impact of an active management approach to the postdate fetus with a reactive nonstress test and FHR decelerations. Obstet Gynecol 1987;70:1987.
61. Clark SL, Sabey P, Jolley K. Nonstress testing with acoustic stimulation and amniotic fluid volume assessment: 5,973 tests without unexpected fetal death. Am J Obstet Gynecol 1989;160:694.
62. Ingemarsson I, Arulkumaran S, Ingemarsson E, et al. Admission test: a screening test for fetal distress in labor. Obstet Gynecol 1986;68:800.
63. Ingemarsson I, Arulkumaran S, Paul RH, et al. Fetal acoustic stimulation in early labor in patients screened with the admission test. Am J Obstet Gynecol 1988;158:70.
64. Phelan JP, Sarno AP, Ahn MO. The fetal admission test. Pre-

sented at the 36th Annual Clinical Meeting of the American College of Obstetricians and Gynecologists. Atlanta: May, 1989.

65. Premature rupture of the membranes. Technical bulletin 115. Washington, DC: American College of Obstetricians and Gynecologists, 1988.
66. Vintzileos AM, Campbell WA, Nochimson DJ, Weinbaum PJ. Degree of oligohydramnios and pregnancy outcome in patients with premature rupture of the membranes. Obstet Gynecol 1985;66:162.
67. Vintzileos AM, Campbell WA, Nochimson DJ, Weinbaum PJ, Escoto DT, Mirochnick MH. Qualitative amniotic fluid volume versus amniocentesis in predicting infection in preterm premature rupture of the membranes. Obstet Gynecol 1986;67:579.
68. Vintzileos AM, Campbell WA, Nochimson DJ, Weinbaum PJ. The use of the nonstress test in patients with premature rupture of the membranes. Am J Obstet Gynecol 1986;155:149.
69. Garite TJ, Freeman RK, Linzey EM, Braly P. The use of amniocentesis in patients with premature rupture of the membranes. Obstet Gynecol 1979;54:226.
70. Smith CV, Greenspoon J, Phelan JP, Platt LD. The clinical utility of the nonstress test in the conservative management of patients with preterm spontaneous premature rupture of the membranes. J Reprod Med 1987;32:1.
71. Vintzileos AM, Feinstein SJ, Lodeiro JG, Campbell WA, Weinbaum PJ, Nochimson DJ. Fetal biophysical profile and the effect of premature rupture of the membranes. Obstet Gynecol 1986;67:818.
72. Clark SL. Managing PROM: a continuing controversy. Contemp OB/GYN 1989;33:49.
73. Sadovsky Y, Amon E, Bade ME, Petrie RH. Prophylactic amnioinfusion during labor complicated by meconium: a preliminary report. Am J Obstet Gynecol 1989;161:613.
74. Nageotte MP, Freeman RK, Garite TJ, Dorchester W. Prophylactic intrapartum amnioinfusion in patients with preterm premature rupture of the membranes. Am J Obstet Gynecol 1985;153:557.
75. Ogita S, Imanaka M, Matsumoto M, Oka T, Sugawa T. Transcervical amnioinfusion of antibiotics: a basic study for managing premature rupture of membranes. Am J Obstet Gynecol 1988;158:23.
76. Miyazaki FS, Taylor NA. Saline amnioinfusion for relief of variable or prolonged decelerations: a preliminary report. Am J Obstet Gynecol 1983;146:670.
77. Miyazaki FS, Nevarez F. Saline amnioinfusion for relief of repetitive variable decelerations: a prospective randomized study. Am J Obstet Gynecol 1985;153:301.
78. Strong TH, Hetzler G, Sarno AP, Paul RH. Prophylactic intrapartum amnioinfusion: a randomized clinical trial. Am J Obstet Gynecol 1990;162:1370.
79. Sarno AP, Ahn MO, Phelan JP. Intrapartum amniotic fluid volume at term: association of ruptured membranes, oligohydramnios and increased fetal risk. J Reprod Med 1990;35:719.
80. Hickok DE, Hollenbach KA, Reilly SF, Nyberg DA. The association between decreased amniotic fluid volume and treatment with nonsteroidal anti-inflammatory agents for preterm labor. Am J Obstet Gynecol 1989;160:1525.
81. Kirshon B, Mari G, Moise KJ Jr. Indomethacin therapy in the treatment of symptomatic polyhydramnios. Obstet Gynecol 1990;75:202.

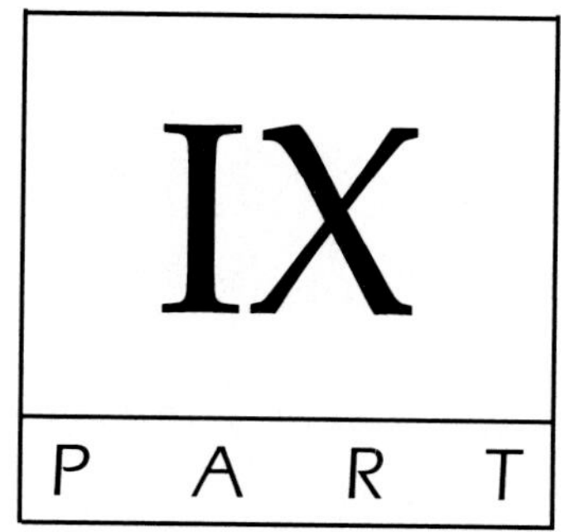

PART IX

FETAL THERAPY

51

CHAPTER

THE FETUS AT SURGERY

N. Scott Adzick and Michael R. Harrison

Routine obstetrical sonography has changed the surgical management of many congenital anomalies. Most correctable malformations that can be diagnosed in utero are best managed by appropriate medical and surgical therapy after maternal transport and planned delivery at term. Prenatal diagnosis may also influence the timing (Table 51-1) or the mode (Table 51-2) of delivery, and in some cases may lead to elective termination of the pregnancy (Table 51-3). In rare cases, various forms of in utero therapy may be possible, either currently or in the future (Table 51-4).

The perinatal management of these patients involves many different medical disciplines, including obstetricians, sonographers, neonatologists, geneticists, pediatric surgeons, and pediatricians. It is essential that the affected family be managed by a team approach, and that information and experience be exchanged freely.

Prenatal detection and serial sonographic study of fetuses with anatomic lesions now make it possible to define the natural history of these abnormalities, determine the pathophysiologic features that affect clinical outcome, and plan management based on prognosis. Prenatal diagnosis has defined a "hidden mortality" for some lesions, such as congenital diaphragmatic hernia, bilateral hydronephrosis, sacrococcygeal teratoma, and cystic hygroma. These lesions, when first evaluated and treated postnatally, demonstrate a favorable selection bias. The most severely affected fetuses often die in utero or immediately after birth, before an accurate diagnosis has been made. Consequently, such a condition detected prenatally may have a worse prognosis than the same condition first diagnosed after delivery.[1]

In recent years, there have been attempts to treat prenatally diagnosed fetal medical conditions in utero; some of these are discussed in more detail in Chapters 53 and 54. The earliest and most successful examples involve the treatment of fetal deficiencies. Fetal anemia secondary to isoimmunization-induced hemolysis can be treated by intraperitoneal or intravascular transfusion of red blood cells.[2] Fetal arrhythmias can be treated by administering appropriate medications to the mother, and various vitamin deficiencies have been treated by maternal vitamin ingestion. Medications can also be injected into the amniotic fluid, where they are swallowed and absorbed by the fetus. An example of this is the treatment of congenital hypothyroidism with intra-amniotic thyroid hormone. In addition, it may be possible in the near future to treat hematopoietic stem cell and hepatic enzyme deficiencies by in utero stem cell and hepatocyte transplantation.[3]

Certain prenatally diagnosed anatomic malformations have been treated with in utero tube decompression. Despite the experimental nature of these procedures, an extensive experience has been accumulated. Examples of these conditions include hydrothorax, hydrocephalus, and obstructive uropathy. A relatively large worldwide experience with in utero drainage of hydrocephalus has been generally disappointing,[4] and our current approach to fetal ventriculomegaly remains conservative.[5] The issue of urinary tract shunts and thoracoamniotic shunts will be discussed below.

There remain a number of congenital anomalies that are frequently diagnosed prenatally, are potentially lethal or disabling, and cannot or may not best be treated by catheter drainage. The possibility of open fetal intervention, although a formidable undertaking, may be the only solution for many fetuses. This approach is only justifiable, however, if the natural history and pathophysiology of the disease are well understood, in utero correction is shown to be efficacious in animal models, and maternal risk is proven to be acceptably low. Over the past 10 years, we have investigated the rationale and feasibility of in utero repair for a number of fetal anomalies, including congenital hydronephrosis, congenital diaphragmatic hernia, sacrococcygeal teratoma, cystic adenomatoid malformation, chylothorax, cleft lip and palate, and simple types of congenital heart disease.

TABLE 51–1. DEFECTS THAT MAY LEAD TO INDUCED PRETERM DELIVERY

Obstructive hydronephrosis
Gastroschisis or ruptured omphalocele
Intestinal ischemia and necrosis secondary to volvulus, meconium ileus, etc.

DEVELOPMENT OF TECHNIQUES FOR OPEN FETAL SURGERY

There is a great deal of experience with open fetal surgery in lower animals such as sheep and rabbits. These animals are ideal for research because of the relatively low risk of premature labor associated with hysterotomy. Primates, however, have a longer period of gestation and a much more responsive uterus. It was therefore imperative to develop anesthetic and operative techniques in nonhuman primates prior to attempting human open fetal intervention. Our experience with open fetal surgery in over 200 nonhuman primates led to the development of a satisfactory system for maternal and fetal monitoring, and a regimen for the control of premature labor.[6,7] In addition, techniques for hysterotomy and uterine closure,[8] as well as fetal urinary tract exteriorization,[9] diaphragmatic hernia repair,[10] and pulmonary resection,[11] were developed. Maternal mortality and morbidity were minimal in the nonhuman primate model, and future fertility after midgestation hysterotomy did not appear to be affected.[7] Clinical application was first successful in the management of fetal bilateral hydronephrosis, and we will review our experience in this area in detail.

CONGENITAL HYDRONEPHROSIS

The fetus with bilateral hydronephrosis presents a difficult diagnostic and therapeutic challenge. Obstetric ultrasonography has permitted the frequent prenatal detection of fetal urologic obstruction. These patients represent a spectrum of pathophysiology and severity that requires an individual approach to evaluation and management.

Optimal clinical management of both patients, mother and fetus, requires a thorough understanding of the natural history, pathophysiology, and sequelae of obstructive uropathy in the developing fetus. The pathophysiologic rationale for early decompression of the obstructed urinary tract is straightforward: unrelieved obstruction causes progressive damage to the developing kidneys and lungs, which compromises survival at birth.[12] The challenge in management is how to select from the large number of fetuses with dilated urinary tracts those few for whom intervention is appropriate; that is, those with obstruction severe enough to compromise renal and pulmonary function at birth but not so severe that the damage is irreversible.

TABLE 51–2. DEFECTS THAT MAY LEAD TO CESAREAN DELIVERY

Giant omphalocele
Large sacrococcygeal teratoma, cervical cystic hygroma, or cervical teratoma
Malformations requiring preterm delivery in the presence of inadequate labor or fetal distress

TABLE 51–3. DEFECTS USUALLY MANAGED BY SELECTIVE ABORTION

Anencephaly
Severe anomalies associated with chromosomal abnormalities (eg, trisomy 13)
Bilateral renal agenesis, infantile polycystic kidney disease
Severe, untreatable, inherited metabolic disorders (eg, Tay-Sachs)

The theoretical basis for in utero decompression of bilateral fetal hydronephrosis has been established by numerous experimental studies.[13–16] These studies demonstrate that potentially fatal pulmonary hypoplasia caused by oligohydramnios resulting from obstructive uropathy may be ameliorated by decompression in utero. In utero decompression, in addition, may arrest dysplastic morphogenesis of the kidney and preserve renal function, depending on the timing and the duration of the obstruction.

Two major controversies surround the management of the fetus with severe congenital bilateral hydronephrosis: accuracy in predicting outcome and efficacy of decompression in utero. Appropriate selection of patients for prenatal intervention can now be performed based on an improved understanding of the natural history and pathophysiology of the disease, as well as qualitative and quantitative tests of fetal renal function.

Diagnostic Methods

Ultrasonography. In many cases, ultrasonography is the only study needed for fetal urologic evaluation.[17] The findings of bilateral renal agenesis, severe renal hypoplasia, or bilateral multicystic dysplasia are uniformly fatal, and the family may be counseled and allowed to choose expectant management or termination. In cases of unilateral obstruction with normal amniotic fluid production, the patient may be observed by serial ultrasound with no further diagnostic evaluation. In cases of urologic abnormality with associated life-threatening anomalies, the evaluation of the urinary tract may assume secondary importance.

In cases of bilateral dilatation with oligohydramnios or decreasing amniotic fluid volume on serial ultrasound examinations, the fetus should undergo a complete prognostic evaluation to determine residual renal function and the potential for normal renal and pulmonary function at birth.[18] The initial step in the assessment of fetal renal function is the determination of the quantity of amniotic fluid. Because the majority of amniotic fluid in middle and late pregnancy is a product of fetal urination, the presence of a normal amount of am-

TABLE 51-4. DEFECTS THAT MAY REQUIRE IN UTERO TREATMENT

MALFORMATION	EFFECT ON DEVELOPMENT		IN UTERO TREATMENT
Urethral obstruction	Hydronephrosis, lung hypoplasia renal, respiratory failure	→	Vesicostomy
Congenital diaphragmatic hernia	Pulmonary hypoplasia Respiratory failure	→	CDH closure
Fetal chylothorax	Pulmonary hypoplasia Respiratory failure	→	Thoraco-amniotic shunt
Sacrococcygeal teratoma	Massive arteriovenous shunting placentomegaly, hydrops	→	Excision

niotic fluid usually implies the presence of at least one functioning kidney. However, amniotic fluid status is predictive only in the extremes, ie, normal volume late in gestation suggests adequate function, whereas severe oligohydramnios early in gestation suggests poor function.

The fetal bladder can be visualized easily by 15 weeks gestation. Normally, the fetal bladder cyclically increases in size and empties. In the setting of distal urinary tract obstruction, we have found that evaluative tests using either urine reaccumulation after bladder aspiration or Lasix stimulation of urine output are unreliable.

Similarly, the ultrasonographic appearance of the fetal kidneys lacks the sensitivity and specificity to be used as the sole test for predicting function.[19] Our ultrasonographers previously have correlated the renal ultrasound appearance with the histopathology of 49 fetal kidneys. They found the presence of renal cortical cysts to be highly predictive of renal dysplasia (sensitivity, 44%; specificity, 100%), but the absence of cysts did not preclude the presence of renal dysplasia. The presence of increased renal echogenicity had a sensitivity of 73% and a specificity of 80%, and the presence of hydronephrosis was least predictive (sensitivity, 41%; specificity, 73%).

It is clear that ultrasound can accurately delineate the gross anatomy of the dilated urinary tract, as well as provide qualitative information about renal function. However, it cannot accurately determine the degree of irreversible dysfunction or dysplasia, or give accurate prognostic information in the majority of cases.

Analysis of Fetal Urine. Analysis of the fetal urine represents a more direct and quantitative method of evaluating fetal renal function. Fetal urine is produced by the 13th gestational week and is an ultrafiltrate of fetal serum made hypotonic by selective tubular reabsorption of sodium and chloride in excess of free water. Fetal urine composition remains constant throughout gestation until just before term. Thus, changes in fetal urine composition might reflect changes in renal function. Total urine output is a combination of glomerular filtration and tubular reabsorption and secretion.

To evaluate the prognostic value of these factors in predicting which fetuses have the potential for normal renal and pulmonary function at birth, we reviewed the management of 40 fetuses with bilateral hydronephrosis and oligohydramnios.[20] Early in our experience, the fetal urinary tract was exteriorized by the percutaneous placement of a balloon-tipped catheter into the dilated fetal bladder under ultrasound guidance, but more recently single fetal bladder aspirations have been performed. Based on these results, six prognostic criteria to identify the fetus with good function and poor function were generated (Table 51-5). The development of prognostic criteria that predict the potential for recovery has greatly simplified counseling of the families and selection of appropriate management. The prognostic criteria (urine Na < 100 mEq/L, Cl < 90 mEq/L, Osm < 210 mOsm, and normal fetal kidneys by ultrasonography) have proven to reliably predict neonatal and long-term outcome after in utero urinary tract decompression, and the urine studies can be obtained by single fetal bladder aspiration.

CLINICAL MANAGEMENT

Using the methods described previously, we have derived guidelines for the evaluation and management of the fetus with congenital hydronephrosis (Fig. 51-1). Initial evaluation should include ultrasonography to confirm the diagnosis, delineate the anatomy of the obstruction, define the status of the amniotic fluid, and

TABLE 51-5. PROGNOSTIC CRITERIA FOR THE FETUS WITH BILATERAL OBSTRUCTIVE UROPATHY—FETAL URINE COMPOSITION AND VOLUME

PREDICTED FUNCTION	SODIUM (mEq/mL)	CHLORIDE (mEq/mL)	OSMOLARITY (mOsm)	OUTPUT (mL/hr)
Poor	>100	>90	>210	<2
Good	<100	<90	<210	>2

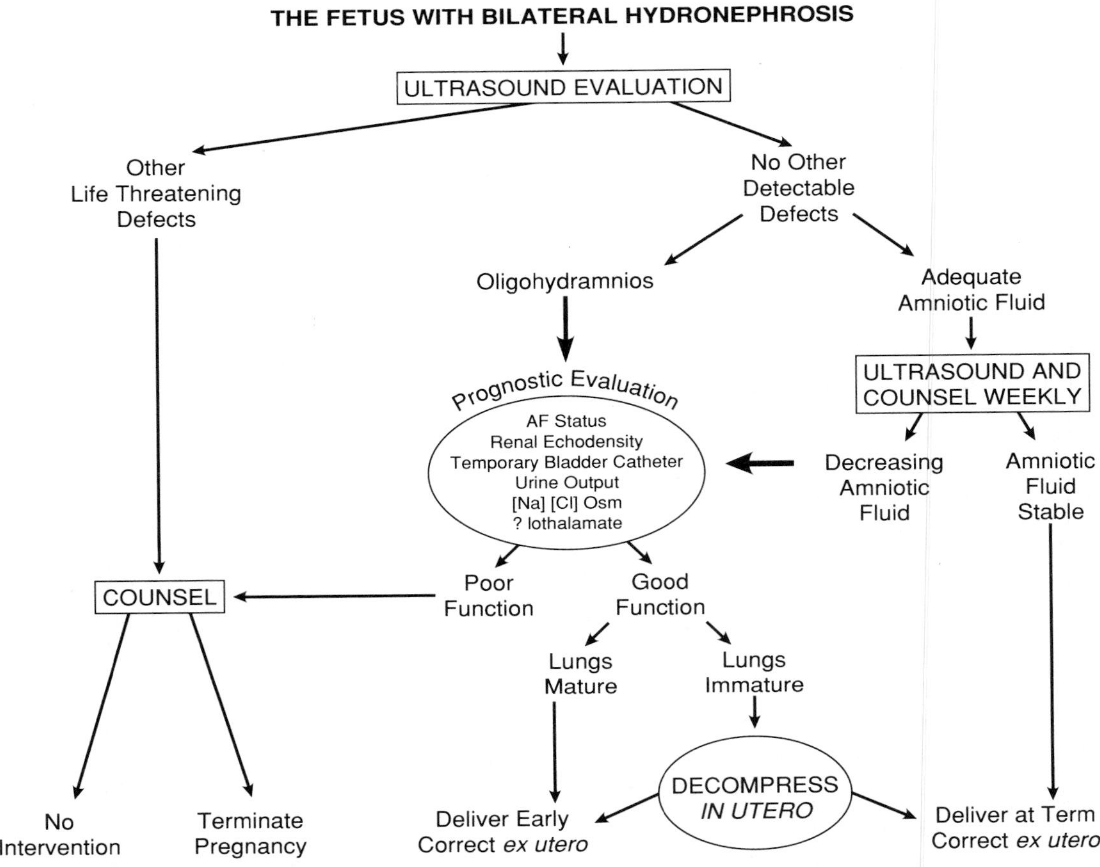

FIGURE 51–1. Management scheme for the fetus with bilateral hydronephrosis.

rule out associated life-threatening anomalies. If no associated anomaly is detected and the amniotic fluid is normal, the pregnancy should be followed by serial ultrasonography. If amniotic fluid remains adequate, the mother should receive routine obstetric care, and the fetus can be treated postnatally. If amniotic fluid decreases and oligohydramnios develops, a prognostic evaluation should be performed, including (1) amniotic fluid status at presentation; (2) sonographic appearance of the renal parenchyma; and (3) fetal bladder aspiration to determine urine Na, Cl, and osmolarity. Although we have only preliminary clinical experience with fetal creatinine clearance, laboratory data suggest that fetal creatinine clearance studies will allow an additional simple, quantitative estimate of fetal renal function.[13]

Prenatal intervention should be reserved for those fetuses with adequate renal function for postnatal survival and pulmonary immaturity precluding early delivery. Alternatives for decompression include percutaneous catheter placement or fetal surgery. Vesicoamniotic shunts have been successfully placed in more than 80 human fetuses worldwide, but due to the high incidence of catheter clogging and displacement and the associated risk of chorioamnionitis, vesicoamniotic shunts are not satisfactory for long-term fetal urinary tract decompression.[4] We currently favor surgical decompression by bladder marsupialization or bilateral ureterostomies for the appropriate fetus with obstructive uropathy.

Fetal Surgery

The indications for prenatal intervention are narrow, and open fetal surgery is appropriate only for a select group of fetuses diagnosed in the late first and early second trimester, with associated oligohydramnios, favorable fetal urine electrolytes and osmolarity, and normal renal parenchyma on ultrasound. Open fetal surgery is preferable to catheter decompression if a prolonged period (greater than 2 to 3 weeks) remains until lung maturity, to allow reliable long-term decompression and restoration of amniotic fluid dynamics.

More than 200 cases of fetal hydronephrosis have been referred to the Fetal Treatment Program at the University of California, San Francisco Medical Center from 1978 to 1988. Five patients were found suitable for open intervention. One fetus had bilateral ureterostomies, and the subsequent four had marsupialization of the bladder at 18 to 24 weeks gestation. All pregnancies proceeded to cesarean delivery at 32 to 35 weeks gestation. There was no long-term maternal morbidity, and two mothers have since carried normal pregnancies.[21]

Three fetuses had return of normal amniotic fluid dynamics, and all three had adequate pulmonary function at birth, suggesting that fatal pulmonary hypoplasia associated with early severe oligohydramnios had been reversed. Two neonates died at birth with pulmonary hypoplasia. One had no amniotic fluid even after decompression, due to our inability to predict fetal renal function early in our experience. The other had some amniotic fluid after decompression, but also had a tiny chest cavity due to the long period of severe oligohydramnios before decompression. Of the three surviving infants, one had normal renal function when she died of unrelated causes at 9 months of age. One has normal renal function at 16 months. The third developed failing renal function by 3 years, has grown and developed normally, and subsequently has received a successful kidney transplant. Our current selection criteria would now accurately exclude from treatment the two fetuses who died of pulmonary hypoplasia.

Fetal Surgical Technique. In brief, anesthetic and tocolytic techniques include preoperative indomethacin, halothane for uterine relaxation and fetal and maternal anesthesia intraoperatively, and postoperative tocolytic therapy with ritodrine or terbutaline. The uterus is exposed by a low transverse abdominal incision, and intraoperative sonography confirms the fetal position and the placental location. The uterus is opened with either cautery or a newly developed resorbable stapling device, and the lower part of the fetal body is delivered through the hysterotomy. A transcutaneous oximeter placed around the fetal thigh allows continuous monitoring of fetal oxygen saturation and heart rate. The distended and thick-walled bladder is opened and marsupialized to the fetal skin with interrupted sutures (Fig. 51-2). Fetal heart rate has proven to be a very sensitive monitor of fetal condition: any episodes of fetal bradycardia are easily reversed by changing the fetal position to minimize compression of the umbilical cord. The fetal surgical procedure takes 15 minutes or less; the monitoring devices are then removed and the fetus returned to the uterine cavity. Amniotic fluid volume is restored with warm Ringer's lactate containing oxacillin. The uterus is closed with two layers of running PDS suture, making certain to include both the amniotic membranes and the myometrium in the inner layer. After uterine closure, intraoperative sonography can determine fetal heart rate and confirm bladder decompression. Maternal epidural morphine is used postoperatively for analgesia, and perioperative antibiotics are continued for 3 days. Ritodrine hydrochloride is given intravenously for 3 days and then orally to control uterine activity and prevent preterm labor. Mother and fetus usually leave the hospital within a week, are followed weekly thereafter by ultrasonography, and undergo cesarean delivery weeks later.

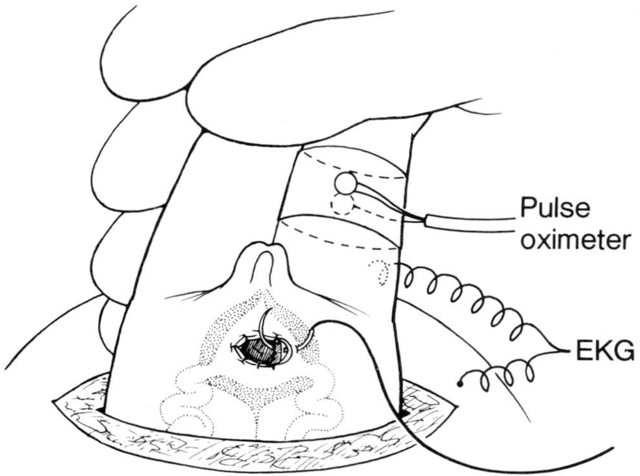

FIGURE 51–2. Technique of fetal bladder marsupialization in utero. EKG, electrocardiogram.

The maternal risks of open fetal surgery remain a principal concern in electing this experimental treatment. Prior to offering fetal surgery to our patients, the efficacy of fetal decompression was established in sheep,[9,13–16,22] and the feasibility and safety of open fetal surgery were established in the more rigorous nonhuman primate model.[6,7] The tocolytic, anesthetic, and surgical techniques were all developed and extensively tested in the nonhuman primate prior to this successful clinical application. We believe that the paucity of complications in these five patients, as well as nine others with open fetal procedures performed for other reasons, is a direct result of our extensive preparation in experimental fetal animals, which should be a requisite for anyone considering these inherently dangerous procedures. We know of only one other human open fetal surgical case that was performed at a medical center where the investigators chose not to do preparatory work in nonhuman primates, and that procedure failed.

Our initial limited experience suggests that:

1. Our prognostic criteria for predicting outcome and selecting management for fetuses with obstructive uropathy have proven accurate.
2. Open fetal surgery is safe in experienced hands, and the risks of open fetal surgery can be minimized by extensive preparatory experimental work.
3. In a few highly selected cases, open decompression can restore amniotic fluid dynamics and is efficacious in preventing pulmonary hypoplasia at birth.

The effect of decompression on long-term renal function remains unknown.

CONGENITAL DIAPHRAGMATIC HERNIA

Congenital diaphragmatic hernia (CDH) is an anatomically simple defect that is easily correctable after birth. However, despite optimal postnatal medical management and surgical repair, 50% to 80% of all infants with CDH die of pulmonary hypoplasia.[23,24] Because the pulmonary hypoplasia appears to be a developmental consequence of compression by the herniated viscera, removal in utero of this space-occupying lesion should allow lung development to proceed so that pulmonary function will be adequate to support life at birth.

In the fetal lamb model, we have shown that compression of the lungs during the last trimester, either with an intrathoracic balloon[25] or by creation of a diaphragmatic hernia,[26,27] results in fatal pulmonary hypoplasia. In addition, removal of the compressing lesion allows the lung to grow and develop sufficiently to permit survival at birth. In addition, a technique for successful surgical correction in utero has been developed experimentally.[8]

Correct management of the fetus with a prenatal diagnosis of CDH is dependent on a knowledge of the natural history of the disease. The reported mortality among prenatally diagnosed fetuses with this lesion is approximately 80%[28,29]; this is significantly higher than the 50% mortality generally reported for neonates without a prenatal diagnosis.[30] In addition, a number of poor prognostic indicators have been identified that are evident on prenatal sonography,[31,32] including diagnosis prior to 25 weeks, polyhydramnios, associated anomalies, and liver in the chest. Our ability to diagnose these fetuses early in gestation, and to predict which will have the worst outcome without intervention, suggests that prenatal repair may offer great hope to the highly selected fetus with CDH.

We attempted to salvage eight highly selected fetuses with severe CDH by open fetal surgery.[33] The first three fetuses died at operation because attempts to reduce the friable incarcerated liver from the fetal chest were unsuccessful. In the fourth case, a Gore-tex diaphragm was constructed around the liver, but lung decompression was ineffective and the baby died at birth. The last four fetuses were successfully repaired. All four demonstrated rapid growth of the lung in utero, and had surprisingly good lung function after birth. Two subsequently died of nonpulmonary problems (an unrelated nursery accident in one and intestinal complications in the other), but the last two babies have done well.

Diaphragmatic hernia remains the best studied and most compelling example of a defect requiring correction before birth. However, we continue to believe that in utero repair of this defect in humans represents a formidable challenge that should not be attempted under any but the most rigorous conditions.

SACROCOCCYGEAL TERATOMA

Sacrococcygeal teratoma (SCT) is the most common tumor of newborns. The majority of these are diagnosed in newborns when the malignant potential is low and the prognosis is good. Prenatal diagnosis, however, has identified cases of SCT that die in utero. These findings have elucidated the natural history of SCT and have implications for management.

The gestational age at diagnosis has important prognostic significance. We have reported a series where six out of eight cases survived when the diagnosis was made after 30 weeks gestation. In cases diagnosed before 30 weeks gestation, only 1 of 14 survived.[28] Recent cases have elucidated the pathophysiology of these lethal cases. When diagnosed earlier than 30 weeks gestation, invariably there has been development of massive tumor enlargement, fetal hydrops, and placentomegaly. In each of six cases diagnosed at 14 to 23 weeks gestation, the mothers developed a severe preeclampsia syndrome with vomiting, hypertension, edema, and proteinuria. Two of the six affected mothers required treatment in the intensive care unit for pulmonary edema.

We have recently demonstrated by Doppler ultrasound that the tumor in these severe cases behaves as a large arteriovenous fistula, with markedly increased distal aortic blood flow and shunting of blood away from the placenta to the tumor.[29] Fetal demise presumably occurs because of high-output cardiac failure. The cause of the severe maternal preeclampsia state is less clear, but may be an example of "mirror syndrome," described for severe hemolytic disease of the newborn, where the maternal condition mirrors the fetal illness.[30] This phenomenon may be mediated by the release of chorionic gonadotropin or vasoactive compounds from the placenta.

These findings have important implications for management. Fetuses with lesions greater than 5 cm should be delivered by cesarean section to avoid dystocia, tumor rupture, or hemorrhage into the tumor, which might occur with vaginal delivery.[3] Cases with hydrops diagnosed after 30 weeks gestation should be delivered when pulmonary maturity is attained. Lesions diagnosed prior to 30 weeks gestation usually have a poor outcome. Prenatal excision at 21 weeks gestation was successful in decreasing the distal aortic flow with subsequent reversal of hydrops.[34] Despite improvement in the fetal condition, the maternal preeclampsia did not improve, and the fetus had to be delivered for maternal considerations. The infant died due to pulmonary immaturity when delivered 2 weeks after surgery. In utero surgery remains an experimental approach to SCT that is diagnosed early in gestation and accompanied by hydrops. Prenatal tumor excision or elective termination should be considered, especially when the fetal condition causes serious maternal illness.

CONGENITAL CYSTIC ADENOMATOID MALFORMATION

Congenital cystic adenomatoid malformation (CCAM) can present as a fatal lesion in a fetus or neonate, or as a relatively mild lesion causing respiratory difficulty or recurrent infections in an infant or child. CCAM represents a spectrum of disease characterized by cystic lesions of the lung. The macrocystic type has cysts larger than 5 mm in diameter. These may be solitary cysts that grow to several centimeters in diameter. Microcystic disease has multiple cystic lesions less than 5 mm in diameter. Prenatal ultrasound can generally distinguish individual cysts in macrocystic disease, while microcystic lesions usually have the appearance of an echogenic, solid lung mass.[35]

Polyhydramnios is a frequent accompanying finding in more than 50% of cases.[35] Although the precise pathogenesis of polyhydramnios is unknown, two possible explanations are decreased fetal swallowing of amniotic fluid due to esophageal compression by the thoracic mass, or increased fetal lung fluid production by the abnormal lung tissue. The differential diagnosis includes congenital diaphragmatic hernia (CDH) and other lung lesions, such as extralobar pulmonary sequestration, bronchogenic cyst, and mediastinal cysts. Although associated lethal anomalies and chromosomal abnormalities are unusual, amniocentesis for karyotyping and careful sonographic survey to rule out other lesions should be performed. The prenatal diagnosis of CCAM should prompt referral to a tertiary center with a pediatric surgeon available. Normal vaginal delivery can usually be carried out with prompt resuscitation and postnatal surgery.

Differences in survival rate of patients with CCAM have been previously ascribed to the histologic type of the lesion, but our experience and that of others demonstrates that an unfavorable outcome is most closely associated with hydrops. Hydrops is probably secondary to vena cava obstruction or cardiac compression from the extreme mediastinal shift caused by these lesions, and hydrops has been documented in association with other space-occupying thoracic lesions.[35] However, loss of protein from the CCAM into the amniotic fluid may be a contributing factor, because the amniotic fluid protein concentration has been shown to be elevated in some cases. There has been only one reported survivor when CCAM was associated with hydrops, regardless of lesion type.[36] The almost invariably fatal outcome seen with microcystic lesions is related to several factors, including development of fetal hydrops, hypoplasia of normal lung tissue secondary to prolonged compression in utero, and lack of early diagnosis and immediate postnatal surgery. Macrocystic lesions may resolve spontaneously when followed by serial ultrasound throughout the course of pregnancy.[37]

It is possible that in utero surgical decompression or removal of the CCAM will reverse the hydrops and allow sufficient lung growth to permit survival in these severe cases. We have demonstrated experimentally that in utero pulmonary resection is feasible, and that compensatory growth of the opposite lung occurs.[11]

Thoracentesis of macrocystic lesions in utero does not provide lasting decompression of normal lung tissue. However, percutaneous placement of a double pigtail catheter shunt between a large lung cyst and the amniotic space in a 20-week fetus with CCAM resulted in sustained cyst decompression, and resolution of hydrops with successful delivery and postnatal surgery 17 weeks later, at the time of delivery.[38]

In utero resection of a huge CCAM has been performed in a 23-week fetus with ascites but no placentomegaly.[39] The ascites resolved, good lung growth occurred in utero, and the child survived. Early diagnosis, the large size of the tumor, and the early onset of hydrops indicated a dismal prognosis. Appropriately selected cases of CCAM are now amenable to fetal surgical therapy.

CONGENITAL HYDROTHORAX

Congenital pleural effusions are often due to fetal chylothorax (FCT), and can be diagnosed as early as 16 weeks gestation.[40] Although small effusions may be harmless, large effusions may result in pulmonary compression, pulmonary hypoplasia, and hydrops.

We recently reported a series of 32 cases.[41] The overall mortality was 53%. Polyhydramnios was present in 22 cases, and was not associated with a higher mortality. Early diagnosis (less than 32 weeks gestation) and hydrops were associated with a higher mortality. Pleural fluid was available in 12 patients, all of whom had more than 80% lymphocytes on cell count, which confirmed the diagnosis of FCT.

Small effusions diagnosed late in gestation often have a satisfactory outcome without treatment, and some resolve spontaneously. In these cases, serial ultrasound should be performed, with appropriate postnatal follow-up. For large effusions causing hydrops, in utero decompression may offer the only hope for survival. Although success with repeated aspirations in utero has been reported,[40] we have used a thoracoamniotic shunt to successfully decompress the FCT after multiple attempts at aspiration had been unsuccessful. Rodeck reported the successful placement of a thoracoamniotic shunt in eight fetuses with FCT.[42] Six of these infants survived, five without postnatal respiratory difficulty. Lung reexpansion was seen in all of the survivors, but not in the two who died.

CLEFT LIP AND PALATE

Cleft lip and palate are the most common congenital facial anomalies, with an incidence of 1 in 800 live births in whites. The inheritance is multifactorial, with genetic predisposition and environmental factors both playing a role. Cleft lip and palate are associated with multiple progressive abnormalities as the child grows:

1. Abnormal speech, requiring a secondary operation on the palate and speech therapy, in 25% to 35%
2. Nasal deformity consisting of depression of the alar base and tip and deviation of the septum (unilateral cleft lip/palate) and bilateral widening of the alar base and short columella (bilateral)
3. Midface growth deficiency resulting in maxillary retrusion and relative mandibular prognathism
4. Recurrent otitis media (in cases of cleft palate) secondary to abnormal eustachian tube function
5. Dental anomalies consisting of missing, extra, and malpositioned teeth.[43]

Experimental models for the study of cleft lip and palate have existed for many years.[44–46] These have been used primarily to document the embryologic events leading to development of the deformity. In addition, cleft lip and palate models have been used to document the secondary growth effects of postnatal cleft lip and palate repair. More recently, investigators have examined the feasibility of fetal cleft lip repair.[43]

It is well known that midface retrusion and deficiency in maxillary width are often the result of surgically induced scar formation. Bardach has demonstrated that increased lip pressure following postnatal repair of cleft lip in animals is associated with progressive midface hypoplasia.[47] Several studies in animal models have shown that fetal wound healing is fundamentally different from that in adults. The fetal process does not involve inflammation or scarring.[48–50] Hallock has demonstrated that in utero repair of cleft lip is possible in mice.[43] Our fetal surgery laboratory is currently developing techniques for in utero cleft lip repair in larger animals with a longer gestation.

A simple linear repair of cleft lip in utero might result in healing without scar formation. The resultant oral sphincter, with intact muscle, would provide a normal "functional matrix" for the growing fetus. The esthetic result would be greatly improved. The major advantage, however, would be unimpaired facial growth without the adverse effect of the lip or palate scar.

It is not known whether fetal healing without scar occurs throughout gestation. Our preliminary studies indicate that by the third trimester fetal wounds heal in a more adult fashion. This is important, because in utero repair of cleft lip should be performed at a time in gestation when fetal morbidity would be low but also when there would be healing without scar. This developmental "window" has not been established. However, it is likely that the median human fetal gestational age of 24 weeks in the initial series of open fetal surgery at our institution would fall in such a window.

Cleft lip and palate are craniofacial anomalies where fetal intervention may be applicable. The genetics, epidemiology, and predicted recurrence risk for these malformation are known. Women who are at risk for subsequent pregnancies may undergo fetal ultrasound. Fortunately, ultrasound is a reliable technique to diagnose fetal cleft lip and palate as early as 15 to 20 weeks gestation. Thus, a mother who is carrying a fetus with a cleft lip may be referred to a fetal treatment program. In the future, an in utero repair could potentially be offered as a therapeutic option. Clearly, further laboratory investigation, including work in the nonhuman primate model, is necessary before fetal craniofacial surgery can be applied clinically.

CONGENITAL HEART DISEASE

Many types of congenital cardiac disease are now readily diagnosable in utero, with a great degree of accuracy. Although the pathophysiology of many of these lesions is not completely understood, it appears that decreased blood flow during fetal life may result in secondary hypoplasia of vessels or cardiac chambers. An example of this may include the hypoplastic pulmonary arteries seen with pulmonic stenosis. In utero correction may allow for normal development of the pulmonary arteries, with a markedly improved postnatal prognosis. Techniques have been described for operating on the fetal heart,[51] and with further experimental work on both pathophysiology and techniques, open fetal cardiac surgery may become a possibility.

THE FUTURE OF OPEN FETAL INTERVENTION

Prenatal diagnosis offers new hope for improved management of the fetus with a congenital defect. However, the more invasive diagnostic and therapeutic procedures involve significant risks for both fetus and mother, raising difficult ethical questions about risks versus benefits and about the rights of the fetus and the mother. It is imperative that all who consider embarking on this type of treatment be committed to continuously developing the enterprise through ongoing research and responsible reporting of all clinical experience. Because prenatal intervention carries such risk, we believe that it should not be considered for any given condition until the following criteria have been met:

1. The physiologic rationale, efficacy, and feasibility are demonstrated experimentally.
2. The prenatal diagnosis is shown to be accurate, capable of excluding other anomalies, and able to predict which fetuses have sufficiently bad prognosis to justify in utero intervention.
3. The natural history and outcome of the untreated condition in the human fetus is defined by serial observations.
4. The safety of hysterotomy and control of preterm labor are established.

Our ability to diagnose fetal birth defects has achieved considerable sophistication. With continuing research efforts and responsible, cautious clinical experience, the indications for open fetal intervention will undoubtedly continue to expand.

REFERENCES

1. Harrison MR, Golbus MS, Filly RA. The unborn patient. Philadelphia: WB Saunders, 1991.
2. Liley AW. Intrauterine transfusion of foetus in haemolytic disease. Br Med J 1963;2:1107.
3. Flake AW, Harrison MR, Adzick NS, et al. Transplantation of fetal hematopoietic stem cells in utero: the creation of hematopoietic chimeras. Science 1986;233:776.
4. Manning FA, Harrison MR, Rodeck C, et al. Catheter shunts for fetal hydronephrosis and hydrocephalus. N Engl J Med 1986;315:336.

5. Glick PL, Harrison MR, Nakayama DK, et al. Management of ventriculomegaly in the fetus. J Pediatr 1984;105:97.
6. Harrison MR, Anderson J, Rosen M, et al. Fetal surgery in the primate. I: anesthetic, surgical, and tocolytic management to maximize fetal–neonatal survival. J Pediatr Surg 1982;17:115.
7. Adzick NS, Harrison MR, Anderson JV, et al. Fetal surgery in the primate. III: maternal outcome after fetal surgery. J Pediatr Surg 1986;21:477.
8. Adzick NS, Harrison MR, Flake AW, et al. Automatic uterine stapling device in fetal surgery: experience in a primate model. Surg Forum 1985;36:476.
9. Harrison MR, Nakayama DK, Noall R, et al. Correction of congenital hydronephrosis in utero. II: decompression reverses the effects of obstruction on the fetal lung and urinary tract. J Pediatr Surg 1982;17:965.
10. Harrison MR, Ross NA, deLorimier AA. Correction of congenital diaphragmatic hernia in utero. III: development of a successful surgical technique using abdominoplasty to avoid compromise of umbilical blood flow. J Pediatr Surg 1981;16:934.
11. Adzick NS, Harrison MR, Hu LM, et al. Compensatory lung growth after pneumonectomy in fetal lambs: a morphometric study. Surg Forum 1986;37:309.
12. Harrison MR, Golbus MS, Filly RA. Management of the fetus with a urinary tract malformation. JAMA 1981;246:635.
13. Adzick NS, Harrison MR, Flake AW, et al. Development of a fetal renal function test using endogenous creatinine clearance. J Pediatr Surg 1985;20:602.
14. Adzick NS, Harrison MR, Flake AW, Glick PL. Fetal urinary tract obstruction: experimental pathophysiology. Semin Perinatol 1985;9:79.
15. Glick PL, Harrison MR, Noall R, et al. Correction of congenital hydronephrosis in utero. III: early mid-trimester urethral obstruction produces renal dysplasia. J Pediatr Surg 1983;18:681.
16. Glick PL, Harrison MR, Adzick NS, et al. Correction of congenital hydronephrosis in utero. IV: in utero decompression prevents renal dysplasia. J Pediatr Surg 1984;19:649.
17. Harrison MR, Golbus MS, Filly RA, et al. Management of the fetus with congenital hydronephrosis. J Pediatr Surg 1982; 17:728.
18. Glick PL, Harrison MR, Adzick NS, et al. Management of the fetus with congenital hydronephrosis. II: prognostic criteria and selection for treatment. J Pediatr Surg 1985;20:376.
19. Mahony BS, Filly RA, Callen PW, et al. Sonographic evaluation of fetal renal dysplasia. Radiology 1984;152:143.
20. Crombleholme TM, Harrison MR, Golbus MS, et al. Fetal intervention in obstructive uropathy: Prognostic indicators and efficacy of intervention. Am J Obstet Gynecol 1990;162:1239.
21. Crombleholme TM, Harrison MR, Anderson RL, et al. Early experience with open fetal surgery for congenital hydronephrosis. J Pediatr Surg 1988;23:1114.
22. Harrison MR, Ross NA, Noall R, et al. Correction of congenital hydronephrosis in utero. I: the model: fetal urethral obstruction produces hydronephrosis and pulmonary hypoplasia in fetal lambs. J Pediatr Surg 1983;18:247.
23. Nguyen L, Guttman FM, de Chadarevian JP, et al. The mortality of congenital diaphragmatic hernia: is total pulmonary mass inadequate, no matter what? Ann Surg 1983;198:766.
24. Harrison MR, Bjordal RI, Landmark F, et al. Congenital diaphragmatic hernia: the hidden mortality. J Pediatr Surg 1979;13:227.
25. Harrison MR, Jester JA, Ross NA. Correction of congenital diaphragmatic hernia in utero. I: the model: intrathoracic balloon produced fetal pulmonary hypoplasia. Surgery 1980;88:174.
26. Harrison MR, Bressack MA, Churg AM. Correction of congenital diaphragmatic hernia in utero. II: simulated correction permits fetal lung growth with survival at birth. Surgery 1980;88:260.
27. Adzick NS, Outwater KM, Harrison MR, Reid LM. Correction of congenital diaphragmatic hernia in utero. IV: an early gestational model for pulmonary vascular morphometic analysis. J Pediatr Surg 1985;20:673.
28. Flake AW, Harrison MR, Adzick NS, et al. Fetal sacrococcygeal teratoma. J Pediatr Surg 1986;21:563.
29. Bond SJ, Harrison MR, Schmidt KG, et al. Death from high output cardiac failure in fetal sacrococcygeal teratoma. J Pediatr Surg 1990;25:1287.
30. Nicolay KS, Gainey HL. Pseudotoxemic state associated with severe Rh-isoimmunization. Am J Obstet Gynecol 1964;89:41.
31. Adzick NS, Harrison MR, Glick PL, et al. Diaphragmatic hernia in the fetus: prenatal diagnosis and outcome in 94 cases. J Pediatr Surg 1985;20:357.
32. Adzick NS, Vacanti JP, Lillehei CW, et al. Fetal diaphragmatic hernia: ultrasound diagnosis and clinical outcome in 38 cases from a single medical center. J Pediatr Surg 1989;24:654.
33. Harrison MR, Adzick NS, Longaker MT, et al. Successful repair in utero of a fetal diaphragmatic hernia after removal of herniated viscera from the left thorax. N Engl J Med 1990;322:1582.
34. Langer JC, Harrison MR, Schmidt KG, et al. Fetal hydrops and demise from sacrococcygeal teratoma: rationale for fetal surgery. Am J Obstet Gynecol 1989;160:1145.
35. Adzick NS, Harrison MR, Glick PL, et al. Fetal cystic adenomatoid malformation: prenatal diagnosis and natural history. J Pediatr Surg 1985;20:483.
36. Golladay ES, Mollitt DL. Surgically correctable fetal hydrops. J Pediatr Surg 1984;19:59.
37. Saltzman DH, Adzick NS, Benacerraf BR. Fetal cystic adenomatoid malformation of the lung: apparent improvement in utero. Obstet Gynecol 1988;71:1000.
38. Clark SL, Vitale DJ, Minton SD, et al. Successful fetal therapy for cystic adenomatoid malformation associated with second trimester hydrops. Am J Obstet Gynecol 1987;157:294.
39. Harrison MR, Adzick NS, Jennings RW, et al. Antenatal intervention for congenital cystic adenomatoid malformation. Lancet 1990;336:965.
40. Benacerraf BR, Frigoletto FD, Wilson M. Successful midtrimester thoracentesis with analysis of the lymphocyte population in the pleural effusion. Am J Obstet Gynecol 1986;155:398.
41. Longaker MT, Laberge JM, Dansereau J, et al. Primary fetal hydrothorax: natural history and management. J Pediatr Surg 1989;24:573.
42. Rodeck CH, Fisk NM, Fraser DI, Nicolini U. Long-term in utero drainage of fetal hydrothorax. N Engl J Med 1988;319:1135.
43. Hallock GG. In utero cleft lip repair in A/J mice. Plast Reconstr Surg 1985;75:785.
44. McClure HM, Wilk AL, Horigan EA, et al. Induction of craniofacial malformations in rhesus monkeys (Macaca mulatta) with cyclophosphamide. Cleft Palate Journal 1979;16:248.
45. Gibson JE, Becker BA. The teratogenicity of cyclophosphamide in mice. Cancer Res 1968;28:475.
46. Sulik KK, Johnson MC, Ambrose LJH, et al. Phenytoin (Dilantin)-induced cleft lip and palate in A/J mice: a scanning and transmission electron microscopic study. Anat Rec 1979;195:243.
47. Bardach J, Bakowska J, McDermott-Murray J, et al. Lip pressure changes following lip repair in infants with unilateral clefts of the lip and palate. Plast Reconstr Surg 1984;74:476.
48. Burrington JD. Wound healing in the fetal lamb. J Pediatr Surg 1971;6:523.
49. Robinson BW, Goss AN. Intrauterine healing of fetal rat cheek wounds. Cleft Palate Journal 1987;18:251.
50. Roswell A. The intrauterine healing of foetal muscle wounds: experimental study in the rat. Br J Plast Surg 1984;37:635.
51. Adzick NS, Harrison MR, Slate RK, et al. Surface cooling and rewarming the fetus: a technique for experimental fetal cardiac surgery. Surg Forum 1984;35:313.

52

CHAPTER

IN UTERO CARDIAC THERAPY

Charles S. Kleinman and Joshua A. Copel

In this chapter we focus on the potential for in utero therapy of functional and structural fetal heart disease. During the course of the past dozen years increasing attention has been paid to the potential for diagnosing cardiovascular abnormalities in the human fetus during the second and third trimesters of gestation. Through the use of M-mode, two-dimensional, pulsed, and color Doppler echocardiographic imaging, it has become commonplace for major forms of structural heart disease to be diagnosed before delivery.

In the vast majority of cases the fetal cardiovascular system has undergone a gradual adaptation to the abnormal flow patterns attending the structural abnormalities within the central circulation. The developing fetus is rarely compromised by such structural heart disease, and in utero therapies, with their attendant risks to both mother and fetus, would clearly be inappropriate. In rare situations, however, structural heart disease may be associated with progressive compromise of the fetus's well-being. The common denominator in such cases is usually the development of nonimmune hydrops fetalis. This is most frequently associated with severe volume overload of the fetal heart. Such volume overload is often associated with atrioventricular valve regurgitation, as, for instance, in Ebstein malformation of the tricuspid valve, severe right ventricular outflow tract obstruction at the level of the pulmonic valve, severe mitral regurgitation in association with left ventricular outflow tract obstruction at the aortic valve, or the presence of severe semilunar valve insufficiency (as in absent pulmonary valve syndrome). The potential for providing either in utero medical therapy aimed at improving fetal myocardial performance to enable the fetal heart to cope with such volume-overloading or potential surgical therapies on the fetal heart is discussed later in this chapter.

Such treatment, despite dramatic successes, remains innovative at best and continually "walks the line" between innovative therapy and clinical investigation. It is incumbent on the physician who is treating the pregnant woman and her sick fetus to guard against the temptation to provide even the best-intentioned therapy without explaining the innovative nature of such treatment, the unknown effects that could be experienced by both mother and fetus, and the potential alternatives that could be available. We are reminded of the recommendations that have been made by Harrison and colleagues when considering the development of in utero surgical treatments.[1] The ethical grounds for a new therapy cannot be judged solely on the basis of its success or failure. It is essential that before a new therapy is offered some groundwork be done to define the frequency with which one might expect to encounter such abnormalities in the future (in part to determine the cost effectiveness of developing a new treatment protocol) and that the pathophysiology and the feasibility of the treatment be studied in advance of human therapy. In most cases this involves an experimental animal model. It is essential to define the natural history of the disease in question by serial follow-up studies of untreated fetuses.[2]

THERAPY OF FETAL CARDIAC ARRHYTHMIAS

Although most disturbances of fetal cardiac rhythm represent isolated extrasystoles of little clinical importance to the human fetus, sustained arrhythmias may sometimes be associated with nonimmune hydrops fetalis (fetal cardiac failure). In such cases in utero antiarrhythmic therapy may be life-saving. Such therapy should be provided only if the electrophysiologic mechanism of the arrhythmia is known. Such information guides the selection of antiarrhythmic agents. In addition, a means of monitoring both maternal and fetal hemodynamic responses to such therapy is essential. For the purposes of this discussion a fetal arrhythmia is defined as any irregularity of fetal cardiac rhythm unassociated with uterine contraction or a sustained regular rhythm outside the range of 100 to 160 beats per minute.

ECHOCARDIOGRAPHIC ANALYSIS OF FETAL CARDIAC RHYTHM

Using tomographic real-time imaging techniques, a sequential analysis of segmental cardiac anatomy is performed. Thereafter the two-dimensional image is used to orient the position of the M-mode sampling line. Hard-copy recordings of cardiac motion against time are made using a strip-chart recorder (Fig. 52-1). These recordings are used to time the electromechanical events of the fetal cardiac cycle. It would be preferable to perform rhythm diagnosis using an accurate electrocardiographic signal from the fetal heart. However, multiple studies have demonstrated that although it is feasible to obtain fetal QRS complexes with a transabdominal electrocardiographic recording system, 60-cycle interference and interference from the maternal electrocardiographic signal obscure electrical activity of the fetal atria, making detailed analysis of cardiac rhythm impossible from the recordings.

Using the M-mode echocardiographic information, the electrical events of the cardiac cycle are deduced on the basis of the mechanical responses of both atrial and ventricular structures recorded on the M-mode echocardiographic recording. Such recordings may provide sufficient information to allow accurate timing of atrial and ventricular electrical events. On occasion, however, the fetal heart may be oriented in a position that precludes obtaining a single M-mode echocardiographic line of information that intersects both atrial and ventricular structures simultaneously. In such cases the use of "dual M-mode" sampling capability that is available on some phased array scanners allows simultaneous recording of atrial and ventricular wall motion. A "ladder-diagram" analysis of atrioventricular contraction sequence may then be constructed to provide accurate analysis of cardiac rhythm.[3–8] Using the two-dimensional image, the sample volume of a duplex pulsed Doppler scanner may be placed within the cardiac chambers and great vessels to provide further information about the timing of mechanical events and their influence on ventricular filling and great arterial flow.[9,10]

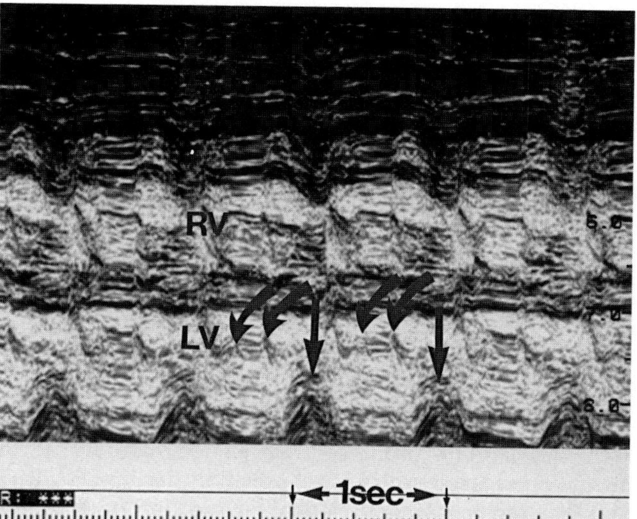

FIGURE 52–1. M-mode echocardiogram in 32-week fetus with 2:1 atrioventricular block. The M-mode sampling line transects the fetal ventricles, demonstrating atrioventricular valve motion within the fetal left and right ventricles (LV and RV). The mitral valve motion pattern demonstrates two atrial "a wave" undulations (*curved arrows*) for each ventricular wall contraction (*bold vertical arrows*). These undulations represent the mechanical responses to the electrical events in the fetal cardiac cycle. At the lower portion of the figure the paper speed is calibrated to allow atrial and ventricular rates to be measured.

EVALUATION AND MANAGEMENT OF FETAL CARDIAC ARRHYTHMIAS

The existence of a technique for the accurate diagnosis of fetal cardiac rhythm disturbances is not sufficient to justify the administration of potent antiarrhythmic agents to both a pregnant woman and her fetus. The appropriate decisions for managing a fetal arrhythmia are even more complex than those for managing a neonatal arrhythmia. Appropriate management requires an understanding of the natural history of the arrhythmia, a precise definition of its electrophysiologic mechanism, a firm understanding of the pharmacology and pharmacokinetics of the antiarrhythmic agents in the maternal–fetal environment, and a detailed risk:benefit analysis that includes an in-depth understanding of the natural history if the arrhythmia is left untreated.

The frequent association of hydrops fetalis with sustained fetal supraventricular tachyarrhythmias is well described.[11] It has also become evident in many studies that the mortality rate for severely hydropic neonates is very high, regardless of the underlying cause of the edema.[12] It therefore appears reasonable that severely hydropic fetuses with sustained supraventricular tachyarrhythmias are at extremely high risk and that vigorous efforts at in utero therapy would be warranted if they could be applied with a reasonable expectation of success and at low risk to the mother. Even a moderate risk to the mother could be acceptable in the light of the extremely poor prognosis for the fetus if the arrhythmia and the hydrops remain unresolved. The risk to the fetus increases proportionately with the degree of prematurity at the time of diagnosis.

Conversely, it follows in the fetus with sustained tachycardia without hydrops fetalis that the approach must be dictated by an estimation of the risk:benefit ratio to the fetus and mother. If the fetus is encountered at a gestational age when pulmonary maturity is likely (and this is documented by amniotic fluid analysis for markers of surfactant production), delivery with provision of therapy postnatally is preferable.[13] With increasing degrees of prematurity, immediate delivery may not be a viable option. In this setting the decision regarding the provision of therapy must depend on considerations that include the potential risk of hydrops fetalis (admittedly difficult to ascertain), the potential risks of antiarrhythmic therapy to both mother and fetus, and individual considerations, including the feasibility of providing medical follow-up to the mother and fetus. The risks of antiarrhythmic therapy largely depend on the electrophysiologic mechanism of the arrhythmia, because this will determine which antiarrhythmic agents are to be used, and on individual responses to each agent. It is important to remember that virtually every antiarrhythmic agent, with the possible exception of digoxin, carries with it the potential for significant negative inotropic effects on both the maternal and fetal cardiovascular system. In addition, various agents differ in their pro-arrhythmic effect (ie, the potential for precipitating potentially dangerous arrhythmias). Thus, it is incumbent on the treating physician to provide careful monitoring of the hemodynamic responses of both the mother and fetus under therapy.

In the presence of sustained arrhythmia without associated hydrops fetalis, it may be difficult or impossible to determine the likelihood of the subsequent development of hydrops fetalis in a given patient. In our own series of 39 patients with supraventricular tachycardia, hydrops fetalis was manifest in 30 out of 39 patients at the time of presentation and therefore warranted in utero therapy. Two additional patients with sustained tachycardia before the 34th week of gestation were observed, without therapy, for 24 to 48 hours after presentation. Each of these fetuses received antiarrhythmic therapy after pleural, pericardial, or ascitic effusions developed. Two additional patients received digoxin for supraventricular tachycardia, despite the absence of fetal hydrops, after a detailed risk:benefit analysis was discussed with the parents.

Observation of two patients who developed effusions after 24 to 48 hours of incessant tachycardia led the authors to believe that the risk of development of hydrops fetalis is relatively high despite the presence of normal cardiac structure. Recent studies by Nimrod and colleagues, using a fetal lamb model of supraventricular tachycardia, demonstrated the development of hydrops fetalis in all fetal animals within 18 to 48 hours of the onset of rapid atrial pacing.[14] The development of hydrops fetalis was preceded by a marked elevation of systemic venous pressure and the rapid development of hypoalbuminemia. Of note is the finding that the hydrops fetalis in these fetal animals resolves rapidly (within 48 hours) after restoration of normal sinus rhythm, a finding that parallels our clinical experience.

The fact that not all fetuses with supraventricular tachycardia develop hydrops fetalis is well known. It has been suggested that the "parallel" circuitry of the fetal cardiovascular system might impart some protection against the development of hydrops fetalis. However, the unique properties of the fetal cardiovascular system, including a physiologic "volume overload" on the right atrium and ventricle as well as the intrinsic diastolic properties of the ventricular myocardium that render the fetal ventricular cavity less distensible than the neonatal myocardium, make the fetal heart more susceptible to systemic edema in response to a variety of hemodynamic disturbances. Kallfelz has suggested that even a brief interlude of sinus rhythm interposed into an incessant tachycardia will provide the fetus with protection against the development of hydrops fetalis.[15] That there is some threshold beyond which fetal heart failure will develop appears virtually certain, but this threshold is probably highly individual, related in part to such intangibles as intrinsic myocardial reserve, making blanket recommendations regarding medical therapy in the absence of already manifest hydrops fetalis unjustifiable.

Experience strongly suggests that the hydropic fetus with sustained tachycardia in utero should be treated, and we consider such a situation a potential medical emergency. Unless no evidence of hydrops exists in the fetus and there is no doubt regarding pulmonary maturity, in utero therapy should be considered seriously in the management of this arrhythmia. A rational approach to treatment requires accurate identification of the electrophysiologic mechanism of the arrhythmia.

ELECTROPHYSIOLOGY OF FETAL ARRHYTHMIAS

Supraventricular Tachycardia

Sustained tachyarrhythmias appear to carry the greatest clinical import for the involved fetus. Most of the tachycardiac patients treated by our group have been identified as having supraventricular tachycardia (SVT). Supraventricular tachyarrhythmias may be reentrant (reciprocating; related to a "circus movement" of electrical activity), automatic (arising in an irritable ectopic focus above the bundle of His), or a manifestation of atrial flutter or fibrillation.[16–19]

In the neonate and in our experience in the fetus, the most common electrical mechanism underlying SVT involves a reciprocating electrical wave front that reenters the atrium from the ventricle, resulting in a circular movement of repeated electrical stimulation that is faster than and usurps the normal sinus nodal pacemaker. Because the heart responds to the fastest intrinsic pacemaker, this electrical stimulus drives it at a tachycardic rate. Such a reentrant mechanism may occur within the sinus nodal tissue (very rarely) or within the atrium itself. It occurs much more frequently within the atrioventricular node itself because of a dissociation of conduction tissue within the AV node or, alternatively, a discrete accessory conduction pathway outside the AV node (eg, the "Kent bundle" encountered in the

Wolff-Parkinson-White [WPW] syndrome), which directly connects atrial and ventricular myocardium without interposing the delay to conduction that is intrinsic in atrioventricular nodal tissue. AV nodal reentrant tachycardia (AVNRT) is the most common type of fetal and neonatal SVT.

Reentrant tachycardias of this type depend on the existence of an available pathway, with fibers that differ in conduction velocities and effective refractory periods, and require as a substrate appropriately timed extrasystoles. Reentrant tachycardias can be recognized by their tendency toward sudden onset and sudden termination, with both events associated with precipitating extrasystoles occurring at critical "coupling intervals" to the previous normal beats. These tachycardias usually have very typical rates. (For fetal SVT the typically encountered heart rate is so regularly within the range of 220 to 260 beats per minute that we strongly recommend that if a tachycardia outside this range is encountered that one consider this a rhythm other than supraventricular tachycardia until proved otherwise.)

Atrioventricular reentrant tachycardia (AVRT) is similar in many ways to AVNRT, in that both involve a reentrant circuit at the atrioventricular junction, requiring two electrical "limbs" with discrete electrical properties. Both may result in reentrant SVT of sudden onset and cessation following atrial or ventricular extrasystoles that occur with a critical "coupling interval" to the preceding sinus beat. In AVRT a discrete accessory conduction pathway bypasses the usual delay within the atrioventricular node. This pathway directly connects atrial to ventricular muscle (in the WPW syndrome) and serves as the fast limb in the circus movement of electrical energy resulting in SVT. Four of 39 patients with reentrant SVT, two patients with atrial flutter, and one patient with atrial bigeminy in utero were subsequently diagnosed on the neonatal electrocardiogram as having Wolff-Parkinson-White syndrome. These patients represent the only fetuses in the group who have had protracted tachyarrhythmias postnatally, requiring multidrug therapy. In both forms of reciprocating SVT the arrhythmia depends on a critical relationship between conduction velocities and refractory periods within the two pathways for impulse conduction. Therapeutic interventions are logically aimed at a perturbation of the delicate electrical timing balance between the two limbs of the electrical reentrant circuit needed to support the tachycardia.

Postnatal maneuvers that increase vagal tone, which in turn slows atrioventricular nodal conduction, may abruptly terminate reentrant tachycardia involving the AV node as part of the reentrant circuit. Such maneuvers have been employed in the fetus. Several patients in our series, who presented near term with intermittent supraventricular tachycardia in the absence of hydrops fetalis, demonstrated that increased vagal tone caused by cord or head compression during uterine contraction will result in "breaks" in the sustained periods of SVT.[20] Such maneuvers can hardly be recommended as a standard fetal therapy and provide no means of prophylaxis against repeated episodes of tachycardia. Antiarrhythmic agents that depress conduction and prolong refractory periods in AV nodal or accessory conduction tissue can disturb the reentrant circuit and may be useful for the termination of, as well as the prevention of, AVNRT or AVRT. Such agents may include the cardiac glycosides (digoxin), type I-A antiarrhythmics (quinidine, procainamide, disopyramide), type I-C antiarrhythmics (flecainide or encainide), beta blockers (propranolol), calcium channel blocking agents (verapamil), and type III antiarrhythmics (amiodarone).[21,22,23,24]

Atrial Flutter–Fibrillation

The incidence of atrial flutter and fibrillation in this series (Table 52-1) suggests that these arrhythmias are rarer than SVT in fetal life. This series also demonstrates that patients with atrial flutter may present with hydrops fetalis. The relatively high mortality rate in this subgroup of patients (Table 52-2) attests to the difficulties encountered in controlling these arrhythmias in utero and to the high association with congenital heart malformations.

Atrial flutter appears to result from a circus movement of electrical energy within the body of the atrium itself. The atrial rate in atrial flutter in the postnatal period is typically in the range of 300 beats per minute, whereas in the fetus monotonous atrial flutter rates of 400 to 500 beats per minute are the rule (Fig. 52-2). Varying degrees of atrioventricular block may be seen in association with fetal atrial flutter, resulting in varying ventricular response rates, which may be fixed and unresponsive to fetal activity (in the case of fixed 2:1 AV block) or irregular (in cases with varying degrees of AV block). The almost invariable association of atrial flutter with some degree of atrioventricular block is important evidence that this arrhythmia does not involve atrioventricular reentry through the AV node as the underlying electrophysiologic mechanism (inducing AV block in the presence of AV reentry tachycardia would "break" the circus movement tachycardia).

Clinical experience demonstrates that digoxin and/or verapamil rarely "break" atrial flutter, although they may increase the degree of atrioventricular block, resulting in a slower ventricular response rate. Alternatively, these agents may precipitate the development of atrial fibrillation when given to a patient with atrial

TABLE 52-1. FETAL CARDIAC ARRHYTHMIAS (*n* = 923)

Isolated extrasystoles	826
Supraventricular tachycardia	41
Atrial flutter	9
Atrial fibrillation	2
Sinus tachycardia	6
Junctional tachycardia	1
Ventricular tachycardia	4
Second-degree AV block	6
Complete heart block	26

Data collected at Yale Fetal Cardiovascular Center, 1977–1990.

TABLE 52–2. FETAL CARDIAC ARRHYTHMIAS—ATRIAL FLUTTER (n = 9)

Gestational ages	24–29 weeks
Sustained	9
Hydrops fetalis	7
In utero therapy	9
In utero control	4
Postnatal control	3
Congenital heart disease	4
Deaths	4
Wolff-Parkinson-White	2

Data collected at Yale Fetal Cardiovascular Center, 1977–1990.

flutter. The resulting arrhythmia is associated with a slower ventricular response rate because of the presence of "concealed conduction" into the atrioventricular node. Unlike the experience with the postnatal therapy of atrial flutter, in which decreasing the ventricular response rate per se may lead to a decrease in the degree of heart failure, we have been disappointed to find that mere control of ventricular response rate in the fetus with severe hydrops fetalis secondary to atrial flutter has not resulted in an improvement in the fetal hemodynamic status with a subsequent resolution of third-spaced fluid. We believe that this results from the unique cardiovascular dynamics of the fetus in which the relatively "restrictive" ventricular myocardium and the relatively "volume loaded" right heart place the fetal cardiovascular system in a precarious situation. We believe that much of the fetal cardiovascular decompensation that accompanies sustained supraventricular tachyarrhythmias reflects diastolic, rather than systolic, dysfunction. Therefore, unless the atrial flutter is controlled, there will continue to be atrial contractions against a closed or partially closed atrioventricular valve, which results in atrial pressure waves that keep the systemic venous pressure high, retarding the resolution of fetal edema and effusions. Nimrod's work has suggested that there is the rapid development of hypoalbuminemia in the presence of sustained tachyarrhythmia.[14] The low resultant oncotic pressure compounded by the high mean hydrostatic pressure related to the continued atrial flutter waves retards the resolution of fetal edema and effusions. This makes it imperative that the therapeutic end point of antiarrhythmic therapy be the restoration of normal sinus rhythm, with resumption of a 1:1 atrioventricular contraction sequence. This may well require the use of a type I antiarrhythmic agent such as quinidine, procainamide, or flecainide in the antiarrhythmic protocol for atrial flutter, following control of ventricular response rate with digoxin, verapamil, or both.

Atrial fibrillation appears to be even rarer in the fetus than atrial flutter. We have encountered only two patients in our series with this arrhythmia, and both responded to digoxin therapy alone. If, however, the arrhythmia had persisted despite the control of the ventricular response rate and if there had been associated prematurity and/or hydrops fetalis, a type I-A or I-C antiarrhythmic agent would have been used for the same reasons that were outlined for atrial flutter. The high (four out of 11 cases) morality rate in our patients with atrial flutter–fibrillation reflects the difficulty that may be encountered in controlling this arrhythmia, but it also reflects the association with congenital heart disease (four of 11 cases). In these cases (two with critical pulmonary outflow obstruction and tricuspid insufficiency, one with Ebstein malformation of the tricuspid valve, and one with atrioventricular septal defect with AV valve insufficiency and complete AV block), marked atrial dilation was associated with the development of atrial flutter. The four deaths in this series included those patients with associated congenital heart disease. Of interest is the fact that the only patient in the series of 39 cases with fetal reciprocating supraventricular tachycardia with a congenital cardiac malformation had premature closure of the foramen ovale, and that fetus was the only one in this group who died, despite restoration of normal sinus rhythm for several days prior to the fetal demise. It should be noted that the association of congenital heart disease with sustained fetal arrhythmias and hydrops fetalis appears to

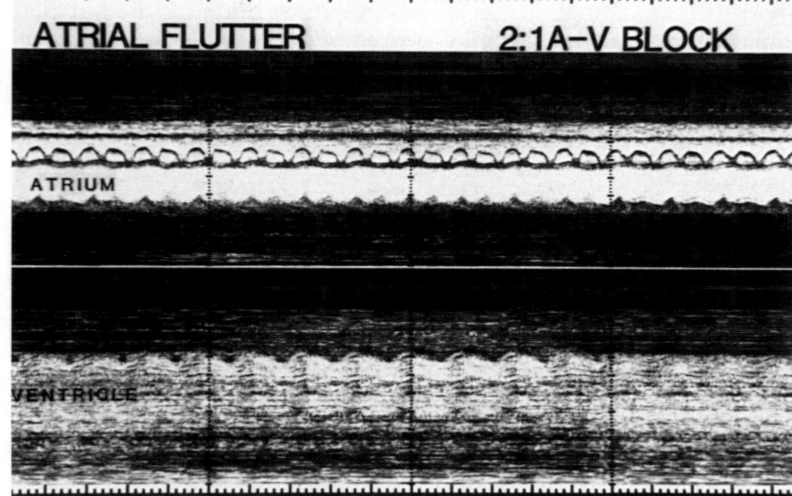

FIGURE 52–2. M-mode echocardiogram in a 30-week fetus with atrial flutter with 2:1 atrioventricular block. In this fetus two simultaneous M-mode echocardiograms are inscribed one on top of the other. The upper tracing demonstrates atrial wall and foramen ovale undulations. The vertical hatched lines are spaced at 1-second intervals. The atrial rate is approximately 480 beats per minute. The simultaneously inscribed ventricular wall undulation rate is exactly one half of the atrial rate.

be an ominous one, imparting an extremely poor prognosis for survival with or without vigorous in utero and postnatal therapy. We have encountered two fetuses with sinus tachycardia. Both had baseline heart rates of approximately 180 to 190 beats per minute with normal variations in fetal heart rate associated with fetal activity. In the first of these fetuses no explanation for the tachycardia was found even following birth, despite careful monitoring and screening for abnormalities such as thyroid and adrenal dysfunction. This fetus remained well throughout the last 6 weeks of gestation and was noted to have a significant sinus tachycardia for the first several months after birth. This baby ultimately manifested evidence of severe congestive cardiomyopathy and, despite negative results from viral titers on both mother and fetus, we strongly suspect that the sinus tachycardia was the manifestation of an unknown form of viral myocarditis.

The second fetus with sinus tachycardia was the offspring of a mother with poorly controlled thyrotoxicosis. This fetus was noted in utero to have a larger goiter and marked sinus tachycardia. Although the goiter resolved as maternal thyroid function was controlled with propylthiouracil, sinus tachycardia persisted. Hydrops fetalis never developed. Although administration of propranolol was considered, it was not given until the neonatal period, when the neonate was thought to be in impending thyroid storm. Beta blockade during the neonatal period was associated with the onset of severe congestive cardiac failure, despite the use of a relatively modest dose of propranolol. The sensitivity of this neonate's myocardium to the beta-blocking agents was impressive, and we can only speculate that a similar response would have occurred if there had been fetal exposure to the beta-blocking agents.

Ventricular Tachycardia

Ventricular tachycardias are much less common than those of supraventricular origin. In our series the heart rate during tachycardia ranged from 190 beats per minute to 240 beats per minute. As previously noted, the usual range of 220 to 260 beats per minute encountered in fetuses with atrioventricular reciprocating tachycardia may be of use in considering the nature of the origin of a sustained tachycardia. All of the patients we have encountered with ventricular tachycardia were initially thought to have supraventricular tachycardia. In three of these patients the tachycardiac rate was between 190 and 210 beats per minute, engendering a high level of suspicion about the accuracy of our initial diagnosis. Further careful evaluation demonstrated the presence of atrioventricular dissociation (the lack of a 1:1 relationship between atrial and ventricular contraction). This is an important finding to suggest that the arrhythmia does not result from atrioventricular reentry. AV dissociation may also be found in junctional tachycardia but is not found in atrioventricular reciprocating tachycardia.

Not all neonates with ventricular tachycardia are ill, which means that not all require antiarrhythmic therapy. Three patients in our series were free of hydrops fetalis and had normal cardiac structural scans and were therefore not treated in utero. These fetuses did not receive antiarrhythmic therapy as neonates, and in light of the infrequency of episodes of tachycardia after birth, the lack of symptoms during tachycardia, and the lack of structural heart disease, it was believed that the decision not to offer treatment prenatally was indeed a correct one. A fourth fetal patient developed tachycardia during labor associated with marked right ventricular and right atrial dilation. Therapy was not administered until after delivery. This patient had a marked degree of right ventricular dilation with congestive cardiac failure associated with prolonged episodes of ventricular tachycardia. A diagnosis of arrhythmogenic right ventricular dysplasia was established, and the neonate was successfully treated with intravenous lidocaine followed by the administration of oral mexiletine. A fifth fetus was initially thought to have supraventricular tachycardia with associated congenital heart disease. Careful evaluation demonstrated a heart rate of 210 beats per minute during tachycardia. On further evaluation clear-cut episodes of atrioventricular dissociation with a faster ventricular than atrial rate were documented (Fig. 52-3). On this basis a diagnosis of probable ventricular versus junctional tachycardia with atrio-

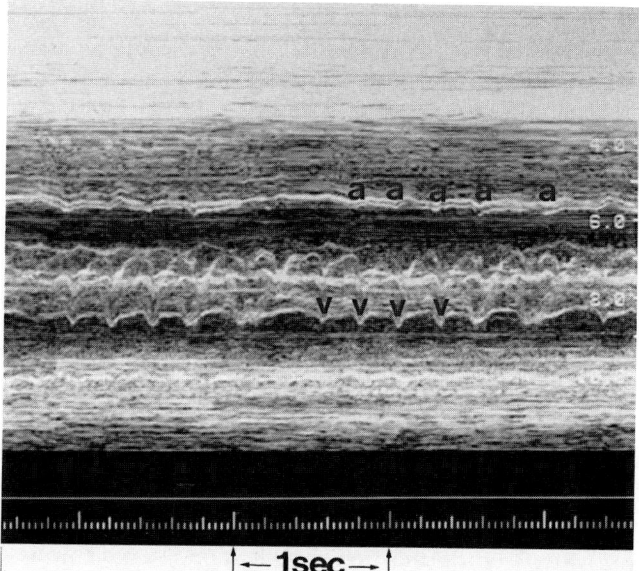

FIGURE 52–3. M-mode echocardiogram in a 34-week fetus who was evaluated due to paroxysms of fetal tachycardia. The fetal ventricular undulations (v) occasionally occur at a rate that differs from the atrial undulation (a) rate and exceeds the atrial rate. This demonstrates that the tachycardia is associated with atrioventricular dissociation. This virtually rules out atrial tachycardia or atrial flutter as the underlying basis of the arrhythmia. Atrioventricular dissociation is a characteristic of junctional or ventricular tachycardia. This fetus also manifested episodes of ventricular tachycardia during the neonatal period.

ventricular dissociation was established. Careful structural evaluation demonstrated evidence of marked right ventricular dilation without the initially suspected interventricular septal defect. Again a strong suspicion existed of either arrhythmogenic right ventricular dysplasia or, alternatively, marked right ventricular dilation resulting from sustained ventricular or junctional tachycardia. Because this fetus was thought to be previable, based on the presence of immature L–S ratio on the amniocentesis in this 35-week fetus of a diabetic mother, digoxin was withheld and flecainide therapy administered. The fetal response to flecainide was favorable, with resolution of the tachycardia within 3 days of the onset of therapy. Right ventricular dilation improved and the patient was delivered at term. Only after delivery at term did the electrocardiogram demonstrate the true nature of the underlying rhythm. The patient apparently had long episodes of junctional tachycardia, but of interest was the presence of a marked right bundle branch block with QRS duration of greater than 0.15 seconds. In addition, the patient's corrected QT interval was in excess of 0.5 seconds. The presence of such a remarkable conduction disturbance continued to be manifest after withholding of flecainide therapy, and the patient resumed having episodes of wide QRS complex tachycardia with atrioventricular dissociation. The markedly prolonged QRS duration was an absolute contraindication to the use of flecainide, and the patient responded to beta blockade therapy. This cause underlines the potential dangers associated with the use of potent antiarrhythmic agents in the fetus, in which the echocardiogram is used as the sole means of attaining an electrical diagnosis. The misdiagnosis of a ventricular arrhythmia as a supraventricular arrhythmia could lead to exposure of this fetus to digoxin with the potential risk of precipitation of ventricular fibrillation. Alternatively, we were lulled into a false sense of security by the use of flecainide, which resulted in normal sinus rhythm. For it was only after birth that we were able to obtain electrocardiographic documentation of a severe intraventricular conduction disturbance that could easily have resulted in a fatal outcome due to the concomitant application of flecainide. This case therefore underscores the potential for disaster that exists even when fetal diagnosis and monitoring are done by a relatively experienced group. It clearly reaffirms our resolve to identify such therapy as innovative–bordering on investigational and emphasizes the importance of obtaining truly "informed" consent before administration of therapy.

Fetal Antiarrhythmic Agents

The greatest volume of experience that has been achieved in the in utero therapy of fetal cardiac abnormalities is treatment directed at supraventricular tachyarrhythmias. Although there have been isolated reports involving the use of a number of antiarrhythmic agents in this setting,[25,26,27,28,29,30,31,32,33,34,35,36] the pharmacology and pharmacokinetics of the most frequently used fetal antiarrhythmic agents are discussed later. When m-mode or pulsed Doppler echocardiography demonstrates sudden onset and sudden termination of episodes of tachycardia with induction of arrhythmias by extrasystoles with a 1:1 atrioventricular relationship, this has been considered as diagnostic of reentrant supraventricular tachycardia. The onset and termination of the arrhythmia may not be observed until after a trial of antiarrhythmic therapy has begun. If therapy aimed at slowing conduction and increased refractoriness in the slow atrioventricular conduction pathways results in AV nodal block without termination of the arrhythmia, one can rule out AVNRT or AVRT with the AV node serving as one limb of the reentrant circuit as the mechanism of the arrhythmia (see Fig. 52-4). Further therapy should be guided by this information.

Digoxin

Digoxin is the drug of first choice in the treatment of in utero supraventricular tachycardia. Experience has suggested that fetal and maternal serum levels of this agent can be similar, although the ratio of fetal to maternal levels may vary from 0.3 to 1.0. It is well documented that pregnant women and neonates (and fetuses) may have serum digoxin immunoreactivity even in the absence of exogenous digoxin administration.[37] This finding may account for the suggestion that neonates may tolerate, or even require, higher serum levels of this agent than older children and adults without developing clinical evidence of digoxin toxicity.[38] Although exogenous digoxin and endogenous immunoreactive substance may be additive in serum assays for digoxin, there does not appear to be added risk of digoxin toxicity in fetuses and mothers receiving digoxin therapy.[39] Although it may be of interest to monitor serum levels of digoxin, even before initiation of digoxin therapy, this has been found to be of no clinical value. The authors monitor both mother and fetus carefully for evidence of digoxin toxicity (which is a clinical rather than a laboratory diagnosis) while striving to attain maternal serum digoxin levels toward the upper end of the therapeutic range for the laboratory (2 ng/mL), in the absence of clinical evidence of digoxin toxicity. To attain these levels, in light of the limited oral absorption of digoxin during pregnancy, the intravenous route has been used for digoxin loading over the first 24 hours, followed by the use of rather large oral maintenance doses (usually in the range of 0.50 to 0.75 mg/day). The use of digoxin for treatment of SVT in the setting of the Wolff-Parkinson-White syndrome is being reexamined in many centers because of the potential for digoxin-induced shortening of the effective refractory period within the accessory conduction pathway. This may serve as the substrate for potentially fatal rapid conduction of atrial fibrillation resulting in ventricular fibrillation.[40] Because some of these fetuses may well be expected to manifest evidence of Wolff-Parkinson-White syndrome on the postnatal electrocardiogram and because it is difficult, if not impossible, to establish such a diagnosis on the basis of a fetal m-mode echocardiogram, it is imperative to obtain informed consent from the parents of these fetuses before administering any antiarrhythmic medications. All patients who are being considered for transplacental therapy of SVT with digoxin should be informed about the potential risks associated with digoxin and the WPW syndrome, acknowledging the inability, to date, of diagnosing this syndrome from fetal echocardiographic tracings. We believe that the risk:benefit analysis is heavily weighted in favor of such therapy in previable fetuses with sustained SVT and hydrops fetalis. This analysis becomes somewhat less obvious with advancing fetal maturity and in the absence of florid hydrops fetalis.

Recent studies have suggested that the hydropic fetus may be very inefficient in absorbing digoxin through the maternal uterine circulation, and failures of therapy may well be encountered in the presence of adequate maternal serum levels of digoxin. We believe that there is a potential use, therefore, for obtaining umbilical blood samples to determine fetal serum digoxin levels, and in the setting of poor absorption there is the potential for administration of digoxin to the fetus either directly through the umbilical vein or intramuscularly.

Verapamil

Verapamil was added to the antiarrhythmic treatment protocol after a futile effort to control SVT in a 29-week fetus with severe hydrops fetalis using digoxin, propranolol, and procainamide therapy. As a blocker of slow inward calcium and sodium currents, verapamil is a potent agent for blocking AV nodal conduction. It is useful for the treatment and prophylaxis of reciprocating tachycardias involving AV nodal conduction as one limb of the reentry circuit.

It is important to note that the use of intravenous verapamil for the acute treatment of neonatal SVT has been strongly discouraged, because of the significant risk of hemodynamic collapse that appears to relate to the increased dependence of immature myocardium on slow calcium channels for contraction.[41] For this reason we have used oral, rather than intravenous, administration of this medication when it is needed for the pregnant woman in whom digoxin alone has not controlled the fetal arrhythmia adequately. Nonetheless there must be concern over the potential for hemodynamic deterioration in the face of such therapy, and this must be included in discussions with the parents and physicians before this drug is added to the treatment regimen. Verapamil is used only in treating extremely immature and severely hydropic fetuses whose arrhythmias have been unresponsive to digoxin. A rational risk:benefit analysis does not allow the use of this drug in the treatment protocol of the fetus who is less than critically ill. Before verapamil was included in our treatment protocol, an extensive experience with the use of intravenous verapamil in pregnancy in Europe was researched. Verapamil had been included in the "tocolytic cocktail" for control of premature labor as an agent to prevent cardiovascular side effects (predominantly tachycardia) associated with the use of beta agonists for control of uterine contractions. Although the use of verapamil for this purpose has been reexamined, this experience documented the safety of its use for both the mother and fetus during the third trimester of pregnancy.[42] Postnatal studies of verapamil effects in the normal heart suggest that despite the potential for negative inotropic effect associated with calcium channel blockage, the drug appears to be well tolerated. Cardiac output remains in the normal range because the decreased contractility is counterbalanced by afterload reduction attending the arterial dilation caused by the drug.[43]

Although an early report of oral verapamil administration during active labor suggested transplacental passage with a ratio of maternal to cord levels of the drug of 4:1 to 6:1, our experience suggests variable absorption of the agent (levels of 155 to 210 ng/mL in one woman receiving 120 mg orally every 8 hours, whereas another woman of similar size and gestational age attained levels of only 17 to 29 ng/mL on the same oral dose). At a steady state after 6 to 12 weeks of therapy, levels of verapamil and norverapamil in cord serum approximate 35% to 40% of maternal levels 6 to 8 hours after the last oral dose.

Although dysfunctional labor or excessive postpartum hemorrhage attributable to verapamil-induced impairment of uterine contraction has not been encountered in our experience, oral verapamil administration during active labor has been routinely discontinued.

Because of the potential for an additive negative inotropic effect and an additive effect on AV nodal conduction, the authors have been reluctant to administer verapamil to patients who are already receiving beta-blocking agents.

Verapamil is generally added to digoxin therapy if the latter agent has not controlled the fetal arrhythmia. One must be aware of the potential for digoxin accumulation due to impaired drug excretion when verapamil therapy is started, even after a digoxin steady state has been reached.[44] This effect on digoxin clearance has been described by others and has required a 33% to 50% decrease in digoxin dosage in the cases in which this combination has been used.

Quinidine

Quinidine is the oldest agent in the antiarrhythmic armamentarium. It is one of the drugs of choice for control of rapid ventricular response to atrial fibrillation and flutter in the presence of an AV bypass tract and should be considered for early inclusion in the treatment protocol when m-mode echocardiography demonstrates atrial flutter–fibrillation. In this setting digoxin, verapamil, or propranolol should be administered first, to prevent the rapid ventricular response that may occur if quinidine's vagolytic action enhances AV nodal conduction at the onset of therapy or if the atrial refractory period is increased, therefore slowing the atrial flutter rate enough to allow for AV conduction of more of the atrial beats. Quinidine may prolong PR, QRS, and QT intervals postnatally and may precipitate ventricular tachycardia, which may be associated with excessive QT prolongation (which must be carefully sought in mothers taking the drug but which cannot be monitored in the fetus in utero). This "pro-arrhythmic" potential is cause for alarm when agents in this class are used and must be discussed with parents when informed consent is obtained for its use in the treatment regimen.

Quinidine may result in noncardiac side effects, including gastrointestinal upset, fever, skin rash, cinchonism, and autoimmune thrombocytopenia and hemolytic anemia.

The addition of quinidine to the treatment regimen of a patient receiving digoxin may lead to a twofold or greater increase in the serum digoxin level. When this combination is used, digoxin serum levels should be watched and the patients must be monitored closely for clinical evidence of digoxin toxicity. We have routinely divided the digoxin maintenance dose in half when quinidine has been added to the regimen.

Anecdotal reports of fetal thrombocytopenia, retinal damage, and in utero death associated with maternal quinidine administration have led to a sparing use of this agent.[45] Recent reports from other laboratories have documented the effective use of this agent either alone or in combination with digoxin for the therapy of fetal SVT and fetal atrial flutter. We have recently included this agent as our drug of second choice in place of verapamil for the treatment of fetal SVT and flutter–fibrillation unresponsive to digoxin alone. Transplacental passage of this agent appears to be highly variable (with cord levels varying from less than 25% to as high as 94% of the maternal serum level).[46] Quinidine cannot be administered intravenously because of its tendency to cause hemodynamic collapse when used by this route.

Procainamide

The pharmacologic activity of procainamide is similar to that of quinidine. Our clinical experience with procainamide is limited to three occasions when digoxin alone was unsuccessful in controlling in utero SVT in two cases and a resistant atrial flutter in a third case. In all three situations the response was disappointing. The lack of success may have been related to low therapeutic maternal serum levels of procainamide plus its active metabolite *n*-acetylprocainamide that were attained in two cases, despite high intravenous infusion rates. In the third case atrial flutter persisted despite IV administration of procainamide directly via the fetal umbilical vein.

We remain reluctant to include this agent in our treatment protocol.

Nonetheless on the basis of the high fetal wastage, especially with atrial flutter, one must consider the fact that hydrops fetalis in the presence of arrhythmia has a poor enough prognosis to warrant therapy with type I agents, and in the event that oral treatment cannot be tolerated by the mother, procainamide may well be considered early in the treatment protocol. If, in response to digoxin, there is an acceleration of ventricular response rate in the presence of atrial flutter or fibrillation suggesting the possibility of enhanced atrioventricular conduction with the Wolff-Parkinson-White syndrome, one should consider adding this agent intravenously.

Propranolol

Modest success has resulted from the combination of digoxin and the beta-blocking agent propranolol. Transplacental transfer of propranolol has been demonstrated in the past, although the degree of transfer has been disputed. The broad therapeutic index of propranolol allows for an increase in maternal dosage without development of untoward maternal effects while attempting to attain therapeutic fetal drug levels. The risks of maternal propranolol therapy have been well described and the potential for causing low birth weight, hypoglycemia, and sinus node depression must be weighed against the therapeutic goal of conversion of the in utero tachycardia.[47,48,49,50]

Amiodarone

Amiodarone is a class III agent that has recently been released in the United States for use as an antiarrhythmic agent for treatment of life-threatening arrhythmias. This agent has an unusual spectrum of toxicity, the most serious being pneumonitis, which can lead to fatal pulmonary fibrosis. This complication has been reported in 1% to 5% of patients in some series and up to 10% of patients in one series. This appears to be a dose-related phenomenon, and recent reports suggest that its incidence in the pediatric age group is lower than that in adults. A pro-arrhythmic effect may result from QT prolongation. This agent also has a complex effect on the metabolism of thyroid hormone. (It contains iodine in its molecule and has a molecular similarity to thyroxine.) Hypothyroidism or hyperthyroidism may develop in 3% to 5% of patients

Recent reports from France and Montreal demonstrated successful conversion of fetal supraventricular tachycardia using orally administered amiodarone, with resolution of hydrops.[25,33] These fetuses were, however, documented to have hypothyroidism in the neonatal period. Although the hypothyroidism reportedly resolved spontaneously, this has caused us grave concern because of the well-described long-term sequelae on intellectual attainment in neonates born with hypothyroidism, despite administration of thyroid supplementation early in life.[51]

A recent report has suggested that multiple intravenous administrations of amiodarone directly infused into the umbilical vein may be life-saving in cases of resistant atrial tachycardia or flutter. The intravenous form of this medication is investigational at this time in the United States.

The potentially severe side effects of this medication are compounded by the extraordinarily prolonged half-life (25 to 110 days). As of this writing the authors do not recommend the use of this drug to control fetal arrhythmias.

Flecainide

Flecainide acetate is a new antiarrhythmic agent whose primary action is to depress membrane responsiveness by inhibiting the influx of sodium through its ion channel. It is several times more potent than procainamide and quinidine in depressing cardiac conduction. It has been classified as a type I-C local anesthetic agent and has been shown to be of value in the treatment of a broad spectrum of atrial, junctional, and ventricular arrhythmias. Flecainide prolongs the PR, QRS, and QTc intervals. The prolongation of the QTc interval is largely a result of QRS prolongation. Flecainide can decrease the degree of preexcitation on the electrocardiogram in patients with the WPW syndrome. Although adverse effects are relatively common with this medication, they are frequently self-limited and disappear with a decrease in dosage or by altering the frequency of administration from twice to three times daily. Unlike quinidine, gastrointestinal side effects such as nausea are rare. This agent is very successful in treating supraventricular tachycardia of the reentrant type. It is useful for the treatment of automatic supraventricular tachycardia, for the chemical conversion of atrial fibrillation, and for the treatment of ventricular arrhythmias. At first blush one would consider this to be almost an ideal antiarrhythmic agent. Unfortunately, however, the provocation of serious ventricular arrhythmias is of great concern. Morganroth and colleagues have studied this problem and have found that the most serious pro-arrhythmic effect is found in patients who have undergone therapy for the most severe arrhythmia (most commonly in patients being treated for sustained ventricular tachycardia), the associated presence of structural heart disease, and the presence of preexisting sinus node dysfunction.[52] Flecainide therapy should be initiated carefully, if at all, in patients with abnormalities of cardiac conduction. Flecainide may facilitate incessant supraventricular tachycardia. In addition, the agent appears to have a significant negative inotropic effect, precipitating heart failure in patients with diminished cardiac contractile performance. In summary, although this agent is one with great potential, the initial flush of excitement that attended its introduction to the clinical armamentarium has been tempered by the fear of substantial side effects. The pro-arrhythmic impact is believed to be so significant that a recent recommendation of the NIH and Food and Drug Administration has suggested that this agent not be administered unless it is used for treatment of life-threatening ventricular arrhythmias. This recommendation resulted from a recent study in which the agent was used for prophylaxis of ventricular arrhythmias in a group of postmyocardial infarction patients. Although pediatric cardiologists are reassessing the use of this agent in patients in the pediatric age group who differ markedly from the patient population in the CAST study,[53] one must be aware of the controversy surrounding the use of this medication and the, at least theoretical, issues that may surround its administration both to fetus and to presumably healthy mother. It is also important to reemphasize the experience that we have had recently with the administration of this agent. The one case in which we used flecainide was in a patient who subsequently was found to have junctional tachycardia. Although the agent had the desired effect, it was only after the infant was born that we detected the presence of severe intraventricular conduction disturbances that, had they been known prenatally, would have been an absolute contraindication to the use of this agent.

In summary, although we have enjoyed a flush of success in the treatment of sustained supraventricular tachyarrhythmias with a variety of antiarrhythmic agents, it is clear that our understanding of the natural history of these arrhythmias is still evolving. In addition, the unnatural history of the arrhythmias is in the process of being appreciated. The agents being administered are potent and have significant potential side effects that must be factored into any equation evaluating a risk:benefit ratio for both mother and fetus.

Bradydysrhythmias

Sinus Bradycardia. During the last several years we have encountered four fetuses with sinus bradycardia. Two of these were subsequently diagnosed to have associated congenital heart disease with left atrial isomerism and normal atrioventricular conduction. Both were diagnosed postnatally to have wandering supraventricular pacemakers. Neither patient had associated hydrops fetalis. One of the two required emergency systemic to pulmonary artery shunting in the neonatal period due to the presence of severe pulmonary outflow obstruction. Our other two patients had sinus bradycardia with baseline rates in the range of 80 to 90 beats per minute with normal heart rate variability on nonstress tests performed near term. Both of these tolerated labor and delivery well and remain in normal condition. In the presence of normal cardiac structure with normal heart rate responses to fetal activity in the absence of hydrops fetalis, moderate (heart rates between 80 and 100 beats per minute) sinus bradycardia does not appear to be an ominous fetal arrhythmia.

Block Atrial Bigeminy. Five fetuses in our series were found to have atrial bigeminy with block of the extrasystolic beat. Both had been referred for evaluation of severe (rates of 60 to 70 beats per minute) bradycardia. The referring obstetricians in each case had considered each fetus to have congenital complete atrioventricular block. In each case every second beat was very early and was so closely coupled to the previous normal sinus beat that it encountered the AV node while it was still refractory, therefore resulting in every second beat being blocked. Alternatively, if the atrioventricular node was no longer refractory, the early extrasystole resulted in the ventricle contracting before there had been adequate diastolic filling. In this latter situation each extrasystolic beat resulted in a ventricular response that resulted in a ventricular output that was inadequate to create enough forward flow to result in a detectable pulse on the Doppler listening devices. One of these fetuses subsequently developed sustained supraventricular tachycardia after birth and was diagnosed to have Wolff-Parkinson-White syndrome following electrical cardioversion to normal sinus rhythm.

Second-Degree Atrioventricular Block. Three fetuses with Mobitz type II atrioventricular block have been studied. Two of these had 3:2 and 2:1 atrioventricular block prenatally. One of these fetuses remained in second-degree block until birth. A second was born with varying degrees of Mobitz type I (Wenckebach) and Mobitz type II atrioventricular block but subsequently developed complete heart block by 1 month of age. Neither of these fetuses had structural heart disease and neither mother had a positive autoimmune antibody screen. The third patient was noted to have 2:1 and 3:1 atrioventricular block prenatally. There was no evidence of hydrops fetalis or structural heart disease, but the mother was noted to have a markedly positive anti-Ro antibody titer. Reasoning that this fetus was developing progressive damage to the atrioventricular node on an autoimmune basis, an attempt was made to ameliorate the inflammatory autoimmune-mediated response by application of absorbable anti-inflammatory steroid therapy administered to the mother. This was to no avail and this fetus developed complete atrioventricular block prior to delivery.

Complete Heart Block. Clinical experience with fetal complete heart block suggests that these fetuses may be divided into two discrete groups. It appears that in the majority of cases one can consider either that these fetuses have complex congenital heart disease associated with heart block or, if cardiac structure is normal, that the heart block is highly likely to be associated with immune complex related damage to fetal conduction tissue, secondary to the presence of maternal autoantibodies.[54] Of the 21 patients encountered with congenital complete heart block, 10 have been found to have associated congenital heart disease. Eight of these fetuses have had atrioventricular septal defects (six with left atrial isomerism) and two had associated Down syndrome with complete atrioventricular septal defect. The remaining two patients had atrioventricular inversion (corrected transposition of the great arteries). Of note is the fact that one fetus was diagnosed to have polysplenia with left atrial isomerism at a time when the fetus was in normal sinus rhythm without associated hydrops fetalis. Previous experience with this lesion led the authors to counsel the parents that there was significant risk of the development of complete heart block and that if the latter rhythm disturbance developed, it was likely that the fetus would become hydropic and that in utero demise would be probable. This was, in fact, the clinical course in this case. The case was instructive in several ways. It demonstrated that these fetuses may initially have established electrical communication from atrium to ventricle with subsequent deterioration of AV nodal function. It also suggested that atrioventricular block per se may impart enough hemodynamic compromise to result in severe fetal hydrops. The latter probably occurs secondary to a further increase in systemic venous pressure attending the slow heart rate and "cannon" A waves associated with atrial contraction against the closed atrioventricular valve. All the fetuses with congenital heart block and associated AV septal defects became severely hydropic, and there were no survivors in this group. Of the remaining 11 fetuses in the series who had no evidence of associated congenital heart disease, none developed hydrops fetalis. Eight of the 11 mothers had positive autoantibody screens (fluorescent antinuclear antibodies, anti-Ro titers, or anti-La titers). Only two of the mothers in this group had clinically diagnosed systemic lupus erythematosus. All fetuses survived to delivery and all these children remain alive. Three have required pacemaker insertion for a variety of clinical indications that included extreme bradycardia (one), ventricular arrhythmias (one), or congestive cardiac failure (one).

The association between maternal autoimmune disease and fetal congenital heart block has been well established. Recent reports have demonstrated selective binding of immune complexes to His Purkinje tissue and to fetal myocardium. This has been associated with the presence of inflammatory infiltrates and fibrosis in the region of the atrioventricular node and bundle of His. The immune complex binding to fetal myocardium may also account for the clinical finding of congestive cardiomyopathy that has been reported by some groups.

Maternal administration of beta agonists such as Ritodrine or Terbutaline may be associated with as much as a 50% increase in fetal heart rate. This increase in ventricular rate has not been associated, in our experience, with an improvement in the fetal edema in patients with heart block, hydrops fetalis, and structural heart disease. We are not aware of a drug-induced improvement in the hemodynamic state of other investigators' patients with hydrops fetalis and congenital heart block in the absence of structural heart disease. Again, we believe that this relates to the necessity of restoring a 1:1 atrioventricular contraction sequence in these fetuses so that systemic venous pressure can be reduced sufficiently to allow resolution of the hydrops. For this reason, although the report of external pacing of the fetal ventricle via the maternal transabdominal and fetal transthoracic route is of interest,[55] the authors do not believe that such therapy is warranted unless studies of animal models demonstrate that ventricular pacing per se may have a positive therapeutic effect. We strongly suspect, however, that atrioventricular sequential pacing will be necessary in such situations.

Recently, it has been demonstrated that echocardiographic monitoring techniques may be used in conjunction with continuous-wave Doppler fetal heart rate monitoring to track atrial responses to the variations in vagal tone that are associated with uterine contraction during the vaginal delivery of patients with varying degrees of AV block. Although cesarean sections for these fetuses may well be needed, especially if intrapartum fetal monitoring proves impossible, the authors believe that the combination of echocardiographic and Doppler monitoring with scalp electrode monitoring of fetal ECG and scalp pH may allow some of these fetuses to be delivered safely via the vaginal route.[56]

Congestive Cardiac Failure

During the first several years of our experience using fetal echocardiography for the assessment of pregnancies deemed to be at higher than normal risk for cardiovascular disease in the fetus, we were impressed with the frequency with which cardiac dilation was seen in association with nonimmune hydrops fetalis.[11] From this evolved the concept that nonimmune hydrops fetalis represents end-stage cardiovascular decompensation. In the course of many discussions concerning the fetal heart that have been held at international meetings it has become clear to these authors that nonimmune hydrops fetalis–congestive cardiac failure in the fetus has been interpreted by many people to be synonymous with impaired systolic pump performance. We have, in fact, become increasingly impressed with the fact that the edema attending the development of fetal congestive cardiac failure represents, in large part, diastolic rather than systolic dysfunction of the fetal heart. Fetal animal research laid the groundwork for our understanding of the impaired diastolic reserve of the fetal heart.[57] These studies, in the lamb fetus, demonstrated that isolated fetal ventricular muscle strips and whole ventricular preparations derived from fetal lambs were relatively "stiffer" in diastole than similar preparations in the neonatal or adult sheep. This restriction to ventricular filling was attributed to the relative paucity of myocardial contractile elements and the increased amount of interstitial fibrous tissue that exists in the fetal heart. For this reason any given increment in diastolic filling volume is associated with an increase in hydrostatic venous pressure. This, in association with the relative volume overload of the right ventricle attending normal fetal flow pathways, makes the fetal heart especially susceptible to the development of profound systemic edema in the presence of increases in either pre- or afterload on the fetal heart. Although it is almost certain that there are clinical states in which the human fetus suffers from inadequate forward output, it is unclear that these situations manifest in a manner that we are currently able to recognize. Our postnatal experience suggests that patients with chronically decreased forward flow can be expected to have poor systemic perfusion and, in the long run, poor somatic growth.

It is not surprising, therefore, that attempts to treat nonimmune hydrops fetalis with the administration of digoxin, in an effort to improve myocardial systolic performance, have not been met with resounding success. We are not even aware of a significant body of literature that has laid the groundwork that would convince us that digoxin, administered either via maternal administration or by direct fetal intravenous infusion, has a profoundly positive inotropic effect on the fetal heart. Despite the lack of such fundamental information, we will readily admit to having administered this agent orally to several pregnant women whose fetuses we believed were suffering from a dilated form of congestive cardiomyopathy. In one such case severe ascites was found in association with marked biventricular dilation and bilateral atrioventricular valve regurgitation. We subsequently learned that the mother's cytomegalovirus (CMV) titer increased remarkably during the last trimester of pregnancy, suggesting that our clinical supposition of an infectious myocarditis was probably correct. After administering digoxin orally to this woman, a gradual improvement in fetal myocardial performance was apparent, based on improvement in biventricular shortening fraction as measured on the m-mode echocardiogram. There was a gradual diminution of atrioventricular valve regurgitation and, ultimately, resolution of ascites prior to delivery of a child who, despite clinical evidence of moderate pulmonary hypoplasia, survived the neonatal period and subsequently thrived. This case represented our first such experience with the use of digoxin. For this reason, despite a case series of only one, we were enthusiastic in our embrace of digoxin as a treatment for congestive cardiomyopathy. Several months later, a similar case was encountered, but despite considerable urging on our part the parents of this fetus chose to decline digoxin therapy. Much to our surprise this fetus followed a similar course to our index case and gradually improved systolic shortening, resolved the atrioventricular valve regurgitation, and resolved the hydropic state spontaneously. Thus our initial assumption, that digoxin treatment was responsible for our initial success, remains unproved.

Significant ventricular dilation and atrioventricular valve regurgitation have been encountered in the presence of severe ventricular outlet obstruction in utero. The combination of marked left ventricular dilation and mitral regurgitation was described in a study in which we collaborated with our colleagues from the University of California–San Francisco.[58] The presence of an echodense subendocardium with marked left ventricular dilation and mitral regurgitation in the presence of little, if any, forward flow into the ascending aorta and poor systolic excursion of the aortic valve with a diminutive ascending aorta were thought to represent evidence of critical aortic outlet obstruction with secondary endocardial fibroelastosis, papillary muscle dysfunction, and subsequent mitral regurgitation. It should be noted, in truth, that although this has been interpreted as evidence of critical aortic stenosis with secondary myocardial dysfunction, it is completely feasible that such fetuses present with a primary myocardial process with small aorta relating to poor forward flow into the left ventricular outflow tract. This association has been reported to have a high mortality rate. We have applied the use of digoxin to the treatment of one such fetus and have seen a remarkable, and surprising, improvement in left ventricular systolic shortening with resolution of hydrops fetalis. Nonetheless, the patient was born with exceedingly poor left ventricular function and aortic hypoplasia and did not survive the neonatal period. This single experience has led us to apply such therapy for the treatment of three subsequent fetuses with left ventricular dilation and aortic hypoplasia in association with severe hydrops fetalis and secondary polyhydramnios that resulted in premature labor in pregnancies in which the fetus with ventricular dysfunction represented one of a pair of twins in which the opposite member was normal. It has been our approach to believe that administration of digoxin to attempt to improve the hydropic state could help to stabilize or resolve the polyhydramnios and associated premature labor in an effort to allow the normal fetus the opportunity to develop to the point of adequate maturity. This has proved to be successful in each such case, although none of the fetuses with ventricular dysfunction have survived the neonatal period. We have been able to salvage the three normal twins. As we increase the vigor of neonatal surgical interventions in the presence of left ventricular or aortic hypoplasia (the Norwood operation versus neonatal cardiac transplantation) it may well be found that fetuses treated with positive inotropic agents in the presence of left ventricular endocardial fibroelastosis may ultimately be salvaged.

Although as of the time of this writing the information regarding this case is sketchy, a similar case has been reported recently in the popular literature to have been subjected to an aggressive interventional catheterization approach in utero. The popular press has reported a case of a fetus in Great Britain who presented with severe left ventricular dilation, mitral regurgitation, and poor aortic forward flow who apparently was subjected to balloon aortoplasty for presumed critical aortic stenosis with secondary left ventricular dilation, fibroelastosis, and mitral regurgitation. As described in the newspapers, a transabdominal puncture of the maternal abdomen and uterus with transthoracic puncture of the fetus, introduction of a trocar into the ascending aorta, subsequent passage of a balloon angioplasty catheter across the aortic valve into the left ventricle, and balloon dilation of the aortic valve were performed on two separate occasions. It was reported on the front page of the local New Haven newspaper that this fetus was liveborn and was subjected to yet another aortic angioplasty in the neonatal period. This was hailed as the first successful cardiac surgical procedure in a human fetus. It is our understanding that this infant subsequently succumbed. This approach should be judged not on the outcome of the case but on the appropriateness of the procedure, based on the criteria that were discussed earlier for the application of any in utero therapy. It is unfortunate that this infant apparently did not survive. It is more unfortunate, however, that many months have passed since this case was reported in the popular press, and to our knowledge has not yet been reported in the scientific literature. It is impossible to judge the appropriateness of this therapy, which obviously involved considerable invasion of both the maternal and fetal autonomy, and it is imperative that the data on this case and the animal and natural history studies that served as the foundation for the development of this new therapy be presented to the scientific community.

Fetal Open-Heart Surgery

The entire medical community has been impressed in recent years by the prodigious effort of the surgical group at the University of California at San Francisco in which extensive animal studies have been performed to lay the groundwork for the subsequent development of surgical procedures on the human fetus. Investigation has progressed along several fronts, including diagnosis, surgical technique, and effective tocolysis. After appropriate groundwork was laid, these workers were the first to exteriorize a human fetus successfully to perform surgery on obstructive uropathy. Recent reports have demonstrated the feasibility of prenatal surgical repair of diaphragmatic hernia.[59] Recently, Verrier and colleagues, working in the same laboratory, have demonstrated the feasibility of exteriorizing the lamb fetus and placing the fetus on cardiopulmonary bypass (Verrier E, personal communication). Speculation has centered on the potential for performing open-heart relief of certain cardiac malformations. For example, it has been suggested that fetuses with pulmonary atresia and intact interventricular septum who, subsequently, are found to have exceedingly poor salvage rates that relate to inadequate development of right ventricular cavity and inadequate development of distal pulmonary arteries. Such fetuses could profit by early diagnosis in utero and performance of pulmonary valvotomy and patch reconstruction of the right ventricular outflow tract. It is likely that the first human surgery will focus on this lesion. It is also true that a considerable body of research still needs to be done before the first human cardiac surgery can be considered.

In conclusion, we believe that the era of in utero cardiac therapy has begun. The greatest body of experience has been in the area of fetal antiarrhythmic therapy. It is likely that further efforts will be made to affect therapy for congestive cardiac failure. Ultimately, the potential for in utero surgical palliation exists. Rather than focusing on the development of a "magic bullet" to treat all arrhythmias or to improve myocardial performance, the challenge for physicians caring for such patients is to ensure that we do not allow our enthusiasm for new treatment modalities and our genuine desire to "do good" to cloud our judgment. None of the agents currently available for cardiac therapy are without significant side effects, to both mother and fetus. The surgical interventions under consideration likewise carry significant potential for harm. It is our responsibility to ensure that such therapies are offered in a safe and ethical fashion. The administration of cardiac therapy requires an integrated approach involving, at the very least, specialists from several disciplines, including obstetrics/gynecology, pediatric cardiology, and, in many cases, radiology, pharmacology/laboratory medicine, and pediatric/fetal surgery. It is essential as well that there be a free and complete sharing of information concerning the application of these new therapies. Negative as well as positive results must be reported. The initial flush of enthusiasm for some fetal surgical techniques, such as in utero shunts for hydrocephaly and obstructive uropathy, has been tempered over the course of the last several years as it has become apparent that the "unnatural history" did not necessarily improve on the natural history of these lesions. If those of us involved in the evolution of in utero cardiac therapies do not learn from the mistakes of our predecessors, then we are doomed to repeat them.

REFERENCES

1. Harrison MR, Golbus MS, Filly RA. The unborn patient: prenatal diagnosis and treatment. Orlando: Grune & Stratton, 1984:437.
2. Blandon R, Leandro I, Fetal heart arrhythmia: clinical experience with antiarrhythmic drugs. In: Doyle EF, Engle MA, Gersony WM, Rashkind WJ, Talner NS, eds. Pediatric cardiology: proceedings of the second world congress. New York: Springer-Verlag, 1985:483.
3. Kleinman CS, Hobbins JC, Jaffe CC, et al. Echocardiographic studies of the human fetus. Prenatal diagnosis of congenital heart disease and cardiac dysrhythmias. Pediatrics 1980;65:1059.
4. Allan LD, Anderson RH, Sullivan ID, et al. Evaluation of fetal arrhythmias by echocardiography. Br Heart J 1983;50:240.
5. Crowley DC, Dick M, Rayburn WF, Rosenthal A. Two-dimensional and m-mode echocardiographic evaluation of fetal arrhythmia. Clin Cardiol 1985;8:1.
6. DeVore GR, Siassi B, Platt LD. Fetal echocardiography. III. The diagnosis of cardiac arrhythmias using real-time-directed M-mode ultrasound. Am J Obstet Gynecol 1983;146:792.
7. Kleinman CS, Donnerstein RL, Jaffe CC, et al. Fetal echocardiography. A tool for evaluation of in utero cardiac arrhythmias and monitoring of in utero therapy: analysis of 71 patients. Am J Cardiol 1983;51:237.
8. Kleinman CS, Donnerstein RL. Ultrasonic assessment of cardiac function in the intact human fetus. J Am Coll Cardiol 1985;5:84S.
9. Wladimiroff JW, Struyk P, Stewart PA, et al. Fetal cardiovascular dynamics during cardiac dysrhythmia. Case report. Br J Obstet Gynaecol 1983;90:573.
10. Kleinman CS, Valdes-Cruz LM, Weinstein EM, Sahn DJ. Two-dimensional Doppler echocardiographic analysis of fetal cardiac arrhythmias. Ped Res 1984;18:124A.
11. Kleinman CS, Donnerstein RL, DeVore GR, et al. Fetal echocardiography for evaluation of in utero congestive heart failure: a technique for study of nonimmune fetal hydrops. N Engl J Med 1982;306:568.
12. Andersen HM, Hutchison AA, Fortune DW. Nonimmune hydrops fetalis: changing contribution to perinatal mortality. Br J Obstet Gynaecol 1983;90:636.
13. Gluck L, Kulovich MV, Borer RC, Keidel WN. The interpretation and significance of the lecithin/sphingomyelin ratio in amniotic fluid. Am J Obstet Gynecol 1974;120:142.
14. Nimrod C, Davies D, Harder J, et al. Ultrasound evaluation of tachycardia-induced hydrops in the fetal lamb. Am J Obstet Gynecol 1987;157:655.
15. Kallfelz HC. Cardiac arrhythmias in the fetus—diagnosis, significance, and prognosis. In Goodman MJ, Marquis RM, eds. Paediatric cardiology. Vol 2. New York: Churchill Livingstone, 1979.
16. Ludomirsky A, Garson A Jr. Supraventricular tachycardia. In Garson A Jr, Bricker JT, McNamara DG, eds. The science and practice of pediatric cardiology. Philadelphia: Lea & Febiger, 1990:1809.
17. Gillette PC. The mechanisms of supraventricular tachycardia in children. Circulation 1976;54:133.
18. Reder RF, Rosen MR, Basic electrophysiologic principles: application to treatment of dysrhythmias. In: Gillette PC, Garson A Jr, eds. Pediatric cardiac dysrhythmias. New York: Grune & Stratton, 1981.
19. Sapire D. Supraventricular tachycardias in the young. Cardiology 1985;11:165.
20. Martin CB, Jr., Nijhuis JG, Weijer AA. Correction of fetal supraventricular tachycardia by compression of the umbilical cord: report of a case. Am J Obstet Gynecol 1984;150:324.
21. Singh et al., 1987.
22. Antman et al., 1980.
23. Lie KI, Duren DR, Manger CV, et al. Long-term efficacy of verapamil in the treatment of paroxysmal supraventricular tachycardias. Am Heart J 1983;105:688.
24. Rotmensch HH, Belhassen B. Ferguson RK. Amiodarone: benefits and risks in perspective. Am Heart J 1982;104:1117.
25. Arnoux P, Seyral P, Llurens M, Djiane P, Potier A, Unal D, Cano JP, Serradimigni A, Rouault F. Amiodarone and digoxin for refractory fetal tachycardia. Am J Cardiol 1987;59:166.
26. Bergmans MGM, Jonker GJ, Kock HCLV. Fetal supraventricular tachycardia. Review of the literature. Obstet Gynecol Surv 1985;40:61.
27. Dumesic DA, Silverman NH, Tobias S, Golbus MS. Transplacental cardioversion of fetal supraventricular tachycardia with procainamide. N Engl J Med 1982;307:1128.
28. Given BD, Phillippe M, Sanders SP, Dzau VJ. Procainamide cardioversion of fetal supraventricular tachyarrhythmia. Am J Cardiol 1984;53:1460.
29. Golichowski AM, Caldwell R, Hartsough A, Peleg D. Pharmacologic cardioversion of intrauterine supraventricular tachycardia. A case report. J Reprod Med 1985;30:139.
30. Johnson WH Jr, Dunnigan A, Fehr P, Benson DW Jr. Association of atrial flutter with orthodromic reciprocating fetal tachycardia. Am J Cardiol 1987;59:374.
31. Kerenyi TD, Gleicher N, Meller J, et al. Transplacental cardioversion of intrauterine supraventricular tachycardia with digitalis. Lancet 1980;2:393.
32. Lingman G, Ohrlander S, Ohlin P. Intrauterine digoxin treatment of fetal paroxysmal tachycardia. Br J Obstet Gynaecol 1980;87:340.
33. Lasson JR, Beytout M, Jacquetin B, Lamaison D, Cassagnes J. Traitement d'une tachycardie supraventriculaire foetale: association digoxine-amiodarone. Coeur 1985;15:315.
34. Spinnato JA, Shaver DC, Flinn GS, et al. Fetal supraventricular tachycardia: in utero therapy with digoxin and quinidine. Obstet Gynecol 1984;64:730.
35. Teuscher A, Bossi E, Imhof P, et al. Effect of propranolol on fetal tachycardia in diabetic pregnancy. Am J Cardiol 1978;42:304.

36. Wolff F, Breuker KH, Schlensker KH, Bolte A. Prenatal diagnosis and therapy of fetal heart rate anomalies: with a contribution on the placental transfer of verapamil. J Perinat Med 1980;8:203.
37. Valdes R Jr. Endogenous digoxin—immunoreactive factor in human subjects. Fed Proc 1985;44:2800.
38. Rogers MC, Willerson JT, Goldblatt A, Smith TW. Serum digoxin concentrations in the human fetus, neonate and infant. N Engl J Med 1972;287:1010.
39. Ringel R, Hamlyn J, Pinkas G. Is the plasma digoxin immunoreactivity of pregnancy associated with digitalis-like (Na^+K^+) ATPase inhibition? Pediatr Res 1987;21:193A.
40. Wellens HJJ, Durrer D. Effect of digitalis on atrioventricular conduction and circus movement tachycardia in patients with the Wolff-Parkinson-White syndrome. Circulation 1973;47:1229.
41. Garson A Jr. Medicolegal problems in the management of cardiac arrhythmias in children. Pediatrics 1987;79:84.
42. Strigl R, Pfeiffer U, Erhardt W, et al. Does the administration of the calcium antagonist verapamil in tocolysis with beta sympathomimetics still make sense? J Perinat Med 1981;9:235.
43. Stone PH, Antman EM, Muller JE, Braunwald E. Calcium channel blocking agents in the treatment of cardiovascular disorder. Part II. Hemodynamic effects and clinical applications. Ann Intern Med 1980;93:886.
44. Klein HO, Lang R, Segni ED, Kaplinsky E. Verapamil-digoxin interaction. N Engl J Med 1980;303:160.
45. Hill LM, Malkasian GD Jr. The use of quinidine sulfate throughout pregnancy. Obstet Gynecol 1979;54:366.
46. Rotmensch HH, Elkayem U, Frishman W. Antiarrhythmic drug therapy during pregnancy. Ann Intern Med 1983;98:487.
47. Gladstone GR, Hordof A, Gersony WM. Propranolol administration during pregnancy: effects on the fetus. J Pediatr 1975;86:9962.
48. Habib A, McCarthy JS. Effects on the neonate of propranolol administered during pregnancy. J Pediatr 1977;91:808.
49. Rubin PC. Beta-blockers in pregnancy. N Engl J Med 1981;305:1323.
50. Wu D, Denes P, Dhingra R, et al. The effects of propranolol on induction of AV nodal reentrant paroxysmal tachycardia. Circulation 1974;50:665.
51. Rovet J, Ehrlich R, Sorbac D. Intellectual outcome in children with fetal hypothyroidism. J Pediatr 1987;110:700.
52. Morganroth J, Anderson JL, Gentzkow GD. Classification by type of ventricular arrhythmia predicts frequency of adverse cardiac events from flecainide. J Am Coll Cardiol 1986;8:607.
53. The Cardiac Arrhythmia Suppression Trial (CAST) Investigators. Preliminary report: effect of encainide and flecainide on mortality in a randomized trial of arrhythmia suppression after myocardial infarction. N Engl J Med 1989;321:386.
54. Litsey et al., 1985.
55. Carpenter et al., 1986.
56. Kleinman et al., 1987.
57. Romero et al., 1972.
58. Silverman et al., 1984.
59. Harrison MR, Adzick NS, Longaker MT, Goldberg JD, Rosen MA, Filly RA, et al. Successful repair in utero of a fetal diaphragmatic hernia after removal of herniated viscera from the left thorax. N Engl J Med 1990;32:1952.

53

CHAPTER

FETAL METABOLIC AND GENE THERAPY

Mark I. Evans and Mark Paul Johnson

Recent developments in surgical fetal therapy have received international attention. The first successful repair of a diaphragmatic hernia in utero was the culmination of over a decade of hard, tedious, and meticulous work.[1,2]

Despite the recent attention, fetal therapy is not new. The first thoughts of ameliorating fetal hemolytic disease came in the 1960s.[3] Intraperitoneal transfusions were attempted, and by the 1970s transfusions had become a common form of intervention. In the late 1970s and throughout the 1980s attempts at other surgical interventions of fetal disease by shunting obstructed bladders and hydrocephalus and the first forays into open fetal surgery have been made.[2] Despite the popularity of surgeries in the popular press, some of the most significant advances in fetal therapy have been pharmacologic, and the future will include the correction of genetic defects.[4,5] Pharmacologic cardiac therapy is considered in Chapter 52. In this chapter we shall review the spectrum of pharmacologic interventions that provide documented reversals of pathophysiology, prevention of structural anomalies, biochemical alterations of questionable clinical significance, and strategies for gene therapy. With the evolving sophistication of diagnostic techniques, there is increased confidence almost daily about our abilities to put agents into the fetus. The debate now moves to when and whom to treat, and the best way to treat the fetus pharmacologically (ie, either indirectly through the mother and placenta, or now directly into the fetus). Gene therapy that requires direct entry into the fetus, embryo, or preembryo will be a major focus of research for the end of this millennium.

PHARMACOLOGIC MANAGEMENT OF METABOLIC DEFECTS

The potential effects of drugs or maternal metabolites on the fetus are well known. In many cases, as with known teratogens, the effects are adverse and may be in part genetically determined. Furthermore, some maternal metabolic diseases may have profound fetal effects, as is perhaps best demonstrated by the extensive fetal damage seen secondary to maternal phenylketonuria and resultant fetal hyperphenylalaninemia.

For decades drugs and other agents have been administered to pregnant women for treatment of fetal disorders not usually classified as metabolic in the hope of improving the capacity for postnatal adaptation. Well-known examples include exchange transfusions in Rh disease, the administration of corticosteroids for the prevention of respiratory distress syndrome in premature infants, and the administration of phenobarbital prior to birth in the hope of inducing liver enzymes for postnatal reduction of serum bilirubin concentration. However, there are only a very few examples of attempted prenatal treatment for genetically determined metabolic defects.

The Rh-isoimmunization model provides a successful illustration of medical intervention in the developing fetus. Until the introduction of RhoGAM in the early 1970s, thousands of infants died in utero or in the early neonatal period with acute hemolytic disease secondary to Rh-isoimmunization. Many of the surviving affected infants suffered from mental retardation, incapacitating neurologic disability, or deafness. The first prenatal transfusion was performed by Liley in the early 1960s and was complemented by the development of postnatal transfusions.[3] Finally, early complete prevention of hydrops by passive isoimmunization was made possible by RhoGAM. Unlike other surgical and medical fetal interventions that are still technically experimental, exchange transfusions have clearly moved into the realm of standard practice for Rh-isoimmunization.

CONGENITAL ADRENAL HYPERPLASIA

The fetal adrenal gland can be pharmacologically suppressed by maternal replacement doses of dexamethasone.[6] In congenital adrenal hyperplasia (CAH) caused by 21-hydroxylase deficiency, impaired metabolism of cholesterol to cortisol creates excess 17-OH progesterone, which becomes androstenedione and androgens. Consequently, genetic females are exposed to excess androgens and can be masculinized. The abnormal differentiation can vary from clitoral hypertrophy to complete formation of a phallus and apparent scrotum.

In an attempt to prevent this birth defect, Evans and colleagues administered dexamethasone, a fluorinated steroid, to an at-risk mother beginning in the 10th week of gestation.[6] Maternal estriol and cortisol values indicated rapid and sustained fetal and maternal adrenal gland suppression. This fetus ultimately turned out to be a carrier.

Following the initial observation of Evans and colleagues, Forrest and David used the same protocol of 0.25 mg of dexamethasone qid beginning at 9 weeks to treat several fetuses and demonstrated that fetuses known to be clinically affected with the severe form of 21-hydroxylase deficiency CAH were prevented from external congenital masculinization.[7,8] To date, several infants with classic CAH, who clearly would have been masculinized, have been born with normal genitalia. In a few cases some masculinization has still been observed following this regimen beginning at 9 weeks. Our current protocol, therefore, is to begin at 7 weeks, although there have been too few cases to assess this modification.[9,10] These events represent the first prevention of a birth defect and may serve as a model for other attempts at pharmacologic fetal therapy. One interesting element of the first case was the fact that therapy had to begin long before a diagnosis was possible. With the autosomal recessive genetics of CAH, only one of eight pregnancies would be expected to benefit (females with CAH). Now, with the availability of a probe for the gene,[11,12] a nearly definitive diagnosis would be possible by DNA analysis of chorionic villi in the first trimester but still after therapy has to be started. If the fetus is an affected female, therapy continues throughout gestation and is tapered slowly postpartum. If the fetus is male or unaffected, then therapy can be discontinued at the time of diagnosis.

The fundamental principles addressed in such attempted prevention of masculinization are logically extended to other medical fetal therapies. The concepts of a thorough informed consent procedure, thorough documentation of progress, and high-risk obstetric management have generally been followed by investigators in these fields.

METHYLMALONIC ACIDEMIA

Methylmalonic acidemia is related to a functional vitamin B_{12} deficiency. Coenzymatically active B_{12} is required for the conversion of methylmalonyl-coenzyme A to succinyl-coenzyme A. Several genetically determined etiologies for methylmalonic acidemia include defects in methylmalonyl-coenzyme A mutase or in the metabolism of vitamin B_{12} to the coenzymatically active form, adenosylcobalamin by the converting enzyme. Some patients may respond to administration of large doses of B_{12}, which can enhance the amount of active holoenzyme (mutase apoenzyme plus adenosylcobalamin).

Ampola and colleagues were the first to attempt prenatal diagnosis and treatment of a B_{12}-responsive variant of methylmalonic acidemia.[13] They followed the pregnancy of a patient who had previously suffered the loss of a child to severe acidosis and dehydration at the age of 3 months. The diagnosis of methylmalonic acidemia was only made posthumously by chemical analysis of blood and urine. In the pregnancy they followed, an amniocentesis was performed at 19 weeks gestation. An elevated methylmalonic acid content was documented in the cell-free amniotic fluid. Cultured amniotic fluid cells had defective propionate oxidation, undetectable levels of adenosylcobalamin, and normal succinate oxidation and methylmalonyl-coenzyme A mutase activity in the presence of added adenosylcobalamin. These studies established by approximately 23 weeks gestation that the fetus suffered from methylmalonic acidemia seemingly due to deficient synthesis of adenosylcobalamin.

It was already known that fetal methylmalonic acidemia is associated with increased methylmalonic acid excretion in maternal urine. Ampola and colleagues documented increased methylmalonic acidemia in a maternal urine sample first collected at 23 weeks gestation; the methylmalonic acid excretion per milligram of creatinine was approximately twice the upper normal limit and demonstrated a further rise by 25 weeks. Urinary methylmalonate excretion is not abnormal in heterozygous females carrying a normal fetus, as shown subsequently by these same investigators.

At 32 weeks gestation, cyanocobalamin (10 mg/day) was administered orally to the mother in divided doses. The treatment only marginally altered the maternal serum B_{12} level; however, there was a slight reduction of urinary methylmalonic acid excretion that remained severalfold above normal. At approximately 34 weeks gestation, 5 mg of cyanocobalamin per day intramuscularly was begun. The maternal serum B_{12} level then rose gradually to more than sixfold above normal and was accompanied by a progressive decrease in urinary methylmalonic acid excretion. Maternal urinary methylmalonate was only slightly above the normal range when delivery occurred at 41 menstrual weeks. Amniotic fluid methylmalonic acid concentrations were three times the normal mean at 19 menstrual weeks and four times the normal mean at term, despite prenatal treatment.

Postnatally, the diagnosis of methylmalonic acidemia was confirmed. The infant suffered no acute neonatal complications and had an extremely high serum B_{12} level. Long-term postnatal management involved protein restriction; however, no continuous B_{12} treatment was required.

In this instance prenatal treatment certainly improved the fetal and, secondarily, the maternal biochemistry. Whether there was any significant clinical benefit to the fetus by in utero treatment cannot be assessed adequately. It seems likely that reducing the fetal burden of methylmalonic acid should have some beneficial effect on fetal development and could reduce the risks in the neonatal period. However, this is only speculation.

Nyhan has suggested that an increased frequency of minor anomalies may be associated with untreated fetal methylmalonic acidemia.[14] Thus, very early or perhaps even prophylactic treatment with B_{12} prior to prenatal diagnosis in at-risk cases might be indicated for optimal therapy of B_{12}-responsive methylmalonic acidemia.

The report by Ampola and colleagues was the first example of treatment of a vitamin-responsive inborn error of metabolism in utero.[13] A subsequent report of prenatal treatment of methylmalonic acidemia revealed similar results, and other pregnancies have been monitored by the authors. However, a number of important questions raised by the study are still unresolved and may ultimately require many years to treat enough patients to establish the risk-to-benefit ratio of this approach.

MULTIPLE CARBOXYLASE DEFICIENCY

Biotin-responsive multiple carboxylase deficiency is an inborn error of metabolism in which the mitochondrial biotin-dependent enzymes, pyruvate carboxylase, propionyl-coenzyme A carboxylase, and β-methylcrotonyl-coenzyme A carboxylase have diminished activity. Affected patients present as newborns or in the early childhood period with dermatitis, severe metabolic acidosis, and a characteristic pattern of organic acid excretion. Metabolism in patients or in their cultured cells can be restored toward normal levels by biotin supplementation. There have been two reports of prenatal administration of biotin to fetuses affected with this disorder.

Roth and colleagues treated a fetus without the benefit of prenatal diagnosis in a case in which two siblings of the fetus had died of multiple carboxylase deficiency.[15] The first sibling had died within 3 days of birth, and in the second the diagnosis of biotin-responsive carboxylase deficiency was made posthumously.

The patient was first seen at 34 weeks gestation. Prenatal diagnosis was not attempted because of the late stage of pregnancy. The maternal urinary organic acid profile was normal throughout the final 4 weeks of pregnancy. Because of severe neonatal manifestations in the previous siblings and the probable harmlessness of biotin, oral administration of this compound to the mother was begun at a dose of 10 mg/day. There were no apparent untoward effects; maternal urinary biotin excretion increased by a factor of approximately 100 during biotin administration.

Nonidentical twins were subsequently delivered at term. Cord blood and urinary organic acid profiles were normal, and cord blood biotin concentrations were four to seven times greater than normal. The neonatal course for both twins was unremarkable. Subsequent study of the cultured fibroblasts of both twins compared under biotin-rich and biotin-depleted growth conditions indicated that in biotin-depleted medium, the cells of twin B (but not of twin A) had virtually complete deficiency of all three carboxylase activities. Genetic complementation studies confirmed that despite the normal clinical presentation during the newborn period, twin B was homozygous for the disease mutation.

Packman and colleagues have also reported prenatal diagnosis and treatment of biotin-responsive multiple carboxylase deficiency for a mother who had previously given birth to a male with the neonatal-onset form of this disease.[16] In the next pregnancy, maternal urine organic acid profiles were normal. The three carboxylase activities were assayed in cultured amniotic fluid cells obtained by amniocentesis at 17 menstrual weeks. In biotin-restricted medium, the amniotic cells demonstrated the characteristic severe reduction in carboxylase activities.

At 23.5 menstrual weeks, the mother started receiving 10 mg/day of oral biotin. After birth, the term female exhibited no clinical or gross chemical abnormalities. Postnatal biotin administration was begun postnatally on day 4. The diagnosis of multiple carboxylase deficiency was confirmed employing fibroblasts derived from the neonate. Postnatal development of the infant was normal.

The preceding two cases provide compelling evidence that biotin administration effectively prevents neonatal complications in certain patients with biotin-responsive multiple carboxylase deficiency. No toxicity from treatment was observed. At this time, it is not possible to assess definitively the relative advantages or disadvantages of prenatal treatment, although such therapy appears both effective and logical.

ABNORMALITIES OF MINERAL METABOLISM

Specific prenatal mineral supplementation has yet to be reported for prevention of human fetal disease. However, such additives have been used in animals with genetic deficiencies. Animal studies are of considerable interest and suggest the possibility of analogous human treatment.

Manganese

The effects of prenatal manganese supplementation on the prevention of otolith defects in mice affected with the pallid mutation have been investigated. Pallid mice have defective pigmentation, including an absence of pigment from the membranous labyrinth. This pigmentary characteristic is fully penetrant in the pallid homozygous recessive; whereas another manifestation, impaired otolith formation, is variably expressed. A significant correlation between litter size and the expression of the otolith abnormalities in the offspring have been known for decades; the otolith defect may be influenced by competition in utero for an unidentified substance.

Hurley and colleagues reported that development of the inner ear in normal rats and mice was affected by decreased manganese.[17] In mice, experimental manganese deprivation in utero induced a defect of the inner ear that was morphologically and behaviorally indistinguishable from pallid, although manganese deficiency did not mimic the effect of the mutant gene on pigmentation. Subsequently, these investigators observed that manganese supplementation of pallid mice throughout gestation with a diet containing from 45 to 2000 parts per million of manganese yielded a dose-dependent decrease in the percentage of abnormal otoliths.

These data have been extended to a genetic basis for susceptibility. In several studies on prenatal manganese restriction, the percentage of otolith abnormalities was influenced by the strain of mice studied. Thus, interactions of manganese intake and genetic predisposition influence otolith development in several strains. These observations suggest that at low or borderline levels of dietary intake of many nutrients, the genotype of the fetus can substantially alter fetal responses.

There are a number of genetic defects in animals with associated pigmentary and inner ear abnormalities. Some data suggest that manganese may play a role in modifying the expression of such defects. Hurley and colleagues have suggested that a sex-linked form of ocular albinism in humans, associated with labyrinthine dysfunction, may be analogous to some of these animal models. We are unaware of any studies of manganese metabolism in human ocular albinism, or of attempts to administer manganese prenatally in the hope of ameliorating expression of any associated labyrinthine defects.

Copper

Hurley and colleagues have investigated possible deleterious effects of prenatal copper administration on mice with the recessive mutant "crinkled" gene.[17] These investigators have suggested that the "crinkled" gene produces many phenotypic characteristics common to patients with Menkes' kinky-hair syndrome. Dietary supplementation of pregnant mice with copper sulfate partially ameliorated the effects of the crinkled gene in the offspring. Different prenatal copper regimens have resulted in varying degrees of success. Copper nitrilotracete appeared to be superior to copper sulfate in increasing postnatal survival and body copper content of the mutant offspring of heterozygous dams. Postnatal supplementation with copper did not increase survival of the mutants.

These studies may lead to insights relevant to prenatal treatment of Menkes' syndrome, a sex-linked disorder characterized by progressive degeneration of neurologic function in infants. Alterations suggestive of functional copper deficiency are present in affected infants. Fibroblasts from patients with Menkes' disease accumulate excess copper probably present in an abnormally bound form. Howell feels that Menkes' syndrome can be reliably diagnosed in utero by demonstrating abnormally increased copper uptake in Menkes cultured amniotic fluid cells incubated in a high-copper medium. Menkes' disease has been refractory to postnatal therapy with copper; and it is conceivable that by analogy to the crinkled mutation, prenatal treatment might be of benefit.[4]

Despite apparent responses to prenatal mineral administration of pallid and crinkled mutations, the relationships of these mutants, if any, to ocular albinism and Menkes' disease, respectively, remain speculative. Although animal studies have proved encouraging, they have not yet led to trials of prenatal mineral supplementation in genetically defective human beings.

Galactosemia

Galactosemia is an inborn error of metabolism caused by diminished activity of the enzyme galactose-1-phosphate uridyltransferase. It is inherited in an autosomal recessive manner and results in cataracts, growth deficiency, and ovarian failure. Galactosemia can be diagnosed prenatally by study of cultured amniocytes and chorionic villi. Clinical symptoms appear in the neonatal period and can be largely ameliorated by elimination of galactose from the diet. However, oocytes have already been damaged irreversibly long before birth. Cellular damage in galactosemia is thought to be mediated by accumulation of galactose-1-phosphate intracellularly and of galactitol in the lens.

There are suggestions that even the early postnatal treatment of galactosemic individuals with a low-galactose diet may not be sufficient to ensure normal development. Some have speculated that prenatal damage to galactosemic fetuses could contribute to subsequent abnormal neurologic development and to lens cataract formation. Furthermore, it has been recognized recently that female galactosemics, even when treated from birth with galactose deprivation, have a high frequency of primary or secondary amenorrhea because of ovarian failure. There also may be some subtle abnormalities of male gonadal function.

Exposure to a high-galactose diet has been considered to represent an animal model for human galactosemia. Chen and colleagues have observed a reduction in the oocyte content of rat ovaries after prenatal exposure to a 50% galactose diet.[18] No analogous alterations in the testes were observed in prenatally treated males. Experiments in rats suggest that toxicity to the female gonads from galactose or its metabolites is most obvious during the premeiotic stages of ovarian development.

These observations in animals and human beings have led to speculation that galactose restriction during pregnancy may be desirable if the fetus is affected with galactosemia. In the human female, ovarian meiosis begins at 12 and is complete by 28 menstrual weeks. Thus, ovarian damage, and perhaps neurologic or lens abnormalities, might occur prior to the usual time when prenatal diagnosis by amniocentesis can be accomplished. Thus, anticipatory treatment in pregnancies at risk for having a galactosemic fetus might best be initiated very early in gestation or even preconceptually.

Despite these experiments and speculations, we are

unaware of studies that adequately assess the impact of prenatal administration of a low-galactose diet to galactosemic infants. For obvious reasons such data, especially controlled, will be difficult to obtain. Nevertheless, prenatal galactose restriction is probably desirable in galactosemia and should be harmless. There is little reason to suppose that galactose restriction would have adverse consequences, since galactosemic and normal fetuses are both capable of some endogenous galactose synthesis.

FUTURE DEVELOPMENTS

Only the most preliminary steps have been taken toward the therapy of genetic metabolic disorders in the fetus. Certain categories of diseases may be particular candidates for future attempts at treatment, especially if some newer approaches are developed.

Vitamins

Prenatal therapy has been reported for two vitamin-responsive genetic errors of metabolism. A significant number of other vitamin-responsive defects are known and have responded to postnatal treatment. Antenatal treatment of some of these may be anticipated, especially for those with neonatal manifestations.

We also speculate that in addition to the usual vitamin-responsive errors, there may be genetic defects for which prenatal vitamin E administration may be justifiable. Postnatally, vitamin E administration prevents abnormalities of leukocyte function and improves the shortened red cell survival in glutathione synthetase deficiency. Because grossly lowered intracellular glutathione levels in this mutant state seem to predispose to oxidant-mediated cellular damage, it might be desirable to consider prenatal antioxidant therapy with vitamin E. Most patients with glutathione synthetase deficiency have neurologic impairment, which can be progressive. Functioning as an antioxidant, vitamin E might inhibit the development of neurologic abnormalities. Such speculations can only be confirmed or denied by future clinical studies.

In abetalipoproteinemia, which is associated with very low serum vitamin E levels, progressive and fatal neurologic impairment gradually develops. It is now known that high-dose vitamin E supplementation can retard or prevent neurologic damage. Although patients with abetalipoproteinemia, like glutathione synthase-deficient patients, appear not to manifest gross neurologic abnormalities at birth, prenatal damage could be occurring. Prenatal treatment with vitamin E might be justifiable on an experimental basis.

Pharmacologic and Nutritional Approaches

It might be appropriate to consider suppressing excessive cholesterol production prenatally in severe hypercholesterolemia if a safe and effective agent for accomplishing this were available (although there is no clear evidence for hypercholesterolemic prenatal damage).

If cysteamine or related agents were to prove an effective treatment for lethal variants of cystinosis, prenatal therapy might be considered, because excessive and possibly harmful cystine accumulation is evident in cystinotic fetuses. Cysteamine levels have been detected in chorionic villi, and significant elevations even at 10 weeks gestation have been hypothesized.

Inhibitors of gamma-glutamyl transpeptidase, if safe, would elevate intracellular glutathione levels and inhibit oxoproline production in glutathione synthase deficiency, thereby averting the characteristic neonatal acidosis.

In theory, it would be desirable to minimize copper accumulation in Wilson disease as early as possible. If and when reliable prenatal diagnosis of Wilson disease is possible, cautious administration of penicillamine prenatally might be considered. This would be a double-edged sword, however, as the teratogenic and lathyritic potential of penicillin would demand careful evaluation.

Batshaw and colleagues have treated certain urea cycle defects by administering arginine and benzoate. Since hyperammonemia in some of these entities develops very acutely after birth, it might be desirable to consider pretreating the fetus with these compounds just prior to or during labor to minimize postnatal hyperammonemia.[19]

Conversely, it may be desirable to consider drug avoidance as an approach to fetal treatment. For example, fetuses with glucose-6-phosphate dehydrogenase deficiency are sensitive to a variety of drugs that induce hemolysis. It would probably be appropriate to avoid administering such agents to women carrying or known to be at risk for carrying fetuses deficient in glucose-6-phosphate dehydrogenase.

Umbilical cord catheterization under ultrasound guidance may lead to the development of other types of fetal treatment.[20] Systems such as gene replacement are being developed for certain lysosomal storage disorders. Progress is being made in postnatal experimental models on administration of thymic cells for certain immune deficiency states, bone marrow transplantation for a variety of genetic disorders, and gene transfer. The development of better and earlier techniques for prenatal treatment will be complex, especially with regard to gene transfer; but progress will be made, and access to the fetal vasculature may be required for these methods to have a chance for success.

Bone marrow transplantation or thymic cell infusion is actually only a specialized example of organ transplantation. In the future, fetal organ transplantation may become possible and may open many prospects for surgical treatment of certain biochemical genetic disorders.

One can also speculate about the therapeutic possibilities involving compounds administered directly into the amniotic fluid or into the fetal intestinal tract. It might be possible, for example, to administer thyroid hormone in this fashion or to prevent meconium ileus in cystic fibrosis by instilling not yet determined enzymes into the fetal intestinal tract.

MULTIFACTORIAL DISORDERS

CARDIAC FETAL THERAPY

Although great strides have been made in the diagnosis of fetal cardiac anatomical and functional abnormalities, in utero cardiac therapy currently is limited to the treatment of significant arrhythmias. In the future, treatment of some congenital anomalies, particularly valvular anomalies, may be attempted prenatally. Treatment of fetal arrhythmias is discussed in Chapter 52.

NEURAL TUBE DEFECTS

Animal studies suggest that neural tube defects (NTDs) can arise from a variety of vitamin or mineral deficiencies. There are historical data in humans suggesting increased NTD frequencies in subjects with poor dietary histories or with intestinal bypasses. Biochemical evidence of suboptimal nutrition is present in some women bearing infants with NTDs. The studies of Smithells and colleagues and Milunsky suggested that vitamin supplementation—and perhaps folate alone—can reduce the frequency of NTD recurrence in families with one or more prior affected children.[21,22] Pooled data from investigations in different centers using Smithell's mixture of vitamins and minerals show that NTD recurrence in offspring of women treated with vitamin supplements was about 0.7% but was about 4.6% in women who did not receive supplements. These data suggest a beneficial effect. In other studies with folate treatment alone, no effect has been seen.[22] If studies are considered together, a reasonable case can be made that folate supplementation is of value in preventing recurrent NTDs. However, there are conflicting data concerning a possible decrease in the pregnancy risk of occurrence of NTDs by folate supplementation.[23–27]

GENE THERAPY

Advances in molecular genetics and recombinant DNA technology in the past decade have been dramatic and have led to the development of sensitive diagnostic techniques for a continuously increasing number of single-gene disorders. Cutting DNA with restriction endonucleases and analysis of restriction fragment length polymorphisms (RFLP), sequence-specific DNA isolation techniques, and cloning of single-stranded DNA have allowed the formation of highly specific gene probes. These have increased not only the accuracy of diagnosis of abnormal conditions, but also our basic understanding of normal gene function and regulation, with specific emphasis on the understanding of the development of mechanisms of cancer and its treatment.[28,29] The next natural step in this evolving technology was the development of techniques to introduce purified or cloned gene sequences into cultured cells and living animals to correct single-gene defects. Once established, attention could then be directed to their application to treatment and care of single-gene disorders in the human.

Gene therapy has attracted the attention of the medical community and the lay media. The possibility of treating severe disorders that are not amenable to any other mode of treatment is obviously appealing to the medical community, especially when these disorders affect children. However, public acceptance is limited by valid concerns about ethical issues surrounding still undeveloped methods and endangered by pseudoscientific publications on the potential to change traits, appearance, behavior, and other "Frankensteinian" connotations. As a result, controversy persists over the advantages and dangers of gene therapy. However, gene therapy is not one uniform issue, and different levels of gene therapy will have definite and different potential advantages and dangers.

Approaches to gene therapy can be divided initially into three concepts: modification of existing material, removal of material, and addition of material.

Modification has been used with initial success in hemoglobinopathies. Ley and colleagues have demonstrated that 5-azacytidine and other demethylating agents can induce the expression of fetal hemoglobin in baboons and humans with beta-thalassemia and sickle cell anemia.[30] The genes for hemoglobin F and A are adjacent on chromosome 11. 5-Azacytidine removes the methyl group attached to cytosine (C) in some CG sequences that acts normally as an inhibitor of transcription. Demethylation results in increased production of hemoglobin F, and some clinical improvement has been documented. Unfortunately, the effects have been short-lived and currently available drugs are otherwise quite toxic.

Recently, a technique known as "site-directed homologous recombination" has been used to modify the expression of a specific gene in a mouse model.[31] The process involves construction of a "targeting gene" that carries homologous sequences at each of its ends with an intervening nonfunctional or marker gene region to assess integration into the host genome. Once introduced into the target nucleus, this gene aligns itself to the homologous regions of the target gene. When somatic recombination, which is analogous to meiotic crossing over, occurs, insertion into or replacement of the target gene by the incoming DNA segment results. This technique can be used to disrupt a normal gene or to replace it by a mutant copy. Alternatively, it can be used to replace a mutant gene by a normal copy (ie, gene therapy). Subsequent assay of successful integration can be easily accomplished by RFLP or polymerase chain reaction (PCR) probing for the original gene or an inserted segment. In gene therapy applications, the return of a function absent before therapy would be a sign of successful integration. This approach may someday prove useful for the specific modification of specific genetic disorders, and again could in principle be done not only in somatic cells (eg, erythroid, lymphoid, or liver) but even at a preimplantation embryonic level.

Removal of genetic material is theoretically possible in conjunction with in vitro fertilization. Multiple phenotypic abnormalities, such as those seen with Down syndrome, are caused by the extra copy of chromosome 21. If it were possible to remove or destroy the expression of the extra material, development should occur normally. By birth, the baby will have only 5% of adult body weight but 90% of total cell number, and the additional chromosome will appear in all of them. Attempt at any removal would have to be applied extremely early in pregnancy—probably at the single-cell stage. Although irrelevant for most couples, for those at extremely high risk (eg, balanced translocation carriers), fertilization by IVF with immediate karyotype analysis and potential ablation or removal of extra material may someday be feasible, although it is far beyond existing technology.

Addition of material is the most promising approach for stable correction of defects. Anderson defines three potential levels of genetic engineering and therapy[32,33]:

1. Somatic cell gene therapy: when a gene is inserted into body cells of an affected individual to correct a genetic disorder in this individual only
2. Germ line gene therapy: insertion of a gene into the germ cells of an affected individual to correct a disorder in the patient and his or her future offspring
3. Enhancement genetic engineering: insertion of a gene into a normal individual, intended to enhance a desirable known characteristic.

Active workers in the field now agree that human gene therapy will be feasible and should be applied to at least some serious genetic disorders.[34] It is also generally held that human gene therapy should not be applied at this time to germ cells but only to somatic cells that cannot transmit the altered genetic material to subsequent generations.[35] The first target to human gene therapy would, therefore, be the somatic cell.

SOMATIC CELL GENE THERAPY

Gene products are required for normal growth and development, homeostasis and metabolism, complex organ function, immunity, and reproduction. Abnormal gene function causes diseases such as the hemoglobinopathies, inborn errors of metabolism, coagulopathies, or endocrine disorders. Somatic gene therapy for such diseases would involve the introduction of a normal recombinant gene into the body cells of an individual to reconstitute specific gene products and their functions.[36] From this definition evolve a few requirements about those disorders likely to be attempted for somatic cell gene therapy:

1. The disorder should be severe and crippling enough to justify offering experimental treatment.
2. The symptoms of the disorder should be reversible with treatment.
3. The disease should be correctable by gene insertion into bone marrow cells, which is the only tissue that can be extracted, treated in vitro, and successfully returned at this time.
4. The defect should be a single-gene alteration with simple regulation, most probably an enzymatic defect that can be corrected by relatively low expression of the inserted gene.
5. The deficiency must be known to be caused by a known, identified, and cloned gene.
6. A safe and effective method of introducing the cloned gene into the treated cells must be available.

Three diseases are among the most likely to be first treated by gene therapy (Table 53-1): Lesch-Nyhan syndrome, an X-linked disorder caused by hypoxanthine-guanine phosphoribosyltransferase (HGPRT) deficiency; severe combined immunodeficiency syndrome (SCID), caused by adenosine deaminase (ADA) deficiency; and immunodeficiency resulting from purine nucleoside phosphorylase (PNP) abnormalities.[37] These conditions meet most of the criteria. Moreover, heterologous bone marrow transplantation has been found to be beneficial for some of these patients.[38] Diseases correctable by bone marrow transplantation[39] are the natural candidates for human somatic cell gene therapy. The problems associated with allogenic bone marrow transplantation (availability of histocompatible bone marrow donors, graft versus host disease, and the need for complete lymphoid and hematopoietic ablation in the recipient before transplant) would be avoided by use of autologous bone marrow treated by gene insertion.

Techniques for Gene Insertion

The several techniques of gene insertion into mammalian cells have been summarized recently (Table 53-2).[35-37,40] The most common method, transfection, uses calcium-phosphate precipitation to facilitate the uptake

TABLE 53–1. DISEASES POTENTIALLY TREATABLE BY HUMAN GENE THERAPY

DISORDER	INHERITANCE
Lesch-Nyhan syndrome	X-linked
Severe combined immune deficiency (SCID)	Autosomal recessive
Isolated T-cell deficiency	Autosomal recessive
Hemoglobinopathies	
Thalassemia	Autosomal recessive
Sickle cell anemia	Autosomal recessive
Agammaglobulinemia	X-linked
Wiskott-Aldrich syndrome	X-linked

TABLE 53–2. METHODS OF GENE TRANSFER INTO CELLS

PHYSICAL	BIOLOGICAL
Transfection	DNA viruses
Cell fusion	RNA viruses
Electroporation	Stem cell transplants
Microinjection	

and stable integration of microprecipitates of exogenous DNA. The advantages of this procedure include technical simplicity and the ability to manipulate highly purified gene sequences.[35] It is, however, relatively inefficient and unstable, and even in the best recipient cell lines, overall efficiency is minimal.[37] Other physical methods of gene insertion include cell fusion, electroporation, and microinjection. This last method seems to be ideal in terms of efficiency, but only a few cells may be injected with soluble DNA at a time and many of these subsequently die. Consequently, microinjection has limited value in somatic cell gene therapy but is the ideal method of treatment for germ cell therapy—injecting the purified DNA in solution into the pronucleated embryo. The incorporated genetic material would subsequently appear in all cells derived from multiplication of the injected one-cell embryo, including the germ cells.

A still more efficient way of inserting exogenous DNA into cells is the use of biological vectors—DNA and RNA viruses. Several DNA viruses have been used, such as the simian virus 40 (SV40), bovine papilloma virus, and adenovirus.[37] Experiments with SV40 were limited by the amount of foreign DNA the virus can carry, and the bovine papilloma virus was not successful in integrating the DNA into chromosomes of replicating cells. Adenoviruses may be of the greatest use, as they infect a wide range of host cells; however, the systems for their use are still poorly defined and the potential risk of neoplastic transformation of the infected cells exists.[35,41]

RNA viruses of the retrovirus type are currently the center of most interest as biological vectors for gene insertion in animal models. These are simple viruses with small and well-defined viral genomes. For purposes of expression and replication, they insert a reverse transcript of their viral RNA into host DNA that is integrated as a single copy at a single site. If portions of the viral genome are replaced by exogenous sequences, the virus will often lose its ability to replicate. However, if the recombinant retroviral genome containing the gene of interest is transfected into cells previously infected with a wild virus, complementation of functions can occur, giving rise to new retroviral particles containing the defective recombinant genome, and being infectious to suitable target cells.[37] Using this method, a large number of proliferating cells can be effectively infected and the recombinant DNA introduced into their genome. As long as target cells are proliferating, retroviruses demonstrate little tissue specificity and only minimal species specificity.[36]

Several problems and potential dangers are associated with the use of retroviral delivery systems (Table 53-3). The site of integration of the retrovirus is random, leading to potential problems of stability and expression of the inserted gene. It may occasionally integrate into the middle of an otherwise normal gene, creating new mutations by insertional mutagenesis.[42] The strong promoter usually encoded in the viral long terminal repeat (LTR) could accidentally activate protooncogenes adjacent to the insertion site, thus leading to damage of the cell (and the organism).[43] Excision and mobilization to a new location in the genome may further increase the risk for loss of function and for mutagenesis.[37]

Retroviruses have been used in animal studies to introduce human intact genes that were subsequently expressed in vitro by the cultured cells. Mouse primary hepatocytes, NIH 3T3, and hepatoma cells were infected successfully using human phenylalanine hydroxylase (PAH) genes.[44,45] Human betaglobin genes have been introduced into mouse erythroleukemia cells.[46] Although they were inserted in foreign positions, the gene maintained normal regulation. Expression was roughly comparable to that of endogenous mouse betaglobin genes. Canine hematopoietic progenitor cells in culture were infected using retrovirus packaging cell lines, and the genes inserted conferred resistance to antibiotics and methotrexate.[47]

In human cells cultured in vitro, the retrovirus delivery system has been used for infection and integration of glucocerebrosidase into type 2 Gaucher fibroblasts.[48] Secretion of fully active factor IX has also been demonstrated in human skin fibroblasts.[49] The introduction of the adenosine deaminase (ADA) gene into ADA-deficient skin fibroblasts[50] and correction of ADA-deficiency have been achieved in cultured human T and B cells by retrovirus insertion of the ADA gene.[51] Retrovirus-mediated transfer and expression of drug-resistant genes were achieved in human hematopoietic progenitor cells,[52] and thioguanine-resistant human leukemia cells were sensitized by retroviral insertion of the human HGPRT gene.[53] Efficient introduction of plasmid DNA into human hematopoietic cells has also been demonstrated for DNA viruses.[54]

Another important principle for gene transfer is selectivity. To increase the number of cells taking up and expressing the gene, that gene must convey some advantage during cell proliferation. Cellular transformation by drug-resistant genes and cell growth in media containing the antiproliferative drug will favor the proliferation of genetically transformed cells. The combina-

TABLE 53–3. PROBLEMS AND POTENTIAL DANGERS ASSOCIATED WITH GENE INSERTION USING RETROVIRUSES

Random integration
Insertional mutagenesis
Activation of oncogenes adjacent to insertion site
Recombination of viral genome to form replicating infectious particles

tion of methotrexate and methotrexate-resistant genes was the first such selective system used in gene transfer in vivo and is still the most practical for clinical use.[35,55] Other systems include selection by resistance to antibiotics (aminoglycoside G-418) and 6-thioguanine.[56] One must choose a selection system carefully, as conferred resistance to some drugs will eliminate the potential therapeutic use of that agent to treat disease in that organism.

Current Status

Although much progress has been made in gene transfer into cultured cells, studies extending this technology into live animals are still in preliminary stages. It is possible to infect the whole animal with viral vectors leading to transformation of cells with the recombinant gene product in vivo, although the loss of target specificity may entail greater risks.[36] A safer approach would involve the introduction of the recombinant gene in vitro and then transplanting the transformed cells into live animals. This method is applicable only to tissues that are able to proliferate in vitro, such as bone marrow, skin fibroblasts, or liver cells. Bone marrow infected with recombinant retroviruses containing the bacterial neomycin resistance gene and transplanted into live mice will express the product of the recombinant gene in vivo.[36,57] Recombinant mouse fibroblast clones transplanted into the peritoneal cavity of nude mice express human alpha$_1$-antitrypsin gene in vivo, with enzymatic activity in both sera and epithelial surface of the lungs.[58] An advantage in proliferation of the recombinant bone marrow cells is conveyed by total body irradiation with ablation of endogenous bone marrow cells. However, more limited skeletal irradiation (300 rad to the femur) appears to allow engraftment.[59]

Hematopoietic stem cell (HS-cell) transplantation offers another approach. Fetal derived early hematopoietic stem cells can be isolated from fetal liver preparations. These stem cells would possess the potential to differentiate into any of the hematologic cell lines and as such could carry their genetic information for gene product synthesis with them. The impact of this in such disorders as beta-thalassemia, ADA, or SCID is obvious. Being of fetal origin, HS-cells would also be devoid of antigenic cell surface markers and could be transplanted early into fetuses by intra-abdominal or umbilical artery injection, where they would colonize the fetal marrow, producing a chimera. If transplanted early, tolerance may occur to any cell-specific surface antigenic markers that might develop on these cells later in the fetus or neonate and thereby circumvent the problems of graft rejection or graft-versus-host disease.

A recently developed technique for creating transgenic animals uses embryonic stem cells (ES-cells) as carriers of genetic information. ES-cells are derived from the inner cell mass component of the early blastocyst. These cells are pluripotential and give rise to the endodermal, ectodermal, and mesodermal compartments.[60] This stage of development is therefore the ideal time for introduction of genetically manipulated material.

ES-cells have been shown to remain in undifferentiated form in vitro if maintained on embryonic fibroblast feeder-cell layers. If placed into cell suspension culture they will begin differentiation and eventually form embryoid bodies with elements of glandular, heart and skeletal smooth muscle, nerve cells, keratin-producing cells, and even melanocytes.[61]

ES-cells "in vitro" can be modified by any of the aforementioned techniques and then microinjected back into the blastocyst cavity of a developing embryo, where they integrate into the inner cell mass to form a chimera. The earlier in development this procedure is done, the higher the percentage of chimera cells and the greater the chance of incorporation into germ cell lines and subsequent transmission to future generations of offspring.

Gossler and colleagues used the transfection technique to introduce a circular plasmid containing neomycin resistance gene into mouse ES-cells.[62] The successfully transfected cells were injected back into mouse blastocysts, where they incorporated into the developing inner cell mass, resulting in chimeric animals.

Other approaches to gene introduction have included injection of retroviruses carrying a specific gene sequence into ES-cell nuclei or into preimplantation embryos, with nonspecific genome integration of these genes.[63] Culturing ES-cells on embryonic fibroblast feeder layers that have been transfected with retrovirus carrying an inserted gene sequence has resulted in successful transfection and incorporation of that sequence into these cells. The nonspecific integration into the host genome, the inability to select or screen before implantation, and the additional possibility of insertional mutagenesis are the major drawbacks of these methods.

Embryonic stem cell transplants offer a unique system in which to introduce modified genetic information into early pluripotential embryonic cells with successful integration and expression of this information in the resulting chimeric animal. Very early transplants carry the possibility of integration of this new material into germ cell lines and transmission onto subsequent generations. This system further allows the selection and screening of pretransplanted cells to ensure the appropriate gene number and orientation prior to introduction back into the embryo. We have recently attempted stem cell transplantation for β thalassemia diagnosed by chorionic villus sampling in the first trimester. Unfortunately the fetus miscarried before information about engraftment could be obtained.

GERM LINE GENE THERAPY

Insertion of genetic material can be accomplished via micromanipulation of a pronucleus in the single-cell embryo. The resultant incorporated material would be duplicated in every cell of the organism, including germ cells for future generations. Two methods—microinjection of purified DNA into one of the two pronuclei,[64,65] and nuclear transplantation[66]—have proved successful in animal studies, producing transgenic mice, rabbits, sheep, and pigs. Following appropriate gene insertion into the pronucleus, murine hereditary dwarfism[67] and thalassemic mice[68] have been cured. The HGPRT gene has been introduced in mouse embryos and expressed in the central nervous system of such transgenic mice.[69] Since the possibility of diagnosing HGPRT deficiency in the preimplantation mouse embryo has been reported recently,[70] a putative scenario can be developed on this model. Women at risk for having children with Lesch-Nyhan syndrome would be referred to a center for in vitro fertilization and preimplantation diagnosis. Maternal eggs would be obtained after adequate hormonal stimulation and fertilized in vitro. Male and female embryos would be differentiated by means of a Y-DNA probe. Female embryos would be returned to the uterus by the usual methods of embryo transfer either in the treatment cycle or in a natural cycle after cryopreservation. In male fetuses HGPRT-deficiency tests would be employed. In those found to be deficient, HGPRT gene microinjection could be used, and gene expression assessed in culture as an index of the success of treatment. About one in five cells could be expected to be permanently transfected by microinjection.[33] Embryos for whom treatment was successful could then be cryopreserved and transferred in a later cycle.

The arguments in favor of germ line gene therapy include efficiency and expression of the gene in all organs, including some that are not accessible to somatic cell gene therapy (ie, the brain). Disadvantages of the germ line modality are the yet undefined risks of embryonic and fetal death, tumors and malformation that may occur, the absence of control over the site of insertion of the injected DNA in the recipient genome (with implications in terms of tissue specificity and expression of the inserted gene and insertional mutagenesis), and the current high failure rate of the procedure. The available data suggest that 10% to 20% of transgenic mice may carry recessive mutations of essential genes.[71] In animal studies involving microinjection of an immunoglobulin gene into mouse eggs, only 64% of the injected eggs were considered to be healthy enough to be transferred to surrogate mothers. Only 3.7% proceeded to live birth, and only 2% carried the injected gene. In a cumulative study from in vitro fertilization centers in the United States, a 12.6% clinically confirmed pregnancy rate (per egg retrieval) was reported, about half of them resulting in live births.[72] Based on current data and the potential problems, the arguments for germ line therapy are not as compelling as those for somatic cell experiments, and therefore, clinical trials need to await further basic advancement. Accumulation of data and experience from basic biological research and animal studies may render human germ line therapy feasible in the future.

ENHANCEMENT GENETIC ENGINEERING

Genetic engineering (for eugenics) is considerably different from the previously discussed approaches. Here the attempt is not to try to correct a genetic abnormality but to insert additional genetic material into the normal individual in order to change or enhance a specific characteristic, such as linear growth.

The body exists in a very complex and delicate homeostasis, on the cellular as well as the whole organism level. The intricate pathways of interaction are as yet only poorly defined. Insertion of additional genetic information can alter this delicate balance, with consequences that cannot be appreciated at our present state of knowledge. These consequences are probably justifiable if a normal gene is inserted to replace a faulty one. As emphasized by Anderson, we know too little about the human body to attempt inserting a gene designed for "improvement" in the normal individual.

Fletcher underlined a moral distinction between the use of human gene therapy in cases where it may relieve severe morbidity or mortality and in cases where the intent is to alter characteristics that have nothing to do with disease.[73] In the first situation, accepting some risks, even if poorly defined, is in the best interest of the affected individual. In the latter cases the benefit obtained may be very slight, if any, and the potential wrong done to the individual may be severe. It should also be remembered that although the technical possibility exists today to insert a gene into a cell population, we do not have methods yet to extract or inactivate a specific gene once it is inserted. Therefore, a gene, once inserted, even if it is later found to be harmful, will continue to act until the death of the cell, or the individual.

The principles of justice are also violated by applying gene therapy to normal individuals. When resources are scarce and precious, they should be used to alleviate suffering and early death and not to promote special interests of normal persons. Moreover, enhancement genetic experiments would probably be more susceptible to the control of interested societies and governments.[73]

Changes of traits like appearance, intelligence, and character are not possible in the foreseeable future. These traits are influenced by interactions between numerous genes, in pathways not presently clear. Environmental factors also influence these traits. In time, however, the genes and their interactions may be discovered and the technical availability of enhancement genetic engineering may become a reality. The scientific community and the public should cooperate in evaluating the medical, ethical, and philosophical aspects of this issue. Such debate and resolution should be done well before such procedures are technically possible.

Ethical Issues

From animal studies we have learned that most problems associated with somatic cell gene therapy (definition of target disorders, mode of delivery for the gene, expression, and safety) can be overcome and that human somatic gene therapy is at our doorstep. As with every experimental procedure, before transferring it from the laboratory to clinical treatment in humans, the ethical implications should be considered. One of the main questions involves "risk assessment"[74]: morbidity and mortality rates associated with the disease, existing therapy and its effectiveness, and the possibility of therapy to stop or reverse clinical deterioration. The safety of the protocol for gene insertion and the effectiveness of gene expression in the treated cells should be judged on the basis of well-controlled animal studies, including fairness in patient selection and informed consent—as with other "first of their kind" experiments, such as artificial organ and xenograft transplantations.[75] Questions of privacy and confidentiality may also arise in this matter.

The Working Group on Human Gene Therapy, an interdisciplinary subgroup of the NIH Recombinant DNA Advisory Committee, has published a guiding document representing a framework to review in each specific case the most important areas of concern affected by human gene therapy.[76] The major areas discussed in this document were:

1. Objectives and rationale of proposed research
2. Research design, anticipated risks, and benefits
3. Selection of patients
4. Informed consent
5. Privacy and confidentiality.

In addition to the professional review suggested by these guidelines, a special public review mechanism has been established to evaluate proposals to perform gene therapy in humans. In early experiments, however, the information given to the patients and family for informed consent or for review would be based only on animal studies. Therefore, long-term consequences and results, as well as safety levels, can only be speculative.

SUMMARY

Genetic therapy has the potential to offer a cure to individuals affected by serious disorders that are the cause of severe disability and early death. Somatic cell gene therapy is technically possible and ethically permissible; human treatment in these aspects is ready to be applied. The first attempts to treat adenosine deaminase deficiency have been made in children at the National Institutes of Health. Problems of control of insertion site and regulation of gene expression in specific tissues still need to be solved when specific genes are being transplanted. Hematologic stem cell and embryonic stem cell transplant therapy are technically possible and in use with animal models, and first attempts in humans are occurring. Isolation and propagation of cell lines for human transplantation are problems presently being addressed. Long-term immunologic consequences of stem cell transplants remain the major concern. Germ line gene therapy is technically possible, but the high loss rate of the procedure and the possibility of inducing malformation and tumors in the offspring cause this procedure to be unacceptable at this time. Once these technical problems are solved, this procedure will be potentially applicable. Enhancement genetic engineering may in the future be technically possible, but it remains ethically unacceptable, because the consequences of inserting additional genetic material into the normal genetically balanced individual may be severe and the scientific basis for such engineering does not at present exist.

REFERENCES

1. Harrison MR, Longaker MT, Adzick NS, Goldberg JD, Rosen MA, Filly FA, et al. Repair of diaphragmatic hernia in utero. N Engl J Med 1990;322:1582.
2. Evans MI, Drugan A, Manning FA, Harrison MR. Fetal surgery in the 1990's. Am J Dis Child 1989;143(12):1431.
3. Liley AW. Intrauterine transfusion of foetus in haemolytic disease. Br Med J 1963;2:1107.
4. Evans MI, Pinsky WW, Johnson MP, Schulman JD. Medical fetal therapy. In: Evans MI, ed. Reproductive risks and prenatal diagnosis. Norwalk, CT: Appleton & Lange, 1992:236.
5. Anderson WF. Gene therapy. In: Evans MI, Fletcher JC, Dixler AO, Schulman JC, eds. Fetal diagnosis and therapy: science, ethics, and the law. Philadelphia: JB Lippincott, 1989:421.
6. Evans MI, Chrousos GP, Mann DL, Larsen JW Jr, Green I, McCluskey J, et al. Pharmacologic suppression of the fetal adrenal gland in utero: attempted prevention of abnormal external genital masculinization in suspected congenital adrenal hyperplasia. JAMA 1985;253:1015.
7. Forrest M, David M. Prenatal treatment of congenital adrenal hyperplasia due to 21 hydroxylase deficiency. 7th International Congress of Endocrinology, Abstract y11, Quebec, Canada, 1984.
8. David M, Forest MG. Prenatal treatment of congenital adrenal hyperplasia resulting from 21-hydroxylase deficiency. J Pediatr 1984;105(5):799.
9. Shulman DI, Mueller OT, Gallardo LA, Stiff D, Ostrer H. Treatment of congenital adrenal hyperplasia in utero. Pediatr Res 1989;25(4):2.
10. Pang S, Pollack MS, Marshall RN, Immken L. Prenatal treatment of congenital adrenal hyperplasia due to 21-hydroxylase deficiency. N Engl J Med 1990;22(2):111.
11. Phillips JA III, Burr IM, Orlando P, et al. DNA analysis of human steroid 21-hydroxylase genes on congenital hyperplasia. Am J Hum Genet 1985;37:A171.
12. White PC, Grossberger D, Onufer BJ, Chaplin DD, New MI, Dupont B, Strominger JL. Two genes encoding steroid 21-hydroxylase are located near the genes encoding the fourth component of complement in man. Proc Natl Acad Sci USA 1985;82:1089.
13. Ampola MG, Mahoney MJ, Nakamura E, et al. Prenatal therapy of a patient with vitamin B responsive methylmalonic acidemia. N Engl J Med 1975;293:313.
14. Nyhan WL. Prenatal treatment of methylmalonic aciduria. N Engl J Med 1975;293:353.
15. Roth KS, Yang W, Allen L, et al. Prenatal administration of biotin: biotin responsive multiple carboxylase deficiency. Pediatr Res 1982;16:126.
16. Packman S, Cowan MJ, Golbus MS, et al. Prenatal treatment of biotin responsive multiple carboxylase deficiency. Lancet 1982;1:1435.
17. Hurley LS, Bell LT. Genetic influence on response to dietary manganese deficiency in mice. J Nutr 1974;104:133.
18. Chen YT, Mattison DR, Feigenbaum L, et al. Reduction in oocyte number following prenatal exposure to a high galactose diet. Science 1981;314:1145.
19. Batshaw M, Brusilow S, Waber L, et al. Treatment of inborn

errors of urea synthesis: activation of alternative pathways of waste nitrogen synthesis and excretion. J Engl J Med 1982;306:1387.
20. Nicolaides KH, Thorpe-Beeston JG, Noble P. Cordocentesis. In: Eden RD, Boehm FH, eds. Assessment and care of the fetus: physiological, clinical and medicolegal principles, Norwalk, CT: Appleton & Lange, 1990:291.
21. Smithells RW, Nevin NC, Seller MJ, Sheppard S, Harris R, Read AP, et al. Further experience of vitamin supplementation for prevention of neural tube defect recurrences. Lancet 1983;1:1027.
22. Milunsky A. The prenatal diagnosis of neural tube and other congenital defects. In: Milunsky A, ed. Genetic disorders and the fetus: diagnosis, prevention and treatment. New York: Plenum Press, 1986:453.
23. Younis JS, Granat M. Insufficient transplacental digoxin transfer in severe hydrops fetalis. Am J Obstet Gynecol 1987;157:1268.
24. Mills JL, Rhoads GG, Simpson JL, Cunningham GC, Conley MR, Lassman MR, et al. The absence of a relation between the periconceptional use of vitamins and neural-tube defects. N Engl J Med 1989;321:430.
25. Mulinare J, Cordero JF, Erickson JD, Berry RJ. Periconceptional use of multivitamins and the occurrence of neural tube defects. JAMA 1988;260:3141.
26. Milunsky A, Jick H, Jick SS, Bruell CL, MacLaughlin DS, Rothman KJ, Willett W. Multivitamin/folic acid supplementation in early pregnancy reduces the prevalence of neural tube defects. JAMA 1989;262:2847.
27. Schulman JD. Treatment of the embryo and the fetus in the first trimester: current status and future prospects. Am J Med Genet 1990;35:197.
28. Miller WL.Recombinant DNA and the pediatrician. J Pediatr 1981;99:1.
29. Antonarakis SE, Phillips JA, Kazazian HH. Genetic disease: diagnosis by restriction endonuclease analysis. J Pediatr 1982; 100:845.
30. Ley TJ, DeSimone J, Anagnou NP, et al. 5-Azacytidine selectively increases gamma-globin synthesis in a patient with beta-thalassemia. N Engl J Med 1982;307:1469.
31. Doetschman T, Maeda N, Smithies O. Targeted mutation of the Hprt gene in mouse embryonic stem cells. Proc Natl Acad Sci USA 1988;85:8583.
32. Anderson WF. Human gene therapy—scientific and ethical considerations. J Med Philos 1985;10:275.
33. Anderson WF. Prospects for human gene therapy in the born and unborn patient. Clin Obstet Gynecol 1986;29(3):586.
34. Human Genetic Engineering, Hearings Before the Subcommittee on Investigations and Oversight of the Committee on Science and Technology (US House of Representatives 97th Congress No 170) Washington, DC: US Government Printing Office, 1983.
35. Cline MJ. Gene therapy: current status. Am J Med 1987;83:291.
36. Ledley FD. Somatic gene therapy for human disease: background and prospects. J Pediatr 1987;110(1):1.
37. Shapiro LJ, Comings DE, Jones OW, et al. New frontiers in genetic medicine. Ann Int Med 1986;104:527.
38. Markert ML, Hershfield MS, Schiff RI, et al. Adenosine deaminase and purine nucleoside phosphorylase deficiencies: evaluation of therapeutic intervention in eight patients. J Clin Immunol 1987;7(5):389.
39. Milewski EA. Discussions on human gene therapy. Recomb DNA Tech Bulletin 1986;9:88.
40. Griffin JA. Recombinant DNA—Potential for gene therapy. Am J Med Sci 1985;289(3):98.
41. Lacey M, Alpert S, Hanahan D. Bovine papillomavirus genome elicits skin tumours in transgenic mice. Nature 1986;322:609.
42. Ling W, Patel MD, Lobel LI, et al. Insertion mutagenesis of embryonal carcinoma cells by retroviruses. Science 1985;228:554.
43. Hayward WS, Neel BG, Astrin SM. Activation of a cellular oncogene by promoter insertion in ALV induced lymphoid leukosis. Nature 1981;290:475.
44. Ledley FD, Grenett HE, McGinnis Shelnott M, et al. Retroviral mediated gene transfer of human phenylalanine hydroxylase into NIH 3T3 and hepatoma cells. Proc Natl Acad Sci USA 1986;83:409.
45. Ledley FD, Darlington GJ, Hahn T, et al. Retroviral gene transfer into primary hepatocytes: implications for genetic therapy of liver-specific functions. Proc Natl Acad Sci USA 1987;84:5335.
46. Rund D, Dobkin C, Bank A. Regulated expression of amplified B globin genes. Blood 1987;70(3):733.
47. Kwok WW, Schuening F, Stead RB, et al. Retroviral transfer of genes into canine hemopoietic progenitor cells in culture: a model for human gene therapy. Proc Natl Acad Sci USA 1986;83:4552.
48. Choudary PV, Tsuji S, Martin BM, et al. The molecular biology of Gaucher disease and the potential for gene therapy. Cold Spring Harbor Symposia on Quantitative Biology 1986;51:1047.
49. Anson DS, Hock RA, Austen D. Towards gene therapy for hemophilia B. Mol Biol Med 1987;4:11.
50. Palmer TD, Hock RA, Osborne WRA, et al. Efficient retrovirus mediated transfer and expression of a human adenosine deaminase gene in diploid skin fibroblasts from an adenosine deaminase deficient human. Proc Natl Acad Sci USA 1987;84:1055.
51. Kantoff PW, Kohn DB, Mitsuya D, et al. Correction of adenosine deaminase deficiency in cultured human T and B cells by retrovirus-mediated gene transfer. Proc Natl Acad Sci USA 1986;83:6563.
52. Hock RA, Miller AD. Retrovirus-mediated transfer and expression of drug resistant genes in human haematopoietic progenitor cells. Nature 1986;320:275.
53. Howell SB, Murphy MP, Johnson J, et al. Gene therapy for thioguanine-resistant human leukemia. Mol Biol Med 1987;4:157.
54. Oppenheim A, Peleg A, Fibach E, et al. Efficient introduction of plasmid DNA into human hemopoietic cells by encapsidation in simian virus 40 pseudovirions. Proc Natl Acad Sci USA 1986;83:6925.
55. Robertson M. Gene therapy—desperate appliances. Nature 1986;320:213.
56. Woo SLC, DiLella AG, Marvit J, et al. Molecular basis of phenylketonuria and potential somatic gene therapy. Cold Spring Harbor Symposia on Quantitative Biology 1986;51:395.
57. Dick JE, Magli MC, Haszar D, et al. Introduction of a selectable gene into primitive stem cells capable of long term reconstitution of the hematopoietic system in W/WV mice. Cell 1985;42:71.
58. Garver RI, Chytil A, Courtney M, et al. Clonal gene therapy: transplanted mouse fibroblast clones express human alpha-1 antitrypsin gene in vivo. Science 1987;237:762.
59. Cline MK. Perspectives for gene therapy. Inserting new genetic information into mammalian cells by physical technique and viral vectors. Pharmacol Ther 1985;29:69.
60. Doetschman TC, Eistetter H, Katz M, Schmidt W, Kemier R. The in vitro development of blastocyst-derived embryonic stem cell lines: formation of visceral yolk sac, blood islands and myocardium. J Embryol Exp Morphol 1985;87:27.
61. Doetschman T, Williams P, Meada N. Establishment of hamster blastocyst-derived embryonic stem (ES) cells. Dev Biol 1988;127:224.
62. Gossler A, Doetschman T, Korn R, Serfline E, Kemler R. Transgenesis by means of blastocyst-derived embryonic stem cell lines. Proc Natl Acad Sci USA 1986;83:9065.
63. Rubenstein JLR, Nicolas JF, Jacob F. Introduction of genes into preimplantation mouse embryos by use of a defective recombinant retrovirus. Proc Natl Acad Sci USA 1986;83:366.
64. Gordon JW, Ruddle FH. Gene transfer into mouse embryos: pro-

duction of transgenic mice by pronuclear injection. Methods Enzymol 1983;101:411.
65. Hammer RE, Pursel VG, Rexroad CE, et al. Production of transgenic rabbits, sheep and pig by microinjection. Nature 1985;315:680.
66. Willadsen SM. Nuclear transplantation in sheep embryos. Nature 1986;320:63.
67. Hammer RE, Palmiter RD, Brinster RL. Partial correction of murine hereditary growth disorder by germ line incorporation of a new gene. Nature 1984;311:65.
68. Costantini F, Chada K, Magraw J. Correction of murine beta thalassemia by gene transfer into the germ line. Science 1986;233:1192.
69. Stout JT, Chen HY, Brennand J, et al. Expression of human HPRT in the central nervous system of transgenic mice. Nature 1985;317:250.
70. Monk M, Hardy K, Handyside A, et al. Preimplantation diagnosis of deficiency of hypoxantine phosphoribosyl transferase in a mouse model for Lesh-Nyhan syndrome. Lancet 1987;2:423.
71. Muller H. Human gene therapy: possibilities and limitations. Experientia 1987;43(4):375.
72. Seibel MM. A new era in reproductive technology. N Engl J Med 1988;318(13):828.
73. Fletcher JC. Ethical issues in and beyond prospective clinical trials of human gene therapy. J Med Philos 1985;10:293.
74. Walters L. The ethics of human gene therapy. Nature 1986;320:225.
75. Drugan A, Evans WJ, Evans MI. Fetal organ and xenograft transplantation. Am J Obstet Gynecol 1989;160:288.
76. National Institutes of Health/Recombinant DNA Advisory Committee. Points to Consider in the Design and Submission of Human Somatic-Cell Gene Therapy Protocols. Recomb DNA Techn Bulletin 1985;8:116.

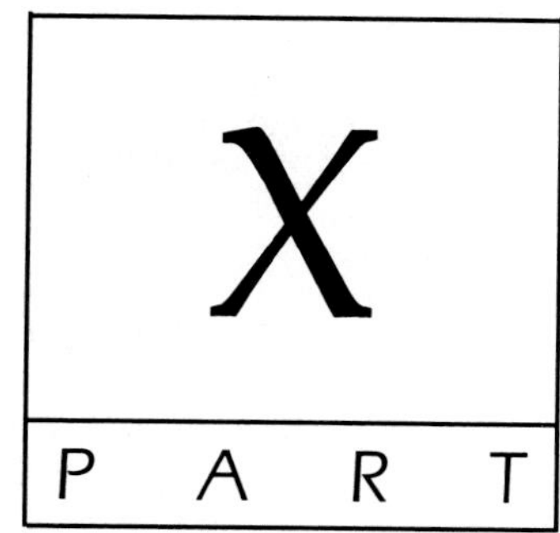

MATERNAL BIOLOGIC ADAPTATIONS TO PREGNANCY

54

CHAPTER

MATERNAL BIOLOGIC ADAPTATIONS TO PREGNANCY

Valerie M. Parisi and Robert K. Creasy

Remarkable anatomic and physiologic changes begin to occur in the female shortly after conception. Some appear prior to any recognizable need of the mother or fetus, such as early breast fullness and tenderness (see Chapter 91), others occur seemingly to benefit the growth and development of the fetus, and still others occur as a result of the growth of the uterus and contents. These profound changes come about quickly, and in the main are totally reversible. The maternal–fetal interaction is the prime basis for these alterations, and it is necessary to have a thorough understanding of these changes in order to properly interpret normality and pathology during the gestation. Indeed, many of the biological adaptations could be considered major disease states if pregnancy was not present.

THE REPRODUCTIVE TRACT

THE UTERUS

Because the fetus, placenta, and amniotic fluid must grow and function within the uterus, it is necessary for the uterus to undergo some dramatic changes. The uterus in the non-pregnant state weighs approximately 40 to 70 g, depending on parity. The majority of uterine growth occurs as a result of myometrial cellular hypertrophy, although some hyperplasia is seen, particularly in the first trimester. The non-pregnant myometrial cell of 50 to 90 μm in length reaches 500 to 800 μm by term.[1] By term, the uterine weight approaches 1200 g. In addition to myometrial cellular changes, there is also an increase in collagenous connective, vascular, and nervous tissue, again by hyperplasia or hypertrophy. Early in pregnancy, the increase in cell size and number is probably related to sex steroid stimulation,[2] but later in pregnancy it is thought that the increasing size of the conceptual mass plays a role as well. Myometrial growth is most marked in the fundal portion.

In the first trimester, uterine wall thickness increases, only to become thinner as the conceptual mass increases. In addition, the uterus becomes softer in pregnancy, in comparison to the non-pregnant state, with the fetus readily palpable, and fetal movements able to be observed through the abdominal wall in the latter half of gestation.

Initially, the uterus maintains its pear shape. It becomes more spherical by 12 to 16 weeks gestation, and then becomes ovoid as length increases more than width. Another important change occurs in the isthmus of the uterus, or that portion of the uterus between the uterine cavity and the largely fibrous connective tissue of the cervix. By 12 weeks of gestation, this area has elongated to become part of the uterine cavity. Finally, this portion of the lower uterine segment becomes relatively thin, with decreased myometrial cellular content.[3]

The uterus is known to contract in both the non-pregnant and pregnant state. Early in gestation, the uterus is relaxed, with sporadic contractions occurring. These may involve the entire uterus or only a segment, and are usually of low amplitude in pressure. These sporadic contractions occur occasionally with higher amplitude as the gestation advances, and may at times be rhythmical for short periods. As term approaches, the frequency of these contractions increases.

In parallel fashion to the increase in uterine growth is a progressive increase in uterine perfusion. Although various approaches to indirect measurements in the human have been made, all with potential errors, uterine blood flow values in the range of 500 to 700 mL/min have been estimated in late gestation.[4,5] Although absolute uterine blood flow increases dramatically in pregnancy, the blood flow per gram of uterus and contents is probably relatively constant. Animal experiments and human studies indicate that at least 80% of the blood flow is to the placental implantation site, thus providing for the increased oxygen and nutrient needs of the developing fetal tissues.

The majority of information relative to the regulation of uterine blood flow is available from animal experimentation. Estradiol administration into the uterine artery of the non-pregnant or pregnant sheep results in increased blood flow by vasodilatation, probably mediated by vasoactive agents. Decreased sensitivity to angiotensin II is probably more pronounced in the uterine vasculature than in the systemic vessels, at least in normal gestation. In general, catecholamine activity of the uterus is reduced as the gestation advances. In addition, vasodilator prostaglandins such as prostacyclin and prostaglandin E can vasodilate uterine vessels in sheep. It is obvious that a complex interplay of hormonal factors, neurotransmitters, and prostaglandins probably controls the uterine circulation during pregnancy by mechanisms that remain to be determined.[6]

THE CERVIX

The cervix undergoes increased softening during pregnancy. This is due to a number of different factors, including a marked increase in vascularity, a change in connective tissue with decreased association of collagen fibers, edema, and a marked change in the endocervical glands. Significant proliferation of the endocervical glands occurs to such a degree that they account for approximately one half of the cervical mass. These glands produce thick, tenacious mucus that obstructs the canal; this mucus plug is sloughed off prior to labor. This proliferation of the endocervical glands results in an eversion of the external os over the portio vaginalis and an inflamed appearance.

The changes in the isthmus have been discussed previously, but assist to set the final stage for labor. The explanation of parturition must include an understanding of the ripening process of the cervix, which permits the cervix to be withdrawn in back of the presenting part at term, after previously being an obstruction to the conceptus for many months. Although the exact etiologic mechanisms of cervical ripening remain to be defined, near term there is an increase in hyaluronic acid and increased collagen dissociation. It is thought that relaxin and arachidonic acid metabolites play a role in this ripening process.

THE VAGINA

The vagina also participates in the prominent increase in vascularity during pregnancy. This increased vascularity lends a bluish purple color to the mucosa, the so-called Chadwick's sign of early pregnancy. In addition, there is a marked thickening of the vaginal mucosa, hypertrophy of the underlying smooth muscle, and a general loosening of the abundant surrounding connective tissue. All of these changes facilitate marked distensibility of the vaginal canal prior to parturition. The tissues of the vulva share in these changes as well. The vaginal mucosa is rich in glycogen, and increased vaginal secretions (and cervical secretions) result in a more pronounced white, somewhat thick, acidotic discharge.

THE ADNEXA

The fallopian tubes generally undergo minimal change in pregnancy.

A significant change in the ovaries is that ovulation ceases and the corpus luteum of pregnancy persists. This corpus luteum is of major importance in the production of progesterone and maintenance of early pregnancy for the first 5 weeks after conception.[7] The corpus luteum also secretes relaxin throughout pregnancy, although the role of this hormone remains to be clearly defined.[8]

A decidual reaction also occurs at the surface of the ovaries, forming tissue that can bleed easily upon irritation.

CARDIOVASCULAR SYSTEM

Profound alterations in both cardiovascular anatomy and functional physiology occur from early in the first trimester of pregnancy, and allow the gravida to support the markedly increased oxygen and nutrient demands of the growing fetus. Although the cardiovascular hemodynamic changes of pregnancy are well tolerated by normal women, a complete understanding of the basic principles of cardiovascular physiology allows the clinician to appropriately assess and predict which women with medically complicated pregnancies may undergo a significant deterioration as the normal adaptation mechanisms come into play.

PLASMA VOLUME

Plasma volume rises progressively throughout pregnancy, beginning at approximately 6 to 8 weeks of gestation and tapering off at about 30 to 32 weeks of gestation.[9] The normal primigravid woman can expect a total increase in plasma volume of about 40% to 50%, with the increase in subsequent pregnancies being slightly greater.[10] This increase in plasma volume is positively correlated with the size of the fetus,[10] so that women carrying multiple pregnancies have proportionally higher increases in plasma volume.

RED CELL VOLUME

Total red cell volume increases by about 20% to 30% during normal gestation, depending on the use of iron supplementation.[11] This increase in red cells progresses steadily between the end of the first trimester and term.[10] The disproportionately larger increase in plasma volume relative to red cell volume results in a significant drop in maternal hematocrit, which is evident at the beginning of the third trimester. This normal mechanism has been inappropriately dubbed "the physiologic anemia of pregnancy," because it does not in fact represent a true anemia, but rather a normal physiologic hemodilution. Red cell volume decreases dramatically at delivery as a result of blood loss, and the return to normal, non-pregnant blood volumes is accomplished by 3 weeks after delivery.[12,13]

PERIPARTUM CHANGES IN BLOOD VOLUME

Vaginal delivery of a singleton infant at term is associated with an average blood loss of 500 mL, and uncomplicated cesarean delivery results in an average blood loss of 1000 mL.[13] The preexisting hypervolemia modifies the gravida's response to blood loss at delivery. Unless there is massive postpartum hemorrhage accounting for at least 25% of total blood volume, there is no physiologic compensatory increase in blood volume postpartum, and the normal postpartum diuresis will result in a gradual fall in plasma volume. The normal gravida with a prepartum hemoglobin of a least 12 g/dL can tolerate the loss of 1000 mL of blood without a significant fall in hemoglobin concentration. A significant drop in hemoglobin or hematocrit by 5 days after delivery is indicative of either inappropriate total blood volume expansion during pregnancy, or increased total blood loss at the time of delivery.[14]

The massive increase in total blood volume that occurs during pregnancy serves several purposes in the protection of both the maternal and fetal condition. The reserves in intravascular volume manifested by term offer some maternal protection against prepartum hemorrhage, as well as from late pregnancy hypotension, when an increased proportion of blood volume is entrapped by the lower extremities. The disproportionate increase in plasma volume over red cell volume results in a decrease in viscosity and, subsequently, a decreased resistance to blood flow. This mechanism allows the maternal increase in cardiac output to occur with a smaller proportionate increase in cardiac work. Much of the increased cardiac output of normal pregnancy is distributed to the skin, to allow for heat loss, and to the kidneys, to allow for excretion of both maternal and fetal metabolic waste. These excretory functions depend on an increase in plasma volume rather than red cell volume. The increase in red cell volume during pregnancy approximates the increase in oxygen requirement to support both maternal cardiovascular function and fetal growth.

ANATOMIC CHANGES OF THE HEART AND GREAT VESSELS

The heart and great vessels undergo anatomic alterations during pregnancy in order to adapt to the marked increase in blood volume that begins at the end of the first trimester. Myocardial hypertrophy has been documented histologically as well as by echocardiographic evidence of increased muscle mass in the ventricular wall and an increase in end diastolic volume.[15] Myocardial contractility is also increased during gestation.[15,16] The progressive upward displacement of the diaphragm during pregnancy results in superior, lateral, and anterior displacement of the heart. This anatomic alteration, along with the finding of a small amount of benign pericardial effusion during pregnancy,[17] increases the width of the cardiac silhouette on chest radiograph, making the diagnosis of cardiomegaly by non-pregnant standards inappropriate.

Both left and right ventricular end-diastolic dimensions increase in the second and third trimesters.[16] However, there is no change in the left ventricular end-systolic dimension.[16] Several significant auscultatory changes are also evident during pregnancy. The first heart sound becomes louder and develops an exaggerated split between the mitral and tricuspid valvular closures.[18] The second heart sound remains essentially unchanged throughout pregnancy. An audible third heart sound is present in close to 90% of gravidas by midgestation, while a fourth heart sound is audible in fewer than 5%,[18] and is an indication of pathologic cardiac function. The ubiquitous systolic ejection murmur of pregnancy is best heard along the left lateral sternal border and is present in almost all women.[18] These early to midsystolic murmurs may be increased on inspiration (right side), increased on expiration (left side), or be unchanged by respiration.

It is thought that the entire vascular system undergoes a general softening of collagen and smooth muscle hypertrophy during gestation.[19] The increased blood volume and blood flow through the great vessels result in the anatomically prominent appearance of both the pulmonary artery and its vasculature on chest radiograph during pregnancy.

CARDIAC OUTPUT

Cardiac output rises 30% to 50% during normal pregnancy, with the majority of this change occurring in the late first trimester, and a small but continued rise until approximately 32 weeks of gestation.[20,21] Stroke volume and heart rate determine cardiac output, with increased stroke volume the predominant factor in the rise during the first half of pregnancy. Stroke volume then decreases near term, whereas heart rate rises progressively throughout pregnancy and is responsible for the continued rise of cardiac output through most of the second half of gestation.[20] Maternal position is critical in the assessment of cardiac output in the third trimester of pregnancy. Vena caval compression by the enlarging uterus causes cardiac output to fall in the supine position, whereas measurements made in the lateral position show a 22% increase over those measurements made in the supine position.[22] Assumption of the standing position results in a significant drop in cardiac output.[23] Easterling recently completed a longitudinal study of hemodynamic parameters in normotensive pregnant women and reported a fall in mean cardiac output from 32 weeks to term when measured by Doppler echocardiography.[24]

Systemic vascular resistance is calculated as mean arterial pressure divided by cardiac output. Normal pregnancy results in both a fall in blood pressure and a rise in cardiac output, resulting in a decreased systemic vascular resistance. However, as blood pressure rises toward term and cardiac output most likely falls somewhat, vascular resistance subsequently rises.

Although the blood volume expansion of normal pregnancy is approximately equal to the increase in cardiac output, it does not seem that these two parameters are related as cause and effect, when one considers that the majority of the increase in blood volume does not occur until well after the increase in cardiac output is established. The decreased systemic vascular resistance seen in normal pregnancy represents a decrease in afterload and, according to Starling's law of the heart, should result in an increased cardiac output from an increase in ejection fraction.[24] The 50% increase in cardiac output seen in normal pregnancy would mandate an associated increase in ejection fraction of more than 90%.[25] The previously described anatomical changes of pregnancy provide an additional mechanism responsible for the marked increase in cardiac output. Compliance of the heart is increased, evidenced by the fact that end diastolic volume is increased without an increase in end diastolic pressure.[15,16] Therefore, the normal pregnant heart is physiologically dilated while maintaining ejection fraction with a small increase in contractile force.[24]

The peripartum period represents a time of acute hemodynamic stress for the gravid patient. Although the normal gravida will adapt to this condition, the woman with even mild underlying cardiac dysfunction may deteriorate because of the increased hemodynamic demands of active labor. Maternal cardiac output in late labor is additionally increased by approximately 13% over the resting output.[26] This additional increase in cardiac output is thought to be primarily due to a further increase in stroke volume. At the peak of uterine contractions, approximately 500 mL of blood is acutely returned to the systemic circulation, which serves to increase preload and further increase cardiac output by one third above the baseline value for labor. The anxiety and pain associated with labor may produce increased catecholamine release and tachycardia, creating an additional slight increase in cardiac output. It is clear that these mechanisms will contribute to the potential rapid deterioration of the gravida with even minimal underlying cardiac dysfunction in the face of active labor, because pulmonary artery wedge pressure will be increased acutely during uterine contractions and may contribute to the development of pulmonary edema in these patients.

The choice of anesthetic for labor and delivery also affects cardiac output. The initiation of epidural anesthesia results in a 37% increase in cardiac output over baseline, whereas the induction of general anesthesia results in a 26% increase in cardiac output.[27] These increases are associated with elevations in both heart rate and stroke volume and are transient, returning to baseline within 60 to 90 minutes. The massive increases in cardiac output associated with normal pregnancy, labor, and delivery abate rapidly postpartum, as evidenced by a 25% decrease in cardiac output when measured 2 weeks postpartum.[28]

BLOOD PRESSURE

As with other cardiovascular hemodynamic parameters in pregnancy, the position in which blood pressure is measured is of critical importance. In the sitting or standing positions, there is only a slight decrease in systolic and diastolic arterial pressure from non-pregnant values. This slight decrease is evident from the first trimester of pregnancy and remains unchanged through pregnancy in the sitting and standing positions.[29] Both systolic and diastolic blood pressures are approximately 10 mm Hg higher standing and sitting than in the left lateral recumbent position.[30] Followed longitudinally throughout normal pregnancy, the systolic and diastolic arterial blood pressure, measured in the left lateral recumbent position, is decreased, reaching its lowest level at approximately 28 to 32 weeks.[29] The systolic and diastolic arterial pressures slowly return to normal levels during the third trimester, approximating nonpregnant levels by 40 weeks gestation. It should be noted that when blood pressures are taken with the gravida in the left lateral position, there will be significant differences between the upper and lower arm blood pressure reading due to hydrostatic forces.[31] After mid-pregnancy, the supine position may result in vena caval compression and a significant increase in both systolic and diastolic blood pressures over those values measured in the left lateral position. Although the maximal fall of systolic blood pressure during pregnancy is approximately 12 mm Hg, diastolic pressures fall between 10 and 20 mm Hg, resulting in an increased pulse pressure.[29] Figure 54-1 graphically depicts the longitudinal evaluation of systolic and diastolic blood pressure throughout pregnancy and the postpartum period, as well as the relationship of these values to positional changes. Diastolic blood pressures higher than 90 mm Hg at any time during pregnancy represent abnormal values. It has been postulated that diastolic blood pressures greater than 80 mm Hg in the second half of pregnancy are not normal and may represent latent hypertension.[24]

DISTRIBUTION OF INCREASED CARDIAC OUTPUT

The increase in cardiac output observed during normal gestation is distributed among several maternal organ systems. The low-resistance uteroplacental circulation manifests a tenfold increase in blood flow, and receives

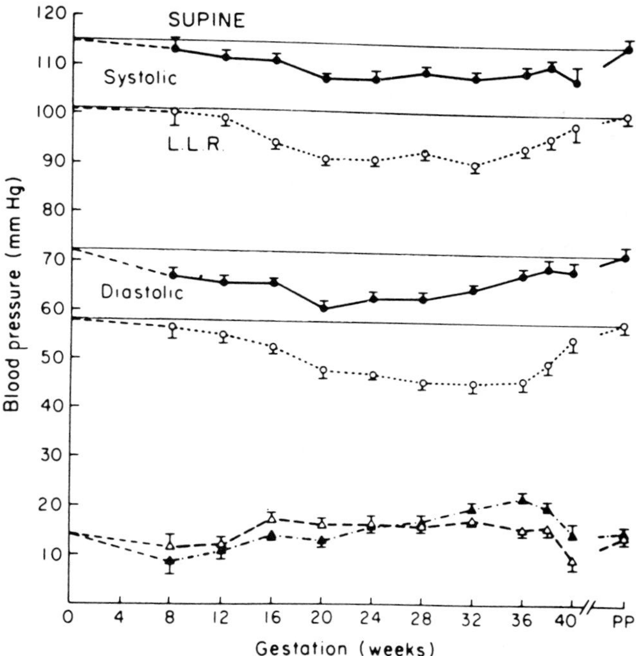

FIGURE 54–1. Longitudinal changes in systolic and diastolic blood pressure in both supine and left lateral recumbent (LLR) position during pregnancy and postpartum (PP). The bottom graph represents the increase in systolic (open triangles) and diastolic (closed triangles) pressure noted when the gravida's position is changed from left lateral to supine. (From Wilson M, Morganti AA, Zervoudakis J, et al. Blood pressure, the reninaldosterone system and sex steroids throughout normal pregnancy. Am J Med 1980; 68: 97.)

approximately 17% to 20% of total maternal cardiac output or 500 to 800 mL/min at term. Limited data obtained from humans are summarized by Gant and Worley,[26] and agree with more invasive techniques used in animal studies.[33] The renal circulation also receives a significant percentage of maternal cardiac output, because renal blood flow increases approximately 50% over non-pregnant levels by mid-pregnancy (see the renal section of this chapter). The breasts and skin also receive an increased percentage of cardiac output during pregnancy, representing a marked increase in total organ blood flow over the non-pregnant state.[34] Figure 54-2 graphically represents the redistribution of maternal cardiac output during pregnancy.

SUMMARY

Normal maternal physiologic adaptation to pregnancy results in a hyperdynamic state characterized by elevations in cardiac output, heart rate, and stroke volume, accompanied by significant decreases in systemic vascular resistance and mean arterial pressure. These hemodynamic changes maintain stroke work within a normal range, are evident by the end of the first trimester of pregnancy, and are clearly out of proportion to the needs of the growing fetus at that time. The precise cause for the timing and magnitude of the normal hemodynamic alterations of pregnancy remains unclear at present.

HEMOSTASIS DURING PREGNANCY

The normal process of hemostasis depends on vascular integrity, normal number and function of platelets, coagulation factors, and the process of fibrinolysis. The normal physiological adaptation to pregnancy is marked by an increase in the hepatic production of coagulation factors (see the section on liver function). The dramatic increase in the production of fibrinogen results in an increase in fibrin, which is subsequently deposited in the vessel walls of the uteroplacental circulation. These changes are accompanied by a significant depression in fibrinolysis. Teleologically, one supposes that these changes, in combination with the increased blood volume of pregnancy, serve to protect the gravida from the potential catastrophe of severe postpartum hemorrhage. These mechanisms render pregnancy a hypercoagulable state.

Maintenance of normal vascular integrity is a complex process. Production of prostacyclin by the vascular endothelium not only prevents aggregation of platelets, but also has the capability of disaggregating platelets that are already clumped together.[35] The normal number and function of platelets allows for adhesion to small defects in the vasculature and the formation of small fibrin clots, which are removed from the circulation by fibrinolysis. The generation of prostacyclin by the vascular endothelium allows platelet adhesion, but prevents pathologic aggregation and thrombus formation. The disruption of the normal production and function of prostacyclin within vessels in diseases such as preeclampsia, hemolytic uremic syndrome, and thrombocytopenic purpura will make the vascular environment conducive to thrombus formation.[36]

Although previous data have been conflicting, a recent review of all information on platelet counts during normal pregnancy would suggest that, if anything, there is a slight decrease in platelet count as normal pregnancy progresses toward term, although each value still falls within the normal non-pregnant range.[37,38] There is also evidence of increased turnover of platelets, as well as low-grade platelet activation during pregnancy.[37,38] Subsequently, the normal gravida has a population of relatively young platelets, whose mean platelet volume is increased over that of the non-pregnant woman. It is generally accepted that the normal physiologic adaptation to pregnancy includes a chronic, low-grade intravascular coagulation within the uteroplacental vasculature. Further evidence for the low-grade activation of platelets during the last two trimesters of normal pregnancy comes from reports that plasma levels of the platelet agranular secretory protein B-thromboglobulin are increased at this time.[39]

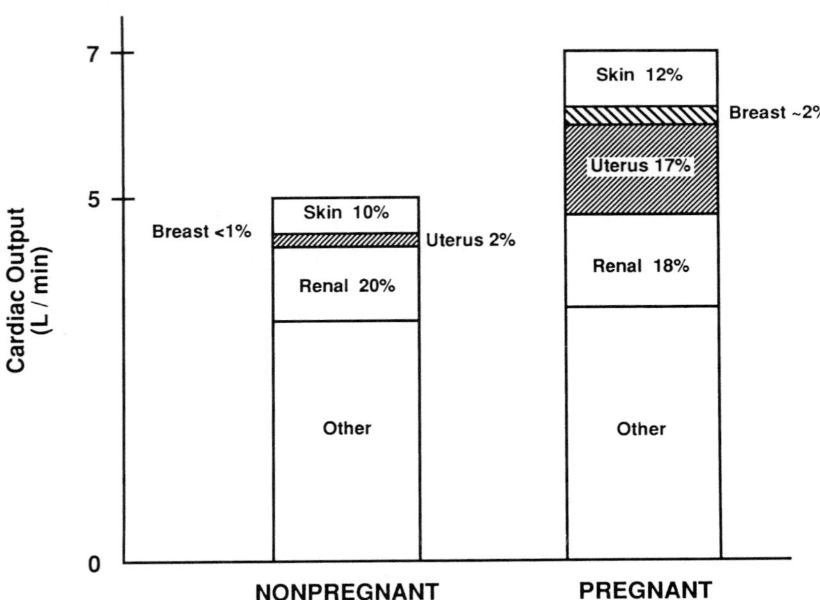

FIGURE 54–2. Distribution of maternal cardiac output in the non-pregnant and term pregnant state. Note that although the percentage of renal, skin, and breast blood flow does not increase, the absolute blood flow to these organs increases during pregnancy because of the large increase in cardiac output. (Data from references 13, 32, 34, 65, and 66.)

INTRINSIC/EXTRINSIC CASCADE CHANGES

Both activated partial thromboplastin time (aPTT) and prothrombin time (PT) have been reported to be reduced in pregnant women when compared with non-pregnant controls.[40] The aPTT and PT are direct measures of the functionality of both the intrinsic and extrinsic mechanisms of coagulation. When a blood vessel sustains an injury, the process of coagulation is initiated both by activation of factor VII via tissue thromboplastin release (extrinsic pathway) and by activation of factor XII by collagen (intrinsic mechanism). Both of these pathways are necessary for normal coagulation and the ultimate formation of an insoluble fibrin clot. These two pathways merge to a final pathway following the activation of factor X (Fig. 54-3). The intrinsic pathway evolves slowly, requiring approximately 5 to 20 minutes to result in visible fibrin formation. However, the lipoprotein thromboplastin, which is present in all tissues, markedly accelerates the rate at which blood clots. Thromboplastin is present in high concentrations in lung, brain, and placenta. Placental thromboplastin activation will produce the formation of fibrin within 12 seconds by bypassing the intrinsic pathway of coagulation. Figure 54-3 shows changes in the coagulation system during pregnancy, which are characterized by an increase in factors VII, VIII, X, and plasma fibrinogen.[41] These coagulation factors are increased from the end of the first trimester of pregnancy.

Although pregnancy has been described as a hypercoagulable state protecting the gravida from massive hemorrhage, mechanisms are also in place that normally limit clot formation at the site of vascular injury in order to prevent generalized thrombosis. These mechanisms involve complex interactions between procoagulants and the naturally occurring anticoagulants. Antithrombin III (AT III), synthesized in the liver, is the major physiologic inhibitor of coagulation factors II, IX, X, XI, XII, and thrombin. To date, there is no information to indicate that pregnancy produces an alteration in AT III levels,[42] although total synthesis must be increased during gestation in order to maintain equivalent serum concentrations in the face of the expanded plasma volume. Peripartum alterations of AT III concentrations have been reported to be decreased at delivery and increased in the postpartum period, potentially increasing puerperal thrombosis development.[42] Familial AT III deficiency results in an increased risk of thrombosis.[43] The protein C-thrombomodulin-protein S system also exerts natural anticoagulant activity. Factors X and XIII are inactivated by protein C, which is a vitamin K-dependent substance also produced in the liver. Protein C must be activated by two cofactors, endothelial cell-produced thrombomodulin and protein S. Familial inherited deficiency of protein C[44] or protein S[45] results in increased risk of thromboembolic disease. Limited information is currently available on longitudinal measurements of this system throughout pregnancy, although the data available seem to indicate small fluctuations within the normal non-pregnant range throughout pregnancy.[46]

FIBRINOLYSIS

The physiologic adaptation to normal pregnancy includes a decrease in plasma fibrinolytic activity that persists through the process of parturition and then returns rapidly to normal within a short time after delivery of the placenta.[47] The placental production of fibrinolytic inhibitors is responsible for this rapid alteration.

In summary, hemostatic changes in normal pregnancy are characterized by an ongoing, low-grade activation of the coagulant system. The deposition of fibrin has been documented in the uteroplacental vasculature (both spiral arteries and intervillous space). The smooth

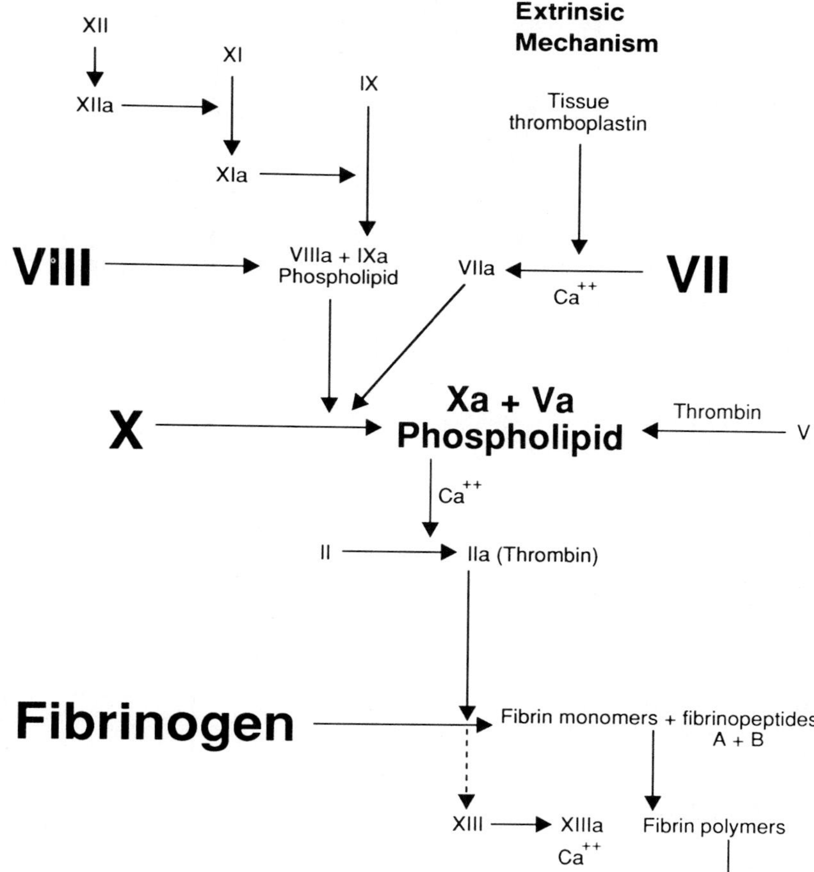

FIGURE 54–3. Both the extrinsic and intrinsic pathways of coagulation are depicted. The boldface factors (**VII, VIII, X, X_a, V_a, fibrogen,** and **fibrin**) are markedly increased in pregnancy. The subscript **a** indicates the activated form of factors. (Adapted from Letsky EA. Coagulation defects. In: deSwiet M, ed. Medical disorders in obstetric practice. Oxford, Blackwell Scientific Publications, 1990: 110.)

muscle and elastic lamina of the spiral arteries are eroded by the trophoblast and replaced partially by fibrin. These anatomic changes allow for increased vessel diameter, which accommodates the tenfold increase in uteroplacental blood flow by producing a decreased vascular resistance in the uteroplacental circulation. Increased levels of coagulation factors and fibrinogen allow the normal gravida to successfully coagulate the placental separation site at delivery. These changes result in a hypercoagulable state during normal pregnancy that places even the normal gravida at increased risk for thromboembolic disease during pregnancy and the puerperium.

THE RESPIRATORY SYSTEM

ANATOMICAL/MECHANICAL CHANGES

During pregnancy, the configuration of the thorax changes before there is any increase in uterine size that could exert a mechanical pressure. The level of the diaphragm rises by approximately 4 cm, the transverse diameter of the thorax increases by 2 cm, and the thoracic circumference increases by approximately 6 cm.[48,49] The actual excursion of the diaphragm, despite the enlarging conceptual mass, is increased by 1.5 cm.

The upper airway also participates in the increased vascularity of pregnancy, leading to mucosal hyperemia and edema. The result is increased nasal stuffiness, and nasal bleeding is not rare.

LUNG VOLUMES

Although the basic respiratory rate is unchanged during pregnancy, some rather major changes occur in various components of ventilation (Fig. 54-4). The resting tidal volume, or the volume of air exchange with each breath, is increased by approximately 40%, with a similar rise in minute ventilation.[50,51] These changes occur in the first trimester, and they remain essentially unchanged for the remainder of gestation.[52]

The residual volume (both the expiratory reserve volume and the residual volume) is decreased by approximately 20%.[50,51] Because the alveolar volume is re-

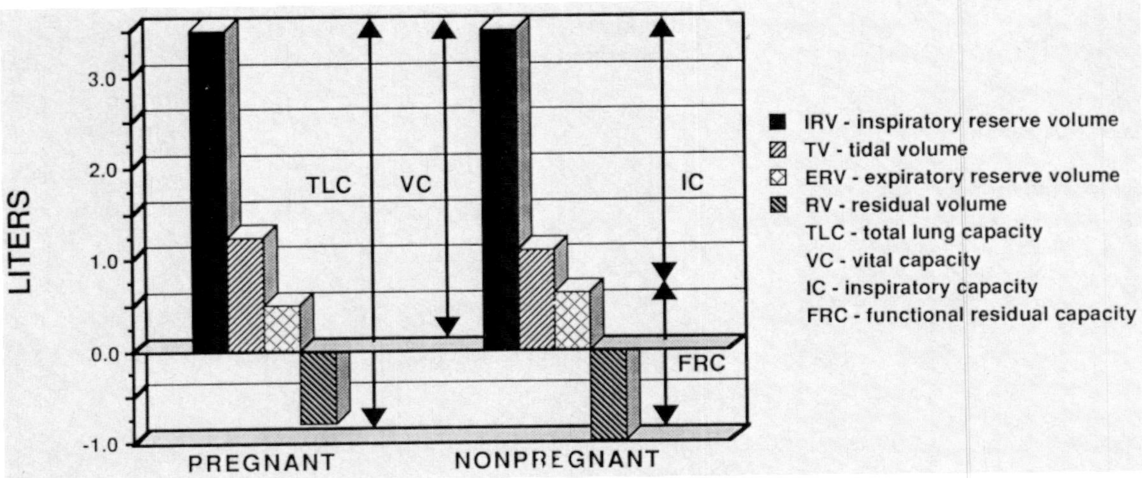

FIGURE 54–4. Comparison of lung capacities during pregnancy and the non-pregnant state. (Data from references 50, 51, and 52.)

duced, and the tidal volume increased, the effective alveolar ventilation is increased even further. The vital capacity, the sum of the inspiratory reserve volume, the tidal volume, and the expiratory reserve volume, which equates with the maximal amount of air that can be forcefully ventilated, is essentially not changed. Due to the decrease in functional residual volume, the total lung volume is decreased about 5%.

PULMONARY FUNCTION

Resistance of large airways is more important than small airway resistance when considering work expended in breathing. Indirect measurements that reflect large airway resistance, such as forced expiratory flow in 1 minute, indicate there is no significant change during gestation in large airway resistance. The point at which small airways close during expiration has been controversial, but is probably not altered in a major way.

Oxygen consumption during pregnancy is increased by approximately 20% due to the presence of the fetus and placenta, the increased cardiac and ventilatory work, the extra breast and uterine tissues, etc. The increase in minute ventilation of 40% is thus far greater than is necessary to meet the demands of oxygen. The partial pressure of arterial oxygen (P_aO_2) is minimally changed, perhaps rising slightly to 103 to 107 mm Hg, and the arteriovenous oxygen difference decreased.[53–55] Due to the increase in minute ventilation, the partial pressure of arterial carbon dioxide (P_aCO_2) falls to approximately 30 mm Hg very early in gestation.[54] This decrease in P_aCO_2 is compensated by an equivalent increase in renal excretion of bicarbonate and a resultant decrease in plasma bicarbonate concentration.

The increase in ventilation and the resultant decrease in P_aCO_2 is due to progesterone, in part acting on the central respiratory center.[56] In addition, carbonic anhydrase in red cells, which facilitates carbon dioxide transfer, is increased in pregnant patients and in patients receiving oral contraceptives.[57] Despite, if anything, an improvement in ventilation during gestation, at least half of pregnant women experience a sense of breathlessness or dyspnea.[58] The basis of this symptom has not been delineated.

THE URINARY SYSTEM

ANATOMIC ALTERATIONS

Both kidneys increase in overall size during pregnancy, increasing in length by 1 to 1.5 cm. In part, this increase in size is thought to be secondary to an increase in renal vascular volume. In addition, there is a dilatation of the renal pelvis, and the calyceal system as well as the ureters above the pelvic brim. The dilatation of the urinary collecting system becomes quite obvious by midgestation, with the right ureter more frequently involved than the left (in three fourths of gravidas the right is dilated; in one third, the left is dilated) and more dilated than the left ureter.[59] The portion of the ureters below the pelvic brim are rarely dilated. In addition to the dilatation, the ureters frequently elongate, become more tortuous, and may be displaced laterally.

The cause of the hydroureter and hydronephrosis in pregnancy is usually ascribed to obstruction or compression, with progesterone possibly playing a role in adding to the compliance of the system. The difference in the incidence and degree of dilatation between the right and left collecting systems may result from a cushion effect provided the left ureter by the sigmoid colon, and dextrorotation of the uterus and the right ovarian vein, which crosses over the right ureter. The increase in dead space of the collecting systems may predispose to urinary tract infection, and alters interpretation of functional evaluation of the urinary system and intravenous pyelography. Ureteral peristalsis in regard to frequency and intensity of contractions is probably not altered. Ureteral tone above the pelvic brim has been reported to be increased in the latter half of pregnancy, becoming normal shortly after delivery.[60,61]

Urodynamic studies have shown that bladder pressure is doubled from the first trimester to late pregnancy, indicating a reduction in bladder capacity and increased demand on the ability of the urethra to close.[62] Cystometric studies had previously shown that the capacity of the bladder increases during pregnancy.[63] At the end of pregnancy, with the fetus occupying the pelvis, this capacity is reduced. A compensatory feature is that the absolute and functional lengths of the urethra are increased at the end of pregnancy by approximately 20%, along with a similar percentage increase in intraurethral closure pressure.[62] These latter features tend to counteract the possibility of stress incontinence, which has been reported to be present to some degree in two thirds of pregnant women.[64]

RENAL FUNCTION

Renal plasma flow, coincident with cardiac output, increases early in the first trimester. Increases in effective renal plasma flow of approximately 50% over non-pregnant flow rates are present by mid-pregnancy and remain elevated until late pregnancy, when a slight decline occurs.[65,66] The assumption of the supine position may markedly decrease venous return, as discussed earlier in this chapter, which may in turn lead to a decrease in effective renal plasma flow in some patients. However, the late pregnancy decrease in effective renal plasma flow is not merely due to studying patients in the supine position.[66,67]

The glomerular filtration rate (GFR) also increases in the first trimester. GFR as measured by inulin clearance (which is cleared only by the glomerulus) is elevated by 50% by mid-pregnancy, which persists until term. GFR as measured by creatinine clearance (creatinine being both cleared by the glomerulus and to a variable degree excreted by the tubules) also increases by approximately 50% at midgestation, only to decrease from its elevation by approximately 15% in the late third trimester.[65,66] Thus, normal creatinine clearances in the pregnant patient in mid-pregnancy approximate 140 to 160 mL/min, and near term approximate 120 mL/min (Fig. 54-5). Due to the increase in GFR without a significant change in the production of urea or creatinine, the plasma serum concentrations of these substances decrease. Serum creatinine concentrations of 0.8 to 1.0 mg/dL in the non-pregnant state approximate 0.7 mg/dL by the end of the first trimester and 0.5 to 0.6 mg/dL by midgestation. Blood urea nitrogen concentrations approximate 8 to 9 mg/dL by midgestation. Serum uric acid concentrations decrease by at least 25% in the first trimester, only to rise back to normal, non-pregnant levels by mid-pregnancy, reaching similar non-pregnant concentrations by term.[68,69] Urate is freely filtered, but is then actively reabsorbed, the amount of reabsorption increasing in late pregnancy.

One of the most dramatic alterations in renal function pertains to tubular sodium reabsorption in pregnancy. Sodium excretion is favored by the increase in GFR (an increase of 5000 to 10,000 mEq of sodium/24 hrs), increases in progesterone, and decreased plasma albumin. Despite this increased filtered load of sodium, there is an overall net retention of approximately 1000 mEq of sodium distributed among the maternal extracellular space and the fetus. This positive sodium balance occurs gradually over the gestation. Increased tu-

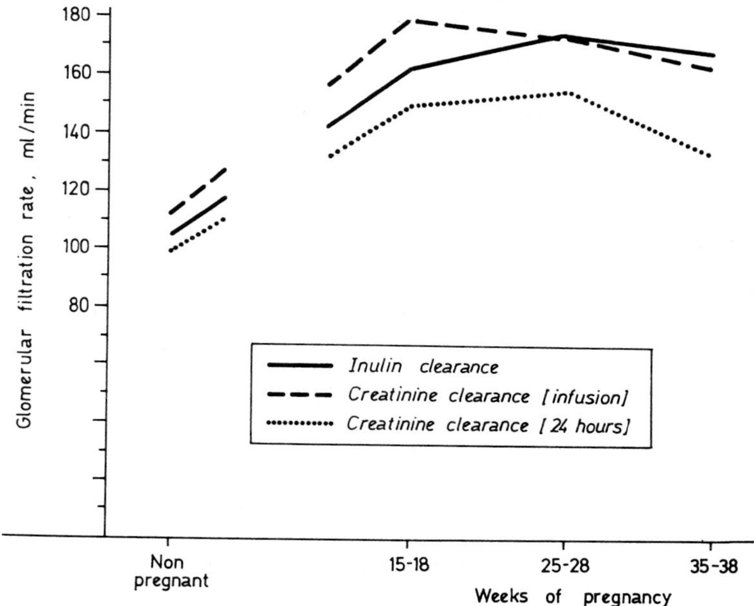

FIGURE 54–5. Mean glomerular filtration rate measured by three methods in ten healthy women during pregnancy and 8 to 12 weeks after delivery. (From Davison JM, Hytten FE. Glomerular filtration during and after pregnancy. J Obstet Gynaecol Br Commonw 1974; 81: 588.)

bular reabsorption is promoted by the increase in plasma aldosterone as well as other hormones, such as estrogen, deoxycortisone, and placental lactogen. Plasma osmolality, as a result of water retention in slight excess of solute, is markedly reduced by 8 to 10 mOsm/L to approximately 280 mOsm/L, beginning in the first trimester.[70] Although one would expect this decrease to promote a diuresis, this does not occur, probably due to a resetting of osmotic control thresholds.

All three components of the renin–angiotensin–aldosterone system are elevated in pregnancy, beginning in the first trimester.[71] It is currently unknown whether these elevations are a response to the volume expansion that occurs, but they do play a role in protecting against the natriuretic effect of an increase in filtration and progesterone. There is also an increased vascular refractoriness to the increased levels of angiotensin in normal pregnancy.

A number of nutritional substrates are also affected by the increase in glomerular filtration. Glucosuria may occur due to a combination of an increase in the filtered amount of glucose and some impairment of tubular reabsorption, despite normal blood glucose.[72] At least 10% of an unselected obstetrical population may have random glucosuria, but less than 1% of these have abnormal glucose tolerance tests.[73] There is a very slight increase of urinary albumin excretion of 7 to 18 ng/24 hours.[74] Aminoaciduria also occurs in pregnancy, presumably due in part to an increased filtered load of various amino acids, but little is known about mechanisms. Glycine, histidine, threonine, serine, and alanine excretion increases early and continues to rise until term.[75] Lysine, cystine, taurine, tyrosine, leucine, valine, and phenylalanine excretion increases in the first half of gestation, but then decreases slightly thereafter. Excretion of asparagine, glutamic acid, methionine, isoleucine, ornithine, and arginine is unaffected. Excretion of some vitamins, such as folate and vitamin B_{12}, is also increased.

ORAL/ESOPHAGEAL/ GASTROINTESTINAL SYSTEM

A number of symptoms and signs relative to the entire alimentary system occur during pregnancy. Some symptoms, such as nausea and vomiting, occur early and are suggestive signs of early pregnancy. Others, such as constipation, also occur early, and unlike nausea and vomiting persist throughout the gestation. The basis for the increase in first trimester of nausea and emesis, which typically occurs in the morning and tends to abate during the day, is unknown. It has been postulated that chorionic gonadotropins may play a role, because the nausea tends to parallel the rise and fall in human chorionic gonadotropin, and in pregnancies with unusually elevated concentrations, such as trophoblastic disease, the nausea and emesis may persist. Most women experience an increase in appetite by the end of the first trimester, and although quantitation is lacking, pica, defined as an abnormal craving for unnatural foods, is reportedly increased.

ORAL CAVITY

The gingiva become softer and hyperemic during pregnancy, with the result that gingival bleeding increases in frequency. A specific pregnancy-related lesion, the epulis of pregnancy, may occur at any time. This is a localized vascular growth that is frequently pedunculated and is benign. It will usually regress after delivery, but may need excision for excessive bleeding.

The production of saliva is probably unchanged during gestation, although some reports suggest some electrolyte changes from specific glands. Excessive salivation or ptyalism is an uncommon complication of pregnancy that can lead to loss of 2 liters of saliva a day. The cause or ptyalism is unknown.

Although some have suggested that tooth disease is increased, there is no evidence that the incidence or progression of dental caries is altered by the presence of gestation.

ESOPHAGUS AND STOMACH

Pregnant women have decreased lower intraesophageal pressures and higher intragastric pressures than non-pregnant women.[76] In addition, esophageal peristaltic amplitudes and speed are decreased. Thus, there is an increased potential for gastric reflux and esophagitis, giving rise to a high incidence of heartburn (pyrosis) experienced by pregnant women. The reported increased incidence of hiatus hernia during pregnancy could also contribute to the symptom of heartburn. However, not all women with hiatus hernias have symptoms.[77]

The stomach also has decreased tone and motility, which leads to delayed gastric emptying. It has been suggested that decreased gastric acid secretions in the first two trimesters are the basis for a reduced incidence of peptic ulcer disease. Acid secretion is higher in the last trimester than in non-pregnant women.[78] These features also predispose the pregnant patient to regurgitation and aspiration during inhalation anesthesia used for delivery.

INTESTINES

There is also decreased tone and motility of the small and large bowel, with resultant decreased transit times.[79,80] There is approximately a 60% increase in water absorption in the large bowel which, combined with the decreased tone, leads to a high incidence of constipation during pregnancy. Constipation and increased circulating blood volume and venodilatation result in higher rates of hemorrhoidal formation.

The cause of the overall decrease in muscle tone in

the gastrointestinal tract is thought to be secondary to the significant rise in progesterone during gestation or decreased levels of the smooth muscle-stimulating hormone motilin during pregnancy.[81]

LIVER AND GALLBLADDER

THE LIVER

The overall size and histology of the liver is, in essence, not altered during pregnancy.[82,83] Although there is a significant increase in cardiac output during pregnancy, hepatic blood flow has been reported in one small study to be relatively unchanged.[84]

Normal pregnancy is frequently associated with tests of hepatic function that would be considered abnormal results from the non-pregnant woman. The clinical findings of an increased incidence of spider angiomata and palmar erythema, discussed elsewhere in this chapter, are secondary to the hormonal changes of a normal gestation and can also erroneously support a diagnosis of hepatic dysfunction.

The bromosulfophthalein (BSP) test, when performed in pregnancy, shows reduced clearance of the injected dye. The ability of the liver to remove and store the dye is actually increased, but the maximal tubular excretory rate decreases.[85] The same changes have been observed by administering estrogen to non-pregnant women.[86] Various hepatic enzymes and protein synthesized in the liver are also altered in pregnancy, and partially summarized in Table 54-1.

Serum alkaline phosphatase concentrations are at least twice as high during normal pregnancy as they are in non-pregnant women, and therefore cannot be used as a reflection of hepatic function during pregnancy. This rise is due in part to placental production of a heat-stable alkaline phosphatase isoenzyme, which can account for up to two thirds of the enzyme activity. There may also be an increase from hepatic sources as well, because the administration of estrogen to non-pregnant women increases serum alkaline phosphatase activity.[87] The serum levels of aspartate aminotransferase and alanine aminotransferase are unchanged. Serum bilirubin concentrations are unchanged or minimally elevated.

TABLE 54–1. CHANGES IN LIVER FUNCTION EVALUATIONS IN PREGNANCY

Test	Change
Alkaline phosphatase	↑ 2×
Alanine aminotransferase (SGPT)	↔
Albumin	↓ 20%
Albumin/globulin	↓
Aspartate aminotransferase (SGOT)	↔
α and β globulin	sl↑
Bilirubin	→
Bromosulphalein clearance	sl↓
Ceruloplasmin	↑ 2×
Cholesterol	↑ 2×
Prothrombin	→
Fibrinogen	↑ 50%

Serum concentrations of various proteins and lipids that relate to hepatic function also change in pregnancy. Serum albumin and total protein concentrations decrease in pregnancy. Serum albumin concentration is approximately 25% to 30% lower in pregnancy, or about 3 gm/dL.[88] There is a slight increase in the alpha and beta fractions of globulins, and an overall decrease in albumin/globulin. Serum concentrations of fibrinogen increase by approximately 50%, and clotting factors VII, VIII, IX, and X are elevated. Levels of prothrombin are unchanged (see the hemostasis section in this chapter). There is also a major increase in the serum concentrations of various lipids. Serum cholesterol concentrations rise linearly throughout gestation until near term, when they have approximately doubled.

THE GALLBLADDER

The gallbladder also participates in the decrease in motility observed in other sites. Ultrasonographic studies show that both fasting and residual volumes are increased in mid- and late pregnancy to twice that observed in non-pregnant women.[89] It is again believed that increased progesterone concentrations are the basis of the observed decreased motility and decreased emptying. Minimal information is available on the composition of bile. Because the occurrence of gall stones is at least twofold greater in women than in men, and the decreased motility in pregnancy would predispose to stone formation, it is thought that repetitive pregnancy may increase the probability of cholelithiasis.

ENDOCRINE SYSTEM

PANCREATIC FUNCTION AND CARBOHYDRATE METABOLISM

Normal pregnancy is characterized by hyperplasia of the insulin-producing beta cells in the pancreatic islets of Langerhans. There is documented increased insulin secretion and greater sensitivity to a lower dose of glucose.[90] Normal human pregnancy is characterized by an exaggerated plasma glucose response and plasma insulin response to a given oral glucose load.[91] Although there is no difference in the decay curve of injected insulin between normal non-pregnant and normal term pregnant women, there is a much reduced hypoglycemic response to injected insulin in women at term with normal pregnancies.[92] Fasting blood glucose in normal pregnancy decreases by 10% to 20% in the first trimester, long before fetal demands are significant.[90] This fasting hypoglycemia is a result of pancreatic beta cell hyperplasia, increased insulin secretion, and an increased peripheral glucose usage. As pregnancy progresses and the growing fetus has greater nutrient demands, maternal glucose stores are mobilized and hepatic glycogenolysis occurs. Increasing insulin resistance during pregnancy is mediated by ever-increasing placental production of human placental lactogen and, to a lesser extent, prolactin and cortisol.[90]

In contradistinction to fasting hypoglycemia, postprandial glucose levels in normal pregnancy are elevated to approximately 130 to 140 mg/dL, likely due to the effect of placentally produced anti-insulin hormones. Mean maternal plasma glucose values stay relatively constant throughout pregnancy at 80 to 90 mg/dL, which is essentially unchanged from non-pregnant values.[90]

Plasma concentrations of glucose in the postabsorptive state decrease as pregnancy advances. This is due to an increase in placental uptake of glucose to meet both the fetal demands and placental metabolic demands as well. Gluconeogenesis seems to be limited in pregnancy as the major substrate, alanine, is increasingly taken up by the placenta and therefore unavailable for uptake by the maternal liver.

Insulin is an anabolic hormone whose metabolic effects in the adult include increased peripheral glucose uptake, glycogen synthesis, protein synthesis, and inhibition of lipolysis. Insulin resistance is part of the normal physiologic adaptation to pregnancy. During the first half of pregnancy, increased insulin levels allow excess maternal calories to be directed to lipid stores and tissue glycogen, while blood glucose levels remains low. However, in the second half of pregnancy, as the placenta produces increasing amounts of human placental lactogen and other anti-insulin hormones, the insulin response is blunted at the postreceptor level, increasing maternal circulatory glucose, which is then available for transfer to the fetus. Insulin degradation is unaltered during normal pregnancy.

Inpaired glucose tolerance during normal pregnancy is the result of both increasing insulin resistance *and* a relative paucity of circulating insulin. Most normal pregnant women are able to increase their insulin secretion appropriately to counteract the physiologically produced insulin resistance. However, gestational diabetes can result in those women with limited ability to secrete insulin.

MATERNAL–PLACENTAL–FETAL TRANSFER OF NUTRIENTS

The interrelationships of glucose, insulin, amino acids, and free fatty acid transfer across the placenta are schematically shown in Figure 54-6. Glucose is transported to the fetus by carrier-mediated diffusion, which equilibrates fetal blood glucose levels with maternal levels. Extensive metabolic studies in the pregnant ewe have documented that both the uterine and placental tissues take up and use glucose from the maternal circulation.[93,94] The fetus also uses amino acids as primary building blocks for growth. Fetal concentrations of most amino acids are actually higher than those of maternal concentrations, and are subsequently maintained against a concentration gradient within the placenta.[95] There is rapid transfer of the essential branched-chain neutral amino acids across the placenta, while straight-chained amino acids such as alanine and glycine are slowly transferred. There is essentially no transport of the acidic amino acids glutamate and aspartate, whose fetal requirements need to be satisfied by fetal synthesis.[96] The placenta is responsible for the de novo synthesis of nonessential amino acids, which are then transported to the fetus. Free fatty acids cross the placenta by gradient dependent diffusion and are used by the fetus.[97]

The placenta acts not only as a transporter of nutrients to the fetus, but as a modulator of this transport system. The increase of human placental lactogen in the second half of pregnancy also stimulates lipolysis, which subsequently allows the availability and transfer of increased amounts of both glucose and amino acids to the fetus during the period of maximal fetal growth.

THYROID FUNCTION

The thyroid gland undergoes noticeable enlargement during normal gestation, attributable to the combination of increased vascularity and cellular hyperplasia. It was once thought that goiter itself was a normal consequence of pregnancy; however, this is not the case when one examines the physiology of thyroid metabolism during pregnancy. During the first trimester, as glomerular filtration rate increases, there is a decrease in renal tubular absorption of iodide and a resultant increase in urinary excretion of iodide. This results in a fall in the plasma iodide level, so that the thyroid gland markedly increases its uptake of iodine from blood.[98] In parts of the world where there may be iodine deficiency in the diet, the thyroid gland must hypertrophy in order to respond to the normal demands of pregnancy for increased thyroid hormone. Under these circumstances, a great majority of pregnant women will develop goiter during pregnancy.[99] However, in parts of the world where dietary intake of iodine is high, particularly in the United States, where salt is routinely iodized, this compensatory hypertrophy of the thyroid gland does not occur and the incidence of goiter is no higher than that in the non-pregnant female population.[100]

The secretion of thyroid-binding globulin (TBG) by the liver is doubled by the 12th week of pregnancy and is attributable to estrogen's effect on hepatic metabolism.[101] Subsequently, pregnancy is characterized by a significant increase in the amount of both thyroxine (T_4) and triiodothyronine (T_3) bound to TBG. Despite this increase in the total concentrations of both T_4 and T_3, the amounts of circulating free (unbound) hormone are not significantly increased over the non-pregnant state.[102] Mean plasma concentrations of T_4 during pregnancy range from 9 to 16 mg/dL, as compared with 5 to 12 mg/dL in the non-pregnant woman.[103]

Thyroid-stimulating hormone (TSH) is produced by the pituitary gland, circulates unbound in the blood, and does not cross the placenta, and its concentration in maternal plasma does not appear to be elevated during

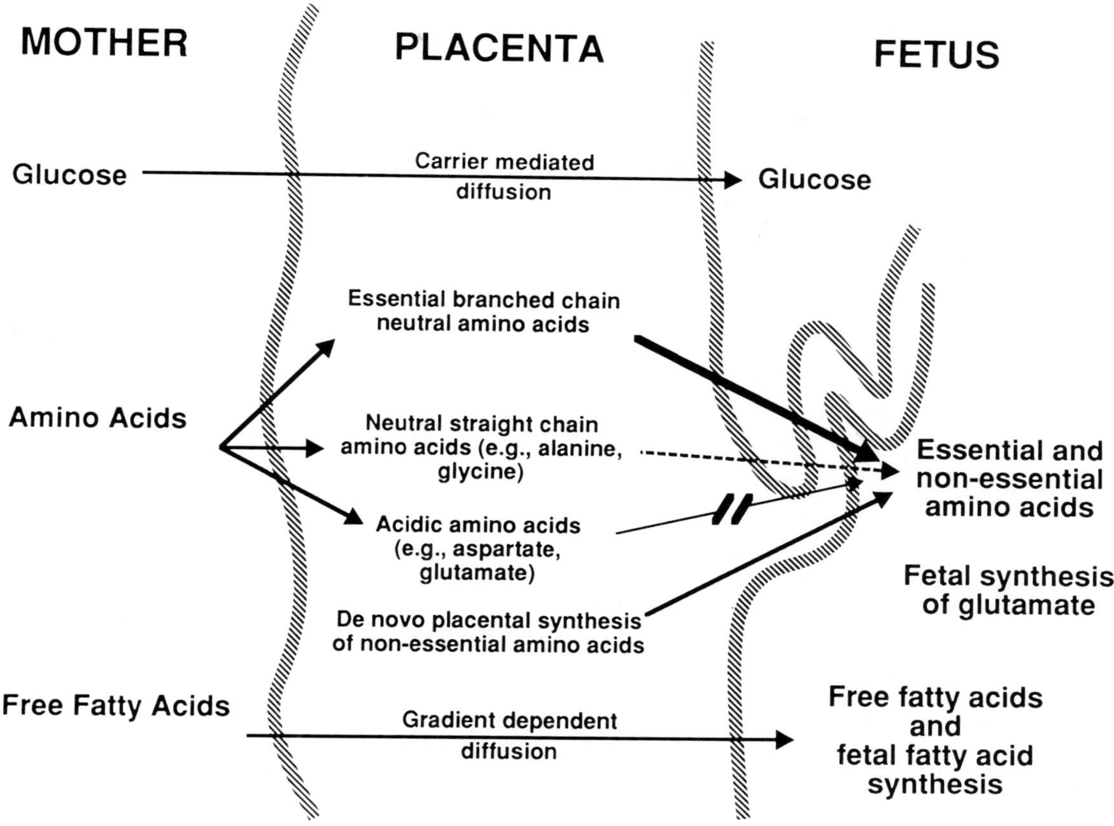

FIGURE 54–6. Maternal to fetal transport of glucose, amino acids, and free fatty acids. Note that the placental synthesizes nonessential amino acids, and that the fetus must synthesize its own supply of glutamate. The fetus is also able to synthesize fatty acids in addition to those provided by maternal transport. (Adapted from Hollingsworth DR, Moore TR. Diabetes and pregnancy. In: Creasy RK, Resnik R, eds. Maternal-fetal medicine: principles and practice. Philadelphia, WB Saunders, 1989: 933.)

pregnancy.[103,104] Chorionic thyrotropin has been identified as a second thyroid-stimulating substance that is produced by the placenta and transported to the maternal circulation.[105] Placental production of human chorionic gonadotrophin (hCG) also results in stimulation of maternal thyroid activity, particularly in women with pregnancies complicated by hydatidiform mole.[106] Thyrotropin-releasing hormone (TRH) is a hypothalamic neurotransmitter that regulates both synthesis and release of TSH from the pituitary.[106] Although the levels of TRH during normal pregnancy are not altered, TRH does in fact cross the placenta with ease, and can stimulate the production of TSH by the fetal pituitary, as well as prolactin, thereby playing a regulatory role in fetal thyroid homeostasis.

FETAL–MATERNAL THYROID FUNCTION INTERACTION

Due to the relative inability of TSH, T_4, and T_3 to cross the placenta, thyroid function in mother and fetus remain independently regulated (Fig. 54-7). Maternal TRH is the only thyroid-related hormone that crosses the placenta in significant amounts. Although the regulation of fetal thyroid function seems to be fairly independent from maternal control, the fetus is dependent on the gravida for its supply of iodine. It should also be noted that because iodine readily crosses the placenta, any abnormal increase in maternal ingestion of iodine-containing products may result in fetal goiter and hypothyroidism.

PARATHYROID FUNCTION AND CALCIUM HOMEOSTASIS DURING PREGNANCY

By term, the fetus has accumulated 30 gm of calcium and approximately 15 gm of phosphorus, all of which has been supplied by the gravida.[107] The majority of the calcium requirement for the fetus occurs in the third trimester of pregnancy, when fetal skeletal growth reaches an accelerated phase. This large demand on the part of the fetus mandates an anticipatory increase in maternal calcium absorption from early pregnancy onward, for if this did not occur, the necessary calcium would be extracted

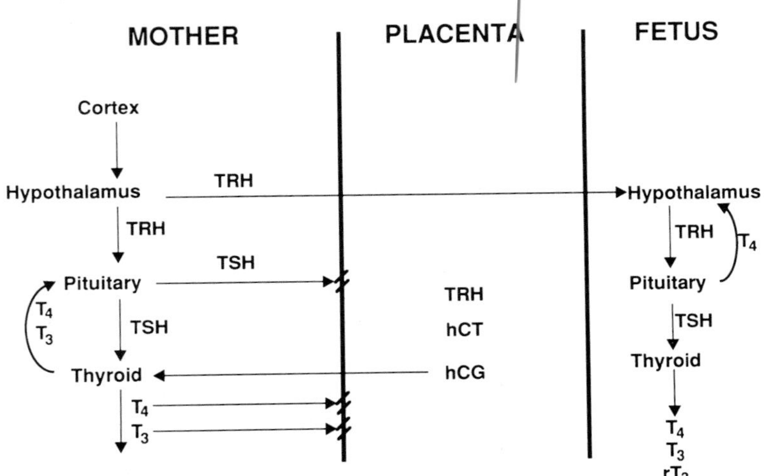

FIGURE 54–7. Maternal–placental–fetal thyroid hormone interactions. Note that thyrotropin-releasing hormone (TRH) is synthesized in the placenta to some degree, and is the only hormone capable of crossing the placenta from mother to fetus. hCT, human chorionic thyrotrophin; hCG, human chorionic gonadotrophin; rT_3, reverse triiodothyronine. (Adapted from Hollingsworth DR. Endocrine disorders of pregnancy. In: Creasy RK, Resnik R, eds. Maternal-fetal medicine: principles and practice. Philadelphia, WB Saunders, 1989: 998.)

from maternal bone. Breast-feeding mothers have prolonged requirements for increased intake of calcium. Maternal concentrations of serum calcium during pregnancy are dependent on a complex interaction of parathyroid hormone (PTH), calcitonin, and vitamin D and its metabolites. Total serum calcium and phosphorus actually decrease in pregnancy.[108] The decrease in serum calcium is accompanied by a similar decrease in serum proteins such as albumin during pregnancy, lending evidence to the concept that the fall in serum proteins accounts for the decline in measured serum calcium. Further evidence for this concept lies in the fact that ionized calcium has been reported to either remain stable or rise very slightly throughout pregnancy.[109]

Calcitonin is a calcium-lowering 32-amino acid hormone secreted by the C-cells of the thyroid gland. Plasma levels of calcitonin in the non-pregnant state are quite low, and are increased markedly during both pregnancy and lactation.[110] Calcitonin acts in opposition to both parathyroid hormone and vitamin D in order to maintain skeletal calcification. Calcium, magnesium, gastrin, and glucagon are known to increase calcitonin levels.[103]

The release of parathyroid hormone is stimulated by decreases in plasma calcium or magnesium. Conversely, increases in plasma calcium and magnesium levels suppress parathyroid hormone. PTH exerts an effect on calcium, phosphorus, and magnesium metabolism, and plays a role in bone resorption, intestinal absorption, and kidney reabsorption of these minerals, ultimately resulting in increased calcium and decreased phosphate in the extracellular fluid compartment. There has been some controversy as to the pregnancy-induced change in PTH concentration, although recent evidence indicates that plasma PTH levels fall during the first trimester and then increase progressively until term.[111] Plasma volume expansion, increased glomerular filtration rate, and increased transfer of calcium to the fetus collectively result in decreased maternal calcium concentrations during normal pregnancy, and may subsequently act as the trigger for increased parathyroid hormone levels. Despite the significant decrease in total calcium concentration during pregnancy, it seems to be the small decrease in ionized calcium that regulates the feedback mechanism for the secretion of PTH. Estrogen may also play a role in calcium homeostasis by interfering with the action of PTH on bone resorption. Thus, the normal adaptation to pregnancy involves the development of a mildly hyperparathyroid state, most likely in order to assist the gravida in meeting the high fetal demands for calcium.

Maternal concentrations of vitamin D during pregnancy depend on diet, exposure to sunshine, and the use of oral supplements. Vitamin D undergoes hydroxylation in the liver to produce 25-hydroxyvitamin D_3. This metabolite then reaches the proximal convoluted tubule of the kidney, where it undergoes 1_α hydroxylation to produce 1,25-dihydroxyvitamin D_3. Both the decidua and the placenta also appear to be capable of 1_α hydroxylase activity.[112] The kidney and placenta are also capable of 24 hydroxylation to produce 24,25-dihydroxyvitamin D, which then may undergo 1_α hydroxylation.[113] Of all the reported metabolites of vitamin D, 1,25 dihydroxyvitamin D_3 seems to be the biologically active compound. The marked increase in 1,25-dihydroxyvitamin D_3 activity during pregnancy may be a result of a parathyroid hormone-induced increase in maternal 1_α hydroxylase activity. Some have questioned this postulate based on the fact that the demonstrated rise in parathyroid hormone during pregnancy does not coincide with the onset of enhanced calcium absorption.[104] An even more attractive hypothesis, proposed by Ramsay,[104] invokes the stimulation of renal 1_α hydroxylase activity by estrogen in the presence of progesterone,[114] lowered plasma phosphate, and potentially even prolactin or human placental lactogen (HPL). There is some evidence to suggest that 1,25-dihydroxyvitamin D_3 may in fact be synthesized by the placenta itself.[112] In summary, the activation of renal 1_α hydroxylase activity during pregnancy results in increased concentrations of 1,25-dihydroxyvitamin D_3 and, eventually, increased calcium absorption. The precise initiating mechanism for this process awaits further elucidation.

The calcium-stimulated placental ATPase pump allows transfer of calcium from mother to fetus, and results in increased fetal plasma concentrations of calcium. Parathyroid tissue is present in the fetus as early as six weeks of gestation,[115] and at term fetal PTH levels are decreased and calcitonin concentration increased compared with values during infancy.

The net result of pregnancy-induced changes in calcium metabolism is an increase in total maternal calcium with resultant transfer of calcium to the fetus without depleting the maternal skeleton.

SKIN AND MUSCULOSKELETON

THE SKIN

Increased pigmentation occurs in at least 90% of pregnant women to some degree.[116] Although most patients have a mild generalized hyperpigmentation, specific areas are more involved. Melasma gravidarum (the mask of pregnancy) involves the forehead and cheeks; the bridge of the nose can be pronounced. This usually regresses after pregnancy, but can persist for months. Similar changes have been reported in non-pregnant women taking oral contraceptives. The areola of the breast, the linea alba (becomes the linea negra), axillae, and genital skin are other areas affected.

The mechanisms responsible for this hyperpigmentation are poorly understood. They occur more frequently in dark-skinned women than in fair- or blond-skinned women. Melanocyte-stimulating hormone (MSH) is increased in pregnancy, and sex steroids can effect the melanocytes in the epidermis, but some believe that increased MSH is not the source of the melasma.[116,117]

A number of changes occur in the skin as a result of vascular dilatation and proliferation, most likely caused by the hyperestrogenic state of pregnancy. Dilatation of capillary vessels and small arteries leads to a variety of angioma. Spider angiomata are particularly common in white women, characterized by a central red elevation (central arteriole) with radiating thin vessels, most common in exposed areas of the body. Redness of the palms or palmar erythema can occur in a blotching distribution. Usually these vascular changes regress after completion of the pregnancy.

Connective tissue changes, presumably induced by estrogens, lead to the development of striae gravidarum in approximately half of all pregnancies. These represent linear tears in dermal skin and appear reddish in the current pregnancy. Common areas of involvement are the abdomen, breasts, thighs, and buttocks. The degree of skin distention does not appear to be the etiologic mechanism, leading to the concept of genetic susceptibility.[118] There is no known method of prevention, and although they become less pronounced after pregnancy, and lose coloration, they do not completely regress.

Estrogen is known to decrease the rate of hair growth. In late pregnancy, the number of hair follicles in the telogen phase (resting phase) is approximately 5% to 10%, rising two- to fourfold in the puerperium, which results in a transient hair loss at about 3 to 4 months after birth.[119] However, normal growth recurs by 6 to 9 months without any therapy.

THE MUSCULOSKELETON

Ligaments of the sacroiliac joints and pubic symphysis are reported to soften in pregnancy, leading to some separation of joints. Widening of the pubic symphysis of 3 to 4 mm can occur. In addition, there is progressive lordosis of the spine as the uterus enlarges, leading frequently to low back discomfort for the remainder of the gestation. There is accompanying flexion of the neck, and downward movement of the shoulders. This latter feature may place more traction on the ulnar and median nerves, contributing to aching and numbness. The numbness may also be due to edema increasing the carpal tunnel syndrome.

CONCLUSION

Pregnancy produces marked physiologic alterations in every organ system in order to support the nutritional needs of the developing fetus and to protect the gravida from the negative effects of her potentially parasitic fetus. This chapter has focused on providing a summary of these major pregnancy-induced changes and their interrelationship with fetal growth and development, in order that maternal and fetal physiologic conditions may be better understood.

REFERENCES

1. Reynolds SRM. Physiology of the uterus. New York: Hafner Publishing, 1965.
2. Katzenellenbogen BS, Bhakoss HS, Ferguson ER, et al. Estrogen and anti-estrogen action in reproductive tissues and tumors. Recent Prog Horm Res 1979;34:259.
3. Danforth DN. The fibrous nature of the human cervix and its relation to the isthmic segment in the gravid and non-gravid uteri. Am J Obstet Gynecol 1947;53:541.
4. Metcalfe J, Romney SL, Ramsey LH, et al. Estimation of uterine blood flow in women at term. J Clin Invest 1955;34:1632.
5. Rekonen A, Luotola H, Pitkanen M, et al. Measurement of intervillous and myometrial blood flow by an intravenous 133_{Xe} method. Br J Obstet Gynaecol 1976;83:723.
6. Rosenfeld CR. Consideration of the uteroplacental circulation in intra-uterine growth. Semin Perinatol 1974;8:12.
7. Csapo AI, Pulkkinen MO, Wiest WG. Effects of hysterectomy and progesterone replacement in early pregnant patients. Am J Obstet Gynecol 1973;115:759.
8. Eddie LW, Bell RJ, Lester A, et al. Radioimmunoassay of relaxin

in pregnancy with an analogue of human relaxin. Lancet 1986;1:1344.
9. Hytten H, Paintin BD. Increase in plasma volume during normal pregnancy. J Obstet Gynaecol Br Commonwealth 1963;70:402.
10. Hytten F, Leitch I. The physiology of human pregnancy. 2nd ed. Oxford: Blackwell Scientific Publications, 1971:1.
11. Pritchard JA. Changes in the blood volume during pregnancy and delivery. Anesthesiology 1965;26:393.
12. de Leevw NKM, Lowenstein L, Tucker EC, et al. Correlation of red cell loss at delivery with changes in red cell mass. Am J Obstet Gynecol 1968;100:1092.
13. Letsky EA. Blood volume, haematinics, anaemia. In: De Swiet M, ed. Medical disorders in obstetric practice. Oxford: Blackwell Scientific Publications, 1990:48.
14. Peck TN, Arias F. Hematologic changes associated with pregnancy. Clin Obstet Gynecol 1979;22:785.
15. Laird-Meeter K, Vande Lay G, Bom TH, et al. Cardiocirculatory adjustments during pregnancy and echocardiographic study. Clin Cardiol 1979;2:328.
16. Rubler S, Damani P, Pinto E. Cardiac size and performance during pregnancy estimated with echocardiography. Am J Cardiol 1977;49:534.
17. Enein M, Zina AAA, Kassem M, El-Tabbakh G. Echocardiography of the pericardium in pregnancy. Obstet Gynecol 1987;69:851.
18. Cutforth R, MacDonald CD. Heart sounds and murmurs in pregnancy. Am Heart J 1966;71:741.
19. Marazita AJD. The action of hormones on varicose veins in pregnancy. Med Rec 1946;159:422.
20. Ueland K, Novy M, Peterson E, et al. Maternal cardiovascular dynamics. IV: the influence of gestational age on the maternal cardiovascular response to posture and exercise. Am J Obstet Gynecol 1969;104:856.
21. Lees M, Taylor S, Scott D, et al. A study of cardiac output at rest throughout pregnancy. J Obstet Gynecol Br Commonwealth 1967;74:319.
22. Ueland K, Hansen JM. Maternal cardiovascular dynamics: II. Posture and uterine contractions. Am J Obstet Gynecol 1969;103:1.
23. Easterling TR, Schmucker BC, Benedetti TJ. The hemodynamic effects of orthostatic stress during pregnancy. Obstet Gynecol 1988;72:550.
24. Easterling TR. Cardiovascular physiology of normal pregnancy. In: Maternal-fetal physiology. Society of Perinatal Obstetricians 10th Annual Meeting, Houston, Texas, January 1991.
25. Morton M, Metcalfe J. Changes in maternal hemodynamics during pregnancy. In: Artal R, Wiswell R, ed. Exercise in pregnancy. Baltimore: Williams & Wilkins, 1986:113.
26. Ueland K, Metcalf J. Circulatory changes in pregnancy. Clin Obstet Gynecol 1975;18:41.
27. James C, Banner T, Caton D. Cardiac output in women undergoing cesarean section with epidural or general anesthesia. Am J Obstet Gynecol 1989;160:1178.
28. Robson SC, Dunlop W, Boys RJ, et al. Cardiac output during labour. Br Med J 1987;295:1169.
29. Wilson M, Morganti AA, Zervoudakis J, et al. Blood pressure, the reninaldosterone system and sex steroids throughout normal pregnancy. Am J Med 1980;68:97.
30. Gallery E, Ross M, Hunyor S, et al. Predicting the development of pregnancy associated hypertension: the place of standardized blood pressure measurement. Lancet 1977;1:1274.
31. Benedetti T, Read J. The effect of hydrostatic pressure on interpretation of the supine pressor test. J Reprod Med 1982;27:161.
32. Gant NF, Worley RJ. Measurement of uteroplacental blood flow in the human. In: Rosenfeld CR, ed. The uterine circulation. Ithaca: Pernatology Press, 1989:53.
33. Rosenfeld CR. Distribution of cardiac output in ovine pregnancy. Am J Physiol 1977;232:H231.
34. Brinkman CR III. Biologic adaptation to pregnancy. In: Creasy RK, Resnik R, eds. Maternal-fetal medicine: principles and practice. Philadelphia: WB Saunders, 1989:739.
35. Moneada MD, Vane JR. Arachidonic acid metabolites and the interaction between platelets and blood vessel walls. N Engl J Med 1979;300:1142.
36. Lewis PJ. The role of prostacyclin in preeclampsia. Br J Hosp Med 1982;62:1048.
37. Sell PR, Lind T, Walker W. Platelet values during normal pregnancy. Br J Obstet Gynaecol 1985;92:480.
38. Fay RA, Hughes AO, Farron NT. Platelets in pregnancy: hyperdestruction in pregnancy. Obstet Gynecol 1983;61:238.
39. Ingles JCM, Stuart J, George AJ, et al. Haemostatic and rheologic changes in normal pregnancy and preeclampsia. Br J Haematol 1981;50:461.
40. Nossel HL, Langkowsky P, Levy S, et al. A study of coagulation factor levels in women during labor and their newborn infants. Thromb Haemost 1966;16:185.
41. Bonnar J. Hemostasis and coagulation disorders in pregnancy. In: Bloom AL, Thomas DP, eds. Haemostasis and thrombosis. Edinburgh: Churchill Livingston, 1981:454.
42. Hellgren M, Blomback M. Blood coagulation and fibrinolysis in pregnancy, during delivery and in the puerperium. Gynecol Obstet Invest 1981;12:141.
43. Winter JH, Fenech A, Ridley W, et al. Familial antithrombin III deficiency. Q J Med 1982;204:373.
44. Horellou MH, Cinard J, Bertua RM, et al. Congenital protein C deficiency and thrombotic disease in nine French families. Br Med J 1984;289:1285.
45. Comp PC, Esmon CT. Recurrent venous thromboembolism in patients with a partial deficiency of protein S. N Engl J Med 1984;311:1525.
46. Letsky EA. Coagulation defects. In: DeSwiet M, ed. Medical disorders in obstetric practice. Oxford: Blackwell Scientific Publications, 1990:104.
47. Bonnar J, Prentice CRM, McNicol GP, et al. Haemostatic mechanism in uterine circulation during placental separation. Br Med J 1971;2:564.
48. Klaften E, Palugvay J. Zur physiologie der Atmung in der Schwangerschaft. Arch Gynakol 1926;129:414.
49. Mobius WV. Abrung und Schwangerschaft. Munchener Medizinsche Worchenschrift 1961;103:1389.
50. Cugell DW, Frank NR, Gaensler EA, et al. Pulmonary function in pregnancy. Serial observations in normal women. American Review of Tuberculosis 1953;67:568.
51. Lehmann V, Fabel H. Lungenfunktionsuntersuchungen and Schwangergen I: lungenvolumina. Z Geburtshilfe Perinatol 1973;177:387.
52. Milne JA, Mills RJ, Howie AD, et al. Large airway functions during normal pregnancy. Br J Obstet Gynaecol 1977;84:448.
53. Templeton AA, Kelmon GR. Maternal blood-gases, (PAO_2 — P_aO_2) physiological shunt and V_d/V_t in normal pregnancy. Br J Anaesth 1976;48:1001.
54. Eng M, Butler J, Bonick JJ. Respiratory function in pregnant obese women. Am J Obstet Gynecol 1975;123:241.
55. Bader RA, Bader ME, Rose DJ, et al. Haemodynamics at rest and during exercise in normal pregnancy as studied by cardiac catheterization. J Clin Invest 1955;34:1524.
56. Lyons HA, Antonio R. The sensitivity of the respiratory centre in pregnancy and after the administration of progesterone. Trans Assoc Am Physicians 1959;72:173.

57. Schenker JC, Ben-Yoseph Y, Shapira E. Erythrocyte carbonic anhydrase B levels during pregnancy and use of oral contraceptives. Obstet Gynecol 1972;39:237.
58. Milne JA, Howie AD, Pack AI. Dyspnea during normal pregnancy. Br J Obstet Gynaecol 1978;84:448.
59. Shulman A, Herlinger H. Urinary tract dilatation in pregnancy. Br J Radiol 1975;48:638.
60. Sala NL, Rubi RA. Ureteral function in pregnant women. II: ureteral contractility during normal pregnancy. Am J Obstet Gynecol 1967;99:228.
61. Rubi RA, Sala NL. Ureteral function in pregnant women. III: effect of different positions and of fetal delivery upon ureteral tonus. Am J Obstet Gynecol 1968;101:230.
62. Iosif S, Ingermarsson I, Ulmsten U. Urodynamics studies in normal pregnancy and in puerperium. Am J Obstet Gynecol 1980;137:696.
63. Youssef AF. Cystometric studies in gynecology and obstetrics. Obstet Gynecol 1956;8:181.
64. Beck RP, Hsu N. Pregnancy, childbirth and the menopause related to the development of stress incontinence. Am J Obstet Gynecol 1965;91:820.
65. Davison JM, Hytten FE. Glomerular filtration during and after pregnancy. J Obstet Gynaecol Br Commonwealth 1974;81:588.
66. Dunlop W. Serial Changes in renal haemodynamics during normal human pregnancy. Br J Obstet Gynaecol 1981;88:1.
67. Ezimokhai M, Davison JM, Phillips PR, Dunlop W. Non-postural serial changes in renal function during the third trimester of normal human pregnancy. Br J Obstet Gynaecol 1981;88:465.
68. Lind T, Godfrey KA, Otun H, et al. Changes in serum uric acid concentrations during normal pregnancy. Br J Obstet Gynaecol 1984;91:128.
69. Dunlop W, Davidson JM. The effect of pregnancy upon the renal handling of uric acid. Br J Obstet Gynaecol 1977;84:13.
70. Davison JM, Shiells EA, Phillips PR. Serial evaluation of vasopression release and thirst in human pregnancy: the role of human chorionic gonadotropin in the osmoregulatory changes of gestation. J Clin Invest 1988;81:798.
71. Chesley LC. Renin, angiotensin and aldosterone in pregnancy. In: Chesley LC, ed. Hypertensive disorders in pregnancy. New York: Appleton-Century-Crofts, 1978:236.
72. Davison JM, Hytten FE. The effect of pregnancy on the renal handling of glucose. J Obstet Gynaecol Br Commonwealth 1975;82:374.
73. Sutherland HW, Stowers JM, McKenzie C. Simplifying the clinical problem of glycosuria in pregnancy. Lancet 1970;1:1069.
74. Lopez-Espinona I, Dhar H, Humphreys S, et al. Urinary albumin excretion in pregnancy. Br J Obstet Gynecol 1986;93:176.
75. Hytten FE, Cheyne GA. The aminoaciduria of pregnancy. J Obstet Gynaecol Br Commonwealth 1972;79:424.
76. Ulmsten U, Sundstrom G. Esophageal manometry in pregnant and nonpregnant women. Am J Obstet Gynecol 1978;132:260.
77. Sutherland CG, Atkinson JC, Brogdon BG, et al. Esophageal hiatus hernia in pregnancy. Obstet Gynecol 1956;8:261.
78. Hunt JN, Murray FA. Gastric function in pregnancy. J Obstet Gynaecol Br 1958;65:78.
79. Parry E, Shields R, Turnbull AC. Transit time in the small intestine in pregnancy. J Obstet Gynaecol Br Commonwealth 1970;77:900.
80. Parry E, Shields R, Turnbull AC. The effect of pregnancy on the colonic absorption of sodium, potassium and water. J Obstet Gynaecol Br Commonwealth 1970;77:616.
81. Christofides ND, Ghatei MA, Bloom SR, et al. Decreased plasma motilin concentrations in pregnancy. Br Med J 1982;284:1453.
82. Combes B, Adams RH. Pathophysiology of the liver in pregnancy. In: Assali NS, ed. Pathophysiology of gestation. New York: Academic Press, 1971:479.
83. Ingerslev M, Teilum G. Biopsy studies of the liver in pregnancy II. Liver biopsy on normal pregnant women. Acta Obstet Gynecol Scand 1946;24:352.
84. Munnel EW, Taylor HC Jr. Liver blood flow in pregnancy hepatic vein catheterization. J Clin Invest 1947;26:952.
85. Combes B, Shibata J, Adams R, et al. Alterations in bromsulphalein sodium-removal mechanisms from blood during normal pregnancy. J Clin Invest 1963;42:1431.
86. Mueller MN, Kappas A. Estrogen pharmacology. I: the influence of estradiol and estriol on hepatic disposal of sulfobromophthalein (BSP) in man. J Clin Invest 1964;43:1905.
87. Song CS, Kappas A. The influence of estrogens, progestins and pregnancy on the liver. Vitam Horm 1968;26:147.
88. Mendenhall SW. Serum protein concentrations in pregnancy. I: concentrations in maternal serum. Am J Obstet Gynecol 1970;106:388.
89. Braverman, DZ, Johnson ML, Kern F. Effects of pregnancy and contraceptive steroids on gallbladder function. N Engl J Med 1980;302:363.
90. Dickinson JE, Palmer SM. Gestational diabetes: pathophysiology and diagnosis. Semin Perinatol 1990;14:2.
91. Hollingsworth DR. Maternal metabolism in normal pregnancy and pregnancy complicated by diabetes mellitus. Clin Obstet Gynecol 1985;28:457.
92. Yen SSC. Metabolic homeostasis during pregnancy. In: Yen SSC, Jaffe RF, eds. Reproductive endocrinology. Philadelphia: WB Saunders, 1978:537.
93. Battaglia FC, Meschia G. Principal substrates of fetal metabolism. Physiol Rev 1978;58:499.
94. Meschia G, Battaglia FC, Haw WW, et al. Utilization of substrates by the ovine placenta in vivo. Fed Proc 1980;39:245.
95. Hollingsworth DR, Moore TR. Diabetes and pregnancy. In: Creasy RK, Resnik R, eds. Maternal-fetal medicine: principles and practice. Philadelphia: WB Saunders, 1989:925.
96. Shambaugh GE III. Carbohydrate, fat and amino acid metabolism in the pregnant woman and fetus. In: Falkner F, Tanner JM, eds. Human growth, a comprehensive treatise. 2nd ed. Vol 1. New York: Plenum Press, 1986:291.
97. Knopp RH, Warth MR, Charles D, et al. Lipoprotein metabolism in pregnancy, fat transport to the fetus and the effects of diabetes. Biol Neonate 1986;50:297.
98. Aboul-Khair SA, Crooks J, Turnbull AC, et al. The physiologic changes in thyroid function during pregnancy. Clin Sci 1964;27:195.
99. Crooks J, Aboul-Khair SA, Turnbull AC, et al. The incidence of goiter during pregnancy. Lancet 1964;2:334.
100. Long TJ, Felice ME, Hollingsworth DR. Goiter in pregnant teenagers. Am J Obstet Gynecol 1985;152:670.
101. Man EB, Reid WA, Hellegers AF, et al. Thyroid function in human pregnancy. III: serum thyroxine-binding prealbumin (TBPA) and thyroxine binding globulin (TBG) of pregnant women aged 14 through to 43 years. Am J Obstet Gynecol 1969;103:338.
102. Parker JH. Amerlex free triiodothyroxine and free thyroxine levels in normal pregnancy. Br J Obstet Gynaecol 1985;92:1234.
103. Cunningham FG, MacDonald PC, Gant NF, eds. Maternal adaptation to pregnancy. In: Williams obstetrics. Norwalk, CT: Appleton and Lange, 1989:153.
104. Ramsay I. Thyroid disease. In: deSwiet M, ed. Medical disorders in obstetrics practice. Oxford: Blackwell Scientific Publications, 1990:633.
105. Hershman JM, Starnes WR. Extraction and characterization of a

thyrotropic material from the human placenta. J Clin Invest 1969;48:923.
106. Roti E, Gnudi A, Braverman LE. The placental transport, synthesis and metabolism of hormones and drugs which affect thyroid function. Endocrinol Rev 1983;4:131.
107. Hytten FE, Leitch I. The physiology of human pregnancy. 2nd ed. Oxford: Blackwell Scientific Publications, 1971:383.
108. Gertner JM, Coustan DR, Kliger AS, et al. Pregnancy as a state of physiologic absorptive hypercalciuria. Am J Med 1986; 81:451.
109. Fogh-Anderson N, Schultz-Larsen P. Free calcium ion concentration in pregnancy. Acta Obstet Gynecol Scand 1981;60:309.
110. Whitehead M, Lane G, Young O, et al. Interrelations of calcium-regulating hormones during normal pregnancy. Br Med J 1981;283:10.
111. Allgrove J, Adami S, Manning RM, et al. Cytochemical bioassay of parathyroid hormone in maternal and cord blood. Arch Dis Child 1985;60:110.
112. Weisman Y, Harrell A, Edelstein S, et al. 1,25 Dihydroxyvitamin D_3 and 24,24-dihydroxyvitamin D in vitro synthesis by human decidua and placenta. Nature 1979;281:317.
113. Aurback GD, Marx SJ, Spiegel AM. Parathyroid hormone, calcitonin and the calciferols. In: Williams RH, ed. Textbook of endocrinology. Philadelphia: WB Saunders, 1981:922.
114. Tanaka Y, Castillo L, Wineland MJ, et al. Synergistic effect of progesterone, testosterone and estradiol in the stimulation of chick renal 25-hydroxyvitamin D-1 alpha hydroxylase. Endocrinology 1979;103:2035.
115. Anast CS. Disorders of the parathyroids. In: Kelley VC, Limbeck GA, eds. Metabolic endocrine and genetic disorders of children. New York: Harper & Row, 1974:531.
116. Ances JG, Pomerantz SH. Serum concentration of beta-MSH in human pregnancy. Am J Obstet Gynecol 1974;119:1062.
117. Thody AJ, Plummer NA, Buron JL, et al. Plasma beta-melanocyte stimulating hormone levels in pregnancy. J Obstet Gynaecol Br Commonwealth 1974;81:875.
118. Poidevin LOS. Striae gravidarum: their relationship to adrenal cortical hyperfunction. Lancet 1959;2:436.
119. Schiff BL, Kern AB. A study of postpartum alopecia. Arch Dermatol 1963;87:609.

55

CHAPTER

BIOMECHANICAL AND BIOCHEMICAL CHANGES OF THE UTERUS AND CERVIX DURING PREGNANCY

Niels Uldbjerg, Axel Forman, Lone K. Petersen, Kristjar Skajaa, and Danny Svane

Labor is the end result of coordinated myometrial contractions and cervical dilatation. The basis of this process is the functional changes that take place in the cervix and myometrium during late pregnancy and labor. There is abundant evidence that these alterations result from local processes within the two areas and the fetoplacental unit. The cervix is primarily composed of connective tissue elements, and cervical ripening during pregnancy is characterized by decreased resistance to dilatation due to changes in the collagen and the proteoglycans. Likewise, a ripening process takes place within the myometrium. Thus, improved cell-to-cell communication due to formation of gap junctions and enhanced sensitivity to endogenous agents like oxytocin and prostanoids are essential for the development of coordinated labor activity. These changes are a prerequisite for successful induction of labor, and knowledge of the mechanisms involved is crucial for rational application of the therapeutic principles for inhibition or stimulation of the labor process. In this chapter, we review these basic properties of the cervix and myometrium.

In several species, the fetal pituitary–adrenal system determines the onset of labor through changes in estrogen and progesterone secretion, which controls the release of prostaglandins. The role of these fetal mechanisms is less obvious in humans, but the importance of prostaglandins in controlling the labor process is widely accepted.[1] The synthesis of these compounds is therefore briefly summarized. The subsequent sections will focus on the cervical and myometrial changes involved in the onset and maintenance of labor and the therapeutic possibilities to influence these mechanisms. Finally, the clinical application of these therapeutic principles is briefly reviewed.

PROSTAGLANDIN SYNTHESIS IN THE UTERUS

Prostaglandins are locally active hormone-like substances that are synthesized by nearly every tissue in the body. The biosynthesis of prostaglandins and related compounds proceeds via a series of reactions controlled by enzymes known collectively as prostaglandin synthetases.

The precursors of prostaglandins are 20-carbon fatty acids, which are converted to prostaglandins with one, two, or three double bonds, the 1, 2, and 3 series, depending on the initial substrate available to the synthesis system.[2] The fatty acids are liberated from cell membrane constituents, the phospholipids, by means of phospholipases, which constitute the rate-limiting step. Arachidonic acid and the subsequent 2-series of prostaglandins represent the predominant pathway (Fig. 55-1), but substrate competition through enhanced intake of the long-chain n-3 fatty acids may influence the relative formation of prostaglandins of the 2 and 3 series. Through this mechanism, enhanced intake of marine fat has been suggested to prolong gestation by inhibiting the production of prostaglandins important for the initiation of labor.[3]

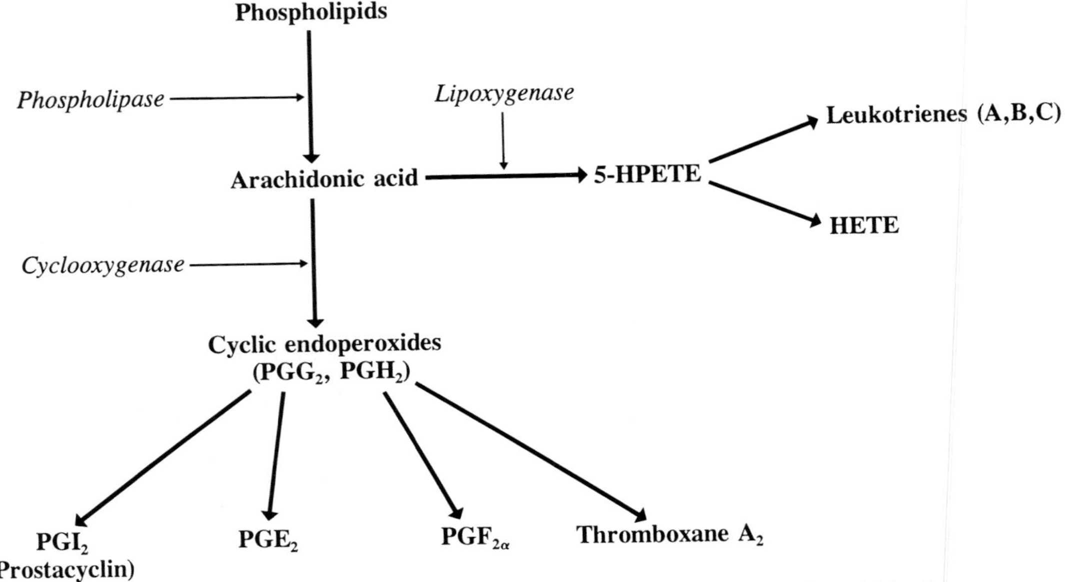

FIGURE 55–1. Schematic presentation of prostaglandin synthesis. Release of arachidonic acid from phospholipids is the rate-limiting step. Prostaglandins of the 2 series are then formed through the intermediate endoperoxide step. Arachidonic acid may alternatively be transformed into leukotrienes and lipoxins, such as Hydroxy-eicosatetraenoic acid (HETE) through a lipoxygenase.

The initial control of arachidonic acid release (Fig. 55-2) is exerted by changes in the activity of phospholipase A_2, or phospholipase C and diacylglycerol (DAG) lipase.[4] Which pathway is more important is uncertain. Phospholipase C is activated through agonist–receptor interaction at the cell membrane level by various agonists, resulting in the release of inositol phosphates.[5] Inositol phosphates seem to mediate the release of intracellular calcium for contractile activation.[6] In the rat myometrium, part of the oxytocin response seems to be mediated through this pathway,[7] but data on the human myometrium are so far not available. The inositol phosphate pathway further liberates arachidonic acid through the breakdown of DAG, which may represent a link between contractile activation following membrane receptor activation and intracellular prostaglandin synthesis.[5]

Phospholipase A_2 is activated by a varity of physical and chemical agents (eg, infection, trauma) and initiates prostaglandin synthesis by directly liberating arachidonic acid from phospholipids.[1]

The activity of phospholipases is influenced by the intracellular Ca^{++} concentration, but whether the ion actually has a regulatory role is uncertain. Local factors that might promote calcium influx for phospholipase activity in amnion cells include leukotriene B4 and platelet-activating factor.[8]

The synthesis of prostaglandins from arachidonic acid proceeds via the formation of the short-lived cyclic intermediates, endoperoxides. Cyclic endoperoxides such as prostaglandin G_2 and H_2 are potent vasoconstrictors and uterotonic agents.[9,10] By an enzymatic mechanism, other prostaglandin compounds, such as prostacyclin (PGI_2), thromboxane A2, PGE_2, PGD_2, and PGF2α, are synthesized from these compounds.

Alternative pathways for arachidonic acid include metabolization to lipoxygenase products, particularly leukotrienes, as well as reincorporation into phospho-

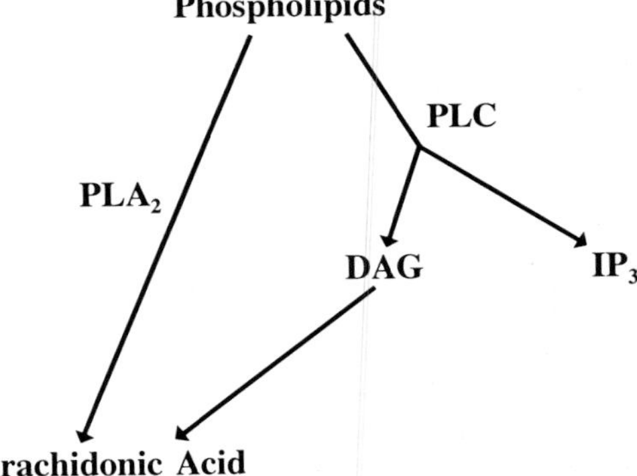

FIGURE 55–2. Phospholipase pathways. Arachidonic acid is released through phospholipase A_2 (PLA_2) action on phosphatidylinositol (PI). This represents the rate-limiting step in prostaglandin synthesis. Phospholipase C (PLC) produces two compounds with second-messenger function from PI: inositol triphosphate (IP_3), which serves to release calcium from intracellular stores, and diacylglycerol (DAG), which enhances the sensitivity of the contractile proteins for Ca^{++} DAG may subsequently be degraded to arachidonic acid.

lipids.[1] The role of leukotrienes in the parturition process is, however, unclear.

MODULATION OF SYNTHESIS IN PREGNANCY

Although no firm correlation between the levels of estrogen and progesterone and prostaglandin synthesis has been demonstrated in man, a role for steroid hormones in the control of these mechanisms is still possible.[1] Thus, in vitro data suggest that prostaglandin synthesis in human endometrium is stimulated by estrogen, and this effect can be blocked by progesterone.[8,11] Moreover, progesterone inhibits phospholipase A2 activity in human endometrial cells pulse-labelled with tritiated arachidonic acid.[12]

Oxytocin stimulates release of arachidonic acid and $PGF_{2\alpha}$ by decidual tissue.[13,14] Administration of $PGF_{2\alpha}$ in rats near term stimulates the formation of oxytocin and prostaglandin receptors,[15] and the concentrations of myometrial and possible decidual oxytocin receptors increase with the onset of labor.[16] Prostaglandins further seem to enhance gap junction formation.[17] Taken together, these mechanisms might provide part of the cascade process needed for the initiation of labor.

Platelet-activating factor (PAF) is a phospholipid that increases $Ca^{2}+$ concentrations in platelets, from which its name is derived, and seems to act on amniotic cells as well.[17a] Increased $Ca^{2}+$ activates phospholipase A_2 and phospholipase C, both of which promote arachidonic acid and prostaglandin synthesis.[1] The preimplantation human embryo secretes PAF, and this may have relevance to the local maternal recognition of pregnancy. The suggestion that PAF takes part in the initiation of labor is, however, controversial.

Systemic infection, whether acute or chronic, is strongly associated with preterm labor.[18] Preterm labor caused by chorioamnionitis is associated with the presence of substances in amniotic fluid (such as PAF and leukotrienes) with the capacity for stimulating prostaglandin synthesis. The microorganisms most strongly associated with preterm labor have a high phospholipase A2 activity, and there is good reason to suggest that local infection may initiate preterm labor by activating the prostaglandin synthetase system.[19]

A likely mediator of parturition following amniotomy is the production of prostaglandin F. An immediate rise in the concentration of the metabolite of prostaglandin F (PGFM) has been demonstrated,[20,21] and the concentration of PGFM 2 hours after the procedure does seem to be related to the induction–delivery interval.[21] Moreover, the concentration of the major metabolite of $PGF_{2\alpha}$ has been shown to be doubled 5 minutes after vaginal examination that included sweeping of the membranes, as well as after amniotomy.[8]

Human seminal fluid contains a number of prostaglandins (PGE and PGF compounds) in amounts that are less than the vaginal dose required to induce an apparent uterine response. However, an effect on uterine contractility is still possible, because during intercourse uterine reactivity to prostaglandins may be increased by different hormonal and neuronal stimuli associated with sexual stimulation.[22]

DIFFERENT COMPOSITION OF CERVICAL AND MYOMETRIAL TISSUES

The maximum contractile ability of cervical biopsies from non-pregnant women is only 3% to 10% of that in the fundus (Fig. 55-3). This difference probably does not change during pregnancy.[23] This is in accordance with histological studies that have shown that smooth muscle cells constitute less than 8% of the distal cervix and 30% of the uterine body.[24] Furthermore, the collagen concentration in the cervix is comparable to that found in skin, tendons, and other fibrous connective tissues, whereas the concentration in the fundus is only 50% of this amount.

CERVICAL CONNECTIVE TISSUE DURING PREGNANCY

Mechanical properties of the cervical tissues change markedly during pregnancy. Thus, the force needed to rupture cervical tissue taken from biopsies from term

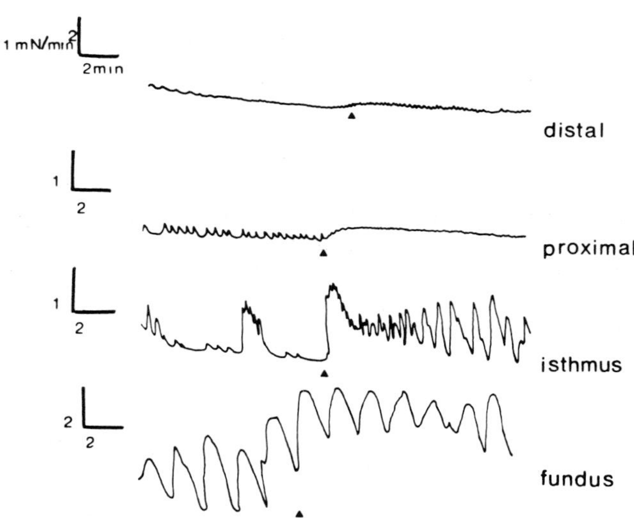

FIGURE 55–3. Maximum muscular contractions of tissue specimens from the distal cervix, proximal cervix, isthmus, and fundus in a non-pregnant woman. Tissue strips were mounted under physiological conditions in organ baths, and maximum contractions were induced by vasopressin 3×10^{-8} M.

pregnant women is only 8% of the force needed to rupture similar tissue obtained from non-pregnant women (Fig. 55-4).[25] A special instrument that determines the force needed to dilate the cervical canal has been used to measure the cervical consistency in vivo. This cervical distensibility index is 1 cm/kg in non-pregnant women, 3 cm/kg at a gestational age of 22 weeks, and 8 cm/kg at term.[26] These figures explain why dilatation of the cervical canal by means of Hegar's stents is less difficult in pregnant women compared to non-pregnant women. Furthermore, they reflect the so-called "ripening process" of the cervix, which takes place during pregnancy and which can be detected to some extent by palpation. In early pregnancy, the signs of Goodell and Hegar represent the softening of the cervix and the isthmus. At term, the Bishop score is often used to describe the ripeness of the cervix.[27] This score includes the length of the collum, the dilatation of the cervical canal, and the consistency of the tissue (Table 55-1). A low Bishop score indicates that the cervix is not yet prepared to dilate and that induction of labor will be associated with a high risk for prolonged duration of labor, instrumental delivery, and eventually cesarean section.

Collagen dominates fibrous connective tissues and constitutes 85% of the dry weight in cervical biopsies from non-pregnant women.[28] The collagen fibrils are made up by tropocollagen molecules, which are linked together by covalent cross links. The number of cross links is rather low in newly synthesized collagen, but increases with the age of the fibril. On electron micrographs, the fibrils are cross-striated due to a characteristic staggering of the tropocollagen molecules. The dermatan sulfate proteoglycans, which belong to the glycosaminoglycans/acid mucopolysaccharides, constitute another family of macromolecules in the cervix. They are made up of different core proteins, to which one to 15 long, negatively charged dermatan sulfate chains are attached.[29] Each dermatan sulfate is composed of about 50 sugar residues linked together in a long chain. One of these proteoglycans, called PG-S2 or decorin, has only one side chain per core protein and a high affinity for collagen. It covers the surfaces of the collagen fibrils and seems to influence the fibril formation and to bind the fibrils together into thicker bundles or fibers (Fig. 55-5). This proteoglycan is quantitatively dominating in the non-pregnant cervix, where it constitutes 85% of the dermatan sulfate proteoglycans.[30] Another proteoglycan is named PG-S1 or biglycan because it contains two dermatan sulfate chains. It has no affinity for collagen but occupies the space between the fibrils and tends to disorganize them.

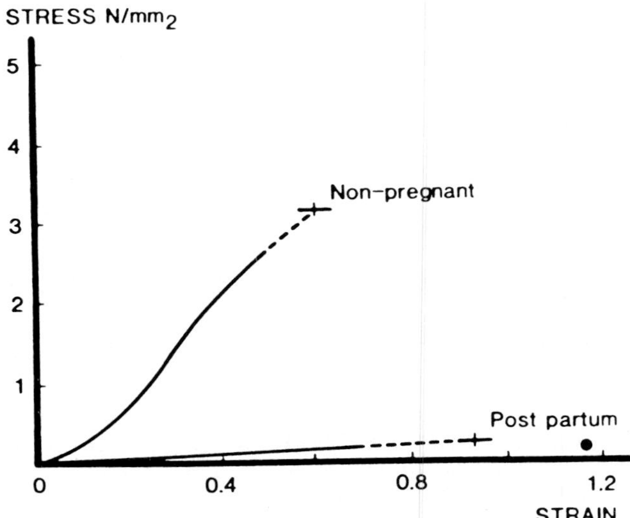

FIGURE 55-4. Stress–strain relationship in cervical specimens from non-pregnant and postpartum women. Tissue strips were gradually extended until rupture occurred. The strain (relative elongation) and the stress (force applied to the biopsy) were recorded. SEM for stress values are marked by bars. Solid circles represent a biopsy from a woman at 18 weeks gestation with cervical incompetence. (Rechberger T, Uldbjerg N, Oxlund H. Connective tissue changes in the cervix during normal pregnancy and pregnancy complicated by cervical incompetence. Obstet Gynecol 1988;71:563.)

TABLE 55-1. BISHOP SCORE FOR ASSESSMENT OF CERVICAL RIPENING

	POINTS AWARDED			
CRITERION	0	1	2	3
Cervical dilatation (cm)	0	1–2	3–4	5–6
Cervical effacement (%)	0–30	40–50	60–70	≥80
Cervical consistency	Firm	Medium	Soft	
Cervical position	Posterior	Central	Anterior	
Station (in relation to the spines)	3 cm above	2 cm above	1–0 cm above	1–2 cm below

Bishop EH. Pelvic scoring for elective induction. Obstet Gynecol 1964;24:266.

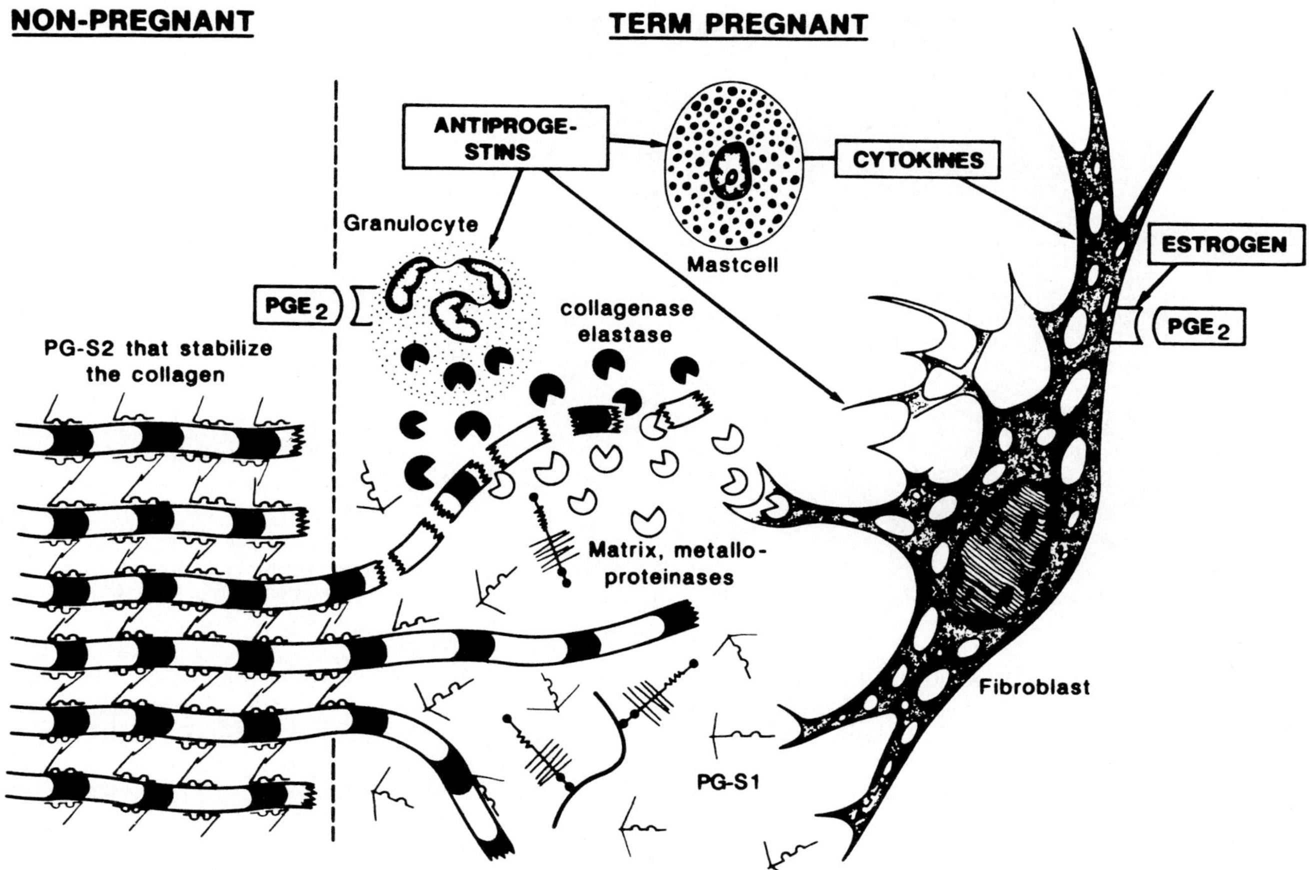

FIGURE 55–5. Aspects of changes in collagen during cervical ripening. In the non-pregnant woman, the collagen concentration is high and the collagen is stabilized by PG-S2 proteoglycans. At term of pregnancy, the collagen concentration has decreased due to high activities of collagenolytic enzymes secreted by fibroblasts and inflammatory cells. Furthermore, the collagen fibrils become disorganized by PG-S1 proteoglycans. Estrogens sensitize the fibroblasts to prostaglandin, perhaps by increasing the number of receptors and mast cells, macrophages, and other inflammatory cells, which influence the system by secretion of leukotriene and other cytokines.

Although the interactions between collagen and proteoglycans are not fully understood, it can be concluded that the mechanical properties of the cervix are determined by the concentration of collagen, by the number of cross links between the tropocollagen molecules, and by the presence of different dermatan sulfate proteoglycans. Therefore, most efforts to explain the mechanical aspects of the ripening process have focused on these components.

Histological examinations have shown that cervical biopsies taken at term seem to contain much less collagen than similar biopsies from non-pregnant women.[31] In addition, the collagen fibers appear to be dissociated into their fibrillar components (Fig. 55-6), and in some areas they have almost disappeared and been replaced by an unidentified amorphous substance.[32]

The cervical collagen concentration has also been determined by biochemical techniques.[33] In accordance with the mechanical and histological changes described above, it decreases in early pregnancy, and at term it is only 35% of the non-pregnant value (Fig. 55-7). At the same time, the number of cross links are reduced, leaving fewer stable collagen fibrils. The clinical importance of the cervical collagen concentration at term is shown in Figure 55-8, demonstrating that, in normal women, the duration of cervical dilatation during labor is directly proportional to the concentration of collagen. It has also been shown that women with prolonged duration of labor have both a pathologically high concentration of collagen and an increased number of cross links.[34] Of course, even these women have much lower collagen concentrations than non-pregnant women.

The concentration of cervical collagen in non-pregnant women depends on parity. In nulligravidae it

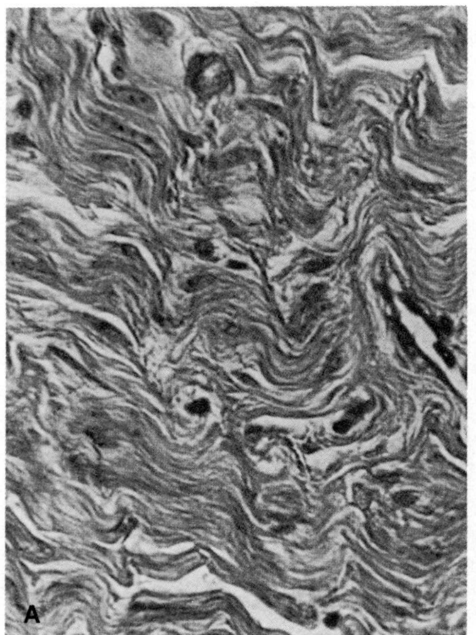

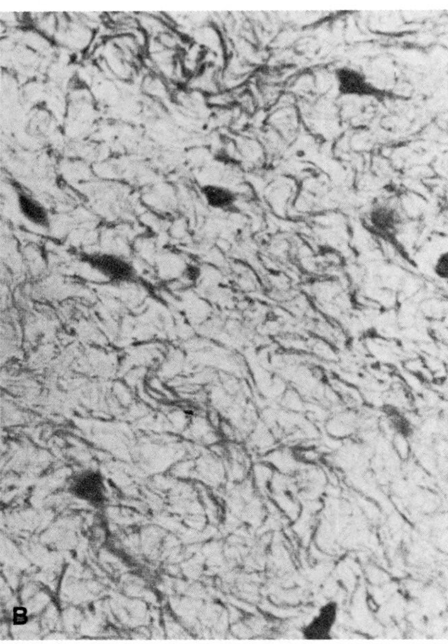

FIGURE 55–6. Histological changes in cervical collagen during pregnancy. (**A**) Non-pregnant. (**B**) Immediately postpartum. Note the dissociation of the collagen fibrils and the appearance of clear spaces between the fibers postpartum (Milligan's tricrome stain for collagen, magnified ×835). (Danforth DN, Buckingham JC, Roddick JW. Connective tissue changes incident to cervical effacement. Am J Obstet Gynecol 1960;80:939.)

has been found to be 195 μg/mg wet tissue weight, whereas it is 166 μg/mg in nulliparae with one previous abortion, and 128 μg/mg in women with previous labor.[35] Thus, it is obvious that the regeneration of the cervix after delivery is only partial, a factor that might explain why the course of labor differs between primi- and multiparous women. Furthermore, the positive correlation between cervical collagen concentration at term and the duration of labor is much more apparent in primiparae than in multiparae.[25]

The role of proteoglycans has been discussed, suggesting they form the amorphous substance that appears during pregnancy and increase the water-binding capacity of cervical tissue. However, these hypotheses have been rejected. Today, it is well established that an increase in the ratio between the concentrations of dermatan sulfate proteoglycans and collagen is essential for the mechanical characteristics of the tissue.[36] This increased ratio is due not only to the decreased collagen concentration, but also to an increased synthesis of PG-S1 (see Fig. 55-5), the dermatan sulfate proteoglycan that seems to disorganize the collagen.[37] Because research in rats has not been able to demonstrate a decrease in the amount of collagen, this increased ratio might be the only fact that explains the ripening process. Also, in the early postpartum period, there exists a close temporal relationship between the changes in the mechanical properties and the dermatan sulfate proteoglycan-to-collagen ratio.[36]

The turnover of both collagen and proteoglycan in the cervix is very high at term. This explains why the mechanical properties can change within hours, eg,

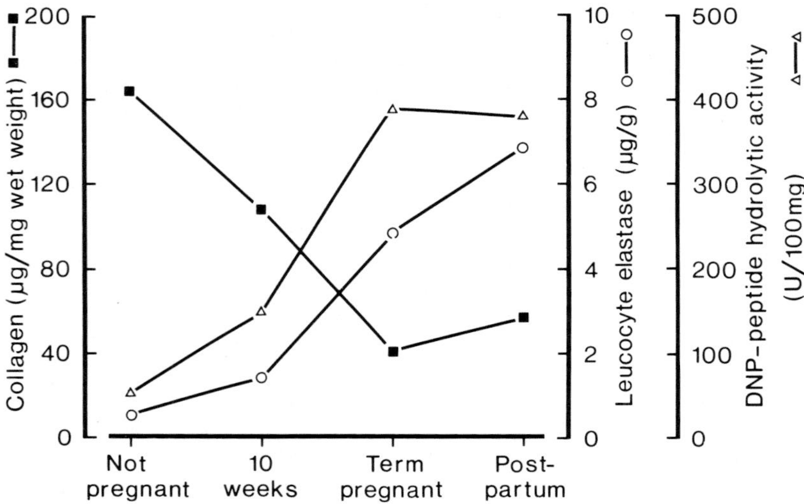

FIGURE 55–7. Collagen concentration, collagenolytic activity given as DNP-peptide hydrolytic activity and leukocyte elastase in cervical biopsies from non-pregnant and pregnant women, as well as immediately after delivery. (Uldbjerg N, Ulmsten U, Ekman G. The ripening of the human uterine cervix in terms of connective tissue biochemistry. Clinical Obstetrics and Gynecology 1983;26.)

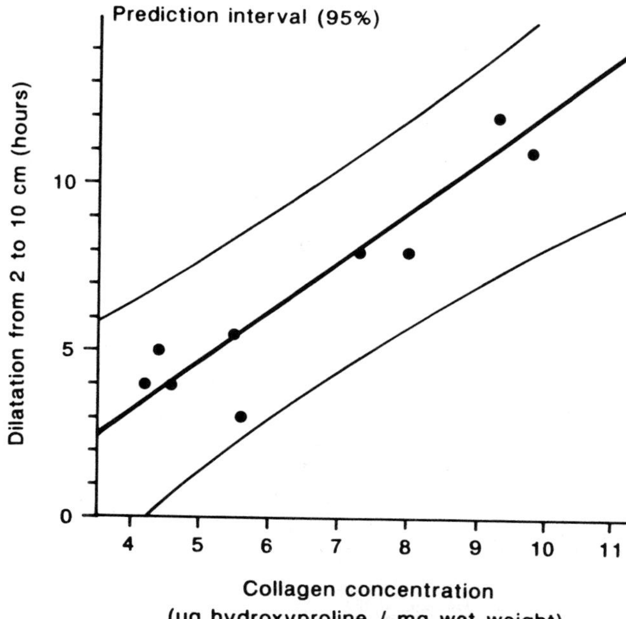

FIGURE 55–8. Cervical dilatation time in active labor as a function of the cervical collagen concentration. (Uldbjerg N, Ekman G, Malmstrøm A, Olsson K, Ulmsten U. Ripening of the uterine cervix related to changes in collagen, glycosaminoglycans, and collagenolytic activity. Am J Obstet Gynecol 1983;147:662.)

after treatment with prostaglandin E_2. The increased synthesis has been studied in vitro, where the incorporation of labelled precursors in cervical biopsies has been followed.[37,38] The catabolism has been evaluated by determinations of concentrations and activities of various collagenolytic enzymes from fibroblasts and inflammatory cells: matrix metalloproteinase 1 or fibroblast collagenase, the intracellular enzyme cathepsin D, leukocyte elastase, and leukocyte collagenase. The changes in fibroblast-derived collagenase activity are not well established. Most authors, however, agree that it is increased by a factor of 5 to 10 at term, as demonstrated in Figure 55-5, whereas some discrepancies concerning the demonstration of a further increase during labor exist. Also, the activity of the collagenolytic enzymes from leukocytes increases (see Fig. 55-5). Furthermore, histological studies have shown that the degradation and the disorganization of collagen is most pronounced in those areas where an infiltration and degranulation of polymorphonuclear and eosinophilic leukocytes can be demonstrated.[31] Thus, cervical ripening involves many elements of inflammatory reactions[39]; and mast cells, macrophages, interleukins, and other growth factors might also be of importance (see Fig. 55-5).

It is difficult to evaluate the relative importance of proteoglycans and collagenolytic enzymes in cervical ripening, but it seems to differ between species. As mentioned above, there is no need to invoke collagenolysis in explaining the dilatation of the rat cervix. However, collagenase may play an important role in cervical dilatation in spherical uteri, such as that of humans, where extensive effacement is required.[36]

CERVICAL INCOMPETENCE

The diagnosis of cervical incompetence is based on a history of repeated spontaneous abortions after the 12th week of pregnancy or spontaneous preterm labor without significant myometrial contractions. Clinically, the cervix is soft and unable to restrain the increasing pressure from the growing fetus. This reduced strength has been demonstrated in both pregnant and non-pregnant women with a history of cervical incompetence.[25,40] The condition is caused by an abnormal composition of the cervix, having an increased number of smooth muscle cells and a decreased number of cross links, such giving a weak collagen.[41]

The aim of treatment is to reinforce the cervix and prevent dilatation. Several methods, including that described by McDonald,[42] use different techniques that apply a tight, nonabsorbable suture around the cervix in the first trimester.

HORMONAL CONTROL OF CERVICAL RIPENING

PROSTAGLANDINS

It is well established that prostaglandins E_2 and $F_{2\alpha}$ are involved in cervical ripening.[43] Thus, cervical tissue homogenates produce these two prostaglandins together with prostacyclin and lipoxygenase, and free PGE_2 and $PGF_{2\alpha}$ receptors have been demonstrated in the microsome fraction. Furthermore, prostaglandin treatment induces a cervical softening within hours in women with unfavorable cervical states. Clinically, this pharmacologically induced cervical ripening is similar to the physiological ripening of the cervix that normally occurs over several weeks in late pregnancy.

The mechanical properties of cervical biopsies taken after PGE_2-induced cervical ripening are comparable to those observed after the physiological ripening.[44] This effect on the cervix is present even when myometrial contractions are not induced by the treatment, ie, it is independent of myometrial activity. It has been suggested that PGE_2 might have a higher cervical specificity than $PGF_{2\alpha}$.[45] This difference is only marginal, however, if present at all. The mechanism of this action is not completely understood. Electron microscopic examinations have shown that PGE_2 treatment in the first trimester induces changes in cervical stromatic tissue similar to those normally seen in late pregnancy.[46] At term, collagen concentration decreases to normal levels when unripe cervices with pathologically high collagen concentrations are treated with PGE_2.[34] The collagenase activity is doubled, but this increase can hardly account for the striking clinical effect of the treatment; therefore, alterations in the concentration of protease inhibitors such as tissue inhibitor of metalloprotease (TIMP) might be of importance. The most pronounced biochemical change has been demonstrated in proteoglycan synthesis, where PGE_2 induced a very marked increase of the synthesis of PG-S1 (which disorganizes the collagen), while that of PG-S2 (which stabilizes the collagen) is decreased (see Fig. 55-5).

RELAXIN

The hormone relaxin is a polypeptide with a structure very similar to that of insulin. It is produced during pregnancy in the corpus luteum, as well as in the decidua and placenta. The physiological importance of relaxin is well established in several species, where it induces cervical softening, loosening of the pelvic girdle, and decreased myometrial activity during pregnancy.[47] In women, however, the role of relaxin is uncertain, because the highest serum relaxin concentration is found during the first trimester, contrary to many other species, where the concentration rises continuously during pregnancy and often shows an abrupt fall immediately prior to parturition.[48] Also, the inhibitory action on the myometrial activity in vitro is less pronounced in women.[49]

Relaxin-induced cervical ripening has been studied extensively in rats, where histological and biochemical changes have been found to be very similar to those found in physiological ripening: the collagen fibrils split up, the concentration of collagen decreases, and the concentration of dermatan sulfate increases, ie, the ratio of dermatan sulfate to collagen increases.[50] Pharmacological induction of cervical ripening in term pregnant women by means of local application of porcine relaxin has shown promising results, because it caused a significant increase in Bishop scores and a reduction in the duration of labor.[49,51]

Cervical priming by relaxin may be advantageous compared to prostaglandins, because relaxin does not stimulate myometrial contractions. This is of special importance in patients with a distressed fetus, ie, cases of intrauterine growth retardation or preeclampsia, where the fetus is susceptible to further reduction in the fetoplacental circulation induced by contractions.

STEROIDS

Estrogens seem to be involved in physiological cervical ripening, because during pregnancy serum concentrations of estrogens rise simultaneously with the softening of the uterine cervix and after treatment with dehydroepiandrosterone sulfate (DHAS). DHAS is metabolized in the placenta, producing 178β-estradiol, which in turn induces cervical ripening.[52] However, normal vaginal delivery can be obtained in most pregnancies with very low 17β-estradiol levels due to placental steroid sulfatase deficiency.[53] However, at-term estrogen treatment causes only limited cervical ripening.[54,55]

Intravenous infusion of 17β-estradiol induces histological changes similar to those of physiological cervical ripening.[56] This is associated with an increased collagenolytic activity,[57] which might be mediated by an increased prostaglandin synthesis.[58,59] Furthermore, estrogens sensitize the cervix to prostaglandins, perhaps by increasing the number of prostaglandin receptors (see Fig. 55-5). This explains why PGE_2 has no effect on the cervix in non-pregnant women, in whom the estrogen levels are low, and why the initiation of labor by PGE_2 at term is most successful in women with high estrogen levels.[60] Clinically, this principle has been used in prostaglandin-induced second-trimester abortions, where estrogen pretreatment shortened the induction–abortion interval.[61]

The "progesterone block" hypothesis suggested by Csapo suggested that parturition was initiated by a sudden fall in serum progesterone concentration. Although this fall has not been demonstrated in women, local changes of the progesterone-to-estrogen ratio in the amniotic fluid may be of importance in the initiation of parturition.[62]

Antiprogestins, which block progesterone at the receptor level, induce cervical ripening in the first trimester,[63] and the resulting histological changes are similar to those described in late pregnancy.[64] Although antiprogestins increase the myometrial activity by increasing the number of gap junctions,[65,66] cervical ripening seems to be independent of myometrical activity.[67]

Clinically, antiprogestins have been introduced as a nonsurgical method for termination of early pregnancies. When used alone for 3 to 4 days, abortion is achieved in 70% of the women; whereas the addition of a single, relatively small dose of prostaglandin at the end of treatment improves the outcome to more than 95%.[68] This treatment seems less successful after 49 days of gestation.

FETAL MEMBRANES

The collagen concentration of fetal membranes is comparable to that of the pregnant cervix. There might be some decrease in this concentration during the last weeks of pregnancy. After normal vaginal delivery, the thickness at the rupture site is less than 50% of that at other locations. It is unknown whether this thinning is due to a degradation of the membranes or whether it is secondary to the forces of labor.[69] There is no marked histological change in the collagen of the membranes at term, but the presence of inflammatory cells and leukocyte elastase in high concentrations at the rupture site suggests that a ripening process may also exist in the fetal membranes.[70] Preterm, prelabor rupture of membranes is associated with a reduced collagen concentration, a reduced number of cross links, and increased collagenolytic activity.[71,72] These characteristics may be determined by subclinical infections with bacteria that either secrete collagenolytic enzymes or change the arachidonic acid metabolism of the membranes. Alternatively, they may be caused by a structural deficiency that is also found in the intracranial arteries of some newborns, placing them at risk for intracranial hemorrhage.[73]

ENDOGENOUS CONTROL OF MYOMETRIAL ACTIVITY AT TERM

Myometrial contractile activity is controlled by a variety of endogenous mechanisms, which show profound changes during pregnancy. Moreover, the fetus, the fetal membranes, and the decidua participate in controlling myometrial activity through the synthesis of agents such as steroids and prostanoids. Finally, evidence is accumulating that circulating oxytocin is involved in the labor process. In this section, we will review the endogenous mechanisms involved in the control of myometrial activity and the pharmacological possibilities that may influence labor contractions.

Among the multiple structural changes of the myometrium during pregnancy, some specific characteristics are important in understanding the endogenous mechanisms involved in the control of labor. In several species, including humans, pregnancy seems to involve a progressive degeneration of the myometrial,[74–77] but not of the cervical autonomous neuronal supply.[75] Thus, a neuronal influence on the labor process is possible through effects on the cervix,[78] while direct sympathetic influence on myometrial contractile activity seems of minor importance at term.

Another specialized property of the term myometrium is the development of cell-to-cell adhesions known as gap junctions. These structures represent opposed membrane areas of low resistance for transmission of membrane events and form the basis for rapid propagation of contractile activation with subsequent coordinated myometrial contractions.[17,79] Although low concentrations of gap junctions are found in the quiescent myometrium, term as well as preterm labor are associated with markedly increased levels.[79] The hormonal control of the formation of these gap junctions includes stimulation by estrogens and inhibition by progesterone. Moreover, prostanoids enhance gap junction formation.[17,66,80] The appearance of these ultrastructural changes is an important part of what might be described as myometrial ripening, because these changes accompany the cervical ripening presenting to the clinician at vaginal examination.

MYOMETRIAL EXCITATION–CONTRACTION COUPLING

Human myometrial smooth muscle displays spontaneous depolarization of the cell membrane with subsequent spike activity, leading to contractile activation.[81] These events are myogenic, ie, they occur in the absence of stimulation. Myometrial contractile activation induced by endogenous agonists and drugs is preceded by enhancement of the depolarization and spike activity.[82–84] This spike activity is sensitive to removal of external calcium and calcium-entry blockade by the organic calcium antagonists,[81,82,85] suggesting the involvement of transmembrane calcium influx through so-called voltage-operated channels (VOCs), ie, membrane channels activated by membrane depolarization (Fig. 55-9).[83,86] This type of contractile activation is often designed electromechanical coupling.[87] The transmembrane influx of calcium may directly influence the contractile proteins (see below), but more likely "triggers" further release of calcium from intracellular stores such as the sarcoplasmatic reticulum.[83]

Agonists and drugs further produce contractile activation through other membrane mechanisms, the receptor-operated channels (ROCs), and may further effect calcium release from intracellular calcium stores.[83] These mechanisms are also called pharmacomechanical coupling.[87] The membrane channels involved are intimately connected with the phosphatidylinositol pathway, which provides IP_3 as the secondary messenger needed to release calcium from the intracellular stores, most notably the endoplasmic reticulum.[88] Furthermore, the breakdown of phosphatidylinositol results in formation of DAG, which seems to increase the calcium sensitivity of the contractile proteins. The latter mechanism may be essential for sustained contractile activation, because Ca^{++} mobilized from the internal stores seems to be rapidly expelled through the plasma membrane by mechanisms discussed below. Compounds like oxytocin and prostaglandins are further suggested to directly effect release of calcium from intracellular calcium stores.[6]

The relative importance of the various sources of calcium for contractile activation has traditionally been evaluated by the in ability to contract in calcium-free medium and by testing the effects of organic calcium antagonists. This is a heterogenous group of drugs believed to act preferentially through inhibition of transmembrane calcium influx. Among the most potent are the dihydropyridines, such as nifedipine, nitrendipine, and isradipine, which seem to selectively affect the VOC-type calcium channels.[89] In fact, a dihydropyridine receptor seems to be located on these channels, allowing for agonist–receptor-binding studies. Subtypes of VOCs with different sensitivities for dihydropyridines exist; variations in the tissue density, functional state and relative amounts of these subtypes imply marked regional differences in the effects of calcium antagonists such as nifedipine.[89]

Human isolated myometrium shows marked dependency on extracellular calcium for contractile activation (see Fig. 55-9).[84] Although this might support the importance of transmembrane calcium influx in excitation–contraction coupling, an alternative explanation could be rapid depletion of calcium from intracellular stores into the extracellular medium. Of importance,

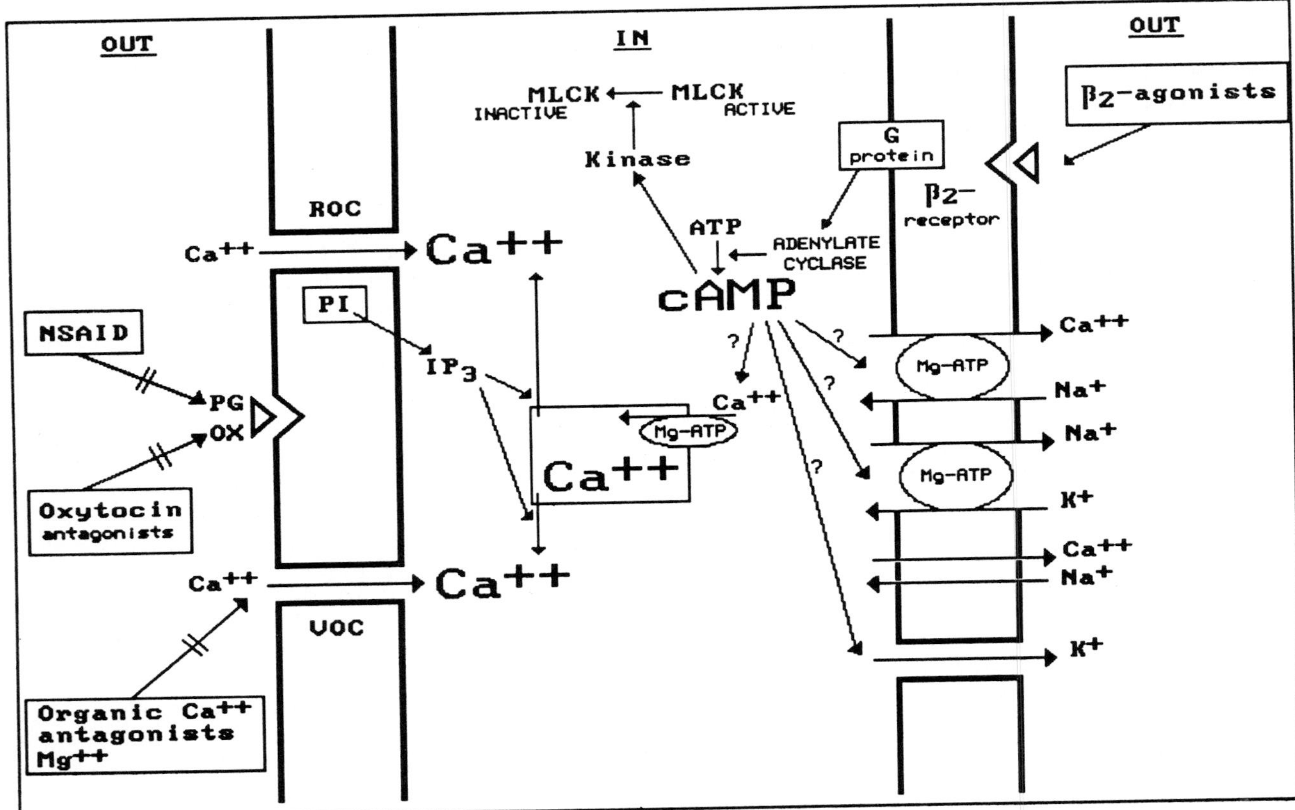

FIGURE 55–9. Mechanisms involved in mobilization of calcium for contractile activation and principles for myometrial relaxation. The left part of the figure shows factors that tend to increase the intracellular Ca^{++} concentration, and the right part shows factors that tend to lower the Ca^{++} concentration. Ca^{++} enters the cell through voltage-operated calcium channels (VOC) or receptor-operated channels (ROC). In the myometrium, ROCs are activated by oxytocin (OX) or prostaglandins (PG). The activation of ROCs is associated with a breakdown of certain membrane constituents, ie, phosphoinositides (PI). Inositoltriphosphate (IP_3) is a product of this breakdown and serves as a second messenger for the receptor activation in mobilizing Ca^{++} from intracellular stores. Mechanisms for lowering the intracellular Ca^{++} concentration include extrusion of Ca^{++} through the plasma membrane or re-uptake into the sarcoplasmatic reticulum by an Mg^{++}–ATP-dependent Ca^{++} pump, a Ca^{++}-Na exchange mechanism coupled to activation of the Mg^{++}–ATP-dependent Na^+-K^+ pump or an increase in membrane K^+ conductance. cAMP is produced by adenylate cyclase as a result of adrenoreceptor occupation and seems to stimulate the Ca^{++}-extrusion mechanisms. Moreover, cAMP activates a proteinkinase that deactivates the myosine light chain kinase (MLCK). The possible influences of contractile activation include organic calcium-channel antagonists and Mg^{++}, which inhibit the Ca^{++} flux through VOCs. In addition, oxytocin antagonists and inhibitors of the cyclooxygenase-dependent prostaglandin synthesis, NSAIDs, may decrease myometrial activity. Finally, stimulation of the adrenoreceptors by β_2-agonists increases the intracellular level of cAMP.

however, is that spontaneous contractions as well as the predominant, phasic component of responses to oxytocin and $PGF_{2\alpha}$ show marked sensitivity to dihydropyridine calcium antagonists.[90] This supports the view that calcium influx through VOCs is an important event during contractile activation of the human myometrium. The tonic component of responses to oxytocin and $PGF_{2\alpha}$ is unaffected by dihydropyridine calcium antagonists and may reflect activation of ROCs, as well as intracellular mobilization of calcium.[91]

CONTRACTILE PROTEINS IN MYOMETRIAL SMOOTH MUSCLE

As in skeletal muscle, the contractile proteins in smooth muscle cells consist of thin and thick filaments, referred to as actin and myosin, and the sliding filament hypothesis[92] is valid for both types of muscle.[93] Although the contraction in skeletal muscle is regulated by Ca^{++} binding to the troponin–tropomyosin complex located on the actin filament, contraction of smooth muscle is dependent on phosphorylation of the light chain of the myosin filament catalyzed by the enzyme myosine light-chain kinase (MLCK) (Fig. 55-10). When intracellular Ca^{++} concentration rises, Ca^{++} combines with the protein calmodulin, and this complex activates the myosine light-chain kinase in the presence of ATP and Mg^{++}. When the light chain of the myosin is phosphorylated by MLCK, it is able to interact with the actin filament to cause a contraction of the muscle cell.

Besides the Ca^{++}–calmodulin complex, the MLCK activity is influenced by cyclic adenosine 3′-5′-monophosphate cAMP, because this compound activates a protein kinase, which phosphorylates the MLCK to an inactive enzyme.[94] Accordingly, factors that tend to increase intracellular cAMP levels may cause a desensitization of the contractile proteins for Ca^{++}. cAMP may further interfere with myometrial excitation–contraction coupling by decreasing the Ca^{++}-binding capacity of calmodulin.[94]

At the same time in which the intracellular Ca^{++} concentration is increased, several mechanisms are involved in order to decrease the intracellular Ca^{++} concentration. Extrusion of Ca^{++} through the plasma membrane or reuptake into the sarcoplasmatic reticulum by an ATP-dependent Ca^{++} pump seems to be the most important mechanism, but also a Ca^{++}-Na exchange mechanism is probably present.[95] An intracellular Ca^{++} concentration below 0.1 μM results in relaxation of the muscle cell.

INFLUENCE OF ESTROGEN AND PROGESTERONE ON THE MYOMETRIUM

Progesterone and estrogen have various direct or indirect effects on the myometrial activity.[96] Both hormones influence protein synthesis, including the contractile proteins, enzymes, and receptors involved in the processes of contractile activation. In general, estrogen has stimulatory effects, whereas progesterone mainly has inhibitory effects on these factors. Thus, progesterone was found to reduce and estrogen to increase the activity of MLCK in rat myometrium.[97] Moreover, the formation of gap junction is stimulated by estrogen and

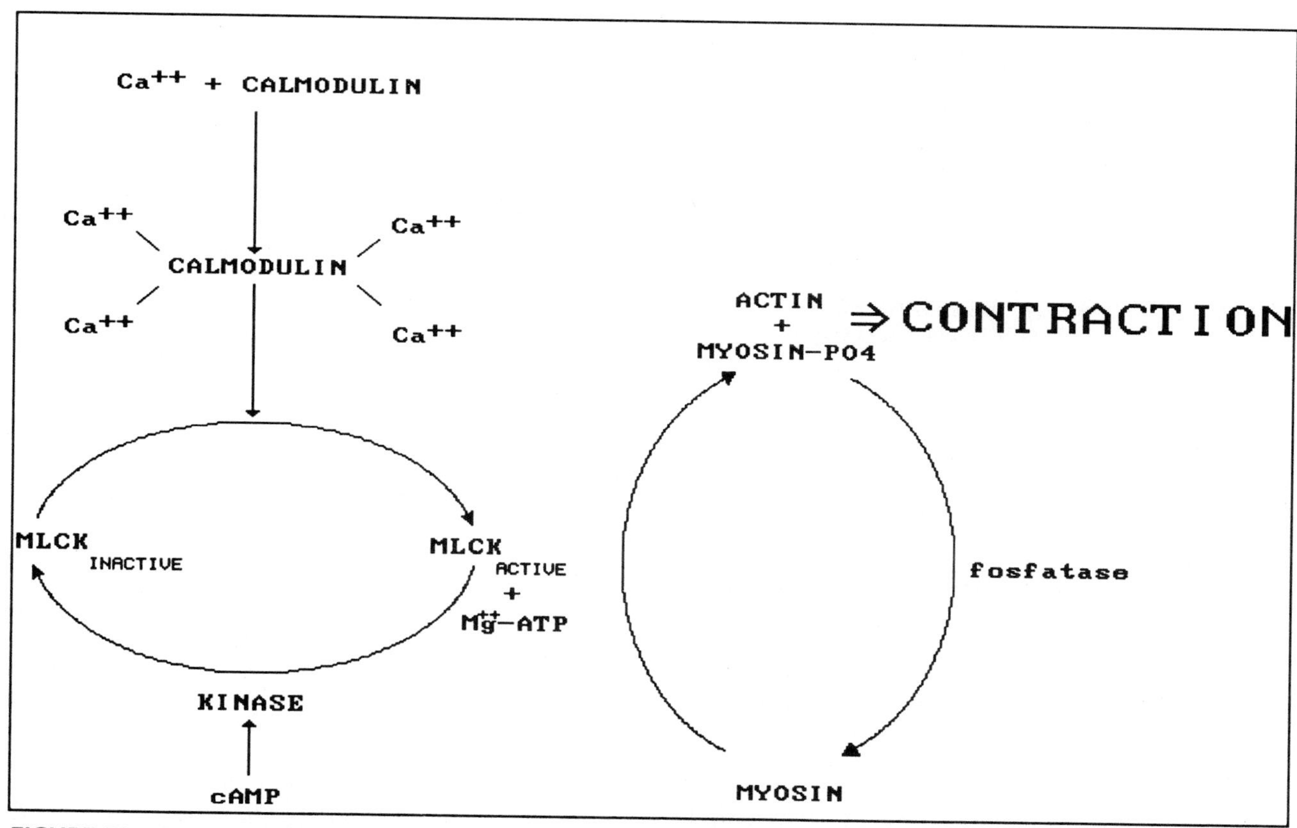

FIGURE 55–10. Activation of contractile proteins. Ca^{++} combines with the protein calmodulin, and this complex activates the enzyme myosin light chain kinase (MLCK). MLCK catalyzes the phosphorylation of the myosin molecule, and the phosphorylated myosin molecule is then able to interact with the actin molecule to produce contractions. Cyclic AMP (cAMP) is able to inactivate MLCK and, therefore, tends to relax the cell. When the intracellular Ca^{++} concentration is below 0.1 μM, a phosphatase dephosphorylates the myosin molecule. Relaxation is produced because the dephosphorylated myosin molecule is unable to interact with actin.

inhibited by progesterone.[17,66,80] Besides, progesterone seems to be responsible for the depletion of noradrenaline seen in sympathetic nerve terminals during pregnancy.[98] These aspects suggest that progesterone is important for the quiescence of the uterus during pregnancy, while estrogen may be responsible for some of the functional changes that precede initiation of labor.[17,96]

Studies in animal models have demonstrated that tissue and plasma progesterone levels decline prior to labor, with subsequently increased myometrial activity. These observations formed the basis for the progesterone-block theory by Csapo,[99] which stated that progesterone was responsible for uterine quiescence during pregnancy and that a decline in the levels of progesterone enhanced myometrial activity, culminating in labor contractions. In man, the levels of progesterone do not, however, decline prior to labor. Moreover, progesterone administration has not been able to reduce the risk for miscarriage, premature labor, stillbirth, or neonatal death, and there is no scientific basis for prescribing progesterone in pregnancy.[100] A role for progesterone in the maintenance of pregnancy is, however, supported by studies on the effects of antiprogesterones, which are antagonists of progesterone at the receptor level. These agents increase the myometrial activity by increasing the number of gap junctions[101] and are effective in terminating early pregnancies.[17,68] The data available therefore suggest a modified progesterone-block theory, because a functional decline of progesterone activity at the myometrial receptor level may be involved in initiation of labor.[17,96]

POSSIBILITIES FOR ACTIVATION OF THE HUMAN MYOMETRIUM

OXYTOCIN

The role of oxytocin in parturition has long been anticipated from the selective and potent effects of the hormone on the myometrium. More direct evidence for the importance of this peptide in the labor process has eventually developed. Thus, oxytocin released from the maternal and fetal pituitaries participates in a complex interplay between the sensitivity of the myometrium (governed by factors such as the number of receptors and of gap junctions mediating the coordination of the contractile response) and effects on prostanoid synthesis.[96]

Pituitary release of oxytocin is characterized by short spurts.[102] In line with this pattern, pulsatile administration of oxytocin reduces the total dose needed for induction of labor.[103] The peptide shows no protein binding in peripheral plasma,[104] and data on the half-life vary from about 3 to 17 minutes.[105] Side effects are minimal during standard use for induction or enhancement of labor. However, bolus injections of 5 to 10 IU produce transient hypotension due to peripheral vasodilatation, and care should be taken in cases of heavy postpartum bleeding.[106,107] Moreover, the antidiuretic effect should be taken into account when high doses are infused in cases of postpartum atonia.[108]

Cervical and vaginal stretching are believed to represent an important stimulus of pituitary release of oxytocin through the Ferguson reflex,[104] and increasing levels have been detected during labor.[96]

The concentration and location of oxytocin receptors and their subsequent effects on prostaglandin production and contractile activation seem of central importance for the role of the peptide during initiation and maintenance of labor. Thus, enhanced sensitivity to the effects of circulating oxytocin, rather than increased secretion, may constitute the mechanism by which the hormone participates in the initiation of labor.[96] Myometrial oxytocin receptor levels show a marked rise during pregnancy,[96] with a further increase during labor.[109] Data from animal models suggest a regulatory role for estrogen and progesterone, with increasing effects of estrogen and decreasing effects of progesterone.[110–112] In parallel to the rise in oxytocin receptor levels, increased concentrations of gap junctions are found.[113–117] Apart from direct stimulation of myometrial contractile activation, oxytocin further seems to enhance local synthesis of prostanoids. This may be effected through formation of IP3 with release of arachidonic acid and subsequent prostaglandin synthesis, which by itself enhances the sensitivity to oxytocin.[95] The importance of prostanoid synthesis for the effects of oxytocin is further supported by the finding that successful labor induction with the hormone is characterized by increased peripheral levels of $PGF_{2\alpha}$ metabolites.

Taken together, these changes are probably of importance for the ripening of the myometrium that occurs in parallel to the cervical ripening process. These changes present to the clinician during vaginal examination and are characterized by enhanced sensitivity to infused oxytocin with subsequent development of coordinated uterine contractile activity.

PROSTAGLANDINS

The effects of prostaglandins such as PGE_2 and $PGF_{2\alpha}$ in term pregnancy are of two different types. The first includes the changes involved in cervical and myometrial ripening, ie, remodeling of the cervical connective tissues and formation of myometrial gap junctions and oxytocin receptors, which provide the basis for coordinated labor contractions and cervical dilatation (see the section on Hormonal Control of Cervical Ripening earlier in this chapter). These alterations partly explain the markedly enhanced sensitivity to oxytocin after initial treatment with $PGF_{2\alpha}$ or PGE_2. The structural changes take some time to develop and are probably achieved through the steady absorption of low doses that seems to take place during local application of the agents within or near the cervix (see the section on Induction of Labor later in this chapter). By this use of prostaglandins, mainly PGE_2, the frequency of systemic side effects is low, although accidental rapid absorption might occur.

Direct stimulation of myometrial contractile activity is another type of response to agents like $PGF_{2\alpha}$ and PGE_2. This is achieved through high-dose systemic administration or through escape of locally applied prostaglandin through the extraamniotic space to the myometrium. This response develops immediately and is mediated through interaction with specific receptors for PGE_2 and $PGF_{2\alpha}$.[118] Early studies on systemic administration of prostaglandins for induction or enhancement of labor mainly intended to rapidly produce effective uterine contractions, in parallel to the common use of oxytocin. By this approach, induction of labor with prostaglandins showed no significant advantage as compared with oxytocin, while the incidence of uterine hypertonus and other side effects seemed to be higher with prostaglandins.[119] The potent contractile effects of prostaglandins are, however, of interest in the treatment of postpartum atony, where intramyometrial injection of $PGF_{2\alpha}$ or intramuscular administration of the analogue 15-methyl $PGF_{2\alpha}$ are increasingly used.[120] Systemic side effects have occurred, however, especially in cases of accidental intravascular administration.

The main uterine side effect during labor induction with prostaglandins is hypertonic contractions. This can be effectively treated with β_2-adrenoceptor agonists such as terbutaline.[121] Major systemic side effects of $PGF_{2\alpha}$ and 15-methyl $PGF_{2\alpha}$ are mainly related to peripheral and pulmonal vasoconstriction.[122–124] These drugs should be used with caution in cases of pregnancy-induced hypertension or cardiac disease. Moreover, both drugs may induce bronchoconstriction and should not be used in patients with bronchial asthma.[122,125] Other side effects include diarrhea and hot flashes, and venous erythema when intravenous infusion is used.[119]

The systemic side effects of PGE_2 differ from those of $PGF_{2\alpha}$; thus, peripheral vasodilatation is seen during intravenous infusion of up to 15 μg/min. Pulmonary vascular resistance remains unchanged,[124] while the agent induces bronchodilatation.[125] Other symptoms of clinical significance include diarrhea and local venous erythema at the intravenous infusion site.[119]

ERGOMETRINE AND METHYLERGOMETRINE

Ergometrine and methylergometrine belong to the ergot alkaloid group of drugs and are derived from lysergic acid. The effects of these compounds are complex and include contraction of vascular and myometrial smooth muscle, as well as an influence on the central nervous system.[126]

Ergometrine and methylergometrine selectively produce contraction of the uterus. Although the effects on peripheral vessels are of minor importance in normotensive patients, these drugs should be avoided during pregnancy in patients with hypertensive disorder.[124] The exact site of action is unknown but may involve the influence of several receptor systems.[126] An important step in contractile activation seems to be calcium influx through VOCs, because methylergometrine-induced contractions in human myometrium can be inhibited by nifedipine both in vitro and in vivo.[128]

The marked, irregular myometrial contractions induced by ergometrine and methylergometrine make these drugs unsuited for induction or enhancement of labor. These effects are, however, useful in the puerperium, where intravenous injection of 0.1 to 0.2 mg methylergometrine produces a sustained increase in uterine activity.[129–131] Uterine activity remains elevated for several hours and declines gradually in normal puerperal patients.[128] A second dose has less pronounced effects, suggesting the development of tachyphylaxis, and some patients do not respond to these drugs at all.

POSSIBILITIES FOR INHIBITION OF THE HUMAN MYOMETRIUM

β_2-ADRENOCEPTOR AGONISTS

The presence of β_2-adrenergic receptors in human myometrium is an established fact.[132–136] Experimental studies on human myometrium[133,137,138] and clinical studies[139] have unquestionably demonstrated the ability of selective β_2-adrenoceptor agonists to inhibit uterine contractions. Treatment is given as intravenous infusion, and the rate is limited mainly by the maternal systemic side effects. These include tachycardia mediated by stimulation or cardiac β-adrenoceptors and by a reflex response to peripheral vasodilation. Cardiac output and myocardial contractility is increased. This increased cardiac load is probably a main cause of the pulmonary edema, which has been reported during this treatment.[139] The metabolic effects include hyperglycemia, increases in free fatty acids, and hypokalemia.[139,140] Diabetic patients are at risk for altered glycemic control. Despite these multiple side effects, serious fetal or maternal complications are rare. Thus, the drugs of this class are widely used clinically to inhibit or suppress abnormal or unwanted uterine activity.

The exact mechanism for the action of the β-adrenoceptor agonists has yet to be established. It is common belief that the receptor occupation results in activation of adenylate cyclase through some intermediate steps involving stimulus of specific signal-transducing proteins, termed G-proteins because of their ability to hydrolyze the guanine nucleotide guanosine triphosphate (GTP).[141] The activation of adenylate cyclase increases the intracellular content of cAMP, and the relaxant effect of β-adrenoceptor agonists is assigned the intracellular effects of cAMP.[142] However, the direct correlation between the myometrial level of cAMP and the relaxant effects of β-adrenoceptor agonists on myometrial activity found by some investigators have been questioned by others.[137,143]

Many intracellular actions of cAMP have been suggested in the myometrium, as well as in other types of smooth muscle. The increased level of cAMP may initiate a series of enzymatic reactions, providing energy for Ca^{++} extrusion from the cell and re-uptake in cellular compartments, resulting in a lowering intracellular Ca^{++} concentration. CAMP may also activate a cAMP-dependent kinase, which deactivates MLCK.[94] It has further been proposed that the increased level of cAMP caused by the β-adrenoceptor agonist directly stimulates Na^+-K^+ ATPase activity.[144–147] This would lead to increased Ca^{++} extrusion by the Na^+,Ca^{++}-exchange mechanism.[145] Moreover, cAMP might decrease Ca^{++} entry through VOCs as a result of the hyperpolarization of the cell membrane caused by the increased activity of the Na^+,K^+ ATPase.[147] However, no evidence has been found to show that the relaxant effect of β-adrenoceptor agonist on isolated myometrial from rats[148] or from man[138] should be effected through stimulation of the Na^+,K^+ ATPase activity. Instead, the increased level of cAMP may increase potassium conductance of the cell membrane[149] or promote active extrusion of Ca^{++} by stimulation of a Ca^{++} pump.[150] Both mechanisms would lead to hyperpolarization of the cell membrane and, hence, relaxation.

MAGNESIUM

Since the late 1950s when it was recognized that magnesium sulfate possesses tocolytic effects,[151] the use of this agent has increased in the treatment of premature contractions.[152,153] Several clinical studies have compared the effectiveness of terbutaline and magnesium sulfate in treatment of preterm labor.[154–156] No major differences have been found between the two agents concerning their ability to inhibit uterine contractions, whereas magnesium sulfate seems to produce fewer maternal side effects.[95]

In human uteroplacental vasculature, Mg^{++}-inhibited Ca^{++} responses probably by interfering with Ca^{++} influx through voltage-operated calcium channels.[157,158] In addition, Mg^{++} inhibited both resting and K^+-stimulated $^{45}Ca^{++}$ influx in isolated human nonpregnant myometrial strips.[159] In isolated human pregnant myometrium, Mg^{++} caused relaxation by a mechanism independent of stimulation of the Na_1K-ATPase.[138] In animal vasculature, Mg^{++} and Ca^{++} were found to elicit reciprocal antagonistic effects on endothelium-relaxing factor formation and on smooth muscle contraction.[160,161] Furthermore, it has been demonstrated[162] in cat vascular preparations that Mg^{++} interfered with Ca^{++} release from intracellular depots without involvement of cAMP. Taken together, these data suggest that Mg^{++} competitively antagonizes the mobilization and the effects of Ca^{++} at several membrane and intracellular sites.[163] Thus, the observation that Mg^{++} augmented the β-adrenoceptor-mediated actions in rat myometrium may be a result of different sites of action for Mg^{++} and β-adrenoceptor agonists.[164]

CALCIUM ANTAGONISTS

The early finding of potent inhibitory effects in isolated human myometrium of dihydropyridine calcium antagonists has suggested the use of these agents for treatment of preterm labor.[165,166] In further support of this therapeutic principle, nifedipine effectively reduced prostaglandin-induced uterine activity in second-trimester pregnancy[167] and myometrial contractions induced by methylergometrine, oxytocin, and $PGF_{2\alpha}$ in the early puerperium.[128,168] According to these results, transmembrane calcium influx sensitive to dihydropyridine calcium antagonists is an important mechanism for contractile activation of the human pregnant uterus in vivo. Results from clinical studies are encouraging, but experience is still limited.[169,170] However, data from in vivo animal models have suggested the possibility of negative fetal effects during such therapy.[171] Although no fetal morbidity has been encountered so far, further studies are needed to clarify the clinical potential of these drugs in treatment of preterm labor.

OXYTOCIN ANTAGONISTS

The suggested role for oxytocin in the initiation and maintenance of labor has called for the development of oxytocin-receptor antagonists. Several compounds have been developed and show marked selectivity for the myometrial responses to oxytocin in vitro and in vivo.[172,173] Data on its effects on spontaneous labor are, however, sparse; pilot studies have suggested that these drugs may represent a new principle for treatment of preterm labor.[173]

PROSTAGLANDIN–SYNTHETASE INHIBITORS

Because prostaglandins are so intimately involved in the initiation of labor, treatment with inhibitors of prostaglandin synthesis is an attractive principle for treatment of preterm labor. Thus, arrest or even regression of the cervical and myometrial structural changes associated with premature initiation of the labor process might be expected during such treatment.

Of the drugs available for inhibition of prostaglandin synthesis, the cyclooxygenase inhibitor indomethacin has been most extensively tested for treatment of premature labor. The data available on this therapeutic approach have been thoroughly reviewed by Witter and Niebyl.[174] Since the initial report by Zuckerman and coworkers in 1974, a large number of patients have been treated with this or similar drugs.[174,175] Although there is no doubt that arrest of preterm labor can be achieved without major maternal side effects, indomethacin readily passes the placenta,[176] causing concern as to the possible fetal side effects.

Intrauterine patency of the ductus arteriosus is probably maintained through fetal synthesis of PGE_2. There is much evidence to suggest that partial constriction occurs in some cases resulting from cyclooxygenase inhibition for preterm labor, as recently verified in human pregnancy.[177] Other possible side effects include pulmonary hypertension and oligohydramnios secondary to inhibition of renal PG synthesis. Interference with fetal platelet function may also occur.[174] In spite of these potential concerns, no major morbidity has been reported, and the principle may be applied in selected cases.

CLINICAL APPLICATIONS

In this section we will comment briefly on the clinical applications of the therapeutic possibilities of influencing the cervical state and myometrial activity. These include treatment of preterm labor, induction of labor at term, inhibition of unwanted uterine activity during labor, and treatment of postpartum uterine hemorrhage.

PRETERM LABOR

Preterm labor is characterized by premature ripening of the cervix and myometrium with subsequent initiation of the labor process. This condition may be secondary to pregnancy complications, such as partial placental ablation; in these patients, pharmacological treatment aimed at labor arrest is contraindicated. In other cases, however, preterm labor occurs in otherwise normal pregnancies with an assessed fetal weight appropriate for gestational age. Ascending colonization with group B streptococci may account for about 25% of such cases; the cause is otherwise unknown, even though specific social factors seem associated with an increased risk.

The cervical and myometrial functional changes that precede the preterm labor process seem to be similar to those occurring at term. Thus, cervical ripening can be found at vaginal examination, and the myometrial changes include increased formation of gap junctions that allow for coordinated myometrial contractions. Treatment is traditionally directed at myometrial relaxation, but principles like inhibition of prostaglandin synthesis might provide the possibility of arresting or even attenuating these cervical and myometrial functional changes.

Treatment with penicillin has been shown to increase the time to delivery in patients with cervical colonization of group B streptococci, while other patients with preterm labor do not seem to benefit from such treatment. Therefore, penicillin treatment should not be instituted until a diagnosis of the cervical culture has been obtained.

Subsequent therapy is directed at arresting the labor process, mainly until sufficient glucocorticoid treatment for prevention of respiratory distress syndrome (RDS) has been given. Because prostaglandin synthesis seems intimately involved in both myometrial activation and cervical softening, treatment with prostaglandin-synthesis inhibitors, ie, indomethacin, is a logical approach. Possible fetal side effects restrict the use of this principle in selected cases, but labor inhibition may be achieved by indomethacin as short-term treatment before 34 weeks of gestation.

The main treatment for labor inhibition is with β_2-adrenoceptor agonists such as ritodrine and terbutaline, which act through stimulation of myometrial β_2-adrenoceptors and increased intracellular cAMP levels.[139,178] These drugs are administered by increasing intravenous infusion until myometrial quiescence is achieved. Although such treatment seems effective for the short-term tocolysis needed for glucocorticoid RDS prophylaxis, long-term oral treatment has not proven of value in delaying labor.[179]

Parenteral administration of magnesium is a further principle for treatment of preterm labor that is widely used in the United States. The myometrial relaxation achieved is partly based on inhibition of membrane calcium influx, but the ion may further influence intracellular mechanisms for activation of contractions. The therapeutic effect seems comparable to that of terbutaline.[180] Treatment of preterm labor with magnesium is associated with relatively few side effects, which makes the principle attractive when compared to β_2-adrenoceptor agonists.[152]

Apart from these agents, calcium antagonists of the dihydropyridine type have been applied for inhibition of myometrial contractile activity.[90,170] Although effective in experimental models and in open clinical studies, the possible fetal side effects of such treatment need further investigation before common clinical use can be recommended.

SHORT-TERM UTERINE RELAXATION

Transient uterine relaxation is indicated in fetal distress due to hypertonic contractions, most commonly secondary to hyperstimulation. When occurring in normal labor, the possibility of placental ablation should, however, be considered. β_2-adrenoceptor agonists are used for uterine relaxation of hypertonic contractions,[139] but magnesium sulfate seems effective as well.[180] Magnesium has further been shown to be effective in providing the uterine relaxation necessary to perform internal version and mobilization of locked twins.[181] In cases of puerperal inversion, reposition can be achieved by the use of a β-agonist, with subsequent uterine contractions through intramyometrial application of $PF_{2\alpha}$.[182] prostaglandin-synthesis inhibitors are often used to contract surgical trauma during cervical cerclage procedures; however, β-adrenoceptor agonists are more commonly used for this purpose.

INDUCTION OF LABOR

Depending on local clinical practice, induction of labor is indicated in 2% to 15% of all pregnancies. This includes cervical priming, stimulation of endogenous prostaglandin synthesis, and pharmacological stimulation of myometrial contractions.

Induction of myometrial contractions in women with unfavorable cervical states is associated with increased risk for prolonged duration of labor and subsequent instrumental delivery or cesarean section. Therefore, cervical priming is indicated before induction of labor in women with Bishop scores below 4 to 6 (see Table 55-1). Clinical experiences with relaxin and antiprogestins for this purpose are very limited, whereas the effect of PGE_2 is well established. Today, it is usually administered by vaginal pessaries containing 3 to 5 mg PGE_2 or in a viscous gel with 0.5 mg PGE_2 applied within the cervical canal.[183] An improved cervical state can usually be detected after 4 to 24 hours; in some women, two treatments are necessary. The intracervical application might be superior to the vaginal application in women with very low Bishop scores, but the maternal discomfort experienced during the application of a pessary is less than that from gel application.

Although the main purpose of local PGE_2 application is to induce cervical ripening, about one third of these women will go into active labor without further treatment. Thus, there exists a mechanism by which PGE_2 ripens not only the cervix but also the myometrium. In women with favorable cervical states but without regular myometrial contractions after PGE_2 treatment, labor can be induced by amniotomy or by intravenous infusion of oxytocin, as in women with spontaneous high Bishop scores. Uterine hyperstimulation before or during oxytocin administration after PGE_2 gel occurs in $<1\%$ of the pregnant women and is reversible with use of β_2-adrenoceptor agonists.

POSTPARTUM ATONIA

Effective uterine contraction is a main therapeutic objective in the puerperium, and atonia requires immediate measures for stimulation of myometrial activity.[184] Initial therapy usually includes intravenous administration of ergometrine or methylergometrine, which produce a sustained increase in myometrial activity in the normal puerperium.[130] When needed, subsequent treatment involves oxytocin given intravenously in doses exceedingly higher than those used for labor induction. Bolus injections may however cause a transient drop in blood pressure,[185] and the risk of water intoxication at prolonged infusion of high doses should be borne in mind.[108,186]

Despite these measures, persistent uterine atony can require drastic procedures, such as internal iliac artery ligation or hysterectomy.[187] Most of these cases may, however, be effectively treated with prostaglandins, as initially suggested by Bygdeman et al.[188] Thus, local administration of $PGF_{2\alpha}$[189] or intramuscular administration of analogues like 15-methyl $PGF_{2\alpha}$[184,190,191] have been shown to be highly effective; this approach should invariably be tried prior to more invasive measures.

REFERENCES

1. Liggins GC, Wilson T. Phospholipases in the control of human parturition. Am J Perinatol 1989;6:153.
2. Green K. Structure, biosynthesis and metabolism. In: Bygdeman, M, Berger GS, Keith LG, eds. Prostaglandins and their inhibitors in clinical obstetrics and gynecology. Lancaster: MTP Press Ltd, 1989:13.
3. Olsen SF, Hansen SF, Sorensen TI, et al. Intake of marine fat, rich in (n-3) -polyunsaturated fatty acids, may increase birthweight by prolonging gestation. Lancet 1986;2:367.
4. Irvine RF. How is the level of free arachidonic acid controlled in mammalian cells? Biochem J 1982;204:3.
5. Liggins GC. Initiation of labour. Biol Neonate 1989;55:366.
6. Reimer RK, Roberts JM. Activation of the uterine smooth muscle contraction. Implication for eicosanoid action and interaction. Semin Perinatol 1986;10:276.
7. Kanmura Y, Missiaen L, Casteels R. Properties of intracellular calcium stores in pregnant rat myometrium. Br J Pharmacol 1988;95:284.
8. Mitchell MD. Regulation of eicosanoid biosynthesis during pregnancy and parturition. In: Hillier K, ed. Eicosanoids and reproduction. Lancaster: MTP Press, 1987:108.
9. Wilhelmsson L, Wikland M, Wiqvist N. PGH2, TxA2 and PGI2 have potent and differentiated actions on human uterine contractility. Prostaglandins 1981;21:227.
10. Bunting S, Moncada S, Vane JR. The effects of prostaglandin endoperoxides and thromboxane A_2 on strips of rabbit coeliac artery and other smooth muscle preparations. Br J Pharmacol 1978;57:462.
11. Abel M, Baird DT. The effect of 17β-estradiol and progesterone on prostaglandin production by human endometrium maintained in organ culture. Endocrinology 1980;106:1599.
12. Wilson T, Liggins GC, Aimer GP, Watkin EJ. The effect of progesterone on the release of arachidonic acid from human endometrial cells stimulated by histamine. Prostaglandins 1986;31:343.
13. Fuchs AR, Husslein P, Fuchs F. Oxytocin and the initiation of human parturition. II: stimulation of prostaglandin production in human decidua by oxytocin. Am J Obstet Gynecol 1981;141:694.
14. Wilson T, Liggins GC, Whittaker DJ. Oxytocin stimulates the release of arachidonic acid and prostaglandin F2a from human decidual cells. Prostaglandins 1988;35:771.
15. Chan WY. Enhanced prostaglandin synthesis in the parturient rat uterus and its effects on myometrial oxytocin receptor concentrations. Prostaglandins 1987;34:889.
16. Fuchs AR, Fuchs F, Husslein P, Soloff MS, Fernström MJ. Oxytocin receptors and human parturition: a dual role for oxytocin in the initiation of labor. Science 1982;215:1396.
17. Garfield RE. Control of myometrial function in preterm versus term labor. Clin Obstet Gynecol 1984;27:572.
17a. Billah MM, Johnston JM. Identification of phospholipid platelet-activating factor (1-0-alhyl-2-acetyl-sn-glycero-3-phosphocholine) in human amniotic fluid and urine. Biochem Biophys Res Commun 1983;113:5.
18. Curbello V, Bejar R, Benirschke K, Gluck L. Prostaglandin precursors in human placental membranes. Obstet Gynecol 1981;57:473.
19. Bejar R, Curbello V, Davis C, Gluck L. Preterm labor and bacterial sources of phospholipase. Obstet Gynecol 1981;57:479.
20. Sellers SM, Hodgson HT, Mitchell MD, Anderson ABM, Turnbull AC. Release of prostaglandins after amniotomy is not mediated by oxytocin. Br J Obstet Gynaecol 1980;87:43.
21. Huslein P, Kofler E, Rasmussen AB, Sumulong L, Fuchs AR, Fuchs F. Oxytocin and the initiation of human parturition. IV:

plasma concentrations of oxytocin and 13, 14-dihydro-15-keto-prostaglandin F_2 alpha during induction of labor by artificial rupture of the membranes. Am J Obstet Gynecol 1983;147:503.
22. Bygdeman M. Male fertility. In: Bygdeman M, Berger GS, Keith LG, eds. Prostaglandins and their inhibitors in clinical obstetrics and gynaecology. Lancaster: MTP Press, 1986:131.
23. Danforth DN, Evanston MD. The distribution and functional activity of the cervical musculature. Am J Obstet Gynecol 1954;68:1261.
24. Schwalm H, Dubrauszky V. The structure of the musculature of the human uterus-muscles and connective tissue. Am J Obstet Gynecol 1966;94:391.
25. Rechberger T, Uldbjerg N, Oxlund H. Connective tissue changes in the cervix during normal pregnancy and pregnancy complicated by cervical incompetence. Obstet Gynecol 1988;71:563.
26. Cabrol D, Jannet D, Le Houezec R, Dudzik W, Bonoris E, Cedard L. Mechanical properties of the pregnant human uterine cervix. Use of an instrument to measure the index of cervical distensibility. Gynecol Obstet Invest 1990;29:32.
27. Bishop EH. Pelvic scoring for elective induction. Obstet Gynecol 1964;24:266.
28. Uldbjerg N, Ekman G, Malmström A, Olsson K, Ulmsten U. Ripening of the human uterine cervix related to changes in collagen, glycosaminoglycans, and collagenolytic activity. Am J Obstet Gynecol 1983;147:662.
29. Ruoslahti E. Structure and biology of proteoglycans. Ann Rev Cell Biol 1988;4:229.
30. Uldbjerg N, Danielsen CC. A study of the interaction in vitro between type-I collagen and a small dermatan sulphate proteoglycan. Biochem J 1988;251:643.
31. Junqueira LCU, Zugaib M, Montes GS, Toledo, OMS, Krisztán RM, Shigihara KM. Morphologic and histochemical evidence for the occurrence of collagenolysis and for the role of neutrophilic polymorphonuclear leukocytes during cervical dilation. Am J Obstet Gynecol 1980;138:273.
32. Danforth DN, Buckingham JC, Roddick JW. Connective tissue changes incident to cervical effacement. Am J Obstet Gynecol 1960;80:939.
33. Ito A, Kitamura K, Mori Y, Hirakawa S. The change in solubility of type I collagen in human uterine cervix in pregnancy at term. Biochem Med 1979;21:262.
34. Ekman G, Malmström A, Uldbjerg N, Ulmsten U. Cervical collagen. An important regulator of cervical function in term labor. Obstet Gynecol 1986;67:633.
35. Petersen LK, Uldbjerg N. Cervical hydroxyproline concentration in relation to age and parity (abstract). In: Leppert P, Woessner F, eds. The extracellular matrix and the reproductive tract. Rochester, NY: Perinatology Press (in press).
36. Kokenyesi R, Woessner JF. Relationship between dilatation of the rat uterine cervix and a small dermatan sulfate proteoglycan. Biol Reprod 1990;42:87.
37. Norman M, Ekman G, Ulmsten U, Barchan K, Malmström A. Proteoglycan metabolism in the connective tissue of pregnant and non-pregnant human cervix — an in vitro study. Biochem J (in press).
38. Norström A. Influence of prostaglandin E_2 on the biosynthesis of connective tissue constituents in the pregnant human cervix. Prostaglandins 1982;23:361.
39. Liggins GC. Cervical ripening as an inflammatory reaction. In: Ellwood DA, Anderson ABM, eds. The cervix in pregnancy and labour: clinical and biochemical investigations. Edinburgh: Churchill Livingstone, 1981:1.
40. Anthony GS, Calder AA, MacNaughton MC. Cervical resistance in patients with previous spontaneous mid-trimester abortion. Br J Obstet Gynaecol 1982;89:1046.
41. Buckingham JC, Buethe RA, Danforth DN. Collagen-muscle ratio in clinically normal and clinically incompetent cervices. Am J Obstet Gynecol 1965;91:232.
42. McDonald IA. Suture of the cervix for inevitable miscarriage. J Obstet Gynaecol Br Emp 1957;64:346.
43. Uldbjerg N, Ulmsten U, Ekman G. The physiological role of eicosanoids in controlling the form and function of the cervix. In: Hillier K, ed. Eicosanoids and reproduction. Lancaster: MTP Press, 1987;163.
44. Conrad JT, Ueland K. Reduction of the stretch modulus of human cervical tissue by prostaglandin E_2. Am J Obstet Gynecol 1976;126:218.
45. MacKenzie IZ, Embrey MP. A comparison of PGE_2 and PGF_2 vaginal gel for ripening of the cervix before induction of labour. Br J Obstet Gynaecol 1979;86:167.
46. Theobald PW, Rath W, Kühnle H, Kuhn W. Histological and electron-microscopic examinations of collagenous connective tissue of the non-pregnant cervix, the pregnant cervix, and the pregnant prostaglandin-treated cervix. Arch Gynecol 1982;231:241.
47. Sherwood OD. Relaxin. In: Knobil E, Neill, et al, eds. The physiology of reproduction. New York: Raven Press, 1988:585.
48. Bell RJ, Eddie LE, Lester AR, Wood EC, Johnston PD, Niall HD. Level of relaxin in human pregnancy measured with a homologous radioimmuno assay for human relaxin. Obstet Gynecol 1987;69:585.
49. MacLennan AH, Green C, Bryant-Greenwood GD, Greenwood FC, Seamark RF. Ripening of the uterine cervix and induction of labour with purified porcine relaxin. Lancet 1980;i:220.
50. Downing JS, Sherwood OD. The physiological role of relaxin. IV: the influence of relaxin on cervical collagen and glycosaminoglycans. Endocrinology 1986;118:471.
51. Evans MI, Dougan MB, Moawad AH, Evans W, Bryant-Greenwood GD, Greenwood C. Ripening of the human cervix with porcine ovarian relaxin. Am J Obstet Gynecol 1983; 147:410.
52. Sasaki K, Nakano R, Kadoya Y, Shima IK, Sowa M. Cervical ripening with dehydroepiandrosterone sulphate. Br J Obstet Gynecol 1982;89:195.
53. Lykkesfeldt G, Damkjær Nielsen M, Lykkesfeldt AE. Placental steroid sulfatase deficiency: biochemical diagnosis and clinical review. Obstet Gynecol 1984;64:49.
54. Peedicayil A, Jasper P, Balasubramaniam N, Jairaj P. A randomized controlled trial of extraamniotic ethinylestradiol in ripening of the cervix at term. Br J Obstet Gynaecol 1989;96:973.
55. Thiery M, De Gezelle H, van Kets H, et al. The effect of local administrated estrogens on human cervix. Zeitschrift für Geburtshilfe und Perinatologie 1979;183:448.
56. Pinto RM, Rabow W, Votta RA. Uterine cervix ripening in term pregnancy due to the action of estradiol-17β. Am J Obstet Gynecol 1965;92:319.
57. Mochizuki M, Honda T, Tojo S. Collagenolytic activity and steroid levels after administration of dehydroepiandrosterone sulphate. Int J Obstet Gynecol 1978;16:248.
58. Fitzpatrick RJ, Dobson H. Softening of the ovine cervix at parturition. In: Ellwood DA, Anderson ABM, eds. The cervix in pregnancy and labour: clinical and biochemical investigations. Edinburgh: Churchill Livingstone, 1981:40.
59. MacKenzie IZ. Clinical studies on cervical ripening. In: Ellwood DA, Anderson ABM, eds. The cervix in pregnancy and labour: clinical and biochemical investigations. Edinburgh: Churchill Livingstone, 1981:163.
60. MacKenzie IZ, Jenkin G, Bradley S. The relation between plasma oestrogen, progesterone and prolactin concentrations and the efficacy of vaginal prostaglandin E_2 gel in initiating labour. Br J Obstet Gynaecol 1979;86:171.

61. Allen J, Uldbjerg N, Petersen LK, Secher NJ. Intracervical 17β-oestradiol before induction of second trimester abortion with a prostaglandin E_1 analouge. Eur J Obstet Gynecol Reprod Biol 1989;32:123.
62. Romero R, Scoccia B, Mazor M, Wu YK, Benveniste R. Evidence for a local change in the progesterone/estrogen ratio in human parturion at term. Am J Obstet Gynecol 1988:159:657.
63. Radestad A, Christensen NJ, Stromberg L. Induced cervical ripening with mifepristone in first trimester abortions. Contraception 1988;38:310.
64. Hegele-Hartung C, Chwalisz K, Beier HM, Elger W. Ripening of the uterine cervix of the guinea-pig after treatment with the progesterone antagonist onapristone (ZK 98, 299): an electron microscopic study. Hum Reprod 1989;4:369.
65. Bygdeman M, Swahn ML. Uterine contractility and abortifacient drugs. Baillieres Clin Obstet Gynaecol 1990;4:249.
66. Garfield RE, Baulieu EE. The antiprogesterone steroid RU 486: a short pharmacologic and clinical review, with emphasis on the interruption of pregnancy. Baillieres Clin Endocrinol Metab 1987;1:207.
67. Chwalisz K, Shi Shao Q, Neef G, Elger W. The effect of antigestagen ZK 98,299 on the uterine cervix. Acta Endocrinol 1987;283:113.
68. Swahn ML, Bygdeman M. Medical methods to terminate early pregnancy. Baillieres Clin Obstet Gynaecol 1990;4:293.
69. Oxlund H, Helmig R, Halaburt JT, Uldbjerg N. Biomechanical analysis of human chorioamniotic membranes. Eur J Obstet Gynecol Reprod 1990;34:247.
70. Yoshida Y, Manabe Y. Different characteristics of amniotic and cervical collagenous tissue during pregnancy and delivery: a morphologic study. Am J Obstet Gynecol 1990;162:190.
71. Kanayama N, Terao T, Kawashima Y, Horiuchi K, Fujimoto D. Collagen types in normal and prematurely ruptured amniotic membranes. Am J Obstet Gynecol 1985;153:899.
72. Vadillo-Ortega F, González-Avila G, Karchmer S, Cruz NM, Ayala-Ruiz A, Lama MS. Collagen metabolism in premature rupture of amniotic membranes. Obstet Gynecol 1990;75:84.
73. Hegedüs K, Molnar P. On the pattern of reticular fibers in the intracranial arteries of mature newborn with and without intracranial hemorrhage. Childs Nerv Syst 1986;2:2.
74. Nakanishi H, McLeans J, Wood C, Burnstock G. The role of sympathetic nerves in control of the non-pregnant and pregnant human uterus. J Reprod Med 1969;1:20.
75. Thorbert G. Regional changes in structure and function of adrenergic nerves in guinea-pig uterus during pregnancy [thesis]. Acta Obstet Gynecol Scand 1979;suppl 79:5.
76. Wikland M, Lindblom B, Dahlström A, Haglid KG. Structural and functional evidence for the denervation of human myometrium during pregnancy. Obstet Gynecol 1984;64:503.
77. Lundberg LM, Alm P, Thorbert G. Local mechanical effects and humoral factors evoke degeneration of guinea pig uterine innervation. Acta Obstet Gynecol Scand 1989;68:487.
78. Wilhelmsson L, Norström A, Hamberger L, Wikland M, Lindblom B, Wiqvist N. Interaction between PGs and catecholamines on cervical collagen synthesis. Acta Obstet Gynecol Scand 1983;su113:171.
79. Miller SM, Garfield RE, Daniell EE. Improved propagation in myometrium associated with gap junctions during parturition. Am J Physiol 1989;256:C130.
80. Garfield RE, Kannan MS, Daniell EE. Gap junction formation in myometrium: control by estrogens, progesterone and prostaglandins. Am J Physiol 1980;238:C81.
81. Inoue Y, Nakao K, Okabe K, et al. Some electrical properties of human pregnant myometrium. Am J Obstet Gynecol 1990;162:1090.
82. Reiner O, Marshall JM. Action of D-600 on spontaneous and electrically induced activity of the partuirent rat uterus, Naunyn Schmiedebergs Arch Pharmacol 1976;292:21.
83. Bolton TB. Mechanisms of action of transmitters and other substances on smooth muscle. Physiol Rev 1979;59:606.
84. Forman A. Calcium entry blockade as a therapeutic principle in the female urogenital tract. Acta Obstet Gynecol Scand 1984;suppl 121:7.
85. Tritthart H, Grün G, Byon KY, Fleckenstein A. Influence of Caantagonistic inhibitors of excitation-contraction coupling in isolated uterine muscle studied with the sucrose gap method. Pflügers Arch 1970;319:R117.
86. Nayler WG. Classification of calcium antagonists. In: Nayler WG, ed. Calcium antagonists. London: Academic Press, 1988:101.
87. Somlyo AV, Somlyo AP. Electromechanical and pharmacomechanical coupling in vascular smooth muscle. J Pharmacol Exp Ther 1968;159:129.
88. Daniell EE, Grover AK, Kwan CY. Calcium. In: Stephens NL, ed. Biochemistry of smooth muscle. Vol III. Boca Raton, FL: CRC Press, 1983:2.
89. Nayler WG. Tissue selectivity. In: Nayler WG, ed. Calcium antagonists. London: Academic Press, 1988:113.
90. Forman A, Andersson KE, Maigaard S. Effects of calcium channel blockers on the female genital tract. Acta Pharm Toxicol 1986;58:183.
91. Maigaard S, Forman A, Andersson KE, Ulmsten U. Comparison of the effects of nicardipine and nifedipine on isolated human myomterium. Gynecol Obstet Invest 1984;16:354.
92. Huxley HE. The double array of filaments in cross striated muscle. J Biophys Biochem Cytosol 1957;3:631.
93. Mulvany MJ. Crossbridges in smooth muscle. In: Stephens NL, ed. Smooth muscle contraction. New York: Marcel Dekker, 1984:145.
94. Roberts JM. Current understanding of pharmacologic mechanisms in the prevention of preterm birth. Clin Obstet Gynecol 1984;27:592.
95. Carsten ME, Miller JD. A new look at uterine muscle contraction. Am J Obstet Gynecol 1987;157:1303.
96. Fuchs AA, Fuchs F. Endocrinology of human parturition: a review. Br J Obstet Gynecol 1984;91:948.
97. Badia E, Nicolas JC, Haiech J, Crastes-de-Paulet A. Effects of steroid hormones on the regulation of uterine contractility. Pflugers Arch 1986;407:670.
98. Bell C, Malcolm SJ. Neurochemistry of the sympathetic innervation to the uterus. Clin Exp Pharmacol Physiol 1988;15:667.
99. Csapo AI. Progesterone block. Am J Anat 1956;98:273.
100. Goldstein PA, Sacks HS, Chalmers TC. Hormone administration for the maintenance of pregnancy. In: Chalmers I, Enkin M, Keirse MJNC, eds. Effective care in pregnancy and childbirth. New York: Oxford University Press, 1989:612.
101. Garfield RE, Gasc JM, Baulieu EE. Effects of the antiprogesterone RU 486 on preterm birth in the rat. Am J Obstet Gynecol 1987;157:1281.
102. Gibbens CD, Chard T. Observations on maternal oxytocin release during human labor and the effect of intravenous alcohol infusion. Am J Obstet Gynecol 1976;126:243.
103. Randolph GW, Fuchs AR. Pulsatile administration enhances the effect and reduces the dose of oxytocin required for induction of labor. Am J Perinatol 1989;6:159.
104. Ginsburg M. Production, release, transportation and elimination of the neurohypophysical hormones. In: Berde B, ed. Neurohypophyseal hormones and similar polypeptides. Handbook of experimental pharmacology. Vol 23. Berlin: Springer-Verlag, 1968:286.
105. Chard T. Fetal and maternal oxytocin in human parturition. Am J Perinatol 1989;6:145.

106. Hendricks CH, Brenner WE. Cardiovascular effects of oxytocic drugs used post partum. Am J Obstet Gynecol 1970;108:751.
107. Secher NJ, Arnsbo P, Wallin L. Haemodynamic effects of oxytocin and methyl ergometrine on the systemic and pulmunary circulations of pregnant anaesthetized women. Acta Obstet Gynecol Scand 1978;57:97.
108. Abdul-Karim R, Assali NS. Renal function in human pregnancy. V: effects of oxytocin on renal hemodynamics and water and electrolyte excretion. J Lab Clin Med 1961;57:522.
109. Fuchs AR, Fuchs F, Husslein P, Soloff MS. Oxytocin receptors in the human uterus during pregnancy and parturition. Am J Obstet Gynecol 1984;150:734.
110. Nissensson R, Flouret G, Hechter O. Opposing effects of estradiol and progesterone on oxytocin receptors in rabbit uterus. Proc Natl Acad Sci USA 75:2044.
111. Alexandrova M, Soloff MS. Oxytocin receptors and parturition. I: control of oxytocin receptor concentration in the rat myometrium at term. Endocrinology 1980;106:730.
112. Fuchs AR, Periyasamy S, Alexandrova M, Soloff MS. Correlation between oxytocin receptor concentration and responsiveness to oxytocin in pregnant rat myometrium: effects of ovarian steroids. Endocrinology 1983;113:742.
113. Garfield RE, Sims S, Daniel EE. Gap junctions: their presence and necessity in myometrium during parturition. Science 1977;198:958.
114. Garfield RE, Merrett D, Grover AK. Studies on gap junction formation and regulation in myometrium. Am J Physiol 1980;239:C217.
115. Garfield RE, Hayashi RH. Appearance of gap junctions in the myometrium of women during labor. Am J Obstet Gynecol 1981;140:254.
116. Puri CP, Garfield RE. Changes in hormone levels and gap junctions in the rat uterus during pregnancy and parturition. Biol Reprod 1982;27:967.
117. Garfield RE, Puri CP, Csapo AI. Endocrine, structural and functional changes in the uterus during premature labor. Am J Obstet Gynecol 1982;142:21.
118. Giannopoulos G, Jackson K, Kredentser J, Tulchinsky D. Prostaglandin E and F2a receptors in human myometrium during the menstrual cycle and in pregnancy and labor. Am J Obstet Gynecol 1985;153:904.
119. Thiery M, Amy J-J. Induction of labour with prostaglandins. In: Karim SMM, ed. Prostaglandins and reproduction. New York: MTP Press Limited, 1975:149.
120. Toppozada MK. Post partum haemorrhage. In: Bygdeman M, Berger G, Keith G, eds. Prostaglandins and their inhibitors in clinical obstetrics and gynecology. London: MTP Press, 1986:233.
121. Andersson KE, Bengtsson LP, Ingemarsson I. Terbutaline inhibition of midtrimester uterine activity induced by prostaglandin $F_{2\alpha}$ and hypertonc saline. Br J Obstet Gynaecol 1975;82:745.
122. Andersen HL, Secher NJ. Pattern of total and regional lung function in subjects with bronchoconstriction induced by 15-ME-PGF2α. Thorax 1976;31:685.
123. Secher NJ, Andersen HL. Changes in the pattern of regional pulmunary blood flow after PGF20 infusion in pregnant women. Cardiovasc Res 1977;11:26.
124. Secher NJ, Thayssen P, Arnsbo P, Olsen J. Effects of prostaglandin F2α and E2 on the systemic and pulmunary circulation in pregnant anaesthetized women. Acta Obstet Gynecol Scand 1982;61:213.
125. Smith AP. The effects of intravenous infusion of graded doses of prostaglandin F^{20} and E2 on lung resistance in patients undergoing termination of pregnancy. Clin Sci 1973;44:17.
126. Rall TW, Schleifer LS. Oxytocin, prostaglandins, ergot alkaloids and other drugs: tocolytic agents. In: Gilmann AG, Goodman LS, Rall TW, Murad F, eds. The pharmacological basis of therapeutics. New York: MacMillan, 1985:926.
127. Müller Schweinitzer E, Weidmann H. Basic pharmacological properties. In: Berde B, Schild HO, eds. Ergot alkaloids and related compounds. Handbuch der Experimentellen Pharmakologie. Vol 49. erlin: Springer Verlag, 1978:87.
128. Forman A, Gandrup P, Andersson KE, Ulmsten U. Effects of nifedipine on oxytocin and prostaglandin F2α-induced activity in the post partum uterus. Am J Obstet Gynecol 1982;144:665.
129. Gill RC. The effect of methylergometrine on the human puerperal uterus. J Obstet Gynaecol Br 1947;54:482.
130. Hendricks CH. Uterine contractility changes in the early puerperium. Clin Obstet Gynecol 1968;2:125.
131. Saameli K. Effects on the uterus. In: Berde B, Schild HO, eds. Ergot alkaloids and related compounds. Handbuch der Experimentellen Pharmakologie. Vol 49. Berlin: Springer Verlag, 1978:233.
132. Wansborough H, Nakanishi H, Wood C. Effect of epinephrine on human uterine activity in vitro and in vivo. Obstet Gynecol 1967;30:779.
133. Andersson KE, Ingemarsson I, Persson CGA. Relaxing effects of β-receptor stimulators in isolated, gravid human myometrium. Life Sci 1973;13:335.
134. Hayashida DN, Leung R, Goldfien A, Roberts JM. Human myometrial adrenergic receptors: identification of the beta-adrenergic receptor by [3H]dihydroalprenolol binding. Am J Obstet Gynecol 1982;142:389.
135. Berg G, Andersson RGG, Ryden G. Alpha-adrenergic receptors in human myometrium during pregnancy. Am J Obstet Gynecol 1986;154:601.
136. Breuiller M, Rouot B, Leroy MJ, Blot P, Kaplan L, Ferre F. Adrenergic receptors in inner and outer layers of human myometrium near term: characterization of beta-adrenergic receptor sites by [125I] iodocyanopindolol binding. Gynecol Obstet Invest 1987;24:28.
137. Andersson RGG, Berg G, Johansson SRM, Ryden G. Effects of nonselective and selective beta-adrenergic agonists on spontaneous contractions and cyclic AMP levels in myometrial strips from pregnant women. Gynecol Obstet Invest 1980;11:286.
138. Skajaa K, Everts ME, Forman A, Clausen T. Effects of magnesium and terbutaline on contractility and K^+ uptake in isolated human uterine muscle. Am J Obstet Gynecol (in press).
139. Ingemarsson I. Use of β-receptor agonists in obstetrics. Acta Obstet Gynecol Scand 1982;suppl 108:29.
140. Bengtsson B, Andersson KE. Metabolic effects of beta-adrenoceptor agonists on mother and fetus. Acta Pharmacol Toxicol 1979;suppl 11:76.
141. Raymond JR, Hnatowich M, Lefkowitz RJ, Garon MG. Adrenergic receptors. Models for regulation of signal transduction processes. Hypertension 1990;15:119.
142. Krall JF, Fortier M, Korenman SG. Smooth muscle cyclic nuclotide biochemistry. In: Stephens NL, ed. Biochemistry of smooth muscle. Vol III. Boca Raton, FL: CRC Press, 1983:89.
143. Marshall JM, Fain JN. Effects of forskolin and isoproterenol on cyclic AMP and tension in the myometrium. Eur J Pharmacol 1985;107:25.
144. Webb RC, Bohr DF. Relaxation of vascular smooth muscle by isoproterenol, dibutyryl-cyclic AMP and theophyllin. J Pharmacol Exp Ther 1981;217:26.
145. Scheid CR, Fay FS. β-adrenergic stimulation of 42K influx in isolated smooth muscle cells. Am J Physiol 1984;246:C415.
146. Somlyo AP, Somlyo AV, Smiesko V. Cyclic AMP and vascular smooth muscle. Advances in cyclic nucleotide research 1972;1:175.
147. Gunst SJ, Stropp JQ. Effect of Na-K adenosinetriphosphatase

activity on relaxation of canine tracheal smooth muscle. J Appl Physiol 1988;64:635.
148. Sanborn BM. Rat myometrial Na/K ATPase is increased by serum but not by isoproterenol and relaxin. Comp Biochem Physiol 1989;93C:341.
149. Kroeger EA, Marshall JM. Beta-adrenergic effects on rat myometrium: Mechanisms of membrane hyperpolarization. Am J Physiol 1973;225:1339.
150. Bulbring E, Tomita T. Catecholamine action on smooth muscle. Pharmacol Rev 1987;39:49.
151. Hall DG, McGaughey HS, Corey EL, et al. The effects of magnesium therapy on the duration of labor. Am J Obstet Gynecol 1959;78:27.
152. Elliot JP. Magnesium sulfate as a tocolytic agent. Am J Obstet Gynecol 1983;147:277.
153. Dudley D, Gagnon D, Varner M. Long-term tocolysis with intravenous magnesium sulfate. Obstet Gynecol 1989;73:373.
154. Beall MH, Edgar BW, Paul RH, et al. A comparison of ritrodine, terbutalin and magnesium sulfate for the suppression of preterm labor. Am J Obstet Gynecol 1985;153:854.
155. Cotton DB, Strassner HT, Hill LM, Schifrin BS, Paul RH. Comparison of magnesium sulfate, terbutaline and a placebo for inhibition of preterm labor. A randomized study. J Reprod Med 1984;29:92.
156. Hollander DI, Nagey DA, Pupkin MJ. Magnesium sulfate and ritrodine hydrochloride: a randomized comparison. Am J Obstet Gynecol 1987;156:631.
157. Skajaa K, Forman A, Andersson K-E. Effects of magnesium on isolated human fetal and maternal vessels. Acta Physiol Scand 1990;139:551.
158. Skajaa K, Svane D, Andersson K-E, Forman A. Effects of magnesium and isradipine on contractile activation induced by the TxA_2 analogue U46619 in human uteroplacental vessels in term pregnancy. Am J Obstet Gynecol 1990;163:1323.
159. Popper LD, Batra SC, Akerlund M. The effect of magnesium on calcium uptake and contractility in the human myometrium. Gynecol Obstet Invest 1989;28:78.
160. Ku D, Ann HS. Magnesium deficiency produces endothelium dependent vasorelaxation in canine coronary arteries. J Pharm Exp Ther 1987;241(3):961.
161. Gold M, Buga G, Wood KS, Byrns RE, Chaudhuri G, Ignarro LJ. Antagonistic modulatory roles of magnesium and calcium on release of endothelium-derived ralaxing factor and smooth muscle tone. Circ Res 1990;66:355.
162. Sjögren A, Edvinsson L. The influence of magnesium on the release of calcium from intracellular depots in vascular smooth muscle cells. Pharmacol Toxicol 1988;62:17.
163. Isery LT, French JH. Magnesium: nature's physiological calcium blocker. Am Heart J 1984;108:188.
164. Marata K, Osa T. Augmentation by external Mg ions of β-adrenoreceptor-mediated actions in the longitudinal muscle of rat uterus. Br J Pharmacol 1989;96:707.
165. Fleckenstein A. Specific pharmacology of calcium in myometrium, cardiac pacemakers and vascular smooth muscle. Ann Rev Pharmacol Toxicol 1977;149:149.
166. Forman A, Andersson KE, Persson CGA, Ulmsten U. Relaxant effects of nifedipine on isolated human myometrium. Acta Pharmacol Toxicol 1979;45:81.
167. Andersson KE, Ingemarsson I, Ulmsten U, Wingerup L. Inhibition of prostaglandin induced uterine activity by nifedipine. Br J Obstet Gynaecol 1979;86:175.
168. Forman A, Gandrup P, Andersson KE, Ulmsten U. Effects of nifedipine on spontaneous and methylergometrine-induced activity post partum. Am J Obstet Gynecol 1982;144:237.
169. Ulmsten U, Andersson KE, Wingerup L. Treatment of premature labor with the calcium antagonist nifedipine. Arch Gynecol 1980;229:1.
170. Read MD, Welby DE. The use of a calcium antagonist (nifedipine) to suppress preterm labour. Br J Obstet Gynaecol 1986;93:933.
171. Harake B, Gilbert RD, Ashwal S, Power GG. Nifedipine: effects on fetal and maternal haemodynamics in pregnant sheep. Am J Obstet Gynecol 1987;157:1003.
172. Chan WY, Hruby VJ, Rockway TW, Hlavacek J. Design of oxytocin antagonists with prolonged action: potential tocolytic action for the treatment of preterm labor. J Pharmacol Exp Ther 1985;239:84.
173. Demarest KT, Hahn DW, Ericson E, Capetola RJ, Fuchs AR, McQuire JL. Profile of an oxytocin antagonist RWJ 22164 for treatment of preterm labor in laboratory models for uterine contractility. Am J Perinatol 1989;6:200.
174. Witter FR, Niebyl JR. Inhibition of arachidonic acid metabolism in the perinatal period: pharmacology, clinical application, and potential adverse effects. Semin Perinatol 1986;10:316.
175. Zuckerman H, Reiss U, Rubenstein I. Inhibition of human premature labour by indomethacin. Obstet Gynecol 1974;44:787.
176. Traeger A, Noschel H, Zaumseil J. The pharmacokinetics of indomethacin in pregnant and parturient women and in their newborn infants. Zentralbl Gynakol 1973:95:635.
177. Moise KJ, Giancarlo M, Kirshon B, Huhta JC, Walsh SW, Cano L. The effect of indomethacin on the pulsatility index of the umbilical artery in human fetuses. Am J Obstet Gynecol 1990;162:199.
178. Keirse MJNC, Grant A, King JF. Preterm labour. In: Chalmers I, Enkin M, Keirse MJNC, eds. Effective care in pregnancy and childbirth. New York: Oxford University Press, 1989:694.
179. Miller J, Keane M, Horger E. A comparison of magnesium sulfate and terbutaline for the arrest of preterm labor. J Reprod Med 1982;27:348.
180. Fougner AC, Wilson SJ. The use of magnesium sulphate in the management of fetal distress. Am J Obstet Gynecol 1984;149:587.
181. Reece EA, Chervenak FA, Romero R, Hobbins JC. Magnesium sulphate in the management of acute intrapartum fetal distress. Am J Obstet Gynecol 1984;148:104.
182. Thiery M, Gerris J, Baele G. Management of acute puerperal inversion of the uterus with betamimetic drugs and prostaglandins. Eur J Obstet Gynecol Reprod Biol 1978;8:359.
183. Rayburn WF. Prostaglandin E2 gel for cervical ripening and induction of labor. A critical analysis. Am J Obstet Gynecol 1989;160:529.
184. Toppozada MK, ElBossaty M, ElRahman HA, Shams AH. Control of intractable tonic uterine post partum hemorrhage by 15-methyl prostaglandin F2α. Obstet Gynecol 1981;58:327.
185. Nakano J. Cardiovascular effects of oxytocin. Obstet Gynecol Surv 1973;28:75.
186. Gupta DR, Cohen NH. Oxytocin salting out and water intoxication. JAMA 1972;220:681.
187. Gibbs CE, Locke WE. Maternal deaths in Texas 1969 to 1973. Am J Obstet Gynecol 1976;126:687.
188. Bygdeman M, Kwon SU, Murkherjee T, Wiquist N. Effect of intravenous infusion of prostaglandin E1 and E2 on motility of the pregnant human uterus. Am J Obstet Gynecol 1968;102:317.
189. Takagi T, Yoshida T, Togo Y, et al. The effects of intramyometrial injection of prostaglandin F2α on severe post partum hemorrhage. Prostaglandins 1976;12:565.
190. Corson ST, Bolognese RJ. Post partum uterine atony treated with prostaglandins. Am J Obstet Gynecol 1977;129:918.
191. Hayashi RH, Castillo MS, Noah MI. Management of severe post partum haemorrhage due to uterine atony using an analogue of prostaglandin F. Obstet Gynecol 1981;58:426.

56

CHAPTER

MATERNAL NUTRITION

Barbara Luke

HISTORICAL PERSPECTIVE

And the angel of the Lord appeared to the woman and said to her, "Behold, you are barren and have no children: but you shall conceive and bear a son. Therefore beware, and drink no wine or strong drink, and eat nothing unclean, for lo, you shall conceive and bear a son."

–Judges 13:2

From Biblical times and earlier, women have been advised about what to eat and what not to eat during pregnancy. The preceding passage refers to the prospective mother of the legendary Samson, renowned for his unsurpassed strength, the foundation of which may have been in sound antepartum nutrition! Throughout history, records are replete with advice to pregnant women, most often reflecting the religious, scientific, medical, and social beliefs of that era. Most medical knowledge and practice before the seventeenth century was based on the ideas expressed by Hippocrates, Aristotle, and Galen. Diet therapy was used to sustain pregnancy and produce a healthy baby and mother. Diet was believed to be related directly to the prevention of abortion through its role in the nourishment of the embryo. The nutritive quality of the blood from the mother to the fetus was thought to depend not only on the amount of food ingested by the mother, but also on the kinds of foods and their effects on her humoral balance. The inability of the maternal circulation to provide adequate nourishment to the fetus was therefore believed to initiate parturition. In other words, when the fetus could not obtain sufficient nutriment in the womb, it came out to seek sustenance.

RICKETS AND THE CONTRACTED PELVIS

During this time the prevailing philosophy regarding diet during pregnancy was very liberal, based on the concept that, "when the child is bigger, let her diet be more, for it is better for women with child to eat too much than too little, lest the child should want nourishment."[1] Maternal and infant mortality was high during this period and later, because of a variety of factors, including widespread infantile rickets, which resulted in a rachitic or contracted pelvis in the adult woman. William Smellie, the famed British obstetrician and founder of pelvimetry, was one of the first to associate infantile rickets with pelvic deformities in adults, saying that ". . .most of those who have been rickety in their infancy, whether they continue little and deformed, or, recovering of that disease, grow up to be tall, stately women, are commonly narrow and distorted in the pelvis and consequently subject to tedious and difficult labours for, as the pelvis is more or less distorted, the labour is more or less dangerous and difficult."[2] A contracted pelvis was a very common obstetric problem in the United States as recently as 50 years ago, and particularly before surgical delivery became a practical alternative to vaginal delivery. In a 1926 study by J. Whitridge Williams of 11,630 women delivering at the Johns Hopkins Hospital from 1896 to 1924, there was a 27% overall incidence of contracted pelvis, 14% in white women and 43% among black women.[3]

OPTION OF LIMITING THE MATERNAL DIET

Other options for delivery in the presence of a distorted pelvis were "destructive operations": craniotomy, embryotomy, evisceration, or decapitation of the unborn child; or induction of premature delivery of a live but smaller child. This latter option was often unsuccessful, with infant mortality rates for premature infants of 85% or even higher as recently as 1916.[4] Another option was developed as a more humane alternative to destructive operations or premature or surgical delivery, that of manipulating the maternal diet to produce a much smaller child at term who could be delivered vaginally, even in the presence of a contracted pelvis. This technique was devised in 1788 by the British surgeon James Lucas and published in the second volume of the *Memoirs of the Medical Society of London* in 1794. He proposed "temperance in diet, a diminution in the usual quantity and a change in the quality of the food, an increase in exercise, the occasional loss of a few ounces of blood, and the moderate use of cooling asperients. The regimen was more strictly enjoined in the last months of pregnancy."[5]

The idea of manipulating the maternal diet was further refined and popularized by the German obstetrician Ludwig Prochownick in 1889 and 1901. Based on a total of 48 cases, Prochownick demonstrated that the maternal diet can influence the size, weight, and osseous development of the fetus, making it possible for it to be born vaginally at full term, whereas in previous pregnancies instrumental means or the induction of premature labor had been necessary.[6,7] The Prochownick diet was high in protein and fat and restricted in calories, fluids, and carbohydrates. This diet provided the foundation of maternal nutrition for nearly a century, long outliving its original intent, which had never been conclusively demonstrated in the first place. It was not only accepted but embraced by generations of obstetricians for its therapeutic effects in facilitating easier deliveries, reducing the incidence of preeclampsia, and treating obesity and diabetes during pregnancy, along with a wide range of other potential obstetric complications.

THE FETUS-AS-PARASITE PHILOSOPHY

The concept of limiting maternal weight gain while avoiding any adverse effects on the fetus became an obstetric axiom during the twentieth century, to the point where the fetus was regarded as a "parasite" that effectively abstracted its needed nutrients from the mother during intrauterine development, making maternal nutrition during pregnancy a nonissue.[8] This simplistic thinking, although widespread and nearly universally accepted by practitioners during this century, was in direct contrast to the most prevalent obstetric problems of the day: low birth weight and prematurity. Such restrictive practices, based on little scientific evidence, soon found their way into numerous textbooks. For example, in the first edition of Williams's *Obstetrics* (1903), it is suggested that patients normally gain weight only during the last 3 months of pregnancy, totaling about 3–5 pounds.[9] It is further stated that "this is not entirely due to the increased size of the uterus and its contents, but to a considerable extent results from an additional deposit of fat in the other portions of the body."

Although clearly in the minority, some obstetricians at this time opposed the fetus-as-parasite theory and believed very strongly that the nutritional state of the mother affected fetal development and subsequent birth weight. In 1916, G. F. D. Smith, a London obstetrician, published his study of 6162 cases from Dublin and London, examining the effects of the mother's nutritional status during pregnancy and at the time of delivery on the condition of her child at birth and during the first few days of life.[10] Smith concluded that a state of poor nutrition at the time of labor caused by insufficient food increased the rate of stillbirths and premature births, decreased mean birth weight, and increased postnatal infant mortality. A state of good nutrition was associated not only with an increase in mean birth weight, but with an improved ability to breast-feed.

MATERNAL MALNUTRITION: WAR STUDIES

The fetus-as-parasite theory persisted through the 1950s and 1960s, despite evidence of the adverse effects of maternal malnutrition on the course and outcome of pregnancy. Such evidence included studies of the influence of wartime conditions on perinatal mortality and birth weights. Two of these studies reported on maternal and infant morbidity and mortality in Holland and Russia: Antonov described the effects of the 1942 siege of Leningrad, and Smith reported on the consequences of semistarvation from 1942 to 1945 in Holland.[11,12] Antonov indicated that during the 18-month period of starvation, the infant mortality rate doubled, including 9% of full-term infants and 31% of low–birth-weight infants.[11] Smith found that Dutch women who had severely restricted diets during 6 months of their pregnancies (<1000 calories and 30–40 g of protein/day) gave birth to infants 10% lighter in birth weight.[12] Smith also reported a decrease in the incidence of preeclampsia during the Dutch famine; future obstetricians would misinterpret this as further evidence to restrict weight gain in pregnancy.

During World War II the British government instituted a policy under which all expectant and nursing mothers and children under 5 years of age received a pint of milk daily at reduced cost or free, as well as vitamin supplements, black currant syrup (or orange juice), and cod liver oil.[13] In 1944, the infant mortality rate, neonatal mortality rate, maternal mortality rate, and stillbirth rates were the lowest on record, and the birth rate was the highest in 15 years. Improved nutrition was at least partially responsible.

The Recommended Dietary Allowances (RDAs), issued by the Food and Nutrition Board of the National Academy of Sciences, also followed this restrictive philosophy for many years. In its first edition, published in 1945, it advised no increase in caloric intake during pregnancy.[14] By the fourth edition (1953), the recommendation had changed to 400 additional calories per day, but for the third trimester only.[15]

CURRENT RESEARCH AND RECOMMENDATIONS

With the publication of two landmark studies in 1968, a major change occurred in the philosophy of maternal nutrition in this country. First, the Eastman and Jackson study of 25,154 pregnancies observed at the Johns Hopkins Hospital between 1954 and 1961 found that both an increase in weight gain and an increase in prepregnancy weight independently and together were associated with progressive increases in birth weight.[16] For women of pregravid weight less than 120 pounds, they recommended liberal gains, especially during the first half of pregnancy. Preliminary analysis of 10,000 births in the Collaborative Study of Cerebral Palsy was also published in 1968.[17] This was one of the first studies to document the influence of antepartum weight gain on infant growth and development at 1 year of age. The highest maternal weight gains (>36 pounds) were associated with higher birth weights, lower prematurity rates, and better growth and development in the infant's first year of life.

Numerous other studies since 1968 have confirmed these findings that improved maternal nutrition benefits both mother and infant. A recent analysis from the 1980 National Natality Survey reported that a low weight gain during pregnancy was associated with a lower average birth weight and a higher risk of low birth weight (<2500 g) or fetal death outcome.[18] This study also reported that a low prepregnancy weight combined with a small weight gain was associated with a 29% incidence of low birth weight. The risk of fetal death outcome was also lowered with added weight gain, up to 35 pounds. For the gestational periods of 32–40 weeks, the risk of fetal death dropped by about half as weight gain increased from less than 16 to 26–35 pounds.

EVALUATION OF MATERNAL NUTRITION

CRITERIA FOR REFERRAL AND ADMISSION

Although every woman should have the opportunity to have a thorough nutritional evaluation by a nutritionist or registered dietitian specially trained in maternal nutrition, this is not always practical or feasible. When resources are limited, antepartum patients should be screened during the first prenatal visits and those women with a history of a previous low–birth-weight infant or who currently have a pregnancy with intrauterine growth retardation or SGA should be referred to nutrition counseling (Table 56-1). Other indications for referral include maternal pregravid weight 20% or more above ideal weight for her height or excessive weight gain during pregnancy (7 pounds or more per month); 10% or more below ideal weight for height or inadequate weight gain during pregnancy (less than 2 pounds per month after the first trimester); or excessive vomiting, sufficient to cause weight loss or ketonuria. Additional indications for nutrition counseling include the possibility of diet-related anemias (iron deficiency, pica, or vegetarianism), any medical problems that existed before conception, and gestational diabetes, lactose intolerance, alcoholism, or drug use. These guidelines for referral are summarized in Table 56-1.

TABLE 56–1. CRITERIA FOR REFERRAL FOR NUTRITION COUNSELING

- **I.** Weight or growth problems
  - **A.** Infant
    - **1.** Previous low-birth-weight infant
    - **2.** Present intrauterine growth retardation or SGA
  - **B.** Mother
    - **1.** Overweight
      - **a.** Pregravid obesity (≥20% above ideal weight for height)
      - **b.** Excessive weight gain (>7 pounds/month)
    - **2.** Underweight
      - **a.** Low pregravid weight (≥10% below ideal weight for height)
      - **b.** Inadequate weight gain (<2 pounds/month after first trimester)
      - **c.** Excessive vomiting (sufficient to cause weight loss or ketonuria)
- **II.** Diet-related anemias
  - **A.** Iron deficiency anemia
  - **B.** Pica
  - **C.** Vegetarian
- **III.** Medical problems
  - **A.** Gestational diabetes
  - **B.** Lactose intolerance
  - **C.** Alcoholism
  - **D.** Drug use

In some instances the nutrition-related problems during pregnancy become severe enough to retard fetal growth and seriously threaten maternal health and well-being. In these cases the antepartum patient should be admitted for intensive hydration, elemental alimentation, and monitoring of her own health status and that of her unborn child. Guidelines for admission for maternal malnutrition, as developed in 1978 at the Columbia-Presbyterian Medical Center by Barbara Luke, Edward T. Bowe, and Samuel Bruce, are given in Table 56-2. These guidelines include a weight loss of 10% or more of pregravid weight during the first trimester; inadequate net weight gain (less than 10 pounds) by 30 weeks gestation; hyperemesis gravidarum; and discrepancy between size and dates of 2 weeks or more at 20 weeks gestation or later with weight loss or failure to gain.

TABLE 56–2. GUIDELINES FOR ADMISSION FOR MATERNAL MALNUTRITION

1. Weight loss of 10% or more of pregravid weight during the first trimester
2. Inadequate net weight gain (less than 10 pounds) by 30 weeks gestation
3. Hyperemesis gravidarum: as defined by meeting two of the following criteria:
   - **a.** Inability to retain any solid or liquid food
   - **b.** Abnormal electrolytes (especially chlorides); acidosis
   - **c.** Acetonuria
   - **d.** Weight loss or no gain by 12 weeks gestation or later
   - **e.** Failure of drug therapy
4. Discrepancy between size and dates of 2 weeks or more at 20 weeks gestation or later with weight loss or failure to gain

PREGRAVID WEIGHT

The two strongest predictors of infant birth weight, after length of gestation, are maternal pregravid weight and gestational weight gain.[19] In view of the findings of the Collaborative Study of Cerebral Palsy, the 1980 National Natality Survey and the most current recommendations from the National Academy of Sciences,[20] pregravid weight should be average for height, or even higher to include a margin of safety for variations in weight gain during gestation. Those women at either extreme, underweight or overweight, before conception are at increased risk for prematurity or low birth weight, as well as other complications. Underweight is defined as 10% or more below a standard or ideal weight for height, or a body mass index [BMI = weight (kg)/height (m^2)] < 19.8; overweight is 20% or more above standard weight for height, or a BMI > 26.0. Optimal range for pregnancy, therefore, is ideal or standard to about 15% above, or a BMI of 19.8–26.0 (Table 56-3).

MATERNAL AGE

JUVENILE GRAVIDAS

Extremes of maternal age have been associated with poor course and outcomes of pregnancy, although the exact etiology remains unclear. According to national statistics, as shown in Table 56-4, more low–birth-weight infants (<2500 g) are born to mothers under the age of 15 years than to any other age group, followed by women over age 45 years.[21] Research has shown that pregnant teenagers, especially those under age 15, have higher rates of complications, maternal morbidity and mortality, and premature or low–birth-weight babies.[22] The most frequently cited reasons for such poor outcomes among adolescent gravidas are physiologic immaturity and poor nutrition.[23,24] However, her physical growth is nearly complete by the time she has the ability to reproduce, and postmenarcheal girls have not been shown to have poorer diets than their older counterparts.[25,26] Recent research has suggested that adolescents are at greater risk not because of their age but because of their poor sociodemographic and prenatal care status.[27,28]

ELDERLY GRAVIDAS

Studies of pregnancy course and outcomes among elderly gravidas (≥35 years of age) have also documented an increase in medical complications (eg, diabetes, chronic hypertension, and antepartum bleeding) and preterm delivery as compared to younger gravidas.[29] Researchers suggest that the outcome of pregnancy in this age group is affected by multiple confounding variables and that medical complications, parity, and age play major roles.

OBSTETRIC HISTORY

In addition to maternal pregravid weight, height, and age, obstetric history may contribute adversely to a woman's nutritional risk during pregnancy. Research has shown that there is a tendency to repeat low–birth-weight and small-for-gestational-age (SGA) deliveries in subsequent births.[30] The relative risk of a second birth also being SGA was found to be 3.4; similar results were found for repeat low–birth-weight or preterm deliveries. Other research has shown that the recurrence rate of fetal growth retardation was nearly 50%.[31] Stein and Susser suggest that the "most widespread environmental cause of IUGR (intrauterine growth retardation) is probably maternal undernutrition."[32] The nutritional status of a woman both before and during pregnancy is therefore an important influence on both the adequacy of intrauterine growth and the length of gestation.

TABLE 56-3. IDEAL AND DEVIATIONS OF PREGRAVID WEIGHT FOR HEIGHT

HEIGHT	IDEAL WEIGHT	UNDERWEIGHT (<10%)	NORMAL RANGE (−9% TO +19%)	OPTIMAL RANGE (IDEAL TO +15%)
4′9″	104	94	95–124	104–120
4′10″	107	96	97–127	107–123
4′11″	110	99	100–131	110–127
5′0″	113	102	103–135	113–130
5′1″	116	104	105–138	116–133
5′2″	118	106	107–141	118–136
5′3″	123	111	112–147	123–141
5′4″	128	115	116–153	128–147
5′5″	132	119	120–157	132–152
5′6″	136	122	123–162	136–156
5′7″	140	126	127–167	140–161
5′8″	144	130	131–172	144–166
5′9″	148	133	134–177	148–170
5′10″	152	137	138–181	152–175

(Adapted from Luke B. Maternal nutrition. Boston: Little, Brown, 1980.)

TABLE 56-4. MATERNAL AGE AND PERCENTAGE OF INFANTS LESS THAN 2500 GRAMS (1976)

MATERNAL AGE (YEARS)	WHITE (%)	BLACK (%)
<15	11.8	17.1
15–19	8.1	14.7
20–24	6.0	12.6
25–29	5.3	11.3
30–34	5.8	11.6
35–39	7.0	13.1
40–44	8.3	12.8
45–49	9.4	16.3

(Adapted from National Center for Health Statistics, Factors Associated With Low Birthweight, 1976. Vital and Health Statistics, Series 21, No 37. DHEW No (PHS) 80–1915. Public Health Service. Washington, DC: US Government Printing Office, April, 1980.)

DIETARY RECOMMENDATIONS

THE RDAs AND RINs

Table 56-5 lists the recommended dietary allowances (RDAs) for non-pregnant and pregnant adolescents and adult women, developed by the Food and Nutrition Board of the National Research Council, and the recommended intakes of nutrients (RINs), formulated by the Food and Agriculture Organization. The RDAs suggest higher protein; calcium; iron; vitamins A, B_{12}, D, C; and thiamine than the RINs, whereas the RINs suggest generally more calories for females 19 years of age and younger. The RDAs provide the most current standard for the United States for prescribing a balanced diet during gestation and will be the basis of this section.

Table 56-6 gives a summary of the changes in RDAs for women aged 22 years and older from the non-pregnant to the pregnant state, as well as food sources for each nutrient. Contrary to popular belief, nutrient requirements generally do not double during gestation. As shown in Table 56-6, only iron, folic acid, and vitamin D requirements increase 100% over non-pregnant requirements, whereas other nutrients, such as calcium, phosphorus, thiamine, and vitamin B_6 increase between 33% and 50%. Requirements for protein, zinc, and riboflavin increase about 20% to 25%, whereas those for energy, magnesium, iodine, niacin, and vitamins A, B_{12}, and C increase by 17% or less. These increases are translated into a daily food plan in Table 56-7, based on the RDAs during pregnancy for adult women aged 22 or older.

CALORIC INTAKE

As recommended in the National Academy of Sciences 1990 report on nutrition during pregnancy,[20] caloric intake should be based on the pregnant woman's pregravid weight and best rate of weight gain to achieve the optimal total gestational weight gain. For women who begin pregnancy within the optimal weight range for height (BMI 19.8–26.0), a good total gestational gain would be 25–35 pounds. This weight should be gained at the rate of about 3.5 pounds during the first trimester and about 1 pound per week for the second and third

TABLE 56-5. RECOMMENDED DIETARY ALLOWANCES (RDAs) AND RECOMMENDED INTAKE OF NUTRIENTS (RINs) FOR ADOLESCENT AND ADULT WOMEN

	NONPREGNANT						PREGNANT	
NUTRIENT	RIN 13–15 YR	RDA 15–18 YR	RIN 16–19 YR	RDA 19–24 YR	RIN ADULT	RDA 25–50 YR	RDA	RIN (LATTER HALF)
Energy (kcal)	2900	2200	3070	2200	2200	2200	+300*	+350
Protein (g)	31	44	30	46	29	50	60	38
Calcium (g)	0.6–0.7	1.2	0.5–0.6	1.2	0.4–0.5	0.8	1.2	1.0–1.2
Iron (mg)	12–24	15	14–28	15	14–28	15	30	†
Vitamin A (μg)	725	800	750	800	750	800	800	750
Vitamin D (μg)	2.5	10	2.5	10	2.5	5	10	10
Vitamin C (mg)	30	60	30	60	30	60	70	30
Thiamin (mg)	1.0	1.1	0.9	1.1	0.9	1.1	1.5	+0.1
Riboflavin (mg)	1.5	1.3	1.4	1.3	1.3	1.3	1.6	+0.2
Niacin (mg)	16.4	15	15.2	15	14.5	15	17	+2.3
Folate (μg)	200	180	200	180	200	180	400	400

Adapted from National Research Council, Food and Nutrition Board. Recommended dietary allowances. 10th ed Washington, DC: National Academy Press, 1989, and R. Passmore et al. Handbook on human nutritional requirements. FAO Nutritional Studies No. 28, WHO Monograph Series No. 61, Rome, Italy: Food and Agriculture Organization of the United Nations, 1974.

* Increase of 300 kcal/day is for the last two trimesters only.

† For women whose iron intake throughout life has been at the level recommended in this table, the daily intake of iron during pregnancy and lactation should be the same as that recommended for nonpregnant, nonlactating women of childbearing age. For women whose iron status is not satisfactory at the beginning of pregnancy, the requirement is increased, and in the extreme situation of women with no iron stores, the requirement can probably not be met without supplementation. (Passmore R et al, cited above)

TABLE 56-6. SUMMARY OF RDAS FOR WOMEN AGES 24 AND OLDER, CHANGES FROM NONPREGNANT TO PREGNANT, AND FOOD SOURCES

NUTRIENT	NONPREGNANT	PREGNANT	PERCENT INCREASE	DIETARY SOURCES
Folic acid	180 μg	400 μg	+122	Leafy vegetables, liver
Vitamin D	5 μg	10 μg	+100	Fortified dairy products
Iron	15 mg	30 mg	+100	Meats, eggs, grains
Calcium	800 mg	1200 mg	+50	Dairy products
Phosphorus	800 mg	1200 mg	+50	Meats
Pyridoxine	1.6 mg	2.2 mg	+38	Meats, liver, enriched grains
Thiamin	1.1 mg	1.5 mg	+36	Enriched grains, pork
Zinc	12 mg	15 mg	+25	Meats, seafood, eggs
Riboflavin	1.3 mg	1.6 mg	+23	Meats, liver, enriched grains
Protein	50 g	60 g	+20	Meats, fish, poultry, dairy
Iodine	150 μg	175 μg	+17	Iodized salt, seafood
Vitamin C	60 mg	70 mg	+17	Citrus fruits, tomatoes
Energy	2200 kcal	2500 kcal	+14	Proteins, fats, carbohydrates
Magnesium	280 mg	320 mg	+14	Seafood, legumes, grains
Niacin	15 mg	17 mg	+13	Meats, nuts, legumes
Vitamin B_{12}	2.0 μg	2.2 μg	+10	Animal proteins
Vitamin A	800 μg	800 μg	0	Dark green, yellow, or orange fruits and vegetables, liver

trimesters. For women who are overweight when they begin pregnancy (20% or more above ideal, or BMI > 26.0), the total gestational weight gain should be about 15–25 pounds, at the rate of about 2 pounds during the first trimester and about two thirds of a pound per week during the second and third trimesters. For women who begin pregnancy underweight (10% or more under ideal, or BMI < 19.8), the total gain should be about 28–40 pounds, depending on the severity of their pregravid weight deficit. For these women, much of the initial weight gain goes to correcting their own weight, with little remaining for the developing fetus. Research has shown that only after the mother's own weight has been brought up to within a normal range for her height can any additional nutrients be effectively utilized for normal growth of the fetus.[33,34] For this reason weight gain for the underweight woman should be about 5 pounds during the first trimester and slightly more than a pound per week during the second and third trimesters.

PROTEIN

As shown in Tables 56-5 and 56-6, protein requirements increase from 50 g for the non-pregnant woman to 60 g during pregnancy, equivalent to about 0.95 g/kg/day. Amino acids supplied by the maternal diet

TABLE 56-7. RDA-BASED DAILY FOOD PLAN DURING PREGNANCY

FOOD	SERVING SIZE	NUMBER OF SERVINGS: FIRST HALF OF PREGNANCY	NUMBER OF SERVINGS: SECOND HALF OF PREGNANCY
Dairy products			
Whole, skim, or buttermilk	8 oz.		
Yogurt	8 oz.		
Cottage cheese	12 oz.	2–4	4
Ice cream	6 oz.		
Processed cheese	1.5 oz.		
Hard (aged) cheese	1 oz.		
Meats			
Lean meat, fish, poultry	1 oz.	3–4	6–8
Eggs	1 medium/large	1	1–2
Vegetables			
Dark green or deep yellow	.5 cup	1	1
Citrus fruits	.5 cup	1–2	2
Other fruits and vegtables	.5 cup	1	2
Breads and grains			
Whole grain or enriched	1 oz. (1 slice)	3	4–5

(Adapted from Luke B. Maternal nutrition, Boston: Little, Brown, 1980:92.)

augment the accelerated protein synthesis needed for the expansion of the maternal blood volume, uterus, breasts, and fetal and placental tissues. This allowance must provide for maternal physiologic adjustments as well as growth and development of the fetus and placenta. The RDA for protein during pregnancy is generous because of uncertainties about efficiency of protein storage and utilization during gestation, as well as the possibility of adverse effects on both mother and fetus from an inadequate intake.

IRON

Iron deficiency has been found to be the most common nutritional disorder and the most important cause of anemia in the world.[35–37] As a constituent of hemoglobin, myoglobin, and a number of enzymes, iron is an essential nutrient for humans. The requirement for iron is greatest when there is rapid expansion of tissue and red cell mass, such as during infancy, childhood, and pregnancy. During gestation the greatest blood volume expansion and, therefore, the greatest iron need is in women of low pregravid weight with large weight gains.[38] During pregnancy, iron needs average about 3.5 mg/day, with a range of 2–4 mg.[38] Iron requirements may reach 4 mg/day during the latter half of pregnancy. During pregnancy, demands are made on iron stores because of the needs of the growing fetus and placenta and the expanding maternal blood volume and red cell mass; additional demands are created by the blood losses at delivery.[36,39–41] These requirements are superimposed on the non-pregnant baseline needs. Although the increased demands are in part offset by amenorrhea and increased iron absorption, it is doubtful that needs can be met by dietary sources alone.[42] Total demands during a singleton pregnancy average 1000–1100 mg.[43] Iron absorption from food ranges from 1% with some vegetable sources to 10% to 25% with meats.[44] Nonanimal dietary sources of iron are also adversely affected by other dietary components, such as tea, calcium, phytates in wheat bran, and yolk phosphoprotein.[45–49] The RDA during pregnancy of 30 mg assumes that women have a mixed diet (animal and vegetable sources of iron) and that most women in the United States cannot meet this increased requirement without supplementation.

CALCIUM

During gestation calcium requirements increase to 1200 mg/day, 50% higher than non-pregnant needs. Calcium accretion during pregnancy totals approximately 30 g, mostly in the fetal skeleton and is deposited during the last trimester.[50] Based on this need, the RDA during pregnancy is 400 mg/day above non-pregnant levels, which allows for a margin of 100 mg/day for individual variation. Although calcium absorption increases during pregnancy and excretion decreases, additional dietary requirements are still needed to meet the demands of pregnancy. Calcium-deficient diets during gestation have been associated with decreased bone density in the newborn infant.[51]

Milk and milk products provide the majority of calcium in the American diet, with an average consumption of 116 quarts per year.[52] The majority of the world's adult population, however, is unable to digest varying quantities of milk due to a low level of activity of the enzyme lactase.[53–55] Lactase is located in the brush border of the small intestine and is responsible for the hydrolysis of the disaccharide lactose, which is found exclusively in milk and milk products, into its component monosaccharides, glucose and galactose. Lactose, the main synergistic agent in milk, enhances the body's use of minerals and protein.[56] Research has shown that lactose enhances animal protein absorption and utilization as well as improving the digestibility and utilization of vegetable proteins.[57] Inadequate dietary calcium and vitamin D have been shown to result in biochemical changes tending toward osteomalacia in the mother and relative hypothyroidism in the infant.[58,59] For these reasons, pregnant women with lactose intolerance should include ample amounts of low-lactose, high-calcium foods in their diets, such as yogurt, aged cheeses, or specially treated milks.

OTHER VITAMINS AND MINERALS, INCLUDING MEGADOSES

As outlined in Tables 56-5 and 56-6, the requirements for the remaining vitamins are also increased, in proportion to their need during gestation. Their requirements can be met easily through a mixed diet, as described in Table 56-7. Vitamin and mineral deficiencies are rare in the United States, since most commonly used foods are either fortified or enriched (eg, vitamins A and D in milk; iodine in table salt; iron and B vitamins in breads and breakfast cereals). In the United States, the easy accessibility of large doses of vitamins without prescriptions is much more of a problem. The Food and Drug Administration's National Clearinghouse for Poison Control Centers estimates that 4000 cases of vitamin poisonings are reported to them each year.[60]

The fat-soluble vitamins, particularly vitamins A and D, are the most potentially toxic during pregnancy. Birth defects have been produced experimentally in animals given doses equivalent in humans to 500,000 IU.[61] Among the congenital anomalies observed were ear and eye malformations, as well as cleft palate.[61–64] The pediatric and obstetric literature includes case reports of kidney malformations in children whose mothers took between 40,000 and 50,000 IU of this vitamin during gestation.[65–67] Even at lower doses, excessive amounts of vitamin A may cause subtle damage to the developing nervous system, resulting in serious behavioral and learning disabilities in later life.[68] Large doses of vitamin A, in the range of 50,000–150,000 IU/day, are sometimes prescribed by dermatologists for various skin disorders. Women who are planning to become pregnant or who think they may have just conceived should avoid this type of treatment.

Vitamin D, if it is taken in large doses, can have toxic effects during pregnancy. The margin of safety is smaller for this vitamin than for any other. Birth defects of the heart, particularly aortic stenosis, have been reported in both human newborns and experimental animals with doses as low as 4000 IU (10 times the RDA) during pregnancy.[69-71] Infants who were oversupplemented in England during World War II developed a syndrome known as infantile hypercalcemia, characterized by cerebral, cardiovascular, and renal damage.[72]

Megadoses (10 times the RDA or greater) of vitamin C have resulted in a variety of adverse effects, including kidney stones in individuals susceptible to gout; possible damage to the insulin-producing cells of the pancreas; diarrhea; difficulties with fertility; and inactivation of vitamin B-12.[73] Large doses of vitamin C cause the urine to become acidic, leading to the possible formation of kidney stones in some individuals and interfering with urine tests for the presence of sugar.[74,75] Case reports of scurvy have appeared in the literature among infants of women who took megadoses of vitamin C during pregnancy.[76,77] The effects of large doses of other vitamins during pregnancy remain unclear.

SPECIAL CONSIDERATIONS

ALCOHOL USE DURING PREGNANCY

The adverse effects of maternal alcohol use on the developing fetus have been known empirically since ancient times. It was not until 1968 that a formal description appeared in the scientific literature when Lemoine and associates reported a set of abnormalities that were consistently observed in children born to alcoholic women: prenatal growth deficiency, an unusual facies, psychomotor retardation (IQ 70), and a 25% incidence of congenital anomalies (especially cleft palate and cardiac malformations).[78] This pattern of abnormalities was also reported by other investigators, and in 1973, Jones and Smith designated this pattern of altered growth and dysmorphogenesis the fetal alcohol syndrome (FAS).[79] Since Jones and Smith's original description of the characteristic features of FAS, many other clinicians and investigators have added their cases and additional clinical findings. It has been estimated that the worldwide incidence of FAS is 1.9 per 1000 live births (full characteristics),[80] and of fetal alcohol effects is 2.5–5 per 1000 live births (partial characteristics).[81,82] Among alcoholic women, the incidence of FAS is estimated at 25 per 1000 live births, whereas fetal alcohol effects are estimated at 90 per 1000.[82] It is the leading cause of mental retardation in the Western world, surpassing Down syndrome and cerebral palsy.[80]

Many experimental animal models (including primates) demonstrating the teratogenicity of alcohol have been developed and have shown a clear dose–response effect between maternal alcohol consumption and fetal risk.[82,83] For example, the characteristic midfacial abnormalities and many of the midline brain abnormalities can be produced in the mouse by one brief period of maternal alcohol intoxication during gastrulation.[84,85] Epidemiological studies have also demonstrated that maternal alcohol consumption presents a significant risk for adverse fetal development[86,87] and that risk increases with increasing alcohol intake.[88] Central to the characterization of this syndrome is retarded and deviant growth, manifested in nearly every organ system in proportion to timing and amount of alcohol exposure in utero. These effects may be the result of direct or indirect consequences of alcohol metabolism. Both alcohol and its major metabolite, acetaldehyde, readily cross the placenta, and both can be directly teratogenic.[89] Both alcohol and acetaldehyde have been shown to impair nucleic acid and protein synthesis directly in vitro.[90] The pharmacologic effects of ethyl alcohol result from cell membrane narcosis and cause a general depression of cell function.[89] All cells are affected, but the effects are most pronounced in those with excitable membranes.[89]

The mother metabolizes alcohol very differently from the way the developing fetus metabolizes it. Because alcohol is both water and lipid soluble, it passes readily through all biological membranes, equilibrating rapidly throughout the entire water volume of the maternal–placental–fetal unit. The amniotic fluid acts as a reservoir for unchanged alcohol and acetaldehyde, and because the fetus lacks the necessary enzymes to degrade these substances,[90] it is exposed to them long after they have been cleared from the maternal system.[89,91] It has also been suggested that alcohol or acetaldehyde may be toxic to the placenta as well as to the fetus and that ethanol-associated placentotoxicity could result in "selective" fetal malnutrition, independent of maternal nutritional status.[92]

Maternal undernutrition or malnutrition often accompanies alcohol abuse, and exacerbating its effects. For example, protein malnutrition is known to increase alcohol's hepatotoxicity, and alcohol itself impairs the absorption, utilization, and metabolism of nutrients.[93] Although moderate to severe alcohol intake can be complicated by some degree of undernutrition, current evidence strongly suggests that primary malnutrition is not solely responsible for FAS.[86,94] For example, in studies of the malnourished infants born during the post–World War II famine in Holland, microcephaly at birth did not result in mental retardation in later development.[95] By contrast, in children with FAS, the severity of the physical abnormalities present at birth (including microcephaly) was highly predictive of intellectual development in later years.[96,97] Poor nutritional status of the mother, plus the toxic effects of alcohol, may be more detrimental to the developing fetus than either factor alone. In addition, impairment of placental transport of amino acids by alcohol may result in transient or chronic deprivation of essential amino acids, resulting in intrauterine growth retardation, as well as potentially compounding any toxic effects of ethanol on embryogenesis. Reduced placental transfer of zinc and folic acid have also been demonstrated in animal models of alcohol-induced teratogenesis.[92,98]

In addition to the nutritional implications of alcohol abuse, alcohol can impair fetal development in a wide variety of other ways. Alcohol-related hypothermia, dehydration, fetal hypoxia and acidosis, placental pathology and dysfunction, and endocrine disturbances have all been shown to occur with increasing maternal alcohol intake.[99–103] Genetic factors, including individual variation in the metabolism of alcohol and the possibility of paternal influence on the susceptibility of the fetus to alcohol's teratogenic actions, may also be important in the expression of this disorder.[80,92,104]

In 1978 Clarren and Smith summarized the prenatal risk of maternal alcohol intake. These findings are equally relevant today, more than a decade later:

> . . .the variability of phenotype probably results from variable dose exposure at variable gestational timings offset by the genetic background of the individual fetus. Nearly all patients recognized as having the full fetal-alcohol-syndrome phenotype have been born to daily heavy alcohol users or relatively frequent heavy intermittent alcohol users. The evidence to date suggests that chronic consumption of 89 ml of absolute alcohol or more per day—the equivalent of about six hard drinks—constitutes a major risk to the fetus. Lower levels of consumption or less frequent use of alcohol carries an unknown risk and may be shown to be associated with less seriously affected children. No absolutely safe level of ethanol consumption has yet been established.[105]

MATERNAL PHENYLKETONURIA

Phenylketonuria (PKU) was the first metabolic disorder to be screened for on a national basis. Newborns were screened for this genetic disorder of amino acid metabolism starting in 1961 and treated with diet therapy until 6 years of age. After this age, many of the affected individuals were lost to medical follow-up because further treatment was unnecessary. As a result of this screening and treatment program, many of these individuals are now of childbearing age, and affected females pose a special problem during their pregnancies, that of screening for and treatment of maternal PKU to prevent the development of mental retardation in utero. The unique clinical challenge today is to develop an approach that would assure an improved course and outcome for women with PKU.[106]

It has been known for many years that excess maternal phenylalanine levels have a teratogenic effect on the developing fetus. During pregnancy there is a positive gradient of phenylalanine from mother to fetus. Maternal blood phenylalanine levels above 20 mg/dL during pregnancy are associated with a 90% incidence of mental retardation, microcephaly, congenital heart defects, and low birth weight among the surviving offspring; maternal blood phenylalanine levels below 16 mg/dL result in a 20% incidence of these adverse outcomes.[107–111] Spontaneous abortion is also more common among women with PKU, thought to be due to the possible toxic effects of high levels of phenylalanine or its related metabolites on the fetus.[108,109,112,113] It has been estimated that if each woman with PKU were to have two offspring, within one generation the prevalence of mental retardation related to PKU could rebound to the level present in the population before the advent of mass screening and treatment of this disorder.[114]

Clinical studies have found that initiation of dietary therapy prior to conception results in the most favorable outcomes.[115–117] Specific dietary guidelines have been developed to provide adequate prenatal nutrition while restricting dietary phenylalanine sufficiently to lower and maintain blood phenylalanine levels in the range of 2–8 mg/dL.[118]

MULTIPLE BIRTHS

Multiple births increased in the 1980s, mainly because women were delaying childbirth and older women have a higher incidence of twins: for example, mothers 30 years of age or older accounted for 20% of all births in 1980, compared to 25% in 1985.[119] The use of fertility drugs and in vitro fertilization during the 1980s may also have contributed to this increase. Multiple births are becoming a larger proportion of total births, as reflected by the multiple birth ratio (MBR), the number of multiple births per 1000 live births. In 1980, the MBR was 19.3; by 1985 it had risen to 21.0, including 20.4 for whites and 25.3 for blacks.[119]

The mortality rate for twin births is four to eight times higher than that for singletons, and most of this excess has been attributed to low birth weight, resulting from prematurity, and to intrauterine growth retardation, resulting from monozygosity and maternal nutrition.[120–123] In a study of 7001 live-born twins in Georgia born between 1974 and 1978, it was found that twins had a sixfold increase in neonatal mortality rate compared to that of singletons.[122] The twins in this study, though, had a weight-specific mortality rate equivalent to or less than that for singletons after adjustment for birth weight. Other studies have confirmed low birth weight as the major factor increasing perinatal and neonatal death rates in twin pregnancies.[124] This poor outcome is magnified an additional threefold when the mortality rates for monozygotic versus dizygotic twins are compared.[121,123,125]

There are no current standardized dietary recommendations for the woman with a multiple gestation. A recent monograph on twins recommended that the maternal caloric intake be increased an additional 300 kcal/day above the recommendations for singleton pregnancies, for a projected total weight gain of about 48 pounds.[126] Preliminary research indicates that both higher maternal pregravid weight for height and greater rates of gestational gain and total weight gain augment intrauterine growth in twins and increase length of gestation.[127] Recent studies on term twin births suggest that higher pregravid weight and gains of about 45 pounds are associated with better birth weights.[128,129]

CONCLUSION

Technological advances during the twentieth century will continue to push back the limits of viability. In future decades the nutrition–fertility link will be expanded at the opposite end of the spectrum, and nutrition in utero will emerge as a powerful tool with which to augment growth, development, and vitality. Careful evaluation and aggressive therapy will help ensure the most positive outcomes during gestation as a foundation of childhood health.

REFERENCES

1. Culpepper N. A directory for midwives. Book IV. London: 1684:156.
2. Smellie W. Treatise on the theory and practice of midwifery. London: D. Wilson, 1752 (facsimile printing by Scolar Press, London, 1974).
3. William JW. A statistical study of the incidence and treatment of labor complicated by contracted pelvis in the obstetrical service of the Johns Hopkins Hospital from 1896 to 1924. Am J Obstet Gynecol 1926;11:735.
4. LaFetra LE. The hospital care of premature infants. Trans Am Pediatr Soc 1916;28:90.
5. Spencer HR. An address on some changes in obstetrical practice since the foundation of the Medical Society of London. Br Med J 1923;2:639.
6. Prochownick L. Ein Versuch zum Ersatze der Kunstlichen Fruhgeburt. Centralblatt Gynakologie 1889;33:577.
7. Prochownick L. Ueber Ernahrungscuren in der Schwangerschaft. Ther Monatsh 1901;15:446.
8. Burke BS, Stuart HC. Nutritional requirements during pregnancy and lactation. JAMA 1948;137:119.
9. William JW. Obstetrics: a textbook for the use of students and practitioners. New York: D Appleton, 1903.
10. Smith GFD. An investigation into some of the effects of the state of nutrition of the mother during pregnancy and labour on the condition of the child at birth and for the first days of life. Lancet 1916;2:54.
11. Antonov AM. Children born during the siege of Leningrad in 1942. J Ped 1947;30:250.
12. Smith CA. Effects of maternal undernutrition upon newborn infants in Holland (1944–1945). J Ped 1947;30:229.
13. Oakley A. The captured womb: a history of the medical care of pregnant women. Oxford: Basil Blackwell, 1984.
14. Food and Nutrition Board, National Academy of Sciences, National Research Council. Recommended dietary allowances. 2nd ed. Washington, DC: National Academy Press, 1945.
15. Food and Nutrition Board, National Academy of Sciences, National Research Council. Recommended dietary allowances. 4th ed. Washington, DC: National Academy Press, 1953.
16. Eastman NJ, Jackson E. Weight relationships in pregnancy: the bearing of maternal weight gain and pre-pregnancy weight on birth weight in full term pregnancies. Obstet Gynecol Surv 1968;23:1003.
17. Singer JE, Westphal M, Niswander K. Relationship of weight gain during pregnancy to birth weight and infant growth and development in the first year of life. Obstet Gynecol 1968;31:417.
18. National Center for Health Statistics, S. Taffel. Maternal weight gain and the outcome of pregnancy, United States, 1980. Vital and Health Statistics. Series 21, No. 44, DHHS Publication No. (PHS) 86–1922. Public Health Service. Washington, DC: US Government Printing Office, 1986.
19. Luke B. Maternal Nutrition. Boston: Little, Brown, 1980.
20. National Academy of Sciences. Nutrition during pregnancy. Washington, DC: National Academy Press, 1990.
21. National Center for Health Statistics. Factors Associated With Low Birthweight, 1976. Vital and Health Statistics, Series 21, No. 37. DHEW No. (PHS) 80–1915. Public Health Service. Washington, DC: US Government Printing Office, April 1980.
22. National Research Council. Risking the future: adolescent sexuality, pregnancy, and childbearing. Washington, DC: National Academy Press, 1987.
23. Osofsky HJ. The pregnant teenager. Springfield, IL: Charles C Thomas, 1968.
24. Stepto RC, Keith L, Keith D. Obstetrical and medical problems of teenage pregnancy. In: Zackler J, Brandstadt W, eds. The pregnant teenager. Springfield, IL: Charles C Thomas, 1975.
25. Ancri G, Morse EH, Clarke RP. Comparison of the nutritional status of pregnant adolescents with pregnant women. III. Maternal protein and caloric intake and weight gain in relation to size of infant at birth. Am J Clin Nutr 1963;30:568.
26. Hegsted DM. Current knowledge of energy, fat, protein, and amino acid needs of adolescents. In: McKigney JI, Munro JN, eds. Nutrient requirements in adolescence. Cambridge, MA: MIT Press, 1976.
27. Horon IL, Strobino DM, MacDonald HM. Birth weights among infants born to adolescent and young adult women. Am J Obstet Gynecol 1983;146:444.
28. Lee K-S, Ferguson RM, Corpuz M, Gartner LM. Maternal age and incidence of low birth weight at term: a population study. Am J Obstet Gynecol 1988;158:84.
29. Yasin SY, Beydoun SN. Pregnancy outcome at ≥20 weeks' gestation in women in their 40s: a case-control study. J Reprod Med 1988;33:209.
30. Bakketeig LS, Hoffman HJ, Harley EE. The tendency to repeat gestational age and birth weight in successive births. Am J Obstet Gynecol 1979;135:1086.
31. Visser GHA, Huisman A, Saathof PWF, Sinnige HAM. Early fetal growth retardation: obstetric background and recurrence rate. Obstet Gynecol 1986;67:40.
32. Stein ZA, Susser M. Intrauterine growth retardation: epidemiological issues and public health significance. Semin Perinatol 1984;8:5.
33. Luke B, Jonaitis MA, Petrie RH. A consideration of height as a function of prepregnancy nutritional background and its potential influence on birth weight. J Am Dietet Assoc 1984;84:176.
34. Luke B, Dickinson C, Petrie RH. Intrauterine growth: correlations of maternal nutritional status and rate of gestational weight gain. Eur J Gynecol Reprod Biol 1981;12:113.
35. Control of nutritional anaemia with special reference to iron deficiency. WHO Technical Report Series No. 580. Geneva, Switzerland: WHO, 1975.
36. Finch CA. Iron deficiency anemia. Am J Clin Nutr 1969;22:512.
37. Beaton GH. Epidemiology of iron deficiency. In: Jacobs A, Worwood M, eds. Iron in biochemistry and medicine. London: Academic Press, 1974:477.

38. American Medical Association Committee on Iron Deficiency. Iron deficiency in the United States. JAMA 1968;203:407.
39. DeLeeuw NRM, Lowenstein L, Hsieh YS. Iron deficiency and hydremia in normal pregnancy. Medicine 1966;45:291.
40. Goltner E. Iron requirement and deficiency in menstruating and pregnant women. In: Kief H, ed. Iron metabolism and its disorders. New York: American Elsevier, 1975:159.
41. Pritchard JA, Scott DE. Iron demands during pregnancy. In: Hallberg L, Harwerth HG, Vannatti A, eds. Iron deficiency. London: Academic Press, 1970:173.
42. Food and Nutrition Board, National Research Council. Recommended dietary allowances. 9th ed. Washington, DC: National Academy Press, 1980.
43. Jacobs A. Transferrin and transferrin iron. In: Jacobs A, Worwood M, eds. Iron in biochemistry and medicine. London: Academic Press, 1974.
44. Nutritional anaemias: report of a WHO scientific group. WHO Technical Report Series No. 405, Geneva, Switzerland, 1968.
45. Bjorn-Rausmussen E. Iron absorption from wheat bread: influence of various amounts of bran. Nutr Metab 1974;16:107.
46. Callender ST, Marney SR Jr, Warner GT. Eggs and iron absorption. Br J Haematol 1970;19:657.
47. Conrad ME. Factors affecting iron absorption. In: Hallberg L, Harwerth HG, Vannotti A, eds. Iron deficiency. London: Academic Press, 1970:87.
48. Turnbull A. Iron absorption. In: Jacobs A, Worwood M, eds. Iron in biochemistry and medicine. London: Academic Press, 1974:369.
49. Disler PB, et al. The effect of tea on iron absorption. Gut 1975;16:193.
50. Pitkin RM. Calcium metabolism in pregnancy: a review. Am J Obstet Gynecol 1975;121:724.
51. Krishnamachari KAVR, Iyengar L. Effect of maternal malnutrition on the bone density of the neonates. Am J Clin Nutr 1975;28:482.
52. Bunch KL. Food consumption, prices, expenditures 1985. National Economics Division, Economic Research Service, US Department of Agriculture, Statistical Bulletin No. 749. Washington, DC: US Government Printing Office, 1987.
53. Bayless TM, et al. Lactose intolerance and milk drinking habits. Gastroenterology 1971;60:605.
54. McCracken RD. Lactase deficiency: an example of dietary evolution. Curr Anthropol 1971;12:479.
55. Simoons FJ. New light on ethnic differences in adult lactose intolerance. Am J Digest Dis 1972;18:595.
56. National Dairy Council. The role of lactose in the diet. Dairy Council Digest 1974;45:25.
57. Sewell RF, West JP. Some effects of lactose on protein utilization in the baby pig. J Anim Sci 1965;24:239.
58. Watney PJ, Rudd BT. Calcium metabolism in pregnancy and in the newborn. J Obstet Gynaecol Br Commonw 1974;81:210.
59. Liu SH, et al. Calcium and phosphorus metabolism in osteomalacia: XI. The pathogenetic role of pregnancy and relative importance of calcium and vitamin D supply. J Clin Invest 1941;20:255.
60. Myths of vitamins. FDA Consumer, March 1974.
61. Arnich L. Toxic effects of megadoses of fat-soluble vitamins. In: Hathcock JN, Coon J, eds. Nutrition and drug interrelations. New York: Academic Press, 1978.
62. Pick JB, Evans CA. Growth inhibition and occurrence of cleft palate due to hypervitaminosis A. Experientia 1981;37:1189.
63. Padmanabhan R, Singh G, Singh S. Malformations of the eye resulting from maternal hypervitaminosis A during gestation in the rat. Acta Anat 1981;110:291.
64. Weidenbecher M. Vitamin A-induced ear malformations in rats as a model for analysis of atresia auris congenita. Ann Otol Rhinol Laryngol (Suppl) 1981;90:3.
65. Bernhardt IB, Dorsey DJ. Hypervitaminosis A and congenital renal anomalies in a human infant. Obstet Gynecol 1974;43:750.
66. Geelen JAG. Hypervitaminosis A induced teratogenesis. CRC Crit Rev Toxicol 1979;6:351.
67. Pilotti G. Ipervitaminosis A gravidanza e malforazioni dell'apparato urinario nel feto. Minerva Pediatr 1975;27:682.
68. American Academy of Pediatrics Committee on Drugs and Nutrition. The use and abuse of vitamin A. Nutr Rev 1974;32:541.
69. Dalerup LM, Stockman VA, Rechsteiner de Vos H, et al. Survey on coronary heart disease in relation to diet in physically active farmers. Voeding 1965;26:245.
70. Dalderup LM. Vitamin D, cholesterol, and calcium. Lancet 1968;1:645.
71. Seelig MS. Vitamin D and cardiovascular, renal, and brain damage in infancy and childhood. Ann NY Acad Sci 1969;147:537.
72. Taussig HB. Possible injury to the cardiovascular system from vitamin D. Ann Intern Med 1966;65:1195.
73. Herbert V, Jacobs F. Destruction of B-12 by ascorbic acid. JAMA 1974;230:241.
74. Ringsdorf WM, Cheraskin E. Nutritional aspects of urolithiasis. So Med J 1981;74:41.
75. Toxicity of vitamin C megadoses. Nutr MD 1980;6(10).
76. Cochrane WA. Over-nutrition in prenatal and neonatal life: a problem? Can Med Assoc J 1965;931:893.
77. Bean WB. Some aspects of pharmacologic use and abuse of water-soluble vitamins. In: Hathcock NJ, Coon J, eds. Nutrition and drug interrelations. New York: Academic Press, 1978.
78. Lemoine P, Harrousseau H, Borteyru JP, Menuet J. Les enfants de parents alcooliques: anomalies observées. A propos de 127 cas. Quest Medical 1968;25.476.
79. Jones KL, Smith DW, Ulleland CN, et al. Pattern of malformation in offspring of chronic alcoholic mothers. Lancet 1973;1:1267.
80. Stressiguth AP, Sampson PD, Barr HM, Clarren SK, Martin DC. Studying alcohol teratogenesis from the perspective of the fetal alcohol syndrome: methodological and statistical issues. Ann NY Acad Sci 1986;477:63.
81. Abel EL, Sokol RJ. Incidence of fetal alcohol syndrome and economic impact of fas-related anomalies. Drug Alcohol Depend 1987;19:51.
82. Streissguth AP, Landesman-Dwyer S, Martin JC, Smith DW. Teratogenic effects of alcohol in humans and laboratory animals. Science 1980;209:353.
83. Clarren SK, Bowden DM. Fetal alcohol syndrome: a new primate model for binge drinking and its relevance to human ethanol teratogenesis. J Pediatr 1982;101:819.
84. Sulik KK, Johnston MC, Webb MA. Fetal alcohol syndrome: embryogenesis in a mouse model. Science 1981;214:936.
85. Sulik KK, Lauder JM. Brain malformations in fetal mice resulting from acute maternal alcohol exposure during the gastrulation stage of embryogenesis. Int J Dev Neurosci (abstract) 1983;1(3).
86. Kaminsky M, Rumeau C, Schwartz D. Alcohol consumption in pregnant women and the outcome of pregnancy. Alcohol Clin Exp Res 1978;2:155.
87. Sokol RJ, Miller SI, Reed G. Alcohol abuse during pregnancy: an epidemiological study. Alcohol Clin Exp Res 1980;4:135.
88. Smith DW. The fetal alcohol syndrome. Hosp Pract October 1979;121.
89. Kennedy LA. The pathogenesis of brain abnormalities in the fetal alcohol syndrome: an integrating hypothesis. Teratology 1984;29:363.

90. Pikkarainen PH, Raiha NC. Development of alcohol dehydrogenase activity in the human liver. Pediatr Res 1967;1:165.
91. Brien JF, Loomis CW, Tranmer J, McGrath H. Disposition of ethanol in human maternal venous blood and amniotic fluid. Am J Obstet Gynecol 1983;146:181.
92. Fisher SE. Ethanol: effect on fetal brain growth and development. In: Tarter RE, Van Thiel DH, eds. Alcohol and the brain: chronic effects. New York: Plenum Press, 1985:265.
93. Shaw S, Lieber CS. Effects of ethanol on nutritional status. In: Hodges RE, ed. Human nutrition: metabolic and clinical applications. New York: Plenum Press, 1979:223.
94. Weiner SG, Shoemaker WJ, Koda LY, Bloom FE. Interaction of ethanol and nutrition during gestation: influence on maternal and offspring development in the rat. J Pharmacol Exp Ther 1981;216:572.
95. Stein Z, Susser M, Saenger G, Marolla F. Chapter IV. Mental performance after prenatal exposure to famine. Famine and human development: the Dutch hunger winter of 1944/45. New York: Oxford University Press, 1975:197.
96. Streissguth AP, Herman CS, Smith DW. Intelligence, behavior and dysmorphogenesis in the fetal alcohol syndrome. J Pediatr 1978;92:363.
97. Streissguth AP, Clarren SK, Jones KL. Natural history of the fetal alcohol syndrome: a 10-year follow-up of eleven patients. Lancet 1985;2:85.
98. Ghishan FK, Patwardhan R, Greene HL. Fetal alcohol syndrome: failure of zinc supplementation to reverse the effect of ethanol on placental transport of zinc. Pediatr Res 1983;17:529.
99. Henderson GI, Hoyumpa AM, Schenker S. Effect of chronic and acute maternal alcohol consumption on fetal growth parameters and protein synthesis in fetal tissues. In: Abel EL, ed. Fetal alcohol syndrome: animal studies. Vol 3. Boca Raton, FL: CRC Press, 1982:151.
100. Henderson GI, Turner D, Patwardhan RV, et al. Inhibition of placental valine uptake after acute and chronic maternal alcohol ingestion. J Pharmacol Exp Ther 1981;216:465.
101. Mukherjee AB, Hodgen GD. Maternal ethanol exposure induces transient impairment of umbilical circulation and fetal hypoxia in monkeys. Science 1982;218:700.
102. Wunderlich SM, Boliga S, Munro HN. Rat placental protein synthesis and peptide secretion in relation to malnutrition from protein deficiency in alcohol administration. J Nutr 1979;109:1534.
103. Clarren SK, Alvord CA, Sumi S, Streissguth AP, Smith DW. Brain malformations related to prenatal exposure to ethanol. J Pediatr 1978;92:64.
104. Chernoff GF. The fetal alcohol syndrome in mice: maternal variables. Teratology 1980;22:71.
105. Clarren SK, Smith DW. The fetal alcohol syndrome. N Engl J Med 1978;298:1063.
106. Luke B, Keith L. The challenge of maternal phenylketonuria screening and treatment. J Reprod Med 1990;35:667.
107. Fisch RO, Doeden D, Lansky LL, Anderson JA. Maternal phenylketonuria: detrimental effects on embryogenesis and fetal development. Am J Dis Child 1969;118:847.
108. Stevenson RE, Huntley CC. Congenital malformations in offspring of phenylketonuria mothers. Pediatrics 1967;40:33.
109. Lenke RR, Levy HL. Maternal phenylketonuria and hyperphenylalanemia: an international survey of the outcome of untreated and treated pregnancies. N Engl J Med 1980;303:1202.
110. Koch R, Friedman EG, Wenz E, et al. The maternal PKU collaborative study. J Inher Metab Dis (Suppl) 1986;9(2):159.
111. MacCready RA, Levy HL. The problem of maternal phenylketonuria. Am J Gynecol 1972;113:121.
112. Kerr GR, Chamove AS, Harlow HF, Waisman HA. "Fetal PKU": the effect of maternal hyperphenylalanemia during pregnancy in the rhesus monkey (Macaca mulatta). Pediatrics 1968;42:27.
113. Menkes JH, Aeberhard E. Maternal phenylketonuria: the composition of cerebral lipids in an affected offspring. J Ped 1969;74:924.
114. Cartier L, Clow CL, Lippman-Hand A, Morissette J, Scriver CR. Prevention of mental retardation in offspring of hyperphenylalanemia mothers. Am J Public Health 1982;72:1386.
115. Levy HL, Waisbren SE. Effects of untreated maternal phenylketonuria and hyperphenylalanemia on the fetus. N Engl J Med 1983;309:1269.
116. Drogari E, Beasley M, Smith I, Lloyd JK. Timing of strict diet in relation to fetal damage in maternal phenylketonuria. Lancet 1987;2:927.
117. Lenke RR, Levy HL. Maternal phenylketonuria—results of dietary therapy. Am J Obstet Gynecol 1982;142:548.
118. Acosta PB, Blaskovics M, Cloud H, et al. Nutrition in pregnancy of women with hyperphenylalanemia. J Am Dietet Assoc 1982;80:443.
119. Advance report of final natality statistics, 1985. Monthly Vital Statistics Report (Suppl) July 17, 1987;36.
120. Ho SK, Wu PYK. Perinatal factors and neonatal morbidity in twin pregnancy. Am J Obstet Gynecol 1975;122:979.
121. Naeye RL, Tafari N, Judge D, Marboe CC. Twins: causes of perinatal death in 12 United States cities and one African city. Am J Obstet Gynecol 1978;131:267.
122. McCarthy BJ, Sachs BP, Layde PM, et al. The epidemiology of neonatal death in twins. Am J Obstet Gynecol 1981;141:252.
123. Keith L, Ellis R, Berger GS, et al. The Northwestern University multihospital twin study. Am J Obstet Gynecol 1980;138:781.
124. Medearis AL, Jonas HS, Stockbauer JW, Domke HR. Perinatal deaths in twin pregnancy. Am J Obstet Gynecol 1979;134:413.
125. Nylander PPS. Perinatal mortality in twins. Acta Genet Med Gemellol 1979;28:363.
126. Ahn MO, Phelan JP. Multiple pregnancy: antepartum management. Clin Perinatol 1988;15:55.
127. Luke B. Twin births: influence of maternal weight on intrauterine growth and prematurity. Fed Proc 1987;46:1015.
128. Pederson AL, Worthington-Roberts B, Hickok DE. Weight gain patterns during twin gestations. J Am Dietet Assoc 1989;89:642.
129. Brown JE, Schloesser PT. Prepregnancy weight status, prenatal weight gain, and the outcome of term twin gestations. Am J Obstet Gynecol 1990;162:182.

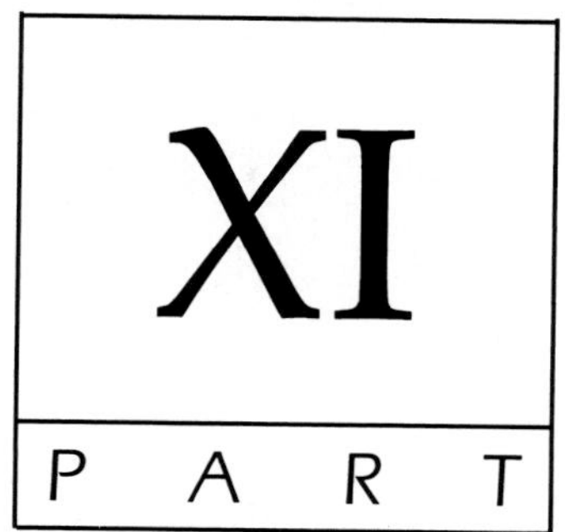

MATERNAL DISEASES COMPLICATING PREGNANCY

57

CHAPTER

TRAUMA, SHOCK, AND CRITICAL CARE OBSTETRICS

Gary A. Dildy and David B. Cotton

DEFINITION OF SHOCK

"Shock is a condition in which circulation fails to meet the nutritional needs of the cell and fails to remove metabolic wastes."[1] This condition may result from hypovolemia (absolute or relative) or cardiac dysfunction. When the circulating blood volume is less than the capacity of its vascular bed, hypotension with diminished tissue perfusion results, leading to cellular hypoxia and, ultimately, cell death.[2] Depending on the duration and severity of the insult, irreversible organ damage or even death of the individual may ensue.

HISTORICAL ASPECTS OF SHOCK

In reviewing the origin of the word *shock,* Simeone[3] attributes the first use of the word in the English medical literature to a 1743 translation of Henry-François Le Dran's second French edition of *A Treatise or Reflexions Drawn from Experiences with Gunshot Wounds.* The French words *saisissement, se cousse, commotion, coup,* from which the English was derived meant "violent impression, jolt, commotion, and a blow."[3]

Over the years, much of the insight that has contributed to the understanding of shock has been gained on the battlefields during the American Civil War, World War I, World War II, and the Korean and Vietnam conflicts.[1] During the Vietnam conflict, respiratory distress syndrome was recognized as a distinct entity.[4] Later, development of the pulmonary artery catheter helped resolve the controversy surrounding the etiology of respiratory distress syndrome. This syndrome develops following shock and conditions that activate the coagulation and inflammatory responses, resulting in damage to the pulmonary microvasculature and increased vascular permeability.[1,5] In obstetrics, shock has played a major role in maternal morbidity and mortality. One of the most frequent causes of maternal death in the United States is hemorrhagic shock.[6,7] The knowledge and technology acquired partly from medical experience on the battlefield have also led to reductions in maternal morbidity and mortality.

INCIDENCE OF SHOCK IN THE OBSTETRIC POPULATION

The actual incidence of shock in obstetric patients is unclear. However, by extrapolating mortality data, we can obtain an indication of the relative incidence of shock severe enough to result in death of the patient. A steady decline in maternal mortality has been noted since 1915, when national vital statistics in the United States first were recorded (Fig. 57-1).[8–10] Of 321 maternal deaths in 1978, 19% were due to toxemia, 19% to sepsis, 12% to ectopic pregnancies, and 11% to hemorrhage.[9] Kaunitz and colleagues reviewed the causes of maternal mortality in the United States between 1974 and 1978.[7] Of 2475 maternal deaths, 2067 were pregnancy-related without abortive outcomes. The most frequent causes of death were embolism, hypertensive disease, obstetric hemorrhage, and infection; and the most common cause in the abortive-related group was ectopic pregnancy (Table 57-1). This study indicated that all causes of maternal death have been decreasing with time except for embolism, which may be less preventable and possibly overreported. In a review of 501 consecutive maternal deaths in Texas between 1969 and 1973, Gibbs and Locke demonstrated that most deaths occurred in the postpartum period (297 postpartum deaths versus 155 antepartum deaths).[11] Of the

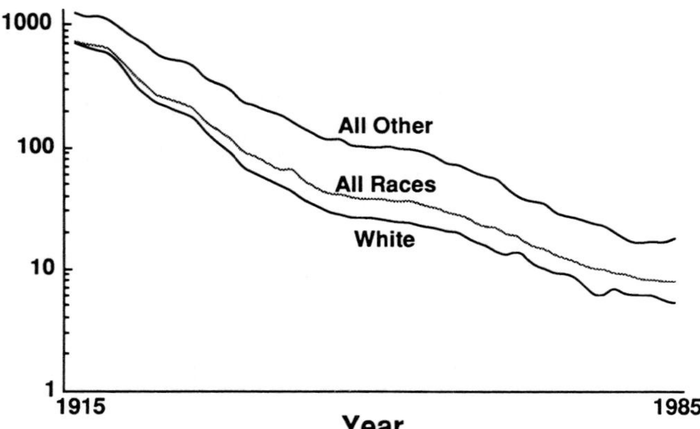

FIGURE 57-1. Maternal deaths in United States per 100,000 live births, 1915–1985.

309 maternal deaths secondary to direct obstetric causes, 36% were secondary to hemorrhage, 24% to toxemia, 21% to infection, 7% to amniotic fluid embolism, and 5% to anesthesia. Several studies have shown a markedly increased risk of death with advancing maternal age.[12–14] Retrospective determination of preventability has varied between 19%[14] and 65%.[15]

Anesthesia-related maternal mortality was studied in Michigan between 1972 and 1984.[16] Of 292 direct and indirect maternal deaths, anesthesia was considered a primary cause in 15 and a contributing factor in four. In more recent years, the failure to secure an airway was identified as the predominant factor. Patient risk factors included obesity, emergent nature of surgery, and hypertension. As with other causes of maternal mortality, an overall decline in anesthesia-related deaths has occurred. Reports from other developed countries show a similar decline in maternal mortality.[12,14]

TABLE 57-1. SELECTED CAUSES OF MATERNAL DEATHS IN THE UNITED STATES FROM 1974 TO 1978

CLASSIFICATION	NO.	%
Pregnancies not associated with abortive outcomes	2067	83.5
Embolism	491	19.8
Thrombotic	271	
Amniotic fluid	189	
Air	25	
Other/unspecified	6	
Hypertensive disease	421	17.0
Preeclampsia/eclampsia	396	
Other	25	
Obstetric hemorrhage	331	13.4
Postpartum	114	
Uterine rupture	71	
Abruptio placentae	55	
Nonuterine	39	
Retained placenta	33	
Placenta previa	19	
Obstetric infection	199	8.0
Upper genital tract	135	
Chorioamnionitis	18	
Postpartum intestinal rupture/ischemia	12	
External genitalia/perineum	4	
Other/unspecified	30	
Cerebrovascular accident	107	4.3
Postpartum	55	
Ante- or intrapartum	19	
Other/unspecified	33	
Anesthesia/analgesia complication	98	4.0
Aspiration of gastric contents	28	
Other/unspecified	70	
Other and unspecified causes of maternal death	420	17.0
Pregnancies with abortive outcomes	408	16.5
Ectopic	254	
Abortion	141	
Hydatidiform mole	13	
Total maternal deaths	2475	100.0

(From Kaunitz AM, Hughes JM, Grimes DA, Smith JC, Rochat RW, Kafrissen ME. Causes of maternal mortality in the United States. Reprinted with permission of the American College of Obstetrics and Gynecologists. Obstet Gynecol 1985;65:605.)

ETIOLOGY OF SHOCK

Shock in the obstetric patient may be categorized as either hypovolemic, septic, neurogenic, or cardiogenic. Although these etiologies are different, they often can share common pathophysiologic pathways and ultimately lead to hypoperfusion at the tissue and cellular levels. This decreased perfusion, secondary to hypovolemia or cardiac pump failure, leads to hypoxia and acidosis, which results in the clinical shock picture (Fig. 57-2).

Hypovolemic shock is usually the result of hemorrhage. Profound vasodilation and movement of intravascular fluids into the extravascular space result in hypoperfusion in anaphylactic shock. Hemorrhage is secondary either to disruption of a closed cardiovascular circuit or to coagulopathy. Causes of the former include uterine atony, abnormal placentation or development, and trauma. Uterine atony can occur in association with several conditions. Abnormalities of placentation and abnormal development of the placenta usually refer to conditions such as placenta previa, abruptio placentae, placenta accreta, ectopic pregnancy, spontaneous abortion, and hydatidiform mole. Trauma secondary to obstetric causes can be categorized as spontaneous or surgical. Spontaneous trauma refers to lacerations of the cervix, vagina, and perineum, as well as rupture of the uterus and rupture of the liver. Surgical trauma can be associated with episiotomy, forceps delivery, cesarean section, dilatation and curettage, and legal abortion. Non-obstetric trauma can be categorized as blunt trauma or penetrating trauma. The former may result from falls or motor vehicle accidents, and the latter is usually associated with gunshot wounds or stab wounds.

Coagulopathies leading to hemorrhage can be acquired or hereditary. Acquired coagulopathies, although not common, may be secondary to induced

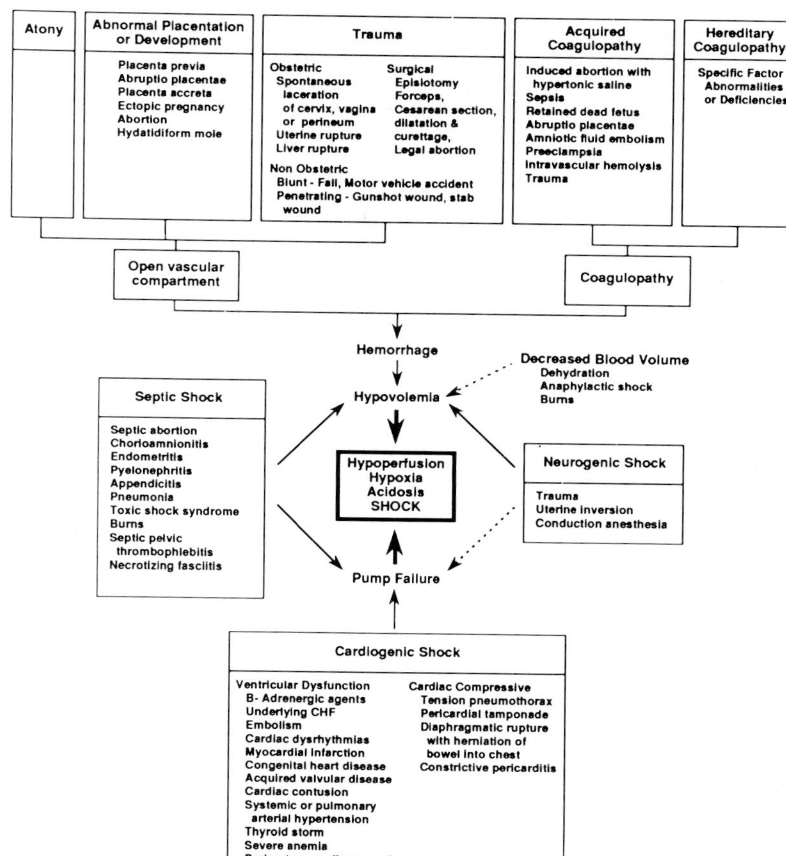

FIGURE 57–2. Etiology of shock in the obstetric patient.

abortion by hypertonic saline,[17–19] sepsis,[20–24] retained dead fetus syndrome,[25–31] abruptio placentae,[32–34] amniotic fluid embolism,[35–47] preeclampsia or eclampsia,[48–52] intravascular hemolysis,[23] or trauma.[53] Hereditary coagulopathies are secondary to a congenital lack of the coagulation factors required to activate or promote the coagulation cascade. Coagulopathy may also be precipitated by hemorrhage in conjunction with massive volume replacement with crystalloid and packed red blood cells and concomitant utilization of circulating clotting factors, with exacerbation of the initial condition.

Sepsis may lead to shock as the result of several pathophysiologic mechanisms, usually related to intravascular volume depletion and myocardial depression. Septic shock in obstetrics can occur in association with many conditions, some of which are unique to obstetrics. Chorioamnionitis,[54–58] pyelonephritis,[59–63] appendicitis,[64–74] septic abortion,[75] toxic shock syndrome,[76–80] and septic pelvic thrombophlebitis[81–87] are all well described in the obstetric literature. Septic shock secondary to chorionic villus sampling has also been reported.[88,89]

Cardiogenic shock occurs secondary to ventricular dysfunction or cardiac compression (see Fig. 57-2). Unique to the obstetric patient are such conditions as amniotic fluid embolism and peripartum cardiomyopathy. Certain structural cardiac defects can be lethal during the peripartum period.

Neurogenic shock may be associated with uterine inversion at the time of delivery, conduction anesthesia, or central nervous system trauma. Other miscellaneous causes of shock, such as anaphylactic shock and insulin shock, may be seen in the obstetric patient but are rarely reported.

GENERAL SUPPORTIVE MEASURES

INITIAL TREATMENT

Several important initial steps should be performed when the diagnosis of shock is made in the obstetric patient. Placement of two large-bore intravenous lines, preferably 16-gauge, for rapid expansion of intravascular volume is the first step. One liter of normal saline or lactated Ringer's solution should be infused over the first 15 minutes while other measures are taken. An indwelling catheter is placed for hourly determination of urine output. An arterial line allows continuous measurement of systemic blood pressure, as well as easy access for laboratory investigations. Oxygen should be administered via nasal prongs or face mask at 6–8 L/min and the F_IO_2 adjusted according to arterial blood gas results. If the ability to maintain an adequate tidal volume or arterial oxygenation is impaired or if the airway is obstructed, endotracheal intubation with positive pressure ventilation may be required.

Initial laboratory investigation should include blood type and cross-match, complete blood count, platelets, prothrombin time, partial thromboplastin time, fibrinogen, electrolytes, blood urea nitrogen and creatinine, and arterial blood gases. Urine postcatheterization should be sent for analysis and microscopic evaluation. When the patient is stabilized, cultures from blood, urine, sputum, amniotic fluid, endometrial cavity, and stool are taken, as indicated, if sepsis is suspected.

VOLUME REPLACEMENT

Whether to give crystalloids or colloid solutions for initial treatment is controversial.[90] Rackow and colleagues showed that two to four times as much 0.9% saline was required to reach the same hemodynamic end points as 6% hetastarch and 5% albumin.[91] Colloid osmotic pressure (COP) rose when albumin and hetastarch were administered and fell when saline was given. Resuscitation with normal saline resulted in a higher incidence of pulmonary edema, probably related to the fall in COP.

Standard dextran with a molecular weight averaging 75,000 may initiate intravascular coagulation. Low-molecular-weight dextran, with a molecular weight averaging 40,000, carries a smaller risk of initiating disseminated intravascular coagulopathy (DIC), but also has less tendency to pull fluid into the intravascular space.[92] A 1984 American College of Obstetricians and Gynecologists technical bulletin entitled "Hemorrhagic Shock" recommends avoidance of dextran because of its anticoagulant effects and risks of anaphylaxis.[93]

Correction of metabolic acidosis may be aided by adding sodium bicarbonate to intravenous fluids. Lactated solutions are not used because aerobic metabolism is required for the conversion of lactate to bicarbonate.[2]

If initial crystalloid therapy does not result in the desired clinical improvement, the administration of colloids for further volume expansion should be strongly considered.

In the case of hemorrhagic hypovolemic shock and in cases of disseminated intravascular coagulation, blood component therapy will be indicated, mostly by laboratory parameters. An obvious exception is profuse hemorrhagic shock for which immediate blood components—specifically, packed red blood cells—are indicated. It must be remembered that, grossly, the degree of hemorrhage is often underestimated by as much as 50%.[94] "Relative bradycardia," a sign of acute intraperitoneal bleeding, may occur when hypotension is accompanied by a normal pulse rate, as opposed to the expected tachycardia produced by blood loss.[95]

Packed red blood cells (PRBC) are administered through an 18-gauge or larger intravenous line in order to increase blood volume and oxygen-carrying capacity to the tissues. The term *massive blood replacement* is used when one total volume is replaced over a 24-hour period.[94] In those patients whose red cells are typed and serums are screened for antibodies, the risks of abbreviating the major cross-match in urgent or massive transfusion after an "immediate spin" phase of the cross-match are low.[96]

The use of fresh-frozen plasma (FFP) is now under scrutiny and requires specific indications: replacement of isolated factor deficiencies, reversal of warfarin effect with active bleeding or requiring emergency surgery, antithrombin-III deficiency, immunodeficiencies, thrombotic thrombocytopenia purpura, and massive blood transfusion in cases in which factor deficiencies are presumed to be the sole or principal derangement.[97,98] Besides containing the components of the coagulation, fibrinolytic, and complement systems, FFP also contains proteins that maintain oncotic pressure and modulate immunity. Because of risks, including disease transmission, anaphylactoid reactions, alloimmunization, and volume overload, alternative therapy with crystalloids and colloids is encouraged. Because pathologic hemorrhage in the patient receiving massive transfusion is usually due to thrombocytopenia rather than depletion of coagulation factors, empiric administration of FFP should be allowed only in those patients in whom factor deficiencies are presumed to be the sole or principal derangement.[97] In these cases, concentrated platelet infusions are appropriate. No evidence exists that, in massively transfused patients, prophylactic transfusion of FFP per certain number of units of PRBC decreases transfusion requirements unless coagulation factor defects have been documented.[99] The most useful tests for predicting abnormal bleeding and guiding therapy in massively transfused trauma patients are the platelet count and fibrinogen level.[100]

Thrombocytopenia may be secondary to dilution effect or to consumption of platelets. Adults have a limited mobilizable platelet pool and a limited ability to increase production acutely.[101] Moreover, platelets in refrigerated blood quickly become nonviable.[102]

Platelet transfusion should be performed when the platelet count falls below 20,000/μL, or below 50,000/μL in preparation of a surgical procedure or in the face of active bleeding. Minimization of blood product transfusion can be effected by correcting thrombocytopenia and specific coagulation factor defects.[94] In trauma patients, platelets are usually required after a patient receives over 20 units of blood in a 12-hour period.[100] However, in obstetric patients who experience thrombocytopenia secondary to other causes, such as preeclampsia, platelet transfusion may be indicated much earlier in the course of treatment.

Cryoprecipitate should be administered instead of FFP when the calculated coagulation factor defect based on blood fibrinogen levels may result in volume overload. Table 57-2 demonstrates the therapeutic contents per volume of each blood product.[103]

TABLE 57–2. SUMMARY CHART OF BLOOD COMPONENTS

COMPONENT	CONTENT	INDICATIONS FOR USE	AMOUNT OF ACTIVE SUBSTANCE PER UNIT	VOLUME (mL)
Red blood cells	Red blood cells, some plasma, some white blood cells and platelets or their degradation products	Increase red blood cell mass for symptomatic anemia	200 mL packed red blood cell mass	250–350
Leukocyte-poor red blood cells	Red blood cells, some plasma, few white blood cells	Prevent febrile reactions due to leukocyte antibodies, and increase red blood cell mass	185 mL packed red blood cell mass	200–250
Frozen–thawed washed red blood cells	Red blood cells, no plasma, minimal white blood cells and platelets	Increase red blood cell mass Prevent sensitization to HLA antigens Prevent febrile or anaphylactic reactions to white blood cells, platelets, and proteins (IgA) Provide rare blood cells	170–190 mL packed red blood cells	300
Platelet concentrations	Platelets, few white blood cells, some plasma	Bleeding due to thrombocytopenia or thrombocytopathia	At least 5.5 $\times 10^{10}$ platelets	30–50
Fresh-frozen plasma	Plasma, all coagulation factors, no platelets	Treatment of coagulation disorders	0.7–1.0 U Factors II, V–VI, VIII–XIII, 500 mg fibrinogen	220–250
Cryoprecipitated AHF	Fibrinogen, Factor VIII, Factor XIII, von Willebrand factor	Factor VIII deficiency (hemophilia A) von Willebrand's disease Factor XIII deficiency FIbrinogen deficiency	80 U Factor VIII 200 mg fibrinogen	10–25
Albumin	Albumin	Plasma volume expansion		
5%			12.5 g	250
25%			12.5 g	50

(Modified from Borucki, DT, ed. Blood component therapy: a physician's handbook. 3rd ed. Washington, DC: American Association of Blood Banks, 1981:25.

INOTROPIC AGENTS

If adequate intravascular volume replacement is not successful in supporting blood pressure (ie, a systolic blood pressure of at least 80 mm Hg), an advanced stage of shock should be suspected and inotropic therapy instituted (Table 57-3). Dopamine is considered the first-line inotropic agent. Dopamine is an endogenous catecholamine, structurally similar to norepinephrine and epinephrine. Dopamine increases myocardial contractility and heart rate via β-adrenergic receptors and releases norepinephrine from myocardial storage sites. Its action on blood vessels is dose dependent, resulting in vasodilation of renal, mesenteric, coronary, and intracerebral vessels via dopamine receptors, and vasoconstriction of all vascular beds in higher doses via α-adrenergic receptors.[104] Dopamine should be started at 2–5 μg/kg/min and titrated to desired clinical parameters.[104] Doses between 2 and 5 μg/kg/min result in vasodilation of renal and mesenteric vasculature via B_2 and dopaminergic receptors, whereas doses between 5 and 10 μg/kg/min result in increased myocardial contractility and cardiac output via B_1 receptors.[105] Doses beyond 20 μg/kg/min result in generalized vasoconstriction via α-adrenergic receptors.

If satisfactory hemodynamic parameters are not achieved, dobutamine should be added to the dopamine regimen at 2–10 μg/kg/min (Fig. 57-3).[106] Dobutamine increases cardiac output with minimal tachycardia by acting as a myocardial β-receptor stimulant. If dobutamine does not provide adequate improvement, isoproterenol, a β-adrenergic agonist, may be added. Increased heart rate and contractility are achieved at the risk of ventricular ectopy, excessive tachycardia, and peripheral vasodilation. Other inotropic agents, such as digoxin and amrinone (Inocor), may also be utilized to improve myocardial contractility.[90] Digoxin is usually administered with continuous electrocardiographic monitoring by giving an initial bolus of 0.5 mg IVP, followed by 0.25-mg doses every 4 hours for a total loading dose of 1.0 mg. The maintenance dosage in pregnant patients is usually 0.25–0.37 mg/day, de-

TABLE 57–3. INOTROPIC AGENTS

INOTROPIC AGENT	MECHANISM OF ACTION	DOSAGE
Dopamine	Dopaminergic (0.5–5.0 μg/kg/min) vasodilation of renal and mesenteric vasculature β_1-adrenergic (5.0–10.0 μg/kg/min) increased myocardial contractility, SV, CO α-adrenergic (15–20 μg/kg/min) increased general vasoconstriction	2–5 μg/kg/min and titrate to BP & CO
Dobutamine	Myocardial β_1-receptor stimulant increased CO, minimal tachycardia	2–10 μg/kg/min
Isoproterenol	β-adrenergic receptors increased contractility and heart rate, but ventricular ectopy, tachycardia, vasodilation	1–20 μg/min
Digoxin	Improved contractility of myocardium	0.5 mg IV push and 0.25 mg q 4 h × 2, then 0.25–0.37 mg/day

(Modified from Lee W, Clark SL, Cotton DB, et al. Septic shock during pregnancy. Am J Obstet Gynecol 1988;159:410.)

pending on plasma levels.[106] Amrinone, an inotropic agent with vasodilatory activity, is indicated for the short-term management of cardiac failure.[90] A bolus of 0.75 mg/kg over 2–3 minutes is given, and an infusion of 5–10 μg/kg/min should follow. Vasodilation may be undesirable in septic shock and thus may be contraindicated.

VASOPRESSOR AGENTS

If blood pressure does not respond to inotropic therapy, a peripheral vasoconstrictor should be started to maintain systemic vascular resistance (Table 57-4). Phenylephrine, an α-adrenergic agonist, may be initiated at 1–5 μg/kg/min. Norepinephrine, a mixed alpha and beta agonist with powerful vasoconstrictive properties, may be added to provide generalized vasoconstriction and increased systemic vascular resistance. This agent should be used only in situations where blood pressure is dangerously low despite other therapy, because perfusion to vital organs, such as the kidneys and lungs, may be reduced by the vasoconstriction.

Caution must be exercised with use of these agents in gravid patients. The primary goal is stabilization of the mother; however, consideration must be given to the fetus. Dopamine administered to the normotensive pregnant ewe at less than 10 μg/kg/min resulted in no change in uterine blood flow; higher doses resulted in decreased blood flow.[107] In pregnant ewes subjected to spinal hypotension, dopamine administered in sufficient doses to maintain blood pressure resulted in further diminishment of uterine blood flow and increased uterine vascular resistance in comparison to controls.[108] Greiss and others noted a marked increase in uterine vascular resistance that exceeded the increase in blood pressure, thus decreasing uterine blood flow in pregnant ewes.[109] They concluded that these vasopressors were only indicated in cases in which they were essential for maternal survival.

INVASIVE MONITORING

Since the introduction in 1970 by Swan, Ganz, and colleagues of the pulmonary artery catheter for the determination of pressures in the right side of the heart and pulmonary capillary wedge pressure, the uses of the Swan-Ganz catheter have become increasingly important in managing critically ill patients.[110] Many clinical indications exist for use of the Swan-Ganz catheter,[111] some of which are unique to obstetrics (Table 57-5).[93,112–116]

The pulmonary artery catheter provides a direct means of measuring central venous pressure, pulmonary capillary wedge pressure, cardiac output, systemic

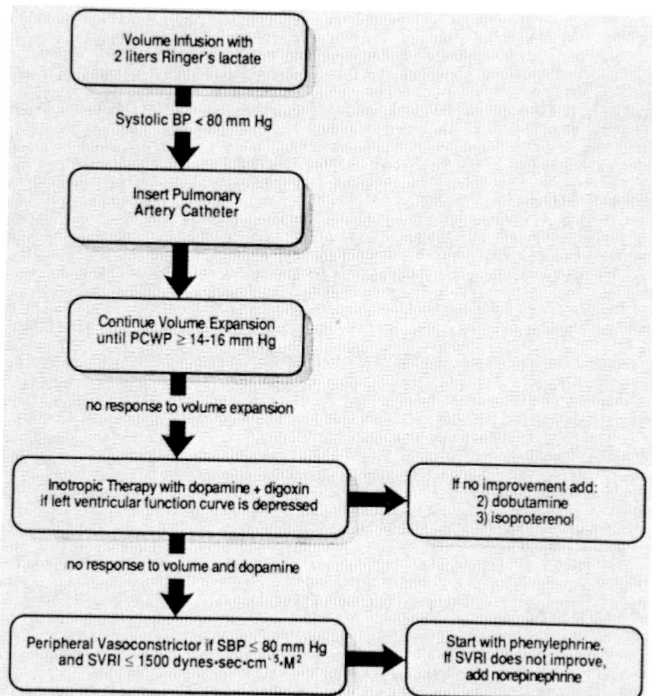

FIGURE 57–3. Hemodynamic algorithm for obstetric septic shock. BP = blood pressure; PCWP = pulmonary catheter wedge pressure; SBP = systolic blood pressure; SVRI = systemic vascular resistance index. (From Lee W, Clark SL, Cotton DB, et al. Septic shock during pregnancy. Am J Obstet Gynecol 1988; 159: 414.)

vascular resistance, and mixed venous oxygen saturation[112] and may be used to initiate atrioventricular pacing and fluid challenge.

Furthermore, pathophysiologic conditions secondary to or in association with the pregnant state may be diagnosed and treated appropriately with the Swan-Ganz catheter. The differentiation between pulmonary edema secondary to high pulmonary capillary wedge pressure versus low pulmonary capillary wedge pressure can be determined with the pulmonary artery catheter. Kirshon and Cotton found that the development of hydrostatic pulmonary edema may occur at lower pulmonary capillary wedge pressures during pregnancy secondary to a lower colloid osmotic pressure.[112] Cotton and Benedetti indicate that central venous pressure inaccurately reflects pulmonary capillary wedge pressure in patients with myocardial infarction, peritonitis, ischemic ST-T EKG changes, and severe pregnancy-induced hypertension.[113] Benedetti, Cotton, and others demonstrated that in three of nine patients with severe pregnancy-induced hypertension, the central venous pressure did not correlate with pulmonary capillary wedge pressure.[115] In a later study of 18 patients with severe pregnancy-induced hypertension, Cotton and others reported that central pressure is not a reliable predictor of pulmonary capillary wedge pressure.[117] Packman and Rackow found that changes in central venous pressure and wedge pressure during fluid loading in patients with hypovolemia and septic shock did not correlate and stated that left heart filling pressure during fluid resuscitation should not exceed 12 mm Hg.[118] Clark, Horenstein, and others[114] suggest that the Swan-Ganz catheter is particularly helpful in managing patients with severe preeclampsia and patients who have structural cardiac defects during the peripartum period.

Upon insertion of the Swan-Ganz catheter, advancement to the right side of the heart demonstrates characteristic pressure tracings through the right atrium, right ventricle, pulmonary artery, and pulmonary capillary wedge positions (Fig. 57-4).[119] From these wave forms, specific hemodynamic and ventilatory parameters can be determined (Table 57-6).[112] Cardiac output may then be used to construct a ventricular function curve (Fig. 57-5).[113] Hemodynamic subsets of ventricular function can be evaluated by plotting stroke index against left ventricular filling pressure (Fig. 57-6). A knowledge of pulmonary capillary wedge pressure, pulmonary artery diastolic-wedge gradient, and the AV-02 difference make it possible to ascertain the precise etiology of cardiopulmonary compromise (Fig. 57-7).

After placement of the Swan-Ganz catheter, a chest x-ray should be obtained to rule out pneumothorax and to confirm the catheter's position. Complications of Swan-Ganz catheter placement range from 0.4% to 9.9%.[112,120] Specific complications include those occurring at the time of insertion, such as cardiac arrhythmias, pneumothorax, hemothorax, injury to vascular and neurologic structures, pulmonary infarction, and pulmonary hemorrhage. Later complications, such as

TABLE 57–4. VASOPRESSOR AGENTS

VASOPRESSOR AGENT	MECHANISM OF ACTION	DOSAGE
Phenylephrine (Neo-Synephrine)	α-adrenergic increased SVR	1–5 μg/kg/min
Norepinephrine (Levarterenol)	Mixed adrenergic alpha and beta generalized vasoconstriction, increased SVR	1–4 μg/min

(Modified from Lee W, Clark SL, Cotton DB, et al. Septic shock during pregnancy. Am J Obstet Gynecol 1988;159:410.)

TABLE 57–5. INDICATIONS FOR PULMONARY ARTERY CATHETERIZATION DURING PREGNANCY

1. Massive blood loss with large transfusion requirements, particularly in the face of oliguria or pulmonary edema
2. Septic shock, especially when accompanied by hypotension or oliguria, required volume resuscitation or vasopressor therapy
3. Cardiac failure or pulmonary edema of uncertain etiology
4. Severe pregnancy-induced hypertension complicated by pulmonary edema, oliguria unresponsive to initial fluid challenge, or severe hypertension refractory to conventional therapy (hydralazine)
5. Labor and delivery in patients with significant cardiovascular disease (New York Heart Association Functional Class III and IV patients)
6. Intraoperative cardiovascular decompensation (eg, pulmonary hypertension with shunting secondary to amniotic fluid embolism)
7. During peripartum period in patients with severe preeclampsia and structural cardiac defects
8. Thyroid storm with evidence of high output failure
9. Diabetic ketoacidosis with severe hypovolemia and oliguria

(Data from references 93,112–116.)

catheter migration into the pericardial and pleural space with subsequent cardiac tamponade and hydrothorax, as well as balloon rupture, thromboembolism, catheter knotting, and pulmonary valve rupture, may occur.[112,113,120]

An alternate approach to invasive monitoring is pulse-Doppler ultrasound.[121] Pulse-Doppler ultrasound correlates closely with thermodilution-derived estimations for stroke volume and cardiac output and may be beneficial when invasive monitoring is not feasible, such as in maternal thrombocytopenia, or where hemodynamic monitoring capabilities are not available. It may also prove beneficial in patients in whom cardiac output measurements are misleading by thermodilution technique, as in the case of tricuspid insufficiency or pulmonic insufficiency.[121]

SURGICAL THERAPY

Surgical therapy, in conjunction with medical therapy and support, is an integral part of managing obstetric

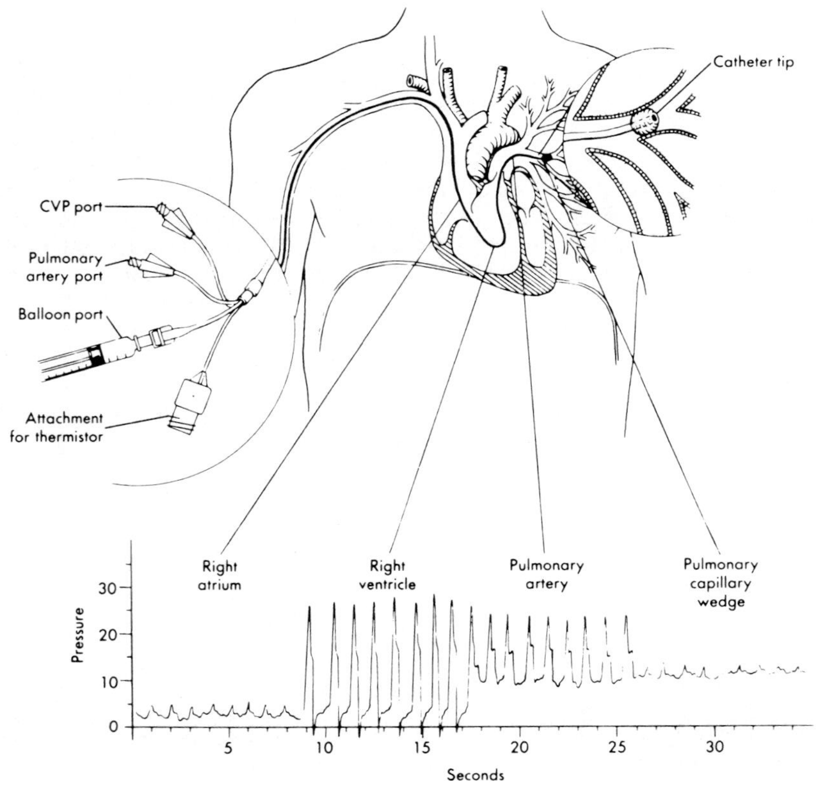

FIGURE 57–4. Swan-Ganz catheter placement. Swan-Ganz catheter (7 French) depicting CVP port, PA and balloon port, and attachment for thermistor. During advancement through right side of heart, characteristic pressure tracings are recorded from right atrial, right ventricular, PA, and PCW positions. (From Gibson RS, Kistner JR. In: Suratt PM, Gibson RS, eds. Manual of medical procedures. St Louis: CV Mosby, 1982: 61.)

TABLE 57–6. HEMODYNAMIC AND VENTILATORY PARAMETERS

	NONPREGNANT	PREGNANT
Central venous pressure (mm Hg)	1–7	Unchanged
Pulmonary capillary wedge pressure (mm Hg)	6–12	Unchanged
Mean pulmonary artery pressure (mm Hg)	9–16	Unchanged
Systemic vascular resistance (dynes · sec · cm^5)	800–1200	Decreased 25%
Pulmonary vascular resistance (dynes · sec · cm^5)	20–120	Decreased 25%
Cardiac output (L/min)	4–7	Increased 30% to 45%
Arterial pO_2 (mm Hg)	90–95	104–108
Arterial pCO_2 (mm Hg)	38–40	27–32
Arterial pH	7.35–7.40	7.40–7.45
Oxygen consumption (mL/min)	173–311	249–331

(From Kirshon B, Cotton DB. Invasive hemodynamic monitoring in the obstetric patient. Clin Obstet Gynecol 1987;30:579.)

patients in shock. Obstetric patients in shock may require surgical intervention, which, above all, must be well timed.

Uterine bleeding at the time of delivery requires prompt management and planning. As in the case of uterine atony, although medical therapy is being initiated, plans for surgical intervention should also be considered. Uterine artery ligation, initially described by Waters,[122] is performed by grasping the uterine wall and broad ligament and passing a single No. 1 chromic catgut suture anteroposteriorly through the lower uterine segment. The ascending uterine vessels are encompassed and the suture exited through the avascular area at the base of the board ligament.[123] This method also has been reported to be successful in uterine hemorrhage secondary to septic incomplete abortion.[124] Several cases of a transvaginal approach have been reported, but this is not widely used or promoted.[125,126] If hemorrhage persists after uterine artery ligation, the hemodynamic stability of the patient should determine if one proceeds with a hypogastric artery ligation or hysterectomy. Clark, Phelan, and others feel that hypogastric artery ligation should be reserved for stable patients of low parity who strongly desire further childbearing, as they found a high complication rate and a low success rate with hypogastric artery ligation in obtaining control of uterine hemorrhage.[127] They also advocate that the ligation be performed distal to the posterior division of the hypogastric artery and that a second suture be placed beneath the ovarian ligament at its junction with the uterus. Cesarean hysterectomy is clearly indicated for profound intractable hemorrhage if the patient is unstable, multiparous, or not desirous of future childbearing.[128]

Profuse bleeding secondary to placenta previa requires immediate cesarean section and, in some cases, especially if complicated by placenta accreta, progression to hysterectomy after less radical surgical maneuvers, such as uterine artery ligation and hypogastric artery ligation, have failed. On the other hand, bleeding secondary to abruptio placentae, depending on the severity, may be treated by expectant management or by immediate cesarean section according to the status of the mother and the fetus. Patients with previous cesarean sections and placenta previa are also more

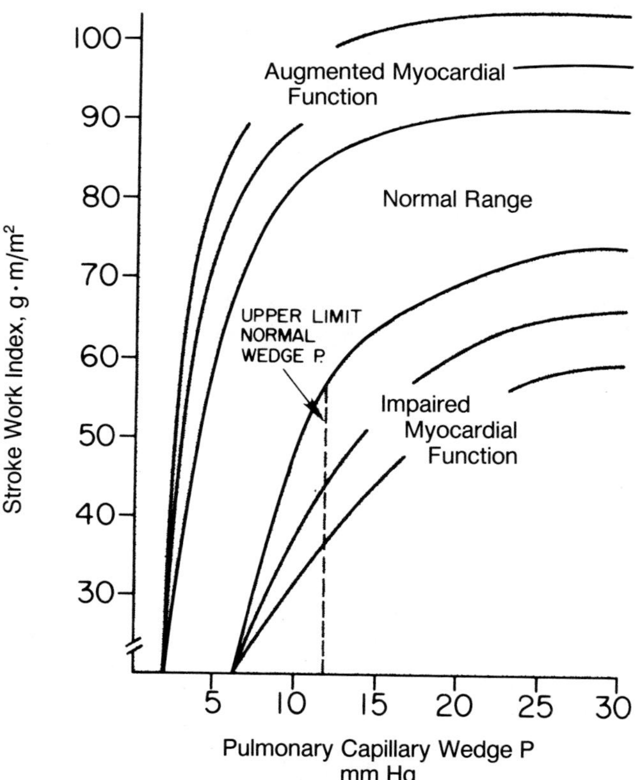

FIGURE 57–5. Normal ventricular function curve. (From Cotton DB, Benedetti TJ. Use of the Swan-Ganz catheter in obstetrics and gynecology. Obstet Gynecol 1980; 56: 644.)

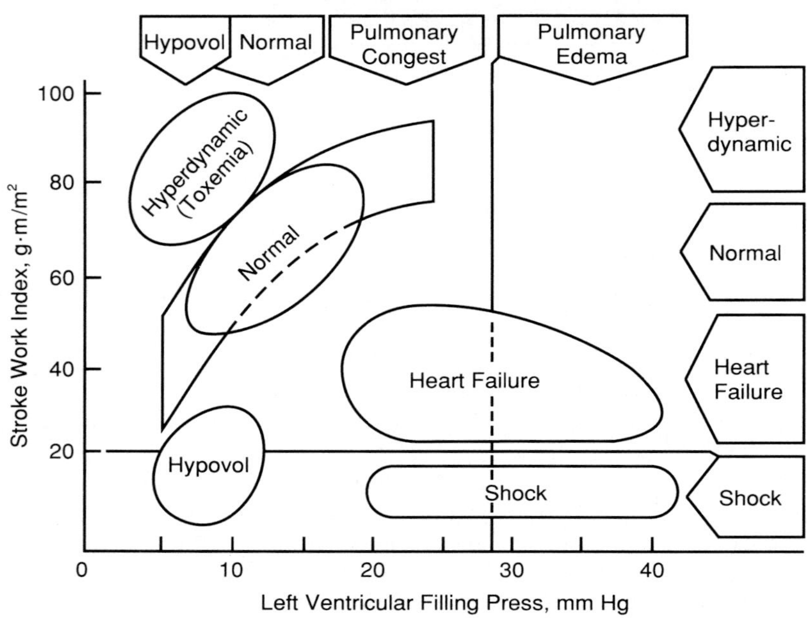

FIGURE 57–6. Hemodynamic subsets of ventricular function. (From Cotton DB, Benedetti TJ. Use of the Swan-Ganz catheter in obstetrics and gynecology. Obstet Gynecol 1980; 56: 644.)

likely to have a coexisting placenta accreta, which, in a significant number of cases, ultimately requires hysterectomy.[129]

Ectopic pregnancy is typically managed surgically by laparoscopy or exploratory laparotomy. Although severe blood loss secondary to spontaneous abortion is rare, timely intervention with dilatation and curettage can minimize the effect of further blood loss.

Molar pregnancies, which may bleed profusely, require careful evacuation by suction curettage and aggressive medical management of uterine muscular tone.

Bleeding secondary to obstetric trauma, such as that occurring during vaginal delivery with episiotomy, vaginal lacerations, or cervical lacerations, or during cesarean section with uterine extensions, is usually managed by direct repair of the damaged tissues with appropriate suture materials. Maternal trauma, depending on the anatomical location, may require surgical intervention, such as thoracotomy for chest injuries, laparotomy for intra-abdominal injuries, and orthopedic surgery for limb fractures.

In some cases of septic shock, surgical intervention is required to remove the source of infection. In the case of chorioamnionitis, delivery of the products of concep-

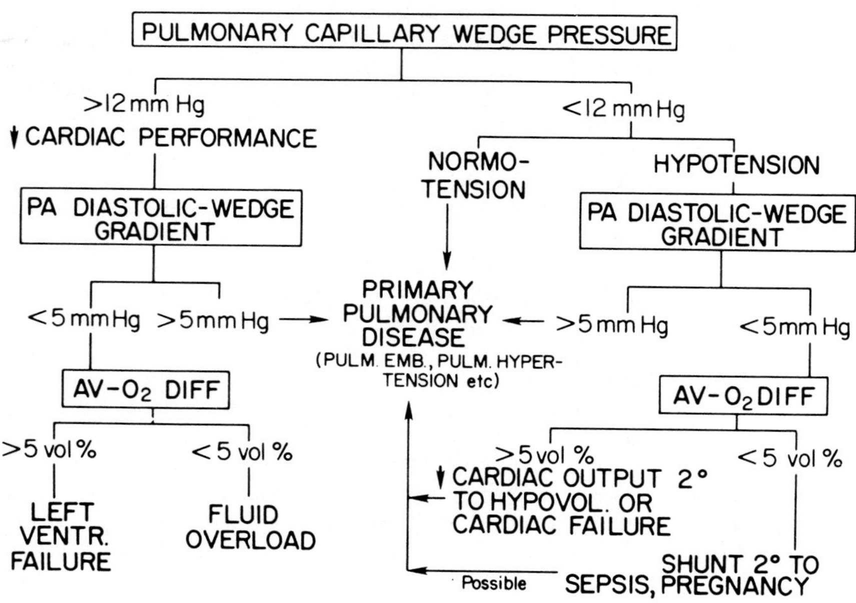

FIGURE 57–7. Flow diagram for interpretation of Swan-Ganz catheter. (From Cotton DB, Benedetti TJ. Use of the Swan-Ganz catheter in obstetrics and gynecology. Obstet Gynecol 1980; 56: 644.)

tion achieves this goal. Factors related to the maternal and fetal well-being play an integral role in determining the timing and mode of delivery.

In cases of suspected appendicitis, exploratory laparotomy with removal of the appendix is mandated. Pregnant patients are at increased risk for misdiagnosis or late diagnosis of appendicitis, with subsequent increased maternal and fetal morbidity and mortality. A high index of suspicion and a low threshold for laparotomy are required to avoid the potential maternal and fetal hazards of late diagnosis.[65] The risks of negative laparotomy are felt to be not as significant as those of a late laparotomy with positive findings.[68]

Cases of septic abortion are managed by supportive medical therapy, broad coverage with antibiotics, and early removal of the products of conception by dilatation and curettage. Most cases of endometritis are managed by antibiotic therapy alone; however, some cases require laparotomy with hysterectomy in order to remove the abscessed tissues that are the source of persistent, refractory sepsis.

Septic pelvic vein thrombophlebitis that does not respond to antibiotics and intravenous heparin therapy requires surgical therapy with exploratory laparotomy and ligation of the inferior vena cava and the ovarian vessels.

Cardiogenic shock demanding surgical intervention is rare in obstetrical experience. However, diaphragmatic rupture with herniation of bowel contents into the thoracic cavity requires prompt diagnosis and therapy to avoid catastrophic consequences.[130] Cardiac valvular replacement at the time of cesarean section has also been reported in the literature.[131,132]

Neurogenic shock secondary to uterine inversion is usually treated simply with manual replacement of the uterus in its proper anatomical position with simultaneous shock therapy.[133] However, cases not amenable to the usual conservative method of manual replacement of the uterus necessitate exploratory laparotomy with transabdominal maneuvers aimed at reducing the inverted uterus.[134–136]

CONTROVERSIAL AND EXPERIMENTAL REGIMENS

Most of the controversy surrounding the medical treatment of shock involves the treatment specifically of septic shock. One of the most investigated class of drugs creating controversy is the corticosteroids.

Corticosteroids are believed to be useful in the treatment of septic shock by correcting hypoadrenalism, reversing cardiovascular system depression, stabilizing cell membrane and lysosomal membranes, preventing complement-induced activation of polymorphonuclear leukocytes, inhibiting endorphin release, and eliciting metabolic effects, such as secretion of glucagon, gluconeogenesis, and increased liver protein syntheses.[137]

Numerous animal model studies and a few human studies have produced conflicting results. Studies in nonhuman primates have demonstrated that survival is improved in septic shock following treatment with a corticosteroid and antibiotic regimen, even if treatment is delayed until sustained systemic hypotension results.[138–142]

Human clinical studies have been criticized for flaws in study design and nonstandardization of regimens.[143] In 1976, Schumer published the results of a two-part clinical study that involved prospective and retrospective groups. The prospective study of 172 patients who were treated with dexamethasone, methylprednisolone, or saline showed an overall mortality rate in the steroid-treated group of 10.4%, with somewhat better results with dexamethasone. A 38.4% mortality rate was seen in the saline-treated group. The retrospective study involving 328 patients showed similar results, with a 42.5% mortality rate in the control group and a 14% morality rate in the steroid-treated group.[144]

In 1984, Sprung demonstrated in a prospective, randomized study of 56 patients that corticosteroids may improve survival if administered early in septic shock but did not improve overall survival in patients with severe, late septic shock.[145]

Hoffman reported in 1984 that the mortality rate of patients with severe typhoid fever could be decreased by treatment with corticosteroids.[146]

In 1987, the Methylprednisolone Severe Sepsis Study Group published data from a prospective, randomized, double-blind, placebo-controlled trial of 382 patients, concluding that the use of high-dose corticosteroids provided no benefit in the treatment of septic shock. They also reported an increased mortality secondary to infections.[143]

Known potential side effects from the administration of corticosteroids include gastrointestinal bleeding, hyperglycemia, superinfection, and altered monocyte activity.[137,147]

Currently, in our institution (Baylor College of Medicine), corticosteroids are rarely used for treatment of septic shock in obstetric patients.

Naloxone, an opiate antagonist, has been studied in animals[148–151] and humans[152–154] for the reversal of opiate-induced hypotension in endotoxic shock. The rationale for use of naloxone is that the endogenous opiate β-endorphin is stored with ACTH and both seem to be released simultaneously under physical stress.[155,156] Studies using the rat endotoxic shock model have suggested that naloxone both prophylactically blocks and rapidly reverses endotoxin-induced hypotension, which appears to be partially mediated by endogenous opiates.[151]

Canine studies demonstrated improved cardiovascular parameters and survival in animals treated with naloxone in endotoxic shock.[148–150]

Data published so far on humans have been controversial. Roberts and colleagues[152] suggest that earlier studies found no positive effects secondary to short observation periods.[153,154] Their data suggested that continuous intravenous infusion of naloxone resulted in decreased inotrope and vasopressor requirements in patients with septic shock. Positive hemodynamic effects (decreased heart rate with increased stroke volume) were observed more than 4 hours after an initial naloxone bolus, and no side effects were identified.

In the absence of narcotics, naloxone is supposed to be devoid of side effects.[157] However, treatment of patients with naloxone who have received opiates for chronic pain relief could precipitate opiate withdrawal and possibly cardiovascular collapse.[158]

Further controlled clinical studies are required before the general usage of naloxone for endotoxic shock can be recommended.

Nonsteroidal anti-inflammatory drugs (NSAIDs) are also thought to protect against the many deleterious effects of prostaglandins on the cardiovascular, pulmonary, and coagulation systems during endotoxic shock. Each agent acts at specific points in the prostaglandin synthesis pathway. Aspirin, ibuprofen, indomethacin, and meclofenamate are cyclo-oxygenase inhibitors, whereas imidazole is a selective inhibitor of thromboxane synthetase (Fig. 57-8).

Current data regarding the effects of NSAIDs on humans are lacking. Studies in sheep have shown that administration of *Escherichia coli* endotoxin causes respiratory distress, pulmonary hypertension, systemic arterial hypoxemia, and increased levels of systemic and pulmonary prostaglandins, specifically $PGF_{2\alpha}$ and PGE. Prostaglandin synthesis inhibitors given before administration of endotoxin prevented the rise in prostaglandins and subsequent development of respiratory distress.[159]

In the primate model, pretreatment with aspirin prevented decreased renal arterial blood flow and thrombocytopenia in female baboons who were administered *E. coli* endotoxin.[160] Future clinical investigation in humans appears warranted.

Antilipopolysaccharide (anti-LPS) immunoglobulin G (IgG) is found in freeze-dried human plasma obtained from blood donors. Plasma found to have high titers of IgG is used for therapy.[161] IgG has been found to bind to LPS from a wide range of gram-negative bacteria.[162] Early studies in humans have demonstrated a decreased mortality from septic shock.[163] Ziegler and colleagues treated bacteremic patients with human antiserum to a mutant *E. coli* during the onset of the illness and observed a significant reduction in deaths from gram-negative bacteremia and septic shock.[163] Lachman and others recently have shown that anti-LPS immunotherapy for the treatment of septic shock of obstetric and gynecologic origin in humans decreases complications, hospital stay, and mortality.[164] Control patients demonstrated a mortality rate of 47.4% (9/19), compared to a mortality rate of 7.1% (1/14) in the treated group.

PERIMORTEM CESAREAN SECTION

"Postmortem cesarean section is a procedure shrouded in mystique and antiquity, overshadowed by fear, religion, and law."[165] Mythological and historical accounts of this procedure date back to antiquity.[166] The term

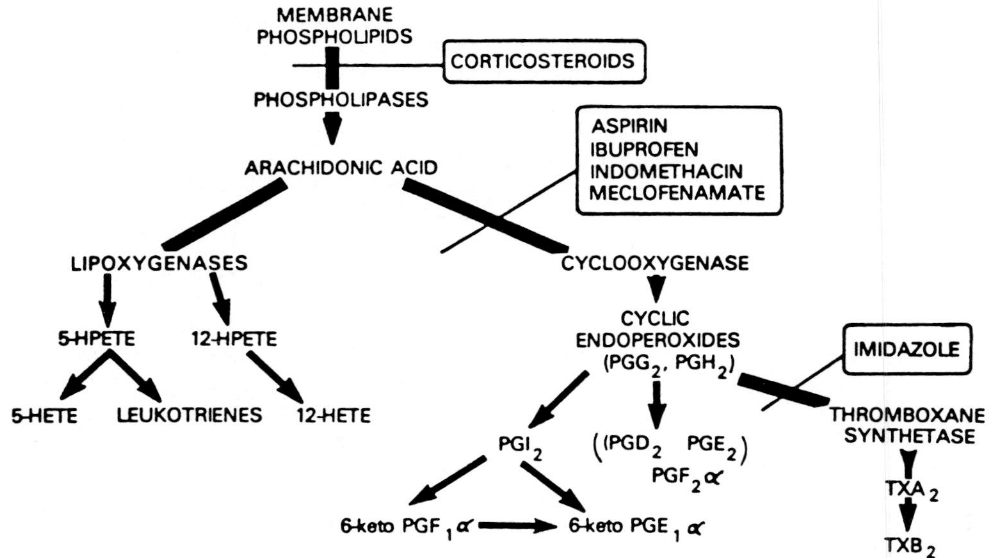

FIGURE 57–8. Scheme of arachidonic acid metabolism showing proposed sites of actions of some specific enzyme inhibitors and major stable metabolites. (From Schein RMH, Long WM, Sprung CL. Controversies in the management of sepsis and septic shock: corticosteroids, naloxone and nonsteroidal anti-inflammatory agents. In: Sibbald WJ, Sprung CL, eds. Perspectives on sepsis and septic shock. Fullerton, CA: Society of Critical Care Medicine, 1986: 350.)

cesarean section dates back to 715 BC, when the Roman king Numa Pompilius decreed that a woman who died while pregnant should have the fetus cut out of her abdomen. This was part of the *Lex Regia* (King's Law), which became part of the *Lex Caesare* (Emperor's Law).[167]

Maternal mortality has become rare, and its causes have changed. Behney's 1961 review of the 1950–1957 Michigan Mortality Study showed polio and toxemia to be the leading causes of death in these cases.[168] Ritter's 1961 review of the world literature showed eclampsia and tuberculosis to be the most common causes of maternal death in 120 successful postmortem cesarean sections.[167]

Katz and others stress that today most maternal deaths occur acutely and that chances of fetal survival when perimortem cesarean section is initiated are improved if maternal death is sudden.[166] Also of importance is timing of the operation. If initiation of the procedure is begun within 4 minutes of maternal cardiac arrest, fetal outcome is improved and the mother may survive.[166] The longest documented time interval from maternal death to delivery with fetal survival is 25 minutes.[169] In cases of moribund patients suffering from chronic disease, preparation for perimortem cesarean section should be planned well in advance. Rare cases in which the operation is performed electively before death of the mother should address the appropriate medico-legal questions.[165,166,169]

Recent case reports have indicated an increased success rate of delivering live infants, which may be related to changing causes of maternal death and improved neonatal resuscitation. Most important, fetal outcome is related to fetal gestational age and the amount of time that has elapsed between maternal death and delivery.[170] However, underreporting of unsuccessful cases may prohibit an establishment of the actual success rate.

Katz and others have concluded that there is minimal legal risk for the physician in performing a perimortem section.[166] The benefits include a chance for infant survival and improved maternal cardiopulmonary resuscitation.

Removal of the placenta at the time of delivery is encouraged, as postoperative placental expulsion has been known to occur.[165]

SPECIFIC ETIOLOGIES AND THEIR DIAGNOSES, PATHOPHYSIOLOGIES, AND TREATMENTS

HYPOVOLEMIC SHOCK

Hypovolemia may result from hemorrhage or solely from loss of intravascular fluids. The causes of hemorrhage in obstetrics are numerous (see Fig. 57-2). The most common cause of hemorrhage is uterine atony following delivery of the placenta. The second most frequent occurrence is obstetric trauma, followed by other causes, such as uterine inversion, amniotic fluid embolism, retroperitoneal extension of bleeding from birth trauma, and various coagulopathies.[94]

Hemorrhagic shock is often easy to control and reverse; however, hemorrhage is still one of the leading causes of death in the obstetric population.[7]

Pritchard has shown that the average amount of blood volume expansion induced by pregnancy is around 1500 mL.[171] The average amount of blood lost during a vaginal delivery is 500 mL and 1000 mL at elective repeat cesarean section. No physiologic compromise should be encountered so long as the volume of blood lost at delivery does not exceed the amount added during pregnancy. When this balance is exceeded, hypovolemia results in decreased venous return and decreased cardiac output. The sympathoadrenal reaction with the release of catecholamines results in peripheral vasoconstriction and tachycardia in an effort to increase cardiac output to the vital organs, such as the brain and heart. This often occurs at the expense of the skin, subcutaneous tissues, and splanchnic organs. If hypoperfusion is prolonged, ischemia leads to anoxia and anaerobic metabolism. Normal metabolic pathways are blocked and cellular energy production is reduced, resulting in failure of the Na^+–K^+ pump and cellular damage.[172] Lysosomal enzymes are released with the generation of vasoactive substances, such as histamine, bradykinin, and serotonin. As lactate production increases from anaerobic metabolism, lactate clearance by the liver decreases secondary to decreased liver perfusion, resulting in further acidosis. Acidosis affects vasodilation, increased capillary permeability, and depressed myocardial performance, exacerbating the process by allowing venous pooling and extravasation of fluid into the extravascular space.[172] If the process is not halted and enters a refractory state, death will result.

Treatment of hemorrhagic shock involves correcting the initiating process as well as instituting general supportive measures, as previously discussed in this chapter. If medical therapy is unsuccessful, surgical procedures,[128] such as uterine artery ligation,[122–124,126,173] internal iliac artery ligation,[127,174] and emergency hysterectomy,[175] are required. Over the years, uterine atony and placenta accreta have replaced uteroplacental apoplexy (Couvelaire uterus) and simple dehiscence of a uterine scar as major indications for hysterectomy at the time of cesarean section.[128] Other modalities, such as percutaneous transcatheter hypogastric artery embolization[176] and the use of the gravity suit,[177] may have their place in certain situations but are not without their own risks.

External pressure created by the gravity suit results in autotransfusion from the lower extremities and abdomen to the vital organs and provides pressure to bleeding sites, thus improving hemostasis.

Response to therapy is reflected by hemodynamic parameters and laboratory values. Blood products should be administered after identifying the underlying disorder by laboratory indices.[99] While quantitative laboratory tests are pending, the clot observation test may be performed by drawing maternal venous blood into a clean, dry test tube and observing for clot formation.

In patients with acute blood loss who respond to fluid therapy but in whom blood transfusion either is undesirable or is refused by the patient, iron dextran (Imferon) may be administered to restore red blood cell mass. Dudrick and colleagues were able to increase hemoglobin levels from an average of 5.0 g/dL to 10.6 g/dL over a 23-day period with replacement doses of intravenous iron dextran.[178]

UTERINE ATONY

Uterine atony, occurring in one of 20 deliveries, is the most common cause of postpartum hemorrhage.[93] Factors associated with atony include precipitous or prolonged labor, use of oxytocin augmentation, use of magnesium sulfate, chorioamnionitis, overdistention of the uterus, and operative deliveries.[179] Clark and colleagues noted that atony was the most common indication for emergency hysterectomy and was associated with chorioamnionitis, oxytocin augmentation, cesarean section for arrest of labor, magnesium sulfate administration, and increased fetal weight.[175]

The diagnosis is made following delivery of the placenta when excessive bleeding is noted per vaginam. The uterine fundus is boggy. Examination of the birth canal reveals no lacerations that may account for bleeding. The uterine cavity should be explored to rule out retained placenta, retained blood clots, and disruption of the uterine wall. Initial management includes bimanual fundal massage and administration of oxytocin (Pitocin, Syntocinon), 20–30 U/L at a rapid intravenous rate or via intramyometrial injection. Methylergonovine maleate (Methergine), 0.2 mg, may be given intramuscularly but should be avoided in hypertensive patients.

Prostaglandin derivatives have been shown to be effective in treating postpartum uterine atony where other modalities have failed. Takagi and associates showed that intramyometrial injection of $PGF_{2\alpha}$ was superior to intravenous or intramuscular administration.[180] They noted that administration of intramyometrial $PGF_{2\alpha}$ was associated with increased oxytocin levels, possibly via the Ferguson reflex, with enhanced release of oxytocin from the pituitary. Hayashi and others evaluated the 15-methyl analog of prostaglandin $F_{2\alpha}$, (15-S)-15-methyl prostaglandin $F_{2\alpha}$-tromethamine (Prostin 15/M), in the management of postpartum hemorrhage secondary to uterine atony that was unresponsive to conventional therapy.[179] Successful control was obtained in 86% (44 of 51) of the patients, and four of the seven patients who failed therapy were noted to have chorioamnionitis. The intramyometrial route of administration may be preferred to peripheral intramuscular injection, especially in patients who are in shock with compromised circulation. Side effects were noted to be infrequent and mild in degree. However, Hankins and colleagues reported marked transient maternal arterial oxygen desaturation secondary to intrapulmonary shunting in five women with severe uterine atony and postpartum hemorrhage who were treated with 15-methyl prostaglandin $F_{2\alpha}$.[181] If hemorrhage persists despite medical therapy, surgical intervention is mandated.

PLACENTA PREVIA

Placenta previa may be classified as marginal, partial, or total, depending on the relationship of the placenta to the internal os of the cervix. The overall incidence near term is one in 200 pregnancies.[182] By using diagnostic ultrasound, the incidence of placenta previa at 16–18 weeks has been found to be 5.3%, decreasing by 90% to 0.58% at the time of delivery.[183]

The major hazards associated with placenta previa are profound maternal hemorrhage and shock, with significant perinatal morbidity and mortality. Risk factors associated with the development of placenta previa include high parity, advanced maternal age, previous history of abortions, and previous history of cesarean section.[184] Clark and colleagues noted that the incidence of placenta previa was 0.26% with an unscarred uterus, with a linear increase to 10% in patients with four or more cesarean sections.[129]

Diagnosis is best made by ultrasound, which may also be useful in predicting, during the early second trimester, which patients will be at risk for total placenta previa at term.[185] If the diagnosis based on ultrasound is in question, a double set-up examination should be performed, with preparations made for blood transfusion and cesarean section.

Since the conservative management of placenta previa was described by Macafee in 1945,[186] marked improvement in perinatal survival has occurred. With further advances in perinatal medicine, the "conservative aggressive management" of placenta previa, using expectant management, has resulted in further reduction of perinatal mortality to approximately 12.6%.[187] This approach includes antenatal transfusions, tocolytic agents for preterm labor, and elective termination of pregnancy based on amniotic fluid maturity studies.

Placenta previa is also associated with placenta accreta, increta, and percreta, especially in the presence of a previous cesarean section.[129]

PLACENTA ACCRETA, INCRETA, AND PERCRETA

When Nitabuch's membrane is deficient and trophoblastic tissue attaches directly to the myometrium, placenta accreta is said to occur. If the trophoblast invades the myometrium or penetrates the myometrium, placenta increta and placenta percreta exist. When the placenta detaches, areas of adherence prevent the normal mechanism of myometrial contraction and compression of vascular channels from occurring, resulting in hemorrhage.

Recent clinical studies reveal an apparent increasing trend in incidence, perhaps secondary not only to a true increase in incidence, but also to better case reporting. In a review of 56,381 deliveries at the Los Angeles County/University of Southern California Medical Center between 1975 and 1979, a clinical diagnosis of placenta accreta of one per 2562 deliveries was noted, and pathologically confirmed cases were noted in one per 4027 deliveries.[188] Cases were reviewed of 22 patients, of whom 14 (64%) underwent hysterectomy and eight underwent conservative treatment, with one maternal death occurring intraoperatively secondary to massive hemorrhage and coagulopathy. A significant improvement in maternal mortality from the 37% reported prior to 1934 was noted.[189] There were no perinatal deaths, compared to a 25% rate reported in 1976.[190] Read and colleagues state that the hallmark of placenta accreta is multiparity.[188] The most common associated factor was placenta previa, found in 14 (63.6%) patients, of whom six had previous cesarean sections. Improved maternal and fetal outcomes are felt to be secondary to improved antenatal surveillance, increased use of cesarean section, and better neonatal care.

Kistner and others reported in 1952 the association of previous cesarean section and placenta previa with placenta accreta.[191] Clark and associates demonstrated a linear increase in risk of placenta accreta in patients with placenta previa and previous uterine scars.[129] These investigators noted that patients presenting with placenta previa and an unscarred uterus had a 5% risk of having placenta accreta. The risk of placenta accreta increased to 24% in patients with a placenta previa and one previous cesarean section. Those patients with placenta previa and four previous cesarean sections experienced a 67% incidence of placenta accreta.[129]

Treatment generally involves hysterectomy; however, conservative management may be appropriate in certain cases. McHattie's 1972 review of the literature showed a maternal mortality of 41.9% with conservative management and a maternal mortality of 6.5% with hysterectomy.[192] In Clark and colleagues' review of patients treated between 1977 and 1983, no maternal deaths were observed in the 28% of those patients treated with conservative methods. They recommend individualized treatment and conservative procedures, such as curettage, local repair, and uterine artery ligation, in selected patients.[129]

Rare cases of invasion into extrauterine structures, such as the bladder, requiring bladder resection and massive transfusion, have been reported in the literature.[193]

ABRUPTIO PLACENTAE

Abruptio placentae is estimated to occur in one of 120 deliveries.[194] The exact etiology is unknown, but associated conditions include hypertensive disorders, parity, and history of previous abruption.[195] Although the incidence is relatively low, abruption accounts for 15% to 25% of all perinatal mortality and is associated with its own perinatal mortality rate of 25% to 50%.[194,196]

The patient often presents with painful vaginal bleeding. Amniotomy may reveal bloody amniotic fluid. In patients who present with uterine and lower back pain with or without vaginal bleeding and fetal demise or fetal distress, abruption should be strongly considered. Antenatal ultrasonographic evidence of a retroplacental blood clot or subchorionic hematoma is rarely seen. At the time of delivery, however, adherent hematoma and compression of placental tissue are usually noted. In some cases, complete detachment of the placenta with free blood in the uterine cavity is encountered.

Abdella and associates studied the relationship of hypertensive disease to abruptio placentae.[197] Of 265 cases of abruption, 26.8% were complicated by a hypertensive disorder. A distinct correlation was noted between the incidence of abruption and the severity of hypertension, with a 2.3%, 10.0%, and 23.6% incidence of abruption among preeclamptics, chronic hypertensives, and eclamptics, respectively.

Pritchard and Brekken noted an incidence of abruption resulting in fetal death in one per 433 deliveries (0.2%) between 1956 and 1965.[32] They estimated that at least 2 L of blood must be lost to result in fetal death. In 38% of the patients, the fibrinogen level was below 150 mg/100 mL and in 28% it was below 100 mg/100 mL.

Another possible risk factor for abruption is cocaine abuse during pregnancy.[198] Cocaine can cause placental vasoconstriction, decreased blood flow to the fetus, and increased uterine contractility.[199] In a comparison of cocaine users with methadone users, a significant difference in complications of labor and delivery was noted, with cocaine-using mothers experiencing a 17.3% abruption rate and methadone-using mothers a 1.3% abruption rate.[199] With more common usage of this drug today, an increased prevalence would be expected during pregnancy. Little and others reported a 9.8% prevalence of cocaine abuse during pregnancy in an indigent population.[200] The exact impact on the incidence of abruption is not known.

Other causes of abruption, such as trauma or sudden decompression of the uterus, as occurs with rupture of the membranes in polyhydramnios, have been noted.[195,201]

Management of abruption has long been controversial. Initial treatment includes placement of large-bore intravenous access, oxygen supplementation, type and crossmatch for red blood cells, hematologic and coagulation laboratory studies, fetal heart rate monitoring, maternal urinary output via indwelling catheter, and amniotomy with use of oxytocin in selective cases.[202] Simultaneous correction of anemia and coagulation defects should be instituted. The decision about whether to allow vaginal delivery or to proceed with cesarean section with a live fetus has been somewhat facilitated by the advent of electronic fetal monitoring. In most situations, consideration of maternal hemodynamic and coagulation status coupled with fetal well-being will guide clinical decision making, with cesarean section reserved for usual obstetric indications as well as severe hemorrhage or worsening coagulopathy developing at a time remote from expected delivery. Anemia and infection are commonly encountered during the postpartum period.[202]

A rare case of fetal survival following abruption and DIC with resolution during the second trimester has been reported.[203]

ECTOPIC PREGNANCY

Ectopic pregnancy continues to play a major role in maternal morbidity and mortality in the United States. Of 292 maternal deaths in 1982, 43 were attributable to ectopic pregnancies.[8] The incidence is said to be one per 100 pregnancies.[204] Over the last 30 years, a steady rise has occurred in the ectopic rate, with a fall in the death-to-case rate (Fig. 57-9).[205] This increased incidence may be secondary to an increase in the presence of risk factors, such as acute salpingitis, or secondary to methods of reporting and improved methods of diagnosis.

Acute salpingitis is probably the most important factor associated with ectopic pregnancy. Other factors, such as tubal surgery and adhesion formation, intrauterine device use, and history of infertility, have been identified as causative agents.[206] Recent technological advances in infertility, such as tubal surgery and ovulation induction, have been implicated as causative factors.[207]

The usual symptoms associated with ectopic pregnancy include abdominal pain, amenorrhea or irregular vaginal bleeding, pregnancy symptoms, and sometimes syncope and shoulder pain secondary to intraperitoneal bleeding. Common signs include adnexal tenderness, adnexal mass, slightly enlarged uterus, and, in patients who have sustained significant blood loss, tachycardia and hypotension.

The diagnosis is made by further evaluation using urine or serum β-hCG testing, culdocentesis, and ultrasound. When positive, culdocentesis is very accurate in predicting the presence of ectopic pregnancy. Quantitative β-hCG levels usually double over a 48-hour period. If a rise of less than 66% occurs over a 2-day period, a high probability of ectopic pregnancy is considered.[208] Ultrasonography has advanced our ability to diagnose ectopic pregnancies at an early stage; an intrauterine sac should be observed at a β-hCG level of 6500 mIU using transabdominal ultrasonography and at 3600 mIU by transvaginal ultrasound.[209] If no gestational sac is seen at these levels, then ectopic pregnancy should be strongly considered.

Depending on available information, dilatation and curettage, laparoscopy, and laparotomy may be indicated. If an ectopic pregnancy is confirmed, many surgical routes, ranging from conservative to radical, may be taken. In rare instances, hysterectomy is indicated for an ectopic pregnancy. The main goals of treatment are to remove the trophoblastic tissue, control bleeding, and minimize damage to the reproductive tract, especially in patients of low parity.

Ovarian, interstitial, and abdominal pregnancies are much more dangerous from the standpoint of hemorrhage than tubal pregnancies, with the latter making up the vast majority (97.7%) of ectopic pregnancies.[210,211]

Currently, methotrexate is being evaluated as a potential chemotherapeutic treatment for ectopic preg-

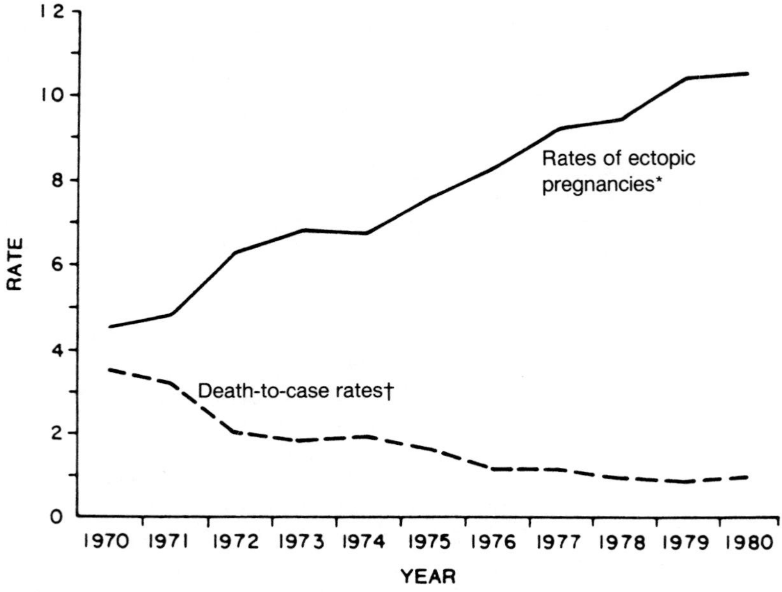

FIGURE 57–9. Rates of ectopic pregnancies and death-to-case rates, by year, United States 1970–1980.

nancies.[212] Even with improved early diagnosis and a decreased death-to-case rate, the overall number of maternal deaths secondary to hemorrhage would not be expected to fall as long as the overall incidence of ectopic pregnancy continues to increase. A high index of suspicion is needed to rule out ectopic pregnancy in reproductive-age women who present with lower abdominal pain, abnormal vaginal bleeding, and other associated signs and symptoms.

TRAUMA

For the purpose of categorization, trauma may be described as obstetric-related or non–obstetric-related. Obstetric trauma may occur spontaneously, as with laceration of the lower genital tract during the second stage of labor, spontaneous uterine rupture, and spontaneous rupture of the liver, which may occur in patients with pregnancy-induced hypertension. Obstetric trauma may also occur as a result of surgical procedures (eg, during episiotomy, forceps operations, cesarean section, dilatation and curettage, and induced abortion). Non–obstetric-related trauma may, for practical purposes, be subdivided into blunt trauma, as occurs during a fall or motor vehicle accident, and penetrating trauma, such as that sustained from gunshot and stab wounds.

The pathophysiologic significance of trauma is usually related to hypovolemia; however, tissue damage and necrosis may play an integral role in the pathophysiologic process as well.

SPONTANEOUS OBSTETRIC TRAUMA

Lacerations of the Lower Genital Tract

Spontaneous lacerations of the lower genital tract may occur with resultant blood loss. The amount of blood loss is related to the degree and depth of the laceration and the time elapsed before repair. The primary surgical goals are to begin the suture line above the apex of the laceration in order to control retracted vessels and to restore anatomy.

Uterine Rupture

Spontaneous rupture of the gravid uterus still carries a significant maternal and fetal mortality rate. The incidence is approximately one in 2000 deliveries.[94] Earlier studies demonstrated maternal and fetal mortality in the ranges of 2.3% to 28%, and 48% to 66%, respectively.[213–215] More recent figures demonstrate a 9.7% maternal mortality rate and a fetal wastage of 56%.[216]

Uterine rupture may be spontaneous, secondary either to trauma or to rupture of a previous uterine scar. In a study published in 1962, 57.8% of uterine ruptures were found to be spontaneous, 23.1% were secondary to scar rupture, and 18.8% were secondary to trauma. Prolonged or obstructed labor was felt to be the causative factor for spontaneous rupture.[214]

Conditions associated with uterine rupture include use of oxytocin, cephalopelvic disproportion, grand multiparity, and abruption.[216] Some older studies identified previous cesarean section scars to be the most important etiologic factor.[217]

The most common clinical presentation is that of mild vaginal bleeding, shock, and lower abdominal pain.[216] In some instances, the area that fetal heart tones can be observed from will be shifted. Sometimes, acute bradycardia is noted. In cases of catastrophic rupture and fetal demise, inability to detect fetal heart tones may occur concomitant with acute abdominal pain and hypotension.

Treatment of uterine rupture should be individualized. Abdominal hysterectomy is no longer advocated in all cases. If the fetus is still undelivered or if uterine bleeding is felt to be secondary to a uterine or cervical defect, prompt laparotomy is indicated. In many cases, the diagnosis is made only at the time of repeat cesarean section. If the patient desires future childbearing and surgical repair is possible, hysterectomy should be avoided. In cases in which the tear extends either laterally into the broad ligament or in which damage is extensive, hysterectomy is indicated for control of blood loss. Sometimes, removal of the adnexa on the involved side is required to control broad-ligament bleeding. If a defect is found at the time of postpartum examination but no bleeding is noted and the patient is otherwise stable, close observation without laparotomy may be warranted.

Golan and colleagues noted that rupture of an unscarred uterus bore a worse prognosis for the mother and fetus than rupture of a scarred uterus.[216] Tears associated with previous scars tended to be transverse, whereas those involving previously unscarred uteri were often longitudinal and more extensive. An overall fetal wastage of 56% was noted, 74% if associated with a previously unscarred uterus and 22% with a previously scarred uterus. The 9.7% maternal mortality rate involved only patients with unscarred uteri.

Spontaneous Hepatic Rupture

Spontaneous rupture of the liver during pregnancy was first described in 1844 by Abercrombie.[218] Cases reported since then have usually been associated with pregnancy-induced hypertension and have occurred in multiparous patients.[219,220]

The patient, often diagnosed with preeclampsia, develops epigastric or right upper quadrant pain associated with nausea and vomiting. Occasionally, upper abdominal tenderness is present on examination. If subcapsular hepatic hemorrhage has extended beyond Glisson's capsule and intraperitoneal bleeding occurs, signs and symptoms of shock follow.

Laboratory values may show evidence of a falling hematocrit, elevated liver enzymes and serum bilirubin, and developing coagulopathy.

The diagnosis is often made on clinical grounds; however, paracentesis,[220] liver scan,[221] ultrasonography, and computed tomography may be helpful in establishing the diagnosis. Liver biopsy usually reveals fibrin thrombi in the hepatic arterioles, extending to the periportal sinusoids and periportal hemorrhagic necrosis.[222]

Expedient exploratory laparotomy is mandated for a patient in shock with evidence of intraperitoneal bleeding, as delay in laparotomy has been associated with increased mortality. Packing the liver and adequate drainage are recommended.[223] Death is usually secondary to massive, uncontrollable hemorrhage. In cases where bleeding was controlled by hepatic artery ligation or lobectomy, death usually followed postoperatively secondary to hepatic failure and multisystem organ failure. It is postulated that the preexisting hepatic damage may not allow sufficient hepatic reserve following arterial occlusion or partial liver resection to sustain life.[223]

Also of note is the occasional finding of a right pleural effusion in patients with spontaneous liver rupture.[222]

SURGICAL OBSTETRIC TRAUMA

Forceps Operations

Complications of forceps deliveries resulting in hemorrhage include uterine rupture, cervical lacerations, vaginal lacerations, pelvic hematomas, and episiotomy extensions. The significance of associated bleeding is relative to preexisting cardiovascular status, extent of injury, and quantity of active bleeding and time elapsed before surgical repair. These complications are usually not of major clinical significance, and major complications can usually be prevented by good judgment and the avoidance of excessive force.[224]

Legal Abortion

Maternal death resulting from legal abortion still remains a problem in modern obstetrics. Information regarding this problem has been reported by the Centers for Disease Control in Atlanta. This report revealed 24 deaths from hemorrhage and 132 deaths from other causes among 7.298 million legal abortions performed between 1972 and 1979.[75] The most common cause of death was infection (23%), followed by complications of anesthesia (17%) and hemorrhage (15%). Hemorrhage may result from uterine perforation, retained products of conception, consumptive coagulopathy related to use of chemical abortifacients,[19] or uterine rupture during midtrimester-induced abortion.[225] Clinical features common to these cases of lethal hemorrhage included uterine trauma, inadequate postoperative monitoring, delayed surgical intervention, and delayed blood transfusions. Recommendations to avoid trauma to the uterus included accurate assessment of estimated gestational age; local rather than general anesthesia[226,227]; gradual, careful cervical dilatation; careful curettage technique; and avoidance of overstimulation of the uterus during abortion by labor induction with oxytocin.[228]

Management of overt bleeding includes early recognition, surgical intervention, and volume replacement, utilizing blood components as necessary.[75]

If unusual postabortal bleeding does not resolve, diagnostic laparoscopy or exploratory laparotomy should be performed without delay.[75,229–231]

In cases of suspected uterine perforation, close attention must be paid to the site of perforation.[229,230] Some authors recommend conservative monitoring of a patient who is suspected of having a perforation in the fundal region with no obvious bleeding or pain and hospitalization with laparoscopy in a patient with a suspected lateral perforation.[230] At our institution, any patient with evidence of a lateral perforation is admitted for observation with serial hematocrits and examinations. Laparoscopy or laparotomy is performed in a patient in whom persistent bleeding is suspected or cannot be ruled out, damage to intraperitoneal organs is suspected, or pain is felt to be excessive or worsening.

Other Surgery-Related Causes of Bleeding

Dilatation and curettage for missed abortion or incomplete abortion is not usually associated with significant blood loss unless uterine perforation, usually lateral, occurs. Cesarean section, in general, is associated with approximately 1000 mL of blood loss unless associated with extensions of postpartum atony. Extensions are managed by identifying anatomical landmarks and reapproximating the separated tissue edges. Often the bladder must be dissected inferiorly to identify the apical margin of a lower uterine segment extension. Hysterectomy is rarely required for control of extensions associated with cesarean section. The management of uterine atony has previously been described.

NON-OBSTETRIC TRAUMA

The subject of trauma during pregnancy has been documented comprehensively in the literature.[170,232–237] The incidence of accidental injury during pregnancy is estimated to be 6% to 7%.[170] In most cases, injury is minimal and is not associated with a significant increase in perinatal mortality.[233,238] An increased incidence of minor trauma has been observed as pregnancy progresses.[238] Major trauma, however, may place the mother and infant at severe risk.

The initial management of a pregnant woman who has sustained severe or major trauma is essentially the same as that of a non-pregnant person.[239] Crosby has described in detail the initial evaluation of the gravid trauma patient.[232] Maternal stabilization often leads to fetal stabilization. Delivery of the fetus prior to stabilization of the mother may worsen the mother's condition and result in delivery of a premature fetus. Electronic fetal monitoring during maternal evaluation will provide information regarding fetal and maternal well-being because deteriorating maternal cardiovascular status may be reflected early via fetal distress.[232]

Animal studies have shown that maternal hypoxia results in a reduction of uterine and placental blood flow via liberated catecholamines.[240] Signs of fetal well-being reflect maternal cardiovascular stability.

Blunt trauma sustained from falls and motor vehicle accidents is often managed differently from penetrating trauma caused by stab wounds and projectiles, such as bullets.

Blunt Trauma

Rothenberger and colleagues reviewed 103 cases of blunt maternal trauma.[233] The etiological classification consisted of four groups: automobile accidents, pedestrian accidents, falls, and assaults. The majority of the cases were categorized as minor (17%) or insignificant (63%); however, the group sustaining major trauma (20%) demonstrated a 24% mortality rate, usually succumbing to hemorrhagic shock. Blaisdell, however, defines traumatic shock as a separate entity from hypovolemic, neurogenic, and cardiogenic shock because the soft-tissue injury itself leads to pulmonary, coagulation, and renal complications.[53] Fetal injuries, usually skull fractures and intracranial hemorrhage, occur later in gestation because of a reduced amniotic fluid–fetal ratio, fixation of the fetal head in the bony pelvis, and placement of the fetal body outside the bony pelvis. Fetal death was related to maternal death, maternal hypotension, fetal injury, and injuries of the pelvic viscera, uterus, and placenta.

Case reports have described fetal and neonatal death secondary to in utero traumatic splenic rupture,[241] placental laceration,[242] and contusion with hemorrhage of the liver, adrenal gland, and kidney.[243] Rose and associates identified evidence of fetal–maternal hemorrhage in 28% of pregnant trauma patients.[244] They recommend a protocol consisting of electronic fetal monitoring, Kleihauer-Betke analysis (with repeat analysis, if positive, to rule out chronic fetal–maternal hemorrhage), and Rh determination of the mother, with appropriate dosage of Rh-immune globulin therapy for the Rh-negative mother.

Crosby and Costiloe reviewed accident and medical reports of 208 pregnant victims of severe motor vehicle accidents.[245] They found that maternal death was the leading cause of fetal death. Among maternal survivors, premature separation of the placenta was the most frequent cause of fetal death. Fetal and maternal death was significantly higher when the mother was ejected from the vehicle; thus, lap belts to prevent ejection were recommended for pregnant travelers. Crosby and others, however, demonstrated, in a series of pregnant baboons, that a shoulder harness restraint was superior to a lap belt restraint alone in preventing fetal death.[246]

Simple falls that do not result in loss of consciousness or bruises are unlikely to produce significant injury to the mother or the fetus.[232] We recommend some type of fetal assessment (NST or biophysical profile) to provide reassurance to a concerned mother and her physician. Maternal Rh status should be checked and the Kleihauer-Betke test should be considered. Clotting studies are indicated if placental abruption is suspected.

Serious falls are associated with multiple bone fractures and internal injury. Diagnostic peritoneal lavage for blunt trauma in pregnant women has been found to be both safe and accurate in diagnosing intra-abdominal injuries.[247] Physical examination of the abdomen is felt to be less reliable in the pregnant patient.[234]

Splenic rupture has been postulated to occur more frequently in pregnant than in non-pregnant women.[248] Buchsbaum noted a 15.4% mortality rate of splenic rupture.[249] A clinical pattern of "biphasic rupture" or "delayed hemorrhage," with a prolonged latent period prior to massive hemorrhage, mandates close prolonged surveillance in suspected cases.[248,249]

Pelvic fractures are usually associated with motor vehicle accidents. Serious complications are related to urologic and vascular damage. Retroperitoneal hemorrhage may be massive, resulting from minor pelvic fractures with minimal bony displacement.[234] Nonexpanding retroperitoneal hematomas found at laparotomy should probably be left alone to prevent further hemorrhage.[232] The most common site of fracture occurs through the anterior half of the pelvic ring, at the horizontal pubic rami.[250] Fewer than 10% of patients with pelvic fractures require cesarean section secondary to pelvic deformity.[251]

Penetrating Trauma

The gravid uterus becomes the most frequently injured organ in cases of penetrating abdominal trauma.[237] As the uterus expands, the bowel is compartmentalized into the upper abdomen. Because of the physical forces involved, gunshot wounds carry a substantially higher mortality rate than stab wounds. Nance and others reported a 12.5% mortality rate related to gunshot wounds, as compared to a 1.4% mortality rate related to stab wounds in the civilian population.[252] Gunshot wounds are also the most common type of penetrating injury during pregnancy.[235]

A review by Buchsbaum indicated a lower than expected mortality rate in association with gunshot wounds to the uterus, as reflected by no reported deaths between 1912 and 1979.[235] An 89% incidence of fetal injury and a 66% perinatal mortality rate were noted in one series reported by Buchsbaum.[236] Prematurity contributed significantly to perinatal mortality. In all cases of gunshot wounds to the abdomen, exploratory laparotomy should be performed to determine the extent of visceral injury.[236,253] However, exploratory laparotomy is not a reason to perform a cesarean section.[170,232–234] Maternal indications for delivery include severely compromised maternal cardiovascular status (see the section on perimortem cesarean section) and obstruction of the operating field by the gravid uterus that limits surgical exposure of damaged vital structures. Fetal indications for delivery include fetal hemorrhage and distress and intra-amniotic infection.[235] Such factors as suspected fetal injury and fetal distress must be balanced against those of fetal maturity. Even if labor has begun, some authors feel that vaginal delivery following exploratory laparotomy is preferable to hysterotomy.[232]

Stab wounds of the abdomen are somewhat more complicated in management. Determination of whether the peritoneal cavity has been violated can be difficult. Fistulograms using Hypaque and peritoneal lavage have been promoted in the management of stab wounds.[235,247,254] Stab wounds only require surgical repair in about one half of reported cases.[235] As with gunshot wounds, if the wound is confined to the lower abdomen, the uterus usually sustains most injuries, whereas other viscera are spared. Because of a high incidence of upper abdominal wounds, treatment and consideration for exploratory laparotomy should be individualized.[235]

A rare but lethal complication of blunt or penetrating trauma to the chest or upper abdomen is delayed traumatic rupture of the diaphragm.[130] Mortality is related to the number of herniated organs, strangulation of herniated organs, and elapse of time from rupture to surgical intervention. Most of these hernias occur on the left side, probably a result of the liver providing protection against herniation on the right side. The patient presents with pain, fever, and dyspnea. The diagnosis is made on radiologic grounds. Treatment is surgical via a thoracotomy incision. Some authors recommend routine baseline chest x-ray of all prenatal patients with a history of penetrating wounds and suggest that cesarean section be performed if labor begins within 4 weeks of reparative surgery.[130]

ACQUIRED COAGULOPATHY

Acquired coagulation defects in pregnancy are not uncommon. Familiar clinical states that may be associated with or causes of coagulopathy include sepsis, retained dead fetus syndrome, abruptio placentae, amniotic fluid embolism, preeclampsia–eclampsia, intravascular hemolysis, trauma, and induced abortion by hypertonic saline. Other cases involving afibrinogenemia secondary to a degenerating leiomyoma,[255] placenta previa accreta with afibrinogenemia,[256] hydatidiform mole,[257,258] and ovarian vascular accidents secondary to anticoagulation therapy[259] have been reported.

INDUCED ABORTION BY HYPERTONIC SALINE

Prior to the development of prostaglandin derivatives, midtrimester abortion was commonly induced with intra-amniotic infusion of hypertonic saline. Case reports of consumptive coagulopathy surfaced in the early 1970s.[17] Laros and others observed decreased platelets, decreased fibrinogen, elevated prothrombin time, and detection of fibrin degradation products in a prospective study of 25 patients undergoing intra-amniotic instillation of hypertonic (20%) saline for pregnancy termination.[18] Cohen and Ballard retrospectively reviewed 4919 midtrimester abortions induced with hypertonic saline, some of which were augmented with intravenous oxytocin.[19] Five cases of coagulopathy developed among the 4112 women (1/823) who aborted with hypertonic saline alone and five cases of coagulopathy were identified among 807 women (1/161) who aborted after receiving intra-amniotic saline plus intravenous oxytocin. The average instillation-to-abortion time was generally shorter in those patients who received oxytocin and in those who developed coagulopathy. The use of intravenous oxytocin in saline-induced abortions was associated with a fivefold increase in incidence of coagulopathy.

SEPSIS AND DIC

DIC may be triggered in patients with septic shock; however, the exact mechanism remains to be elucidated.[23] The role of platelets is felt to be significant in the development of DIC secondary to sepsis.[20] Endotoxins administered to baboons have been shown to lead to a hypercoagulable state, followed by depletion of platelets and clotting factors, resulting in DIC.[21]

Although the first organism associated with DIC was meningococcus, many other organisms have been isolated in obstetric patients with sepsis.[24] Obstetric infections are usually of the mixed polymicrobial variety.[22] Gram-negative enteric organisms, such as *Escherichia coli, Klebsiella–Enterobacter, Pseudomonas,* and *Serratia,* have been the most common isolated organisms.[20] Gram-negative anaerobes (ie, *Bacteroides*), gram-positive organisms, viremias (ie, *Varicella*), and fungal infections may all lead to septic shock and DIC.[20,23] Therefore, the factors triggering DIC may not always be endotoxins; they can be exotoxins, antigen–antibody complexes, or other mediators.[23]

Treatment includes general supportive measures, antibiotic coverage, correction of coagulopathy, and, if possible, removal of the source of infection.

RETAINED DEAD FETUS SYNDROME

With the advent of ultrasonography, improved methods of labor induction, and aggressive management, the retained dead fetus syndrome is rarely encountered in obstetric practice today.[26] Weiner and others reported a case of coagulation defects in a patient with intrauterine death from Rh isosensitization in 1950.[27] The actual association of fetal death, not Rh sensitization, was made in 1953 after identifying a coagulopathy in an Rh-positive patient with a longstanding fetal demise.[28] Data published in 1955 revealed the process to be slowly progressive.[29] Further data from Pritchard in 1959 revealed that coagulopathy was unlikely to develop earlier than 5 weeks following fetal death; after 5 weeks, an incidence of 26% was noted if delivery did not occur.[25]

The cause of coagulopathy is postulated to be the release of tissue thromboplastin from the fetus or placenta, activating the extrinsic pathway and resulting in DIC and secondary activation of the fibrinolytic system.[26]

The patient may present in a compensated or decompensated hemostatic state, as manifested by clinical evidence of bleeding and laboratory studies. Romero and associates stress the need for coagulation screening of all patients with intrauterine fetal demise prior to attempts to deliver the fetus in order to detect a potentially lethal coagulopathy.[26] Laboratory studies should include a complete blood count, platelet count, fibrinogen, fibrin split products, prothrombin time, and partial thromboplastin time. Thrombin time (TT) is prolonged when (1) fibrinogen is less than 100 mg/dL; (2) qualitative disorders of fibrinogen are present; (3) fibrin split products are elevated, resulting in inhibition of fibrin polymerization; or (4) the thrombin inhibitor heparin has been exogenously administered.[26]

If the patient is found to have DIC and is in labor, fibrinogen is replaced by administration of cryoprecipitate, as the volume of fresh-frozen plasma may be excessive and result in volume overload. If the patient is not in labor, heparin may be administered by continuous intravenous infusion until fibrinogen levels rise to between 200 and 300 mg/dL and platelets are greater than 60,000/μL. Heparin is then discontinued and induction of labor is instituted 6 hours after discontinuation of heparin.[26]

Cases of single fetal death in multiple gestations with resultant coagulopathy that were treated with heparin have been reported.[30,31] Romero and colleagues have reported a case of intrauterine death of a single twin complicated by DIC that was successfully treated with intravenous heparin.[30] Coagulopathy resumed after the first time heparin was discontinued, but not after the second discontinuation, suggesting that the coagulopathy may not be irreversible.

In modern obstetrics, prompt termination of a fetal demise by prostaglandin agents should avoid the dead fetus syndrome.

ABRUPTIO PLACENTAE AND DIC

Abruptio placentae and its relationship to hemorrhagic shock has been discussed previously. Twenty-six percent of all cases of abruption are associated with signs of shock.[33] Pritchard noted a 38% incidence of hypofibrinogenemia complicating abruption severe enough to result in fetal death.[32] DIC probably results from the release of an unidentified thrombogenic substance into the circulation. Hypofibrinogenemia and the presence of fibrin-split products correlate closely with postpartum hemorrhage.[34]

Treatment consists of prompt blood transfusion, replacement of clotting factors, and delivery of the products of conception.

AMNIOTIC FLUID EMBOLISM AND DIC

The clinical diagnosis of amniotic fluid embolism is rare, estimated to be one in 20,000 to one in 80,000 deliveries.[39,260] Of great significance is an overall mortality rate of approximately 80%.[39,260] First described in 1926 by Meyer,[40] it was not delineated as a distinct pathologic entity until Steiner and Lushbaugh reported a case series in 1941.[41]

Risk factors include advanced maternal age, multiparity, vigorous uterine contractions, meconium presence in amniotic fluid, large fetal size, and fetal demise.[39] Fetal death prior to the acute episode occurs in 40% of cases, and abruptio placentae may accompany 50% of cases.[45]

Passage of amniotic fluid into the maternal vasculature results in cardiopulmonary compromise mimicking pulmonary hypertension and cor pulmonale. Later, DIC results from the coagulant activity of amniotic fluid.[35] Microemboli may pass through the pulmonary capillary bed and into the systemic vessels.[36]

The patient classically develops chills, restlessness, dyspnea, cyanosis, nausea, vomiting, altered mental status, and then hypotension and tachycardia.[41] Cardiorespiratory arrest follows.

Hemodynamic findings in humans with documented amniotic fluid embolism show a mild-to-moderate rise in mean pulmonary artery pressure, a variable rise in central venous pressure, and a high pulmonary capillary wedge pressure with evidence of left ventricular failure.[42,47] Clark proposes a biphasic hemodynamic alteration in which the initial episode of hypoxia is secondary to a transient pulmonary artery vasospasm. This event is followed by left ventricular and pulmonary capillary injury, possibly secondary to the initial episode of hypoxia or a direct effect of amniotic fluid on the myocardium.[45] The mortality rate in the first hour is 25% to 50%.[39,46]

In a patient surviving this initial episode, coagulopathy subsequently develops in 40% of cases and hemorrhagic shock may ensue.[39,260] Uterine atony may accompany coagulopathy.

Coagulopathy is thought to result from release of thromboplastin or a powerful anticoagulant into the maternal circulation.[39]

Diagnosis traditionally is made at autopsy, with fetal squames, mucin, and amorphous debris found in arteries under 1 mm in diameter, arterioles, and capillaries of the pulmonary vasculature.[41] Recent evidence suggests that the presence of trophoblastic or squamous cells in maternal pulmonary circulation may not be pathognomonic of clinically significant amniotic fluid embolism.[43,44] Gregory and Clayton proposed the use of lung scans in the diagnosis of amniotic fluid embolism.[38] It appears that diagnosis of amniotic fluid embolism will be made on clinical grounds in survivors and on both clinical and histologic grounds in nonsurvivors.

Treatment includes cardiovascular resuscitation, respiratory support, and correction of the abnormal coagulation state. Intravenous heparin has been reported in the treatment of amniotic fluid embolism, but is not in widespread use.[37] Inotropic support is warranted in the face of left ventricular failure and pulmonary edema.[42]

PREGNANCY-INDUCED HYPERTENSION

In 1954, Pritchard and colleagues described a syndrome of intravascular hemolysis, thrombocytopenia, and other hematologic abnormalities associated with preeclampsia.[52] Pritchard and others studied coagulation changes in 95 cases of eclampsia and found a 29% incidence of thrombocytopenia, a 50% incidence of prolonged thrombin time, a 3% incidence of elevated serum fibrinogen–fibrin degradation products, and a 2% incidence of overt hemolysis.[48] At the present time, our clinical understanding of coagulopathy related to preeclampsia–eclampsia revolves around the HELLP syndrome, characterized by microangiopathic hemolytic anemia, elevated liver enzymes, and thrombocytopenia.[49,50] Thrombocytopenia is thought to be secondary to an increased consumption of platelets, possibly resulting from adherence to exposed collagen in damaged vascular endothelium. Hemolytic anemia is also thought to occur secondary to red blood cell destruction in small blood vessels. Burr cells, schistocytes, and polychromasia are seen on peripheral blood smear. Serum haptoglobin may help identify cases of hemolytic anemia in patients with HELLP syndrome.[51]

Delivery of the products of conception is the only known treatment for patients with preeclampsia and HELLP syndrome. Replacement of fluids, blood products, and other supportive measures are instituted as indicated.

INTRAVASCULAR HEMOLYSIS

DIC can be triggered by intravascular hemolysis, perhaps via release of red cell ADP or red cell membrane phospholipoprotein.[23] Intravascular hemolysis of any etiology, including frank hemolytic transfusion reactions and minor hemolysis secondary to multiple transfusions of banked whole blood, may initiate activation of the coagulation cascade and result in DIC.

TRAUMA AND DIC

DIC may result from trauma in several ways. Massive crushing injuries cause release of substances, probably from damaged tissue, into the circulation, activating the coagulation cascade.[53] Massive hemorrhage from injury may result in depletion of coagulation factors. Trauma to the uterus may result in abruption or amniotic fluid embolism, which are both known to cause DIC. Treatment includes replacement of blood and coagulation products, general supportive care, and measures directed to correcting the inciting factors.

INHERITED COAGULOPATHIES

Hereditary disorders of coagulation occur in approximately one to two per 10,000 persons and therefore are rarely encountered in obstetric practice.[46] A deficiency of any factor in the intrinsic, extrinsic, or common pathways of blood coagulation may result in a clotting disorder.[46,261–280]

Screening tests include platelet count, prothrombin time (PT), partial thromboplastin time (PTT), bleeding time, thrombin clotting time (TCT), and clot stability test (Table 57-7). Depending on the results of these studies, specific clotting factor assays may be indicated.[46]

Von Willebrand's disease is the most common coagulation defect encountered by obstetricians.[263] It is typically an inherited autosomal dominant disorder of

TABLE 57–7. SCREENING TESTS IN PATIENTS WITH HEREDITARY COAGULOPATHIES

ABNORMALITY	BLEEDING TIME	PLATELET COUNT	PROTHROMBIN TIME (PT)	PARTIAL THROMBOPLASTIN TIME (PTT)	THROMBIN CLOTTING TIME (TCT)	CLOTTING STABILITY TEST
Von Willebrand's disease	A	N	N	N or A	N	N
Deficiency of fibrinogen	N or A	N	A	A	A	N or A
Prothrombin (II)	N	N	A	A	N	N
Factor V	N or A	N	A	A	N	N
Factor VII	N	N	A	N	N	N
Factor VIII	N	N	N	A	N	N
Factor IX	N	N	N or A	A	N	N
Factor X	N	N	A	A	N	N
Factor XI	N or A	N	N	A	N	N
Factor XII	N	N	N	A	N	N
Contact factors	N	N	N	A	N	N
Factor XIII	N	N	N	N	N	A

(From Caldwell DC, Williamson RA, Goldsmith JC. Hereditary coagulopathies in pregnancy. Clin Obstet Gynecol 1985;28:53.).
N, normal; A, abnormal.

hemostasis, manifested by mucocutaneous, posttraumatic, and postoperative bleeding.[261] Close monitoring for a rise in Factor VIII-related activities (Factor VIII coagulant activity, Factor VIII-related antigen, and Factor VIII ristocetin co-factor) during the antepartum period will predict developing coagulopathy.[261] Cryoprecipitate, containing all forms of the Factor VIII macromolecular complex, is preferred over commercial Factor VIII concentrates, which do not provide the high-molecular-weight forms of the macromolecular complex.[46,261,262,281] Management of cryoprecipitate transfusion in pregnancy is outlined by Caldwell and colleagues[46] and Lipton and colleagues.[261]

Increased risk of thromboembolic events is associated with antithrombin-III deficiency,[279,282,283] Factor XII deficiency,[266,284] and the dysfibrinogenemias.[46] Recurrent abortion is associated with Factor XIII deficiency[274] and Factor I (fibrinogen) abnormalities.[276,277]

Inheritance of coagulation factor defects may be autosomal dominant, autosomal recessive, or X-linked recessive. Diagnosis is based on screening tests and specific factor assays. Treatment, specific for each entity, may require cryoprecipitate, fresh-frozen plasma, factor concentrates, DDAVP, ϵ-amino-caproic acid, or heparin.

OTHER CAUSES OF HEMORRHAGIC SHOCK

Spontaneous abortion very rarely is associated with hemorrhage great enough to result in shock. Prompt evacuation of the uterus by curettage and administration of uterotonic agents allow myometrial contraction resulting in hemostasis.

Bleeding associated with the evacuation of a hydatidiform mole may be significant enough to require transfusion. Schlaerth and others reported a 35.4% incidence of blood transfusion (mean 2.47 units) among women undergoing elective termination by suction curettage.[285] Accepted treatment options include curettage and hysterectomy. Uterotonic agents and blood products should be readily available, as the likelihood of profuse bleeding is considerable.

ANAPHYLACTIC SHOCK

Anaphylactic reactions may be fatal in as many as 10% of cases.[286] Obstetric patients are especially at risk, as they will, at some point during pregnancy, probably receive some form of pharmacologic therapy. Antibiotics, nonsteroidal anti-inflammatory agents, narcotics, local anesthetics, iodinated radiocontrast agents, hormones, blood products, colloid solutions, and antivenoms are all known to have the potential to cause anaphylactic reactions.[286–288] Few reports exist in the current obstetric literature regarding this subject. Hofmann and others reported a case of anaphylactic shock secondary to chlorobutanol in chlorobutanol-preserved oxytocin, and Entman and Moise reported a case of anaphylactic shock resulting from administration of a horse serum–based antivenom following a snake bite.[289,290]

The difference between an anaphylactic reaction and an anaphylactoid reaction is that the former is mediated by an IgE class immunoglobulin; both may be clinically identical. It is thought that exposure to certain chemical agents results in direct release of primary and secondary mediators, without antigen–antibody interaction, producing the anaphylactoid reaction.[286]

Exposure to the triggering agent results in release of primary mediators, such as histamine, prostaglandins, leukotrienes, eosinophil chemotactic factor of anaphylaxis, neutrophil chemotactic factor, and platelet-activating factor.[286] These initiate release of the secondary mediators via the complement, intrinsic coagulation, fibrinolytic, and kallikrein–kinin enzyme systems. Multiple products, such as leukotrienes, prostaglandins, vasoactive amines, and oxygen radicals, are then released from white blood cells, platelets, and eosinophils.[286]

Clinical manifestations may be mild to severe (Table 57-8). Life-threatening events include airway obstruction and cardiovascular collapse.

The first priority of management is ventilation, oxygenation, and external cardiac massage, which, in general, is followed by the subcutaneous administration of epinephrine in 0.2-mg increments up to a total dose of 1.0 mg.[291] In obstetric patients, ephedrine, 25–50 mg by IV push, has been recommended because other vasoactive agents carry detrimental uteroplacental ef-

TABLE 57-8. CLINICAL SPECTRUM OF ANAPHYLACTIC REACTIONS

MILD	MODERATE	SEVERE
Local erythema/itching	Dizziness	Hypotension/cyanosis
Pruritus/urticaria	Generalized skin reactions	Angioedema
Coryza	Hoarseness	Stridor/wheezes
Nausea/vomiting	Swelling of lips/tongue	Cardiac arrhythmias
Diarrhea	Tachypnea	Syncope/seizures
Conjunctival suffusion	Tachycardia	Altered mental status
Anxiety	Increasing respiratory distress and anxiety	Shock
		Cardiopulmonary arrest

(From Carlson RW, Bowles AL, Haupt MT. Anaphylactic, anaphylactoid, and related forms of shock. Crit Care Clin 1986;2:347.)

fects.[109,290,292] However, failure to achieve clinical response with ephedrine should not contraindicate the use of other, more potent agents, such as epinephrine, dopamine, norepinephrine, and isoproterenol, in patients with unresponsive shock.

Other drugs, such as aminophylline, antihistamines, and corticosteroids, have been recommended to enhance clinical response.[286,288]

Aggressive fluid replacement is required. In severe cases of anaphylactic shock, colloid volume expanders are required, as crystalloids have been observed to be ineffective in volume replacement.[288,291]

If cardiopulmonary resuscitation (CPR) is not successful, Fisher recommends consideration of cardiopulmonary bypass as a last resort.[288]

SEPTIC SHOCK

Septic shock is rare in obstetrics; however, it is one of the most frequent causes of maternal mortality in the United States.[11] Many infections may result in septic shock in obstetric patients (see Fig. 57-2), but endometritis, chorioamnionitis, and pyelonephritis are the most common causes.[112] Before legalization of abortion, septic shock resulting from criminal abortion was common.[15,293–296]

Significant risk factors for septic shock include prolonged rupture of membranes, retained products of conception, and instrumentation of the genitourinary tract.[106] A significant increase in post-cesarean section infection is seen in indigent patients compared to affluent patients.[297] Other infections that develop in obstetric patients include pneumonia,[298] appendicitis,[64–74] septic abortion,[75] toxic shock syndrome,[76–80] septic pelvic thrombophlebitis,[81–87] and endocarditis.[299]

Bacteremia has been shown to occur in 7.5 of 1000 obstetric admissions and in 9.7% of patients suspected of having infection in whom blood cultures were obtained.[300] Mortality from septic shock in the general population is reported to be as high as 40% to 90%, as opposed to 3% in obstetric and gynecologic patients.[301,302] This may be explained by the relative good health and youth of obstetric patients, prompt vigorous treatment, and infrequency of underlying disease processes.[300] Animal studies, nonetheless, demonstrate an increased susceptibility to complications in pregnant versus non-pregnant subjects following intravenous injection of endotoxin.[303] Endotoxin administered to pregnant baboons causes increased uterine activity and severe fetal distress, with intrauterine death.[304]

Obstetric infections are usually caused by organisms normally found in the genital tract and thus are often polymicrobial.[22,305,306] Common organisms include *Escherichia coli, Klebsiella–Enterobacter, Pseudomonas,* and *Serratia*.[20] Most cases of bacterial infection complicated by shock are caused by gram-negative enteric organisms.[307] Gram-negative infections are usually systemic, whereas gram-positive infections tend to be suppurative.[147]

Shock secondary to sepsis results from a combination of events. The release of bacterial endotoxins and intracellular mediators causes increased capillary permeability with fluid shifts, creating intravascular hypovolemia. Endotoxin itself may cause myocardial depression.[21] Endotoxin has been shown to cause metabolic and membrane transport abnormalities in the lungs at the cellular level, resulting in pulmonary edema.[308] Renal, gastrointestinal, metabolic, and coagulation involvement are all well documented.[20,142,304,309]

Septic shock has classically been described in three phases: the early warm-hypotensive phase, the late cold-hypotensive phase, and the irreversible phase.[20,310] Flushed warm skin, fever, chills, diaphoresis, and tachycardia are manifest in the early warm-hypotensive phase, which is reversible. Pulse pressure and urine output remain stable. The late cold-hypotensive phase is characterized by cool and clammy skin, a drop in body temperature, and diminished mental status. Hypotension, tachycardia, and oliguria develop. This phase is reversible with treatment. If medical intervention is not begun and cellular hypoxia and anaerobic metabolism continue, the irreversible phase of septic shock will develop. Metabolic acidosis, anuria, respiratory distress, cardiac distress, and coma are ominous signs.

Lee and colleagues found that 80% of pregnancies complicated by septic shock occurred during the postpartum period.[106] Significant hemodynamic observations included decreased peripheral vascular resistance with decreased left ventricular function.

Diagnosis requires identification of the source of infection. This source is usually found to be the genital or urinary tract in obstetric patients.[82] Clinical signs include fever, tachycardia, warm–flushed or cool–clammy skin, and tenderness elicited over the affected tissues. Routine laboratory evaluation of patients with suspected septic shock include complete blood count (CBC) with differential, platelets, coagulation studies, electrolytes, BUN, creatinine, lactate, urinalysis, and arterial blood gasses. Laboratory evidence of infection may include leukocytosis on peripheral blood smear, pyuria and bacteriuria on urinalysis, and blood gas aberrations, such as a metabolic acidosis with compensatory respiratory alkalosis. In some patients, evidence of coagulopathy is manifested by abnormalities in platelet count, fibrinogen, prothrombin time, partial thromboplastin time, and the presence of fibrin-split products.

Cultures should be obtained in all patients from the urine, blood, and, if possible, the amniotic fluid or the endometrium. The technique of endometrial culture may affect bacteriologic findings.[311] Other specific sources, such as stool, wound, and sputum, are cultured as indicated. Lumbar puncture should be considered in patients with altered mental status.[147]

Chest x-ray should be obtained to rule out infiltrates, evidence of pulmonary edema, and adult respiratory distress syndrome (ARDS). Abdominal x-rays should be obtained to rule out free air under the diaphragm or a foreign body.[310]

Treatment of septic shock requires general supportive measures, including restoration of intravascular volume and often inotropic support (see the section on general supportive measures). Adequate oxygenation is essential. Antibiotic therapy for sepsis should be tailored directly to the suspected source guided by information obtained by gram stain. In cases of septic stock, however, we usually institute intravenous broad-spectrum antibiotic coverage with ampicillin, 2 g every 6 hours; clindamycin, 900 mg every 8 hours; and gentamicin, 1.5 mg/kg every 8 hours. Gentamicin dosage is guided by serum peak and trough levels.

Failure of the patient to respond promptly to simple volume resuscitation warrants transfer to an intensive care setting.[296] If response to treatment is not satisfactory, close examination for abscessed or necrotic tissue must be carried out and surgical intervention instituted.[312] Timely drainage of abscesses and removal of necrotic tissue, sometimes via hysterectomy, are required for clinical improvement. In postpartum patients with refractory fevers, septic pelvic vein thrombophlebitis must be ruled out. Computed tomography scan may be helpful in making the diagnosis.[20,87] In a patient who does not respond to medical therapy with antibiotics and heparin, exploratory laparotomy with ligation of the inferior vena cava and ovarian veins may be mandated.[81] Isolation in blood cultures of *Clostridium perfringens* does not warrant surgical intervention unless myonecrosis is present.[300]

Therapeutic regimens for septic shock that are currently controversial have been discussed previously.

SEPTIC ABORTION

Before the availability of legalized abortions, septic shock and death following criminal abortion were common. In 1970, Santamarina and Smith stated that more than 95% of septic abortions and septic shock cases were secondary to illegal, or nonmedical abortions.[313] Septic abortion rarely complicates spontaneous incomplete abortion. Sepsis is still the most common complication of legal abortion resulting in maternal death in the United States.[75]

Treatment includes general supportive measures, antibiotics, and removal of the infected necrotic tissue. Broad coverage with an aminoglycoside, clindamycin, and penicillin or ampicillin is recommended because the infection is usually of a mixed aerobic–anaerobic type. Dilatation and curettage is performed to remove the infectious nidus in the uterus. Antibiotic therapy and evacuation of uterine contents will successfully control approximately 95% of all cases.[313] If the infection has progressed beyond the endometrium and is not responsive to conservative therapy, exploratory laparotomy, hysterectomy, and possibly removal of the adnexa are required.

Chorionic villus sampling (CVS), a relatively new procedure used in the prenatal diagnosis of genetic abnormalities, carries a small risk of both fetal loss and maternal infection.[88] Barela and others have reported septic shock complicated by renal failure following CVS, unresponsive to uterine evacuation, antibiotics, and vasopressor therapy.[89] Clinical improvement followed exploratory laparotomy, total abdominal hysterectomy, and bilateral salpingo-oophorectomy.

CHORIOAMNIONITIS

Uterine infections in pregnancy may be grouped into three categories. Septic abortion occurs prior to 20 weeks' gestation, chorioamnionitis occurs after the twentieth week, and puerperal sepsis (postpartum endometritis) begins after delivery.[54] Chorioamnionitis occurs in approximately 1% of deliveries.[306] Although maternal and fetal complications are significant, the overall clinical outcome is usually good.[55] In a series of 212 patients diagnosed with amnionitis, Clark and Anderson found that the most common predisposing factor to chorioamnionitis was premature rupture of membranes.[56] Prematurity was noted in 55% of 216 infants. A 15.3% incidence of breech presentation was found, probably related to prematurity. A retrospective review of 171 cases between 1974 and 1978 revealed a 35% incidence of cesarean section, probably related to dysfunctional labor and malpresentations.[58]

The diagnosis is usually made on clinical grounds based on evidence of leakage of fluid from the vagina, fever, maternal or fetal tachycardia, leukocytosis, uterine tenderness, and foul-smelling amniotic fluid.[55,56,58] Gram stain of amniotic fluid obtained by transabdominal amniocentesis or through intrauterine pressure catheters may be helpful.

Bacteremia was documented in 12% of patients with the diagnosis of chorioamnionitis in one series.[55] Septic shock occurs, but rarely.[55,58] Today maternal death is rare; however, earlier reviews have demonstrated significant mortality associated with chorioamnionitis.[11,57] Maternal morbidity was more significant in those patients who delivered by cesarean section than in those who delivered vaginally.[55] Perinatal mortality is increased six-fold in near-term fetuses of mothers with chorioamnionitis.[56] Increased perinatal mortality may be related more to prematurity than to sepsis.[58]

Treatment consists of hydration, administration of parenteral antibiotics, and prompt delivery of the fetus. Diagnosis-to-delivery time limits should not be set.[58] Vaginal delivery is preferable to cesarean section in the presence of chorioamnionitis except when the maternal condition deteriorates, fetal distress ensues, or the usual obstetric indications for cesarean section are present.

ENDOMETRITIS

Endometritis following vaginal delivery is very rare. It is more often encountered after cesarean section, with a wide range of incidence depending on the patient population studied. After blood, urine, and endometrial cultures are obtained, broad-spectrum antibiotic coverage is instituted to cover aerobic and anaerobic organisms.

Although most cases respond to antibiotic therapy, hysterectomy may be necessary in those cases that do not respond because of formation of intramyometrial abscesses. Consideration of the diagnosis of septic pelvic thrombophlebitis must also be made in patients who do not respond to medical therapy. Gas gangrene of the uterus, caused by *Clostridium perfringens*, requires supportive medical therapy, surgical removal of infected tissue, and broad antibiotic coverage.[314] Abdominal radiography may reveal physometra (gas in the uterus), aiding in the diagnosis of gas gangrene.

PYELONEPHRITIS

Acute pyelonephritis complicates 1% to 2% of all pregnancies and usually occurs in the latter half of pregnancy.[59,61] The incidence of asymptomatic bacteriuria in pregnancy is 5% to 6%. Untreated asymptomatic bacteriuria will progress to pyelonephritis in 30% of patients.[61]

Presenting symptoms include back pain, fever, chills, lower urinary tract symptoms, nausea, and vomiting. The usual clinical findings are fever and costovertebral angle tenderness. Diagnosis is confirmed by urinalysis with findings of bacteriuria and pyuria, and urine cultures, which are positive in 90% of cases. *Escherichia coli* is isolated in the majority of cases.[59]

Duff found that 7.2% of patients with pyelonephritis developed bacteremia.[61] Septic shock occurs in 1.3% to 3% of patients hospitalized for acute pyelonephritis.[60,61] Cunningham and others reported four cases of respiratory insufficiency with multisystem derangement associated with pyelonephritis in pregnancy, thought to be secondary to endotoxin effects.[62]

Treatment of pyelonephritis necessitates early administration of an antibiotic to which the organism is susceptible. If urosepsis is suspected, broad-spectrum coverage is recommended.[63] The choice of antibiotics should be based on known bacterial drug resistance at each individual hospital.[61] Because of a high incidence of *E. coli* resistance to ampicillin, therapy at our institution is begun with cefazolin, 1 g intravenously every 8 hours. If severe infection or urosepsis is suspected, we provide wider coverage by administering an aminoglycoside plus ampicillin. Hydration with crystalloid solutions is another crucial aspect of therapy. After the patient has been afebrile for 24 hours, intravenous antibiotics are discontinued and an oral antibiotic to which the organism is known to be sensitive is started.

Gilstrap and colleagues demonstrated significant transient renal dysfunction in 21% of women with pyelonephritis they tested.[59] Therefore, therapy with nephrotoxic drugs and intravenous fluids should be closely monitored.

If the patient is still febrile after 72 hours of starting therapy, antibiotic resistance, urinary tract obstruction, or misdiagnosis must be suspected. An intravenous pyelogram should be performed to rule out renal or ureteral stones and obstruction.[61]

APPENDICITIS

Appendicitis is the most common non-obstetric indication for exploratory laparotomy in the obstetric patient.[72] The incidence of appendicitis is one per 1500 deliveries.[67] The incidence of pregnancy in women found to have appendicitis is 2%.[74] Appendicitis may occur at any age, but 90% of patients have been found to be younger than 30 years of age and 75% of patients have been found to be between the ages of 20 and 30.[67] As pregnancy progresses, the diagnosis becomes more difficult secondary to anatomical and physiologic changes associated with pregnancy.[66] Associated with this delay in diagnosis and treatment is an increase in fetal–maternal mortality and morbidity.[69] As the risk of a negative laparotomy to the mother and fetus is not significant, especially in relationship to a neglected diagnosis of appendicitis, exploratory laparotomy is mandated in all cases of suspected appendicitis.[67,69,72,315] "The mortality of appendicitis complicating pregnancy is the mortality of delay."[71] Delay in diagnosis is related to gestational age and has been found to be 0%, 18%, and 75% in the first, second, and third trimesters, respectively.[69]

The classic signs and symptoms of appendicitis are present less frequently in the pregnant patient.[69] Cunningham's retrospective review of 34 cases demonstrated that abdominal pain and nausea were reliably present symptoms, whereas diarrhea and urinary symptoms were not.[69] Anorexia was common early in pregnancy, but occurred less frequently as pregnancy advanced. Reliable signs included direct abdominal tenderness and low-grade fever. Rebound tenderness and rectal tenderness were common early in pregnancy, but became less frequent as pregnancy advanced. Localization of abdominal tenderness may change as gestation progresses, as described by Baer (Fig. 57-10).[74]

Useful laboratory values include leukocytosis in the range of 10,000–15,000/μL, with a quarter of patients having a WBC count of less than 10,000/μL and a quarter of patients having a WBC count greater than 15,000/μL.[67] Urinalysis may reveal pyuria without bacteriuria. Urinalysis is normal in 91% of cases.[69]

Differential diagnoses include cholecystitis, adnexal torsion, degenerating myoma, ruptured corpus luteum cyst, ruptured dermoid, infarction of the ovary, preterm labor, abruptio placentae, and pneumonia.[66] Pyelonephritis is the most commonly confused diagnosis.[65]

Treatment is surgical.[64] Exploratory laparotomy is performed through an incision that will allow access to other suspect anatomical regions, as diagnostic accuracy is around 75% at best.[64,67] The choice of abdominal incision should be individualized. Some authors recommend a midline vertical incision for adequate exposure of the abdomen[69]; others recommend a right paramedian incision[68] or a right horizontal muscle-splitting incision over the point of maximal tenderness.[67,70]

When a normal-appearing "lily-white" appendix is encountered, most authorities recommend removal of the appendix, as some appendices are found to be histo-

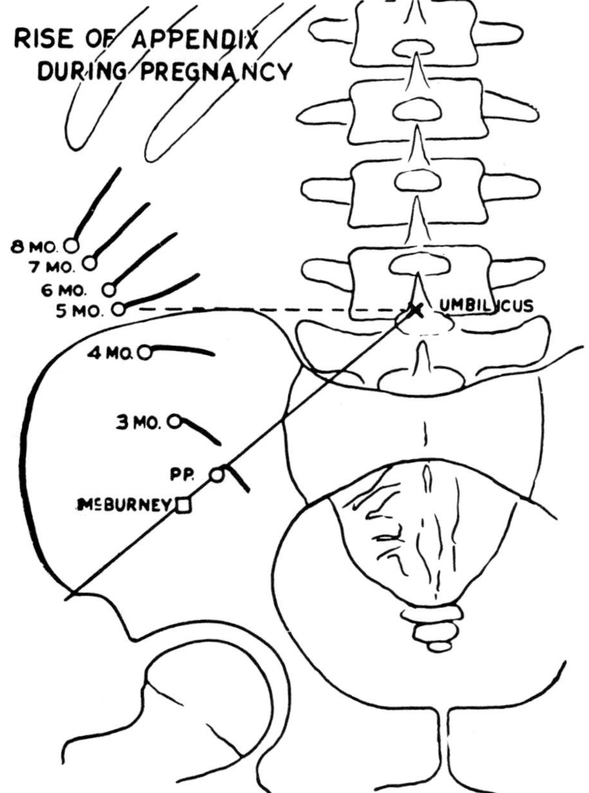

FIGURE 57–10. Changes in position and direction of appendix during pregnancy. After the fifth month of pregnancy the appendix lies at the crest level and rises above this level during the last trimester. The postpartum position of the appendix (pp) corresponds to its position in the nonpregnant state. Roentgenologically, the base of the appendix is usually found medial to McBurney's point. The average position of the umbilicus corresponds to the point at which a line extended horizontally from the iliac crest crosses the spine. (From Baer JL, Reis RA, Arens RA. Appendicitis in pregnancy, with changes in position and axis of the normal appendix in pregnancy. JAMA 1932; 98: 1363.)

logically abnormal, suggesting early appendicitis, and future diagnostic dilemmas may be avoided.[67,69]

Routine postoperative antibiotic therapy is controversial and may depend on the visual appearance of the appendix.[67] Maternal mortality was found to be 2% overall and 7.3% in the last trimester.[70] This high mortality rate is related to gestational age and delay in diagnosis.[69,70] Perinatal mortality is 8.7% to 17.3%[67–70] and is related to prematurity in 29% to 37.5% of cases.[68,69] The perforated appendix is felt to take a more pathologic course in the pregnant patient because the omentum, which lies in the upper abdomen, is not able to wall off the ruptured appendix. The appendix itself may lie outside the pelvic cavity in a location more amenable to general peritoneal contamination. Uterine contractions may also inhibit the localization process.[70] Furthermore, elevated maternal adrenocorticosteroids may decrease inflammatory response and mask signs of infection.[73]

In conclusion, appendicitis is not rare in pregnancy and is a difficult diagnosis to confirm.[64] Confirmation relies on surgical exploration, which, if delayed, may result in severe maternal and fetal consequences. The risks of anesthesia and surgery are less than those of a missed diagnosis of appendicitis in the pregnant patient.[65,68]

TOXIC SHOCK SYNDROME

Toxic shock syndrome (TSS) has been reported to occur in association with vaginal delivery, spontaneous abortion, cesarean section, and mastitis.[76–79] The exact incidence of nonmenstrual TSS is unknown.[78] Mortality may be as high as 5%.

TSS is defined by a fever greater than 102°F, diffuse macular erythrodermal rash with desquamation, hypotension, and evidence of multiple organ system involvement caused by systemic absorption of exotoxin produced by certain strains of *Staphylococcus aureus.*[80] Vasodilation and egress of intravascular fluid and serum proteins into the extravascular compartment result in oliguria, hypotension, edema, low central ve nous pressure, hypoproteinuria, and hypoalbuminemia.[80]

Initial clinical management requires aggressive fluid replacement to correct systemic hypotension. Invasive monitoring in an intensive care unit is necessary in many instances. Cultures should be obtained from the usual sources, such as blood and urine, as well as from the genital tract and other suspected areas (eg, surgical wound, cutaneous lesion, or throat). β-lactamase-resistant antistaphylococcal antibiotics (oxacillin, dicloxacillin, nafcillin), first-generation parenteral cephalosporins, and aminoglycosides may be used for treatment, although they usually do not have a significant effect on the course of the acute disease. Dopamine administration was required to maintain a low-normal blood pressure in seven of 22 patients with TSS reported by Chesney and colleagues.[80] If the diagnosis is in question, an aminoglycoside should be added to cover gram-negative organisms. Irrigational washing of the vagina or other suspected sources of bacteria and exotoxins would appear helpful but has not been proven beneficial.

SUPPURATIVE PELVIC THROMBOPHLEBITIS

Septic or suppurative pelvic thrombophlebitis (SPT) describes a condition of the pelvic veins in which septic thrombosis occurs.[83] Trauma along the surfaces of the genital tract is felt to be the inciting factor preceding thrombosis and infection.[83] In addition to bacteremia and sepsis, thromboembolism may occur, with pulmonary infarction occurring in 45.7% of patients.[84]

Presenting symptoms include fever up to 106°F, chills, and tachycardia of the plateau type. Pelvic examination is essentially normal except for palpation of tender thrombosed veins in 30% of cases.[81] Chest x-ray may reveal pulmonary shadows suggestive of infarction.[84] A 35% incidence of positive blood cultures is reported.[81]

Diagnosis may be difficult and is often one of exclusion. Recently, computed tomography scan of the pelvis for detection of venous thrombosis has been proposed.[20,87]

Medical therapy with broad-spectrum antibiotics (eg, gentamicin, clindamycin, and ampicillin) for suspected endometritis is often instituted before the diagnosis of SPT is made. Institution of intravenous heparin is then begun and clinical improvement within 48 hours is anticipated. In the absence of pulmonary emboli, heparin may be continued for 10 days.[82] Surgical therapy, which was once the mainstay, is still indicated if medical therapy is unsuccessful, if pulmonary infarction develops during medical therapy or if the patient presents prior to therapy with pulmonary infarction.[85] Surgical therapy of SPT, as emphasized by Collins and his associates, involves ligation of the inferior vena cava and both ovarian veins.[81,85,86] Collins recommended discontinuation of all medical therapy on completion of surgical therapy.[81]

Mortality has been reported to be 52% in the early part of this century and 10% in a series of 202 cases collected between 1941 and 1969.[81] Mortality is more often from thromboembolic than septic complications.

BURNS

Approximately 2.2 million people each year in the United States suffer burns significant enough to present for medical treatment.[316]

Most burns are minor. Minor burns are superficial or partial-thickness injuries covering less than 10% of the total body surface. Major burns are partial-thickness or full-thickness injuries covering more than 10% of the total body surface. Major burns may be further classified as moderate (10% to 19% total body burn), severe (20% to 39% total body burn), or critical (40% or greater total body burn).[317]

Early complications of burns include severe hypovolemia secondary to fluid and electrolyte shifts resulting from vascular damage.[318] Hypovolemia, hypotension, and shock are prevented by aggressive fluid and electrolyte replacement. Electrolytes must be monitored carefully, as sodium and potassium values may fluctuate widely.[317]

Hypoxemia may occur in conjunction with hypovolemia or secondary to upper and lower respiratory damage as a result of inhalation of noxious fumes. Oxygenation warrants close monitoring, and supplemental oxygen should be administered as required, occasionally via endotracheal intubation.

Later complications include wound infection and sepsis. Hospital-acquired resistant organisms may complicate therapeutic management. Septicemia and pneumonia are reported to contribute to nearly one half of all deaths in burn patients.[319]

Wound scarring may cause local discomfort and pruritus.[320] Rai and Jackson reported no increase in difficulties during labor or cesarean section from severe abdominal scarring secondary to burns.[321]

Maternal mortality, fetal mortality, and the incidence of premature labor are all directly proportional to the extent of maternal injury.[318,322] Maternal mortality was found to be 3% and fetal mortality was from 17% to 27% if the burn involved less than 40% of the total body surface.[317]

Because experience with pregnant burn patients is limited, few specific treatment guidelines beyond electrolyte and fluid replacement, adequate ventilatory support, and antibiotic therapy have been proposed. Tocolytic therapy must be managed carefully. β-mimetic therapy may result in further electrolyte imbalance and cardiopulmonary complications. Magnesium sulfate may produce unwanted vasodilative effects. Indomethacin has been proposed as an acute temporary method of managing premature labor, which may be managed expectantly or by conventional means after the patient's condition has stabilized.[323] As in other instances of maternal injury, maternal stability, fetal well-being, and fetal maturity must all be considered in making decisions about delivery. The route and timing of delivery should be based on obstetric indications.[320]

NECROTIZING FASCIITIS

Necrotizing fasciitis, a suppurative bacterial infection of the superficial and deep fasciae, is a rare but deadly complication in obstetrics.[324] Only two of four cases reported by Golde and Ledger survived.[325] Treatment requires prompt diagnosis, wide surgical debridement of necrotic tissue, drainage, and parenteral antibiotics with emphasis on anaerobic coverage.[324,325]

CARDIOGENIC SHOCK

A review of maternal mortality in California between 1960 and 1968 has revealed heart disease to be a significant contributor to non-obstetric maternal mortality.[326] Cardiac disease was the most common non-obstetric cause of maternal death, constituting 77 of 348 (22%) non-obstetric deaths. Rheumatic heart disease was the most common cardiac lesion, with congenital heart disease, peripartum cardiomyopathy, and coronary heart disease contributing significantly to mortality.

As in other areas of medicine, the causes and relative frequencies of disease entities change with advancing technology. The ratio of rheumatic heart disease to congenital heart disease is narrowing with time, as the incidence of rheumatic fever is decreasing and patients with congenital heart disease are surviving into their reproductive years as a result of surgery.[327,328] Nevertheless, rheumatic heart disease is still sufficiently prevalent, and complications such as pulmonary congestion, pulmonary edema, right heart failure, dysrhythmias, and embolism may occur in pregnancy.[329]

Cardiogenic shock may be secondary to ventricular dysfunction or extrinsic cardiac compression, both of which result in diminished cardiac output and hypoperfusion at the cellular level (see Fig. 57-2).[1] Many of these processes may develop in the non-pregnant state; however, amniotic fluid embolism and peripartum cardiomyopathy are unique to the obstetric population.

VENTRICULAR DYSFUNCTION

β-ADRENERGIC AGENTS

Ventricular dysfunction, as manifested by arrhythmias, angina pectoris, pulmonary edema, or cardiovascular collapse, has been reported with the use of terbutaline, salbutamol, hexoprenaline, and ritodrine in the tocolytic therapy of premature labor.[330–335] Early cessation of the tocolytic agent, close monitoring, and treatment of associated maternal arrhythmias and cardiopulmonary derangements are essential in preventing further serious complications.

EMBOLISM

Thrombotic Pulmonary Embolism

Obstruction of the pulmonary vessels may result in pulmonary hypertension and right heart failure, leading to cardiogenic shock and death. Massive embolization, defined as greater than 40% to 50% obstruction, may result in depression of cardiac output in normal patients.[336] Kaunitz and others found embolism to be the leading cause of maternal death in the United States.[7] Thrombotic, amniotic fluid, and air embolism constituted 55%, 39%, and 5% of cases, respectively.

Treatment of thrombotic pulmonary embolism consists of cardiopulmonary support and heparin anticoagulation to prevent progressive thrombus formation. The efficacy and safety of thrombolytic agents, such as streptokinase, urokinase, and tissue plasminogen activator, remain unproven, especially in obstetrics.[337] However, urokinase has been used successfully in pregnancy.[338] Additionally, urokinase and streptokinase do not cross the placenta. Recent surgery or delivery is a contraindication to thrombolytic therapy.[339] Surgical embolectomy is indicated in rare cases.[337,339]

Amniotic Fluid Embolism

Amniotic fluid embolism (AFE) has been described in this chapter with respect to its relationship to acquired coagulation defects that result in hemorrhage. Hemodynamic observations derived from pulmonary artery catheterization in humans reveal evidence of left ventricular failure and pulmonary edema, rather than pulmonary artery vasospasm and cor pulmonale, which have been the main observations in experimental animal models.[42,47] On this basis, Clark and others suggest that inotropic support may be the critical therapeutic modality in patients diagnosed with AFE.[42]

HYPERTHYROIDISM

Forfar and colleagues demonstrated a significant fall in left ventricular ejection fraction (LVEF) during exercise in non-pregnant hyperthyroid patients with high LVEF at rest.[340] These same patients were then tested in the euthyroid state and found to have higher LVEF during exercise. These findings were felt to represent a reversible functional cardiomyopathy manifested during exercise or stress. Clark and others observed a reversible decline in left ventricular function in a pregnant patient with thyrotoxicosis undergoing cesarean section.[341] Consideration for invasive monitoring, fluid restriction, and beta blockade should be given to patients with thyrotoxicosis who are to undergo the stress of surgery.[341] Propylthiouracil is the antithyroid drug of choice for pregnant patients in "thyroid storm."[342]

SEVERE ANEMIA

When chronic blood loss results in a drop in hemoglobin to 4.4 g/dL or hematocrit to 14%, profound circulatory changes develop and cardiac failure may follow.[343] Patients with chronic severe anemia will require slow transfusion with packed red blood cells in combination with potent, rapidly acting diuretics. In emergency situations, such as labor or surgery, rapid correction of severe anemia may be performed via partial exchange transfusion in order to avoid volume overload.[343]

CARDIAC COMPRESSION

Extrinsic cardiac compression decreases venous return and impairs optimal pumping of the heart. Decreased cardiac output can result in shock. Tension pneumothorax, pericardial tamponade, and rupture of the diaphragm with herniation of the abdominal contents into the thoracic cavity may cause significant cardiac compression.

Placement of a chest tube will alleviate compression secondary to a tension pneumothorax. Pericardiocentesis will relieve the high intrapericardial pressure produced by cardiac tamponade.[337] Diaphragmatic rupture with herniation of abdominal viscera is a surgical emergency.[130]

Maternal death secondary to constrictive pericarditis following thoracic radiotherapy has been reported.[344]

OTHER CAUSES OF CARDIOGENIC SHOCK

Other potential causes of cardiogenic shock include cardiac dysrhythmias, myocardial infarction,[345,346] congenital heart disease,[347–350] acquired heart disease,[131,132,329,351–353] and peripartum cardiomyopathy.[354–360] These entities are described elsewhere in this text.

NEUROGENIC SHOCK

Neurogenic shock is said to occur when generalized vasodilation causes venous pooling, resulting in decreased filling of the right heart and diminished cardiac output. Neurogenic shock in obstetrics may accompany conduction anesthesia, central nervous system trauma, and puerperal uterine inversion.

CENTRAL NERVOUS SYSTEM TRAUMA

Spinal shock, characterized by hypotension and bradycardia, results from loss of peripheral sympathetic vascular tone with intact cardiac vagal tone in patients with cervical or high thoracic spinal cord injuries.[361] It is a very rare cause of shock in obstetrics. Management of spinal cord injuries is beyond the scope of this chapter.

PUERPERAL UTERINE INVERSION

Shock resulting from puerperal uterine inversion traditionally has been thought to be secondary to a combination of reflex parasympathetic stimulation and acute blood loss. Although classically described as "shock out of proportion to blood loss," some authors believe that blood loss is often grossly underestimated.[362] Earlier reports showed significant maternal mortality ranging from 13% to 41%,[363] with recent reports demonstrating no maternal mortality, perhaps a result of early recognition and aggressive treatment.[362,364]

Most authorities recommend that shock be corrected prior to manual replacement of the inverted uterus.[364] The inverted uterine fundus may be manually replaced by the technique described by Johnson.[365] It is also suggested that, if the placenta is still attached, removal of the placenta should follow replacement of the uterus.[364] Shock is corrected by the usual means, including oxygenation, volume replacement, and sometimes vasopressors. Once the uterus is manually replaced, uterotonic agents should be administered to assure complete contraction of the uterus. The operator's hand should not be removed from the uterine cavity until contraction of the uterus is assured. If the cervix has contracted around the uterus, rendering replacement impossible, uterine relaxation should be achieved by administration of halothane. If manual methods are not successful, surgical techniques, as described by Spinelli,[134] Haultain,[135] or Huntington,[136] should be employed. Prophylactic antibiotics should be considered, depending on the degree of blood loss, hypotension, and manual manipulation.

CONDUCTION ANESTHESIA

Conduction anesthesia may result in hypotension and shock via sympathetic blockade, resulting in venous pooling, decreased venous return, and decreased cardiac output. Shnider and colleagues found that a 40% or greater decrease in arterial blood pressure resulted in fetal hypoxia, hypercapnia, and acidosis in pregnant ewes subjected to maternal hypotension during obstetric spinal anesthesia.[366]

Hypotension and shock secondary to regional anesthesia are treated by rapid fluid replacement, cardiovascular support, and ventilatory support. Placement of the patient in the Trendelenburg position and alleviating uterine aortocaval compression may be helpful. Vasopressors should be carefully used if the preceding methods are unsuccessful. Ephedrine is preferred to other vasopressors that correct hypotension at the expense of decreasing uteroplacental blood flow.[108,366,367] Mechanical ventilatory support may be required when large doses of local anesthetics are injected into the subarachnoid space when intended for the peridural space.[291] Hypotension may be prevented by intravenous fluid preloading, Trendelenburg positioning, and left uterine displacement.[367] Additional caution should be taken in patients with hypertensive disorders, as greater drops in mean arterial blood pressure have been demonstrated as compared to normotensive subjects.[368]

COMPLICATIONS OF SHOCK

In states of profound or prolonged shock, any organ system may become temporarily or permanently damaged. In the 1940s and 1950s, acute renal failure was the leading cause of death in shock patients. With improved renal support, respiratory failure, specifically the adult respiratory distress syndrome (ARDS), became the survival-limiting factor.[4] With the development of pulmonary support, patients began to survive respiratory failure but then succumbed to a sequential failure of organ systems. In the early 1970s, the syndrome of multisystem organ failure (MSOF) emerged. Infection is thought to be the etiology of MSOF.[369] However, positive blood cultures were detected in only 50% of patients with established MSOF.[370] Sepsis and organ failure are produced by any process that activates the inflammatory response, including microorganisms and necrotic tissue.[371,372] Many inflammatory mediators have been identified in the pathogenesis of MSOF.[373] Specific-organ failure in MSOF is summarized in Table 57-9.[374]

Mortality rates in MSOF are reported in a wide range. The number of organ systems involved correlates directly with mortality. Fry and associates demonstrated an 80% mortality rate with involvement of three organ systems and a 100% mortality rate with four.[375] An-

TABLE 57–9. SPECIFIC ORGAN FAILURE IN MULTISYSTEM ORGAN FAILURE

ORGAN	PATHOPHYSIOLOGY	RESULT
Lung	Increased permeability and ventilation–perfusion mismatch	Decreased compliance and hypoxemia
	Decreased metabolism of vasoactive substances	Hemodynamic instability
	Antimicrobial dysfunction and impaired lung defenses	Nosocomial pneumonia
Liver synthesis	Early increase	Acute-phase protein synthesis and hypermetabolism
	Late decrease	Jaundice and coagulopathy
	Decreased IgA production	Increased gastrointestinal tract bacteria
	Decreased bile salts	Increased gastrointestinal tract endotoxin
Immunologic	Kupffer's cell activation	Hepatocyte depression and peripheral catabolism
	Decreased fibronectin and decreased phagocytosis	Bacteremia, endotoxemia, and microvascular emboli
Kidney	Hypovolemia, redistribution of renal blood flow, and nephrotoxic drugs	Azotemia with or without oliguria
Gastrointestinal tract	Decreased IgA and use of antibiotics and antacids	Increased luminal bacteria and endotoxin
	Mucosal atrophy and increased permeability	Leaks bacteria and endotoxin, stress bleeding
Heart	Circulating myocardial depressant factor	Decreased ejection fraction
Central nervous system	Circulating false neurotransmitters	Altered mental status
	Endogenous opioid-mimetics	Hemodynamic stability

(From DeCamp MM, Demling RH. Posttraumatic multisystem organ failure. JAMA 1988;260:530.)

other study reported a mortality rate of 40% with respiratory failure alone; when respiratory failure coexisted with one, two, three, or four organ systems, mortality rates of 56%, 73%, 82%, and 100%, respectively, were noted.[376] The mortality rate of MSOF has fallen with time, partly as a result of emphasis placed on nutritional support.[377,378]

Established, experimental, and disproved methods of treatment for MSOF are outlined in Table 57-10.[374]

NEUROLOGIC COMPLICATIONS

Cerebral blood flow is maintained by autoregulation, but once mean arterial pressure falls below 60 mm Hg, cerebral blood flow falls in a linear fashion[379] and hypoxic encephalopathy occurs. This condition is usually reversible if circulatory collapse is corrected. At worst, a mild state of confusion and memory loss persists unless a cerebrovascular accident secondary to hypotension or intracranial bleeding secondary to DIC occurs.[337] Except in advanced states of septic shock, the autonomic nervous system produces peripheral vasoconstriction in the face of decreased tissue perfusion in order to maintain perfusion to the vital organs. This may result in further tissue hypoxia and accumulation of anaerobic metabolites.

PULMONARY COMPLICATIONS

Respiratory failure following any form of shock may be secondary to multiple causes, such as pulmonary edema, aspiration of gastric contents, pneumonia, and obstruction. A separate clinical entity, the adult respiratory distress syndrome (ARDS), may occur alone or in conjunction with these other causes of respiratory failure.[5] ARDS is a result not only of increased capillary permeability, but of complement activation, leukocyte aggregation, superoxide-induced injury, protease release, platelet aggregation, prostaglandins, and oxygen toxicity.[337,380] A triad of clinical findings—intrapulmonary shunting with hypoxemia, decreased pulmonary compliance, and radiologic findings consistent with diffuse bilateral pulmonary edema—develops within 24 hours after the initial hypotensive episode, reaching a peak after 24–48 hours, with death ensuing in 48–72 hours if untreated.[381,382] Clinically, the patient becomes tachypneic after the hypotensive crisis. As respiratory effort increases, the patient may complain of dyspnea. Arterial blood gases may demonstrate hypoxemia and a respiratory alkalosis. Initially, the lungs are clear to auscultation, and chest x-ray is negative for infiltrates. After 24 hours, radiologic signs, such as fine reticular infiltrates, may progress to complete consolidation. Therapy consists of mechanical ventilation with intermittent positive-pressure ventilation at the minimal inspired oxygen concentration sufficient to maintain a pO_2 of at least 60 mm Hg. After 4 days of ventilatory support, some authors recommend that a tracheostomy be placed if an imminent discontinuation of ventilatory support is impossible.[382] As the mortality rate from renal failure is greater than that from respiratory failure, protection of the lungs by restricting fluids, thus risking renal shutdown, is ill advised.[53]

GASTROINTESTINAL COMPLICATIONS

Generalized systemic illness and hypoperfusion of the gastrointestinal tract may lead to hypersecretion of gas-

TABLE 57–10. THERAPEUTIC OPTIONS IN MULTISYSTEM ORGAN FAILURE

Established Methods
- Prevention and support
  - Aggressive fluid resuscitation
  - Early cardiopulmonary support
    - Invasive monitoring
    - Mechanical ventilation
    - Inotropic support
  - Early excision of burn wounds
  - Early fracture fixation
  - Aggressive surveillance and treatment/drainage of infection
  - Aggressive and early nutritional support
    - Combination of enteral and parenteral routes
    - Attention of protein and caloric needs

Experimental Methods
- Prevention and support
  - Maximize oxygen delivery and consumption
    - Prostaglandin E_1 or prostacyclin infusion
    - Red blood cell transfusions to increase oxygen delivery
  - Optimize nutrition and modify the inflammatory response
    - Protein—branched-chain amino acid solutions
    - Lipid—decrease linoleic acids and increase fish oils
  - Stimulate wound healing with growth hormone and growth factors
  - Eliminate sources of infection by gut sterilization with nonabsorbable antibiotics
- Immunotherapy
  - Nonspecific modifications
    - Replete fibronectin (purified fibronectin or cryoprecipitate)
    - Nonspecific immune enhancement (muramyl dipeptide)
  - Specific immunotherapy
    - Anti–lipid A antibodies to block endotoxin activity
    - Lipid X treatment to block lipid A activity
- Mediator-specific treatment
  - Arachidonic acid metabolite inhibitors and antagonists
    - Cyclo-oxygenase inhibitors (ibuprofen)
    - Thromboxane synthetase inhibitors
    - Lipoxygenase inhibitors and leukotriene antagonists
  - Platelet-activating factor antagonists
  - Oxygen radical scavengers
    - Superoxide dismutase and/or catalase
  - Anti–tumor necrosis factor antibody
  - Endorphin antagonists (naloxone)

Disproved Methods
- Corticosteroid therapy

(From DeCamp MM, Demling RH. Posttraumatic multisystem organ failure. JAMA 1988;260:530.)

tric acid and ulceration of gastric mucosa, resulting in massive upper gastrointestinal bleeding. Prior to the advent of H-2 blockers, surgical treatment was often utilized and morbidity and mortality were significant.[383] In animal models, hemorrhagic shock has been shown to cause injury to gastrointestinal mucosa, leading to subepithelial edema and focal areas of necrosis, resulting in translocation of bowel bacteria, notably *E. coli* and *Enterococcus*, to the mesenteric lymph nodes, liver, and spleen.[384,385] These findings are significant, as many patients with bacteremia who die of sepsis and multiple-organ failure are found to have no identifiable septic focus clinically or at autopsy. Third-spacing of fluids in the gut also leads to further cardiovascular compromise. Endoscopy is the best technique to identify these lesions. Surgical intervention is usually reserved for 30% loss of blood volume over the first 24 hours, transfusion requirement of 1500 mL per 24 hours, gastrointestinal hemorrhage resulting in hypotension or shock, and rebleeding during medical therapy.[386]

HEPATIC COMPLICATIONS

Hypotension and hypoxia may result in liver damage with elevation of the transaminases and sometimes serum bilirubin. Central lobular necrosis of the liver may result in impaired processing of heme pigments and jaundice.[387] Release of bacteria and other substances from the gastrointestinal tract may further hepatic damage. Impaired liver function further predisposes the patient to sepsis.[337] In those patients who survive, resolution of the jaundice is observed with no obvious residual liver damage.[387]

ENDOCRINOLOGIC COMPLICATIONS

Massive hemorrhage or shock during parturition may be associated with infarction of the anterior pituitary gland, resulting in panhypopituitarism.[388] Evidence for hypothalamic involvement in Sheehan's syndrome has been submitted by Whitehead.[389]

During the postpartum period, the patient fails to lactate and later fails to resume a normal menstrual cycle. Some patients do not demonstrate any evidence of pituitary deficiency until several years later, when atrophy of the genital organs, hypothyroidism, and adrenal cortical insufficiency become evident.

DiZerega and associates have proposed a sequential stimulation test to aid in the diagnosis of Sheehan's syndrome.[390]

IMMUNOLOGIC COMPLICATIONS

"Sepsis is unquestionably the most common cause of late death in shock patients."[1] With control and prevention of early renal and pulmonary complications that would result in early death, sepsis often ultimately occurs and initiates multiple organ system failure leading to death.[369] The immunologic depression secondary to shock is not yet completely understood; however, loss of plasma fibronectin and impairment of the reticuloendothelial system phagocyte function, T-cell function, and neutrophil migratory response are known to occur.[172]

RENAL COMPLICATIONS

When perfusion to the kidneys becomes diminished, urine output drops and blood is shunted to the renal medulla. Cortical ischemia and damage result if this condition persists.[391,392] Hypoperfusion of the kidneys may cause prerenal failure, followed by acute tubular necrosis or renal cortical necrosis.[393] If shock is successfully treated, renal damage may be averted. If hypoperfusion is prolonged or severe, renal failure may occur and persist for days or weeks, requiring dialysis. In most cases, renal function ultimately recovers.[337]

Lordon and Burton observed high mortality rates in Vietnam casualties with posttraumatic renal failure, despite early dialysis, probably related to the severe nature of combat trauma.[394]

CARDIAC

Myocardial perfusion is under autoregulatory control via coronary artery vasodilation until a drop in mean arterial pressure below 60–70 mm Hg, where perfusion is solely dependent on arterial blood pressure.[395] Coronary hypoperfusion leads to myocardial metabolic derangements, followed by decreased contractility and decreased systemic and coronary blood flow. If this vicious cycle continues, ventricular function worsens and becomes irreversible, with death soon following.

PROGNOSIS OF SEVERE SHOCK

As technology has developed and changed the clinical course of critically ill patients, many clinical observations have been reported and attempts at devising systems to predict outcome of severe illness have been made.

In 1968, Freid and Vosti demonstrated the importance of underlying disease in patients with gram-negative bacteremia in relationship to mortality.[396] Wilson and colleagues observed in 1969 that the presence and the degree of physiologic shunting in the lung is a sensitive indicator of impending respiratory failure and mortality in patients following shock or trauma.[397] In 1973, Shoemaker and colleagues described physiologic patterns relating to hemodynamics, oxygen transport, acid–base balance, temperature, hemoglobin, and blood volume in surviving and nonsurviving critically ill postoperative patients.[398] Studies published in 1979 and 1980 demonstrated the relationship of the number of organ systems involved in MSOF to survival.[375,376] Kraus and colleagues described the APACHE system, which used 34 laboratory or physical parameters to create a scale to predict mortality risks in ICU patient populations.[399] This system was followed by the APACHE II system, which required only 12 readily available laboratory values.[400]

Hardaway studied 29 consecutive patients in severe states of refractory shock admitted to a special shock research unit.[401] He found a high mortality associated with a partial thromboplastin time above 100 seconds, elevated lactic dehydrogenase above 500 U/mL, elevated serum glutamic–oxalacetic transaminase above 60 U/mL, elevated serum glutamic–pyruvate transaminase above 60 U/mL, and elevated lactate above 52 mg/mL. An arterial pO_2/alveolar pO_2 ratio below 15% was associated with 100% mortality, between 15% and 30% associated with 50% mortality, and greater than 30% associated with 0% mortality. The presence and intensity of DIC were effective indices of mortality in patients with severe shock.

Shoemaker and others prospectively evaluated an algorithm for prediction of outcome in acute circulatory failure.[402] Cardiorespiratory variables developed from previous retrospective data were used to develop a predictive index that was found useful in objectively measuring severity of illness and aiding in clinical decision making.

Gonik outlined prognostic indicators found in the literature that were associated with poor outcome in septic shock.[22] Delay in initial diagnosis, underlying debilitating disease, and end-organ failure worsen the prognosis.

In a review of scoring systems designed to assess patients with surgical sepsis, Dellinger noted that such systems are better at predicting death than survival and that they are accurate for populations of patients but have no place in making individual therapeutic decisions. He noted that all these systems simply describe how far from homeostasis the patient has strayed in response to sepsis.[403]

PREVENTIVE MEASURES

In many cases, the development of shock is unforeseeable and unavoidable. However, clinical suspicion and advanced preparation may decrease the severity and subsequent morbidity and mortality of a developing event. All obstetric patients should be considered potential victims of hemorrhage. Certain patients present with conditions placing them in a high-risk category, such as placenta previa, multiple previous cesarean sections, intrauterine fetal demise near term, and pregnancy-induced hypertension. Preparation by ensuring good venous access, availability of volume expanders and blood products, anesthesia, and uterotonic agents may allow prompt and effective treatment in the event of acute blood loss, which may intercept further blood loss and prevent subsequent complications. Recently, autologous blood donation in obstetrics has come to the attention of researchers. Concern over risks of homologous blood transfusion have prompted new interest. Currently, it is estimated that transmission of non-A, non-B hepatitis occurs 1:100 per unit; hepatitis B, 1:200 to 1:300 per unit; and HIV between 1:40,000 and 1:1,000,000 per unit. The risk of fever, chills, or urticaria is 1:100; of hemolytic transfusion reaction, 1:6,000; and of fatal hemolytic reactions, 1:100,000.[404] Transmission of the HIV virus in screened blood products may occur.[405] In November, 1986, the Council on Scientific Affairs of the American Medical Association stated that pregnant patients may participate in autologous blood donations.[406] However, in May, 1987, the

Committee on Obstetrics: Maternal and Fetal Medicine of the American College of Obstetricians and Gynecologists stated that data in pregnant patients were insufficient to allow general endorsement of such programs.[407] Kruskall and others found that autologous blood donation during pregnancy was safe for both the mother and the fetus; however, the use of postpartum transfusion was low (7.7%), possibly secondary to the fact that risk factors were present in only 17 of 48 women.[408] Herbert and others found that 50% of obstetric patients with risk factors for hemorrhage were transfused, and more than 85% of these were able to avoid homologous blood.[407] They found autologous blood donation safe for the mother and her fetus. Although data seem to support the safety and benefit of autotransfusion programs in pregnancy, widespread endorsement is currently lacking. High-risk patients, such as those with placenta previa, previous cesarean sections, and rare blood types, may benefit by avoiding transfusion reactions, antibody development, and disease transmission associated with homologous transfusion.

Potentially grave consequences of sepsis and septic shock may be curtailed by early diagnosis and aggressive treatment of patients at risk. Early resuscitation of intravascular volume, treatment with broad-spectrum antibiotics after obtaining cultures, and removal of the infectious source, if possible, will result in optimal outcome. Chorioamnionitis may be prevented by induction of labor with oxytocin in patients with premature rupture of membranes.[310] The risks of infection must be weighed against the risks of prematurity.

Close hemodynamic monitoring during the peripartum period, especially in patients with severe pregnancy-induced hypertension and in those with serious structural cardiac defects, may help diminish or prevent impending cardiovascular collapse. Pulmonary artery catheterization is very useful in specific clinical situations.

Rare occasions of neurogenic shock may sometimes be prevented with advanced preparation. Adequate volume preloading in obstetric patients undergoing conduction anesthesia is essential in preventing maternal hypotension and fetal distress. Basic clinical maneuvers and technique will avoid some, but not all, episodes of uterine inversion.

In general, preparedness and identification of patients at risk for shock may minimize or prevent maternal and fetal life-threatening events.

REFERENCES

1. Holcroft JW, Blaisdell FW. Shock: causes and management of circulatory collapse. In: Sabiston DC, ed. Textbook of surgery. 13th ed. Philadelphia: WB Saunders, 1986:38.
2. Cavanagh D, Knuppel RA, Shepherd JH, Anderson R, Rao PS. Septic shock and the obstetrician/gynecologist. South Med J 1982;75:809.
3. Simeone FA. Shock, trauma, and the surgeon. Ann Surg 1963;158:759.
4. Webb WR. Pulmonary complications of non-thoracic trauma: summary of the National Research Council Conference. J Trauma 1969;9:700.
5. Blaisdell FW, Lewis FRJ. Etiologic factors in the respiratory distress syndrome. In: Respiratory distress syndrome of shock and trauma. Philadelphia: WB Saunders, 1977:49.
6. Cavanagh D, Knuppel RA, Marsden DE. Hemorrhagic shock in obstetrics. In: Queenan JT, ed. Managing Ob/Gyn emergencies. 2nd ed. Oradell, NJ: Medical Economics, 1985:100.
7. Kaunitz AM, Hughes JM, Grimes DA, Smith JC, Rochat RW, Kafrissen ME. Causes of maternal mortality in the United States. Obstet Gynecol 1985;65:605.
8. National Center for Health Statistics. Vital statistics of the United States, 1982. Vol II, Mortality, Part A. DHHS Publication No (PHS) 86–1122. Public Health Service. Washington, DC: US Government Printing Office, 1986:64.
9. National Center for Health Statistics. Vital statistics of the United States, 1978. Vol II, part A. DHHS Publication No (PHS) 83–1101. Public Health Service. Washington, DC: US Government Printing Office, 1982:1.
10. US Bureau of the Census. Statistical Abstract of the United States: 1988. 108th ed. Washington, DC, 1987:75.
11. Gibbs CE, Locke WE. Maternal deaths in Texas, 1969 to 1973. Am J Obstet Gynecol 1976;126:687.
12. Parazzini F, LaVecchia C, Mezzanotte G. Maternal mortality in Italy, 1955 to 1984. Am J Obstet Gynecol 1988;159:421.
13. Hansen JP. Older maternal age and pregnancy outcome: a review of the literature. Obstet Gynecol Surv 1986;41:726.
14. Hogberg U. Maternal deaths in Sweden, 1971–1980. Acta Obstet Gynecol Scand 1986;65:161.
15. OSMA Committee on Maternal Health. Maternal mortality report for Ohio: a 10-year survey, 1955–1964. Ohio State Med J 1967;63:323.
16. Endler GC, Mariona FG, Sokol RJ, Stevenson LB. Anesthesia-related maternal mortality in Michigan, 1972 to 1984. Am J Obstet Gynecol 1988;159:187.
17. Beller FK, Rosenberg M, Kolker M, Douglas GW. Consumptive coagulopathy associated with intra-amniotic infusion of hypertonic salt. Am J Obstet Gynecol 1972;112:534.
18. Laros RK, Collins J, Penner JA, Hage ML, Smith S. Coagulation changes in saline-induced abortion. Am J Obstet Gynecol 1973;116:277.
19. Cohen E, Ballard CA. Consumptive coagulopathy associated with intraamniotic saline instillation and the effect of intravenous oxytocin. Obstet Gynecol 1974;43:300.
20. Knuppel RA, Rao PS, Cavanagh D. Septic shock in obstetrics. Clin Obstet Gynecol 1984;27:3.
21. Cavanagh D, Rao PS, Sutton, DMC, Bhagat BD, Bachmann F. Pathophysiology of endotoxin shock in the primate. Am J Obstet Gynecol 1970;108:705.
22. Gonik B. Septic shock in obstetrics. Clin Perinatol 1986;13:741.
23. Bick RL. Disseminated intravascular coagulation and related syndromes: etiology, pathophysiology, diagnosis, and management. Am J Hematol 1978;5:265.
24. McGehee WG, Rapaport SI, Hjort PF. Intravascular coagulation in fulminant meningococcemia. Ann Intern Med 1967;67:250.
25. Pritchard JA. Fetal death in utero. Obstet Gynecol 1959;14:573.
26. Romero R, Copel JA, Hobbins JC. Intrauterine fetal demise and hemostatic failure: the fetal death syndrome. Clin Obstet Gynecol 1985;28:24.
27. Weiner AE, Reid DE, Roby CC, Diamond LK. Coagulation defects with intrauterine death from Rh isosensitization. Am J Obstet Gynecol 1950;60:1015.
28. Reid DE, Weiner AE, Roby CC, Diamond LK. Maternal afibrinogenemia associated with long-standing intrauterine fetal death. Am J Obstet Gynecol 1953;66:500.
29. Pritchard JA, Ratnoff OD. Studies on fibrinogen and other he-

mostatic factors in women with intrauterine death and delayed delivery. Surg Gynecol Obstet 1955;101:467.
30. Romero R, Duffy TP, Berkowitz RL, Chang E, Hobbins JC. Prolongation of a preterm pregnancy complicated by death of a single twin in utero and disseminated intravascular coagulation: effects of treatment with heparin. N Engl J Med 1984;310:772.
31. Skelly H, Marivate M, Norman R, Kenoyer G, Martin R. Consumptive coagulopathy following fetal death in a triplet pregnancy. Am J Obstet Gynecol 1982;142:595.
32. Pritchard JA, Brekken AL. Clinical and laboratory studies on severe abruptio placentae. Am J Obstet Gynecol 1967;97:681.
33. Douglas RG, Buchman MI, MacDonald PA. Premature separation of the normally implanted placenta. J Obstet Gynaecol Br Emp 1955;62:710.
34. Basu HK. Fibrinolysis and abruptio placentae. Br J Obstet Gynaecol 1969;76:481.
35. Schneider CL. Coagulation defects in obstetric shock: meconium embolism and heparin; fibrin embolism and defibrination. Am J Obstet Gynecol 1955;69:758.
36. Schneider CL, Henry MM. Meconium embolism in vivo. Am J Obstet Gynecol 1968;101:909.
37. Chung AF, Merkatz IR. Survival following amniotic fluid embolism with early heparinization. Obstet Gynecol 1973;42:809.
38. Gregory MG, Clayton EM Jr. Amniotic fluid embolism. Obstet Gynecol 1973;42:236.
39. Courtney LD. Amniotic fluid embolism. Obstet Gynecol Surv 1974;29:169.
40. Meyer JR. Brasil-medico 1926;2:301.
41. Steiner PE, Lushbaugh CC. Maternal pulmonary embolism by amniotic fluid. JAMA 1941;117:1245.
42. Clark SL, Montz FJ, Phelan JP. Hemodynamic alterations associated with amniotic fluid embolism: a reappraisal. Am J Obstet Gynecol 1985;151:617.
43. Lee W, Ginsburg KA, Cotton DB, Kaufman RH. Squamous and trophoblastic cells in the maternal pulmonary circulation identified by invasive hemodynamic monitoring during the peripartum period. Am J Obstet Gynecol 1986;155:999.
44. Plauche WC. Amniotic fluid embolism. Am J Obstet Gynecol 1983;147:982.
45. Clark SL. Amniotic fluid embolism. In: Clark SL, Phelan JR, Cotton DB, eds. Critical care obstetrics. Oradell, NJ: Medical Economics Books, 1987:315.
46. Caldwell DC, Williamson RA, Goldsmith JC. Hereditary coagulopathies in pregnancy. Clin Obstet Gynecol 1985;28:53.
47. Clark SL, Cotton DB, Gonik B, Greenspoon J, Phelan JP. Central hemodynamic alterations in amniotic fluid embolism. Am J Obstet Gynecol 1988;158:1124.
48. Pritchard JA, Cunningham FG, Mason RA. Coagulation changes in eclampsia: their frequency and pathogenesis. Am J Obstet Gynecol 1976;124:855.
49. Weinstein L. Syndrome of hemolysis, elevated liver enzymes and low platelet count: a severe consequence of hypertension in pregnancy. Am J Obstet Gynecol 1982;142:159.
50. Weinstein L. Preeclampsia/eclampsia with hemolysis, elevated liver enzymes, and thrombocytopenia. Obstet Gynecol 1985;66:657.
51. Poldre PA. Haptoglobin helps diagnose the HELLP syndrome. Am J Obstet Gynecol 1987;157:1267.
52. Pritchard JA, Weisman R Jr, Ratnoff OD, Vosburgh GJ. Intravascular hemolysis, thrombocytopenia and other hematologic abnormalities associated with severe toxemia of pregnancy. N Engl J Med 1954;250:89.
53. Blaisdell FW. Traumatic shock: the search for a toxic factor. ACS Bulletin 1983;68:2.
54. Busing CM, Bleyl U. Shock in pregnancy: pathophysiology and morphologic findings. Pathol Res Pract 1979;165:253.
55. Yoder PR, Gibbs RS, Blanco JD, Castaneda YS, St Clair PJ. A prospective, controlled study of maternal and perinatal outcome after intra-amniotic infection at term. Am J Obstet Gynecol 1983;145:695.
56. Clark DM, Anderson GV. Perinatal mortality and amnionitis in a general hospital population. Obstet Gynecol 1968;31:714.
57. Russell KP, Anderson GV. Aggressive management of ruptured membranes. Am J Obstet Gynecol 1962;83:930.
58. Gibbs RS, Castillo MS, Rodgers PJ. Management of acute chorioamnionitis. Am J Obstet Gynecol 1980;136:709.
59. Gilstrap LC, Cunningham FG, Whalley PJ. Acute pyelonephritis in pregnancy: an anterospective study. Obstet Gynecol 1981;57:409.
60. Cunningham FG, Morris GB, Mickal A. Acute pyelonephritis of pregnancy: a clinical review. Obstet Gynecol 1973;42:112.
61. Duff P. Pyelonephritis in pregnancy. Clin Obstet Gynecol 1984;27:17.
62. Cunningham FG, Leveno KJ, Hankins GDV, Whalley PJ. Respiratory insufficiency associated with pyelonephritis during pregnancy. Obstet Gynecol 1984;63:121.
63. Bahnson RR. Urosepsis. Urol Clin North Am 1986;13:627.
64. King RM, Anderson GV. Appendicitis and pregnancy. Calif Med 1962;97:158.
65. Lowthian J. Appendicitis during pregnancy. Ann Emerg Med 1980;9:431.
66. DeVore GR. Acute abdominal pain in the pregnant patient due to pancreatitis, acute appendicitis, cholecystitis, or peptic ulcer disease. Clin Perinatol 1980;7:349.
67. Babaknia A, Parsa H, Woodruff JD. Appendicitis during pregnancy. Obstet Gynecol 1977;50:40.
68. Townsend JM, Greiss FC. Appendicitis in pregnancy. South Med J 1976;69:1161.
69. Cunningham FG, McCubbin JH. Appendicitis complicating pregnancy. Obstet Gynecol 1975;45:415.
70. Brant HA. Acute appendicitis in pregnancy. Obstet Gynecol 1967;29:130.
71. Babler EA. Perforative appendicitis complicating pregnancy. JAMA 1908;51:1310.
72. Sarason EL, Bauman S. Acute appendicitis in pregnancy: difficulties in diagnosis. Obstet Gynecol 1963;22:382.
73. Black WP. Acute appendicitis in pregnancy. Br Med J 1960;1:1938.
74. Baer JL, Reis RA, Arens RA. Appendicitis in pregnancy, with changes in position and axis of the normal appendix in pregnancy. JAMA 1932;98:1359.
75. Grimes DA, Kafrissen ME, O'Reilly KR, Binkin NJ. Fatal hemorrhage from legal abortion in the United States. Surg Gynecol Obstet 1983;157:461.
76. Gibney RTN, Moore A, Muldowney FP. Toxic-shock syndrome associated with post-partum staphylococcal endometritis. Irish Med J 1983;76:90.
77. Tweardy DJ. Relapsing toxic shock syndrome in the puerperium (letter). JAMA 1985;253:3249.
78. Petitti D, D'Agostino RB, Oldman MJ. Nonmenstrual toxic shock syndrome. Methodologic problems in estimating incidence and delineating risk factors. J Reprod Med 1987;32:10.
79. Vergeront JM, Evenson ML, Crass BA, et al. Recovery of staphylococcal enterotoxin F from the breast milk of a woman with toxic-shock syndrome. J Infect Dis 1982;146:456.
80. Chesney PJ, Davis JP, Purdy WK, Wand PJ, Chesney RW. Clinical manifestations of toxic shock syndrome. JAMA 1981; 246:741.
81. Collins CG. Suppurative pelvic thrombophlebitis: a study of 202 cases in which the disease was treated by ligation of the vena cava and ovarian vein. Am J Obstet Gynecol 1970;108:681.

82. Gibbs RS. Treatment of refractory postpartum fever. Clin Obstet Gynecol 1976;19:83.
83. Collins CG, MacCallum EA, Nelson EW, Weinstein BB, Collins JH. Suppurative pelvic thrombophlebitis. I. Incidence, pathology and etiology. Surgery 1951;30:298.
84. Collins CG, Nelson EW, Collins JH, Weinstein BB, MacCallum EA. Suppurative pelvic thrombophlebitis. II. Symptomatology and diagnosis. Surgery 1951;30:311.
85. Collins CG, Ayers WB. Suppurative pelvic thrombophlebitis. III. Surgical technique. Surgery 1951;30:319.
86. Collins CG, Jones JR, Nelson EW. Surgical treatment of pelvic thrombophlebitis. New Orleans M&S J 1943;95:324.
87. Puerperal infection. In: Pritchard JA, MacDonald PC, Gant NF, eds. Williams' obstetrics. 17th ed. Norwalk, CT: Appleton-Century-Crofts, 1985:728.
88. Cowart V. NIH considers large-scale study to evaluate chorionic villi sampling. JAMA 1984;252:11.
89. Barela AI, Kleinman GE, Golditch IM, Menke DJ, Hogge WA, Golbus MS. Septic shock with renal failure after chorionic villus sampling. Am J Obstet Gynecol 1986;154:1100.
90. Kirshon B, Cotton DB. Fluid replacement in the obstetric patient. In: Sciarra JJ, ed. Gynecology and obstetrics. Vol. 3. Hagerstown, MD: Harper & Row, 1989:1.
91. Rackow EC, Falk JL, Fein IA, et al. Fluid resuscitation in circulatory shock: a comparison of the cardiorespiratory effects of albumin, hetastarch, and saline solutions in patients with hypovolemic and septic shock. Crit Care Med 1983;11:839.
92. Hardaway RM. Coagulation disorders and hemorrhagic shock in the parturient. Int Anesthesiol Clin 1968;6:743.
93. Hemorrhagic Shock. In: ACOG Technical Bulletin 82. Washington, DC: ACOG, 1984;1.
94. Hayashi RH. Hemorrhagic shock in obstetrics. Clin Perinatol 1986;13:755.
95. Jansen RPS. Relative bradycardia: a sign of acute intraperitoneal bleeding. Aust NZ J Obstet Gynaecol 1978;18:206.
96. Oberman HA, Barnes BA, Friedman BA. The risk of abbreviating the major crossmatch in urgent or massive transfusion. Transfusion 1978;18:137.
97. Consensus Conference: Fresh-frozen plasma. Indications and risks. JAMA 1985;253:551.
98. Oberman HA. Uses and abuses of fresh frozen plasma. In: Garratty A, ed. Current concepts in transfusion therapy. Arlington, VA: American Association of Blood Banks, 1985:109.
99. Mannucci PM, Federici AB, Sirchia G. Hemostasis testing during massive blood replacement: a study of 172 cases. Vox Sang 1982;42:113.
100. Counts RB, Haisch C, Simon TL, Maxwell NG, Heimbach DM, Carrico CJ. Hemostasis in massively transfused trauma patients. Ann Surgery 1979;190:91.
101. Shulman NR, Watkins SP, Itscoits SB, Students AB. Evidence that the spleen retains the youngest and hemostatically most effective platelets. Trans Assoc Am Physicians 1968;81:302.
102. Murphy S, Gardner FH. Platelet preservation: effect of storage temperature on maintenance of platelet viability—deleterious effect of refrigerated storage. N Engl J Med 1969;280:1094.
103. Borucki DT, ed. Blood component therapy: a physician's handbook. 3rd ed. Washington, DC: American Association of Blood Banks, 1981:25.
104. Goldberg LI. Dopamine—clinical uses of an endogenous catecholamine. N Engl J Med 1974;291:707.
105. Abboud FM. Shock. In: Wyngaarden JB, Smith LH, eds. Cecil textbook of medicine. 17th ed. Philadelphia: WB Saunders, 1985:211.
106. Lee W, Clark SL, Cotton DB, et al. Septic shock during pregnancy. Am J Obstet Gynecol 1988;159:410.
107. Callender K, Levinson G, Shnider SM, Feduska NJ, Biehl DR, Ring G. Dopamine administration in the normotensive pregnant ewe. Obstet Gynecol 1978;51:586.
108. Rolbin SH, Levinson G, Shnider SM, Biehl DR, Wright RG. Dopamine treatment of spinal hypotension decreases uterine blood flow in the pregnant ewe. Anesthesiology 1979;51:36.
109. Greiss FC, Van Wilkes D. Effect of sympathomimetic drugs and angiotensin on the uterine vascular bed. Obstet Gynecol 1964;23:925.
110. Swan HJC, Ganz W, Forrester J, Marcus J. Diamond G, Chonette D. Catheterization of the heart in man with use of a flow-directed balloon-tipped catheter. N Engl J Med 1970;283:447.
111. Swan HJC, Ganz W. Use of balloon flotation catheters in critically ill patients. Surg Clin North Am 1975;55:501.
112. Kirshon B, Cotton DB. Invasive hemodynamic monitoring in the obstetric patient. Clin Obstet Gynecol 1987;30:579.
113. Cotton DB, Benedetti TJ. Use of the Swan-Ganz catheter in obstetrics and gynecology. Obstet Gynecol 1980;56:641.
114. Clark SL, Horenstein JM, Phelan JP, Montag TW, Paul RH. Experience with the pulmonary artery catheter in obstetrics and gynecology. Am J Obstet Gynecol 1985;152:374.
115. Benedetti TJ, Cotton DB, Read JC, Miller FC. Hemodynamic observations in severe pre-eclampsia with a flow-directed pulmonary artery catheter. Am J Obstet Gynecol 1980;136:465.
116. Strauss RG, Keefer JR, Burke T, Civetta JM. Hemodynamic monitoring of cardiogenic pulmonary edema complicating toxemia of pregnancy. Obstet Gynecol 1980;55:170.
117. Cotton DB, Gonik B, Dorman K, Harrist R. Cardiovascular alterations in severe pregnancy-induced hypertension: relationship of central venous pressure to pulmonary capillary wedge pressure. Am J Obstet Gynecol 1985;151:762.
118. Packman MI, Rackow EC. Optimum left heart filling pressure during fluid resuscitation of patients with hypovolemic and septic shock. Crit Care Med 1983;11:165.
119. Gibson RS, Kistner JR. In: Suratt PM, Gibson RS, eds. Manual of medical procedures. St Louis: CV Mosby, 1982:59.
120. Mitchell SE, Clark RA. Complications of central venous catheterization. AJR 1979;133:467.
121. Lee W, Rokey R, Cotton DB. Noninvasive maternal stroke volume and cardiac output determinations by pulsed Doppler echocardiography. Am J Obstet Gynecol 1988;158:505.
122. Waters EG. Surgical Management of postpartum hemorrhage with particular reference to litigation of uterine arteries. Am J Obstet Gynecol 1952;64:1143.
123. O'Leary JL, O'Leary JA. Uterine artery litigation in the control of intractable postpartum hemorrhage. Am J Obstet Gynecol 1966;94:920.
124. Deere JL, Jacobs WM. Profuse uterine hemorrhage associated with septic incomplete abortion managed by ligation of uterine arteries. Am J Obstet Gynecol 1963;86:136.
125. Faier E. Atonic hemorrhage after manual separation of a low-situated placenta arrested by ligation of the uterine vessels through the vagina. Akush Ginekol 1962;6:28.
126. Fuchs K. Afibrinogenemia treated by ligation of uterine arteries. Gynaecologia 1959;148:407.
127. Clark SL, Phelan JP, Yeh S-Y, Bruce SR, Paul RH. Hypogastric artery ligation for obstetric hemorrhage. Obstet Gynecol 1985;66:353.
128. Clark SL, Phelan JP. Surgical control of ob hemorrhage. Contemp Ob/Gyn 1984;24:70.
129. Clark SL, Koonings PP, Phelan JP. Placenta previa/accreta and prior cesarean section. Obstet Gynecol 1985;66:89.
130. Dudley AG, Teaford H, Gatewood TS Jr. Delayed traumatic rupture of the diaphragm in pregnancy. Obstet Gynecol 1979;53:25s.
131. Shemin RJ, Phillippe M, Dzau V. Acute thrombosis of a composite ascending aortic conduit containing a Bjork-Shiley valve

during pregnancy: successful emergency cesarean section and operative repair. Clin Cardiol 1986;9:299.

132. Bernal JM, Miralles PJ. Cardiac surgery with cardiopulmonary bypass during pregnancy. Obstet Gynecol Surv 1986;41:1.

133. Gauwerky JFH, Heinrich D, Kubli F. Puerperal uterine inversion. Z Geburtshilfe Perinatol 1987;191:238.

134. Spinelli PG. Cura chirurgica conservatrice dell'inversione cronica dell'utero col processo Kehrer. Arch Ital Ginecol 1899;2:7.

135. Haultain FWN. The treatment of chronic uterine inversion by abdominal hysterectomy, with a successful case. Br Med J 1901;2:974.

136. Huntington JL. Acute inversion of the uterus. Boston Med Surg J 1921;184:376.

137. Schein RMH, Long WM, Sprung CL. Controversies in the management of sepsis and septic shock: corticosteroids, naloxone and nonsteroidal anti-inflammatory agents. In: Sibbald WJ, Sprung CL, eds. Perspectives on sepsis and septic shock. Fullerton, CA: Society of Critical Care Medicine, 1986:339.

138. Hinshaw LB, Archer LT, Beller-Todd BK, et al. Survival of primates in LD_{100} septic shock following steroid/antibiotic therapy. J Surg Res 1980;28:151.

139. Hinshaw LB, Archer LT, Beller-Todd BK, et al. Survival of primates in LD_{100} septic shock following steroid-antibiotic therapy. J Surg Res 1980;28:151.

140. Hinshaw LB, Archer LT, Beller-Todd BK, Benjamin B, Flournoy DJ, Passey R. Survival of primates in lethal septic shock following delayed treatment with steroid. Circ Shock 1981;8:291.

141. Hinshaw LB, Beller-Todd BK, Archer LT, et al. Effectiveness of steroid/antibiotic treatment in primates administered LD_{100} Escherichia coli. Ann Surg 1981;194:51.

142. Hinshaw LB, Beller-Todd BK, Archer LT. Current management of the septic shock patient: experimental basis for treatment. Circ Shock 1982;9:543.

143. Bone RC, Fisher CJ, Clemmer TP, Slotman GJ, Metz CA, Balk RA. A controlled clinical trial of high-dose methylprednisolone in the treatment of severe sepsis and septic shock. N Engl J Med 1987;317:653.

144. Schumer W. Steroids in the treatment of clinical septic shock. Ann Surg 1976;184:333.

145. Sprung CL, Caralis PV, Marcial EH, et al. The effects of high-dose corticosteroids in patients with septic shock. A prospective, controlled study. N Engl J Med 1984;311:1137.

146. Hoffman SL, Punjabi NH, Kumula S, et al. Reduction of mortality in chloramphenicol treated severe typhoid fever by high-dose dexamethasone. N Engl J Med 1984;310:82.

147. Rackow EC. Clinical definition of sepsis and septic shock. In: Sibbald WJ, Sprung CL, eds. Perspectives on sepsis and septic shock. Fullerton, CA: The Society of Critical Care Medicine, 1986:1.

148. Thijs LG, Balk E, Tuynman HARE, Koopman PAR, Bezemer PD, Mulder GH. Effects of naloxone on hemodynamics, oxygen transport, and metabolic variables in canine endotoxin shock. Circ Shock 1983;10:147.

149. Reynolds DG, Gurll NJ, Vargish T, Lechner RB, Faden AI, Holaday JW. Blockade of opiate receptors with naloxone improves survival and cardiac performance in canine endotoxic shock. Circ Shock 1980;7:39.

150. Raymond RM, Harkema JM, Stoffs WV, Emerson TE Jr. Effects of naloxone therapy on hemodynamics and metabolism following a superlethal dosage of *Escherichia coli* endotoxin in dogs. Surg Gynecol Obstet 1981;152:159.

151. Holaday JW, Faden AI. Naloxone reversal of endotoxin hypotension suggests role of endorphins in shock. Nature 1978;275:450.

152. Roberts DE, Dobson KE, Hall KW, Light RB. Effects of prolonged naloxone infusion in septic shock. Lancet 1988; 2(8613):699.

153. Bonnet F, Bilaine J, Lhoste F, Mankikian B, Kerdelhue B, Rapin M. Naloxone therapy of human septic shock. Crit Care Med 1985;13:972.

154. DeMaria A, Heffernan JJ, Grindlinger GA, Craven DE, McIntosh TK, McCabe WR. Naloxone versus placebo in treatment of septic shock. Lancet 1985;i:1363.

155. Guillemin R, Vargo T, Rossier J, et al. Beta-endorphin and adrenocorticotropin are secreted concomitantly by the pituitary gland. Science 1977;197:1367.

156. Rossier J, French ED, Rivier C, Ling N, Guillemin R, Bloom FE. Foot-shock induced stress increases beta-endorphin levels in blood but not brain. Nature 1977;270:618.

157. Physicians' desk reference. 4th ed. Oradell, NJ: Medical Economics, 1987:903.

158. Holaday JW, Faden AI. Naloxone treatment in shock. Lancet 1981;ii:201.

159. Cefalo RC, Lewis PE, O'Brien WF, Fletcher JR, Ramwell PW. The role of prostaglandins in endotoxemia: comparisons in response in the nonpregnant, maternal, and fetal models. Am J Obstet Gynecol 1980;137:53.

160. Rao PS, Cavanagh D, Gaston LW. Endotoxic shock in the primate: effects of aspirin and dipyridamole administration. Am J Obstet Gynecol 1981;140:914.

161. Gaffin SL, Badsha N, Brock-Utne J, Vorster B, Conradie J. An ELISA procedure for detecting human anti-endotoxin antibodies in serum. Ann Clin Biochem 1982;19:191.

162. Badsha N, Vorster B, Gaffin SL. Properties of human LPS specific gamma globulin. Circ Shock 1983;10:248.

163. Ziegler EJ, McCutchan JA, Fierer J, et al. Treatment of gram-negative bacteremia and shock with human antiserum to a mutant *Escherichia coli*. N Engl J Med 1982;307:1225.

164. Lachman E, Pitsoe SB, Gaffin SL. Anti-lipopolysaccharide immunotherapy in management of septic shock of obstetric and gynaecological origin. Lancet 1984;i:981.

165. Weber CE. Postmortem cesarean section: review of the literature and case reports. Am J Obstet Gynecol 1971;110:158.

166. Katz VL, Dotters DJ, Droegemueller W. Perimortem cesarean delivery. Obstet Gynecol 1986;68:571.

167. Ritter JW. Postmortem cesarean section. JAMA 1961;175:715.

168. Behney CA. Cesarean section delivery after death of the mother. JAMA 1961;176:617.

169. Buchsbaum HJ. Traumatic injury in pregnancy. In: Barber HRK, Garber EA, eds. Surgical disease in pregnancy. Philadelphia: WB Saunders, 1974:184.

170. Patterson RM. Trauma in pregnancy. Clin Obstet Gynecol 1984;27:32.

171. Pritchard JA. Changes in the blood volume during pregnancy and delivery. Anesthesiology 1965;26:393.

172. Shamji FM, Todd TRJ. Hypovolemic shock. Crit Care Clin 1985;1:609.

173. O'Leary JL, O'Leary JA. Uterine artery ligation for control of postcesarean section hemorrhage. Obstet Gynecol 1974;43:849.

174. Burchell RC. Internal iliac artery ligation: hemodynamics. Obstet Gynecol 1964;24:737.

175. Clark SL, Yeh S-Y, Phelan JP, Bruce S, Paul RH. Emergency hysterectomy for the control of obstetric hemorrhage. Obstet Gynecol 1984;64:376.

176. Smith DC, Wyatt JF. Embolization of the hypogastric arteries in the control of massive vaginal hemorrhage. Obstet Gynecol 1977;49:317.

177. Gunning JE. For controlling intractable hemorrhage: the gravity suit. Contemp Ob/Gyn 1983;22:23.

178. Dudrick SJ, O'Donnell JJ, Raleigh DP, Matheny RG, Unkel SP.

Rapid restoration of red blood cell mass in severely anemic surgical patients who refuse transfusion. 1985;120:721.
179. Hayashi RH, Castillo MS, Noah ML. Management of severe postpartum hemorrhage with a prostaglandin $F_2\alpha$ analogue. Obstet Gynecol 1984;63:806.
180. Takagi S, Yoshida T, Togo Y, et al. The effects of intramyometrial injection of prostaglandin $F_2\alpha$ on severe postpartum hemorrhage. Prostaglandins 1976;12:565.
181. Hankins GDV, Berryman GK, Scott RT Jr, Hood D. Maternal arterial desaturation with 15-methyl prostaglandin $F_{2\alpha}$ for uterine atony. Obstet Gynecol 1988;72:367.
182. Hibbard LT. Placenta previa. Am J Obstet Gynecol 1969;104:172.
183. Rizos N, Doran TA, Miskin M, Benzie RJ, Ford JA. Natural history of placenta previa ascertained by diagnostic ultrasound. Am J Obstet Gynecol 1979;133:287.
184. Bender S. Placenta previa and previous lower segment cesarean section. Surg Gynecol Obstet 1954;98:625.
185. Wexler P, Gottesfeld KR. Early diagnosis of placenta previa. Obstet Gynecol 1979;54:231.
186. Macafee CHG. Placenta previa—a study of 174 cases. J Obstet Gynaecol Br Commonw 1945;52:313.
187. Cotton DB, Read JA, Paul RH, Quilligan EJ. The conservative aggressive management of placenta previa. Am J Obstet Gynecol 1980;137:687.
188. Read JA, Cotton DB, Miller FC. Placenta accreta: changing clinical aspects and outcome. Obstet Gynecol 1980;56:31.
189. Irving FC, Hertig AT. A study of placenta accreta. Surg Gynecol Obstet 1937;64:178.
190. Breen JL, Neubecker R, Gregori CA, Franklin JE Jr. Placenta accreta, increta, and percreta: survey of 40 cases. Obstet Gynecol 1977;49:43.
191. Kistner RW, Hertig AT, Reid DE. Simultaneously occurring placenta previa and placenta accreta. Surg Gynecol Obstet 1952;94:141.
192. McHattie TJ. Placenta previa accreta. Obstet Gynecol 1972;40:795.
193. Aho AJ, Pulkkinen MO, Vaha-Eskeli K. Acute urinary bladder tamponade with hypovolemic shock due to placenta percreta with bladder invasion. Case report. Scand J Urol Nephrol 1985;19:157.
194. Knab DR. Abruptio placentae: an assessment of the time and method of delivery. Obstet Gynecol 1978;52:625.
195. Pritchard JA. Genesis of severe placental abruption. Am J Obstet Gynecol 1970;108:22.
196. Golditch IM, Boyce NE. Management of abruptio placentae. JAMA 1970;212:288.
197. Abdella TN, Sibai BM, Hays JM Jr, Anderson GD. Relationship of hypertensive disease to abruptio placentae. Obstet Gynecol 1984;63:365.
198. Acker D, Sachs BP, Tracey KJ, Wise WE. Abruptio placentae associated with cocaine use. Am J Obstet Gynecol 1983;146:220.
199. Chasnoff IJ, Burns KA, Burns WJ. Cocaine use in pregnancy: perinatal morbidity and mortality. Neurotoxicol Teratol 1987;9:291.
200. Little BB, Snell LM, Palmore MK, Gilstrap LC. Cocaine use in pregnant women in a large public hospital. Am J Perinatol 1988;5:206.
201. Hibbard BM, Jeffcoate TNA. Abruptio placentae. Obstet Gynecol 1966;27:155.
202. Hurd WW, Miodovnik M, Hertzberg V, Lavin JP. Selective management of abruptio placentae: a prospective study. Obstet Gynecol 1983;61:467.
203. Monteiro AA, Inocencio AC, Jorge CS. "Placental abruption" with disseminated intravascular coagulopathy in the second trimester of pregnancy with fetal survival. Case report. Br J Obstet Gynaecol 1987;94:811.
204. American College of Obstetricians and Gynecologists. Ectopic pregnancy. ACOG Technical Bulletin 126. Washington, DC, ACOG, 1989.
205. Centers for Disease Control. Ectopic pregnancies—United States, 1979–1980. MMWR 1984;33:201.
206. Marchbanks PA, Annegers JF, Coulam CB, Strathy JH, Kurland LT. Risk factors for ectopic pregnancy. A population-based study. JAMA 1988;259:1823.
207. Taylor RN. Ectopic pregnancy and reproductive technology. JAMA 1988;259:1862.
208. Kadar N, Caldwell BV, Romero R. A method of screening for ectopic pregnancy and its indications. Obstet Gynecol 1981;58:162.
209. Shapiro BS, Cullen M, Tayler KJ, DeCherney AH. Transvaginal ultrasonography for the diagnosis of ectopic pregnancy. Fertil Steril 1988;50:425.
210. Dorfman SF, Grimes DA, Cartes W Jr, Binkin NJ, Kafrissen ME, O'Reilly KR. Ectopic pregnancy mortality, United States, 1979 to 1980: Clinical aspects. Obstet Gynecol 1984;64:386.
211. Breen JL. A 21 year survey of 654 ectopic pregnancies. Am J Obstet Gynecol 1970;106:1004
212. Ory SJ, Villanueva AL, Sand PK, Tamura RK. Conservative treatment of ectopic pregnancy with methotrexate. Am J Obstet Gynecol 1986;154:1299.
213. Donnelly JP, Franzoni KT. Uterine rupture. A thirty year survey. Obstet Gynecol 1964;23:774.
214. Krishna Menon MK. Rupture of the uterus: a review of 164 cases. J Obstet Gynaecol Br Commonw 1962;69:18.
215. Margulies D, Crapanzano JT. Rupture of the intact uterus. Obstet Gynecol 1966;27:863.
216. Golan A, Sandbank O, Rubin A. Rupture of the pregnant uterus. Obstet Gynecol 1980;56:549.
217. Ferguson RK, Reid DE. Rupture of the uterus: a twenty-year report from the Boston Lying-In Hospital. Am J Obstet Gynecol 1958;76:172.
218. Abercrombie J. Case of hemorrhage of the liver. London Med Gaz 1844;34:792.
219. Owen A, Kandalaft E. Spontaneous subcapsular hematoma and rupture of the liver during pregnancy. Br J Obstet Gynaecol 1973;80:852.
220. Jewett JF. Eclampsia and rupture of the liver. N Engl J Med 1977;297:1009.
221. Castaneda H, Garcia-Romero H, Canto M. Hepatic hemorrhage in toxemia of pregnancy. Am J Obstet Gynecol 1970;107:578.
222. Mokotoff R, Weiss LS, Brandon LH, Camillo MF. Liver rupture complicating toxemia of pregnancy. Arch Intern Med 1967;119:375.
223. Aziz S, Merrell RC, Collins JA. Spontaneous hepatic hemorrhage during pregnancy. Am J Surg 1983;146,680.
224. O'Grady JP. Complications and birth injuries. In: Modern instrumental delivery. Baltimore: Williams & Wilkins, 1988:187.
225. Propping D, Stubblefield PG, Golub J, Zuckerman J. Uterine rupture following midtrimester abortion by laminaria, prostaglandin $F_{2\alpha}$, and oxytocin. Report of two cases. Am J Obstet Gynecol 1977;128:689.
226. Grimes DA, Schulz KF, Cates W Jr, Tyler CW Jr. Local versus general anesthesia: which is safer for performing suction curettage abortions? Am J Obstet Gynecol 1979;135:1030.
227. Peterson HB, Grimes DA, Cates W Jr, Rubin GL. Comparative risk of death from induced abortion at $\leq$12 weeks' gestation performed with local versus general anesthesia. Am J Obstet Gynecol 1981;141:763.
228. Grimes DA, Cates W Jr, Petitti DB, Pakter J. Fatal uterine rup-

ture during oxytocin-augmented, saline-induced abortion. Am J Obstet Gynecol 1978;130:591.
229. Berek JS, Stubblefield PG. Anatomic and clinical correlates of uterine perforation. Am J Obstet Gynecol 1979;135:181.
230. Freiman SM, Wulff GJL Jr. Management of uterine perforation following elective abortion. Obstet Gynecol 1977;50:647.
231. Hern WM. First trimester abortion: complications and their management. In: Sciarra JJ, ed. Gynecology and obstetrics. Philadelphia: Harper & Row, 1982.
232. Crosby WM. Traumatic injuries during pregnancy. Clin Obstet Gynecol 1983;26:902.
233. Rothenberger D, Quattlebaum FW, Perry JF, Zabel J, Fischer RP. Blunt maternal trauma: a review of 103 cases. J Trauma 1978;18:173.
234. Buchsbaum HJ. Accidental injury complicating pregnancy. Am J Obstet Gynecol 1968;102:752.
235. Buchsbaum HJ. Penetrating injury of the abdomen. In: Buchsbaum HJ, ed. Trauma in pregnancy. Philadelphia: WB Saunders, 1979:82.
236. Buchsbaum HJ. Diagnosis and management of abdominal gunshot wounds during pregnancy. J Trauma 1975;15:425.
237. Crosby WM. Trauma during pregnancy: maternal and fetal injury. Obstet Gynecol Surv 1974:29:683.
238. Fort AT, Harlin RS. Pregnancy outcome after noncatastrophic maternal trauma during pregnancy. Obstet Gynecol 1970;35:912.
239. Jacobson M, Mitchell R. Trauma to the abdomen in pregnancy. S Afr J Surg 1983;21:71.
240. Karlsson K. The influence of hypoxia on uterine and maternal placental blood flow, and the effect of alphaadrenergic blockade. J Perinat Med 1974;2:176.
241. Rothenberger DA, Horrigan TP, Sturm JT. Neonatal death following in utero traumatic splenic rupture. J Pediat Surg 1981;16:754.
242. Civil ID, Talucci RC, Schwab CW. Placental laceration and fetal death as a result of blunt abdominal trauma. J Trauma 1988;28:708.
243. Connor E, Curran J. In utero traumatic intra-abdominal deceleration injury to the fetus—a case report. Am J Obstet Gynecol 1976;125:567.
244. Rose PG, Strohm PL, Zuspan FP. Fetomaternal hemorrhage following trauma. Am J Obstet Gynecol 1985;153:844.
245. Crosby WM, Costiloe JP. Safety of lap-belt restraint for pregnant victims of automobile victims of automobile collisions. N Engl J Med 1971;284,632.
246. Crosby WM, King AI, Stout LC. Fetal survival following impact: improvement with shoulder harness restraint. Am J Obstet Gynecol 1972;112:1101.
247. Rothenberger DA, Quattlebaum FW, Zabel J, Fischer RP. Diagnostic peritoneal lavage for blunt trauma in pregnant women. Am J Obstet Gynecol 1977;129:479.
248. Sparkman RS. Rupture of the spleen in pregnancy: a report of two cases and review of the literature. Am J Obstet Gynecol 1958;76:587.
249. Buchsbaum HJ. Splenic rupture in pregnancy. Obstet Gynecol Surv 1967;22:381.
250. Golan A, Sandbank O, Teare AJ. Trauma in late pregnancy: a report of 15 cases. S Afr Med J 1980;57:161.
251. Eastman NJ. Editorial comment. Obstet Gynecol Surv 1958;13:69.
252. Nance FC, Wennar MH, Johnson LW, Ingram JC, Cohn I. Surgical judgment in the management of penetrating wounds of the abdomen: experience with 2,212 patients. Ann Surg 1974;179:639.
253. Kobak AJ, Hurwitz CH. Gunshot wounds of the pregnant uterus: review of the literature and two case reports. Obstet Gynecol 1954;4:383.
254. Smithwick III W, Gertner Jr HR, Zuidema GD. Injection of hypaque (sodium diatrizoate) in the management of abdominal stab wounds. Surg Gynecol Obstet 1968;127:1215.
255. Glueck HI, Burket RL, Sutherland JM, Garber ST. Afibrinogenemia in pregnancy apparently due to a degenerating leiomyoma. Obstet Gynecol 1961;18:285.
256. Koren Z, Zuckerman H, Brzezinski A. Placenta previa accreta with afibrinogenemia: report of three cases. Obstet Gynecol 1961;18:138.
257. Henderson SR, Lund CJ. Severe preeclampsia, disseminated intravascular coagulopathy and hydatidiform mole complicating a 20-week pregnancy with a fetus. Obstet Gynecol 1971;37:722.
258. Talbert LM, Easterling WE, Flowers CE, Graham JB. Acquired coagulation defects of pregnancy—including a case of a patient with hydatidiform mole. Obstet Gynecol 1961;18:69.
259. Goldman JA, Dekel A, Peleg D. Ovarian vascular accidents: a complication of anticoagulant therapy. Eur J Obstet Gynecol Reprod Biol 1978;8:163.
260. Morgan M. Amniotic fluid embolism. Anesthesia 1979;34:29.
261. Lipton RA, Ayromlooi J, Coller BS. Severe von Willebrand's disease during labor and delivery. JAMA 1982;248:1355.
262. Weinstein M, Deykin D. Comparison of factor VIII-related von Willebrand factor proteins prepared from human cryoprecipitate and factor VIII concentrate. Blood 1979;53:1095.
263. Silwer J. Von Willebrand's disease in Sweden. Acta Paediatr Scand (Suppl) 1973;238:5.
264. Osterud B, Bouma BN, Griffin JH. Human blood coagulation Factor IX: purification, properties, and mechanism of activation by activated Factor XI. J Biol Chem 1978;253:5946.
265. Bennett B, Ratnoff OD, Hold JB, Roberts HR. Hageman trait (Factor XII deficiency): a probable second genotype inherited as an autosomal dominant characteristic. Blood 1972;40:412.
266. McPherson RA. Thromboembolism in Hageman trait. Am J Clin Pathol 1977;68:420.
267. Saito H, Ratnoff OD, Waldmann R, Abraham JP. Fitzgerald trait. J Clin Invest 1975;55:1082.
268. Wuepper KD. Prekallikrein deficiency in man. J Exp Med 1973;138:1345.
269. Broze GJ, Majerus PW. Purification and properties of human coagulation Factor VII. J Biol Chem 1980;255:1242.
270. Seeler RA. Parahemophilia: Factor V deficiency. Med Clin North Am 1972;56:119.
271. Rush B, Ellis H. The treatment of patients with Factor-V deficiency. Thromb Diath Haemorrh 1965;14:74.
272. Graham JB, Barrow EM, Hougie C. Stuart clotting defect. II. Genetic aspects of a "new" hemorrhagic state. J Clin Invest 1957;36:497.
273. White GC, Roberts HR, Kingdon HS, Lundblad RL. Prothrombin complex concentrates. Potentially thrombogenic materials and clues to the mechanism of thrombosis in vivo. Blood 1977;49:159.
274. Kitchens CS, Newcomb TF. Factor XIII. Medicine 1979;58:413.
275. Mammen EF. Fibrinogen abnormalities. Semin Thromb Hemost 1983;9:1.
276. Hahn L, Lundberg PA. Congenital hypofibrinogenaemia and recurrent abortion. Br J Obstet Gynaecol 1978;85:790.
277. Gralnick HR, Coller BS, Fratantoni JC, Martinez J. Fibrinogen Bethesda III: a hypodysfibrinogenemia. Blood 1979;53:28.
278. Mammen EF. 2-antiplasmin deficiency. Semin Thromb Hemost 1983;9:52.
279. Nelson DM, Stempel LE, Brandt JT. Hereditary antithrombin III deficiency and pregnancy: report of two cases and review of the literature. Obstet Gynecol 1985;65:848.

280. Mammen EF. Factor X abnormalities. Surg Thromb Hemost 1983;9:31.
281. Mammen EF. Factor VIII abnormalities. Semin Thromb Hemost 1983;9:22.
282. Bleich HL, Boro ES. Actions and interactions of antithrombin and heparin. N Engl J Med 1975;292:146.
283. Hellgren M, Tengborn L, Abildgaard U. Pregnancy in women with congenital antithrombin III deficiency: experience of treatment with heparin and antithrombin. Gynecol Obstet Invest 1982;14:127.
284. Ratnoff OD, Busse RJ Jr, Sheon RP. The demise of John Hageman. N Engl J Med 1968;279:760.
285. Schlaerth JB, Morrow CP, Montz FJ, d'Ablaing G. Initial management of hydatidiform mole. Am J Obstet Gynecol 1988;158:1299.
286. Carlson RW, Bowles AL, Haupt MT. Anaphylactic, anaphylactoid, and related forms of shock. Crit Care Clin 1986;2:347.
287. Hanzlik PJ, Karsner HT. Anaphylactoid phenomena from the intravenous administration of various colloids, arsenicals and other agents. J Pharmacol Exp Ther 1920;14:379 and 1924;23:173.
288. Fisher M. Anaphylaxis. Sem Respir Med 1982;3:257.
289. Hofmann H, Goerz G, Plewig G. Anaphylactic shock from chlorobutanol-preserved oxytocin. Contact Dermatitis 1986;15:241.
290. Entman SS, Moise KJ. Anaphylaxis in pregnancy. South Med J 1984;77:402.
291. Smith BE. Anesthetic emergencies. Clin Obstet Gynecol 1985;28:391.
292. Ladner C, Brinkman CR, Weston P, Assali NS. Dynamics of uterine circulation in pregnant and nonpregnant sheep. Am J Physiol 1970;218:257.
293. Maternal deaths due to sepsis with septic shock. Ohio State Med J 1970;66:589.
294. Gordon M, Horowitz A. Septic shock in obstetrics and gynecology. Postgrad Med 1969;46:144.
295. McKay DG, Jewett JF, Reid DE. Endotoxin shock and the generalized Schwartzman reaction in pregnancy. Am J Obstet Gynecol 1959;78:546.
296. Hawkins DF. Management and treatment of obstetric bacteraemic shock. J Clin Pathol 1980;33:895.
297. Sweet RL, Ledger WJ. Puerperal infectious morbidity: a two-year review. Am J Obstet Gynecol 1973;117:1093.
298. Benedetti TJ, Valle R, Ledger WJ. Antepartum pneumonia in pregnancy. Am J Obstet Gynecol 1982;144:413.
299. Seaworth BJ, Durack DT. Infective endocarditis in obstetric and gynecologic practice. Am J Obstet Gynecol 1986;154:180.
300. Blanco JD, Gibbs RS, Castaneda YS. Bacteremia in obstetrics: clinical course. Obstet Gynecol 1981;58:621.
301. Ledger WJ, Norman M, Gee C, Lewis W. Bacteremia on an obstetric gynecologic service. Am J Obstet Gynecol 1975;121:205.
302. Parker MM, Parrillo JE. Septic shock: hemodynamics and pathogenesis. JAMA 1983;250:3324.
303. Beller FK, Schmidt EH, Holzgreve W, Hauss J. Septicemia during pregnancy: a study in different species of experimental animals. Am J Obstet Gynecol 1985;151:967.
304. Morishima HO, Niemann WH, James LS. Effects of endotoxin on the pregnant baboon and fetus. Am J Obstet Gynecol 1978;131:899.
305. Duff P. Pathophysiology and management of septic shock. J Reprod Med 1980;24:109.
306. Gibbs RS, Blanco JD, St Clair PJ, Castaneda YS. Quantitative bacteriology of amniotic fluid from women with clinical intraamniotic infection at term. J Infect Dis 1982;145:1.
307. Weil M. Current understanding of mechanisms and treatment of circulatory shock caused by bacterial infections. Ann Clin Res 1977;9:181.
308. Sayeed MM. Pulmonary cellular dysfunction in endotoxin shock: metabolic and transport derangements. Circ Shock 1982;9:335.
309. Marx GF. Anesthetic management of the parturient in septic shock. Int Anesthesiol Clin 1968;6:813.
310. Cavanagh D. Septic shock in a pregnant or recently pregnant woman. Postgrad Med 1977;62:62.
311. Duff P, Gibbs RS, Blanco JD, St Clair PJ. Endometrial culture techniques in puerperal patients. Obstet Gynecol 1983;61:217.
312. Roberts JM, Laros RK. Hemorrhagic and endotoxic shock: a pathophysiologic approach to diagnosis and management. Am J Obstet Gynecol 1971;110:1041.
313. Santamarina BAG, Smith SA. Septic abortion and septic shock. Clin Obstet Gynecol 1970;13:291.
314. Mariona FG, Ismail MA. Clostridium perfringens septicemia following cesarean section. Obstet Gynecol 1980;56:518.
315. Gomez A, Wood M. Acute appendicitis during pregnancy. Am J Surg 1979;137:180.
316. Feller I, Crane K. Planning and designing a burn care facility. National Institute for Burn Medicine, Ann Arbor, MI, 1971:1.
317. Smith BK, Rayburn WF, Feller I. Burns and pregnancy. Clin Perinatol 1983;10:383.
318. Rayburn W, Smith B, Feller I, Varner M, Cruikshank D. Major burns during pregnancy: effects on fetal well-being. Obstet Gynecol 1984;63:392.
319. Feller I, Archambeault C. Nursing the burned patient. National Institute for Burn Medicine, Ann Arbor, MI, 1975.
320. Deitch EA, Rightmire DA, Clothier J, Blass N. Management of burns in pregnant women. Surg Gynecol Obstet 1985;161:1.
321. Rai YS, Jackson D. Childbearing in relation to the scarred abdominal wall from burns. Burns 1974;1:167.
322. Amy BW, McManus WF, Goodwin CW, Mason A, Pruitt BA. Thermal injury in the pregnant patient. Surg Gynecol Obstet 1985;161:209.
323. Gonik B. Intensive care monitoring of the critically ill pregnant patient. In: Creasy RK, Resnik R, eds. Maternal-fetal medicine: principles and practice. 2nd ed. Philadelphia: WB Saunders, 1989:845.
324. Lowthian JT, Gillard LJ. Postpartum necrotizing fasciitis. Obstet Gynecol 1980;56:661.
325. Golde S, Ledger WJ. Necrotizing fasciitis in postpartum patients. Obstet Gynecol 1977;50:670.
326. Hibbard LT. Maternal mortality due to cardiac disease. Clin Obstet Gynecol 1975;18:27.
327. Ullery JC. Management of pregnancy complicated by heart disease. Am J Obstet Gynecol 1954;67:834.
328. Niswander KR, Berendes H, Deutschberger J, Lipko N, Westphal MC. Fetal morbidity following potentially anoxigenic obstetric conditions: V. Organic heart disease. Am J Obstet Gynecol 1967;98:871.
329. Szekely P, Turner R, Snaith L. Pregnancy and the changing pattern of rheumatic heart disease. Br Heart J 1973;35:1293.
330. Michalak D, Klein V, Marquette GP. Myocardial ischemia: a complication of ritodrine tocolysis. Am J Obstet Gynecol 1983;146:861.
331. Tye KH, Desser KB, Benchimol A. Angina pectoris associated with use of terbutaline for premature labor. JAMA 1980;244:692.
332. Carpenter RJ, Decuir P. Cardiovascular collapse associated with oral terbutaline tocolytic therapy. Am J Obstet Gynecol 1984;148:821.
333. Smythe AR, Sakakini J. Maternal metabolic alterations secondary to terbutaline therapy for premature labor. Obstet Gynecol 1981;57:566.

334. Chew WC, Lew LC. Ventricular ectopics after salbutamol infusion for preterm labor. Lancet 1979;22:1383.
335. Frederiksen MC, Toig RM, Depp R. Atrial fibrillation during hexoprenaline therapy for premature labor. Am J Obstet Gynecol 1983;145:108.
336. McIntyre KM, Sasahara AA. Hemodynamic and ventricular responses to pulmonary embolism. Prog Cardiovasc Dis 1974;17:175.
337. Billhardt RA, Rosenbush SW. Cardiogenic and hypovolemic shock. Med Clin North Am 1986;70:853.
338. Delclos GL, Davila F. Thrombolytic therapy for pulmonary embolism in pregnancy. Am J Obstet Gynecol 1986;155:375.
339. Bonnar J. Venous thromboembolism and pregnancy. Clin Obstet Gynaecol 1981;8:455.
340. Forfar JC, Muir AL, Sawers SA, Toft AD. Abnormal left ventricular function in hyperthyroidism: evidence for a possible reversible cardiomyopathy. N Engl J Med 1982;307:1165.
341. Clark SL, Phelan JP, Montoro M, Mestman J. Transient ventricular dysfunction associated with cesarean section in a patient with hyperthyroidism. Am J Obstet Gynecol 1985;151:384.
342. Cooper DS. Which anti-thyroid drug? Am J Med 1986;80:1165.
343. Harrison KA. Anaemia, malaria and sickle cell disease. Clin Obstet Gynaecol 1982;9:445.
344. Gray SF, Muers MF, Scott JS. Maternal death from constrictive pericarditis 15 years after radiotherapy. Case report. Br J Obstet Gynaecol 1988;95:518.
345. Iung B, Squara P, Fruchaud J, et al. Postpartum myocardial infarction with normal coronary arteries. Apropos of a case. Arch Mal Coeur 1986;79:1951.
346. Hankins GDV, Wendel GD, Leveno KJ, Stoneham J. Myocardial infarction during pregnancy: a review. Obstet Gynecol 1985:65:139.
347. Shime J, Mocarski EJM, Hastings D, Webb GD, McLaughlin PR. Congenital heart disease in pregnancy: short- and long-term implications. Am J Obstet Gynecol 1987;156:313.
348. Whittemore R, Hobbins JC, Engle MA. Pregnancy and its outcome in women with and without surgical treatment of congenital heart disease. Am J Cardiol 1982;50:641.
348. Homans J. Thrombosis of the deep veins of the lower leg causing pulmonary embolism. N Engl J Med 1934;211:993.
349. Schaefer G, Arditi LI, Solomon HA, Ringland JE. Congenital heart disease and pregnancy. Clin Obstet Gynecol 1968; 11:1048.
350. Gleicher N, Midwall J, Hochberger D, Jaffin H. Eisenmenger's syndrome and pregnancy. Obstet Gynecol Surv 1979;34:721.
351. Ibarra-Perez C, Arevalo-Toledo N, Alvarez-de la Cadena O, Noriega-Guerra L. The course of pregnancy in patients with artificial heart valves. Am J Med 1976;61:504.
352. Barrett JM, Van Hooydonk JE, Boehm FH. Pregnancy-related rupture of arterial aneurysms. Obstet Gynecol Surv 1982; 37:557.
353. Clark SL, Phelan JP, Greenspoon J, Aldahl D, Horenstein J. Labor and delivery in the presence of mitral stenosis: central hemodynamic observations. Am J Obstet Gynecol 1985; 152:984.
354. Veille J-C. Peripartum cardiomyopathies: a review. Am J Obstet Gynecol 1984;148:805.
355. Walsh JJ, Burch GE. Postpartal heart disease. Arch Intern Med 1961;108:817.
356. Demakis JG, Rahimtoola SH, Sutton GC, et al. Natural course of peripartum cardiomyopathy. Circulation 1971;XLIV:1053.
357. Sanderson JE, Adesanya CO, Anjorin FI, Parry EHO. Postpartum cardiac failure—heart failure due to volume overload? Am Heart J 1979;97:613.
358. Burch GE, McDonald CD, Walsh JJ. The effect of prolonged bed rest on postpartal cardiomyopathy. Am Heart J 1971;81:186.
359. Homans DC. Peripartum cardiomyopathy. N Engl J Med 1985;312:1432.
360. Cunningham FG, Pritchard JA, Hankins GDV, Anderson PL, Lucas MJ, Armstrong KF. Peripartum heart failure: idiopathic cardiomyopathy or compounding cardiovascular events? Obstet Gynecol 1986;67:157.
361. Soderstrom CA, McArdle DQ, Ducker TB, Militello PR. The diagnosis of intra-abdominal injury in patients with cervical cord trauma. J Trauma 1983;23:1061.
362. Shah-Hosseini R, Evrard JR. Puerperal uterine inversion. Obstet Gynecol 1989;73:567.
363. Das P. Inversion of the uterus. Br J Obstet Gynaecol 1940;47:525.
364. Watson P, Besch N, Bowes WA. Management of acute and subacute puerperal inversion of the uterus. Obstet Gynecol 1980;55:12.
365. Johnson AB. A new concept in the replacement of the inverted uterus and a report of nine cases. Am J Obstet Gynecol 1949;57:557.
366. Shnider SM, DeLorimier AA, Holl AW, Chapler FK, Morishima HO. Vasopressors in obstetrics. I. Correction of fetal acidosis with ephedrine during spinal hypotension. Am J Obstet Gynecol 1968;102:911.
367. James III FM, Greiss FC Jr, Kemp RA. An evaluation of vasopressor therapy for maternal hypotension during spinal anesthesia. Anesthesiol 1970;33:25.
368. Kleinerman J, Sancetta SM, Hackel DB. Effects of high spinal anesthesia on cerebral circulation and metabolism in man. J Clin Invest 1958;37:285.
369. Fry DE, Pearlstein L, Fulton RL, Polk HC. Multiple system organ failure. The role of uncontrolled infection. Arch Surg 1980;115:136.
370. Meakins JL, Wicklund B, Forse RA, McLean APH. The surgical intensive care unit: current concepts in infection. Surg Clin North Am 1980;60:117.
371. Goris RJA, te Boekhorst TPA, Nuytinck JKS, Gimbrere JSF. Multiple-organ failure. Generalized autodestructive inflammation? Arch Surg 1985;120:1109.
372. Wiles JB, Cerra FB, Siegel HJ, Border JR. The systemic response: does the organism matter? Crit Care Med 1980;8:55.
373. Fry DE. Multiple system organ failure. Surg Clin North Am 1988;68:107.
374. DeCamp MM, Demling RH. Posttraumatic multisystem organ failure. JAMA 1988;260:530.
375. Fry DE, Garrison RN, Heitsch RC, Calhoun K, Polk HC. Determinants of death in patients with intraabdominal abscess. Surgery 1980;88:517.
376. Extracorporeal support for respiratory insufficiency. A collaborative study in response to RFP-NHLI-7320. National Heart, Lung, and Blood Institute, 1979.
377. Cerra FB. The systemic septic response: multiple systems organ failure. Crit Care Clin 1985;1:591.
378. Cerra FB, Shronts EP, Konstantinides RN, et al. Enteral feeding in sepsis: a prospective randomized, double-blind trial. Surgery 1985;98:632.
379. Harper AM. Autoregulation of cerebral blood flow: influence of the arterial blood pressure on the blood flow through the cerebral cortex. J Neurol Neurosurg Psychiatry 1966;29:398.
380. Rinaldo JE, Rogers RM. Adult respiratory distress syndrome: changing concepts of lung injury and repair. N Engl J Med 1982;306:900.
381. Sladen A. Methylprednisolone: pharmacologic doses in shock lung syndrome. J Thorac Cardiovasc Surg 1976;71:800.
382. Blaisdell FW, Schlobohm RM. The respiratory distress syndrome: a review. Surgery 1973;74:251.

383. Wilson WS, Gadacz T, Olcott C, Blaisdell FW. Superficial gastric erosions. Am J Surg 1973;126:133.
384. Baker JW, Deitch EA, Li M, Berg RD, Specian RD. Hemorrhagic shock induces bacterial translocation from the gut. J Trauma 1988;28:896.
385. Deitch EA, Winterton J, Li M, Berg R. The gut as a portal of entry for bacteremia. Ann Surg 1987;205:681.
386. Larson DE, Farnell MB. Upper gastrointestinal hemorrhage. Mayo Clin Proc 1983;58:371.
387. Nunes G, Blaisdell FW, Margaretten W. Mechanism of hepatic dysfunction following shock and trauma. Arch Surg 1970;100:546.
388. Sheehan HL, Murdoch R. Postpartum necrosis of the anterior pituitary: pathological and clinical aspects. Br J Obstet Gynecol 1938;45:456.
389. Whitehead R. The hypothalamus in post-partum hypopituitarism. J Pathol Bacteriol 1963;86:55.
390. DiZerega G, Kletzky OA, Mishell DR. Diagnosis of Sheehan's syndrome using a sequential stimulation test. Am J Obstet Gynecol 1978;132:348.
391. Humphreys MH, Sheldon G. Acute renal failure in trauma patients (Trauma Rounds). West J Med 1975;123:148.
392. Lucas CE. The renal response to acute injury and sepsis. Surg Clin North Am 1976;56:953.
393. Emmanouel DS, Katz AI. Acute renal failure in obstetric septic shock. Current views on pathogenesis and management. Am J Obstet Gynecol 1973;117:145.
394. Lordon RE, Burton JR. Post-traumatic renal failure in military personnel in Southeast Asia. Am J Med 1972;53:137.
395. Mosher P, Ross J Jr, McFate PA, Shaw RF. Control of coronary blood flow by an autoregulatory mechanism. Circ Res 1964;14:250.
396. Freid MA, Vosti KL. The importance of underlying disease in patients with gram-negative bacteremia. Arch Intern Med 1968;121:418.
397. Wilson RF, Kafi A, Asuncion Z, Walt AJ. Clinical respiratory failure after shock or trauma: prognosis and methods of diagnosis. Arch Surg 1969;98:539.
398. Shoemaker WC, Montgomery ES, Kaplan E, Elwyn DH. Physiologic patterns in surviving and nonsurviving shock patients. Arch Surg 1973;106:630.
399. Knaus WA, Zimmerman JE, Wagner DP, et al. APACHE-acute physiologic and chronic health evaluation: a physiologically based classification system. Crit Care Med 1981;9:591.
400. Knaus WA, Draper EA, Wagner DP, Zimmerman JE. APACHE II: a severity of disease classification system. Crit Care Med 1985;13:818.
401. Hardaway RM. Prediction of survival or death of patients in a state of severe shock. Surg Gynecol Obstet 1981;152:200.
402. Shoemaker WC, Appel PL, Bland R, Hopkins JA, Chang P. Clinical trial of an algorithm for outcome prediction in acute circulatory failure. Crit Care Med 1982;10:390.
403. Dellinger EP. Use of scoring systems to assess patients with surgical sepsis. Surg Clin North Am 1988;68:123.
404. Consensus Conference. Perioperative red blood cell transfusion. JAMA 1988;260:2700.
405. Ward JW, Holmberg SD, Allen JR, et al. Transmission of human immunodeficiency virus (HIV) by blood and transfusions screened as negative for HIV antibody. N Engl J Med 1988;318:473.
406. Council on Scientific Affairs. Autologous blood transfusions. JAMA 1986;256:2378.
407. Herbert WNP, Owen HG, Collins ML. Autologous blood storage in obstetrics. Obstet Gynecol 1988;72:166.
408. Kruskall MS, Leonard S, Klapholz H. Autologous blood donation during pregnancy: analysis of safety and blood use. Obstet Gynecol 1987;70:938.

58

CHAPTER

HYPERTENSIVE DISEASES IN PREGNANCY

Fiona M. Fairlie and Baha M. Sibai

Approximately 10% of pregnancies are complicated by hypertension. The incidence varies according to the population studied and the criteria used for diagnosis. Apart from being the most common medical complication of pregnancy, hypertensive disorders are associated with significant maternal, fetal, and neonatal morbidity and mortality.[1,2] Preeclampsia accounts for 70% of hypertension in pregnancy, and chronic essential hypertension accounts for most of the remaining 30%.

HYPERTENSION

The American College of Obstetricians and Gynecologists Committee on Terminology defines hypertension in pregnancy as either a systolic pressure of ≥140 mm Hg or an increment of ≥30 mm Hg (from a baseline in the first half of pregnancy) or a diastolic pressure of ≥90 mm Hg or an increment of ≥15 mm Hg. The pressures or increases in pressure must be observed on at least two occasions 6 hours apart.[3] If blood pressure in the first half of pregnancy is unknown, readings of 140/90 mm Hg after 20 weeks are considered sufficiently elevated to diagnose preeclampsia. The committee also regards an increase in mean arterial blood pressure of 20 mm Hg or, if previous blood pressure is unknown, a mean arterial pressure of 105 mm Hg as diagnostic of hypertension.

The validity of using increments of >15 mm Hg diastolic and >30 mm Hg systolic pressure to define hypertension has been questioned. It requires a baseline reading in the first half of pregnancy that may be unavailable. Furthermore, blood pressure normally falls during the second trimester and rises again toward term.[4,5] MacGillivary and colleagues observed that 73% of primigravid patients with normotensive pregnancies demonstrated a rise in diastolic blood pressure of >15 mm Hg at some stage during their pregnancy.[5]

The measurement of blood pressure is subject to many inaccuracies. Faulty equipment and a careless technique are obvious sources of error. It is more difficult to assess the influence of differences in equipment, cuff size, position of the arm, duration of rest period before measurement, and patient characteristics, particularly race, obesity, smoking, and anxiety.[6,7] Blood pressure is a continuous variable, and a single recording may not reflect the true state of the patient. It has been recommended that at least two abnormal measurements are made 4 to 6 hours apart before diagnosing hypertension.

There has been considerable controversy over whether Korotkoff phase 4 (muffling of sound) or phase 5 (disappearance of sound) should be used to measure the diastolic blood pressure. American obstetricians usually use phase 5, whereas Europeans and Australians favor phase 4. Phase 4 measures about 5 to 10 mm Hg higher than phase 5. In pregnancy the standard deviation in diastolic pressure at phase 5 is considerable because of the hyperdynamic circulation. It has been suggested that both phases should be measured but that phase 4 reading should be used for diagnosis and clinical trials.[8,9]

PROTEINURIA

The concentration of urinary protein is highly variable. It is influenced by several factors, including contamination with vaginal secretions, blood, or bacteria; urine specific gravity and pH; exercise; and posture. Protein excretion in the urine increases in normal pregnancy from approximately 5 mg/100 mL in the first and second trimesters to 15 mg/100 mL in the third trimester. These low levels are not detected by dipstick. Significant proteinuria is defined as >0.3 g in a 24-hour urine collection or 0.1g/L (>2+ on the dipstick), in at least two random samples collected 6 hours or more apart.

EDEMA

Preeclampsia has been described traditionally as a triad of edema, proteinuria, and hypertension. Although excessive weight gain (>2 pounds per week in the third trimester) may be the first sign of preeclampsia, moderate edema is a feature of 80% of normotensive pregnancies.[10] Preeclampsia with edema has been reported to have a lower perinatal mortality when compared with the equivalent disorder without edema.[11] In addition, 39% of a series of eclamptic patients were noted to have no edema, and generalized edema was evident in only 22%.[12] The assessment of edema is subjective. It should be considered pathologic only if it is generalized, involving the hands, face, and legs. This is not always made clear in the literature and has led to confusion. Consequently, it is now generally accepted that edema or weight gain should not be included in the definition of preeclampsia.

PREECLAMPSIA

Preeclampsia is the most common hypertensive complication of pregnancy. It can be classified as mild or severe. Mild preeclampsia is diagnosed by a blood pressure of 140/90 mm Hg on two occasions 6 hours apart (with or without proteinuria). According to the American College of Obstetricians and Gynecologists Committee on Terminology, severe preeclampsia is diagnosed when any one of the criteria listed in Table 58-1 is present.

ECLAMPSIA

Eclampsia is defined as the development of convulsions or coma or both in a patient with signs and symptoms of preeclampsia. Other causes of seizures must be excluded (Table 58-2). Although eclampsia is usually associated with significant proteinuria, this sign will be absent in 20% of cases.[13] Eclampsia may present antepartum, intrapartum, or postpartum. Approximately 50% of cases occur antepartum, usually during the third trimester. A few occur between 21 and 27 weeks of gestation, and rare cases have been reported before 20 weeks gestation.[14] Late-onset postpartum eclampsia (convulsions more than 48 hours after delivery) is a controversial entity. Sibai and colleagues reported six cases[15] and have subsequently increased their experience to 33 cases.[13] All patients reported having headaches with or without visual disturbances for 1 to 4 days before the onset of convulsions. Physical and laboratory findings immediately after convulsions were consistent with eclampsia in all cases.

TABLE 58–1. CRITERIA FOR THE DIAGNOSIS OF SEVERE PREECLAMPSIA

1. Blood pressure ≥160 mm Hg systolic or ≥110 mm Hg diastolic on two occasions at least 6 hours apart with the patient at bedrest
2. Proteinuria ≥ 5 g in a 24-hour urine collection or ≥3+ on dipstick in at least two random clean-catch samples at least 4 hours apart
3. Oliguria (≤400 mL in 24 hours)
4. Cerebral or visual disturbances
5. Epigastric pain
6. Pulmonary edema or cyanosis

Data from Hughes EC, ed. Obstetric-gynecologic terminology. Philadelphia: FA Davis, 1972:442.

TABLE 58–2. DIFFERENTIAL DIAGNOSIS OF ECLAMPSIA

- Cerebrovascular accidents
  - Cerebrovenous thrombosis
  - Cerebroarterial occlusion
  - Cerebroarterial embolism
  - Intracerebral hemorrhage
- Hypertensive disease
  - Hypertensive encephalopathy
  - Pheochromocytoma
- Space-occupying central nervous system lesions
  - Tumor
  - Abscess
- Infectious disease
  - Meningitis
  - Encephalitis
- Metabolic disease
  - Hypoglycemia
  - Hypocalcemia
  - Water intoxication
  - Epilepsy

From Villar MA, Sibai BM. Eclampsia. In: Arias F, ed. High risk pregnancy. Obstetrics and gynecology clinics of North America. Philadelphia: WB Saunders, 1988:358.

HELLP SYNDROME

Recently, a syndrome of hemolysis, elevated liver enzymes, and low platelets was described as a variant of preeclampsia.[16] However, Goodlin maintained that this clinical presentation had been reported in the obstetric literature a century earlier.[17] There is considerable controversy about the definition, diagnosis, incidence, etiology, and management of HELLP syndrome. In terms of diagnosis, the most consistent finding in the literature is thrombocytopenia (platelet count < 100,000/μL).

CHRONIC HYPERTENSION

Chronic hypertension is diagnosed if there is persistent elevation of blood pressure to at least 140/90 mm Hg on two occasions more than 24 hours apart before 20 weeks gestation. Hypertension that persists for more than 42 days postpartum is also classified as chronic hypertension. Other factors that may suggest the presence of chronic hypertension include

Retinal changes on funduscopic examination
Radiologic and electrocardiographic evidence of cardiac enlargement
Compromised renal function or associated renal disease
Multiparity with a previous history of hypertensive pregnancies
Presence of hypertension more than 6 weeks postpartum.[18]

It may be difficult to be certain of a diagnosis of chronic hypertension because of significant changes in blood pressure that occur during midpregnancy. Sibai and colleagues noted that women with mild chronic hypertension showed greater decreases in their blood pressure during pregnancy than did normotensive women.[9] Furthermore, blood pressure was within the normal range during midpregnancy.

Chronic hypertension may be classified as mild or severe. Mild chronic hypertension implies a systolic blood pressure of less than 160 mm Hg and a diastolic of less than 110 mm Hg. Severe chronic hypertension is diagnosed if either the systolic or diastolic pressure exceeds these limits.

SUPERIMPOSED PREECLAMPSIA

Chronic hypertension may be complicated by superimposed preeclampsia (or eclampsia). Superimposed preeclampsia is diagnosed when there is an exacerbation of hypertension (elevation of 30 mm Hg systolic and 15 mm Hg diastolic or 20 mm Hg mean arterial pressure) and the development of proteinuria or generalized edema that was not previously apparent. About 15% to 30% of chronically hypertensive women develop this complication.

LATENT OR TRANSIENT HYPERTENSION

Latent or transient hypertension is defined as hypertension occurring antepartum, in labor, or in the first 24 hours postpartum without generalized edema or proteinuria and with a return to normotension within 10 days of delivery.

CLASSIFICATION OF HYPERTENSIVE DISORDERS IN PREGNANCY

Numerous attempts have been made to classify hypertensive disorders of pregnancy. The American College of Obstetricians and Gynecologists (ACOG) suggested four categories—preeclampsia and eclampsia, chronic hypertension, chronic hypertension with superimposed preeclampsia, and late or transient hypertension.[5] However, it is frequently difficult to differentiate among preeclampsia, chronic hypertension, and chronic hypertension with superimposed preeclampsia. The normal midtrimester fall in blood pressure may conceal the presence of underlying chronic hypertension, and unless the patient presents in the first trimester or has a well-documented history of chronic hypertension, accurate classification will be impossible. The ACOG does not insist on proteinuria as a diagnostic sign of preeclampsia, since it often appears late. However, many members of the British Commonwealth use the Nelson classification, which includes proteinuria in the definition of severe preeclampsia.[19] Furthermore, the ACOG criteria for severe preeclampsia do not include other findings that also indicate severe disease, such as hemoconcentration, abnormal hepatic function, low platelets, and fetal growth retardation.

In 1988, Davey and MacGillivary proposed a new clinical classification that is based only on signs of hypertension and proteinuria and that disregards etiology and pathology.[20] Compared with previous classifications, it appears to be more relevant and applicable to clinical practice.

In this chapter the pathophysiology of pregnancy-related hypertension will be considered according to underlying etiology. The discussion of management will focus on the control of blood pressure and the assessment of fetal and maternal well-being.

PATHOPHYSIOLOGY

PREECLAMPSIA

Preeclampsia is a disorder peculiar to human pregnancy. Reported incidence ranges from 2% to 35%, depending on the diagnostic criteria and the population studied. It is principally a disease of young primigravidas and rarely presents before 20 weeks gestation. Early presentation is more likely to be associated with unrecognized renal disease,[21] whereas onset at term or intrapartum is more often associated with transient or latent hypertension. Although geographic and racial differences in incidence have been reported, it is difficult to be certain that other influences (eg, socioeconomic status) are not involved. Several risk factors have been identified as predisposing to the development of preeclampsia (Table 58-3). The pathophysiology of preeclampsia has been well described.[22,23] The underlying abnormality is general arteriolar constriction and increased vascular sensitivity to pressor peptides and amines.[24] Despite extensive investigation, the etiology of this disease is unknown.

Histopathology

Kidney. A distinct renal lesion has been described and widely accepted as pathognomonic for preeclampsia. It is characterized by swelling of the endothelial and at times the mesangial cells. The glomerulus enlarges, the

TABLE 58-3. RISK FACTORS FOR PREECLAMPSIA

Nulliparity
Multiple gestation
Family history of preeclampsia–eclampsia
Preexisting hypertension–renal disease
Previous preeclampsia–eclampsia
Diabetes
Nonimmune hydrops fetalis
Molar pregnancy

From Sibai BM, Moretti MM. Pregnancy induced hypertension. Contemporary Ob/Gyn 1988;31:57.

capillary lumen narrows, and the basement membrane, tubules, and vasculature are usually not altered.[25] This renal lesion is almost never seen in the absence of proteinuria.[26] Changes in renal function include a reduced glomerular filtration rate and renal plasma flow that may progress to renal ischemia. Intravascular volume falls while interstitial fluid accumulates.

Liver. Sheehan and Lynch described periportal fibrin deposition and zonal necrosis.[26] These lesions are often but not always present in fatal cases of eclampsia. Sheehan and Lynch believed that periportal fibrin deposition is specific to fatal cases of eclampsia, but identical lesions have been reported in the livers of pregnant women dying from infections, placental abruption, or postpartum hemorrhage. Areas of liver necrosis in fatal cases of eclampsia are very similar to necrotic lesions seen in the livers of patients dying from shock of any cause.

Placenta. In normal pregnancy, the trophoblast migrates down the intima of the spiral arteries. The musculoelastic tissue of the vessel wall is gradually eroded and replaced by fibrinoid material. The spiral arteries are converted from small muscular end arteries to wide, tortuous uteroplacental arteries that empty into the intervillous space. Brosens and colleagues termed this process *physiologic changes.*[27] It has been suggested that the formation of uteroplacental arteries occurs in two stages. Conversion of the decidual segments takes place in the first trimester, whereas the myometrial segments are transformed by a second wave of trophoblast invasion in the second trimester.[28]

Brosens and colleagues observed that in pregnancies complicated by preeclampsia, physiologic vascular changes were restricted to the decidual segments.[29] Khong and colleagues confirmed this finding and showed that in about one third to one half of spiral arteries from hypertensive pregnancies there was no evidence of trophoblastic invasion.[30] Furthermore, these placental abnormalities were present in a proportion of normotensive pregnancies complicated by fetal growth retardation.

It is important to appreciate that the vascular changes seen in the liver, kidneys, and placenta in preeclampsia and eclampsia are characteristic of but not specific to the disease. They are compatible with intravascular coagulation and vasoconstriction but are secondary phenomena and do not indicate the primary cause of preeclampsia.

Proposed Etiologies

Prostacyclin–Thromboxane Imbalance. It has been suggested that an imbalance of prostaglandins is central to the pathophysiology of preeclampsia.[31] Prostacyclin (PGI_2) is synthesized by the vascular endothelium and the renal cortex. It is a vasodilator and inhibits platelet aggregation. Thromboxane A_2 (TxA_2) is produced primarily by platelets and is a potent vasoconstrictor and aggregator of platelets. Reproductive tissues produce large quantities of prostanoids. During normal pregnancy there is increased production of prostanoids by maternal, fetal, and placental tissues.[23]

A decrease in PGI_2 production and plasma PGI_2 concentration and an increase in the TxA_2–PGI_2 ratio have been demonstrated in preeclampsia.[32,33] Prostacyclin has a half-life of 3 minutes in blood at 37°C. It is usually quantified by measuring its stable degradation product, 6-keto-$PGF_{1\alpha}$. The plasma concentration and urinary excretion of 6-keto-$PGF_{1\alpha}$ has been found to be decreased in patients with preeclampsia.[34,35] The defective PGI_2 action does not appear to be due to changes in tissue responsiveness. Platelet prostacyclin receptors have the same affinity and binding capacity in normal and hypertensive pregnancy.[36] Thromboxane A_2 has a half-life of about 30 seconds at 37°C, and it is usually quantified by assaying its stable hydrolysis product thromboxane B_2. Makila and colleagues have shown an increased rate of TxA_2 production by the placenta in hypertensive pregnancies.[32]

Preeclampsia is associated with vasospasm and activation of the coagulation system. Saleh and colleagues demonstrated high fibronectin, low antithrombin III, and increased β-thromboglobulin in patients with preeclampsia (ie, findings suggestive of endothelial injury, enhanced clotting, and increased platelet activation and consumption).[37] In preeclampsia, vascular endothelial damage may cause decreased prostacyclin production and activation of clotting and fibrinolysis, with subsequent generation of thrombin and plasmin. Thrombin consumes antithrombin III, resulting in fibrin deposition. Platelet activation leads to the release of thromboxane A_2 and serotonin, causing further vasospasm, platelet aggregation, and endothelial injury. Although this hypothesis may explain some of the hematologic and biochemical abnormalities associated with preeclampsia, it does not reveal the underlying etiology.

Genetic Susceptibility. A familial factor in the pathogenesis of preeclampsia has been recognized for many years. Chesley and Cooper referred to an account by Elliot in 1883 of eclampsia occurring in a mother and four daughters.[38] Despite the accumulation of evidence to suggest a genetic etiology, the exact mode of inheritance and the interaction between maternal and fetal genotype have not been elucidated. Maternal genotype alone was implicated by Sutherland and colleagues, who reported an increased frequency of preeclampsia in the mothers but not in the mothers-in-law of preeclamptic women.[39] Chesley and Cooper observed an increased frequency of preeclampsia in the daughters and granddaughters, but not the daughters-in-law, of women who themselves had a history of eclampsia.[38] These data suggest a recessive inheritance dependent on the maternal genotype.

Evidence to support a fetal genetic contribution to the pathogenesis of preeclampsia came from reports of an apparent increase in HLA homozygosity in the mother,[40] an increase in the HLA compatibility between preeclamptic women and their partners,[41] and a higher incidence if the fetus is male[42] and in pregnancies conceived by partners of dissimilar race. However, later studies have failed to confirm these observations.[43]

Cooper and colleagues reported a high incidence of eclampsia in the daughters of eclamptic mothers.[44] The frequency of eclampsia was greatest in daughters who themselves had been a product of an eclamptic pregnancy. Three- and four-generation involvement was described that was more suggestive of a dominant or multifactorial inheritance than an autosomal recessive mechanism. Recent studies have shown an association between eclampsia and trisomy 13.[45] Although genetic factors appear to have a role in the etiology of preeclampsia, it is clear that neither a single gene theory nor multifactorial inheritance can explain all the manifestations of this disease.

Immunology. Speculation that the cause of preeclampsia may be found within the immune system has stimulated considerable interest and research over the last 10 to 15 years. The data that have implicated activation of the immune system in preeclampsia were critically reviewed by Stirrat.[46]

1. Women with proteinuric preeclampsia have low levels of serum IgG. However, this finding is not specific to preeclampsia and similar changes have been reported in nephrotic syndrome.
2. Some women with preeclampsia have immune complexes in their serum, whereas others show deposits of immunoglobulin and complement components in cutaneous blood vessels. However, immune complexes are difficult to assay. Some workers have failed to confirm these findings, but others have found immune complexes in all pregnant women.
3. There is no consensus about whether HLA antibodies are present or absent in severe preeclampsia.
4. Some studies have shown activation of the complement system in proteinuric preeclampsia. However, this is not a constant finding. Furthermore, preeclampsia stimulates an acute-phase reaction that may explain altered serum concentrations of complement components.

Stirrat concluded that although there is some suggestion that the humoral immune system and complement activation are involved in the preeclamptic process, there is no evidence that immunologic factors cause the condition. At present there are no data to support a role for cell-mediated immunity.

Renin–Angiotensin–Aldosterone. The renin–angiotensin–aldosterone system (RAAS) plays an important role in the control of vascular tone and blood pressure. In this system, angiotensinogen secreted by the liver is cleaved by renin to produce angiotensin I. Inactive angiotensin I is then converted into biologically active angiotensin II by an angiotensin-converting enzyme that is bound to vascular endothelium. Circulating angiotensin II interacts with specific receptors to induce smooth muscle contraction, stimulate aldosterone production and sodium retention, facilitate norepinephrine release and inhibit norepinephrine reuptake by sympathetic nerve terminals, and potentiate vascular smooth muscle reactivity to norepinephrine.

In normal pregnancy, concentrations of the components of the RAAS are increased.[47] However, the vascular response to most pressor substances is impaired.[48] Conversely, in preeclampsia, some of the components of the RAAS are lower than those in normal pregnancy and there is a markedly increased sensitivity to pressor peptides and catecholamines. Gant and colleagues found that the pressor response to angiotensin II was significantly increased by 18 weeks gestation in women who went on to develop preeclampsia.[49]

The regulation of angiotensin II sensitivity appears to be closely linked to prostanoid synthesis. Everett and colleagues showed that prostaglandin synthetase inhibitors augmented the pressor response to angiotensin II in normal pregnancy.[50] Studies by Broughton-Pipkin and colleagues demonstrated that the infusion of prostaglandin E_2, prostaglandin E_1, and prostacyclin all reduced the pressor response to angiotensin II in the second trimester of pregnancy, whereas indomethacin increased vascular sensitivity.[51,52] A deficiency in prostanoid synthesis in preeclampsia may predispose toward increased vascular tone and hypertension. Although this hypothesis could account for increased vascular resistance and reactivity in preeclampsia, it does not explain the etiology of the disease.

ECLAMPSIA

Why some patients with symptoms of preeclampsia develop convulsions and/or coma and others do not is unknown. Several mechanisms have been suggested as predisposing factors:

Cerebral vasospasm
Cerebral hemorrhage
Cerebral ischemia
Cerebral edema
Hypertensive encephalopathy
Metabolic encephalopathy.

Most patients with eclamptic seizures have an abnormal electroencephalogram (EEG).[53] However, EEG changes are almost always transient and resolve completely. Furthermore, they give no clue to the underlying pathophysiology. Computed tomography is also unhelpful and is rarely abnormal.[53] Whether the newer technique of nuclear magnetic resonance imaging will prove more illuminating remains to be seen.

CHRONIC HYPERTENSION

The most common etiology of chronic hypertension is essential hypertension. Other causes are listed in Table 58-4. Most of these other causes require specific medication in addition to antihypertensive therapy. Early diagnosis is important, because, if untreated, many of these disorders are associated with significant maternal and fetal morbidity and mortality. Mild to moderate hypertension is associated with a normal cardiac output and increased total peripheral resistance. With time, signs of cardiac strain become evident, with progressive thickening of the left ventricular wall. In the absence of renal disease, plasma volume contraction is proportionate to the increase in diastolic blood pressure. Severe essential hypertension is characterized by end-organ damage. Total peripheral resistance continues to rise and cardiac output may begin to fall. The intravascular volume decreases further and plasma renin activity rises. These changes increase left ventricular tension and reduce myocardial contractility. Without treatment, pulmonary edema will occur.

MANAGEMENT OF HYPERTENSION IN PREGNANCY

The management of a pregnancy complicated by hypertension is determined by the effects of the disorder on maternal and fetal well-being rather than by the pathophysiology. In a minority of cases, the hypertension will have a treatable cause (eg, pheochromocytoma). In this situation the appropriate management is that of the underlying disease.

TABLE 58–4. ETIOLOGY OF CHRONIC HYPERTENSION

1. Renal factors
   - a. Acute and chronic glomerulonephritis
   - b. Acute and chronic pyelonephritis
   - c. Polycystic renal disease
   - d. Renovascular disease
2. Collagen disease with renal involvement
   - a. Lupus erythematosus
   - b. Periarteritis nodosa
   - c. Scleroderma
3. Endocrine factors
   - a. Diabetes with vascular involvement
   - b. Thyrotoxicosis
4. Coarctation of the aorta
5. Pheochromocytoma

Data from Sibai BM. Chronic hypertension during pregnancy. In: Sciarra JJ, ed. Gynecology and obstetrics. Philadelphia: JB Lippincott, 1988.

PREECLAMPSIA

Prediction of Preeclampsia

Numerous clinical and biochemical tests have been reported as predicting the future development of preeclampsia. Chesley and Sibai summarized 39,876 cases of preeclampsia and 207 cases of eclampsia and investigated the predictive value of elevated mean arterial pressure in the second trimester.[54] The sensitivity ranged from 0 to 92%, and the specificity varied from 53% to 97%. They concluded that if increased second-trimester mean arterial blood pressure predicts anything, it is transient hypertension rather than preeclampsia or eclampsia.

The "roll-over test" was first described by Gant and colleagues.[55] They claimed a high sensitivity and specificity for the prediction or exclusion of subsequent preeclampsia. Kuntz reviewed its accuracy as a predictor of preeclampsia.[56] Contrary to Gant and colleagues, most investigators have reported a significant incidence of false-negative and false-positive results. The significance of the angiotensin II infusion test[50] for the prediction of preeclampsia was studied by Nakamura and colleagues.[57] The test has a specificity of 90% to 95%, but the sensitivity is very variable. Furthermore, it is an invasive procedure and therefore not suitable for screening purposes.

Table 58-5 lists some of the components of maternal blood and urine that have been reported to be useful predictors of preeclampsia. These reports often differ in their methodology and use heterogeneous populations

TABLE 58–5. BIOCHEMICAL TESTS USED TO PREDICT FUTURE PREECLAMPSIA

- Uric acid
- Plasma volume
- Prostaglandin metabolites
- Coagulation parameters
  - Platelet count
  - Fibrinogen
  - β-thromboglobulin
  - Fibronectin
  - Antithrombin-III
- α-Fetoprotein
- Hormones
  - Estriol
  - HPL
  - Prolactin
- Cations
  - Iron
  - Zinc
  - Magnesium
  - Calcium in blood and urine excretion

From Sibai BM, Moretti MM. Pregnancy induced hypertension. Contemp Ob/Gyn 1988;31:57.

with all forms of hypertension, parity, and gestational ages. Comparison and evaluation are therefore limited, but none of the substances in Table 58-5 has proved sufficiently reliable to use as a clinical test to predict preeclampsia.

Preeclampsia is associated with reduced uteroplacental blood flow as measured by metabolic clearance of dehydroepiandrosterone sulfate[58] and functional placental scintigraphy.[59] By the time a patient presents with clinical signs of preeclampsia, uteroplacental blood flow is already reduced by 50%. It has been postulated that in women destined to develop preeclampsia, the conversion of high-resistance spiral arteries to low-resistance uteroplacental arteries does not occur.[29,60] If this is true, it is possible that failure of this conversion may be detected by Doppler ultrasound—a noninvasive method of measuring changes in blood flow velocity. Campbell and colleagues screened 126 consecutive pregnancies between 16 and 18 weeks.[61] An abnormal uteroplacental waveform pattern predicted preeclampsia and intrauterine growth retardation with a sensitivity of 68% and a specificity of 69%. The positive and negative predictive values were 42% and 87%, respectively. A similar study by Steel and colleagues screened primigravida women at 24 weeks gestation.[62] The sensitivity for any degree of hypertension in pregnancy was 29%. However, for severe preeclampsia with intrauterine growth retardation, the sensitivity of this screening test rose to 100%. Although these results are encouraging, further assessment is necessary to know whether this technique offers any clear advantage over other methods of predicting the risk of preeclampsia

The Prevention of Preeclampsia

Preeclampsia is associated with vasospasm, activation of the coagulation system, and prostacyclin–thromboxane imbalance. Various attempts have been made to correct these abnormalities in the hope of ameliorating or preventing the disease. There is no evidence that diuretics alter the incidence of preeclampsia.[63] Diets low in salt and high in protein have been suggested to prevent preeclampsia. However, the efficacy of these regimes has never been proved.

Kawasaki and colleagues compared 22 women given calcium supplementation (600 mg calcium aspartate daily) from 20 weeks to delivery with 72 women who did not receive supplementation.[64] All 94 women were at risk for preeclampsia. Calcium supplementation was associated with a significant reduction in vascular sensitivity to angiotensin II infusions. The incidence of preeclampsia was 4.5% in the calcium-supplemented group and 21.2% in the nonsupplemented group. This is a surprising result, since the amount of elemental calcium ingested by the supplemented group (156 mg daily) would hardly meet normal daily requirements. It is difficult to understand how it could alter the incidence of preeclampsia. Villar and colleagues reported a double-blind controlled trial involving 52 pregnant women.[65] Calcium supplementation (1.5 g of elemental calcium daily) was given to 25 women after 26 weeks gestation, and 27 received a matching placebo. The incidence of preeclampsia was 4% in the calcium group and 11.1% in the placebo group. Although this is an interesting finding, the small number of patients makes it difficult to draw any conclusions.

Preeclampsia is associated with platelet consumption and a deficiency in prostacyclin. Aspirin binds irreversibly with the cyclooxygenase enzymes within the platelets and inhibits aggregation. Dipyridamole increases peroxidase activity within platelets, which indirectly increases prostacyclin production and discourages platelet aggregation. It has been suggested that aspirin with or without dipyridamole may avert or ameliorate the development of preeclampsia. Aspirin also interferes with prostacyclin production by the vascular endothelium. However, platelets cannot recover from the effect of aspirin, because they have no nucleus. The endothelial cell has a nucleus and will recover the ability to produce prostacyclin within about 6 hours.[66] It was postulated that the use of low-dose aspirin would inhibit the majority of platelets but would leave the endothelium relatively unharmed. There have been two recent studies on the use of aspirin in patients at risk of developing preeclampsia or intrauterine growth retardation. Beaufils and colleagues treated 52 patients with a combination of aspirin 150 mg/day and dipyridamole 300 mg/day from 12 weeks gestation until delivery and compared outcome with a control group of 50 patients.[67] There was no incidence of preeclampsia or fetal deaths in the treatment group, although the control group had a 13% incidence of preeclampsia and 11% perinatal deaths. Fetal growth retardation occurred in 29% of the control group compared with 8% of the treated group. The patients studied by Beaufils and colleagues were selected on the basis of a past history of pregnancy loss (ie, not just preeclampsia). Furthermore, the two groups were not comparable with regard to preexisting renal disease or chronic hypertension. Wallenburg and colleagues studied 46 primigravidas selected on the basis of a positive angiotensin II infusion test at 28 weeks gestation.[68] Half the group received aspirin 60 mg/day and the other half was given a placebo. The control group had significantly more cases of preeclampsia and intrauterine growth retardation compared with the treated group. However, there were no differences between the two groups in average gestational age or birth weight at delivery or the incidence of fetal loss. The long-term benefits of aspirin therapy have yet to be proved and will require large multicenter trials with clear selection criteria and end points.

Management of Preeclampsia

The most effective therapy for preeclampsia is delivery of the fetus and placenta. In pregnancies at or near term where the cervix is favorable, labor should be induced. Intravenous magnesium sulfate should be administered during labor to reduce the risk of convulsions. Preeclampsia remote from term presents a much more difficult management problem. The decision of whether to intervene and deliver a preterm infant that may require prolonged intensive care or to institute expectant management is usually governed by disease severity and the length of gestation.

Mild Preeclampsia. Mild preeclampsia remote from term can be managed on an ambulatory basis, or the patient can be admitted to the hospital. Ambulatory management is applicable in the early stages of the disease. The patient is allowed to remain at home but advised to spend most of the day resting. The attending obstetrician must evaluate maternal and fetal well-being every second day. If there is any evidence of disease progression and or if acute hypertension develops, then prompt hospitalization is indicated.

Once a patient has been admitted to the hospital, intensive maternal and fetal monitoring should be instituted. Table 58-6 summarizes the measures used, at the University of Tennessee, Memphis to evaluate maternal and fetal well-being. The frequency of testing depends on the severity of the disease. In many cases of mild preeclampsia the disease does not progress and pregnancy can be managed conservatively until the fetus reaches maturity. Gilstrap and colleagues reported the results of treating 545 primigravidas with singleton pregnancies complicated by preeclampsia.[69] Patients with mild disease were hospitalized and intensively monitored. Duration of hospital admission averaged 24 days. Eighty-one percent of the study group became normotensive after admission, 13% were intermittently hypertensive, and 6% had persistent hypertension and were delivered within a week of admission. Forty-two percent of the women who became normotensive had recurrent hypertension before labor, and 45% became hypertensive during labor. However, 87% of the total were delivered at or beyond 37 weeks gestation. This study suggested that early and prolonged hospitalization for patients with mild preeclampsia remote from term improves perinatal survival, reduces maternal morbidity, and is cost effective.

If a patient becomes normotensive after hospitalization and is remote from term with no evidence of fetal compromise, outpatient surveillance may be considered. This requires a minimum of twice-weekly maternal and fetal assessment. There is no place for conservative management if there are signs of progression to severe preeclampsia or if fetal monitoring tests become abnormal.

Conservative management of mild disease beyond term is not beneficial to the fetus, because uteroplacental blood flow is suboptimal. After 37 weeks gestation, labor should be induced as soon as the cervix is favorable.

TABLE 58-6. MATERNAL-FETAL EVALUATION OF MILD PREECLAMPSIA REMOTE FROM TERM

Maternal Evaluation

1. Blood pressure (four times daily)
2. Presence of generalized edema (particularly facial and abdominal edema) and/or excessive weight gain (daily)
3. Patellar reflexes (daily)
4. Symptoms of persistent occipital headache, visual symptoms, or epigastric pain (daily)
5. Urinalysis (daily). (A dipstick test will provide only a crude estimate of proteinuria. A 24-hour urine collection should be analyzed for protein and creatinine clearance—twice a week.)
6. Hematocrit and platelet count (every 2 days)
7. Serum uric acid, creatinine (twice a week)
8. Liver function tests (SGOT, LDH, serum bilirubin) (weekly)

Fetal Evaluation

1. Daily fetal movement records
2. Nonstress test (twice weekly)
3. Biophysical profile, if nonstress test is unreactive
4. Untrasound assessment of fetal growth (every 2 weeks)

The Role of Antihypertensive Therapy. Antepartum use of antihypertensive therapy for mild preeclampsia remote from term is controversial. Rubin and colleagues compared atenolol beta$_1$-selective adrenoreceptor blocking agent) against placebo in a randomized study.[70] The mean gestation at entry was 33.8 weeks and the mean blood pressure was 140/95. A similar study by Walker and colleagues compared labetalol (a nonselective beta blocker with some alpha$_1$-blocking effects) with bedrest.[71] The mean gestation at entry was 34.8 weeks and the mean blood pressure was 141/96. Both studies showed a significant improvement in stabilization of diastolic pressure to <90 mm Hg prior to delivery, a significant reduction in the incidence of patients who progressed to severe disease, and a significant decrease in the development of proteinuria. These studies suggested that in mild preeclampsia, bedrest alone has little effect on blood pressure or disease progression, whereas antihypertensive therapy appeared to reduce the incidence of progression to severe disease as measured by increasing blood pressure and development of proteinuria. There was no benefit to mother or fetus apart from a reduction in hospitalization. Sibai and colleagues compared labetalol plus hospitalization with hospitalization alone in the management of 200 mild preeclamptics remote from term.[72] There was no difference between the two groups in gestational age or birth weight at delivery, cord blood gases, or incidence of admission to the special care nursery. However, there were significantly more small-for-gestational-age infants in the labetalol group. Both groups showed a significant deterioration in proteinuria, creatinine, and uric acid. The authors concluded that perinatal outcome was not improved by lowering blood pressure in mild preeclampsia.

In the past, diuretics were widely used to treat hypertension in pregnancy. Collins and colleagues reviewed nine randomized controlled trials of diuretics in pregnancy and concluded that there is no evidence to indicate any worthwhile effect of diuretic therapy on perinatal outcome.[63] These drugs may be harmful to both mother and fetus,[73] and since they have no proven beneficial effect they should not be used.

Severe Preeclampsia. There is considerable evidence to show the deleterious effects of severe hypertension in non-pregnant humans and in experimental animals.[74] In treating severe preeclampsia, blood pressure should be maintained below 160/110 mm Hg. The most widely used antihypertensive agent in pregnancy is methyldopa. An adequate therapeutic response may be expected within 12 hours. If blood pressure cannot be controlled with a single agent, combination therapy (usually methyldopa and hydralazine) is usually effective. Intravenous hydralazine administered as a bolus of 5 mg at 15- to 20-minute intervals is the treatment of choice for acute rises in blood pressure > 160/100 mm Hg. The aim is to reduce diastolic pressure gradually to the range of 90 to 100 mm Hg. Intermittent therapy with hydralazine rarely produces a dramatic fall in blood pressure, but the level must be carefully and frequently monitored. An alternative regime is to use boluses of intravenous labetalol 20 to 50 mg. Unlike hydralazine, labetalol does not cause maternal tachycardia, flushing, or headaches.

In most studies of eclampsia, 20% of women had only a minimal rise in blood pressure. Consequently, all patients who meet the blood pressure criteria for preeclampsia should be given intravenous magnesium sulfate to minimize the risk of eclampsia. In Memphis this drug is administered by a controlled continuous intravenous infusion with a loading dose of 6 g in 100 mL. Maintenance therapy is given at a rate of 2 g in 100 mL of fluid per hour. Serum magnesium levels are obtained 4 to 6 hours later, and the rate of infusion is adjusted to keep serum magnesium levels between 4.8 and 9.6 mg/dL. Treatment is continued for 24 hours postpartum. Intramuscular magnesium injections should be avoided. Not only is this a very painful regime, but it is much more difficult to control magnesium levels compared with the intravenous route.

Magnesium is excreted in the urine. In the therapeutic range it slows neuromuscular conduction and depresses CNS irritability. Maternal respiratory rate, deep tendon reflexes, and level of consciousness must be frequently monitored to detect magnesium toxicity. If respiratory depression does occur, 1 g of calcium gluconate should be given intravenously over 3 minutes. Magnesium sulfate may also decrease beat-to-beat variability of the fetal heart rate,[75] and signs of neonatal hypermagnesemia have been reported after only 24 hours intravenous therapy.[76] The mode of action of magnesium ions is uncertain and there is disagreement as to whether it has a predominantly central or peripheral effect.

The effectiveness of magnesium sulfate as an anticonvulsant is controversial.[77,78] As a consequence, interest has focused on other anticonvulsants, particularly on phenytoin. This drug is cleared rapidly from the brain and must be given by continuous infusion to maintain therapeutic levels. Slater and colleagues reported no maternal or fetal side effects after intravenous administration of phenytoin for anticonvulsant prophylaxis in severe preeclampsia.[79] Whether this agent is superior to magnesium sulfate in seizure prophylaxis requires further investigation. Meticulous attention to fluid balance is an important aspect of the management of severe preeclampsia. Input and output should be assessed hourly, and a Foley catheter should be inserted to permit accurate measurement of urine output. The aim is to maintain urine output at 30 mL/h. If output is less than 100 mL in 4 hours, fluid input (including magnesium sulfate infusion) should be reduced accordingly. For patients in active labor, urine output often increases after 2 or 3 hours, and specific therapy is unnecessary.

Satisfactory maternal analgesia can be achieved intrapartum with intermittent use of small doses (25 to 50 mg) of meperidine. Local anesthesia is used for vaginal deliveries and general anesthesia is used for cesarean sections. Continuous epidural anesthesia has been advocated in preeclampsia and eclampsia in the belief that it not only controls pain but also aids in stabilizing blood pressure and increases renal and uterine blood flow.[80] However, this procedure requires an arterial line and central hemodynamic monitoring (both invasive procedures), and the contracted blood volume characteristic of preeclampsia makes the risk of hypotension high. If a significant fall in blood pressure does occur following epidural anesthesia, attempts to achieve normotension by fluid loading can precipitate pulmonary edema. For these reasons, the authors would advocate the use of epidural analgesia in preeclampsia or eclampsia only if it is administered by personnel skilled in obstetric anesthesia. There should be no evidence of fetal distress, maternal platelet count should be greater than 100,000/μL, and bleeding time should be less than 12 minutes.

Blood loss at delivery in severe preeclampsia may be greater than that for a normal pregnancy. Magnesium sulfate may inhibit uterine contraction, and tolerance to blood loss is reduced by the contracted blood volume. Cross-matched blood should therefore be available in the labor and delivery area. The mode of delivery should be determined by gestational age and by fetal and maternal condition. For gestations less than 32 weeks, cesarean section is the route of choice in the absence of labor or a ripe cervix. The preterm fetus is at significant risk of intrapartum asphyxia, and the presence of severe preeclampsia increases this risk. Intrapartum electronic fetal monitoring at this gestation is often technically difficult. Furthermore, induction of labor before 32 weeks is often a prolonged process that increases the likelihood of fetal asphyxia.

Experience based on the management of 303 cases of severe preeclampsia[81] has led the authors to conclude that the management of choice for almost all patients who are beyond 28 weeks gestation is prompt delivery. In Memphis these patients are usually admitted to the labor and delivery area for evaluation. They all receive intravenous magnesium sulfate. If there is evidence of

25–28 Weeks ≤ Intensive Maternal–Fetal Management	24 Weeks Termination of Pregnancy
IV magnesium sulfate for 24 hours	PGE vaginal suppository
Antihypertensive if diastolic BP ≥ 110 mmHg	IV magnesium sulfate
Daily evaluation of fetal well-being	Hydralazine if required
Daily evaluation of maternal status	
Cesarean section if there is evidence of	
Fetal lung maturity	
Fetal distress	
Maternal distress	

FIGURE 58–1. Management of severe midtrimester preeclampsia. (from Sibai BM. Preeclampsia–eclampsia. In: Sciarra JJ, ed. Gynecology and obstetrics. Philadelphia: JB Lippincott, 1988, 8.)

acute fetal compromise or it is impossible to stabilize the maternal condition, delivery is the treatment of choice, regardless of the gestational age or fetal lung maturity. In a minority of patients with severe preeclampsia, diastolic pressure stabilizes below 100 mm Hg within 24 hours of admission. These pregnancies may be managed conservatively until fetal maturity is achieved, provided they are followed closely in a tertiary care center with daily maternal and fetal monitoring. Most will require delivery within 3 to 10 days of admission. Hence, amniocentesis should be performed for lecithin–sphingomyelin (L–S) ratio; if the fetal lung is immature, the patient should be given steroids to accelerate maturity.

The management of severe preeclampsia at less than 28 weeks gestation is a difficult problem. A review by Sibai and colleagues of conservative management in 60 patients over a 7-year period suggested a poor maternal and perinatal outcome.[82] The perinatal mortality was 87%, and 74% of the stillbirths occurred in patients presenting at or before 25 weeks gestation. Figure 58-1 details the recommended management of severe midtrimester preeclampsia based on the Memphis experience.

HELLP Syndrome

The reported incidence of HELLP syndrome in preeclampsia has ranged from 2% to 12%.[83] White women are more commonly affected than black women, and there appears to be a higher incidence in preeclamptic patients managed conservatively.[84] It is sometimes difficult to distinguish between HELLP syndrome and other disorders associated with liver dysfunction or hemolytic anemia (eg, idiopathic thrombocytopenic purpura, thrombotic thrombocytopenic purpura, hemolytic uremic syndrome, gallbladder disease, and viral hepatitis). Consequently, the diagnosis of HELLP syndrome is often confused and delayed by inappropriate medical or surgical treatment. The criteria used in Memphis to diagnose HELLP syndrome are shown in Table 58-7.

Management. Patients with a diagnosis of HELLP syndrome should be considered as having severe preeclampsia. They should be managed as such and referred to a tertiary care center. The method of management is controversial. Some recommend immediate delivery[16,85]; others favor a conservative approach in pregnancies remote from term.[17,86] A recent report by Van Dam and colleagues, based on data from 18 patients with HELLP, found that patients with clinical disseminated intravascular coagulation (DIC) at delivery developed significantly more life-threatening maternal complications than did patients with suspected DIC.[87] The authors suggested that conservative management can be considered in patients who present without laboratory evidence of DIC.

ECLAMPSIA

The reported incidence of eclampsia varies between 0.5% and 0.2% of all deliveries. In Memphis the incidence is one in 300, and this figure has not changed over the past 30 years. Eclampsia is associated with multiple organ dysfunction. Factors determining the degree of dysfunction include a delay in the treatment of preeclampsia and the presence of complicating obstetric and medical factors. Eclampsia is associated with a wide spectrum of signs and symptoms, ranging from extreme hypertension, hyperreflexia, 4+ proteinuria, and generalized edema to isolated mild hypertension. Laboratory findings also vary. Serum uric acid and creatinine are usually elevated, and creatinine clearance is reduced. Hemoconcentration reflected by an increased hematocrit and reduced plasma volume is common. Elevated liver function tests are found in 11% to 74% of

TABLE 58–7. LABORATORY VALUES USED TO DIAGNOSE HELLP SYNDROME

Hemolysis
Abnormal peripheral blood smear (with burr cells and schistocytes)
Increased bilirubin ≥ 1.2 mg/dL*
Increased lactic dehydrogenase > 600 IU/L*
Elevated liver enzymes
Increased SGOT ≥ 72 IU/L*
Increased lactic dehydrogenase as above
Low platelets
Platelet count < 100,000/μL

Data from Sibai BM, Taslimi MM, El-Nazar A, Amon E, Mabie WC, Ryan G. Maternal–perinatal outcome associated with the syndrome of hemolysis, elevated liver enzymes, and low platelets in severe preeclampsia–eclampsia. Am J Obstet Gynecol 1986;155:501.

* These values are more than four standard deviations above the mean for the Memphis population.

TABLE 58-8. FACTORS INVOLVED IN UNAVOIDABLE ECLAMPSIA

FACTOR	ALL CASES OF ECLAMPSIA (*n* = 232)	UNAVOIDABLE ECLAMPSIA (*n* = 84)
Abrupt onset	45	36
Late postpartum onset	38	27
Convulsion of magnesium sulfate	26	10*
Mild preeclampsia with good response†	117	7
Early onset (<21 weeks)	6	4

* Adequate serum levels.
† Normal blood pressure after hospitalization.

eclamptic patients. HELLP syndrome complicates about 10% of eclampsia and usually occurs in longstanding disease and in patients with medical complications. Disseminated intravascular coagulopathy may develop if treatment is delayed or abruptio placentae with fetal demise has occurred.

The question of whether eclampsia is a preventable complication is controversial. Although the incidence can be significantly lowered by adequate antenatal care, some cases present without warning signs or symptoms. Zuspan believes that the key to prevention is appropriate prenatal care.[88] However, Campbell and Templeton studied factors leading to the development of eclampsia in 66 women.[89] They concluded that convulsions were not preventable in 42% of the cases they studied. This agrees with the Memphis experience (Table 58-8).

Management

The protocol used to manage eclampsia in Memphis is outlined in Table 58-9. The first priority is to control convulsions. Magnesium sulfate is the anticonvulsant of choice. It is important to remember that the maximum dose when given over a short time should not exceed 8 g. Once convulsions have been abolished, arterial blood gas measurements and a chest radiograph should be obtained to ensure adequate maternal oxygenation and exclude aspiration. Hypoxemia and acidemia should be corrected. The next step is to treat maternal hypertension. Hydralazine administered as intermittent boluses (5 to 10 mg) is a safe and effective antihypertensive in this situation.

TABLE 58-9. AUTHORS' PROTOCOL FOR MANAGING ECLAMPSIA

1. Convulsions are controlled or prevented with a loading dose of 6 g magnesium sulfate in 100 mL 5% dextrose in Ringer's lactated solution, given over 15 minutes, followed by a maintenance dose of 2 g/h.
2. Serum magnesium level is obtained 4 to 6 hours later, and the rate of infusion is adjusted to maintain magnesium levels between 4.8 and 9.6 mg/dL. If serum magnesium levels are not available, the dose is adjusted according to patellar reflexes and urine output in the previous 4-hour period.
3. Diuretics, plasma volume expanders, and invasive hemodynamic monitoring are not used.
4. Induction and/or delivery is initiated within 4 hours after maternal stabilization
5. Magnesium sulfate is continued for 24 hours after delivery or, if postpartum, 24 hours after the last convulsion. In some cases, the infusion is continued for 72 hours as needed.

Following stabilization of maternal condition, steps should be taken to deliver the fetus. This is the definitive treatment for eclampsia. Induction of labor with oxytocin is often successful after 32 weeks gestation. The fetal heart rate and uterine activity must be closely monitored. Fetal bradycardia is a common finding during an eclamptic fit,[90] but the rate usually returns to normal once convulsions cease. If bradycardia persists or the uterus is hypertonic, placental abruption should be suspected. For gestations of less than 32 weeks, cesarean section is advocated. This recommendation is based on the experience of Sibai and colleagues, who found that eclampsia prior to 32 weeks gestation was associated with a high incidence of fetal growth retardation (30%), abruption (23%), and intrapartum fetal distress (65%).[91]

Some authors have suggested that eclampsia indicates hemodynamic monitoring with Swan-Ganz catheters. This question was reviewed by Hankins and colleagues, who concluded that such intensive monitoring is rarely necessary.[92] This agrees with the experience in Memphis, where over an 8-year period, Swan-Ganz catheters have only been used in four of 186 eclamptic patients.

OUTCOME OF PREGNANCIES COMPLICATED BY PREECLAMPSIA OR ECLAMPSIA

The outcome of studies by Gilstrap and colleagues and Sibai and colleagues of hospitalized patients with mild preeclampsia remote from term is summarized in Table 58-10.[69,72] Maternal and perinatal morbidity and mortality in this group of patients are extremely low and approach those of normotensive pregnancies. This contrasts sharply with the outcome of severe preeclampsia. Sibai and colleagues reported on 303 pregnancies complicated by severe preeclampsia.[81] There were 28 still-

TABLE 58–10. MATERNAL–PERINATAL OUTCOME IN HOSPITALIZED PATIENTS WITH MILD PREECLAMPSIA REMOTE FROM TERM

	GILSTRAP et al (*n* = 545)	SIBAI et al (*n* = 200)
Gestation ≤ 36 weeks	373 (68.5%)	200 (100%)
Significant proteinuria	44 (8%)	200 (100%)
Average pregnancy prolongation (days)	24	21
Mean birth weight (in grams)	2824	2258
Fetal growth retardation	46 (8.4%)	27 (13.5%)
Perinatal deaths	5 (1.0%)	1 (0.5%)
Abruptio placentae	5 (1%)	2 (1%)
Eclampsia	1 (0.2%)	0

From Sibai BM. Preeclampsia–eclampsia. Contemp Ob/Gyn 1988;32:109.

births and 15 neonatal deaths, giving a corrected perinatal mortality rate of 135 in 1000. Perinatal survival was zero when preeclampsia developed before 28 weeks but rose to 100% when disease developed after 36 weeks gestation. The severity and incidence of neonatal complications were also closely linked to gestational age at delivery. Maternal morbidity was common. Seventeen percent had thrombocytopenia (platelet count < 150,000/μL) and 8.5% had HELLP syndrome. Disseminated intravascular coagulation occurred in 7.3%, and pulmonary edema developed in 2% of cases.

Reported perinatal mortality for preeclampsia with HELLP syndrome has ranged from 7.7% to 60%,[83] and maternal mortality has ranged from 0 to 24%.[86,93] There is a high incidence of abruptio placentae and disseminated intravascular coagulation. Multiple transfusions of blood and blood products are usually necessary, and patients are at risk of developing acute renal failure, pulmonary edema, ascites, and hepatic rupture. Sibai and colleagues reported on the maternal–perinatal outcome of 112 cases of HELLP syndrome studied over an 8-year period.[83] Maternal and perinatal outcome is summarized in Table 58-11. Based on this extensive experience, they recommend prompt delivery after stabilizing maternal condition.

Maternal mortality resulting from eclampsia is usually associated with mismanaged or complicated cases. Lopez-Llera reviewed 365 cases of eclampsia occurring in Mexican women between 1964 and 1973.[93] There were 49 deaths. The risk of maternal mortality was significantly increased if eclampsia presented before 28 weeks gestation, maternal age was >25 years, and the pregnancy was a multiple gestation. In Memphis there has been one maternal death in 250 cases of eclampsia between 1977 and 1988 (Sibai, unpublished data). Maternal morbidity was greater in multigravidas than in primigravidas. This difference may be due to a higher incidence of chronic hypertension and underlying renal disease in the multigravida. The complication rate was also higher in patients who had no prenatal care or who were transferred from other hospitals (Table 58-12). The fetus of the eclamptic woman is particularly at risk from abruptio placentae, preterm delivery, intrauterine growth retardation, and acute hypoxia during maternal convulsions.[91,94] The reported perinatal mortality rate varies between 10% and 28%. Neonatal mortality for fetuses alive on admission to perinatal centers is about 4%. Follow-up data for up to 50 months on 28 preterm infants and 14 full-term infants of eclamptic women were reported by Sibai and colleagues.[91] Twelve infants were small for dates at birth. Only two remained growth retarded by weight, height, and head circumference. Both were mentally retarded. Three other infants were diagnosed as having cerebral palsy. Among the premature infants, there was significant morbidity, especially related to pulmonary and neurologic complications. Maternal and neonatal morbidity and mortality can be reduced by early transfer of eclamptic patients to tertiary care centers with neonatal intensive care units.

TABLE 58–11. PREGNANCY OUTCOME IN HELLP SYNDROME

	NUMBER	(%)
Maternal Outcome (*n* = 112)		
Abruptio placentae	22	20.0
DIC	42	38.0
Acute renal failure	9	8.0
Pleural effusions	8	7.1
Pulmonary edema	5	4.5
Ruptured liver hematoma	2	1.8
Maternal deaths	2	1.8
Fetal Outcome (*n* = 114 births)		
Perinatal deaths	38	33.3
Gestational age (wk)		
≤30	47	41.2
31–36	46	40.4
≥36	21	18.4
SGA	36	31.6

Data from Sibai BM, Taslimi MM, El-Nazer A, Amon E, Mabie WC, Ryan G. Maternal–perinatal outcome associated with the syndrome of hemolysis, elevated liver enzymes, and low platelets in severe preeclampsia–eclampsia. Am J Obstet Gynecol 1986;155:501.

DIC = disseminated intravascular coagulation.

SGA = small for gestational age.

TABLE 58-12. MATERNAL COMPLICATIONS FROM ECLAMPSIA: 1977–1988

COMPLICATION	MATERNAL TRANSFER AND NO PERINATAL CARE (*N* = 135; % = 58)	PRENATAL CARE AT UNIVERSITY (*N* = 97; % = 42)	TOTAL (*N* = 232; % = 100)
Abruptio placentae	19 (14)	4 (4)	23 (10.0)
Pulmonary edema	6 (4)	4 (4)	10 (4.3)
Cardiorespiratory arrest	6 (4)	2 (2)	10 (4.3)
Acute renal failure	9 (6)	1 (1)	8 (3.4)
Aspiration	4 (3)	1 (1)	5 (2.1)
Maternal death	1 (0.7)	0 0	1 (0.4)

COUNSELING WOMEN WHO HAVE HAD PREECLAMPSIA OR ECLAMPSIA

Byrans and colleagues, in a long-term follow-up study of women who had eclampsia, concluded that preeclampsia–eclampsia did not cause hypertensive disease and was not a manifestation of underlying essential hypertension.[95] Chesley and colleagues followed 187 eclamptic women.[96] They found no evidence to indicate that eclampsia causes hypertension and reported that the prognosis for future pregnancies after eclampsia was good. Sibai and colleagues found that primigravidas developing severe preeclampsia or eclampsia were at much higher risk of mild and severe preeclampsia in a subsequent pregnancy than women who remained normotensive in their first pregnancy.[97] This risk was particularly high if preeclampsia–eclampsia developed before 30 weeks. This study also showed that severe preeclampsia or eclampsia in a first pregnancy was associated with a significant incidence of subsequent chronic hypertension compared with normotensive first pregnancies.

The sisters and daughters of eclamptic and preeclamptic women are at increased risk of developing this disease. Sutherland and colleagues reported a 13.8% incidence of severe preeclampsia for women whose sisters had severe preeclampsia during their first pregnancy.[39] This compared with an incidence of only 4.5% in primigravidas whose sisters had no history of preeclampsia. The incidence of severe preeclampsia was also higher in primigravidas whose mothers had a history of severe preeclampsia compared with primigravidas who had no maternal history of preeclampsia. Chesley and colleagues reviewed the incidence of preeclampsia in the first pregnancies of daughters of eclamptic women.[96] Table 58-13 summarizes the outcome of these pregnancies.

Sibai and colleagues recommend that all pregnant women should be asked about a history of severe preeclampsia in their mothers or sisters. If this is positive, renal function should be determined early in pregnancy and antenatal visits should be increased to every 2 weeks from 28 weeks gestation. Patients with a history of preeclampsia or eclampsia occurring before 34 weeks are at significant risk of severe preeclampsia, eclampsia, and fetal growth retardation in a subsequent pregnancy. Weekly fetal–maternal monitoring is indicated from 28 weeks onward.

CHRONIC HYPERTENSION

Patients with hypertension secondary to renal disease, pheochromocytoma, endocrine disease, and coarctation of the aorta are relatively uncommon in pregnancy. Their management is that of the underlying disease. Most patients with chronic hypertension have essential hypertension, and the discussion that follows will be directed toward this group of patients. The presence of chronic hypertension in pregnancy increases maternal and perinatal morbidity and mortality.[98] Most of the morbidity and mortality is related to the development of superimposed preeclampsia and abruptio placentae. Maternal and fetal risk can be reduced by proper antepartum surveillance.

TABLE 59-13. THE RISK OF ECLAMPSIA IN RELATIVES OF WOMEN WITH ECLAMPSIA

RELATIONSHIP TO ECLAMPTIC WOMEN	NO. WITH PREGNANCIES >20 WEEKS	PRECLAMPSIA		ECLAMPSIA	
		N	%	*N*	%
Eclamptic women (all future pregnancies)	340	70	20.6	3	0.9
Sister (all future pregnancies)	147	54	37.6	6	4.1
Daughter (first pregnancy)	257	63	24.9	7	2.7
Daughter-in-law (first pregnancy)	75	6	8.0	—	—

From Villar MA, Sibai BM. Eclampsia. In: Arias F, ed. High risk pregnancy. Obstetrics and gynecology clinics of North America. Philadelphia: WB Saunders, 1988:373.

In the last decade, over 1000 pregnancies complicated by chronic hypertension have been delivered in Memphis. The following plan of management is based on this extensive experience. Ideally, patients with chronic hypertension should be seen before conception so that full investigation and assessment of their disease can be carried out and the potentially harmful effects of antihypertensive drugs can be discussed. The following evaluation should be initiated as soon as the patient attends for antepartum care:

- General physical examination, including funduscopy
- Measurement of blood pressure in four extremities
- Effect on blood pressure of changes in physical activity and posture.

Laboratory investigations should include:

- Urinalysis and culture, 24 hour-urine collection for protein, electrolytes, and creatinine clearance
- SMAC-20.

In selected patients antinuclear antibodies, urine catecholamines and vanillylmandelic acid (VMA), chest x-ray, and electrocardiogram are indicated.

On the basis of this assessment patients are classified as either high or low risk. Some of the factors that classify the patient as high risk are:

- Maternal age > 40 years
- Duration of hypertension > 15 years
- Blood pressure > 160/110 mm Hg early in pregnancy
- Diabetes (class B-F)
- Cardiomyopathy
- Renal disease
- Connective tissue disease.

Most patients are hospitalized at the time of their first prenatal visit. They are seen by a nutritionist and given dietary advice. Daily sodium intake should be restricted to 2 g. The harmful effects of smoking, stress, and caffeine on maternal blood pressure and fetal well-being are stressed and frequent rest periods are encouraged.

Patients are seen every 2 weeks up to 28 weeks and then weekly until delivery. At each visit systolic and diastolic blood pressure should be recorded and the urine tested for the presence of glucose and protein. Urine culture should be performed every trimester. Evaluation of maternal status includes serial measurements of hematocrit, serum creatinine, uric acid, creatinine clearance, and 24-hour urinary excretion of protein and sodium. Prompt hospitalization is indicated if there is an exacerbation of hypertension, development of pyelonephritis, significant proteinuria, or an elevation of uric acid. An elevation of uric acid > 6 mg/dL is often an early warning sign of superimposed preeclampsia.

Fetal evaluation includes serial ultrasound measurements of growth and antepartum fetal heart rate testing from 34 weeks. For those considered high risk, nonstress testing may commence as early as 26 weeks. Daily fetal-movement counts and biophysical profiles are also used in some patients to determine the optimum time for delivery.

Antihypertensive therapy is restricted to patients with severe hypertension. Diuretics are rarely used. Low-risk pregnancies are allowed to continue to 42 weeks gestation with close monitoring. High-risk pregnancies and patients receiving antihypertensive drugs are delivered at or before 40 weeks gestation. Superimposed preeclampsia or fetal growth retardation are considered indications for delivery, regardless of gestation. If preterm delivery is contemplated, amniocentesis is performed and steroids are administered if the L–S ratio indicates the fetal lung is immature.

Antihypertensive Therapy

There is considerable disagreement among obstetricians worldwide about antihypertensive therapy in pregnancy, particularly about what drugs are most appropriate and at what level of blood pressure treatment should be commenced. Maternal mortality associated with chronic hypertension in pregnancy is usually due to a malignant rise in blood pressure with subsequent congestive cardiac failure or cerebrovascular accidents. There is no evidence to suggest any maternal benefits from treating mild to moderate hypertension during pregnancy.[9] Treatment of severe hypertension, on the other hand, is associated with a reduction in maternal mortality and morbidity.[99] Fetal and perinatal outcome is closely linked to the incidence of superimposed preeclampsia and abruption. Antihypertensive therapy does not alter the incidence of these two complications and thus confers no perinatal benefit. The drugs most commonly used in pregnancy are adrenoreceptor blocking agents, thiazide diuretics, and hydralazine.

Adrenoreceptor Blocking Agents. Two classes of adrenoreceptors are recognized—alpha and beta. Alpha and beta receptors are subdivided into types 1 and 2 and into presynaptic or postsynaptic, according to their location at the adrenergic nerve terminals. The action and side effects of adrenoreceptor blocking agents depend on how selective the drug is for a particular receptor type. In addition, adrenoreceptors are located peripherally and centrally. Stimulation or blockade of the receptors at different sites will produce opposite effects.

Methyldopa. Methyldopa is the most commonly used antihypertensive agent worldwide. It acts by stimulating central $alpha_2$ receptors. It may also be an $alpha_2$ blocker acting by a false neurotransmitter effect. The drug is given orally with a loading dose of 1 g followed by maintenance therapy of 1 to 2 g daily in four divided doses. Peak plasma levels occur within 2 hours of an oral dose, and the fall in blood pressure is maximal 4 hours after tablet ingestion. Side effects include drowsiness and a dry mouth. Hepatitis, hemolytic anemia, and a positive Coomb's test have been reported in association with long-term usage.

Four independent controlled trials of treating hypertension in pregnancy have compared methyldopa with no medication. Leather and colleagues and Redman and colleagues reported an improved perinatal outcome (mainly due to a reduction in midtrimester loss) but no difference in the incidence of superimposed preeclampsia.[100,101] However, Arias and colleagues and Weitz and colleagues observed no reduction in perinatal mortality.[102,103] Gallery and colleagues and Fidler compared methyldopa with the beta blocker oxprenolol.[104,105] Gallery's study reported greater plasma volume expansion, greater neonatal weights, and improved perinatal outcome in the oxprenolol group. Fidler and colleagues found no difference in perinatal outcome or birth weight comparing the two drugs but observed a higher incidence of intrapartum fetal heart rate abnormalities in the oxprenolol group. Adverse perinatal effects of methyldopa remain unproved, and follow-up studies on infants exposed to methyldopa in utero have shown no untoward effects at the age of 7.5 years.[106]

Clonidine. Clonidine is a powerful $alpha_2$ central stimulant. The usual oral dose in pregnancy is 75 to 150 μg twice daily. Rebound hypertension has been reported following abrupt cessation of the drug. Horvath and colleagues compared clonidine and methyldopa in 100 pregnant women with hypertension at a mean gestation of 32 weeks.[107] There was no difference in perinatal outcome, and neither drug was associated with significant maternal or neonatal side effects. Horvath and colleagues concluded that clonidine was a safe and effective drug for treating hypertension in pregnancy.[107]

A variety of beta-blocking agents have been used to treat hypertension in pregnancy. These drugs have different actions, depending on their receptor selectivity and the presence of intrinsic sympathomimetic activity. Their use has been associated with neonatal bradycardia, hypoglycemia, fetal growth retardation, altered adaptation to perinatal asphyxia, and neonatal respiratory depression.[108] However, there is no evidence to suggest an increase in fetal or neonatal mortality or severe morbidity, and it is likely that most of these reported side effects are due to maternal disease rather than to a drug effect. Rubin reviewed the use of beta blockers in pregnancy and concluded that these agents are safe in pregnancy and in fact are associated with a better fetal outcome than either methyldopa or hydralazine.[109] It is difficult to compare the results of studies using beta blockers, since they usually involve heterogeneous groups of patients with both chronic hypertension and preeclampsia. Furthermore, beta blockers were often used in combination with other antihypertensive agents, and the blood pressure at the onset of treatment and the duration of therapy varied considerably.

Thiazide Diuretics. Although thiazide diuretics are commonly used to treat hypertension in the nonpregnant population, their role in pregnancy is highly controversial. If diuretic therapy is discontinued during pregnancy, additional hypertensive drugs are rarely required. Several harmful maternal and fetal effects of diuretics have been reported.[110] Gant and colleagues found that their short-term use in pregnancy was accompanied by a reduction in uteroplacental blood flow.[111] Sibai and colleagues observed a marked reduction in plasma volume in pregnant patients treated with diuretics compared with a control group receiving no medication.[73] Although this effect was reversed after discontinuing the diuretic therapy, plasma volume depletion is associated with a poor perinatal outcome: In view of their potential detrimental effects and no proven benefits, diuretics should be avoided in pregnancy.

Hydralazine. Hydralazine is the drug most commonly used to control severe hypertension in pregnancy. It is usually given as intermittent injections or as a continuous infusion. Hydralazine is a potent vasodilator, with its a peak hypotensive effect occurring 20 minutes after intravenous administration. Side effects include fluid retention, tachycardia, facial flushing, and headache. Chronic administration may be associated with a maternal lupus syndrome and neonatal thrombocytopenia. Oral hydralazine is a weak antihypertensive when used alone and is usually combined with methyldopa or a diuretic.

Calcium Channel Blockers. Calcium channel blockers have been used successfully to manage hypertension in non-pregnant patients. To date, there have been few studies relating to their use in human pregnancy. Allen and colleagues studied the acute effects of oral nitrendipine (20 mg) in 10 women with pregnancy-induced hypertension.[112] Blood pressure fell by 10–15 mm Hg within 1 hour and remained stable for 4 hours after medication. There were no significant fetal or maternal side effects. Nifedipine has been used in pregnancy both as a single agent[113] and as a second-line drug in combination with other antihypertensives.[114] Although these initial studies have suggested that nifedipine is an effective antihypertensive in pregnancy with few maternal side effects, further study is required to be certain of fetal safety and to determine whether this agent has any advantages over the antihypertensives in current use.

At present, it seems likely that methyldopa will remain the most widely used antihypertensive in pregnancy until another agent can be proved to be more beneficial, particularly in terms of improving fetal outcome.

Outcome

Chronic hypertension in pregnancy is usually associated with a good maternal and fetal outcome unless complicated by maternal renal disease or superimposed preeclampsia. Patients with mild "low-risk" chronic hypertension have a perinatal outcome similar to the general obstetric population. Antihypertensive therapy is often not required and the pregnancy can be safely prolonged to term.

Patients with severe "high-risk" chronic hypertension have a significant risk of fetal and maternal morbidity and perinatal mortality. Outcome is closely related to the development of superimposed preeclampsia. Sibai and Anderson studied the pregnancies of 44 women with severe hypertension in the first trimester.[115] Fifty-two percent developed superimposed preeclampsia. There were 10 stillbirths and one neonatal death. All the perinatal deaths occurred in the patients with superimposed preeclampsia. Patients with severe chronic hypertension in early pregnancy or underlying renal disease require early referral for antenatal care, intensive fetal and maternal monitoring as described earlier, and delivery in a tertiary care center. Antihypertensive therapy is indicated and should maintain blood pressure between 140 to 150 mm Hg systolic and 90 to 100 mm Hg diastolic. Persistent blood pressure levels below these ranges in patients who have previously been very hypertensive may jeopardize placental perfusion.

CONCLUSIONS AND PROSPECTS FOR THE FUTURE

Maternal morbidity and mortality related to preeclampsia are principally associated with eclampsia and HELLP syndrome. Fetal mortality and morbidity are associated mainly with midtrimester severe preeclampsia and preterm delivery. Greater understanding of the pathophysiology of preeclampsia is the key to improving both fetal and maternal outcome. In the present state of knowledge, patients with severe disease should be referred to a tertiary center with the experience and facilities to manage maternal complications and to provide intensive care for a preterm infant. In the future it may be possible to identify factors that clearly distinguish between pregnant women at low risk of developing hypertensive complications and those at high risk. This would allow rationalization of antenatal care and maternal–fetal monitoring. The ultimate goal is to be able to detect the disease in its early stages and to have available a therapy that either is curative or at least ameliorates progression and allows the fetus to reach maturity.

REFERENCES

1. Quilligan EJ, Little AB, Oh W. Pregnancy, birth and the infant. Washington, DC: US Department of Health and Human Services, Public Health Services, National Institutes of Health, 1981:11.
2. Department of Health and Social Security. Report on confidential inquiries into maternal deaths in England and Wales in 1979–81. London: HM Stationery Office, 1986.
3. Hughes EC, ed. Obstetric-gynecologic terminology. Philadelphia: FA Davis, 1972:442.
4. Schwartz R. The behaviour of the circulation in normal pregnancy. 1. Arterial blood pressure. Arch Gynaek 1964;199:549. Quoted by Hytten FE, Leitch I. In: The physiology of human pregnancy. 2nd ed. Oxford: Blackwell Scientific Publications, 1971.
5. MacGillivary I, Rose GA, Rowe D. Blood pressure survey in pregnancy. Clin Sci 1969;37:395.
6. Sibai BM. Pitfalls in the diagnosis and management of preeclampsia. Am J Obstet Gynecol 1988;159:1.
7. Murnaghan GA. Methods of measuring blood pressure and blood pressure variability. In: Sharp F, Symonds EM, eds. Hypertension in pregnancy. Ithaca, New York: Perinatalogy Press 1986:19.
8. Reiss RE, Tizzano TP, O'Shaughnessy RW. The blood pressure course in primiparous pregnancy. A prospective study of 383. J Reprod Med 1987;32:523.
9. Sibai BM, Abdella TN, Anderson GD. Pregnancy outcome in 211 patients with mild chronic hypertension. Obstet Gynecol 1983;61:571.
10. Robertson EG. The natural history of oedema during pregnancy. J Obstet Gynaecol Br Commonw 1967;74:1.
11. Vosburgh GJ. Blood pressure, edema and proteinuria in pregnancy. 5. Edema relationships. Prog Clin Biol Res 1976;7:155.
12. Sibai BM, McCubbin JH, Anderson GD, Lipshitz J, Dilts PV. Eclampsia 1. Observations from 67 recent cases. Obstet Gynecol 1981;58:609.
13. Villar MA, Sibai BM. Eclampsia. In: Arias F, ed. High risk pregnancy. Obstetrics and gynecology clinics of North America. Philadelphia: WB Saunders, 1988:355.
14. Sibai BM, Abdella TH, Taylor HA. Eclampsia in the first half of pregnancy. A report of three cases and review of the literature. J Reprod Med 1982;27:706.
15. Sibai BM, Schneider JM, Morrison JC, Lipshitz J, Anderson GD, Shier RW. The late postpartum eclampsia controversy. Obstet Gynecol 1980;55:74.
16. Weinstein L. Syndrome of hemolysis, elevated liver enzymes, and low platelet count: a severe consequence of hypertension in pregnancy. Am J Obstet Gynecol 1982;142:159.
17. Goodlin RC. Hemolysis, elevated liver enzymes, and low platelets syndrome. Obstet Gynecol 1984;64:499.
18. Sibai BM. Chronic hypertension during pregnancy. In: Sciarra JJ, ed. Gynecology and obstetrics. Philadelphia: JB Lippincott, 1988.
19. Nelson TR. A clinical study of pre-eclampsia. J Obstet Gynaecol Br Emp 1955;62:48.
20. Davey D, MacGillivary I. The classification and definition of the hypertensive disorders of pregnancy. Am J Obstet Gynecol 1988;158:892.
21. Ihle J, Long P, Oats J. Early onset preeclampsia—recognition of underlying renal disease. Br Med J 1987;294:78.
22. Lindheimer MD, Katz A. Current concepts: hypertension in pregnancy. N Engl J Med 1985;313:675.
23. Ylikorkala O, Makila U-M. Prostacyclin and thromboxane in gynecology and obstetrics. Am J Obstet Gynecol 1985;152:318.
24. Brinkman CR. Hypertensive disorders of pregnancy. In: Hacker NF, Moore JG, eds. Essentials of obstetrics and gynecology. Philadelphia: WB Saunders, 1986:125.
25. Lindheimer MD, Chesley LC, Taylor JR, Spargo BH, Katz AI. Renal function and morphology in the hypertensive disorders of pregnancy. In: Sharp F, Symonds EM, eds. Hypertension in pregnancy. Ithaca, New York: Perinatalogy Press, 1986:73.
26. Sheehan HL, Lynch JB. Pathology of toxaemia of pregnancy. London: Churchill Livingstone, 1973.
27. Brosens I, Robertson WB, Dixon HG. The physiological response to the vessels of the placental bed to normal pregnancy. J Pathol Bacteriol 1967;93:569.
28. Pijnenborg R, Bland JM, Robertson WB, Brosens I. Uteroplacental arterial changes related to interstitial trophoblast migration in early human pregnancy. Placenta 1983;4:397.

29. Brosens I, Robertson WB, Dixon HG. The role of the spiral arteries in the pathogenesis of pre-eclampsia. Obstet Gynecol Annu 1972;1:177.
30. Khong TY, De Wolf F, Robertson WB, Brosens I. Inadequate maternal vascular response to placentation in pregnancies complicated by pre-eclampsia and by small-for-gestational-age infants. Br J Obstet Gynaecol 1986;93:1049.
31. Walsh SW. Preeclampsia: an imbalance in placental prostacyclin and thromboxane production. Am J Obstet Gynecol 1985;152:335.
32. Makila UM, Viinikka L, Ylikorkala O. Increased thromboxane A_2 production but normal prostacyclin by the placenta in hypertensive pregnancies. Prostaglandins 1984;27:87.
33. Downing L, Shepherd GL, Lewis PJ. Reduced prostacyclin production in pre-eclampsia. Lancet 1980;2:1374.
34. Fitzgerald DJ, Entman SS, Mulloy K, Fitzgerald GA. Decreased prostacyclin biosynthesis preceding the clinical manifestations of pregnancy-induced hypertension. Circulation 1987;75:956.
35. Goodman RP, Killam AP, Brash AR, Branch RA. Prostacyclin production during pregnancy: a comparison of production during normal pregnancy and pregnancy complicated by hypertension. Am J Obstet Gynecol 1982;142:817.
36. Shephard GL, Lewis PJ, deMey C, Blair IA, MacDermot J. Platelet prostacyclin receptors in pregnancy. In: Lewis PJ, Moncada S, O'Grady J, eds. Prostacyclin in pregnancy. New York: Raven Press, 1983:199.
37. Saleh AA, Bottoms SF, Welch RA, Abdelkarim AM, Mariona FG, Mammen EF. Preeclampsia, delivery and the hemostatic system. Am J Obstet Gynecol 1987;157:331.
38. Chesley LC, Cooper DW. Genetics of hypertension in pregnancy: possible single gene control of pre-eclampsia and eclampsia in the descendants of eclamptic women. Br J Obstet Gynaecol 1986;93:898.
39. Sutherland A, Cooper DW, Howie PW, Liston WA, MacGillivary I. The incidence of severe pre-eclampsia amongst mothers and mothers-in-law of pre-eclamptics and controls. Br J Obstet Gynaecol 1981;88:785.
40. Redman CWG, Bodmer JG, Bodmer WF, Beilin LJ, Bonnat J. HLA anitgens in severe pre-eclampsia. Lancet 1978;2:397.
41. Jenkins DM, Need JA, Scott JS, Morris H, Pepper M. Human leucocyte antigens and mixed lymphocyte reaction in severe pre-eclampsia. Br Med J 1978;1:542.
42. Toivanen P, Hirvonen T. Sex ratio of newborns: preponderance of males in toxemia of pregnancy. Science 1970;170:187.
43. Liston WA. Genetic factors and longterm prognosis. In: Sharp F, Symonds EM, eds. Hypertension in pregnancy. Ithaca, New York: Perinatalogy Press, 1986:51.
44. Cooper DW, Hill JA, Chesley LC, Bryans Cl. Genetic control of susceptibility to eclampsia and miscarriage. Br J Obstet Gynaecol 1988;95:644.
45. Boyd PA, Lindenbaum RH, Redman C. Pre-eclampsia and trisomy 13. Lancet 1987;2:794.
46. Stirrat GM. The immunology of hypertension in pregnancy. In: Sharp F, Symonds EM, eds. Hypertension in pregnancy. Ithaca, New York: Perinatalogy Press, 1986:249.
47. Nolten WE, Ehrlich EN. Sodium and mineralocorticoids in normal pregnancy. Kidney Int 1980;18:162.
48. Talledo OE. Renin-angiotensin system in normal and toxemic pregnancies. I. Angiotensin infusion test. Am J Obstet Gynecol 1966;96:141.
49. Gant NF, Daley GL, Chand S, Whalley PJ, MacDonald PC. A study of angiotensin II pressor response throughout primigravid pregnancy. J Clin Invest 1973;52:2682.
50. Everett RB, Worley RJ, MacDonald PC, Gant NF. Effect of prostaglandin synthetase inhibitors on pressor response to angiotensin II in human pregnancy. J Clin Endocrinol Metab 1978;46:1007.
51. Broughton Pipkin F, Hunter JC, Turner SR, O'Brien PMS. Prostaglandin E_2 attenuates the pressor response to angiotensin II in pregnant, but not non-pregnant humans. Am J Obstet Gynecol 1982;142:168.
52. Broughton Pipkin F, Hunter JC, Turner SR, O'Brien PMS. The effect of prostaglandin E_2 upon the biochemical response to infused angiotensin II in human pregnancy. Clin Sci 1984;66:399.
53. Sibai BM, Spinnato JA, Watson DL, Lewis JA, Anderson GD. Eclampsia IV. Neurological findings and future outcome. Am J Obstet Gynecol 1985;152:184.
54. Chesley LC, Sibai BM. Clinical significance of elevated mean arterial pressure in the second trimester. Am J Obstet Gynecol 1988;159:275.
55. Gant NF, Chand S, Worley RJ, Whalley PJ, Crosby UD, MacDonald PC. A clinical test useful for predicting the development of acute hypertension of pregnancy. Am J Obstet Gynecol 1974;120:1.
56. Kuntz WD. Supine pressor (roll-over) test: an evaluation. Am J Obstet Gynecol 1980;1367:764.
57. Nakamura T, Masaharu I, Matsui K, Yoshimura T, Kawasaki N, Maeyama M. Significance of angiotensin sensitivity test for prediction of pregnancy-induced hypertension. Obstet Gynecol 1986;67:388.
58. Worley RL, Everett RB, Madden JD. Fetal considerations. Metabolic clearance rate of maternal plasma dehydroepandrosterone sulfate. Semin Perinatol 1979;2:15.
59. Lunell NO, Nylund L, Lewander R, Sardy B. Uteroplacental blood flow in preeclampsia. Clin Exp Hypertens 1982;B1:105.
60. Gerretsen G, Huisjes HJ, Elema JD. Morphological changes of the spiral arteries in the placental bed in relation to pre-eclampsia and fetal growth retardation. Br J Obstet Gynaecol 1981;88:876.
61. Campbell S, Pearce JMF, Hackett G, Cohen-Overbeck T, Hernandez CJ. Qualitative assessment of uteroplacental blood flow: an early screening test for high risk pregnancies. Obstet Gynecol 1986;68:649.
62. Steel SA, Pearce MJ, Chamberlain G. Doppler ultrasound of the uteroplacental circulation as a screening test for severe pre-eclampsia with intrauterine growth retardation. Eur J Obstet Gynecol Rep Biol 1988;28:279.
63. Collins R, Yusuf S, Peto R. Overview of randomized trials of diuretics in pregnancy. Br Med J 1985;290:17.
64. Kawasaki N, Matsui K, Masaharu I, Nakamura T, Yoshimura T, Hidetaka U. Effect of calcium supplementation on the vascular sensitivity to angiotensin II in pregnant women. Am J Obstet Gynaecol 1985;153:576.
65. Villar J, Repke J, Belizan J, Pareja G. Calcium supplementation reduced blood pressure during pregnancy: results from a randomized controlled trial. Obstet Gynecol 1987;70:317.
66. Heavey DL, Barrow SE, Hickling ME, Ritter JM. Aspirin causes short-lived inhibition of bradykinin-stimulated prostacyclin production in man. Nature 1984;318:186.
67. Beaufils M, Uzan S, Donsimoni R, Colau JC. Prevention of pre-eclampsia by early anti-platelet therapy. Lancet 1985;1:840.
68. Wallenburg HCS, Dekker GA, Makovitz JW, Rotmans P. Low dose aspirin prevents pregnancy induced hypertension and pre-eclampsia in angiotensin sensitive primigravidae. Lancet 1986;1:1.
69. Gilstrap LC, Cunningham FG, Whalley PJ. Management of pregnancy-induced hypertension in the nulliparous patients remote from term. Semin Perinatol 1978;1:73.
70. Rubin PC, Clark DM, Sumner DJ, Steedman D, Low RA, Reid

JL. Placebo controlled trial of atenolol in treatment of pregnancy associated hypertension. Lancet 1983;1:413.
71. Walker JJ, Crooks A, Erwin L, Calder AA. Labetalol in pregnancy induced hypertension: fetal and maternal effects. In: Riley A, Symonds EM, eds. The investigation of labetalol in the management of hypertension in pregnancy. Proceedings of Symposium No 591. International Congress Series, Excerpta Medica, 1982:148.
72. Sibai BM, Gonazalez AR, Mabie WC, Moretti M. A comparison of labetalol plus hospitalization versus hospitalization alone in the management of preeclampsia remote from term. Obstet Gynecol 1987;70:323.
73. Sibai BM, Abdella TN, Anderson GD, Dilts PV. Plasma volume findings in pregnant women with mild hypertension. Am J Obstet Gynecol 1983;145:539.
74. McRae RP, Liebson PR. Hypertensive crisis. Med Clin North Am 1986;70:749.
75. Stallworth JC, Yeh SY, Petrie RH. The effect of magnesium sulfate on fetal heart rate variability and uterine activity. Am J Obstet Gynecol 1981;140:702.
76. Lipsitz PJ. The clinical and biochemical effects of excess magnesium in the newborn. Pediatrics 1971;47:501.
77. Dinsdale HB. Does magnesium sulfate treat eclamptic seizures? Yes. Arch Neurol 1988;45:1360.
78. Kaplan PW, Fisher RS. No, magnesium sulfate should not be used in treating eclamptic seizures. Arch Neurol 1988;45:1361.
79. Slater RM, Smith WD, Patrick J, et al. Phenytoin infusion in severe preeclampsia. Lancet 1987;1:1417.
80. Jones MM, Joyce T. Anesthesia for the parturient with pregnancy induced hypertension. Clin Obstet Gynecol 1987;30:591.
81. Sibai BM, Spinnato JA, Watson DL, Hill GA, Anderson GD. Pregnancy outcome in 303 cases with severe preeclampsia. Obstet Gynecol 1984;64:319.
82. Sibai BM, Taslimi M, Abdella T, Brooks TF, Spinnato JA, Anderson GD. Maternal and perinatal outcome of conservative management of severe preeclampsia in midtrimester. Am J Obstet Gynecol 1985;152:32.
83. Sibai BM, Taslimi MM, El-Nazer A, Amon E, Mabie WC, Ryan G. Maternal-perinatal outcome associated with the syndrome of hemolysis, elevated liver enzymes, and low platelets in severe preeclampsia-eclampsia. Am J Obstet Gynecol 1986;155:501.
84. Goodlin RC. Beware the great imitator—severe preeclampsia. Contemp Obstet Gynecol 1984;20:215.
85. Killam AP, Dillard SH, Patton RC, Pederson PR. Pregnancy-induced hypertension complicated by acute liver disease and disseminated intravascular coagulation. Am J Obstet Gynecol 1975;123:823.
86. MacKenna J, Dover NL, Brame RG. Preeclampsia associated with hemolysis, elevated liver enzymes and low platelets—an obstetric emergency? Obstet Gynecol 1983;62:751.
87. Van Dam PA, Renier M, Baekelandt M, Buytaert P, Uyttenbroeck F. Disseminated intravascular coagulation and the syndrome of hemolysis, elevated liver enzymes and low platelets in severe preeclampsia. Obstet Gynecol 1989;73:97.
88. Zuspan FP. Problems encountered in the treatment of pregnancy induced hypertension. Am J Obstet Gynecol 1978; 131:591.
89. Campbell DM, Templeton AA. Is eclampsia preventable? In: Bonnar J, MacGillivary EM, Symonds EM, eds. Pregnancy hypertension. Baltimore: University Park Press, 1980:483.
90. Paul RH, Koh KS, Bernstein SG. Changes in fetal heart rate–uterine contraction patterns associated with eclampsia. Am J Obstet Gynecol 1978;130:165.
91. Sibai BM, Anderson GD, Abdulla TN, McCubbin JH, Dilts PV. Eclampsia III. Neonatal outcome, growth and development. Am J Obstet Gynecol 1983;146:307.
92. Hankins GDV, Wendel GD, Cunningham FG, Leveno KJ. Longitudinal evaluation of hemodynamic changes in eclampsia. Am J Obstet Gynecol 1984;150:506.
93. Lopez-Llera M, Linares GR, Horta JL. Maternal mortality rates in eclampsia. Am J Obstet Gynecol 1976;124:149.
94. Brazy JE, Grimm JK, Little VA. Neonatal manifestations of severe maternal hypertension occurring before the thirty-sixth week of pregnancy. J Pediatr 1982;100:165.
95. Byrans Cl, Southerland WL, Zuspan FP. Eclampsia: a long-term follow-up study. Obstet Gynecol 1963;21:6.
96. Chesley LC, Cosgrove RA, Annitto JE. A followup study of eclamptic women. Am J Obstet Gynecol 1962;83:1360.
97. Sibai BM, El-Nazer A, Gonzalez-Ruiz AR. Severe preeclampsia-eclampsia in young primigravidas: subsequent pregnancy outcome and remote prognosis. Am J Obstet Gynecol 1986; 155:1011.
98. Page EW, Christianson R. The impact of mean arterial pressure in the middle trimester upon the outcomes of pregnancy. Am J Obstet Gynecol 1975;125:740.
99. Redman CWG. Treatment of hypertension in pregnancy. Kidney Int 1980;18:267.
100. Leather HM, Humphreys DM, Baker PB, Chadd MA. A controlled trial of hypertensive agents in hypertension in pregnancy. Lancet 1968;1:488.
101. Redman CWG, Beilin LJ, Bonnar J, Ounsted MK. Fetal outcome in a trial of antihypertensive treatment in pregnancy. Lancet 1976;2:753.
102. Arias F, Zamora J. Antihypertensive treatment and pregnancy outcome in patients with mild chronic hypertension. Obstet Gynecol 1979;53:489.
103. Weitz C, Khauzami V, Maxwell K, Johnson J. Treatment of hypertension in pregnancy with methyldopa: a randomized double blind study. Int J Gynecol Obstet 1987;25:35.
104. Gallery EDM, Saunders DM, Hunyor SN, Gyory AZ. Randomized comparison of methyldopa and oxyprenolol for treatment of hypertension in pregnancy. Br Med J 1979;1:1591.
105. Fidler J, Smith V, Fayers P, De Swiet M. Randomized controlled comparative study of methyldopa and oxyprenolol in treatment of hypertension in pregnancy. Br Med J 1983;286:1927.
106. Cockburn J, Ounsted M, Moar VA, Redman CWG. Final report of study on hypertension during pregnancy: the effects of specific treatment on the growth and development of the children. Lancet 1982;1:647.
107. Horvath JS, Phippard A, Korda A, Henderson-Smart, Child A, Tiller DJ. Clonidine hydrochloride: a safe and effective antihypertensive agent in pregnancy. Obstet Gynecol 1985;66:634.
108. Court DJ, Parer JT. Ob risks and benefits of propranolol and other beta blockers. Contemp Obstet 1984;20:179.
109. Rubin PC. Beta-blockers in pregnancy. N Engl J Med 1981;305:1323.
110. Berkowitz RL. Antihypertensive drugs in the pregnant patient. Obstet Gynecol Surv 1980;35:191.
111. Gant NF, Madden JD, Siiteri PK, MacDonald PC. The metabolic clearance rate of dehydroisandrosterone sulfate. Am J Obstet Gynecol 1975;123:159.
112. Allen J, Maigaard S, Forman A, et al. Acute effects of nitrendipine in pregnancy-induced hypertension. Br J Obstet Gynecol 1987;94:222.
113. Walters BNJ, Redman CWG. Treatment of severe pregnancy-associated hypertension with the calcium antagonist nifedipine. Br J Obstet Gynecol 1984;91:330.
114. Constantine G, Beevers DG, Reynolds AL, Tuesley DM. Nifedipine as a second line antihypertensive drug in pregnancy. Br J Obstet Gynecol 1987;94:1136.
115. Sibai BM, Anderson GD. Pregnancy outcome of intensive therapy in severe hypertension in first trimester. Obstet Gynaecol 1986;67:517.

59

CHAPTER

CARDIAC DISEASE IN PREGNANCY

Steven L. Clark

Pregnancy causes many significant alterations in the maternal cardiovascular system. The pregnant patient with normal cardiac function accommodates these physiologic changes without difficulty. However, in the presence of significant cardiac disease, pregnancy may be extremely hazardous, resulting in decompensation and even death. Despite advances in the diagnosis and treatment of maternal cardiovascular disease, such conditions remain a significant cause of non-obstetric maternal deaths, even in Western countries.[1] This chapter will focus on the interaction between structural cardiac disease and pregnancy.

COUNSELING THE PREGNANT CARDIAC PATIENT

Prior to 1973, the Criteria Committee of the New York Heart Association recommended a classification of cardiac disease based on clinical function (classes I to IV). Although such a classification was useful in discussing the pregnant cardiac patient, up to 40% of patients developing congestive heart failure and pulmonary edema during pregnancy were functional class I prior to pregnancy, and in one review, the majority of maternal deaths during pregnancy occurred in patients who were initially class I or II.[2] Today the older functional classification has been replaced by a more complex descriptive system encompassing etiological, anatomical, and physiologic diagnosis.[3] Despite this reclassification, the functional classification remains useful when comparing the performance of individuals with uniform etiological and anatomical diagnosis.[4] Counseling the pregnant cardiac patient regarding her prognosis for successful pregnancy is further complicated by recent advances in medical and surgical therapy, fetal surveillance, and neonatal care. Such advances render invalid many older estimates of maternal mortality and fetal wastage.

Table 59-1 represents a synthesis of current maternal mortality estimates for various types of cardiac disease. Counseling of the pregnant cardiac patient and general management approaches are based on this classification.[5] Category I includes conditions that, with proper management, should have negligible maternal mortality (<1%). Cardiac lesions in category II carry with them a 5% to 15% risk of maternal mortality; in individual cases, and after appropriate counseling, this risk may prove acceptable to some women. Patients with cardiac lesions in group III are subject to a mortality risk exceeding 25%. In all but exceptional cases, this risk will prove unacceptable to the patient, and prevention or interruption of pregnancy should be recommended strongly. When the severity of disease is in question, the measurement of oxygen consumption during exercise has been suggested as an indicator of functional reserve.[6] When pulmonary hypertension is suspected, pulmonary artery catheterization and assessment of pulmonary artery pressures may allow more precise counseling either prior to conception or early in pregnancy.

CONGENITAL CARDIAC DISEASE

The relative frequency of congenital as opposed to acquired heart disease is changing.[2,4] Rheumatic fever is uncommon in the United States, and more patients with congenital cardiac disease now survive to reproductive age. In a review in 1954, the ratio of rheumatic to congenital heart disease seen during pregnancy was 16:1; by 1967, this ratio had changed to 3:1.[7,8] In the subsequent discussion of specific cardiac lesions, no attempt will be made to duplicate existing comprehensive texts regarding physical diagnostic, electrocardiographic, and radiographic findings of specific cardiac lesions. (For a comprehensive discussion of diagnostic findings, see Braunwald E, ed. Heart disease: a textbook of cardiovascular medicine. 2nd ed. Philadelphia: WB

TABLE 59–1. MORTALITY RISK ASSOCIATED WITH PREGNANCY

Group I: Mortality < 1%
Atrial septal defect*
Ventricular septal defect*
Patent ductus arteriosus*
Pulmonic–tricuspid disease
Corrected tetralogy of Fallot
Bioprosthetic valve
Mitral stenosis, NYHA classes I and II
Group II: Mortality 5% to 15%
Mitral stenosis with atrial fibrillation
Artificial valve
Mitral stenosis, NYHA classes III and IV
Aortic stenosis
Coarctation of aorta, uncomplicated
Uncorrected tetralogy of Fallot
Previous myocardial infarction
Marfan syndrome with normal aorta
Group III: Mortality 25% to 50%
Pulmonary hypertension
Coarctation of aorta, complicated
Marfan syndrome with aortic involvement

From Clark SL, ed. Critical care obstetrics. Oradell, NJ: Medical Economics Books, 1987.
* Uncomplicated.

Saunders, 1984.) Instead the discussion here will focus on aspects of cardiac disease that are unique to pregnancy.

ATRIAL SEPTAL DEFECT

Atrial septal defect (ASD) is the most common congenital lesion seen during pregnancy and is generally asymptomatic.[9–11] The two significant potential complications seen with ASD are arrhythmias and heart failure. Although atrial arrhythmias are not uncommon in patients with ASD, their onset generally occurs after the fourth decade of life. Thus, such arrhythmias are unlikely to be encountered in the pregnant woman. In patients with ASD, atrial fibrillation is the most common arrhythmia encountered; however, supraventricular tachycardia and atrial flutter also may occur.[12] Initial therapy is with digoxin; less commonly, propranolol, quinidine, or even cardioversion may be necessary. The hypervolemia associated with pregnancy results in an increased left-to-right shunt through the ASD, and thus a significant burden is imposed on the right ventricle. Although this additional burden is tolerated well by most patients, congestive failure and death with ASD have been reported.[13–16] In contrast to the high-pressure–high-flow state seen with ventricular septal defect (VSD) and patent ductus arteriosus (PDA), ASD is characterized by high pulmonary blood flow associated with normal pulmonary artery pressures. Because pulmonary artery pressures are low, pulmonary hypertension is unusual. The vast majority of patients with ASD tolerate pregnancy, labor, and delivery without complication. Neilson and colleagues reported 70 pregnancies in 24 patients with ASD; all patients had an uncomplicated ante- and intrapartum course.[13] During labor, avoidance of fluid overload, oxygen administration, labor in the lateral recumbent position, and pain relief with epidural anesthesia, as well as prophylaxis against bacterial endocarditis, are the most important considerations (Tables 59-2 and 59-3).

TABLE 59–2. PATIENTS AT HIGH RISK FOR BACTERIAL ENDOCARDITIS

Prosthetic heart valves (including bioprostheses)
Most congenital cardiac malformations
Surgical systemic–pulmonary shunts
Rheumatic and other acquired valvular dysfunction
Idiopathic hypertrophic subaortic stenosis (IHSS)
Previous history of bacterial endocarditis
Mitral valve prolapse with insufficiency

VENTRICULAR SEPTAL DEFECT

Ventricular septal defect (VSD) may occur as an isolated lesion, or in conjunction with other congenital cardiac anomalies, including tetralogy of Fallot, transposition of the great vessels, and coarctation of the aorta. The size of the septal defect is the most important determinant of clinical prognosis during pregnancy. Small defects are tolerated well, whereas larger defects are associated more frequently with congestive failure, arrhythmias, or the development of pulmonary hypertension. In addition, a large VSD often is associated with some degree of aortic regurgitation, which may add to the risk of congestive failure. Pregnancy, labor, and delivery generally are tolerated well by patients with uncomplicated VSD.[16] Schaefer and colleagues compiled a series of 141 pregnancies in 56 women with VSD.[14] The only two maternal deaths were in women whose VSD was complicated by pulmonary hypertension (Eisenmenger syndrome). Although very rarely indicated, successful primary closure of a large VSD during pregnancy has been reported.[17] Intrapartum management considerations for patients with uncomplicated VSD or PDA are similar to those outlined for

TABLE 59–3. BACTERIAL ENDOCARDITIS PROPHYLAXIS*

I.	Ampicillin 2 g/IV
	plus
	Gentamicin 1.5 mg/kg/IM or IV
II.†	Vancomycin 1 g/IV
	plus
	Gentamicin 1.5 mg/kg/IM or IV

* Administer 0.5 to 1 hour prior to delivery. May be repeated 8 hours later.
† For patients allergic to penicillin.
From Clark SL, ed. Critical care obstetrics. Oradell, NJ: Medical Economics Books, 1987, with permission.

ASD. In general, invasive hemodynamic monitoring is unnecessary. Management considerations for patients with uncomplicated VSD, without pulmonary hypertension, are similar to those outlined for ASP.

PATENT DUCTUS ARTERIOSUS

Although patent ductus arteriosus (PDA) is one of the most common congenital cardiac anomalies, its almost universal detection and closure in the newborn period make it uncommon during pregnancy.[18,19] As with uncomplicated ASD and VSD, most patients are asymptomatic, and PDA is generally tolerated well during pregnancy, labor, and delivery. As with a large VSD, however, the high-pressure–high-flow left-to-right shunt associated with a large, uncorrected PDA can lead to pulmonary hypertension. In such cases, the prognosis becomes much worse. In one study, of 18 pregnant women who died of congenital heart disease, three had PDA; however, all these patients had secondary severe pulmonary hypertension.[15] Management considerations for patients with uncomplicated PDA, without pulmonary hypertension, are similar to those outlined under ASD.

EISENMENGER SYNDROME

Eisenmenger syndrome develops when, in the presence of congenital left-to-right shunt, progressive pulmonary hypertension leads to shunt reversal or bidirectional shunting. Although this syndrome may occur with ASD, VSD, or PDA, the low-pressure–high-flow shunt seen as ASD is far less likely to result in pulmonary hypertension and shunt reversal than is the condition of high-pressure and high-flow symptoms seen with the VSD and PDA. Whatever the etiology, pulmonary hypertension carries a grave prognosis during pregnancy. During the antepartum period, the decreased systemic vascular resistance associated with pregnancy increases the likelihood or degree of right-to-left shunting. Pulmonary perfusion then decreases; this decrease results in hypoxemia and deterioration of maternal and fetal condition. In such a patient, systemic hypotension leads to decreased right ventricular filling pressures. In the presence of fixed pulmonary hypertension, such decreased right heart pressures may be insufficient to perfuse the pulmonary arterial bed. This insufficiency may result in sudden, profound hypoxemia. Such hypotension can result from hemorrhage or complications of conduction anesthesia and may result in sudden death.[20–23] Avoidance of such hypotension is the principal clinical concern in the intrapartum management of patients with pulmonary hypertension of any etiology.

Maternal mortality in the presence of Eisenmenger syndrome is reported as 30% to 50%.[21,22] In a review of the subject, Gleicher and colleagues reported a 34% mortality associated with vaginal delivery and a 75% mortality associated with cesarean section.[21] Eisenmenger syndrome associated with VSD appears to carry a higher mortality risk (65%) than that associated with PDA or ASD (33%). In addition to the previously discussed problems associated with hemorrhage and hypovolemia, thromboembolic phenomena have been associated with up to 43% of all maternal deaths in Eisenmenger syndrome.[21] However, Pitts and colleagues reported an increased mortality associated with prophylactic peripartum heparinization.[24] Sudden delayed postpartum death, occurring 4 to 6 weeks after delivery, also has been reported.[21,25] Such deaths may involve a rebound worsening of pulmonary hypertension associated with the loss of pregnancy- associated hormones.

Because of the high mortality associated with continuing pregnancy, abortion is the preferred management of choice for the woman with pulmonary hypertension of any etiology. Therapeutic abortion in either the first or second trimester appears to be safer than allowing the pregnancy to progress to term.[6] Dilatation and curettage in the first trimester or dilatation and evacuation in the second trimester is the method of choice. Hypertonic saline and F-series prostaglandins are contraindicated. Although E-series prostaglandins may be safer from a theoretical standpoint, the safety of such agents in clinical practice has yet to be documented. For the patient with a continuing gestation, hospitalization for the duration of pregnancy is often appropriate. Continuous administration of oxygen, the pulmonary vasodilator of choice, is mandatory and may improve perinatal outcome. In cyanotic heart disease of any etiology, fetal outcome correlates well with maternal hematocrit, and successful pregnancy is unlikely with a hematocrit > 65%.[26] Maternal paO_2 should be maintained at a level of 60 to 70 mm Hg or above.[27] Third-trimester fetal surveillance with antepartum testing is important because at least 30% of the fetuses will be growth retarded.[21] Overall fetal wastage with Eisenmenger syndrome is reported to be up to 75%.

Pulmonary artery catheterization is recommended during the intrapartum period. Placement and maintenance of the pulmonary artery catheter often are difficult in the presence of pulmonary hypertension. In such cases, we have successfully used a catheter with an accessory lumen. Following placement, a guidewire is introduced to provide the necessary rigidity to maintain the catheter in place. In a number of cases, simultaneous cardiac imaging with ultrasound also has been helpful in catheter placement. If the possibility of right-to-left shunting exists, balloon inflation with carbon dioxide is preferable to that with air, to avoid systemic air embolus associated with occasional balloon rupture. During labor, uterine contractions are associated with a decrease in the ratio of pulmonary to systemic blood flow (Qp/Qs).[28] Pulmonary artery catheterization and serial arterial blood gas determinations allow the clinician to detect and treat early changes in cardiac output, pulmonary artery pressure, and shunt fraction. We have used a fiberoptic pulmonary artery catheter in conjunction with an oximeter to detect early changes in mixed venous oxygen saturation during the successful intrapartum management of patients with pulmonary hypertension. Because the primary concern in such patients is the avoidance of hypotension, any attempt to preload reduction (ie, diuresis) must be undertaken with great caution, even in the face of initial fluid overload. We prefer to manage such patients on the "wet" side, maintaining a preload margin of safety against unexpected blood loss, even at the expense of some degree of pulmonary edema.[29]

Anesthesia for patients with pulmonary hypertension is controversial. Theoretically, conduction anesthesia, with its accompanying risk of hypotension, should be avoided. However, there are several reports of its successful use in patients with pulmonary hypertension of different etiologies.[28,30] The use of epidural or intrathecal morphine sulfate, a technique devoid of effect on systemic blood pressure, has been described by Aboud and colleagues and represents perhaps the best approach to anesthetic management of these difficult patients.[31]

Bedrest and the administration of oxygen to maintain a PO_2 of more than 60 mm Hg are essential during the antepartum period. Fetal assessment with serial ultrasound examinations and antepartum fetal heart rate assessment are also important. Careful monitoring of maternal oxygenation and symptoms is essential to detect clinical deterioration. At times, such deterioration may respond to hospitalization and increased concentrations of oxygen. At other times, however, a worsening maternal cardiovascular status may mandate delivery even prior to term.

Ideally, if the patient has reached a point where fetal pulmonary maturity can be documented and the cervix is favorable for induction, she would be admitted to the hospital the night prior to induction. Pulmonary artery catheterization should be performed to optimize hemodynamics prior to the initiation of labor. Because decreased cardiac output will be most hazardous for such patients, an attempt is made to maintain a high cardiac output and wedge pressure, even at the risk of incurring some pulmonary edema. A recommended therapeutic goal would be to maintain a wedge pressure in the 16- to 18-mm Hg range. Any hemodynamic manipulation must be carried out with careful attention to cardiac output, blood pressure, and other maternal cardiovascular indices. A patient should labor on her side with both continuous administration of oxygen and continuous electronic fetal heart rate monitoring. Narcotic epidural anesthesia is the anesthetic method of choice for pain relief during labor and delivery and, if necessary, cesarean section. Because of the increased risk of significant blood loss and hypotension associated with operative delivery, cesarean section should be reserved exclusively for obstetric indications. Similarly, midforceps delivery is not warranted to shorten the second stage but should be reserved for standard obstetric indications only.

If surgery is necessary, meticulous attention to hemostasis and surgical technique with an experienced surgical team will serve to minimize the risk of blood loss, hypotension, and death in these patients. Despite expert management, a substantial risk of maternal mortality remains during labor and delivery.

A significant portion of pregnancy-associated deaths in patients with pulmonary hypertension is associated with thromboembolic phenomenon. Although prophylactic heparinization might be considered, the only study examining this issue showed an increased risk of maternal mortality associated with prophylactic anticoagulation. However, this study was performed before the advent of modern techniques for management of such patients. Thus, the use of prophylactic anticoagulation for patients with pulmonary hypertension remains controversial.

Sudden postpartum cardiovascular deterioration and death are not unusual in the first 2 to 4 weeks postpartum in patients with pulmonary hypertension. Although it has been suggested that prolonged hospitalization or observation in an intensive care unit may allow the clinician to detect and treat this condition early, no evidence exists in the literature to suggest that prolonged hospitalization or any other therapeutic maneuver can prevent the occurrence of sudden postpartum death in patients with pulmonary hypertension.

COARCTATION OF THE AORTA

Coarctation of the aorta accounts for approximately 9% of all congenital cardiac disease.[32] The most common site of coarctation is the origin of the left subclavian artery. Associated anomalies of the aorta and left heart, including VSD and PDA, are common, as are intracranial aneurysms in the Circle of Willis.[33] Coarctation is usually asymptomatic. Its presence is suggested by hypertension confined to the upper extremities, although Goodwin cites data suggesting a generalized increase in peripheral resistance throughout the body.[32] Resting cardiac output may be increased; however, increased left atrial pressure with exercise suggests occult left ventricular dysfunction. Aneurysms also may develop below the coarctation, or involve the intercostal arteries, and may lead to rupture. In addition, ruptures without prior aneurysm formation have been reported.[34]

Over 400 patients with coarctation have been reported during pregnancy, with maternal mortality ranging from none to 17%.[14,34–36] Half of the fatalities occur during the first pregnancy. In a review of 200 pregnant women with coarctation of the aorta before 1940, Mendelson reported 14 maternal deaths and recommended routine abortion and sterilization of these patients.[37] Deaths in this series were from aortic dissection and rupture, congestive heart failure, cerebrovascular accidents, and bacterial endocarditis. Six of the 14 deaths occurred in women with associated lesions. In contrast to this dismal prognosis, a more recent series by Deal and Wooley reported 83 pregnancies in 23 women with uncomplicated coarctation of the aorta.[35] All were NYHA class I or II prior to pregnancy. In these women, there were no maternal deaths or permanent cardiovascular complications. In one review, aortic rupture was more likely to occur in the third trimester, prior to labor and delivery.[38] Thus, it appears that today patients having coarctation of the aorta uncomplicated by aneurysmal dilatation or associated cardiac lesions who enter pregnancy as class I or II have a good prognosis and a minimal risk of complications or death. Even if uncorrected, uncomplicated coarctation carries with it a risk of maternal mortality of only 3% to 4%.[32] Maternal risk is increased if preeclampsia develops.[4] In the presence of aortic or intervertebral aneurysm, known aneurysm of the circle of Willis, or associated cardiac lesions, however, the risk of death may approach 15%; therefore, therapeutic abortion must be strongly considered.[5]

TETRALOGY OF FALLOT

Tetralogy of Fallot refers to the cyanotic complex of VSD, overriding aorta, right ventricular hypertrophy, and pulmonary stenosis. Most cases of tetralogy of Fallot are corrected during infancy or childhood. Several published reports attest to the relatively good outcome of pregnancy in patients with corrected tetralogy of Fallot.[4,39–41] In a review of 55 pregnancies in 46 patients, there were no maternal deaths among nine patients with correction prior to pregnancy. However, in patients with an uncorrected lesion, maternal mortality ranges from 4% to 15%, with a 30% fetal mortality due to hypoxia.[4,40] In patients with uncorrected VSD, the decline in SVR that accompanies pregnancy can lead to worsening of the right-to-left shunt.[4] This condition can be aggravated further by systemic hypotension as a result of peripartum blood loss. A poor prognosis has been related to prepregnancy hematocrit exceeding 65%, history of syncope or congestive failure, electrocardiographic evidence of right ventricular strain, cardiomegaly, right ventricular pressure in excess of 120 mm Hg, and peripheral oxygen saturation below 80%.[39]

PULMONIC STENOSIS

Pulmonic stenosis is a common congenital defect. Although obstruction can be valvular, supravalvular, or subvalvular, the degree of obstruction, rather than its site, is the principal determinant of clinical performance. A transvalvular pressure gradient exceeding 80 mm Hg is considered severe and mandates surgical correction.[5] A compilation (totaling 106 pregnancies) of three series of patients with pulmonic stenosis revealed no maternal deaths.[13–15] With severe stenosis, right heart failure can occur; fortunately, this is usually less severe clinically than is the left heart failure associated with mitral or aortic valve lesions.

FETAL CONSIDERATIONS

Perinatal outcome in patients with cyanotic congenital cardiac disease correlates best with hematocrit; successful outcome in patients with a hematocrit exceeding 65% is unlikely.[26] Such patients have an increased risk of spontaneous abortion, intrauterine growth retardation, and stillbirth. Maternal pO_2 below 60 mm Hg results in decreased fetal oxygen saturation; thus, paO_2 should be kept above this level during pregnancy, labor, and delivery.[27] In the presence of maternal cardiovascular disease, the growth-retarded fetus is especially sensitive to intrapartum hypoxia, and fetal decompensation may occur sooner.[42] During the antepartum period, serial antepartum sonography for the detection of growth retardation and antepartum fetal heart rate testing are mandatory in any patient with significant cardiac disease. Fetal activity counting may also be of value in patients with severe disease.[43] Of equal concern in patients with congenital heart disease is the risk of fetal congenital cardiac anomalies. Although this risk was previously felt to be on the order of 5%, recent data suggest the actual risk may be as high as 10%, or even higher in women whose congenital lesion involves ventricular outflow obstruction.[44] In such patients, fetal echocardiography is indicated for prenatal diagnosis of congenital cardiac defects. Of special interest is the fact that affected fetuses appear to be concordant for the maternal lesion in only 50% of cases.

ACQUIRED CARDIAC LESIONS

Acquired valvular lesions generally are rheumatic in origin, although endocarditis secondary to intravenous drug abuse may be involved occasionally, especially with right heart lesions. During pregnancy, maternal morbidity and mortality with such lesions result from congestive failure or arrhythmias. Pulmonary edema is the leading cause of death in rheumatic heart disease patients during pregnancy.[2] Szekely and colleagues found the risk of pulmonary edema in pregnant patients with rheumatic heart disease to increase with increasing age and with increasing length of gestation.[2] The onset of atrial fibrillation during pregnancy carries with it a higher risk of right and left ventricular failure (63%) than does fibrillation with onset prior to gestation (22%). In addition, the risk of systemic embolization after the onset of atrial fibrillation during pregnancy appears to exceed that associated with onset in the non-pregnant state.[2] In counseling the patient with severe rheumatic cardiac disease on the advisability of initiating or continuing pregnancy, the physician must also consider the long-term prognosis of the underlying disease. Chesley followed 134 women, who had functionally severe rheumatic heart disease and who had completed pregnancy, for up to 44 years.[45] He reported a mortality of 6.3% per year but concluded that in patients who survived the gestation, maternal life expectancy was not shortened by pregnancy. Thus, in general, pregnancy has no long-term sequelae for patients who survive the pregnancy.[6]

Intrapartum management of patients with valvular disease or pulmonary hypertension has been facilitated by the use of the pulmonary artery catheter.[46] In determining which patients may benefit from such invasive monitoring, we have found the older NYHA functional classification to be useful. Patients who reach term as class I or II usually tolerate properly managed labor without invasive monitoring. Patients who are or have been class III or IV, or those in whom pulmonary hypertension is present or suspected, often benefit from pulmonary artery catheterization during the intrapartum period.[5,46]

PULMONIC AND TRICUSPID LESIONS

Isolated right-sided valvular lesions of rheumatic origin are uncommon; however, such lesions are seen with increased frequency in intravenous drug abusers, where they are secondary to valvular endocarditis. Pregnancy-associated hypervolemia is far less likely to be symptomatic with right-sided lesion than with those involving the mitral or aortic valves. In a review of 77 maternal cardiac deaths, Hibbard reported none associated with isolated right-sided lesions.[15] In a recent review, congestive heart failure occurred in only 2.8% of women with pulmonic stenosis.[44] Even following complete tricuspid valvectomy for endocarditis, pregnancy, labor, and delivery are generally well tolerated. Cautious fluid administration is the mainstay of labor and delivery management in such patients. In general, invasive hemodynamic monitoring during labor and delivery is not necessary.

MITRAL STENOSIS

Mitral stenosis is the most common rheumatic valvular lesion encountered during pregnancy.[25] It can occur as an isolated lesion, or in conjunction with aortic or right-sided lesions. The principal hemodynamic aberration involves ventricular diastolic filling obstruction, resulting in a relatively fixed cardiac output. Marked increases in cardiac output accompany normal pregnancy, labor, and delivery. If the pregnant patient is unable to accommodate such volume fluctuations, pulmonary edema will result.

Cardiac output in patients with mitral stenosis depends largely on two factors.[25] First, these patients depend on adequate diastolic filling time. Thus, although in most patients tachycardia is a clinical sign of underlying hemodynamic instability, in patients with mitral stenosis, the tachycardia itself, regardless of etiology, may contribute significantly to hemodynamic decompensation. During labor, such tachycardia may accompany the exertion of pushing or be secondary to pain or anxiety.[46] Such a patient may exhibit a rapid and dramatic fall in cardiac output and blood pressure in response to tachycardia. This fall compromises maternal as well as fetal well-being. To avoid hazardous tachycardia, the physician should consider oral beta-blocker therapy for any patient with severe mitral stenosis who enters labor with a pulse exceeding 90 beats per minute. In patients who are not initially tachycardiac, acute control of tachycardia with an intravenous beta-blocking agent is only rarely necessary.[25]

A second important consideration in patients with mitral stenosis is left ventricular preload. In the presence of mitral stenosis, pulmonary capillary wedge pressure is not an accurate reflection of left ventricular filling pressures. Such patients often require high-normal or elevated pulmonary capillary wedge pressure to maintain adequate ventricular filling pressure and cardiac output. Any preload manipulation (ie, diuresis) therefore must be undertaken with extreme caution and careful attention to maintenance of cardiac output.[25]

Potentially dangerous intrapartum fluctuations in cardiac output can be minimized by using epidural anesthesia[47]; however, the most hazardous time for these women appears to be the immediate postpartum period. Such patients often enter the postpartum period already operating at maximum cardiac output and cannot accommodate the volume shifts that follow delivery. In a series of patients with severe mitral stenosis, we found that a postpartum rise in wedge pressure of up to 16 mm Hg could be expected in the immediate postpartum period.[25] Because frank pulmonary edema generally does not occur with wedge pressures below 28 to 30 mm Hg,[48] it follows that the optimal predelivery wedge pressure for such patients is 14 mm Hg or lower, as indicated by pulmonary artery catheterization.[25] Such a preload may be approached by cautious intrapartum diuresis and with careful attention to the maintenance of adequate cardiac output. Active diuresis is not always necessary in patients who enter with evidence of only mild fluid overload. In such patients, simple fluid restriction and the associated sensible and insensible fluid losses that accompany labor can result in a significant fall in wedge pressure prior to delivery.

In a patient with functional class II or III mitral stenosis, many of the same management considerations apply to those discussed under the section dealing with pulmonary hypertension. Bedrest and, at times, the administration of oxygen to maintain the therapeutic goal of a PO_2 greater than 60 mm Hg are essential. Under ideal circumstances, the patient would be admitted at term with a favorable cervix. Pulmonary artery catheterization allows the hemodynamic condition to be optimized prior to the stress of labor. The patient should labor on her side with the administration of oxygen. Epidural anesthesia will also assist in minimizing hemodynamic fluctuations during labor and delivery.[25,29] Because pulmonary edema is the major concern in these patients, we recommend that diuresis be carried out in order to approach a wedge pressure of 12 to 14 mm Hg. Such manipulation, however, must be performed with careful attention to cardiac output maintenance. It is important to realize that many patients with mitral stenosis will not tolerate a normal wedge pressure. In some cases, wedge pressures of 20 mm Hg or more are necessary to maintain cardiac output and blood pressure. If the pulse rises above 90 mm Hg, we recommend the administration of a beta-blocking agent such as propranolol to avoid tachycardia and subsequent falls in cardiac output.

Previous recommendations for delivery in patients with cardiac disease have included the liberal use of midforceps to shorten the second stage of labor. In cases of severe disease, cesarean section with general anesthesia also has been advocated as the preferred mode of delivery.[49,50] If intensive monitoring of intrapartum cardiac patients cannot be carried out in the manner described here, such recommendations for elective cesarean delivery may be valid. However, with the aggressive management scheme presented, our experience suggests that vaginal delivery is safe even in patients with severe disease and pulmonary hypertension.[25] Additionally, we have found it unnecessary to resort routinely to midforceps deliveries.

MITRAL INSUFFICIENCY

Hemodynamically significant mitral insufficiency is usually rheumatic in origin and most commonly occurs in conjunction with other valvular lesions. This lesion generally is tolerated well during pregnancy, and congestive failure is unusual. A more significant risk is the development of atrial enlargement and fibrillation. There is evidence to suggest that the risk of developing atrial fibrillation is increased during pregnancy.[2] Because of this increased risk, some authors have recommended prophylactic digitalization during pregnancy for patients with significant mitral insufficiency.[51] In Hibbard's review of 28 maternal deaths associated with rheumatic valvular lesions, no patient died with complications of mitral insufficiency unless there was coexisting mitral stenosis.[15]

Congenital mitral valve prolapse is much more common during pregnancy than is rheumatic mitral insufficiency and can occur in up to 17% of young healthy women. This condition is generally asymptomatic.[52] The midsystolic click and murmur associated with congenital mitral valve prolapse are characteristic. However, the intensity of this murmur, as well as that associated with rheumatic mitral insufficiency, may decrease during pregnancy because of decreased systemic vascular resistance.[53] Endocarditis prophylaxis during labor and delivery is recommended for rheumatic mitral insufficiency as well as for the more common mitral valve prolapse syndrome, if associated with a click or murmur.[54]

AORTIC STENOSIS

Aortic stenosis is most commonly of rheumatic origin and usually occurs in conjunction with other lesions. Less often it occurs congenitally and represents 5% of all congenital cardiac lesions. There appears to be a higher maternal mortality associated with rheumatic as opposed to congenital aortic stenosis. In one recent series of pregnancies in 15 women with congenital aortic stenosis, no maternal deaths were observed.[4] In contrast to mitral valve stenosis, aortic stenosis generally does not become hemodynamically significant until the orifice has diminished to one third or less of normal. The major problem experienced by patients with valvular aortic stenosis is maintenance of cardiac output. Because of the relative hypervolemia associated with gestation, such patients generally tolerate pregnancy well. However, with severe disease, cardiac output will be relatively fixed and during exertion may be inadequate to maintain coronary artery or cerebral perfusion. This inadequacy can result in angina, myocardial infarction, syncope, or sudden death. Thus, marked limitation of physical activity is vital to patients with severe disease. If activity is limited and the mitral valve is normal, pulmonary edema will be rare during pregnancy.

Delivery and pregnancy termination appear to be the times of greatest risk for patients with aortic stenosis.[55] The maintenance of cardiac output is crucial; any factor leading to diminished venous return will cause an increase in the valvular gradient and diminished cardiac output. The literature suggests that pregnancy termination may be especially hazardous in this regard and carries a mortality of up to 40%.[55] Hypotension resulting from blood loss, ganglionic blockade from epidural anesthesia, or supine vena caval occlusion by the pregnant uterus may result in sudden death. Such problems are similar to those encountered in patients with pulmonary hypertension, discussed previously.

The cardiovascular status of patients with aortic stenosis is complicated further by the frequent coexistence of ischemic heart disease. Thus, death associated with aortic stenosis can occur secondary to myocardial infarction rather than as a direct complication of the valvular lesion itself.[55] The overall reported mortality associated with aortic stenosis in pregnancy is 17%. Patients with shunt gradients exceeding 100 mm Hg are at greatest risk. Pulmonary artery catheterization may allow precise hemodynamic assessment and control during labor and delivery. Management considerations for the patient with aortic stenosis are similar to those in women with pulmonary hypertension, in that decreases in cardiac preload and output may result in sudden death. In addition, pulmonary edema is rare in the presence of a competent mitral valve. Thus, we prefer to manage these patients on the wet side, attempting to maintain a wedge pressure of 16 to 18 mm Hg during labor. Once again, midforceps or cesarean delivery should be reserved for standard obstetric indications only, assuming that continuous invasive monitoring during labor and delivery is available.

AORTIC INSUFFICIENCY

Aortic insufficiency is most commonly rheumatic in origin and as such is associated almost invariably with mitral valve disease. The aortic insufficiency generally is tolerated well during pregnancy because the increased heart rate seen with advancing gestation decreases time for regurgitant flow during diastole. In Hibbard's series of 28 maternal rheumatic cardiac deaths, only one was associated with aortic insufficiency in the absence of concurrent mitral stenosis.[15] Endocarditis prophylaxis during labor and delivery is indicated.

PERIPARTUM CARDIOMYOPATHY

Peripartum cardiomyopathy is defined as cardiomyopathy developing in the last month of pregnancy or the first 6 months postpartum in a woman without previous cardiac disease and after exclusion of other causes of cardiac failure.[56] It is therefore a diagnosis of exclusion that should not be made without a concerted effort to identify valvular, metabolic, infectious, or toxic causes of cardiomyopathy. Much of the current controversy surrounding this condition is the result of many older reports in which these causes of cardiomyopathy were not investigated adequately. Other peripartum complications, such as amniotic fluid embolism, severe preeclampsia, and corticosteroid or sympathomimetic-induced pulmonary edema, must also be considered before making the diagnosis of peripartum cardiomyopathy. Sympathomimetic agents may also unmask underlying peripartum cardiomyopathy.[57]

The incidence of peripartum cardiomyopathy is estimated at between one in 1500 and one in 4000 deliveries in the United States.[58] An incidence as high as 1% has been suggested in women of certain African tribes. However, idiopathic heart failure in these women may be primarily a result of unusual culturally mandated peripartum customs involving excessive sodium intake and may represent, as such, simple fluid overload.[58–60] In the United States, the peak incidence of peripartum cardiomyopathy occurs in the second postpartum month and appears most frequently among older, multiparous black females.[60] Other suggested risk factors include twinning and pregnancy-induced hypertension.[60,61] In some cases, a familial recurrence pattern has been reported. The condition is manifest clinically by increasing fatigue, dyspnea, and peripheral or pulmonary edema. Physical examination reveals classic evidence of congestive heart failure, including jugular venous distention, rales, and an S_3 gallop. Cardiomegaly and pulmonary edema are found on chest x-ray, and the electrocardiogram often demonstrates left ventricular and atrial dilation and diminished ventricular performance. In addition, up to 50% of patients with peripartum cardiomyopathy may manifest evidence of pulmonary or systemic embolic phenomena. Overall mortality ranges from 25% to 50%.[58,60]

The histologic picture of peripartum cardiomyopathy involves nonspecific cellular hypertrophy, degeneration, fibrosis, and increased lipid deposition. Although some reports have documented the presence of a diffuse myocarditis, it must be questioned whether such cases represent the same syndrome.

Because of the nonspecific clinical and pathologic nature of peripartum cardiomyopathy, its existence as a distinct entity has been questioned.[62] Its existence as a distinct entity is supported primarily by epidemiologic evidence suggesting that 80% of cases of idiopathic cardiomyopathy in women of childbearing age occur in the peripartum period.[58,60] Such an epidemiological distribution could also be attributed to an exacerbation of underlying subclinical cardiac disease related to the hemodynamic changes accompanying normal pregnancy.[62] However, as such changes are maximal in the third trimester of pregnancy and return to normal within a few weeks postpartum, such a pattern does not explain the peak incidence of peripartum cardiomyopathy occurring, in most reports, during the second month postpartum. Nevertheless, the diagnosis of peripartum cardiomyopathy remains primarily a diagnosis of exclusion and cannot be made until underlying conditions, including chronic hypertension, valvular disease, and viral myocarditis, have been excluded.

Although nutritional, hormonal, and autoimmune etiologies all have been suggested, substantial backing for any of these theories is lacking. In one case, an autoimmune phenomenon clearly seemed to be involved, because of transplacental passage of antibody and subsequent stillbirth.[63]

Therapy includes digitalization, diuretics, sodium restriction, and prolonged bedrest.[5] In refractory cases, concomitant afterload reduction with hydralazine or nitrates may be useful. Early endomyocardial biopsy to identify a subgroup of patients who have a histologic picture of inflammatory myocarditis and who may be responsive to immunosuppressive therapy has been suggested.

A notable feature of peripartum cardiomyopathy is its tendency to recur with subsequent pregnancies. Several reports have suggested that prognosis for future pregnancies is related to heart size. Patients whose cardiac size returned to normal within 6 to 12 months had an 11% to 14% mortality in subsequent pregnancies; those patients with persistent cardiomegaly had a 40% to 80% mortality.[56] Thus, pregnancy is definitely contraindicated in all patients with persistent cardiomegaly; the 11% to 14% risk of maternal mortality with subsequent pregnancy seen in patients with normal heart size would seem, in most cases, to be unacceptable as well.

IDIOPATHIC HYPERTROPHIC SUBAORTIC STENOSIS (IHSS)

IHSS is an autosomal dominantly inherited condition with variable penetrance. IHSS most commonly becomes clinically manifest in the second or third decade of life; thus, it often may be first manifest during pregnancy. Detailed physical and echocardiographic diagnostic criteria have been described elsewhere. IHSS involves primarily left ventricular hypertrophy typically involving the septum to a greater extent than the free wall. The hypertrophy results in obstruction to left ventricular outflow and secondary mitral regurgitation, the two principal hemodynamic concerns of the clinician.[64] Although the increased blood volume associated with normal pregnancy should enhance left ventricular filling and improve hemodynamic performance, this positive effect of pregnancy is counterbalanced by the fall in arterial pressure and vena caval obstruction that are found in late pregnancy. In addition, tachycardia resulting from pain or fear in labor diminishes left ventricular filling and aggravates the relative outflow obstruction, an effect also resulting from second-stage Valsalva maneuver.

The keys to successful management of the peripartum period in patients with IHSS involve avoidance of hypotension (resulting from conduction anesthesia or blood loss) and tachycardia, as well as conducting labor in the left lateral recumbent position. The use of forceps to shorten the second stage also has been recommended. As with most other cardiac disease, cesarean section of IHSS patients should be reserved for obstetric indications only.

Despite the potential hazards, maternal and fetal outcome in IHSS patients is generally good. In a recent report of 54 pregnancies in 23 patients with IHSS, no maternal or neonatal deaths occurred.[65] Although beta-blocking agents once were used routinely in patients with IHSS, currently they are reserved for patients with angina, recurrent supraventricular tachycardia, or occasional beta-blocker–responsive arrhythmias. Although fetal bradycardia and growth retardation have been reported in patients receiving beta-blockers, a cause-and-effect relationship is not clear; in general, the benefits of such therapy outweigh potential fetal effects.[66] Antibiotic prophylaxis against subacute bacterial endocarditis is recommended.

MARFAN SYNDROME

Marfan syndrome is an autosomal dominant disorder characterized by generalized weakness of connective tissue; the weakness results in skeletal, ocular, and cardiovascular abnormalities. The increased risk of maternal mortality during pregnancy stems from aortic root and wall involvement, which may result in aneurysm formation, rupture, or aortic dissection. Fifty percent of aortic aneurysm ruptures in women under age 40 occur more frequently during pregnancy.[34] Rupture of splenic artery aneurysms also occurs more frequently during pregnancy.[34] Sixty percent of patients with the Marfan syndrome have associated mitral or aortic regurgitation.[67] Although some authors feel pregnancy is contraindicated in any woman with documented Marfan syndrome, prognosis is best individualized and should be based on echocardiographic assessment of aortic root diameter and postvalvular dilatation. It is important to note that enlargement of the aortic root is not demonstrable by chest x-ray until dilatation has become pronounced.[67] Women with an abnormal aortic valve or aortic dilatation may have up to a 50% pregnancy-associated mortality; women without these changes and having an aortic root diameter less than 40 mm have a mortality of less than 5%.[68] Even in patients meeting these echocardiographic criteria, however, special attention must be given to signs or symptoms of aortic dissection because even serial echocardiographic assessment is not invariably predictive of complications.[69] In counseling women with Marfan syndrome, the genetics of this condition and the shortened maternal lifespan must be considered, in addition to the immediate maternal risk.[4] The routine use of oral beta-blocking agents to decrease pulsatile pressure on the aortic wall has been recommended.[70] If cesarean section is performed, retention sutures should be used because of generalized connective tissue weakness.

MYOCARDIAL INFARCTION

Coronary artery disease is uncommon in women of reproductive age; therefore, myocardial infarction in conjunction with pregnancy is rare. In a review of 68 reported cases, myocardial infarction during pregnancy was associated with a 35% mortality rate.[71] Only 13% of patients were known to have had coronary artery disease prior to pregnancy. Two thirds of the women suffered infarction in the third trimester; mortality for these women was 45%, as compared to 23% in those suffering infarction in the first or second trimesters. Thus, it appears that the increased hemodynamic burden imposed on the maternal cardiovascular system in late pregnancy may unmask latent coronary artery disease in some women and worsen the prognosis for patients suffering infarction. Fetuses from surviving women appear to have an increased risk of spontaneous abortion and unexplained stillbirth.

Women with class H diabetes mellitus face risks beyond those imposed by their cardiac disease alone. Although successful pregnancy outcome may occur, maternal and fetal risks are considerable. Such considerations, as well as the anticipated shortened lifespan of these patients, make special counseling of such women of major importance.[72]

Antepartum care of women with prior myocardial infarction includes bedrest to minimize myocardial oxygen demands. Diagnostic radionuclide cardiac imaging during pregnancy results in a fetal dose of no more than 0.8 rads and thus does not carry the potential for teratogenesis.[6] If cardiac catheterization becomes necessary, the simultaneous use of contrast echocardiography may reduce the need for cineangiography and thus reduce radiation exposure to the fetus.[73] In women with angina, nitrates have been used without adverse fetal effects. Delivery within 2 weeks of infarction is associated with increased mortality; therefore, if possible, attempts should be made to allow adequate convalescence prior to delivery. If the cervix is favorable, cautious induction under controlled circumstances after a period of hemodynamic stabilization is optimal. Labor in the lateral recumbent position, the administration of oxygen pain relief with epidural anesthesia, and, in some cases, hemodynamic monitoring with a pulmonary artery catheter are important management considerations.

PROSTHETIC VALVES AND ANTICOAGULATION

The proper drug for anticoagulation in the patient with an artificial heart valve during pregnancy is controversial.[54] The teratogenic effects of oral anticoagulants must be weighed against a potential increased risk of thrombosis and thromboembolism incurred by using heparin rather than warfarin.[74] Today a few authorities favor using the potentially more effective warfarin in pregnant patients with an artificial heart valve.[75] This practice is based on both a belief that the actual fetal risks of warfarin are less than have been reported (Oakley estimates the chance of a liveborn abnormal baby to be less than 10% following Coumadin exposure) and anecdotal experience in which heparin failed to prevent thrombosis of an artificial heart valve during pregnancy.[76,77] However, most physicians in the United States favor the use of heparin.[78,79]

Indications for antithrombotic therapy recently were reviewed at a national conference sponsored by the American College of Chest Physicians and the National Heart, Lung, and Blood Institute.[80] The recommendation of this committee was to treat pregnant women who have prosthetic heart valves with adjusted-dose subcutaneous heparin from conception until delivery. Sodium heparin, 8000 to 14,000 U, is injected every 8 to 12 hours to achieve an activated partial thromboplastin time of 1.5 to 2 times control 6 hours after injection.

A small series of patients with nonbiological prosthetic heart valves has been treated during pregnancy with antiplatelet agents, including aspirin and dipyridamole. Although maternal outcome was good, a high rate of spontaneous abortion was encountered in one study, and the size of these series makes it difficult to draw conclusions about the safety and efficacy of these regimens.[74,81,82]

Patients with bioprosthetic or xenograft valves usually are not treated with anticoagulants during pregnancy.[74] This fact makes the bioprosthetic valve the ideal choice of prosthesis for young women of childbearing age.[54,83] Patients with a bioprosthetic valve who are in atrial fibrillation or have evidence of thromboembolism, however, should be anticoagulated.

Two anticoagulation regimes have been assessed sufficiently to determine that they should not be used during pregnancy: subcutaneous "minidose" heparin (because of an unacceptable rate of thromboembolic complications) and heparin administered by continuous subcutaneous pump (because of major bleeding complications that occurred despite a therapeutic partial thromboplastin time).[54,84–86]

ARRHYTHMIAS

The use of antiarrhythmic therapy in pregnancy has been reviewed extensively by Rotmensch and colleagues.[87] Digoxin, quinidine, and procainamide may be used for the usual indications and, in therapeutic doses, have not been shown to be harmful to the fetus. Disopyramide has been associated with preterm labor in one patient.[88] The use of beta-blockers is appropriate in some tachyarrhythmias, in idiopathic hypertrophic subaortic stenosis, and for the control of hyperthyroid symptoms. Despite earlier concerns, it is now apparent that beta-blocker therapy is not associated with adverse fetal outcomes.[89] Although neonatal hypoglycemia and bradycardia may occur, they are not usually serious, and intrauterine growth retardation appears to be a function of the disease for which beta-blockers are prescribed rather than a complication of therapy itself. Verapamil is a calcium-entry-blocking drug that is effective in converting a supraventricular tachycardia to a sinus rhythm. There are no reports of its adverse effects on the fetus, and it has been used specifically to treat fetal supraventricular arrhythmias.[90]

Pregnant patients with atrial fibrillation should be anticoagulated with the subcutaneous adjusted-dose heparin regimen if they meet the criteria accepted for non-pregnant patients.[54] These include atrial fibrillation with a history of thromboembolic complications, in the presence of valvular disease, cardiomyopathy, or thyrotoxic heart disease. Anticoagulation is recommended for 3 weeks prior to cardioversion of atrial fibrillation and 4 weeks after conversion to a sinus rhythm. Anticoagulation may also be considered in a patient with atrial fibrillation and congestive heart failure.

Maternal cardioversion has been reported and appears safe for the fetus.[91]

CARDIOVASCULAR SURGERY

There are numerous reports of cardiovascular surgery during pregnancy, most of which are favorable; they include successful correction of most types of congenital and acquired cardiac disease.[6,92] Early reports of closed mitral valve commissurotomy during pregnancy were also favorable and indicated a maternal death rate of 1% to 2% and perinatal loss in the range of 10%.[93] Subsequently, this procedure has been replaced by open valvuloplasty with equally good results.

Initial reports of cardiopulmonary bypass during pregnancy were not nearly as favorable, indicating a fetal wastage of up to 33%.[5,6] Initiation of cardiopulmonary bypass generally is followed by fetal bradycardia, which may be correctable by high flow rates.[94,95] With the use of continuous electronic fetal heart rate monitoring, flow rate can be adjusted to avoid or correct fetal hypoperfusion and bradycardia, thus reducing fetal mortality to less than 10%. High-flow–high-pressure normothermic perfusion and continuous electronic fetal heart rate monitoring appear to be optimal for the fetus.[92] Maternal mortality is highly dependent on the specific nature of the procedure being performed and does not appear increased significantly by pregnancy. Successful pregnancy following heart transplantation has been reported. Principles of counseling and management for these complex patients have recently been summarized.[96]

REFERENCES

1. Steinberg WM, Farine D. Maternal mortality in Ontario from 1970 to 1980. Obstet Gynecol 1985;66:510.
2. Szekely P, Turner R, Snaith L. Pregnancy and the changing pattern of rheumatic heart disease. Br Heart J 1973;35:1293.
3. The Criteria Committee of the New York Heart Association. Nomenclature and criteria for diagnosis of diseases of the heart and great vessels. 8th ed. New York: New York Heart Association, 1979.
4. Shime J, Mocarski EJM, Hastings D, et al. Congenital heart disease in pregnancy: short- and long-term implications. Am J Obstet Gynecol 1987;156:313.
5. Clark SL. Structural cardiac disease in pregnancy. In: Clark SL, Cotton DB, Phelan JP, eds. Critical care obstetrics. Oradell, NJ: Medical Economics Books, 1987:92.
6. Elkayam V, Gleicher N. Cardiac problems in pregnancy. I. Maternal aspects: the approach to the pregnant patient with heart disease. JAMA 1984;251:2838.
7. Ullery JC. Management of pregnancy complicated by heart disease. Am J Obstet Gynecol 1954;67:834.
8. Niswander KR, Berendes H, Dentschberger J, et al. Fetal morbidity following potential anoxigenic obstetric conditions. V. Organic heart disease. Am J Obstet Gynecol 1967;98:871.
9. Rush RW, Verjans M, Spraklen FH. Incidence of heart disease in pregnancy. S Afr Med J 1979;55:808.
10. Etheridge MJ, Pepperell RJ. Heart disease and pregnancy at the Royal Women's Hospital. Med J Aust 1971;2:277.
11. Veran FX, Cibes-Hernandez JJ, Pelegrina I. Heart disease in pregnancy. Obstet Gynecol 1968;34:424.
12. Ellison CR, Sloss CJ. Electrocardiographic features of congenital heart disease in the adult. In: Roberts WC, ed. Congenital heart disease in adults. Philadelphia: FA Davis, 1979:119.
13. Neilson G, Galea EG, Blunt A. Congenital heart disease and pregnancy. Med J Aust 1970;30:1086.
14. Schaefer G, Arditi LI, Solomon HA, et al. Congenital heart disease and pregnancy. Clin Obstet Gynecol 1968;11:1048.
15. Hibbard LT. Maternal mortality due to cardiac disease. Clin Obstet Gynecol 1975;18:27.
16. Mendelson CL. Cardiac disease in pregnancy. Philadelphia: FA Davis, 1960:151.
17. Zitnick RS, Brandenburg RO, Sheldon R, et al. Pregnancy and open heart surgery. Circulation 1969;39:157.
18. Szekely P, Julian DG. Heart disease and pregnancy. Curr Probl Cardiol 1979;4:1.
19. Kelly DT. Patent ductus arteriosus in adults. In: Roberts WC, ed. Congenital heart disease in adults. Philadelphia: FA Davis, 1979:321.
20. Knapp RC, Arditi LI. Pregnancy complicated by patent ductus arteriosus with reversal of flow. NY J Med 1967;67:573.
21. Gleicher N, Midwall J, Hochberger D, et al. Eisenmenger's syndrome and pregnancy. Obstet Gynecol Surv 2979;34:721.
22. Pirlo A, Herren AL. Eisenmenger's syndrome and pregnancy. Anesth Rev 1979;6:9.
23. Sinnenberg RJ. Pulmonary hypertension in pregnancy. S Med J 1980;73:1529.
24. Pitts JA, Crosby WM, Basta LL. Eisenmenger's syndrome in pregnancy. Does heparin prophylaxis improve the maternal mortality rate? Am Heart J 1977;93:321.
25. Clark SL, Phelan JP, Greenspoon J, et al. Labor and delivery in the presence of mitral stenosis: central hemodynamic observations. Am J Obstet Gynecol 1985;152:984.
26. Clark SL. Shock in the pregnant patient. Seminar Perinatol 1990;14:52.
27. Sobrevilla LA, Cassinelli MT, Carcelen A, et al. Human fetal and maternal oxygen tension and acid-base status during delivery at high altitude. Am J Obstet Gynecol 1971;111:1111.
28. Midwall J, Jaffin H, Herman MV, et al. Shunt flow and pulmonary hemodynamics during labor and delivery in the Eisenmenger syndrome. Am J Cardiol 1978;42:299.
29. Clark SL. Labor and delivery in the patient with structural cardiac disease. Clin Perinatol 1986;13:695.
30. Spinnato JA, Kraynack BJ, Cooper MW. Eisenmenger's syndrome in pregnancy: epidural anesthesia for elective cesarean section. N Engl J Med 1981;304:1215.
31. Abboud JK, Raya J, Noueihed R, et al. Intrathecal morphine for relief of labor pain in a parturient with severe pulmonary hypertension. Anesthesiology 1983;59:477.
32. Goodwin JF. pregnancy and coarctation of the aorta. Clin Obstet Gynecol 1961;4:645.
33. Taylor SH, Donald KW. Circulatory studies at rest and during exercise in coarctation, before and after correction. Br Heart J 1960;22:117.
34. Barrett JM, VanHooydonk JE, Boehm FH. Pregnancy-related rupture of arterial aneurysms. Obstet Gynecol Surv 1982;37:557.
35. Deal K, Wooley CF. Coarctation of the aorta and pregnancy. Ann Intern Med 1973;78:706.
36. Szekely P, Snaith L. Heart disease and pregnancy. London: Churchill Livingstone, 1974:167.
37. Mendelson CL. Pregnancy and coarctation of the aorta. Am J Obstet Gynecol 1940;39:1014.
38. Barash PG, Hobbins JC, Hook R, et al. Management of coarctation of the aorta during pregnancy. J Thorac Cardiovasc Surg 1975;69:781.
39. Jacoby WJ. Pregnancy with tetralogy and pentalogy of Fallot. Am J Cardiol 1964;14:866.
40. Meyer EC, Tulsky AS, Sigman P, et al. Pregnancy in the presence of tetralogy of Fallot. Am J Cardiol 1964;14:874.
41. Loh TF, Tan NC. Fallot's tetralogy and pregnancy: a report of a successful pregnancy after complete correction. Med J Aust 1975;2:141.
42. Block BSB, Llanos AJ, Creasy RK. Responses of the growth-retarded fetus to acute hypoxemia. Am J Obstet Gynecol 1984;148:878.
43. Simon A, Sadovsky E, Aboulatia Y, et al. Fetal activity in pregnancies complicated by rheumatic heart disease. J Perinat Med 1986;14:331.
44. Whittemore R, Hobbins JC, Engle MA. Pregnancy and its outcome in women with and without surgical treatment of congenital heart disease. Am J Cardiol 1982;50:641.
45. Chesley LC. Severe rheumatic cardiac disease and pregnancy: the ultimate prognosis. Am J Obstet Gynecol 1980;126:552.

46. Clark SL. How labor and delivery influence mitral stenosis. Contemp Ob/Gyn 1986;27:127.
47. Ueland K, Akamatsu TJ, Eng M, et al. Maternal cardiovascular dynamics. VI. Cesarean section under epidural anesthesia without epinephrine. Am J Obstet Gynecol 1972;114:775.
48. Forrester JS, Swan HJC. Acute myocardial infarction: a physiological basis for therapy. Crit Care Med 1974;2:283.
49. Ueland K, Hansen J, Eng M, et al. Maternal cardiovascular dynamics v. section under thiopental, nitrous oxide and succinylcholine anesthesia. Am J Obstet Gynecol 1970;108:615.
50. Bonica JJ. Obstetric analgesia and anesthesia. 2nd ed. Amsterdam: World Federation of Societies of Anesthesiologists, 1980:152.
51. Ueland, K. Rheumatic heart disease and pregnancy. In: Elkayam Y, Gleicher N, eds. Cardiac problems in pregnancy. New York: Alan R Liss, 1982:82.
52. Markiewicz W, Stoner J, London E, et al. Mitral valve prolapse in one hundred previously healthy young females. Circulation 1976;53:464.
53. Haas JM. The effect of pregnancy on the midsystolic click and murmur of the prolapsing posterior leaflet of the mitral valve. Am Heart J 1976;92:407.
54. Greenspoon J. Prosthetic valves, arrhythmias and anticoagulation in pregnancy. In: Clark SL, ed. Critical care obstetrics. Oradell, NJ: Medical Economics Books, 1987:114.
55. Arias F, Pineda J. Aortic stenosis and pregnancy. J Reprod Med 1978;20:229.
56. Demakis JG, Rahimtoola SH, Sutton GC, et al. Natural course of peripartum cardiomyopathy. Circulation 1971;44:1053.
57. Blickstein I, Zalel Y, Katz Z, et al. Ritodrine-induced pulmonary edema unmasking underlying peripartum cardiomyopathy. Am J Obstet Gynecol 1988;159:332.
58. Homans DC. Peripartum cardiomyopathy. N Engl J Med 1985;312:1432.
59. Seftel H, Susser M. Maternity and myocardial failure in African women. Br Heart J 1961;23:43.
60. Veille JC. Peripartum cardiomyopathies: a review. Am J Obstet Gynecol 1984;148:805.
61. Pierce JA, Price BO, Joyce JW. Familial occurrence of postpartal cardiomyopathy. Arch Intern Med 1963;111:651.
62. Cunningham FG, Pritchard JA, Hankins GDV, et al. Peripartum heart failure: idiopathic cardiomyopathy or compounding cardiovascular events? Obstet Gynecol 1986;67:157.
63. Rand RJ, Jenkins DM, Scott DG. Maternal cardiomyopathy of pregnancy causing stillbirth. Br J Obstet Gynecol 1975;82:172.
64. Kolibash AJ, Ruiz DE, Lewis RP. Idiopathic hypertrophic subaortic stenosis in pregnancy. Ann Intern Med 1975;82:791.
65. Oakley GDG, McGarry K, Limb DG, et al. Management of pregnancy in patients with hypertrophic cardiomyopathy. Br Med J 1979;1:1749.
66. Briggs GB, Bodendorfer JW, Freeman RK, Yaffe SJ, eds. Drugs in pregnancy and lactation. Baltimore: Williams & Wilkins, 1983:310.
67. Pyeritz RE, McKusick VA: The Marfan syndrome: diagnosis and management. N Engl J Med 1979;300:772.
68. Pyeritz RE. Maternal and fetal complications of pregnancy in the Marfan syndrome. Am J Med 1984;71:784.
69. Rosenblum NG, Grossman AR, Gabbe SG, et al. Failure of serial echocardiographic studies to predict aortic dissection in a pregnant patient with Marfan's syndrome. Am J Obstet Gynecol 1983;146:470.
70. Slater EE, DeSanctis RW. Dissection of the aorta. Med Clin North Am 1979;63:141.
71. Hankins GDV, Wendel GD, Leveno KJ, et al. Myocardial infarction during pregnancy: a review. Obstet Gynecol 1985;65:139.
72. Gast MJ, Rigg LA. Class H diabetes and pregnancy. Obstet Gynecol 1985;66:5(s).
73. Elkayam U, Kawanishi D, Reid CL, et al. Contrast echocardiography to reduce ionizing radiation associated with cardiac catheterization during pregnancy. Am J Cardiol 1983;52:213.
74. Deviri E, Levinsky L, Yechezkel M, et al. Pregnancy after valve replacement with porcine xenograft prosthesis. Surg Gynecol Obstet 1985;160:437.
75. Oakley C. Pregnancy in patients with prosthetic heart valves. Br Med J 1983;286:1680.
76. Oakley CM, Doherty P. Pregnancy in patients after heart valve replacement. Br Heart J 1976;38:1140.
77. Antunes MJ, Myer IG, Santos LP. Thrombosis of mitral valve prosthesis in pregnancy: management by simultaneous caesarean section and mitral valve replacement. Case report. Br J Obstet Gynaecol 1984;91:716.
78. Eden RE. Disorders of blood coagulation factors, in Gleicher N, ed. Principles of medical therapy in pregnancy. New York: Plenum Press, 1985:1201.
79. Noller KL. Cardiac surgery and pregnancy. In: Gleicher N, ed. Principles of medical therapy in pregnancy. New York: Plenum Press, 1985:713.
80. Dalen E, Hirsh J (co-chairmen). American College of Chest Physicians and the National Heart, Lung, and Blood Institute National Conference on Antithrombotic Therapy. Chest (Suppl 2) 1986;89:1S.
81. Biale Y, Cantor A, Lewenthal H, et al. The course of pregnancy in patients treated with artificial heart valves treated with dipyridamole. Int J Gynaecol Obstet 1980;18:128.
82. Nunez L, Larrea JL, Aguado MG, et al. Pregnancy in 20 patients with bioprosthetic valve replacement. Chest 1983;84:26.
83. Starr A, Grunkemeier GL. Selection of a prosthetic valve. JAMA 1984;251:1739.
84. Wang RYC, Lee PK, Chow JSF, et al. Efficacy of low-dose subcutaneously administered heparin in treatment of pregnant women with artificial heart valves. Med J Aust 198;2:126.
85. Salazar E, Zajarias A, Gutierrez N, et al. The problem of cardiac valve prostheses, anticoagulants, and pregnancy. Circulation (Suppl I) 1984;70:I-169.
86. Baras VA, Schwartz PA, Greene MF, et al. Use of the subcutaneous heparin during pregnancy. J Reprod Med 1985;30:899.
87. Rotmensch HH, Elkayam U, Frishman W. Antiarrhythmic therapy during pregnancy. Ann Intern Med 1983;98:487.
88. Leonard RF, Braun TE, Levy AM. Initiation of uterine contractions by disopyramide during pregnancy. N Engl J Med 1978;299:84.
89. Rubin PC. Beta-blockers in pregnancy. N Engl J Med 1981; 305:1323.
90. Kleinman CS, Copel JA, Weinstein EM, et al. In-utero diagnosis and treatment of fetal supraventricular tachycardia. Semin Perinatol 1985;9:113.
91. Schroeder JS, Harrison DC. Repeated cardioversion during pregnancy: treatment of refractory paroxysmal atrial tachycardia during three successive pregnancies. Am J Cardiol 1971;27:445.
92. Bernal JM, Miralles PJ. Cardiac surgery with cardiopulmonary bypass during pregnancy. Obstet Gynecol Surv 1986;41:1.
93. Ueland K. Cardiovascular surgery and the OB patient. Contemp Ob/Gyn, Oct 1984:117.
94. Koh KS, Friesen RM, Livingstone RA, et al. Fetal monitoring during maternal cardiac surgery with cardiopulmonary bypass. CMAJ 1975;112:1102.
95. Werch A, Lambert HM, Cooley D, et al. Fetal monitoring and maternal open heart surgery. South Med J 1977;70:1024.
96. Kossoy LR, Herbert CM, Wentz AC. Management of heart transplant recipients: guidelines for the obstetrician-gynecologist. Am J Obstet Gynecol 1980;159:490.

60

CHAPTER

MATERNAL PULMONARY DISORDERS COMPLICATING PREGNANCY

Mark J. Clinton, Michael S. Niederman, and Richard A. Matthay

Pregnant women are afflicted by the same respiratory ailments as non-pregnant women, but these conditions are complicated by the physiologic alterations of pregnancy. Certain lung diseases, such as asthma, are common in women of childbearing age and may be seen frequently in pregnant women. However, asthma and other pulmonary diseases may first manifest during pregnancy or change their course during gestation. In this chapter we first review diagnostic techniques for lung disease, including history and physical examination, pulmonary function tests, arterial blood gases, and radiographic tests. Then we summarize the physiologic alterations of the respiratory system during pregnancy. Specific respiratory illnesses, including those found in women with chronic disease as well as those found in women who were previously normal, are discussed. Special attention has been given to the following areas:

1. How women with chronic respiratory illness can be recognized, followed, and managed to prevent complications to the fetus and to avoid progression to extreme illness
2. How pregnancy alters the course of chronic respiratory disease
3. How respiratory illness can affect both maternal and fetal outcomes during pregnancy
4. How pharmacologic treatment of lung disease can be undertaken to minimize adverse effects to both mother and fetus
5. How adult respiratory distress syndrome (ARDS), a common cause of acute respiratory failure, can be recognized and managed.

Pulmonary tuberculosis and thromboembolic disease are discussed elsewhere and are omitted from detailed discussion here.

DIAGNOSTIC TECHNIQUES

HISTORY AND PHYSICAL EXAMINATION

Most common respiratory disorders lead to symptoms such as shortness of breath, exercise intolerance, cough, sputum production, wheezing, chest tightness, fever, chills, night sweats, or hemoptysis. A careful history should elicit information about medications, smoking history, and prior respiratory illness. Physical exam should be done with particular attention to the duration of the expiratory phase, the use of accessory muscles, and the presence of rales, rhonchi, wheezing, pleural rubs, signs of pleural effusions, consolidation, and chest wall abnormalities. Taken together, these aspects of the history and physical examination provide the necessary data base for the care of patients with pulmonary disease during pregnancy. If the patient has been pregnant in the past, the presence of respiratory symptoms during the prior pregnancy should be noted and compared to the patient's usual respiratory symptoms when not pregnant.

Dyspnea is the most common respiratory complaint during pregnancy, with as many as 60% to 70% of previously normal women having this symptom at some time during pregnancy. The complaint usually begins in the first or second trimester but is most prevalent at term.[1–3] It is not usually due to underlying lung disease but probably results from the subjective perception of hyperventilation that normally accompanies pregnancy. In pregnancy, as a result of increased progesterone levels, the volume of air taken into the lungs with each breath (tidal volume), increases, giving a sensation of hyperventilation despite a lack of change in breathing frequency. As the woman acclimates to this new sensation, her perception of dyspnea is reduced and there is stabilization of dyspnea as the pregnancy progresses. Unlike pathologic dyspnea, symptoms do not increase with exertion. Maximum dyspnea seems to correlate with the time of lowest arterial carbon dioxide tension, suggesting a role for hypocarbia in mediating this symptom.

ARTERIAL BLOOD GASES

Arterial blood sampling provides valuable data about maternal oxygenation and acid–base status. Because of the well-documented risks of fetal hypoxia and the good response of umbilical vein oxygen tension to maternal oxygen administration, arterial blood gas data should be obtained when any acute respiratory complaint is present. Interpretation of acid–base abnormalities is greatly aided by reference to any of the widely available acid–base nomograms, such as the one shown in Figure 60-1.[4] In a normal pregnant female, arterial blood gas measurements will usually show a compensated respiratory alkalosis due to maternal hyperventilation. The pH generally ranges from 7.40 to 7.47, and the partial pressure of arterial carbon dioxide is 25–32 mm Hg.[5–8] The partial pressure of arterial oxygen may be as high as 106 mm Hg in early pregnancy, decreasing during pregnancy but remaining at 100 mm Hg, or slightly higher, at term.[5]

The measured arterial oxygen tension represents the partial pressure of oxygen dissolved in blood but is only an indirect reflection of the blood's oxygen content. Calculating the oxygen content of blood requires a knowledge of the amount of oxygen dissolved in the blood, the maximum amount of oxygen able to be carried per gram of hemoglobin, the hemoglobin concentration, and the oxygen saturation of hemoglobin.

$$\text{Oxygen content} = [(\text{Hb (gms/dL)} \times 1.39 \text{ mL } O_2/\text{gm Hb}) \times (\text{oxygen saturation})] + [(0.003 \text{ mL } O_2/100 \text{ mL of blood}) \times PaO_2 \text{ (mm Hg)}]$$

As the equation shows, 1 g of fully saturated Hb can combine with 1.39 mL of oxygen. Since normal blood has about 15 g of Hb/100 mL, the maximal oxygen-carrying capacity is usually about 20.8 mL O_2/100 mL of blood. The oxygen saturation of Hb is usually taken from the oxyhemoglobin dissociation curve (Fig. 60-2)[9] and is affected by such variables as pH, PCO_2, temperature, and the amount of 2,3-diphosphoglycerate (DPG) present. The amount of dissolved oxygen (O_2) is calculated by applying Henry's law, which states that the amount of dissolved gas is proportional to its partial pressure. For each 1 mm Hg of partial pressure of oxygen, 0.003 mL of oxygen is dissolved per 100 mL of blood (0.003 mL O_2/100 mL of blood). Thus, the dissolved oxygen content of arterial blood with a PaO_2 of 100 mm Hg is 0.3 mL O_2/100 mL of blood.

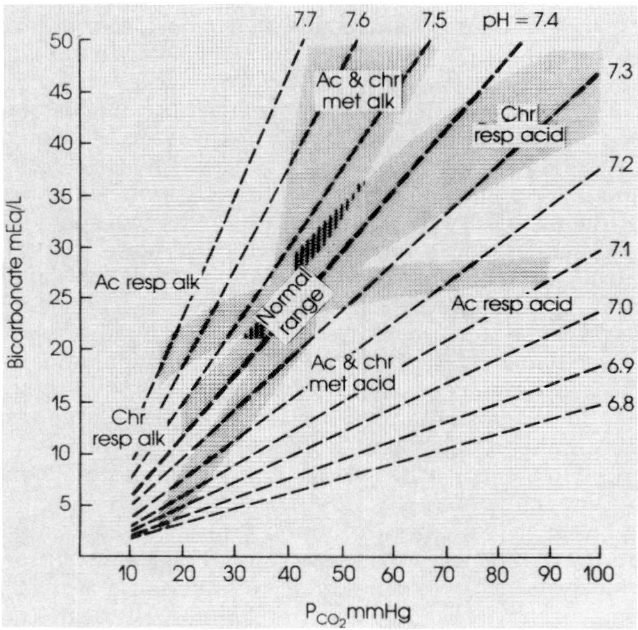

FIGURE 60–1. Nomogram showing bands for uncomplicated respiratory or metabolic acid–base disturbances in intact subjects. Each "confidence" band represents the mean ± standard deviation for the compensatory response of normal subjects or patients to a given primary disorder. Ac, acute; chr, chronic; resp, respiratory; met, metabolic; acid, acidosis; alk, alkalosis. (Modified from Arbus.) (Reproduced with permission from Levinsky, NG. Acidosis and alkalosis. 11th ed. In: Braunwald E, Isselbacher KJ, Petersdorf RG, et al, eds. Harrison's principles of internal medicine. New York: McGraw-Hill: 1987; 209.)

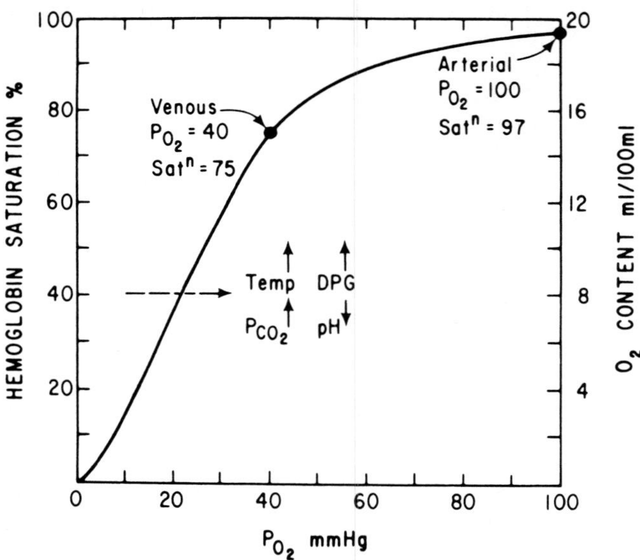

FIGURE 60–2. Anchor points of the oxygen dissociation curve. The curve is shifted to the right by an increase in temperature, PCO_2, and 2,3-DPG and a fall in pH. The oxygen content scale is based on a hemoglobin concentration of 14.5 g/100 mL. (Reproduced with permission from West JB. Pulmonary pathology—the essentials. 3rd ed. Baltimore: Williams & Wilkins, 1987: 21.)

The adequacy of alveolar gas exchange is dependent on the matching of ventilation and blood perfusion within various regions of the lung. Mismatching of ventilation and perfusion is responsible for most of the defective gas exchange in pulmonary diseases. The adequacy of alveolar gas exchange can be assessed by calculating the alveolar–arterial oxygen tension gradient, and if the alveolar oxygen tension (PAO_2) greatly exceeds the measured arterial oxygen tension (PaO_2), then alveolar gas exchange is abnormal. Ideal alveolar oxygen tension (PAO_2) is calculated as follows:

$$PaO_2 = FIO_2 \times (PB - 47) - PaCO_2/0.8$$

where

FIO_2 = fractional percentage of inspired oxygen

PB = barometric pressure

47 = water vapor pressure

$PaCO_2$ = arterial blood tension of carbon dioxide

0.8 = respiratory quotient

This equation states that a patient's alveolar oxygen tension equals the tension of oxygen in inspired air minus the amount of oxygen taken up in the lung in exchange for carbon dioxide. This latter exchange relationship, the respiratory quotient, is equal to 0.8 volume of carbon dioxide released in exchange for every volume of oxygen delivered. PaO_2, obtained from blood gas measurement is subtracted from PAO_2 to obtain a measure of the $(A - a)O_2$ gradient.

In the non-pregnant patient, the $(A - a)O_2$ gradient varies with age, but a prediction formula for the expected range of normal is not applicable during pregnancy. In one study, the mean $(A - a)O_2$ gradient in normal pregnant women in the supine position during the third trimester was 20 mm Hg, whereas in the sitting position it decreased to 14.3 mm Hg.[10] In another study of normal obstetric patients, PaO_2 increased by 13 mm Hg when changing from a supine to a sitting position, and arterial PCO_2 decreased by 2 mm Hg, leading to a net decrease in the $(A - a)O_2$ gradient of 10 mm Hg.[11] The increased gradient noted in the supine position may be the result of decreased cardiac output attributable to decreased venous return from compression of the inferior vena cava by the uterus.[10,12] Since most acute lung diseases are accompanied by an increased $(A - a)O_2$ gradient, the gradient should be assessed with the pregnant patient in the upright position and should be considered abnormal if it exceeds 25 mm Hg. It is important to emphasize that blood gas analysis should be accompanied by calculation of the gradient, because on casual observation, with the usual decreased PCO_2 of pregnancy, a "normal" PaO_2 can be seen even with an abnormally increased $(A - a)O_2$ gradient.

PULMONARY FUNCTION TESTS

Normal respiratory physiology is altered in pregnancy, and these changes must be considered when evaluating tests of lung function. In the terminology of pulmonary function testing (Table 60-1), a "volume" is a single discrete component of the lung. Four such volumes exist: tidal volume (TV), residual volume (RV), inspiratory reserve volume (IRV), and expiratory reserve volume (ERV). The term *capacity* refers to a sum of volumes. Except for RV, each of the volumes defined can be recorded and measured by simple spirometry. Residual volume, the volume of gas remaining in the thorax at the end of a maximal exhalation, can be measured only by indirect methods (eg, helium dilution, nitrogen washout, or body plethysmography).

The enlarging fetus and the increased concentration of circulating hormones during pregnancy account for the changes in pulmonary function seen with gestation. The hyperventilation of pregnancy is characterized by an increased depth of breathing (tidal volume increases from 450 to 600 mL) and not a higher respiratory rate.[7,13] Minute ventilation is increased in excess of the rise in oxygen consumption associated with pregnancy and is thought to be due to a progesterone-mediated increase in sensitivity to carbon dioxide. In one study, at term, minute ventilation was 48% above normal, whereas oxygen consumption increased only 21%.[14] Vital capacity generally remains unchanged because there is an increase in inspiratory capacity but a decrease in expiratory reserve volume. In the second half of pregnancy a slight reduction in functional residual capacity (FRC) (18%), RV, and total lung capacity (TLC) occurs, caused by compression of the resting lung by the elevated intra-abdominal pressure secondary to uterine enlargement.[15] Typical pulmonary volumes and

TABLE 60–1. PULMONARY PARAMETERS

Lung Volumes

Tidal volume (TV): The volume of air inhaled or exhaled with each normal breath

Residual volume (RV): The volume of air remaining in the lungs after a vital capacity maneuver

Inspiratory reserve volume (IRV): The maximal additional volume of gas that can be inhaled after a tidal breath is inhaled

Expiratory reserve volume (ERV): The maximal volume of gas that can be exhaled after a tidal breath is exhaled

Lung Capacities

Total lung capacity (TLC): The volume of air in the lungs at maximal inspiration

Vital capacity (VC): The maximum amount of air that can be exhaled after a maximal inspiration to TLC

Inspiratory capacity (IC): The maximal volume of gas that can be inspired from the resting expiratory level

Functional residual capacity (FRC): The volume of air remaining in the lungs after a tidal volume exhalation

Forced vital capacity (FVC): The volume of air exhaled during a rapid forced expiration starting at full inspiration

Other Measurements Made By Spirometry

Forced expiratory volume in one second (FEV_1): The volume of air expelled in one second during a forced expiration starting at full inspiration

Minute ventilation (MV): The amount of air exhaled per minute. It is measured under resting conditions

Peak expiratory flow rate (PEFR): The peak rate (L/min) of a forceful expiration of a vital capacity capacities and the modifications caused by pregnancy are schematically diagrammed in Figure 60-3.

Abnormal spirometry usually is classified as fitting a pattern of either obstruction or restriction. Normal spirometric lung values are within 20% of a predicted normal, which is based on a patient's age, sex, height, and weight. Flow rates are preserved in both large and small airways during a normal pregnancy. A restrictive pattern is present when total lung capacity is below 80% of the predicted normal. With restrictive disease, air flow rate, expressed by FEV_1 as a percentage of FVC (FEV_1/FVC), can be increased to greater than 85%. Restrictive ventilatory defects are caused by skeletal, neuromuscular, pleural, interstitial, and alveolar diseases that lead to a reduction in lung volume or chest wall expansion. Sarcoidosis and chest wall deformity are the most common restrictive lung diseases seen in women of childbearing age.

An obstructive pattern is present when the FEV_1/FVC ratio is less than 75% and FEV_1 is less than 80% of the predicted value, indicating a reduction in airflow rates. Lung volumes may be normal, or they may be increased if air is trapped as a result of early airway closure. Asthma is the most common obstructive airway disease encountered in pregnancy. Other obstructive lung diseases include cystic fibrosis, bronchiectasis, and emphysema.

The diffusing capacity of the lung, which reflects the amount of oxygen that can be taken up by the pulmonary capillary blood, is either unchanged or increased during pregnancy. Diffusing capacity has been reported to be most elevated in the first trimester[16–18] as a result of the increase in capillary blood volume that accompanies pregnancy. Diffusing capacity may also be increased in asthmatic patients because relative pulmonary hypertension, secondary to hypoxemia, results in redistribution of pulmonary blood flow to the upper lobes, where alveoli have higher ventilation-to-perfusion ratios.[19]

When a patient with known lung disease seeks advice about the risks of pregnancy, pulmonary function studies should be obtained. In combination with other clinical data, an objective assessment of the patient's risks during pregnancy can be made. However, no strict guideline can be given as to the level of pulmonary function that will prohibit a safe pregnancy. In general, although there has been a report of a well-tolerated pregnancy in a patient with a vital capacity of 800 mL,[20] a patient with a vital capacity less than 1 L will have significant difficulties. If the FEV_1 exceeds 1 L, the woman will not ordinarily experience dyspnea at rest, even at term. As further protection for the patient with respiratory insufficiency, resting ventilation during pregnancy is increased less in patients with lung disease than in normals.[20] Although patients with obstructive lung disease vary widely in their tolerance of pregnancy, those with restrictive disease tolerate pregnancy well.[21,22] Studies in patients with lung disease due to

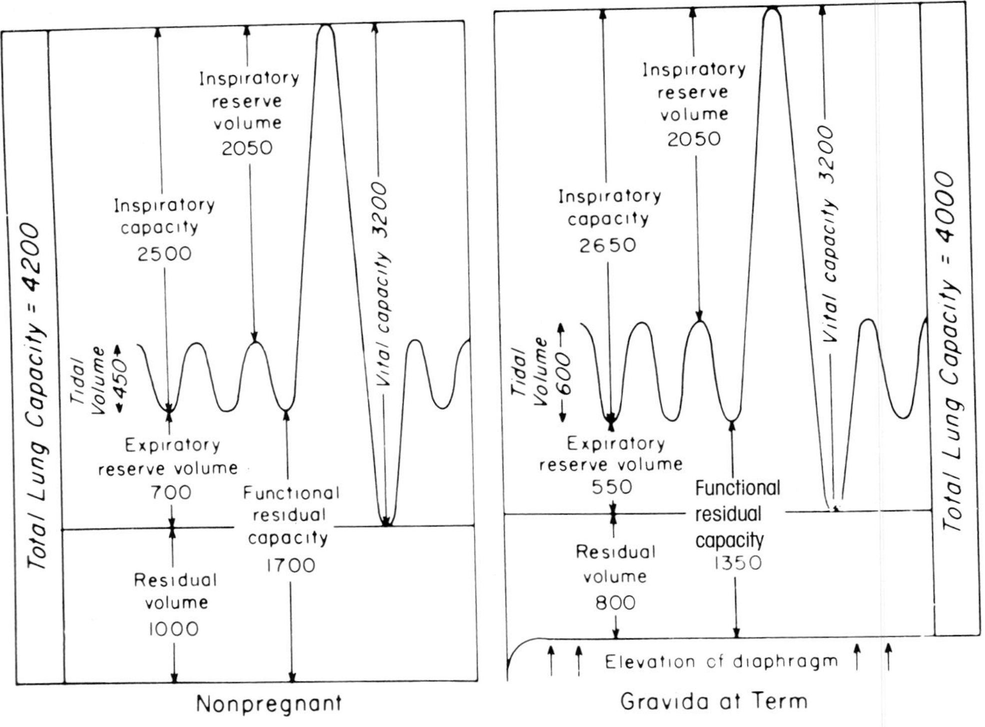

FIGURE 60–3. Alterations in pulmonary volumes and capacities associated with pregnancy (Reproduced with permission from Leontic EA. Respiratory disease in pregnancy. Med Clin North Am 1977; 61: 114.)

lung resection have shown the potential for normal pregnancy and fetal development.[23] Indeed, even intrapartum lung resection has been done when necessary without adverse outcome.[24] In view of these data, a woman with a respiratory disease that is unlikely to deteriorate during pregnancy, an FEV_1 greater than 1 L, and no dyspnea at rest can undertake pregnancy safely.

When a pregnant patient must undergo general anesthesia and lung disease is suspected, pulmonary function should be assessed. Postoperative respiratory complications of atelectasis, inadequate secretion clearance, infection, or respiratory failure are more likely to occur when the FEV_1 is less than 2 L. A higher FEV_1 is required to undergo uncomplicated surgery than is needed to tolerate pregnancy alone, because of an expected reduction of lung function in the immediate postoperative period.

RADIOGRAPHIC TESTING

Radiologic evaluation is a cornerstone of pulmonary medicine. Chest radiography inadvertently performed on a pregnant patient may expose the fetus to 8 to 36 mrads.[25,26] Chest fluoroscopy exposes the fetus to approximately 70 mrads, an estimate that will vary, depending on the operator, shielding, and reason for fluoroscopy.[25] Technetium-99m, a radionuclide frequently used in lung scanning, has a short half-life (6 h), is rapidly excreted, emits no beta rays, and is attached to macroaggregates of human albumin with a particle size of approximately 20 μm, which does not cross the placenta. Its use in pregnancy has not been subjected to direct studies,[26] and the biologic effects may differ from those secondary to x-radiation exposure. Nevertheless, fetal radiation exposure has been estimated to range between 500 mrads and 1 rad.[25]

If at any time during pregnancy, the health of the mother or fetus would be compromised by failure to perform a radiologic examination, the examination should be performed and every care should be taken to shield the fetus from scatter radiation and from the direct beam when appropriate. Although available data are not conclusive, both epidemiologic and laboratory studies indicate that some levels of radiographic exposure can be harmful to the developing human. Irradiation in utero may increase the risk of childhood leukemia and other malignancies by 40% to 50%.[27] Experimental studies show that doses as low as 5 rads can kill the early embryo, cause neural and skeletal malformations, and impair several aspects of behavior, including learning ability and emotional response to varied stimuli.[27] Obvious malformations are particularly associated with irradiation during the period of major organogenesis, which extends from approximately week 2 through week 9 after conception.[28] Taking into account the greatest oncogenic risk, the overall risk of any adverse effect from exposure to 1 rad is estimated to be 0.1%,[29] a risk that is thousands of times smaller than the risks of spontaneous abortion, malformation, or genetic disease.[25] Fetal exposure to less than 5 rads is considered insufficient reason to recommend termination of a desired pregnancy.[25,26,30,31]

When chest radiographs are performed in the pregnant patient, normal findings differ from those seen in non-pregnant women of childbearing age.[15] The diaphragm may be elevated 4 cm at term, but there will be a compensatory increase in anteroposterior diameter. There is an increase in the subcostal angle from 68.5° to 103.5° from early to late pregnancy.[32] Also, lung markings may be increased, giving a false impression of mild congestive heart failure. Hughson and colleagues reported that pleural effusions frequently occurred in the first 24 hours following delivery[33] and that in the absence of symptoms or signs of illness, no intervention was necessary. A subsequent prospective ultrasound study of 50 women within 1 to 45 hours of delivery found only one patient with a pleural effusion, a patient who was also in pulmonary edema.[34] The results of this study suggest that postpartum pleural effusions may not be a normal occurrence.

MATERNAL–FETAL OXYGEN EXCHANGE

Fetal oxygen delivery depends on maternal respiratory function, hemoglobin concentration, and cardiac output. During pregnancy, plasma volume increases by 30 mL/kg (from 40 to 70 mL/kg), and red cell volume increases from 25 mL/kg to 30 mL/kg.[35] As a result, even though erythrocyte mass is increased, there is a decrease in hemoglobin concentration to a value as low as 10.5 to 11.0 g/dL.[25] Maternal cardiac output, however, is enhanced by 30% to 40%, early in the second trimester,[25] because of an increase in stroke volume, left ventricular compliance, and heart rate, along with a reduced systemic vascular resistance (Table 60-2).[35] The net result of these physiologic changes is to ensure a high rate of oxygen delivery to the gravid uterus.

In a woman with no pulmonary disease breathing room air, arterial blood typically has a Pao_2 of 91 mm Hg and a Pco_2 of 36 mm Hg. In the fetal umbilical vein a simultaneous blood gas would typically show a Po_2 of 32 mm Hg and a Pco_2 of 50 mm Hg. The same woman breathing 100% oxygen would raise her Pao_2 to 583

TABLE 60–2. HEMODYNAMIC ALTERATIONS IN PREGNANCY

Plasma volume	++
Red cell volume	+
Hemoglobin	−−
Hematocrit	−−
Stroke volume	+
Left ventricular compliance	+
Heart rate	+
Systemic vascular resistance	−
Cardiac output	+++

++, increased; +, slightly increased; −, slightly decreased; −−, decreased.

mm Hg while the P_{O_2} of the umbilical vein would increase from 32 to 40 mm Hg, illustrating a large shunt effect.[36] Experimental data in sheep demonstrate that the oxygen tension in the fetal umbilical vein is always less than that in the uterine arteries, over all levels of maternal oxygenation.[37] Increases in the concentration of inspired oxygen result in the expected rise in oxygen tension in the maternal arteries but not in large increases in the oxygen tension of the fetal umbilical veins.[37] Nevertheless, even a small increase in uterine oxygen content can result in a significant increase in oxygen transfer to the fetus. This occurs because of the high maternal perfusion rate of the uterus, the enhanced avidity of fetal hemoglobin for oxygen, and the leftward shift of the fetal oxyhemoglobin dissociation curve. These adaptations allow the fetus to tolerate small changes in oxygen delivery, such as a reduction in maternal inspired oxygen to as low as 15%.[36] However, the fetus is sensitive to large shifts in oxygen delivery, caused by a fall in cardiac output, and with complete interruption of oxygen supply to the umbilical vein, the fetus has only a 2- to 4-minute oxygen reserve.[38]

Blood pH is an important determinant of uterine blood flow, and the finding of an acute, uncompensated respiratory alkalosis in a pregnant female signals possible compromise of fetal oxygenation. In one study of women at term, hyperventilation during inspiration of room air was associated with an increase in maternal oxygen tension from 91 to 100 mm Hg, but fetal scalp oxygen tension fell from 25 to 19 mm Hg because of a reduction in maternal carbon dioxide tension from 25 to 19 mm Hg. Maternal inhalation of 95% oxygen and 5% carbon dioxide restored the fetal oxygen tension to a normal level.[39] These data and studies in sheep have suggested that maternal alkalosis can result in decreased fetal oxygen tensions because of reduced uterine blood flow due to hypocarbia-induced vasoconstriction of uterine arteries, because of the mechanical effects of hyperventilation causing decreased maternal venous return and because of a shift in the maternal oxyhemoglobin dissociation curve to the left, thereby impairing oxygen transfer to the fetus.[37,39] In the studies of Wulf and colleagues fetal oxygen delivery was compromised when maternal pH exceeded 7.6 and P_{CO_2} was 15 mm Hg, values unlikely to be reached in acute asthma.[36,40]

ASTHMA

Asthma, or reversible narrowing of large or small airways, is the most common obstructive lung disease affecting women of childbearing age, occurring in 0.4% to 1.3% of pregnant women.[21,41]

THE EFFECT OF ASTHMA ON THE OUTCOME OF PREGNANCY

One large Norwegian study of pregnant women concluded that hyperemesis, vaginal hemorrhage, and toxemia were found to be more frequent in asthmatics than in nonasthmatics.[42] However, most asthmatics experience pregnancy with few ill effects, and in general there are no striking differences between the outcome of pregnancy in asthmatics compared with a control population. Nevertheless, severe and inadequately managed asthma can be associated with increased maternal and fetal complications, such as enhanced maternal and fetal mortality; a slight increase in the incidence of premature births, stillbirth, low–birth-weight babies; and subsequent neurologic abnormalities in the offspring.[42] No differences in the frequency of multiple births or congenital malformations or in the infants' Apgar scores have been seen in the children of asthmatic mothers.[43] In one study of 277 asthmatics during pregnancy, perinatal infant mortality was 5.9%,[44] but one quarter of these infant deaths came from a small group of mothers with severe asthma. These data contrast with a series of 55 corticosteroid-treated asthmatics, under close medical supervision, who had no increase in maternal or fetal mortality compared to a control population, although there was a slight increase in the incidence of premature births.[45] These contrasting outcomes suggest that with good control of asthmatic exacerbations in pregnancy, fetal outcome can be excellent.

THE EFFECT OF PREGNANCY ON THE COURSE OF ASTHMA

It is impossible to predict accurately how a specific patient's asthma will act during pregnancy. Retrospective studies have shown that asthma worsens during pregnancy in slightly more than one third of patients, improves in slightly more than one fourth of patients, and remains unchanged in one third of patients.[46,47] The change in asthma course associated with pregnancy usually reverts to the prepregnancy course within 3 months after delivery, and the course of asthma tends to be similar in a given woman during subsequent pregnancies. In a prospective analysis, Schatz and colleagues reported that in women whose asthma worsened during pregnancy, there was an increase in total asthma symptoms, and severe asthma symptoms, during weeks 29 to 36 of gestation. Asthma improved in all subjects in the final 4 weeks of pregnancy, and symptoms appeared to be rare during labor and delivery.[47]

Improvement in asthma during pregnancy may result from the net effect of several hormonal changes leading to increased levels of progesterone, causing bronchodilatation; serum-free cortisol levels; maternal histaminase; serum cyclic adenosine 3′, 5′-monophosphate (cAMP) levels, serum prostaglandin E (during the last weeks of pregnancy), and serum epinephrine (during labor and delivery).[41,47] Mechanical factors (ie, the "dropping" of the baby in the final weeks of pregnancy) may cause improvement in asthma by decreasing the mechanical impingement of the gravid uterus on the lungs, leading to improved ventilation–perfusion ratios. Offsetting these beneficial effects are alterations that can worsen asthma: antigenicity of the fetus, increased mouth breathing due to nasal congestion, increased susceptibility to viral infections, and hyperventilation.[46]

CLINICAL PRESENTATION

Classically, two clinical patterns of asthma have been recognized. One group, the so-called extrinsic asthmatics, develops asthma at a young age, has a family history of atopy, may have other atopic manifestations (skin and nasal allergies), and has evidence of IgE-mediated responses along with blood and sputum eosinophilia. Attacks are often seasonal and precipitated by well-defined allergens.[19,48] Interestingly, recent studies have shown that atopic patients (extrinsic asthmatics) have both immediate and late-phase responses to allergens.[49] The second group, the "intrinsic asthmatics," develops asthma later in life, has no family history of asthma or atopy, has no evidence of IgE-mediated bronchospasm, uncommonly has eosinophilia, but may have severe asthma that is difficult to treat. The intrinsic asthmatic is sensitive to environmental irritants, and acute exacerbations are often triggered by viral respiratory illness.[19,48] Many patients do not fit easily into either of these two groups. Other clinical patterns include the triad of chronic asthma, a history of nasal polyps and pansinusitis, and the development of significant reductions in airflow rates following ingestion of aspirin or nonsteroidal anti-inflammatory drugs.[19] In these patients, bronchospasm develops within minutes to hours, and symptoms may be severe or even life-threatening. Exercise-induced asthma is another common variant and is characterized by the development of bronchospasm following discontinuation of exercise in patients who may or may not have chronic asthmatic symptoms.[19]

An acute attack of asthma is usually heralded by the clinical triad of cough, wheezing, and dyspnea. Dyspnea may be interpreted as a tightness in the chest. Attacks often occur at night, perhaps related to fluctuations in airway receptor thresholds resulting from circadian variations in the circulating levels of endogenous catecholamines and histamine.[50] Usually, there is a history of exposure to a specific allergen, physical exertion, a viral respiratory tract infection, or emotional excitement preceding the onset of an exacerbation, and the patient will often have a history of similar episodes in the past. In some patients, asthma is manifested as a nonproductive cough unrelieved by antibiotics or cough suppressants.[19] Occasionally, asthma can evolve insidiously, without well-defined attacks, and the gradual increase in the degree of bronchospasm eventually leads to breathlessness during exertion.

Physical examination during an exacerbation reveals audibly harsh respirations, inspiratory and expiratory wheezing with a prolonged expiratory phase, tachypnea, tachycardia, and mild systolic hypertension. The lungs are overinflated and the anterior–posterior diameter of the thorax is increased beyond that typically expected in pregnancy. With increased duration and severity of an attack, the accessory respiratory muscles become visibly active and the patient may develop a paradoxical pulse, both signs of severe respiratory compromise.

The chest radiograph during an acute attack usually shows hyperinflation of the lungs with a small, elongated heart. It is not often necessary to obtain a chest radiograph in a pregnant asthmatic, during an exacerbation, especially if she is a known chronic asthmatic. One study found that chest radiography during acute asthma did not reveal pathology that was unsuspected by an adequate history and physical examination.[51] The chest film may be necessary to exclude complications such as pneumothorax, pneumomediastinum, cardiomegaly, pneumonia, mucoid impaction, or bronchopulmonary aspergillosis, but only when these conditions are suspected on clinical grounds.

Laboratory studies are nonspecific during an acute attack. The electrocardiogram may show sinus tachycardia or, occasionally, right axis deviation, clockwise rotation, right ventricular dominance, right bundle branch block, or ventricular ectopic beats. A complete blood count often displays a mild to moderate eosinophilia that may be reduced or absent if the patient has been taking corticosteroids.

The differential diagnosis of wheezing is large (Table 60-3), but with a typical history and presentation, an acute asthma attack is usually easy to recognize. Acute left heart failure, perhaps secondary to unrecognized

TABLE 60–3. DIFFERENTIAL DIAGNOSIS OF WHEEZING

Upper Respiratory Tract
Amyloid
Angioedema
Foreign body
Goiter
Infection
Neuromuscular disease
Relapsing polychondritis
Tracheal stenosis
Tumor
Vocal cord paralysis
Lower Respiratory Tract
Adenopathy
Amyloid
Asthma
Aspiration
Bronchiolitis
Chronic obstructive pulmonary disease
Cystic fibrosis
Foreign body
Pulmonary infiltrates with eosinophilia
Sarcoidosis
Vascular
Adult respiratory distress syndrome
Congestive heart failure
Pulmonary embolism
Vasculitis
Extrathoracic
Carcinoid
Factitious

(From Hollingsworth, HM, Pratter MR, Irwin RS. Acute respiratory failure in pregnancy. *J Intensive Care Med* 1989;4:11.)

critical mitral stenosis, may present with a similar clinical picture, but the presence of cardiomegaly and signs of left heart dysfunction should help to make the distinction. Patients with pulmonary embolism can occasionally present with wheezing or chest tightness, and pregnant women can develop this condition with increased frequency. Acute bronchitis may be difficult to differentiate from asthma, but the absence of a prior history of asthma, the presence of upper respiratory tract symptoms (pharyngitis, coryza, and so on), and occurrence during a community-wide epidemic should help to make the distinction. Upper airway obstruction by a tumor, foreign body, or edema can occasionally be confused with asthma, but the presence of stridor and a lack of widespread wheezing will usually allow the physician to suspect these problems.

In the initial phase of an asthma exacerbation, the small airways become narrowed. If the patient has had long-standing asthma, the total amount of bronchial smooth muscle may be increased, leading to a reduction in the cross-sectional diameter of the airways, even when the patient is asymptomatic. Bronchial smooth muscle spasm occurs acutely during an attack and may be reversible, whereas mucus plugging and inflammation play an increasingly important role in a prolonged attack and in status asthmaticus.[52]

As airway narrowing increases, the patient begins to increase ventilation and the chronic respiratory alkalosis, normal in pregnancy, acutely worsens. With increasing airway obstruction air can enter smaller bronchi but may not be fully expired, and as a result of air trapping, FRC increases and ventilation–perfusion mismatching occurs, leading to significant hypoxemia. As the attack progresses, airway resistance increases, further air trapping occurs, the work of breathing goes up, oxygen consumption increases, and ventilation becomes very difficult. With sufficient airway obstruction, the energy required to do the work of breathing may exceed the body's capacity to deliver oxygen to the respiratory muscles, and anaerobic metabolism can occur, leading to a lactic acidosis. The pathophysiologic relationships in severe asthma are diagrammed in Figure 60-4.

Life-threatening risks can be avoided by careful and routine medical attention during pregnancy and by early pharmacologic intervention during an exacerbation. The clinical hallmarks of cough, wheezing, and dyspnea do not correlate in any predictable way with lung function. Thus, if the patient can perform a forced expiration, the FEV_1 or the peak expiratory flow rate (PEFR) should be used to assess the severity and progress of airway obstruction. Carbon dioxide retention begins to occur at an FEV_1 of approximately 750 mL (about 25% of the predicted value),[53] and a PEFR of less than 100 L/min is thought to be associated with an increased risk of a potentially fatal attack.[52] With severe asthma, accessory muscle use and pulsus paradoxicus may be seen, suggesting that the FEV_1 is less than 25% of normal.[54] Recent studies of patients who died from asthma both in and out of the hospital have consis-

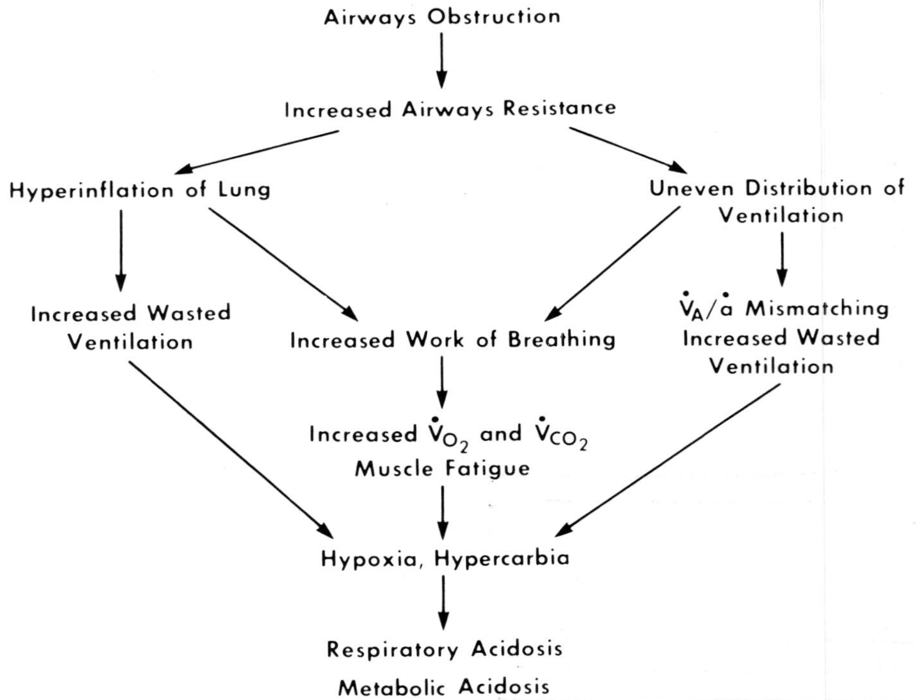

FIGURE 60–4. Pathophysiologic relationships in severe asthma (Reproduced with permission from Hopewell PC, Miller TM. Pathophysiology and management of severe asthma. Clin Chest Med, 1984; 5(4): 626.)

tently shown that the patient or the physician was unaware of the severity of the attack, because the status of the patient had been inadequately assessed.[53,55] In extreme exacerbations, wheezing may markedly lessen or even disappear completely, cough may become extremely ineffective, and the patient may begin a gasping type of respiratory pattern.[49] These findings imply extensive mucus plugging and impending suffocation.

PHARMACOLOGY OF ASTHMA THERAPY

Ideally, the management of asthma should begin prior to conception so as to avert, or suppress, acute episodes of asthma and incidents of status asthmaticus. Most of the agents that are used in controlling asthma can be used safely in pregnant women when given in recommended dosages (Table 60-4). The dangers of inadequately controlled asthma are far greater than the small risks posed by pharmacotherapy. Nevertheless, common sense dictates that when medication is required, the minimum number of medications necessary to control symptoms should be used.

The normal bronchial smooth muscle cell has adrenergic receptors. Beta agonists produce bronchodilation by directly stimulating $beta_2$ receptors in airway smooth muscle, whereas alpha receptor stimulation causes bronchoconstriction.[50] $Beta_1$ receptors are present in the cardiovascular system, and their stimulation by nonselective beta-mimetic agents does not improve pulmonary function but does lead to the cardiac side effects (especially tachycardia) of these drugs.[50] $Beta_2$ receptor

TABLE 60–4. ASTHMA MEDICATION SAFETY IN PREGNANCY AND POSTPARTUM

ROUTE	AGENT	PREGNANCY	BREAST-FEEDING	COMMENTS
Sympathomimetics*				
Aerosol	Epinephrine Isoproterenol	yes	yes	Short-acting Side effects: tachycardia, nervousness, muscle tremor
	Metaproterenol Albuterol	yes	yes	Less side effects Useful as pretreatment for exercise-induced asthma
	Terbutaline	yes	yes	Associated with pulmonary edema near term
Oral	Ephedrine Metaproterenol Albuterol Terbutaline	yes	yes	Patient intolerance due to tachyphylaxis resulting in hypertension and anxiety
Subcutaneous	Epinephrine	yes	yes	Concerns about use in first trimester—see test
	Terbutaline	yes	yes	
Theophyllines				
Oral		yes	yes	May exacerbate morning nausea and vomiting and gastroesophageal reflex Need to monitor serum levels Various drug interactions—see text Possible infantile irritability and insomnia with breast-feeding
Intravenous		yes	yes	
Corticosteroids				
Aerosol	Beclomethasone	yes	yes	Aerosols may replace or reduce oral steroid requirements
Oral	Prednisone Prednisolone Methylprednisolone	yes	yes	Corticosteroids may increase responsiveness to beta-adrenergics
Intravenous	Hydrocortisone Methylprednisone	yes	yes	
Cromolyn Sodium†				
Aerosol		yes	yes	A 4–6 week trial is recommended Useful as pretreatment for exercise-induced asthma
Ipratropium Bromide†				
Aerosol		probable	probable	Limited indications

* Terbutaline and inhaled beta agonists are thought to be safe in the first trimester but documentation is lacking.

† Ipratropium bromide and cromolyn sodium are not absolutely contraindicated in the first trimester but because of "newness," there is still an unknown teratogenic risk.

stimulation leads to intracellular activation of bronchial smooth muscle cell adenylate cyclase that increases intracellular cyclic amp (cAMP) and leads to reduced smooth muscle tone. Beta agonists also prevent the development of bronchial smooth muscle edema after exposure to mediators such as histamine. They also tend to increase mucus secretion from submucosal glands and ion transport across airway epithelium, possibly leading to enhanced mucociliary clearance.[50] Generally, beta agonists are effective in treating an immediate asthmatic reaction but have less effect on the late-phase response.[56]

Intracellular cAMP is broken down by a cytoplasmic enzyme, phosphodiesterase, which can be inhibited by methylxanthines. This inhibition had commonly been thought to be the mechanism of action of theophylline. However, with the dosages of theophylline currently being used, phosphodiesterase cannot be significantly affected and there is no evidence that airway smooth muscle cells concentrate theophylline to achieve higher intracellular than circulating concentrations.[57] Rather, theophylline may function as an adenosine antagonist. Adenosine is a natural bronchoconstrictor and theophylline is a potent inhibitor of adenosine receptors at therapeutic concentrations.[57–59] Unquestionably, although theophylline's mechanism is controversial, its efficacy and its safety in pregnancy are not. In addition to causing bronchodilatation, theophylline can stimulate respiration, increase cardiac inotropy and chronotropy, stimulate diaphragmatic contraction, and cause a mild diuresis. The beneficial and undesirable effects of theophylline can be enhanced by caffeine.

Corticosteroids are important pharmacologic agents that act through mechanisms different from those of the bronchodilators. They are transported into the target cells and conveyed to the nucleus, where they affect the DNA transcription of specific messenger RNA and subsequently of specific proteins. This sequence of events may take several hours and explains the delay in onset of most corticosteroid effects. Their actions are multiple and include vasoconstriction of the bronchial vasculature with reduction in edema formation and dilation of bronchial smooth muscle,[60] inhibition of antibody formation, reduction in the accumulation of neutrophils and macrophages, eosinopenia, and inhibition of antigen penetration of the bronchial mucosa. In addition, they block the formation of many inflammatory mediators and increase beta-adrenergic responsiveness (thus reversing or preventing tolerance to nebulized beta agonists).[60,61] Recently, studies suggest that corticosteroids may decrease airway reactivity and that they can block the late-phase asthmatic response,[62] while having only a variable effect on the immediate reaction.[63]

Atropine, atropine methylnitrate, and ipratropium bromide are topically active specific antagonists of muscarinic receptors. Muscarinic receptors may mediate resting bronchomotor tone, probably through tonic vagal nerve impulses. Considerable evidence exists in animals that cholinergic pathways may also play an important role in regulating acute bronchomotor responses by eliciting reflex bronchoconstriction via vagal pathways. Thus, muscarinic antagonists have been postulated to have a role as bronchodilators in acute asthma. Multiple controlled studies have since documented that, although muscarinic antagonists may be somewhat effective against acute challenges by agents such as sulfur dioxide, cold air, and psychogenic stress, they are less effective against antigenic challenge.[64,65] Conversely, anticholinergic drugs have been found to be at least as effective as beta agonists in the symptomatic treatment of emphysema. Their greater efficacy in chronic obstructive pulmonary disease (COPD) may be attributed to the greater contribution of vagal tone to airway obstruction in those diseases.[64,65]

Cromolyn sodium, a prophylactic medication for asthma, was originally thought to act solely by stabilizing the mast cell membrane and thereby inhibiting the release of inflammatory mediators in response to allergen. Further research has suggested that cromolyn actually has a low potency in stabilizing human lung mast cells and that it may have effects on neurotransmission.[66,67] Cromolyn sodium may also indirectly block mast cell calcium channels and the phosphorylation of a membrane protein necessary for mediator release. Because it prevents mast cell degranulation, it is effective in preventing both the immediate and late-phase allergic responses.[67]

MEDICATION SAFETY IN PREGNANCY

Beta-Adrenergic Agents

Beta$_2$-adrenoceptor agonists are extremely effective bronchodilators in asthma (see Table 60-4). They should be given as an aerosol and are probably the drugs of choice for treating episodic wheezing and acute asthma attacks during pregnancy.[68,69] There are minimal maternal side effects, such as tachycardia, nervousness, and muscle tremor. The newer beta$_2$-specific agents, such as metaproterenol, albuterol, or terbutaline, have fewer of these unpleasant side effects than the less specific agents, such as isoproterenol and ephedrine. In animal studies, sympathomimetic drugs have caused teratogenic effects, such as cleft palate, craniostenosis, hydrocephalus, and other bony abnormalities.[70] Comparatively high doses are required to produce these effects, and there is little evidence that similar deformities are produced in humans by conventional doses.[38] In Europe, inhaled beta agonists have become the therapy of choice for acute asthma.[68]

Metaproterenol or albuterol, given as a metered-dose inhaler, can be used as pretreatment for exercise-induced asthma. Metaproterenol, ephedrine, and albuterol are also available in oral forms. Terbutaline is available in both oral and parenteral forms. These agents should be used cautiously near term because of an association with pulmonary edema in patients receiving both beta agonists and corticosteroids to treat premature labor.[40] Ephedrine has a history of extensive use during pregnancy, suggesting that it has no detrimental effects on the fetus or placenta. There may be problems with patient tolerance, as it appears to induce tachyphylaxis readily and may result in hypertension and anxiety.[38] Similarly, terbutaline has a long history of use as a tocolytic agent and is thought to be free of teratogenic effects.[43]

Epinephrine

Epinephrine given subcutaneously has primarily a beta-adrenergic effect and is commonly used in the emergent treatment of acute bronchospasm. Its use as the treatment of choice in pregnant women, especially during the first trimester, continues to provoke controversy. Advocates favor it because it is an endogenous chemical, is readily available, is rapidly metabolized, has not been associated with tocolysis, and has generally not been associated with long-term sequelae in the fetus.[37,40] Critics point out that studies have linked epinephrine to congenital malformations and decreased uterine blood flow.[68,71] Epinephrine administered intravenously or intra-aortically has been associated with decreased uterine blood flow in the rhesus monkey. Whether a correlation to subcutaneous administration in the human female exists is controversial.[72] The conclusions of a study linking epinephrine to teratogenic effects have also been questioned.[72,73] Although epinephrine should probably be avoided in the first trimester, its ready availability, the fact that it is an endogenous chemical that is rapidly metabolized, its lack of tocolytic effects, and the considerable risk that an acute asthmatic attack represents to the fetus may justify its use.

Theophylline

Although theophylline readily crosses the placenta, it is customarily felt to be safe throughout pregnancy because it has not been demonstrated to be teratogenic. Theophylline and its derivatives are a mainstay of asthma therapy and have additive bronchodilator effects when given with a beta agonist.[60,61] Fixed combinations of theophylline, ephedrine, antihistamines, and barbiturates should not be used during pregnancy. In the first trimester theophylline may be poorly tolerated because it may exacerbate morning nausea and vomiting, whereas later it may exacerbate gastroesophageal reflux.

If given in excessive doses, theophylline can lead to both maternal and fetal toxicity. Neonatal toxic reactions include jitteriness, tachycardia, gagging, vomiting, and opisthotonos, all of which can occur at neonatal theophylline blood levels that are considered therapeutic in the adult.[74] Adult reactions can include seizures, in addition to the preceding findings. One study showed that fetal toxicity can occur in the absence of maternal toxicity, owing to increased fetal sensitivity to and slower elimination of the drug.[74] Another study showed that, although the fetus may have higher heelstick theophylline levels than maternal blood levels, side effects that frequently occur are minor and transient, making maternal theophylline use safe for the fetus at term.[75] To avoid toxic complications, the physician should aim for blood levels of theophylline between 5 and 14 μg/mL.[76] Smoking and phenytoin increase theophylline clearance, whereas erythromycin, cimetidine, viral infections, and pneumonia decrease it. A recent study of the pharmacokinetics of theophylline in pregnancy demonstrated that the distribution volume and half-life of theophylline increased significantly in the third trimester, but clearance was reduced to an even greater extent. The study concluded that third-trimester theophylline levels could increase by 40% unless dosage reductions were made.[77] Based on these considerations, it is necessary to monitor serum levels closely during pregnancy, especially near term.

Corticosteroids

When managing severe or mild asthma unresponsive to bronchodilators and theophylline, steroids can be added and can result in a significant reduction in disease morbidity and mortality. Human studies have not confirmed the increased risk of cleft palate seen in offspring of corticosteroid-treated animals,[45] and both inhaled beclomethasone and prednisone appear to be safe, even when given during the first trimester.[68,78,79] Neonatal adrenal suppression has been seen only rarely, probably because of rapid conversion of prednisone to its active form, prednisolone, in the mother and because of poor placental passage of prednisolone. Additionally, the fetus may be unable to convert prednisone, which can cross the placenta, to prednisolone. Neonatal recovery from corticosteroid-induced adrenal suppression is rapid and does not appear to present a significant clinical risk.

Atropine

It is not yet clear whether atropine, which has been shown to be safe in early pregnancy, will be a valuable addition to current asthma therapy.[40] Atropine itself is not recommended for aerosol administration during late pregnancy because it has maternal systemic side effects and can cross the placenta, theoretically causing fetal tachycardia.[80] Ipratropium, a muscarinic antagonist, has not been adequately studied in pregnancy but is poorly absorbed when given via the aerosol route and presumably is less likely to reach or affect the fetus. In patients with significant vagally mediated bronchospasm, such as those with asthma exacerbated by emotional stress or those who have bronchitis accompanied by marked wheezing, ipratropium may be a useful alternative.[38] This use has not, however, been approved by the FDA.

Cromolyn Sodium

Cromolyn sodium, like ipratropium, has not been specifically approved by the Food and Drug Administration for use in pregnancy. Cromolyn sodium has been shown to prevent asthmatic reactions to antigen, exercise, cold air, hyperventilation, aspirin, and sulfur dioxide. Children apparently respond better than adults, and younger adults respond better than older adults, but there are no obvious differences between intrinsic and extrinsic asthmatics.[50,81,82]

Large intravenous doses of sodium cromoglycate in rats and rabbits do not have any teratogenic effects,[40] and a study in 296 asthmatic women, using recommended inhaled dosages of cromolyn sodium throughout pregnancy, did not document an increased risk of fetal malformations.[83] Because it is poorly absorbed after inhalation, the amount available for transfer across the placenta is probably insignificant, although this has not been specifically studied.[68] Notable systemic side effects are limited to irritation caused by the dry powder.[84] When cromolyn is used, a 4- to 6-week trial of therapy is indicated, because it may take from 2 to 4 weeks for the effects to become apparent. A single dose, administered 20 minutes prior to exercise, may prevent exercise-induced asthma.

Other Agents

Drugs to be specifically avoided in the pregnant asthmatic are the antihistamines brompheniramine (fetal malformations); hydroxyzine and cyproheptadine (insufficient data); tetracycline (damage to fetal teeth, bone, and liver); iodide expectorants (life-threatening fetal goiter); amobarbital, an agent used in some combination medications (cardiovascular malformations); and aspirin or tartrazine dye in sensitive patients (precipitates asthma) (Table 60-5).[85] Oral products containing alpha-adrenergic agents, such as those used to clear nasal obstruction, should be avoided. Theoretically, at any time during pregnancy, they could cause constriction of placental vessels, thereby endangering the fetus.[38] Antitussives, especially those containing codeine, should be avoided because they may have a teratogenic effect when used in the first trimester and may affect the breathing of the neonate at term. Mucokinetic agents, such as guaifenesin, have limited value, and although they are probably harmless to the fetus, they have been associated with increased vomiting and therefore are not recommended in the pregnant woman with asthma. Likewise, acetylcysteine, a mucolytic agent, is poorly tolerated by many bronchospastic patients when given by aerosol and is rarely indicated in pregnancy.[38]

TABLE 60–5. MEDICATIONS RELATIVELY OR ABSOLUTELY CONTRAINDICATED IN THE PREGNANT ASTHMATIC

Antihistamines
Brompheniramine
Hydroxyzine
Cyproheptadine
Tetracycline
Amobarbital
Iodide expectorants
Aspirin
Tartrazine dye
Oral and topical decongestants
Alpha-adrenergic agonists
Antitussives
Codeine
Mucokinetic agents
Guaifenesin
Mucolytic agents
Acetylcysteine

Medications in Labor and Delivery

Beta-mimetic agents should be discontinued if possible during labor and delivery because of the risk of tocolysis and postpartum uterine atony. Antiasthmatic medications should be administered intravenously, and women who have received systemic or inhaled corticosteroids during pregnancy should be given hydrocortisone (100 mg intravenously or intramuscularly) upon admission in labor, followed by the same dose every 8 hours thereafter for 24 hours; then the patient should be returned to her previous corticosteroid regimen.[37] If general anesthesia is necessary for delivery, halogenated gases are broncholytic and are preferable to nonhalogenated agents.

Medications During Lactation

Breast feeding is safe for the children of asthmatics, including those taking antiasthmatic medications (see Table 60-4). Although theophylline is secreted into the breast milk in significant quantities, the infant usually receives less than 10% of the mother's dose. Occasionally, this may be associated with irritability and insomnia in the infant, requiring temporary withdrawal or a decrease in the mother's dose.[84] Inhaled beta agonists and oral or inhaled corticosteroids are safe for the mother and baby.[68] It is not known whether cromolyn sodium or ipratropium bromide are excreted in breast milk.[86]

EVALUATION AND THERAPY OF THE OUTPATIENT ASTHMATIC DURING PREGNANCY

Once pregnancy is contemplated or realized, a thorough evaluation of the asthmatic is warranted (Table 60-6). A careful history should be performed to characterize the severity of a patient's asthma and to identify any recognizable precipitants of bronchospasm. Chronic and as-needed medications should be reviewed with the aim of optimizing dosage and frequency of administration. Aspirin and aspirin-containing medications should be avoided because of the association of these medications with bronchospasm in up to 25% of asthmatics.[43] If the patient wishes to engage in safe but vigorous exercise, proper medication given prior to exertion will effectively block exercise induced asthma. Swimming is customarily

TABLE 60-6. PROPHYLACTIC EVALUATION AND MANAGEMENT OF THE OUTPATIENT ASTHMATIC

1. Take a careful history to determine the severity of asthma and to identify precipitants.
2. Discourage use of aspirin, antihistamines, decongestants, etc.
3. Optimize dosage and frequency of medications.
4. Patient counseling:
   a. Appropriate exercise with prophylactic modifications if needed
   b. Advice on how to avoid precipitants
   c. Instruction in early recognition of wheezing and need for prompt intervention
5. Take baseline PFTs including vital capacity, FEV_1, and PEFR with repetition as disease activity warrants.
6. Obtain serial serum theophylline levels.
7. Vaccinate against influenza in the autumn or after the first trimester
8. Immunotherapy may be continued but should not be started, nor should the dose be increased in large increments because of the risk of anaphylaxis

thought to be a good cardiovascular exercise and, because of the humid environment, is generally well tolerated by asthmatics. Instruction in the early recognition of wheezing and the need for prompt intervention should be given.

Pulmonary function studies, which include the vital capacity, FEV_1, and PEFR, should be performed early to provide a baseline and then repeated throughout pregnancy as warranted by disease activity. The serum level of theophylline should be measured and repeated periodically. Influenza vaccination should be given in the autumn but should be delayed if possible until after the first trimester.[38] Immunotherapy, if begun prior to pregnancy, should be continued, but it should not be started during pregnancy, nor should doses be raised in large increments, because of the risk of maternal anaphylaxis.[87]

If symptoms are not well controlled, therapy is begun with beta-agonist inhalation, alone or in combination with an oral theophylline preparation. If symptoms persist, the patient should be tried on a short course of oral steroids (prednisone, hydrocortisone). Corticosteroids should be given in an effective dose initially (30 to 60 mg of prednisone) and then tapered gradually over the course of approximately 4 to 7 days.[37] A patient who requires repeated short courses of oral steroids or who requires chronic doses of steroids should probably be started on an inhaled corticosteroid in an attempt to eliminate, change to alternate day, or decrease the dose of oral corticosteroids.

THERAPY OF ACUTE ASTHMA ATTACKS

An acute attack of asthma should be aggressively managed and the patient should be evaluated carefully for possible hospital admission (Fig. 60-5). In approximately 10% to 15% of pregnancies complicated by asthma, the patient may require hospitalization for sta-

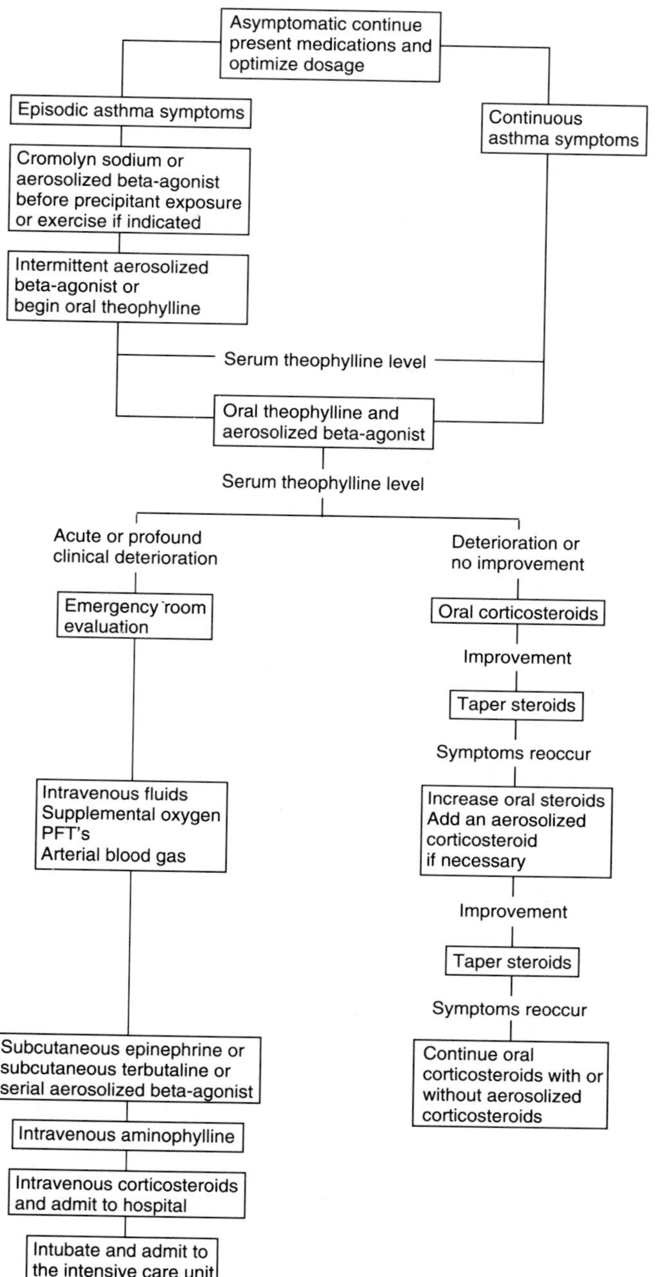

FIGURE 60-5. Therapy of acute asthma exacerbations.

tus asthmaticus,[43] a condition characterized by refractory airway obstruction, with failure to resolve after appropriate treatment. A quick search for a precipitating event and questioning about prior and current corticosteroid use are part of the initial history. Then examination of pulse, blood pressure, respiratory rate, pulsus paradoxus, and FEV_1 and/or peak expiratory flow is indicated. A pulse of more than 120/min, respiratory rate of more than 30/min, pulsus paradoxus more than 18 mm Hg, peak expiratory flow less than 120 L/min, moderate to severe dyspnea, accessory muscle use, and severe wheezing at the time of presentation are all signs of potentially life-threatening disease and probably indicate a need for acute hospitalization.[88] Additional warning signs of a fatal attack are listed in Table 60-7. In assessing the degree of wheezing present, the combination of inspiratory and expiratory wheezes signifies more obstruction than if expiratory wheezes alone are present. In the most severe cases of asthma, relatively few wheezes are heard because very little air is moved through the markedly narrowed airways.

The most reliable guides to the severity of an attack are the blood gas tensions, especially if the patient is too distressed to perform a forced expiration.[89,90] In mild asthma, arterial carbon dioxide tension is normal (for pregnancy) or slightly reduced. In the more severe stages of asthma, normocarbia or hypercarbia develops and arterial hypoxemia becomes more marked. Administration of oxygen is safe and is indicated to alleviate hypoxemia and minimize respiratory alkalosis. Bedside spirometry and measurement of FEV_1/FVC and peak expiratory flow rate are also useful, especially when compared with previous values and when followed serially through an attack.

In an emergency setting, epinephrine (0.3 mL of 1:1000 dilution) can be given subcutaneously with serial injections leading to cumulative improvements in airway function that may persist for up to 4 hours.[91,92] Subcutaneous epinephrine should be avoided in patients with marked hypertension (systolic pressure above 200 mm Hg) or an irregular pulse.[52] Acceptable alternatives to the use of epinephrine are subcutaneous terbutaline and nebulized, inhaled beta-adrenergic agonists. If inhaled beta agonists are used, sequential inhalations can produce a greater improvement than an equivalent dose administered as a single inhalation.[91] In an emergent setting, nebulized, inhaled beta-adrenergic agonists can be given in reduced dosages every 20 minutes for at least the first hour after presentation.

Concurrent administration of intravenous aminophylline should be started during a severe acute attack. If the patient is already taking a theophylline preparation, no loading dose is necessary; if the patient is not taking such a preparation, aminophylline 5 to 6 mg/kg (up to 400 mg) is given intravenously over 30 minutes with dosage calculations based on lean body mass. Partial loading doses can be used for patients with subtherapeutic serum theophylline concentrations. Then a continuous aminophylline infusion is given at 0.5 mg/kg/h, preferably via an infusion pump, and a theophylline blood level is checked in 10 to 12 hours to assure that the concentration is in the safe, effective range of 5 to 14 μg/mL. When the attack resolves, intravenous aminophylline is replaced with oral theophylline, given in divided doses, starting with 85% of the total dose (in milligrams) of aminophylline given over the previous 24 hours. The intravenous aminophylline should not be discontinued until 3 to 4 hours after the first dose of oral theophylline is given.

TABLE 60-7. STATUS ASTHMATICUS: WARNING SIGNS OF FATAL ATTACK

Previous or recurrent episodes of status asthmaticus, especially previous intubation
FVC < 1.0 L; FEV_1 < 0.5 L; PEFR < 100 L/min
Little or no response to bronchodilator therapy at one hour (ΔFEV_1 < 400 mL; Δ PEFR < 60 mL/min)
Altered consciousness
Unequivocal central cyanosis; arterial Po_2 < 50 mm Hg
Pco_2 > 45 mm Hg
Pulsus paradoxus
ECG abnormalites
Presence of pneumothorax or pneumomediastinum

(From Summer WR. Status asthmaticus. Chest (Suppl) 1985;87:895.)

Simultaneous supportive management in the form of supplemental oxygen and intravenous fluids should be given. Oxygen is given by nasal cannula beginning at a rate of 2 to 3 L/min and titrated to maintain an arterial $Po_2 \geq 70$ mm Hg. Some patients with asthma may be dehydrated because of marked hyperventilation, diaphoresis, and decreased oral intake, and intravenous fluids should be used to restore normovolemia, which will aid the expectoration of sputum. Sedation to treat the anxiety associated with severe asthma is never indicated. In one study of patients requiring mechanical ventilation for status asthmaticus, 8 out of 21 patients received large doses of sedatives that were ordered by house physicians, suggesting that sedative use was related to the ensuing respiratory failure.[93]

If the clinical examination and serial spirometries show that the patient is not responding adequately despite aggressive therapy over the course of 2 to 4 hours, if the patient has a long history of corticosteroid use for prior exacerbations, if the attack has been present for several days before the patient seeks help, or if the patient is already taking corticosteroids, then corticosteroid therapy is indicated. The recommended dose of corticosteroids for the first 24 hours of a severe attack varies between 100 and 3000 mg (average, 300 mg/24 h) of hydrocortisone or its equivalent.[52] High-dose corticosteroid therapy has been associated with altered host defense mechanisms and has not been shown to be superior in the treatment of acute asthma.[52,94] We recommend a regimen of 30 to 60 mg of Solu-Medrol every 4 to 6 hours as initial therapy.

If corticosteroids are used, the patient should be admitted to the hospital and this regimen should be continued until the attack resolves. Corticosteroids are then continued orally at a starting dose of 60 mg of prednisone daily and tapered as tolerated by 20 mg at 4-day intervals until a daily dose of 20 mg is reached. From this point, the dose is tapered weekly by 5 mg until corticosteroids are stopped or the patient reaches the lowest dose that keeps her free of symptoms. It has been suggested that the elimination of peripheral eosinophilia may give some indication that adequate systemic corticosteroids are being given.[52] If corticosteroids cannot be withdrawn completely, then inhaled beclomethasone can be added or therapy with alternate-day oral corticosteroids may be initiated. Because adequate control of asthma is essential for optimizing fetal and maternal outcome, there should be no hesitation about continuing corticosteroids indefinitely throughout pregnancy, if needed, to control the asthma.

Antibiotics are used in an acute asthma attack if pneumonia is present or if bacterial respiratory infection appears to have played a precipitating role. For therapy of infectious bronchitis, oral erythromycin or an oral cephalosporin can be used until the results of a sputum culture are available and a full 10-day course of therapy is given. Antibiotic therapy of bacterial pneumonia is discussed later.

THERAPY OF RESPIRATORY FAILURE DUE TO ASTHMA

Adherence to the preceding treatment program will manage most episodes of acute asthma (see Fig. 60-5). There remains a small population of patients who will continue to deteriorate despite aggressive, appropriate therapy. Documentation of a persistently normal or elevated arterial P_{CO_2} during an asthma attack, rather than the expected hypocarbia, warrants admission to an intensive care unit. In a patient who is near term, external fetal monitoring can be employed to assure adequate oxygen delivery to the fetus.

Mechanical ventilation is required if, in spite of bronchodilator therapy, the patient cannot maintain a Pa_{O_2} of 70 mm Hg or greater with supplemental oxygen. Other grounds for early endotracheal intubation include the presence of significant mental status changes, acute respiratory acidosis, life-threatening cardiac arrhythmias, and evidence of myocardial ischemia.[53]

A volume-cycled ventilator should always be used and a continuous mechanical ventilation (CMV) mode should be used initially, to allow the respiratory muscles to rest completely and thus relieve the work of breathing and reduce oxygen consumption. Adjustment of the ratio of inspiration to expiration is the most difficult aspect of respirator management in the severely obstructed patient. A balance must be found between the marked slowing of the expiratory phase because of airway obstruction and the preference for a slow inspiratory time so as to minimize peak airway pressures.[53] Sedation to the point of apnea is one means of obtaining better control of pulmonary mechanics, but this may be risky to the fetus, especially near term. Alternatively, milder sedation combined with muscular paralysis by pancuronium bromide can be employed. Pancuronium does not cause histamine release and is approved for operative obstetrics because very little crosses the placental barrier and there have been no known sequelae after short-term administration.[95] Vercuronium, a newer muscle relaxant, also has not generally been associated with histamine release, but it has not been approved for operative obstetrics and is probably contraindicated in pregnant patients.[96] Sedation is achieved with morphine because it is easily titratable and reversible with naloxone. Theoretically, morphine can release histamine and increase bronchoconstriction, but this has not proven to be of practical importance.

If mechanical ventilation is unable to correct the hypoxemia and the patient is near term, consideration should be given to delivering the baby via cesarean section. Desperate efforts to ease refractory hypoxemia include fiberoptic bronchoscopy to remove inspissated secretions from the larger airways and bronchoalveolar lavage in an attempt to clear smaller airways. General halogenated anesthesia may be tried for its broncholytic effects.

Mechanical ventilation is an important life-saving form of support for the severe asthmatic, but it is associated with a high incidence of complications and a 38% mortality in one series.[93] This difficulty arises because the severely obstructed asthmatic requires high airway pressures to achieve an adequate tidal volume, and barotrauma, in the form of pneumothorax or pneumomediastinum, may follow.[97] Recently, it has been suggested that this risk may be reduced by ventilating asthmatics with lower tidal volumes and respiratory rates, so as to reduce the peak airway pressure, and by treating the resulting acidosis with intravenous bicarbonate,[98] but this approach has not been tried in pregnant patients. With the use of positive pressure ventilation, even a small pneumothorax can quickly transform to a tension pneumothorax, and thus therapy with a chest tube is necessary. Pneumothorax should be suspected whenever an abrupt increase in peak airway pressure is accompanied by hypotension and tachycardia, and the diagnosis can be confirmed by chest radiography.

Although mechanical ventilation can quickly correct altered blood gas values, weaning from the ventilator should not begin until the airway obstruction significantly improves. During mechanical ventilation the peak airway pressure provides a rough indication of airway obstruction, and once peak airway pressure declines below 30 cm H_2O, weaning can be considered. The mean duration of mechanical ventilation for status asthmaticus in one study was 3 days, whereas in another it was 113 hours.[55,93]

Mucus plugging is common in severe asthma and contributes to the bronchospasm, hypoxemia, and atelectasis found in this disease. With the institution of mechanical ventilation, the presence of central airway plugging may result in a one-way ball valve, as air becomes trapped beyond inspissated mucus. This may lead to a tension shift of the mediastinum and associated cardiopulmonary compromise. In one such case, the diagnosis was made via chest radiography that demonstrated the presence of a mediastinal shift with bilateral lung markings present, thus eliminating the possibility of a tension pneumothorax. Treatment consisted of bedside bronchoscopy and lung lavage.[99]

Mediastinal emphysema can occur not only with asthma but also during the second stage of labor, with hyperemesis of early pregnancy, or after a bout of coughing. It may or may not accompany pneumothorax in severe exacerbations of asthma. Clinically, the patient presents with sharp retrosternal pain, which can radiate to the arms and shoulders. On examination, subcutaneous emphysema is present and a crunching noise, Hamman's sign, can be heard with each heartbeat at the left sternal edge. Pneumothorax, often on the left, is associated in some cases. Treatment involves analgesia and oxygen, drainage by chest tube of an associated pneumothorax, and careful observation.

OTHER OBSTRUCTIVE LUNG DISORDERS

Severe emphysema due to α_1-antitrypsin deficiency and cystic fibrosis (CF) can occur in women of childbearing age. Care of these patients is primarily supportive, with attention to the physiologic parameters of lung function and oxygenation discussed earlier. As noted, the effect of pregnancy on these diseases and the effect of these diseases on fetal outcome are more variable than with restrictive lung disorders. This is primarily because pulmonary function can deteriorate rapidly as a result of the respiratory infections that frequently complicate these diseases.

A National Institutes of Health study followed 129 pregnancies in CF patients and found only 86 viable infants, leading the investigators to conclude that CF patients have greatly increased fetal wastage.[100] In the study there were six spontaneous abortions, 25 therapeutic abortions, and 11 perinatal deaths. Ten of the perinatal deaths occurred in infants born at less than 37 weeks gestation, whereas premature labor occurred in 26 of the 129 pregnancies and infant mortality was 18% within 24 months of delivery. The authors recommended that pregnancy be avoided unless the potential CF mother was clinically healthy, a suggestion supported by other studies that have found that pregnancy outcome was more related to the severity of maternal disease at the onset of pregnancy than to the effects of CF on pregnancy.[101,102] Any woman with cor pulmonale and pulmonary hypertension should probably not undertake pregnancy because of her inability to tolerate the increased cardiac load and circulating blood volume.[100] A reasonable set of guidelines is to advise against pregnancy in any CF patient with a VC less than 50% of that predicted, hypoxemia, cor pulmonale, or pancreatic insufficiency. The absence of pancreatic insufficiency may identify a subgroup more able to tolerate pregnancy.[103]

Bronchial drainage, antibiotic therapy, prophylactic immunization (including annual influenza vaccine administration), and optimal nutritional and psychosocial care are essential components in the care of the CF patient contemplating pregnancy. Respiratory infections may be responsible for increased fetal and maternal mortality during pregnancy. Although the use of continuous antibiotic prophylaxis is controversial, therapy for acute exacerbations accompanied by a change in sputum character is effective.[104] Therapy is often given intravenously with antibiotics directed against *Pseudomonas aeruginosa* and *Staphylococcus aureus*, which commonly infect CF patients. Antibiotic therapy can be guided further by results of sputum cultures, but intravenous aminoglycosides should be avoided because of potential fetal toxicity.

Patients with α_1-antitrypsin deficiency or bronchiectasis are managed using these same principles. All should be regarded as high-risk patients and serial spirometries and blood gas analyses are indicated. Using these principles, a woman with α_1-antitrypsin deficiency was successfully managed and gave birth to a healthy infant.[105]

ASPIRATION OF STOMACH CONTENTS

Mendelson's syndrome, the aspiration of low-pH liquid stomach contents into the tracheobronchial tree, with subsequent chemical pneumonitis, was first described in women undergoing labor and delivery.[106] This syndrome is most likely to develop if aspirated material has a pH less than 2.5, but some reports suggest that respiratory dysfunction can occur even if the pH of the aspirate is higher.[107,108] Other syndromes that can result from aspiration are bronchial obstruction by an aspirated foreign body and bacterial pneumonia from aspiration of oropharyngeal bacteria. Foreign-body aspiration is managed by bronchoscopic removal whereas aspiration pneumonia is treated with antibiotics, chosen on the basis of whether the event occurred out of hospital, shortly after admission, or during a prolonged hospital stay.[109]

In the pregnant patient, the acid aspiration syndrome is more frequently encountered and can lead to maternal mortality.[110] The pregnant woman is vulnerable to this problem because increased circulating progesterone levels tend to relax the esophageal sphincter and because the gravid uterus can compress the stomach and elevate intragastric pressure. Labor itself delays gastric emptying, and in one study 55% of intrapartum patients had more than 40 mL of liquid gastric juice and 42% had a pH of less than 2.5.[110] Alcohol can stimulate gastric acid secretion and lead to obtundation, thus facilitating aspiration.[111] Forceful abdominal manipulation and obtundation during anesthesia also add to the risk of aspiration.

If the aspiration is massive, immediate clinical illness may appear, but usually there is a delay of 6 to 8 hours before the appearance of bronchospasm, tachycardia, hypotension, tachypnea, cyanosis, and frothy pink sputum production. The latter finding appears if noncardiogenic pulmonary edema and capillary leak develop. Diagnosis is facilitated by having a high index of suspicion in the postpartum patient with respiratory distress.

Treatment of acid aspiration is supportive with oxygen and mechanical ventilation if needed. If aspiration is observed, endotracheal suctioning should be performed, but saline lavage is not indicated and may even serve to spread the acid to uninvolved areas.[106,111]

Bronchodilators may be used to control bronchospasm, but antibiotic therapy should be withheld until the patient develops signs of infection. Corticosteroids have been used in the treatment of witnessed gastric aspiration in the past, but they are of unproven benefit and have no role in current therapy.

Prophylaxis of aspiration should always be undertaken, with antacids given during labor to raise the gastric pH above 2.5 and thus reduce the chance of a dangerous aspiration. One study found that the risk of serious aspiration of gastric fluid with a pH of more than 2.5 could be reduced with the use of 30 mL of antacid given every 3 hours after the onset of labor.[112] Gibbus and colleagues have demonstrated that adverse pulmonary reactions may result from aspirating antacid particles; thus, the use of nonparticulate agents is preferred.[113] Recently, various combinations of oral nonparticulate antacids and H_2-receptor blockers have been advocated as a convenient prophylactic regimen for patients about to undergo elective or emergency cesarean section, but no particular combination appears to be clearly superior.[114] Additional prophylactic measures include limiting oral intake to essential medications once labor has begun, nasogastric evacuation of a distended stomach, selection of regional anesthesia when possible, use of a cuffed endotracheal tube, and use of cricoid pressure during intubation.

RESPIRATORY INFECTIONS

The upper respiratory tract infections include acute and chronic rhinitis, sinusitis, acute pharyngitis, and acute otitis media. These maladies are common in pregnant patients. Except for infections caused by the influenza viruses, they do not tend to complicate pregnancy seriously and are omitted from discussion here except to point out that treatment is modified in pregnancy. In the pregnant patient, the physician should avoid decongestants and antihistamines and should select antibiotics such as the penicillins, cephalosporins, and those erythromycins that are generally considered to be safe in pregnancy.

Acute bronchitis is characterized by upper respiratory tract symptoms, productive cough, and the absence of a significant fever. Physical examination of the chest may reveal scattered rhonchi and occasional wheezes, but there are no signs of pulmonary consolidation. Acute bronchitis is usually caused by a virus, and antibiotic treatment is not generally indicated except in patients who suffer from chronic obstructive pulmonary disease. Chest radiography is not indicated unless there are localizing signs on the physical examination.

BACTERIAL PNEUMONIA

Pneumonia of all etiologies is the second most common cause of maternal mortality. It has been reported in 0.1% to 0.84% of all pregnancies, with a mortality rate of 3.5% to 8.6%,[115] although antibiotics and modern obstetric care seem to have improved the prognosis.[116] *Streptococcus pneumoniae* is the most common infectious agent implicated in antepartum pneumonia, and other common bacterial pathogens include *Mycoplasma pneumonia* and *Haemophilus influenzae.*[116] *Legionella* pneumonia and *Listeria monocytogenes* have rarely been reported to cause respiratory failure in pregnancy.[29,117,118]

Pneumococcal pneumonia classically begins with the abrupt onset of shaking chills, fever, pleuritic chest pain, cough productive of purulent sputum, and shortness of breath. The physical examination often shows signs of consolidation, such as dullness to percussion, tactile fremitus, and egobronchophony. A chest radiograph usually reveals evidence of lobar consolidation but bronchopneumonia may also occur. Laboratory examination may reveal a polymorphonuclear leukocytosis in the range of 12,000 to 25,000 cells/mm^3, but a normal white blood cell count can be seen in patients with overwhelming infection and bacteremia. A sputum specimen for culture and gram stain should always be obtained and may demonstrate gram-positive encapsulated cocci in pairs and short chains. Blood cultures are positive in approximately 20% to 30% of patients and should be collected prior to the administration of antibiotics. Penicillin G is still the antibiotic of choice and will lead to defervescence within 24 hours in half of the patients and within 3 to 4 days in the rest. An acceptable alternative for a patient who is allergic to penicillin is erythromycin.

Mycoplasma pneumoniae produces symptoms similar to a viral infection, with a flulike syndrome and interstitial infiltrates and alveolar filling. Small pleural effusions are common, and approximately 50% of affected patients have cold agglutinins in their serum. Because tetracycline is contraindicated in pregnancy, erythromycin is the drug of choice.

Haemophilus influenzae pneumonia may have a gradual rather than an abrupt onset and may be clinically indistinguishable from *Streptococcus pneumoniae.* It is infrequently seen in young adults unless the patient has a history of chronic obstructive lung disease or is an alcoholic. Sputum gram stain will usually show abundant neutrophils and pleomorphic cocco-bacillary gram-negative organisms. The chest radiograph may show either bronchial or lobar consolidation, and pleural effusions are common. In pregnancy, despite the occurrence of significant ampicillin resistance,[119,120] ampicillin remains the drug of choice, but susceptibility testing should be performed on all culture isolates.

INFLUENZA

Although the magnitude of the maternal fatality rate from influenza is not known, during the 1918 influenza epidemic, maternal mortality with the illness varied from 30% to 50%.[121] In one study of the 1957 epidemic, pregnancy increased mortality ninefold in the 20- to

29-year age group,[122] and in a review of all deaths due to influenza from 1957 through 1960, 1% to 11% occurred in pregnant patients.[123] These deaths were concentrated late in the third trimester and early puerperium and were more likely to occur with increased maternal age. In more recent studies, 39% to 60% of asymptomatic pregnant women had serologic evidence of recent influenza infection, and up to 35% of pregnant symptomatic women had no serologic evidence of recent influenza infection.[121,124,125] Since earlier studies were based on the clinical diagnosis of influenza, the conclusion that pregnancy predisposes to infection or to an enhanced severity of illness is controversial.[121]

Influenza usually begins abruptly with systemic symptoms, such as headache, fever, chills, myalgia, and malaise accompanied by an upper respiratory illness. In an uncomplicated case, complaints of a sore throat and cough may persist for a week or more. Physical findings may be minimal, but injection of the mucous membranes and a postnasal discharge can be seen along with mild cervical adenopathy. The chest examination may be normal but can reveal rhonchi, wheezes, and scattered rales. Occasionally, the disease can progress rapidly to fulminant cardiopulmonary failure, or it can be complicated by secondary bacterial or mixed viral–bacterial pneumonia involving streptococcus, staphylococcus, or *Haemophilus influenzae*.

Amantadine, an oral antiviral agent active against influenza A, can be used therapeutically and can prevent 70% to 90% of experimentally produced and natural infections. It is not effective in treating infections due to influenza B. If used within 48 hours of the onset of symptoms, amantadine will shorten the duration of the illness by up to 50%, reduce fever, and hasten the resumption of normal activities.[126] If given concomitantly with an influenza vaccine it can protect the patient for the 2 to 3 weeks necessary for immunity to develop during exposure to an epidemic. Its safety during pregnancy has not been adequately established, but at least one patient has received it during pregnancy without ill effects.[127]

Although influenza virus can cross the placenta, it has not been isolated from fetal blood,[121] and transplacental passage does not appear to cause congenital defects. Although fetal abnormalities such as circulatory defects, central nervous system malformations, cleft lip, and childhood cancer have been attributed to influenza, most investigators have found that no definite influenza-induced congenital syndrome exists.[121,128] Although influenza vaccination is available, it is of unproven safety in pregnancy and is recommended only during an anticipated pandemic. Since increased mortality from infections usually occurs late in pregnancy, vaccination can be delayed until the middle of the second trimester.[129]

VIRAL PNEUMONIA

Other life-threatening viral pneumonias can develop in the pregnant patient, including varicella pneumonia, which may accompany chickenpox and can range from a mild to a rapidly fatal illness. In pregnancy, varicella is rare, but if pneumonia develops, mortality is high, ranging from 30% to 40% in some series.[130,131] In addition, varicella pneumonia has been associated with an increased incidence of premature labor.[131] The pneumonia can be completely asymptomatic, but in its severe form, it is accompanied by tachypnea, high fever, cough, dyspnea, and pleuritic chest pain. The chest examination may be unimpressive and correlates poorly with the severity of the pneumonia, but the chest radiograph usually shows extensive bilateral peribronchial fluffy, nodular infiltrates, which are more prominent when the skin eruption is maximal.[132] In severe cases, rapid pulmonary deterioration requiring intubation can occur within a matter of hours. Maternal varicella infection in any trimester of pregnancy can be associated with infrequent, but possibly lethal, congenital anomalies. If the maternal infection occurs within 5 days of delivery, the infant is at risk of fatal disseminated infection. Despite its classification as a pregnancy risk category C drug, there are at least four case reports of acyclovir usage in pregnancy, in the third trimester, without evidence of fetal toxicity.[133] Given the high mortality rate associated with varicella pneumonia occurring in pregnancy and lack of demonstrated human fetal toxicity, consideration should be given to acyclovir use, particularly in the latter half of pregnancy. Some authors have recommended administration of varicella-zoster immune globulin, if available, to both mother and fetus exposed to peripartum varicella.[134]

FUNGAL PNEUMONIA

Cryptococcus neoformans, Blastomyces dermatitidis, and *Sporothrix schenckii* have rarely been reported as causing serious respiratory infection in pregnancy. The clinical course and outcome are generally the same in pregnant and non-pregnant patients.[135] It has been estimated that coccidioidomycosis occurs in less than one of every 1000 pregnancies.[135] However, infection in pregnancy, particularly during the second and third trimesters, increases the rate of disseminated infection from 0.2% to above 20%.[136] It has been suggested that 17-beta-estradiol has a stimulatory effect on the fungus and may be responsible for the increased risk of dissemination associated with pregnancy.[135] The maternal mortality rate from disseminated coccidioidomycosis approaches nearly 100%, a rate approximately twice that seen in non-pregnant patients,[136] and dissemination is associated with increased fetal prematurity and mortality.[136]

Symptomatic pulmonary coccidioidomycosis manifests as cough, fever, chest pain, malaise, and occasionally hypersensitivity reactions. Chest radiography may show an infiltrate, hilar adenopathy, or pleural effusions. The peripheral blood count may show eosinophilia. The diagnosis is made by serologic testing and by culture and wet smear examination of sputum, urine, and pus. Dissemination should be suspected in the setting of rapidly progressive respiratory failure with a clinical picture similar to miliary tuberculosis.[29]

Amphotericin B has been used to treat cryptococcosis, blastomycosis, and disseminated coccidioidomycosis in pregnancy.[29,135,136] It crosses the placenta and can be found in both amniotic fluid and fetal blood. Although use in pregnancy has not been well studied, normal, full-term infants have been born to patients who received amphotericin B in the first trimester.[29] Its use is associated with anemia; thus, serial hematocrits need to be followed.

PNEUMOCYSTIS CARINII PNEUMONIA

Pneumocystis carinii pneumonia is the most common opportunistic infection affecting the lungs of patients with acquired immunodeficiency syndrome (AIDS).[137,138] It can be confused with atypical mycobacterial infection, cryptococcosis, and histoplasmosis. Clinically, *P. carinii* pneumonia manifests with fever, dyspnea, and nonproductive cough, which may have an insidious onset followed by a rapid progressive deterioration. Arterial blood gases usually demonstrate hypoxemia, with an increased alveolar–arterial gradient, and respiratory alkalosis, and the chest radiograph classically shows bilateral diffuse infiltrates beginning in the perihilar regions and lower lung fields that progress to involve the entire parenchyma. Diagnosis is made by specific staining of sputum, bronchial aspirates, or material obtained by bronchoscopically performed bronchoalveolar lavage or biopsy.

There are only a few case reports of *P. carinii* pneumonia complicating pregnancy.[139,140] However, because a cumulative AIDS case total of 365,000 is predicted by the end of 1992, with 263,000 cumulative deaths,[141] and because women of childbearing age represent a significant portion of some of the groups at risk for AIDS, the number of infected mothers will surely increase. The treatment of choice in pregnant women with AIDS and *P. carinii* pneumonia is trimethoprim-sulfamethoxazole, even though trimethoprim is a folate antagonist and sulfamethoxazole is a sulfonamide. Recent studies of in utero exposure to sulfadiazine failed to show an increase in prematurity, hyperbilirubinemia, or kernicterus.[142] Patients should be monitored for drug toxicity, such as rash, fever, neutropenia, thrombocytopenia, and hepatitis. Nausea and vomiting may occur and can exacerbate hyperemesis gravidarum. Pentamidine is an alternative therapy, but its use has not been studied in pregnancy. In patients who cannot tolerate trimethoprim-sulfamethoxazole, pentamidine may be required because of the life-threatening risk of withholding treatment from the mother.[138] If pentamidine is used, the mother should be closely monitored for hypoglycemia. Aerosolized pentamidine, because of poor systemic absorption and decreased systemic side effects, has been advocated as safe, effective prophylaxis for *P. carinii* pneumonia.[143] Treatment of even mild cases of *P. carinii* pneumonia with aerosolized pentamidine may be effective, but some investigators have discouraged this therapy because of a concern about treatment failure.[143] Pyrimethamine-sulfadoxine has been used as prophylaxis, and no fetal malformations have been associated with its use, although it is a folate antagonist and thus should be used cautiously.[138]

AMNIOTIC FLUID EMBOLISM

Although the true incidence and mortality associated with amniotic fluid embolism is difficult to establish, amniotic fluid embolism has been estimated to complicate from one per 8000 to one per 80,000 live births.[144] This disease accounts for 11% to 13% of all maternal deaths in the United States,[145] and fetal mortality may exceed 40%.[146] Complications leading to maternal death include uncontrolled disseminated intravascular coagulation (DIC) and cardiorespiratory failure due to severe pulmonary hypertension and right ventricular failure. Clinically, one may see excessive bleeding, especially uterine bleeding, bronchospasm, respiratory distress, pulmonary hypertension, pulmonary edema, cyanosis, frank DIC, bradycardia, shock, and cardiovascular collapse.[21,29,145] The differential diagnosis includes conventional causes of thromboembolic disease, toxemia of pregnancy, peripartum cardiomyopathy, Mendelson's syndrome, and fulminant pneumonia.[147]

Amniotic fluid can enter the maternal vascular space through small endocervical veins, uterine or cervical tears, or iatrogenic uterine trauma.[145] Tumultuous labor, use of uterine stimulants, presence of meconium in the amniotic fluid, advanced maternal age, multiparity, and intrauterine fetal death are some of the risk factors for this catastrophic event.[21] Although most episodes occur during labor (90%), amniotic fluid embolism can occur at any time throughout pregnancy.[144] Once access to the maternal circulation is gained, the embolus travels to the lungs, usually resulting in cardiovascular collapse. The embolized material can include amniotic fluid, fetal squames, lanugo hairs, meconium, fat, mucin, and bile.[21] These materials can be recovered in pulmonary artery catheter aspirates, sampled as long as 3 days after the precipitating event, and sampling by this means may help establish the diagnosis.[147] The pulmonary physiologic changes probably result from a combination of occlusive emboli, vasospasm, and possibly increased permeability pulmonary edema.[29,144,145,148] Prostaglandin $F_{2\alpha}$, present in the amniotic fluid in late pregnancy, has been implicated as being at least partially responsible for the vasospastic component.[149] Fetal lipids and mucin circulating freely in the maternal circulation may be responsible for the onset of DIC.[69]

Treatment is supportive and includes oxygen, mechanical ventilation with or without the use of positive end-expiratory pressure (PEEP), fluid, vasopressors, reduction of uterine bleeding via mechanical massage, oxytocin infusion, and when necessary, methylergonovine maleate; blood products should be replaced as indicated.[29,144] Emergency cesarean section, performed either to salvage a viable fetus or to attempt to save the mother's life, is controversial.[144]

VENOUS AIR EMBOLISM

Venous air embolism may account for as many as 1% of maternal deaths, [29] with risk factors being the performance of surgery, intravenous infusions, and central venous catheter placement. However, because the venous sinuses of the uterus are particularly susceptible to the entry of air during pregnancy,[150] air embolism can occur during normal labor, delivery of a placenta previa, criminal abortions using air, orogenital sex, and insufflation of the vagina during gynecological procedures.[29] Maternal mortality associated with a clinically significant event exceeds 90% in untreated cases.[151] The severity of a venous air embolism depends on the amount and rate of air entry. Small amounts of venous air may be clinically undetectable, but accidental bolus injections of 100 mL to 300 mL of air have been reported to be fatal.[150] However, there are reports of patients surviving infusions of up to 1600 mL.[151,152]

Embolization of a large bolus of venous air to the right ventricle results in mechanical obstruction to the forward flow of blood in the pulmonary artery outflow tract.[153] In addition, the pumping action of the right ventricle acting on blood and air may produce platelet damage and fibrin formation, resulting in fibrin emboli that lodge in the pulmonary vascular bed. Maldistribution of pulmonary blood flow may result in ischemia or hyperperfusion, with the hyperperfused areas being susceptible to developing interstitial and alveolar edema. Areas that are initially ischemic may also become abnormally permeable once perfusion is restored.[153] In animal models, the permeability pulmonary edema following venous air embolism has been related to leukocyte production and the release of toxic oxygen metabolites.[154] Paradoxical embolization can occur if there is an atrial septal defect, resulting in arterial ischemia or occlusion.[150]

The patient initially presents with a feeling of faintness, dizziness, fear of impending doom, dyspnea, cough, diaphoresis, and substernal chest pain. Physical examination may reveal a state of altered consciousness, cyanosis, tachypnea, wheezing, tachycardia, hypotension, elevated jugular venous pressure, gallop rhythm, and an evanescent "mill wheel" or "waterwheel" murmur heard over the precordium.[29,150] Paradoxical embolism may be evidenced by bubbles in the retinal arterioles, marblelike skin (air in superficial dermal vessels), and possibly stroke or myocardial infarction.[150] A blood gas will characteristically reveal hypoxemia, and there may be an associated metabolic acidosis. Chest radiography may occasionally demonstrate air in the right side of the heart or the main pulmonary artery, and the electrocardiogram may show signs of right heart strain, ischemia, or arrhythmia.[29,150] Therapy must be instituted promptly, and the patient should be placed in the left lateral decubitus position to minimize obstruction to the right ventricular outflow tract. Administration of 100% oxygen will promote removal of nitrogen from the air bubble and result in more rapid absorption of the embolus. Nitrous oxide is highly soluble, and in a patient receiving general anesthesia, it should be discontinued, since it can increase the size of the air embolus.[152] In the presence of cardiovascular collapse, closed chest compression and aspiration of air from the right side of the heart, via venous catheterization or transthoracic puncture, are probably warranted. Hyperbaric oxygen may be useful in the setting of cerebral venous air embolism, anticoagulation has been suggested to minimize the formation of fibrin microemboli,[152] and mechanical ventilation may be necessary to treat permeability pulmonary edema.

ADULT RESPIRATORY DISTRESS SYNDROME (ARDS)

Adult respiratory distress syndrome (ARDS) is the final common pathway of pathophysiologic changes occurring in the lungs as a consequence of a variety of acute bodily insults that reach the lung directly or via the vasculature (Table 60-8). Clinically, patients present with marked respiratory distress, tachypnea, hypoxemia refractory to oxygen therapy, "stiff" non-compliant lungs that require high pressures to achieve inflation, and diffuse bilateral interstitial and alveolar infiltrates on chest radiograph.[155] The central pathophysiologic event in ARDS is injury to the alveolar-capillary membrane, either directly or via mediators delivered by the pulmonary vasculature resulting in increased vascular permeability and noncardiogenic pulmonary edema. Severe hypoxemia results from both increased shunting of unoxygenated blood and impaired ventilation and perfusion matching in the al-

TABLE 60–8. CAUSES OF ARDS IN PREGNANT WOMEN

Abruptio placentae
Air embolism
Amniotic fluid embolism
Aspiration
Bacterial pneumonia
Blood transfusion
Carcinomatosis
Dead fetus syndrome
Diabetic ketoacidosis
Drugs (narcotics, barbiturates)
Fat embolism
Fractures
Fungal and *Pneumocystis carinii* pneumonia
Head trauma
Inhaled toxin
Intra-abdominal abscess
Lung contusion
Nonthoracic trauma
Pancreatitis
Preeclampsia, eclampsia
Seizure
Septic abortion
Septicemia
Shock
Tocolytic therapy with sympathomimetics and glucocorticoids
Tuberculosis
Uremia

veoli, with an arterial Po_2 typically less than 50 to 60 mm Hg, despite an inspired oxygen concentration of 60% or more.[156] To make the diagnosis of ARDS, chronic pulmonary disease and left heart failure (cardiogenic pulmonary edema) must be excluded, and an appropriate precipitating event should be present. Right heart catheterization is often required to demonstrate that the pulmonary capillary hydrostatic pressure is not elevated,[157] but these data should be assessed in light of the expected decrease in colloid oncotic pressure during pregnancy and in the immediate postpartum period.[158] Mortality in patients with ARDS continues to exceed 50%, a figure that has remained fairly constant over the last 20 years.[159]

In the pregnant patient, ARDS can be associated with many of the factors that complicate pregnancy and delivery, including septicemia, amniotic fluid embolism, aspiration of stomach contents, eclampsia, septic abortion, air embolism, abruptio placentae, blood transfusion (with white cell agglutination in the pulmonary circulation), dead fetus syndrome (with disseminated intravascular coagulation), drug overdose (narcotics, barbiturates, aspirin), fat embolism (after long bone fracture), hemorrhagic shock, seizures, and overwhelming pneumonia.[156,160] The incidence of ARDS in pregnancy is unknown, but in one general hospital respiratory care unit 9.5% of all patients carried this diagnosis, and it is estimated that over 150,000 cases occur annually in the United States.[157]

PATHOPHYSIOLOGY OF ARDS

Except in cases of direct damage to the alveolar-capillary membrane (inhaled toxins, aspiration, invasive organisms), the specific mechanisms that initiate lung injury in ARDS are generally unknown. Multiple humoral and cellular mediators contribute to the intense inflammatory response that characterizes ARDS. These mediators include polymorphonuclear leukocytes, alveolar macrophages, platelets, free fatty acids, arachidonic acid metabolites (prostaglandins, leukotrienes, thromboxane A_2), fibrin-derived peptides, and tumor necrosis factor.[156,161,162] Initial injury to the alveolar-capillary membrane results in increased endothelial cell permeability and noncardiogenic pulmonary edema.[156,163] This capillary leak is the earliest finding in ARDS and results in the accumulation of protein-rich fluid in the extravascular space of the lung,[164] initially in the interstitium, and later in the alveolar sacs. Alveolar type 1 epithelial cells are injured, the alveolar basement membrane is denuded, and the alveolar space fills with red blood cells, leukocytes, macrophages, and cell debris. Damage to the epithelium results in the loss of surfactant and alveolar collapse. Early hyaline membranes composed of protein, fibrin, and cellular debris can be seen.[165] Morphologically, epithelial cell injury is more obvious than endothelial cell injury, which may indicate a greater reparative capacity of the endothelial cells.[165] After 24 to 96 hours, the early exudative phase of injury is followed by a cellular proliferative phase, with repopulation of the alveolar basement membrane by alveolar type 2 cells. The hyaline membrane begins to organize, and morphologic evidence of endothelial injury is more obvious.[165] This phase is present from the third to the tenth day and is followed by a fibrotic proliferative phase as the hyaline membranes undergo fibrosis.

CLINICAL PRESENTATION

Clinically, the patient with ARDS of any etiology may go through four clinical stages: (1) injury, (2) apparent stability, (3) respiratory insufficiency, and (4) terminal stage.[18] The initial injury may occur without outward clinical signs and may last for up to 6 hours. Next, the patient develops dyspnea associated with rapid shallow breathing and a persistent cough. Approximately 12 to 24 hours after injury, the chest radiograph shows bilateral infiltrates that coalesce into a diffuse haze, representing perivascular fluid accumulation, interstitial edema, and alveolar edema.

As the disease progresses, mechanical ventilation is usually required because the pulmonary edema and localized atelectasis have resulted in ventilation–perfusion mismatching and an increased alveolar–arterial oxygen gradient, resistant to high inspired oxygen concentrations.[156] Other physiologic derangements include an increase in physiologic dead space, frequently exceeding 60% of each breath and resulting in significant carbon dioxide retention, despite the presence of a very high minute ventilation. Narrowing and obstruction of the pulmonary vessels, primarily caused by edema fluid, results in "stiff lungs" and is often associated with a high pulmonary arterial pressure despite a low or normal capillary hydrostatic pressure.

THERAPY OF ARDS

Corticosteroids, in doses up to several grams of methylprednisone over 24 hours, have been widely used in the treatment of full-blown ARDS without a clear demonstration that they are effective.[166] An exception is in the use of corticosteroids and mineralocorticoids to treat patients who are in shock that might be caused by or accompanied by adrenal insufficiency.[166] Prophylactic corticosteroid therapy for ARDS is also considered unproven and controversial.[167] Potential adverse effects far outweigh any putative, unproven benefit. Efforts to identify pharmacologic agents effective in enhancing lung repair or blocking mediators of lung injury in ARDS have been largely unsuccessful. Recently, nonsteroidal anti-inflammatory drugs (NSAIDs), such as ibuprofen, meclofenamate, and indomethacin, have been studied in vitro and in animals and have shown some promise.[167]

The care of a patient with ARDS is primarily supportive, with the mainstays of therapy being supplemental oxygen and the application of PEEP. Despite the lack of any clear evidence that its use improves mortality rates, PEEP is almost universally employed because it improves oxygenation and can reduce oxygen needs below potentially toxic concentrations.[167] Pepe and colleagues have demonstrated that the early application of PEEP (prophylactic PEEP) cannot prevent the development of ARDS.[168]

Reversible causes of ARDS, such as occult intra-abdominal or pelvic abscesses, should be sought because early surgical intervention and antimicrobial therapy may be life-saving. Patients with eclampsia, severe preeclampsia, abruptio placentae, dead fetus syndrome, and septic abortion often have accompanying disseminated intravascular coagulation (DIC) and should undergo delivery of the fetus, or evacuation of the uterus as soon as the coagulopathy is corrected and the patient is surgically stable.[160]

MECHANICAL VENTILATION IN ARDS

Ventilator therapy should be instituted when refractory hypoxemia is present and should be considered at the earliest recognition of ARDS, to ensure fetal well-being. With correction of hypoxemia and respiratory alkalosis, fetal oxygen delivery can be maintained at an adequate level. Pregnant patients with ARDS should be placed in the left lateral decubitus position, with the right buttock and hip elevated approximately 15°, or with the uterus manually displaced to the left, to maximize venous return.[27] Continuous external fetal heart monitoring should be instituted when appropriate and pulse oximetry can permit continuous monitoring of arterial oxygenation, and periodic blood gas determinations should be obtained to check acid–base status.

When indicated, volume-cycled mechanical ventilation is begun using 100% oxygen, a respiratory rate of 10 to 12 breaths per minute, and a tidal volume of 10 to 15 mL/kg. The maternal pH should be maintained in the normal pregnancy range of 7.4 to 7.47 with an arterial CO_2 between 25 and 32 mm Hg. Under normobaric conditions, the fraction of inspired oxygen (FIO_2), initially set at 1.0, can be continued for up to 24 hours without the threat of pulmonary oxygen toxicity,[169] although an FIO_2 of 0.5 can be administered indefinitely without adverse sequelae. In ARDS, the increased work of breathing caused by the noncompliance of the lungs and the increased airway resistance caused by bronchial edema and possibly bronchospasm[167] can be relieved using the CMV mode of mechanical ventilation that will allow the respiratory muscles to rest completely, thereby reducing oxygen consumption. Use of the CMV mode may require sedation or paralysis to maximize ventilation and minimize patient oxygen requirements and discomfort. Should a vaginal delivery of the fetus be contemplated while the patient is intubated, withdrawal of sedation and a change of respirator mode to intermittent mandatory ventilation is probably warranted to allow the patient to assist in the delivery effort. Using these principles a patient underwent vaginal delivery of a viable infant while on a respirator.[170]

If the maternal arterial oxygen saturation cannot be maintained at or above 90%, with an FIO_2 of 0.6 or less, then PEEP should be added. PEEP recruits atelectatic areas for gas exchange, which would otherwise collapse during expiration and which are difficult to expand due to the loss of surfactant and structural derangements. The result is an increase in systemic arterial oxygen tension and in the lung's FRC and compliance.[171] The use of PEEP is not without pitfalls, however, as it can overdistend alveoli, thereby decreasing compliance and increasing the risk of pneumothorax. Its most important adverse effect is to decrease cardiac output by impeding venous return to the right side of the heart, particularly when the blood volume is low.[171] Application of PEEP is accomplished by titrating upward from levels of 5 cm H_2O and checking PaO_2 15 to 30 minutes later. By following serial arterial blood gases or by using a pulse oximeter, PEEP can be increased until either the required FIO_2 is less than 0.6 or cardiac output declines. Generally, levels above 15 cm H_2O are not required, but values as high as 20 cm H_2O may occasionally be necessary to provide an appreciable increase in arterial oxygen. Applying PEEP at high levels may lead to retention of excessive lung water.[89] If PEEP is then decreased, this lung water can flood alveoli and lead to a deterioration in gas exchange, which is not easily reversible by simply raising levels of PEEP.[172] This problem can be avoided by starting PEEP at low levels and then gradually increasing as needed.

An optimal PEEP has been defined as a level that increases oxygenation without significantly reducing cardiac output, and consequently oxygen delivery. Studies have shown that this level correlates with maximal pulmonary compliance.[171] Use of a pulmonary artery catheter will permit calculation of maximal pulmonary compliance or "best PEEP" by direct sampling of the mixed venous oxygen saturation (SvO_2) and measurement of the cardiac output by the thermodilution method. The SvO_2 reflects the balance between tissue oxygen delivery and tissue oxygen utilization and declines with inadequate tissue perfusion.[173] The normal average value for SvO_2 is 73%, with saturations below 60% being considered low.[173] Because of the altered pulmonary capillary permeability inherent in ARDS, an increase in pulmonary capillary blood pressure that would be well tolerated by a healthy individual may cause life-threatening pulmonary edema in a patient suffering with ARDS. Therefore, the ultimate goal of fluid management in ARDS is to maintain adequate maternal and fetal tissue oxygen delivery while keeping pulmonary microvascular pressures as low as possible, a task made easier with the use of a pulmonary artery catheter to measure pulmonary capillary wedge pressure and cardiac output serially. Units of packed red cells are given to patients who are anemic and who would benefit from the increased oxygen-carrying capacity provided by blood transfusion.

Therapy of ARDS in the pregnant patient is complicated because a cardiac output sufficient to supply maternal needs may not be adequate for placental perfusion. Additionally, vasopressor drugs often used to increase cardiac output may have deleterious effects on uterine blood flow.[170] In an uncomplicated patient, placental reserve is judged to be approximately 50%. However, given the lack of information regarding the effects of hemodynamic and pharmacologic manipulation on uterine blood flow in the critically ill patient, it seems prudent to lower intravascular volume only to a level tolerated by the circulation and to avoid pharmacologic manipulation. External fetal heart rate monitoring is a useful adjunct in assessing fetal oxygen delivery.[170]

After the initiation of therapy for ARDS, the patient may begin to show signs of improvement, with less impairment of gas exchange and increases in lung compliance and $S\bar{v}O_2$. If the FIO_2 can be reduced to less than 0.5 and PEEP can be reduced to 5 cm H_2O, consideration should be given to weaning from mechanical ventilation. Most patients who are successfully weaned will require supplemental oxygen for several days or more after mechanical ventilation is discontinued.

COMPLICATIONS OF ARDS

Therapy of ARDS requires knowledge not only of the disease process and its management, but also of associated complications. Table 60-9 lists complications resulting from intubation and mechanical ventilation and emphasizes that this severe disease can involve many organ systems in addition to the lungs. Two specific complications, pulmonary barotrauma and infection, merit special attention.

Pulmonary barotrauma is common and in one series of ARDS patients, 38% of the group was found to have pneumomediastinum or pneumothorax.[174] Pneumothorax may cause further deterioration in gas exchange, and tension pneumothorax may produce life-threatening pulmonary and cardiovascular deterioration. Factors that have been implicated as predisposing to these complications include high inflation pressures resulting from poor lung compliance, large tidal volumes, and high levels of PEEP.

Approximately two thirds of all critically ill patients have respiratory tract colonization with gram-negative bacteria, and Brodie and colleagues found concurrent pneumonia in a majority of patients with ARDS.[175] Intravenous catheters, endotracheal tubes, bladder catheters, and intra-arterial cannulae can all be sources of infection. Respiratory assistance devices and medical personnel are other potential sources of infection.[176,177]

Infection can be both an important etiological factor in ARDS and a secondary complication that increases mortality. Ashbaugh and Petty, in a retrospective review of 51 patients with ARDS, reported a mortality of 70% in patients who acquired respiratory infection, in contrast to a fatality rate of 40% in patients without respiratory tract infection.[178] Seidenfeld found a mortality of more than 70% in ARDS patients with infection, whereas mortality was only 20% when patients were infection-free.[179]

TABLE 60–9. COMPLICATIONS ASSOCIATED WITH THE ADULT RESPIRATORY DISTRESS SYNDROME

Pulmonary
Pulmonary emboli
Pulmonary barotrauma
Pulmonary fibrosis
Pulmonary complications of ventilatory and monitoring procedures
Mechanical ventilation
Right main stem intubation
Alveolar hypoventilation
Swan-Ganz catheterization
Pulmonary infarction
Pulmonary hemorrhage
Gastrointestinal
Gastrointestinal hemorrhage
Ileus
Gastric distention
Pneumoperitoneum
Renal
Renal failure
Fluid retention
Cardiac
Arrhythmia
Hypotension
Low cardiac output
Infection
Sepsis
Nosocomial pneumonia
Hematologic
Anemia
Thrombocytopenia
Disseminated intravascular coagulation
Other
Hepatic
Endocrine
Neurologic
Psychiatric

(From Balk RB, Bone RC. The adult respiratory distress syndrome. Med Clin N am 1983;67:685.)

Pneumonia in the setting of ARDS is notoriously difficult to diagnose. In one study, although 58% of patients with ARDS had histologic evidence of pneumonia,[180] 36% of these cases were not clinically detected and 20% of those without pneumonia were incorrectly given this diagnosis. Fever, leukocytosis, and focal infiltrates may be present in ARDS patients, independent of the presence of pneumonia. The relatively recent development of the bronchoscopically directed protected specimen brush may help make this diagnosis in complicated patients.[181]

In addition to pneumonia, other infections may complicate the course of ARDS. Nasotracheal and large nasogastric tubes predispose to bacterial sinusitis by blocking ventilation and drainage of the sinuses. Sinus infections are particularly likely to occur in patients who have underlying disorders of the nasal passages and in those who have sustained either facial trauma or trauma due to instrumentation. Parenteral empiric antibiotics should cover both gram-positive and nosocomial gram-negative organisms, and patients may benefit from a topical nasal decongestant.[182] Other complications of ARDS include airway trauma from translaryngeal intubation,[183] and persistent pulmonary function abnormalities (both small-airways disease and reduced diffusion).[183,184]

REFERENCES

1. Cugell DW, Frank NR, Gaensler EA, et al. Pulmonary function in pregnancy. I. Serial observations in normal women. Am Rev Tuberc 1953;67:568.
2. Gilbert R, Auchincloss JH Jr. Dyspnea of pregnancy: clinical and physiological observations. Am J Med Sci 1966;252:270.
3. Milne JA, Howie AD, Pack AI. Dyspnea during normal pregnancy. Br J Obstet Gynaecol 1978;85:260.
4. Levinsky NG. Acidosis and alkalosis. Harrison's principles of internal medicine. 11th ed. In: Braunwald E, Isselbacher KJ, Petersdorf RG, et al, eds. New York: McGraw-Hill, 1987:209.
5. Andersen GJ, James GB, Mathers, et al. The maternal oxygen tension and acid-base status during pregnancy. J Obstet Gynecol [Br Commonw] 1969;76:16.
6. Lim VS, Katz AI, Lindheimer MD. Acid-base regulation in pregnancy. Am J Physiol 1976;231:1764.
7. Lucius H, Gahlenbeck H, Kleine HO, et al. Respiratory functions, buffer system, and electrolyte composition of blood during human pregnancy Respir Physiol 1970;9:311.
8. Templeton A, Kelman GR. Maternal blood gases, (PAo_2-Pao_2), physiological shunt and Vd/Vt in normal pregnancy. Br J Anesth 1976;48:1001.
9. West JB. Pulmonary pathology—the essentials. 3rd ed. Baltimore: Williams & Wilkins, 1987:21.
10. Awe RJ, Nicotra MB, Newsom TD, Viles R. Arterial oxygenation and alveolar-arterial gradients in term pregnancy. Obstet Gynecol 1979;53:182.
11. Ang CK, Tan TH, Walters WAW, Wood C. Postural influence on maternal capillary oxygen and carbon dioxide tension. Br Med J 1969;4:201.
12. Lees MM, Scott DB, Kerr MG, Taylor SH. The circulatory effects of recumbent postural change in late pregnancy. Clin Sci 1967;32:453.
13. Turner ES, Greenberger PA, Patterson R. Management of the pregnant asthmatic patient. Ann Intern Med 1980;6:905.
14. Prowse CM, Gaensler EA. Respiratory and acid-base changes during pregnancy. Anesthesiology 1965;26:381.
15. Leontic EA. Respiratory disease in pregnancy. Med Clin North Am 1977;61:111.
16. Milne JA, Mills RJ, Coutts JRT, et al. The effect of human pregnancy on the pulmonary transfer factor for carbon monoxide as measured by the single breath method. Clin Sci Mol Med 1977;53:271.
17. Milne JA. The respiratory response to pregnancy. Postgrad Med J 1979;55:318.
18. Novy MJ, Edwards MJ. Respiratory problems in pregnancy. Am J Obstet Gynecol 1967;99:1024.
19. Greenberger PA. Asthma in pregnancy. Clin Perinatol 1985;12(3):571.
20. Hung CT, Pelosi M, Langer A, Harrington JT. Blood gas measurements in the kyphoscoliotic gravida and her fetus: report of a case. Am J Obstet Gynecol 1975;121:287.
21. Gaensler EA, Patton WE, Verstraeten JM, et al. Pulmonary function in pregnancy. III. Serial observations in patients with pulmonary insufficiency. Am Rev Tuberc 1953;67:779.
22. Weinberger, SE Weiss ST, Cohen WR, et al. Pregnancy and the lung. Am Rev Respir Dis 1980;121:559.
23. Laros KD. The postpneumonectomy mother. Respiration 1980;39:185.
24. Tarnoff J, Lees WM, Fox RT. Major thoracic surgery during pregnancy. Am Rev Respir Dis 1967;96:1169.
25. Barron WM. The pregnant surgical patient: medical evaluation and management. Ann Intern Med 1984;101:683.
26. Swartz HM, Reichling BA. Hazards of radiation exposure for pregnant women. JAMA 1978;239:1907.
27. Amatuzzi R. Hazards to the human fetus from ionizing radiation at diagnostic dose levels: review of the literature. Perinatology-Neonatology 1980;4(6):23.
28. Committee on the Biological Effects of Ionizing Radiations. Division of Medical Sciences, Assembly of Life Sciences, National Research Council. Somatic effects: effects other than cancer. The effects on populations of exposure to low levels of ionizing radiation. Washington, DC: National Academy Press, 1980:477.
29. Hollingsworth HM, Pratter MR, Irwin RS. Acute respiratory failure in pregnancy. J Intensive Care Med 1989;4:11.
30. Brent RL. The effects of embryonic and fetal exposure to x-ray, microwaves, and ultrasound. Clin Obstet Gynecol 1983;26:484.
31. Mole RH. Radiation effects on pre-natal development and their radiological significance. Br J Radiol 1979;52:89.
32. Thompson KJ, Cohen ME. Studies on the circulation in pregnancy. II. Vital capacity observations in normal pregnant women. Surg Gynecol Obstet 1938;66:591.
33. Hughson WG, Friedman PJ, Feigin DS, et al. Postpartum pleural effusion: a common radiologic finding. Ann Intern Med 1982;97:856.
34. Udeshi UL, McHugo JM, Crawford JS. Postpartum pleural effusion. Br J Obstet Gynecol 1988;95:894.
35. Cheek TG, Gutsche BB. Maternal physiologic alterations during pregnancy. In: Shnider SH, Levinson G, eds. Anesthesia for obstetrics. Baltimore: Williams & Wilkins, 1984:3.
36. Wulf KH, Kunzel W, Lehmann V. Clinical aspects of gas exchange. In: Longo LD, Bartels H, eds. Respiratory gas exchange and blood flow in the placenta. Bethesda, MD: Public Health Service, 1972:505.
37. Greenberger PA, Patterson R. Management of asthma during pregnancy. N Engl J Med 1985;312(14):897.
38. Ziment I, Au JP. Managing asthma in the pregnant patient. J Respir Dis 1988;9(6):66.
39. Quilligan EJ. Maternal physiology. In: Danforth DN, ed. Obstetrics and gynecology. Philadelphia: JB Lippincott, 1982:326.
40. Greenberger PA. Pregnancy and asthma. Chest (Suppl) 1985;87:85.
41. Weinstein AM, Dubin BD, Podleski WK, et al. Asthma and pregnancy. JAMA 1979;241:1161.
42. Bahna SL, Bjerkedal T. The course and outcome of pregnancy in women with bronchial asthma. Allergy 1972;27:397.
43. Holbreich M. Asthma and other allergic disorders in pregnancy. Am Fam Physician 1982;25(3):187.
44. Gordon M, Niswander KR, Berendes H, Kantor AG. Fetal morbidity following potentially anoxygenic obstetric conditions. VII. Bronchial asthma. Am J Obstet Gynecol 1970;106:421.
45. Schatz M, Patterson R, Zeitz S, et al. Corticosteroid therapy for the pregnant asthmatic patient. JAMA 1975;233:804.
46. Gluck JC, Gluck PA. The effects of pregnancy on asthma: a prospective study. Ann Allergy 1976;37:164.
47. Schatz M, Harden K, Forsythe A, et al. The course of asthma during pregnancy, postpartum, and with successive pregnan-

cies: a prospective analysis. J Allergy Clin Immunol 1988;81(3):509.
48. Schwartz DB. Medical disorders in pregnancy. Emerg Med Clin North Am 1987;5(3):509.
49. Kallinger MA. The late phase reaction and its clinical implications. Hosp Pract 1987;15 Nov:73.
50. Woolcock AJ. In: Murray JF, Nadel JA, eds. Asthma textbook of respiratory medicine. Vol 1. Philadelphia: WB Saunders, 1988:1030.
51. Findley LJ, Sahn SA. The value of chest roentgenograms in acute asthma in adults. Chest 1981;80:535.
52. Summer WR. Status asthmaticus. Chest (Suppl) 1985;87:88S.
53. Hopewell PC, Miller TM. Pathophysiology and management of severe asthma. Clin Chest Med 1984;5(4):623.
54. Rebuck AS, Read J. Assessment and management of severe asthma Am J Med 1971;51:788.
55. Westerman DE, Benatar SR, Potgieter PD, Ferguson AD. Identification of the high-risk asthmatic patient: experience with 39 patients undergoing ventilation for status asthmaticus. Am J Med 1979;66:565.
56. Wilson MC, Larsen GL. Gaining control over the late asthmatic response. J Respir Dis 1986;7(8):51.
57. Fredholm BB, Persson CGA. Xanthine derivatives as adenosine receptor antagonists. Eur J Pharmacol 1982;81:673.
58. Lunell E, Svedmyr N, Anderson KE, Persson CGA. A novel bronchodilator xanthine apparently without adenosine receptor antagonism and tremoragenic effect. Eur J Respir Dis 1983;64:333.
59. Perrson CGA. Universal adrenoreceptor antagonism is neither necessary nor desirable with xanthine anti-asthmatic. Med Hypotheses 1982;8:515.
60. Webb-Johnson DC, Andrews JL. Bronchodilator therapy. N Engl J Med 1977;297:476.
61. Hui KKP, Conolly ME, Tashkin DP. Reversal of human lymphocyte beta-adrenoceptor desensitization by glucocorticoids. Clin Pharmacol Ther 1982;32:566.
62. Larsen GL. The pulmonary late phase response. Hosp Pract 1987;22(11):155.
63. Cockcroft DW. The bronchial late phase response in the pathogenesis of asthma and its modulation by therapy. Ann Allergy 1985;55:857.
64. Gross NJ, Skorodin MS. Anticholinergic, antimuscarinic bronchodilators. Am Rev Respir Dis 1984;129:856.
65. Mann JS, George CF. Anticholinergic drugs in the treatment of airways disease. Br J Dis Chest 1985;79:209.
66. Church MK, Gradidge CF. The activity of sodium cromoglycate analogues in human lung in vitro: a comparison with rat passive cutaneous anaphylaxes and clinical efficacy. Br J Pharmacol 1980;70:307.
67. Harries MG, Parkes PEG, Lessof MH. Role of bronchial irritant receptors in asthma. Lancet 1981;i:5.
68. Chung KF, Barnes PJ. Treatment of asthma. Br Med J 1987;294:104.
69. Taenaka N, Shimada Y, Kawai M, et al. Survival from DIC following amniotic fluid. Anaesthesia 1981;36:389.
70. Briggs GC, Freman RK, Yaffe SJ. Drugs in pregnancy and lactation. 2nd ed. Baltimore: Williams & Wilkins, 1986.
71. Altenberger KM. Letter to the editor. N Engl J Med 1985;313(8):517.
72. Greenberger PA, Patterson R. Letter to the editor. N Engl J Med 1985;313(8):518.
73. Slone D, Shapiro S. Drugs and pregnancy. Ann Intern Med 1979;90:275.
74. Arwood LL, Dasta JF, Friedman C. Placental transfer of theophylline: two case reports. Pediatrics 1979;63:844.
75. Labovitz E, Spector S. Placental theophylline transfer in pregnant asthmatics. JAMA 1982;247:786.
76. Vann Dellen RG. Intravenous aminophylline. Chest 1979;76:2.
77. Fredericksen MC, Ruo TI, Chow MJ, et al. Theophylline pharmokinetics in pregnancy. Clin Pharmacol Ther 1986;40:321.
78. Greenberger PA, Patterson R. Beclomethasone dipropionate for severe asthma during pregnancy. Ann Intern Med 1983;98:478.
79. Heinonen OP, Slone D, Shapiro S. Birth defects and drugs in pregnancy. Littleton, MA: Publishing Science Group, 1977:388.
80. Onnen I Barrier, G, d'Athis PH, et al. Placental transfer of atropine at the end of pregnancy. Eur J Clin Pharmacol 1979;15:443.
81. Bernstein IL. Cromolyn sodium in the treatment of asthma: coming of age in the United States. J Allergy Clin Immunol 1985;76:381.
82. Brompton Hospital MRC Collaborative Trial. Long-term study of disodium cromoglycate in treatment of severe extrinsic or intrinsic bronchial asthma in adults. Br Med J 1972;4:383.
83. Wilson J. Utilisation du cromoglycate de sodium au cours de la grossesse. Acta Therapeutica (Suppl) 1982;8:45.
84. Mawhinny H, Spector SL. Optimum management of asthma in pregnancy. Drugs 1986;32:178.
85. Greenberger PA, Patterson R. Safety of therapy for allergic symptoms during pregnancy. Ann Intern Med 1978;89:234.
86. Barnhart ER. Physicians' desk reference. Oradell, NJ: Medical Economics, 1989:684, 937.
87. Metzger WJ, Turner E, Patterson R. The safety of immunotherapy during pregnancy. J Allergy Clin Immunol 1978;61:268.
88. Fischl MA, Pitchenik A, Gardner LB. An index predicting relapse and need for hospitalization in patients with acute bronchial asthma. N Engl J Med 1981;305:783.
89. Gong H, Tierney DF. Respiratory distress syndrome: use of positive end-expiratory pressure and outcome. In: Simmons DH, ed. Current pulmonology. Vol 2. Boston: Houghton Mifflin, 1980:103.
90. Rees HA, Millar JS, Donald KW. A study of the clinical course and arterial blood gas tensions of patients with status asthmaticus. Q J Med 1968;37:541.
91. Kattan M. Emergency management of acute asthma. Hosp Pract 1986;21(11):81.
92. Sly RM, Badiei B, Faciane J. Comparison of subcutaneous terbutaline with epinephrine in the treatment of asthma in children. J Allergy Clin Immunol 1977;59:128.
93. Scoggin CH, Sahn SA, Petty TL. Status asthmaticus: a nine year experience. JAMA 1977;238(11):1158.
94. Tanaka RM, Santiago SM, Kuhn GJ, et al. Intravenous methylprednisone in adults in status asthmaticus (comparison of two dosages). Chest 1982;84:438.
95. Roizen MF, Feeley TW. Pancuronium bromide. Ann Intern Med 1978;88:64.
96. O'Callaghan AC, Scadding G, Watkins J. Bronchospasm following the use of vercuronium. Anaesthesia 1986;41:940.
97. Anthonisen NR, Filuk RB. Pneumothorax. In: Fishman AP, ed. Pulmonary diseases and disorders. 2nd ed. New York: McGraw-Hill, 1988:2175.
98. Menitove SM, Goldring RM. Combined ventilator and bicarbonate strategy in the management of status asthmaticus. Am J Med 1983;74:898.
99. Niederman MS, Gambino A, Lichter, et al. Tension ball valve mucus plug in asthma. Am J Med 1985;79:131.
100. Cohen LF, DiSant'Agnese PA, Friedlander J. Cystic fibrosis and pregnancy: a national survey. Lancet 1980;2:842.
101. Huang NN. Special features, survival rate and prognostic factors in young adults with cystic fibrosis. Am J Med 1987;82:871.
102. Pittard WB III, Sorenson RU, Schnatz PT. Pregnancy outcome

in mothers with cystic fibrosis: normal neonatal immune responses. South Med J 1987;80(3):344.
103. Corky CWB, Newth CJL, Corey M, Levison H. Pregnancy in cystic fibrosis: a better prognosis in patients with pancreatic function. Am J Obstet Gynecol 1981;140:737.
104. Hyatt AC, Chipps BE, Kumor KM, et al. A double-blind controlled trial of anti-*Pseudomonas* chemotherapy for acute respiratory exacerbations in patients with cystic fibrosis. Pediatrics 1981;99:307.
105. Howie AD, Milne JA. Pregnancy in patients with bronchiectasis. Br J Obstet Gynecol 1978;85:197.
106. Wynne JW, Modell JH. Respiratory aspiration of stomach contents. Ann Intern Med 1977;87:466.
107. Bond VK, Stoelting RK, Gupta CO. Pulmonary aspiration syndrome after inhalation of gastric fluid containing antacid. Anesthesiology 1979;51:452.
108. Schwartz DJ, Wynne JW, Gibbs CP, et al. The pulmonary consequences of aspiration of gastric contents at pH values greater than 25. Am Rev Respir Dis 1980;121:119.
109. Bartlett JG, Borach SL. The triple threat of aspiration pneumonia. Chest 1975;68:560.
110. Baggish MS, Hopper S. Aspiration as a cause of maternal death. Obstet Gynecol 1979;53:182.
111. Greenhouse BS, Hook R, Hehre FW. Aspiration pneumonia following intravenous administration of alcohol during labor. JAMA 1969;210:2393.
112. Roberts RB, Shirley MA. The obstetrician's role in reducing the risk of aspiration pneumonitis, with particular reference to the role of oral antacids. Am J Obstet Gynecol 1976;124:611.
113. Gibbus CP, Schwartz DJ, Wynne JW, et al. Antacid pulmonary aspiration in the dog. Anesthesiology 1979;51:380.
114. Sweeny A, Wright I. The use of antacids as a prophylaxis against Mendelson's syndrome in the United Kingdom. A survey. Anesthesia 1986;41:419.
115. Hopwood HG. Pneumonia in pregnancy. Obstet Gynecol 1965;25:875.
116. Benedetti TJ, Valle R, Ledger WJ. Antepartum pneumonia in pregnancy. Am J Obstet Gynecol 1982;144(4):413.
117. Boucher M, Yonekura ML, Wallace RJ, Phelan JP. Adult respiratory distress syndrome: a rare manifestation of *Listeria monocytogenes* infection in pregnancy. Am J Obstet Gynecol 1984;149(6):687.
118. Soper DE, Melone PJ, Conover WB. Legionnaire disease complicating pregnancy. Obstet Gynecol 1986;67:10S.
119. Schlech WF, Band JD, Hightower AW, et al. Bacterial meningitis in the United States. 22nd interscience conference on antimicrobial agents and chemotherapy. Miami: American Society of Microbiology, 1982.
120. Schwartz RH, Goldenberg RI, Park C, et al. The increasing prevalence of bacteremic ampicillin-resistant *Haemophilus influenza* infections in a community hospital. Pediatr Infect Dis 1982;1:242.
121. Korones SB. Uncommon virus infections of the mother, fetus, and newborn: *Influenza*, mumps and measles. Clin Perinatol 1988;15(2):261.
122. MacKenzie JS, Houghton M. *Influenza* infections during pregnancy: association with congenital malformations and with subsequent neoplasms in children and potential hazards of live virus vaccines. Bacteriol Rev 1974;38:356.
123. Eikoff TC, Sherman IL, Serling RE. Observations on excess mortality associated with epidemic influenza JAMA 1961;176:776.
124. Walker WM, McKee AM. 633 women with Asian flu antibodies. No congenital malformations (retrospective study). Obstet Gynecol 1959;13:394.
125. Wilson MG, Stein AM. Teratogenic effects of Asian influenza. JAMA 1971;216:1022.
126. Mostow SR. Prevention, management, and control of *influenza*: role of amantadine. Am J Med (Suppl 6A) 1987;82:35.
127. Kirshon B, Faro S, Zurawin RK, et al. Favorable outcome after treatment with amantadine and ribavirin in a pregnancy complicated by influenza pneumonia: a case report. J Reprod Med 1988;33(4):399.
128. Coffey VP, Jessop WJE. Congenital abnormalities. Ir J Med Sci 1955;349:30.
129. Schoenbaum SC, Weinstein L. Respiratory infections in pregnancy. Clin Obstet Gynecol 1979;22:293.
130. Fleischer G, Henry W, McSorley M, et al. Life-threatening complications of varicella. Am J Dis Child 1981;135:896.
131. Harris RE, Rhoades ER. Varicella pneumonia complicating pregnancy: case report and review of the literature. Obstet Gynecol 1965;25:734.
132. Hockberger RS, Rothstein RJ. Varicella pneumonia in adults: a spectrum of disease. Ann Emerg Med 1986;15(8):931.
133. Hankins GDV, Gilstrap LC, Patterson AR. Acyclovir treatment of varicella pneumonia in pregnancy. Letter to the editor. Critical Care Med 1987;15(4):336.
134. DeNicola LK, Hanshaw JB. Congenital and neonatal varicella. J Pediatr 1979;94:175.
135. Catanzaro A. Pulmonary mycosis in pregnant women. Chest (Suppl) 1984;86(3):14S.
136. Harris RE. Coccidioidomycosis complicating pregnancy. Obstet Gynecol 1966;28:401.
137. Coolfont report: a PHS plan for prevention and control of AIDS and the AIDS virus. Public Health Report 1986;101:341.
138. Feinkind L, Minkoff HL. HIV in pregnancy. Clin Perinatol 1988;15(2):193.
139. Jensen LP, O'Sullivan MJ, Gomez-del-Rio M, et al. Acquired immunodeficiency (AIDS) in pregnancy. Letter to the editor. Am J Obstet Gynecol 1984;148(8):1145.
140. Minkoff H, Haynes deRegt R, Landesman S, Schwarz R. *Pneumocystis carinii* pneumonia associated with acquired immunodeficiency syndrome in pregnancy: a report of three maternal deaths. Obstet Gynecol 1986;67(2):284.
141. Quarterly report to the Domestic Policy Council on the prevalence and rate of spread of HIV and AIDS—United States. MMWR 1988;37(36):552.
142. Baskin CG, Law S, Wenger NK. Sulfadiazine rheumatic fever prophylaxis—Does it increase the risk of kernicterus in the newborn? Cardiology 1980;65:222.
143. Armstrong D, Bernard E. Aerosol Pentamidine. Letter to the editor. Ann Intern Med 1988;109:852.
144. Sterner S, Campbell B, Davies S. Amniotic fluid embolism. Ann Emerg Med 1984;13:343.
145. Turner R, Gusack M. Massive amniotic fluid embolism. Ann Emerg Med 1984;13:359.
146. Peterson EP, Taylor HB. Amniotic fluid embolism: an analysis of 40 cases. Obstet Gynecol 1970;35:787.
147. Masson RG, Ruggieri J, Siddiqui M. Amniotic fluid embolism: definitive diagnosis in a survivor. Am Rev Respir Dis 1979;120:187.
148. Duff P, Engelsgjerd B, Zingery LW. Hemodynamic observations in a patient with intrapartum amniotic fluid embolism. Am J Obstet Gynecol 1983;146(1):112.
149. Morgan M. Amniotic fluid embolism. Anaesthesia 1979;34:20.
150. Fyke III FE, Kazmier FJ, Harms RW. Venous air embolism: life-threatening complications of orogenital sex during pregnancy. Am J Med 1985;78:333.
151. Gottlieb JD, Ericsson JA, Sweet RB. Venous air embolism. Anesth Analg 1965;44:773.
152. O'Quinn RJ, Lakshminarayan S. Venous air embolism. Arch Intern Med 1982;142:2173.

153. Ence TJ, Gong H Jr. Adult respiratory distress syndrome after venous air embolism. Am Rev Respir Dis 1979;119:1033.
154. Clark MC, Flick MR. Permeability pulmonary edema caused by venous air embolism. Am Rev Respir Dis 1984;129:633.
155. Petty TI, Asbaugh DG. The adult respiratory distress syndrome: clinical features, factors influencing prognosis and principles of management. Chest 1971;60:233.
156. Balk RB, Bone RC. The adult respiratory distress syndrome. Med Clin N Am 1983;67:685.
157. Hansen-Flaschen J, Fishman AP. Adult respiratory distress syndrome: clinical features and pathogenesis. In: Fishman AP, ed. Pulmonary diseases and disorders. 2nd ed. New York: McGraw-Hill, 1988:2201.
158. Berkowitz RL. The Swan-Ganz catheter and colloid osmotic pressure determinations. In: Berkowitz RL, ed. Critical care of the obstetric patient. New York: Churchill Livingstone, 1983:1.
159. Maunder RJ. Clinical prediction of the adult respiratory distress syndrome. Clin Chest Med 1985;6(3):413.
160. Anderson HF, Lynch JP, Johnson TRB. Adult respiratory distress syndrome in obstetrics and gynecology. Obstet Gynecol 1980;55:291.
161. Andreadis N, Petty TL. Adult respiratory distress syndrome: problems and progress. Am Rev Respir Dis 1985;132:1344.
162. Rinaldo JE, Rogers RM. Adult respiratory distress syndrome: changing concepts of lung injury and repair. N Engl J Med 1982;306:900.
163. Snapper JR. Lung mechanics in pulmonary edema. Clin Chest Med 1985;6(3):399.
164. Fein A, Grossman RF, Jones JG, et al. The value of edema fluid protein measurement in patients with pulmonary edema. Am J Med 1979;67:32.
165. Bachofen M, Weibel ER. Structural alterations of lung parenchyma in the adult respiratory distress syndrome. Clin Chest Med 1982;3(1):35.
166. Flick MR, Murray JF. High-dose corticosteroid therapy in the adult respiratory distress syndrome. JAMA 1984;251(8):1054.
167. Bernard GR, Brigham KL. Pulmonary edema: pathophysiologic mechanisms and new approaches to therapy. Chest 1986;89(4):598.
168. Pepe PE, Hudson LD, Carrico CJ. Early application of positive end-expiratory pressure in patients at risk for the adult respiratory distress syndrome. N Engl J Med 1984;311:281.
169. Winter PM, Smith G. The toxicity of oxygen. Anesthesiology 1972;37:210.
170. Sosin D, Krasnow J, Moawad A, Hall JB. Successful spontaneous vaginal delivery during mechanical ventilatory support for the adult respiratory distress syndrome. Obstet Gynecol (Suppl) 1986;68:19.
171. Suter PM, Fairley HB, Isenberg MD. Optimum end-expiratory airway pressure in patients with acute pulmonary failure. N Engl J Med 1975;292:284.
172. Lynch JP, Mhyre JG, Dantzker DR. Influence of cardiac output on intrapulmonary shunt. J App Physiol 1979;46:315.
173. Hankins GDV. Principles of invasive hemodynamic monitoring. Clin Perinatol 1986;13(4):772.
174. De Latorre FJ, Tomasa A, Klamburg J, et al. Incidence of pneumothorax and pneumomediastinum in patients with aspiration pneumonia requiring ventilatory support. Chest 1977;72:141.
175. Brodie DA, Deane R, Shinozaki T, et al. Adult respiratory distress syndrome, sepsis, and extracorporeal membrane oxygenation. J Trauma 1977;17:579.
176, Albert RK, Condie F. Hand washing patterns in medical intensive care units. N Engl J Med 1981;304:1465.
177. Cross AS, Roup B. Role of respiratory assistance devices in endemic nosocomial pneumonia. Am J Med 1981;70:681.
178. Ashbaugh DG, Petty TL. Sepsis complicating the acute respiratory distress syndrome. Surg Gynecol Obstet 1972;135:865.
179. Seidenfeld JL, Pohl DF, Bell RC, et al. Incidence, site, and outcome of infections in patients with the adult respiratory distress syndrome. Am Rev Respir Dis 1986;134:12.
180. Andrews CP, Coalson JJ, Smith JD, Johanson WG. Diagnosis of nosocomial bacterial pneumonia in acute diffuse lung injury. Chest 1981;80:254.
181. Niederman MS, Fein AF. The interaction of infection and the adult respiratory distress syndrome. Crit Care Clin 1986;2(3):471.
182. Hansen-Flaschen J, Fishman AP. Adult respiratory distress syndrome: management. In: Fishman AP, ed. Pulmonary diseases and disorders. 2nd ed. New York. McGraw-Hill, 1988:2230.
183. Ingbar DH, Matthay RA. Pulmonary sequelae and lung repair in survivors of the adult respiratory distress syndrome. Crit Care Clin 1986;2(3):629.
184. Ghio AJ, Elliot CG, Crapo RO, et al. Impairment after adult respiratory distress syndrome. An evaluation based on American Thoracic Society Recommendations. Am Rev Respir Dis 1989;139:1158.

61

CHAPTER

DIABETES MELLITUS IN PREGNANCY

Zion J. Hagay and E. Albert Reece

Diabetes mellitus is a heterogeneous disorder characterized by hyperglycemia, which is a result of relative or absolute insulin deficiency. It is estimated that diabetes mellitus affects approximately 1.5 million women of childbearing age in the United States.

Peel, in an excellent historical review of diabetes and pregnancy, noted that before 1856 there were few reports of pregnancy-complicated diabetes.[1] At that time, diabetes was a disease with a dismal prognosis and infertility was common in women with diabetes. The advent of insulin brought about a dramatic change in the overall outlook for diabetics and their reproductive potential. A dramatic fall in maternal mortality from 45% to just over 2% was observed shortly after the introduction of insulin in 1922.[2] A decline in perinatal mortality, however, has been achieved more gradually over time and must be credited to a number of developments, including a better understanding of metabolism in diabetic patients, a recognition of the need for stringent metabolic control to achieve glucose levels as close as possible to nondiabetic values to ensure better pregnancy outcome, the improvement in neonatal intensive care units, the spread of new techniques for fetal surveillance, and the spread of devices for self-monitoring blood glucose. In fact, perinatal mortality rates have been reduced remarkably, from approximately 15% to 20% in the 1960s to about 4% to 5% at present.[2–4] Furthermore, if mortality secondary to major congenital malformations is excluded, then perinatal mortality rates in well-controlled diabetics approximates that of nondiabetics. There are, however, still some unresolved problems, such as macrosomia and congenital anomalies.

At present, there is no doubt that the goal in treating diabetic patients is not only a reduction of perinatal mortality, but also a decrease in perinatal morbidity.

CLASSIFICATION

Recently, a new classification system has been proposed by the Diabetes Data Group of the National Institutes of Health.[5] This classification is based on etiologic factors and insulin dependency (Table 61-1).

Another classification proposed almost 40 years ago by White is still generally accepted and remains a useful prognostic guide.[6] White's classification relates the onset of diabetes, its duration, and the degree of vasculopathy to the outcome of pregnancy. Since there were differences and some confusion in the interpretation of class A diabetes, particularly when the patient required insulin for therapy, a revision made by White and her group proposed that class A diabetes include women known to have diabetes before pregnancy and who are treated with diet alone.[7] Thus, White's class A classification includes only patients with pregestational diabetes and defines gestational diabetes as a completely separate group.

Practically speaking, women with pregnancies complicated by diabetes mellitus may be separated into one of two groups:

Gestational diabetes. Women with carbohydrate intolerance of variable severity, with onset or first recognition during the present pregnancy.

Pregestational diabetes. Women known to have diabetes before pregnancy.

Table 61-2 presents the classifications that include these two groups.[8]

In general, it is true that the more severe the degree of vasculopathy in pregnancy, the worse the prognosis. There are data to show that when metabolic control is stringently maintained during pregnancy, the perinatal outcome does not appear to be significantly different

TABLE 61–1. CLASSIFICATION OF GLUCOSE INTOLERANCE

	NOMENCLATURE	OLD NAMES
Type I.	Insulin-dependent diabetes mellitus (IDDM)	Juvenile-onset diabetes
Type II.	Non–insulin-dependent diabetes mellitus	Maturity-onset diabetes
Type III.	Gestational diabetes or carbohydrate intolerance	
Type IV.	Secondary diabetes	

Based on recommendations of the National Diabetes Data Group. Classification and diagnosis of diabetes mellitus. Washington, DC: National Institutes of Health, 1986.

between various classes.[9] The White classification of pregestational diabetes is still important for descriptive purposes and for identifying pregnancies that may be at increased risk for fetal and maternal complications. Since pregestational and gestational diabetes pose different risks to the mother and her fetus, different programs of care are needed, and therefore the two categories will be discussed separately.

EPIDEMIOLOGY, ETIOLOGY, AND GENETICS

Significant advances in the understanding of genetic features of diabetes mellitus have been achieved in the last 20 years.[10] Since diabetes mellitus is a heterogeneous disorder rather than a single disease, the different types of diabetes should be distinguishable from each other. To improve differentiation of the various forms of diabetes, the National Diabetes Data Group introduced a new method of classification in 1979 (see Table 61-1).[5]

Ninety percent of all pregnant diabetic patients have gestational diabetes mellitus (GDM), whereas insulin-dependent diabetes mellitus (IDDM, type I) and non-insulin-dependent diabetes mellitus (NIDDM, type II) account for the remaining 10%.[11] The clinical distinction between the ketosis-prone IDDM and the nonketosis-prone NIDDM has been recognized by clinicians for many years, but the two types were thought to represent differences in expression of a single disease.[12] Twenty years ago it was discovered that IDDM is an HLA-linked disorder, whereas NIDDM is not, making them two different diseases genetically.[13–15] In general, IDDM and NIDDM can be distinguished from each other using clinical criteria and/or islet-cell antibody studies (Table 61-3).

IDDM accounts for 6% to 10% of all cases of diabetes in the general population.[16,17] It has an increased prevalence rate in Caucasians but is rare in certain ethnic groups (eg, Japanese, Chinese, and Eskimos).[18,19] The prevalence of IDDM in Europe and the United States is estimated to be in the range of 0.1% to 0.4% in various age groups under 30 years of age.[20]

By contrast, NIDDM (formerly known as maturity or adult-onset diabetes) is the most common form of diabetes observed in the general population. It has a peak incidence at age 65, with 80% of cases appearing after 40 years of age.[18,19] The prevalence of NIDDM is estimated to be 69 out of 1000 in the United States,[19] and 50 to 150 per 1000 in other Western populations.[21]

TABLE 61–2. CLASSIFICATION OF DIABETES IN PREGNANCY

		Pregestational Diabetes		
Class	Age of Onset (year)	Duration (year)	Vascular Disease	Therapy
A	Any	Any	No	Diet only
B	>20	<10	No	Insulin
C	10–19	10–19	No	Insulin
D	Before 10 or after 20	>20	Benign retinopathy	Insulin
F	Any	Any	Nephropathy	Insulin
R	Any	Any	Proliferative retinopathy	Insulin
H	Any	Any	Heart disease	Insulin

		Gestational Diabetes	
Class	Fasting Glucose Level		Postprandial Glucose Level
A-1	<105 mg/dL	and	<120 mg/dL
A-2	>105 mg/dL	and/or	>120 mg/dL

Based on the American College of Obstetricians and Gynecologists (ACOG), Technical Bulletin No. 92 (Chicago), May 1986, with modifications.

TABLE 61-3. PREDOMINANT CHARACTERISTICS OF IDDM AND NIDDM

CHARACTERISTICS	IDDM	NIDDM
Prevalence	0.1–0.5%	5–10%*
Weight at onset	Nonobese	Often obese
Age at onset	Usually young, <30 years	Usually older, >40 years
Seasonal variations	Yes	No
Insulin level	Low or absent	Variable
Ketosis	Most often	Unusual
MHC† gene associations	HLA DR_4, HLA DR_3, HLA DQ	No
Twin studies	30%–50% concordance	80–100% concordance
Anti–islet-cell antibodies	Positive in 70% of new IDDM or prediabetic IDDM	No

* Prevalence in Western countries.
† MHC: Major histocompatibility complex.

GENETIC FACTORS IN IDDM (TYPE I)

In the past few years it has become increasingly clear that autoimmunity plays a key role in type I diabetes.[22,23] It is currently believed that type I diabetes mellitus is actually a slow process in which insulin-secreting cells are gradually destroyed, leading to islet-cell failure and hyperglycemia. The development of type I diabetes can be divided conceptually into six stages, beginning with genetic susceptibility and ending with complete B-cell destruction (Table 61-4).[22]

The total genetic basis of IDDM cannot exceed 50%, since this is the maximum estimate of the rate of its concordance in identical twins. As much as 60% to 70% of genetic susceptibility is attributable to genes located in the HLA region on the short arm of chromosome 6. Another 30% to 40% of genetic susceptibility is accounted for by genes on non–HLA-associated chromosomes (see Table 61-4, stage I).[21] In fact, this may indicate that the genetic susceptibility is polygenic, ie, involves many genes in the HLA and non-HLA regions.

The association of HLA and disease may have important implications for diagnosis, prognosis, and possible pharmacologic prophylaxis. In many cases, this association has helped to clarify the disease heterogeneity. It should be stressed that in IDDM the disease is not inherited per se; it is the susceptibility to the disease that is inherited, and the development of the disease is dependent on other genetic factors, and possibly on environmental factors as well.

In IDDM, the first association between HLA and disease was observed with the HLA-B group of class I antigens (HLA-B_7, HLA-B_{15}). When "D-typing" was introduced (class II antigens), however, HLA-DR showed a stronger association with IDDM than did HLA-B. In fact, 60% of IDDM patients possessed HLA-B_8 or B_{15}, but over 90% possessed DR_3 and/or DR_4.[24] Individuals who co-inherited both DR_3 and DR_4 have the highest risk (about 15 times) for developing type I diabetes.[10,25] It is possible to calculate the absolute risk for inheriting IDDM according to various HLA phenotypes and genotypes.[10,26] For example, individuals with DR_2 have a lower absolute risk for IDDM (1:2500) than does the general population (1:500). On the other hand, individuals with DR_3/DR_4 have the highest risk (1:42) of developing IDDM.[26] However, this association with the HLA-D region is not pathognomonic for IDDM, since DR_3 and/or DR_4 are also found in approximately 50% of healthy individuals.[12] Studies using genetic probes for the HLA-region and monoclonal antibodies against distinct allelic products have recently indicated that HLA-DQ may be more closely linked to the disease loci than the HLA-DR region.[20,24,27] However, HLA linkage does not account for all the genetic susceptibility to IDDM.

Although it is anticipated that non-HLA loci play some role in the genetics of IDDM, the precise details are as yet unknown, in large part due to conflicting findings. It is possible that manifestations of IDDM require the interaction of at least five different genes (on chromosomes 2, 6, 7, 11, and 14) together with environmental factors.

The exact mechanism of the inheritance of IDDM is not known. Formerly, it was suggested that the risk to offspring with one affected parent of inheriting diabetes was in the range of 1% to 6%.[28,29] Based on recent information,[30] it has become clear that IDDM is transmitted less frequently to the offspring of diabetic mothers than to those of diabetic fathers: 1.3% versus 6%, respectively. This higher preferential paternal transmission rate may be related to the higher transfer of DR_4 alleles to the offspring of DR_4 fathers than that observed to the offspring of DR_4 mothers.[31] Family studies have shown that the estimated risk of recurrence of IDDM to offspring in a family with one already affected sibling, but with unaffected parents, is 5% to 6%.[32,33]

GENETICS OF NIDDM

There are clear genetic and immunologic differences between IDDM and NIDDM. The latter is not linked with HLA, and no specific genetic markers have been found. Furthermore, NIDDM does not seem to be an autoimmune or endocrine disease. Currently available information indicates that NIDDM occurs when there is both impaired insulin secretion and insulin antagonism.[34]

Although the genetic markers for NIDDM are not yet defined, it is evident from family and twin studies that the genetic component of NIDDM is much stronger than that of IDDM. Indeed, monozygotic twins have a much higher rate of concordance for type II diabetes (almost 100%) than for type I diabetes (20% to 50%).[35,36] It is likely that there is a genetic heterogeneity

TABLE 61–4. PROPOSED STAGES IN THE PATHOGENESIS OF IDDM

STAGE AND OCCURRENCE	COMMENTS
Stage I	
Genetic susceptibility	Most likely polygenic *HLA association with IDDM* Chromosome 6 90% of Caucasians with IDDM express HLA DR3 or DR4 or both. *Non-HLA association with IDDM* Immunoglobulin loci (encoded on chromosomes 2, 14) Polymorphic region 5′ of the insulin gene (chromosome II) T cell receptor (chromosomes 7, 14)
Stage II	
Triggering factors	Environmental factors: toxic chemicals (?); viruses such as coxsackie B, rubella, mumps; stress (?).
Stage III	
Active autoimmunity	Many immunologic abnormalities may precede overt DM by more than 9 yrs; anti-islet-cell antibodies may be present in up to 70% of pre-DM patients.
Stage IV	
Progressive loss of antibodies.	Reduction in β-cell mass, evidenced by abnormal IV GTT in ≥50% of first-degree relatives (IDDM) with islet-cell glucose-stimulated insulin secretion.
Stage V	
Early onset of overt DM	≥10% of β-cells remain. Trials of immunotherapy (ie, steroids and cyclosporin) have been attempted.
Stage VI	
Overt DM w/complete β-cell destruction	Several years may elapse between Stages V and VI.

DM, diabetes mellitus; GTT, glucose tolerance test.

in NIDDM. It has been shown, for example, that there is a special subgroup of NIDDM in which the disease develops, not at midlife, but much earlier—in adolescence or young adulthood.[16,37] This subgroup is referred to as maturity-onset diabetes of the young (MODY) and is transmitted in an autosomal dominant fashion, with as many as 50% of offspring inheriting the disease or manifesting glucose intolerance.[37]

Another example of the genetic heterogeneity of NIDDM is the discovery of differences in familial aggregations. Fifteen percent of siblings of nonobese diabetics are affected, compared to 7.3% of siblings of obese diabetics (Table 61-5).[38]

For NIDDM relatives, the empirical risk of developing the disease is much higher than it is for IDDM relatives. The risk of transmitting NIDDM to first-degree relatives is almost 15%, and as many as 30% will have impaired glucose tolerance.[16] When both parents have type II diabetes, the chance of developing the disease is much higher, reaching 60% to 75%.[19]

TABLE 61–5. EMPIRICAL RISK FOR OFFSPRING OF IDDM AND NIDDM DEVELOPING DIABETES

AFFECTED PARENT(S)	EMPIRICAL RISK ESTIMATE OF OFFSPRING
IDDM	
Diabetic mother	1%
Diabetic father	6%
Parents unaffected Sibling affected	Overall: 5–6% No. of haplotypes shared: 1 Haplotype = 5% 2 Haplotypes = 13% No haplotypes = 2%
Both parents affected	33%
NIDDM	
MODY	50%
Obese	7%
Nonobese	15%
Both parents affected	60%–75%

MODY, maturity-onset diabetes of the young.

GENETICS OF GESTATIONAL DIABETES MELLITUS

Gestational diabetes mellitus (GDM) is defined as carbohydrate intolerance of variable severity discovered (or perhaps arising) during pregnancy. Glycemic control is often achieved by diet or insulin therapy,[5] but 15% of these patients will require insulin treatment during pregnancy, because of either fasting or postprandial hyperglycemia.[39] These differences in disease severity demonstrate that the degree of metabolic disturbances may vary among patients with GDM. Until recently, GDM was believed to be a variant of NIDDM; however, available data now support the concept that GDM is a heterogeneous disorder representing, at least in part, patients who are destined to develop either IDDM or NIDDM in later life.[39,40] The exact percentage difference of each subgroup is unknown, but it appears that most GDM cases represent a preclinical state of NIDDM. Immunologic studies have shown that as many as 30% of GDM patients may have circulating islet-cell antibodies (ICA),[40] and anti–islet-cell antibodies have been found in many patients with pre-IDDM.[41–44] Furthermore, it has been shown that GDM patients who were ICA positive had a higher prevalence of HLA-DR_3 or DR_4 than those who were ICA negative. More than half the patients who were ICA positive developed IDDM within an 11-year period after the diagnosis of GDM.

It is noteworthy that in a recent study of Pima Indians (a group in which the incidence of NIDDM is high), there was a greater prevalence of diabetes in the offspring of women who had NIDDM during pregnancy than in the offspring of women who developed diabetes only after the pregnancy (45% versus 8.6% at age 20 to 24 years).[44] The authors suggested that the intrauterine environment is an important determinant of the development of diabetes in the offspring, and its effect is additive to genetic factors.

The previously mentioned data support the concept that GDM is clearly heterogeneous and composed of patients who are prone to develop either IDDM or NIDDM later in life. Further studies are needed to clarify this heterogeneity.

TABLE 61-6. SUMMARY OF THE METABOLIC EFFECTS OF INSULIN

Target tissue	Enhances glucose and amino acid uptake Increases glycogen synthesis Converts glucose into fatty acids Inhibits glyconeogenesis
Muscle	Enhances glucose and amino acid uptake Increases glycogen synthesis
Adipose tissue	Increases glucose and amino acid transport Increases fatty acid synthesis Inhibits release of fatty acids from fat stores "Fat-sparing effect" be enhanced glucose utilization in many tissues
Central nervous system	Has little or no effect on uptake or metabolism of glucose
All tissues	Increases protein synthesis Inhibits protein catabolism

Reprinted with permission from Brumfield C, Huddleston JF. The management of diabetic ketoacidosis in pregnancy. Clin Obstet Gynecol 1984;27(1):50.

METABOLIC CHANGES IN NORMAL AND DIABETIC PREGNANCIES

An understanding of the metabolic changes in normal pregnancy may provide the basis for better management of pregnant diabetic patients. For this reason it will be useful to describe these normal changes and then to examine the metabolic adjustments that occur in the pregnant diabetic.

INSULIN SECRETION AND INSULIN RESISTANCE IN NORMAL PREGNANCY

Insulin is the major hormonal signal regulating metabolic responses to feeding and tissue use of carbohydrates; it is also the major glucose-lowering hormone. It is produced by the B-cell of the pancreas and is secreted into the hepatic portal circulation, from which it reaches and acts on the liver and on other peripheral tissues (ie, muscle and fat). Insulin suppresses endogenous glucose production by inhibition of hepatic glycogenolysis and gluconeogenesis. On the other hand, it stimulates glucose uptake and fuel storage of glycogen and triglyceride in the liver, muscle, and adipose tissue (Table 61-6).[45]

The effect of insulin on tissue is determined by the following factors:

The amount of insulin secretion
The rate of insulin clearance
The degree of insulin binding to its receptors and its ability to produce postreceptor effects.

In normal pregnancy, basal insulin levels are almost unchanged in the first and second trimesters but are increased by as much as 50% in the third trimester, suggesting insulin resistance at that time (Fig. 61-1).[46,47] During pregnancy, fasting values of insulin rise from roughly 5 mU/L to about 8 mU/L until term.[48,49] The increase in insulin release in response to a glucose load from early pregnancy becomes pronounced by the third trimester.[46,48,50–52] Data show that the release of insulin in response to a challenge with oral or intravenous glucose in the last trimester of pregnancy is about 1.5 to 2.5 times greater than it is in non-pregnant women.[47,50] In the first trimester of pregnancy, insulin action is enhanced by estrogen and progesterone; thus, an increase in peripheral glucose use leads to lower fasting plasma glucose levels,[53] a decrease that may explain the clinical observation of increased episodes of hypoglycemia ex-

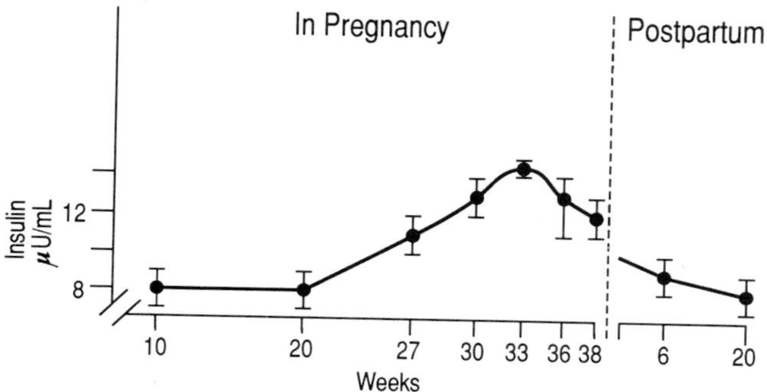

FIGURE 61-1. Plasma insulin in normal pregnancy and postpartum after overnight fast. Basal insulin levels are increased in the last half of pregnancy. (Modified from Knopp RH et al. Metabolic Adjustment in Normal and Diabetic Pregnancy. Clin Obstet Gynecol 1981;24:29.)

perienced by pregnant diabetic patients in early pregnancy.

The increase in levels of progesterone and estrogen that begins in early pregnancy leads to pancreatic B-cell hyperplasia and increased insulin response to a glucose load.[53] The exact mechanism by which estrogen and progesterone affect carbohydrate metabolism is unknown. However, it has been shown that estrogen can increase the insulin sensitivity in some diabetic states.[54,55] On the other hand, studies in rats have indicated that progesterone decreases insulin receptor response,[56] whereas progesterone enhances insulin secretion.[57]

Human placentas contain insulin-degrading enzymes (insulinases). No evidence exists to show that insulinase increases insulin clearance from the placenta.[58,59]

Insulin resistance in pregnancy has been demonstrated by several authors, who showed that hypoglycemic response to intravenous insulin is impaired progressively as gestation proceeds.[46,60] Furthermore, it has been shown that insulin sensitivity in pregnancy is decreased by as much as 80% when compared to the nonpregnant state. This fact has been demonstrated by studying the hypoglycemic effectiveness of insulin during a constant plasma level of glucose.[61]

Data from many workers have indicated that pregnancy has a diabetogenic effect on the mother, as demonstrated by glucose intolerance during pregnancy.[46,48,62,63] O'Sullivan documented an increase in the upper limit of "normal" in the two-hour blood glucose levels during oral glucose tolerance tests.[64] Freinkel has shown that in pregnancy there is an increased level of glucose, insulin, and triglyceride after an oral glucose load but an enhanced suppression of glucagon.[65]

Several authors have studied the role of insulin receptors during pregnancy in the production of insulin resistance.[66–70] The results, however, are inconsistent, since insulin binding may vary from time to time and according to the metabolic state of the subject.[71] Some investigators have found increased insulin binding to circulating monocytes,[66,67] whereas others have found it to be decreased.[68] In human pregnancy, adipose tissue insulin binding is diminished,[70] but it is increased in erythrocytes.[64] Therefore, the available data indicate that insulin resistance is not significantly related to diminished insulin binding. The possibility of reduced postreceptor response in intracellular pathways needs further investigation.

Elevated insulin concentrations during human pregnancy can be attributed to a variety of hormonal changes that promote insulin resistance or directly increase pancreatic islet B-cell mass. Rising levels of maternal plasma progesterone,[53] human placental lactogen,[72–74] free cortisol,[75] and prolactin[76] have been implicated in this process.

Human placental lactogen (HPL) is a single-chain polypeptide secreted by the syncytiotrophoblast. The levels of HPL in maternal blood rise steadily during the first and second trimesters, and the concentration is proportional to placental mass. During the last 4 weeks of pregnancy, HPL levels reach a plateau. Late in the second trimester of pregnancy, when HPL levels rise to a peak value, HPL has a major role in the diabetogenic effect of pregnancy. The principal metabolic action of HPL is mobilization of lipids as free fatty acids. It has also been shown that HPL is elevated during hypoglycemia and decreased during hyperglycemia. HPL, which increases lipolysis in the fasting state, provides free fatty acids as a source of energy for maternal metabolism; thus, glucose and amino acids are available to the fetus. The mechanism for the insulin antagonism by HPL may be explained by the fact that this hormone has a similar structure to human growth factor and, as such, may reduce insulin binding to specific high-affinity receptors.[77] It is also possible that the increase in maternal free fatty acid levels caused by HPL action interferes with insulin action and the uptake of glucose by the cells.

Free cortisol levels are also increased during pregnancy.[78,79] Cortisol stimulates endogenous glucose production and glycogen storage and decreases glucose utilization.[80] Thus, cortisol reduces the effectiveness of insulin.

Prolactin is increased five- to 10-fold during late pregnancy.[81] Gustafson and colleagues have shown that glucose tolerance curves, basal insulin levels, and postchallenge plasma insulin responses were significantly higher in non-pregnant women with hyperprolactinemia than in a control group.[76] The profiles in non-pregnant women with hyperprolactinemia were similar to those observed in normal pregnant patients with physiologic hyperprolactinemia of the same magnitude. These data suggest that prolactin has a significant influence on pancreatic islet-cell insulin secretion during late gestation.

Glucagon is secreted from the A-cells of the pancreatic islet and acts predominantly on the liver. It is a potent activator of glycogenolysis and gluconeogenesis: it increases hepatic glucose production within a few minutes. Glucagon release is stimulated when plasma glucose levels are decreased to fasting levels. Suppression of glucagon is caused by hyperglycemia, by the administration of glucose, or by the ingestion of protein.[81]

Several studies have shown that glucagon levels in the fasting state during the third trimester are higher than those in the second trimester.[49,82] It has therefore been postulated that glucose intolerance and insulin resistance could be mediated through increased secretion of glucagon. However, studies by Kühl and Holst have demonstrated that the insulin–glucagon ratio in pregnancy increases significantly as compared to that in the non-pregnant state.[49] In the fasting state, basal insulin levels are increased proportionally more than glucagon levels. Thus, the insulin–glucagon ratio may explain the low fasting glucose levels observed during normal pregnancy. When glucagon levels are studied following glucose administration, it has been shown that glucagon levels are suppressed to a greater degree in pregnant women than in non-pregnant women (Fig. 61-2).[65] Therefore, it can be concluded that changes in glucagon secretion during pregnancy cannot explain the insulin resistance of late pregnancy.

MATERNAL GLUCOSE HOMEOSTASIS IN THE FASTING STATE

During normal pregnancy, the fasting blood glucose level decreases.[83] Lind and Aspillaga have shown that during normal pregnancy, plasma fasting glucose levels decrease in the first few weeks of gestation, reaching a nadir by the 12th week of gestation and remaining unchanged thereafter until delivery (Fig. 61-3).[84] This finding is in agreement with that of Felig and Lynch, who have reported a decrease of glucose levels in pregnancy of 15 mg/100 mL after overnight fasting as compared to non-pregnant controls.[85]

RESPONSE TO GLUCOSE LOAD

In normal pregnancy it has been shown that during late gestation, there is an increase in the 1- and 2-hour

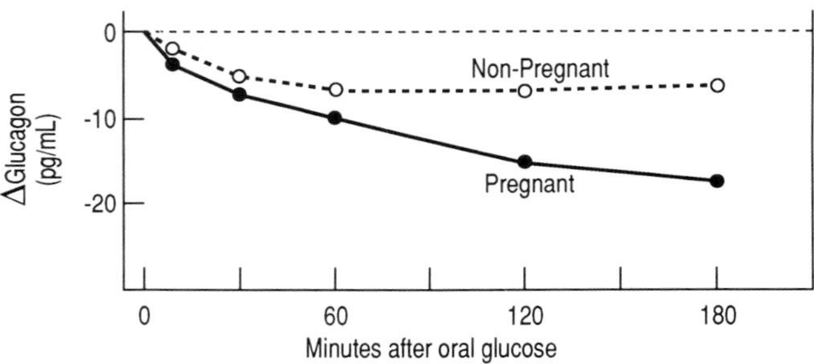

FIGURE 61–2. The response of plasma glucagon to oral glucose administration in late pregnancy and in non-pregnant patients. Values have been expressed as changes from basal concentration. (Freinkel N. Of pregnancy and progeny. Diabetes 1980;29:1026.)

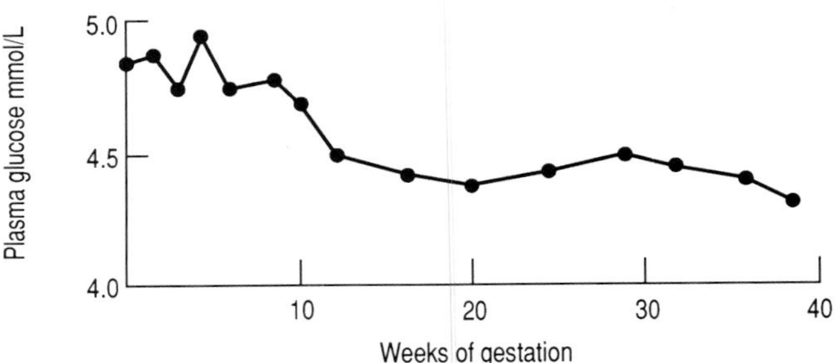

FIGURE 61–3. Plasma fasting glucose concentrations throughout normal pregnancy; mg/dL = mmol/L × 18. (Lind T., Aspillaga M. Metabolic Changes During Normal and Diabetic Pregnancies, p. 77. In: Reece EA, Coustan D. (eds). Diabetes mellitus in pregnancy; Principles and practice. Edinburgh: Churchill Livingstone, 1988:77.)

blood glucose levels after glucose tolerance testing as compared to non-pregnant controls.[64] Moreover, postprandial glucose levels are higher in pregnancy after a standard meal.[86] As previously reported by O'Sullivan and Mahan,[64] Fitch and King have recently demonstrated that oral glucose elicits a greater increase in plasma glucose during late pregnancy than that elicited in non-pregnant women at 60, 120, and 180 minutes after the glucose load, but this difference was significant only after 60 minutes.[87] Insulin plasma levels were significantly higher in pregnant than in non-pregnant women at all time points studied (15, 30, 60, 120, and 180 minutes after glucose load) (Fig. 61-4).

Freinkel postulated that this greater and more prolonged hyperglycemia may indicate "facilitated anabolism" during feeding periods.[65] The prolonged hyperglycemia after a glucose load or meal would "facilitate" access of ingested glucose to the fetus. Moreover, since triglycerides cross the placenta poorly, the increased rise in plasma triglycerides could abet this objective further by replacing some of the circulating glucose as ma-

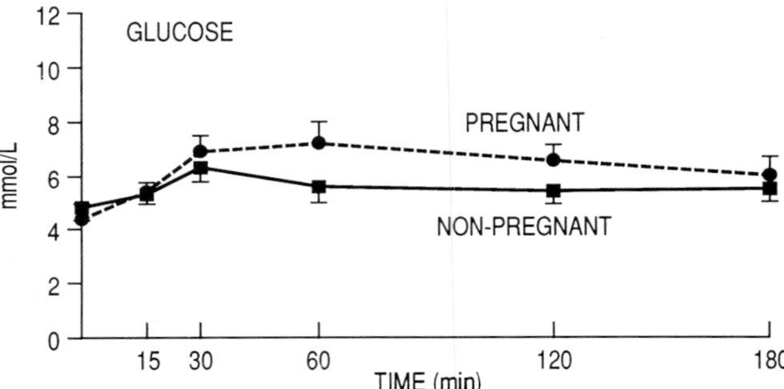

FIGURE 61–4. Plasma glucose and insulin responses to oral glucose tolerance test, ±SEM in late pregnancy and in non-pregnant women; mg/dL = mmol/L × 18. (Modified from Fitch WL, King J. Plasma amino acids, glucose and insulin responses to moderate-protein and high-protein test meals in pregnant, nonpregnant, and gestational diabetic women. Am J Clin Nutr 1987;46:243.)

ternal oxidative fuel, sparing glucose for transplacental flux.

THE EFFECT OF PREGNANCY ON DIURNAL VARIATION OF PLASMA GLUCOSE DURING MIXED-MEAL FEEDING

Several years ago, Freinkel described the effect of normal late pregnancy on the diurnal changes in plasma glucose and insulin.[88] All patients received 2.11 kcal/day of liquid formula diet in three equal feedings and had regular blood sampling over a 24-hour period. This study demonstrated that in normal late pregnancy there is a greater postmeal increment and premeal decrement in plasma glucose than there is in non-pregnant controls and that the concurrent excursions in insulin are of far greater amplitude (Fig. 61-5).

Cousins and colleagues performed a longitudinal study in normal pregnant women and studied the progressive effect of second and third trimesters on the level of plasma glucose, measured at hourly intervals throughout the 24-hour day.[86] The mean 24-hour glucose concentrations were significantly reduced during the second trimester (85.6 ± 2.9 mg/dL) and the third trimester (87.3 mg/dL ± 1.7 mg/dL) compared to the postpartum control values (93.4 mg/dL ± 1.9 mg/dL). A significant elevation of the 2-hour postprandial value was clearly evident in the third trimester compared to both second-trimester and postpartum values. However, it was noted that there is a progressive decrease of plasma glucose during sleeping hours from the second to the third trimester of pregnancy, and this may contribute to the decreased 24-hour glucose concentration.

It is interesting to note that the anabolic glucose excursions (maximal increments above the 24-hour mean) during the feeding hours of the day in pregnancy were very similar to the postpartum state (ranging between 30 mg/dL and 35 mg/dL).

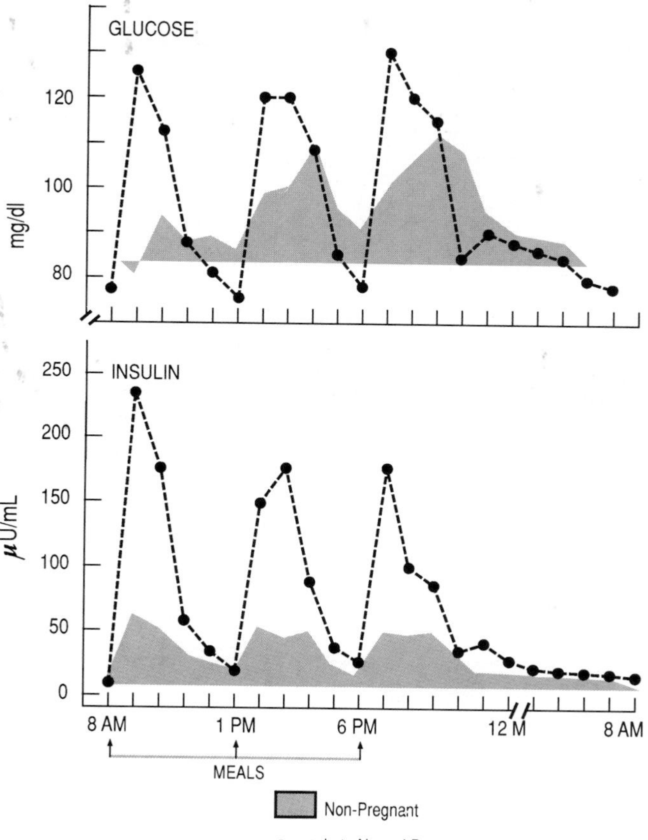

FIGURE 61–5. The effect of normal late pregnancy on the diurnal changes in plasma glucose and insulin. All patients received three equal feedings. (For details, see text.) (Reproduced with permission from Freinkel N, Phelps NL, Metzger BE. Intermediary metabolism during normal pregnancy. In: Sutherland HW, Stowers JM, eds. Carbohydrate metabolism in pregnancy and the newborn. New York: Springer-Verlag, 1979:1.)

LIPID METABOLISM

Knopp and colleagues have proposed two phases of adipose tissue metabolism in pregnancy: an increase in storage until midgestation, and diminished storage with enhanced mobilization (lypolysis) in late gestation.[89] It has been well documented that in pregnancy there is a tendency for accelerated fat mobilization and ketone body formation, particularly with prolonged periods of starvation.[89] As mentioned previously, human placental lactogen is depressed by hyperglycemia and increased by hypoglycemia.[85,90] In the fasting state, glucose levels are decreased, leading to decreased insulin levels, but are associated with increased levels of HPL. HPL increases lypolysis, so free fatty acids may serve as a source of energy for maternal metabolism to maintain an adequate supply of plasma glucose and amino acid for the fetus. Freinkel has termed this "accelerated starvation." Ravnikar and colleagues found that in pregnancy at 32 to 38 weeks of gestation, plasma concentrations of FFA and b-hydroxybutyrate were significantly higher than they were in the nongravid state only after at least 12 hours of fasting.[91] In prolonged periods of fasting, ketone bodies are transferred to the fetus, and this may serve as an alternative to the decreased glucose supply.

Since ketone bodies may be used by the fetal brain for energy, some consideration has been given to the effect of ketones on normal fetal brain development.[92] Maternal hyperketonemia was initially reported to be associated with lower intelligence quotient in the offspring.[93,94] However, subsequent work has not corroborated these findings. Therefore, at present it is unknown what effect, if any, hyperketonemia has on the fetal brain.

In normal pregnancy, total lipids increase in all three lipoprotein fractions (very-low-density lipoproteins, low-density lipoproteins, and high-density lipoproteins). Triglyceride and cholesterol content of the three lipoproteins are increased throughout pregnancy. Third-trimester human pregnancy is characterized by a two- to threefold increase in plasma triglycerides and a lesser increase in cholesterol and phospholipids.[95] The increase of triglycerides during pregnancy is mainly due to increases in both VLDLs and LDLs. The HDL triglycerides increase toward the end of the second trimester; no further increases are observed after that.[96]

Cholesterol is increased during pregnancy, mainly due to the VLDL and LDL fractions. HDL cholesterol increases slowly until midpregnancy and then declines as pregnancy progresses (Fig. 61-6).

PROTEIN METABOLISM

The concentration of most amino acids is lower among pregnant women than among non-pregnant women.[97] Young found that most amino acid levels are lower in maternal plasma than in fetal blood.[98] Following the ingestion of food, the increase in plasma levels of amino acids is smaller in normal pregnancy than in the non-pregnant state.[99] It has been suggested that this is a result of a higher transfer of amino acids to the fetus or an increase in maternal gluconeogenesis.[84]

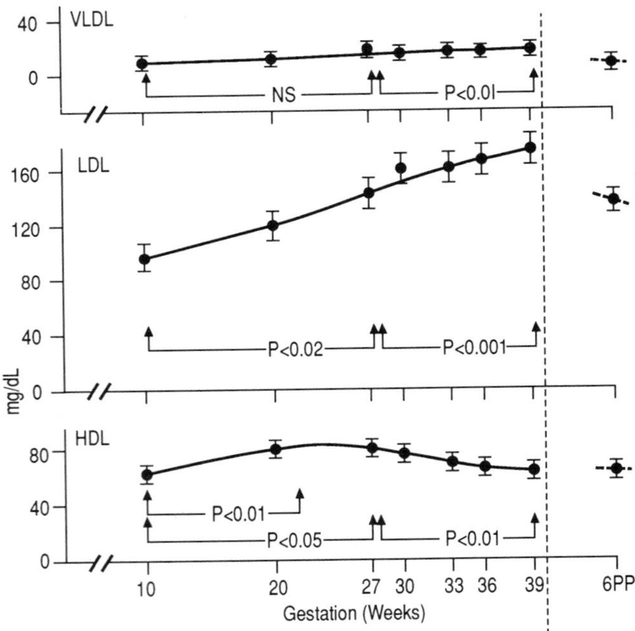

FIGURE 61–6. Serial changes in lipoprotein cholesterol in pregnancy. Cholesterol increases slowly in VLDL and rapidly in LDL throughout gestation. The HDL-cholesterol concentration peaks mid-pregnancy and then decreases as pregnancy progresses. (Knopp RH, Montes A, Childs M, Li JR, Mabuchi H. Metabolic adjustments in normal and diabetic pregnancy. Clin Obstet Gynecol 1981;24:36.)

PLACENTAL TRANSFER OF NUTRIENTS

The placenta is a complex organ that has an important function in the transfer of gases and nutrients between the mother and the fetus. Fetal growth is controlled by various factors and depends on the uptake of nutrients and oxygen by the placenta and on their transfer to the fetus. The availability of nutrients to the fetus depends principally on the maternal metabolic state. Placental transfer of the principal nutrients is discussed briefly here (Fig. 61-7).

Glucose

Experimental studies have provided evidence that the process of transplacental glucose transfer involves a carrier-mediated active transport system.[100,101] In this process of facilitated diffusion, the net result is that fetal blood glucose levels are 15% to 20% lower than maternal levels. It is believed that this difference in blood glucose levels between maternal and fetal blood is a result of placental use of glucose. It has been shown that the placenta contains insulin receptors; however, their role is not yet clear.[102] The fetus seems to be "protected" from very high maternal glucose levels. In fact, it has been found that the placental transport system of glucose is saturated when maternal glucose levels are maintained up to about 250 mg/dL. It is not possible to increase fetal plasma glucose levels above this threshold.[103,104]

Amino Acids

Placental transfer of amino acids is an active process. Amino acids are transferred against a concentration gradient; in the fetus, amino acid levels are three to four times higher than those in the maternal blood. However, the concentration of amino acids in the placenta is higher than that in either fetal or maternal blood.[105]

METABOLISM IN THE DIABETIC PREGNANCY

Islet cells function completely differently in IDDM than in NIDDM. It is therefore unsurprising that there is a

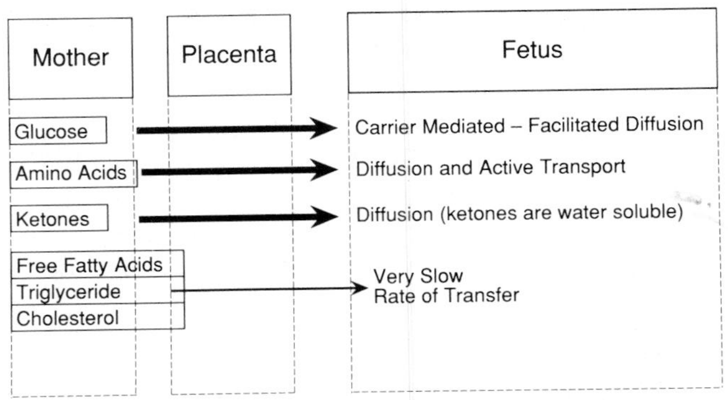

FIGURE 61–7. Transplacental transfer of maternal fuels to the fetus (for details, see text).

difference in insulin secretion between the two forms of diabetes. C-peptide, which is the connecting peptide between the a and b chains of insulin, was found to be higher in NIDDM pregnant women than in normal controls. However, C-peptide release in NIDDM was lower following meals.[106] This may indicate impaired effectiveness of insulin in target tissues and pancreatic B-cell dysfunction in patients with NIDDM.

In IDDM, C-peptide levels were found to be very low or almost undetectable, which may indicate no residual B-cell function. It has also been shown that in IDDM patients the increase in insulin requirement is almost 40%, whereas in NIDDM it can be much higher, reaching as high as 100%.[71] For several years it has been known that maternal fuel levels other than that of glucose can be abnormal in diabetic pregnant patients. Metzger and colleagues have shown that plasma triglyceride levels are elevated in obese pregnant patients with gestational diabetes or NIDDM.[107] Skryten and colleagues reported higher plasma triglyceride concentrations in IDDM pregnant patients during the third trimester.[108] This, however, has not been confirmed in more recent studies.[109]

Metzger and associates reported that plasma FFA tends to be higher in patients with gestational diabetes compared to normal pregnant patients.[107] Furthermore, FFA was also found to be elevated in IDDM pregnant patients. A correlation between these concentrations and neonatal birth weight was reported.[110] In yet another study, HDL cholesterol concentrations were found to be low in NIDDM and not significantly changed in IDDM compared to nondiabetic pregnant controls.[109]

In summary, the metabolic disturbances in diabetic pregnant patients are expressed in increased concentrations of circulating metabolic fuels, including carbohydrate, protein, and fat. This increased circulating maternal level can be transferred to the fetus and may contribute to the development of fetal macrosomia.[108,111]

GESTATIONAL DIABETES MELLITUS

DEFINITION

Gestational diabetes mellitus is defined as carbohydrate intolerance of variable severity with onset or first recognition during the present pregnancy.[10] This means the glucose intolerance may have antedated the pregnancy but was not recognized by the patient or physician. Although this is infrequent, patients who actually have diabetes mellitus type I or II may therefore initially be classified as having gestational diabetes.

INCIDENCE

The incidence of gestational diabetes mellitus varies in different study populations and is estimated to occur in 3% to 5% of pregnant women.[112]

SCREENING FOR GESTATIONAL DIABETES

In the past, patient selection for an oral glucose tolerance test (GTT) (100 g) was based on historic and clinical risk factors. High-risk groups included patients with one of the following: obesity, glycosuria, previous macrosomic infants, previous history of fetal or neonatal death or congenital anomalies, family history of diabetes, and hypertension during current pregnancy. It has been shown that if risk factors only are used as an indication for oral glucose tolerance testing, only 63% of patients with gestational diabetes will be identified.[113] The Second International Workshop–Conference on Gestational Diabetes Mellitus recommended that all pregnant women receive screening for glucose intolerance, because selective screening based on risk factors has been found to be inadequate and ineffective.[113] Pregnant women who have not been identified as having glucose intolerance before the 24th week of gestation should have a screening glucose challenge test between the 24th and 28th weeks consisting of 50 g oral glucose given without regard to time of the last meal or time of day. A value of plasma venous glucose of 140 mg/dL or more has been recommended as a threshold to indicate the need for a full diagnostic GTT.

Diagnosis of gestational diabetes is based on the results of the 100 g oral GTT. This method of screening has a sensitivity of 79%, and specificity for all pregnant women is 87%.[114] There is almost general agreement in the United States that pregnant patients should be screened with a 50 g oral glucose load.

The American Diabetes Association has recommended universal screening for all pregnant women. The American College of Obstetrics and Gynecology recommended screening all pregnant women over 30 years of age as well as women with any risk factor.[115] Others have recommended screening patients who are at least 24 years old[116] or 25 years or older.[114] This strategy, instead of the universal screening, may reduce costs without significant reduction in diagnostic accuracy. For example, Marguette and colleagues have shown, in a prospective study of 1012 pregnant women screened for gestational diabetes, that by limiting the screening age to 24 years old and older, only two cases out of 24 diagnosed to have gestational diabetes will be misdiagnosed.[117] They have also shown that by limiting the screening test to patients of 24 years or older, costs can be reduced by almost 50% without a significant decrease in the diagnostic accuracy of screening for gestational diabetes mellitus (GDM), which approaches 91%.

Coustan and Carpenter have proposed decreasing plasma glucose screen values to >130 mg/dL following a 50-g glucose load.[118] By using this lower threshold, they have increased sensitivity to almost 100%, although there was a decrease of specificity approaching 80%.

The same investigators have shown that with increasing increments of glucose screen values, there is a sharp increase in the incidence of gestational diabetes,[119] and when the plasma glucose screening test results are >185 mg/dL, patients are gestational diabetics and no further testing is required (Table 61-7).

The necessity for diagnostic testing (GTT) is increased from 17% to 25% of the screened population when one uses a threshold of 135 mg/dL instead of 140 mg/dL. However, this lower threshold may help to detect an additional 16% of gestational diabetics.

Marguette and colleagues have demonstrated that a higher threshold of 150 mg/dL limited to gravidas over 24 years old could be a reasonable alternative to universal screening,[117] since the incidence of gestational diabetes in the group of patients with plasma screening test results between 130 and 149 mg/dL is very low (<0.7%) in their population.

Different racial and social groups seem to be predisposed to different rates of gestational diabetes. It is therefore possible that different thresholds may be required for adequate sensitivity in different obstetric populations. Most authorities recommend testing at 24 to 48 weeks gestation, at a time when there is an increase in insulin resistance.[115] Since, in patients with risk factors for GDM, the diagnosis can be made earlier, some investigators recommend screening for GDM at the first prenatal visit for all patients with risk factors.[120] A negative screening test is repeated at 24 to 28 weeks. In patients with positive screening and a normal oral GTT at early gestation, the oral GTT should be repeated later in pregnancy.

Watson has studied the changes in 50-g oral glucose testing in 55 pregnant patients.[121] Patients were screened serially at 20, 28, and 34 weeks gestation. As expected, a significant increase in plasma glucose values after a 50-g oral GTT was observed as pregnancy advanced. The author has shown that 8% of patients with negative screening at 28 weeks had a subsequent positive test at 34 weeks. It is suggested, therefore, that patients with screen test values of 120 to 139 mg/dL at 24 to 28 weeks be retested at 34 weeks. In fact, 11% of GDM patients in Watson's study would have been undetected if patients were screened only at 24 to 28 weeks.

Glycosylated hemoglobin and fructosamine levels have been investigated as possible screening tests for gestational diabetes.[122,123] Their use for this purpose is limited because of low sensitivity and specificity.[124,125]

TABLE 61-7. INCIDENCE OF A POSITIVE GLUCOSE TOLERANCE TEST AMONG 96 GRAVIDAS WITH 50-G, 1-HOUR SCREENING TEST VALUES >134 mg/dL (PLASMA, GLUCOSE OXIDASE)

SCREENING TEST RESULT	INCIDENCE OF GESTATIONAL DIABETES (%)
135–144	14.6
145–154	17.4
155–164	28.6
165–174	20.0
175–184	50.0
>185	100.0

From Carpenter MW, Coustan DR. Criteria for screening tests for gestational diabetes. Am J Obstet Gynecol 1982;144:768. By permission.

DIAGNOSIS

The diagnosis of gestational diabetes is, in most cases, based on an abnormal result of an oral GTT during pregnancy. A minority of cases will be diagnosed on the basis of high fasting glucose levels during pregnancy, in which case the oral glucose tolerance test will not have to be performed. The GTT is administered under standard conditions: 100 g of glucose is given orally in at least 400 mL of water after an overnight fast of 8 to 14 hours. The patient should have at least 3 days of unrestricted diet with more than 150 g carbohydrate and should be at rest during the study. Diagnosis requires that at least two of four glucose levels of the oral GTT meet or exceed the upper limits of normal values. The normal upper limit was determined by O'Sullivan and Mahan as 2 SD above the mean for each of four glucose values of 752 pregnant patients undergoing 100 g oral GTTs.[64] Their criteria for the oral GTT in pregnancy are the most widely used in the United States. O'Sullivan and Mahan studied whole blood using the Somogyi-Nelson method, which has been shown to identify other saccharides in addition to glucose.[64] The National Diabetes Data Group[126] has modified O'Sullivan's data for plasma values by increasing whole blood values by 15% because plasma glucose values are approximately 15% higher than those in whole blood.[119]

Further modifications of O'Sullivan's criteria were proposed by Carpenter and Coustan, who took into consideration not only the change in the medium tested (whole blood versus plasma), as had been done by the NDDG, but also the changes in methodology.[119] Currently, the most widely used methods of glucose measurement in plasma are the glucose oxidase, or hexokinase, assay. These new methodologies are more specific for glucose and have been shown to result in approximately 5 mg/dL lower values as compared to the less specific Somogyi-Nelson method. Thus, the criteria of Carpenter and Coustan for oral glucose tolerance testing are stricter.[119] Whole blood and plasma glucose criteria of the oral GTT used for the diagnosis of gestational diabetes are presented in Table 61-8.

Recent data have shown that criteria even more stringent than those currently used may be necessary to define gestational diabetes. Tallarigo and colleagues have demonstrated that even a limited degree of maternal hyperglycemia is related to adverse pregnancy outcome.[127] They have shown that pregnant patients with normal glucose tolerance according to O'Sullivan's criteria with 2-hour glucose levels in the range of 120 to 164 mg/dL have a significant increase in the incidence of macrosomia, congenital anomalies, tox-

TABLE 61–8. ORAL GLUCOSE TOLERANCE TEST (100 g) VALUES FOR THE DIAGNOSIS OF GESTATIONAL DIABETES (mg/dL)

	O'SULLIVAN (1964)[64]	NDDG (1979)[126]	CARPENTER AND COUSTAN[119]
Fasting	90	105	95
1 Hour	165	190	180
2 Hour	145	165	155
3 Hour	125	145	140

emia, and cesarean section. Further studies are needed to establish the degree of risk, if any, in patients with a minimal degree of hyperglycemia during pregnancy.

MANAGEMENT

GDM has been associated with increased perinatal mortality, an increased rate of cesarean sections, significant risk of macrosomia, and other neonatal morbidities, including serious birth trauma, hypoglycemia, hypocalcemia, polycythemia, and hyperbilirubinemia.[123,128] Without adequate screening, GDM may remain unrecognized. Several investigators have strongly supported screening for gestational diabetes and have demonstrated improved pregnancy outcomes in GDM patients identified through screening.[113,129–132] Management of GDM is directed toward reducing perinatal mortality and morbidity, a goal that may be achieved by maintaining close surveillance of the mother and fetus. Maternal surveillance includes close monitoring of glucose levels.

After the diagnosis of gestational diabetes has been made, patients receive nutritional counseling—the mainstay of therapy in this group of patients. Since as many as 15% to 20% of patients will have deterioration of glucose homeostasis as gestation proceeds, it is mandatory to identify this group early and to initiate insulin therapy. It is our practice to monitor glucose levels in gestational diabetics once or twice weekly. If fasting plasma glucose levels are ≥105 mg/dL or 2-hour postprandial glucose levels are ≥120 mg/dL on two or more occasions within a 2-week interval, insulin therapy is initiated.[113] The offspring of mothers with fasting plasma glucose levels ≥105 mg/dL and postprandial levels ≥120 mg/dL are at greatest risk of intrauterine death and neonatal mortality.[113] This group of patients is encouraged to self-monitor glucose levels more frequently. Glycemic control may be assessed with glycosylated hemoglobin periodically.

The majority of women with gestational diabetes will be in good control—that is, fasting plasma glucose levels ≤105 mg/dL or postprandial levels ≤120 mg/dL—with dietary therapy. It has been shown that prophylactic insulin may be of some benefit in reducing neonatal morbidity in this group of patients.[129]

Coustan and Imarah studied the effect of prophylactic insulin in gestational diabetes.[129] The incidence of babies weighing over 4000 g at birth was reduced from 18% in 184 gestational diabetics treated with diet to 7% in 115 treated with prophylactic insulin. In addition, the incidence of operative delivery was 30% in the diet-treated group compared to 16% in the prophylactic insulin–treated group. In another clinical trial of prophylactic insulin, in which lower doses of insulin were used as prophylaxis, there was no significant difference in the incidence of macrosomia between treated and untreated groups.[129] Further studies are needed to determine the benefits of prophylactic insulin treatment in gestational diabetes.

Antenatal testing is recommended in some patients with gestational diabetes. The gestational age at which this testing should begin and the best method of antepartum testing have not been determined. Landon and Gabbe recommend that antepartum testing with weekly nonstress tests and maternal surveillance of fetal movements begin at 32 weeks gestation only in selected groups of patients.[133] Such groups would include insulin-requiring gestational diabetics and those who are not being treated with insulin but who have additional risk factors, such as chronic hypertension, preeclampsia, or a previous stillbirth. Gabbe and colleagues have shown that this group of patients may be safely allowed to go until 40 weeks, as long as fasting euglycemia is maintained, before fetal surveillance is initiated.[134]

In our medical centers, we still use antepartum fetal testing in all gestational diabetes. Beginning at 28 weeks, all patients record fetal activity daily, and from 34 weeks, weekly nonstress tests are performed. Delivery may be delayed until spontaneous labor or 42 weeks in well-controlled patients. In poorly controlled patients, induction of labor as soon as there is pulmonic maturity is recommended. For unfavorable cervixes, methods of cervical ripening may be employed prior to labor induction.

Because fetal macrosomia is frequent in gestational diabetes, fetal weight estimation is prudent prior to an attempted vaginal delivery. As in overt diabetes, cesarean section will be performed on most patients with estimated fetal weight of >4500 g in order to prevent shoulder dystocia and birth trauma.

In patients with estimated fetal weight between 4000 g and 4500 g, management should be individualized based on the size of the pelvis and the patient's previous obstetric history. In addition, and most importantly, the use of midpelvic operative delivery should be discouraged in patients with suspected macrosomia. In patients with prolonged second stage labor in which the head is still in midpelvis, cesarean section should be seriously considered to reduce the risk of shoulder dystocia.[135]

During labor and delivery, it is important, as in overt diabetes, to monitor maternal glycemia. To maintain euglycemia, glucose tests are performed in insulin-requiring gestational diabetics at 1- to 2-hour intervals.

LONG-TERM MATERNAL OUTCOME OF GESTATIONAL DIABETES

Several investigators have shown that patients with gestational diabetes mellitus are at increased risk for developing diabetes years after pregnancy.[132,136] O'Sullivan, in a long-term study of the outcome of women with gestational diabetes, has shown the development of overt diabetes beyond 20 years following pregnancy to be as high as 20%, and 50% had impaired glucose tolerance.[137]

It is recommended, therefore, that women with GDM be followed postpartum to detect diabetes early in its course. They should be evaluated at the first postpartum visit by a fasting plasma glucose test and by a 2-hour oral GTT (30, 90, and 120 minutes) using a 75-g glucose load.[32] The criteria of the National Diabetes Data group[126] for the diagnosis of diabetes mellitus in non-pregnant adults include a fasting plasma glucose level of >140 mg/dL on more than one occasion, or a 75-g, 2-hour oral GTT in which the 2-hour value and at least one other value are >200 mg/dL. The criteria for the diagnosis of impaired glucose tolerance are the following: fasting plasma glucose below 140 mg/dL and 2-hour value between 140 and 200 mg/dL, and at least one other value of 200 mg/dL or more.

The risk of developing diabetes later in life in GDM is greatly influenced by body weight, with the highest rate occurring in obese patients. Therefore, obese GDM patients should be advised to control their weight.[138]

PREGESTATIONAL DIABETES MELLITUS

PERICONCEPTIONAL CARE

Management of the pregnant diabetic woman is a complex task that should start before conception. Prepregnancy clinics were first initiated in Edinburgh in 1976. In such clinics, physicians have the opportunity to explain to the patient and her partner the practice of diabetes care during pregnancy, in particular the need for stringent glycemic control. At the initial visit, the patient is assessed as to her general medical status, and signs of retinopathy, nephropathy, hypertension, and ischemic heart disease are looked for. The patient undergoes ophthalmologic evaluation, electrocardiography, and kidney function tests.[139] Thus, patients with severe retinopathy can be identified and treatment with laser coagulation performed before pregnancy, if necessary. In patients with coronary artery disease, termination of the pregnancy should be seriously considered. A patient taking oral hypoglycemic drugs should discontinue them and begin insulin treatment.

An increasing body of evidence shows that the incidence of congenital anomalies is related to hyperglycemia in early pregnancy.[140] One of the first goals of the prepregnancy clinic is to achieve optimum diabetic control even before the time of conception. Several studies have shown significant reduction of congenital malformations following such a prepregnancy treatment program. In one study, 7.5% of the infants of diabetic patients (n = 292) who had begun strict metabolic control after their eighth week of pregnancy had congenital anomalies, as compared to only 0.8% fetal anomalies in the offspring of a group of 128 diabetics in whom intensive treatment began before conception.[140] Other studies, albeit with less dramatic results, have all shown reductions in the rates of congenital malformation with prepregnancy treatment.

CONGENITAL ANOMALIES IN INFANTS OF DIABETIC MOTHERS

The frequency of major congenital anomalies among infants of diabetic mothers has been estimated as 6% to 10%, which represents a two- to fivefold increase over the frequency observed in the general population.[141] In Copenhagen, Jorgen Pedersen, one of the pioneers in the study of diabetes in pregnancy, has studied 1452 IDDM patients seen between 1926 and 1977—one of the largest series reported in the literature.[142] Dealing only with the malformations identified in the first week of life, he found that 8% of infants of diabetic mothers had congenital anomalies, as compared to 2.8% in nondiabetic controls. Kucera reviewed the world literature and described 340 (4.7%) malformations in 7111 infants of diabetic mothers, representing a 2.7-fold increase of malformations in children of diabetic mothers as opposed to nondiabetic mothers.[143] Congenital malformations in fetuses of diabetic patients are now responsible for approximately 40% of all perinatal deaths, replacing respiratory distress syndrome as the leading cause of infant death.[3,144] These malformations usually involve multiple organ systems (Table 61-9), with cardiac anomalies being the most common, followed by central nervous system and skeletal malformations.[143]

Cardiovascular Abnormalities

Kucera reported cardiac anomalies as the most frequent malformation, occurring four times more often in children of diabetic mothers than in those of nondiabetic controls.[143] Rowland and colleagues reported the incidence of congenital heart disease to be 4% in the offspring of 470 IDDM patients, a rate five times higher than that seen in the general population.[145] In diabetic pregnancies, the major cardiac anomalies include transposition of the great vessels, ventricular septal defects, coarctation of the aorta, and situs inversus.[143,145]

The Central Nervous System

Infants of diabetic mothers are at higher risk for neural tube defects, with anencephaly being the most frequent, followed by spina bifida. This increased risk of neural tube defects in diabetic pregnancy varies in dif-

TABLE 61–9. CONGENITAL ANOMALIES OF INFANTS OF DIABETIC MOTHERS

Skeletal and CNS
Caudal regression syndrome
Neural tube defects excluding anencephaly
Anencephaly with or without herniation of neural elements
Microcephaly
Cardiac
Transposition of the great vessels with or without ventricular septal defect
Ventricular septal defects
Coarctation of the aorta with or without ventricular septal defect or patent ductus arteriosus
Atrial septal defects
Cardiomegaly
Renal anomalies
Hydronephrosis
Renal agenesis
Ureteral duplication
Gastrointestinal
Duodenal atresia
Anorectal atresia
Small left colon syndrome
Other
Single umbilical artery

Reprinted by permission from Reece EA, Hobbins JC. Diabetes embryopathy, pathogenesis, prenatal diagnosis and prevention. Obstet Gynecol Surv 1986;41:325.

ferent reports, ranging between two and 19 times greater than nondiabetic controls.[143,146]

The Skeletal System

Skeletal anomalies most frequently involve the vertebrae and limbs.[147,148] Kucera reported that vertebral anomalies occur five times as frequently in offspring of diabetics as in those of controls.[143] Hemivertebra is reported to be the most common vertebral defect.[149] The caudal regression syndrome is characterized by osseous deficiencies, particularly of the sacrum, coccyx, and lower limbs. Associated anomalies include, among others, cleft lip and palate, congenital heart disease, microcephaly, and renal malformations.[150] This syndrome of caudal regression is very rare and affects about 0.2% to 0.5% of infants of diabetic mothers. However, in diabetic offspring there is about a 200-fold increase in the rate of caudal regression syndrome over that seen in nondiabetic controls.[151] Nevertheless, since this lesion is also seen in nondiabetics it cannot be considered pathognomonic for diabetes.

Other Anomalies

An increased rate of renal malformations and genitourinary anomalies among diabetic offspring has been observed. (For further details, the reader is referred to a review by Reece and Hobbins.[152])

Pathogenesis of Diabetes-Associated Congenital Anomalies

Both clinical and experimental studies are in agreement that diabetes-associated birth defects occur following disruption of developmental processes during organogenesis and are associated with abnormal metabolism, thought to be related mostly to hyperglycemia.[104,153,154] In vivo studies in which rats were made diabetic by streptozotocin or alloxan therapy resulted in fetal anomalies.[155,156] These studies suggest a cause-and-effect relationship between altered glucose metabolism and congenital anomalies; however, the target site of action remains unknown. Studies in our laboratory at Yale on diabetes-related teratogenesis focused on the mechanism and possible target site of action.[156,157] Using the in vitro rodent conceptus culture system, we conducted studies of glucose-induced embryopathy. In all cases of embryopathy, there were concomitant characteristic yolk sac changes observed by both gross and microscopic examinations. These findings support our hypothesis that the yolk sac is the primary target site for the adverse metabolic effect of diabetes and that embryonic malformations occur as a secondary phenomenon to the primary yolk sac damage. Factors other than hyperglycemia have been implicated in diabetes-associated birth defects, including ketone bodies, hypoglycemia, low levels of trace metals, and somatomedin-inhibiting factors.[158,159] This subject has been reviewed recently.[141]

In laboratory studies in chickens, rabbits, and rats there is evidence that insulin has a teratogenic effect; however, its effect in humans is still controversial.[141] The fundamental question, still unresolved, is the "barrier" property of the human placenta to the passage of insulin. Some investigators reported that the human placenta is impermeable to insulin.[160] Others found that insulin readily crosses it.[161] Pitkin and Reynolds, using rhesus monkey preparations, showed limited transfer of insulin from mother to fetus and vice versa.[162]

In summary, there is not enough evidence to incriminate insulin in diabetes-associated embryopathy in humans, since the fetal compartment is virtually free of insulin. It seems that only limited transfer of maternal insulin is possible, and the fetal pancreas does not produce insulin until after organogenesis.[163] What influence circulating maternal insulin has on extraembryonic membranes and how the potential damage to this organ may influence embryogenesis remain unknown.

Prevention of Fetal Anomalies

Clinical studies suggest that euglycemia during organogenesis is critical in the prevention of congenital anomalies.[141] Several investigators have recruited diabetic women before pregnancy and attempted to place them under tight glycemic control before conception.[140,164,165] These studies are summarized in Table 61-10.

From Edinburgh, Steel reported a malformation rate of 3.9% in 78 subjects treated intensively before conception, as compared to a rate of 9.2% in 65 pregnancies in which the women did not attend the prepregnancy clinics.[168] In this study, a lower malformation rate was observed in the group treated intensively before conception, but the difference in rates was not significant. Goldman and colleagues reported no major malformations in 44 pregnancies in which good glycemic control was achieved before conception, as compared to three major malformations in 31 pregnancies in which patients had not sought antenatal care.[169]

The most recent and most extensive clinical study on the subject is that by Mills and colleagues, at the U. S. National Institute of Child Health and Human Development.[165] In this study 347 diabetic women and 389 controls were enrolled within the first 24 days of conception (early-entry group), and 279 diabetic women entered later (late-entry group). Major malformations were detected in 4.9% of the offspring of the early-entry diabetic women, in 2.1% of nondiabetic controls, and in 9.0% of the late-entry diabetic women. These results reveal that the malformation rates were significantly higher among the offspring of late-entry and so-called "untreated" diabetics than among early-entry or treated diabetic women ($p = 0.03$). It is noteworthy that when the early-entry data were analyzed critically, there was no correlation between the risk of congenital abnormalities in the infant and mean blood glucose, glycosylated hemoglobin, or hypoglycemia. This study is the only one that failed to show a correlation between hyperglycemia and the rate of malformations. It has been argued that this relationship was not observed, since the range of hyperglycemia was narrow and probably did not exceed the threshold above which an exponential dose effect would be expected. In this light, it is recommended that diabetic women contemplating pregnancy be encouraged to delay conception until satisfactory metabolic control is achieved so that embryogenesis can occur in an optimal metabolic milieu.

Diagnostic Evaluation for Diabetic Embryopathy

All patients with pregestational diabetes are evaluated for possible fetal anomalies. Patients are routinely evaluated by maternal serum α-fetoprotein (MSAFP), an early glycosylated hemoglobin determination, ultrasonography for a general fetal anatomical survey, and fetal echocardiography.

Glycosylated Hemoglobin. Glycosylated hemoglobins (HbA_1), or the minor hemoglobins, are postsynthetic transformations of native hemoglobin A_0 in which a sugar moiety is attached to the N-terminal valine of each b-chain. The largest fraction of the glycosylated hemoglobins is HbA_{1c}, which constitutes up to 80% of the minor hemoglobins. HbA_{1c} is formed when glucose is slowly and irreversibly linked to hemoglobin A_0.[171]

HbA_1 is expressed as a percentage of total hemoglobin and provides an integrated retrospective reflection of glycemic status over the 4 to 8 weeks preceding its determination.[172] Two groups of investigators have re-

TABLE 61–10. SUMMARY OF SELECTED CLINICAL STUDIES USING A PROGRAM OF PERICONCEPTUAL METABOLIC CONTROL TO PREVENT DIABETES-ASSOCIATED BIRTH DEFECTS

INVESTIGATOR	NO. PATIENTS	MALFORMATION RATE (%)	GLUCOSE CONTROL ACHIEVED	NO. PATIENTS	MALFORMATION RATE (%)	GLUCOSE CONTROL ACHIEVED
Pedersen et al[164]	284	14.1	Inadequate glucose control	363	7.4	Improved glucose control
Miller et al[166]	58	22.4	$HbA_1C > 8.5\%$	58	3.4	$HbA_1C \leq 8.5\%$
Fuhrmann et al[140]	292	7.5	Mean daily plasma glucose was ≤110 mg/dL in 88.3% of patients	128	0.8	Mean daily plasma glucose was ≤110 mg/dL in 20.7% of patients
Fuhrmann et al[167]	144	6.2	87% blood glucose readings between 2.3 and 7.7 mmol/L achieved by only 9.7% of patients	56	1.7	87% blood glucose readings were between 2.3 and 7.7 mmol/L achieved by 69.6% of patients
Steel[168]	65	9.2		78	3.9	
Goldman et al[169]	31	9.6	MBG = 163 ± 10.2 mg/dL HbA_1C = 10.42 + 0.47%			MBG = 110 ± 6.5 mg/dL HbA_1C = 7.39 + 0.34%
Kitzmiller et al[170]	53	15.1	$HbA_1C < 9.0\%$ in 47% of patients	46	2.2	$HbA_1C < 9.0\%$ in 87% of patients
Mills et al[165]	279	9.0		397	4.9	

Reprinted with permission from Reece EA, Gabrielli S, Abdellah M. The prevention of diabetes-associated birth defects. Semin Perinatol 1988;12(4):292.

ported a significant correlation between elevated HbA_{1c} levels in early pregnancy (<14 weeks of gestation) and an increased rate of fetal anomalies.[166,173] Miller and colleagues divided their diabetic patients into groups on the basis of HbA_{1c} values.[166] When HbA_{1c} levels were less than or equal to 8.5%, the malformation rates were low, approaching 3.4%. However, in patients with HbA_{1c} levels above 9.5%, a significantly higher malformation rate was observed that approached 22%. Similar results were obtained by Ylinen and colleagues.[173]

To compare Miller's study with that of Mills and colleagues,[165] one should convert HbA_1 data to standard deviations from the normal control mean. Applying the same 7-SD cutoff to Miller's study, 93% of their study population fell into Miller and colleagues' low-risk group. This fairly narrow range of reasonably well-controlled diabetics might represent the lower end of the curvilinear slope, so that a lack of correlation between glycemia and malformations would not be observed, thereby explaining why the study of Mills and colleagues failed to show a correlation between glycemic control and malformation rate.[141]

Based on the preceding data, it seems that the risk for delivering anomalous infants cannot be fully determined by HbA_1 levels, especially at low levels. It should be emphasized that diabetic embryopathy may be present even in patients with a normal HbA_1 level, and further evaluation is still necessary.

Maternal Serum α-Fetoprotein

Routine screening for the diabetic patient is essential for prenatal evaluation in view of the reported 20-fold increase in neural tube defects.[141] It has been suggested that the maternal serum α-fetoprotein (MSAFP) values should be interpreted with caution in diabetic pregnancy, since they are lower per gestational age than in the nondiabetic pregnancy.[174] Milunsky and colleagues have suggested a correction of 2 weeks in diabetic pregnancy.[175] However, in a study by Reece and colleagues, this finding was not confirmed.[176] They reported that when MSAFP was associated with euglycemia, the lower level among diabetics disappeared. Therefore, in well-controlled diabetics there is no need for adjustment of MSAFP values prior to interpretation.[176] The Connecticut AFP program stationed at Yale reports MSAFP corrected by HbA_1 obtained at the same time with the MSAFP.

Ultrasonic Evaluation

Routine screening of all diabetic pregnancies with ultrasonic evaluation should be made at approximately 20 weeks of gestation. This evaluation includes a general anatomical survey and fetal echocardiography. Sonographic examination of the fetal heart may be useful not only in the detection of malformations, but also to exclude diabetes-related cardiac hypertrophy. The finding of cardiac enlargement may indicate poor glycemic control. However, Kleinman has found no significant statistical differences in interventricular thickness between well-controlled pregnant diabetics and nondiabetic controls.[177]

One important observation by a single investigator that challenges the accuracy of crown–rump length (CRL) for dating diabetic pregnancies deserves comment. Pedersen and Molsted-Pedersen have reported that early growth delay (measured by CRL) occurs in almost 30% of diabetic pregnancies.[178] Of 38 embryos with early growth delay, seven (27%) were later found to have congenital anomalies.[179] These data, however, used previous menstrual history to estimate gestational age; thus, one cannot preclude the possibility that the smaller CRL ratios found in the fetuses of diabetics were a function of late ovulation. In fact, it is noteworthy that subsequent studies by our group at Yale (unpublished data) and that of Cousins and colleagues failed to show evidence of early growth delay in diabetic pregnancies when the date of conception was established by basal body temperature or day of ovulation.[180]

INSULIN ADMINISTRATION AND GLUCOSE EVALUATION

Over the last two decades perinatal mortality and morbidity have decreased significantly. In the past, the perinatal mortality rate in diabetic pregnant patients was in the range of 14% to 35%, depending on the duration and severity of the disease.[181] Most centers currently report perinatal mortality rates in the range of 3% to 5%. The critical factor contributing to this improvement has been the discovery that a stringent program of glucose control results in better fetal outcome.[3,134,182]

In an elegant pioneering study in 1972, Karlsson and Kjellmer showed a linear relationship between glycemic control and perinatal mortality.[3] In their retrospective study of 167 diabetics, they demonstrated that the lowest perinatal mortality rate was associated with mean blood glucose levels below 100 mg/dL. In patients with mean third-trimester blood glucose higher than 150 mg/dL, the perinatal mortality rate was 23.6%, whereas, in patients with mean blood glucose levels between 100 and 150 mg/dL and less than 100 mg/dL, the associated perinatal death rates were 15.3% and 3.4%, respectively.

Several other studies have also emphasized the beneficial effect of establishing euglycemia to improve pregnancy outcome.[182–184] It should be stressed that a cause-and-effect relationship between euglycemia and reduction in perinatal mortality has not been documented by appropriate randomized clinical trials, but there is a large body of evidence to support the current belief that normalization of blood glucose levels can reduce perinatal mortality rates. Other factors have certainly contributed to the reduction in perinatal death rates (eg, fetal surveillance, assessment of lung maturity, and advances in maternal and neonatal care). These factors, although important, are believed to be less crucial than the optimization of metabolic control. This conclusion is supported by the fact that immediate delivery necessitated by evidence of deteriorating fetoplacental function accounts for less than 3% of cases in well-controlled diabetic patients.[9]

The criteria for satisfactory metabolic control vary widely between reports.[3,148,183] Most authorities, however, recommended that maternal plasma glucose levels during normal pregnancy be the goal when treating pregnancies complicated by diabetes mellitus.[185,186] Gillmer and colleagues, and other investigators, have determined that in normal pregnancy, fasting plasma levels are generally 60 to 80 mg/dL, mean diurnal glucose is 85 mg/dL, and postprandial values rarely exceed 120 mg/dL.[185,187] These data serve as therapeutic objectives for treating diabetics in pregnancy (see Table 61-11).[188]

The feasibility of achieving normal glucose profiles in IDDM patients has been demonstrated by several investigators.[9,188,189] Furthermore, it was demonstrated that normalization of glucose levels in pregnant diabetic women also results in normalization of other metabolic fuels, such as free fatty acids, branched-chain amino acids, triglycerides, and cholesterol.[190]

Insulin Preparations

Advances in insulin delivery and monitoring of glucose have made the goal of stringent glycemic control feasible. Whenever insulin is used, dosages must be individualized and balanced with diet and exercise.[189,191] A variety of insulin preparations exists, marketed by different manufacturers.

In the past, insulin was prepared only from animal sources (pork, beef, and beef–pork combinations). In recent years, new types of insulin have been developed, called "human insulin,"[192] produced either by the conversion of pork insulin to human insulin (semisynthetic human insulin) or by recombinant DNA technology (biosynthetic human insulin).

Animal Source Insulin. Earlier insulin preparations from pork and beef pancreases have the disadvantage of containing various contaminants; therefore, it is not surprising that in some patients these preparations cause unacceptable side effects, such as systemic anaphylactic reactions, urticaria, lipoatrophy, and immunogenic insulin resistance due to antibody formation.[193] A marked reduction in the incidence of these side effects was clearly noted when highly purified insulin of animal origin was introduced.[194] These insulins, even when highly purified, are still different in their composition from human insulin. For example, the amino acid sequence of beef insulin differs in three positions from human insulin, whereas pork insulin differs in only one. This might explain why porcine insulin is less immunogenic than beef insulin.

Insulin antibodies produced by the mother are able to cross the placenta. Some investigators have shown that neonatal morbidity is higher in infants of mothers with high insulin antibody titers.[195–197] However, the effect of these antibodies on the fetal B-cell function and their contribution to the hyperinsulinism in the fetus are still controversial.[191,197,198]

Human Insulin. Human insulin preparations are identical in amino acid sequences to natural insulin in humans. There are two kinds of human insulin: semisynthetic and biosynthetic.

The semisynthetic human insulin is produced by substitution of the single nonhomologous amino acids of the porcine insulin. Biosynthetic human insulin is

TABLE 61–11. GENERAL GUIDELINES FOR INSULIN ADMINISTRATION

REGIMEN NO.	PREBREAKFAST INSULIN	PRELUNCH INSULIN	PREDINNER INSULIN	BEDTIME INSULIN	COMMENTS
I 2-injection scheme	NPH + Regular 2:1	— —	NPH + Regular 1:1	— —	Give ²/₃ of the total dose as prebreakfast dose and ¹/₃ as a predinner dose. • Disadvantage: Predinner NPH may cause nocturnal hypoglycemia (1–3 AM) and may not be effective in controlling the early morning glucose level.
II 3-injection scheme	NPH + Regular 2:1	— —	Regular	NPH (or Lente)	This regimen may be more effective than Regimen I. By changing the administration of NPH to bedtime, nocturnal hypoglycemia may be prevented and early morning glucose control may be achieved.
III 4-injection scheme	NPH + Regular	Regular	Regular	NPH (or Lente)	This is the most effective regimen. We use it as an alternative to Regimen II. Here the dose of insulin given at bedtime replaces basal daily insulin requirements. In some cases, ultralente is given at predinner times to replace the administration of NPH.

synthesized in bacteria with the use of recombinant DNA technology.

Human insulin very rarely causes allergy or lipoatrophy. However, it has been shown to stimulate the production of antibodies, because of polymerization of insulin.[199] These antibodies remain at low levels and are of no clinical significance. Since human insulin has very low immunogenicity, it is recommended for use in patients who have not received insulin previously. It should be noted that intermittent exposure to an antigen stimulates antibody formation, and this is an important consideration in the insulin treatment of gestational diabetic patients. Based on the preceding data, the American Diabetes Association recently made recommendations for the use of human insulin for the following indications:

Pregnant women with diabetes and diabetics considering pregnancy
Individuals with allergies or immune resistance to animal-derived insulins
All patients receiving insulin for the first time
Patients expected to use insulin only intermittently (ie, gestational diabetes).

It should be stressed that human insulins have a more rapid onset and shorter duration of activity than animal-source insulin, and this should be taken into consideration before transferring the patient from animal-source insulin to human insulin.[200] Insulin is available in three forms that may be injected separately or mixed in the same syringe:[200]

1. *Short-acting insulins:* regular and semi-Lente, with a peak activity of 2 to 4 hours
2. *Intermediate-acting insulins:* Lente and NPH with 5- to 12-hour span of peak activity
3. *Long-acting insulins:* protamine zinc insulin (PZI) and ultra-Lente with 12- to 24-hour-span of maximum activity.

Insulin is injected into the subcutaneous tissue. In selecting a site, the variable absorption rates should be taken into consideration. The abdomen has the fastest rate of absorption, followed by the arms, thighs, and buttocks. Rotation of the injection site is recommended to prevent lipohypertrophy or lipoatrophy.

Insulin Administration

In general, regimens that intend to achieve stringent metabolic control of diabetics must simulate the normal diurnal profile of endogenous insulin release. In nondiabetics, there is a diurnal basal insulin secretion accompanied by an abrupt insulin level rise at mealtimes. The patient's need for insulin is dramatically changed during pregnancy. In the first trimester, maternal insulin requirement is 0.7 U/kg body weight/day, and this is increased in late pregnancy to 1.0 U/kg.[201] The method of insulin administration may either be by multiple subcutaneous injections or by continuous subcutaneous insulin infusion (CSII).

Multiple Daily Subcutaneous Injections. There are several approaches to insulin administration to obtain meticulous control (see Table 61-11). In general, plasma glucose levels must be measured several times each day, and appropriate doses of insulin must be supplied. In our practice, we have found it most useful to observe a few days of a new insulin regimen before changing the insulin dose again.

Regimen I: Two-Injection Scheme. Regimen I (two-injection scheme) is in wide use for IDDM patients before pregnancy and has been demonstrated to be effective during pregnancy as well.[196] The initial distribution of insulin in the two-injection scheme is to give two thirds of the total daily dose in the morning and one third in the evening. The prebreakfast insulin is given in a 2:1 ratio of NPH and regular insulin, and the predinner insulin is given in a ratio of 1:1. We have found that this regimen may cause frequent episodes of nocturnal hypoglycemia between 1:00 and 3:00 AM. This may be avoided by the administration of predinner NPH or Lente insulin at bedtime, as illustrated in Regimen II.

Regimen II: Three-Injection Scheme. Regimen II has been demonstrated to be more effective in pregnancy. We prefer this regimen, since administration of NPH or Lente insulin just before bedtime prevents nocturnal hypoglycemia and results in better control of prebreakfast plasma glucose values.

Regimen III: Four-Injection Scheme. In Regimen III regular insulin is given before each meal, and basal insulin administration is provided by intermediate-acting insulin (NPH or Lente) at bedtime. Recently, human ultra-Lente insulin became available, and this can be used together with regular insulin at predinner times, replacing the bedtime injection. This permits the use of three injections per day. Ultra-Lente insulin given in this method may account for 50% to 60% of the total daily insulin requirement.

Continuous Subcutaneous Insulin Infusion Continuous subcutaneous insulin infusion (CSII)—open-loop subcutaneous insulin infusion (insulin pump)—has theoretical advantages compared to conventional insulin therapy (multiple subcutaneous injections), since it most closely simulates the normal physiology of insulin delivery. The pump system delivers regular insulin in continuous amounts to maintain basal blood glucose levels and a bolus at each meal. The device is usually attached to the patient's abdominal wall. Many investigators have demonstrated that the CSII can be a safe and effective means of glucose control in diabetic pregnant patients.[201–203]

Coustan and colleagues recently examined whether the method of insulin administration influences the degree of metabolic control.[204] In a randomized clinical trial, 22 IDDM pregnant patients were selected to receive conventional therapy or CSII. No significant difference between the two forms of insulin administration was observed with regard to glucose control or mean amplitude of glycemic excursions. Furthermore, the frequency of adverse effects, such as hypoglycemia, was comparable in both groups. The results of this study indicate that, in compliant and motivated pregnant patients, although CSII offers a very effective means of glycemic control, the use of intensified regimens of three or four daily insulin injections could be equally effective. CSII remains a valuable method of achieving euglycemia, especially in patients with very erratic eating schedules.

In converting to pump therapy, the same total dose of insulin that the patient had been receiving with conventional therapy is used. Fifty percent of the dose is administered at a basal rate and the remainder is given as a bolus before each meal. Breakfast requires a larger bolus than the other meals (eg, 20% at breakfast, 15% at lunch, and 15% at dinner) (Table 61-12).

Although the use of CSII is usually safe, specific complications, including severe hypoglycemia, ketoacidosis, and skin abcesses, have been reported.[205,206] Another new method of insulin delivery, the closed-loop subcutaneous insulin infusion, deserves comment. In this system, a glucose sensor measures glucose levels and their rate of change over the previous few minutes. Consequently, the amount of insulin or dextrose to be delivered is calculated and infused. However, this system is still primarily a research tool.[207]

Self-Monitoring of Blood Glucose

The introduction of portable blood glucose meters has made it possible for diabetics to evaluate blood glucose several times per day in their homes. These devices have led to a decrease in hospital admissions, improved glucose control, and enhanced motivation among patients to achieve and maintain euglycemia.

Currently, several methods are available for testing blood glucose. All these methods use glucose oxidase–impregnated reagent strips on which a drop of blood is placed to be read either by visual comparison with a color chart or by a reflectance meter. The reaction of the drop of blood on the reagent strip must be carefully timed.

Visual interpretation has an element of subjectivity, and many patients express their blood glucose readings as a range between values. Because of this limitation, glucose reflectance meters are preferred, and they are widely used during pregnancy when it is necessary to ascertain a precise glucose level. These meters determine the glucose values by transforming a signal that is dependent on the amount of light reflected from the test strip. The capillary whole-blood values obtained by this method show a close correlation with venous plasma determinations and with automated laboratory methods.[208,209]

New generations of glucose meters have a memory capacity. Recent studies suggest that the memory capacity of the meters improves accurate reporting and thus affects the overall achievement of euglycemia.[210] Blood glucose determinations should be obtained six to eight times a day every day. Patients are instructed to test their blood for glucose whenever they feel symptoms of hypoglycemia. The patient and family members should be taught how to treat hypoglycemia, including the use of glucagon.

Several authors have reported that self-monitoring of blood glucose achieves control that is equivalent to or better than monitoring in the hospital.[201,203] This technique of home blood glucose monitoring has become the mainstay of outpatient management of pregnancies complicated by diabetes mellitus.

TABLE 61–12. GUIDELINES FOR INSULIN SCHEDULE FOR PATIENTS CONVERTING TO PUMP THERAPY

1. Use the same total daily dose of insulin that the patient received with conventional therapy.
2. Fifty percent of the daily insulin dose is given as a constant basal rate.
3. The remaining 50% is divided into three doses, each administered as a bolus 15–30 minutes before each meal:
   20% before breakfast
   15% before lunch
   15% before dinner

Diet

Diet therapy is considered a standard treatment of diabetes mellitus. All patients are seen by the dietitian in the clinic, and individual meal plan adjustments are made. The American Diabetes Association (ADA) recommends 35 kcal/kg of ideal body weight, and a diet composed of 20% protein, 30% fat, and 50% carbohydrate.[211] Restricted saturated fats and cholesterol and increased dietary fiber are suggested. Most patients are instructed on how to maintain a diet that consists of three meals and one to three snacks, the last snack usually being taken at bedtime. The bedtime snack should be composed of complex carbohydrates with proteins to maintain adequate blood glucose levels during the night, thereby avoiding nocturnal hypoglycemia.

Patient weight gains are assessed at each visit to the clinic, and caloric intake is adjusted accordingly. The aim is to prevent weight reduction and its associated ketogenic risk while ensuring optimal weight gain. It is desirable to increase weight by 2 to 4 lb (0.9 to 1.7 kg) in the first trimester and 0.5 to 1.0 lb (200 to 450 g) per week thereafter until term. A total weight gain of 22 to 30 lb (10 to 13 kg) during normal and diabetic pregnancy is recommended.[212]

It is generally agreed that pregnancy is not the time for weight reduction; however, excessive weight gain must be firmly discouraged. Dietary advice to the obese pregnant diabetic patient is a matter of controversy. Several authors have indicated that caloric restriction in obese pregnant patients is contraindicated.[212] However, there are data to show that modest caloric restriction (25 to 30 kcal/day), especially for the morbidly obese patient, is not associated with ketonuria or elevated plasma ketone concentrations.[213,214]

Many recent studies in non-pregnant diabetic patients have shown an improvement in overall diabetic control with various types of fiber-enriched diets.[215,216] Investigators who studied the beneficial effect of these diets in non-pregnant diabetic patients have found decreased postprandial hyperglycemia and lower insulin requirements.[214,217] Although the role of fiber in the management of non-pregnant diabetic patients has been extensively studied in the last few years, few data are available on the use of fiber in pregnancy. Gabbe and associates have shown an improvement in oral glucose tolerance tests in four GDM patients following the administration of high-fiber diets.[218] Ney and colleagues studied the effect of high-fiber diets in 10 IDDM and 10 NIDDM pregnant patients.[219] In the latter study, mean plasma glucose levels improved in patients on both the high-fiber diet and the control diet. However, the magnitude of the decrease was not significantly different between the two groups. The most important observation noted by these investigators was the decrease in insulin requirement following the intake of high dietary fiber. Recently, a randomized clinical trial was conducted at Yale–New Haven Hospital to assess the efficiency of high-fiber diets compared with the standard American Diabetes Association (ADA) diet.[220] In this study, we were unable to show that an increase in consumption of dietary fiber by pregnant diabetic patients was associated with reduced blood glucose levels and decreased insulin requirements. However, the fiber-enriched diet appears to be associated with a lower frequency of hypoglycemic reactions as compared to the ADA diet. The reason for this may be related to the slower rate of absorption of food in the presence of high-fiber diets, resulting in a smoother glucose curve with fewer glycemic excursions. This study, however, did not find the beneficial effects of improved glycemic control, as reported previously for non-pregnant diabetic patients.

MATERNAL COMPLICATIONS

Diabetic women have a markedly higher risk of a number of pregnancy complications. Because of a paucity of data regarding maternal complications during diabetic pregnancy, the exact relative risk for each complication is not known. Complications that have been reported to be more frequent in diabetic pregnancy include spontaneous abortion, preterm labor, pyelonephritis, hydramnios, and hypertensive disorders. Also directly related to metabolic control are hypoglycemia and diabetic ketoacidosis (DKA). These complications, together with the vascular alterations and the higher cesarean section rate, contribute to the higher maternal morbidity and mortality among diabetic pregnant patients.

Maternal Mortality

The advent of insulin in 1922 brought about a dramatic fall in the maternal mortality from 45% to just over 2% shortly after the widespread introduction of insulin in 1935.[2] Together with improved medical and obstetric care, maternal mortality has decreased to as low as 0.5%.[221] More recently, a mortality rate of 0.11% was reported among 2614 pregnant diabetic patients.[222] Although improved medical and obstetric care has reduced the maternal diabetic mortality rate, it is still very high—an estimated eight to 10 times higher than that of normal nondiabetic patients.

Causes of maternal deaths have shifted from mainly diabetic ketoacidosis to cardiorenal complications. In fact, at the Joslin Clinic between 1966 and 1968, 74% of maternal deaths were related to vascular complications and only 1% were associated with maternal DKA.[223]

Causes or events related to maternal death among diabetics include acute myocardial infarction during cesarean section,[224] sepsis, hemorrhage, ketoacidosis, hypoglycemia, and anesthetic and hypertensive complications.[221] Maternal mortality seems to be highest (approaching 65%) among patients with coronary artery diseases.[225]

Diabetic Ketoacidosis

In recent years, the incidence of diabetic ketoacidosis (DKA) during pregnancy has decreased significantly. Cousins, in a review of a large number of studies, has found an incidence of 9.3% of DKA among 1508 diabetics.[222] Ketoacidosis has been reported to occur in pregnant diabetic patients more rapidly and at lower blood glucose levels than in non-pregnant patients. It may be precipitated by stress, infection (eg, urinary tract), or omission of insulin because of patient neglect. The use of B-sympathomimetic agents in pregnant diabetics may induce DKA.[226]

Omission of insulin or insulin deficiency in IDDM pregnant patients results in hyperglycemia and glucosuria. Osmotic diuresis results in urinary potassium, sodium, and water losses. Hyperglycemia is aggravated, since, as a consequence of hypovolemia, there is an increase in the secretion of glucagon and cathecolamines.[227,228] Lipolysis consequent to insulin deficiency leads to increased hepatic oxidation of fatty acids with the formation of ketone bodies (acetone, b-hydroxybutyrate, and acetoacetate), which leads, in turn, to the production of metabolic acidosis (Fig. 61-8). In addition, serum hyperosmolality may cause tissue damage because of intracellular dehydration. This situation is life-threatening to both the mother and her fetus. Common clinical presentation is abdominal pain, nausea and vomiting, polyuria, and polydypsia. The initial examination usually suggests the diagnosis: an odor of acetone, rapid and deep respiration, hypotension, and impaired mental status that varies from drowsiness to profound lethargy. Diagnosis is confirmed by the

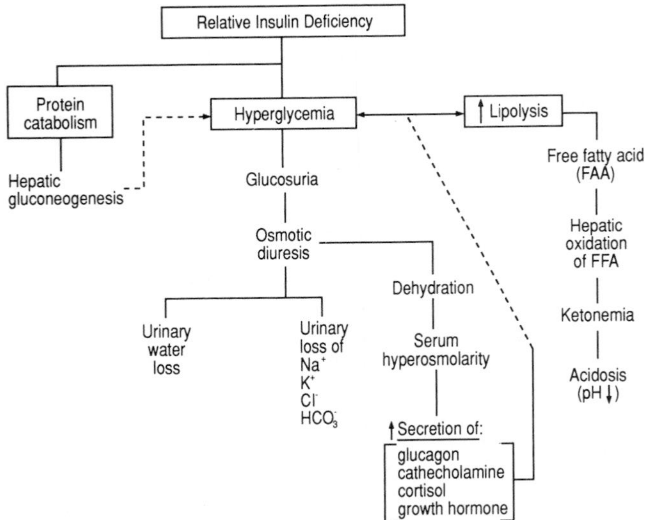

FIGURE 61–8. Metabolic alterations in diabetic ketoacidosis.

documentation of hyperglycemia, ketonemia, and ketonuria.

Ketoacidosis is defined as plasma glucose of more than 300 mg/dL, plasma bicarbonate of less than 15 mEg/L ,and arterial pH of less than 7.3.[229] However, it should be stressed that ketoacidosis in pregnancy may develop at glucose levels below 300 mg/dL.[227] On admission, serum electrolytes usually show hyperkalemia as a consequence of acidosis. Therefore, normal or low potassium levels in a patient with DKA may indicate severe potassium deficiency and mandate replacement therapy. The sodium level is usually normal or low, and the relative hyponatremia usually reflects hypertriglyceridemia and dilution of extracellular space due to hyperglycemia. Arterial blood gases on admission will indicate metabolic acidosis. Prompt and vigorous treatment in an obstetric intensive care unit is necessary in this serious situation to reduce the high maternal and fetal mortality that may accompany acidosis. Treatment of diabetic ketoacidosis in pregnancy is directed toward correcting volume deficit, electrolyte imbalance, hyperglycemia, and infection, if present.[230]

In recent years, treating DKA with a constant, low-dose insulin infusion regimen, and not with high-dose bolus therapy, has been recommended. The advantage of a low-dose regimen is its simplicity, which reduces complications, such as hypoglycemia and hypokalemia, observed with the traditional high-dose bolus therapy. The following are some general guidelines for the treatment of diabetic ketoacidosis:

1. Insert two IV lines; obtain blood to assess levels of glucose, serum electrolytes and ketones, and arterial blood gases; administer oxygen by face mask. Frequently assess the clinical status and follow urinary output. Repeat blood and urinary test often.
2. Patients with DKA require simultaneous correction of fluid and electrolyte imbalance and treatment of hyperglycemia and acidosis.
   - a. *Replacement of fluid.* The average fluid deficit is 3 to 5 L. It is therefore necessary to administer 1000 to 2000 mL of isotonic saline rapidly during the first hour. If hypernatremia is present, 0.45% sodium chloride is preferred. After the first hour, 300 to 500 mL/h is given, depending on hemodynamic status. Normal saline is given to hypotensive patients in larger amounts. In these cases, a central line may be necessary.
   - b. *Insulin therapy.* Administer an initial bolus of 10 to 20 U of regular insulin intravenously. Follow this with a constant infusion of about 10 U/h. (Add 50 U of regular insulin per 500 mL of normal saline.) Larger doses of constant regular insulin infusion of 12 to 20 U/h may be required if acidosis does not begin to respond within 3 hours or if plasma glucose level does not fall by 30%.
   - c. *Glucose administration.* To reduce the risk of hypoglycemia and cerebral edema, change the intravenous solution to 5% dextrose when the plasma glucose level reaches 200 to 250 mg/dL and simultaneously decrease the rate of the insulin infusion.
   - d. *Potassium administration.* On admission, hyperkalemia is usually present. At this point, potassium administration is not required, and, in fact, may be dangerous or even lethal, since hyperkalemia may rapidly reach cardiotoxic levels. Potassium administration is usually started after 3 to 4 hours of insulin therapy, when potassium begins to fall to normal or low levels. It is given by adding 40 mEq of potassium chloride per 1000 mL normal saline at a rate of 10 to 20 mEq/h, as needed. It should be stressed that when potassium is administered, it is given with extreme caution, and that potassium and urinary output are monitored carefully.
   - e. *Bicarbonate administration.* Add 44 mEq sodium bicarbonate to 1 L 0.45% saline and administer intravenously only if arterial pH is less than 7.1 or serum bicarbonate is less than 5 mEq. If the pH is less than 7, the sodium bicarbonate dose should be doubled (88 mEq). Bicarbonate administration should be terminated if arterial pH has been corrected to 7.2. Alkali administration in DKA is still controversial, because this therapy might aggravate tissue hypoxia.

Today maternal death is rare in properly treated patients with DKA. Fetal mortality is still high and ranges from 50% to 90% after one episode of ketoacidosis.[227] The mechanism by which maternal ketoacidosis affects the fetus is not completely clear, but several explanations have been offered. In animal models, it has been shown that ketoacidosis may lead to a decrease in uterine blood flow and thus to fetal hypoxemia.[231,232] In addition, maternal phosphate deficits that accompany DKA seem to contribute further to fetal hypoxia. Phosphate deficiency causes depletion of the red blood cells' 2,3-diphosphoglycerate (2,3-DPG), resulting in impaired red cell oxygen delivery to the fetus.[233] Another explanation of the danger to the fetus observed during maternal DKA is that the same maternal metabolic disturbances, such as acidosis and potassium depletion, are induced in the fetus.

Fetal potassium deficit may lead to fetal cardiac arrest.[227] During the maternal treatment of DKA, it is important to monitor the fetal heart rate continuously, particularly in late gestation. Pathologic fetal heart rate patterns may improve following maternal intensive care treatment.[234] Because of the serious effect of DKA on both the mother and the fetus, prevention of DKA in pregnancy is an important goal for the physician caring for diabetic pregnant patients. Efforts should be directed toward patient education, instructing patients to report any episodes of ketonuria or suspected infection so that treatment can be started promptly.

Hypoglycemia

The goal of very stringent glycemic control during diabetic pregnancy places the patient at increased risk for hypoglycemic episodes. Coustan and associates observed a high frequency of both symptomatic and biochemical hypoglycemia.[204] Forty-five percent of IDDM patients treated with multiple daily insulin injection had severe hypoglycemia requiring hospitalization or emergency room care. The main symptoms of hypoglycemic reactions in patients with IDDM include sweating, tremors, blurred or double vision, weakness, hunger, confusion, paresthesia of lips and tongue, anxiety, palpitation, nausea, headache, and stupor.[235] The increased risk of hypoglycemia in pregnant IDDM patients may be related to defective glucose counterregulatory hormone mechanisms.

In non-pregnant IDDM patients, the glucagon response to hypoglycemia is lost early in the disease and patients are dependent on epinephrine to promote recovery from hypoglycemia.[236] Some non-pregnant IDDM patients with long-standing disease may develop deficient epinephrine secretory responses to hypoglycemia and may experience severe hypoglycemic episodes without the warning symptoms that allow the patient time to eat before hypoglycemia becomes severe.

Recently, we studied glucose counterregulatory systems in pregnant IDDM patients.[237] In this study, maternal and fetal responses to induced maternal hypoglycemia were evaluated. Using the insulin clamp technique, glucose was lowered from fasting levels to 90, 80, 70, 60, 50, and 40 mg/dL at intervals of 40 minutes. At each step, anti-insulin hormones were determined and fetal well-being was assessed. We studied nine IDDM women at 26 to 34 weeks gestation, and seven non-pregnant healthy women as controls. Reductions in glucose from 107 ± 6 to 44 ± 2 mg/dL in pregnant diabetic women failed to produce an increase in glucagon levels. Epinephrine, a key anti-insulin hormone, was also markedly suppressed in the pregnant diabetic patients during hypoglycemia (96 ± 29 pg/mL in diabetics versus 265 ± 27 pg/mL in controls; $p < 0.01$). During hypoglycemia, there was no significant alteration in fetal heart rate (FHR) reactivity or in fetal movements. Fetal breathing temporarily increased, then significantly decreased, especially at glucose levels below 70 mg/dL. It would therefore appear that hypoglycemic episodes of short duration are well tolerated by the developing fetus. Hypoglycemia in animal studies and during organogenesis may be a teratogen in early pregnancy. The spectrum of potential adverse effects of maternal hypoglycemia on the human fetus has not been clearly established and awaits further investigation.

Pyelonephritis

Pederson reported a 6% incidence of pyelonephritis in diabetic pregnant patients, which he includes as one of the "prognostic bad sign[s] of pregnancy" because it is associated with higher perinatal mortality and morbidity.[238] Cousins reported an incidence of pyelonephritis of 2.2% among 356 class B and C diabetics, and 4.9% of 264 class D, F, and R diabetics in an extensive literature review.[222] However, in no study was a nondiabetic control group used for comparison. It appears that in recent years there has been a reduction in the frequency of pyelonephritis in diabetic pregnancy.[239] This reduction, however, has not been confirmed statistically.[222] Nevertheless, it is our practice to perform serial urine cultures at least once in each trimester of pregnancy and to treat asymptomatic bacteriuria vigorously in diabetic pregnant patients, since if left untreated it may result in frank pyelonephritis.

Polyhydramnios

Polyhydramnios occurs commonly in diabetics, with a reported incidence that varies from 3% to 32%.[222] Differences between reports are attributed to different criteria used by authors to define polyhydramnios. Lufkin and associates found that polyhydramnios is 30 times more frequent in pregnant diabetics than in nondiabetic controls (29% versus 0.9%, respectively).[240] Although this condition can be associated with central nervous system and gastrointestinal abnormalities, in almost 90% of diabetics with polyhydramnios, no etiology can be found.[240]

The etiology of polyhydramnios in diabetics is not clear. Suggested mechanisms include increases in amniotic fluid osmolality caused by increases in glucose load, decreased fetal swallowing, high gastrointestinal tract obstruction, and fetal polyuria secondary to fetal hyperglycemia. Experimental work, however, has not provided strong evidence for any of these explanations.[152] Although the most likely reason for the higher fluid volume is increased fetal urine production in diabetics, this was not demonstrated by sequential estimation of bladder volume over time.[241]

Polyhydramnios complicating diabetes in pregnancy is associated with a higher perinatal mortality and morbidity rates than can be attributed to the higher rates of preterm delivery and congenital anomalies caused by this condition.[240] In one report, the preterm delivery rate among diabetics with hydramnios was twice as high as that in diabetics without polyhydramnios (13% versus 6.1%, respectively).

Preterm Labor

Earlier studies have found that the incidence of prematurity in diabetic pregnancies is three times higher than that in nondiabetics.[242] This high rate was attributed in part to the higher rate of iatrogenic preterm delivery. In a recent study by Miodovnik and colleagues, it was reported that the rate of spontaneous preterm labor was 31.1% in IDDM patients, a rate that is three to four times more than that reported in the general obstetric population.[243] The authors found these factors to be significantly associated with premature labor: premature rupture of membrane and previous history of preterm labor and delivery. Furthermore, patients with poor glycemic control during the second trimester of pregnancy had increased rates of preterm delivery. Interestingly, polyhydramnios was not significantly associated with preterm labor in this study.

Magnesium sulfate therapy is considered the drug of choice in diabetic patients with premature labor, since this drug has no effect on diabetic control. In contrast, B-sympathomimetic tocolytic agents or glucocorticosteroids have been reported to induce hyperglycemia and ketoacidosis.[239] Therefore, treatment with both medications in diabetics requires great caution, intensive monitoring of glucose levels, and treatment with intravenous insulin infusion as needed.

Spontaneous Abortions

The rate of spontaneous abortion in pregestational pregnant diabetic patients varies considerably between reports, ranging from 6% to 29%.[244] Most studies are retrospective and do not have nondiabetic control groups for comparison. Kalter, in an extensive literature review of the years 1950 to 1986, concluded that the incidence of spontaneous abortion in diabetic women is similar to that of nondiabetic women, approaching 10%.[245] However, the single prospective study reported so far, from Cincinnati, Ohio, showed a significantly higher rate of spontaneous abortions among pregnant IDDM patients than among pregnant nondiabetic women (30% versus 15%, respectively).[246] Furthermore, the same group in another study demonstrated that the higher rate of spontaneous abortions in IDDM women was associated with poor glycemic control in the early postconceptional period, as reflected by high levels of glycohemoglobin A1 early in pregnancy.[247] The latter findings were confirmed by the results of the most recent Diabetes in Early Pregnancy study.[247a]

Diabetic Retinopathy

Diabetic retinopathy is considered the most common form of vascular disease in diabetics and is one of the leading causes of adult blindness in the United States.[248] There is a large body of evidence to show that diabetic retinopathy is a direct consequence of hyperglycemia. This observation is based on clinical and experimental studies that have demonstrated that with increased duration of diabetes there is an increase in the prevalence and severity of retinopathy.[249–251] Furthermore, retinopathy has been reported to develop in patients with secondary diabetes and has been induced in diabetic animal models.[249]

The mechanisms by which high glucose levels cause microvascular lesions are unknown, but there are several possible explanations. High glucose levels are believed to decrease retinal blood flow and to induce ischemia and hypoxia through the following mechanisms[252]:

1. Hyperglycemia increases platelet and red blood cell aggregation, decreases oxygen release from red blood cells, and may cause thickening of retinal capillary walls.
2. Hyperglycemia leads to the accumulation of significant levels of sorbitol and fructose in tissues such as nerves and lenses in which intracellular glucose levels are not regulated by insulin. Increase in this metabolic pathway (polyol pathway) is believed to lead to alteration in tissue function by impairment in myoinositol metabolism and to lead to narrowing of capillaries due to basement membrane thickening.[253]
3. Hyperglycemia is also believed to induce the production of high levels of plasma proteins, fibrinogen, and α-globulin. This plasma protein in high concentrations may lead to higher plasma viscosity and, thus, to a decrease in retinal blood flow.

Diabetic retinopathy is usually classified as background simple diabetic retinopathy and proliferative diabetic retinopathy. The characteristic lesions of diabetic retinopathy are presented in Table 61-13.

Microaneurysms alone are not usually associated with severe loss of vision, but when maculopathy is present with either macular edema or macular ischemia, serious loss of vision can occur. The most serious condition, however, is proliferative retinopathy, which carries a high risk of blindness. It is believed that background retinopathy represents an early stage of the disease: as it worsens, it leads to proliferative retinopathy that, when developed, is usually associated with the characteristic lesions of background retinopathy.[254]

In the Wisconsin Epidemiologic Study of Diabetic Retinopathy, the prevalence of any retinopathy was found to be 2% within 2 years of the onset of IDDM and 98%

TABLE 61–13. CHARACTERISTIC LESIONS OF DIABETIC RETINOPATHY

Background Diabetic Retinopathy
Microaneurysms
Small vessel obstruction, soft exudate, intraretinal microvascular abnormalities
Venous abnormalities
Retinal hemorrhages
Hard exudate
Disk edema
Maculopathy
Proliferative Diabetic Retinopathy
Neovascularization
Fibrous deposition
Vitreous hemorrhage
Retinal detachment

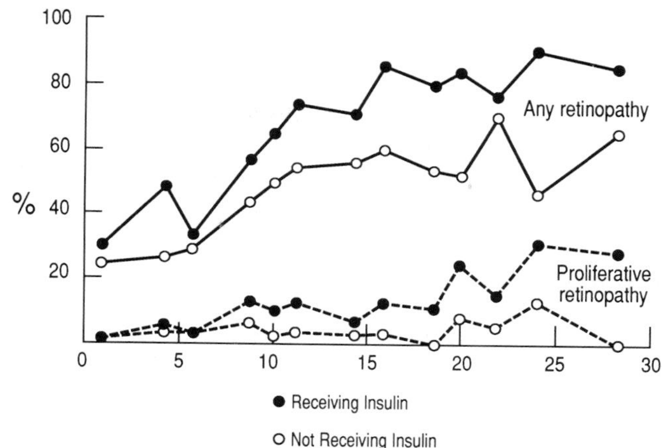

FIGURE 61–9. Frequency of retinopathy or proliferative retinopathy by duration of diabetes (in years) in persons taking insulin who were diagnosed to have diabetes prior to 30 years of age and who participated in the Wisconsin Epidemiologic Study of Diabetic Retinopathy, 1980–1982. (From: Klein R, Klein BEK, Moss SE, et al. The Wisconsin Epidemiologic Study of Diabetic Retinopathy: III. Prevalence and risk of diabetic retinopathy when age at diagnosis is less than 30 years. Arch Ophthalmol 1984;102:527.)

in individuals with 15 or more years of disease.[255] Proliferative retinopathy was observed in 20% to 25% of patients with IDDM of 15 years' duration. Hence, the severity of diabetic retinopathy is clearly related to the duration of diabetes. This is supported by the fact that proliferative retinopathy is very rare (indeed, is almost nonexistent) in IDDM patients of 5 years' duration or less, whereas the rate for diabetics of 20 years' duration or more is higher than 50% (Fig. 61-9).

In contrast to IDDM patients, those with NIDDM may have retinopathy during the first few years of known diabetes or even at the time of their diagnosis.[256]

The effect of pregnancy on diabetic retinopathy is still controversial. Perhaps the most important question concerns whether pregnancy in diabetic patients influences either the development or the progression of established retinopathy. Another important question, raised in the last few years, is what effect the current obstetric practice of rapid and stringent glycemic control during pregnancy may have on the progression of retinopathy in pregnancy.

Pregnancy and Progression of Diabetic Retinopathy. Investigators have reported controversial findings regarding the role of pregnancy in the development and progression of diabetic retinopathy. Most recent reports have shown that in some diabetic patients pregnancy is associated with progression of diabetic retinopathy, from minimal to marked deterioration of the retina.[257–260] However, many changes during pregnancy have proved to be reversible, and many patients have experienced regression of their lesion after delivery.

Moloney and Drury showed that in a group of pregnant IDDM patients in a case-control study, 15% developed background retinopathy during pregnancy—a much higher rate than that observed in non-pregnant controls.[261] However, in patients with background retinopathy present before conception, progression occurred during pregnancy in 29% of the patients. Background retinopathy progressed to proliferative disease in only one pregnant woman.

In another large study, similar observations were made.[260] In a third of White's class C patients in whom there was no evidence of retinopathy before pregnancy, background retinopathy developed during the second and third trimesters. Half of the patients who had background retinopathy before pregnancy experienced retinal deterioration during pregnancy, and 10% developed proliferative retinopathy.

Both of these last two studies found that in most patients retinal deterioration had regressed postpartum. In one of the studies, even patients who experienced progression to proliferative retinopathy showed regression to background retinopathy a few months after delivery.[260] Carefully controlled prospective clinical trials are needed to determine the influence of pregnancy on diabetic retinopathy.

Tight Metabolic Control in Pregnancy and Diabetic Retinopathy. Studies in non-pregnant IDDM patients investigated the effect of glycemic control on progression of diabetic retinopathy.[262,263] These studies have shown that progression of diabetic retinopathy was significantly higher over an 8-month period when compared to a control group with proper metabolic control.[262,263] After 2 years of follow-up, no statistical significance was found between the rates of progression of retinopathy in the two groups. The authors suggest that caution should be used and that one should avoid achieving good glycemic control too rapidly in IDDM patients with retinopathy and poor glycemic control.

Phelps and colleagues have reported similar findings recently in pregnant IDDM patients.[264] These authors emphasized that retinal changes were relatively minor and that the benefits of careful diabetic control during gestation outweighed the retinal changes noted. The conclusion must be that the increased risk for progression of diabetic retinopathy by rapid glycemic control should not suggest that less rigid control is appropriate.

Principal Management of Diabetic Retinopathy in Pregnant Diabetics. Diabetic retinopathy occurring during pregnancy should be treated in essentially the same manner as in the non-pregnant state.[254] Laser treatment can be used safely during pregnancy when indicated. It is recommended that diabetic patients undergo careful retinal examination before conception and be treated with laser photocoagulation before pregnancy if necessary. It is our practice to perform ophthalmoscopy every trimester in pregnant IDDM patients and even more frequently in patients with documented retinopathy prior to pregnancy.

The preferred mode of delivery in patients with active proliferative retinopathy remains controversial. In the past, the performance of cesarean sections was suggested to avoid the Valsalva maneuver and the risk of vitreous hemorrhage.[252,265–267] Today, however, most investigators do not recommend cesarean delivery in patients with active neovascularization because it has been found that vitreous hemorrhages during childbirth are extremely rare.[267] Furthermore, there are no data to show any advantage of cesarean section over vaginal delivery in patients with proliferative retinopathy.

Diabetic Nephropathy

Diabetic nephropathy is a disease that develops slowly and appears on an average of 17 years after the onset of IDDM. Background retinopathy complicates almost all these pregnancies, and proliferative retinopathy affects about 35% to 65% of patients.[268,269]

The prevalence of diabetic nephropathy in IDDM pregnant patients is estimated at 6%.[238] Five evolutionary stages of nephropathy in diabetics have been described for type I:[270]

1. Early hypertrophy–hyperfunction
2. Glomerular lesions without clinical disease
3. Incipient nephropathy characterized by microproteinuria
4. Overt nephropathy characterized by macroproteinuria
5. End-stage diabetic renal disease.

In type I diabetes, renal insufficiency eventually occurs in all patients who exhibit macroproteinuria, whereas in type II diabetes, deterioration occurs in only 10% of the cases.[271] A diagnosis of diabetic nephropathy in pregnancy is made if there is persistent proteinuria of greater than 300 mg/day in the first half of pregnancy in the absence of urinary tract infection.[269]

Several studies examining fetal outcome and maternal risks in women with diabetic nephropathy suggest that during the course of pregnancy most patients will have an increase in proteinuria.[268,272] Reece and colleagues reported an increase in the third-trimester proteinuria that exceeded 3.0 g/day in 70% of the pregnancies studied.[269] Kitzmiller and colleagues, in a similar group of patients to that reported by Reece and colleagues, also found increasing proteinuria in the third trimester, with almost 60% exceeding 6.0 g/day in the third trimester.[268]

Acute worsening of hypertension is very common in patients with diabetic nephropathy and occurs in almost 60% of cases. In the report by Reece and colleagues, hypertension during pregnancy developed in 32% of women who began pregnancy with normal blood pressure levels.[269] However, following delivery, changes in renal function, proteinuria, and/or hypertension returned to values observed in the first trimester. Based on a 9-year follow-up study, the long-term maternal course was judged consistent with the expected course of diabetic nephropathy in non-pregnant women.

Many investigators have shown that the likelihood of a successful fetal and neonatal outcome in patients with diabetic nephropathy is comparable to that of IDDM patients without overt renal disease.[268,272] Fetal survival has been reported to exceed 90% when contemporary methods of fetal and maternal care are applied.[268,269,272] Perinatal mortality and morbidity in patients with diabetic nephropathy may be attributed to the higher incidence of early delivery (31%), a higher incidence of low–birth-weight infants (21%),[268] an increased incidence of fetal distress, and preeclampsia. Therefore, pregnant patients with diabetic nephropathy require an intensive program of maternal and fetal evaluation; adequate bedrest during pregnancy; assessment of renal function and retinal status at regular intervals; blood pressure monitoring; and treatment of hypertension when required using methyldopa, arteriolar vasodilator, or beta blockers. In patients on antihypertensive medications prior to pregnancy, the same regimen is continued during pregnancy (with the exception of diuretics, which should be discontinued). A modest sodium restriction (1500 mg Na) in all patients with significant proteinuria (>500 mg/dL) is suggested to reduce the rate of edema formation.

Although we assume that all patients will go to term, early delivery would obviously be indicated for maternal complications or fetal compromise.

ANTEPARTUM ASSESSMENT

Maternal Assessment

As indicated in an earlier section, intensive insulin therapy should begin before conception or as soon as possible thereafter. In the past, liberal hospitalization of diabetic patients was employed in early pregnancy, with routine readmission in the third trimester. In recent years, however, it has been demonstrated that there is no significant difference in maternal blood glucose control, fetal hyperinsulinemia, and perinatal mortality and morbidity between an outpatient approach and long-term hospitalization.[273] In fact, hospitalization of diabetic patients is currently the exception, rather than the rule, and most of our patients are seen as outpatients, generally at 1- to 2-week intervals. In most cases, telephone contacts are made between visits to review blood glucose levels and suggest adjustment in insulin dosage. Hospitalization is currently reserved for those who are poorly controlled, often noncompliant and in the third trimester, or with evidence of infection-induced hyperglycemia, worsening diabetic nephropathy, or frank preeclampsia.

Ophthalmologic and renal function tests, including creatinine clearance and total urinary protein excretion, are performed in each trimester, or more often if indicated. In patients with vasculopathy, an electrocardiogram is performed at the initial visit and repeated if clinically indicated. In patients in White's class H, the electrocardiogram is performed routinely in each trimester. The echocardiogram is performed at enrollment and repeated in the pregnancy, depending on the initial findings. It is extremely important to detect early signs of pregnancy-induced hypertension; therefore, assessment of blood pressure, signs of proteinuria, and edema formation is essential. It is estimated that approximately 25% of all diabetics will develop preeclampsia during pregnancy. The highest incidence is seen among patients with vasculopathy.[274] In many cases differentiation between pregnancy-induced hypertension and chronic hypertension is very difficult. In addition, in patients with diabetic nephropathy, the diagnosis of preeclampsia may be challenging. We have used a number of factors as adjunctive clues—namely, acute increase in blood pressure, the elevation of fibrin split products, liver function test abnormality, or thrombocytopenia. Most helpful is the increase in fibrin split product as a reasonably sensitive marker of underlying consumptive coagulopathy. We recognize this is less than ideal, but at the present time it is the best that is available.

Fetal Surveillance

All pregnancies complicated by diabetes require extra assessment. The use of ultrasonography provides essential information about the fetus. A first-trimester scan is used to date the pregnancy, and to establish viability and fluid volume status. A second-trimester scan is repeated at 18 to 20 weeks of gestation to rule out fetal anomalies. Subsequent ultrasound evaluations are then performed at 4- to 6-week intervals to assess fluid volume and fetal growth. Since diabetic patients are at risk for growth aberrations (IUGR and macrosomia), this frequency is recommended to identify states of altered growth.

Fetal Macrosomia. Macrosomia, arbitrarily defined as fetal weight in excess of 4000 g, or as a birth weight above the 90th percentile for gestational age, occurs in about 10% of all pregnancies. Almost 30% of all diabetics will deliver infants weighing over 4000 g.[275] Gabbe and colleagues reported an incidence of macrosomia of 20% and 25% in gestational diabetes and IDDM patients, respectively.[276]

Fetal macrosomia is thought to be related to maternal hyperglycemia that induces fetal hyperglycemia and hyperinsulinemia. Fetal hyperinsulinemia results in enhanced glycogen synthesis, lipogenesis, increased protein synthesis, and, thus, fetal organomegaly and fat deposition. Experimental studies in rhesus monkeys have demonstrated that insulin administration induces macrosomia, supporting the belief that insulin is the primary growth promoter.[277] Macrosomia is much more frequent in IDDM patients without vasculopathy than in those with vasculopathy. Furthermore, infants delivered of patients with diabetic nephropathy are of significantly lower birth weight than those of controls.[238]

Macrosomic fetuses have higher perinatal morbidity and mortality—a result caused mainly by the traumatic delivery. These fetuses are at increased risk of severe fetal asphyxia due to head and neck birth trauma. Shoulder dystocia is more common in macrosomic fetuses; therefore, infants of diabetics experience more shoulder dystocia than those of nondiabetics. Disproportional growth of the body compared with the head is believed to be the cause of shoulder dystocia. Acker and associates reported the incidence of shoulder dystocia in nondiabetic offspring weighing 4000 g to 4499 g and that in those weighing 4500 g or more to be 10% and 22%, respectively.[278] Among the offspring of diabetics, the incidence is much higher, and in infants with birth weights of 4000 g to 4499 g and of 4500 g or more, the incidence is doubled, reaching 23.1% and 50%, respectively.

Several labor abnormalities have been suggested as possible markers for shoulder dystocia. These include prolonged second stage, protracted descent, arrest of descent, failure of descent, abnormal first stage, molding, and the need for midpelvic delivery.[279] Unfortunately, Aker and colleagues found that in offspring of diabetic patients only 27% of shoulder dystocia could be predicted on the basis of an abnormal labor.[278] In more recent studies, similar results were obtained, confirming that shoulder dystocia cannot be predicted from clinical characteristics or labor abnormalities in most cases.[279]

Ultrasound examination for fetal weight estimation before planned delivery is highly recommended for diabetics to detect macrosomic fetuses. Even though the accuracy of ultrasound measurement to predict macrosomia is less than satisfactory with fetuses weighing over 4000 g, this method is the most accurate available and therefore should be used for clinical decision making.

It has been suggested that cesarean section should be employed to deliver diabetic mothers of babies of 4000 g or more.[278] In our institutions, primary cesarean section is performed if the estimated fetal weight is 4500 g or more. In cases of estimated fetal weight of 4000 to 4500 g, the mode of delivery is determined individually for each patient and is based on the clinical assessment of the pelvis and the past history (eg, birth weight of previous babies). In such cases, midpelvic instrumental delivery should be avoided as much as possible.

Finally, the question of whether macrosomia is preventable by using metabolic control of diabetic patients is still controversial.[9,280] Coustan and colleagues reported no correlation among well-controlled IDDM patients between mean maternal glucose values and the incidence of macrosomia.[9] It is therefore believed that the increased adiposity of infants of diabetic mothers in well-controlled patients is related to the increased transfer of placental free fatty acids and amino acids to the fetus of the diabetic mother.[281]

Antepartum Fetal Testing. In pregnant diabetic patients, stillbirth occurs with increased frequency, particularly in the third trimester.[282] Therefore, a program of fetal monitoring should be initiated, usually at 32 to 33 weeks. Currently, in most medical centers, outpatient protocols for antepartum fetal surveillance are used that include either once- or twice-weekly nonstress tests (NSTs) or a once-weekly oxytocin challenge test (OCT), or biophysical profiles.[283] What is the best test to be used remains controversial, since controlled, prospective randomized studies comparing the various methods of antepartum fetal assessment are lacking. Many investigators have concluded that the NST is simple, inexpensive, and reasonably reliable. Therefore, the NST is most widely used for pregnancies complicated by diabetes mellitus.[283,284]

In a series of 107 diabetic patients assessed by NST twice weekly, no perinatal loss was observed.[275] Freeman, however, has indicated that OCT is a better test for fetal reserve than the NST.[285]

Gabbe and colleagues observed no intrauterine fetal death within 1 week of a negative contraction stress test (CST) in 211 metabolically well-controlled IDDM patients.[37,134] This observation suggests that negative CST in metabolically controlled patients predicts fetal survival for 1 week. The high incidence of false-positive CST (50%) and the potential unnecessary intervention as a result of these false-positive findings are major disadvantages.

Recently, the biophysical profile has been shown to have a lower false-abnormal test rate than either CST or NST.[286] Golde and Platt have demonstrated that a biophysical score of 8 is reliable in predicting good fetal outcome in diabetics, which is comparable to the reliability of reactive NST.[283]

Sadovsky has shown that maternal evaluation of fetal movements has a very low false-negative rate and that patients with decreased fetal movements of less than 10 in 12 hours may show severe fetal compromise.[287] Therefore, further testing is necessary in cases of decreased fetal movements. Maternal assessment of fetal activity not only seems to be a practical approach toward evaluation of fetal condition but a simple, inexpensive, and valuable screening technique. Patients with diabetes are instructed to count fetal movements, beginning as early as 28 to 29 weeks of gestation, and to report any decrease in fetal movements so that further testing can be initiated if necessary.

There is a large body of evidence to show that maternal glucose control is the most important factor in improved perinatal mortality and morbidity rates. Therefore, any method of fetal surveillance will be ineffective unless strict control of maternal diabetes is performed.[283] In fact, the need for elective intervention resulting from abnormal antepartum fetal testing in diabetics in good metabolic control is very low as compared to patients in poor metabolic control.[288] Several investigators reported an intervention rate of 1% to 5%, based on abnormal fetal testing in pregnant IDDM patients.[273,288,289] In one report, no intervention for abnormal fetal testing was required in 82 IDDM patients.[290] Drury and colleagues have shown that when strict maternal metabolic control is achieved, antepartum fetal testing can be used less frequently and that despite limited use of antepartum testing, the perinatal mortality was low and approached 3%.[289]

In summary, in recent years, management protocols using strict metabolic control consistent with various techniques of antepartum surveillance have allowed more diabetic patients to deliver at term and to achieve good fetal outcome similar to that of the general obstetric population.

Doppler Ultrasound. Many investigators studied the utility of Doppler ultrasonography as a means of assessing potential alteration of vascular resistance prior to fetal compromise. At present, however, the clinical utility of Doppler ultrasound has not been proved conclusively.[291] Most recently, antenatal assessment of uteroplacental and fetoplacental blood flow using Doppler ultrasonography has been applied in diabetic pregnancies.[292,293] Reece and colleagues studied umbilical artery waveform velocity in 56 insulin-requiring diabetic patients beginning at 17 to 20 weeks gestation and every 4 weeks thereafter.[292] The investigators who performed these Doppler examinations were not involved in the clinical management of the patients, and results were not available to the clinician caring for the patients. An increase was seen in the systolic–diastolic ratio (S/D), the Pourcelot index, and the resistance index of the fetal umbilical artery, as compared to nondiabetic controls. These data indicate an increased resistance circuit among diabetics, which may reflect a relative reduction in uteroplacental blood flow. Additionally, a tendency toward adverse outcome was observed in patients with S/D ratios exceeding 3.5.

TIMING AND MODE OF DELIVERY

In recent years there has been a significant change in the attitude of obstetricians and perinatologists toward the mode of timing of delivery of IDDM and NIDDM pregnant patients. In the past, a policy of early delivery in pregnancies complicated by diabetes was almost the rule in most medical centers.[294] At that time, because of the observation of an increased rate of intrauterine fetal death after 36 weeks of gestation, many authorities recommended delivery of diabetic patients at 36 to 37 weeks.[295] This practice resulted in a very high elective cesarean section rate and a higher rate of infants suffering from RDS.

It is now recognized worldwide that if the pregnant diabetic patient and her fetus are under stringent metabolic control and antepartum surveillance, delivery may be safely delayed in most cases until term or the onset of spontaneous labor.[186,296]

Drury and colleagues found excellent pregnancy outcomes in a group of 129 IDDM patients in Dublin who were allowed to go to term with no significant maternal or fetal problems.[289] In this group 84% were delivered after 38 weeks gestation. Jonanovic and colleagues have also reported a mean gestational age at delivery of 39 weeks with excellent results in a group of uncomplicated IDDM patients.[297] This new approach—to allow diabetic women to go to term—has increased the incidence of spontaneous labor among diabetics, resulting in a significant decrease in delivery by cesarean section. Despite these efforts, the cesarean section rate remains high in diabetics. Kitzmiller and colleagues reported a high cesarean section rate in 1978 of 72%, and Roversi and colleagues reported a low rate of 25% in a very large series of 479 diabetics.[298,299] The lowest cesarean section rate (19%) was reported from the Dublin group.[300]

Selecting the time of delivery is individualized in patients with diabetes and should take into account the following three factors:

1. Degree of glycemic control
2. Maternal complications
3. Fetal well-being.

In pregnancy complicated by diabetes mellitus, delivery is delayed until term if good glycemic control has been maintained, with no signs of fetal compromise or other maternal pregnancy complications. If patients at term have a favorable cervix for induction of labor, it is reasonable to induce labor. However, induction is usually not attempted if estimated fetal weight is 4500 g or more. In these cases, elective cesarean section is preferred to prevent traumatic vaginal delivery. If the cervix is unfavorable at term, it is ripened before induction of labor with prostaglandin gel, laminaria, or an intracervical balloon. In certain cases, when cervical ripening has not been achieved, it is preferable to wait for either spontaneous cervical change or spontaneous labor when antepartum surveillance is normal. Patients without vasculopathy and who are in good glycemic control may be allowed to go beyond the due date, but never beyond 42 weeks.

Some diabetics are electively delivered at 38 weeks after fetal lung maturity has been confirmed by amniotic fluid studies. The following might be included in this group:

1. Patients in poor metabolic control
2. Patients with worsening hypertensive disorders of pregnancy
3. Patients with suspected fetal macrosomia, growth retardation, or polyhydramnios.

In certain rare cases, preterm delivery may be necessary in spite of immaturity of the fetal lungs. These cases include situations such as severe preeclampsia that does not respond to conventional therapy or signs of severe fetal compromise.

Other relative indications will depend on severity and gestational age. These include worsening diabetic nephropathy leading to renal failure and worsening retinopathy not responding to laser therapy.

Management During Labor and Delivery. During labor and delivery, it is necessary to maintain maternal euglycemia to avoid neonatal hypoglycemia. Induced maternal hyperglycemia during labor in diabetics is associated with neonatal hypoglycemia.[301,302] Soler and associates have demonstrated that mean glucose levels above 90 mg/dL during labor are associated with higher rates of neonatal episodes of hypoglycemia.[301] Therefore, the goal should be to maintain glucose levels of 70 to 90 mg/dL during labor.

Caloric and insulin requirements in diabetic patients during labor have been studied extensively.[303] Investigators have documented a decrease in insulin requirements, particularly in the first stage of labor, with constant glucose requirement during this time. Jovanovic and Peterson, using an artificial pancreas (Biostator) for 12 IDDM patients during labor, have demonstrated the lack of insulin requirement during the first stage of labor, despite a constant and continuous glucose infusion rate of 2.5 mg/kg/min.[303] In another study by Golde and colleagues, 48% of IDDM patients undergoing induction of labor required no insulin therapy.[304]

Therefore, in patients undergoing induction of labor, the morning insulin doses should be withheld and glucose levels determined once every hour with a home glucometer. In well-controlled patients, 1 unit of insulin per hour and 3 to 6 g of glucose per hour are usually required to maintain a glucose level of 70 to 90 mg/dL. If the initial glucose level is between 80 and 120 mg/dL, 10 units of regular insulin can be added to 1000 mL of 5% dextrose in 0.5 normal saline or D5RL and administered at an infusion rate of 125 mL/h. However, if initial glucose levels are below 70 mg/dL, it is recommended that initially 5% dextrose in water without insulin at a rate of 100 to 120 mL/h be administered throughout labor.

If the patient presents in spontaneous labor and has already taken her morning intermediate-acting insulin, additional insulin may not be required throughout labor and delivery, but a continuous glucose infusion will be necessary (125 mL/h of 5% dextrose in water).

When an elective cesarean section is planned for a

diabetic patient, the procedure should be scheduled early in the morning, when glucose levels are usually in the normal range because of the action of the intermediate-acting insulin dose given the night before. Infusion without glucose is preferred (ie, normal saline), and glucose levels are monitored frequently. If the patient is under regional anesthesia, it is easier to detect signs of hypoglycemia.

After delivery, a dramatic decrease in the insulin requirement is almost the rule because of a significant decrease in the level of placental hormones that have anti-insulin action. At this time there is no need for stringent glucose control, and glucose levels below 200 mg/dL are satisfactory. In the first few days after delivery, it is preferable to give regular insulin subcutaneously before each meal on the basis of plasma glucose levels. After the patient is able to eat regular meals, she may receive one half of the prepregnancy dosage of insulin, usually divided into two daily injections.

Breast feeding should not be discouraged, but the mother should be instructed to increase her caloric intake just before nursing (eg, drink a glass of milk), since insulin requirements are lower after breast feeding and may result in hypoglycemia.

MORBIDITY OF THE INFANT OF THE DIABETIC MOTHER

In the last decade the perinatal morbidity rate in pregnancies complicated by diabetes mellitus has been remarkably reduced. However, severe neonatal morbidity in infants of diabetic mothers is still a problem that may affect even infants delivered at term.[305,306]

Neonatal morbidity is frequent in both gestational and pregestational diabetes mellitus but is much higher in the latter group. The exact etiology of many of these disorders remains unclear. However, there is evidence to show that neonatal morbidity is related to poor maternal metabolic control during pregnancy and that tight maternal glycemic control may prevent several major forms of morbidity.[305,307] Landon and colleagues studied the relationship between glycemic control and neonatal morbidity in 75 IDDM patients.[305] The study group included only patients from White's classes B, C, and D. It was found that in patients with excellent control of diabetes (mean capillary blood glucose <110 mg/dL) during the second and third trimesters, there was less neonatal morbidity than among diabetics with less stringent metabolic control (mean capillary blood glucose >110 mg/dL). The latter group had higher rates of macrosomia (34.3% versus 9.3%), respiratory distress syndrome (21.8% versus 2.3%), neonatal hyperbilirubinemia (40.6% versus 23.2%), and hypoglycemia (40.6% versus 18.6%) than patients under better metabolic control.

Other investigators were unable to show a relationship between the degree of glycemic control and perinatal morbidity.[299,308] These differences in results may be attributed at least in part to the fact that these studies included diabetic patients with different degrees of severity and relatively limited data on long-term glycemic control during pregnancy. In a recent study significant correlation was demonstrated between amniotic fluid C-peptide and insulin levels with maternal metabolic control.[309] High levels of insulin and C-peptide in the amniotic fluid seem to reflect hyperplasia of fetal islet cells with greater secretion of fetal insulin and may indicate poorly controlled maternal diabetes. The authors have found that high levels of this marker in the amniotic fluid are associated with higher rates of fetal macrosomia, neonatal hypoglycemia, and hypocalcemia.

In summary, current evidence suggests that many of the neonatal morbidities in infants of diabetic mothers are preventable by tight maternal glycemic control during pregnancy. The following sections will briefly discuss each of these neonatal morbidities.

Hypoglycemia

Hypoglycemia is diagnosed when plasma glucose levels are less than 35 mg/dL and 25 mg/dL in term and preterm infants, respectively. Infants of diabetic mothers in unsatisfactory glycemic control often develop hypoglycemia during the first few hours of life. The reported incidence ranges from 25% to 40% of infants of diabetic mothers. Poor glycemic control during pregnancy and high maternal plasma glucose levels at the time of delivery increase the risk of occurrence, particularly if the patients have been delivered by cesarean section.[309]

The neonatal hypoglycemia in infants of diabetic mothers is probably related to the overproduction of insulin by the fetal pancreas that has been stimulated in utero by significant hyperglycemia. At birth, the transplacental source of glucose is stopped abruptly, and since there is higher plasma insulin levels in neonates of diabetic mothers during the first 24 hours of life, there is an increased risk of developing neonatal hypoglycemia.[310] It was demonstrated in a series of 53 IDDM patients that only infants of mothers who had plasma glucose levels above 7.0 mmol/L at the time of delivery had an increased risk of developing neonatal hypoglycemia.[311]

In normal infants, the decrease in plasma glucose after delivery is associated with a rapid increase in plasma glucagon, which reaches a peak in the first few hours of life. However, in neonates of diabetic mothers, glucagon remains unchanged during the first few hours, and thereafter no significant increase was observed.[312] These data support the conclusion that neonatal hypoglycemia in neonates of diabetic mothers is a result of hyperinsulinemia in combination with decreased glucagon response.

It has been shown that catecholamine response among infants of diabetic mothers is blunted in response to hypoglycemia. These studies, however, used urinary levels of catecholamines, which is less accurate than the use of plasma in the first 24 hours of life.[309] In fact, it was demonstrated that plasma adrenaline and noradrenaline are increased in newborns of diabetic mothers who became severely hypoglycemic.[313] Therefore, adrenaline and noradrenaline in infants of diabetic mothers seem to counteract the lowering effect of insulin on blood glucose.

Clinical signs of neonatal hypoglycemia include tremor, apathy, episodes of cyanosis, convulsions, weak or high-pitched cry, and episodes of sweating. Since prolonged and severe hypoglycemia may be associated with neurologic sequelae, initiation of treatment is advised in all neonates of diabetic mothers with plasma glucose levels of less than 40 mg/dL.

The most efficient means of therapy for hypoglycemia is continuous dextrose infusion at the rate of 4 to 6 mg/kg/min. The use of a bolus of a hypertonic glucose infusion should be avoided to prevent later rebound hypoglycemia.[310] Occasionally, hypoglycemia may persist beyond the second day of life and may require the use of glucocorticoids. Glucagon administration does not seem to be an efficient treatment of neonatal hypoglycemia, since the short rise in blood glucose levels may be followed by rebound hypoglycemia.[314,315]

Epinephrine has also been used for the treatment of neonatal hypoglycemia. It has the disadvantage of producing untoward cardiovascular side effects and lactic acidosis.[314] In rare cases, when hypoglycemia persists and does not respond to therapy, other pathologic conditions should be ruled out, such as nesidioblastosis (B-cell hyperplasia) or islet-cell tumor.

Hypocalcemia and Hypomagnesemia

There is a significant increase in the incidence of hypocalcemia and hypomagnesemia in infants of diabetic mothers.[316,317] The incidence of neonatal hypocalcemia, defined as calcium levels at or below 7 mg/dL, has been reported to approach 20% in a group of infants with mean gestational age at delivery of 38 ± 0.2 weeks.[307] Serum calcium levels in infants of diabetic mothers are lowest in the second to the third day of life. The etiology of hypocalcemia in neonates of diabetic mothers is not yet clear. However, there is some evidence to show that neonatal hypocalcemia in neonates of diabetic mothers is associated with "relative" neonatal hypoparathyroidism.[318] It has also been postulated that magnesium deficiency may contribute to hypoparathyroidism and hypocalcemia in infants of diabetic mothers.[310]

Polycythemia

Polycythemia is diagnosed when venous hematocrit exceeds 65%. This condition has been reported to affect a third of neonates of diabetic mothers in the first few hours of life.[319] The mechanism responsible for polycythemia in these babies may be related to chronic intrauterine hypoxia that leads to an increase in erythropoietin and a consequent increase in red cell production.

Usually, polycythemia is associated with hyperviscosity of the blood, which may impede the velocity of blood flow and increase the risk of microthrombus formation in multiple organs.[320,321] Kidneys, adrenals, and lungs are the most commonly affected organs. Clinically, infants with polycythemia appear plethoric. Some of these infants have convulsions, respiratory distress, tachycardia, congestive heart failure, and hyperbilirubinemia. The treatment of polycythemia consists of partial exchange transfusion with a volume expander (ie, plasma) to reduce the hematocrit to about 55%.[322]

Respiratory Distress Syndrome

Respiratory distress syndrome (RDS) is considered a common neonatal morbidity in the infants of diabetic mothers. Factors contributing to the development of RDS in these infants are preterm deliveries, delayed fetal lung maturation, and high rate of elective cesarean section. Fortunately, elective preterm delivery of diabetics is becoming less common, and there is an increased tendency to deliver more diabetics vaginally. This trend is expected to lead to a reduction in the incidence of RDS.[310,322]

Several investigators have reported delayed fetal lung maturation in classes A, B, and C and accelerated maturation in classes D, F, and R.[323,324] Others have not found differences in lung maturity between the different White's classes.

Recent studies have demonstrated a low incidence of RDS in neonates of diabetic mothers whose glycemic control was stringently regulated during pregnancy.[297,310,325] In one study, the incidence of RDS in tightly controlled diabetic pregnancies was not different from that of nondiabetic controls.[326] These results have not been consistently found by other investigators. Hence, the influence of tight glucose control on the incidence of RDS remains unsettled.

In the poorly controlled diabetic patients, the reason for the increased risk for RDS seems to be related to the inhibitory effect of high fetal insulin levels on surfactant phospholipid synthesis and secretion and possibly through decreased prolactin levels.[327,328]

The value of the lecithin–sphingomyelin (L/S) ratio as a predictor in lung maturation in pregnancies complicated by diabetes is still controversial.[325,329] Several authors have reported the development of RDS in neonates of diabetic mothers despite mature L/S ratios (≥2).[305,330–332] Phosphatidylglycerol (PG) seems to have a stabilizing effect on pulmonary surfactant. The finding of PG in amniotic fluid is almost always associated with the absence of RDS in normal and complicated pregnancies.[324,333] In pregnancies complicated by diabetes, the appearance of PG in amniotic fluid is often delayed when compared to normal controls of similar gestational age.[334,335]

Because a significant number of infants may develop RDS despite L/S ratio of ≥2, the use of an L/S ratio of more than 3.5 or at least 3.0 has been recommended as an indicator of fetal lung maturity in infants of diabetic mothers.[335–337] Most authorities, however, prefer to analyze both L/S ratios and PG in the amniotic fluid before undertaking elective delivery.[305,332] Burtos and colleagues have reported that no neonate develops RDS when PG is found in the amniotic fluid.[338]

Reduction of the rate of RDS in IDMs is expected if delivery is planned at term whenever possible and assessment of fetal lung maturation is performed prior to delivery. Some have suggested that after 39 weeks in well-controlled diabetics, elective induction may be considered without amniocentesis.[305,339] We disagree with that position as a general principle, since we have observed severe RDS in well-controlled, well-dated pregnancies delivered at 40 weeks. In patients without vasculopathy in whom prolongation of the gestation would be acceptable, amniocentesis would be well advised. Conversely, in patients at term for whom the results of the amniotic fluid analysis would not influence management, amniocentesis may be deleted.

Occasionally, premature delivery in pregnancy complicated by diabetes may be necessary because of maternal or fetal complications before fetal lung maturation has occurred. Under these circumstances pharmacologic acceleration of fetal lung maturation should be considered. The beneficial effect of steroid administration for fetal lung maturity in diabetic pregnancies is unclear, and its use has been associated with an increase in maternal insulin requirement.[340]

Hyperbilirubinemia

Infants of diabetic mothers have a higher incidence of hyperbilirubinemia when compared to infants of nondiabetic mothers matched for gestational age.[341] The mechanism for this increased risk of jaundice is not clear, but several possible factors have been proposed[342,343]:

1. Infants of diabetic mothers have a higher rate of polycythemia. This may lead to hyperbilirubinemia because of the increased breakdown of red blood cells.
2. Macrosomia may be associated with higher rates of birth trauma, hematoma formation, and increased red cell breakdown.
3. In infants of diabetic mothers, oral feedings may be delayed because of different medical problems. This may decrease intestinal motility and increase enterohepatic circulation of unconjugated bilirubin.

Prevention of hyperbilirubinemia in IDMs may be possible by reducing the incidence of prematurity, improvement of maternal metabolic control, and possibly reducing macrosomia by even more stringent glucose control. Finally, early treatment of polycythemia may further reduce the risk of hyperbilirubinemia.

Birth Asphyxia

Birth asphyxia in neonates of diabetic mothers is much more common than that observed in the general obstetric population. Poorly controlled diabetics have an increased risk of macrosomia and chronic intrauterine hypoxia and therefore a greater risk of intrauterine or neonatal asphyxia.[344]

Birth injuries in the macrosomic infants of diabetic mothers include Erb's palsy, fractured clavicle, facial paralysis, phrenic nerve injury, and intracranial hemorrhage. Severe birth injuries may result in permanent neonatal morbidity and sometimes in neonatal death.

Cardiomyopathy

Infants of diabetic mothers have a higher risk of hypertrophic types of cardiomyopathy and congestive heart failure.[345] The incidence of neonates of diabetic mothers cardiomyopathy is not known. According to one study, 10% of infants of diabetic mothers may have evidence of myocardial and septal hypertrophy. The characteristic findings in echocardiography are generalized myocardial hypertrophy with disproportionate hypertrophy of the interventricular septum. Infants of diabetic mothers with severe cardiomyopathy may develop left ventricular outflow tract obstruction with reduced cardiac output and congestive heart failure.[346–348] The natural history of cardiomyopathy in infants of diabetic mothers is different from other types of cardiomyopathy in that there is a complete regression of hypertrophic changes to normal after several months.[345,349] Several studies have demonstrated a strong correlation between the risk of cardiomyopathy in infants of diabetic mothers and poor maternal diabetic control.[346,348,350] Experimental studies in animals have demonstrated that fetal hyperinsulinemia will lead to macrosomia and cardiomyopathy characteristics of infants of diabetic mothers.[277] These data indicate that tight diabetic control may also reduce the risk of cardiomyopathy in infants of diabetic mothers.

REFERENCES

1. Peel J. A historical review of diabetes and pregnancy. J Obstet Gynaecol Br Commonw 1972;79:385.
2. Reece EA. The history of diabetes mellitus. In: Reece EA, Coustan DR, eds. Diabetes mellitus in pregnancy, principles and practice. Edinburgh: Churchill-Livingstone, 1988:10.
3. Karlsson K, Kjellmer I. The outcome of diabetic pregnancies in relation to the mother's blood sugar level. Am J Obstet Gynecol 1972;112:213.
4. Martin FIR, Health P, Mountain KR. Pregnancy in women with diabetes mellitus: fifteen year's experience 1970–1985. Med J Aust 1987;146:187.
5. National Diabetes Data Group. Classification and diagnosis of diabetes mellitus. Washington, DC: National Institute of Health, 1986.
6. White P. Pregnancy complicating diabetes. Am J Med 1949;7:609.
7. Hare JW, White P. Gestational diabetes and the White classification. Diabetes Care 1980;3:394.
8. The American College of Obstetricians and Gynecologists. ACOG Technical Bulletin No. 92 (Chicago), May 1986.
9. Coustan DR, Berkowitz RL, Hobbins JC. Tight metabolic control of overt diabetes in pregnancy. Am J Med 1980;68:845.

10. Hitman GA. Progress with the genetics of insulin-dependent diabetes mellitus. Clin Endocrinol 1986;25:463.
11. Freinkel N. Gestational diabetes 1979: philosophical and practical aspects of a major health problem. Diabetes Care 1980;3:399.
12. Barnett AH, ed. Immunogenetics of insulin-dependent diabetes. Lancaster, UK: MTP Press Ltd, 1987:11.
13. Singal DP, Blajchman MA. Histocompatibility (L-A) antigens, lymphocytotoxic antibodies and tissue antibodies in patients with diabetes mellitus. Diabetes 1973;22:429.
14. Nerup J, Platz P, Anderson OO, et al. ALA-antigens and diabetes mellitus. Lancet 1974;ii:864.
15. Cudworth AG, Woodrow JC. HLA system and diabetes mellitus. Diabetes 1975;24:245.
16. Rotter JI, Rimoin DL. The genetics of diabetes. Hosp Pract 1987;22:79.
17. Ekoe JM. Diabetes Mellitus. Aspects of world-wide epidemiology of diabetes mellitus and its long-term complications. Amsterdam: Elsevier, 1988:34.
18. Zimmet P, Taylor RR, Whitehouse S. Prevalence rates of impaired glucose tolerance and diabetes mellitus in various Pacific populations according to the new WHO criteria. WHO Bull 1982;60:279.
19. Zimmet P, Taft P. The high prevalence of diabetes mellitus in Nauru, a central Pacific Island. Adv Metab Discord 1978;9:225.
20. Thompson G, Robinson WP, Kuhner MK, et al. Genetic heterogeneity, modes of inheritance, and risk estimates for a joint study of Caucasians with insulin-dependent diabetes mellitus. Hum Genet 1988;43:799.
21. Radder JK, Lemkes HHPJ, Krans HMJ, eds. Pathogenesis and Treatment of diabetes mellitus. Dordrecht: Martinus Nijhoff, 1986:18.
22. Eisenbarth GS. Type I diabetes mellitus. A chronic autoimmune disease. N Engl J Med 1986;314(21):1360.
23. Srikanta S, Ganda OP, Gleason RE, et al. Pre-type I diabetes: linear loss of B-cell response to intravenous glucose. Diabetes 1984;33:717.
24. Todd JA, Bell JI, McDevitt HO. A molecular basis for genetic susceptibility to insulin-dependent diabetes mellitus. Trends Genet 1988;4:129.
25. Wolf W, Spencer KM, Cudworth AG. The genetic susceptibility to type I (insulin dependent) diabetes: analysis of the HLA-DR association. Diabetologia 1984;24:224.
26. Maclaren NK, Henson V. The genetics of insulin-dependent diabetes. Growth Genet Horm 1986;2:1.
27. Field LL. Insulin-dependent diabetes mellitus: a model for the study of multifactorial disorders. Am J Hum Genet 1988; 43:793.
28. Kobberling J, Bruggeboes B. Prevalence of diabetes among children of insulin-dependent diabetic mothers. Diabetologia 1980;18:459.
29. Wagener DK, Sacks JM, Laporte RE, et al. The Pittsburgh study of insulin-dependent diabetes mellitus: risk for diabetes among relatives of IDDM. Diabetes 1982;31:136.
30. Warram JH, Krolewski AS, Gottlieb MS, et al. Differences in risk of insulin-dependent diabetes in offspring of diabetic mothers and diabetic fathers. N Engl J Med 1984;311:149.
31. Vadheim CM, Rotter JI, Maclaren NK, et al. Preferential transmission of diabetic alleles within the HLA gene complex. N Engl J Med 1986;315:1314.
32. Gamble DR. An epidemiological study of childhood diabetes affecting two or more sibling. Diabetologia 1980;19:341.
33. Tillil H, Kobberling J. Age-corrected empirical genetic risk estimates for first-degree relatives of IDDM patients. Diabetes 1987;36:93.
34. Cahill GF Jr. Heterogeneity in type II diabetes (editorial). West J Med 1985;142:240.
35. Pyke DA. Diabetes: the genetic connections. Diabetologia 1979;17:333.
36. Barnett AH, EFF C, Leslie DRG, et al. Diabetes in identical twins. Diabetologia 1981;20:87.
37. O'Rahilly S, Spivey RS, Holman RR, et al. Type II diabetes of early onset: a distinct clinical and genetic syndrome? Br Med J 1987;294:923.
38. Permutt MA, Andreone T, Chirgwin J, et al. The genetics of type I and type II diabetes: analysis by recombinant DNA methodology. Adv Exp Med Biol 1985;189:89.
39. Ober C, Wason CJ, Andrew K, et al. Restriction fragment length polymorphisms of the insulin gene hypervariable region in gestational onset diabetes mellitus. Am J Obstet Gynecol 1987;157:1364.
40. Ginsberg-Fellner F, Mark EM, Nechemias C, et al. Islet cell antibodies in gestational diabetics. Lancet 1980;ii:362.
41. Freinkel N, Metzger BE. Gestational diabetes: problems in classification and implications for long-range prognosis. In: Vranic M, Hollenberg CH, Steiner G, eds. Comparison of type I and type II diabetes. Similarities and dissimilarities in etiology, pathogenesis, and complications. New York: Plenum, 1985:47.
42. Vardi P, Dib SA, Tuttlemen M, et al. Competitive insulin autoantibody assay. Prospective evaluation of subjects at high risk for development of type I diabetes mellitus. Diabetes 1987;36:1286.
43. Ginsberg-Fellner F, Witt ME. Franklin BH, et al. Triad of markers for identifying children at high risk of developing insulin-dependent diabetes mellitus. JAMA 1985;254:1469.
44. Pettit DJ, Aleck KA, Baird HR, et al. Congenital susceptibility to NIDDM. Role of intrauterine environment. Diabetes 1988; 37(5):622.
45. Brumfield C, Huddleston JF. The management of diabetic ketoacidosis in pregnancy. Clin Obstet Gynecol 1984;27(1):50.
46. Knopp RH, Montes A, Wrath MR. Carbohydrate and lipid metabolism in normal pregnancy. In: Food and nutrition board, eds. Laboratory indices of nutritional status in pregnancy. Washington, DC: National Academy of Sciences, 1978.
47. Kühl C. Glucose metabolism during and after pregnancy in normal and gestational diabetic women: I. Influence of normal pregnancy on serum glucose and insulin concentration during basal fasting conditions and after a challenge with glucose. Acta Endocrinol 1975;79:709.
48. Lind T, Billewicz WZ, Brown G. A serial study of changes occurring in the oral glucose tolerance test during pregnancy. J Obstet Gynaecol Br Commonw 1973;80:1033.
49. Kühl C, Holst JJ. Plasma glucagon and insulin:glucagon ratio in gestational diabetes. Diabetes 1976;25:16.
50. Spellacy WN, Goetz FC. Plasma insulin in normal late pregnancy. N Engl J Med 1963;268:988.
51. Kalkhoff R, Schalch DS, Walker JL, Beck P, Kipnis SM, Daughaday WH. Diabetogenic factors associated with pregnancy. Trans Assoc Am Physicians 1964;77:270.
52. Bleicher SJ, O'Sullivan JB, Freinkel N. Carbohydrate metabolism in pregnancy. V. The interrelations of glucose, insulin, and free fatty acids in late pregnancy and postpartum. N Engl J Med 1964;271:866.
53. Kalkhoff RK, Kissebah AH, Kim H-J. Carbohydrate and lipid metabolism during normal pregnancy: relationship to gestational hormone action. Semin Perinatol 1978;12:291.
54. Houssay BA, Foglia VG, Rodriguez RR. Production or prevention of some types of experimental diabetes with estrogen or corticosteroids. Acta Endocrinol 1954;17:146.
55. Rodriquez RR. Influence of estrogens and androgens on production of diabetes. In: Leibel BS, Wrenshall GA, eds. On the na-

ture and treatment of diabetes. New York: Excerpta Medica Foundation, 1965.
56. Krauth MC, Schillinger E. Changes in insulin receptor concentration in rat fat cells following treatment with the gestagens clomegestone acetate and cyproterone acetate. Acta Endocrinol (Kbh) 1977;86:667.
57. Costrini NV, Kalkhoff RK. Relative effects of pregnancy estradiol and progesterone on plasma insulin and pancreatic islet insulin secretion. J Clin Invest 1971;50:992.
58. Freinkel N. The effect of pregnancy on insulin homeostasis. Diabetes 1964;13:260.
59. Goodner CJ, Freinkel N. Carbohydrate metabolism in pregnancy: the turnover of I131 insulin in the pregnant rat. Endocrinology 1960;67:862.
60. Burt RL. Peripheral utilization of glucose in pregnancy: III. Insulin tolerance. Obstet Gynecol 1956;7:658.
61. Fisher PM, Sutherland HW, Bewsher PD. The insulin response to glucose infusion in gestational diabetes. Diabetologia 1980;19:10.
62. Hurwits D, Jensen D. Carbohydrate metabolism in normal pregnancy. N Engl J Med 1946;234:327.
63. O'Sullivan JB. Gestational diabetes and its significance. In: Camerini-Davalos RA, ed, Early diabetes. New York: Academic Press, 1970.
64. O'Sullivan JB, Mahan CM. Criteria for the oral glucose tolerance test in pregnancy. Diabetes 1964;13:278.
65. Freinkel N. Of pregnancy and progeny. Diabetes 1980;29:1023.
66. Neufeld ND, Braunstein CD, Grataos J, Artal R, Mestman J. Insulin receptor studies in normal and diabetic pregnancies: correlations with placental hormones. Endocrine Society, 62nd Annual Meeting (Abstr 152), 1980:112.
67. Soman V. Coustan DR, Felig P. Dissociation between insulin binding to monocytes and insulin sensitivity in normal pregnancy. Endocrine Society, 61st Annual Meeting (Abstr. 184), 1979:118.
68. Beck-Nielsen H, Kuhl C, Pedersen O, Bjerre-Christensen C, Nielsen TT, Klebe JG. Decreased insulin binding to monocytes from normal pregnant women. J Clin Endocrinol Metab 1979;49:810.
69. Flint DJ, Sinnett-Smith PA, Clegg RA, Vernon RG. Role of insulin receptors in the changing metabolism of adipose tissue during pregnancy and lactation in the rat. Biochem J 1979;182:421.
70. Pagano G, Cassoder M, Massobri M, Bozzo C, Tossare GF, Menato G, Lenti G. Insulin binding to human adipocytes during late pregnancy in healthy, obese, and diabetic states. Hormone Metab 1980;12:177.
71. Knopp R, Montes A, Childs M, Li JR, Mabuchi H. Metabolic adjustments in normal and diabetic pregnancy. Clin Obstet Gynecol 1980;24(1):21.
72. Beck P, Daughaday WH. Human placental lactogen: studies of its acute metabolic effects and disposition in normal man. J Clin Invest 1967;46:103.
73. Samaan N, Yen SCC, Gonzalez D, Pearson OH. Metabolic effects of placental lactogen (HPL) in man. J Clin Endocrinol Metab 1968;28:485.
74. Kalkhoff RK, Richardson BL, Beck P. Relative effects of pregnancy, human placental lactogen and prednisolone on carbohydrate tolerance in normal and subclinical diabetic subjects. Diabetes 1969;18:153.
75. Burke CW, Roulet F. Increased exposure of tissues to cortisol in late pregnancy. Br Med J 1970;1:657.
76. Gustafson AB, Banasiak MF, Kalkhoff RK, Hagen TC, Kim H-J. Correlation of hyperprolactinemia with altered plasma insulin and glucagon: similarity to effects of late human pregnancy. J Clin Endocrinol Metab 1980;51:242.
77. Soman V, Tamborlane W, Defrenzo R, et al. Insulin binding and insulin sensitivities in isolated growth hormone deficiency. N Engl J Med 1978;299:1025.
78. Clerico A, Del Chicca MG, Ghione S, et al. Progressively elevated levels of biologically active (free) cortisol during pregnancy by a direct radioimmunological assay of cortisol in an equilibrium dialysis system. J Endocrinol Invest 1980;3:185.
79. Nolten WE, Lindheimer MD, Rueckert PA, et al. Diurnal patterns and regulation of cortisol secretion in pregnancy. J Clin Endocrinol Metab 1980;51:466.
80. Rizza RA, Mandarino L, Gerich JE. Cortisol induced insulin resistance in man: impaired suppression of glucose production and stimulation of glucose utilization due to a postreceptor defect of insulin action. J Clin Endocrinol Metab 1981;54:131.
81. Unger RH, Orci L. Glucagon and the A cell; physiology and pathophysiology. N Engl J Med 1981;304:1518.
82. Daniel RR, Metzger BE, Freinkel N, Faloona GR, Unger RH, Nitzan M. Carbohydrate metabolism in pregnancy: XI. Response of plasma glucagon to overnight fast and oral glucose during normal pregnancy in gestational diabetes. Diabetes 1974;23:771.
83. Fischer PM, Hamilton PM, Sutherland HW, et al. The effect of gestation on intravenous glucose tolerance in women. J Obstet Gynaecol Br Commonw 1974;81:285.
84. Lind T, Aspillaga M. Metabolic changes during normal and diabetic pregnancy. In: Reece AS, Coustan DR, eds. Diabetes mellitus in pregnancy. Edinburgh: Churchill-Livingstone, 1988:75.
85. Felig P, Lynch V. Starvation in human pregnancy: hypoglycemia, hypoinsulinemia, and hyperketonemia. Science 1970;170:990.
86. Cousins L, Rigg L, Hollingsworth D, Brink G, Aurand J, Yen SSC. The 24-hour excursion and diurnal rhythm of glucose, insulin and c-peptide in normal pregnancy. Am J Obstet Gynecol 1980;136:483.
87. Fitch WL, King JC. Plasma amino acids, glucose and insulin responses to moderate-protein and high-protein test meals in pregnant, nonpregnant, and gestational diabetic women. Am J Clin Nutr 1987;46:243.
88. Freinkel N, Phelps RL, Metzger BE. Intermediary metabolism during normal pregnancy. In: Sutherland HW, Stowers JM, eds. Carbohydrate metabolism in pregnancy and the newborn 1978. New York: Springer-Verlag, 1979:1.
89. Knopp RH, Saudek CD, Arky RA, O'Sullivan JB. Two phases of adipose tissue metabolism in pregnancy: maternal adaptations for fetal growth. Endocrinology 1973; 92:984.
90. Freinkel N, Metzger BE, Nitzan M, Daniel R, Surmaczynska B, Nagel T. Facilitated anabolism in late pregnancy: some novel maternal compensations for accelerated starvation. In: Malaise WJ, Pirart J, eds. Proceedings of the VIIIth Congress of the International Diabetes Federation. Amsterdam, Excerpta Medica, International Congress Series No. 312, 1974:474,
91. Ravnikar V, Metzger BE, Freinkel N. Is there a risk of "accelerated starvation" in normal human pregnancy? Diabetes (Abstr.) 1978;27:463.
92. Shambaugh GE, Mrozak SC, Freinkel N. Fetal fuels: I. Utilization of ketones by isolated tissues at various stages of maturation and maternal nutrition during late gestation. Metabolism 1977;26:623.
93. Naeye RL, Chez RA. Effects of maternal acetonuria and low pregnancy weight gain on children's psychomotor development. Am J Obstet Gynecol 1981;139:139.
94. Stehbens JA, Baker GL, Kitchell M. Outcome at age 1, 3 and 5 years of children born to diabetic women. Am J Obstet Gynecol 1977;127:408.
95. Warth M, Arky RA, Knopp RH. Lipid metabolism in pregnancy. III. Altered lipid composition in intermediate, very low, low,

and high-density lipoprotein fractions. J Clin Endocrinol Metab 1975;41:649.

96. Darmady JM, Postle AD. Lipid metabolism in pregnancy. Br J Obstet Gynaecol 1982;89:211.
97. Hytten FE, Cheyne GA. The aminoaciduria of pregnancy. J Obstet Gynaecol Br Commonw 1972;79:424.
98. Young M. The accumulation of protein by the fetus. In: Beard RW, Nathanielsz PW, eds. Fetal Physiology and medicine. Philadelphia: WB Saunders, 1976:59.
99. Metzger BE, Unger RH, Freinkel N. Carbohydrate metabolism in pregnancy. XIV. Relationships between circulating glucagon, insulin, glucose and amino acids in response to a "mixed meal" in late pregnancy. Metabolism 1977;26:151.
100. Rice PA, Rourke JE, Nesbitt REL. Some characteristics of the glucose transport. Gynecol Invest 1976;7:213.
101. Johnson LW, Smith CH. Monosaccharide transport across microvillous membrane of human placenta. Am J Physiol 1980;238:160.
102. Battaglia FC, Meschia G. An introduction to fetal physiology. New York: Academic Press, 1986.
103. Cordero L, Yea S-Y, Grunt JA, et al. Hypertonic glucose infusion during labor. Maternal-fetal blood glucose relationships. Am J Obstet Gynecol 1970;107:295.
104. Oakley NW, Beard RW, Turner RC. Effect of sustained maternal hyperglycaemia on the fetus in normal and diabetic pregnancies. Br Med J 1972;1:466.
105. Young M. Techniques for studying placental metabolism and transfer. In: Beaconsfield P, Villee C, eds. Placenta, a neglected experimental animal. Oxford: Pergamon Press, 1979:96.
106. Hollingsworth DR. Alterations of maternal metabolism in normal and diabetic pregnancies. Differences in insulin-dependent, non-insulin-dependent and gestational diabetes. Am J Obstet Gynecol 1983;146:417.
107. Metzger BE, Phelps RL, Freinkel N, et al. Effects of gestational diabetes on diurnal profiles of plasma glucose, lipids, and individual amino acids. Diabetes Care 1980;3:402.
108. Skryten A, Johnson G, Samisøe G, et al. Studies in diabetic pregnancy: I. Serum lipids. Acta Obstet Gynecol Scand 1976;55:211.
109. Knopp RH, Chapman M, Bergelin R, et al. Relationships of lipoprotein lipids to mild fasting hyperglycemia and diabetes in pregnancy. Diabetes Care 1980;3:416.
110. Molsted-Pedersen L, Wagner L, Klebe G, et al. Aspects of carbohydrate metabolism in newborn infants of diabetic mothers. IV. Neonatal changes in plasma free fatty acid concentration. Acta Endocrinol 1972;71:338.
111. Szabo AJ, Opperman W, Hanover B, et al. Fetal adipose tissue development: relationship to maternal free fatty acid levels. In: Camerini-Davalos RA, Cole HS, eds. Early diabetes in early life. New York: Academic Press, 1975.
112. Sepe SJ, Connell FA, Geiss LS, et al. Gestational diabetes. Incidence, maternal characteristics, and perinatal outcome. Diabetes (Suppl 2) 1985;34:13.
113. Frienkel N, Hadden D. Summary and recommendations of the Second International Workshop-Conference on Gestational Diabetes Mellitus. Diabetes 1985;34:123.
114. O'Sullivan JB, Mahan CM, Charles D, et al. Screening criteria for high-risk gestational diabetic patients. Am J Obstet Gynecol 1973;116:895.
115. American College of Obstetrics and Gynecology. Management of diabetes mellitus in pregnancy. ACOG Technical Bulletin (Chicago) No. 92, 1986:1.
116. Marquette GP, Klein VR, Niebyl JR. Efficacy of screening for gestational diabetes. Am J Perinatol 1985;2:7.
117. Marquette GP, Klein VR, Repke JT, et al. Cost-effective criteria for glucose screening. Obstet Gynecol 1985;66:181.
118. Coustan D, Carpenter M. Detection and treatment of gestational diabetes. Clin Obstet Gynecol 1985;28:507.
119. Carpenter MW, Coustan DR. Criteria for screening tests for gestational diabetes. Am J Obstet Gynecol 1982;144:768.
120. Sacks D, Abu-Fadil S, Karten G, et al. Screening for gestational diabetes with the one-hour 50 g glucose test. Obstet Gynecol 1987;70:89.
121. Watson W. Serial changes in the 50 g oral glucose test in pregnancy: implications for screening. Obstet Gynecol 1989;74:40.
122. Roberts AB, Baker JR. Serum fructosamine: a screening test for diabetes in pregnancy. Am J Obstet Gynecol 1986;154:1027.
123. Cousins L, Dattel BJ, Hollingsworth DR, et al. Glycosylated hemoglobin as a screening test for carbohydrate intolerance in pregnancy. Am J Obstet Gynecol 1984;150:455.
124. Baxi L, Barad D, Reece EA, et al. Use of glycosylated hemoglobin as a screen for macrosomia in gestational diabetes. Obstet Gynecol 1984;64:347.
125. Gyves MT, Schulman PK, Merkatz IR. Results of individualized intervention in gestational diabetes. Diabetes Care 1980;3:495.
126. National Diabetes Data Group. Classification and diagnosis of diabetes mellitus and other categories of glucose intolerance. Diabetes 1979;28:1039.
127. Tallarigo L, Giampietro O, Penno G, et al. Relation of glucose tolerance to complications of pregnancy in non-diabetic women. N Engl J Med 1986;315:989.
128. Persson B, Stangenberg M, Hansson U, et al. Gestational diabetes mellitus (GDM): comparative evaluation of two treatment regimens, diet versus insulin and diet. Diabetes (Suppl 2) 1985;34:101.
129. Coustan DR, Imarah J. Prophylactic insulin treatment of gestational diabetes reduces the incidence of macrosomia, operative delivery, and birth trauma. Am J Obstet Gynecol 1984;150:836.
130. Coustan DR, Lewis SB. Insulin therapy for gestational diabetes. Obstet Gynecol 1978;51:306.
131. American Diabetes Association, Inc. Gestational diabetes mellitus. Ann Intern Med 1986;105:461.
132. Metzger BE, Bybee DE, Freinkel N, et al. Gestational diabetes mellitus. Correlations between the phenotypic and genotypic characteristics of the mother and abnormal glucose tolerance during the first year postpartum. Diabetes (Suppl 2) 1985;34:111.
133. Landon MB, Gabbe SG. Antepartum fetal surveillance in gestational diabetes mellitus. Diabetes (Suppl 2) 1985;34:50.
134. Gabbe SG, Mestman JH, Freeman RK, et al. Management and outcome of pregnancy in diabetes mellitus, classes B to R. Am J Obstet Gynecol 1977;129:723.
135. Benedetti TJ, Gabbe SG. Shoulder dystocia. Obstet Gynecol 1978;52:526.
136. Stowers JM, Sutherland HW, Kerridge DF. Long-range implications for the mother. The Aberdeen experience. Diabetes (Suppl 2) 1985;34:106.
137. O'Sullivan JB, Charles D, Mahan CM, et al. Gestational diabetes and perinatal mortality rate. Am J Obstet Gynecol 1973; 116:901.
138. O'Sullivan, JB. Body weight and subsequent diabetes mellitus. JAMA 1982;248:949.
139. Steel JM, Johnstone FD, Smith AF, et al. Five years' experience of a "pre-pregnancy" clinic for insulin-dependent diabetics. Br Med J 1982;285:353.
140. Fuhrmann K, Risker H, Semmler K, et al. Prevention of congenital malformations in infants of insulin-dependent diabetic mothers. Diabetes Care 1983;6:219.
141. Reece EA, Gabrielli S, Abdalla M. The prevention of diabetes-associated birth defects. Semin Perinatol 1988;12(4):292.
142. Pedersen JF. Congenital malformations. In: The pregnant dia-

betic and her newborn. 2nd ed. Copenhagen: Munksgaard, 1977:191.

143. Kucera J. Rate and type of congenital anomalies among offspring of diabetic women. J Reprod Med 1971;7:61.

144. Mills JL. Malformations in infants of diabetic mothers. Teratology 1982;25:385.

145. Rowland TW, Hubbell JP, Nadas AS. Congenital heart disease in infants of diabetic mothers. J Pediatr 1973;83:815.

146. Milunsky A. Prenatal diagnosis of neural tube defects. The importance of serum alpha-fetoprotein screening in diabetic pregnant women. Am J Obstet Gynecol 1982;142:1030.

147. Farquhar JW. Prognosis for babies born to diabetic mothers in Edinburgh. Arch Dis Child 1969;44:36.

148. Leveno KJ, Hauth JC, Gilstrap LC, et al. Appraisal of "rigid" blood glucose control during pregnancy of the overtly diabetic woman. Am J Obstet Gynecol 1979;135:853.

149. Grix A. Malformations in infants of diabetic mothers. Am J Med Genet 1982;13:131.

150. Dignan PJ. Teratogenic risk and counseling in diabetes. Clin Obstet Gynecol 1981;24(1):149.

151. Mills JL, Baker L, Goldman AS. Malformations in infants of diabetic mothers occur before the seventh gestational week. Implications for treatment. Diabetes 1979;28:292.

152. Reece EA, Hobbins JC. Diabetes embryopathy, pathogenesis, prenatal diagnosis and prevention. Obstet Gynecol Surv 1986;41:325.

153. Goldman AS, Baker L, Piddington R, et al. Hyperglycemia-induced teratogenesis is mediated by a functional deficiency of arachidonic acid. Proc Natl Acad Sci USA 1985;82:8277.

154. Pinter E, Reece EA, Leranth C, et al. Arachidonic acid prevents hyperglycemia-associated yolk sac damage and embryopathy. Am J Obstet Gynecol 1986;155:691.

155. Mintz DH, Chez RA, Hutchinson DL. Subhuman primate pregnancy complicated by streptozotocin-induced diabetes mellitus. J Clin Invest 1972;51:837.

156. Pinter E, Reece EA, Leranth C, et al. Yolk sac failure in embryopathy due to hyperglycemia. Ultrastructural analysis of yolk sac differentiation of rat conceptuses under hyperglycemic culture conditions. Teratology 1986;33:363.

157. Pinter E, Reece EA, Leranth C, et al. Ultrastructural analysis of malformations of the embryonic neural axis induced by in vitro hyperglycemic culture conditions. 5th Annual Scientific Meeting of the Society of Perinatal Obstetricians (Abstr.), 1985.

158. Horton WE Jr, Sadler TW. Effects of maternal diabetes on early embryogenesis: alternations in morphogenesis produced by the ketone body, b-hydroxybutyrate. Diabetes 1983;32:610.

159. Sadler TW, Horton WE, Hunter ES. Mechanisms of diabetes-induced congenital malformations as studied in mammalian embryoculture. In: Jovanowic L, Petersen CM, Fuhrmann K, eds. Diabetes and pregnancy: teratology, toxicity and treatment. New York: Praeger, 1986:51.

160. Buse MG, Roberts WJ, Buse J. The role of the human placenta in the transfer and metabolism of insulin. J Clin Invest 1962;41:29.

161. Josimovich JB, Knobil E. Placental transfer of I-131 insulin in the Rhesus monkey. Am J Physiol 1961;200:471.

162. Pitkin RM, Reynolds WA. Insulin transfer across the hemochorial placenta. Obstet Gynecol 1969;33:626.

163. Gitlin D, Kumate J, Morales C. On the transport of insulin across the human placenta. Pediatrics 1965;35:65.

164. Pedersen JF, Pedersen-Molsted L. Congenital malformations: the possible role of diabetes care outside pregnancy. Ciba Foundation Symposium, 1979:265.

165. Mills JL, Knopp RH, Simpson JL, et al. Lack of relation of increased malformation rates in infants of diabetic mothers to glycemic control during organogenesis. N Engl J Med 1988;318:671.

166. Miller E, Hare JW, Cloherty JP, et al. Elevated maternal hemoglobin A1c in early pregnancy and major congenital anomalies in infants of diabetic mothers. N Engl J Med 1981;304:1331.

167. Fuhrmann K, Reiber H, Semmler K, et al. The effect of intensified conventional insulin therapy before and during pregnancy on the malformation rate in offspring of diabetic mothers. Exp Clin Endocrinol 1984;83:173.

168. Steel JM. Preconception, conception and contraception. In: Reece EA, Coustan DR, eds. Diabetes mellitus in pregnancy: principles and practice. New York: Churchill-Livingstone, 1988:601.

169. Goldman A, Dicker D, Feldberg D, et al. Pregnancy outcome in patients with insulin-dependent diabetes mellitus with preconceptional diabetic control: a comparative study. Am J Obstet Gynecol 1986;155:293.

170. Kitzmiller J, McCoy D, Grin F, et al. A regional perinatal program to present congenital anomalies in infants of diabetic mothers. Proc Soc Gynecol Invest (Abstr.), 1986:56.

171. O'Shaughnessy R. Role of the glycohemoglobins in the evaluation and management of the diabetic pregnancy. Clin Obstet Gynecol 1981;24(1):65.

172. Bunn HF, Haney DN, Kamin S, et al. The biosynthesis of human hemoglobin A1c: slow glycosylation of hemoglobin in vivo. J Clin Invest 1976;57:1652.

173. Ylinen K, Aula P, Stenman Y-H, Kesaniemi-Kuokkanen T, Teramo K. Risk of minor and major fetal malformations in diabetics with high haemoglobin A1c values in early pregnancy. Br Med J 1984;289:345.

174. Wald NJ, Cuckle HS. Open neural tube defects. In: Wald NJ, ed. Antenatal and neonantal screening. Oxford: Oxford University Press, 1984:25.

175. Milunsky A, Alpert E, Kitzmiller JL, et al. Prenatal diagnosis of neural tube defects. VIII. The importance of serum alpha-fetoprotein screening in diabetic pregnant women. Am J Obstet Gynecol 1982;142:1030.

176. Reece EA, David N, Mahoney MJ, Baumgarten A. Maternal serum alpha-fetoprotein in diabetic pregnancy: correlation with glycemic controls. Lancet 1987;i:275.

177. Kleinman CS. Fetal echocardiography. In: Sanders R, ed, Ultrasound annual. New York: Raven Press, 1982:321.

178. Pedersen JF, Molsted-Pedersen L. Early growth retardation in diabetic pregnancy. Br Med J 1979;1:18.

179. Pedersen JF, Molsted-Pedersen L. Early fetal growth delay detected by ultrasound marks increased risk of congenital malformation in diabetic pregnancy. Br Med J 1981;283:261.

180. Keys, TC, Cousins L, Moore TR. Early fetal growth in insulin-dependent diabetics. In: Proceedings of the 32nd Annual Meeting of the Society for Synecological Investigation, 1 March 1985.

181. Pedersen J, Molsted-Pedersen L, Anderson B. Assessors of fetal perinatal mortality in diabetic pregnancy. Diabetes 1974;23:302.

182. Gyves MT, Rodman HM, Little AB, et al. A modern approach to management of pregnant diabetics: a two-year analysis of perinatal outcomes. Am J Obstet Gynecol 1977;128:606.

183. Seeds AE, Knowles HC. Metabolic control of diabetic pregnancy. Clin Obstet Gynecol 1981;24:51.

184. Artal E, Golde SH, Dorey F, et al. The effect of plasma glucose variability on neonatal outcome in the pregnant diabetic patient. Am J Obstet Gynecol 1983;147:537.

185. Gillmer MDG, Beard RW, Brooke FM, et al. Carbohydrate metabolism in pregnancy. I. Diurnal plasma glucose profile in normal and diabetic women. Br Med J 1975;3:399.

186. Gabbe SG. Management of diabetes mellitus in pregnancy. Am J Obstet Gynecol 1985;153:824.

187. Cousins L, Rigg L, Hollingsworth D, et al. The 24-hour excur-

sion and diurnal rhythm of glucose, insulin, and C-peptide in normal pregnancy. Am J Obstet Gynecol 1980;136:483.

188. Adashi EY, Pinto H, Tyson JE. Impact of maternal euglycemia on fetal outcome in diabetic pregnancy. Am J Obstet Gynecol 1979;133:268.

189. Jovanovic L, Peterson CM, Sacena BB, et al. Feasibility of maintaining normal glucose profiles in insulin-dependent pregnant diabetic women. Am J Med 1980;68:105.

190. Reece EA, Coustan D, Sherwin R, et al. Does intensive glycemic control in diabetic pregnancies result in normalization of other metabolic fuels. Diabetes Anaheim, California (Abstr.), 1986.

191. Persson B, Heding LG, Lunell NO, et al. Foetal β-cell function in diabetic pregnancy. Amniotic fluid concentrations of proinsulin, insulin and C-peptide during the last trimester of pregnancy. Am J Obstet Gynecol 1982;144:455.

192. Goeddel DV, Kleid DG, Bolivar F, et al. Expression in Escherichia coli of chemically synthesized genes for human insulin. Proc Natl Acad Sci USA 1979;76:106.

193. Fireman P, Fineberg SE, Galloway JA. Development of IgE antibodies to human (rDNA), porcine and bovine insulins in diabetic subjects. Diabetes Care (Suppl 2) 1982;5:119.

194. Kurtz AB, Matthews JA, Mustaffa BE, et al. Decrease of antibodies to insulin, proinsulin and contaminating hormones after changing therapy from conventional beef to purified pork insulin. Diabetologia 1980;18:147.

195. Jovanovic L, Peterson CM. Optimal insulin delivery for the pregnant diabetic patient. Diabetes Care (Suppl 1) 1982;5:24.

196. Vaughan NJA, Oakley NW. Treatment of diabetes in pregnancy. Clin Obstet Gynecol 1986;13(2):291.

197. Mylvaganam R, Stowers JM, Steel JM, et al. Insulin immunogenicity in pregnancy: maternal and fetal studies. Diabetologia 1983;24:19.

198. Bauman WA, Yalow RS. Placental passage of antibody and insulin-antibody complexes. Diabetes (Suppl 2) 1982;31:154a, 589.

199. Fineberg SE, Galloway JA, Fineberg NS, et al. Immunogenicity of recombinant DNA human insulin. Diabetologia 1983;25:465.

200. American Diabetes Association. Insulin administration. Diabetes Care 1990;13(1):28.

201. Potter JM, Reckless JPD, Cullen DR. Subcutaneous continuous insulin infusion and control of blood glucose concentration in diabetics in third trimester of pregnancy. Br Med J 1980; 28:1099.

202. Kitzmiller JI, Younger MD, Hare JW, et al. Continuous subcutaneous insulin therapy during early pregnancy. Obstet Gynecol 1985;66:606.

203. Rudolf MCJ, Coustan DR, Sherwin RS, et al. Efficacy of the insulin pump in the home treatment of pregnant diabetics. Diabetes 1981;30:891.

204. Coustan DR, Reece RA, Sherwin R, et al. A randomized clinical trial of insulin pump vs. intensive conventional therapy in diabetic pregnancies. JAMA 1986;255:631.

205. Unger RH. Meticulous control of diabetes: benefits, risks and precautions. Diabetes 1982;34:479.

206. Mecklenburg RS, Benson JW Jr, Becker NM, et al. Clinical use of the insulin infusion pump in 100 patients with Type I diabetes. N Engl J Med 1982;307:513.

207. Santiago JV, Clarke WL, Arias F. Studies with a pancreatic beta-cell simulator in third trimester pregnancies complicated by diabetes. Am J Obstet Gynecol 1978;132:455.

208. Landon MB, Gabbe SG. Glucose monitoring and insulin administration in the pregnant diabetic patient. Clin Obstet Gynecol 1985;28:496.

209. Skyler JS. Self-monitoring of blood glucose. Med Clin North Am 1982;66:1227.

210. Mazze RS, Shamson H, Pasmantier R, et al. Reliability of blood glucose monitoring by patients with diabetes mellitus. Am J Med 1984;77:211.

211. American Diabetes Association. Principles of nutrition and dietary recommendations for individuals with diabetes mellitus. Diabetes Care 1979;2:520.

212. Pitken RM. Nutritional influences during pregnancy. Med Clin North Am 1977;61:3.

213. Coetzee EJ, Jackson WP, Berman PA. Ketonuria in pregnancy, with special reference to calorie-restricted food intake in obese diabetics. Diabetes 1980;29:177.

214. Kay RM, Grobin W, Track NS. Diets rich in natural fiber improve carbohydrate tolerance in maturity-onset, non-insulin-dependent diabetics. Diabetologia 1981;20:18.

215. Hagander B. Fiber and diabetic diet: an evaluation of metabolic response to standardized meals. Acta Med Scand (Suppl) 1987;716:1.

216. Vinkin A, Jenkins DJA. Dietary fiber in management of diabetes. Diabetes Care 1988;11:160.

217. Jenkins DJA, Leeds AR, Gassull MA, et al. Decrease in postprandial insulin and glucose concentrations by guar and pectin. Ann Intern Med 1977;86:20.

218. Gabbe SG, Cohen AW, Herman GD, et al. Effect of dietary fiber on the oral glucose tolerance test in pregnancy. Am J Obstet Gynecol 1982;143:514.

219. Ney D, Hollingsworth DR, Cousins L. Decreased insulin requirement and improved control of diabetes in pregnant women given a high-carbohydrate, high-fiber, low-fat diet. Diabetes Care 1982;5(5):529.

220. Reece EA, Hagay Z, Gay LJ, et al. A randomized clinical trial of a fiber-enriched diabetic diet vs the standard American Diabetes Association recommended diet in the management of diabetes mellitus in pregnancy. (Submitted for publication.)

221. Gabbe S, Mestman J, Hibbard L. Maternal mortality in diabetes mellitus. An 18 year survey. Obstet Gynecol 1976;48:549.

222. Cousins L. Pregnancy complications among diabetic women: review 1965–1985. Obstet Gynecol Surv 1987;42(3):140.

223. Marble A, White P, Bradley RF, et al. Joslin's diabetes mellitus. 11th ed. 1971.

224. Olofsson P, Liedholm H, Sartor G, et al. Diabetes and pregnancy. A 21-year Swedish material. Acta Obstet Gynecol Scand 1984;122:3.

225. Reece EA, Egan JFX, Coustan DR, et al. Coronary artery disease in diabetic pregnancies. Am J Obstet Gynecol 1986;154:150.

226. Thomas D, Gill B, Brown P, et al. Salbutamol-induced diabetic ketoacidosis. Br Med J 1977;2:438.

227. Kitzmiller JL. Diabetes ketoacidosis and pregnancy. Contemp Obstet Gynecol 1982;20(1):141.

228. Schade DS, Eaton RP. The pathogenesis of diabetes ketoacidosis: a reappraisal. Diabetes Care 1979;2:296.

229. Kreisberg RA. Diabetic ketoacidosis: new concepts and trends in pathogenesis and treatment. Ann Intern Med 1978;88:681.

230. Brumfield C, Huddleston JF. The management of diabetic ketoacidosis in pregnancy. Clin Obstet Gynecol 1984;27(1):50.

231. Hay WW. Fetal metabolic consequences of maternal diabetes. In: Jovanovic L, Peterson CM, Fuhrmann K, eds. Diabetes and pregnancy. New York: Praeger, 1986:185.

232. Miodovnik M, Skillman C, Hertzberg V, et al. Effects of hyperketonemia on hyperglycemic pregnant ewes and their fetuses. Am J Obstet Gynecol 1986;154:394.

233. Ditzel J, Standl E. The oxygen transport system of red blood cells during diabetic ketoacidosis and recovery. Diabetologia 1975;11:255.

234. LeBue C, Goodlin RC. Treatment of fetal distress during diabetic ketoacidosis. J Reprod Med 1978;20:201.

235. Goldgenicht C, Slama G, Papoz L, et al. Hypoglycemic reaction

in 172 type 1 (insulin dependent) diabetes patients. Diabetologia 1983;24:95.
236. Gerich JE, Langlois M, Noacco C, et al. Lack of glycagon response to hypoglycemia in diabetes: evidence for an intrinsic pancreatic alpha cell defect. Science 1973;182:171.
237. Reece EA, Roberts A, Hagay Z, et al. Induced hypoglycemia in pregnant women (insulin clamp technique) and the assessment of maternal and fetal responses. Proceedings, 11th Annual Meeting of the Society of Perinatal Obstetricians (Abstr.), 1991.
238. Pedersen J. The pregnant diabetic and her newborn. 2nd ed. Copenhagen: Munksgaard, 1977.
239. Diamond M, Vaughn W, Salyer S. Efficacy of outpatient management of insulin-dependent diabetic pregnancies. J Perinatol 1985;5:2.
240. Lufkin G, Nelson R, Hill L, et al. An analysis of diabetic pregnancies at Mayo Clinic, 1950–79. Diabetes Care 1984;7:539.
241. Wladimiroff JW, Barentsen R, Wallenburg HCS, et al. Fetal urine production in a case of diabetes associated with polyhydramnios. Obstet Gynecol 1975;46:100.
242. Molsted-Pedersen L. Preterm labour and perinatal mortality in diabetic pregnancy: obstetric considerations. In: Sutherland HW, Stowers JM, eds. Carbohydrate metabolism in pregnancy and the newborn, 1978. Berlin: Springer-Verlag, 1979:392.
243. Miodovnik M, Mimouni F, Siddiqi TA, et al. High spontaneous premature labor rate in insulin-dependent diabetic (IDD) pregnant women: an association with poor glycemic control. Scientific Abstracts of the Seventh Annual Meeting of the Society for Perinatal Obstetrics, Lake Buena Vista, Florida, February 5–7, 1987.
244. Miodovnik M, Mimouni F, Siddiqi TA, et al. Periconceptional metabolic status and risk for spontaneous abortion in insulin-dependent diabetic pregnancies. Am J Perinatol 1988;5(4):368.
245. Kalter H. Diabetes and spontaneous abortion: an historical review. Am J Obstet Gynecol 1987;156:1243.
246. Miodovnik M, Lavin JP, Knowles HC, et al. Spontaneous abortion among insulin-dependent diabetic women. Am J Obstet Gynecol 1984;150:372.
247. Miodovnik M, Skillman C, Holroyde JC, et al. Elevated maternal hemoglobin A1 in early pregnancy and spontaneous abortion among insulin-dependent diabetic women. Am J Obstet Gynecol 1985;153:439.
247a. Mills JL, Knopp RH, Simpson JL et al. Lack of relationship of increased malformation rates in infants of diabetic mothers to glycemic control during organogenesis. N Engl J Med 1988;318:671.
248. Diabetic Retinopathy Study Group. Photocoagulation treatment of proliferative diabetic retinopathy: clinical application of Diabetic Retinopathy Study (DRS) findings (DRS Report 8). Ophthalmology 1983;88:583.
249. Engerman RL, Bloodworth JMB, Nelson S. Relationship of microvascular disease in diabetes to metabolic control. Diabetes 1977;26:760.
250. Skyler JS. Complications of diabetes mellitus: relationship to metabolic dysfunction. Diabetes Care 1977;2:499.
251. Sinclair S, Nesler C, Schwartz S. Retinopathy in the pregnant diabetic. Clin Obstet Gynecol 1985;28(3):536.
252. Klein R. Recent developments in the understanding and management of diabetic retinopathy. Med Clin North Am 1988;72(6):1415.
253. Frank RN. On the pathogenesis of diabetic retinopathy. Ophthalmology 1984;91:626.
254. Puklin J. Diabetic retinopathy. In: Reece EA, Coustan D, eds. Diabetes mellitus in pregnancy. Edinburgh: Churchill-Livingstone, 1988.
255. Klein R, Klein BEK, Moss SE, et al. The Wisconsin Epidemiologic Study of Diabetic Retinopathy: II. Prevalence and risk of diabetic retinopathy when age at diagnosis is less than 30 years. Arch Ophthalmol 1984;102:520.
256. Klein R, Klein BEK, Moss SE, et al. The Wisconsin Epidemiologic Study of Diabetic Retinopathy: III. Prevalence and risk of diabetic retinopathy when age at diagnosis is less than 30 years. Arch Ophthalmol 1984;102:527.
257. Klein R, Klein BEK, Moss SE, et al. Effect of pregnancy on progression of diabetic retinopathy. Diabetes Care 1990;13:34.
258. Laatikainen L, Teramo K, Hieta-Heikurainen H, et al. A controlled study of the influence of continuous subcutaneous insulin infusion treatment on diabetic retinopathy during pregnancy. Acta Med Scand 1987;221:367.
259. Price JH, Hadden DR, Archer DB, et al. Diabetic retinopathy in pregnancy. Br J Obstet Gynaecol 1984;91:11.
260. Serup L. Influence of pregnancy on diabetic retinopathy. Acta Endocrinol (Copenh) 1986;277:122.
261. Moloney JBM, Drury MI. The effect of pregnancy on the natural course of diabetic retinopathy. Am J Ophthalmol 1982;93:745.
262. Kroc Collaborative Study Group. The Kroc study patients at 2 years: a report on further retinal changes. Diabetes (Suppl 1) 34:39A, 1985.
263. Lauritzen T, Frost-Larsen K, Larsen HW, et al. Two year experience with continuous subcutaneous insulin infusion in relation to retinopathy and neuropathy. Diabetes (Suppl 3) 1985;34:74.
264. Phelps RL, Sakol P, Metzger BE, et al. Changes in diabetic retinopathy during pregnancy: correlations with regulation of hyperglycemia. Arch Ophthalmol 1986;104:1806.
265. Kitzmiller JL, Aiello LM, Kaldany A, et al. Diabetic vascular disease complicating pregnancy. Clin Obstet Gynecol 1981;24:107.
266. Elman K, Welch RA, Frank RN, et al. Diabetic retinopathy in pregnancy: a review. Obstet Gynecol 1990;75:119.
267. Sunness JS. The pregnant women's eye. Surv Ophthalmol 1988;32:219.
268. Kitzmiller JL, Brown ER, Phillippe N, et al. Diabetic nephropathy and perinatal outcome. Am J Obstet Gynecol 1981;141:741.
269. Reece EA, Coustan DR, Hayslett JP, et al. Diabetic nephropathy: pregnancy performance and fetomaternal outcome. Am J Obstet Gynecol 1988;159:56.
270. Mogensen CE. Renal function changes in diabetes. Diabetes 1976;25:871.
271. Deckert T, Andersen AR, Christiansen JS, et al. Course of diabetic nephropathy. Factors related to development. Acta Endocrinol 1981;97:242.
272. Redman CWG. Controlled trials of treatment of hypertension during pregnancy. Obstet Gynecol Surv 1982;37:523.
273. Golde SH, Montoro M, Good-Anderson B, et al. The role of NST, fetal biophysical profile and CST in the outpatient management of insulin-requiring diabetic pregnancies. Am J Obstet Gynecol 1984;148:269.
274. Simonson DC. Etiology and prevalence of hypertension in diabetic patients. Diabetes Care 1988;11:821.
275. Elliot JP, Garite TJ, Freeman RK, et al. Ultrasonic prediction of fetal macrosomia in diabetic patients. Obstet Gynecol 1982;60:159.
276. Gabbe SG, Mestman JH, Freeman RK, et al. Management and outcome of class A diabetes mellitus. Am J Obstet Gynecol 1977;127:465.
277. Susa JB, McCormick KL, Widness JA, et al. Chronic hyperinsulinemia in the fetal Rhesus monkey. Effects on fetal growth and composition. Diabetes 1979;28:1058.
278. Acker D, Sachs BP, Friedman EA. Risk factors for shoulder dystocia. Obstet Gynecol 1985;66:762.
279. O'Leary JA, Leonetti HB. Shoulder dystocia: prevention and treatment. Am J Obstet Gynecol 1990;162:5.
280. Willman SP, Lereno KJ, Guzick DS, et al. Glucose threshold for

macrosomia in pregnancy complicated by diabetes. Am J Obstet Gynecol 1986;154:470.

281. Szabo AJ, Szabo O. Placental free fatty acid transfer and fetal adipose tissue development. Lancet 1974;2:498.
282. North AF, Mazumdar S, Logrillo VM. Birth weight, gestational age, and perinatal death in 5,471 infants of diabetic mothers. J Pediatr 1977;90:444.
283. Golde S, Platt L. Antepartum testing in diabetes. Clin Obstet Gynecol 1985;28(3):516.
284. Phelan JP. The nonstress test: a review of 3000 tests. Am J Obstet Gynecol 1981;139:7.
285. Freeman RK. Contraction stress testing for primary fetal surveillance in patients at high risk for uteroplacental insufficiency. Clin Perinatol 1982;9:265.
286. Manning FA, Morrison I, Lange IR, et al. Fetal assessment based on fetal biophysical profile scoring: experience in 12,260 referred high-risk pregnancies. Am J Obstet Gynecol 1985; 151:343.
287. Sadovsky E. Fetal movements and fetal health. Semin Perinatol 1981;5:131.
288. Teramo K, Ammala P, Ylinen K, et al. Pathologic fetal heart rate associated with poor metabolic control in diabetic pregnancies. Obstet Gynecol 1983;61:559.
289. Drury MI, Stronge JM, Foley ME, et al. Pregnancy in the diabetic patient: timing and mode of delivery. Obstet Gynecol 1983;62:279.
290. Jovanovic R, Jovanovic L. Obstetric management when normoglycemia is maintained in diabetic pregnant women with vascular compromise. Am J Obstet Gynecol 1984;149:617.
291. Copel JA, Grannum PA, Hobbins JC, et al. Doppler ultrasound in obstetrics. Williams Suppl No. 16. Appleton and Lange, Jan/Feb 1988.
292. Reece EA, Hagay Z, Assimakopoulos E, et al. Diabetes mellitus in pregnancy and the assessment of feto-placental blood flow using pulsed Doppler ultrasonography. I. The umbilical artery. Am J Obstet Gynecol (in press)
293. Landon MB, Gabbe ST, Bruner JP, et al. Doppler umbilical artery velocimetry in pregnancy complicated by insulin-dependent diabetes mellitus. Obstet Gynecol 1989;73(6):961.
294. Usher RM, Allen AC, Maclean FH. Risk of respiratory distress syndrome related to gestational diabetes, route of delivery and maternal diabetes. Am J Obstet Gynecol 1971;111:826.
295. Duhring JL. Discussion on: A modern approach to management of pregnant diabetics. Am J Obstet Gynecol 1977;128:614.
296. Coustan DR. Delivery: timing, mode and management. In: Reece EA, Coustan DR, eds. Diabetes mellitus in pregnancy. Edinburgh: Churchill-Livingstone, 1988:525.
297. Jovanovic L, Druzin M. Peterson C. Effect of euglycemia on the outcome of pregnancy in insulin-dependent women as compared with normal control subjects. Am J Med 1981;71:921.
298. Kitzmiller JL, Cloherty JP, Younger MD, et al. Diabetic pregnancy and perinatal morbidity. Am J Obstet Gynecol 1978;131:560.
299. Roversi GD, Gargiulo M, Nicolini U, et al. A new approach to the treatment of diabetic pregnant women. Am J Obstet Gynecol 1979;135:567.
300. Stronge JM, Foley ME, Drury MI. Diabetes mellitus and pregnancy. New Engl J Med 1986;58:314.
301. Soler NG, Soler SM, Malins JM. Neonatal morbidity among infants of diabetic mothers. Diabetes Care 1978;1:340.
302. Grylack LJ, Chu SS, Scanlon JW. Use of intravenous fluids before cesarean section: effect on perinatal glucose insulin and sodium hemostasis. Obstet Gynecol 1984;63:654.
303. Jovanovic L, Peterson CM. Insulin and glucose requirements during the first stage of labor in insulin-dependent diabetic women. Am J Med 1983;75:605.
304. Golde SH, Good-Anderson B, Montoro M, et al. Insulin requirements during labor: a reappraisal. Am J Obstet Gynecol 1982;144:556.
305. Landon MB, Gabbe SG, Piana R, et al. Neonatal morbidity in pregnancy complicated by diabetes mellitus: predictive value of maternal glycemic profiles. Am J Obstet Gynecol 1987; 156:1089.
306. Kitzmiller JL, Younger MD, Tabatabaii A, et al. Diabetic pregnancy and perinatal morbidity. Am J Obstet Gynecol 1978;131:560.
307. Fallucca F, Gargiulo P, Troili F, et al. Amniotic fluid insulin, c-peptide concentrations, and fetal morbidity in infants of diabetic mothers. Am J Obstet Gynecol 1985;153:534.
308. Engle M, Langan SM, Sanders RL. The effects of insulin and hyperglycemia on surfactant phospholipid biosynthesis in organotypic cultures of type II pneumocytes. Biochem Biophys Acta 1983;753:6.
309. Hertel J, Kühl C. Metabolic adaptations during the neonatal period in infants of diabetic mothers. Acta Endocrinol (Copenh) 1986;277:136.
310. Tsang RC, Ballard J, Colleen B. The infant of the diabetic mother: Today and tomorrow. Clin Obstet Gynecol 1981;24(11):125.
311. Anderson O, Hertel J, Schmølker L, et al. Impact of maternal plasma glucose at deliver on the risk of hypoglycemia of infants of insulin-treated diabetic mothers. Acta Paediatr Scand 1985;74:268.
312. Sperling MA, DeLamater PV, Phelps D, et al. Spontaneous and amino acid-stimulated glucagon secretion in the immediate postnatal period. J Clin Invest 1974;53:1159.
313. Hertel J, Kuhl C, Christensen NJ, et al. Plasma noradrenaline and adrenaline in infants of diabetic mothers: relation to plasma lipids. Acta Paediatr Scand 1985;74:521.
314. Haworth JC, Dilling LA, Vidyasagar D. Hypoglycemia in infants of diabetic mothers. Effect of epinephrine therapy. J Pediatr 1973;82:94.
315. Wu PYK, Modanlou H, Karelitz M. Effect of glucagon on blood glucose homeostasis in infants of diabetic mothers. Acta Paediatr Scand 1975;64:441.
316. Tsang RC, Kleinman L, Sutherland JM, et al. Hypocalcemia in infants of diabetic mothers: studies in Ca, P and Mg metabolism and in parathormone responsiveness. J Pediatr 1972;80:384.
317. Tsang RC, Strub R, Steichen H, et al. Hypomagnesemia in infants of diabetic mothers. Perinatal studies. J Pediatr 1976;89:115.
318. Noaguchi A, Eren M, Tsang RC. Parathyroid hormone in hypocalcemic and normocalcemic infants of diabetic mothers. J Pediatr 1980;97:112.
319. Gamsu HR. Neonatal morbidity in infants of diabetic women. J R Soc Med 1978;71:211.
320. Nichols MM, Laharopoulos P. Thrombosis of superior mesenteric artery in a newborn infant. Am J Dis Child 1969;117:599.
321. Oh W. Neonatal outcome and care. In: Reece EA, Coustan DR, eds. Diabetes mellitus in pregnancy. Edinburgh: Churchill-Livingstone, 1988:547.
322. Nogee L, McMahan M, Witsett JA. Hyaline membrane disease and surfactant protein, SAP-35, in diabetes in pregnancy. Am J Perinatol 1988;5(4):374.
323. Kulovich M, Gluck L. The lung profile. II. Complicated pregnancy. Am J Obstet Gynecol 1979;135:64.
324. Tsai M, Shultz E, Nelson J. Amniotic fluid phosphatidylglycerol in diabetic and control pregnant patients at different gestational lengths. Am J Obstet Gynecol 1984;149:388.
325. Dudley D, Black D. Reliability of lecithin/sphingomyelin ratios in diabetic pregnancy. Obstet Gynecol 1985;66:521.

326. Mimouni F, Miodovnik M, Whitsett JA, et al. Respiratory distress syndrome in infants of diabetic mothers in the 1980s: no direct adverse effect of maternal diabetes with modern management. Obstet Gynecol 1987;69:191.
327. Bourbon JR, Farrell PM. Fetal lung development in the diabetic pregnancy. Pediatr Res 1985;19:253.
328. Saltzman DH, Barbieri RL, Frigoletto FD. Decreased fetal cord prolactin concentration in diabetic pregnancy. Am J Obstet Gynecol 1986;154:1035.
329. Tabash K, Brinkman C, Bashore R. Lecithin/sphingomyelin ratio in pregnancies complicated by insulin-dependent diabetes mellitus. Obstet Gynecol 1982;59:353.
330. Duhring J, Thompson S. Amniotic fluid phospholipid analysis in normal and complicated pregnancies. Am J Obstet Gynecol 1975;121:218.
331. Cruz A, Buhi W, Birk S, et al. Respiratory distress syndrome with mature lecithin/sphingomyelin ratios: diabetes mellitus and low Apgar scores. Am J Obstet Gynecol 1976;126:78.
332. Cunningham M, Desai N, Thompson S, et al. Amniotic fluid phosphatidylglycerol in diabetic pregnancies. Am J Obstet Gynecol 1978;131:719.
333. Ferroni K, Gross T, Sokol R, et al. What affects fetal pulmonary maturation during pregnancy? Am J Obstet Gynecol 1984;150:270.
334. Hallman M, Teramo K. Amniotic fluid phospholipid profile as a predictor of fetal lung maturity in diabetic pregnancies. Obstet Gynecol 1979;54:703.
335. Whittle M, Wilson A, Whitfield C, et al. Amniotic fluid phosphatidylglycerol and lecithin/sphingomyelin ratio in the assessment of fetal lung maturity. Br J Obstet Gynaecol 1982;89:727.
336. Meuller-Beubach E, Caritis SN, Edelstone DI, et al. Lecithin/sphingomyelin ratio in amniotic fluid and its value for the prediction of neonatal respiratory distress syndrome in pregnant diabetic women. Am J Obstet Gynecol 1978;130:28.
337. Cunningham MD, Desai NS, Thompson SA, et al. Amniotic fluid phosphatidylglycerol in diabetic pregnancies. Am J Obstet Gynecol 1978;131:719.
338. Burtos R, Kulovich M, Gluck L, et al. Significance of phosphatidylglycerol in amniotic fluid in complicated pregnancies. Am J Obstet Gynecol 1979;133:899.
339. Dudley DKL, Black DM. Reliability of lecithin/sphingomyelin ratios in diabetic pregnancy. Obstet Gynecol 1985;66:521.
340. Borberg C, Gillmer M, Beard R, et al. Metabolic effects of betasympathomimetic drugs and dexamethasone in normal and diabetic pregnancies. Br J Obstet Gynaecol 1978;85:184.
341. Taylor PM, Wofson JH, Bright NH, et al. Hyperbilirubinemia in infants of diabetic mothers. Biol Neonate 1963;5:289.
342. Gross GP, Hathaway WE, McGaughey HR. Hyperviscosity in the neonate. J Pediatr 1973;82:1004.
343. Poland RL, Odell GB. Physiologic jaundice: the enterohepatic circulation of bilirubin. N Engl J Med 1971;284:1.
344. Whitsett J, Brownscheidle CM. Aspects of placental structure and function in maternal diabetes. In: Merkatz JR, Adam PAJ, eds. The diabetic pregnancy: a perinatal perspective. New York: Grune & Stratton, 1979.
345. Breitweser JA, Meyer RA, Sperling MA, et al. Cardiac septal hypertrophy in hyperinsulinemic infants. J Pediatr 1980; 96:535.
346. Mace S, Hirschfeld SS, Riggs T, et al. Echocardiographic abnormalities in infants of diabetic mothers. J Pediatr 1979;95:1013.
347. Gutgesell HP, Speer ME, Rosenburg HS. Characterization of the cardiomyopathy in infants of diabetic mothers. Circulation 1980;61:441.
348. Leslie J, Shen SC, Strauss L. Hypertrophic cardiomyopathy in a midtrimester fetus born to a diabetic mother. J Pediatr 1982;100:631.
349. Way GL, Wolfe RR, Eshaghpour E, et al. The natural history of hypertrophic cardiomyopathy in infants of diabetic mothers. J Pediatr 1979;95:1020.
350. Reller MD, Tsang RC, Meyer RA, et al. Relationship of prospective diabetes control in pregnancy to neonatal cardiorespiratory function. J Pediatr 1985;106:86.

62

CHAPTER

ENDOCRINE DISORDERS IN PREGNANCY

A. B. Galway and G. N. Burrow

HYPOTHALAMUS AND PITUITARY GLAND

Hypothalamic neuropeptides act directly on the pituitary gland to regulate the biosynthesis, processing, and secretion of its hormones, thereby modulating the endocrine function of the entire body. Although these dynamic relationships remain largely intact during pregnancy, the absolute hormone concentrations change. Functional pituitary integrity is necessary for conception, and pregnancy is uncommon in women with pituitary abnormalities. Hypophysectomized women on full hormone replacement therapy are capable of normal conception, gestation and parturition, indicating that an intact hypothalamic-pituitary axis per se is not required.[1–4] Inadequate treatment of pituitary disorders during pregnancy may result in preterm labor, stillbirth, or neonatal death; therefore, a knowledge of normal physiological relationships is essential to the management of any pregnant woman.

ANATOMY AND HISTOLOGY

The pituitary gland is composed of three lobes—the anterior pituitary (adenohypophysis), the intermediate lobe (pars intermedia), and the posterior pituitary (neurohypophysis). The anterior pituitary comprises the bulk of the gland (75%) and enlarges up to three times during pregnancy.[5,6] There are five cell types in the adenohypophysis that have hormone-secreting capacity: gonadotrophs (luteinizing hormone [LH] and follicle-stimulating hormone [FSH]), lactotrophs (prolactin), thyrotrophs (thyroid-stimulating hormone [TSH]), somatotrophs (growth hormone [GH]), and corticotrophs (adrenocorticotropic hormone [ACTH] and B-lipotrophin [BLPH]). It is the increased cell number and size of lactotrophs that accounts for most of the pituitary enlargement in pregnancy.[5,6] The intermediate lobe of the pituitary occupies a very small area in the adult and has an uncertain role in neuroendocrine function. The neurohypophysis (posterior pituitary) is a direct extension of cell bodies in the hypothalamic supraoptic and paraventricular nuclei responsible for the synthesis and secretion of the hormones oxytocin and vasopressin, and their carrier proteins neurophysin I and II.

PHYSIOLOGIC ADAPTATIONS TO PREGNANCY

Serum prolactin rises during pregnancy secondary to the increasing serum estrogen and progesterone concentrations. Levels increase from approximately 20 ng/mL at 5 to 8 weeks gestation to up to 200 to 400 ng/mL at term (Fig. 62-1).[7–12] The normal circadian rhythm of nocturnal rise in prolactin release is sustained during pregnancy, despite the elevated levels.[13] At parturition an acute decrease occurs, followed by a postpartum increase lasting 1 to 3 weeks in nonlactating women.[14] Menses resume after normalization of prolactin levels, expected by 4 to 6 months postpartum. A failure of menstrual periods to return by this time in a nonlactating mother may indicate underlying pathology such as a pituitary prolactinoma, primary hypothyroidism, or Sheehan's syndrome (pituitary necrosis).[15,16] Hypothalamic control of pituitary prolactin release is exerted by the inhibiting factor dopamine and the stimulating factor thyrotropin-releasing hormone (TRH). The physiologic significance of the TRH–prolactin interaction, however, remains unclear. During pregnancy, a normal or enhanced prolactin response to TRH or antidopaminergic agents occurs—contrary to the blunted responses seen in pathologic states of hyperprolactinemia.[17–21]

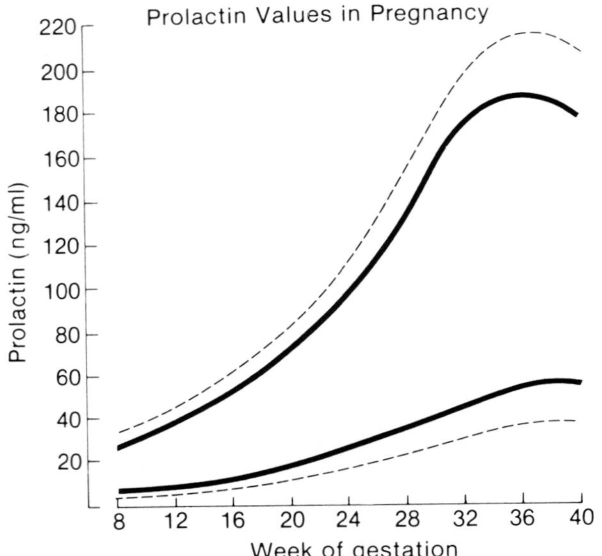

FIGURE 62–1. Prolactin values in pregnancy (10th and 90th percentiles in solid lines, range in broken lines). (From Biswas S, Rodeck CH. Plasma prolactin levels during pregnancy. Br J Obstet Gynaecol 1976; 83: 683.)

The gonadotrophins, luteinizing hormone (LH), and follicle-stimulating hormone (FSH) are suppressed from very early in pregnancy, and by mid-pregnancy do not respond normally to exogenous gonadotropin-releasing hormone (GnRH) (Fig. 62-2).[22–27] This blunted or absent response to GnRH is presumably due to a feedback inhibitory effect of the high circulating estrogen and progesterone levels.[28] Postpartum levels return gradually, with FSH occurring earliest, at 2 to 3 weeks. As prolactin levels decline to non-pregnant levels in nonlactating women, a rise in estradiol occurs, with an accompanying increase in plasma LH.[27,29]

Although basal growth hormone concentrations remain comparable to the non-pregnant state, a blunted rise of growth hormone to the usual physiologic stimuli is noted during the third trimester.[30–32] Thus, impaired responses to insulin-induced hypoglycemia and 1-argininine infusion are observed.[33–35] Because attempted stimulation of growth hormone secretion by hypoglycemia is undesirable in pregnancy, use of growth hormone-releasing hormone (GHRH) is probably the best choice, if absolutely necessary. For screening purposes, a plasma growth hormone can be determined 60 to 90 minutes after nocturnal sleep or 20 minutes after vigorous exercise. Concentrations greater than 5 ng/mL are expected and therefore make further testing unnecessary. The rise of human placental lactogen and cortisol during pregnancy may be responsible for the blunted growth hormone release observed.[36,37]

Hypothalamic TRH controls pituitary TSH release which, in turn, stimulates the biosynthesis and secretion of thyroxine (T4) and triiodothyronine (T3) from the thyroid gland. TSH levels are slightly decreased during the first trimester and return to normal during the second and third trimesters.[38,39] This may be explained by the high levels of human chorionic gonadotropin (hCG) early in pregnancy (Fig. 62-3).[38] hCG may interact with and activate the TSH receptor when present at such high concentrations, owing to the common alpha subunit structure.[40] Although increased TSH responses to TRH have been reported in some women between 16 and 20 weeks of pregnancy, many women demonstrate TSH responses comparable to the non-pregnant state.[18,41,42] Despite these alterations, normal levels of free thyroid hormones are usually evident throughout gestation, although variations within the normal range have been reported.[38,39,43]

Adrenocorticotrophic hormone (ACTH) is derived from a larger precursor hormone—pro-opiomelanocortin (POMC)—following exposure to hypothalamic corticotropin-releasing hormone (CRF). ACTH, in turn, stimulates adrenal steroidogenesis, resulting in production of glucocorticoids, sex steroids, and mineralocorticoids. ACTH concentrations rise during pregnancy despite the concomitant rise of free cortisol; furthermore, ACTH itself may be incompletely suppressed following exogenous glucocorticoid administration.[44–47] The failure of cortisol to suppress the high levels of ACTH may be explained by the elevated progesterone concentrations occurring simultaneously. Progesterone binding to intracellular receptors may compete with cortisol, and thereby render the pituitary relatively insensitive to negative feedback by cortisol.[48,49]

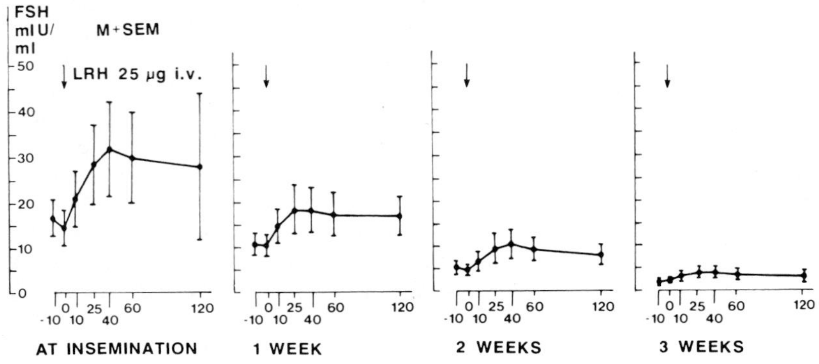

FIGURE 62–2. Effects of 25 μg of luteinizing hormone-releasing hormone (LHRH or GnRH) given intravenously on basal levels of FSH in four women during pregnancy. Each woman was tested on the day of insemination and then once a week. Data are mean ± SEM. (From Jeppsson S, Rannevik G, Liedholm P, Tharell JI. Basal and LRH-stimulated secretion of FSH during early pregnancy. Am J Obstet Gynecol 1977; 127: 32.)

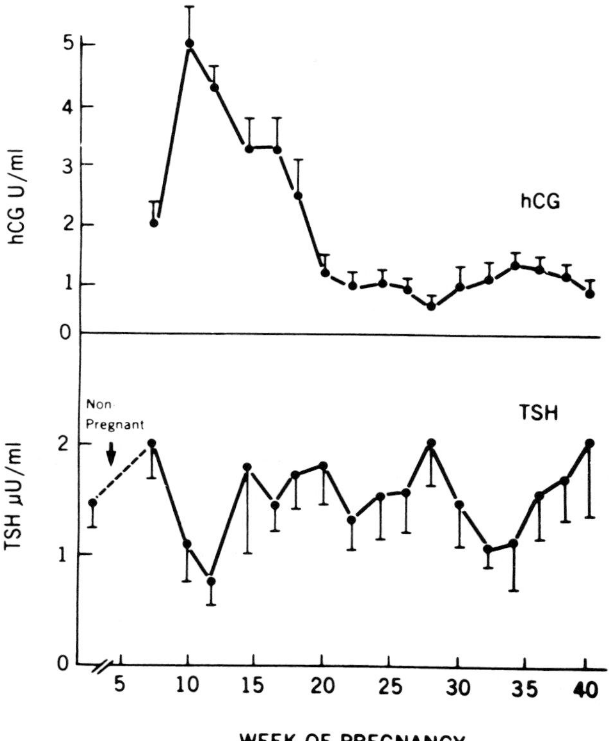

FIGURE 62–3. Serum hTSH and hCG concentrations during pregnancy. Non-pregnant control values are at left. Values are based on samples obtained from 339 women; each point represents mean ± SEM. (From Harada A, Hershman JM, Reed AW, et al. Comparison of thyroid stimulators and thyroid hormone concentrations in the sera of pregnant women. J Clin Endocrinol Metab 1979; 48: 793.)

The posterior pituitary hormones oxytocin and vasopressin (antidiuretic hormone) are normally released from cell bodies in the hypothalamic supraoptic and paraventricular nuclei, along with their carrier proteins, neurophysin I and II. These hormones travel along axons to nerve terminals in the medial eminence and posterior pituitary, where they await release following exposure to the appropriate physiologic stimuli. The plasma levels of neurophysins are elevated during pregnancy, apparently because of the increased estrogen concentrations.[50,51] Vasopressin release is regulated by changes in either blood osmolarity or volume, with a normal set point of 285 mOsm/kg. During pregnancy, a decrease in the set point for osmoregulation occurs, such that the normal plasma osmolarity is 5 to 10 mOsm/kg lower than during the non-pregnant state.[52,53] There is a concomitant rise in plasma volume and a decline in serum sodium during normal pregnancy.[54] Despite these alterations of basal hormone secretion, normal dynamic feedback interactions exist with suppression of vasopressin upon water loading and stimulation with water deprivation.[53] These tests are not recommended during pregnancy. Oxytocin is released in response to suckling and thereby mediates myoepithelial reflex contraction with milk let-down. Oxytocin levels increase in maternal plasma during pregnancy from approximately 10 pg/mL at the end of the second month to about 74 pg/mL at 38 weeks gestation.[55] A further rise to approximately 124 pg/mL occurs during the second stage of labor, although it is unclear how essential this is to normal labor progression.[56,57] Hypophysectomized women may have spontaneous normal labor, albeit sometimes delayed in onset.[58,59]

PATHOPHYSIOLOGY

Disorders resulting in either hyperfunction or hypofunction of the pituitary gland may occur during pregnancy—most commonly hyperprolactinemia secondary to a pituitary microadenoma, or panhypopituitarism from postpartum ischemic necrosis (Sheehan's syndrome). Pituitary tumors may involve any of the five cell types normally present in the pituitary. These may be microadenomas (<10 mm in size) or macroadenomas (>10 mm). Macroadenomas, by virtue of their compressive effects on the surrounding nontumorous pituitary gland, may impair the remainder of pituitary function while hypersecreting one or more hormones. Microadenomas, in contrast, are usually unassociated with hypopituitarism.

DISORDERS OF HYPERSECRETION

Prolactin-secreting microadenomas are the most common pituitary tumors (40%) and are often associated with the syndrome of amenorrhea and galactorrhea. The elevation of prolactin that occurs with adenomatous tissue is often below 200 ng/mL for microadenomas and above 250 ng/mL for macroadenomas.[60] Furthermore, pathological hyperprolactinemia is associated with loss of the normal circadian pattern of prolactin release, resulting in sustained levels throughout the day and night.[61] During normal pregnancy, the nocturnal rise of prolactin still occurs, albeit higher than in the non-pregnant state.[12,13] The infertility that occurs in about one third of affected women is largely a result of impaired GnRH pulsatile secretion.[62,63] A direct ovarian inhibitory effect of prolactin may also contribute. The dopamine agonist bromocriptine will restore ovulatory cycles in over 80% of such women.[64] Its use has been approved for ovulation induction in the presence of either a microadenoma (<1 cm size) or a macroadenoma (>1 cm size) confined to the sella turcica. Macroadenomas with suprasellar expansion should, however, probably be treated surgically prior to attempted pregnancy. Bromocriptine is the only dopamine agonist currently marketed in the United States. The usual adult oral dose of bromocriptine is 1.25 mg every 12 hours starting with an initial dose of 1.25 mg at bedtime. Total doses up to 30 mg per day have been administered to less responsive tumors. Longer-acting dopamine agonist preparations are also under investigation; these include injectable forms (Parlodel LA), as well as oral preparations (pergolide mesylate).[65,66] At least one study revealed promising results with pergolide treatment, showing more stable lower prolactin levels and fewer side effects than bromocriptine.[66] Other classes of compounds (the synthetic 8-alpha-amino ergolines) are also under investigation for potentially fewer side effects and longer durations of action.[67] There is a risk of tumor expansion during pregnancy secondary to the rising estrogen and progesterone levels—1.6% for microadenomas and 15.5% for macroadenomas.[68] Therefore, patients who become pregnant should be carefully followed by monthly visual field examinations by Goldman perimetry. Symptoms or signs of expansion, such as headaches, blurred vision, visual field or funduscopic changes, should be investigated with an imaging examination, preferably magnetic resonance imaging (MRI). Bromocriptine crosses the placenta and should be discontinued as soon as possible after conception has occurred and reinstated only with evidence of tumor expansion. Large numbers of women have successfully undergone pregnancy with normal outcomes while receiving bromocriptine throughout gestation, but long-term studies have not yet been performed.[69–76] Postpartum suckling does not further increase prolactin secretion in the presence of a prolactinoma and is not significantly associated with risks of tumor expansion.[77] Therefore, patients who wish to breast-feed should not be discouraged from doing so. Eventually, postpartum nonlactating mothers should have the bromocriptine resumed, because chronic hyperprolactinemia is associated with hypoestrogenism and its attendant risks of bone loss.

Growth hormone hypersecretion is usually secondary to a pituitary macroadenoma and results in the syndrome of acromegaly with its attendant bony overgrowth, visceromegaly, and hyperhidrosis. Hypertension and impaired glucose tolerance are often manifest, further complicating the success of pregnancy occurring simultaneously. Acromegaly is also associated with infertility via impaired pulsatile gonadotropin secretion and the hyperprolactinemia (<100 ng/mL) that may occur in 50% of patients.[78,79] Therefore, pregnancy is uncommon in this disease. When it does occur, growth hormone levels are elevated (>7 ng/mL) and inadequately suppressed following an oral glucose tolerance test (normal suppression <2 ng/mL). Growth hormone does not cross the placenta, and therefore high maternal levels do not disrupt the fetal hypothalamic–pituitary axis. Pregnancy has also been reported in acromegaly after treatment with bromocriptine, which suppresses the secretion of biologically active growth hormone in some patients.[72,80] The treatment modality chosen—medical or surgical—depends on associated symptoms, with surgery recommended when visual changes or headaches suggest tumor expansion. Although bromocriptine may lower growth hormone levels in up to 50% of patients, it usually has minimal impact on tumor size.[81–83] If bromocriptine is chosen, it can be continued until fetal lung maturation is assured, at which time induction of labor may be performed if necessary.

DISORDERS OF HYPOSECRETION

Impaired pituitary hormone secretion may result from space-occupying lesions, head trauma, ischemic damage, or as a sequel to surgery or irradiation. Syndromes of hypopituitarism uniquely associated with pregnancy include lymphocytic hypophysitis and Sheehan's syndrome.

Lymphocytic hypophysitis is an autoimmune disorder associated with pituitary enlargement and functional insufficiency. There have been several case reports of women with apparent pituitary tumors who were found to have lymphocytic hypophysitis on biopsy. In about half of the cases, the disease was detected in the postpartum period, and in two cases the onset was during gestation.[84] This disorder occurs with increased frequency in association with multiple autoimmune glandular disease (diabetes mellitus, Hashimoto's thyroiditis, hypoparathyroidism), raising the possibility that it may be related to changes in autoimmunity during pregnancy and the postpartum period. The resultant inflammation may mimic a pituitary adenoma, and should be suspected with appearance of pituitary enlargement more than normal for pregnancy.

Before clinical manifestations of pituitary hypofunction become evident, about three quarters of the entire pituitary must be destroyed. The most common cause of anterior pituitary insufficiency in the adult woman is Sheehan's syndrome.[16] This syndrome of postpartum pituitary necrosis is associated with postpartum hemorrhage; however, cases with minimal known blood loss have been described. It is presumably the hypersensitive pituitary of pregnancy with its increased size and vascular demand that accounts for this unique association, because this syndrome is distinctly uncommon in other conditions associated with shock and vascular collapse. Patients may follow a predictable pattern of hormone loss with consecutive loss of gonadotropins, growth hormone, TSH, and ACTH. Only rarely does the functional impairment approach that seen with large macroadenomas; in fact, approximately 50% of women may resume menses and lactate normally postpartum.[85] Thirty-nine pregnancies have occurred after the onset of hypopituitarism in 19 women with Sheehan's syndrome.[86] Of these women, eight were able to conceive without hormonal therapy. Furthermore, patients have been known to develop impaired anterior pituitary function following a subsequent uncomplicated pregnancy.

Posterior pituitary involvement is distinctly uncommon in this disorder. An increased risk of pituitary necrosis also occurs in diabetics, heralded by a deep midline headache and falling insulin requirements in the third trimester.[87,88] Investigation of suspected patients should include dynamic testing of pituitary reserve, because normal baseline hormone levels will not exclude the diagnosis. Combined anterior pituitary function testing with the hypothalamic releasing factors GnRH, TRH, GHRH, and CRF provides a thorough approach (Fig. 62-4).[89–92] Treatment with replacement doses of adrenal glucocorticoids (cortisone acetate 20 to 25 mg each morning and 10 to 12.5 mg each evening) and thyroid hormone (L-thyroxine 0.1 to 0.15 mg per day) is usually adequate to maintain well-being. It is important to recognize that increased cortisol requirements occur during intercurrent illness or stress, such as infection, surgery, or labor. Furthermore, when hormone replacement is initially begun, the glucocorticoid administration should be started before thyroid hormone in order to avoid precipitation of hypoadrenal crisis. Estrogen replacement is also recommended for hypogonadotrophic women, who may eventually have exogenous gonadotropin induction of ovulation when pregnancy is desired. There do not appear to be any ill effects of growth hormone deficiency, other than a slightly greater risk of hypoglycemia during pregnancy. It is not recommended that growth hormone be replaced in these patients. Sexually ateliotic dwarfs have no growth hormone, nor may their offspring in utero. In such cases, not only the birth weight, but also the birth length, is normal.[93] There is speculation that human placental lactogen takes over the role of growth hormone in these cases.

Diabetes insipidus (DI), which may be either centrally or peripherally mediated, occurs when there is either insufficient secretion or action of the hormone vasopressin. Central loss of vasopressin secretion may occur with space-occupying lesions, head trauma, surgery or, rarely, genetic disease (autosomal dominant in <1% of all cases). About one third of all patients have an idiopathic type for which no definite cause can be found. One type of peripheral DI uniquely associated with pregnancy that has been described is mediated by an increase in the enzyme vasopressinase (possibly placental), resulting in enhanced breakdown of vasopressin.[94] Patients with diabetes insipidus typically complain of polyuria and polydipsia, and have urine specific gravity levels less than 1.005. The diagnosis is established by standard tests of water deprivation that reveal a failure to concentrate urine to levels above plasma osmolarity. These tests are not, however, recommended during pregnancy. A return toward normal following exogenous administration of vasopressin usually occurs in central diabetes insipidus. Treatment is best accomplished with 1-desamino-8-d-arginine vasopressin (DDAVP), a synthetic analog of vasopressin.[95] This drug can be administered either intranasally (for daily maintenance) or parenterally when intranasal administration is not practical. The usual intranasal dose is 5 to 20 μg per nostril twice daily. The onset of effect occurs within 1 hour and lasts 6 to 20 hours. The vasopressinase-mediated DI of pregnancy will also respond to the preparation DDAVP, but is typically unsuccessfully treated with arginine vasopressin (AVP) due to enzyme-mediated inactivation.

DI is of particular interest during pregnancy because of the relation to the other neurohypophyseal hormone oxytocin. There is no substantial evidence to suggest that labor is inadequate in women with central DI.[96] Indeed, direct measurement of oxytocin in one pregnant woman with diabetes insipidus demonstrated a surge of oxytocin during labor.[97] Patients with DI have no impairment of fertility, and pregnancy is not adversely affected by the disease. Although vasopressin may cause uterine contractions, there have been no consistent reports of abortion or premature labor. DDAVP does have decreased pressor activity compared to vasopressin itself, and therefore can be used safely during pregnancy.

THYROID GLAND

Thyroid disorders are the most common endocrinopathies encountered during pregnancy—both hyperthyroidism and hypothyroidism are five to ten times more common in women than in men. The symptoms of hy-

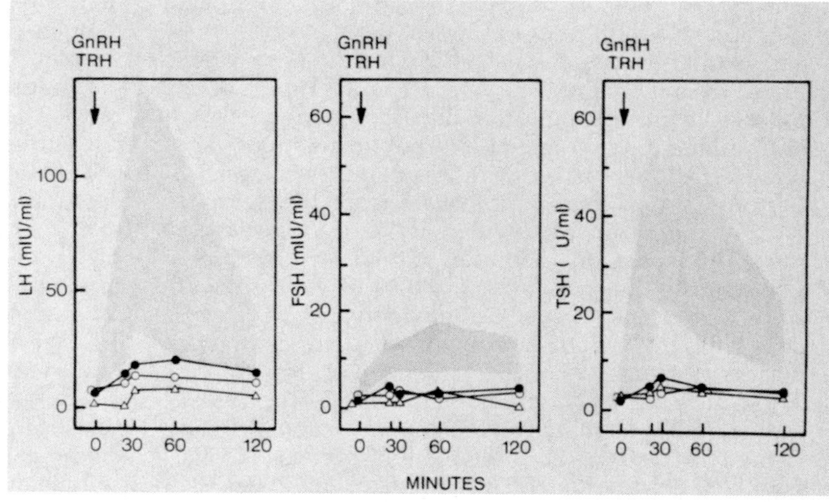

FIGURE 62–4. Luteinizing hormone FSH and TSH responses to GnRH-TRH administration in control subjects (shaded area) and in three patients with Sheehan's syndrome. (From Dizerega G, Kletzky DA, Mishell DR. Diagnosis of Sheehan's syndrome using a sequential pituitary stimulation test. Am J Obstet Gynecol 1978; 132: 348.)

perthyroidism may mimic the normal hypermetabolic state of pregnancy, and therefore a high index of suspicion is necessary to make the diagnosis. This is further complicated by the altered thyroid function tests that occur during normal pregnancy—most notably, a rise in thyroxine-binding globulin and total thyroxine levels. The free thyroid hormone levels remain normal, however, and therefore a state of euthyroidism state exists. Treatment of thyroid disorders is complicated by the presence of the fetus, because pharmacologic therapy beneficial to the mother may be harmful to the fetal thyroid. A knowledge of both normal and abnormal thyroid physiology will aid treatment of these affected women.

ANATOMY

The normal adult thyroid gland weighs 15 g to 20 g and is comprised of two encapsulated lateral lobes as well as a variably present pyramidal lobe extending superiorly in the midline. Embryological development begins as a pouch in the pharyngeal floor, which becomes the thyroglossal duct during its descent through the neck. Ultimately, the thyroid becomes a bilobar structure that sits on the thyroid cartilage just inferior to the cricoid cartilage. Aberrant descent of the thyroid may result in appearance of tissue anywhere from the base of the tongue (lingual) to a substernal location adjacent to the thymus. The thyroid gland is palpable in many normal individuals, with a smooth surface and soft texture. Goitrous enlargement of the thyroid may be associated with a euthyroid, hyperthyroid, or hypothyroid state. The thyroid gland may enlarge during pregnancy due to relative deficiency of iodine, a phenomenon that is distributed geographically in accordance with dietary intake of iodine.

PHYSIOLOGY IN THE NON-PREGNANT STATE

The biosynthesis of the thyroid hormones—thyroxine (T4) and triiodothyronine (T3)—involves a series of reactions that involve the colloidal glycoprotein prohormone, thyroglobulin. Iodine uptake and trapping occur followed by its organification (incorporation) into tyrosine residues on thyroglobulin. Coupling of mono- and diiodotyrosines ensues with resultant formation of thyronines, and finally proteolysis leads to release of both T4 and T3 into the circulation. The thyroid gland is the only source of T4 under normal circumstances, whereas the majority (70% to 80%) of T3 is derived from peripheral tissue deiodination of T4 by 5′ de-iodinase.[98,99] Both hormones circulate bound to plasma proteins—99.97% for T4 and 99.9% for T3. These include thyroid-binding globulin (TBG), thyroxine-binding prealbumin (TBPA), and albumin. Although T4 binds to all three binding proteins, T3 has very little avidity for TBPA, binding primarily to TBG and albumin.[100] Overall, approximately 85% of thyroid hormone is transported in serum bound TBG, and 15% by TBPA. TBG is the major binding protein, and its production is increased in the presence of high estrogen levels, such as during pregnancy.[101]

PHYSIOLOGIC ADAPTATIONS TO PREGNANCY

An increased glomerular filtration rate during pregnancy results in an early rise in renal iodine clearance and a subsequent decrease in the plasma inorganic iodine concentration.[102] The thyroid responds by increasing its uptake of iodine and thus usually maintains euthyroid levels of thyroid hormone production. Dietary iodine may therefore be limiting in certain geographic locations, and result in formation of an iodine-deficient goiter. In a study done in Scotland, 70% of pregnant women were diagnosed as having a goiter in contrast to 38% of non-pregnant women.[103] Previous pregnancies did not appear to affect this incidence, because goiters were found in 39% of nulliparous women and 35% of non-pregnant parous women. These investigators subsequently failed to find increased incidence of goiter during pregnancy in Iceland[104]; other investigators have not found this phenomenon in the United States.[105] These geographic variations can be explained on the basis of dietary iodine intake and resultant plasma iodine concentrations. Iodine-deficient goiter is unlikely to occur at plasma iodine concentrations above 0.08 μg/100 mL.[106] Residents of North America or Iceland have plasma inorganic iodine concentrations of approximately 0.30 μg/100 mL, whereas most Europeans have levels ranging from 0.10 to 0.15 μg/100 mL.[107] Supplemental iodine in order to achieve an intake of 250 μg/day is recommended during pregnancy and easily attained with prenatal vitamin supplements. Care must be taken to avoid excessive intake (>2000 μg/day), because this may also be harmful to the mother and fetus.

A rise of thyroxine-binding globulin (TBG) to approximately twice normal occurs during pregnancy, from 12 to 30 μg/L to 30 to 50 μg/L, measured by radioimmunoassay.[108] This increase reflects increased hepatic biosynthesis secondary to estrogenic stimulation.[109] Because approximately 85% of thyroid hormone circulates are bound to TBG, an increased total T4 and T3 will occur. Despite the rising total thyroid hormone levels, free thyroid hormone concentrations remain normal.[38,39,43] The contribution of the increased TBG to the high total thyroxine levels in pregnancy has been studied by examining pregnant patients with partial or total TBG deficiency.[110] In these women a rise in total T4 does not occur, confirming that this elevation is secondary to the rising TBG in normal pregnancy.

The basal metabolic rate (BMR) slowly increases from the fourth month of pregnancy, primarily due to increasing uterine demands.[111] Measurement of the BMR is difficult and impractical, because separation from total metabolism—including oxygen consumption from digestive and muscular activity—is necessary.

LABORATORY INVESTIGATIONS

Radioiodine Thyroid Uptake

The thyroid radioiodine uptake test is contraindicated during pregnancy, because radioisotopes cross the placenta and may be concentrated in the fetal thyroid (after 10 weeks gestation).[112] However, when inadvertently done, the uptake is usually increased, largely due to the reduced plasma iodine pool.[113] Despite the elevated uptake, limited reports suggest that normal suppression by T3 occurs.

Thyroid Hormones

The rise of TBG that occurs during pregnancy can be measured directly by radioimmunoassay. Indirect methods of its estimation, although imperfect, are readily available. The T3 uptake test (RT_3U) measures uptake of exogenous ^{123}I-T3 by a binding resin, such that higher serum TBG levels result in a decreased ^{123}I-T3 resin uptake, and lower TBG levels have opposite effects. Thus, the RT_3U is lower during pregnancy than non-pregnancy and tends to be in the hypothyroid range (Fig. 62-5). This test does not always accurately reflect absolute levels of TBG, because other serum proteins may affect the binding of ^{123}I-T3 to the resin, and thus result in misinterpretation of TBG levels. T4 and T3 concentrations measured by radioimmunoassay measure the total T4 and T3 (bound plus free fractions) and are therefore elevated during pregnancy (Fig. 62-6). Despite this, levels of free thyroid hormones are usually within the normal range.[43] An indirect estimate of free hormone concentrations may be made by determination of the free thyroxine index (FT_4I) $= T4 \times RT_3U/100$. However, due to failure of the RT_3U test to accurately determine TBG concentrations, this estimate may not provide a true index of free T4 levels. In most cases, however, a normal FT_4I and TSH level will exclude significant underlying thyroid pathology. More accurate determination of free T4 and T3 may be made with tracer amounts of ^{125}I-T4 and equilibrium dialysis of the patient's serum. A percentage of dialyzable fraction is found and, when multiplied by the serum thyroxine determination, yields the free thyroxine concentration. This method is the only direct method of determination of thyroid functions that accounts for alterations in TBG levels and capacity, but it is technically difficult to perform. Another method of determination of free thyroxine concentration using the kinetics of binding to glass beads has been developed, but this procedure may prove inaccurate due to altered binding in the presence of elevated TBG concentrations, depending on the particular test.[114]

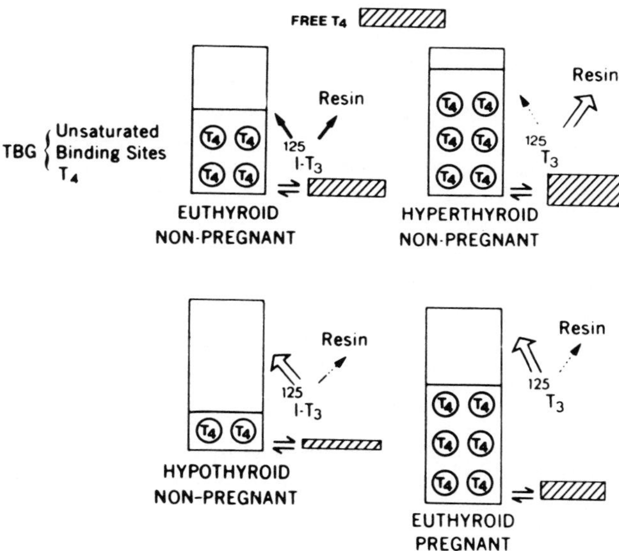

FIGURE 62–5. Resin triiodothyronine uptake. The clear area represents the unsaturated binding sites on thyroid-binding globulin (TBG). In a hypothyroid non-pregnant woman, there is less bound thyroid hormone and more available binding sites. Conversely, in hypothyroidism there are fewer unsaturated binding sites, and more ^{125}-T3 binds to the resin. In a pregnant woman, the increase in TBG results in an increase in bound thyroid hormone, but there are also an increased number of unsaturated binding sites compared to the non-pregnant state, and less ^{125}-T3 binds to the resin. (From Burrow GN. Thyroid diseases. In: Meier A, ed. Medical complications during pregnancy. Philadelphia: WB Saunders, 1988: 227.)

Hypothalamic–Pituitary–Thyroid Axis

The TRH test is performed by injecting 200 to 400 μg TRH intravenously and monitoring the change in TSH

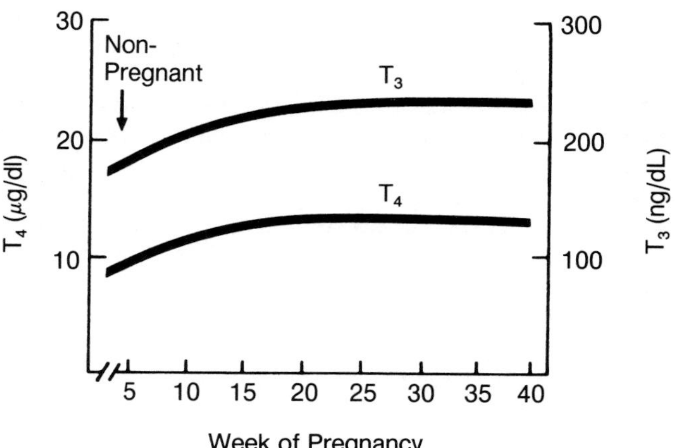

FIGURE 62–6. Serum thyroid hormone concentrations increase during pregnancy. Serum T4 and T3 are expressed in different units. (From Burrow GN. Thyroid diseases. In: Meier A, ed. Medical complications during pregnancy. Philadelphia: WB Saunders, 1988: 227.)

20 and 60 minutes after injection. TRH crosses the placenta when administered in such pharmacologic doses, and may affect the fetal pituitary–thyroid axis. This test is therefore not recommended in pregnancy. Traditionally, the TRH test was performed to elucidate the presence of primary hyperthyroidism, where a blunted or absent TSH response occurs. The newer, more sensitive TSH assays are capable of differentiating normal from suppressed levels, and therefore should replace the TRH test as the best mode to diagnose hyperthyroidism in pregnancy.[115] TSH levels are largely unchanged by normal pregnancy (minimal decrease in the first trimester),[38,39] and the suppression that occurs with primary hyperthyroidism during pregnancy will be detectable by a sensitive TSH assay. Conventional TSH radioimmunoassays exhibit a normal range of 1 to 2 μU/mL up to 6 μU/mL, with up to 20% of random samples from normal subjects failing to yield detectable levels. In contrast, the newer assays exhibit a normal range of 0.3 to 6 μU/mL, with values below 0.1 μU/mL commonly encountered in hyperthyroidism. A useful rule is to suspect the presence of hyperthyroidism in pregnancy if the RT_3U is normal for the non-pregnant state. A T4 >14 μg/100 mL or T3 >250 ng/100 mL should also raise suspicion. In such cases, the sensitive TSH assay should be used. In fact, this assay may turn out to be useful in screening for thyroid disease during pregnancy.

Thyroid Autoantibodies

Thyroid-stimulating immunoglobulins may be detectable in the serum of women with either active or inactive Graves' disease (hyperthyroidism). These antibodies may cross the placenta and rarely (1%) induce a state of fetal or neonatal thyrotoxicosis.[116] Thus, determination of the levels of these stimulating immunoglobulins (TSI) is recommended in women with evidence of past or present Graves' disease, especially in the presence of fetal tachycardia greater than 140 beats per minute. The recent cloning of the TSH receptor may give rise to accurate TSI assays.[117] Antimicrosomal and antithyroglobulin antibodies may also be elevated in certain forms of thyroiditis, although deleterious fetal effects have only rarely been described. The levels of maternal thyroid autoantibodies tend to decline as pregnancy advances, and thus it is not uncommon to see amelioration of the thyroid hyperfunction with advancing gestation.[118,119]

PLACENTAL–FETAL THYROID PHYSIOLOGY

The placenta is relatively impermeable to the thyroid hormones T4 and T3 as well as TSH; hence fetal thyroid function is independent of maternal influences under normal circumstances.[120] The placenta contains deiodinase enzymes that degrade T4 and T3, and this may account for the failure of these hormones to cross from the maternal to fetal circulation in an active form. Hyperthyroidism due to maternal Graves' disease may, however, result in fetal hyperthyroidism due to the placental transfer of thyroid-stimulating immunoglobulins. Furthermore, drugs used in treatment of such hyperfunction (thiouracils, propranolol, iodine) readily cross the placenta and may thus impair fetal thyroid function. Placental hCG, which shares a common alpha subunit with TSH,[40] has a weak thyroid-stimulating capacity and may therefore account for minimal thyroid stimulation early in pregnancy, when its endogenous levels are high (Fig. 62-3).[38] When hCG levels are abnormally high, as in trophoblast disease, frank hyperthyroidism may rarely occur. Levels of 300,000 mIU/mL hCG are necessary to induce clinical hyperthyroidism.[121–123] hCG has an activity in the TSH bioassay of 0.2 μU TSH/μ hCG.[38]

Fetal Thyroid Function

The human fetal thyroid gland is capable of concentrating iodine by the 10th to 12th week of gestation, at which time TSH can be detected in the fetal pituitary and TRH in the hypothalamus. Serum TSH is first detectable in fetal serum at 10 weeks of age, and progressively rises from 20 to 30 weeks, reaching a peak of 15 μU/mL. Thereafter, levels decline to approximately 7 μU/mL.[124] Fetal serum total T4 concentrations increase, secondary to the rising TSH concentrations, from 2 to 3 μg/100 mL at 10 weeks to 5 to 10 μg/mL at 30 weeks. After 30 weeks the T4 level continues to increase despite declining TSH levels.[125] The reciprocal relationship of serum free T4 and TSH in the normal fetus after 30 weeks suggests that the fetal hypothalamic–pituitary–thyroid axis is fully operational then. Total and free serum T3 levels are very low prior to 28 to 30 weeks, and although a rise occurs thereafter during gestation, the absolute levels remain well below adult values through labor and delivery. However, high levels of reverse T3 (rT3) are present in fetal serum after 28 weeks. At parturition, fetal thyroid function undergoes profound alterations, with a marked rise in TSH from 7.5 μU/mL to 30 μU/mL within 3 hours (Fig. 62-7).[126,127] A surge in T3 > T4 then occurs in the neonatal serum, reaching a maximum by 24 hours and returning toward baseline by the end of the first week of life.[128] Neonatal radioactive iodine uptake by the thyroid is elevated at 10 hours postpartum, reaching a peak by day 2 and returning toward adult normal limits by day 5 of life.[129]

Amniotic Fluid

During the first half of pregnancy, amniotic fluid thyroid hormone concentrations increase progressively, reaching peak concentrations at 25 to 30 weeks, although levels of thyroxine are higher and rise more rapidly than triiodothyronine (Fig. 62-8).[130] During the latter half of pregnancy, the T4 levels decrease while T3 levels continue to increase. Reverse T3 concentrations are also elevated in the amniotic fluid, reaching peak

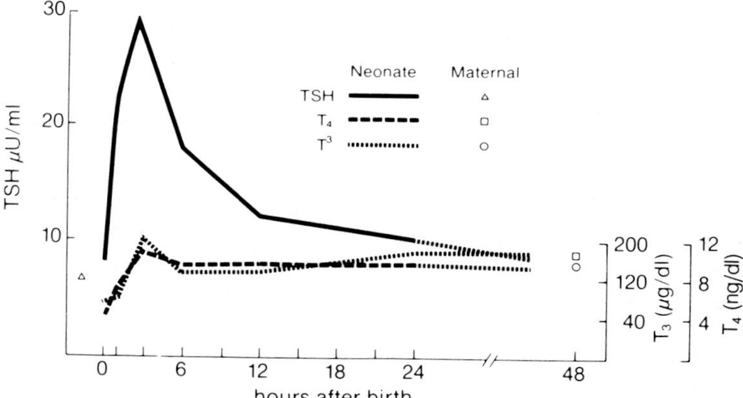

FIGURE 62–7. Serum (TSH), thyroid-stimulating hormone T4 and T3 concentrations during the first 48 hours in the neonate. (From Stubbe P, Gatz J, Heidemann P, Muhlen A, Hesch R. Thyroxine-binding globulin, triiodothyroxine, thyroxine and thyrotropin in newborn infants and children. Horm Metab Res 1978; 19: 58.)

levels at 17 to 20 weeks. Although the source of these thyroid hormones may be the fetus, the absolute levels of amniotic fluid thyroid hormones does not necessarily correlate with fetal thyroid status. For this reason, it is necessary to be cautious when diagnosing fetal thyroid dysfunction on this basis. Treatment of fetal thyroid hypofunction has been successfully performed by administration of thyroxine directly into the amniotic fluid, although this procedure is unpredictable with respect to thyroid hormone exposure to the fetus.[131,132]

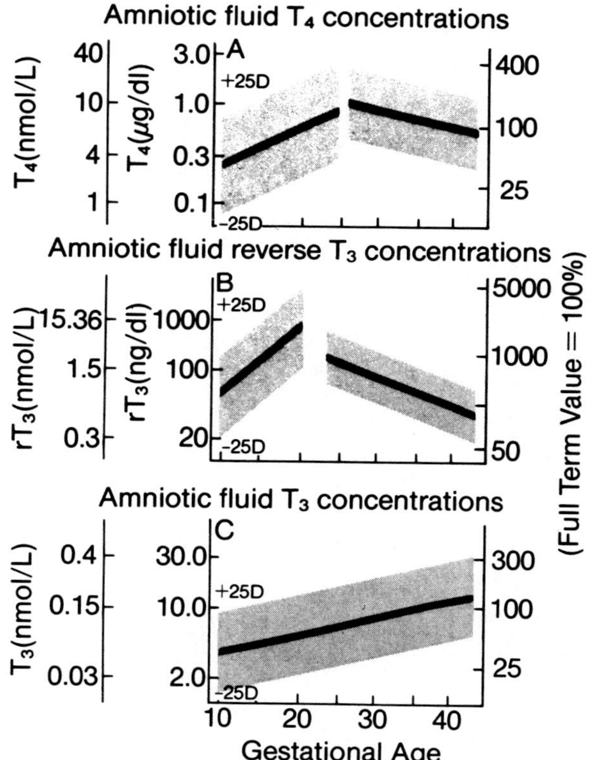

FIGURE 62–8. Amniotic fluid T4, T3, and reverse T3 concentrations during pregnancy. (**A**) Amniotic fluid T4 concentrations. The vertical axis on the left is a logarithmic scale of standard concentrations, and the one on the right is the percentage of the term mean value ± 2 SD calculated form the regression lines, which are also plotted. (**B**) Amniotic fluid reverse T3 concentrations plotted in the same manner. (**C**) Amniotic fluid T3 concentrations plotted in the same manner. (From Klein AH, Murphy BEP, Artal R, Oddie TH, Fisher DA. Amniotic fluid thyroid hormone concentration during human gestation. Am J Obstet Gynecol 1980; 136: 626.)

DISORDERS OF HYPOSECRETION

Maternal Hypothyroidism

Although decreased thyroid function is not rare in women of reproductive age, its association with pregnancy is unusual.[133] This most likely stems from the amenorrhea, menorrhagia, and anovulatory cycles, which frequently coexist and thus impair fertility.[134,135] Hypothyroidism may be primary, with failure of the thyroid gland itself or secondary to loss of pituitary TSH stimulation. The latter usually occurs with either space-occupying lesions, such as macroadenomas and craniopharyngiomas, or ischemic necrosis. Primary hypothyroidism is much more common, and usually results from Hashimoto's thyroiditis, idiopathic myxedema, or ^{131}I ablation of the thyroid gland. Idiopathic myxedema is insidious in onset and related to Hashimoto's thyroiditis. An interesting association has been noted in that mothers of children with Down syndrome have sometimes been found to have high titers of thyroid antibodies.[136] It has been suggested that maternal thyroid autoimmunity predisposes to aneuploidy and thus may be involved in the pathogenesis of Down syndrome in younger mothers. Hashimoto's thyroiditis is more common in patients with diabetes mellitus and other autoimmune disorders, such as Addison's disease, pernicious anemia, vitiligo, hypoparathyroidism, and chronic active hepatitis. Cold intolerance, fatigability, constipation, dry skin, and weight gain accompany hypothyroidism in both the pregnant and nonpregnant state. Paresthesias are an early symptom in about 75% of patients. The thyroid gland is enlarged, firm, nontender, and bosselated (irregular) in Hashimoto's thyroiditis, whereas in idiopathic myxedema it is markedly atrophic and therefore impalpable. Physical examination may otherwise reveal a delayed relaxation phase of the deep tendon reflexes and, less commonly, frank myxedema with periorbital edema and vocal cord thickening may be observed.

Diagnosis. The laboratory diagnosis of primary hypothyroidism rests on the demonstration of an elevated serum TSH concentration, usually in association with a lower serum T4 concentration. As TBG levels are elevated during pregnancy, the total T4 may remain within normal limits for the non-pregnant state. The corrected T4 (determined by the free T4 index) may be decreased in these cases. Thyroid antimicrosomal and antithyroglobulin antibodies may be elevated, and further substantiate autoimmune destruction of the thyroid gland.

Course. Hypothyroid women who are inadequately treated during pregnancy have higher risks of spontaneous abortion, stillbirth, and abnormal offspring, with congenital defects and developmental retardation in some cases.[137,138] Because maternal thyroid hormones and TSH do not cross the placenta in significant amounts, the fetal pituitary–thyroid axis develops normally under these circumstances. Any thyroid hormone necessary for fetal growth before the onset of fetal thyroid hormone secretion in the second trimester must come from the maternal side, and in severely hypothyroid mothers this hormone would be lacking. Although the offspring have not been subjected to extensive developmental testing, they have been reported as normal.[135]

TREATMENT

As soon as the diagnosis of primary hypothyroidism is established, L-thyroxine should be instituted in full replacement doses. Most patients require 125 to 150 μg per day of oral levothyroxine. The normal steady state production of T4 by the thyroid gland in pregnancy is 80 μg/day, and expected absorption of 50% to 75% of exogenous thyroxine should result in physiological levels. Follow-up determination of serum TSH levels every 3 weeks should reveal levels <6 μU/mL, and T4 concentrations should also return to the normal range for pregnancy. If the values are still abnormal, the dose of L-thyroxine should be increased by 50 μg increments. It is usually unnecessary to adjust the dose for the remainder of gestation once euthyroid levels have been achieved.

Congenital and Neonatal Hypothyroidism

Most infants with congenital hypothyroidism appear clinically normal at birth, although thyroid hormone deficiency during the fetal and neonatal periods may be associated with developmental retardation.[139] The severity of associated abnormalities depends, in part, on the time of occurrence and degree of thyroid hormone deficiency. If hypothyroidism is diagnosed and treated before 3 months of age, four fifths of affected children will have an intelligence quotient (IQ) above 90. Appearance of hypothyroidism after 2 years of age appears to have minimal effect on mental development.

Etiology. The most common cause of congenital primary sporadic hypothyroidism is thyroid dysgenesis, occurring approximately once in every 4000 births (Table 62-1). In this condition, about two thirds of children have ectopic thyroids and one third have complete thyroid agenesis.[140] This disorder has a hereditary predisposition, and it is speculated that thyrotoxic factors are transferred across the placenta in some affected infants.[141–143] Uncommon causes of hypothyroidism in utero include inborn errors of thyroid hormone biosynthesis transmitted as an autosomal recessive trait, iodine-induced hypothyroidism, and pituitary TSH deficiency.

Diagnosis. Cretinism is a syndrome of severe mental retardation, abnormal growth, deaf-mutism, spasticity, strabismus, and abnormal sexual maturation secondary to iodine deficiency occurring in utero. It occurs with higher frequency in regions of endemic goiter, such as the South American Andes, New Guinea, and Central Africa. Other causes of hypothyroidism are usually not apparent at birth, but may be associated with umbilical hernia, a large posterior fontanel, dry skin, hypothermia, constipation, and respiratory difficulties. A high index of suspicion will prevent many of the irreversible sequelae, if left untreated. Laboratory findings include a low serum T4 (<4 μg/100 mL) with a high TSH (>80 μU/mL), which should be determined after the peak TSH surge that normally occurs at 24 hours of life (Fig. 62-7). Infants with borderline T4 (4–7 μg/100 mL) or TSH levels (20 to 80 μU/mL) require further testing with TRH. An ^{123}I uptake and thyroid scan can be performed to investigate the presence of either ectopic thyroid tissue or inborn errors of thyroid hormone synthesis. Bone age determination may reveal the decreased maturation associated with deficiency of thyroid hormone. In particular, the lack of ossification of the distal femoral epiphysis suggests fetal hypothyroidism.

Treatment. Replacement therapy should begin as soon as the diagnosis of hypothyroidism is made in the neonatal period. The usual initial dose is 10 μg/kg per day of oral thyroxine as a single dose, which is then adjusted to maintain the serum T4 levels within the normal range (8 to 12 μg/100 mL). Bone age should be

TABLE 62–1. ETIOLOGY AND INCIDENCE OF CONGENITAL HYPOTHYROIDISM

Primary hypothyroidism	
Thyroid dysgenesis	1 in 4,000
Inborn errors of thyroid function	1 in 30,000
Drug-induced	1 in 10,000
Endemic hypothyroidism	1 in 7
Secondary and tertiary hypothyroidism	1 in 60,000

closely followed for signs of either excessive or inadequate thyroxine treatment. The requirements gradually decrease to approximately 5 μg/kg at the age of 12 months. At this time, cessation of thyroxine may be attempted with close follow-up of thyroid function tests. Although intra-amniotic administration of thyroid hormone has been successfully attempted for treatment of hypothyroidism in utero, it is difficult to determine the exact absorption and hence appropriate dose.[131,132,144]

DISORDERS OF HYPERSECRETION

Maternal Thyrotoxicosis

Although there is an increased incidence of menstrual irregularities in thyrotoxic patients, it is evident that women who suffer from mild hyperthyroidism may become pregnant. Indeed, there is no proof that fertility is impaired in mild to moderate hyperthyroidism. The incidence of thyrotoxicosis during pregnancy is approximately 0.2%, with most women (95%) suffering from Graves' disease.[138,145] Other causes of primary hyperthyroidism include toxic multinodular goiter (Plummer's disease), toxic uninodular goiter, subacute thyroiditis and, very rarely, metastatic follicular cancer. Ectopic sources of thyroid hormone excess exclusively associated with pregnancy include trophoblastic tumors and hydatiform moles. These gestational tumors should be considered when thyrotoxicosis first appears early in pregnancy, although they usually cause biochemical rather than clinical hyperthyroidism.

Symptoms and Signs. The clinical features of hyperthyroidism may closely mimic the normal pregnant state, because both conditions are associated with a hyperdynamic state. Heat intolerance, increased appetite, increased cardiac output with systolic flow murmurs and widened pulse pressure, skin warmth, and resting tachycardia occur in normal pregnancy. A resting heart rate above 100 beats per minute, which does not slow with the Valsalva maneuver, increases the suspicion of concurrent thyrotoxicosis. Other features specific to Graves' disease may include infiltrative eye signs (proptosis, disordered movement) and pretibial myxedema, although these signs do not necessarily indicate that thyrotoxicosis per se is present. Thyrotoxicosis during pregnancy may also present with hyperemesis gravidarum, resulting in rapid weight loss early in pregnancy.[146–148] This generally resolves following successful treatment of the hyperthyroidism.

Diagnosis. Hyperthyroidism during pregnancy may be confirmed by the finding of elevated free T4 hormone level. The newer, more sensitive TSH assays, if available, provide the best test for confirmation of hyperthyroidism where values are often below 0.1 μU/mL.[115] This may be directly measured by either equilibrium dialysis or nonequilibrium dialysis methods, or indirectly estimated by measuring the free T4 index. Serum T4 levels above 15 μg/dL coincident with RT_3U values within the euthyroid or hypothyroid nonpregnant range are likely to occur in hyperthyroidism. The free T3 index = T4 × $RT_3U/100$ is usually elevated in such cases. Unfortunately, because of elevated TBG in pregnancy, the free thyroxine index is not an accurate measure of the actual free thyroxine concentration.[149] Occasionally the free T4 or free T4 index are normal when the T3 is elevated—so-called T3 toxicosis. This is more likely to occur with a toxic nodular goiter, and should be excluded if thyrotoxic symptoms are present with normal T4 values. Furthermore, determination of thyroid autoantibodies (especially thyroid-stimulating immunoglobulins) are important when Graves' disease is suspected, because high levels may warn of increased fetal risk. Ectopic sources of thyroid hormone excess (through hCG stimulation from gestational tumors) may be excluded by determination of hCG, which would be inappropriately elevated for the gestational age.[38]

Course. Untreated hyperthyroidism does not increase maternal mortality unless preeclampsia occurs, although there is an increase in neonatal morbidity (low birth weight, congenital malformations) and mortality in some reports.[138,150–151] Down syndrome has also been reported to occur more frequently in the offspring of thyrotoxic mothers, but these studies were not well-controlled.[152] There is no evidence that pregnancy makes hyperthyroidism more difficult to control; in fact, the severity of Graves' disease tends to decrease as pregnancy progresses. Furthermore, postpartum exacerbations can occur within weeks, presumably due to increasing thyroid-stimulating immunoglobulin (TSI) levels. It is speculated that rising fetal T-cell suppressor function during pregnancy and the subsequent decline postpartum results in parallel changes in TSI, and hence disease activity.[153]

Treatment. Therapeutic intervention is recommended in all but the mildest forms of hyperthyroidism during pregnancy. Because radioactive iodine is contraindicated, treatment usually involves either antithyroid drugs (thionamides) or surgery. If pregnancy occurs after onset of thionamide treatment, the medication should be continued and thyroid hormone levels closely monitored.

The thionamide drugs propylthiouracil (PTU) and methimazole inhibit iodination of tyrosine and hence decrease thyroid hormone biosynthesis. PTU also decreases the peripheral conversion of T4 and T3, and this further enhances its efficacy in treatment. Methimazole has been reported to cause aplasia cutis (scalp) in some offspring, and therefore is contraindicated in pregnancy (Fig. 62-9).[154–156] Because PTU inhibits formation of new thyroid hormone, but does not prevent release of previously formed hormone, its effect is slow in onset and requires 4 to 6 weeks to achieve a maximal effect. The dose of PTU should start at 100 to 150 mg three times daily, but may require 200 mg three times per day. Once clinical and biochemical improvement are evident, the dose should be decreased to 50 mg four times per day. If the patient remains euthyroid, the PTU could be decreased to 50 mg three times per day after 3 weeks. With monthly determination of the T4 level, the goal should be a serum level in the range of upper normal at a dose of less than 100 mg per day of PTU if possible.[157] If thyrotoxicosis recurs, the PTU should again be increased to 300 mg per day. This should be especially noted in the postpartum period.

COMPLICATIONS OF PTU

Approximately 2% of patients taking PTU will experience a mild, occasionally purpuric, skin rash, usually within the first 4 weeks of therapy. If this occurs, PTU should be stopped and may be replaced with methimazole. Pruritus, drug fever, and nausea may also occur in a small number of patients. More serious complications include the blood dyscrasias—leukopenia and agranulocytosis. Agranulocytosis usually occurs after 4 to 8 weeks of therapy in approximately 0.3% of those treated, leading to a fatal outcome in less than 1 of 10,000 treated patients. The development of agranulocytosis should be treated with cessation of PTU (and no substitution with methimazole or other thioamides), and surveillance cultures should be obtained. Antibiotic therapy should be administered if signs of infection coexist.

Antithyroid drugs cross the placenta and may block thyroid hormone biosynthesis in the fetal gland (Fig. 62-10).[158] The resultant rise in fetal TSH may result in goiter formation.[159] When treatment is closely monitored to avoid excessive dosing, there does not appear to be any impairment of intellectual function in these children.[156] Approximately 1% to 5% of children exposed to PTU develop transient hypothyroidism; usually sufficient maternal thyroid hormone crosses the placenta to prevent fetal goiter. Furthermore, because fetal loss is markedly reduced by treatment of maternal hyperthyroidism, and the long-term risks to offspring exposed in utero to propylthiouracil are minimal, these drugs should be the first line of treatment of thyrotoxicosis. Thionamides are secreted in breast milk, although in sufficiently small amounts to have little effect on neonatal thyroid function.[160,161] It appears that the amount of propylthiouracil transferred to the suckling infant is less than the amount of methimazole, although in each case a small theoretical risk of neonatal drug reaction still exists. In any case, if a mother desires to breast feed, it is recommended that close monitoring of neonatal thyroid function be performed.

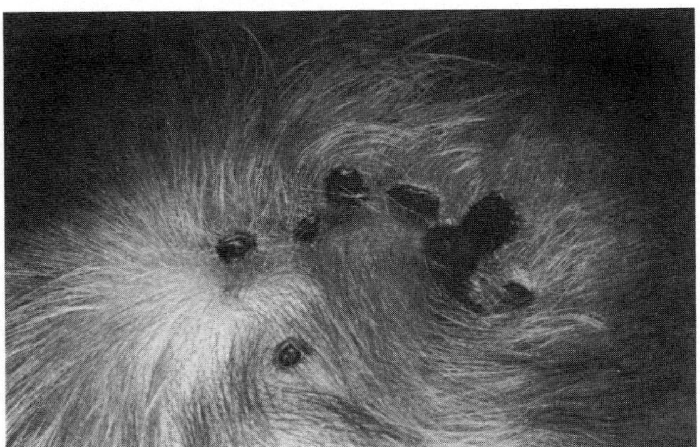

FIGURE 62–9. Aplasia cutis in a child whose mother had received methimazole. (From Mujtaba Q, Burrow GN. Treatment of hyperthyroidism in pregnancy with propylthiouracil and methimazole. Obstet Gynecol 1975; 46: 282.)

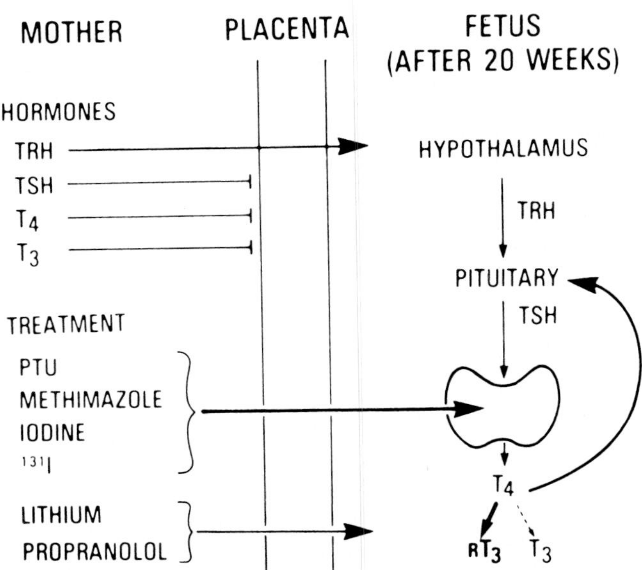

FIGURE 62–10. Maternal–fetal thyroid relationships at 20 weeks of gestation. The fetus has an autonomous hypothalamic–pituitary thyroid endocrine system. (From Hollingsworth D. Endocrine disorders. In: Hollingsworth DR, Resnik R, eds. Medical counseling before pregnancy. New York: Churchill-Livingstone, 1988: 334.)

SEVERE HYPERTHYROIDISM

Addition of the beta-blocking drug propranolol to thionamide therapy may be considered in cases where hyperthyroidism is severe. Although reports of intrauterine growth retardation, small placental size, and neonatal bradycardia, hypoglycemia, and respiratory depression have been associated with maternal beta-blocker ingestion,[162–164] other investigators have reported successful outcomes.[165,166] The recommended oral dose of propranolol is 40 mg every 6 hours. Cardioselective beta-blockers such as atenolol may also be used (50 to 100 mg per day), although a clear advantage over propranolol has not been demonstrated.

Iodide treatment may also be instituted for not more than 1 week, because iodides readily cross the placenta and impair fetal thyroid function. It seems justifiable to use them only when temporary measures of control are necessary, such as preoperative preparation where subtotal thyroidectomy is planned or in cases of thyroid storm. The recommended dose of five drops of Lugol's solution twice daily represents 100 mg of iodide and far surpasses the amount necessary to block fetal thyroid function (12 mg). This dose, however, is necessary to adequately inhibit maternal iodide uptake and thyroid hormone secretion.

THYROID STORM

This dramatic presentation of hyperthyroidism leads to a clinical picture of fever, dehydration, and cardiac decompensation, and has a mortality rate as high as 25%. An underlying cause should be sought and treated in order to gain control of the hyperthyroid state. Often, an infection or surgery may be the precipitating event, especially in a previously undiagnosed individual. Prompt treatment with intravenous fluids (losses may be as high as 5 L), oxygen, antipyretics, and antithyroid drugs are necessary. Propylthiouracil 400 mg orally every 8 hours or methimazole 30 to 40 mg via rectal suppository every 8 hours should be initiated. PTU is preferred because of its peripheral inhibition of T4 conversion to T3, an effect that is not mediated by methimazole. Sodium iodide 1 g intravenously in 500 mL of fluid may be administered once every 24 hours during the critical disease phase. This will sufficiently block thyroid hormone secretion. Lithium 300 mg orally every 8 hours will also block thyroid hormone secretion. Propranolol 40 mg orally every 6 hours should be administered, unless cardiac failure is present. Intravenous administration of small doses of 1 to 2 mg may be used if necessary, but should be done only with cardiac monitoring. Dexamethasone 2 mg orally or intramuscularly every 6 hours will block peripheral conversion of T4 to T3. Hypothermia treatment for malignant hyperthermia may rarely be necessary in addition to acetaminophen, the preferred antipyretic.[167] Aspirin is not recommended, because it can increase the percent of free T4 and theoretically worsen the hyperthyroid state. Plasma exchange has been successfully used in life-threatening situations during pregnancy, such as severe Rh isoimmunization without harm to the fetus.[168] It has also been used along with antithyroid drugs in three pregnant hyperthyroid women,[169] and thus remains a potential therapy in cases where hyperthyroidism is refractory to the standard treatment.

SURGERY

Although medical treatment with thionamides is considered to be the mainstay of treatment for hyperthyroidism occurring during pregnancy, occasional patients may become surgical candidates. Large doses of antithyroid drugs (PTU 300 to 600 mg per day) may impair fetal thyroid function, and if such requirements continue throughout gestation, surgery may be recommended. Patient compliance should be considered when such apparent drug resistance is present. Serious complications of thionamide use, such as agranulocytosis, may also lead to surgical management of hyperthyroidism during pregnancy. Surgery does have risks whether performed during pregnancy or not and, although relatively uncommon, these complications are quite significant. When surgery is deemed necessary, it seems reasonable to continue thionamides until surgery is performed, if the patient is not experiencing side effects from their use. Further preoperative disease control may be attained by the use of propranolol 40 mg orally every 6 hours and Lugol's solution (iodide) 3 to 5 drops twice daily for a maximum of 1 week. Iodides reduce the vascularity of the thyroid gland and thereby may make surgery easier, in addition to their beneficial inhibitory effect on thyroid hormone secretion. When surgery is required, it seems best to perform a subtotal thyroidectomy after medical disease control has been established. Although the risk of spontaneous abortion is greatest during the first trimester, it is reasonable to perform surgery during the first trimester when absolutely necessary. Ideally, however, surgery is best done during the second trimester. Reports of satisfactory surgical outcomes exist for all trimesters.[170–172] However, the usual complications of thyroid surgery still exist during pregnancy. These include rarely a postoperative life-threatening hematoma, and an approximate 1% risk of recurrent laryngeal nerve damage or hypoparathyroidism. Thyroid hormone replacement (0.125 to 0.2 mg orally of daily L-thyroxine) should be begun immediately on detection of subnormal thyroid hormone levels, which should be followed closely postoperatively (every 3 weeks).

RADIOACTIVE IODINE

Although radioactive iodine (I^{131}) ablation of the thyroid is a therapeutic option in treatment of hyperthyroidism in the non-pregnant state, it is never considered justifiable to use radioactive isotopes of iodine for either diagnostic or therapeutic use during pregnancy. The fetal thyroid will concentrate I^{131} after the 10th to 12th week of gestation, and therefore any radioactive iodine administered after that time is expected to result in congenital hypothyroidism. If a patient is given I^{131} treatment for hyperthyroidism and discovered within 1 week of administration to be 10 or more weeks pregnant, then propylthiouracil 100 mg orally every 8 hours for 10 days is recommended to block recycling of the radioactive iodine within the fetal thyroid. Inadvertent maternal exposure to a thyroid scan of I^{123} or a pertechnetate exposes the fetal thyroid to approximately 5 to 20 mrad, whereas maternal treatment with 5 to 10 mCi I^{131} for hyperthyroidism exposes the fetal thyroid to 0.75 to 1.5 rads.[173,174] The amount of exposure experienced with scanning is much less severe, and does not require intervention with PTU. Fetal tissues are more radiosensitive than maternal tissues and complications such as microcephaly, mental retardation, and malignancies have been described in children irradiated in utero.[175–177] These serious complications usually are associated with doses much higher than that experienced following I^{131} treatment of hyperthyroidism, and therefore pregnancy termination need not necessarily be recommended.

Fetal and Neonatal Thyrotoxicosis

Etiology. Transplacental passage of thyroid-stimulating immunoglobulins (TSI) in mothers with either active or apparently inactive Graves' disease may rarely result in fetal thyrotoxicosis.[178–180] This disease entity may first become evident in women who have had thyroid ablation with either surgery or I^{131} and continue to have circulating TSI, and then present with either fetal tachycardia (>160 beats per minute) or intrauterine growth retardation (IUGR). This paradox is important to remember and emphasizes the need to monitor closely all women with past or present Graves' disease with TSI levels if possible. Neonatal thyrotoxicosis also results from maternal TSIs, but usually in the setting of maternal PTU ingestion. When the PTU is withdrawn at birth, the neonate remains under the influence of the abnormal circulating TSIs. Although the half-life of these abnormal stimulating antibodies is 4 to 10 days, disease activity may continue up to 2 to 3 months.[181,182] The incidence of neonatal thyrotoxicosis is approximately 1% of all pregnant patients with Graves' disease.[183]

Symptoms and Signs. Fetal tachycardia (>160 beats per minute) and IUGR are typical manifestations of intrauterine thyrotoxicosis. Neonatal thyrotoxicosis may be evident at birth with jaundice, tremulousness, diarrhea, tachycardia (>200 beats per minute), cardiac failure, hepatosplenomegaly, goiter, and eye signs of Graves' disease. However, when maternal PTU treatment has been used, the neonate may not demonstrate clinical signs of thyrotoxicosis until 2 to 14 days after birth. This is because the continued effects of maternal PTU in the newborn's circulation take up to 2 weeks to subside. Both males and females are affected equally with this disorder, in contrast to the striking female predominance of adult Graves' disease.[183] There are, however, a small number of cases of true congenital Graves' disease, which does have a female predisposition and is transmitted as an autosomal dominant trait.

Diagnosis. The diagnosis of fetal thyrotoxicosis must be made based on strong clinical suspicion in the presence of maternal Graves' disease. Ideally, elevated circulating maternal TSI levels are detected, but these assays are not always readily available and may take several weeks to get results. Neonatal thyrotoxicosis likewise rests on strong likelihood when faced with the typical constellation of symptoms and signs. Elevated serum thyroxine will confirm the diagnosis, but it must be remembered that both T4 and T3 are elevated in the normal neonate up to 5 days of life.

Course. The mortality of this disease is high, approaching 15% to 25% in spite of treatment.[184,185] For those infants who survive, the disease is usually transient, lasting up to 2 to 3 months. Neonatal thyrotoxicosis may result in long-term complications, such as craniosynostosis and minimal brain dysfunction.[184]

Treatment. PTU in doses of 50 to 100 mg orally daily administered to the mother may ameliorate fetal thyrotoxicosis. The dose may be adjusted based on the fetal heart rate. Neonatal thyrotoxicosis should be treated with Lugol's iodide 1 drop orally every 8 hours (1 mg every 8 hours) and propranolol 2 mg/kg orally daily in divided doses if the disease severity is such that intervention is required. Additional measures include PTU 5 to 10 mg/kg per day in divided doses and digitalis if heart failure is present.

Disordered Hyper- and Hyposecretion—Postpartum Thyroiditis

Postpartum autoimmune thyroiditis is a disorder known to occur in approximately 5.5% of women.[186,187] It may present initially with symptoms of hyperthyroidism occurring 3 to 6 months after delivery and lasting typically 1 to 3 months. The subsequent hypothyroid phase is also transient, lasting usually up to 3 months as well. Patients may have a history of painless goiter prior to pregnancy, unassociated with the systemic symptoms typically accompanying subacute (de Quervain's) thyroiditis. The underlying disease is thought to be autoimmune in nature, with lymphocytic thyroid infiltration and high titers of thyroid autoantibodies.[187] The diagnosis may be established by finding an elevated serum thyroxine level in the presence of a low thyroid radioiodine uptake (1% to 2% or less at 24 hours), which contrasts with the elevated uptake seen with Graves' disease (>30%). A woman who is breast feeding should stop for 5 days after the test (and discard the pumped breast milk during this time) and then may safely resume. Treatment of postpartum thyroiditis depends largely on the stage and severity of the disease. Mild hyperthyroidism may be treated with propranolol, and hypothyroidism with L-thyroxine replacement. Spontaneous recovery occurs 90% of the time, although the disease tends to recur in future pregnancies.

Thyroid Cancer

The occurrence of thyroid cancer in 15% to 20% of single thyroid nodules means that investigation and treatment of all such nodules is warranted during pregnancy. Features such as hardness and associated lymphadenopathy, histories of previous head and neck irradiation or familial multiple endocrine neoplasia, or rapid growth all increase the likelihood that a nodule is malignant. In any event, a fine needle aspiration biopsy of the nodule is necessary, and if cytologic diagnosis of malignancy is made, surgical resection is recommended. A benign lesion should be suppressed with L-thyroxine 0.2 mg orally daily for the remainder of pregnancy. Thyroid scanning should not be performed during pregnancy.

There is no evidence that pregnancy alters the natural course of thyroid carcinoma, and women previously treated for this disease may become pregnant without apparent sequelae.[188,189] Furthermore, there is no evidence that benign lesions are affected adversely by the pregnant state.

ADRENAL GLAND

Adrenal glucocorticoids are essential for survival, and disordered production has profound effects on the mother or her fetus. Maternal disease is most commonly found at the hypothalamic–pituitary level (ACTH), whereas fetal and neonatal disruption usually involves impaired adrenal steroidogenesis. Fortunately, adrenal diseases are not common during pregnancy, and when they do occur a high index of suspicion is necessary. Laboratory investigations are complicated by the normal rise of both ACTH and free cortisol known to occur in pregnancy. A precise knowledge of adrenal function during pregnancy is necessary for satisfactory management of disease.

ANATOMY AND HISTOLOGY

The adult adrenals are subdivided into an outer cortex and inner medulla, each with different embryonic origins. The cortex is further divided into three zones: the zona glomerulosa, zona fasciculata, and zona reticularis (outer, middle, and inner), each of which secrete different classes of steroid hormones. The zona glomerulosa secretes aldosterone and other mineralocorticoids, the zona fasciculata primarily secretes cortisol and other glucocorticoid intermediates, and the zona reticularis is responsible for sex steroid production. The adrenal medulla is derived from chromaffin cells and secretes the hormones norepinephrine and epinephrine. The cortical zona fasciculata is the only portion of the adult adrenal that enlarges during pregnancy, although overall gland weight does not significantly increase over the non-pregnant weight (5 g).[190]

PHYSIOLOGY IN THE NON-PREGNANT STATE

Glucocorticoids

The normal adrenal gland responds to episodic pituitary ACTH release in a diurnal manner, such that cortisol secretion is highest in the early morning and lowest in the late evening hours. Presumably, this variation in ACTH release reflects a similar pattern of hypothalamic CRF secretion. The mechanism whereby ACTH stimulates the adrenal to produce glucocorticoids first involves stimulation of adenylcyclase, with subsequent production of cAMP and thereby activated cAMP-dependent protein kinase. Ultimately, the enzymes cholesterol ester hydrolase (which mobilizes cholesterol from the cytoplasmic lipid storage sites) and cholesterol side-chain cleavage enzyme (a cytochrome P450 enzyme that allows formation of pregnenolone) are phosphorylated by cAMP-dependent protein kinase, and hence activated. Once formed, pregnenolone becomes a substrate for 3-β-hydroxylation to progesterone, and subsequent 17, 21, and 11 hydroxylations yield cortisol. Pregnenolone may also directly become 17-hydroxylated prior to conversion by 3-β-hydroxysteroid dehydrogenase to 17-hydroxyprogesterone, which is then 21- and 11-hydroxylated to cortisol as well. Each step of biosynthesis is regulated by ACTH, which enhances the activity of essential enzymes in the steroidogenic pathway.

Cortisol circulates primarily in a bound form, with 70% bound to cortisol-binding globulin and approximately 20% to albumin, but with lower affinity. Between 5% to 10% of cortisol remains unbound and physiologically active in a nonstressed individual. Metabolites of cortisol are derived primarily from reducing reactions, and are generally conjugated with either glucuronic acid or sulfate prior to urinary excretion.

Mineralocorticoids

The main hormonal product of the zona glomerulosa is aldosterone, a mineralocorticoid that is regulated by the renin–angiotensin axis. ACTH can stimulate aldosterone production, but this response is minimal under normal circumstances. Renin is a product of cells in the juxtaglomerular apparatus of the kidney and is secreted in response to volume depletion or hypotension. It subsequently converts the α-2-globulin angiotensinogen to angiotensin I. Angiotensin I is acted on by the ubiquitous antiotensin-converting enzyme to become angiotensin II. This hormone is responsible for general vasoconstriction as well as stimulation of aldosterone secretion. Aldosterone in turn stimulates renal sodium reabsorption and potassium losses, and thereby reexpands plasma volume and raises blood pressure.

PHYSIOLOGIC ADAPTATIONS TO PREGNANCY

Glucocorticoids

A rise of both total (bound) and free (unbound) cortisol occurs during normal pregnancy. The cortisol-binding globulin (CBG) level rises steadily to reach levels that stabilize at approximately twice the upper limit of normal by the end of the second trimester (Figs. 62-11 and 62-12).[191,192] This rise in CBG results in a prolonged circulating half-life of cortisol in maternal plasma,[193] an effect that can be mimicked by estrogen administration to non-pregnant women.[194] Furthermore, the maternal cortisol production rate more than doubles and may thereby partly account for the higher maternal free cortisol that occurs simultaneously. In spite of these elevations of bound and free cortisol, a normal diurnal secretion remains, in contrast to the persistently elevated levels without diurnal variation typically seen in pathologic states of hypercortisolism.[195,196] ACTH secretion also tends to be elevated during pregnancy, although varied reports of increased or decreased levels exist depending on the assay method used.[44–46] It is generally believed that a state of clinical hypercortisolism does not exist, in spite of the elevated ACTH and free cortisol levels. This may be explained in part by the coincident elevated progesterone levels, which may compete with cortisol for intracellular binding sites, and thereby render the pituitary relatively insensitive to the expected inhibitory effects of the high circulating cortisol levels. In addition, this theoretical diminished intracellular cortisol binding would reduce expected peripheral signs of true hypercortisolism. This explanation, however, remains to be conclusively demonstrated. A further explanation for the high ACTH levels may be a placental source of this peptide, which remains unresponsive to the inhibitory effects of peripheral cortisol concentrations.[197]

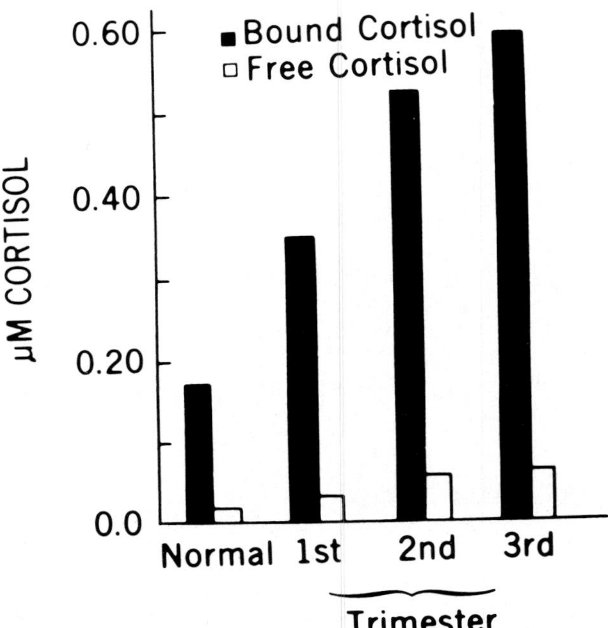

FIGURE 62–12. Free and bound cortisol concentrations during pregnancy. (From Rosenthal HE, Slaunwhite WR, Sandberg AA. Transcortin: a corticosteroid-binding protein of plasma. X: cortisol and progesterone interplay and unbound levels of these steroids in pregnancy. J Clin Endocrinol Metab 1969; 29: 352.)

Mineralocorticoids

The renin–angiotensin–aldosterone axis is activated during pregnancy, and levels of all three hormones increase from early gestation. Renin levels peak at approximately the end of the first trimester, reaching levels twice that of the non-pregnant state.[198,199] The site of this renin production remains unclear, and it is possible that a uterine source is responsible.[200] A simultaneous increase of both angiotensin II and aldosterone occurs, reaching values several-fold higher than before pregnancy by the third trimester.[199,201] By this time, renin levels are declining, possibly in response to these high angiotensin II and aldosterone levels. In spite of the high mineralocorticoid levels during this stage of gestation, normal electrolytes are maintained. It is the high progesterone levels, which have endogenous antialdosterone effects, that protect from inordinate losses of potassium.[202,203] Furthermore, blood pressure is actually lower during pregnancy than postpartum, suggesting that factors other than the absolute levels of these hormones are important. The mineralocorticoid deoxycorticosterone (DOC), formed from corticosterone by 21 hydroxylation, is increased during pregnancy.[204] The peripheral tissues have an estrogen-stimulated 21-hydroxylase, which is responsible for this increased production.[205,206] In spite of these high levels, however, DOC has minimal apparent effect on sodium retention. It has been suggested that maternal sulfotransferase activity also increases during pregnancy, and the resultant DOC-sulfate has less activity.

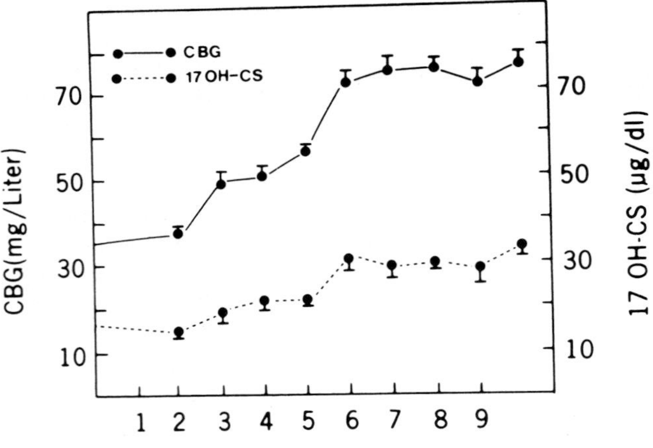

FIGURE 62–11. Cortisol-binding globulin concentration during pregnancy. (From Doe RP, Fernandez R, Seal US. Measurement of corticosteroid binding globulin in man. J Clin Endocrinol Metab 1964; 24: 1029.)

Sex Steroids

Pregnancy is associated with a rise in sex hormone-binding globulin, secondary to the elevated estrogen concentrations. A rise of total serum testosterone occurs because of the higher percentage of bound hormone.[207,208] The percentage of free testosterone is therefore reduced. Androstenedione also rises during normal pregnancy, providing an increased substrate for estrogen production. In contrast, the plasma levels of dehydroepiandrosterone (DHEA) do not normally increase in maternal serum, and in fact the levels of DHEA-sulfate actually decline. Both of these hormones are important substrates for maternal production of estrogen.[209–212]

LABORATORY INVESTIGATIONS

Basal Hormone Determination (Glucocorticoids)

When glucocorticoid excess is suspected clinically, simple determination of plasma electrolytes and glucose should be performed. Although 24-hour urinary free cortisol is elevated in normal pregnancy, levels higher than 225 μg are more often associated with Cushing's syndrome.[213] The usual range of normal pregnancy is 68 to 252 μg.[214,215] In addition, the measured morning and late evening cortisol levels in serum are higher, but retain the normal diurnal evening decline during pregnancy.[216] Therefore, measurements that show an absent or blunted diurnal pattern are consistent with abnormal glucocorticoid production. The more specific diagnostic tests are dynamic in nature (see below).

Glucocorticoid deficiency also manifests abnormalities in serum electrolytes (hyponatremia, hyperkalemic acidosis) and glucose homeostasis (hypoglycemia), but effective testing requires dynamic testing because basal cortisol levels may appear normal despite disease. Typically, ACTH rises in adrenocortical failure (Addison's disease), but the already elevated ACTH levels of pregnancy make this feature difficult to assess.

Dynamic Tests (Glucocorticoids)

In order to establish a state of hormone excess, it is necessary to assess the degree of adrenal suppression following exogenous dexamethasone administration. Normally in pregnancy, the expected response is suppression to ≤ 5 μg/dL of plasma cortisol drawn at 8 A.M. following 1 mg of dexamethasone orally at 11 P.M. the evening before.[204,217] For those subjects who fail to suppress this dose of dexamethasone, a longer, low-dose test should be performed. This consists of administration of 0.5 mg dexamethasone orally every 6 hours for 48 hours, during which time urine is collected for determination of free cortisol. It must also be remembered to collect a basal urine for free cortisol determination before administration of the dexamethasone (UFC). The normal response is suppression of UFC to ≤ 19 to 25 μg/day.[213,217] A further step may be taken if this test proves abnormal, with ingestion of a higher dose of dexamethasone—2 mg orally every 6 hours for 48 hours. If the UFC fails to suppress to 50% of baseline, then an adrenal or ectopic source of glucocorticoid excess is likely. A modification of the high-dose dexamethasone suppression test consists of administration of 8 mg oral dexamethasone at 11 P.M. with a plasma cortisol determination the following morning at 8 A.M.[218] In adrenal or ectopic sources of ACTH excess, a less than 50% decline in plasma cortisol is expected. A more dramatic suppression is typically seen in pituitary ACTH excess (Cushing's disease).

Tests of glucocorticoid reserve to diagnose adrenal cortical failure include the rapid ACTH stimulation test performed over 60 minutes, and a more prolonged test over 3 days. For the rapid test, 250 μg of a synthetic ACTH derivative is injected for determination of a baseline plasma cortisol. Blood is collected at 30 and 60 minutes for determination of cortisol, and normally increases by 23 ± 3.3 (SEM) μg/dL in the second trimester and 26 ± 5.5 (SEM) μg/dL in the third trimester.[204,213] For the longer test, ACTH is infused over 8 hours each day (250 μg per day) for 3 consecutive days. In nonpregnant patients with primary adrenal failure, no rise in either UFC or plasma cortisol is seen, even at the end of 3 days infusion. In contrast, those subjects with pituitary ACTH deficiency show a gradual adrenal response with low cortisol production on day 1, but approximately threefold increases by day 3.[219] Comparative testing in pregnant subjects has not yet been reported.

Basal Hormone Determination (Mineralocorticoids)

Due to the high circulating levels of renin and aldosterone normally present during pregnancy, the basal determination of these hormones is of minimal value in cases of suspected overproduction.

Dynamic Hormonal Evaluation (Mineralocorticoids)

In order to assess the ability to suppress elevated aldosterone levels in cases of suspect primary hyperaldosteronism, it is important to regulate both salt and potassium intake. A steady diet of 100 to 150 mEq sodium for 3 to 5 days is recommended before testing. Furthermore, potassium supplementation is important to eliminate any deficits. Normally, volume expansion with either oral or intravenous sodium chloride will inhibit renin production and thereby decrease plasma aldosterone concentrations.[220–222] It is important to evaluate carefully the volume status of any pregnant patient, however, before administration of any sodium-containing fluids.

Basal Hormone Determination (Catecholamines)

The adrenal medulla normally produces the catecholamines epinephrine and norepinephrine. Their metabolites include total metanephrines and vanillylmandelic acid (VMA). In cases where overproduction is suspected, plasma determination of catecholamines may be performed. The best initial test for diagnosis of pheochromocytoma is the 24-hour urinary estimation of VMA and metanephrines.[223] Dietary modification may be necessary depending on the laboratory, but generally includes avoidance of bananas, coffee and tea, and vanilla.[224] The n-methylating enzyme responsible for conversion of norepinephrine to epinephrine is confined to the adrenal and organ of Zuckerkandl,[225] and hence urinary elevations of both catecholamines is compatible with disease in either location.[226,227] Although not specific, the exclusive presence of elevated norepinephrine levels points to an extraadrenal source one third of the time. Dynamic testing with clonidine suppression or various provocative agents (glucagon, phentolamine) are generally not recommended during pregnancy.

PLACENTAL–FETAL ADRENAL PHYSIOLOGY

The fetal adrenal plays an important role in maintenance of the necessary placental steroid hormone (estrogen) production. Its formation begins by the fourth week of gestation and has differentiated into an outer and inner fetal cortical zone by the eighth week. The outer zone will eventually become the adult adrenal cortex, whereas the inner zone largely regresses after birth and is virtually absent by 1 year of life.[228] An important role of the inner fetal zone is to convert placental substrates (progesterone and pregnenolone) to DHEA, using cytochrome P450 enzymes (17-hydroxylase and 17, 20-lyase) that are not present in the placenta. This fetal-derived DHEA then becomes a substrate for placental production of estrone. The fetal adrenal also has sulfokinase, and thereby may produce DHEAs.

In addition to its role in placental estrogen biosynthesis, the fetal adrenal independently functions under the influence of pituitary ACTH. The full complement of steroidogenic enzymes allows production of glucocorticoids, mineralocorticoids, and sex steroids before birth. Disordered activity of the enzymes in this pathway of steroid biosynthesis leads to profound disturbances characteristic of congenital adrenal hyperplastic syndromes. The fetus is not dependent on maternal cortisol; in fact, most of the maternal cortisol is converted to cortisone (inactive) in crossing the placenta.[229–231] ACTH does not cross the placenta,[232] and therefore the maternal–fetal hypothalamic–pituitary axes remain separate. Although aldosterone does cross the placenta, adrenal androgens normally do not.[208,233]

DISORDERS OF HYPERSECRETION

Maternal Cushing's Syndrome

The occurrence of glucocorticoid excess during pregnancy is rare and, when present, is associated with adverse fetal effects.[234,235] The accompanying hyperglycemia and hypertension further increase the obstetrical risk of these patients. Two thirds of cases are caused by pituitary ACTH secretion in excess of normal (Cushing's disease), which results in bilateral adrenal hyperplasia. Approximately one third are due to either adrenal or ectopic causes.[236]

Symptoms and Signs. Certripedal weight gain with a buffalo hump, moon facies and supraclavicular fat pads, thin fragile easy bruising skin, purple striae, and hirsutism or acne may all manifest in the presence of glucocorticoid excess. The presence of virilizing signs such as male pattern hair loss, voice changes, and clitoromegaly should alert one to the possibility of an underlying adrenal tumor. Complaints of muscle weakness and easy fatiguability may be inadvertently dismissed as features expected during normal pregnancy. Indeed, many of the clinical signs may be masked by the pregnant state.

Diagnosis. The diagnosis of Cushing's syndrome rests on demonstration of elevated plasma or urinary cortisol that fails to suppress after exogenous dexamethasone (see Laboratory Investigations). Typically, pituitary sources of ACTH excess (Cushing's disease) fail to suppress after the overnight or low-dose dexamethasone suppression tests, but do suppress after high-dose dexamethasone administration. The higher baseline UFC levels and plasma cortisol levels that occur during pregnancy must be remembered when interpreting these diagnostic tests. MRI of suspected sites of abnormal ACTH or cortisol excess may be done if necessary.

Course and Treatment. If the results of dexamethasone testing indicate that a pituitary source of excess ACTH is likely, then transphenoidal resection is recommended, and results in successful treatment 85% to 95% of the time.[237–239] Postoperative hypocortisolism must be anticipated and treated with replacement glucocorticoids. Cyproheptadine, a serotonin antagonist, has been used successfully in two cases of Cushing's disease, but remains a largely untested form of treatment.[240] When hormone testing reveals a pattern of steroid excess compatible with an adrenal or ectopic source of disease, it is important to localize the site prior to surgery. In this case, MRI scanning is probably the best choice. When the situation does not allow for surgical treatment, such as with disseminated disease, it may be worthwhile to try an inhibitor of adrenal steroidogenesis such as aminoglutethimide or metyrapone.[241] Metyrapone use for diagnosis testing, however, is not recommended in pregnancy. Other adrenal cytolytic compounds (O,P′-DDD) have also been used to control steroid excess during pregnancy.[242]

Although maternal cortisol is largely converted to inactive cortisone on passage through the placenta, a theoretical risk of fetal pituitary ACTH suppression exists when such high levels of endogenous maternal cortisol exist. However, it is extremely rare that infants born to such mothers experience any adrenal dysfunction.[234]

Primary Hyperaldosteronism

This disorder is rare even in the non-pregnant state, and when present usually results in hypertension and electrolyte disturbances—hypernatremia and hypokalemic alkalosis. The most common cause is an adrenal aldosteronoma (85%), with the remainder of cases usually caused by adrenal hyperplasia. Symptoms and signs are mild, including headaches, fatigue and polyuria. Hypokalemia impairs insulin secretion and may thereby impair glucose homeostasis. The diagnosis is made by demonstrating failure of renin and aldosterone to suppress on salt loading (see Laboratory Investigations), and the treatment is surgical if possible. Control of blood pressure is important for successful outcome of pregnancy, but the use of antialdosterone agents (spironolactone) to do so is contraindicated in pregnancy. Antiandrogenic effects of these drugs on developing gonadal tissue have been found in animal studies.[243]

Pheochromocytoma

This tumor usually occurs in the adrenal medulla (10% extraadrenal) and secretes the catecholamines norepinephrine and epinephrine. The resultant clinical picture of sporadic hypertension, palpitations, flushing, and sweating attacks may easily be dismissed as anxiety attacks. A careful search for the associated features of hypoglycemia and postural hypotension may lead one to suspect this diagnosis. Familial syndromes associated with a higher incidence of pheochromocytoma include von Hippel-Lindau, neurofibromatosis, and multiple endocrine neoplasia type II. Diagnostic elevations of urinary catecholamines and their metabolites (see Laboratory Investigations) occur, and subsequent treatment recommended is surgical if diagnosed before 24 weeks gestation.[244,245] It is important to localize the site of disease with imaging studies, preferably MR scanning. Patients must be adequately alpha-blocked (phenotolamine or phenoxybenzamine) prior to beta-blockade (with propranolol) in order to prevent exacerbation of alpha-adrenergic symptoms and thus hypertensive crisis. The pharmacologic blockade so performed will decrease surgical mortality. For women diagnosed after 24 weeks gestation, the treatment of choice is alpha-blockage alone until the fetus is sufficiently mature to be delivered by cesarean section. At this time, tumor removal should also be performed. Barbiturate anesthesia is preferred over other forms of general or local anesthesia.[246] Both maternal (11%) and fetal (46%) mortality are high in this disorder, even when diagnosed during pregnancy. Indeed, maternal mortality reaches extraordinary rates of 55% when diagnosis is not made until the postpartum period.[227] Catecholamines do not cross the placenta, and therefore any effects on fetus are indirect through the adverse maternal environment. Once born, the neonate does not suffer further risks long term.

DISORDERS OF HYPOSECRETION

Maternal Adrenal Insufficiency

Adrenal cortical insufficiency may be either primary, resulting from failure of the adrenal tissue itself, or secondary to loss of pituitary ACTH stimulation. Primary failure impairs adrenal production of all three classes of steroid hormones (glucocorticoids, mineralocorticoids, sex steroids), whereas secondary insufficiency leads to significant losses of glucocorticoid production only. The most common underlying cause of primary failure is autoimmune destruction, and this disease is also associated with other organ-specific autoimmune diseases: Hashimoto's thyroiditis, diabetes mellitus, hypoparathyroidism, and premature ovarian failure.[247–249] Other causes include tuberculosis, fungal infections, metastatic carcinoma (especially breast), lymphomas, and infiltrative disorders (sarcoidosis and amyloidosis). These are, however, far less common than autoimmune destruction. Secondary adrenal failure most often results from large macroadenomas of the pituitary, which impair function of the surrounding tissue. Generally, in such cases the loss of ACTH secretion occurs late and is preceded by signs of loss of the other anterior pituitary hormones. It is important to note in this regard that thyroid hormone insufficiency secondary to decreased TSH secretion may coexist with ACTH deficiency. This is especially relevant during treatment, because thyroid hormone supplementation is critical before steroid replacement in order to avoid precipitation of acute adrenal crisis (see below).

Symptoms and Signs. The rather vague and nonspecific complaints that accompany diminished adrenal glucocorticoid and mineralocorticoid secretion may easily go undetected. These include prominent anorexia, nausea, vomiting, and weight loss. Similar complaints occur during pregnancy and may be misdiagnosed as hyperemesis gravidarum. Other features include generalized weakness, postural hypotension, skin hyperpigmentation (especially in recent scars or pressure points), and areas of vitiligo.

Diagnosis. A definitive diagnosis rests on the demonstration of impaired glucocorticoid production in response to exogenous ACTH (see Laboratory Investigations). The serum electrolytes show hyponatremia and hyperkalemic acidosis, with a tendency to hypoglycemia.

Treatment. Once diagnosed, immediate replacement with glucocorticoids (cortisone acetate 25 mg orally in the morning and 12.5 mg in the evening) and mineralocorticoids (0.05 to 0.10 mg 9-alpha-fluro-hydrocortisone daily) is necessary. If the patient is significantly dehydrated or unable to take medications by mouth, then intravenous saline with glucose supplementation and intravenous cortisol 25 mg every 6 hours is recommended. It should be noted that requirements are significantly increased in times of stress, and the cortisol should thus be increased. If a patient with well-controlled Addison's disease is in labor or having a cesarean section, then an additional 100 mg cortisol may be infused over several hours. With addisonian crisis the requirements are higher, and initial administration of 200 mg of intravenous cortisol hemisuccinate followed by 100 mg of intravenous cortisol in each liter of intravenous fluids for the first 24 hours is recommended. Intravenous fluid losses may be as high as 6 L, and replacement with isotonic saline is usually appropriate. Due to the initially high levels of serum potassium, no supplementation is recommended. Careful follow-up of serum levels is necessary during the first 6 to 8 hours of treatment, because total body potassium is often low (even though serum levels may initially be high) due to the associated nausea and vomiting. Once serum levels reach the normal range, then 20 mEq potassium should be placed in each liter of intravenous fluids. Furthermore, because hypoglycemia tends to occur, the first liter of intravenous fluids should be supplemented with 50 g of glucose. Secondary adrenal insufficiency will rarely present such profound disturbances of fluid and electrolytes, because mineralocorticoid secretion is maintained due to an intact renin–angiotensin–aldosterone axis. For this reason, glucocorticoid replacement usually suffices.

Course. Patients with pregnancy and Addison's disease in whom treatment is begun before pregnancy have no ill apparent effects. If a pregnant patient with undiagnosed Addison's disease manages to complete a pregnancy successfully, then the neonate appears to suffer no serious effects either. However, a significant risk of maternal postpartum adrenal crisis exists in this setting.[250,251] Furthermore, although maternal autoantibodies do cross the placenta, there does not appear to be any subsequent fetal or neonatal adrenal destruction.[252] Finally, although a small proportion of maternal steroids do cross the placenta and could theoretically suppress fetal adrenal function, it is rarely necessary to administer glucocorticoids to the newborn.

DISORDERED FETAL ADRENAL STEROIDOGENESIS

Congenital Adrenal Hyperplasia

The congenital adrenal hyperplasias result from inherited defects in enzymes required in the biosynthetic pathways of steroid hormones of all three groups (gluco- and mineralocorticoids and sex steroids). Due to variable sites of blockade in the enzymatic pathway, the clinical features will be different for each disorder. Build-up of metabolic precursors as well as deficiency of necessary hormones distal to the defects leads to abnormal developmental and metabolic parameters. The most common abnormality is in the enzyme 21-hydroxylase, which is responsible for conversion of 17-hydroxyprogesterone to 11-deoxycortisol. Other enzymes that may be affected include 11-β-hydroxylase, 17-α-hydroxylase, 3-β-hydroxysteroid dehydrogenase, cholesterol desmolase, and 18-hydroxylase (Fig. 62-13).[253]

Symptoms and Signs. Over 90% of patients with congenital adrenal hyperplasia have defective 21-hydroxylase, which may present as severe salt-wasting, simple virilizing, attenuated, or cryptic disease. Severe salt-wasting disease is manifest at birth with ambiguous genitalia in the female and normal genitalia in the male. The synthetic block at 21-hydroxylase is almost complete, and thereby markedly diminishes both cortisol and deoxycorticosterone (mineralocorticoid) production, leading to severe salt-wasting disease. The excess steroid precursors that are shunted along the adrenal androgen pathway are responsible for the ambiguous female genitalia. Simple virilizing disease lacks the degree of mineralocorticoid deficiency seen with more severe disease, but results in similar ambiguity of the female genitalia. Attenuated (late onset) disease may first become manifest clinically with precocious appearance of pubertal signs in a child or hirsutism and irregular cyclicity in a postpubertal individual. The disease is present at birth, but the biochemical detection not made until after signs become apparent. Finally, cryptic 21-hydroxylase deficiency refers to entirely asymptomatic individuals who are discovered to have abnormal 17-hydroxyprogesterone responses to ACTH stimulation (accentuated), usually in the course of family investigations. 21-hydroxylase deficiency is inherited as an autosomal recessive disorder, and the severity of the disease is based on allelic variation at the P450 c21 locus.[254]

11-β-hydroxylase deficiency accounts for approximately 5% of cases of congenital adrenal hyperplasia.[255] This defect results in diminished cortisol but elevated levels of deoxycorticosterone (DOC) and adrenal androgens. For this reason, hypertension may be a feature of this disorder, along with masculinization of the female fetus.[255] This condition is also inherited as an autosomal recessive disorder.

The other forms of congenital adrenal hyperplasia are quite rare. It is noteworthy that 17-α-hydroxylase deficiency and 3-β-hydroxysteroid dehydrogenase deficiency produce hypogonadal ambiguity of male genitalia, with minimal (3BHD) or no adverse effects on the development of the female genitalia.

Diagnosis. Because these disorders (21-hydroxylase and 11-β-hydroxylase deficiencies) may present later in

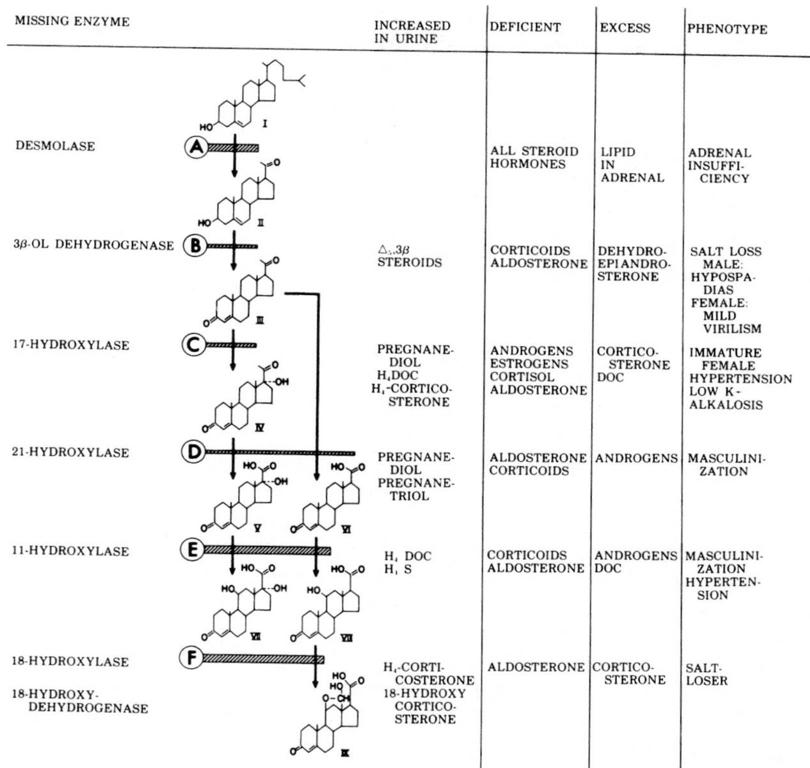

MISSING ENZYME
INCREASED IN URINE
DEFICIENT
EXCESS
PHENOTYPE
DESMOLASE
ALL STEROID HORMONES
LIPID IN ADRENAL
ADRENAL INSUFFICIENCY
3β-OL DEHYDROGENASE
Δ5,3β STEROIDS
CORTICOIDS ALDOSTERONE
DEHYDROEPIANDROSTERONE
SALT LOSS MALE: HYPOSPADIAS FEMALE: MILD VIRILISM
17-HYDROXYLASE
PREGNANEDIOL H,DOC H,-CORTICOSTERONE
ANDROGENS ESTROGENS CORTISOL ALDOSTERONE
CORTICOSTERONE DOC
IMMATURE FEMALE HYPERTENSION LOW K-ALKALOSIS
21-HYDROXYLASE
PREGNANEDIOL PREGNANETRIOL
ALDOSTERONE CORTICOIDS
ANDROGENS
MASCULINIZATION
11-HYDROXYLASE
H, DOC H, S
CORTICOIDS ALDOSTERONE
ANDROGENS DOC
MASCULINIZATION HYPERTENSION
18-HYDROXYLASE
18-HYDROXY-DEHYDROGENASE
H,-CORTICOSTERONE 18-HYDROXY CORTICOSTERONE
ALDOSTERONE
CORTICOSTERONE
SALT-LOSER

FIGURE 62–13. Steroid pathway for cortisol synthesis and possible metabolic blocks (From Bondy PK, Rosenberg LE. Metabolic control and disease. 8th ed. Philadelphia: WB Saunders, 1980: 1480.)

life with menstrual irregularities, hirsutism, and acne, it is possible that a minority of individuals suffering from disturbances of fertility are actually undiagnosed patients. In 21-hydroxylase deficiency the 17-hydroxyprogesterone response to ACTH injection is accentuated, whereas 11-β-hydroxylase deficiency is associated with elevated serum levels of DOC and 11-deoxycortisol, which can be further increased by ACTH.[256]

Prenatal diagnosis of 21-hydroxylase deficiency is possible by HLA typing of amniotic cells in high-risk individuals.[257] Both 17-hydroxyprogesterone and 11-deoxycortisol levels can be determined in amniotic fluid, and elevations suggest the presence of abnormal fetal adrenals.[258–260]

Treatment. Replacement of glucocorticoids with 25 mg orally of cortisone acetate in the morning and 12.5 mg orally in the evening is adequate for maintenance both before and during pregnancy in the mother with CAH. This dose will suppress elevated ACTH levels and thereby diminish the excess adrenal androgen (21-hydroxylase and 11-β-hydroxylase) and DOC (11-β-hydroxylase) production. In times of stress, the amount will need to be increased temporarily. Mineralocorticoid replacement in cases of salt-wasting congenital adrenal hyperplasia likewise does not require dose adjustment unless problems with maternal blood pressure supervene. Attempts to prenatally treat female offspring with congenital adrenal hyperplasia have been made in order to prevent virilization.[261] Ambiguous genitalia will occur, however, unless maternal dexamethasone ingestion is begun before the end of the ninth week.

Course. If maternal disease is adequately treated during pregnancy, then no untoward fetal or maternal effects are anticipated. However, the typically narrow android maternal pelvis often results in poor labor progression and thus cesarean section.[262,263] Furthermore, hypertension appears commonly during these pregnancies and should be appropriately managed. Spontaneous abortion rates as high as 20% have been reported.

CALCIUM AND PARATHYROID GLANDS

Calcium homeostasis is critical for normal development of the fetal skeleton, and maternal ingestion should be increased during pregnancy in order to accommodate these elevated demands. The fetal skeleton acquires approximately 30 mg of calcium by term, compared to the average adult female skeleton content of 1000 g. These enormous requirements by the fetus mean that calcium must be actively transported across the placenta from mother to fetus.

PHYSIOLOGY IN THE NON-PREGNANT STATE

The serum calcium is normally regulated by both parathyroid hormone and vitamin D. Parathyroid hormone mobilizes calcium from bone and is also responsible for activation of 25-hydroxyvitamin D to 1,25-dihydroxyvitamin D through stimulation of the 1-α-hydroxylase enzyme within the kidney. 1,25-dihydroxyvitamin D is the biologically active form of vitamin D, which enhances intestinal calcium absorption. Calcitonin is secreted by the parafollicular C cells of the thyroid, and can inhibit bone resorption, thereby decreasing serum levels of calcium. Calcium exists in three forms within the plasma: free, bound (primarily to albumin), and chelated. The free form is that which is biologically active.

PHYSIOLOGY IN THE PREGNANT STATE

Total serum calcium falls from the second or third month of gestation, along with declining levels of albumin (Fig. 62-14).[264] The free fraction of calcium actually remains relatively stable. Parathyroid hormone levels are elevated in the mother (Fig. 62-15), such that a state of "physiologic hyperparathyroidism" exists.[264] Variable reports of elevated calcitonin levels have also been published.[265,266] Of importance is the increase in 1,25-dihydroxyvitamin D noted in pregnant women, which is presumably responsible for the increased maternal calcium absorption.[267]

LABORATORY INVESTIGATIONS

Evaluation of the serum calcium level must be done in conjunction with serum albumin, the major binding protein. It is estimated that approximately 1 g of albumin binds to 0.8 mg of calcium. Therefore, 0.8 mg can be added to the measured total calcium determination for every 1 g the serum albumin is below normal. Ionized (free) calcium determinations remain within the normal range, despite disturbances of protein concentrations. Levels of parathyroid hormone may be determined when disease is suspected, and the nephrogenic cAMP levels also are indicative of PTH biologic activity.

FETAL PHYSIOLOGY

The fetus remains in positive calcium balance through gestation, and in doing so receives its calcium from the mother. Calcium levels are relatively high in the fetus, whereas the fetal parathyroid hormone levels are either low or normal. Maternal PTH, calcitonin, and 25-hydroxyvitamin D do not cross the placenta, whereas the placenta is capable of 1-α-hydroxylating maternal 25-hydroxyvitamin D to 1,25-dihydroxyvitamin D. Fetal calcitonin levels are high, and presumably stimulate uptake of calcium into bone. At birth, a sudden withdrawal from maternal calcium sources occurs, and thus neonatal levels decline for the first 1 to 2 days of life. Thereafter, the neonatal parathyroids increase PTH production and calcium levels stabilize.

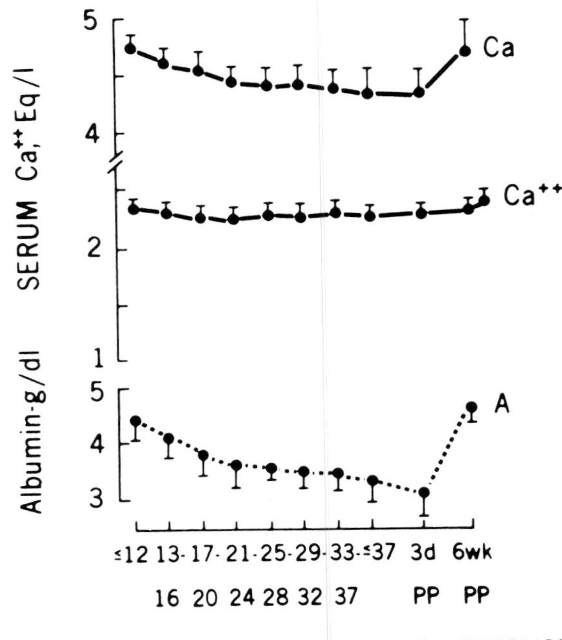

FIGURE 62–14. Serum calcium, ionized calcium, and albumin concentrations during pregnancy. (From Pitkin RM, Reynolds WA, Williams GA, Hargis GK. Calcium metabolism in normal pregnancy: a longitudinal study. Am J Obstet Gynecol 1979; 133: 781.)

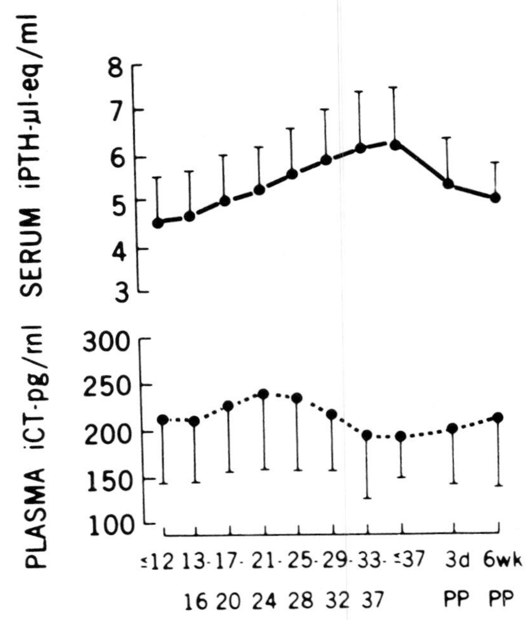

FIGURE 62–15. Serum parathyroid hormone and calcitonin concentrations during pregnancy. (From Pitkin RM, Reynolds WA, Williams GA, Hargis GK. Calcium metabolism in normal pregnancy: a longitudinal study. Am J Obstet Gynecol 1979; 133: 781.)

DISORDERS OF HYPERSECRETION

Maternal Hyperparathyroidism

Hyperparathyroidism may be quite insidious in its presentation, with such nonspecific complaints as fatigue, polyuria, and bone pain. It is usually caused by a single adenoma, but adenomatous hyperplasia of all four glands may also occur, especially in familial syndromes. Pregnancy may exacerbate preexisting hyperparathyroidism, and when this does occur, spontaneous abortion and late fetal deaths occur much more commonly than normal.[268–270]

Diagnosis. The diagnosis is confirmed by finding elevated serum calcium levels (free), low serum phosphorous levels, and inappropriately normal (nonsuppressed) or high levels of parathyroid hormone. Localization studies may be necessary and, if done, attention to minimization of radiation exposure should be sought.

Treatment. The preferred treatment is surgical removal of the adenomatous parathyroid tissue; successful results are often obtained.[271–273] If surgery is contraindicated for other reasons, then serum calcium may be controlled by thiazide diuretics and oral phosphate therapy.[274,275]

Fetal Effects. A high percentage of neonates born to women with hyperparathyroidism experience subnormal calcium levels after birth. This is likely due to the prolonged exposure to elevated levels of maternal calcium in utero, and thus suppression of the fetal parathyroid gland. The effects are transient and often appear from 1 to 2 weeks of life.[276] Controversy exists, however, regarding the underlying mechanism, as reports of normal or even elevated neonatal PTH levels have been described.[277,278]

DISORDERS OF HYPOSECRETION

Maternal Hypoparathyroidism

Hypoparathyroidism usually results from inadvertent removal at the time of thyroid surgery, but rarely autoimmune destruction may occur. Pseudohypoparathyroidism is a term used to describe peripheral resistance to the effects of PTH, and this is a quite rare entity.

Symptoms and Signs. Most symptoms are related to the subnormal serum calcium that occurs in this condition, and include paresthesias, numbness and tingling, muscle cramps, and even tetany. Alkalosis increases calcium binding and thereby decreases the biologically active free calcium level. For this reason, tetany is more likely to occur when alkalosis coexists.

Diagnosis and Treatment. The diagnosis of hypoparathyroidism is made by demonstration of a subnormal serum calcium level with a low PTH serum determination. Treatment with calcium supplementation and vitamin D (either 100,000 units of vitamin D_2 or 0.25 to 1.0 μg of 1,25-dihydroxyvitamin D daily) should return the serum calcium to the normal range. Calcium supplementation is not always necessary in the nonpregnant state, but seems justifiable during gestation.

Pregnancy is associated with increasing fetal calcium demands with advancing gestation, and therefore it is not surprising that dosages of calcium and vitamin D may need to be increased over time.[279] If hypoparathyroidism is poorly controlled during pregnancy, then the fetus suffers from hypocalcemia and skeletal undermineralization. At birth, such neonates may exhibit elevated PTH levels with widespread osteitis fibrosa cytica.[280] Furthermore, treated mothers of such infants should not breast-feed because transmission of maternal 25-hydroxyvitamin D may occur.[281] In addition, maternal calcium supplementation is difficult when such losses are occurring in breast milk (approximately 400 mg/L).

REFERENCES

1. Little B, Smith OW, Jessiman AG, et al. Hypophysectomy during pregnancy in a patient with cancer of the breast: case report with hormone studies. J Clin Endocrinol Metab 1958;18:425.
2. Kaplan NM. Successful pregnancy following hypophysectomy during the twelfth week of gestation. J Clin Endocrinol Metab 1961;21:1139.
3. Gemzell CA, Kjessler G. Treatment of infertility after partial hypophysectomy with human pituitary gonadotropins. Lancet 1964;1:644.
4. Corral J, Caldern J, Goldzieher JW. Induction of ovulation and term pregnancy in a hypophysectomized woman. Obstet Gynecol 1972;39:397.
5. Floderus S. Changes in the human hypophysis in connection with pregnancy. Acta Anat (Basel) 1949;8:329.
6. Goluboff LG, Ezrin C. Effect of pregnancy on the somatotroph and the prolactin cell of the human adenohypophysis. J Clin Endocrinol Metab 1969;29:1533.
7. Tyson JE, Hwang P, Guyda H, Friesen HG. Studies of prolactin secretion in human pregnancy. Am J Obstet Gynecol 1972;113:14.
8. Barberia JM, Abu-Fadil S, Kletzky OA, Nakamura RM, Mishell DR. Serum prolactin patterns in early human gestation. Am J Obstet Gynecol 1975;121:1107.
9. Schenker JG, Ben-David M, Polishuk WZ. Prolactin in normal pregnancy: relationship of maternal, fetal and amniotic fluid levels. Am J Obstet Gynecol 1975;123:834.
10. Biswas S, Rodeck CH. Plasma prolactin levels during pregnancy. Br J Obstet Gynecol 1976;83:683.
11. Sadorsky E, Weinstein D, Ben-David M, Polishuk WZ. Serum prolactin in normal and pathologic pregnancy. Obstet Gynecol 1977;50:559.
12. Rigg LA, Lein A, Yen SSC. Pattern of increase in circulating prolactin levels during human gestation. Am J Obstet Gynecol 1977;129:454.
13. Boyar RM, Finkelstein JW, Kapen S, Hellman L. Twenty-four

hour prolactin secretory pattern during pregnancy. J Clin Endocrinol Metab 1975;40:1117.
14. Rigg LA, Yen SSC. Multiphasic prolactin secretion during parturition in human subjects. Am J Obstet Gynecol 1977;128:215.
15. Kinch RA, Plunkett ER, Devlin MC. Postpartum amenorrheagalactorrhea of hypothyroidism. Am J Obstet Gynecol 1969; 105:766.
16. Sheehan HL. The frequency of postpartum hypopituitarism. J Obstet Gynecol Br Commonwealth 1965;72:103.
17. Sialy R, Rastogi GK, Gupta AN. Serum prolactin and its response to thyrotropin releasing hormone in normal pregnancy. Indian J Med Res 1977;65:519.
18. Ylikorkala O, Kivenen S, Reinila M. Serial prolactin and thyrotropin responses to thyrotropin-releasing hormone throughout normal human pregnancy. J Clin Endocrinol Metab 1979; 48:288.
19. Guiterman A, Aparicio NJ, Mancini A, Debeljuk L. Release of prolactin during pregnancy: effect of sulpiride. Fertil Steril 1978;30:42.
20. Brandes JM, Itskovitz J, Fisher M, Shen-orr Z, Barzilai D. The acute effect of metoclopramide on plasma prolactin during pregnancy. Acta Obstet Gynecol Scand 1981;60:243.
21. Zarate A, Canales ES, Villalobos H, et al. Pituitary hormonal reserve in patients presenting hyperprolactinemia, intrasellar masses and amenorrhea without galactorrhea. J Clin Endocrinol Metab 1975;40:1034.
22. Jeppsson S, Rannevik G. Studies on the gonadotropin response after administration of LH-FSH releasing hormone (LRH) during pregnancy and after therapeutic abortion in the second trimester. Am J Obstet Gynecol 1976;125:484.
23. Jeppsson S, Rannevik G, Thorell JI. Pituitary gonadotropin secretion during the first weeks of pregnancy. Acta Endocrinol (Copenh) 1977;85:177.
24. Jeppsson S, Rannevik, G, Liedholm P, Thorell JI. Basal and LRH-stimulated secretion of FSH during early pregnancy. Am J Obstet Gynecol 1977;127:32.
25. Miyake A, Tanizawa O, Aono T, et al. LH concentration in human maternal and cord serum. Clin Endocrinol (Tokyo) 1977;24:105.
26. Miyake A, Tanizawa O, Aono T, Kurachi K. Pituitary responses in LH secretion to LHRH during pregnancy. Obstet Gynecol 1977:49:549.
27. Marrs RP, Kletzky OA, Mishell DR. Functional capacity of the gonadotrophs during pregnancy and the puerperium. Am J Obstet Gynecol 1981;141:658.
28. Thompson IE, Arfania J, Taymor ML. Effects of estrogen and progesterone on pituitary response to stimulation by luteinizing releasing factor. Endocrinol Jpn 1973;37:152.
29. Rollard R, Lequin RM, Schellekens LA. The role of prolactin in the restoration of ovarian function during early postpartum period in the human. I: a study during physiological lactation. Clin Endocrinol (Oxf) 1975;4:15.
30. Kaplan SL, Grumbach MM. Serum chorionic "growth hormone-prolactin" and serum pituitary growth hormone in mother and fetus at term. J Clin Endocrinol Metab 1965;21:1370.
31. Board JA. Plasma human growth hormone in the puerperim. Am J Obstet Gynecol 1968;100:1106.
32. Samaan NA, Bradbury JT, Goperlund CP. Serial hormonal studies in normal and abnormal pregnancy. Am J Obstet Gynecol 1969;104:781.
33. Yen SSC, Vela P, Tsai CC. Impairment of growth hormone secretion in response to hypoglycemia during early and late pregnancy. J Clin Endocrinol Metab 1970;31:29.
34. Tyson JE, Rabinowitz D, Merimee TJ, Friesen H. Response of plasma insulin and human growth hormone to arginine in pregnant and postpartum females. Am J Obstet Gynecol 1969;103:313.
35. Samaan NA, Goperlund CP, Bradbury JT. Effect of arginine infusion on plasma levels of growth hormone, insulin and glucose during pregnancy and puerperium. Am J Obstet Gynecol 1970;107:1002.
36. Doe RP, Dickinson P, Zinneman HH, Seal US. Elevated nonprotein-bound cortisol (NPC) in pregnancy, during estrogen administration and carcinoma of the prostate. J Clin Endocrinol Metab 1969;29:757.
37. Varma SK, Son Ksen PH, Varma K, Soeldner JS, Selenkow HA, Emerson K. Measurement of human growth hormone in pregnancy and correlation with human placental lactogen. J Clin Endocrinol Metab 1971;32:328.
38. Harada A, Hershman JM, Reed AW, et al. Comparison of thyroid stimulators and thyroid hormone concentrations in the sera of pregnancy women. J Clin Endocrinol Metab 1979;48:793.
39. Yamamoto T, Amino N, Tanizawa O, et al. Longitudinal study of serum thyroid hormones, chorionic gonadotropin and thyrotropin during the after normal pregnancy. Clin Endocrinol 1979;10:459.
40. Matzuk MM, Biome I. Mutagenesis and gene transfer define site-specific roles of the gonadotropin oligosaccharides. Biol Reprod 1989;40:48.
41. Burrow GN, Polackwich R, Donabedian R. The hypothalamic-pituitary-thyroid axis in normal pregnancy. In: Fisher DA, Burrow GN, eds. Perinatal thyroid physiology and disease. New York: Raven Press, 1975:1.
42. Vandalem JL, Pirens G, Hennen G. Gaspard V. Thyroliberin and gonadoliberin tests during pregnancy and the puerperium. Acta Endocrinol (Copenh) 1977;86:695.
43. Osathanondh R, Tulchinsky D, Chopra IJ. Total and free thyroxine and triiodothryonine in normal and complicated pregnancy. J Clin Endocrinol Metab 1976;42:98.
44. Genazzani AR, Frioli F, Hurlimann J, Fioretti P, Felber JP. Immunoreactive ACTH and cortisol plasma levels during pregnancy. Detection and partial purification of corticotropin-like placental hormone: the human chorionic corticotropin (hCC). Clin Endocrinol 1975;4:1.
45. Genazzani RA, Felber JP, Fioretti P. Immunoreactive ACTH, immunoreactive human chorionic somatomammotropin (HCS) and 11-OH steriods plasma levels in normal and pathological pregnancies. Acta Endocrinol (Copenh) 1977;83:800.
46. Carr BR, Parker CR Jr, Madden JD, MacDonald PC, Porter J. Maternal plasma adrenocorticotropin and cortisol relations throughout human pregnancy. Am J Obstet Gynecol 1981; 139:416.
47. Beck P, Eaton CJ, Young IS, Kupperman HS. Metyrapone response in pregnancy. Am J Obstet Gynecol 1968;100:327.
48. Baxter JD, Forsham PH. Tissue effects of glucocorticoids. Am J Med 1972;53:573.
49. Ogawa K, Sueda K, Matsui N. The effect of cortisol progesterone and transcortin on phytohemaglutinin-stimulated human blood mononuclear cells and their interplay. J Clin Endocrinol Metab 1983;56:121.
50. Robinson AG, Archer DF, Tolstoi LF. Neurophysin in women during oxytocin-related events. J Clin Endocrinol Metab 1973;37:645.
51. Robinson AG. Elevation of plasma neurophysin in women on oral contraceptives. J Clin Invest 1974;54:209.
52. Davison JM, Vallotton MB, Lindheimer MD. Plasma osmolality and urinary concentration and dilution during and after pregnancy: evidence that lateral recumbency inhibits maximal urinary concentrating ability. Br J Obstet Gynaecol 1981;88:472.
53. Davison JM, Gilmore EA, Durr J, Robertson GL, Lindheimer

MD. Altered osmotic thresholds for vasopressin secretion and thirst in human pregnancy. Am J Physiol 1983;246:F105.
54. Barron WM, Lindheimer MD. Renal sodium and water handling in pregnancy. Obstet Gynecol Ann 1984;13:35.
55. Dawood MY, Ylikorkala O, Trivedi D, Fuchs F. Oxytocin in maternal circulation and amniotic fluid during pregnancy. J Clin Endocrinol Metab 1979;49:429.
56. Gibbens GLD, Chard T. Observations on maternal oxytocin release during human labor and the effect of intravenous alcohol administration. Am J Obstet Gynecol 1976;126:243.
57. Dawood MY, Raghaven KS, Pociask C, Fuchs F. Oxytocin in human pregnancy and parturition. Obstet Gynecol 1978; 51:138.
58. Fisher C, Magoun HW, Ranson SW. Dystocia in diabetes insipidus. Am J Obstet Gynecol 1938;36:1.
59. Nibbelink KDW. Paraventricular nuclei, neurophypophysis and parturition. Am J Physiol 1961;200:1229.
60. Hardy J. Le prolactiname. Neurochirurgie 1981;27:1s.
61. Malarkey WB, Johnson JC. Pituitary tumors and hyperprolactinemia. Arch Intern Med 1976;136:40.
62. Kilbanski A, Beitins IZ, Merriam GR, McArthur JW, Zervas NT, Ridgway EC. Gonadotropin and prolactin pulsations in hyperprolactinemic women before and during bromocriptine therapy. J Clin Endocrinol Metab 1984;58:1141.
63. Sauder SE, Frager M, Case GD, Kelch RP, Marshall JC. Abnormal patterns of pulsatile luteinizing hormone secretion in women with hyperprolactinemia and amenorrhea: responses to bromocriptine. J Clin Endocrinol Metab 1984;59:941.
64. Vance ML, Evans WS, Thorner MO. Bromocriptine. Ann Intern Med 1984;100:78.
65. Bronstein MD, Cardim CS, Marino R Jr. Short-term management of macroprolactinomas with a new injectable form of bromocriptine. Surg Neurol 1987;28:31.
66. Mattox JH, Bernstein J, Buckman MT. Control of hyperprolactinemia with pergolide. Int J Fertil 1986;30:39.
67. Dallabonzana D, Liuzzia A, Oppizzi G, et al. Chronic treatment of pathological hyperprolactinemia and acromegaly with the new ergot derivative terguride. J Clin Endocrinol Metab 1986;63:1002.
68. Molitch M. Pregnancy and the hyperprolactinemic woman. N Engl J Med 1985;312:1364.
69. Modena G, Portioli I. Delivery after bromocriptine therapy. Lancet 1977;2:558.
70. Espersen T, Ditzel J. Pregnancy and delivery under bromocriptine therapy. Lancet 1977;2:985.
71. Yuen BH. Bromocriptine pituitary tumors and pregnancy. Lancet 1978;2:1314.
72. Bigazzi M, Ronga R, Lancranjan I, et al. A pregnancy in an acromegalic woman during bromocriptine treatment: effects on growth hormone and prolactin in the maternal, fetal, and amniotic compartments. J Clin Endocrinol Metab 1979;48:9.
73. Canales ES, Garcia IC, Ruiz JE, Zarate A. Bromocriptine as prophylactic therapy in prolactinoma during pregnancy. Fertil Steril 1981;36:524.
74. Konopka P, Raymond JP, Merceron RE, Seneze J. Continuous administration of bromocriptine in the prevention of neurological complications in pregnant women with prolactinomas. Am J Obstet Gynecol 1983;146:935.
75. Ruiz-Velasco V, Tolis G. Pregnancy in hyperprolactinemic women. Fertil Steril 1984;41:793.
76. Raymond JP, Goldstein E, Konopka P, Leleu MF, Merceron RE, Loria Y. Follow-up of children born of bromocriptine-treated mothers. Horm Res 1985;22:239.
77. Andersen AN, Tabor A, Hertz JB, Schioler V. Abnormal prolactin levels and pituitary-gonadal axis in the puerperium. Obstet Gynecol 1981;57:725.
78. Putnam TJ, Davidoff LM. Cited in: Abelove WA, Rupp JJ, Paschkis KE. Acromegaly and pregnancy. J Clin Endocrinol Metab 1954;14:32.
79. Franks S, Jacobs HS, Nabarro ON. Prolactin concentrations in patients with acromegaly: clinical significance and response to surgery. Clin Endocrinol 1976;5:63.
80. Luboshitzky R, Dickstein G, Bazilai D. Bromocriptine induced pregnancy in an acromegalic patient. JAMA 1980;244:574.
81. Sachdev Y, Tunbridge WMG, Weightman DR, et al. Bromocriptine therapy in acromegaly. Lancet 1975;2:1164.
82. Wass JAH, Thorner MD, Moffis DV, et al. Long-term treatment of acromegaly with bromocriptine. Br Med J 1977;1:875.
83. Corenblum B. The medical treatment of the hypersecreting pituitary gland. Can J Neurol Sci 1985;12:243.
84. Asa SL, Bilbao JM, Kovacs K, Josse RE, Kreines K. Lymphocytic hypophysitis of pregnancy resulting in hypopituitarism: a distinct clinicopathologic entity. Ann Intern Med 1981;95:166.
85. Drury MI, Keelan DM. Sheehan's syndrome. J Obstet Gynecol Br Commonwealth 1966;73:802.
86. Grimes HG, Brooks MA. Pregnancy in Sheehan's syndrome. Report of a case and review. Obstet Gynecol Surv 1980;35:481.
87. Schalch DS, Burday SZ. Antepartum pituitary insufficiency in diabetes mellitus. Ann Intern Med 1971;74:357.
88. Dorfman SG, Dillaplain RP, Gambrell RD Jr. Antepartum pituitary infarction. Obstet Gynecol 1979;53(Suppl):21S.
89. Lufkin EG, Kao PC, O'Fallon WM, Mangan MA. Combined testing of anterior pituitary gland with insulin, thyrotropin-releasing hormone, and luteinizing hormone-releasing hormone. Am J Med 1983;75:471.
90. Holl R, Fink P, Hetzel WD. Combined pituitary stimulation test with releasing hormones. Acta Endocrinol (Copenh) 1985;267 (Suppl 108):18.
91. Sheldon WR, DeBold CR, Evans WS, et al. Rapid sequential intravenous administration of four hypothalamic-releasing hormones as combined anterior pituitary function test in normal subjects. J Clin Endocrinol Metab 1985;60:623.
92. DiZerega G, Kletzky DA, Mishell DR. Diagnosis of Sheehan's syndrome using a sequential pituitary stimulation test. Am J Obstet Gynecol 1978;132:348.
93. Tyson JE, Barnes AC, McKusick VA, Scott CL, Jones GS. Obstetric and gynecologic considerations of dwarfism. Am J Obstet Gynecol 1970;108:688.
94. Durr JA, Hoggard JG, Hunt JM, Schrier RW. Diabetes insipidus in pregnancy associated with abnormally high vasopressionase activity. N Engl J Med 1987;316:1070.
95. Robinson AG. DDAVP in the treatment of central diabetes insipidus. N Engl J Med 1976;294:507.
96. Hime MC, Richardson JA. Diabetes insipidus and pregnancy. Obstet Gynecol Surv 1978;33:375.
97. Sende P, Pantelakis N, Suzuki K, Facog, Bashore R. Plasma oxytocin determinations in pregnancy with diabetes insipidus. Obstet Gynecol 1976;48:38s.
98. Schimmez M, Utiger RD. Thyroidal and peripheral production of thyroid hormones: review of recent findings and their clinical implications. Ann Intern Med 1977;87:760.
99. Cavalieri RR. Peripheral metabolism of thyroid hormones. Thyroid Today 1980;3:7.
100. Oppenheimer JH. Role of plasma proteins in binding, distribution and metabolism of the thyroid hormones. N Engl J Med 1968;278:1153.
101. Oppenheimer JH, Volpe R. Measurement of thyroid function. In: Meier A, ed. Thyroid function and disease. Philadelphia: WB Saunders, 1990:124.

102. Aboul-Khair SA, Crooks J, Turnbull AC, Hytten FE. The physiological changes in thyroid function during pregnancy. Clin Sci 1964;27:195.
103. Crooks J, Aboul-Khair SA, Turnbull AC, Hytten FE. The incidence of goiter during pregnancy. Lancet 1964;2:334.
104. Crooks J, Tulloch MI, Turnbull AC, et al. Comparative incidence of goitre in pregnancy in Iceland and Scotland. Lancet 1964;2:625.
105. Levy RP, Newman DM, Rejali LS, Barford DAG. The myth of goiter in pregnancy. Am J Obstet Gynecol 1980;137:701.
106. Alexander WD, Koutras DA, Crooks J, et al. Quantitative studies of iodine metabolism in thyroid disease. Q J Med 1962;31:281.
107. Koutras DA, Pharmakoitis AD, Koliopoulos N, Tsoukalos J, Souvatzoglou A, Sfontouris J. The plasma inorganic iodine and the pituitary thyroid axis in pregnancy. J Endocrinol Invest 1978;1:227.
108. Burr WA, Ramsden DB, Evans SE, Hogan T, Hoffenberg R. Concentration of thyroxine-binding globulin: value of direct assay. Br Med J 1977;1:485.
109. Glinoer D, Gershengorn MC, Dubois A, Robbins J. Stimulation of thyroxine-binding globulin synthesis by isolated rhesus monkey heptocytes after in vivo beta-estradiol administration. Endocrinology 1977;100:807.
110. Premachandra BN, Gossain VV, Perlstein IB. Effect of pregnancy on thyroxine binding globulin (TBG) in partial TBG deficiency. Am J Med Sci 1977;274:189.
111. Mussey RD. The thyroid gland and pregnancy. Am J Obstet Gynecol 1938;36:529.
112. Sternberg J. Irradiation and radiocontamination during pregnancy. Am J Obstet Gynecol 1970;108:490.
113. Halnan KE. The radioiodine uptake of the human thyroid in pregnancy. Clin Sci 1958;17:281.
114. Witherspoon LR, Shuler SE, Garcia MM, Zollinger LA. An assessment of methods for the estimation of free thyroxine. J Nucl Med 1980;21:529.
115. Ross DS. New sensitive immunoradiometric assays for thyrotropin. Ann Intern Med 1986;104:718.
116. Munro DS, Dirmikis SM, Humphries H, Smith T, Bradhead GD. The role of thyroid stimulating immunoglobulins of Graves' disease in neonatal thyrotoxicosis. Br J Obstet Gynaecol 1978;85:837.
117. Parmentier M, Libert F, Maenhaut C, et al. Molecular cloning of the thyrotropin receptor. Science 1989;246:1620.
118. Amino N, Kuro R, Tanizawa O, et al. Changes of serum antithyroid antibodies during and after pregnancy in autoimmune thyroid diseases. Clin Exp Immunol 1978;31:30
119. Froelich EJ, Goodwin JS, Bankhurst AD, Williams RC. Pregnancy, a temporary fetal graft of suppressor levels in autoimmune disease. Am J Med 1980;69:329.
120. Grumbach MM, Werner SC. Transfer of thyroid hormone across the human placenta at term. J Clin Endocirnol Metab 1956;16:1392.
121. Higgins HP, Hershman JM, Kenimer JG, Patillo RA, Bayley A, Walfish P. The thyrotoxicosis of hydatidiform mole. Ann Intern Med 1975;83:307.
122. Hershman JM. Hyperthyroidism caused by trophoblastic tumors. Thyroid Today 1981;4:1.
123. Soutter WP, Norman R, Green-Thompson RW. The management of choriocarcinoma causing severe thyrotoxicosis. Br J Obstet Gynaecol 1981;88:938.
124. Oddie TH, Fisher DA, Bernard B, Lam RW. Thyroid function at birth in infants of 30 to 45 weeks' gestation. J Pediatr 1977;90:803.
125. Fisher DA, Hobel CJ, Gazara R, Pierce CA. Thyroid function in the preterm fetus. Pediatrics 1970;46:208.
126. Fisher DA, Odell WD. Acute release of thyrotropin in the newborn. J Clin Invest 1969;48:1670.
127. Stubbe P, Gatz J, Heidemann, P, Muhlen A, Hesch R. Thyroxine-binding globulin, triiodothyroxine, thryoxine and thyrotropin in newborn infants and children. Horm Metab Res 1978;10:58.
128. Sack J, Beaudry M, DeLamater PV, et al. Umbilical cord cutting triggers hypertriiodothyroninemia and nonshivering thermogenesis in the newborn lamb. Pediatr Res 1976;10:169.
129. Fisher DA, Oddie TH, Burroughs JC. Thyroidal radioiodine uptake rate measurement in infants. Am J Dis Child 1962;103:738.
130. Klein AH, Murphy BEP, Artal R, Oddie TH, Fisher DA. Amniotic fluid thyroid hormone concentration during human gestation. Am J Obstet Gynecol 1980;136:626.
131. Lightner ES, Fismer DA, Giles H, Woolfenden J. Intraamniotic injection of thyroxine (T_4) to a human fetus. Am J Obstet Gynecol 1977;127:487.
132. Landau H, Sack J, Frucht H, Palti Z, Hochner-Celnikier D, Rosenmann A. Amniotic fluid 3, 3;pr5;pr-triiodothyronine in the detection of congenital hypothyroidism. J Clin Endocrinol Metab 1980;50:799.
133. Echt CR, Doss JF. Myxedema in pregnancy. Obstet Gynecol 1963;22:615.
134. Goldsmith RE. Sturgis SH, Lerman J, Stanbury JB. The menstrual pattern in thyroid disease. J Clin Endocrinol 1952;12:846.
135. Potter JD. Hypothyroidism and reproductive failure. Surg Gynecol Obstet 1980;150:251.
136. Fialkow PJ. Autoimmunity and chromosomal aberrations. Am J Hum Genet 1966;18:93.
137. Greer MA, Meihoff WC, Studer H. Treatment of hyperthyroidism with a single daily dose of propylthiouracil. N Engl J Med 1965;272:888.
138. Niswander KR, Gordon M, Berendes HW. The women and their pregnancies. Philadelphia: WB Saunders, 1972.
139. Hetzel BS, Hay ID. Thyroid function, iodine nutrition and fetal brain development. Clin Endocrinol 1979;11:445.
140. Dussault JH, Coulombe P, Laberge C, Letarte J, Guyda H, Khoury K. Preliminary report on a mass screening program for neonatal hypothyroidism. J Pediatr 1975;86:670.
141. Miyai K, Fukunishi T, Mizuta H, Amino N, Nose O, Tsuruhara T. HLA-A and -B antigens in Japanese patients with congenital hypothyroidism and their parents. Tissue Antigens 1984; 23:210.
142. Sutherland JM, Esselborn VM, Burket RL, Skillman TB, Bensen JT. Familial nongoitrous cretinism apparently due to maternal antithyroid antibody. Report of a family. N Engl J Med 1960;263:336.
143. Chandler JW, Blizzard RM, Hung W, Kyle M. Thyroid antibodies pass to fetus. N Engl J Med 1962;267:376.
144. Van Herle AJ, Young RT, Fisher DA, Uller RP, Brinkman CR III. Intra-uterine treatment of a hypothyroid fetus. J Clin Endocrinol Metab 1975;40:474.
145. Van de Spuy AM, Jacobs HS. Management of endocrine disorders in pregnancy. I: thyroid and parathyroid disease. Postgrad Med 1984;60:245.
146. Rosenthal FD, Jones C, Lewis SI. Thyrotoxic vomiting. Br Med J 1976;2:209.
147. Valentine BH, Jones C, Tyack AJ. Hyperemesis gravidarum due to thyrotoxicosis. Postgrad Med J 1980;56:746.
148. Dozeman R, Kaiser FE, Cass O, Pries J. Hyperthyroidism appearing as hyperemesis gravidarum. Arch Intern Med 1983; 143:2202.
149. Souma JA, Niejadlik DC, Cottrel S, Rankle S. Comparison of thyroid function in each trimester of pregnancy with the use of triiodothyronine uptake, thyroxine, free thyroxine and free thyroxine index. Am J Obstet Gynecol 1973;116:905.

150. Mussey RD. Hyperthyroidism complicating pregnancy. Mayo Clin Proc 1939;14:205.
151. McLaughlin CW Jr, McGoogan LS. Hyperthyroidism complicating pregnancy. Am J Obstet Gynecol 1943;45:591.
152. Myers CR. An application of the control group method to the problem of the etiology of mongolism. Proc Am Assoc Mental Def 1938;62:142.
153. Davis TF, Weiss L. Autoimmune thyroid disease and pregnancy. Am J Reprod Immunol Microbiol 1981;1:187.
154. Mujtaba Q, Burrow GN. Treatment of hyperthyroidism in pregnancy with propylthiouracil and methimazole. Obstet Gynecol 1975;46:282.
155. Stephan MJ, Smith DW, Ponzi JW, Alden ER. Origin of scalp vertex aplasic cutis. J Pediatr 1982;101:850.
156. Burrow GN, Klatskin EH, Genel M. Intellectual in children with mothers who received propylthiouracil during pregnancy. Yale J Biol Med 1978;51:151.
157. Momotani N, Ito K, Hamada N, et al. Maternal hyperthyroidism and congenital malformation in the offspring. Clin Endocrinol 1984;20:695.
158. Marchant B, Brownlie BEW, Hart DM, et al. The placental transfer of propylthiouracil, methimazole and carbimazole. J Clin Endocrinol Metab 1977;45:1187.
159. Refetoff S, Ochi Y, Selenkow HA, Rosenfield RL. Neonatal hypothyroidism and goiter in one infant of each of two sets of twins due to maternal therapy with antithyroid drugs. J Pediatr 1974;85:240.
160. Kampmann JP, Hansen JM, Johansen K, Helweg J. Propylthiouracil in human milk. Lancet 1980;1:736.
161. Cooper DS, Bode HH, Nath B, Saxe U, Maloof F, Ridgway EC. Methimazole pharmacology in man: studies using an newly developed radioimmunoassay for methimazole. J Clin Endocrinol Metab 1984;58:473.
162. Gladstone GR, Hordof A, Gersony WM. Propranolol administration during pregnancy: effects on the fetus. J Pediatr 1975;86:962.
163. Habib A, McCarthy JS. Effects on the neonate of propranolol administered during pregnancy. J Pediatr 1977;91:808.
164. Pruyn SC, Phelan JP, Buchanan GC. Long-term propranolol therapy in pregnancy: maternal and fetal outcome. Am J Obstet Gynecol 1979;135:485.
165. Bullock JL, Harris RE, Young R. Treatment of thyrotoxicosis during pregnancy with propranolol. Am J Obstet Gynecol 1975;121:242.
166. Rubin PC. Beta-blockers in pregnancy. N Engl J Med 1983;18:73.
167. Ingbar SH. Management of emergencies. IX: thyrotoxic storm. N Engl J Med 166;274:1252.
168. Ashkar FS, Katims RB, Smoak WM, Gilson AJ. Thyroid storm treatment with blood exchange and plasmapheresis. JAMA 1970;214:1275.
169. Derksen RHWM, van der Wiel A, Poortman J, der Kunderens PJ, Kater L. Plasma exchange in the treatment of severe thyrotoxicosis in pregnancy. Eur J Obstet Gynecol Reprod Biol 1984;18:139.
170. Piper J, Rosen J. Management of hyperthyroidism during pregnancy. Acta Med Scand 1954;150:215.
171. Bell GO, Hall J. Hyperthyroidism in pregnancy. Med Clin North Am 1960;44:363.
172. Howe P, Francis HH. Pregnancy and thyrotoxicosis. Br Med J 1962;2:817.
173. Smith EM, Warner GG. Estimates of radiation doses to the embryo from nuclear medicine procedures. J Nucl Med 1976;17:836.
174. Husak V, Wiedermann M. Radiation absorbed dose estimates to the embryo from some nuclear medicine procedures. Eur J Nucl Med 1980;5:202.
175. Goldstein L, Murphy DP. Etiology of the ill-health in children born after maternal pelvic irradiation. II: defective children born after postconception pelvic irradiation. AJR 1929;22:322.
176. Stewart A, Webb J, Hewitt D. A survey of childhood malignancies. Br Med J 1958;1:1495.
177. MacMahon B. Prenatal x-ray exposure and childhood cancer. J Natl Cancer Inst 1962;28:1173.
178. Dirmikis SM, Munro DS. Placental transmission of thyroid stimulating immunoglobulins. Br Med J 1975;2:665.
179. Munro DS, Dirmikis SM, Humphries H, Smith T, Broadhead GD. The role of thyroid stimulating immunoglobulins of Graves' disease in neonatal thyroxtoxicosis. Br J Obstet Gynaecol 1978;85:837.
180. McKenzie JM, Zakarija M. Pathogenesis of neonatal Graves' disease. J Endocrinol Invest 1978;2:182.
181. Maisey MN, Stimmler L. The role of long acting thyroid stimulator in neonatal thyrotoxicosis. Clin Endocrinol 1972;1:81.
182. Munro DS, Cooke ID, Dirmikis SM, et al. Neonatal thyrotoxicosis. Q J Med 1976;45:689.
183. Fisher DA. Pathogenesis and therapy of neonatal Graves' disease. Am J Dis Child 1976;130:133.
184. Hollingsworth DR, Mabry CC. Congenital Graves' disease. Four familial cases with long-term follow-up and perspective. Am J Dis Child 1976;130:148.
185. Kaplan MM. Thyroid diseases in pregnancy. In: Gleicher N, ed. Principles of medical therapy in pregnancy. New York: Plenum Publishing, 1985:192.
186. Amino N, Mori H, Iwatani Y, et al. High prevalence of transient post-partum thyrotoxicosis and hypothyroidism. N Engl J Med 1982;306:849.
187. Jansson R, Bernander S, Karlsson A, Levin K, Nilsson G. Autoimmune thyroid dysfunction in the postpartum period. J Clin Endocrinol Metab 1984;58:681.
188. Rosvoll RV, Winship T. Thyroid carcinoma and pregnancy. Surg Gynecol Obstet 1965;121:1039.
189. Hill CS Jr, Clark RL, Wolf M. The effect of subsequent pregnancy on patients with thyroid carcinoma. Surg Gynecol Obstet 1966;122:1219.
190. Whiteley HJ, Stoner HB. The effect of pregnancy on the human adrenal cortex. J Endocrinol 1957;14:325.
191. Doe RP, Fernandez R, Seal US. Measurement of corticosteroid binding globulin in man. J Clin Endocrinol Metab 1974;24:1029.
192. Rosenthal HE, Slaunwhite WR, Sandberg AA. Transcortin: a corticosteroid-binding protein of plasma. X: cortisol and progesterone interplay and unbound levels of these steroids in pregnancy. J Clin Endocrinol Metab 1969;29:352.
193. Christy NP, Wallace EZ, Gordon WEL, Jailer JW. On the rate of hydrocortisone clearance from plasma in pregnant women and in patients with Laennec's chirrhosis. J Clin Invest 1959;38:299.
194. Peterson RE, Nokes G, Chen PS Jr, Black RL. Estrogen and adrenocortical function in man. J Clin Endocrinol Metab 1960;20:495.
195. Migeon CJ, Kenny FM, Taylor FH. Cortisol production rate. VIII: pregnancy. J Clin Endocrinol Metab 1968;28:661.
196. Nolten WE, Lindheimer MD, Rueckert PA, Oparil S, Ehrlich EN. Diurnal patterns and regulation of cortisol secretion in pregnancy. J Clin Endocrinol Metab 1980;51:466.
197. Rees LH, Burke CW, Chard T, Evans SW, Letchworth AT. Possible placental origin of ACTH in normal human pregnancy. Nature 1975;254:620.
198. Gordon RD, Symonds EM, Wilmshurst EG, et al. Plasma renin activity, plasma angiotensin and plasma and urinary electro-

lytes in normal and toxaemic pregnancy, including a prospective study. Clin Sci 1973;45:115.
199. Weir RJ, Jehoiada, Brown J, et al. Relationship between plasma renin, renin-substrate, angiotensin II, aldosterone and electrolytes in normal pregnancy. J Clin Endocrinol Metab 1975; 40:108.
200. Ferris TF, Stein JH, Kauffman J. Uterine blood flow and uterine renin secretion. J Clin Invest 1972;51:2827.
201. Watanabe M, Meeker CI, Gray MJ, Sims EAH, Soloman S. Secretion rate of aldosterone in normal pregnancy. J Clin Invest 1963;42:1619.
202. Landau RL, Luigibihl K. Inhibition of the sodium-retaining influence of aldosterone by progesterone. J Clin Endocrinol Metab 1958;18:1237.
203. Ledoux F, Genest J, Nowaczynski W, Kuchel O, Lebel M. Plasma progesterone and aldosterone in pregnancy. CMAJ 1975;112:943.
204. Nolten WE, Lindheimer MD, Oparil S, Ehrlich EN. Desoxycorticosterone in normal pregnancy. Am J Obstet Gynecol 1978;132:414.
205. Winkel CA, Milewich L, Parker CR, Gant NF, Simpson ER, MacDonald PC. Conversion of plasma progesterone to deoxycorticosterone in men, nonpregnant and pregnant women, and adrenalectomized subjects: evidence for steroid 21-hydroxylase activity in nonadrenal tissues. J Clin Invest 1980;66:803.
206. Casey ML, MacDonald PC. Extradrenal formation of a mineralocorticosteroid: deoxycorticosterone and deoxycorticosterone sulfate biosynthesis and metabolism. Endocr Rev 1982;3:396.
207. Rivarola MA, Forest MG, Migeon CJ. Testosterone, androstenedione and dehydroepiandrosterone in plasma during pregnancy and at delivery: concentrations and protein binding. J Clin Endocrinol Metab 1968;28:34.
208. Forest MG, Ances IG, Tapper AJ, Migeon CJ. Percentage binding of testosterone, androstenedione, and dehydroepiandrosterone in plasma at the time of delivery. J Clin Endocrinol Metab 1971;32:417.
209. Nieschlag E, Walk T, Schindler AE. Dehydroepiandrosterone (DHA) and DHA-sulfate during pregnancy in maternal blood. Horm Metab Res 1974;6:170.
210. Gandy HM. Estrogens and androgens. In: Fuchs F, Klopper A, eds. Endocrinology pregnancy. 2nd ed. New York: Harper & Row, 1977:73.
211. Bolte E, Mancuso S, Eriksson G, Wiqvist N, Diczfalusy E. Studies on the aromatization of neutral steroids in pregnant women. Aromatization of dehydroepiandrosterone and of its sulphate administered simultaneously into a uterine artery. Acta Endocrinol (Copenh) 1964;45:560.
212. MacDonald PC, Siiteri PK. Origin of estrogen in women pregnant with an anencephalic fetus. J Clin Invest 1965;44:465.
213. Vagnucci A, Lee P. Diseases of the adrenal cortex in pregnancy. In: Brody SA, Ueland K, eds. Endocrine disorders in pregnancy. East Norwalk, CN: Appleton and Lange, 1989:177.
214. Lindholm J, Schultz-Moller N. Plasma and urinary cortisol in pregnancy and during estrogen-gestagen treatment. Scand J Clin Lab Invest 1973;31:119.
215. Murphy BEP, Okouneff LM, Klein GP, Ngo SC. Lack of specificity of cortisol determinations in human urine. J Clin Endocrinol Metab 1981;53:91.
216. Nolten WE, Lindheimer MD, Rueckert PA, Oparil S, Ehrlich EN. Diurnal patterns and regulation of cortisol secretion in pregnancy. J Clin Endocrinol Metab 1980;51:466.
217. Crapo L. Cushing's syndrome. A review of diagnostic tests. Metabolism 1979;28:955.
218. Tyrrell JB, Findling JW, Aron DC, Fitzgerald PA, Forsham PH. An overnight high-dose dexoamethasone suppression test for rapid differential diagnosis of Cushing's syndrome. Ann Intern Med 1986;104:180.
219. Irvine WJ, Barnes EW. Adrenocortical insufficiency. Clin Endocrinol Metab 1972;1:549.
220. Rodriguez JA, Lopez JM, Biglieri EG. DOCA test for aldosteronism: its usefulness and implications. Hypertension 1981;3:102.
221. Williams GH, Moore TJ. The renin-angiotensin-aldosterone axis. In: Tulchinsky D, Ryan KY, eds. Maternal-fetal endocrinology. Philadelphia: WB Saunders, 1980:84.
222. Bravo EL, Tarazi RC, Dustan HP, et al. The changing clinical spectrum of primary aldosteronism. Am J Med 1983;74:641.
223. Melmon KL. The endocrinologic function of selected autacoids: catecholamines, acetylcholine, serotonin, and histamine. In: Williams RH, ed. Textbook of endocrinology. Philadelphia: WB Saunders, 1981:515.
224. Hendee AE, Martin RD, Waters WC. Hypertension in pregnancy: toxemia or pheochromocytoma? Am J Obstet Gynecol 1969;105:64.
225. Axelrod J. Purification and properties of phenylethanolamide-N-methyltransferase. J Biol Chem 1962;237:1657.
226. Crout JR, Pisano JJ, Sjoerdsma A. Urinary excretion of catecholamines and their metabolites in pheochromocytoma. Am Heart J 1961;61:375.
227. Schenker JG, Granat M. Phaecochromocytoma and pregnancy — an updated appraisal. Aust NZ J Obstet Gynaecol 1982;22:1.
228. Johannisson E. The foetal adrenal cortex in the human. Acta Endocrinol (Suppl) (Copenh) 1968;130:7.
229. Beitins IZ, Bayard F, Ances IG, Kewarski A, Migeon CJ. The metabolic clearance rate, blood production, interconversion and transplacental passage of cortisol and cortisone in pregnancy near term. Pediatr Res 1973;7:509.
230. Campbell AL, Murphy BEP. The maternal-fetal cortisol gradient during pregnancy and at delivery. J Clin Endocrinol Metab 1977;45:435.
231. Dancis J, Jansen V, Levitz M, Rosner W. Effect of protein binding on transfer and metabolism of cortisol in perfused human placenta. J Clin Endocrinol Metab 1978;46:863.
232. Allen JP, Cook DM, Kendall JW, McGilvra R. Maternal ACTH relationship in man. J Clin Endocrinol Metab 1973;37:230.
233. Bayard F, Ances IG, Tapper AJ, Weldon VV, Kowarski A, Migeon CJ. Transplacental passage and fetal secretion of aldosterone. J Clin Invest 1970;49:1389.
234. Kreines K, DeVaux WD. Neonatal adrenal insufficiency associated with maternal Cushing's syndrome. Pediatrics 1971; 47:516.
235. Koerten JM, Morales WJ, Washington SR III, et al. Cushing's syndrome in pregnancy: a case report and literature review. Am J Obstet Gynecol 1986;154:626.
236. Gold EM. The Cushing syndromes: changing views of diagnosis and treatment. Ann Intern Med 1979;90:829.
237. Tyrrell JB, Brooks RM, Fitzgerald PA, Cofoid PB, Forsham PH, Wilson CB. Cushing's disease. Selective transsphenoidal resection of pituitary microadenomas. N Engl J Med 1978;298:753.
238. Bigos ST, Somma M, Rasio E, et al. Cushing's disease. Management by transsphenoidal pituitary microsurgery. J Clin Endocrinol Metab 1980;50:348.
239. Boggan JE, Tyrell JB, Wilson CB. Transsphenoidal microsurgical management of Cushing's disease. Report of100 cases. J Neurosurg 1983;59:195.
240. Kasperlik-Zaluska A, Migdalska B, Hartwig W. Two pregnancies in a woman with Cushing's syndrome treated with cyproheptadine. Br J Obstet Gynaecol 1980;87:1171.
241. Gormley MJ, Hadden DR, Kennedy T, Montgomery DAD, Murnaghan GA, Sheridan B. Cushing's syndrome in pregnancy — treatment with metyrapone. Clin Endocrinol 1982;16:283.
242. Leiba S, Kaufman H, Winkelsberg G, Bahary CM. Pregnancy in

a case of Nelson's syndrome. Acta Obstet Gynecol Scand 1978;57:373.

243. Messina M, Biffignandi P, Ghigo E, Jeantet MG, Molinatti GM. Possible contraindication of spironolactone during pregnancy. J Endocrinol Invest 1979;2:222.
244. Smith AM. Phaechromocytoma and pregnancy. J Obstet Gynaecol Br Commonwealth 1973;80:848.
245. Griffith MI, Felts JH, James FM. Successful control of pheochromocytoma in pregnancy. JAMA 1974;229:437.
246. Burgess GE, Cooper JR, Marino RJ, Peuler MJ. Anesthetic management of combined cesarean section and excision of pheochromocytoma. Anesth Analg 1978;57:276.
247. Irvine WJ, Barnes EW. Addison's disease, ovarian failure and hypoparathyroidism. Clin Endocrinol Metab 1975;4:379.
248. Poonai A, Jelercic F, Pop-Lazic B. Pregnancy with diabetes mellitus, Addison's disease, and hypothyroidism. Obstet Gynecol 1977;49(Suppl):86s.
249. Hadi HA, Fadel HE, Huff TA. Pregnancy in a patient with type II polyendocrinopathy. J Reprod Med 1983;28:547.
250. Brent F. Addison's disease and pregnancy. Am J Surg 1950:79:645.
251. Drucker D, Shumak S, Angel A. Schmidt syndrome presenting with intrauterine growth retardation and post partum addisonian crises. Am J Obstet Gynecol 1984;149:229.
252. Gamlen TR, Aynsley-Green A, Irvine WJ, McCallum CJ. Immunological studies in the neonate of a mother with Addison's disease and diabetes mellitus. Clin Exp Immunol 1977;28:192.
253. Bondy PK, Rosenberg LE. Metabolic control and disease. 8th ed. Philadelphia: WB Saunders, 1980:1480.
254. Holler W, Scholz S, Knorr D, Bidlingmaier F, Keller E, Albert ED. Genetic differences between the salt-wasting, simple virilizing, and nonclassical types of congenital adrenal hyperplasia. J Clin Endocrinol Metab 1985;60:757.
255. Zachmann M, Tassanari D, Prader A. Clinical and biochemical variability of congenital adrenal hyperplasia due to 11-B-hydroxylase deficiency. A study of 25 patients. J Clin Endocrinol Metab 1983;56:222.
256. New MI, Dupont B, Pang S, et al. Metabolic errors of adrenal steroidogenesis. In: Martin L, James BHT, eds. Current topics in experimental endocrinology. Vol 5. New York: Academic Press, 1983;309.
257. Pollack MS, Levine LS, Pang S, et al. Prenatal diagnosis of congenital adrenal hyperplasia (21-hydroxylase deficiency) by HLA typing. Lancet 1979;1:1107.
258. Rosler A, Leiberman E, Rosenmann A, Ben-Uzilio R, Weidenfeld J. Prenatal diagnosis of 11-beta-hydroxylase deficiency congenital adrenal hyperplasia. J Clin Endocrinol Metab 1979; 49:546.
259. Hughes IA, Laurence KM. Antenatal diagnosis of congenital adrenal hyperplasia. Lancet 1979;2:7.
260. Schumert Z, Rosenmann A, Landau H, Rosler A. 11-deoxycortisol in amniotic fluid: prenatal diagnosis of congenital adrenal hyperplasia due to 11B-hydroxylase deficiency. Clin Endocrinol 1980;12:257.
261. David M, Maguelone GF. Prenatal treatment of congenital adrenal hyperplasia resulting from 21-hydroxylase deficiency. J Pediatr 1984;105:799.
262. Speroff L. The adrenogenital syndrome and its obstetrical aspects. A review of the literature and case report. Obstet Gynecol Surv 1965;20:185.
263. Mori N, Miyakawa I. Congenital adrenogenital syndrome and successful pregnancy. Obstet Gynecol 1970;35:394.
264. Pitkin RM, Reynolds WA, Williams GA, Hargis GK. Calcium metabolism in normal pregnancy: a longitudinal study. Am J Obstet Gynecol 1979;133:781.
265. Samaan NA, Hill CS Jr, Beceiro JR, Schultz PN. Immunoreactive calcitonin in medullary carcinomas of the thyroid and in maternal and cord serum. J Lab Clin Med 1973;81:671.
266. Samaan NA, Anderson GD, Adam-Mayne ME. Immunoreactive calcitonin in the mother, neonate, child, and adult. Am J Obstet Gynecol 1975;121:622.
267. Steichen JJ, Tsant RC, Gratton TL, Hamstra A, DeLuca HF. Vitamin D homeostasis in the perinatal period. N Engl J Med 1980;302:315.
268. Pellegrino SV. Primary hyperparathyroidism exacerbated by pregnancy. J Oral Maxillofac Surg 1977;35:915.
269. Johnstone RE II, Kreindler T, Johnstone RE. Hyperparathyroidism during pregnancy. Obstet Gynecol 1972;40:580.
270. Delmonico FL, Neer RM, Cosimi AB, Barnes AB, Russell PS. Hyperparthyroidism during pregnancy. Am J Surg 1976; 131:328.
271. Croom RD III, Thomas CG Jr. Primary hyperparathyroidism during pregnancy. Surgery 1984;96:1109.
272. Gershberg H, Young BK. Primary hyperparathyroidism in pregnancy. NY State J Med 1984;84:323.
273. Kristoffersson A, Dahlgren S, Lithner F, Jarhult J. Primary hyperparathyroidism in pregnancy. Surgery 1985;97:326.
274. Montoro MN, Collea JV, Mestman JH. Management of hyperparathyroidism in pregnancy with oral phosphate therapy. Obstet Gynecol 1980;55:431.
275. Levy HA, Pierucci L, Stroup P. Oral phosphate treatment of hypercalcemia in pregnancy. J Med Soc NJ 1981;78:113.
276. Watney PJ, Chance GW, Scott P, Thompson JM. Maternal factors in neonatal hypocalcaemia: a study in three ethnic groups. Br Med J 1971;2:432.
277. Monteleone JA, Lee JB, Tashijan AH, Cantor HE. Transient neonatal hypoclacemia, hypomagnesemia, and high serum parathyroid hormone with maternal hyperparathryoidism. Ann Intern Med 1975;82:670.
278. Jacobson BB, Terslev E, Lund B, Sorensen OH. Neonatal hypocalcemia associated with maternal hyperparathyroidism. Arch Dis Child 1978;53:308.
279. Sadeghi-Nejad A, Wolfsdorf JI, Senior B. Hypoparathyroidism and pregnancy: treatment with calcitriol. JAMA 1980;243:254.
280. Bronsky D, Weisbery MG, Gross MC, Barron JJ. Hyperparathyroidism and acute postpartum pancreatitis with neonatal tetany in the child. Am J Med Sci 1970;260:160.
281. Goldberg LD. Transmission of a vitamin-D metabolite in breast milk. Lancet 1972;2:1258.

63

CHAPTER

GASTROINTESTINAL DISEASES COMPLICATING PREGNANCY

Washington Clark Hill

Pregnancy can complicate almost any gastrointestinal disease. The pregnant woman may enter pregnancy with a gastrointestinal disorder, or it may develop during the pregnancy. The physiologic effects of pregnancy may cause gastrointestinal disturbances such as nausea, vomiting, hyperemesis gravidarum, and esophageal reflux. Conversely, gastrointestinal disorders such as ruptured appendix and inflammatory bowel disease may effect the course of pregnancy. This chapter discusses the various gastrointestinal diseases complicating pregnancy and their effect on the fetus and its mother. The chapter is organized into three parts: (1) diseases within the gastrointestinal tract—nausea, vomiting, hyperemesis gravidarum, oral cavity complications of pregnancy, reflux esophagitis, peptic ulcer disease, acute intestinal obstruction, inflammatory bowel disease, appendicitis, pregnancy following operation for morbid obesity, and constipation; (2) diseases outside the gastrointestinal tract—gallbladder disease and pancreatitis; and (3) total parenteral nutrition in pregnancy.

DISEASES WITHIN THE GASTROINTESTINAL TRACT

NAUSEA, VOMITING, AND HYPEREMESIS GRAVIDARUM

Nausea with or without vomiting is an especially common symptom during early pregnancy. It usually occurs during the first trimester of pregnancy, and by mid-pregnancy most women no longer complain of these symptoms. The incidence has not been well studied, but it occurs in approximately 60% to 80% of pregnancies in the United States. In its mildest form, it is referred to as "morning sickness," which is unpleasant and distressing, both physically and psychologically, but requires no particular therapy. About 1 to 2 per 1000 pregnant patients may experience some morning sickness throughout their entire pregnancy. It is unknown why some patients experience no morning sickness and others are bothered by it all of the time.

The cause of nausea and vomiting during pregnancy is unknown. The smooth muscle of the stomach does relax during pregnancy, and this physiologic change may play some role. The role of human chorionic gonadotropin has been studied by Soules and coworkers.[1,2] These authors, however, were unable to demonstrate a clear correlation between the maternal serum hCG levels and the severity of morning sickness. Patients with high levels of hCG, as in twin gestations or hydatidiform moles, may or may not experience exaggerated nausea and vomiting throughout pregnancy. Other less-studied theories include a deficiency in progesterone and hyperthyroidism.[2]

The management of nausea and vomiting during pregnancy is primarily supportive. Therapeutic regimens include reassurance, physical and psychological support, frequent small meals, the avoidance of foods that are unpleasant or that may initiate symptoms, adequate hydration and fluid intake, and selective, occasional use of antiemetics. There is no ideal antiemetic currently available for the treatment of morning sickness. Until 1983, Bendectin was available; this drug was a combination of doxylamine succinate (10 mg) and pyridoxine (10 mg). Bendectin, which had been approved by the Food and Drug Administration (FDA) for the treatment of nausea and vomiting in pregnancy, was removed from the market by the pharmaceutical company in 1983, primarily because of litigation. There is no evidence that Bendectin was teratogenic.[3–7] When symptoms require treatment, both pyridoxine and doxylamine are still available over-the-counter as Unisom (25 mg). Antiemetic therapy should be used when supportive measures are not effective. Other antiemetics that have also been used successfully in the treatment of nausea and vomiting of pregnancy include the phenothiazines, trimethobenzamide, metoclopramide, and diphenhydramine.

Hyperemesis gravidarum is the abnormal condition of pregnancy associated with pernicious nausea and vomiting. Hyperemesis is both infrequent and uncommon. These patients experience persistent intractable nausea and vomiting associated with weight loss, fluid and electrolyte imbalance, ketonuria, and ketonemia. Electrolyte imbalance may include decreased sodium, potassium, and chloride, and metabolic alkalosis. The patient usually becomes clinically dehydrated and may even develop jaundice, hyperpyrexia, and peripheral neuritis. Recurrent hyperemesis gravidarum has caused recurrent first trimester jaundice.[8] Wernicke's encephalopathy has even been reported in patients with hyperemesis gravidarum.[9,10] If the patient is not appropriately treated, there may be a failure of the mother and fetus to increase their weight. A patient with hyperemesis gravidarum who has abnormal electrolyte, renal, or liver tests should be promptly hospitalized for fluid management. Outpatient therapy consisting of intravenous fluid hydration is usually sufficient, along with supportive therapy. Intravenous pyridoxine 100 mg/L of intravenous fluid has also been included as a part of the intravenous therapy. However, when the patient's condition does not improve, hospitalization with appropriate electrolyte, caloric, and fluid management is necessary.

Levine and Esser have reported the safe and effective use of first trimester total parenteral nutrition in the management of hyperemesis gravidarum, which was initiated in the hospital was continued in the patient's home.[11] Using a standard method of indirect calorimetry, the basal metabolic expenditure and adjusted metabolic expenditure were determined. Appropriate calories were calculated for each of their ten patients. After being on total parenteral nutrition, these patients showed improved nutritional status. The authors report no evidence of placental insufficiency during labor, placental emboli on pathologic examination, and no evidence of preterm labor. Stellato and coworkers have also reported the successful use of total parenteral nutrition in treating hyperemesis gravidarum in the hospital and at home.[12] Maternal and fetal death have been reported as a result of this therapy by Greenspoon and colleagues.[13]

The role of psychosocial stressors, such as an undesired pregnancy, in the etiology of nausea, vomiting, and hyperemesis gravidarum has been only partially studied. A report by Callahan and associates emphasizes the importance of behavioral treatment of hyperemesis gravidarum.[14] These investigators studied patients and devised a problem-solving approach that provided the patients with alternative strategies for dealing with critical stressors other than pernicious nausea and vomiting. Their stress management techniques led to decreased nausea and vomiting in each patient. Their approach enlisted the patient's interest in environmental manipulation to improve their social situation. Henker used adjunctive psychotherapeutic measures in treating ten consecutive women referred to his psychiatric service because of severe intractable vomiting.[15] In addition to customary medical measures, these patients received three types of psychotherapy: supportive psychotherapy, hypnotherapy, and behavior modification. Nine patients recovered and completed normal pregnancies, while one improved but later aborted due to other complications. When compared with a control group of routinely treated patients, recovery was more rapid. These approaches require further study, but certainly social and psychological evaluation of the patient with severe hyperemesis gravidarum is indicated.

Although most patients with pernicious nausea and vomiting of pregnancy have hyperemesis gravidarum, other gastrointestinal diseases must be ruled out. These include bowel obstruction, pancreatitis, biliary colic, and peptic ulcer disease, which are discussed elsewhere in this chapter.

Some patients with hyperemesis gravidarum have transient hyperthyroidism.[16,17] Thyroid evaluation should be a part of the work-up of these patients. Whether the hyperthyroidism is a cause of hyperemesis or is present because of the condition is a difficult differential diagnosis. Drug-induced nausea by antibiotics or other medications must also be considered a cause of pernicious nausea and vomiting. Rarely do these patients have other signs of hyperthyroidism such as tremor, hyperreflexia, temperature elevation, or intestinal hypermotility. They have in one study required or been given antithyroid treatment.[18] Whether or not antithyroid is necessary in the treatment of transient hyperthyroidism occurring in hyperemetic pregnancies remains controversial.

Most patients with hyperemesis gravidarum improve with appropriate medical therapy. Maternal mortality is rare, but has been reported when severe metabolic abnormalities go untreated, esophageal tears (Mallory-Weiss syndrome) occur, or hematemesis develops. The exact cause and role of stress in the development of hyperemesis gravidarum remains to be defined.

The association of nausea and vomiting in pregnancy with pregnancy outcome has been investigated by several authors. A recent study by Weigel and Weigel reviewed the pregnancy outcome in 903 women who had experienced nausea and vomiting early in pregnancy.[19] Their analysis showed that vomiting was associated with a decreased risk of miscarriage. Women with nausea but no vomiting had a miscarriage rate equal to that in the sample overall. Among the subsample of women with signs of threatened miscarriage, those who had experienced vomiting also had a decreased risk of miscarriage. The authors had no explanation for these findings, which had also been reported previously by Klenbanoff and colleagues.[20] In the Weigel study, nausea and vomiting of pregnancy was not associated significantly with any other factor such as postdate pregnancy, preterm labor, low infant birth weight, fetal anomalies, placental weight, head circumference, or body length. Other earlier studies have suggested various associations.[19,20] Weigel and Weigel, in a subsequent meta-analytical review of 11 previous studies evaluating nausea and vomiting of pregnancy and pregnancy outcome, concluded that there was a strong significant association of nausea and vomiting of pregnancy with decreased risk of miscarriage, but could define no consistent association with perinatal mortality.[21] Their analysis also confirmed the association of nausea and vomiting of early pregnancy with decreased fetal mortality during the first 20 weeks of pregnancy. Although nausea and vomiting of early pregnancy may be a bothersome and common symptom, there appears to be no consistent or significant effect from this gastrointestinal disorder on pregnancy outcome, good or bad.

ORAL CAVITY COMPLICATIONS OF PREGNANCY

Many pregnant women enter pregnancy with poor dental care. They may not have seen a dentist since their own childhood. Their teeth are in poor condition, and numerous cavities and gingivitis are present due to poor dental hygiene. They should be referred and encouraged to see a dentist, because dental care is not prohibited during pregnancy. Pregnant women should be urged to practice good oral hygiene.[22]

In 1926, Ziskin studied the incidence of dental caries in pregnant and nulliparous women and concluded that they were no more susceptible to tooth decay than the non-pregnant patient.[23] No relation was found between dental caries experience and pregnancy or between caries and the number of pregnancies. There was actually a slightly lower number of caries in the pregnant group, and it was postulated that pregnancy might even be protective against caries. Later, Liskin and Hotelling again raised this possibility.[24] There is no agreement that normal pregnancy causes decreased or increased caries. Rather, the worsening of dental caries during pregnancy is due to poor dental hygiene.[25,26]

This may not be true for the diabetic pregnancy. Albrecht and colleagues recently studied the dental and oral changes of 271 pregnant and non-pregnant diabetic and nondiabetic women.[27] One hundred and thirty-two pregnant diabetics under care showed a 96% prevalence of gingivitis higher than in any of the other three groups. This is also higher than most other reports of nondiabetic pregnant women.[22–24] The intensity of the gingivitis in the diabetic women was most marked in weeks 11 to 15 and 24 to 26 of pregnancy. The severity of diabetes had no effect on the degree of gingivitis. As for caries, the mean number of carious, filled, and extracted teeth increased during diabetic pregnancies more than in the diabetic non-pregnant women. Oral hygiene was significantly worse at all stages of pregnancy in the diabetics than in the nondiabetic pregnant women.

The chemical and mineral composition of human teeth has not been shown to be changed by pregnancy or lactation.[28,29] The endocrine changes of pregnancy may affect the oral cavity, resulting in increased blood supply to the gingivae, hyperplastic gingivae, and a thin, smooth, shiny surface epithelium.[22,25] The color may not change at all or may become deeply reddened. Pregnancy does not cause gingivitis; it is caused by bacteria.[26] The increase in gingival vascularity can result in accentuated gingival hyperplasia or enlargement, which is commonly referred to as "pregnancy gingivitis." The incidence of this common oral condition during pregnancy is unknown, but probably occurs in at least 50% of pregnant women. Once the hormonal changes of pregnancy decline, the exaggerated gingivitis due to pregnancy decreases.[30] Pregnancy does not increase the amount of oral calculus present on the teeth. Calculus, however, may, when oral hygiene is poor, lead to mild, moderate, or severe gingivitis and other periodontal disease (Figs. 63-1, 63-2, and 63-3). Although it is universally accepted that pregnancy gingivitis is due to increased vascularity of the gingivae, studies are not in agreement whether these changes are due to progesterone, estrogen, or neither hormone.[31–33]

Bleeding from the gingivae, a common complaint of pregnant women, due to pregnancy gingivitis, requires no treatment.[22] Gingivitis that is due to poor dentition and hygiene is treated by a good cleaning of the teeth and by meticulous dental care.[22,26] There is no basis for delaying dental care during pregnancy, and patients who require treatment should obtain it promptly. Prenatal care should include a good examination of the teeth by a dentist who may then consult with the obstetrician about the best treatment plan.

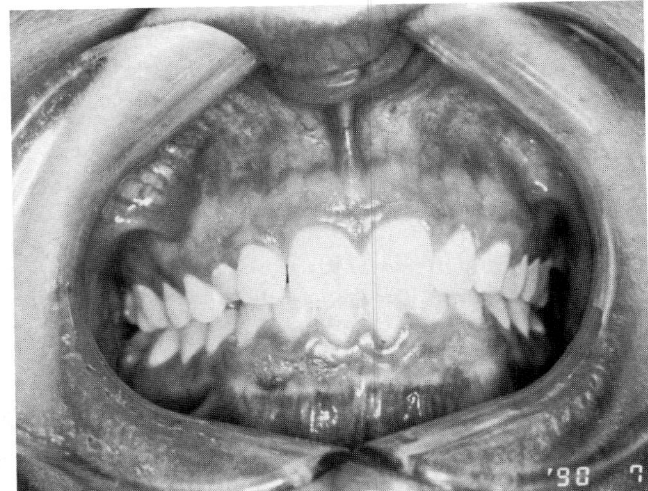

FIGURE 63–1. Mild gingivitis in 10-week pregnant patient due to poor dental hygiene that resolved with improved dental hygiene. (Courtesy of Dr. John Marley)

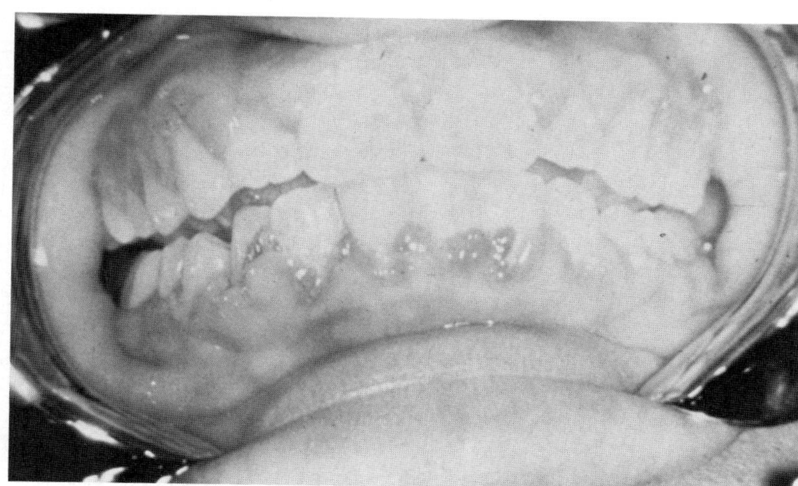

FIGURE 63–2. Moderate gingivitis of pregnancy at 20 weeks gestation. (Courtesy of John Francis and Dr. Carole Brenniese)

Pregnancy tumor is a granuloma that forms as a result of exaggerated gingival enlargement during pregnancy.[25,26,34] It appears as a localized enlargement of the hyperplastic gingivae or pedunculated growth (Fig. 63-4). Pregnancy tumors are pyogenic granulomas because they result from nonspecific inflammatory gingivitis secondary to poor oral hygiene, associated with deposits of plaque and calculus on the teeth. The poor teeth and gums adjacent to these lesions are responsible for the local irritation resulting in the pregnancy tumor. These predisposing inflammatory factors, along with the hormonal effects of pregnancy on the gingival tissues, predispose to the development of pregnancy tumors. These lesions are usually present on the anterior maxillary gingivae. They vary in size, but are usually not larger than 2 to 3 cm in diameter. Setia reported the case of a large pregnancy tumor that resulted in hemorrhage from the palate.[35] This is usually not the case, but these tumors can sometimes produce significant bleeding. Pregnancy tumors occur in approximately 1% to 5% of pregnant women,[36,37] and have been reported to have a race predominance in white patients.[38,39] The tumors are typically pedunculated, lobulated, red due to their vascularity, and soft with a smooth surface. The lesion is painless and is first noticed by the patient as a mass, unless it is so large that it interferes with mastication. Consultation with a dentist is indicated. Biopsy is not usually necessary. Histology on the surgically removed tumor is always benign (Fig. 63-5). The treatment for pregnancy tumor is complete surgical excision.[25,26] The adjacent teeth should be cleaned aggressively to remove debris, plaque, and calculus. If the tumor is not completely removed, it may recur, and recurrence during a future pregnancy is not uncommon. Some authors suggest the term "pregnancy tumor" should be dropped, because these tumors are identical to pyogenic granulomas, which occur in men and non-pregnant women.[25]

The treatment of dental problems associated with pregnancy is rarely contraindicated and, when several guidelines are used, may be performed safely.[22] If the treatment is necessary but elective, it is best delayed until the second trimester, when there is the least risk for teratogenesis. Emergency treatment should be obtained whenever indicated. Sweet suggests that dental

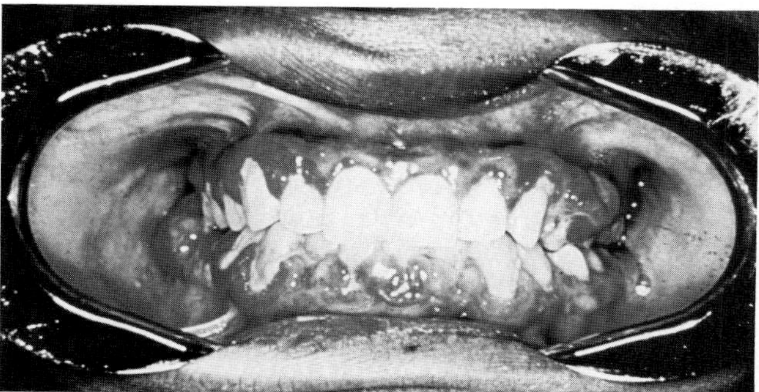

FIGURE 63–3. Severe gingivitis of pregnancy made worse by poor dental hygiene. (Courtesy of Dr. John Marley)

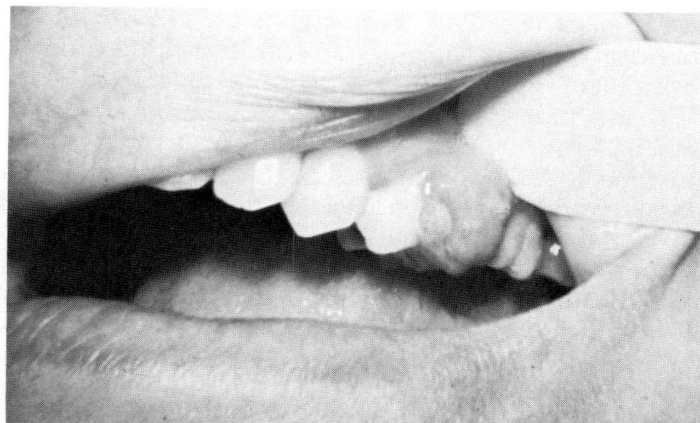

FIGURE 63–4. Gross appearance of pregnancy tumor that was soft, red, smooth, and friable in a patient at 16 weeks gestation, which was removed 10 days later because of repeated episodes of significant bleeding. (Courtesy of Dr. John Marley)

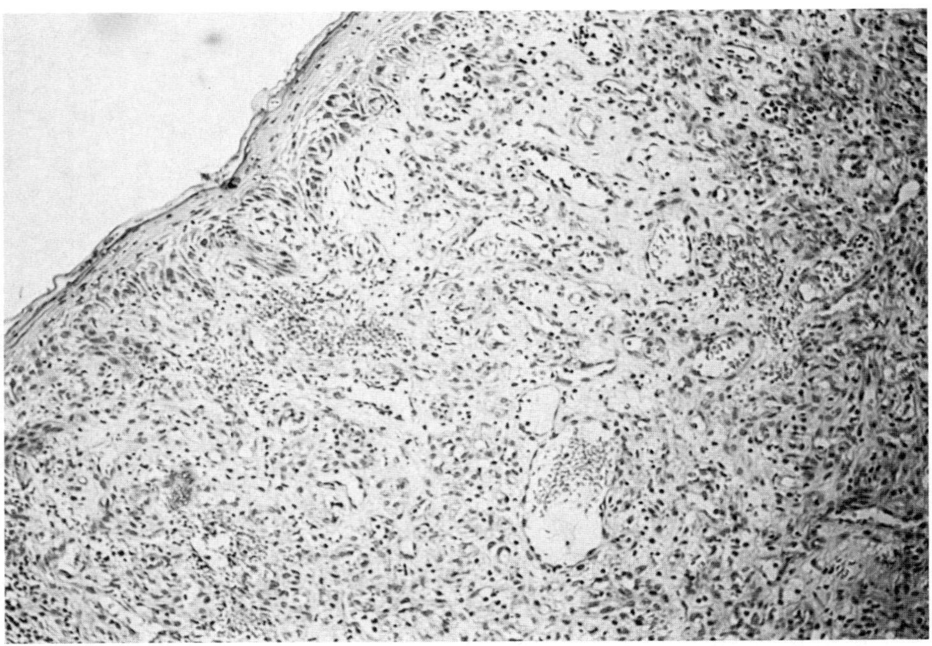

FIGURE 63–5. Microscopic appearance of pregnancy tumor histopathology (see Fig. 63–4), demonstrating the stratified squamous epithelium covering the mass, benign connective tissue, numerous thin-wall blood vessels, and inflammatory infiltrate. (Courtesy of Dr. John Marley)

procedures during the last two months of pregnancy could precipitate premature labor, although there are no studies to support this opinion.[40] Construction of prostheses such as permanent bridges and other restorative dentistry should be postponed until after pregnancy. Dental procedures such as fillings, extractions, and crowns can be safely performed during pregnancy. The supine hypotensive syndrome, which occurs most frequently during the third trimester, can be avoided by keeping the patient turned toward her side while she is in the dental chair.[41]

Radiographs, which are often necessary to establish a proper dental diagnosis, may be safely taken during any stage of pregnancy. The maternal abdomen should be shielded with a lead apron. Using fast x-ray film, the exposure time is minimized. There is little or no harm to the fetus when dental radiographs are taken with the necessary precautions, good techniques, and modern equipment.[34,42–44]

Dental procedures may cause pain. Efforts should be made by the dentist to reduce the pain and stress of the treatment. Although there is concern by the dentist, a local or topical anesthetic is usually recommended and is safe for both mother and fetus.[34,40] The smallest amount necessary to achieve satisfactory anesthesia should be used. When incorporated with a vasoconstrictor such as epinephrine, the anesthetic's effect is prolonged, blood loss decreased, and the dosage of anesthesia is minimized. Lidocaine (Xylocaine) and mepivacaine (Carbocaine) combined with 1:100,000 epinephrine have become the local anesthetics of choice for dental work during pregnancy. Low doses of intravenous medications may be used, but should be titrated to an acceptable level before administrating the local anesthesia.[22,40,45] Inhalation or general anesthesia should be reserved for those patients who are hospitalized and require extensive dental surgery. The anesthesia should be administered by an anesthetist or anesthesiologist who is familiar with the risks of the procedure.[46] It is best whenever possible to avoid the use of an inhalational anesthetic for dental procedures during pregnancy.

Most dental procedures require no antibiotics. When antibiotics are necessary, tetracycline should not be given to the pregnant woman.[47] Erythromycin and penicillin, frequently used by the dentist for treatment or prophylaxis therapy, are safe to use during pregnancy and would be the drugs of choice.[48]

REFLUX ESOPHAGITIS

The esophagus is a fibromuscular tube that connects the oral pharynx and the stomach.[49,50] It is predominantly an interthoracic organ, although a small portion (1 to 2 cm) of the esophagus is located beneath the diaphragm. It is the absence of this portion that causes hiatal hernia. The function of the esophagus is to move food from the oral pharynx to the stomach. The esophagus also prevents or helps to prevent the movement of air from the oral pharynx into the stomach and the movement of food from the stomach into the oral pharynx, called gastroesophageal reflux. Peristalsis carries food into the stomach. This wave of smooth muscle activity is initiated by swallowing. At the distal end of the esophagus is the lower esophageal sphincter, consisting of circular muscle fibers of approximately 2 cm in length. Normally, the lower esophageal sphincter is in a state of tonic contraction, thus preventing gastroesophageal reflux.

Heartburn or pyrosis is really a symptom of reflux esophagitis. Reflux esophagitis is the pathophysiologic process in the esophagus that causes the symptom of heartburn.[49,50] Heartburn is a very common, bothersome complaint during pregnancy and occurs in as many as 70% of pregnant patients. A quarter of pregnant patients experience some degree of heartburn daily.[51] The symptoms of heartburn include burning and substernal discomfort radiating to the back of the neck. Heartburn usually is more severe after meals and is aggravated by recumbent positions.[50] The pain is not limited to being substernal in nature, but may also be epigastric, between the shoulders or, rarely, generalized chest pain. Usually, the symptoms of reflux esophagitis occur in the last trimester, but they can occur at any time during pregnancy.[52] They subside after 36 weeks of gestation and improve, as expected, postpartum with the decrease in the size of the uterus.

The exact cause of heartburn and reflux esophagitis of pregnancy remains unknown and controversial.[52,53] It probably occurs due to some degree of gastroesophageal reflux. Pregnancy, perhaps as a result of progesterone, results in slower esophageal peristalsis with lessened wave amplitude and increased motor nonpropulsive activity of the esophagus.[54] There is limited evidence that physiologic changes of the esophagus during pregnancy result in gastroesophageal reflux or reflux esophagitis.[55] Van Thiel and coworkers concluded from a small study of volunteer pregnant women that the progressive increase in plasma progesterone alone, or in combination with estrogen, is responsible for the reduction of lower esophageal sphincter pressure, allowing for esophageal reflux to occur with the resultant development of heartburn.[56] This is supported by another Van Thiel study, where lower esophageal sphincter pressure was measured in women using sequential oral contraceptives and found to decrease significantly during the phase of the cycle when volunteers took their progestational agent.[57] The hormones of pregnancy, particularly progesterone and perhaps estrogen, appear to play a role in the development of reflux esophagitis in pregnant women. This hypothesis appears to be the one most accepted as the cause of heartburn during pregnancy.[52] Intragastric pressure increases as pregnancy advances, also increasing the possibility of gastroesophageal reflux. When a pregnant patient performs the Valsalva maneuver, she may provoke symptoms of heartburn. Another possible cause for heartburn is the presence of an incompetent lower esophageal sphincter. This can be demonstrated in some, but not all, patients with these symptoms.[54] The development of gastroesophageal reflux is favored also by the decreased gastric emptying time during pregnancy and by the increased intra-abdominal pressure created by the enlarged uterus. The differential diagnosis of esophageal reflux includes dysphasia, achalasia, cardiac symptoms, peptic ulcer disease, and hiatal hernia.

Treatment of reflux esophagitis during pregnancy consists primarily of neutralizing the acid material that is being refluxed into the esophagus, thereby decreasing gastroesophageal reflux.[50,52,53] Symptomatic strategies include dietary modification. Foods and drinks such as chocolate, caffeine, peppermint, and alcohol may actually decrease the lower esophageal sphincter pressure. Fatty or spicy foods aggravate the symptoms and are to be avoided. The avoidance of recumbency, particularly immediately after eating a meal, is likewise to be avoided. Elevation of the head of the bed while reclining may provide symptomatic relief. A variety of antacids have been prescribed for heartburn. All of these over-the-counter preparations neutralize gastric acid, which is responsible for the symptoms. In the non-pregnant patient, the lower esophageal sphincter pressure has been elevated with a variety of medications, including metoclopramide.[58–60] The use of this and similar drugs during pregnancy has not been studied, is usually not necessary, and should be avoided except in severe cases.[7] Anticholinergic drugs used in the treatment of other gastrointestinal symptoms have not been found effective in the management of reflux esophagitis.

Prolonged esophageal reflux can result in complications such as peptic esophageal stricture, hemorrhagic esophagitis, gastrointestinal bleeding, and hemorrhage. Ulceration of the esophageal mucosa can also occur with significant bleeding. The symptoms of reflux esophagitis can be so severe or difficult to treat that esophagoscopy, parenteral hyperalimentation, and parenteral nutrition are necessary.[61,62] These procedures may be performed safely during pregnancy.

PEPTIC ULCER DISEASE

An ulcer is a defect that occurs in the gastrointestinal mucosa and extends through the muscularis mucosa. The stomach, pyloris, or duodenum are the usual sites for ulcers. However, they may occur, as pointed out elsewhere in this chapter, in the esophagus as a result of gastroesophageal reflux. Benign ulcers of the upper gastrointestinal tract are caused primarily by the action of hydrochloric acid and pepsin on the gastrointestinal mucosa.[50,63] Because of the action of acid and pepsin, these defects are called "peptic ulcers." This discussion will be limited to ulcers of the stomach and duodenum.

Ulcerations of the stomach affect both sexes equally and are less common than duodenal ulcer disease, which is two times more common in men than in women.[50,63] The development of peptic ulcer disease during pregnancy is uncommon and rare. Patients who have peptic ulcers before pregnancy frequently experience fewer symptoms during pregnancy and may even become totally asymptomatic.[64] This is the primary reason why complications of ulcer disease, such as perforation, bleeding, and pyloric stenosis, are rare during pregnancy.

Clark studied pregnant women with peptic ulcer disease.[64] His investigation showed that the majority of women became asymptomatic or have a marked decrease in symptoms. There was a recurrence in 50% of the patients by 3 months and in 75% of patients by 6 months postdelivery.

There are no conclusive studies regarding gastric acid secretion changes during pregnancy. Studies to date have shown conflicting data, with some showing no change and others a slight decrease in gastric acid secretion.[56,65–70] Some investigators[70] have suggested that peptic ulcer disease may improve during pregnancy, not from a change in gastric acid secretion, but because of an increase in histaminase, an enzyme produced by the placenta. There is increased histaminase activity during pregnancy.[70] The elevation in this placental enzyme could cause a decrease in histamine production and therefore a decrease in gastric acid output. It has been theorized that estrogen and progesterone may also play a role in the amelioration of peptic ulcer disease during pregnancy by decreasing gastric acid secretion and increasing the production of gastric mucous.[67] Warzecha and associates reported that the gastric and duodenal mucosa during pregnancy has an increased ability to regenerate and heal, resulting from the hyperplasia of the mucosa taking place in pregnancy, which is the effect of an increase in the level of endogenous epidermal growth factor I.[71] However, these theoretic possibilities have yet to be proven, and the exact cause of a decrease in symptoms remains unknown.

The symptoms of peptic ulcer disease are quite similar to those of reflux esophagitis.[50,63] The diagnosis during pregnancy may therefore be delayed. The most common symptom of peptic ulcer disease is complaints of heartburn or dyspepsia. The patient may experience nausea and vomiting, which is a common complaint of pregnancy. She may also have anorexia, bloating, or epigastric pain and discomfort. Patients with duodenal ulcer disease more frequently have epigastric pain than those with gastric ulcers. There are no typical physical findings.[50] When presenting to her obstetrician, the patient may have already taken antacids and found that they may have helped her symptoms. Peptic ulcer disease is diagnosed by the visualization of the ulcer by radiography or endoscopy. Although the upper gastrointestinal series is frequently used to diagnose peptic ulcer disease in a non-pregnant patient, esophagoscopy when necessary should be used in the pregnant patient. This is usually not necessary except in the patient who has symptoms that do not respond to antacids.

Complications of peptic ulcer disease rarely occur during pregnancy, because in most cases the disease does not worsen. Complications that can occur include perforation, hemorrhage or other bleeding, pyloric stenosis, and gastrointestinal obstruction.[72–74] One report suggests that perforation occurs more frequently in pregnancies complicated by preeclampsia or renal disease.[75] When serious complications occur, they should be managed as in the non-pregnant patient. There will be less maternal and fetal mortality.[76] There is disagreement in the literature as to whether or not a cesarean section should be performed at the time of an emergency gastric resection. The decision to perform a cesarean section would depend on the gestational age of the fetus. The experience of most clinicians is not to perform an emergency cesarean prior to the peptic ulcer surgery.[73,77,78] Patients who have had previous peptic ulcer disease surgery are at no increased risk for complications during future pregnancies.[79]

Lewis and Weingold have extensively reviewed the use of gastrointestinal drugs during pregnancy and lactation.[7] The treatment of peptic ulcer disease consists primarily of the use of antacids, which are safe to use during pregnancy.[7] Fifteen to 30 mL 1 to 3 hours after meals and at bedtime is usually recommended. Antacids neutralize acid that has been secreted by the gastrointestinal lining. In most cases, it will improve symptoms. A combination of magnesium trisilicate and aluminum hydroxide is found in most antacid preparations. Sodium bicarbonate should not be used as an antacid during pregnancy, because it can lead to the absorption of large amounts of sodium. Patients with peptic ulcer disease should avoid a diet of foods that cause their discomfort. Some authorities suggest that milk, which is frequently included in the diet of the pregnant patient, stimulates acid secretion and should be taken in moderation. Smoking, which should be avoided in both the pregnant and non-pregnant woman, and alcohol should certainly be eliminated from the diets of these patients. Aspirin and the nonsteroidal anti-inflammatory drugs such as indomethacin can produce gastric irritation and, with prolonged use, gastric ulcers. Their use should be avoided in a patient with peptic ulcer disease. Other dietary modification is not necessary, although bedtime snacks are to be avoided. Indomethacin, which has been used for tocolysis, should be avoided in patients with active or a history of peptic ulcer disease.[80]

Cimetidine is an H_2-receptor antagonist. H_2-receptors are located on parietal cells of the gastrointestinal lining. Their stimulation results in the production of histamine. H_2-receptor antagonists decrease the production of histamine. It is a mainstay in the medical therapy of peptic ulcer disease. There are several concerns about the use of cimetidine during pregnancy. It is an antiandrogen and has produced gynecomastia and impotence in a small number of male animals and male users.[81,82] Cimetidine does cross the placenta. Its effect on the H_2-receptors in the uterine myometrium has not been well studied, but no adverse effect on uterine activity has been reported. No teratogenicity has been linked to the use of cimetidine during pregnancy.[7] However, its use should be reserved for those patients who have symptoms refractory to antacid therapy. There are no data to support the discontinuation of cimetidine during pregnancy.

Ranitidine is another H_2-receptor antagonist that has been used for ulcer therapy. It possesses no antiandrogen activity, but its use during pregnancy has been limited.[7] However, Armentano and coworkers report the use of ranitidine in the treatment of reflux esophagitis without maternal or neonatal complication.[83] Sucralfate is a mucosal-protective aluminum hydroxide salt that has been used in the non-pregnant patient to "enhance mucosal defense." Some investigators have suggested that sucralfate forms a shield over the ulcer crater. There has been limited use of this new drug during pregnancy, and although it may have theoretic advantages, its use during pregnancy cannot be recommended.[7]

ACUTE INTESTINAL OBSTRUCTION

Intestinal obstruction is a serious complication of pregnancy that is occurring with increasing frequency. The incidence is approximately 1 in 2500 to 1 in 3500 pregnancies.[84–86] Older reports suggested that the incidence was rare, but there has recently been a rising incidence due to the increasing number of abdominal surgeries performed on women.[87] Matthews and Mitchell noted three time periods during pregnancy when obstruction is likely to occur: (1) during the fourth and fifth months, when the enlarging uterus is no longer a pelvic organ; (2) during the eighth and ninth months, when the fetal head descends into the pelvis; and (3) during the puerperium, when there is a marked change in the size of the uterus.[88] Beck thought these were periods during pregnancy when normal intra-abdominal relationships are most likely to be disturbed.[89] Acute intestinal obstruction is most common in the third trimester, less common in the second, and least likely in the first trimester.[89–92]

The most common cause for intestinal obstruction in the pregnant and non-pregnant woman is adhesions.[84,86] More than half of intestinal obstructions are secondary to adhesions that usually, but not always, are due to prior abdominal surgery. Previous laparotomy for appendectomy or gynecologic surgery is the most frequent preceding operation.[84,86] Intussusception and hernias are less common causes for intestinal obstruction during pregnancy.[93–95] Adhesions may also form as the result of pelvic inflammatory disease or may rarely be congenital in origin.[96]

A number of authors have reported volvulus as a cause of intestinal obstruction during pregnancy.[97–101] Volvulus usually involves the sigmoid colon rather than the small intestine or cecum and is the second most common cause of intestinal obstruction during pregnancy.[102] Although sigmoid volvulus is usually treated by surgery, Allen reported a case that was successfully treated conservatively.[103] The combination of an overdistended uterus caused by multiple gestation with bed rest has been reported by Dan and colleagues as an uncommon cause of mechanical ileus.[104] Small bowel obstruction occurring during pregnancy after surgery for morbid obesity has been reported by Graubard and associates.[105] Rachagan and coworkers reported an unusual case of intestinal obstruction following previous myomectomy and the use of betasympathomimetics.[106] The authors suggested that the use of tocolytic agents to suppress premature uterine contractions following myomectomy may be a predisposing factor and probably intensifies the obstruction by decreasing peristalsis.

Goldthorp determined that 80% of intestinal obstruction cases caused by past appendectomy adhesions occurred during the first pregnancy after the operation.[98] Spontaneous small bowel obstruction associated with a spontaneous triplet gestation has been reported by Ludmir and coworkers.[107] Their patient had no predisposing factors, delayed diagnosis, delivered preterm, and required surgery to alleviate the obstruction. The authors emphasize the importance of considering the diagnosis of intestinal obstruction when nausea, vomiting, and an overdistended abdomen occur during pregnancy.

The diagnosis of intestinal obstruction in pregnancy is not easy.[86,96] As with appendicitis, delay in diagnosis is not uncommon. This can result in perforated or strangulated bowel, preterm labor, and increased maternal and fetal mortality. The classic triad of presenting symptoms in intestinal obstruction are abdominal pain, vomiting, and constipation. All of these are common symptoms during the normal pregnancy. The physician must have a high index of suspicion for the presence of acute intestinal obstruction. Pain, although usually present, may be constant, colicky, mild, severe, diffuse, or localized. Morris reported abdominal pain to be present in over 85% of cases of intestinal obstruction in pregnancy.[91] Uterine contraction may be present. Physical examination may or may not reveal guarding or rebound tenderness. Abdominal distention can easily be missed in late pregnancy because of the normally large uterus and abdomen. When present, it usually indicates large bowel rather than small bowel obstruction. Bowel sounds may be normal, absent, or high pitched with rushes. Physical examination, however, can be completely nondiagnostic. The white count is usually not helpful because it is elevated normally in pregnancy. If there is considerable delay in diagnosis and the patient is not appropriately treated, then third spacing of fluids occurs. This results in dehydration, electrolyte imbalance, hypotension, oliguria, fever, tachycardia and, eventually, shock and death.

Diagnosis, once expected clinically, can be made by radiographic studies showing bowel distention, intraluminal fluid levels, and decreased gas in the large bowel.[86,96] The concern of obtaining radiographic studies during pregnancy should be tempered by the increased maternal and fetal mortality associated with delayed or misdiagnosis. X-ray or serial studies showing dilated, gas-filled loops of bowel with air-fluid levels is diagnostic.

Treatment of intestinal obstruction during pregnancy is the same as in the non-pregnant patient.[96] Exploratory laparotomy is the treatment of choice. Prior to surgery, close attention must be paid to correction of fluid and electrolyte imbalance, maintenance of adequate urinary output, administration of blood and blood products, and fetal monitoring. Antibiotics may be indicated.

A vertical abdominal incision should be made to provide adequate exposure. Care should be taken by the operating surgeon to avoid manipulating, touching, or tugging on the pregnant uterus, because this could result in preterm labor. If labor occurs while the patient in surgery, tocolysis should be initiated. The prophylactic use of tocolytic therapy before, during, or after surgery has not been proved and is debatable.[86] When surgery occurs at term, a well-repaired abdominal incision will tolerate labor without difficulty. At the time of surgery, a cesarean section should be performed only for obstetrical reasons. Vaginal delivery can occur without difficulty following abdominal surgery. There do not appear to be many, if any, clinical indications for the use of a long intestinal tube rather than surgery to treat obstruction.

Maternal and fetal mortality from undiagnosed cases of intestinal obstruction have decreased over the years.[87,89,96] Because this is a disease of the third trimester, preterm labor and neonatal death can cause significant fetal mortality.[84] This should be reduced with early diagnosis and aggressive operative treatment. It is well, therefore, for the clinician to remember that an abdominal scar on a pregnant woman with abdominal pain should raise the suspicion of acute intestinal obstruction.[88,89]

INFLAMMATORY BOWEL DISEASE

The term inflammatory bowel disease refers to a group of idiopathic chronic inflammatory diseases of the intestinal tract.[50] The two most commonly seen during pregnancy are ulcerative colitis and Crohn's disease, also called regional enteritis. Both of these disorders are not uncommon in women during their reproductive years and are frequently seen, therefore, either before or during pregnancy.[49,50,108–110]

The pathologic features of these two diseases distinguish and differentiate them.[49,50] Ulcerative colitis is an inflammatory ulcerative pathologic process primarily of the mucosal lining of the left colon or rectum. It is characteristically not transmural. A typical biopsy of ulcerative colitis lesions shows diffuse mucosal ulceration and a chronic inflammatory response consisting of polymorphonuclear cells, lymphocytes, and plasma cells. There may be abscesses of the mucosa. The mucosal lining is edematous and replaced by a chronic inflammatory infiltrate. As this chronic process continues over time, the bowel may become thickened. Areas of stricture, fibrosis, and stenosis develop. Intestinal obstruction and toxic dilatation of the colon with resultant perforation can complicate ulcerative colitis.[111] Crohn's disease is an inflammatory disease that may involve any area of the gastrointestinal tract, but the distal small intestine, colon, and anal rectal regions are most often affected. The pathologic process is transmural; ie, the granulomatous enteritis involves all layers of the bowel, mesentery, and lymph nodes. The inflammatory process consists primarily of plasma cells and lymphocytes. The bowel that is affected is edematous, thickened, hyperemic, and ulcerated. There may be adhesions of the involved portion with other loops of intestine. Intestinal obstruction, perforation, and fistula formation between loops of bowel can result. The nearby mesentery may also be thickened and involved. Mesenteric lymphadenopathy is present. The chronic inflammatory process is more granulomatous than ulcerative colitis. Granulomas, multinucleated giant cells, and chronic ulcerations are present. Skip areas are characteristically found in removed bowel affected by regional enteritis. These are unaffected areas of the bowel located next to diseased areas. Skip areas are uncommon in ulcerative colitis.

These two disorders share a common cause, clinical findings, and management.[49,50] Ulcerative colitis and Crohn's disease may be so similar clinically that a specific diagnosis of the type of inflammatory disease present cannot be made. They can be characterized as chronic disorders that go through periods of quiescence and exacerbation, making differentiation even more difficult. Ulcerative colitis primarily affects females, while both sexes are equally affected with Crohn's disease.[108–110]

The effect of inflammatory bowel disease on fertility has been studied by several authors.[112–118] Most reports show that ulcerative colitis does not affect or alter female fertility.[112,113] The conception rate in women with ulcerative colitis is therefore the same as those in women not affected by this disease.[113] Numerous reports have shown and there is general agreement that fertility is decreased in patients with Crohn's disease.[114–117] This is probably due to the chronic pelvic adhesions that occur as a result of the inflammatory process. The activity of the disease process also affects fertility. Although it is decreased during exacerbations, there is also a decrease in fertility when the disease is quiescent. Improved fertility after the removal of intestine affected by regional enteritis has been reported by DeDombal and colleagues.[117] In a recent study, however, by Wikland and coworkers, conventional proctocolectomy and ileostomy for ulcerative colitis or Crohn's disease was associated with reduced fertility.[118] These authors reported that fertility was significantly reduced after surgery, because only 37% of the women who attempted to become pregnant succeeded within 5 years, whereas 72% have become pregnant before surgery. Those who conceived went through pregnancy and parturition without any incident. The study concluded that the operations seems to decrease the chances of a woman becoming pregnant, but the decrease in fertility could also be caused by pelvic adhesions that have developed as a result of the inflammatory bowel disease.[109,110]

Ulcerative colitis and regional enteritis can affect pregnancy. The earliest and most extensive report is by Abramson, who reviewed the effect of ulcerative colitis on pregnancy.[119] Patients were divided into four groups: Group 1 consisted of those patients with a history of ulcerative colitis, *inactive* at conception; Group 2 consisted of those with ulcerative colitis that was *active* at the time of conception; Group 3 consisted of those with the development of ulcerative colitis *during* pregnancy; Group 4 consisted of those with the development of ulcerative colitis *postpartum*. Pregnancy outcome was best in Group 1, in which 18 to 20 patients had a full-term pregnancy and exacerbation of the disease occurred in 7 patients. All of the 12 patients in Group 2 had term pregnancies; however, they also experienced exacerbations of their disease both during pregnancy and postpartum. Pregnancy outcome worsened in Groups 3 and 4, in which the disease developed during pregnancy or during the puerperium. This report suggests that the best prognosis for pregnancy is in those patients who had inactive disease at the time of conception or whose active disease is limited to early pregnancy. Later reports, occurring over the past 40 years, during which time there has been a change in the medical management of these patients, consistently show that patients with inactive ulcerative colitis that becomes active during early pregnancy do not have an increased risk of spontaneous abortion; and that patients who develop active disease later in pregnancy or postpartum are at increased risk for spontaneous abortion, stillbirth, and preterm labor.[112,120,121] This is true whether it is reactivation of quiescent disease or the development of new disease. In general, a good prognosis can be expected and ulcerative colitis does not adversely affect fetal outcome. Brostrom recently suggested that pregnancy, if planned, should be encouraged when the patient is in remission, although the disease or its standard treatment does not seem to dangerously affect the patient, fetus, or the newborn infant.[122] The more inactive the disease at the time of conception, the better the prognosis for a more favorable pregnancy outcome.

The effect of Crohn's disease on pregnancy is similar. Numerous investigators have concluded that there is little or no decrease on the live birth rate.[110,115–117,123,124] Adverse pregnancy outcome, as reflected by prematurity, stillbirths, spontaneous abortion, or congenital anomalies, does not appear to be increased.

The route of delivery may be affected by inflammatory bowel disease. Cesarean section has been recommended if severe perineal fistulas or perineal scarring, which can occur as a complication of Crohn's disease, is present. Patients who have recently had a proctocolectomy performed to promote healing of perineal disease should also be delivered by cesarean section. Cesarean section is not indicated in patients who have had successful restorative surgery for inflammatory bowel disease.[125]

The clinical manifestations of inflammatory bowel disease will depend on the area of the gastrointestinal tract involved.[49,50] Some symptoms occur with both diseases or are more common with one or the other. Symptoms occurring with *both* of these diseases may include soft stools, rectal bleeding, diarrhea, abdominal pain, weight loss, and urgency of defecation. Rectal bleeding is more common in ulcerative colitis. Abdominal pain, diarrhea, weight loss, fever, and rectal bleeding are the most frequent symptoms occurring in ulcerative colitis. The symptoms of Crohn's disease are most frequently episodic abdominal pain, fever, diarrhea, and weight loss. Perineal fistulas and scarring are more commonly present with regional enteritis and occur in one third to one half of the patients with this disease.

The clinical features and presentations of these two disorders can be quite similar, requiring sigmoidoscopy, colonoscopy, radiography, and histologic examination of a biopsy to tell the difference.[49,50] Endoscopic techniques have replaced radiography in making the diagnosis during pregnancy.[108–110]

Extraintestinal manifestations of the inflammatory bowel diseases occur in both the pregnant and non-pregnant patient.[49,50,109] These include nutritional and metabolic abnormalities, hematologic abnormalities, skin and mucous membrane lesions, arthritis, and eye and renal complications. Hepatic and biliary complications can also occur with the development of hepatitis and gallstones. Systemic complications and manifestations have been reported to occur all over the body.[49] Local complications requiring surgical and gastroenterological intervention can occur depending on the severity of the disease. These include stricture, stenosis, bleeding, malignancy, abscess formation, perforation, fistulas, and perineal problems. A case of pregnancy and toxic dilatation of the colon has been reported by Becker.[111] This serious complication of ulcerative colitis occurred in a pregnant patient who was gravely ill. The patient improved with intensive medical therapy, including intravenous steroids.

There is little evidence to suggest that pregnancy has an effect on inflammatory bowel disease. DeDombal and coworkers followed patients with ulcerative colitis during pregnancy and determined there is no higher rate of relapse in pregnant patients when compared with a similar group of non-pregnant female patients.[121] Another report by Willoughby and Truelove showed that almost two thirds of patients who conceived while in remission remained inactive.[112] The clinical course of the ulcerative colitis was worsened when pregnancy occurred when the disease was active. The risk of exacerbation in pregnant patients of their ulcerative colitis is approximately 50%, not dissimilar from that in the non-pregnant patient. One third of patients who conceive while their colitis is inactive will have an exacerbation during their pregnancy. The worst prognosis for the pregnant woman, according to Nielsen and colleagues, occurs when the patient develops ulcerative colitis for the first time during pregnancy.[126] The maternal mortality rate under those circumstances was 15%. Pregnancy should be avoided if possible while the disease is active. One third of these patients will have worsening of their disease, and less than half will show a remission or improvement.

Crohn, in an early investigation, reported that when pregnancy occurred, there was an unfavorable effect on the course of the disease when regional enteritis was active.[115] Another report by Fielding and Cooke showed minimal adverse effect on the disease's course during pregnancy.[117] During the postpartum period, 25% to 40% of the patients in this study relapsed. Recent studies by Norton and Patterson[124] and DeDombal and associates[117] support the general impression that pregnancy has little or no effect on Crohn's disease and the overall maternal prognosis is good. When an exacerbation in inflammatory bowel disease occurs during pregnancy, it most frequently happens during the first trimester or the postpartum period. This may be due to a correlation with levels of circulating corticosteroids during pregnancy.[121,127] It must be kept in mind, however, that the clinical course of inflammatory bowel disease is one of exacerbations and remissions. Inflammatory bowel disease is treated by both medical and surgical measures during pregnancy. In general, the treatment is the same as in the non-pregnant patient,[49,50] with several special considerations.[109,128] The mainstay of the medical therapy for both ulcerative colitis and Crohn's disease is the use of sulfasalazine and corticosteroids. Sulfasalazine is more efficacious in the treatment of ulcerative colitis than in regional enteritis. The steroids most frequently used are prednisone, hydrocortisone, and prednisolone. Metronidazole, azathioprine, and 6-mercaptopurine have also been used in the medical therapy of inflammatory bowel disease. These three agents have possible teratogenic effects, and their use during pregnancy cannot be recommended.[129] Metronidazole has been shown effective in the management of inflammatory bowel disease, particularly Crohn's disease for perineal fistula. Although efficacious, it should be used during pregnancy and postpartum only in severe and unusual cases, because teratogenesis has been reported in animals.[7]

Sulfasalazine is the most commonly used drug in the treatment of inflammatory bowel disease. It is a combination of sulfonamide, sulfapyridine, and 5-aminosalicylic acid. It is usually prescribed in 1 to 1.5 g every 6 hours for active disease. The use of this drug has caused folic acid deficiency, and patients who are on it long-term should receive supplemental folic acid. The dose used for prophylaxis after the patient has been controlled on the initial treatment of active disease is usually 0.5 g every 6 hours. The question frequently arises whether sulfasalazine can be continued during pregnancy. Several studies have shown that sulfasalazine can be safely used both during pregnancy and while the mother is breast-feeding.[7,130] The drug should be started as soon as possible after delivery to prevent the possibility of a postpartum exacerbation. Although there is the theoretic possibility that sulfasalazine could bind to fetal albumin with the displacement of bilirubin and the development of hyperbilirubinemia, this does not appear to be a real clinical risk.[130]

Corticosteroid therapy has been used in both of these diseases to suppress the inflammatory response present in the bowel.[49,50,109] It is frequently used also in treating exacerbations of Crohn's disease. Doses of prednisone range from 40 to 60 mg daily for a period of several weeks to a month. Some pregnant patients who have been unable to be weaned from corticosteroids may enter pregnancy on a low dose. The continuation of their medication or even the institution of corticosteroid therapy during pregnancy is not contraindicated.[7,109,128] The mother may experience the usual side effects of steroid therapy, but there are no proven adverse effects on the fetus from the use of steroids during pregnancy. Breast-feeding likewise is not contraindicated in the mother on corticosteroid therapy.[7,108–110]

Medical management should include nutritional assessment and treatment, as in any patient with a chronic disease.[49,50,109] Adequate calories should be provided to help in the prevention of weight loss. Parenteral nutrition, sometimes required in the management of some of the other gastrointestinal complications of pregnancy, is infrequently needed in these patients. If medically necessary to provide adequate caloric intake, total parenteral nutrition may be safely used during pregnancy.[109] General therapeutic measures used include antidiarrheal drugs such as codeine, opium, paregoric, and diphenoxylate with atropine (Lomotil). As in the treatment of hyperemesis gravidarum, the patient should have the opportunity to discuss the psychological factors of pregnancy or other aspects of her life, which may be playing a part in the precipitation of inflammatory bowel disease.

Inflammatory bowel disease may require surgical treatment. The procedure most frequently used in the treatment of ulcerative colitis is total proctocolectomy with construction of an ileostomy.[49,50] This procedure is curative. Indications for partial or total colectomy and ileostomy include perforation (with or without abscess formation), massive bleeding, and carcinoma of the colon. Patients who develop toxic megacolon and do not respond to other therapy may also be candidates for this surgical therapy. The procedure should not be done during pregnancy, because the surgery would not only be difficult to perform as the pregnant uterus enlarges, but could precipitate preterm labor.[111] Patients with ulcerative colitis who have been treated before pregnancy with proctocolectomy and ileostomy have no increased risk during their pregnancy. Care of the ileostomy is not hampered by pregnancy. There is no evidence that the enlarging uterus will interfere with the function of the ileostomy. Vaginal delivery is not contraindicated, but should be encouraged. The performance of a cesarean section for obstetrical indications is recommended, with draping of the ileostomy out of the surgical site.

Surgical therapy for Crohn's disease or regional enteritis is the same as for ulcerative colitis.[49,50] Intractability of symptoms is the most frequent indication for surgery. Perianal complications such as fistulas may also lead to total proctocolectomy with ileostomy or some other variance of this surgery. As with ulcerative colitis, there is a high recurrence rate of the disease with an internal anastomosis. Unlike ulcerative colitis, Crohn's disease is not cured by total proctocolectomy, because there is a recurrence rate as high as 80% in 5 years. Surgery for both of these disorders should only be performed during pregnancy after intensive medical therapy has failed.[131]

A recent review of pregnancy and inflammatory bowel disease by Zeldis made suggestions about the medical management of inflammatory bowel disease during pregnancy, with the following conclusions:

1. Judicious medical therapy is effective in controlling inflammatory bowel disease during pregnancy.
2. Sulfasalazine or steroid therapy should not be withdrawn in a patient who needs it to achieve or maintain a quiescent state of inflammatory bowel disease during the course of pregnancy.
3. Immunosuppressive therapy should be avoided.
4. Aggressive medical therapy with total parenteral nutrition and a team approach with a gastroenterologist, surgeon, and perinatologist usually will avoid the need for surgical intervention during pregnancy, with a good fetal outcome in a patient whose disease is active.
5. Contraception against pregnancy need only be considered in those patients whose disease is so severe that operative therapy is imminent.[132]

The interested reader is referred to several other extensive reviews of inflammatory bowel disease in pregnancy.[108–110]

APPENDICITIS

Appendicitis remains the most common cause of an acute abdomen during pregnancy. The incidence during pregnancy has been reported to vary from 1 per 1000 to 1 per 2000 pregnancies, with an average incidence of 1 per 1500 deliveries. There appears to be no increased frequency during any particular trimester.[133] Appendicitis occurring postpartum is particularly difficult to diagnose, because peritonitis is a less prominent finding. During pregnancy, the usual symptoms and physical changes may delay the diagnosis or confuse the clinical picture of appendicitis. This delay in diagnosis can be further compounded by the commonly experienced nausea, vomiting, and abdominal discomfort of pregnancy and the displacement of the appendix upward by the enlarging uterus. Additionally, the usual elevation of the white blood count during pregnancy and the elevated sedimentation rate may also delay the diagnosis. Unfortunately, pregnant women have a higher mortality when they develop appendicitis. This is primarily due to procrastination in diagnosis and treatment with resultant perforation of the appendix and peritonitis.[134] Appendicitis in pregnancy is therefore frequently associated with peritonitis due to a delay in diagnosis.

The pregnant woman with appendicitis has symptoms and signs similar to those in the non-pregnant patient, but may not experience abdominal rigidity, rebound, or similar signs of peritonitis. Abdominal pain is present, but usually not at McBurney's point. This is due to the change in the position and direction of the appendix during pregnancy.[135] As pregnancy advances, the cecum is displaced toward the iliac crest, thus moving the appendix laterally, superiorly, and posteriorly (Fig. 63-6). The abdominal pain of appendicitis typically is mild at its onset. During pregnancy it is even less severe. It may be intermittent or colicky, due to a fecalith within the appendix. The pain is followed within an hour or two by anorexia, nausea, and vomiting, symptoms frequently seen during a normal pregnancy. The temperature may be normal or there may be a low-grade fever. An increasing left shift may be helpful in making the diagnosis. The urinalysis is usually not helpful other than in excluding the diagnosis of urinary tract infection.

In order to reduce both maternal and perinatal mortality associated with appendicitis during pregnancy, the diagnosis must be made promptly. A delay in diagnosis appears to increase with gestational age.[136] The diagnosis must be suspected in the pregnant patient who experiences persistent right-sided abdominal pain and atypical gastrointestinal symptoms. The removal of a normal appendix may occur in half of the cases and should not be criticized, because such an operation rate may be necessary to detect the case with minimal or

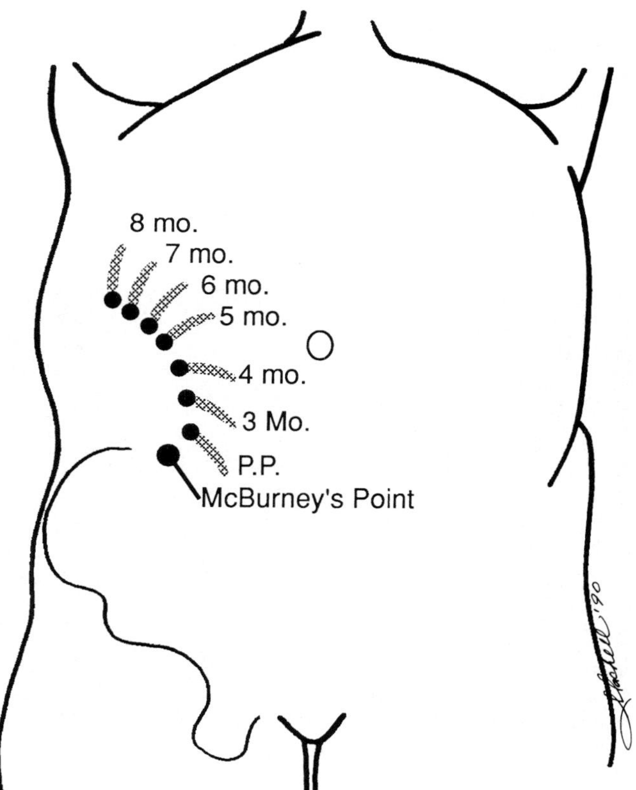

FIGURE 63–6. Change in the position of the appendix during pregnancy.

unusual symptoms, thus decreasing fetal and maternal mortality.[137] An uncomplicated appendectomy does not increase the risk for preterm labor. However, the presence of peritonitis and a perforated appendix more frequently results in preterm labor and preterm birth.[138] If in doubt, the appendix should be removed, especially during pregnancy.[139]

The differential diagnosis of appendicitis during pregnancy includes threatened abortion, ectopic pregnancy, pelvic inflammatory disease, pyelonephritis, placental accidents, twisted ovarian cyst, pancreatitis, gallbladder disease, degenerating fibroids, ruptured corpus luteum, chorioamnionitis, infarcted omentum, and the difficult-to-diagnose "round ligament syndrome." The use of laparoscopy and graded compression sonography in the differential diagnosis of acute appendicitis in the non-pregnant patient has been studied by several authors.[140–143] Although these diagnostic techniques have been helpful in gynecologic cases, they have not been well studied in the pregnant patient. Sonography can be helpful in the diagnosis of a postappendectomy abscess (Fig. 63-7). The diagnosis of appendicitis in pregnancy must always be considered when a pregnant patient presents with abdominal pain. Babaknia and coworkers, in an extensive review of appendicitis during pregnancy, pointed out 16 conditions that were frequently misdiagnosed as appendicitis in 43 cases.[133] The most frequent condition was pyelonephritis.

Appendectomy is the treatment of choice for appendicitis during pregnancy. It is the most frequent nonobstetric procedure performed during pregnancy. Surgeons suggest the use of a transverse muscle-splitting incision directly over the point of maximum tenderness. When necessary, this incision can be extended without much difficulty. During the operation, the uterus should be manipulated as little as possible. The left lateral position with uterine displacement should be used to minimize the chance for the development of supine hypotension. There is no need for drainage of the incision if the appendix is unruptured and the incision can be primarily closed. Antibiotics are indicated when the appendix is perforated or there is extensive inflammation. There are no data to indicate that tocolysis reduces the incidence of uterine contractions or premature labor.[138] Therefore, the routine usage of such agents in these circumstances cannot be supported. When the diagnosis is made in the third trimester, there are few, if any, indications for a simultaneous cesarean delivery, except in the presence of obstetrical indications. On occasion, a patient will present in labor with appendicitis. Vaginal delivery is not precluded, with minilaparotomy and appendectomy immediately postpartum. This scenario presumes the patient is not in acute distress from a possible perforation. Ammerman and Toffle reviewed the concurrence of appendicitis and pregnancy at term concluding the fetus should be monitored, delivery should be immediate, induction of labor may be indicated, and appendectomy should be promptly performed.[144]

The complication rate with rupture of the appendix can be very high, including fetal loss and maternal morbidity.[145,146] When the diagnosis is made promptly and procrastination in treatment does not occur, fetal loss is lowered.[147–149] Prophylactic appendectomy at the time of cesarean section has been studied prospectively by Parsons and coworkers[150] and Tungphaisal and colleagues,[151] who found that this procedure does not add to the risk of elective cesarean section. Nevertheless, most elective cesarean sections performed today are not accompanied by an incidental appendectomy, even though they may be safe.

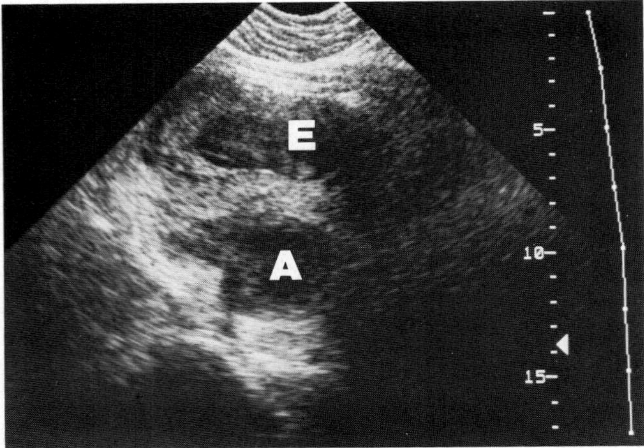

FIGURE 63–7. Transverse ultrasound scan 12 days postappendectomy demonstrating embryo (E) at 6 weeks and showing echogenic fluid in the retrouterine cul-de-sac suspicious for abscess (A) in a patient with persistent postoperative fevers. The abscess resolved with intravenous antibiotic therapy. (Courtesy of Dr. Joseph C. Anderson)

PREGNANCY FOLLOWING OPERATION FOR MORBID OBESITY

Over the past 25 years, patients who are morbidly obese have been undergoing a variety of surgical bypass operations to induce weight loss.[152] Seventy-five percent of these patients are female and therefore can be seen following their bypass for pregnancy.[153] There are basically two types of bypass operations: the older jejunoileal and the more recently developed gastric techniques.

The jejunoileal bypass results in weight loss by bypassing approximately 90% of the small bowel, which decreases the area of the bowel available for absorption of food.[152–155] In performing the jejunoileal shunt, an end-to-end or end-to-side anastomosis of the jejunum is accomplished.

A newer procedure is the gastric bypass, which involves altering the stomach in some manner to produce a slower, as well as a physiologically better-tolerated, weight loss. This can be accomplished by a variety of techniques.[152,153] The gastric procedures have less long-term morbidity and mortality, making the jejunoileal bypass operation now obsolete.[53,152]

Successful pregnancy following jejunoileal bypass continues to occur and has been reported by a number of investigators.[53,153–163]

Knudsen and Kallen studied delivery of 77 women who, prior to pregnancy, had undergone an intestinal bypass operation.[154] The infants born to these women had an increased rate of low birth weight, short gestation, and also growth retardation. In their study, there was no distinct difference between these infants, whether they were conceived less than 24 months or more than 24 months after the operation. A previous report by Stenning had suggested that pregnancy not long after the procedure could result in fetal loss and a complicated maternal course.[157]

Most pregnant women with a jejunoileal bypass tolerate pregnancy quite well. It has been recommended that they receive supplemental iron, folic acid, vitamin B_{12}, and a prenatal vitamin–mineral preparation.[53] An occasional patient appears to do poorly, developing intrauterine growth retardation and metabolic disorders.[53] Pregnancy is not contraindicated after jejunoileal bypass,[53,158,159] but a 2-year interval before pregnancy is undertaken has been suggested so the patient will not become pregnant during the highest phase of weight loss and to allow the weight loss to plateau.[152,158,160–162] The longer the interval from surgery to pregnancy, the better the prognosis for both mother and newborn.[156] In a report by Savel, there was a higher incidence of severe congenital anomalies, but this has not been confirmed by other studies.[53,154,158,159]

Gray and Cabaniss recently reported that pregnancy after jejunoileal bypass for obesity is generally well tolerated without serious complications.[163] A diabetic patient who had previously had a jejunoileal bypass procedure was successfully treated with home total parenteral nutrition. Other authors have also suggested that total parenteral nutrition may be necessary in some patients who have previously undergone a jejunoileal bypass when they have evidence of intrauterine growth retardation and inadequate absorption of nutrients.[155,164]

Because of long-term complications, including persisting electrolyte abnormalities, the jejunoileal bypass procedure is no longer performed.[152] Gastric-restrictive operations have now developed as the operations of choice for the patient who is morbidly obese.[152] These include gastroplasty, gastric stapling, and gastric bypass techniques. Deitel has recommended that a woman undergoing one of these procedures not become pregnant for at least 1 year afterward, because during that year significant postoperative metabolic changes occur in the patient.

Printen and Scott reported 45 patients who had 54 pregnancies following gastric bypass.[153] Forty-six infants were delivered. The results of the study showed that neither the mother nor the developing fetus was unduly endangered by a pregnancy that developed after the 6-month period of rapid postoperative weight loss. There was no higher incidence of preterm births or intrauterine growth retardation. However, these authors suggested that the patient should be counseled not to become pregnant within the first year after the procedure. The timing of pregnancy after these procedures has also been studied by other authors. Deitel has suggested that pregnancy be deferred for 1 year following gastroplasty, to the period beyond massive loss of weight and when lean tissue (protein) is no longer lost.[152]

Following gastroplasty, there is also a substantial change in sex hormones with the weight loss, with return of regular periods occurring in many women.[152] This results in a return of ovulation, with an increased chance of pregnancy. It has been suggested, therefore, that pregnancy early after gastroplasty may be particularly hazardous to mother and child because of rapid weight loss and poor nutrition at that time. Pregnancy within 6 months after the initial surgery has required parenteral nutrition because of decreased albumin and anemia.[165] Grace recommends that women be warned about the possibility of pregnancy and use appropriate contraception during the first year after gastroplasty.[166] The patient who has surgery for morbid obesity and becomes pregnant soon after the therapy is still at risk for the main antenatal complications of obesity during pregnancy. These include eclampsia, hypertension, and diabetes.[53] Pregnancy after 1 year has been uncomplicated and the patient may actually benefit from the weight loss that has occurred before conception.[152,166]

CONSTIPATION

It is difficult to define constipation in the pregnant or non-pregnant patient. A decrease in the frequency of stools, painful defecation, increased straining, or increased consistency of the stool is usually thought of as constipation. A patient will complain of being constipated if she experiences any of these symptoms, but a patient's perception of being constipated may differ considerably from that of her physician. Constipation is a common symptom of pregnancy, but its frequency has not been well studied. Levy and coworkers interviewed 1000 healthy postpartum women about their bowel habits before and during pregnancy.[167] In 54.6%, there was no change in the bowel frequency during pregnancy. Increased frequency occurred in 34.4%, and only 11% experienced a decreased frequency. Five percent of the subjects actually reported diarrhea of 2 to 8 weeks' duration in the last trimester. Ninety percent of the women interviewed experienced either no change or an increase of bowel frequency during pregnancy, contrary to the generally accepted view that constipation is frequent in pregnancy. These findings are supported by Greenhalf and Leonard, who found in a similar study that only 30% of pregnant women reported constipation in pregnancy.[168]

Why pregnancy may cause constipation remains unclear and unknown, but several interesting theories exist. Attempts have been made to demonstrate slow transit of feces through the colon during pregnancy and increased fluid absorption by the colon as a cause of constipation during pregnancy. Hormonal influences may play a role, because progesterone has an inhibitory effect on intestinal smooth muscle, which can therefore result in prolonged gastrointestinal transit time.[169–172] Christofides and coworkers studied plasma motilin in pregnancy, a hormonal peptide that has gastrointestinal smooth muscle–stimulating effects.[173] In 37 women studied during the second and third trimesters of pregnancy and for 1 week after delivery, plasma motilin concentrations were found to be decreased. Plasma motilin concentrations were significantly reduced during pregnancy, but returned to the normal range postpartum. Their study concluded that pregnancy appears to have a profound inhibitory effect on plasma motilin, and that this may in part be responsible for the gastrointestinal hypomotility associated with pregnancy.

It has been hypothesized that the enlarged uterus pressing on the large colon may also be responsible for constipation by slowing transit of feces, especially in the third trimester. However, this remains speculative, because an increased frequency of constipation in the third trimester has not been found consistently by all investigators.[167,168] Perry and colleagues studied the effect of pregnancy on colonic absorption of sodium, potassium, and water.[174] Using a technique of colon perfusion, they demonstrated that pregnancy resulted in a significantly increased absorption of sodium and water across the colonic mucosa. These findings have been implicated as a cause of constipation in pregnancy. Iron preparations taken by the pregnant woman may also contribute to the development of constipation during gestation.

Colonic diseases, including chronic obstructive lesions of the large colon, rectosigmoid colon, and Hirschsprung's disease, have been rare but serious causes of constipation during pregnancy.[175–179]

Several authors have recently shown that the treatment of constipation during pregnancy should consist mainly of nutrition counseling, increasing fluid intake, and dietary modification.[180–182] If these measures are unsuccessful, then laxatives and stool softeners may be used. These preparations should be used sparingly and are usually not necessary. Laxatives most commonly recommended are Metamucil, magnesium hydroxide, castor oil, and other nonprescription drugs. The use of excess laxatives by patients to induce labor should not be condoned. The stool softener dioctyl sulfosuccinate may be used to make the stool softer and able to be passed with less straining. No teratogenic effects have been reported from the use of these common laxatives and stool softeners.[7,183,184] Lewis and Weingold have suggested that they be used cautiously in the breastfeeding patient because they may be transmitted to the infant.[7]

Constipation may result in the development of hemorrhoids. These can usually be treated by topical ointments or sprays, stool softeners, sitz baths, and over-the-counter preparations such as Preparation H. When hemorrhoids develop during the puerperium after vigorous pushing, they may become thrombosed. Incision after local anesthesia may be necessary and beneficial.

DISEASES ADJACENT TO THE GASTROINTESTINAL TRACT

GALLBLADDER DISEASE

Classically, the female patient with gallbladder disease has been described as "fair, fat, forty, and fertile."[185] Gallbladder disease is uncommon during pregnancy. It may occur as cholelithiasis or acute cholecystitis.

Cholelithiasis

Pregnancy predisposes to gallstones. Gerdes and Boyden, in an early study, concluded that the rate of emptying of the human gallbladder in pregnancy was decreased.[186] Braverman and associates studied gallbladder function during pregnancy and during treatment with contraceptive steroids.[187] Using real-time ultrasonography, gallbladder kinetics were studied in 11 non-pregnant women, 17 women using steroid contraceptives, and 33 pregnant women. They found that after the first trimester of pregnancy, the gallbladder volume during fasting and residual volume after contraction were twice as large as in the control subjects. The rate of gallbladder emptying and the percentage emptied was reduced. Although there is an increased incidence of gallstones associated with contraceptive steroids, this study showed they had no effect on gallbladder function. The authors concluded that pregnancy increases the risk of cholesterol gallstones by causing incomplete emptying of the gallbladder, particularly in late pregnancy, leaving a large residual volume due to decreased gallbladder contractility. In this way, pregnancy increases the risk of gallstone formation. The decreased gallbladder motility is theorized to be due to the high progesterone levels present in the second and third trimesters of pregnancy. Sex hormone receptors, estrogen and progesterone, have been found in gallbladder tissue.[188] The function of cholecystokinin, the hormone responsible for causing contraction of the gallbladder, is impaired by progesterone.

Oral contraceptives do not appear to be associated with the formation of gallstones, except in women less than 29 years of age.[189,190] The risk of developing gallstone disease increases in association with increasing parity, particularly among younger women. Older women had a decreased risk of developing gallstones.

The exact incidence of cholelithiasis in male or nonpregnant female patients is unknown, because many gallstones are asymptomatic. The same is true during pregnancy. Chesson and coworkers[191] and Stauffer and associates[192] reported 2% to 4% of asymptomatic women undergoing routine obstetrical ultrasound examinations have cholecystolithiasis. When asymptomatic gallstones are found incidentally during a prenatal ultrasound examination, no therapy is indicated. We advise the patient that she has cholelithiasis and to seek follow-up evaluation after her pregnancy. There is no evidence that asymptomatic gallstones become symptomatic at a higher or lower frequency rate during pregnancy. Gallstones create a problem by passing through or becoming impacted in the biliary tract, producing colic. It has been estimated that one-half of asymptomatic silent stones will cause a problem during a patient's life. The most common complication of cholelithiasis is choledocholithiasis. This occurs in about 15% to 25% of patients with gallstones. The incidence of choledocholithiasis and biliary colic does not appear to be affected by pregnancy. The presence of gallstones may also lead to the development of acute and chronic cholecystitis.

Biliary colic, which is due to choledocholithiasis, is a form of chronic cholecystitis where the gallstones become impacted or pass through the biliary tract (Fig. 63-8), and is the most common symptom that gallstones produce during pregnancy. It affects 15% of patients with cholecystolithiasis.[50] The pain is due to the passage of the gallstones from the gallbladder into the cystic duct or the common bile duct. This produces a spasm of the gallbladder or the biliary duct involved. The pain is right upper quadrant and moderate to severe. It may be cramping or steady. The pain may come on abruptly, particularly after eating a fatty meal. It usually does not last more than a few hours. Although biliary colic is most frequently present in the right upper quadrant, it may also be epigastric, colicky, or steady in intensity. Unlike appendicitis, the pain of biliary colic is not altered in location or character. The patient may also experience nausea, vomiting and, if cholangitis is present, fever. Jaundice may be present, although gallstones account for only 5% of the causes for jaundice during pregnancy. Depending on where the stone becomes impacted in the biliary tree, obstructive jaundice (common bile duct) or acute pancreatitis (ampulla of Vater) may occur (see Fig. 63-8). The symptoms of cholelithiasis may cease spontaneously once the stone is passed through the biliary tract or may persist, requiring surgical removal.

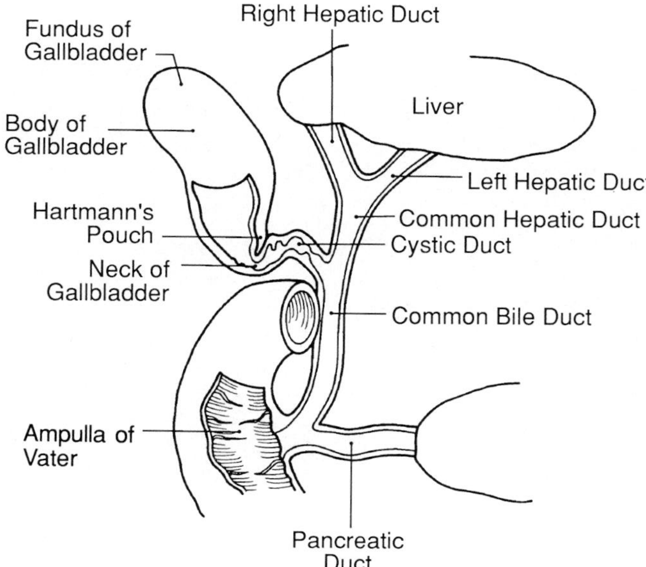

FIGURE 63–8. Diagram of biliary ducts. (Courtesy of Charter Lakeside Hospital, Memphis, TN.)

Laboratory diagnosis of gallstones in pregnancy is the same as during non-pregnancy. The leukocyte count and differential may be normal or slightly elevated, depending on the degree of cholangitis. Slight hyperbilirubinemia and slight elevation in the aspartate aminotransferase (AST, formerly SGOT) may be present. The serum alkaline phosphatase is elevated by biliary colic. This is not helpful during pregnancy because elevated serum alkaline phosphatase is normal in the pregnant patient as a result of placental production. The presence of acute pancreatitis as a result of common duct stones may cause pancreatitis and elevated serum amylase.

Real-time ultrasound has revolutionized the diagnosis of biliary tract disease during pregnancy (Figs. 63-9A and B). Several studies have shown ultrasound to be 95% to 98% sensitive in diagnosing both solitary and multiple gallstones in the gallbladder or biliary tract (Fig. 63-10, 63-11, and 63-12).[193–197] The technique used in the pregnant and non-pregnant patient is the same and has been well described.[197] Ultrasonography, which has been used in all trimesters to identify gallstones, is completely safe during pregnancy and should be a part of the evaluation of any pregnant woman with right upper quadrant pain.[193,198]

The treatment of cholelithiasis during pregnancy is the same as in the non-pregnant patient. Accurate diagnosis should be made as previously described. Therapy should be tailored to the patient's symptoms, physical examination, gestational age, duration of illness, and clinical condition. Asymptomatic gallstones do not require any therapy. Most patients who have silent gallstones will never develop symptoms. Cholecystectomy is recommended for the patient with gallstones who has recurrent episodes of biliary colic, common bile duct gallstones, and gallstone pancreatitis.[199] The development of gallstone pancreatitis that does not improve promptly with nonoperative therapy requires cholecystectomy. Increased maternal and fetal morbidity and mortality occurs if complications of biliary tract disease are not promptly treated during pregnancy. Cholecystectomy is the second most frequent nonobstetrical abdominal surgical procedure performed in pregnancy. Nonoperative therapy consisting of hospitalization, antibiotics, analgesia, non per os, and nasogastric suction may be all that is necessary in patients who have mild illness. Patients with symptoms that do not improve with observation and medical therapy require prompt cholecystectomy. Many authors have demonstrated that a delay in surgery for biliary tract disease complications results in increased maternal and fetal morbidity and mortality.[84,200,201] Cholecystectomy during preg-

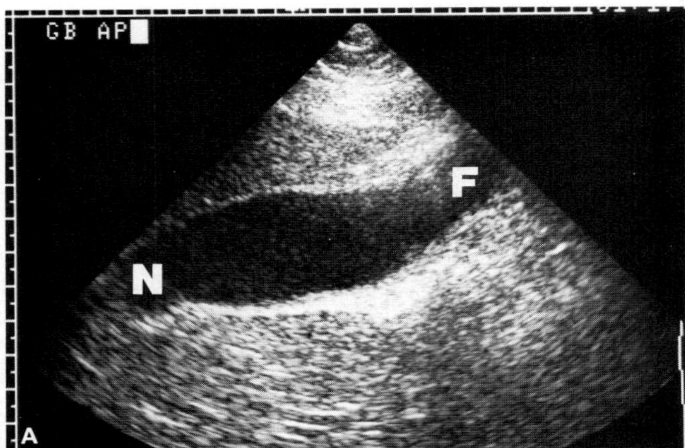

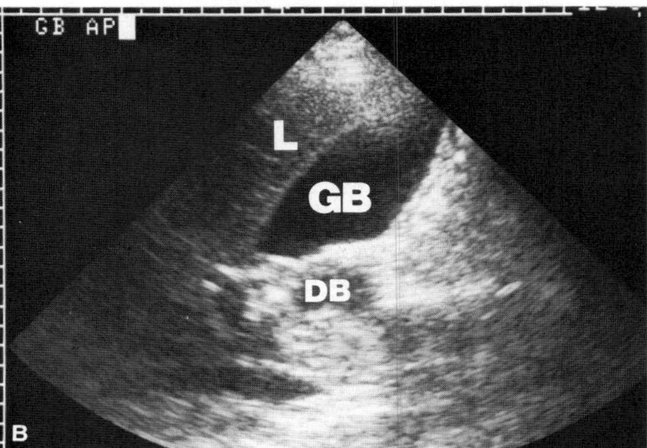

FIGURE 63–9. (**A**) Longitudinal ultrasound scan of normal gallbladder at 16 weeks gestation demonstrating no stones, anechoic bile, normal gallbladder fundus (F), neck (N), and wall thickness (less than 4 mm). (**B**) Longitudinal ultrasound scan of the same patient, showing relationship of gallbladder (GB) to liver (L) and duodenal bulb (DB). (Courtesy of Margaret Colwell, RDMS)

nancy should be performed during the second trimester if possible. This recommendation was made by Hill, who found in 20 patients undergoing elective cholecystectomy at the Mayo Clinic that the best pregnancy outcome was when the surgery was performed in the late second trimester.[199] Several recommendations should be kept in mind when a patient requires cholecystectomy in the second half of pregnancy:

Tocolytic therapy may be necessary and should be instituted if preterm labor occurs.

There are no data to support or condemn the use of prophylactic tocolysis around the time of surgery.

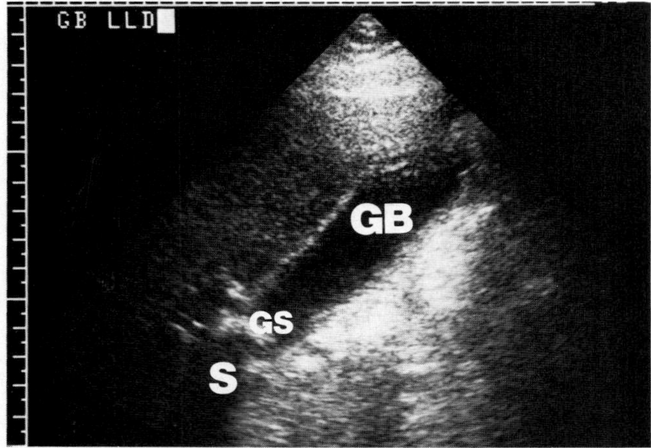

FIGURE 63–10. Longitudinal ultrasound scan of solitary stone (GS) in the gallbladder (GB) in asymptomatic patient at 20 weeks gestation. The gallstone is stuck in the neck of the gallbladder and produces acoustic shadowing (S). False positives are uncommon. A small percentage of false negatives occur. (Courtesy of Jolene Snell, RDMS, BS, and Dr. John D. Terry)

Surgery should be delayed until after delivery if possible if symptoms arise in the third trimester.

Agents to dissolve gallstones such as chenodeoxycholic acid (CDCA) are contraindicated during pregnancy.[7]

Acute Cholecystitis

Acute cholecystitis is a rare gastrointestinal disorder during pregnancy. The incidence is not well known. Friley and Douglas[202] reported an incidence of 1 per 10,000 births, but in a more recent study, Landers,[193] investigating patients at two hospitals in San Francisco, reported a higher incidence of 1 per 1000 births. The rate of acute cholecystitis in pregnancy in their report is

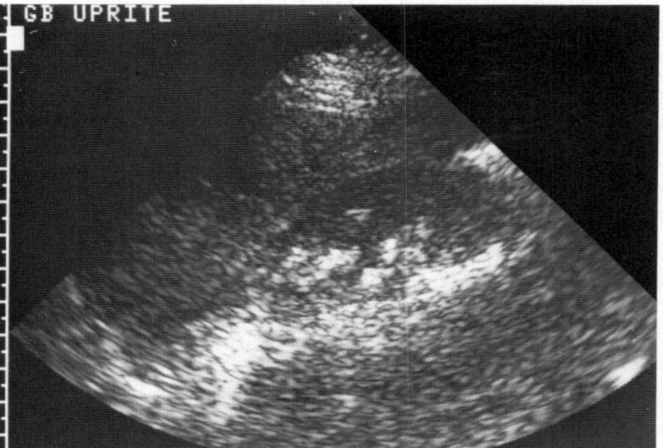

FIGURE 63–11. Longitudinal ultrasound scan of multiple gallstones, some floating in the gallbladder, at 30 weeks gestation in patient with recurrent episodes of biliary colic. A cholecystectomy was performed 7 days postpartum. (Courtesy of Jolene Snell, RDMS, BS)

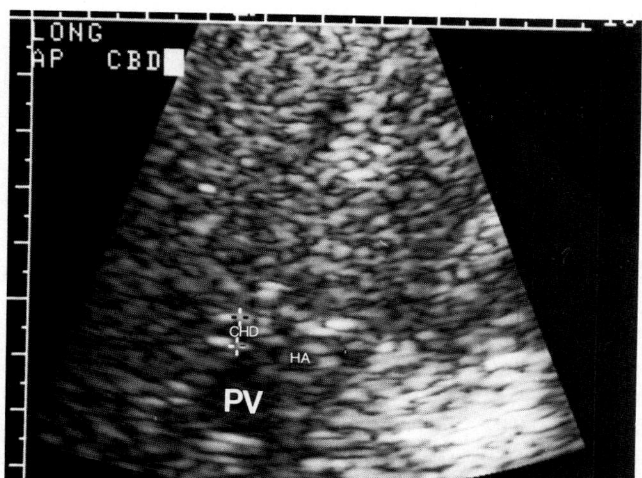

FIGURE 63–12. Transverse ultrasound scan showing the common hepatic duct (CHD) measuring 5.2 mm (less than 6 mm is normal) in patient with right upper quadrant pain at 20 weeks gestation. A normal portal vein (PV) and hepatic artery proper (HA) are also seen. No stones are visible in any of the biliary ducts. (Courtesy of Susan Crouch and Dr. John D. Terry)

higher than the 6 to 20 per 100,000 expected from other series. Fewer pregnant women developed acute cholecystitis than appendicitis during pregnancy.

After appendectomy, cholecystectomy is the most frequently performed nonobstetrical operation during pregnancy. Acute cholecystitis and appendicitis must be included frequently in the differential diagnosis of the pregnant patient presenting with right upper quadrant pain. As has already been pointed out, the appendix may after midgestation be located in the right upper quadrant, thus confusing the clinical picture. Acute pancreatitis must also be considered in the differential diagnosis and may coexist with acute pancreatitis. The incidence of acute cholecystitis does not change through all three trimesters.

The clinical manifestations of acute cholecystitis during pregnancy are the same as in the non-pregnant patient. An attack usually begins with abdominal pain, which may increase in severity. The pain is in the right upper quadrant or epigastrium. Between 70% and 80% of patients have had a previous episode of biliary colic. The pain may radiate to the back and be associated with low-grade fever and chills. A history of previous fatty food intolerance can usually be obtained. The pain may be associated with nausea, vomiting, and anorexia. As with other intra-abdominal inflammation, peritoneal signs may be absent. The pain may radiate to the back. A positive Murphy's sign (right upper quadrant tenderness that is increased while taking a deep breath) is elicited.

The leukocyte count may be normal or mildly elevated. If gallstone pancreatitis is present, there is an elevation in the serum amylase. When common bile duct obstruction occurs, there will be hyperbilirubinemia and liver enzyme elevation. Only 5% of jaundice in pregnancy is due to choledocholithiasis.[203] The evaluation of laboratory data is rarely diagnostic.

Ultrasound has revolutionized the accuracy and safety of diagnosing biliary tract disease during pregnancy.[202,204] The technique of gallbladder sonography can be used throughout pregnancy without harm to the fetus. In Landers's series, 96% of the patients scanned had evidence of gallstones. This technique is over 95% sensitive and equally specific. Sali and coworkers performed an ultrasound study on 137 pregnant women during and immediately after pregnancy.[205] Their study suggests that pregnancy does not affect the size of the gallbladder or the frequency of gallstones. There is no evidence that the ultrasonographic appearance of the gallbladder changes during pregnancy (see Figs. 63-9 through 63-12). Gallstones within the gallbladder or biliary tract are easily seen with sonography and appear as an echodense area within the gallbladder or biliary tract (see Figs. 63-10 and 63-11). They usually cast a shadow and move with a change in position of the patient. The gallbladder wall may be thickened due to chronic cholecystitis, and the biliary ducts dilated due to an impacted stone. Conservative medical management is the mainstay in the treatment of the pregnant patient with acute cholecystitis. This consists of nasogastric suction when necessary, analgesia, intravenous hydration, and antibiotics. Intravenous ampicillin or a cephalosporin are the drugs of choice. Most patients will respond to this medical management. Cholecystectomy should be reserved for those patients who have gallstone pancreatitis, jaundice, repeated attacks, or who fail medical management. When necessary, it should be performed during the second trimester. In Landers's recent series, 84% of the patients were successfully treated conservatively.[193] Favorable pregnancy outcomes occurred when those patients who failed conservative management had their cholecystectomy during the second trimester. As has been pointed out by Hill[199] and supported by the study of Landers,[193] surgery during the first trimester can result in spontaneous abortion. Third trimester cholecystectomy can precipitate preterm labor, which should be managed aggressively with tocolysis. Patients who require cholecystectomy in their third trimester should have it delayed if possible until fetal viability or during the puerperium. Maternal morbidity is not increased when cholecystectomy is performed during pregnancy. Fetal loss after cholecystectomy during pregnancy has been reported to occur in 15% of all procedures performed during pregnancy, but in less than 5% of cholecystectomies performed during the first trimester.[206] When necessary (gallstone pancreatitis, worsened maternal condition with medical therapy, or other complications), cholecystectomy should not be delayed because of pregnancy.

The new technique of laparoscopic laser cholecystectomy, which has been recently performed successfully on the non-pregnant patient, has not been performed during pregnancy.[207–210] It may have a role in treating patients, however, during the puerperium when the uterus is involuted and the abdomen easy to distend.

PANCREATITIS

The exact incidence of acute pancreatitis during pregnancy has been difficult to determine. It is not common and has been reported to occur in 1 per 1000 to 1 per 12,000 pregnancies in an extensive review by Wilkinson.[211] Montgomery and colleagues[212] reported pancreatitis to be more common in primigravida than multipara women, while Crohn and coworkers[115] did not find this to be the case. Although acute pancreatitis may occur in any stage of gestation, it is a disease of late pregnancy, particularly the third trimester, or the early postpartum period.[212,213] Pancreatitis can reoccur during the same or subsequent pregnancy or the puerperium.[214,215] When pancreatitis develops in women less than age 30 years, half of them are pregnant.[213]

Pregnancy probably predisposes a woman to the development not of pancreatitis but of cholelithiasis.[216] It is the most common cause of acute pancreatitis in the pregnant patient. Young[215] and Key[52] have reviewed the many other factors that predispose to the development of acute pancreatitis during pregnancy: alcoholism, acute infections, abdominal surgery, abdominal trauma, pyelonephritis, tetracycline or thiazide use during pregnancy and, rarely, pregnancy-induced hypertension. Hyperlipidemia and hyperparathyroidism have also been reported by several investigators to cause acute pancreatitis.[217–222] However, biliary disease is at least present in, if not responsible for, 90% of pancreatitis in pregnancy.[213] In a study by Block and Kelly, all 21 pregnant patients reported had cholelithiasis.[223] The gallstone can block the ampulla of Vater (see Fig. 63-8), causing active pancreatic proteolytic enzymes to cause autodigestion. The most common predisposing factor in the non-pregnant patient is alcoholism.[16]

The clinical picture of acute pancreatitis is characteristic and has been summarized by numerous authors.[50,211,213,215,224] The symptoms and signs include a rapid onset of constant, central mid-epigastric pain that may radiate to the chest and back, and can be quite severe. In mild cases of pancreatitis, pain may be the only symptom that the patient experiences. Not infrequently, however, nausea and severe vomiting may occur alone or with pain. Low-grade fever and absent or decreased bowel sounds also aid in the diagnosis. The classic clinical presentation of a patient with pancreatitis is an individual rocking in the bed with her knees drawn up and trunk flexed in agony.[224] The pain may also radiate to the flanks or shoulders due to the development of peritoneal irritation. Other symptoms include tachycardia in response to the pain, hypotension, ascites, pleural effusion, hypotonic bowel sounds or ileus, tenderness over the epigastrium, and generalized peritonitis. An adynamic ileus may be demonstrated on radiographic examination. The severity of the clinical features will depend on the severity of the pancreatitis and whether or not complications occur, such as pseudocyst or abscess formation.[225,226] Fortunately, the pregnant patient usually experiences only a mild attack of the disease; however, the clinical picture is unchanged.[50,215]

Laboratory evaluation of the patient suspected to have pancreatitis may be helpful.[50,215,224] Rarely is the white blood cell count above 30,000 cells/mm^3. It may even be within the range for normal pregnancy, 10,000 to 20,000 cells/mm. The serum amylase is the specific test used to diagnose pancreatitis and is usually elevated to at least 100 to 200 units/100 mL. However, it is elevated in other conditions, causing an acute abdomen such as perforation of a peptic ulcer, cholecystitis, intestinal bowel obstruction, hepatic trauma, and ruptured ectopic pregnancy.[224] The rise occurs rather quickly after the onset of the illness, usually within 12 to 24 hours, but values do not correlate with the severity of the disease. A serum amylase above 1000 units/100 mL almost always is indicative of pancreatitis or an obstruction of the pancreatic duct.[215] Serum amylase has been reported both increased and unchanged in the normal pregnancy.[227,228] Kaiser and associates studied serum amylase activity in 200 normal pregnant women in various stages of pregnancy.[227] These investigators concluded that serum amylase rises gradually during pregnancy until reaching a peak of 200 units/100 mL during the 25th week, and thereafter falls slightly. Serum amylase values of this level may therefore be found in normal pregnant women, particularly during the second and third trimesters, exceeding those in normal non-pregnant women. The renal clearance rate of amylase increases throughout pregnancy. However, there is also an increase in the production of pancreatic enzymes. These mild changes result in fluctuations in the serum amylase, but not to the degree that would cause confusion in the diagnosis of acute pancreatitis.

The amylase/creatinine clearance ratio has been used in making the diagnosis of pancreatitis in pregnancy. As a result of an increased creatinine clearance during pregnancy, the amylase/creatinine clearance ratio is normally decreased. DeVore and coworkers demonstrated that patients who were diagnosed accurately with pancreatitis had an increased ratio.[229]

Other abnormal laboratory data seen in acute pancreatitis include slight elevation of the liver function tests, elevated serum lipase, hemoconcentration, hyperglycemia, hypocalcemia, and acidemia due to abnormal pancreatic function.[50,211,215,224] Diagnostic ultrasound can be used to visualize the pancreas for the presence of infection, pseudocyst, or abscess (Fig. 63-13).[225,226,230–233] When inflamed, the pancreas can appear normal, swollen, or enlarged (Fig. 63-14). At the same time, the gallbladder and biliary ducts can be visualized to rule out the presence of gallstones. The pancreas can also be evaluated during pregnancy by a computed tomography (CT) scan. This procedure is safe to perform during pregnancy, because the dose of radiation to the fetus is low.[53,231]

Treatment for acute pancreatitis is primarily nonoperative.[215,224,234] Management includes intravenous fluid

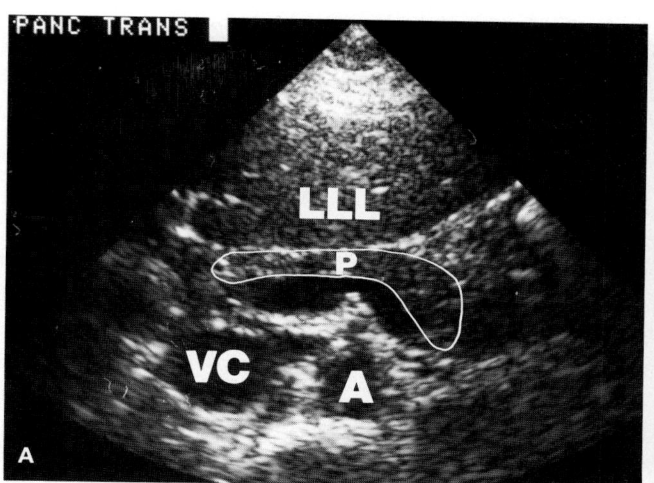

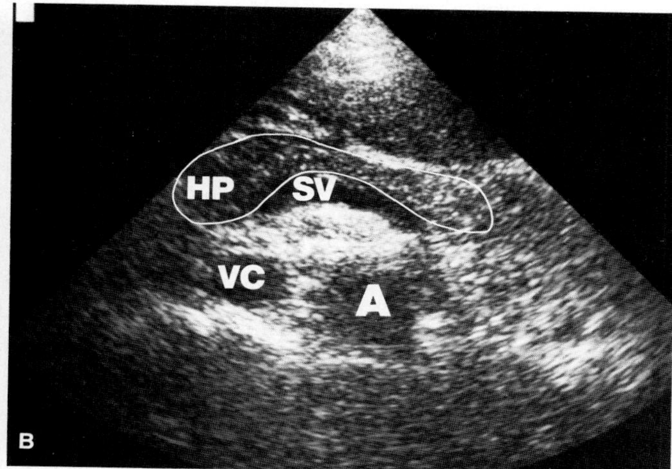

FIGURE 63–13. (**A**) Transverse ultrasound scan of the normal body of the pancreas (P) less than 2.5 cm at 20 weeks gestation, also demonstrating a normal appearing vena cava (VC), aorta (A), and left lobe of the liver (LLL). (**B**) Transverse ultrasound scan of another patient at 18 weeks gestation showing normal head of the pancreas (HP) less than 3.0 cm. The normal relationship of the pancreas to the aorta (A), vena cava (VC), and splenic vein (SV) is also seen. (Courtesy of Margaret Targy and Dr. Joseph C. Anderson)

hydration to correct hypovolemia and electrolyte imbalance, correction of hyperglycemia, enteric rest with nasogastric suction, broad spectrum antibiotics, and adequate analgesia. Insulin may be necessary to reduce the blood sugar. Acute pancreatitis, when managed appropriately, usually subsides in 2 to 3 days. Cholecystectomy or other operative procedures are reserved for the patient with abscess formation, recurrent attacks of pancreatitis, biliary duct obstruction, or a prolonged or nonresponsive attack of pancreatitis.[213] This would increase the patient's risk for preterm labor. Because of peritoneal irritation, if the patient is in the second half of pregnancy, an attempt should be made to detect preterm labor early and to treat it once diagnosed. Magnesium sulfate would be the tocolytic drug of choice, because hyperglycemia could be worsened if the betamimetic drugs were used.[80] Theoretically, the prostaglandin antagonists may be effective, because animal experiments have shown an elevation of prostaglandin-like activity in the pancreatic venous drainage and peritoneal exudate with induced pancreatitis.[235] The clinician should be concerned about maintaining adequate volume replacement, electrolyte balance, and be vigilant for the formation of pancreatic pseudocyst or abscess formation in the patient who does not rapidly improve. Blood coagulation disorders, thrombophlebitis, pulmonary embolus, and vitamin K deficiency have all occurred as a complication of management.[211,215] The most feared complications of acute pancreatitis are hypocalcemia, pancreatic abscess, and pseudocyst formation, but they occur rarely during pregnancy or postpartum.[225,226] Total parenteral nutrition can be safely and effectively used in the management of pancreatitis during pregnancy, when there is concern for the nutritional status of the mother or the development of IUGR.[215,221,236–239]

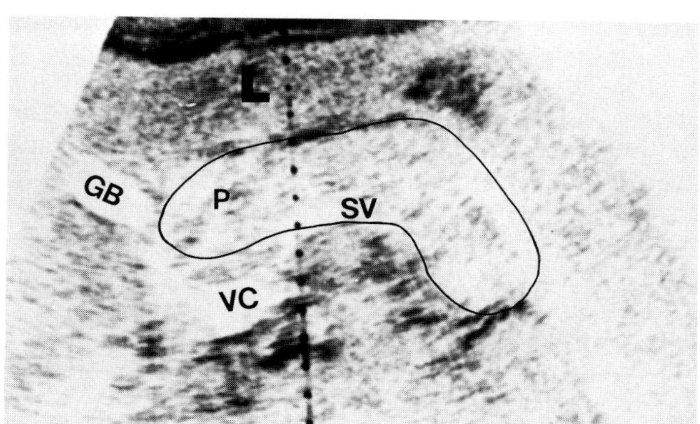

FIGURE 63–14. A 31-year-old G6 P4014 with history of alcohol and heroin abuse who at 35 weeks gestation developed severe vomiting, abdominal pain, and distention. Laboratory evaluation: serum amylase, 250; lipase, 290; LDH, 127; SGOT, 55; alkaline phosphatase, 66; WBC, 4,400; and increased amylase/creatinine clearance ratio. Transverse ultrasound scan showing a 3.5 cm hypoechoic enlarged (normal is <2.5 cm) body of the pancreas (P) due to acute pancreatitis. The liver (L) echogenicity is increased due to fatty infiltration of liver from alcoholism. The gallbladder (GB) was normal. The vena cava (VC) and splenic vein (SV) are also seen. A clinical, laboratory, and ultrasonographic diagnosis was made of acute pancreatitis. The patient improved with conservative medical therapy; however, the full-term infant weighed 4 lb, 3 oz and demonstrated the fetal alcohol syndrome. (Courtesy of Dr. Joseph C. Anderson)

As has been pointed out by Corlett and colleagues[214] and Young,[215] maternal mortality is low when diagnosis is made promptly and appropriate management instituted. Pancreatitis is now a rare cause for maternal death unless the diagnosis is either delayed or missed entirely.[214] The prognosis for the fetus is also good unless severe peritonitis occurs, which predisposes the patient to spontaneous abortion or preterm birth.[215] Preterm labor occurs in 60% of patients when pancreatitis develops late in pregnancy. The mode of delivery is not affected by pancreatitis and, unless contraindicated for obstetric reasons, vaginal delivery is recommended.[211,214,215]

TOTAL PARENTERAL NUTRITION IN PREGNANCY

Pregnant patients unable to consume sufficient nutrients orally require an effective method of feeding. Alternative forms of nutrition are being used more frequently in obstetrics.[240] This may be particularly necessary to maintain maternal nutrition when a gastrointestinal disease complicates pregnancy and can be given as enteral nutrition (tube feeding) or as total parenteral nutrition.[241] Total parenteral nutrition (TPN), parenteral nutrition, hyperalimentation, intravenous hyperalimentation (IVH), and intravenous feedings are used synonymously and interchangeably to describe the various methods of providing all required nutrients intravenously.[241] Supplemental nutrition, eg, Ringer's lactate or saline solutions, can be administered by accessing a peripheral vein. However, TPN, in order to meet basal, maintenance, and the additional demands of growth and development of the patient and fetus, is hyperosmolar and requires jugular or subclavian venous catheterization.[240–248] Subclavian venous catheterization is now the preferred technique for long-term inpatient TPN.[243]

Recently, numerous authors have reported long-term TPN being provided with good results to a variety of hospitalized or outpatient pregnant patients at significant risk for malnutrition and poor fetal outcome (Table 63-1).[9,11–13,53,63,243–258] Patients at high risk for malnutrition during pregnancy may also benefit from TPN (Table 63-2). Silberman and Eisenberg discuss in detail, but succinctly, therapeutic nutrition in the hospitalized patient and principles applicable to the outpatient and pregnant patient.[241]

TABLE 63–1. DISEASES TREATED WITH INPATIENT OR OUTPATIENT TOTAL PARENTERAL NUTRITION DURING PREGNANCY

Hyperemesis gravidarum
Reflux esophagitis
Peptic ulcer disease
Intestinal obstruction or failure
Inflammatory bowel disease
Pregnancy following operation for morbid obesity
Gallbladder disease
Pancreatitis
Malignancy
Diabetes mellitus with gastroenteropathy
Cystic fibrosis with marasmus
Anorexia nervosa
Maternal brain damage
End-stage renal disease

TABLE 63–2. PATIENTS AT HIGH RISK FOR MALNUTRITION DURING PREGNANCY

1. Pregnancy weight 10% below ideal body weight
2. Adolescents: the younger the patient, the greater the nutritional risk
3. Neuropsychiatric problems
   a. Depression
   b. Dietary faddism
   c. Pica
   d. Eating disorder (anorexia nervosa, bulimia)
4. Prolonged dysfunction of the gastrointestinal tract
   a. Postoperative ileus
   b. Diabetic gastroenteropathy
   c. Inflammatory bowel disease
   d. Infectious gastrointestinal disease
   e. Hyperemesis gravidarum
   f. Cystic fibrosis with marasmus
5. Obstetrical conditions
   a. Rapid reproduction with short intervals between conceptions
   b. Repeated delivery of low birthweight infants
6. Low socioeconomic status

Adapted from Lee RV, Rodgers BD, Young C, Eddy E, Cardinal J. Total parenteral nutrition during pregnancy. Obstet Gynecol 1986;68:563, with permission.

Although convenient and less expensive, peripheral parenteral nutrition (PPN) can only be used for short periods of time. It is commonly used in the postoperative patient who is pregnant or during the puerperium. PPN provides an inadequate long-term caloric supply for patient maintenance. Another major disadvantage of PPN is that it requires large fluid volumes to decrease the osmolality of the solution and to prevent thrombophlebitis.[240]

TPN, whether in the pregnant or non-pregnant patient, can be complicated by maternal death. Other complications include accidental pneumothorax or hemothorax, catheter infection, various metabolic disorders, glycosuria, hypoglycemia and, rarely, clinical sepsis (Table 63-3).[13,240,242,243,247,254] Wernicke-

TABLE 63–3. PREGNANT PATIENTS' MAJOR RISK FROM PARENTERAL NUTRITION

1. Complications of catheter placement
   a. Superficial thrombophlebitis (for PPN)
   b. Pneumothorax
   c. Mediastinal disturbances
   d. Catheter-related infection (for TPN)
   e. Hydrothorax
   f. Cardiac tamponade
2. Metabolic complications
   a. Hyperglycemia
   b. Hypoglycemia
   c. Hypophosphatemia
   d. Electrolyte derangements
3. Hepatocellular abnormalities
   a. Increased SGOT
   b. Increased SGPT
4. Vitamin and trace element deficiency syndromes

Adapted from data from Catanzarite VA, Argubright K, Mann BA, Brittain VL. Malnutrition during pregnancy? Consider parenteral feeding. Contemp Obstet Gynecol 1986;27:110, with permission.

Korsakoff syndrome, with irreversible neurologic abnormalities, has occurred after institution of TPN and has been reported by various authors.[9,240,249] Catanzarite concludes that this syndrome, although a disturbing complication of TPN, is not unique to pregnancy, but may occur in any severely malnourished patient given hypertonic glucose.[240]

Heller has suggested that lipid solutions might precipitate premature labor.[242] His studies found an increase in uterine activity when infusing linoleic acid and caused him to theorize that this could lead to an increased synthesis of arachidonic acid, a precursor of prostaglandins.[242,243] Although interesting, these findings in animals have not occurred clinically in humans, and linoleic acid is no longer used in TPN solutions.[11,240,245,248] There is general agreement, therefore, that TPN does not cause preterm labor or small-for-gestational-age infants. However, the disease process for which parenteral nutrition is being given may be the cause of this adverse perinatal outcome.

It has been demonstrated that enteral or TPN can be safely and effectively administered during pregnancy.[11,63,240–248] A team of qualified, knowledgeable individuals who are familiar with the technique being used should explain it to the patient, obtain a written consent, and manage the administration of the parenteral nutrition.[240,243,259,260] Landon and coworkers have also suggested that TPN be administered in hospitals with an intensive care nursery, because many of the infants of the mothers who are receiving this therapy deliver preterm.[243]

TABLE 63–4. CRITERIA FOR SELECTION OF PREGNANT PATIENTS FOR TOTAL PARENTERAL NUTRITION

- **I.** Inaccessible or inadequate gastrointestinal nutrition route for any reason
- **II.** Maternal malnutrition
  - **A.** Weight loss greater than 1 kg/wk for 4 wk consecutively
  - **B.** Total weight loss of 6 kg or failure to gain weight
  - **C.** Underlying chronic disease which increases basal nutritional requirements, including preconception malnutrition
  - **D.** Biochemical markers of malnutrition
    - **1.** Severe hypoalbuminemia less than 2.0 g/dL
    - **2.** Persistent ketosis
    - **3.** Hypocholesterolemia
    - **4.** Lymphocytopenia
    - **5.** Macrocytic anemia: diminished folic acid
    - **6.** Microcytic anemia and decreased serum Fe
    - **7.** Negative nitrogen balance
  - **E.** Anthropometric markers of malnutrition
    - **1.** Weight and height
    - **2.** Growth rate
      - **a.** Poor weight gain
      - **b.** Delayed growth of adolescent
    - **3.** Skin fold thickness
    - **4.** Head, chest, waist, and arm circumference
  - **F.** Intrauterine growth retardation of fetus

Adapted from Lee RV, Rodgers BD, Young C, Eddy E, Cardinal J. Total parenteral nutrition during pregnancy. Obstet Gynecol 1986;68:563, with permission.

REFERENCES

1. Soules MR. Nausea and vomiting of pregnancy: role of human chorionic gonadotropin and 17-hydroxyprogesterone. Obstet Gynecol 1980;55:696.
2. Rubin PH, Janourtz HD. The digestive tract. In: Cherry SH, Berkowitz RL, Kase NG, eds. Rovinsky and Guttmacher's medical, surgical, and gynecologic complications of pregnancy. 3rd ed. Baltimore: Williams and Wilkins, 1985:196.
3. US Department of Health and Human Services. Indications for Bendectin narrowed. FDA Drug Bulletin 1981;11:1.
4. Cordero JF, Oakley GP, Greenberg F, et al. Is Bendectin a teratogen? JAMA 1981;245:2307.
5. Shapiro S, Heinonen OP, Siskind V, et al. Antenatal exposure to Bendectin in relation to congenital malformations, perinatal mortality rate, birth weight, and intelligence quotient score. Am J Obstet Gynecol 1977;128:480.
6. Holmes LB. Teratogen update: Bendectin. Teratology 1983; 27:277.
7. Lewis JH, Weingold AB. The use of gastrointestinal drugs during pregnancy and lactation. Am J Gastroenterol 1985;80:912.
8. Larrey D, Rueff B, Feldmann G, Degott C, Danan G, Benhamou JP. Recurrent jaundice caused by recurrent hyperemesis gravidarum. Gut 1984;25:1414.
9. Lavin PJM, Smith D, Kori SH, Elinburger C. Wernicke's encephalopathy: a predictable complication of hyperemesis gravidarum. Obstet Gynecol 1983;62(suppl):13.
10. Fairweather DV. Nausea and vomiting in pregnancy. Am J Obstet Gynecol 1968;102:135.
11. Levine MG, Esser D. Total parenteral nutrition for the treatment of severe hyperemesis gravidarum: maternal nutritional effects and fetal outcome. Obstet Gynecol 1988;72:102.
12. Stellato TA, Danziger LH, Burkons D. Fetal salvage with maternal total parenteral nutrition: the pregnant mother as her own control. JPEN, Journal of Parenteral and Enteral Nutrition 1988; 12:412.
13. Greenspoon JS, Masaki DI, Kurz CR. Cardiac tamponade in pregnancy during central hyperalimentation. Obstet Gynecol 1989;73:465.
14. Callahan EJ, Burnett MM, DeLawyer D, Brasted WS. Behavioral treatment of hyperemesis gravidarum. Journal of Psychosomatic Obstetrics and Gynaecology 1986;5:187.
15. Henker FO. Psychotherapy as adjunct in treatment of vomiting during pregnancy. South Med J 1976;69:1585.
16. Dozeman R, Kaiser FE, Cass O, Pries J. Hyperthyroidism appearing as hyperemesis gravidarum. Arch Intern Med 1983; 143:2202.
17. Juras N, Banovack K, Sekso M. Increased reverse trilodothyronine in patients with hyperemesis gravidarum. Acta Endocrinol 1983;102:284.
18. Lao TT, Chin RKH, Change AMZ. The outcome of hyperemetic pregnancies complicated by transient hyperthyroidism. Aust NZ J Obstet Gynaecol 1987;27:99.
19. Weigel MM, Weigel RM. Nausea and vomiting of early pregnancy and pregnancy outcome. An epidemiological study. Br J Obstet Gynaecol 1989;96:1304.
20. Klebanoff MA, Koslowe PA, Kaslow R, Rhoads GG. Epidemiology of vomiting in early pregnancy. Obstet Gynecol 1985;66:612.
21. Weigel RM, Weigel MM. Nausea and vomiting of early pregnancy and pregnancy outcome. A meta-analytical review. Br J Obstet Gynaecol 1989;96:1312.
22. Carranza F. Glickman's clinical periodontology. 7th ed. Philadelphia: WB Saunders, 1990.
23. Ziskin DE. The incidence of dental caries in pregnant women. Am J Obstet Gynecol 1926;12:710.

24. Ziskin DE, Hotelling H. Effect of pregnancy, mouth acidity, and age on dental caries. J Dent Res 1937;16:507.
25. Shafer WG, Hine MK, Levy BM. A textbook of oral pathology. 4th ed. Philadelphia: WB Saunders, 1983.
26. Regezi JA, Sciubba JJ. Oral pathology: clinical pathologic correlations. Philadelphia: WB Saunders, 1989.
27. Albrecht M, Banoczy J, Baranyi E, et al. Studies of dental and oral changes of pregnant diabetic women. Acta Diabetol Lat 1987;24:1.
28. Dargiff DA, Karsham M. Effect of pregnancy on the chemical composition of human dentin. J Dent Res 1943;2:26.
29. Deakins M, Looby J. Effects of pregnancy on the mineral content of human teeth. Am J Obstet Gynecol 1943;6:265.
30. Silness J, Loe H. Periodontal disease in pregnancy. Acta Odontol Scand 1967;22:122.
31. Gedalia I. Placental transfer of fluoride in the human fetus at low and high intake. J Dent Res 1963;43:669.
32. Linde J, Branemark PI. The effects of sex hormones on vascularization of granulation tissue. J Periodont Res 1968;3:6.
33. O'Neil TC. Plasma female sex hormone levels in gingivitis in pregnancy. J Periodontol 1979;50:279.
34. Klaytell J, Kaplin AS. Dental complications of pregnancy. In: Cherry SH, Berkowitz RL, Kase NG, eds. Rovinsky and Guttmacher's medical, surgical, and gynecologic complications of pregnancy. 3rd ed. Baltimore: Williams and Wilkins, 1985:820.
35. Setia AP. Severe bleeding from a pregnancy tumor. Oral Surg Oral Med Oral Pathol 1973;36:192.
36. Hatziotis JC. The incidence of pregnancy tumors and their probable relation to the embryo's sex. J Periodontol 1972;43:447.
37. Zarka FL, Stark MM. Gingival tumors of pregnancy: review of "pregnancy tumors" and a report of two cases. Obstet Gynecol 1956;8:597.
38. Bhaskar SN, Jacoway JR. Pyogenic granuloma-clinical features, incidence, histology and result of treatment. J Oral Surg 1966;24:391.
39. Angelopoulos AP. Pyogenic granuloma of the oral cavity: statistical analysis of its clinical features. J Oral Surg 1971;29:840.
40. Sweet JB. Pregnancy-associated dental problems. Contemp Obstet Gynecol 1980;16:33.
41. Howard B, Goodson J, Mengert W. Supine hypotensive syndrome in late pregnancy. Obstet Gynecol 1953;1:371.
42. Lloyd P. Pregnancy and dentistry. Journal of the Dental Association of South Africa 1979;34:763.
43. Lyon LZ, Wisham MA. Management of pregnant dental patients. Dent Clin North Am 1965(Nov);623.
44. Schwartz H, Reichling B. Hazards of radiation exposure for pregnant women. JAMA 1978;239:1907.
45. Grant DA, Stern IB, Listgarten MA. Periodontics. 6th ed. St. Louis: CV Mosby, 1988.
46. Levinson G, Shnider SM. Anesthesia for surgery during pregnancy. In: Shnider SM, Levinson G, eds. Anesthesia for obstetrics. 2nd ed. Baltimore: Williams and Wilkins, 1987:188.
47. Cohlan S. Tetracycline staining of teeth. Teratology 1977; 15:127.
48. Hamod KA, Khouzami VA. Antibiotics in pregnancy. In: Niebyl JR, ed. Drug use in pregnancy. 2nd ed. Philadelphia: Lea and Febiger, 1988:29.
49. Wyngaarden JB, Smith LH. Cecil textbook of medicine. 18th ed. Philadelphia: WB Saunders, 1988.
50. Sleisenger MH, Fordtran JS. Gastrointestinal disease — pathophysiology, diagnosis, management. 4th ed. Philadelphia: WB Saunders, 1989.
51. Nebel OT, Fonres MF, Castell DO. Symptomatic gastroesophageal reflux: incidence and precipitating factors. Am J Dig Dis 1976;21:953.
52. Key T. Gastrointestinal diseases. In: Creasy RK, Resnik R, eds. Maternal-fetal medicine. 2nd ed. Philadelphia: WB Saunders, 1989:1032.
53. Cunningham FG, MacDonald PC, Gant NF. Williams obstetrics. 18th ed. Norwalk: Appleton and Lange, 1989.
54. Ulmsten U, Sundstrom G. Esophageal manometry in pregnant and nonpregnant women. Am J Obstet Gynecol 1978;132:260.
55. Dodds, WJ, Dent J, Hogan WJ. Pregnancy and the lower esophageal sphincter itorial;cb. Gastroenterology 1978;74:1334.
56. Van Thiel DH, Gavaler JS, Joshi SN, et al. Heartburn of pregnancy. Gastroenterology 1977;72:666.
57. Van Thiel DH, Gavaler JS, Stremple J. Lower esophageal sphincter pressure in women using sequential oral contraceptives. Gastroenterology 1976;71:232.
58. Brock-Utne JG, Dow GB, Welman S, et al. The effect of metoclopramide on the lower esophageal sphincter in late pregnancy. Anaesth Intensive Care 1978;6:26.
59. Hey VM, Cowley DJ, Ganguli PC, et al. Gastroesophageal reflux in late pregnancy. Anaesthesia 1977;32:372.
60. Winnan J, Auella J, Callachan C, et al. Double blind trial of metoclopramide versus placebo antacid in symptomatic gastroesophageal reflux [abstract]. Gastroenterology 1980;78:1292.
61. Swinhoe JR, Cochrane GO, Wishart R. Esophageal stricture due to reflux esophagitis in pregnancy: case report. Br J Obstet Gynaecol 1981;88:1249.
62. Palmer ED. Upper gastrointestinal hemorrhage during pregnancy. Am J Med Sci 1961;242:223.
63. Connon J. Gastrointestinal Complications. In: Burrow GN, Ferris TF, eds. Medical complications during pregnancy. 3rd ed. Philadelphia: WB Saunders, 1988:303.
64. Clark DH. Peptic ulcer disease in women. Br Med J 1953;1:1254.
65. Spiro HM, Schwartz ED, Pilot ML. Peptic ulcer in pregnancy. A serial study of gastric secretion during pregnancy. Am J Dig Dis 1959;4:289.
66. Labate JS. The effect of pregnancy on gastric secretion. Am J Obstet Gynecol 1939;38:650.
67. O'Sullivan GM, Bullingham RES. The assessment of gastric acidity and antacid effect in pregnant women by a non-invasive radiotelemetry technique. Br J Obstet Gynaecol 1984;91:973.
68. Hornnes PJ, Kuhl C, Lauritsen KB. Gastroentero-pancreatic hormones in normal pregnancy: response to a protein rich meal. Eur J Clin Invest 1981;11:345.
69. Murray FA, Erskine JP, Fielding J. Gastric secretion in pregnancy. J Obstet Gynaecol Br Empire 1957;64:373.
70. Clark DH, Tankel HI. Gastric acid and plasma histaminase during pregnancy. Lancet 1954;2:886.
71. Warzecha Z, Dembinski A, Konturek SJ, Zdebski Z. Influence of pregnancy on the healing of chronic gastric and duodenal ulcers. Role of endogenous epidermal growth factor I. Ginekol Pol 1989;60:166.
72. Becker-Andersen H, Husfelt V. Peptic ulcer in pregnancy. Acta Obstet Gynecol Scand 1971;50:391.
73. Burkitt R. Perforated peptic ulcer in late pregnancy. Br Med J 1961;2:938.
74. Dilts PV, Coopersmith B, Sweitzer C. Perforated peptic ulcer in pregnancy. Am J Obstet Gynecol 1967;99:293.
75. Langmade CF. Epigastric pain in pregnancy toxemias. West J Surg 1956;64:540.
76. Jones PF, McEwan AB, Bernard RM. Haemorrhage and perforation complicating peptic ulcer in pregnancy. Lancet 1969;2:350.
77. Paul M, Tew WL, Holliday RL. Perforated peptic ulcer in pregnancy with survival of mother and child: case report and review of the literature. Can J Surg 1976;19:427.
78. Tew WL, Holliday RL, Phibbs G. Perforated duodenal ulcer in pregnancy with double survival. Am J Obstet Gynecol 1976;125:1151.

79. Peck DA, Welch JS, Waugh JM, et al. Pregnancy following gastric resection. Am J Obstet Gynecol 1964;90:517.
80. Besinger RE, Niebyl JR. The safety and efficacy of tocolytic agents for the treatment of preterm labor. Obstet Gynecol Surv 1990;45:415.
81. Parker S, Schade RR, Pohl CR, et al. Prenatal and neonatal exposure of male rats to cimetidine but not ranitidine adversely affect subsequent adult sexual functioning. Gastroenterology 1984;86:675.
82. Spence RW, Gelestine LR. Gynaecomastia associated with cimetidine. Gut 1979;20:154.
83. Armentano G, Bracco PL, Di Silverio C. Ranitidine in the treatment of reflux oesophagitis in pregnancy. Clin Exp Obstet Gynecol 1989;16:130.
84. Kammerer WS. Non-obstetric surgery during pregnancy. Med Clin North Am 1979;63:1157.
85. Lewis G. Intestinal obstruction complicating pregnancy. JAMA 1974;74:113.
86. Davis MR, Bohon CJ. Intestinal obstruction and pregnancy. Clin Obstet Gynecol 1983;26:832.
87. Smith JA, Barlett MK. Acute surgical emergencies of the abdomen in pregnancy. N Engl J Med 1944;223:529.
88. Matthews S, Mitchell PR. Intestinal obstruction in pregnancy. J Obstet Gynaecol Br Emp 1948;55:653.
89. Beck WW. Intestinal obstruction in pregnancy. Obstet Gynecol 1974;43:374.
90. Anderson GV, Ball A. Acute abdominal problems in pregnancy. Contemp Obstet Gynecol 1981;18:27.
91. Morris ED. Intestinal obstruction in pregnancy. J Obstet Gynaecol Br Commonwealth 1965;72:36.
92. Kohn SG, Briele HA, Douglas LH. Volvulus in pregnancy. Am J Obstet Gynecol 1944;48:398.
93. Moore DT, Watts CD, Wilbanks GD. Intussusception complicating pregnancy: report of a case. J Natl Med Assoc 1967;59:20.
94. Holbert TR. Intussusception in pregnancy. A case report. J Tenn Med Assoc 1987;80:409.
95. Watson R, Quayle AR. Intussusception in pregnancy. Case report and review of the literature. Br J Obstet Gynaecol 1986;93:1093.
96. Hill LM, Symmonds RE. Small bowel obstruction in pregnancy. A review and report of 4 cases. Obstet Gynecol 1977;49:170.
97. Hammonde AA. Acute intestinal obstruction during pregnancy. A brief review and report of 2 cases. Aust NZ J Obstet Gynaecol 1967;7:101.
98. Goldthorp WO. Intestinal obstruction during pregnancy and the puerperium. Br J Clin Pract 1966;20:367.
99. Charles D, Stronge J. Special problems of the colon and rectum encountered in obstetric practice. Clin Obstet Gynecol 1972;15:522.
100. Wenetick LH, Roschen FP, Dunn JM. Volvulus of the small bowel complicating pregnancy. J Reprod Med 1975;14:82.
101. Glinter KP. Intestinal obstruction complicating pregnancy. JAMA 1972;72:979.
102. Graubard Z, Graham KM, van der Merwe FJ, Koller AB. Caecal volvulus in pregnancy. A case report. S Afr Med J 1988;73:188.
103. Allen JC. Sigmoid volvulus in pregnancy. J R Army Med Corps 1990;136:55.
104. Dan U, Rabinovici J, Koller M, Barkai G, Mashiach S. Iatrogenic mechanical ileus due to over-distended uterus. Gynecol Obstet Invest 1988;25:143.
105. Graubard Z, Graham KM, Schein M. Small-bowel obstruction in pregnancy after Scopinaro weight reduction operation. A case report. S Afr Med J 1988;73:127.
106. Rachagan SP, Raman S, Silvanesaratnam V, Sinnathuray TA. Intestinal obstruction following previous myomectomy and the use of beta-sympathomimetics in pregnancy. Eur J Obstet Gynecol Reprod Biol 1986;22:99.
107. Ludmir J, Samuels P, Armson BA, Torosian MH. Spontaneous small bowel obstruction associated with a spontaneous triplet gestation. A case report. J Reprod Med 1990;34:985.
108. Sorokin JJ, Levine SM. Pregnancy and inflammatory bowel disease: a review of the literature. Obstet Gynecol 1983;62:247.
109. Hanan IM, Kirsner JB. Inflammatory bowel disease in the pregnant woman. Clin Perinatol 1985;12:669.
110. Warsof, SL. Medical and surgical treatment of inflammatory bowel disease in pregnancy. Clin Obstet Gynecol 1983;26:822.
111. Becker IM. Pregnancy and toxic dilatation of the colon. Am J Dig Dis 1972;17:79.
112. Willoughby CP, Truelove SC. Ulcerative colitis and pregnancy. Gut 1980;21:469.
113. Webb MJ, Sedlack RE. Ulcerative colitis in pregnancy. Med Clin North Am 1974;58:823.
114. Homan WP, Thorbjarnarson B. Crohn's disease and pregnancy. Arch Surg 1976;111:545.
115. Crohn BB, Yarnis H, Korelitz BI. Regional ileitis complicating pregnancy. Gastroenterology 1956;31:615.
116. Fielding JF, Cooke WT. Pregnancy and Crohn's disease. Br Med J 1970;2:76.
117. DeDombal FT, Burton IL, Goligher JC. Crohn's disease and pregnancy. Br Med J 1972;3:550.
118. Wikland M, Jansson I, Asztely M, et al. Gynecological problems related to anatomical changes after conventional proctocolectomy and ileostomy. Int J Color Dis 1990;5:49.
119. Abramson D, Jankelson IR, Milner LR. Pregnancy in idiopathic ulcerative colitis. Am J Obstet Gynecol 1951;6:121.
120. Crohn BB, Yarnis H, Cohen EB, Crohn EB, Walter RI, Gabrilove LJ. Ulcerative colitis and pregnancy. Gastroenterology 1956; 30:391.
121. DeDombal FT, Watts JM, Watkinson G, Goligher JC. Ulcerative colitis and pregnancy. Lancet 1965;2:599.
122. Brostrom O. Prognosis in ulcerative colitis. Med Clin North Am 1990;74:201.
123. Khosla R, Willoughby CP, Jewell DP. Crohn's disease and pregnancy. Gut 1984;25:52.
124. Norton RA, Patterson JF. Pregnancy and regional enteritis. Obstet Gynecol 1972;40:711.
125. Pezim ME. Successful childbirth after restorative proctocolectomy with pelvic ileal reservoir. Br J Surg 1984;71:292.
126. Nielson OH, Andreasson B, Bondesen S, Jacobsen O, Jarnum S. Pregnancy in Crohn's disease. Scand J Gastroenterol 1984; 19:724.
127. Bayliss RIS, Brown JCM, Round BP, Steinbeck AW. Plasma 17-hydroxycorticosteroids in pregnancy. Lancet 1955;1:62.
128. Vanagunas A, Marshall S. Gastrointestinal complications of pregnancy. In: Sciarra JJ, Depp R, Eschenbach DA, eds. Gynecology and obstetrics. Revised ed. Philadelphia: JB Lippincott, 1988;3:1.
129. Mogadam M, Dobbins WO, Korelitz BI, Ahmed SW. Pregnancy in inflammatory bowel disease: effect of sulfasalazine and corticosteroids on fetal outcome. Gastroenterology 1981;80:72.
130. Jarnerot G, Into-Malmberg MD. Sulfasalazine treatment during breast feeding. Scand J Gastroenterol 1979;14:869.
131. Mogadam M, Korelitz BI, Ahmed SW, Dobbins W, Baiocco PJ. The course of inflammatory bowel disease during pregnancy and postpartum. Am J Gastroenterol 1981;75:265.
132. Zeldis JB. Pregnancy and inflammatory bowel disease. West J Med 1989;151:168.
133. Babaknia A, Parsa H, Woodruff J. Appendicitis during pregnancy. Obstet Gynecol 1977;50:40.
134. Babler EA. Perforative appendicitis complicating pregnancy. JAMA 1908;51:1310.

135. Baer JL, Reis RA, Arens RA. Appendicitis in pregnancy with changes in position and axis of the normal appendix in pregnancy. JAMA 1932;98:1359.
136. Cunningham FG, McCubbin JH. Appendicitis complicating pregnancy. Obstet Gynecol 1975;45:415.
137. Dornhoffer JL, Calkins JW. Appendicitis complicating pregnancy. Kans Med 1988;89:139.
138. Hunt MG, Martin JN, Martin RW, Meeks GR, Wiser WL, Morrison JC. Perinatal aspects of abdominal surgery for nonobstetric disease. Am J Perinatol 1989;6:412.
139. McGee TM. Acute appendicitis in pregnancy. Aust N Z J Obstet Gynaecol 1989;24:378.
140. Bongard F, Landers DV, Lewis F. Differential diagnosis of appendicitis and pelvic inflammatory disease: a prospective analysis. Am J Surg 1985;150:90.
141. Spirtos NM, Eisenkop SM, Spirtos TW, Poliakin RI, Hibbard LT. Laparoscopy — a diagnostic aid in cases of suspected appendicitis: its use in women of reproductive age. Am J Obstet Gynecol 1987;156:90.
142. Abu Yousef MM, Franken EA. An overview of graded compression sonography in the diagnosis of acute appendicitis. Seminars in Ultrasound, CT and MR 1989;10:352.
143. Marn CS, Bree RL. Advances in pelvic ultrasound: endovaginal scanning for ectopic gestation and graded compression sonography for appendicitis. Ann Emerg Med 1989;18:1304.
144. Ammerman KS, Toffle RC. Concurrent appendicitis and pregnancy at term. W V Med J 1987;83:63.
145. McComb P, Laimon H. Appendicitis complicating pregnancy. Can J Surg 1980;23:92.
146. Saunders P, Milton PJD. Laparotomy during pregnancy: an assessment of diagnostic accuracy and fetal wastage. Br Med J 1973;3:165.
147. Frisenda R, Roty AR, Kilway JB, Brown AL, Peelan M. Acute appendicitis during pregnancy. Am Surg 1979;45:503.
148. Zaitoon MM, Mrazek RG. Acute appendicitis associated with pregnancy, labor, and the puerperium. Am Surg 1977;43:395.
149. Weingold AB. Appendicitis in pregnancy. Clin Obstet Gynecol 1983;26:80.
150. Parsons AK, Sauer MV, Parsons MT, Tunca J, Spellacy WN. Appendectomy at cesarean section: a prospective study. Obstet Gynecol 1986;68:479.
151. Tungphaisal S, Pinjaroen S, Chandeying V, Sutthycinroon S. Incidental appendectomy at cesarean section: a prospective study. J Med Assoc Thai 1989;72:633.
152. Deitel M. Surgery for the morbidly obese patient. Philadelphia: Lea and Febiger, 1989.
153. Printen KJ, Scott D. Pregnancy following gastric bypass for the treatment of morbid obesity. Am Surg 1982;48:363.
154. Knudsen LB, Kallen B. Intestinal bypass operation and pregnancy outcome. Acta Obstet Gynecol Scand 1986;65:831.
155. Ayromlooi J, Parsa H. Pregnancy following jejunoileal bypass for obesity. Am J Obstet Gynecol 1977;129:921.
156. McCarthy PJ. Pregnancy following jejuno-ileal bypass. Obstet Gynecol 1974;43:455.
157. Stenning H, Campbell R, Brake I, et al. Pregnancy after jejunoileal shunt. Med J Aust 1977;1:781.
158. Savel LE, Simon SR, Maxon WS. Pregnancy after jejunoileal bypass. Obstet Gynecol 1978;52(suppl):58.
159. Woods JR. Brinkman CR. The jejunoileal bypass and pregnancy. Obstet Gynecol Surv 1978;33:697.
160. Ingardia CJ, Fischer JR. Pregnancy after jejunoileal bypass and the SGA infant. Obstet Gynecol 1978;52:215.
161. Olow B, Akesson BA, Dencker H, et al. Pregnancy after jejunoileostomy because of obesity. Acta Chir Scand 1976;142:82.
162. Taylor JL, O'Leary JP. Pregnancy following jejunoileal bypass. Obstet Gynecol 1970;48:425.
163. Gray DS, Cabaniss ML. Home total parenteral nutrition in a pregnant diabetic after jejunoileal bypass for obesity. JPEN, Journal of Parenteral and Enteral Nutrition 1989;13:214.
164. Karamatsu JT, Boyd AT, Cooke J, Vinall PS, McMahon MJ. Intravenous nutrition during a twin pregnancy. JPEN, Journal of Parenteral and Enteral Nutrition 1987;11:499.
165. Holian DK. Biliopancreatic bypass. In: Deitel M, ed. Surgery for the morbidly obese patient. Philadelphia: Lea and Febiger, 1989:105.
166. Grace DM. Metabolic complications following gastric restrictive procedures. In: Deitel M, ed. Surgery for the morbidly obese patient. Philadelphia: Lea and Febiger, 1989:339.
167. Levy N, Lenberg E, Sharf M. Bowel habit in pregnancy. Digestion 1971;4:216.
168. Greenhalf JO, Leonard HSD. Laxatives in the treatment of constipation in pregnant and breast-feeding mothers. Practitioner 1973;210:259.
169. Kumar D. In vitro inhibitory effect of progesterone on extrauterine human smooth muscle. Am J Obstet Gynecol 1962;84:1300.
170. Hytten FE, Chamberlain T. Clinical physiology in obstetrics. Oxford: Blackwell Scientific Publications, 1981.
171. Lawson M, Kern F, Everson GT. Gastrointestinal transit time in human pregnancy. Prolongation in the second and third trimesters followed by postpartum normalization. Gastroenterology 1985;89:996.
172. Wald A, VanThiel DH, Hoechstetter L, et al. Gastrointestinal transit: the effect of the menstrual cycle. Gastroenterology 1981;80:1497.
173. Cristofides ND, Ghatia NA, Bloom SR, Borberg C, Gillberg MDG. Decreased plasma motilin concentrations in pregnancy. Br Med J 1982;285:1453.
174. Parry E, Shields R, Turnbull AC. The effect of pregnancy on the colonic absorption of sodium, potassium, and water. J Obstet Gynaecol Br Commonwealth 1970;77:616.
175. Nash AG. Perforated large bowel carcinoma in late pregnancy. Proc R Soc Med 1967;60:504.
176. O'Leary JA, Pratt JH, Symmonds RE. Rectal carcinoma and pregnancy: a review of 17 cases. Obstet Gynecol 1967;30:862.
177. Rothman LA, Cohen CJ, Astarloa J. Placental and fetal involvement by maternal malignancy: a report of rectal carcinoma and review of the literature. Am J Obstet Gynecol 1973;116:1023.
178. Clement PB. Perforation of the sigmoid colon during pregnancy: a rare complication of endometriosis. Case report. Br J Obstet Gynaecol 1977;84:548.
179. Balfour RP, Burke M. Hirschsprung's disease complicating pregnancy. Br J Clin Pract 1976;30:70.
180. Brucker MC. Management of common minor discomforts in pregnancy. III: managing gastrointestinal problems in pregnancy. J Nurse Midwifery 1988;33:67.
181. Anderson AS. Dietary factors in the aetiology and treatment of constipation during pregnancy. Br J Obstet Gynaecol 1986;93:245.
182. Anderson AS, Whichelow MJ. Constipation during pregnancy: dietary fibre intake and the effect of fibre supplementation. Human Nutrition: Applied Nutrition 1985;39:202.
183. Briggs GG, Freeman RK, Yaffe SJ. Drugs in pregnancy and lactation. 2nd ed. Baltimore: Williams & Wilkins, 1986.
184. Schad RF, Rayburn WF: Antiemetics, iron preparations, vitamins, and OTC drugs. In: Rayburn WF, Zuspan FP, eds. Drug therapy in obstetrics and gynecology. 2nd ed. Norwalk: Appleton-Century-Crofts, 1986:24.
185. Deaver JB. Sequelae of biliary tract infection. JAMA 1950;95:1644.
186. Gerdes MM, Boyden EA. The rate of emptying of the human gallbladder in pregnancy. Surg Gynecol Obstet 1938;66:145.
187. Braverman DZ, Johnson ML, Kern F Jr. Effects of pregnancy

and contraceptive steroids on gallbladder function. N Engl J Med 1980;302:362.
188. Singletary BK, Van Thiel DH, Eagon PK. Estrogen and progesterone receptors in human gallbladder. Hepatology 1986;6:574.
189. Royal College of General Practitioners. Oral contraceptive study. Lancet 1982;2:957.
190. Scragg, RKR, McMichael AJ, Seamark RF. Oral contraceptives, pregnancy and endogenous estrogen in gallstone disease. Br Med J 1984;288:1795.
191. Chesson RR, Gallup DG, Gibbs RL, Jones BE, Thomas B. Ultrasonographic diagnosis of asymptomatic cholelithiasis in pregnancy. J Reprod Med 1985;30:921.
192. Stauffer RA, Adams A, Wygal J, Lavery JP. Gallbladder disease in pregnancy. Am J Obstet Gynecol 1982;144:661.
193. Landers D, Carmona R, Crombleholme W, Lim R. Acute cholecystitis in pregnancy. Obstet Gynecol 1987;69:131.
194. Leopold G, Amberg J, Gosink B, et al. Gray scale ultrasonic cholecystography: a comparison with conventional radiographic techniques. Radiology 1976;121:445.
195. Bolondi L, Bazzocchi R, Arienti V, et al. Sonographic evaluation of gallbladder wall thickening. Clinical and pathological correlation with particular regard to acute cholecystitis. Italian Journal of Gastroenterology 1982;14:7.
196. Bartrum RJ, Crow HCC, Foote SR. Ultrasound and radiographic cholecystography. N Engl J Med 1977;296:538.
197. Harned RK, Williams SM, Anderson JC. Gallbladder disease. In: Eisenberg RL, ed. Diagnostic imaging — an algorithmic approach. Philadelphia: JB Lippincott, 1987:154.
198. Reece EA, Assimakopoulous E, Zheng X, Hagay Z, Hobbins JC. The safety of obstetrical ultrasonography: concern for the fetus. Obstet Gynecol 1989;76:139.
199. Hill LM, Johnson CE, Lee RA. Cholecystectomy in pregnancy. Obstet Gynecol 1975;46:291.
200. Thorbjarnarson B. Inflammatory diseases of the biliary tract. In: Thorbjarnarson B, ed. Surgery of the biliary tree. Philadelphia: WB Saunders, 1986:126.
201. Printen JK, Ott RA. Cholecystectomy during pregnancy. Am Surg 1978;44:432.
202. Friley MD, Douglas G. Acute cholecystitis in pregnancy and the puerperium. Am Surg 1972;38:314.
203. Haemmerli UP. Jaundice during pregnancy with special reference to recurrent jaundice during pregnancy and its differential diagnosis. Acta Med Scand 1966;444(suppl):1.
204. DeGraff CS, Grade M. Gallstones, pregnancy and ultrasound. Conn Med 1979;43:424.
205. Sali A, Dats JN, Acton CM, Elzarka A, Vitettal. Effect of pregnancy on gallstone formation. Aust NZ J Obstet Gynaecol 1989;29:36.
206. Greene J, Rogers A, Rubin L. Fetal loss after cholecystectomy during pregnancy. Can Med Assoc J 1963;88:576.
207. Reddick EJ, Olsen DO. Laparoscopic laser cholecystectomy. Surg Endosc 1989;3:131.
208. Reddick EJ, Olsen DO, Daniell JF. Laparoscopic laser cholecystectomy. Laser Med Surg News 1989;7:38.
209. Dubois F, Icard P, Berthelot G, Levard H. Coelioscopic cholecystectomy. Ann Surg 1990;211:60.
210. Fitzgibbons RJ, Schmid S, Hinder R, et al. Laparoscopic cholecystectomy: the beginning of a new era in general surgery. Surgery (submitted for publication).
211. Wilkinson EJ. Acute pancreatitis in pregnancy: a review of 98 cases and a report of 8 new cases. Obstet Gynecol Surv 1973;28:281.
212. Montgomery WH, Miller FC. Pancreatitis and pregnancy. Obstet Gynecol 1970;35:658.
213. McKay AJ, O'Neill J, Imrie CW. Pancreatitis, pregnancy and gallstones. Br J Obstet Gynaecol 1980;87:47.
214. Corlett RC, Mishell DR. Pancreatitis in pregnancy. Am J Obstet Gynecol 1972;113:281.
215. Young KR. Acute pancreatitis in pregnancy: two case reports. Obstet Gynecol 1982;60:653.
216. Cohen S. The sluggish gallbladder of pregnancy. N Engl J Med 1980;302:397.
217. Nies BM, Dreiss RJ. Hyperlipidemic pancreatitis in pregnancy: a case report and review of the literature. Am J Perinatol 1990;7:166.
218. DeChalain TM, Michell WL, Berger GM. Hyperlipidemia, pregnancy and pancreatitis. Surg Gynecol Obstet 1988;167:469.
219. Rajala B, Abbasi RA, Hutchinson HT, Taylor T. Acute pancreatitis and primary hyperparathyroidism in pregnancy. Obstet Gynecol 1987;70:460.
220. Fabrin B, Eldon K. Pregnancy complicated by concurrent hyperparathyroidism and pancreatitis. Acta Obstet Gynecol Scand 1986;65:651.
221. Weinberg RB, Sitrin MD, Adkins GM, Lin CC. Treatment of hyperlipidemic pancreatitis in pregnancy with total parenteral nutrition. Gastroenterology 1982;83:1300.
222. Levine G, Tsin D, Risk A. Acute pancreatitis and hyperparathyroidism in pregnancy. Obstet Gynecol 1979;54:246.
223. Block P, Kelly TR. Management of gallstone pancreatitis during pregnancy and the postpartum period. Surg Gynecol Obstet 1989;168:426.
224. Levitt MD. Pancreatitis. In: Wyngaarden JB, Smith LH, eds. Cecil textbook of medicine. 18th ed. Philadelphia: WB Saunders, 1988:774.
225. Strickland N. Acute pancreatitis with pseudocyst formation during pregnancy; report of a case. Obstet Gynecol 1966; 27:347.
226. Winship D, et al. Pancreatitis: pancreatic pseudocysts and their complications. Gastroenterology 1977;73:593.
227. Kaiser R, Berk JE, Fridhandler L, Montgomery K, Wong D. Serum amylase changes during pregnancy. Am J Obstet Gynecol 1975;122:283.
228. Strickland DM, Hauth JC, Widish J, Strickland K, Perez R. Amylase and isoamylase activities in serum of pregnant women. Obstet Gynecol 1984;63:389.
229. DeVore GR, Bracken M, Berkowitz RL. The amylase/creatinine clearance ratio in normal pregnancy and pregnancies complicated by pancreatitis, hyperemesis gravidarum, and toxemia. Am J Obstet Gynecol 1980;136:747.
230. Bolondi L, LiBassi S, Gaiani S, Barbara L. Sonography of chronic pancreatitis. Radiol Clin North Am 1989;27:815.
231. Jeffrey RB. Sonography in acute pancreatitis. Radiol Clin North Am 1989;27:5.
232. Sarti DA. Ultrasonography of the pancreas. In: Sarti DA, ed. Diagnostic ultrasound — text and cases. 2nd ed. Chicago: Yearbook Medical Publishers, 1987:214.
233. Hagen-Ansert SL. Pancreas. In: Hagen-Ansert SL, ed. Textbook of diagnostic ultrasonography. 3rd ed. St. Louis: CV Mosby, 1989:246.
234. Ettien JT, Webster PD III. The management of acute pancreatitis. Adv Intern Med 1980;25:169.
235. Glazer G, Bennett A. Elevation of prostaglandin-like activity in the blood and peritoneal exudate of dogs with acute pancreatitis. Br J Surg 1974;61:922.
236. Stowell JC, Bottsford JE Jr, Rubel HR. Pancreatitis with pseudocyst and cholelithiasis in third trimester of pregnancy: management with total parenteral nutrition. South Med J 1984;77:502.
237. Gineston JL, Capron JP, Delcenserie R, Delamarre J, Blot M, Boulanger JC. Prolonged total parenteral nutrition in a pregnant woman with acute pancreatitis. J Clin Gastroenterol 1984;6:249.
238. Rivera-Alsina ME, Saldana LR, Stringer CA. Fetal growth sus-

tained by parenteral nutrition in pregnancy. Obstet Gynecol 1984;64:138.

239. Kirby DF, Fiorenze V, Craig RM. Intravenous nutritional support during pregnancy. JPEN, Journal of Parenteral and Enteral Nutrition 1988;12:72.
240. Catanzarite VA, Argubright K, Mann BA, Brittain VL. Malnutrition during pregnancy? Consider parenteral feeding. Contemp Obstet Gynecol 1986;27:110.
241. Silberman H, Eisenberg D. Parenteral and enteral nutrition for the hospitalized patient. Norwalk: Appleton-Century-Crofts, 1982.
242. Heller L. Parenteral nutrition in obstetrics and gynecology. In: Greep JM, Soefers PB, Westdorp RC, eds. Current concepts in parenteral nutrition. The Hague: Martinus-Nijheff Medical Publishers, 1977:179.
243. Landon MB, Gabbe SG, Mullen JL. Total parenteral nutrition during pregnancy. Clin Perinatol 1986;13:57.
244. Lee RV, Rodgers BD, Young C, Eddy E, Cardinal J. Total parenteral nutrition during pregnancy. Obstet Gynecol 1986;68:563.
245. Hatjis CG, Meis PJ. Total parenteral nutrition in pregnancy. Obstet Gynecol 1985;66:585.
246. Hew LR, Deitel M. Total parenteral nutrition in gynecology and obstetrics. Obstet Gynecol 1980;55:464.
247. Martin R, Blackburn GL. Principles of hyperalimentation during pregnancy. In: Berkowitz RL, ed. Critical care of the obstetric patient. New York: Churchill Livingstone, 1983:133.
248. Seifer DB, Silberman H, Catanzarite VA, Conteas CN, Wood R, Ueland K. Total parenteral nutrition in obstetrics. JAMA 1985;253:14.
249. Wood P, Murray A, Sinha B, Godley M, Goldsmith HJ. Wernicke's encephalopathy induced by hyperemesis gravidarum. Br J Obstet Gynaecol 1983;90:583.
250. Nuutinen LS, Alahuhta SM, Heikkinen JE. Nutrition during ten-week life support with successful fetal outcome in a case with fatal maternal brain damage. JPEN, Journal of Parenteral and Enteral Nutrition 1989;13:432.
251. Brookhyser J. The use of parenteral nutrition supplementation in pregnancy complicated by end-stage renal disease. J Am Diet Assoc 1989;89:93.
252. Gatenby SJ. Maintenance of pregnancy in Crohn's disease by parenteral nutrition: a case study. Human Nutrition: Applied Nutrition 1987;41:345.
253. Lockwood C, Stiller RJ, Bolognese RJ. Maternal total parenteral nutrition in chronic cholecystitis. A case report. J Reprod Med 1987;32:785.
254. Breen KJ, McDonald IA, Panelli D, Ihle B. Planned pregnancy in a patient who was receiving home parenteral nutrition. Med J Aust 1987;146:215.
255. Nugent FW, Rajala M, O'Shea RA, et al. Total parenteral nutrition in pregnancy: conception to delivery. JPEN, Journal of Parenteral and Enteral Nutrition 1987;11:424.
256. Cole BN, Seltzer MH, Kassabian J, Abboud SE. Parenteral nutrition in a pregnant cystic fibrosis patient. JPEN, Journal of Parenteral and Enteral Nutrition 1987;11:205.
257. Jacobson LB, Clapp DH. Total parenteral nutrition in pregnancy complicated by Crohn's disease. JPEN, Journal of Parenteral and Enteral Nutrition 1987;11:93.
258. Mughal MM, Shaffer JL, Turner M, Irving MH. Nutritional management of pregnancy in patients on home parenteral nutrition. Br J Obstet Gynaecol 1987;94:44.
259. Heller L. Guidelines for the dosage and application of the intravenous provision of nutrient substances in obstetrics and gynecology. In: Ahnefeld FW, ed. Parenteral nutrition. Berlin: Springer, 1976:167.
260. Rayburn W, Wolk R, Mercer N, Roberts J. Parenteral nutrition in obstetrics and gynecology. Obstet Gynecol Surv 1986; 41:200.

64

CHAPTER

LIVER DISEASES IN PREGNANCY

Caroline A. Riely

Despite its central role in physiology, the liver rarely complains. It is a vigorous organ, able to carry out its tasks even if 70% to 80% is removed. Because the only sensory nerves serving the liver are those to the capsule, pain is a rare symptom. As a result, symptoms of hepatic dysfunction do not become evident until major, life-threatening injury has occurred. Because the liver is so silent, liver disease is often overlooked. This is particularly true in the pregnant woman, who is usually healthy and young. In this chapter we discuss the spectrum of liver disorders in pregnancy, starting with those that are unique to pregnancy, continuing with those exacerbated by the pregnant state, and ending with a discussion of the significance of common liver diseases complicating pregnancy. We also deal with that relative rarity, pregnancy in a patient with preexisting liver disease. The reader is referred to several previously published reviews of this topic.[1–3]

LIVER DISEASES UNIQUE TO PREGNANCY

Several liver diseases occur only in the pregnant woman and are considered to be associated etiologically with the pregnant state. As a rule, the obstetrician is more familiar with these disorders than is the consulting gastroenterologist. The major problem is that of differential diagnosis (Table 64-1). It is important to confirm the diagnosis if one of these conditions is being considered in the differential, as therapy may hinge on removal of the inciting cause—more specifically, on termination of the pregnancy.

HYPEREMESIS GRAVIDARUM

Early-morning nausea is an extremely common symptom of pregnancy, indeed often the first.[4] When the nausea is associated with intractable vomiting leading to dehydration and ketosis, hospitalization is required and the diagnosis of hyperemesis gravidarum is made. The usual clinical setting for hyperemesis gravidarum includes onset in the first 10 weeks of pregnancy. Even severe vomiting usually resolves at the end of the first trimester, although in some cases it may persist up to term. Affected women often have ptyalism, excessive production of saliva requiring frequent spitting as distinct from vomiting.

This syndrome has been considered psychogenic, associated with conflicted emotions about the pregnancy,[5] but there are epidemiologic data that suggest that it has a physical rather than a psychic basis. Patients affected with hyperemesis gravidarum are more likely to be younger than age 20, nulliparous, obese, and nonsmokers.[6] They are more likely to have a multiple gestation or a molar pregnancy[5] and are more likely to go to term without fetal wastage than are unaffected women.[4,7] Transient hyperthyroidism during the time of the excessive vomiting has been reported.[8]

Liver dysfunction in patients with hyperemesis gravidarum has been reported.[9,10] In our own experience, abnormal liver tests (primarily elevated transaminases [AST or SGOT, AST or SGPT]) are present in close to one half of patients requiring hospitalization for hyperemesis gravidarum. Usually these are modest elevations, less than 250 units, but rarely they may approach 1000 units. The transaminase elevations parallel the vomiting, with the highest levels seen in the worst vomiters and with the levels falling as the patient is rehydrated and begins to resume oral intake. In the most severe cases, the bilirubin and prothrombin times may also be abnormal. Liver biopsy shows no inflammation, as would be characteristic of hepatitis, but rather central hepatocyte ballooning and vacuolization, as well as bile-stained Kupffer cells, suggestive of a cholestatic toxin (Fig. 64-1).

Treatment of the liver dysfunction associated with hyperemesis gravidarum does not differ from that for

TABLE 64–1. DIFFERENTIAL DIAGNOSIS OF LIVER DISEASE IN PREGNANCY

USUAL TRIMESTER	DISORDER	SYMPTOMS	LAB	LIVER BIOPSY
First	Hyperemesis gravidarum	Vomiting	+ Ketones, ↑ transaminases	Central vacuolization
Second	Cholestasis of pregnancy	Pruritus	↑ GGTP, bile acids	Cholestasis
Third	HELLP	Abdominal pain	↓ Plts, ↑ transaminase	Periportal hemorrhage
	Rupture	Abdominal pain, fever	↑↑ Transaminases, + CT scan	
	Acute fatty liver of pregnancy	Nausea, vomiting	↑ Protime	Microvesicular fat
Any	Viral hepatitis	Nausea, vomiting	↑ Transaminase	Inflammation and necrosis

+, positive findings; ↑, elevated; ↑↑, markedly elevated; ↓, decreased.

the underlying disorder, namely, rehydration and antiemetic therapy. In severe cases, total parenteral nutrition is necessary. It is not unusual for severely affected patients to lose a significant percentage of their body weight. There are no known (or suspected) hepatic residua.

The pathogenesis of this disorder, and its attendant liver dysfunction, is unknown. It is associated temporally with the rapid rise in chorionic gonadotropin levels in early pregnancy, but no correlation has been found between the severity of the vomiting and the level of β-HCG in affected patients.[6,11] In one study affected patients did have higher levels of estradiol and sex hormone binding globulin than nonvomiting patients at the same gestational age.[6] Thus, the pathogenic mechanism underlying the liver disorder of hyperemesis gravidarum remains incompletely understood, as does the syndrome itself. Further exploration of the associated liver disease may lead to a better understanding of this common disorder.

CHOLESTASIS OF PREGNANCY

Cholestasis of pregnancy is the most common of the liver disorders unique to pregnant women. The clinical hallmark of this syndrome is pruritus, which, by definition, is present in all affected patients. Indeed, cholestasis of pregnancy should be considered in the differential diagnosis of generalized itching in any pregnant patient. Any liver dysfunction in pregnancy associated with itching should be considered to be cholestasis of pregnancy until proved otherwise. In severe cases, the cholestasis progresses to jaundice. Jaundice of pregnancy and itching of pregnancy are terms used in the

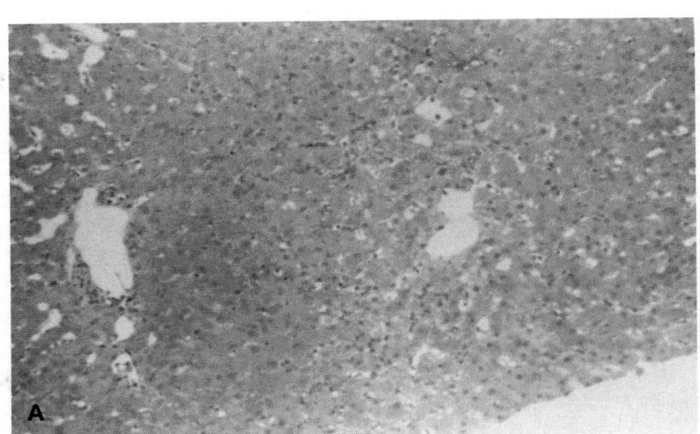

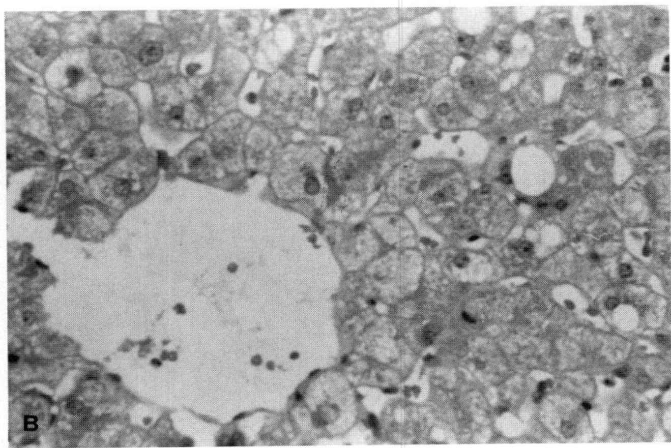

FIGURE 64–1. Liver biopsy in hyperemesis gravidarum. This is the biopsy of an 18-year-old G1P0 woman in her 15th week of gestation who had a peak transaminase elevation of 800 units. (**A**) The hepatocytes around the central vein (on the right) are pale, whereas those around the portal triad (on the left) are not (hematoxylin and eosin stain, ×10). (**B**) The pericentral hepatocytes are pale, ballooned, and vacuolated (hematoxylin and eosin stain, ×25).

past for parts of the syndrome now known as cholestasis of pregnancy.

The clinical characteristics of this syndrome, other than the associated pruritus, are variable. It may begin at almost any point in gestation, from early in the second trimester to late in the third.[12] Itching is the first, and usually the only, symptom. Typical itching of cholestasis is generalized over all the body but worse on the palms and soles and worse at night. This symptom, when severe, is almost intolerable, and patients will beg to be delivered.

Laboratory tests show elevations in the serum bile acid levels, most conveniently measured as serum cholylglycine, a test that is widely available commercially.[13] The "cholestatic" enzymes—alkaline phosphatase, γ-glutamyl transpeptidase, and 5′-nucleotidase—are elevated. The levels of transaminases (AST and ALT) vary but may rise above 1000 units in rare cases.[14] The urine may be positive on dipstick for bilirubin, even in the presence of a normal serum level. Only rarely does the serum level climb into the range associated with visible jaundice (above 3 mg/dL). Both the itching and the laboratory abnormalities may wax and wane during the pregnancy. All abnormalities resolve after delivery, but rarely this resolution may be delayed by several months.

Therapy for this condition is limited. Efforts to relieve the symptom of pruritus usually meet with little success. Treatment with cholestyramine, a bile acid–binding resin, may help but will also exacerbate the steatorrhea associated with cholestasis. Phenobarbital therapy may help, presumably as a centrally acting sedative but perhaps also as a choleretic.[15] Therapy with S-adenosylmethionine (SAM) has been suggested but has not been widely advocated.[16] All affected patients should be assumed to be malabsorbing fat and should be supplemented with vitamin K via the parenteral route prior to delivery.

Generally, the outcome of this condition is benign, with resolution of the pruritus promptly after delivery and with no hepatic residua for the mother. Some reports have documented an increase in both prematurity and stillbirths, and all affected pregnancies should be monitored with increased vigilance as term approaches.[12,17,18] Very rarely, the cholestasis will recur outside of pregnancy, and it will be recognized that the woman is affected with some other cholestatic disorder, such as primary biliary cirrhosis or benign recurrent cholestasis, which happened to have its presentation during pregnancy. There is an increased incidence of gallstones in women previously affected with cholestasis of pregnancy.[19]

Patients affected in one pregnancy may have a recurrence of symptoms, either more or less severe, in subsequent pregnancies. And affected patients may have a history of cholestasis while on birth control pills, or a family member (mother, sisters) may have had it. Thus, it appears that this syndrome is related pathogenically to the hormonal changes of pregnancy, and affected patients are sensitive to the cholestatic effects of exogenously administered ethinyl estradiol.[12,20] Estrogens are known to cause cholestasis in experimental animals.[21] Presumably, in humans this is an inherited sensitivity, and the syndrome has been traced through a large sibship, with demonstration of inheritance as a sex-limited dominant trait through an unaffected male.[22] This is a condition that is most common in certain ethnic groups, most notably Scandinavians and the Indians of Chile,[19,23] but it has been reported in American blacks as well.[14]

LIVER INVOLVEMENT IN PREECLAMPSIA

Preeclampsia is a very common disorder of pregnancy. Although conventionally defined by the presence of hypertension and proteinuria, it is better understood as a multisystem disease that is associated exclusively with pregnancy and thus is related to it etiologically.[24] This syndrome may begin anytime during the second half of pregnancy or may even have its onset after delivery, but it is most commonly encountered close to term. Hepatic involvement in preeclampsia is increasingly recognized to be common and to have serious implications about the severity of this poorly understood systemic disorder.

Given that preeclampsia exists as a broad spectrum, including normotensive preeclampsia, it is easy to comprehend that the spectrum of liver disease is also broad. It ranges from subclinical involvement, with the only manifestation of liver disease being deposition of fibrinogen along the hepatic sinusoids[25] to rupture of the liver, usually associated with maternal and fetal demise.[26] Within these extremes fall the HELLP syndrome[27] and hepatic infarction.[28] The gross and microscopic pathology of the liver in preeclampsia has been well characterized.[29]

Acute fatty liver of pregnancy is also associated with preeclampsia. Like the other liver disorders of preeclampsia, it begins to resolve with delivery. There may well be an overlap between these disorders, and patients with both HELLP syndrome and acute fatty liver of pregnancy have been reported[30] Fat has been found histologically in patients who presumably had preeclamptic liver disease.[29,31,32] Nevertheless, these two syndromes are different clinically and will be discussed separately, although the separation may be arbitrary.

By far the most commonly encountered of these disorders is the syndrome dubbed the HELLP syndrome (for *hemolysis, elevated liver enzymes,* and *low platelets*) or some variant thereof.[33] Affected patients can present with a variety of clinical pictures. HELLP may be present in a patient hospitalized with hypertension who, over the course of several days in the hospital, begins to show a dropping platelet count with rising transaminases in the absence of any complaints such as bleeding or abdominal pain. Or it may be present in the patient who comes to the emergency room because of severe mid-epigastric or right upper quadrant pain, waking her from sleep, perhaps with a pleuritic component. Or the patient may present with nausea, vomiting, and generalized malaise, with or without obvious preeclampsia, as defined by hypertension and proteinuria. In any such patient, the combination of thrombocytopenia with abnormal transaminases implies hepatic involvement, and this in turn implies serious disease, with a potentially fatal outcome. Indeed, elevated transaminases alone in the later half of pregnancy can presage the onset of preeclampsia. Thus, the combination of elevated transaminases and a platelet count that is known to be falling, even though still within the range of normal, has serious implications.

On physical examination, affected patients may have tenderness to palpation or to shock over their right upper quadrant or right lower chest. Jaundice is unusual and rarely occurs except in the most severely affected patients. The transaminase elevations may be modest or may exceed 1000 to 2000 units. Usually, coagulation studies other than platelet count, including prothrombin time and fibrinogen, are normal. The liver biopsy may be normal or may show the periportal hemorrhage and fibrin deposition typical of preeclampsia (Fig. 64-2).

In mild cases, in which patients have only borderline abnormalities of transaminases and platelet count and very mild hypertension, some time may be bought by bed rest, hydration, and careful monitoring. Almost invariably, however, these patients require delivery, often because of fetal distress. If these signs are overlooked, disaster may ensue for both mother and fetus. Therefore, screening liver function tests and platelet count should be part of the initial assessment of any woman with preeclampsia, abdominal or chest pain, or nausea and vomiting and should be repeated frequently in any patient being followed with preeclampsia.

Definitive treatment is identical to that for the underlying disorder—namely, termination of the pregnancy. The timing and route are obstetrical judgments. Platelet transfusion is advisable if the count is severely depressed (<50,000). Recurrent HELLP syndrome has been reported, and any woman affected should be followed in subsequent pregnancies as a patient at increased risk. There are no hepatic sequelae.

Hepatic infarction is presumably a very severe, and fortunately very rare, extension of the HELLP syndrome.[2,28] Affected patients complain of abdominal or chest pain and are febrile without an obvious source. There is often accompanying leukocytosis, and the transaminase values are extremely high, often above 5000 units. Severely affected women may have enough hepatic injury to experience true hepatic failure, with coagulopathy, encephalopathy, and jaundice. The infarcts are best visualized on CT scanning (Fig. 64-3), as ultrasonography may fail to demonstrate the extensive areas of infarct.[34] Despite the obviously extensive liver damage, most patients recover without sequelae, although there may be a fever of unknown etiology that lasts for several weeks.

Subcapsular hematoma and frank rupture of the liver are further extensions of this preeclamptic liver disease. When the rupture is contained within the capsule, the patient experiences severe pain but is hemodynamically stable.[35] Again, the CT scan is the most reliable way to make this diagnosis. Patients who have hepatic rupture present in shock, with hemoperitoneum, and have a high mortality. Optimal therapy for this rare condition is unclear. Most patients are taken to emergency laparotomy and the liver is resected and packed off. The capsule may be ruptured in several locations, and suturing to the underlying necrotic and infarcted liver can be difficult.[31] Some authors have recommended arterial embolization via angiography as a means of gaining control over the hemorrhage.[36]

ACUTE FATTY LIVER OF PREGNANCY

Recent reports have expanded our knowledge of this once dreaded complication of late pregnancy. It is evi-

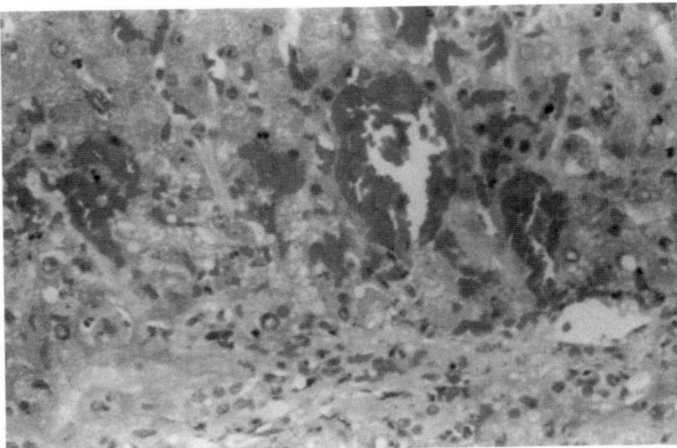

FIGURE 64–2. Liver biopsy in HELLP syndrome. The portal triad running along the bottom of the figure is surrounded by areas of hemorrhage and hepatocyte necrosis (hematoxylin and eosin stain, ×25).

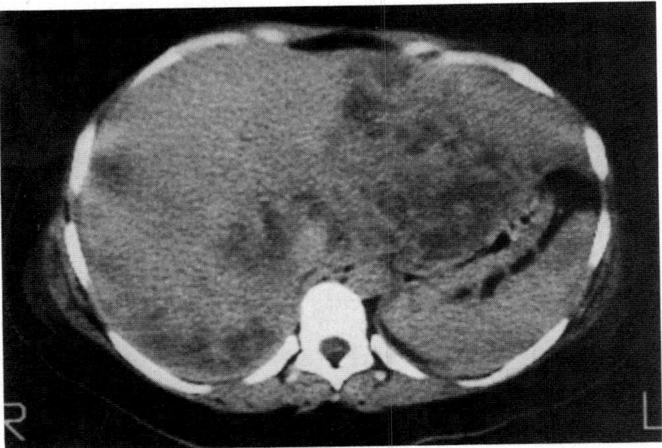

FIGURE 64–3. CT scan of the liver in preeclampsia with hepatic infarction. The liver contains multiple areas, particularly prominent in the left lobe, of geographic infarction.

dent that this disorder is more common and less frequently fatal than previously thought.[30,37–43] It also appears that acute fatty liver usually occurs in the setting of preeclampsia. This diagnosis is often difficult to make in affected patients, as acute fatty liver is a syndrome of fulminant hepatic failure, and hepatic failure is associated, almost invariably, with relative hypertension. Thus, affected patients have "normotensive preeclampsia."[24] Interestingly, acute fatty liver of pregnancy is usually distinct clinically from the other liver conditions of preeclampsia discussed earlier. There may, however, be overlap between these syndromes, and fat in the liver has been reported in typical preeclamptic liver disease[29] and in rupture of the liver.[31] HELLP syndrome also has been reported in patients with typical acute fatty liver of pregnancy.

The clinical characteristics typical of acute fatty liver of pregnancy include presentation in the third trimester, near term, with signs and symptoms typical of both acute hepatitis and preeclampsia. Patients often have nausea, vomiting, and severe malaise and fatigue. Jaundice occurs frequently, but not invariably. Patients also complain of headache, thirst, and midepigastric or right upper quadrant pain. Rarely, a patient has no symptoms and is identified because of abnormal liver function tests. As the disease progresses, the patient can manifest typical hepatic failure, with agitation followed by stupor and coma, and severe coagulopathy with attendant bleeding. Like the other conditions associated with preeclampsia, acute fatty liver of pregnancy usually has its onset before delivery, but it may not be recognized until after delivery. Physical examination demonstrates a small, nonpalpable liver and normal to low blood pressure.

Laboratory tests confirm the presence of hepatic failure, with elevations in prothrombin time, a decrease in serum fibrinogen below the usually elevated levels in pregnancy, hyperammonemia, and often hypoglycemia. The transaminase levels are elevated, but they are usually below 1000 units, and normal values at presentation have been reported.[2] Typical severe cases show elevation in the serum bilirubin. In keeping with their preeclampsia, most patients have hyperuricemia. In severe cases, the patients may develop oliguric renal failure (the so-called hepatorenal syndrome) and may have complicating pancreatitis, both seen frequently in fulminant hepatic failure of any etiology.

Transient diabetes insipidus has been reported to be associated with preeclampsia and with acute fatty liver of pregnancy.[44–47] Typical patients are hypernatremic and have an inappropriate diuresis and are often resistant to vasopressin. Indeed, hypernatremia, polyuria, and abnormal liver function tests at term should suggest the diagnosis of acute fatty liver of pregnancy with accompanying diabetes insipidus.

The diagnosis of acute fatty liver of pregnancy should be suggested by the typical clinical picture and should be considered in the differential diagnosis of all patients with abnormal liver function tests in the third trimester. It can be a difficult diagnosis to confirm. The abdominal CT scan may be helpful if it shows a decrease in Houndsfield units in the liver, suggesting fatty infiltration.[48] Unfortunately, the CT scan may not be helpful. In cases of diagnostic uncertainty, liver biopsy is indicated. Using special stains, the typical microvesicular fatty infiltration can be seen (Fig. 64-4). Light microscopy may be misleading, however, in the absence of stains for fat, and the biopsy appearance may suggest viral hepatitis.[30,49] The periportal hemorrhage and fibrin deposition typical of preeclamptic liver disease have not been reported in association with typical acute fatty liver of pregnancy.

The course, in typical patients, is toward recovery, beginning with delivery. If the hepatic failure is severe, the patient may be in coma for several days prior to improvement. During this time, maximal support by a multispecialty team in an intensive care unit is indicated. One case of a patient undergoing liver transplantation for acute fatty liver of pregnancy has been reported.[50] With early recognition and prompt delivery, such heroic therapy should not be necessary.

Affected patients are left with no hepatic residua. There have been many reports of subsequent normal pregnancy in such patients.[37,51] One affected patient is known to have had acute fatty liver of pregnancy on her subsequent gestation.[52] Patients with a history of acute fatty liver of pregnancy need not be dissuaded from becoming pregnant again but should be followed with care as high-risk pregnancies.

The pathogenesis of this fascinating syndrome remains unclear. It is strikingly similar to the fatal fatty liver seen in pregnant patients with a history of tetracycline administration.[53] It is also similar clinically to the microvesicular fatty infiltrative disorders of Reye's syndrome and valproic acid toxicity.[54,55] These similarities suggest some circulating toxin, one that is induced by preeclampsia and is cleared by delivery.

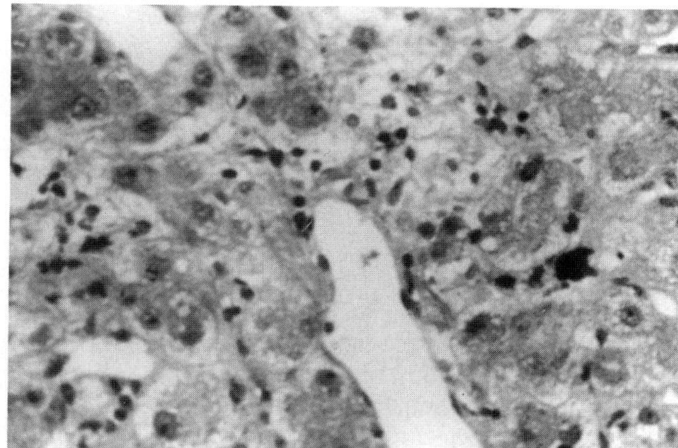

FIGURE 64–4. Liver biopsy in typical acute fatty liver of pregnancy. The hepatocytes surrounding this central vein are pleomorphic and vacuolated. There has been hepatocyte necrosis and there are scattered darkly stained pigment-laden macrophages (PAS with diastase stain, ×25).

LIVER DISEASES EXACERBATED BY OR PRECIPITATED BY PREGNANCY

The pregnant state, in and of itself, can make the woman more susceptible to certain diseases. In each case, this increased susceptibility is related to the altered physiology of pregnancy, although the pathogenesis for these disorders remains incompletely understood.

BUDD-CHIARI SYNDROME

Veno-occlusive disease of the hepatic veins of the liver has been reported in patients taking oral contraceptives.[56] This devastating disease is also reported to occur following pregnancy, primarily in India but rarely in the United States.[57,58] The onset is usually in the weeks following delivery and is marked by abdominal pain and the abrupt onset of ascites and hepatomegaly. Liver function deteriorates, sometimes rapidly. Although this condition is usually fatal, successful pregnancy after Budd-Chiari syndrome has been reported.[59]

Presumably, this condition results from the normal increase in coagulability that occurs in pregnancy as term approaches. In a recently observed case, the patient had been started on oral contraceptives 2 weeks after delivery and developed veno-occlusive disease several weeks thereafter.

CHOLELITHIASIS

Gallstone disease is conventionally thought of as a disorder of fertile women; occasionally, a woman presents during pregnancy with biliary colic, acute cholecystitis, or gallstone pancreatitis. If the patient does not respond promptly to conservative management, then cholecystectomy should be done and can be accomplished in pregnancy without undue risk.[60] A recent study suggests that small stones may resolve after pregnancy.[61]

Normal pregnancy is lithogenic. Gallbladder motility, like motility of other gut smooth muscle, is depressed during pregnancy. The usual enterohepatic cycling of bile acids, which solubilize cholesterol in bile, is decreased, and the bile becomes more lithogenic.[62,63]

HEPATITIS E

Reports from developing nations have suggested an increased morbidity and mortality from viral hepatitis among pregnant women.[64] Most of these reports did not include viral serologies, but epidemiology suggested that the hepatitis in question was a water-borne non-A, non-B hepatitis. It has been known that chronic viral hepatitis, both B and presumably C, is not associated with excess mortality in pregnant women in the United States.[65]

Recently, the virus associated with these water-borne epidemics has been identified. It is known as hepatitis E and is an RNA virus that is found throughout the world in water contaminated with stool; so far it has not been seen in the United States.[66] Why this virus should be so particularly lethal in pregnancy is unclear. Pregnant women should be discouraged from traveling to endemic areas, particularly India, Africa, Southeast Asia, and parts of Mexico and the Soviet Union, where outbreaks of this infection have been documented.

HERPES SIMPLEX HEPATITIS

Like hepatitis E, infection with herpes simplex can cause fulminant hepatitis in pregnant women.[67–71] Affected patients present with a viral syndrome, often including upper respiratory tract symptoms, followed by fever, and associated with abnormal liver function tests. The transaminase elevations are often elevated out of proportion to the bilirubin, which is normal or only modestly elevated. There is usually an accompanying genital eruption. The diagnosis can be made by cultures of the lesions or by liver biopsy; in one case, suggestive "holes" were seen in the liver on CT scan. Therapy with acyclovir has been successful, but there is a high mortality rate among untreated women. Early diagnosis is crucial for both mother and infant.

LIVER DISEASES OCCURRING CONCURRENT WITH PREGNANCY

Pregnant women are, of course, not immune to usual liver diseases that can affect anyone at any time. These conditions can occur in pregnancy with no increased morbidity or mortality but may lead to diagnostic confusion, or correct diagnosis may be delayed because of the pregnant state.

HEPATITIS A, B, AND C

Acute viral hepatitis due to one of the primary hepatotrophic viruses is not associated with increased morbidity or mortality in pregnant women, with the exception of hepatitis E (see the earlier discussion).[72] But diseases of pregnancy—namely, preeclamptic liver disease (HELLP, hepatic infarction) and acute fatty liver of pregnancy—can mimic acute viral hepatitis and are often mistaken for it. Such a misdiagnosis can have serious consequences, as pregnancy-associated disease is treated with delivery, whereas acute viral hepatitis is not improved by, and does not indicate, delivery.

DRUG-INDUCED HEPATOTOXICITY

Women are also susceptible to acute drug or toxin-induced liver disease during pregnancy.[73] Luckily, as most women do not take medications during pregnancy, such instances are rare. Nevertheless, drug-induced hepatotoxicity should always be considered in the differential diagnosis of liver disease, and a careful history for drug ingestion should be obtained.

METASTATIC MALIGNANCY

Rarely, malignant disease metastatic to the liver presents during pregnancy. Affected patients have palpable hepatomegaly, a very unusual finding during pregnancy and one that should prompt immediate evaluation.[74] Rarely, as in the non-pregnant state, such patients can present with fulminant hepatic failure.[75] Unfortunately, the prognosis in pregnant patients is as dismal as it is in the non-pregnant.

PREGNANCY IN PATIENTS WITH PREEXISTING LIVER DISEASE

Chronic liver disease is associated with decreased fertility, and such women rarely ovulate. Amenorrhea or premature menopause is a common symptom of chronic liver disease. As a consequence, the physician is rarely faced with a pregnant patient with chronic liver disease, with several special exceptions.

CHRONIC HEPATITIS B

The hepatitis B virus may exist in a chronic carrier state, not associated with any clinical disease but still highly infectious. Indeed, this is probably the most common chronic viral disease in humans, and it is perpetuated by mother–infant spread, transmission of the virus from the healthy carrier mother to the infant at birth. This transmission can only be interrupted by appropriate immunoprophylaxis of the infant at birth. It is now the standard of care for all pregnant women to be screened for chronic hepatitis B early in gestation by testing them for hepatitis B surface antigen (HBsAg).[76] If the mother is positive for this infection, then the infant is given hepatitis B hyperimmune globulin at birth and is begun on a three-dose regimen of vaccination with hepatitis B vaccine prior to discharge from the hospital. Cesarean section can lower the incidence of transmission but is not necessary if the infant is given correct immunoprophylaxis.[77] Breast-feeding does not increase the risk of transmission and is not contraindicated. It should be recognized that infected women pose a risk to their sexual partners and are themselves at increased risk for developing hepatocellular carcinoma. Such women should be referred for long-term follow-up.

CHRONIC HEPATITIS C

The hepatitis C virus, now known to be the most common cause of posttransfusion non-A, non-B hepatitis, also exists in the population in a chronic carrier state, affecting approximately 1% of healthy blood donors.[78] This virus appears to be less infectious than the hepatitis B virus and has less sexual and mother–infant transmission. Nevertheless, mother–infant transmission has been documented.[79] As there is no known way to interrupt transmission of this virus, routine screening in pregnant women is not yet of value. Nevertheless, this is a common infection, and all women with abnormal transaminases of unexplained etiology should be tested for it. Infected persons are positive for anti–hepatitis C antibody.

STEROID-RESPONSIVE CHRONIC ACTIVE HEPATITIS

Steroid-responsive chronic active hepatitis, called autoimmune or lupoid chronic active hepatitis, occurs primarily in young women and is not rare. Affected patients respond (by definition) to immunosuppression with corticosteroids, often augmented with azathioprine. When treated, affected women go into remission and regain their fertility. Pregnancy in such women can be successful, but is known to be associated with an increased incidence of stillbirths, prematurity, and obstetric complications such as preeclampsia.[80] The immunosuppression must be continued, or the disease will recur. Despite its potential teratogenicity, azathioprine in the low doses used in these patients has not been associated with problems in their offspring.

WILSON'S DISEASE

Wilson's disease, a disorder of copper metabolism, is associated with chronic liver disease, as well as chronic neurologic disease, and leads to death if untreated. Treatment with copper chelation, with either D-penicillamine or trientene, leads to a return to normal of hepatic function and to resumption of ovulation in affected young women. Such women may have successful pregnancies but must be maintained on their chelation therapy for the duration of the pregnancy. In this setting, there has been no associated teratogenicity of D-penicillamine.[81]

PORTAL HYPERTENSION

It is rare for patients with cirrhosis and portal hypertension to get pregnant. On the other hand, patients with noncirrhotic portal hypertension have normal fertility. Such women may sustain variceal hemorrhage while pregnant but tolerate it well. Patients with cirrhosis fare less well. Optimal therapy for variceal hemorrhage in pregnancy is probably sclerosis of the esophageal varices. If this fails, such women can successfully undergo shunting procedures. Fetal wastage and prematurity are more common in cirrhotic patients.[82,83]

REFERENCES

1. Riely CA. The liver in pregnancy. In: Schiff L, Schiff ER, eds. Diseases of the liver. 6th ed. Philadelphia: JB Lippincott, 1987:1059.
2. Riely CA. Case studies in jaundice of pregnancy. Semin Liver Dis 1988;8:191.
3. Wilkinson ML. Diagnosis and management of liver disease in pregnancy. Adv Intern Med 1990;35:289.
4. Klebanoff MA, Koslowe PA, Kaslow R, et al. Epidemiology of vomiting in early pregnancy. Obstet Gynecol 1985;66:612.
5. Fairweather DVI. Nausea and vomiting in pregnancy. Am J Obstet Gynecol 1968;102:135.
6. Depue RH, Berstein L, Ross RK, et al. Hyperemesis gravidarum in relation to estradiol levels, pregnancy outcome, and other maternal factors: a seroepidemiologic study. Am J Obstet Gynecol 1987;156:1137.
7. Brandes JM. First-trimester nausea and vomiting as related to outcome of pregnancy. Obstet Gynecol 1967;30:427.
8. Borber SA, McGill AC, Tunbridge WMG. Thyroid function in hyperemesis gravidarum. Acta Endocrinol (Copenh) 1986; 111:404.
9. Adams RH, Gordon J, Combes B. Hyperemesis gravidarum. I. Evidence of hepatic dysfunction. Obstet Gynecol 1968;31:659.
10. Larrey D, Rueff B, Feldman G, et al. Recurrent jaundice caused by recurrent hyperemesis gravidarum. Gut 1984;25:1415.
11. Soules MR, Hughes CL Jr, Garcia JA, et al. Nausea and vomiting of pregnancy: role of human chorionic gonadotropin and 17-hydroxyprogesterone. Obstet Gynecol 1980;55:696.
12. Reyes H, Radrigan ME, Gonzalez MC, et al. Steatorrhea in patients with intrahepatic cholestasis of pregnancy. Gastroenterology 1987;93:584.
13. Lunzer M, Barner P, Byth K, et al. Serum bile acid concentrations during pregnancy and their relationship to obstetric cholestasis. Gastroenterology 1986;91:825.
14. Wilson JAP. Intrahepatic cholestasis of pregnancy with marked elevation of transaminases in a black American. Dig Dis Sci 1987;32:665.
15. Laatikainen T. Effect of cholestyramine and phenobarbital on pruritus and serum bile acid levels in cholestasis of pregnancy. Am J Obstet Gynecol 1978;132:501.
16. Frezza M, Pozzato G, Chilsa L, et al. Reversal of intrahepatic cholestasis of pregnancy in women after high dose S-adenosyl-L-methionine administration. Hepatology 1984;4:274.
17. Reid R, Ivey KJ, Rencoret RH, et al. Fetal complications of obstetric cholestasis. Br Med J 1974;1:870.
18. Heikkinen J. Serum bile acids in the early diagnosis of intrahepatic cholestasis of pregnancy. Obstet Gynecol 1983;61:581.
19. Samsioe G, Svendsen P, Johnson P, et al. Studies in cholestasis of pregnancy. V. Gallbladder disease, liver function tests, serum lipids and fatty acid composition of serum lecithin in the non-pregnant state. Acta Obstet Gynecol Scand 1975;54:417.
20. Kreek MJ. Female sex steroids and cholestasis. Semin Liver Dis 1987;7:8.
21. Vore M. Estrogen cholestasis: membranes, metabolites, or receptors? Gastroenterology 1987;93:643.
22. Holzbach RT, Sivak DA, Braun WE. Familial recurrent intrahepatic cholestasis of pregnancy: a genetic study providing evidence for transmission of a sex-limited, dominant trait. Gastroenterology 1983;85:175.
23. Reyes H. The enigma of intrahepatic cholestasis of pregnancy: lessons from Chile. Hepatology 1982;2:87.
24. Redman CWG. Platelets and the beginnings of preeclampsia. N Engl J Med 1990;323:478.
25. Arias F, Mancilla-Jimenez R. Hepatic fibrinogen deposits in pre-eclampsia. Immunofluorescent evidence. N Engl J Med 1976;295:578.
26. Copas P, Dyer M, Akin H, Linton R. Rupture of the liver in preeclampsia. A review and report of two cases. J Tenn Med Assoc 1985;78:419.
27. Sibai BH. The HELLP syndrome (hemolysis, elevated liver enzymes, and low platelets): much ado about nothing? Am J Obstet Gynecol 1990;162:311.
28. Krueger KJ. Hoffman BJ, Lee WM. Hepatic infarction associated with eclampsia. Am J Gastroenterol 1990;85:588.
29. Rolfes DB, Ishak KG. Liver disease in toxemia of pregnancy. Am J Gastroenterol 1986;81:1138.
30. Riely CA, Latham PS, Romero R, et al. Acute fatty liver of pregnancy: a reassessment based on observations in 9 patients. Ann Intern Med 1987;106:703.
31. Minuk GY, Lui RC, Kelly JK. Rupture of the liver associated with acute fatty liver of pregnancy. Am J Gastroenterol 1987;82:457.
32. Minakami H, Oka N, Sato T, et. al. Preeclampsia: a microvesicular fat disease of the liver? Am J Obstet Gynecol 1988;159:1043.
33. Weinstein L. Syndrome of hemolysis, elevated liver enzymes, and low platelet count: a severe consequence of hypertension in pregnancy. Am J Obstet Gynecol 1982;142:159.
34. Dammann HG, Hagemann J, Runge, M, Klöppel G. In vivo diagnosis of massive hepatic infarction by computed tomography. Dig Dis Sci 1982;27:73.
35. Manas KJ, Welsh JD, Rankin RA, Miller DD. Hepatic hemorrhage without rupture in preeclampsia. N Engl J Med 1985;312:424.
36. Herbert WNP, Brenner WE. Improving survival with liver rupture complicating pregnancy. Am J Obstet Gynecol 1982;142:530.
37. Riely CA. Acute fatty liver of pregnancy. Semin Liver Dis 1987;7:47.
38. Burroughs AK, Seong NY, Dojcinov DM, et al. Idiopathic acute fatty liver of pregnancy in 12 patients. Q J Med 1982;204:481.
39. Bernuau J, Degott C, Nouel O, et al. Non-fatal acute fatty liver of pregnancy. Gut 1983;24:340.
40. Pockros PJ, Peters RL, Reynolds TB. Idiopathic fatty liver of pregnancy: findings in 10 cases. Medicine 1984;63:1.
41. Hou SH, Levin S, Ahola S, et al. Acute fatty liver of pregnancy: survival with early cesarean section. Dig Dis Sci 1984;29:449.
42. Ebert EC, Sun EA, Wright SH, et al. Does early diagnosis and delivery in acute fatty liver of pregnancy lead to improvement in maternal and infant survival? Dig Dis Sci 1984;29:453.
43. Ahola SJ, Lyman BT, Hogan AF, Schmid RE. Acute fatty liver of pregnancy. Increased survival by early recognition and aggressive therapy. Diagn Gynecol Obstet 1982;4:69.
44. Barron WN, Cohen LH, Ulland LA, et al. Transient vasopressin-resistant diabetes insipidus of pregnancy. N Engl J Med 1984;310:442.
45. Durr JA, Hoggard JG, Hunt JM, Schrier RW. Diabetes insipidus in pregnancy associated with abnormally high circulating vasopressinase activity. N Engl J Med 1987;316:1070.
46. Cammu H, Velkeniers B, Charels K, et al. Idiopathic acute fatty liver of pregnancy associated with transient diabetes insipidus. Case report. Br J Obstet Gynecol 1987;94:173.
47. Harper M, Hatjis CG, Appel RG, Austin WE. Vasopressin-resistant diabetes insipidus, liver dysfunction, hyperuricemia and decreased renal function. A case report. J Reprod Med 1987;32:862.
48. Mabie WC, Dacus JV, Sibai BM, et al. Computed tomography in acute fatty liver of pregnancy. Am J Obstet Gynecol 1988;158:142.
49. Rolfes DB, Ishak KG. Acute fatty liver of pregnancy: a clinicopathologic study of 35 cases. Hepatology 1985;5:1149.
50. Ockner SA, Brunt EM, Cohn SM, et al. Fulminant hepatic failure caused by acute fatty liver of pregnancy, treated by orthotopic liver transplantation. Hepatology 1990;11:59.

51. Breen KJ, Perkins KW, Schenker S, et al. Uncomplicated subsequent pregnancy after idiopathic fatty liver of pregnancy. Obstet Gynecol 1972;40:813.
52. Barton JR, Sibai BM, Mabie WC, Shanklin DR. Recurrent acute fatty liver of pregnancy. Am J Obstet Gynecol 1990;163:534.
53. Allen ES, Brown WE. Hepatic toxicity of tetracycline in pregnancy. Am J Obstet Gynecol 1966;95:12.
54. Weber FL, Snodgrass PJ, Powell DE, et al. Abnormalities of hepatic mitochondrial urea-cycle enzyme activities and hepatic ultrastructure in acute fatty liver of pregnancy. J Lab Clin Med 1979;94:27.
55. Sherlock S. Acute fatty liver of pregnancy and the microvesicular fat diseases. Gut 1983;24:265.
56. Hoyumpa AM. Budd-Chiari syndrome in women taking oral contraceptives. Am J Med 1971;50:137.
57. Khurro MS. Budd-Chiari syndrome following pregnancy. Am J Med 1980;68:113.
58. Covillo FV, Nyong O AO, Axelrod JL. Budd-Chiari syndrome following pregnancy. Missouri Med 1984;81:356.
59. Vons C, Smadja C, Franco D, et al. Successful pregnancy after Budd-Chiari syndrome. Lancet 1984;ii:975.
60. Hill LM, Johnson CE, Lee RA. Cholecystectomy in pregnancy. Obstet Gynecol 1975;48:291.
61. Valdivieso V, Covarrubias C, Siegel F, Cruz F. Natural history of gallstones diagnosed after pregnancy. Gastroenterology 1990;97:A132.
62. Everson GT, McKinley C, Lawson M, et al. Gallbladder function in the human female: effect of the ovulatory cycle, pregnancy, and contraceptive steroids. Gastroenterology 1982;82:711.
63. Kern F Jr, Everson GT, DeMark B, et al. Biliary lipids, bile acids and gallbladder function in the human female: effects of pregnancy and the ovulatory cycle. J Clin Invest 1981;68:1229.
64. Khurroo MS. Study of an epidemic of non-A, non-B hepatitis: possibility of another hepatitis virus distinct from post-transfusion non-A, non-B type. Am J Med 1980;68:818.
65. Hieber JP, Dalton D, Shorey J, Combes B. Hepatitis and pregnancy. J Pediatr 1977;91.545.
66. Zuckerman AJ, Hepatitis E. The main cause of enterically transmitted non-A, non-B hepatitis. Br Med J 1990;300:1475.
67. Klein NA, Mabie WC, Shaver DC, et al. Herpes simplex virus hepatitis in pregnancy: two patients successfully treated with acyclovir. Gastroenterology 1991;100:239.
68. Young EJ, Killam AP, Greene JF Jr. Disseminated herpesvirus infection. Association with primary genital herpes in pregnancy. JAMA 1976;235:2731.
69. Hillard P, Seeds J, Cefalo R. Disseminated herpes simplex in pregnancy: two cases and a review. Obstet Gynecol Surv 1982;37:449.
70. Wertheim RA, Brooks BJ Jr, Rodriguez FH Jr, et al. Fatal herpetic hepatitis in pregnancy. Obstet Gynecol 1983;62:38S.
71. Goyert GL, Bottoms SJ, Sokol RJ. Anicteric presentation of fatal herpetic hepatitis in pregnancy. Obstet Gynecol 1985;65:585.
72. Adams RH, Combes B. Viral hepatitis during pregnancy. JAMA 1965;192:195.
73. Aneckstein AG, Weingold AB. Chlorthiazide-induced hepatic coma in pregnancy. Am J Obstet Gynecol 1966;95:136.
74. Gamberdella FR. Pancreatic carcinoma in pregnancy: a case report. Am J Obstet Gynecol 1984;149:15.
75. Friedman E, Moses B, Engelberg S, et al. Malignant insulinoma with hepatic failure complicating pregnancy. South Med J 1988;81:86.
76. Stevens CE. Perinatal hepatitis B virus infection: screening of pregnant women and protection of the infant. Ann Intern Med 1987;107:412.
77. Lee S-D, Lo K-J, Tsai Y-T, et al. Role of caesarean section in prevention of mother-infant transmission of hepatitis B virus. Lancet 1988;ii:833.
78. Alter HJ, Purcell RH, Shih JW, et al. Detection of antibody to hepatitis C virus in prospectively followed transfusion recipients with acute and chronic non-A, non-B hepatitis. N Engl J Med 1989;321:1494.
79. Wejstål R, Hermodsson S, Iwarson S, Norkrams G. Mother to infant transmission of hepatitis C virus infection. J Med Virol 1990;30:178.
80. Steven MM, Buckley JD, Mackay IR. Pregnancy in chronic active hepatitis. Quart J Med 1979;48:519.
81. Scheinberg IH, Sternlieb I. Wilson's disease. Philadelphia: WB Saunders, 1984.
82. Schreyer P, Caspi E, El-Hindi JM, et al. Cirrhosis—pregnancy and delivery: a review. Obstet Gynecol Surv 1982;37:304.
83. Cheng Y-S. Pregnancy in liver cirrhosis and/or portal hypertension. Am J Obstet Gynecol 1977;128:812.

65

CHAPTER

PREGNANCY COMPLICATED BY RENAL DISORDERS

John P. Hayslett

Reduction in renal function during pregnancy, resulting from primary renal disease or systemic disorders, may threaten fetal development as well as the health of the mother. Because assessment of renal function must account for the significant and unique functional and morphological changes that occur in normal gestation, this review provides a summary of the main features of renal physiology during pregnancy, as well as a description of the more common clinical disorders.

RENAL FUNCTION AND VOLUME HOMEOSTASIS DURING PREGNANCY

Normal pregnancy is characterized by a gradual cumulative retention of 500 to 900 mEq of sodium and 6 to 8 L of water, which are distributed between maternal extracellular fluid and the products of conception. Maternal plasma volume increases 30% to 45%; the incremental rise is most marked in the second trimester and is sustained until term. Renal plasma flow increases by 80% between conception and the second trimester, and subsequently falls to a level about 60% greater than the non-pregnant norm. The glomerular filtration rate (GFR) achieves an incremental increase of 30% to 50% by the 12th week, which is sustained until term, after which the rate rapidly falls to non-gravid levels (Fig. 65-1). Davison has shown that the 24-hour creatinine clearance increased from 117 ± 18 to 136 ± 11 mL/min between early and mid-pregnancy.[1] The mechanism responsible for this remarkable alteration in renal function probably relates to the generalized vasodilation that characterizes pregnancy, because micropuncture studies indicate that GFR correlates solely with the increase in glomerular plasma flow, and not with a rise in intraglomerular capillary pressure.[2] Studies in experimental animals also demonstrated hypertrophy of renal parenchyma during pregnancy, characterized by an increase in tubular length.[3]

In health, the volume of body water is regulated within narrow limits by the kidney through the action of antidiuretic hormone (ADH), which maintains serum osmolality at about 280 mOsm/kg H_2O in the non-gravid state. A rise above that level induces a release of the hormone, while a fall inhibits ADH release. In pregnancy, the plasma osmolality falls to approximately 270 mOsm/kg H_2O. Studies in experimental animals demonstrated that the gestation-induced change in osmolality is secondary to a resetting of the osmostat, the mechanism responsible for release of ADH.[4] The physiological response to changes in osmolality above or below the new level is comparable with that in the non-pregnant state. The mechanism that regulates total body sodium is expressed by variation in the fraction of filtered sodium that is reabsorbed by renal tubules, in such a way that urinary sodium excretion parallels sodium intake. In pregnancy, a resetting of this mechanism permits the gradual increase in body sodium, and a corresponding rise in extracellular fluid volume, to a new level that is maintained until term. The mechanism preserving the extracellular volume setting in pregnancy, through changes in renal tubular sodium reabsorption, is dynamic, because reactions to further increases or decreases in sodium intake are similar to the non-pregnant state,[5] despite high levels of plasma aldosterone associated with pregnancy.

Besides changes in GFR and renal plasma flow, studies in normal gravidas suggest alterations in the renal tubular absorption of non-electrolyte solutes. The fractional reabsorption of glucose,[6] amino acids,[7] and B_2 microglobulin[8] is decreased, resulting in higher rates of urinary excretion, consistent with the notion that reab-

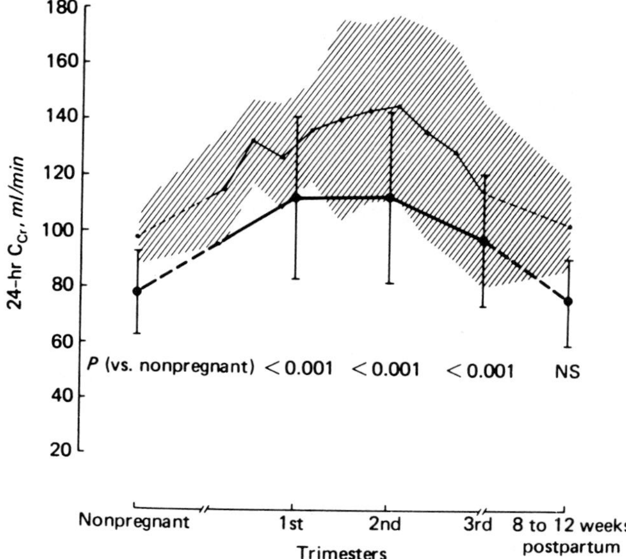

FIGURE 65–1. Alterations in 24-hour creatinine clearance determinations before conception, during each trimester, and 8 to 12 weeks postpartum, in 10 normal gravidas (mean ± 1 SD), shown in the shaded area and in 33 gravidas with primary renal disease and normal or near normal renal functions, shown by solid line. (Katz AI, Davison JM, Hayslett JP, et al. Pregnancy in women with kidney disease. Kidney Int 1980;18:192.)

sorption of non-electrolyte solutes by the proximal tubule is reduced. This phenomenon may have clinical relevance in some patients who exhibit glucosuria during pregnancy, in the absence of hyperglycemia. Total urinary protein excretion also rises in normal pregnancy, from a first trimester value of 103 ± 49 mg/24 hr (mean ± SD), to 151 ± 40 in the second trimester, and to 180 ± 50 in the third trimester.[9] Although the permselective properties of the glomerular capillary wall tend to retain the bulk of albumin within the vascular space, a small quantity of plasma albumin, perhaps amounting to 1 to 2 gm per day, is filtered and subsequently reabsorbed by the proximal tubule. The increase in urinary protein excretion during normal pregnancy may, therefore, primarily reflect a decrease in proximal tubular reabsorption of non-electrolyte solutes. This mechanism may explain the common observation that protein excretion usually increases further during gestation among individuals with overt proteinuria before conception due to glomerular disease, which increases the filtration of plasma protein.

In clinical practice, simple screening techniques for estimating the level of GFR usually rely on measurements of serum levels of urea nitrogen and creatinine. Because of the expansion of extracellular fluid and increased GFR, levels of these substances are substantially lower during gestation than in non-pregnant women. Compared to non-pregnant values of 13 ± 3 mg/dL (mean ± SD) of serum urea nitrogen and 0.67 ± 0.14 mg/dL of plasma creatinine, levels fall to 8.7 ± 1.5 mg/dL and 0.46 ± 0.13 mg/dL, respectively, in pregnancy.[5] Concentrations that exceed 13 mg/dL of urea nitrogen and 0.8 mg/dL of creatinine suggest the possibility of renal insufficiency. In patients with known or suspected renal insufficiency, formal estimates of GFR are required. In non-pregnant individuals and in early pregnancy, GFR can be estimated from the clearance of creatinine (C_{cr}) obtained from 24-hour collections of urine. In the latter half of pregnancy, however, the 24-hour estimate of C_{cr} underestimates the maximal capacity for filtration because of the pooling of fluid in the lower extremities. In the latter half of pregnancy, therefore, C_{cr} should be measured with the subject lying on her side after hydration with water in such a manner that urine flow exceeds 5 to 6 mL/min. Two to three timed collections of urine of at least 30 minutes are obtained, along with a plasma sample, for the determination of creatinine clearance. Based on measurements obtained in normal gravidae, under this condition a $C_{cr} < 100$ mL/min is considered to be abnormal.

EFFECT OF RENAL DISEASE ON PREGNANCY

Renal disease may be caused by many different types of tissue injury. Regardless of the type of injury, the functional consequences that result in morbidity usually take one or two non-exclusive forms—namely, the nephrotic syndrome and renal insufficiency. In this discussion, therefore, I will orient the analysis to these common clinical expressions.

NEPHROTIC SYNDROME

The nephrotic syndrome is defined as heavy proteinuria of at least 3.0 gm/1.73 m^2/24 hours and a serum albumin level < 3.0 gm/dL. Patients with this syndrome inevitably have a reduced capacity to excrete sodium and will retain salt and water as edema fluid if sodium intake exceeds their maximum excretory capacity. The nephrotic syndrome, therefore, represents symptomatic proteinuria, in contrast to lesser rates of proteinuria, which are not associated with clinical symptoms, although the type and severity of renal injury may be similar. In addition, and apparently as a consequence of hypoalbuminemia, these patients usually exhibit elevated cholesterol and triglyceride levels, due to increased lipid production. The GFR may be reduced, depending on the severity of the renal injury. Table 65-1 provides an overall classification of renal parenchymal diseases, but it should be emphasized that nephrotic syndrome always results from an injury reaction that affects the glomerulus, either in primary or in systemic diseases, which increases the rate of filtration of plasma proteins.

The nephrotic syndrome in pregnancy may be caused by preexisting renal disease, renal disease that first de-

TABLE 65–1. CLASSIFICATION OF RENAL PARENCHYMAL DISEASE

- I. Glomerular
  - A. Primary renal disease
    - 1. Epithelial disease
      - a. Minimal-change disease
      - b. Focal glomerulosclerosis
    - 2. Membranous nephropathy
    - 3. Proliferative glomerulonephritis
    - 4. Chronic glomerulonephritis
  - B. Systemic disease
    - 1. Diabetic glomerulosclerosis
    - 2. Systemic lupus erythematosus
    - 3. Systemic vasculitis
    - 4. Amyloidosis
    - 5. Preeclampsia
- II. Interstitial
  - A. Acute interstitial nephritis
  - B. Chronic interstitial nephritis
  - C. Pyelonephritis
- III. Vascular
  - A. Arterionephrosclerosis
  - B. Vasculitis
  - C. Arterial emboli

(From Hirch DJ, Hayslett JP. Renal disease during pregnancy. In: Berkowitz RL, ed. Critical care of the obstetric patient. New York: Churchill Livingstone, 1983:443.)

velops during pregnancy, or preeclampsia. This distinction between intrinsic renal disease and preeclampsia has important clinical implications because of differences in patient management. In patients with established renal disease before pregnancy or in whom proteinuria is documented before the 20th week of gestation, diagnosis of renal disease as the cause of nephrotic syndrome is readily made. The onset of proteinuria in the latter part of pregnancy, however, presents certain diagnostic problems because of the similarities in clinical features to preeclampsia. In this case, it may not be possible to determine the diagnosis of preeclampsia in the absence of coagulation and liver function disturbances that may suggest preeclampsia.

The difficulty in distinguishing between primary renal disease and preeclampsia is highlighted in a report by Fisher and associates, who analyzed 176 patients with proteinuria and hypertension and in whom the underlying renal injury was documented by renal biopsy within 6 days of delivery.[10] Among primigravidas, the incidence of preeclampsia, primary renal disease, and hypertensive glomerulosclerosis were 83%, 12%, and 5%, respectively. Although the nephrotic syndrome is not a common complication of preeclampsia, preeclampsia was the most common cause of nephrotic syndrome in this series. In contrast, in multiparous patients preeclampsia occurred in only 38%, while renal disease accounted for 26% of cases, and hypertensive renal disease accounted for 24%. Because a clinical diagnosis of preeclampsia was made in nearly all of these patients during pregnancy, this study demonstrates that, in primigravidas and especially in multiparous women, primary renal disease can present clinically with the same features as preeclampsia.

Important practical questions that arise when pregnancy and renal disease coexist are:

1. Does pregnancy adversely affect the course of the underlying renal disease?
2. Is the outcome of pregnancy reduced?
3. What are the maternal complications?

In patients with nephrotic syndrome due to primary renal disease or preeclampsia, several analyses of relatively large numbers of patients have concluded that, in the absence of moderate or severe renal insufficiency, pregnancy does not seem to affect the natural course of the underlying renal disease in either the presence or the absence of nephrotic syndrome.[11–13] In patients with isolated severe preeclampsia, the long-term outlook is not complicated by either hypertension or signs of renal dysfunction.[14] Regarding outcome for the product of conception, Studd and Blainey reported that low birth weight correlated with low serum albumin levels,[11] but this relationship was not observed in other series.[12] Although the analysis of published series of patients with nephrotic syndrome due to primary renal disease is complicated by some patients with moderately severe renal insufficiency or hypertension, the fetal survival rate appears to reach normal expected levels when neither complication is present. Fetal outcome in patients with nephrotic syndrome due to preeclampsia, however, is reported to be reduced, compared to preeclamptic patients with lesser amounts of proteinuria, probably because high rates of proteinuria represent a more severe form of preeclampsia.[10] In regard to maternal morbidity, the progressive accumulation of edema formation may cause massive edema, especially near term, that may increase the risk of thromboembolic disease, may aggravate or cause hypertension, and has been reported to complicate vaginal delivery because of vulvar edema.

The clinical management of patients with nephrotic syndrome should aim to mitigate the severity of edema formation. Because proteinuria in patients with preexisting renal disease often increases during pregnancy to nephrotic levels, we suggest initiating a low sodium intake in early pregnancy (1.5 gm Na) to reduce the rate of edema formation. In addition, frequent periods of bed rest with the subject lying on her side to promote a higher GFR, especially in late pregnancy, will enhance the rate of sodium excretion. In most patients, these conservative measures will suffice to prevent massive edema. In cases of primary renal disease where dietary salt restriction does not prevent massive symptomatic edema formation, we employ diuretic agents, such as furosemide, on an intermittent basis, to reduce edema to more tolerable levels. In the absence of significant hypertension or renal insufficiency, pregnancy is carried to term with the expectations of a vaginal delivery. In preeclamptic patients, the usual approach in the management of this condition is employed.

Most patients experience a spontaneous diuresis, associated with a gradual fall in urinary protein and rise in serum albumin, within 2 to 4 weeks of delivery. In patients in whom the cause of nephrotic syndrome has not been established, we advocate renal biopsy within 1 week of delivery to determine the type of underlying lesion.

RENAL DISEASE WITH NORMAL OR NEAR-NORMAL RENAL FUNCTION

Even before the introduction of effective oral antihypertensive agents and modern techniques for monitoring fetal growth and development, some authors reported that the course of pregnancy was relatively uneventful in patients with preserved renal function.[15] The first of several large series involving patients with primary renal disease with normal or near-normal renal function was reported in 1980. In that study by Katz and associates,[13] 121 pregnancies in 89 gravidae were analyzed. Criteria for inclusion were continuation of pregnancy beyond the first trimester and sufficient data to evaluate its impact on the underlying renal disease. In all patients, a histological diagnosis was established. At onset of pregnancy, the serum creatinine was ≤1.4 mg/dL, proteinuria was present in one third of women, and hypertension was observed in 20%. During pregnancy, hypertension increased or occurred de novo in about one quarter; renal function decreased in 16%, most often in women with diffuse glomerulonephritis; and protein excretion rose in one half and exceeded 3.0 g/24 hr in 39 of 57 pregnancies. These changes generally resolved after delivery, and during long-term follow-up the decline in renal function was judged to be similar to the expected natural history of the underlying types of renal disease. The live birthrate was 94.3%, and perinatal mortality (stillbirths plus neonatal deaths) was 9%, compared to a level of 2% in the general population. The incidences of preterm deliveries (20%) and small-for-gestational-age infants (24.3%) were substantially above corresponding rates for all gravidae (13.3% and 5.7%, respectively). These results, which indicate a moderate incidence of reversible maternal complications and a moderate decrease in fetal survival, have in general been confirmed by other large series, which have also concluded that pregnancy does not appear to affect the course of the underlying disease.[16,17] It should be noted that because hypertension was present in a large fraction of patients in each of these reports, it is difficult to determine whether the high incidence of fetal growth retardation and preterm deliveries was due to hypertension or some other factor related to renal disease.

The management of this group of patients requires the skills of physicians trained in high-risk pregnancies and pediatric facilities designed to care for preterm and growth-retarded infants. Because recent experimental data suggest that accelerated glomerular injury correlates with elevated glomerular hydrostatic pressure, a condition expected in both systemic hypertension and chronic renal disease, hypertension during pregnancy should be controlled to obviate further renal damage.[18] Efforts to control edema formation in patients with nephrotic syndrome have been discussed. Anemia, sometimes of significant proportions, may also require direct intervention, and intermittent transfusions are advocated to maintain hematocrit levels above 25%. It should also be noted that patients with reduced renal function have a reduced capacity to excrete water and electrolytes. Therefore, they are at increased risk of developing dilutional hyponatremia when large amounts of solute-free water are administered, or hypernatremia, hyperkalemia, and metabolic acidosis after treatment with various types of electrolyte-containing intravenous solutions. Appropriate restrictions in the use of parenterally administered fluids are required during treatment of severe hypertension, prolonged labor, and other conditions requiring intensive therapy. As in other types of high-risk pregnancies, careful fetal monitoring is indicated in all cases.

RENAL DISEASE WITH MODERATE RENAL INSUFFICIENCY

The effect of pregnancy on the course of renal disease in women with serum creatinine ≥ 1.5 mg/dL but <5.0 mg/dL is less certain because of the paucity of data and lack of information on levels of renal function before conception in reported patients. Based on published reports and our personal experience, women with GFR levels between 15% and 40% of normal are likely to experience a hectic clinical course during pregnancy, due in large part to severe hypertension, and a successful pregnancy outcome of 50% to 75%. Because there are few patients in this category who do not exhibit significant hypertension, it is not possible to distinguish between elevated blood pressure and the metabolic consequences of renal insufficiency as the primary cause of impaired fetal development and fetal mortality. Table 65-2, prepared by Davison and Lindheimer, illustrates the general correlations between functional renal status and maternal complications–fetal outcome derived from the recent literature; in this analysis, categories of renal insufficiency were based on serum creati-

TABLE 65-2. PREGNANCY AND RENAL DISEASE: FUNCTIONAL RENAL STATUS AND PROSPECTS

PROSPECTS	CATEGORY		
	MILD	MODERATE	SEVERE
Pregnancy complications	22%	41%	84%
Successful obstetric outcome	95%	90%	47%
Long-term sequelae	<5%	25%	53%

Estimates are based on 804 women/1162 pregnancies (1973–1987) and do not include collagen diseases.

(From Davison JM, Lindheimer MD. Renal disorders. In: Creasy K, Risnik R, eds. Maternal-fetal medicine: principles and practice. 2nd ed. Philadelphia: WB Saunders, 1989:828.)

nine levels in mg/dL, ie, mild, <1.4; moderate, >1.4 and <2.5; and severe, >2.5.[19]

On the basis of an analysis of 23 patients with moderately severe renal insufficiency (serum creatinine ≥ 1.4 mg/dL), largely drawn from a questionnaire, Hou and associates reported that in seven women the decline in GFR was greater than expected from the natural course of the renal disease, and they suggest that pregnancy may accelerate the rate of functional deterioration.[20] Clearly, this is a category of patients that represents a challenge to the perinatalogist and where more information is needed.

RENAL DISEASE WITH SEVERE RENAL INSUFFICIENCY

The term "severe" is used to classify a level of GFR less than 15% to 20% of normal. Because women with severe renal failure are generally infertile, this condition in pregnancy results from either acute renal failure or a rapid progression of renal parenchymal disease acquired prior to conception or during gestation. This complication of pregnancy is associated with a high incidence of intrauterine death and fetal growth retardation.

Acute Renal Failure

Acute renal failure is defined as a rapid decline in GFR toward a value that approaches zero. Hallmark clinical features include a near linear increase in serum creatinine at a rate of 0.5 to 1.5 mg/dL/day, a progressive rapid rise in serum urea nitrogen, and usually a fall in urine flow rate to less than 400 to 500 mL/day. Sustained severe renal failure for more than a few days results in the manifestations of uremia and marked metabolic acidosis, hyperkalemia, and anemia. The general classification of acute renal failure is shown in Table 65-3.

TABLE 65-3. CLASSIFICATION OF CAUSES OF ACUTE RENAL FAILURE

Prerenal
Renal hypoperfusion due to
1. Hypotension
2. Decreased circulating plasma volume
3. Decreased cardiac output

Renal Parenchymal
Acute tubular necrosis—reversible
Cortical necrosis—irreversible
Caused by
1. Renal hypoperfusion due to
    a. Hypotension
    b. Decreased circulating plasma volume
    c. Decreased cardiac output
    d. Disseminated intravascular coagulation (DIC)
2. Nephrotoxins

Postrenal
Obstruction of ureters or bladder outlet
Extravasation of urine from urinary collecting system

The term *prerenal* implies that GFR is reduced because of renal hypoperfusion without renal histopathological changes or impaired tubular function. After renal blood flow falls, fractional sodium excretion is reduced to less than 1%, calculated as $(U_{Na} \times P_{Cr}/U_{Cr} \times P_{Na}) \times 100$, where U_{Na} and P_{Na} are the sodium concentrations of urine and plasma, respectively, and urine osmolality rises to ≥450 mOsm/kg H_2O. As noted in Table 65-3, renal hypoperfusion can result from hypotension, volume contraction, and heart failure. Common causes of renal hypoperfusion in pregnancy are hyperemesis gravidarum, septic shock, and preeclampsia, which cause volume contraction, and abruptio placentae, which causes hypotension. Correction of renal hypoperfusion in these conditions promptly restores GFR and reverses the metabolic consequences of renal failure.

Acute renal failure can result from *renal parenchymal* injury that results in acute tubular necrosis or cortical necrosis. Acute tubular necrosis occurs when the renal insult from severe ischemia or the action of nephrotoxins causes severe but reversible damage to renal tubular cells. The histopathological lesion is characterized by interstitial edema and necrotic, often sloughed, tubular cells; glomeruli appear normal by light microscopy, although in disseminated intravascular coagulation (DIC), fragments of red blood cells and fibrin deposits are commonly seen in glomerular capillaries. In contrast to prerenal acute failure, tubular transport function is markedly impaired and results in increased fractional sodium excretion (>1% to 2%) and impaired concentrating ability (<400 mOsm/kg H_2O). The same factors that cause prerenal hypoperfusion also cause acute tubular necrosis in pregnancy. In addition, hemoglobinuria due to hemolysis and disseminated vascular coagulation in septic patients and the specific nephrotoxic effects of some abortifacients are sufficient to cause renal shutdown. Restoration of renal function usually becomes clinically evident within 5 to 21 days of onset, and requires another 1 to 2 weeks to return to normal, which depends at least in part on regeneration of tubular epithelial cells.

Renal cortical necrosis is a pathological entity characterized by tissue death throughout the cortex in a diffuse or patchy pattern, with sparing of the medullary portions of the kidney. The causes and clinical characteristics of cortical necrosis are the same as those of acute tubular necrosis, except for the lack of morphological and functional recovery. Cortical necrosis is uncommon in non-pregnant individuals, but is relatively common in obstetric complications. Although the reason for the higher susceptibility to irreversible renal injury in pregnancy is not established, it is postulated that increased reactivity to vasoactive amines and the local activation of coagulation may play an important role.

Lastly, *postrenal* causes are listed as causes of acute renal failure, and in pregnancy include bilateral obstruction of ureters in polyhydramnios and ureteral obstruction from renal stones in patients with one functioning kidney, as well as ureteral tears caused by operative procedures. It should be noted that acute renal failure does not occur when only one kidney is obstructed in a patient with two functioning kidneys.

The approach to a patient with the clinical findings of acute renal failure begins by determining the category of the most likely cause for the sudden decline in renal function. Postrenal causes are evaluated by simple straight catheterization of the urinary bladder and assessment of ureteral diameter by renal ultrasound. Evaluation of the urine for fractional sodium excretion and concentrating ability is helpful in distinguishing prerenal from acute tubular necrosis as a cause of acute renal failure. The presence of hypotension or clinically evident cardiac failure or dehydration demands prompt corrective measures to restore renal perfusion. Because effective plasma volume is often difficult to evaluate at the bedside, especially in edematous patients, Swan-Ganz catheterization to determine pulmonary wedge pressure is the most reliable means of evaluating volume status. In the presence of reduced filling pressures, isotonic fluids, or packed red blood cells (RBCs) when hemorrhage has occurred, should be administered until filling pressures are normalized.

Restoration of plasma volume in the absence of tubular injury should increase renal perfusion and GFR. The absence of functional improvement after correction of volume status or cardiac output indicates the presence of acute tubular necrosis or cortical necrosis. In our judgment, potent diuretic agents should not be administered because they do not stimulate recovery of renal function and are associated with the risk of ototoxicity.

If the diagnosis of acute tubular necrosis or cortical necrosis seems likely after exclusion of pre- and postrenal factors, therapy is begun to minimize the consequences of severe renal insufficiency. Fluid administration is restricted, after restoring volume status to normal, to match urine volume plus insensible losses of water (400 to 500 mL/day); calories are provided in the form of carbohydrates or lipids at a minimum of 2000 kcal/day; and the administration of sources of sodium, potassium, and metabolic acid are avoided. The hematocrit should be maintained at at least 25% with transfusion of packed RBCs, and hypertension should be controlled. After the patient is stabilized, a decision should be made regarding delivery. If delivery is performed, dialysis therapy should be instituted after the procedure. In the event that delivery is impractical because of fetal immaturity, dialysis therapy should be instituted within a few days to minimize the functional consequences of renal failure. Early dialysis also has the advantage of permitting the administration of protein and calories in the large amounts that are often required in severely catabolic patients.

Severe Progressive Renal Failure

This entity may occur with any type of glomerular or interstitial disease shown in Table 65-1. In contrast to acute renal failure, in which GFR falls rapidly, the decline in GFR in progressive renal failure usually occurs over days or weeks. There is a progressive rise in serum creatinine to 5 mg/dL and above, a fall in plasma HCO_3 to values < 20mEq/L, a rise in plasma potassium and phosphate levels, and worsening anemia. Severe hypertension is usually present. In most cases, the specific cause of renal failure will have been established before conception or in early pregnancy, or will be evident from the clinical signs of a systemic disorder. Changes in the rate of a decline of GFR during pregnancy or the finding of progressive renal insufficiency for the first time during pregnancy, however, require exclusion of pre- and postrenal causes of renal failure.

Disturbances in acid–base balance and electrolytes should be managed by conservative means when they occur, and dialysis therapy should be instituted when the GFR reaches the level of 10 to 15 mL/min. The timing of delivery is a paramount concern in these patients and should be delayed until there is reasonable evidence of fetal maturity.

There is a paucity of data on fetal survival in severe renal failure, but from reports on small series of patients, fetal wastage is high and growth retardation is common. The adverse effect of hypertension is probably of major importance in regard to impairment of fetal development, and vigorous efforts should be made to control hypertension.

SYSTEMIC DISEASE AND RENAL DISEASE

A number of systemic diseases that involve the kidney can occur in women of reproductive age. When pregnancy occurs in these women, the potential risks to the mother and fetus may include the additive factors of the systemic disease and renal insufficiency. Our discussion will focus on two common systemic diseases—diabetes mellitus and systemic lupus erythematosus (SLE)—and will consider these questions:

1. Does pregnancy aggravate the systemic process and alter its natural course?
2. What are the common maternal complications?
3. How is fetal outcome affected?

DIABETES MELLITUS AND RENAL DISEASE

The maternal and fetal risks for women with diabetes and the major metabolic complications in the diabetic pregnancy are discussed in Chapter 62. Recent experience has shown that advances in perinatal and neonatal care have eliminated maternal mortality and reduced the perinatal death rate in diabetics in general to levels that approach the general population. The outlook, however, for patients with diabetes complicated by vascular disease has not improved in parallel with the general diabetic population. A 1977 report on the Joslin Clinic experience, for example, demonstrated a fetal survival of 84% in Class R, 72% in Class F, and 81% in

Class FR, representing women with retinopathy (R), nephropathy (F), or a combination of both vascular complications (FR).[21] Recently, two studies with a total of 57 patients with diabetic nephropathy have described a more favorable outlook for this group of patients, managed with optimal perinatal technique and modern methods of fetal monitoring. Reece and associates studied 31 continuing pregnancies managed at the Yale–New Haven Hospital between 1975 and 1984.[22] At the initial visit, 26% of cases were complicated by nephrotic syndrome and 33% had proteinuria > 0.5 g/24 hr. Renal insufficiency was present in 48%, and 68% had proliferative retinopathy. During pregnancy, renal function worsened in 45%, and blood pressure increased in 29%. Most patients had significant increases in proteinuria, and nephrotic syndrome occurred during gestations in 71%. Following delivery, changes in renal function, blood pressure, and protein excretion returned to values similar to that observed in the first trimester. The long-term maternal course was viewed as not differing from the expected course of diabetic nephropathy in subjects who had not become pregnant. These maternal complications and the postpartum course were similar to the observations reported by Kitzmiller and associates from the Joslin Clinic in 26 patients.[23]

The fetal outcomes reported in these two studies are shown in Table 65-4, and are compared to results in a large series of patients with primary renal disease. Inspection of Table 65-4 shows that perinatal survival in the two groups of diabetic patients averaged 91%, a value that was not different from patients with primary renal disease and normal or near normal renal function. Because the data taken together indicate similar rates of fetal survival, preterm deliveries, and small-for-gestational age infants, it seems likely that fetal complications in the diabetic population were primarily caused by renal injury or associated hypertension. In contrast, the high incidence of large-for-gestational age infants, neonatal complications, and major congenital anomalies were confined to the groups with diabetes, suggesting that these complications were caused by metabolic factors induced by diabetes. Recent studies have demonstrated that the latter group of complications can be prevented or markedly reduced by normalizing maternal blood glucose levels from the inception of pregnancy through term.[24,25]

In summary, recent experience in patients with diabetic nephropathy managed with modern perinatal techniques suggests that pregnancy does not accelerate the course of diabetic glomerulosclerosis. Additional complications during pregnancy may occur in this group, however, as in non-diabetic patients with renal disease, due to the development of nephrotic syndrome with associated peripheral edema, transient renal insufficiency, and worsening of hypertension. Fetal outcome is related to a summation of factors related to diabetes and renal insufficiency and hypertension. In the management of this group of patients in the future, efforts will be required to reduce and possibly eliminate the diabetic-induced complications by normalization of maternal blood glucose levels from the first few weeks of gestation. Because hypertension during pregnancy (in the absence of renal disease) is associated with reduced fetal growth and a higher perinatal death rate, it is possible that efforts to provide better control of hypertension will reduce the fetal complications associated with renal disease.[26]

TABLE 65-4. PERINATAL OUTCOME OF PATIENTS WITH NONSYSTEMIC RENAL DISEASE AND PATIENTS WITH DIABETES-ASSOCIATED RENAL DISEASE

	PREGNANT NONDIABETIC PATIENTS WITH RENAL DISEASE	PREGNANT DIABETIC PATIENTS WITH RENAL DISEASE (WHITE CLASS F OR FR)	
No. of patients	121*	26†	31‡
Fetal death	7 (5.7%)	2 (7.7%)	2 (6.4%)
Preterm deliveries	24 (20.0%)	8 (30.8%)	3 (9.6%)
Small for gestational age	27 (24.3%)	5 (20.8%)	5 (16.0%)
Large for gestational age	6 (5.4%)	3 (12.5%)	4 (12.9%)
Appropriate for gestational age	78 (70.2%)	18 (69.2%)	22 (72.0%)
Major congenital anomalies	—	3 (11.1%)	3 (9.6%)
Neonatal			
Respiratory distress syndrome	—	6 (23.0%)	6 (19.3%)
Hypoglycemia	—	11 (44.0%)	2 (6.5%)
Hyperbilirubinemia phototherapy	—	11 (44.0%)	8 (25.8%)
Death	6 (4.9%)	1 (4.0%)	0 (0.0%)
Perinatal survival	90.0%	88.9%	93.6%

* Data from Katz AI, Davison JM, Hayslett JP, et al.[13].
† Data from Kitzmiller JL, Brown ER, Phillippe M, et al.[23]
‡ Data from Reece EA, Coustan DR, Hayslett JP, et al.[22]
(From Reece EA, Coustan DR, Hayslett JP, et al. Diabetic nephropathy: pregnancy performance and fetomaternal outcome. Am J Obstet Gynecol 1988;159:56.)

SLE AND LUPUS NEPHROPATHY

Because SLE has a female predominance and experimental studies have demonstrated that estrogens activate an animal model of SLE, it is not unexpected that pregnancy may aggravate this autoimmune disorder. Two studies that used patients as self-controls reported an increase in the rate of exacerbations during pregnancy in women with SLE.[27,28] One recent prospective analysis that compared pregnant SLE patients with mild disease with non-pregnant women with SLE who were matched for age, race, and severity of disease, failed to find more frequent flares during pregnancy.[29] The opposite findings in these reports probably reflect differences in patient selection, because recent findings show that disease activity before conception has a major influence on the activity of SLE during pregnancy.

Hayslett and Lynn reported the first large series of patients with lupus nephropathy in 1980.[30] In an analysis of 65 pregnancies of 47 patients in whom clinical renal disease was present before pregnancy in 80%, they found that the rate and severity of exacerbations correlated with disease activity during the 6 months prior to conception. In 31 patients in clinical remission for at least 6 months, the relapse rate during pregnancy was 35%, and clinical flares were usually mild and resolved after delivery. In contrast, in 25 women with evidence of disease activity when pregnancy began, the exacerbation rate was 48%, and clinical manifestations were often more severe and did not always resolve postpartum. Table 65-5 is a summary of recent reports on patients with lupus nephropathy and, in general, confirms the relationship between the level of disease activity at the onset of pregnancy and the subsequent course (see reference 36 for a detailed discussion).

Regarding outcome for the product of conception, the overall fetal survival was 76% in eight studies published since 1980, shown in Table 65-6. Inspection of these data, however, shows a relatively good outcome in some patients, especially in women who were in clinical remission at the time of conception, and fewer, mild flares during gestation. In patients who exhibited clinical remission prior to pregnancy, fetal survival varied between 88% and 100%. In contrast, when pregnancy occurred in women with active SLE, survivorship was reduced to 50% to 75% in the same series. Not surprisingly, the worst outcomes were reported in pregnancies characterized by the onset of SLE during pregnancy or the puerperium; in these pregnancies, analyzed in Table 65-6, fetal survival was markedly decreased to 50% to 64%.

In summary, these data, reviewed by Hayslett and Reece,[36] suggest that the likelihood for a successful pregnancy is reduced in women with SLE and lupus nephropathy, especially in those with signs of active disease at the onset of pregnancy, because the occurrence of clinical flares, or concurrence of hypertension or renal insufficiency, was associated with an increase in fetal wastage, preterm deliveries and small-for-gestational-age infants. In contrast, the outlook was relatively good in women in clinical remission, regardless of severity or complications in the remote past.

TABLE 65–5. EFFECT OF PREGNANCY ON THE CLINICAL COURSE OF SYSTEMIC LUPUS ERYTHEMATOSUS IN PATIENTS WITH ESTABLISHED DISEASE

		STATUS OF SLE		
	NO. OF PREGNANCIES	UNCHANGED OR IMPROVED	EXACERBATION IN PREGNANCY OR POSTPARTUM	MATERNAL DEATHS
Hayslett and Lynn[30]		SLE Inactive at Onset of Pregnancy		
	31	21 (68%)	10 (32%)	
		SLE Active at Onset of Pregnancy		
	25	13 (52%)	12 (48%)	1
Jungers et al[31]		SLE Inactive at Onset of Pregnancy		
	11	9 (82%)	2 (18%)	
		SLE Active at Onset of Pregnancy		
	15	10 (66%)	5 (35%)	
Houser et al[32]		SLE Inactive at Onset of Pregnancy		
	10	8 (80%)	2 (20%)	
		SLE Active at Onset of Pregnancy		
	8	4 (50%)	4 (50%)	
Tozman et al[33]		SLE Inactive at Onset of Pregnancy		
	11	10 (91%)	1 (9%)	
		SLE Active at Onset of Pregnancy		
	13	9 (69%)	4 (31%)	
Varner et al[34]	30	21 (70%)	9 (30%)	1
Imbasciati et al[35]	22	5 (23%)	17 (77%)	2
Zulman et al[28]	22	10 (45%)	12 (55%)	4

(From Hayslett JP, Reece EA. Systemic lupus erythematosus in pregnancy. Clin Perinatol 1985;12:539.)

TABLE 65–6. EFFECT OF SYSTEMIC LUPUS ERYTHEMATOSUS

	FETAL SURVIVAL	FULL-TERM LIVE DELIVERY	PRETERM DELIVERY	PERINATAL DEATH	STILLBIRTH	SPONTANEOUS ABORTION
Hayslett and Lynn[30]		**SLE Inactive at Onset of Pregnancy**				
	21 (88%)	20	1			3
		SLE Active at Onset of Pregnancy				
	14 (64%)	13	1		4	3
		Onset of SLE During Pregnancy or Puerperium				
	5 (63%)	4	1		1	2
Jungers et al[31]		**SLE Inactive at Onset of Pregnancy**				
	11 (100%)	9	2			
		SLE Active at Onset of Pregnancy				
	9 (75%)	7	2			3
		Onset of SLE During Pregnancy or Puerperium				
	4 (57%)	3	1		1	2
Houser et al[32]		**SLE Inactive at Onset of Pregnancy**				
	10 (100%)	10				
		SLE Active at Onset of Pregnancy				
	4 (50%)	1	3			4
Tozman et al[33]		**SLE Inactive at Onset of Pregnancy**				
	9 (90%)	7	2			1
		SLE Active at Onset of Pregnancy				
	6 (86%)	6			1	
Varner et al[34]		**Onset of SLE Before Pregnancy**				
	23 (88%)	20	3			3
		Onset of SLE During Pregnancy or Puerperium				
	4 (50%)	3	1	2	2	
Imbasciati et al[35]		**Onset of SLE Before Pregnancy**				
	15 (63%)	12	3		3	6
Fine et al[46]		**Onset of SLE Before Pregnancy**				
	32 (71%)	18	14		10	3
Zulman et al[28]		**Onset of SLE Before Pregnancy**				
	21 (84%)	20	1	1		2

(From Hayslett JP, Reece EA. Systemic lupus erythematosus in pregnancy. Clin Perinatol 1985;12:539.)

It should be noted that infants born to women with SLE have additional risks besides impaired development in utero and preterm delivery. Transmission of autoantibodies to the fetus from maternal circulation is known to result in two types of disorders that are either transient or result in permanent tissue injury. Antinuclear antibodies and a positive lupus erythematosus (LE) cell test have been described in cord blood, but maternal antibodies disappear from neonatal blood within about 4 months.[37] Although clinical involvement of the newborn with maternal SLE is uncommon, a few cases of discoid lupus, and of hemolytic anemia, neutropenia, and thrombocytopenia have been reported.[39,39] These clinical episodes have been transient. A more important complication involves transmission of antibody to a soluble tissue ribonucleoprotein antigen called Ro (SS-A). Transmission of this antibody in utero has been associated with complete heart block in infants born to women with established SLE and to women with this circulating antibody in the absence of clinical features of connective tissue disease.[40,41] At autopsy, a diffuse and extensive endocardial fibrosis has been described that involved all four cardiac chambers and replaced septal musculature in the area of the atrioventricular node. Because the presence of this antibody is not associated with cardiac conduction defects in adults and disappears from the blood of infants within 6 months of birth, it seems likely that fetal tissue is uniquely susceptible to the cytotoxic action of this antibody. Tissue–antigen variation in the child may be important, because not all children born to anti-Ro (SS-A) positive women develop heart block. Nevertheless, pregnant women with SLE should be screened for anti-Ro (SS-A) and, if positive, fetal electrocardiac monitoring should be performed.

DIALYSIS IN PREGNANCY

Because severe renal insufficiency is associated with infertility, the issue of renal dialysis usually arises in patients with acute renal failure or severe progressive renal failure who conceived before the appearance of renal failure. Pregnancy has occurred, however, in women on dialysis, and in most cases was diagnosed late in gestation because it was unexpected and menstrual irregularities are common under this condition. A comprehensive understanding of maternal and fetal complications incurred by this group of patients is not available, because information is based on case reports and small series, and probably tends to favor successful gestation (see reference 42 for review). In 1978, the European Dialysis and Transplantation Association reported 115 pregnancies in 13,000 woman of child-bearing age. Of 70 women who did not abort therapeutically, there was a successful outcome in 23%. On the basis of case reports and small series of patients that were described in some detail, the incidence of viable births was about 50% among patients who conceived before dialysis. As expected, there was a high rate of preterm deliveries and intrauterine growth retardation. Early delivery most commonly occurred because of premature labor, fetal distress, abruptio placentae, or maternal bleeding.

Recently, a small series of eight pregnancies treated with peritoneal dialysis and six with hemodialysis was reported.[43] It was of interest that peritoneal dialysis was started in late pregnancy in some cases and was not associated with complications of hernia formation, peritonitis, or respiratory distress. Although spontaneous labor occurred in some cases, contractions were suppressed by adding $MgSO_4$ to the dialysate to achieve plasma levels of 5 mEq/L for periods of a week or more. Among patients treated with peritoneal dialysis, the survival rate was 63%, with 8 of 10 infants born preterm. Because this form of treatment tends to avoid dramatic changes in fluid volume, does not include use of anticoagulants, and provides a more constant metabolic milieu, it promises to be the preferred form of dialysis for those cases that require such treatment during pregnancy.

Among patients who develop severe renal failure after the onset of pregnancy, the aim of dialysis is to prevent uremic complications in the mother and provide a more favorable environment for the fetus until the likelihood of extrauterine viability reaches a reasonable level. Because of limited experience with this procedure in pregnancy, guidelines for management have not been established. It is common practice, however, to initiate dialysis treatment earlier than is usually prescribed in non-pregnant individuals, when the blood urea nitrogen level reaches a value of about 100 mg/dL. When hemodialysis is selected as the mode of therapy, an arteriovenous fistula should be formed early in gestation of patients with a progressive decline in renal function to permit maturation. In acute renal failure, vascular access can be achieved rapidly at any time during pregnancy with a subclavian catheter. In cases where peritoneal dialysis is selected, the surgical placement of a permanent catheter can be performed when the decision to begin dialysis is made, even, as noted, in the later stages of gestation.

It is also common practice to employ frequent hemodialysis, on a daily or alternating day basis, to maintain the blood urea nitrogen level below 50 mg/dL, and to reduce large changes in fluid volume and plasma electrolyte levels. A bicarbonate-containing dialysate, rather than acetate, is preferred, and efforts are recommended to maintain free calcium levels within the normal range by administration of oral calcium and 1,25 $(OH)_2$ D_3, along with appropriate adjustments in the dialysate level of calcium. It is further recommended to minimize heparin doses to reduce the risk of bleeding. Specific recommendations for management with peritoneal dialysis are provided by Redow and associates, and include a reduction in the volume of dialysate in late pregnancy in association with more frequent exchanges.[43] Regardless of the mode of dialysis therapy, we consider control of hypertension as critical in the preservation of fetal development, and aim to maintain diastolic blood pressure at a level of 90 mm Hg or less.

The occurrence of severe renal failure in pregnancy represents a significant threat to fetal viability. Close cooperation among patient, perinatologist, and nephrologist is essential, and is likely to be achieved most successfully in centers experienced in the management of high-risk pregnancy. We regard the recent report in the use of peritoneal dialysis[43] as an important advance in the management of these uncommon and challenging cases.

RENAL TRANSPLANTATION AND PREGNANCY

Because a successful renal transplant restores fertility as well as renal function, it is not surprising that some women have become pregnant after transplantation or desire to do so after their sense of well-being returns. In 1980, Penn reviewed the course of 56 pregnancies in 37 such women.[44] Of 21 patients with impaired graft function or hypertension before conception, 10 developed presumptive evidence of preeclampsia. In 5 other transplant recipients, preeclampsia occurred despite good graft function, and 3 of these developed persistent renal impairment. Of 56 pregnancies, there were 1 ectopic pregnancy and 8 abortions, 7 of which were therapeutic. Of the 44 live births, 70% were normal and 30% had complications, including respiratory distress, seizures, and anomalies. Four infants had congenital abnormalities. Labor and delivery were uncomplicated. Because these patients were routinely treated with immunosuppressive agents, sterile precautions were followed during vaginal examinations, and premature rupture of membranes was an indication for early induction of labor.

In a recent review, Davison reports a complication rate of 46% in pregnancies continuing beyond the first trimester, including uncontrolled hypertension, renal deterioration, and rejection.[45] Clinical differentiation between rejection of the graft and preeclampsia is difficult. The rate of successful obstetric outcome was 73% in women with complications before 28 weeks gestation and 92% in patients without early complications. The incidence of preterm delivery was 45% to 60%, and growth retardation was observed in 20%. The potential side effects of prednisone and azathioprine are described, and it is noted that no serious congenital abnormalities have been reported. Cyclosporin A is a new immunosuppressive agent that is now commonly employed. There is little known about either the maternal or fetal effects of this drug in pregnancy. It is important to stress the need for counseling at the time of transplantation, because women who were previously infertile may not be aware of the possible change in their fertility status. In addition, women desirous of pregnancy should be advised to avoid pregnancy for at least 18 months after surgery because of the higher incidence of rejection, infection, and permanent loss of graft function in this early postoperative interval.

REFERENCES

1. Davison JM, Hytten FE. Glomerular filtration during and after pregnancy. J Obstet Gynaecol Br Commonwealth 1974;81:588.
2. Baylis C. The mechanism of the increase in glomerular filtration rate in the 12 day pregnant rat. J Physiol 1980;305:405.
3. Garland HO, Green R, Moriarty RJ. Changes in body weight, kidney weight, and proximal tubule length during pregnancy in the rat. Renal Physiol 1978;1:42.
4. Durr JA, Stamoutsos B, Lindheimer MD. Osmoregulation during pregnancy in the rat. J Clin Invest 1981;68:337.
5. Lindheimer MD, Katz AI. Kidney function and disease in pregnancy. Philadelphia: Lea & Febiger, 1977:337.
6. Davison JM, Hytten FE. The effect of pregnancy on the renal handling of glucose. Br J Obstet Gynaecol 1975;82:374.
7. Hytten FE, Cheyne GA. The aminoaciduria of pregnancy. J Obstet Gynaecol Br Commonwealth 1972;79:424.
8. Pedersen B, Rasmussen AB, Johannesen P, et al. Urinary excretion of albumin, beta-2-microglobulin and light chains in preeclampsia, essential hypertension in pregnancy and normotensive pregnant and non-pregnant control subjects. Scand J Clin Invest 1981;41:777.
9. Davison JM. The effect of pregnancy on kidney function in renal allograft recipients. Kidney Int 1985;25:74.
10. Fisher KA, Luger A, Spargo BH, Lindheimer MD. Hypertension in pregnancy: clinical-pathological correlations and remote prognosis. Medicine 1981:60:267.
11. Studd JWW, Blainey JD. Pregnancy and the nephrotic syndrome. Br Med J 1969;1:276.
12. Strauch BS, Hayslett JP. Kidney disease and pregnancy. Br Med J 1974;2:278.
13. Katz AI, Davison JM, Hayslett JP, Singson E, Lindheimer MD. Pregnancy in women with kidney disease. Kidney Int 1980;18:192.
14. Chesley LC. Remote prognosis. In: Chesley LC, ed. Hypertensive disorders of pregnancy. New York: Appleton-Century-Crofts, 1978:421.
15. Oken DE. Chronic renal diseases and pregnancy. Nephron 1966;94:1023.
16. Surian N, Imbasciate E, Cosci P, et al. Glomerular disease and pregnancy: a study of 123 pregnancies in patients with primary and secondary glomerular disease. Nephron 1984;36:101.
17. Jungers P, Forget D, Houillier P, Henry-Amar M, Grunfeld JP. Pregnancy in IgA nephropathy, reflux nephropathy and focal glomerular sclerosis. Am J Kidney Dis 1987;9:334.
18. Meyer TW, Anderson S, Rennke HG, et al. Control of glomerular hypertension retards progression of established glomerular injury in rats with renal ablation. Kidney Int 1985;27:247.
19. Davison JM, Lindheimer MD. Renal disease during pregnancy. In: Creasy K, Resnick R, eds. Maternal-fetal medicine: principles and practice. 2nd ed. Philadelphia: WB Saunders, 1989:828.
20. Hou SH, Grossman SD, Madeas NE. Pregnancy in women with renal disease and moderate renal insufficiency. Am J Med 1985;78:185.
21. Hare JW, White P. Pregnancy in diabetics complicated by vascular disease. Diabetes 1977;26:953.
22. Reece EA, Coustan DR, Hayslett JP, et al. Diabetic nephropathy: pregnancy performance and fetomaternal outcome. Am J Obstet Gynecol 1988;159:56.
23. Kitzmiller JL, Brown ER, Phillippe M, et al. Diabetic nephropathy and perinatal outcome. Am J Obstet Gynecol 1981;141:741.
24. Fuhrmann K, Reiher H, Semmler K, Fischer F, Fischer M, Glockner E. Prevention of congenital malformations in infants of insulin-dependent diabetic mothers. Diabetes Care 1983;6:219.
25. Jovanovic R, Jovanovic L. Obstetric management when normoglycemia is maintained in diabetic pregnant women with vascular compromise. Am J Obstet Gynecol 1984;149:6178.
26. Lin C, Lindheimer MD, River R, Moa Wad AH. Fetal outcome in hypertensive disorders of pregnancy. Am J Obstet Gynecol 1982;142:255.
27. Garsenstein M, Pollak VE, Kark RM. Systemic lupus erythematosus and pregnancy. N Engl J Med 1962;267:165.
28. Zulman JI, Talal N, Hoffman GS, et al. Problems associated with the management of pregnancies in patients with systemic lupus erythematosus. J Rheumatol 1980;7:37.
29. Lockskin ND, Reintz E, Druzin NL, et al. Lupus pregnancy: case control prospective study demonstrating absence of lupus eracerbation during and after pregnancy. Am J Med 1984;77:893.
30. Hayslett JP, Lynn RI. Effect of pregnancy in patients with lupus nephropathy. Kidney Int 1980;18:207.
31. Jungers P, Dougados M, Pelissier C, et al. Lupus nephropathy and pregnancy: report of 104 cases in 36 patients. Arch Intern Med 1982;142:771.
32. Houser NT, Fish AJ, Tagatz GE, et al. Pregnancy and systemic lupus erythematosus. Am J Obstet Gynecol 1980;138:409.
33. Tozman ECS, Urowitz NB, Gladman DD. Systemic lupus erythematosus and pregnancy. J Rheumatol 1980;7:624.
34. Varner MW, Meehan RT, Syrop CH, et al. Pregnancy in patients with systemic lupus erythematosus. Am J Obstet Gynecol 1983;145:1025.
35. Imbasciati E, Surian N, Bottino S, et al. Lupus nephropathy and pregnancy: a study of 26 pregnancies in patients with lupus erythematosus and nephritis. Nephron 1984;36:46.
36. Hayslett JP, Reece EA. Systemic lupus erythematosus in pregnancy. Clin Perinatol 1985;12:539.
37. Bridge RG, Foley FE. Placental transmission of the lupus erythematosus factor. Am J Med Sci 1954;227:1.
38. Seip M. SLE in pregnancy with hemolytic anemia, leukopenia, and thrombocytopenia in mother and her newborn infant. Arch Dis Child 1960;35:364.
39. Sefanine M, Mele RH, Skinner D. Transitory congenital neutropenia. A new syndrome. Am J Med 1958;25:749.
40. Chameides L, Truex RC, Vetter V, et al. Association of maternal systemic lupus erythematosus with congenital complete heart block. N Engl J Med 1977;297:1204.
41. Scott JS, Maddison PJ, Taylor PV, et al. Connective-tissue disease, antibodies to ribonucleoprotein, and congenital heart block. N Engl J Med 1983;309:209.
42. Hou S. Peritoneal dialysis and hemodialysis in pregnancy. Baillieres Clin Obstet Gynecol 1987;1:1009.
43. Redrow M, Cherem L, Elliot J, et al. Dialysis in the management of pregnant patients with renal insufficiency. Medicine 1988;67:199.
44. Penn I, Makowski EL, Harris P. Parenthosal following renal transplantation. Kidney Int 1980;18:221.
45. Davison JM. Pregnancy in renal allograft recipients: prognosis and management. Baillieres Clin Obstet Gynecol 1987;1:1027.
46. Fine LG, Barnett EV, Donovitch GM, et al. Systemic lupus erythematosus in pregnancy. Ann Intern Med 1981;94:667.

66

CHAPTER

NEUROLOGIC DISORDERS OF PREGNANCY

James O. Donaldson

Obstetricians often care for patients with headache and nocturnal acroparesthesias. Approximately once per year, almost all obstetricians care for a pregnant woman with epilepsy. Less frequently encountered is any one of a broad array of conditions, some incidental, others life-threatening. This chapter will summarize the various neurologic diseases in pregnancy—their pathogenesis, manifestations and treatment.

CEREBROVASCULAR DISEASE

Cerebrovascular disease is a major cause of maternal mortality, especially spontaneous subarachnoid hemorrhage and stroke associated with systemic diseases, and would be even greater if eclamptic deaths attributed to brain lesions were added. Because cerebrovascular disease in young pregnant and puerperal women can be caused by a variety of unusual conditions, each case needs to be thoroughly investigated. Angiography is usually required to make a firm diagnosis and prognosis.

SUBARACHNOID HEMORRHAGE

Spontaneous subarachnoid hemorrhage commonly results from rupture of an aneurysm and an arteriovenous malformation (AVM).[1] Approximately one third of instances are symptomatic of bleeding disorders, endocarditis, sickle cell disease, vasculitis and, rarely, choriocarcinoma. Subarachnoid hemorrhage in gravidas under the age of 25 years is more likely to be from an AVM, whereas in gravid women over age 25 years, often multiparas, the likely cause would be a ruptured congenital berry aneurysm. AVMs are more likely to initially bleed in the second trimester and during labor. The incidence of the initial rupture of aneurysms increases with each trimester of pregnancy. Intrapartum rebleeding is common for both conditions, and is probably related to the Valsalva maneuver, which almost irresistibly accompanies strong uterine contractions.

If possible, the offending aneurysm should be surgically clipped or the AVM excised during pregnancy so that the woman may be delivered vaginally with no special risk. Surgery can be done as usual with hypothermia and controlled hypotension.[2] Surgery for unruptured aneurysms can be postponed, with the exception of aneurysms with diameters more than 10 mm.

If the lesion cannot be cured, vaginal delivery is a risk, although some physicians try vaginal delivery for multiparous women whose aneurysms bled in early pregnancy if bearing down can be prevented by panting and regional anesthesia. Almost all women known to have an AVM and multiparas with aneurysms are delivered by elective cesarean section.

ARTERIAL ISCHEMIA

Pregnancy increases the risk of a cerebral ischemic event approximately tenfold. As many arterial occlusions occur during the first week postpartum as during the second and third trimesters combined.[3] Almost all will be in the carotid territory. Approximately one quarter of these strokes are caused by premature vascular disease accompanying diabetes mellitus, chronic hypertension, and familial hypercholesterolemia. For another quarter, no explanation will be found. Fully one half are caused by a long list of conditions including mitral valve prolapse, atrial fibrillation, paradoxical emboli, bacterial endocarditis, cardiomyopathies, thrombotic thrombocytopenic purpura, metastatic choriocarcinoma, syphilis, and moya moya disease.

Management and prognosis depend on the underlying disease. Prophylactic anticoagulation is indicated for atrial fibrillation, cardiomyopathy, and the hypercoagulable state associated with antiphospholipid antibodies. The management of unexplained transient ischemia attacks (TIAs) during pregnancy is controversial. I recommend anticoagulation after the second TIA. The risk of having another unexplained cerebral ischemic episode during a subsequent pregnancy is undetermined, but probably is so rare that anticoagulation is not recommended. Heparin is the preferred anticoagulant during pregnancy, because it is a large molecule that does not cross the placenta, while warfarin crosses the placenta easily.[4]

CEREBRAL VENOUS THROMBOSIS

Puerperal aseptic cerebral phlebothrombosis is now uncommon in Western industrialized nations, with an incidence of 1 to 4 per 10,000 deliveries. These cases occur from 4 days to 4 weeks postpartum, 80% in the second and third weeks. A few cases have occurred in the first trimester.[5] In India the incidence is much higher—40 to 50 per 10,000 deliveries—and cases occur sooner after childbirth.[6] Almost all of these women were delivered at home, and by custom had been severely fluid restricted in a hot climate. Other puerperal cases have been attributed to sickle cell crises, minor head trauma, paroxysmal nocturnal hemoglobinuria, and hyperviscosity due to leukemia, polycythemia, and cryofibrinoginemia. Deep vein thrombosis in the leg and pelvis coexists for approximately 10%.

The presentation depends on which veins are involved. A thrombosis of the superior sagittal sinus may present with headache and increased intracranial pressure. If a cortical vein is thrombosed, a focal seizure at the height of the headache's intensity is usually followed by weakness and aphasia. Intermittently progressive deficits, often punctuated by seizures, connote propagation of the clot. A quickly propagating clot prevents adequate drainage by collateral veins, increases the likelihood of hemorrhagic venous infarction, and predicts a poor prognosis. The presence of intracerebral bleeding, which can be detected by computed tomography (CT) scan, is a strong but not absolute contraindication to anticoagulation. Thus, rapid diagnosis by magnetic resonance imaging (MRI) and angiography can allow anticoagulation early enough to prevent clot propagation. Historically, mortality has been approximately 30% in Western and Indian series; however, early anticoagulation decreases mortality to 20% or less. Those who survive usually have little residual disability.

EPILEPSY

Although the effect of pregnancy on epilepsy is unpredictable for any patient, the best indicator is the degree of control beforehand.[7] Almost all women experiencing at least one convulsion per month can expect a worsening seizure state during pregnancy, whereas only 25% of those gravidas who were seizure-free for the 9 months before becoming pregnancy will have a seizure while pregnant. Those seizure-free for 2 years have only a 10% chance of convulsing during pregnancy.[8]

The major factor responsible for an increased seizure frequency is an increased apparent plasma clearance (daily dose divided by blood level) of anticonvulsant.[9] This is especially true in the case of phenytoin, for which gastrointestinal absorption can markedly decrease. For almost all drugs, the hepatic metabolism and volume of distribution increases. For phenobarbital, renal excretion increases due to the mild chronic respiratory alkalosis of pregnancy. Other factors that can lower seizure thresholds include high estrogen levels and, in late pregnancy, insomnia.

The outcome of pregnancy depends more on socioeconomic status, regular prenatal care, and maternal factors such as age, parity, and other diseases, than on maternal epilepsy. A single maternal grand mal seizure may be followed by fetal bradycardia for 20 minutes or more.[10] Although there is every reason to believe that transient hypoxemia and acidemia are of potential danger to the fetus, there is usually no apparent harm caused by isolated seizures. Conversely, status epilepticus is a real threat: one half of fetuses and one third of mothers do not survive.

Infants of epileptic women do have a higher risk of major birth defects. The risk is present whether or not the fetus is exposed to an anticonvulsant, and increases with the severity of maternal epilepsy and the number of anticonvulsants used. The best controlled study found that the absolute risk increased from 3.5% to 4.4%.[11] That Norwegian study did not find the risk of orofacial clefts to be significantly increased, although many other surveys find that risk to be a fivefold increase.[12] The incidence of congenital heart disease is not increased, except among infants exposed in utero to trimethadione, which is considered a human teratogen.[13] The only malformation specifically related to an anticonvulsant is a defect in neural tube closure, which occurs in 1% to 2% of fetuses exposed to valproic acid in the first trimester.[14,15]

Dysmorphic facial features have been described with various fetal anticonvulsant syndromes and are not specific to any one anticonvulsant. Distal digital hypoplasia occurs in 15% to 30% of infants exposed in utero to phenytoin and, in one unconfirmed report, in 26% of infants exposed to carbamazepine.[16,17] Usually these "minor" malformations become less recognizable as the child grows.

The first goal of the management of epilepsy is to keep the patient seizure-free.[10,18] This applies to pregnant epileptics, too. Epilepsy should be treated with the fewest drugs in the lowest dose needed to prevent convulsions. This is especially true for women who may become pregnant. Single-drug therapy is recommended if possible. Although I do not prefer any one agent just because pregnancy is contemplated, I rely on carbamazepine and phenytoin in my practice, and this is reflected in the drugs used by my patients during pregnancy.

The use of valproate during pregnancy is a special problem because it is associated with a 1% to 2% risk of a neural tube defect, which can usually be detected by ultrasonography and amniocentesis early enough to induce abortion, if desired. If a patient contemplating pregnancy understands this risk and accepts its consequences, I recommend valproate be continued for patients with a specific type of epilepsy for which valproate is the first choice, for those for whom valproate as monotherapy is more successful then any combination of polytherapy, and for those requiring valproate as a second drug.[5]

I recommend maintaining during pregnancy what had been determined to be a therapeutic blood level beforehand. Blood levels can be checked monthly and doses adjusted accordingly. Other physicians keep their patients on the same dose, check blood levels, and alter doses only if a convulsion occurs. Anticonvulsants should not be changed or added during pregnancy unless therapeutic doses of the previously proven regimen are no longer effective.

I recommend dietary supplementation with folic acid before and during pregnancy because it may decrease birth defects and third trimester bleeding. Inhibition of folate absorption by phenytoin and other anticonvulsants has been proposed as a teratogenic mechanism. An improved outcome of pregnancy in epileptic women has been associated with adequate progestational folate levels.[19] Thus, starting a multivitamin tablet with folic acid, 0.5 or 1.0 mg, when a women stops using contraception seems reasonable.

Although mothers taking phenytoin, phenobarbital, and primidone have normal coagulation, about one half of their newborns will have a deficiency of vitamin K-dependant clotting factors. A few newborns will demonstrate hemorrhage. This can be prevented by maternal administration of vitamin K near term. The lowest effective dose has not been determined, but vitamin K, 20 mg per day for 2 weeks before term, results in normal clotting of cord blood. A parenteral dose of 10 mg during early labor may be an adequate alternative.

MULTIPLE SCLEROSIS

Multiple sclerosis rarely affects fertility, but it does alter family patterns. More women with multiple sclerosis remain unmarried, elect to have fewer children, have more elective abortions, and become divorced. The course of multiple sclerosis is unpredictable. It is a consistent observation that the rate of exacerbations decreases with each successive trimester of pregnancy, only to rebound in the puerperium, when approximately 40% will have a relapse.[20] The rate is the same for women who breast-feed and those who bottle feed their babies.[21] For the entire pregnancy year, which includes the first three postpartum months, the exacerbation rate is at least as high as for a non-pregnancy year. An abortion during a relapse does not induce a remission.

For most women with mild multiple sclerosis, the management and outcome of pregnancy is unaffected. Spinal anesthesia is usually avoided. Epidural anesthesia, regional blocks, and general anesthesia can be administered as usual. The gravid uterus can complicate bladder control and increases the risk of cystitis. More seriously disabled women can have increased difficulty walking as weight increases. The incidence of congenital malformations among infants of women with multiple sclerosis is not increased.

HEADACHE

Pregnancy can modify the frequency and severity of an established headache syndrome. A change in the quality of headache and the onset of headache during pregnancy may be symptomatic of an underlying condition, and should be evaluated accordingly just as for a nonpregnant woman. A thorough neurological examination including ophthalmoscopy is essential. Papilledema may be the only abnormality found in a patient with pseudotumor cerebri.

CLASSIC MIGRAINE

Pregnancy usually improves classic migraine.[22] Migraine can begin during pregnancy, usually in the first trimester, a time when focal or complicated migraine is also likely to occur.

The treatment of an acute migraine in a pregnant or lactating puerperal woman is complicated, because ergot alkaloids should not be used. Reliance is placed on analgesics (acetaminophen and, if needed, codeine or meperidine) and an antiemetic. If episodes are frequent and disabling, prophylactic therapy with a beta-adrenergic blocker is indicated.[23] Both propranolol at 40 to 160 mg/day and atenolol at 50 or 100 mg/day are effective. An alternative is amitriptyline.

TENSION HEADACHE

The effect of pregnancy on chronic muscle contraction/tension headache has not been systematically studied, although in my experience it is the most common headache during pregnancy and can be symptomatic of difficult psychological adjustments.[5]

An occasional headache can be treated with a simple analgesic, muscle massage, and either hot or cold packs to the neck. Regular use of aspirin should be avoided because aspirin can increase intrapartum blood loss and impair neonatal hemostasis. Acetaminophen also crosses the placenta but has not been found to cause problems in 40 years of use. Recalcitrant tension headaches often respond to tricyclic antidepressants. Both amitriptyline and imipramine have an extensive record of reasonably safe use during pregnancy. The usual dose for either drug is 75 mg/day, with a range of 50 to 150 mg/day. Benzodiazepine tranquilizers should be avoided. Diazepam is poorly metabolized by the fetus and may cause neonatal depression.

PSEUDOTUMOR CEREBRI

The typical patient with idiopathic pseudotumor cerebri is an overweight, fertile woman with headache and papilledema. Women with established pseudotumor cerebri worsen when they become pregnant. Gestational pseudotumor cerebri begins in the third, fourth, or fifth months of pregnancy and usually lasts 1 to 3 months, although for a few it persists until the puerperium.[24] Pseudotumor cerebri may recur with subsequent pregnancies. The outcome of pregnancy is good; labor and delivery are normal. Epidural anesthesia may be used.

Treatment may be necessary to preserve vision. Visual acuity, visual fields, and optic discs should be evaluated regularly. I recommend a diet sufficient for maternal and fetal requirements but restrictive enough to curb excessive weight gain. If this is unsuccessful or if vision is already impaired, repeated lumbar punctures to drain cerebrospinal fluid and dexamethasone, 2 or 4 mg per day, are options. Shunting may be necessary for recalcitrant cases.

BRAIN TUMOR

The coexistence of brain tumors and pregnancy is coincidental, if not less frequent then expected. All types of primary brain tumors have occurred during pregnancy, usually presenting during the second half.[25] A cerebral mass may be the signal lesion of metastatic choriocarcinoma. The treatment of the tumor and the management of pregnancy and delivery must be considered on a case-by-case basis. Surgery for meningiomas, some acoustic neuromas, and other slowly growing benign tumors can often be postponed until several weeks postpartum, when estrogen-induced tumor growth has regressed and the operative field can be expected to be drier. Supratentorial malignant tumors and many posterior fossa tumors are operated on during pregnancy to avoid the risk of tentorial herniation during delivery.

PITUITARY ADENOMAS

Pituitary tumors may cause primary or secondary amenorrhea.[26] Before fertility drugs are prescribed for a hyperprolactinemic woman, a neurological examination and imaging of the region with CT or MRI is indicated. If a woman with a prolactinoma becomes pregnant, the tumor will enlarge. Only 5% of microadenomas measuring less than 10 mm in diameter become symptomatic during pregnancy, whereas 15% to 35% of macroadenomas and extrasellar adenomas can be expected to do so. Women whose macroadenomas are excised before pregnancy revert to the low-risk group.[27] Thus, patients with intrasellar macroadenomas commonly have transphenodial hypophysectomy before attempting pregnancy.

Headache routinely precedes visual deficits by 1 month. Visual acuity and visual fields can be done monthly by standard bedside techniques. CT or MRI is indicated if visual deficits develop and during the puerperium. Following prolactin levels is not helpful. If vision is impaired, bromocriptine therapy can be instituted. If corrected visual acuity becomes less than 20/50, or if the bitemporal hemianopia encroaches upon nasal sectors, more definitive treatment is indicated. One must recall that hypopituitarism may be developing. Surgery can be managed in any trimester; nevertheless, if the fetus has adequate pulmonary maturity, labor is often induced. A pituitary mass that is first noticed in the postpartum period may be lymphocytic hypophysitis.[28]

NEUROPATHY

BELL'S PALSY

Idiopathic unilateral facial paralysis is prone to occur in the third trimester and the first 2 weeks postpartum.[29,30] The closer the onset to childbirth, the better the prognosis for complete spontaneous recovery. A brief course of high-dose corticosteroid therapy is indicated for patients with complete weakness, but may not improve cosmetic outcome for patients with partial weakness. In endemic areas, Lyme disease must be considered.

CARPAL TUNNEL SYNDROME

Approximately 20% of pregnant women complain of nocturnal acroparesthesias. Most have a postural obstruction of blood flow. A few develop a carpal tunnel syndrome, commonly in the dominant hand, during the second half of pregnancy, which can be expected to remit within a few weeks postpartum.[29,31] Most women respond to nocturnal splinting with the wrist in mid-position or slightly flexed. Surgical division of transcarpal ligaments entrapping the median nerve is indicated during pregnancy if weakness exists and the diagnosis is confirmed by electromyography.

MERALGIA PARESTHETICA

Meralgia paresthetica is a painful nuisance of the third trimester, which is presumably caused by an enlarged abdomen entrapping the purely sensory lateral femoral cutaneous nerve as it passes beneath the inguinal ligament. Symptoms typically resolve within 3 months after delivery.[29]

MATERNAL OBSTETRIC PALSY

The fetal head and forceps may compress intrapelvic peripheral nerves.[5,29] The typical patient is a short woman carrying a large baby whose labor is prolonged by cephalopelvic disproportion. The most common maternal obstetric palsy is foot drop caused by the fetal brow pressing against the lumbosacral trunk as it crosses the pelvic brim. This neuropathy is almost always unilateral and contralateral to the presentation of the vertex (ie, right occipital anterior = left brow posterior). Foot drop may also be caused by compression of the lateral peroneal nerve between the fibular head and a leg holder.

Femoral neuropathy, sometimes coexisting with an obturator neuropathy, may be unilateral or bilateral and is associated with labor arrested in a transverse lie. Around 1900, 3% of deliveries were followed by femoral neuropathy. Now this problem is rare, with probable prevention by cesarean section.

The prognosis of neuropractic lesions due to distortion of myelin sheaths is excellent, with full recovery within 6 weeks. If axons have been crushed, recovery is slower and may not be complete. During a subsequent pregnancy, women with previous neuropraxia may have a cautious trial of labor but should expect a cesarean section should dystocia develop. Women who had axonal degeneration from a previous delivery probably should be delivered by cesarean section in subsequent pregnancies.

GESTATIONAL POLYNEUROPATHY

A distal symmetric axonal polyneuropathy during pregnancy can be caused by malnutrition, specifically by a deficiency of thiamine. It may present in early pregnancy as a mild neuropathy associated with hyperemesis gravidarum and sometimes Wernicke's encephalopathy, or later as an insidious subacute polyneuropathy.

GUILLAIN-BARRÉ SYNDROME

Acute inflammatory demyelinating polyneuritis occurs randomly during pregnancy and runs its course seemingly independent of pregnancy. The Guillain-Barré syndrome affects neither pregnancy, labor, nor the fetus.[32] Early plasmapheresis decreases severity, and can be done during any trimester of pregnancy. Patients with autonomic dysfunction, especially pregnant women, can be sensitive to rapid changes in plasma volume. Fluid loading before plasmapheresis may prevent hypovolemia and hypotension. Transient postexchange deficiency of clotting factors is a potential risk.

CHRONIC INFLAMMATORY DEMYELINATING POLYNEUROPATHY

Chronic inflammatory demyelinating polyneuropathy is approximately three times more likely to relapse during the third trimester and postpartum than expected.[33] Some relapses have been associated with use of oral contraceptives. The infants are normal.

MUSCLE DISEASE

MYASTHENIA GRAVIS

Pregnancy has a profound but unpredictable effect on myasthenia gravis.[32] In pregnant women with this disorder almost equal thirds will be strengthened, weakened, and remain static.

Pregnancy has little effect on the treatment of myasthenia gravis. Previous thymectomy decreases the risk of pregnancy-associated exacerbations.[34] Pyridostigmine does not cross the placenta. Corticosteroid therapy has been used throughout pregnancy, but cytotoxic agents should be avoided. Thymectomy has been performed during pregnancy. In crisis, a series of plasmaphereses is certainly of less risk than prolonged immobilization with assisted ventilation. Postpartum presentations of myasthenia gravis are not infrequent, and postpartum relapses occur in at least 40% of myasthenic women.

Myasthenia gravis does not affect the myometrium. Labor and delivery are normal. Magnesium sulfate will precipitate a myasthenic crisis. Regional anesthesia is preferred. Lidocaine is recommended for patients taking pyridostigmine and neostigmine, which would inhibit the hydrolysis of procaine by cholinesterase.

Maternal myasthenia gravis appears not to affect the fetus because intrauterine movements are forceful and polyhydramnios does not develop. At least 12% of infants of mothers with generalized myasthenia gravis develop neonatal myasthenia due to maternal anti-acetylcholine receptor IgG that has crossed the placenta.[35] Feeding problems, floppy limbs, and a feeble cry usually appear at birth or during the first day of life, but need not appear until the fourth day. Weakening during the first few days is typical. Thus, neonates at risk must be carefully watched for 4 days before leaving the hospital. The delayed neonatal onset and the absence of fetal myasthenia are presumably caused by fetal produced α-fetoprotein, which in vitro blocks binding of antibody to receptors.[36] Remission occurs spontaneously as the neonate's level of antibody declines, usually in 2 to 4 weeks.

MYOTONIC DYSTROPHY

Women with myotonic muscular dystrophy usually weaken during the third trimester, and their myotonia can become more prominent. Breathing may be impaired.

Myotonic muscular dystrophy affects myometrium in addition to skeletal and smooth muscle.[37] Spontaneous abortion, premature labor, and uterine inertia during and after labor are common. Oxytocin stimulates uterine contractions. Regional anesthesia is preferred. Depolarizing muscle relaxants (eg, succinylcholine) can provoke rigor and hyperthermia.

The fetus can be affected, as manifested by polyhydramnios and arthrogryposis multiplex congenita. Affected neonates are floppy with facial diplegia and suck poorly. Women with mild, often overlooked, disease can have severely affected babies.

POLYMYOSITIS

Polymyositis is a subacute or chronic inflammatory myopathy that in young women is frequently a manifestation of systemic lupus erythematosus and other collagen-vascular disorders.[32,38] This disease is more virulent during pregnancy, and remission need not occur after abortion or parturition. Aggressive corticosteroid therapy and perhaps plasmapheresis is warranted. Fetal wastage is high, approximately 50%. However, there is no clinical or pathologic evidence that the fetus is affected. After birth these neonates thrive.

REFERENCES

1. Wiebers DO. Subarachnoid hemorrhage in pregnancy. Semin Neurol 1988;8:226.
2. Willoughby JS. Sodium nitroprusside, pregnancy and multiple intracranial aneurysms. Anaesth Intensive Care 1984;12:351.
3. Wiebers DO. Ischemic cerebrovascular complications of pregnancy. Arch Neurol 1985;42:1106.
4. Hiilesmaa VK, Bardy A, Teramo K. Obstetric outcome in women with epilepsy. Am J Obstet Gynecol 1985;152:499.
5. Donaldson JO. Neurology of pregnancy. 2nd ed. London: WB Saunders, 1989.
6. Srinivasan K. Puerperal cerebral venous and arterial thrombosis. Semin Neurol 1988;8:222.
7. Holmes GL. Effects of menstruation and pregnancy on epilepsy. Semin Neurol 1988;8:234.
8. Schmidt D, Canger P, Ayanzini G. Change in seizure frequency in pregnant epileptic women. J Neurol Neurosurg Psychiatry 1983;46:751.
9. Leppik IE, Rask CA. Pharmacokinetics of antiepileptic drugs during pregnancy. Semin Neurol 1988;8:240.
10. Yerby MS. Problems and management of the pregnancy woman with epilepsy. Epilepsia 1987;28(suppl 3):S29.
11. Bjerkedal T. Outcome of pregnancy in women with epilepsy, Norway, 1966 to 1978: congenital malformations. In: Janz D, Dam M, Richens A, eds. Epilepsy, pregnancy, and the child. New York: Raven Press, 1982:289.
12. Friis ML, Holm NV, Sindrop EH. Facial clefts in sibs and children of epileptic patients. Neurology 1986;30:346.
13. Friis ML, Hauge M. Congenital heart defects in liveborn children of epileptic parents. Arch Neurol 1985;42:374.
14. Källen B, Robert E, Mastroiacovo P. Anticonvulsant drugs and malformations. Is there a drug specificity? Eur J Epidemiol 1989;5:31.
15. Lammer EJ, Sever LE, Oakley GP. Teratogen update: valproic acid. Teratology 1987;35:465.
16. Gaily E, Granström M-L, Hiilesmaa V. Minor anomalies in offspring of epileptic mothers. J Pediatr 1988;112:520.
17. Jones KL, Lacro RV, Johnson DA. Pattern of malformations in the children of women treated with carbamazepine during pregnancy. N Engl J Med 1989;320:1661.
18. Saunders M. Epilepsy in women of childbearing age. Br Med J 1989;299:581.
19. Dansky LV, Andermann E, Rosenblatt D. Anticonvulsant, folate levels, and pregnancy outcome: a prospective study. Ann Neurol 1987;21:176.
20. Birk K, Rudick R. Pregnancy and multiple sclerosis. Arch Neurol 1986;43:719.
21. Nelson LM, Franklin GM, Jones MC. Risk of multiple sclerosis exacerbation during pregnancy and breast-feeding. JAMA 1988;259:2441.
22. Reik L. Headaches in pregnancy. Semin Neurol 1988;8:187.
23. Fishman H, Chesner M. Beta-adrenergic blockers in pregnancy. Am Heart J 1988;155:147.
24. Dirge EB, Varner MW, Corbett JJ. Pseudotumor cerebri and pregnancy. Neurology 1984;31:877.
25. Roelvink NCA, Kamphorst V, van Alphen HSM. Pregnancy-related primary brain and spinal cord tumors. Arch Neurol 1987;44:209.
26. Molitch MD. Pregnancy and the hyperprolactinemic women. N Engl J Med 1985;312:1364.
27. Toffle RC, Webb SM, Tagatz GE. Pregnancy-induced changes in prolactinomas as assessed with computed tomography. J Reprod Med 1988;33:821.
28. Cosman F, Post KD, Holub DA. Lymphocytic hypophysitis. Medicine 1989;68:240.
29. Massey EW. Mononeuropathies in pregnancy. Semin Neurol 1988;8:193.
30. McGregor JA, Guberman A, Amer J. Idiopathic facial nerve paralysis (Bell's palsy) in late pregnancy and the puerperium. Obstet Gynecol 1987;69:435.
31. Ekman-Ordenberg G, Salgeback S, Ordeberg G. Carpal tunnel syndrome in pregnancy, a prospective study. Acta Obstet Gynecol Scand 1987;676:133.
32. Parry GJ, Heiman-Patterson TD. Pregnancy and autoimmune neuromuscular disease. Semin Neurol 1988;8:197.
33. McCombe PA, McManis PG, Frith JA. Chronic inflammatory demyelinating polyradiculoneuropathy associated with pregnancy. Ann Neurol 1987;21:102.
34. Eden RD, Gall SA. Myasthenia gravis and pregnancy: a reappraisal of thymectomy. Obstet Gynecol 1983;62:328.
35. Morel E, Eymard B, Vernet-der Garbedian B. Neonatal myasthenia gravis: a new clinical and immunologic appraisal of 30 cases. Neurology 1988;38:138.
36. Abramsky O, Brenner T, Lisak RP. Significance in neonatal myasthenia gravis of inhibitory effect of amniotic fluid on binding of antibodies to acetylcholine receptor. Lancet 1979;2:1333.
37. Jaffe R, Mock M, Abramowicz J. Myotonic dystrophy and pregnancy: a review. Obstet Gynecol Surv 1986;31:272.
38. Rosenzeig BA, Rotmensch S, Binette SP. Primary idiopathic polymyositis and dermatomyositis complicating pregnancy: diagnosis and management. Obstet Gynecol Surv 1989;44:162.

67

CHAPTER

THROMBOEMBOLIC DISORDERS OF PREGNANCY

J. S. Ginsberg and J. Hirsh

Thromboembolism is a common cause of maternal mortality.[1] Its management is difficult and controversial because most recommendations about the proper management of thromboembolic disorders during pregnancy are based on imperfect evidence.

INCIDENCE OF VENOUS THROMBOEMBOLISM DURING PREGNANCY

The true incidence of deep vein thrombosis (DVT) and pulmonary embolism (PE) during pregnancy is unknown, but a recent retrospective study, in which women with suspected DVT underwent contrast venography, estimated the risk of acute antepartum DVT at 0.13 per 1000, whereas the risk of puerperal DVT was estimated as 0.61 per 1000.[1] Women were at higher risk after a cesarean section than after a vaginal delivery. (This study did not address the incidence of asymptomatic DVT, because only symptomatic women were investigated.)

DIAGNOSIS OF DEEP VEIN THROMBOSIS AND PULMONARY EMBOLISM

The diagnosis of DVT and PE during pregnancy presents special problems, because the clinical diagnosis is inaccurate and a number of key diagnostic tests expose the fetus to ionizing radiation.

POTENTIAL HAZARDS OF DIAGNOSTIC RADIATION TO THE FETUS

The adverse effects of radiation on the fetus can be broadly classified into oncogenicity and teratogenicity. Teratogenicity includes congenital malformations, intrauterine growth retardation, and embryonic death. Only data on the adverse effects of radiation in doses similar to those used in diagnostic radiology (less than 5000 mrad) will be reviewed in this chapter.

Oncogenicity

It is not entirely clear if the risk of childhood cancers is increased in individuals exposed to less than 5000 mrad of radiation in utero. There are, however, a number of studies suggesting such an association. The Oxford Survey data suggest a relative risk of approximately 2 following in utero radiation exposure from maternal abdominal radiographs (average radiation dose, 200 to 300 mrad).[2] The data used were based on reviewing childhood deaths from malignancy in the United Kingdom between 1953 and 1967. Critics of these studies state that the crude dose–response curves used are faulty and the methods used to calculate relative risk are erroneous.[3]

In a case control study of over 37,000 twins, Harvey and coworkers found a relative risk of childhood malignancies of 2.4 after in utero exposure to pelvimetry or abdominal plain radiographs (estimated radiation dosage, 160 to 4000 mrad).[4] Because of the small number of cases (31), the 95% confidence intervals of the relative risk of 2.4 are wide (1.0 to 5.9). Subgroup analysis reveals that the relative risk of leukemia is 1.6, whereas it is 3.2 for other cancers. One criticism of this study is the possibility that postnatal x-ray exposure could have been a confounding factor, because infants exposed to radiation in utero may have been more likely to have had obstetrical complications (eg, twins).[5] Therefore, they may have required more intensive postnatal care, including more exposure to radiation.

Lilienfeld reviewed several studies that investigated the risk of leukemia following in utero radiation exposure and found that most of the studies show an increased frequency of leukemia of 1.3- to 1.8-fold.[6] Although these studies have been criticized because of lack of matching for a number of possible confounders, there is no evidence that these confounders were present more frequently in the mothers of the children who developed cancer. On balance, therefore, it is likely that fetal exposure to radiation doses of even less than 5000 mrad is associated with a small increase in the risk of childhood cancer to the exposed individuals.

Teratogenicity

Most experts agree that fetal exposure to less than 5000 mrad of radiation is *not* associated with an increased risk of abortions, congenital malformations, or intrauterine growth retardation.[7] The teratogenic potential increases with increasing doses of radiation, but there is likely a threshold dose (approximately 25,000 mrad) below which no increase in teratogenicity is demonstrable. This is supported by animal experiments that show a similar threshold. Although no gross changes are demonstrable, this does not rule out subtle biochemical or central nervous system abnormalities that could escape detection. Nevertheless, if they do occur, they are likely to be rare.

RADIATION DOSES TO FETUS WITH PROCEDURES USED TO DIAGNOSE THROMBOEMBOLIC DISEASE

The doses of fetal radiation with venography and pulmonary angiography are calculations based on data obtained from the equipment used to perform these diagnostic procedures at McMaster University Medical Centre (Table 67-1). The dose of a given x-ray projection and for a given procedure is influenced by the equipment and techniques used, and therefore can vary considerably between different institutions (up to tenfold or more), and even between different x-ray rooms in the same institution.[8] It is essential, therefore, that an accurate determination of the expected absorbed dose to the fetus be made for each facility in which x-ray procedures on pregnant patients are being contemplated.

TABLE 67–1.

PROCEDURE	ESTIMATED FETAL RADIATION (mrad)
Bilateral venography without abdominal shield	610
Unilateral venography without abdominal shield	305
Limited venography	<50
Pulmonary angiography via femoral route	405
Pulmonary angiography via brachial route	<50
Perfusion lung scan	
^{99m}TcMAA	
3 mCi	18
1–2 mCi	6–12
Ventilation lung scan	
1 ^{33}Xe	3–20
^{99m}TC-DTPA	7–35
^{99m}TC-SC	1–5
Radioisotope venography	205
^{125}I fibrinogen leg scanning	2,000

From Ginsberg JS, Hirsh J, Ranbow A, Coates G. Risks to the fetus of radiological procedures used in the diagnosis of maternal thromboembolic disease. Thromb Haemost 1989;61:189, with permission.

Contrast Venography

Contrast venography is the most definitive method available for diagnosing DVT in the non-pregnant patient.[9] If adequately performed and interpreted, this test can be used to either confirm or exclude the diagnosis of DVT. Interpretation of venography during pregnancy may be difficult because of extrinsic compression of pelvic vessels by the gravid uterus.[10–13] Typical venography at our institution consists of six spot films and 1 minute of fluoroscopy for each leg. Based on measurements performed on water phantoms at McMaster University, the total absorbed dose to the fetus for bilateral venography *without* shielding of the abdomen is approximately 610 mrad. Unilateral venography halves the fetal exposure to approximately 305 mrad. A limited venogram, which is performed by shielding the abdomen, is associated with fetal radiation exposure of well under 50 mrad.

Lung Scanning

The perfusion lung scan is the pivotal test for the investigation of patients with suspected pulmonary embolism.[14] A normal perfusion lung scan excludes PE, and a segmental or greater perfusion defect with normal ventilation (high probability scan) reliably diagnoses PE. Conversely, subsegmental perfusion defects or segmental perfusion defects with matching ventilation defects are inconclusive and require pulmonary angiography.

The radiopharmaceuticals used to perform perfusion lung scans (^{99m}Tc-MAA or microspheres) remain in the lung or are broken down and phagocytosed by the reticuloendothelial system in the liver and spleen. The radiation dose to the embryo or fetus arises almost entirely from gamma rays emitted from lung, liver, or spleen. Using the usual dose of ^{99m}Tc-MAA of 3 mCi, the dose absorbed by the fetus would be approximately 18 mrad.[15] Use of 1 to 2 mCi of ^{99m}Tc-MAA, which still gives good quality scans, reduces the dose to 6 to 12 mrad.

The radiation dose from a ventilation study depends on the radiopharmaceutical used. For ^{133}Xe with 3 minutes of rebreathing from a closed system and 1 mCi of ^{133}Xe per liter of air, the fetal absorbed dose is 3.7 mrad.[15] Some laboratories use 20 mCi of ^{133}Xe in 4 liters of air, giving a fetal absorbed dose of 18.5 mrad. Many nuclear medicine departments are now using radio aerosols of ^{99m}Tc-diethylene triamine penta-acetic acid (DTPA). Fetal radiation exposure would arise primarily from isotope in the mother's bladder, because this material is freely diffusible and is filtered by the kidneys. This radiopharmaceutical also crosses the placenta into the fetal circulation. The absorbed dose to the fetus from ^{99m}Tc-DTPA is 35 mrad/mCi of injected isotope.[16] In a typical ventilation study, 0.2 to 1 mCi of ^{99m}Tc-DTPA is inhaled and subsequently absorbed into the blood stream, with a half-time of 80 minutes. The fetal absorbed dose is less when the isotope is inhaled than when it is injected intravenously, and therefore is less than 7 to 35 mrad. In the case of inhaled ^{99m}Tc sulfur colloid (SC) aerosol, the radiation dose to the fetus is less because the isotope does not leave the lungs. The fetal absorbed dose is 1 to 5 mrad for a ventilation scan done with ^{99m}Tc-SC. Therefore, using 1 mCi of ^{99m}Tc-MAA for the perfusion scan and ^{99m}Tc-SC for the ventilation scan, lung scanning can be done with fetal absorbed radiation of 11 mrad or less. Even performing full-dose perfusion lung scans and using a radiopharmaceutical other than ^{99m}Tc-SC for the ventilation scan, it should be possible to do a full ventilation–perfusion lung scan with a fetal absorbed dose of less than 50 mrad.

Pulmonary Angiography

Pulmonary angiography is the most definitive method for diagnosing pulmonary embolism.[17] It may be required when lung scanning does not provide a definitive answer, such as when a matched segmental defect in perfusion and ventilation is seen or with any subsegmental perfusion defect.

Pulmonary angiography is generally performed using 2 to 5 minutes of fluoroscopy and between 21 and 31, 14 × 14-inch spot films coned to one lung. Based on measurements performed on water phantoms at McMaster University, the total dose to the fetus is approximately 405 mrad for the entire examination. If performed by the brachial route and with appropriate abdominal shielding, the amount of radiation exposure should be well under 50 mrad. Therefore, every effort should be made either to use the brachial route or to use the femoral route with abdominal shielding and minimize the fluoroscopy used.

Fibrinogen Leg Scanning

The estimated fetal dose after 100 μCi of ^{125}I-fibrinogen is 2000 mrad. In addition, any free ^{125}I crosses the placenta and accumulates in the fetal thyroid. This technique is contraindicated in pregnancy.

SUMMARY OF RADIATION HAZARDS OF DIAGNOSTIC PROCEDURES

There is an understandable reluctance to expose the developing embryo or fetus to radiation. Although every effort should be made to minimize radiation exposure, failure to make the correct diagnosis has important implications. The unreliability of the clinical diagnosis of venous thrombosis and pulmonary embolism is well established. Treating all women with symptoms compatible with deep vein thrombosis or pulmonary embolism exposes a large proportion of patients to the potential hazards of anticoagulant therapy. Conversely, the consequences of untreated venous thromboembolism can be disastrous. Therefore, the best approach is the judicious selection of diagnostic procedures combined with efforts to minimize fetal radiation doses; ie, lead shielding of the abdomen, reduction of doses of radioisotope for perfusion scanning, and pulmonary angiography by the brachial vein.

If bilateral venography is performed in a patient with suspected venous thrombosis, the fetal radiation exposure should not exceed 1000 mrad. If modified perfusion and ventilation lung scanning plus pulmonary angiography via the brachial route are performed, the fetal radiation exposure should again be well under 1000 mrad. The current evidence suggests that the only likely adverse effect of in utero exposure to these doses of radiation is a small increase in the frequency of childhood cancers. Even assuming a doubling of childhood cancers, given a frequency of malignancy of approximately 1 per 1000 children, this level of exposure would give a frequency of childhood cancer of 0.2%. Our estimate of this low degree of risk is supported by a study of pregnancy in women radiologists, which showed that the frequency of children without childhood cancers was 99.93% when they were not exposed to radiation, compared to 99.84% when they absorbed 1000 mrem of radiation. Furthermore, the percentage of children without cancer or a malformation was 95.93% when absorbing no radiation, compared with 95.83% when 1000 mrem of radiation were absorbed.[18]

OTHER TECHNIQUES USED FOR THE DIAGNOSIS OF VENOUS THROMBOEMBOLISM

Impedance Plethysmography

Impedance plethysmography (IPG) is a noninvasive method used for the diagnosis of proximal DVT. In the non-pregnant patient, this test is sensitive and specific for proximal vein thrombosis, but is insensitive to calf vein thrombosis.[19–23] Although there are no apparent reasons why false negative tests would occur more frequently in pregnant than in non-pregnant patients, there is the potential for false positive tests in the latter part of the third trimester due to compression of the iliac veins by the enlarged uterus.[10] This may be corrected by repeating the IPG with the patient lying on one side.[10]

Duplex Ultrasonography

Duplex ultrasonography is a new technique that is accurate for the detection of proximal DVT in non-pregnant patients.[24] However, it has not yet been validated in pregnant patients. One potential disadvantage is the inability to consistently visualize the iliac veins, which can be the site of isolated thrombosis in pregnant patients.

APPROACH TO THE DIAGNOSIS OF VENOUS THROMBOSIS DURING PREGNANCY

Our current approach to the diagnosis of suspected DVT during pregnancy favors the use of IPG as the initial test for this disorder. If the initial IPG is abnormal in patients during the first two trimesters of pregnancy, a diagnosis of proximal deep vein thrombosis is made, and the patient is treated with anticoagulants. If the IPG is abnormal during the third trimester, two options are available: (1) perform a venogram to differentiate between proximal deep vein thrombosis and compression of the iliac veins by the enlarged uterus, or (2) treat the patient with anticoagulants. A limited venogram can be performed first and the patient anticoagulated if this test is abnormal. If the limited venogram is normal, serious consideration should be given to performing a complete venogram to visualize the iliofemoral veins, because false-positive IPG results occur more commonly in the last trimester of pregnancy. Although this approach has the disadvantage of exposing the fetus to the hazards of radiation, in absolute terms the risk of childhood cancer is minor and must be weighed against the risks, inconvenience, and expense of unnecessary heparin treatment in patients with false-positive IPG results in the latter part of pregnancy.

If the initial IPG is normal, isolated calf DVT cannot be excluded, so the IPG is repeated the day following referral (day 1) and then at days 3, 5, 7, 10, and 14. Patients are treated with anticoagulants if the test becomes abnormal during repeated testing, whereas therapy is withheld if it remains normal.[21]

If IPG is not available, a limited venogram should be performed; if the result is negative, the lead-lined apron should be removed and a complete venogram should be performed.

It is highly likely that duplex ultrasonography will complement the IPG for the diagnosis of DVT during pregnancy. In particular, if both noninvasive tests are negative, it further reduces the likelihood that the patient has proximal vein thrombosis. Conversely, if the duplex ultrasound is clearly abnormal and demonstrates noncompressibility of a venous segment, a diagnosis of venous thrombosis can be made (even if the IPG is normal).[24] Finally, it is likely that when the duplex ultrasound is normal and the IPG is abnormal, the patient has iliac vein thrombosis or external compression of the iliac vein.

APPROACH TO THE DIAGNOSIS OF PULMONARY EMBOLISM DURING PREGNANCY

It is our opinion that the potential risks of the tests used for the diagnosis of pulmonary embolism are less than the risks of not treating pulmonary embolism, or of treating patients with anticoagulants when the clinical symptoms and signs are not caused by pulmonary embolism. Our approach to the diagnosis of suspected pulmonary embolism in pregnancy is similar to the approach used in the non-pregnant patient. If the clinical features are compatible with pulmonary embolism, perfusion lung scanning is performed. If this test is normal, the diagnosis of pulmonary embolism can be excluded. If the perfusion lung scan shows one or more segmental defects, a ventilation scan is performed and, if the perfusion defect(s) is mismatched, the patient is treated with anticoagulants. Patients with segmental matched defect(s), subsegmental perfusion defect(s), or indeterminate lung scans are candidates for pulmonary angiography because these scan patterns do not exclude pulmonary embolism.

JUSTIFICATION FOR TREATMENT OF VENOUS THROMBOEMBOLISM DURING PREGNANCY

The treatment of venous thromboembolism during pregnancy is complicated because of the potential risks to the fetus and the inconvenience and possible side effects in the mother. However, these risks must be weighed against the dangers of not treating patients who have venous thromboembolism during pregnancy. There are several descriptive studies in the literature that suggest that the risks of not treating venous thromboembolism during pregnancy are substantial. In a retrospective analysis of 297 pregnant women with antepartum venous thrombosis, of 163 who were not given anticoagulant therapy 26 developed a complicating pulmonary embolism that was lethal in 21, for an overall mortality of 12.8%. In contrast, only 1 death occurred in the 134 patients who were treated with anticoagulants.[25] Several other retrospective studies strongly suggest that patients with venous thromboembolism fare much better if treated with anticoagulants.[26,27] Although all of these studies can be criticized on methodologic grounds, they strongly suggest that there is a substantial risk of fatal pulmonary embolism if patients with venous thrombosis during pregnancy are left untreated.

ANTICOAGULANTS

The pharmacology and clinical use of anticoagulants are reviewed comprehensively elsewhere and will not be reviewed in this chapter.[28–33]

SIDE EFFECTS OF ANTICOAGULANTS IN PREGNANCY

Anticoagulants have the potential to produce adverse effects in mother and fetus, and the safety of their use in pregnancy remains a subject of debate. Heparin does not cross the placenta and therefore might not be expected to produce fetal complications, whereas oral anticoagulants cross the placenta, enter the fetal circulation and have the potential to produce adverse effects in the fetus.[34,35] Nevertheless, in a recent review of anticoagulant use in pregnancy, it was concluded that the use of anticoagulants was associated with an adverse fetal outcome in approximately one third of pregnancies, regardless of whether heparin or coumarin derivatives were used.[36] The implication of the findings of the review is that the use of heparin during pregnancy is not safer for the fetus than oral anticoagulants. However, two recent studies suggest that heparin therapy is relatively safe to the fetus.[37,38] The first study reviewed published studies through 1986 and demonstrated that, when pregnancies associated with comorbid maternal conditions that could independently cause adverse fetal outcomes were excluded, the rate of adverse fetal outcomes in heparin-treated patients was similar to a normal population. Thus, the high rate of adverse fetal outcomes previously reported is largely due to the practice of treating toxemia, glomerulonephritis, and recurrent abortions, all of which are independent causes of adverse fetal outcomes, with heparin therapy. The second study reviewed 100 consecutive pregnancies associated with heparin therapy and demonstrated that the rate of adverse fetal/neonatal outcomes was comparable to a normal population. Thus, to summarize, it is likely that heparin therapy is safe for the fetus, whereas oral anticoagulants may not be, particularly during the first trimester.

The reported fetopathic effects of warfarin include the warfarin embryopathy and central nervous system abnormalities.[36] Warfarin embryopathy consists of nasal hypoplasia or stippled epiphyses after in utero exposure to oral anticoagulants in the first trimester of pregnancy. Central nervous system abnormalities that have been associated with oral anticoagulant use include dorsal midline dysplasia characterized by agenesis of the corpus callosum, Dandy-Walker malformations, and midline cerebellar atrophy; ventral midline dysplasia characterized by optic atrophy; and hemorrhage.

The report by Iturbe-Alessio and coworkers, which documented warfarin use in 72 pregnancies, is the only prospective study that looked for congenital malformations following warfarin.[39] Warfarin embryopathy occurred in 10 of 35 (28.5%) infants after warfarin exposure during the 7th to the 12th week of gestation, and in none of the infants in whom warfarin was discontinued between 6 and 12 weeks of gestation. There were no central nervous system abnormalities reported.

Although the interpretation of the above data is limited by the design of the reported studies, it is very likely that heparin use in pregnancy is much safer for the fetus than is the use of oral anticoagulants.

MATERNAL COMPLICATIONS

The most common maternal complication is hemorrhage. A recent study of 100 consecutive pregnancies associated with heparin therapy reported a bleeding rate of 2%—a rate that is comparable to the bleeding rate reported in a non-pregnant cohort of heparin-treated patients.[38,40]

HEPARIN-INDUCED OSTEOPOROSIS

There have been 22 patients reported with heparin-associated osteoporosis. With the exception of one randomized trial with only 40 patients,[41] all other studies examining the relationship between heparin and osteoporosis have been descriptive series or case reports. Seven patients with heparin-associated osteoporosis received long-term subcutaneous heparin for ischemic heart disease,[42,43] six patients received continuous infusion heparin by implantable pump for recurrent thromboembolic disease,[44,45] one 15-year-old male was heparinized for pulmonary veno-occlusive disease,[46] one patient received heparin for peripheral arterial disease,[47] and seven pregnant women were heparinized for venous thromboembolic disease.[48–54] Patients on heparin who developed osteoporosis commonly presented with bone pain and radiologic findings that included rib fractures, vertebral collapse, and asymptomatic osteopenia of thoracolumbar vertebrae. In all patients, serum calcium, phosphorus, and alkaline phosphatase were within the normal range.

Except for one report, the daily dose of heparin was 15,000 U or more.[49] In three patients, the duration of treatment was 5 months or less, whereas in all other reports treatment was in excess of 6 months.[47,48,52]

In the descriptive study by Griffith and coworkers, six of ten patients who received between 15,000 and 20,000 U daily for longer than 6 months developed clinical osteoporosis.[42] None of 107 patients receiving lower doses developed this complication. This important study, which drew attention to a possible association between heparin and osteoporosis, suffered from a lack of a clear inception cohort and a lack of description of the methods used to exclude osteoporosis.

In a randomized controlled trial by Howell and associates, 1 out of 20 women randomized to receive long-term antenatal heparin prophylaxis (10,000 U twice daily) developed clinical osteoporosis, while none of the control patients developed this complication.[41] The number of patients in this trial was too small to provide a reliable estimate of the true incidence. Thus, the 95% confidence intervals on the observed incidence of 5% ranged from 0.13% to 24.87%, implying that the true incidence could be lower than 1% or higher than 20%.

Two recent studies suggest that although symptomatic fractures are a rare complication of heparin therapy, a subclinical reduction in bone density occurs more commonly.[55,56] Ambrus and colleagues demonstrated that the administration of heparin for 3 months to female mice can lead to significant loss of body calcium.[57,58] The mechanism for heparin-associated osteoporosis is unknown, although several mechanisms have been suggested.[59]

In summary, it is likely that osteoporosis is an uncommon but real complication of heparin therapy, but the true risk of developing heparin-induced osteoporosis is unknown. There may be a dose effect, and it is unlikely that 3 months of treatment with moderate doses of heparin (approximately 20,000 units per 24 hours) is associated with symptomatic osteoporosis. Nevertheless, a subclinical reduction in bone density may be a relatively common sequel to long-term heparin therapy.[55,56] This should be considered before heparin therapy is started in pregnant women with previous venous thromboembolism.

TREATMENT OF VENOUS THROMBOEMBOLISM IN PREGNANCY

Because of the inaccuracy of clinical diagnosis of venous thromboembolism and the potential risks of anticoagulant therapy during pregnancy, a decision to treat a patient should be made only after the diagnosis has been confirmed objectively.

ANTICOAGULANT THERAPY DURING PREGNANCY

For reasons previously discussed, heparin is probably safe to use in pregnant women and is the anticoagulant of choice during pregnancy. Oral anticoagulants are probably contraindicated at all times during pregnancy unless heparin cannot be given, in which case the risk of oral anticoagulant therapy to the fetus must be weighed against the risk of not treating the mother.

USE OF ANTICOAGULANTS IN THE NURSING MOTHER

Heparin is not secreted into breast milk and can be safely administered to nursing mothers. There have been two convincing reports that warfarin does not induce an anticoagulant effect in the breast-fed infant when the drug is administered to a nursing mother.[61,62] In the first report, warfarin was not detected in the breast milk of 13 nursing mothers using a very sensitive and specific warfarin assay. Seven of these mothers were breast-feeding their infants, and warfarin was not detected in the plasma in any of these infants. In the second study, detailed investigations were performed on the plasma and breast milk of two nursing mothers who were being treated with warfarin and on the plasma of their breast-fed infants. Coagulation tests in each mother performed over a period of 56 days and 132 days of warfarin treatment revealed that the prothrombin time was between 20% and 30% of control and that Factor II, Factor VII, and Factor X levels were approximately 20%. No warfarin could be detected in the breast milk. In contrast to the effects seen in the mothers, the prothrombin time of both infants was 100% of control activity and the Factor II, Factor VII, and Factor X assays were 100% (even though the results in the mother's plasma were approximately 20%). The results of these two studies indicate that treatment of a nursing mother with warfarin does not induce an anticoagulant effect in the breast-fed infant.

A SUGGESTED APPROACH TO THE TREATMENT OF VENOUS THROMBOEMBOLISM IN PREGNANCY

Patients who develop deep vein thrombosis or pulmonary embolism during pregnancy should be treated by continuous intravenous infusion of heparin for 5 to 14 days to maintain the activated partial thromboplastin time (aPTT) at 1.5 to 2 times control (equivalent to a heparin level of 0.2 to 0.5 U/mL). This should be followed by subcutaneous heparin given in moderate therapeutic doses for the duration of the pregnancy. Subcutaneous heparin is administered every 12 hours in a dose that maintains the mid-interval aPTT (6 hours after the morning dose) between 1.5 and 2 times control. The efficacy and safety of this approach is suggested by two studies, one performed in non-pregnant patients and the other in pregnant patients.[38,40]

Patients with a past history of deep vein thrombosis or pulmonary embolism have a risk of recurrence that has been estimated at 5% to 12%.[41,62] Thus, some form of prophylaxis or surveillance seems reasonable. One option is to administer low-dose heparin in subsequent pregnancies during the first two trimesters and adjusted-dose subcutaneous heparin in therapeutic doses during the last trimester. The other option is to withhold anticoagulant prophylaxis and follow-up the patient with serial impedance plethysmography or duplex ultrasonography at weekly intervals.

APPROACH TO THE PATIENT WHO IS BEING TREATED WITH LONG-TERM ANTICOAGULANTS AND PLANNING PREGNANCY

Long-term or life-long anticoagulant therapy is indicated in patients with recurrent venous thrombosis and in most patients with mechanical heart valve prostheses. The correct approach to patients who are being treated with long-term oral anticoagulants and wish to become pregnant is problematic. Ideally, oral anticoagulant therapy should be replaced with heparin before conception. However, in practice this may expose the patient to months of subcutaneous heparin therapy before conception. Results of a recently published cohort study suggest that there may be an alternative strategy that is more practical and reasonably safe.[39] In this report, 12 patients with prosthetic heart valve replacements who were being treated with oral anticoagulants at the time of conception discontinued anticoagulant therapy at 6 weeks of pregnancy and none gave birth to children with warfarin embryopathy. It may therefore be reasonable to advise patients to have a diagnostic test for pregnancy performed frequently at appropriate times while they are attempting to conceive, and to replace oral anticoagulants with heparin when the test for pregnancy becomes positive, provided that pregnancy can be diagnosed within 6 weeks of conception.

REFERENCES

1. Kierkegaard A. Incidence and diagnosis of deep vein thrombosis associated with pregnancy. Acta Obstet Gynecol Scand 1983;62:239.
2. Bithell JF, Stewart AM. Prenatal irradiation and childhood malignancy: a review of British data from the Oxford Survey. Br J Cancer 1975;31:271.
3. Totter JR, MacPherson HG. Do childhood cancers result from prenatal x-rays? Health Phys 1982;40:511.
4. Harvey EB, Boice JD Jr, Hareyman M, Flannery JT. Prenatal x-ray exposure and childhood cancers in twins. N Engl J Med 1985;312:541.
5. DeSwiet M. Letter to the editor. N Engl J Med 1985;312:1574.
6. Lilienfeld AM. Epidemiological studies of the leukemogenic effects of radiation. Yale J Biol Med 1966;39:143.
7. Brent RL. The effects of embryonic and fetal exposure to x-ray, microwave and ultrasound. Clin Obstet Gynecol 1983;26:484.
8. Rainbow AJ. Survey of some factors affecting patient exposure in radiography. Phys Med Biol 1977;22:585.
9. Rabinov K, Paulin S. Roentgen diagnosis of venous thrombosis in the leg. Arch Surg 1972;104:134.
10. Ginsberg JS, Turner C, Brill-Edwards P, Harrison L, Hirsh J. Pseudothrombosis in pregnancy. Can Med Assoc J 1988; 1399:409.
11. Fogarty TJ, Wood JA, Krippaehne WW, Dennis DL. Management of iliofemoral venous thrombosis in the antepartum state. Surg Gynecol Obstet 1969;123:546.
12. Samuel E. The inferior vena cavogram in pregnancy. Proc R Soc Med 1964;57:702.
13. Kerr MG, Scott DB, Samuel E. Studies of the inferior vena cava in late pregnancy. Br Med J 1964;1:532.
14. Biello DR, Mattar AG, McKnight RC. Ventilation perfusion studies in suspected pulmonary embolism. AJR 1979;133:1033.
15. Roedler HD, Kaul A, Hine GJ. Internal radiation dose in diagnostic nuclear medicine. Berlin: Verlag H. Hoffmann, 1978:76.
16. Husak V, Wiedermann M. Radiation absorbed dose estimates to the embryo from some nuclear medicine procedures. Eur J Nucl Med 1980;35:205.
17. Sasahara AA, Stein M, Simon M, et al. Pulmonary angiography in the diagnosis of thromboembolic disease. N Engl J Med 1964;270:1075.
18. Wagner LK, Hayman LA. Pregnancy in women radiologists. Radiology 1982;145:559.
19. Wheeler HB, O'Donnell JH, Anderson FA, et al. Occlusive impedance plethysmography. A diagnostic procedure for venous thrombosis and pulmonary embolism. Prog Cardiovsc Dis 1974;17:19.
20. Hirsh J, Hull R. Comparative value of tests for the diagnosis of venous thrombosis. World J Surg 1978;2:27.
21. Hull RD, Hirsh J, Carter C, et al. Diagnostic efficacy of impedance plethysmography for clinically suspected deep-vein thrombosis: a randomized trial. Ann Intern Med 1985;102:21.
22. Hull R, Hirsh J, Sackett D, et al. Combined use of leg scanning and impedance plethysmography in suspected venous thrombosis. An alternative to venography. N Engl J Med 1977;296:1497.
23. Hull R, Hirsh J, Sackett D. Replacement of venography in suspected venous thrombosis by impedance plethysmography and ^{125}I-fibrinogen leg scanning. Ann Intern Med 1981;94:12.
24. Appelman P, De Jong T, Lampmann L. Deep venous thrombosis of the leg: US findings. Radiology 1987;163:743.
25. Villasanta V. Thromboembolic disease in pregnancy. Am J Obstet Gynecol 1985;93:142.
26. Aaro L, Johnson T, Jvergery J. Acute deep vein thrombosis associated with pregnancy. Obstet Gynecol 1966;28:553.
27. Ullery JD. Thromboembolism diseases complicating pregnancy and puerperium. Am J Obstet Gynecol 1954;67:1243.
28. Hirsh J. Marder VJ, Salzman EW, et al. Treatment of venous thromboembolism. In: Colman RW, Hirsh J, Mardec VJ, Salzman EW, eds. Hemostasis and thrombosis. 2nd ed. Philadelphia: JB Lippincott, 1987:1266.
29. O'Reily RA. Therapeutic modalities for thrombotic disorders. In: Colman RW, Hirsh J, Mardec VJ, Salzman EW, eds. Hemostasis and thrombosis. 2nd ed. Philadelphia: JB Lippincott, 1987:1367.
30. Rosenberg RD. The heparin-antithrombin system: a natural anticoagulant mechanism. In: Colman RW, Hirsh J, Mardec VJ, Salzman EW, eds. Hemostasis and thrombosis. 2nd ed. Philadelphia: JB Lippincott, 1987:1373.
31. Hirsh J, Deykin D, Poller L. Therapeutic range for oral anticoagulant therapy. Chest 1986;89:11.
32. Levine M, Raskob G, Hirsh J. Hemorrhagic complications of long-term anticoagulant therapy. Chest 1986;89:16.
33. Levine HJ, Pauker G, Salzman EW. Antithrombotic therapy in valvular heart disease. Chest 1986;89:26.
34. Flessa HC, Kapstrom AB, Glueck MJ, et al. Placental transport of heparin. Am J Obstet Gynecol 1965;93:570.
35. Becker MH, Genvesser NB, Finegold M, et al. Chondrodysplasia punctata. Is maternal warfarin a factor? Am J Dis Child 1975;129:356.
36. Hall JAG, Paul RM, Wilson KM. Maternal and fetal sequelae of anticoagulation during pregnancy. Am J Med 1980;68:122.
37. Ginsberg J, Hirsh J, Turner DC, Levine M, Burrows R. Risks to the

fetus of anticoagulant therapy during pregnancy. Thromb Haemost 1989;61:197.

38. Ginsberg J, Kowalchuk G, Hirsh J, Brill-Edwards P, Burrows R. Heparin therapy during pregnancy: risks to the fetus and mother. Arch Int Med 1989;149:2233.
39. Iturbe-Alessio I, del Carmen Fonseca M, Mutchinik O, et al. Risks of anticoagulant therapy in pregnant women with artificial heart valves. N Engl J Med 1986;315:1390.
40. Hull R, Delmore T, Carter C, et al. Adjusted subcutaneous heparin versus warfarin sodium in the long-term treatment of venous thrombosis. N Engl J Med 1982;306:189.
41. Howell R, Fidler J, Letsky E, et al. The risks of antenatal subcutaneous heparin prophylaxis: a controlled trial. Br J Obstet Gynaecol 1983;90:1124.
42. Griffith GC, Nichols G Jr, Asher JD, et al. Heparin osteoporosis. JAMA 1965;193:85.
43. Jaffe MD, Willis PW. Multiple fractures associated with long term sodium heparin therapy. JAMA 1965;193:152.
44. Buchwald H, Rhode TD, Schneider PD, et al. Long-term, continuous intravenous heparin administration by an implantable infusion pump in ambulatory patients with recurrent venous thrombosis. Surgery 1980;88:507.
45. Rupp WM, McCarthy HB, Rhode TD, et al. Risk of osteoporosis in patients treated with long-term intravenous heparin therapy. Curr Surg 1982;39:419.
46. Sackler JP, Liu L. Heparin-induced osteoporosis. Br J Radiol 1973;46:548.
47. Miller WE, DeWolfe VG. Osteoporosis resulting from heparin therapy. Report of a case. Cleve Clin Q 1986;33:31.
48. Aarskog D, Aksnes L, Lehmann L. Low 1,125-dihydroxyvitamin D in heparin-induced osteopenia [letter]. Lancet 1980;2:650.
49. Griffiths HT, Liu DTY. Severe heparin osteoporosis in pregnancy. Postgrad Med J 1984;60:424.
50. Hellgren M, Hygards EB. Long-term therapy with subcutaneous heparin during pregnancy. Gynecol Obstet Invest 1982;13:76.
51. Megard M, Cuche M, Grapeloux A, et al. Analyse histomophometrique de la biopsie osseuse. Une observation. Nouv Presse Med 1982;11:261.
52. Squires JW, Pinch LW. Heparin-induced spinal fractures. JAMA 1979;241:2417.
53. Wise PH, Hall AJ. Heparin-induced osteopenia in pregnancy. Br Med J 1980;281:110.
54. Zimran A, Shilo S, Fisher D, Bab I. Histomorphometric evaluation of reversible heparin-induced osteoporosis in pregnancy. Arch Intern Med 1986;146:380.
55. De Swiet, Ward PD, Fidler J, et al. Prolonged heparin therapy in pregnancy causes bone demineralization. Br J Obstet Gynaecol 1983;90:11.
56. Ginsberg J, Kowalchuk G, Brill-Edwards P, et al. Heparin effect on bone density. Thromb Haemost 1990;64:286.
57. Ambrus JL Jr, Robin JC, Kelly RS, et al. Studies on osteoporosis. I: experimental models. Effect of age, sex, genetic background, diet, steroid and heparin treatment on calcium metabolism of mice. Res Commun Chem Pathol Pharmacol 1978;22:3.
58. Robin JC, Ambrus JL, Ambrus CM. Studies on osteoporosis. X: effect of estrogen-progestin combination on heparin-induced osteoporosis. Steroids 42:669.
59. Avioli LV. Heparin-induced osteoporosis: an appraisal. Adv Exp Med Biol 1975;52:375.
60. Orme L, Lewis M, DeSwiet M, et al. May mothers given warfarin breast-feed their infants? Br Med J 1977;1:1564.
61. McKenna R, Cale ER, Vasan V. Is warfarin sodium contraindicated in the lactating mother? J Pediatr 1983;103:325.
62. Badaracco MA, Vessey M. Recurrence of venous thromboembolic disease and use of oral contraceptives. Br Med J 1974;1:215.

68

CHAPTER

COAGULATION DISORDERS IN PREGNANCY

Susan L. Sipes and Carl P. Weiner

Abnormal clotting may be identified when an unexpected aberration is noted on a routine laboratory bleeding profile or in association with a catastrophic event. Clotting abnormalities are commonly encountered in obstetrics and hemorrhage remains a leading cause of maternal death. Timely administration of the correct therapy significantly improves the likelihood of patient survival. It is imperative that the physician have a working knowledge of both coagulation physiology and pathology in order to select the optimal procedures to establish a timely diagnosis and to direct therapy.

PHYSIOLOGY OF COAGULATION

The circulatory system depends on the interaction of platelets, the soluble coagulation components, and the vascular endothelium for both integrity and patency. An acquired or inherited abnormality affecting any subdivision can produce hypo- or hypercoagulability.

Hemostasis is commonly divided into two phases. First, a platelet plug forms at the site of endothelial disruption, effectively sealing the defect. Second, a fibrin cap forms over the platelet plug, strengthening and stabilizing it. Multiple regulatory systems exist to prevent extension of the clot past the site of endothelial damage.

THE PLATELET

When the vascular endothelium is disrupted, a complicated chain of events stimulates platelet adherence to the exposed subendothelial collagen layer. Platelet adhesion refers to the reaction between the platelets and the subendothelial collagen. This reaction is mediated by a plasma protein, the von Willebrand factor. Platelet adhesion triggers a conformational change associated with degranulation and secretion of platelet granule contents. Initially, the platelet plug is loose, so that blood continues to flow over and through it. Further platelet aggregation is promoted by the collision of arriving platelets and by platelet release of adenosine diphosphate (ADP), platelet factors 3 and 4, serotonin, and thromboxane A_2 (TxA_2).[1] The plug becomes progressively more dense as additional platelets aggregate and adhere to the site. Within minutes, the fibrin cap forms over the platelet plug and bloodflow through the defect is no longer possible. The platelet contractile elements cause clot retraction, a process mediated by platelet fibrinogen, whereby the platelet attaches to fibrin strands.[2,3] The size of the thrombus is limited laterally by the adjacent normal vascular endothelium, which releases endothelium-derived relaxing factors (EDRF) and prostacyclin in response to platelet released ADP, TxA_2, and serotonin.

THE SOLUBLE COMPONENTS

Fibrin is the end result of a sequence of enzyme-mediated steps. Tissue thromboplastin and contact activation are distinct but interacting mechanisms that initiate enzymatic reactions that converge on a common pathway. The result is thrombin formation with fibrin generation (Fig. 68-1).

Contact activation begins a series of reactions along one of two pathways: *intrinsic* and *extrinsic*. Contact

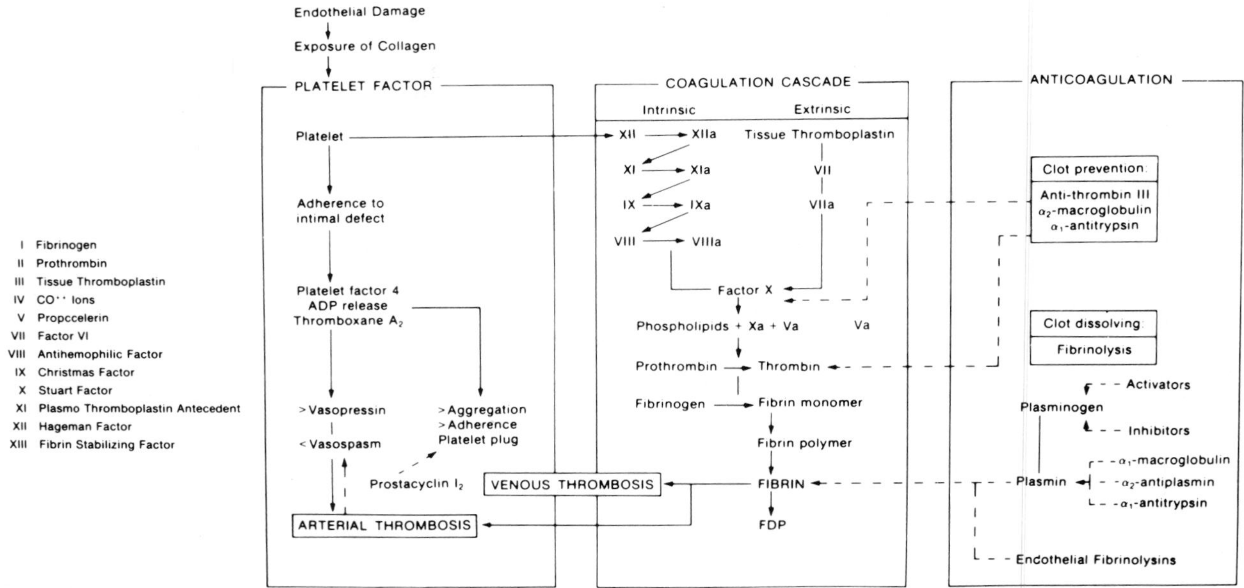

FIGURE 68–1. Integrated relationship among platelet activity, coagulation, and fibrinolysis (------, inhibitory; ——, stimulatory). (From Notelovitz M. Oral contraception and coagulation. Clin Obstet Gynecol 1985; 28: 77.)

activation is initiated by a variety of biological surfaces: bacterial lipopolysaccharides (endotoxin), long-chain fatty acids, unbroken skin, vascular basement membrane, and possibly fibrin and elastin.[4] The intrinsic pathway, so called because all necessary components circulate, involves factors XII, XI, IX, and VIII, high molecular weight kinogen, platelet factor 3, and prekallikrein. A minimum concentration of each of these moderate-size enzymes (80,000 to 160,000 daltons) is necessary for normal pathway function. Most proenzymes are synthesized in the liver. Although factor IX is vitamin K dependent, its half-life is such that a vitamin K deficiency exerts little influence on the intrinsic cascade. The final product of the intrinsic pathway is activated factor X: the beginning of the common pathway. The partial thromboplastin time (PTT) reflects the integrity of the intrinsic and common pathways. Deficiencies of factor XII, prekallikrein, or high molecular weight kinogen do not cause clotting abnormalities. However, the kinin pathway is important in disorders that are associated with excess clotting, such as septic shock.

Factor VIII has been extensively studied due to its association with hemophilia A and von Willebrand's syndrome. Circulating factor VIII is a complex composed of at least two proteins: VIII:C and VIII:RCoF. Factor VIII:RA may be part of the same protein as VIII:RCoF. Factor VIII:C accelerates the activation of factor X by factor IXa. Hemophilia A results from a deficiency of factor VIII:C. Von Willebrand's syndrome results from a deficiency of factor VIII:RCoF, which is synthesized by the vascular endothelium and megakaryocytes. Factor VIII:RCoF functions as a carrier for factor VIII:C in plasma and mediates platelet adhesion with collagen surfaces.

The role of the kinin system remains unclear, although some interactions are known. Factor XII catalyzes the conversion of prekallikrein to kallikrein.[5] Kallikrein accelerates the intrinsic pathway by amplifying factor XII activity and may also act directly on factor IX and plasminogen.[6–8] High molecular weight kinogen plays a similar role, enhancing the activation of factor XI and prekallikrein and amplifying the effect of kallikrein on factor XII.[9] Bradykinin, the product of high molecular weight kinogen, has no known function in clot formation but generates the hypotension associated with septic shock.

Exposure of *tissue thromboplastin* initiates the *extrinsic pathway* (see Fig. 68-1). Although intrinsic pathway cofactors are unnecessary for these reactions, kallikrein, factor XIIa, and factor IXa each enhance factor VII activation.[10,11] Pregnancy promotes this interaction.[12] Tissue thromboplastin is not found in plasma but has been found in every tissue examined to date. The prothrombin time (PT) is the laboratory measurement used to evaluate the extrinsic pathway.

The common pathway leads to thrombin generation by the interaction of factor V, factor X, prothrombin, and calcium on a phospholipid matrix provided by the membranous platelet factor 3 (see Fig. 68-1). Platelet factor 3 is also necessary for the interaction of factors IXa and VIII.[13] Attachment of these factors to platelet factor 3 concentrates and orients them with respect to each other as well as protecting them from the action of antithrombin III.[14]

Clotting cofactors, like platelet factor 3, are not enzymes. Rather, they are proteins that facilitate the interaction between the active enzyme and its substrate protein. The plasma cofactors are all large proteins

(>300,000 daltons) and, except for factor VIII:C, are synthesized in the liver. The cofactors bind to the phospholipid surface to become part of the receptor complex for the active enzyme and its substrate. The presence of the cofactor greatly enhances the rate of the reaction. Cofactors V and VIIIC must be activated by thrombin in order to express full cofactor activity.

In the final step of the cascade, thrombin cleaves fibrinogen to generate soluble fibrin monomer. Two peptides, fibrinopeptide A and fibrinopeptide B, are released during this reaction.

THE VASCULATURE

The vascular smooth muscle aids hemostasis only by retraction and spasm. However, the vascular endothelium plays a key role in hemostasis. Normal intact endothelium neither activates the soluble components nor attracts platelets, but it does bind and synthesize von Willebrand factor.[15,16] The endothelium is the primary source of tissue plasminogen activator and prostacyclin, and the sole source of EDRF. The latter two are potent inhibitors of platelet adhesion and aggregation.[17] The production and release of each is increased during pregnancy. Prostacyclin deficiency has been reported in pathologic obstetric conditions such as preeclampsia.[18,19]

COAGULATION MODULATORS

The platelet, the soluble components, and the vascular endothelium interact with the coagulation modulators to maintain homeostasis. Pathologic thrombosis is prevented by both plasma-clotting inhibitors and the plasma fibrinolytic system. α_2-plasmin inhibitor prevents pathologic fibrinolysis. A deficiency or excess of any of these coagulation modulators may lead to either excess clot formation or breakdown, respectively. Both local and humoral modulators exist.

Local modulators include blood flow, fibrin, endothelial cell receptors, and endothelium-derived factors. Blood flow removes activated coagulants, thus limiting clot extension. Fibrin and the platelet plug limit enzyme activation by blocking access to the initiating stimuli. Fibrin neutralizes large quantities of thrombin by reversibly adsorbing it.[20] A specific protein receptor on the endothelial cell surface called thrombomodulin also binds thrombin. After thrombin binds to thrombomodulin, it is unable to cleave fibrinogen or activate factor V. The thrombin-thrombomodulin complex also activates protein C, a humoral inhibitor of thrombin.

Humoral modulators regulate fibrin generation and degradation. All of these coagulation enzymes are serine proteases with the exception of factor XIII. Antithrombin III, one of a group of inhibitors that includes α_1-antitrypsin, α_2-antiplasmin, and C1-esterase inhibitor, is the major physiologic in vivo inhibitor of thrombin and factor Xa.[21] These inhibitors are quite similar in sequence and are moderately cross-reactive. Lethal hemorrhage has resulted from a single amino-acid substitution in the α_1-antitrypsin molecule, converting it to a thrombin inhibitor.[22] Antithrombin III also inactivates factors IXa, XIa, XIIa, as well as plasmin and kallikrein.[23] Deficient antithrombin III activity leads to excess thrombosis. Heparin-bound antithrombin III accelerates the rate of enzyme-inhibitor complex formation, which explains why heparin is ineffective in the absence of antithrombin III.[24] The variable response of patients with disseminated intravascular coagulopathy to heparin therapy may result from a variable antithrombin III concentration. PAPP-A, a pregnancy-specific protein, functions like heparin and facilitates the interaction between antithrombin III and thrombin. However, it does not aid the interaction between antithrombin III and factor Xa.[25]

The second important modulator of thrombin generation is the vitamin K-dependent protein C. Activated protein C promotes fibrinolysis and limits coagulation both by degrading factors Va and VIIIa and by stimulating endothelial cell release of plasminogen activator.[26] The concentration of protein C is stable during normal pregnancy.[27,28] The heterozygous deficiency state is associated with venous thrombosis during young adult life, while the homozygous deficiency state is incompatible with life.[29,30] Protein S, a protein C cofactor, is also vitamin K–dependent. In contrast to antithrombin III and protein C, it is markedly decreased during normal pregnancy.[27,28] Recurrent protein S deficiency is associated with thrombosis.[31] Increased protein C and protein S levels are found in women with mild to moderate preeclampsia.[27]

The plasmin system is responsible for fibrinolysis (fibrin removal), which begins as soon as the hemostatic task of fibrin has been completed. The proenzyme plasminogen binds to both fibrin and fibrinogen. Large amounts of plasminogen are incorporated inside the fibrin mass during clot formation. The activators of plasminogen are found in greatest concentration in the walls of the microvasculature, but also are present in blood, urine (urokinase), and other vascular endothelium.[32]

Although the exact mechanism for plasmin activation is unknown, its importance is clear. Vasospasm occurs in response to such physiologic and pathologic challenges as exercise, stress, epinephrine, bacterial pyrogens, ischemia, and shock.[33–36] Fibrin generation is associated with each of these. In vitro study suggests that plasminogen activation involves the interaction of factor XIIa with proactivators, although factor XIIa may act directly.[37] Because the plasmin-binding site for fibrin is shared with α_2-antiplasmin, free plasmin is rapidly neutralized by circulating antiplasmins while fibrin-bound plasmin is protected. Fibrinogen degradation probably occurs only when the concentration of free plasmin exceeds the supply of inhibitor.

Fibrin degradation products or *fibrin split products* (FSP) are the result of plasmin activity. These products have a half-life of approximately 9 hours and are cleared by the reticuloendothelial system. The Y and D fragments are especially potent antithrombins and impair platelet aggregation.[38] Although fibrinolysis occurs slowly within large blood vessels, it is rapid within the microvasculature.[39] FSP are thought to contribute to the hemorrhage that can accompany disseminated intravascular coagulation (DIC).

PREGNANCY-ASSOCIATED CHANGES IN COAGULATION

Pregnancy has a significant impact on the clotting system, presumably through enhanced hormonal synthesis (Table 68-1). Current theory holds that pregnancy is a state of chronic compensated DIC where component synthesis equals or exceeds consumption. In support of this theory, fibrinopeptide A, the first peptide cleaved from fibrinogen during thrombin-mediated fibrin generation, increases before the end of the first trimester.[40] Presumably a reflection of increased thrombin generation, it is the earliest documented pregnancy-mediated alteration in coagulation. Antithrombin III activity is not significantly altered by pregnancy, but the "reserve" of antithrombin III is diminished. A minor illness during pregnancy, such as a viral upper respiratory infection, can cause a dramatic decline in plasma antithrombin III activity.[41] Fibrin deposition does not occur in the maternal microvasculature to a great extent during normal pregnancy, because fibrinolytic activity increases during the first and second trimester (although it decreases in the early third trimester).[42] The concentrations of other coagulation factors change during pregnancy (see Table 68-1). Many of the soluble components originate in the liver and are estrogen sensitive. Some of the changes observed during pregnancy occur in women taking oral contraceptives.

The elevation of fibrinopeptide A and thrombin-antithrombin complexes later in gestation confirms that pregnancy is a "hypercoagulable state." This, coupled with the venous stasis present in the dependent limbs throughout pregnancy and the vascular damage that occurs during delivery, presumably accounts for the high incidence of thromboembolic disease in the peripartum period.

TABLE 68–1. CHANGES IN COAGULATION DURING PREGNANCY

INCREASED	UNCHANGED	DECREASED
Fibrinogen (I)	II [↑]	XI
VII	V [↑]	XIII
VIII RC	IX [↑]	platelets [→, ↑]
VIII RAg	Antithrombin III [↓]	
VIII RvWF		
X		
XII		
Fibrinopeptide A		

[ ], controversial.

From Weiner CP. Evaluation of clotting disorders during pregnancy. In: Sciarra JJ, ed. Gynecology and obstetrics. Vol. 3. Philadelphia: JB Lippincott, 1988:5, with permission.

CLINICAL EVALUATION OF A BLEEDING DISORDER

HISTORY AND PHYSICAL EXAMINATION

The more common acquired bleeding disorders are addressed in this section. A complete bleeding history and physical examination should be included as part of the routine prenatal evaluation and any suspicious findings pursued. A mild bleeding disorder may be missed unless specific inquiries are made in addition to the standard questions concerning a family history of "bleeding" or past transfusions. For example, was the patient informed that either persistent or excessive bleeding occurred from her umbilical cord stump (factor XIII deficiency)? Patients with hereditary bleeding disorders rarely have problems shedding deciduous teeth. The question to ask is whether she bled briskly for more than 1 hour after a dental extraction or oozed for more than 2 days, as might occur if she had von Willebrand's syndrome or was a symptomatic factor VIII deficiency carrier? Inquire specifically about any recent medications taken, because numerous drugs are associated with either qualitative or quantitative platelet disorders (Table 68-2).

TABLE 68–2. COMMON DRUGS CAUSING PLATELET FUNCTION DEFECTS

Anti-inflammatory Drugs
Aspirin
Ibuprofen
Indomethacin
Mefenamic acid
Psychiatric Drugs
Cardiovascular Drugs
Dipyridamole
Propranolol
Theophylline
Antibiotic Drugs
Ampicillin
Gentamicin
Nitrofurantoin
Penicillin G
Carbenicillin
Anesthetic Drugs
Procaine
Gaseous anesthetics
Miscellaneous
Antihistamines
Furosemide
Glyceryl guaiacolate (cough syrup)

From Weiner CP. Evaluation of clotting disorders during pregnancy. In: Sciarra JJ, ed. Gynecology and obstetrics. Vol. 3. Philadelphia: JB Lippincott, 1988:6, with permission.

The timing of the hemorrhage is important. A delayed onset is common in a patient with a soluble component disorder, while immediate onset is associated with platelet abnormalities. Spontaneous bleeding from a body orifice occurs equally in patients suffering from soluble component or platelet disorders. In rare cases, menorrhagia may be the initial presenting complaint of a woman with von Willebrand's syndrome or mild thrombocytopenia.

The initial step in the evaluation of abnormal bleeding is to determine whether it results from local pathology, a generalized defect in the clotting system or, as is frequent in obstetrics, both. Several signs and symptoms can be virtually diagnostic and save costly laboratory evaluation. Petechiae are characteristic of either a platelet or vascular disorder. They appear in crops and are more common on the dependent parts of the body. Deep dissecting hematomas and hemarthroses are more characteristic of a soluble component disorder.

Unexplained, easy bruising may be the result of a vascular abnormality. Although not usually associated with spontaneous hemorrhage, these disorders are important because the frequency of hemorrhage and thrombosis is increased after operative or traumatic stress. The most common acquired defects result from collagen disorders, Cushing's syndrome, diabetes, and infections. Autoimmune evaluation, tissue biopsy, or evaluation of the kinin system are often necessary to make this challenging diagnosis.

BASIC LABORATORY EVALUATION

The four components of a basic clotting screen include the prothrombin time (PT), the partial thromboplastin time (PTT), the platelet count, and the bleeding time. The bleeding time is of limited benefit in an obstetric emergency and is best replaced by a fibrinogen level.

The PTT evaluates the intrinsic and common pathways, and as such is often used to monitor heparin therapy. However, prolongation of the PTT does not necessarily correlate with "clinical" anticoagulation and, in fact, correlates poorly with the plasma heparin level. The latter may or may not be important, because the therapeutic level of heparin remains poorly defined and clinical experience confirms that a 50% increase in the PTT is associated with a marked reduction in subsequent thrombotic events. Prolongation of the PTT implies an intact heparin–antithrombin III pathway. A reduction in antithrombin III, as seen in DIC, increases the heparin requirement.

The PT evaluates the extrinsic and common pathways. It is most sensitive to deficiencies of factors V, VII, and X. Because factor VII has the shortest half-life of the vitamin K-dependent factors (II, VII, IX, and X), the PT is a useful monitor of warfarin therapy. It is unaltered by hypofibrinogenemia until the fibrinogen concentration is below 100 mg/dL. Eventually, automated tests for specific components of the extrinsic and intrinsic pathways may replace the PT and PTT.

The platelet count is a first step in evaluating the platelet contribution to hemostasis. The incidence of thrombocytopenia is increased during pregnancy.[43] Thrombocytopenia is not a diagnosis, but rather a symptom of an underlying disease. Although there is no absolute cut-off point, a count below 120,000/mm^3 is clearly atypical. Excessive bleeding is rare when the platelet count exceeds 40,000/mm^3. Should bleeding occur when the count is above this level, a functional platelet disorder should be considered. Spontaneous bleeding may occur when the platelet count is below 40,000/mm^3, but rarely is severe when the count is above 10,000/mm^3. A low count should always be confirmed by a manual count, because the anticoagulant EDTA does not always prevent platelet clumping. These clumps are not recognized by the automated counters, which then erroneously report a low count.

The bleeding time is measured from a series of standardized stab wounds and reflects both platelet number and function. The bleeding time can be prolonged by a qualitative platelet disorder such as that which occurs in association with von Willebrand's syndrome, Glanzmann's thromboasthenia, the ingestion of antiprostaglandin drugs (ie, aspirin, ibuprofen), and preeclampsia. It may also be associated with a vascular abnormality, but this possibility is much less common and should be pursued last.

Platelet function can also be evaluated by the in vitro response of platelets to aggregating agents as measured by the change in optical density of a light beam passed through platelet-rich plasma. The aggregating agents most commonly employed include ADP, serotonin, epinephrine, collagen, arachidonic acid, and ristocetin. Diseases associated with acquired platelet dysfunction include autoimmune disorders, preeclampsia, anemia, drug-induced disorders, uremia, and myeloproliferative syndromes.

A decline in the fibrinogen level unassociated with overwhelming liver disease suggests that consumption is exceeding production and a cause should be sought. A bedside clotting test is invaluable in the emergent situation. Five mL of blood in a silicone-coated tube (red top) is obtained. The absence of clot after 10 minutes indicates a fibrinogen concentration below 50 mg/dL. Rapid clot breakdown suggests the present of excess circulating FSP.

The interpretations of the various screening tests are listed in Table 68-3. An isolated prolongation of the PTT is quite common. If the patient has been and is currently asymptomatic, the prolongation may be due to an acquired inhibitor (most often an antibody) or to a deficiency of either prekallikrein, factor XII, or high molecular weight kinogen. If the abnormality is due to an antibody, the PTT will not correct when the patient's plasma is mixed 1:1 with normal plasma. Inhibitors are not usually associated with hemorrhage, except when directed against factor VIII or IX.

An isolated prolongation of the PT is uncommon. More often, both PT and PTT are prolonged. DIC with fibrin-fibrinogenolysis is the most common cause of a

TABLE 68-3. LABORATORY TESTS IN BLEEDING DISORDERS

CLINICAL BLEEDING	PTT	PT	BLEEDING TIME	PLATELET COUNT	FIBRINOGEN	COMMON CAUSES	
						ACQUIRED	HEREDITARY
−	P	N	N	N	N	Lupus anticoagulant	High molecular weight kinogen, prekallikrein, factor XII deficiencies
+	P	N	N	N	N	Heparin, factor VIII inhibitors	Hemophilia A and B, factor XI deficiency
+	P	P	N	N	N	Heparin, coumarin, vitamin K deficiency, antibiotics	Deficiency in factors V, X, and II and dysfibrinogenemia
+	N	P	N	N	N		Factor VII deficiency
+	P	N	P	N	N	Lupus-like anticoagulant, factor VIII complex inhibitor	von Willebrand's syndrome
+	P	P	P	N			Afibrinogenemia
+	N	N	P		N	Thrombocytopenia secondary to immune thrombotic thrombocytopenia [ITP], drugs, etc.	Aldrich's syndrome, others
+	N	N	P	N	N	Aspirin, uremia, etc.	Thrombasthenia, deficient platelet release, Bernard-Soulier syndrome
+	N	N	N	N	N		Factor XIII deficiency
+	P	P				DIC, liver disease	

−, absent; +, present; N, normal; P, prolonged.

Modified from Colman RW, Hirsh J, Marder VJ, Salzman EW. Approach to the bleeding patient. In: Colman RW, Hirsh J, Marder VJ, Salzman EW. Hemostasis and thrombosis. Philadelphia: JB Lippincott, 1982:700, with permission.

prolonged PT and PTT in the obstetric patient. Other acquired causes include isolated deficiencies or inhibitors of the common pathway clotting factors, hypofibrinogenemia, liver disease, massive transfusion of banked blood, and vitamin K deficiency. Vitamin K deficiency may be due to either warfarin ingestion or prolonged broad-spectrum antibiotic therapy. A woman with a clinical bleeding disorder characterized by a normal coagulation screen has either a factor XIII deficiency or a vascular abnormality.

SPECIALIZED TESTS

Fibrin split products (FSP) result from plasmin catabolism of fibrinogen and fibrin. Fragments X and Y are generated early in the degradation process; fragment Y is a particularly potent anticoagulant. FSP can be measured directly by several techniques. Prolongation of both the thrombin and reptilase times indicates FSP concentrations above 5 mg/dL.

Fibrinopeptide A (FPA) is the first peptide cleaved from fibrinogen during thrombin-mediated fibrin generation. With a 3-minute half-life, the concentration of FPA directly reflects fibrin generation. FPA is measured by radioimmunoassay and is elevated during normal pregnancy. Significantly higher concentrations are found during pregnancies complicated by preeclampsia, sepsis, and thromboembolic disease.[40,44,45] A normal FPA during pregnancy is inconsistent with an acute thrombosis of any size.

Antithrombin III (AT III) inhibits most active soluble clotting components. Because of its function and the availability of rapid chromogenic substrate assays, AT III activity measurement has become one of the most useful laboratory parameters for monitoring the effect of therapy on DIC.[46] Cessation of AT III consumption implies therapy has eliminated or blunted the causative process. Infection, preeclampsia, and thromboembolic disease are associated with a reduction in AT III activity during pregnancy, suggesting a low reserve.[41] The finding of a normal AT III value during pregnancy would be inconsistent with the diagnosis of DIC.

Euglobulin lysis time is a crude but practical measure of plasminogen activator and plasmin activity.

DIAGNOSIS AND MANAGEMENT OF COAGULATION DISORDERS

DISSEMINATED INTRAVASCULAR COAGULATION

A number of diseases unique to pregnancy or complications of pregnancy are associated with intravascular clotting abnormalities. These include abruptio placentae, the preeclampsia/eclampsia syndrome, amniotic fluid embolus, saline abortion, the dead fetus syndrome, and

TABLE 68–4. CONDITIONS ASSOCIATED WITH DIC

Obstetrical Accidents
Abruptio placentae
Dead fetus syndrome
Amniotic fluid embolus
Saline abortion
Preeclampsia eclampsia syndrome
Septicemia
Gram-negative (endotoxin)
Gram-positive (mucopolysaccharides?)
Viremia (varicella)
Intravascular Hemolysis
Multiple transfusions (banked whole blood)
Hemolytic transfusion reaction
Vascular Disorders
Acid-Base Imbalance
Hypoxic-Ischemic Endothelial Damage

Modified from Weiner CP. Treatment of clotting disorders during pregnancy. In: Sciarra JJ, ed. Gynecology and obstetrics. Vol. 3. Philadelphia: JB Lippincott, 1988:2, with permission.

septic abortion/shock. DIC is not a single clinical entity but an intermediate mechanism of a well-defined disease (Table 68-4).[47] It exists whenever there is abnormal, intravascular activation of the clotting cascade, causing excess consumption of at least the soluble components. DIC is a continuum in which a variety of symptoms may appear. Its multiple presentations include hemorrhage, thrombosis, and laboratory abnormalities.

The clinical presentation of DIC provides insight into the laboratory abnormalities, because plasmin generation occurs simultaneously with cascade activation. Diffuse thrombosis is the presentation when the intravascular clotting process dominates and secondary fibrinogenolysis is minimal (eg, malignancy).[48] Hemorrhage is the clinical presentation when secondary fibrinogenolysis dominates and FSP are present in a high concentration (eg, abruptio).[48] Sometimes, hemorrhage and thrombosis may occur concurrently. Finally, as is common in the obstetric patient, DIC may be present as a chronic disorder without clinical signs, but only manifested by laboratory abnormalities.

Pathophysiology

The clinical disorders that trigger DIC produce excess systemic generation of thrombin and plasmin (Fig. 68-2). Once abnormal coagulation has begun, the pathophysiology becomes intricate (Fig. 68-3). Normally, fibrin monomer polymerizes as insoluble fibrin. The fibrin-bound plasminogen begins controlled fibrin degradation and free plasmin is rapidly inactivated by inhibitors. However, if excess plasmin is generated, fibrin *and* fibrinogen are degraded. These FSP bind to fibrin monomer, preventing polymerization and inhibiting the platelet-mediated primary phase of coagulation.[49] The soluble fibrin–FSP complexes are the basis for paracoagulation tests such as protamine sulfate and ethanol gelation.[50] A high concentration of circulating plasmin can inactivate/degrade factors V, VII, IX, and

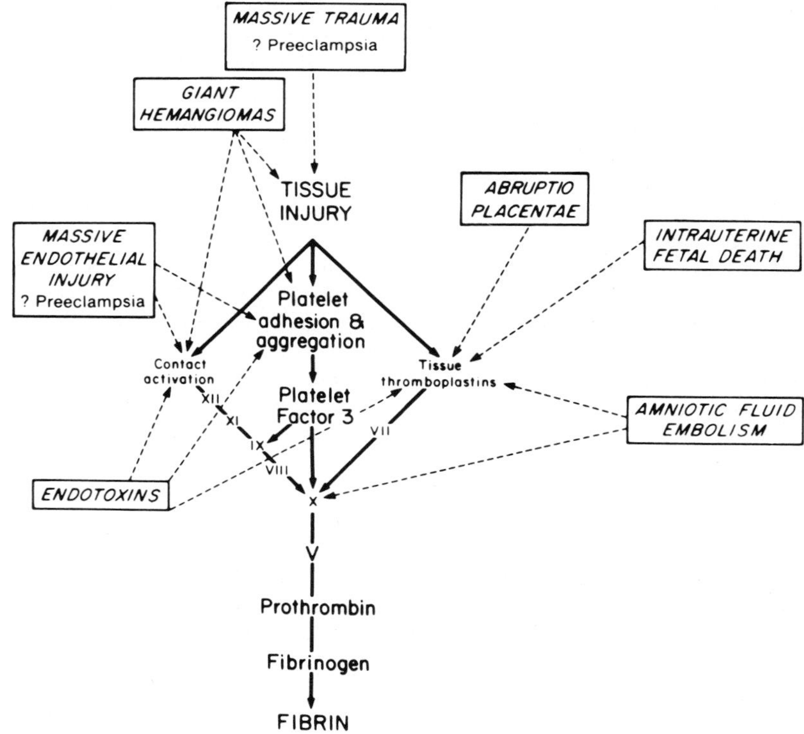

FIGURE 68–2. Factors that initiate disseminated intravascular coagulation (DIC). The processes illustrated are theoretical in many ways. (Modified from Wintrobe MM. Acquired coagulation disorders: diffuse intravascular coagulation. In: Wintrobe MM, Lee GR, Boss DR, et al, eds. Clinical hematology. 8th ed. Philadelphia: Lea & Febiger, 1981:1216.)

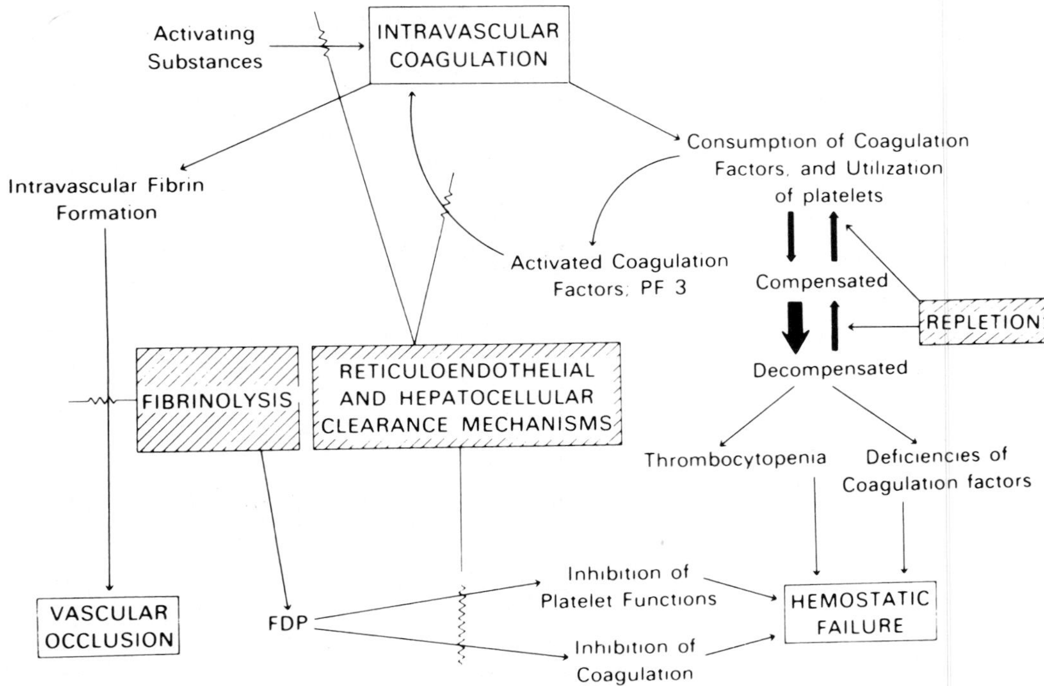

FIGURE 68–3. Outline of pathophysiology after abnormal coagulation has been triggered. (From Wintrobe MM. Acquired coagulation disorders: diffuse intravascular coagulation. In: Wintrobe MM, Lee GR, Boggs DR, et al, eds. Clinical hematology. 8th ed. Philadelphia: Lea & Febiger, 1981:1215.)

XI, ACTH, growth hormone, insulin, complement, and other plasma proteins. Fibrin monomer, which does polymerize within the free circulation, is ultimately filtered out by the microvasculature, forming "plugs" that restrict blood flow. The resulting tissue hypoxia leads to ischemic necrosis of multiple end organs. Thrombocytopenia results from platelet entrapment within the fibrin-webbed microvasculature. RBC contact with fibrin produces hemolysis, releasing components capable of propagating the DIC cycle. If factor XII activation occurs, the kinin system will be activated. Excess bradykinin produces several common clinical manifestations of DIC such as systemic hypotension and increased vascular permeability.[51,52] Plasmin activates the first and third complement components, causing cell lysis, immunoadherence, and other immune phenomena.[53] It is easy to see that, once begun, the cycle of DIC is self-propagating.

Diagnosis

A patient who hemorrhages secondary to acute DIC has multiple hemostatic defects and bleeds from at least three sites at once (ie, melena, hematuria, epistaxis, hemoptysis, oozing from puncture wounds, purpura, or petechiae). Shock associated with acute DIC is often out of proportion to the volume of blood loss. Renal failure is common. In contrast, patients with chronic DIC rarely have significant bleeding or other clinical findings. These patients are more likely to present with minor mucosal bleeding, hematuria, epistaxis, or easy bruisability. They are at greater risk to decompensate with an additional hemostatic stress.[47] Settings for chronic DIC include malignancy, preeclampsia, and intrauterine fetal demise.

Laboratory confirmation of the clinical diagnosis should be obtained. Characteristic findings include prolongation of the PT, prolongation of the PTT, an abnormal platelet count (low and high), abnormal clotting factor concentrations, elevated FSP, abnormal clot retraction, reduced antithrombin III activity, a positive protamine sulfate test, leukocytosis, and schistocytosis on a smear of peripheral blood. In acute DIC, each parameter can be abnormal. In chronic DIC, only individual factor consumption rates may be elevated, while many of the previously noted tests remain normal.

Over 50% of the patients with acute DIC have both a prolonged PT and PTT. Rarely, these times are shortened in a patient with chronic DIC. Fifteen percent of patients with acute DIC have normal FSP levels. Ten percent of acute DIC patients have negative paracoagulation tests.[47] It is possible that the FSP are degraded past the point of detection for commercially available assays. Due to changes in renal clearance, the actual FSP titer may have little clinical relevance.

AT III is the major in vivo inhibitor of thrombin production and is the most sensitive laboratory parameter for the diagnosis of DIC.[54] Abnormal consumption of

AT III by either thrombin or another activated serine protein must occur for DIC to be present. Usually, the level of AT III declines as consumption exceeds production. However, in patients with malignancy and diabetes, AT III can behave as an acute phase reactant and may be normal or slightly increased despite rapid consumption. Thus, sensitivity of the test is reduced. In contrast, the sensitivity of AT III measurement to excess clotting activity seems to increase. During normal pregnancy, plasma AT III activity is essentially unchanged.[55] AT III activity declines in the presence of systemic illnesses during pregnancy, such as pyelonephritis, viral infection, and bacterial pneumonia.[41] In the non-pregnant patient, a decrease in AT III activity with infection is unusual unless overwhelming sepsis occurs.

Treatment

Therapy must be tailored to fit the pathophysiology and the clinical manifestations. Mortality from DIC can result from either the coagulopathy or the underlying disease. The primary therapeutic goal is to treat the underlying disorder and remove the triggering event (Table 68-5). When accompanied by hemorrhage, treatment must be accompanied by aggressive support of blood volume and pressure (ie, volume replacement with crystalloids and colloids, antibiotic therapy, pressor medications). Hypoxic ischemia due to hypotension and hypoperfusion damages the microvascular endothelium, providing a new trigger for the DIC cycle. Underreplacement is a common error. In the vast majority of obstetric-related DIC syndromes, these steps alone constitute adequate therapy. Component replacement (platelets, cryoprecipitate, or fresh frozen plasma) may occasionally be helpful to aid oozing from a wound associated with laboratory abnormalities. Replacement does not add "fuel to the fire" if the underlying cause of the DIC has been treated and the cycle broken.[56]

TABLE 68–5. SUGGESTED THERAPY FOR ACUTE DIC

Treatment or Removal of the Triggering Event
Evacuation of the uterus
Antibiotics
Volume replacement and expansion (crystalloid, Plasmanate, albumin)
Component Therapy
Packed red cells
Platelets
Fresh frozen plasma
Prothrombin complex
Anticoagulant Therapy
Low dose heparin
Heparin
Antiplatelet drugs (chronic DIC)
Antithrombin III concentrates
Inhibition of Residual Fibrinolysis
e-Amino caproic acid
Caution: ventricular arrhythmias, hypotension, hypokalemia

From Weiner CP. Treatment of clotting disorders during pregnancy. In: Sciarra JJ, ed. Gynecology and obstetrics. Vol. 3. Philadelphia: JB Lippincott, 1988:4, with permission.

Anticoagulation should be initiated only when the aforementioned measures fail to correct a clinically significant DIC. This situation is exceedingly rare in the obstetric patient. Observation for at least 4 hours after treatment of the underlying disease (if the hemorrhage is not severe) is recommended prior to starting anticoagulants. This allows adequate time for laboratory evaluation to identify the precise clotting defect.

In the past, large quantities of heparin have been given for anticoagulation. Its efficacy was unpredictable. The unpredictable response to heparin may be partially caused by the variable AT III concentration at the time of anticoagulation.[57,58] AT III activity should be determined during the observational period if heparin therapy is contemplated.

In many instances, low-dose heparin appears to be as effective as the larger dose of heparin for the treatment of DIC and minimizes the possibility of exacerbating the hemorrhage. A reasonable approach consists of the subcutaneous administration of heparin (5000 U) every 8 to 12 hours. The PTT should normalize with treatment. AT III concentrate alone has been used successfully to treat acute DIC secondary to obstetric complications.[59,60] This concentrate has recently become available in the United States.

After the above therapy, a rare patient may continue to bleed secondary to residual fibrinogenolysis. This is one of two instances in obstetrics when antifibrinolytic agents (epsilon-amino caproic acid) may be of value for the treatment of DIC (see Amniotic Fluid Embolus).

Obstetric Causes

Pregnancy is a well documented hypercoagulable condition.[40] There is solid clinical and experimental evidence that pregnancy predisposes young women to develop DIC.[61,62] Six major pregnancy-related entities can be associated with DIC.

Preeclampsia/Eclampsia Syndrome. Overt DIC is uncommon in women with preeclampsia. Although thrombocytopenia is present in some 10% of women with severe preeclampsia/eclampsia, only a small percentage develop symptomatic bleeding.

However, there is now overwhelming evidence that a subclinical, consumptive coagulopathy is typical in women with the clinical diagnosis of preeclampsia. A decline in platelet number is one of the earliest laboratory signs of preeclampsia.[63] Platelet factor 4 and B-thromboglobulin are elevated.[64] These changes often occur prior to clinical onset of disease.[65] Fibrin-like material is often identified in renal and liver biopsy specimens from preeclamptic women.[66–68] A significant and pathologic decrease in AT III occurs in women with preeclampsia proportional to severity, which is secondary to increased consumption.[41,69,70] Factor VIII consumption increases by an amount that correlates with disease severity. These changes occur before clinical manifestations of the disease appear.[71–73] Fibrinopeptide A concentration is significantly elevated in women with preeclampsia.[45,74] The fibrinolytic activity of whole blood normally decreases between 30 and 32 weeks' gestation, but is further decreased in women with preeclampsia.[42] This coincides with the time preeclampsia most often manifests clinically. Women with chronic hypertension but no evidence of preeclampsia have none of these coagulation abnormalities. The observation that some women with the clinical diagnosis of preeclampsia do not show these changes is consistent with the reported 15% to 65% error in the clinical diagnosis of preeclampsia (definitive diagnosis based on renal biopsies).[75]

Clotting studies may help resolve diagnostic dilemmas in hypertensive women. Management decisions are often difficult in the preterm, hypertensive multipara suspected of having preeclampsia. Over 50% of the clinical diagnoses of preeclampsia are wrong in this instance if the findings on renal biopsy are taken as the ultimate arbitrator. Such errors may lead to a preterm delivery on the assumption that pharmacologic therapy is inappropriate. The measurement of plasma AT III activity may be helpful, because normal activity is uncommon in women with significant preeclampsia.[76] A trial of oral antihypertensive therapy may be a reasonable approach in a hospitalized patient whose AT III activity is normal in the absence of maternal or fetal distress.

All hypertensive women in labor should have a platelet count, because the degree of thrombocytopenia does not necessarily correlate with disease severity. No other studies are needed for vaginal delivery. A PT and PTT on admission would also be justified because of the increased likelihood of cesarean delivery in this population. If conduction anesthesia is planned, a bleeding time should be performed to evaluate platelet function. Measurement of FSP is unnecessary in the absence of significant hemorrhage. In the presence of DIC, AT III concentrate reportedly normalizes consumption.[60] In the absence of AT III concentrate, fresh frozen plasma should be used because of its high concentration of AT III. No other anticoagulation is needed. Rarely, a bleeding diathesis can develop in a preeclamptic woman based on component depletion. The effect of preeclampsia on the fetal/neonatal clotting system is unclear, although most investigations employing sensitive assays found no abnormalities in the absence of a compromised fetus. From the standpoint of prophylaxis in high-risk patients, low-dose aspirin may be effective when begun in the early to mid-second trimester.[77]

Abruptio Placentae. Abruptio placentae complicates approximately 0.8% of deliveries, yet accounts for 15% to 20% of perinatal mortality.[78] About 20% of women with abruptio placentae have a gross defect in clotting.[79] Thus, placental abruption is probably the most common obstetric cause of acute DIC. One fourth of patients with a gross clotting defect will hemorrhage postpartum. This excludes the women whose clotting disorder is based on massive blood loss and tissue hypoxia. These will be discussed later.

Massive extravascular clot formation with secondary component consumption does not explain the alterations in coagulation seen in women with placental abruption. The activation of the fibrinolytic system and consumption of the soluble components are out of proportion to the blood loss. Postpartum hemorrhage is most often preceded by hypofibrinogenemia, and FSP concentration has the greatest correlation with postpartum hemorrhage of any parameter.[80] This contrasts with placenta previa which, although associated with major blood loss, is rarely associated with elevated FSP in the absence of concurrent abruption.

The source of circulating FSP in patients with abruption is unclear. When both placenta and fetus are healthy, the fibrinolytic activity is similar in both uterine artery and vein.[80] FSP (and presumably plasminogen activator) increase significantly in the uterine vein effluent following normal delivery. A similar increase occurs following an abruption, even if the fetus and placenta remain in utero.[80] Thus, it appears that the process of placental separation itself contributes to the FSP elevation. The concentration of FSP continues to rise during labor if the placenta has only partially separated, and peaks shortly after complete placental separation. The response to delivery is dramatic, resulting in FSP clearance from the circulation within 12 to 24 hours.[81]

A partial understanding of abruptio and its associated postpartum hemorrhage has resulted from the investigation of the relationship between postpartum hemorrhage and FSP concentration. In vitro, a concentration of FSP higher than that usually found in the peripheral circulation inhibits myometrial contractility.[80] Due to the high concentration necessary, FSP would seem an unlikely cause of postpartum hemorrhage. However, evidence does exist to support a direct role for FSP. First, the concentration of FSP is higher in the uterine vein after placental separation than it is systemically. Second, the FSP concentration in the lochia of women with abruptio placentae is significantly higher than that in the lochia of women following a normal delivery.[80] Third, uterine inertia is uncommon unless the FSP exceed 330 μg/mL. Fourth, intravenous infusion of an antifibrinogenolytic agent reverses uterine inertia secondary to placental abruption, even when that inertia had previously been resistant to amniotomy and pitocin.[82]

The basic tenets of therapy for abruptio placentae follow the general guidelines for management of DIC. The uterus should be emptied and the blood volume vigorously supported with crystalloid, colloid, or blood products as necessary. Although coagulation components are rarely required antepartum for vaginal delivery, their use may be prudent if surgical intervention is contemplated. Oxytocin remains an effective stimulant of labor in most cases. Antifibrinolytic drugs have been reported to reverse uterine inertia resistant to oxytocin.

However, further experience with these potentially dangerous antifibrinolytic drugs is necessary before recommending them.[82] Once emptied, even the Couvelaire uterus responds well to oxytocin.

A chronic placental abruption is as difficult to manage as it is to diagnose. Accurate sonographic diagnosis is difficult. Patients with a suspected small abruption remote from term may be managed expectantly if their symptoms resolve, laboratory abnormalities do not exist, and fetal surveillance tests remain normal. With this possible exception, the diagnosis of placental abruption usually necessitates some type of intervention. The perinatal morbidity and mortality from abruptio placentae increase with delay. One large study observed that if the fetus was alive when the mother was admitted but subsequently died in utero, 75% of these deaths occurred more than 90 minutes after admission. Seventy percent of the perinatal mortality occurred 2 or more hours after the diagnosis of placental abruption was entered into the record.[78] Diagnostic error may be ultimately unavoidable if no significant abruption is to be missed. However, a cesarean section is not always necessary. If the labor progresses appropriately, the laboratory coagulation parameters are normal, the fetus is not in distress, and an emergency cesarean section can be performed, a closely observed labor is preferred. If any of these abnormalities are present, delivery should be effected immediately. An abnormal clotting profile unassociated with either fetal demise or distress is uncommon. The obstetrician should not be deceived by the normal fetal heart rate tracing.

Fetal Death Syndrome. The association between intrauterine fetal demise (IUFD) and a subsequent coagulopathy is well established. This syndrome may occur following the death of a singleton fetus or of a fetus in a multiple gestation. The onset of fetal death syndrome (FDS) is gradual. Most laboratory abnormalities are not detectable until 3 to 4 weeks after the demise,[83] although the concentration of fibrinopeptide A rises within days. Manifestations of the coagulopathy include varying degrees of hypofibrinogenemia, decreased plasminogen, decreased AT III activity, increased generation of both fibrinopeptide A and FSP, and thrombocytopenia.[84] The laboratory picture is consistent with a true chronic DIC condition.[85] Its cause is unknown. One unsubstantiated theory suggests that tissue thromboplastin leaks from the decaying fetus into the maternal circulation. Fibrinolysis does not appear to contribute significantly to FDS, because antifibrinolytics are of little benefit.[84]

Approximately 80% of women with an IUFD labor spontaneously within 2 to 3 weeks. This is the basis for the traditional recommendation to await spontaneous labor. One third of undelivered patients (6% of all pregnancies with an IUFD) will develop a progressive hemostatic defect 4 to 5 weeks after the demise if left undelivered. The incidence of coagulopathy increases with the duration of the delay, but only 1% to 2% of these women suffer a significant hemorrhagic complication. The advent and availability of prostaglandin E_2 has simplified management considerably. The treatment of a medically stable patient with an intrauterine, singleton fetal demise is now delivery.

A dilemma arises when the fetus who has died is part of a preterm multiple gestation. This may become a more common problem as the incidence of selective feticide increases. It had been held that chronic DIC secondary to an IUFD is irreversible, unless either heparin is given or delivery is effected. However, delivery would put the surviving fetus at risk for complications of prematurity. Several recent reports document a limited duration of the coagulopathy secondary to the death of one fetus in a multiple gestation.[86–88]

There are also fetal implications in multiple gestations with FDS. If the pregnancy was allowed to continue and the gestations were monozygotic with vascular anastomoses, "thromboplastic" material might theoretically embolize to the surviving fetus, producing fetal DIC, multicystic encephalomalacia, or other structural anomalies. Whether this actually occurs is unclear.[89–92] Chronic heparin therapy would not protect the fetus because heparin does not cross the placenta.

Heparin is the treatment of choice for the mother whose coagulopathy is associated with FDS. Most women require 5000 to 10,000 U subcutaneously twice a day rather than a larger dose of heparin, which would prolong the PTT. There is one report of a triplet gestation in which 20,000 U/day of heparin was inadequate to reverse the laboratory abnormalities.[88] This resistance to heparin may reflect a decreased concentration of AT III. Theoretically, it should be possible to titrate the heparin dose based on normalization of the fibrinopeptide A level. A prompt increase in plasma fibrinogen should follow.

Septic Abortion. Another well documented obstetric cause of DIC is septic abortion.

Pathophysiology. Most patients with septic abortion and probably all patients with septic shock have altered coagulation if tested thoroughly.[93] The coagulopathy is consistent with true DIC accompanied by various degrees of fibrinolysis.[94] There is a high correlation between the severity of the disease and the degree of coagulopathy. Bacterial endotoxin is likely the initiating mechanism. Animal and clinical studies demonstrate an increased sensitivity to bacterial endotoxin during pregnancy.[95–98] The shock syndrome has been described as an endotoxin-mediated Shwartzman's reaction. It results from a complex interaction between endotoxin, the vascular endothelium, platelets, and complement, ultimately generating histamines, kinins, and serotonin. The net result is hypotension, hypoxia, and acidosis, which perpetuate the cycle of kinin activation.

The main clinical findings of septic shock are attributable to DIC. Kinin activation occurs early in the clotting cascade. The amount of kallikrein generated correlates directly with the severity of the shock.[51] Massive perfusion disturbances are created within the microvasculature by fibrin emboli that exacerbate the effects of blood stasis and hypotension. Although the kidney is rarely unaffected, death most often results from pulmonary complications.[99,100]

Treatment. The two goals of therapy are prevention and treatment of the underlying disease. The general protocol for the treatment of DIC applies with a few minor modifications. Aggressive antibiotic therapy and evacuation of the uterus in the absence of shock are the foundation of treatment.

A high index of suspicion is needed for early detection of developing shock. When septic shock is present, crystalloid or colloid fluid replacement should be guided by a pulmonary artery catheter. The pulmonary capillary wedge pressure is nearly always low. Pulmonary edema resulting from pulmonary capillary permeability defects render the central venous pressure (CVP) erroneously high. It should not be used alone to determine volume replacement.[97] Lactated Ringer's solution should also be avoided because it might potentiate the metabolic acidosis.[101] The hematocrit should be maintained above 36% with packed red blood cells. High doses of corticosteroids (30 mg/kg) may be of use stabilizing biomembranes, exerting a positive inotropic effect upon the heart, dilating the vasculature and preventing beta-endorphin release by the pituitary.[102–104] In reference to the latter, pretreatment with naloxone may reduce the severity of septic shock.[105,106] Survival of an episode of septic shock correlates well with estimated survival time from the underlying disease. The mortality from septic shock in an otherwise healthy patient is 20%, compared to 80% in cancer patients.[102]

Eradication of the septic source leads to rapid resolution of the coagulopathy. The application of anticoagulation is controversial. Because sepsis is associated with widespread activation of the clotting cascade, and microvascular fibrin thrombi would further disrupt flow, heparin would seem logical to prevent further fibrin generation. However, it neither prevents kinin activation nor eliminates platelet aggregation.

The published clinical experience with septic shock does not resolve this controversy. One review concluded that survival was significantly increased after the first 24 hours if the patient received heparin, while a similar report (covering many of the same studies) noted no difference in survival.[107,108] The heterogeneity of both the underlying diseases and the AT III concentration may be responsible for the differences in patient response to heparin. In the absence of a definitive study, heparin therapy in septic shock becomes a matter of physician choice. Heparin therapy has also been suggested in the setting of profound hypofibrinogenemia and thrombocytopenia in conjunction with factor replacement. In this instance, the therapeutic goal is a PTT 1.5 to 2 times baseline. Coagulation factor replacement is best done with fresh frozen plasma, because cryoprecipitate has little AT III. However, in one situation, heparin administration does seem indicated. Prophylactic administration of heparin to women with septic abortions decreases the incidence of subsequent septic shock and reduces the level of soluble fibrin monomer to normal; 5000 U of subcutaneous heparin given two or three times daily is sufficient.[93,109]

Saline Abortion. Increased consumption of intrinsic clotting cascade factors, increased FSP, and decreased platelet count occur during saline abortion.[110–114] The syndrome is usually subclinical and the cause is unknown. Clotting abnormalities precede both the onset of uterine contractions and the occurrence of fetal death and may occur within 1 to 3 hours of saline administration. They may then resolve prior to delivery of the abortus. Hypertonic saline crosses the chorioamnion into the maternal circulation.[110,111] Presumably, this accounts for the increase in maternal intravascular volume and urinary sodium excretion observed in women undergoing saline abortion.[111] Yet intravascular volume expansion alone is inadequate to account for the decrease in platelets and soluble clotting components. Low-dose heparin prevents the development of DIC.[115]

Occasionally, clinical bleeding occurs. If one defines a significant hemorrhage as requiring a transfusion, 1% to 2% of women undergoing a saline abortion experience hemorrhage.[116] In contrast, only 0.3% of women aborted with intra-amniotic urea and prostaglandin F_2 alpha hemorrhage.

Amniotic Fluid Embolus. Amniotic fluid embolus (AFE) complicates between 1 per 7000 and 1 per 300,000 deliveries. Despite the small numbers of AFE cases, 5% to 10% of the maternal mortality in industrialized countries is attributed to AFE. The associated mortality rate approximates 80%. Case reports without mortality may be misleading, because many reported survivors of AFE have findings equally consistent with other diagnoses.[117–119] As a result of its rarity, there are no large therapeutic trials to guide the treatment of AFE.

Diagnosis. An AFE may occur at any time during the peripartal period, although the classic description involves an elderly multiparous woman with a large, term, meconium-stained infant, in the midst of or just having completed a vigorous labor with intact membranes when profound cardiovascular collapse occurs. This is Phase 1. Phase 2 begins 0.5 to 4 hours after the first phase, with the onset of uterine bleeding refractory to oxytocin, bleeding from old puncture sites, and easy bruisability.[120] There are few adequately documented cases of hemorrhage associated with AFE without preceding cardiovascular symptoms.

From the diagnostic standpoint, it is difficult to document an AFE without a postmortem examination. It had been stated that the presence of fetal debris in a blood sample drawn from a right-sided cardiac catheter is diagnostic of AFE.[121] The minimum volume of an AFE necessary to evoke the syndrome or to be detectable in plasma by histologic techniques is not known.

The conclusion was based on a unique and unrepeated study of the transfer of radiolabeled red blood cells from the amniotic cavity into the maternal circulation.[122] There is now clear evidence that fetal debris can be found in samples obtained from the right heart of asymptomatic women.[123] Therefore, the finding of fetal squames in a right-sided cardiac blood sample is consistent with but not diagnostic of AFE.

Pathophysiology. The pathophysiology of AFE is not completely understood. Phase 1 involves occurrence of the AFE with associated pulmonary vasospasm and interstitial edema. The result is myocardial necrosis with characteristic electrocardiographic (ECG) changes.[124] It was once thought that the pulmonary arterial pressure was increased and cardiac output decreased secondary to increased afterload. But recent studies with Swan-Ganz catheters reveal left ventricular failure without pulmonary hypertension.[125] A mixed respiratory–metabolic acidosis results. The appearance of pulmonary edema and shock is evidence of worsening clinical status.

Only 45% of patients survive Phase 1. The survivors are at risk to develop severe coagulopathy and uterine atony during Phase 2. There are few hematologically well-studied cases of AFE in the literature.[126–128] Each reports a profound excess of fibrinolytic activity as demonstrated by decreased plasminogen levels, increased plasmin activator, or a very high concentration of FSP. Laboratory abnormalities precede the clinical manifestation by 30 to 60 minutes.[124,126] Numerous soluble clotting factors are decreased, and in most cases there is hypofibrinogenemia. Excessive plasmin activation results in nonspecific proteolysis of various proenzymes. Because fibrinopeptide A has yet to be studied during AFE, it is difficult to predict how much of the reduced clotting component concentration represents proenzyme degradation versus thrombin-mediated consumption. This information would impact on therapy.

As noted above, the amniotic fluid volume necessary to cause the syndrome is unknown. If 20% of the total amniotic fluid volume were to enter the circulation as an intravascular bolus, a 1:20 to 1:30 dilution would occur within minutes. The resulting concentration of amniotic fluid is much less than that necessary to disturb coagulation in vitro. In addition, the number of fetal squames in the maternal pulmonary vasculature does not correlate with clinical findings. Therefore, the AFE syndrome may not be the result of the volume of intravascular amniotic fluid per se, because it is the result of an abnormal substance within the amniotic fluid.[129]

The cause of the coagulopathy remains controversial. When amniotic fluid is added to human plasma, it accelerates clotting along both the extrinsic and intrinsic pathways through factor X.[130] This procoagulant effect persists after filtering the amniotic fluid and correlates with both gestational age and phospholipid content.[131,132] Parenteral administration of unfiltered but not filtered amniotic fluid to the dog evokes the syndrome, showing that there are species differences.[133] Human amniotic fluid collected during labor is much more toxic to the cat than amniotic fluid from nonlaboring women.[134] Prostaglandins and leukotrienes, each present in increased concentrations during labor, can mimic some of the hemodynamic and procoagulant effects of the AFE syndrome.[135] In the rabbit, pretreatment with an inhibitor of the lipoxygenase system (including leukotrienes) prevents death following intravascular injection of amniotic fluid.[136]

Controversy exists over the cause of hypofibrinogenemia in AFE syndrome. Some investigators favor primary fibrinogenolysis as the mechanism rather than a consumptive coagulopathy with secondary fibrinolysis.[127,128] The finding of fibrin thrombi scattered through the pulmonary vascular bed argues against primary fibrinogenolysis as the sole explanation. Alternatively, cardiovascular collapse coupled with endothelial abrasion from particulate emboli might produce sufficient damage to initiate fibrin generation. In this instance, fibrinopeptide A would be elevated. Thrombin-mediated fibrin generation secondary to pulmonary endothelial damage would activate both plasmin and kinins. In the absence of antiplasmin, these substances perpetuate their own generation. Thus, if thrombin generation occurred in the setting of excess plasmin proactivator (supplied by the amniotic fluid), a coagulopathy dominated by fibrin-fibrinogenolysis could result.[137] Any recent fibrin thrombi within the uterine spiral arteries and at previous puncture sites would lyse, and oozing would result. As discussed under placental abruption, the high level of FSP could inhibit uterine contractility, leading to frank hemorrhage.

Treatment. A well-documented, successful therapeutic protocol does not exist, due to the rarity of AFE. The known pathophysiology suggests a few minor changes to the protocol used to treat DIC.

During Phase 1, therapy is directed toward cardiovascular and ventilatory support. A pulmonary artery catheter should be placed without delay. A clotting profile and heparinized sample for histologic study, as well as several extra tubes of citrated blood for later study, should next be drawn from the catheter. Liberal use of dopamine (or similar agent) and colloids as dictated by the information obtained from the pulmonary artery catheter is recommended for cardiovascular support. Fluid overload must be carefully avoided. Rapid digitalization may help.

Intubation is the key to ventilatory support. Positive end-expiratory pressure (PEEP) has been suggested, but its use too should be guided by parameters obtained from the pulmonary artery catheter. If, for example, the contributions of interstitial edema and capillary permeability abnormalities to pulmonary edema are minimal, the lungs may remain compliant. With compliant lungs, PEEP could increase right ventricular afterload, produce bulging of the interventricular septum into the left ventricle, and decrease stroke volume and cardiac output. Such an event would more than offset any ventilatory gain from PEEP.[102] Both corticosteroids and aminophylline have been used to treat coexistent bronchospasm.

It is unclear whether the AFE-associated coagulopathy can be prevented. In one report, a patient survived a presumed AFE after administration of a small dose of heparin. Although laboratory evidence of a clotting abnormality occurred, the patient did not hemorrhage.[138] Heparin would be the logical choice to blunt cascade activation and the resulting plasmin generation. The quantity of heparin necessary is as yet unknown. Knowledge of the fibrinopeptide A level would again be helpful here. If the fibrinopeptide A concentration was high, it would indicate massive thrombin generation and the need for large quantities of heparin. Based on this one case report, a single intravenous heparin bolus of 3000 to 5000 U as soon as the diagnosis is made would appear to be an option.[136]

Once fibrin-fibrinogenolysis is well established, component replacement alone may be adequate.[119,126,139] Should the patient fail to respond to this plan, the administration of an antifibrinolytic agent (epsilon-amino caproic acid or aprotonin) should be considered. The dose of e-amino caproic acid is 4 g to 6 g every 4 to 6 hours.

Other Obstetrically Related Causes. Other purported causes of DIC include placenta previa, placenta accreta, degenerating leiomyomas, and hydatidiform mole.[140–143] Some of the data are consistent with DIC and secondary fibrinolysis, while other reports merely reflect extravascular consumption with associated intravascular depletion.

Nonobstetric Causes

Antibiotics. A continually growing number of broad spectrum antibiotics are associated with hypoprothrombinemia (Table 68-6). Malnourished patients are at highest risk. There are two mechanisms known.[144,145] First, a vitamin K deficiency results from depletion of the bowel flora that synthesize the vitamin K. Second, a cephalosporin metabolite, methyltetrazolethiol, directly inhibits hepatic prothrombin synthesis. A prothrombin time should be obtained periodically on patients at risk and prior to surgery. The administration of vitamin K reverses the abnormalities. These same antibiotics augment warfarin anticoagulation by depleting bowel flora and by displacing warfarin from albumin.[144]

Some antibiotics (see Table 68-6) inhibit platelet function. The primary mechanism of action is decreased adenosine diphosphate (ADP) mediated platelet aggregation.[146,147] One metabolite of penicillin is thought to bind the platelet membrane ADP receptor. Antiplatelet effects are dose-related and are detectable 12 to 24 hours after first administering the drug. They may persist for up to 12 days, suggesting that the megakaryocytes are affected. These problems are usually seen in the setting of high-dose penicillin or cephalosporin administration for severe gram-negative infections.

TABLE 68-6. ANTIBIOTICS AND HEMOSTASIS

Hypoprothrombinemic
Ampicillin
Cephamandole
Cefoperazone
Moxalactam
Penicillin G
Tetracycline
Chloramphenicol
Inhibit Platelet Function
Carbenicillin
Sulbenicillin
Ticarcillin
Piperacillin
Mezlocillin
Azlocillin
Cephalothin (asymptomatic)
Moxalactam
Cefazolin (with uremia)
Coumadin Effect
Nalidixic acid
Sulfonamides
Metronidazole
Chloramphenicol
Rifampin

From Weiner CP. Treatment of clotting disorders during pregnancy. In: Sciarra JJ, ed. Gynecology and obstetrics. Vol. 3. Philadelphia: JB Lippincott, 1988:12, with permission.

Acquired Inhibitors. Specific inhibitors of individual clotting factors have been identified in previously healthy women during pregnancy. These frequently are antibodies. Inhibitors of factors V, VIII:C, VIII:RCoF, IX, XI, and XIII have all been reported in previously healthy women.[148–154] The two most common inhibitors are a lupus anticoagulant and an antifactor VIII antibody.

A factor deficit is most easily differentiated from an inhibitor by performing a 1:1 mix of the patient's plasma with normal plasma. If the clotting time remains prolonged, an inhibitor is present. However, a low titer inhibitor may become apparent only after incubating the plasma mix. An antibody inhibitor usually shows progressive, time-dependent prolongation of the clotting time.

Lupus-like inhibitors, or antiphospholipid antibodies, were first found in patients with systemic lupus erythematosus. They have now been identified in association with a wide variety of diseases and drugs, including chlorpromazine and penicillin.[154–156] An anticardiolipin antibody is one type of antiphospholipid antibody. It blocks the binding of phospholipid and interferes with the action of the preformed prothrombinase complex.[157,158] As a result, both the PT and PTT may be prolonged. The addition of phospholipid corrects the abnormality. Incubation of lupus anticoagulant with normal plasma does not decrease clotting time further.

The presence of a lupus anticoagulant has significant obstetric implications. It is associated with recurrent fetal demise, congenital heart block, and intrauterine growth retardation.[149,159–161] The fetal heart block is secondary to an associated antibody, anti-SS-A (Ro), which binds RNA in the right atrial wall.[162] Women with lupus and an inhibitor have a worse perinatal prognosis than those with lupus and no inhibitor. A history of a prior fetal demise, when combined with an inhibitor, is associated with the highest perinatal death rate.[163] Factor VIII is not decreased and bleeding is uncommon. Rather, these women are at highest risk for thrombosis.

During pregnancy, there is general agreement that treatment is beneficial, but the optimal regimen is unclear. Several regimens have been tried judging outcome on the basis of pre- and post-pregnancy loss rates.[164,165] Treatment is begun after organogenesis has been completed (12w). The most frequently tried combination has been prednisone, 30 mg to 60 mg/day, in order to reduce the inhibitor titer in most patients, and aspirin, 75 mg to 81 mg/day. If the inhibitor titer does not decline on this regimen, azathioprine 75 mg/day has been suggested. Therapy is continued until delivery. However, caution is needed. Recently, prednisone therapy has been reported to worsen the outcome of pregnancies complicated by prior fetal demise, and low-dose aspirin was not beneficial.[163]

Factor VIII inhibitors are associated with hemorrhage indistinguishable clinically from hemophilia.[152] These inhibitors are usually an IgG class antibody that therefore may cross the placenta. Only the PTT is prolonged. This syndrome frequently presents as a catastrophic, delayed postpartum hemorrhage.[148,150–152] The diagnosis of a factor VIII inhibitor is usually missed or made after surgical intervention for presumed uterine atony. The inhibitor may disappear within 18 months of delivery. Once gone, there are no reports of recurrence during a subsequent pregnancy.

The treatment available for patients with factor VIII inhibitor is unsatisfactory.[166] Factor VIII replacement is usually ineffective and may actually increase the antibody titer. Three other treatment options exist. First, bovine or porcine factor VIII concentrate, which may have a lower affinity for the antibody, can be used. Second, a continuous, slow infusion of concentrate might be more effective than bolus administration based on the time dependency of the antibody–antigen interaction. Neither of these two options has been documented to be clinically effective. A third option is administration of activated vitamin K-dependent concentrates. Corticosteroids, immunosuppressants, exchange transfusion, and plasmapheresis are ineffective.

HEREDITARY COAGULOPATHIES

The hereditary coagulopathies comprise the smallest group of patients suffering a clotting abnormality seen by the practicing obstetrician. A genetically determined defect has been identified at most points in the coagulation cascade. This discussion focuses on the more common of these defects.

Von Willebrand's Syndrome

Von Willebrand's syndrome (VWS) is a heterogeneous group of disorders usually inherited as an autosomal dominant trait. One especially severe form is inherited as an autosomal recessive trait.[167] Clinically, VWS involves mucocutaneous, post-traumatic, and postoperative bleeding. It may occasionally present as menorrhagia or postpartum hemorrhage. VWS can be difficult to diagnose, because only moderate to severe forms are characterized by a prolonged bleeding time. Inconsistently abnormal bleeding times are common in patients with milder forms. Therefore, a single normal factor VIII level or bleeding time does not exclude the diagnosis of VWS.

Factor VIII is a multimer. The VIII related cofactor (VIII:RCoF) protein serves as a carrier plate for the factor VIII related antigen (VIII:RA) and factor VIII coagulant (VIII:C) protein. It is, however, possible that VIII:RCoF and VIII:RA are parts of the same protein. VWS is identified by a qualitative or quantitative deficiency of VIII:RCoF. This is the portion of the factor VIII complex necessary for in vitro ristocetin-mediated platelet aggregation as well as for platelet adherence to the endothelium. The two most common forms of VWS are classic (Type I) and variant I (Type IIA). Each is associated with a prolonged bleeding time, decreased platelet adhesiveness, and decreased levels of VIII:C, VIII:RA, and VIII:RCoF. The lack of the carrier protein may cause decreased production or increased destruction of VIII:C and VIII:RA. The variant is a qualitative VIII:RA disorder, while the classic is a deficiency state.[168,169] Selective replacement of VIII:C does not correct the bleeding time. VIII:RCoF administration not only corrects the bleeding time, but also stimulates a transient increase in VIII:RA and VIII:C out of proportion to the amount of VIII:RCoF infused. The clinical risk of hemorrhage in patients with VWD correlates best with either the VIII:RCoF concentration or bleeding time.[170]

Patients with either classic and variant VWS have been investigated during pregnancy.[169,171–178] Labor and delivery often proceeds uneventfully, because VIII:C, VIII:RA, and VIII:RCoF usually increase to hemostatic levels during pregnancy. This gradual increase (when it occurs) starts after 11 to 12 weeks gestation. However, bear in mind that the increase is neither uniform in occurrence nor degree.[174,177] Therefore, it should not be assumed that factor VIII complex is increasing. Further, the individual components decrease postpartum at a varying rate, which could account for the 20% incidence of postpartum hemorrhage.[169,174,176,177] Patients who spontaneously or electively abort are at significant risk for hemorrhage. A baseline VIII:RCoF should be obtained early in pregnancy and again once or twice in the third trimester should the initial value be abnormal.

The need for transfusion support is determined by the degree to which the VIII:RCoF normalizes during pregnancy. In the absence of a significant surgical challenge, a 50% level of VIII:RCoF is sufficient for most hemostatic stresses.[174] But delivery constitutes a profound hemostatic challenge. In women with clinically mild disease whose indices normalize antepartum, prophylactic transfusion of cryoprecipitate is not needed for vaginal delivery, although an episiotomy should be avoided, as should the deep injection of a local anesthetic and conduction anesthesia. Cryoprecipitate should be available in case of emergency. Prophylactic transfusion of cryoprecipitate is indicated for vaginal delivery if the VIII:RCoF level fails to reach 80% by term. Postpartum, serial VIII:RCoF levels/bleeding times are obtained and cryoprecipitate therapy given for 7 days to prevent delayed hemorrhage. Cryoprecipitate should be given regardless of the laboratory parameters to all but the mildest cases of VWD if cesarean section is contemplated. Enough cryoprecipitate should be given to raise the VIII:RCoF level above 100%. Postoperatively, the VIII:RCoF level is maintained at 100% until the abdominal sutures are removed.[174] Additional cryoprecipitate transfusions may not be necessary due to the associated increases in VIII:RA and VIII:C that occur in response to the first transfusion of cryoprecipitate or fresh frozen plasma. The cryoprecipitate dose is empiric. Fifteen to 20 units are usually necessary twice daily in severe disease. Antiplatelet drugs and intramuscular injections should be avoided.

The fetus is assumed affected unless proven otherwise. The use of a scalp electrode is precluded. Fetal hemorrhage during labor due to VWS is rare, although intracranial hemorrhage during labor has been reported. Circumcision should be avoided until the diagnosis is ruled out. Prenatal diagnosis is possible from fetal blood. Fetal factor VIII:RCoF can be measured by the technique of Weiss and coworkers.[179] Type I is usually a mild condition, so that cordocentesis can usually be performed without significant risk of maternal hemorrhage. Type IIA, however, can be severe and maternal transfusion of cryoprecipitate may be necessary prior to cordocentesis.[180]

Hemophilia A and B

Hemophilia A and B are characterized, respectively, by low levels of either factor VIII coagulant (VIII:C) or factor IX coagulant (IX:C) activity, and a normal to increased level of the factor-related antigen (RA). Both are X-linked and cannot be distinguished clinically from each other. Hemophilia affects 20/100,000 males; thus, an estimated 1/5,000 women are carriers.[181,182] Eighty-five percent of hemophilia is hemophilia A. One third of men with hemophilia have no family history of a bleeding disorder, suggesting their illness is the result of a spontaneous mutation.[183]

The smallest unit in the factor VIII complex is VIII:C. It contains the locus responsible for the coagulation activity of factor VIII. Coagulant activity can also be determined immunologically, using an antibody directed against this section of the multimer (VIII:CA).[184] The high molecular weight portion of the complex can be measured by an immunoassay of the factor VIII-related antigen (VIII:RA). This portion also contains the receptor site responsible for ristocetin-mediated platelet aggregation, VIII:RCoF or VIII:vWF, the von Willebrand's factor. An antibody exists for this receptor site as well. Factor IX may also be measured both by its coagulant activity (IX:C) and its immunologic presence (IX:RA).

The task of the obstetrician in reference to hemophilia includes carrier identification, treatment of the symptomatic pregnant women, and prenatal diagnosis. Because one X chromosome is randomly inactivated in each cell (lyonization), the average ratio of the related antigen to coagulant activity is 2:1. Measurement of this ratio allows the diagnosis of 80% to 90% of non-pregnant carrier women.[185–189] The application of an immunoassay for the coagulant activity has enhanced diagnostic accuracy. Although the ratio of antigen to coagulant activity increases with increasing gestational age to a variable degree, pregnant women should not be denied carrier analysis if prior to 20 weeks gestation. A higher percentage of carrier identification has been reported in the second trimester than in the non-pregnant state, for reasons unknown.[190]

Rarely, carriers of hemophilia are symptomatic. Those women whose VIII:C activity is less than 50% at delivery and who undergo cesarean section should be given cryoprecipitate adequate to elevate the VIII:C level above 80% prior to surgery and to keep it above 30% to 40% for 3 to 4 days postoperatively.[191] If the VIII:C level is less than 30%, cryoprecipitate should be given prior to delivery regardless of the type. In contrast to hemophilia A, fresh frozen plasma rather than cryoprecipitate is given to women with hemophilia B. Cryoprecipitate contains little active factor IX. Prothrombin complex concentrates are given only to patients with severe disease because of the risk of thrombosis.

Hemophilia A and B may be diagnosed prenatally by either DNA analysis or direct study of fetal blood. The method depends on the gestational age at which the patient is first seen and the degree to which the patient's family has been studied. The first step is to determine the karyotype. Prior to 10 weeks gestation, chorion villus sampling may be done and thereafter amniocentesis may be done. Because there seems to be a variety of possible deletions and point mutations involved, family members should be investigated. If the restriction fragment length polymorphism linkage studies of the family are informative, they can be applied for a definitive diagnosis. For diagnosis of hemophilia A, intragenic and extragenic probes (such as the recombinant DNA ST or DX13 probes) are used. Extragenic probes have a 4% risk of error due to recombination. Intragenic probes have a negligible risk of error from recombination.[192] All normal results should later be confirmed by coagulation studies of fetal blood.[180] By the midsecond trimester, definitive diagnosis of fetal hemophilia A is possible by measuring the ratio of VIII:RA to VIII:CA in a blood sample obtained by cordocentesis.[182,193,194] Prenatal diagnosis of an affected fetus changes intrapartum and early postnatal management. Intrapartum use of scalp electrodes, the vacuum extractor, forceps, and prolonged labor should be avoided.[180] Six to ten percent of hemophiliac neonates suffer a perinatal hemorrhagic complication.

Antithrombin III Deficiency

AT III is the major in vivo inhibitor of thrombin activity. The incidence of AT III deficiency in the general population is about 1 per 2000.[195] This makes AT III deficiency the most common clotting disorder in women. Forty to 70% of people with this autosomal dominant trait develop symptomatic thrombi.[195] Among those patients hospitalized for recurrent thrombi, 2% to 3% have an AT III deficiency.[196] An abnormality of tissue plasminogen activator release frequently accompanies AT III deficiency. Although this is a heterogeneous disorder on the molecular level, the defect tends to remain constant within families.[197] Therefore, prenatal diagnosis using linkage techniques is theoretically possible.

Pregnancy exponentially increases the risk of thrombosis in women with AT III deficiency.[198–201] AT III activity is not significantly altered by pregnancy. Approximately two-thirds of pregnant women with congenital AT III deficiency suffer thrombosis; 75% of these occur antepartum.[201] The risk of thrombosis increases if the patient has a history of thromboembolism, and can occur even after a first trimester abortion.

The ideal regimen for thrombosis prophylaxis during pregnancy of women with an AT III deficiency has until recently been somewhat controversial. One regimen employs subcutaneous heparin prior to conception through the first trimester, changes to oral anticoagulants from 13 until 36 weeks gestation, and then reinstitutes subcutaneous heparin. The use of oral anticoagulants makes this regimen undesirable. Another regimen employs subcutaneous heparin throughout the pregnancy and is the one we currently favor.[202] AT III concentrate can be given during labor or if a thrombosis develops. Fresh frozen plasma is less helpful than AT III concentrate. Recent series substantiate these recommendations.[198,201,203–205] The participants at the First World Symposium on Antithrombin III Deficiency in West Berlin in 1987 concluded that oral anticoagulation was unnecessary.[206]

Patients with AT III deficiency are resistant to heparin, so that a quantity of heparin required for a given effect is usually larger than in the nondeficient patient. Preliminary evidence suggests that effective prophylaxis requires enough heparin administered subcutaneously to prolong the activated partial thromboplastin time 5 to 10 seconds above the patient's baseline throughout the pregnancy and puerperium.[201] The PTT should be measured just prior to the next dose. When functional AT III activity is 40% to 50%, 20,000 to 45,000 IU/day of heparin is required. During an acute thrombotic episode, 40,000 to 80,000 IU/day is usually required to prolong the activated partial thromboplastin time 1.5 to 2 times above baseline.[201] AT III concentrate may also be of benefit. Heparin therapy is continued at least 4 weeks after completion of the pregnancy or the patient is converted over to chronic warfarin anticoagulation postpartum.[23] Danazol in a dose of 400 to 600 mg/day may increase the AT III activity so that anticoagulation is no longer necessary.[207–209] Warfarin, which is not known to affect AT III concentrations, may be used with the danazol to provide anticoagulation. The dose of warfarin may need to be reduced with continuing danazol therapy to prevent excessive anticoagulation.[209]

The newborn delivered to a woman with AT III deficiency is at risk for inheriting the disease. Possible neonatal complications include fatal thrombosis. The newborn's plasma AT III activity should be measured and, if less than 10%, fresh frozen plasma administered.

Protein C And Protein S And Other Inherited Coagulation Disorders

A number of other inherited coagulation disorders have implications for management in pregnancy. In general, small patient numbers preclude prospective trials of the recommended interventions, although some observations may be made.

Protein C is a serine protease that inactivates factors Va and VIIIa and stimulates endothelial cell release of plasminogen activator. Protein C deficiency is an autosomal dominant trait with incomplete penetrance. The heterozygous disorder is associated with a propensity for venous thrombosis in early adulthood.[28] The homozygous disorder can result in massive thrombosis during the neonatal period.[29] Intrauterine central nervous system infarction has been described in homozygous fetuses.[210] Pregnant patients may exhibit manifestations of protein C deficiency, presenting with thromboembolism.[211,212] Warfarin is the treatment of choice for this deficiency state, but during pregnancy full anticoagulation with heparin is advised.[212] A deficiency of protein S, a protein C cofactor, is also associated with outcomes similar to protein C.[213] Prenatal diagnosis is possible for each of these disorders, using cordocentesis.[214]

Factor V deficiency is an autosomal recessive disorder commonly associated with menorrhagia and easy bruisability, and rarely with hemarthrosis and intramuscular bleeding. The few reports suggest that factor V levels increase to near normal concentrations during pregnancy. The major risk to the pregnant patient is postpartum hemorrhage.[215–217] Fresh frozen plasma is the treatment of choice. A report of severe fetal central nervous system hemorrhage at birth and in utero exists.[218]

Factor XI deficiency is an autosomal recessive disorder most common among Jewish families. The severity of the effect varies in a manner unrelated to the factor XI level. Despite the slight decline in factor XI that occurs during normal pregnancy, these women tend to have pregnancies marked only by increased bleeding from lacerations.[219,220] Fresh frozen plasma to maintain the activity level above 20% during the labor, delivery, and postpartum periods is recommended.

Factor XII deficiency is an autosomal dominant trait, and affected women tolerate pregnancy well.[221] This deficiency does not result in clinically significant hemostatic abnormalities.

Factor XIII deficiency is an autosomal recessive disorder. Factor XIII declines during normal pregnancy, although women with a factor XIII deficiency reportedly tolerate pregnancy well. The risk of postpartum hemorrhage seems increased.[220] Case reports suggest the patient's factor XIII activity should be maintained above 1% to 2% by an intermittent infusion of 300 to 450 mL of fresh frozen plasma every 14 days or 500 units of concentrate every 21 days. Classically, a factor XIII deficiency firsts manifests in the neonate as delayed bleeding from the umbilical cord stump. The disorder has also been associated with increased fetal wastage.

PLATELET DISORDERS

Quantitative or qualitative platelet disorders are common causes of abnormal coagulation in a pregnant woman. Platelet disorders often manifest as bleeding from mucous membranes or into the skin. Other findings include easy bruising, epistaxis, gastrointestinal or gingival bleeding, hematuria, menorrhagia, and petechiae. Maternal or fetal central nervous system hemorrhage is the most serious complication.Because the maternal and fetal implications are serious, a thorough understanding of these platelet disorders is essential.

Thrombocytopenia

Thrombocytopenia is defined as a platelet count less than 150,000 platelets/mm^3. Primary bone marrow disorders such as leukemia, lymphomas, megaloblastic anemia, and metastatic malignancies can cause thrombocytopenia. However, this review will concentrate on the most likely and significant causes of isolated thrombocytopenia during pregnancy.

Thrombocytopenia may result from either decreased platelet production or increased platelet consumption/destruction. This distinction is based on measurement of the mean platelet volume and a bone marrow evaluation. When production is down, megakaryocytes are decreased; when production is up, megakaryocytic hyperplasia is found. Platelets may pool in the spleen, causing a relative but not an absolute thrombocytopenia. In this case, the bone marrow sample might appear normal. Bone marrow biopsy is also helpful in ruling out a primary marrow dyscrasia.

Environmental causes of thrombocytopenia include drugs, chemicals, and ionizing radiation (Table 68-7). Almost all medications have been implicated in one or more cases of thrombocytopenia. Because this is a very common cause of thrombocytopenia, a careful search for drug exposure should be made. Medication should be changed or stopped completely if possible. Even a tiny amount of a drug can cause a profound thrombocytopenia in a previously sensitized individual with drug-related, immune-mediated thrombocytopenia. Heparin-induced thrombocytopenia is a potentially serious example of this phenomenon; it is associated with heparin-resistance, thromboembolism, heparin-related platelet aggregation, and even DIC. If this condition develops, the heparin must be discontinued. Because heparin is not a single substance and its molecular make-up varies with each preparation, another manufacturer's lot of heparin or low molecular weight heparin can often be substituted.[222,223] The small amounts of quinine in some soft drinks can trigger a similar response.[224] Drug-induced thrombocytopenia usually resolves once the drug exposure ceases.

TABLE 68–7. DRUGS THAT MAY PRODUCE THROMBOCYTOPENIA

Drugs That Suppress The Marrow
Cytotoxic agents such as those used in cancer chemotherapy (nitrogen mustard, cyclophosphamide, 5-fluorouracil, methotrexate, and many others)
Drugs That By Immune Mechanisms Accelerate Platelet Destruction
Chlorothiazides
Chlorpropamide
Diazepam
Diphenylhydantoin
Gold salts
Quinidine
Quinine
Sulfisoxazole
Drugs Whose Mechanism of Antiplatelet Activity Is Unknown
Acetaminophen
Aminopyrine
Chlorpromazine
Cimetidine
Furosemide
Heparin
Heroin
Penicillamine
Penicillin
Phenylbutazone
Various sulfonamides
Tolbutamide

From Anderson HM. Maternal hematologic disorders. In: Creasy RK, Resnik R, eds. Maternal-fetal medicine: principles and practice. Philadelphia: WB Saunders, 1989:908, with permission.

Immune Thrombocytopenic Purpura. The diagnosis of immune thrombocytopenic purpura (ITP) is made by demonstration of a platelet-associated antibody and the exclusion of all the other causes of thrombocytopenia. A bone marrow smear reveals megakaryocyte hyperplasia and the mean platelet volume is increased. In common with other autoimmune diseases, ITP is common in young women. Patients with this disorder have IgG antibody directed against the platelet. The coated platelets are then removed from the circulation by reticuloendothelial cells. Survival of autologous platelets transfused to ITP patients ranges from a few minutes to 3 days, compared to the normal platelet lifespan of 9 to 12 days.[224] Abnormal skin and mucous membrane bleeding appear when the platelet count declines below 100,000 cells/mm^3. Counts below 20,000 cells/mm^3 are associated with spontaneous bleeding. Specific complications and bleeding severity vary greatly between patients.

Because the platelet count has been included in the automated complete blood count (CBC), an increased incidence of mild thrombocytopenia (platelet count between 100,000 and 150,000 cells/mm^3) has been recognized during pregnancy. Many of these women have been treated perhaps unnecessarily as having ITP. The mechanism seems to differ from ITP in that C3, rather than IgG, binds to the platelets.[225] When an underlying medical disorder such as ITP, lupus, or DIC is ruled out, the outcome is good. In none of these patients, in whom another platelet disorder was ruled out, was there any maternal or neonatal complications associated with the thrombocytopenia.[226] Mild thrombocytopenia unassociated with other abnormalities needs no treatment. A recommendation for cesarean delivery or even a routine fetal scalp platelet count in labor for all thrombocytopenic women would expose these pregnancies to unnecessary interventions.[226]

Epidural anesthesia is felt to be safe during the labor of a patient with an unexplained thrombocytopenia if the platelet count is at least 100,000 cells/mm^3.[227] A maternal bleeding time is neither a necessary nor useful test in this setting. Epidural anesthesia has been given to women with a platelet count between 50,000 to 100,000 cells/mm^3 without evidence of an epidural hematoma.[227] However, experience with these more severely thrombocytopenic patients is limited and the safety of epidural anesthesia in this circumstance must be considered unknown.

Treatment. Corticosteroid therapy should be initiated when the platelet declines below 100,000/mm^3 secondary to an immune mechanism. Prednisone 80 to 100 mg/day in divided doses is given. Corticosteroids increase platelet production without any change in the platelet lifespan.[228] Patient activity should be restricted if the count is below 50,000/mm^3 to avoid hemorrhage secondary to trauma. The platelet count should begin to improve within 3 to 10 days of initiating therapy. The steroid dose is tapered to the minimum value that permits a stable count once the platelet count exceeds 100,000/mm^3. Other immunosuppressive medications such as azathioprine, vincristine, and cyclophosphamide have been employed successfully for the treatment of ITP, but should be avoided during pregnancy if possible.[224] In drug-related cases, the steroids can usually be discontinued completely. In immune-mediated cases, 5 to 40 mg of prednisone per day may be necessary for the long term to prevent relapse. Steroid treatment may only be needed during periods of high risk, such as near term. Splenectomy during pregnancy may precipitate abortion and has been virtually replaced by steroid and other medical treatments.[229] Postpartum, splenectomy may well be preferable to chronic steroid treatment. Platelet transfusion is only transiently effective in immune-mediated disorders, because the antiplatelet IgG binds to donor platelets as well, and is only recommended to treat a life-threatening emergency.

Intravenous gamma globulin (400 mg/kg/day for 5 days) recently has been employed to treat immune thrombocytopenia during pregnancy. Most women respond to therapy with an increased platelet count within a few days of the initiation. The improvement may last from a few days to a few weeks.[222,228] The neonatal response is more variable. Some reports have demonstrated severe neonatal thrombocytopenia despite the recommended intravenous gamma globulin regimen.[230,231] This may be a dose-related phenomena that could be overcome by increasing the dose and frequency of gamma globulin. Therapeutic fetal blood levels of gamma globulin have been demonstrated by Hammarstrom and Smith following repeated, semiweekly maternal intravenous infusions.[231] Although effective, this therapy is very expensive.

Fetal Considerations. The treatment of maternal ITP during pregnancy with steroids, splenectomy, or intravenous gamma globulin is successful. However, to date treatment has had no beneficial effect on the circulating antiplatelet IgG titers that cross the placenta to the fetus. In fact, splenectomy may enhance the fetal risk. Currently recommended steroid and gamma globulin regimens have not been shown to cross the placenta well.[230] Neither maternal platelet count, platelet-associated IgG, or free antiplatelet antibody are useful in predicting neonatal thrombocytopenia.[232,233]

Perhaps the key issue is the antenatal risk to the fetus of an ITP-affected pregnancy. A literature review indicates that fetal in utero hemorrhage is a reportable event despite the commonness of the disorder.

Cesarean section delivery was, in the past, recommended for all patients with thrombocytopenia. This was unnecessary for most pregnancies.[234] Fetal scalp blood sampling permits a fetal platelet count early in labor (about 3 to 4 cm dilation). This technique is safe, with a low incidence of false-negative results.[235] There is a modest false-positive rate secondary to platelet aggregation in the sample if it is contaminated by amniotic fluid or vernix.[180,236]

Cordocentesis has been used to diagnose fetal thrombocytopenia in women with ITP. It is clearly effective and the risk of cordocentesis is fairly low, 0.1% to 2%. However, because the likelihood of antenatal hemorrhage is much lower, it is very unlikely that the risk of cordocentesis is exceeded by its benefit. Therefore, a scalp platelet count is preferred.

The infant should be watched closely after birth. Infants not thrombocytopenic at birth may become so within the first few days of life.

Alloimmune Thrombocytopenia in the Fetus. Alloimmune thrombocytopenia is the platelet equivalent of Rh sensitization. The diagnosis is most often made following the birth of an affected sibling. Fifty percent of affected women are affected during their first pregnancy; 88% to 97% of fetuses in subsequent pregnancies are affected. The sensitized mother produces IgG antibodies to a foreign platelet antigen. There are six known platelet antigens: PLA 1, Zwb, Koa, Kob, PLE, and Duzo, as well as several leukoplatelet antigens: HLA-5, HLA-9, PLGrLyC1, and PLGrLyB1.[237] The majority of cases of alloimmune thrombocytopenia are caused by PLA 1, PLGrLyC1, and PLGrLyB1, with greater than 50% of cases related to PLA 1.[238] High-risk groups for alloimmunization include HLA types B8 and DR3.[239] PLA 1 occurs in 98% of the population. PLA 1, PLGrLyB1, and PLGrLyC1 are inherited as autosomal dominant traits.[240] PLA 1 is the most potent of the isoantigens. By present laboratory methods, there is no correlation between the maternal antiplatelet antibody titers and the severity of the disease.[240]

The neonate presents with varying symptoms, such as a petechial rash, hematemesis, melena, hematochezia, hematuria, a cephalohematoma, or the most severe: intracranial hemorrhage. About 90% of children present with only mild bleeding, which resolves without residual deficits within 1 to 4 weeks after birth.[40] However, there is still a high rate of perinatal morbidity and 10% incidence of perinatal mortality, usually due to intracranial hemorrhage (ICH). About a third of ICHs occur in utero.[241–244] The risk of early neonatal bleeding is 20%.[180]

Treatment. Antepartum maternal therapy has met with varying success until recently. Corticosteroid therapy often has no affect on the fetal platelet count.[245] Intravenous gamma globulin to the mother had been unsuccessful in treating fetal thrombocytopenia in doses used for the treatment of ITP (400 mg/kg/day) over 5 days.[239] However, repetitive weekly high doses of intravenous gamma globulin have been more successful. Bussel and coworkers treated seven patients with intravenous gamma globulin 1.0 g/kg body weight, infused over 4 to 7 hours once a week.[246,247] All had a prior child with severe alloimmune thrombocytopenia and were PLA 1 negative. Six patients had serial fetal blood samples performed prior to delivery (second sample 4 to 6 weeks after start of treatment), and all had improvement of the fetal platelet count. The addition of dexamethasone to this treatment regimen did not seem to improve the results. The mean increase (± SD) in fetal platelet count between the first and second samples was $72.5 \pm 62 \times 10^9$ cells/L. This promising treatment requires further investigation.

Other authors have been concerned that the incidence of fetal ICH increases markedly after 30 weeks gestation and recommended intravenous fetal transfusion of maternal washed platelets (PLA 1 negative) to alleviate thrombocytopenia and prevent ICH.[248] Several different regimens have been recommended. Because platelet lifespan following transfusion is only 4 to 6 days, weekly in utero fetal transfusions have been recommended until the age of fetal lung maturity. One final platelet transfusion is carried out, followed by elective cesarean section.[248,249] Certainly, medical therapy is more desirable.

In a middle ground approach, Daffos and associates developed a management plan for patients at risk for neonatal alloimmune thrombocytopenia.[180,239,250] A cordocentesis is performed at 20 weeks gestation for fetal PLA 1 typing and platelet count. If the fetus is PLA 1 negative, the pregnancy can continue normally. If the fetus is PLA 1 positive and already thrombocytopenic, the patient is counseled to avoid any risk of trauma (rest, no driving, etc). Serial ultrasounds are performed in search of ICH. A second cordocentesis is performed at approximately 37 weeks gestation (time of expected fetal pulmonary maturity). If the fetal platelet count is less than 100×10^9 cells/L, maternal platelets are transfused to the fetus.[180] Several authors now believe that a normal vaginal delivery can be attempted without risk to the fetus if the fetal platelet count at the end of this final transfusion is $>100 \times 10^9$ cells/L.[180,236]

We believe a combination of these approaches seems prudent. When an affected fetus is documented, intravenous gamma globulin therapy should be initiated. In the authors' hands, the addition of dexamethasone has benefited select fetuses. Only when the fetus was unresponsive to medical therapy would transfusion be necessary. This sequence would reduce the number of fetal platelet transfusions needed. Further investigation continues.

Thrombotic Thrombocytopenic Purpura. Classically, thrombotic thrombocytopenic purpura (TIP) is characterized by a diagnostic pentad of fever, microangiopathic hemolytic anemia, thrombocytopenia, central nervous system (CNS) symptoms, and renal impairment.[251] Bukowski suggested three major criteria in the non-pregnant patient: platelet count less than 75,000, hemoglobin less than 10 mg/dL, and CNS symptoms, and several minor criteria: temperature >38.3°C, blood urea nitrogen ≥40 mg/dL, serum creatinine ≥3 mg/dL, positive tissue biopsy for microthrombi, no evidence of DIC, and no autoantibodies.[252,253] An increase in the ratio of thromboxane to prostacyclin is thought to contribute to the development of widespread microvascular thrombi in TTP.[253] The thrombi in TTP represent aggregated platelets without fibrin. DIC is uncommonly associated with TTP. The AT III level is normal in TTP.[254] Unless treatment is successful, the usual course of this disease is progressive deterioration followed by death within 3 months.

The presentation and management of this disorder during pregnancy has recently been reviewed.[254] Distinctive clotting abnormalities found in TTP may enable easier, earlier diagnosis of this disorder. Rather than being another condition associated with DIC, multiple studies have now shown that although TTP manifests as increased platelet destruction and decreased platelet survival similar to DIC, fibrinogen turnover is normal in TTP.[255] No substantial evidence for primary endothelial damage exists. Serum fibronectin concentration has usually been normal when measured in patients with TTP, in contrast to the elevated levels found in preeclampsia.[256] Coagulation tests or factors such as the PT/PTT, AT III, protein C, fibrinogen, the ratio of factor VIII antigen to activity, and FSP are almost always normal in patients with TTP.[257]

In a compilation of published cases, TTP preceded delivery in 89% (40/45) of the patients.[254] The mean maternal age was 23 years ± 6.8 years, and 58% (23/40) of patients initially presented at or before 24 weeks. Although the clinical definition of preeclampsia was fulfilled in 38% of women who developed TTP after 24 weeks, clear-cut preeclampsia occurred simultaneously with TTP only three times.

TTP places both mother and fetus at extreme jeopardy. Only 25% (10/40) of maternal–infant pairs survived when antepartum TTP was present. Eighty percent (32/40) of the infants died directly or indirectly as a result of maternal disease.

Treatment. The treatments that have shown some therapeutic efficacy for TTP include corticosteroids, aspirin, dextran, dipyridamole, and plasmapheresis.[253,254] The latter is the treatment of choice. Plasmapheresis with donor plasma replacement (30 to 40 mL/kg) has increased survival up to 90%.[258,259] In a review of published cases associated with pregnancy, the overall maternal mortality rate was 44% (20/45).[254] But when split by mode of treatment, the mortality rate was 68% (19/28) if plasma therapy was not used and 0% (0/17) if it was ($p < 0.05$).[254]

Life-threatening anemia is treated by infusion of packed red blood cells. Renal failure is treated by dialysis. Splenectomy is rarely of use during pregnancy. Immunosuppressive agents and heparin have not been effective. Platelet transfusion can have disastrous results, actually increasing intravascular thrombi formation and thus exacerbating the disease.[253]

Based on literature review, the following treatment protocol for TTP in pregnancy is suggested.[254] Plasma exchange with donor plasma should be initiated promptly, exchanging one plasma volume during the first 24 hours. The concentration of lactic dehydrogenase (LDH) levels is monitored as an indicator of ongoing hemolysis and ischemic tissue damage. If there is no or inadequate response, glucocorticoids (the equivalent of 1 to 2 mg/kg/day of prednisone) and antiplatelet agents are added. Splenectomy during pregnancy should be considered only as a last resort.

Fetal Considerations. Fetal survival has been reported when TTP develops in the late second and third trimester.[254,258,259] Maternal TTP does not improve with delivery.[254] Successful treatment may allow the pregnancy to be lengthened by 4 weeks or more.[254] Preterm delivery may be necessary because of fetal compromise. When TTP presents in the first trimester, the fetus typically does not survive.

Other Disorders. Other pregnancy-associated disorders may present similarly to TTP (Table 68-8).

Preeclampsia. There is approximately a 10% incidence of thrombocytopenia in women with severe preeclampsia. In some cases, thrombocytopenia precedes the clinical manifestations of preeclampsia.[260] Preeclampsia associated thrombocytopenia is due to accelerated platelet destruction. Bone marrow compensation accelerates marrow platelet production, resulting in younger, larger platelets on the peripheral smear. The platelet distribution width is increased.[261] Platelet aggregation is probably secondary to damaged vascular endothelium.[261] Abnormal antiplatelet immunoglobulin G (IgG), immu-

TABLE 68–8. DIFFERENTIATING CAUSES OF THROMBOCYTOPENIA IN PREGNANCY

	TTP	HUS	PREECLAMPSIA	ITP
Clinical features				
CNS	+	−	+	−
Fever	+	−	−	−
Hypertension	−	−	+	−
Petechiae	+	−	+	+
Laboratory				
Hemolytic anemia	+	+	+	−
Lactate dehydrogenase	↑	↑	↑	N
SGOT/SGPT	N	N	↑	N
Antithrombin III activity	N	N	↓	N
Autoantibodies	−	−	−	+
Proteinuria	+	+	+	−
Serum creatinine	↑	↑	↑	N
Blood urea nitrogen	↑	↑	↑	N

CNS, central nervous system symptoms; HUS, hemolytic uremic syndrome; ITP, idiopathic thrombocytopenic purpura; N, normal; SGOT, serum glutamic-oxalacetic transaminase; SGPT, serum glutamic-pyruvic transaminase; TTP, thrombotic thrombocytopenia purpura; +, present; −, absent; ↑, increased; ↓, decreased.

noglobulin M (IgM), or C3 titers that do not correlate with either the maternal or fetal platelet count were found in one study in the majority of preeclamptic patients.[262] Antiplatelet IgG is found most often. The significance of the increased antiglobulin titers in preeclampsia is unclear.[234,262,263]

Preeclampsia can be confused with TTP, especially when its manifestations include thrombocytopenia, microangiopathic hemolysis, and renal failure. TTP may also be mistakenly diagnosed as severe preeclampsia. The differences in maternal serum AT III activity may aid in the diagnosis. AT III activity is decreased in women with severe preeclampsia, but remains stable in TTP and hemolytic uremic syndrome.

The following management protocol is suggested when the differential diagnosis is TTP versus severe atypical preeclampsia. If the gestational age is 34 weeks or greater, AT III activity should be measured and the patient delivered. If the correct diagnosis was preeclampsia, the AT III activity level will be decreased and the patient will start to recover soon after delivery. If the AT III level was normal and the patient does not recover soon after delivery, the correct diagnosis is likely TTP, and plasma therapy should be initiated. If the patient is <28 weeks gestation, AT III activity should be measured prior to delivery. When the fetal condition is satisfactory, a trial of plasma therapy is recommended. Rapid maternal clinical improvement supports the diagnosis of TTP. If there is no improvement with treatment, the diagnosis is most likely preeclampsia and the patient should be delivered. There is little evidence that preeclampsia is altered by plasma therapy in the absence of such confounding variables as delivery. Between 28 and 34 weeks, treatment should be individualized. If the AT III activity level is normal, the fetus is not compromised, and the amniotic fluid studies are incompatible with fetal lung maturity, a trial of plasma therapy should be instituted and continued until the postpartum period, when a remission has been achieved. It should not be discontinued during the pregnancy. The likelihood of relapse is increased during pregnancy. If the patient does not respond, she should be delivered.

Postpartum Hemolytic Uremic Syndrome. Hemolytic uremic syndrome (HUS) is often confused with TTP. It too can present with microangiopathic anemia, thrombocytopenia, and renal failure. HUS may be associated with seizures due to renal failure or hypertension, but is rarely associated with neurologic changes. Other distinguishing features of HUS include the following:

- History of a prodromal gastrointestinal disorder with diarrhea
- Early, severe renal failure with anuria and hypertension
- Milder bleeding and thrombocytopenia than in TTP
- Onset 48° after a normal delivery.[224]

The primary coagulation defect in HUS involves the platelet. Thrombocytopenia is often but not always present. AT III activity is usually normal.[254] In contrast to TTP, FSP are frequently increased, possibly due to fibrinogen rather than fibrin degradation. Urinary free hemoglobin is common secondary to hemolysis.[254]

Treatment recommendations for HUS are similar to those for TTP, with the addition of dialysis. Heparin has not been shown to be effective. In a literature review of postpartum HUS, the outcomes were worse than for pregnancy-associated TTP.[254] The overall maternal mortality rate was 55% (34/62). Furthermore, almost half of the survivors required long-term dialysis (13/28), five others underwent kidney transplantation, and one died following organ rejection. Plasma therapy is apparently beneficial, although the numbers are small. Fifty-eight percent (34/59) of women who did not receive plasma therapy died, in contrast to zero (0/3) women who received plasma therapy.[254]

Thrombocytopenia in pregnancy can also be caused by systemic lupus erythematosus and variant von Wilebrand's disease (Type IIB). The latter disorder may produce thrombocytopenia by binding of the abnormal von Willebrand factor (VWF) to the patient's platelets. This is followed by platelet aggregate formation and clearance.[264] Variant VWF synthesis increases in pregnancy.[265,266]

Functional Platelet Defects

Acquired disorders of platelet function can occur in conjunction with medical illnesses such as uremia, myeloproliferative disorders, and congestive heart failure. Drug-induced platelet dysfunction is much more common in pregnancy.

Aspirin and other nonsteroidal anti-inflammatory agents are the most important of the drugs affecting platelet function because they are so commonly used. Aspirin is the longest acting of these drugs. It irreversibly acetylates platelet cyclooxygenase, inhibiting thromboxane synthesis. This results in decreased platelet aggregation in the presence of collagen. The bleeding time can be prolonged. Usually, any bruisability or bleeding is mild in someone who has recently taken aspirin. Although otherwise normal pregnant women who ingest aspirin within 10 days of delivery are reported to have increased blood loss both intrapartum and postpartum, and their infants have an increased incidence of abnormal coagulation, these effects are rarely clinically significant.[267] Other nonsteroidal anti-inflammatory agents have similar effects on platelet function, although they are less potent and of shorter duration. None of these medications are recommended during pregnancy.

Acetaminophen should be the antipyretic and analgesic drug of choice for pregnant women.

Carbenicillin can impair platelet function, resulting in severe hemorrhage. Some other antibiotics can have similar but much milder effects on platelets. Glyceryl guaiacolate, used in over-the-counter cold medications, can also affect platelet activity.[224]

Congenital disorders of platelet function are extremely rare and there is little experience with them in pregnancy. A discussion of these disorders is beyond the scope of this chapter, although good reviews exist in the hematology and pathology literature.[268]

REFERENCES

1. Sixma JJ, Wester J. The hemostatic plug. Semin Hematol 1977;14:265.
2. Bettex-Galland M, Trescher EF. Thrombosthenin, the contractile protein from blood platelets and its relation to other contractile proteins. Adv Protein Chem 1965;20:1.
3. Erichson RB, Katz AJ, Cintron JR. Ultrastructural observations on platelet adhesion reactions: platelet fibrin interaction. Blood 1967;29:385.
4. Wintrobe WM, Lee GR, Boggs DR, et al. Blood coagulation. In Wintrobe WM, Lee GR, Boggs DR, et al, eds. Clinical hematology. 8th ed. Philadelphia: Lea & Febiger, 1981:418.
5. Bagdasarian A, Talano RC, Dolman RW. Isolation of high molecular weight activators of human plasma prekallikrein. J Biol Chem 1973;248:3456.
6. Weiss AS, Gallin JI, Kaplan AP. Fletcher factor deficiency. J Clin Invest 1974;53:622.
7. Osterud B, Laake K, Prydz H. The activation of human factor IX. Thromb Haemost 1975;33:553.
8. Mandle RJ, Kaplan AP. Hageman factor substrates. J Biol Chem 1977;252:6097.
9. Griffin SH, Cochmane CG. Mechanisms for the involvement of high molecular weight kinogens in surface dependent reactions of Hageman factor. Proc Natl Acad Sci USA 1976;73:2554.
10. Nemerson Y. Biological control of factor VII. Thromb Haemost 1976;35:96.
11. Sauto H, Ratnoff OD. Alterations of factor VII activity by activated Fletcher factor (a plasma kallikrein): a potential link between intrinsic and extrinsic clotting systems. J Lab Clin Med 1975;85:405.
12. Gjonnaess H, Fagerhol MK, Stormorken H. Studies on coagulation and fibrinolysis in blood from puerperal women with and without estrogen treatment. Br J Obstet Gynaecol 1975;82:151.
13. Schick P. The role of platelet membranes in platelet hemostatic activities. Semin Hematol 1979;16:221.
14. Walsh PN. Platelet coagulant activities and hemostasis: a hypothesis. Blood 1974;43:597.
15. Jaffe EA, Hoyer LW, Nachman RL. Synthesis of antihemophilic factor antigen by cultured human endothelial cells. J Clin Invest 1973;52:2757.
16. Ischopp TB, Weiss JH, Baumgartner HR. Decreased adhesion of platelets to subendothelium in von Willebrand's disease. J Lab Clin Med 1974;83:296.
17. Moncada S, Vane JR. The role of prostacyclin in vascular tissue. Fed Proc 1979;38:66.
18. Goodman RP. Prostacyclin production during pregnancy: comparison of production during normal pregnancy and pregnancy complicated by hypertension. Am J Obstet Gynecol 1982; 142:817.
19. Dadak C, Kefalides A, Sinzinger H, Weber G. Reduced umbilical artery prostacyclin formation in complicated pregnancies. Am J Obstet Gynecol 1982;144:792.
20. Ogston D, Bennett B. Naturally occurring inhibitors of coagulation. In Ogston B, Bennett B, eds. Haemostasis: biochemistry, physiology and pathology. London: John Wiley & Sons, 1977:230.
21. Bick RL. Clinical relevance of antithrombin III. Semin Thromb Hemost 1982;4:276.
22. Owen MC, Brennan SO, Lewis JH, Carrell RW. Mutation of antitrypsin to antithrombin: alpha-1 antitrypsin Pittsburgh (358 Met-Arg), a fatal bleeding disorder. N Engl J Med 1983; 309:684.
23. Gallus AS. Familial venous thromboembolism and inherited abnormalities of the blood clotting system. Aust NZ J Med 1984;14:807.
24. Gruenberg JC, Smallridge RC, Rosenberg RD. Inherited antithrombin III deficiency causing mesenteric thrombosis: a new clinical entity. Ann Surg 1975;181:791.
25. Bischof P, Meisser A, Sizonenko PC, Herrmann WL. Pregnancy-associated plasma protein A inhibits thrombin-induced coagulation. Washington, DC: Proceedings of the Society for Gynecologic Investigation, 1984:abstract ;ns321.
26. Comp PC, Esmon CT. Evidence for multiple roles of activated protein C in fibrinolysis. In Mann KG, Taylor FB Jr, eds. The regulation of coagulation. New York: Elsevier/North-Holland, 1980:583.
27. Hopmeier P, Halbmayer M, Schwarz HP, Heuss F, Fischer M. Protein C and protein S in mild and moderate preeclampsia [letter]. Thromb Haemost 1987;58:794.
28. Malm J, Laurell M, Dahlback B. Changes in the plasma levels of vitamin K-dependent proteins C and S and C4b-binding protein during pregnancy and oral contraception. Br J Haematol 1988;68:437.
29. Griffin JH, Evatt B, Zimmerman TS, et al. Deficiency of protein C in congenital thrombotic disease. J Clin Invest 1980;68:1370.
30. Seligsohn U, Berger A, Abend M, et al. Homozygous protein C deficiency manifested by massive venous thrombosis in the newborn. N Engl J Med 1984;310:559.
31. Comp PC, Esmon CT. Recurrent venous thromboembolism in patients with a partial deficiency of protein S. N Engl J Med 1984;311:1525.
32. Holemans R, Mann LS, Cope C. Fibrinolytic activity of renal venous and arterial blood. Am J Med Sci 1967;254:330.
33. Cash JD. Effect of moderate exercise on the fibrinolytic system in normal young men and women. Br Med J 1966;2:502.
34. Deutsch E, Elsner P. The mechanism of fibrinolysis induced by bacterial pyrogens. Thromb Haemost 1959;3:286.
35. Kwaan HC. On the inhibition of plasma fibrinolytic activity by exercised ischaemic muscles. Clin Sci 1958;17:361.
36. Sawyer WD, Fletcher AP, Alkjaersig N, Sherry S. Studies on the thrombolytic activity of human plasma. J Clin Invest 1960; 39:426.
37. Kaplan AP, Austen KF. The fibrinolytic pathway of human plasma: Isolation and characterization of the plasminogen proactivator. J Clin Invest 1973;52:2591.
38. Larrieu MJ, Rigollot C, Marder VJ. Comparative effects of fibrinogen degradation fragments D & E on coagulation. Br J Haematol 1972;22:719.
39. Ogston D, Ogston CM, Fullerton HW. The plasminogen content of thrombi. Thromb Haemost 1966;15:220.
40. Weiner CP, Kwaan H, Hauck WW, Duboe FJ, Paul M, Wallemark CB. Fibrin generation in normal pregnancy. Obstet Gynecol 1984;64:46.
41. Weiner CP, Brandt J. Plasma antithrombin III activity: an aid in the diagnosis of preeclampsia-eclampsia. Am J Obstet Gynecol 1982;142:275.
42. Arias F, Andrenopoulos G, Zamora J. Whole blood fibrinolytic activity in normal and hypertensive pregnancies and its relation to placental concentration of urokinase inhibitor. Am J Obstet Gynecol 1979;133:624.
43. Freedman J, Musclow E, Garvey B, Abbott D. Unexplained periparturient thrombocytopenia. Am J Hematol 1986;21:397.

44. Weiner CP, Kwaan H, Duboe F. Diagnosis of septic pelvic vein thrombophlebitis by measurement of fibrinopeptide A. Am J Perinatol 1985;2:93.
45. Weiner CP, Sabbagha RE, Vaisrub N. Distinguishing preeclampsia from chronic hypertension using antithrombin III. Washington, DC: Proceedings of the Society for Gynecologic Investigation, 1983:abstract ;ns29.
46. Bick RL. Disseminated intravascular coagulation: clinical and laboratory characteristics in 48 patients. Ann NY Acad Sci 1981;370:843.
47. Bick RL. Disseminated intravascular coagulation and related syndromes: etiology, pathophysiology, diagnosis, and management. Am J Hematol 1978;5:265.
48. Mersky C. Defibrination syndrome. In Biggs R, ed. Human blood coagulation, hemostasis and thrombosis. London: Blackwell Scientific, 1976:492.
49. Kopec M, Wegrzynowiczy Z, Budzynski A, et al. Interaction of fibrinogen degradation products with platelets. Exp Biol Med 1968;3:73.
50. Gurewich V, Hutchinson E. Detection of intravascular coagulation by a serial dilution protamine sulfate test. Ann Intern Med 1971;75:895.
51. Mason JW, Kleeberg U, Dolan P, Colman RW. Plasma kallikrein and Hageman factor in gram-negative bacteremia. Ann Intern Med 1970;73:545.
52. Kaplan A, Meier H, Mandle R. The Hageman factor. Dependent pathways of coagulation, fibrinolysis, and kinin generation. Semin Thromb Hemost 1976;3:6.
53. Ratnoff OD, Naff GB. The conversion of CiLS to Cl esterase by plasmin and trypsin. J Exp Med 1961;125:337.
54. Bick RL, Dukes ML, Wilson WL, Fekete LF. Antithrombin III as a diagnostic aid in disseminated intravascular coagulation. Thromb Res 1977;10:721.
55. Weiner CP, Brandt J. Plasma antithrombin III activity in normal pregnancy. Obstet Gynecol 1980;56:601.
56. Wintrobe WM, Lee GR, Boggs DR, et al, eds. Clinical hematology. 8th ed. Philadelphia: Lea & Febiger, 1981:1223.
57. Turpie AGG, Hirsh J. When and how to use heparin prophylaxis and treatment. Geriatrics 1979;34:59.
58. Yin ET. Effect of heparin on neutralization of factor X and thrombin by the plasma alpha-2 globulin inhibitor. Thromb Haemost 1974;33:43.
59. Brandt P, Jespersen J, Gregersen G. Postpartum hemolytic-uremic syndrome successfully treated with antithrombin III. Br Med J 1980;280:449.
60. Buller HR, Weenink AH, Treffers PE, Kahle LH, Otten HA, TenCate JW. Severe antithrombin III deficiency in a patient with preeclampsia: observations on the effect of human AT III concentrate transfusion. Scandinavian Journal of Haematology 1980;25:81.
61. Mueller-Eckhardt C, Heene D, Muller-Berghaus G, Lasch HG. Hamolytische Transfusion-szwischenfalle mit Verbrauschkoagulopathie durch seltene Blutgruppenatikorper. Thromb Haemost 1969;22:336.
62. Woodfield DG, Cole SK, Allan AG, Cash JD. Systemic fibrinolysis during and following elective cesarean section and gynecologic operations. J Obstet Gynaecol Br Commonwealth 1972;79:538.
63. Redman CWG, Bonnar J, Berlin L. Early platelet consumption in preeclampsia. Br Med J 1978;1:467.
64. Socol ML, Weiner CP, Louis G, Rehnberg K, Ross EC. Platelet activation in preeclampsia. Am J Obstet Gynecol 1985;151:494.
65. Romero R, Snyder E, Rickles F, et al. The clinical significance and mechanism of thrombocytopenia in pregnancy-induced hypertension. Dallas: Proceedings, Society for Gynecologic Investigation, 1982:abstract ;ns69.
66. Kincaid-Smith P. Participation of intravascular coagulation in the pathogenesis of glomerular and vascular lesions. Kidney Int 1975;7:242.
67. Morris RH, Vassalli P, Beller FK, McCluskey RT. Immunofluorescent studies of renal biopsies in the diagnosis of toxemia of pregnancy. Obstet Gynecol 1964;24:32.
68. Anas F, Mancilla-Jimenez R. Hepatic fibrinogen deposits in preeclampsia: immunofluorescent evidence. N Engl J Med 1976;295:578.
69. Weenink GH, Borm JJJ, TenCate JW, Treffers PE. Antithrombin III levels in normotensive and hypertensive pregnancy. Gynecol Obstet Invest 1983;16:230.
70. Elyan A, Abdelhady M, Halim HA, Altohamy S, Goubran F. Antithrombin III levels in normal pregnancy and preeclampsia. Proceedings, 4th World Congress of the International Society for the Study of Hypertension in Pregnancy. Nottingham, England, 1984:211.
71. Redman CW, Denson KW, Berlin LJ, Bolton FG, Stirrat GM. Factor VIII consumption in preeclampsia. Lancet 1977;2:1249.
72. Howie PW, Begg CB, Purdie DW, Prentice CR. The use of coagulation tests to predict the clinical progress of preeclampsia. Lancet 1976;2:323.
73. Fournie A, Monrozies M, Pontonnier T, Boneu B, Bierme R. Factor VIII complex in normal pregnancy, preeclampsia and fetal growth retardation. Br J Obstet Gynecol 1981;88:251.
74. Douglas JT, Shah M, Lowe GD, Belch JJ, Forbes CD. Plasma fibrinopeptide A and beta-thromboglobulin levels in preeclampsia and hypertensive pregnancy. Thromb Haemost 1982;47:54.
75. Fisher KA, Luger A, Spango BH, Linheimer MD. Hypertension in pregnancy: clinical-pathological correlations and late prognosis. Medicine 1981;60:267.
76. Weiner CP, Kwaan HC, Xu C, Paul M, Burmeister L, Hauck W. Antithrombin III activity in women with hypertension during pregnancy. Obstet Gynecol 1985;65:301.
77. Wallenburg HCS, Makovitz JW, Dekker GA, Rotmans P. Low-dose aspirin prevents pregnancy-induced hypertension and preeclampsia in angiotensinsensitive primigravidae. Lancet 1986; 1:1.
78. Knab DR. Abruptio placentae: an assessment of the time and method of delivery. Am J Obstet Gynecol 1978;52:625.
79. Douglas RG, Buckman MI, MacDonald PF. Premature separation of the normally implanted placenta. J Obstet Gynaecol Br Emp 1955;62:710.
80. Basu HK. Fibrinolysis and abruptio placentae. Br J Obstet Gynaecol 1969;76:481.
81. Sutton DMC, Hauser R, Kulapongs P, Bachmann F. Intravascular coagulation in abruptio placentae. Am J Obstet Gynecol 1971;109:604.
82. Sher G. Pathogenesis and management of uterine inertia complicating abruptio placentae with consumption coagulopathy. Am J Obstet Gynecol 1977;129:164.
83. Pritchard JA. Fetal death in utero. Obstet Gynecol 1959;14:573.
84. Jimenez JM, Pritchard JA. Pathogenesis and treatment of coagulation defects resulting from fetal death. Obstet Gynecol 1968;32:449.
85. Waxman B, Gambrill R. Use of heparin in disseminated intravascular coagulation. Am J Obstet Gynecol 1972;112:434.
86. Levine W, Rosengart M, Siegler A. Spontaneous correction of hypofibrinogenemia with fetal death in utero. Obstet Gynecol 1962;19:551.
87. Romero R, Duffy TP, Berkowitz RL, et al. The use of heparin to prolong a preterm gestation complicated by maternal DIC due to the death of a single twin in utero. N Engl J Med 1984;310:772.
88. Skelly H, Marivate M, Norman R, Kenoyer G, Martin R. Con-

sumptive coagulopathy following fetal death in a triplet pregnancy. Am J Obstet Gynecol 1982;142:595.

89. Moore CM, McAdams AJ, Southerland J. Intrauterine disseminated intravascular coagulation: a syndrome of multiple pregnancy with a dead twin fetus. J Pediatr 1969;74:523.
90. Benirschke K. Twin placenta and perinatal mortality. NY J Med 1961;61:1499.
91. Reisman LE, Pathak A. Bilateral renal cortical necrosis in the newborn. Am J Dis Child 1966;111:541.
92 Yoshioka H, Kadomoto Y, Mino M, Morikawa Y, Kasubuchi Y, Kusunoki T. Multicystic encephalomalacia in live-born twin with a stillborn macerated co-twin. J Pediatr 1979;95:798.
93. Graeff H, Ernst E, Bocaz R, von Hugo R, Hafter R. Evaluation of hypercoagulability in septic abortion. Hemostasis 1976;5:285.
94. Phillips LL, Margaretten W, McKay DG. Changes in the fibrinolytic enzyme system following intravascular coagulation induced by thrombin and endotoxin. Am J Obstet Gynecol 1968;100:319.
95. Kuhn W, Graeff H. Prophylaktische massnahmen beim septischen abort. In Zander J, ed. Septischer Abort und Bakterieller Schock. Heidelburg: Springer, 1968:74.
96. McKay DG. Disseminated intravascular coagulation. New York: Harper & Row, 1965.
97. McKay DG, Jewett JF, Reid DE. Endotoxin shock and the generalized Shwartzman reaction in pregnancy. Am J Obstet Gynecol 1959;78:546.
98. Beller FK, Schoendorf T. Augmentation of endotoxin-induced fibrin deposits by pregnancy and estrogen-progesterone treatment. Gynecol Obstet Invest 1972;3:176.
99. Beller FK, Uszynski M. Disseminated intravascular coagulation in pregnancy. Clin Obstet Gynecol 1974;17:250.
100. Duff P. Pathophysiology and management of septic shock. J Reprod Med 1980;24:109.
101. Margulis RR, Dustin RW, Lovell JR, Robb H, Jabs C. Heparin for septic abortion and the prevention of endotoxic shock. Obstet Gynecol 1971;37:474.
102. McLees BD. Critical care medicine. In Wyngaarden JB, Smith LH, eds. Cecil textbook of medicine. Philadelphia: WB Saunders, 1982:2186.
103. Schumer W. Steroids in the treatment of clinical septic shock. Ann Surg 1976;184:333.
104. Glenn TM, Leffer AM. Role of lysosomes in the pathogenesis of splanchnic ischemic shock in cats. Circ Res 1970;27:783.
105. Gahhos FN, Chiu RC, Hinchey EJ, Richards GK. Endorphins in septic shock: hemodynamic and endocrine effects of an opiate receptor antagonist and agonist. Arch Surg 1982;117:1053.
106. Peters WP, Johnson MW, Friedman PA, Mitch WE. Pressor effect of naloxone in septic shock. Lancet 1981;1:529.
107. Colman RW, Robboy SJ, Minna JD. Disseminated intravascular coagulation: a reappraisal. Annu Rev Med 1979;30:359.
108. Corrigan JJ Jr. Heparin therapy in bacterial septicemia. J Pediatr 1977;91:695.
109. Kuhn W, Graeff H. Gerinnungsstorungen in der Geburtshilfe. Stuttgart: Thieme, 1970.
110. Talbert LM, Adcock DF, Weiss AE, Easterling WE Jr, Odom MH. Studies on the pathogenesis of clotting defects during salt-induced abortions. Am J Obstet Gynecol 1973;115:656.
111. Easterling WE, Weiss AE, Odom MH, Talbert LM. Plasma volume, electrolyte, and coagulation factor changes following intra-amniotic hypertonic saline infusion. Am J Obstet Gynecol 1972;113:1065.
112. Shaw ST, Ballard CA. Subclinical coagulopathy following amnioinfusion with hypertonic saline. Am J Obstet Gynecol 1974;118:1081.
113. Laros RK, Collins J, Penner JA, Hage ML, Smith S. Coagulation changes in saline-induced abortion. Am J Obstet Gynecol 1973;116:271.
114. Stander RW, Flessa HC, Glueck HI, Kisker CT. Changes in maternal coagulation factors after intra-amniotic injection of hypertonic saline. Obstet Gynecol 1971;37:660.
115. Cohen E, Ballard CA. Consumptive coagulopathy associated with intra-amniotic saline instillation and the effect of intravenous oxytocin. Obstet Gynecol 1974;43:300.
116. Binkin NJ, Schultz KF, Grimes DA, Cates W Jr. Urea-prostaglandin versus hypertonic saline for instillation abortion. Am J Obstet Gynecol 1983;146:947.
117. Courtney LD. Amniotic fluid embolism. Obstet Gynecol Surv 1974;29:169.
118. Scott MM. Cardiopulmonary considerations in nonfatal amniotic fluid embolism. JAMA 1963;183:989.
119. Pritchard JA, Dugan RJ. Presumed amniotic fluid embolism with recovery. Ohio State Med J 1956;52:379.
120. Steiner PE, Lushbaugh CC. Maternal pulmonary embolism by amniotic fluid as a cause of obstetrical shock and unexpected deaths in obstetrics. JAMA 1941;117:1245.
121. Resnik R, Swartz WH, Plumer MH, Benirschke K, Stratthaus ME. Amniotic fluid embolism with survival. Obstet Gynecol 1976;47:295.
122. Sparr RA, Pritchard JA. Studies to detect the escape of amniotic fluid into the maternal circulation during parturition. Surg Gynecol Obstet 1958;107:560.
123. Kuhlman K, Hidvegi D, Tamura RK, Deep R. Is amniotic fluid material in the central circulation of peripartum patients pathologic? Am J Perinatol 1985;2:295.
124. Graeff J, Kuhn W. Coagulation disorders in obstetrics—pathobiochemistry, pathophysiology, diagnosis, treatment. Philadelphia: WB Saunders, 1980.
125. Clark SL, Montz PJ, Phelan JP. Hemodynamic alterations associated with amniotic fluid embolism: a reappraisal. Am J Obstet Gynecol 1985;151:617.
126. Skjodt P. Amniotic fluid embolism: a case investigated by coagulation and fibrinolysis studies. Acta Obstet Gynecol Scand 1965;44:437.
127. Beller FK, Douglas GW, Debrovner CH, Robinson R. The fibrinolytic system in amniotic fluid embolism. Am J Obstet Gynecol 1963;87:48.
128. Albrechtsen OK, Storm O, Trolle D. Fibrinolytic activity in circulating blood following amniotic fluid infusion. Acta Haematol (Basel) 1955;14:309.
129. Clark SL, Pavlova Z, Greenspoon J, Horenstein J, Phelan JP. Squamous cells in the maternal pulmonary circulation. Am J Obstet Gynecol 1986;154:104.
130. Phillips LL, Davidson EC. Procoagulant properties of amniotic fluid. Am J Obstet Gynecol 1972;113:911.
131. Yaffe H, Bar-On H, Eldor A, Ron M, Sadovsky E. Correlation between thromboplastin activity and lecithin/sphingomyelin ratio in amniotic fluid: preliminary report. Br J Obstet Gynecol 1977;84:354.
132. Weiner CP, Brandt J. A modified activated partial thromboplastin time with the use of amniotic fluid. Am J Obstet Gynecol 1982;144:234.
133. Attwood HD, Downing SE. Experimental amniotic fluid in meconium embolism. Surg Gynecol Obstet 1965;120:255.
134. Kitzmiller JL, Lucas WE. Studies on a model of amniotic fluid embolism. Obstet Gynecol 1972;39:626.
135. Karim SMM, Devlin J. Prostaglandin content of amniotic fluid during pregnancy and labor. J Obstet Gynecol Br Commonwealth 1979;74:230.
136. Azegami M, Mori N. Amniotic fluid embolism and leukotrienes. Am J Obstet Gynecol 1986;155:1119.

137. Albrechtsen OK, Trolle D. A fibrinolytic system in human amniotic fluid. Acta Haematol (Basel) 1955;14:376.
138. Maki M, Tachita K, Kawasaki Y, Nagasawa K. Heparin treatment of amniotic fluid embolism. Tohoku J Exp Med 1969; 97:155.
139. Lalos O, von Schoultz B. Amniotic fluid embolism: a review of the literature with two case reports. Int J Gynaecol Obstet 1977;15:48.
140. Henderson SR, Lund CJ. Severe preeclampsia, disseminated intravascular coagulopathy and hydatiform mole complicating a 20 week pregnancy with a fetus. Obstet Gynecol 1971;37:722.
141. Talbert LM, Easterling WE, Flowers CE, Graham JB. Acquired coagulation defects of pregnancy — including a case of a patient with hydatiform mole. Obstet Gynecol 1961;18:69.
142. Glueck HI, Burket RL, Sutherland JM, Garber ST. Afibrinogenemia in pregnancy apparently due to a degenerating leiomyoma. Obstet Gynecol 1961;18:285.
143. Koren Z, Zuckerman H, Brzezinski A. Placenta previa accreta with afibrinogenemia: report of three cases. Obstet Gynecol 1961;18:138.
144. Antimicrobials and haemostasis itorial;cb. Lancet 1983;1:510.
145. Neu HC. The in vitro activity, human pharmacology and clinical effectiveness of new beta-lactam antibiotics. Annu Rev Pharmacol Toxicol 1982;22:599.
146. Brown CH, Natelson EA, Bradshaw MW, Williams TW Jr, Alfrey CP Jr. The hemostatic defect produced by carbenicillin. N Engl J Med 1974;291:265.
147. Ikeda Y, Kikuchi M, Matsuda S, et al. Inhibition of platelet function by sulbenicillin and its metabolite. Antimicrob Agents Chemother 1978;5:881.
148. Margolius A, Jackson DP, Ratnoff OD. Circulating anticoagulants: a study of 40 cases and a review of the literature. Medicine 1961;40:145.
149. Carreras LO, Defreyn G, Machin SJ, et al. Arterial thrombosis, intrauterine death and "lupus" anticoagulant: detection of immunoglobulin interfering with prostacyclin formation. Lancet 1981;1:244.
150. Marengo-Rowe AJ, Murff G, Leveson JE, Cook J. Hemophilia-like disease associated with pregnancy. Obstet Gynecol 1972;40:56.
151. Greenwood RJ, Rabin SC. Hemophilia-like postpartum bleeding. Obstet Gynecol 1967;30:362.
152. Voke J, Letsky E. Pregnancy and antibody to factor VIII. J Clin Pathol 1977;30:928.
153. Fischer DS, Clyne LP. Circulating factor XI antibody and disseminated intravascular coagulation. Arch Intern Med 1981; 141:515.
154. Lechner K. Acquired inhibitors in nonhemophiliac patients. Hemostasis 1974;3:65.
155. Boxer M, Elleman L, Carvalho A. The lupus anticoagulant. Arthritis Rheum 1976;19:1244.
156. Canoso RT, Hutton RA. A chlorpromazine-induced inhibitor of blood coagulation. Am J Hematol 1977;2:183.
157. Feinstein DI, Rapaport SI. Acquired inhibitors of blood coagulation. Prog Hemost Thromb 1972;1:75.
158. Feinstein DI, Rapaport SI. Anticoagulants in systemic lupus erythematosus. In Dubois EL, ed. Lupus erythematosus. Supplement 2. Los Angeles: University of Southern California Press, 1974:438.
159. De Wolf F, Carreras LO, Moerman P, Vermylen J, Van-Assche A, Renaer M. Decidual vasculopathy and extensive placental infarction in a patient with repeated thromboembolic accidents, recurrent fetal loss, and a lupus anticoagulant. Am J Obstet Gynecol 1982;142:829.
160. Stephensen O, Cleland WP, Hallidie-Smith K. Congenital complete heart block and persistent ductus arteriosus associated with maternal systemic lupus erythematosus. Br Heart J 1981;46:104.
161. Chameides L, Truex R, Vetter V, Rashkind WJ, Galioto FM, Jr., Noonan JA. Association of maternal systemic lupus erythematosus with congenital complete heart block. N Engl J Med 1977;297:1204.
162. Scott JS, Maddison PJ, Taylor PV, Esscher E, Scott O, Skinner RP. Connective tissue disease, antibodies to ribonucleoprotein, and congenital heart block. N Engl J Med 1983;309:209.
163. Lockshin MD, Druzin ML, Qamar T. Prednisone does not prevent recurrent fetal death in women with antiphopholipid antibody. Am J Obstet Gynecol 1989;160:439.
164. Lubbe WF, Butler WS, Palmer SJ, Wiggins GC. Fetal survival after prednisone suppression of maternal lupus-anticoagulant. Lancet 1983;1:1361.
165. Prednisone and maternal lupus anticoagulant blood;cb. Lancet 1983;2:576.
166. Feinstein DI. Acquired inhibitors against factor VIII and other clotting proteins. In Coleman RW, Hirsch J, Marder VJ, Salzman EW, eds. Hemostasis and thrombosis. Philadelphia: JB Lippincott, 1982:567.
167. Von Willebrand EA. Hereditar psudohemofili. Finska Lakaresalleskapets Handlinger 1926;68:87.
168. Bloom AL. The von Willebrand syndrome. Semin Hematol 1980;17:215.
169. Hanna W, McCarroll D, McDonald T, et al. Variant von Willebrand's disease and pregnancy. Blood 1981;58:873.
170. Weiss HJ. Relation of von Willebrand's factor to bleeding time. N Engl J Med 1974;291:420.
171. Punnonen R, Nyman D, Gronroos M, Wallen O. Von Willebrand's disease in pregnancy. Acta Obstet Gynecol Scand 1981;60:507.
172. Evans PC. Obstetric and gynecologic patients with von Willebrand's disease. Obstet Gynecol 1971;38:38.
173. Sorosky J, Klatsky A, Nobert GF, Burchell RC. Von Willebrand's disease complicating second trimester abortion. Obstet Gynecol 1980;55:253.
174. Lipton RA, Ayromlooi J, Coller BS. Severe von Willebrand's disease during labor and delivery. JAMA 1982;248:1355.
175. Krishnamurthy M, Miotti AB. Von Willebrand's disease in pregnancy. Obstet Gynecol 1977;49:244.
176. Noller KL, Bowie EJW, Kempers RD, Owen CA Jr. Von Willebrand's disease in pregnancy. Obstet Gynecol 1973;41:865.
177. Adashi EY. Lack of improvement in von Willebrand's disease during pregnancy. N Engl J Med 1980;303:1178.
178. Levine NM. Von Willebrand's disease during pregnancy: review and case report. JAMA 1980;79:520.
179. Weiss HJ, Rogers J, Brand H. Defective ristocetin-induced aggregation in von Willebrand's disease: its correction by factor VIII. J Clin Invest 1973;52:2697.
180. Daffos F, Forestier F, Kaplan C, Cox W. Prenatal diagnosis and management of bleeding disorders with fetal blood sampling. Am J Obstet Gynecol 1988;158:939.
181. Ramgren O. A clinical and medical social study of hemophilia in Sweden. Acta Med Scand 1962;171:759.
182. Department of Health, Education and Welfare: National Heart, Lung and Blood Institute study to evaluate the supply–demand relationships for AHF and PTC through 1980. Washington, DC: US Government Printing Office, 1977.
183. Barrai I, Cann HM, Cavalli-Sforza LL, DeNicola P. The effect of parental age on rates of mutation for hemophilia and evidence for differing mutation rates for hemophilia A and B. Am J Hum Genet 1968;20:175.
184. Firshein SI, Hoyer LW, Lazarchick J, et al. Prenatal diagnosis of classic hemophilia. N Engl J Med 1979;300:937.
185. Elston RC, Graham JB, Miller CH, Reisner HM, Bouma BN.

Probabilistic classification of hemophilia A carriers by discriminant analysis. Thromb Res 1976;8:683.
186. Seligsohn U, Zivelin A, Perez C, Modan M. Detection of hemophilia A carriers by replicate factor VIII activity and factor VIII antigenicity determinations. Br J Haematol 1979;42:433.
187. Ratnoff OD, Steinberg AG. Detection of the carrier state of classic hemophilia. NY Acad Sci 1975;240:95.
188. Klein HG, Aledort LM, Bouma BN, Hoyer LW, Zimmerman TS, DeMets DL. Cooperative study for detection of the carrier state of classic hemophilia. N Engl J Med 1977;296:959.
189. Orstavik KH, Veltkamp JJ, Bertina RM, Hermans J. Detection of carriers of hemophilia B. Br J Haematol 1979;42:293.
190. Hoyer LW, Carta CA, Mahoney MJ. Detection of hemophilia carriers during pregnancy. Blood 1982;60:1407.
191. Levine PH. The clinical manifestations and therapy of hemophilias A and B. In Coleman RW, Hirsch J, Marder VJ, Salzman EW, eds. Hemostasis and thrombosis. Philadelphia: JB Lippincott, 1982:85.
192. Sampietro M, Camerino G, Romano M, et al. Combined use of DNA probes in first-trimester prenatal diagnosis of hemophilia A. Thromb Haemost 1987;58:988.
193. Mibashan RS, Peake IR, Rodeck CH, et al. Dual diagnosis of prenatal hemophilia A by measurement of fetal factor VIII C and VIII C antigen (VIII C Ag). Lancet 1980;2:994.
194. Holmberg L, Gustavii B, Cordesius E, et al. Prenatal diagnosis of hemophilia B by an immunoradiometric assay of factor IX. Blood 1980;56:397.
195. Thaler E, Lechner K. Antithrombin III deficiency in thromboembolus. Clinics in Haematology 1981;10:369.
196. Rosenberg RD. Actions and interactions of antithrombin III and heparin. N Engl J Med 1975;292:146.
197. Prochownik EV, Antonarakis S, Bauer KA, Rosenberg RD, Fearon ER, Orkin SH. Molecular heterogeneity of inherited antithrombin III deficiency. N Engl J Med 1983;308:1549.
198. Brandt P, Stembjerg S. Subcutaneous heparin for thrombosis in pregnant women with hereditary antithrombin deficiency. Br Med J 1980;1:449.
199. Egeberg O. Inherited antithrombin deficiency causing thrombophilia. Thromb Haemost 1965;13:516.
200. Johansson L. Hedner U, Nilsson IM. Familial antithrombin III deficiency as pathogenesis of deep venous thrombin. Acta Med Scand 1978;204:491.
201. Hellgren M, Tengborn L, Abildgaard U. Pregnancy in women with congenital antithrombin III deficiency: experience of treatment with heparin and antithrombin. Gynecol Obstet Invest 1982;14:127.
202. Weiner CP. Thromboembolic disease in the obstetric patient: evaluation, diagnosis, and treatment. In Kwaan HC, ed. Clinical thrombosis, vol 2. Boca Raton, FL: CRC Press, 1989:291.
203. Vellenga E, Van Imhoff GW, Aarnoudse JG. Effect of prophylaxis with oral anticoagulants and low dose heparin during pregnancy in an antithrombin III deficient woman. Lancet 1983;2:224.
204. Samson D, Stirling Y, Woolf L, Howarth D, Seghatehian MJ. Management of planned pregnancy in a patient with congenital antithrombin III deficiency. Br J Haematol 1984;56:243.
205. LeClerc JR, Geerts W, Panju A, Nguyen P, Hirsh J. Management of antithrombin III deficiency during pregnancy without administration of anti-thrombin III. Thromb Res 1986;41:567.
206. Weiner CP. Unpublished data.
207. Fairfax AJ, Ibbotson RM. Danazol raises antithrombin III levels in cases of familial deficiency. Lancet 1984;2:1272.
208. Wautier JL, Caen JP. Treatment of antithrombin III deficiency with danazol. Lancet 1984;2:599.
209. Fairfax AJ, Ibbotson RM. Effect of danazol on the biochemical abnormality of inherited antithrombin III deficiency. Thorax 1985;40:646.
210. Manco-Johnson MJ, Marlar RA, Jacobson CJ, Hays T, Warody BA. Severe protein C deficiency in newborn infants. J Pediatr 1988;113:359.
211. Morrison AE, Walker ID, Black WP. Protein C deficiency presenting as deep venous thrombosis in pregnancy. Case report. Br J Obstet Gynaecol 1988;95:1077.
212. Vogel JJ, de Moerloose A, Bounameaux H. Protein C deficiency and pregnancy: a case report. Obstet Gynecol 1989;73:455.
213. Comp PC, Esmon CT. Recurrent venous thromboembolism in patients with a partial deficiency of protein S. N Engl J Med 1984;311:1525.
214. Melissari E, Nicolaides KH, Scully MF, Kakkar VV. Protein S and C4b-binding protein in fetal and neonatal blood. Br J Haematol 1988;70:199.
215. Stahlman F, Herrington WJ, Maloney WC. Parahemophilia: report of a case in a woman with studies on other members of her family. J Lab Clin Med 1951;38:842.
216. Field JB, Ware AG. Studies on parahemophilia. J Clin Invest 1954;33:932.
217. Philips LL, Little WA. Factor V deficiency in obstetrics. Obstet Gynecol 1962;19:507.
218. Whitelaw A, Haines ME, Bolsover W, Harris E. Factor V deficiency and antenatal intraventricular haemorrhage. Arch Dis Child 1984;59:997.
219. Purcell G, Nossel HL. Factor XI (PTA) deficiency: surgical and obstetric aspects. Obstet Gynecol 1970;35:69.
220. Czapek EE. Coagulation problems. Int Anesthesiol Clin 1973;11:175.
221. Saidi P, Siegelman M, Mitchell VB. Effect of factor XII deficiency on pregnancy and parturition. Thromb Haemost 1979;41:523.
222. Coppleston A. Oscier DG. Heparin-induced thrombocytopenia in pregnancy ;obletter;cb. Br J Haematol 1987;65:248.
223. Meytes D, Ayalon H, Virag I, Weisbort Y, Zakut H. Heparin-induced thrombocytopenia and recurrent thrombosis in pregnancy: a case report. J Reprod Med 1986;31:993.
224. Anderson HM. Maternal hematologic disorders. In Creasy RK, Resnick R, eds. Maternal–fetal medicine: principles and practice. Philadelphia: WB Saunders, 1989:890.
225. Freedman J, Musclow E, Garvey B, Abbott D. Unexplained perparturient thrombocytopenia. Am J Hematol 1986;21:397.
226. Burrows RF, Kelton JG. Incidentally-detected thrombocytopenia in healthy mothers and their infants. N Engl J Med 1988;319:142.
227. Rolbin SH, Abbott D, Musclow E, Papsin F, Lie LM, Freedman J. Epidural anesthesia in pregnant patients with low platelet counts. Obstet Gynecol 1988;71:918.
228. Gernsheimer T, Stratton J, Ballem PJ, Slichter SJ. Mechanisms of response to treatment in autoimmune thrombocytopenic purpura. N Engl J Med 1989;320:974.
229. Tancer LM. Idiopathic thrombocytopenic purpura and pregnancy. Am J Obstet Gynecol 1960;79:148.
230. Davies SV, Murray JA, Gee H, Giles HM. Transplacental effect of high-dose immunoglobulin in idiopathic thrombocytopenia (ITP) ;obletter;cb. Lancet 1986;1:1098.
231. Hammarstrom L, Smith CI. Placental transfer of intravenous immunoglobulin ;obletter;cb. Lancet 1986;1:681.
232. Kelton JG. Management of the pregnant patient with idiopathic thrombocytopenic purpura. Ann Intern Med 1983;99:796.
233. Kelton JG, Inwood MJ, Barr RM. The prenatal prediction of thrombocytopenia in infants of mothers with clinically diagnosed immune thrombocytopenia. Am J Obstet Gynecol 1982;144:449.
234. Pritchard JA, Cunningham FG, Pritchard SA, Mason RA. How

often does maternal preeclampsia-eclampsia incite thrombocytopenia in the fetus? Obstet Gynecol 1987;69:292.
235. Christiaens GCML, Helmerhorst FM. Validity of intrapartum diagnosis of fetal thrombocytopenia. Am J Obstet Gynecol 1987;157:864.
236. Weiner CP. Cordocentesis. Obstet Gynecol Clin North Am 1988;15:283.
237. Pearson H, Schulman N, Marder V, Cone T. Immune neonatal thrombocytopenic purpura: clinical and therapeutic considerations. Blood 1964;23:154.
238. Schulman NR, Marder VJ, Hiller MC, Collier EM. Platelet and leukocyte antigens and their antibodies. Serologic, physiologic, and clinical studies. Prog Hematol 1964;4:222.
239. Kaplan C, Daffos F, Forestier F, et al. Management of alloimmune thrombocytopenia: antenatal diagnosis and in utero transfusion of maternal platelets. Blood 1988;72:340.
240. Patriarco M, Yeh SY. Immunologic thrombocytopenia in pregnancy. Obstet Gynecol Surv 1986;41:661.
241. Zalneraitis E, Richard Y, Krischnamoorthy K. Intracranial hemorrhage in utero, a complication of isoimmune thrombocytopenia. J Pediatr 1979;95:611.
242. DeVries LS, Connell J, Bydder GM, et al. Recurrent intracranial haemorrhages in utero in an infant with alloimmune thrombocytopenia. Case report. Br J Obstet Gynaecol 1988;95:299.
243. Burrows RF, Caco CC, Kelton JG. Neonatal alloimmune thrombocytopenia: spontaneous in utero intracranial hemorrhage. Am J Hematol 1988;28:98.
244. Herman JH, Jumbelic MI, Ancona RJ, Kickler TS. In utero cerebral hemorrhage in alloimmune thrombocytopenia. Am J Pediatr Hematol Oncol 1986;8:312.
245. Donner M, Aronsson S, Holmberg L, Olofsson P. Corticosteroid treatment of maternal ITP and risk of neonatal thrombocytopenia. Acta Paediatr Scand 1987;76:369.
246. Bussel JB, Berkowitz RL, McFarland JG, Lynch L, Chitkara U. Antenatal treatment of neonatal alloimmune thrombocytopenia. N Engl J Med 1988;319:1374.
247. Bussel J, Berkowitz R, McFarland J, Lynch L, Chitkara U. In-utero platelet transfusion for alloimmune thrombocytopenia ;obletter;cb. Lancet 1988;2:1307.
248. Mueller-Eckhardt C, Kiefel V, Jovanovic V, et al. Prenatal treatment of fetal alloimmune thrombocytopenia. Lancet 1988; 2:910.
249. Management of alloimmune neonatal thrombocytopenia ;obreview article;cb. Lancet 1989;1:137.
250. Daffos F, Forrestier F, Kaplan C. Prenatal treatment of fetal alloimmune thrombocytopenia [letter]. Lancet 1988;2:910.
251. Moschowitz E. An acute febrile pleiochromic anemia with hyaline thrombosis of terminal arterioles and capillaries. An undescribed disease. Arch Intern Med 1925;36:89.
252. Bukowski RM. TTP, a review. Prog Hemost Thromb 1982; 6:287.
253. Pinette MG, Vintzileos AM, Ingardia CJ. Thrombotic thrombocytopenic purpura as a cause of thrombocytopenia in pregnancy. Literature review. Am J Perinatol 1989;6:55.
254. Weiner CP. Thrombotic microangiopathy in pregnancy and the postpartum period. Semin Hematol 1987;24:119.
255. Harker LA, Slichter SJ. Platelet and fibrinogen consumption in man. N Engl J Med 1972;287:999.
256. Byrnes JJ, Moake JL. Thrombotic thrombocytopenic purpura and the haemolytic-uraemic syndrome. Evolving concepts of pathogenesis and therapy. Clin Haematol 1986;15:413.
257. Jaffe EA, Nachman RL, Herskey C. Thrombotic thrombocytopenic purpura: coagulation parameters in twelve patients. Blood 1973;42:499.
258. Ambrose A, Welham RT, Cefalo RC. TTP in early pregnancy. Obstet Gynecol 1985;66:267.
259. Vandekerchove F. TTP mimicking toxemia. Am J Obstet Gynecol 1984;150:320.
260. Romero R, Mazor M, Lockwood CJ, et al. Clinical significance, prevalence, and natural history of thrombocytopenia in pregnancy-induced hypertension. Am J Perinatol 1989;6:32.
261. Stubbs TM, Lazarchick J, Van Dorsten P, Cox J, Loadholt CB. Evidence of accelerated platelet production and consumption in nonthrombocytopenic preeclampsia. Am J Obstet Gynecol 1986;155:263.
262. Samuels P, Main EK, Tomaski A, Mennuti MT, Gabbe SG, Cines D. Abnormalities in platelet antiglobulin tests in preeclamptic mothers and their neonates. Am J Obstet Gynecol 1987;157:109.
263. Hart D, Dunetz C, Nardi M, Porges RF, Weiss A, Karpatkin M. An epidemic of maternal thrombocytopenia associated with elevated antiplatelet antibody: platelet count and antiplatelet antibody in 116 consecutive pregnancies. Relationship to neonatal platelet count. Am J Obstet Gynecol 1986;154:878.
264. Rick ME, Williams SB, Sacher RA, McKeown LP. Thrombocytopenia associated with pregnancy in a patient with type IIB von Willebrand's disease. Blood 1987;69:786.
265. Giles AR, Hoogendoorn H, Benford K. Type IIB von Willebrand's disease presenting as thrombocytopenia during pregnancy. Br J Haematol 1987;67:349.
266. Conti M, Mari D, Conti E, Muggiasca ML, Mannucci PM. Pregnancy in women with different types of von Willebrand disease. Obstet Gynecol 1986;68:282.
267. Stuart MJ, Gross SJ, Elred H, Graeber JE. Effects of acetylsalicylic acid ingestation on maternal and neonatal hemostasis. N Engl J Med 1982;307:909.
268. White JG. Inherited abnormalities of the platelet membrane and secretory granules. Hum Pathol 1987;18:123.

69

CHAPTER

HEMATOLOGIC DISORDERS OF PREGNANCY

Russell K. Laros, Jr.

Anemia is usually defined as a hemoglobin (Hgb) value below the lower limits of normal that is not explained by the state of hydration. The normal hemoglobin level for the adult woman is 14.0 ± 2.0 g/dL.[1,2] The above definition has physiologic validity in that it is the amount of Hgb per unit volume of blood that determines the O_2 carrying capacity of blood. Using the above normal, 20% to 60% of prenatal patients will be found to be anemic at some time during pregnancy. Some centers have chosen to use slightly lower Hgb values (11.0 or 10.5 g/dL) to define anemia during pregnancy. Although this practice will decrease the number of gravidas found to be anemic, it does so by calling some mildly anemic patients normal and thus delaying additional hematologic evaluation. Such a decision is practical and appropriate as long as the practitioner remembers to obtain a follow-up hemogram to be sure that there is not a progression of the anemia.

CLINICAL PRESENTATION

Symptoms due to anemia are those of tissue hypoxia, those of the cardiovascular system's attempts to compensate for the anemia, or those due to an underlying disease. Tissue hypoxia produces fatigue, light-headedness, weakness, and exertional dyspnea. Cardiovascular compensation leads to symptoms of a hyperdynamic circulation, such as palpitations and tachycardia. Clinical situations commonly associated with anemia include multiple pregnancy, trophoblastic disease, chronic renal disease, arthritis, chronic liver disease, and chronic infection. However, in obstetric patients anemia is most commonly discovered because a complete blood count (CBC) is obtained as part of routine laboratory evaluation, either at the initial prenatal visit or at 28 to 32 weeks gestation.

Additional history of value is the use of "tonics," a family history of anemia or splenectomy, a history of gastrointestinal bleeding or melena, genitourinary bleeding, or exposure to oxidant drugs in individuals at risk for glucose-6-phosphate dehydrogenase (G6PD) deficiency. Such agents include antimalarials, sulfonamides, sulfones, nitrofurans, various analgesics, fava beans, moth balls, para-aminosalicyclic acid (PAS), probenecid, and isoniazid (INH).

USE OF THE COMPLETE BLOOD COUNT

Anemia is not a diagnosis, but rather a sign, such as fever or edema. The key issue in the evaluation of anemia is to define the mechanism or disease process. Although a mild anemia during pregnancy caused by iron deficiency is of little consequence to either the mother or the fetus, a similarly mild anemia caused by a carcinoma of the colon has grave implications. One must also keep in mind the genetic implications of many anemias, such as the hemoglobinopathies or hereditary spherocytosis.

Table 69-1 presents a classification of anemia based on the pathophysiologic mechanism involved. Although a mechanistic classification of anemia provides an exhaustive catalog of diagnoses, it does not lend itself to a systematic investigation of an individual patient.[3] Rather one wants to know the following:

Is the patient anemic?
What is the morphology of the anemia?
What is the reticulocyte count?

TABLE 69-1. ANEMIA CLASSIFIED BY PATHOPHYSIOLOGIC MECHANISM

- **I.** Dilutional (expansion of the plasma volume)
  - **A.** Pregnancy
  - **B.** Hyperglobulinemia
  - **C.** Massive splenomegaly
- **II.** Decreased red blood cell production
  - **A.** Bone marrow failure
    - **1.** Decreased building blocks or stimulation
      - **a.** Iron, protein
      - **b.** Chronic infection, chronic renal disease
    - **2.** Decreased erythron
      - **a.** Hypoplasia (hereditary, drugs, radiation, toxins)
      - **b.** Marrow replacement (tumor, fibrosis, infection)
  - **B.** Ineffective production
    - **1.** Megaloblastic (B_{12} and folate deficiency, myelodysplasia, erythroleukemia)
    - **2.** Normoblastic (refractory anemia, thalassemia)
- **III.** Increased red cell loss
  - **A.** Acute hemorrhage
  - **B.** Hemolysis
    - **1.** Intrinsic RBC disorders
      - **a.** Hereditary
        - **i.** Hemoglobinopathies
        - **ii.** RBC enzyme deficiency
        - **iii.** Membrane defects
        - **iv.** Porphyrias
      - **b.** Acquired
        - **i.** Paroxysmal nocturnal hemoglobinuria
        - **ii.** Lead poisoning
    - **2.** Extrinsic RBC disorders
      - **a.** Immune
      - **b.** Mechanical
      - **c.** Infection
      - **d.** Chemical agents
      - **e.** Burns
      - **f.** Hypersplenism
      - **g.** Liver disease

RBC; red blood cell.

Developing the answers to the above questions allows one to make a first approximation of a specific diagnosis and answer the following questions:

What is the mechanism of the anemia?
Is there an underlying disease?
What is appropriate treatment?

The CBC and the reticulocyte count provide the answers to the first three questions and are really the hematologist's "critical biopsy." These data allow a morphologic classification of the anemia and define whether the marrow is hyper- or hypoproliferative. Table 69-2 presents normal values for women. The Hgb is determined by converting the pigment to cyanmethemoglobin and quantitating the amount spectrophotometrically. The remainder of the values are obtained by flow cytometry with an electronic cell counter. Based on the size of the red blood cells (RBCs), anemia can be classified as microcytic, normocytic, or macrocytic. The appearance of the RBCs may also provide a clue as to the mechanism of anemia. For example, hypochromic microcytic cells associated with a low reticulocyte count suggest iron deficiency, thalassemia trait, sideroblastic anemia, or lead poisoning. Oval macrocytes combined with a low reticulocyte count and hypersegmented polymorphonuclear leukocytes suggest megaloblastic anemia (B_{12} or folate deficiency). Oval microcytes and an elevated reticulocyte count are characteristic of hereditary spherocytosis. Various poikilocytes, such as sickle cells, acanthrocytes, target cells, and schistocytes, suggest sickle cell disease, acanthrocytosis, hemoglobin C disease, and mechanical RBC destruction, respectively.

TABLE 69-2. NORMAL VALUES FOR RED BLOOD CELLS

Erythroid values	
Hemoglobin (Hgb)	12–16 gm/dL
Hematocrit (Hct)	36–46%
Red cell count (RBC)	$4.0–5.2 \times 10^{12}$/L
Erythroid indices:	
Mean corpuscular volume (MCV)	80–100 fL
Mean corpuscular hemoglobin concentration (MCHC)	31–36 g/dL
Red cell morphology	
Anisocytosis	Variation in cell size
Poikilocytosis	Variation in cell shape
Polychromatophilia	Amount of 'blueness'
Hypochromia	Amount of central pallor
Platelet estimate	5–10 platelets per oil immersion field
Reticulocyte count	$48–152 \times 10^9$/L
White blood cell count	$5–14 \times 10^9$/L

The peripheral blood smear also allows evaluation of the white blood cells (WBCs). In most cases of leukemia, abnormal granulocytes or lymphocytes appear. The presence of nucleated RBCs in association with marked poikilocytosis suggests erythroleukemia, myeloid metaplasia or marrow infiltration with solid tumor, or granulomatous infection.

ADDITIONAL LABORATORY STUDIES

Although use of the CBC allows one a excellent first approximation at the diagnosis of anemia, additional studies are usually necessary to confirm the diagnosis.[1-3] Table 69-3 details laboratory studies frequently used in the evaluation of an anemic patient.

Serum hemoglobin and serum haptoglobin levels are useful in defining intravascular hemolysis. When a low or absent serum haptoglobin is associated with an elevated serum hemoglobin, intravascular hemolysis is established. Further studies are necessary to rule in or out specific causes of intravascular hemolysis, such as severe autoimmune hemolytic anemia (direct Coombs' test), paroxysmal nocturnal hemoglobinuria (osmotic fragility), and hemoglobinopathies such as sickle cell disease and thalassemia major (hemoglobin electrophoresis).

The total bilirubin is elevated modestly in hemolytic anemia (rarely >4 mg/dL). The increase is due predominantly to an increase in the indirect fraction. However,

TABLE 69-3. LABORATORY STUDIES USEFUL IN EVALUATION OF ANEMIA

STUDY	NORMAL VALUE
Serum hemoglobin	<1.0 mg/dL
Serum haptoglobin	30–200 mg/dL
Total bilirubin	0.1–1.2 mg/dL
Direct Coombs's test	Negative
G-6-PD	
Electrophoresis	B+ (A+, A−, B−, 150 others are abnormal)
Quantitative study	4–8 U/g of Hgb
Hemoglobin electrophoresis	>98% A <3.5% A2 <2% F
RBC enzymes	Multiple types; pyruvate kinase most common
Osmotic fragility	Preincubation: 0.40–0.46% NaCl Postincubation: 0.48–0.60% NaCl
Serum ferritin	>10 μg/L
Free erythrocyte protoporphyrine (FEP)	<3.0 μg/g
Plasma iron	40–175 μg/dL
Plasma total iron-binding capacity	216–400 μg/dL
Transferrin saturation	16–60%
Stool guaiac	Negative
Serum folate	6–12 μg/L
RBC folate	165–760 μg/L
Serum B_{12}	190–950 ng/L
Anti-intrinsic factor antibody (AIF)	Negative
Bone marrow	Normal distribution of erythroid and myeloid precursors

RBC; red blood cell.

significant hemolysis can occur without an elevation in the bilirubin. Thus, the bilirubin level is helpful only when elevated.

The direct Coombs's test uses antihuman globulin to detect globulins attached to the surface of RBCs. A positive test indicates an immune cause for a hemolytic anemia. In such cases, it is important to search for underlying causes for autoimmunity, such as connective tissue disease, lymphoma, carcinoma, and sarcoidosis.

Inherited as a sex-linked recessive disorder, G6PD deficiency is rare in females and therefore will not be discussed further. The diagnosis and management of the various hemoglobinopathies and red cell enzyme deficiencies are discussed in Chapter 32.

The free erythrocyte protoporphyrine (FEP),[4] plasma iron, plasma total iron-binding capacity,[5] and the serum ferritin level[6,7] are all useful in establishing a diagnosis of iron deficiency. Iron is transported in the plasma bound to transferrin. In the iron-deficient state, the plasma iron decreases, the iron-binding capacity increases, and the percent saturation decreases. In contrast, with chronic infection both the plasma iron and the iron-binding capacity are decreased and the percent saturation remains normal. Serum ferritin correlates very closely with body iron stores; in the iron-deficient state, the serum ferritin level is <20 μg/L. Both the plasma iron and serum ferritin levels are increased following the ingestion of iron.[8,9] Thus, iron therapy must be discontinued for 24 to 48 hours before these studies are carried out. In iron deficiency, the FEP increases approximately fivefold. Which of the above studies is the most sensitive and specific for making the diagnosis of iron deficiency is still debated.

Whenever a diagnosis of iron deficiency anemia is made, it is essential to rule out gastrointestinal bleeding as the cause for the iron deficit. This is accomplished by testing the stool for the presence of occult blood with guaiac or some other equally sensitive reagent.

Serum folate, RBC folate, and serum B_{12} levels are useful in defining the cause of a macrocytic anemia. Because the RBC folate more accurately depicts the body's folate stores, many laboratories no longer offer the serum folate determination. The presence of serum intrinsic factor antibodies is very specific for pernicious anemia. Because they are absent in approximately 40% of cases, the absence of these antibodies does not rule out a diagnosis of pernicious anemia.

Examination of the bone marrow by aspiration or biopsy can add much useful information. In addition to providing a ratio of myeloid to erythroid production (normally approximately 3:1), it provides a measure of iron stores, allows a differential count of myeloid and erythroid precursors, provides evidence of infiltration with neoplasm, and allows histologic and bacteriologic confirmation of infection.

NORMAL HEMATOLOGIC EVENTS ASSOCIATED WITH PREGNANCY

BLOOD VOLUME CHANGES

During pregnancy there is normally an increase of 36% in the blood volume, with the maximum being reached at 34 weeks gestation.[10] The plasma volume increases 47% and the RBC mass only 17%. The latter reaches its maximum at term. As shown in Figure 69-1, there is relative hemodilution throughout pregnancy, which is at its maximum from 28 to 34 weeks gestation. Although this dilutional effect will lower the Hgb, hematocrit (Hct), and RBC count, it causes no change in the mean corpuscular volume (MCV) or in the mean corpuscular hemoglobin concentration (MCHC). Thus, serial evaluation of these two indices is useful in differentiating dilutional anemia from progressive iron deficiency anemia during pregnancy. In the former, the indices do not change, while in the latter they decrease progressively.

IRON KINETICS

The classic study by Scott and Pritchard shows that iron stores in healthy women are marginal at best.[11] Figure 69-2 shows the iron stores found in the bone marrows

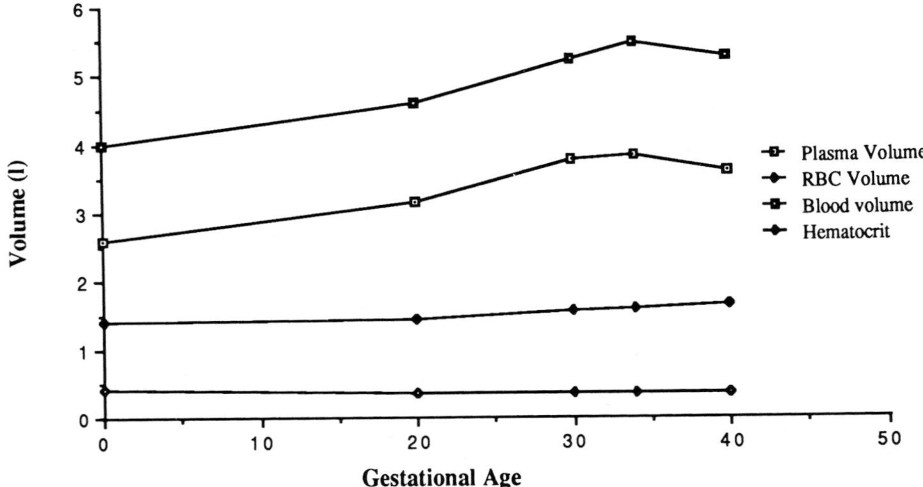

FIGURE 69–1. Hematologic changes during pregnancy.

of healthy, white college students who had never been pregnant or donated blood. Approximately two thirds had minimal iron stores. The same authors also demonstrated that almost 50% of healthy primagravidas had minimal iron stores in their marrow during the first trimester of pregnancy.[12]

The major reason for poor iron stores is thought to be menstrual loss. Monsen's studies confirm that the usual menstrual loss is 25 to 30 mL of whole blood.[13] This is equivalent to 12 to 15 mg of elemental iron, because each mL of blood contains 0.5 mg of iron. To meet the iron loss for menses alone, a woman requires 1.5 to 2.0 mg of elemental iron to be absorbed from her diet each day. Because only 10% of dietary iron is usually absorbed and the average diet contains only 6 mg per 1000 kcal, a woman's iron balance is precarious at best.

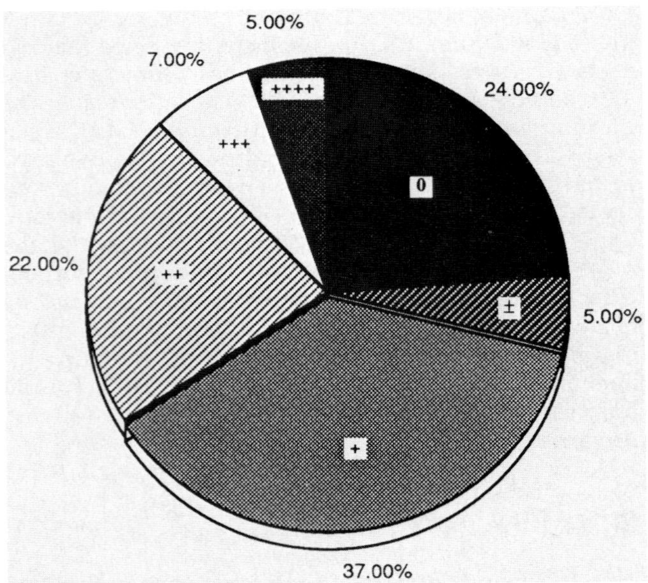

FIGURE 69–2. Distribution of iron stores in healthy college students.

Pregnancy presents substantial demands on iron balance above and beyond what is saved by 9 months of amenorrhea.[12] Table 69-4 lists the iron requirements for pregnancy. If there is insufficient iron available to meet the demands of pregnancy, iron-deficient erythropoiesis will result. Fenton and colleagues used the serum ferritin level to evaluate iron stores in pregnant women.[14] Figure 69-3 shows the difference in ferritin levels in those receiving iron supplementation as compared to an unsupplemented group.

Thus, most young women enter their first pregnancy with marginal stores. Pregnancy places a large demand on iron balance that cannot be meet with the usual diet. In the absence of supplementation, iron deficiency develops. The usual sequence of events with iron deficiency is an absence of iron in the marrow followed by the development of abnormal plasma iron studies (transferrin, ferritin, or free red cell protoporphyrin). The RBCs first become microcytic, then hypochromic. Finally, anemia develops.

FOLATE

Folic acid is a water soluble vitamin that is generally widely available in the diet. Dietary folates are in fact a family of compounds and generally appear as polyglutamates. In humans, the only source of folate is the diet, and absorption is primarily in the proximal jejunum. Before folate can be absorbed, it must be reduced to the monoglutamate form.[15] Pancreatic conjugases within the intestine are responsible for this process. The activity of conjugase is decreased by anticonvulsants, oral contraceptives, alcohol, and sulfa drugs.[16] Thus, in addition to an absolute diminution in the dietary intake, the combination of increased need (as in multiple pregnancy and hemolytic anemia) coupled with decreased absorption can lead to folate deficiency.[17–19]

TABLE 69–4. IRON REQUIREMENTS FOR PREGNANCY

REQUIRED FOR	AVERAGE (mg)	RANGE (mg)
External iron loss	170	150–200
Expansion of RBC mass	450	200–600
Fetal iron	270	200–370
Iron in placenta and cord	90	30–170
Blood loss at delivery	150	90–310
Total requirement	980	580–1340
Requirement less RBC expansion	840	440–1050

RBC; red blood cell.

During pregnancy, there is a significant increase over the non-pregnant folate requirement of 50 μg/day to 800 to 1000 μg/day.[12,20] When folate depletion occurs, the usual sequence of events is a decreased serum folate, hypersegmentation of polymorphonuclear leukocytes, a decrease in RBC folate, the appearance of ovalocytes in the blood, development of an abnormal marrow and, finally, anemia.[15]

VITAMIN B_{12}

Vitamin B_{12} is also abundantly available in the diet, bound to animal protein. Absorption requires hydrochloric acid and pepsin to free the cobolamine molecule from protein. Intrinsic factor is also essential for absorption. Once absorbed, transport occurs by binding to transcobalamin II. The majority of storage is in the liver, and most humans have a 2- to 3-year store available.[5]

MORPHOLOGIC CLASSIFICATION OF ANEMIA

As discussed above, a CBC allows placement of a given case of anemia into one of three major groups, based on size and hemoglobin content of the RBCs. The classification is augmented by the reticulocyte count, which adds information about the bone marrow's activity.[2,3]

MICROCYTIC ANEMIA

This group of anemias is characterized by abnormal Hgb synthesis with normal RBC production. Figure

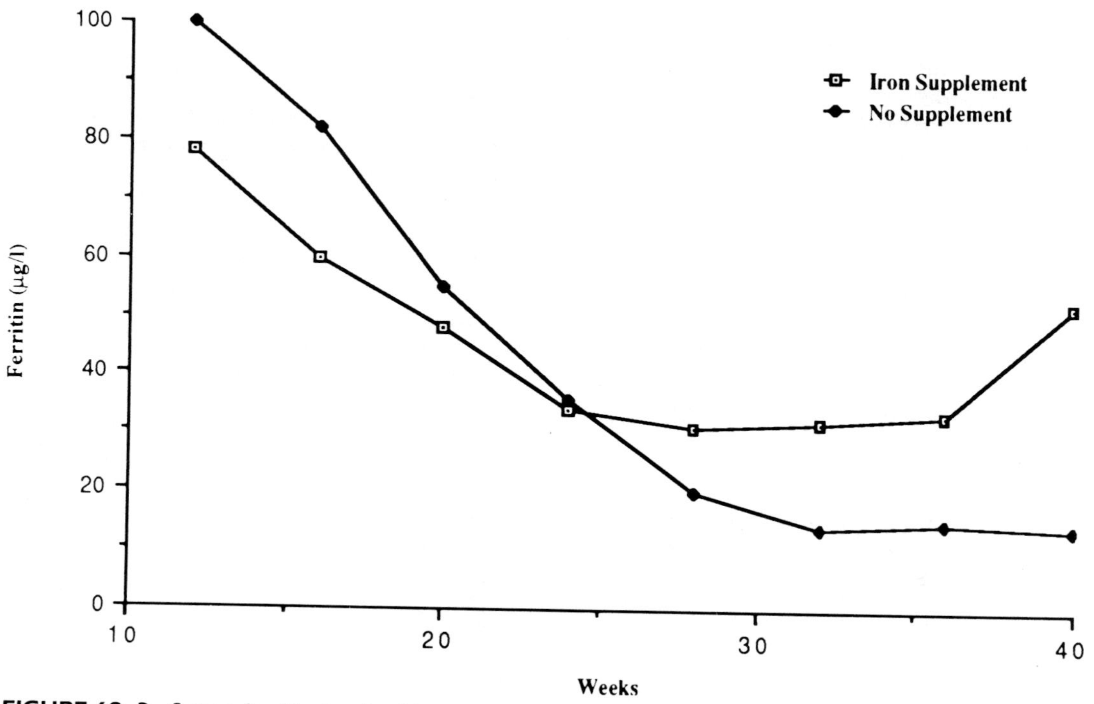

FIGURE 69–3. Serum ferritin level with and without supplementation.

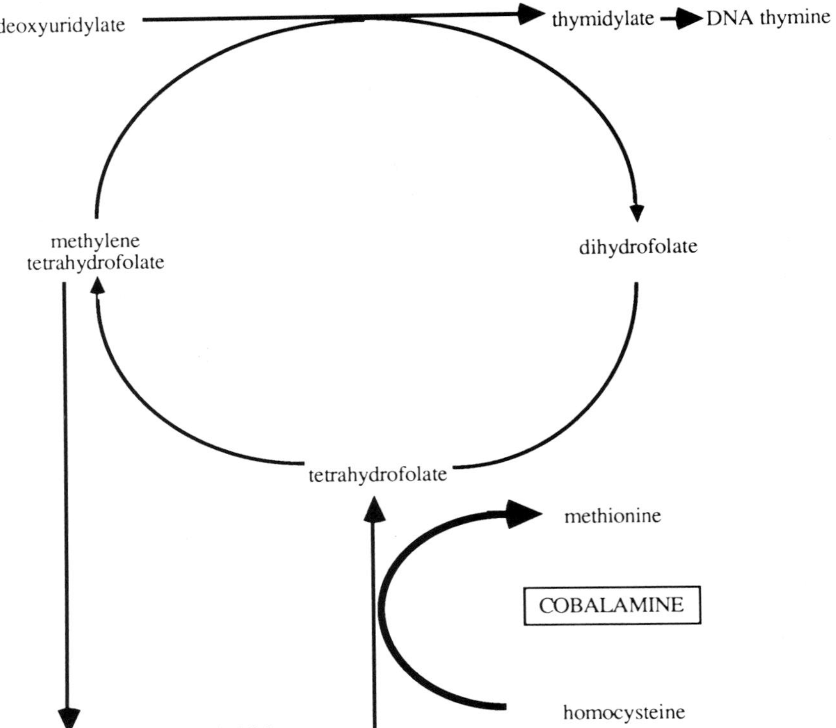

FIGURE 69–4. Folate and B_{12} interact in thymidylate synthesis.

69-5 presents a logical progression of diagnostic steps for evaluation of a microcytic anemia. The first step is to rule in or out iron deficiency. If present, it is also essential to consider whether or not chronic blood loss from the gastrointestinal or genitourinary tracts is a factor in the cause.

When a microcytic anemia is not due to iron deficiency, one must then differentiate between cases due to a hemoglobinopathy, chronic infection, or the various sideroblastic anemias. This differentiation is made based on the plasma iron and iron-binding capacity, the FEP, a hemoglobin electrophoresis, DNA probing for α-genes, and bone marrow examination.

NORMOCYTIC ANEMIA

Evaluation of a normocytic anemia is the most difficult. The difficulty is due to the diverse nature of this group. Figure 69-6 presents a diagnostic algorithm for normocytic anemias and macrocytic anemias with normoblastic erythropoiesis. The reticulocyte count differentiates between cases with increased versus normal or decreased RBC production. If erythropoiesis is increased, one must then differentiate between hemorrhage and an increased rate of destruction. The blood smear may reveal a type of RBC that is virtually diagnostic. Fragmented cells are seen in microangiopathic hemolysis (the HELLP syndrome of preeclampsia/eclampsia and thrombotic thrombocytopenic purpura) and in association with prosthetic heart valves. Other types of named poikilocytes include sickle cells, target cells, stomatocytes, ovalocytes, spherocytes, elliptocytes, and acanthrocytes.

Coombs' test will differentiate immune from nonimmune causes of hemolysis. Immune hemolysis is related to alloantibodies, drug-induced antibodies, and autoantibodies. Nonimmune causes of hemolysis include various hemoglobinopathies, hereditary disorders of the RBC membrane (spherocytosis and elliptocytosis), hereditary deficiency of a RBC enzyme, and the porphyrias. Acquired, nonimmune hemolysis is due either to paroxysmal nocturnal hemoglobinuria or lead poisoning.

Bone marrow examination is essential for evaluation of patients with hypoproliferative anemias with normal iron studies. If erythropoiesis is megaloblastic, folate or B_{12} deficiency is a likely cause. If sideroblastic, both acquired and hereditary forms of sideroblastic anemia must be considered. Finally, if erythropoiesis is normoblastic, causes fall into two major categories. The first group shows myeloid:erythroid (M:E) ratios of >4:1 and includes aplasia, infiltration, the effects of chronic diseases, and endocrine disorders such as hypothyroidism and hypopituitarism. Ineffective erythropoiesis, usually associated with an M:E ratio of <2:1, marks the second group.

MACROCYTIC ANEMIA

Macrocytic anemia is associated either with an increased rate of RBC production with release of less than fully mature RBCs or with disorders of impaired DNA

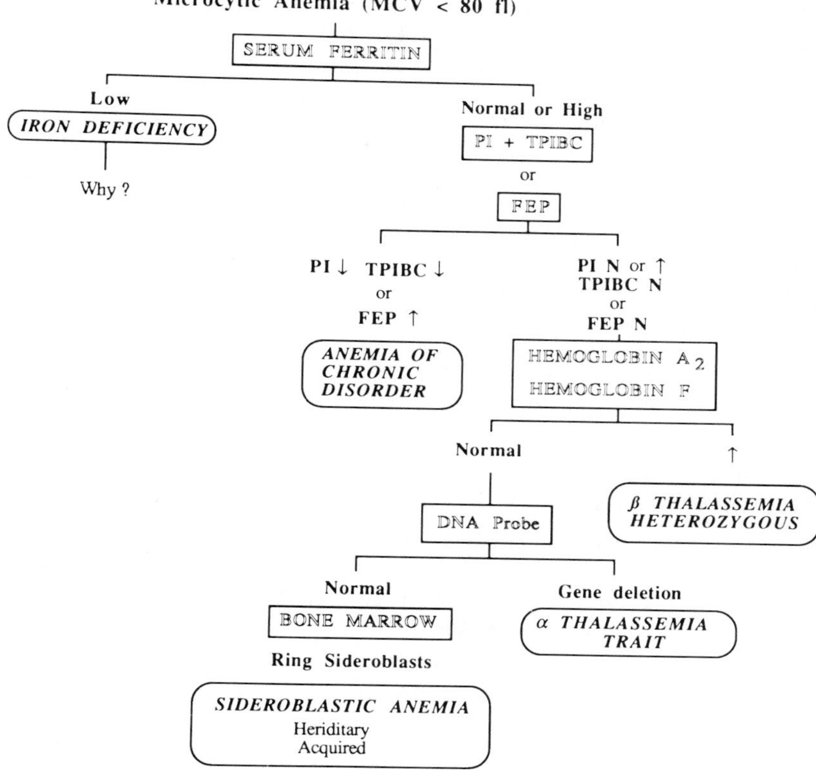

FIGURE 69–5. Diagnostic algorithm for microcytosis. PI, plasma iron; TPIBC, total plasma iron-binding capacity; FEP, free erythrocyte protoporphyrin.

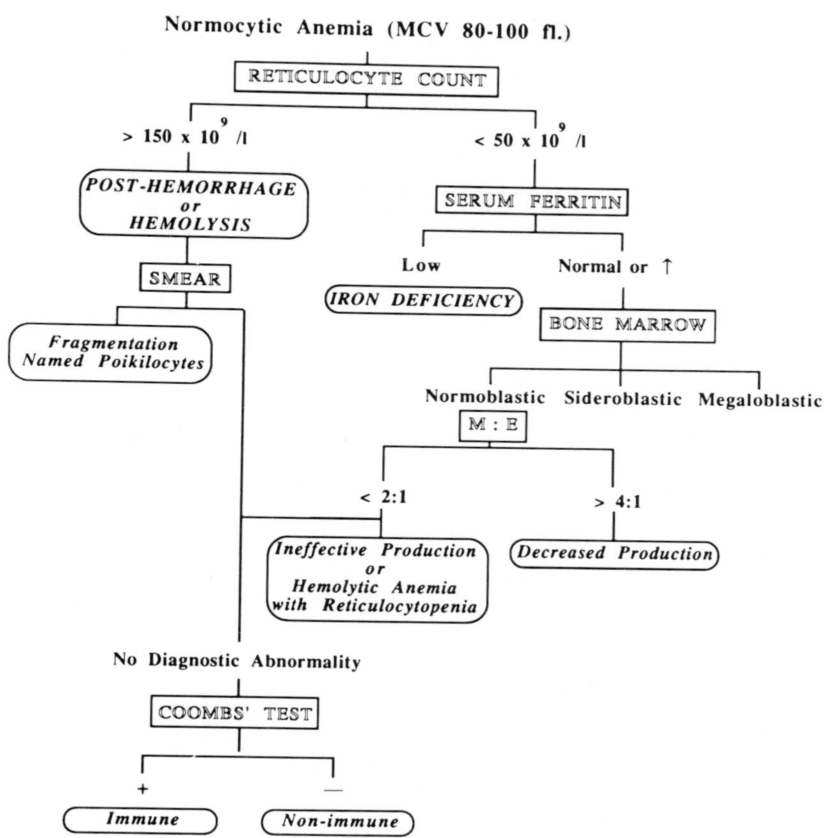

FIGURE 69–6. Diagnostic algorithm for normocytic anemia. M:E, myeloid/erythroid ratio.

synthesis. Figure 69-7 outlines an algorithm for evaluation of macrocytosis. One quickly notes that there are substantial areas of overlap between the evaluation of a normocytic and a macrocytic anemia. Early use of a bone marrow examination is very helpful in pointing the investigation in the correct direction.

When maturation is megaloblastic, serum B_{12} and RBC folate levels will allow a diagnosis of B_{12} or folate deficiency. When folate deficiency is diagnosed, the various causes of decreased deconjugation of the polyglutamate and malabsorption must be considered. If anti-intrinsic factor antibodies are present, a diagnosis of pernicious anemia (PA) is assured. If absent, a Schilling test is required to differentiate between PA and a small bowel malabsorption syndrome.

ANEMIA AND PERINATAL MORBIDITY AND MORTALITY

THE EFFECTS OF ANEMIA

Although it has been traditionally taught that significant maternal anemia is associated with suboptimal fetal outcome, the data supporting this concept are scarce. There are several studies, carried out in developing countries, that compare fetal outcome in groups of women with hemoglobins above and below 6 to 7 g/dL. Although these studies show improved reproductive function in those women with higher hemoglobin levels, they do not control for protein malnutrition and chronic parasitic infestation.

Maternal anemia has been reported in association with placental gigantism (>900 g), and maternal anemia is frequently associated with low plasma estriol values.[21,22] Sagen's study showed an inverse relation between placental weight, fetal weight, and maternal Hct.[23] These data are interpreted as evidence of chronic hypoxia.

Studies in sheep show that fetal O_2 consumption is maintained until the maternal Hct is reduced by >50%.[24] Furthermore, there are several anecdotal reports where fetal distress, noted in a fetal heart rate tracing, was completely relieved by correction of maternal anemia. Thus, while profound maternal anemia can have adverse effects on the fetus, the margin of safety appears to be large.

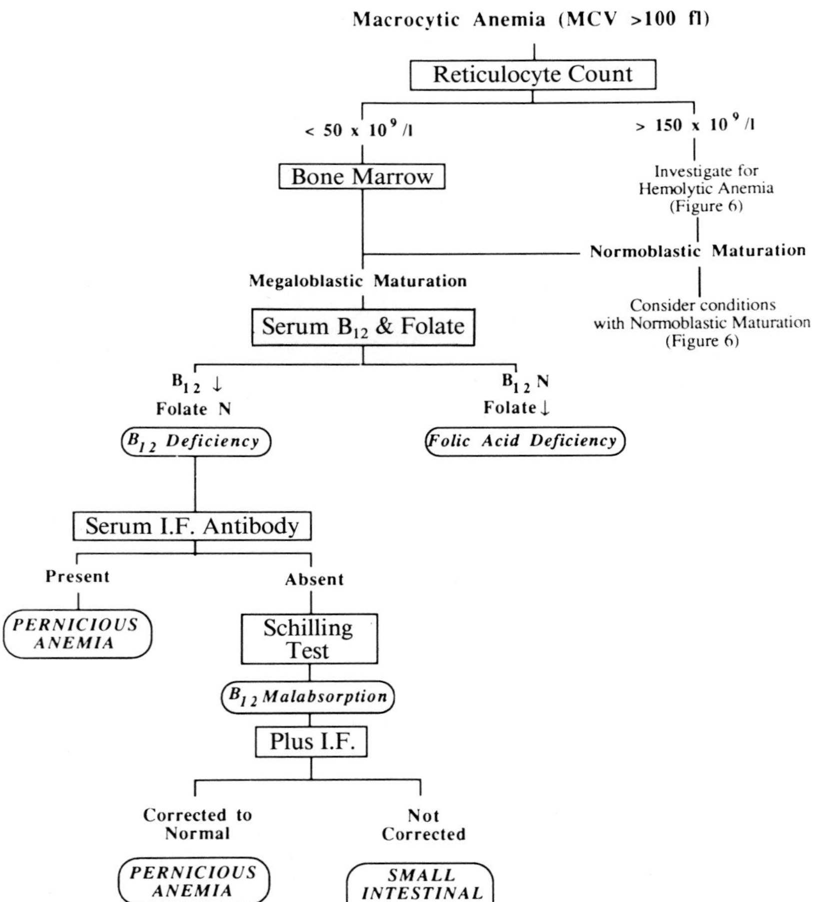

FIGURE 69–7. Diagnostic algorithm for macrocytic anemia. I.F., intrinsic factor.

THE EFFECTS OF SPECIFIC NUTRITIONAL DEFECTS

Fortunately, the fetal compartment preferentially obtains iron,[25,26] folate, and B_{12}[19] from and at the expense of the mother. In Fenton's study, the cord blood ferritin levels of infants whose mothers were iron deficient were reduced below that of infants whose mothers were not iron deficient.[14] However, the infants whose ferritins were low were not anemic, had normal iron kinetics, and their serum ferritin values were not in the iron-deficient range. In a study of newborns of women with severe folate deficiency, Pritchard and colleagues found normal neonatal levels of folate.[12,19]

GENETIC IMPLICATIONS

It is important to remember that many of the hemolytic anemias are inherited as either autosomal dominant or recessive traits. Thus, once the correct diagnosis has been made, the genetic implications should be thoroughly discussed with the patient and her partner. Where appropriate, the discussion should include antenatal diagnosis.

SPECIFIC ANEMIAS

Space does not allow a detailed discussion of the diagnosis and treatment of literally hundreds of different anemias. Instead, we have presented a scheme of diagnostic studies useful in evaluating any anemia and will limit discussion of specific anemias to only a few that are commonly seen during the course of pregnancy.

IRON DEFICIENCY ANEMIA

Iron deficiency is one of the most common causes of anemia during pregnancy. We have already discussed the demands placed on iron metabolism by both menstruation and pregnancy. Clinical symptoms include easy fatigue, lethargy, and headache. Pica involving clay, dirt, ice, or starch is a classic manifestation of iron deficiency. Clinical findings include pallor, glossitis, and cheilitis. Koilonychia has been associated with iron deficiency anemia, but is a rare finding.

The laboratory characteristics of iron deficiency anemia have been discussed above. In summary, one finds a microcytic, hypochromic anemia with evidence of depleted iron stores. The plasma iron is low and the total iron-binding capacity high, the serum ferritin is low, or the free erythrocyte protoporphyrin is elevated. If a bone marrow examination is done, stainable iron is markedly depleted or absent.

The specific treatment is oral iron. Most commonly, ferrous sulfate in a dose of 320 mg three times daily is used. Although a variety of other iron preparations are available, most are more expensive and do not offer any advantage over ferrous sulfate if equal amounts of elemental iron are given. Reticulocytosis should be observed after 7 to 10 days of therapy, and the Hgb can rise by as much as 1 g per week in severely anemic individuals. Absorption from the gastrointestinal tract can be enhanced by administration of 500 mg of ascorbic acid with each dose of iron. Once the anemia has resolved, the patient should continue receiving iron therapy for an additional 6 months in order to replace iron stores.

Gastrointestinal symptoms associated with iron therapy include nausea, vomiting, abdominal cramps, diarrhea, or constipation. These symptoms relate to the dose of elemental iron ingested and, if troublesome, the dose of iron should be reduced. Ferrous sulfate syrup is an effective way of tailoring the dose to the patient's tolerance.

Parenteral administration of iron dextran is rarely indicated and should be reserved for patients with a malabsorption syndrome or patients who absolutely will not take oral iron and who are significantly anemic (Hgb <8.5 g/dL).[27] We prefer administration of the total calculated dose by the intravenous route. Because severe anaphylaxis can occur, a test dose should be administered first. In the absence of any reaction, the full dose then can be administered over approximately 30 minutes. The required dose of iron dextran to correct anemia and replenish stores can be calculated as:

$$\text{Iron required (grams)} = \frac{(14 - \text{pt Hgb})(\text{pt wt in lbs})(0.124)}{100} + 0.05$$

where pt = patient, wt = weight.

MEGALOBLASTIC ANEMIA

Megaloblastic anemia is the second most common nutritional anemia seen during pregnancy. Most commonly, folate deficiency is the cause, but a deficiency in vitamin B_{12} also must be considered.

Patients with folate deficiency present with the typical symptoms of anemia plus roughness of the skin and glossitis. The CBC reveals a macrocytic, normochromic or normocytic, normochromic anemia with hypersegmentation of the polymorphonuclear leukocytes. The reticulocyte count is normal or low, and the WBC and platelet counts are frequently decreased. Bone marrow examination is usually not necessary to make the diagnosis, but if done shows megaloblastic erythropoiesis. The RBC folate is decreased to <165 μg/dL and the vitamin B_{12} level is normal.

Treatment consists of the administration of oral folic acid in a dose of 1 mg three times daily. Parenteral folic acid may be indicated in individuals with malabsorption. A reticulocyte response should be seen in 48 to 72 hours, and the platelet count will normalize within a few days. The neutrophils will normalize after 1 to 2 weeks.

In addition to anemia, individuals with B_{12} deficiency may also evidence neurologic defects relating to damage to the posterior columns of the spinal cord. It is critical that individuals with B_{12} deficiency not be treated with folic acid alone. Such treatment may well improve the anemia, but will have absolutely no salutary effect on the neuropathy and, in fact, may make it worse. As with folate deficiency, vitamin B_{12} deficiency is associated with either dietary deficiency, an increased requirement, or both. Except in strict vegetarians who avoid all animal products, dietary deficiency is very rare. The most common causes are inadequate production of intrinsic factor (pernicious anemia), inadequate production of intrinsic factor after gastrectomy, or the presence a malabsorption syndrome.

The morphologic features of B_{12} deficiency are similar to those of folate deficiency. In this instance, the serum B_{12} level is low and the folate normal. Because ineffective erythropoiesis is a prominent feature, evidence of low-grade hemolysis may be present (increased bilirubin and decreased haptoglobin). The Schilling test and measurement of anti-intrinsic factor antibodies are useful. Because the Schilling test requires ingestion of a radionuclide, its performance is not advised during pregnancy.

Treatment consists of 1000 μg of vitamin B_{12} administered parenterally weekly for 6 weeks, followed by monthly administration for life in cases of pernicious anemia. Again, a prompt reticulocyte response is anticipated after 3 to 5 days of therapy.

HEREDITARY SPHEROCYTOSIS AND ELLIPTOCYTOSIS

Spherocytosis is the most common form of inherited hemolytic anemia. The inheritance is as an autosomal dominant with variable penetrance. The exact defect in the RBC leading to the anemia is unknown, but is most likely a structural defect in the cell wall. The classic characteristic is an increased RBC osmotic fragility. The prevalence of the gene is 2.2×10^{-4}, indicating that there are over 650 pregnancies nationally per year in women with spherocytosis. A hemolytic crisis can be precipitated by many conditions, including infection, trauma, or pregnancy itself.[28] A relationship between increased hemolysis and increased maternal blood volume and splenic blood flow has been suggested. An alternative suggestion is an increased osmotic fragility during the third trimester of pregnancy.[29]

The diagnosis is suspected on the basis of family history and by findings in the CBC and reticulocyte count that suggest the hyperproliferative branches of the diagnostic algorithms in Figures 69-6 and 69-7. Confirmation is obtained with the osmotic fragility test.

Prenatal care of women with hereditary spherocytosis who have not had a splenectomy requires vigilance for hemolytic crisis and folate supplementation to ensure adequate marrow function. A hemolytic crisis can be treated conservatively with replacement transfusions or with splenectomy. Splenectomy is mechanically difficult to accomplish during the third trimester of pregnancy unless preceded by cesarean section. In the absence of severe, untreated anemia, spherocytosis does not contribute to perinatal morbidity or mortality.

Hereditary elliptocytosis, also inherited as an autosomal dominant trait, is a milder hemolytic state also caused by a structural defect in the RBC wall. The signs and symptoms are similar to spherocytosis, but not as severe. Most cases diagnosed during pregnancy have been successfully treated with supportive therapy alone.[30]

AUTOIMMUNE HEMOLYTIC ANEMIA

There are two major types of antibodies responsible for autoimmune hemolytic anemia (AIHA), warm-reactive and cold-reactive. Most warm-reactive antibodies are of the IgG class and are directed against some component of the Rh system on the surface of the red cell. In contrast, most cold-reactive antibodies are IgM and usually are specific for anti-I or anti-i. AIHA with warm-reactive antibodies is frequently seen in association with various hematologic malignancies (chronic lymphocytic leukemia, lymphoma), lupus erythematosus, viral infections, and drug ingestion. Penicillin, stibophen, and α-methyldopa all have been reported to cause AIHA. Cold-reacting antibodies can be seen in association with mycoplasma infections, infectious mononucleosis, and lymphoreticular neoplasms. Unfortunately, in a large number of cases no specific inciting event can be identified.[31]

Diagnosis is suspected by identifying a hyperproliferative, macrocytic anemia. The stained smear of the peripheral blood often reveals microcytes, polychromatophilia, poikilocytosis, and the presence of normoblasts. Leukocytosis is frequently seen and is a result of marrow hyperactivity. The critical study to confirm the diagnosis is a positive direct Coombs' test.

Treatment of AIHA is directed toward both the hemolytic process and the underlying disease. Blood transfusion, corticosteroid therapy, immunosuppression, and splenectomy are the most frequently used measures. In cases with warm-reactive antibodies, corticosteroids should be tried initially, because approximately 80% of patients will respond dramatically. Splenectomy is an effective form of treatment in approximately 60% of patients with warm-reactive antibodies. If the patient is refractory to both corticosteroid therapy and splenectomy, a trial of immunosuppression is warranted.

The treatment of cold-reactive antibodies depends on the severity of the hemolytic process. In patients with mild anemia, avoidance of cold temperatures is all that is required. Corticosteroid therapy and splenectomy are usually not effective if the majority of RBC breakdown occurs intravascularly. In patients with severe anemia, a trial of immunosuppression or plasmapheresis should be considered.

APLASTIC AND HYPOPLASTIC ANEMIA

Aplastic anemia is characterized by a reduction in the number of circulating RBCs, neutrophils, and platelets, and by the presence of a hypocellular bone marrow. Three mechanisms have been postulated to explain the development of aplastic anemia:

- Insufficient stem cells, either because of an intrinsic defect or a reduction in number after exposure to some noxious agent
- The presence of some suppressor substance that inhibits the maturation of the myeloid precursors
- The development of autoimmune reaction that causes death of the stem cells.

Table 69-5 lists various agents that have been reported to be associated with aplastic anemia. In the first group are agents, such as benzene, that predictably lead to marrow aplasia. In the second category are agents, such as chloramphenicol, that induce aplasia only in an occasional patient. Finally, there are literally hundreds of agents of various types that have been implicated in several cases as causes of aplastic anemia. Unfortunately, in about half of all cases, careful search does not reveal any causative agent.

In 1953, Holly described eight patients with hypoplastic anemia diagnosed during pregnancy who remitted spontaneously after delivery.[32] The bone marrow was described as hypocellular with an increase in megakaryocytes. To date, approximately 50 cases have been reported.[33] However, these cases present a spectrum of clinical and bone marrow findings that make it difficult to substantiate that a hypoplastic anemia specifically related to pregnancy does in fact exist. Support for such a hypothesis is found only in those cases in which recovery occurred after delivery, an entirely normal marrow is documented between pregnancies, and relapse occurs with a subsequent pregnancy.

Patients with aplastic anemia seek medical attention because of symptoms relating to either a profound anemia, bleeding, or infection. The CBC reveals pancytopenia with a hypoproliferative reticulocyte count. Examination of the bone marrow reveals hypoplasia with normoblastic erythropoiesis.

Severe aplastic anemia is fatal for more than 50% of affected patients.[34] Bone marrow transplantation is now the treatment of choice, and long-term survival of 50% to 70% can be expected. Several survivors have had successful pregnancies following transplantation.[35–37] During pregnancy, supportive therapy remains the major objective.

Several reports summarize the results of aplastic anemia during pregnancy. In recent years, with modern supportive therapy, the maternal mortality rate has been only 15%, and more than 90% of patients survive in remission.

Treatment consists of maintenance of hemoglobin levels by periodic transfusion, prevention and treatment of infection, stimulation of hematopoiesis with androgens, splenectomy, therapeutic abortion and premature delivery, intravenous gamma globulin, and marrow transplantation.[38]

Androgen therapy can be effective in stimulating erythropoiesis. However, androgens are contraindicated during pregnancy unless the fetus is known to be male. Agents commonly used include fluoxymesterone (0.25 mg/kg/day), oxymetholone (3–5 mg/kg/day); nandrolone decanate (3–4 mg/kg weekly), or testosterone ethanate (1–3 mg/kg/week). Adrenocorticosteroids have also been widely used with some benefit. Unfortunately, the remission rate with steroids is only 12%.

Bone marrow transplantation is now the treatment of choice for patients with severe aplastic anemia. Another therapy that shows promise is administration of antihuman thymocyte globulin. Unfortunately, neither of these modalities can be used safely during pregnancy.

Because of the anecdotal reports of complete remission following pregnancy termination, it is tempting to consider therapeutic abortion. However, thorough examination of the available literature indicates that abortion or premature termination of pregnancy is not associated with a more favorable outcome. The only reason to terminate pregnancy prematurely is the inability to support the patient satisfactorily with transfusion alone and thus the need to proceed to either marrow transplantation or antithymocyte globulin therapy.

TABLE 69–5. AGENTS ASSOCIATED WITH APLASTIC ANEMIA

CONSISTENTLY ASSOCIATED	OCCASIONALLY ASSOCIATED	RARELY ASSOCIATED
Benzene and related agents Ionizing radiation Nitrogen mustard and related agents Antimetabolites Antimitotic agents Certain antibiotics Other toxic chemicals	Certain antibiotics Anticonvulsants Analgesics Gold salts	More than 100 described

PAROXYSMAL NOCTURNAL HEMOGLOBINURIA

Hemolysis occurs in paroxysmal nocturnal hemoglobinuria (PNH) due to an unexplained structural defect in the RBC. There are distinct cohorts of long-lived and short-lived cells. The inherent defect makes the RBCs unusually susceptible to lysis by complement.

PNH usually begins insidiously and there is no familial tendency. There is considerable variability in severity of the disease, and the classic presentation of hemoglobinuria is seen in only 25% of patients. Exacerbations of the hemolytic process are precipitated by infection, menstruation, transfusion, surgery, and ingestion of iron.

The most serious complications associated with PNH are marrow aplasia, thrombosis, and infection. Thrombosis accounts for 50% of deaths and is of particular concern during pregnancy. Although anemia is the most prominent hematologic feature of PNH, leukopenia and thrombocytopenia also occur frequently. The diagnosis of PNH is based on a series of special tests that demonstrate the sensitivity of the patient's RBCs to complement.

The ideal treatment for PNH is replacement of the abnormal stem cell with cells capable of producing the normal cellular components. This has been accomplished by bone marrow transplantation. The major therapeutic modalities during pregnancy are iron therapy, androgen treatment, corticosteroids, and transfusions.[39–41] As discussed above, androgen therapy is useful but can only be used during pregnancy if the presence of a male fetus is documented. Iron can be administered orally to replace the considerable amount lost in the urine. Unfortunately, in significantly iron-deficient patients, such treatment may lead to a burst of erythropoiesis with delivery of a cohort of cells susceptible to the lytic action of complement. If a hemolytic episode follows iron therapy, it should be treated with either suppression of erythropoiesis by transfusion or suppression of hemolysis with corticosteroids. Prednisone in a dose of 1 mg/kg/day is an effective regimen.

When acute hemolytic episodes occur, treatment is aimed at diminishing hemolysis and preventing complications. Because patients with PNH have frequent episodes of venous thrombosis, this must be watched for carefully. In cases of acute deep venous thrombosis, anticoagulation should be begun. Care must be taken in the use of heparin, because hemolytic episodes clearly can be related to its use. During pregnancy heparin is the anticoagulant of choice; however, during the puerperium or non-pregnant state, warfarin is preferred. Only a few pregnancies have been reported in women with PNH, and both spontaneous abortion and thrombolic events appear to be increased in frequency.

REFERENCES

1. Laros RK, ed. Blood disorders in pregnancy. Philadelphia: Lea & Febiger, 1986.
2. Thorup OA, ed. Fundamentals of clinical hematology. Philadelphia: WB Saunders, 1987.
3. Horowitz JJ, Laros RK. Anemia and pregnancy: a review of the pathophysiology, diagnosis and treatment. Obstet Gynecol 1979;1:9.
4. Schifman RB, Thomasson JE, Evers JM. Red blood cell zinc protoporphyrin testing in iron-deficiency anemia in pregnancy. Am J Obstet Gynecol 1987;157:304.
5. Ho CH, Yuan CC, Yeh SH. Serum ferritin, folate and coabalamin levels and their correlation with anemia in normal full-term pregnant women. Eur J Obstet Gynecol Reprod Biol 1987;26:7.
6. Foulkes J, Goldie DJ. The use of ferritin to assess the need for iron supplements in pregnancy. Obstet Gynecol 1982;3:11.
7. Puolakka A, Janne O, Pararinen A, et al. Serum ferritin in the diagnosis of anemia during pregnancy. Acta Obstet Gynecol Scand (Suppl) 1980;95:57.
8. Seligman PA, Caskey JH, Frazier JL, et al. Measurements of iron absorption from prenatal multivitamin-mineral supplements. Obstet Gynecol 1983;61:356.
9. Taylor DJ, Mallen C, McDougall N, et al. Effect of iron supplement on serum ferritin levels during and after pregnancy. Br J Obstet Gynaecol 1982;89:1011.
10. Peck TM, Arias F. Hematologic changes associated with pregnancy. Clin Obstet Gynecol 1979;22:785.
11. Scott DE, Pritchard JA. Iron deficiency in healthy young college women. JAMA 1967;199:147150.
12. Pritchard JA, Whalley PJ, Scott DE. The influence of maternal folate and iron deficiency on intrauterine life. Am J Obstet Gynecol 1969;104:388.
13. Monsen ER, Kuhn JH, Finch CA. Iron status of menstruating females. Am J Clin Nutr 1967;20:842.
14. Fenton V, Cavill J, Fisher J. Iron stores in pregnancy. Br J Haematol 1977;37:145.
15. Herbert V, Colman N, Spivack M. Folic acid deficiency in the United States: folate assays in a prenatal clinic. Am J Obstet Gynecol 1975;123:175.
16. Shojania AM, Hornady GJ. Oral contraceptives and folate absorption. J Lab Clin Med 1973;82:869.
17. Iyengar L. Folic acid absorption in pregnancy. Br J Obstet Gynaecol 1975;82:20.
18. Johan E, Magnus EM. Plasma and red blood cell folate during normal pregnancy. Acta Obstet Gynecol Scand 1981;60:247.
19. Pritchard JA, Walley, PJ, Scott DE. Infants of mothers with megaloblastic anemia due to folate deficiency. JAMA 1969;211:1982.
20. Kitay DZ. Folic acid deficiency in pregnancy. Am J Obstet Gynecol 1969;104:1067.
21. Beischer NA, Holsman M, Kitchen WH. Relation of various forms of anemia to placental weight. Am J Obstet Gynecol 1968;101:801.
22. Beischer NA, Townsend L, Holsman M, et al. Urinary estriol excretion in pregnancy anemia. Am J Obstet Gynecol 1968; 102:819.
23. Sagen N, Nilsen ST, Kim HC, et al. Maternal hemoglobin concentration is closely related to birth weight in normal pregnancies. Acta Obstet Gynecol Scand 1984;63:245.
24. Paulone ME, Edelstone DI, Shedd A. Effects of maternal anemia on utroplacental and fetal oxidative metabolism in sheep. Am J Obstet Gynecol 1987;156:230.
25. Galbraith GMP, Galbraith RM, Temple A, et al. Demonstration of transferrin receptors on human placental trophoblast. Blood 1980;55:240.
26. Okuyama T, Tawada T, Furuya H, et al. The role of transferrin and ferritin in the fetal-maternal-placental unit. Am J Obstet Gynecol 1985;152:344.
27. Hamstra RD, Block MH, Schocket AL. Intravenous iron dextran. JAMA 1980;1726.

28. Moore A, Sherman MM, Strongin MJ. Hereditary spherocytosis with hemolytic crisis during pregnancy. Obstet Gynecol 1976;47(s):19.
29. Magid MS, Perkins M, Gottfried EL. Increased erythrocyte osmotic fragility in pregnancy. Am J Obstet Gynecol 1982;144:910.
30. Breckenridge RL, Riggs JA. Hereditary elliptocytosis with hemolytic anemia complicating pregnancy. Am J Obstet Gynecol 1968;101:861.
31. Sacks DA, Platt L, Johnson CS. Autoimmune hemolytic anemia during pregnancy. Am J Obstet Gynecol 1981;140:942.
32. Holly RG. Hypoplastic anemia in pregnancy. Obstet Gynecol 1953;1:533.
33. Fleming AF. Hypoplastic anaemia in pregnancy. Clin Haematol 1973;2:477.
34. Lynch RE, Williams DM, Reading JC, et al. The prognosis in aplastic anemia. Blood 1975;45:517.
35. Deeg HJ, Kennedy MS, Sanders JR, et al. Successful pregnancy after marrow transplantation for severe aplastic anemia and immunosuppression with cyclosporine. JAMA 1983;250:647.
36. Schmidt H, Ehninger G, Dopfer R, et al. Pregnancy after bone marrow transplantation for severe aplastic anemia. Bone Marrow Transplant 1987;2:329.
37. Doney K, Storb R, Buckner CD, et al. Marrow transplantation for treatment of pregnancy-associated aplastic anemia. Exp Hematol 1985;13:1080.
38. McGuire WA, Yang HH, Bruno E, et al. Treatment of antibody-mediated pure red-cell aplasia with high-dose intravenous gammaglobulin. N Engl J Med 1987;317:1004.
39. Frakes JT, Burmeister RE, Giliberti JJ. Pregnancy in a patient with paroxysmal nocturnal hemoglobinuria. Obstet Gynecol 1976;47(s):22.
40. Hurd WW, Miodovnik M, Stys SJ. Pregnancy associated with paroxysmal nocturnal hemoglobinuria. Obstet Gynecol 1982;60:742.
41. Solal-Celigny P, Tertian G, Fernandez H, et al. Pregnancy and paroxysmal nocturnal hemoglobinuria. Arch Intern Med 1988;148:593.

70

CHAPTER

MATERNAL ALLOIMMUNIZATION AND FETAL HEMOLYTIC DISEASE

John M. Bowman

Although fetal hemolytic disease was first described in twins in 1609, one dying a hydropic death shortly after birth, the other dying of kernicterus at a few days of age, its pathogenesis and the relation between hydrops and kernicterus remained unknown until 1932. In that year, Diamond and colleagues showed that hydrops fetalis, severe jaundice, and anemia of the newborn were different manifestations of the same disease, characterized by marked hepatosplenomegaly, hepatosplenic erythropoiesis, and the presence of immature nucleated red cells (erythroblasts) in the fetal and neonatal circulation.[1] The postulate that fetal hemolysis was due to the development of a blood group antibody in the mother directed against a blood group antigen present on the red cells of her fetus was proved in 1941 by Levine and colleagues, following the discovery of the Rh blood group system in 1940 by Landsteiner and Wiener.[2,3] Although the blood group antigen (LW) discovered by Landsteiner and Wiener is not quite the same as the human red cell Rh antigen, this in no way reduces the importance of their discovery, which laid the foundations for safe blood transfusion practice, the science of human anthropology, and the elucidation of the etiology, pathogenesis, treatment, and ultimately the prevention of Rh immunization and fetal hemolytic disease.

THE Rh BLOOD GROUP SYSTEM

Although other blood group systems, which will be discussed later in this chapter, are assuming greater importance as the prevalence of maternal Rh immunization diminishes, the Rh blood group system is still the most common system causing serious alloimmunization and fetal hemolytic disease.

There are three different nomenclatures for the Rh blood group system. Although the theory of Wiener and Wexler[4] of a single locus occupied by a pair of complex agglutinogens may be the most accurate and the numbering system of Rosenfield and colleagues[5] the most logical (favored by geneticists), the nomenclature and theories of inheritance put forward by Fisher and Race[6] are simple and work well in practice.

According to Fisher and Race, there are three pairs of antigens—commonly Dd, Cc, Ee—which are inherited in two sets of three, one from each parent. The presence or absence of the antigen D determines whether an individual is Rh-positive or Rh-negative (its hypothetical allele "d" has never been demonstrated).

Some sets of Rh antigens are more common than others (Table 70-1), with CDe(R^1),c(d)e(r),cDE(R^2) being the most common. About 45% of D-positive individuals are homozygous for D, having inherited a D-containing set from both parents; the remaining 55% are heterozygous, having inherited a D-containing set from only one parent. If the Rh-positive husband of an Rh-negative woman is homozygous, all his children will be D-positive; if he is heterozygous, in each pregnancy there is an equal chance that the fetus will be D-negative or D-positive. Only D-positive fetuses provoke Rh immunization and only D-positive fetuses will be affected by the Rh antibody provoked.

Because anti-d has never been found (and probably does not exist), the zygosity of an Rh-positive husband can only be determined if he fathers two infants who have inherited two different sets of Rh antigens from him. Because certain sets are more common, the determination of his C, c, E, e status will determine his most likely zygosity (Table 70-2).

The Rh blood group system is very complex. Forty antigens other than the five already mentioned have

TABLE 70–1. Rh GENE FREQUENCIES IN A WHITE CANADIAN POPULATION OF 2000 UNRELATED ADULTS

GENE COMPLEX	FREQUENCY (%)
CDe(R^1)	41
c(d)e(r)	39
cDE(R^2)	16
cDe(R^o)	2.2
C(d)e(r′)	1.1
c(d)E(r″)	0.6
CDE(R^z)	0.08
C(d)E(r^Y)	0.00

(From Lewis M, Kaita H, Chown B. The inheritance of the Rh blood groups: Frequencies in 1000 unrelated Caucasian families consisting of 2000 parents and 2806 children. Vox Sang 1971;20:502.)

been described.[7] C^w, an allele for C, is not uncommon. D^u replacing D is also not rare. D^u positivity (ie, an incomplete D antigen or "D variant") is commoner in blacks. Six subgroups of D variant have been described by Tippett and Sanger (1962).[8] On very rare occasions, a D^u mother may become D immunized, which on at least one occasion caused hydrops fetalis.[9]

Rh-negativity is primarily a Caucasian trait. In most Caucasian populations, the incidence of Rh-negativity is 15% to 16%. In Finland it is 10% to 12%. In the Basques it is 30% to 35%. In Chinese and Japanese it is less than 1%. About 1% to 2% of North American Indians and Inuit are Rh-negative, as are about 2% of Indo-Eurasians. In blacks the incidence ranges from 4% to 8%, being higher in North American than in African blacks. Rh-negativity, millennia ago, was probably confined to the Basques. The present-day incidence in other Caucasians and in non-Caucasians is related to the intermingling of Basque genes into other Caucasian groups and now the intermingling of Caucasian genes into other races.

The Rh(D) antigen is a protein with a molecular weight of 28 to 32 kd.[7] Unlike the ubiquitous ABO antigens, the Rh antigens are confined to the red cell membrane, although there is disputed evidence that they may also be present in human trophoblast.[10] Rh antigens are essential red cell membrane components. The rare Rh-null individuals, who lack all Rh antigens, have defective red cell membranes and suffer from mild to moderate hemolytic anemia.

PATHOGENESIS OF MATERNAL ALLOIMMUNIZATION

Before the discovery of the Rh blood group system, blood transfusion was a common cause of Rh immunization. It is still a very common cause of non–D blood group immunization. Although many non–D blood group antibodies are of no clinical significance, others may produce erythroblastosis as severe as that caused by anti-D.

Following the discovery of the Rh blood group system and the introduction of transfusion of Rh(D) compatible blood, the prevalence of Rh immunization diminished only very slightly. Wiener's postulate,[11] that fetal transplacental hemorrhage (TPH) into the mother caused Rh immunization, was proved by Chown in 1954.[12]

The Kleihauer acid elution test[13] is an accurate and very sensitive method of determining the incidence and size of TPH (Fig. 70-1). Seventy-five percent of women

TABLE 70–2. ZYGOSITY FOR Rh(D) OF D-POSITIVE HUSBAND (D-NEGATIVE WIFE)

ANTIGENS PRESENT IN HUSBAND	A (MOST LIKELY Rh GENOTYPE)	B (LESS LIKELY Rh GENOTYPE)	C (LEAST LIKELY Rh GENOTYPE)
1. CDe	CDe/CDe(R^1R^1)* Homozygous	CDe/Cde(R^1r′) Heterozygous	
2. CDce	CDe/cde(R^1r) Heterozygous	CDe/cDe(R^1R^o) Homozygous	cDe/Cde(R^or′) Heterozygous
3. CDEce	CDe/cDE(R^1R^2) Homozygous	cDE/Cde(R^2r′) CDe/cdE(R^1r″) Heterozygous	CDE/cDe(R^zR^o) Homozygous
4. DEc	cDE/cDE(R^2R^2)* Homozygous	cDE/cdE(R^2r″) Heterozygous	
5. DEce	cDE/cde(R^2r) Heterozygous	cDE/cDe(R^2R^o) Homozygous	cDe/cdE(R^or″) Heterozygous
6. Dce	cDe/cde(R^or) Heterozygous	cDe/cDe(R^oR^o) Homozygous	

* Genotypes 1A and 4A can very infrequently be proved because the infant will usually be of only one paternal genotype (CDe in 1A and cDE in 4A). The remainder of the husband's possible genotypes can be proved only if he produces children of two different genotypes. (From Bowman JM, Friesen RF. Rh-isoimmunization. In: Goodwin JW, Godden JO, Chance G, eds. Perinatal medicine. Baltimore: Williams & Wilkins, 1976:92–107.)

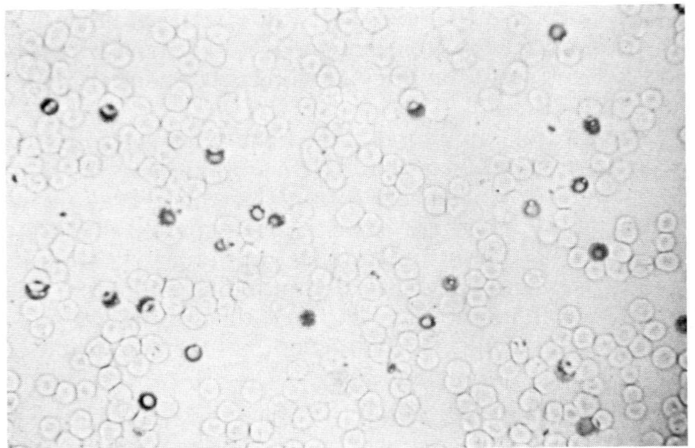

FIGURE 70–1. Acid elution technique of Kleihauer. Fetal red blood cells stain with eosin (they appear dark). Adult red blood cells do not stain (they appear as ghosts). This maternal blood smear contained 11.2% fetal red blood cells, representing a transplacental hemorrhage of about 450 mL of blood. (From Bowman JM. Hemolytic disease of the newborn. In: Conn HF, Conn RB, eds. Current diagnosis 5. Philadelphia: WB Saunders, 1977:1103.)

have evidence of fetal TPH at some time during pregnancy or at the time of delivery.[14] The size of the hemorrhage is usually small, but about 1% of women will have as much as 5 mL and 0.25% will have 30 mL or more of fetal blood in their circulation. Antepartum hemorrhage, toxemia of pregnancy, cesarean section, manual removal of the placenta, and external version increase both the risk and size of TPH. As might be expected, the incidence and size of TPH increase as pregnancy progresses, from 3% (0.03 mL) in the first trimester, to 12% (usually less than 0.1 mL) in the second trimester, to 45% (occasionally up to 25 mL) in the third trimester.[14] Abortion carries a risk of TPH, usually of less than 0.1 mL. After a therapeutic abortion, the risk may be as high as 20% to 25%, with volumes exceeding 0.2 mL in 4% of such abortions. Contrary to the weak expression of the ABO antigens on fetal red cells, the Rh antigens are well developed by 30 days gestation.

THE Rh IMMUNE RESPONSE

The initial (primary) Rh immune response is slow to develop, usually requiring 6 to 12 weeks and sometimes as long as 6 months to appear. The primary response is usually (but not invariably) weak, and frequently is predominantly IgM in nature at first. IgM antibody (mol wt 900,000) does not cross the placenta. However, most, but not all, immunized women quickly convert to IgG anti-D (mol wt 160,000) production. IgG anti-D readily crosses the placenta, coats Rh-positive fetal red cells, and causes hemolysis.

A second fetal TPH, which may be very small, produces a very different (secondary) immune response. The response is rapid (days) and is usually predominantly IgG in nature. It may be very strong. Further TPH may produce further increases in antibody titer. Long periods between Rh-positive red cell exposure are often associated with marked increases in Rh antibody, with an increase in its avidity (the binding constant) for the D antigen. The greater the avidity, the more severe will be the degree of erythroblastosis.

ANTIBODY DETECTION AND MEASUREMENT METHODS

The following are some of the methods used to measure and detect antibodies:

1. *Saline.* Rh-positive erythrocytes suspended in isotonic saline are agglutinated only by IgM anti-D. IgG anti-D cannot bridge the gap between red cells suspended in saline. In the early 1940s, when only saline-suspended red cell antibody screening methods were available, many women giving birth to severely affected erythroblastotic babies could not be shown to be Rh-immunized because they had only IgG anti-D in their sera.
2. *Colloid.* In 1945 it was observed that Rh-positive red cells suspended in more viscous colloid media such as albumin were agglutinated by IgG anti-D.[15,16] Bovine serum albumin is the most frequently used colloid medium. Because IgM anti-D also agglutinates colloid-suspended Rh-positive red cells, if saline and colloid anti-D levels (titers) are about the same, the albumin titer may not be an accurate measurement of IgG anti-D. Mixing such a serum with dithiothreitol disrupts IgM sulfhydryl bonds, destroying IgM but leaving IgG intact. Subsequent retitration in colloid medium allows a true measurement of the IgG anti-D level.
3. *Indirect antiglobulin (IDAT).*[17] Antihuman globulin antibody (Coombs serum, AHG) is produced by injection of human serum (or specific human IgG) into other animal species. Following incubation of Rh-positive red cells with serum being screened for Rh antibody, anti-D, if present, adheres to the red cells. The red cells are then washed with isotonic saline and suspended in the AHG serum. If the red cells are coated with antibody, they agglutinate, a positive indirect antiglobulin test (IDAT or indirect Coombs test). The reciprocal of the highest dilution causing agglutination is the indirect antiglobulin titer. IDAT screening is more sensitive than albumin screening. IDAT titers are usually one to three dilutions higher than albumin titers.
4. *Enzyme.* Incubation of red cells with enzymes (papain, trypsin, or bromelin) reduces the negative electrical potential of the red cells. Red cells so treated, suspended in saline, lie closer together and are agglutinated by IgG anti-D. Enzyme techniques are the most sensitive available manual methods for detecting Rh immunization.[18]

5. *AutoAnalyzer.* AutoAnalyzer (AA) methods, bromelin,[19] and low-ionic methods[20] are the most sensitive techniques for the detection of Rh antibody. They are so sensitive that if manual methods fail to confirm the presence of Rh antibody, the mother may not be Rh-immunized. A modification of the bromelin method[21] is used to measure accurately (in micrograms per milliliter) the amount of serum anti-D.

THE PREVALENCE OF Rh IMMUNIZATION

Quite small amounts of Rh-positive blood, in some instances as little as 0.3 mL, will produce Rh immunization in Rh-negative volunteers.[22] The incidence of Rh immunization is antigen-dose dependent, 15% after 1 mL, 33% after 10 mL, and 65% after 50 to 250 mL of Rh-positive red cells.[23] A secondary immune response may occur after very small doses (as little as 0.05 mL of Rh-positive red cells). In pregnant Rh-negative women, if serial Kleihauer examinations never detect a TPH as great as 0.1 mL, the incidence of Rh immunization detected up to 6 months after delivery is 3%; if the volume is greater than 0.1 mL, the incidence is 14%[22]; if the volume is greater than 0.4 mL, the incidence is 22%.[24]

The risk of Rh immunization appearing within 6 months after delivery of the first Rh-positive ABO-compatible baby is 8% to 9%. However, an equal number of women will demonstrate that they also were immunized by the first pregnancy, but at an undetectable antibody level, until they mount a secondary immune response in the next Rh-positive pregnancy.[25] Nevalinna called this phenomenon "sensibilization." Therefore, the overall risk of Rh immunization occurring as a result of the first Rh-positive ABO-compatible pregnancy is about 16%. An unimmunized Rh-negative woman faces about the same risk in a second such pregnancy. However, as parity increases and the ratio of good immune responders to poor immune responders decreases, the risk becomes less. Nevertheless, after a woman has undergone five Rh-positive ABO-compatible pregnancies, there is a 50% likelihood that she will be Rh-immunized. About 30% of Rh-negative women are nonresponders and will not become Rh-immunized despite exposure to repeated doses of Rh-positive red cells.

ABO INCOMPATIBILITY

ABO incompatibility between the Rh-positive fetus and the Rh-negative mother reduces her risk of becoming Rh-immunized to 1.5% to 2%.[24] Partial protection is probably produced by rapid intravascular hemolysis of the fetal ABO-incompatible Rh-positive red cells and the sequestration of the red cell stroma in the liver, where there are much fewer potential antibody-forming lymphocytes than there are in the spleen. However, once Rh immunization has developed, ABO incompatibility of the Rh-positive fetus confers no protection at all against the development of severe fetal hemolytic disease.[26]

A significant incidence of Rh immunization occurs during pregnancy. In one study,[27] five of 3533 Rh-negative women carrying Rh-positive fetuses (0.14%) were Rh-immunized before 28 weeks gestation; 57 (1.61%) were Rh-immunized between 28 weeks gestation and 3 days after delivery (total 1.8%). Since the total incidence of Rh immunization as a result of an Rh-positive pregnancy is about 13% (16% in the 80% carrying ABO-compatible babies, 1.5% to 2.0% in the 20% carrying ABO-incompatible babies), 13% to 14% of all instances of Rh immunization $\left(1.8 \times \frac{100}{13}\right)$ occur during pregnancy or within 3 days after delivery. This important observation will be considered in detail in the section on Rh prophylaxis.

Rh IMMUNIZATION CAUSED BY ABORTION

Since fetal red cells have been found in the maternal circulation as early as the tenth week of gestation,[14] the woman who has an abortion is at risk of becoming Rh-immunized. The risk is about 2% after spontaneous abortion and is 4% to 5% after therapeutic abortion. The woman who becomes Rh-immunized after abortion is a "good responder." She frequently has very severely affected babies subsequently.

PATHOGENESIS OF FETAL HEMOLYTIC DISEASE

Blood production in the fetus begins as early as the third week of gestation. Rh antigen is present in the red cell membrane by the sixth week. Erythropoiesis is predominantly in the liver and spleen in early gestation, shifting to the bone marrow by the sixth month. If fetal anemia resulting from chronic blood loss or hemolysis occurs, extramedullary erythropoiesis will persist and may become extreme.

Maternal IgG anti-D traverses the placenta and coats the D-positive fetal red cells (the reason for the direct positive antiglobulin or Coombs test). Anti-D does not fix complement. The fetal red cells are destroyed extravascularly, primarily in the spleen. The resulting anemia stimulates erythropoietin production and increased erythropoiesis. When marrow red cell production cannot compensate for the increased hemolysis, extramedullary erythropoiesis recurs primarily in liver and spleen. Hepatomegaly may be extreme (Fig. 70-2).

Control of erythrocyte maturation in this situation is poor. Nucleated red cell precursors from normoblasts to very primitive erythroblasts are released into the circulation (Fig. 70-3). Because of this finding, Diamond coined the initial name for this disease, erythroblastosis fetalis.

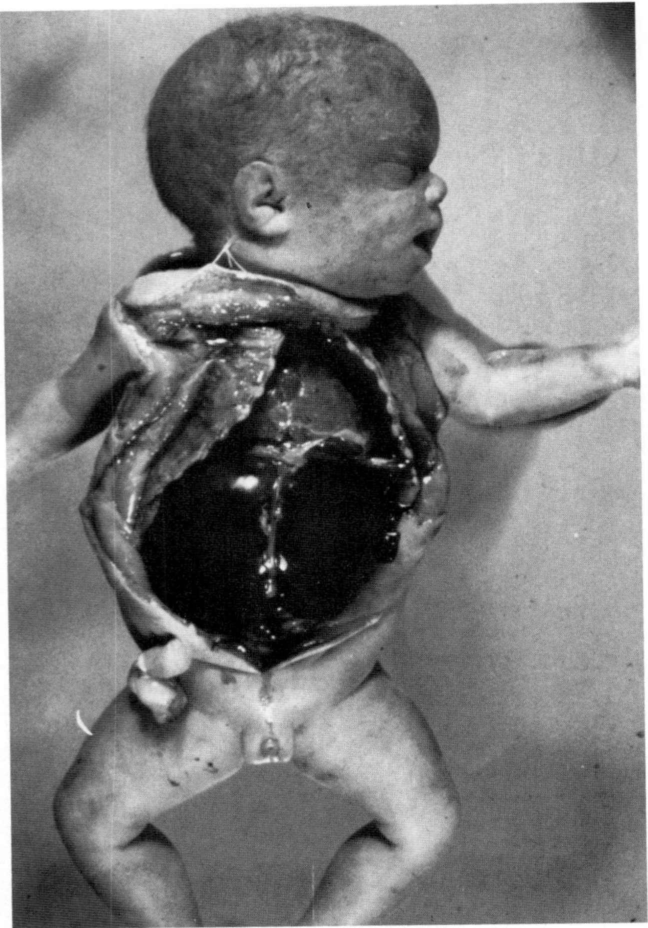

FIGURE 70–2. Hydropic neonate who died a few minutes after birth. Note extreme enlargement of the liver and moderate enlargement of the spleen. (From Bowman JM. Blood-group incompatibilities. In: Iffy L, Kaminetzky HA, eds. Principles and practice of obstetrics and perinatology. New York: John Wiley, 1981:1200.)

DEGREES OF Rh HEMOLYTIC DISEASE

Severity of hemolytic disease is determined by the amount of maternal IgG anti-D (the titer), its affinity or avidity for the fetal red cell membrane D antigen (the binding constant) and the ability of the fetus to keep up with the red cell destruction without becoming hydropic.

MILD DISEASE—NO TREATMENT

About one half of all affected fetuses do not require treatment after birth (Table 70-3). They are only modestly anemic (cord blood hemoglobin level no less than 120 g/L) and are not severely hyperbilirubinemic (cord serum bilirubin levels ≤68 μmol/L [≤4 mg/100 mL]). Their cord blood red cells are coated with anti-D, making them strongly direct antiglobulin (Coombs) positive, the hallmark of all alloimmune (except ABO) fetal hemolytic disease. The hemoglobin levels do not drop below 110 g/L, nor do the serum indirect bilirubin levels exceed 340 μmol/L (20 mg/dL) in the neonatal period; 260 to 300 μmol/L (15 to 17.5 mg/dL) in premature infants. Post–hospital discharge hemoglobin levels never drop below 75 to 80 g/L. These babies are normal and survive without treatment now, just as they did 50 years ago, before any treatment was available.

INTERMEDIATE DISEASE—KERNICTERUS

About 25% to 30% of affected fetuses have intermediate disease. They are born at term or near term in good condition, without severe anemia (cord blood hemoglobin levels greater than 90 g/L). Hepatosplenic erythropoiesis is not so excessive that hepatic function is compromised. Prior to birth, products of blood destruction are metabolized and excreted by the mother. After delivery, the baby must use his own resources.

When red cells are destroyed, globin is split from hemoglobin, leaving heme pigment, which is converted by heme oxygenase to biliverdin and then by biliverdin reductase to neurotoxic indirect bilirubin. In fetal hemolytic disease, there is increased production of indirect bilirubin. The newborn liver is deficient in glucuronyl transferase and Y transport protein. Thus, in the presence of increased indirect bilirubin production and the inability of the newborn infant to conjugate and excrete it as water-soluble bilirubin diglucuronide, indirect bilirubin increases in the infant's intravascular and extravascular fluid compartments.

Indirect bilirubin is water-insoluble and can remain in the plasma only when bound to albumin. When the

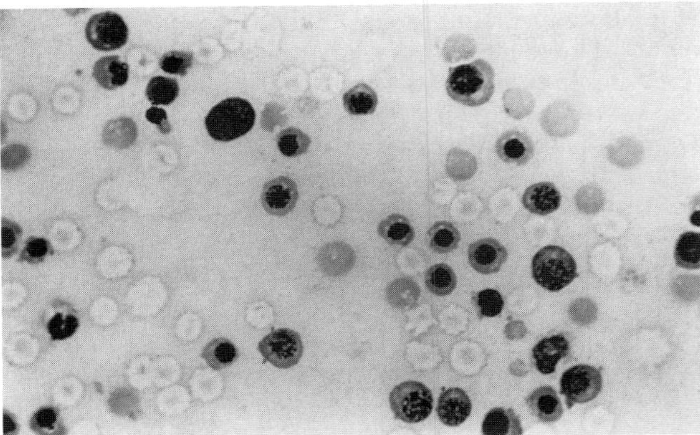

FIGURE 70–3. Cord blood of baby with severe Rh erythroblastosis fetalis who required multiple fetal transfusions and exchange transfusions. Smear treated by Kleihauer technique and Wright's stain. Note adult donor ghost red cells, dark fetal red cells, and early fetal erythroid series from erythroblasts through to normoblasts. (From Bowman JM. The management of Rh-isoimmunization. Obstet Gynecol 1978; 52:3.)

TABLE 70–3. CLASSIFICATION OF SEVERITY OF Rh HEMOLYTIC DISEASE

DEGREE OF SEVERITY	DESCRIPTION	INCIDENCE (%)
Mild	Indirect bilirubin does not exceed 16–20 mg/100 mL. No anemia. No treatment needed.	45–50
Moderate	Fetal hydrops does not develop. Moderate anemia. Severe jaundice with risk of kernicterus unless treated after birth.	25–30
Severe	Fetal hydrops develops in utero	20–25
	Before 34 weeks gestation	10–12
	After 34 weeks gestation	10–12

(From Bowman JM. Maternal blood group immunization. In: Creasy R, Resnik R, eds. Maternal-fetal medicine: principles and practice. Philadelphia: WB Saunders, 1984:561–602.)

albumin-binding capacity of the neonate's plasma is exceeded, "free" indirect bilirubin appears. Being water-insoluble and lipid-soluble, it cannot remain in the plasma but diffuses into fatty tissues. The neuron membrane has a high lipid content. "Free" indirect bilirubin traverses the lipid neuron membrane. Within the neuron it interferes with vital cellular metabolism. Mitochondrial swelling, ballooning, and then neuron death occurs. The dead neurons with accumulated bilirubin appear yellow at autopsy (kernicterus).

Babies who develop bilirubin encephalopathy (kernicterus) become deeply jaundiced. On the third to the fifth day they become lethargic and then hypertonic. They lie in a position of opisthotonos with neck hyperextended, back arched, and knees, wrists, and elbows flexed (Fig. 70-4). They suck poorly; vegetative reflexes disappear; apneic spells develop. Death occurs in about 90% of babies with kernicterus.

In the remaining 10%, jaundice fades and spasticity becomes less. However, as time passes, they show evidence of severe central nervous system dysfunction. Most have profound neurosensory deafness and choreoathetoid spastic cerebral palsy. Intellectual retardation may be relatively mild, but learning and functioning are very difficult because of the deafness and spastic choreoathetosis.

SEVERE-HYDROPS FETALIS

The 20% to 25% of most severely affected fetuses, despite maximal red cell production, become progressively more anemic. Ascites with anasarca (generalized edema) occurs (Fig. 70-5). Half of these fetuses become hydropic between 18 and 34 weeks gestation; the other half, between 34 weeks and term (see Table 70-3).

Although heart failure may develop in hydropic infants after birth (Fig. 70-6), it is not commonly the underlying cause of hydrops fetalis caused by fetal hemolytic disease.[28] Hepatic circulatory obstruction and hepatocellular damage are the probable causes of alloimmune hydrops fetalis.[29]

With progressive blood destruction and increasing hepatic erythropoiesis, expanding islets of erythropoiesis distort hepatic cords and obstruct portal venous blood flow, causing portal hypertension. Placental edema and retention of cytotrophoblast interfere with placental perfusion. Ascites develops. As hepatocellular damage increases, because of obstruction of portal blood flow and increasing anemia, albumin production diminishes, hypoalbuminemia occurs, and anasarca appears. Pleural and pericardial effusions develop. The fetus usually dies. If the fetus is liveborn, compression hypoplasia of the lungs may make oxygenation impossible.

The hepatic obstruction and damage hypothesis explains the variable relationship of hydrops to severity of

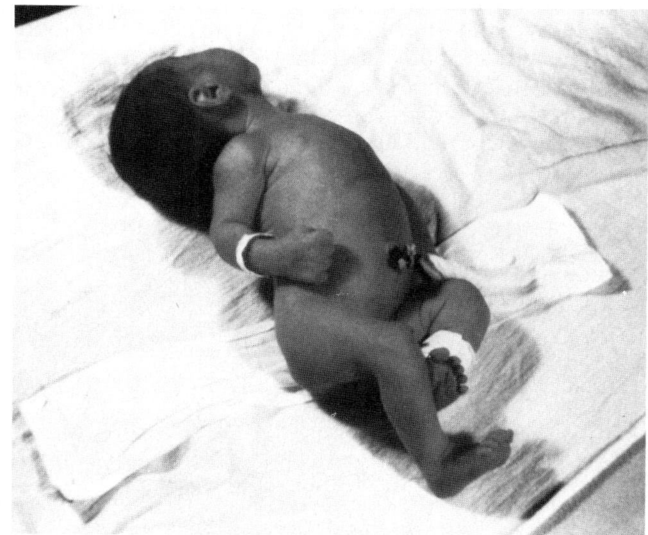

FIGURE 70–4. Infant with kernicterus; note spasticity and opisthotonos. (From Bowman JM. Rh-isoimmunization 1977. Mod Med Can 1977;32:18.)

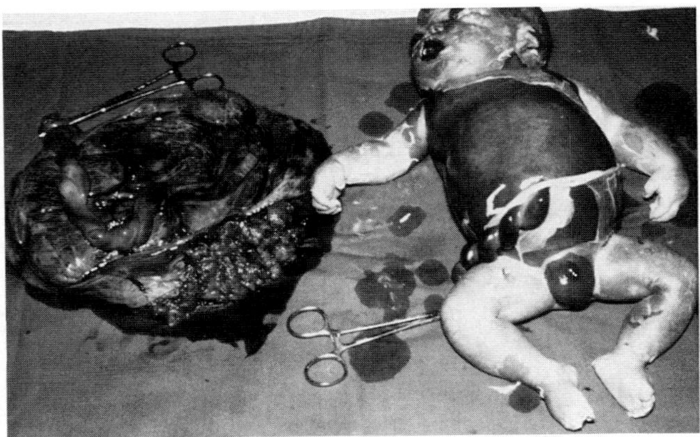

FIGURE 70–5. Stillborn fetus with hydrops fetalis. Note the edema and markedly enlarged placenta. (From Bowman JM. Rh-isoimmunization 1977. Mod Med Can 1977;32:19.)

anemia. Although most hydropic fetuses are severely anemic, with hemoglobin levels well below 60 g/L, we have on occasion seen hydrops with hemoglobin levels well above 70 g/L. Conversely, we have seen nonhydropic fetuses with hemoglobin levels well below 50 g/L (in one instance 25 g/L).

MONITORING THE MOTHER AND HER FETUS AT RISK

PRENATAL BLOOD TESTING

Unless prenatal blood grouping and antibody screening tests are carried out, the physician will not know which of his patients are Rh-negative and at risk of Rh immunization and which already have Rh or atypical blood group antibodies and are carrying fetuses at risk for hemolytic disease. A blood sample must be obtained from every woman at her first prenatal visit for blood grouping and antibody screening. There must be no deviation from this policy, which must be universal no matter what the woman's parity or what screening tests showed in her previous pregnancies. Mistyping of an Rh-negative woman may have occurred in a prior pregnancy. An Rh-positive woman, particularly if she has been transfused, may have developed a dangerous atypical blood group antibody.

THE UNIMMUNIZED PREGNANT WOMAN

The Rh-positive woman without demonstrable blood group antibodies at her first prenatal visit is not likely to develop dangerous atypical blood group antibodies later in her pregnancy. For this reason, frequent retesting is not cost effective and is not recommended. Since, on occasion (albeit rarely), significant atypical antibodies may develop, we do recommend repeat screening at 34 to 38 weeks gestation. This policy has recently been condemned as not cost effective.[30]

The Rh-negative woman without Rh antibodies should be ABO grouped and the Rh status of her husband should be determined. If he is Rh-negative, her fetus should be Rh-negative, putting her at no risk of Rh immunization. Since extramarital pregnancies do occur, we recommend rescreening at 32 to 36 weeks gestation and cord blood Rh testing at delivery. If the father is Rh-positive, his ABO group and Rh phenotype should be determined. Depending on his Rh phenotype, the likelihood of his Rh zygosity can be determined (see Table 70-2). If he is heterozygous, there is a 50% chance that the fetus will be Rh-negative, halving the risk of Rh immunization. If the husband is ABO incompatible with his wife, there is about a 60% chance that the baby will be ABO incompatible. If the fetus is ABO incompatible, the risk of Rh immunization is reduced from 16% to 1.5% to 2%. When the ABO blood group of the mother and father and the Rh phenotype of the father are known, the risk of Rh immunization can be estimated (Table 70-4).

The Rh-negative pregnant woman whose husband is Rh-positive must have further screening tests during her pregnancy. A second test should be carried out at 18 weeks gestation. It is recommended that she be rescreened every 4 weeks thereafter. Labor and delivery must be managed with care. Cesarean section and man-

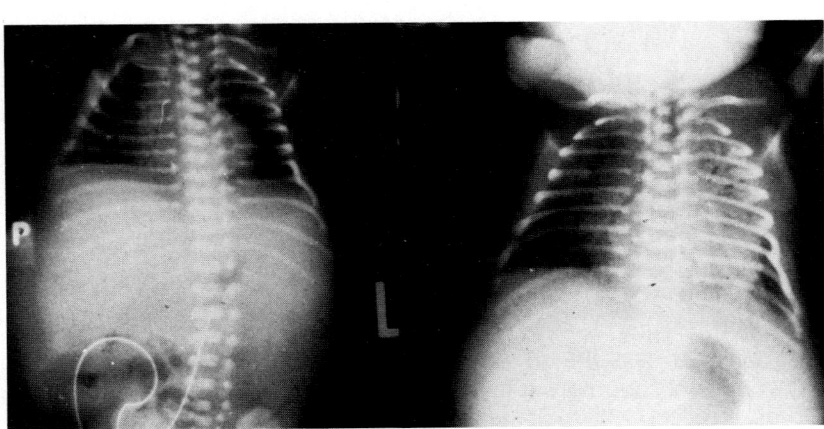

FIGURE 70–6. X-ray of a hydropic newborn at birth and 6 hours later after exchange transfusion. Note the small heart at the time of birth, with a very marked increase in heart size and evidence of pulmonary congestion denoting heart failure 6 hours later. The fetus has extreme ascites. (From Bowman JM. Blood group incompatibilities. In: Iffy L, Kaminetzky HA, eds. Principles and practice of obstetrics and perinatology. New York: John Wiley, 1981: 1203.)

TABLE 70–4. APPROXIMATE RISK OF Rh IMMUNIZATION

HUSBAND	BABY	RISK (%)
D-negative	D-negative	0
D-positive Homozygous ABO-compatible	D-positive ABO-compatible	16
D-positive Homozygous ABO incompatible	D-positive ABO-unknown	7
	D-positive ABO-incompatible	2
D-positive Heterozygous ABO-compatible	D status unknown ABO-compatible	8
D-positive Heterozygous ABO-incompatible	D status unknown ABO unknown	3.5

ual removal of the placenta increase the frequency and size of fetal–maternal TPH, increasing the risk of Rh immunization if the fetus is Rh-positive. Amniocentesis carried out for genetic purposes or for determination of pulmonary maturity carries a risk of TPH. If carried out under ultrasound guidance, the risk is about 2%.[31]

At delivery, cord and maternal blood must be tested —cord blood for the ABO and Rh type of the infant and the direct antiglobulin (Coombs) status of the infant's red cells, and maternal blood for the presence of Rh antibody and fetal red cells (TPH). Although most instances of Rh immunization occur after small or undetectable fetal TPH, maternal Rh prophylaxis being readily provided by one dose of Rh-immune globulin (120 to 300 μg), about one woman in 400 will have a fetal TPH greater than 30 mL of blood and may not be protected by a single prophylactic dose.

THE IMMUNIZED PREGNANT WOMAN

The physician caring for the Rh-immunized woman and her atypical blood group–immunized Rh-positive counterpart must be able to predict the severity of fetal hemolytic disease and, if severe, the gestation at which hydrops is likely to occur. Only fetuses in whom there is a risk of hydrops developing should be subjected to intrauterine diagnostic and management procedures.

PREDICTING SEVERITY OF Rh HEMOLYTIC DISEASE

HISTORY

Disease may remain of about the same degree of severity from baby to baby (mild, moderate, or severe), but it is just as likely to become progressively more severe from pregnancy to pregnancy. Infrequently, but not rarely, disease may become less severe. Occasionally, after having two or three mildly affected babies, a woman may have a very severely affected one. If a woman has had a hydropic baby, there is about a 90% chance that the next affected fetus will also become hydropic. In a first sensitized pregnancy, where there is no history, the risk of hydrops is 8% to 10%. When hydrops has developed in a prior pregnancy and the father is heterozygous, the physician is in a dilemma—the fetus may be Rh-negative and unaffected or Rh-positive and severely affected. Usually, but not invariably, hydrops develops in a subsequent affected fetus at the same time or earlier in gestation.

Rh ANTIBODY TITERS

If Rh antibody titers are measured in the same laboratory by the same experienced personnel using the same methods and test red cells, the results are reproducible and of some value in predicting the risk of severe hemolytic disease. Because the binding constant of the Rh antibody will vary, as may the amount of Rh antigen on the red cell membrane and the ability of the fetus to compensate for red cell hemolysis without developing portal hypertension and hepatocellular damage, the titer indicates only which fetus is at risk. The maternal antibody titer that puts the fetus at risk must be determined for each laboratory. Generally speaking, an albumin titer of 16 or an indirect antiglobulin titer of 32 to 64 puts the fetus at about a 10% risk of becoming hydropic.

Because it is the Rh antibody titer that selects the immunized woman who has a fetus at risk, titers should be repeated after measurement at the first prenatal visit at 16 to 18 weeks gestation, at 22 weeks gestation, and at 2-week periods thereafter.

Maternal history and antibody titer alone are inadequate to allow proper management of the Rh-immunized woman and her fetus. In a study of 426 Rh-immunized women managed at one hospital between 1954 and 1961,[32] there were 67 perinatal deaths and 54 infants who survived only because they were delivered prematurely, some as early as 32 weeks gestation. In only 62% of the 121 fetuses was severity of disease predicted accurately. If prediction of severity of hemolytic disease had been completely accurate, up to 50% of the 67 deaths could have been prevented by treatment measures available at that time.

Ultrasound has added a new noninvasive dimension to the monitoring of the Rh-sensitized pregnancy. Today it is possible to assess indirectly the size of the fetal liver and to measure directly placental thickness, both of which are often enlarged prior to full-blown hydrops. Also, one can assess the amount of amniotic fluid, which often increases in hydrops. In a sequence of events leading to frank fetal ascites, increased bowel echogenicity, probably resulting from the presence of fluid between individual bowel loops, leading to a small rim of fluid around the periphery of the abdomen has been described. Although these ultrasound findings are helpful, it must be emphasized that ultrasound cannot be used as the sole instrument for monitoring the status of the isoimmunized pregnant patient.

AMNIOTIC FLUID SPECTROPHOTOMETRY

Amniotic fluid surrounding severely affected fetuses is stained yellow. The pigment, which absorbs visual light at 450 nm, is bilirubin. Amniotic fluid is predominantly fetal in origin. The bilirubin present in the fluid is probably derived from fetal tracheal and pulmonary secretions.

Although Liley was not the first to use amniotic fluid spectrophotometry in predicting severity of hemolytic disease, in 1961 he published a method that allows comparisons from one laboratory to another.[33] Amniotic fluid, protected from light that destroys bilirubin, after centrifugation and filtration has optical density readings made over the visual wavelength spectrum 700 to 350 nm. The readings are plotted on semilogarithmic graph paper (wavelength the horizontal linear coordinate, optical density the vertical logarithmic coordinate). The readings are joined. The deviation from linearity at 450 nm (the ΔOD 450 reading; Fig. 70-7) is directly related to severity of disease. A further rise at 405 nm, if present, is due to heme. If the fluid has not been contaminated with blood, the heme peak is a further indication of severe disease.

The ΔOD 450 reading must be plotted according to gestation, since early in gestation unaffected fetuses produce bilirubin. Liley, from a study of single amniotic fluid ΔOD 450 readings, all after 28 weeks gestation, in 101 pregnancies, was able to divide the graph into three zones (see Fig. 70-7; Fig. 70-8). Readings in zone 3 indicate severe disease, usually hydrops within 7 to 10 days. Readings falling into zone 1 indicate mild or no disease but do not exclude the possibility that treatment after birth will be required. Readings in zone 2 indicate intermediate disease, increasing in severity as the zone 3 boundary is approached.

The zone boundaries slope downward because of the diminishing amount of bilirubin normally produced as

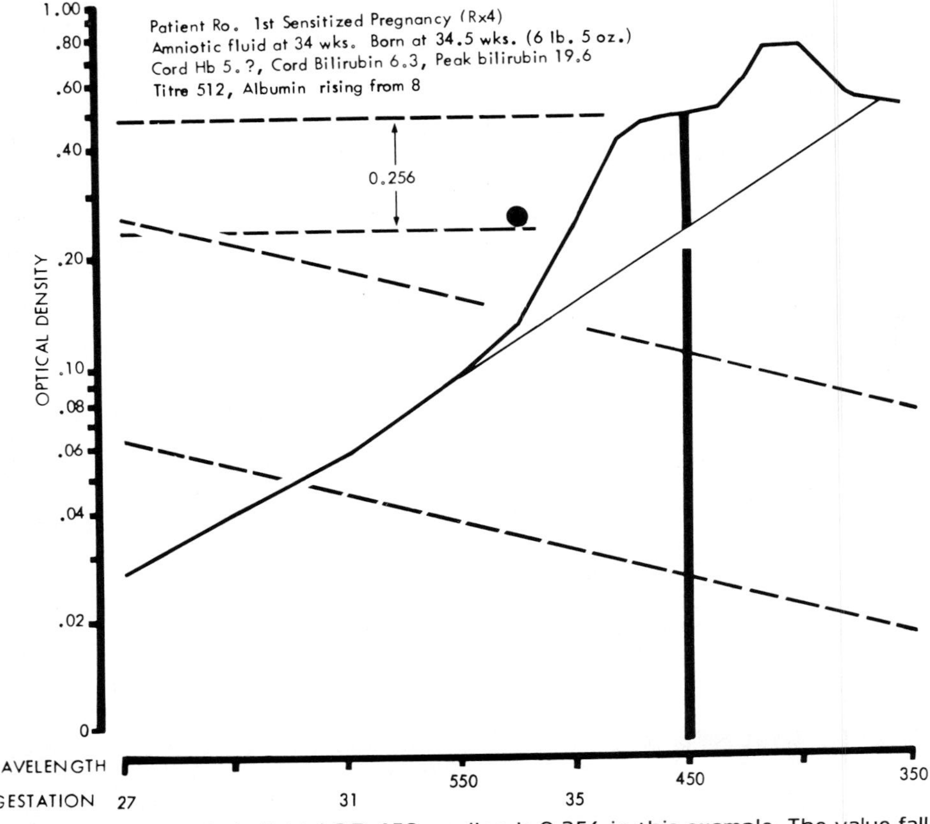

FIGURE 70–7. Amniotic fluid ΔOD 450 reading is 0.256 in this example. The value falls into zone 3, indicating impending fetal death. A further rise at 405 nm is due to heme pigment, further evidence of severe hemolytic disease. This first affected infant induced and delivered at 34.5 weeks gestation was prehydropic and edematous with a cord hemoglobin of 50 g/L and required four exchange transfusions. The child is alive and well. (From Bowman JM, Pollock JM. Amniotic fluid spectrophotometry and early delivery in the management of erythroblastosis fetalis. Pediatrics 1965;35:822.)

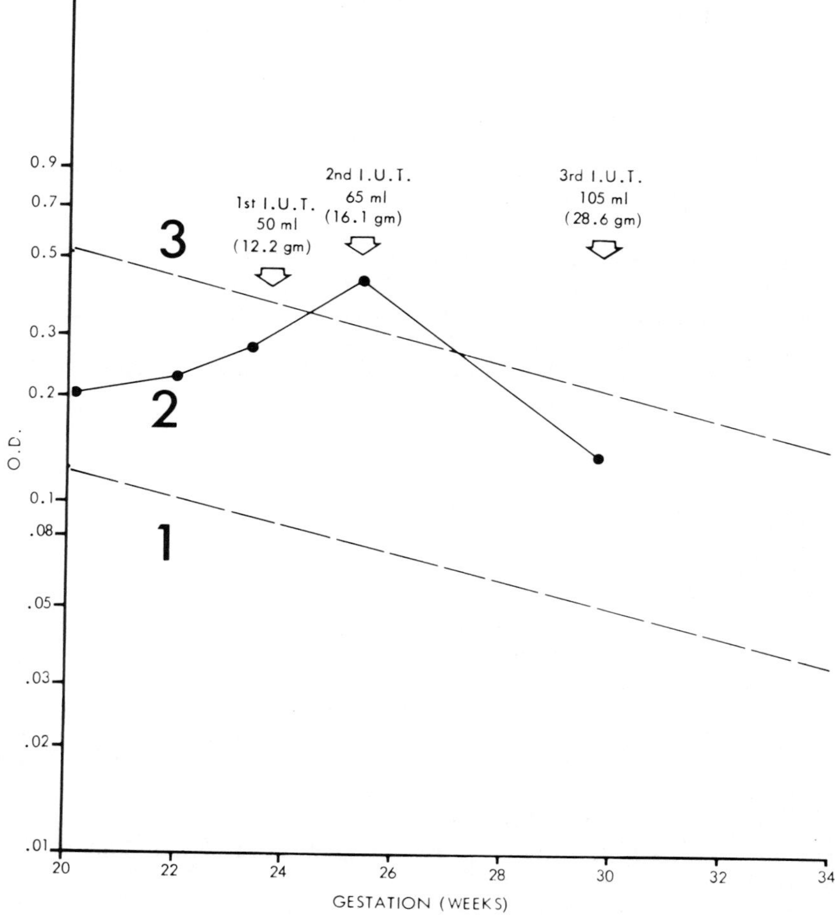

FIGURE 70–8. Serial spectrophotometric readings (Liley method) in a gravida with a history of two hydropic fetal deaths at 38 and 32 weeks gestation. First IPT was given when reading was at 80% level in zone 2 at 24 weeks gestation. The fetus required three transfusions and was delivered at 33.5 weeks gestation. Only donor red cells were found in the neonatal circulation. Birth weight was 2000 g; cord hemoglobin was 12.5 g/100 mL; and cord bilirubin was 4.5 mg/100 mL. The neonate required three exchange transfusions to survive. (From Bowman JM. Maternal blood group immunization. In: Creasy R, Resnik R, eds. Maternal-fetal medicine: principles and practice. Philadelphia: WB Saunders, 1984:576.)

pregnancy progresses. This may not be true before 25 weeks gestation, since the zone boundaries are almost certainly parabolic rather than linear, probably reaching their highest levels at 22 to 24 weeks gestation. Early in gestation (between 18 and 25 weeks) Nicolaides and colleagues could find little relationship between ΔOD 450 measurements and fetal circulating hemoglobin concentrations.[34] For this reason, to predict severity of hemolytic disease before 26 weeks gestation, they recommended direct fetal blood sampling, without amniotic fluid ΔOD 450 measurements.

Although single ΔOD 450 measurements before 26 weeks gestation may be misleading unless they are very high (≥0.400), serial measurements, often as frequent as every 5 to 7 days, do give a reasonable prediction of severity of hemolytic disease in the second trimester. Nevertheless, since 1986, in the face of rising ΔOD 450 readings, direct fetal blood sampling (if possible) is strongly recommended prior to undertaking fetal treatment measures.

Serial ΔOD 450 readings have increased the accuracy of determination of severity of hemolytic disease very substantially. From examination of 3177 amniotic fluids obtained from 1027 immunized women (Table 70-5) the following observations can be made:

1. A ΔOD 450 reading ≥0.400 at any gestation is associated with hydrops fetalis in 65% of instances.
2. On occasion, hydrops may be present with readings of 0.200 to 0.250 at 28 weeks gestation.
3. Once serial readings reach the 80% to 85% level in zone 2, if treatment is not undertaken, hydrops may be present by the time the reading reaches zone 3.

TABLE 70–5. ACCURACY OF AMNIOTIC FLUID ΔOD 450 SPECTROPHOTOMETRY (Liley Method)*

ZONE OF LAST SAMPLE	NUMBER OF WOMEN	RATE OF INACCURATE PREDICTIONS (%)
1	253	2.4
2	530	8.9
3	314	1.6
Total	1097	5.3

The number of samples examined between December 15, 1961, and July 3, 1981 was 3177.

4. Disease may be fulminant. For example, readings of 0.160 at 23 weeks and 0.240 at 27 weeks were followed in 2 weeks by readings of 0.385 and 0.370, respectively, with hydrops found at the time of the second amniocentesis.
5. Conversely, rarely, readings of 0.200 to 0.250 at 20 to 22 weeks may occur in the presence of a negative unaffected fetus.

Other spectrophotometric measurements of amniotic fluid have been developed. Bartsch has concluded that none are better than the Liley method and some are worse.[35] The experience and judgment of the individual assessing the amniotic fluid findings are more important than the method of measurement used.

AMNIOCENTESIS TECHNIQUES

Amniocentesis must be preceded by ultrasound placental localization. If the placenta is anterior, amniocentesis should be carried out under direct ultrasound guidance. Every effort must be made to avoid traversing the placenta with the amniocentesis needle. Without ultrasound placental localization, amniocentesis carries with it a 10% likelihood of causing placental trauma, TPH, and a rising antibody titer.[36]

Amniotic fluid aspiration is carried out under careful aseptic technique. A clotted maternal blood sample is obtained before and 5 minutes after the procedure. A 20- or 22-gauge spinal puncture needle is introduced into the amniotic cavity to the depth at which ultrasonography has determined fluid to be present and 10 to 15 mL of fluid are aspirated gently. If fluid is not obtained, the needle may be cautiously advanced or withdrawn slightly, or rotated to obtain fluid. The fluid will have a varying degree of yellow pigmentation and will be slightly to moderately turbid later in gestation. The fluid, protected from light, is sent for a ΔOD 450 measurement and for fetal pulmonary maturity measurements if the pregnancy is past 32 weeks gestation. The maternal blood samples are sent for antibody measurement and fetal red cell screening.

HAZARDS OF AMNIOCENTESIS

When carried out by an experienced perinatal obstetrician with prior ultrasound placental localization, amniocentesis is a relatively benign procedure. Maternal risks are negligible. Infection should never occur. Rarely, precipitation of labor and placental abruption have been reported.

Fetal hazards are also not great, but they are not negligible. Direct needle trauma has occurred,[37] as (very rarely) has fetal exsanguination. The major risk is placental trauma causing TPH, rising titers, and increasing severity of fetal hemolytic disease.

SOURCES OF ERROR

Maternal or fetal blood produces sharp 580-, 540-, and 415-nm oxyhemoglobin peaks, which obscure the ΔOD 450 readings, making the fluid valueless (Fig. 70-9). Smaller amounts of blood will not mask the ΔOD 450 reading, but small amounts of plasma, particularly fetal plasma, will increase the ΔOD 450 reading, giving a falsely high reading. Heme produces a 405-nm peak, which may obscure the 450-nm peak but is in itself indicative of severe hemolytic disease. Meconium in amniotic fluid distorts and increases the 450-nm peak. Exposure of the sample to light (particularly fluorescent light) decolorizes bilirubin, reducing the ΔOD 450 peak.

Maternal urine produces no 450-nm peak. Ascitic fluid is clear, bright yellow and more viscous due to a higher protein level. It has a much higher ΔOD 450 level.

Congenital anomalies such as anencephaly, open meningomyelocele, and upper gastrointestinal obstruction produce hydramnios and markedly elevated ΔOD 450 readings, which may be misleading if the mother is immunized.

INDICATIONS AND APPROPRIATE GESTATION FOR AMNIOCENTESIS

The following represents our approach to the management of the sensitized patient. Amniocentesis should be carried out only when the history or titer is such that the fetus is at risk of hydrops and death. Amniocentesis is required in only about one half of Rh-immunized pregnancies. If a previously affected perinate has died or required fetal transfusion or exchange transfusion after birth, fetal assessment and amniocentesis are required at 18 to 19 weeks gestation. If the placenta is anterior and cannot be avoided, fetal blood sampling is a better alternative than amniocentesis. Failing such a history, amniocentesis is carried out only if the antibody titer ($\geq$16 in albumin, $\geq$32 to 64 by indirect antiglobulin) indicates a risk of fetal hydrops. If this titer is present before 20 weeks gestation, the initial amniocentesis is carried out at 18 to 19 weeks gestation; otherwise, the initial amniocentesis is done within 7 days after the titer has reached the critical level. Amniocenteses are repeated at 5- to 28-day intervals, with the interval depending on the ΔOD 450 measurement of the immediately preceding fluid sample.

FETAL ULTRASONOGRAPHY

The introduction of ultrasound linear array B scan imaging techniques has been a major advance in management in many areas of maternal blood group immunization. Because ultrasound is noninvasive, it can be used serially (often daily) to determine severity of hemolytic disease and to monitor fetal condition over time

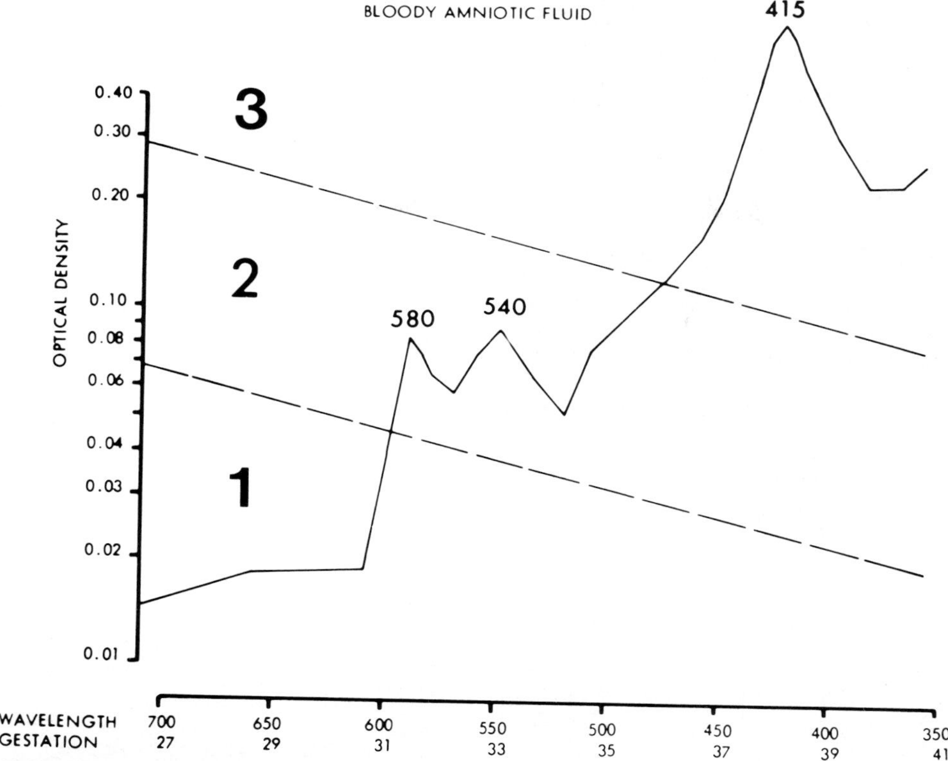

FIGURE 70–9. Spectrophotometric curve (Liley method) of amniotic fluid grossly contaminated with blood. Note sharp peaks at 580, 540, and 415 nm that obscure the 450-nm rise. (From Bowman JM. Hemolytic disease of the newborn. In: Conn HF, Conn RB, eds. Current diagnosis 5. Philadelphia: WB Saunders, 1977:1107.)

and in relation to specific treatment measures. Ultrasound allows a determination of placental and hepatic size and the presence or absence of edema and effusions (hydrops fetalis; Figs. 70-10, 70-11). Unfortunately, it may not give as accurate a prediction of impending hydrops as do serial amniotic fluid ΔOD 450 readings.

Ultrasonography has improved the accuracy and reduced the trauma from needle insertion at intraperitoneal fetal transfusion and is essential when direct intravascular fetal transfusions are being carried out. Following intraperitoneal transfusions, serial ultrasound examinations confirm the presence of blood in the peritoneal cavity and its rate of absorption. Following both intraperitoneal and intravascular transfusions, ultrasound biophysical profile scoring provides an accurate assessment of fetal well-being and whether improvement or deterioration in fetal condition is occurring.

FETAL BLOOD SAMPLING

With the development of very sophisticated ultrasound equipment and perinatologists skilled in its use, percutaneous umbilical blood sampling (PUBS) has become available in tertiary-level perinatal centers.[38] This procedure, which usually precedes direct intravascular transfusion, allows a measurement of all blood parameters that can be measured after birth (hemoglobin, hematocrit, serum bilirubin, direct and indirect platelet count, leukocyte count, serum proteins, and blood gases). Fetal blood sampling is by far the most accurate means of determining degree of severity of hemolytic disease, in the absence of hydrops fetalis.

Fetal blood sampling is a surprisingly benign procedure, carrying with it a fetal mortality rate of a fraction of 1%.[38] Since it carries with it a very high risk of fetal transplacental hemorrhage (much higher than amniocentesis), its use is recommended in two situations: (1) where serial amniotic fluid ΔOD 450 readings are rising into the upper 75% level of zone 2; and (2) where an anterior placenta cannot be avoided at amniocentesis and maternal history and antibody titer put the fetus at risk. Direct fetal blood sampling may be possible as early as 16 to 18 weeks gestation; it is usually feasible by 20 to 21 weeks gestation. It may not be possible if the placenta is posterior and the fetal body completely overlies the cord insertion. In this situation, some authorities carry out a blood-sampling procedure at the insertion of the cord into the fetal abdomen.[39,40]

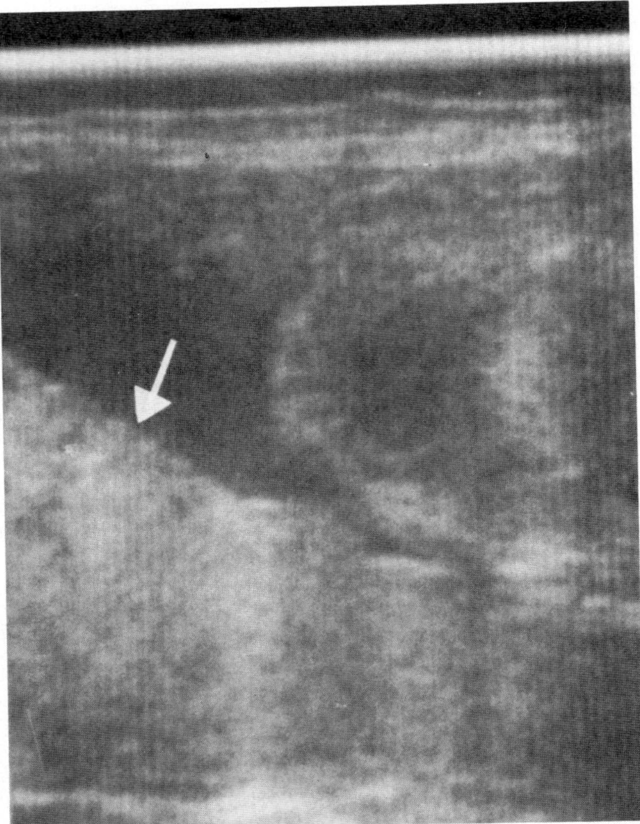

FIGURE 70–10. Ultrasound examination of fetus with hydrops fetalis. Placenta is enormously thickened and edematous (white arrow). Fetal abdomen, grossly distended with ascitic fluid, appears to the right of the arrow. (From Bowman JM. Maternal blood group immunization. In Creasy R, Resnik R, eds. Maternal-fetal medicine: principles and practice. Philadelphia: WB Saunders, 1984:589.)

MANAGEMENT OF THE Rh-IMMUNIZED WOMAN AND HER FETUS

In the 50% of pregnancies not requiring amniocentesis (or fetal blood sampling) and in those where the Δ450 reading has been consistently below the middle of zone 2, spontaneous delivery at term may be allowed to occur. If the expected date is firm and conditions are favorable, induction and delivery at 38.5 to 39 weeks gestation may be carried out. If there is a bad history or a high titer, a heterozygous husband and serial readings in zone 1 or low zone 2, the fetus is Rh-negative. Again, delivery should be allowed to take place spontaneously. If the readings rise into the 50% to 75% level of zone 2 by 35 to 37 weeks gestation, delivery should be carried out at 36 to 38 weeks gestation, provided that there is evidence of pulmonary maturity. If pulmonary maturity is not demonstrated and if the fluid reading is in the 70% to 75% level of zone 2, a fetal blood-sampling procedure may be considered. These fetuses should not be left undelivered after 38 weeks gestation. Although not hydropic, they may be significantly anemic and require prompt treatment.

About one half of the 20% to 25% of fetuses who will become hydropic do so after 34 weeks gestation. If the ΔOD 450 reading falls in the 80% to 85% level of zone 2 at 34 weeks gestation or later, prompt delivery should be undertaken, provided again that there is evidence of pulmonary maturity. Failing this evidence, a blood-sampling procedure should be carried out, followed by a direct intravascular transfusion, if fetal blood parameters indicate the need for it. If fetal blood sampling in this situation is not feasible, if the fetus appears appropriate for gestational age (≥34 weeks gestation), administration of corticosteroids for 48 hours followed by delivery is recommended.

INTRAUTERINE FETAL TRANSFUSION (IUT)

Induced delivery too early in gestation carries with it a high neonatal mortality rate. Prior to 1963, induction as

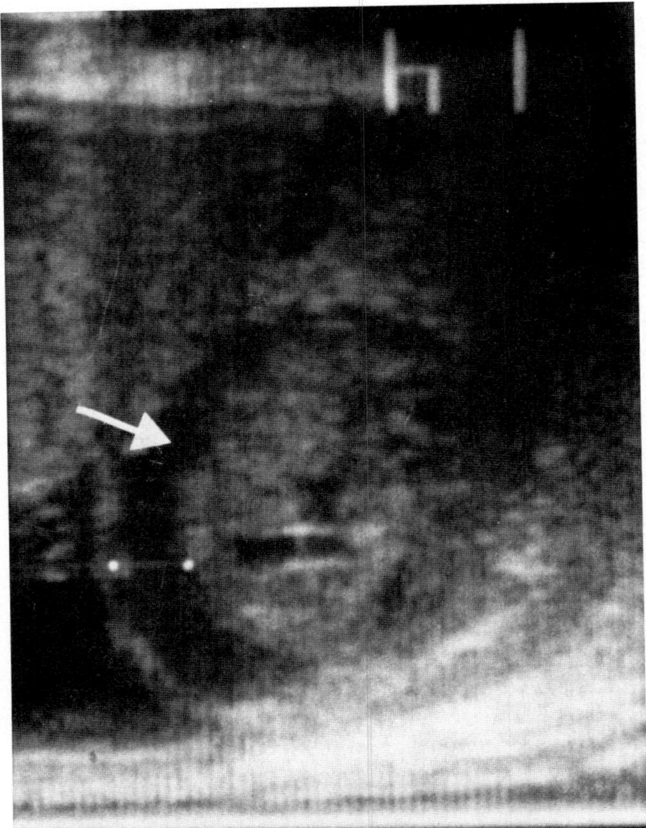

FIGURE 70–11. Ultrasound examination of fetus with hydrops fetalis. Fetal abdomen encloses a large volume of ascitic fluid (under white arrow) and a large liver with a dilated ductus venosus. (From Bowman JM. Maternal blood group immunization. In Creasy R, Resnik R, eds. Maternal-fetal medicine: principles and practice. Philadelphia: WB Saunders, 1984:589.)

early as 31 to 32 weeks gestation was carried out (mortality rate 25%), because no other management measures were available. Eight percent of affected fetuses become hydropic before 32 weeks gestation. In 1963, Liley's introduction of intraperitoneal fetal transfusion (IPT) completely altered the outlook for these most severely affected fetuses.[41]

Liley's IPT technique has to a great extent been supplanted by fetal blood sampling and direct intravascular transfusion (IVT) first carried out via fetoscopy in 1981,[42] and followed in 1982 by ultrasound-directed IVT.[39]

INTRAPERITONEAL FETAL TRANSFUSIONS (IPT)

It has been known for the past 80 years that red cells placed in the peritoneal cavity of any animal with a diaphragm are absorbed intact into the circulation. They are absorbed via the subdiaphragmatic lymphatics and the right thoracic duct into the venous circulation. Diaphragmatic contractions are necessary for the absorption of these red cells.[43]

In the absence of fetal hydrops, 10% to 12% of transfused red cells are absorbed during each 24 hours following the transfusion. In the presence of hydrops, absorption is very capricious. It may be very reasonable,[44] or it may be very poor. When the fetus is moribund (not breathing), little or no absorption will occur. The volume of blood injected is limited by the size of the peritoneal cavity. If the volume transfused is such that intraperitoneal pressure exceeds umbilical venous pressure, blood flow from the placenta to the fetus will stop and the fetus will die.[45] Our laboratory has found that fetuses usually tolerate IPT volumes calculated by the following formula:

$$\text{IPT volume} = (\text{weeks gestation} - 20) \times 10 \text{ mL},$$

(ie, 50 mL at 25 weeks, 90 mL at 29 weeks). Calculation of residual donor hemoglobin concentration is necessary to space IPT optimally so that the fetus can be brought to reasonable maturity—34 to 35 weeks gestation—with as few procedures as possible. Following IPT, 80% of the infused red cells will be in the fetoplacental circulation (based on a fetoplacental blood volume of 125 mL/kg fetal body weight). The residual donor hemoglobin concentration is calculated according to the following formula:

$$\text{residual hemoglobin concentration (g/L)} = \frac{0.80 \times a}{125 \times b} \times \frac{120 - c}{120},$$

where a is the amount of donor red cell hemoglobin transfused in grams, b is the estimated fetal weight according to gestation (eg, 1 kg at 27 weeks gestation, 1.5 kg at 30 weeks gestation), c is the interval in days after the IPT, and 120 days is the lifespan of the donor red cell. For example, 10 days after IPT of 55 mL of blood with a hemoglobin concentration of 280 g/L, a fetus of 27 weeks gestation (weight 1 kg) would have a residual donor hemoglobin concentration of

$$\frac{0.80 \times 55 \times 280}{125 \times 1} \times \frac{120 - 10}{120} = 90.3 \text{ g/L}.$$

Since the aim is to raise the donor hemoglobin concentration into the range of 150 to 160 g/L and since one cannot raise the donor hemoglobin concentration to that level with one IPT, a second IPT is carried out as soon as the red cells from the first IPT have been absorbed (9 to 12 days). Subsequent IPT intervals are about 4 weeks, the last one rarely after 32 weeks gestation. The aim is delivery 3.5 to 4 weeks after the last IPT at greater than 33.5 to 34 weeks gestation.

DIRECT INTRAVASCULAR FETAL TRANSFUSION (IVT)

Pioneering attempts at direct intravascular transfusion (IVT) into either a fetal vessel[46,47] or a placental vessel[48] approached through a hysterotomy incision were carried out in the mid-1960s. These procedures were discontinued because survival rates were only 17% (5 of 29 fetuses transfused). Deaths for the most part were due to the prompt precipitation of premature labor by the hysterotomy. In 1981, Rodeck introduced direct fetal blood sampling and IVT through a needle introduced down a fetoscope.[42] He salvaged 18 of 25 fetuses (72%) with his fetoscopic method.[49] Blood sampling and IVT via fetoscopy require very special equipment and skills. The presence of blood (common after a first IVT), meconium, or turbidity (common in later gestation), in amniotic fluid creates major problems with visualization of fetal vessels through the fetoscope.

Fetal blood sampling and direct intravascular transfusion are now carried out in most, if not all, tertiary-level centers by the insertion of the tip of a 20- or 22-gauge spinal needle, under careful ultrasound guidance, into an umbilical blood vessel (preferably the umbilical vein, preferably at its insertion into the placenta). Although fetal blood sampling and direct intravascular transfusion are considered in detail in Chapters 42 and 70, they are such an integral part of treatment of fetal hemolytic that further reference must be made to them here.

SELECTION OF PATIENTS FOR IUT

Only fetuses at risk of hydrops or hydropic before 33 to 34 weeks gestation are candidates for IUT. Patients are selected based on history or titer (or both) for either amniocentesis or direct blood sampling, the procedure chosen being dependent on placental site and ultrasound findings. If a pregnant woman meets the history or titer criteria for further investigation, she is assessed by ultrasound at 16 to 18 weeks gestation or as soon (later in gestation) as she meets the criteria.

If the fetus looks well, without ultrasound evidence of hydrops or prehydrops, and if the placenta is not anterior and can be avoided at amniocentesis, an initial amniocentesis is carried out. The interval between further amniocenteses will be determined by the prior ΔOD 450 reading. If the placenta is anterior and the amniotic cavity cannot be reached without traversing it, amniocentesis is not carried out. Depending on the gestation of the assessment and the size and accessibility of the umbilical vein placental insertion, if the fetus looks well, nothing may be done at that time (16 to 20 weeks gestation), with reassessment in 7 to 14 days, or a direct blood-sampling procedure may be carried out. If there is ultrasound evidence of prehydrops or hydrops, immediate fetal blood sampling and IVT are carried out no matter what the gestation or placental site. If the fetus continues to look well but serial amniotic fluid ΔOD 450 measurements rise into the 75th percentile of zone 2, prompt fetal blood sampling is carried out followed by IVT, if there is significant fetal anemia (a fetal circulating hemoglobin concentration of less than 110 g/L at any gestation).

Because of the availability of fetal blood sampling, we no longer recommend IUT based on serial amniotic fluid ΔOD 450 readings or a very high single zone 3 reading, but would use these criteria to have blood available for immediate transfusion if fetal blood sampling indicates its need. Only if fetal blood sampling is not possible due to fetal vessel inaccessibility would we now carry out IUT (an IPT in this circumstance), based on amniotic fluid findings alone (a single high zone 3 fluid or ΔOD 450 readings rising into the 80th to 85th percentile of zone 2).

Because the number of candidates for IUT is diminishing as a result of the success of Rh prophylaxis, the ability to maintain adequate experience with the carrying out of IPT and IVT in individual centers is decreasing. IPT and IVT techniques are not simple. Comprehensive management of the mother and her severely affected fetus and infant requires a coordinated team approach, combining skills of the highest order of the perinatal ultrasonographer, perinatal obstetrician, neonatologist, and immunohematologist. Only through such an approach will a tertiary-level center achieve high success rates with IUT, leading to the intact survival of very sick fetuses with hemolytic disease. To maintain such expertise, the transfusion team must deal with a minimum of four or five fetuses annually in whom 15 to 20 IUT will be carried out. To attain these numbers, the team must receive all IUT transfusion candidates from an annual delivery base of 30,000 to 40,000 per year (a population of 2 or 3 million).

SUITABLE BLOOD FOR IUT

Blood for IUT (either IPT or IVT) should be drawn from the donor no more than 3 days before the transfusion is planned. It should be group O and missing the antigen (or antigens) to which the mother is sensitized (D-negative if the mother is Rh-negative with anti-D). It should be remembered that highly Rh-immunized Rh-negative women with very sick erythroblastotic fetuses are hyperresponders. They frequently have other blood group antibodies, such as M, S, s, Jk^a, Fy^a, and so on. Careful crossmatch of the donor red cells with the mother's serum, by the most sensitive techniques, is imperative immediately prior to each transfusion. A second antibody may become manifest after one or two IUT, jeopardizing the lifespan of the donor red cells infused at the previous IUT.

The blood unit should be centrifuged, the red cells tightly packed, and the supernatant plasma with buffy coat expressed and discarded. Although x-ray irradiation of the donor red cells is recommended and carried out by many centers to prevent donor lymphocyte engraftment and graft versus host disease, we believe it to be unnecessary, since we would expect that the immune-competent fetus would destroy viable donor lymphocytes and resist engraftment well before 20 weeks gestation. In Winnipeg, in the past 25 years, during which 1039 fetal transfusions have been carried out on 398 fetuses with nonirradiated red cells, of the 263 surviving infants, children, and now young adults, not one has shown any evidence of graft versus host disease. Conversely, since irradiation does not shorten the lifespan of the donor red cell, there is no contraindication to donor red cell irradiation prior to IUT.

Immediately prior to the IUT, sterile isotonic saline should be added to the packed red cells (10 to 12 mL in the case of IVT, 12 to 18 mL in the case of IPT). The resulting hemoglobin and hematocrit of the donor unit will be 280 to 300 g/L and 0.85 to 0.90, respectively. The entire aim at IUT is to transfuse the largest possible number of compatible donor red cells in the smallest possible volume.

TECHNIQUE OF IUT

IVT has almost completely replaced IPT in Winnipeg (79 IVT and only six IPT were carried out in the year ending October 31, 1988). Nevertheless, on occasion, particularly after 30 to 32 weeks gestation, in the situation where a growing fetus completely obscures the cord vessel insertion into a posteriorly implanted placenta, IPT may be the preferable alternative to the placement of a needle tip into a cord blood vessel inserted into the fetal abdomen. For this reason, IUT teams must continue to be experienced and competent in carrying out IPT. Since IPT preceded IVT and have now been performed for more than 25 years, the IPT technique will be described first.

Technique of IPT

Although there have been many modifications of Liley's original IPT method, the Winnipeg team continues to use his method with excellent results.[50] The only modifications have been elimination of intra-amniotic radiopaque contrast injections, amniograms, and pretransfusion radiograms and addition of the use of real-time ultrasonography to assess fetal well-being and fetal position and to facilitate introduction of the IPT needle and catheter.

Whereas, in the past, IPTs were carried out in the radiology department because of the need for pre- and posttransfusion radiograms, they are now carried out in the fetal assessment unit. The mother is premedicated with an analgesic and muscle relaxant but is not anesthetized. The perinatal ultrasonographer, using real-time scan, localizes the target area, the fetal abdomen. The maternal abdomen is painted with an appropriate antiseptic agent and is then draped. Meticulous asepsis is observed. The maternal abdomen directly over the target area is infiltrated with a local anesthetic. Under ultrasound guidance, the perinatal obstetrician directs a 16-gauge, 18-cm Tuohy needle into the fetal abdomen. Ideally, the fetus should be lying in a lateral position so that the needle insertion is in the lower lateral area, avoiding liver, spleen, and posterior retroperitoneal structures. If the fetal abdomen is in an anterior position (Fig. 70-12), care should be taken to insert the needle well below the mid-abdomen, to avoid the umbilical area through which the cord vessels travel. If the fetal back is anterior, IPT is too hazardous and should not be undertaken until the fetus has assumed a more favorable position. If the placenta is anterior and the fetal abdomen cannot be approached without traversing it, we do not carry out IPT, since the risk of the procedure is tripled (7% per procedure). In this situation, the cord vessel insertion into the placenta is readily accessible. Fetal blood sampling and IVT are the procedures of choice.

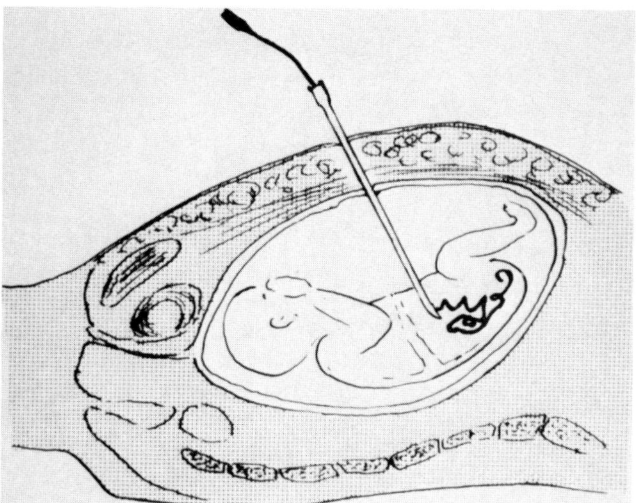

FIGURE 70–12. IPT diagram. The Tuohy needle has been inserted across the maternal abdominal wall and uterine wall into the fetal peritoneal cavity, and the epidural catheter has been threaded into the peritoneal cavity of the fetus. The safest position for the fetus at IPT is not with the abdomen anterior (as shown in this diagram), because the umbilical fetal vessels then lie in the center of the target area. (From Bowman JM. Blood-group incompatibilities. In: Iffy L, Kaminetzky HA, eds. Principles and practice of obstetrics and perinatology. New York: John Wiley, 1981:1213.)

As the IPT needle reaches the depth of the fetal abdomen and is then advanced into the abdomen, usually, but not always, the needle tip can be seen (by ultrasonography), indenting the abdomen and then penetrating the fetal peritoneal cavity. Frequently the obstetrician feels resistance as the needle tip indents the fetal abdomen, which disappears as the tip enters the abdomen. The needle stylet is withdrawn and a size 16 epidural catheter, with the blind tip and side holes removed, is threaded down the needle. If it threads past the needle tip, it is in a cavity—the peritoneal cavity, one hopes (see Fig. 70-12). As the catheter is threaded through the needle, its tip often may be seen ultrasonographically moving around the peritoneal cavity. After about 30 cm of catheter have been threaded down the needle, the needle is withdrawn over the catheter to lie on the maternal abdomen. Under very careful ultrasonographic observation, 0.5 to 1 mL of well-shaken saline, with dissolved air, is then injected down the catheter. If the saline and air bubbles produce a sonographic opacity rising promptly and freely to lie under the most upper part of the fetal abdominal cavity, indicating beyond doubt that the tip of the catheter is indeed free in the peritoneal cavity, the transfusion is continued. If the tip, by the preceding ultrasonographic observation and maneuver, cannot be demonstrated with certainty to be lying free in the peritoneal cavity, the woman is transferred to the radiology department. Two milliliters of radio contrast (76% meglumine diatrizoate) are injected through the catheter, and an anteroposterior x-ray is taken. If the catheter tip is free in the peritoneal cavity, in the absence of ascites, semilunes of contrast outline fetal bowel and contrast can be seen around the liver (Fig. 70-13). If ascites is present, contrast can be seen diffusing into the ascitic fluid (Fig. 70-14).

Although ultrasonography has improved the accuracy of insertion of needle and catheter into the fetal peritoneal cavity, success on the first attempt is not always possible. If the catheter cannot be threaded past the needle tip, the needle is embedded in fetal soft tissue. It must be removed and redirected. If ultrasonography cannot guarantee correct placement of the catheter tip, and injection of radio contrast reveals nothing, the tip is in the amniotic cavity. Conversely, the tip may be in any abdominal hollow viscus (eg, stomach, bowel, and bladder). Injection of contrast readily determines where the tip is and that it is not free in the peritoneal cavity. In all the preceding situations, the catheter must be removed, the needle redirected, and the catheter reinserted.

When the catheter tip has been shown to be lying free in the peritoneal cavity, the transfusion is begun. The donor-packed red cell unit with added saline has a blood infusion set attached, the other end of which is inserted into the side arm of a three-way metal stopcock. The IPT catheter is cut off 8 to 10 cm from the

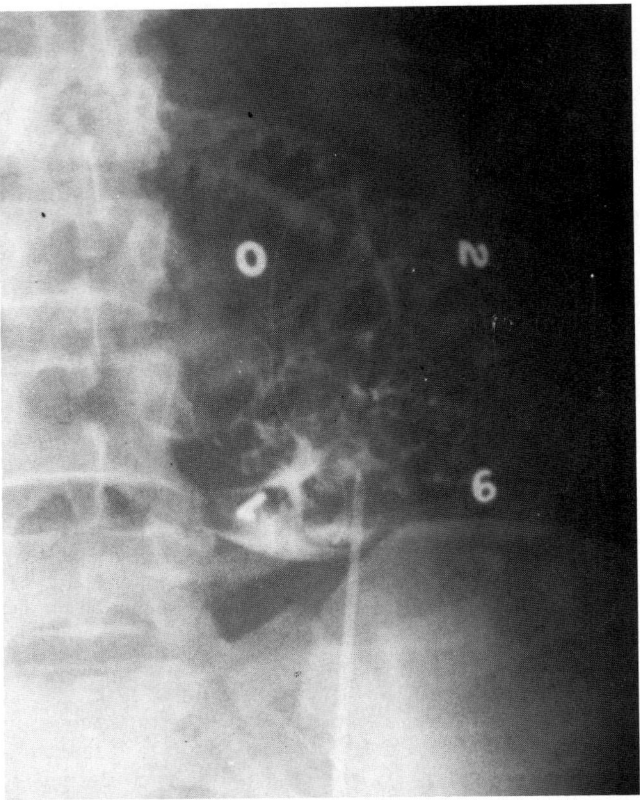

FIGURE 70–13. Successful catheterization of fetal peritoneal cavity at IPT, as shown by radiopaque contrast agent in the peritoneal cavity, outlining negative shadows of small bowel and the liver. (From Bowman JM. Haemolytic disease of the newborn. In: Roberton NRC, ed. A textbook of neonatology. Edinburgh: Churchill Livingstone, 1986:474.)

maternal abdomen, and a blunted 22-gauge needle is inserted into the cut end. The needle hub is attached to the stopcock, as is a 10-mL glass syringe. Plastic syringes and stopcocks may not withstand the pressures required to inject the red cells down the catheter.

The red cells are infused in 10-mL aliquots, each 10 mL taking 3 to 6 minutes, to a total volume calculated according to the IPT transfusion formula already outlined. The fetal heart rate is monitored by Doppler ultrasound at the end of each 10-mL infusion and continuously for the last 10 to 15 mL. If the fetus is in good condition, with an intact autonomic nervous system, the heart rate increases to 160 to 190 beats per minute. Early bradycardia is rare but very ominous. Late bradycardia, also rare, is an indication for prompt termination of the IPT, since intraperitoneal pressure may be approaching umbilical venous pressure. As intraperitoneal red cells increase in volume, real-time ultrasound will reveal an enlarging crescent of sonar lucency between the diaphragm and liver, further confirming the successful placement of the catheter tip.

At the end of the procedure, the catheter is removed slowly with continuous Doppler fetal heart rate monitoring, since vagal reflex–induced bradycardia may occur. Both fetal heart rate and fetal movements are monitored at regular intervals after IPT. The fetus may move very little for the first 12 to 24 hours; the mother should be reassured that this is to be expected. The mother is discharged about 24 hours after the IPT and is examined every 3 to 7 days by real-time ultrasound to assess both fetal condition and the adequacy of absorption of the intraperitoneal red cells.

Technique of IVT

Neither fetoscopic nor intracardiac IVT will be discussed in this chapter. Only IVT, as carried out in Winnipeg, under ultrasound direction will be considered. Although some transfusion teams prefer IVT into the fetal abdominal end of the umbilical vein,[39,40] most teams prefer to insert the needle tip into an umbilical vessel at its insertion into the placenta (usually a vein but occasionally an artery).[51–54] In the same manner as for IPT, the mother is given full analgesic and muscle-relaxant premedication. The same transfusion sets, metal stopcocks, and glass syringes are used as for IPT.

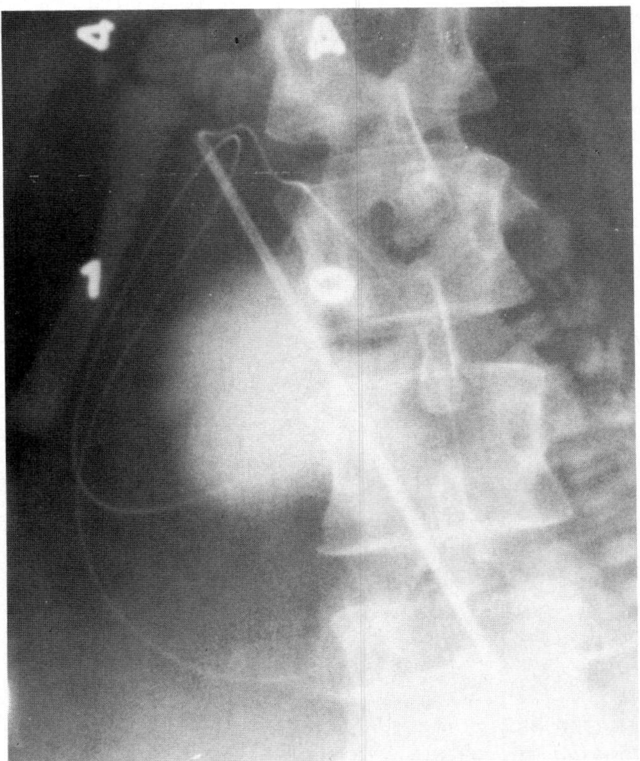

FIGURE 70–14. Hydrops fetalis at IPT. Gross ascites at first IPT (31.5 weeks' gestation) and second IPT given 4 days later (shown). Severe residual hydrops at emergency cesarean section (33.5 weeks' gestation). At birth, cord hemoglobin was 6.2 g/100 mL (99% of donor origin), and cord bilirubin was 5.4 mg/100 mL. Neonate required five exchange transfusions, respiratory care for 4 days, and intensive nursery care for 3 weeks to survive.

To the stopcock end to which, in the case of IPT, the epidural catheter is attached, a length of extension tubing is attached and filled with donor red cells, taking great care to ensure that no bubbles of air are in the extension tubing, stopcock or syringe.

Prior to preparation of the maternal abdomen, the peritoneal ultrasonographer takes considerable time and great care in identifying the cord vessel insertion, the target for the IVT needle (Fig. 70-15). The ultrasonographer is the most important member of the team. The success of IVT depends primarily on his or her skill and experience.

After careful aseptic preparation of the maternal abdomen and local anesthetic infiltration over the target area, the obstetrician-venipuncturist, under real-time ultrasound guidance (the transducer being enclosed in sterile plastic), directs a spinal puncture needle (22 gauge if the fetus is between 20 and 30 weeks gestation; 20 gauge if between 30 and 34 weeks gestation), toward the target vessel. The transducer is positioned in such a plane that there can be simultaneous identification of the target vessel and the needle tip. Because the needle tip is being advanced in a three-dimensional plane, under the direction of the ultrasonographer using a two-dimensional instrument, repeated small, delicate corrections of needle direction are required to get the needle tip into the fetal vessel. In most instances the needle tip can be seen indenting and then penetrating the fetal vessel.

When the needle appears to be in the vessel, the stylet is withdrawn and aspiration of fetal blood (0.8 mL) into a lightly heparinized 1-mL tuberculin syringe is attempted. If free-flow blood is obtained, confirmation that the needle is correctly placed is determined in two ways:

1. A small aliquot of the blood is tested immediately for fetal hemoglobin by alkaline denaturation. If the hemoglobin solution resists alkaline denaturation (remains pink), the blood is fetal and the needle is correctly placed. An immediate hemoglobin examination of the fetal blood sample also is carried out (HemoCue). Subsequently, the fetal red cells are blood-grouped and direct antiglobulin tested. The hemoglobin is repeated and hematocrit, serum bilirubin, serum protein, platelet, and blood gas measurements are carried out in the laboratory.
2. Further confirmation of the proper placement of the needle is obtained by injecting 0.5 to 1.0 mL of sterile isotonic saline down the needle and observing characteristic ultrasound turbulence as the saline courses down the vein. If fetal movements are likely to disturb the needle insertion, pancuronium is injected into the fetal vessel to stop fetal movement temporarily. If the circulating red cell hemoglobin criterion ($\leq$110 g/L) is met, the blood-filled extension tubing, connected via the stopcock to the unit of donor red cells, is attached to the hub of the spinal needle, which is held very firmly, without any needle movement, by the obstetrician venipuncturist. The third member of the team then injects the donor red cells in aliquots of 10 mL, the injection of each aliquot taking 1 to 2 minutes. The transfusion is monitored continuously by the perinatal ultrasonographer. Stream-

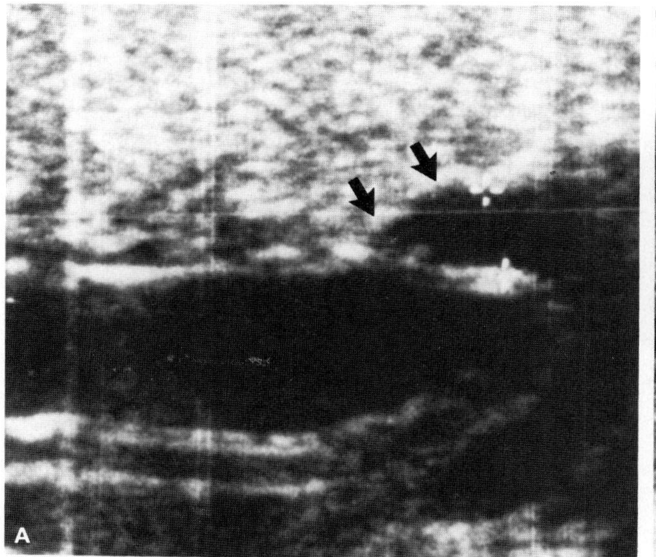

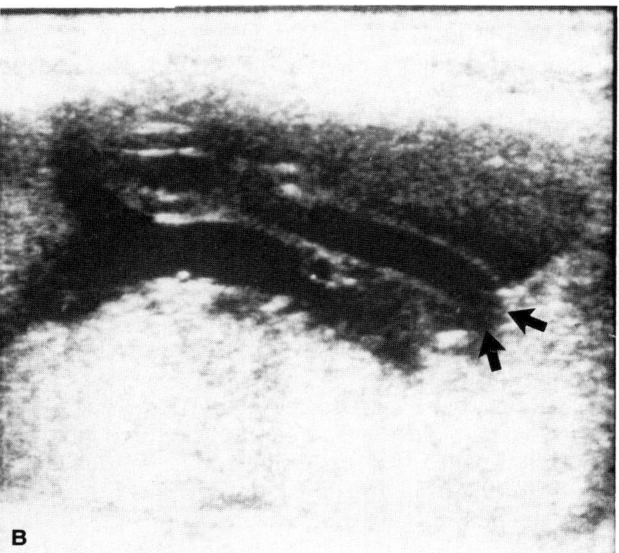

FIGURE 70–15. Real-time scan ultrasound view of insertion of the umbilical vein into the placenta (arrows). (**A**) anterior placenta; (**B**) posterior placenta. The lumen of the umbilical vein is sonar lucent. (From Bowman JM. Maternal blood group immunization. In: Creasy R, Resnik R, eds. Maternal-fetal medicine: principles and practice. 2nd ed. Philadelphia: WB Saunders, 1989:637.)

ing turbulence is seen as the donor red cells pass down the vein. Conversely, if the needle tip is in an umbilical artery, turbulence is seen coursing in the opposite direction onto the fetal surface of the placenta. If characteristic turbulence is not seen, no blood should be transfused. If turbulence, once present, disappears, the transfusion must be stopped at once. Since only 2 to 3 mm of needle are in the fetal vessel, there is a significant risk of dislodgment, either into the amniotic cavity (easily recognized and not hazardous—the needle needs to be promptly reinserted into the vessel) or into the cord substance. The latter is potentially very dangerous, since further infusion of blood will produce a cord hematoma with great risk of umbilical venous compression, interference with venous blood flow, and serious fetal compromise.

As the experience of the Winnipeg IVT team has increased (163 IVT in 45 fetuses, from May 26, 1986 to February 27, 1989), it has become apparent that the fetus, connected to its expansile placental vascular bed, can tolerate large volumes of blood (up to 60 mL per estimated kilogram nonhydropic fetal weight). The actual volume infused varies from 40 mL/kg to 60 mL/kg, depending on the pretransfusion hemoglobin concentration and fetal condition. If the pretransfusion hemoglobin concentration is greater than 90 g/L or if the fetus is severely hydropic with a hemoglobin of 40 g/L or less, the initial IVT volume is 40 mL/kg of estimated nonhydropic fetal weight. Thereafter, transfusion volumes are usually of the order of 50 mL/kg body weight but on occasion may be as great as 60 mL/kg, again depending on pretransfusion donor-recipient hemoglobin concentration. The aim is to reach, but not exceed, a donor-recipient circulating hemoglobin concentration of 200 to 210 g/L. A transfusion of 50 mL per estimated kg body weight of packed red cells, with a hemoglobin concentration of 280 g/L, will raise the circulating donor-recipient hemoglobin concentration 112 g/L (if the estimated fetal body weight is accurate).

The ultrasonographer monitors the fetal heart rate and size of the right ventricle periodically during the IVT, more frequently as transfusion volumes increase beyond 40 mL/kg. On the very rare occasions when the fetal heart rate slows (under 110 beats per minute) or there is evidence of significant right ventricular dilation before the planned transfusion volume is reached, the IVT is discontinued.

When the desired packed red cell volume has been transfused, the needle is cleared of packed red cells by the injection of 0.5 mL of sterile isotonic saline. Then two 0.8-mL posttransfusion blood samples are withdrawn. The first, slightly diluted with saline (which was in the needle), is sent for blood gas measurements. The second sample is tested for hemoglobin, hematocrit, platelet, serum bilirubin, serum protein, and Kleihauer acid elution adult donor fetal red cell ratio estimations. All the preceding tests are done on all subsequent pre- and post-IVT blood samples.

By raising the donor-recipient hemoglobin concentration to about 200 g/L, we aim to stop fetal erythropoiesis altogether. This donor-recipient hemoglobin level can be attained with two IVT spaced 2 to 7 days apart (the actual interval depending on the condition of the fetus and the initial pretransfusion circulating fetal hemoglobin level). Thereafter, transfusion intervals are determined by the donor-recipient red cell hemoglobin attrition rate (4 g/L/day), the posttransfusion donor-recipient hemoglobin concentration, and our desire not to let the circulating hemoglobin concentration in the fetus fall below 90 g/L.

Because of the rapid expansion of fetoplacental blood volume by the large volumes of blood given at IVT (30% to 40% of the pretransfusion fetoplacental blood volume), the measured posttransfusion hemoglobin level is an underestimate of the true circulating hemoglobin concentration when the fetoplacental blood volume has reequilibrated. The true circulating donor hemoglobin concentration can be more accurately calculated from the following formula:

$$\text{post-IVT donor-recipient Hb (g/L)} = \text{pre-IVT donor-recipient Hb (g/L)} + \frac{\text{g of donor red cell Hb infused}}{\text{fetoplacental blood volume}}.$$

Fetoplacental blood volume is estimated to be 0.125 L/kg nonhydropic fetal weight, which is the average fetal weight for that gestation. For example, if at 28 weeks gestation a fetus of average weight (1.15 kg) with a pretransfusion hemoglobin concentration of 90 g/L is transfused with 55 mL of donor red cells, with a hemoglobin concentration of 280 g/L (15.4 g donor hemoglobin transfused), the posttransfusion hemoglobin concentration will be

$$90 + \frac{15.4}{0.125 \times 1.15} = 90 + 107 = 197 \text{ g/L}$$

Knowing from past experience that the donor-recipient hemoglobin attrition rate is about 4 g/L/day, and with the aim to transfuse the fetus again when fetal hemoglobin drops to 90 g/L, the next IVT would be carried out in 27 days:

$$\left(\frac{197 - 90}{4}\right) = 27.$$

Because IVT volumes are smaller than IPT volumes and because we deliver IVT fetuses after 36 weeks gestation because of the greater safety of IVT (Table 70-6), the numbers of IVT per fetus are greater than the numbers of IPT (4 versus 2.7).

IUT IN THE PRESENCE OF HYDROPS FETALIS

Doctors try to predict impending hydrops in order to commence IUT before hydrops develops. Unfortunately, in the past 9 years, because of late referral, hy-

TABLE 70–6. INTRAUTERINE TRANSFUSIONS WINNIPEG ULTRASOUND ERA

	204 IPT (JULY 1980–OCTOBER 1986)	163 IVT* (MAY 1986–FEBRUARY 1989)
Total Fetuses	75	44
Survivors	57 (76.0%)	41 (93.2%)
Nonhydrops	45	28
Survivors	39 (86.7%)	27 (96.4%)
Hydrops	30	16
Incidence of hydrops	40.0%	35.6%
Survival of hydrops	18 (60.0%)	14 (87.5%)
Moribund hydrops	8	6
Survival	0 (0.0%)	5 (83.3%)
Nonmoribund hydrops	22	10
Survival	18 (81.8%)	9 (90.0%)
IUT per fetus	2.7	4
Traumatic deaths	7 (10.0%)	1 (2.3%)
Risk of death per IUT	3.5%	0.62%

* Fourteen IPT were carried out on the 44 IVT fetuses whose management was primarily IVT.

drops has been encountered in 35% to 40% of fetuses undergoing IUT in Winnipeg (see Table 70-6).

In the pre-IVT era the occasional fetus not hydropic at first IPT would develop gross ascites (early hydrops) in the 9 to 12 days between the first and second IPT because of the slow rate of red cell absorption following IPT (Fig. 70-16). This does not occur with IVT. A fetus not hydropic at first IVT will not become hydropic if appropriately transfused. In the pre-IVT era, if a hydropic fetus was not moribund and survived following one or two transfusions, reversal of hydrops frequently, but not invariably, occurred (see Fig. 70-16). After serial IVT, the hydropic fetus, unless dying at the time of the first IVT, nearly always becomes nonhydropic unless delivery occurs too soon after the first or second IVT to allow the hydrops to resolve. As donor-recipient red cell hemoglobin is maintained at normal, or above-normal levels, fetal erythropoietin production ceases, erythropoiesis stops, the liver shrinks in size, intrahepatic blood flow improves, portal and umbilical venous pressures drop, hepatic function improves, albumin levels rise, and fetal ascites and edema disappear; the hydrops has reversed.

If gross ascites is present, IVT is the procedure of choice; indeed it is the only hope for the fetus so severely affected that no breathing movements are present. Without diaphragmatic movement, no absorption of intraperitoneal blood occurs.[43] Only if venous access is impossible (a very rare occurrence) and the fetus is not moribund should IPT be carried out in the hydropic fetus. When the IPT needle is inserted, if possible a volume of ascitic fluid 50% greater than the normal IPT transfusion volume should be aspirated before the catheter is inserted. The IPT transfusion volume should then be increased by 20% to 25%.

If feasible, subsequent procedures should be IVTs. If further IPTs must be carried out, a second IPT should be given in 4 to 12 days, with the interval depending on

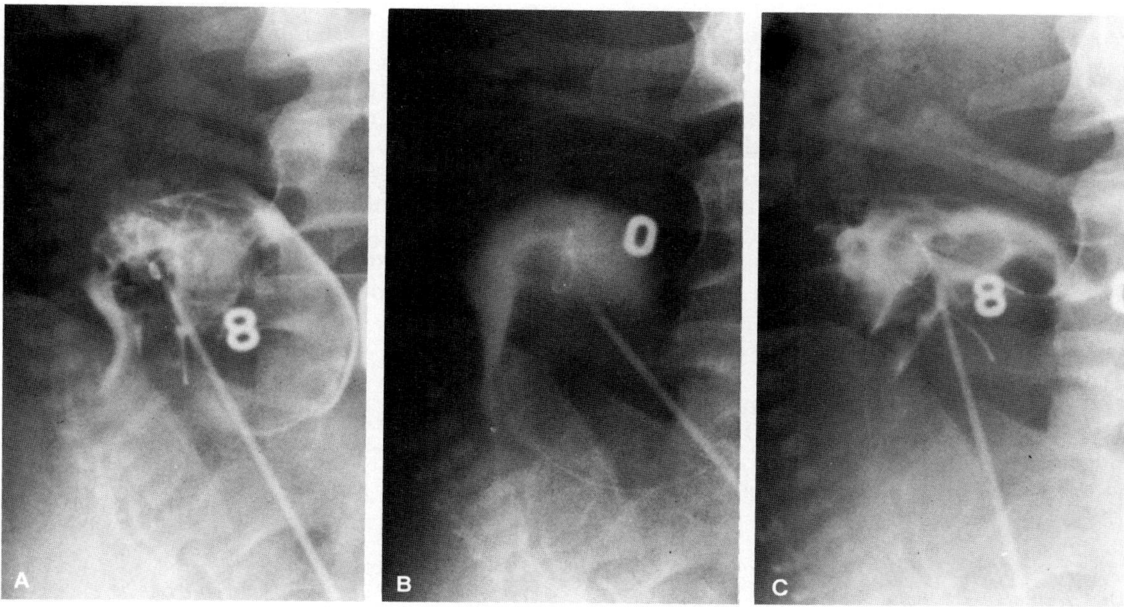

FIGURE 70–16. Reversed hydrops. (**A**) No ascites at first IPT (25 weeks' gestation); (**B**) gross ascites (hydrops fetalis) at second IPT (27 weeks' gestation); (**C**) no residual hydrops at third IPT (30 weeks' gestation). Baby was delivered at 34 weeks gestation with no evidence of hydrops. Cord hemoglobin was 9.9 g/100 mL (99.9% of donor origin); cord bilirubin was 5.0 g/100 mL. Baby required only one exchange transfusion and is alive and well. (From Bowman JM. Maternal blood group immunization. In: Creasy R, Resnik R, eds. Maternal-fetal medicine: principles and practice. Philadelphia: WB Saunders, 1984:586.)

ultrasound assessment of fetal condition and whether the hydrops is becoming more severe (increasing ascites, the appearance of pleural and pericardial effusions, increasing edema). At the second procedure, as much as possible of the ascitic fluid diluted with the residual blood from the first IPT should be removed and replaced with compatible, highly concentrated donor red cells, to a volume equal to 80% of the ascitic fluid removed. At one time we instilled digoxin into the peritoneal cavities of hydropic fetuses and placed their mothers on maintenance digoxin and a diuretic. Because of the evidence that alloimmune hydrops fetalis is not caused by fetal heart failure, we have discontinued this practice.

If IVTs are feasible in the hydropic fetus, and they nearly always are, 40 to 60 mL of red cells per estimated kilogram of dry fetal weight for gestation should be transfused. The actual volume administered depends on the ultrasonographer's assessment of fetal condition (heart rate, myocardial contractility, and ventricular size). Severely hydropic, nonmoribund fetuses with hemoglobin levels as low as 20 to 22 g/L have tolerated transfusions up to 60 mL/kg dry fetal weight, further evidence that fetal heart failure is not the cause of this type of hydrops fetalis. When the fetus is hydropic and moribund, we restrict the volume of the first IVT to 40 mL/kg, increasing to 50 mL to 60 mL/kg thereafter. The very anemic hydropic fetus may be very thrombocytopenic (platelet counts below 20,000/mm^3) and at risk of exsanguinating hemorrhage. On several occasions, faced with this situation, transfusions of platelet concentrate have been required (3 to 8 mL, depending on gestation), at the first IVT or at a second IVT, carried out a few hours after the first IVT because of intractable bleeding.[55] Platelet transfusions are given following IVT or using platelet concentrates as a diluent rather than saline whenever platelet concentrations are expected or known to be less than 30,000/mm^3. If used in the first manner, the volume (3 to 8 mL) must be considered and subtracted from the proposed total transfusion volumes to arrive at the red cell volume to be transfused.

Since again our aim is to raise the total donor-recipient circulating hemoglobin to 200 g/L as quickly as possible, the second IVT is carried out within 1 to 7 days, at a time when the calculated donor-recipient hemoglobin level will be in the range of 90 to 100 g/L. Subsequent transfusion intervals do not differ from those in nonhydropic fetuses and are calculated in the same manner.

SURVIVAL AFTER FETAL TRANSFUSION

Reported IPT survival rates have varied from 49%[56] and 84%[57] (no hydropic fetuses were transfused in this series) to 86%.[58] In Winnipeg, from January 2, 1964 to October 21, 1986, of 353 fetuses treated with 862 IPT, 222 (62.7%) survived. Winnipeg IPT experience in the ultrasound era is shown in Table 70-6, column 1. The overall IPT survival rate was 76.0% (86.7% when the fetus was not hydropic, 60% when the fetus was hydropic). Of the eight moribund nonbreathing hydropic fetuses, none survived; whereas 81.8% (18 of 22) nonmoribund hydropic fetuses survived. Survival rates were 43% and 60% when IPT was required before 23 and 26 weeks gestation, respectively. Survival with IPT begun as early as 21 weeks gestation has been achieved.

Survival rates with IVT vary from an unacceptably low figure of 11%,[59] to 75%,[40,52] 82%,[51] and 94%.[53] The Winnipeg experience is set out in Table 70-6, column 2. Overall IVT survival rates were 93.2% (41 of 44 fetuses transfused and delivered). Of the 28 nonhydropic fetuses transfused, 27 (96.4%) survived. The one nonhydropic death was not IVT related (neonatal death at 7 days of age, following elective cesarean section at 36 weeks gestation, cord hemoglobin concentration of 100 g/L, and weight of 2600 g). Fourteen of 16 hydropic fetuses (87.5%) survived; six of the 16 were moribund and five survived. Only one of the three deaths after IVT was due to trauma at IVT (exsanguination because of failure to keep the tip of the needle in the vein of a severely hydropic fetus at 22.5 weeks gestation). Three of the 45 fetuses required IVT before 20.5 weeks gestation; all three survived.

RISKS OF IUT

Maternal risks with either IPT or IVT are very low. Both carry some risk to the fetus (see Table 70-6; Table 70-7). In Winnipeg, traumatic death at IPT occurred in 10% of fetuses (3.5% per IPT); traumatic death at IVT occurred in only 2.3% of fetuses (one fetus; 0.62% per IVT). However, three other fetuses were put at very serious risk. Fortunately, the hazard was recognized by ultrasound monitoring (cord hematoma in one, fetal bleeding in two). Two survived following emergency cesarean section; the other, by further IVT supplemented with platelet concentrate infusions.[55] If the placenta is implanted anteriorly and must be traversed by the 16-gauge IPT needle that is used in Winnipeg, the traumatic fetal death rate is 20% (7% per IPT). Conversely,

TABLE 70–7. HAZARDS OF IUT

IPT–IVT
Maternal or fetal infection
Maternal or fetal tissue trauma
Exsanguination
Precipitation of labor
Fetal–maternal transplacental hemorrhage
Graft versus host disease
Transient susceptibility to infection
IPT
Overtransfusion, increased intraperitoneal pressure, obstruction to umbilical venous circulation
IVT
Overtransfusion with fetal heart failure
Umbilical cord hematoma, obstruction to umbilical venous circulation

if the placenta can be avoided at IPT, the traumatic death rate is 6.4% per fetus (2.2% per IPT).

There should be very little risk of either maternal or fetal infection if careful aseptic technique is maintained. Although we realize that antibacterial prophylaxis is controversial, we do administer ampicillin and cloxacillin for 24 to 48 hours after IUT, provided that the mother is not allergic to penicillin. We have had no reactions to this regimen, nor have we had any maternal or fetal infections. It is of course axiomatic that the blood used for IUT should be from healthy, carefully screened, low-risk volunteer donors who are HIV antibody and HB_sAg negative.

With the use of real-time ultrasound, there should be no risk of inadvertent maternal tissue trauma. In the pre-ultrasound era, IPT carried a small but definite risk of maternal trauma, including one instance of abruptio placentae and maternal shock, with disseminated intravascular coagulation.[60] Fortunately, the mother survived; however, the fetus died. At present, the only fetal tissue trauma risk, exsanguination, is vascular in origin. It may occur after either IPT or IVT.

Precipitation of labor, a real risk, is more common after IPT (30%) than after IVT. Fortunately, it usually occurs well after 30 weeks gestation, and the majority of the resulting infants survive.

The risk of fetal–maternal transplacental hemorrhage with increasing maternal antibody titer is great with IVT, because of needle insertion into the fetal vessel at its placental end, fetal TPH occurring in at least 50% of cases. TPH at IPT will occur only if the placenta is inadvertently transfixed.

Graft versus host disease caused by the engraftment of donor lymphocytes has been reported.[61] For this reason, as already discussed, many centers x-irradiate blood before IUT. As already stated, we do not irradiate blood for IUT and have not observed graft versus host disease in any of our 263 IUT survivors. With the almost exclusive use of ultrasound, the hazards of exposure of the fetus to x-ray radiation have disappeared. No radiation sequelae have been observed in any of our older IPT survivors, who are now in their early to middle 20s. Many of them received as much as 3.5 to 4.0 rads.

We have noted, following IPT, transient susceptibility to infection in the first few months of life. Acute gram-negative sepsis has occurred, as have acute severe adenoviral and syncytial viral infections.[50] We do not know the underlying cause, nor has it been reported to us in our IVT survivors. Fortunately, this hazard is transient, disappearing before 1 year of age.

There is a risk of overtransfusion with specific different hazards, such as intraperitoneal pressures exceeding umbilical venous pressures at IPT compromising umbilical venous blood flow and hypervolemia at IVT precipitating fetal heart failure. The IPT problem can be circumvented by not exceeding the IPT volume formula already outlined and by discontinuing the transfusion at the first sign of fetal bradycardia. Hypervolemia at IVT, precipitating fetal heart failure, will undoubtedly occur if excessive volumes are transfused. We have been pleasantly surprised by the large volumes that the fetus will tolerate without going into heart failure. We never exceed 60 mL/kg estimated nonhydropic fetal weight and usually restrict the volume to 50 mL/kg. We discontinue the transfusion at smaller volumes if fetal bradycardia or marked cardiac dilation occurs, but the situation rarely arises.

A potentially serious and never-to-be-forgotten hazard at IVT, which has already been referred to, is the risk of producing a cord hematoma if the needle tip inadvertently is in the cord substance. Such a hematoma may cause interference with venous blood flow and compromise the fetus. A skilled, experienced perinatal ultrasonographer will forestall such an accident by quickly having the transfusion stopped at the first sign of a cord hematoma forming (visible by ultrasound) or if the turbulence produced by the infused blood disappears.

THE ADVANTAGES AND DISADVANTAGES OF IVT VERSUS IPT

The ability to sample fetal blood directly and infuse blood into the fetal circulation is a major advance in the management of the fetus with severe erythroblastosis. Because diagnosis of severity of disease is rendered much more accurate and because the response to direct transfusion occurs immediately, not over an 8- to 10-day period as it is with IPT, IVT is unquestionably the superior procedure and is the transfusion method of choice wherever possible.

If the placenta is anterior and unavoidable at IPT, IVT should be the only procedure considered, since the risk of IPT is more than 10 times greater (7% versus 0.62%). Similarly, if the fetus is moribund and not breathing, only IVT is capable of fetal rescue and survival (83.3% survival, versus zero survival with IPT).

There are, however, certain situations in which IPT may be the only feasible procedure. On rare occasions in very early pregnancy (before 20 to 22 weeks gestation), the fetal vessels may be too small to access, although this is uncommon. In such a situation, if there is an ominous amniotic fluid reading and ultrasound evidence of early but not severe hydrops, an initial IPT as a temporizing measure, until venous access is possible, is indicated. More frequently, after serial IVT early in gestation—when the placenta and cord insertion are posterior and venous access is obstructed by the fetus (32 to 33 weeks)—we will elect a final IPT to carry the fetus to 36 to 37 weeks gestation, unless access to the umbilical vein at its insertion into the fetal abdomen appears very easy. In the year ending October 31, 1988, during which 79 IVTs were carried out, one IPT was carried out for the first reason and five for the second.

Therefore, although IVT is now the procedure of choice, there is still a place for IPT, albeit small, in the management of the alloimmunized mother and her severely affected fetus.

Although the intravascular route is essential in getting the packed cells to a dying fetus, some advocate combining an intravascular procedure (providing immediate help to the fetus) with the intraperitoneal approach. The latter would add a later infusion of absorbed red cells from the peritoneal cavity. The rationale is that this added "delayed release" would lengthen the time required between transfusions and would decrease the number of transfusions necessary. This approach awaits further study.

DELIVERY OF THE FETUS FOLLOWING IUT

The severely affected infant who has undergone IUT may be delivered in excellent condition. Nevertheless, since the infant may have to be delivered prematurely, and on occasion may still be hydropic, delivery should be carried out only in a tertiary-level perinatal–neonatal center.

The availability of fetal blood sampling and IVT with surprisingly low risk (0.62% in our hands) has altered the gestation at which delivery is recommended. Where IVT is feasible, the fetus should not be delivered before 36 weeks gestation. An IVT at 34 weeks gestation will allow delivery at 37.5 to 38 weeks gestation. If IVT is not possible and IPT must be used (invariably with a posterior placenta; the risk per procedure is 2.2% in our hands), we would not carry out IPT after 31 to 31.5 weeks gestation, preferring delivery at 34.5 to 35 weeks gestation. These delivery times may be modified by the presence in amniotic fluid of evidence of pulmonary maturity. Nevertheless, even with such evidence, we would not recommend delivery before 32 to 33 weeks gestation, and if IVT were feasible, we would not deliver the infant before 36 weeks gestation.

Provided that the mother has not undergone previous cesarean section and that the fetus is in good condition and is in a vertex position, we recommend induction, with very careful fetal monitoring. Vaginal delivery is successful about 80% of the time.

If the mother has had a prior cesarean section, if the fetus is in a breech position, if labor has not begun within 24 hours following rupture of membranes, or if fetal heart rate monitoring reveals fetal distress, cesarean section should be carried out promptly.

During labor and delivery every effort should be made to keep the baby well oxygenated. Epidural anesthesia is the anesthetic of choice. Immediately after delivery, thorough, gentle suction of the baby's nasopharynx and oropharynx should be carried out. After prompt clamping and division of the cord, the baby is handed to a neonatologist experienced in the care of such infants. Ten to 15 mL of blood are drained from the placental end of the cord into a heparinized tube. The blood is sent for appropriate testing.

Management of such infants is usually surprisingly easy, easier than before the era of IUT, since they usually are born after 34 weeks gestation and have reasonably good hemoglobin levels (≥90 g/L). However, if earlier delivery is required and the infant is hydropic, management may require all the resources of the most experienced tertiary-level neonatal intensive care unit.

SUPPRESSION OF Rh IMMUNIZATION

Since the mid-1940s, efforts have been made to suppress Rh immunization. Rh hapten proved valueless.[62] Administration of promethazine chloride has been touted by Gusdon and Rh stroma by Bierme,[63,64] but neither has proved to be effective.[65,66] Following treatment with promethazine in two cases known to the author, one fetus died and the other required IUT.

PLASMA EXCHANGE

Intensive plasma exchange—whereby large amounts of maternal antibody-containing plasma (3 L/day, 5 days/week) are removed and replaced with saline, 5% albumin, and small amounts of fresh-frozen plasma—will reduce circulating maternal blood group antibody levels by 75% to 80%. Such reductions, in the author's experience, are always transient and at best may delay the need for IUT by 2 or 3 weeks. The procedure is very costly, both in professional time and resources. With the advent of fetal blood sampling and IVT as early as 18 to 20 weeks gestation, intensive plasmapheresis, which carries minor risks to the mother, including the need for transfusion of small amounts of plasma, is only very rarely indicated. We would recommend its use only for the woman with an extremely high antibody level (≥256), with a documented history of prior hydropic fetal death before 22 to 24 weeks gestation, and with a husband homozygous for the antigen to which she is sensitized. If plasma exchange is decided on, based on the preceding criteria, it should be started at 12 to 14 weeks gestation; 15 L of plasma should be removed each week. Twice-weekly fetal assessments should be started at 16 weeks gestation, with amniocentesis and/or fetal blood sampling as early as possible (18 to 20 weeks gestation).

INTRAVENOUS IMMUNE SERUM GLOBULIN

Intravenous immune serum globulin (IVIG) administration has been reported to reduce severity of hemolytic disease.[67] Doses required are 400 mg/kg maternal body weight administered for 5 days and repeated every 4 to 6 weeks. IVIG may exert a beneficial effect: by negative feedback reducing maternal antibody levels (by 50% in the author's experience); by saturating trophoblastic FC receptor sites impeding placental transfer of antibody into the fetus; and by saturating fetal FC receptor sites preventing destruction of antibody-coated fetal red cells. High-dose IVIG is extremely expensive and is not of confirmed significant benefit. Again, with the advent of very early fetal blood sampling and IVT, administration of high-dose IVIG is rarely, if ever, indicated. It may be used as an alternative treatment measure to intensive plasma exchange for the type of patient cited in the section on plasma exchange.

PREVENTION OF Rh IMMUNIZATION

The ability to prevent Rh immunization is a major advance in the management of the Rh-negative pregnant woman. In 1900, Von Dungern showed that administration to rabbits of antibody to ox red cells with ox red cells prevented the development of ox red cell antibodies.[68] He proved the axiom that the presence of antibodies to an antigen, if in sufficient amount, will suppress active immunization to the antigen.

This information was used 60 years later in New York[69] and Liverpool[70] and shortly thereafter in Winnipeg.[22] Initial experiments, carried out on Rh-negative male volunteers, in which the volunteers were given Rh-positive red cells and Rh antibody in the form of Rh-immune globulin (RhIG, anti-D IgG), showed that the anti-D prevented Rh immunization from developing.

Clinical trials followed, in which Rh-negative unimmunized women after delivery of Rh-positive infants and therefore at risk of Rh immunization were give RhIG. All such trials were uniformly successful. One such trial is set out in Table 70-8.[71] In 1968, as a result of these trials, RhIG was licensed for use in North America. The standard dose in the United States is 300 μg given intramuscularly (IM). Smaller doses of 100 to 125 μg IM are used in Europe and Australia; 120 μg either IM or IV is the standard postpartum dose in Canada. All these doses appear about equally effective.

RhIG will always prevent Rh immunization, with two provisos: it must be given in adequate amount, and it must be given before Rh immunization has begun. RhIG administration will not suppress Rh immunization once it has begun, no matter how weak the immunization.[72]

STANDARD Rh PROPHYLAXIS RECOMMENDATIONS

Standard Rh prophylaxis recommendations are that one prophylactic dose of RhIG should be given to the Rh-negative unimmunized mother as soon as her baby has been determined to be Rh-positive, and in no event later than 72 hours after delivery. If the Rh status of the baby is not known within 72 hours, the mother should be given RhIG regardless of the fact that in one third of such instances the baby will be Rh-negative and she will not be at risk. It is obviously better to treat unnecessarily than to fail to treat a mother who is at risk. Rh-negative mothers of all Rh-positive babies should be protected irrespective of the ABO status of the mother and baby. ABO incompatibility of the baby with its mother is only partially protective. If there is inadvertent failure to administer RhIG within the 72-hour deadline, Rh prophylaxis should still be administered up to 28 days after delivery. There is experimental evidence that RhIG provides some protection up to 13 days after exposure to Rh-positive red cells.[73]

Rh PROPHYLAXIS PROBLEMS

In the past 21 years, standard postdelivery Rh prophylaxis programs have greatly reduced but have not entirely eliminated Rh immunization. Residual problems are outlined in Table 70-9.[74,75]

Failure of Compliance After Delivery

Occasional failures to provide protection to the Rh-negative woman after delivery of an Rh-positive infant arise. There are three reasons:

1. The mother may not have attended for prenatal care.

TABLE 70–8. WESTERN CANADIAN Rh IMMUNIZATION PREVENTION TRIAL (MARCH 1, 1967, TO JANUARY 31, 1968)

TREATMENT AND PARITY	NUMBER OF PATIENTS IN TRIAL*	PATIENTS Rh-IMMUNIZED 6–9 MONTHS LATER	
		NUMBER	%
RhIG, 145–435 μg, given within 72 hours postpartum			
Primiparas	481	0	0
Multiparas	735	0	0
TOTAL	1216	0	0
No treatment			
Primiparas	203	18	8.9
Multiparas	297	18	6.1
TOTAL	500	36	7.2

* Only Rh-negative women who had just produced ABO-compatible, Rh-positive babies were entered in the trial. (Adapted from Chown B, Duff AM, James J, et al. Prevention of primary Rh immunization: first report of the Western Canadian Trial. Can Med Assoc J 1969;100:1021.)

TABLE 70–9. RESIDUAL PROBLEMS IN Rh PROPHYLAXIS

1. Failure of compliance after delivery
2. Failure to give prophylaxis after abortion
3. Failure to give prophylaxis after amniocentesis
4. Failure of protection after massive fetal TPH
5. Failure to protect against Rh immunization during pregnancy
6. The question of augmentation of the risk of Rh immunization
7. The question of Rh immunization during infancy
8. The question of the D^u mother
9. The question of suppression of weak Rh immunization
10. Reactions to IM RhIG–ion exchange and RhIG–monoclonal RhIG

2. The physician may not have had prenatal blood samples tested.
3. The hospital obstetric unit may not have sent cord and maternal samples for testing.

Women should be educated to seek prenatal care early in pregnancy. Obstetricians and obstetrical units must know who their Rh-negative patients are and develop fail-safe methods of adequate screening during pregnancy and after delivery, so that every unimmunized Rh-negative woman delivering an Rh-positive baby can be given Rh prophylaxis.

Failure to Give Prophylaxis After Abortion

Therapeutic abortion carries with it a 4% to 5% risk of Rh immunization; spontaneous abortion carries a 2% risk. It is mandatory that the Rh-negative woman who aborts or is aborted be given Rh prophylaxis. Therapeutic abortion should not be carried out without knowledge of a woman's Rh status. Universal Rh prophylaxis after spontaneous abortion is more difficult, since the woman may not be admitted to hospital or hospitalization may be very brief. If minidoses of RhIG (50 μg) are available, they will provide protection for first-trimester spontaneous abortions. The woman who has antepartum bleeding (threatened abortion) should be given 300 μg of RhIG. If the pregnancy continues, this dose should be repeated every 12 weeks until delivery.

Failure to Give Prophylaxis After Amniocentesis

If the placenta is situated on the anterior uterine wall, there is a risk that it will be traversed by the amniocentesis needle. Although this risk has been very much reduced by prior ultrasonographic placental localization, it still occurs in about 2% of amniocenteses.[31] It follows, therefore, that the unimmunized Rh-negative woman undergoing genetic amniocentesis or later amniocentesis for determination of pulmonary maturity should be given RhIG. The dose should be 300 μg, repeated in 12 weeks if she remains undelivered. Although there are very few data on the exact risk of fetal TPH following chorionic villus sampling, there is a risk, since chorionic villi are being removed. For this reason, prophylaxis after chorionic villus sampling should be carried out in exactly the same manner as after amniocentesis. RhIG given to the pregnant woman, for any reason at any gestation, will not harm her Rh-positive conceptus.[27]

Failure of Protection After Massive Fetal TPH

Protection against Rh immunization is dose dependent. It has been shown experimentally that 300 μg of RhIG administered IM will prevent Rh immunization up to an exposure to 30 mL of Rh-positive blood (12 to 15 mL of red cells).[23] If the volume of blood is greater, protection is only partial. Rh immunization occurred in about 30% of Rh-negative male volunteers given up to 450 mL of blood with 300 μg of RhIG IM.[76] Since only about one woman in 400 will be exposed to greater than 30 mL of blood, Rh immunization due to failure to diagnose massive fetal TPH and therefore failure to give more than 300 μg of RhIG will occur very rarely (one in 1400 Rh-negative women carrying Rh-positive babies). Nevertheless, screening the Rh-negative woman for massive fetal TPH after delivery is recommended.

If massive TPH is diagnosed after delivery of an Rh-positive baby, 300 μg of RhIG should be given IM if the TPH is 25 mL or less, 600 μg (two vials) if the TPH is greater than 25 mL but less than 50 mL, 900 μg (three vials) if the TPH is greater than 50 mL but less than 75 mL, and so on. Up to 1200 μg (four vials) IM should be given every 12 hours until the total dose has been administered.

On the very rare occasion where massive TPH is diagnosed prior to delivery (nearly always in the third trimester), not only is there a risk of Rh immunization, but there is also a risk of fetal exsanguination if the TPH exceeds 100 mL. Moreover, there is a risk of fetal red cell hemolysis from the large amounts of RhIG required to be given before delivery. If the TPH does not exceed 50 mL of blood, the dose required (600 μg) will not cause significant fetal red cell hemolysis.

If the TPH exceeds 50 mL, the fetus should be delivered if gestation is ≥33 weeks and there is evidence of pulmonary maturity. If the baby is Rh-positive, the mother should be given an appropriate amount of RhIG. The baby should be examined immediately, and, if he or she is pale and shocky or has significant anemia, an immediate transfusion should be given.

If a fetal TPH greater than 50 mL is diagnosed early in pregnancy, at a time when there is no evidence of fetal lung maturity, a fetal blood-sampling procedure, to determine fetal pH and hemoglobin status, should be carried out. If significant anemia is present (less than 100 g/L) an intravascular transfusion of compatible, group O, Rh negative red cells, 50 mL/kg estimated fetal body weight, should be given. If the fetus is Rh-positive, 600 μg of RhIG should be given to the mother. The fetus should be followed carefully with ultrasound and with amniotic fluid measurements of lung maturity. If gestation and lung maturity are such that delivery is not feasible within 10 to 14 days of a blood-sampling procedure, a second fetal blood-sampling procedure should be carried out. As soon as delivery is feasible, management should be carried out as described in the previous paragraph.

RH IMMUNIZATION DURING PREGNANCY —ANTENATAL Rh PROPHYLAXIS

Rh immunization during pregnancy constitutes about 13% of all instances of Rh immunization if no prophylaxis is carried out. In the Manitoba experience, 1.8% (62) of 3533 mothers carrying Rh-positive fetuses, without evidence of Rh immunization at the beginning of their pregnancies, were Rh-immunized during pregnancy or within 3 days after delivery.[27] Similar findings have been reported from Hamilton, Ontario[77] and Sweden.[78] A somewhat lower incidence has been reported from Finland,[79] which overall has both a lower incidence of Rh-negativity and of Rh immunization. Rh immunization during pregnancy has also been reported in the United States.[80]

A clinical trial of antenatal Rh prophylaxis, whereby 300 μg of RhIG was given IM at 28 and again at 34 weeks gestation, was successful and reduced the incidence of Rh immunization from 1.8% to 0.1%.[27] As a result of this trial, antenatal Rh prophylaxis is now the rule in Manitoba and is the accepted practice elsewhere in North America. Antenatal prophylaxis consists of one injection of 300 μg of RhIG at as close to 28 weeks gestation as possible. The single dose at 28 weeks gestation has been highly successful.[81] Universal antenatal prophylaxis combined with universal postpartum, postabortion, and postamniocentesis prophylaxis will reduce the prevalence of Rh immunization from the preprophylaxis incidence of about 13% to 0.27% (ie, by about 97%).[82]

Administration of RhIG during pregnancy will not harm the fetus. When 300 μg are given at 28 weeks gestation and 34 weeks gestation, one third of babies will have red cells that are weakly direct antiglobulin positive. However, none will show any evidence of anemia or hyperbilirubinemia. Only very rare babies, after their mothers have received 300 μg just once, at 28 weeks gestation, will have direct antiglobulin-positive red cells.

THE QUESTION OF AUGMENTATION OF THE RISK OF Rh IMMUNIZATION

Whether the risk of Rh immunization increases when the level of circulating passive anti-D drops below a critical level has been debated. The observation of an increased incidence of Rh immunization when Rh-negative volunteers were given only 4.5 μg of RhIG for each milliliter of Rh-positive red cells injected[83] could not be confirmed.[84] However, there was strong evidence of augmentation of Rh immunization when Rh-negative volunteers were given only 1 μg of RhIG for each milliliter of Rh-positive red cells injected.[85] For this reason, it is strongly recommended that a further 300-μg dose of RhIG be given if a woman given RhIG antepartum, for any reason, has not delivered within 12 weeks after her first 300-μg injection. If she then delivers within 3 weeks after administration of a second (or a third) dose, postdelivery RhIG need not be given if she has no evidence of a fetal TPH greater than 0.1 mL of fetal red cells.

THE QUESTION OF Rh IMMUNIZATION DURING INFANCY (THE GRANDMOTHER THEORY)

It has been hypothesized that reverse maternal TPH of Rh-positive red cells into an Rh-negative fetus at the time of delivery will cause Rh immunization (60% of the mothers of Rh-negative babies are Rh-positive).[86] The true incidence of maternal reverse TPH is 2% and the volumes are usually minute, equivalent to 0.005 mL fetal TPH.[87] Reports of an extremely high prevalence of Rh immunization in infancy (11% to 22%)[88,89] have been refuted.[90] If these reports were true, antenatal prophylaxis would not be as successful as it is (residual Rh immunization 0.27%).[82] Rh immunization during infancy does occur;[91] however, it is exceedingly rare. Administration of RhIG to Rh-negative infants born of Rh-positive mothers is not indicated.

THE QUESTION OF THE D^u MOTHER

The great majority of "D^u" mothers are genetically Rh(D)-positive, the weakened expression of D being "environmental," because of the presence of C on the other chromosome [ie, C(d)ecDe]. They are not at risk of Rh immunization and do not require RhIG. The less common D variant (genetic D^u) mother is missing part of the D antigen and is at risk of Rh immunization, but very much less so than the true Rh(D)-negative woman. If the genetic D^u mother can be differentiated from the "environmental" D^u mother, we recommend that she be given postpartum RhIG, although the risk of Rh immunization is very small. There is one well-documented instance of a D^u mother developing Rh immunization so severe that her fetus became hydropic.[9]

THE QUESTION OF SUPPRESSION OF WEAK Rh IMMUNIZATION

Not infrequently, an Rh-negative woman will be determined to have a very weak Rh antibody. If the antibody can be detected only by an AutoAnalyzer (AA) technique and not by any manual method, she should be given Rh prophylaxis, since in about 85% of cases she is not Rh-immunized (the AA technique is so sensitive that frequently it is nonspecific). Conversely, if the Rh antibody is demonstrable, even if only very weakly, by the most sensitive manual technique (enzyme), she is truly Rh-immunized, and RhIG administration will not prevent progression of her Rh immunization. Attempts to suppress such weak Rh immunization by administration of 300 μg of RhIG every 6 weeks were completely unsuccessful.[72] Two thirds of women so treated and two thirds of untreated control women had progression of their Rh immunization and delivered babies with hemolytic disease.[72] Nevertheless, if there is any question about the specificity of such an antibody, it should be given, because RhIG will do no harm.

REACTIONS TO IM RhIG—NEWER FORMS OF RhIG

Ion Exchange RhIG

RhIG is predominantly prepared by the Cohn cold ethanol precipitation process. Cohn-prepared RhIG is effective and has a low incidence of adverse reactions. However, it does contain small amounts of IgA, IgM, and other plasma proteins. Because it is anticomplementary, it may be given IM only. The efficiency of yield of anti-D from the starting plasma is quite low (35% to 45%). On one occasion, a severe anaphylactic reaction occurred after its use.[92]

Following Hoppe's preparation of RhIG by ion exchange chromatography,[93] his method was adapted for use in North America. An ion exchange–prepared RhIG has been licensed for use in Canada since 1980.[94] RhIG processed by this method is very pure, with a low total protein content, no demonstrable IgM, and an IgA content only 0.3% of that found in Cohn-prepared RhIG. It has very low anticomplementarity and can be given safely IV. The efficiency of yield from starting plasma is 85% to 90%.

When it is given IV it is twice as effective, and therefore it may be given in half the dose after delivery (120 μg). However, since its half-life, when given IV, is no greater than the half-life of Cohn RhIG given IM, the antenatal prophylaxis dose must be the same (300 μg).

Clinical trials and service programs in which hundreds of thousands of doses of ion exchange RhIG have been given (either IV or IM) have shown that it is at least as successful in preventing Rh immunization as Cohn-prepared RhIG. The observed prevalence of Rh immunization in 9295 Rh-negative women carrying Rh-positive babies, given ion exchange–prepared RhIG both antepartum and postpartum was reduced from the expected 601 to 25, a reduction of 95.9%.[82] If the eight are excluded who had evidence of primary Rh immunization before antenatal Rh prophylaxis was given, the protection rate was 97.1%.[82]

The advantages of ion exchange–prepared RhIG are the following: greater purity, less likelihood of an adverse reaction, greater efficiency of yield (and, therefore, lower cost), lower dose, and less discomfort when given IV.

Monoclonal RhIG

At present, RhIG is manufactured from the plasma of hyperimmunized Rh-negative donors, either from the plasma of sterile women initially immunized by pregnancy or from the plasma of Rh-negative immunized male volunteers. The former, the best source of Rh-immune plasma, are decreasing in number, because of the success of Rh prophylaxis. Deliberate Rh immunization of male volunteers has been questioned on moral and ethical grounds, since the majority exposed to Rh-positive red cells will not produce acceptable Rh antibody levels.

Within the next few years, RhIG will be produced in tissue culture. Monoclonal anti-D has been produced by Epstein-Barr virus transformation of lymphoblastoid cell lines taken from Rh-immunized donors[95,96] and by fusion of similar transformed cell lines with mouse–human heteromyelomas (hybridomas).[97,98] Once sufficient stable monoclonal anti-D's are produced, tissue culture RhIG will become a reality and will replace plasma-prepared RhIG.

CURRENT RECOMMENDATIONS FOR Rh PROPHYLAXIS

The following are the current recommendations for Rh prophylaxis:

1. Every Rh-negative unimmunized woman who delivers an Rh-positive baby must be given one prophylactic dose of RhIG as soon as possible after delivery.
2. Every Rh-negative unimmunized woman, unless her husband is known to be Rh-negative, who aborts or threatens to abort must be given RhIG.
3. Every Rh-negative unimmunized woman who undergoes amniocentesis or chorionic villus sampling, unless her husband is known to be Rh-negative, must be given 300 μg of RhIG at the time of the procedure, with subsequent doses at 12-week intervals until delivery.
4. Every Rh-negative unimmunized woman whose husband is either Rh-positive or Rh-unknown should be given 300 μg of RhIG at 28 weeks gestation. A second dose should be given in 12.5 weeks if delivery has not taken place and need not be repeated postpartum if delivery occurs within 3 weeks.
5. If massive TPH is diagnosed, 300 μg of RhIG should be given IM for every 25 mL of blood or fraction thereof in the maternal circulation; the dose may be halved if RhIG is given IV.
6. One prophylactic dose of RhIG should be given antepartum to the mother who has an AA-only detectable Rh antibody and again after delivery if she delivers an Rh-positive baby. If the antibody is detectable by a manual enzyme method, administration of RhIG will not prevent progression of her

immunization. However, it should be given if there is any question about the specificity of the enzyme reactions.

NON-Rh(D) BLOOD GROUP IMMUNIZATION

ABO HEMOLYTIC DISEASE

Although ABO-incompatible hemolytic transfusion reactions are intravascular and much more serious than extravascular Rh-incompatible hemolytic transfusion reactions, ABO hemolytic disease is much milder than Rh hemolytic disease. Kernicterus due to hyperbilirubinemia in ABO hemolytic disease may occur, but the author has never seen hydrops caused by ABO hemolytic disease. The rare reports of hydrops due to ABO hemolytic disease do not bear close scrutiny and are more likely due to nonimmune hydrops associated with ABO incompatibility—for example, (1) fetal death and hydrops fetalis in an ABO-incompatible fetus whose red cells were direct antiglobulin negative[99]; or (2) neonatal death due to hydrops fetalis in an ABO-incompatible newborn with direct antiglobulin-positive red cells but whose cord blood hematocrit was 43%, equivalent to a hemoglobin level of 145 g/L, a normal hemoglobin level unlikely to be associated with alloimmune hydrops fetalis.[100]

ABO hemolytic disease is mild because A and B antigens are not well developed on the fetal red cell membrane, most anti-A and anti-B is IgM and does not cross the placenta, and most of the small amounts of IgG anti-A and anti-B that do cross the placenta become attached to the numerous other tissue and fluid A or B antigens. Only a small amount of the small amount of A or B antibody that does traverse the placenta binds to red cell antigenic sites. This explains why the cord blood direct antiglobulin test is only weakly positive and may be negative unless a sensitive test is used. Even with the most sensitive test, red cells taken from a 1- or 2-day-old baby with ABO hemolytic disease may be direct antiglobulin negative.

Serologically, ABO hemolytic disease is by far the most common hemolytic disease. In the period 1954 to 1965, out of 45,000 deliveries at the Winnipeg General Hospital, 9000 ABO-incompatible babies were born. Of the 9000, 2500 had weakly direct antiglobulin-positive cord blood red cells and therefore had serologic ABO erythroblastosis. Of those 2500, only 41 (<2%) required exchange transfusion.[101] Management of ABO erythroblastosis is entirely pediatric. Amniocentesis and other fetal investigative measures are not required in the ABO-incompatible pregnancy.

HEMOLYTIC DISEASE CAUSED BY ATYPICAL BLOOD GROUP ANTIBODIES

With the reduction in incidence of Rh(D) immunization, the increased prevalence of blood transfusion, and the greater screening of Rh-positive pregnant women, hemolytic disease due to other blood group antibodies is becoming relatively and absolutely more common. In the 26-year period from November 1, 1962, to October 31, 1988, the numbers of Rh(D)-immunized pregnant women and the numbers of Rh(D)-positive fetuses with hemolytic disease in Manitoba annually dropped from a mean of 194 and 149 in the first 5 years to a mean of 28 and 12.5 in the final 6 years. Conversely, the mean numbers of pregnant women with atypical blood group antibodies and fetuses affected by their antibodies rose from a mean of 14 and 10 annually in the first 5 years to a mean of 88 and 17 in the final 6 years. Therefore, at the present time pregnant women with atypical blood group antibodies outnumber pregnant women with Rh(D) antibodies by three to one, and fetuses with hemolytic disease due to atypical antibodies outnumber their Rh-affected counterparts by four to three.

Many atypical blood group antibodies are without consequence. Others are potentially as hazardous as anti-D. A survey of non-Manitoba patients referred for consultation and or management with IPT or PUBS and IVT over the 25-year period January 1, 1964, to December 31, 1988, revealed that in the first 15 years, 140 Rh-immunized women were referred and only three with atypical blood group antibodies were referred. Conversely, in the last 10-year period, 83 Rh-immunized women were referred and 19 with atypical antibodies were referred. The atypical blood group antibodies in the referred women, which produced very severe disease (hydrops) in either a prior or the current pregnancy, were anti-Kell 9, anti-c or anti-cE 8, and one each of the following: anti-Fy^a, anti-Jk^a, anti-CC^w, anti-k, and anti-E.

The 26-year Manitoba experience with atypical blood group antibodies and the referred experience indicate that anti-c and anti-Kell are potentially as lethal as anti-D. However, whereas the woman with anti-c (183 examples in 26 years) has a 65% likelihood of having an affected baby and a 9% likelihood that the affected baby will become hydropic or will require IUT to prevent hydrops, the woman with anti-Kell (337 examples in 26 years) has only a 4.5% likelihood of having an affected fetus. Although anti-Kell has been benign in Manitoba fetuses (only 8 of 337 fetuses affected, only two requiring exchange transfusion after birth, none at risk of hydrops), this has certainly not been the case with referred anti-Kell patients, four of whom had severely hydropic fetuses at 21 to 23 weeks gestation. Anti-E is usually very benign. Of the 350 examples of anti-E in the past 26 years, only 31% (108) of fetuses were affected, and of these only 12 required exchange transfusion at birth. Although no Manitoba patients were severely affected, one of our referred patients had anti-E and lost her fetus at IPT.

From the preceding experience and isolated case reports, Table 70-10 lists four categories of atypical blood group antibodies and their potential for hemolytic disease. Pregnant women with atypical antibodies listed in the common and uncommon group should be managed in exactly the same manner as if they were Rh-negative

TABLE 70–10. ASSOCIATION OF HEMOLYTIC DISEASE WITH ATYPICAL MATERNAL BLOOD GROUP ANTIBODIES

Common
c(cE): incidence high, disease common, may be severe
Kell: incidence high, disease uncommon but if present may be severe
E: incidence high, disease common, usually mild, rarely may be severe
C(Ce, C^w): incidence moderate, disease common, usually mild, rarely may be severe
Uncommon
k: rarely present but when present may be very severe
$Kp^a(Kp^b)$: rare, disease may require treatment, very rarely severe
Jk^a: uncommon, may require treatment, rarely may be severe
Fy^a: uncommon, usually mild, may require treatment, rarely severe
S: uncommon, usually mild, may require treatment, rarely severe
Rarely, if Ever, Cause Hemolytic Disease
s, U, M, Fy^b, N, Do^a, Di^a, Di^b, Lu^a, Yt^a, Jk^b
Never Cause Hemolytic Disease
Le^a, Le^b, P

and Rh(D) immunized. Although some of these antibodies are common and only occasionally (or rarely) cause dangerous hemolytic disease (eg, anti-Kell and anti-E) and others are very rare but if present may cause severe disease (ie, anti-k), the potential for severe disease resides in them all. Antibodies that never cause hemolytic disease may be disregarded, as for the most part may those that rarely, if ever, cause hemolytic disease. However, if in the latter group, the antibody appears very potent and of high titer, amniocentesis and/or fetal blood sampling is indicated. For example, although none of 82 Manitoba pregnant women with anti-M produced affected babies, there are at least two reports of severe anti-M erythroblastosis.[102,103]

A recent report has questioned the value of amniotic fluid ΔOD 450 readings in assessing severity of anti-Kell hemolytic disease.[104] This is not the Manitoba experience, although it should be noted that occasionally in patients referred to us, the disease has been so fulminant that a very high zone 2 or zone 3 fluid was not present until hydrops was present. As with Rh hemolytic disease, interpretation of atypical hemolytic disease is based on history, titer, amniotic fluid measurements, and ultrasound assessment. If these parameters indicate severe disease, fetal blood sampling, if possible, and IUT (IVT if possible) should be carried out.

REFERENCES

1. Diamond LK, Blackfan KD, Baty JM. Erythroblastosis fetalis and its association with universal edema of the fetus, icterus gravis neonatorum and anemia of the newborn. J Pediatr 1932;1:269.
2. Levine P, Katzin EM, Burnham L. Isoimmunization in pregnancy: its possible bearing on the etiology of erythroblastosis fetalis. JAMA 1941;116:825.
3. Landsteiner K, Wiener AS. An agglutinable factor in human blood recognized by immune sera for rhesus blood. Proc Soc Exp Biol Med 1940;43:223.
4. Wiener AS, Wexler IB. Heredity of the blood groups. New York: Grune & Stratton, 1958.
5. Rosenfield RE, Allan FH Jr, Swisher SN, Kochwa S. A review of Rh serology and presentation of a new terminology. Transfusion 1962;2:287.
6. Race RR. The Rh genotype and Fisher's theory. Blood (Special Issue No. 2) 1948;3:27.
7. Issitt PD. The Rh blood group system, 1988: eight new antigens in nine years and some observations on the biochemistry and genetics of the system. Transfus Med Rev 1989;3:1.
8. Tippett P, Sanger R. Observations on subdivisions of the Rh antigen D Vox Sang 1962;7:9.
9. Lacey PA, Caskey CR, Werner DJ, Moulds JJ. Fatal hemolytic disease of the newborn due to anti-D in an RH positive D^u variant mother. Transfusion 1983;23:91.
10. Goto S, Nishi H, Tomoda A. Blood group Rh-D factor in human trophoblast determined by immunofluorescent method. Am J Obstet Gynecol 1980;137:707.
11. Wiener AS. Diagnosis and treatment of anemia of the newborn caused by occult placental hemorrhage. Am J Obstet Gynecol 1948;56:707.
12. Chown B. Anemia from bleeding of the fetus into the mother's circulation. Lancet 1954;1:1213.
13. Kleihauer E, Braun H, Betke K. Demonstration von fetalem haemoglobin in den erythrozyten eines blutausstriches. Klin Wochenschr 1957;35:637.
14. Bowman JM, Pollock JM, Penston LE. Fetomaternal transplacental hemorrhage during pregnancy and after delivery. Vox Sang 1986;51:117.
15. Wiener AS. Conglutination test for Rh sensitization. J Lab Clin Med 1945;30:662.
16. Lewis M, Chown B. A short albumin method for the determination of isohemagglutinins, particularly incomplete Rh antibodies. J Lab Clin Med 1957;50:494.
17. Coombs RRA, Mourant AE, Race RR. A new test for the detection of weak and "incomplete" Rh agglutinins. Br J Exp Pathol 1945;26:255.
18. Lewis M, Kaita H, Chown B. Kell typing in the capillary tube. J Lab Clin Med 1958;52:163.
19. Rosenfield RE, Haber GV. Detection and measurement of homologous human hemagglutinins. Automation in Analytical Chemistry-Technicon Symposia, 1965:503.
20. Lalezari P. A Polybrene method for the detection of red cell antibodies. Fed Proc 1967;26:756.
21. Moore BPL. Automation in the blood transfusion laboratory. I. Antibody detection and quantitation in the Technicon AutoAnalyzer. Can Med Assoc J 1969;100:381.
22. Zipursky A, Israels LG. The pathogenesis and prevention of Rh immunization. Can Med Assoc J 1967;97:1245.
23. Pollack W, Ascari WQ, Kochesky RJ, O'Connor RB, Ho TY, Tripodi D. Studies on Rh prophylaxis. I. Relationship between doses of anti-Rh and size of antigenic stimulus. Transfusion 1971;11:333.
24. Woodrow JC. Rh immunization and its prevention. Series Hematologia. Vol III. Copenhagen: Munksgaard, 1970.
25. Nevanlinna HR. Factors affecting maternal Rh immunization. Ann Med Exp Biol (Fenn Suppl 2) 1953;31:1.
26. Bowman JM. Fetomaternal ABO incompatibility and erythroblastosis fetalis. Vox Sang 1986;50:104.
27. Bowman JM, Chown B, Lewis M, Pollock JM. Rh-immunization during pregnancy: antenatal prophylaxis. Can Med Assoc J 1978;118:623.
28. Phibbs RH, Johnson P, Tooley WH. Cardio-respiratory status of erythroblastotic infants. II. Blood volume, hematocrit and serum albumin concentration in relation to hydrops fetalis. Pediatrics 1974;53:13.
29. James LS. Shock in the newborn in relation to hydrops. In: Rob-

ertson JG, Dambrosio F, eds. International Symposium on the Management of the Rh Problem. Annali Obstet Ginec 1970; Special Number 193.

30. Barss VA, Frigoletto FD, Konugres A. The cost of irregular antibody screening. Am J Obstet Gynecol 1988;159:428.
31. Bowman JM, Pollock JM. Transplacental fetal hemorrhage after amniocentesis. Obstet Gynecol 1985;66:749.
32. Bowman JM, Pollock JM. Amniotic fluid spectrophotometry and early delivery in the management of erythroblastosis fetalis. Pediatrics 1965;35:815.
33. Liley AW. Liquor amnii analysis in management of pregnancy complicated by rhesus immunization. Am J Obstet Gynecol 1961;82:1359.
34. Nicolaides KH, Rodeck CH, Mibashan MD, Kemp JR. Have Liley charts outlived their usefulness? Am J Obstet Gynecol 1986;155:90.
35. Bartsch FK. Bilirubin in the amniotic fluid: a review. In: Robertson JG, Dambrosio F. eds. International Symposium on the Management of the Rh Problem. Annali Obstet Ginec Milano 1970; Special Number 73.
36. Peddle LJ. Increase of antibody titer following amniocentesis. Am J Obstet Gynecol 1968;100:567.
37. Rehder H, Weitzel H. Intrauterine amputation after amniocentesis. Lancet 1978;1:832.
38. Daffos F, Capella-Pavlovsky M, Forestier F. Fetal blood sampling during pregnancy with use of a needle guided by ultrasound: a study of 606 consecutive cases. Am J Obstet Gynecol 1985;153:655.
39. Bang J, Bock JE, Trolle D. Ultra-sound guided fetal intravenous transfusion for severe rhesus haemolytic disease. Br Med J 1982;284:373.
40. De Crespigny LC, Robinson HP, Quinn M, Doyle L, Ross A, Cauchi M. Ultrasound-guided fetal blood transfusion for severe rhesus isoimmunization. Obstet Gynecol 1985;66:529.
41. Liley AW. Intrauterine transfusion of fetus in hemolytic disease. Br Med J 1963;2:1107.
42. Rodeck CH, Holman CA, Karnicki J, Kemp JR, Whitmore DN, Austin MA. Direct intravascular fetal blood transfusion by fetoscopy in severe rhesus isoimmunization. Lancet 1981;1:652.
43. Menticoglou SM, Harman CR, Manning FA, Bowman JM. Intraperitoneal fetal transfusion: paralysis inhibits red cell absorption. Fetal Therapy 1987;2:154.
44. Lewis M, Bowman JM, Pollock JM, Lowen B. Absorption of red cells from the peritoneal cavity of an hydropic twin. Transfusion 1973;13:37.
45. Crosby WM, Brobmann GF, Chang ACK. Intrauterine transfusion and fetal death: relationship of intraperitoneal pressure to umbilical vein flow. Am J Obstet Gynecol 1970;108:135.
46. Adamsons K Jr, Freda VJ, James LS, Towell ME. Prenatal treatment of erythroblastosis fetalis following hysterotomy. Pediatrics 1965;35:848.
47. Asensio SH, Figueroa-Longo JG, Pelegrina A. Intrauterine exchange transfusion. Am J Obstet Gynecol 1966;95:1129.
48. Seelen J, Van Kessel H, Eskes T, et al. A new method of exchange transfusion in utero: cannulation of vessels on the fetal side of the human placenta. Am J Obstet Gynecol 1966;95:872.
49. Rodeck CH, Nicolaides KH, Warsof SL, Fysh WS, Gamsu HR, Kemp JR. The management of severe rhesus isoimmunization by fetoscopic intravascular transfusion. Am J Obstet Gynecol 1984;150:769.
50. Bowman JM. Management of Rh-isoimmunization. Obstet Gynecol 1978;52:1.
51. Grannum PAT, Copel JA, Moya FR, et al. The reversal of hydrops fetalis by intravascular intrauterine transfusion in severe isoimmune fetal anemia. Am J Obstet Gynecol 1988;158:914.
52. Berkowitz RL. Chitkara U, Goldberg JD, Wilkins I, Chervenak FA. Intrauterine intravascular transfusions for severe red blood cell isoimmunization: ultrasound-guided percutaneous approach. Am J Obstet Gynecol 1986;155:574.
53. Nicolaides KH, Soothill PW, Clewell W, Rodeck CH, Campbell S. Rh Disease: intravascular fetal blood transfusion by cordocentesis. Fetal Therapy 1986;1:185.
54. Seeds JW, Bowes WA. Ultrasound-guided intravascular transfusion in severe rhesus immunization. Am J Obstet Gynecol 1986;154:1105.
55. Harman CR, Bowman JM, Menticoglous SM, Pollock JM, Manning FA. Profound fetal thrombocytopenia in Rhesus disease: serious hazard at intravascular transfusion. Lancet 1988;2:741.
56. Frigoletto FD, Umansky I, Birnholz J, et al. Intrauterine fetal transfusion in 365 fetuses during fifteen years. Am J Obstet Gynecol 1981;139:781.
57. Hamilton EG. Intrauterine transfusion. Safeguard or peril? Obstet Gynecol 1977;50:255.
58. Watts DH, Luthy DA, Benedetti TJ, Cyr DR, Easterling TR, Hickok D. Intraperitoneal fetal transfusion under direct ultrasound guidance. Obstet Gynecol 1988;71:84.
59. MacKenzie IZ, Bowell PJ, Ferguson J, Castle BM, Entwistle CC. In-utero intravascular transfusion of the fetus for the management of severe Rhesus isoimmunization—a reappraisal. Br J Obstet Gynaecol 1987;94:1068.
60. Barnes PH, McInnis AC, Friesen RF, Bowman JM. Maternal mishap following fetal transfusion. Can Med Assoc J 1965; 92:1277.
61. Parkman R, Mosier D, Umansky I, Cochran W, Carpenter CB, Rosen FS. Graft versus host disease after intrauterine and exchange transfusions for hemolytic disease of the newborn. N Engl J Med 1974;290:359.
62. Carter BB. Preliminary report on a substance which inhibits anti-Rh serum. Am J Clin Pathol 1947;17:646.
63. Gusdon JP Jr, Caudle MR, Herbst GA, Iannuzzi NP. Phagocytosis and erythroblastosis. I. Modification of the neonatal response by promethazine hydrochloride. Am J Obstet Gynecol 1976;125:224.
64. Bierme SJ, Blanc M, Arbal M, Fournie A. Oral Rh treatment for severely immunised mothers (letter). Lancet 1979;1:604.
65. Stenchever MA. Promethazine hydrochloride: use in patients with RH isoimmunization. Am J Obstet Gynecol 1978;130:665.
66. Gold WR Jr, Queenan JT, Woody J, Sacher RA. Oral desensitization in Rh disease. Am J Obstet Gynecol 1983;146:980.
67. Berlin G, Selbing A, Ryden G. Rhesus haemolytic disease treated with high-dose intravenous immunoglobulin (letter). Lancet 1985;i:1153.
68. Von Dungern F. Beitrage zur immunitatslehr. Munch Med Wochenschr 1900;47:677.
69. Freda VJ, Gorman JG, Pollack W. Successful prevention of experimental Rh sensitization in man with an anti-Rh gamma-2-globulin antibody preparation: a preliminary report. Transfusion 1964;4:26.
70. Clarke CA, Donohoe WTA, McConnell RB, et al. Further experimental studies in the prevention of Rh-haemolytic disease. Br Med J 1963;1:979.
71. Chown B, Duff AM, James J, et al. Prevention of primary Rh immunization: first report of the Western Canadian Trial. Can Med Assoc J 1969:100:1021.
72. Bowman JM, Pollock JM. Reversal of Rh alloimmunization. Fact or fancy? Vox Sang 1984;47:209.
73. Samson D, Mollison PL. Effect on primary Rh-immunization of delayed administration of anti-Rh. Immunology 1975;28:349.
74. Bowman JM. Controversies in Rh prophylaxis: who needs Rh immune globulin and when should it be given? Am J Obstet Gynecol 1985;151:289.
75. Bowman JM. The prevention of Rh immunization. Transfus Med Rev 1988;2:129.
76. Pollack W, Ascari WQ, Crispin JF, O'Connor RR, Ho TY. Stud-

ies on Rh prophylaxis. II. Rh immune prophylaxis after transfusions with Rh-positive blood. Transfusion 1971;11:340.

77. Zipursky A, Blajchman M. The Hamilton Rh prevention studies. Presented at McMaster Conference on Prevention of Rh Immunization, 28–30 September, 1977, Vox Sang 1979;36:50.
78. Bartsch F, Sandberg L. Incidence of anti-D at delivery in previously non-immunized Rh-negative mothers with Rh-positive babies. Presented at McMaster Conference on Prevention of Rh Immunization, 28–30 September, 1977. Vox Sang 1979;36:50.
79. Eklund J, Nevanlinna HR. Rh antibody appearance during pregnancy in Finland. Presented at McMaster Conference on Prevention of Rh Immunization, 28–30 September, 1977. Vox Sang 1979;36:50.
80. Scott JR, Beer AE, Guy LR, Liesch M, ELbert G. Pathogenesis of Rh immunization in primigravidas. Fetomaternal versus maternofetal bleeding. Obstet Gynecol 1977;49:9.
81. Bowman JM, Pollock JM. Antenatal Rh prophylaxis: 28 week gestation service program. Can Med Assoc J 1978;118:627.
82. Bowman JM, Pollock JM. Failures of intravenous Rh immune globulin prophylaxis: an analysis of the reasons for such failures. Transfus Med Rev 1987;1:101.
83. Pollack W, Gorman JG, Hager HJ, Freda VJ, Tripodi D. Antibody-mediated immune suppression to the Rh factor: animal models suggesting mechanism of action. Transfusion 1968; 8:134.
84. Contreras M. Mollison PL. Failure to augment primary Rh immunization using a small dose of "passive" IgG anti-Rh. Br J Haematol 1981:49:371.
85. Mollison PL. Can primary Rh immunization be augmented by passively administered antibody? In: Frigoletto FD Jr, Jewett JF, Konugres AA, eds. Rh hemolytic disease—new strategy for eradication. Boston: Hall, 1982:161.
86. Taylor JF. Sensitization of Rh-negative daughters by their Rh-positive mothers. N Engl J Med 1967;276:547.
87. Cohen F, Zuelzer WW. The transplacental passage of maternal erythrocytes into the fetus. Am J Obstet Gynecol 1965;93:566.
88. Bowen FW, Renfield M. The detection of anti D in Rh (D)-negative infants born of Rh (D)-positive mothers. Pediatr Res 1976;10:213.
89. Carapella-de Luca E, Casadei AM, Pascone R, Tardi C, Pacioni C. Maternofetal transfusion during delivery and sensitization of the newborn against Rhesus D-antigen. Vox Sang 1978;34:241.
90. Bernard B, Presley M, Caudillo G, Clauss B, Roualt CL, McGregor J. Maternal fetal hemorrhage: incidence and sensitization (abstract). Pediatr Res 1977;11:467.
91. Biggins KR, Bowman JM. Rh(D) alloimmunization in the absence of exposure to Rh(D) antigen. Vox Sang 1986;51:228.
92. Rivat L. Rivat C, Parent M, Ropartz C. Accident survenu après injection de gamma-globulines anti-Rh dû à la présence d'anticorps anti-λ A. Presse Med 1970;78:2072.
93. Hoppe HH, Mester T, Hennig W, Krebs HJ. Prevention of Rh-immunization: modified production of IgG anti Rh for intravenous application by ion exchange chromatography(IEC). Vox Sang 1973;25:308.
94. Bowman JM, Friesen AD, Pollock JM, Taylor WE. WinRho: Rh immune globulin prepared by ion exchange for intravenous use. Can Med Assoc J 1980;123:1121.
95. Crawford DH, Barlow MJ, Harrison JF, Winger L, Huehns ER. Production of human monoclonal antibody to Rhesus D antigen. Lancet 1983;1:386.
96. Crawford DH, McDougall DCJ, Mulholland N, Zanders ED, Tippett P, Huehns ER. Further characterisation of a human monoclonal antibody to the Rhesus D antigen produced in vitro. Behring Inst Mitt 1984;74:55.
97. Bron D, Feinberg MB, Teng NNH, Kaplan HS. Production of human monoclonal IgG antibodies against Rhesus (D) antigen. Proc Natl Acad Sci USA 1984;81:3214.
98. MacDonald G, Primrose S, Biggins K, et al. Production and characterization of human-human and human-mouse hybridomas secreting Rh(D)-specific monoclonal antibodies. Scand J Immunol 1987;25:477.
99. Miller DF, Petrie SJ. Fatal erythroblastosis fetalis secondary to ABO incompatibility—report of a case. Obstet Gynecol 1963;22:773.
100. Gilja BK, Shah VP. Hydrops fetalis due to ABO incompatibility. Clin Pediatr 1988;27:210.
101. Bowman JM. In: Queenan JT, ed. Neonatal management in modern management of the Rh problem. 2nd ed. New York: Harper & Row, 1977;209.
102. MacPherson CR, Christiansen MJ, Newton WA, Wheeler WE, Zartman ER. Anti-M antibody as a cause of intrauterine death. Am J Clin Pathol 1961;35:31.
103. Yoshida H, Yoshida Y. Tatsumi K, Asoh T. A new therapeutic antibody removal method using antigen positive red cells: application to M-incompatible pregnant women. Vox Sang 1982;43:35.
104. Caine ME, Mueller-Heubach E. Kell sensitization in pregnancy. Am J Obstet Gynecol 1986;154:85.

71

CHAPTER

MATERNAL INFECTIONS DURING PREGNANCY

William Ledger

The altered immune state of pregnancy increases the risk of infection for the adult host. This is a paradox. The blunting of the immunologic response in a pregnancy is beneficial, because it permits the maintenance of a foreign protein graft—the placenta and the fetus. Without this, humanity could not perpetuate itself. At the same time, it can be detrimental to the pregnant woman when she is exposed to such foreign antigens as viruses and bacteria. Both the frequency and severity of infection can be increased.

There are conflicting laboratory data about a reduced immunologic response during pregnancy. For purposes of discussion, any evaluation of immunity is divided into two categories: humoral and cellular. Most of the studies of humoral immune response in pregnancy show reactions similar to those found in non-pregnant women.[1] This equivalence has been confirmed in several studies that evaluated different schedules of immunization in pregnant women; all showed acceptable antibody responses.[1] In contrast, the cellular immune response has generally been diminished. There are a number of changes seen in the neutrophils of pregnant women that resemble those seen in neutrophils of non-pregnant women with infections. These include neutrophilia, increased levels of alkaline phosphatase, reduced myeloperoxiadase levels, and increased granular staining.[1] Despite these observations, there have been discordant reports on neutrophil function in pregnancy. One study demonstrated enhanced neutrophil activity in pregnancy.[2] In contrast, other studies showed impaired neutrophil function, although one observer has suggested this response could be due to subclinical infection during pregnancy.[1] Although the mechanism remains in question, pregnancy generally has been associated with a depressed cell-mediated immunity.

The most important test of the hypothesis of diminished cell-mediated immunity in pregnancy is clinical observation. If infection in pregnant women is more frequent or severe, this should settle the issue. There have been many studies with a multitude of varied pathogens that document a diminished host response in pregnant women. For example, Finland's detailed study, published in 1939, of a large number of Boston women who had pneumococcal pneumonia documented a death rate higher than in non-pregnant women with the same disease, particularly when the disease was contracted in the third trimester.[5] The increased severity of infection in pregnant women is not limited to bacterial infections. Viruses are also a problem. In the influenza pandemic of 1957, death was much more common among pregnant women.[6] Fortunately, these unfavorable responses in pregnant women have been modified by medical advances. The introduction of safe, effective systemic antibiotics has diminished the risk of pneumococcal pneumonia, as well as the risk of the superimposed staphylococcal pneumonias seen in influenza pandemics. Influenza vaccines also help. Fortunately, in the United States death from these illnesses is so infrequent that it is no longer an important measure of the pregnant woman's altered cellular immune response to bacteria and viruses. Protozoal disease and systemic fungal disease can also be serious. For example, pregnant women have an increase in both the incidence and complications of malaria, and in endemic regions, coccidioidomycosis is a leading cause of maternal death.[8] All of these different disease entities, caused by bacteria, viruses, protozoa, and fungi, share two similar traits—they are normally held in check by cell-mediated immune mechanisms, and all are more serious in pregnancy.

Poverty is an important factor in maternal infection during pregnancy. Poor women have more frequent and severe infections than middle class or upper class women, for many reasons. The first, which should be obvious to any concerned physician, is that poor women in America do not have the same access to antepartum medical care as women of higher economic levels. Less than adequate sanitary conditions in lower class neighborhoods; the lack of support groups for women, especially affordable day care facilities, which prevents many women from getting jobs and escaping the cycle of poverty and illness; and the tremendous inroads of illicit drug use all play a role. In addition, there is good experimental evidence that malnutrition can diminish the immune response.[9] Clinically, in the underdeveloped countries of the tropics, malnutrition in pregnancy is the major factor in the higher death rate with hepatitis A.[10] In contrast, increased mortality rates with hepatitis A have not been reported in the United States, presumably because nutritional deprivation is seen less frequently. Although this is encouraging, the morbidity associated with all infections is greater in the pregnant poor than in women of higher economic levels in the United States.

The rest of this chapter will address problems of maternal infection during pregnancy with an emphasis on organ systems.

URINARY TRACT INFECTIONS

Increased stasis of urine during pregnancy makes the urinary tract the most common site of infection. This altered state is caused by the convergence of a number of normal pregnancy changes. The capacity of the urinary tract is usually increased. Although there are few radiologic observations of the urinary tract in normal pregnant women, the available data indicate that dilation is mild in the first half of pregnancy, although this dilation is not a uniform phenomenon. After mid-pregnancy, the right side is dilated in three quarters of cases, and the left side is dilated in a third.[11] In addition, there is expansion of the renal pelves and calyces; there is also an increase in bladder capacity. At the same time, the collecting capacity is increased, and more urine is delivered to this dilated urinary excretion system in pregnancy as renal blood flow and glomerular filtration rate increase. Increased progesterone production effects urinary tract function. Ureteral peristalsis slows, and transit time from kidneys to bladder is prolonged. The impact on the bladder is hypotonia with an increase in the residual volume of urine. All of these changes increase the risk of urinary tract infection. Urine is an excellent growth medium for bacteria, and the stagnant urine provides an environment that encourages overgrowth of bacteria and subsequent clinical infection. The bacterial nidus for infection is present in the 2% to 10% of pregnant women with asymptomatic bacteriuria.[12] It is small wonder that urinary tract infections are seen so frequently in pregnant women.

Prevention is the appropriate starting place for any discussion of therapy of urinary tract infections in pregnancy. Prevention will eliminate the morbidity of symptomatic infections. This can be achieved in some instances.

PREVENTION OF PYELONEPHRITIS

It is estimated that 25% to 30% of women with asymptomatic bacteriuria at the time of their first antepartum visit will develop pyelonephritis later in pregnancy.[13] This is the group that is the focus for programs of detection and therapeutic intervention. Probably 80% of all cases of pyelonephritis in pregnancy could be eliminated if this population was identified and treated.[14] To support this contention, Harris documented the experience of the Wilford Hall United States Air Force Medical Center over a 20-year period. In that hospital, a conscious effort was made to identify and then treat pregnant women with asymptomatic bacteriuria. With this program in place, the annual incidence of acute antepartum pyelonephritis fell from 4% to 0.8%, a fivefold decrease.[15]

These results support the idea of a standardized approach for pregnant women seen for the first time by the obstetrician. All should have a culture of voided urine to test for significant bacteriuria. The health team caring for these women should be skilled in patient instruction to get a clean voided urine sample, and the specimens should be processed immediately or refrigerated until they can be transported to the laboratory. (This prevents bacterial overgrowth and false-positive urine cultures.)

A variety of screening tests are available, but Lenke has noted difficulties with the nitrite test. Although it is much cheaper than the screening culture, it is not sensitive enough to detect all cases of significant bacteriuria.[16] When urine culture tests are used to detect asymptomatic bacteriuria, a significant colony count is >100,000 colonies of one bacterial species. If multiple bacterial isolates are obtained, the specimen was probably contaminated at the time of collection and the test should be repeated. If the test is positive with a single bacterial species, it should be repeated, because a single positive test has only an 80% chance of reflecting the reality of bacteria in the bladder urine. A second positive test for the same bacterial species increases the accuracy to 96%.[17] Women in high-risk categories for pyelonephritis should be rescreened during pregnancy. These include patients with a past history of pyelonephritis, those with sickle cell trait or disease, and those with diabetes. Any asymptomatic patient with two consecutive positive cultures should be treated. Any plan for therapeutic intervention in these patients must be based on solid microbiologic data. For example, at least one study demonstrated an increasing incidence of gram-positive aerobes recovered from urine cultures, particularly Group B β-hemolytic streptococcus, and this finding has been my experience as well.[18] The types of bacterial isolates in asymptomatic bacteriuria can vary from hospital to hospital. It is important for obstetricians to have some idea of the frequency of bacterial isolates in their own patients with asymptomatic bacteriuria.

For treatment, one choice is the use of a nitrofurantoin for 10 days after the 12th week of pregnancy. This family of drugs is chosen because there is minimal alteration in the fecal flora of the women taking them, which minimizes the risk of subsequent infections with some resistant organisms. There are many safe and effective alternative antibiotics that can be prescribed. Harris has demonstrated similar cure rates with ampicillin, the cephalosporins, or sulfas.[19] If a high percentage of the bacterial isolates in any individual practice are Klebsiella, ampicillin could be a bad choice, because so many of these strains are resistant. Similarly, if Enterococcus is a frequent isolate, a cephalosporin often is inappropriate. Following treatment, the patient should have another urine culture to determine if the bacteriuria has been eliminated. If the repeat urine culture is positive for the same bacterial species and it is not resistant, treatment should be done with an antibiotic effective against the isolate. In those women who are culture negative after treatment, clean voided urine cultures should be repeated in each subsequent trimester of pregnancy, because many patients will have a recurrence of bacteriuria later in pregnancy.

CYSTITIS AND PYELONEPHRITIS

Cystitis during pregnancy is a confusing disease. Despite universal screening and treatment of women with asymptomatic bacteriuria, the incidence of cystitis has remained the same, even though the frequency of pyelonephritis diminished fivefold.[15] There is no scientific explanation for this. It is possible that cystitis develops more rapidly than pyelonephritis. Pyelonephritis in pregnancy frequently occurs after a period of time in a patient with asymptomatic bacteriuria, before symptoms and kidney infection develop. A rapid onset of cystitis is suggested by Harris's data.[15] In his study, 38 of 89 (43%) patients with cystitis were seen for the first time when they were symptomatic. Clearly, screening was not possible for this group. Of the remaining 51, 48 (94%) had a negative screening urine culture at their first prenatal visit. Only 3 (6%) of the population of women who developed cystitis after their first prenatal visit had asymptomatic bacteriuria when initially seen. The first prenatal visit screening did not identify a population at risk for the subsequent development of cystitis. This probably reflects the rapid de novo development of an acute cystitis during pregnancy. There is an alternative explanation. Stamm has shown that fewer than 10^5 *Escherichia coli* in voided urine samples reflect bladder bacterial contamination in symptomatic women with cystitis.[20] Perhaps fewer bacteria are needed to initiate cystitis.

The diagnosis of cystitis should be suspected in any pregnant woman with frequency and dysuria, with or without a fever. Patients with these symptoms can have other problems, such as a vaginitis or urethritis. Because of this, they should have a hanging drop examination of vaginal secretions to determine whether or not the patient has candida vaginitis, trichomonas vaginitis, or bacterial vaginosis. An endocervical culture for *Neisseria gonorrhoeae* and *Chlamydia trachomatis* should also be obtained in these patients to rule out those infections. Cooperation between the clinician and the laboratory is needed for accurate microbiology reports in women with cystitis. An agreement must be reached. If the clinician notes on the request slip that the clinical diagnosis is cystitis, the laboratory must agree to continue to work up any *E. coli* isolates, even when more than one species is recovered, and do antibiotic susceptibility studies. Colony counts of less than 100,000 have meaning in these women. These reports will guide appropriate therapy. A 10-day regimen with a nitrofurantoin is my choice; alternatively, ampicillin, cephalosporins, or sulfas can be used. Although there is a theoretical concern about the use of sulfas in a woman about to deliver a premature baby, this class of drugs can be prescribed and then discontinued if there is any evidence of labor. There have been reports of effective single-dose antibiotic treatment of lower urinary tract infection in a non-pregnant population,[21] but the poor success of single-dose treatment of asymptomatic bacteriuria in pregnancy makes this an unacceptable therapeutic alternative at present.[22] All of these patients require a posttreatment culture. If positive, long-term suppression with the nitrofurantoins is often used.

The treatment of patients with pyelonephritis during pregnancy is much more intense. These patients are sicker and will usually benefit from in-patient therapy so that problems of fever, hydration, and electrolyte imbalance, as well as the infection, can be treated. In addition, premature labor can occur in these women. This increase in uterine activity can be due to actions of the bacterial products causing the pyelonephritis, fever, or decreased intravascular volume. Therapy can modify these changes, and the uterus can be monitored to see if a contraction pattern is becoming established. If necessary, tocolytic therapy may be indicated in addition to the antibiotics. Occasionally, some of these women become critically ill. In a series with a large number of pregnant women with pyelonephritis, 3 of 99 (3%) had evidence of septic shock.[23] In addition, adult respiratory distress syndrome has been reported in pregnant women with pyelonephritis.[24–26] These women require close medical supervision.

All of these potential problems require a broad therapeutic approach to the pregnant patient with pyelonephritis. The diagnosis is usually obvious clinically. These patients look ill, are febrile, and usually have flank pain. The uterus should be assessed immediately to be sure there is not a pattern of uterine contractions, and there should be immediate fetal heart rate monitoring to ascertain the health of the fetus. A vaginal examination should be done to be sure there is no cervical dilatation, and cultures obtained to rule out maternal colonization with Group B β-hemolytic streptococcus,

C. trachomatis and *N. gonorrhoeae*. As soon as a voided urine sample can be obtained from the patient, a portion should be examined microscopically for the presence of bacteria. Uncentrifuged urine samples have been used by the author, but a recent survey of laboratory studies in patients with bacteriuria recommended oil immersion microscopy of a gram-stained centrifuged urine.[27] A portion of the urine should be sent for culture. If the clinical diagnosis has been made, treatment should begin. Fluid replacement should be an important part of therapy. Many of these women are dehydrated, which is further aggravated because they are febrile with an increased insensible fluid loss. This probably is the reason that some investigators have noted diminished renal function in the first 24 hours of treatment of pregnant women with pyelonephritis.[28] They need sufficient intravenous fluid replacement with a balanced electrolyte solution to ensure a urine output of at least 50 mL/hour. Because septic shock and respiratory distress have been reported in these women, they should be frequently observed with regular monitoring of vital signs. In addition, these patients must be monitored for premature labor. If it occurs, tocolytic agents can be employed. Because respiratory distress can occur when these agents are used, an electrocardiogram (ECG) should be obtained before treatment begins.[29] If the patient has unrelenting flank pain, an ultrasound evaluation for the presence of urinary tract calculi should be done. At least one study had good results in eight women with persistent flank pain who had internal ureteral stents put in place.[30] This avoided any further intervention during pregnancy. If electrolyte abnormalities are noted in the initial screening blood chemistries, these can be corrected and repeat electrolyte determinations done until they are normal. Intravenous antibiotics should be given for treatment. Either ampicillin or one of the cephalosporins is acceptable. Both are usually well tolerated during pregnancy. The cephalosporins are an excellent choice if Klebsiella is frequently isolated from the cultures of women with pyelonephritis on a service, while ampicillin is the best bet if Enterococcus is recovered. Both of these antibiotics achieve high levels in urine. Because of this, a laboratory report of bacterial resistance can still be associated with a clinical cure. If such a report is obtained in a patient who has shown a good clinical response, the culture should be repeated. Only if the culture is positive with an organism resistant to the antibiotic should the regimen be changed. These are the asymptomatic patients who can have a recurrence within a few weeks if this is not done. If the patient is allergic to penicillin, an aminoglycoside can be given. All patients should have a repeat culture done at 48 hours after the initiation of treatment. If bacteria are still recovered, consideration should be given to switching antibiotics to an agent more effective against the organism to avoid later recurrence of infection. When patients have been afebrile for 24 to 48 hours, they can be switched to an oral penicillin or cephalosporin to complete 10 days of therapy. (In the case of aminoglycosides, there is no alternative oral antibiotic.) All of these women should have a posttreatment culture obtained, and if it is positive, they should be treated with a different agent that is effective against the isolates. In these women who remain culture positive after a full course of treatment, it would be appropriate to get an ultrasound examination to check for the presence of urinary tract calculi. If the follow-up culture is negative, there is controversy about the subsequent care of these women for the rest of the pregnancy. Harris has championed antibiotic suppression of these women for the remainder of the pregnancy.[19] I favor this approach and use the nitrofurantoins, 50 to 100 mg/day. Lenke and his coworkers had poor results with this regimen, however; they favored routine urine culturing with short courses of treatment in women who are culture positive.[31] Lenke's urban poor population had many patients lost to follow-up. In this setting, treatment compliance for long-term suppression was not good. Assessment of the patient population under care should influence the treatment decisions about follow-up in these women.

ACQUIRED IMMUNE DEFICIENCY SYNDROME

Acquired immune deficiency syndrome (AIDS) is the most serious infection found in pregnancy, because it can be lethal for the mother and the fetus, and there are currently no cures. AIDS can take many forms in pregnancy. The presentations can range from a seemingly healthy woman who delivers a newborn subsequently found to have AIDS in the nursery, to a critically ill patient dying of an infection with unusual pathogens.

The clinical suspicion of AIDS should be highest in an urban poor population, in which there is a history of intravenous drug use among either these women or their sexual partners. Uncommon organisms causing infection, such as *Pneumocystis carinii* pneumonia or central nervous system infection with *Toxoplasmosis gondii*, tuberculosis, or herpes virus, should increase the suspicion that AIDS is the underlying problem; initiate appropriate blood testing with the patient's permission. Therapy should be directed toward the offending pathogens, and the medical care team should use appropriate precautions while drawing blood and in the operating room.

There is still controversy about routine antepartum testing for human immunodeficiency virus (HIV) antibodies. The arguments against it usually reflect concerns about cost effectiveness, the possibility of false-positive tests in populations with low incidence of the disease, and the fact that no treatment is available for these patients. There obviously are variations in incidence figures depending on the hospital site and its clientele. In an urban setting, I agree with Minkoff and favor routine antibody testing with consent, confidentiality, and counseling.[32] The information obtained would guide health team members and the patient in this setting, for there are preventive treatments that can prolong quality living.

RESPIRATORY TRACT INFECTION

UPPER RESPIRATORY TRACT

Upper respiratory infections occur frequently in the wintertime. Most are viral in origin and antibiotics will not be beneficial. Women with these infections should be examined and, if the throat is inflamed or if tonsillitis is present, a culture for the Group A β-hemolytic streptococcus should be obtained. If there is clinical suspicion of a Group A β-hemolytic streptococcus infection, penicillin should be prescribed. If the patient is allergic to penicillin, erythromycin can be started. Because both of these antibiotics increase the risk of a *Candida albicans* vulvovaginitis, it is appropriate to give these women concomitant local vaginal antifungal therapy. If the clinician suspects a viral cause for a sore throat, it is appropriate to wait for the culture report before starting therapy.

LOWER RESPIRATORY TRACT

Although uncommon, pneumonia is a serious disease for a pregnant woman. In one recent 7.5-year review of an urban poor population of women in which there were 89,219 deliveries, 39 pregnant women satisfied the criteria for pneumonia (0.04%).[33]

The prognosis for pregnant women with pneumonia has markedly improved in the last 20 years. In the preantibiotic era (before World War II), maternal death from pneumococcal pneumonia occurred in approximately one third of the patients.[5] The first major advance in the care of pneumonia in pregnancy was the introduction of antibiotics, which resulted in a reduction in the maternal death rate to less than 10%.[34] Further improvement was noted in a 1982 report, in which there were no maternal deaths among the 39 patients.[33] Part of this improvement was due to early diagnosis and less severe disease (ie, no patients had bacteremia.)[33] Important added factors include the availability of better ventilatory aids and more precise techniques to monitor fluid requirements and vital signs, so that a comprehensive therapeutic response can be mounted against the systemic effects of sepsis.

The key to the care of these women is early diagnosis. Patients with respiratory symptoms need a meticulous evaluation to determine if they have a lower respiratory tract infection. The evaluation begins with careful percussion and auscultation. A sputum sample should be obtained for Gram's stain and culture. Careful microscopic examination of the expectorate is important. The presence of polymorphonuclear leukocytes and the absence of squamous epithelial cells indicate that the specimen is expectorate and not saliva. A chest radiograph should be obtained, as well as an arterial pO_2. Blood studies, including a complete blood count and electrolytes, can be helpful. In most cases, the diagnosis is established by the roentgen findings.

The most frequent organism causing pneumonia in pregnant women is *Streptococcus pneumoniae*. This pathogen should be suspected in the febrile patient with lobar consolidation on chest radiograph and with white cells with gram-positive diplococci present on microscopic examination of a smear of the expectorate. Although there have been scattered reports of the isolation of penicillin-resistant strains of pneumococci, penicillin remains the drug of choice in the treatment of these women.[35] Premature labor can be a problem. Adequate hydration and close monitoring of uterine activity is important. Because cardiopulmonary problems can occur with ritodrine, the use of magnesium sulfate is the best choice if tocolytic therapy is indicated in such patients.

A wide variety of other organisms can be implicated in the pneumonia in pregnancy in which the patient is febrile with an elevated white count. The initial examination of the patient must be carefully done to determine the cause, because this will influence the choice of antibiotics. There are three pathogens other than *S. pneumoniae* that cause pneumonia and should be considered by the clinician: *Haemophilus influenzae*, Group A β-hemolytic streptococcus, and the coagulase-positive Staphylococcus. *H. influenzae* should be suspected if gram-negative rods are seen on Gram's stain of the expectorate. If this organism is suspected, ampicillin is usually the treatment of choice, although physicians should be aware of the frequency of *H. influenzae* resistance to ampicillin in their region.[36] Pneumonia due to Group A β-hemolytic streptococcus is quite rare, but it should be suspected if chains of gram-positive cocci are seen on the Gram's stain of the expectorate and if a pleural effusion is seen on the chest radiograph which, when aspirated, is found to be an empyema.[37] The antibiotic of choice for these patients is penicillin, but the clinical response often takes many days for improvement and resolution of symptoms, despite the susceptibility of Group A streptococci to minute concentrations of penicillin. Pneumonia caused by the coagulase-positive staphylococcus can be serious. Fortunately, it is rare but it should be considered by the clinician as a complication in women with influenza.[38] It should be suspected when clumps of gram-positive cocci are seen on Gram's stain. In this situation, the drug of choice is a cephalosporin.

Another category of patients, which constitutes a large segment of pregnant women with pneumonia, is made up of those with an atypical clinical presentation. These are the patients with roentgen evidence of pneumonia who may not be febrile. The most important diagnostic clue to these atypical pneumonias is the microscopic examination of the expectorate. If few or no bacteria are found, *Legionella pneumophila* and Mycoplasma are prime concerns.[39,40] Although culture is the most sensitive diagnostic test for Legionella, it requires invasive procedures to get the appropriate culture material.[39] In these women, blood should be drawn for serologic testing for Legionella and Mycoplasma, and repeat titers should be drawn in 4 weeks. The antibiotic of choice for both of these organisms is erythromycin. Fortunately, this antibiotic is safe to use during pregnancy, although it can give pregnant women abdominal discomfort and bloating when given by the oral route.

There are other uncommon pneumonias that will tax the diagnostic and therapeutic skills of the obstetrician. Chickenpox is a serious disease for pregnant women, and a Varicella pneumonia can be life threatening. This diagnosis can be confirmed by roentgen examination of the lungs of a very ill patient with cutaneous manifestations of chickenpox.[41] Fortunately, acyclovir, a potent antiviral agent, is available for the treatment of these women. In addition, assisted ventilation can be necessary in some women with extensive pulmonary involvement. The fetus will receive passive immunity from the transplacental passage of IgG antibodies from the mother, as long as delivery occurs at an interval long enough for maternal antibody formation to occur. First trimester Varicella can result in the fetal varicella syndrome,[42] and this concern can be the rationale for termination of the pregnancy. There are other pneumonias that are not as immediate a threat to the mother but have serious implications. The first is tuberculosis. The incidence increased in the United States in the 1980s.[43] This should be part of the differential diagnosis in the patient with apical changes on radiograph who has no resolution of lung findings on treatment, particularly in the patient from an urban poor population or part of a population of recent immigrants to the United States from the Caribbean or the Far East. Skin testing should be done and sputum sent for *Mycobacterium tuberculosis* culture. Another atypical pneumonia is caused by *P. carinii*. These patients usually have high fever, a lowered pO_2, and may have no changes initially on chest radiograph, but subsequently have diffuse bilateral alveolar disease. Diagnosis is made definitively by isolation of the organism from material from the lung. This should be obtained by the pulmonary specialist and consultation for these cases is indicated. If this diagnosis is made, appropriate testing for antibodies to HIV should be done. Although this is most frequently seen in urban poor minority groups who have used intravenous drugs or whose sexual partners have used intravenous drugs, heterosexual transmission of the virus is also a possibility. If the pulmonary infection lingers in a pregnant woman, and an unexpected pathogen or no pathogen is recovered, this remains a diagnostic possibility. In endemic areas, pulmonary infection due to yeast can occur. The most common pathogens in these patients are *Coccidioides immitis* and *Histoplasma capsulatum*. The diagnosis can be determined by specific culture techniques. In the case of Coccidioides, systemic treatment with antifungal agents such as amphotericin B can be life saving.[8]

MENINGITIS

Primary meningitis in pregnancy is very uncommon, but when it occurs, it is life-threatening. A major problem, caused by the infrequency with which the disease is seen by obstetricians, is the failure to make a diagnosis at an early stage of the disease when the prognosis for cure is the best. The possibility of meningitis should be considered in any patient who has had generalized malaise for a period of time, followed by headache, nausea, vomiting, and hyperthermia. If a patient has convulsions in addition to these other signs, the concern about meningitis should be high.

The diagnosis should be arrived at in a logical manner. The febrile patient who has nuchal rigidity is a candidate for a spinal tap, with cultures, Gram's stain, and chemical studies of the spinal fluid performed. If the Gram's stain of the spinal tract reveals bacteria, consideration should be given to possible pathogens and then antibiotic therapy. In adults, *Neisseria meningitidis* and *S. pneumoniae* are the most common causes, while *H. influenzae* is rarely seen. A presumptive diagnosis can be made of *N. meningitidis* by the presence of gram-negative cocci on Gram's stains and for *S. pneumoniae* by the presence of gram-positive diplococci.

There are some cases in which the spinal fluid examination is not diagnostic, because bacteria are not present and the glucose level is not reduced. In these situations, the major diagnostic concern is a viral meningitis such as coxsackievirus B2.[44] Viral cultures should be done on the cerebrospinal fluid (CSF) and antibiotics discontinued if studies of the spinal fluid are positive for a virus. Listeria meningitis can be confused with a viral meningitis. Many such patients will have no bacteria seen on Gram's stain and normal or borderline CSF glucose levels are found.[45] A positive culture for *Listeria monocytogenes* will confirm the diagnosis. The treatment of choice for most women is penicillin. This agent is effective against the two most common pathogens, *N. meningitidis* and *S. pneumoniae*. In addition, it is effective against most strains of *L. monocytogenes*. In the case of Listeria, the addition of aminoglycoside seems to improve results. If the patient is allergic to penicillin, chloramphenicol is probably the drug of choice.

In endemic areas, cryptococcal meningitis should be considered. The diagnosis should be suspected if encapsulated organisms are present on India ink preparation and confirmed by culture. The treatment of choice is amphotericin B given intravenously.[46]

BACTERIAL ENDOCARDITIS

Bacterial endocarditis is another rare but serious infection for a pregnant woman. It is infrequently seen. In 1983, Pastorek and coworkers reported three cases and estimated an incidence of 1 in 4000 deliveries.[47] In 1988, Cox and associates reported seven cases, of whom four were from their clinic population, with an incidence of 1 per 16,500 deliveries.[48] Both of these reports stress the increasing frequency of this disease in urban pregnant women with an increasing number of intravenous drug abusers.

This is a different population than in the past, where our focus was on women with rheumatic or congenital heart disease. Although bacterial endocarditis occurs infrequently, it can be life-threatening, because maternal death has been reported in pregnant women with this infection.[48] This is a difficult diagnosis for the obstetrician. It is an uncommon disease, and the clinical and laboratory findings can be subtle. It should be considered in a febrile patient who is lethargic with no localizing signs of infection. There are clues that this could be the problem. The patient should be questioned and examined for evidence of intravenous drug abuse. Cutaneous manifestations can be seen, particularly splinter hemorrhages under the fingernails or nontender purpuric spots on the heels or palms. The most diagnostic clinical sign is a changing heart murmur. A number of laboratory tests can be used to confirm the diagnosis if there is clinical suspicion this is the case. At least three blood cultures should be drawn 30 to 60 minutes apart. An ECG should be obtained and an echocardiograph done to determine if there is vegetation on any of the valves.

The treatment of these women varies from most of our antibiotic treatment experience in pregnancy. They should be treated with intravenous bactericidal antibiotics for at least 28 days. The choice of antibiotics will be guided by the susceptibilities of blood culture isolates, but penicillin and an aminoglycoside usually suffice. In penicillin-allergic patients, vancomycin is another option. In those rare patients with a *Staphylococcus aureus* endocarditis, a semisynthetic penicillin or cephalosporin should be used. Women with bacterial endocarditis are at risk for preterm labor with the delivery of premature infants.[48] Careful monitoring of uterine activity and meticulous attention to fluid balance is important in this population.

GASTROINTESTINAL INFECTIONS

Gastrointestinal infections have a broad range of presentation in a pregnant population. Physicians can be asked to evaluate cases such as a patient with chronic diarrhea or, at the other end of the spectrum, a woman with an acute life-threatening emergency, such as a ruptured appendix.

APPENDICITIS

Acute appendicitis illustrates how pregnancy can modify many of the clinical manifestation of intra-abdominal disease. The large uterus and immunologic suppression of pregnancy change patient symptomatology. For example, appendicitis in pregnancy usually presents with no fever, no leukocytosis, and right mid-quadrant pain,[49] which is not the same picture seen in non-pregnant women. The obstetrician has to take the responsibility for making the diagnosis, because many internists and general surgeons are not familiar with pregnancy changes. If the obstetrician makes the diagnosis of appendicitis in pregnancy, a surgical exploration of the abdomen should be carried out. It is better to explore a few patients who do not have appendicitis than to observe one patient with inconclusive signs and subsequently discover that she has a ruptured appendix.

CHOLECYSTITIS

Acute cholecystitis is another gastrointestinal problem seen in pregnant women. It should be suspected in the patient with nausea, vomiting, and right upper quadrant pain. New sophisticated imaging techniques that do not use radiation can be used to detect the presence of stones in the gall bladder or the collecting ducts. An important differential diagnosis in urban poor patients is the presence of an amoebic liver abscess (Druzin M. Personal communication, 1983). This abscess will respond to medical treatment with metronidazole, which should be given to avoid intra-abdominal rupture of the abscess.

PERITONITIS

Primary bacterial peritonitis is a rare but life-threatening condition in pregnant women. In non-pregnant women, such problems usually are secondary to a bacteremia with gram-positive aerobic cocci such as Group A β-hemolytic streptococcus or pneumococcus. In pregnant women, it has been associated with underlying disease or acute salpingitis.[50,51] The diagnosis should be considered in any pregnant woman with fever and abdominal tenderness. If more common entities such as chorioamniotis and appendicitis have been ruled out, and if the patient has evidence of liver disease, primary peritonitis should be considered as a diagnosis. Paracentesis and microscopic examination of peritoneal fluid should confirm this diagnosis, and the treatment should be with systemic antibiotics. Some of these women are critically ill, and they should be monitored closely for evidence of premature labor.

DIARRHEA

Diarrhea is seen with some frequency in any large obstetrical practice. Fortunately, it is usually self-limited and without complication. If it is explosive in nature or persists beyond 24 hours, the associated dehydration can be accompanied by premature labor. Close lines of communication with these patients must be kept.

I take a wait-and-see approach to pregnant patients who notify me that they have diarrhea. The patient is advised to take adequate oral fluids and to limit the use of medications in the first 24 hours to Kaopectate, a non-absorbed local medicine that does not alter intestinal motility. Acute diarrhea in these women can be caused by rotaviruses or by Norwalk-like viruses. These infections are usually self-limited, and the diarrhea represents the response of the host's gastrointestinal tract to eliminate pathogens and toxins. The use of medication to diminish gastrointestinal activity is not indicated, because it simply prolongs the exposure of the gut to the microbiologic agents causing disease. If the diarrhea persists beyond 24 hours, the patient should be seen, evaluated for dehydration and uterine activity, and a stool specimen obtained. A portion of stool should be examined in the laboratory for ova, parasites, and fecal leukocytes.[52] Another portion will be sent for culture to see if such organisms as *E. coli*, Campylobacter, *Yersinia enterocolitis*, Salmonella, or Shigella are recovered. The treatment of these isolates will be guided by antibiotic susceptibility studies. In the United States, it is rare for the diarrhea to be so severe that the patient requires admission and treatment with intravenous fluids for the dehydration.

CHRONIC DIARRHEA

There is another category of women who require evaluation of the gastrointestinal tract. These are women with chronic diarrhea. They need to be evaluated for ova and parasites, particularly *Giardia lamblia* and *Entamoeba histolytica*. These symptomatic women should be treated with quinacrine and metronidazole, respectively, after the 12th week of pregnancy.[52] The influx of refugees from Southeast Asia, the Caribbean and Central America, plus immigrants from South America, have increased the pool of pregnant patients in the United States with intestinal parasites.[53,54] In one evaluation of 97 Southeast Asian refugees in Philadelphia, 65% were colonized with gastrointestinal parasites. The most common isolates in the study were hookworm, *Trichuris trichiura, Clonorchis sinensis, Ascaridia lumbricoides, Strongyloides stercoralis, E. histolytica, G. lamblia, Endolimax nana*, Taenia, and *Plasmodium vivax*.[53] Despite the high infection rate, this population had uncomplicated pregnancy outcomes with the usual pregnancy care and treatment of symptomatic patients. Lee counsels therapeutic conservatism if obstetricians discover intestinal parasites in their pregnant patients.[54] He suggests two major indications for therapy: gastrointestinal problems that persist and interfere with maternal health, and parasite-related extraintestinal abnormalities.[54] Table 71-1 is a suggested scheme for the treatment of parasitic infections during pregnancy.[53]

TABLE 71–1. TREATMENT OF PARASITIC INFECTIONS DURING PREGNANCY

	TREAT DURING PREGNANCY?	THERAPY	BREAST FEEDING ALLOWED?
Malaria			
Plasmodium vivax	Yes	Chloroquine phosphate, 1 g initially, 500 mg at 6, 24, and 48 hr, continued 500 mg weekly until end of pregnancy. Postpone primaquine until after pregnancy for radical cure	Yes
P. malariae	Yes	If sensitive to chloroquine, treat with same regimen as for *P. vivax*	Yes
P. falciparum			
P. falciparum resistant to chloroquine or if severe infection	Yes	Quinine. If necessary, pyrimethamine and sulfadoxine (Fansidar). If Fansidar-resistant, then tetracycline	
Entamoeba histoylica			
Asymptomatic	No	Treat an asymptomatic cyst carrier postpartum with diloxanide furoate (Furamide)	Yes
Symptomatic	Yes	Paromomycin (Humatin) if no intestinal ulcerations	
		Metronidazole for severe cases or if paromomycin unsuccessful	No
Chlonochis sinensis (liver fluke)	No	Treat with praziquantel if complicated by cholecystitis, preferably postpartum	No
Enterobious vermicularis (pinworm)	No	Pyrantel pamoate (Antiminth)	Yes
Giardia lamblia			
Asymptomatic or mild	No		
Symptomatic (poor weight gain)	Yes	Paromomycin; if fails, then metronidazole	Yes
Hookworm (*Necator*	Yes	Iron therapy; if fails, or heavy worm burden then, pyrantel pamoate	Yes
americanus, Ancyclostoma duodenale)	Yes		
Taenia solium	No	Quinacrine, postpone until after delivery	Yes
T. saginata	No	Niclosamide	
Strongyloides stercoralis			
Asymptomatic	No		
Symptomatic	Yes	After first trimester, thiabendazole (known teratogen)	No
Tricuris trichuria (whipworm)	No	Severe disease rare, mebendazole (known teratogen)	No
Hymenolepsis nana (tapeworm)	No	Niclosamide	No
Ascaris lumbricoides	Yes	Pyrantel pamoate in the late third trimester	Yes

From Roberts NS, Copel JA, Bhutani V, et al. Intestinal parasites and other infections during pregnancy in Southeast Asian refugees. J Reprod Med 1985;30:720, with permission.

MALARIA

Fortunately, malaria is rare in the United States. In the tropics it is a common and serious infection. There are reported data that indicate that pregnant women living in areas endemic for malaria are more susceptible to *Plasmodium falciparum*.[55] There are drugs available to treat patients with this diagnosis. Some treatment guidelines are noted in Table 71-1.[53]

LYME DISEASE

Lyme disease is a new infection for obstetricians. It was first described in 1975, because of clustering of children with suspected juvenile rheumatoid arthritis in Lyme, Connecticut.[56] It is caused by a tickborne spirochete, *Borrelia burgdorferi* and is spread by the bite of infected ticks, *Ixodes dammini*, or related ixodid ticks.[57] It is a multisystem disorder that usually begins in the summer with a spreading skin eruption, to be followed weeks to months later with cardiac, neurologic, or arthritic abnormalities. Unfortunately for the obstetrician, this is a transplacental infection that can result in intrauterine fetal death or impairment of cerebral function because of in utero acquired central nervous system infection.[58,59] Fortunately, this pathogen is susceptible to antibiotics, so that cure can be achieved, particularly when an early diagnosis is made.

The diagnosis of Lyme disease will depend on the clinical awareness of the obstetrician, backed up by appropriate laboratory testing. In the United States, most of the cases to date have been clustered in three areas: the Northeast from Massachusetts to Maryland, the Midwest in Wisconsin and Minnesota, and in the West in California and Oregon.[60] Recent studies suggest that cases are extending beyond these boundaries.[61] Clinically, the disease begins as a red macule or papule at the site of the tick bite, and this lesion spreads. Concomitant with this, the patient complains of malaise, fatigue, headache, chills, and fever. This is not the "flu," to be dismissed by physician admonitions "to take fluids and acetaminophen, get to bed, and let nature take its course." These women need to be examined meticulously for skin lesions. Blood should be drawn for IgM antibodies. One recent study indicated that immunoblotting was superior to indirect ELISA tests for diagnosing early Lyme disease.[62] Patients with Lyme disease will not have a positive reagin test for syphilis (for example a VDRL), but they can cross-react with other treponemal tests, and have a positive FTA-ABS.[63] In non-pregnant women, the treatment of choice would seem to be tetracycline, which gives superior results to erythromycin, particularly in the prevention of the major late complications, myocarditis, meningitis, and arthritis.[64] In pregnancy, phenoxymethyl penicillin would seem to be the drug of choice for early disease. For patients who are first diagnosed with late disease, arthritis, ceftriaxone seems to be the drug of choice, because of its long half-life.[65]

CONCLUSIONS

This has been an overview of problems of maternal infection during pregnancy. In any evaluation of a sick pregnant woman, the physician has two responsibilities: to do a thorough evaluation of the gravida to determine the exact site of infection, and to assess the health of the fetus and to keep fetal needs in mind when planning therapy.

REFERENCES

1. Brabin BJ. Epidemiology of infection in pregnancy. Rev Infect Dis 1985;7:579.
2. Mitchell GW Jr, Jacobs AA, Haddad V, et al. The role of the phagocyte in host-parasite interactions. XXV: metabolic and bactericidal activity of leukocytes from pregnant women. Am J Obstet Gynecol 1970;108:805.
3. El-Maallem H, Fletcher J. Impaired neutrophil function and myeoloperoxidase deficiency in pregnancy. Br J Haematol 1980;44:375.
4. Weinberg ED. Pregnancy associated depression of cell mediated immunity. Rev Infect Dis 1984;6:814.
5. Finland M, Dublin TD. Pneumococcal pneumonias complicating pregnancy and the peurperum. JAMA 1939;122:1027.
6. Greenberg M, Jacobziner H, Pakter J, et al. Maternal mortality in the epidemic of Asian influenza, New York City, 1957. Am J Obstet Gynecol 1958;76:897.
7. Bray RS, Anderson MJ. Falciparum malaria and pregnancy. Trans R Soc Trop Med Hyg 1979;73:427.
8. Smale LE, Waechter KG. Dissemination of coccidiodomycosis in pregnancy. Am J Obstet Gynecol 1970;107:356.
9. Salvaraj RJ, Bhat KS. Metabolic and bactericidal activities of leukocytes in protein-calorie malnutrition. Am J Clin Nutr 1971;25:166.
10. Morrow RH Jr, Smetana HF, Sai FT, et al. Unusual features of viral hepatitis in Accra, Ghana. Ann Intern Med 1968;68:1250.
11. Schulman A, Herlinger H. Urinary tract dilatation in pregnancy. Br J Radiol 1975;48:638.
12. Harris RE, Thomas VL, Shelokov A. Asymptomatic bacteriuria in pregnancy. Antibody coated bacteria, renal function and intrauterine growth retardation. Am J Obstet Gynecol 1976;126:20.
13. Monif GRG. UTI in pregnancy: part 1. Inf Dis Letter for Obstet Gynecol 1984;6:7.
14. Whalley PJ. Bacteriuria of pregnancy. Am J Obstet Gynecol 1967;97:723.
15. Harris RE. The significance of eradication of bacteriuria during pregnancy. Obstet Gynecol 1979;53:71.
16. Lenke RR, Von Dorsten JP. The efficacy of the nitrite test and microscopic urinalysis in predicting urine culture results. Am J Obstet Gynecol 1981;140:427.
17. Norden CW, Kass EH. Bacteriuria of pregnancy: a critical appraisal. Annu Rev Med 1968;19:431.
18. Mead PJ, Harris RE. Incidence of group B beta hemolytic streptococcus in antepartum urinary tract infections. Obstet Gynecol 1978;51:412.
19. Harris RE. The treatment of urinary tract infections during pregnancy. In Ledger WJ, ed. Antibiotics in obstetrics and gynecology. Boston: Martinus Nijhoff, 1982.
20. Stamm WE, Counts CW, Running KR, et al. Diagnosis of coliform infection in acutely dysuric women. N Engl J Med 1982;307:463.
21. Ronald AR, Boutros P, Mourtada II. Bacteriuria localization

and response to single dose treatment in women. JAMA 1976; 235:1854.

22. Whalley PJ, Cunningham FG. Short term versus continuous antimicrobial therapy for asymptomatic bacteriuria in pregnancy. Obstet Gynecol 1977;49:262.
23. Cunningham FG, Morris GB, Mickal A. Acute pyelonephritis of pregnancy: a clinical review. Obstet Gynecol 1973;42:112.
24. Cunningham FG, Leveno KJ, Hankins GOV, et al. Respiratory insufficiency associated with pyelonephritis during pregnancy. Obstet Gynecol 1984;63:121.
25. Pruett K, Faro S. Pyelonephritis associated with respiratory distress. Obstet Gynecol 1987;69:444.
26. Elkington KW, Greb LC. Adult respiratory distress syndrome as a complication of acute pyelonephritis during pregnancy: case report and discussion. Obstet Gynecol 1986;67:18S.
27. Jenkins RD, Fenn JP, Matson JM. Review of urine microscopy for bacteriuria. JAMA 1986;255:3397.
28. Whalley PJ, Cunningham FG, Martin F. Transient renal dysfunction associated with acute pyelonephritis of pregnancy. Obstet Gynecol 1975;46:174.
29. Benedetti TJ. Maternal complications of parenteral beta-sympathomimetic therapy for premature labor. Am J Obstet Gynecol 1983;145:1.
30. Loughlin KR, Bailey RB Jr. Internal ureteral stents for conservative management of ureteral calculi during pregnancy. N Engl J Med 1986;315:1647.
31. Lenke RR, Van Dorsten JP, Schifrin BS. Pyelonephritis in pregnancy: a prospective randomized trial to prevent recurrent disease evaluating suppressive therapy with nitrofurantoin and close surveillance. Am J Obstet Gynecol 1983;146:953.
32. Minkoff HL. Universal screening for acquired immunodeficiency syndrome. Obstet Gynecol Rep 1988;1:78.
33. Benedetti TJ, Valle R, Ledger WJ. Antepartum pneumonia in pregnancy. Am J Obstet Gynecol 1982;144:413.
34. Hopwood HG. Pneumonia and pregnancy. Obstet Gynecol 1965;25:875.
35. Cooksey RC, Facklam RR, Thornsberry C. Antimicrobial susceptibility patterns of Streptococcus pneumoniae. Antimicrob Agents Chemother 1978;13:645.
36. Smith AL. Current concepts: antibiotics and invasive hemophilus influenzae. N Engl J Med 1976;294:1329.
37. Henschke C, Liberman L. Streptococcal empyema: the role of cross-sectional diagnostic imaging. Inf in Surg 1989;8:11.
38. Robertson L, Caley JP, Moore J. Importance of Staphylococcus aureus in pneumonia in the 1957 epidemic of influenza A. Lancet 1958;2:233.
39. Soper DE, Melone PJ, Conover WB. Legionnaire disease complicating pregnancy. Obstet Gynecol 1986;67:10S.
40. Couch RB. Mycoplasma pneumonia (primary atypical pneumonia). In Mandell GL, Douglas RG Jr, Bennett JE, eds. Principles and practices of infectious diseases. 2nd ed. New York: John Wiley and Sons, 1985.
41. Landsberger EJ, Hager WD, Grossman JH. Successful management of varicella pneumonia complicating pregnancy. A report of three cases. J Reprod Med 1986;31:311.
42. Preblud S, Cochi SL, Orenstein W. Varicella-zoster infection in pregnancy. N Engl J Med 1986;315:1416.
43. Tuberculosis–United States, 1985. MMWR 1986;35:699.
44. McKernan PD, Schare MB. Type B-2 Coxsackie virus meningitis in pregnancy. J Reprod Med 1988;33:667.
45. Louria DB, Hensle T, Armstrong D, et al. Listerosis complicating malignant disease, a new association. Ann Intern Med 1967; 67:261.
46. Stafford CR, Fisher JF, Fadel HE, et al. Cryptococcal meningitis in pregnancy. Obstet Gynecol 1983;62:355.
47. Pastorek JG, Plauche WC, Faro S. Acute bacterial endocarditis in pregnancy. A report of three cases. J Reprod Med 1983;28:611.
48. Cox SM, Hankins GDV, Leveno KJ, et al. Bacterial endocarditis. J Reprod Med 1988;33:671.
49. Reed C, Killackey M. The acute surgical abdomen in pregnancy. Inf in Surg 1982;1:26.
50. Stauffer RA, Wygal J, Lavery JP. Spontaneous bacterial peritonitis in pregnancy. Am J Obstet Gynecol 1982;144:104.
51. Browne MK, Cassie R. Spontaneous bacterial peritonitis during pregnancy. Br J Obstet Gynaecol 1981;88:1158.
52. Monif GRG. Infectious diarrheas. Inf Dis and Med Letter for Obstet Gynaecol 1986;8:7.
53. Roberts NS, Copel JA, Bhutani V, et al. Intestinal parasites and other infections during pregnancy in Southeast Asian refugees. J Reprod Med 1985;30:720.
54. Lee RV. G.I. parasites: how hazardous in pregnancy? Contemp Gynecol Obstet 1987;29:137.
55. Brabin BJ. An analysis of malaria in pregnancy in Africa. Bull WHO 1983;61:1005.
56. Steere AC, Malawista SE, Snydman DR, et al. Lyme arthritis: an epidemic of oligoarticular arthritis in children and adults in three Connecticut communities. Arthritis Rheum 1977;20:7.
57. Burgdorfer W, Barbour AG, Hayes SF, et al. Lyme disease — a tick borne spirochetosis? Science 1982;216:1317.
58. Schlesinger PA, Duray PH, Burke BA, et al. Maternal-fetal transmission of the Lyme disease spirochete, Borrelia burgdorferi. Ann Intern Med 1985;103:67.
59. Markowitz LE, Steere AC, Benach JL. Lyme disease during pregnancy. JAMA 1986;255:3394.
60. Steere AC, Malawista SE. Cases of Lyme disease: locations correlated with distribution of Ixodes dammini. Ann Intern Med 1979;91:730.
61. Schmid GP, Horsley R, Steere AC, et al. Surveillance of Lyme disease in the United States, 1982. J Infect Dis 1985;151:1144.
62. Grodzicki RL, Steere AC. Comparison of immunoblotting and indirect enzyme linked immunosorbent assay using different antigen preparations for diagnosing early Lyme disease. J Infect Dis 1988;157:790.
63. Magnarelli LA, Anderson JF, Johnson RC. Cross-reactivity in serological tests for Lyme disease and other spirochetal infections. J Infect Dis 1987;156:183.
64. Steere AC, Hutchinson GW, Rahn DW, et al. Treatment of the early manifestations of Lyme disease. Ann Intern Med 1983; 99:22.
65. Dattwyler RJ, Halperin JJ, Pass H, et al. Ceftriaxone as effective therapy in refractory Lyme disease. J Infect Dis 1987;155:1322.

72

CHAPTER

HIV AND OTHER SEXUALLY TRANSMITTED DISEASES IN PREGNANCY

Cheryl K. Walker and Richard L. Sweet

Although sexually transmitted diseases (STDs) have been recognized for over three millennia and have played major roles in the history of civilization, the last two decades have brought the greatest progress in our understanding of this rapidly expanding field.[1] Advances in the basic sciences of microbiology and immunology have made our comprehension of their pathogenesis and amplified treatment options more sophisticated. Simultaneously, cooperation between clinicians in internal medicine, pediatrics, and obstetrics and gynecology, and specialists in the fields of epidemiology, public health, and community medicine has facilitated dissemination and implementation of these new ideas.

Despite these breakthroughs, the epidemic of STDs remains unabated in America. Increasing numbers of sexually active adults, both men and women, are at risk for acquiring STDs. In particular, this trend has had far-reaching implications on the reproductive health of women.

Not only is there a resurgence of traditional agents such as gonorrhea, syphilis, and chancroid, but also new ones have been added to the list (Table 72-1). Some of the new additions, like hepatitis B virus, have long been recognized, but only recently have been understood to have a sexual mode of transmission. Unfortunately, many of these new STDs are either incurable or associated with serious sequelae in women. *Chlamydia trachomatis* has been associated with infertility,[2–4] ectopic pregnancy,[2,5–9] and a host of adverse perinatal outcomes[10]; human papilloma virus (HPV) is associated with genital squamous cell carcinomas[11–14]; herpes simplex virus (HSV) becomes a chronic infection; and human immunodeficiency virus (HIV) is ultimately fatal, and had become one of the five leading causes of death in women of reproductive age by 1991.[15] Many of these infections have been associated with abortion, preterm delivery, premature ruptured membranes, and amnionitis. Finally, many of these agents, including HIV, HSV, gonorrhea, chlamydia, and syphilis, can be transmitted to the fetus or newborn.

As might be expected, all of the STDs regularly occur in pregnancy, with varying effects on mother, fetus, and neonate. This chapter will focus on issues related to HIV, gonorrhea, syphilis, chlamydia, HPV, HSV, trichomonas, and chancroid infections in pregnant women and their fetuses.

HUMAN IMMUNODEFICIENCY VIRUS

Infection with HIV results in a systemic, degenerative, and ultimately fatal disease that assaults the immune and central nervous systems. Its pathognomonic finding is a selective depletion of $CD4^+$ helper T lymphocytes. The final stage of infection, called the acquired immunodeficiency syndrome (AIDS), is characterized by complete derangement of the immune system, with occurrence of opportunistic infections (OIs) or neoplasms.

Although this syndrome first appeared in humans in 1976, it was not recognized as a disease until 5 years later.[16–18] In 1979, an immunodeficiency illness in homosexual men was described, called gay-related immune deficiency (GRID). In July of 1981, the first cases of *Pneumocystis carinii* pneumonia (PCP) and Kaposi's sarcoma (KS) were reported by the CDC, and 5 months later these opportunistic infections were associated with immunodeficiency.[16,17] The name acquired immunodeficiency syndrome (AIDS) was attached to the disease in 1982.

TABLE 72–1. SEXUALLY TRANSMITTED PATHOGENS

Bacterial Agents	Viral Agents
Neisseria gonorrhoeae	Human papilloma virus
Chlamydia trachomatis	Herpes simplex virus
Gardnerella vaginalis	Hepatitis B virus
Haemophilus ducreyi	Cytomegalovirus
Shigella sp.	*Molluscum contagiosum* virus
Group B Streptococcus	Human immunodeficiency virus
Treponema pallidum	**Protozoan Agents**
Mycoplasma Agents	*Trichomonas vaginalis*
Mycoplasma hominis	*Entamoeba histolytica*
Ureaplasma urealyticum	*Giardia lambia*
	Fungal Agents
Ectoparasites	*Candida albicans*
Phthirius pubis	
Sarcoptes scabiei	

Although homosexual and bisexual men still account for the majority of cases in the United States, the leading mode of transmission worldwide is heterosexual activity. The rate of heterosexual transmission in the United States is growing steadily, from 4% in 1988[19] to 10% in September of 1990.[20] Given that 80% of women with AIDS currently are in their reproductive years, primary care and reproductive health care providers will likely be taking a more prominent role in the war against this disease.

EPIDEMIOLOGY

From early in the epidemic, the transmission of HIV was well understood. Modes of acquisition include contact with blood or blood products, intimate sexual contact, and vertical transmission from mother to fetus or neonate.

By August of 1990, 146,746 cases of AIDS had been reported to the Centers for Disease Control (CDC), with 144,221 of these in adults.[20] Of the women with AIDS, 51% were intravenous drug users (IVDUs), 32% were at risk of heterosexual transmission from male IVDUs or bisexual men, 10% had been transfused with blood or blood products, and 7% admitted no risk behaviors (Table 72-2). Of the 13,807 cumulative AIDS cases in women, over 80% were in their reproductive years, and 83% of cases in children were acquired through vertical transmission.

Unfortunately, the number of reported AIDS cases is misleading. There are an estimated 1 to 2 million asymptomatic HIV-infected individuals in the United States, many of whom are unaware of their status.[21] It has been estimated that the epidemic will continue, with approximately 270,000 AIDS cases diagnosed in the United States by 1991. Of the 74,000 cases expected during 1991 alone, approximately 7200 will be women and 1000 children.[22]

It is not surprising that the majority of AIDS cases in women have occurred in the large metropolitan areas of New York, New Jersey, Florida, and California, which have high rates of IVDU or large populations of homosexual and bisexual men. The major risk indicators for HIV infection in women include geographic location, urban residence, IVDU and needle sharing, heterosexual activity with an IVDU, age, and race/ethnicity. The ratio of AIDS cases in black and Hispanic to white women is reportedly 10:1.[23]

Intravenous Drug Use

Although as of May 1990, IVDU transmission was reported in 21% of AIDS cases, a disproportionate share of female AIDS patients were either IVDUs (52%) or heterosexual partners of IVDUs (20%).[20] The predominant source of spread in IVDUs is the sharing of needles contaminated with HIV-infected blood.

Heterosexual Sexual Activity

Although the vast majority (60%) of AIDS cases in the United States have occurred in homosexual or bisexual men, heterosexual transmission is more common worldwide and is increasing in the United States. Although this mode of acquisition accounts for only 5% of AIDS cases overall, it ranks second after IVDU as a risk behavior for American women, currently accounting for 32% of female AIDS cases.[20]

TABLE 72–2. EXPOSURE CATEGORIES OF ADULT/ADOLESCENT AIDS CASES REPORTED TO THE CDC AS OF AUGUST 1990

	MALES	FEMALES	TOTAL
Homosexual/Bisexual Male	86,113 (66%)	—	86,113 (60%)
IV Drug Abuser	24,045 (18%)	7069 (51%)	31,114 (22%)
Homosexual Male & IVDA	9776 (7%)	—	9776 (7%)
Hemophilia/Coagulation Disorder	1258 (1%)	30 (0%)	1288 (1%)
Heterosexual	2993 (2%)	4425 (32%)	7418 (5%)
Transfusion	2097 (2%)	1320 (10%)	3417 (2%)
Undetermined	4132 (3%)	963 (7%)	5095 (4%)
Totals	130,414 (91%)	13,807 (9%)	144,221 (100%)

IV, intravenous; IVDA, intravenous drug abuser.

HIV appears to be much less contagious than most other STDs. The chance of acquiring HIV infection per sexual contact in the general population ranges from 1:1,000,000 to 1:100,000,000. This risk rises to 1:10,000 for a single heterosexual contact with an HIV-infected person using a condom, and to 1:1000 for a single instance of unprotected intercourse with an infected partner.[24]

Studies following the steady heterosexual partners of HIV-infected persons have documented seroconversion in 7% to 68%.[25,26] The risk of male-to-female transmission has ranged from 9% to 47%,[26–37] while rates of female-to-male transmission, although not as well studied, run 19% to 40%.[34,38] The use of condoms has been associated with lower transmission rates.[39] Infectivity is highest for male partners of female IVDUs and Haitian or Central African women.

Other factors appear to govern the rates of heterosexual infectivity. Both anal intercourse and a higher number of sexual contacts are associated with increased risk of transmission.[26] Also, increased duration of infection, low absolute CD_4 counts, p 24 antigenemia, the presence of coexistent STDs (especially those manifesting genital ulcers), lack of circumcision, and nonuse of barrier methods of contraception all correlated with elevated risk of transmission.[28]

Coinfection with other STDs carries a higher risk for heterosexual acquisition of HIV. Genital ulcer disease, caused predominantly by chancroid, syphilis, and HSV, is associated with heterosexual spread of HIV in Africa.[40–42] This association has also been made for homosexual men in the United States.[43] In theory, the ulcer provides an ideal port of entry for the virus, and the state of acute inflammation with localized infiltration of activated lymphocytes and macrophages enhances HIV infection and virus proliferation.[44,45]

Transfusion

Transfusion-associated HIV infection occurred as the result of the parenteral administration of infected whole blood, blood cellular components, plasma, or clotting factors between 1978 and 1985, at which time routine screening practices for HIV antibody were instituted. The current risk of infection after receiving a unit of blood ranges from 1:100,000 to 1:1,000,000.

There have been three discernible shifts thus far in the AIDS epidemic in the United States. The initial wave involved homosexual and bisexual men, and was closely followed by a surge of IVDUs acquiring AIDS. The most recent increase is among the female partners of male IVDUs and bisexual men. Over 80% of these women are of childbearing age, and they represent a growing challenge to providers of reproductive health care. It is not hard to predict a fourth and fifth wave, composed respectively of the general heterosexual population followed by the infants born to HIV-infected women.

PATHOGENESIS

HIV-1 is one of the more complex members of the retrovirus family. It is composed of core (p 18, p 24, and p 27) and surface (gp 120 and gp 41) proteins, genomic RNA, and the reverse transcriptase enzyme, surrounded by a lipid bilayer envelope. The virion contains three structural genes (*gag, pol,* and *env*), and an intricate set of regulatory genes that control, among other things, each other and the rate of HIV production.[46,47] Two of these genes (*tat* and *vif*) speed viral replication,[47–50] while two more (*nef* and *vpu*) restrain growth.[47,51] One last gene (*rev*) appears to operate as a switch, promoting protein expression and viral replication.[52–54] It may direct the progression from latent to active infection.

HIV gains access to host cells via the binding of its surface protein gp 120 to CD4 receptors on helper T lymphocytes, B lymphocytes, macrophages, lymph nodes, Langerhans' cells of the skin, and some brain cells.[55,56] The virion then fuses directly with the host cell membrane, an action apparently mediated by the gp 41 surface protein. Once inside, its reverse transcriptase converts its RNA genome to DNA, which is incorporated into the host genome.

A latent period of variable length ensues, during which HIV replication is restricted. The triggers for activation are poorly understood, and may include mitogenic, antigenic, or allogenic stimulation. An interesting finding is that in vitro HIV infection of resting helper T cells results in latent viral behavior, while infection of activated helper T cells, usually a very small percentage of the total T-cell population, leads to prolific HIV replication.[44,57] Multiple infections (eg, cytomegalovirus [CMV], HBV, HSV) and inflammatory processes (eg, contact with semen, blood, allografts) induce T cell activation and may play a role in activating the virus.

Once activated, the infected host genome transcribes mRNA and virion RNA, the latter of which is packaged and transported to the cell surface for exocytosis. The host cell is killed during HIV replication.[55,58] It is this latter phenomenon that results in the depletion of helper T lymphocytes and the subsequent immunodeficiency associated with clinical disease.

CLINICAL MANIFESTATIONS

The spectrum of HIV infection continues to broaden as advances in treatment transform it into a chronic disease. The first CDC definition for AIDS in 1982 required proof of cell-mediated immune deficiency in the form of KS or an opportunistic infection, such as PCP.[59] In 1985, direct proof of HIV infection, such as antibody, antigen, or culture, was added to the diagnostic qualifications.[60] The last modifications were published in 1987.[61]

The average incubation time from HIV exposure to primary infection is 2 to 4 weeks, with a range from 3

TABLE 72-3. CENTERS FOR DISEASE CONTROL HIV INFECTION CLASSIFICATION SCHEME

Group I: Acute HIV Infection
Group II: Asymptomatic HIV seropositivity
Group III: Persistent generalized lymphadenopathy (PGL)
Group IV: Severe AIDS-related diseases
A: Constitutional symptoms (formerly called AIDS-related complex or ARC)
B: Neurologic disease
C-1: Opportunistic infections listed in CDC surveillance definition
C-2: Other recurrent infections
D: Opportunistic malignancies listed in CDC surveillance definition
E: Other serious conditions

days to 3 months. When patients are symptomatic, most report the sudden onset of a flu-like syndrome with fever, malaise, lassitude, headache, myalgias, arthralgias, diarrhea, sore throat, lymphadenopathy, and a maculopapular rash on the trunk. Less frequent findings are elevated liver function tests and neurologic abnormalities. Symptoms can persist for 2 weeks. Patients suffering from primary infection will not have circulating antibodies to HIV, although viral cultures and tests identifying antigen or viral DNA should be positive.[62]

Following this, the infection enters a latent phase of variable duration. Most HIV-infected persons fall into this category. Dormant HIV infection has been reported to last longer than 10 years in some individuals, although progression to symptomatic disease and death appear inevitable.[63,64]

A common sign of disease progression is the development of persistent generalized lymphadenopathy (PGL), a condition involving at least 2 extragenital sites.[65,66] In the mid-1980s, PGL was considered to be part of the AIDS-related complex (ARC) syndrome, a designation which has fallen into disuse. Individuals with PGL who exhibit constitutional symptoms, oral candidiasis, or hairy leukoplakia are likely to develop AIDS within 14 months.[67]

TABLE 72-4. OPPORTUNISTIC INFECTIONS INCLUDED IN THE CDC DEFINTITION OF AIDS (GROUP IV-C_1)

Pneumocystis carinii pneumonia
Chronic cryptosporidiosis
Extraintestinal strongyloidiasis
Cytomegalovirus infection (other than liver, spleen, or lymph nodes)
Mycobacterium avium complex or *M. kansasi* disease, disseminated
Candidiasis of esophagus, trachea, bronchi or lungs
Herpes simplex virus infection, disseminated or chronic mucocutaneous
Toxoplasmosis of the brain
Cryptococcosis, extrapulmonary
Histoplasmosis, extrapulmonary
Isosporiasis
Progressive multifocal leukoencephalopathy

TABLE 72-5. RECURRENT INFECTIONS COMMONLY COMPLICATING HIV INFECTION (CDC GROUP IV-C_2)

Recurrent Salmonella bacteremia
Multidermatomal *Herpes zoster*
Nocardiosis
Tuberculosis
Oral candidiasis
Oral hairy leukoplakia

Evidence of more substantial immunocompromise can take many forms. Constitutional symptoms such as weight loss, fevers, night sweats, and diarrhea are worrisome. Neurologic involvement either from direct HIV infection or opportunistic infection or neoplasm is common. Histologic central nervous system involvement has been documented in 40% to 80% of those dying of AIDS.[68,69] Opportunistic infections included in the CDC surveillance definition of AIDS are listed in Table 72-3, while other recurrent infections associated with HIV disease progression are listed in Table 72-4. Finally, a number of opportunistic malignancies characteristic of HIV infection have been included in Table 72-5.

To introduce some order into the chaos of HIV-related illnesses, classification schemes have been proposed recently by both the CDC[61] and the Walter Reed Army Hospital.[70] With the CDC scheme (see Table 72-3), HIV-infected persons are separated into four groups. Group I consists of those with acute primary HIV infection; patients in Group II are seropositive but asymptomatic; those in Group III have persistent generalized lymphadenopathy; and Group IV is reserved for those with more serious disease manifestations. The subgroups of group IV are (A) constitutional symptoms, (B) neurologic disease, (C_1) opportunistic infection (see Table 72-4), (C_2) other severe, recurrent infection (see Table 72-5), (D) opportunistic malignancies (Table 72-6), and (E) other serious diseases, including thrombocytopenia or Hodgkin's disease. Clustering these serious illnesses into Group IV places them on an equal footing, and reminds the clinician that neurologic manifestations carry the same prognosis as opportunistic infection.

The Walter Reed (WR) system for staging HIV infection (Table 72-7) is composed of seven progressive levels of immune dysfunction, numbered 0 through 6. WR0 designates exposure to the virus; seropositive asymptomatic patients are placed in WR1; people with persistent generalized lymphadenopathy belong in WR2; in WR3, helper T cell counts fall below 400; patients in WR4 exhibit asymptomatic partial defects in

TABLE 72-6. OPPORTUNISTIC MALIGNANCIES COMMONLY COMPLICATING HIV INFECTION (CDC GROUP IV-D)

Kaposi's sarcoma
B-cell non-Hodgkin's lymphoma

TABLE 72–7. WALTER REED HIV INFECTION CLASSIFICATION SCHEME

	HIV ANTIBODY OR ANTIGEN	CHRONIC LYMPHADENOPATHY	T-HELPER CELLS	DELAYED HYPERSENSITIVITY	THRUSH	OIS
WR0	–	–	>400	Normal	–	–
WR1	+	–	>400	Normal	–	–
WR2	+	+	>400	Normal	–	–
WR3	+	+	<400	Normal	–	–
WR4	+	+	<400	Partial	–	–
WR5	+	+	<400	Complete cutaneous anergy or thrush	–	
WR6	+	+	<400	Partial to complete	+	+

delayed hypersensitivity; complete cutaneous anergy or oral candidiasis develops in WR5; and WR6 is reserved for those who develop opportunistic infection.

MATERNAL AND FETAL RISKS

The essential issues in HIV infection and pregnancy concern both the effect of pregnancy on HIV infection and that of HIV infection on pregnancy, including vertical transmission.

Effects of Pregnancy on HIV Infection

Initial reports suggested that gestational changes in the immune system fostered more rapid progression of HIV infection to symptomatic disease.[71] Studies by Scott and coworkers[72] and Minkoff and colleagues[73] reported a high percentage of progression to ARC or AIDS among asymptomatic HIV-infected women during or shortly following pregnancy. This seems logical in light of our understanding of gestational immune function: CD_4 counts fall slightly during pregnancy,[74] and the host response appears to be altered in a number of infections —depressed with CMV and rubella,[75,76] and amplified with certain viral diseases such as varicella, poliomyelitis and influenza.[77,78] In retrospect, both studies were biased in that their populations consisted of women identified through prior vertical transmission. More recent prospective controlled studies have failed to discern an alteration in the progression of HIV infection during pregnancy.[79,80]

Effects of HIV Infection on Pregnancy Outcomes

Preliminary data suggested a number of adverse perinatal outcomes in pregnancies complicated by HIV infection. They indicated an increase in the rates of preterm delivery and intrauterine growth retardation.[81–84] Subsequent studies that controlled for IVDU failed to support this contention.[85–89] Another retrospective study reported no variation in the rates of spontaneous abortion, ectopic pregnancy, PROM, preeclampsia, anemia, low weight gain, oligohydramnios, chorioamnionitis, or intrapartum fetal distress.[85] The most common cause of AIDS-related deaths during pregnancy was *Pneumocystis carinii* pneumonia.[90]

Perinatal HIV Transmission

Although it is accepted that perinatal transmission occurs, little is understood about the rate, timing, mode of spread, or cofactors involved in the process. First trimester transplacental infection has been hypothesized, based on the description of an AIDS embryopathy syndrome and viral antigen identification from electively aborted fetuses.[91,92] Intrapartum transmission resulting from exposure to infected bodily secretions seems plausible, but has not been proved. HIV infection has developed in infants born by cesarean section with intact membranes.[84,93] Transmission of HIV through breast-feeding has been documented in a limited number of cases. This has prompted authorities to recommend breast-feeding only for HIV-infected mothers in undeveloped countries; bottle-feeding is advocated for women living in industrialized countries.[94,95]

Vertical transmission rates were initially thought to be 36% to 65%,[72,73,96–98] but current estimates are much lower, ranging from 17% to 41%.[87,88,93,99] The major difficulty in assessing vertical transmission is that infants will carry passively acquired HIV IgG antibody for up to 15 months. Because our mainstay tests involve antibody recognition, the diagnosis must be delayed in many children. Experimental use of polymerase chain reaction techniques for earlier diagnosis of HIV infection in neonates is promising.[100]

The search continues for a tool to predict the probability of transmission to the fetus or neonate. Factors that appear to foreshadow disease progression, such as depressed helper T cell counts, elevated suppressor T cell count, anemia, lymphocytopenia, p 24 antigenemia, and elevated levels of $\beta 2$ microglobulin, may also portend vertical transmission. There is some suggestion that a low maternal absolute CD_4 count predisposes to neonatal infection.[101] Stage and virulence of maternal HIV infection may also affect transmission. The most encouraging data emanate from studies correlating high levels of maternal antibody to HIV envelope glycoprotein gp 120 with uninfected children.[102]

PHYSICAL DIAGNOSIS

Close attention and thoroughness are necessary in the antepartum assessment of HIV-infected women. Periodic review of systems should uncover constitutional symptoms such as weight loss, malaise, fatigue, persistent fevers, chills, and night sweats; respiratory symptoms; and neurologic abnormalities. Physical examination should be meticulous. Ocular hallmarks include cotton-wool spots in PCP and diffuse hemorrhages in CMV. Mucous membranes may harbor candidal infection or KS lesions. Skin lesions in the form of seborrheic dermatitis, herpes zoster, tinea, molluscum, or KS are typical, and generalized lymphadenopathy is common. A dry cough with rales is the rule with PCP; hepatosplenomegaly is often encountered in hepatitis, ideopathic thrombocytopenic purpura, and PGL. Neurologic abnormalities can be remarkably subtle. Gynecologic manifestations include candidal vaginitis, rapidly growing condylomata acuminata, secondary syphilis, HPV, and KS lesions.

LABORATORY DIAGNOSIS

Common laboratory abnormalities during HIV infection include the following:

- Decreased CD_4 levels
- Decreased helper/suppressor T cell ratio
- Absolute leukopenia, lymphopenia, anemia, or thrombocytopenia
- Elevated serum globulins
- Abnormal delayed cutaneous hypersensitivity.

Numerous researchers have attempted to identify markers foreshadowing progression to AIDS. The most suggestive are:

- Elevated levels of $\beta 2$ microglobulin
- HIV p 24 antigenemia
- Anemia
- Low helper T cell count
- High proportion of suppressor T cells
- Absolute lymphocytopenia
- Reduced level of HIV antibody
- Elevated level of CMV antibody
- Sexual contact with someone in whom AIDS has developed.[103,104]

The most common tests for HIV infection include detection of antibody or antigen and direct culture. Antibody tests include enzyme-linked immunoabsorbent assay (ELISA), immunofluorescent antibody (IFA), or Western blot. ELISA testing is highly sensitive and specific. False-negative ELISA results have been obtained in the brief window of time during early infection, before antibody production has occurred. Given the implication of a positive test result, it is recommended that confirmatory testing be done using the more specific Western blot, which isolates the core protein p 24 and the surface protein gp 41. Viral culture is expensive, slow, and relatively insensitive. Finally, there is great enthusiasm for polymerase chain reaction (PCR), the new rapid technique for the detection of viral DNA.[105,106]

TREATMENT

Zidovudine

Zidovudine (AZT) functions as an inhibitor of the reverse transcriptase enzyme of HIV, thus preventing viral DNA incorporation into the host genome. It has been shown to reduce opportunistic infections and prolong survival in AIDS patients.[107] The initial patient selection criteria for AZT therapy include the criterion that the patient must carry the diagnosis of PCP or have an absolute CD_4 count of $<200/mm^3$.

Treatment trials have been conducted in asymptomatic HIV infection to restrain progression to AIDS, and early results are promising. Current indications for AZT include asymptomatic HIV infection with CD_4 cell count $<500\ mm^3$, symptomatic HIV infection, and evidence of HIV-associated infection or immunocompromise in children over the age of 3 months.

The current recommendation is a dosage of 500 to 600 mg/day (much lower than the original dose of 1500 mg). This lower dose has significantly reduced the toxicity associated with AZT use.

Sulfamethoxazole-Trimethoprim

This is the first-line drug of choice for PCP. Although many patients are treated orally, reduced gastric absorption during pregnancy favors parenteral administration.[77] Both elements of this therapy cross the placenta, and while sulfa use is usually not recommended in the third trimester, the morbidity associated with PCP outweighs the minimal risk to the fetus.[108–110]

Pentamidine

There are two main uses for pentamidine in HIV disease. The first is in patients who have failed first-line treatment for PCP. Although its use in pregnancy has not been well studied, the hazards of untreated PCP override concern for the fetus. Aerosolized pentamidine is also being used for its prophylactic ability against the development of PCP, although its effects in pregnancy are unknown.

PREVENTION

No vaccine or antiviral treatment against HIV exists. Therefore, prevention is our only means of controlling this infection. At this time, universal screening is not advocated. However, counseling and testing for women at high risk for HIV infection are warranted in order to provide them with the information and resources necessary to reduce acquisition and transmission and to make informed decisions about reproduction. Early diagnosis in the asymptomatic phase of infection may allow for prophylactic therapy that could slow the disease progression.

GONORRHEA

Gonorrhea is perhaps the oldest known STD, with references to its symptoms dating back to numerous ancient civilizations.[111] The term gonorrhea, meaning "flow of seed" in Greek, first appeared in the writings of Galen, circa AD 150. It was not until relatively recent times that the disease's effects in women were first described.

Neisseria gonorrhoeae infects both columnar and transitional epithelium, including the endocervix, urethra, anal canal, pharynx, and conjunctivae. Local spread in women results in endometritis, salpingitis, and bartholinitis, while systemic manifestations include arthritis, dermatitis, endocarditis, meningitis, myocarditis, and hepatitis. It is estimated that 2 to 3 million cases occur annually in the United States, with an incidence in pregnancy reported at 0.6% to 7.5%.[112]

EPIDEMIOLOGY

Humans are the only natural host for this organism, and the only known forms of transmission are sexual and vertical. Widespread reporting of gonorrhea in many parts of the industrialized world is a phenomenon of the 20th century, and has expanded our understanding of its behavior.

A number of risk markers for gonorrhea have been identified. These include age less than 30 years, male sex, nonwhite race, early onset of sexual activity, low socioeconomic status, unmarried status, urban dwelling, illicit drug use, and prostitution. All of these markers influence sexual behavior, response to illness, or accessibility of health care. In 1987, 82% of patients with gonorrhea were aged 15 to 29 years, with higher rates among sexually active teens.[113,114] Ethnic minorities have reported case rates that are ten times those in whites, which in part may be due to under-reporting of white patients by private doctors.[115] The use of condoms, diaphragms, and spermicidal foams all have been shown to decrease the rate of sexual transmission of gonorrhea.[116,117]

Women appear to be at higher risk than men for contracting gonorrhea. The chance of becoming infected as the result of a single sexual encounter with an infected heterosexual partner is estimated to be 20% to 25% for men and 80% to 90% for women.[118]

In the 1960s, *Neisseria gonorrhoeae* strains in the United States developed increasing resistance to penicillin and tetracycline, largely as the result of subcurative treatment regimens. Then, in 1976, the first β-lactamase or penicillinase-producing *N. gonorrhoeae* (PPNG) strains were noted. They are plasmid-mediated and appear to have been imported from Africa to the United Kingdom and from the Philippines to the United States. Nearly 2% of reported cases in the United States are penicillinase-producing.[119]

Two other forms of resistance have materialized recently. Chromosomal resistance to penicillin, tetracycline, cephalosporins, spectinomycin, and aminoglycosides (CMRNG) first appeared in 1983, and plasmid-mediated resistance to tetracycline (TRNG) has also been reported.

PATHOGENESIS

Four distinct morphologic variants of this gram-negative diplococcus have been described: T_1 and T_2, now called P^+ and P^{++}, both retain their virulence in subculture and are covered by surface projections called pili; T_3 and T_4, now collectively called P^-, are less virulent and do not possess pili. The best ways to differentiate strains, however, is either by nutritional requirement (auxotype) or surface antigen variation.

The organism attaches to mucosal cells with the aid of its pili, and enters the cell by endocytosis. It releases endotoxins, causing widespread cell damage. A vigorous host response ensues, compounding mucosal injury.[120,121]

CLINICAL MANIFESTATIONS

The clinical presentation depends on the site of inoculation, duration of infection, and whether the infection has remained local or has spread systemically. The percentage of women with asymptomatic infection ranges between 25% and 80%.[122,123] Gonococcal infections in pregnant patients are commonly asymptomatic.

Anogenital Gonorrhea

Acute symptomatic anogenital infections in women are characterized by dysuria, increased urinary frequency, increased vaginal discharge secondary to an exudative endocervicitis, abnormal menstrual bleeding, or anorectal discomfort. Most women who become symptomatic do so within 3 to 5 days of inoculation, or during menstruation. Inflammation of the Skene's or Bartholin's glands is usually unilateral and acute in nature. Only 15% of all women with gonorrhea will have extension of infection to the upper genital tract, although this is rarely seen during pregnancy.

Localized Extragenital Gonorrhea

The majority of patients with pharyngeal infections are asymptomatic. The most common signal is a mild sore throat, while erythema, lesions, and a tonsilar/pharyngeal exudate may be present. Pharyngeal infection is more common during gestation.[124]

Gonococcal conjunctivitis, as the result of direct sexual contact or indirect autoinoculation, is rare and heralded by the acute onset of severe inflammation and purulent exudate.

Disseminated Gonococcal Infection

Disseminated gonococcal infection (DGI) occurs in 1% to 3% of adult infections, and 80% of these cases are in women.[125,126] Most women with DGI develop symptoms either during pregnancy or while menstruating. The majority of *N. gonorrhoeae* isolates recovered from patients with DGI are sensitive to antibiotics but resistant to complement-mediated bactericidal activity in normal serum. Further support for this perception derives from the finding that people with complement deficiencies are more prone to DGI.[127]

There are two distinct clinical syndromes found in DGI: an early bacteremic and a later arthritic stage. Patients with disseminated infection rarely complain of genital symptoms. Bacteremic patients complain of fever, chills, malaise, and skin lesions. The initial dermatologic manifestation most frequently involves distal extremities, including the palms and soles, with up to 20 lesions. Lesions are characterized as small vesicles that become first pustular, then necrotic, and finally heal spontaneously. Endocarditis, meningitis, and toxic hepatitis are infrequent complications of this phase. The arthritic phase typically is asymptomatic and involves the knees, ankles, and wrists, with purulent tenosynovitis. The pain is thought to be secondary to deposition of immune complexes. Without treatment, symptoms usually resolve in about a week's time; the infection may either become chronic, or progress to septic arthritis and joint destruction.

MATERNAL AND FETAL RISKS

The association between maternal gonorrheal infection and ophthalmia neonatorum has been appreciated for over a century. Before routine administration of silver nitrate, this disease occurred in 10% of newborns. The institution of routine neonatal prophylaxis reduced this rate dramatically, although recently there has been a resurgence. Gonococcal infection is transmitted to 30% to 35% of babies who pass through an infected cervix.[128] After an incubation period of between 4 and 21 days, bilateral purulent conjunctivitis is the usual manifestation, with rapid progression to corneal ulceration, scarring, and blindness in the absence of treatment. Although they have been described, neonatal infections of the pharynx, respiratory tract, anal canal, and sepsis are uncommon.

More recently, gonococcal infection during gestation has been linked with a wide variety of perinatal complications. Postabortal and postpartum endometritis occur more frequently in women with untreated gonococcal cervicitis at the time of delivery. Intra-amniotic infection (IAI) has also been described.[129–132] Characterized by inflammation of the fetal membranes, placenta, and umbilical cord, it results in maternal fever, leukocytosis, and fetal infection. A chronic, low-grade infection may ensue, with resultant intrauterine growth retardation.[132] Whether infection predisposes to or is the result of premature rupture of the membranes remains controversial. Preterm delivery is the customary outcome, and both mother and infant are at risk for continued infection and sepsis. The incidence of preterm delivery in women with untreated cervical gonorrhea has been recorded as high as 67%.[129]

LABORATORY DIAGNOSIS

While Gram's stain of urethral discharge is both sensitive and specific in men, it has two major disadvantages in women: asymptomatic patients will not be tested, and the test has poor sensitivity in women. Thus, the diagnosis of gonococcal infection in women requires a positive culture.

Selective plates, such as Thayer-Martin, provide optimal conditions for isolation of the organism. *N. gonorrhoeae* forms oxidase-positive colonies that can be differentiated from other Neisseria by their ability to dissimilate glucose but not maltose, sucrose, or lactose.

If one relies on urine culture, only 50% of infected women will have organism counts $\geq 10^5$ col/mL. Massage of the urethra through the anterior vagina or of the Skene's or Bartholin's glands may express exudate suitable for culture. In DGI, the incidence of positive blood cultures declines precipitously after 48 hours of symptoms. Positive synovial fluid cultures are more frequently obtained after extended duration of symptoms.

The most reliable method of gonorrhea detection in women is culture of the cervix and any other symptomatic site. Given the high percentage of asymptomatic gonococcal infection in sexually active women under the age of 30 years, routine annual endocervical screening is advocated. During pregnancy, cultures should be obtained from all patients at the first antenatal visit and again in the third trimester in those at high risk for infection. Factors identifying those at high risk include sex with a symptomatic partner, bleeding induced by cervical swab, Medicaid as a method of payment, age at first intercourse ≤ 16 years, and low abdominal or pelvic pain.[133]

Proper collection techniques ensure the highest possible yield of organisms. A dry cotton swab should be used to sample the endocervical canal; it should be turned to achieve contact with all surfaces of the canal and then allowed to soak up organisms for 30 seconds. The swab should immediately be plated, and the plate placed in a candle jar or incubator with 5% CO_2 awaiting expeditious transport to the laboratory.

TREATMENT

Anogenital and Pharyngeal Infection

The factors to consider in the treatment of uncomplicated anogenital gonococcal infection are (1) the incidence in many urban areas of resistant strains of *N. gonorrhoeae,* (2) the availability of effective single-dose agents against *N. gonorrhoeae,* (3) the coexistence of chlamydial infection in up to 50% of patients, and (4) the absence of a rapid, reliable, inexpensive means of making the diagnosis of *C. trachomatis.*[134] With these in mind, patients with gonococcal infections should be treated with regimens effective against both pathogens. The CDC has recently updated their recommendations.[135] For pregnant women, ceftriaxone plus erythromycin is suggested (Table 72-8). Ceftriaxone has a long serum half-life, is effective against PPNG and CMRNG, and is effective in both anogenital and pharyngeal infections.

Alternatives to ceftriaxone for the pregnant patient include spectinomycin, cefuroxime, cefotaxime, and ceftizoxime. Spectinomycin is the preferred alternative because it is covers resistant strains of *N. gonorrhoeae;* unfortunately, it is ineffective against pharyngeal infection. Both doxycycline and the quinolones are contraindicated during pregnancy because of their effects on the fetus. In women who develop gastrointestinal complaints with erythromycin, a reduced dose may be given for 14 days.

The incidence of treatment failure among those treated with ceftriaxone/doxycycline is extremely rare, obviating the need for test-of-cure cultures for *N. gonorrhoeae.* These women should be tested for reinfection in 2 to 3 months. Women undergoing other treatment regimens should have follow-up cultures performed 7 to 14 days after completion of therapy. These cultures should be obtained from the rectum as well as the cervix, because 25% of female treatment failures harbor organisms only in the rectum. Any gonococcal isolate recovered after treatment failure should be tested for antibiotic sensitivity, because the incidence of resistance is high. These patients should be treated with a single dose of ceftriaxone.

All women diagnosed with gonorrhea should undergo serologic testing for syphilis, be offered confidential counseling and testing for HIV infection, and have a Papanicolaou (Pap) smear 6 weeks following completion of treatment to screen for cervical dysplasia and carcinoma.

TABLE 72–8. CENTERS FOR DISEASE CONTROL 1989 RECOMMENDED TREATMENT GUIDELINES FOR UNCOMPLICATED ANOGENITAL GONORRHEA DURING PREGNANCY

Recommended Regimen
Ceftriaxone 250 mg intramuscularly once
plus
Erythromycin 500 mg orally 4 times daily for 7 days
or
Erythromycin ethylsuccinate 800 mg orally 4 times a day for 7 days
Alternatives to Ceftriaxone
Spectinomycin 2 g intramuscularly once
Cefuroxime axetil 1 g orally once with probenecid 1 g orally
Cefotaxime 1 g intramuscularly once
Ceftizoxime 500 mg intramuscularly once

TABLE 72–9. CENTERS FOR DISEASE CONTROL 1989 RECOMMENDED TREATMENT GUIDELINES FOR DISSEMINATED GONOCOCCAL INFECTION DURING PREGNANCY

Recommended Inpatient Regimens
Ceftriaxone 1 g IM or IV every 24 hrs
or
Ceftizoxime 1 g IV every 8 hrs
or
Cefotaxime 1 g IV every 8 hrs
or
Spectinomycin 2 g IM every 12 hrs
or
Ampicillin 1 g IV every 6 hrs, for strains known to be penicillin-sensitive
Recommended Ambulatory Follow-up Regimens
Cefuroxime axetil 500 mg orally 2 times daily
or
Amoxicillin 500 mg plus clavulanic acid orally 3 times daily

Extragenital Disseminated Infection

Inpatient treatment is advisable for patients with DGI, particularly those with endocarditis, meningitis, synovial effusions, or compliance problems. CDC recommendations for treatment include ceftriaxone, ceftizoxime, cefotaxime, or spectinomycin (Table 72-9).[135] Once an organism has been shown to be sensitive to penicillin, treatment may be changed to ampicillin. Inpatient treatment should continue until 48 hours following resolution of all symptoms. Therapy should continue on an outpatient basis in compliant patients to complete a week's course of antibiotics. Although the value of continued inpatient observation of pregnant patients to reduce the risk of adverse perinatal outcomes has not been demonstrated, it may be advisable.

The treatment of meningitis and endocarditis infections due to *N. gonorrhoeae* involves high-dose intravenous treatment with ceftriaxone (1 to 2 g every 12 hours) for 2 and 4 weeks, respectively.

PREVENTION

Efforts to reduce the incidence of gonococcal infections rest with screening programs to identify asymptomatic cases; careful tracing of the sexual contacts of infected persons; rapid, adequate treatment strategies; education in safe sexual practices; and the neonatal use of prophylactic silver nitrate ointment or eyedrops containing either erythromycin or tetracycline.

SYPHILIS

Syphilis is a chronic, debilitating systemic infection, characterized by infrequent but severe and varied exacerbations, caused by the spirochete *Treponema palli-*

dum. This infection has played a fascinating role in history during the last four centuries. Pre-antibiotic era autopsy studies have shown that 5% to 10% of the general population had evidence of advanced syphilis, while the prevalence among those of low socioeconomic status was 25%.[136–138]

When untreated, the natural history of this infection may encompass several decades. Two major stages are designated, early and late, and each of these is further separated. The phases of early syphilis are incubating, primary, secondary, and early latent. Late syphilis progresses from late latent to tertiary.

EPIDEMIOLOGY

Globally, there has been a steady decline in the incidence of syphilis since 1960. Both the United States and Europe experienced syphilis epidemics during World War II. Since 1982, there has been an overall reduction in its incidence, which is due primarily to the fear of HIV and use of safer sexual practices in the male homosexual community.[139] Alarmingly, the incidence among inner-city heterosexuals, particularly in New York City, Florida, Texas, and California, has risen since 1987; a disproportionate number of these cases have been in women and have led to a dramatic rise in the prevalence of congenital syphilis.[140–142]

Gestational and congenital syphilis tend to occur in young, nonwhite, unmarried, poor, inner-city dwellers with insufficient antenatal care. The CDC reported that of 437 infants with congenital syphilis born from 1983 to 1985, only 48% had any prenatal care, and of those who had care, the average gestation at first visit was 22 weeks.[140]

PATHOGENESIS

Syphilis is efficiently transmitted during sexual contact, with 60% of partners acquiring the infection after a single sexual encounter.[143] Spirochetes require a break in the integument in order to gain access to the host. Microscopic tears in genital mucosa occur almost universally during sexual intercourse. There follows a mean incubation period of 21 days, with a range of 10 to 90 days. The organism sets up a local infection and eventually disseminates widely via lymphatic drainage. Wherever it lodges, it stimulates an immune response.

CLINICAL MANIFESTATIONS

The manifestations of syphilis are wide ranging, involving nearly every organ system. The degree of clinical expression clearly reflects the immune status of the host. With an intact immune system, 60% of patients remain in the latent phase. Among patients coinfected with HIV, however, early syphilis can be life-threatening.

Primary

The first sign of primary infection is the development of a single, nontender lesion at the site of entry. The most customary sites of infection in the female include the vulva, introitus, or cervix. Extragenital sites include the lips, tongue, tonsils, breasts, and fingers. The lesion is a painless, dull red macule, which becomes a papule and then ulcerates. Ulcers are rounded with a well-defined margin and a rubbery, indurated, weeping base. The ulcer persists for 3 to 6 weeks without treatment and then heals spontaneously.

Painless unilateral or bilateral inguinal lymphadenopathy often develops a week after the appearance of the lesion. Nodes are small, rubbery and nonsuppurative. Worth noting is that both ulcers and lymph nodes may become tender in the face of secondary infection.

Secondary

The symptoms of secondary syphilis typically emerge 3 to 6 weeks later. By this time, the infection is widely disseminated and most symptoms are due to immune complex deposition. Nonspecific complaints include fever, malaise, sore throat, headache, musculoskeletal pains, and weight loss.

A classic faint macular rash develops over the trunk and flexor surfaces in the vast majority of infected individuals. Its lesions are pink, rounded, and ordinarily less than 1 cm in diameter. The rash spreads over the whole body, including the palms and soles, and becomes first dull red and papular, then squamous. Superficial ulcerations called mucous patches appear in the mucous membranes in 30% of patients. Also, generalized lymphadenopathy is present in the majority.

Less than 10% of patients have other manifestations. They include arthritis, bursitis, osteitis,[144] hepatitis,[145–147] glomerulonephritis,[148–150] gastritis,[145] hypersplenism, and iritis.[137]

Latent

By definition, this stage lacks clinical manifestations. The early latent phase (<1 year) has been associated with recurrence of secondary mucocutaneous lesions, and these lesions are infectious. Although late latent syphilis (>1 year) cannot be transmitted sexually, vertical transmission persists.

Tertiary

In the absence of appropriate treatment, one third of patients develop tertiary syphilis. This is characterized by involvement of the cardiovascular, central nervous, or musculoskeletal systems. The presence of gummas in various tissues designate late benign tertiary syphilis. Aortic aneurysms and aortic insufficiency are characteristic cardiovascular lesions, while generalized paresis, tabes dorsalis, and optic atrophy with the Argyll Robertson pupil that accommodates but does not react to light are all features of neurosyphilis.

LABORATORY DIAGNOSIS

The gold standard for diagnosis of early syphilis is the detection of treponemes on dark-field examination of ulcer scrapings or tissue samples. It is inexpensive and easy, and provides immediate results. The reliability of this test is proportional to the skill of the person performing it. The lesion should be cleansed thoroughly with saline and scraped firmly to collect serum. If no spirochetes are apparent, the test should be repeated twice to increase sensitivity. Although a positive test is diagnostic, a negative one does not preclude the possibility of infection.

Indirect diagnosis of syphilis can be made with the use of two types of serologic tests. Nontreponemal tests such as the Venereal Disease Research Laboratory (VDRL), which has been available since 1943, and rapid plasma reagin (RPR) become reactive approximately 2 weeks following development of the initial lesion. Both measure anticardiolipin antibody. The VDRL is positive in 50% to 70% of patients with primary syphilis.[151] If more than one specimen has been drawn, a rising titer is also evidence of primary infection. In secondary syphilis, the VDRL titer is usually ≥1:16. Following successful treatment, the VDRL should decrease fourfold in 3 months and eightfold in 6 months. It should be nonreactive 1 year after therapy for primary infection, and 2 years for secondary disease.

Treponemal tests include the fluorescent treponemal antibody absorbed (FTA-ABS) and microhemagglutination assay for antibody to *T. pallidum* (MHA-TP). More sensitive (70% to 90%) than nontreponemal tests, these tests become reactive at about the same time as the primary lesion develops and are used to confirm the serologic diagnosis of syphilis.[152] Unfortunately, these tests remain positive for life.

The diagnosis of latent syphilis is made on the basis of two elevated nontreponemal serologic tests taken at least 1 year apart. A further diagnostic work-up includes evaluation of the cerebrospinal fluid (CSF) and a chest radiograph to screen for calcification of the ascending aorta.

The diagnosis of neurosyphilis is challenging, because no one test is reliable. The CSF should be tested for cell count, protein, and VDRL. An elevated count of >5 white blood cells (WBC) per mm^3 is a relatively sensitive indicator of active infection. A positive CSF VDRL is diagnostic for neurosyphilis. Alternatively, a negative result cannot be used to rule out syphilis. In such cases, an FTA-ABS may be ordered; although less specific, it is highly sensitive, meaning that a negative result rules out the diagnosis of syphilis.

TREATMENT

In 1943, penicillin was found to be effective in treating syphilis. To date, no resistance has developed. The goal in therapy is to provide continuous, low-level concentrations of penicillin in infected tissues. It is still the preferred drug in gestational and congenital syphilis, as well as neurosyphilis, despite concern over its level of CNS penetration. Women with history of a penicillin allergy should undergo skin testing to validate the sensitivity, and proceed with desensitization and penicillin therapy for optimal results.[153,154]

Treatment regimens in pregnancy are listed in Table 72-10. Alternative regimens in non-pregnant patients include tetracycline and doxycycline, both contraindicated during pregnancy. Erythromycin carries a high risk of treatment inadequately in the fetus, with risk for congenital infection.[140,155–159]

The Jarisch-Herxheimer reaction is an acute reaction, apparently provoked by the release of prostaglandins during the initiation of treatment for primary or secondary infection.[160] The reaction must be differentiated from penicillin allergy. It occurs within 24 hours of receiving the first dose of antibiotic, and is characterized by fever, malaise, headache, musculoskeletal pain, nausea, tachycardia, and exacerbation of skin lesions. Although the reaction is more common in primary disease, its symptoms are more severe with secondary. Fluids and antipyretics are recommended for symptomatic relief. Pregnant women are at risk for preterm labor and intrauterine fetal demise (IUFD).

MATERNAL AND FETAL RISKS

Pregnancy does not appear to alter the course of syphilis; however, *T. pallidum* adversely affects pregnancy. It crosses the placenta and has been associated with preterm delivery, stillbirth, congenital infection, and neonatal death, depending on the timing of infection. The majority of infants with congenital syphilis are born to mothers with early syphilis, particularly recent or current secondary infection. Fetal infection during the first and second trimesters carries significant morbidity, while third trimester exposure results in asymptomatic infection.[161]

TABLE 72-10. CENTERS FOR DISEASE CONTROL 1989 RECOMMENDED TREATMENT GUIDELINES FOR SYPHILIS IN PREGNANCY

Early Syphilis Recommended Regimen
Benzathine penicillin G 2.4 million units IM once (1.2 million units in each buttock)
Late Latent, Gummas, and Cardiovascular Syphilis Recommended Regimen
Benzathine penicillin G 7.2 million units total administered as three doses of 2.4 million units IM given 1 week apart for 3 consecutive weeks
Neurosyphilis Recommended Regimen
Aqueous crystalline penicillin G 12–24 million units administered 2–4 million units IV every 4 hours for 10–14 days
Neurosyphilis Alternative Regimens
Procaine penicillin 2–4 million units IM daily *with* Probenecid 500 mg orally 4 times daily, both for 10–14 days

Infants with early congenital syphilis are usually asymptomatic at birth, but develop symptoms at 10 to 14 days of life. A maculopapular rash arises and often desquamates or becomes vesicular. Many develop a flu-like syndrome with a copious nasal discharge, commonly referred to as "snuffles." Other symptoms include oropharyngeal mucous patches, lymphadenopathy, hepatosplenomegaly, jaundice, osteochondritis, iritis, and chorioretinitis.[162,163] Untreated early congenital syphilis progresses to the late phase, marked by Hutchinson teeth, mulberry molars, deafness, saddle nose, saber shins, mental retardation, hydrocephalus, general paresis, and optic nerve atrophy.

Pregnant women undergoing treatment for syphilis are at minimal risk for IUFD. Those who develop Jarisch-Herxheimer reactions are at increased risk for preterm labor.

PREVENTION

As noted above, the accessibility of early and complete antenatal care with routine screening and adequate treatment for this infection is critical for prevention.

Careful post-treatment follow-up is essential for controlling the spread of syphilis. Treatment failure is difficult to distinguish from reinfection. Patients should be examined and serologically tested at 3 and 6 months. If signs and symptoms persist or if nontreponemal antibody tests have not fallen appropriately after appropriate therapy, patients should undergo evaluation of their CSF and be retreated as warranted.

Partner tracing is particularly important in syphilis, given its prolonged course and multiple asymptomatic phases. In women with primary syphilis, all partners in the last 3 months should be evaluated; this time period should extend to 12 months for those diagnosed with secondary syphilis.

All patients with syphilis should be screened for other STDs, including confidential counseling and testing for HIV. Patients with coexistent HIV infection should be evaluated more frequently, and treated for neurosyphilis in the event of any signs of persistent infection.

CHLAMYDIAL INFECTIONS

Chlamydia trachomatis is probably the most frequently diagnosed sexually transmitted disease in the United States today,[164] with an estimated prevalence of over 4 million cases,[165–168] and an annual cost of over $1 billion.[169] Lower genital tract infection predisposes in non-pregnant women to pelvic inflammatory disease (PID) and in pregnant women to a variety of maternal and neonatal infections.

EPIDEMIOLOGY

C. trachomatis is the causative agent of trachoma, perhaps the leading preventable cause of blindness in the developing world.[170] In the United States, *C. trachomatis* is most frequently manifested as genital tract infections in the adult and inclusion conjunctivitis and pneumonia in the neonate.

It has been estimated that between 20% and 40% of sexually active women in the United States have been exposed to *C. trachomatis*. Cervical infection rates range from 5.5% to 22.5% of asymptomatic women attending family planning clinics to 34% to 63% of women with mucopurulent cervicitis.[171,172] The prevalence among pregnant women depends on the population sampled, varying from 2% to 37%.[173–181]

Chlamydial infections tend to occur in women at high risk for other STDs, with infection rates proportional to the number of sexual partners[182,183] and inversely proportional to age.[182,184] Risk markers in pregnant women include age <20 years, unmarried status, low socioeconomic status, residence in inner cities, late presentation for prenatal care, the presence of other STDs, and the findings of mucopurulent endocervicitis or bacteriuric pyuria.[182,184–186] The greatest risk factor is sexual contact with men with nongonococcal urethritis.[185,187–189] Up to two thirds of women with cervical chlamydial infection are asymptomatic, creating a large reservoir for both horizontal and vertical transmission.[184]

PATHOGENESIS

There are 15 recognized serotypes of *C. trachomatis*, eight of which appear to cause oculogenital infection.[182] The organism is classified as an obligate intracellular bacterium, requiring viable columnar or pseudostratified columnar epithelial cells for survival and multiplication. The bacterium has an interesting life cycle: the elementary body (EB) is the form of the organism capable of infecting cells, while the reticulate body (RB) is the metabolically active, multiplying form responsible for producing the characteristic inclusions.

CLINICAL MANIFESTATIONS

The incubation period for genital chlamydial infections ranges from 6 to 14 days. A variety of clinical manifestations, from bartholinitis to PID with peritonitis and perihepatitis, have been described. The most common perinatal syndromes are briefly described below.

Endocervicitis

The most commonly infected site in the female genital tract is the endocervix. As mentioned above, the majority of infected women are asymptomatic. Findings on physical examination extend from normal to cervical erosion and mucopurulent cervicitis (MPC). Requisite components of the diagnosis of MPC include endocervical friability; erythema or edema; the presence of yellow or green endocervical mucopus; and >10 polymorphonuclear leukocytes (PMNs) per high-power field of a cervical Gram's stain.

Acute Urethral Syndrome

Chlamydial infection has also been implicated in the etiology of 25% of patients with acute urethral syndrome. Such women present with dysuria and increased urinary frequency in the face of sterile urine or low level bacteriuria. Also, many report oral contraceptive use, recent contact with a new sexual partner, and a prolonged symptom duration of up to 14 days.[190] Although *C. trachomatis* can sometimes be cultured from the urethra, it is more frequently recovered from the endocervix of these patients.

Endometritis

It has been well established that the incidence of postabortion endometritis is higher among women with chlamydial cervicitis.[191–195] Because up to 35% of women with chlamydial cervical infection who undergo elective termination develop endometritis, antibiotic prophylaxis is recommended for high-risk women.

The association between chlamydial infection and postpartum endometritis is more controversial. Although some authors have found such an association,[196–199] others have not.[200–202] The answer to this question awaits further prospective, well-controlled studies.

Acute Pelvic Inflammatory Disease

The association between maternal lower genital tract *C. trachomatis* infection, neonatal inclusion conjunctivitis, and the subsequent development of postpartum pelvic inflammatory disease (PID) has been recognized for over half a century.[203] Chlamydial PID can also occur during pregnancy, although its incidence appears to be extremely rare.[204–210] Pregnancy confounds the diagnosis, given the frequency of adverse gastrointestinal complaints and a physiologic leukocytosis among normal pregnant women, and the low prevalence of gestational PID. Because the rate of fetal wastage approximates 50% in pregnancies complicated by PID, prompt administration of appropriate broad-spectrum antibiotic coverage should be initiated once the diagnosis has been entertained.[211]

MATERNAL AND FETAL RISKS

Vertical transmission rates secondary to passage through an infected cervix are as high as 60% to 70%.[171,185,187,212] Inclusion conjunctivitis develops during the first 2 weeks of life in 25% to 50% of these neonates, while another 10% to 20% will develop chlamydial pneumonia within 4 months of birth. Although the use of erythromycin eye prophylaxis has markedly decreased the incidence of conjunctivitis, this topical preparation has no protection against pneumonia.

The role of endocervical *C. trachomatis* infection in the development of spontaneous abortion, fetal death, premature rupture of the membranes (PROM), preterm delivery (PTD), and intrauterine growth retardation is hotly debated. A strong association between spontaneous abortion, preterm delivery, and perinatal mortality was noted by Martin and associates.[178] These contentions have remained unsubstantiated in subsequent larger studies by numerous authors.[200,201,213,214] Interestingly, however, both Harrison and colleagues[201] and Sweet and associates[202] have identified a subgroup of pregnant women with chlamydial infection, those with IgM seropositivity, who may be at increased risk for PROM and preterm delivery. One recent retrospective study compared the pregnancy outcomes of women with chlamydial infection who underwent successful treatment with both untreated infected and non-infected women and found a higher incidence of PROM and PTD in the untreated infected group.[215] Well-designed, placebo-controlled prospective studies are needed to further our understanding of this issue.

LABORATORY DIAGNOSIS

Culture remains the optimal means of making the diagnosis of chlamydial infection. Isolation of *C. trachomatis* remains challenging, because the organism requires a susceptible tissue culture cell line. The McCoy cell is most commonly employed, using a technically arduous procedure whereby these cells are inoculated with specimen and then examined 24 to 72 hours later for the development of inclusions. Recent improvements that have increased the sensitivity of culture include the performance of a second passage for specimens initially negative, and the use of a cytobrush for sample collection.[168]

Two chlamydial antigen detection products have become available recently. One uses fluorescent monoclonal antibody staining of chlamydial EBs (MicrotracSyva Company, Palo Alto, CA), and the other is an enzyme-linked immunosorbent assay (ELISA) (Chlamydiazyme, Abbott Laboratories, Chicago, IL). The sensitivities and specificities of both products are comparable at over 90%.[216–222] Their most appropriate use is in populations with a high prevalence of chlamydial infection, because their positive predictive value decreases markedly in low-prevalence populations.

Two common diagnostic techniques have little applicability in chlamydial infection. Cytology has both poor sensitivity and specificity, and serologic testing is hampered by the high proportion of previous exposure among sexually active women.[223,224] However, those with high levels of IgM can be considered to have had a recent infection. The microimmunofluorescent (Micro-IF) test is relatively sensitive and differentiates between IgG and IgM, although its use is primarily reserved for research.

TREATMENT

The optimal treatment for uncomplicated chlamydial infection during pregnancy remains debatable. The CDC recommends erythromycin base or ethylsuccinate, given its good performance in multiple treatment trials, and reserves amoxicillin, which has been shown in limited trials to reduce vertical transmission, for an alternative regimen (Table 72-11).[225,226] Erythromycin estolate can cause hepatotoxicity and is thus contraindicated during pregnancy.

PREVENTION

The risks of vertical transmission to newborns, horizontal transmission to sexual partners, and possible adverse perinatal outcomes underscore the need for large-scale screening programs to detect and eradicate cervical chlamydial infections. The CDC recommends diagnostic testing for *C. trachomatis* at the first prenatal visit and, for those at high risk for contracting this infection, again during the third trimester. Finally, as with other STDs, it is important to emphasize the importance of partner screening and treatment, as well as education about safe sexual practices to avert reinfection.

HUMAN PAPILLOMA VIRUS

Among women in the United States today, genital warts caused by human papilloma virus (HPV) is the most common viral STD. Difficulties in deciphering the molecular biology of HPV slowed our progress in understanding of this infection. Since the 1970s, however, the association of HPV with genital intraepithelial neoplasias and squamous cell carcinomas has been publicized widely, resulting in an increased public awareness of the problem.

EPIDEMIOLOGY

Sexual transmission of venereal warts results in urogenital and anorectal lesions. The highest risk groups are sexually active teenagers and young adults. Transmission rates are high, with 65% of sexual contacts becoming infected.[227] Although sexual transmission predominates, vertical transmission can occur, particularly with HPV types 6 and 11.

Because of extensive publicity about this infection and its association with genital cancers, there has been a significant increase in outpatient visits for this complaint. Estimates of its prevalence range from 2% to 20% depending on the population studied and the means used to identify infection.[228–232] Host immunity plays an important role in development of this infection. Immunosuppressed patients, such as renal transplant recipients and pregnant women, have a higher incidence of genital warts and their symptoms are more severe.[233]

TABLE 72–11. CENTERS FOR DISEASE CONTROL 1989 RECOMMENDED TREATMENT GUIDELINES FOR CHLAMYDIAL INFECTIONS IN PREGNANCY

Recommended Regimen
Erythromycin base 500 mg orally 4 times a day for 7 days
Alternative Regimens
Erythromycin base 250 mg orally 4 times a day for 14 days
or
Erythromycin ethylsuccinate 800 mg orally 4 times a day for 7 days
or
Erythromycin ethylsuccinate 400 mg orally 4 times a day for 14 days
or, if erythromycin cannot be tolerated,
Amoxicillin 500 mg orally 3 times a day for 7 days (limited data)

PATHOGENESIS

HPV is a member of the papovavirus family, and is composed of double-stranded DNA. Over 50 types have been identified. The HPV type correlates with site of infection and virulence; types 6 and 11 are associated with condyloma accuminata,[234–237] while types 16 and 18 are strongly associated with cervical and vulvar carcinomas.[243,235,238,239]

CLINICAL MANIFESTATIONS

The majority of HPV lesions are subclinical, identified only with the use of colposcopy, cytology, tissue examination, or in situ hybridization techniques. They can be found on the vulva, vagina, cervix, and anorectal region. Exophytic warts, also called condyloma acuminata, are typically caused by HPV types 6 and 11. They appear as friable, pink, fleshy skin appendages that vary greatly in size and are either broad based or pedunculated. Many lesions, however, are not visible to the naked eye. These flat endophytic condylomata are found with the use of colposcopy on the cervix, vagina, and vulva.

Colposcopy uses a lighted, magnification system to view genital epithelium. A 3% to 5% solution of acetic acid is applied to the area to be examined and allowed to absorb. Common colposcopic findings in HPV infection are irregularly defined patches that appear shiny and white and are not confined to the transformation zone. Any suspicious lesion should be biopsied.

LABORATORY DIAGNOSIS

The diagnosis of condyloma acuminata is usually made on clinical grounds. Given the high prevalence of subclinical disease, cytology, tissue biopsy, and in situ hybridization techniques are often necessary to make the diagnosis.

In the least sensitive of laboratory methods available to us, cytologic evidence in the form of koilocytosis has been found in approximately 2% of women receiving Pap smears.[228] Cervical biopsies tested for both koilocytosis and HPV antigen found that 20% were positive by both methods.[230] To date, the most sensitive detection method for HPV is DNA in situ hybridization. One study tested routine Pap smears using this technique and found that 16% had evidence of HPV types 6, 11, 16, or 18.[231] Although there appears to be a strong association between HPV and abnormal cervical cytology,[231,232] one worrisome study of 3000 cytologically normal smears found that 5% or more carried the DNA for HPV types 16 or 18.[234] Although these HPV-DNA tests are now widely available, their clinical usefulness has not been established.

Biopsy to rule out dysplasia and other pathology should be used liberally to evaluate any lesion that appears atypical, pigmented, or persists despite treatment. Histologic evidence of HPV infection includes koilocytosis, occasional normal-appearing mitotic figures, epidermal hyperplasia and parakeratosis, and prominent microvasculature. Two findings are peculiar to HPV infection: asperites, tiny spicules only visible with magnification,[240] and reverse punctation, minute slightly-raised white dots.[241]

TREATMENT

The most critical concept in HPV treatment is that none of our currently used regimens eradicates the virus. Remedies that are expensive, toxic, or scarring are of no known benefit to patients. Thus, therapy must be aimed at the removal of visible or dysplastic warts and symptomatic improvement.

External Genital and Perianal Warts

Cryotherapy using liquid nitrogen or a cryoprobe is preferred in the treatment of external genital and perianal warts (Table 72-12). Topical application of trichloroacetic acid (TCA) and electrodessication or electrocautery are recommended as alternatives. These remedies are inexpensive, nontoxic and, when used correctly, do not harm normal surrounding tissue. TCA should be applied only to warts and unreacted acid should be removed by powdering the affected area with talc or sodium bicarbonate (baking soda). This procedure may be repeated weekly. The use of podophyllin is contraindicated in pregnancy. Electrodessication cannot be used in patients with cardiac pacemakers, or on lesions proximal to the anal verge. The carbon dioxide laser is most useful in patients with extensive lesions.

Cervical Warts

For women with cervical warts, dysplasia must be ruled out as discussed above. Cryotherapy, laser, and surgical approaches must be carried out in consultation with someone trained in the treatment of dysplasia.

TABLE 72–12. CENTERS FOR DISEASE CONTROL 1989 RECOMMENDED TREATMENT GUIDELINES FOR HPV IN PREGNANCY

External Genital or Perianal Warts

Recommended Regimen
Cryotherapy with liquid nitrogen or cryoprobe

Alternative Regimens
Trichloroacetic acid (TCA) (80%–90%): Applied to warts weekly.

or

Electrodessication/electrocautery

Cervical Warts

Dysplasia must be ruled out prior to the institution of any therapy. Treatment should be performed with the aid of one trained in the treatment of dysplasia.

Vaginal or Anal Warts

Recommended Regimen
Cryotherapy with liquid nitrogen

Alternative Regimen
TCA as above

Vaginal and Anal Warts

Warty lesions in the vagina and anus can be treated using liquid nitrogen cryotherapy. The use of a cryoprobe for vaginal lesions is not recommended. The only alternative during pregnancy is TCA, using the same technique as for external lesions. Extensive or persistent lesions should be treated by an expert.

MATERNAL AND FETAL RISKS

Warty lesions have a tendency to grow and become more vascularized during pregnancy. The only contraindications to a vaginal delivery are extensive lesions that might result in dystocia and lesions that might bleed heavily with birth trauma. Although some suggest removal of large warts during pregnancy, this practice is of uncertain benefit. Vertical transmission of HPV is rare, but can result in respiratory papillomatosis in the exposed infant. The exact mode of spread is unknown.

PREVENTION

Given the fact that transmission rates are low, and adverse perinatal outcome unknown, it is not recommended that pregnant patients be routinely screened for HPV. Sex partners of infected women should be examined for the presence of warts, and those infected should be schooled in safe sexual practices to avoid transmission to uninfected partners.

HERPES SIMPLEX VIRUS

Genital herpes is an infection caused by sexual transmission of herpes simplex virus types 1 and 2 (HSV-1 and HSV-2).

EPIDEMIOLOGY

The prevalence of genital herpes in the obstetric population has been estimated at 0.1% to 4%.[242–245] The incidence of HSV infection rose sharply between 1966 and 1979,[246] with a concomitant rise in the incidence of neonatal herpes infections.[247] Risk markers for herpes describe a population much different from the ones at risk for other STDs; this infection tends to occur in older, well educated, married white individuals.

Efforts have been made to identify those women at high risk for vertical transmission. Although primary maternal HSV bestows the highest risk for perinatal infection, it has been noted that 70% of neonates with severe HSV infection are born to mothers with asymptomatic disease.[248] The risk of contracting neonatal herpes from an asymptomatic mother with a history of recurrent genital HSV appears to be less than 1:1000. The targeting of this population has proven difficult, leading to the current opinion that neonatal exposure to asymptomatic maternal HSV infection is neither predictable nor preventable.[249]

PATHOGENESIS

The majority of genital herpetic infections are caused by HSV-2, although up to 15% may be due to HSV-1.[250,251] HSV is a double-stranded DNA virus that infects susceptible mucosal surfaces. It has an incubation period of 2 to 10 days, which is followed by a primary infection characterized by focal vesicle formation and a pronounced cellular immune response. The infection enters a latent phase, with the virus ascending peripheral sensory nerves and coming to rest in nerve root ganglia. Recurrent exacerbations occur intermittently, stimulated by poorly understood mechanisms.

CLINICAL MANIFESTATIONS

There are three types of herpetic episodes. Primary infections occur in previously unexposed hosts, and are characterized by multiple painful vesicular lesions that ulcerate, with inguinal lymphadenopathy, and flu-like symptoms including fever, malaise, nausea, headaches, and myalgias. Symptoms usually persist for about 2 weeks, with viral shedding for about 12 days. Nearly 4% will progress to viral meningitis.[250]

First episode nonprimary genital herpes occurs in an individual with previous nongenital exposure to HSV-1 or HSV-2. Its presentation is generally much milder than primary infections.

Recurrent HSV is more frequent following HSV-2 infection. Approximately one half of infected individuals will experience a recurrence within 6 months.[252] Most of these episodes are prefaced by a 1- or 2-day prodrome consisting of localized pruritus, pain, and paresthesias. Systemic manifestations are absent. The episode usually lasts about half as long as the primary outbreak, with only 4 to 5 days of viral shedding.

LABORATORY DIAGNOSIS

The diagnosis can be made using a number of laboratory techniques. Culture remains the gold standard. Results are typically available within 72 hours. Its sensitivity ranges from 70% to 95%, and is highest early in the course of primary infection.[253]

Until recently, the collection of weekly viral cultures late in the third trimester from women with a history of herpes was advocated. A number of well-designed studies proved that these cultures failed both to predict maternal viral shedding at delivery and to prevent neonatal infection.[254–256]

Although classic findings of intranuclear inclusions and multinucleated giant cells can be found on Pap smear, its sensitivity in HSV infection is only about 50%.[250]

Monoclonal antibody testing compares well with culture in high prevalence populations, although the positive predictive value falls as the HSV prevalence falls.[257] For this reason, culture is still preferred. ELISAs are not recommended for the same reason, although further testing is indicated.[258]

MATERNAL AND FETAL RISKS

Maternal HSV infection does not seem to confer any deleterious effect on pregnancy itself. The infection may be vertically transmitted, however, either transplacentally or perinatally. Fortunately, transplacental transmission is rare. Neonatal symptoms typically arise during the first 7 days of life. The infection is characterized by vesicular skin lesions and CNS abnormalities such as microcephaly, hydranencephaly, and microphthalmia. Death occurs in approximately one third of infants, and neurologic sequelae are noted in most survivors.[259] Perinatal acquisition occurs either with passage through an infected birth canal or from contact with orolabial lesions in the parents or hospital workers.[260]

Infectivity appears to be enhanced during maternal primary infection.[261,262] Also, the severity of perinatal morbidity is worsened in primary maternal infection; spontaneous abortion secondary to herpetic chorioamnionitis, preterm delivery, intrauterine growth retardation, neonatal infection, and death have all been described.[262]

Because weekly maternal vaginal cultures in the third trimester do not predict viral shedding at the time of delivery, they are no longer indicated. The Infectious Disease Society for Obstetrics and Gynecology developed a position paper on the peripartum management of women with a history of HSV.[263] They made the following suggestions:

Weekly antenatal cultures should be abandoned.
In the absence of genital lesions, cesarean sections should be performed for obstetric considerations only.
A culture should be obtained from mother or neonate at delivery in order to identify exposed infants.
Women with genital lesions should undergo cesarean section, preferably within 6 hours of membrane rupture, to prevent HSV exposure in the neonate.
The mother should not be isolated from her infant.

Limited experience with active herpetic lesions in the face of preterm premature ruptured membranes suggest that expectant management may be successful.

TREATMENT

Because there is no known cure for this virus, HSV becomes a chronic and usually recurrent infection. Acyclovir (Zovirax) is an antiviral agent that inhibits viral DNA synthesis. It has been shown to ameliorate the symptoms of primary infections, and when given prophylactically, may reduce the frequency and intensity of recurrences.

The drug is available in three forms: topical, oral, and intravenous. The oral preparation is considerably more effective than its topical counterpart. Oral acyclovir is recommended by the CDC for primary genital herpes.[264] Intravenous treatment should be reserved for severe infection or immunocompromised hosts.

The safety of acyclovir in pregnancy has not been fully established. However, experience to date has not identified adverse fetal effects. In nonpregnant patients oral acyclovir has safely been used to suppress severe recurrent HSV for up to 3 years.

PREVENTION

As with other STDs, the use of safe sexual practices is essential in the control of genital herpes spread.

TRICHOMONAS VAGINALIS

Trichomoniasis is a localized genitourinary infection caused by the protozoon *Trichomonas vaginalis*. It was first described in 1836 by Donne as a nonpathogenic resident of the genital tract.[265] Its pathogenicity was recognized during the early part of this century in a novel set of experiments in which healthy male and female volunteers were inoculated with organisms and followed to described the natural history of the infection.[266,267]

One of the most prevalent parasites in humans, it has been found in nearly 10% of healthy women and up to 50% of patients screened at STD clinics. It has been estimated that 2 to 3 million women in the United States contract the infection annually.[268]

EPIDEMIOLOGY

Sexual contact is the primary mode of transmission for *T. vaginalis*, although the infection can be passed from mother to female infants during vaginal delivery.

Because trichomoniasis is not a reportable infection, its epidemiology is difficult to ascertain. Screening studies comparing various populations have discerned that prevalence parallels degree of sexual activity: 5% of women who attend family planning clinics; 13% to 25% from gynecology clinics; and 50% to 75% of prostitutes.[268,269] As might be expected, barrier contraception has a protective effect, as do oral contraceptives.[269]

It appears that asymptomatic infected men may serve as reservoirs for their female partners. Although only 30% to 40% of male partners of infected women carried *T. vaginalis*, it was recovered in 85% of female partners of infected men.[270] Finally, carriage of this STD is a risk marker for other STDs, especially gonorrhea, which is 1.4 to 3 times more frequent among women with trichomoniasis.[269,271]

PATHOGENESIS

T. vaginalis is an oval-shaped, moderately anaerobic protozoon. The presence of four flagellae and an undulating membrane render it motile. Multiple serotypes, which may correlate with virulence, have been identified. The parasite attaches to mucous membranes, but neither enters nor kills the cells. Instead, it induces a moderate cellular immune response.

CLINICAL MANIFESTATIONS

It appears that this pathogen confines itself to the genitourinary system. Although most men are asymptomatic, anywhere from 50% to 90% of infected women will become symptomatic at some time. Host factors, such as vaginal pH, circulating hormonal levels, the integrity of the normal vaginal flora, and the presence of menstrual blood, appear to play important roles in the development of symptoms. In most women, symptoms materialize shortly following menstruation.[272]

An abnormal vaginal discharge is noted by 50% to 75% of symptomatic women. In only 10% of these women is the exudate malodorous. Pruritus, dysuria, and dyspareunia are experienced in up to half of them. Low abdominal pain and lymphadenitis are relatively uncommon complaints.[270,273,274]

Physical examination findings will be normal in 15% of infected patients. Vaginal erythema and an excessive vaginal discharge is present in up to 75%, while vulvar inflammation is much less common. The so-called "classic" findings of a yellowish-green frothy discharge and strawberry cervix are relatively uncommon, seen in 25% and 2%, respectively.[275]

LABORATORY DIAGNOSIS

Because clinical manifestations are so nonspecific, the clinician must rely on laboratory parameters to make the diagnosis. The vaginal pH is ≥4.5 in the majority of patients. Performance of a Pap smear makes the diagnosis nearly 70% of the time.[269,274,276]

Collection of a sample of vaginal discharge for wet mount or culture is the diagnostic procedure of choice. Because the organism attaches only to squamous cells, evaluation of the endocervical columnar epithelium is positive in only 13% of women. A cotton swab should be used to wipe both anterior and posterior fornices. In the preparation of a wet mount, the swab should then be rubbed across a slide containing a drop of sodium chloride and immediately overlaid with a cover slip. Low to medium (100 to 400×) magnification with a light or dark field microscope should be used to examine the material. Large numbers of PMNs are generally present. The organisms can be seen as motile ovoids that appear slightly larger than PMNs. The sensitivity of the wet mount ranges between 40% and 80%, matching that of the Pap smear.[269,275,277–279] Anaerobic culture, using a number of selective media, promotes growth in 2 to 7 days, and is 95% sensitive.[269,277,280]

T. vaginalis can be isolated from the vagina in 95% of infected women, while recovery from the urethra is possible in only 5%.[281] Rare reports have described the isolation of *T. vaginalis* from kidney and perinephric abscess cultures.[282]

TREATMENT

Until two decades ago, trichomoniasis was a chronic, relapsing urogenital infection. In the 1960s, the 5-nitroimidazoles, including metronidazole, were developed and found to be effective in the treatment of this infection.[283] Recent years have seen the development of isolated clusters of resistant organisms.[284–287]

Given the colonization of both genital and urinary tracts, a systemic agent is needed. The original regimen for metronidazole therapy lasted 7 days. This has been shortened to a single oral dose in order to improve compliance, decrease the total dose, and deal with the problems of alcohol use during treatment (Table 72-13). Cure with this regimen is achieved in 82% to 88%, and this increases to 95% when partners are treated empirically.[288–291] Treatment failures or patients who get reinfected should be given the 7-day alternative regimen of metronidazole.

Metronidazole freely crosses the placenta and has unknown teratogenic potential. Although studies of limited numbers of pregnant women have shown no increased risk of spontaneous abortion or adverse perinatal outcomes,[266,267,292] it is recommended that first trimester use of this drug be avoided. Instead, local symptomatic treatments are advocated at least until the first trimester is completed. Vaginal creams or gentle vinegar douches typically provide some symptomatic relief. Because of the urethral reservoir of organisms, local therapy is rarely curative.

TABLE 72–13. CENTERS FOR DISEASE CONTROL 1989 RECOMMENDED TREATMENT GUIDELINES FOR TRICHOMONIASIS IN PREGNANCY

Recommended Regimen
Metronidazole* 2 g orally in a single dose
Alternative Regimen
Metronidazole* 500 mg twice daily for 7 days

* Metronidazole cannot be recommended for use in the first trimester.

MATERNAL AND FETAL RISKS

Maternal infection with *T. vaginalis* probably results in little or no effect during pregnancy, although at least one study has indirectly associated it with PROM and preterm rupture of the membranes.[293] Approximately 5% of female infants delivered vaginally of infected women will develop trichomoniasis. This manifests as a neonatal or infantile vaginal discharge. Preliminary results from a large collaborative study sponsored by the NIH on the role of vaginal infections in preterm delivery suggest that *T. vaginalis* increases the risk for preterm delivery and PROM (Ronald Gibbs, personal communication).

PREVENTION

Because this infection is sexually transmitted, its diagnosis should serve as a reminder to test carefully for the coexistence of other, more dangerous STDs.

CHANCROID

Chancroid is a localized ulcerative STD, traditionally differentiated from syphilis by its appearance as a "soft" sore. It is often complicated by the appearance of an inguinal bubo. The offending organism is a gram-negative facultative anaerobic bacillus *Haemophilus ducreyi*.

EPIDEMIOLOGY

Worldwide, chancroid is more common than syphilis,[294,295] and in some tropical areas more common than gonorrhea.[396,297] It can be found primarily among uncircumcised heterosexual men of low socioeconomic status who frequent prostitutes.[298,299] The case report ratio of men to women with this disease is 10:1, perhaps because women with chancroid typically have few or no symptoms, and therefore are not evaluated. Its only known route of transmission is sexual contact, and female prostitutes with asymptomatic chancres may serve as a reservoir.

The annual incidence of chancroid fell steadily from 1950 to 1978, at which time there were fewer than 1000 cases reported annually in the United States. During that time, the majority of outbreaks occurred at seaports, or involved isolated cases in travellers returning from the tropics. This decline ended abruptly in 1985 with an epidemic largely confined to large urban areas, most notably New York, Boston, Dallas, and several cities in Florida.[300,301]

Numerous reports from Africa have associated genital ulcers with HIV.[302–305] Among women in Africa and other Third World countries, the presence of genital ulcers appears to be the major risk for heterosexual spread of HIV.

PATHOGENESIS

Penetration of the epidermis by chancroid organisms appears to require prior trauma or fresh abrasions. Multiple strains of the organism exist, with varying levels of virulence. The more virulent strains are resistant to phagocytosis by PMNs and complement-mediated killing by normal serum.[306,307] The host immune response is dynamic, resulting in inguinal lymph node suppuration, leading to the formation of buboes in 50% of patients. The contents of these buboes is viscous pus with sheets of PMNs and rare microorganisms.

CLINICAL MANIFESTATIONS

The normal incubation period for chancroid is 4 to 7 days, with a range of 2 to 10 days. There does not appear to be a prodrome. The chancre appears as a papule surrounded by an erythematous halo. In men, the lesion is usually singular and painful,[308] while in women 4 to 5 painless lesions is the average.[309] Symptoms depend on the location of lesions.[310] Most lesions occur at the entrance to the vagina, including the posterior forchette, labia, vestibule, and clitoris. Less common genital sites include the periurethra, perianus, vagina, and cervix; extragenital lesions on the breasts, fingers, thighs, and mouth, although rare, do occur.

After 24 to 48 hours, the papules become pustular, eroded, and ulcerated, with sharply defined borders and no induration; hence the so-called "soft" chancre. The ulcer base is friable, granulomatous, and usually covered by a gray or yellow necrotic exudate. Without treatment, some ulcers resolve, but most recur or become chronic ulcers.

Bubo formation, or inguinal adenitis, develops 7 to 10 days after appearance of the genital lesion. The process is usually unilateral, with erythema of the overlying skin. It can become fluctuant and rupture. Buboes are much less common in women.

LABORATORY DIAGNOSIS

Culture of *H. ducreyi* remains the definitive diagnostic criterion. This can be obtained by stroking the purulent base of a chancre with a cotton or calcium alginate swab. Careful handling of the culture is important, because organisms can survive for only 2 to 4 hours without refrigeration. Growth of the organism is difficult, and several have recommended use of nutritionally rich agar base fortified with hemoglobin and serum and made selective by the addition of antibiotics.[311,312] Colonies usually appear within 2 to 4 days. Immunologists are working to perfect an enzyme-linked immunosorbent assay (ELISA), which is reported to have high sensitivity and specificity.[313]

If culturing techniques are not available, the diagnosis can be made on clinical grounds, once syphilis and HSV have been ruled out.

TREATMENT

Since the development of antibiotics several decades ago, a wide array of agents, including penicillin, sulfonamides, tetracycline, streptomycin, and chloramphenicol, has been employed in the treatment of chancroid. In the 1970s, resistance to tetracycline and chloramphenicol was first reported, and since then, plasmid-mediated resistance has been reported with most of the rest.

The 1989 CDC recommendations include erythromycin for 7 days or ceftriaxone in a single dose (Table 72-14). Alternative regimens include trimethoprim/sulfamethoxazole for 7 days, amoxicillin/clavulanic acid for 7 days, and ciprofloxacin for 3 days (CDC-1989). Quinolones, such as ciprofloxacin, are contraindicated during pregnancy.

TABLE 72–14. CENTERS FOR DISEASE CONTROL 1989 RECOMMENDED TREATMENT GUIDELINES FOR CHANCROID IN PREGNANCY

Recommended Regimen
Erythromycin base 500 mg orally 4 times daily for 7 days
or
Ceftriaxone 250 mg IM in a single dose
Alternative Regimens
Trimethoprim/sulfamethoxazole 160/800 mg (one double-strength tablet) orally twice a day for 7 days
or
Amoxicillin/clavulanic acid 500/125 mg orally 3 times a day for 7 days

Symptomatic improvement can be seen approximately 3 days after beginning treatment, and ulcers should heal within 7 days. Lymphadenitis is slower to resolve and may require multiple aspirations through healthy adjacent skin to prevent rupture. Treatment failure can be the result of any of a number of sources: (1) the treatment was not taken as prescribed, (2) the strain of *H. ducreyi* was resistant to the antibiotic, (3) reinfection by an untreated partner has occurred, (4) the diagnosis was incorrect, or (5) another STD, including HIV, may be present. There is a high incidence of treatment failure in HIV-infected individuals with chancroid.

MATERNAL AND FETAL RISKS

Due to the paucity of cases among women, this STD has not been well described in pregnancy. There are no reports to date of adverse perinatal outcomes or vertical transmission associated with chancroid.

PREVENTION

The greatest deterrent to prevention of this STD is that most women have minor symptoms or are asymptomatic. Therefore, they do not seek treatment and continue to be sexually active.[314] Programs aimed at eradicating chancroid should include education in the routine use of condoms, regular gynecologic examinations of prostitutes, early treatment of infections, and routine testing for other STDs once the diagnosis of chancroid has been made.

REFERENCES

1. Rosebury T. Microbes and morals. New York: Viking, 1971.
2. Westrom L. Incidence, prevalence and trends of acute pelvic inflammatory disease and its consequences in industrialized countries. Am J Obstet Gynecol 1980;38:880.
3. Westrom L. Effect of acute pelvic inflammatory disease on fertility. Am J Obstet Gynecol 1975;122:707.
4. McCormack WM, Nowroozi K, Alpert S, et al. Acute pelvic inflammatory disease: characteristics of patients with gonococcal and non–avegonococcal infection and evaluation of their response to treatment with aqueous procaine penicillin G and spectinomycin hydrochloride. Sex Transm Dis 1977;4:125.
5. Chow JM, Yonekura ML, Richwald GA, et al. The association between *Chlamydia trachomatis* and ectopic pregnancy: a matched-pair, case-control study. JAMA 1990;263:3164.
6. Rubin GL, Peterson HB, Dorfman SF, et al. Ectopic pregnancy in the United States: 1970 through 1978, JAMA 1983;249:1725.
7. Weinstein L, Morris MB, Dotters D, et al. Ectopic pregnancy — a new surgical epidemic. Obstet Gynecol 1983;61:698.
8. Svensson L, Mardh P-A, Ahlgren M, et al. Ectopic pregnancy and antibodies to *Chlamydia trachomatis*. Fertil Steril 1985; 44:313.
9. Brunham RC, Binns B, McDowell J, et al. *Chlamydia trachomatis* infection in women with ectopic pregnancy. Obstet Gynecol 1986;67:722.
10. Martin DH, Koutsky L, Eschenbach DA, et al. Prematurity and perinatal mortality in pregnancies complicated by maternal *Chlamydia trachomatis* infections. JAMA 1982;247:1585.
11. Gissmann L, Schwarz E. Persistence and expression of HPV in genital cancer. Ciba Found Symp 1986;120:190.
12. Gross G, Ikenberg H, Gissman L, et al. Papillomavirus of the anogenital region: correlation between histology, clinical picture and virus type. Proposal of a new nomenclature. J Invest Dermatol 1985;85:147.
13. Reid R, Laverty CR, Copplesson M, et al. Noncondylomatous cervical wart virus infection. Obstet Gynecol 1980;55:476.
14. zur Hausen H, Schneider A. The role of papillomaviruses in human anogenital cancer. In: Salzmann NP, Howley PM, eds. The papovaviridae, the papillomaviruses. Vol 2. New York: Plenum, 1987:245.
15. Chu SY, Buehler JW, Berkelman RL. Impact of the human immunodeficiency virus epidemic on mortality in women of reproductive age, United States. JAMA 1990;264:225.
16. Centers for Disease Control. Pneumocystis pneumonia—Los Angeles. MMWR 1981;30:250.
17. Centers for Disease Control. Kaposi's sarcoma and pneumocystis pneumonia among homosexual men—New York and California. MMWR 1981;30:305.
18. Gottlieb MS, Schroff R, Schanker HM, et al. *Pneumocystis carinii* pneumonia and mucosal candidiasis in previously healthy homosexual men: evidence of a new acquired cellular immunodeficiency. N Engl J Med 1981;305:1425.
19. AIDS and human immunodeficiency virus infection in the United States: 1988 update. MMWR 1989;38(Suppl 4):1.
20. Centers for Disease Control. HIV/AIDS surveillance. U.S. Department of Health and Human Services, September, 1990.
21. Curran JW, Morgan WM, Hardy AM, et al. The epidemiology of AIDS: current status and future prospects. Science 1985;229:1352.
22. Coolfont report: a PHS plan for prevention and control of AIDS and the AIDS virus. Public Health Rep 1986;101:341.
23. Centers for Disease Control. Acquired immunodeficiency syndrome (AIDS) among blacks and Hispanics—United States. MMWR 1986;35:655.
24. Padian N, Wiley J, Winkelstein W. Male to female transmission of human immunodeficiency virus: current results, infectivity rates, and San Francisco population seroprevalence estimates. Presented at the Third International Conference on AIDS, Washington, DC, June, 1987.
25. Friedland GH, Klein RS. Transmission of the human immunodeficiency virus. N Engl J Med 1987;317:1125.
26. Padian N, Marquis L, Francis DP, et al. Male-to-female transmission of human immunodeficiency virus. JAMA 1987; 258:788.
27. Haverkos HW, Edelman R. The epidemiology of acquired immunodeficiency syndrome among heterosexuals. JAMA 1988;260:1922.
28. Goedert JJ, Eyster ME, Biggar RJ. Heterosexual transmission of human immunodeficiency virus (HIV): association with severe T_4-cell depletion in male hemophiliacs (abstract W.2.6). Presented at the Third International Conference on AIDS, Washington, DC, June, 1987.
29. Kreiss JK, Kitchen LW, Prince HE, et al. Antibody to human T-lymphotropics virus type III in wives of hemophiliacs: evidence for heterosexual transmission. Ann Intern Med 1985; 102:623.
30. Lawrence DN, Jason JM, Bouhasin JD, et al. HTLV-III/LAV antibody status of spouses and household contacts assisting in home infusion of hemophilia patients. Blood 1986;66:703.
31. Jason JM, McDougal JS, Dixon G, et al. HTLV-III/LAV antibody and immune status of household contacts and sexual partners of persons with hemophilia. JAMA 1986;255:212.

32. Allain J-P. Prevalence of HTLV-III/LAV antibodies in patients with hemophilia and in their sexual partners in France [letter]. N Engl J Med 1986;315:517.
33. Redfield RR, Markham PD, Salahuddian SZ, et al. Frequent transmission of HTLV-III among spouces of patients with AIDS-related complex and AIDS. JAMA 1985;253:1571.
34. Peterman TA, Stoneburner RI, Allen JR, et al. Risk of HIV transmission from persons with transfusion-associated infections. JAMA 1988;259:55.
35. Saltzman BR, Friedland GH, Vileno JL, et al. Epidemiologic and clinical features of heterosexual men and women with AIDS (abstract 189). Abstracts of the Second International Conference on AIDS, Paris, June 1986.
36. Stewart GH, Tyler JPP, Cunningham AL, et al. Transmission of human T-cell lymphotropic virus type III (HTLV-III) by artificial insemination by donor. Lancet 1985;2:581.
37. Padian N. Heterosexuals and AIDS: what is the risk? San Francisco: Focus AIDS Health Project, University of California, February, 1988.
38. Luzi G, Ensoli B, Turbessi G, et al. Transmission of HTLV-III infection by heterosexual contact [letter]. Lancet 1985;2:1018.
39. Fischl MA, Dickinson GM, Scott GM, et al. Evaluation of heterosexual partners, children and household contacts of adults with AIDS. JAMA 1987;257:640.
40. Quinn TC, Mann JM, Currant JW, Piot P. AIDS in Africa: an epidemiologic paradigm. Science 1986;234:955.
41. Kreiss JK, Koech D, Plummer FA, et al. AIDS virus infection in Nairobi prostitutes: spread of the epidemic in East Africa. N Engl J Med 1986;314:414.
42. Greenblatt RM, Lukehart SA, Plummer FA, et al. Genital ulceration as a risk factor for human immunodeficiency virus infection in Kenya. Aids 1988;2:47.
43. Stamm WE, Handsfield HH, Rompalo AM, et al. The association between genital ulcer disease and acquisition of HIV infection in homosexual men. JAMA 1988;260:1429.
44. Popovic M, Sarngadharan MG, Read E, Gallo RC. Detection, isolation, and continuous production of cytopathic retroviruses (HTLV-III) from patients with AIDS and pre-AIDS. Science 1984;224:497.
45. Folks T, Posell DM, Lightfoote MM, et al. Induction of HTLV-III/LAV from a nonvirus-producing T-cell line: implications for latency. Science 1986;231:600.
46. Haseltine WA, Wong-Staal F. The molecular biology of the AIDS virus. Sci Am 1986;259:52.
47. Haseltine WA. Replication and pathogenesis of the AIDS virus. J Acquired Immune Deficiency Syndrome 1988;1:217.
48. Sodroski J, Rosen C, Wong-Staal F, et al. Trans-acting transcriptional regulation of human T-cell leukemia virus type III long terminal repeat. Science 1985;227:171.
49. Lee TH, Coligan, JE, Allan JS, et al. A new HTLV-III/LAV protein encoded by a gene found in cytopathic retroviruses. Science 1986;231:1546.
50. Sodroski J, Goh WC, Rosen C, et al. Replicative and cytopathic potential for HTLV-III/LAV with *sor* gene-deletions. Science 1986;231:1549.
51. Cohen E, Terwilliger EF, Sodroski JG, Haseltine WA. Identification of a protein encoded by the *vpu* gene of HIV-1. Nature 1988;334:532.
52. Sodroski JG, Goh WC, Rosen CR, et al. A second post-transcriptional transactivator gene required for HTLV-III replication. Nature 1986;321:412.
53. Feinberg MB, Jarrett RF, Aldovini A, et al. HTLV-III expression and production involve complex regulation at the levels of splicing and translation of viral RNA. Cell 1986;46:807.
54. Terwilliger EF, Sodroski JG, Haseltine WA, Rosen CR. The art gene product of human immunodeficiency virus is required for replication. J Virol 1988;62:655.
55. Levy JA. The human immunodeficiency virus and its pathogenesis. Infect Dis Clin North Am 1988;2:285.
56. Weber JN, Weiss RA. HIV infection: the cellular picture. Sci Am 1988;259:101.
57. Barre-Sinoussi F, Chermann JC, Rey F, et al. Isolation of a T-lymphotropic retrovirus from a patient at risk for acquired immune deficiency syndrome (AIDS). Science 1983;220:868.
58. Ho DD, Pomerantz RJ, Kaplan JC. Pathogenesis of infection with human immunodeficiency virus. N Engl J Med 1987; 317:278.
59. Centers for Disease Control. Update on acquired immunodeficiency syndrome (AIDS)—United States. MMWR 1982; 31:507.
60. Centers for Disease Control. Revision of the case definition of acquired immunodeficiency syndrome for national reporting — United States. MMWR 1985;34:372.
61. Centers for Disease Control. Revision of the CDC surveillance case definition for acquired immunodeficiency syndrome. MMWR 1987;36(S):3.
62. Cooper DA, Gold J, Maclean P, et al. Acute AIDS retrovirus infection. Definition of a clinical illness associated with seroconversion. Lancet 1985;1:547.
63. Hessol NA, Rutherford GW, O'Malley PM, et al. The natural history of human immunodeficiency virus infection in a cohort of homosexual and bisexual men: a 7-year prospective study [abstract]. Proceedings of the Third International Conference of AIDS, Washington DC, June 1987:1.
64. Jaffe HW, Darrow WW, Echenberg DF, et al. The acquired immunodeficiency syndrome in a cohort of homosexual men: a six year follow-up study. Ann Intern Med 1985;103:210.
65. Abrams DI, Lewis BJ, Beckstead JH, et al. Persistent diffuse lymphadenopathy in homosexual men: endpoint or prodrome? Ann Intern Med 1984;100:801.
66. Metroka CE, Cunningham-Rundles S, Pollack MS, et al. Persistent generalized lymphadenopathy in homosexual men. Ann Intern Med 1983;99:585.
67. Greenspan D, Greenspan JS, Hearst NG, et al. Oral history leukoplakia: human immunodeficiency virus status and risk for development of AIDS. J Infect Dis 1987;55:475.
68. Petito CK, Cho Es, Lemann W, et al. Neuropathology of acquired immunodeficiency syndrome (AIDS): an autopsy review. J Neuropathol Exp Neurol 1988;45:635.
69. Price RW, Brew B, Sidts J, et al. The brain in AIDS: central nervous system. Science 1988;259:586.
70. Redfield RR, Wright DC, Tramont EC. The Walter Reed staging classification for HTLV-LAV infection. N Engl J Med 1986; 314:131.
71. Minkoff HL. Care of pregnant women infected with human immunodeficiency virus. JAMA 1987;258:2714.
72. Scott GB, Fischl MA, Klimas N, et al. Mothers of infants with the acquired immunodeficiency syndrome: evidence for both symptomatic and asymptomatic carriers. JAMA 1985;253:363.
73. Minkoff H, Nanda D, Menez R, et al. Pregnancies resulting in infants with acquired immunodeficiency syndrome or AIDS-related complex. Follow-up of mothers, children, and subsequently born siblings. Obstet Gynecol 1987;69:288.
74. Sridama V, Pacini F, Yang SL, et al. Decreased levels of helper T-cells—a possible cause of immunodeficiency in pregnancy. N Engl J Med 1982;307:352.
75. Gehrz RC, Christianson WR, Linner KM, et al. Cytomegalovirus — specific humoral and cellular immune responses in human pregnancy. J Infect Dis 1981;143:391.
76. Thong YH, Steele RW, Vincent MM, et al. Impaired in-vitro cell mediated immunity. N Engl J Med 1973;289:604.

77. Feinkind L, Minkoff HL. HIV in pregnancy. Clin Perinatol 1988;15:189.
78. Paryani SG, Arvin AM. Intrauterine infection with varicella-zoster virus after maternal varicella. N Engl J Med 1986; 314:1542.
79. Selwyn PA, Schoenbaum EE, Davenny K, et al. Prospective study of human immunodeficiency virus infection and pregnancy outcomes in intravenous drug users. JAMA 1989;261:1289.
80. Landesman SH. Human immunodeficiency virus infection in women: an overview. Semin Perinatol 1989;13:2.
81. Rubenstein A, Sicklick M, Gupta A, et al. Acquired immunodeficiency with reversed T_4/T_8 ratios in infants born to promiscuous and drug-addicted mothers. JAMA 1983;249:2350.
82. Thomas PA, Jaffe HW, Spira TJ, et al. Unexplained immunodeficiency in children: a surveillance report. JAMA 1984;252:639.
83. Scott GB, Buck BE, Leterman JG, et al. Acquired immunodeficiency syndrome in infants. N Engl J Med 1984;310:638.
84. Minkoff H, Nanda D, Menez R, Fikrig S. Pregnancies resulting in infants with acquired immunodeficiency syndrome or AIDS-related complex. Obstet Gynecol 1987;69:285.
85. Selwyn PA, Schoenbaum EE, Davenny K, et al. Prospective study of human immunodeficiency virus infection and pregnancy outcomes in intravenous drug users. JAMA 1989;261:1289.
86. Johnston FD, MacCallum L, Brettle R, et al. Does infection with HIV affect the outcome of pregnancy? Br Med J 1988;296:467.
87. The European Collaborative Study. Mother-to-child transmission of HIV infection. Lancet 1988;2:1039.
88. Italian Multicentre Study. Epidemiology, clinical features, and prognostic factors of pediatric HIV infection. Lancet 1988;2:1043.
89. Minkoff H, Willoughby A, Mendez S, et al. Human immunodeficiency virus in pregnant women and their offspring (abstract 159). Society of Perinatal Obstetricians, Las Vegas, February 1988.
90. Koonin LM, Ellerbrock TV, Atrash HK, et al. Pregnancy-associated deaths due to AIDS in the United States. JAMA 1989;261:1306.
91. Marion RW, Wiznia AA, Hutcheon RG, Rubinstein A. Human T cell lymphotropic virus type III (HTLV-III) embryopathy: a new dysmorphic syndrome associated with intrauterine HTLV-III infection. Am J Dis Child 1986;140:638.
92. Peutherer JF, Rebus S, Aw D, et al. Detection of HIV in the fetus: a study of six cases (abstract 7235). Fourth International Conference on AIDS, Stockholm, June 1988.
93. Mok JQ, Rossi A, DeAdes A, et al. Infants born to mothers seropositive for human immunodeficiency virus: preliminary findings from a multicenter European study. Lancet 1987; 1:1164.
94. Ziegler JB, Cooper DA, Johnson RO, Gold J. Postnatal transmission of AIDS-associated retrovirus from mother to infant. Lancet 1985;1:896.
95. Weinbreck P, Loustand V, Denis F, Liozon F. Breast feeding and HIV transmission (abstract 5102). Fourth International Conference on AIDS, Stockholm, June 1988.
96. Scott GB, Mastrucci M, Hutto S, et al. Pediatric HIV infections: factors influencing case identification and prognosis. Pediatr Res 1987;27:334A.
97. Abrams EJ, New York City Collaborative Study Group. Perinatal transmission of the human immunodeficiency virus: a longitudinal study of the children (abstract WP62). Third International Conference on AIDS, Washington, DC, June 1987.
98. Mendez H, Willoughby A, Hittelman J, et al. Human immunodeficiency virus (HIV) infection in pregnant women and their offspring. Pediatr Res 1987;21:1466A.
99. Braddick M, Kreiss J, Quinn T, et al. Congenital transmission of HIV in Nairobi, Kenya (abstract TH 7.5). Third International Conference on AIDS, Washington, DC June, 1987.
100. Rogers MF, et al. Use of the polymerase chain reaction for early detection of the proviral sequences of human immunodeficiency virus in infants born to seropositive mothers. N Engl J Med 1989;320:1649.
101. Landers DV, Sweet RL. Perinatal infections. In: Scott J, ed. Danforth's obstetrics and gynecology. 6th ed. Philadelphia: JB Lippincott, 1990:535.
102. Rossi P, Moschese V, Broliden PA, et al. Presence of maternal antibodies to human immunodeficiency virus 1 envelope glycoprotein gp120 epitopes correlates with the uninfected status of children born to seropositive mothers. Proc Natl Acad Sci 1989;86:8055.
103. Goedert JJ, Mendex H, Drummond JE, et al. Mother-to-infant transmission of HIV Type 1: association with prematurity or low anti-gp120. Lancet 1989;2:1351.
104. Moss AR, Bacchetti P, Osmond D, et al. Seropositives for HIV and the development of AIDS or AIDS related condition: three year follow-up of the San Francisco General cochort. Br Med J 1988;296:745.
105. Polk BF, Fox R, Brookmeyer R, et al. Predictors of the acquired immunodeficiency syndrome developing in a cohort of seropositive homosexual men. N Engl J Med 1987;316:61.
106. Laure F, Rouziox C, Veber F, et al. Detection of HIV, DNA in infants and children by means of the polymerase chain reaction. Lancet 1988;2:538.
107. Hart C, Spira T, Moore J, et al. Direct detection of HIV RNA expression in seropositive subjects. Lancet 1988;2:596.
108. Fischl MA, Richman DD, Grieco MH, et al, and the AZT Collaborative Working Group. The efficacy of azidothymidine (AZT) in the treatment of patients with AIDS and AIDS-related complex; a double blind placebo-controlled trial. N Engl J Med 1987;317:185.
109. Human immune deficiency virus infections. ACOG Technical Bulletin 123. December, 1988.
110. Ocho PG. Trimethoprim and sulfamethoxazole in pregnancy. JAMA 1976;217:1244.
111. Rosebury T. Microbes and morals. New York: Viking, 1971.
112. Kampmeier RH. Identification of the gonococcus by Albert Neisser. Sex Transm Dis 1978;5:71.
113. Centers for Disease Control. Sexually Transmitted Disease Statistics, Calendar Year 1987 (No. 136). Atlanta: US Public Health Service, 1988:1.
114. Rice RJ, Aval SO, Blount JH. Gonorrhea in the United States 1975–84: is the giant only sleeping? Sex Transm Dis 1987;14:83.
115. Barnes RC, Holmes KK. Epidemiology of gonorrhea: current perspectives. Epidemiol Rev 1984;6:1.
116. Cates W Jr, Weisner PJ, Curran JW. Sex and spermicides: preventing unintended pregnancy and infection. JAMA 1982;248:1636.
117. Louv WC, Austin J, Alexander WJ, Stagno S, Cheeks J. A clinical trial of nonoxynol-9 for preventing gonococcal and chlamydial infections. J Infect Dis 1988;158:518.
118. Dans PE. Gonococcal anogenital infection. Clin Obstet Gynecol 1975;18:103.
119. Centers for Disease Control. Antibiotic-resistant strains of *Neisseria gonorrhoeae*. Policy guidelines for detection, management and control. MMWR 1987;36(S):1.
120. Pierce WA, Buchanan TM. Attachment role of gonococcal pili: optimum conditions and quantitation of adherence of isolated pili to human cells in vitro. J Clin Invest 1978;61:931.
121. King GL, Swanson J. Studies on gonococcus infection. XV: iden-

tification of surface proteins of *Neisseria gonorrhoeae* correlated with leukocyte association. Infect Immun 1978;21:575.

122. Pedersen AHB, Bonin P. Screening females for asymptomatic gonorrhea infection. Northwest Med 1971;70:255.
123. McCormack WM, Stumacher RJ, Johnson K, Donner A. Clinical spectrum of gonococcal infection in women. Lancet 1977;2:1182.
124. Corman LC, Levison ME, Knight R, Carrington ER, Kaye D. The high frequency of pharyngeal gonococcal infection in a prenatal clinic population. JAMA 1974;230:568.
125. Holmes KK, Counts GW, Beaty HN. Disseminated gonococcal infection. Ann Intern Med 171;74:979.
126. Suleiman SA, Grimes EM, Jones HS. Disseminated gonococcal infections. Obstet Gynecol 1983;61:48.
127. Peterson BH, Lee TJ, Snyderman R, Brooks GF. Neisseria meningitis and *Neisseria gonorrhoeae* bacteremia associated with C_6, C_7, C_8 deficiency. Ann Intern Med 1979;90:917.
128. Holmes KK. Gonococcal infection. In: Remington JS, Klein JO, eds. Infectious diseases of the fetus and newborn infant. Philadelphia: WB Saunders, 1983:616.
129. Amstey MS, Steadman KT. Symptomatic gonorrhea and pregnancy. J Am Vener Dis Assoc 1976;3:14.
130. Sarrel PM, Pruett KA. Symptomatic gonorrhea during pregnancy. Obstet Gynecol 1968;32:670.
131. Handsfield HH, Hodson A, Holmes KK. Neonatal gonococcal infection. I: orogastric contamination with *Neisseria gonorrhoeae*. JAMA 1973;225:697.
132. Edwards LE, Barrada MI, Hamann AA, Hakanson EY. Gonorrhea in pregnancy. Am J Obstet Gynecol 1978;132:637.
133. Phillips RS, Hanff PA, Wertheimer A, Aronson MD. Gonnorhea in women seen for routine gynecologic care: criteria for testing. Am J Med 1988;85:177.
134. Sweet RL, Schachter J, Landers DV. Chlamydial infections in obstetrics and gynecology. Clin Obstet Gynecol 1983;26:143.
135. 1989 Sexually transmitted diseases treatment guidelines 1989. MMWR 1989;38(suppl):21.
136. Stokes JH. Modern clinical syphilology. 3rd ed. Philadelphia: WB Saunders, 1945.
137. King A, et al. Venereal diseases. 4th ed. London: Bailliere Tindall, 1980.
138. Hudson EH. Non-venereal syphilis. Edinburgh: Livingston, 1958.
139. Moore JE. Penicillin in syphilis. Springfield, IL: Charles C Thomas, 1946.
140. Centers for Disease Control. Congenital syphilis, United States, 1983-1985. MMWR 1986;35:625.
141. Centers for Disease Control. Increases in primary and secondary syphilis, United States. MMWR 1987;36:393.
142. Centers for Disease Control. Publication 9.688. Atlanta: Public Health Service, CDC, 1987.
143. Shroeter AL, Turner RM, Lacas JB, Brown NJ. Therapy for incubating syphilis: effectiveness of gonorrhoea treatment. JAMA 1971;218:711.
144. Chapel TA. The signs and symptoms of secondary syphilis. Sex Transm Dis 1980;7:161.
145. Harris JRW. Recent advances in sexually transmitted diseases. 3rd ed. Edinburgh: Churchill Livingston, 1981:73.
146. Campisi D, Whitcomb C. Liver disease in early syphilis. Arch Intern Med 1978;139:365.
147. Feher J, Somogyi T, Timmer N, Jozsa L. Early syphilitic hepatitis. Lancet 1975;2:896.
148. Bhorade MS, Carag HB, Potter EV, Dunea G. Nephropathy of secondary syphilis: a clinical and pathological spectrum. JAMA 1971;216:1159.
149. Gamble CN, Reardon JB. Immunopathogenesis of syphilitic glomerulonephritis: elution of antitreponemal antibody from glomerular immune-complex deposits. N Engl J Med 1975; 292:449.
150. O'Regan S, Fong JS, de Chadarevian JF, et al. Treponemal antigen in congenital and acquired syphilitis nephritis? Demonstration by immunofluorescense studies. Ann Intern Med 1976;85:325.
151. Wende RB, Wende RD, Mudd RL, Knox JM, Holden WR. The VDRL slide test in 322 cases of dark field positive primary syphilis. South Med J 1971;64:5.
152. Duncan WC, Knox JM, Wende RD. The FTA-ABS test in dark field positive primary syphilis. JAMA 1974;228:859.
153. Ziya PR, Hankins DV, Gilstrap LC, Halsey AB. Intravenous penicillin desensitization and treatment during pregnancy. JAMA 1986;256:2561.
154. Wendel GD, Stark BJ, Jamison RB, et al. Penicillin allergy and desensitization in serious maternal/fetal infections. N Engl J Med 1985;312:1299.
155. Fenton LJ, Irwin JL. Congenital syphilis after maternal treatment with erythromycin. Obstet Gynecol 1976;47:492.
156. Hashisaki P, Wertzberger GG, Conrad CR, et al. Erythromycin failure in the treatment of syphilis in a pregnant woman. Sex Transm Dis 1983;10:36.
157. Mascola L, Pelosi R, Blount JH, et al. Congenital syphilis: why is it still occurring? JAMA 1984;252:1719.
158. Mamunes P, Cave UG, Budell JW, et al. Early diagnosis of neonatal syphilis: evaluation of a gamma M-fluorescent treponemal antibody test. Am J Dis Child 1970;120:17.
159. South MA, Knox JM, Short DH. Failure of erythromycin estolate therapy in in utero syphilis. JAMA 1964;190:182.
160. Cox SM, Klein VR, Wendel GD. The Jarisch-Herxheimer reaction in pregnancy (abstract 106). Society of Perinatal Obstetricians, San Antonio, February 1987.
161. Fiumara NJ, Fleming WL, Downing JG, et al. The incidence of prenatal syphilis at the Boston City Hospital. N Engl J Med 1952;247:48.
162. Ingall D, Musher D. Syphilis. In: Remington JS, Klein JO, eds. Infectious diseases of the fetus and newborn infant. Philadelphia: WB Saunders, 1983:335.
163. Fiumara NJ, Fleming WL, Downing JG, Good FL. The incidence of prenatal syphilis at the Boston City Hospital. N Engl J Med 1952;247:48.
164. Schachter J. Chlamydial infections. N Engl J Med 1978; 298:428.
165. Centers for Disease Control. *Chlamydia trachomatis* infections: policy guidelines for prevention and control. MMWR 1985;34(suppl 3S):535.
166. Schacter J, Hanna L, Hill EC, et al. Are chlamydial infections the most prevalent venereal disease? JAMA 1975;231:1252.
167. National Institute of Allergy and Infectious Diseases. Summary and recommendations of the National Institute of Allergy and Infectious Diseases Study Group on Sexually Transmitted Diseases. Washington, DC, 1980.
168. Schachter J, Grossman M. Chlamydial infections. Annu Rev Med 1981;32:45.
169. Washington AE. Chlamydia: a major threat to reproductive health. Research highlights. San Francisco: Institute for Health Policy Studies, University of California, 1984;2:1.
170. Jones BR. Laboratory tests for chlamydial infection: their role in epidemiological studies of trachoma and its control. Br J Ophthalmol 1974;58:438.
171. Hobson D, Johnson FWA, Rees E, et al. Simplified method for diagnosis of genital and ocular infections with Chlamydia. Lancet 1974;2:555.
172. Kuo C-C, Wang S-P, Wentworth BB, et al. Primary isolation of TRIC organisms in HeLa 229 cells treated with DEAE-dextran. J Infect Dis 1972;125:665.

173. Hammerschlag MR, Anderka M, Semine DZ, McComb D, McCormack WM. Prospective study of maternal and infantile infection with *Chlamydia trachomatis*. Pediatrics 1979;64:142.
174. Schachter J, Holt J, Goodner E, Grossman M, Sweet R, Mills J. Prospective study of chlamydial infection in neonates. Lancet 1979;2:377.
175. Frommel GT, Rothenberg R, Wang S-P, et al. Chlamydial infection of mothers and their infants. J Pediatr 1979;95:28.
176. Chandler JW, Alexander ER, Pheiffer TA, Wang S-P, Holmes KK, English M. Ophthalmia neonatorum associated with maternal chlamydial infections. Trans Am Acad Opthalmol Otolaryngol 1977;83:302.
177. Heggie AD, Lumicao CG, Stuart LA, Gyues MT. *Chlamydia trachomatis* infection in mothers and infants. A prospective study. Am J Dis Child 1981;135:507m.
178. Martin DH, Koutsky L, Eschenbach DA, et al. Prematurity and perinatal mortality in pregnancies complicated by maternal *Chlamydia trachomatis* infections. JAMA 1982;247:1585.
179. Thompson S, Lopez B, Wong KH, et al. The relationship of low birthweight and infant mortality to vaginal microorganisms. Presented at the 3rd International Meeting on Sexually Transmitted Diseases, Antwerp, Belgium, October 1980.
180. Grossman M, Schachter J, Sweet R, Bishop E, Jordan C. Prospective studies of Chlamydia in newborns. In: Mardh P-A, Holmes KK, Oriel JD, Piot P, Schachter J, eds. Chlamydia infections. Vol 2. Fernstrom Foundation series. Amsterdam: Elsevier, 1982:213.
181. Alexander ER, Harrison R. Role of *Chlamydia trachomatis* in perinatal infection. Rev Infect Dis 1983;5:713.
182. Thompson SE, Washington AE. Epidemiology of sexually transmitted *Chlamydia trachomatis* infections. Epidemiol Rev 1983;5:96.
183. Washington AE, Gove S, Schachter J, Sweet RL. Oral contraceptives *Chlamydia trachomatis* infection and pelvic inflammatory disease: a word of caution about protection. JAMA 1985;253:2246.
184. Schachter J, Stoner E, Moncoda J. Screening for chlamydial infections in women attending family planning clinics: evaluations of presumptive indicators for therapy. West J Med 1983;138:375.
185. Arya OP, Mallinson H., Goddard AD. Epidemiological and clinical correlates of chlamydial infection of the cervix. British Journal of Venereal Disease 1981;57:118.
186. Chacko MR, Louchik JC. *Chlamydia trachomatis* infection in sexually active adolescents: prevalence and risk factors. Pediatrics 1984;73:836.
187. Tait IA, Rees E, Hobson D, et al. Chlamydial infection of the cervix in contacts of men with nongonococcal urethritis. British Journal of Venereal Disease 1980;56:37.
188. Dunlap EMC, Jones BR, Darougar S. Chlamydial and non-specific urethritis. Br Med J 1972;2:575.
189. Oriel JD, Reeve P, Powis P, et al. Chlamydial infection: isolation of *Chlamydial* from patients with non-specific genital infection. British Journal of Venereal Disease 1972;48:419.
190. Stamm WE, Wagner KF, Ansel R, et al. Causes of the acute urethral syndrome in women. N Engl J Med 1980;303:409.
191. Moller BR, Ahorns S, Laurin J, Mardh P-A. Pelvic infection after elective abortion associated with *Chlamydial trachomatis*. Obstet Gynecol 1982;59:210.
192. Westergard L, Philipson T, Scheibel J. Significance of cervical *Chlamydia trachomatis* infection in postabortal pelvic inflammatory disease. Obstet Gynecol 1982;60:322.
193. Quigstad E, Skaug K, Jerve F, et al. Pelvic inflammatory disease associated with *Chlamydia trachomatis* infection after threrapeutic abortion. Br J Vener Dis 1983;59:189.
194. Osser S, Persson K. Postabortal pelvic infection associated with *Chlamydia trachomatis* and the influence of humoral immunity. Am J Obstet Gynecol 1984;150:699.
195. Barbacci MB, Spence MR, Kappus EW, et al. Postabortal endometritis and isolation of *Chlamydia trachomatis*. Obstet Gynecol 1986;68:686.
196. Ismail MA, Chandler AE, Beem MO, Moawad AH. Chlamydial colonization of the cervix in pregnant adolescents. J Reprod Med 1985;30:549.
197. Wager GP, Martin DH, Koutsky L, et al. Puerperal infectious morbidity: relationship to route of delivery and to antepartum *Chlamydia trachomatis* infection. Am J Obstet Gynecol 1980;138:1028.
198. Cytryn A, Sen P, Haingsub R, et al. Severe pelvic infection from *Chlamydia trachomatis* after cesarean section. JAMA 1982;247:1732.
199. Hoyme UB, Kiviat N, Eschenbach DA. Microbiology and treatment of late postpartum endometritis. Obstet Gynecol 1986;68:226.
200. Thompson S, Lopez B, Wong KG, et al. A prospective study of chlamydial and mycoplasmal infections during pregnancy. In: Mardh P-A, Holmes KK, Oriel JD, Piot P, Schachter J, eds. Chlamydial infections. Vol 2. Fernstrom Foundation series. Amsterdam: Elsevier, 1982:155.
201. Harrison HR, Alexander ER, Weinstein L, et al. Cervical *Chlamydia trachomatis* and mycoplasmal infections in pregnancy. Epidemiology and outcomes. JAMA 1983;250:1721.
202. Sweet RL, Landers DV, Walker C, Schachter J. *Chlamydia trachomatis* infection and pregnancy outcome. Am J Obstet Gynecol 1987;156:824.
203. Thygeson, P, Mengert WF. The virus of inclusion conjunctivitis: further observations. Arch Ophthalmol 1936;15:377.
204. Lennon GG. Acute salpingitis during pregnancy. J Obstet Gynaecol Br Commonwealth 1949;56:1035.
205. McCord M, Simmons CM. Acute prurulent salpingitis during pregnancy. Am J Obstet Gynecol 1953;65:1136.
206. Scott TM, Hay D. Acute salpingitis and surgery. J Obstet Gynaecol Br Commonwealth 1954;61:788.
207. Lancet M, Cohen A. Acute prurulent salpingitis in late pregnancy. Obstet Gynecol 1957;14:426.
208. Acosta AA, Mabray CR, Kaurman RH. Intrauterine pregnancy and coexistent pelvic inflammatory disease. Obstet Gynecol 1971;37:282.
209. Jafari K, Vilovic-Kos J, Webster A, et al. Tuboovarian abscess in pregnancy. Acta Obstet Gynecol Scand 1977;56:1.
210. Fuselier P, Alam A. Pregnancy complicated by pelvic abscess. J Reprod Med 1978;21:257.
211. Blanchard AC, Pastorek JG II, Weeks T. Pelvic inflammatory disease during pregnancy. South Med J 1987;80:1363.
212. Burns DCM, Darougar S, Thin RN, et al. Isolation of *Chlamydia* from women attending a clinic for sexually transmitted disease. British Journal of Venereal Disease 1975;51:314.
213. Martin DH, Faro S, Pastorek G. High prevalence of chlamydial infections in an inner city obstetric population. Program and abstracts of the 21st Interscience Conference on Antimicrobial Agents and Chemotherapy. Chicago: American Society for Microbiology, 1981.
214. Hardy PH, Hardy JB, Nell EE, et al. Prevalence of six sexually transmitted disease agents among pregnant inner-city adolescents and pregnancy outcome. Lancet 1984;2:333.
215. Cohen I, Veille JC, Calkins BM. Improved pregnancy outcome following successful treatment of chlamydial infection. JAMA 1990;263:3160.
216. Tam MR, Stamm WE, Handsfield HH, et al. Culture-dependent diagnosis of *Chlamydia trachomatis* using monoclonal antibodies. N Engl J Med 1984;310:1146.
217. Amortegui AJ, Meyer MP. Enzyme immunoassay for detection

of *Chlamydia trachomatis* from the cervix. Obstet Gynecol 1985;65:523.
218. Uyeda CT, Welborn PP, Ellison-Birang N, et al. Evaluation of Micro Frak direct specimen test for identification of *Chlamydia trachomatis* in clinical specimens [abstract]. Presented at the Annual Meeting of the American Society for Microbiology, St. Louis, March 1984:254.
219. Graber CD, Williamson O, Pike J, et al. Detection of *Chlamydia trachomatis* infection in endocervical specimens using direct immunofluorescence. Obstet Gynecol 1985;66:727.
220. Quinn TC, Warfield P, Kappus E, et al. Screening for *Chlamydia trachomatis* infection in an inner-ciy population. A comparison of diagnostic methods. J Infect Dis 1984;152:419.
221. Stamm WE, Harrison HR, Alexander ER, et al. Diagnosis of *Chlamydia trachomatis* infections by direct immunofluorescent staining of genital secretions: a multi-center trial. Ann Intern Med 1984;101:683.
222. Howard LV, Coleman PF, England BJ, et al. Evaluation of chlamydiazyme for the detection of genital infection caused by *Chlamydia trachomatis*. J Clin Microbiol 1986;23:329.
223. Schachter J, Dawson CR. Comparative efficiency of various diagnostic methods for chlamydial infection. In: Hobson D, Holmes KK, eds. Nongonococcal urethritis and related infections. Washington, DC: American Society for Microbiology, 1977:337.
224. Spence MR, Barbacci M, Kappus E, Quinn T, eds. Nongonococcal urethritis and related infections. Washington, DC: American Society for Microbiology, 1977:337.
225. Podgore JK, Belts R, Alden E, Alexander ER. Effectiveness of maternal third trimester erythromycin in prevention of infant *Chlamydia trachomatis* infection (abstract 524). In Programs and Abstracts of the 20th Interscience Conference on Antimicrobial Agents and Chemotherapy. Washington, DC: American Society for Microbiology, 1980.
226. Schachter J, Sweet RL, Grossman M, et al. Experience with the routine use of erythromycin for chlamydial infections in pregnancy. N Engl J Med 1986;314:276.
227. Oriel JD. Natural history of genital warts. British Journal of Venereal Disease 1971;47:1.
228. Meisels A, Morin C. Human papillomavirus and cancer of the uterine cervix. Gynecol Oncol 1981;12:5111.
229. Byrne P, Woodman C, Meanwell C, et al. Koilocytes and cervical human papillomavirus infection. Lancet 1986;1:205.
230. Singer A, Wilter J, Walker P, et al. Comparison of prevalence of human papillomavirus antigen in biopsies from women with cervical intraepithelial neoplasia. J Clin Pathol 1985;38:855.
231. Lorinez AT, Temple GF, Patterson JA, et al. Correlation of cellular atypia and human papillomavirus DNA in exfoliated cells of the uterine cervix. Obstet Gynecol 1986;68:508.
232. Coleman DV, Wickendon C, Malcolm ADB. Association of human papillomavirus with squamous carcinoma of the uterine cervix. Ciba Found Symp 1986;120:175.
233. Halpert R, Fruchter RG, Sedlis A, et al. Human papillomavirus and lower genital neoplasia in renal transplant patients. Obstet Gynecol 1986;68:251.
234. Gissmann L, Schwarz E. Persistence and expression of HPV in genital cancer. Ciba Found Symp 1986;120:190.
235. Gross G, Ikenberg H, Gissman L, et al. Papillomavirus of the anogenital region: correlation between histology, clinical picture and virus type. Proposal of a new nomenclature. J Invest Dermatol 1985;85:147.
236. Gissman L, zur Hausen H. Partial characterization of viral DNA from human genital warts (condyloma acuminata). Int J Cancer 1980;25:605.
237. Staguet MJ, Viac J, Bustamante R, Thivolet J. Human papillomavirus type I purified from human genital warts. Dermatologica 1981;162:213.
238. Reid R, Laverty CR, Copplesson M, et al. Noncondylomatous cervical wart virus infection. Obstet Gynecol 1980;55:476.
239. zur Hausen H, Schneider A. The role of papillomaviruses in human anogenital cancer. In: Salzmann NP, Howley PM, eds. The papovaviridae, the papillomaviruses. Vol 2. New York: Plenum, 1987:245.
240. Paavonen J. Colposcopic findings associated with human papillomavirus infection of the vagina and cervix. Obstet Gynecol Surv 1985;40:185.
241. Roy M, Meisels A, Fortier M, et al. Vaginal condylomata: a human papillomavirus infection. Clin Obset Gynecol 1981; 24:461.
242. Bolognese RJ, Cosen SL, Fuccillo DA, et al. Herpes virus hominis type II infections in asymptomatic pregnant women. Obstet Gynecol 1976;48:507.
243. Tejani N, Klein SW, Kaplan M. Subclinical herpes simplex genitalis infections in the perinatal period. Am J Obstet Gynecol 1979;135:547.
244. Scher J, Bottone E, Desmond E, Simons W. The incidence and outcome of asymptomatic herpes simplex genitalis in an obstetric population. Am J Obstet Gynecol 1982;144:906.
245. Nahmias AJ, Roczman B. Infection with herpes simplex virus I and II. N Engl J Med 1973;289:781.
246. Baker DA. Herpes virus. Clin Obstet Gynecol 1983;26:165.
247. Sullivan-Bolyai J, Hull HF, Wilson C, Corey L. Neonatal herpes simplex infection in King County, Washington. Increasing incidence and epidemiological correlates. JAMA 1983;250:3059.
248. Whitley RJ, Nahmias AJ, Visintine AM, et al. The natural history of herpes simplex virus infection of mother and newborn. Pediatrics 1980;66:489.
249. Rooney JF, Felser JM, Ostrove JM, et al. Medical intelligence: acquisition of genital herpes from an asymptomatic sexual partner. N Engl J Med 1986;314:1561.
250. Corey L. Herpes simplex virus. In: Holmes KK, Mardh PA, eds. International perspectives on neglected sexually transmitted diseases. Washington, DC: Hemisphere Publishing, 1983:63.
251. Corey L. The diagnosis and treatment of genital herpes. JAMA 1982;258:1041.
252. Adam E, Kaufman RH, Mirkovic RR, et al. Persistence of virus shedding in asymptomatic women after recovery from herpes genitalis. Obstet Gynecol 1979;54:171.
253. Lafferty WE, Coombs RW, Benedetti J, et al. Recurrences after oral and genital herpes simplex virus infection: influence of site on infection and viral type. N Engl J Med 1987;316:1444.
254. Arvin AM, Hensleigh PA, Prober CG, et al. Failure of antepartum maternal cultures to predict the infant's risk of exposure to herpes simplex virus at delivery. N Engl J Med 1986;315:796.
255. Growdon WA, Apodaca L, Cragun J, et al. Neonatal herpes simplex virus infection occurring in second twin of an asymptomatic mother. JAMA 1987;257:508.
256. Binkin NJ, Koplan JP, Cates W. Preventing neonatal herpes: the value of weekly viral cultures in pregnant women with recurrent genital herpes. JAMA 1984;251:2816.
257. Lafferty WE, Krofft S, Remington M, et al. Diagnosis of herpes simplex virus by direct immunofluorescence and viral isolation from samples of external genital lesions in a high-prevalence population. J Clin Microbiol 1987;25:323.
258. Alexander I, Ashley CR, Smith KJ, et al. Comparison of ELISA with virus isolation for the diagnosis of genital herpes. J Clin Pathol 1985;38:554.
259. Hutto C, Arvin A, Jacobs R, et al. Intrauterine herpes simplex virus infections. J Pediatr 1987;110:97.
260. Gibbs RS. Infection control of herpes simplex virus infections in obstetrics and gynecology. J Reprod Med 1986;31:395.

261. Nahmias AJ, Josey WE, Naib ZM, et al. Perinatal risk associated with maternal genital herpes simplex virus infection. Am J Obstet Gynecol 1971;110:285.
262. Brown AZ, Vontver LA, Benedetti J, et al. Effects on infants of a first episode of genital herpes during pregnancy. N Engl J Med 1987;317:1246.
263. Gibbs RS, Amstey MS, Sweet RL, et al. Management of genital herpes infection in pregnancy. Obstet Gynecol 1988;71:779.
264. Sexually transmitted diseases treatment guidelines 1989. MMWR 1989;38(suppl):21.
265. Kampmeier RH. Description of *Trichomonas vaginalis* by MA Donne. Sex Transm Dis 1978;5:119.
266. Hesseltine HC, et al. Experimental human vaginal trichomoniasis. J Infect Dis 1942;71:127.
267. Lancely F, MacEntegart MC. Trichomonas vaginalis in the male: the experimental infection of a few volunteers. Lancet 1953;4:668.
268. Rein MF, Chapel TA. Trichomoniasis, candidiasis, and the minor venereal disease. Clin Obstet Gynecol 1975;18:73.
269. Wolner-Hanssen P, Krieger JN, Stevens CE, et al. Clinical manifestations of vaginal trichomoniasis. JAMA 1989;264:571.
270. Honigberg B. Trichomonads of importance in human medicine. In: Kreier JP, ed. Parasitic protozoa. Vol 2. New York: Academic Press, 1978:275.
271. Rein MF. Epidemiology of gonococcal infection. In: Roberts RB, ed. The gonococcus. New York: Wiley, 1977:1.
272. Catterall RD. Trichomonal infection of the genital tract. Med Clin North Am 1972;56:1203.
273. Wisdom AR, Dunlop EMC. Trichomoniasis: study of the disease and its treatment in women and men. British Journal of Venereal Disease 1965;41:90.
274. Rein MF. Clinical manifestations of urogenital trichomoniasis in women. In: Honigberg BM, ed. Trichomonads parasitic in humans. New York: Springer, 1989:227.
275. Fouts AC, Kraus SJ. *Trichomonas vaginalis*: reevaluation of its clinical presentation and laboratory diagnosis. J Infect Dis 1980;141:137.
276. Spence MR, Hollander DH, Smith J, McCaig L, et al. The clinical and laboratory diagnosis of *Trichomonas vaginalis* infection. Sex Transm Dis 1980;7:168.
277. Krieger JM. Diagnosis of trichomoniasis. Comparison of conventional wetmount preparation with cytologic studies, cultures, and monoclonal antibody staining of direct specimens. JAMA 1988;259:1223.
278. Hipp SS, Kirkwood MW, Gaafar HA. Screening for *Trichomonas vaginalis* infection by use of acridine orange fluorescent microscopy. Sex Transm Dis 1979;6:235.
279. Schou M, et al. *Trichomonas vaginalis* is now a very rare disease in Sweden. Scandinavian Society for Genitourinary Medicine, Fifth Meeting, 1988:37.
280. Lossick JG. The diagnosis of vaginal trichomoniasis [editorial]. JAMA 1988;259:1230.
281. Grys E. Topography of trichomoniasis in the reproductive organ of the woman. Wiad Parazytol 1964;10:122.
282. Suriyanon V, et al. *Trichomonas vaginalis* in a perinephric abscess: a case report. Am J Trop Med Hyg 1975;24:776.
283. Lossick JG. Treatment of *Trichomonas vaginalis* infections. Rev Infect Dis 1982;4:801.
284. Smith RF, DiDomenico A. Measuring the in vitro susceptibility of *Trichomonas vaginalis* to metronidazole. Sex Transm Dis 1980;7:120.
285. Meingassner JG, Thurner J. Strain of *Trichomonas vaginalis* resistant to metronidazole and other 5-nitroimidazoles. Antimicrob Agents Chemother 1979;15:254.
286. Lossick JG, Muller M, Gorrell TE. In vitro drug susceptibility and doses of metronidazole required for cure in cases of refractory vaginal trichomoniasis. J Infect Dis 1986;153:948.
287. Krajden S, Lussick JG, Wilk E, et al. Persistent *Trichomonas vaginalis* infection due to a metronidazole-resistant strain. Can Med Assoc J 1986;134:1373.
288. Underhill RA, Peck JE. Causes of therapeutic failure after treatment of trichomonal vaginitis with metronidazole: comparison of single dose treatment with a standard regimen. Br J Clin Pract 1974;28:134.
289. Hager WD, Brown ST, Kraus SJ, et al. Metronidazole for vaginal trichomoniasis: seven day vs single dose regimens. JAMA 1980;244:1219.
290. Dykers JR. Single dose metronidazole for trichomonal vaginitis. N Engl J Med 1975;293:23.
291. Fleury FS. A single dose of two grams of metronidazole for *Trichomonas vaginalis* vaginitis. Am J Obstet Gynecol 1977;128:320.
292. Rodin P, Hass G. Metronidazole and pregnancy. British Journal of Venereal Disease 1966;42:210.
293. Minkoff H, Grunebaum A, Feldman J, et al. Relationship of vaginal pH and papanicolaou smear results to vaginal flora and pregnancy outcome. Int J Gynaecol Obstet 1987;25:17.
294. Ronald AR, Wilt JC, Albritton WL. *Haemophilus ducreyi*. In: Holmes KK, Mardh P-A, eds. International perspectives on neglected sexually transmitted diseases. Washington, DC: Hemisphere Publishing, 1983:93.
295. Kibukamusoke JW. Venereal disease in East Africa. Trans R Soc Trop Med Hyg 1965;59:642.
296. Gaisin A, Heaton CL. Chancroid: alias the soft chancre. Int J Dermatol 1975;14:188.
297. Marmar JL. The management of resistant chancroid in Vietnam. J Urol 1972;107:807.
298. Blackmore CA, Limpakarnjanarat K, Rigau-Perez JG, et al. An outbreak of chancroid in Orange County, California: descriptive epidemiology and disease-control measures. J Infect Dis 1985;151:840.
299. Hart G. Venereal disease in a war environment: incidence and management. Med J Aust 1975;1:808.
300. Centers for Disease Control. Summary of notifiable diseases 1986. MMWR 1987;35:1.
301. Schmid GP, Sanders LL Jr, Blount JH, Alexander ER. Chancroid in the United States, reestablishment of an old disease. JAMA 1987;258:3265.
302. Piot P, Plummer FA, Rey MA, Ngugi EN, et al. Retrospective seroepidemiology of AIDS virus infection in Nairobi populations. J Infect Dis 1987;155:1108.
303. Greenblatt RM, Lukehart SA, Plummer FA, et al. Genital ulceration as a risk factor for human immunodeficiency virus infection. Aids 1988;2:47.
304. Simonsen JN, Cameron DW, Gakinya MN, et al. Human immunodeficiency virus infection in men with sexually transmitted diseases. N Engl J Med 1988;319:274.
305. Melbye M, Njelesani EK, Bayley A, et al. Evidence of heterosexual transmission and clinical manifestation of human immunodeficiency virus infection and related conditions in Lusaka, Zambia. Lancet 1986;2:1113.
306. Odumeru JA, Wiseman GM, Ronald AR. Role of lipopolysaccharide and complement in susceptibility of *Haemophilus ducreyi* to human serum. Infect Immun 1985;50:495.
307. Odumeru JA, Wiseman GM, Ronald AR. Virulence factors of *Haemophilus ducreyi*. Infect Immnun 1984;43:607.

308. Hammond GW, Slutchuk M, Scatliff J, et al. Clinical, epidemiological, laboratory and therapeutic features of an urban outbreak of chancroid in North America. Rev Infect Dis 1980;2:867.

309. Asin J. Chancroid: a report of 1402 cases. Am J Syph Gon Vener Dis 1952;36:483.

310. Plummer FA, D'Costa LJ, Nsanze H, et al. Clinical and microbiologic studies of genital ulcers in Kenyan women. Sex Transm Dis 1985;12:193.

311. Hammond GW, Chang JL, Wilt JC, Ronald AR. Comparison of specimen collection and laboratory techniques for isolation of *Haemophilus ducreyi*. J Clin Microbiol 1978;7:39.

312. Dylewski J, Nsanzett H, Maitha G, et al. Laboratory diagnosis of *Haemophilus ducreyi*: sensitivity of culture media. Diagn Microbiol Infect Dis 1986;4:241.

313. Museyi K, Van Dyck E, Vervoot T, Taylor D. Use of an enzyme immunoassay to detect serum IgG antibodies to *Haemophilus ducreyi*. J Infect Dis 1988;157:1039.

314. D'Costa LJ, Plummer FA, Bowner I, et al. Prostitutes are a major reservoir of sexually transmitted diseases in Nairobi, Kenya. Sex Trans Dis 1985;12:64.

73 CHAPTER

ARTHRITIS AND PREGNANCY

David Trock and Joe Craft

APPROACH TO THE PREGNANT PATIENT WITH ARTHRITIS

Musculoskeletal complaints are common among pregnant patients. The physician should attempt to classify these problems as either structural or inflammatory. Certain *structural* changes are secondary to hormonal changes (sacroiliac relaxation), due to alteration in weight (postural back pain), or related to redistribution of body fluid (entrapment neuropathy), while common overuse syndromes and minor trauma unrelated to pregnancy may be responsible for tendinitis or bursitis.

Inflammatory arthritis should be classified as monoarticular, migratory, or polyarticular, with each pattern offering helpful clues to diagnosis. For example, bacterial infection should be excluded during acute monoarticular arthritis, while rheumatoid arthritis, systemic lupus erythematosus (SLE), and viral syndromes should be considered if the presentation is polyarticular. A migratory arthritis raises the suspicion of gonococcal infection, Lyme disease, and others. Even in the presence of underlying conditions such as rheumatoid arthritis, new joint complaints require prompt attention, because associated infectious, vasculitic, and neoplastic conditions can pose a risk to the fetus.

RHEUMATOID ARTHRITIS AND PREGNANCY

GENERAL ASPECTS

Rheumatoid arthritis (RA), a systemic inflammatory disorder, causes pain and swelling of synovial joints in a symmetrical distribution. The smaller, peripheral joints (metacarpophalangeal, proximal interphalangeal, wrist, and metatarsophalangeal) are typically affected, and the arthritis is associated with morning stiffness and fatigue. The disease may be complicated by extra-articular manifestations, including rheumatoid nodules, serositis, interstitial lung disease, Sjögren's syndrome, Felty's syndrome, and vasculitis. RA occurs in all races worldwide, affecting women three times as often as men. The prevalence of RA (0.5% to 2.0%, depending on criteria used) increases with age, but its onset is generally during the childbearing years. The socioeconomic implications of RA abound, with estimates of $1 billion of lost wages and annual health expenses, increased mortality, and incalculable discomfort.[1,2]

In addition to chronic peripheral joint swelling, the diagnosis of RA is supported by the presence of serum rheumatoid factor (an autoantibody which binds the Fc portion of IgG), normochromic normocytic anemia, and elevated sedimentation rate. In RA, synovial fluid is yellow and turbid, with low glucose and decreased viscosity due to degradation of hyaluronic acid by lysosomal enzymes. The cell count of such synovial fluid varies, but is generally between 3,000 and 20,000 white blood cells (WBCs) per mm^2, with a predominance of neutrophils. Initial radiographs reveal juxta-articular osteopenia and soft tissue swelling, with subsequent marginal joint erosions, joint-space narrowing, and subluxation (Fig. 73-1). The 1987 American Rheumatism Association Criteria for RA (Table 73-1) allow proper diagnosis with greater than 90% sensitivity and specificity.[3]

With a proper stepwise approach to management, patients with RA can lead active lives with varying degrees of restriction. The treatment of RA in non-pregnant women includes resting and splinting of swollen joints, often combined with physical therapy to maintain muscle tone and preserve function. Pharmacologic therapy in non-pregnant women includes analgesics, nonsteroidal anti-inflammatory agents (salicylates and other nonsteroidal anti-inflammatory agents), and

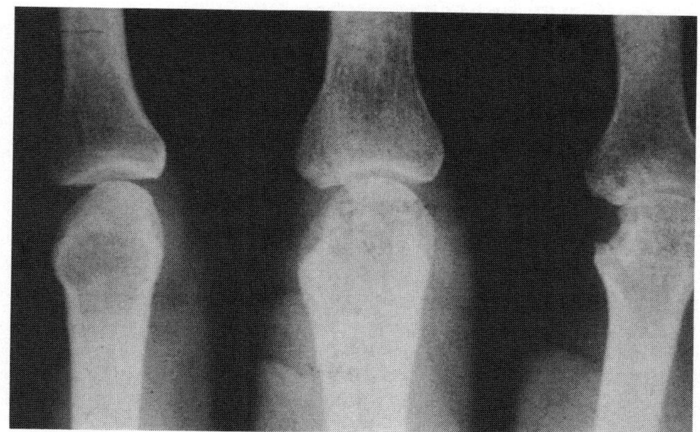

FIGURE 73–1. Serial radiographs of a metacarpophalangeal joint of a patient with rheumatoid arthritis. The left panel shows soft tissue swelling; the middle panel shows cortical thinning of the medial aspect of the metacarpal head, as well as narrowing of the joint space secondary to diffuse cartilage loss; and the right panel reveals a marginal erosion on the medial aspect of the joint. (From the Revised Clinical Slide Collection on the Rheumatic Diseases. The American College of Rheumatology, 1981, with permission.)

sometimes steroids (oral and intra-articular). Remittive therapy (gold salts, auranofin, hydroxychloroquine, sulfasalazine, methotrexate, penicillamine, and azathioprine) is used in those patients unresponsive to anti-inflammatory agents or those with progressive or erosive disease. Surgery (synovectomy, arthrodesis, and joint replacement) can be beneficial in selected individuals.

EFFECT OF PREGNANCY ON RHEUMATOID ARTHRITIS

Since the earliest description of RA, physicians and pregnant women have observed gestational remission of symptoms. In 1938, Hench reported the first series of 22 pregnant women, 20 of whom enjoyed remission of their inflammatory arthritis.[4] This observation was disputed in a survey of 732 women with RA, with disease onset occurring in 70 women within 6 months of delivery, raising the suspicion and continued controversy that pregnancy might actually be a risk factor in the causation of RA.[5,6] Still, Hench's original report has been confirmed by several investigators, and the ameliorating effect of pregnancy on RA is generally accepted.[7–9]

Improvement usually begins early in pregnancy, with a gradual reduction of pain, swelling and stiffness, a decrease in the requirement for analgesics, and a sense of well-being that peaks near term. Both Persellin[8] and Ostensen[10] have observed gestational remission among 75% of women with RA. Of these patients, 75% improve during the first trimester, 20% during the second trimester, and 5% during the third trimester. Persellin and coworkers have also illustrated gestational improvement of experimental adjuvant arthritis in rats.[11]

It is difficult to determine which women will improve, because gestational remission of RA is independent of rheumatoid factor, the type of joint involvement, disease duration, number of children, or sex of the fetus.[10] One study suggests a more likely chance of remission among women who had elevated serum IgG and IgM when compared to controls.[12] A remission during one pregnancy usually predicts further remission during subsequent pregnancies.[13] If RA develops or worsens during one pregnancy, remission may still occur in subsequent pregnancies.

MECHANISMS OF REMISSION

During the early part of the 20th century, attempts at inducing remission in RA included prolonged starvation diets, induction of febrile reactions with typhoid vaccines, tonsillectomy, and even hysterectomy.[14] Hench's 1938 report of pregnancy-induced remission of inflammatory arthritis inspired an enthusiastic search for the effect of pregnancy-related hormones on RA. This search led to the eventual use of corticosteroids for RA and other rheumatic diseases. Although cortisol levels are raised during pregnancy, the levels return to normal within 5 days of delivery, and the pattern of disease exacerbation many weeks later does not correspond to that of steroid withdrawal.[15] Accordingly, remission cannot be explained on this basis alone, nor is remission in RA confined to women with high plasma cortisol levels. Additionally, the administration of estrogens has been unsuccessful at inducing remission of active RA, although prolonged use of oral contraceptives may be associated with a delay in disease onset, or protection against the development of RA.[16,17]

Rather than a hormonal cause for disease remission, recent studies have focused on immunologic changes during pregnancy. The mother should have the potential to reject the fetus by mounting a cell-mediated immune response; however, several changes in both cellular and humoral immune function occur during pregnancy that are perhaps responsible for prevention of fetal rejection. Amelioration of RA may be a fortuitous byproduct of these changes.

There is evidence for depressed cellular immunity during pregnancy, such as increased virulence and susceptibility to viral, fungal, and intracellular protozoal infections, delayed rejection of skin allografts, and decreased reactivity to tuberculin skin testing.[8,18,19] An increase in suppressor T-cell subpopulations during pregnancy may cause inversion of T-cell subsets, and contribute to weakening of maternal cellular immunity.[20,21]

During the past decade, much attention also has been focused on a pregnancy-associated globulin (PAG), known as α-2 PAG, which is believed to be beneficial in RA. Persellin called this α-2 globulin PZP (pregnancy

TABLE 73–1. THE 1987 REVISED CRITERIA FOR THE CLASSIFICATION OF RHEUMATOID ARTHRITIS (TRADITIONAL FORMAT)*

CRITERION	DEFINITION
1. Morning stiffness	Morning stiffness in and around the joints, lasting at least 1 hour before maximal improvement
2. Arthritis of 3 or more joint areas	At least 3 joint areas simultaneously have had soft tissue swelling or fluid (not bony overgrowth alone) observed by a physician. The 14 possible areas are right or left PIP, MCP, wrist, elbow, knee, ankle, and MTP joints
3. Arthritis of hand joints	At leat 1 area swollen (as defined above) in a wrist, MCP, or PIP joint
4. Symmetric arthritis	Simultaneous involvement of the same joint areas (as defined in **2**) on both sides of the body (bilateral involvement of PIPs, MCPs, or MTPs is acceptable without absolute symmetry)
5. Rheumatoid nodules	Subcutaneous nodules, over bony prominences, or extensor surfaces, or in juxta-articular regions, observed by a physician
6. Serum rheumatoid factor	Demonstration of abnormal amounts of serum rheumatoid factor by any method for which the result has been positive in <5% of normal control subjects.
7. Radiographic changes	Radiographic changes typical of rheumatoid arthritis on posteroanterior hand and wrist radiographs, which must include erosions or unequivocal bony decalcification localized in or most marked adjacent to the involved joints (osteoarthritis changes alone do not qualify)

* For classification purposes, a patient shall be said to have rheumatoid arthritis if he/she has satisified at least 4 of these 7 criteria. Criteria 1 through 4 must have been present for at least 6 weeks. Patients with 2 clinical diagnoses are not excluded. Designation as classic, definite, or probable rheumatoid arthritis is *not* to be made.

PIP, proximal interphalangeal; MCP, metacarpophalangeal; MTP, metatarsophalangeal.

From Arnett FC, Edworthy SM, Bloch DA, et al. The American Rheumatism Association 1987 revised criteria for the classification of rheumatoid arthritis. Arthritis Rheum 1988;31:315, with permission.

zone protein), which is detectable in the non-pregnant state, but rises markedly during the first trimester, coincident with disease remission.[22] PAG levels normalize during lactation, when most women experience reactivation of RA. PAG can inhibit both lymphocyte mitogenesis and lymphokine release, and suppress the inflammation of experimentally induced arthritis in rats.[11] Kasukawa observed a significant correlation between PAG levels in rheumatoid plasma and suppression of cellular immunity, but no associated change in acute phase reactants (C-reactive protein, sedimentation rate, complement levels, or haptoglobin).[23] The association of PAG and disease activity was supported by Unger and associates, who studied 14 pregnant women with RA. The mean PAG level was significantly higher ($P < 0.001$) among women whose RA improved, while levels of another pregnancy-specific protein, β-1 glycoprotein (SP1), did not correlate with disease activity.[24] By contrast, Ostensen's group found no correlation between improvement of RA and α-2 PAG levels, but markedly elevated PAG levels occurred in all of six women (three with RA and three with ankylosing spondylitis) taking oral contraceptives, without demonstrable changes in disease activity during an 8-month period. This latter study demonstrated that PAG is a marker for pregnancy, but not necessarily an inducer of remission of RA.[25]

There is growing evidence that circulating factors are responsible for alteration of antigen recognition and suppression of the maternal immune response. Circulating immune complexes, detectable during pregnancy, can bind to cells that express Fc receptors, and act as "blocking factors," affording the rheumatoid synovium similar protection to that which is received by the placental allograft.[26] Additionally, placental immunoglobulins contain alloantibodies directed against transplacental antigens. Sany and colleagues explored the ameliorating effect of pregnancy on RA by administering placenta-eluted antibodies to 11 patients with active, severe RA.[27] When compared to pooled gamma globulin given intravenously, placenta-eluted antibodies were able to suppress certain clinical features of RA in 7 of 11 patients. The authors suggested a polyspecific anti-HLA DR activity of placenta-eluted gamma globulins, possibly responsible for their favorable effect.

Recently, attention has been focused on the alteration of carbohydrate composition of IgG during pregnancy. Generally, IgG from patients with RA contain less galactose, potentially increasing its autoaggregation.[28,29] Conversely, Pekelharing and associates have demonstrated increased galactosylation of IgG during normal pregnancy.[30] It would be of interest to demonstrate a normalization of IgG galactosylation among pregnant women with RA, which would correlate with disease activity.

In summary, the cause for gestational remission in RA appears multifactorial. All of the proposed mechanisms of remission can serve as a springboard toward our better understanding of the pathogenesis of RA. Because oral contraceptives do not induce remission in RA, women taking oral contraceptives could serve as a control group for further investigation.

POSTPARTUM

". . .well, here they go again, my rheumatism and my monthlies."—1932, one of Phillip Hench's patients.

At least 90% of women will have an exacerbation of RA, generally between 2 and 10 weeks after delivery.[31] The rest (10%) may enjoy a prolonged postpartum remission, which rarely exceeds 8 months. Breastfeeding provides no protection against this postpartum flare.[10] Likewise, abortion, either spontaneous or therapeutic, is often followed by exacerbation of RA; however, RA does not generally induce spontaneous abortion.[32] Five of 31 women evaluated by Ostensen had fever in conjunction with their postpartum flare, but there were no other systemic, extra-articular manifestations of RA during pregnancy, or in the 12 months following delivery.[9]

EFFECT OF RA ON PREGNANCY

RA patients usually deliver healthy newborns of normal birth weight.[7,33] When compared to healthy pregnant women, those with RA have no increased frequency of spontaneous abortion, premature labor, or complications at delivery.[9,10,33] One recent evaluation of 96 women with RA differed from previous reports, however, showing a higher ratio of spontaneous abortion among women with RA (0.33%) when compared to a control group (0.20%).[34] This discrepancy requires further investigation.

In the unusual setting of RA with rheumatoid vasculitis, one author reported intrauterine growth retardation at 36 weeks with premature rupture of membranes, and a placenta that showed multiple calcified infarcts, presumably due to insufficient uterine blood flow.[35] Complications in both the mother and fetus are more likely to arise with antirheumatic drugs, which are not withdrawn in 25% of cases due to activity of disease.

FERTILITY IN RA

An early report suggesting decreased fertility among women with RA, even before disease onset, was inspired by the observation that married women attending an arthritis clinic had fewer children than nondisease controls.[36] The findings of fewer live births to women with RA might have been more related to decreased parity (due to chronic illness or diminished sexual activity) than fertility. More recent surveys have shown no decrease of fertility among women with RA.[34,37]

ANTIRHEUMATIC DRUG THERAPY

The symptoms of RA usually improve during pregnancy, and the need for drug treatment is often reduced. However, the patient whose disease does not improve presents an interesting and difficult problem for the clinician. Although the fetus is largely unaffected by its mother's synovial inflammation, it remains susceptible to the side effects of many anti-inflammatory and remittive agents, which commonly cross the placenta. To minimize any harmful effects on the fetus, only well-known drugs with short elimination half-lives should be used, in the lowest possible dose for limited periods.

In this section, the approach to drug therapy is primarily directed at the 25% of women whose RA remains active, the 2% of women who experience the *onset* of RA during pregnancy, and the 90% of women whose disease flares postpartum during lactation (Table 73-2).

Acetaminophen

Acetaminophen, although not necessarily effective for symptoms of acute inflammation in rheumatoid arthritis, is nevertheless commonly prescribed for pain relief in patients with rheumatic diseases. It freely crosses the placenta, although there is no clear evidence that it causes congenital anomalies.[38]

Salicylates

Aspirin is inexpensive and efficacious, and remains the initial drug of choice for RA. It exerts an anti-inflammatory effect via decreased prostaglandin synthesis; this drug also stabilizes lysosomal membranes, inhibits leukocyte function, and decreases histamine release. Its role, and that of other nonsteroidal anti-inflammatory agents (see below) in the inhibition of prostaglandin synthesis, has an obvious effect on fetal development. Most notably, it inhibits the synthesis of prostaglandin E_2, which maintains pulmonary and systemic vessel relaxation, as well as patency of the ductus arteriosus.[31,87]

Toxicity of aspirin is often dose-related, including tinnitus, respiratory alkalosis, gastrointestinal erosion, and elevation of transaminases. Other side effects that are less dose-dependent include asthma, head-

TABLE 73–2. Antirheumatic Drug Therapy During Pregnancy

DRUG	POTENTIAL SIDE EFFECTS IN MOTHER	REPORTED SIDE EFFECTS IN FETUS	SAFETY IN LACTATION	REMARKS
Salicylates	Prolonged gestation and labor, anemia, elevated transaminases, maternal bleeding during delivery and postpartum	Neonatal intracranial hemorrhage, platelet dysfunction, respiratory distress, fetal salicylism/metabolic acidosis, decreased birth weight, hypoglycemia	No; high levels in breast milk	Stop aspirin 4–6 weeks prior to delivery. Can be given in low doses; less than 3 grams/day
Glucocorticoids	Avascular necrosis and osteoporosis, glucose intolerance, infection	Intrauterine growth retardation, adrenal insufficiency, cleft palate, thymic suppression	Yes; up to 30 mg prednisone	Should attempt the lowest possible oral dose; i.e., 10 mg/day or less if possible. Prednisone and prednisolone are usually safe if prescribing less than 30 mg/day. Intra-articular route is safe. During chronic use, stress doses should be used during delivery. Dexamethasone crosses the placenta.
NSAIDs	Prolonged gestation and labor, decreased uteroplacental circulation, gastrointestinal toxicity, renal dysfunction	Premature closure of the ductus arteriosus, pulmonary hypertension, oligohydramnios, renal dysfunction	Indomethacin is contraindicated due to high levels in milk; ibuprofen, naproxen, and ketoprofen are allowed.	Should be given in the smallest possible dose Stop NSAIDs 4 weeks prior to delivery.
Gold (intramuscular)	Bone marrow suppression, proteinuria, dermatitis	Congenital malformation in one case report, renal dysfunction in a breastfed infant	Yes; only trace amounts in milk	If used, the longest possible dosing interval should be used. Should not be started if RA develops during pregnancy
Auranofin (oral gold)	Diarrhea; otherwise similar to IM gold, with less dermatitis	None reported	Unknown	May be safely withdrawn
Hydroxychloroquine	Retinal pigment deposition, gastrointestinal upset, thrombocytopenia	Retinal and uveal tract pigmentation, sensorineural hearing loss, chromosome damage	Unknown	May be safely withdrawn
Penicillamine	Proteinuria, dysgeusia, marrow suppression, rash	Cutis laxa in the neonate (reversible), impaired wound healing, myasthenia gravis in the newborn, vitamin B_6 deficiency	No	Not recommended for RA during pregnancy or lactation
Azathioprine	Leukopenia, gastrointestinal intolerance	Intrauterine growth retardation, pancytopenia in one case	No	No proven risk of teratogenesis May be safely withdrawn at the onset of pregnancy
Methotrexate	Hepatotoxicity, leukopenia, stomatitis	May induce spontaneous abortion, may induce congenital malformations, particularly if used in early pregnancy	No	Contraindicated in RA, use with contraception Stop 1–3 months prior to pregnancy Termination of pregnancy should be discussed if pregnancy ensues
Cyclophosphamide	Hemorrhagic cystitis, leukopenia, alopecia, ovarian failure	Congenital malformations, particularly if used in early pregnancy	No, high levels achieved in breast milk	Should be used with contraception, not recommended for RA

NSAIDs, nonsteroidal anti-inflammatory drugs; RA, rheumatoid arthritis.

ache, interstitial nephritis, and inhibition of platelet aggregation.

Salicylates freely cross the placenta, causing craniovertebral abnormalities in rats when given at five times the normal dosage.[38,39] Similar defects have been demonstrated in mice injected with 500 mg/kg of sodium salicylate.[40] Dogs given toxic doses of aspirin between days 23 and 30 after mating had a 50% malformation rate in their offspring.[41]

The teratogenic potential of a prolonged therapeutic salicylate blood level in humans is unknown. The inhibited synthesis of prostaglandin E_2 and F_2 from arachidonic acid may be responsible for the delayed onset and prolonged duration of labor, while blockage of the enzyme cyclooxygenase, which is essential for platelet aggregation via the synthesis of thromboxane and prostacyclin, can lead to a prolonged bleeding time for up to 1 week after the last dose of aspirin. This mechanism may be responsible for the significant increase in blood loss at delivery among women taking aspirin, when compared to controls.[38,42,43] Additionally, maternal use of aspirin has been associated with a reduced mean birth weight, and neonatal intracranial hemorrhage, as illustrated in one study of premature infants.[44,45] Infants born with high salicylate levels (>30 mg/dL) may experience withdrawal symptoms, including generalized hypertonia and agitation lasting several weeks.[46] Learning difficulties, seen in rats exposed to aspirin in utero, have not been observed or studied in humans.[47]

Early reports suggesting that salicylates are teratogenic in humans may be biased because they consisted of questionnaires given to mothers of malformed infants, inquiring retrospectively about aspirin use.[48,49] Two more recent prospective studies, observing the casual use of aspirin during pregnancy, showed that it is not a significant cause of fetal malformation.[44,50] In fact, 64% of pregnant women admit to casual aspirin use.[50]

As RA improves during pregnancy, women may find adequate relief from 650 mg twice or three times daily. Full anti-inflammatory doses of aspirin (3 to 4 g/day), which are often necessary to achieve a therapeutic salicylate blood level of 15 to 25 mg/dL during active synovitis, however, are best avoided if possible. Aspirin should be given in the lowest effective dose and should be withdrawn late in pregnancy, preferably 4 weeks prior to delivery. Aspirin accumulates in breast milk, and should not be resumed until the cessation of breast-feeding; alternatively, a proprionic acid nonsteroidal can be substituted. Despite the potential adverse effects outlined, aspirin remains one of the safest and most useful drugs for RA during pregnancy.

Nonsteroidal Anti-Inflammatory Drugs

There are many new nonsteroidal anti-inflammatory drugs (NSAIDs) that have enjoyed popularity as alternatives to aspirin, due to their longer half-lives and reasonable side-effect profile. Even though there have been no reports of NSAID-related teratogenicity in humans, the reluctance to use them routinely during pregnancy has stemmed largely from the lack of controlled trials and a suitable alternative in aspirin. In the last decade, indomethacin was used as a prostaglandin inhibitor for the prevention of premature labor, with reports of infantile gastrointestinal hemorrhage, hyperbilirubinemia, transient renal dysfunction, premature closure of the ductus arteriosus, and primary pulmonary hypertension.[51,52]

It is unknown if the other indole derivatives (sulindac, tolmetin) and the newer NSAIDs share the same side-effect potential as indomethacin. For this reason, NSAIDs should be held during mild disease, and replaced with aspirin. When NSAIDs become necessary, as in severe ankylosing spondylitis or in patients who are allergic or intolerant to aspirin, the propionic acid derivatives (ibuprofen, naproxen, ketoprofen) may be the safest alternatives, when used intermittently in the lowest possible doses, and withdrawn 4 weeks prior to delivery.[10] Only trace amounts of these three agents are found in mother's milk, suggesting that it is safe to use these agents during lactation.[53] Unlike other NSAIDs, indomethacin attains *high* levels in breast milk, and should be avoided if breast-feeding is desired, to prevent neonatal morbidity.

Gold

Intramuscular gold salts have been the standard of RA therapy for over 50 years, inducing remission in roughly 70% of patients by an unclear mechanism. Gold inhibits phagocyte function, stabilizes lysosomal membranes, and decreases titers of rheumatoid factor, immunoglobulin, and the third component of complement.[54] The two types of intramuscular gold commonly employed are the water-soluble aurothioglucose (Solganal), and the oil-based gold sodium thiomalate (Myochrysin). Potential side effects of these agents include dermatitis, membranous nephropathy, bone marrow suppression, hepatotoxicity, and interstitial pneumonitis. Gold has a serum half-life of 5½ days, and remains in the body long after it is discontinued. For this reason, a blood count and urinalysis are performed just prior to each gold injection. Most untoward effects are reversible upon the discontinuance of gold, and in some cases gold can be restarted at a lower dose. The risk–benefit analysis of gold therapy for non-pregnant patients with active RA clearly favors its use, and the drug should not be discontinued when remission is achieved, because the results of a second trial of gold can be disappointing.[55] This observation is particularly relevant for the woman who sustains her gold-induced remission into pregnancy.

Placental transfer of gold has been established.[56,57] A case report of a healthy infant born with a therapeutic gold level (225 μg/dL) suggests the possible safe use of gold in selected patients, as supported by other cases.[10,57,58] Although this neonate sustained no untoward effect of gold, it should be pointed out that a therapeutic serum gold level theoretically subjects an infant to the same potential toxicity (nephropathy, marrow suppression), without the ability to perform reliable screening in utero. Renal dysfunction has been reported in an infant who was breastfed by a woman receiving gold.[59] There is also one case report of a possible teratogenic effect of gold, in which biweekly gold injections into the second trimester were associated with an occipital encephalocele, cerebral degeneration, marked hypertelorism, cleft lip, cleft palate, and bilateral simian creases.[60] Chromosome analysis was normal. This phenotype has not been reported elsewhere, and its relationship to gold therapy is speculative. A prospective study of seven children exposed to gold compounds in utero revealed normal physical, psychomotor, and intellectual development at a mean 7.4 years of age.[61]

Because RA is likely to improve during pregnancy, some would argue that gold treatment should be withheld for this reason alone, while others remind us that the clinical decision to discontinue gold in pregnant women should not be made with haste.[10] Due to the potential for teratogenicity, as evidenced by one case report, the decision to continue gold should be made along with both partners, accompanied by informed consent.

Oral Gold. In animal studies, oral gold has been demonstrated to freely cross the placenta, and is associated with fetal abnormalities, including edema, low birth weight, and induced abortion, varying according to dosage.[62–64] In humans, 13 women with RA who continued oral gold therapy during pregnancy reportedly developed healthy infants.[53] This report is encouraging, but further investigation is needed before oral gold can be considered safe during pregnancy and lactation.

Corticosteroids

Corticosteroids are commonly used during a flare of rheumatoid synovitis and during serious extra-articular manifestations of RA. Prednisone is a popular choice because it is inexpensive and well absorbed when given orally, and remains a useful adjunct to the remittive agents, particularly for short-term use. When used on a long-term basis, the side-effect profile of high-dose prednisone, including glucose intolerance, osteopenia, posterior subcapsular cataracts, infection, myopathy, and cushingoid features, becomes unfavorable. Adrenal suppression may occur in doses greater than 5 mg to 7.5 mg per day (prednisone or equivalent), especially when administered in divided doses. Therefore, corticosteroids are best given as a once-daily dose, and should be tapered slowly when adrenal-suppressive doses are given for longer than 14 days. The control of rheumatoid synovitis is often disappointing if steroids are used on an alternate-day basis, or if they are tapered too quickly. Corticosteroids do not affect the long-term course of RA, nor do they prevent erosions or eventual joint destruction.

Corticosteroids are generally safe in pregnancy. Those used in RA, including prednisone, prednisolone, and dexamethasone, all cross the placenta, with variable levels found in the fetus.[65] However, the placenta provides an effective barrier to prednisone and prednisolone due to placental 11-β dehydrogenase,[66] which partially inactivates cortisone. Dexamethasone, conversely, is not reliably deactivated in the placenta, and is not recommended during pregnancy.[67] Dexamethasone can cause fetal adrenal suppression when administered within 12 hours of delivery, and is thus best avoided.[68]

Reports of adverse fetal outcomes attributed to corticosteroids have included premature birth, growth retardation, impaired immunologic responses to thymic suppression, masculinization of the female infant, adrenal suppression, and one early report of stillbirth with cleft palate.[70–72] Earlier work in animals raised concern about the high risk of cleft palate, but the experience with humans has not supported these findings. Larger series of pregnant women with asthma who require steroids have been encouraging, showing no evidence of increased malformations.[73] The plasma cortisol levels may be reduced in infants born of mothers taking steroids during pregnancy, but the response to ACTH is normal in most.[74] Nevertheless, the infant should still be observed for signs of adrenal insufficiency.

Ideally, the daily dose of prednisone should be 5 to 10 mg, and should not exceed 20 mg for rheumatoid synovitis. Higher doses may be required to control rheumatoid vasculitis and other extra-articular manifestations of RA, although the risk/benefit is not clear. For localized synovitis, selected intra-articular injections with 20 to 40 mg of triamcinolone or methylprednisolone may be a useful measure in active RA, and should be dispensed by experienced hands. The serum level attained after an intra-articular corticosteroid injection is not known to be harmful to the fetus.[75] At parturition, stress doses of steroids should be considered in patients who have been receiving adrenal suppressive doses, particularly when a cesarean section is planned.

During lactation, low-dose corticosteroids are acceptable. Less than 1% of an oral dose of 5 mg prednisolone accumulates in mother's milk, but the effect of higher doses in the nursing infant has not been fully studied.[76] When high doses (>30 mg) of cortisone or equivalent are required in the setting of a postpartum flare, consideration may be given to discontinuation of breast-feeding.

Penicillamine

Toxicity to penicillamine occurs in 40% of patients, including dysgeusia, skin rash, nephritis, pneumonitis, and gastrointestinal intolerance. Several untoward effects have been reported in infants of mothers receiving penicillamine for Wilson's disease, cystinuria, and RA, including an Ehlers-Danlos–like syndrome, with generalized connective-tissue laxity leading to hypotonia and poor wound healing.[77] Despite a prior report of 19 normal infants delivered to mothers taking penicillamine for RA, the more current and conservative posture recommends withdrawal of penicillamine when a pregnancy is being planned.[10,78]

Sulfasalazine

Sulfasalazine, widely used for inflammatory bowel disease, was originally formulated for treating RA, and is now enjoying increased use as a disease-modifying agent. Both the 5-amino salicylic acid and sulfapyridine components of sulfasalazine cross the placenta, without a known increase in congenital abnormalities.[79,80] In patients with ulcerative colitis taking sulfasalazine, there may be a slight increase in spontaneous abortion, possibly due to underlying active bowel disease.[79] Theoretically, the sulfa component can complete with bilirubin for binding sites on plasma proteins, leading to kernicterus, although this has not been a significant clinical problem. Reversible azoospermia and infertility have been reported in men receiving sulfasalazine, although infertility is not known to be a side effect among women. Until further reports of the risks/benefits of sulfasalazine in pregnant women with RA become clear, this useful agent should probably be withheld during pregnancy and lactation.

Hydroxychloroquine

Antimalarials such as hydroxychloroquine (Plaquenil) are commonly used in women with RA, with occasional toxicity such as skin rash, gastrointestinal intolerance, and transient visual blurring. There is also the rare consequence of permanent retinal deposition (more associated with chloroquine, rather than hydroxychloroquine), which requires routine ophthalmologic surveillance.

When given during pregnancy, individual case reports of toxicity with antimalarials have included retinal and uveal pigmentation, ototoxicity, and chromosome damage.[81,82] Alternatively, there is longstanding testimony to the safe use of these drugs given to pregnant women for malaria prophylaxis.[83] Even with the remote risks and potential benefit derived by these agents, there are ample alternative therapies for pregnant women with RA. If a woman on hydroxychloroquine becomes pregnant, the drug should be withdrawn.

IMMUNOSUPPRESSIVE THERAPY

Methotrexate and azathioprine are useful in RA, but should be avoided during pregnancy. Neither has been proven to impair fertility.[67]

Methotrexate has caused craniovertebral congenital malformations, with an incidence of 3.4% in a recent review of 290 live births.[67,84] It can potentially induce abortion, and should be discontinued at least one menstrual cycle before planning a pregnancy. If a woman taking methotrexate becomes pregnant, the risk to the fetus and termination of pregnancy should be discussed. Additionally, women whose male partner is receiving methotrexate should not plan a pregnancy until he has avoided the drug for 3 months.[85]

Azathioprine is largely deactivated in the placenta to 6-thioguanine, and is safely used in pregnant patients with renal allografts.[86,87] However, reports of impaired fetal growth, neonatal immunosuppression, and pancytopenia warrant the withdrawal of azathioprine when used by the pregnant RA patient, without the need to consider terminating the pregnancy.

PLASMAPHERESIS

Plasmapheresis has been used in the non-pregnant state, providing a short-lived reprieve of symptoms, presumably by reducing the load of immune complexes bound for the reticuloendothelial system.[88] However, the decreased levels of immunoglobulin may also raise susceptibility to infections, especially herpes zoster. During pregnancy, this treatment remains experimental for autoimmune diseases such as Goodpasture's syndrome. In RA, plasmapheresis is best used in conjunction with high-dose corticosteroids and cyclophosphamide, and is not recommended during pregnancy.

SURGERY

Surgery, including synovectomy, arthrodesis, and prosthetic joint replacement, has greatly contributed to the preservation of ambulation and performance of activities of daily living for patients with severe RA. When possible, surgery should be deferred until the postpartum state.

ADDITIONAL MANAGEMENT CONCERNS

When the diagnosis of RA is unclear, treatment problems arise, or if extra-articular manifestations occur, a rheumatologic consultation is recommended. Several disorders require differentiation from RA, such as reactive and infectious arthritis, systemic lupus, immune complex disease (serum sickness, hepatitis B viremia, endocarditis), and others. The clinician should entertain the possibility of infection in all patients with RA who complain of a single, isolated swollen joint. Patients on steroids with acute hip or knee pain should be evaluated for avascular necrosis, joint infection, transient regional osteoporosis, or active RA. If imaging becomes necessary in this region, magnetic resonance imaging (MRI) is preferred, because it precludes exposure of the fetus to ionizing radiation.[89] The patient with severe hip arthritis or artificial hip joints can still have a vaginal delivery if the stirrups are modified to minimize abduction.[13]

Flexion films of the cervical spine are important for women with RA, even in the absence of neck pain, to search for atlantoaxial (C1–C2) subluxation. Greater than 3 mm of subluxation should alert the anesthesiologist to avoid excessive neck manipulation. These women should arrive in the delivery room wearing a soft cervical collar. If there is no subluxation, the anesthesiologist should still be aware of the presence of RA due to the potential exacerbation of temporomandibular joint arthritis, or the possibility of a narrowed trachea if cricoarytenoid arthritis is present.

If remission is achieved, this is an ideal time for muscle strengthening, toning, and joint mobility exercises, preferably through the physiotherapy department. A balance between rest and exercise is preferred, with at least two daily rest periods of 1 hour each. Exercise in a heated swimming pool is ideal, allowing muscle toning without undue stress on joints. In preparation for the post-delivery period, mothers should be informed about the likelihood of arthritis exacerbation, fatigue, and postpartum depression.[90,91] Baby clothes should have Velcro ties or zippers instead of buttons, and occupational therapy should be specifically geared toward bathing and holding the infant. Reassurance with regard to self-esteem, body image, sexuality, and independence requires particular sensitivity in dealing with the woman with RA and other disabilities.[92]

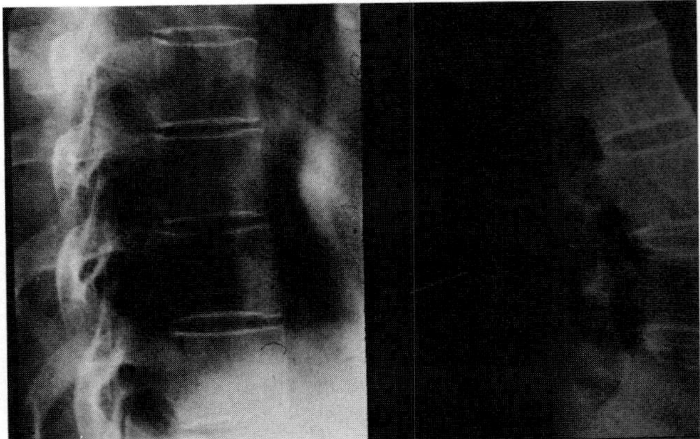

FIGURE 73–2. The left panel reveals a lateral view of the lower thoracic spine of a patient with ankylosing spondylitis. The vertebrae are osteopenic with preserved joint spaces. Most notably, there is squaring of the vertebral bodies secondary to inflammatory changes at ligament insertions. The right panel is a radiograph of the lateral view of the lumbar spine of a second patient with ankylosing spondylitis. There is osteopenia and calcification of the anterior longitudinal ligaments. (From the Revised Clinical Slide Collection on the Rheumatic Diseases. The American College of Rheumatology, 1981, with permission.)

ANKYLOSING SPONDYLITIS AND OTHER SPONDYLOARTHROPATHIES

Ankylosing spondylitis is characterized by progressive stiffness and discomfort of the spine, often beginning during the childbearing years. There is uniform sex distribution and a striking association with HLA-B27.[93] Symptoms often begin in the lumbar spine, which may be seen radiographically as squaring of the vertebral bodies (Fig. 73-2), progressing to calcification of the outer fibers of the annulus fibrosus, giving a "bamboo spine" appearance (see Fig. 73-2). The resulting loss of spinal mobility is characterized by flattening of the normal lordosis, poor chest expansion, and increased susceptibility to spinal fractures. Sacroiliitis, when present, is initially painful, and may lead to fusion of the sacroiliac joints. Painful laxity and subluxation of the sacroiliac joints were reported in a multiparous woman with spondylitis.[94] Peripheral arthritis occurs in up to 20% to 30%, often involving the hips, shoulders, and knees.[95] Other manifestations of spondylitis include uveitis, pulmonary fibrosis, aortic insufficiency, and cardiac conduction defects. The above features, as well as the New York criteria for ankylosing spondylitis, support the clinical and radiographic diagnosis of spondylitis.[96] Several other conditions, including Reiter's syndrome, psoriatic arthritis, and ulcerative colitis-associated arthritis, belong to the spondyloarthropathy family, and can present like ankylosing spondylitis. Sclerosis of the lateral aspect of the sacroiliac joint, or *osteitis condensans ilii*, is an occasional postpartum phenomenon that is not necessarily associated with spondylitis.

The long-term goals of therapy for spondylitis include preservation of chest expansion and posture with spinal extension exercises and swimming. NSAIDs are helpful in diminishing pain and morning stiffness, but do not alter the radiographic progression of the disease. The short-term goals of therapy include analgesics when needed, and intra-articular steroid injection of involved peripheral joints. The patient and physician should be aware of potential emergencies, including uveitis, spondylodiscitis, spinal fracture, cardiac conduction disturbance, and adverse reaction to NSAIDs.

ANKYLOSING SPONDYLITIS AND PREGNANCY

Ankylosing spondylitis differs markedly from RA with regard to its gestational course, in that pregnancy does not usually induce remission in women with the former illness.[97] Early reports were contradictory because they were written at a time when spondylitis was seldom diagnosed in females. In addition, certain features of normal pregnancy such as low back pain and elevation of sedimentation rate made activity of spondylitis difficult to discern in retrospective studies. The first prospective look at spondylitis during pregnancy by Ostenses and Husby comprised 13 patients, most of whom experienced aggravated disease during the second and third trimester, including spinal tenderness, morning stiffness, nocturnal pain, and increased need for NSAID therapy.[33] Among spondylitis patients whose disease is active during gestation, relief of symptoms is typically not felt until a few days after delivery, lasting 4 to 8 weeks, after which an exacerbation of spinal disease may be accompanied by peripheral arthritis in up to 50% of patients, and anterior uveitis in up to 20%.[33,98]

Scattered reports of complications due to spondylitis include complete ankylosis of the sacroiliac and hip joints in one patient, making vaginal delivery unfeasible, and with associated neck disease making it difficult to maintain her airway during cesarean section. Despite transient cyanosis, the mother delivered a healthy infant.[99] Complications also may arise from caudal anesthesia in spondylitis, because one author reported hypotension and seizure activity associated with intraosseous puncture.[100]

Interestingly, patients whose disease *improves* during pregnancy may have underlying arthropathy associated with spondylitis, such as psoriatic arthritis or ulcerative colitis-associated spondylitis.[33] Women with psoriatic arthritis are similar to those with RA in that they enjoy improvement during the first trimester, and typically throughout the pregnancy.[101] As in RA, the postpartum period may be difficult for those women with psoriatic arthritis.[102]

Despite maternal difficulties during gestation, it should be noted that in a recent survey of pregnancy in 50 women with spondylitis, all 50 had uneventful pregnancies and gave birth to 120 healthy children.[103] This confirmed previous observations that ankylosing spondylitis does not influence fertility or fetal welfare. There appears to be no increased tendency toward spontaneous abortion, premature labor, or stillbirth.

INFECTIOUS ARTHRITIS

GENERAL CONCEPTS

Several types of infectious arthritis may complicate pregnancy, including gonococcal arthritis, Lyme disease, and parvoviral infections. Additionally, certain pregnancies at high risk for fetal complications, including patients with syphilis, rubella, hepatitis B virus, endocarditis, or human immunodeficiency virus (HIV) infection, may *first* present with arthritis.[104] Alternatively, an acute presentation of RA or systemic lupus may include fever, giving the false appearance of underlying infection; however, the presence of underlying RA does not rule out the possibility of joint sepsis. Indeed, the pregnant woman with arthritis and fever presents a multidisciplinary challenge. As a rule, all patients with acute monoarticular arthritis should have the joint aspirated for Gram's stain and culture and, particularly if accompanied by tenosynovitis, must be considered to have gonococcal arthritis until proven otherwise.

GONOCOCCAL ARTHRITIS AND TENOSYNOVITIS

Gonococcal arthritis is the most frequent form of pyogenic arthritis in young adults, with a predilection for women during menstruation or pregnancy, particularly in the third trimester.[105] A migratory polyarthritis and tenosynovitis typically affects large joints such as the knees, wrists, or ankles, and occasionally the hip or shoulder.[106] Fever is often present, but other systemic manifestations are generally mild. One third of patients develop skin lesions, frequently on the palms or soles, appearing as an erythematous patch with a necrotic, central pustule (Fig. 73-3). The organism is labile and difficult to culture, yielding positive results from synovial or pustular fluid in only 40% to 50% of individuals. Blood and cervical cultures may help confirm the diagnosis. Radiographs and other tests are nonspecific, and antibiotic selection is often based on clinical grounds.

Parenteral penicillin therapy provides a dramatic response and is safe for the fetus. In certain areas, ceftriaxone has been recommended for genital gonococcal infection due to increasing penicillin resistance, and has been used safely in pregnancy with sufficient concentration into placenta and fetal tissues.[107] Although disseminated gonococcal infection is usually penicillin-sensitive, inquiry regarding local penicillin resistance is desirable. Untreated, gonococcal infection has been associated with premature rupture of membranes, fetal sepsis with meningitis arthritis, and ophthalmia neonatorum. These complications have been treated satisfactorily with parenteral penicillin, and the latter with topical silver nitrate.[108]

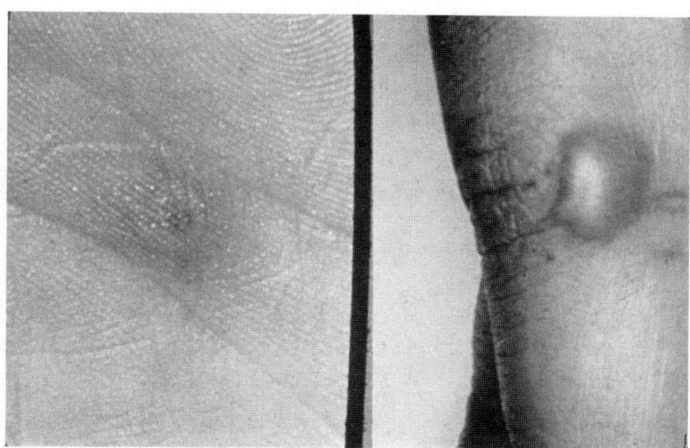

FIGURE 73–3. The rash of disseminated gonococcal infection is shown in both panels. A pustule with necrosis is shown on the left, and a hemorrhagic bulla is on the right. (From the Revised Clinical Slide Collection on the Rheumatic Diseases. The American College of Rheumatology, 1981, with permission.)

LYME DISEASE

Lyme disease is a tick-borne infection caused by the spirochete *Borrelia burgdorferi,* with endemic foci in the United States and abroad, particularly in central Europe from Scandinavia to Switzerland and from England to the Soviet Union. The major areas of disease in the United States include the Northeast, from Maryland to Massachusetts, the Midwest in Wisconsin and Minnesota, and the Far West in northern California and Oregon. The Southeast is also becoming a frequent site of Lyme disease, from eastern Texas to North Carolina.

Lyme disease is a multisystem disorder that occurs in stages, similar to other spirochetal infections. The onset of symptoms peaks during the summer months when the small deer tick, *Ixodes dammini,* is most likely to bite. A characteristic expanding skin lesion, erythema migrans (Fig. 73-4), evolves over days to weeks at the site of the tick bite. It typically has a red border with central clearing, and reaches a median diameter of 15 cm. This lesion may be warm and pruritic, and occurs in 60% to 80% of patients with Lyme disease. An accompanying flu-like syndrome is common, including fever, fatigue, headache, arthralgia, and upper respiratory infection symptoms.[109] Days to weeks later patients may develop secondary skin lesions via hematogenous spread of the organism, followed by later manifestations such as aseptic meningitis, Bell's palsy, and cardiac conduction disturbances.[110] If left untreated, chronic intermittent arthritis occurs in up to 60% of patients, with the potential for joint destruction in about 10%. Chronic neurologic sequelae, including cognitive impairment, behavioral change, and fatigue syndromes, have also been reported.

The clinical diagnosis of Lyme disease is supported by the presence of serum antibodies to *B. burgdorferi.* However, days after the tick bite, during the rash of erythema migrans or during the initial flu-like symptoms, antibody serologies are usually negative. The specific IgM antibody response begins to rise 2 weeks after the tick bite, and peaks at 6 weeks. IgG antibody levels begin to rise 3 to 6 weeks after the tick bite, and may remain elevated for months to years despite successful treatment, although titers may gradually fall as well. Laboratory confirmation is not required for a diagnosis of Lyme disease if a patient has erythema migrans, or has an ixodid tick bite in an endemic area followed by a flu-like illness during the summer months.

The treatment of early Lyme disease in the nonpregnant state is tetracycline 250 to 500 mg orally four times a day, or doxycycline 100 mg orally twice a day for 10 to 21 days, depending on the persistence of symptoms.[111] Later stages of Lyme disease may require more prolonged courses (4 to 6 weeks) of oral antibiotics, or parenteral antibiotics such as penicillin (20 million units intravenously daily in divided doses) or ceftriaxone (2 g intravenously once daily) for 10 to 14 days.

Lyme Disease and Pregnancy

The implications of contracting Lyme disease prior to and during pregnancy are still uncertain with incomplete predictive data, but available reports do provide a useful foundation upon which clinical decisions can be based. Other spirochetal infections, including leptospirosis and relapsing fever due to borreliosis, may predispose to fetal demise, and syphilis during pregnancy is associated with spontaneous abortion, stillbirths, and congenital malformations.[112,113] Likewise, there have been several reports of adverse fetal outcome in the setting of Lyme disease,[114–116] but unlike syphilis, there does not appear to be a uniform congenital malformation or distinct phenotype as a result of exposure to *B. burgdorferi* in utero.

Several incidents of fetal demise associated with cardiac anomalies presumed due to Lyme disease (including poor left ventricular function, valvular aortic stenosis, atrioventricular canal-ventricular septal defect, atrial septal defect, and coarctation of the aorta) have been reported, but there has been no uniform cardiac

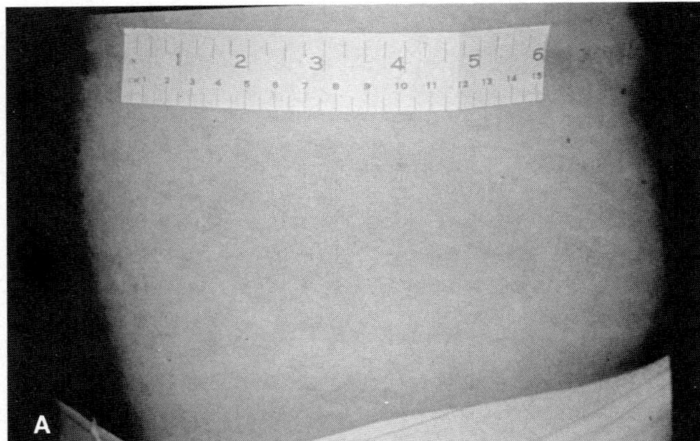

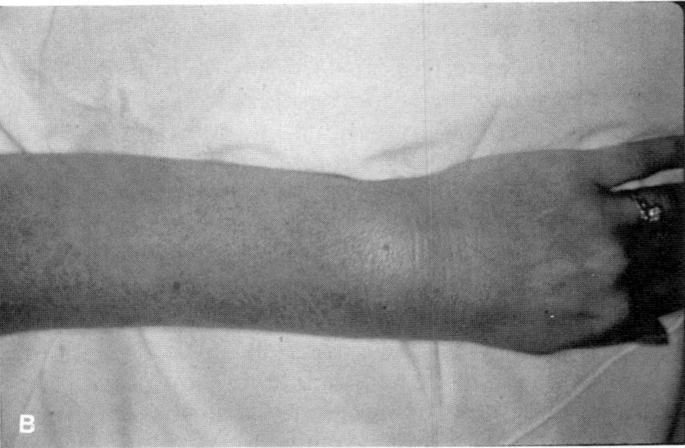

FIGURE 73–4. (**A**) Erythema migrans, the hallmark of Lyme disease. (**B**) An atypical presentation of erythema migrans. (From Steere A, Bartenhagen N, Craft J, et al. The early clinical manifestations of Lyme disease. Ann Intern Med, 1983; 99:76.)

defect.[115] These reports suggest that there may be an increased risk of harm to the fetus when maternal Lyme disease is contracted during the first trimester, coincident with cardiac organogenesis. In addition, MacDonald encountered four cases of fetal borreliosis (*B. burgdorferi* isolated from fetal liver), suggesting that *B. burgdorferi* may be an etiologic agent in fetal demise of uncertain cause.[117] Finally, a series of pregnant women with Lyme disease revealed several adverse outcomes despite therapy, including cortical blindness, fetal wastage, and syndactyly, although culture and serology of the placenta and fetal tissues were negative for *B. burgdorferi* and it was unclear if these outcomes were a result of congenital infection.[114]

Of equal importance, this latter study showed that the vast majority of pregnancies associated with maternal Lyme disease remained normal. Moreover, follow-up studies of maternal Lyme disease have shown no association with fetal malformations and no association between cord blood anti-*B. burgdorferi* antibodies of the IgG class and congenital malformations.[118] At this time, routine prenatal screening for antibodies to *B. burgdorferi* is not recommended. Current research efforts will help determine the risk of ixodid tick bites in endemic areas, and the optimal treatment for affected women.

Although spirochetes have been identified in the placenta by modified silver stain or monoclonal antibody immunofluorescence, the placenta in Lyme disease is grossly normal. Additionally, the placental histology is typically normal, without inflammatory cells, in striking contrast to that which is seen in syphilis.[119]

Treatment of Lyme Disease in Pregnancy

Due to the insidious nature of Lyme disease, primary emphasis should be placed on prevention of the illness. Pregnant women in endemic areas should exercise caution by avoiding areas where ticks are commonly found, such as high grass or wooded areas, although it should be noted that well-mowed lawns may also harbor these organisms. They should check their body surfaces for ticks prior to retiring each night, and gently remove any embedded ticks with a forceps or tweezer. If an ixodid tick bite is documented, pregnant women may receive empiric antibiotic coverage with penicillin VK 250 to 500 mg orally four times a day for 14 days. There are no clinical studies to support this position, however, and antibiotics are not routinely prescribed following asymptomatic ixodid tick bite in the non-pregnant individual.[120] Penicillin-allergic women can receive erythromycin 250 to 500 mg orally four times a day for 14 days.

For uncomplicated erythema migrans, the same dosage of oral antibiotics may be extended to 21 days. However, based on one case report of fetal demise after treatment of erythema migrans with low-dose oral penicillin (lower than current recommendations), parenteral therapy for mild disease could be considered.[121] All additional manifestations are best treated with parenteral penicillin 10 to 20 million units daily given intravenously in divided doses for 14 days; ceftriaxone (2 g daily intravenously) is an alternative.

RUBELLA-ASSOCIATED ARTHRITIS

Transient arthralgias lasting up to 1 month develop in 30% of women during rubella infection or after rubella vaccination.[122] Less commonly, women may develop an acute symmetric polyarthritis involving the fingers, wrists, and knees, typically several days after the onset of the morbilliform rash, sometimes with notable tenosynovitis and painful stiff hands.[123] Rarely, the arthritis precedes the rash. Rheumatoid factor may be positive, and synovial fluid is moderately inflammatory, with 15,000 to 60,000 WBC/mm^3.[124] In several cases, rubella antigen has been demonstrated in synovial fluid mononuclear cells using immunofluorescence.[125] The characteristic rash and posterior cervical lymphadenopathy, seen 14 to 21 days after exposure to the virus, serve to distinguish rubella arthritis from new-onset RA. Serologic confirmation is essential in pregnant women with such a presentation due to the potential for congenital deafness, blindness, or cardiac defects, particularly during the first trimester.[126] Although arthritis may result when the rubella vaccine is inadvertently given during pregnancy, there have been no reports of vaccine-induced congenital malformation.[127] Rubella-associated arthritis is treated with analgesics, and generally lasts several weeks, rarely if ever progressing to chronic arthritis.

PARVOVIRUS-ASSOCIATED ARTHRITIS

Human parvovirus B19, the etiologic agent in erythema infectiosum or fifth disease, causes transient, symmetric polyarthritis in adults. The illness typically occurs during the winter, 4 to 14 days after exposure, and is characterized by a mild upper respiratory infection accompanied by a bright red rash on the face and followed by a lace-like eruption over the arms and legs. During this time, moderate synovitis of the small joints of the hands, wrists, and knees lasting several weeks to months may occur; occasionally, arthritis may appear in the absence of a viral prodrome.[128] Positive serology for human parvovirus-specific IgM antibody helps confirm the diagnosis. Otherwise, radiographs and synovial fluid are nonspecific, and rheumatoid factor is negative. Treatment of the arthritis is supportive with analgesics.

Although there are no congenital malformations associated with intrauterine parvovirus infection, there is increased risk of fetal death and aplastic anemia, particularly if exposure is during the first 18 weeks of pregnancy.[129] These complications are monitored by ultrasound (hydrops fetalis and ascites), and maternal serum α-fetoprotein levels.[130,131] During the course of monitoring, women should be reassured that the vast majority of pregnancy outcomes will be normal.

MISCELLANEOUS CAUSES OF REGIONAL PAIN

FIBROMYALGIA

On occasion, women with musculoskeletal pain who have no objective abnormalities will describe sleep disturbance, tiredness, and typical trigger points indicative of fibromyalgia syndrome.[132] This remains a diagnosis of exclusion, and is best treated with reassurance and gentle conditioning during pregnancy.

TRANSIENT OSTEOPOROSIS

The first report of transient osteoporosis in 1959 described three pregnant women in their third trimester with painful demineralization of one or both hips, and recovery over 3 to 12 months.[133] The cause remains unknown, although a neurovascular cause related to reflex sympathetic dystrophy is likely.[134] The hip, knee, or ankle may be involved, sometimes in a migratory fashion, with severe pain upon motion or weight bearing lasting several months before gradually resolving completely. Erythema and swelling may be present, and synovial fluid is clear or straw-colored with 300 to 700 mononuclear cells/mL, with no organisms.[135] Radiographs may be initially normal, but within 4 to 8 weeks severe osteopenia of subchondral cortical bone is seen, with normal overlying cartilage.[136] ^{99}Technetium bone scanning reveals uptake, but does not rule out infection, avascular necrosis, or inflammatory arthritis; thus, a positive result is not diagnostic. Bone biopsy is likewise nondiagnostic, and is only required if systemic features raise the suspicion of osteomyelitis or neoplasm.

Treatment is conservative, with rest and protected weight bearing for pain relief and prevention of fracture. Ibuprofen or naproxen can be used until 4 weeks prior to term. Low-dose prednisone is commonly used, although it does not always hasten recovery.[135] Recurrences have been reported, and symptoms may worsen over 1 to 4 months, but the mother should be reassured that transient osteoporosis is not harmful to the fetus, and her prognosis for recovery is excellent.

SCOLIOSIS AND PREGNANCY

Scoliosis, usually present during adolescence, can lead to discomfort, fatigability, and susceptibility to respiratory infection.[137] Exercise and orthotics are useful treatments, particularly in younger women with curvatures less than 40 degrees, although surgical correction is becoming more common for children and adolescents. In pregnancy, scoliosis may be associated with increased breathlessness and back pain, neither of which are correlated with the severity of the spinal curve. In a study of 118 pregnancies in 64 women with scoliosis (two thirds in excess of 60 degrees), there were no serious cardiorespiratory complications attributed to the spinal deformity,[138] and the majority had normal vaginal deliveries.

LOW BACK PAIN AND PELVIC ARTHROPATHY

Back pain is a frequent complaint among pregnant women, usually due to an exaggerated lumbosacral lordosis with decreased abdominal tone, causing undue stress of the ligaments and muscles of the lower spine. This condition is more common among those with underlying back disease such as spondylitis or scoliosis, prior trauma of disc disease, poor posture, and perhaps among older pregnant women. Conservative treatment with rest on a firm mattress, acetaminophen, and periodic moist heat are usually adequate. Prolonged sitting is associated with increased disc pressure, and should be avoided. The natural history of associated back strain and disc disease (without neurologic compromise) is also favorable, and should be approached similarly. When pain is localized and fever is present, MRI is useful to rule out pyogenic infection of the sacroiliac joint, particularly if the pregnant patient is an intravenous drug abuser.[139–141]

Pelvic relaxation, or pelvic arthropathy, occurs during the second or third trimester due to excess hormone-induced relaxation of the sacroiliac joints and pubic symphysis.[142] The patient experiences pain and instability of these joints, particularly on weight bearing. Point tenderness and excessive movement of the pubic bone can be demonstrated by pelvic examination. Radiographs may reveal greater than 2 cm of widening and malalignment of the joint space. Rest and analgesia usually suffice, and delivery can proceed vaginally. Severe instability may require a sturdy fitted girdle, securing the sacrum and symphysis for several months until joint stability returns to normal.

Several weeks after delivery, laxity of the pubic symphysis, coupled with the trauma of childbirth, may lead to osteitis pubis.[143] These patients develop pain over the symphysis pubis, radiating down the inner aspect of the thigh, often aggravated by coughing or straining. Radiographs may be normal initially, but osteolysis and irregular joint margins develop with 2 to 4 weeks. There may be associated periostitis or erosion if there is underlying spondylitis or rheumatoid arthritis.[144] Treatment is similar to that for pelvic relaxation, and remission occurs in several months.

Coccydynia, seen after a difficult delivery, is associated with pain and soreness of the coccyx radiating to the low back, aggravated by climbing stairs or during a bowel movement.[145] A careful bimanual examination and radiographs should be performed to rule out abscess or bony lesion. A ring-cushion may relieve pressure while sitting, and stool softeners may prove invaluable. Some patients find relief from a local injection of anesthetic with steroids. Spontaneous recovery over weeks to months can be expected.

REGIONAL PAIN DUE TO ENTRAPMENT NEUROPATHY

Carpal tunnel syndrome due to compression of the median nerve may cause episodic numbness, wrist or forearm pain, and weakness of grasp.[146] During pregnancy, in the absence of local trauma to the wrist, the diagnosis of carpal tunnel syndrome can be made clinically, without the use of electrodiagnostic testing. Neural irritability and paresthesia of the second and third digits is reproduced by percussion over the volar carpal ligament (Tinel's sign), or by holding the wrist in maximal flexion (Phalen's sign). The examiner may also check for weakness of the opponens pollicis muscle by measuring pinch strength. Splinting of the wrist in a neutral position usually provides adequate relief until delivery, and low-dose salicylates, if given, should be stopped several weeks prior to expected delivery. If pain is severe, a carefully placed steroid injection into the carpal tunnel may help, particularly when there is underlying inflammatory arthritis. Surgical release and evaluation for underlying endocrine or inflammatory conditions should be considered if symptoms persist beyond delivery.

Compression of the lateral femoral cutaneous nerve as it emerges from the inguinal ligament may cause a burning dysesthesia or hypesthesia over the anterior and lateral thigh. This phenomenon, known as a meralgia paresthetica, is exacerbated by direct palpation of the superficial perineural tissue in the anterolateral thigh.[147] Pregnant women with meralgia should wear loose clothing, and avoid further compressive trauma to the nerve by resting with the hips semiflexed. Acetaminophen, salicylates, and moist heat offer relief of symptoms. When necessary, a local steroid injection, targeting the region of greatest discomfort, is useful. The contents of the syringe should be injected as the needle is slowly withdrawn, avoiding direct injection into the nerve. Compression and symptoms abate on delivery.

BIBLIOGRAPHY

1. McDuffie FC. Morbidity impact of rheumatoid arthritis on society. Am J Med 1985;78(suppl1A):1.
2. Scott DL, Symmons DPM, Coulton BL, Porort AJ. The long–term outcome of treating rheumatoid arthritis: results after 20 years. Lancet 1987;1:1108.
3. Arnett FC, Edworthy SM, Bloch DA, et al. The American Rheumatism Association revised criteria for the classification of rheumatoid arthritis. Arthritis Rheum 1988;31:315.
4. Hench PS. The ameliorating effect of pregnancy on chronic atrophic (infectious rheumatoid) arthritis, fibrositis, and intermittent hydrarthrosis. Proc Mayo Clin 1938;13:161.
5. Oka M. Effect of pregnancy on the onset and course of rheumatoid arthritis. Ann Rheum Dis 1953;12:227.
6. Silman AJ. Is pregnancy a risk factor in the causation of rheumatoid arthritis? Ann Rheum Dis 1986;45:1031.
7. Kaplan D, Diamond H. Rheumatoid arthritis and pregnancy. Clin Obstet Gynecol 1965;8:286.
8. Persellin RH. The effect of pregnancy on rheumatoid arthritis. Bull Rheum Dis 1977;27:922.
9. Ostensen M, Aune B, Husby G. The effect of pregnancy and hormonal changes on the activity of rheumatoid arthritis. Scand J Rheumatol 1983;12:69.
10. Ostensen M, Husby G. Ensuring a healthy pregnancy for the woman with severe rheumatoid arthritis. Journal of Musculoskeletal Medicine 1988;13.
11. Persellin RH, Vance SE, Peery A. Effect of pregnancy serum on experimental inflammation. Br J Exp Pathol 1973;55:26.
12. Ostensen M. The influence of pregnancy on blood parameters in patients with rheumatic disease. Scand J Rheumatol 1984;13:203.
13. Thurnau GR. Rheumatoid arthritis. Clin Obstet Gynecol 1983;26:558.
14. Hench P. The potential reversibility of rheumatoid arthritis. Proc Mayo Clin 1949;24:167.
15. Pinals RS. Remission in rheumatoid arthritis. Postgrad Adv Rheumatology 1988;3:1.
16. Gilbert M, Kotstein J, Cunningham C. Norethynodrel with mestranol in the treatment of rheumatoid arthritis. JAMA 1964;190:235.
17. Vandenbroucke JP, Witteman JCM, Valkenburg HA, et al. Noncontraceptive hormones and rheumatoid arthritis in perimenopausal and postmenopausal women. JAMA 1986;10:1299.
18. Andresen RH, Monroe CW. Experimental study of the behavior of adult human skin homografts during pregnancy. Am J Obstet Gynecol 1962;84:1096.
19. Lichtenstein MR. Tuberculin reaction in TB during pregnancy. Am Rev Tuberculosis 1942;46:89.
20. Hirahara F, Gorai I, Tanaka K, Matsuzaki Y, Sumiyoshi Y, Shiojima Y. Cellular immunity in pregnancy. Clin Exp Immunol 1980;41:353.
21. Froelich CJ, Goodwin JS, Bawkhurst AD, Williams RC. Pregnancy: a temporary fetal graft of suppressor cells in autoimmune disease? Am J Med 1980;69:329.
22. Persellin RH. Inhibitors of inflammatory and immune responses in pregnancy serum. Clin Rheum Dis 1981;7:769.
23. Kasukawa R, Ohara M, Yoshida H, Yoshida T. Pregnancy-associated alpha glycoprotein in rheumatoid arthritis. Int Arch Allergy Appl Immunol 1979;58:67.
24. Unger A, Kay A, Griffin AJ, Panayi GS. Disease activity and pregnancy associated alpha-2 glycoprotein in rheumatoid arthritis during pregnancy. Br Med J 1983;286:750.
25. Ostensen M, Von Schoultz B, Husby G. Comparison between serum alpha-2 pregnancy associated globulin and activity of rheumatoid arthritis and ankylosing spondylitis during pregnancy. Scand J Rheumatol 1983;12:315.
26. Masson PL, Delire M, Cambiaso CL. Circulating immune complexes in normal human pregnancy. Nature 1977;266:542.
27. Sany J, Clot J, Bonneau M, Andary M. Immunomodulating effect of human placenta-eluted gamma globulins in rheumatoid arthritis. Arthritis Rheum 1982;25:17.
28. Stanworth DR. A possible immunochemical explanation for pregnancy associated remissions in rheumatoid arthritis? Ann Rheum Dis 1988;47:89.
29. Mannik M, Nardella FA. IgG rheumatoid factors and self-association of these antibodies. Clinics in the Rheumatic Diseases 1985;11:551.
30. Pekelharing JM, Hepp E, Kamerling JP, Gerwig GJ, Leijnse B. Alterations in carbohydrate composition of serum IgG from patients with rheumatoid arthritis and from pregnant women. Ann Rheum Dis 1988;47:91.
31. Cecere FA, Persellin RH. The interaction of pregnancy and the rheumatic diseases. Clinics in the Rheumatic Diseases 1981;7:747.
32. Felbo M, Snorranson E. Pregnancy and the place of therapeutic

abortion in rheumatoid arthritis. Acta Obstet Gynecol Scand 1961;40:116.

33. Ostensen M, Husby G. A prospective clinical study of the effect of pregnancy on rheumatoid arthritis and ankylosing spondylitis. Arthritis Rheum 1983;26:1155.
34. Kaplan D. Fetal wastage in patients with rheumatoid arthritis. J Rheumatol 1986;13:875.
35. Duhring JL. Pregnancy, rheumatoid arthritis, and IUGR. Am J Obstet Gynecol 1970;108:325.
36. Kay A, Bach F. Subfertility before and after the development of rheumatoid arthritis in women. Ann Rheum Dis 1965;24:169.
37. Siamopoulou-Mavridou A, Manoussakis MN, Mavridis AK, Moutsopoulos HM. Outcome of pregnancy in patients with autoimmune rheumatic disease before the disease onset. Ann Rheum Dis 1988;47:982.
38. Collins E. Maternal and fetal effects of acetaminophen and salicylates in pregnancy. Obstet Gynecol 1981;58(suppl 5):57s.
39. Warkany J, Takacs E. Experimental production of congenital malformations in rats by salicylate poisoning. Am J Pathol 1959;35:315.
40. Larsson KS, Ericksson M. Salicylate-induced fetal death and malformation in two mice strains. Acta Paediatr Scand 1966;55:569.
41. Robertson RT, Allen HL, Bokelman DL. Aspirin: teratogenic evaluation in the dog. Teratology 1979;20:313.
42. Lewis RB, Schulman JD. Influence of acetylsalycilic acid, an inhibitor of prostaglandin synthesis, on the duration of human gestation and labor. Lancet 1973;2:1159.
43. Collins E, Turner G. Maternal effects of regular salicylate ingestion in pregnancy. Lancet 1975;2:335.
44. Turner G, Collins E. Fetal effects of regular salicylate ingestion. Lancet 1975;2:338.
45. Rumack CM, Guggenheim MA, Rumack BH, Peterson RG, Johnson ML, Braithwaite WR. Neonatal intracranial hemorrhage and maternal use of aspirin. Obstet Gynecol 1981; 58(suppl 5):52s.
46. Lynd PA, Andreasen AC, Wyatt RJ. Intrauterine salicylate intoxication in a newborn. Clin Pediatr 1976;15:912.
47. Butcher RE, Vorhees CV, Kimmel CA. Learning impairment from maternal salicylate treatment in rats. Nature 1972; 236:211.
48. Richards ID. Congenital malformations and environmental influences in pregnancy. British Journal of Preventive and Social Medicine 1969;23:218.
49. Nelson MM, Forfar JO. Associations between drugs administered during pregnancy and congenital abnormalities of the fetus. Br Med J 1971;1:523.
50. Slone D, Siskind V, Heinonen OP, Monson RR, Kaufman DW, Shapiro S. Aspirin and congenital malformations. Lancet 1976;1:1373.
51. Goudie BM, Dossetor JFB. Effect on the fetus of indomethacin given to suppress labor. Lancet 1979;2:1187.
52. Manchester D, Margolis HS, Sheldon RE. Possible association between maternal indomethacin therapy and primary pulmonary hypertension of the newborn. Am J Obstet Gynecol 1976;126:467.
53. Ostensen M, Husby G. Antirheumatic drug treatment during pregnancy and lactation. Scand J Rheumatol 1985;14:1.
54. Gottlieb NL. Crysotherapy. Bull Rheum Dis 1977;27:912.
55. Evers AE, Sundstrom WR. Second course gold therapy in rheumatoid arthritis. Arthritis Rheum 1981;24(abstract):s82.
56. Rocker I, Henderson WJ. Transfer of gold from mother to fetus. Lancet 1976;2:1246.
57. Cohen DL, Orzel J, Taylor A. Infants of mothers receiving gold therapy. Arthritis Rheum 1981;24:104.
58. Gibbons RB. Complications of chrysotherapy. Arch Intern Med 1979;139:343.
59. Committee on drugs. Transfer of drugs and other chemicals into breast milk. Pediatrics 1983;72:375.
60. Rogers JG, Anderson RM, Chow CW, Gillam GL, Markman L. Possible teratogenic effects of gold. Aust Paediatr J 1980; 16:194.
61. Tarp U, Graudal H. A follow up study of children exposed to gold compounds in utero. Arthritis Rheum 1985;28:235.
62. Szabo KT, Guenriero J, Kang YJ. The effects of gold-containing compounds on pregnant rats and their fetuses. Vet Pathol 1978;(suppl 5)15:89.
63. Szabo KT, DiFebbo ME, Phelan DG. The effects of gold-containing compounds on pregnant rabbits and their fetuses. Vet Pathol 1978;(suppl 5)15:97.
64. Committee on drugs. Auranofin: a preliminary review. Drugs 1984;27:392.
65. Blanford AT, Murphy BEP. In vitro metabolism of prednisolone, dexamethasone, betamethasone, and cortisol by the human placenta. Am J Obstet Gynecol 1977;127:264.
66. Osinski PA. Steroid 11 β01-dehydrogenase in human placenta. Nature 1960;187:177.
67. Roubenoff R, Hoyt J, Petri M, Hochberg MC, Hellmann DB. Effects of anti-inflammatory and immunosuppressive drugs on pregnancy and fertility. Semin Arthritis Rheum 1988;18:88.
68. Taeusch HW Jr, Kamali H, Hehre A, et al. Dexamethasone and its effect on adrenal function in prematures [abstract]. Pediatr Res 1977;11:432.
69. Taeusch HW Jr, Frigoletto F, Kitzmiller J, et al. Risk of respiratory distress syndrome after prenatal dexamethasone treatment. Pediatrics 1979;63:64.
70. Schatz M, Patterson R, Zeitz S, O'Rourke J, Melam H. Corticosteroid therapy for the pregnant asthmatic patient. JAMA 1975;233:804.
71. Reinisch JM, Simon NG. Prenatal exposure to prednisone in humans and animals retards intrauterine growth. Science 1978;202:436.
72. Harris JWS, Lond MB, Ross IP, et al. Cortisone therapy in early pregnancy: relation to cleft palate. Lancet 1956;2:1045.
73. Snyder RD, Snyder D. Corticosteroid for asthma during pregnancy. Ann Allergy 1978;41:340.
74. Lee P. Anti-inflammatory therapy during pregnancy and lactation. Clin Invest Med 1985;8:328.
75. Koehler BE, Urowitz MB, Killinger DW. The systemic effects of intra-articular corticosteroid. J Rheumatol 1974;1:117.
76. McKenzie SA, Selley JA, Agnew JE. Secretion of prednisolone into breast milk. Arch Dis Child 1975;50:894.
77. Solomon L, Abrams G, Dinner M, et al. Neonatal abnormalities associated with D-penicillamine treatment during pregnancy. N Engl J Med 1977;296:55.
78. Lyle WH. Penicillamine in pregnancy. Lancet 1978;1:1064.
79. Willoughby CP, Truelove SC. Ulcerative colitis and pregnancy. Gut 1980;21:469.
80. Mogadan M, Dobbins WO, Korelitz BI, Ahmed SW. Pregnancy in inflammatory bowel disease: effect of sulfasalazine and corticosteroids on fetal outcome. Gastroenterology 1981;80:72.
81. Ullberg S, Lindquist NG, Sjostrand SE. Accumulation of chorioretinotoxic drugs in the fetal eye. Nature 1970;227:1257.
82. Neill WA, Panay GS, Duthie JJR, Prescott RJ. Action of chloroquine sulfate in rheumatoid arthritis: chromosome damaging effect. Ann Rheum Dis 1973;32:547.
83. Lewis R, Lauersen NH, Birnbaum S. Malaria associated with pregnancy. Obstet Gynecol 1973;42:696.
84. Milunsky A, Graef JW, Gaynor MF. Methotrexate-induced congenital malformations. J Pediatr 1968;72:790.

85. Physician's desk reference. Oradell, NJ: Medical Economics, 1989:1131.
86. Saarikoski S, Seppala M. Immunosuppression during pregnancy: transmission of azathioprine and its metabolites from the mother to the fetus. Am J Obstet Gynecol 1973;115:1100.
87. Brooks PM, Needs CJ. The use of antirheumatic medication during pregnancy and in the puerperium. Rheum Dis Clin North Am 1989;15:789.
88. Hoshes GR. Plasma exchange. Agents Actions 1980;(suppl)7:62.
89. Weinrib JC, Lowe TW, Rigoberto SR, Cunningham FG, Parkey R. Magnetic resonance imaging in obstetric diagnosis. Radiology 1985;154:157.
90. Conine TA, Carty EA, Wood-Johnson F. Nature and source of information received by primiparas with rheumatoid arthritis on preventive maternal and child care. Can J Public Health 1987;78:393.
91. Carty EA, Conine TA, Wood-Johnson F. Rheumatoid arthritis and pregnancy: helping women to meet their needs. Midwives Chronicle of Nursing 1986;254.
92. Carty EA, Conine TA. Disability and pregnancy: a double dose of disequilibrium. Rehabilitation Nursing 1988;13:85.
93. Calin A, Fries JF. Striking prevalence of ankylosing spondylitis in healthy B27 positive males and females: a controlled study. N Engl J Med 1975;293:835.
94. Inman RD, Mani VJ. Subluxation of the SI joints in a black female with ankylosing spondylitis. J Rheumatol 1979;6:300.
95. Calin A. Seronegative spondylarthropathies. Med Clin North Am 1986;70:323.
96. Bennett PHJ, Burch TA. New York symposium on population studies in the rheumatic diseases. Bull Rheum Dis 1967;7:453.
97. Ostensen M, Husby G. Pregnancy and rheumatic disease. Klin Wochenschr 1984;62:891.
98. Ostensen M, Romberg O, Husby G. Ankylosing spondylitis and motherhood. Arthritis Rheum 1982;25:140.
99. Hart FD, Bell ACH, Organe GSW. Pregnancy in ankylosing spondylitis. Ann Rheum Dis 1951;9:54.
100. Weber S. Caudal Anesthesia complicated by intraosseous injection in a patient with ankylosing spondylitis. Anesthesiology 1985;63:716.
101. Ostensen M. Pregnancy in psoriatic arthritis. Scand J Rheumatol 1988;17:67.
102. McHugh NJ, Laurent MR. The effect of pregnancy on the onset of psoriatic arthritis. Br J Rheumatol 1989;28:50.
103. Husby G, Ostensen M. Presented at the Eleventh European Congress of Rheumatology, 1988. Athens, Greece.
104. Rynes RI. Acquired immunodeficiency syndrome and rheumatology. Postgraduate Advances in Rheumatology 1988;3:1.
105. Chapman DR, Fernandez-Rocha L. Gonococcal arthritis in pregnancy: a ten-year review. South Med J 1975;68:1333.
106. Mehta A, Wright TA. Gonococcal arthritis in pregnancy. Can Med Assoc J 1977;117:1190.
107. Kafetzis DA, Brater DC, Fanourgakis JE, Voyatzis J, Georgakopoulus P. Ceftriaxone distribution between maternal blood and fetal blood and tissues at parturition, and between blood and milk post-partum. Antimicrob Agents Chemother 1983;23:87.
108. Lossick JG. Prevention and management of neonatal gonorrhea. Sex Transm Dis 1979;6:192.
109. Steere AC, Bartenhagen NH, Craft JE, et al. The early clinical manifestations of Lyme disease. Ann Intern Med 1983;99:76.
110. Steere AC, Batsford WP, Weinberg M, et al. Lyme carditis: cardiac abnormalities of Lyme disease. Ann Intern Med 1980;93:8.
111. Treatment of Lyme disease. Medical Letter July, 1988.
112. Fuchs PC, Oyama AA. Neonatal relapsing fever due to transplacental transmission of borrelia. JAMA 1969;208:690.
113. Wendel GD. Gestational and congenital syphilis. Clin Perinatol 1988;15:287.
114. Markowitz LE, Steere AC, Benach JL, Slade JD, Broome CV. Lyme disease during pregnancy. JAMA 1986;255:3394.
115. Schlesinger PA, Duray PH, Burke BA, Steere AC, Stillman T. Maternal-fetal transmission of the Lyme disease spirochete, Borrelia burgdorferi. Ann Intern Med 1985;103:67.
116. MacDonald AB, Benach JL, Burgdorfer W. Stillbirth following maternal Lyme disease. NY State J Med 1987;87:615.
117. MacDonald AB. Human fetal borreliosis, toxemia of pregnancy, and fetal death. Zentralbl Bakteriol Mikrobiol Hyg [A] 1986;263:189.
118. Williams CL, Benach JL, Curran AS, Spierling P, Medici F. Lyme disease during pregnancy: a cord blood serosurvey. Ann NY Acad Sci 1988;539:504.
119. Russell P, Altshuler G. Placental abnormalities of congenital syphilis. Am J Dis Child 1974;128:160.
120. Costello CM, Steere AC, Pinkerton RE, Feder HM. A prospective study of tick bites in an endemic area for Lyme disease. Conn Med 1989;53:338.
121. Weber K, Bratcke HJ, Neubert U, Wilske B, Duray PH. Borrelia burgdorferi: in a newborn despite oral penicillin for Lyme borreliosis during pregnancy. Pediatr Infect Dis J 1988;7:286.
122. Freij BJ, South MA, Sever JL. Maternal rubella and the congenital rubella syndrome. Clin Perinatol 1988;15:247.
123. Chambers RJ, Bywaters EGL. Rubella synovitis. Ann Rheum Dis 1963;22:263.
124. Johnson RE, Hall AP. Rubella arthritis: report of cases studied by latex tests. N Engl J Med 1958;258:743.
125. Fraser JRE, Cunningham AL, Hayes K, Leach R, Lunt R. Rubella arthritis in adults: isolation of virus, cytology and other aspects of the synovial reaction. Clinical and Experimental Rheumatology 1983;1:287.
126. Shirley JA, Revill S, Cohen BJ et al. Serological study of rubella-like illness. J Med Virol 1987;21:369.
127. Center for Disease Control. Rubella vaccination during pregnancy — United States 1971–1986. MMWR 1987;36:457.
128. White DG, Mortimer PP, Blake DR, Woolf AD, Cohen BJ, Bacon PA. Human parvovirus arthropathy. Lancet 1985;1:419.
129. Anderson LJ, Hurwitz ES. Human parvovirus B19 and pregnancy. Clin Perinatol 1988;15:273.
130. Anand A, Gray ES, Brown T, et al. Human parvovirus infection in pregnancy and hydrops fetalis. N Engl J Med 1987;316:183.
131. Carrington D, Gilmore DH, Whittle MJ, et al. Maternal serum alpha-fetoprotein: a marker of fetal aplastic crisis during intrauterine human parvovirus infection. Lancet 1987;1:433.
132. Goldenberg DL. Fibromyalgia syndrome: an emerging but controversial condition. JAMA 1987;257:2782.
133. Curtiss PH JR, Kincaid WE. Transitory demineralization of the hip in pregnancy. J Bone Joint Surg [Am] 1959;41:1327.
134. Lequesne M. Transient osteoporosis of the hip: a non-traumatic variety of Sudek's atrophy. Ann Rheum Dis 1968;27:463.
135. Lakhanpal S, Ginsburg WW, Luthra HS, Hunder GG. Transient regional osteoporosis. Ann Intern Med 1987;106:444.
136. Bramlett KW, Killian JT, Nasca RJ, Daniel WW. Transient osteoporosis. Clin Orthop 1987;222:197.
137. Kane WJ. Scoliosis: a review for the generalist. Bull Rheum Dis 1987;37:1.
138. Siegler D, Zorab PA. Pregnancy in thoracic scoliosis. British Journal of Diseases of the Chest 1981;75:367.
139. Wilbur AC, Langer BG, Spigos DG. Diagnosis of scroiliac joint infection in pregnancy by magnetic resonance imaging. Magn Reson Imaging 1988;6:341.
140. Delbarre F, Rondier J, Delrieu F, et al. Pyogenic infection of the

sacroiliac joint: report of 13 cases. J Bone Joint Surg [Am] 1975;57:819.

141. Gomar C, Luis M, Nalda MA. Sacroiliitis in a (pregnant) heroin addict: a containdication to spinal anesthesia. Anaesthesia 1984;39:167.

142. Sequeira W. Diseases of the pubic symphysis. Semin Arthritis Rheum 1986;16:11.

143. Wiltse LL, Frantz CH. Non-suppurative osteitis pubis in the female. J Bone Joint Surg [Am] 1956;38:500.

144. Scott DL, Eastmond CJ, Wright V. A comparative radiological study of the pubic symphysis in rheumatic disorders. Ann Rheum Dis 1979;38:529.

145. Bucknill TM. Disorders of the sacrum and coccyx. Practitioner 1979;222:77.

146. Dehaan MR, Wilson RL. Diagnosis and management of carpal tunnel syndrome. Journal of Musculoskeletal Medicine 1989;Feb:47.

147. Deese JM JR, Baxter DE. Compressive neuropathies of the lower extremity. Journal of Musculoskeletal Medicine 1988;Nov:68.

74

CHAPTER

SELECTED IMMUNOLOGIC AND CONNECTIVE TISSUE DISORDERS IN PREGNANCY

Michael de Swiet

SYSTEMIC LUPUS ERYTHEMATOSUS

Systemic lupus erythematosus (SLE) is a multisystem disease that most frequently presents in young women. It is therefore relatively common in pregnancy, and it is certainly the connective tissue disease that has been studied most intensively. The apparent prevalence has increased as more mild forms of the disease are recognized. In 1974 Fesse found a prevalence of one in 700 women aged 15 to 64 years.[1] In black women the prevalence was one in 245. Women in "minority" races have a risk fivefold of that in white women.[2] The diagnosis may be based on the patient having at least four of the features noted by the American Rheumatism Association, either simultaneously or following each other (Table 74-1).However, the necessity of having four rather than three criteria has been challenged.[3]

Since the publication of the American Rheumatism Association Criteria, the measurement of antinuclear factor and of anti-DNA antibodies has replaced the LE cell test in the diagnosis of SLE.

In pregnancy, proteinuria and thrombocytopenia can lead to confusion with preeclampsia. The clinical features of preeclampsia—which usually run a much more acute course, remit after delivery and are not associated with other features summarized in Table 74-1—normally distinguish the two conditions. In preeclampsia, however, proteinuria may occasionally appear early in pregnancy, and the process may not be so acute. In this situation, measurement of antinuclear factor helps to distinguish SLE from other renal conditions and preeclampsia.

Systemic lupus erythematosus runs a fluctuating course. In the advanced forms, with severe nephritis or nervous system involvement, the overall prognosis is bad. However, when less severe forms are recognized, the prognosis is improved, so that centers should report a greater than 95% survival at 5 years. If treatment is required, the drugs most commonly used are aspirin, prednisone, and antimalarials such as hydroxychloroquine and azathioprine (see sections later in this chapter for treatment in pregnancy. For other reviews of SLE in pregnancy see references 4–7.)

EFFECT OF PREGNANCY ON SLE

As with most illnesses that run a fluctuating course, such as asthma or disseminated sclerosis, it is difficult to document any special effect of pregnancy on SLE. Certainly a simple comparison of the prevalence of autoantibodies in a normal population has shown no difference between pregnancy and the non-pregnant state.[8] The general consensus is that pregnancy does not affect the long-term prognosis of SLE[9] but that pregnancy itself may be associated with more "flare-ups," particularly in the puerperium.[10,11] Since patients are usually observed more closely in pregnancy, this is not surprising. Also, patients with SLE are normally advised against conceiving during an active phase of the disease and therefore conceive when they are well.[12] If the effect of pregnancy is judged by a comparison of the state of pregnancy with that before conception,[13] their condition can only stay unchanged, if they were well before pregnancy, or deteriorate; this is a further cause of bias. However, in a comparison with the prepregnancy period, Garsenstein and coworkers[9] found that the exacerbation rate was three times greater in the first half of

TABLE 74-1. CRITERIA FOR THE DIAGNOSIS OF SLE AS SUGGESTED BY THE AMERICAN RHEUMATISM ASSOCIATION

1. Facial butterfly rash
2. Discoid lupus
3. Photosensitivity—skin rash as a result of unusual reaction to sunlight
4. Oral or nasopharyngeal ulceration
5. Nonerosive arthritis involving two or more peripheral joints
6. Pleurisy or pericarditis
7. Proteinuria > 0.5 g/day or cellular casts
8. Psychosis or convulsions
9. One of the following:
   a. Hemolytic anemia
   b. Leukopenia, WBC < 4000 μL on two or more occasions
   c. Lymphopenia < 1500/μL on two or more occasions
   d. Thrombocytopenia <100,000 μL
10. Immunologic disorder:
   a. Positive LE preparation
   b. Antibody to native DNA in abnormal titer
   c. Antibody to SM nuclear antigen
   d. Chronic false-positive syphilis serology for 6 months
11. Antinuclear antibody in abnormal titer

From Tan EM, Cohan AS, Aries JF, Masi AT, McShane DJ, Rothfield N, et al. The 1982 revised criteria for the classification of systemic lupus erythematosus. Arthritis Rheum 1982;25:1271.

pregnancy, one and one half times greater in the second half, and at least six times greater in the puerperium—the time when the majority of maternal deaths occur.[13] These deaths, which are not uncommon, have been due to pulmonary hemorrhage[14] or lupus pneumonitis.[15,16] However, successive pregnancies do not necessarily affect an individual in the same way.[12]

Chorea gravidarum is a rare complication of SLE in pregnancy.[17,18]

EFFECT OF SLE ON PREGNANCY

SLE affects pregnancy and its outcome in three main ways. First, it increases the risks of late pregnancy losses due to hypertension and renal failure. Second, it is an important cause of heart block and other cardiac defects in the newborn. This effect may be part of a more general neonatal lupus syndrome. Third, it increases the risk of abortion. Although technically most of the latter cases, being pregnancy losses before 28 weeks, should be classified as abortions, it is clear that they are quite different from most abortions, which occur at about 12 weeks. The losses in association with SLE may occur at gestations up to and even after 28 weeks with a bias toward the later part of pregnancy. Even if the fetus does not die, it is at risk of developing fetal distress as judged by abnormal fetal heart rate traces.[19]

Hypertension and Renal Failure

As indicated earlier, patients with trivial SLE, or even no clinical evidence of SLE, have a much higher risk of abortion. The other group of patients at risk of fetal morbidity are those with renal involvement who may also have hypertension. For example, Houser and colleagues studied 18 pregnancies in patients with SLE.[20] Ten occurred in patients with no evidence of renal disease and were uncomplicated. The remaining eight occurred in patients with renal disease. There were four abortions (one elective), three premature deliveries, and only one normal-term delivery. It is difficult to be precise as to what level of renal impairment is significant, but a creatinine clearance of less than 65 mL/min/m^3 or proteinuria greater than 2.4 g in 24 hours would be ominous. Hayslett and Lynn noted a 50% fetal loss rate in mothers with a serum creatinine in excess of 132 mmol/L (1.5 mg/dL).[21]

The Neonatal Lupus Syndrome[22]

The neonatal lupus syndrome includes hematologic complications, cardiac abnormalities, babies in whom skin lesions are present[23] or are the only abnormalities, and neonates who develop SLE in the absence of any involvement in the mother.[24] Maternal IgG antibodies have been shown to cross the placenta,[24] and it is likely that SLE is one of the conditions—such as rhesus disease, Graves' disease, or myasthenia gravis—where transplacental passage of antibodies harms the fetus. However, in SLE the precise antibody that affects the fetus has not been identified, and the fetal outcome cannot be correlated with fetal (or maternal) antibody levels apart from the relationship between congenital heart block and certain maternal antibodies (see below).

The hematologic abnormalities are hemolytic anemia, leukopenia, and thrombocytopenia. They are usually transient and not a major problem.[25]

The cardiac pathology has been best defined by McCue[26] and Scott.[27] By far the most common abnormality is complete heart block, which may be present and detected antenatally.[28] Although the majority of infants born to mothers with SLE are normal, about one in three mothers (38%) who deliver babies with isolated congenital heart block have, or will have, a connective tissue disease.[27] Most frequently, the disease is SLE, but in 16% of cases the mother had rheumatoid arthritis, and 25% have a less well-defined form of connective tissue disease.

About 60% of mothers who deliver a child with congenital heart block have antibodies to soluble tissue ribonucleoprotein antigen (anti-Ro and anti-La antibodies). Since the production of anti-Ro and anti-La antibodies is correlated with the presence of HLA antigen DR3 and is more common in patients with Sjögren's syndrome,[29] Sjögren's syndrome is a particular risk factor for having an infant with congenital heart block.[30,31] In one series, these autoantibodies were invariably present in the mothers with SLE who delivered an affected child, but they were also present in some of those asymptomatic women who had a child with congenital heart block.[32] There is therefore strong circumstantial evidence to implicate antibodies to soluble tissue ribonucleoprotein directly or indirectly in the pathogenesis of congenital heart block. Antibody has been found in the site of the conducting tissue in the heart of a fetus that died with complete heart block.[33] The antibody was both IgG and IgA and, since IgA does not cross the placenta, the IgA antibody was presumably derived from the fetus. More recently, it has been shown that the mothers and their offspring may also have an IgG antibody that reacts with fetal cardiac tissue.[34] This antibody may also be involved in the pathogenesis of congenital heart block, and the presence of this and other autoantibodies may explain why the fetal prognosis is not invariably good even in the absence of well-established markers for fetal death such as anticardiolipin antibodies (see Abortion and the Cardiolipin Syndrome). Thus, although the baby usually survives the perinatal period and often does not require pacing, in a few cases with congenital heart block and without cardiolipin antibodies the fetus dies antenatally or in labor.[35] Perhaps the antibodies directed against cardiac muscle are causing a fetal cardiomyopathy.[36] This would certainly be in keeping with the finding of diffuse IgG antibody in all cardiac tissue of a fetus that died in association with high maternal titers of anti-Rho in early pregnancy.[37] In addition, fatal cases may be associated with endomyocardial fibrosis[27] or pericarditis.[38] Of course, fetuses may have congenital heart block because of a primary fetal abnormality, frequently an atrioventricular canal defect.[39] Under these circumstances there is usually no association with maternal connective tissue disease, but of the 26 cases reviewed by Shenker and colleagues, all but one were dead within 2 years of birth.[39]

McCuistion and Schoch first described discoid skin lesions in a neonate whose mother subsequently developed SLE.[40] The lesions are usually on the face or the scalp and are present at birth. They have normally disappeared by 1 year of life and are associated only rarely with other organ involvement.[41] Some skin lesions have been associated with maternal and fetal antibodies to U_1 RNP (nRNP), a protein found in normal human skin cells.[42]

Abortion and the Cardiolipin Syndrome[43]

The incidence of abortion in patients with SLE may be as high as 40%.[10] On reviewing previous pregnancies, even those occurring before the onset of SLE, Fraga and colleagues found that the incidence of abortion was 23%—about twice as high as that in a group of control patients.[10] Chesley also analyzed the outcome of 630 pregnancies in mothers with SLE and found that there was a 36% failure rate.[44]

The risk of abortion is not related to the severity of the condition. In SLE, abortion often occurs later than the usual 12 to 14 weeks' gestation and indeed may occur at any gestation up to 28 weeks. The risk of abortion is not shared by other connective tissue diseases such as rheumatoid arthritis[45] or scleroderma.[46] Baesnihan and colleagues showed a high titer of lymphocytotoxic antibodies in three of four patients with SLE whose pregnancies ended in abortion.[47] These antibodies can be absorbed by trophoblast, which suggests some interference with placental function. For example, Abramowsky and colleagues have described necrotizing decidual vascular lesions with immunoglobulin deposition in placentas of women whose pregnancies were complicated by SLE.[48]

However, in the last 5 years it has been realized that the presence of lupus anticoagulant and cardiolipin antibodies may be very closely related to the risk of abortion and later fetal loss.[49–56] It is probable that those women with clinical lupus who do not have significant cardiolipin antibodies or lupus anticoagulant do not have excess fetal risk[56] apart from the slight excess that may be present in association with anti-Ro or anti-La antibodies (see section on Neonatal Lupus Syndrome). The lupus anticoagulant is an inhibitor of the coagulation pathway found in 5% to 10% of patients with SLE and causes prolongation of the kaolin clotting time.[57] In contrast to the situation in coagulopathies, this prolongation is not corrected by mixing the patient's plasma with control plasma. There are increasingly complicated hematologic tests to detect lupus anticoagulant.[58–60] Paradoxically, the lupus anticoagulant is associated with an increased risk of thromboembolism, both arterial and venous,[61] and excessive bleeding is very rare.[60,62] Lupus anticoagulant acts by preventing the formation of prothrombin activator, a complex of a phospholipid called platelet factor 3, factors Xa and V, and calcium ions.[63]

Anticardiolipin antibodies are active against certain phospholipid components of cell walls. They are responsible for the "false-positive" Wasserman reaction, which has been known to occur in SLE. The higher the titer of anticardiolipin antibodies, the greater the risk to the fetus.[64] Even in the absence of known lupus and without knowledge of cardiolipin antibody status, a retrospective study of patients with biologically false-positive tests for syphilis showed an increased fetal loss rate,[65] 24% in comparison with 8% in matched controls.[66] The preceding and other clinical features of the "anticardiolipin syndrome" are summarized in Table 74-2.[43]

In patients with SLE who have a bad obstetric history, both antibodies are often present in high titer. Patients who have cardiolipin antibodies in high titer usually have high levels of lupus anticoagulant.[67,68] If they do not, the level of cardiolipin antibodies is usually considered to be a better predictor of fetal outcome,[56,69] probably because it is subject to less variability.[64] Cardiolipin antibodies may belong to both IgG and IgM subtypes. The IgG antibodies seem to be better predictors of fetal outcome, although the presence of IgM antibodies is not without risk to the fetus.[69] The levels of these antibodies may be elevated disproportionately to the clinical severity of lupus. Indeed, some patients have a bad obstetric history with high titers of cardiolipin antibodies or lupus anticoagulant and almost no clinical evidence of lupus.[56,70,71] Careful questioning, however, will often elicit a history of mild joint pains,

TABLE 74–2. CLINICAL FEATURES OF THE ANTICARDIOLIPIN SYNDROME

1. Abortion: Recurrent IUD, placental thrombosis, and infarction
2. Thrombosis
   a. Venous: Recurrent DVT (also axillary, IVC, and retinal vein thrombosis)
   b. Arterial: Cerebrovascular accidents, peripheral arterial gangrene, coronary thrombosis, retinal artery thrombosis
   c. Other: Pulmonary hypertension, ? avascular necrosis
3. Thrombocytopenia: intermittent, often acute
4. Other occasional features: Coombs' positivity, livedo reticularis, migraine, chorea, epilepsy, ?endocardial disease, ? progressive dementia due to repeated cerebrovascular thromboses

From Hughes GRV, Harris EN, Gharavi AE. The anticardiolipin syndrome. *J Rheumatol* 1986;13:486.

"growing pains" as a child, or vitiligo or livido reticularis. The risk to the fetus if the mother has lupus anticoagulant has been put at 85%[53] to 92%[51] mortality. However, the series of Lubbe and Liggins[51] was derived from the literature and represents patients where the lupus anticoagulant was often measured because of the patient's bad obstetric history. In a group of women attending a rheumatology clinic for SLE who have the lupus anticoagulant or cardiolipin antibodies, the risk to the fetus may be much less, although Lockshin's retrospective study of cardiolipin antibodies in patients with SLE does not support this concept.[56] The problem is compounded by considerable methodological variation in assay procedures.[67,72,73] In the general obstetric population the incidence of lupus anticoagulant is very low, probably less than 1%. In patients presenting with unexplained recurrent abortion the incidence of subclinical autoimmune disease varies between 1% (Beard, personal communication, 1987) and 29%.[74,75]

It is therefore clear that the fetus of the woman who has lupus anticoagulant or cardiolipin antibodies is at risk, but it is difficult to quantify that risk[52] and difficult to state what its excess risk is over that of the normal population.[76–78] This is of particular relevance when considering treatment options, some of which are not without maternal risk (see Fetal Considerations). In addition, lupus anticoagulant levels show spontaneous variation between non-pregnancy and pregnancy[78] and even within the same pregnancy.

The mechanism(s) by which these agents might affect the fetus is unknown. The placenta is usually severely infarcted and the fetus is often growth retarded. Even in the pregnancies of those fetuses that survive, severe preeclampsia is very common. Current theories center around the damage to placental vascular endothelium caused by cardiolipin antibodies, platelet deposition, and imbalance in thromboxane–prostacylin production directed toward too much thromboxane and too little prostacyclin.[79,80] Inhibition of protein C has been postulated as the mechanism whereby lupus anticoagulant may cause thrombosis.[81,82]

MANAGEMENT OF SLE IN PREGNANCY

Maternal Considerations

The drugs most frequently used for the treatment of SLE are simple analgesics, such as acetaminophen, and nonsteroidal anti-inflammatory drugs, including aspirin.[83] In more severe cases antimalarial drugs, corticosteroids, and cytotoxic agents are used.

Acetaminophen (paracetamol) has been used widely in pregnancy with no adverse effects in normal therapeutic doses. Aspirin has been extensively studied. Three large prospective studies, including the Perinatal Collaborative Project of over 14,000 women exposed to aspirin in the United States, have shown no teratogenic risk.[84–86] However, salicylate and other nonsteroidal anti-inflammatory agents have been associated with neonatal hemorrhage because of their action in inhibiting platelet function.[86,87] In addition, there is the risk that prostaglandin synthetase inhibitors will cause premature closure of the ductus arteriosus and pulmonary hypertension.[88] This appears to be more a theoretical than a practical risk.[89] So far, only occasional cases have been reported following maternal indomethacin treatment.[90] There were no such complications in over 200 infants exposed to indomethacin in studies of its effect in preterm labor.[91,92] Chloroquine causes choroidoretinitis and should be avoided.[93] Prednisone, at least in doses up to 30 mg/day, and hydrocortisone should be considered safe in pregnancy.[94,95] Although an association between steroid therapy and facial clefts in the fetus has been claimed,[96] the only data to support this are in rabbits.[97] There is always concern that steroid hormones may cross the placenta, suppressing the fetal hypothalamus–pituitary–adrenal axis, and predisposing the fetus to Addisonian collapse after delivery.[98] In practice, this occurs very rarely, if at all, probably because these steroids, in contrast to dexamethasone and betamethasone, are metabolized by the placenta[99] and therefore do not enter the fetal circulation in significant quantities.[100] If a woman has taken regular glucocorticoid therapy for more than 1 month in the year before delivery, parenteral steroids such as hydrocortisone (100 mg every 6 hours) should be given to prevent Addisonian collapse at this time. Azathioprine is the cytotoxic agent most commonly used in rheumatic conditions and the only cytotoxic agent that can be considered for use in pregnancy. Azathioprine has been used rather widely in pregnancy, chiefly in patients with renal transplants. There have not been any specific ill effects reported in the fetus.[101] The worry concerning azathioprine is that it induces chromosome breaks. These have been observed in peripheral blood leukocytes in neonates exposed to maternal azathioprine therapy. They disappear as the infants grow older and the cells are replaced by others that have not been in contact with azathioprine. But the female fetus contains all the ova that the woman will ever shed during ovulation. It is therefore possible that these ova may be affected and that azathioprine will have impaired the future reproductive capacity of the female fetus.[101]

In summary, acetaminophen is the best agent to use as an analgesic and an antirheumatic in pregnancy. Nonsteroidal anti-inflammatory agents are best avoided in normal therapeutic doses in the last trimester; if a patient requires extra therapy for this relatively short time, corticosteroids should be used. Since the ESR is elevated in normal pregnancy, it cannot be taken as an index of disease activity, and reduction of C_3 complement may be used instead.[102] In patients taking long-term corticosteroids, parenteral steroid cover should be given in labor (see previous paragraph). Because of the risk of dangerous exacerbation of SLE in the puerperium, steroid dosage should only be reduced with great care after delivery. The use of azathioprine should be reserved for cases where steroid therapy has failed or is contraindicated.

Plasmapheresis has been successfully used in pregnancy for maternal reasons in patients with severe proximal myopathy induced by steroids[103] and with a very bad obstetric history.[104] A single successful case raises the possibility that plasmapheresis and steroid therapy may decrease the risk of the development of complete heart block in the fetus of a patient who is anti-Ro positive.[105] However, a subsequent attempt at this form of therapy has not been successful.[37] In breast-feeding women the nonsteroidal anti-inflammatory drugs with short half-lives and rapidly eliminated or inactive metabolites are best (ie, ibuprofen, flurbiprofen, and diclofenac).[38] Salicylates and antimalarial drugs should be avoided for the reasons given earlier. Minute quantities of prednisolone are secreted in breast milk, and this drug should therefore be considered safe.

Fetal Considerations

It was originally hoped that the use of corticosteroids would decrease the high abortion rate associated with SLE. In general, this has not been the case.[10] However, more recently it has been reported that aggressive treatment with aspirin 75 to 300 mg/day and prednisone in doses increasing to 60 mg/day can suppress lupus anticoagulant and anticardiolipin antibodies and consequently improve fetal outcome. Lubbe and colleagues[50] and Branch and colleagues[53] have reported two series of 10 and eight patients in which the outcome (50% and 62% survival) was much superior to that expected in untreated patients (see section on Abortion and the Cardiolipin Syndrome). In addition, there have been several case reports of similar successes.[106,107] However, the dose of prednisone often makes the patients Cushingoid[50] and induces diabetes that requires further treatment. Even with such treatment the pregnancies are usually complicated by hypertension or growth retardation and require very careful monitoring of both mother and fetus.[53] Since many laboratories do not run lupus anticoagulant or cardiolipin assays frequently, there is often delay in getting the results of these tests. In cases where the dose of prednisone is being increased rapidly in an attempt to reduce anticardiolipin and lupus anticoagulant activity, the physician needs an easily available test to know whether to increase prednisone further. The kaolin clotting time (KCT) should be available within a few hours from most coagulation laboratories. When the KCT is normal, the patient probably no longer has significant lupus anticoagulant.[108] Removal of anticardiolipin antibodies and lupus anticoagulant is not a guarantee of success,[53,56] nor is failure to remove the antibodies a guarantee of fetal death.[58,77,78] Furthermore, we still do not know the significance in fetal terms of these antibodies in an unselected population (see section on Abortion and the Cardiolipin Syndrome). Therefore, controlled clinical trials of this aggressive form of therapy are urgently required.[107,109]

At present I reserve steroid therapy for patients who have antibodies and a bad obstetric history. Patients who have antibodies but a good obstetric history or no obstetric history (primigravidas) are treated with aspirin 75 mg/day only. In patients where steroid and aspirin therapy has been unsuccessful, a variety of additional therapies have been tried, including azathioprine,[110,111] heparin,[50] and plasmapheresis. However, at this juncture I prefer to use intravenous gamma globulin that has been well tried in pregnancy complicated by immune thrombocytopenic purpura (see Chap. 68) and that is potentially less harmful than any of the preceding additional therapies. If gamma globulin works it may do so by suppression of antibody production[112] or inhibition of its action.[113] This makes monitoring of therapy difficult. In practice, we have given Sandoglobulin by IV infusion every 3 to 6 weeks from 12 weeks of pregnancy in patients with a bad obstetric history and where there has been persisting lupus anticoagulant activity despite low-dose aspirin and maximal steroid therapy. Gamma globulin may also be used for a steroid-sparing effect. The place of these therapies is even less clear than the place of aspirin and steroid therapy. Monitoring of the fetus of the mother with cardiolipin syndrome requires all the resources that can be mustered in each department, since delivery may be necessary from 26 weeks' gestation onward. Such monitoring should include clinical judgment, ultrasound measurement of growth, and cardiotocography. Even nonspecific bradycardia at the end of the second trimester may be an indication for elective delivery.[114] In addition, many departments will use Doppler estimation of maternal uterine and fetal umbilical blood flows.

Patients who also have a history of thromboembolism, arterial or venous, should be treated with subcutaneous heparin throughout pregnancy in addition to any aspirin and prednisone therapy that might be considered necessary. The heparin is given as described for patients with thromboembolism in pregnancy (see Chaps. 67 and 68). Although this treatment will exacerbate any bone loss associated with steroid therapy, I believe it to be necessary in view of the dire consequences, particularly of cerebral arterial thrombosis.[106]

Patients with lupus anticoagulant or cardiolipin antibodies and no history of thromboembolism are treated with low-dose aspirin alone (75 mg/day) unless it is judged that they also require steroids for fetal reasons.

The timing of delivery in patients with SLE without the cardiolipin syndrome depends on the severity of the condition and whether the patients have renal involvement or hypertension. If there are none of these complications, the patient should be delivered at term. Increasing degrees of renal failure or hypertension will necessitate early delivery, either for these reasons alone or because of evidence of fetal compromise, as judged earlier. With the advent of cardiotocography and widespread use of ultrasound to measure fetal growth, there is far less emphasis on estriol levels. But it should be noted that these can also be depressed purely by corticosteroid therapy, although usually only in dosages greater than 75 mg of cortisol per day.[115]

Congenital heart block should be diagnosed before delivery from routine auscultation of the fetal heart and subsequent cardiotocography when bradycardia is discovered. If possible, a detailed ultrasound examination of the fetal heart should then be performed. This will show atrioventricular dissociation confirming complete heart block and also demonstrates any structural heart disease that is present in 15% to 20% of cases[116] and that may occur in the absence of maternal connective tissue disease.[39] If the fetus has complete heart block, it is difficult to assess its general condition in utero, since accurate assessment usually depends on measurement of fetal heart rate and its variability. Measurement of umbilical blood flow by Doppler ultrasound can be of value, and antenatal fetal blood sampling to measure fetal blood gases could be of real value.[117,118] In this situation the fetus can be monitored by repeated fetal blood gas estimation during labor,[30] but many such fetuses are understandably delivered by elective cesarean section.

SCLERODERMA AND OTHER CONNECTIVE TISSUE DISORDERS

SCLERODERMA, POLYARTERITIS, DERMATOMYOSITIS

Scleroderma is a connective tissue disease affecting skin, gastrointestinal tract (esophagus), kidneys, and lungs. The cause is unknown, and there is no known cure or disease-modifying therapy. There have been four series of 87 patients,[46,119–121] several case reports,[122] and a review[123] describing the interaction of scleroderma and pregnancy. Scleroderma has been divided into localized cutaneous and diffuse cutaneous forms. In the localized cutaneous form, the scleroderma process is localized usually to the hands; it is associated with Raynaud's phenomenon and without organ involvement. The prognosis is good in general and particularly good in pregnancy. Diffuse cutaneous scleroderma has more widespread cutaneous manifestations and is a much more aggressive illness.

Raynaud's phenomenon is less common and the patient may have SCL-70 antibodies. Organ involvement is frequent, affecting heart, lungs, and kidneys, and is the cause of death. The prognosis in general, and in pregnancy in particular, is far worse than that for scleroderma. Since many patients deteriorate, their physicians often advise against pregnancy,[122] particularly since they may not be able to look after their children even if they survive pregnancy. However, it is not clear whether pregnancy itself accelerates the inevitable deterioration in these patients.

The fetal outcome is also poor. In a review of 17 pregnancies reported in the literature, Karlen and Cook documented five perinatal deaths and five instances of premature delivery.[122] Involvement of the cervix has been implicated as a cause of dystocia.[124] These patients often have sclerotic skin and blood vessels, making venipuncture, venous access, and blood pressure measurement difficult. Both regional and general anesthesia are associated with technical problems, particularly the difficulty of endotracheal intubation.[125] Such patients should see an anesthetist early in their pregnancy so that anesthetic management can be planned rather than guessed at in an emergency. Captopril has been advocated as treatment for crises in patients with scleroderma.[126] It is usually used as an antihypertensive drug but should be avoided in pregnancy because of concern about the fetus.

Other connective tissue diseases that rarely complicate pregnancy are polyarteritis nodosa,[127] dermatomyositis,[14] and Wegener's granulomatosis. In all these conditions there is insufficient experience to be confident of the effect of pregnancy. Since some patients have deteriorated in pregnancy, termination has been suggested for cases of polyarteritis nodosa,[128] but this may not be justified.

WEGENER'S GRANULOMATOSIS

Wegener's granulomatosis is a rare condition in which necrotizing granulomatous lesions affect the upper respiratory tract (particularly the nose—causing perforation of the septum) and the lungs and in which the kidneys are affected by glomerulonephritis. It presents with nasal symptoms, hemoptysis, general malaise, or renal failure. Untreated, it is rapidly fatal, but the condition is now being diagnosed more frequently in[129] or before[130] pregnancy as less severe cases are recognized and are treated with prednisone and cyclophosphamide. The latter drug, an alkylating agent, is teratogenic; at least three case reports have documented various abnormalities following first-trimester use.[131–133] Therefore, patients who conceive while taking cyclophosphamide should be offered termination, and patients who have Wegener's granulomatosis should wait until they are in remission so that cyclophosphamide can be stopped before pregnancy. Cyclophosphamide has been used in the latter half of pregnancy in Wegener's granulomatosis[129] and other conditions.[134] The only fetal abnormality noted was leukopenia,[135] but this was of concern in view of the potential of alkylating agents to induce leukemia.[136] However, at present, lack of experience makes it difficult to comment whether the course of Wegener's granulomatosis is affected by pregnancy.

REFERENCES

1. Fessel WJ. Systemic lupus erythematosus in the community. Incidence, prevalence, outcome and first symptoms; the high prevalence in black women. Arch Intern Med 1974;134:1027.
2. Grimes DA, LeBolt SA, Grimes KR, Wingo PA. Systemic lupus erythematosus and reproductive function: a case-control study. Am J Obstet Gynecol 1985;153:179.
3. Manu P. Serial provability analysis of the 1982 revised criteria for the classification of systemic lupus erythematosus. N Engl J Med 1983;309:1460.
4. Boelaert J, Ryckaert R, Tser Kezoglou A, Daneels R. Systemic lupus erythematosus and pregnancy. Acta Clin Belg 1980;35:183.
5. Devoe LD, Taylor RL. Systemic lupus erythematosus in pregnancy. Am J Obstet Gynecol 1979;135:473.
6. Scott JS. Systemic lupus erythematosus and allied disorders in pregnancy. Clin Obstet Gynecol 1979;6:461.
7. Syrop CM, Varner MW. Systemic lupus erythematosus. Clin Obstet Gynecol 1983;26:547.
8. Patton PE, Coulam CB, Bergstralh E. The prevalence of autoantibodies in pregnant and nonpregnant women. Am J Obstet Gynecol 1987;157:134.
9. Garsenstein M, Pollak VE, Karik RM. Systemic lupus erythematosus and pregnancy. N Engl J Med 1962;267:165.
10. Fraga A, Mintz G, Orozco J, Orozco JH. Sterility and fertility rates, fetal wastage and maternal morbidity in systemic lupus erythematosus. J Rheumatol 1974;1:1293.
11. Mund A, Simson J, Rothfield N. Effect of pregnancy on course of systemic lupus erythematosus. JAMA 1963;183:917.
12. Estes D, Larson DL. Systemic lupus erythematosus and pregnancy. Clin Obstet Gynecol 1965;8:307.
13. Zulman JI, Talal N, Hoffman GS, Epstein WV. Problems associated with the management of pregnancies in patients with systemic lupus erythematosus. J Rheumatol 1980;7:37.
14. Spiera H. Connective tissue disease in pregnancy. Mt Sinai J Med 1980;47:438.
15. Ainslie WH, Britt K, Moshipur JA. Maternal death due to lupus pneumonitis in pregnancy. Mt Sinai J Med 1979;46:494.
16. Leung ACT, Bolton Jones M. Why do patients with lupus nephritis die? Br Med J 1985;290:937.
17. Donaldson LM, Espiner EA. Disseminated lupus erythematosus presenting as chorea gravidarum. Arch Neurol 1971;25:240.
18. Lubbé WF, Walker EB. Chorea gravidarum associated with lupus anticoagulant: successful outcome of pregnancy with prednisone and aspirin therapy. Br J Obstet Gynaecol 1983;90:487.
19. Lockshin MD, Druzin ML, Goei S, Qamar T, Magid MS, Jovanovic L, Ferenc M. Antibody to cardiolipin as a predictor of fetal distress or death in pregnant patients with systemic lupus erythematosus. N Engl J Med 1985;313:152.
20. Houser MT, Fish AJ, Tagatz GE, Williams PP, Michael AF. Pregnancy and systemic lupus erythematosus. Am J Obstet Gynecol 1980;138:409.
21. Hayslett JP, Lynn RI. Effect of pregnancy in patients with lupus nephropathy. Kidney Int 1980;18:207.
22. Lee LA, Bias WB, Arnett FC, Huff C, Norris DA, Harmon C, et al. Immunogenetics of the neonatal lupus syndrome. Ann Intern Med 1983;99:592.
23. Lockshin MD, Gibofsky A, Peebles CL, Gigli I, Fotino M, Hurwitz S. Neonatal lupus erythematosus with heart block: family study of a patient with anti-SS-A and SS-B antibodies. Arthritis Rheum 1983;26 210.
24. Hardy JD, Solomon S, Banwell GS, Beach R, Wright V, Howard FM. Congenital complete heart block in the newborn associated with maternal systemic lupus erythematosus and other connective tissue disease. Arch Dis Child 1979;54:7.
25. Nathan DJ, Snapper I. Simultaneous placental transfer of factors responsible for L E cell formation and thrombocytopenia. Am J Med 1958;25:647.
26. McCue CM, Matakas ME, Tinglesrad JB, Ruddy S. Congenital heart block in newborns of mothers with connective tissue disease. Circulation 1977;56:82.
27. Esscher E, Scott JS. Congenital heart block and maternal systemic lupus erythematosus. Br Med J 1979;1:1235.
28. Altenburger KM, Jedziniak M, Roper WL, Hernandez J. Congenital complete heart block with hydrops fetalis. J Pediatr 1977;91:618.
29. Hughes GRV. Autoantibodies in lupus and its variants: experience in 1000 patients. Br Med J 1984;289:339.
30. Paredes RA, Morgan M, Lachelin GCL. Congenital heart block associated with maternal Sjorgren's syndrome. Case report. Br J Obstet Gynaecol 1983;90:870.
31. Veille JC, Sunderland C, Bennett RM. Complete heart block in a fetus associated with maternal Sjögren's syndrome. Am J Obstet Gynecol 1985;151:660.
32. Maddison PJ, Skinner RP, Esscher E, Taylor PV, Scott O, Scott JS. Serological studies in congenital heart block. Ann Rheum Dis 1983;42:218.
33. Litsey SE, Noonan JA, O'Connor WM, Cottrill CM, Mitchell B. Maternal connective tissue disease and congenital heart block. Demonstration of immunoglobulin in cardiac tissue. N Engl J Med 1985;312:98.
34. Taylor PV, Scott JS, Gerlis LM, Essecher E, Scott O. Maternal autoantibodies against fetal cardiac antigens in congenital complete heart block. N Engl J Med 1986;315:667.
35. Singsen BM, Arhter SZ, Weinstein MW, Sharp GC. Congenital complete heart block and SSA antibodies: obstetric implications. Am J Obstet Gynecol 1985;152:655.
36. Herreman G, Galelowski N. Maternal connective tissue disease and congenital heart block. N Engl J Med 1985;312:1329.
37. Venning ME, Burn DS, Ward RM, Henry SA, Davison JM. Neonatal lupus syndrome: optimism justified? Lancet 1988;i:640.
38. Doshi N, Smith B, Klionsky B. Congenital pericarditis due to maternal lupus erythematosus. J Pediatr 1980;96:699.
39. Shenreer L, Reed KL, Anderson CF, Marx GR, Sobonya LE, Graham AR. Congenital heart block and cardiac anomalies in the absence of maternal connective tissue disease. Am J Obstet Gynecol 1987;157:248.
40. McCuistion CH, Schoch EP. Possible discoid lupus erythematosus in a newborn infant: report of case with subsequent development of acute systemic lupus erythematosus in mother. Arch Dermatol Syphilol 1954;70:782.
41. Vonderheid EC, Koblenzer PJ, Ming P, Ming L, Burgoon CF. Neonatal lupus erythematosus, report of four cases with a review of the literature. Arch Dermatol 1976;112:698.
42. Provost TT, Watson R, Gammon WR, Radowsky M. Harley JB,

Reichlin M The neonatal Lupus syndrome associated with V_1RNP (nRNP) antibodies. N Engl J Med 1987;316:1135.
43. Hughes GRV, Harris EN, Gharavi AE. The anticardiolipin syndrome. J Rheumatol 1986;13:486.
44. Chesley LC. Hypertensive disorders in pregnancy. New York: Appleton-Century-Crofts, 1978:504.
45. Kaplan D, Diamond H. Rheumatoid arthritis and pregnancy. Clin Obstet Gynecol 1965;8:286.
46. Johnson TR, Banner EA, Winkelmann RK. Scleroderma and pregnancy. Obstet Gynecol 1964;23:467.
47. Baesnihan B, Grigor RR, Oliver M, Lewkonia RM, Hughes GRV, Lovins RE, Fault WP. Immunological mechanism for spontaneous abortion in systemic lupus erythematosus. Lancet 1977;2:1205.
48. Abramowsky CR, Vegas ME, Swinehart G, Gyves MT. Decidual vasculopathy of the placenta in lupus erythematosus. N Engl J Med 1980;303:668.
49. Lubbé WF, Butler WS, Palmer SJ, Liggins GC. Fetal survival after prednisone suppression of maternal lupus-anticoagulant. Lancet 1983;1:1361.
50. Lubbe WF, Butler WS, Palmer SJ, Liggins GC. Lupus anticoagulant in pregnancy. Br J Obstet Gynaecol 1984;91:357.
51. Lubbe WF, Liggins GC. Lupus anticoagulant and pregnancy. Am J Obstet Gynecol 1985;153:322.
52. Ros JO, Tarres MV, Baucells MV, Maired JJ, Solano JT. Prednisone and maternal lupus anticoagulant. Lancet 1983;ii:576.
53. Branch WD, Scott JR, Kochenour NK, Hershgold E. Obstetric complications associated with the lupus anticoagulant. N Engl J Med 1985;313:1322.
54. Derue GJ, Englert MJ, Harris EN, Charavl AE, Morgan SM, Hull RG, Elder MG, Hawkins DF, Hughes GRV. Fetal loss in systemic lupus: association with anticardiolipin antibodies. J Obstet Gynaecol 1985;5:207.
55. Englert H, Derve GM, Loizou S, Hawkins DF, Elder MG, de Swiet M, et al. Pregnancy and lupus: prognostic indicators and response to treatment. Q J Med 1987;66:125.
56. Lockshin MD, Druzin ML. Antiphospholipid antibodies and pregnancy. N Engl J Med 1985;313:1351.
57. Schlieder MA, Nachman RL, Jaffe EA, Colman M. A clinical study of the lupus anticoagulant. Blood 1976;48:499.
58. Reece EA, Romero R, Clyne LP, Kriz NS, Hobbins JC. Lupus titre anticoagulant in pregnancy: Lancet 1984;1:344.
59. Exner T, Rickard KA, Kronenberg H. A sensitive test demonstrating lupus anticoagulant and its behavioural patterns. Br J Hematol 1978;40:143.
60. Boxer M, Ellman L, Carvalho A. The lupus anticoagulant. Arthritis Rheum 1976;19:1244.
61. Lancet editorial. Anticardiolipin antibodies: a risk factor for venous and arterial thrombosis. Lancet 1985;1:912.
62. Ordi J, Vilardel M, Oristrell M, Valdes M, Knobel A, Alijotas J, et al. Bleeding in patients with lupus anticoagulant. Lancet 1984;ii:868.
63. Thiagarajav P, Shapiro SS, DeMarco L. Monoclonal immunoglobin MT coagulation inhibitor with phospholipid specificity: mechanism of a lupus anticoagulant. J Clin Invest 1980;66:397.
64. Harris EN, Chan J, Asherson R, Chavari A, Hughes GRV. Predictive value of the antocardiolipin antibody for thrombosis, fetal loss and thrombocytopaenia. Clin Sci 1986;70:56P.
65. Thornton JR, Scott JS, Tovey LAD. Anticardiolipin antibodies in pregnancy. Br Med J 1984;289:697.
66. Thornton JG, Foote GA, Page CE, Clayden AD, Tovey LAD, Scott JS. False positive results of tests for syphilis and outcome of pregnancy: a retrospective case conclusive study. Br Med J 1987;295:355.
67. Harris EN, Gharavi AE, Boey ML, Patel BM, Mackworth-Young CG, Loizou S, Hughes GRV. Anticardiolipin antibodies: detection by radioimmunoassay and association with thrombosis in systemic lupus erythematosus. Lancet 1983;2:1211.
68. Harris EN, Loizou S, Englert M, Derue G, Chan JK, Gharavi AE, Hughes GRV. Anticardiolipin antibodies and lupus anticoagulant. Lancet 1984;ii:1099.
69. Lockwood CJ, Reece EA, Romero R, Hobbins JC. Antiphospholipid antibody and pregnancy wastage. Lancet 1986;ii:742.
70. Firkin BG, Howard MA, Radford N. Possible relationship between lupus inhibitor and recurrent abortion in young women. Lancet 1980;2:366.
71. Gardlund B. The lupus inhibitor in thromboembolic disease and intrauterine death in the absence of systemic lupus. Acta Med Scand 1984;215:293.
72. Harris EN, Hughes GRV. Standardizing the anti-carciolipin antibody test. Lancet 1987;i:277.
73. Lockshin MD. Anticardiolipin antibodies in pregnant patients with systemic lupus erythematosus. N Engl J Med 1986; 314:1392.
74. Unander AM, Norberg R, Hahn L, Arfors L. Anticardiolipin antibodies and complement in ninety-nine women with habitual abortion. Am J Obstet Gynecol 1987;156:114.
75. Cowchock S, Dehoratius RD, Wapner RJ, Jackson LG. Subclinical autoimmune disease and unexplained abortion. Am J Obstet Gynecol 1984;150:367.
76. Scott JS. Immunological factors and recurrent fetal loss. Lancet 1984;i:1122.
77. Prentice RL, Gatenby PA, Loblay RM, Shearman RP, Kronenberg M, Basten A. Lupus anticoagulant in pregnancy. Lancet 1984;2:464.
78. Kilpatrick DC. Anti-phospholipid antibodies and pregnancy wastage. Lancet 1986;ii:980.
79. Carreras LO, Defreyn G, Machin SJ, Vermylen J, Deman R, Spitz B, Van Assch A. Arterial thrombosis, intrauterine death and "lupus" anticoagulant: detection of immunoglobulin interfering with prostacyclin formation. Lancet 1981;1:244.
80. de Castellarnau C, Vila L, Sancho MJ, Borrell M, Fontcuberta J, Rutllant ML. Lupus anticoagulant, recurrent abortion, and prostacyclin production by cultured smooth muscle cells. Lancet 1983;ii:1137.
81. Comp PC, De Bault LE, Esmon NL, Esmon CT. Human thrombomodulin is inhibited by IgG from two patients with non-specific anticoagulants. Blood (Suppl) 1983;1:1099.
82. Cariou R, Tobelem G, Soria C, Caen J. Inhibition of protein C activation by endothelial cells in the presence of lupus anticoagulant. N Engl J Med 1986;314:1193.
83. Byron MA. Treatment of rheumatic diseases. Br Med J 1987;293:236.
84. Slone D, Sisilind V, Heinonen OP, Monson RR, Kaufman DW, Shapiro S. Aspirin and congenital malformations. Lancet 1976;1:1373.
85. Buckfield P. Major congenital faults in newborn infants: a pilot study in New Zealand. NZ Med J 1973;78:159.
86. Turner G, Collins E. Fetal effects of regular salicylate ingestion in pregnancy. Lancet 1975;2:338.
87. Stuart MJ, Gross SJ, Elrad H, Graeber JE. Effects of acetylsalicylic-acid ingestion on maternal and neonatal hemostasis. N Engl J Med 1982;307:902.
88. Lancet editorial. PG-synthetase inhibition in obstetrics and after. Lancet 1980;2:185.
89. Heymann MA. Nonsteroidal anti-inflammatory agents. In: Eskes TKAB, Finster M, eds. Drug therapy during pregnancy. London: Butterworths, 1985:85.
90. Goudie BM, Dossetor JFB. Effect on the fetus of indomethacin given to suppress labour. Lancet 1979;ii:1187.
91. Dudley DKL, Hardie MJ. Fetal and neonatal effects of indo-

methacin used as a tocolytic agent. Am J Obstet Gynecol 1985;151:181.

92. Niebyl JR, Witter FR. Neonatal outcome after indomethacin treatment for preterm labour. Am J Obstet Gynecol 1986;155:747.

93. Rees RB, Maibach HH. Chloroquine: a review of reactions and dermatologic indications. Arch Dermatol 1963;88:96.

94. Schatz M, Patterson R, Zeitz S. Corticosteroid therapy for the pregnant asthmatic patient. JAMA 1975;233 804.

95. Turner ES, Greenberger PA, Patterson R. Management of the pregnant asthmatic patient. Ann Intern Med 1980;6:905.

96. Francis HH, Smellie J. General diseases in pregnancy. Br Med J 1964;1:887.

97. Fainstall T. Cortisone-induced congenital cleft palate in rabbits. Endocrinology 1954;55:520.

98. Warrell DW, Taylor R. Outcome for the fetus of mother receiving prednisolone during pregnancy. Lancet 1968;1:117.

99. Levitz M, Jansen V, Dancis J. The transfer and metabolism of corticosteroids in the perfused human placenta. Am J Obstet Gynecol 1978;132:363.

100. Beitins R, Baynard F, Ances IG, Kowarsk A, Migeon CJ. The transplacental passage of prednisone and prednisolone in pregnancy near term. J Pediatr 1972;81:936.

101. Davison J. Renal disease. In: de Swiet M, ed. Medical disorders in obstetric practice. Oxford: Blackwell, 1984:226.

102. Zurier RB, Argyros TG, Urman JD, Warren J, Rothfield NF. Systemic lupus erythematosus. Management during pregnancy. Obstet Gynecol 1978;51:178.

103. Thomson BJ, Watson ML, Liston WA, Lambie AT. Plasmapheresis in a pregnancy complicated by acute systemic lupus erythematosus. Case report. Br J Obstet Gynaecol 1985;92:532.

104. Frampton G, Cameron JS, Thom M, Jones S, Raferty M. Successful removal of anti-phosopholipid antibody during pregnancy using plasma exchange and low-dose prednisolone. Lancet 1987;ii:1023.

105. Barclay CS, French MAH, Ross LD, Sokol RJ. Successful pregnancy following steroid therapy and plasma exchange in a woman with anti-Ro (SS-A) antibodies. Case report. Br J Obstet Gynaecol 1987;94:369.

106. Farquharson RG, Compston A, Bloom AL. Lupus anticoagulant: a place for pre-pregnancy treatment? Lancet 1985;ii:842.

107. Spitz B, Van Assche FA, Vermylen J. Lupus anticoagulant and pregnancy. Am J Obstet Gynecol 1986;154:1169.

108. DeBoer FC, Chu P. Pregnancy complicated by lupus anticoagulant. Immunosuppression monitored by the Kaolin clotting time. J Obstet Gynecol 1988;9:37.

109. Feinstein DI. Lupus anticoagulant, thrombosis and fetal loss. N Engl J Med 1985;313:1348.

110. Chan JKM, Marris EN, Mughes GRV. Successful pregnancy following suppression of cardiolipin antibodies and lupus anticoagulant with azathioprine in systemic lupus erythematosus. J Obstet Gynaecol 1986;7:16.

111. Gregorini G, Setti G, Remuzzi G. Recurrent abortion with lupus anticoagulant and preeclampsia: a common final pathway for two different diseases? Case report. Br J Obstet Gynaecol 1986;93:194.

112. Carreras LO, Perez GN, Vega HR, Casavilla F. Lupus anticoagulant and recurrent fetal loss: successful treatment with . Lancet 1988;ii:393.

113. Barbui T, Finazzi G, Falanga A, Cortellazo S. Intravenous gamma globulin, antiphospholipid antibodies and thrombocytopenia. Lancet 1988;ii:969.

114. Druzin ML, Lockshin M, Edersheim TG, Hutson JM, Krauss AL, Kogut E. Second-trimester fetal monitoring and preterm delivery in pregnancies with systemic lupus erythematosus and/or circulating anticoagulant. Am J Obstet Gynecol 1987;157:1503.

115. Oakey RE. The interpretation of urinary oestrogen and pregnanediol excretion in women receiving corticosteroids. J Obstet Gynaecol Br Commonw 77:922.

116. Stephensen O, Cleland WP, Mallidie-Smith K. Congenital heart block and persistent ductus arteriosus associated with maternal systemic lupus erythematosus. Br Heart J 1981;46:104.

117. Nicolaides KH, Soothill PW, Rodeck CH, Campbell S. Ultrasound-guided sampling of umbilical cord and placental blood to assess fetal wellbeing. Lancet 1986;i:1065.

118. Soothill PW, Nicolaides KH, Rodeck CH, Campbell S. The effect of gestational age on blood gas and acid-base values in human pregnancy. Fetal Ther 1986;1:166.

119. Leinwald I, Durgee AW. Scleroderma. Ann Intern Med 1954;41:1033.

120. Slate WG, Graham AR. Scleroderma and pregnancy. Am J Obstet Gynecol 1968;101:335.

121. Haynes DM. In: Haynes MM, ed. Medical complications during pregnancy. New York: McGraw-Hill, 1989.

122. Karlen JG, Cook WA. Renal scleroderma and pregnancy. Obstet Gynecol 1974;44:349.

123. Gopelrud CP. Scleroderma. Clin Obstet Gynecol 1983;26:587.

124. Bellucci MJ, Coustan DR, Plotz RD. Cervical scleroderma: a case of soft tissue dystocia. Am J Obstet Gynecol 1984;150:891.

125. Thompson J, Conklin KA. Anesthetic management of a pregnant patient with scleroderma. Anesthesiology 1983;59:69.

126. McKenna F, Martin MFR, Bird MA, Wright V. Captopril. Br Med J 1983;287:1299.

127. Debeukelaer MM, Travis LB, Roberts DK. Polyarteritis and pregnancy: report of a successful outcome. South Med J 1973;66:613.

128. Nagey DA, Fortier KJ, Linder J. Pregnancy complicated by pericarditis nodosa: induced abortion as an alternative. Am J Obstet Gynecol 1983;147:103.

129. Talbot SF, Main DM, Levinson AI. Wegener's granulomatosis: first report of a case with onset during pregnancy. Arthritis Rheum 1984;27:109.

130. Cooper K, Stafford J, Turner Warwick M. Wegener's granuloma complicating pregnancy. Br J Obstet Gynaecol 1970;77:1028.

131. Toledo TM, Harper RC, Moser RH. Fetal effects during cyclophosphamide and radiation therapy. Ann Intern Med 1971;74:87.

132. Coates A. Cyclophosphamide in pregnancy. Aust NZ J Obstet Gynaecol 1970;10:33.

133. Greenberg LH, Tanaka KR. Congenital anomalies probably induced by cyclophosphamide. JAMA 1964;188:423.

134. Gilland J, Weinstein L. The effects of cancer chemotherapeutic agents on the developing fetus. Obstet Gynecol Surv 1983;38:6.

135. Wheeler GE. Cyclophosphamide associated leukaemia in Wegner's granulomatosis. Ann Intern Med 1981;94:161.

136. Casciato J. Leukaemia following cytotoxic therapy. Med 1979;58:32.

137. Tan EM, Cohan AS, Aries JF, Masi AT, McShane DJ, Rothfield N, et al. The 1982 revised criteria for the classification of systemic lupus erythematosus. Arthritis Rheum 1982;25:1271.

75

CHAPTER

DERMATOLOGIC DISORDERS OF PREGNANCY

Pravit Bisalbutra and Kim B. Yancey

Skin changes in pregnancy include alterations common to most gestations as well as unique cutaneous eruptions specific to pregnancy. These alterations usually raise questions regarding the skin (eg, scarring and hair loss), the possibility of recurrence in subsequent pregnancies, and concerns for associated maternal or fetal morbidity. An overview of various physiologic changes and dermatologic disorders of pregnancy will be presented in this chapter. It should also be kept in mind that other skin diseases that are not related to pregnancy may develop coincidentally during gestation.

CUTANEOUS CHANGES IN PREGNANCY

PIGMENTARY CHANGES

Hyperpigmentation

Darkening of skin during pregnancy is common, occurring in up to 90% of women. It is more pronounced in women with brown eyes and darker complexions.[1] The areas commonly affected are the areolae of the breasts (so-called secondary areolae),[2] the abdominal midline (darkening of the linea alba to form the linea nigra), and the axillae, perineum, perianal area, and genitalia. Freckles, nevi, and scars may also darken during gestation.[3] Hyperpigmentation usually appears during the first trimester of pregnancy, progresses until delivery, and regresses postpartum.[4] However, it may persist in the areolae and the linea nigra.[5] Persistent, but possibly less severe, involvement may be seen in other sites as well. Melasma, a specific facial hyperpigmentation that frequently develops during pregnancy, will be discussed later.

It is hypothesized that pregnancy-associated hyperpigmentation is due to an increase in ovarian, placental, and pituitary hormones. Although the exact physiologic basis of this hyperpigmentation is unknown, estrogen and progesterone are believed to be mainly responsible for these alterations. Preferred sites of hyperpigmentation may have greater numbers of melanocytes (ie, pigment-producing epidermal cells) or unique melanocytes that are susceptible to hormonal stimulation.[6]

Melasma (Chloasma Gravidarum, the Mask of Pregnancy)

Melasma affects 50% to 75% of pregnant women and up to one third of non-pregnant women exposed to oral contraceptives.[7] Its onset is usually in the second half of gestation. Melasma is characterized by blotchy, brownish macules or patches on the cheeks, forehead, chin, upper lip, or mandible (Fig. 75-1). Histologically, two patterns of hyperpigmentation are recognized in patients with melasma. In the epidermal type, melanin is found within basal and suprabasal keratinocytes; in dermal melasma, melanin is present within macrophages (so-called melanophages) in the dermis. As expected, some patients demonstrate both patterns of melasma. Clinically, epidermal melasma is accentuated when patients are examined in a dark room with a Wood's lamp (ie, ultraviolet light source), whereas dermal melasma is not.[4]

Melasma in pregnancy is probably caused by a combination of hormonal changes, a genetic predisposition, and sun exposure. Melasma is not specific to pregnancy or oral contraceptive exposure. Similar patterns of facial hyperpigmentation may develop in non-pregnant women without associated exposure to oral contraceptives or in some men. Patients with this condition should use photoprotective measures (ie, sunscreens)

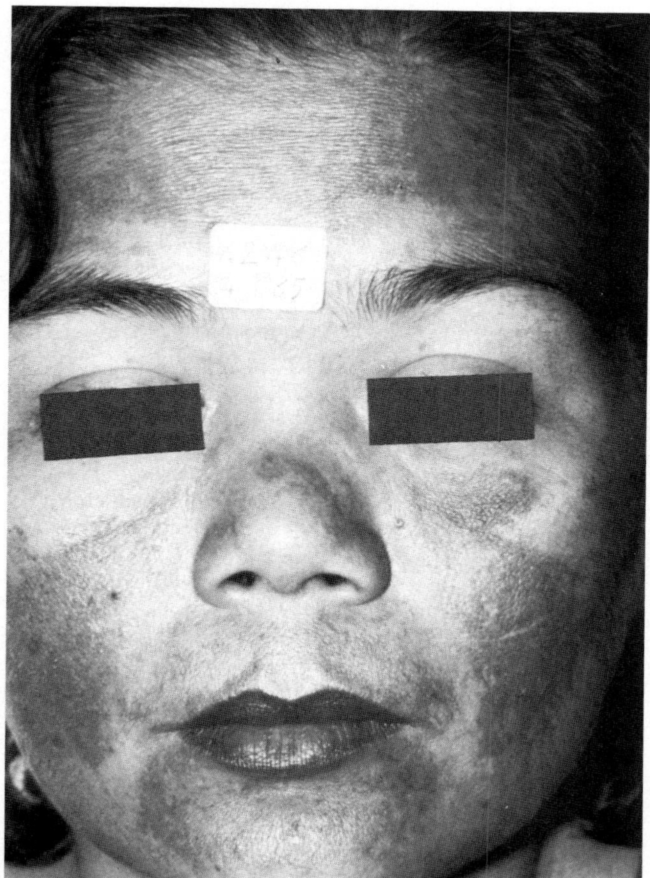

FIGURE 75–1. This patient demonstrates melasma over the forehead, cheeks, chin, nose, and upper lip. This hyperpigmentation is noninflammatory and nonpalpable.

and avoid exposure to oral contraceptives. Specific topical treatments may be employed postpartum to lighten sites of pronounced hyperpigmentation.

VASCULAR CHANGES

Spider Angiomas (Spider Nevi)

Spider angiomas are characterized by a pulsatile central red punctum and radiating branches. These lesions are a common vascular abnormality associated with pregnancy. Spider angiomas usually begin to appear during the second to the fifth month of pregnancy and may increase in size and number until delivery.[6] They are seen in approximately two thirds of whites and 10% of blacks by the third trimester.[8]

Pregnancy-associated spider angiomas usually occur in areas drained by the superior vena cava, such as the neck, throat, face (especially the periorbital area), and arms.[8] Spider angiomas can also be seen in normal healthy individuals as well as in patients with liver diseases. However, in the latter group, spider angiomas are usually larger and more numerous.[6] Three fourths of these lesions fade by the seventh week postpartum[9] and require no specific treatment. However, some lesions may persist, and in these cases the therapeutic options are opaque creams or electrodesiccation of the central vascular punctum. Electrodesiccation is best reserved for lesions that persist several months postpartum.

Palmar Erythema

Palmar erythema is a frequent finding in pregnancy. Bean states that approximately 60% of whites and 35% of blacks develop palmar erythema during pregnancy.[10] Its onset usually begins in the first trimester. Clinically, there are two forms of this disorder—specifically, erythematous areas that are sharply separated from adjacent normal skin or a diffuse erythematous mottling of the entire palm.[6] The latter form is more common. Because both palmar erythema and spider angiomas often occur together in the same patient, a similar pathogenesis is suggested.[10] Increased levels of estrogen, a marked rise in blood volume, increased blood flow in pregnancy, and a genetic predisposition are possible etiologies of this problem. This finding usually resolves postpartum and requires no specific therapy.

Varicosities

Varicosities occur in approximately half of pregnant women and frequently involve the saphenous and hemorrhoidal veins as well as vessels in the vulvar region. Despite this incidence, symptomatic thromboses in these lesions are relatively rare.[11] Varicosities may develop as early as the first trimester in response to a combination of factors, including increased intrapelvic pressure due to a gravid uterus, hormonally induced vascular relaxation, or predisposing genetic factors. Treatment consists of frequent elevation of the legs, sleeping in Trendelenburg's position, avoidance of clothing that interferes with venous return, and elastic support for the legs. Varicosities tend to regress after delivery.[1]

Hemangioma

Small, superficial or subcutaneous cavernous hemangiomas occur in a few pregnant women. These lesions usually appear at the end of the first trimester and enlarge slowly until delivery.[8] They usually regress after delivery. Persistent lesions may require surgical treatment.

Purpura

Purpura on the legs is common during the final trimester. This may be due to increased capillary permeability and/or fragility.[12]

Hyperemia, Hypertrophy of the Gingiva, and Granuloma Gravidarum

Hyperemia and hypertrophy of the gingiva occur in up to 80% of pregnant women. Proliferation of capillaries within such hypertrophic gingiva can result in the formation of granuloma gravidarum (also known as pregnancy tumor). These lesions clinically and histologically resemble pyogenic granulomas—dull red, vascular nodules that grow rapidly in size to 0.5 to 1.0 cm in diameter. Granuloma gravidarum is found in approximately 2% of pregnant women and commonly appears between the second and fifth months of gestation. These lesions are usually located in the gingival papillae between adjacent teeth or on the buccal or lingual surface of the marginal gingival mucosa.[8] Like pyogenic granulomas, they bleed and ulcerate easily when traumatized. These lesions usually regress after delivery. Proper dental hygiene and avoidance of trauma are appropriate therapy for most patients; selected cases may require surgical treatment.

Congestion of the Vestibule, Vaginal Mucosa, and Cervix

Vascular distention and congestion of the vestibule and vaginal mucosa occur early in gestation and constitute a diagnostic feature of pregnancy itself (Chadwick's sign). Bluish discoloration of cervical tissue (Goodell's sign) occurs in the same way and is seen in early pregnancy, sometimes as early as the fourth week.[13]

Nonpitting Edema of Eyelids, Face, and Extremities

Nonpitting edema of the eyelids, face, and extremities is a common feature of pregnancy.[8] Fluid and sodium retention in these patients is thought to be related in part to increased levels of circulating adrenocortical, ovarian, and placental hormones.[12,14] Moreover, the gravid uterus increases the hydrostatic pressure within lower-extremity vessels and contributes to increased capillary permeability in dependent regions. However, it is important that cardiac and renal abnormalities as well as preeclampsia–eclampsia be excluded as causes of this problem. This finding is most commonly seen in the third trimester and resolves after delivery.

Vasomotor Instability (Flushing, Hot and Cold Sensations, Cutis Marmorata)

Vasomotor instability accounts for such symptoms as pallor, facial flushing, hot and cold sensations, and cutis marmorata (a transitory bluish-red mottling of the skin occurring on exposure to cold) during pregnancy. These changes may be secondary to increased estrogen levels. They resolve upon delivery and usually require no specific therapy. Transient vasomotor instability should be distinguished from persistent livedo reticularis, which warrants a search for an underlying connective tissue disease, neoplasm, or blood dyscrasia.

HAIR CHANGES

Postpartum Telogen Effluvium

Postpartum telogen effluvium is a rapid hair loss that begins roughly 4 to 20 weeks after delivery and often continues for several months. The pathophysiology of this nonscarring form of hair loss is as follows. Under normal circumstances, approximately 85% to 90% of all scalp hairs are in what is called the anagen or growth phase. During the second and third trimesters, a greater percentage of follicles remains in the anagen phase. Following delivery, there is a rapid conversion of anagen hairs to telogen (resting) hairs, which are then shed. Factors contributing to postpartum telogen effluvium include the stress of delivery (eg, fever, surgery, emotional factors, and hormonal changes).[6] This condition requires no specific treatment, and hair regrowth within 6 to 15 months is the rule.

Increased Hair Growth

The growth of coarse, terminal, male-patterned hair is sometimes seen during pregnancy. A common site of this problem is the face, especially the upper lip, chin, and cheeks; the arms, legs, and back may also be affected. Increased suprapubic and abdominal midline hair growth[15] as well as acne may also be found in these patients.[16] Excessive body hair usually regresses within 6 months of delivery, but coarse terminal hair may persist. Endocrine factors (increased adrenocorticotropic hormone, adrenocorticosteroids, as well as ovarian androgens) may account for this increased hair growth. Patients with evidence of a substantial increase in numbers of coarse, terminal hairs may need to be evaluated for evidence of hirsutism, virilizing tumors, or virilizing syndromes.

CONNECTIVE TISSUE CHANGES

Striae Gravidarum (Stretch Marks, Striae Distensae, Linear Striae)

Striae gravidarum develop in a large percentage of pregnant women and appear to have a familial tendency.[8] They are more common in whites than in blacks or Asians. Their onset is usually during the second half of pregnancy. Striae gravidarum appear as irregular, linear, pink-to-violet lesions that are initially edematous and pruritic. They eventually become atrophic and hypopigmented. Although these lesions commonly occur in areas of maximal stretch (ie, on the abdomen, breasts, and thighs), there is no direct correlation between their severity and enlargement of body size during pregnancy.[6] Although their exact etiology is unknown, stretching of the skin, adrenocortical hormones, and a genetic predisposition have been suggested to play roles in their pathogenesis. The lesions fade gradually after delivery but do not completely resolve.

Molluscum Fibrosum Gravidarum

Molluscum fibrosum gravidarum, which clinically and histologically resembles a skin tag, often develops during the second or the third trimester of pregnancy. These lesions are commonly found on the sides of the face, neck, upper portion of the chest, and beneath the breasts.[7] Their size ranges from 1 to 5 mm in diameter. They are pedunculated, skin-colored or slightly pigmented, and soft. Their pathogenesis is unknown, but endocrinologic changes have been implicated. These lesions may or may not regress after delivery. Persistent, unsightly, or irritated lesions may be treated with shave excision or light electrodesiccation.

MISCELLANEOUS CHANGES

Nail Changes

Nail changes during pregnancy develop in selected patients and may begin as early as the sixth week of gestation. These changes consist of transverse grooving, brittleness, and onycholysis (ie, distal separation of the nail plate from the nail bed). The pathogenesis of these changes is unknown. Patients should be advised to keep their nails short if they are brittle and prone to separate from the nail bed. Other possible causes of nail abnormalities should be considered in these patients.

Changes in Eccrine Sweat Glands

Eccrine sweat gland activity increases progressively in pregnancy and may lead to an increased incidence of miliaria (heat rash), hyperhidrosis (increased sweating), and dyshidrotic eczema. The precise etiology of this alteration is unknown.[1]

Changes in Apocrine Sweat Glands

Apocrine sweating, which occurs mainly in the axillae and groin, tends to decrease during pregnancy. This may contribute to an improvement in preexisting Fox-Fordyce disease (an occlusive disorder involving apocrine pilosebaceous units) or hidradenitis suppurativa (a chronic, recurrent, deep-seated pyoderma of apocrine pilosebaceous units).[8]

Changes in Sebaceous Glands

Sebaceous glands on the areolae of the breasts tend to enlarge during pregnancy and appear as small brown papules. These papules are called Montgomery's tubercles and are considered a common manifestation of pregnancy. These papules may appear as early as 6 weeks of gestation; they tend to regress postpartum.[4,8]

DERMATOSES OF PREGNANCY

HERPES GESTATIONIS

Herpes gestationis (HG) is a rare, pruritic, nonviral, blistering eruption of pregnancy and the immediate postpartum period.[17] It may also occur in association with hydatidiform mole or choriocarcinoma.[18] It is perhaps the most well defined of all the dermatoses of pregnancy. *Herpes* is derived from the Greek word meaning "to creep" and has often been used to describe skin conditions characterized by the formation of small, clustered vesicles.[17] This disorder is not related to an active or prior herpes virus infection. Herpes gestationis was proposed to be a distinct bullous skin disease with characteristic immunopathologic findings by Provost and Tomasi in 1973.[19]

The estimated incidence of HG ranges from one in 3000 to one in 60,000 gestations.[20,21] The most recent estimate of its incidence is one in 50,000 Caucasian births.[17,22] HG is less common among blacks. HG usually begins in the second or third trimester[17] but may develop as early as the ninth week of gestation or as late as 1 week postpartum.[23] HG tends to recur in subsequent pregnancies; in those instances of recurrent disease, the onset tends to be at an earlier phase of the gestation.

HG is a polymorphous (ie, many forms of lesions) eruption characterized by intense pruritus. Pruritus may precede skin lesions by days or weeks.[17,24] Besides pruritus, other prodromal symptoms include malaise, fever, nausea, and headache. The morphology of lesions in these patients may include urticarial papules and plaques, vesicles, bullae, and excoriations. Vesicles or bullae rimming inflammatory, urticarial plaques is a classic (but not specific) morphologic feature of HG (Fig. 75-2). In some patients, bullae are found on noninflamed skin. Patients often demonstrate a variety of morphologic lesions. In 50% to 90% of cases, lesions initially appear within the umbilicus[17,25] and then spread over the abdomen. The chest, back, buttocks, and extremities are also frequently involved in a generalized, sometimes symmetric pattern.[24,26,27] Lesions may also develop on the palms and soles (Fig. 75-3). Facial or mucosal lesions are unusual and occur in less than 10% of cases.[17] Because HG is quite pruritic, numerous crusts and excoriations are commonly seen in these patients.[3] Healing usually proceeds without scar formation unless bacterial infection or severe excoriation has occurred. Postinflammatory hyperpigmentation at lesional sites is common and typically resolves with time. The differential diagnosis of HG includes bullous pemphigoid, erythema multiforme, pruritic urticarial papules and plaques of pregnancy (PUPPP), and other inflammatory skin diseases.

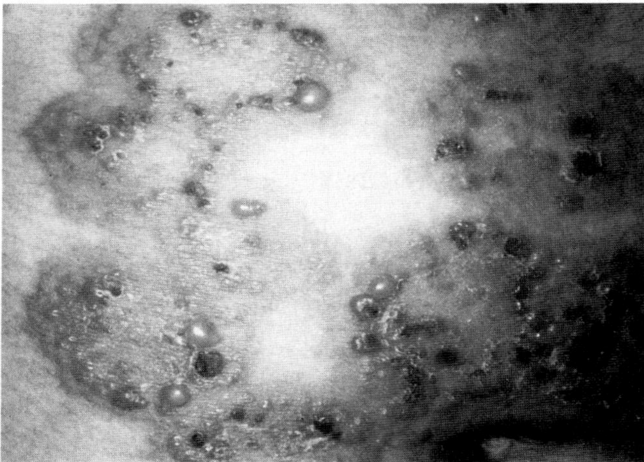

FIGURE 75–2. A patient with herpes gestationis demonstrates polymorphic lesions on the abdomen and within the umbilicus (lower right corner of the photograph). Lesions consist of urticarial inflammatory plaques rimmed by vesicles, bullae, and crusts. (From Yancey KB, Lawley TJ. Herpes gestationis. In: Thiers B, Dobson RL, eds. Pathogenesis of skin diseases. New York: Churchill Livingstone, 1986:185.)

HG often improves somewhat during the latter portion of gestation only to flare at the time of delivery.[3,17] In fact, postpartum flares (or onset of disease) are seen in roughly 50% of patients with HG.[3,28] Clearing of skin lesions in patients with HG generally occurs within 3 months of delivery but may be later if the disease is late in onset.[3,6] Temporary exacerbations or recurrences may also be noted when menses resume during the first few months postpartum. Flares can also occur if patients with a prior history of HG are exposed to oral contraceptives (both estrogens and progestins). Although there is no increased risk of maternal mortality in HG, maternal morbidity may be substantial because of severe pruritus, generalized malaise, fever, cutaneous erosions, or secondary bacterial infections.

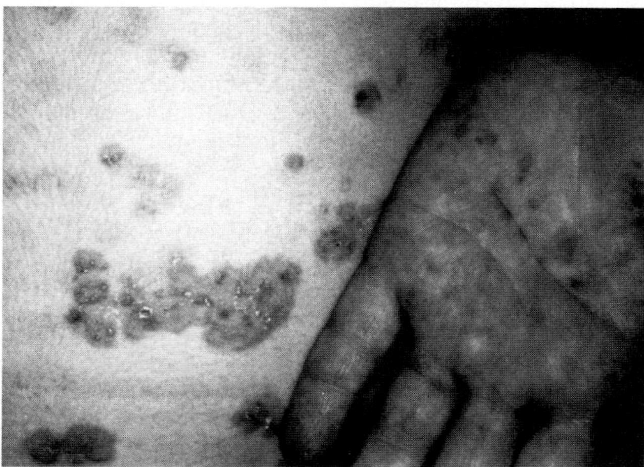

FIGURE 75–3. Lesions on the palm and abdomen of a patient with herpes gestationis. (From: Yancey KB, Lawley TJ. Herpes gestationis. In: Thiers B, Dobson RL, eds. Pathogenesis of skin disease. New York: Churchill Livingstone, 1986: 185.)

The incidence of fetal morbidity and mortality in patients with HG is controversial. Lawley and colleagues reviewed the fetal outcome in 40 immunologically confirmed cases of HG and found nine premature deliveries, three stillbirths, and one spontaneous abortion.[28] Holmes and Black reported a 26% incidence of low birth weight (ie, <2.5 kg) and small-for-date (ie, below the 10th percentile) infants in 50 gestations associated with herpes gestationis.[29] They believed that infants born to mothers with HG may be at risk of increased morbidity and should be delivered in units that have neonatal intensive care facilities.[29] However, Shornick and colleagues could not demonstrate an increased risk of fetal complications in 28 previously unreported cases of immunologically confirmed HG.[22] Although the exact interpretation of these various findings is currently debated, there is general agreement that these patients should be carefully followed by obstetricians and dermatologists for evidence of disease progression or complications.

Cutaneous lesions in newborns are occasionally seen and may consist of urticarial, vesicular, or bullous eruptions. These lesions are usually mild and transient, and resolve spontaneously during the first several weeks of life.[3,30,31] In general, lesions in newborns of affected mothers require no specific therapy.[32]

The histopathologic features of herpes gestationis are distinctive yet not entirely specific or diagnostic.[3] Biopsies of early vesicular lesions in patients with HG show a subepidermal blister, eosinophils within blister cavities and the upper dermis, dermal edema, and a mixed but eosinophil-rich, perivascular lymphohistiocytic infiltrate (Fig. 75-4).[33] Urticarial lesions in HG patients are characterized by a moderately dense, perivascular, mixed inflammatory-cell infiltrate composed of lymphocytes, histiocytes, and eosinophils around blood vessels in both the superficial and mid dermis, marked upper dermal edema, spongiosis (intercellular edema between epidermal cells), and focal necrosis of epidermal basal keratinocytes.[33] Because similar findings may be seen in other inflammatory subepidermal blistering skin diseases, it is not possible to distinguish HG completely from these other disorders histologically.

Direct immunofluorescence microscopy of normal-appearing, perilesional skin from patients with HG reveals linear deposits of C3 (the third component of complement) in the epidermal basement membrane zone.[34] This immunopathologic finding is universal among HG patients and should be demonstrated before the diagnosis is made. Approximately 30% to 50% of these patients also demonstrate deposits of IgG in this same location.[35] Rare cases may also demonstrate deposits of IgA or IgM.[23,34,35] Alternative pathway complement components (eg, properdin and factor B) as well as classical pathway complement components (eg, Clq, C4, and C5) can sometimes be demonstrated in this

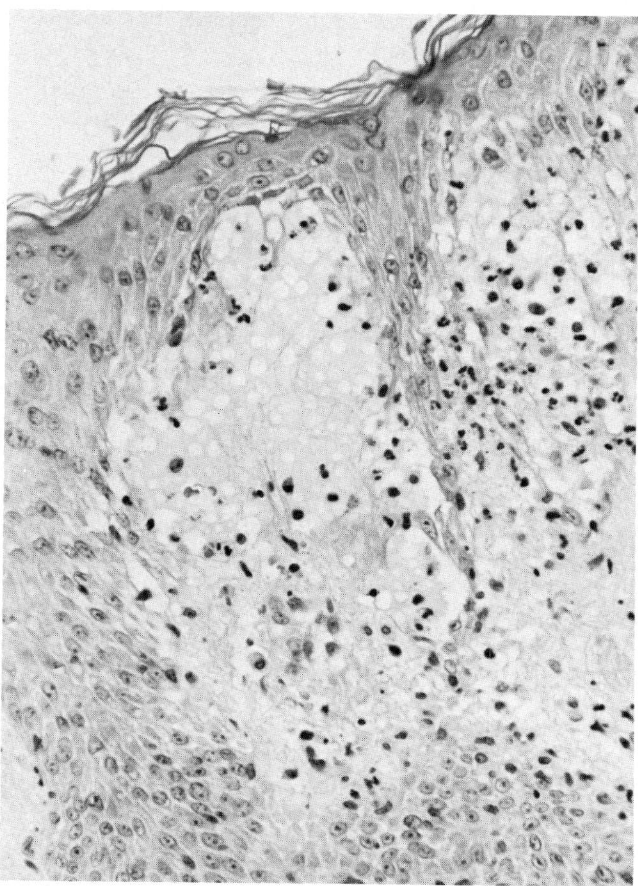

FIGURE 75–4. A biopsy from early lesional skin of a patient with herpes gestationis demonstrates papillary dermal edema resulting in microvesicle formation. A granulocyte-rich infiltrate is present in the upper dermis.

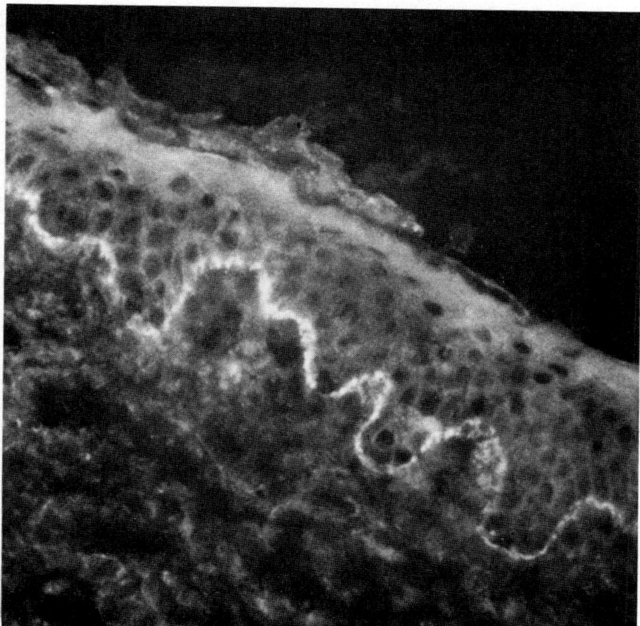

FIGURE 75–5. This section of normal human skin was treated with serum from a patient with herpes gestationis and followed by the addition of normal human serum containing functionally active complement components. The presence of C3 in this test substrate (depicted as white continuous deposits at the junction between the epidermis and dermis) provides evidence of a complement-fixing, antiepidermal basement membrane zone autoantibody in this HG patient's serum.

same distribution.[19,34] By immunoelectron microscopy, these immunoreactants are found just beneath basal keratinocytes within the lamina lucida of the epidermal basement membrane zone.[36,37] Similar deposits of C3 and other immunoreactants have also been found in the skin of infants born of affected mothers.[34,38]

Conventional indirect immunofluorescence microscopy uses a normal human skin substrate to test patient serum for the presence of a circulating autoantibody against the epidermal basement membrane zone. Utilizing this technique, circulating IgG antiepidermal basement membrane zone antibody is found in only 25% to 40% of HG patients.[28,34] However, when these same patients' sera are tested in indirect immunofluorescent microscopy studies that employ complement fixation, roughly 75% show evidence of a circulating IgG antiepidermal basement membrane zone autoantibody[3,38,39] (Fig. 75-5). Similar tests of cord sera demonstrate that this low-titer, avid-complement-fixing autoantibody can be transmitted across the placenta. Hence, it is possible for this autoantibody to deposit in fetal skin and produce tissue damage. Given the fact that specialized immunopathologic tests are required for the demonstration of these circulating antiepidermal basement membrane zone autoantibodies (as well as the fact that they are not demonstrable in all HG patients), it is critical to study patient skin for in situ deposits of C3 for the diagnosis of this disease.

The antiepidermal basement membrane zone autoantibodies in patients with HG bind a distinct site within the lamina lucida. Recent studies have shown that sera from the majority of HG patients with complement-fixing antiepidermal basement membrane zone autoantibodies recognize a 180,000-Da protein in epidermal cell extracts.[40] Interestingly, this same protein is also recognized by autoantibodies in the sera of a number of patients with bullous pemphigoid, thus suggesting a degree of relatedness of target antigens in these bullous skin diseases.

Immunogenetic studies have demonstrated that individuals with selected haplotypes have an increased relative risk of HG.[17] Specifically, 61% to 85% of patients with HG express the HLA-DR3 haplotype, and 43% to 45% express the paired-haplotype HLA-DR3, -DR4.[41,42] Despite these associations, these haplotypes alone are neither sufficient nor required for the development of this disease. In addition to the immunogenetic observations presented earlier, a recent study demonstrated that 85% of 26 patients with HG showed evidence of anti-HLA antibodies (in contrast to 25% of normal multiparous controls). Moreover, in 58% of these serum samples reactivity of these antibodies were specific to paternal antigens.[43] This laboratory finding has relevance to the accepted clinical observation that selected patients first develop HG coincident with a change in sexual partner.[41] Shornick and colleagues found laboratory support of such a role of paternal antigens by demonstrating an increased frequency of the HLA-DR2 haplotype among consorts of patients with HG (and especially among HG patients with the HLA-DR3, -DR4 paired-haplotype).[43]

Selected patients with HG demonstrate peripheral eosinophilia.[3,28] Moreover, one study has suggested that patients with very high peripheral blood eosinophil counts generally have higher titers of antiepidermal basement membrane zone autoantibodies and more severe maternal disease.[28] Further study of these associations is of interest.

The exact etiology of HG is unknown. However, the association of HG with pregnancy, oral contraceptives, and menstruation suggests that a hormonal influence in a genetically predisposed individual may result in this disease. Interestingly, a well-documented case of herpes gestationis has never been reported from use of oral contraceptives in an individual with no prior history of pregnancy-associated HG.[34] HG is considered an immunologically mediated skin disease in which a complement-fixing, IgG antiepidermal basement membrane zone autoantibody deposits in skin, activates complement, and produces an influx of leukocytes that causes tissue damage. The formation of these IgG autoantibodies may be initiated in response to an antigenic stimulus peculiar to pregnancy, parturition, or oral contraceptives. The skin lesions in newborns of affected mothers are explained by placental passage of IgG antiepidermal basement membrane zone autoantibodies that similarly deposit in situ and initiate tissue damage.

Treatment of mild cases of HG may require only frequent applications of topical glucocorticosteroids. For more extensive and symptomatic disease, systemic glucocorticosteroids are often required.[32] Moderate doses of daily prednisone (ie, 20 to 40 mg) usually control this eruption and relieve pruritus.[28,32,41] Some patients respond faster to divided daily doses of glucocorticosteroids that may be consolidated to single morning doses once the disease is under control. Severe cases of HG may require higher doses of systemic glucocorticosteroids. All patients should be continually monitored to ensure that they are receiving the lowest possible dose of glucocorticosteroids for control of the disease. In fact, some degree of disease activity in these patients is acceptable. It is important to keep in mind that HG often flares at the time of delivery, and it may be necessary to increase (or reinstitute) doses of glucocorticosteroids at that time. Rare, severe cases have required combination therapy with systemic glucocorticosteroids and immunosuppressives for control of postpartum exacerbations. Infants of mothers exposed to systemic glucocorticosteroids should be evaluated at birth for evidence of adrenal insufficiency.

PRURITIC URTICARIAL PAPULES AND PLAQUES OF PREGNANCY (PUPPP)

PUPPP is a distinct dermatosis of pregnancy first defined in 1979 by Lawley and colleagues.[44] This pruritic eruption has characteristic clinical features that separate it from other dermatoses of pregnancy.[44,45] These clinical findings are important because no specific laboratory abnormality has been demonstrated in these patients. For this reason, the diagnosis of PUPPP is best restricted to a clinically homogeneous group of patients. More specific diagnostic measures may someday allow differentiation of this disorder from other pregnancy-associated dermatoses with similar clinical features.

The exact incidence of PUPPP is unknown. However, it is probably underreported because of its benign nature and its transient occurrence very late in pregnancy. It is reasonable to believe that it is a relatively common disorder because several large series have been reported (eg, Callen and Hanno's series of 15,[46] Nogeuera and colleagues's series of 15,[47] Yancey and colleagues's series of 25,[45] and Alcalay and colleagues's series of 21).[48]

PUPPP is most frequently seen in primigravidas; in fact, these patients have accounted for 80% of cases in two large series.[45,46]. In addition, PUPPP most often develops during the latter part of the third trimester.[45,46] One large series found that the average time of onset of PUPPP was the 36th week of gestation and that the most frequent week of onset was the 39th.[45] Clinically, this eruption consists of pruritic, erythematous urticarial papules and plaques that initially develop on the abdomen, especially within periumbilical striae distensae (Fig. 75-6).[45,46,48] Subsequent lesions often involve

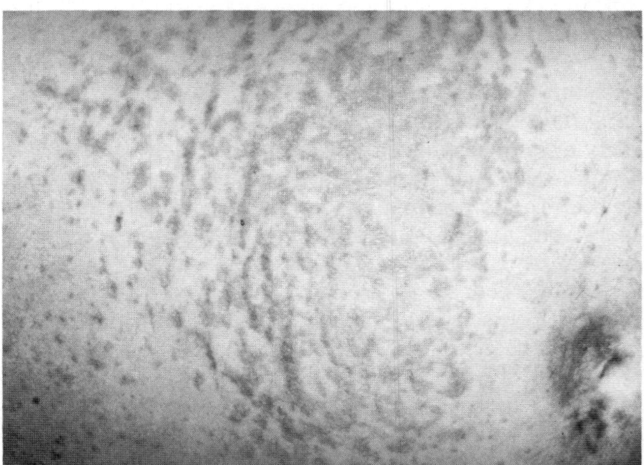

FIGURE 75–6. A patient with PUPPP demonstrates erythematous, urticarial papules and plaques on the abdomen and within striae distensae.

the thighs, buttocks, upper inner arms, and lower back; lesions occasionally develop on the hands or feet. Lesions on or above the breasts in patients with PUPPP are rare[3]; facial involvement is extremely rare.[44,45] Lesions in these patients are characterized by severe pruritus that often interferes with sleep. Interestingly, despite intense pruritus, excoriations are unusual in these patients.

PUPPP usually resolves within 1 week of delivery and may abate prior to parturition. To date, PUPPP has not been associated with an increased risk of fetal morbidity or mortality. One case of urticarial lesions resembling PUPPP in an infant of an affected mother has been reported.[49] However, the specific diagnosis of HG was not conclusively ruled out in that patient. In general, PUPPP does not recur in subsequent pregnancies, though anecdotal reports of recurrent disease have been made.

It is important to distinguish PUPPP from the urticarial form of HG. Direct immunofluorescence microscopy of normal-appearing skin from patients with PUPPP shows no evidence of immunoreactants, in contrast to the linear deposits of C3 in the epidermal basement membrane zone of HG patients. The differential diagnosis of PUPPP includes other skin diseases not associated with pregnancy. Erythema multiforme, drug eruptions, contact dermatitis, urticaria, insect bites, and viral infections can all coincidentally occur during pregnancy and may resemble PUPPP. These other disorders usually can be distinguishable by history, laboratory tests, or biopsies.[3]

Histologic study of lesional skin from patients with PUPPP reveals consistent but not specific alterations. In general, two histopathologic patterns have been documented in these patients. Although both patterns demonstrate a dermal, perivascular lymphohistiocytic infiltrate, they are distinguished by the presence of mild epidermal changes (eg, thickening of the epidermis, presence of leukocytes in the epidermis, edema between epidermal cells) in one pattern but not in the other.[44,45] As mentioned earlier, direct immunofluorescence microscopy of perilesional skin from patients with PUPPP shows no evidence of specific immunoreactants.

Other laboratory studies in patients with PUPPP are generally within expected limits for the patients' respective stage of pregnancy. Studies have shown that these patients' complete blood count, liver function tests, urinary chorionic gonadotropin levels, and serum levels of estrogen and progesterone are normal.[44,45,50,51] Moreover, Alcalay and colleagues recently reported that patients with PUPPP have normal levels of serum beta subunit human chorionic gonadotropin, estradiol, and cortisol as well as normal urinary estriol levels.[52] Yancey and colleagues studied HLA determinations in 10 randomly selected PUPPP patients and found that they were not different from a normal North American control population.[45] Furthermore, none of these PUPPP patients demonstrated the paired-haplotype -DR3, -DR4 reported to be of increased frequency in patients with herpes gestationis.[45]

The precise etiology of PUPPP is unknown. However, one clinical impression is that this disorder tends to develop in gestations associated with a substantial weight gain. In support of this hypothesis has been the finding of an increased incidence of twinning among PUPPP patients in one large series.[45] However, additional study is necessary to confirm this preliminary clinical impression.

Most patients with PUPPP respond to frequent applications of potent topical glucocorticosteroids.[3,53] With this approach, lesions usually stop appearing within 2 to 3 days; most patients can then begin to taper their frequency of treatment. Brief tapering courses of systemic glucocorticosteroids (in moderate doses of 20 to 40 mg/day) are reserved for severe or refractory cases. Antihistamines and emollients are usually less effective than topical or systemic glucocorticosteroids in relief of symptoms and control of the eruption.[45]

IMPETIGO HERPETIFORMIS

Impetigo herpetiformis is the nosologic designation for a rare form of pustular psoriasis that develops during pregnancy.[3,54] Only approximately 100 cases of impetigo herpetiformis have been reported. This disorder is accompanied by significant constitutional symptoms, including fever, chills, nausea, vomiting, diarrhea, and in severe cases, tetany secondary to hypocalcemia. This disease has been considered a life-threatening dermatosis.

Clinically, impetigo herpetiformis is characterized by erythematous plaques surmounted at their margins by tiny superficial sterile pustules. The plaques expand peripherally with new pustules forming at their leading edges. Lesions commonly begin in flexural areas but may extend to involve a substantial portion of the body surface area. In advanced cases, involvement of mucous membranes and nails (ie, subungual pustules and onycholysis, separation of the nail plate from the nail bed) occurs.

Biopsies of early lesional skin from patients with this disorder reveal changes identical to those seen in cases of pustular psoriasis. In brief, these alterations include elongation of epidermal rete ridges, parakeratosis, and neutrophil-rich microabscesses within the epidermis. Additional laboratory abnormalities in these patients include elevated peripheral blood leukocyte counts and elevated erythrocyte sedimentation rates. Selected patients may also demonstrate hypoalbuminemia and hypocalcemia. Patients require careful monitoring, supportive treatment, and specific therapy for their skin disease.[3,55–57] Some reports have suggested an increased risk of fetal morbidity and mortality in these patients. Impetigo herpetiformis tends to remit promptly after delivery but may recur in subsequent gestations.[55] Interestingly, patients may or may not have a personal or family history of psoriasis.

PRURIGO GRAVIDARUM/RECURRENT CHOLESTASIS OF PREGNANCY

Prurigo gravidarum (also called intrahepatic cholestasis of pregnancy or benign recurrent intrahepatic cholestasis) is a hepatic disorder with associated cutaneous features.[3,54] Clinically, it is characterized by severe pruritus that may be followed by jaundice in selected patients. It usually first presents in the third trimester but may begin earlier. The initial manifestation of recurrent cholestasis of pregnancy is pruritus. Pruritus in these patients is often localized initially and then becomes generalized.[58] Although no specific skin lesions are associated with this pruritus, excoriations may be seen. In general, pruritus in patients with recurrent cholestasis of pregnancy precedes the onset of jaundice by 2 to 4 weeks. In addition, selected patients may develop malaise, fatigue, anorexia, nausea, or vomiting. Liver function tests in these patients often demonstrate elevated alkaline phosphatase, leucine aminopeptidase, and bilirubin. Recurrent cholestasis of pregnancy tends to remit soon after delivery, but as its name suggests it usually recurs in subsequent gestations. Although the exact etiology of this disorder is not known, it is believed to be hormonally induced in susceptible patients. Moreover, some patients with a history of this disorder have developed cholestatic jaundice when exposed to oral contraceptives.[59]

Current data suggest that there is an increased incidence of prematurity and postpartum hemorrhage in these patients.[3,60] Although controversial, several studies have suggested that there is an increased incidence of fetal loss in these patients.[54,61] It is important to rule out other causes of generalized pruritus (eg, scabies, drug reactions, underlying lymphoma) in patients suspected of having recurrent cholestasis of pregnancy. Similarly, it is important to determine that no underlying, non–pregnancy-associated liver disease (eg, hepatitis) is present in such patients.

Dermatologic therapy in these patients is entirely symptomatic. Emollients, topical antipruritics, and in selected cases systemic antihistamines with or without cholestyramine may be beneficial.

OTHER ERUPTIONS REPORTED IN ASSOCIATION WITH PREGNANCY

A number of different cutaneous eruptions have been reported to be associated with pregnancy.[3,4] However, most of these eruptions have been incompletely characterized clinically, histologically, and immunopathologically. Moreover, the existence of some of these disorders is controversial. Some probably refer to the same clinical problem. Several major types of these eruptions will be briefly reviewed.

Prurigo Gestationis of Besnier

In 1904, Besnier described prurigo gestationis as a series of grouped, pruritic, papular lesions distributed over the proximal, exterior surface of the extremities and upper trunk.[3,4] The lesions in this disorder are typically excoriated and crusted. This eruption is reported to begin within the second or third trimester and resolve promptly after delivery. Healed lesions demonstrate postinflammatory hyperpigmentation. Prurigo gestationis of Besnier is not thought to be associated with an increased risk of fetal morbidity or mortality. Also, it is thought not to recur in subsequent gestations. Histologic, immunopathologic, and laboratory studies on patients with this disorder have not been performed. Hence, it is not possible to distinguish it critically from other pruritic, papular eruptions of pregnancy except by clinical findings.

Spangler's Papular Dermatitis of Pregnancy

Spangler's papular dermatitis of pregnancy is a rare eruption whose existence is currently controversial.[3,4,62] As originally described, this disorder is a generalized, extremely pruritic, papular eruption that may develop during any trimester of pregnancy. Lesions appear in small numbers in a nongrouped distribution. Morphologically, Spangler described these lesions as papules, 3 to 5 mm in diameter, that are surmounted by a smaller central papule that is often excoriated.[62] Lesions last 7 to 10 days and then resolve with postinflammatory hyperpigmentation. Pruritus in this disorder is severe. Spangler's papular dermatitis is reported to resolve promptly after delivery but to recur in subsequent pregnancies. Spangler described three patients with persistent postpartum disease that abated with removal of retained placental fragments.[62] However, histologic and immunopathologic studies of patients with this diagnosis were not performed by Spangler or his colleagues.

A number of different laboratory abnormalities in these patients have been described. Specifically, these patients demonstrate elevated levels of urinary chorionic gonadotropin and reduced determinations of plasma cortisol, plasma cortisol half-life, and urinary estriol.[62,63] Moreover, Spangler reported that patients with this disorder develop inflammatory responses following intradermal challenge with placental extracts from patients with papular dermatitis of pregnancy but not following skin tests with placental extracts from normal controls.[62]

Historically, there has been considerable attention devoted to the high estimates of fetal mortality in this disorder.[62] Based on Spangler's review of 37 pregnancies in 12 patients, he estimated that the incidence of fetal death in this disorder is approximately 27%. However, a number of cases of fetal loss in these patients were confined to gestations in which papular dermatitis of pregnancy was not observed. When data were reevaluated within this context, 12% of these gestations were associated with fetal mortality—a figure not significantly different from the generally accepted rate of 10% for spontaneous abortions in the healthy population.[3,4]

Spangler's papular dermatitis of pregnancy has been reported to respond to systemic glucocorticosteroids.[62]

Recommendations for diethylstilbestrol therapy in these patients have been withdrawn.[63,64] Topical glucocorticosteroids have been tried by others.[65] Additional reports and studies of these rare patients would be informative.

Autoimmune Progesterone Dermatitis of Pregnancy

In 1973, Bierman described a single patient with a cutaneous eruption that developed in two successive pregnancies, each of which was complicated by spontaneous abortion in the first trimester.[66] The lesions in this patient were characterized as an acneiform papulopustular eruption distributed over the extremities and buttocks in association with arthritis. Intradermal challenge with aqueous progesterone produced reactions that were histologically similar to naturally occurring lesions. Interestingly, this patient did not develop similar lesions premenstrually when endogenous progesterone levels were elevated. It is important to distinguish this patient from those with autoimmune progesterone dermatoses unassociated with pregnancy. In the latter, pruritic urticarial or vesiculobullous lesions develop cyclically, 7 to 10 days prior to each menses.[54]

Pruritic Folliculitis of Pregnancy

Zoberman and Farmer have described a distinctive eruption in pregnancy in which hair follicles show intrafollicular pustule formation.[67] These cases are further characterized by onset in the fourth to the ninth month of gestation, a distribution that is usually generalized, negative findings on direct immunofluorescence microscopy, and resolution without associated fetal morbidity or mortality.

Miscellaneous Disorders

A variety of other dermatoses of pregnancy have been described and likely overlap or are essentially identical to those described earlier.[3,4,68,69] Also, new disorders continue to be reported and merit further study as additional cases become available.[70]

CONCLUSION

This chapter has summarized the physiologic changes that occur in the skin during pregnancy and has presented an overview of the major dermatoses of pregnancy. In addition to these disorders, it should also be kept in mind that pregnancy may either exacerbate or improve various preexisting or underlying dermatologic diseases.[54,71] Although this topic is beyond the scope of this chapter, several recent reviews have addressed this subject and interested readers are referred to these specific references.[54,71]

REFERENCES

1. Sodhi VK, Sausker WF. Dermatoses of pregnancy. Am Fam Physician 1988;37:131.
2. Cummings K, Derbes VJ. Dermatoses associated with pregnancy. Cutis 1987;3:120.
3. Lawley TJ. Skin changes and diseases in pregnancy. In: Fitzpatrick TB, Eisen AZ, Wolff K, Freedberg IM, Austen KF, eds. Dermatology in general medicine. 3rd ed. New York: McGraw-Hill, 1987:2082.
4. Winton GB, Lewis CW. Dermatoses of pregnancy. J Am Acad Dermatol 1982;6:977.
5. Vander Ploeg DE. Skin changes and diseases of pregnancy. In: Pauerstein CF, ed. Clinical obstetrics. New York: John Wiley & Sons, 1987:555.
6. Wade TR, Wade SL, Jones HE. Skin changes and diseases associated with pregnancy. Obstet Gynecol 1978;52:233.
7. McKenzie AW. Skin disorders in pregnancy. Practitioner (London) 1971;206:773.
8. Wong RC, Ellis CN. Physiologic skin changes in pregnancy. J Am Acad Dermatol 1984;10:929.
9. Bean WB, Cogswell RC, Dexter M, Embick JF. Vascular changes of the skin in pregnancy. Surg Gynecol Obstet 1949;88:739.
10. Bean WB. Vascular spiders and related lesions of the skin. Springfield, IL: Charles C Thomas, 1958:59.
11. Scoggins RB. Skin changes and diseases in pregnancy. In: Fitzpatrick TB, Eisen AZ, Wolff K, Freedberg IM, Austen KF, eds. Dermatology in general medicine. 2nd ed. New York: McGraw-Hill, 1979:1363.
12. Hellreich PD. The skin changes of pregnancy. Cutis 1974;13:82.
13. Taylor CM, Pernoll ML. Normal pregnancy and prenatal care. In: Pernoll ML, Benson RC, eds. Current obstetric and gynecologic diagnosis and treatment. 6th ed. Norwalk, CT: Appleton and Lange, 1987:161.
14. Benson RC. Medical and surgical complications during pregnancy. In: Benson RC, ed. Current obstetric and gynecologic diagnosis and treatment. 5th ed. Los Altos, CA: Lange Medical Publications, 1984:869.
15. Demis DJ. Skin conditions during pregnancy. In: Demis DJ, Dobson RL, McGuire, eds. Clinical dermatology. New York: Harper & Row, 1975:(2)12.
16. Rook A. The ages of man and their dermatoses. In: Rook A, Wilkinson DS, Ebling FJG, eds. Textbook of dermatology. 3rd ed. Oxford: Blackwell, 1979:213.
17. Shornick JK. Herpes gestationis. J Am Acad Dermatol 1987;17:539.
18. Tillman WG. Herpes gestationis with hydatidiform mole and chorion epithelioma. Br Med J 1950;1:1471.
19. Provost TT, Tomasi TB. Evidence for complement activation via the alternative pathway in skin diseases: herpes gestationis, systemic lupus erythematosus, and bullous pemphigoid. J Clin Invest 1973;53:1779.
20. Russell B, Thorne NA. Herpes gestationis. Br J Dermatol 1957;69:339.
21. Kolodny RC. Herpes gestationis: a new assessment of incidence, diagnosis, and fetal prognosis. Am J Obstet Gynecol 1969;104:39.
22. Shornick JK, Bangert JL, Freeman RG, Gilliam JN. Herpes gestationis: clinical and histologic features of twenty-eight cases. J Am Acad Dermatol 1983;8:214.
23. Holmes RC, Black MM, Dann T, James DCO, Bhogal B. A comparative study of toxic erythema of pregnancy and herpes gestationis. Br J Dermatol 1982;106:499.
24. Dacus JV, Muram D. Pruritus in pregnancy. South Med J 1987;80:614.
25. Holmes RC, Black MM. The specific dermatoses of pregnancy. J Am Acad Dermatol 1983;8:405.

26. Holmes RC, Black MM. Herpes gestationis. Dermatol Clin 1983;1(2):195.
27. Winton GB. Dermatoses of pregnancy. J Assoc Military Dermatol 1981;7:20.
28. Lawley TJ, Stingl G, Katz SI. Fetal and maternal risk factors in herpes gestationis. Arch Dermatol 1978;114:552.
29. Holmes RC, Black MM. The fetal prognosis in pemphigoid gestationis (herpes gestationis). Br J Dermatol 1984;110:67.
30. Chorzelski TP, Jablonska S, Beutner EH, Marciejowska E, Jarzabek-Chorzelska M. Herpes gestationis with identical lesions in the newborn. Arch Dermatol 1976;112:1129.
31. Katz A, Minta JO, Toole JWP, Medwidsky W. Immunopathologic study of herpes gestationis in mother and child. Arch Dermatol 1977;113:1069.
32. Yancey, KB. Herpes gestationis. In: Lichtenstein LM, Fauci AS, eds. Current therapy in allergy, immunology, and rheumatology. 3rd ed. Toronto: BC Decker, 1988:176.
33. Hertz KC, Katz SI, Maize J, Ackerman AB. Herpes gestationis—a clinicopathologic study. Arch Dermatol 1976;112:1543.
34. Katz SI, Provost TT. Herpes gestationis. In: Fitzpatrick TB, Eisen AZ, Wolff K, Freedberg IM, Austen KF, eds. Dermatology in general medicine. 3rd ed. New York: McGraw-Hill. 1987:586.
35. Yancey KB, Lawley TJ. Herpes gestationis. In: Thiers B, Dobson R, eds. Pathogenesis of skin disease. New York: Churchill Livingstone, 1986:185.
36. Holubar K, Konrad K, Stingl G. Detection by immunoelectron microscopy of immunoglobulin G deposits in skin of immunofluorescence negative herpes gestationis. Br J Dermatol 1977;96:569.
37. Jurecka W, Holmes RC, Black MM, McKee P, Das AK, Bhogal B. An immuno electron microscopy study of the relationship between herpes gestationis and polymorphic eruption of pregnancy. Br J Dermatol 1983;108:147.
38. Katz SI, Hertz KC, Yaoita H. Herpes gestationis. Immunopathology and characterization of the HG factor. J Clin Invest 1976;57:1434.
39. Jordon RE, Heine KG, Tappeiner G, Bushkell LL, Provost TT. The immuno pathology of herpes gestationis. Immunofluorescent studies and characterization of the "HG factor." J Clin Invest 1976;57:1426.
40. Morrison LH, Labib RS, Zone JJ, Diaz LA, Anhalt GJ. Herpes gestationis autoantibodies recognize a 180-kD human epidermal antigen. J Clin Invest 1988;81:2023.
41. Holmes RC, Black MM, Jurecka W, Dann J, James DCO, Timlin D, Bhogal B. Clues to the aetiology and pathogenesis of herpes gestationis. Br J Dermatol 1983;109:131.
42. Shornick JK, Stastny P, Gilliam JN. High frequency of histocompatibility antigens HLA-DR3 and DR4 in herpes gestationis. J Clin Invest 1981;68:553.
43. Shornick JK, Stastny P, Gilliam JN. Paternal histocompatibility (HLA) antigens and maternal anti-HLA antibodies in herpes gestationis. J Invest Dermatol 1983;81:407.
44. Lawley TJ, Hertz KC, Wade TR, Ackerman AB, Katz SI. Pruritic urticarial papules and plaques of pregnancy. JAMA 1979;241:1696.
45. Yancey KB, Hall RP, Lawley TJ. Pruritic urticarial papules and plaques of pregnancy. Clinical experience in 25 patients. J Am Acad Dermatol 1984;10:473.
46. Callen JP, Hanno R. Pruritic urticarial papules and plaques of pregnancy (PUPPP). A clinicopathologic study. J Am Acad Dermatol 1981;5:401.
47. Noguera J, Moreno A, Moragas JM. Pruritic urticarial papules and plaques of pregnancy (PUPPP). Acta Dermatovenerol (Stock) 1983;63:35.
48. Alcalay J, Ingber A, David M, Hazaz B, Sandbank M. Pruritic urticarial papules and plaques of pregnancy. A review of 21 cases. J Reprod Med 1987;32:315.
49. Uhlin SR. Pruritic urticarial papules and plaques of pregnancy: involvement in mother and infant. Arch Dermatol 1981;117:238.
50. Schwartz RA, Hansen RC, Lynch PJ. Pruritic urticarial papules and plaques of pregnancy. Cutis 1981;29:425.
51. Ahmed AR, Kaplan R. Pruritic urticarial papules and plaques of pregnancy. J Am Acad Dermatol 1981;4:679.
52. Alcalay J, Ingber A, Kafri B, Segal J, Kaufman H, Hazaz B, Sandbank M. Hormonal evaluation and autoimmune background in pruritic urticarial papules and plaques of pregnancy. Am J Obstet Gynecol 1988;158:417.
53. Yancey KB. Skin diseases of pregnancy. In: Rakel RE, ed. Conn's current therapy. Philadelphia: WB Saunders, 1986:679.
54. Braverman IM. Pregnancy and the menstrual cycle. In: Skin signs of systemic disease. Philadelphia: WB Saunders, 1981:761.
55. Beveridge GW, Harkness RA, Livingstone JR. Impetigo herpetiformis in two successive pregnancies. Br J Dermatol 1966;78:106.
56. Sauer G. Impetigo herpetiformis. Arch Dermatol 1961;83:119.
57. Oosterling RJ, Nobrega RE, Du Boeuff JAD, Van Der Meer JB. Impetigo herpetiformis or generalized pustular psoriasis? Arch Dermatol 1978;114:1527.
58. Holzbach RT. Jaundice in pregnancy. Am J Med 1976;61:367.
59. De Pagter AGF, Van Berge Henrgouwen GP, Ten Bokkel Huinink JA, Brandt KH. Familial benign recurrent intrahepatic cholestasis. Gastroenterology 1976;71:202.
60. Johnston WG, Baskett TF. Obstetric cholestasis: a 14-year review. Am J Obstet Gynecol 1979;133:299.
61. Rencoret R, Aste H. Jaundice during pregnancy. Med J Aust 1973;1:167.
62. Spangler AS, Reddy W, Bardawil WA, Roby CC, Emerson K. Papular dermatitis of pregnancy. JAMA 1962;181:577.
63. Spangler AS, Emerson K. Estrogen levels and estrogen therapy in papular dermatitis of pregnancy. Am J Obstet Gynecol 1971;110:534.
64. Spangler AS. Letter to the editor. Am J Obstet Gynecol 1972;113:570.
65. Michaud RM, Jacobson D, Dahl MV. Papular dermatitis of pregnancy. Arch Dermatol 1982;118:1003.
66. Bierman SM. Autoimmume progesterone dermatitis. Arch Dermatol 1973;107:896.
67. Zoberman E, Farmer E. Pruritic folliculitis of pregnancy. Arch Dermatol 1976;112:1534.
68. Bourne G. Toxemic rash of pregnancy. Proc R Soc Med 1962;55:462.
69. Nurse DS. Prurigo of pregnancy. Aust J Dermatol 1968;9:258.
70. Alcalay J, Ingber A, Hazaz B, David M, Sandbank M. Linear IgM dermatosis of pregnancy. J Am Acad Dermatol 1988;18:412.
71. Winton GB. Skin diseases aggravated by pregnancy. J Am Acad Dermatol 1989;20:1.

76 CHAPTER

CANCER IN PREGNANCY

Peter E. Schwartz

Cancer during pregnancy is unusual. Limited experience has suggested that cancer is more aggressive when it develops during pregnancy and that termination of pregnancy might favorably influence the rate of progression of the disease. Recent observation suggests that, as a result of physiologic changes that normally occur in pregnancy, cancer during pregnancy may become more advanced because the diagnosis is not recognized as early as it otherwise might have been. In other words, stage-for-stage, cancer during pregnancy is no more virulent than cancer occurring in the non-pregnant state. Furthermore, the routine interruption of pregnancy to influence cancer progression has not been established.

Bold new advances are necessary to successfully manage patients with cancer diagnosed in pregnancy. Chemotherapy experiences have been reported in a sufficient number of patients to state that congenital malformations will not routinely occur in patients treated in the second or third trimesters of pregnancy, and selective use of chemotherapy in the first trimester of pregnancy may obviate congenital malformations previously reported when patients had been exposed to alkylating and antifolate agents. However, prematurity and low birth weight remain problems in a substantial number of infants exposed in utero to chemotherapeutic agents during any trimester of pregnancy. The pregnant woman and her family should have the most experienced physicians involved in managing the cancer and the pregnancy. Physicians must assess the risk to the patient and the fetus, both from continuing the pregnancy and from treating the cancer in pregnancy, taking into account the stage of the pregnancy and the likelihood of spontaneous abortion, prematurity, and low infant birth weight, and they must counsel the patient in this highly emotionally charged time of her life.

INCIDENCE

Data reflecting the incidence of cancers during pregnancy are scant because of a lack of information accrued by population-based tumor registries. Estimates of cancer during pregnancy vary considerably (Table 76-1). The uterine cervix remains the most common site for neoplasia to develop in pregnancy. It is estimated that one in 770 pregnancies will be associated with cervical intraepithelial neoplasia and that invasive cervical cancer will occur in one of every 2200 pregnancies.[1] The breast is the second most common site for malignancy that occurs during pregnancy, with an estimated incidence of one in 3000.[2] The frequency distribution of other cancers during pregnancy—such as leukemia, lymphoma, and cancers of the ovary, vulva, vagina, skin (melanoma), brain, and gastrointestinal tract—reflects that of cancer occurring in all women in the reproductive years.[3] The tendency to delay childbearing may lead to a higher future incidence of cancer in pregnant women.

Haas's study reporting the incidence of cancer during pregnancy as compared to that in control non-pregnant women suggested that there may be a significantly reduced incidence of cancer in pregnancy.[4] These data were based on a population-based epidemiologic study in the German Democratic Republic. As women grew older, the 5-year age group observed-to-expected ratios of pregnancy-associated cancers increased from 0.22 for women 15 to 19 years old (1.9 cancers per 100,000 live births) to 1.40 (232.4 cancers per 100,000 live births) for those 40 to 44 years old (Fig. 76-1). The frequency of occurrence, in descending order, was cervical cancer, breast cancer, ovarian cancer, lymphoma, melanoma, brain cancer, and leukemia. Incomplete reporting might be an explanation of the low incidence of cancer during pregnancy in this series.

TABLE 76-1. ESTIMATES OF CANCER OCCURRING IN PREGNANCY

SITE	ESTIMATED INCIDENCE	AUTHORS
Cervix		
Carcinoma in situ	1/767	Sokal and Lessmann[1]
Invasive	1/2205	Sokal and Lessmann[1]
Breast	1/3000	Benedet et al[2]
	10–39/100,000	Wallack et al[14]
	1/1008	Potter & Schoeneman[5]
Vulva	1/8000	Nugent & O'Connell[65]
Ovary	1/9000	Nugent & O'Connell[65]
	1/25,000	Rubeiro & Palmer[71]
Leukemia	<1/75,000	Applewhite et al[56]
	1/100,000	Haas[4]
Hodgkin's disease	1/1000	Riva et al*
	1/6000	Morgan et al†
		Stewart & Monto††
Colorectal	1/100,000	Fisher et al[134]
		Clark et al[136]
Skin–melanoma	2.8/1000	Smith & Randal§

* Riva HL, Anderson PS, Grady JW. Pregnancy and Hodgkin's disease: a report of 8 cases. Am J Obstet Gynecol 1953;66:866.

† Morgan DS, Hall SE, Gibbs WN. Hodgkin's disease in pregnancy: a report of three cases. West Indian Med J 1976;25:121.

†† Stewart HL, Monto RW. Hodgkin's disease and pregnancy. Am J Obstet Gynecol 1952;63:570.

§ Smith RS, Randal P. Melanoma during pregnancy. Obstet Gynecol 1969;34:825.

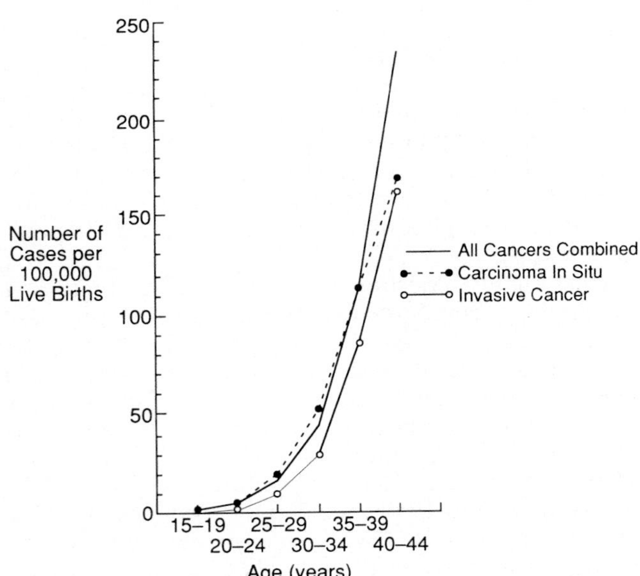

FIGURE 76-1. Overall incidence of cancer occurring in pregnancy by age and incidence of carcinoma in situ and invasive cervical cancer. (Modified from Haas JF. Pregnancy in association with a newly diagnosed cancer: A population-based epidemiologic assessment. Int J Cancer 1984; 34: 229.)

A fear expressed by pregnant patients is that the cancer might spread to the fetus. Similar concerns have been expressed by physicians. Information collected during the past two decades suggests that transplacental metastasis is extremely unusual, and metastases to the fetus are so rare as to preclude this as an indication for termination of a pregnancy complicated by cancer. The most common malignancy to be associated with fetal metastases is malignant melanoma. The reported number of cases in the literature of such an event is less than 30.[5]

SURGERY IN PREGNANCY

Patients may undergo successful surgical procedures when they are pregnant without interfering with the fetus. In general, surgery should be delayed until the second trimester, which seems to be the safest time in terms of avoiding patients going into labor. Spontaneous abortion frequently occurs when surgery is performed in the first trimester, and premature labor has been associated with surgery in the third trimester. Corpus luteum function is replaced by the placenta after the 12th week of gestation. Pathologic ovaries may be safely removed once the patient has entered into the second trimester.[6]

In preparing the patient for a surgical procedure, simple technical considerations may have an important impact on the success of the operation. For example, placing the patient in a lateral position to avoid vena cava and aortic compression is an important factor in considering anesthetic consequences of surgery.[7] To displace the uterus off the inferior vena cava, a 15° wedge may be placed under the right hip when the patient is lying supine. This will help avoid fetal complications of hypoxemia or hypertension.[8] The gastroesophageal junction in pregnancy tends to be relaxed, and its ability to control regurgitation is diminished. The patient should be operated on only after being certain that her stomach is emptied. Anesthesiologists must always act as if a pregnant woman has a full stomach, as progesterone relaxes the gastroesophageal sphincter and pyloric displacement by the gravid uterus impedes gastric emptying.[9]

RADIATION IN PREGNANCY

Radiation is commonly employed in the routine management of cancers that may occur in pregnancy. Deleterious effects that the fetus may experience from being exposed to radiation therapy have been recognized for many years.[10,11] Production of genetic mutations by radiation in the laboratory was documented as early in 1927, but data directly applicable to humans are scant.[12] Three phases of pregnancy must be considered with regard to radiation damage.[13] The preimplantation phase lasts for approximately 7 to 10 days and represents the time from fertilization to the implantation of the blastocyst into the uterine wall. Spontaneous abortion is the most likely consequence of an embryo being exposed to radiation in the preimplantation phase. For many patients the pregnancy may not be clinically recognized.[14]

Organogenesis, the period from the first to 10th week of gestation, represents the most sensitive time for the fetus with regard to radiation injury.[13] This is the time of major organ formation and the time the fetus is most susceptible to teratogenic agents. However, the central nervous system, the eyes, and the hematopoietic system remain highly sensitive to the effect of radiation throughout the entire pregnancy. Radiation has been associated with microcephaly—the most common malformation observed in humans exposed to high-dose radiation during pregnancy—and mental retardation.[15] In general, such effects are seen in fetuses exposed to amounts greater than 50 rads (0.5 cGy) of low-energy-transfer (LET) radiation.[15] Embryonic exposure to 5 rads (0.05 cGy) or less is rarely associated with anomalies.[15] The actual radiation dose rates are extremely important in assessing the risks to the fetus for developing growth retardation, malformations, or death.

Pregnant women exposed to radiation therapy of 250 rads or greater during the first 2 to 3 weeks of gestation have an increased risk of spontaneous abortion but not a dramatic risk of severe congenital anomalies.[16] However, once patients are exposed to such radiation during the third to 10th week of gestation, multiple congenital anomalies—including low birth weight, microcephaly, mental retardation, retinal degeneration, cataracts, and genital and skeletal malformations—have been reported.[16] Radiation exposure between the 11th and 20th weeks has been associated with a significant decline in anomalies. Exposure after the 20th week of gestation is usually limited to anemia, skin pigmentation changes, and dermal erythema. The risks of growth retardation and abnormalities of the eye and central nervous system increases throughout the later period of fetal radiation exposure. It has been suggested that fetuses exposed to radiation doses higher than 10 rads should be considered for therapeutic abortion.[13]

Pelvic irradiation for the management of malignancies, particularly cervical lesions in pregnancy, will result in fetal demise and will usually lead to spontaneous abortion. The fetus may receive only minor exposure when supradiaphragmatic irradiation is given, particularly if such radiation is tapered so that the internal scatter is minimal during the first trimester of pregnancy. However, as the fetus grows, its exposure to supradiaphragmatic radiation increases. Such radiation may not be appropriate in the more advanced stages of pregnancy.

CHEMOTHERAPY AND PREGNANCY

Prior experience supported the concept that cytotoxic chemotherapy should not be administered to patients, especially during the first trimester of pregnancy. This was due to the high incidence of spontaneous abortion following exposure to chemotherapy and the teratogenic effects of these agents on the developing fetus.[17,18] However, as anecdotal and small series reports have accumulated, it appears that although certain drugs must be avoided during early pregnancy, others might be life-saving and might not cause congenital anomalies in the fetus.[19–22] The reports of such experiences are limited at present and should be viewed with caution, as prematurity and low birth weight are frequent complications of chemotherapy exposure in any trimester of pregnancy. However, the fear of exposure in the second and third trimesters of pregnancy resulting in congenital anomalies no longer appears to be a major concern, provided that the selection of drugs is appropriate.[17,18] The long-term neurologic consequences of intrauterine exposure to chemotherapeutic agents has yet to be established. The National Cancer Institute in Bethesda, Maryland, is maintaining a record to determine what the consequences to children of in utero exposure to chemotherapy might be. The data are limited, but those children who have been born after in utero exposure to chemotherapeutic agents during the second and third trimesters have not been noted to have significant congenital abnormalities. One study of 17 children exposed in utero to chemotherapy for the management of maternal acute leukemia revealed no fetal malformations. The children's growth and development, school performance, intelligence tests, neurologic examinations, and hematologic evaluations (with a follow-up period ranging from 4 to 22 years) were normal.[22] Another study of 16 pregnant women treated for non-Hodgkin's lymphoma reported similar results.[20]

Physiologic effects of pregnancy may have an impact on the efficacy and toxicity of chemotherapeutic agents. For example, renal blood flow, glomerular filtration rate, and creatinine clearance increases may lead to increased clearance of drugs from the body.[23] It has been suggested that amniotic fluid may act as a pharmacologic third space for such drugs as methotrexate, in a fashion somewhat analogous to ascites or pleural effusions that may then increase methotrexate toxicity.[24] Gastrointestinal absorption of drugs may be decreased due to delayed gastric motility. The distribution and kinetics of antineoplastic agents may be substantially affected by the physiologic increase of body water in a pregnant woman in association with a 15% increase in plasma volume and changes in plasma protein concentrations.[25] Drugs that cross the placenta have low molecular weight, have high lipid solubility, are nonionized, and are loosely bound to plasma proteins.[24,26,27] However, knowledge regarding transplacental passage of chemotherapeutic agents is extremely limited.

In assessing the teratogenic effects of chemotherapeutic agents administered in pregnancy it must be kept in mind that up to 3% of children have associated major congenital anomalies and 9% have minor anomalies in pregnancies not complicated by cancer treatments or exposure to a chemotherapeutic agent.[28]

Alkylating agents are cell cycle nonspecific drugs that form cross linkages with DNA therapy, preventing the DNA from dividing. These agents may also interfere with normal intracellular mechanisms. Melphalan, chlorambucil, cyclophosphamide, triethylene thiophosphoramide, *cis*-diamminedichloroplatinum, streptozotocin, BCNU, CCNU, methyl-CCNU, and busulfan are common alkylating agents. Congenital anomalies have been noted in patients treated in the first trimester of pregnancy with these agents but not in the second and third trimesters.[17] A chlorambucil syndrome has been characterized by renal aplasia, cleft palate, and skeletal abnormalities following exposure in the first trimester of pregnancy.[29]

Antimetabolites are structural analogs of precursor purine bases that, when incorporated into DNA molecules, lead to nonfunctional DNA and cell death. These agents include amethopterin (methotrexate), aminopterin, 5-fluorouracil (5FU), cytosine arabinoside, 6-mercaptopurine, imidazole carboxamide, 6-thioguanine, 5-azacytodine, hydroxyurea, hexamethylmelamine, and L-asparaginase. These agents are cell cycle–specific and interfere with DNA, RNA, and some coenzymes. Aminopterin and methotrexate act as abortifacients for patients when administered during the first trimester.[1,17] An aminopterin syndrome characterized by cranial dysostosis, hypertelorism, anomalies of the external ears, micrognathia, and cleft palate has been described secondary to first-trimester exposure in pregnancy.[30,31] Only one congenital anomaly was observed in 56 patients exposed to other antimetabolites during pregnancy.[18] Second- and third-trimester exposure to a variety of antimetabolites resulted in no congenital anomalies in 37 fetuses. Thus, antimetabolites other than amethopterin and aminopterin may be relatively safely employed in the management of cancer during pregnancy.

Antibiotics are cell cycle–nonspecific agents that interfere with DNA-dependent RNA syntheses. Cell death occurs as a result of a lack of RNA and an inability to produce cell proteins. Actinomycin D, doxorubicin, daunorubicin, bleomycin, mitomycin C, and mithramycin have been used relatively safely in the second and third trimesters of pregnancy. Recent data suggest that doxorubicin and daunorubicin may be relatively safely used in the first trimester of pregnancy, but the follow-up information on children exposed in utero remains extremely limited.[32,33]

Vinca alkaloids are cell phase–specific agents that act predominantly in the end phase of the cell cycle on the microtubular protein involved in spindle formation during mitosis. They cause mitotic arrest. These agents include vincristine, vinblastine, VP-16, and VM-26. A limited experience with exposure to vinca alkaloids suggests that only one of 15 pregnancies exposed during the first trimester was associated with a congenital anomaly. No anomalies were seen in 11 patients treated later in pregnancy.[17,18]

Corticosteroids have been used as part of combination chemotherapy for lymphomas and Hodgkin's disease in pregnancy.[34] An extensive review by Sindu and Hawkins revealed that cleft lips and palates were a consequence of such therapy.[34] It was not clear that the occurrence of these anomalies, which were observed only during first-trimester exposure, was statistically significant. A risk of hypoadrenalism caused by exogenous steroid hormone administration in pregnancy may lead to infant death.

The reported rate of fetal malformations when exposed to combination chemotherapy in the first trimester (7 of 45 [16%]) is similar to that of single-agent therapy.[19,35–37] Theoretically, the incidence could be reduced to 6% by removing folate antagonists in common with radiation therapy.[19] Doll and colleagues summarized the findings of 71 patients treated with single-agent therapy in the last two trimesters and of 79 patients treated with combination therapy; they identified one child in each treatment group with a congenital anomaly.[19] Thus, second and third trimester chemotherapy appears safe with regard to teratogenicity in the fetus.[19] Nevertheless, a 40% incidence of low birth weight was reported by Nicholson when fetuses were exposed to chemotherapy in utero.[17]

Other complications may occur in the fetus exposed to cytotoxic chemotherapy in addition to teratogenicity, death, and stunted growth.[38] Anemia, leukopenia, and thrombocytopenia may occur in the fetus as a result of bone marrow suppression and leukopenia, or immune suppression may lead to secondary infection.[21] Timing of chemotherapy in relation to the anticipated delivery must be carefully assessed. Deliveries should occur when the patient is not bone marrow suppressed. Breast feeding is discouraged in patients who are receiving cytotoxic chemotherapy, although the data supporting this are weak.[38] To date there have been no reports of children developing leukemia subsequent to in utero exposure to chemotherapeutic agents.

ASSESSING FETAL MATURITY

The early delivery of a child has been incorporated into the management strategy in treating pregnant cancer patients. This strategy requires that highly sophisticated newborn special care units be available for maintaining such infants. The survival rate for infants treated in the newborn special care unit at Yale–New Haven Hospital for the years 1984 through 1988 is presented in Figure 76-2. Infants born after 30 weeks of gestation have a definite survival advantage. The data presented are typical of experiences in other newborn special care units throughout the United States (Gross I, personal communication, 1990).

Premature delivery results in an increased risk for respiratory distress syndrome, the single most important factor in determining the quality of a premature infant's life. The use of the lecithin-to-sphingomyelin (L/S) ratio in amniotic fluid is extremely important. Corticosteroid therapy may hasten fetal lung maturation and avoid respiratory distress syndrome, provided the fetus is at least 30 weeks gestation.[39] The available data suggest that female infants respond better to dexamethasone therapy than male infants. Black infants have shown the most marked response to corticosteroid therapy. Infants in multiple births apparently show no benefit from this treatment. Dexamethasone therapy administered to the mother between 24 hours and 7 days prior to delivery appears to be most beneficial to infants.

CERVICAL CANCER

Invasive cervical cancer is on the decline in the United States. Effective Pap smear screening techniques in combination with colposcopy for directed biopsies have allowed physicians to recognize the presence of malignancy early and to treat patients with simple office procedures. However, worldwide, cancer of the cervix is the most common cancer in women. Squamous cell cancer of the cervix, the most common histologic type of cervical malignancy, appears to be a sexually transmitted disease and is highly significantly associated with the presence of human papilloma virus infection.[40] Although the decline of invasive cancer is evident in the United States, an increase in cervical intraepithelial neoplasia has occurred as a result of wide-scale cytologic screening.[41,42] The cervix remains the most common site for precancerous and cancerous changes in pregnancy (see Table 76-1 and Fig. 76-1). Epidemiologic studies suggest that women who develop cervical intraepithelial neoplasia and invasive cancer in pregnancy tend to be married at an earlier age, have an earlier age of diagnosis of cervical intraepithelial neoplasia and invasive cancer, and have a higher parity than a control population.[43–45]

The most common histologic types of cancer occurring in the cervix are squamous cell (93.1%), adenocarcinoma (3%), anaplastic carcinoma (2.6%), adenosquamous carcinoma (1.1%), adenoacanthoma (0.1%), and sarcoma (0.1%).[46] Four case reports of a small-cell neuroendocrine carcinoma arising in the uterine cervix in pregnancy have recently been reported.[47]

CERVICAL INTRAEPITHELIAL NEOPLASIA

The presence of cervical intraepithelial neoplasia (CIN) in pregnancy is usually identified by Pap smear and confirmed by colposcopically directed biopsies. It is the policy at Yale–New Haven Hospital to use colposcopy

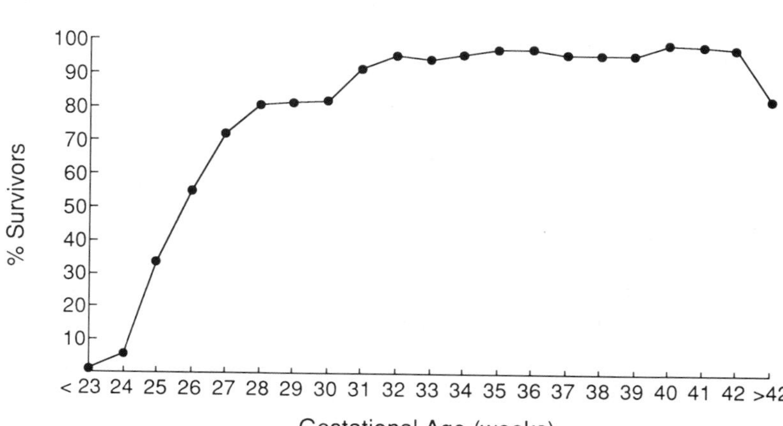

FIGURE 76–2. Newborn Special Care Unit survival statistics, Yale–New Haven Hospital, 1984–1988 (*N* = 3477). (Courtesy Dr I Gross.)

to evaluate patients with abnormal Pap smears in pregnancy and to limit the biopsy to one site, the one that has the worst colposcopic appearance. The reason for this is that the cervix is highly vascularized in pregnancy, so that biopsying the cervix may be associated with significant bleeding. In general, colposcopy will show the entire transformation zone, as the squamocolumnar junction tends to be present well out on the exocervix during pregnancy. If the entire transformation zone is not seen in early pregnancy, it is usually safe to wait a few weeks and repeat the colposcopy before making any definitive decisions regarding additional patient management, provided the Pap smear is consistent with cervical intraepithelial neoplasia and not invasive cancer. The latter diagnosis requires immediate evaluation. Cone biopsies of the cervix are avoided, as they are associated with hemorrhage, abortion, and premature labor.[48]

It has been a successful policy at Yale–New Haven Hospital to biopsy the worst colposcopically identified site, and if the cervical biopsy and Pap smear are consistent, simply to follow the patient throughout the pregnancy with Pap smears every 3 months. Patients are reevaluated at approximately 36 weeks gestation with repeat colposcopy and Pap smears to be as certain as possible that the lesion has not progressed. Cotton-tip applicator sticks are used to obtain endocervical cytologic specimens in pregnancy as opposed to the nonpregnant state, where cytobrushes are used. The preference for the cotton-tip applicator stick is to avoid disrupting the fetal membranes with the wirelike tip of the cytobrush. Adenocarcinomas arising in association with carcinoma in situ of the exocervix are easily visualized in pregnancy and may be readily biopsied.[49] In the 15 years that this policy has been practiced only one case of a stage IB cancer of the cervix has occurred in a patient assessed initially to have a precancerous lesion. That patient was recognized at delivery to have an invasive lesion and was subsequently successfully managed with a type III radical hysterectomy and bilateral deep pelvic lymphadenectomy.

If the assessment at 36 weeks remains consistent with cervical intraepithelial neoplasia, the patient and her physician are advised that the patient may deliver vaginally, if obstetrical indications are appropriate. No attempt is routinely made to perform cesarean hysterectomies in the management of cervical intraepithelial neoplasia, as most patients consulted on at Yale–New Haven Hospital in the past decade have desired further pregnancies. Assessment of precancerous changes can be readily done 8 to 12 weeks following delivery. In general, regression rather than progression is observed when one assesses patients postpartum for cervical intraepithelial neoplasia.

MICROINVASIVE CANCER OF THE CERVIX

Microinvasive cancer of the cervix is defined as a lesion that has only microscopically penetrated through the basement membrane. The current International Federation of Gynecologists and Obstetricians (FIGO) staging system is seen in Table 76-2. Confirmation of the presence of stage Ia1 of stage Ia2 microinvasive cancer is important in distinguishing it from frankly invasive cancer. In general, patients with microinvasive cancer are found to have abnormal Pap smears and undergo routine colposcopic assessment. The confirmation of extent of disease is extremely important in pregnancy and may require more than a simple colposcopically

TABLE 76–2. INTERNATIONAL FEDERATION OF GYNECOLOGISTS AND OBSTETRICIANS (FIGO) CERVICAL CANCER STAGING CLASSIFICATION

0	Carcinoma in situ, intraepithelial carcinoma; cases of stage 0 should not be included in any therapeutic statistics for invasive carcinoma
I	The carcinoma is strictly confined to the cervix (extension to the corpus should be disregarded)
Ia	Preclinical carcinoma of the cervix; that is, those diagnosed only by microscopy
Ia1	Minimal microscopically evident stromal invasion
Ia2	Lesions detected microscopically that can be measured; the upper limit of the measurement should not show a depth of invasion of >5 mm taken from the base of the epithelium, either surface or glandular, from which it originates; a second dimension, the horizontal spread, must not exceed 7 mm; larger should be staged as Ib
Ib	Lesions of greater dimension than stage Ia2, whether seen clinically or not; preformed space involvement should not alter the staging but should be specifically recorded so as to determine whether it should affect treatment decisions in the future
II	The carcinoma extends beyond the cervix but has not extended onto the pelvic wall; the carcinoma involves the vagina, but not as far as the lower third
IIa	No obvious parametrial involvement
IIb	Obvious parametrial involvement
III	The carcinoma has extended onto the pelvic wall; on rectal examination there is no cancer-free space between the tumor and the pelvic wall; the tumor involves the lower third of the vagina; all cases with a hydronephrosis or nonfunctioning kidney should be included, unless they are known to be due to other cause
IIIa	No extension onto the pelvic wall, but involvement of the lower third of the vagina
IIIb	Extension onto the pelvic wall or hydronephrosis or nonfunctioning kidney
IV	The carcinoma has extended beyond the true pelvis or has clinically involved the mucosa of the bladder or rectum
IVa	Spread of the growth to adjacent organs
IVb	Spread to distant organs

From Gynecol Oncol 1986;25:383.

directed biopsy. It may require a more extensive biopsy in the form of a hemicone biopsy or a cone biopsy of the cervix. If surgical margins are histologically free of disease on the cervical biopsy, patients may safely continue with the pregnancy as long as they are willing to be assessed with frequent Pap smears and colposcopy. Stage Ia2 patients have more extensive microinvasive cancer. Once again, the issue is related to the margins of the biopsy used to establish the diagnosis and the patient's desire to preserve the pregnancy and her fertility. Those patients with microinvasive cancer who wish to undergo prompt therapy are usually successfully managed with a simple hysterectomy and leaving the ovaries in place. Patients who wish to have definitive surgery performed following completion of pregnancy may be delivered vaginally and have a subsequent hysterectomy or may be delivered by cesarean section followed by an extrafascial hysterectomy.

The prognostic significance of vascular space involvement associated with microinvasive cervical cancer is debatable. Anecdotal experience at Yale–New Haven Hospital suggests that such findings in pregnancy are of concern for the management of the mother. However, a large series of pregnant women with microinvasive cervical cancer and vascular space involvement treated in a conservative fashion is not available. Our general treatment recommendation is for a modified or type II radical hysterectomy and lymph node sampling. However, individual decisions have to be made with each patient, taking into account considerations for the patient's health and for her pregnancy. There is definitely a role for attempting to preserve the pregnancy until fetal viability is evident and then performing definitive surgery for the cervical lesion at the time of a cesarean section.

INVASIVE CANCER

The identification of invasive cancer of the cervix requires prompt treatment, except for patients in the third trimester, when one may briefly delay therapy until fetal viability is established. Patients with stage IB and stage IIA cervical cancer recognized in the first trimester of pregnancy are routinely recommended to be treated with a type III radical hysterectomy and bilateral deep pelvic lymphadenectomies. This approach affords the patient the opportunity to preserve ovarian function and have a more pliable vagina as compared to patients treated with radiation therapy.

The surgical approach to the management of invasive cancer of the cervix in pregnancy has had mixed reviews in the literature. Some physicians believe that there is an increase in complications secondary to major blood loss and that postoperative complications, such as fistulae, are more likely.[50] Other investigators have not found this to be as significant a problem.[42,44,51] My personal experience suggests that for most patients radical hysterectomy in pregnancy is not particularly difficult, as there is substantial tissue edema and tissue planes are easy to establish.

Patients with more advanced cervical cancer are routinely recommended to be treated with radiation therapy. External beam radiation therapy has generally been employed first and will induce spontaneous abortion. Intracavitary radiation follows completion of the external beam radiation regimen. Radiation therapy is a known abortifacient when treating pelvic malignancies. Abortion following initiation of radiation exposure occurs more rapidly in the first trimester than in the second.[52] In the first trimester, the average time to abortion was 32.7 days (range 27 to 50 days).[52] In the second trimester, the average time interval is approximately 43.9 days, with a range of 33 to 60 days.[52] Some physicians have recommended that a hysterotomy and termination of pregnancy be performed prior to initiating radiation therapy in second-trimester cervical cancer patients, rather than waiting until the onset of labor secondary to the radiation.[52] In general, the plan of management at Yale–New Haven Hospital for cervical cancer management is to use external beam radiation first and not to attempt to deliver the fetus prior to initiation of therapy. There are no data to suggest that delivering the fetus through an irradiated cervix affects the course of the disease. However, four cases of pregnant women with squamous cell carcinoma who delivered vaginally and were diagnosed to have the same type of malignancy subsequently in episiotomy sites have been reported.[53]

Advanced-stage cervical cancer has a particularly poor response to standard radiation therapy. A major effort in the past few years has resulted in the development of neoadjuvant chemotherapy protocols for the management of such disease.[54] The role for neoadjuvant chemotherapy in the control and treatment of patients with cervical cancer in pregnancy has yet to be assessed. In part, this is due to the lack of availability of any long-term studies showing the efficacy of such treatment and due in part to the fear of injury to the fetus. However, many of the agents used in the therapeutic treatment of noncervical cancers occurring in pregnancy have been incorporated into short-term successful regimens in the management of cervical cancer. Thus, it may be appropriate to consider a role for neoadjuvant chemotherapy in the management of locally advanced cervical cancer, particularly in situations where definitive treatment will be excessively delayed in order for the fetus to reach viability. In reviewing the 5-year survival for pregnant women with stage I and II cancers treated in pregnancy compared to those patients not pregnant at diagnosis, the survivals were 74.5% and 47.8%, respectively, as compared with 76.5% and 55% for overall 5-year survival in the FIGO annual report.[46] Stage III and IV disease did more poorly in pregnancy, with 16.2% as compared to 27.9% survival in FIGO annual report.[46] Thus, the treatment for cervical cancer remains unsatisfactory in the advanced stage, particularly in pregnancy, and bold new initiatives will be necessary for managing the most common cancer in pregnant women.

BREAST CANCER

The breast is the second most common site for invasive cancers in pregnant women. It is estimated that approximately one in 3000 pregnancies will be associated with breast cancer.[2,55] It is likely that the incidence of breast cancer will increase as women delay pregnancy because of career choices. The average age for patients to develop breast cancer in pregnancy is between 32 and 38 years.[14] Breast self-examination as well as physician examinations should be a routine part of prenatal care. The diagnosis of cancer in pregnancy is complicated by the physiologic enlargement of the breast and associated hyperemia. This can confuse the patient as well as the physician examiner. There is no evidence to confirm that breast cancer progresses more rapidly in pregnancy. Breast cancer diagnosed in pregnancy tends to be more advanced because of the misinterpretation of the significance of the mass and the ascription of that lesion to being part of normal pregnancy changes.[56,57] Mammography may be employed safely in pregnancy, provided the abdomen is shielded. However, interpretation of mammograms may be difficult because of the increased water density of the breast during pregnancy. Indeed, 52% of mammograms in non-pregnant women below the age of 35 with a palpable malignant breast mass had normal mammograms in one report.[58] A similar finding occurred in six to eight pregnant women. Thus, suspicious breast masses in pregnancy must be biopsied.

Seemingly prolonged delays between the recognition of a mass and the diagnosis of breast cancer in pregnancy have been reported.[56,57] The upper outer quadrants of the breasts are the most likely sites to identify breast cancer, as 50% of breast cancer will arise in these quadrants. Fine-needle-aspiration biopsy techniques have now been perfected and should be liberally used to separate benign masses from malignancy. Most malignant breast masses occurring in pregnancy are first discovered by the patient.

Excisional biopsy is the best way to confirm the nature of a breast mass. The biopsy can be done either under local anesthesia or under general anesthesia. One series of 134 patients undergoing a general anesthetic for excisional biopsy of a breast mass experienced only one pregnancy loss following that surgery.[59] The frequencies of the histologic types of breast cancer occurring in pregnancy are similar to the non-pregnant state.[60] However, an occasional lactational mastitis can be confused with an inflammatory breast carcinoma. The differential diagnosis of neoplastic diseases occurring in breast masses in pregnancy include Hodgkin's disease,[57] Burkitt's lymphoma,[61,62] acute myelogenous leukemia,[63] and sarcomas.[64]

It is routine to send a piece of the excised breast mass for estrogen and progestin receptor protein analysis. However, 23 of 32 patients with diagnosed breast cancer in pregnancy had cancer specimens that were negative for estrogen receptor, and the three cancers assayed for progestin receptors also were lacking that receptor.[14,58,65,66] Although it is possible that the receptors were already saturated by the endogenous high levels of hormones in pregnancy, these findings were also compatible with an earlier report suggesting that breast cancer arising in pregnancy is not hormonally sensitive, because no objective response occurred in 32 pregnant breast cancer patients following oophorectomy.[14,67] The best success in treating pregnant patients with breast cancer is achieved in early-stage cancers. However, stage-for-stage, the prognosis for breast cancer patients in pregnancy is similar to that in the non-pregnant state.[68,69] The current staging system for breast cancer is presented in Table 76-3.

It has been suggested that women who develop breast cancer in pregnancy have a poor prognosis because circulating hormone levels stimulate the breast cancer to grow rapidly and at the same time decrease cellular and humoral immunity.[14] Indeed, it had been suggested that breast cancer occurring in pregnancy was uniformly associated with a poor prognosis. Peters' study revealed considerable variation in the growth of breast cancer in pregnancy, with no obvious discernible pattern.[70] Nugent and O'Connell ascribed the worst prognosis to cancers developing in women under 40 years of age and hormonally insensitive based on a lack of estrogen and progestin receptors in the tumor specimen.[65] Ribeiro and Palmer reported an overall five-year survival of 70% for women with breast cancer developing in pregnancy and noted that advanced cancer was more likely to be diagnosed late in pregnancy than in early pregnancy.[71]

A team approach to the management of a patient found to have breast cancer in pregnancy should routinely be employed. A social worker or psychologist should participate in the counselling of such patients due to the intense emotional impact that a mastectomy might have on a pregnant woman. The patient should be aware that there is no objective evidence to demonstrate that terminating the pregnancy would favorably influence prognosis.[70,72,73]

Breast cancer occurring in pregnancy should be treated in a manner similar to the non-pregnant state.[74] Early-stage breast cancer in pregnancy is treated with a modified radical mastectomy.[14] Additional chemotherapy and radiation therapy are based on the findings of the axillary node dissection. Lumpectomy and radiation therapy play a very limited role in pregnancy due to the significant internal radiation scatter to the fetus.[75] Surgery should not be delayed until fetal viability, as there is no evidence to demonstrate a benefit to the patient or the fetus.[68,71] The chance of aborting the pregnancy as a result of mastectomy is approximately 1%.[59]

Locally advanced disease without lymph node spread, for instance T4 NO, requires chemotherapy or radiation therapy to prevent recurrence at the mastectomy site. It has been recommended that in the first

TABLE 76–3. INTERNATIONAL UNION AGAINST CANCER (UICC) AND THE AMERICAN JOINT COMMISSION ON CANCER STAGING AND END RESULTS REPORTING (AK) BREAST CANCER STAGING CLASSIFICATION

T — Primary tumors
T1 — Tumor 2 cm or less in its greatest dimension
  a. No fixation to underlying pectoral fascia or muscle
  b. Fixation to underlying pectoral fascia or muscle
T2 — Tumor more than 2 cm but not more than 5 cm in its greatest dimension
T3 — Tumor more than 5 cm in its greatest dimension
  a. No fixation to underlying pectoral fascia or muscle
  b. Fixation to underlying pectoral fascia or muscle
T4 — Tumor of any size with direct extension to chest wall or skin. Note: Chest wall includes ribs, intercostal muscles, and serratus anterior muscle, but not pectoral muscle
  a. Fixation to chest wall
  b. Edema (including peau d'orange), ulceration of the skin of the breast, or satellite skin nodules confined to the same breast
  c. Both of the above
  d. Inflammatory carcinoma

Dimpling of the skin, nipple retraction, or any other skin changes except those in T4b may occur in T1, T2, or T3 without affecting the classification.

N — Regional lymph nodes
N0 — No palpable homolateral axillary nodes
N1 — Movable homolateral axillary nodes
  a. Nodes not considered to contain growth
  b. Nodes considered to contain growth
N2 — Homolateral axillary nodes containing growth and fixed to one another or to other structures
N3 — Homolateral supraclavicular or infraclavicular nodes containing growth or edema of the arm
M — Distant metastasis
M0 — No evidence of distant metastasis
M1 — Distant metastasis present, including skin involvement beyond the breast area

Clinical Stage Grouping

Stage	T	N	M
Stage I	T1a or T1b	N0 or N1a,	M0
Stage II	T0	N1b	M0
	T1a or T1b	N1b	M0
	T2a or T2b	N0, N1a or N1b	M0
Stage III	T1a or T1b	N2	M0
	T2a or T2b	N2	M0
	T3a or T3b	N0, N1, or N2	M0
Stage IV	T4,	Any N	Any M
	Any T	N3	Any M
	Any T	Any N	M1

DeVita VT Jr, Hellman S, Rosenberg SA, eds. Cancer: principles and practice of oncology. 3rd ed. Philadelphia: JB Lippincott, 1989;1211.

trimester, therapeutic abortion followed by radiation to the breast and regional lymph nodes or chemotherapy be employed as the routine method of management. Six weeks following completion of this treatment, a mastectomy and regional lymph node sampling should be performed. During the second trimester, a hysterectomy should be performed, followed by radiation or chemotherapy and then mastectomy. In the third trimester, treatment for massive local disease may be delayed until fetal viability is achieved.[76]

The survival for patients with breast cancer is influenced by the presence of metastases to the axillary lymph nodes. Patients with metastatic disease to these lymph nodes benefit from adjuvant cytotoxic chemotherapy in the non-pregnant state.[77] Because chemotherapy has teratogenic effects, pregnant women in the first trimester should be counseled regarding the possibility of a pregnancy termination. Patients in the third trimester may wish to delay chemotherapy until fetal maturity is achieved and the baby is delivered. Anecdotal experience has been reported regarding women receiving chemotherapy in pregnancy for breast cancer. Long-term effects on the children exposed in utero remain to be determined. Data currently available suggest that terminating a pregnancy in the presence of breast cancer has no effect on patient survival.[70,72,73] Similarly, prophylactic castration of the pregnant woman with breast cancer does not influence her survival.[68]

Disseminated breast cancer is routinely treated in the non-pregnant state with systematic chemotherapy and possibly additional radiation or hormonal therapy. The effects of such treatment on the fetus are particularly obvious in the first trimester. In the third trimester, delaying systematic treatment until fetal maturity is achieved appears reasonable. However, Willemse and colleagues have recently reported a 42-year-old woman at 25 weeks gestation with stage IV breast cancer treated with two cycles of doxorubicin, methotrexate, and vincristine.[32] The patient delivered a normal infant at 33 weeks gestation. The child initially had sepsis and mild respiratory distress syndrome but was functioning normally at 2 years of age. Thus, there may be a role for systemic chemotherapy in pregnant women willing to accept the risk of premature delivery or low-birth-weight infants.

Previously, it was recommended that patients who developed cancer in pregnancy not become pregnant again. It now seems that delaying 3 to 5 years before conceiving might be wise, as most patients with breast cancer in whom the cancer recurs have those recurrences within the first few years of the diagnosis.[78] Such patients may be placed on birth control pills without incurring a risk of reactivating the cancer.[76]

OVARIAN CANCER

Ovarian cancer is slowly rising in the United States, with an estimated incidence of 20,500 new cases in 1990 and approximately 12,500 deaths anticipated in that same year.[3] Most ovarian cancers in the United States are epithelial in origin and occur in women over age 35. Most ovarian cancers complicating pregnancy are either borderline malignant potential epithelial cancers or germ cell malignancies. Invasive epithelial cancers are rare in pregnancy, and sex cord stromal tumors occur extremely infrequently.

It can be expected that the incidence of ovarian neoplasms recognized in pregnancy will be increasing with the routine use of diagnostic ultrasound in pregnancy. As a result, more patients are now being seen in our institution with ovarian masses. A recent series of adnexal masses reported from the Yale–New Haven Hospital suggests that ultrasound evaluation is a very successful way of assessing the nature of an ovarian tumor.[48] Magnetic resonance imaging (MRI) is useful in further delineating the nature of the ovarian neoplasm.[48,79] Our experience suggests, however, that for most patients an ultrasound assessment of an adnexal mass is likely to establish the benign nature of the lesion, with MRI being used in those patients where the ultrasound findings are equivocal or the lesion cannot be distinguished from a uterine neoplasm, in particular a uterine leiomyoma.[48] Figure 76-3 demonstrates an MRI confirming a uterine fibroid that ultrasonographically was indistinguishable from an ovarian tumor associated with a 15-week pregnancy. Figure 76-4 demonstrates a benign cystic teratoma diagnosed in pregnancy by MRI techniques.

Ovarian malignancies occurring in pregnancy are estimated to complicate one in 9000 to one in 25,000 pregnancies.[65,71,80] Ovarian neoplasms are usually observed in the first trimester and are operated upon in the second trimester. These lesions tend to be asymptomatic when recognized. However, torsion is a relatively frequent presentation for a germ cell malignancy of the ovary and requires prompt surgical intervention. Simple cysts of the ovary may be followed with serial ultrasound examinations until the cysts resolve. Lesions greater than 6 cm in diameter, complex cysts (ie, cysts containing both solid and cystic elements), and solid tumors are the usual indications for operative intervention in pregnancy. Figure 76-5 demonstrates a complex

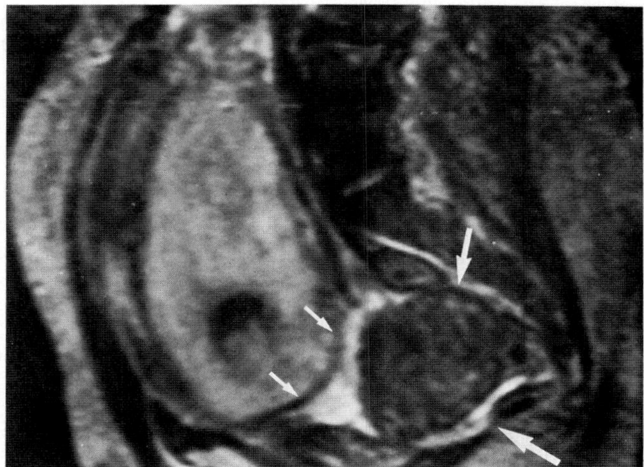

FIGURE 76–3. Uterine leiomyoma, T2-weighted sagittal magnetic resonance image. The low signal intensity of this well-circumscribed mass (large arrows) and origin from the posterior wall of the gravid uterus (small arrows) permit a confident diagnosis of a uterine leiomyoma. (Courtesy Dr R Kier.)

ovarian cyst that proved to be a mucinous carcinoma of the ovary. The patient continued the pregnancy, received chemotherapy, and subsequently delivered a normal infant.

Germ cell ovarian malignancies occur relatively infrequently in younger women but must be considered in the differential diagnosis of solid or solid and cystic pelvic masses occurring in pregnancy.[81] The more rapidly growing tumors (ie, the endodermal sinus tumors and embryonal carcinoma) may be associated with hemorrhage and necrosis, giving a rather inhomogeneous appearance to the mass on ultrasound or magnetic resonance imaging scans. Elevated levels of circulating tumor markers may help distinguish germ cell tumors from other ovarian neoplasms. In the non-pregnant state, serum α-fetoprotein (AFP) elevations and the beta subunit of human chorionic gonadotropin (B-hCG) elevations can be very effective circulating tumor markers for the diagnosis and follow-up of endodermal sinus tumors and nongestational trophoblastic tumors, respectively. The combination of an elevated AFP and B-hCG may be an excellent way for diagnosing and following embryonal carcinoma patients.[81] However, elevated AFP and B-hCG titers are routine in pregnancy, and such assays may be more confusing than informative in the preoperative evaluation of patients with pelvic masses. Similarly, serum lactic dehydrogenase (SLDH) and other liver enzyme levels may be elevated in non-pregnant women with solid adnexal tumors that prove to be dysgerminoma.[83] However, serum LDH and other liver enzymes may be elevated in the pregnant state unrelated to the presence of a dysgerminoma. Similarly, CA 125, an antigenic determinant made by approximately 80% of ovarian cancers, may be elevated in early pregnancy for reasons unrelated to the presence of a malignancy.[83–85]

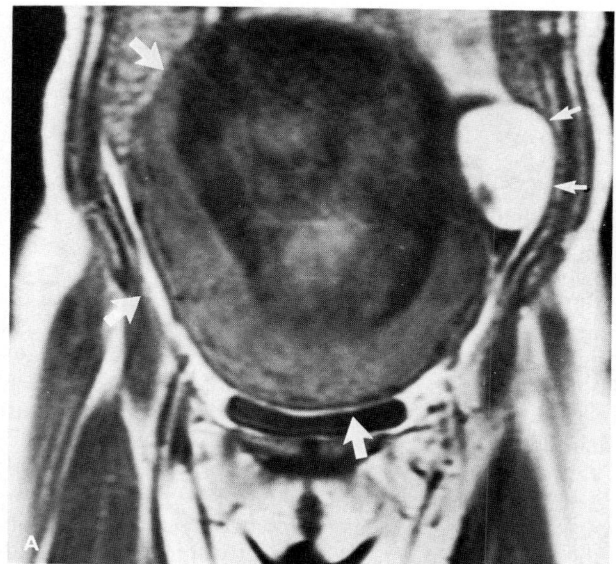

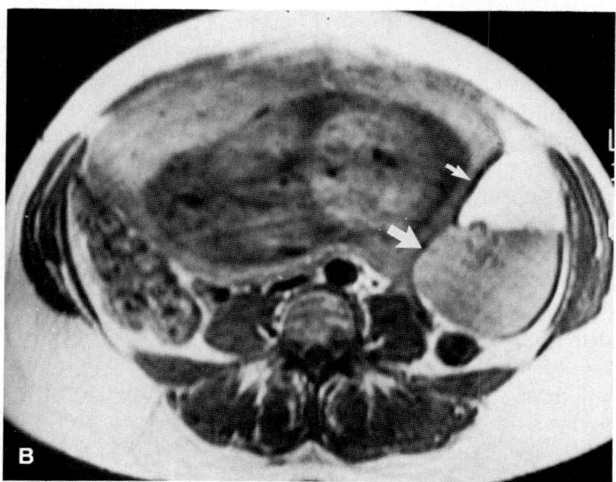

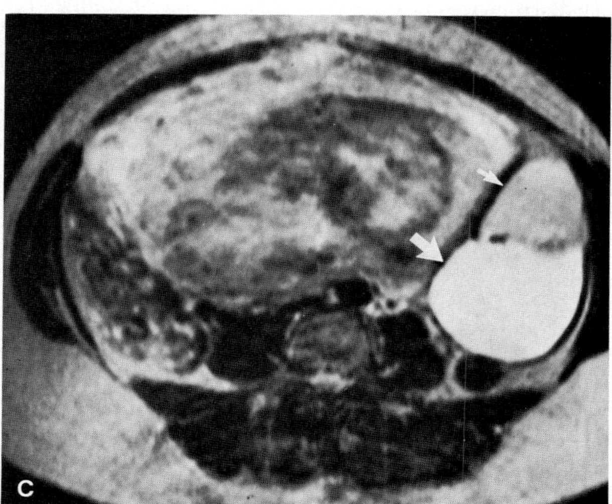

FIGURE 76–4. Mature cystic teratoma of the left ovary. (**A**) Coronal T1-weighted MR image demonstrates a left ovarian mass (small arrows) next to the gravid uterus (large arrows). High signal intensity on T1-weighted images is consistent with the presence of fat within the tumor (**B**). Axial T1-weighted image demonstrates the left ovarian mass next to the gravid uterus. Fat floats in the nondependent portion of the mass (small arrows), whereas fluid within the mass (large arrow) is dependent within the mass (**C**). T2-weighted axial image again demonstrates the fatty component of the tumor (small arrows) floating above fluid (large arrows). On T2-weighted images, the fat becomes of intermediate signal intensity, whereas the serum becomes high signal intensity. (Courtesy Dr R Kier.)

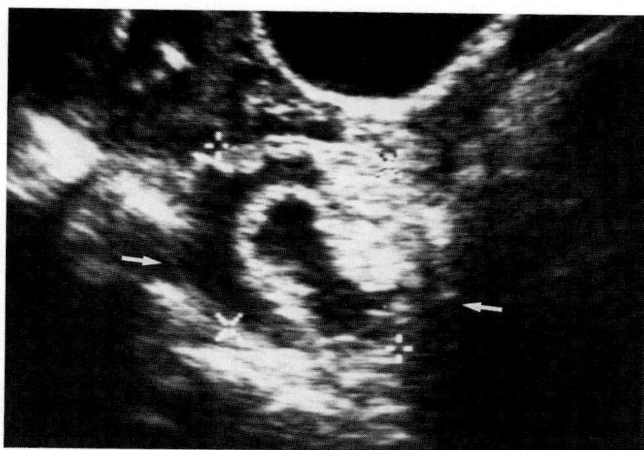

FIGURE 76–5. Mucinous carcinoma of the ovary. Sagittal ultrasonogram demonstrates a complex ovarian mass (arrows) posterior to the lower uterine segment of the gravid uterus. (Courtesy Dr MG Tompkins.)

In general, surgical management of ovarian neoplasms occurring in pregnancy is delayed until the second trimester, provided the patient is asymptomatic and the tumor is not suspicious for malignancy by diagnostic imaging techniques. Symptomatic patients and patients with tumors suspicious for malignancy should promptly undergo surgery to diagnose and initiate the treatment of the cancer. The final decision regarding management must be based on the histologic assessment of the operative specimens.

SURGICAL STAGING

Surgical staging for ovarian cancer in pregnancy should be the same as that recommended for surgical staging in the non-pregnant state. However, the pregnant uterus makes assessment of the retroperitoneum much more difficult, and a vertical incision should be used. On entering the abdomen, any free fluid should be aspirated and sent for cytology. If no free fluid is present, washings of the paracolic spaces, the pelvis, and subdiaphragmatic spaces should be obtained. The ovarian lesion should then be removed and sent for frozen section histologic analysis. Every effort should be made to remove the tumor intact. The remaining ovary should be carefully inspected and biopsied. Any peritoneal abnormalities should be sampled. Any retroperitoneal nodularities should also be sampled. Sampling of periaortic lymph nodes should be attempted. This can be the most difficult part of the procedure in pregnancy because of the bulk of the gravid uterus. It is inappropriate to remove both ovaries when a germ cell ovarian malignancy is diagnosed by frozen section techniques. The most common neoplasm in the contralateral ovary of a woman with a germ cell malignancy is a benign cystic teratoma. However, if both ovaries are involved with malignant growths and the patient is in the second trimester of pregnancy, each ovary should be removed, as the pregnancy will sustain itself in the second and third trimesters without ovaries being present.[49] Germ cell ovarian malignancies are almost invariably unilateral. Removing the contralateral ovary does not affect prognosis for the patient. Recent evidence suggests that occult dysgerminomas may be present in a grossly normal contralateral ovary.[86] In such a circumstance it is not necessary to remove the entire ovary. Non-pregnant women with microscopic dysgerminoma in the contralateral ovary have subsequently been treated with chemotherapy and have gone on to conceive normal healthy children. The current FIGO staging system for ovarian cancer is presented in Table 76-4.

EPITHELIAL OVARIAN CANCER

Borderline malignant potential tumors are the most common epithelial ovarian cancers in pregnancy.[87] In a series of 100 consecutive borderline epithelial cancers treated or consulted on at Yale–New Haven Hospital between 1978 and 1986, two were first diagnosed at cesarean section. One diagnosed at 22 weeks gestation was successfully treated with a unilateral oophorectomy and continued the pregnancy to term. The other patient underwent a bilateral salpingo-oophorectomy at 16 weeks gestation for bilateral serous borderline malignant potential tumors of the ovary.[49,88] The pregnancy of the latter patient was uncomplicated. She delivered a normal, healthy infant.

Stage IA and IB borderline malignant potential tumor patients appeared to be adequately treated with surgery alone. More advanced stage ovarian borderline malignant potential tumors are also treated surgically, chemotherapy being reserved only for the unusual group of patients with invasive metastases in association with borderline malignant potential tumors of the ovary.[88]

Patients found to have stage I invasive cancers of the ovary are generally managed conservatively, and the pregnancy is allowed to go to term. Recent data suggest that in a non-pregnant state, patients with stages Ia and Ib, grades 1 and 2, epithelial cancers of the ovary are adequately treated with surgery alone.[89] Additional adjuvant chemotherapy appears to play no significant role in improving a very high disease-free survival. However, the latter series was performed by gynecologic oncologists who thoroughly surgically staged the patients before they were eligible to participate in a prospective randomized study. Once the cancer is more advanced than stage Ib, aggressive surgical cytoreductive surgery is necessary. In general, a total abdominal hysterectomy and bilateral salpingo-oophorectomy, omentectomy, and para-aortic and pelvic lymph node sampling and resection of all gross tumor is recommended in early-stage ovarian cancer. The patient is subsequently treated with platinum-based combination chemotherapy. Recent studies with germ cell ovarian malignancies suggest that platinum-based chemotherapy may be given successfully in the second and third trimester prior to the fetus reaching viability.[90] Such a strategy may be employed for common epithelial cancers as well, first recognized to be present in the second and third trimesters of pregnancy. Malfetano and Goldkrand treated one patient successfully with *cis*-platinum-based chemotherapy after conservative surgery at 16 weeks gestation confirmed the presence of an

TABLE 76-4. FIGO OVARIAN CANCER STAGING CLASSIFICATION

I	Growth limited to the ovaries
Ia	Growth limited to one ovary; no ascites; no tumor on the external surface; capsule intact
Ib	Growth limited to both ovaries; no ascites; no tumor on the external surfaces; capsule intact
Ic	Tumor either stage Ia or Ib, but with tumor on surface of one or both ovaries; or with capsule ruptured; or with ascites present containing malignant cells; or with positive peritoneal washings
II	Growth involving one or both ovaries with pelvic extension
IIa	Extension and/or metastases to the uterus and/or tubes
IIb	Extension to other pelvic tissues
IIc	Tumor either stage IIa or IIb but with tumor on surface of one or both ovaries; or with capsule ruptured; or with ascites present containing malignant cells; or with positive peritoneal washings
III	Tumor involving one or both ovaries with peritoneal implants outside the pelvis and/or positive retroperitoneal or inguinal nodes; superficial liver metastases equals stage III; tumor is limited to the true pelvis but with histologically proven malignant extension to small bowel or omentum
IIIa	Tumor grossly limited to the true pelvis with negative nodes but with histologically confirmed microscopic seeding of abdominal peritoneal surfaces
IIIb	Tumor involving one or both ovaries with histologically confirmed implants of abdominal peritoneal surfaces none exceeding 2 cm in diameter; nodes are negative
IIIc	Abdominal implants greater than 2 cm in diameter and/or positive retroperitoneal or inguinal nodes
IV	Growth involving one or both ovaries with distant metastases. If pleural effusion present, there must be positive cytology to allot a case to stage IV; parenchymal liver metastasis equals stage IV

Gynecol Oncol 1986:25:383.

advanced-stage epithelial ovarian cancer.[91] That patient went on to a vaginal delivery and a postpartum laparotomy that revealed no evidence of persistent cancer.

GERM CELL OVARIAN MALIGNANCIES

Germ cell ovarian malignancies are infrequently occurring tumors that present in women in their second and third decades of life. Karlen and colleagues suggested that the dysgerminoma was the most common malignancy in pregnancy.[92] However, they were only able to obtain details on 27 such patients reported in English literature between 1937 and 1978. Management of dysgerminoma requires removal of the primary tumor and careful surgical staging, as described earlier. Dysgerminomas are the only germ cell malignancies of the ovary to frequently (5% to 15%) involve both ovaries. Thus, biopsying the contralateral ovary is appropriate even if it grossly appears to be normal. Dysgerminomas also have a tendency to spread to the para-aortic nodes. Every effort should be made to sample the para-aortic lymph nodes surgically at the time of the extirpation for the dysgerminoma.

Dysgerminomas are exquisitely sensitive to radiation therapy. Recent data suggest that they are also exquisitely sensitive to combination chemotherapy.[81] In nonpregnant women we have been very favorably impressed at Yale University School of Medicine with the vincristine, actinomycin D, and cyclophosphamide (VAC) regimen. Bleomycin, etoposide, and platinum (BEP) is also an extremely effective regimen for the chemotherapeutic management of dysgerminomas.[93] Stage Ia dysgerminoma may be very effectively treated with surgery.[81] Advanced-stage dysgerminoma should be treated with chemotherapy.[81] Pregnant women should be given the chance to maintain the pregnancy if a dysgerminoma is present. They may be given chemotherapy in the second or third trimesters to control and possibly cure the patient of the cancer. BEP and VAC chemotherapy regimens require only short-term administration. They are usually administered every 3 to 4 weeks. A cesarean section is used to deliver the fetus at the time of fetal viability. A second-look procedure also may be performed at that surgery. Zinser and colleagues have reported treating a pregnant dysgerminoma patient diagnosed at 27 weeks with two courses of cyclophosphamide, platinum, and doxorubicin therapy, followed by a cesarean section, at which time no disease was evident.[94] At age 4 months the child was reported to be normal.

The endodermal sinus tumor is the most virulent of all the germ cell ovarian malignancies. It was associated with a 2-year survival of 12% to 19% in the prechemotherapy era. Experience at Yale–New Haven Hospital suggests that stage I disease is exquisitely sensitive to the VAC chemotherapy regimen and that more advanced disease is routinely controlled and indeed cured using platinum-based chemotherapy.[81] Our current recommendation for this disease is the BEP regimen. Three case reports have now appeared in the literature in which patients with endodermal sinus tumors diagnosed in pregnancy received combination chemotherapy in pregnancy followed by a planned cesarean section.[90,95,96] In each case the patient delivered a normal, healthy child, and the patient appeared to be clinically free of disease following completion of therapy. No deleterious effects were noted in the offspring of these women.

Other germ cell malignancies include the embryonal carcinoma, the immature teratoma, choriocarcinoma, and mixed germ cell tumors. Their management is based on both the stage of disease and the presence or absence of circulating oncofetal proteins that can be used as markers for response to therapy. In general, these malignancies required aggressive therapy in the form of resection of all viable tumor followed by intense combination chemotherapy.[81] Pregnant women found to have these tumors in the second and third trimesters of pregnancy should be offered the opportunity to receive chemotherapy during pregnancy as a way of being treated and not terminating the pregnancy. However, because of the rarity of these tumors in pregnancy, limited supporting data are available for these recommendations. Christman and colleagues have reported a patient with a stage Ic, grade 3, immature teratoma who was successfully treated with a unilateral salpingo-oophorectomy at 15 weeks gestation and one course of *cis*-platinum, vinblastine, and bleomycin in her 19th week of gestation.[97] The patient delivered a normal-term infant, received four more cycles of therapy postpartum, and is alive and well 61 months from diagnosis. The child has developed normally.

SEX CORD STROMAL TUMORS

Sex cord stromal tumors are rare tumors that may complicate pregnancy. The granulosa theca cell tumor is the most common member of this category and is associated with estrogen production.[98] The Sertoli-Leydig cell tumor is rare and is associated with androgen production. Young and colleagues reported on 36 sex cord stromal tumors diagnosed in pregnancy.[99] All were stage I. Thirteen of the 36 patients presented with pain due to rupture of the tumor; two of the latter patients were in hemorrhagic shock. Treatment was limited to removing the tumor. Only one of these patients has subsequently recurred. Advanced-stage sex cord stromal tumors require more aggressive chemotherapy. Our current recommendation in the non-pregnant state is bleomycin, etoposide, and platinum.[100]

NONSPECIFIC MESENCHYME MALIGNANCIES

Nonspecific mesenchyme malignancies are rare in the non-pregnant state. The most frequent histologic type is the mixed mesodermal tumor that occurs in older women. One would expect to find these lesions mostly in peri- and postmenopausal women. They should not complicate pregnancy. Management is aggressive surgery followed by platinum-based combination chemotherapy.

HODGKIN'S DISEASE

Hodgkin's disease generally occurs during the reproductive years, the peak incidence being between ages 18 and 30.[101] It is estimated that one third of women with Hodgkin's disease are pregnant or have delivered within 1 year of the diagnosis.[102,103] As with almost all malignancies associated with pregnancy, Hodgkin's disease has not been reported to be affected by the pregnancy.[104–106] It is a disease that is extremely sensitive to therapy. The cure rate for localized disease treated with radiation therapy is 80%, and patients with advanced disease treated with chemotherapy can anticipate a long-term disease-free survival of 65%.[107,108] Peripheral lymphadenopathy is the most common presenting symptom for patients with Hodgkin's disease. Between 60% and 80% of Hodgkin's disease patients have enlarged cervical lymph nodes. In addition, patients may be asymptomatic or may have a history of fever, night sweats, weight loss, malaise, and pruritus.[109]

The diagnosis of Hodgkin's disease is based on the histologic demonstration of the Reed-Sternberg cell, a dedifferentiated histiocyte.[109] The most important prognostic factors for Hodgkin's disease are the histologic appearance and the pattern of spread. The lymphocyte-predominant histologic type has the best prognosis, followed by mixed-cellularity, lymphocyte-depleted, and nodular sclerosis Hodgkin's disease. Nodular sclerosis Hodgkin's disease is the most common type in women and usually involves the neck, supraclavicular, anterior, and superior mediastinal regions.[101,109]

Selection of local radiation or systemic chemotherapy is based on the staging system (Table 76-5). Staging studies recommended for a patient with Hodgkin's disease are done in an attempt to identify extranodal disease. If such a finding is made, no further detailed studies are necessary prior to commencing treatment. The minimal studies necessary, in addition to the routine history and physical examination, are identification of the clinical distribution of the nodal disease, a chest x-ray, complete blood count, an erythrocyte sedimentation rate, renal and liver function tests, and a bone marrow aspirate and biopsy. Negative studies require further evaluation in a non-pregnant woman, and such studies would include bipedal lymphangiography, an intravenous urogram, or a computed tomogram (CT). Patients who are being considered for radiation then undergo an exploratory laparotomy, splenectomy, liver biopsy, and mapping of abdominal lymph node involvement as required.[110] Pregnant women may undergo ultrasound or magnetic resonance imaging studies of the liver, spleen, and retroperitoneal lymph nodes to avoid the hazard of diagnostic imaging radiation exposure to the fetus.

Strategies for treating patients with stage I and stage II Hodgkin's disease usually are radiotherapeutic, with reported 5-year survivals of 89% and 67%, respectively.[109] Radiation is the only modality necessary for patients with stage IIIA lymphocyte-predominant or nodular-sclerosing Hodgkin's disease. Stage IIIA disease with other histologic types is treated with radiation and combination chemotherapy. More advanced disease is treated with combination chemotherapy.[111]

The standard mantle field for midline mediastinal radiation to doses of 4000 rads results in fetal exposure to a degree that is greater than acceptable degree.[112] It has been recommended that the fetus in the first trimester of pregnancy should not be exposed to more than 10 rads (0.1 cGy). Internal radiation scatter from standard mantle fields cannot be shielded and would result in a greater exposure rate to the fetus than the dose recommended for continuation of the pregnancy.[111] Patients with pelvic disease or disease localized to the inguinal or abdominal region should undergo therapeutic abortion prior to radiation therapy. Similar disease first recognized in the third trimester would be treated with localized radiation therapy once fetal maturity was achieved and the infant delivered. Patients found to have rapidly progressing disease routinely receive chemotherapy, with the decision for initiating treatment based on the trimester of pregnancy and the patient's desires.

Advanced (stage III and stage IV) Hodgkin's disease has been successfully treated with the MOPP regimen —Mustargen (nitrogen mustard), Oncovin (vincristine), procarbazine, and prednisone.[109] Eighty-one percent of patients in the National Cancer Institute series with previously untreated stage III and stage IV disease were

TABLE 76-5. ANN ARBOR STAGING CLASSIFICATIONS FOR HODGKIN'S DISEASE

Stage I	Involvement of a single lymph node region (I) or a single extralymphatic organ or site (I_E)
Stage II	Involvement of two or more lymph node regions on the same side of the diaphragm (II) or localized involvement of an extralymphatic organ or site (II_e)
Stage III	Involvement of lymph node regions on both sides of the diaphragm (III) or localized involvement of an extralymphatic organ or site (III_E) or spleen (III_s) or both (III_{se})
Stage IV	Diffuse or disseminated involvement of one or more extralymphatic organs with or without associated lymph node involvement. The organ(s) involved should be identified by a symbol: A = Asymptomatic B = Fever, sweats, weight loss >10% of body weight

DeVita VT Jr, Hellman S, Rosenberg SA, eds. Cancer: principles and practice of oncology. 3rd ed. Philadelphia; JB Lippincott, 1989.

successfully managed with only 6 months of treatment.[108] The role for chemotherapy in the management of Hodgkin's disease in the first trimester of pregnancy is only beginning to become defined. Ward and Weiss suggested that patients who must be treated in the first trimester because of infradiaphragmatic disease that is difficult to follow, systemic symptoms, visceral involvement, or disease progression could receive vinblastine during the first trimester with "minimal risk" to the fetus.[106] When the patient enters into the second trimester, a modified mantle radiation field and vinblastine or a change to a combination chemotherapy if disease progresses is possible.[106] Therapeutic abortion should be offered to those patients in the first half of pregnancy who are unwilling to accept an increase in risk of adverse fetal outcome potentially attributable to treatment.

NON-HODGKIN'S LYMPHOMA

Fewer than 50 cases of non-Hodgkin's lymphomas during pregnancy have been published.[20,109,113] The mean age of patients with non-Hodgkin's lymphoma is 42 years, suggesting that most patients are past their childbearing years or are in a subfertile period of their reproductive life. The most important prognostic features for non-Hodgkin's lymphoma are the histologic type and the stage of disease. Histologically, the nodular type is more indolent; untreated, it has a survival period of approximately 4 years. The diffuse type is more virulent and has a life expectancy measured in months.[111] Non-Hodgkin's lymphomas tend to be widely disseminated at the time of diagnosis and therefore require less elaborate staging than Hodgkin's disease. Burkitt's lymphoma appears to be a particularly rapidly progressing form of non-Hodgkin's lymphoma. Breast and ovarian involvement is frequent, and breast metastases have a particularly bad prognosis.[114,115]

Localized non-Hodgkin's lymphoma is treated with radiation and has a 50% cure rate. Chemotherapy may also be curative in this disease.[116] Disseminated nodular lymphoma and chronic lymphocytic leukemia fall into a favorable group of disseminated non-Hodgkin's lymphomas. They tend to be relatively indolent.[111] Palliative treatment results in survivals of about 5 years. The unfavorable types of non-Hodgkin's lymphoma have a much shorter life expectancy, although occasional complete remissions and prolonged survival with chemotherapy have been reported.[117]

Because of the aggressive nature of diffuse non-Hodgkin's lymphoma, aggressive therapy should not be delayed until fetal maturity. Several case reports have been published demonstrating successful treatment of pregnant women who subsequently gave birth to normal children after treatment for diffuse non-Hodgkin's lymphoma. Two patients have been successfully treated in pregnancy with combination chemotherapy consisting of cyclophosphamide, vincristine, prednisone, and bleomycin for diffuse non-Hodgkin's lymphoma; they had successful outcomes and normal infants.[118,119] Nantel and colleagues recently reported on a woman with a B-cell immunoblastic lymphoma diagnosed at the 18th week of a twin gestation.[120] The patient received a 12-week chemotherapy regimen consisting of methotrexate, doxorubicin, cyclophosphamide, vincristine, prednisone, and bleomycin (MACOP-B); went into labor at 28 weeks gestation; and delivered two normal male infants. Non-Hodgkin's lymphomas have been reported to grow rapidly in the postpartum period.[121,122]

Aviles and colleagues published the largest experience treating non-Hodgkin's lymphoma in pregnancy.[20] Three of 19 women died during induction treatment. The other 16 patients received chemotherapy (8 of them in the first trimester) and had no obstetrical difficulties. All 16 children born to these patients were healthy, were at a normal level of growth 3 to 11 years after birth, and showed no congenital anomalies. Eight of the mothers who achieved complete remissions were alive and disease-free 4 to 9 years after delivery. This series provides the strongest support for prompt administration of chemotherapy for management of non-Hodgkin's lymphoma in pregnant women who wish to maintain their pregnancy.

ACUTE LEUKEMIA

Acute leukemia rarely complicates pregnancy, the incidence being less than one case in 75,000 pregnancies.[4,56,123] The disease is usually first recognized in the second or third trimester.[124] A recent review of 72 women with leukemia in pregnancy from 1975 to 1988 revealed that 64 (89%) had acute leukemia. Of these 72 women, 44 had acute myelogenous leukemia, 20 had acute lymphocytic leukemia, five had chronic myelogenous leukemia, one had a hairy cell leukemia, and two had unspecified leukemias.[125] Sixteen (22%) were detected in the first trimester, 26 (36%) were detected in the second trimester, and 30 (42%) were detected in the third trimester of pregnancy. Presenting symptoms are easy fatigability, bleeding diathesis, or recurrent infections that reflect bone marrow failure. Specific physical findings associated with acute leukemia include sternal tenderness, skin pallor, petechiae, ecchymoses, and hepatosplenomegaly. Patients with acute lymphocytic, myelocytic, or monocytic leukemia usually have normocytic anemia, normochromic anemia, mild to marked thrombocytopenia, and leukocytosis.[109] Occasionally, the leukocyte count may be lower than normal. Acute myeloblastic leukemia may be differentiated from acute lymphoblastic leukemias by the presence of Auer rods in the cytoplasm of myeloblasts. High serum and urine lysozyme levels are associated with acute monoblastic leukemias. The clinical impression is confirmed by bone marrow aspiration studies.[109]

Pregnancy does not influence the natural history of acute leukemia.[17,125] Substantial improvement in the survival of women with acute leukemia in pregnancy has occurred with the use of chemotherapy, radiation therapy, and supportive care, including blood products, antibiotics, and autologous bone marrow transplantation.[126] Virtually all women treated with chemotherapy in pregnancy will survive to delivery, and 87% of the fetuses will also survive.[109] Intense combination chemotherapy leads to multiple complications, including severe infections secondary to bone marrow suppression and the risk of central nervous system leukemia. The latter is treated with whole brain radiation, intrathecal methotrexate, or cytosine arabinoside. Hyperuricemia is usually treated with allopurinol.[127]

Roy and colleagues reported that three of five pregnant patients diagnosed in the second or third trimesters to have acute myeloblastic leukemia in pregnancy achieved complete remissions following chemotherapy during pregnancy.[126] Four live births were achieved, but one child had Down syndrome. These authors concluded that increased survival was related to more aggressive chemotherapeutic regimens and improved supportive care. Caliguri and Mayer reviewed 58 patients treated in pregnancy between 1975 and 1988 for acute myelogenous and acute lymphocytic leukemias.[125] Eight of 13 fetuses exposed in the first trimester of pregnancy were born prematurely, two went to term, and three aborted, one spontaneous and two electively. Twenty-three of 45 women treated in the second and third trimester delivered prematurely. Twenty-one patients delivered at term, and one patient had a spontaneous abortion.[125] One infant had an ocular abnormality, and another had polydactyly that had been observed in other family members. Anthracycline antibiotics have been used in pregnancy as single agents or in combination therapy without evidence of fetal malformation. Twenty-eight pregnancies (20 of which were leukemia-associated) resulted in a delivery of 24 live births, two ended in spontaneous abortions, and one was terminated by a therapeutic abortion; there were two maternal and fetal deaths. Three patients receiving first-trimester adriamycin delivered normal children. *Vinca* alkaloids have been used for treating acute leukemia in pregnancy. Only one of 14 children exposed in the first trimester had a congenital anomaly. None of six exposed in the second and third trimesters had congenital anomalies. Long-term follow-up of 26 children born to 23 women with leukemia in pregnancy suggests no long-term sequelae from the chemotherapy.[21,22] Unfortunately, although remission may be achieved in 50% to 80% of treated patients, the median survival is less than 1 year.[109]

CHRONIC MYELOCYTIC LEUKEMIA

Chronic myelocytic leukemia makes up 90% of the chronic leukemias complicating pregnancy.[128,129] Pregnancy does not adversely affect the natural history of chronic myelocytic leukemia. Treatment is palliative. Median survival is 45 months. All patients eventually die, most from an acute blastic crisis resembling myeloblastic leukemia.[111] The median survival is less than 1 year following the development of an acute blastic crisis.[109] Eighty-five percent of chronic myelocytic leukemia patients have a Philadelphia chromosome, a 9:22 translocation.[109] The absence of a Philadelphia chromosome, hyperdiploidy, chromosomal instability, presence of marked lymphadenopathy, basophilia, and gross soft tissue disease are poor prognostic factors.[109] The diagnosis of chronic myelocytic leukemia is based on a leukocytosis with basophilia or eosinophilia that may progress in time to 700,000 white cells per mm^3.[109] Bone marrow examination reveals hypercellularity, with mature forms predominating.

The most useful drugs in the management of this disease are busulfan, hydroxyurea, dibromomannitol, and cyclophosphamide. Approximately 96% of pregnant women with chronic myelocytic leukemia survive to delivery. Fetal survival throughout the gestation is 84%.[109]

MELANOMA

Pigment-producing melanocytes are found in the base layer of the epidermis, the mucosa of the gastrointestinal tract, the vagina, and the pigmented portion of the retina. Malignant melanoma derives from such cells and in 90% of cases originates in the skin in preexisting pigmented nevi.[130] Malignant melanoma localized to superficial layers of the skin may spread to regional lymph nodes and is associated with a 50% to 80% cure rate. Lesions that have infiltrated into the lowest third of the dermis or that have metastasized to regional lymph nodes have a 20% cure rate.[109]

Pregnancy frequently induces a darkening in the appearance of pigmented nevi, but a bluish or slightly gray appearance to a nevus requires immediate excisional biopsy. Indeed, pigmented nevi that have become darker or irregular in outline and elevated should always be promptly excised in pregnancy under local anesthesia. Pregnancy does not change the natural history of melanoma.[131,132] McMammy and colleagues reported on 23 patients pregnant at the time of the diagnosis of melanoma and were unable to show the pregnancy had any significant influence on the survival of those patients.[131] They did recommend that subsequent pregnancies be avoided for the first 3 years following excision of a malignant melanoma. Wong and colleagues reviewed 66 patients with stage I melanoma diagnosed during pregnancy and were unable to identify any significant difference between the pregnant population and a control population with regard to the location of the primary tumor, the age of diagnosis, Clark's level, mean depth of invasion, and histologic type.[132] The 5-year survival for the women with melanoma during pregnancy and for the entire population was 86% and 87%, respectively. Thus, the pregnancy did not influence the survival of the patients.[132] Terminating a pregnancy will not initiate a remission.[133] The clinical significance of estrogen receptor protein found in malignant melanoma has yet to be established. Clinical trials with an estrogen agonist–antagonist has yet to be demonstrated to be beneficial in treatment of malignant melanoma.[109,134,135]

Most patients with malignant melanoma present with stage I disease, disease limited to a primary cutaneous lesion. Stage I disease is pathologically staged according to the Clark's level of deepest anatomic invasion or the Breslow system, which places patients with disease invading to a maximum depth of less than 0.76 mm at a low risk, those with invasion of 0.76 to 1.5 mm at an intermediate risk, and those with invasion of greater than 1.5 mm at a high risk.[136,137] Stage II disease represents patients with metastases to regional lymph nodes or disease in lymphatic channels leading to those regional nodes. Stage III disease involves distant, blood-borne metastases.[130] Stage I lesions are usually treated with wide local excisions. Stage II lesions are treated surgically with complete regional lymph node dissections. Stage III disease is treated with systemic chemotherapy, including agents such as dimethyltriazenoimidazole-carboxamide (DTIC) or nitrosoureas such as chloroethylcyclohexyl nitrosourea (CCNU). Response rates are low (20% to 25%), and the median duration of remission is only 8 to 10 months.[130] Adjuvant immunotherapy for completely resected stage I and stage stage II disease has not shown definite benefit.[130] Intradermal nodules may be partially controlled by local injection of BCG intradermally.[109] Surgery should be performed promptly in patients with stage I and stage II disease, whereas patients with stage III disease can only be palliated. Early delivery of the fetus in the third trimester once fetal lung maturation has been achieved should be routinely considered for stage III patients.

Placental or fetal metastases have only been reported 16 times, with four fetal deaths due to transplacental metastases of malignant melanoma.[133] Although malignant melanoma is the most common malignancy to metastasize to the placenta and fetus, this is such a rare event as to preclude the recommendation of pregnancy termination for the management of the disease to avoid transplacental carcinogenesis or to induce a remission.

GASTROINTESTINAL CANCER

COLORECTAL CANCERS

Cancers of the gastrointestinal tract rarely complicate pregnancy.[138] There is no evidence that pregnancy changes the natural history of colorectal cancer, the most common of these neoplasms.[139–141] Most pregnant patients with gastrointestinal cancers have rectal carcinomas. Approximately 20% of patients have carcinoma presenting in the sigmoid colon.[142] Unfortunately, diagnosis is frequently difficult in pregnancy, and there is a considerable delay in diagnosis. Typical presenting symptoms include severe constipation, abdominal distention, and rectal bleeding. Since most diagnoses can be made by rectal examination, these symptoms should be promptly evaluated. Delay in diagnoses can be associated with intussusception, obstruction, or perforation.[68] Carcinoembryonic antigen (CEA) is routinely elevated in pregnancy and is of little use in diagnosing colorectal cancers in the gravid state.[143] The diagnosis may be established through the use of digital rectal examination, examination of the stool for occult blood, and proctoscopy or flexible sigmoidoscopy.

Early-stage colorectal cancers diagnosed in the first and second trimester should be treated with prompt surgery, and the pregnancy should be allowed to go to term.[68] Patients with large colorectal lesions with metastases suspected or present have been allowed to carry the pregnancy until fetal maturity and then have undergone a cesarean section and bowel resection, provided they remained relatively asymptomatic.[142] Most colorectal cancer patients are delivered by cesarean section, since labor may result in dystocia or hemorrhage. Lesions identified initially in the third trimester usually are not treated until fetal maturity is achieved. Standard therapy for curable lesions is definitive surgery, including standard bowel resections, low anterior resections, or abdominal perineal resections. The Mayo Clinic has reported 10 of 16 pregnant rectal carcinoma patients surviving 5 years from initial diagnosis.[144]

PANCREATIC TUMORS

Pancreatic carcinoma rarely complicates pregnancy and is difficult to diagnose in the presence of pancreatitis.[145,146] The most common presenting symptoms are abdominal pain and gastrointestinal symptoms. The most effective way to make the diagnosis is by endoscopic retrograde pancreatography with cytologic examination of pancreatic secretions.[145] Three cases of pancreatic carcinoma have been diagnosed in pregnancy, with the mothers dying soon after delivery.[145,146] Supportive care in the form of biliary drainage and hyperalimentation may be required to maintain the mother during pregnancy. Eight cases of insulinoma have been reported in pregnancy.[147] Each was recognized in the first trimester as a result of hypoglycemic episodes.

STOMACH TUMORS

Gastrinomas rarely complicate pregnancy.[148,149] They may present with a severe ulcer diathesis postpartum. Gastrinomas are associated with elevated serum gastrin, peptic ulceration, and secretion of gastric acid. Their management is surgical.

Gastric cancers rarely complicate pregnancy, and their symptoms are similar to those normally experienced in pregnancy, including gastrointestinal discomfort, nausea, and vomiting.[150–152] Diagnosis may be made by gastroscopy, which avoids diagnostic radiation exposure. Only one half of reported cases of gastric carcinomas are resectable in women who are not pregnant. The remainder are invariably fatal.

LIVER TUMORS

Hepatocellular carcinomas are rare in women and usually present in postmenopausal women. One case report of a hepatocellular carcinoma resulted in a maternal death in pregnancy.[153] Hepatomas are treated surgically. A single case of an extrahepatic biliary tract carcinoma complicating pregnancy has been reported.[154] Recently, a case of an adenocarcinoma arising in a large choledochal cyst was reported. The cyst was resected at the time of a cesarean section and a focus of adenocarcinoma was recognized.[155] Binstock and colleagues recommended that the routine management of a choledochal cyst, excision, and a Roux-en-Y reconstruction be deferred until after delivery because of the risk of fetal mortality and maternal morbidity associated with the procedure.[155]

GYNECOLOGIC MALIGNANCIES

UTERINE CARCINOMA

Adenocarcinoma of the endometrium is an extremely unusual disease in pregnant women, as only 8% of endometrial cancers have reported to recur in women under age 40.[156] Infertility has been a factor associated with women who develop adenocarcinoma of the endometrium. Ten cases of adenocarcinoma of the endometrium associated with pregnancy have been reported.[157–160] The most recent case report was of a woman found to have an endometrioid ovarian carcinoma in association with a well-differentiated adenocarcinoma of the endometrium. The cases were generally associated with vaginal bleeding and were found to be well-differentiated adenocarcinomas or adenoacanthomas. Only one of the patients has died to date. Standard therapy for patients with adenocarcinoma of the endometrium is a total abdominal hysterectomy and bilateral salpingo-oophorectomy. One patient with a mixed mesodermal tumor of the uterus has also been reported from Yale–New Haven Hospital.[161] That patient unfortunately was thought to have uterine leiomyomas associated with pain and vaginal spotting. The diagnosis was made at the time of a cesarean section. The infant did well but the patient failed to respond to combination chemotherapy and died 6 months after diagnosis.[49,161]

VULVA CANCER

Vulvar carcinoma in situ has been increasing, according to data from the Connecticut Tumor Registry.[162] Forty percent of patients with vulvar carcinoma in situ are under age 40. Thus, it can be anticipated that more women will be diagnosed in pregnancy to have vulvar carcinoma in situ. The management of a vulvar lesion in pregnancy is a local excision. Vulvar carcinoma in situ does not progress rapidly to invasive cancer unless associated with an immune deficiency. Definitive therapy in terms of a wide local excision or vulvectomy can be delayed in most cases until after completion of the pregnancy.

Invasive cancer of the vulva has been reported more frequently in the past. It is usually a disease of peri- and postmenopausal women. Lutz and colleagues reported that 5% of women with carcinoma of the vulva seen at the Medical University of South Carolina were diagnosed in pregnancy or within 2 to 6 months postpartum.[163] Squamous cell carcinoma is the most common type of vulvar malignancy, but sarcomas, melanomas, and adenocarcinomas of the Bartholin's gland have been reported.[163] Invasive cancer is usually treated with a radical vulvectomy. Recently, less extensive surgery has been quite effective if the tumor is only superficially invasive.[164] Bilateral inguinal lymphadenectomies have been reduced to ipsilateral lymphadenectomies for invasive unilateral cancers, provided frozen section analysis reveals no evidence of lymph node metastases. Lymph node sampling is now employed when microinvasive cancer is present. Extensive vulvectomies may be performed in pregnancy, but the current trend in the non-pregnant state is to manage microinvasive cancer with wide local excision and, when possible, to reduce the radicality of the vulvar dissection for small-sized invasive cancers.[164] As surgery becomes more extensive, the chances of a spontaneous abortion or premature labor may increase substantially.

VAGINAL CANCER

Carcinoma of the vagina occurs infrequently and usually is a squamous carcinoma presenting in a peri- or postmenopausal woman. Its management is similar to that of cervical cancer. Senekjian and colleagues reported on 20 patients who developed clear cell adenocarcinomas of the vagina in pregnancy.[165] These women had been exposed in utero to diethylstilbestrol. Four additional patients had clear cell carcinomas of the cervix. All but one of the 15 patients with stage I disease were successfully treated with wide local excision with or without radiation (3), radical hysterectomy with or without radiation therapy (10), and radiation therapy alone (2). As the stage of the disease advanced, the results became poorer. It was noted that the pregnancy did not have an adverse effect on clear cell carcinomas of the vagina or cervix. Perhaps this is due to the fact that in a previous report clear cell carcinomas did not have estrogen and progestin receptors.[166]

SOFT TISSUE SARCOMA

Soft tissue sarcomas rarely complicate pregnancy. The overall prognosis is poor. No evidence suggests that if they were successfully managed, subsequent pregnancies would be deleterious to the patient's health.[167,168] Osteogenic sarcoma is the most frequent sarcoma reported in pregnancy. No survival differences were noted in 18 cases of osteogenic sarcoma managed in pregnancy when they were matched with non-pregnant women for skeletal tumor location, histologic appearance, and age.[169] Therapeutic abortion has been recommended in the first trimester for patients exposed to intense cytotoxic chemotherapy.[170] However, it is usually recommended that patients diagnosed in the third trimester undergo early delivery once fetal maturity has been established.[170] A case of a Ewing's sarcoma involving the iliac wing diagnosed at 25 weeks gestation appears to have been successfully treated with multiagent chemotherapy in pregnancy followed by a cesarean section at 34 weeks gestation. At the time of the report, the mother and child were both alive and well 4 years later.[171]

A case of Kaposi's sarcoma arising in a patient suffering from acquired immune deficiency syndrome (AIDS) has been reported.[172] Combination chemotherapy consisting of doxorubicin, bleomycin, and vinblastine was administered during pregnancy. The patient subsequently delivered vaginally a growth-retarded infant.

ENDOCRINE TUMORS

THYROID CANCER

The thyroid is an infrequent site for cancer to develop in pregnancy. As the population delays childbearing it is possible that more papillary adenocarcinomas of the thyroid will be diagnosed in the future, since the peak distribution for papillary adenocarcinomas occurs in women 30 to 34 years old.[173] Patients at high risk for thyroid cancer include women exposed to radiation therapy to the head, neck, or chest during childhood.[174,175] Most cancers of the thyroid present as solitary nodules. Pregnancy changes should not result in the misdiagnosis of thyroid cancer. Most thyroid nodules appear in the first and third trimester of pregnancy and are benign.[176]

The most frequent histologic types of thyroid cancer are the papillary, follicular, and anaplastic carcinomas, whereas medullary carcinomas account for less than 5% of primary thyroid malignancies. The most common type of thyroid cancer to be diagnosed in pregnancy is the papillary carcinoma or mixed papillary follicular carcinoma. These carcinomas usually present as solitary nodules, but on careful sectioning of the tissue, 30% to 40% of patients will have multifocal disease. Prognosis is not affected by subclinical metastases to regional lymph nodes, which is present in 50% to 70% of patients. Women under age 49 are expected to have a 15-year survival rate of 90% to 95%.[174,175] Follicular carcinoma has a slightly worse prognosis than pure papillary carcinoma. It occurs most frequently in women over age 40, presents as a hard mass, and frequently spreads hematogenously.[173] Anaplastic carcinomas have fulminant courses and rarely complicate pregnancy, as they occur most commonly in women over 50 years of age. Medullary carcinomas can occur in association with the multiple endocrine neoplasia type II syndrome (medullary thyroid carcinoma, pheochromocytoma, and parathyroid adenoma) are bilateral and only once have been reported in pregnancy.[177]

Fine-needle aspiration biopsies are used to diagnose thyroid cancer in pregnancy.[178] Radionuclide scans are contraindicated in pregnancy because of the theoretical risk of destroying the fetal thyroid. Fine-needle aspiration biopsy is associated with a false-negative rate of only 6%.[179]

Since the overwhelming number of thyroid cancers presenting in pregnancy are histologically well differentiated, there is no reason to terminate pregnancy or avoid future pregnancies.[180] Pregnancy does not appear to influence the course of thyroid cancer.[67,181] Thyroid suppression therapy may be administered until delivery, regardless of the trimester in which the cancer was diagnosed.[173] Patients should undergo prompt surgery if metastases develop in regional lymph nodes during suppression therapy or the tumor is fixed to surrounding tissue and enlarges during suppression therapy. A subtotal thyroidectomy is usually performed, and ^{131}I should be administered postpartum to avoid the surgical complication of permanent hypoparathyroidism.[182] Extensive surgery should be avoided during pregnancy, as there is a chance of miscarriage occurring as a result of extensive surgery.[183]

Patients diagnosed in the first two trimesters of pregnancy to have a medullary carcinoma should undergo prompt total thyroidectomy and prophylactic neck dissection, whereas those diagnosed in the third trimester can await fetal maturity before definitive surgery. One must be aware of the risk of having a concurrent pheochromocytoma. Standard therapy for undifferentiated carcinomas is a total thyroidectomy and radiation therapy.[185] Prolonged survival has been achieved by combining chemotherapy, in particular doxorubicin, in combination with radiation therapy.[185]

ADRENAL TUMORS

Pheochromocytoma is the most common tumor rising in the adrenal gland in pregnancy. In the past it has been associated with a high maternal mortality (58%) and fetal mortality (55%).[68] However, Harper and colleagues reviewed the literature from 1980 to 1987 and presented 47 cases with pheochromocytoma diagnosed in pregnancy.[185] The overall mortality was 17% and fetal loss was 26%. The importance of antenatal diagnosis was established, as maternal mortality was zero and fetal loss was 15% when the diagnosis was made in pregnancy. Donegan had previously reported on 128 patients with pheochromocytoma in pregnancy reported through 1980 and found that only three of 128 tumors were malignant.[68] Characteristic symptoms associated with pheochromocytoma are episodic hypertension, headaches, anxiety, palpitations, sweating, and congestive heart failure. Supine hypertension with normal blood pressure in the sitting or erect position is characteristic of pheochromocytoma and may be secondary to the gravid uterus pressing on the tumor.

Computed tomography scans and arteriography have been replaced by magnetic resonance imaging for studying pregnant patients suspected of having a pheochromocytoma, because MRI does not result in fetal exposure to ionizing radiation. Magnetic resonance imaging may be used to confirm the presence, laterality, and location of the tumor.[186] Figure 76-6 shows a pheochromocytoma diagnosed at Yale–New Haven Hospital by magnetic resonance imaging in a 25-week-pregnant patient. The pheochromocytoma was removed surgically without disturbing the pregnancy. Provocative tests should not be performed, because these might lead to maternal fatality.[187] Further laboratory confirmation of the diagnosis of pheochromocytoma can be achieved by confirming elevated 24-hour urine collection levels of catecholamines, vanillylmandelic acid (VMA), and metanephrines.

The management of pheochromocytoma has been surgical in the first two trimesters and delivery by cesarean section followed by tumor resection in the third trimester.[69] Medical management of the disease includes preoperative α-adrenergic blockade with oral phenoxybenzamine, to lower the blood pressure, and propranolol to reduce the heart rate and prevent arrhythmias through the β-adrenergic receptor blockade.[188,189] Stenstrom and Swolin have recommended using alpha receptor blocking agents for the treatment of patients diagnosed to have pheochromocytomas in the second and third trimester and delaying surgery until fetal viability is accomplished.[190] Armaroli and colleagues also reported on the successful management of a mother managed in this fashion.[191] Lyons and Colmorgen managed a patient throughout her entire pregnancy with α-adrenergic blockade.[192] She had been demonstrated to have an extra-adrenal pheochromocytoma prior to conception. The pregnancy itself was successfully carried to 35 weeks gestation, at which time a cesarean section was performed. Thus, successful medical management using α-adrenergic blockade is a possibility for patients with pheochromocytoma diagnosed in pregnancy.

PARATHYROID CARCINOMA

One case of a parathyroid carcinoma complicating pregnancy has been reported.[193] That patient presented with acute pancreatitis at 31 weeks gestation, underwent a left parathyroidectomy, subsequently delivered a viable infant, and then had an additional pregnancy.[193]

URINARY TRACT MALIGNANCIES

KIDNEY TUMORS

Renal cell carcinoma is the most common malignancy rising in the urinary tract in pregnancy. Titings and colleagues reviewed 37 cases of renal tumors, 22 of which were renal cell carcinoma.[194] Hematuria is the most common presenting symptom. Nephrectomy with or without radiation therapy is standard treatment. It is recommended that the nephrectomy be performed promptly in pregnancy except for patients diagnosed in the third trimester when surgery is delayed until fetal maturity is achieved. Renal cell carcinoma confined to the kidney has an associated 5-year survival of 60%,

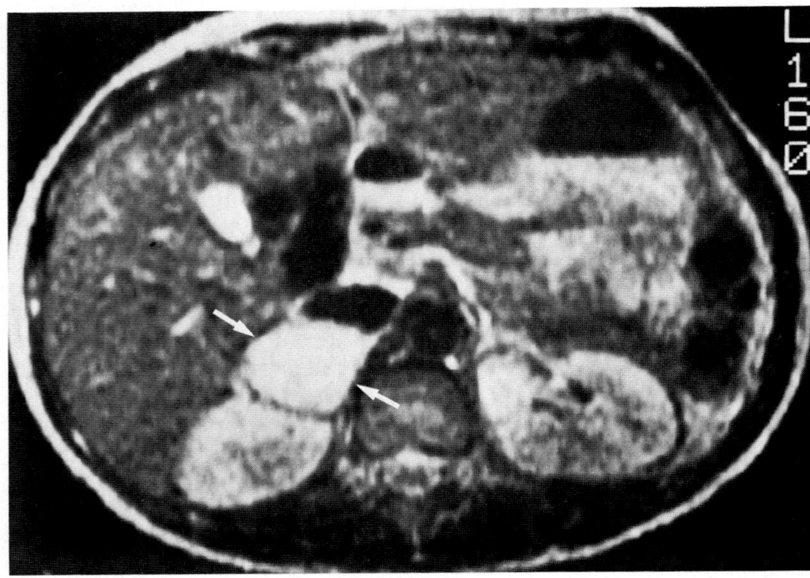

FIGURE 76–6. Pheochromocytoma in a pregnant patient. The right adrenal mass (arrows) is very high signal intensity on this T2-weighted image, consistent with a diagnosis of pheochromocytoma. (Courtesy Dr R Kier.)

whereas the overall survival for renal cell carcinoma is about 30% to 50%.[195] Well-differentiated carcinomas respond much better than anaplastic carcinomas. Spontaneous regression of metastases has not been consistently observed followed nephrectomy.[195] Other malignancies arising in kidneys include tubular adenomas, angioepitheliomas, hamartomas, and Wilms' tumors.[194]

BLADDER CANCERS

Bladder cancers have only infrequently been reported in pregnancy.[196–198] The histologic distribution is similar to that in the non-pregnant state, with an overwhelming majority being transitional cell carcinoma followed by squamous cell and adenocarcinomas. Standard treatment of superficial, well-differentiated bladder cancers is fulguration. Management of deeply invasive cancer requires radiation therapy followed by partial or complete cystectomy. The diagnosis of a bladder cancer in early pregnancy requires therapeutic abortion if radiation therapy is necessary. Patients diagnosed late in pregnancy may delay treatment until fetal viability is achieved. A 54% 3-year survival of early-stage cancer (stages 0, A, and B1) is reported, whereas deep-invasion stages (B2 and C) are associated with a 42% 3-year survival.[199]

URETHRAL CANCERS

A case of a squamous cell carcinoma arising in the urethra has been reported in pregnancy.[200] A case of a low-grade urethral adenocarcinoma diagnosed in the second trimester of pregnancy was managed expectantly.[201] Definitive treatment, radiation therapy, and local excision were not performed until after term and a vaginal delivery,[201] and the patient was alive and disease-free 7 years following diagnosis.

CENTRAL NERVOUS SYSTEM TUMORS

Central nervous system tumors rarely complicate pregnancy.[202] Patients present with headaches and visual disturbances. Magnetic resonance imaging allows for rapid evaluation without radiation exposure. Patients with infratentorial lesions have a particularly poor prognosis. The overall maternal mortality for patients with central nervous system tumors is 60%. Therapeutic abortions have been recommended for patients diagnosed in the first trimester to have malignant brain tumors because of the rapid course of such tumors. Elevated cerebrospinal fluid pressure requires surgical decompression, and steroids are given to reduce cerebral edema. Spinal cord tumors presenting in pregnancy may be diagnosed through magnetic resonance imaging, and decompression procedures should be promptly performed.[203]

REFERENCES

1. Sokal JE, Lessmann EM. Effect of cancer chemotherapeutic agents on the human fetus. JAMA 1960;172:151.
2. Benedet JL, Boyes DA, Nichols TM, et al. Colposcopic evaluation of pregnancy patients with abnormal cervical smears. Br J Obstet Gynecol 1976;84:517.
3. Silverberg E, Boring CC, Squire TS. Cancer statistics, 1990. CA 1990;40:9.
4. Haas JF. Pregnancy in association with a newly diagnosed cancer: a population based epidemiologic assessment. Int J Cancer 1984;34:229.
5. Potter JF, Schoeneman M. Metastasis of maternal cancer to the placenta and fetus. Cancer 1970;25:380.
6. Csapo AI, Pulkkinen MD, Weist WG. Effects of leutectomy and progesterone replacement in early pregnant patients. Am J Obstet Gynecol 1973;115:759.
7. Goodlin RC. Importance of the lateral position during labor. Obstet Gynecol 1971;37:698.
8. Eckstein K, Marx GF. Aortocaval compression and uterine displacement. Anesthesiology 1974;40:92.
9. Roberts RB, Shirley MA. Reducing the risk of acid aspiration during cesarean section. Anesth Analg 1979;53:859.
10. Bailey H, Bragg HJ. Effects of irradiation on fetal development. Am J Obstet Gynecol 1923;5:461.
11. Brill AB, Forgotson EH. Radiation and congenital malformations. Am J Obstet Gynecol 1964;90:1149.
12. Muller HJ. Artificial transmutation of the gene. Science 1927;66:84.
13. Orr JW Jr, Shingleton HM. Cancer in pregnancy. Curr Prob Cancer 1983;8:1.
14. Wallack MK, Wolf JA Jr, Bedwinek J, et al. Gestational carcinoma of the female breast. Curr Prob Cancer 1983;7:1.
15. Brent RC. The effect of embryonic and fetal exposure to x-ray, microwaves, and ultrasound: counseling the pregnant and nonpregnant patient about these risks. Semin Oncol 1989;16:347.
16. Dekaban A. Abnormalities in children exposed to x-irradiation during various stages of gestation: tentative timetable of radiation injury to the human fetus. Part I. J Nucl Med 1968;9:471.
17. Nicholson HD. Cytoxic drugs in pregnancy. J Obstet Gynecol Br Commonw 1968;75:307.
18. Sweet DL, Kinzie J. Consequences of radiotherapy and antineoplastic therapy for the fetus. J Reprod Med 1976;17:241.
19. Doll DC, Ringenberg S, Yarbro JW. Antineoplastic agents and cancer. Semin Oncol 1989;16:337.
20. Aviles A, Diaz-Maqueo JC, Torra V, Garcia EL, Guzman R. Non-Hodgkin's lymphomas and pregnancy: presentation of 16 cases. Gynecol Oncol 1990;37:335.
21. Reynoso EE, Shepherd FA, Messner HA, et al. Acute leukemia during pregnancy: the Toronto leukemia study group experience with long-term follow-up of children exposed in utero to chemotherapeutic agents. J Clin Oncol 1987;5:1098.
22. Aviles A, Niz J. Long-term follow-up of children born to mothers with acute leukemia during pregnancy. Med Pediatr Oncol 1988;16:3.
23. Redmond GP. Physiologic changes during pregnancy and their implications for pharmacologic treatment. Clin Invest Med 1985;8:317.
24. Wan SH, Huffman DH, Azarnoff DL, et al. Effect of route of administration and effusions on methotrexate pharmacokinetics. Cancer Res 1974;34:3487.
25. Pirani BBK, Campbell DM, MacGillivray I. Plasma volume in normal first pregnancy. J Obstet Gynecol Br Commonw 1973;80:884.
26. Muckcow JC. The fate of drugs in pregnancy. Clin Obstet Gynecol 1986;13:161.

27. Powis G. Anticancer drug pharmacodynamics. Cancer Chemother Pharmacol 1985;14:177.
28. Krepart GV, Lotocki RJ. Chemotherapy during pregnancy. In: Allen HH, Nisker JA, eds. Cancer in pregnancy. Mt Kisco, NY: Futura Publishing, 1986:69.
29. Sieber SM, Adamson RH. Toxicity of antineoplastic agents in man: chromosomal aberrations, antifertility effects, congenital malformations, and carcinogenic potential. Adv Cancer Res 1985;22:57.
30. Milunsky A, Graef JW, Gaynor MF. Methotrexate-induced congenital malformation. J Pediatr 1968;72:790.
31. Warkany J. Aminopterin and methotrexate: folic acid deficiency. Teratology 1978;17:353.
32. Willemse PHB, vd Sijde R, Sleijfer DT. Combination chemotherapy and radiation for stage IV breast cancer during pregnancy. Gynecol Oncol 1990;36:281.
33. Garber JE. Long-term follow-up of children exposed in utero to antineoplastic agents. Semin Oncol 1989:16:437.
34. Sindu RK, Hawkins DF. Corticosteroids. Clin Obstet Gynecol 1981;8:383.
35. Mulvihill JJ, McKeen EA, Rosner F, et al. Pregnancy outcome in cancer patients. Cancer 1987;60:1143.
36. Jones RT, Weinterman BH. MOPP (nitrogen mustard, vincristine, procarbazine and prednisone) given during pregnancy. Obstet Gynecol 1979;54:477.
37. Lowenthal RM, Funnell CF, Hope DM, et al. Normal infant after combination chemotherapy including teniposide for Burkitt's lymphoma in pregnancy. Med Pediatr Oncol 1982;10:165.
38. Barber HRK. Fetal and neonatal effects of cytotoxic agents. Obstet Gynecol (Suppl) 1981;58:41.
39. Collaborative Group of Antenatal Steroid Therapy. Effect of antenatal dexamethasone administration on prevention of respiratory distress syndrome. Am J Obstet Gynecol 1981;141:276.
40. Wright JR, Richart RM. Role of human papilloma virus in the pathogenesis of genital tract warts and cancer. Gynecol Oncol 1990;37:151.
41. Stone ML, Weingold AB, Sall S. Cervical carcinoma in pregnancy. Am J Obstet Gynecol 1965;93:479.
42. Sall S, Rini S, Pineda A. Surgical management of invasive carcinoma of the cervix in pregnancy. Am J Obstet Gynecol 1974;118:1.
43. Kinch RA. Factors affecting the prognosis of cancer of the cervix in pregnancy. Am J Obstet Gynecol 1961;82:43.
44. Creasman WT, Rutledge FN, Fletcher GH. Carcinoma of the cervix associated with pregnancy. Obstet Gynecol 1970;36:495.
45. Seltzer V, Sall S, Castadot M, et al. Glassy cell cervical carcinoma. Gynecol Oncol 1979;8:141.
46. Hacker NF, Berek JS, LaGasse LD, et al. Carcinoma of the cervix associated with pregnancy. Obstet Gynecol 1982;59:735.
47. Turner WA, Gallup DG, Talledo OE, et al. Neuroendocrine carcinoma of the uterine cervix complicated by pregnancy. Case report and review of the literature. Obstet Gynecol (Suppl) 1986;67:80.
48. Kier R, McCarthy SM, Scoutt LM, Viscarello RR, Schwartz PE. Pelvic masses in pregnancy: MR imaging. Radiology (in press).
49. Schwartz PE. Cancer in pregnancy. In: Gusberg SB, Shingleton HM, Deppe G, eds. Female genital cancer. New York: Churchill Livingstone, 1988;725.
50. Thompson JD, Caputo TA, Franklin EW, et al. The surgical management of invasive cancer in pregnancy. Am J Obstet Gynecol 1975;121:853.
51. Dudan RC, Yon JF, Ford JR Jr, et al. Carcinoma of the cervix and pregnancy. Gynecol Oncol 1973;1:283.
52. Prem KA, Makowski EL, McKelvey JL. Carcinoma of the cervix associated with pregnancy. Am J Obstet Gynecol 1966;95:99.
53. Gordon AN, Jensen R, Jones HW III. Squamous carcinoma of the cervix complicating pregnancy: recurrence in episiotomy after vaginal delivery. Obstet Gynecol 1989;73:850.
54. Sardi JE, Guillermo R, DiPaola MD, et al. A possible new trend in the management of the carcinoma of the cervix uteri. Gynecol Oncol 1986;25:139.
55. Anderson JM. Mammary cancer and pregnancy. Br Med J 1979;1:1124.
56. Applewhite RR, Smith LR, DiVincenti F. Carcinoma of the breast associated with pregnancy and lactation. Am Surg 1973;39:101.
57. Haagensen CD. Carcinoma of the breast in pregnancy. In: Haagersen CD, ed. Disease of the breast. 2nd ed. Philadelphia: WB Saunders, 1971.
58. Max MH, Klamer TW. Breast cancer in 120 women under 35 years old. Ann Surg 1984;50:23.
59. Byrd BF, Bayer DS, Robertson JC, et al. Treatment of breast tumors associated with pregnancy and lactation. Ann Surg 1962;155:940.
60. Donegan WL. Mammary carcinoma and pregnancy. Major Prob Clin Surg 1967;5:170.
61. Durodola JI. Burkitt's lymphoma presenting during lactation. Int J Obstet Gynecol 1976;14:225.
62. Jones DED, d'Avignon MB, Lawrence R, et al. Burkitt's lymphoma: obstetrics and gynecologic aspects. Obstet Gynecol 1980;56:533.
63. O'Donnell JR, Farrell MA. Acute myelogenous leukemia with bilateral mammary gland involvement. J Clin Pathol 1980;33:547.
64. Peters MV, Meakin JW. The influence of pregnancy in carcinoma of the breast. Prog Clin Cancer 1965;1:471.
65. Nugent P, O'Connell TX. Breast cancer and pregnancy. Arch Surg 1985;120:1221.
66. Holdaway IM, Mason BH, Kay RG. Steroid hormone receptors in breast tumors presenting during pregnancy or lactation. J Surg Oncol 1984;25:38.
67. Bunkers ML, Peters MV. Breast cancer associated with pregnancy or lactation. Am J Obstet Gynecol 1963;85:312.
68. Donegan WL. Cancer in pregnancy. CA 1983;33:194.
69. Greene FL. Gestational breast cancer: a ten-year experience. South Med J 1988;81:1509.
70. Peters MC. The effect of pregnancy in breast cancer. In: Forest APM, Kunkler PB, eds. Prognostic factors in breast cancer. Baltimore: Williams & Wilkins, 1968:65.
71. Ribeiro GG, Palmer MK. Breast carcinoma associated with pregnancy: a clinician's dilemma. Br Med J 1977;2:1524.
72. Rosemond GP, Maier WP. The complication of pregnancy on breast cancer. In: Breast cancer: early and late. Chicago: Year Book Medical Publishers, 1970:227.
73. King RM, Welch JS, Martin JK, et al. Carcinoma of the breast associated with pregnancy. Surg Gynecol Obstet 1985;160:228.
74. Gallenberg MM, Loprinzi CL. Breast cancer and pregnancy. Semin Oncol 1989;16:369.
75. Denoix P. Treatment of malignant breast tumors. Rec Results Cancer Res 1970;31:83.
76. Bush H, McCredie JA. Carcinoma of the breast during pregnancy and lactation. In: Allen HH, Nisker JA, eds. Cancer in pregnancy. Mt Kisco, NY: Futura Publishing, 1986:91.
77. Bonadonna G, Valagussa P. Dose-response effect of adjuvant chemotherapy in breast cancer. Engl J Med 1981;304:10.
78. Donegan WL. Breast cancer and pregnancy. Obstet Gynecol 1977;50:244.
79. Weinreb JC, Lowe TW, Santo-Ramos R, et al. Magnetic resonance imaging in obstetric diagnosis. Radiology 1985;154:157.
80. Chung A, Birnbaum SJ. Ovarian cancer associated with pregnancy. Obstet Gynecol 1973;41:211.

81. Schwartz PE. Combination chemotherapy in the management of ovarian germ cell malignancies. Obstet Gynecol 1984;64:564.
82. Schwartz PE, Morris J Mcl. Serum lactic dehydrogenase, a tumor marker for dysgerminoma. Obstet Gynecol 1988;72:511.
83. Bast RC Jr, Klug TL, St John E, et al. A radioimmuno-assay using a monoclonal antibody to monitor the course of epithelial ovarian cancer. N Engl J Med 1983;309:883.
84. Schwartz PE, Chambers SK, Chambers JT, et al. Circulating tumor markers in the monitoring of gynecologic malignancies. Cancer 1987;60:353.
85. Niloff JM, Knapp RC, Schaetzl E, et al. CA 125 antigen levels in obstetrics and gynecologic patients. Obstet Gynecol 1985; 64:703.
86. Bianchi UA, Sartori E, Favall G, et al. New trends in treatment of ovarian dysgerminoma. Gynecol Oncol 1986;23:246.
87. Dgani R, Shoham Z, Atar E, Zosmer A, Lancet M. Ovarian carcinoma during pregnancy: a study of 23 cases in Israel between the years 1960 and 1984. Gynecol Oncol 1989;33:326.
88. Chamber JT, Merino MJ, Kohorn EI, Schwartz PE. Borderline ovarian tumors. Am J Obstet Gynecol 1988;159:1088.
89. Young RC, Walton LA, Ellenburgss, et al. Adjuvant therapy in stage I and stage III epithelial ovarian cancer: results of two prospective randomized trials. N Engl J Med 1990;322:1021.
90. Malone JM, Gershenson DM, Creasy RK, et al. Endodermal sinus tumor of the ovary associated with pregnancy. Obstet Gynecol (Suppl) 1986;68:86.
91. Malfetano JH, Goldkrand JW. Cis-platinum combination chemotherapy during pregnancy for advanced epithelial ovarian cancer. Obstet Gynecol 1990;75:545.
92. Karlen JR, Akbari A, Cook WA. Dysgerminoma associated with pregnancy. Obstet Gynecol 1979;53:330.
93. Gershensen DM, Morris M, Cangir A, et al. Treatment of malignant germ cell tumors of the ovary with bleomycin, etoposide, and cisplatin. J Clin Oncol 1990;8:715.
94. Zinser JW, Ramirez-Gayton JL, Lara F, Garcia-Rodriguez F, Dominguez-Malagon HR. Ovarian dysgerminoma (D) treated with cisplatin (P) and cyclophosphamide (C). Report of 15 cases. Proceed ASCO 1990;9:163.
95. Metz SA, Day TG, Pursell SH. Adjuvant chemotherapy in a pregnant patient with endodermal sinus tumor of the ovary. Gynecol Oncol 1989;32:371.
96. Kim DS, Park MI. Maternal and fetal survival following surgery and chemotherapy of endodermal sinus tumor of the ovary during pregnancy: a case report. Obstet Gynecol 1989;73:503.
97. Christman JE, Teng NNH, Lebovic GS, Sikic BI. Delivery of a normal infant following cisplatin, vinblastine, and bleomycin (PVB) chemotherapy for malignant teratoma of the ovary during pregnancy. Gynecol Oncol 1990;37:292.
98. Schwartz PE. Sex cord stromal tumors of the ovary. In: Piver S, ed. Ovarian cancer. London: Churchill Livingstone, 1986:251.
99. Young RH, Dudley AG, Scully RF. Granulosa cell, Sertoli-Leydig cell and unclassified sec cord-stromal tumors associated with pregnancy. A clinicopathological analysis of thirty-six cases. Gynecol Oncol 1984;18:181.
100. Colombo N, Sessa C, Landoni F, et al. Cisplatin, vinblastine and bleomycin combination chemotherapy in metastatic granulosa cell tumor of the ovary. Obstet Gynecol 1986;67:265.
101. Desforges JF, Rutherford CJ, Piro A. Hodgkin's disease. N Engl J Med 1979;301:1212.
102. Chapman RM, Sutcliffe SV, Malpas JS. Cytotoxic-induced ovarian failure in women with Hodgkin's disease. I. Hormone function. JAMA 1979;242:1877.
103. Smith RBW, Sheehy TW, Rothberg H. Hodgkin's disease and pregnancy. Arch Intern Med 1958;102:777.
104. Sweet DL, Jr. Malignant lymphoma: implications during the reproductive years and pregnancy. J Reprod Med 1976;17:198.
105. Tawil E, Mercier JP, Dondavino A. Hodgkin's disease complicating pregnancy. J Can Assoc Radiol 1985;36:133.
106. Ward FT, Weiss RB. Lymphoma and pregnancy. Semin Oncol 1989;16:397.
107. Sutcliffe SB, Wrigley PFM, Peto J, et al. MVPP chemotherapy regimen for advanced Hodgkin's disease. Br Med J 1978;1:679.
108. Devita VT, Simon RM, Hubbard SM, et al. Curability of advanced Hodgkin disease with chemotherapy. Ann Intern Med 1980;92:587.
109. Mitchell MS, Capizzi RL. Neoplastic disease. In: Burrow GN, Ferris TF, eds. Medical complications during pregnancy. Philadelphia: WB Saunders, 1982:510.
110. Timothy AR, Sutcliffe SBJ, Lister TA, et al. The management of stage IIIA Hodgkin's disease. Int J Radiat Oncol Biol Phys 1980;6:135.
111. Sutcliffe SB, Chapman RM. Lymphomas and leukemias. In: Allen HH, Nisker JA, eds. Cancer in pregnancy. Mt Kisco, NY: Futura Publishing, 1986:135.
112. Meruk ML, Green JP, Nussbaum H, et al. Phantom dosimetry study of shaped colbalt-60 fields in treatment of Hodgkin's disease. Radiology 1968;91:554.
113. Steiner-Salz D, Yahalon J, Samuelov A, et al. Non-Hodgkin's lymphoma associated with pregnancy. A report of 6 cases with a review of the literature. Cancer 1985;56:2087.
114. Armitages JD, Feagler JR, Skoog DP. Burkitt's lymphoma during pregnancy with bilateral breast involvement. JAMA 1977;237:151.
115. Armon PJ. Burkitt's lymphoma of the ovary in association with pregnancy: two case reports. Br J Obstet Gynaecol 1976;83:169.
116. Miller TP, Jones SE. Chemotherapy of localized histiocytic lymphoma. Lancet 1979;1:358.
117. Devita VT, Jr, Chabner B, Hubbard SP, et al. Advanced diffuse histiocytic lymphoma, a potentially curable disease. 1975; 1:248.
118. Ortega J. Multiple agent chemotherapy including bleomycin for non-Hodgkin lymphoma during pregnancy. Cancer 1977; 40:2829.
119. Falkson HC, Simson IW, Falkson G. Non-Hodgkin's lymphoma in pregnancy. Cancer 1980;45:1679.
120. Nantel S, Parboosingh J, Poon MC. Treatment of an aggressive non-Hodgkin lymphoma during pregnancy with MACOP-B chemotherapy. Med Pediatr Oncol 1990;18:143.
121. Steiner-Salz D, Yahalom J, Samuelov A, et al. Non-Hodgkin's lymphoma associated with pregnancy. A report of six cases, with a review of the literature. Cancer 1985;56:2087.
122. Ioachim HL. Hodgkin's lymphoma in pregnancy. Three cases and review of the literature. Arch Pathol Lab Med 1985;109:803.
123. Yahia C, Hyman GA, Phillips LL. Acute leukemia and pregnancy. Obstet Gynecol Surv 1958;13:1.
124. Hoover BA, Schumacher HR. Acute leukemia in pregnancy. Am J Obstet Gynecol 1966;96:316.
125. Caligiuri MA, Mayer RJ. Pregnancy and leukemia. Semin Oncol 1989;16;388.
126. Roy V, Gutteridge CN, Hysenbaum A, Newliand AC. Combination chemotherapy with conservative obstetric management in the treatment of pregnant patients with acute myeloblastic leukemia. Clin Lab Haematol 1989;11:171.
127. Henderson EJ. Acute leukemia: general considerations. In: Williams WJ, Beutler E, Erslev AJ, Rundles RW, eds. Hematology. 2nd ed. New York: McGraw-Hill, 1977:108.
128. McLain CR Jr. Leukemia in pregnancy. Clin Obstet Gynecol 1974;17:185.
129. Moloney WC. Management of leukemia in pregnancy. Ann NY Acad Sci 1964;114:857.
130. McCulloch PB, Dent PB. Melanoma. In: Allen AA, Nisker JA,

eds. Cancer in pregnancy. Mt Kisco, NY: Futura Publishing, 1986:205.

131. McNamny DS, Moss AL, Pocock PV, Briggs JC. Melanoma and pregnancy: a long-term follow-up. Br J Obstet Gynaecol 1989;96:1419.

132. Wong JH, Sterns EE, Kopald KH, Nizze JA, Mortan DL. Prognostic significance of pregnancy in stage I melanoma. Arch Surg 1989;124:1227.

133. Colbourn DS, Nathanson L, Belilos E. Pregnancy and malignant melanoma. Semin Oncol 1989;16:377.

134. Fisher RI, Neifeld JP, Lippman ME. Estrogen receptors in human malignant melanoma. Lancet 1976:2:337.

135. Houghton A, Flannery J, Viola MV. Malignant melanoma of the skin occurring during pregnancy. Cancer 1981;48:407.

136. Clark WH, From L, Bernardino EA, et al. The histogenesis and biologic behavior of primary malignant melanomas of skin. Cancer Res 1969;29:705.

137. Broslow AL. Tumor thickness, level of invasion and node dissection in stage I cutaneous melanoma. Ann Surg 1975;182:572.

138. Byers T, Graham S, Swanson M. Parity and colorectal cancer risk in women. J Natl Cancer Inst 1982;69:1059.

139. Barber HRK, Brunschwig A. Carcinoma of the bowel. Am J Obstet Gynecol 1968;100:926.

140. Zaridze DG. Environmental etiology of large bowel cancer. J Natl Cancer Inst 1983;70:389.

141. Girard RM, Lamarche J, Baillot R. Carcinoma of the colon associated with pregnancy. Report of a case. Dis Colon Rectum 1981;24:473.

142. Allen HH, Nisker JA. Colorectal cancer in pregnancy. In: Allen HH, Nisker JA, eds. Cancer in pregnancy. Mt Kisco, NY: Futura Publishing, 1986:281.

143. Lamerz R, Ruider H. Significance of CEA determinations in patients with cancer of the colon-rectum and the mammary glands in comparison to physiological states in connection with pregnancy. Bull Cancer 1976;63:575.

144. O'Leary JA, Pratt JH, Symmonds RE. Rectal carcinoma in pregnancy. A review of 17 cases. Obstet Gynecol 1967;30:862.

145. Gamberdella FR. Pancreatic cancer in pregnancy. A case report. Am J Obstet Gynecol 1984;149:15.

146. Boyle JM, McLeod ME. Pancreatic cancer presenting as pancreatitis in pregnancy. Case report. Am J Gastroenterol 1979;70:371.

147. Garner PR, Tsang R. Insulinoma complicating pregnancy presenting with hypoglycemic coma after delivery. A case report and review of the literature. Obstet Gynecol 1989;73:847.

148. Mentgen CN, Moeller DD, Klotz AP. Protection by pregnancy. Zollinger-Ellison syndrome. J Kansas Med Sco 1974;260:56.

149. Waddell WR, Leosons AS, Zuidema GO. Gastric secretory and other laboratory studies on two patients with Zollinger-Ellison syndrome. N Engl J Med 1979;260:56.

150. Skokos CK, Lipshitz J. Adenocarcinoma of the stomach associated with pregnancy. J Tenn Med Assoc 1982;75:103.

151. Sims EH, Schlater TL, Sims M, et al. Obstructing gastric carcinoma complicating pregnancy. J Natl Med Assoc 1980;72;21.

152. Bowers RH, Walters W. Carcinoma of the stomach complicated by pregnancy. Report of an unusual case. Minn Med 1958;41:30.

153. Goncalves CS, Pereira FE, deVargas PR, et al. Hepatocellular carcinoma $HB^{S}A^{S}$ positive in pregnancy. Arq Gastroenterol 1984;21:75.

154. Devoe LD, Moosa AR, Levin B. Pregnancy complicated by an extrahepatic biliary tract carcinoma. J Reprod Med 1983;28:153.

155. Binstock M, Sondak VK, Herd J, Reimnitz C, Lindsay K, Brinkman C, Roslyn JJ. Adenocarcinoma in a choledochal cyst during pregnancy. A case report and guidelines for management. Surgery 1988;103:588.

156. Kempson RL, Pokorny GE. Adenocarcinoma of the endometrium in women aged forty and younger. Cancer 1968;21:650.

157. Sandstrom RE, Welch WR, Green TH Jr. Adenocarcinoma of the endometrium in pregnancy. Obstet Gynecol (Suppl) 1979;53:73.

158. Zirkin HJ, Krugliak L, Katz M. Endometrial adenocarcinoma coincident with intrauterine pregnancy. A case report. J Reprod Med 1983;28:624.

159. Suzuki A, Konishi I, Okamura H, et al. Adenocarcinoma of the endometrium associated with intrauterine pregnancy. Gynecol Oncol 1984;18:261.

160. Hoffman MS, Cavanagh D, Walter TS, Ionata F, Ruffolo EH. Adenocarcinoma of the endometrium and endometrioid carcinoma of the ovary association with pregnancy. Gynecol Oncol 1989;32:82.

161. Scoscia A, Merino MJ, Haas M, Copel JA, Schwartz PE. Malignant mixed mullerian tumor of the uterus arising in associated with a viable gestation. Obstet Gynecol 1988;71:1047.

162. Schwartz PE, Naftolin F. Type 2 herpes simplex virus and vulvar carcinoma in situ. N Engl J Med 1981;305:517.

163. Lutz M, Underwood PB Jr, Rozier JC, et al. Genital malignancy in pregnancy. Am J Obstet Gynecol 1977;129:536.

164. Schwartz PE. Gynecologic cancer. In: Spittell JA Jr, ed. Clinical medicine. Philadelphia: Harper & Row, 1985:1.

165. Senekjian EK, Hubby M, Herbst AL. Clear cell adenocarcinoma (CCA) of the cervix and vagina associated with pregnancy. Gynecol Oncol 1985;20:250.

166. Eisenfeld AJ, Schwartz PE, Morris J Mcl. Estrogen and progesterone receptors in vaginal and uterine adenocarcinomas following estrogen use. Gynecol Oncol 1980;10:63.

167. Cantin J, McNeer GP. The effect of pregnancy on the clinical course of sarcoma of the soft somatic tissues. Surg Gynecol Obstet 1967;125:28.

168. Lysyj A, Berquist JR. Pregnancy complicated by sarcoma. Report of two cases. Obstet Gynecol 1963;21;506.

169. Huvos AG, Butler A, Bretsky SS. Osteogenic sarcoma in pregnant women. Prognosis, therapeutic implications, and literature review. Cancer 1985;56:2326.

170. Simon MA, Phillips WA, Bonfiglio M. Pregnancy and aggressive or malignant bone tumors. Cancer 1984;53:2564.

171. Haerr RW, Pratt AT. Multiagent chemotherapy for sarcoma diagnosed during pregnancy. Cancer 1985;56:1028.

172. Rawlinson KF, Zurbrow AB, Harris MA, et al. Disseminated Kaposi's sarcoma in pregnancy: a manifestation of acquired immune deficiency syndrome. Obstet Gynecol (Suppl) 1984;63:2.

173. Stuart GCE, Temple WJ. Thyroid cancer in pregnancy. In: Allen NH, Nisker JA, eds. Cancer in pregnancy. Mt Kisco, NY: Futura Publishing, 1986;191.

174. Cady B, Sedwick CE, Meissner WA. Changing clinical, pathologic, therapeutic and survival patterns in differentiated thyroid carcinoma. Ann Surg 1976;184:541.

175. Cady B, Sedwick CE, Meissner WA. Risk factor analysis in differentiated thyroid cancer. Cancer 1979;43:810.

176. Rosen IB, Walfish PG. Pregnancy as a predisposing factor in thyroid neoplasia. Arch Surg 1986;121:1287.

177. Chodander CM, Abhyankar SC, Deodhar KP. Sipple's syndrome (multiple endocrine neoplasia) in pregnancy. (Case report) Aust NZ J Obstet Gynecol 1982;22:243.

178. Goldman MH, Tisch B, Chattock AG. Fine needle biopsy of a solitary nodule arising during pregnancy. J Med Soc NJ 1983;80:525.

179. Schwartz AE, Nieburgs HE, Davis TF. The place of fine needle biopsy in the diagnosis of nodules of the thyroid. Surg Gynecol Obstet 1982;155:54.

180. Rosvoll RV, Winship T. Thyroid carcinoma and pregnancy. Surg Gynecol Obstet 1965;121:1039.

181. Hill CS, Clark RL, Wolf M. The effect of subsequent pregnancy in patients with thyroid carcinoma. Surg Gynecol Obstet 1966;122:1219.
182. Farrar WB, Cooperman M, James AG. Surgical management of papillary and follicular carcinoma of the thyroid. Am Surg 1980;192:701.
183. Cunningham MP, Slaughter DP. Surgical treatment of diseases of the thyroid gland in pregnancy. Surg Gynecol Obstet 1970;131:486.
184. Kim JH, Leeper RD. Treatment of anaplastic giant and spindle cell carcinoma of the thyroid gland with combination adriamycin and radiation therapy. Cancer 1983;52:954.
185. Harper MA, Murnaghan GA, Kennedy L, et al. Pheochromocytoma in pregnancy. Five cases and a review of the literature. Brit J Obstet Gynaecol 1989;96:594.
186. Greenberg M, Moawad AH, Wieties BM, et al. Extraadrenal pheochromocytoma: detection during pregnancy using MR imaging. Radiology 1986;161:475.
187. Ellison GT, Mansberger JA, Mansberger AR Jr. Malignant recurrent pheochromocytoma during pregnancy. Case report and review of the literature. Surgery 1988;103:484.
188. Fusge TL, McKinnon WMP, Geary WL. Current surgical management of pheochromocytoma during pregnancy. Arch Surg 1980;115:1224.
189. Leak D, Carroll JJ, Robinson DC, et al. Management of pheochromocytoma during pregnancy. Obstet Gynecol Surv 1977;32:583.
190. Stenstrom G, Swolin K. Pheochromocytoma in pregnancy. Experience of treatment with phenoxybenzamine in three patients. Acta Obstet Gynecol Scand 1985;64:357.
191. Armaroli R, Simoni S, Artuso S, Mattioli G. Pheochromocytoma during pregnancy. Ital J Surg Sci 1989;19:75.
192. Lyons CW, Colmorgan GH. Medical management of pheochromocytoma in pregnancy. Obstet Gynecol 1988;72:450.
193. Hess HM, Dickson J, Fox HE. Hyperfunctioning parathyroid carcinoma presenting as acute pancreatitis in pregnancy. J Reprod Med 1980;25:83.
194. Tydings A, Weiss RR, Lin JH, et al. Renal cell carcinoma and mesangiocapillary glomerulonephritis. NY State J Med 1978;78:1950.
195. Abrams HL. Tumors and cyst of the kidneys. In: Hamburger J, Crosnier J, Grunfeld JP, eds. Nephrology. Vol 2. New York: John Wiley & Sons, 1979:1043.
196. Stanhope CR. Management of the obstetric patient with malignancy. In: Sciarra JJ, ed. Gynecology and obstetrics. Vol 2. New York: Harper & Row, 1984:1.
197. Keegan GT, Forkowitz MJ. Transitional cell carcinoma of the bladder during pregnancy. A case report. Texas Med 1982;78:44.
198. Cruikshank SH, McNellis TM. Carcinoma of the bladder in pregnancy. Am J Obstet Gynecol 1983;145:768.
199. MacKenzie AR. Supervoltage x-ray therapy of bladder cancer. Cancer 1965;18:1255.
200. Smith FR. Effect of pregnancy of malignant tumors. Am J Obstet Gynecol 1937;34:616.
201. Severino LJ, Brockunier A, Davidson MM. Adenocarcinoma of the urethra during pregnancy. Report of a case. Obstet Gynecol (Suppl) 1077;50:22.
202. Carmel PN. Neurologic surgery in pregnancy. In: Barber HRK, ed. Surgical disease in pregnancy. Philadelphia: WB Saunders, 1974:207.
203. Apuzzio J, Pelosi MA, Ganesh W, et al. Spinal cord tumors during pregnancy. Int J Gynecol Obstet 1980;17:608.

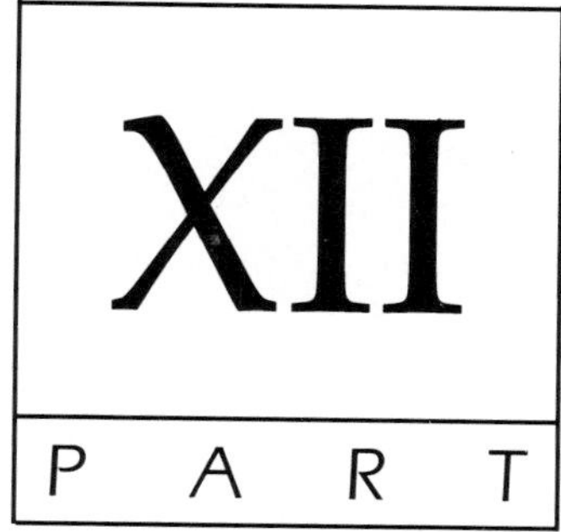

MEDICO-SOCIAL CONSIDERATIONS IN PREGNANCY

77

CHAPTER

SEXUALITY IN PREGNANCY AND THE PUERPERIUM

Philip M. Sarrel and Ulla M. Sellgren

Pregnancy and the puerperium are times of change in sexual function calling for understanding and professional guidance. For the woman herself there are biological changes that affect sexual desire, sexual response, and sexual behavior. Long-established sexual patterns are usually disrupted. Some couples experience sex problems, such as dyspareunia, loss of desire, and nonorgasmic response in the woman as well as erectile difficulties, ejaculatory dysfunction, and desire disorders in the male partner. Such problems can begin or become aggravated during pregnancy or the puerperium and continue permanently thereafter. For many others pregnancy can be the best time in their lives, from a sexual point of view as, freed from the fear of pregnancy and helped by hormonal effects, there may be greater spontaneity and more relaxed and satisfying sex. For these couples the weeks and months following delivery can be a tremendous letdown sexually.

Some investigators report that sex during pregnancy can be harmful to the pregnant woman and the fetus. Others disagree and have shown that sex during pregnancy can be beneficial. Less has been reported on this aspect of sex and pregnancy, but there is some evidence to suggest that sexual activity through pregnancy has psychological benefits and may also benefit pregnancy outcome. In this chapter we shall try to summarize a fairly extensive, albeit nondefinitive, medical literature on the risks and benefits of sex during pregnancy. Our goal will be to develop some reasonable guidelines for behavior that can be recommended to couples.

The role of the health care provider is to understand changes in sexuality that occur in pregnancy and the postpartum period, assess possible risks of sexual activity, offer the opportunity for couples to ask their questions and express their concerns about sex, provide information about sexual function, and help with sexual dysfunction. The information in this chapter should help prepare the health care provider to provide such counseling.

HISTORICAL AND CULTURAL ASPECTS OF SEX AND PREGNANCY

The ways in which different ancient societies and primitive cultures have developed beliefs and attitudes about the pregnant woman are interesting and form a matrix of human understanding from which many of our modern attitudes and behaviors have developed. Most cultures have expressed rules of conduct regarding sex for the pregnant woman. We feel it would be of some interest for us to describe some of these more well-known "nonscientific" understandings.

In primitive cultures there is a wide range of codes for sex during pregnancy. Ford and Beach reviewed more than 60 primitive cultures and found rules ranging from total restriction to none.[1] There are cultures where coition must be restricted during the last two pregnancy months "because semen is thought to impair the eyesight of the unborn child or even choke it to death." Some cultures forbid intercourse once fetal movements are experienced. Alouf and Barglow report that the ancient Hindus believed that semen helped nourish the fetus, and they encouraged intercourse during pregnancy. In ancient Persia women were sexually taboo after the fourth month of pregnancy, and intercourse before the 40th day after delivery was punished by death for both the man and the woman.[2]

Ford and Beach, in their analysis of sexual behavior during pregnancy in different primitive cultures, conclude that "the increasing number of peoples forbidding intercourse towards the end of pregnancy tends to suggest that the majority of societies have become convinced, as a result of centuries of experience, that sexual activities just prior to labor may have unfortunate consequences."[1] It should be noted that when these reflections were made, the frequency of stillbirths and prematurity leading to perinatal deaths was much higher than today, even in developed countries.

In the postpartum period most cultures accept intercourse after 1 to 2 months. In the Talmudic literature a woman was "unclean" 33 days after delivering a male child and 66 days after delivering a female child. Some primitive cultures recommend longer abstinence, but usually as a method for family planning or allowing sufficient nutrition for the newborn.[1]

In Victorian times the ideal situation during pregnancy was sexual "continence," especially for the woman. Sexuality for a pregnant woman was thought to jeopardize the health of the child both physically and mentally. For example, coition during pregnancy was thought to predispose children to epilepsy.[3] There was also the suggestion that abstinence would result in more intelligent children—and that mental retardation would result from a sexually active woman.

The Victorians also expressed concern that the mother would, by her sexual activity, influence the child to develop abnormal sexual instincts. There was a belief that the character, morals, and even physical appearance of the child depended on parental behavior during pregnancy. The Victorians believed that the soul of the fetus was developing while in the womb. The concept of "soul-gardening" evolved in which it was believed that the mother's thoughts and views—whatever was on her mind—would have an effect on the fetus. This passed over to the postpartum period, so that "gratification of passion" would cause "transmission of libidinal tendencies" to the child."[3]

The early 20th-century manuals were part of a social change, a striving to separate middle-class aspirations from those of the working class. One can wonder how the discrepancy between pretensions and reality survived for such an extended period of time. In perhaps the most widely read marriage manual, by Van de Velde, the author forbade "marital embraces" not only for the health of the mother and the fetus but also for the health of marriage—a fact that he later regretted.[3] Still, couples continued to be sexually active. For example, in Sweden, there is a special word for intercourse that could induce or facilitate labor (*faerdknaepp*). Coitus for induction of labor is recommended in a number of manuals for the public.[4]

In Western industrialized cultures there is a lack of codes for sexual behavior in pregnancy and the postpartum period. Before the era of modern contraceptives women were expected to become pregnant once they started having vaginal intercourse. There was no decision making. Young couples could turn to parents or relatives for advice. With rapid changes of attitudes and technology there is a lack of models, and a lack of references for sexual behavior in pregnancy and the postpartum period. Medicine has given arbitrary recommendations without facts to support them. As a result, couples are often confused. With increasing medicalization of normal pregnancies, there is an increased need for the support of nurturing and comforting that physical and psychological intimacy can supply. In this sense, relating sexually is an important part of the means of ensuring that the parents will continue to function as a unit after the child is born.

SEXUAL FUNCTION AND PREGNANCY

Sexual response, sexual behavior, sexual desire, and sexual dysfunction are four aspects of sexual function in which changes during pregnancy may be of clinical significance.

SEXUAL RESPONSE

Human sexual response is a complex function involving the interplay of biological, psychological, interpersonal, and sociocultural factors. The physiology of sex response involves the peripheral and central nervous systems and the cardiovascular and neuromuscular systems. Changes occur in both genital and extragenital tissues and organs. Although the effects of sex response on uterine contractions, uterine blood flow, and cervical dilatation are of greatest interest to the obstetrician, the other changes that occur during sex response are worth knowing, as they may also influence the course of pregnancy and the sense of well-being of the pregnant woman and her partner.

The physiologic changes of sex response can be considered to occur in four sequential phases that together constitute a sex response cycle. The phases, described by Masters and Johnson, are called excitement, plateau, orgasm, and resolution.[5] Within seconds of an arousing stimulus the excitement phase begins with evidence of increased peripheral blood flow and vasocongestion. Alpha wave activity in the brain is increased, and there is a slight increase in heart rate. With continuing stimulation the plateau phase begins, a time of both peripheral vasocongestion and increasing muscle tension. The plateau phase ends with the onset of orgasm, a series of muscle contractions involving the whole body and more specifically the perineal musculature and the uterus. The contractions, in the non-pregnant state, are each 0.8 seconds in duration and may consist of three to eight in a single orgasm. Multiple orgasm can and does occur during which there can be a sequence of contractions that can last for a half hour or more. Specific brain wave discharge during orgasm is thought to derive from the hippocampus, with slow, delta-type wave discharge imposed upon the increased alpha wave activity.[6]

Various chemical changes occur during sex response that can affect uterine blood flow and muscle tension. Serum vasoactive intestinal peptide (VIP) is increased during sexual stimulation, most likely reflecting local release from terminals in the genital tract.[7] The vagina has a very dense innervation of VIP-containing nerve fibers. VIP increases myometrial and vaginal blood flow and inhibits smooth muscle activity in the female reproductive tract.[8] Increased VIP is seen in peripheral venous plasma toward term and during labor and has been related to increased oxytocin near term. Oxytocin has been shown to increase peripheral VIP concentration.[9] The role of VIP in labor and delivery is a subject of continuing research interest. Oxytocin release during sexual stimulation has been reported.[10] In connection with this, it has been shown that intrauterine pressure increases during orgasm.[11]

Effects of sexual stimulation on vaginal fluids are thought to be of significance during the fertilization process.[12] During sexual arousal there is an increase in the quantity of fluid produced; the pH rises; Po_2 in the vaginal wall is elevated; vaginal fluid sodium, glycerol, and stearic acid increase; and chloride decreases. These changes are believed to help maintain a vaginal environment conducive to sperm survival and inhibitory of pathogenic organisms. The most prominent differences are seen in hypoestrogenic states, in which there is an overall decrease in blood flow and diminished vaginal secretion.[13] In addition, progesterone decreases vaginal blood flow and secretion.[14] Because there are such dramatic changes in estrogen and progesterone secretion during pregnancy, one could imagine effects on vaginal blood flow and secretions during sexual stimulation. It is known that vaginal secretions are greater in quantity during sexual stimulation in pregnancy. Whether these secretions are in some way protective is hypothetical. The studies of specific chemical changes seen in nonpregnant women have not repeated on pregnant women.

There are numerous studies in which pregnant women have reported their sexual experience to research investigators. However, we are aware of only one published physiologic study in which direct observations were reported, that of Masters and Johnson.[15]

Masters and Johnson have reported findings from studying sexual physiology in six pregnant women. The women were observed in each trimester and during the postpartum period. Four of the women had been studied previously, before they had become pregnant, providing longitudinal data that could be used for comparison. Of clinical interest are the following observations:

1. In the first trimester
   a. Breast engorgement of pregnancy plus the vasocongestion of sex response can result in severe breast tenderness. Pain is frequently localized in the nipples and areolar tissue.
   b. External and internal genital vasocongestion is much greater than in the non-pregnant state. Vaginal secretions are increased and preorgasmic congestion can narrow the vaginal lumen by 75% or more. Leakage of urine with orgasm was not unusual. The resolution phase was markedly delayed, leaving residual vulvar and vaginal vasocongestion for many hours after sexual activity.
2. In the second trimester
   a. Breast complaints decreased.
   b. Cramping and aching in the lower abdomen and low backache during and after orgasm were noted.
   c. Two of the women had their first experiences of multiple orgasm during the second trimester. The series of orgasms was seen to persist for a half hour or more on two occasions.
3. In the third trimester
   a. Breast and vulvar changes during arousal are not as great because of the already-congested baseline state at this stage of pregnancy.
   b. Vaginal lubrication is at its maximum during these weeks.
   c. With orgasm the uterus can go into spasm lasting as long as a minute and accompanied by a transient decline in fetal heart rate. The resolution stage takes even longer in the third trimester, with residual vasocongestion continuing the sense of sexual arousal.
4. Postpartum
   a. The women were studied at 4 to 5 weeks and at 8 to 9 weeks postpartum. At these times sexual response was slowed, with decreased vaginal lubrication and vasocongestion. Three of the women were nursing. Two nursing women experienced milk ejection in uncontrolled spurts during sexual stimulation. Orgasm was reduced in intensity and duration but was reported to be satisfying. At 3 months postpartum sexual response in these women had returned to the prepregnancy patterns.

Masters and Johnson are the first to agree that a study of only six women is insufficient for drawing conclusions and giving advice. However, for more than 20 years their study has been the only work of its kind available, and several of the observations may prove relevant in individual circumstances. For example, the hypersensitivity of the breasts, the heavy vaginal secretion, the loss of urine, and the uterine contractions that they report to be normal concomitants of sex response during pregnancy could be alarming to a woman or her partner. Knowing about these possibilities could be reassuring. The same could be said about postpartum discomfort and lack of responsiveness, because couples could conclude that their experiences of the early postpartum months could be permanent.

Sex response patterns of pregnancy and the puerperium, in which direct observation was not done, have been reported in quite a few studies since the mid-1960s. In addition to the six women directly observed during sexual activity, Masters and Johnson reported findings from 101 women who volunteered to provide information about their sexual function.[15] Interviews were held during each trimester and postpartum. Nulliparas reported a decrease in sexual responsiveness during the first trimester and an increase during the second trimester. Multiparas also noted increased responsiveness in the second trimester, with little change in responsivity in the first 3 months. In the third trimester both nulliparous and multiparous women reported a decrease in sexual tension, although their capacity to respond sexually appeared unaltered. Falicov interviewed 19 primigravidas prospectively through pregnancy and the puerperium. In a well-controlled and carefully carried out study, her findings appear to confirm those of Masters and Johnson in reporting a decrease in responsiveness in the first trimester, an increase in the second trimester and early third trimester, and an inhibited response in the latter part of the third trimester.[16] Other researchers, however, have reported a steady decrease in frequency of orgasm as pregnancy progresses.[17–19] From these studies it is clear that orgasm does occur during pregnancy and can continue to occur through the third trimester, although it is less frequent as the end of pregnancy draws near. Women can reach previously unattained levels of sexual response during pregnancy but may also experience a decrease from previous experiences.

Sex response during the postpartum period can vary tremendously. In the Masters and Johnson study, most of the women reported decreased responsivity through the third postpartum month. Despite their lack of response, all the women resumed coital activity within 8 weeks of delivery.

Some women experienced rapid return, within 2 to 3 weeks, of non-pregnant sexual responsivity. The 24 women who were breast-feeding reported the highest level of postpartum sexual interest and responsivity. Most of the women reported sexual stimulation induced by suckling their infants. Three women experienced orgasm while breast-feeding.

Ryding's Swedish study is unusual in comparing orgasmic frequency before, during, and after pregnancy.[20] In her study population, the following percentages of the 50 women had been orgasmic with intercourse before pregnancy: always or almost always, 62%; over half the time, 20%; less than half the time, 16%; and never, 26%. During pregnancy 52% were always orgasmic, 20% were so over half the time, and 12% were orgasmic less than half the time; among the women who had never been orgasmic, 40% experienced orgasm for the first time. At 3 months postpartum, only 48% of the women were always orgasmic and 16% were orgasmic over half the time. Over one fourth of the women were once again not having orgasm at all.

These studies give us a much greater data base for sharing sex information with pregnant couples. As a result, it seems reasonable that we inform our patients with regard to expectations of sex response during pregnancy (eg, that some women who have never experienced orgasm may have orgasm for the first time, most likely during the second trimester, that orgasmic frequency and intensity may increase in mid-pregnancy and diminish in the last few weeks, that uterine contractions can persist for hours after sexual activity, and that the postpartum period is naturally a time of diminished responsivity).

SEXUAL DESIRE

Among the more common problems that non-pregnant women and their husbands present for sex therapy are lack of desire or aversion to sexual activity. In a pregnant population, loss of desire or sexual aversion, although troubling, is usually considered normal and transitory. In their studies, Masters and Johnson found that sexual desire fluctuated during the course of pregnancy, with greatest interest occurring during the second trimester.[15] In addition, Masters and Johnson found that almost 20% of husbands lost interest in sex by the third trimester. Reasons cited by the women included fatigue, physical discomfort, and concern about the well-being of the fetus. Husbands' loss of interest reflected concern about the well-being of both mother and child and the antierotic effect of the women's physical appearance. Decline in sexual interest by the third trimester is the most predictable pattern observed in almost every other study we reviewed for this chapter. In Ryding's study, diminished desire was the main reason women stopped having intercourse in the 2 to 3 months prior to birth.[20] She also found that husbands' loss of desire was a significant issue.

Despite the decrease in libido, it is common for pregnant women to desire to be touched. For example, Hollender and McGehee's study at Vanderbilt University explored the issue of "the wish to be held" during pregnancy.[21] Comparing pregnant and non-pregnant patients, they found pregnant women two to three times more likely to report an increase in the wish to be held, a desire that did not correlate with increased sexual desire. Unfortunately, it is easy for the need to be held and an invitation to do so to be misunderstood as initiation of sexual activity. The result can be engaging in sex that is not desired or being unresponsive sexually. This can be confusing both to the partner and to the woman.

Although loss of desire during pregnancy appears to be expected by most, persistence of diminished desire in the postpartum period may not be so readily acceptable. In a prospective study, Ryding found one third of the women to experience significant loss of desire through the third postpartum month. Most often associated with dyspareunia, the problem was seen both in women who had delivered vaginally and in those who had cesarean sections, suggesting that psychological as well as biological factors were involved. Engaging in sexual intercourse despite discomfort, inadequate response, and lack of desire is apparently not unusual and has been cited as a cause of more deeply ingrained sexual dysfunctions later. Ryding cites a Norwegian study by Brudal, who found that one third of couples interviewed 1 year after childbirth were dissatisfied with sex. We will discuss sexual dysfunction and pregnancy later in this chapter.

SEXUAL BEHAVIOR

Coital frequency and alternative sexual behaviors have been the subject of numerous investigations. In a study of 260 women interviewed postpartum, Solberg and colleagues reported a decrease in coital and noncoital (self-stimulation, manual, and oral–genital stimulation by partner) sexual behavior.[18] An increase in the use of the side-by-side position correlated with a decrease in the male-above coital position. Reamy and coworkers also reported increased use of the side-by-side and rear-entry position for intercourse.[19] Although some studies report increased coital activity during the second trimester,[15,16] this activity is rarely as frequent as that before pregnancy. Most studies—for example, those of Lumley,[22] Morris,[23] and Tolor and DiGrazia[24] —show ever-decreasing frequency trimester by trimester. In Ryding's study, prior to pregnancy 30% of the women had intercourse more than three times per week and 70% had intercourse at least one to two times per week. By the second trimester 10% of the women had coital frequencies of three times per week or more, 45% had frequencies of one to two times per week, and the remaining 45% had frequencies of one to two times per month or less. By the third trimester almost 40% of the women were coitally inactive, with another 35% having intercourse only one to two times per month. Still, 5% of the women had coital frequencies of three times per week or more and 20% had frequencies of at least one to two times per week.[20] Ryding cites loss of desire as the predominant factor in sexual abstinence. Included among her study subjects were four women who became averse to sex early in pregnancy and remained inactive throughout. The fear that sex in pregnancy could be harmful kept one woman in Ryding's group from having any intercourse. She had become pregnant after 11 years of infertility. This reaction, especially among previous infertility patients, is represented in most of the studies. It is an issue that emphasizes the need for the health care provider to know and understand the meaning of sexual activity for the individual woman and her partner before making recommendations during pregnancy.

There is little question that the majority of women continue to have sexual intercourse at least one to two times per week during pregnancy, at least through the second trimester. In Ryding's study just over 50% continued intercourse at least one to two times per week until the third trimester. In the Steege and Jelovsek study of 1500 women attending the Duke University Obstetrical Clinic, 55% to 70% of married women and 25% to 45% of unmarried women continued intercourse frequencies of two times a week or more while pregnant.[25] As in the Ryding study, Steege and Jelovsek found just over 25% of the women were abstinent.

Although most studies have not inquired about sexual activity other than coitus, there are some exceptions. Ryding found that 20% of the women and 40% of their husbands responded to orgasm in noncoital sexual activity while practicing coital abstinence during pregnancy.[20] In the Masters and Johnson study "among 77 women abstaining from coitus because of their obstetrician's advice, 49 of the women continued noncoital sexual activity in the last trimester."[15]

The postpartum period can be a difficult time from a sexual viewpoint. Although many obstetricians recommend abstinence only long enough for the episiotomy or cesarean incisions to heal, most couples refrain from intercourse for at least 2 to 3 weeks, if not for the usually suggested 6 weeks. Masters and Johnson found that over half of the women in their study were concerned about an extended period of abstinence and its effects on their husbands. Several women resumed intercourse by 3 weeks, mainly because of their husband's wish. Ryding found that 12% resumed intercourse in the first 4 weeks; 54%, within 5 to 8 weeks; and 16%, after 9 to 12 weeks. One out of six women had not resumed intercourse by 3 months, presenting sex problems that included sexual aversion as well as severe dyspareunia.[20] Fear of repeat pregnancy was also a factor. Before the first postpartum coitus, 40% of the women participated in noncoital sexual activities.

Two problems relating to sexual behavior have been described in the medical literature. Aronson and Nelson reported fatal air embolism as a complication of oral–genital stimulation during which air was blown into the vagina.[26] The second problem is more a social issue—that of husbands having extramarital affairs when faced with male anxieties about sex during pregnancy as well as the restrictions imposed by their wives and their obstetricians or midwives. Of 79 men interviewed by Masters and Johnson, 31 had withdrawn from sexual activity with their pregnant wives for a variety of reasons. Twelve men had extramarital sex during the last part of the pregnancy and another six in the postpartum period.[15] The possibility of extramarital sex should be kept in mind when considering the advisability of sexual relations during pregnancy and when evaluating sexual dissatisfaction.

SEXUAL DYSFUNCTION

As mentioned earlier, pregnancy can be one of the most problem-free and satisfying sexual times in a couple's life. It can also be a time of change in which decreased sexual desire, response, and activity become the norm. Sexual dysfunctions among non-pregnant women are usually categorized as problems of sexual desire (ie, lack of desire and aversion), problems having to do with orgasm (ie, nonorgasmic response or painful orgasms), and problems of dyspareunia. Although desire phase and orgasmic phase changes are normal during pregnancy, it is of some interest that dyspareunia is not common. Ryding reported that five out of 50 women experience pain with penetration during pregnancy.[20] Steege reported a 2.5% incidence of significant dyspareunia, with another 6.9% of the women having an occasional problem. In the Duke study, over 80% had no dyspareunia at all.[25] Masters and Johnson commented primarily on breast pain during sex when pregnant and did not mention dyspareunia.

Males can experience altered sexual function when their partners are pregnant. Loss of desire is the most common occurrence. As already mentioned, Masters and Johnson found that 20% of the men had lost sexual desire by the third trimester, and Ryding's and Falicov's observations are confirmatory. As to the occurrence of other male dysfunctions, such as premature ejaculation, ejaculatory inhibition, erectile difficulty, and dyspareunia, we have been able to find only anecdotal comments and no systematic inquiry.

The major concern with regard to sexual dysfunction is, as previously stated, the continuance of desire and excitement phase disorders and dyspareunia into the postpartum period. We have already mentioned Ryding's comment regarding persistent sexual difficulties in as many as one third of couples a year after pregnancy has been completed. Factors contributing to such dysfunction include the stress of new parenthood, the biological and psychological impact of a time of hormone deficiency, pregnancy and postpartum established patterns of sexual inadequacy, and a variety of fears associated with sex—a woman's fears of internal injury, a man's fear of causing pain, and the fears of both of another pregnancy or of inadequate performance.[27] When the pregnancy, delivery, or postpartum period has been complicated or the baby is not well or is a major source of anxiety, sex can fall among the lowest of priorities.

RISKS AND BENEFITS OF SEXUAL ACTIVITY DURING PREGNANCY

We have already discussed the fact that most pregnant women remain sexually active through a substantial part of their pregnancy, if not all of it. Within medicine there have been diverse opinions about the safety of continuing sexual relations with respect to both mother and fetus. On the one hand, there are a number of published studies in which no detrimental effects could be detected. On the other, there are case reports as well as epidemiological studies that indicate that bleeding, infection, fetal distress, and prematurity can be caused by sexual activities. There are also the rare isolated cases already mentioned, in which air embolus induced by oral–genital stimulation has led to maternal mortality.[26] In that sense there is no question that sex can be harmful. But such instances are extremely rare. What, in fact, are the realities in the vast majority of pregnancies?

Beginning with the Pugh and Fernandez study published in 1953,[28] there are a series of investigations that conclude that coital activity is not associated with unfavorable perinatal outcomes.[18,29–32] The criticism raised against all these studies is that they were carried out retrospectively or involved too small a number of women. In response to this criticism, Klebanoff and colleagues analyzed data from the Collaborative Perinatal Project (CPP).[33] These data represent findings from a multicenter project in which 56,000 pregnant women were enrolled between 1959 and 1966. Information about coital activity was elicited at registration and at each prenatal visit, thus providing data before the outcome of the pregnancy was known. Klebanoff and colleagues studied the data from 39,217 first-study pregnancies, eliminating the repeat pregnancies of women who continued to participate in the CPP study. Data were also eliminated when there were no follow-up prenatal visits and when gestational age could not be determined from the records. Coital frequency decreased with advancing gestation, from 90% of women in the first trimester to 26% at 39 weeks. The authors found a "clear inverse association between coitus and early delivery. Women reporting *no coitus* at 28 to 29 weeks and 32 to 33 weeks were at higher risk of delivery during each week up to 37 weeks, both before and after the elimination of women with complications."[33] Coitus during pregnancy was not associated with either early delivery or increased perinatal mortality. Although it appeared that coitus was protective in some way, the authors did conclude that "coitus may simply be a marker of good general health."[33]

The preceding study as well as the others referred to contrast with reports indicating that sexual activity can cause harm. In a series of thoughtful and provocative papers, Goodlin documents an instance of fetal bradycardia associated with orgasm,[34] reports a case of premature separation of the placenta immediately following orgasm induced by masturbation,[35] and describes the practical difficulties in carrying out a truly scientific study of the risks and benefits of sex during pregnancy. One of the most important issues raised by Goodlin's observations is that any sexual activity that can lead to orgasm could have a negative effect on fetal heart rate and possibly lead to premature placental separation. Masters and Johnson, earlier, had reported fetal bradycardia during orgasm, noting that the effect was transitory and did not appear to affect perinatal outcome. The central issue is the effect of orgasm on fetal and maternal well-being, not the effect of coitus per se. We have cited many studies indicating the prevalence in pregnancy of noncoital as well as coital activity leading to orgasm. Therefore, as Goodlin warns, in situations of high-risk pregnancy where there is any question of compromised fetal oxygenation or of uterine instability or bleeding, one should advise against sexual stimulation of any kind. In the case report of placental separation following orgasm, we are told that the woman had previously been experiencing painful uterine contractions with sexual stimulation.

Goodlin also describes the positive aspects of encouraging sexual behavior in particular as a means of inducing labor near term in a healthy, uncomplicated pregnancy. He writes, "orgasm and breast massage are an effective means of inducing labor. When a patient has a ripe cervix, I continue to recommend either breast message or orgasm for elective induction. I find that if strong uterine contractions occur, the success rate for inducing labor is approximately 60%."[35] Goodlin was concerned that premature labor could result from orgasm and therefore advised abstention between the 28th and 34th weeks of gestation, especially if there was evidence of cervical ripening or a history of prematurity. The study by Klebanoff and colleagues would contradict such advice, as it actually showed that coital activity leads to longer pregnancies. It may be worth mentioning that one of us (PS) has completed an unpublished prospective study comparing pregnancy outcome and labor and delivery among women who remained sexually active through the last days of pregnancy with women who were sexually abstinent for at least a month prior to labor. There were 105 women in the abstinent group and 123 in the sexually active group. In each group there were three premature deliveries, between 28 and 32 weeks' gestation. However, two of the three women in the sexually active group who delivered between 28 and 30 weeks had babies who were in severe distress but did survive. Both women had previous histories of premature deliveries.

Infection caused by sexual intercourse is perhaps the main concern of those who are concerned about the detrimental effects of sex in pregnancy. Javert proposed an association between infection and abortion following coitus.[36] Sarrel and Pruett documented the presence of gonorrheal infection in abortion and premature rupture of membranes.[37] Goodlin also raised the possibility.[35] Perhaps the most controversial study is that of Naeye reported in the *New England Journal of Medicine* in 1979.[38] Analyzing data from the CPP, Naeye found a higher frequency of infection and increased perinatal mortality from infection when coitus once or more per week was reported during the month before delivery. In an editorial in the same issue, Herbst questioned the pathologic criteria for infection used by Naeye.[39] In addition, infection-related deaths were associated with congenital pneumonia and immaturity. These and other difficulties, discussed more fully by Perkins, have challenged the Naeye study.[40] Finally, using the same data base, Klebanoff and colleagues[33] did not find an association between perinatal mortality and coitus. Naeye had studied intercourse frequency in the last month, whereas Klebanoff and colleagues had data from throughout the pregnancy. In a more recent prospective study, Rayburn could not correlate prematurity with either intercourse or orgasm.[41] Mills confirms the Klebanoff finding of a lower incidence of prematurity in sexually active women.[29] In a 1989 report, Nielsen studied twin pregnancies in Zimbabwe and found that prematurity correlated not with intercourse but with the mother's low weight and the number of prenatal visits.[42]

Should we ignore the concern about the possibility of sex-induced infection leading to prematurity and increased perinatal mortality? We do not think so. We live in an age of growing awareness of the significance of both clinical and subclinical pelvic infection. An increasing incidence of teen-age pregnancy means more pregnancies in a population in which pathogenic organisms are more prevalent. In some areas we are facing an increasing HIV-infected population among whom it is extremely important that safe sex measures be taken during pregnancy. The ethical–social problems of advising HIV-risk or already HIV-positive women are presented by Dorfman.[43] In addition, more sophisticated study of amniotic fluid, exemplified in the work of Romero and co-workers, is helping us to understand better the role of subclinical infection in intrauterine growth retardation and prematurity.[44]

For the moment, we believe that the need remains for a prospective study of sexual function combined with technological advances in maternal and fetal evaluation before more definitive conclusions can be reached about the risks of sexual activity. A reliable sexual investigative technique should be coupled with ultrasound determinations of fetal growth and development, bacteriologic and viral studies during pregnancy, and parturition and monitoring of labor and delivery. In addition, the pioneering work of Masters and Johnson, and later of Goodlin, may one day be continued in order to document further the effects of sex response on fetal well-being and the course of labor.

This discussion of the risks of sex and pregnancy should be balanced by mentioning some of the benefits. Alouf and Barglow have discussed the positive psychological meanings of pregnancy with regard to a woman's sense of femininity and the special significance for couples of maintaining sexual intimacy during pregnancy.[2] As we have already mentioned, making love during pregnancy can be among the most satisfying of experiences. Abstinence, on the other hand, can be alienating at a time when it is so important for couples to maintain their bonds with each other and to be mutually supportive. Sex during pregnancy can include some of the most intense sexual responses, and some women experience their first orgasm at this time. Although some authors, most notably Klebanoff and colleagues[33] and Mills,[29] have reported a lower risk of prematurity in sexually active women, the full medical benefits of staying sexually active have yet to be delineated. For example, in this author's (PS) previously mentioned unpublished study, the women who remained sexually active had shorter labors and required less medication than those who had been abstinent.

CONCLUSION

The issues we have considered regarding sex and pregnancy have maintained a traditional focus on understanding the effects of sexual behavior and response on mother and fetus. In addition, we have extended concerns to include the mother's sexual partner. Change in sexual response, desire, and frequency are normal during pregnancy. There is a need to provide information about these changes to pregnant couples to help them enjoy the pleasures of sexual intimacy during pregnancy, understand the adjustments that need to be made, and recognize that most of the "problems" are transitory in nature. Special attention should be paid to explaining natural sexual limitations during the postpartum period. The few risks inherent in sexual activity during pregnancy should be explained and couples should be alerted to signals of sex-induced complications such as uterine pain or vaginal bleeding. Through listening to patients' sexual histories, assessing possible risks, and examining for infection or signs of early cervical dilatation, the health care provider can serve a counseling role that is individualized and helpful. Discussion of the sexuality findings we have presented is important in a time when pregnancy is being medicalized and technicalized. The sense of "my system works" is important for the woman who needs to trust her body in labor. Sexual history is often incomplete during pregnancy and delivery. Because complications may be related, such an omission is not acceptable. When sexual dysfunction is present, specific recommendations may prove helpful. If not, referral to an authority in sexual counseling can be made. We believe the development, in prenatal and postpartum health care, of a protocol to actively consider and deal with sexuality can prove to be helpful to the well-being of the entire family unit—mother, father, and the new child-to-be.

REFERENCES

1. Ford CS, Beach FA. Feminine fertility cycles: effects of pregnancy. In: Patterns of sexual behavior. New York: Harper & Row, 1951:213.
2. Alouf F, Barglow P. Sexual counseling for the pregnant and the postpartum patient. In: Sciarna JJ, ed. Gynecology and obstetrics. Vol 2, Chapter 96. New York: Harper & Row, 1981.
3. Haller JS, Haller RM. Responsibilities of motherhood. In: The physician and sexuality in Victorian America. New York: WW Norton, 1974:131.
4. Kitzinger S. Sex during pregnancy. In: Woman's experience of sex. London: Penguin, 1983:197.
5. Masters HH, Johnson VE. Female sexual response. In: Human sexual response. Boston: Little, Brown, 1966:27.
6. Sarrel PM, Foddy F, McKinnon JB. Investigation of human sexual response using a cassette recorder. Arch Sex Behav 1977;6(4):341.
7. Ottesen B, Ulrichsen H, Fahrenkrug J, et al. Vasoactive intestinal polypeptide and the female genital tract: relationship to reproductive phase and delivery. Am J Obstet Gynecol 1982;143:414.
8. Goodnough JE, O'Dorisio TM, Friedman CI, Kim MH. Vasoactive intestinal polypeptide in tissues of the human female reproductive tract. Am J Obstet Gynecol 1979;134:579.
9. Clark KE, Mills EG, Stys SS, Seeds AE. Effects of vasoactive polypeptides on the uterine vasculature. Am J Obstet Gynecol 1981;139:182.
10. Fox CA, Knaggs GS. Milk-ejection activity (oxytocin) in peripheral venous blood in man during lactation and in association with coitus. J Endocrinol 1969;45:145.
11. Fox CA, Wolff HS, Baker JA. Measurement of intravaginal and intrauterine pressures during human coitus by radio-telemetry. J Reprod Fertil 1970;22:243.
12. Sarrel PM. Human sexuality and infertility. In DeCherney AH, ed. Reproductive Failure. New York: Churchill Livingstone, 1986:73.
13. Semmens J, Wagner G. Estrogen deprivation and vaginal function in postmenopausal women. JAMA 1982;24:445.
14. Sarrel PM. Progestagens and blood flow. Int Proceed J 1989;1:266.
15. Masters HH, Johnson VE. Pregnancy and sexual response. In: Human sexual response. Boston: Little, Brown, 1966:141.
16. Falicov CJ. Sexual adjustment during first pregnancy and postpartum. Am J Obstet Gynecol 1973;117(7):991.
17. Perkins RD. Sexuality in pregnancy: what determines behavior? Obstet Gynecol 1982;59(2):189.
18. Solberg D, Butler BAJ, Wagner NN. Sexual behavior in pregnancy. N Engl J Med 1973;288(21):1098.
19. Reamy K, Daniell WC, White SE, Levine ES. Sexuality and pregnancy. J Reprod Med 1982;27(6):321.
20. Ryding EL. Sexuality during and after pregnancy. Acta Obstet Gynecol Scand 1984;63:679.
21. Hollender MH, McGeheee JB. The wish to be held during pregnancy. J Psychosom Res 1974;18:193.
22. Lumley J. Sexual feelings in pregnancy and after childbirth. Aust NZ J Obstet Gynecol 1978;18:114.
23. Morris NM. The frequency of sexual intercourse during pregnancy. Arch Sex Behav 1975;4(5):507.
24. Tolor A, DiGrazia PV. Sexual attitudes and behavior patterns during and following pregnancy. Arch Sex Behav 1976;5(6):539.
25. Steege JF, Jelovsek FR. Sexual behavior during pregnancy. Obstet Gynecol 1982;60(2):163.
26. Aronson ME, Nelson PK. Fatal air embolism in pregnancy resulting from an unusual sexual act. Obstet Gynecol 1967;30(1):127.
27. Coleman A, Coleman L. Earth father, sky father. Englewood Cliffs, NJ: Prentice-Hall, 1981:132.
28. Pugh WE, Fernandez FL. Coitus in late pregnancy. Obstet Gynecol 1953;2(6):636.
29. Mills JL, Harlap S, Harley EE. Should coitus in late pregnancy be discouraged? Lancet 1981;ii:136.
30. Zlatnik FJ, Burmeister LF. Reported sexual behavior in late pregnancy. J Reprod Med 1982;27(10):627.
31. Perkins RD. Sexual behavior and response in relation to complications of pregnancy. Am J Obstet Gynecol 1979;134(5):498.
32. Georgakopoulos DD, Mechleris D. Sex in pregnancy and premature labour. Br J Obstet Gynecol 1984;91(1):891.
33. Klebanoff MA, Nugent RP, Rhoads GG. Coitus during pregnancy: is it safe? Lancet 1984;ii:914.
34. Goodlin RC, Schmidt W, Creevy DC. Uterine tension and fetal heart rate during maternal orgasm. Obstet Gynecol 1972;39(1):125.
35. Goodlin RC. Can sex in pregnancy harm the fetus? Contemp Ob/Gyn 1976;8:21.
36. Javert CT. Role of the patients activities in the occurrence of spontaneous abortion. Fertil Steril 1960;11(6):550.
37. Sarrel PM, Pruett K. Symptomatic gonorrhea during pregnancy. Obstet Gynecol 1968;32(5):67.
38. Naeye RL. Coitus and associated amniotic-fluid infections. New Engl J Med 1979;301(22):1198.
39. Herbst AL. Coitus and the fetus. N Engl J Med 1979;301(22):1235.
40. Perkins RP. Sexuality during pregnancy. Clin Obstet Gynecol 1984;27(3):706.
41. Rayburn WF, Wilson EA. Coital activity and premature delivery. Am J Obstet Gynecol 1980;137(8):972.
42. Neilson J, Mutambira M. Coitus, twin pregnancy and preterm labor. Am J Obstet Gynecol 1989;160(2):416.
43. Dorfman SF. AIDS and pregnancy. The Female Patient 1989;4:86.
44. Romero R, Quintero R, Oyarzun E et al. Intraamniotic infection and the onset of labor in preterm premature rupture of the membranes. Am J Obstet Gynecol 1988;159(3):662.

78

CHAPTER

IMPORTANT PSYCHIATRIC PROBLEMS DURING PREGNANCY AND THE POSTPARTUM PERIOD

Jennifer I. Downey and Agnes H. Whitaker

Psychiatric problems are important to the obstetrician for three reasons. First, psychiatric disorder may contribute to noncompliance with prenatal care. Second, although pregnancy itself is not associated with excess risk for mental disorder, pregnancy complicates the routine management of psychiatric disorder. Third, during the first month postpartum, women are at markedly increased risk for serious, disabling mental disorder.

This chapter focuses on psychiatric problems that may confront the obstetrician both as primary caretaker of the mother and fetus and as a member of the neonatal care team. The chapter begins with a section on the recognition of psychiatric emergencies and proceeds to separate sections covering important distinctions in psychiatric diagnosis, psychiatric disorders during pregnancy, psychiatric disorders during the postpartum period, breast-feeding, and special management problems. These problems include parental grief following pregnancy loss, parental adjustment to the newborn with special needs, and impaired parenting, including the risk of infanticide. The chapter concludes with a summary of the obstetrician's role in the management of psychiatric problems.

THE RECOGNITION OF PSYCHIATRIC EMERGENCIES

Psychiatric emergencies are most likely to occur in the first month postpartum[1,2] but may arise at any point during the course of obstetric care. Four major conditions should be regarded as emergencies requiring immediate psychiatric consultation: delirium, psychosis, suicidal ideation, and homicidal ideation.

DELIRIUM

The term *delirium* refers to global cognitive impairment of acute onset. The essential features of delirium are disorganized thinking and a reduced ability both to shift and to focus attention. These deficits often manifest themselves as noncooperation with the clinical interview: the examiner must repeat questions and the patient answers in a rambling, irrelevant, or incoherent way or gives the same answer to different questions (perseveration). Other features include disorientation to time (common), place (common), or person (uncommon); perceptual disturbances in the form of misinterpretations, illusions, and hallucinations; memory impairment; increased or decreased psychomotor activity; disturbed sleep–wake cycle; and reduced level of consciousness. The patient typically appears perplexed and frightened and her speech is often pressured. The onset is usually abrupt (over hours to days). Symptoms fluctuate and may recede altogether for minutes or hours (so-called lucid intervals).[3]

Delirium represents a state of acute cerebral insufficiency, frequently confirmed by generalized slowing of background activity on the electroencephalogram[4] and should be regarded as a medical–psychiatric emergency.[5] Delirium may be due to endogenous factors (eg, hepatic encephalopathy) or exogenous factors (eg, drugs). The duration of delirium is usually less than a week. However, unless the underlying disorder is self-limited or is treated immediately, delirium may progress to coma, dementia, or death. Death may be due to the underlying disorder or to injuries incurred by falling out of bed or by attempting to flee from terrifying illusions, hallucinations, or imagined danger from other persons.[3]

PSYCHOSIS

The term *psychosis* refers to "gross impairment in reality testing and the creation of a new reality."[3] The essential features of psychosis are hallucinations and/or delusions. A hallucination is "a sensory perception without external stimulation of the relevant sensory organ." A delusion is "a false personal belief based on an incorrect inference about external reality" that is maintained despite evidence to the contrary.[3]

Psychosis may occur in a number of different psychiatric disorders, associated with delusions and/or hallucinations of characteristic content and organization. The obstetrician is most likely to be concerned with psychosis in five disorders: delirium, organic hallucinosis, organic delusional syndrome, schizophrenia-like psychoses, and affective psychoses (manic and depressive disorders with psychotic features).

In delirium, discussed earlier, delusions are usually fragmentary and based on misinterpretations of events in the environment (eg, physicians consulting at bedside are a murder team); hallucinations are most often visual. Whenever psychosis is accompanied by disorientation, delirium should be suspected.

In organic hallucinations, prominent, persistent, or recurrent hallucinations are present because of a specific organic factor.[3] In women of childbearing age, drug use is most likely to be the organic factor. The type of hallucination may provide a clue to the drug involved. For example, hallucinogens such as phencyclidine (PCP, or angel dust) tend to produce simple visual hallucinations, whereas alcohol tends to produce vivid, persistent visual or auditory hallucinations as well as tactile ones. Essential features of delirium are not present, and the patient may be aware that the hallucinations are not real. The patient usually does not have delusions.[3]

In organic delusional syndrome prominent delusions are present because of a specific organic factor. In women of childbearing age, drug use (eg, of amphetamines, cocaine, cannabis, and hallucinogens) is most likely to be the organic factor. Delusions of persecution are the most common. Essential features of delirium are not present. Hallucinations are not prominent.[3]

In schizophrenia-like psychoses, delusions are bizarre (eg, that one's thoughts are being broadcast; that one's thoughts are under the control of an external agency). Hallucinations are typically auditory (of a voice or voices) and sustained over time. Affect is often flat. Speech may be incoherent or hard to follow because of loosening of associations; however, unlike the delirious patient, the patient is typically oriented to place, time, and person.[3]

In a manic episode with psychotic features, delusions and hallucinations are typically concerned with the manic themes of inflated worth, power, knowledge, or special relationship to a deity or famous person. Persecutory or bizarre delusions may be present. The patient's mood is elevated, expansive, or irritable. Speech is pressured and may be hard to follow because of flight of ideas; unlike the delirious patient, the patient is typically oriented to place, time, and person.[3]

In a depressive episode with psychotic features, delusions and hallucinations are typically concerned with the depressive themes of personal inadequacy, guilt, disease, death, nihilism, or deserved punishment. Persecutory or bizarre delusions may also be present. The patient reports depressed mood and/or loss of all interest or pleasure. Agitation or extreme slowness of thought and action ("psychomotor retardation") may be present. The patient is oriented.[3]

Judgment is so seriously impaired in the presence of delusions or hallucinations that the obstetrician should be concerned about the risk for suicide or homicide. "Command" auditory hallucinations, in which a patient hears a voice directing her actions, are particularly serious.

SUICIDAL IDEATION

Unlike delirium and psychosis, occasional suicidal thoughts are within the realm of ordinary adult experience. However, suicidal ideation accompanied by hopelessness and a sense of foreclosure on other options for solving one's problems should be regarded as a clinical emergency. Suicide is a serious risk in delirium and other psychotic states because the patient is likely to act swiftly and with little or no warning. In patients who are lucid and whose reality testing is intact, suicidal ideation may be expressed passively ("I'd be better off dead") or actively ("I am thinking of ending my life"). It is important to inquire as to whether the patient has envisioned a method by which to take her own life, how long she has been thinking this way, and whether there is any history of suicide attempts. Beyond this the obstetrician should request psychiatric consultation as to the need for medication or hospitalization.

HOMICIDAL IDEATION

Occasional ideas of injuring or killing another person are within the realm of ordinary adult experience. Individuals with obsessive-compulsive disorder often suffer chronically from obsessive thoughts of committing violent acts but regard these thoughts as alien, strongly resist them, and rarely act on them. As with suicide, homicide is a serious risk in delirium and other psychotic states because the patient may act suddenly and without warning, often in response to command hallucinations. In general, the expression of homicidal thoughts should be taken at face value as a plea for immediate help. The obstetrician should request psychiatric consultation as to the need for hospitalization and application of the mandatory duty to warn potential adult victims and to protect potential child victims.[6]

MANAGEMENT OF PSYCHIATRIC EMERGENCIES

The obstetrician who observes or elicits these symptoms should request an immediate evaluation by a psychiatrist and at the same time contact a concerned family member. A delirious, psychotic, or hopeless individual is unlikely to follow through on a verbal referral, and the patient should not be left unsupervised while awaiting psychiatric evaluation. The psychiatrist will make the differential diagnosis of the emergency symptom(s), and advise the obstetrician about the need for hospitalization or psychotropic medication (see the sections on Psychotic Episode, Nonpsychotic Disorders, Postpartum Psychosis, and Nonpsychotic Postpartum Disorders later in this chapter).

IMPORTANT DISTINCTIONS IN PSYCHIATRIC DIAGNOSIS

A mental disorder is defined as "a behavioral or psychological syndrome that is associated with distress or disability."[3] It is useful for the obstetrician to be aware of certain broad distinctions in psychiatric diagnosis (psychotic versus nonpsychotic, organic versus functional) and of the multiaxial method for recording psychiatric diagnoses.

PSYCHOTIC AND NONPSYCHOTIC DISORDERS

Current classification systems recognize a broad division of mental disorders into psychotic and nonpsychotic disorders.[3,7] In psychotic disorders, as discussed earlier, there is a gross impairment in reality testing. In nonpsychotic disorders reality testing is intact. Nonpsychotic disorders of major importance to the obstetrician include major depressive disorder (without delusions or hallucinations), anxiety disorders, substance abuse disorders, and eating disorders.

ORGANIC AND FUNCTIONAL DISORDERS

Current classification systems also divide mental illness into organic and functional (nonorganic) disorders. An *organic* mental disorder is a psychological or behavioral abnormality associated with transient or permanent brain dysfunction,[3] as evidenced on clinical neurologic exam or laboratory tests (eg, EEG, diagnostic brain imaging). The dysfunction may be of primary CNS origin or may be due to medical illness or drug ingestion that secondarily affects brain functioning. Those organic psychotic disorders of most relevance to the obstetrician include delirium, organic hallucinosis, and organic delusional syndrome (discussed earlier). However, nonpsychotic organic mood, anxiety, and personality disorders have been described. A comprehensive review of psychiatric presentations of medical illness is to be found in Lishman.[8]

Functional disorders include distinctive abnormal behavioral and psychological syndromes that are not due to an identifiable organic factor or medical illness. These disorders are no less dependent on brain function.[3] For some disorders, such as schizophrenia, an organic factor is strongly suspected but cannot be demonstrated unequivocally with current technology. Most important, the term *functional* does not mean the disorder is imaginary, under the patient's control, due to weakness of character, or due primarily to psychosocial stress. The phenomenology of these syndromes is the special province of the psychiatrist.

It is important to rule out an identifiable organic basis for any abnormal behavior or psychological symptom. The diagnosis of organic brain syndrome of unknown etiology is appropriate under the following circumstances: the clinical picture is most consistent with that of an organic disorder (eg, delirium, dementia), but no organic etiology can be identified; and the consulting psychiatrist rules out a functional psychiatric disorder on the basis of history and presenting symptoms. A diagnosis of functional psychiatric disorder is made on positive evidence and is not a diagnosis of exclusion.

THE RECORDING OF PSYCHIATRIC DIAGNOSES

Although obstetricians use the International Classification of Diseases (ICD-9)[7] system of classification, psychiatrists in this country use Diagnostic and Statistical Manual of Mental Disorders (DSM III-R).[3] In the multiaxial system of DSM III-R, mental disorders are recorded on Axis I and Axis II. Axis II is limited to developmental disorders (including mental retardation) and personality disorders. Axis III is reserved for any current physical condition or medical disorder. The condition may be etiologic (as for organic psychiatric disorders), or it may not be etiologic but be relevant to the overall management of the case (eg, pregnancy, diabetes). Axis IV is used to rate the severity of psychosocial stressors (the birth of a first child rates as a "severe" stressor). Axis V is used to rate both current level of functioning and the highest level of adaptive functioning for at least a few months in the preceding year.

PSYCHIATRIC DISORDER DURING PREGNANCY

Attention on the part of the obstetrician to the patient's past psychiatric history and prompt referral when psychiatric disorder emerges serve both the mother and fetus well. Untreated psychiatric disorder may contribute to noncompliance with prenatal care, either because of denial of the pregnancy or because of general self-neglect and impaired functioning. Moreover, the more chronic the mother's mental disorder, the greater the incidence of delivery complications.[9] Prenatal maternal stress is also associated with increased incidence of both major and minor anomalies and difficult temperament in the infant.[10] Both obstetrician and patient need to be aware of the implications of pregnancy to the routine management of psychiatric disorder: even well-educated patients may not be aware of the potential teratogenic effects of certain psychotropic agents.

PSYCHOTIC PSYCHIATRIC DISORDER DURING PREGNANCY

Epidemiology of Psychotic Disorders During Pregnancy

The prevalence of psychotic psychiatric disorder among pregnant women does not differ from that among non-pregnant women of childbearing age.[11] Functional psychotic disorders such as schizophrenia and the affective disorders are relatively rare, occurring in less than 2% of women ages 18 to 44.[12] The prevalence of drug-induced psychosis among women in this age group is not known. There is no evidence that pregnancy increases the risk for a first psychotic episode. There is also no evidence that pregnancy protects against psychotic symptoms. In women with a prior history of functional psychosis, symptoms are more likely to worsen than to improve.[11]

Management of the Pregnant Patient With a History of Psychotic Disorder

The woman with a history of psychotic disorder who intends to become pregnant should consult in advance with both an obstetrician and a psychiatrist to evaluate (1) whether she should remain on medication during pregnancy and (2) the indications for prophylaxis against postpartum psychosis, a condition for which she is at increased risk. She should remain under the care of both an obstetrician and a psychiatrist for the duration of the pregnancy and for at least the first 3 months postpartum.

Patients with a history of schizophrenia and schizophrenia-like disorders will most likely have been treated with, and sometimes maintained on, either oral phenothiazine (eg, chlorpromazine, haloperidol, trifluoperazine) or IM injection of depot long-acting phenothiazine (eg, fluphenazine) or thioxanthenes (eg, flupentixol). Because of side effects associated with these medications, the patient may also have been treated with anticholinergic agents such as benztropine (for dystonic movements or extrapyramidal symptoms) or antihistamines such as diphenhydramine (for motor restlessness or akathisia).

When clinically possible, any neuroleptics and medications for side effects should be withdrawn. If there is history of recurrent episodes or chronic residual symptoms, then it may be necessary to continue a neuroleptic, at the minimal possible dosage, throughout the pregnancy. Choice of the specific neuroleptic must be made carefully, based on the patient's history of response and the likelihood of side effects. Because it is associated with a low risk of extrapyramidal side effects, thioridazine has often been chosen for pregnant patients. However, this must be balanced against the higher risk of orthostatic hypotension associated with this medication and the possibility of resultant utero-placental insufficiency.[13] Blood pressure requires close monitoring. Reports on the teratogenic effects of neuroleptics have been contradictory.[14] Neonates whose mothers received a neuroleptic in the 2 weeks prior to delivery show an increased incidence at birth of an extrapyramidal syndrome with tremors, hypertonia, weakness, and poor sucking and other primitive reflexes that may persist up to the age of 10 months.[15]

Because of the known physical and behavioral teratogenic effects of anticholinergics[16] and diphenhydramine,[17,18] it is advisable to withdraw any anticholinergic or antihistamine for the first 12 to 16 weeks of pregnancy and to readminister it only if necessary.

A woman who has recovered from a single episode of mania will usually be taking a neuroleptic, as described earlier, and/or lithium carbonate, either for continued control of manic symptoms or for prophylaxis. If she has had only one episode of mania, then it is reasonable to discontinue the lithium and the neuroleptic prior to conception. However, if she has had more than one episode or if the risk of relapse seems high, then maintenance of a neuroleptic during pregnancy may be indicated.

The use of lithium is usually contraindicated during pregnancy.[19] Lithium is teratogenic in the first trimester and is associated with an increased occurrence of cardiac defects, especially Ebstein's anomaly.[20,21]

Lithium readily equilibrates across the placenta. Maternal lithium plasma concentrations within the therapeutic range during the last trimester can result in signs of neonatal intoxication, including hypotonia and cyanosis. Neonatal euthyroid goiter has also been observed, but this is transient.[22] Therefore, lithium should ideally be withdrawn at least 1 month before conception or immediately after the patient is found to be pregnant. If lithium is necessary to help control otherwise unmanageable manic symptoms, it can be administered beginning in the second trimester. Shifts in fluid balance during pregnancy often require doubling of the lithium dose to achieve therapeutic blood levels. At delivery, however, renal clearance is reduced. To avoid toxicity to both mother and infant, the lithium dose should be decreased by 50% or more in the week prior to the anticipated delivery date[23] or, if the risk of relapse is too high, when labor begins.[22]*

* With their consent, women taking lithium during pregnancy or lactation should be registered with the American Register of Lithium Babies Registry, Langley Porter Neuropsychiatric Institute, 401 Parnassus Avenue, San Francisco, CA 94122.

A woman who has had a single episode of depression with psychosis is most likely to have been treated with tricyclic antidepressants, in conjunction with a neuroleptic, or with electroconvulsive (ECT) therapy. If she has had only one episode and is currently symptom-free, a trial off medications throughout the pregnancy should be considered. If there is a history of recurrent episodes or chronic residual symptoms, it may be necessary to maintain her on medication during the pregnancy.

In this circumstance, the most conservative course of action is to maintain the patient on a phenothiazine alone through the first trimester, adding tricyclic antidepressant only if the phenothiazine does not provide adequate symptom control. Some authorities caution against the use of tricyclic antidepressants during the first trimester,[24,25] primarily because of equivocal data on increased incidence of limb malformations. Tricyclic antidepressants are very slowly metabolized by the newborn, and adverse effects, such as irritability and jitteriness, have been described in newborns whose mothers received tricyclic antidepressants before delivery.[26] It is therefore prudent to reduce the tricyclic antidepressant to a minimum maintenance dose throughout the pregnancy and withdraw it gradually before delivery even if it must be restarted soon afterward.

Monoamine oxidase inhibitors should not be used during pregnancy because of increased rates of fetal malformation.[27] So little is known about the teratogenic effects of the newer agents that they should not be used except under special circumstances and with consultation.

Unlike the psychotic episodes associated with schizophrenia or affective disorders, drug-induced psychoses (organic hallucinosis–delusional syndrome) are usually self-limited. The patient with a history of such an episode is unlikely to be maintained on medication unless she has an additional underlying disorder such as schizophrenia. The history of a drug-induced psychosis, particularly if recent and with an addictive drug such as cocaine, should alert the obstetrician to possible continuing drug use. Pregnant women with positive toxicology studies require careful education by the physician and staff as to the adverse effects of continued drug exposure on both mother and baby. Every effort should be made to admit these women to drug rehabilitation programs while pregnant.

Management of a Psychotic Episode During Pregnancy

Sometimes a patient with a history of psychotic disorder conceives while actively psychotic and taking higher doses of medication. The danger here is that her mental state will continue to worsen with the stress of pregnancy and that she will weave the pregnancy into her delusions. In such a patient the risk to the fetus of deterioration in maternal mental health and possible noncompliance with prenatal care outweighs the hazards to the fetus of neuroleptics. Rapid control of symptoms is of first importance, but the neuroleptic dose should be reduced as soon as possible.[28]

The patient who suffers the onset of a psychotic episode while pregnant requires hospital admission to obtain skilled psychiatric nursing care, the careful observation needed for differential diagnosis, and a thorough work-up for organic factors that might contribute to the illness. Such a work-up is most efficiently accomplished on a psychiatric unit that is part of a general hospital. Since pregnancy per se is not associated with an increased risk of mental disorder, it cannot be assumed to be the etiologic agent. Drug use is probably the most likely organic factor contributing to a psychotic episode during pregnancy, but such conditions as cerebral embolism, pulmonary embolism with hypoxia, autoimmune disorders, and infections of the central nervous system must also be considered.

If physical examination, mental status examination, laboratory studies, and clinical course suggest that the illness is functional, treatment of the patient with the lowest effective dose of phenothiazine is usually the best choice.

Treatment-resistant psychoses may respond to ECT. Several case reports describe the successful use of ECT in pregnant patients for treatment of severe psychotic depression.[29–31] Although no controlled studies are available, the procedure appears to be safe if both mother and fetus are carefully monitored. Guidelines proposed by Wise and colleagues include the following:

- Performing ECT in the presence of an obstetrician
- Endotracheal intubation
- Low-voltage, nondominant ECT with EEG monitoring
- Electrocardiographic monitoring of the mother
- Evaluation of arterial blood gases during and immediately after ECT
- Doppler ultrasonography of fetal heart rate
- Tocodynamometer recording of uterine tone
- Administration of glycopyrrolate as the anticholinergic of choice during anesthesia
- Weekly stress tests.[30]

NONPSYCHOTIC PSYCHIATRIC DISORDER DURING PREGNANCY

Epidemiology of Nonpsychotic Disorders During Pregnancy

With the exception of a slightly increased frequency of depressive disorders during the first trimester,[32] the rate of nonpsychotic psychiatric illness among pregnant women is similar to that of non-pregnant women of childbearing age. Among these disorders, depressive disorders are the most common, with 8% to 26% of women surveyed in community studies reporting at least one episode of past depression.[33] Panic disorder, obsessive-compulsive disorder, and eating disorders, however, are rare, occurring in less than 2% of the population.[12]

Substance abuse during pregnancy is an emergent public health problem on which only preliminary statistics are available. A recent nationwide hospital survey found that 11% of deliveries overall were affected by substance abuse (375,000 newborns affected annually).[34] Variation and rates among hospitals (0.4% to 27.0%) were mainly attributable to differences in the thoroughness of the substance abuse assessment and not to ethnicity, social class, or location. A second hospital survey suggested that the number of drug-exposed births has risen three to four times since 1985.[35]

Management of Nonpsychotic Disorders During Pregnancy

Depressive Episodes. A woman who has recovered from a single major depressive episode (without psychosis) but is still on antidepressants (eg, tricyclics, monoamine oxidase inhibitors) should be advised to withdraw from these antidepressants before conception. If there is a substantial risk of relapse based on multiple past episodes, it may be necessary to continue an antidepressant during pregnancy. This should be a tricyclic on which there is some information as to potential risks (eg, amitriptyline or imipramine).[36] Although lithium has an established role in prophylaxis of recurrent unipolar depression,[37] its use in pregnancy is usually contraindicated for the reasons discussed earlier.

Anxiety, Panic Attacks, and Obsessive Disorders. A more common obstetric problem is the woman who comes for preconception counseling or early in pregnancy and reports that she has been taking a benzodiazepine (such as diazepam, alprazolam, lorazepam) for generalized anxiety symptoms. Benzodiazepines have been associated with an increased incidence of fetal malformations, especially cleft lip or palate. Although the evidence here is controversial,[36] it is probably best to avoid benzodiazepines during the first trimester. Neonatal diazepam withdrawal symptoms similar to neonatal narcotic withdrawal symptoms have been reported after maternal ingestion in the second and third trimester, as have hypothermia and hyperbilirubinemia.[36]

Women with a prior history of panic attacks probably will have been treated with tricyclic antidepressants or benzodiazepines, and these should be withdrawn if at all possible. The woman with a prior history of obsessive-compulsive disorder will probably have been treated with newer agents, such as chlorimipramine or fluoxetine, which also should be withdrawn if at all possible, as there is little or no information on their effects on the fetus.

Psychotropic medication for anxiety, panic, or obsessive symptoms arising during pregnancy should be avoided. Unlike patients with psychosis or severe depression, patients with these symptoms usually retain their insight and judgment. Given the risks involved, only in rare instances will there be compelling reasons for using medication to treat these conditions during pregnancy. Adequate information and reassurance, especially when concerns center around the pregnancy, may be sufficient. Sources of stress, such as family, marital, and social problems, should be treated appropriately. Midwives and physiotherapists can help with relaxation techniques and childbirth education.

Substance Abuse. Women with chronic uncontrolled substance abuse often do not present until they go into labor, whereas women who use drugs only occasionally and heroin-addicted women who are engaged in methadone-maintenance programs are more likely to present for prenatal care. Any woman giving a history of drug abuse or with a positive urine toxicology should be counseled regarding the risks to her and her infant of continued drug use during the pregnancy. Women with addictions to alcohol, heroin, tranquilizers, and pain killers can be referred to established drug detoxification programs with adjunctive use of self-help groups like Alcoholics Anonymous and Pills Anonymous. Although no drug has yet been found that reliably blocks cocaine cravings, and drug rehabilitation programs are presently hard to find for cocaine addicts, every effort should be made to refer pregnant women for the treatment available. The physician should inform himself or herself of the laws requiring reporting of positive urine toxicology results to authorities, since in some states, women with positive urine toxicology at time of delivery are not allowed to take their babies home and it is the physician's legal responsibility to report the situation.

Eating Disorders. Anorexia nervosa and bulimia nervosa are eating disorders with important consequences for weight and reproductive function. Anorexia nervosa is a syndrome characterized by persistent concerns about eating and weight as well as dieting in the face of subaverage weight (85% of expected weight for height). Amenorrhea of at least 3 months' duration is required for the diagnosis. Bulimia nervosa is a syndrome characterized by repeated binge eating and attempts at counteracting weight gain through severe dieting or compulsive laxative use or self-induced vomiting. Oligomenorrhea or amenorrhea are common in bulimia nervosa but are not required for the diagnosis. Anorexia nervosa and bulimia nervosa may be concurrent. Intermediate syndromes are currently called atypical eating disorders.[3]

The world literature on pregnancy in women with eating disorders is small. This probably reflects not only the rarity of the disorders but the lower rates of marriage among these women, infertility related to menstrual disturbance, and decisions not to bear children.[38] Stewart and colleagues found that women in whom anorexia nervosa or bulimia nervosa is in remission at conception had greater maternal weight gain and babies with higher birth weights and 5-minute Apgar scores than women who conceived while they still had

TABLE 78-1. PSYCHIATRIC PROBLEMS DURING THE POSTPARTUM PERIOD

	INITIAL MATERNAL INDIFFERENCE	POSTPARTUM "BLUES"	POSTPARTUM PSYCHOSIS	POSTPARTUM MAJOR DEPRESSIVE DISORDER (NONPSYCHOTIC)
Prevalence	40% (among primiparas)	50% to 70%	0.1% to 0.3%	10% to 15%
Major risk factors	Obstetric (amniotomy and/or unusually painful labor)	Not known	Primiparous, previous postpartum psychosis, history of bipolar affective disorder	History of major depressive disorder, marital instability
Typical onset	Day 1	Day 3 to 1 month	Day 3 to 1 month	6 weeks to 1 year
Typical duration	3 days	Less than 10 days	6–8 weeks (longer without treatment)	6–8 weeks (longer without treatment)
Potential for suicide or infanticide	Rare	Rare	Significant	Possible
Management	Education by physician, support from family	Education by physician, support from family	Hospitalization, medication, social support, psychotherapy	Possible hospitalization, medication, social support, psychotherapy
Prognosis with treatment	Good	Good	Variable, at risk for recurrence	Variable

symptoms of anorexia or bulimia.[39] Women with active anorexia have higher rates of prematurity and low birth weight,[40] attributed to the relationship between low maternal weight and infant weight.[41] Although women with bulimia may experience improvement in their symptoms as pregnancy progresses, most have a return of symptoms in the first postpartum year.[42]

Women with eating disorders may not volunteer their symptoms to their obstetrician. As a general rule, it is advisable to inquire about the symptoms of these disorders in any woman who presents with subaverage weight for height and any woman who casually volunteers that she is dieting or has an eating problem.[43] Women with eating disorders may need special reassurance about the weight gain expected with pregnancy and with postpartum figure changes.[42] Any woman with an active eating disorder should be treated concurrently by a psychiatrist.

The self-induced vomiting in bulimia is to be distinguished from the involuntary emesis seen in up to 32% of pregnant women[44] and from hyperemesis gravidarum, a severe variant occurring in little more than 0.3% of pregnant women.[45] Both conditions are likely to be related to physiologic changes during pregnancy, in particular, delayed gastric emptying due to high levels of cholecystokinin.[46]

PSYCHIATRIC DISORDER DURING THE POSTPARTUM PERIOD

Serious postpartum psychiatric disorder (ie, postpartum psychosis and nonpsychotic depression) casts a long shadow over one of life's most important events. It is important to be aware of the differing symptom patterns of the rare but serious disorders (postpartum psychosis and nonpsychotic major depression) and the common but less disabling disorders (initial maternal indifference and the maternity blues) (Table 78-1).

PSYCHOTIC DISORDERS DURING THE POSTNATAL PERIOD

Historical Overview

Postpartum psychosis has long impressed clinicians as both a disease entity with distinctive clinical features and an entity in which organic factors play an important role.[47] Clinical descriptions dating as far back as Hippocrates in the fourth century B.C. stressed the symptoms of confusion, delirium, hallucinations, and insomnia.[48] In the detailed clinical descriptions of the late 19th century, the condition was variously referred to as *délire triste*,[49] *Verwirrheit* (distressed perplexity),[50] and "miserable sleeplessness."[51] Furstner observed that the delirium of postpartum psychosis differed from that of childbed or milk fever, in that the former was afebrile.[50]

Nonetheless, postpartum psychosis is not accorded status as a distinct entity in current psychiatric classification systems (DSM III-R or ICD-9). This position is based on a number of studies that were unable to find any unique pattern of symptoms in postpartum as compared to nonpostpartum psychiatric disorder.[52–54] However, this "loss of identity" has generated intense controversy (see Hamilton[47] and Meltzer and Kumar[55]).*

* The Marce Society, a scientific society to promote study and the exchange of information on postpartum psychosis, was established in 1982. Information about the society is available from Dr. Beth Alder, Queen Margaret College, Clerwood Terrace, Edinburgh, UK EHIZ 8TS.

Epidemiology of Postpartum Psychosis

Two out of every 1000 women delivered will require admission into a psychiatric unit with a postpartum psychosis.[1] Women in the first month postpartum are 22 times more likely to be admitted with a psychosis than non-pregnant women of childbearing age.[2] Having a first birth, not having a husband at the time of childbirth, perinatal death, and cesarean section are associated with the increased risk of postpartum psychosis.[2] A prior episode of postpartum psychosis increases the risk of a second episode from one in 500 to one in seven or even less.[2] A history of bipolar affective disorder is a major risk factor for postpartum psychosis: among women with bipolar affective disorder, 20% to 30% of pregnancies are followed by postpartum psychosis.[2,56]

Clinical Presentation of Postpartum Psychosis

The vast majority of postpartum psychoses are affective (ie, manic or depressive psychoses).[2,57] A minority are schizophrenia-like conditions, distinguished from schizophrenia by the shorter duration of illness. It is very rare for true schizophrenia to begin during the postpartum period. Most of episodes of postpartum psychosis start very abruptly between day 3 and day 14 of the postpartum period. These psychotic episodes are some of the most severe to be observed in psychiatry and usually present as a mixture of delirium and psychosis, with perplexity, confusion, and prominent delusions and hallucinations. Within a few days of treatment the confusional symptoms lessen, and a picture consistent with depressive, manic, or less commonly, schizophrenia-like psychosis emerges. The onset of symptoms soon after delivery and the prominent features of delirium suggest an organic, most likely hormonal, factor, but this has yet to be conclusively determined.[58,59]

With respect to infant caretaking, mothers with postpartum psychosis show marked disorganization of practical care, raising the specter of accidental injury to the infant. A substantial proportion of mothers (about 25% in the case series described by Margison[60]) do not express abnormal ideas about the infant. When abnormal ideas are present, their content tends to be consistent with the type of psychosis. Manic patients may express grandiose delusions about the child having a special purpose (eg, the Messiah). Depressed patients may express delusional beliefs about the infant's health that are not amenable to reassurance (eg, "the baby is all blue; she is withering away to a skeleton"). Patients with acute schizophrenia may have delusions of special powers ("he can control my thoughts") or of bodily change ("she is turning into a cockroach"). Mothers with postpartum psychosis rarely express predominantly hostile ideas toward the infant[60] and rarely perceive the infant as an active persecutor.[61] Still, the mother may cause injury to the infant because of her psychotic ideas ("he would be better off dead").

Management of Postpartum Psychosis

Women with postpartum psychosis require skilled psychiatric nursing care within a hospital setting and should be admitted with their babies whenever possible. Manic illness often responds very quickly to treatment within 2 weeks, sometimes within days. Most of the severe depressive puerperal psychoses will improve with treatment within 6 to 8 weeks, and the schizophrenia-like conditions will also improve within 6 to 8 weeks.[62]

When postpartum psychosis is first recognized, the first priority is to sedate the patient with phenothiazine or butyrophenones to a level that makes her safe within her environment and allows for adequate hydration and nutrition. Such medication will first sedate, then reduce the perplexity and fear, and over 48 hours it will begin to alleviate hallucinations and delusions.

The psychiatrist is likely to recommend an initial regimen of 50 mg of chlorpromazine or thioridazine periodically together with 75 or 100 mg at night, as frequently the mental state is worse at night. The dose will need to be titrated. Extrapyramidal side effects are rare, so that anticholinergic agents are rarely required. Once the patient is less agitated and the psychotic thought content begins to emerge, the psychiatrist may discontinue chlorpromazine in favor of a less sedating medication such as haloperidol. Lithium may be used if the patient is not responding to phenothiazine or haloperidol. If the clinical picture is that of psychotic depression, patients should be given phenothiazine in preference to a tricyclic.[59] If the patient is not responding with 3 to 7 days of a regimen of phenothiazine medication, then ECT is the treatment of choice. ECT is usually given twice a week for six to eight treatment sessions.[62]

Many early-onset postpartum psychoses respond well to treatment and then relapse. Therefore, continuation of the phenothiazine at a reduced dosage is indicated until the infant is at least 3 months old. In the event of relapse with mania or depression, lithium may be indicated as prophylaxis. There is also some promising evidence that lithium administration immediately after delivery may provide effective prophylaxis against postpartum affective psychosis in women with a history of previous bipolar disorder or postpartum affective psychosis.[63] The only controlled follow-up study to date of infants of mothers with postpartum psychosis finds evidence of continued problems in the mother–child relationship nearly 5 years later, underscoring the importance of prevention, prompt treatment, and follow-up.[64]

NONPSYCHOTIC DISORDERS DURING THE POSTPARTUM PERIOD

There are three types of nonpsychotic disorder in the postpartum period: initial indifference toward the infant, postpartum or maternity blues, and nonpsychotic major depression.

Epidemiology of Nonpsychotic Postpartum Disorders

Robson and Kumar found that 40% of primiparous women experienced indifference toward their infants when they first held them after birth.[65] The best predictors for this condition were amniotomy, painful labor, and pethidine dosage. Transient depressed mood or "postpartum blues" is reported by 50% to 70% of women after delivery.[66–68] The "blues" are not associated with obstetric variables or demographic or psychosocial variables. Far less common is the syndrome of nonpsychotic postpartum depression, occurring in 10% to 15% of women after delivery.[69] Risk factors include a personal and family history of major depression and marital dissatisfaction, whereas obstetric factors, socioeconomic status, and life events do not appear to be risk factors for this disorder.

Clinical Presentation and Management of Nonpsychotic Postpartum Disorders

Initial maternal indifference, most acute on the first postpartum day, has resolved in most instances by the fourth postpartum day. The mother, however, may need reassurance that the symptom is common, probably has a physiologic basis, and does not bode ill for her relationship with her infant.[70]

The postpartum blues often begin with bouts of weeping starting on the third or fourth day after delivery. Symptoms include insomnia (70%), tearfulness (66%), depressed mood (54%), fatigue (54%), anxiety (51%), headaches (35%), poor concentration (29%), and confusion (21%). Elation may also occur, usually on the first day postpartum.[71] The symptoms usually resolve spontaneously by the 10th day after delivery. The complaints of mild cognitive deficit and insomnia have led some investigators to suggest that postpartum blues are a milder variant of postpartum psychosis, related to the same unidentified organic factor.[71] The symptoms of postpartum blues usually resolve without treatment. However, a recent study suggests that women think it would have been helpful to have advance warning from their obstetrician about these feelings and some education as to their common occurrence.[68] There is no evidence that postpartum blues has any long-term adverse effects on the patient or her family.[68]

The syndrome of major depressive disorder is distinguished from postpartum blues by the duration and intensity of the depressed mood as well as other symptoms. The diagnosis of major depressive disorder requires that depression or loss of interest or pleasure be present nearly every day for a period of at least 2 weeks and that functioning at work or at home be impaired. In addition, there must be at least four of the following: change in appetite or weight, insomnia or hypersomnia, psychomotor agitation or retardation, fatigue, feelings of worthlessness, trouble concentrating or making decisions, and thoughts of death.

Mothers with nonpsychotic major depressive disorder most frequently express ideas of rejection of the infant ("I wish that he had never been born; I hate him for ruining my life") or intense feelings of inadequacy that are out of proportion to any actual impairment in parenting skills (eg, "I am just useless as a mother; she won't take any food from me; she'd have starved if the nurses weren't here").[60] Severe nonpsychotic depression will generally require medication such as tricyclics, monoamine oxidase inhibitors, and sometimes lithium. Less severe depressions without marked functional impairment or suicidal ideation may respond to a trial of psychotherapy without the use of medication. The importance of treating a nonpsychotic depressive episode, apart from the relief of maternal suffering, is that depression has been found to interfere with mother–child interaction and to predict later child maladjustment.[72,73]

BREAST-FEEDING

Breast-feeding offers the advantages of maternal antibodies and a mutually gratifying experience for mother and infant. However, extreme caution is warranted in breast-feeding an infant while the mother is taking any psychotropic medication. Deleterious effects of lithium[74] and benzodiazepines[75] are the best established, whereas the evidence for tricyclics and neuroleptics is more equivocal.[75] As a general rule, the concentration of drugs in breast milk is about 10% of the level in the mother's plasma, but there are wide variations,[76] and the effect of even low levels of psychotropic medication on developing infant neurotransmitter systems is not known. The safest approach is to recommend that mothers on any form of psychotropic medication substitute bottle feeding for breast-feeding.[59]

In addition, several other psychological correlates of breast-feeding have been recognized recently and should be considered by the treating obstetrician. In a prospective study, Alder and Bancroft found that women who breast-feed exclusively reported less sexual interest and enjoyment at 3 months postpartum and more dyspareunia at 3 and 6 months postpartum than did women who were not exclusively breast-feeding.[77] Both this study and an earlier retrospective one by Alder and Cox[78] demonstrated that exclusively breast-feeding women had significantly more symptoms of depression. Women who are judged by history at high risk of serious postpartum depression or who are already significantly depressed at the time of delivery should be informed of the risk that depressive symptoms may worsen with intensive breast-feeding and helped to make an informed decision as to whether proceeding with a plan to breast-feed is in their best interest.

SPECIAL MANAGEMENT PROBLEMS

PARENTAL GRIEF AFTER PREGNANCY LOSS

The term *pregnancy loss* encompasses neonatal death, stillbirth, and spontaneous abortion. The loss of an older child or adult usually, although not invariably, involves parents passing through several successive stages of grief[79,80]: denial, anger, bargaining, depression, and finally, acceptance or resignation. When the loss is of a fetus or newborn known to no one except the parents and the medical staff, the grieving process is complicated by the frequent lack of reality that the baby has for the family and friends who would ordinarily assist the parents in the mourning process. The parents themselves may have only vague concepts of the baby, a situation that makes healthy mourning difficult and that is conducive to the development of fearful fantasies, pathologic grief, and impaired emotional status in the next pregnancy. Several investigators have noted in this situation that the development of fixed pathological grief reactions is frequent and may be as high as one fifth to one third of cases.[81,82]

Since these unique hazards of perinatal loss have been recognized, a variety of preventive measures have been found to be helpful. For instance, Cole[83] and Kellner and colleagues[84] describe programs for caretakers that include the following:

1. Establishing the memory of the child by providing pictures, footprints, name bands. Encouraging the parents to view or hold the baby if they wish and to name the baby. Discussing cremation with memorial service or funeral as alternatives to hospital disposal of the remains.
2. Making every effort to ascertain medical conditions that could have contributed to the child's death by means of autopsy and blood tissue samples taken before death. This medical information will later be shared with the family and interpreted.
3. Following the parents by both telephone and scheduled visits. One follow-up visit (for instance, at 8 weeks) should be devoted to meeting with the family to review their questions concerning the child, the results of the autopsy, and their progress in the grieving process. The obstetrician needs to be attentive to such danger signals as drug or alcohol abuse, physical abuse, inability to return to previous life activities, and disabling somatic complaints as well as the declared intention to pursue another pregnancy immediately.

Kellner and colleagues have pointed out that encouraging parents to decide for themselves whether they wish to see, hold, or name the deceased baby or hold a funeral or memorial service is helpful.[84] This process helps parents to regain a sense of mastery over events, and it removes inappropriate responsibility for making these decisions from the medical and nursing staff. In a study of 165 bereaved families experiencing perinatal death, the investigators found that demographic and obstetric features did not predict the choices made by parents. This makes it even more important for the neonatal team to encourage each family's participation in making decisions.

Condon has described pathological grief reactions (excluding postpartum psychotic disorder) as presenting in two typical ways: the absence of any expressed grief or difficulties in bonding to a subsequent baby, or prolonged grief or adjustment disorder with depression.[85] Determining what is "prolonged" is a matter of clinical judgment. Condon judges a grief reaction to be pathological if the stillbirth is still at the center of the patient's emotional life 6 to 9 months later or if there are no signs that resolution is under way. Most patients who present for treatment are women. Men are more likely to indicate disturbance in less direct ways, as with drug or alcohol abuse. Severe sibling reactions require attention.[86] Pathological grief reaction in parent or sibling is an indication for referral to a psychiatrist.

Both Condon and Bourne and Lewis emphasize that the most helpful approach does not stress insight.[85,87] The professional should establish a sympathetic alliance and take a detailed history of the patient's "obstetric genogram" (the births, miscarriages, stillbirths, and terminations of pregnancies occurring in the patient's family of origin); her own experience of being mothered; and a detailed account of the experiences of the pregnancy, especially whether termination was ever considered, as well as the reaction of the other parent. The treatment begins with a focus on everything that is known about the baby, the location of the baby's remains, and a careful review of the circumstances of the death and why it occurred. In the process of this retelling, the woman usually discusses fantasies about the baby and experiences and emotions that can be validated and clarified. Relief results from her lessened guilt and anxiety.

Reports of women who suffered first- and second-trimester spontaneous abortions suggest that these woman are less likely to suffer chronic psychiatric sequelae than women who miscarried when the fetus was more mature.[88,89] However, Leppert and Pahlka reported intense grief in women even when they miscarried in the first trimester.[88] They recommend counseling sessions (at the time of the initial diagnosis and 4 to 6 weeks later, with telephone contacts in between as needed) to inform the couple of any available facts concerning the cause of the miscarriage, to answer their questions, to alleviate their guilt (often for fantasies of having caused the abortion through jogging or lifting heavy objects), and to help them plan for future pregnancies.

A common problem for couples is the different ways and pace at which women and men grieve. Women may be more likely to express sadness, while men may appear to be unaffected, masking feelings of helplessness and depression.[83] The obstetrician and the medical team can assist couples by discussing these differences between mothers and fathers in the follow-up counseling sessions.

Some couples will derive comfort from self-help groups formed by parents who share recent experiences of miscarriage, stillbirth, and infant death.* Self-help groups, however, are not for everyone. Couples who have a great concern about privacy or who tend anxiously to assume that others' problems will also happen to them do not do well in such groups. For this reason we recommend to interested couples that they contact a local chapter and use their own sense of comfort as a guide to whether to pursue involvement.

PARENTAL ADJUSTMENT TO THE NEWBORN WITH SPECIAL NEEDS

The stress associated with the birth of an infant with serious medical problems can cause maladaptive responses in the most well-adjusted of parents. Low birth weight–prematurity is the most common problem, but every obstetrician is familiar with a range of problems that transform a potentially joyous event into one fraught with anxiety.[90,91] Although low birth weight–prematurity is the condition discussed here, the principles of helping parents to adjust to any condition are similar: permission to grieve, the promotion of parental competence and confidence (especially in first-time parents), the enlistment of necessary services prior to discharge, and provision for careful follow-up.

Minde describes the most frequent immediate reaction to birth of a preterm infant as fear that the infant will die.[92] This tends to be most acute when the infant is delivered in a general obstetric unit and then transferred to another neonatal intensive care unit. Minde recommends provision of literature on prematurity right after delivery† as well as frequent visits to the nursery and participation in caretaking routines as soon as possible.

After survival seems ensured, mothers may become almost totally preoccupied with the infant: 40% to 60% of mothers visit daily for many hours, think only about the infant for weeks, and may begin to show signs of self-neglect, fatigue, and irritability.[92] On the other hand, some families rarely visit, and this is not cause for intervention unless an interview with the parents reveals specific psychosocial difficulties. Parents who do not visit their infant often in the intensive care unit or who have been separated during this time for other reasons do not later abuse or neglect their children more often than parents who do not experience such a separation.[93] It is important for the nursery staff to realize that parents may be appropriately tending to other pressing needs, such as siblings at home.

During the first few weeks that the infant is in the nursery, Minde has found that parents often benefit from a group meeting with parents of other prematures.[94] This may be led by a parent who has had personal experience with a premature infant within the last year. The support and comfort afforded by such a group can often permit parents to absorb information more readily that is needed for the practical care of the premature.

Parents of prematures need to be informed that during the first months after discharge premature infants frequently develop feeding, crying, and sleeping problems and are difficult to calm. Parents need to know that these problems are not unusual and to be shown specific techniques for soothing without overstimulating the infant. Minde recommends that parents sleep or "room in" with their infant for one or two nights prior to discharge from the hospital. This will familiarize them with the infant's night and allay parental anxieties commonly encountered after the infant goes home.[92]

Klaus and Kennel sparked intensive research by drawing attention to the often prolonged separation of mother and infant in modern obstetric practice and its possible adverse effects on mother–infant bonding.[95] Subsequent research has found no consistent evidence for a "critical" or "sensitive" period within which "bonding" between parent and child must occur,[70] and parents may need to be reassured of this. On the other hand, this research has led to clinical innovations that promote parental satisfaction, such as early contact after delivery,[96] "rooming in,"[97] and Brazelton demonstrations in the nursery.[98–100] In addition, these interventions have been demonstrated to produce improved early outcomes in infants of mothers from socially disadvantaged backgrounds.[97,98,101] The obstetrician is in a unique position to support neonatal services that promote confidence and competence in mothers whose youth and poverty place them and their babies at high risk.

IMPAIRED PARENTING AND THE RISK OF INFANTICIDE

A very serious risk confronted by the infant during the neonatal period is infanticide. Infanticide is defined as the homicide of a person less than 1 year of age.[102] Homicide is the fifth leading cause of death among persons under the age of 18, and no single age group is at greater risk than infants less than 1 year of age. In the period for which data are available (1976 to 1979) infanticide represented 12% of all child homicide victims, giving an average yearly infanticide rate of 5.6 of 100,000. Over one quarter of these infanticide victims

* Some recommended self-help groups are:

1. Resolve Through Sharing, LaCrosse Lutheran Hospital, 1910 South Ave, LaCrosse, WI 54601 (608) 785-0530, ext 3696.
2. Aiding a Mother Experiencing Neonatal Death (Amend), 4324 Berrywich Terrace, St Louis, MO 63128 (314) 487-7582.
3. Helping Other Parents in Normal Grieving (hoping), Sparrow Hospital, 1215 East Michigan St, Lansing, MI 48909. (517) 483-3873.
4. Resolve, 5 Water St, Arlington, MA 02174. (617) 643-2442.
5. A Source of Help in Airing and Resolving Experiences (Share), St. Elizabeth Hospital, 220 West Lincoln St, Belleville, IL 62220. (618) 234-2415.

† For example, Shosenberg N, Minde K, Swyer P, Fitzhardinge P. The premature infant: a handbook for parents. Toronto: Hospital for Sick Children Foundation, 1980.

were killed in the first week of life, making this a problem of special importance to obstetricians. These infanticide rates are probably underestimates, both because homicide is particularly difficult to ascertain in infants[103] and because of coding changes in the International Classification of Diseases.[104]

Historical,[105] cross-cultural,[106] and epidemiological evidence[107] suggests that infanticide is a separate entity from later child homicide and abuse. The most common cause of death in infanticide is smothering or strangulation; the next most common cause of death is head injury.[108] Christoffel suggests that the precipitants are likely to be universal: parental patience with infant difficult temperament wears thin and when frustration spills over into aggression, infants are particularly vulnerable to fatal injury because of specific biological frailties.[107]

Depressed mothers in particular are more likely to perceive their infants as difficult and irritable.[109] As noted earlier, depressed mothers are more likely to express overt hostility toward their infants and to feel unable to cope. Among mothers who commit infanticide, 62% commit suicide.[110] There is some evidence that this is more common among depressed mothers.[111]

Mothers with postpartum psychosis may be at great risk of accidentally but fatally injuring their child or neglecting the child through practical incompetence or misguided delusions. A difficult area is abandonment of an infant under conditions not likely to permit survival, such as delivery of an otherwise viable infant into a toilet bowl[112] or placement in the garbage. In these instances only detailed investigation of maternal postnatal behavior along with circumstances of the birth and autopsy findings will determine whether willful neglect or denial of psychotic proportions is the main responsible factor.

At present there is no good way to ascertain a particular child's risk for neglect, abuse, or infanticide. Demographic risk factors include single motherhood, mother with less than high school education, very late or no prenatal care, low–birth-weight infants, and out-of-hospital births.[113] Although any parent with a suspected psychiatric disorder should be referred for treatment, the presence of a psychiatric illness does not necessarily imply impaired parenting, and the clinician must be careful not to assume this. Parenting behaviors should be considered independently. Guidelines for identifying parents at risk, based on the literature as well as clinical experience, include the mother (or father) who

1. Either incessantly stimulates or never touches or talks to the baby in the nursery and seems unable to vary his or her ministrations in response to shifts in the infant state of alertness[92]
2. Attributes motives and intentions to the baby that are beyond the infant's developmental abilities (eg, the attribution of hate, revenge, or "being spoiled" to a child less than 12 months of age)[92]
3. Is observed to be delusional or hallucinating
4. By behavior or toxicology screen is actively engaged in substance use
5. Appears consistently depressed in mood and statement
6. Is reluctant to take the baby home
7. Has a family history of child neglect or abuse over several generations[114]
8. Has a history of violence to this child or others. Even minor acts of aggression, when they occur in the context of homicidal thoughts, reflect a significant change from their presence in imagination only.[60] Parents who have obsessional symptoms where aggressive impulses are regarded as foreign to the personality and are strongly resisted probably represent a lesser degree of risk than mothers with other forms of aggressive impulses.[60]

TABLE 78–2. THE PRENATAL ASSESSMENT—ESSENTIAL PSYCHIATRIC INFORMATION

Current state of emotional health
Current social support (finances, housing, presence/absence of spouse and other concerned relatives)
Current and past use of medication for any nervous or mental condition (eg, imipramine for depression, diazepam for anxiety)
Current and past use of alcohol and recreational drugs
History of any emotional difficulties in the year after childbirth (eg, having to have someone else care for the child, psychiatric treatment or hospitalization)
History of bipolar (manic-depressive) or unipolar (depressive) affective disorder

For mothers or fathers thought to be at very high risk, placement of the infant may be necessary. In other cases, frequent postnatal follow-up visits, including home visits, should be arranged so that difficulties can be detected and the appropriate referrals initiated. The obstetrician has an especially important role in providing continuity of care and observation during this period.

SUMMARY

The obstetrician's role in the management of psychiatric disorder begins with the first prenatal visit (see Table 78-2). At this point it is important to elicit history of psychiatric hospitalizations and contacts, history of postpartum affective disorder, history of medications, and current and past substance abuse. The obstetrician is in a unique position to detect psychiatric emergencies at an early point in their evolution and to make appropriate use of psychiatric consultation. As a member of the neonatal care team, the obstetrician often has the special advantages of having known the parents throughout the pregnancy and of being a trusted advisor. This makes him or her uniquely suited to assist in the grieving process and to identify early difficulties in parent–infant interaction.

REFERENCES

1. Paffenbarger RS. Epidemiological aspects of mental illness associated with childbearing. In: Brockington IF, Kumar R, eds. Motherhood and mental illness. New York: Grune & Stratton, 1982.
2. Kendell RE, Chalmers JC, Platz C. Epidemiology of puerperal psychoses. Br J Psychiatry 1987;150:662.
3. American Psychiatric Association. Diagnostic and statistical manual of mental disorders. 3rd ed. rev. Washington, DC: The Association, 1987.
4. Romano J, Engel GL. Physiologic and psychologic considerations of delirium. Med Clin North Am 1944;28:629.
5. Lipowski R. Delirium, clouding of consciousness and confusion. J Nerv Ment Dis 1967;145:229.
6. Simon RI. Clinical psychiatry and the law. Washington DC: American Psychiatric Association, 1986.
7. Commission on Professional and Hospital Activities. International classification of diseases. 9th revision, Clinical modifications (ICD-9 CM). Vol 1. Ann Arbor, MI: The Commission, 1978.
8. Lishman WA. Organic psychiatry: the psychological consequence of cerebral disorder. London: Blackwell Scientific Publications, 1978.
9. Sameroff AJ, Seifer R, Zax M. Early development of children at risk for emotional disorder. Monogr Soc Res Child Dev 1982;47(7, Serial No. 199).
10. Stott DJ. The child's hazards in utero. In: Howells JG, ed. Modern perspective in international child psychiatry. New York: Brunner/Mazel, 1971.
11. McNeil TF, Kaij L, Malmquist-Larsson A. Women with nonorganic psychosis: pregnancy's effect on mental health during pregnancy. Acta Psychiatr Scand 1984;70:140.
12. Robins LN, Helzer JE, Weissman MM, Orvaschel H, Gruenberg E, Burke JD, Regier DA. Lifetime prevalence of specific psychiatric disorders in three sites. Arch Gen Psychiatry 1984;41:949.
13. Spielvogel A, Wile J. Treatment of the psychotic pregnant patient. Psychosomatics 1986;27(7):487.
14. Edlund MJ, Craig TJ. Antipsychotic drug use and birth defects: an epidemiologic reassessments. Compr Psychiatry 1984; 25:32.
15. Hauser LA. Pregnancy and psychiatric drugs. Hosp Community Psychiatry 1985;36:817.
16. Falterman CG, Richardson CJ. Small left colon syndrome associated with maternal ingestion of psychotropic drugs. J Pediatr 1980;97:308.
17. Parkin DE. Probable Benadryl withdrawal manifestations in a newborn infant. J Pediatr 1974;85:580.
18. Saxen I. Cleft palate and maternal diphenhydramine intake. Lancet 1974;1:407.
19. Linden S, Rich CL. The use of lithium during pregnancy and lactation. J Clin Psychiatry 1983;44:358.
20. Weinstein MR, Goldfield MD. Cardiovascular malformations with lithium use during pregnancy. Am J Psychiatry 1975;132:529.
21. Long WA, Willis PW. Maternal lithium and neonatal Ebstein's anomaly: evaluation with cross-sectional echocardiography. Am J Perinatol 1984;1:182.
22. Schou M, Amdisen A, Steenstrup ON. Lithium and pregnancy. II. Hazards to women given lithium during pregnancy and delivery. Br Med J 1973;2:137.
23. Goldfield MD, Weinstein MR. Lithium carbonate in obstetrics: guidelines for clinical use. Am J Obstet Gynecol 1973;116(15):22.
24. Calabrese JR, Gulledge D. Psychotropics during pregnancy and lactation: a review. Psychosomatics 1985;26(5):413.
25. Thiels C. Pharmacotherapy of psychiatric disorder in pregnancy and during breast feeding: a review. Pharmacopsychiatry 1987;20:133.
26. Webster PA. Withdrawal symptoms in neonates associated with maternal antidepressant therapy. Lancet 1973;2:318.
27. Heinonen OP, Slone D, Shapiro, S. Births defects and drugs in pregnancy. Littleton, MA: Publishing Sciences Group, 1977: 336.
28. Oates M. The role of electroconvulsive therapy in the treatment of postnatal mental illness. In: Cox JL, Kumar R, Margison FR, et al, eds. Current approaches: puerperal mental illness. Southampton, England, 1986:1.
29. Levine R, Frost EAM. Arterial blood-gas analyses during electroconvulsive therapy in a parturient. Anesth Analg 1975;54(2):203.
30. Wise MG, Ward SC, Townsend-Parchman W, Gilstrap LC, Hauth JC. Case report of ECT during high-risk pregnancy. Am J Psychiatry 1984;141(1):99.
31. Repke JT, Berger NG. Electroconvulsive therapy in pregnancy. Obstet Gynecol 1984;63(3):395.
32. Kumar R, Robson KM. A prospective study of emotional disorders in childbearing women. Br J Psychiatry 1984;144:35.
33. Weissman MM, Leaf PJ, Tischler GL, Blazer DG, Karno M, Bruce ML, Florio LP. Affective disorders in five United States communities. Psychol Med 1988;18:141.
34. Alcohol, Drug Abuse and Mental Health Administration News, October 1988.
35. US House of Representatives. Placing infants at risk: parental addiction and disease. Hearing before the Select Committee on Children, Youth and Families. Washington, DC: US Government Printing Office, May 21, 1988.
36. Berkowitz RL, Coustan DR, Mochizuki TK. Handbook for prescribing medications during pregnancy. 2nd ed. Boston: Little, Brown, 1986.
37. Schou M. Lithium prophylaxis: myths and realities. Am J Psychiatry 1989;573.
38. Garfinkel PE, Garner DM. Anorexia nervosa: a multidimensional perspective. New York: Brunner/Mazel, 1982.
39. Stewart DE, Raskin J, Garfinkel PE, MacDonald OL, Robinson GE. Anorexia nervosa, bulimia, and pregnancy. Am J Obstet Gynecol 1987;157(5):1194.
40. Brinch M, Isager T, Tolstrup K. Anorexia nervosa and motherhood: reproductional pattern and mothering behavior of 50 women. Acta Psychiatr Scand 1985;77:98.
41. Treasure JL, Russell GFM. Intrauterine growth and neonatal weight gain in babies of women with anorexia nervosa. Br Med J 1988;296:1038.
42. Lacey JH, Smith G. Bulimia nervosa: the impact of pregnancy on mother and baby. Br J Psychiatry 1987;150:777.
43. Willis DC, Rand CS. Pregnancy in bulimic women. Obstet Gynecol 1988;71:708.
44. Vellacott ID, Cooke, EJA, James CE. Nausea and vomiting in early pregnancy. Int J Gynecol Obstet 1988;27:57.
45. Källén B. Hyperemesis during pregnancy and delivery outcome: A registry study. Eur J Obstet Gynecol Reprod Biol 1987;26:291.
46. Uvnas-Moberg K. The gastrointestinal tract in growth and reproduction. Sci Am 1989;(July):78.
47. Hamilton JA. The identity of postpartum psychosis. In: Brockington IF, Kumar R, eds. Motherhood and mental illness. London: Academic Press, 1982:1.
48. Jones WHS. Hippocrates—with an English translation. Vol 1. London: Heinemann, 1923.
49. Marce L, Marce LV. Traité de la folie des femmes enceintes, de nouvelles accouchées et des nourrices. Paris: Ballière, 1858.
50. Furstner C. Veber Schwanngerschaffs—and Puverperal psy-

chosen. Archiv fur Psychiatrie und Neruchkranten 1875; 5:505.
51. Jones R. Puerperal insanity. Br Med J 1902;1:579.
52. Strecker EA, Ebaugh FC. Psychoses occurring during the puerperium. Arch Neurol Psychiatry 1926;15:239.
53. Seager CP. A controlled study of postpartum mental illness. J Ment Sci 1960;106:214.
54. Schopf J, Bryois C, Jonquiere M, Le PK. On the nosology of severe psychiatric post-partum disorders: results of a catamnestic investigation. Eur Arch Psychiat Neurol Sci 1984;234:54.
55. Meltzer ES, Kumar R. Puerperal mental illness, clinical features and classification: a study of 142 mother and baby admissions. Br J Psychiatry 1987;147:647.
56. Reich T, Winokur G. Postpartum psychoses in patients with manic depressive disease. J Nerv Ment Dis 1970;151:60.
57. Brockington IF, Lernik KF, Schofield EM, Downing AR, Francis AF, Keelan C. Puerperal psychosis: Phenomena and diagnosis. Arch Gen Psychiatry 1981;38:829.
58. Brockington IF, Winokur G, Dean C. Puerperal psychosis. In: Brockington IF, Kumar R, eds. Motherhood and mental illness. New York: Grune & Stratton, 1982.
59. Robinson GR, Stewart DE. Postpartum psychiatric disorder. Can Med Assoc J 1986;134(1):31.
60. Margison F. Pathology of the mother-child relationship. In: Brockington IF, Kumark R, ed. Motherhood and mental illness. New York: Grune & Stratton, 1982.
61. Bartschi-Rochaix F. The position of the child in the delusional system of the mother. Z Neurol Psychiatry 1937;159:746.
62. Oates MR. The treatment of psychiatric disorders in pregnancy and the puerperium. Clin Obstet Gynecol 1986;13(2):385.
63. Stewart DE. Prophylactic lithium in post-partum affective psychosis. J Nerv Ment Dis 1988;176(8):485.
64. Uddenberg N, Engelsson I. Prognosis of postpartum mental disturbance: a prospective study of primiparous women and their 4-$^1/_2$ year old children. Acta Psychol (Scand) 1978;58:201.
65. Robson KM, Kumar R. Delayed onset of maternal affection after childbirth. Br J Psychiatry 1980;136:347.
66. Yalom I, Lunde D, Moos R, Hamburg D. Postpartum blues syndrome. Arch Gen Psychiatry 1968;18:16.
67. Pitt B. Maternity blues. Br J Psychiatry 1973;122:431.
68. O'Hara MW, Neunaber DJ, Zekoski EM. Prospective study of postpartum depression: prevalence, course, and predictive factors. J Abnorm Psychol 1984;93(2):158.
69. O'Hara MW. Psychological factors in the development of postpartum depression. In: Inwood DG, ed. Recent advances in postpartum disorders. Washington, DC: American Psychiatric Press, 1985.
70. Robson KM, Powell E. Early maternal attachment. In: Brockington IF, Kumar R, eds. Motherhood and mental illness. New York: Grune & Stratton, 1982.
71. Stein G. The maternity blues. In: Brockington IF, Kumar R, eds. Motherhood and mental illness. New York: Grune & Stratton, 1982.
72. Ghodsian M, Zajickek E, Wolkind S. A longitudinal study of maternal depression and child behavior problems. J Child Psychol Psychiatry 1984;25:91.
73. Billings Af, Moos RH. Children of parents with unipolar depression: a controlled 1-year followup. J Abnorm Child Psychol 1985;14:149.
74. Gelenberg AJ. Psychotropic drugs and the fetus. Biol Mer Psychiatry 1984;7:13.
75. Ananth J. Side effects in the neonate from psychotropic agents excreted through breast feeding. Am J Psychiatry 1978;B5:801.
76. Shurlock B. Human milk may not be ideal for sick babies. Med Post 1983;19:60.
77. Alder E, Bancroft J. The relationship between breast feeding persistence, sexuality and mood in postpartum women. Psychol Med 1988;18:389.
78. Alder EM, Cox JL. Breast feeding and post-natal depression. J Psychosom Res 1983;27(2):139.
79. Lindemann E. Symptomatology and management of acute grief. Am J Psychol 1944;101:141.
80. Kubler-Ross E. On death and dying. New York: Macmillan 1973.
81. Kennell JH, Slyter H, Klaus MH. The mourning response of parents to the death of a newborn. N Engl J Med 1970;238:344.
82. Rowe J, Clyman R, Green C, et al. Follow-up of families who experience a perinatal death. Pediatrics 1978;62:166.
83. Cole FS. Parental grieving. In: Tauesch HW, Yogman MW, ed. Follow-up management of the high-risk infant. Boston: Little, Brown, 1987:307.
84. Kellner KR, Donnelly WH, Gould SD. Parental behavior after perinatal death: lack of predictive demographic and obstetric variables. Obstet Gynecol 1984;43(6):809.
85. Condon JT. Management of established pathological grief reaction after stillbirth. Am J Psychiatry 1986;143(8):987.
86. Reilly TP, Hasazi JE, Bond LA. Children's conceptions of death and personal mortality. J Pediatr Psychol 1983;8:21.
87. Bourne S, Lewis E. Pregnancy after stillbirth or neonatal death;psychological risks and management. Lancet 1984;(July 7):31.
88. Leppert PC, Pahlka BS. Grieving characteristics after spontaneous abortion: a management approach. Obstet Gynecol 1984;64(1):119.
89. Seibel M, Graves, WL. The psychological implications of spontaneous abortions. J Reprod Med 1980;25(4):161.
90. Kaplan DM, Mason EA. Maternal reactions to premature birth viewed as an acute emotional disorder. Am J Orthopsychiatry 1960;30:539.
91. Trause AT, Kramer LI. The effects of premature birth on parents and relationships. Dev Med Child Neurol 1983;25:454.
92. Minde KK. Parenting the premature infant: problems and opportunities. In: Taeush HW, Yogman MW, ed. Follow-up management of the high-risk infant. Boston: Little, Brown, 1987:323.
93. Egeland B, Vaughn B. Failure of "bond formation" as a cause of abuse, neglect and maltreatment. Am J Orthopsychiatry 1981;51:78.
94. Minde K, Shosenberg N, Marton P, et al. Self-help groups in a premature nursery. J Am Acad Child Psychiatry 1980;19:1
95. Klaus MH, Kennell JH. Maternal-infant bonding. St Louis: CV Mosby, 1976.
96. Anisfeld E, Lipper E. Early contact, social support and mother-infant bonding: a joint rebuttal. Pediatrics 1983;72:569.
97. O'Connor S, Vietze PM, Sherrod KB et al. Reduced incidence of parenting inadequacy following rooming-in. Pediatrics 1980; 66:176.
98. Widmayer SM, Field TM. Effects of Brazelton demonstrations for mothers on the development of preterm infants. Pediatrics 1981;67:711.
99. Liptak GS, Keller BB, Feldman AW, Chamberlin RW. Enhancing infant development and parent-practitioner interaction with the Brazelton Neonatal Assessment Scale. Pediatrics 1983;72:71.
100. Sameroff A. Psychologic needs of the parent in infant development. In: Avery GB, Neonatology: pathophysiology and management of the newborn. 3rd ed. Philadelphia: JB Lippincott, 1987.
101. Anisfeld E, Lipper E. Early contact, social support and mother–infant bonding. Pediatrics 1983;72:79.

102. Jason J, Gilliland JC, Tyler CW, Jr. Homicide as a cause of pediatric mortality in the United States. Pediatrics 1983;72(2):191.
103. Norman MG, Newman DE, Smialek JE, Horembala EJ. The postmortem examination on the abused child: pathological, radiographic, and legal aspects. Perspect Pediatr Pathol 1984;8(4):313.
104. Jason J, Carpenter MM, Tyler CW, Jr. Underrecording of infant homicide in the United States. Am J Public Health 1983; 73(2):195.
105. Piers MW. Infanticide: past and present. New York: WW Norton, 1978.
106. Korbin JE. Child abuse and neglect: cross-cultural perspectives. Los Angeles: University of California Press, 1981.
107. Christoffel KK, Liu K, Stamler J. Epidemiology of fatal child abuse: international mortality data. J Chronic Dis 1981;34:57.
108. Spitz WV. Investigation of deaths in childhood. Part I. Infanticide. In Spitz WV, Fisher RS, eds. Medicolegal investigation of death: Guidelines for the application of pathology to crime investigation. 2nd ed. Springfield, IL: Charles C Thomas.
109. Wolkind SN, De Salis W. Infant temperament, maternal mental state and child behavior problems. In: Porter R, Collins GM, eds. Temperamental differences in infants and young children. London: Pitman, 1982.
110. Gibson E. Homicide in England and Wales, 1967–1971. London: HMSO, 1975.
111. West DJ. Murder followed by suicide. London: Heinemann, 1965.
112. Mitchell EK, Davis JH. Spontaneous births into toilets. J Forensic Sci 1983;29(2):591.
113. Emerick SJ, Foster LR, Campbell DT. Risk factors for traumatic infant death in Oregon, 1973 to 1982. Pediatrics 1986; 77(4):518.
114. Oliver JE. Dead children from problem families in NE Wiltshire. Br Med J 1983;286:115.

79
CHAPTER

ETHICAL ISSUES IN PERINATOLOGY

Frank A. Chervenak and Laurence B. McCullough

Maternal–fetal medicine has developed specialized concepts and a technical language to address the scientific and clinical matters of obstetric practice. These have demonstrated their adequacy for many areas of clinical concern, but permit only implicit consideration of the physician's ethical obligations (ie, what the physician ought to do or not do, because it is the right or correct thing). The term *ethical* is used here to distinguish such obligations from legal obligations (ie, what one ought to do or ought not to do because the law requires or forbids it). In ethical theory, ethical obligations are analyzed in terms of ethical principles. Adding the concepts and language of ethical analysis to the concepts and language of perinatal medicine makes it possible for the clinician to identify ethical obligations and to identify and manage conflicts between ethical obligations in obstetric care. The first section of this chapter provides a framework for understanding the physician's ethical obligations in maternal–fetal medicine in concrete, clinical terms. The goal of this section is to describe four types of ethical conflict in maternal–fetal medicine and illustrate them with clinical examples. The next section provides a detailed analysis of the ethical dimensions of two controversies in maternal–fetal medicine: routine obstetric ultrasound and cephalocentesis in the case of fetal hydrocephalus complicated by cephalopelvic disproportion. The goal of this section is to show how in-depth application of the ethical framework described in the first section helps to identify practical, ethically justified clinical management strategies in response to controversies involving conflicting ethical obligations in obstetric practice.

AN ETHICAL FRAMEWORK FOR MATERNAL–FETAL MEDICINE

THE ETHICAL PRINCIPLES OF BENEFICENCE AND RESPECT FOR AUTONOMY

Beauchamp and McCullough argue that the ethical principles of beneficence and respect for autonomy, when applied in clinical practice, generate ethical obligations directing the physician to protect and promote the patient's interests.[1] Beneficence requires the physician to assess as objectively and rigorously as possible available diagnostic and therapeutic options and to implement those that protect and promote the interests of the patient by securing for the patient the greater balance of goods over harms. On this model of clinical judgment the physician evaluates the interests of the patient from medicine's perspective. The principle of beneficence is balanced in clinical judgment by the principle of respect for autonomy. This principle obligates the physician to acknowledge that the patient too has a perspective on his or her interests, which is based on his or her values and beliefs. This model of clinical judgment asserts that the patient should have the freedom to choose alternatives based on these values and beliefs and that, therefore, the clinician is obligated to elicit and act on the value-based preferences of patients. Before application in particular circumstances, these two ethical principles are equally strong. As a matter of ethical theory, both generate serious ethical obligations, which can explain why ethical conflict can occur in clinical practice.

Protecting and promoting the interests of the pregnant woman and the interests of the fetus, and the child it will become, are the basic goals of obstetric care generally and of maternal–fetal medicine in particular. These goals form the basis on which the principles of respect for autonomy and beneficence are applied in maternal–fetal medicine. These principles, in turn, generate ethical obligations to the pregnant woman and fetus. Figure 79-1 illustrates how these obligations work toward goals of protecting and promoting maternal and fetal interests.

Maternal interests are protected and promoted by both autonomy-based and beneficence-based obligations of the physician. The pregnant woman is capable of identifying and expressing value-based preferences, and maternal–fetal medicine has accumulated considerable experience about beneficence-based management strategies that protect and promote maternal health.

The fetus can have no perspective on its interests. Because its central nervous system is insufficiently developed, it has no values or beliefs, which are necessary for an individual to have his or her own perspective on his or her own best interests. Hence, there can be no autonomy-based obligations to the fetus. Fetal interests in maternal–fetal medicine must, therefore, be understood in terms of the principle of beneficence, which grounds ethical obligations to the fetus. Because beneficence and respect for autonomy are, theoretically, equally weighted principles, beneficence-based obligations to the fetus are serious obligations.

The pregnant woman has beneficence-based obligations to the fetus in a pregnancy being taken to term because she is its ethical, although not for that reason alone necessarily legal, fiduciary. She is expected to protect and promote the fetus's interests and, by doing so, those of the child the fetus will become. From medicine's perspective, the goods to be sought for the child the fetus will become and therefore for the fetus are prevention of disease, handicapping conditions, and premature death as well as the cure or amelioration of disease, handicapping conditions, pain, and suffering.[1]

It may be appropriate, therefore, to refer to the fetus as a patient in pregnancies being taken to term.[2,3] In terms of this framework the fetus clearly becomes a patient at viability, because it is capable of surviving ex utero to become a child. Before viability, however, the fetus becomes a patient only as a result of the pregnant woman's decision to take a pregnancy to term. Thus, abortion before viability is not inconsistent with either the physician's or the pregnant woman's possible beneficence-based obligations to the fetus, because before viability such obligations cannot exist independently of the pregnant woman's decision about the disposition of her pregnancy. It is a fundamental feature of obstetric ethics that, before viability, no pregnant woman is ethically obligated to the fetus to regard it as a patient; her decision to confer or withhold such status is entirely a function of her own autonomy.

In pregnancies being taken to term, the ethical obligations of a physician to a pregnant woman and her fetus almost always work in concert because the physician and the woman most often agree on a plan of management that will best serve both the maternal and fetal interests. However, because autonomy-based and beneficence-based obligations to the fetus are a priori equally strong, conflicts among these ethical obligations can occur in maternal–fetal medicine.

CONFLICTS AMONG ETHICAL OBLIGATIONS

These conflicts can be divided into four groups, which will be discussed in the sections to follow:

1. Maternal autonomy-based obligations of the physician and maternal beneficence-based obligations of the physician
2. Fetal beneficence-based obligations of the pregnant woman and fetal beneficence-based obligations of the physician
3. Maternal autonomy-based obligations of the physician and fetal beneficence-based obligations of the physician
4. Maternal beneficence-based obligations and fetal beneficence-based obligations of the physician (see Fig. 79-1).

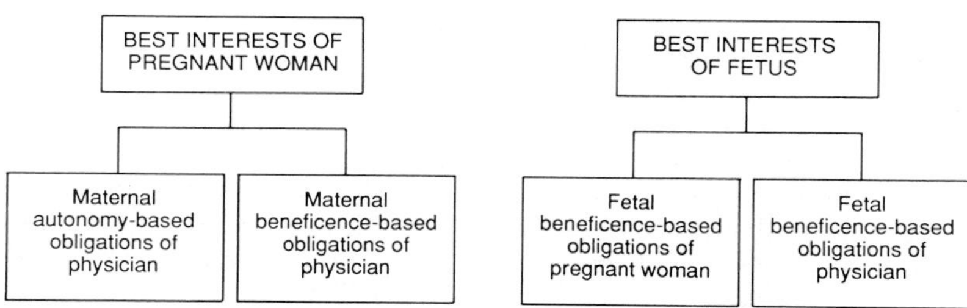

FIGURE 79–1. Ethical obligations in obstetrical care. (Modified from Chervenak FA, McCullough LB. Perinatal ethics. A practical method of analysis of obligations to mother and fetus. Obstet Gynecol 1985; 66: 442.)

Conflicts Between Maternal Autonomy-Based Obligations of the Physician and Maternal Beneficence-Based Obligations of the Physician

Meaningful communication between the physician and the pregnant woman in the form of patient education and eliciting the pregnant woman's values and beliefs and her value-based preferences is essential for a positive synergism between autonomy-based and beneficence-based obligations to her and prevention of potential ethical conflicts. A patient who is well-informed about her condition and therapeutic options has a greater capacity for autonomous decision making. The physician who is knowledgeable about the patient's values and preferences is in a better position to work with the pregnant woman to identify a management plan that would be consistent with her perspective on her best interests.

On occasion, the pregnant woman and her physician identify conflicting management strategies to serve the woman's interests. A Jehovah's Witness, for example, may refuse the administration of life-saving blood products during cesarean delivery because it would jeopardize her eternal salvation; the obstetrician may assess that such refusal would jeopardize her earthly existence.[4] A young woman with her first pregnancy may insist that she have a tubal ligation at the time she has a cesarean delivery because she is certain of her choice and does not desire the risk of a second operation; the physician may believe that such a procedure might lead to irreversible damage to her reproductive capabilities. In such a case the physician faces a conflict between his or her beneficence-based obligations to the pregnant woman (ie, to carry out the management plan that, from medicine's perspective, protects and promotes the best interests of the woman) and autonomy-based obligations to the pregnant woman (ie, to implement the management plan that the patient, on the basis of a voluntary and informed choice, has determined to be in her interests).

In some circumstances, autonomy-based obligations to the pregnant woman justifiably override beneficence-based obligations to her, especially when the basic beliefs and values of the woman are at stake. To override an autonomous decision that is based on such serious matters in a woman's life as her religious beliefs and convictions or her self-determination regarding her reproductive capabilities would constitute an intolerable assault on her autonomy. However, fulfilling such autonomy-based obligations does not obliterate all beneficence-based obligations. The physician is still obligated under beneficence to provide all forms of medical support other than blood products to a Jehovah's Witness who refuses the blood products and to offer to help the patient with a tubal ligation to obtain subsequent tubal reanastomosis if she so desires.

In some cases, beneficence-based obligations justifiably override autonomy-based obligations. This can occur when a woman's decisions are significantly reduced in their autonomy (eg, if there is a seriously reduced ability on her part to understand choices and make voluntary decisions) or when immediate action in an emergency situation is necessary to preserve her health or life. In such circumstances, the physician may be justified in acting in a way that is contrary to what the woman may indicate. A woman in her first pregnancy in labor warrants analgesia and emotional support to help her manage pain. To accede to the infrequent demand for cesarean delivery, when this same woman is in considerable labor pain and is very frightened as a consequence, however, would violate beneficence-based obligations to protect maternal health. Because such a request probably does not reflect her basic values and beliefs, autonomy-based obligations are diminished. Although a woman may strongly desire a low transverse cesarean delivery to permit vaginal delivery in subsequent pregnancies, intraoperatively, the obstetrician may realize that because of a poorly developed lower uterine segment, a vertical uterine incision is necessary to avoid injury to the uterine vessels. Time constraints may not permit the physician to obtain consent for such an incision. Thus, in some cases, a woman's preferences are justifiably overridden in favor of beneficence-based obligations.

In both cases, ethical analysis and judgment conclude that the potential goods of nonintervention (avoidance of cesarean delivery, avoidance of possible hysterectomy) outweigh the potential harms of intervention (maternal discomfort and psychic stress, the necessity of future cesarean deliveries). In all cases in which beneficence-based obligations to the woman justifiably take precedence, there is always an autonomy-based obligation to explain later to the woman what was done and why it was done. This is one important sense in which respect for autonomy helps to prevent dehumanized obstetric care.

Conflicts Between Fetal Beneficence-Based Obligations of the Pregnant Woman and Fetal Beneficence-Based Obligations of the Physician

The pregnant woman and her physician are usually in agreement on the plan of management that provides the greatest balance of fetal goods over harms. However, there is the potential for conflict in matters concerning the diagnosis and management of fetal disorders because the woman and the physician may have well-founded but conflicting views about what is in the interests of the fetus and the child it will become.

Such conflicts can occur in the context of fetal diagnosis and therapy. For example, invasive fetal therapy to place a ventriculoamniotic shunt to alleviate fetal hydrocephalus involves uncertainty about risks of morbidity and mortality resulting from the underlying condition, the efficacy of the therapy to correct the defect, and the risks of morbidity and mortality during and after the intervention.[5] In their analyses of the interests of the fetus, the physician and the pregnant woman may reasonably weigh the various components differently. In such cases, there may be a genuine dilemma (ie, the necessity to choose between two courses of action, both of which are founded on substantial ethical justification). There can be no decisive resolution of the dilemma surrounding experimental invasive fetal therapy until these levels of uncertainty are reduced. That is, the pregnant woman is reasonable to hold that beneficence-based obligations (on her part and the physician's) to perform experimental interventions are minimal in such cases. Thus, to respect a woman's decision concerning experimental, invasive therapies generally is an acceptable way to manage these uncertainties, because no major beneficence-based obligations to the fetus are violated by doing so.

Conflicts Between Maternal Autonomy-Based Obligations of the Physician and Fetal Beneficence-Based Obligations of the Physician

Conflicts between maternal autonomy-based obligations and fetal beneficence-based obligations are probably the most common and challenging ethical conflicts in maternal–fetal medicine. It is especially important that beneficence-based obligations be determined on a careful, objective, and rigorous assessment of the goods and harms of an intervention, so that the fetus's best interests can be established on systematic and therefore reliable grounds. These obligations include such routine matters in obstetric care as providing education about the effects on the fetus of maternal cigarette, alcohol, and drug use and compassionate attempts to modify such maternal behaviors by repeated emphasis on the potential ill effects on the fetus.

In some situations, the fetus stands to benefit from maternal bed rest, hospitalization, or extended fetal heart rate monitoring. In addition, certain drugs administered to the pregnant woman—such as tocolytic agents to prevent premature birth, insulin to prevent macrosomia, digoxin to correct supraventricular tachycardia, or a steroid preparation to induce lung maturity—may provide clear benefit to the fetus. Thus, it is evident that for optimal fetal outcome in some pregnancies maternal participation in the obstetric plan, with subsequent restriction on maternal autonomy, is necessary.

When this cooperation is not present, conflicts arise between autonomy-based obligations to the pregnant woman and beneficence-based obligations to the fetus. The physician should, as a first-line strategy, attempt to discharge fetal beneficence-based obligations by vigorously attempting to persuade the woman to accept the required restrictions or treatment.

This sort of ethical conflict becomes difficult to resolve when more invasive procedures are needed for fetal diagnosis or management, such as amniocentesis to determine lung maturity, intrauterine blood transfusion for erythroblastosis, or cesarean delivery in the event of well-documented fetal distress. This is because a woman may determine that the risks to her well-being are not worth taking, even though the fetus might well benefit from the proposed intervention.

The following guidelines help to negotiate this ethical conflict. The greater the likelihood that a particular intervention will result in a clearly substantial benefit for the fetus (ie, a significant decrease in morbidity and mortality), the stronger are the beneficence-based obligations to the fetus. This is simply the moral logic of beneficence-based obligations. The greater the likelihood that the fetus will be at a substantial risk from the intervention (eg, increased morbidity and mortality), the weaker are fetal beneficence-based obligations, again as a matter of the moral logic of beneficence-based obligations. The greater the risk of harms to the woman (ie, increase in morbidity and mortality), the stronger the maternal autonomy-based obligations in those cases in which the woman refuses the intervention. This is because fiduciary obligations of the pregnant woman to the fetus do not obligate her to accept any and all risks, especially those that she or her physician regard as serious, far-reaching, and irreversible. These guidelines permit fetal diagnosis and treatment, in the authors' view, when the risks to the fetus are minimal, the potential benefit for the fetus is substantial, and the risks to the woman are those she should reasonably accept on behalf of her fetus (ie, they are neither serious, far-reaching, nor irreversible).[6]

Because the outlook for fetal anencephaly is universally dismal, beneficence-based obligations to such a fetus are nonexistent, and termination of pregnancy, even in the third trimester, may be acceptable.[7] By contrast, if maternal brain death were to occur, autonomy-based obligations to her no longer exist and fetal beneficence-based obligations move to the fore, thus possibly justifying sustaining maternal biological life until fetal maturity if there are reliable reasons to think that this is what the pregnant woman would have wanted.[8] Although the two previous paradigms are useful in considering extreme cases, maternal–fetal medicine presents more challenging conflicts, such as whether to perform a cesarean delivery for a breech presentation at 24 to 25 weeks of gestation or whether to use experimental ventriculoamniotic shunting in the management of fetal hydrocephalus. In both instances, the benefits to the fetus of the obstetric intervention would be unclear because the fetus of 24 to 25 weeks' gestation may not survive any mode of delivery[9] and because further clinical studies are necessary before it can be concluded that ventriculoamniotic shunting provides a clearly substantial benefit to the fetus.[10]

By contrast, if intrapartum fetal monitoring reveals severe bradycardia that is subsequently unresponsive to prolonged conservative measures, the beneficence-based obligation to perform a cesarean delivery to preserve fetal life and avoid morbidity and handicapping conditions associated with asphyxial brain damage can become compelling enough to justify overriding maternal autonomy-based obligations that are generated by her refusal of the procedure.

Respect for autonomy in such cases requires the physician again to adapt the first-line strategy of attempting to persuade the woman to permit the procedure by informing her that cesarean delivery is indeed necessary to save her child's life and to avoid potentially serious handicapping conditions, should the fetus survive vaginal delivery. A more coercive approach (eg, threatening to seek or actually seeking a court order) may in very restricted circumstances be morally justifiable. However, this is a matter of considerable controversy in the literature.[11,12] In considering this more serious compromise of maternal autonomy, the benefit to the fetus of such action must be clear and overwhelming and the woman should be accorded respect and compassion, not degradation. Because remedies short of legal action (eg, vigorous persuasion) involve fewer negative consequences for the physician–patient relationship and maternal–infant bonding,[13] the authors believe that such remedies are far better than the resort to court orders. These strategies respect the woman's autonomy while acknowledging beneficence-based obligations to the fetus. Moreover, court orders may not be forthcoming in all cases.[6]

Conflicts Between Maternal Beneficence-Based Obligations of the Physician and Fetal Beneficence-Based Obligations of the Physician

In modern obstetrics, conflicts exist between maternal and fetal beneficence-based obligations. The most difficult of these conflicts involves putting one party at great risk of substantial morbidity and mortality to avoid great risk of similarly grave consequences for the other. These ethical conflicts can sometimes be agonizing in maternal–fetal medicine. Maternal malignancy or abdominal ectopic gestation may necessitate termination of a wanted pregnancy as the only reliable means of saving the woman's life. In other cases, potentially fetotoxic drugs, such as diphenylhydantoin, may be needed to prevent serious maternal disorders such as seizures. The resolution of these sorts of conflicts presents the physician and pregnant woman with tragic choices, because there is no clearly convincing ethical argument in obstetric ethical theory or general philosophical ethical theory that the woman's life is more important than that of the fetus or that one form of serious morbidity and handicap in the pregnant woman is more grave than those in the fetus. Because of the negative consequences for the pregnant woman and for the integrity of the patient–physician relationship that would result from failing to respect the pregnant woman's decisions, respecting them is an acceptable course in these tragic cases.

In summary, when physicians confront ethical conflicts in maternal–fetal medicine, successful clinical management of such conflicts requires identification of the component ethical obligations of the conflict and rigorous judgment about the relative weight or priority of those obligations.[6] This process requires thorough documentation and objective assessment of fetal and maternal interests. An ethically justified decision is consistent with what can be shown to be the weightiest obligations as the result of ethical analysis. At times, however, there is no clear resolution: the competing obligations appear to be of equal weight. It should be recognized that reasonable and conscientious people determine the weight of moral obligations differently. In such cases, respect for the pregnant woman's autonomy is a sound clinical management strategy.

TWO CONTROVERSIES IN MATERNAL–FETAL MEDICINE

ROUTINE OBSTETRIC ULTRASOUND SCREENING

Unfortunately, the present debate in maternal–fetal medicine about the routine use of obstetrical ultrasound has been shaped by two different theories: examine all pregnancies[14] or examine only when indicated.[15] This way of thinking has obscured from view an important and reasonable middle ground: the standard of care in maternal–fetal medicine should include informing all pregnant women who are taking their pregnancies to term about the availability of this technology, including a thorough discussion of its advantages and disadvantages, and permitting the woman to make her own informed decision about whether ultrasound screening will be a routine aspect of her particular pregnancy. Prenatal informed consent for sonogram (PICS), as a middle-ground position on the use of obstetric ultrasound, enhances the autonomy of pregnant women, and thus makes a significant contribution toward the goal of humanizing obstetric care.[16]

There are advantages to routine obstetric ultrasound examinations done once, at about 18 weeks.[14,15,17,18] Dating a pregnancy based on menstrual history or early physical examination is notoriously unreliable. Any improvement in gestational-age assessment might well decrease the morbidity and mortality that accompany an expected premature or postmature birth. Although several age-independent modalities for the detection of intrauterine growth retardation (IUGR) have been described, if information is available concerning an accurate gestational age based on early ultrasound, the diagnosis and, as a result, the management of IUGR at a later age are facilitated.

Major structural anomalies can be diagnosed by ultrasound at 18 weeks in the majority of cases.[14,18,19] This has the good of providing an adequate information base for pregnant women so that they can decide in a thoughtful way about the disposition of their pregnancy. Although some women will choose to terminate a pregnancy when an anomaly is detected, others will continue to term. In these latter cases, outcome can be optimized by appropriate obstetrical management and neonatal care. In addition, one can prevent maternal psychological trauma from an unexpected anomalous birth.

There are other potential goods in pregnancies going to term, such as the detection of multiple gestation or identification of a high-risk group for placenta previa.[14] The value of this information is that it enables more thorough planning for the management of the pregnancy. In addition, in rare cases, an unexpected hydatidiform mole, other tumors, or fetal death could be detected that would greatly benefit a management plan.[4] Moreover, there could be the psychological benefit of increased maternal–fetal bonding by visualization of the fetus.[20]

Besides the preceding benefits there are thought to be harms associated with routine ultrasound. Some harms can occur when false-positive or false-negative ultrasound diagnoses are made. Because all positive diagnoses should generate an appropriate referral, the false-positive rate should thereby be minimized.[21] Nevertheless, maternal anxiety will be caused in the interim. False-negative diagnoses are an inherent risk of all diagnostic interventions. In the case of routine ultrasound, this risk can be minimized by adherence to well-defined standards.[22,23]

Other potential harms could result from routine ultrasound. Kremkau has reviewed four mechanisms by which it is possible theoretically to implicate ultrasound in the causation of fetal anomalies: heat, cavitation, microsteaming, and radiation force.[24] The American Institute of Ultrasound in Medicine, in its safety statement, has assessed these theoretical harms and has concluded that "the benefits to patients of the prudent use of diagnostic ultrasound far outweigh any potential risk."[25] This list of harms might have influenced the NIH consensus panel to not recommend routine ultrasound screening.[15]

One might be tempted to conclude that there is a beneficence-based justification for routine obstetrical ultrasound, if one assumes that its goods can be established. After all, established goods at the present time outweigh harms, because the harms of false-positive and false-negative diagnoses can be minimized and the potential harms described by Kremkau may not exist.[24–26] The problem with this line of reasoning is that there is considerable obstetrical uncertainty about whether the goods of routine obstetric ultrasound have in fact been definitely established.[14,15,17] Elias and Annas's recent admonition that careful validation of the fact that goods do outweigh harms of prenatal screening tests applies here.[27] Thus, even though there is some benefit to ultrasound screening, a clearly decisive beneficence-based argument in favor of routine obstetric ultrasound cannot be established at the present time.

A beneficence-based argument against routine obstetric ultrasound fares no better. Such an argument must assume that the harms of routine ultrasound will outweigh any goods (including new benefits that may be discovered in the future). That is, these harms outweigh the goods of reducing fetal morbidity and mortality. However, the most that can be reasonably assumed at the present time is that some theoretical harms might outweigh some of the goods. Currently, there is no way to know reliably whether, on balance, *all* the harms will come to outweigh *all* the goods. Again, a beneficence-based ethical analysis of the clinical data fails to produce a decisive argument against routine obstetrical ultrasound.

So far our ethical analysis has shown that the principle of beneficence leads to the conclusion that routine ultrasound screening in pregnancies being taken to term might benefit the fetus and the child it will become and that not screening will probably not result in significant harm. Because both alternatives are consistent with the obligation to protect and promote the interests of the fetus, it is reasonable to rely on the ethical principle of respect for autonomy to manage clinical uncertainty.

The informed consent process is the means for implementing the clinical strategy of PICS with every pregnant woman. PICS should be undertaken in several stages. First, shortly after the pregnancy is diagnosed, every pregnant woman should be provided with information about the actual and theoretical benefits of obstetrical ultrasound and about its theoretical harms. Second, the pregnant woman should evaluate this information in terms of her own values and beliefs, something every autonomous patient is qualified to do. It may be helpful to some women to consider, at this point in the process, the physician's scientific evaluation of the clinical data that have been reported in the literature. The third stage in PICS is for the pregnant woman to articulate her preference regarding the use of ultrasound in the management of her pregnancy. The fourth stage is for the physician to provide the pregnant woman with the physician's own recommendation, if he or she has one. The fifth stage is a thoughtful and sensitive discussion of any disagreement that may emerge. Lastly, the woman makes her final decision. This decision should then determine the use of obstetric ultrasound for that pregnant woman. This process provides a significant role for the physician's clinical judgment and experience, as well as any recommendation he or she thinks is in the patient's interest. Thus, respect for the pregnant woman's autonomy does not devalue the physician's role to that of an automaton.

CEPHALOCENTESIS FOR THE INTRAPARTUM MANAGEMENT OF HYDROCEPHALUS

Cephalocentesis has long been accepted as a destructive procedure to avoid intrapartum morbidity and mortality when fetal hydrocephalus occurs with macrocephaly. This procedure performed either transabdominally or transvaginally saved maternal lives prior to the time of safe cesarean delivery.[28] Because cephalocentesis plainly is in conflict with beneficence-based obligations to the fetus, it requires careful ethical justification, if for no other reason than to prevent its unjustified use. Because fetal hydrocephalus presents with varied etiologies that have varied outcomes, ethical analysis must be carried out by respecting the heterogeneity of this condition.[29] Therefore, we will consider resolution strategies for two ends of a continuum: isolated fetal hydrocephalus and fetal hydrocephalus with severe associated abnormalities. We then consider fetal hydrocephalus with other associated abnormalities as a middle ground on the continuum (Fig. 79-2).

Isolated Fetal Hydrocephalus

There is considerable potential for normal, sometimes superior, intellectual function for fetuses with even extreme isolated hydrocephalus.[30–34] However, as a group, infants with isolated hydrocephalus experience a greater incidence of mental retardation and early death than the general population.[30–33] In addition, associated anomalies may go undetected and a fetus may be incorrectly diagnosed as having isolated hydrocephalus.[35–36]

There are compelling ethical reasons, well founded in the beneficence model, for concluding that continuing existence of fetuses with isolated hydrocephalus is in their interests. Because it is impossible to predict that fetuses with isolated hydrocephalus will have mental retardation and because the degree of possible mental retardation cannot be predicted, it cannot be said for any particular fetus with isolated hydrocephalus that cesarean delivery followed by aggressive neonatal management fails to confer a significantly greater balance of goods over harms on the child the fetus will become. Even when performed under optimal therapeutic conditions under sonographic guidance, cephalocentesis, therefore, cannot reasonably be regarded as protecting or promoting the interests of the fetus. Indeed, it is inconsistent with beneficence-based obligations to risk increased mortality and morbidity for the fetus, especially when employed with a destructive intent.

The beneficence-based obligations to the fetus, however, must be balanced against beneficence-based and autonomy-based obligations to the pregnant woman, as required by the ethical framework described in the first section. The physician has a beneficence-based obligation to the woman to avoid performing a cesarean delivery, because the possibility of morbidity and mortality for the woman is higher than that associated with vaginal delivery. The autonomy model obligates the physician to undertake only those interventions or forms of treatment to which the woman has given a voluntary informed consent.[6,37]

If, with informed consent, the woman refuses cesarean delivery, there is a conflict among the physician's obligations to the fetus and to the pregnant woman. On the one hand, the physician has a beneficence-based obligation to the fetus to perform a cesarean delivery. On the other hand, the physician has both a beneficence-based and an autonomy-based obligation to the pregnant woman to perform cephalocentesis followed by vaginal delivery. This conflict should be resolved in favor of the beneficence-based obligations to the fetus, because the benefit to the fetus is very substantial and the risks from cesarean delivery minimal, because cephalocentesis is inconsistent with the obligation to secure that benefit, and because the risks to the woman are those she should reasonably accept on behalf of her fetus. As a first-line strategy, she should be asked to reconsider and consent to cesarean delivery. As a second-line strategy, the physician is justified in recommending this as the intrapartum management of choice, as part of a persistent, vigorous, but respectful attempt to persuade the pregnant woman to change her mind.

If these two strategies fail and the pregnant woman continues to refuse cesarean delivery, the physician confronts tragic circumstances. If neither cesarean delivery nor cephalocentesis is performed, the woman is at risk for uterine rupture and death, and her fetus is at risk for death. The logic of beneficence-based obligations to the fetus is to avoid such total and irreversible harm. The logic of such obligations to the woman is to avoid serious, far-reaching, and possibly irreversible harm. Nonetheless, because of the grave nature of pos-

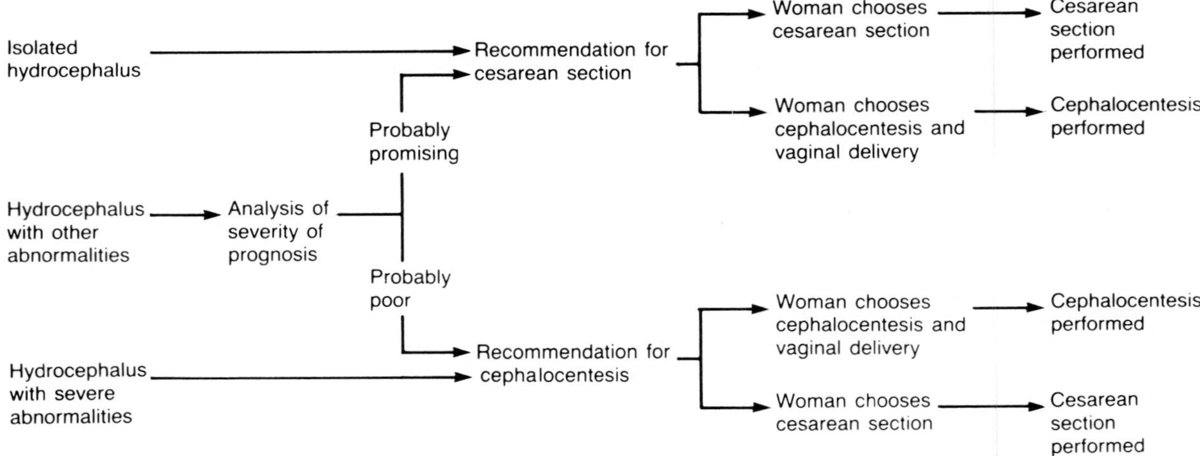

FIGURE 79–2. Resolution strategies for ethical conflicts in the intrapartum management of hydrocephalus with macrocephaly.

sible consequences for the woman and her fetus of performing a surgical procedure on a resistant patient and because of the pitfalls of attempted legal coercion,[11,12] the physician should act on autonomy-based obligations to the woman in such an extreme circumstance. To fail to respect an unwavering, voluntary, and informed refusal of a cesarean delivery constitutes a fundamental assault on the woman's autonomy. The fetus is at high risk for death under either alternative. The woman's death, at least, can be avoided. Serious beneficence-based obligations to the fetus on the part of both the physician and the pregnant woman will probably be violated and a needless death will most probably result, however, by performing a cephalocentesis. Herein lies the tragedy of these circumstances.

Hydrocephalus With Severe Associated Abnormalities

Some abnormalities that occur in association with fetal hydrocephalus are severe for the child afflicted with them. We define "severe" abnormalities as those that either (1) are incompatible with continued existence (eg, bilateral renal agenesis[32] and cloverleaf skull with thanatophoric dysplasia[38]) or (2) although compatible with survival in some cases, result in virtual absence of cognitive function (eg, trisomy 18[35] and alobar holoprosencephaly[39]). Because there is no available intervention to prevent postnatal death in the first group, beneficence-based obligations of the physician and the pregnant woman to attempt to prolong the fetus's life are nonexistent. No ethical theory obligates anyone to attempt the impossible. For the second group, beneficence-based obligations of the physician and the pregnant woman to sustain the fetus's life are minimal. This is because the handicap imposed by the abnormality is severe. In these cases, the potential for cognitive development and, therefore, the achievement of other goods for the child (eg, relationships with others) are virtually absent.

In these circumstances, the woman is released from her fiduciary role to the fetus as a patient because no significant goods can be achieved by cesarean delivery for the fetus or the child it will become. There remain only the autonomy-based and beneficence-based obligations of the physician to the pregnant woman. Because beneficence-based obligations to the fetus are nonexistent or minimal in these cases, we conclude that the physician's overriding moral obligations are to the pregnant woman's voluntary and informed decision. Moreover, because there are no weighty beneficence-based obligations to the fetus, the physician may justifiably recommend cephalocentesis to enable vaginal delivery.

Hydrocephalus With Other Associated Abnormalities

On the continuum between the cases of isolated hydrocephalus and hydrocephalus with severe associated abnormalities, there is found a variety of cases of hydrocephalus associated with other abnormalities of varying degrees of impairment of cognitive and physical function. These range from hypoplastic distal phalanges[32] to spina bifida[40] to encephalocele.[41] Because these conditions involve varying prognoses, it would be clinically inappropriate, and therefore ethically misleading, to treat this third category as homogeneous. Therefore, the authors propose a working distinction, subject to revision in response to new clinical information, between different kinds of prognoses. The first is best called "probably promising," by which it is meant that there is a significant possibility the child will experience cognitive development, with learning disabilities and physical handicaps that may be ameliorated to some extent. The second is called "probably poor," by which it is meant that there is only a limited possibility for cognitive development, because of learning disabilities and physical handicap that cannot be ameliorated to a significant extent.

When the prognosis is probably promising (eg, isolated arachnoid cyst[29]), there are serious beneficence-based obligations to the fetus. However, these are not necessarily on the same order as those that occur in cases of isolated hydrocephalus, especially in light of the possibility that any associated anomaly may increase the possibility of a poor outcome.[32] Therefore, in cases with a prognosis of probably promising, the authors propose that the physician recommend cesarean delivery, although it should not be recommended as vigorously in cases of isolated hydrocephalus. A pregnant woman's informed refusal of cesarean section therefore should be respected.

In cases in which the prognosis, even though uncertain, is probably poor (eg, encephalocele[41]), beneficence-based obligations to the fetus are less weighty than those owed to the fetus with a promising prognosis. Thus, these cases resemble ethically those of hydrocephalus with severe anomalies, with the proviso that some, albeit limited, benefit can be achieved for the fetus by cesarean delivery and aggressive perinatal treatment. Nonetheless, the physician may in these cases justifiably accept an informed voluntary decision by the woman for cephalocentesis followed by vaginal delivery.

CONCLUSION

There are, obviously, other areas of ethical controversy in maternal–fetal medicine that also could be analyzed in depth. Despite the limited scope of this chapter, clinically relevant general lessons can be taken from it. Ethical analysis of a particular controversy in maternal–fetal medicine (1) relies on a clearly articulated framework of ethical obligations to both the pregnant woman and the fetus, (2) applies that framework in a rigorous ethical analysis of conflicts among those obligations, and (3) identifies clinical management strategies that can be justified by reasonable argument, as distinct from what Socrates calls "mere opinion." Mere opinion fails one or more of these tests and is therefore clinically unreliable.

REFERENCES

1. Beauchamp TL, McCullough LB. Medical ethics: the moral responsibilities of physicians. Englewood Cliffs, NJ: Prentice-Hall, 1984pp. 22–51..
2. Pritchard JA, MacDonald PC. Williams obstetrics. 16th ed. New York: Appleton-Century-Crofts, 1980p. vii.
3. Harrison MR, Golbus MS, Filly RA. The unborn patient. New York: Grune & Stratton, 1984.
4. Jewett JF. Report from the Committee on Maternal Welfare: total exsanguination. N Engl J Med 1981;305:1218.
5. Clewell WH, Johnson ML, Meier PR, Newkirk JB, Zide SL, Hendee RW. A surgical approach to the treatment of fetal hydrocephalus. N Engl J Med 1982;306:1320.
6. Chervenak FA, McCullough LB. Perinatal ethics. A practical method of analysis of obligations to mother and fetus. Obstet Gynecol 1985;66:442.
7. Chervenak FA, Farley MA, Walter L, Hobbins JC, Mahoney MJ. When is termination of pregnancy during the third trimester morally justifiable? N Engl J Med 1984;310:501.
8. Dillon WP, Lee RV, Tronolone MJ, Buckwald S, Foote RJ. Life support and maternal brain death during pregnancy. JAMA 1982;248:1089.
9. Hack M, Fanaroff AA. How small is too small? Considerations in evaluating the outcome of the tiny infant. Clin Perinatol 1988;15:773.
10. Manning F, Harrison MR, Rodeck C. Catheter shunts for fetal hydronephrosis and hydrocephalus. Report of the International Fetal Surgery Registry. N Engl J Med 1986;315:336.
11. Annas GJ. Protecting the liberty of pregnant patients. N Engl J Med 1987;316:1213.
12. Nelson LJ, Milliken N. Compelled medical treatment of pregnant women. Life, liberty, and law in conflict. JAMA 1988;259:1060,
13. Engelhardt Jr HT. Current controversies in obstetrics: wrongful life and forced fetal surgical procedures. Am J Obstet Gynecol 1986;151:313.
14. Royal College of Obstetricians and Gynaecologists. Report of RCOG Working Party on Routine Ultrasound Examination in Pregnancy. Royal College of Obstetricians and Gynaecologists. London, December 1984.
15. National Institutes of Health. Diagnostic ultrasound imaging in pregnancy. Report of a Consensus Development Conference Sponsored by the National Institute of Child Health and Human Development, The Office of Medical Applications of Research, The Division Research Resources, and The Food and Drug Administration. February 6–8, 1984. National Institutes of Health, Bethesda, MD.
16. Chervenak FA, McCullough LB, Chervenak JL. Prenatal informed consent for sonogram (PICS): an indication for obstetrical ultrasound. Am J Obstet Gynecol. 1989;161:857.
17. Thacker SB. Quality of controlled clinical trials. The case of imaging ultrasound in obstetrics: a review. Br J Obstet Gynecol 1985;92:437.
18. Sabbagha RE. Diagnostic ultrasound applied to obstetrics and gynecology. Philadelphia: JB Lippincott, 1987.
19. Romero R, Pilu G, Jeanty P, Ghidini A, Hobbins JC. Prenatal diagnosis of congenital anomalies. Norwalk, CT: Appleton and Lange, 1988.
20. Campbell S, Reading AE, Cox DN. Ultrasound scanning in pregnancy: the short term psychological effects of early real time scans. J Psychosom Obstet Gynaecol 1982;1:57.
21. Sabbagha RE, Sheick Z, Tamura RK, Dal Campo S, Simpson JL, Depp R. Predictive value, sensitivity and specificity of ultrasonic targeted imaging for fetal anomalies in gravid women at high risk for birth defects. Am Obstet Gynecol 1985;152:822.
22. American Institute of Ultrasound in Medicine. Official statement of antepartum obstetrical ultrasound examination guidelines. American Institute of Ultrasound in Medicine. Bethesda, MD, October 1985.
23. American Institute of Ultrasound in Medicine. Official statement on guidelines for minimum post-residency training in obstetrical and gynecological ultrasound. American Institute of Ultrasound in Medicine. Bethesda, MD, May 1982.
24. Kremkau FW. Biological effects and possible hazards. Clin Obstet Gynaecol 1983;10:395.
25. American Institute of Ultrasound in Medicine. Bioeffects Committee. J Ultrasound Med 1983;2:R14.
26. Lyons EA, Dyke C, Toms M, Cheang M. In-utero exposure to diagnostic ultrasound: a 6-year follow-up. Radiology 1988;166:687.
27. Elias S, Annas GJ. Routine prenatal genetic screening. N Engl J Med 1987;317:1407.
28. Chervenak FA, Romero R. Is there a role for fetal cephalocentesis in modern obstetrics? Am J Perinatol 1984;1:170.
29. Chervenak FA, McCullough LB. Ethical analysis of the intrapartum management of pregnancy complicated by fetal hydrocephalus with macrocephaly. Obstet Gynecol 1986;68:720.
30. Lorber J. The results of early treatment of extreme hydrocephalus. Med Child Neurol (Suppl) 1981;16:21.
31. McCullough DC, Balzer-Martin LA. Current prognosis in overt neonatal hydrocephalus. J Neurosurg 1982;57:378.
32. Chervenak FA, Duncan C, Ment LR. The outcome of fetal ventriculomegaly. Lancet 1984;2:179.
33. Shurtleff DB, Floz EL, Loeser JD. Hydrocephalus: a definition of its progress and relationship to intellectual function, diagnosis, and complications. Am J Dis Child 1973;125:688.
34. Kovnar EM, Coxe WS, Volpe JJ. Development and marked reconstitution of cerebral mantle after postnatal treatment of intrauterine hydrocephalus. Neurology 1984;34:840.
35. Chervenak FA, Berkowitz RL, Tortora M, Hobbins JC. The management of fetal hydrocephalus. Am J Obstet Gynecol 1985;151:933.
36. Chervenak FA, Berkowitz RL, Romero R, et al. The diagnosis of fetal hydrocephalus. Am J Obstet Gynecol 1983;147:703.
37. Capron AM. Right to refuse medical care. In: Encyclopedia of bioethics. New York: Free Press, 1978:1498.
38. Chervenak FA, Blakemore K, Isaacson G, Mayden K, Hobbins JC. Antenatal sonographic findings of thanatophoric dysplasia with cloverleaf skull. Am J Obstet Gynecol 1983;146:984.
39. Chervenak FA, Isaacson G, Mahoney MJ, Tortora M, Mesologites T, Hobbins JC. The obstetric significance of holoprosencephaly. Obstet Gynecol 1984;63:115.
40. Chervenak FA, Duncan D, Ment LR, Tortora M, McClure M, Hobbins JC. Perinatal management of meningomyelocele. Obstet Gynecol 1984;63:376.
41. Chervenak FA, Isaacson G, Mahoney MJ. The diagnosis and management of fetal cephalocele. Obstet Gynecol 1984;63:376.

80

CHAPTER

LEGAL ISSUES IN MATERNAL–FETAL MEDICINE

Angela R. Holder

Legal issues in maternal–fetal medicine have become at least more newsworthy, if not more frequent, within the past several years. Obstetrical malpractice premiums have risen sufficiently to imperil the availability of medical care for pregnant women, particularly indigent women, in many areas of the country.[1] Newspapers frequently report that a pregnant woman has been criminally prosecuted for "fetus abuse." The issue of abortion remains the most divisive domestic political issue in the country. New developments in prenatal diagnosis impinge upon both the abortion issue and malpractice concerns. From time to time a court orders a cesarean section to be performed upon an unconsenting woman. This chapter attempts a brief survey of some of the current legal issues in maternal–fetal medicine.

MALPRACTICE

The legal definition of *malpractice* was very well explained in an 1898 New York decision (Pike v. Honsinger, 49 NE 760, NY 1898). The court said:

> The law relating to malpractice is simple and well settled, although not always easy of application. A physician and surgeon, by taking charge of a case, impliedly represents that he possesses and the law places upon him the duty of possessing, that reasonable degree of learning and skill that is ordinarily possessed by physicians and surgeons in the locality in which he practices and which is ordinarily regarded by those conversant with the employment as is necessary to qualify him to engage in the business of practicing medicine and surgery. Upon consenting to treat a patient it becomes his duty to use reasonable care and diligence in the exercise of his skill and the application of his learning to accomplish the purpose for which he is employed. He is under the further obligation to use his best judgment in exercising his skill and applying his knowledge.

In other words, an error of judgment is not malpractice. However, failure to use due skill, care, and knowledge, as would be used by the reasonable physician with the same training, is. To cite a simple example, if a physician uses standard and appropriate diagnostic tests, the results are equivocal, and he or she concludes that the patient probably does not have a disease when in fact she does, that is an error of judgment. Failing to do any testing and assuming that the patient does not have the disease is malpractice.

In obstetrics, of course, there are two patients, and negligence toward either may engender successful legal action.[2] Any obstetrician owes the same duty of care to a fetal patient as he or she does to the pregnant woman, and negligent treatment of a fetus if it is to be carried to term constitutes actionable malpractice to the same extent as negligence in the treatment of any other patient (Blake v. Cruz, 698 P 2d 315, Idaho 1984; Martinez v. Long Island Jewish Hillside Medical Center, 504 NYS 2d 693, NY 1986). In particular, failure to diagnose and treat a pregnant woman's illness (such as rubella) with the result that the fetus is deformed is clearly negligent (Harman v. Daniels, 525 F Supp 798, DC Va 1981; Shack v. Holland, 389 NYS 2d 988, NY 1976; Hughson v. St. Francis Hospital, 92 AD 2d 131, NY 1983). The most usual sort of obstetrical malpractice claim involves allegations of negligence during a delivery, with damage to either mother or infant. Damage to a newborn's brain, usually from lack of oxygen, may result in a patient who will be substantially helpless but with a normal lifespan; for that reason the predicted costs of care make this by far the most expensive legal action against a physician of any specialty.

As prenatal diagnosis has become widespread, two sorts of actions have begun to be filed against obstetricians—"wrongful birth" and "wrongful life" suits. Both involve such matters as failing to advise a pregnant woman at risk of having a child with a genetic problem to have amniocentesis or, having advised the test, misinterpreting the results (eg, Karlsons v. Guerinot, 394 NYS 2d 933, NY 1977; Howard v. Lecher, 366 NE 2d 64, NY 1977). Opposition to abortion to the extent that a physician does not tell a patient that she is within a risk group for having a handicapped child and thus should go elsewhere for amniocentesis or another prenatal diagnostic test, lest having the test lead her to have an abortion, would never be defensible in an action of this sort. Other cases involve negligent sterilization when the operation is done in situations in which there is a high probability that the couple will have a child with a genetic problem (eg, Doerr v. Villate, 230 NE 2d 767, Ill 1966; Ochs v. Borelli, 445 A 2d 883, Ct 1982).

"Wrongful birth" suits are brought by parents on their own behalf. They claim either that their handicapped child was crippled by the direct action of the obstetrician (as in negligence during the delivery) or that the reasonably careful obstetrician would have known that the woman was at risk of having a handicapped baby (as, for example, would be the case with a 40-year-old mother) and did not advise proper prenatal testing. If the test had been done and she had known that she was going to have a Down syndrome baby, she would have had an abortion. In either case, the parents ask for the extra costs of caring for the child during its lifetime.

A "wrongful life suit" is one brought by the handicapped infant himself, asking for damages because he would have been better off if he did not exist. Although a few states permit these suits (eg, Curlender v. Bio-Science Laboratories, 165 Cal Rptr 477, Cal 1989; Turpin v. Sortini, 643 P 2d 954, Cal 1982; Harbeson v. Parke-Davis Co., 656 P 2d 483, Wash 1983), the majority do not, since quantifying monetary damages for causing someone to be alive is considered to be beyond the abilities of the judicial system. All states, however, allow parents to recover damages for the extra costs of raising a handicapped child. Since, at least hypothetically, in a state recognizing wrongful life suits there is no reason that a handicapped child could not sue his mother, alleging that she was negligent in failing to have prenatal diagnosis and an abortion so that he would not be alive in his handicapped condition, even if the reason that she did not was that she believed abortion to be immoral, a few states have enacted statutes prohibiting such actions, usually after intensive lobbying by antiabortion groups.

"Wrongful death" actions are brought when a person is killed as the result of another's negligence. At common law, injuries that claimed the life of a fetus were not compensable. The fetus was considered to be a part of the mother's body and in an action arising from an accident that injured both of them, she was the sole plaintiff (eg, Dietrich v. Northampton, 138 Mass 1884). In 1946, however, the courts in the District of Columbia upheld a right of action on behalf of a living child who was seriously handicapped as the result of injuries sustained in an automobile accident while his mother was pregnant (Bonbrest v. Koetz, 65 F Supp 138, DC DC 1946). In all states a living child who was injured before birth now has a cause of action against the tortfeasor who maimed him. Beginning with a decision of the Minnesota Supreme Court in 1949 (Verkennes v. Corniea, 38 NW 2d 838, Minn 1949), some states began to interpret their wrongful death statutes to allow actions to be brought by the families of fetuses who were killed prior to birth but at a time at which they were clearly viable, usually during the last month of pregnancy.[3] Those courts that allow this type of recovery take the position that an automobile driver who runs into a pregnant woman who is nearing delivery should not be able to reduce the judgment against him or her by causing enough injury to kill the fetus instead of damaging it irreparably (eg, Baldwin v. Butcher, 184 SE 2d 428, W Va 1971; Fowler v. Woodward, 138 SE 2d 42, SC 1964).

Some fetal wrongful death suits involve claims against obstetricians or hospitals for negligence during delivery, although in most of these situations, the case is brought with the mother as sole plaintiff and the fact that there was a stillbirth is argued as an element of damages to her (eg, Jones v. Karraker, 440 NE 2d 420, Ill 1982; Mitchell v. Couch, 285 SW 2d 901, Ky 1955; Panagopoulous v. Martin, 295 F Supp 220, DC W Va 1969).

Failure to diagnose pregnancy in time for a woman to have an abortion or failure to perform a sterilization operation correctly so that the couple has an unplanned child in most states will not support a lawsuit as long as the baby is born healthy (eg, Jackson v. Anderson, 230 So 2d 503, Fla 1970; Elliott v. Brown, 361 So 2d 546, Ala 1978).

A number of studies indicate that obstetricians are well aware of the enormous verdicts juries return in malpractice cases against them; as a result, the practice of "defensive medicine" is widespread. For example, several studies indicate that electronic fetal monitoring has had little effect on the incidence of cerebral palsy or other birth problems,[1,4,5] but its application, at whatever increase in the cost of care, is now nearly universal, as is the resulting increase in the number of cesarean deliveries with the resulting discomfort and expense to the mothers. Agreement within the field on standards of practice for the use of technology would in and of itself constitute a defensible legal "standard of care." Thus, those who conformed to it could feel more comfortable knowing that they were protected if they did not apply whatever technology might be at hand, even though it was medically unnecessary. Although the blame for "the malpractice crisis" may be placed variously on lawyers, insurance companies, and physicians, those who are trying to practice in the middle of it should also remember that the patient, not the physician, is the one who may be hurt most seriously by unnecessary surgery or technology.

COMPULSORY TREATMENT AND PROSECUTION FOR FETAL ABUSE

In a number of cases within the past several years, obstetricians have gone to court to ask for judicial orders to treat pregnant women against their will. This treatment may range from blood transfusions for Jehovah's Witnesses to cesarean sections.[6–15]

All surveys of these cases indicate that the patients in all these situations were represented, if at all, by Legal Aid or court-appointed lawyers. Most were minority women, and every one was a clinic patient.[9,12] There is no record of any case in which an obstetrician in private practice has attempted to obtain a court order to treat a patient sufficiently affluent to retain private counsel. As one judge, who had refused to order a cesarean in a case in New York City, said to the press, "Who would ask a judge to order Happy Rockefeller to have a cesarean?"[16]

In six of the 11 known cases of requests for court-ordered cesareans, the woman went on to successful vaginal delivery.[12,16] Moreover, in several of those six, after the court orders were granted on the basis of medical testimony that the fetus could not possibly survive unless a cesarean were performed, the woman escaped from the hospital, went home, and delivered a healthy baby without medical assistance of any sort (Jefferson v. Griffin-Spalding County Hospital Authority, 274 SE 2d 457, Ga 1982; In the Matter of the Application of North Central Bronx Hospital v. Headley, Supreme Court of the State of New York in and for the County of Bronx, January 6, 1986).[12]

It is very likely that whenever a physician asks a judge to order some form of treatment to benefit a child or a fetus, the order will be granted. When the patient is a child, such an order is virtually automatic. Whatever the right of an adult to refuse treatment for religious or other reasons, a parent has no right to allow his or her child to die or to become disabled when medical care can solve the problem.[17–20] The differences, of course, between a court order to treat a 2-week-old baby and a fetus 2 weeks before term is that although the child, once born, is clearly "a person" under the law, the fetus is not "a legal person" until it is born. Even more important, to deliver, transfuse, or operate upon a fetus, it is necessary to do something to the woman's body against her will.

Proponents of legal intervention on behalf of a fetus argue that fetuses have interests protected by law—they may inherit, for example. These advocates for the fetus, however, overlook the fact that for these rights to vest, the fetus must be born alive. For example, if a pregnant woman is beaten so severely that her fetus dies, the assailant may be prosecuted only for the criminal attack on the mother, not for murder of the fetus (eg, New Mexico v. Willis, 652 P 2d 1222, NM 1982; Illinois v. Greer, 402 NE 2d 203, Ill 1980). If, however, a live birth occurs but the newborn dies of the injuries received in the assault, prosecution for murder of the infant will succeed.

There have been numerous attempts in recent years to prosecute women for "fetus abuse" who abused drugs, drank alcohol, or engaged in other detrimental behavior while pregnant (eg, Reyes v. Superior Court, 141 Cal Rptr 912, Cal 1977; In re Steven S., 126 Cal App 3d 23, 1981). It is now clear law—although some prosecutors still attempt such prosecutions, usually shortly before Election Day—that in no state can one abuse a fetus within the meaning of the child abuse law.

Although some courts have ordered cesareans when women refused them, usually as a result of objections involving religious conviction (Jefferson v. Griffin-Spalding County Hospital Authority, 274 SE 2d 457, Ga 1982; Tsai v. Vanderhorst, Family Court, Charleston, S.C., July 13, 1983; In the Matter of the Application of North Central Bronx Hospital v. Headley, Supreme Court of the State of New York in and for the County of Bronx, January 6, 1986), others have refused to order a competent woman's body to be invaded against her will (eg, Taft v. Taft, 446 NE 2d 395 Mass 1983).

Two important principles of Anglo-American law are involved in this issue. First, the right of privacy extends to decisions about one's own body and personal life, including decisions about marriage, abortion, contraception, procreative freedom, and other personal conduct. Second, the requirement of informed consent is based on the competent patient's right to make decisions about his or her own body.[21] Informed consent is defined as "the duty to warn a patient of the hazards and possible complications and expected and unexpected results of the treatment" (Mitchell v. Robinson, 334 SW 2d 11, Mo 1960; Natanson v. Kline, 350 P 2d 1093, 354 P 2d 670, Kansas 1960). The patient must also be told of any alternatives that exist for the proposed treatment. As the probability or severity of risk increases, so does the duty to inform the patient about it. An adult patient (and increasingly, a mature minor) then has the right to refuse treatment, even if such a refusal will lead to certain death (In the Interest of, for example, 161 Ill App 3d 765, 113 Ill Dec 477, 515 NE 2d 286, 1987; In the Matter of Conroy, 457 A 2d 1232, NJ 1983; Satz v. Perlmutter, 362 So 2d 160, Fla 1978). Thus, the patient has the right to agree to or to refuse any recommended therapy and his or her right to such bodily autonomy must be respected. Moreover, the pregnant woman has the right to terminate her pregnancy, even over the objections of her husband (Planned Parenthood Association of Missouri v. Danforth, 428 US 52, 1976).

A widely discussed 1987 case in Washington, DC, resulted in a ruling by a United States Circuit Court of

Appeals on this issue (In re A.C., 533 A 2d 611, DC App 1987).[22] Angela Carder had been treated for cancer since adolescence. When she seemed to be better, she was married and became pregnant. During her sixth month of pregnancy, however, her malignancy returned and it became evident that she was dying. When she was semicomatose, a hospital administrator instructed the hospital's outside counsel to obtain a court order to perform a cesarean in case the baby might be saved. Whatever Mrs. Carder's views on the matter (there was substantial difference of opinion about whether she agreed to the surgery or refused it and, in either case, whether she understood the questions asked her), her husband and her mother (her father was dead) adamantly refused to agree to the surgery. When a judge issued an order to perform the cesarean, her family appealed and the trial judge's order was upheld by telephone and without a hearing. Her own obstetrician and all others on the staff of the university hospital in which she was a patient refused to perform the surgery; an obstetrician had to be brought in from outside to do it. The baby died within hours; Mrs. Carder died 2 days later. Her court-appointed lawyer, however, asked for a rehearing by the appellate court and the court vacated its order. On rehearing, the Court of Appeals reversed its earlier ruling (in re A.C., 573 A 2d 1235, DC App 1990). It held that if a patient is capable of making an informed decision about the course of her medical treatment, her decision will control in virtually all cases. The court continued "we need not decide whether, or in what circumstances, the state's interest can ever previal over the interests of a pregnant patient. . . Indeed, some may doubt that there could ever be a situation extraordinary or compelling enough to justify a massive intrusion into a person's body, such as a cesarean section, against that person's will."

Assuming, however, that a pregnant woman has no right to jeopardize the welfare of her fetus and that the law may require her to protect it, how will such a requirement be enforced? Will pregnant women who drink or use drugs be confined to jails, where hepatitis and tuberculosis are endemic and violence is a way of life? Very few physicians would agree that prison is a healthy environment for a fetus. If the recalcitrant pregnant woman is to be confined in a hospital for a long period of time, who will pay for it? Given the paucity of public funding for prenatal care for indigent women who want it, it seems unlikely that funding at the amounts necessary to house the unwilling for weeks or months will be available. In any case, however, if word spreads in the clinic population that the physicians will get court orders to compel "healthy behavior," women who are Jehovah's Witnesses and would never consent to blood transfusions and alcoholics and drug abusers in fear of prosecution or confinement will simply not appear for prenatal care.

Suppose, for example, that a pregnant physician knows that her work near anesthetic gases, with AIDS patients, in the blood bank, or in radiology could damage her fetus. After investigating the literature, she decides that the risk is insignificant and elects to keep working. Should the state be able to intervene? Hundreds of cases involving the Equal Employment Opportunity laws and federal administrative regulations indicate that pregnant women have the right to make their own decisions about the risks of working; terminating employment to protect a fetus is permitted only under the most extraordinary circumstances (eg, Hayes v. Shelby Memorial Hospital, 726 F 2d 1543, CCA 11, 1984).

In March of 1991 the Supreme Court of the United States ruled that an employer's gender-based fetal protection policy was a violation of women workers' rights (Automobile Workers v. Johnson Controls, 111 S Ct 1196, 1991). The company, Johnson Controls, manufactures batteries. In order to protect fetuses from exposure to lead, Johnson announced a policy barring all women, except those whose infertility was medically documented, from jobs involving actual or potential lead exposure. The court held that the policy violated the Pregnancy Discrimination Act (42 United States Code Section 2000e(k)) and that because fertile men but not fertile women were given choices as to whether they wish to risk their reproductive health for a particular job, the policy also violated the sexual discrimination provisions of the Civil Rights Act (42 United States Code Section 2000e-2(a)). While quite important, this decision did not involve the rights to employment of women who were pregnant—it dealt with the limits of an employer's right to discriminate against women who were capable of becoming pregnant. Other cases (many of which dealt with pregnant airline flight attendants) have established that if a pregnant employee is not able to do her job safely, a company may insist on a layoff or temporary job change, but the Supreme Court has construed "unsafe" very narrowly.

Those who support compulsory treatment to protect fetuses do not seem to be clear about the degree of risk required to justify intervention by the legal system if they wish to confine a drug addict but do not intervene when the patient is an anesthesiologist exposed to gases in the operating room or an oncologist exposed to chemotherapy. What degree of certainty about the risk would be required? Would they extend the intervention of the courts to women who are perfectly compliant with prenatal care but who express a desire to have their babies at home attended by lay midwives? If the woman is at high risk, could she be transferred from her community hospital to a tertiary-care hospital against her will? In the absence of agreement beyond a reasonable doubt among the obstetrical community on these questions, it is not likely that appellate courts will uphold these orders. Only two appellate courts have ruled in these issues, and they reached opposite results.

Additionally, it is quite clear law that neither parent may be compelled to donate bone marrow or to be an organ donor for his or her child. Even if one stipulates that a fetus has the same rights as a 2-year-old child, since the mother could not be legally compelled to have bone marrow removed to save her 2-year-old's life, it is hard to argue that she should be compelled to go to greater risk with a cesarean for a fetus.

However distressing noncompliant pregnant patients are to their physicians and ought to be to society, it may ultimately be impossible to do anything but attempt to educate them. As long as indigent pregnant women who want care have no access to it, it probably does not serve society well to force care on those who do not want it. If a fetus has a legally enforceable right to be protected from harm caused by its mother, might not a child of poverty, born in a shack without running water or heat and delivered by a granny midwife because that is the only health care to which his mother has access, have an equal claim against the government for putting him at such risk?

RESEARCH

Fetal research has once again engendered public debate, most recently because some scientists have wished to use fetal tissue obtained from aborted tissues for implantation in patients suffering from Parkinson's disease. Discussion of the issues involved in research on the fetus ex utero or research in anticipation of abortion is beyond the scope of this chapter. However, research with fetuses in utero to develop new diagnostic procedures and to treat other problems of high-risk pregnancies in order to improve their outcome may also raise both legal and moral issues.[23–31]

The National Research Act of 1974 (PL-93-348, 93rd Congress, July 12, 1974) established the National Commission for the Protection of Human Subjects of Biomedical and Behavioral Research and mandated the commission to make recommendations for federal regulation of fetal research supported by or to be submitted to the federal government. The commission's Recommendations for Research on the Fetus[32] were adopted as federal regulations (45 Code of Federation Regulations, Subpart B).[33–36]

Following the Supreme Court's abortion decisions, many states moved quickly to enact laws that restrict research on live fetuses, in utero or ex utero. These statutes vary widely, with some prohibiting any research on a live fetus, others allowing research that will not harm the fetus or is designed to preserve its life, and some placing no specific limitations on the nature of the research but requiring the consent of the mother. Criminal penalties may be quite severe. An Illinois case indicates that these statutes, or at least the one in Illinois, do not prohibit in vitro fertilization or other infertility treatments (Smith v. Hartigan, 556 F Supp 157, DC Ill 1983). The Louisiana statute was struck down as unconstitutionally restricting the woman's right of privacy (Margaret S. v. Edwards, 488 F Supp 181, DC La 1980, 784 F 2d 994, CCA 5, 1986).[37] As far as can be determined, no other statute has been constitutionally challenged, but it would probably be struck down on the same grounds as the Louisiana statute.

The definition of a fetus accepted by the National Commission was "the human from the time of implantation until a determination is made following delivery that it is viable or possibly viable." The commission concluded that procedures designed to benefit the fetus undertaken as part of research studies should be encouraged and supported by the federal government. These procedures, however, must conform to appropriate medical standards, the mother must consent and the father not object, and the project must have been approved by the appropriate Institutional Review Board (IRB).

Presumably, this recommendation (and now regulation) would preclude, since the mother's informed consent is specifically required, any attempt to obtain a court order to undertake any procedure still considered investigational upon her or her fetus if she refuses to agree. The question of whether the father, by objecting, could refuse to permit a procedure designed to benefit a fetus is one not yet considered by a court, but it is most unlikely that if an intervention is designed to treat a fetal problem and the mother wishes to have it, that father has a right to force her to deliver a deformed or injured child by objecting to potentially useful therapy.

If the research is part of a procedure directed toward the health needs of a pregnant woman, it is permissible under the recommendations as long as it has been evaluated for its impact on the fetus and will place the fetus at risk to the minimum extent consistent with meeting the health needs of the woman, the study has been approved by the IRB, and the woman has given informed consent. Research on the pregnant woman that will confer no benefit on her may be conducted as long as it will impose minimal or no risk to the fetus and special care has been taken to inform the woman of any possible impact on the fetus, the research has been approved by the IRB, and she has given her informed consent. The commission concluded that the father must not object, although his consent does not have to be positively elicited. Finally, procedures directed toward the fetus that will confer no benefit upon it may be conducted if the purpose of the research is the development of important biomedical knowledge that cannot be obtained by other means, investigation on animals and non-pregnant humans has been conducted, minimal or no risk to the fetus will be presented, the research has been approved by the IRB, and the mother consents and the father does not object.

The final federal regulations accepted the commission's recommendations except that paternal consent is required for procedures that confer no benefit on the pregnant woman or her fetus unless "the father's identity or whereabouts cannot be reasonably ascertained, he is not reasonably available or the pregnancy resulted from rape." Nowhere do the regulations indicate what "not reasonably available" means. (Is it out of the room or lost on Mount Everest?) Also, one may not know whether a rape victim's pregnancy resulted from the attack or from consensual intercourse with someone else.

The commission recommended the establishment of Ethics Advisory Boards (EAB) to review on a national level research protocols of this type, and during the short-lived existence of one established by Secretary Joseph Califano, the EAB approved research on the development of fetoscopy. One IRB based its conclusion that amniocentesis, purely for purposes of research, could be permitted on the EAB's opinion. The IRB concluded that the only substantial risk of a properly performed amniocentesis was miscarriage, and since the woman had the right to consent to abortion, it seemed reasonable to allow her to consent to the risk of miscarriage as long as there was no possibility of an injury that could result in a live-born deformed infant.[38]

Thus, at least in terms of studies where attempts are being made to benefit a fetus or the pregnant woman, it is altogether probable that any state statute restricting such activities is very likely to be declared unconstitutional. This would be particularly true in studies designed, for example, to develop new diagnostic technology or technology to aid in surgery or other treatment for a fetus with a life-threatening or permanently disabling condition who might have a chance for a normal life if the procedure is successful.

CONCLUSION

It is unfortunately true that today obstetricians feel threatened by the legal environment in which they practice. Beset with what seems to be a system out to get them if every patient does not have a perfect baby, unsure of how far they can push a noncompliant patient to take care of herself and her fetus, and afraid to depart from the most conservative views of obstetric management, many are just giving up and stopping their obstetrical practices.

Many suggestions for a total overhaul of the legal system have been heard in recent years. Whether these ideas are good or bad, they probably will not occur within the next several years, but some fairly simple suggestions to reduce the risk of legal involvement may be offered:

1. Be courteous and respectful to patients. They are infinitely less likely to sue you if something goes wrong if they like you. Whether justified or not, obstetricians as a group are frequently perceived as being extremely arrogant to their patients. Common courtesy, for example, would preclude calling a patient by her first name without her permission and might, with that permission, mean that she has the right to call the doctor by his or her first name. This sort of unthinking condescension can be enormously annoying to a patient and if a disaster happens later can be the irritant that finally propels her to the lawyer's office.
2. Explain to her what is happening; what will hurt; why you want to do what you want to do; why she should stop smoking, drinking, and using street drugs; and listen to her problems and concerns. Many physicians "can't take the time" to talk to patients themselves and delegate this duty to someone else. That precludes development of the rapport that will calm troubled waters in case of later problems. In short, comply with the law's requirement for *informed* consent. It is the patient's body, not yours.
3. The time spent documenting interactions and discussions with the patient and noting all relevant information in her chart may be a nuisance, but it is considerably less time-consuming than sitting in court throughout a malpractice case that depends for its defense on an accurate medical record.
4. If anything goes wrong, tell the patient the truth. If you do not, another doctor will, and if another doctor does not, the lawyer will do so. The worst possible position a physician (of any specialty) can be in is to have lied to a patient about the cause of a problem. That not only virtually guarantees a successful malpractice suit but may subject him or her to damages for fraud and deceit as well (and those damages are not usually covered by malpractice insurance). In case a baby is born with problems, whether or not it is anyone's "fault," expressing regret and concern and being supportive through the parents' adjustment to the tragedy can deflect anger that might otherwise surface against the physician. "I'm so sorry" is not an admission of guilt.
5. Pursue an unpaid bill only if you are sure that the reason for nonpayment is not anger and that the quality of care the patient received was excellent. Persistent efforts at collection against a patient who is already upset or angry may provoke a lawyer's interest about the quality of the care received if she consults counsel about the collection agency's efforts.

Unless confronted with enormous bills for care of a damaged child that they can pay only with some outside source of income (such as a malpractice award) most patients, obstetrical and otherwise, do not sue physicians unless they are angry. Developing a relationship based on respect with the patient during her pregnancy is the best way to avoid later difficulties if problems occur.

REFERENCES

1. Institute of Medicine, Committee on the Effects of Medical Professional Liability on the Delivery of Maternal and Child Health Care. Medical professional liablity and the delivery of obstetrical care. Washington: National Academy Press, 1989.
2. For an excellent discussion of the law of malpractice as it applies to obstetrics, see Fineberg KS, Peters JD, Willson JR, and Kroll DA. Obstetrics: gynecology and the law. Ann Arbor, MI: Health Administration Press, 1984.
3. Shapiro SR. The right to maintain action or to recover damages

for death of unborn child. American Law Reports (3rd) 1976;84:411.

4. MacDonald D, Grant A, Sheridan-Pereira M. The Dublin randomized control trial of intrapartum fetal monitoring. Am J Obstet Gynecol 1985;152:524.
5. Luthy DA, Shy KK, Van Bell, G. A randomized trial of electronic fetal monitoring in premature labor. Obstet Gynecol 1987;69: 687.
6. Bowers WA, Selegstad B. Fetal versus maternal rights, medical and legal perspectives. Obstet Gynecol 1980;58:209.
7. Finamore E, Jefferson V. To protect the life of an unborn child. Am J Law Med 1983;9:83.
8. Holder AR. Maternal-fetal conflicts and the law. The Female Patient 1985;10(June):80.
9. Kolder VEB, Gallagher J, Parsons M. Court ordered obstetrical interventions. N Engl J Med 1987;316:1192.
10. Loewy EH. The pregnant brain dead and the fetus: must we always try to wrest life from death? Am J Obstet Gynecol 1987;156:1097.
11. Nelson LJ, Milliken N. Compelled medical treatment of pregnant women: life, liberty and law in conflict. N Engl J Med 1988;259:1060.
12. Rhoden NK. The judge in the delivery room: the emergence of court-ordered cesareans. Cal Law Rev 1987;74:1951.
13. Rhoden NK. Cesareans and Samaritans. Law Med Health Care 1987;15:118.
14. Robertson JA. The right to procreate and in utero fetal therapy. J Legal Med 1982;3:333.
15. Robertson JA. Fetal therapy and the legal duties of parents and physicians. The Female Patient 1984;9(July):30.
16. Sandroff R. Invasion of the body snatchers: fetal rights vs. mothers' rights. Vogue, October 1988; p 330.
17. Bennett R. Allocation of child medical care decision-making authority: a suggested interest analysis. U Va Law Rev 1976; 62:285.
18. Holder AR. Parents, courts and refusal of treatment. J Pediatr 1983;103:515.
19. Sher EJ. Choosing for children: adjudicating medical care disputes between parents and the state NYU Law Rev 1983;58:157.
20. Wadlington WJ, Whitebread CH, Davis SM. Children in the legal system. Chapter 13. Mineola, NY: Foundation Press, 1983.
21. Katz J. The silent world of doctor and patient. New York: The Free Press, 1984.
22. Annas GJ. At law: she's going to die. The case of Angela C. Hastings Center Report 1988;18:23.
23. Clapp MJ. State prohibition of fetal experimentation and the fundamental right of privacy. Columbia Law Rev 1988;88:1073.
24. Elias S, Annas GJ. Perspectives on fetal surgery. Am J Obstet Gynecol 1983;145:807.
25. Fletcher J, Ryan KJ. Federal regulations for fetal research: a case for reform. Law Med Health Care 1987;15:126.
26. Lenow J. The fetus as a patient: emerging rights as a person. Am J Law Med 1983;9:1.
27. Ramsey P. The ethics of fetal research. New Haven: Yale University Press, 1975.
28. Reback GE. Fetal experimentation: moral, legal and medical implications, Stanford Law Rev 1874;26:1191.
29. Robertson JA. The right to procreate and in utero fetal therapy. J Law Med 1982;3:333.
30. Terry NP. "Alas! Poor Yorick," I knew him ex utero: the regulation of embryo and fetal experimentation and disposal in England and the United States. Vanderbilt Law Rev 1986;39:419.
31. Warnock M. Moral thinking and government policy: the Warnock Committee on human embryology. Millbank Memorial Fund Q 1985;63:504.
32. National Commission. Report on research involving the fetus. 40 Fed Reg 33526–52, August 8, 1975. Appendix to the Report on Fetal Research, DHEW Publication No. (OS) 76.
33. Lebacqz K. Fetal research: a commissioner's reflection. IRB: a Review of Human Subjects Research 1989;1(3):7.
34. Lebacqz K. Reflections on the report and recommendations of the National Commission: research on the fetus, Villanova Law Rev 1977;22:357.
35. Levine RJ. Ethics and regulation of clinical research. Chapter 12. 2nd ed. Baltimore: Urban and Schwarzenburg, 1987.
36. Levine RJ. The impact on fetal research of the report of the National Commission for the Protection of Human Subjects of Biomedical and Behavioral Research. Villanova Law Rev 1977;22:367.
37. Holder AR. Legal issues in pediatrics and adolescent medicine. Chapter 3. 2nd ed. New Haven: Yale University Press, 1987.
38. Holder AR. Can amniocentesis be performed solely for research? IRB: a Review of Human Subjects Research. 1981;3(6):6.

81

CHAPTER

ESSENTIALS IN BIOSTATISTICS AND PERINATAL EPIDEMIOLOGY

Benjamin P. Sachs and Linda J. Van Marter

STUDY DESIGN

There are two ways to examine the relationship between risk factors and disease. One approach is through a cohort study that measures the frequency of disease occurrence among individuals exposed and unexposed to a particular risk factor of interest. This type of study may be either prospective or retrospective. An alternative approach is the case-control method (another type of retrospective study) that examines the frequency of risk factors among people with and without disease. Table 81-1 contrasts the two types of study design. Lists of definitions and of commonly used rates and ratios appear at the end of this chapter.

COHORT STUDY

An example of a cohort study is the examination of a potential relationship between diabetic control in the first trimester of pregnancy and the incidence of congenital anomalies. For a cohort study, the risk factor is an abnormal glucose level in the first trimester, and the disease outcome is the presence or absence of a congenital anomaly.

CASE-CONTROL STUDY

A relationship between blood sugar control in the first trimester and birth defects can also be examined using the case-control methodology. The cases would be those diabetics who had babies with congenital anomalies; controls are diabetics who deliver normal infants. The outcome measure to be compared would be the rates of poor control in the first trimester in the two groups using, for example, their hemoglobin A1c levels.

Both types of studies have relative strengths and weaknesses that can be summarized as follows. Cohort studies

- Enable direct estimation of disease rates.
- Have less recall bias (eg, a woman who delivers a child with a birth defect is more likely to recall specific exposures).
- Are more likely to be biased in determining disease frequency.
- Require a large study size, particularly if the disease is rare.
- Are more difficult to do if the induction time for development of the disease is long.
- Are more expensive.
- May lead to ethical dilemmas during a study if there is a strong likelihood that an exposure leads to disease and could be removed.
- Are at risk for loss of subjects during the study.

Case-control studies

- Are more economical.
- Are quicker.
- Have more risk of recall bias.

Comparing the two types of studies, the often maligned case-control methodology has, in fact, many advantages. There clearly is a potential for bias in a case-control study. However, if it is well constructed and carried out carefully, it has great potential for economically providing accurate epidemiological data.

TABLE 81–1. STUDY DESIGN

COHORT STUDY				CASE-CONTROL STUDY			
	DISEASE				DISEASE		
Risk factors	Yes	No	Total	Risk factors	Yes		No
Yes	A	B	A + B	Yes	a		b
No	C	D	C + D	No	c		d
				Total	a + c		b + d
Cohort studies compare	$\frac{A}{A + B}$	vs	$\frac{C}{C + D}$	Case control studies compare	$\frac{a}{a + c}$	vs	$\frac{b}{b + d}$

By convention A, B, C, D represent the total population; a, b, c, d represent samples of the population.

EVALUATION OF EPIDEMIOLOGICAL STUDIES

PRECISION AND VALIDITY

Both precision and validity are important in study design and for critical review of the literature. Precision refers to the accuracy with which the outcome measure is estimated. Errors in precision are generally thought to be attributable to the random error that arises from sampling variability or to false statistical inferences about the population parameters that are sampled. Certain aspects of study design that may influence precision include sample size, appropriate and parsimonious selection of variables for control, and variability (statistical variance) of the outcome measured.

Systematic error introduced through imperfections in study design may result in limited study validity. Validity refers to the likelihood that, in the context of the study, the outcome is actually measuring the effect of interest. Kleinbaum and colleagues help to clarify the concepts of precision and validity with a target-shooting analogy: "Validity is concerned with whether or not one is aiming at the correct bull's-eye; precision is concerned with individual variation from shot to shot, given the actual bull's-eye that is being considered."[1]

Validity is often considered on three levels: the study population (the individuals enrolled in the study), the base population (the population from which controls are selected and cases, should they exist, would be ascertained), and the general population (a broader group to which investigators can justify generalizing their results).

"Internal validity" generally refers to validity at the first two levels and is influenced by aspects of study design that include subject selection, quality and appropriateness of exposure and outcome measures, and the presence of confounding factors.

Limitations in internal validity most often result from selection, information, or confounding biases. After determining whether or not a potential bias is likely to exist, it is useful for the critical reviewer to assess the direction in which the anticipated bias would affect the outcome (toward or away from the null value).

"External validity," or applicability, refers to the generalizability of findings to a wider population and is most influenced by the comparability of the base population to the population to whom the generalization is intended for risk factors for the outcome of interest. Some investigators view external validity as nonexistent, believing that little justification exists for generalizing study results beyond the study population.

SELECTION BIAS

Selection bias is common in clinical studies and occurs if recruitment of either cases or comparison groups is skewed with respect to an important risk factor. For example, consider a voluntary study examining the potential benefit of exercise in pregnancy. Such a study could result in a control group that had significantly more obese women. This differential selection could result in a bias toward the control having a poorer pregnancy outcome. The incorrect conclusion would then be drawn that exercise improves pregnancy outcome. This form of bias is called self-selection bias.

Greenland defined selection bias as "a theoretical possibility whenever correlates of the outcome capable of influencing study participation are existent in some individuals at the beginning of the study."[2] He acknowledges that these may be unmeasured or unrecognized by the investigator, but he emphasizes the importance of developing clinical judgment as to the likelihood that such a bias exists. Cohort studies are subject to fewer potential selection biases than case-control studies, as the selection factors can usually be anticipated and controlled prior to measurement of the outcome.

INFORMATION BIAS

Bias can occur when errors are made in obtaining the information required for comparison. A common error is recall bias. An applicable example is a case-control study of the risk of congenital anomalies associated with the use of Bendectin to treat first-trimester hyperemesis. The mothers are interviewed only after delivery. A woman who has delivered a child with a major congenital anomaly is more likely to remember risk exposures than a woman who has had a normal child.

In cohort studies there is often more complete ascertainment of the outcome for the exposed group than for the unexposed group. This could lead to bias. For example, in a prospective study of congenital anomalies associated with the use of retinoic acid in the first trimester, if only those infants who were exposed to retinoic acid were thoroughly examined and tested, ascertainment bias would result.

Another example of information bias occurs when different outcome measures or instruments are used for the two comparison groups. For example, this would occur if the exposed or cases are personally interviewed and their medical records reviewed, but for the comparison or control group information is collected only through a telephone questionnaire.

It is important to recognize that information bias cannot be corrected at the time of analysis.

CONFOUNDING

Confounding is an important form of bias that can profoundly alter the results of a study by either underestimating or overestimating an effect. Confounding can be defined as a risk factor for disease other than the exposure under study that is unequally distributed between the cases and the comparison or control groups. This form of bias can occur in either a case-control or a cohort study. The risk factor is commonly termed a confounding variable.

Rothman describes four characteristics for a potential confounding variable[3]:

A potential confounding variable is a risk factor for disease but does not necessarily have to be an actual cause of the disease.

A confounding variable is linked to the exposure under study.

A confounding variable cannot be an intermediate step in the chain of events between the exposure and the disease outcome.

A potential confounding variable has to be associated with both the disease and the exposure under study.

Many factors, including age, race, and socioeconomic status, are risk factors for prematurity. For example, when these can be linked with the exposure(s) of interest, they may be confounding factors. In an examination of the efficacy of home uterine contraction monitoring to prevent prematurity, such a device is more likely to be used by women who have insurance so that the control group will include more women of lower socioeconomic status. As socioeconomic status is an index of risk for prematurity and, in this study, is linked with the exposure of interest (home monitoring), such a study would be confounded by the distribution of the confounding variable, socioeconomic status.

To reduce the effect of confounding, care should be taken in both the design and the data collection phases to ensure that the confounding variable is evenly distributed between the cases and comparison group. During the study design and the data collection phases the following techniques can be used:

1. Restriction. This limits the admission criteria into the study with respect to known potential confounding factors.
2. Matching. This involves comparison or control groups that are identical to the cases with respect to the matched variables. (This approach may be very costly and requires a specialized matched analysis.)
3. Randomization. This involves assignment of the subjects to different study groups on a random basis, in an effort to distribute known and unknown confounding factors equally among groups. (This technique is most reliable in large studies.)

Confounding is essentially a quantitative problem and can sometimes be addressed in the analytical phase of the study. Techniques that can be used to deal with confounding include multivariate models and stratification of the data.

SCREENING TESTS

Screening tests are the basic tools of the clinician. Whether it is the analysis of the hematocrit or the identification of patients at risk for premature labor, the fundamental concepts are the same. In any population some will suffer from a certain disease and others will not, and the challenge is to identify the diseased individuals at the earliest opportunity.

Sensitivity is defined as the probability of correctly identifying a sick individual. *Specificity* is the probability of correctly identifying a healthy individual. For example, if a normal hematocrit is defined as over 40%, the specificity of the test will be poor because many healthy people will be missed. Conversely, if the abnormal hematocrit is defined as less than 30%, the sensitivity will be poor because many anemic people will be excluded. Thus, defining the normal cut-off value will affect the sensitivity and specificity of a screening test in opposite directions.

More relevant to clinical decision making than sensitivity or specificity is the predictive value of a test. The *predictive value positive* is defined as the proportion of individuals with a specific risk factor who have the disease. The *predictive value negative* is the converse, that is, the proportion of those without the risk factor who are disease-free. The relationship between sensitivity, specificity, and predictive values is shown in Table 81-2.

TABLE 81-2. RELATIONSHIP OF SENSITIVITY, SPECIFICITY, AND PREDICTIVE VALUES

RISK FACTORS	DISEASE YES	DISEASE NO
Yes	a	b
No	c	d

Sensitivity = a/(a + c).
Specificity = d/(d + b).
Predictive value positive = a/(a + b).
Predictive value negative = d/(c + d).

PREDICTIVE VALUE

The predictive value of any screening test is an important assessment. In addition to sensitivity and specificity of the test, this value is dependent on the prevalence of the disease in question. Table 81-3 gives examples of the predictive value of a screening test for various prevalence rates. A good example is screening for AIDS and using the ELISA and Western Blot tests. The joint false-positive rate of these two tests is thought to be in the range of 0.1% to 0.005%.[4] This would mean that the predictive value of HIV testing for female blood donors would be 67% if the joint false-positive rate is 0.005% and only 9% if it is 0.1% (calculated from Table 81-2). The reason for this is simply that the incidence of AIDS among female blood donors is very low.

Another example is the probability of respiratory distress syndrome (RDS) by gestational age and the measurement of the lecithin–sphingomyelin ratio (L/S) in the amniotic fluid (see Table 81-3).[5] This is a very important concept and one that needs to be constantly emphasized.

NULL HYPOTHESIS; TYPE I AND TYPE II ERRORS

The null hypothesis is the focus of statistical testing in biomedical research. This hypothesis stipulates that there is no connection between the two variables. Thus, rejection of the null hypothesis implies that there is an association or that there is a range of association extending from a small effect to a much larger one.

To evaluate the null hypothesis, decision making is used. The common tool is the *P* value, or to put it another way, the probability that the null hypothesis is true. Thus, a *P* value of ≤ 0.05 that is significant indicates that the null hypothesis is rejected. If the *P* value is ≥ 0.05 and, therefore, not significant, the null hypothesis is accepted or "not rejected."

A type I, or alpha, error means that the null hypothesis was incorrectly rejected. With a *P* value of 0.05 this will occur in about 5% of cases.

A type II, or beta, error occurs when the null hypothesis is false but is not rejected.

There is a clear relationship between the type I and type II error. The level of either error depends on the statistical cut-off chosen for the statistical significance. For example, there will be a larger type II error if the type I error is reduced and vice versa.

POWER AND SAMPLE SIZE

The power of a test refers to its ability to detect a difference between the groups being tested at a given level of statistical significance. Stated another way, it is the probability of rejecting the null hypothesis given that the alternative hypothesis is true, or 1 minus the beta (type II) error. Power is influenced by four factors: the significance level chosen, the sample size, the magnitude of the difference in the tested parameter between the comparison groups, and the type of statistical test chosen. The larger the (1) sample size, (2) difference between groups, or (3) alpha error chosen, the greater the power of the statistical test will be.

Because the significance level is conventionally adjusted within a relatively narrow range (*P* = .10 to .05) and the difference between experimental groups is the outcome of interest, the major factor that is under the control of the cohort study investigator is the sample size. In a case-control study, both increasing the sample size and improving the ratio of controls per case enhance study power[6–8]; in the latter case, there is a maximum benefit of approximately a 4:1 control–case ratio.[6]

TABLE 81-3. RELATIONSHIP OF RDS AND L/S BY GESTATIONAL AGE

PREVALENCE OF RDS (%)	GESTATIONAL AGE IN WEEKS	PREDICTIVE VALUE L/H POSITIVE	PREDICTIVE VALUE L/H NEGATIVE
99	—	99	98
90	—	93	85
70	—	78	59
50	30	60	38
30	32	39	21
10	34	14	6
5	36	7	3
1	37	1	1

The failure to consider statistical power is one of the most frequent errors in study design.[9,10] Freiman and colleagues reported an analysis of 71 "negative" randomized controlled clinical trials published in peer review journals and found that 50 (70%) of the trials had insufficient power to detect a 50% improvement in outcome with the treatment.[11] Similarly, DerSimonian and colleagues reported the results of a survey of methods in 67 clinical trials published in four prestigious journals; the statistical power of the trial to detect treatment effects was discussed in only 12% of the articles.[12]

For practical purposes, sample size and power calculations are best derived from commercial computer software programs or existing references.[5,7,8,13–15] For those researchers using measures of effect and confidence intervals, Greenland has reported alternative methods of calculating sample size and power.[16]

COMPARATIVE MEASURES OF EFFECT VERSUS STATISTICAL TESTING

A growing number of researchers advocate an approach to data analysis that focuses on effect measures and their confidence intervals, rather than on the traditional use of formal statistical testing yielding a reported "*P* value."

The *P* value resulting from a statistical comparison may be translated as follows: given 100 independent samples of identical study size from the base population, the *P* value is the proportion of samples that could be expected to reveal a difference as large as or larger than the one observed, given that the null hypothesis is true. For instance, $P = .05$ means that if the null hypothesis was true, given 100 independent samples (of the same study size) from the base population, 5% would show a difference in the outcome measure as large as or larger than the one observed. The calculated *P* value not only reflects the observed difference between experimental groups but also is influenced by the sample size and the appropriateness of the statistical test.

The most common comparative measures of effect include the absolute risk difference, the risk ratio, the odds ratio, and the attributable proportion.

The *risk difference* is the risk of disease in the exposed minus the risk of disease in the unexposed:

$$\frac{\text{No. of diseased and exposed}}{\text{No. of exposed}} - \frac{\text{No. of diseased and unexposed}}{\text{No. of unexposed}}$$

The *risk ratio* is the risk in the exposed divided by the risk in the unexposed:

$$\frac{\text{No. of diseased and exposed/No. of exposed}}{\text{No. of diseased and unexposed/No. of unexposed}}$$

The *odds ratio* or relative odds is the ratio of the odds of disease in exposed individuals relative to the unexposed:

$$\frac{\text{No. of exposed among diseased/No. of exposed among well}}{\text{No. of unexposed among diseased/No. of unexposed among well}}$$

The odds ratio is often used as a surrogate for the risk ratio for case-control studies because the odds ratio is the mathematical equivalent of the *exposure odds ratio:*

$$\frac{\text{No. of exposed among diseased}}{\text{No. of exposed among well}}$$

The *attributable proportion,* also called the etiologic fraction, is an expression of the proportion of the disease among the exposed that is related to the exposure (rather than other risk factors). It is calculated as follows:

$$\frac{\text{Risk ratio} - 1}{\text{Risk ratio}} \times P$$

(P = proportion of exposed among those who develop the disease)

The derivations of the risk ratio for case-control studies, the odds ratio, may be found in Cornfield's landmark reference.[17] The null value for the risk difference and attributable risk is zero; for the risk ratio and odds ratio it is 1. When a confidence interval crosses these values, the null hypothesis is supported at the given level of significance. For example, a relative risk of 3.2 (95% confidence limits from 0.8 to 4) is not statistically significant, at $P < .05$.

Analyses using measures of effect and 95% confidence intervals (consistent with $P = .05$) offer the advantage of being more informative than *P* values alone; the magnitude and precision of the effect and the "significance" of the association are all discernible, given the point estimate and the confidence interval.

Statistical Testing

If statistical testing is chosen as an adjunct to comparative measures of effect and their confidence intervals, a number of factors must be taken into account in selecting the best test or group of tests. All statistical test procedures are founded in probability theory, and the validity of each test is intimately linked to assumptions about how the data relate to the probability distribution underlying the test. Features of the study design and data are also important to statistical testing, including the nature of the exposure and outcome variables, the distribution of values of the variable(s) under study, whether matching was included in the study design, whether measures are independent or repeated for a particular individual, and the potential confounding factors for each association tested.

For the purpose of critical literature review, Table 81-4 gives an outline of categories of statistical tests that are used in examining various combinations of exposure (explanatory) and outcome (response) data. Although Table 81-4 helps to narrow the choice of statistical tests to the appropriate group, the process of selecting the best test requires broader knowledge of the principles of study design and biostatistical testing.

An example of this is found in considering the apparently simple case of testing an association between two binary categorical variables. When examining the proportion of individuals with a particular outcome against a standard value or against another group in a large-sample ($N > 30$) comparison, the z-statistic is the most appropriate test. On the other hand, if the sample is small, and any cell count is ≤ 5, the Fisher's exact test should be used. Otherwise the chi-square test is used.

Stratified categorical tests are more complex: strata may be "standardized" for comparison,[18] summarized by Mantel-Haenszel test, or entered into a multivariate model. If matching has taken place, a matched analysis (McNemar test) is appropriate. In other instances the chi-square goodness-of-fit test is used, except when categories are ordered, in which case the chi-square test-for-trend is used.

Analysis of continuous outcome variables is no more intuitively obvious.[19] The investigator must first choose between parametric and nonparametric tests. The latter are usually selected when the parametrics' assumptions of normal distribution and equal variances are not met. Large sample means between groups or against a standard can be tested using the z-statistics. If a regression model is chosen, comparison analysis may use the t-test, analysis of variance (ANOVA), or correlation coefficient. Finally, matched or repeated measures designs must use a t-test or ANOVA that is adjusted to take pairing into account.[20]

Each cell of Table 81-4 poses a similar dilemma. Choosing the optimal statistical test(s) can only occur when the investigator has considered the question posed, the study design, the nature of the variables, and the assumptions of the optional statistical test procedures.

Because the appropriate use of statistical tests is not a trivial task, we recommend that statistical testing be performed by an individual with expertise in biostatistics. A number of excellent general texts cogently discuss the principles of biostatistics that are relevant to clinical research.[21–25]

The take-home message concerning epidemiologic analyses was well stated by Schoolman and colleagues: "good answers come from good questions not from esoteric analyses."[26]

MULTIPLE COMPARISONS

A frequent criticism relating to the widespread availability of "user-friendly" statistical computer programs is leveled at the tendency of some investigators to approach each epidemiologic study as a series of statistical tests in the quest for a P value $<.05$. These "fishing expeditions" are often characterized by indiscriminate statistical comparisons, often unfounded in prior hypotheses or biological plausibility. The criticism of this approach is based on the probability that a "statistically significant" P value is likely to be obtained by chance alone (ie, in the absence of biological significance) if one performs repetitive statistical tests. This phenomenon is called an alpha or type I error. If the significance level is set at 5% ($P > .05$), the expected frequency of this event is one per 20 tests performed. Incomplete reporting of

TABLE 81–4. ALTERNATIVE UNIVARIATE AND MULTIVARIATE STATISTICAL METHODS USED IN HYPOTHESIS TESTING OF CONTINUOUS AND/OR CATEGORICAL DATA

EXPOSURE (EXPLANATORY) VARIABLES	OUTCOME (RESPONSE) VARIABLES	
	CATEGORICAL	CONTINUOUS
Single		
Categorical	Contingency table (Chi-square or Fisher's exact text) or z-statistic	z-statistic or t-test or ANOVA or nonparametric
Continuous	z-statistic or t-test or ANOVA or nonparametric	Linear Regression Correlation Coefficient
Multiple*		
Categorical	Stratification or loglinear analysis or logistic regression	ANOVA
Continuous	Logistic regression	Multiple regression
Mixed	Logistic regression	ANCOVA

* Adapted from Fineberg[35]
ANOVA, Analysis of variance; ANCOVA, Analysis of covariance.

statistical methods further complicates the interpretation of "significant" *P* values because there exists an apparent publication bias in a direction that reinforces positive results and leads to a reluctance to report the multiple "insignificant" comparisons that sometimes accompany a single statistically significant association.

The "multiple comparison" criticism is best avoided by limiting statistical testing to factors about which a hypothesis has been formulated and for which a biologically plausible relationship to the outcome of interest exists. Other suggestions for improving on current reporting trends are (1) encouraging investigators to include detailed descriptions of the statistical methods and negative results as part of manuscripts that might otherwise focus only on a positive association,[18] or (2) making more stringent requirements for "significance" or adjustments to the *P* value obtained through multiple comparisons.[24]

Although some epidemiologists see multiple statistical comparisons in the absence of well-formulated antecedent hypotheses as absolutely worthless, others, such as Feinstein and Horwitz, see these comparisons as having a role in the generation of new hypotheses[27]: "Although agreement has not been reached on when and how to adjust the statistical levels of significance in a study in which multiple agents have been investigated without preceding hypotheses about them, the results of such studies should be viewed not as conclusions but as tentative hypotheses to be confirmed by further research."

Suggestions for hypothesis testing in the clinical trial offered by Pocock and colleagues may be useful in avoiding the issue of multiple comparisons as well as other statistical considerations[28]:

- It is important to identify a small set of primary end points in advance. In many trials the design should specify a single primary end point.
- Results for secondary end points should be presented as exploratory findings.
- Subgroup analyses should be confined to a limited number of prespecified hypotheses concerning the interaction between treatment and a prognostic factor. If a trial has limited statistical power (ie, not enough patients), subgroup analyses should be avoided.
- Trials with repeated measurements of quantitative end points over time require a prespecified policy for statistical analysis. This should be aimed toward a single specific hypothesis of interest, and repeated significance tests at each time point should be avoided.
- For trials with more than two treatments, the primary treatment contrasts should be specified beforehand and emphasized in the report.
- Authors should use as few significance tests as possible, so that the risk of a type I error is limited. Exact *P* values should be presented, rather than references to arbitrary levels (eg, $P < .05$). The magnitude of treatment differences for primary end points should be stated, along with the confidence limits.
- The intended size of a trial and the mathematical justification of the intended size (eg, power calculations) should be specified in the Methods section.
- If interim analyses of the accumulating data will be undertaken, a policy for the frequency and content of such analyses should be defined in advance.
- The summary or abstract of a trial report should reflect the overall findings fairly. The summary should mention the magnitude of treatment differences rather than their statistical significance.
- All of the preceding recommendations imply that investigators must define a coordinated policy for the statistical aspects of a clinical trial, which reflects a consistency of intent from the design of a trial through its conduct, analysis, interpretation, and reporting.

MULTIVARIATE (MV) ANALYSIS

Stratification is one of the major approaches used in controlling confounding factors in a categorical data analysis. This approach offers the dual advantages of straightforward calculable results and ease of visual inspection of the data. Stratified data may be analyzed by standardization (standardized mortality–morbidity ratios) or summary (Mantel-Haenszel test) methods. Limitations of stratified analyses include their dependence on categorical delineation of the confounders and (given a finite number of subjects) their difficulty accommodating more than a few factors simultaneously without the data becoming too sparse.

Multivariate analyses, most appropriately used as complementary to stratified analysis, offer a number of potential benefits. They can control for a greater number of variables simultaneously, facilitate the exploration of interrelationships between covariates, and provide a model that enables the calculation of the odds of disease for a particular individual.

Four techniques that perform computer-assisted analyses of multiple variables simultaneously are multiple linear regression, logistic regression, log-linear analysis, and proportional hazards modeling.

1. In multiple linear regression, models of multiple covariates—continuous, categorical, or mixed—are used in an attempt to predict one continuous outcome variable.[18] Results are compiled in analysis of variance (ANOVA) tables.
2. A technique gaining popularity, multivariate analysis via logistic regression (LR),[1] is limited to one dichotomous outcome variable and has the advantage of accommodating multiple explanatory variables of a categorical or a continuous nature in its process of maximum likelihood estimation. The summation of the process is expressed mathematically in "logits" whose values are derived from the natural logarithms of the estimated probabilities.

Comparison of probabilities from alternative LR models using the likelihood ratio test yields the significance of a variables contribution at various levels of confounder control. Measures of effect can be compared when the computer-derived coefficients and standard errors for the variables of interest are used to calculate their odds ratios and confidence intervals. One disadvantage of LR is that the program will not tolerate missing values. Data must be imputed or the subject must be entirely omitted from the analysis if even one data point is missing. In addition, the approach to "model building" may influence a variable's significance and/or measure of effect.[29]

3. Log-linear analysis[30,31] uses categorical data in multidimensional contingency tables accommodating multiple categories of both outcome and exposure variables to compare observed and expected cell counts through a process called iterative proportional fitting. The name is derived from the fact that the model is linear on the natural logarithmic scale. Log-linear analysis has the advantage of incorporating terms that evaluate the relationship between the model's covariates. Although statistical testing between log-linear models is straightforward, log-linear modeling and the interpretation of interactions between variables and measures of effect are somewhat more complicated tasks than they are for logistic regression analyses.
4. The proportional hazards model[18] shares some similarities with the logistic regression model but takes a rate-oriented tack: the proportional hazards likelihood is evaluated on the set of subjects who remain under observation after each case occurrence (positive outcome), and the model predicts, for the remaining subjects, the ratio of incidence rates as the outcome variable of interest. Its main disadvantage is that the technique is computationally burdensome even with computer assistance.

Because the results are formulated with iterative processes, a notable disadvantage of the MV approach is that the analyses cannot be performed without the aid of sophisticated computer software. In addition, the investigator is distanced from the data by the "black-box" nature of the process; data are not available for examination during the analysis, there are no clear guidelines regarding the number of variables that may justifiably be introduced in a single data run, and the accuracy of the results of analysis is not easily verifiable. These limitations lead to the recommendation that MV analyses be performed only by experienced operators using well-tested computer programs.

META-ANALYSIS

Meta-analysis is a relatively new concept that uses graphic and statistical methods qualitatively and quantitatively to summarize results from different studies that have explored the same hypothesis. A number of excellent references discuss meta-analysis methods in detail.[32–36]

Furberg and Morgan cite six reasons for conducting meta-analyses:

1. To obtain more stable estimates of treatment effect to guide clinicians
2. To aid in interpreting the generalizability of the results
3. To conduct subgroups analyses for which the individual trials have too few subjects
4. To strengthen submissions to the Food and Drug Administration
5. To aid in the planning of major clinical trials
6. To counterbalance the "overenthusiasm" often seen following the introduction of new technologies.[37]

Figure 81-1 provides an introduction to a common starting point for meta-analysis: the graphic comparison of outcome measures from studies posing the same question. This figure shows the odds ratio (OR) and 95% confidence interval for early neonatal mortality in 10 controlled clinical trials of surfactant therapy for respiratory distress syndrome. This comparison is informative in several ways. First, it is evident that the measures of effect from analyses of all but the one study that achieved statistical significance were accompanied by very wide confidence intervals. However, eight of the 11 studies showed point estimates at or greater than OR = 2.0 in the direction of a benefit of treatment; the three other studies had ORs centered at the null value.

	0 1 10 20 30 40 50
Hallman, 1983[48]	---X-------------------- (60)
Halliday, 1984[49]	---X--
Hallman, 1985[50]	---X--
Wilkinson, 1985[15] Trial I	------X------------------ (117)
Trial II	---X---
Einhorning, 1985[51]	----X------------------ (74)
Kwong, 1985[52]	----X---------
Merritt, 1986[53]	---X---
Gitlin, 1987[54]	----X---
Ten Center Study[5] Group, 1987	--X--

FIGURE 81–1. Odds of early neonatal mortality if untreated in 10 clinical trials of surfactant therapy for respiratory distress syndrome. (Odds ratios and 95% confidence intervals calculated from data presented in original publications. Where cell counts were zero, 0.5 was substituted to allow calculation of the odds ratio.)

TABLE 81–5. HILL'S CAUSAL CRITERIA

Strength of association
Consistency
Temporality
Biologic gradient
Plausibility
Coherence
Experimental evidence
Analogy

None of the studies showed increased mortality with therapy. This analysis provides an incentive for closer examination of the reason for the wide confidence intervals among these studies (question of low study power, uncontrolled confounding factors, or study methods) and for exploration of similarities and differences between studies.

CAUSAL INFERENCE

A widely accepted principle of epidemiology states that "the most one can hope to show, even with several studies, is that an apparent association cannot be explained either by design bias or by confounding effects of other known risk factors."[38] In other words, no matter how well executed and convincing a study is, the closest that the investigator may come to causal inference is to reject the null hypothesis. In so doing the investigator can neither prove an alternative hypothesis nor justifiably make causal inferences.

Despite general agreement on an inability to prove causality, criteria are necessary to assess the likelihood that a given association is causal.

Most students of medicine first become familiar with the concept of assessing causality when they are exposed to Koch's postulates. Partially in response to discussion of Koch's work, Hill proposed the epidemiologic criteria for causality shown in Table 81-5.[39] The merits of these criteria have been subject to considerable academic debate. However, Hill's guidelines provide a reasonable starting point for considering the subject of causal inference.

Breslow and Day's text discusses the derivation of Hill's criteria considered to be most relevant to clinical studies: dose response, specificity of risk to disease subgroups, specificity of risk to exposure subcategories, strength of association, temporal relation or risk to exposure, lack of alternative explanations, and considerations external to the study.[38]

Dose response refers to the likelihood that a causal association will increase with the magnitude and duration of the exposure. Increasing rates of lung cancer seen with increasing exposure to cigarettes per day and years of smoking provide an example of this relationship.[40]

When an association is restricted to certain subcategories of disease, it is said to show *specificity of risk to disease subgroups*. The association of antenatal diethyl-

DEFINITIONS

Description of Disease Occurrence

$$\text{Prevalence } (P) = \frac{\text{Numbers of people having the disease at a specific time}}{\text{Size of population}}$$

The prevalence rate is in effect a proportion that is influenced by the incidence and/or duration of the disease. It is a measure more commonly used to examine chronic diseases.

Incidence

$$(I) = \frac{\text{Number of cases that occur in a population during a time period}}{\text{Numbers of people in the population at risk for acquiring the disease}}$$

The rate expresses the frequency of new cases per unit of time and is useful in investigating acute diseases. The denominator is often calculated by multiplying the size of the population and the length of the period.

Cumulative Incidence

$$(CI) = \frac{\text{Numbers of people that acquire the disease during a defined period}}{\text{Size of population at the beginning of the period } (Z)}$$

This is a measure of the proportion of healthy people who get sick during a defined period.

$P/(Z - P) = I \times D$

(D = duration of the disease.) For rare disease $P = I \times D$

$CI = I \exp(-I \times t)$

($\exp = 2.72$, t = length of period.) For rare disease $CI = I \times t$.

stilbestrol (DES) to a rare adenocarcinoma of the vagina in young women is an example of this kind of association.[41]

Demonstration that an association is stronger for different modes of exposure or groups of individuals is called *specificity of risk to exposure subcategories.*

There is an intuitive appeal to the claim that the *greater the risk of an association,* the less likely that factors other than the association (biases) explain the results. Acceptance of this tenet is inherent in a critical reader's tendency to dismiss a small risk ratio, with a 95% confidence interval that narrowly excludes the null value ("statistically significant") while being intrigued by a larger risk ratio that is accompanied by a confidence interval that just barely includes 1 (not "statistically significant"). As with the association between DES and vaginal adenocarcinoma[42] strong associations have sometimes been demonstrated by studies of very small sample size.

The *temporal relationship* of risk to exposure is often one of the most difficult causal criteria to satisfy. For an infectious disease with a known incubation period this criterion may be easily evaluated: when a susceptible child with an exposure to a friend with varicella develops a vesicular rash within 10 to 21 days of exposure, the presumption is that the child has varicella. However, in other instances the exposure may be difficult to verify or the exposure and disease may be separated by a long "induction" or "incubation" period,[42] as in the case of many cancers. Furthermore, the specific date of disease onset may be difficult to pinpoint, especially for illnesses that are gradually progressive or for which reliable diagnostic tests do not exist.

Considerations external to the study may be used to add perspective to the likelihood of causality. These data may take the form of comparisons with prior studies or examination of population trends in exposure and disease. Examples of the latter include the estimation of association rates of lung cancer and the prevalence of smoking among American men and women,[43,44] the rates of leukemia in children living in high- and low-radiation fallout areas,[45] and the trends in perinatal mor-

COMMONLY USED RATES AND RATIOS

DESCRIPTION OF MEASURE (SPEC. FOR AGE, RACE, SOCIOECONOMIC STATUS)	NUMERATOR	DENOMINATOR	PER 1000 (UNLESS INDICATED)
1. Birth rate	No. of live births during time interval	Est. midinterval	
2. Fertility rate	No. of live births during time interval	Est. no. of women 15–44 at mid interval	
3. Low birth weight ratio	No. live births <2500 g during time interval	No. of live births same time period	100
4. Fetal death rate	No. of fetal deaths ≥28 weeks during time interval	Fetal deaths (numerator) + live births same time interval	
5. Fetal death rate	No. of fetal deaths ≥20 weeks during time interval	Fetal deaths (numerator) + live births same time interval	
6. Neonatal mortality rate	No. of neonatal deaths 0–27 days of age	No. of live births same time interval	
7. Perinatal mortality rate (National Center for Health Statistics)	No. of fetal deaths ≥28 weeks + neonatal deaths 0–6 days of age	No. of live births same time interval	
8. Perinatal mortality rate (WHO National)	No. of fetal deaths ≥500 g > 22 weeks or 25 cm crown–heel + neonatal deaths 0–6 days	No. of live births + these fetal deaths	
9. Perinatal mortality (WHO International)	No. of fetal deaths ≥1000 g or ≥28 wks or 35 cm crown–heel + neonatal deaths 0–6 days	No. of live births + these fetal deaths	
10. Postneonatal mortality rate	No. of infant deaths 28–365 days	No. of life births during period	
11. Infant mortality rate	No. of infant deaths <1 year of age	No. of live births during period	
12. Maternal mortality rates (ACOG)	No. of deaths during pregnancy and 42 days postpartum	No. of terminated pregnancies same time interval	100,000
13. Maternal mortality NCHS and WHO ratio	No. of deaths during pregnancy and 42 days postpartum (excludes nonpregnancy related causes)	No. of live births same period	100,000

tality with changes in the rate of cesarean section births.[46] Other important external considerations relate to the biological plausibility of the hypothesis being tested.

A brief introduction to the casual criteria relevant to clinical studies cannot begin to address the many stimulating historical and contemporary discussions of the subject of causality and causal inference. Some theorists have proposed alternative criteria; others believe that no role exists for causal criteria. For a stimulating debate on causality by contemporary thinkers who refer to "Popperian" (deductivist), "Bayesian" (subjective probabilist), and frequentist (statistical) viewpoints, a recently published text provides interesting reading.[47]

ACKNOWLEDGMENTS

The authors would like to thank Dr. Marcello Pagano, Professor of Statistical Computing at the Harvard School of Public Health, for reviewing the manuscript.

REFERENCES

1. Kleinbaum D, Kupper L, Morgenstern H. Epidemiology research: principles and quantitative methods. Belmont, CA: Lifetime Learning Publications, 1981.
2. Greenland S. Response and follow-up bias in cohort studies. Am J Epidemiol 1977;106:184.
3. Rothman K. A pictorial representation of confounding in epidemiological studies. J Chron Dis 1975;32:101.
4. Burke DS, Brundage JK, Redfield RR, et al. Measurement of the false-positive rate in a screening program for Human Immunodeficiency Virus infections. N Engl J Med 1988;319(15):961.
5. Van Marter LJ, Bowich DM, Torday J, et al. Interpretation of indices of fetal pulmonary maturity by gestational age. Pediatr Perinat Epidemiol 1988;2:360.
6. Lubin J. Some efficiency comments on group size in study design. Am J Epidemiol 1980;111:453.
7. Schlesselman J. Sample size requirements in cohort and case-control studies of disease. Am J Epidemiol 1974;99:381.
8. Ury H. Efficiency of case-control studies with multiple controls per case: continuous or dichotomous data. Biometrics 1975;31:643.
9. Hennekens C, Buring J. Need for large sample sizes in randomized trials. Pediatrics 1987;79:569.
10. Rennie D. Vive la différence. N Engl J Med 1978;299:828.
11. Freiman J, Chalmers T, Smith H, Kuebler R. The importance of beta, the type II error and sample size in the design and interpretation of the randomized control trial. N Engl J Med 1978;299:690.
12. DerSimonian R, Charette L, McPeek B, Mosteller F. Reporting on methods in clinical trials. N Engl J Med 1982;306:1332.
13. Cohen J. Statistical power analysis for the behavioral sciences. New York: Academic Press, 1977.
14. Pasternack B, Shore R. Sample size for group sequential cohort and case-control study designs. Am J Epidemiol 1981;113:182.
15. Walter S. Determination of significant relative risks and optimal sampling procedures in prospective and retrospective comparative studies of various sizes. Am J Epidemiol 1977;105:387.
16. Greenland S. On sample-size and power calculations for studies using confidence intervals. Am J Epidemiol 1988;128:231.
17. Cornfield J. A method of estimating comparative rates from clinical data: applications to cancer of the lung, breast, and cervix. JNCI 1951;11:1269.
18. Rothman K. Modern epidemiology. Boston: Little, Brown, 1986.
19. Godfrey K. Comparing the means of several groups. N Engl J Med 1985;313:1450.
20. Smith E. Analysis of repeated measure designs. J Pediatr 1987;111:723.
21. Bailar III J, Mosteller F. Medical uses of statistics. Waltham, MA: New England Journal Books, 1986.
22. Bland M. An introduction to medical statistics. New York: Oxford University Press, 1987.
23. Glantz S. Primer of biostatistics. New York: McGraw-Hill, 1981.
24. Ingelfinger J, Mosteller F. Thibodeau L, Ware J. Biostatistics in clinical medicine. New York: Macmillan, 1983.
25. Koopmans L. An Introduction to contemporary statistics. Boston: PWS Publishers, 1981.
26. Schoolman H, Becktel J, Best W, Johnson A. Clinical and experimental statistics in medical research: principles versus practices. J Lab Clin Med 1968;71:357.
27. Feinstein A, Horwitz R. Double standards, scientific methods, and epidemiological research. N Engl J Med 1982;307:1611.
28. Pocock S, Hughes M, Lee R. Statistical problems in the reporting of clinical trials. A survey of three medical journals. N Engl J Med 1987;317:426.
29. Greenberg R, Kleinbaum D. Mathematical modeling strategies for the analysis of epidemiologic research. Ann Rev Public Health 1985;6:223.
30. Bishop Y, Fineberg S, Holland P. Discrete multivariate analysis. Cambridge, MA: MIT Press, 1975.
31. Fienberg S. The analysis of cross-classified categorical data. Cambridge, MA: MIT Press, 1980.
32. Chalmers T, Berrier J, Sacks H, Levin H, Reitman D, Nagalingam R. Meta-analysis of clinical trials as a scientific discipline. II: Replicate variability and comparison of studies that agree and disagree. Stat Med 1987;6:733.
33. Chalmers T, Levin H, Sacks H, Reitman D, Berrier J, Nagalingam R. Meta-analysis of clinical trials as a scientific discipline. I: Control of bias and comparison with large co-operative trials. Stat Med 1987;6:315.
34. Light R, Pillemer D. Summing up: the science of reviewing research. Cambridge, MA: Harvard University Press, 1984.
35. Louis T, Fineberg H, Mosteller F. Findings for public health from meta-analyses. Ann Rev Public Health 1985;6:1.
36. Sacks H, Berrier J, Reitman D, Ancona-Berk V, Chalmers T. Meta-analysis of randomized controlled trials. N Engl J Med 1987;316:450.
37. Furberg C, Morgan T. Lessons from overviews of cardiovascular trials. Stat Med 1987;6:295.
38. Breslow N, Day N. Statistical methods in cancer research I: the analysis of case-control studies. Lyon, France, IARC Scientific Publications, 1987.
39. Hill A. The environment and disease: association or causations. Proc R Soc Med 1965;58:295.
40. Cornfield J, Haenszel W, Hammond E, Lilienfeld A, Shimkin M, Wynder E. Smoking and lung cancer: recent evidence and a discussion of some questions. J Nat Can Inst 1959;22:173.
41. Herbst A, Ulfelder H, Poskanzer D. Adenocarcinoma of the vagina: association of maternal stilbesterol therapy with tumor appearance in young women. N Engl J Med 1971;284(16):878.
42. Rothman K. Induction and latent periods. Am J Epidemiol 1981;114:253.
44. Fielding J. Smoking and women. N Engl J Med 1987;317:1343.
45. Lyon J, Klauber M, Gardner J, Udall K. Childhood leukemias associated with fallout from nuclear testing. N Engl J Med 1979;300:397.

46. Pearson J. Cesarean section and perinatal mortality: a nine-year experience in a city/county hospital. Am J Obstet Gynecol 1984;148:155.
47. Rothman K, ed. Causal inference. Epidemiology resources. Boston: Little Brown, 1988.
48. Hallman M, Merritt T, Schneider H, et al. Isolation of human surfactant from amniotic fluid and a pilot study of its efficacy in respiratory distress syndrome. Pediatrics 1983;71:473.
49. Halliday H, Reid M, Meban C, et al. Controlled trial of artificial surfactant to prevent respiratory distress syndrome. Lancet 1984;1:476.
50. Hallman M, Merritt T, Jarvenpaa A, et al. Exogenous human surfactant for treatment of severe respiratory distress syndrome: a randomized prospective clinical trial. J Pediatr 1985;106:963.
51. Einhorning G, Shennan A, Possmayer F, et al. Prevention of neonatal respiratory distress syndrome by tracheal instillation of surfactant: a randomized clinical trial. Pediatrics 1979;145.
52. Kwong M, Egan E, Notter R, et al. Double-blind clinical trial of calf lung surfactant extract for the prevention of hyaline membrane disease in extremely premature infants. Pediatrics 1985;76:585.
53. Merrit T, Hallman M, Bloom B, et al. Prophylactic treatment of very premature infants with human surfactant. N Engl J Med 1986;315:785.
54. Gitlin J, Soll R, Parad R, et al. Randomized controlled trial of exogenous surfactant for the treatment of hyaline membrane disease. Pediatrics 1987;79:31.

82

CHAPTER

MULTIFETAL PREGNANCY REDUCTION

Mark I. Evans and John C. Fletcher

Complications or improper use of fertility drugs such as human menopausal gonadotrophin (Pergonal) or newer agents such as Metrodin, and associated reproductive technologies such as in vitro fertilization (IVF) or gamete intrafallopian transfer (GIFT) have created one of the ultimate ironies in medical care. Usually reserved as the last resort for couples with very significant infertility problems, the overdosage of such drugs or transfer of multiple embryos has led to situations in which women previously infertile now bear more fetuses than they can possibly carry to viability. Spectacular reports, both in the medical literature and in the lay media, have detailed successes such as the Dionne quintuplets of the 1930s, but they have also described equally infamous tragedies, such as the Frustaci septuplets in California in 1985 (Fig. 82-1). Although the successes have touched the public's heart, the reality is that the tragedies of prematurity, with its associated high risks of fetal demise and significant impairment for survivors, have more generally been the rule.[1]

The risks of creating iatrogenic multifetal gestation have been reduced considerably over the past several years, concomitant with the availability of monitoring with high-quality ultrasound as well as monitoring serum estrogen and progesterone levels.[2] Nevertheless, the possibility of inducing multiple gestation is normally expected in about 10% of patients. More than two fetuses have been seen in 1% or more. In some anecdotal instances some programs have substantially higher occurrences of multifetal pregnancies.

Advances in prenatal care and intensive neonatal care have reduced the mortality of multifetal pregnancies. However, neonatal advances have not been equally successful on morbidity.[3,4] Even in the best hands, the obstetric outcome for three or more fetuses is significantly worse than that for singleton or even twin pregnancies.[1,5] The ability to carry quadruplets or more is, by any reasonable definition, significantly compromised, and in grand multiple cases such as sextuplets or more, it has hardly ever been seen.

When faced with such potentially tragic circumstances, couples have had to choose among several unnerving options (Table 82-1). One option is termination of the entire pregnancy with the intent to conceive again. However, because conception is not guaranteed, particularly since most of these patients are infertility cases, this option has generally been very unpalatable. The second option is to continue with all the fetuses. In cases of quadruplets or even quintuplets, survival of some or all is certainly a possibility, but there is significant risk of long-term morbidity. With six or more fetuses, the chance of survival is extremely low, and, for example, in cases of octuplets that we encountered, the chance was certainly zero.

A third option is consideration of selective termination, which over the course of the past few years has become a realistic option in the face of perinatal tragedy from multiple fetuses.[6–10]

TERMINOLOGY

In the literature several terms have been used to describe the procedures discussed in this chapter. A consensus has been reached to use "selective termination" for a procedure performed because of an abnormality diagnosed in one fetus and "multifetal pregnancy reduction" (MFPR) when the indication is solely fetal number without demonstrable fetal defects.

SELECTION OF PATIENTS AND TECHNIQUES

As the awareness of the availability of MFPR becomes more widespread, the number of cases performed will

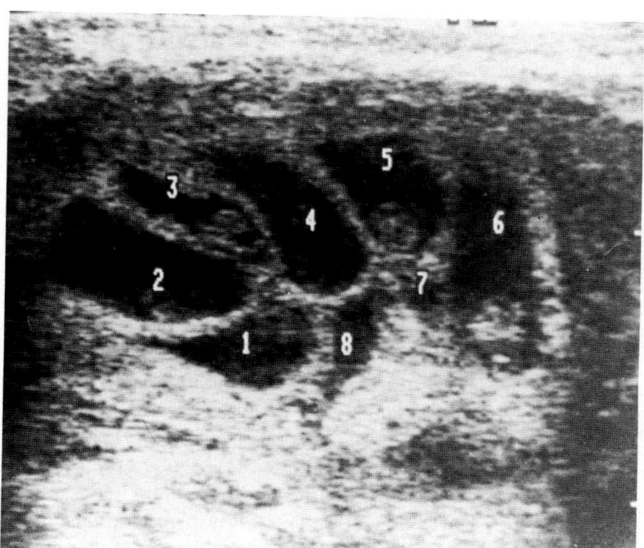

FIGURE 82–1. Ultrasound at 8 weeks showing an octuplet gestation. A ninth sac was empty. (Reprinted with permission from Obstet Gynecol 1988; 71: 290.)

clearly rise. Through 1991, we are aware of approximately 600 cases having been done worldwide. There are undoubtedly others that have not been reported. The largest number of cases have been performed by Dumez, in Paris; Berkowitz, in New York; and Evans, in Detroit.[6–10]

Three different technical procedures have been reported (Table 82-2). Originally, Dumez and Oury reported a technique involving transcervical suction to remove embryos at 8 to 11 weeks.[8] Under ultrasound guidance, a mini-suction curettage was performed. They and others have shown technical success in a majority of cases but with loss of the entire pregnancy in about 50%. This technique is less desirable than transabdominal methods described later because the suction method appears to become more difficult over 9 weeks gestation and because removal of the gestational sac alters intrauterine volume, which could increase the chance of contractions. Another method that has been tried successfully is a transvaginal aspiration of the early embryo, usually at about 6 to 7 weeks. This technique is analogous in many respects to oocyte aspiration for in vitro fertilization and may be useful particularly when the attempt is made very early in gestation. Proponents of transvaginal techniques now believe that delaying the procedure to at least 9 to 10 weeks is desirable to permit at least a rudimentary fetal visualization

TABLE 82–1. OPTIONS IN MULTIFETAL GESTATION

Abortion
Attempt to carry
Multifetal pregnancy reduction

TABLE 82–2. TECHNIQUES OF MULTIFETAL PREGNANCY REDUCTION

Transcervical
Transvaginal
Transabdominal

to look for worrisome signs such as, for example, nuchal folds (I. Timor, personal communication).

The technique that is generally technologically most feasible involves the transabdominal insertion under ultrasound guidance of a spinal needle (usually 22-gauge). The needle is maneuvered into the thorax of the fetus, and a small dose of potassium chloride is injected (Fig. 82-2). This injection (about 0.5–1.0 mL) results in cardiac standstill, usually within 1 to 2 minutes of the injection, with ultimate reabsorption of the sac (Fig. 82-3). On occasion, cardiac motion will continue for a longer time, but a definite slowing, which appears "preterminal," will be apparent.

The decision of which embryo to choose has been strictly a technical issue of which embryos are easiest to reach.[4] Anecdotal experience suggests that it is better not to choose the embryo closest to the cervix, as vaginal discharge is likely. Also, there is concern about removal of amniotic fluid, because a sudden decrease in uterine size might induce contractions and there is concern that devitalization of tissue near the cervix might predispose to ascending infection and increased risk of fetal loss.

Composite data suggest success (defined as the ultimate live birth of babies) in approximately 75% of cases (Table 82-3). In the vast majority of cases, the procedure is technically not very difficult for physicians

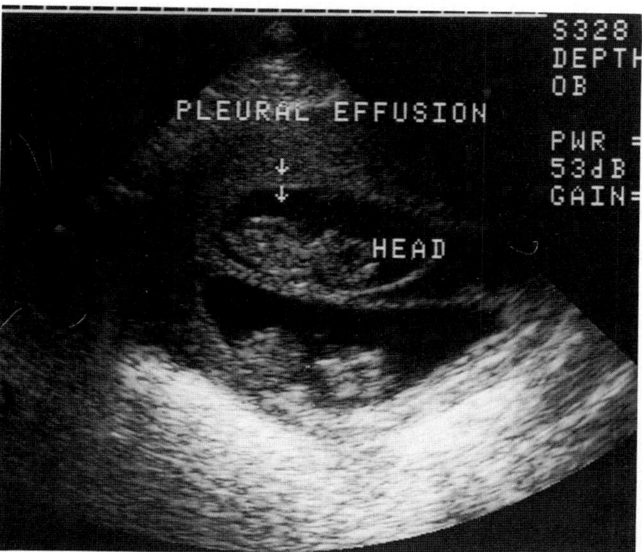

FIGURE 82–2. Pleural effusion in thorax of a fetus at 11 weeks following injection of 0.7 mL KCl. Cardiac standstill was confirmed within 30 seconds.

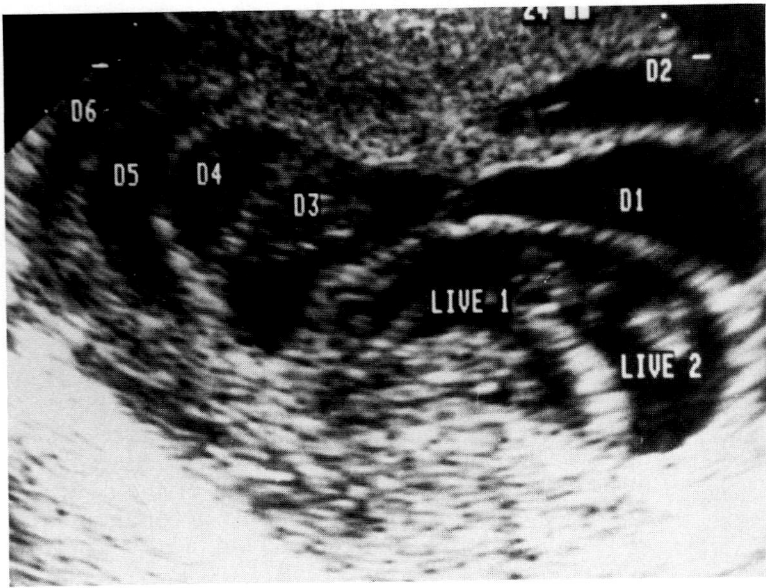

FIGURE 82–3. Ultrasound at 9 weeks following selective termination of three embryos at 8 weeks and three more at 9 weeks (D-1 through D-6). Twins were left (live 1 and live 2), who went 35 weeks and were then delivered—two boys who were healthy at 18 months of age. (Reprinted with permission from Evans MI, Fletcher JL, Zador IE, et al. Selective first trimester termination in octuplet and quadruplet pregnancies: clinical and ethical issues. Obstet Gynecol 1988; 71: 290.)

experienced in performing ultrasound-guided needle procedures.

WHEN?

Most of the transabdominal cases reported to date have been performed at 10 to 12 weeks of pregnancy. Although there are few data, it would seem that transabdominal attempts prior to 8 weeks would be technically more difficult, and the transvaginal approach will probably be best at very early gestational ages. However, the chance at this time of a spontaneous loss of remaining embryos "naturally" is still a considerable possibility and therefore poses a risk of losing the only remaining embryo(s).[11,12] Consequently, even some transvaginal advocates now wait until about 10 weeks. Beyond 12 weeks, the chance of spontaneous loss is minimal, but increased tissue mass left would seem to pose a risk of coagulopathies, such as disseminated intravascular coagulation occasionally seen with the loss of one twin. However, there are no reliable data to show this. Furthermore, uterine size increases dramatically in such cases, risking premature labor.

HOW MANY?

From the beginning our bias, based on existing obstetrical data, was to believe that twins were the best place to stop. Not surprisingly, therefore, the decisions of both the patient and physician have almost always been to leave twins. We felt that by leaving twins there is still some "margin for error." Although the obstetric outcome for twins is not quite as good as that of singleton pregnancies, it is considerably better than that for triplets or more.

In some cases triplets have been left.[7] Obstetrically, the outcome of triplets can be satisfactory, but the risks of prematurity and morbidity are certainly increased above those for twins. Such risks can be justified if the couple understands the high likelihood of alterations of

TABLE 82–3. RESULTS OF MULTIFETAL PREGNANCY REDUCTION

INITIAL NO. FETUSES	NO. PERFORMED	AVERAGE FINAL NO. FETUSES	EARLY LOSS	LATE LOSS	TOTAL LOSS
9	1	2.00	0.00%	0.00%	0.00%
8	2	2.00	0.00%	0.00%	0.00%
7	10	2.20	10.00%	22.20%	30.00%
6	13	2.15	15.38%	22.73%	34.60%
5	29	2.00	13.79%	20.00%	31.03%
4	130	2.00	5.38%	16.14%	21.15%
3	106	1.89	6.60%	12.63%	18.40%
2	19	1.00	0.00%	0.00%	0.00%
	310	1.905	6%	12%	17%

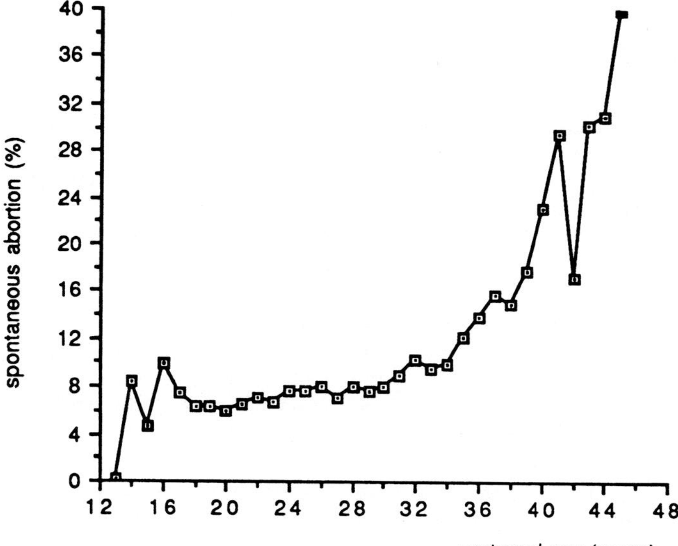

FIGURE 83–5. Risk of spontaneous abortion with age. (Adapted from Naylor AF, Warburton D. Sequential analysis of spontaneous abortion. II. Collaborative study data show that gravidity determines a very substantial rise in risk. Fertil Steril 1979;31:282, with permission.)

acrocentric chromosomes may be particularly prone to the consequences of prolonged meiotic arrest.[102] It has been estimated that the pre-viable pregnancy loss relating to trisomy 21 is 30%.[103] It is thought that older women may be more likely to conceive, and also to abort, a trisomic fetus.[104,105] A collaborative report on chromosome aberrations in 52,965 amniocenteses performed in women over age 35 found an exponential increase, with advancing age, for trisomies 21, 18, and 13 and for XXX and XXY syndromes (Table 83-3). A significant inverse relationship was found with 45 XO cases. Paternal age did not appear to have a significant effect.[104]

Although trisomies account for less than 20% of abortions in women under age 25, they are responsible for 67% of abortions in women over 40. It has been suggested that most conceptions occurring in women over 40 are aneuploid.[105] This might be an exaggeration, because chromosome studies in induced abortion for elective reasons in an otherwise normally progressing pregnancy found much lower rates. In 256 abortions, 2 of 123 cases were aneuploid in women age 35 to 39, 7 of 117 in age 40 to 44, and 4 of 16 over age 45.[106] Of 2404 amniocenteses performed in women over age 35, 2.4% were aneuploid, with 50% trisomy 21.[107]

Trisomies primarily arise from nondisjunction in the first meiotic division.[108] This may be a result of over 35 years of meiotic arrest and the opportunity for structural aging or environmental insults.[109] It may also be due to the greater incidence of delayed ovulation and preovulatory aging that occurs with instability of the endocrine axis, which is more common at the extremes of the reproductive lifespan.[110] Since trisomies arise from the first meiotic division, it is unlikely that delayed fertilization, as might occur with decreased frequency of intercourse, has an effect on the incidence of fertilization, as has been reported.[111]

Although maternal serum alpha-fetoprotein screening provides an additional benefit in screening for trisomy 21, it adds little to the detection of other trisomic disorders. No age-specific difference in maternal alpha-fetoprotein levels has been found.[112]

In a cross-sectional study population of over 8 million births and 88,000 defects, an age association was found in all 16 of the categories of defects.[113] However, when defects due to Down syndrome were excluded, the statistical significance of the age-related incidence was lost (except after age 40, when the rate of defects was 8.8 per 1000). The highest incidence of defects occurred in first births over age 40 (Fig. 83-6). It could be argued that the study period (1961 to 1966) might not reflect current trends, and a more current large-scale study is needed.

TABLE 83–3. MATERNAL AGE-SPECIFIC RATES FOR TRISOMIC CHROMOSOMAL ALTERATIONS OBSERVED BY AMNIOCENTESIS

AGE (yrs)	N	TRISOMY 21	TRISOMY 18	TRISOMY 13	XXX	XXY
35	5409	0.35	0.07	0.05	0.07	0.09
36	6103	0.57	0.08	0.03	0.08	0.08
37	6956	0.68	0.09	0.03	0.07	0.04
38	7926	0.81	0.15	0.04	0.08	0.08
39	7682	1.09	0.19	0.06	0.12	0.16
40	7174	1.23	0.25	0.12	0.06	0.15
41	4763	1.47	0.36	0.17	0.15	0.29
42	3156	2.19	0.63	0.19	0.28	0.35
43	1912	3.24	0.78	0.05	0.31	0.31
44	1015	2.95	0.49		0.49	0.39
45	508	4.53	0.39	0.20	0.39	0.98
46	232	8.19	0.43		0.43	1.29
>46	129	2.33	0.77		1.55	1.55

(From Ferguson-Smith MA, Yates JR. Maternal age-specific rates for chromosome aberrations and factors influencing them: report of a collaborative European study on 52,965 amniocenteses. Prenatal Diagn 1984;4:5.)

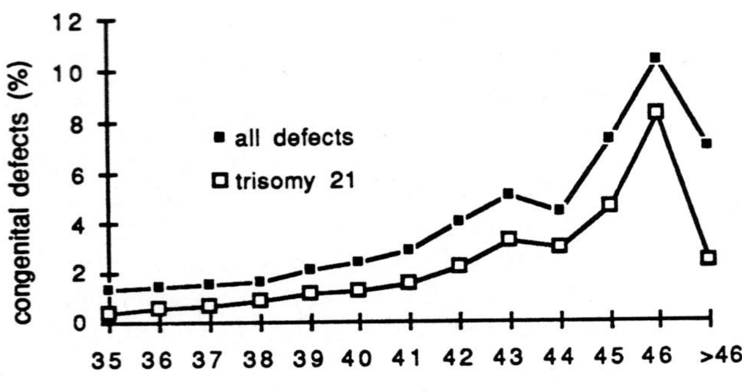

FIGURE 83–6. Risk of congenital defect with age. (Adapted from Hay S, Barbano H. Independent effects of maternal age and birth order on the incidence of selected congenital malformations. Teratology 1972;6:271, with permission.)

Gestational Trophoblastic Disease

In a study of 2202 patients of the Southeastern Regional Trophoblastic Center, a significant increase in trophoblastic disease was seen in women over age 40 and under age 15.[17] The lowest risk of malignancy was found in women under age 15, the highest in those over age 50. It is interesting that this bimodal incidence of trophoblastic disease at the extremes of the reproductive lifespan is similar to that of spontaneous abortion and trisomy 21. This suggests that the polyploidy seen with trophoblastic disease may arise as a result of either preovulatory aging or postovulatory aging, as may occur with delayed fertilization.

PSYCHOLOGICAL CONSIDERATIONS

Most psychological studies have focused on young mothers' adaptation to pregnancy and have ignored the psychological changes that occur in older patients. Negative attitudes during labor have been shown to alter the course of labor.[114] Today, pregnancy after age 35 is usually planned and delivery is prepared for in advance. Robinson and coworkers reported that their study group of older women were less troubled by pregnancy and reported fewer symptoms in the first trimester.[115] Although the level of anxiety increased as the pregnancy progressed, older patients were typically better adjusted as they entered the last trimester. Overall, older mothers may differ psychologically, but show no differences in their adaptability.[116]

HOW OLD IS TOO OLD?

Is there an age at which pregnancy should be definitely discouraged? Although there are scattered reports of pregnancy after age 50, pregnancy in women over age 45 is exceedingly uncommon.[69,117] In a report on 160 births (27 primiparas) to women over age 44, Stanton found that although the pregnancies overall were more complicated than those of younger patients, they were less complicated than those of multiparas.[69] Hansen compiled five studies from long-term studies of 182,252 pregnancies.[118] There were only 3 documented pregnancies to women age 50 (0.0016%) compared with 52 pregnancies at age 46 (0.028%) and 21 pregnancies between ages 47 and 49. These studies take on more importance because many women use no contraception after age 45. Novak reviewed the pathology studies after hysterectomy and bilateral oophorectomy in 200 cases in an attempt to determine the reproductive potential at older ages.[119] He found functional corpora lutea but abnormal uterine histology and concluded that although ovulation was possible after age 50, nidation was impossible.

Between ages 38 and 44 most women lose their capacity to reproduce, but this does not guarantee fertility for the 35-year-old or deny it in the 45-year-old. Whether the loss of fecundity is rapid or slow is unknown; individual variations may be wide. Certainly, much more study is needed on the reproductive potential in this age group. The risk of infertility appears to be the greatest risk that a woman faces in electing pregnancy after age 35. Overall, older patients may show little difference from their younger counterparts except in their decreased fecundity. There is probably no age that a pregnancy is unsafe, nor should age alone ever be a contraindication of pregnancy. Berkowitz and associates reported that although there may be an increased rate of specific pregnancy complications, resulting in increased maternal morbidity and higher health-care costs, a child born to an otherwise healthy private patient in a tertiary-care facility has no increased risk of an adverse neonatal outcome.[120] This is usually the single most important factor to the woman contemplating a pregnancy after age 35.

CONCLUSION

If a representative sample of literature is taken, surprisingly little agreement can be reached about the risks of pregnancy in women under age 20 and over age 35. Composition of study groups, lack of controls, and observer bias call the validity of many previous studies into question. It seems that improved awareness and prenatal care can make a significant difference in both younger and older patients. Younger patients can have excellent outcomes if given good prenatal care. The risks of pregnancy after age 35 seem to have been exaggerated, and the "age 35" obstetric dogma may have little clinical utility. If a gradient of age-dependent risks of pregnancy exists, it may vary with each type of pregnancy complication and certainly will vary among individual women. With good prenatal and neonatal care, age alone is probably never a risk factor for poor perinatal outcome.

REFERENCES

1. Kirz DS, Dorchester W, Freeman RK, Advanced maternal age: the mature gravida. Am J Obstet Gynecol 1985;152:7.
2. Zacharias L, Rand WM, Wurtman R. A prospective study of sexual development and growth in American girls: the statistics of menarche. Obstet Gynecol Surv 1976;31:325.
3. Weir J, Dunn J, Jones E. Race and age at menarche. Am J Obstet Gynecol 1971;111:594.
4. Frisch RE, Revelle R. Height and weight at menarche and a hypothesis of critical body weights and adolescent events. Science 1970;169:397.
5. Johnston FE, Roche AF, Schell LM, Wettenhall NB. Critical weight at menarche: critique of a hypothesis. Am J Dis Child 1975;129:19.
6. Duenhoelter JH, Jimenez JM, Baumann G. Pregnancy performance of patients under 15 years of age. Obstet Gynecol 1975;46:49.
7. Treolar A, Boynton R, Benn B, Brown B. Variation of the human menstrual cycle throughout reproductive life. Int J Fertil 1979;12:77.
8. Erickson JD. Down syndrome, paternal age, maternal age and birth order. Ann Hum Genet 1978;41:289.
9. Gindoff PR, Jewelewicz R. Reproduction potential in the older woman. Fertil Steril 1986;46:989
10. Gosden RG. Biology of menopause: the causes and consequences of ovarian aging. London: Academic Press, 1985.
11. Lee KS, Corpuz M. Teenage pregnancy; trend and impact of rates of low birth weight and fetal, maternal, and neonatal mortality in the United States. Clin Perinatol 1988;15:929.
12. Gale R, Zengen S, Harlap S, et al. Birth out of wedlock and the risk of intrauterine growth retardation. Am J Perinatol 1988;5:278.
13. Machol L. Adoption services for your pregnant patient. Contemp Obstet Gynecol 1989;33:114.
14. Adams MM, Oakley GP Jr, Marks JS. Maternal age and births in the 1980s. JAMA 1982;247:493.
15. Burt MR. Estimates of public costs for teenage childbearing. Washington DC: Center for Population Options, 1986.
16. MMWR 1988;37:19.
17. Bandy LC, Clarke-Pearson BL, Hammond CB. Malignant potential of gestational trophoblastic disease at the extreme ages of reproductive life. Obstet Gynecol 1984;64:395.
18. Cohen BA, Burkman RT, Rosenshein NB, et al. Gestational trophoblastic disease within an elective abortion population. Am J Obstet Gynecol 1979;135:452.
19. Hollingsworth DR. The pregnant adolescent: a sociologic problem with medical consequences. In: Burrow GN, Ferris TF, eds. Medical complications during pregnancy. Philadelphia: WB Saunders, 1982:546.
20. Dott AB, Fort AT. Medical and social factors affecting early teenage pregnancy. Am J Obstet Gynecol 1976;125:532.
21. Zuckerman BS, Walker DK, Frank DA, et al. Adolescent pregnancy: bio-behavioral determinants of outcome. J Pediatr 1984;105:857.
22. Ryan GM Jr, Schneider JM. Teenage obstetric complications. Clin Obstet Gynecol 1978;21:1191.
23. Duenhoelter JH, Jimenez JM, Baumann G. Pregnancy performance of patients under 15 years of age. Obstet Gynecol 1975;46:49.
24. Hutchins, FL Jr, Kendall N, Rubino J. Experience with teenage pregnancy. Obstet Gynecol 1979;54:1.
25. Saller DN, Crenshaw MC Jr. Medical complications in adolescent pregnancy. Maryland Med J 1987;36:935.
26. Oh MK, Feinstein RA, Pass RF. Sexually transmitted diseases and sexual behavior in urban adolescent females attending a family planning clinic. J Adolesc Health Care 1988;9:67.
27. Brown HP. Recognizing common STDs in adolescents. Contemp Obstet Gynecol 1989;33:47.
28. Wetzel AM, Kirz DS. Routine hepatitis screening in adolescent pregnancies: is it cost-effective? Am J Obstet Gynecol 1987;156:166.
29. Pletsch PK. Substance use and health activities of pregnant adolescents. J Adolesc Health Care 1988;9:38.
30. Elster AB. The effects of maternal age, parity, and prenatal care on perinatal outcome in adolescent mothers. Am J Obstet Gynecol 1984;149:845.
31. Spiers PS, Wang L. Short pregnancy interval, low birth weight, and the sudden infant death syndrome. Am J Epidemiol 1975;104:15.
32. Elster AB, McAnarney ER. Medical and psychosocial risks of pregnancy and childbearing during adolescence. Pediatr Ann 1980;9:89.
33. American Dietetic Association. Position of the American Dietetic Association: nutrition management of adolescent pregnancy. J Am Diet Assoc 1989;89:104.
34. Garn SM, Petzold AS. Characteristics of the mother and child in teenage pregnancy. Am J Dis Child 1983;137:365.
35. Sukanich AC, Rogers KD, McDonald HM. Physical maturity and outcome of pregnancy in primiparas younger than 16 years of age. Pediatrics 1986;78:31.
36. Hardy JB, Drage JS, Jackson EC, eds. The first year of life: the collaborative perinatal projects of the WINCDS. Baltimore: Johns Hopkins University Press, 1979:236.
37. Naeye RL. Teenaged and pre-teenaged pregnancies: Consequences of the fetal-maternal competition for nutrients. Pediatrics 1981;67:146.
38. Heald FP, Jacobson MS. Nutritional needs of the pregnant adolescent. Pediatr Ann 1980;9:95.
39. Leppert PC, Nameron PB, Horowitz ED. Cesarean section deliveries among adolescent mothers enrolled in a comprehensive prenatal care program. Am J Obstet Gynecol 1985;152:623.
40. Horon IL, Strobino DM, MacDonald HM. Birth weights among infants born to adolescent and young adult women. Am J Obstet Gynecol 1983;146:444.
41. Scholl TO, Salmon RW, Miller LK. Smoking and adolescent pregnancy outcome. J Adolesc Health Care 1986;7:390.
42. Tietze C. Legal abortions in the United States: rates and ratios by race and age, 1972–1974. Fam Plann Perspect 1977;9:12.
43. Levenson PM, Smith PB, Morrow JR Jr. A comparison of physician-patient views of teen prenatal information needs. J Adolesc Health Care 1986;7:6.
44. Bracken MB, Klerman LV, Bracken M. Abortion, adoption or motherhood: an empirical study of decision-making during pregnancy. Am J Obstet Gynecol 1978;130:251.
45. Gispert M, Falk R. Sexual experimentation and pregnancy in young black adolescents. Am J Obstet Gynecol 1976;126:459.
46. Giblin PT, Poland ML, Sachs BA. Pregnant adolescents' health-information needs: implications for health education and health seeking. J Adolesc Health Care 1986;7:168.
47. Hopfer TW. Teenage pregnancy: an overview. III. Environmental and educational influences. J SC Med Assoc 1988;84:342.
48. World Health Organization Task Force on the Sequelae of Abortion. Gestation, birth-weight and spontaneous abortion in pregnancy after induced abortion. Lancet 1979;i:142.
49. Cates W Jr, Schulz KF, Grimes DA. The risks associated with teenage abortion. New Engl J Med 1983;309:621.
50. Streissguth AP, Darby BL, Barr HM, et al. Comparison of drink-

ing and smoking patterns during pregnancy over a 6-year interval. Am J Obstet Gynecol 1983;145:716.
51. American College of Obstetricians and Gynecologists Task Force on Adolescent Pregnancy. Adolescent perinatal health: a guidebook of services. Author: Chicago, 1979.
52. Wallach EE, Klein L, Repke J, et al. Caring for younger pregnant teenagers: a symposium. Contemp Obstet Gynecol 1987; 30:154.
53. Scholl TO, Miller LK, Salmon RW, et al. Prenatal care adequacy and the outcome of adolescent pregnancy: effects on weight gain, preterm delivery and birth weight. Obstet Gynecol 1987;69:312.
54. Hardy JB, King TM, Repke JT. The Johns Hopkins Adolescent Pregnancy Program: an evaluation. Obstet Gynecol 1987; 69:300.
55. Clark AM, Thompson HD, Mantell CD, Hutton JD. Comprehensive antenatal care and education of young adolescents: beneficial effects on pregnancy and outcome. N Z Med J 1986;99:59.
56. Bloom DE. Delayed childbearing in the United States. Popul Res Policy Rev 1984;3:103.
57. Baldwin WH, Nord CW. Delayed childbearing in the United States: facts and fictions. Popul Bull 1984;39:3.
58. Spenser G. Projections of the population of the United States, by age, sex, and race: 1983–2080. Current Population Reports: Population Estimates and Projections, May 1984.
59. Mansfield PK. Pregnancy for older women: assessing the medical risks. New York: Praeger, 1986:220.
60. Tietze C. Reproductive span and rate of reproduction among Hutterite women. Fertil Steril 1957;8:89.
61. Federation CECOS, Schwartz D, Mayaux MJ. Female fecundity as a function of age. N Engl J Med 1982;306:404.
62. Virro MR, Shewchuk AB. Pregnancy outcome in 242 conceptions after artificial insemination with donor sperm and effects of maternal age on the prognosis for successful pregnancy. Am J Obstet Gynecol 1984;148:518.
63. Dor J, Itzkowic DJ, Mashiach S, Lunenfeld B, Serr D. Cumulative conception rates following gonadotropin therapy. Am J Obstet Gynecol 1980;136:102.
64. Jones GS, Muasher SJ, Rosenwaks Z, Acosta AA, Liu HC. The perimenopausal patient in in vitro fertilization: the use of gonadotropin-releasing hormone. Fertil Steril 1986;46:885.
65. Mosher WD, Pratt WF. Reproductive impairments among married couples. In: Vital and Health Statistics Series 23 (11) National Survey of Family Growth, National Center for Health Statistics, Washington DC.
66. Leridon H. Patterns of fertility at later ages of reproduction. J Biosoc Sci 1979;6:59.
67. Endres J, Dunning S, Poon SW, Welch P, Duncan H. Older pregnant women and adolescents: nutrition data after enrollment in WIC. J Am Diet Assoc 1987;87:1011.
68. Waters EG, Wagner HP. Pregnancy and labor experiences of elderly primigravidas. Am J Obstet Gynecol 1950;59:296.
69. Stanton EF. Pregnancy after 44. Am J Obstet Gynecol 1956;71:270.
70. Kane SH. Advancing age and the primigravida. Obstet Gynecol 1967;29:409.
71. Horger EO III, Smythe SR II. Pregnancy in women over 40. Obstet Gynecol 1977;49:257.
72. Kajanoja P, Widholm O. Pregnancy and delivery in women aged 40 and over. Obstet Gynecol 1978;51:47.
73. Lehmann DK, Chism J. Pregnancy outcome in medical complicated and uncomplicated patients aged 40 years or older. Am J Obstet Gynecol 1987;157:738.
74. Spellacy WN, Miller SJ, Winegar A. Pregnancy after 40 years of age. Obstet Gynecol 1986;68:452.
75. Grimes DA, Gross GK. Pregnancy outcomes in black women aged 35 and older. Obstet Gynecol 1981;58:614.
76. Kaltreider DF. The elderly multigravida. Obstet Gynecol 1959;13:190.
77. Mestman JH. Outcome of diabetes screening in pregnancy and perinatal morbidity in infants of mothers with mild impairment in glucose tolerance. Diab Care 1980;3:447.
78. O'Sullivan JB, Charles D, Mahan CM, Dandrow RV. Gestational diabetes and perinatal mortality rate. Am J Obstet Gynecol 1973;116:901.
79. Gabbe SG, Mestman JG, Freeman RK, Anderson GV, Lowensohn RI. Management and outcome of Class A diabetes mellitus. Am J Obstet Gynecol 1977;127:465.
80. Kessler I, Lancer M, Borenstein R, Steinmetz A. The problem of the older primipara. Obstet Gynecol 1980;56:165.
81. Tuck SM, Yudkin PL, Turnbull AC. Pregnancy outcome in elderly primigravidae with and without a history of infertility. Br J Obstet Gynaecol 1988;95:230.
82. Naeye RL. Maternal age, obstetric complications and the outcome of pregnancy. Obstet Gynecol 1983;61:210.
83. Turner MJ, MacDonald D. Pregnancy after the age of 40 years: are the risks increased? J Obstet Gynaecol 1984;5:1.
84. Morrison I. The elderly primigravida. Am J Obstet Gynecol 1975;121:465.
85. Freidman EA, Sachtleben MR. Relation of maternal age to the course of labor. Am J Obstet Gynecol 1965;91:915.
86. Cohen WR, Newman L, Friedman EA Risk of labor abnormalities with advancing maternal age. Obstet Gynecol 1980;55:414.
87. Booth RT, Williams GL. Elderly primigravidae. J Obstet Gynaecol Br Common 1964;71:249.
88. Posner LB, Chidiac JE, Posner AC. Pregnancy at age 40 and over. Obstet Gynecol 1961;17:194.
89. Martel M, Wacholder S, Lippman A, Brohan J, Hamilton E. Maternal age and primary cesarean section rates: a multivariate analysis. Am J Obstet Gynecol 1987;156:305.
90. Higdon AL. Pregnancy in the woman over 40. Am J Obstet Gynecol 1960;80:38.
91. Forman M, Meirik O, Berendes HW. Delayed childbearing in Sweden. JAMA 1984;252:3135.
92. Peters TJ, Golding J, Butler NR, Fryer JG, Lawrence CJ, Chamberlain G. Predictors of birth weight in two national studies. Br J Obstet Gynaecol 1983;90:1040.
93. Barkan SE, Bracken MB. Delayed childbearing: no evidence for increased risk of low birth weight and preterm delivery. Am J Epidemiol 1987;125:101.
94. Buehler JW, Kaunitz AM, Hogue CJ, Hughes JM, Smith JC, Rochat RW. Maternal mortality in women aged 35 years or older: United States. JAMA 1986;255:53.
95. Kiely JL, Paneth N, Susser M. An assessment of the effects of maternal age and parity in different components of perinatal mortality. Am J Epidemiol 1986;123:444.
96. Naylor AF, Warburton D. Sequential analysis of spontaneous abortion. II. Collaborative study data show that gravidity determines a very substantial rise in risk. Fertil Steril 1979;31:282.
97. Warburton D, Fraser FC. Spontaneous abortion risks in man: data from reproductive histories collected in a medical genetics unit. Am J Human Genet 1964;16:1.
98. Lauritsen JG. Aetiology of spontaneous abortion. Acta Obstet Gynecol Scand 1976;52:1.
99. Kajii T, Ferrier A, Niikawa N, et al. Anatomic and chromosomal abnormalities in 639 spontaneous abortuses. Hum Genet 1980;55:87.
100. Creasy ME, Crolla JA, Alberman ED. A cytogenetic study of

human spontaneous abortions using banding techniques. Hum Genet 1976;31:177.

101. Machin GA. Chromosome abnormality and perinatal death. Lancet 1974;i:549.
102. Mattevi MS, Salzano FM. Effect of sex, age, and cultivation time on number of satellites and acrocentric associations in man. Humangenetik 1975;29:265.
103. Hook EB. Rates of chromosomal abnormalities at different maternal ages. Obstet Gynecol 1981;58:282.
104. Ferguson-Smith MA, Yates JR. Maternal age-specific rates for chromosome aberrations and factors influencing them: report of a collaborative European study on 52,965 amniocenteses. Prenatal Diagn 1984;4:5.
105. Hassold T, Chiu D. Maternal age-specific rates of numerical chromosome abnormalities with special reference to trisomy. Hum Genet 1985;70:11.
106. Tsuji K, Nakano R. Chromosome studies of embryos from induced abortions in pregnant women age 35 and over. Obstet Gynecol 1978;52:542.
107. Golbus MS, Loughman WD, Epstein CJ, Halbasch G, Stephens JD, Hall BD. Prenatal genetic diagnosis in 3000 amniocenteses. N Engl J Med 1979;300:157.
108. Licznerski RL, Lindsten J. Trisomy 21 in man due to maternal nondisjunction during the first meiotic division. Hereditas 1972;70:153.
109. Polani PE, Jagiello GM. Chiasmata, meiotic univalents and age in relation to aneuploid imbalance in mice. Cytogenet Cell Genet 1976;16:505.
110. Butcher RL, Pope RS. Role of estrogen during prolonged estrous cycles of the rat on subsequent embryonic death or development. Biol Reprod 1979;21:491.
111. James WH. Mongolism, delayed fertilization and sexual behavior. Nature 1968;219:279.
112. Ashwood ER, Cheng E, Luthy DA. Maternal serum alpha-fetoprotein and fetal trisomy-21 in women 35 years and older: implications for alpha-fetoprotein screening programs. Am J Med Genet 1987;26:531.
113. Hay S, Barbano H. Independent effects of maternal age and birth order on the incidence of selected congenital malformations. Teratology 1972;6:271.
114. McDonald RL. The role of emotional factors in obstetric complications: a review. Psychosom Med 1968;30:222:108.
115. Robinson GE, Garner DM, Gare DJ, Crawford B. Psychological adaptation to pregnancy in childless women more than 35 years of age. Am J Obstet Gynecol 1987;156:328.
116. Walter CA. The timing of motherhood: is later better? Lexington, Mass.: Lexington Books, 1986:1.
117. Natter CE. Pregnancy after 50. Obstet Gynecol 1964;24:641.
118. Hansen JP. Older maternal age and pregnancy outcome: a review of the literature. Obstet Gynecol Surv 1986;41:726.
119. Novak ER. Ovulation after 50. Obstet Gynecol 1970;36:903.
120. Berkowitz GS, Skovron ML, Lapinski RH, Berkowitz RL. Delayed childbearing and the outcome of pregnancy. N Engl J Med 1990;322:659.

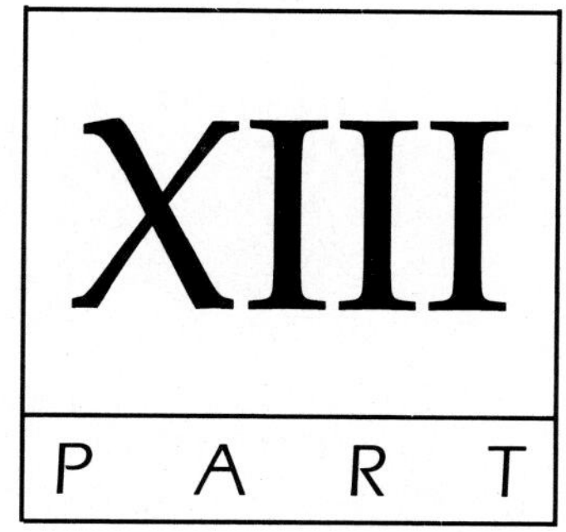

OBSTETRIC AND PERIPARTAL EVENTS

84

CHAPTER

THIRD TRIMESTER BLEEDING

Carl A. Nimrod

Bleeding in the third trimester is a major cause of perinatal morbidity and mortality. Its exact incidence is unclear due to a lack of comprehensive reporting, but community-based studies suggest frequency rates of 3% to 4.8%.[1,2] In 30% of cases definite features of placental abruption exist; placenta previa is responsible for 20% of cases.[3] In about half of these women, no clear reason for the bleeding can be identified, and it is presumed to be from either local lesions in the birth canal, marginal separation, or trauma.[4]

PLACENTAL ABRUPTION

Placental abruption, defined as premature detachment of a normally implanted placenta, recognizably occurs in 1% of pregnancies.[5] Commonly associated with preterm labor and delivery, it accounts for 15% to 25% of all perinatal mortality.[6] Symptoms of abruption include visible maternal hemorrhage in 65% to 80% of patients before delivery; a tense, irritable uterus; fetal distress; and coagulopathy in the most severe situations. More commonly, however, painful vaginal bleeding is the hallmark. This variability of clinical presentation necessitates a high index of suspicion for the diagnosis.

The clinical classification of placental abruption is based on the observation of bleeding at three principal sites (Fig. 84-1). Nyberg and associates described bleeding seen by ultrasound at the following locations:[7]

1. Subchorionic: between the myometrium and the placental membranes
2. Retroplacental: between the myometrium and the placenta
3. Preplacental: between the placenta and amniotic fluid.

The sonographic characteristics of placental hemorrhage change with time. Initially hemorrhage appears to be either hyperechoic or isoechoic with the placenta; after a week the appearance is hypoechoic, and by the end of the second week it is likely to be sonolucent. These factors act as confounding variables when the sensitivity of ultrasound to identify the presence or absence of placental abruption is in question.

This simple ultrasound classification differs from Fox's pathologic description of hemorrhagic sites because the echogenicity of the hemorrhage may be similar to that of the surrounding placental tissue.[8] From a pathologic perspective, blood from a site of vessel damage can:

1. Dissect under the membranes and remain concealed (preplacental or subchorionic bleed)
2. Reach the cervix and become revealed bleeding
3. Rupture the membranes and bleed into the amniotic sac
4. Dissect under the placenta and increase the size of the retroplacental clot
5. Infiltrate into the myometrium and produce a Couvelaire uterus (in severe cases).

Page and coworkers, using a constellation of maternal and fetal signs, devised a classification system based on the degree of morbidity (Table 84-1).[9] The classification, which uses four grades, continues to have practical significance.

Ultrasound visualization of a clot occurs in only about 25% of clinically suspected cases; as a result, the absence of ultrasound findings should not preclude the diagnosis.[10] The difficulty in ultrasound diagnosis is further confounded by the fact that resolving hematomas may be confused with myomas. In addition, an acute retroplacental hemorrhage is likely to be visualized as abnormally thick and heterogenous placenta. Irrespective of the ultrasound appearance or progression of the clot, the clinical, hemodynamic, and hematologic parameters are most important.

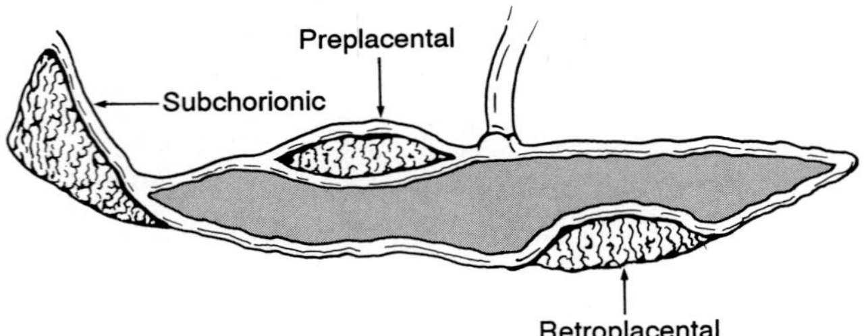

FIGURE 84–1. Sites of periplacental hemorrhage that have been described sonographically. Subchorionic hemorrhage may be remote from the placenta but is thought to arise from marginal abruptions. The term "preplacental" hemorrhage has been chosen to describe both subamniotic hematoma and massive subchorial thrombosis. Intraplacental hemorrhages (intervillous thrombi) also may be identified but are difficult to distinguish from placental lakes or other intraplacental sonolucencies.

Some investigators have suggested that when a clot is visible, its size may be clinically significant. This can be assessed by using Sauerbrei and Pham's method: the volume of the hemorrhage is estimated by multiplying the three perpendicular diameters by 0.52, using the formula for an ellipsoid.[11]

Abruptions may occur throughout gestation. Paterson demonstrated that 18% occur before 32 weeks and 42% occur after 37 weeks.[12]

CLINICAL ASSOCIATIONS

Placental abruption is associated with increasing parity, abdominal trauma, sudden decompression of polyhydramnios, and external cephalic version. The relationship with hypertension is unclear.[13]

In assessing a woman with placental abruption, the possibility of physical abuse or cocaine usage must not be overlooked. Physical abuse may present for the first time during pregnancy, and like cocaine usage it is present in all levels of society. Unless specific questions about these issues are asked, the precipitating cause of the abruption may be missed.

MANAGEMENT PRINCIPLES

The important features of the pregnancy assessment are summarized in Table 84-2.

Mild Abruption

Mild abruption may spontaneously resolve or preterm labor may begin. If the fetus is remote from term and appears healthy, the obstetrician should consider arresting labor. The use of tocolysis in this clinical situation is controversial because theoretically it may promote further bleeding; however, evidence to support this position is lacking. The link between abruption and preterm labor is thought to be due either to the presence of extravasated blood in the myometrium, which triggers uterine activity, or a fetal response to a hostile intrauterine environment.

Moderate to Severe Abruption

In moderate to severe abruption, maternal resuscitation is the priority. The degree of hypovolemia is often underestimated because of the following:

1. The hemorrhage may be concealed.
2. It may have occurred outside of the hospital.
3. An increase in maternal peripheral resistance may occur, giving rise to false reassurance regarding her blood pressure.

Moderate to severe abruption requires aggressive volume replacement. Ideally, fresh whole blood sustains intravascular volume and replaces blood products, but as this is seldom available packed cells in conjunction with fresh frozen plasma are adequate substitutes.

Clotting defects should be sought with a high index of suspicion. A prolonged bedside clotting time serves as a useful marker of the degree of placental separation and coagulopathy. A comprehensive evaluation of the patient's coagulation status in this situation demonstrates a progressive fall in platelet count and fibrinogen, with prolonged prothrombin and partial thromboplastin times. Fibrin degradation products are often increased as well.

TABLE 84–1. CLASSIFICATION OF PLACENTAL ABRUPTION ACCORDING TO MATERNAL AND FETAL SIGNS

GRADE*	CONCEALED HEMORRHAGE	UTERINE TENDERNESS	MATERNAL HYPOTENSION	COAGULOPATHY	FETAL DISTRESS
0	no	no	no	no	no
1	no	no	no	no	no
2	yes	yes	no	rare	yes
3	yes	yes	yes	often	death

* Grade 0 is a retrospective diagnosis from inspection of the placenta. Grade 1 includes "marginal sinus" separation or other limited processes of abruptio placentae. Grades 2 and 3 imply significant hemorrhage requiring immediate therapy with the possibility of maternal complications.

TABLE 84–2. IMPORTANT FEATURES OF THE PREGNANCY ASSESSMENT

FETAL	MATERNAL
• Fetal distress • Fetal demise • Gestational age/size • Size of placental abruption	• Hypovolemia • Coagulation status • Uterine activity and tone • Pain • Rh -ve status

When assessing the fetus, the obstetrician should remember that in 81% of cases the estimated fetal weight is below the mean for gestational age.[4] Signs of fetal distress, including fetal tachycardia and severe variable or late decelerations, may also be present. If fetal demise has occurred, there will be significant alterations in maternal cardiovascular and coagulation status.

Nyberg and associates showed that fetal mortality was significantly increased with retroplacental hemorrhages, particularly those larger than 60 mL.[14] When both of these factors were present, the mortality rate was 75%. Subchorionic hemorrhages in the third trimester appear to carry a much lower risk (7%) of fetal death.

Clinical management decisions in moderate to severe placental abruption must be individualized, and aggressive plans should be made for delivery if there is evidence of hemodynamic or coagulation instability. The state of the cervix is another important variable: in the presence of an otherwise healthy fetus, it may allow vaginal delivery. Caution should, however, be exercised when a prolonged interval from abruption to delivery is expected. Further placental separation and worsening of the coagulopathy may occur without warning.

The use of epidural anesthesia for pain relief is uncommon in moderate to severe abruption, as epidural hemorrhages may occur in situations in which a coagulopathy is evolving. The prudent use of intravenous narcotics is recommended for pain relief.

Rh-immune prophylaxis is recommended in Rh-negative women who do not have antibodies.

PLACENTA PREVIA

In two large series, placenta previa occurred in the third trimester in 0.4% to 0.9% of patients.[15,16] It is a much more common ultrasound diagnosis in the second trimester of pregnancy, with an incidence then of 5.3%.[17] At least 90% of these cases convert by term to a normal placental location, giving rise to the concept of placental migration.[18] Placenta previa is classified as total when it covers the cervical os centrally; partial when it eccentrically covers part of the os; and low-lying when it extends into the lower uterine segment and lies very close to the internal os (Fig. 84-2).

Multiparity, advanced maternal age, multiple pregnancy, and previous cesarean section have been noted in association with placenta previa.[19] A twofold increase in the rate of placenta previa has been seen after a previous section; the risk is greatest in the pregnancy immediately after the section.

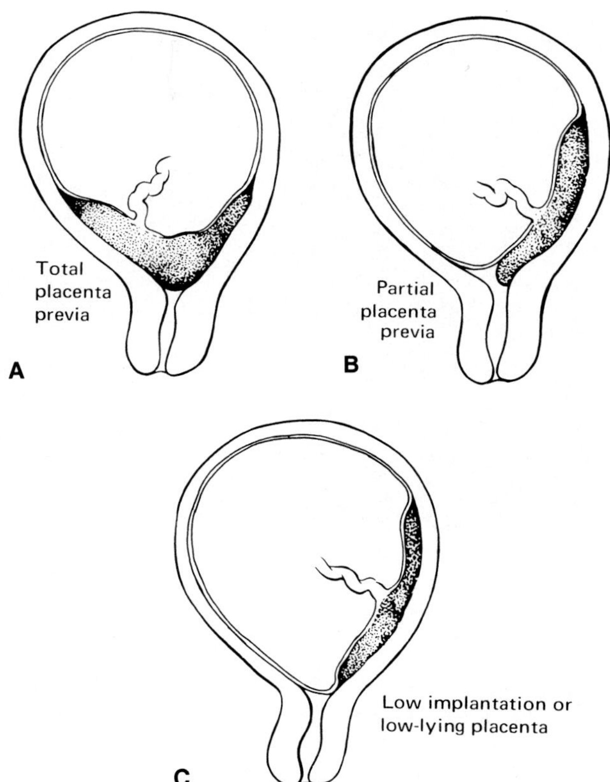

FIGURE 84–2. Classification of placental location. **(A)** Complete placenta previa. **(B)** Partial (marginal) previa. **(C)** Low-lying placenta. (From Goplerud CP. Bleeding in later pregnancy. In Danforth DN, ed. Obstetrics & gynecology. 5th ed. New York: Harper & Row, 1986, with permission.)

DIAGNOSIS

The basis for the diagnosis is the ultrasound demonstration of the placental location relative to the internal cervical os. Using transabdominal ultrasound with a full maternal urinary bladder, the accuracy of this diagnosis ranges from 93% to 97%.[20] Diagnostic errors are due to several factors. Overdistention of the urinary bladder, resulting in apposition of the anterior and posterior walls of the lower uterine segment, is common.[21] Normally the uterine wall is convex toward the bladder; this relationship is reversed when bladder overdistention occurs (Fig. 84-3). Other causes for diagnostic errors include myometrial contractions, fibroids, blood clots, late placental migration, and a posterior placental location, with the calcified fetal head obscuring the exact placental edge.[22]

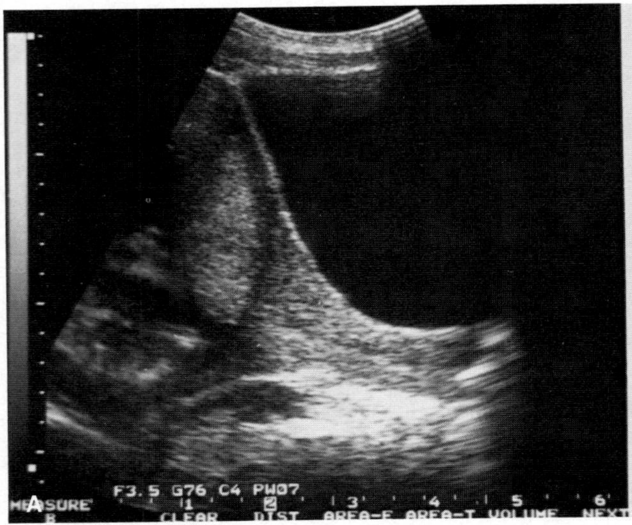

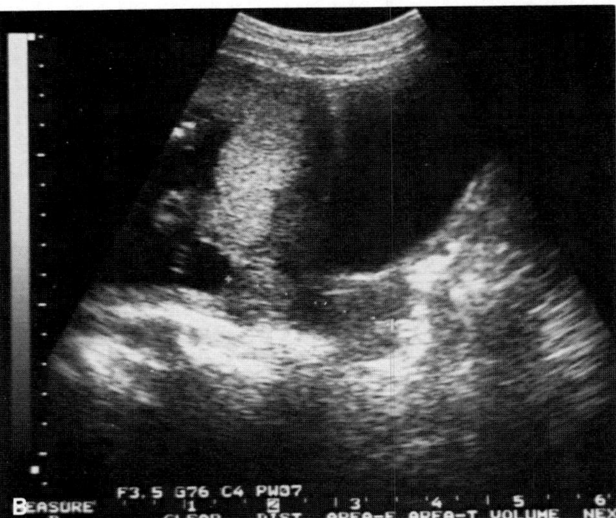

FIGURE 84–3. (**A**) An anteriorly located placenta with a full maternal urinary bladder. A false impression of placenta previa is created. (**B**) The urinary bladder in the same patient has been partially emptied. The placenta is now clear of the cervix.

Farine and colleagues have championed the use of endovaginal sonography to clarify placental location.[23] Closely approximating the probe tip to the site of interest allows the use of a higher-frequency probe, and a higher-resolution image is obtained. This imaging is done under direct sonographic demonstration of the cervix. Since the focal zone of a 5- or 6.5-mHz probe is between 3 and 12 cm or 2 and 7 cm respectively, the best picture is produced when the probe tip is about 3 cm from the cervix.

There have been few published reports of patients with confirmed placenta previa who have been scanned transvaginally, and it appears that the procedure can be conducted safely with no risk of bleeding. No bleeding occurred in a series of 35 patients examined endovaginally; 6 eventually had proven placenta previa (Table 84-3).[22] Further experience is necessary in a large group of patients with total placenta previa.

Guy and colleagues recently reported a small series of patients with placenta previa and lacunar blood flow.[24] This was defined as multiple sonolucent blood lakes that occupied almost the entire thickness of the placenta, with visible blood flowing in these spaces. This sign appeared to act as a marker for abnormally adherent placentas, large blood losses, and the need for extensive operative therapy, including hysterectomy. These observations must be confirmed by independent investigators.

Gillieson and associates demonstrated that anterior wall placentas were more likely to convert than posteriorly positioned ones.[25] The mechanism by which the placenta "migrates" from the cervix with increasing gestational age may be explained by the increased growth of the uterus relative to placental growth in later gestation.

FETAL EVALUATION

Fetal growth retardation may be associated with placenta previa and should be assessed by the usual methods.[26] Continuous wave Doppler ultrasound of the umbilical artery was used to study 100 consecutive patients with placenta previa and a similar number of matched

TABLE 84–3. COMPARISON OF THE DELIVERY DIAGNOSIS WITH TRANSVAGINAL AND TRANSABDOMINAL SONOGRAPHY

SONOGRAPHIC DIAGNOSIS	NO. OF PATIENTS	DELIVERY DIAGNOSIS
No previa by both transabdominal and transvaginal sonography	10	No previa in all patients
No previa by transvaginal and previa by transabdominal sonography	13	No previa in all patients
Previa by both transabdominal and transvaginal sonography	11	Previa in 6 patients, no previa in 5 patients
Previa by transvaginal and no previa by transabdominal sonography	1	Not delivered

controls without previa.[27] The results demonstrated that the incidence of abnormal S/D ratios was higher in patients with placenta previa; in addition, an abnormal S/D ratio was more likely to be associated with adverse perinatal outcome when compared to normal S/D ratios in patients with placenta previa. These adverse outcomes included small for gestational age, the presence of meconium, and low 5-minute Apgar scores.

MANAGEMENT

Management options in the third trimester are based on the existing clinical possibilities and fetal health. These situations may be summarized as follows:

1. The patient has never bled.
2. Heavy bleeding is occurring.
3. Bleeding has stopped in a preterm patient.
4. The fetus is 37 weeks or older.

All third-trimester patients with ultrasound confirmation of complete previa should be admitted to the hospital. For women who have never bled, it is important to note that in over 50% of patients with placenta previa, the first episode of bleeding may occur after 31 weeks.[28] Repeat ultrasound at 2- to 3-week intervals for placental localization may indicate if migration has occurred.

If heavy bleeding is occurring, emergency measures to rapidly stabilize the mother's cardiovascular system are indicated, and delivery should be performed by cesarean section.

Prophylactic Rh immunoglobulin is recommended for all women who are Rh negative without antibodies.

For women whose bleeding has stopped, Macafee's expectant approach continues to be the standard.[29] Its focus is on bed rest and avoiding preterm birth. However, despite Macafee's advocacy, preterm delivery remains a problem: 40% of women with the diagnosis of placenta previa deliver early.[30] Tocolysis may be used with care if premature labor occurs in the presence of a small amount of bleeding.

There is general agreement that there is no place for expectant management in the term patient with placenta previa. An elective cesarean section should be performed if the diagnosis is confirmed.

PLACENTA ACCRETA WITH PLACENTA PREVIA

Placenta accreta, the abnormal adherence of the placenta to the uterine wall, is due to an underdeveloped decidua basalis. The degree of myometrial invasion at histology is used to distinguish placenta accreta (which involves myometrial attachment of villi) from placenta increta (in which the villi extend into the myometrium). In placenta percreta, the entire myometrial wall is penetrated by villi.

Conditions thought to predispose women to placenta accreta include previous dilatation and curettage, uterine scarring due to cesarean section or myomectomy, and manual removal of the placenta. Of these, the most common association of placenta accreta is placenta previa in the presence of a previous cesarean section scar.[31]

Under normal prenatal conditions a thin hypoechoic zone is present between the myometrium and the placenta. This zone is on average 9.5 mm thick, and after 18 weeks gestation it should be seen in all cases throughout the entire placental implantation site.[32] When this hypoechoic zone is breached in whole or in part and is not apparent, placenta accreta, increta, or percreta may be present. The sensitivity and specificity of these observations have not yet been established.

These patients may present with abnormal bleeding in the antenatal period (commonly vaginal or intraperitoneal).[31] Intravesical bleeding has also been reported in placenta percreta.[33]

Management principles are no different from those for patients with placenta previa, except that massive blood transfusions and hysterectomy are quite common because of the profound hemorrhagic shock that may occur. Uterine inversion in the postpartum period may be the first sign of placenta accreta.

OTHER CAUSES OF THIRD-TRIMESTER BLEEDING

CIRCUMVALLATE PLACENTA

This finding occurs in 1% to 2% of pregnancies and may be associated with bleeding and placental abruption. The thickening seen at the placental edge is due to folding of the membranes in conjunction with fibrosis secondary to hemorrhage.

MARGINAL SINUS BLEEDING

Bleeding in this situation occurs at the placental margin, and some clinicians contend that this is a form of placental abruption. The clinical presentation is that of profuse vaginal bleeding that stops as suddenly as it starts. The diagnosis, like that of circumvallate placenta, can be made only after delivery of the placenta. The hallmark is the presence of an adherent clot at the placental edge.

VASA PREVIA

Bleeding from vasa previa is a fetal obstetric emergency. It is primarily associated with velamentous insertion of the umbilical cord or vessels to a succenturiate lobe of the placenta. The hemorrhage in this situation is relatively small by adult standards and usually occurs after spontaneous rupture of the fetal membranes. The sudden fetal heart-rate changes that occur with this fetal hemorrhage must raise a high index of suspicion. There is not always time to confirm the presence of fetal red cells by the Apt test, as prompt delivery is the only management option available.

TRAUMA

Direct trauma to the pregnant uterus may occur due to accidents (eg, motor vehicle or fall) and physical abuse. The maternal and fetal consequences of a fall are generally not as profound as those associated with motor vehicle accidents. Motor vehicle accidents may cause steering wheel trauma, a seat belt injury to the uterus, a sudden deceleration injury to the fetus and placenta, or hemorrhagic shock of the mother (with its consequences to the fetus).

Quite commonly massive placental bleeding is concealed, and even though the clear priority is the assessment and maintenance of maternal health, the fetus and the integrity of the uteroplacental environment should not be ignored. At a minimum, fetal evaluation should include the assessment of fetal–maternal bleeding by the Kleihauer-Betke test and external fetal heart-rate monitoring for several hours. Detailed ultrasound evaluation of the fetus and placenta should occur after maternal resuscitation and stabilization.

Physical abuse occurs in about 8% of pregnant women.[34] This abuse is usually directed to the abdomen, breasts, and genitals. The literature indicates that 25% to 63% of battered women report battering during pregnancy; in some cases, the first episode of abuse occurred during pregnancy. Data are now being accumulated on bleeding and perinatal outcome due to family violence, and only anecdotal reports are currently available.

CERVICAL AND VAGINAL LESIONS

The contribution of lesions in the genital tract to third-trimester bleeding is uncertain. Roberts suggested that 9% of all cases of antepartum hemorrhage may be due to lower genital tract causes.[35] This collective clinical category includes minor unrecognized cases of all types and may have a weak association with premature contractions.

It is important to exclude local lesions (eg, polyps, erosions); this is done by direct visualization of the cervix and genital tract by speculum examination. An expectant management approach is recommended, with monitoring of fetal well-being. Intervention is appropriate if fetal health deteriorates or a reduction in growth is demonstrated.

CONCLUSION

Bleeding in the third trimester, however slight, requires prompt attention and complete evaluation. It is unwise to attempt pelvic examination in a location that is not equipped to manage profuse bleeding. Life-threatening conditions do exist, and professionals who care for pregnant women must be aware of the causes and outcome of such bleeding and must have a clear management plan for this problem when it arises.

REFERENCES

1. Paintin DB. The epidemiology of antepartum hemorrhage: a study of all births in a community. J Obstet Gynaecol Br Common 1962;69;614.
2. Roberts G. Unclassified antepartum hemorrhage: incidence and perinatal mortality in a community. J Obstet Gynaecol Br Common 1970;77:492.
3. Watson R. Antepartum hemorrhage of uncertain origin. Br J Clin Practice 1982;36:222.
4. Hibbard BM, Jeffcoate TNA. Abruptio placentae. Obstet Gynecol 1960;27:155.
5. Green-Thompson RW. Antepartum hemorrhage. Clin Obstet Gynecol 1982;9:479.
6. Knab DR. Abruptio placenta: an assessment of the time and method of delivery. Obstet Gynecol 1978;52:625.
7. Nyberg D, Cyr D, Mack LA, et al. Sonographic spectrum of placental abruption. AJR 1987;148:161.
8. Fox H. Pathology of the placenta. Philadelphia: WB Saunders, 1978:107.
9. Page EW, King EB, Merrill JA. Abruptio placenta: dangers of delay in delivery. Obstet Gynecol 1954;3:385.
10. Sholl JS. Abruptio placentae: clinical management in nonacute cases. Am J Obstet Gynecol 1987;156:40.
11. Sauerbrei EE, Pham DH. Placental abruption and subchorionic hemorrhage in the first half of pregnancy: ultrasound appearance and clinical outcome. Radiology 1986;160:109.
12. Paterson M. The aetiology and outcome of abruptio placentae. Acta Obstet Gynecol Scand 1979;58:31.
13. Naeye RL, Harknes WL, Utts J. Abruptio placentae and perinatal death: a prospective study. Am J Obstet Gynecol 1977;128:701.
14. Nyberg DA, Mack LA, Benedetti TJ, Cyr DR, Shuman WP. Placental abruption and placental hemorrhage: correlation of sonographic findings with fetal outcome. Radiology 1987;164:357.
15. Comeau J, Shaw L, Marcell C, et al. Early placenta previa and delivery outcome. Obstet Gynecol 1983;61:577.
16. Hill DJ, Berscher N. Placenta previa without antepartum hemorrhage. Aust N Z J Obstet Gynecol 1980;20:21.
17. Rizos N, Doran TA, Miskin M, Benzie RJ, Ford JA. Natural history of placenta previa ascertained by diagnostic ultrasound. Am J Obstet Gynecol 1979;133:287.
18. King DL. Placental migration demonstrated by ultrasonography. Radiology 1973;109:167.
19. Singh PM, Rodrigues C, Gupta A. Placenta previa and previous caesarean section. Acta Obstet Gynecol Scand 1981;60:367.
20. Boivie J, Rochester D, Cadkin A, et al. Accuracy of placental localization by ultrasound. Radiology 1978;128:177.
21. Townsend RR, Laing FD, Nyberg DA, et al. Technical factors responsible for "placental migration": a sonographic assessment. Radiology 1986;160:105.
22. Farine D, Fox HE, Jakobson S, Timor-Tritsch IE. Vaginal ultrasound for diagnosis of placenta previa. Am J Obstet Gynecol 1988;159:566.
23. Farine D, Fox HE, Timor-Tritsch I. Vaginal ultrasound for ruling out placenta previa: case report. Br J Obstet Gynaecol 1989;96:117.
24. Guy GP, Peisner DB, Timor-Tritsch IE. Ultrasonographic evalua-

tion of uteroplacental blood flow patterns of abnormally located and adherent placentas. Am J Obstet Gynecol 1990;163:723.

25. Gillieson MS, Winer-Mar HT, Muram D. Low-lying placenta. Radiology 1982;144:577.
26. Varma TR. Fetal growth and placental function in patients with placenta previa. J Obstet Gynaecol Br Common 1973;80:311.
27. Brar HS, Platt LD, DeVore GR, Horenstein J. Fetal umbilical velocimetry for the surveillance of pregnancies complicated by placenta previa. J Reprod Med 1988;33:741.
28. Gabert H. Placenta previa and fetal growth. Obstet Gynecol 1971;38:403.
29. Macafee CHG. Placenta previa: a study of 174 cases. J Obstet Gynaecol Br Common 1945;52:313.
30. Brenner WE, Edelman D, Hendricks CH. Characteristics of patients with placenta previa and results of expectant management. Am J Obstet Gynecol 1978;132:180.
31. de Mendonca LK. Sonographic diagnosis of placenta accreta. J Ultrasound Med 1988;7:211.
32. Callen P, Filly R. The placental/subplacental complex: a specific indication of placental position on ultrasound. J Clin Ultrasound 1980;8:21.
33. Cox S, Carpenter RJ, Cotton D. Placenta percreta: ultrasound diagnosis and conservative surgical management. Obstet Gynecol 1988;71:454.
34. Helton AS, McFarlane J, Anderson ET. Battered and pregnant: a prevalence study. Am J Public Health 1987;77:1337.
35. Roberts G. Unclassified antepartum hemorrhage: incidence and perinatal mortality in a community. J Obstet Gynaecol Br Common 1970;77:492.

85

CHAPTER

NORMAL AND ABNORMAL LABOR

Wayne R. Cohen

Our current understanding of human parturition derives primarily from developments in the clinical and basic sciences during the past 50 years. Because uterine contractions are obviously pivotal in the process of parturition, a primary focus of investigation has been to unravel the complexities of the physiology of myometrial contractility. To this end, we now have a good understanding of the ultrastructure of uterine smooth muscle and of the biochemical intricacies that govern the contractile mechanism.[1] Concomitant with these developments was important work in experimental animals and humans designed to objectify means for characterizing uterine activity.[2,3] Despite the impressive accumulation of knowledge in these areas over the past several decades, the key linking these physiologic and biochemical observations with clinical events during labor remains elusive. Consequently, our management of labor and birth and our approach to the diagnosis of dysfunctional labor depend primarily on observations from clinical research.

A systematic approach to recording and interpreting observations about labor was spawned by the work of Calkins in the United States[4,5] and others in Europe beginning in the late 1920s.[6] These kinds of observations, coupled with the precise and relevant anatomical descriptions of the pelvis by Caldwell and Moloy,[7] constituted the primary basis for labor assessment until the late 1950s.

At that time the work of Emanuel Friedman appeared, which described an accurate and objective method of evaluating labor progress in a clinical setting.[8,9] His introduction of the graphic analysis of labor was revolutionary in that for the first time it elevated the management of labor from a somewhat arbitrary exercise to one in which considerable scientific objectivity could be applied to complement clinical art.

The approach described by Friedman has been modified somewhat and adapted for use in specific circumstances.[10–12] However, the basic notion of evaluating labor progress by determining the relationships among cervical dilatation, descent of the fetus, and elapsed hours in labor has been verified to be a clinical tool of manifest importance. The graphic analysis of labor should form the basis for clinical decision making about dysfunctional labor by all obstetric attendants, but it must be used in conjunction with other kinds of obstetric data. Thus, information about pelvic architecture; uterine contractility; fetal axis, position, and attitude; and state of fetal oxygenation is required to make the most appropriate judgments.

Much information is available about the total duration of labor. For example, Nesheim recently showed that the median duration of labor in nulliparas was 8.2 hours and in multiparas was 5.3 hours.[13] These kinds of data are of interest but are not particularly useful to the clinician who must decide whether an individual patient's labor is normal, even though it may be longer than the median. More complex information, obtainable from graphic displays of progress, is necessary.

Parity has a major effect on the duration and pattern of labor. In general, the labors of multiparas are shorter than those of nulliparas, with shorter latent phase and more rapid rates of dilatation and descent in the active phase and second stage.[14] Multiparous women who have had all previous babies by cesarean section should be judged by nulliparous criteria during labor; if they have had at least one vaginal birth they should be considered multiparas.[15] Labor patterns of multiparas constitute a single population; therefore, criteria for all multiparas are the same, irrespective of how many babies they have had.[13,14]

To a large extent, obstetric decision making with regard to labor aberrations is a process of estimating the probability of a safe vaginal delivery. All the clinical information that is used in reaching decisions about obstetric interventions (especially use of oxytocin, conduction anesthesia, cesarean section, and instrumental delivery) should be viewed with this perspective. In fact, a multiplicity of factors most often must be taken into consideration before decisions are made.

NORMAL CERVICAL DILATATION

The relationship between cervical dilatation and time during labor is described by a sigmoid-shaped curve (Fig. 85-1).[8,9,14] Dilatation is traditionally divided into a *latent phase* and an *active phase*. The latent phase extends from the onset of labor until the upward inflection in the curve and is associated with small (or sometimes no) incremental change in dilatation. Enhancement of the rate of dilatation begins at the onset of the active phase, during which most of the cervical dilatation occurs. A gradual increase in dilatation (the acceleration phase) initiates in the active phase and leads, usually in about 1 hour, to a period of much more rapid and linear dilatation, the phase of maximum slope. During the terminal portion of the active phase dilatation appears to slow. This is more apparent than real, as the cervix is probably continuing to open at a constant rate toward the end of dilatation; but because descent of the head has begun by this time the radial diameter of the cervix measured clinically does not account for the entire extent of cervical change. Because descent is now occurring, the cervix must retract around the head to achieve complete dilatation. Thus, some of the ongoing separation that continues to develop between the lateral borders of the cervix occurs in a cephalolateral direction and cannot be readily appreciated by the examining fingers.

By convention, full cervical dilatation is considered to be 10 cm. This is a clinically useful approximation, but since the cervix does not generally dilate more than the largest diameter of the object passing through it, full dilatation for most term babies is really somewhat less than 10 cm, and for exceptionally large babies it may be more. This issue is of particular importance when interpreting the labor curves of very premature fetuses, in whom the biparietal diameter may be considerably less than 10 cm and the curve of dilatation may be necessarily foreshortened.

LATENT PHASE

From a teleologic standpoint, the latent phase may be considered to constitute a time of preparation of the cervix for the more rapid dilatation that will occur subsequently.[16] Clinically, a number of physical changes in the cervix can be appreciated. These constitute what has been referred to as "ripening" of the cervix and may in some patients (particularly nulliparas) occur largely or completely prior to the onset of labor. The duration of the latent phase is inversely proportional to the degree of prelabor cervical maturation. Palpable softening, effacement, and anterior rotation of the cervix in the pelvic axis often occur during the latent phase and are prerequisites for entering active-phase dilatation.

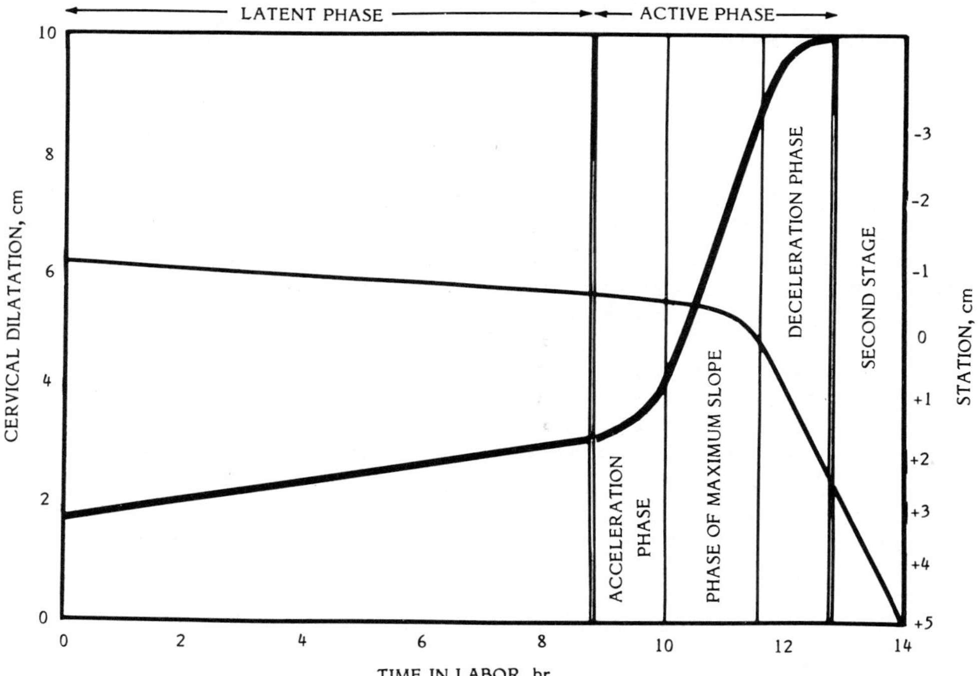

FIGURE 85–1. Composite of normal cervical dilatation and fetal descent curves showing their interrelations and components. (From Cohen WR, Friedman EA, eds. Management of labor. Aspen Publishers, 1983.)

The biochemical and biophysical basis for these clinical changes in the cervix and lower uterine segment is incompletely understood. It is likely that prostaglandins play an important role by altering cervical connective tissue ground substance and stimulating collagen degradation to produce softening.[17] These biochemical developments result in the increase in compliance that characterizes cervical maturation. Endogenous prostaglandins have been employed for their presumed effect as pharmacologic cervical ripening agents prior to the induction of labor.[18]

Precise measurement of the duration of the latent phase requires knowledge of the onset of labor. Obviously, this cannot always be determined with certainty. Generally, the time at which the patient states labor began should be accepted. If she is uncertain, the time at which she began to perceive regular uterine contractions is reasonable to use as an approximation.

The cervix may dilate slowly (maximally 0.5 cm/h) during the latent phase, or not at all. The shift to active phase most often occurs by about 5 cm of cervical dilatation.[19,20] However, it can be misleading to rely on the absolute degree of dilatation to identify this transition. For example, conversion from latent to active phase may be at 3 cm of dilatation, especially in patients who began labor with the cervix closed. Transition to active phase may not occur until 6 to 7 cm in women who began labor with the cervix 4 to 5 cm dilated, particularly among multiparas.

The latent phase indeed tends to be shorter in multiparas than in nulliparas, a consequence, at least in part, of the fact that multiparas tend to begin labor with more cervical dilatation than do nulliparas.[14,19] For the same reason, the latent phase is often short in multiple gestations, in hydramnios, or after removal of a cervical cerclage.

ACTIVE PHASE

Except for the usually brief acceleration and deceleration portions of the active phase, cervical dilatation is linear, and much more rapid than that in the latent phase. Clinical labor assessment takes advantage of this fact by measuring the speed at which the cervix dilates during the active phase to determine normality. When two observations of cervical dilatation have been made during this period of linear change in the active phase (the *phase of maximum slope*), the slope of the dilatation line can be calculated. Once established, this rate tends to be constant for each individual (ie, if the labor is normal, dilatation will continue at the same rate until the deceleration phase is reached). Abnormalities of active phase are defined by deviations from this projected rate of dilatation.

If square-ruled graph paper is used, observation and calculation of slopes are relatively simple.[8] For those who prefer not to perform their own arithmetic, several paradigms have been devised to use the graphic system without the need for any mathematical calculations.[11,12,21]

Full cervical dilatation is diagnosed when the cervix has retracted to the widest portion of the presenting part. Usually the cervix retracts symmetrically, but sometimes a portion of it lingers, particularly anteriorly in the presence of deflexed attitudes of the head. Full dilatation should not be diagnosed until the entire cervix has retracted spontaneously beyond the widest diameter of the leading part of the fetus.

As indicated previously, during the phase of maximum slope of dilatation, descent of the fetus normally begins and tends to accelerate during the terminal portion of dilatation as the widely dilated cervix retracts around the presenting part.

NORMAL FETAL DESCENT

As the cervix dilates in the late active phase, the resistance to fetal descent decreases, and the force of uterine contractions, coupled after complete dilatation with active bearing-down efforts on the part of the mother, begins the expulsion of the fetus from the uterus and birth canal. By the time complete cervical dilatation has been reached, descent has usually become linear and during the second stage normally proceeds in this manner until the presenting part encounters the pelvic floor. As in the active phase of dilatation, the efficiency and normality of the descent mechanism can be judged from the rate of descent. When one plots graphically the relationship between fetal descent and elapsed time in labor, it is apparent that descent also has a latent phase, during which little in the way of descent occurs under most circumstances (see Fig. 85-1). The degree of descent that has occurred before the onset of labor influences the length of the latent phase and has prognostic importance for the probability of vaginal delivery. In fact, the higher in the pelvis one finds the fetal head at the onset of labor, the greater is the likelihood of the need for cesarean delivery. The overall risk of cesarean section for presumed cephalopelvic disproportion when the fetal presenting part is unengaged in nulliparas at the onset of labor may be as high as 30%.[22]

There are circumstances in which considerable descent may occur during the latent phase. In particular, many multiparas, and breech presentations in women of any parity, often commence labor with the presenting part at relatively high stations, and appreciable descent is encountered during the latent phase. Of utmost importance in regard to these issues is that lack of fetal descent prior to active-phase labor is not prima facie evidence of a labor aberration or fetopelvic disproportion.

UTERINE ACTIVITY IN LABOR

Uterine activity in the latent phase is quite variable. In many women contractions begin as mild and somewhat irregular and become progressively more intense, frequent, and regular as the latent phase progresses. However, this is not always so, and a broad range of contraction patterns may be observed in the normal latent phase, including very intense and frequent contractions throughout, which are more generally thought to be characteristic of the active phase. In fact, it is usually impossible to identify the transition from latent to active-phase labor solely on the basis of uterine activity.

During the active phase of labor, contractions are generally more frequent and of greater amplitude and duration than in the latent phase, although this is not necessarily so. Actually, a large spectrum of contractile patterns exists during normal labor,[23] and attempts to classify labor dysfunctions by analysis of information about uterine activity have serious shortcomings. There is no reliable or predictive means by which to identify dysfunctional cervical dilatation or fetal descent by observing uterine activity. Consequently, the clinical identification of dysfunctional labor should be based primarily on aberrations in the graphic patterns of labor. This approach allows continuous online assessment of labor progress and provides an unequivocal language for communication about dysfunctional labor.[24]

Although uterine contractility may not necessarily change during the latter portions of the active phase, the patient's perception of pain is often intensified. This process of "transition," which encompasses the terminal portion of cervical dilatation, reflects the increased discomfort that the patient usually feels as a consequence of maximal distention of the cervix and of other soft parts of the birth canal as descent begins.

TABLE 85–1. PATTERNS OF ABNORMAL LABOR

PATTERN	DIAGNOSTIC CRITERION
Disorders of dilatation	
Prolonged latent phase	
Nulliparas	Latent phase duration 20 h or more
Multiparas	Latent phase duration 14 h or more
Protracted active phase	
Nulliparas	Maximum slope of dilatation of 1.2 cm/h or less
Multiparas	Maximum slope of dilatation of 1.5 cm/h or less
Arrest of dilatation	Cessation of active phase progress for 2 h or more
Disorders of descent	
Failure of descent	Lack of expected descent beginning near full dilatation
Protracted descent	
Nulliparas	Maximum slope of descent of 1.0 cm/h or less
Multiparas	Maximum slope of descent of 2.0 cm/h or less
Arrest of descent	Cessation of descent progression for 1 h or more

Modified from Friedman EA. Labor: clinical evaluation and management. 2nd ed. New York: Appleton-Century-Crofts, 1978.

ABNORMAL LABOR

LATENT PHASE DYSFUNCTION

One abnormality of the latent phase is identifiable, *prolonged latent phase* (Fig. 85-2, Table 85-1). This disorder is diagnosed when the latent phase exceeds 20 hours in nulliparas and 14 hours in multiparas.[14] It is particularly likely to occur when labor begins with the cervix minimally effaced and dilated.[14] The latent phase appears particularly susceptible to the inhibitory qualities of narcotics and anesthetics, and under certain circumstances these agents may predispose to prolongation of this portion of labor.

The diagnosis of prolonged latent phase sometimes lacks precision because of difficulty in ascertaining the exact time of onset of labor. This shortcoming notwithstanding, the simple recognition of the fact that the latent phase may normally be quite long is of special significance in the management of labor. Prolonged latent phase does not appear in and of itself to be associated with an increased need for operative delivery and is not a predictor of more serious labor disorders that have a strong association with cephalopelvic disproportion.[25]

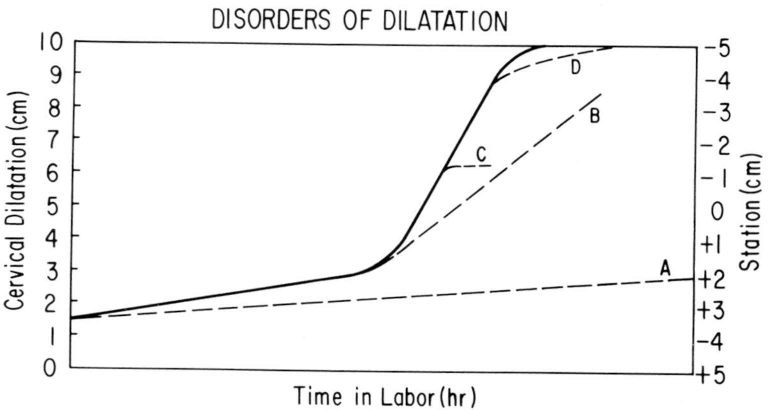

FIGURE 85–2. Schematic showing various disorders of dilatation. [A-prolonged latent phase; B-protracted active phase dilatation; C-arrest of dilatation; D-prolonged deceleration phase (a form of arrest disorder).]

Regrettably, ignorance about the normal course of the latent phase sometimes leads to unnecessary cesarean section under the erroneous assumption that continuous progress should be expected in all phases of labor or that very long labors are always abnormal.

Treatment of a prolonged latent phase may consist of active efforts to stimulate uterine contractility, or heavy maternal sedation. Oxytocin stimulation is effective in 85% of cases in converting latent to active phase. This response generally occurs in less than 3 hours. A similar proportion of patients responds favorably to narcotic sedation ("therapeutic rest"). After a dose of morphine sulfate, the patient often sleeps for several hours and awakens in active-phase labor. Having had a respite from many hours of painful contractions, she may be more eager and better prepared to cope with the rigors of active-phase labor. Another advantage of therapeutic rest is that it permits identification of the approximately 5% of women diagnosed with prolonged latent phase who in fact are in false labor.[14,25] Their contractions abate completely after the narcotic treatment. Oxytocin stimulation is still necessary for the approximately 10% of women who persist in a desultory latent phase after the effects of the narcotic have abated.

The choice between uterine stimulation and therapeutic rest for treatment of prolonged latent phase depends on the clinical situation. Concerns exist about transient fetal deoxygenation occurring with some narcotic drugs,[26] but no adverse outcomes after this kind of treatment for prolonged latent phase have been recognized.[25] The approach does not seem to be associated with an increased rate of neonatal depression, although if the mother delivers unexpectedly early, a narcotic antagonist should be available for administration to the newborn. Whenever a fetal or maternal condition exists that could be jeopardized by prolonging the labor, active intervention should be used, unless there is a clear contraindication to the administration of oxytocin. Similarly, when there is a reason to minimize the duration of labor, it is reasonable to intervene in the latent phase even before it reaches the limit of normal. The presence of prolonged rupture of membranes, preeclampsia, early intrauterine infection, or certain acute maternal illnesses would thus favor an approach of active stimulation of labor. Finally, the mother's wishes should be taken into consideration. Some women prefer oxytocin stimulation; others desire the interposition of some rest into an arduous and stressful experience.

ACTIVE-PHASE DYSFUNCTION

Two abnormalities of active-phase dilatation can be identified (see Fig. 85-2 and Table 85-1). A *protracted active phase* is diagnosed when cervical dilatation progresses linearly after commencement of active phase, but at a rate below the established limits of normal. *Arrest of dilatation* occurs when cervical dilatation ceases for 2 hours during the active phase. Although this is the standard definition, there is evidence that even 1 hour of documented arrest may be of clinical importance and should prompt evaluation.[27,28] Some authorities use the designation of prolonged deceleration phase to describe protracted or arrested labor during the terminal portions of cervical dilatation.[14] The limits for the duration of the deceleration phase are 3 hours in nulliparas and 1 hour in multiparas.

The obstetric conditions associated with protraction and arrest disorders are similar, but the therapeutic approaches to the abnormalities differ.[14,28,29] Both dysfunctions occur commonly in association with cephalopelvic disproportion, minor malpositions (especially persistent occiput posterior or transverse), excessive sedation or anesthesia, and chorioamnionitis. Myometrial dysfunction, which may be primary or a consequence of the preceding factors, also contributes to active-phase dysfunction.

In the evaluation of protracted active phase or arrest of dilatation, thorough examination of the patient to identify any associated or predisposing conditions is necessary. Careful cephalopelvimetry is useful to ascertain the likelihood of disproportion. In addition to determining the architectural characteristics of the pelvis, this examination should confirm fetal position and attitude, the degree of molding of the cranial bones, and caput succedaneum formation. Adequate determination of cephalopelvic relationships is generally ascertainable by proper physical examination by an experienced clinician. This allows evaluation of the dynamic as well as the static aspects of fetopelvic fit. For example, use of the Muller-Hillis maneuver (vaginal examination during the peak of a contraction with gentle fundal pressure applied) provides useful assessment of the degree of descent, rotational tendencies, and attitudinal changes likely to occur with subsequent contractions.[30] If cephalopelvic disproportion seems unlikely and position of the fetal head is normal, then assessment of uterine contractility, a search for chorioamnionitis, and evaluation of the possibility of pharmacologic inhibition of labor are necessary. The risk of dysfunctional active-phase labor may be increased in older mothers,[31] but diagnosis and therapy should not be influenced by maternal age.

The appropriateness of oxytocin use in the presence of protraction abnormalities is controversial. The best available evidence suggests that when these disorders arise de novo, they are not amenable to correction by stimulating uterine contractions.[14,32] Enhancing uterine contractile force in such circumstances probably does not alter the rate of dilatation or descent appreciably. If, however, the protraction disorder appears to have resulted from some inhibitory influence, oxytocin may prove beneficial in overcoming it. For example, if the protraction dysfunction was provoked by conduction anesthesia or by other drugs that have the potential to inhibit contractility, oxytocin infusion may override these inhibitory influences and restore normal dilatation. By contrast, a protraction disorder that has arisen in the absence of these inhibitory factors probably would not be benefited by uterine stimulation, irrespective of the degree of contractility present. A recent randomized trial suggested that oxytocin stimulation can increase the rate of dilatation in what was called "primary dysfunctional labor," a diagnosis that probably includes protraction disorders, but the degree of enhancement was not documented, and many patients responded to placebo infusion.[33] This issue requires further investigation, but current knowledge suggests that the benefits of oxytocin use in protraction abnormalities have not been demonstrated conclusively to exceed the potential risks.

Protraction disorders appear to be sensitive to many inhibitory factors and may be exacerbated or even converted to arrest disorders under some circumstances. An excessively large dose of analgesia or conduction anesthesia may do this. Rupture of the fetal membranes as a treatment for protraction disorders has not proved to be of benefit and may sometimes worsen the situation by precipitating the development of an arrest of dilatation.[14,34]

Arrest of dilatation may evolve during a protracted active phase or during an active phase that had been progressing normally. These dysfunctions require the same kind of evaluation as do protraction abnormalities; but the obstetric attendant must view arrests of labor from the perspective of their more common association with cephalopelvic disproportion. Also, therapeutic considerations differ because arrest disorders have the potential to respond to augmentation of uterine activity by oxytocin. In the presence of an arrest of dilatation, the cephalopelvic relationships must be evaluated carefully and a judgment made about the probability of disproportion. Major degrees of bony disproportion have been reported in at least 40% of women with arrest disorders.[14,34] If the evidence for fetopelvic disproportion is considerable, especially if uterine activity appears normal, it may be appropriate to move directly to cesarean section. If the pelvis is adequate or seems probably adequate, stimulation of uterine activity with close maternal and fetal surveillance is reasonable.

In some women, arrest disorders resolve without the need for oxytocin or for operative intervention. This may result from the abatement of inhibitory factors or may occur spontaneously. The use of maternal ambulation or warm baths has advocates, but the efficacy of these techniques has not been proved. Some obstetric attendants feel that reduction of the patient's anxiety by drugs or psychoprophylactic techniques may help cure these kinds of labor dysfunctions. Proof of the efficacy of this approach is also still lacking, but the techniques bear further evaluation.

Once oxytocin infusion is initiated in the presence of an arrest disorder, three outcomes are possible: absence of further change in dilatation or descent, progress that is as good as or better than that prior to the arrest, or progress at a rate lower than the prearrest rate. Of those patients who respond to the uterotonic infusion, about 85% will have done so by the end of 3 hours, although it may take as long as 7 hours to identify all the responders.[14] Such prolonged administration is appropriate only when extant circumstances speak overwhelmingly for an ultimate safe vaginal delivery. Under most circumstances, if there has been no response to oxytocin stimulation after about 3 hours, cesarean section is necessary.

If oxytocin stimulation of uterine contractions results in cervical dilatation that is at least as rapid as that prior to the arrest, the likelihood of eventual vaginal delivery is high. If dilatation resumes, but at a rate slower than existed prior to the arrest, disproportion or an insurmountable problem with uterine contractility is likely present. A thorough clinical assessment of each individual situation is necessary to determine the most appropriate course of action. The use of an intrauterine pressure catheter is often desirable to document the change in uterine activity in response to oxytocin, and particularly to warn when excessive stimulation is occurring. The goal of treatment must be individualized, but in general firm contractions (about 50 mm Hg in peak intensity) that occur every 2 to 3 minutes indicate sufficient contractility. The use of quantitative measures of contractility, such as Montevideo units, is sometimes helpful, but the relation between these assessments of contractility and the likelihood of change in cervical dilatation or fetal descent is not reliably predictable. Whatever approach to the assessment of contractility is used, it is important to remember that the use of oxytocin may increase the likelihood of fetal hypoxemia. Therefore, continuous fetal heart rate monitoring and close observation of uterine contractility are required when uterotonic drugs are used.

The potential benefit of artificial rupture of membranes in the management of labor is controversial. Although there is no doubt that rupture of the membranes can induce labor in many individuals, its influence on labor already established is less certain. Some studies have shown a modest shortening of active-phase labor in response to rupture of membranes,[35,36] and one randomized trial in a very small sample of mixed parity demonstrated a shortening of the first stage by about 2 hours.[37] Although amniotomy may increase uterine work,[38] its salutary effect on dysfunctional labor has not been proved. Many clinicians feel that rupture of the membranes is effective in terminating arrest disorders, but objective data have failed to verify this.[39] It is nevertheless reasonable to rupture membranes when an arrest disorder has been identified. Those few patients who do respond will do so promptly. It is generally inappropriate, therefore, to wait longer than about 30 minutes to determine whether rupture of membranes has been successful in altering the pattern of labor progress.

When conduction anesthesia is employed, it should generally be initiated during the active phase of dilatation. To have minimal effect on labor progress and provide pain relief when most required, an epidural anesthetic should begin in the acceleration phase of labor. Properly administered, it will have little or no inhibitory effect on the progress of normal cervical dilatation or fetal descent. However, anesthesia is more likely to slow labor progress if administered during the latent phase or in the presence of a protraction or arrest disorder. That is not to imply that conduction anesthesia is contraindicated in such circumstances. To the contrary, it may be beneficial to the parturient who requires pain relief, but it should be employed with full cognizance that it might prolong the latent phase or create an active-phase abnormality, thus requiring concomitant administration of oxytocin.

An alternative approach to some of the management principles outlined earlier has been promulgated at The National Maternity Hospital in Dublin.[40] Termed *active management of labor,* it is designed to minimize the time during which a woman is hospitalized during labor and to ensure that she is not left alone during that interval. This system is unique in several ways. It defines the onset of labor as the time of admission to the hospital, denies the existence (or at least the diagnostic significance) of the latent phase, and works on the principle that true cephalopelvic disproportion does not exist in multiparas. It uses oxytocin and early amniotomy liberally to enhance contractility, with the goal of increasing the likelihood of spontaneous birth, minimizing the need for operative vaginal delivery and cesarean section, and making the whole maternal experience of labor as emotionally satisfying as possible. Although the latter goal is difficult to objectify, this approach has been successful in maintaining very low rates of operative obstetric intervention, and as there is no clear evidence of excess associated risk, it should be considered a reasonable alternative in the conduct of labor.

Whether active management of labor is equally efficacious when applied to other populations than that in which it was developed is a matter of considerable debate. One trial of this approach in North America reported a salutary effect on cesarean and forceps delivery rates.[41] Another, in which patients were randomized, was associated with no changes in the mode of delivery, duration of labor, or perinatal outcome.[42] Comparisons of cesarean section and perinatal mortality rates between North America and Ireland have generated some thought-provoking polemics.[43–45] The most recent analysis does not support the notion that active management per se can safely reduce cesarean section rates.[46]

Many features of a patient population dictate the need for operative delivery and influence the risk of perinatal morbidity. It is difficult, therefore, to know what one's ideal cesarean delivery rate ought to be. This notwithstanding, the cesarean rate of about 25% now extant in the United States is generally agreed to be too high. The disciplined approach to the diagnosis and management of labor disorders presented in this chapter, rigorously applied, will help preclude unnecessary interventions and contribute to minimizing perinatal injury. Primary cesarean rates of 10% or less even in very-high-risk populations can be realized with this approach.[15]

THE SECOND STAGE OF LABOR

The first stage of labor, which extends from the onset of labor to complete cervical dilatation, serves to ready the parturient for expulsion of the fetus from the uterus. Having been prepared by the physical and biochemical changes that result in cervical ripening, uterine contractions produce rapid cervical dilatation. As the cervix retracts around the biparietal diameter to dilate maximally, descent begins. Thus, during the second stage of labor (from complete dilatation to delivery) the focus of interest changes from that of cervical dilatation to descent of the fetus. From the perspective of graphic analysis of labor, the process of fetal expulsion is evaluated from the characteristics of the descent curve. The rate at which active descent occurs is influenced by several factors, including uterine contractile force; voluntary maternal expulsive efforts; fetal size, position, and attitude; the deformability of the fetal head; pelvic architecture; and the characteristics of the pelvic floor.

Three kinds of descent disorders can be identified, namely, *protracted descent, arrest of descent,* and *failure of descent*[14,47,48] (Fig. 85-3; see Table 85-1). All three labor dysfunctions are similar in terms of their associated obstetric conditions, and in many respects they are anal-

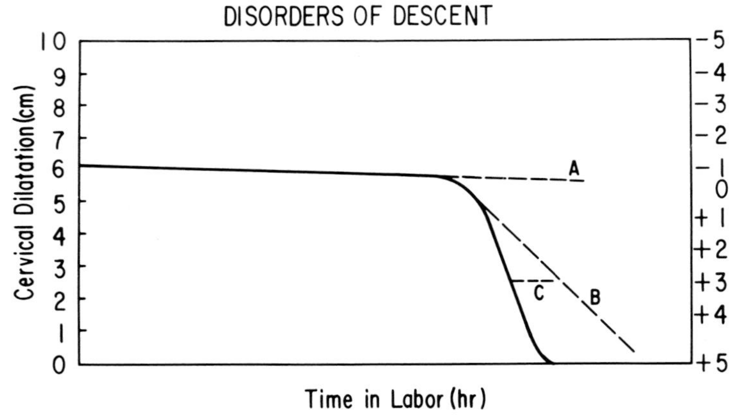

FIGURE 85–3. Schematic showing possible disorders of descent. (A-failure of descent; B-protracted descent; C-arrest of descent.)

ogous to the protraction and arrest disorders of dilatation. Diagnosis of abnormalities in descent requires considerable clinical insight and experience, because assessment must include diagnosis of fetal position and attitude, molding, and determination of the mechanism of labor in relation to the patient's pelvic form. Even identification of the station of the presenting part may be difficult if considerable scalp edema or molding of the head is present. Often suprapubic palpation of the head, as well as vaginal examination, is necessary to determine whether true descent of the head has occurred (as opposed to molding with advancement of the leading edge but no descent of the biparietal diameter).[49]

Careful cephalopelvimetry as well as evaluation for other associated obstetric problems is necessary when descent disorders are diagnosed. Analogous to disorders of active-phase dilatation, the best evidence suggests that oxytocin stimulation of uterine activity is generally not beneficial in the presence of protracted descent, but an arrest or failure of descent will often respond.

CEPHALOPELVIMETRY

To a large degree, emphasis on technological aspects of obstetric diagnosis and treatment has obscured the importance of understanding cephalopelvic relationships. This inattention to a basic clinical skill has been reinforced by reasonable concerns about the safety and efficacy of radiographic pelvimetry. Clinically astute obstetricians and midwives nevertheless take pride in their knowledge of pelvic architecture and its influence on labor. The elegant work of Caldwell and Moloy helped formalize obstetric thinking with regard to the relationship between variations in human pelvic bony architecture and the mechanism of labor.[7,50] The subsequent widespread use of pelvic radiography in the 1940s through the 1960s made an understanding of cephalopelvic relationships a fundamental aspect of clinical management. Although x-ray pelvimetry is now used infrequently, accurate clinical pelvimetry is still required to make proper judgments about labor. As imaging techniques with relatively low doses of radiation (eg, computed tomography) and alternatives such as magnetic resonance imaging evolve, new approaches to pelvimetry may be developed.

The knowledge of pelvic architecture and its relation to labor should be used as a complementary technique to the analysis of labor curves.[47] This kind of interpretation allows one to explain the observed mechanism of labor, to judge the effects of labor on the fetal skull, and thus to assess the probability of the need for operative intervention. When this kind of assessment is interpreted in concert with information from labor curves and uterine activity and assessment of fetal condition, a reasonable judgment can be made concerning the advisability of uterine stimulation or operative intervention.

The value of a keen interpretation of cephalopelvic relationships along with evaluation of the labor curves cannot be overestimated as a means to provide intelligent and safe conduct of dysfunctional labor. Neither kind of information can be used optimally without the other. For example, a narrowed midpelvis with a molded head impinging on the inlet in the presence of a failure of descent makes the probability of safe vaginal delivery remote. Similarly, an arrest of descent with posterior position in a midpelvis with prominent ischial spines (making internal rotation difficult) and a forward lower sacrum (resisting further descent without rotation) also suggests an insurmountable problem. In neither case would oxytocin use be prudent. If these labor disorders occurred in the presence of more favorable pelvic structure, spontaneous delivery would be more likely and uterine stimulation would be safer.

SECOND-STAGE DURATION

It had been assumed for a long time that delivery should be expedited after about 2 hours elapsed during the second stage of labor. This traditional view has recently been challenged, and considerable objective evidence supports the idea that it is not appropriate to terminate labor merely because an arbitrary period of time has passed in the second stage.

The first evidence for this was published in 1977. Cohen evaluated the influence of the duration of second-stage labor on measures of perinatal mortality and immediate morbidity, as well as on maternal puerperal morbidity.[51] No significant trend toward increases in perinatal or neonatal mortality with progressive lengthening of the second stage was observed. A rise in the frequency of low 1-minute Apgar scores did occur among babies born after a long second stage, but this was confined to those women whose labors were managed without continuous electronic fetal heart rate monitoring. Increases in the frequency of maternal hemorrhage and febrile morbidity observed in the study after long second stages were accounted for by the more frequent use of midforceps delivery and cesarean section, respectively, in a long second stage. Other investigators have similarly been unable to demonstrate any direct effect of the duration of second-stage labor on perinatal outcome or maternal morbidity.[52,53] Even in a report that found more metabolic acidosis with longer second stages, almost all babies delivered during the second hour of the second stage had cord artery lactate levels similar to those delivered during the first hour.[54] Much of the observed acidosis was probably accounted for by abnormal heart rate patterns and forceps delivery. As a consequence of these various studies, there has been a documentable trend among practicing obstetricians toward allowing longer second stages before intervention is undertaken.[55] This does not imply that long second stages are always innocuous. They are more commonly associated with dysfunctional descent patterns that often require prompt evaluation and treatment.

Decisions concerning management and intervention in the second stage must be based on careful evaluation of maternal and fetal condition and of the progress of descent. Under some circumstances, a fetus may descend at a normal rate and still take more than 2 hours to encounter the pelvic floor. To subject such patients to potentially traumatic operative procedures merely because they have not delivered within 2 hours after the second stage has begun carries little benefit and considerable risk.

UPRIGHT POSTURE

Maternal posture during the second stage may have important consequences for fetal condition and labor progress. In the United States, some form of recumbency has generally been used for laboring women during most of this century. Recently, the risks of the supine or dorsal lithotomy position have been highlighted, and these are generally avoided during labor to minimize aortocaval compression by the gravid uterus. The lithotomy position is still often used for delivery, although it has several disadvantages. Although many people have advocated the use of upright postures (standing, sitting, or squatting),[56] relatively little information has been available until recently concerning the benefits of this approach.

Upright postures during the second stage may take advantage of the fact that considerable increases in certain pelvic diameters may occur. For example, Russell demonstrated as much as a 1.5-cm increment in the interspinous diameter when a woman moved from supine to a squatting position.[57] Similarly, the sagittal diameter of the outlet may also be improved by certain postures.[58] Also, during squatting posterior rotation of the iliac bones at the sacroiliac joint might increase pelvic diameters. In addition to these anatomical advantages, upright posture may make maternal efforts to bear down maximally effective.[59]

Relatively few controlled studies of the effect of posture on labor have been performed, and results vary. There is evidence that uterine contractility may be greater in upright than in recumbent positions[60] and that overall labor may be shorter.[61] Other investigations have failed to confirm this.[62] Recently, in a randomized trial of the squatting position during labor, Gardosi and colleagues found that in comparison to conventional semirecumbent management, women who squatted during the second stage had fewer forceps deliveries and shorter second stages.[63]

Avoiding the supine position is particularly important. Some investigators have observed a rapid decrease in fetal pH after full dilatation, but it appears that this effect is position-dependent. Humphrey and colleagues and Johnstone and colleagues noted a time-dependent decrease in fetal pH during the second stage in supine patients that did not occur when women labored in the lateral position.[64,65]

Although there is still uncertainty about the importance of maternal posture in providing efficient labor progress, there are much data to support the notion that upright postures may optimize descent in the second stage by enlarging some pelvic diameters and improving the efficiency of voluntary bearing-down efforts. Since there has been no suggestion that these positions have any adverse consequences, they should be encouraged during the second stage of labor, particularly if abnormal descent is present or anticipated.[47,48]

SHOULDER DYSTOCIA

After the descending head extends under the pubic symphysis and crosses the perineum, there is occasionally an obstruction to further descent caused by shoulder dystocia. This dreaded complication is associated with certain risk factors, including arrest and protraction disorders, fetal macrosomia, midcavity delivery, postterm pregnancy, and diabetes mellitus.[66–68] Although the presence of one of these features should encourage the obstetrician to be prepared for the possibility of a disordered shoulder mechanism, the majority of labors with these risk factors are not complicated by shoulder dystocia. In fact, using these traditional criteria, only a small proportion of cases of difficult shoulder delivery can be predicted or prevented.[69] Therefore, the obstetric attendant should always be vigilant and prepared to deal with this complication promptly and efficiently.

It is likely that factors related both to fetal size and morphology and to pelvic architecture and labor progress are important in determining the mechanism of shoulder delivery. During normal descent a process of shoulder "molding" probably occurs.[70] In this manner, the fetal shoulders and trunk gradually accommodate to the conformation of the birth canal during descent, ensuring proper engagement and orientation of the shoulders in the pelvis when the head delivers.

When the fetus is unusually large or the pelvis through which it is descending is contracted, the shoulders may both remain trapped at the inlet. More commonly, the posterior shoulder traverses the inlet, but the anterior one becomes impacted at the pubic symphysis. Although this may occur in any situation in which the fetus is relatively large for the pelvis, it is particularly common in fetuses of diabetic mothers. The explanation for this is that the bisacromial diameter in such babies is disproportionately large in relation to head size in comparison to babies of non-diabetic mothers.[71]

Pelvic architecture may sometimes account for aberrations in the normal mechanism of shoulder engagement and descent. A steeply inclined pubic symphysis favors impaction of the anterior shoulder, particularly if associated with a foreshortened inlet diameter. The influence of patterns of labor progress on the development of shoulder dystocia is not completely understood. Arrest and protraction disorders predispose, perhaps because as concomitants of cephalopelvic disproportion, they may suggest the presence of a fetus too large for the patient's pelvis. In addition, unusually rapid descent confers an increased risk of difficult shoulder delivery.[70,72] Precipitate descent is particularly nettlesome because it is generally not predictable and may preclude adequate preparation for delivery.

Several approaches to the management of shoulder dystocia are effective, and the obstetrician should be prepared to initiate a logical sequence of maneuvers. During all of these the basic principle of avoiding extensive lateral displacement of the cervical spine is important. The most serious consequence in fetuses who survive delivery with shoulder dystocia is permanent brachial plexus injury. Usually, nerve damage occurs when excessive lateral traction is placed on the fetal head in efforts to deliver the obstructed shoulders. Fractures of the clavicle or humerus are also common, but they generally heal without serious sequelae. Sometimes bony and neurologic injury is not preventable, even when adequate precautions and appropriate maneuvers have been used to reduce the shoulder entrapment. To minimize the risk of these injuries, the obstetrician must be prepared to act promptly to solve the problem.[47]

When difficulty with shoulder delivery is encountered, summon the appropriate aid. An obstetric nurse or another experienced attendant should be available, as well as an anesthesiologist. A large episiotomy is often helpful both to relieve any soft tissue obstruction that may be present and to allow sufficient room for the operator to manipulate the shoulders in the vagina. Many obstetricians recommend a large mediolateral episiotomy. A median episioproctotomy may provide even more space and, if repaired correctly, has a very low risk of complications. If gentle downward traction on the head fails to release the shoulders, a vaginal examination should be performed to assess the position of the bisacromial diameter and, in particular, the degree of descent of the posterior shoulder. The presence of an anomalous fetal trunk, although rare, may sometimes be determined at this time.

If the shoulders are in the anteroposterior diameter of the pelvis, they should be shifted promptly to an oblique dimension by rotating the posterior shoulder ventrally with pressure behind the scapula. Sometimes this results in the anterior shoulder stemming under the pubic symphysis. If the anterior shoulder does not descend, the mother's thighs may be flexed against her abdomen. This maneuver sometimes allows delivery of the anterior shoulder by altering the outlet dimensions.[73] If no success has been met, the Woods corkscrew maneuver[74] should be applied if the posterior shoulder is identified below the midplane of the pelvis. This involves rotating the posterior shoulder 180° to the anterior position, at which time it generally moves under the symphysis and can be delivered. If this maneuver fails, one may reach into the birth canal and attempt to deliver the posterior arm by drawing it across the fetal chest. Should this be unsuccessful, the remaining options are to fracture the fetal clavicle intentionally or to perform the Zavenelli maneuver.[75] The latter was recently described and involves pushing the fetal head back into the vagina and delivering the fetus by cesarean section. Limited experience with this approach is available, but it can be successful and should be considered as a last resort.

When initial assessment of the shoulders reveals that the posterior shoulder has not engaged, the situation is serious. The Woods maneuver is not likely to work in this situation, nor are most of the other approaches unless the posterior shoulder can be made to descend. Sometimes direct traction on it with two fingers of the examining hand in the axilla will be successful.

EPISIOTOMY

Episiotomy for a vaginal delivery has been a routine part of obstetric care in North America for the last half century. As trends away from operative deliveries have evolved recently, the necessity for episiotomy has been questioned, and fewer routine episiotomies are being performed.

The debate over use of this technique relates to the potential long-term hazards of failing to perform episiotomy. Most (but not all) evidence suggests that performing episiotomy increases the likelihood of serious perineal lacerations involving the external anal sphincter or rectum.[76,77] Most deliveries, even in nulliparas, can be performed without episiotomy. Often small periurethral lacerations result, and sometimes the perineum tears in the midline; but in general these traumatic injuries are not serious and are easily repaired. At issue is whether episiotomy reduces the likelihood of injury to the pelvic floor and endopelvic fascia, which could result in pelvic relaxation and urinary stress incontinence later in life. There is no unanimity about this and very little in the way of long-term follow-up to prove benefit.[47]

In general, one may view the decision to use episiotomy as a matter of obstetric judgment, a procedure to be performed when the alternative risks of spontaneous laceration or delay in delivery would be more hazardous than the operative incision. The proper timing of episiotomy is important. Many advocate making the incision as the fetal head is crowning, when it becomes obvious that spontaneous delivery would result in lacerations. This approach limits the number of episiotomies performed, but by this time the perineum has been stretched maximally, and most of the damage to the lower vaginal and perineal tissues may already have occurred. Thus, there is some virtue in making the episiotomy prior to extensive distention of the perineum when that is possible.

If episiotomy is used, a thorough knowledge of the functional anatomy of the pelvic floor and proper surgical technique is necessary to provide optimal results. Consequences of poor repair may be prolonged or permanent dyspareunia, or even iatrogenic defects in the fascial supports of the rectum. Rectovaginal fistulae may also occur sometimes as a consequence of improper surgical repair.

CODA

The disciplined approach to the management of labor advocated in this chapter emphasizes the need to objectify clinical information to optimize decision making. It is evident, nevertheless, that the process of assisting women with childbirth requires the practitioner to integrate such objective data with the spectrum of social and psychological features unique to each individual's labor. In so doing, one may aspire to provide the most fulfilling birth experience possible for each patient.

Obviously, each woman's attitudes and expectations concerning pregnancy are conditioned by her own social and cultural background, as well as by her experiences during gestation. Consequently, no universal formula for the provision of emotional support exists; rather, the practitioner must tailor communication to the patient's needs, encouraging her to express her questions, fears, or concerns and discussing them in an honest and reassuring manner.

Although a multiplicity of issues may exist for each parturient, one concern is almost universal during labor —fear of the unknown. To appreciate the degree of anxiety that may occur in this regard, consider that the patient is embarking on a physically taxing and emotionally demanding event that is likely to be painful. She will negotiate this experience nearly naked, in unfamiliar surroundings, and often coached by people she has not previously met (or worse, by no one at all). Her sense of vulnerability may be enhanced if she encounters unanticipated interventions involving high-technology equipment or operative delivery.

Prenatal care plays an important role in this regard, because it is a time during which the patient may be educated about what to expect in labor and delivery. More important, the prenatal visits allow formation of a bond of trust and confidence between practitioner and patient.[78] This bond serves both well, moderating the patient's apprehension through an understanding that her caretakers will be doing their best to make decisions in the interests of the mother and fetus. Moreover, as it is appropriate for the patient to play some role in obstetric decision making, the parameters for this kind of interaction may be set beforehand, tacitly or explicitly. When unexpected events occur that preclude time for detailed discussion, it is the trust the patient has formed previously in her caretakers that provides her with the emotional resources to cope.

It is self-evident that no one should have to endure a momentous and stressful life event alone, and this certainly applies to labor and birth. In addition to the obvious emotional benefits, there is some evidence that appropriate companionship during labor may reduce some complications of labor and enhance the quality of subsequent maternal–infant interaction.[79] To this end, the presence of the patient's husband or other supportive person of her choice should be encouraged during the entire labor and delivery process.

The obstetrician cannot guarantee a good outcome of every childbirth, but through the application of the principles expressed in this chapter he or she can promise to seek the best outcome possible for mother and fetus with the maximal attainable safety. This can occur in the context of a birth experience that is emotionally enriching for the parturient and her family and treats the laboring mother with the requisite gentleness, dignity, and compassion demanded by the process of giving birth.

REFERENCES

1. Bottari S, Thomas JP, Vokaer A, Vokaer R. Uterine contractility. New York: Masson Publishing USA, Inc, 1984.
2. Caldeyro-Barcia R. Uterine contractility in obstetrics. Deux Cong Int Gynecol Obstet 1958;1:65.
3. Poseiro JJ, Noriega-Guerra L. Dose-response relationships in uterine effects of oxytocin infusions. In: Caldeyro-Barcia R, Heller H, eds. Oxytocin. New York: Pergamon Press, 1961.
4. Calkins LA. The value of estimating the length of labor. Clin Obstet Gynecol 1959;2:322.
5. Calkins LA. Second stage of labor: the descent phase. Am J Obstet Gynecol 1944;48:798.
6. Frey E. Die bedeutung der wehentafel fur die physiologie und pathologie der geburt beim vorzeitigen blasensprung. Schweiz Med Wochenschr 1929;59:613.
7. Caldwell, WE, Moloy HC. Anatomical variations in the female pelvis and their effect in labor with a suggested classification. Am J Obstet Gynecol 1933;26:479.
8. Friedman EA. Graphic analysis of labor. Am J Obstet Gynecol 1954;68:1568.
9. Friedman EA. Evolution of graphic analysis of labor. Am J Obstet Gynecol 1978, 132:824.
10. Philpott RH, Castle WM. Cervicographs in the management of labour in primigravidae. II. The action line and treatment of abnormal labour. J Obstet Gynaecol Br Commonw 1972;79:599.
11. Drouin P, Nasah BT, Nkounawa F. The value of the partogramme in the management of labor. Obstet Gynecol 1979; 53:741.
12. Philpott RH, Castle WM. Cervicographs in the management of labour in primigravidae. I. The alert line for detecting abnormal labour. J Obstet Gynaecol Br Commonw 1972;799:592.
13. Nesheim B-I. Duration of labor. An analysis of influencing factors. Acta Obstet Gynecol Scand 1988;67:121.
14. Friedman EA. Labor. Clinical evaluation and management. 2nd ed. New York: Appleton-Century-Crofts, 1978.
15. Chazotte C, Madden R, Cohen WR. Labor patterns in women with previous cesareans. Obstet Gynecol 1990;75:350.
16. Friedman EA. The functional divisions of labor. Am J Obstet Gynecol 1971;109:274.
17. Rath W, Adelmann-Grill BC, Pieper U, Kuhn W. Collagen degradation in the pregnant human cervix at term and after prostaglandin-induced cervical ripening. Arch Gynecol 1987;240:177.
18. Rayburn WF. Prostaglandin E_2 gel for cervical ripening and induction of labor: a critical analysis. Am J Obstet Gynecol 1989;160:529.
19. Peisner DB, Rosen MG. Latent phase of labor in normal patients: a reassessment. Obstet Gynecol 1985;66:644.
20. Peisner DB, Rosen MG. Transition from latent to active labor. Obstet Gynecol 1985;68:448.

21. Friedman EA, Hunt HB, Sachtleben MR. Disordered labor: simplified method for recognition. Ob/Gyn Digest 1975;17:12.
22. Burke L, Rubin HW, Berenberg AL. The significance of the unengaged vertex in a nullipara at thirty-eight weeks' gestation. Am J Obstet Gynecol 1958;76:132.
23. Shulman J, Romney S. Variability of uterine contractions in normal human parturition. Obstet Gynecol 1970;36:215.
24. Schifrin BS, Cohen WR. Labor's dysfunctional lexicon. Obstet Gynecol 1989;74:123.
25. Friedman EA, Sachtleben MR. Dysfunctional labor. I. Prolonged latent phase in the nullipara. Obstet Gynecol 1961;17:135.
26. Baxi L, Petrie RH, James LS. Human fetal oxygenation ($tcPO_2$), heart rate variability and uterine activity following maternal administration of meperidine. J Perinat Med 1988;16:23.
27. Friedman EA, Neff RK. Labor and delivery: impact on offspring. Littleton, MA: PSG Publishing, 1987.
28. Bottoms SF, Sokol RJ, Rosen MG. Short arrest of cervical dilatation: a risk for maternal/fetal/infant morbidity. Am J Obstet Gynecol 1981;140:108.
29. Friedman EA, Sachtleben MR. Station of the fetal presenting part. V. Protracted descent patterns. Obstet Gynecol 1970;36:558.
30. Hillis DS. Diagnosis of contracted pelvis. Ill Med J 1938;74:131.
31. Cohen WR, Neuman L, Friedman EA. Risk of labor abnormalities with advancing age. Obstet Gynecol 1980;55:414.
32. Friedman EA, Sachtleben MR. Dysfunctional labor. II. Protracted active phase dilatation in the nullipara. Obstet Gynecol 1961;17:566.
33. Cardozo L, Pearce JM. Oxytocin in active-phase abnormalities of labor: a randomized study. Obstet Gynecol 1990;75:152.
34. Friedman EA, Sachtleben MR. Dysfunctional labor. III. Secondary arrest of dilatation in the nullipara. Obstet Gynecol 1962;19:576.
35. Schwarcz R, Diaz AG, Belizan JM, Fescina R, Caldeyro-Barcia R. Influence of amniotomy and maternal position on labor. In: Castelazo-Ayala L, MacGregor C, eds. Gynecology and obstetrics. Proceedings of the VIII World Congress of Gynecology and Obstetrics. Amsterdam: Excerpta Medica, 1977:377.
36. Laros RK, Work BA, Witting WC. Amniotomy during the active phase of labor. Obstet Gynecol 1972;39:702.
37. Stewart P, Kennedy JH, Calder AA. Spontaneous labour: when should the membranes be ruptured? Br J Obstet Gynaecol 1982;89:39.
38. Van Praagh I, Hendricks CH. The effect of amniotomy during labor in multiparas. Obstet Gynecol 1964, 24:258.
39. Friedman EA, Sachtleben MR. Amniotomy and the course of labor. Obstet Gynecol 1963;22:755.
40. O'Driscoll K, Meagher D. Active management of labour. Philadelphia: WB Saunders, 1980.
41. Akoury HA, Brodie G, Caddick R, McLaughlan VD, Pugh PA. Active management of labor and operative delivery in nulliparous women. Am J Obstet Gynecol 1988;158:255.
42. Cohen GR, O'Brien WF, Lewis L, Knuppel RA. A prospective randomized study of the aggressive management of early labor. Am J Obstet Gynecol 1987;157:1174.
43. Leveno KJ, Cunningham FG, Pritchard JA. Cesarean section: an answer to the House of Horne. Am J Obstet Gynecol 1985;153:838.
44. O'Driscoll K, Foley M, MacDonald D, Strange J. Cesarean section and perinatal outcome: response from the House of Horne. Am J Obstet Gynecol 1988;158:449.
45. Leveno KJ, Cunningham FG, Pritchard JA. Cesarean section: the House of Horne revisited. Am J Obstet Gynecol 1989;160:78.
46. Iffy L. Cesarean section rate and perinatal mortality. The impact of prematurity and other confounding factors. Abstract, XII European Congress of Perinatal Medicine, Lyon, France, Sept 11–14, 1990.
47. Cohen WR. The pelvic division of labor. In: Cohen WR, Acker DB, Friedman EA, eds. Management of labor. 2nd ed. Rockville, MD: Aspen Publications, 1989.
48. Cohen WR. Labor and delivery. In: Eden RD, Boehm FH, eds. Assessment and care of the fetus: physiological, clinical, and medicolegal principles. Norwalk, CT: Appleton & Lange, 1990:823.
49. Crichton D. A reliable method of establishing the level of the fetal head in obstetrics. S Afr Med 1974;48:784.
50. Caldwell WE, Moloy HC, D'Esopo DA. Studies on pelvic arrests. Am J Obstet Gynecol 1938;36:928.
51. Cohen W. Influence of the duration of second stage labor on perinatal outcome and puerperal morbidity. Obstet Gynecol 1977;49:266.
52. Kadar N. The second stage. In: Studd J, ed. The management of labour. Oxford: Blackwell Scientific Publications, 1985:271.
53. Maresh M, Cheong KH, Beard RW. Delayed pushing with lumbar analgesia in labor. Br J Obstet Gynecol 1983;90:623.
54. Katz M, Lunenfeld E, Meizner I, Bashan N, Gross J. The effect of the duration of the second stage of labor on the acid-base state of the fetus. Br J Obstet Gynaecol 1987;94:425.
55. Reynolds JL, Yudkin PL. Changes in the management of labor. I. Length and management of the second stage. Can Med Assoc J 1987;136:1041.
56. McKay SR. Maternal position during labor and birth. J Obstet Gynecol Neonat Nurs 1980;9:288.
57. Russell JGB. Moulding of the pelvic outlet. J Obstet Gynecol Br Commonw 1969;76:817.
58. Borell U, Fernstrom I. The movements at the sacroiliac joints and their importance to changes in the pelvic dimensions during parturition. Acta Obstet Gynecol Scand 1958;37:54.
59. Chen S-Z, Aisaka K, Mori H, Kigawat. Effects of sitting position on uterine activity in labor. Obstet Gynecol 1987;69:67.
60. Read JA, Miller FC, Paul RH. Randomized trial of ambulation versus oxytocin for labor enhancement. Am J Obstet Gynecol 1981;139:669.
61. Flynn AM, Kelly J, Hollins G, Lynch PF. Ambulation in labor. Br Med J 1978;2:591.
62. McManus TJ, Calder AA. Upright posture and the efficiency of labor. Lancet 1978;1:72.
63. Gardosi J, Hutson N, B-Lynch C. Randomized, controlled trial of squatting in the second stage of labor. Lancet 1989;2:74.
64. Humphrey MD, Chang A, Wood ED, Hounslow D. A decrease in fetal pH during the second stage of labor when conducted in the dorsal position. J Obstet Gynaecol Br Commonw 1974;81:600.
65. Johnstone FD, Abaelmagd MS, Harouny AK. Maternal posture in second stage and fetal acid base status. Br J Obstet Gynaecol 1987;94:753.
66. Acker DB, Sachs BP, Friedman EA. Risk factors for shoulder dystocia. Obstet Gynecol 1985;66:762.
67. Benedetti TJ, Gabbe SG. Shoulder dystocia. A complication of fetal macrosomia and prolonged second stage of labor with midpelvic delivery. Obstet Gynecol 1978;52:526.
68. Hopwood HG. Shoulder dystocia. Fifteen years experience in a community hospital. Am J Obstet Gynecol 1982;144:162.
69. Gross TL, Sokol RJ, Williams T, Thompson K. Shoulder dystocia: a fetal-physician risk. Am J Obstet Gynecol 1987;156:1408.
70. Morris WIC. Shoulder dystocia. J Obstet Gynaecol Br Emp 1955;62:302.
71. Modanlou HD, Komatsu G, Dorchester W, Freeman RK, Bosu Sk. Large-for-gestational age neonates: anthropometric reasons for shoulder dystocia. Obstet Gynecol 1982;60:417.
72. Acker DB, Sachs BP, Friedman EA. Risk factors for shoulder dystocia. Obstet Gynecol 1985;66:762.

73. Gonik B, Stringer CA, Held B. An alternate maneuver for management of shoulder dystocia. Am J Obstet Gynecol 1983; 145:882.
74. Woods CE. A principle of physics as applicable to shoulder delivery. Am J Obstet Gynecol 1943;45:796.
75. Sandberg EC. The Zavanelli maneuver: a potentially revolutionary method for the resolution of shoulder dystocia. Am J Obstet Gynecol 1985;152:479.
76. Bueken P, Lagasse R, Dramaix M, Wollast E. Episiotomy and third degree tears. Br J Obstet Gynaecol 1985;92:820.
77. Borgatta L, Piening S, Cohen WR. Association of episiotomy and delivery position with deep perineal laceration during spontaneous delivery in nulliparous women. Am J Obstet Gynecol 1989;160:294.
78. McRae MG, Mervyn FV. Contemporary issues in childbirth. In: Cohen WR, Acker DB, Fredman EA, eds. Management of labor. 2nd ed. Rockville, MD: Aspen Publications, 1989.
79. Sosa R, Kennell J, Klaus M, Robertson S, Urrutia J. The effect of a supportive companion on perinatal problems, length of labor, and mother-infant interaction. N Engl J Med 1980;303:597.

86

CHAPTER

NORMAL AND OPERATIVE DELIVERIES

David B. Peisner and Mortimer G. Rosen

The delivery of the infant at the end of the gestation is the focus of great concern to the mother. She has had the major responsibility for her health care during the antenatal period, and now she transfers, in part, the responsibility for her health and that of the unborn infant to the hands of an obstetrician or midwife. Although pregnancy is 9 months long, the day of labor is perhaps the most important day in pregnancy after the day of conception. This chapter reviews the implications of normal and operative deliveries for both the mother and fetus. Techniques are described briefly, since the emphasis of this text is on the fetus. The reader is referred to other textbooks for more complete description of techniques.[1–3]

PREPARATION FOR DELIVERY

Delivery of the infant is a continuation of the cardinal movements of the fetal head through the mother's pelvis. Presumably, the fetal head is dipping well into the pelvis and engaged at the beginning of the second stage. However, in primiparous and multiparous women, it is not unusual (in fact, it is normal) for vertex engagement to take place during the second stage. When the head is engaged, it usually is flexed, and this causes the presenting part to be the occiput in most cases. The fetal head then goes through the following cardinal movements: descent, internal rotation, extension, and external rotation (Fig. 86-1). Delivery occurs during the third movement, when the head extends itself as it moves under the symphysis pubis. It is important to remember these movements because they help explain why some deliveries—specifically, shoulder dystocia—are difficult. Prior to the delivery, a note is written in the medical record that describes the findings and expectations for the type of delivery that is anticipated.

The presentation and position of the fetus are confirmed by vaginal exam and Leopold's maneuvers. If necessary, an ultrasound evaluation can be used to erase any doubt of the fetal presentation and size. Fetal weight can be estimated. Both of these evaluations will help the obstetrician determine what type of delivery to do and where to do it.

A normal-term-size (<4000 g) delivery can be done almost anywhere in the delivery suite. However, malpresentations such as occiput posterior, face, or breech deliveries have more potential complications, and when they are anticipated, they should be managed in the delivery room, where additional equipment, including anesthesia, is available. If the estimated fetal weight is high, the chances of fetal morbidity increase. Some researchers have used 4000 g and others have used 4500 g as their cutoff.[4–6] The final decision to attempt a vaginal delivery of a large fetus is based not on absolute numbers but on a clinical judgment that includes the evaluation of the fetus, maternal pelvis, and quality of labor, including patient responses. One of the major problems with large infants is shoulder dystocia, and for extremely large babies weighing more than 4500 to 5000 g, cesarean section may be considered to avoid this increasing risk. As noted, absolute limits are rarely in order. Complete patient evaluation and judgment are needed to determine the route of delivery.

When delivery is imminent, there are some guidelines to management:[7]

1. The patient should not be left unattended.
2. No attempt to delay the birth with restraint or anesthesia should be made.
3. Maternal and fetal monitoring during the second stage of labor should be maintained (fetal heart by electronic means or every 5 minutes by auscultation; maternal pulse and blood pressure every 15 minutes).

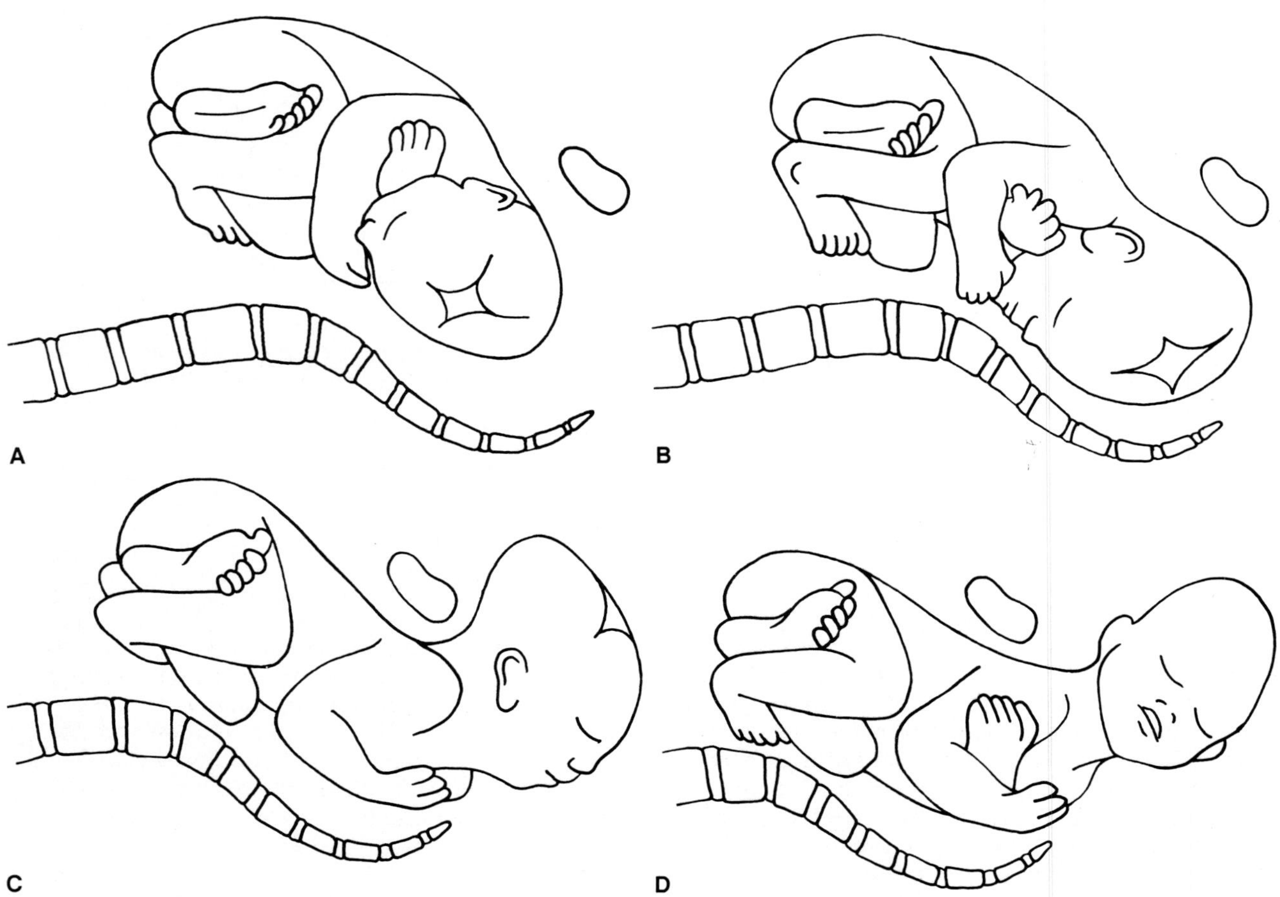

FIGURE 86–1. (**A**) The fetal head usually enters the pelvis flexed and in the transverse position. (**B**) The fetal head undergoes internal rotation in the midpelvis. (**C**) The fetal head delivers by extension. (**D**) The fetal head undergoes external rotation (restitution).

NORMAL VAGINAL DELIVERY

The usual technique of a normal vaginal delivery consists of the following: as the vertex of the fetal head appears at the vaginal introitus, the patient is placed in the lithotomy position, her perineum is cleansed, and she is covered with sterile drapes. Although the delivery itself is not a clean procedure, the drapes are used because the obstetrician often must repair the perineum and occasionally must explore the uterus. To avoid contamination from surrounding skin, the drapes are used. The degree of draping and the patient position may vary, depending on the participants. Only one type of delivery is described here, but others are possible.

Some patients may prefer to deliver from a squatting position, and physiologically this is a reasonable alternative. The uterus of the patient in the supine position compresses the great vessels, which may compromise blood flow to and from the placental circulation. When some patients are placed in the supine position, they may become short of breath. There is decreased blood return to the heart from inferior vena cava compression; in addition, there is aortic compression as noted by the decrease in the pulse pressure of the popliteal artery in the supine gravid patient.[8] In a comparison of patients in the supine and left lateral position in the second stage, Johnstone and colleagues found that although there were no differences in clinical outcome, the infants of the supine group had significantly lower cord pH values.[9] The assistance of gravity in the expulsion of the infant is obvious. It is clear that although the dorsal lithotomy position is the most common, other acceptable choices remain.

Once the patient has been draped and continues to push with contractions, the perineum is allowed to distend gradually. With slow delivery, the mother is less likely to lacerate her perineum. *Crowning* occurs as the largest diameters of the head are passing through the introitus. When it occurs, the birth of the vertex must continue in a controlled manner. On rare occasions, which occur most frequently in the birth of the low–birth-weight infant, too rapid birth and sudden expansion of the cranial bones may lead to laceration of the dural sinuses and development of a subdural hematoma.

Although some may advocate episiotomy as a routine

procedure,[10] more recent studies have advocated selective use of this procedure.[11–14] With each contraction, the fetal head expands the vulva. In certain cases, such as malpresentations or larger infants, an episiotomy is necessary to create more room for the delivery. In some cases, especially during a case of shoulder dystocia, a mediolateral episiotomy may be necessary to make more room for the delivery. If a mediolateral is done, it is usually placed on the right side to avoid the rectum. If the patient has had previous vaginal surgery, an episiotomy may be performed to prevent extensive lacerations because the surgical scar is more likely to tear than the original perineum.

Those who have advocated episiotomies have listed other advantages of the procedure[10]: the perineum is more comfortable the first few days after the delivery, there is less bleeding than with lacerations, the repair is easier, healing is better, and there is less risk of dyspareunia, since there is no loss of elasticity of the sides of the fourchette. Recently, several studies have shown that the degree of perineal lacerations may increase when an episiotomy is performed.[11–14] In a review of the literature, Thorp found an incidence of third- and fourth-degree extensions in 6.5% of patients with an episiotomy and 1.4% of those patients without.[11] Nevertheless, the judgment of the obstetrician determines if an episiotomy is needed as the vertex distends the perineum.

As the fetal head delivers, most obstetricians advocate easing it slowly through the introitus without sudden movements. This certainly helps prevent perineal lacerations, and as noted earlier, this restraint helps to prevent intracranial hemorrhages in the newborn from sudden movements. As the vertex delivers, the flexion of the vertex is maintained with the superior hand, thus avoiding rapid extension of the head and the resulting periurethral lacerations.

After the head has delivered, the obstetrician assesses whether the umbilical cord is wrapped around it. If it is, it should be passed over the head. If the cord is too tight, it can be doubly clamped and cut prior to the birth of the infant's body. Note that if monoamniotic twins are being delivered vaginally, a nuchal cord around the first baby may be the cord of the second infant. Since there is no way to tell if this is the situation, an attempt is made to pass the cord over the body if it is loose enough. If it is cut and it was the cord of the second baby, the next infant obviously must be delivered rapidly.

At this point, the oropharynx and nasopharynx are suctioned. If meconium is present, a flexible catheter is passed into the fetal stomach to empty it, in addition to aspirating meconium from the mouth and nose. Usually, a DeLee catheter or equivalent is used. However, in patients at risk for AIDS, a thin catheter connected to wall suction is safer for the clinician. In the patient without meconium, as the oropharynx is being suctioned, the clinician can feel the biting or sucking reflex of the infant and is reassured of fetal health. During these few moments the clinician allows the shoulders to descend and accommodate to the pelvis, as the head is on the perineum. To attempt to complete the delivery rapidly may aggravate a potential for shoulder dystocia.

After the head has delivered, the obstetrician assesses whether the shoulders will deliver easily or whether dystocia is likely. If dystocia is suspected, an attempt is made to deliver the anterior shoulder before complete external rotation (restitution) occurs. As the normal delivery progresses, the clinician pulls down on the fetal head toward the floor to deliver the anterior shoulder. The head is then lifted to deliver the posterior shoulder and the rest of the body is then delivered. The mouth and nose are once again suctioned as necessary. The cord is then doubly clamped and cut and the infant is passed to the nurse, pediatrician, or mother. At this point, blood samples, if necessary, are obtained from the umbilical cord. One of these may be a doubly clamped length of cord that is sampled at the blood gas laboratory. The blood gases at the time of birth are an indicator of the acid–base status of the infant and reflect recent trends just prior to the delivery. Some hospitals obtain this sample routinely as defensive medicine in today's legal climate; however, its medical value is limited.

FETAL AND NEONATAL EFFECTS OF VAGINAL DELIVERY

When the mother is prepared for delivery, the fetal scalp is often visible at the introitus. Because of molding of the fetal head, the presence of the scalp may be misleading. The mother may have to push for some time in the delivery room.

The vast majority of women have a short second stage. The length of the second stage for normal patients has been studied recently. These intervals do not follow a normal statistical distribution.[15] When the distribution is taken into effect, the median time for the nulliparous patient is 23 minutes and that for the multiparous patient is 9 minutes. However, the 95th percentile for the nulliparous patient ($n = 915$) is 2.5 hours, and that for the multiparous patient ($n = 368$) is 70 minutes. In this study, nonocciput anterior positions and patients with epidural anesthesia were excluded. These factors can prolong the second stage. Since the patient may spend some time in the second stage of labor, it is best not to be in the delivery room if the second stage is likely to be long. This may lead to unnecessary early intervention.

If the second stage of labor is prolonged, the obstetrician attempts to diagnose the reason for the delay in delivery. It may be caused by the size, position, or presentation of the fetus, the expulsive forces, and/or the birth canal. The physician performs a pelvic examination and confirms the presentation and position of the fetus. The type of pelvis is determined and a rough measure of its size is obtained. Several contractions are palpated to feel their strength, and observations of the mother's pushing are made. If the pelvis is too small and even a properly positioned fetal head does not change station in 2 hours of good pushing, a cesarean should be considered. If the pelvis is adequate and the presenting part is descending, there is no arbitrary cut-off time for when a cesarean section should be done. Prudent management by the obstetrician will determine if the second stage should be allowed to continue. For example, if the presentation is occiput posterior, the presenting diameter of the head, the occipitofrontal, is 1 cm larger than the presenting diameter of the occiput anterior presentation, the suboccipitobregmatic diameter. Consequently, it is not surprising that the mother may have to push for a longer time before she is able to deliver a head from the occiput posterior position. The fetal head takes longer to mold when it is in the occiput posterior position.

As the length of the second stage increases, the pH decreases and the umbilical artery lactate levels increase. Katz and colleagues found that the umbilical artery pH decreased from 7.31 to 7.25 in patients with a second stage longer than 30 minutes. This becomes important because many of these patients have variable decelerations during the second stage and may have scalp samples obtained as part of their monitoring in the delivery room. However, fetal distress is usually defined as a pH below 7.2 and there is still some latitude even though these values may decrease during the pushing in the delivery room. In the presence of apparently normal fetal heart rate during labor, brief periods of bradycardias during the last moments of the second stage of labor may cause the cord pH to decrease below 7.2 without necessarily representing fetal distress.

Another reason for the prolonged second stage is the need for the fetal head to mold. Kriewall and colleagues have calculated a molding index[16]:

$$\frac{\text{mentovertical diameter}^2}{\text{biparietal diameter} \times \text{suboccipitofrontal diameter}}$$

Kriewall found that only some of the fetal head diameters changed during the labor and that the head returned to a normal shape within 3 days of the delivery. Sorbe and Dahlgren also studied this and looked at neonatal effects.[17] Although they cited one study where the infants with spontaneous vaginal deliveries from the occiput posterior position had lower Bayley mental scores than those from the occiput anterior position, it was not clear that this was an effect of the molding. There is little information in the literature to indicate a neonatal effect from molding alone.

The heart rate of the infant varies considerably during the end of labor and immediately following the delivery. Klebe and colleagues observed a small number of infants and found that there was an initial bradycardia of 80 to 100 beats per minute (bpm) in vaginally delivered infants.[18] In all infants, there was a tachycardia of 180 bpm associated with the first cry that lasted approximately 10 minutes after the delivery in all infants. Then the heart rate slowed to the predelivery average of 140. By the next day, the heart rate of the infants was 120 bpm.

The changes in the infants' heart rates are a physical sign of stress or adaptation. There are also metabolic signs. Kohno and colleagues studied maternal and umbilical cord cortisol concentrations of patients who underwent spontaneous vaginal, operative vaginal, and cesarean deliveries.[19] Some of the patients who had cesareans had no labor prior to the operation. They found that the highest levels of cortisol in both the mother and infant were in cases of operative vaginal deliveries. The spontaneous vaginal deliveries were intermediate and the lowest levels were in patients who underwent elective cesarean deliveries. Similarly, Tetlow and Pipkin found that renin levels were elevated in mothers and infants who underwent vaginal deliveries when compared to mothers who had cesareans.[20] They also found that the renin substrate concentration in the mother correlated with the length of the second stage of labor.

Immediately after the delivery, the flow of blood in the umbilical cord can markedly alter the blood volume in the infant.[21] If there is a delay in cord clamping, blood will flow from the placenta to the infant. Initially, the infant has about 70 mL/kg of blood volume. After 3 minutes of transfusion from the placenta, this rises to 90 mL/kg. Twenty-five percent to 30% of this transfer occurs in the first 10 to 15 seconds as the uterus contracts. If the infant is held below the table, the entire transfer occurs in 30 seconds instead of 3 minutes. If the infant is held above the mother, the placental transfer can be completely eliminated. Arguments abound as to rapid or delayed cord clamping in the neonate. In general, orderly suctioning involves 1 minute before the cord is clamped. The term infant may be placed on the maternal abdomen and the cutting of the umbilical cord may be shared or performed by the parents. In the at-risk or low-birth-weight infant, more rapid clamping and delivery of the infant for resuscitation and care take place.

COMPLICATIONS OF VAGINAL DELIVERY

Some of the problems after a vaginal delivery include maternal trauma and infant trauma. Infection often occurs from a previously existing condition and is covered elsewhere in this text. Finally, some complications such as meconium aspiration and postpartum hemorrhage may occur after either vaginal or abdominal delivery.

EPISIOTOMY

An episiotomy is a fairly benign procedure but it is not without complications. First, the patient usually loses about 200 mL of blood when it is performed.[22] Although this is not a large amount, it may be significant if the mother is also losing blood for other reasons. Second, an elective episiotomy may predispose the patient to an extension through the rectal sphincter and possibly through the rectum itself.[12] Third, the perineal defect may occasionally rupture in the postpartum period, usually from infection or hemorrhage, and this can cause anal incontinence as well as patient discomfort. Sorensen and colleagues studied the long-term consequences of perineal discomfort and found that even with appropriate immediate repair, most women will have reduced sphincter strength.[23] They also found that rupture occurred more often after operative vaginal delivery. If the rupture occurs due to infection, Monberg and Hammen found that patients who had primary repair with clindamycin for 5 days did better than those patients who had secondary repair.[24]

LACERATIONS

Trauma to the mother may consist of lacerations in the cervix or vagina or, in severe cases, the rectum or urinary tract. If the cervix is lacerated, it should be repaired immediately with absorbable suture with either running or interrupted technique. For treatment of more extensive injuries, the reader is referred to a comprehensive review on the subject.[25] The primary cautions to the physician are to respect the vagina and cervix if increased bleeding is present or if extensions of the episiotomy are seen. It is helpful to palpate the anus and rectum after episiotomy repair before the patient leaves the delivery room to ensure that the mucosa is intact, the sphincter is present, and sutures are not palpated in the rectum.

INFANT TRAUMA

Infant trauma may occur after either spontaneous or operative vaginal delivery. In the term infant, some of the more common problems may include Erb-Duchenne palsy, clavicular fracture, intraventricular hemorrhage, seizures, and meconium aspiration. In a retrospective study of more than 13,000 singleton full-term infants, Levine and colleagues found the following risk factors for birth trauma: weight greater than 3500 g, second stage of labor more than 1 hour, shoulder dystocia, and forceps delivery.[26]

SHOULDER DYSTOCIA

Among these factors, shoulder dystocia itself does not usually cause birth injury. The physical injury may occur when the obstetrician exerts force on the infant's head and neck while trying to deliver the anterior shoulder.[27] Although birth weight may be a factor in injuries following shoulder dystocia,[28] other research has not found a correlation between birth injury and clinical factors.[29] If shoulder dystocia is to occur, the head will literally be sucked back into the perineum immediately after it delivers. At that point, the obstetrician does several things rapidly. First, he or she calls for assistance, including the help of an anesthesiologist and a pediatrician. Although personnel are coming, the obstetrician then tries several maneuvers to deliver the infant. Fundal pressure is not advised, because this will make the dystocia worse by impacting the anterior shoulder behind the pubis.

The management of shoulder dystocia is described in more detail in Chapter 85. Several maneuvers may be attempted to resolve the shoulder dystocia. Classically, the Woods maneuver may be performed. A very effective remedy for shoulder dystocia is the McRoberts maneuver.[30] One technique that has never been proved is the shoulder horn proposed by Chavis.[31] Finally, if all attempts to deliver the infant vaginally fail, the Zavanelli maneuver, which is an abdominal rescue procedure, may be attempted.[32–35]

FRACTURED CLAVICLE

Another infant problem is the fractured clavicle. This will often occur in cases of shoulder dystocia. This is not quite as common (about two in 1000 births) as brachial plexus injury, which occurs in 2.6 in 1000 births.[26] It may also occur without the presence of shoulder dystocia. Ironically, it can be extremely difficult to break the bone when the obstetrician deliberately attempts to fracture the clavicle to make more room in a difficult shoulder dystocia. At the same time, every obstetrician has delivered an infant with little apparent difficulty only to find that the clavicle had spontaneously fractured. Fortunately, most of these fractures resolve without disabilities. Miscellaneous birth injuries not caused by operative vaginal deliveries may occur. The reader is referred to a review for a more complete discussion of the subject.[36]

INTRAVENTRICULAR HEMORRHAGE

Intraventricular hemorrhage may also occur in the peripartum period. It may be associated with operative vaginal delivery (see Chap. 85), but it is more commonly associated with low birth weight, low 5-minute Apgar score, cord pH <7.2, and severe respiratory distress syndrome. Approximately 40% of infants who weigh 500 to 1500 g will develop intraventricular hemorrhages, and as many as 20% of them will die.[37] In Morales's study, the incidence of hemorrhage was not affected by rupture of membranes, length of labor, or route of delivery. Svenningsen and colleagues studied the relationship of fetal head compression to the appearance of retinal hemorrhages in the newborn with pressure transducers on the fetal head during the second stage of labor.[38] Although the pressures from bearing down ranged from 38 to 390 mm Hg, they could not demonstrate that increased pressures correlated with the development of retinal hemorrhages. The development of neonatal seizures is another complication that may be related to intrapartum events. Minchom and colleagues found that the incidence of seizures within 48 hours of birth in term infants was 1.3 per 1000 live births.[39] They found that the following factors were associated with seizures: nulliparity, hydramnios, postterm pregnancy, oxytocin augmentation of labor, abnormal fetal heart tracing or meconium-stained fluid, prolonged second stage of labor, emergency cesarean delivery, operative vaginal delivery, low Apgar score with resuscitation at delivery, and ventilatory support. They concluded that there was no clear pattern among these variables and that a causal relationship for seizures could not be established.

MECONIUM ASPIRATION

Meconium aspiration is a potentially dangerous complication in the newborn. It can cause pneumonitis or pneumonia, persistent fetal circulation, respiratory distress, and long-term complications. Many studies have been done to try to find ways to prevent neonatal problems. Virtually all have advocated suctioning the meconium prior to the infant's first breath to prevent the actual aspiration into the lungs. However, more recent studies, which will be discussed later in this chapter, cast doubt on the ability of such intervention to prevent the problems caused by meconium aspiration.

When meconium is present at the time of birth, it must be suctioned from the infant's mouth and nose immediately. Surprisingly, the method of suctioning (bulb versus deLee) probably does not make much difference. Two recent studies could not demonstrate a difference in outcome between the two techniques.[40,41] Immediately after birth, the infant is handed to the pediatricians. In our institution, these infants undergo immediate intubation to inspect for meconium below the cords and then are suctioned if it is present. However, Falciglia could not demonstrate any difference in the incidence of meconium aspiration in infants born in 1975 when tracheal suctioning was not routinely done versus infants born in 1983 when it was done.[42] Although the mortality from meconium aspiration decreased from 46% to 12% in his study, he felt that this was probably due to advances in neonatal care. He suggested that tracheal suctioning does not prevent aspiration but does lessen its severity. Linder and colleagues reached similar conclusions but also found that 6 of 308 infants who were intubated had complications from the intubation, whereas there were no complications among the 264 infants who were not intubated.[43] Regardless of the methodology, the obstetrician and pediatrician in the delivery room must be experienced in the resuscitation of the newborn when meconium is present. The reader is referred to a recent review for a more detailed discussion of this.[44]

In an attempt to understand how damage is done in meconium aspiration in relation to the birth process, Jovanovic and Nguyen performed experiments on guinea pigs.[45] They infused clear amniotic fluid and meconium-stained fluid into guinea pig fetal lungs in normal and asphyxiating animals. They found that there were no signs of damage to the lungs with or without meconium. The damage was caused by the presence of asphyxia. Since asphyxia and meconium often are present together, this may explain why other researchers have blamed lung damage on meconium. In an attempt to reduce the incidence of aspiration, Wenstrom and Parsons used amnioinfusion in half of the infants in their study of meconium.[46] There were no adverse effects of amnioinfusion, but there was less meconium below the cords and fewer depressed 1-minute Apgar scores in the experimental group. Another aspect of meconium aspiration was presented by Sunoo and colleagues.[47] Of 77 cases of meconium aspiration, seven occurred prior to the onset of labor or during early labor with a normal fetal heart tracing. Their conclusion was that meconium aspiration may occur before labor, which is consistent with the animal experiments that were done by Jovanovic. Thus, it appears that intervention by the obstetrician, operative or otherwise, may make little difference in neonatal outcome in the presence of intrapartum asphyxia and meconium-stained fluid.

After birth, infants who develop meconium aspiration may have long-term problems. Macfarlane and Heaf studied children 6 to 11 years after birth and found that 7 of 18 with previous meconium aspiration had respiratory symptoms.[48] In contrast, Stevens and colleagues found that patients with mild to moderate meconium aspiration did not have any pulmonary sequelae.[49]

POSTPARTUM HEMORRHAGE

Postpartum hemorrhage may be caused by uterine atony, unrecognized pelvic injury, retained placenta or accreta, uterine rupture, or uterine inversion. Although an extensive discussion is beyond the scope of this chapter, appropriate actions for these emergencies are briefly mentioned. First, in the presence of these risks, the patient should have at least one large-bore intravenous line in place and enough physiologic solutions infused to prevent hypovolemia. The patient is moved to the delivery room if she is not already there. A careful and complete pelvic exam should attempt to identify the source of the bleeding. If there is uterine atony, uterine massage is done and additional oxytocin is added to the intravenous solution. A bolus infusion is not used because it may cause hypotension. Ergot alkaloids or prostaglandins may also be used. The uterus is explored and curetted if necessary for additional portions of the placenta that may have been missed. If the uterus still remains atonic, there is an accreta, or there is a rupture that cannot be repaired, a hysterectomy may be necessary. If it is, Plauche and colleagues recommend that all pedicles be clamped and cut before ligatures are placed, to control bleeding as rapidly as possible.[50] If the uterus is inverted, laparotomy is usually not necessary for its replacement if tocolytics are used, followed by prostaglandins when the uterus is in place.[51]

BREECH AND OTHER MALPRESENTATIONS

The majority of presentations other than the cephalic are breech presentations. In a 7-year experience, Brenner and colleagues reported on 1016 breech deliveries and 29,343 nonbreech deliveries in North Carolina (an incidence of 3.3%).[52] More of the breech presentations were premature. Approximately 30% of them delivered prior to 36 weeks gestation, and only about 10% of the nonbreech infants were premature. This may be due to the fact that the head of the fetus is relatively larger than the body until late in the pregnancy and moves to the larger space in the fundus early in the pregnancy. As the body catches up in size late in the pregnancy, the heavier head then moves toward the pelvis. There are still a number of breech deliveries late in pregnancy that are not explained by this theory, however. Fianu and Vaclavinkova suggested that the placement of the placenta may influence the fetal position at or near term.[53] They found that the placenta was located in the cornual region in 73% of the breech presentations but in only 5% of the cephalic presentations. The presence of anomalies or central nervous system disorders affecting fetal movement may also increase the percentage of abnormal positions.

There are other considerations in the breech presentation. Brenner found that regardless of the delivery route, the breech fetus and placenta weighed less than its nonbreech counterpart. There was a higher rate of congenital abnormalities, the perinatal mortality and morbidity rates were higher, the Apgar scores were lower, and there were higher rates of complications in labor for the breech infants. The weight differences of the infant and placenta were not actually very large—only a few hundred grams maximum—but the trend over all birth weights was highly significant. The rate of major congenital anomalies in their study was 6.3% for breech infants and 2.4% for nonbreech infants. When infants greater than 36 weeks were examined, 5.0% of the breeches had anomalies and 2.1% of the nonbreech infants had malformations. It is difficult to compare present morbidity and mortality studies to this older paper. The complications in labor that were increased in the breech infant compared to the nonbreech infant included abruptio placentae (6.0% versus 1.8%), placenta previa (1.6% versus 0.6%), and prolapsed cord (5.2% versus 0.3%). A nuchal cord was less common in the breech infant than in the nonbreech infant (4.3% versus 8.6%).

When the breech of the fetus is in the pelvis, there are three possible presentations. The most common position is the frank breech, when the buttocks are in the pelvis, the hips are flexed, and the knees are extended, placing the legs up against the chest. If the fetus is sitting "cross-legged" with both the hips and knees flexed, this is the complete breech presentation. If the buttocks are higher in the pelvis and one or both of the feet are the presenting part, this is the footling or double-footling presentation. With exceptions, footling breech presentation is usually delivered by cesarean due to the danger of birth trauma from entrapment, since the cervix does not dilate as well with only small parts in the pelvis. The exceptions are a nonviable infant, stillbirth, or a precipitous delivery. Although fewer breech presentations are being delivered vaginally today, this birth route choice is acceptable.

If a vaginal delivery is attempted, it is done in the delivery room with at least one assistant present in case an emergency cesarean needs to be performed. For the same reason, an anesthesiologist and support staff may be helpful. If the fetus is preterm, the delivery may be less traumatic if the membranes are not ruptured until the entire infant has delivered. This delivery "en caul" presents more of a dilating wedge to the cervix and may decrease the potential for trauma as the infant delivers.

Prior to the delivery, the mother and fetus are evaluated. The fetal weight is estimated, either by palpation or by ultrasound. Macrosomic breech infants greater than 4500 g are usually delivered by cesarean. The position of the neck and head may also be evaluated by ultrasound or flat plate of the abdomen, and a cesarean is performed if the head is extended. Finally, clinical pelvimetry is performed to assess the size of the pelvis. Stewart questioned x-ray pelvimetry benefits with regard to the development of childhood leukemia.[54] Her experimental and control groups were not matched. Furthermore, the use of x-rays is not unduly restricted in the nursery for diagnostic purposes. The benefits of x-ray pelvimetry have not been demonstrated.

If possible, as much of the delivery as possible is allowed to progress spontaneously to avoid trauma. Once the body has delivered to the umbilical cord, the pulse may be palpated directly to assess the status of the infant. If the pulse is normal, there is no hurry to extract the rest of the body. Allow the arms and head to adapt to the pelvis. If the presentation is a complete breech, the legs and buttocks will deliver simultaneously. In the case of the frank breech, the infant will usually deliver both the breech and the legs spontaneously. If the mother is unable to push out the legs after the breech has delivered, the Pinard maneuver can be used. In this event, the operator pushes the thigh away from the midline to flex the knee and bring the foot down. The leg is then swept down and out of the vagina.

The legs and body are supported and allowed to deliver spontaneously. As the infant is delivering, an assistant palpates the fetal head through the abdominal wall and maintains pressure to keep it flexed to prevent its entrapment by extension. If a completely spontaneous delivery happens, the outcome is usually good. However, it is often necessary to assist the delivery of the arms and head in the term infant. It is important to try to allow the body to deliver spontaneously. Once the body has delivered, a warm, moist towel may be wrapped around it and the body may be held by an assistant to allow the operator to direct attention to the delivery of the arms and head. If rapid traction is applied to the body, this increases the likelihood that one or both of the arms may become trapped behind the neck (nuchal arms). Nuchal arms are dangerous because they may be difficult to extract and the head cannot be delivered when the arms are above the head. An attempt is made to rotate the body to try to dislodge the nuchal arm. Both directions of rotation are attempted. If the arm(s) cannot be delivered, the patient is anesthetized to relax the pelvis to provide more room for the operator to reach the arms. If the arms are not nuchal, the operator can reach for the upper arm and sweep it across the chest to deliver it. If one arm is still nuchal, draw the delivered arm across the chest and rotate the trunk with traction 180°. This will either spontaneously deliver the remaining nuchal arm or allow the operator to insert one finger along its humerus to provide elbow flexion and bring the hand to a point where it may be grasped and delivered with traction.

When only the head remains in the vagina, it is delivered promptly to prevent the cervix from closing on the neck. The head is delivered by flexing it through the pelvis. Although an assistant applies suprapubic pressure, the obstetrician delivers the head with the Mauriceau maneuver. This is performed by laying the infant's body on the upturned palm of one hand and arm. The fingers of that hand are placed over the fetal maxillae to help flex the head. The fingers of the other hand then grasp the shoulder, and traction is gently applied as the head is flexed. If the head fails to deliver, Piper forceps may be applied to the head to deliver it. These are inserted from below the infant while an assistant holds the body (Fig. 86-2). In applying the Piper forceps, the operator is in a kneeling position well below the patient. The toes of the forceps are introduced into the vagina along the side of the fetal neck, with the handle drawn toward the midline, allowing the forceps blade to move outside the undersurface of the jaw. The maneuver is repeated on the opposite side while an assistant holds the first blade. The application is checked and traction is used to draw the head down and flexed over the perineum. Controlled delivery of the head is critical, and this is often easier with forceps than with spontaneous delivery. In the unlikely event that the cervix has closed on the neck and all attempts to deliver the head have failed, Dührssen incisions can be performed by incising the cervix with a scissors at 10 o'clock and 2 o'clock. This location of the incisions avoids most major vessels and usually provides enough room to deliver the head.

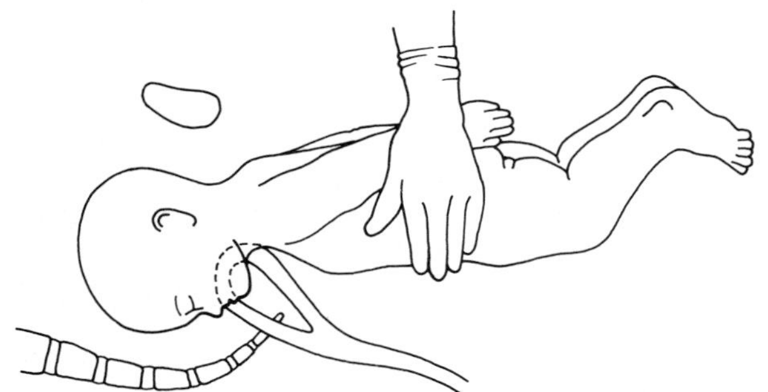

FIGURE 86–2. The Piper's forceps are inserted from beneath the infant while an assistant holds the body.

Today a majority of breech infants are delivered by cesarean, at least in part out of fear of medical malpractice suits.[55] The rationale for this is lacking in the literature. Luterkort and Marsál studied cord pH and blood gas results in 149 consecutive breech term births and found no differences between vaginal and cesarean deliveries.[56] Øian and colleagues studied 580 consecutive breech infants from 1972 to 1979 and analyzed 56 variables for their effect on perinatal mortality.[57] Only four variables—low birth weight, maternal diabetes, congenital malformations, and 5-minute Apgar less than 7—had any effect. During the 8 years of the study, the cesarean rate rose from 8% to 33%, but the mortality statistics did not change. Rosen and Chik did a multiple regression study on breech infants and demonstrated that at all birth weights below 4000 g, delivery route may not affect outcome.[58] Multiple other studies have described the lack of evidence for cesarean superiority over vaginal delivery for the breech infant, including the nonfrank presentation, and several have emphasized the increased maternal morbidity that accompanies cesarean delivery.[59–63]

One area that is controversial in the literature is the best route of delivery for the low–birth-weight breech infant. In a 7-year study, Effer and colleagues documented improved perinatal mortality in this group but concluded that this probably was not due to the increased rate of cesarean sections.[64] Westgren studied infants less than 1500 g and found no difference in mortality when route of delivery was considered.[65] However, Nisell and colleagues studied 110 infants less than 2500 g and concluded that there probably was less morbidity in the low–birth-weight infant between 1000 g and 1500 g.[66] The complication that is of most concern is the presence of intraventricular hemorrhage, since it may be related to traction on the head at the time of the delivery. Tejani and colleagues found that there was no effect of the route of delivery on the incidence of hemorrhage in the infant who weighed less than 1250 g.[67] They did find an effect in infants greater than 1250 g, but there was no breakdown for term infants.

BIRTHS OF MULTIPLE INFANTS

Procedures for delivering multiple infants are somewhat different from those for singletons. First, there must be additional pediatricians, nurses, and equipment for the care of the additional infant(s). Second, regardless of the presentation of the fetuses, an anesthetic support is desirable for the delivery. An ultrasound machine, if desired, may help determine the position of the additional fetus(es) as the infant(s) deliver(s).

If the first fetus is not vertex, some obstetricians will perform a cesarean for delivery except in cases of nonviable infants. Even in the case of frank or complete breech, the primary danger in a nonvertex delivery is the development of interlocking heads, where the head of a second fetus descends into the pelvis before the head of the fetus that is being delivered. If this occurs, a vaginal delivery without injury or death of one or both infants is virtually impossible. The only remedy in this case is an emergency cesarean. If both fetuses of a twin gestation present as breeches, the delivery may be vaginal. An assistant may palpate both heads. As the first infant delivers, one assistant may try to prevent the second head from descending prior to the birth of the first infant. If the first fetus of a multiple gestation is vertex, the delivery may be vaginal unless there are prior contraindications. Once the first infant has been delivered, the succeeding fetus(es) is (are) evaluated as previously indicated and a decision of delivery route can be made prior to each birth. In a 16-year experience at Columbia University, Loucopoulos and colleagues pointed out that if the operator was not confident with vaginal maneuvers in multifetal pregnancies, a cesarean was performed.[68]

In the delivery room, all fetuses are monitored until they are delivered. If a cesarean is performed, the monitoring continues until the delivery room staff is ready and the patient is going to be prepped. The actual monitoring may have technical difficulties. If possible, fetal monitors with different ultrasound frequencies may be used. Often this can be done by using machines from two different manufacturers. If transducers with the same frequency are used, they may interfere with each other and produce strange sounds and readings on both monitors. (This is the same effect as two radio stations trying to transmit on the same frequency at the same time.) If two different transducers are not available, the first fetus can be connected to an internal ECG lead once the membranes are ruptured and the second fetus can be monitored with the ultrasound transducer. If there is a third fetus, an ultrasound imaging machine can usually be used to watch the third heart, because the frequency of these machines is usually higher than those used by the fetal monitors.

Researchers have tried to determine the best route of delivery for multiple gestations by analyzing the outcomes of the infants. However, this is complicated by the fact that labor itself probably affects the outcome. Norman and colleagues studied 57 sets of twins who were delivered by cesarean and found that androstenedione was consistently increased in the first twin compared to the second if the mother had been in either latent or active labor just prior to the cesarean.[69] Laros and colleagues studied the morbidity and mortality of 206 sets of twins with a mean gestational age of 34 weeks from 1976 to 1985 and found that there were no differences between those delivered vaginally and by cesarean, regardless of the effect of labor.[70]

The interval between births has always been of some concern. However, the advent of fetal monitors has allayed some of that concern. If the second or additional fetuses have a good tracing, there is no compelling reason to deliver the next infant in a hurry if both the mother and fetus are in good condition. This was confirmed in two studies that looked at the effects of outcome of second twins with increasing intervals between deliveries. Both studies could find no effect of delivery interval, although Rayburn's work found that there was a higher incidence of cesarean delivery if the interval was greater than 15 minutes.[71,72] Following the delivery of the first infant, the cervix may remain open or may close slightly. Since internal versions are no longer done for singleton deliveries, obstetricians have been reluctant to reach inside to perform an internal version on the second twin if necessary. Nevertheless, it remains an acceptable procedure. Some may prefer an external version instead. Gocke and colleagues performed a retrospective review of 136 twins with weight greater than 1500 g and analyzed the morbidity–mortality of the second nonvertex infant following elective breech extraction, external version, or immediate cesarean.[73] There were no differences.

Following the birth, intraventricular hemorrhage may occur. The effect of birth order has been studied for its effect on this complication in the small infant. Pearlman and Batton studied 29 twins less than 1500 g and found no effect.[74] On the other hand, Morales and colleagues studied 156 twins less than 1500 g and found that the second twin had both an increased incidence of intraventricular hemorrhage and an increased incidence of respiratory distress.[75] They also confirmed previous studies that the difference in weights and not the delivery route was a factor in the incidence of hemorrhage.

OPERATIVE VAGINAL DELIVERY

Operative vaginal delivery can be either a vacuum extraction or a forceps delivery. In the past, these deliveries were used to help shorten the second stage of labor, to avoid a cesarean, and to deal with cases of fetal distress. Today the indications have narrowed considerably because of the decreased morbidity from cesarean delivery and the potential to injure the infant and mother from the delivery instruments. Today appropriate indications for operative vaginal delivery may include inability of the mother to push in the presence of an adequate pelvis and normal size fetus; relative contraindication to pushing, such as cardiac disease or cerebral vascular problem; or development of fetal distress with the fetus at a low station and with an adequate pelvis.

Both vacuum and forceps apply traction to the fetal head, but the vacuum applies its force to the scalp while the forceps pull against the bony parts of the head. In addition, the vacuum cup, especially the modern Silastic version, is not traumatic by itself when it is placed. However, when the vacuum is applied, an increasing amount of force is applied to the fetus. Duchon and colleagues measured the actual force and found that 18 to 20 kg of force could be applied before the cup slips off the head.[76] After the delivery, the primary complication that occurs is a cephalohematoma of the scalp. This is potentially dangerous because a layer of blood 1 cm thick beneath the surface of the scalp over the entire surface of the head, although it may look innocuous, may represent one half of the infant's blood volume. One study found approximately the same incidence—about 4%—of cephalohematomas in vacuum and forceps deliveries.[77] However, most studies report an increased number of hematomas in vacuum extractions—up to 23%—compared to forceps deliveries (6%).[78,79] Berkus and colleagues compared 84 deliveries by vacuum extraction to 84 vaginal deliveries and found no difference in neonatal morbidity.[80] They concluded that the vacuum extractor was a safe instrument for the delivery room.

If an operative vaginal delivery is performed, a number of guides to making this decision should be present. The cervix must be completely dilated and the membranes ruptured. In addition, the mother should be in the delivery room and an anesthesiologist should be available. The bladder is drained just prior to the delivery. The position of the fetal head is identified. The shape of the maternal pelvis is evaluated or known. Finally, the obstetrician should be experienced in the type of delivery to be performed.

If a vacuum delivery is performed, the cup is applied between contractions. However, vacuum and traction are applied only with contractions. As the head delivers, the vacuum is generally lost. The operator attempts to avoid dislodging the vacuum cup in a manner that can cause trauma. The rest of the delivery is then performed as usual.

There are four types of forceps deliveries. An outlet forceps delivery is done when the scalp is at the introitus without separating the labia, the fetal skull has reached the pelvic floor, the sagittal suture is in the anterior–posterior diameter or in the right or left occiput anterior or posterior position, and the fetal head is at or on the perineum. A rotation of the fetal head cannot exceed 45° in an outlet forceps delivery. A low forceps delivery is done when the leading position of the skull is at +2 station or more. Two subdivisions of low forceps are rotation less than 45° and rotation greater than 45°. A midforceps delivery is done when the fetal head is engaged but is above +2 station.[81]

For more information on the techniques of forceps deliveries, the reader is referred to Laufe's book[3] or other textbooks. Only classical forceps at lower stations are described here. If a forceps delivery is indicated, the obstetrician determines the degree of molding of the fetal head and chooses an instrument accordingly. In the presence of molding, a Simpson's forceps or equivalent with its 18-cm blades can be used. If there is no molding, an Elliot or Tucker-McLane, with its 15-cm blades, is the more usual choice for this smaller or rounder head.

In the occiput anterior position, the left branch of the forceps is inserted first (Fig. 86-3). The second and third fingers of the right hand are used to guide the blade along the scalp and inside the cervix while the thumb helps push the blade in. Excessive force need not be used to insert the forceps. If insertion does not go easily, the forceps may be at the wrong angle. Once the blade has been inserted, it is adjusted if necessary (Fig. 86-4). Then the right branch of the forceps is inserted. Once both blades are in, the position is checked for the correct application prior to applying traction.

Traction is then applied in the axis of the vagina. Although the traction does not necessarily need to be done during a contraction, the descent of the fetus may be more effective if traction is applied during a contraction. When the fetal head descends, the blades may be left on until the head is completely outside of the vagina, or they may be removed just as the head starts to deliver. If the blades are left on, the combination of the head and blades may cause more trauma to the perineum. Note that traction includes a vertical force downward on the forceps shanks and a horizontal force on the handles toward the operator. As the vertex descends, the downward force is lowered as the vertex passes under the pubic symphysis and the horizontal traction is increased. When the forceps blades are removed, the vertex will deliver over the episiotomy.

In the last decade, much has appeared in the literature concerning the complications of forceps deliveries, particularly intraventricular hemorrhage. Welch and Bottoms did a multiple regression study on intraventricular hemorrhage and found that forceps and route of delivery were not related to the incidence of intraventricular hemorrhage.[82] Factors that were related included weight less than 1250 g, 1-minute Apgar less

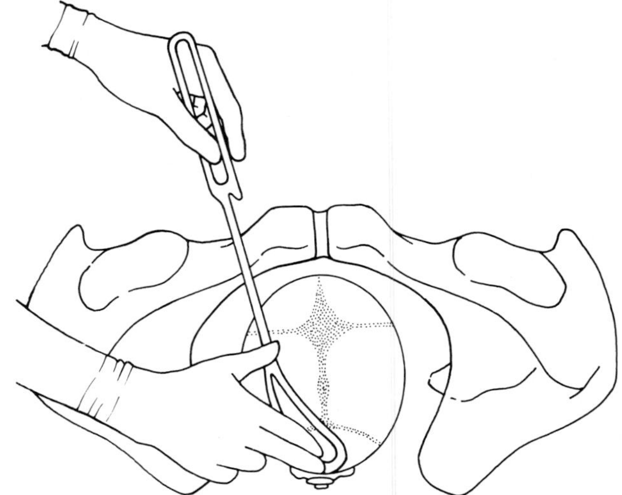

FIGURE 86–3. The left blade of the forceps is inserted. (The vulva is not shown in this drawing so that the relationship between the forceps blade and the fetal head can be seen more clearly.)

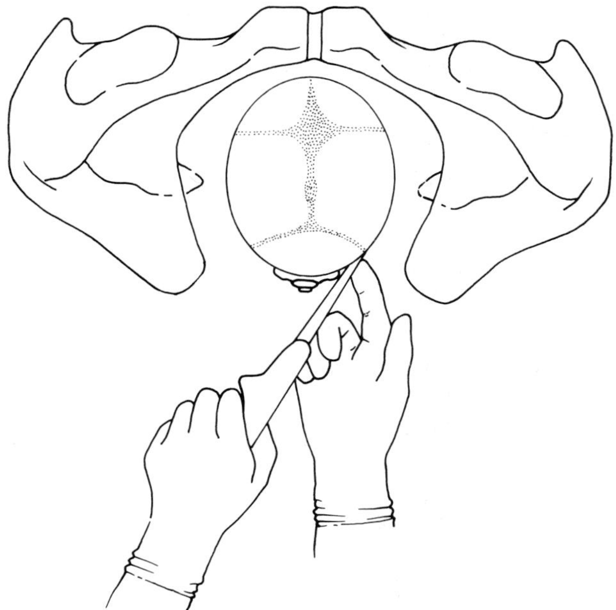

FIGURE 86–4. The position of the forceps is adjusted, if necessary.

than 7, respiratory distress syndrome, and neonatal mortality. Other than cephalohematomas and the resulting neonatal jaundice, several studies also did not find any difference in neonatal outcome between vacuum and forceps deliveries.[83–85] Another question that has been studied is whether a trial attempt at forceps followed by cesarean if the attempt fails is associated with morbidity or mortality. Two recent studies failed to show any increase in fetal or maternal morbidity–mortality.[86,87]

There is no question that the use of forceps may be associated with neonatal morbidity. Chiswick and James found abnormal neurologic behavior in 23% of babies following a Kielland's forcep delivery.[88] This was significantly higher than that in babies from a spontaneous vaginal delivery. O'Driscoll and colleagues found that in autopsies of vertex firstborn infants who died, the only cases where intraventricular hemorrhages were found followed a forceps delivery.[89] However, long-term morbidity is more controversial. Friedman and colleagues matched patients with labor abnormalities and compared the outcomes of midforceps with spontaneous deliveries who had the same labor anomaly. When 7-year-olds were compared, the children who had undergone midforceps delivery had a slightly lower IQ than those from the spontaneous deliveries.[90] However, the patients were not matched for fetal distress or other indications. In Dierker and Rosen's studies, where the indications were matched, there was morbidity in the midforceps group but there was also morbidity in the control group that was delivered with the same indication.[91,92] The differences between the two groups were not significant. In an even longer-term follow-up, Nilsen studied 62 males who were born with forceps and 38 who were born by vacuum extraction.[93] They were studied at age 18, based on the draft records in Norway, and no differences were found between them and the average Norwegian, except that the forceps group had a higher IQ than the national average. From all these studies, we conclude that a midforceps delivery in selected cases is safe when performed by an experienced obstetrician.

CESAREAN DELIVERY

In various situations, a cesarean delivery is performed for necessary reasons. For example, in cases of fetal stress or distress when the scalp pH is less than 7.2 or there is a severe prolonged bradycardia before the cervix is completely dilated, or for other reasons, a cesarean delivery may be indicated. In preparation for the delivery, a patient who has fetal distress may benefit from an intravenous tocolytic to relax the uterus. If the distress is caused by a tetanic contraction or placental insufficiency, the relaxation of the uterus may improve the fetal status. Shekarloo and colleagues studied 36 cases of fetal distress and found that the tracing of 32 fetuses improved after intravenous terbutaline.[94] In the delivery suite, the physician can also be prepared in cases that are more likely to result in a cesarean. For example, placental abruption is fairly rare but is increased in cases of diabetes and preeclampsia.[95] Other cases that may require cesarean deliveries are breech presentations, chorioamnionitis, patients with meconium-stained fluid, and obvious abnormalities of labor that lead to arrest of descent or dystocia.

The type of anesthesia for the cesarean has been covered earlier in this text, and a complete description of the technique of the cesarean operation may also be found elsewhere.[1,96] If the cesarean delivery is an emergency, a vertical incision may be made in the skin to facilitate a more rapid delivery. If speed is not essential, a Pfannenstiehl incision can be made. If more room may be necessary for a large infant or one with a large malformation, a Maylard muscle-cutting incision may be considered, since it will increase the amount of available room for the delivery by about 25%.[97] Once the abdomen has been entered, a bladder flap is created and the uterine incision is made. If the lower uterine segment is well developed, a low transverse incision is recommended, because the potential complications in future pregnancies are lessened with this type of incision. If the lower uterine segment is not well developed or if there is a malpresentation, especially in a premature infant, a vertical incision may be made in the uterus.

In cases of difficult abdominal deliveries or in cases of multiple births by cesarean section, there has been some concern over the length of time from uterine incision to the time of birth. Anderson and colleagues found no effect on Apgar scores or umbilical blood gases from increasing incision-to-birth times.[98] Once the infant has been delivered, a segment of the umbilical cord is obtained for blood gas studies and additional cord blood is obtained if necessary. The location of the placenta is noted and it is then removed. It occasionally will deliver spontaneously from the uterus, but it is usually removed manually. If there is chorioamnionitis, both aerobic and anaerobic cultures are obtained at the time of cesarean.

Much has also been written in the last decade on the use of antibiotics at the time of cesarean, particularly when the mother has been in labor or has had prolonged rupture or membranes. There has been agreement that antibiotics help the patient in labor. However, the type of drug and its duration have been controversial. Recently, McGregor evaluated a regimen that uses only a single dose of cefotetan at the time of delivery and found no difference between it and another multiple-dose regimen.[99] Nevertheless, Duff pointed out that there was no evidence that any regimen from the newer cephalosporins was any better than ampicillin or a first-generation cephalosporin.[100] Prior to the delivery, the use of antibiotics has generally not been recommended because of the fear that a diagnosis of infection in the neonate would be difficult. However, Gibbs studied 45 infants of mothers who had intra-amniotic infections and found that 21% of the infants of mothers without treatment developed neonatal sepsis, whereas none of the infants of mothers who were treated with antibiotics in the intrapartum period developed sepsis.[101]

Perhaps the most controversial aspects of cesarean deliveries are their indications. In the last two decades, the rate of cesareans has increased from about 5% to 25% of deliveries in this country. In 1980, Bottoms and colleagues found that the increase was due to dystocia (33.4%), repeat cesarean (23.1%), breech presentations (18.8%), fetal distress (13.2%), and other causes (11.2%).[102] At the same time, Haesslein and Niswander pointed out that electronic fetal monitoring indications classically thought to be distress were wrong 75% of the time and that some term infants with normal tracings had low 5-minute Apgar scores.[103] They also pointed out that the diagnosis of distress at delivery was less crucial to neurologic outcome than the presence of preexisting chronic fetal distress. These observations make the increase of cesareans due to fetal distress somewhat disturbing.

By 1987, the continued rise in the cesarean rate was due to repeat cesarean (47%), dystocia (19%), fetal distress (16%), breech and other malpresentations (12%), and other causes (4%).[104] The lack of vaginal births after previous cesareans (VBAC) was particularly disturbing, especially with the multitude of articles that have described the safety of VBAC. All the articles have described success rates from 60% to 80%, and uterine ruptures after a low transverse incision have been 1% or less.[105–107] Even cases such as women with multiple gestations or multiple previous low transverse cesarean deliveries may safely deliver vaginally.[108,109] At the same time, clinicians continue to avoid a vaginal delivery after a previous classical uterine incision. One recent report documented up to 13% of the patients with atypical scars and 6% dehiscence with a history of a classical incision.[110]

Unfortunately, even with the documented safety of vaginal births after cesarean births in selected patients, less than half the hospitals in the United States allowed a trial of labor after previous cesarean birth in 1984.[111]

In an attempt to decrease the primary cesarean rate, O'Driscoll and colleagues in Ireland suggested that the cesarean rate in the United States could be decreased by managing labor actively with amniotomy and liberal use of oxytocin.[112] At the time of their article, the cesarean rate in the United States was 15.2%, whereas in Dublin it was 4.8%. At the same time, the perinatal morbidity and mortality did not seem to be improved by the increased cesarean rate. This report stimulated a series of three more articles from both sides of the Atlantic Ocean arguing the merits of that statement.[113–115] The American group argued that the populations in the two hospitals were vastly different, which accounted for the differing cesarean rates. The United States rate continues to rise whereas the Dublin rate has remained about 5%. In Canada, Akoury and colleagues applied O'Driscoll's techniques and were able to reduce the cesarean rate for 552 patients there from 13% to 4.3%.[116] Thus, the increasing cesarean rate in the United States remains controversial.

CONCLUSION

Modern obstetrics has many tools for a safe delivery of the infant. Although there are some instances when operative delivery may be overutilized, the number of options available to the obstetrician has increased with the development of technology. For a healthy infant, the most important points in the care of the mother are the careful monitoring of the patient and her fetus. In the case of a difficult delivery, an experienced obstetrician and an anesthesiologist may be required. A pediatrician is needed in the delivery room to care for a premature or depressed infant.

REFERENCES

1. Cunningham FG, MacDonald PC, Gant NF. Williams obstetrics. 18th ed. Norwalk, CT: Appleton & Lange, 1989.
2. Mattingly RF, Thompson JD. Te Linde's operative gynecology. 6th ed. Philadelphia: JB Lippincott, 1985.
3. Laufe LE. Obstetric forceps. New York: Harper & Row, 1968.
4. Lazer S, Biale Y, Mazor M. Lewenthal H, Insler V. Complications associated with the macrosomic fetus. Journal of Reproductive Medicine 1986;31:501.
5. Acker DB, Sachs BP, Friedman EA. Risk factors for shoulder dystocia. Obstet Gynecol 1985;66:762.
6. Wikstrom I, Axelsson O, Bergstrom R, Meirik O. Traumatic in-

jury in large-for-date infants. Acta Obstet Gynecol Scand 1988;67:259.
7. American College of Obstetricians and Gynecologists. Standards for obstetrics-gynecology services. 7th ed. Washington, DC: American College of Obstetricians and Gynecologists, 1989.
8. Bassell GM, Humayun SG, Marx GF. Maternal bearing down efforts—another fetal risk? Obstet Gynecol 1980;56:39.
9. Johnstone FD, Aboelmagd, Harouny AK. Maternal posture in second stage and fetal acid base status. Br J Obstet Gynecol 1986;94:753.
10. Beynon CL. Midline episiotomy as a routine procedure. Br J Obstet Gynecol 1974;81:126.
11. Thorp JM, Bowes WA, Brame RG, Cefalo R. Selected use of midline episiotomy: effect on perineal trauma. Obstet Gynecol 1987;70:260.
12. Thorp JM, Bowes WA. Episiotomy: can its routine use be defended? Am J Obstet Gynecol 1989;160:1027.
13. Wilcox LS, Strobino DM, Baruffi G, Dellinger WS. Episiotomy and its role in the incidence of perineal lacerations in a maternity center and a tertiary hospital obstetric service. Am J Obstet Gynecol 1989;160:1047.
14. Gass MS, Dunn C, Stys SJ. Effect of episiotomy on the frequency of vaginal outlet lacerations. Journal of Reproductive Medicine 1986;31:240.
15. Peisner DB, Rosen MG. Unpublished data.
16. Kriewall TJ, Stys SJ, McPherson GK. Neonatal head shape after delivery: an index of molding. J Perinat Med 1977;6:260.
17. Sorbe B, Dahlgren S. Some important factors in the molding of the fetal head during vaginal delivery—a photographic study. Int J Gynecol Obstet 1983;21:205.
18. Klebe JG, Espersen T, Poulsen EH. Heart frequency of the fetus at birth. Acta Obstet Gynecol Scand 1986;65:387.
19. Kohno H, Furuhashi N, Fukaya T, Tachibana Y, Shinkawa O, Suzuki M. Serum cortisol levels of maternal vein, umbilical artery, and umbilical vein classified by mode of delivery. Gynecol Obstet Invest 1984;17:301.
20. Tetlow HJ, Pipkin FB. Studies on the effect of mode of delivery on the renin-angiotensin system in mother and fetus at term. Br J Obstet Gynecol 1983;90:220.
21. Yao AC, Lind J. Placental transfusion. JAMA 1974;127:128.
22. Odell LD, Seski A. Episiotomy blood loss. Am J Obstet Gynecol 1947;54:51.
23. Sorensen SM, Bondesen H, Istre O, Vilmann P. Perineal rupture following vaginal delivery. Acta Obstet Gynecol Scand 1988;67:315.
24. Monberg J, Hammen S. Ruptured episiotomia resutured primarily. Acta Obstet Gynecol Scand 1987;66:163.
25. Lieberman BA. Repair to injuries of the genital tract. Clin Obstet Gynecol 1980;7:621.
26. Levine MG, Holroyde J, Woods JR, Siddiqi TA, Scott M, Miodovnik M. Birth trauma: incidence and predisposing factors. Obstet Gynecol 1984;63:792.
27. Acker DB, Gregory KD, Sachs BP, Friedman EA. Risk factors for Erb-Duchenne palsy. Obstet Gynecol 1988;71:389.
28. McFarland LV, Raskin M, Daling JR, Benedetti TJ. Erb/Duchenne's palsy: a consequence of fetal macrosomia and method of delivery. Obstet Gynecol 1986;68:784.
29. Gross TL, Sokol RJ, Williams T, Thompson K. Shoulder dystocia: a fetal-physician risk. Am J Obstet Gynecol 1987;156:1408.
30. Gonik B, Stringer CA, Held B. An alternate maneuver for management of shoulder dystocia. Am J Obstet Gynecol 1983;145:882.
31. Chavis WM. A new instrument for the management of shoulder dystocia. Int J Gynecol Obstet 1979;16:331.
32. Sandberg EC. The Zavanelli maneuver: a potentially revolutionary method for the resolution of shoulder dystocia. Am J Obstet Gynecol 1985;152:479.
33. Sandberg EC. The Zavanelli maneuver extended: progression of a revolutionary concept. Am J Obstet Gynecol 1988;158:1347.
34. Johnson JWC, Porter J, Kellner KR, Bailey HWA, Miller D, Mosely TH. Abdominal rescue after incomplete delivery secondary to large fetal sacrococcygeal teratoma. Obstet Gynecol 1988;71:981.
35. Iffy L, Apuzzio JJ, Cohen-Addad N, Zwolska-Demczuk B, Francis-Lane M, Olenczak J. Abdominal rescue after entrapment of the aftercoming head. Am J Obstet Gynecol 1986;154:623.
36. Gresham EL. Birth trauma. Pediatr Clin North Am 1975;22:317.
37. Morales WJ, Koerten J. Obstetric management and intraventricular hemorrhage in very-low-birth-weight infants. Obstet Gynecol 1986;68:35.
38. Svenningsen L, Lindemann R, Eidal K. Measurements of fetal head compression pressure during bearing down and their relationship to the condition to the newborn. Acta Obstet Gynecol Scand 1988;67:129.
39. Minchom P, Niswander K, Chalmers I. Antecedents and outcome of very early neonatal seizures in infants born at or after term. Br J Obstet Gynecol 1987;94:431.
40. Hageman JR, Conley M, Francis K, et al. Delivery room management of meconium staining of the amniotic fluid and the development of meconium aspiration syndrome. J Perinatol 1988;8:127.
41. Cohen-Addad N, Chatterjee M, Bautista A. Intrapartum suctioning of meconium: comparative efficacy of bulb syringe and De Lee catheter. J Perinatol 1987;7:111.
42. Falciglia HS. Failure to prevent meconium aspiration syndrome. Obstet Gynecol 1988;71:349.
43. Linder N, Aranda JV, Tsur M, et al. Need for endotracheal intubation and suction in meconium-stained neonates. J Pediatr 1988;112:613.
44. McKlveen RE, Ostheimer GW. Resuscitation of the newborn. Clin Obstet Gynecol 1987;30:611.
45. Jovanovic R, Nguyen HT. Experimental meconium aspiration in guinea pigs. Obstet Gynecol 1989;73:652.
46. Wenstrom KD, Parsons MT. The prevention of meconium aspiration in labor using amnioinfusion. Obstet Gynecol 1989;73:647.
47. Sunoo C, Kosasa TS, Hale RW. Meconium aspiration syndrome without evidence of fetal distress in early labor before elective cesarean delivery. Obstet Gynecol 1989;73:707.
48. Macfarlane PI, Heaf DP. Pulmonary function in children after neonatal meconium aspiration syndrome. Arch Dis Child 1988;63:368.
49. Stevens JC, Eigen H, Wysomierski D. Absence of long term pulmonary sequelae after mild meconium aspiration syndrome. Pediatr Pulmonol 1988;5:74.
50. Plauche WC, Gruich FG, Bourgeois MO. Hysterectomy at the time of cesarean section: analysis of 108 cases. Obstet Gynecol 1981;58:459.
51. Catanzarite VA, Moffitt KD, Baker ML, Awadalla SG, Argubright KF, Perkins RP. New approaches to the management of acute puerperal uterine inversion. Obstet Gynecol 1986;68:7S.
52. Brenner WE, Bruce RD, Hendricks CH. The characteristics and perils of breech presentation. Am J Obstet Gynecol 1974;118:700.
53. Fianu S, Vaclavinkova V. The site of placental attachment as a factor in the aetiology of breech presentation. Acta Obstet Gynecol Scand 1978;57:371.

54. Stewart A, Webb J, Giles D, Hewitt D. Malignant disease in childhood and diagnostic irradiation in utero. Lancet 1956; 2:447.
55. Philipson EH, Rosen MG. Trends in the frequency of cesarean births. Clin Obstet Gynecol 1985;28:691.
56. Luterkort M, Marsál K. Umbilical cord acid-base state and Apgar score in term breech neonates. Acta Obstet Gynecol Scand 1987;66:57.
57. Øian P, Skråmm I, Hannisdal E. Bjøro K. Breech delivery an obstetrical analysis. Acta Obstet Gynecol Scand 1988;67:75.
58. Rosen MG, Chik L. The effect of delivery route on outcome in breech presentation. Am J Obstet Gynecol 1984;148:909.
59. Collea JV, Chein C, Quilligan EJ. The randomized management of term frank breech presentation: a study of 208 cases. Am J Obstet Gynecol 1980;137:235.
60. Flanagan TA, Mulchahey KM, Korenbrot CC, Green JR, Laros RK. Management of term breech presentation. Am J Obstet Gynecol 1987;156:1492.
61. Gimovsky ML, Wallace RL, Schifrin BS, Paul RH. Randomized management of the nonfrank breech presentation at term: a preliminary report. Am J Obstet Gynecol 1983;146:34.
62. Ophir E, Oettinger M, Yagoda A, Markovits Y, Rojansky N, Shapiro H. Breech presentation after cesarean section: always a section? Am J Obstet Gynecol 1989;161:25.
63. Schutte MF, van Hemel OJS, van de Berg C, van de Pol A. Perinatal mortality in breech presentations as compared to vertex presentations in singleton pregnancies: an analysis based upon 57,819 computer-registered pregnancies in The Netherlands. Eur J Obstet Gynecol Reprod Biol 1985;19:391.
64. Effer SB, Saigal S, Rand C, et al. Effect of delivery method on outcomes in the very low-birth weight breech infant: is the improved survival related to cesarean section or other perinatal maneuvers? Am J Obstet Gynecol 1983;145:123.
65. Westgren LMR, Songster G, Paul RH. Preterm breech delivery: another retrospective study. Obstet Gynecol 1985;66:481.
66. Nisell H, Bistoletti P, Palme C. Preterm breech delivery. Acta Obstet Gynecol Scand 1981;60:363.
67. Tejani N, Verma U, Shiffman R, Chayen B. Effect of route of delivery on periventricular/intraventricular hemorrhage in the low-birth-weight fetus with a breech presentation. JRM 1987;32:911.
68. Loucopoulos A, Jewelewicz R. Management of multifetal pregnancies: sixteen years' experience at the Sloane Hospital for Women. Am J Obstet Gynecol 1982;143:902.
69. Norman RJ, Deppe WM, Joubert SM, Marivate M. Umbilical artery concentrations of androstenedione increase in early labour in the leading twin fetus. Br J Obstet Gynecol 1984;91:776.
70. Laros RD, Dattel BJ. Management of twin pregnancy: the vaginal route is still safe. Am J Obstet Gynecol 1988;158:1330.
71. Rayburn WF, Lavin JP, Miodovnik M, Varner MW. Multiple gestation: time interval between delivery of the first and second twins. Obstet Gynecol 1984;63:502.
72. Chervenak FA, Johnson RE, Youcha S, Hobbins JC, Berkowitz RL. Intrapartum management of twin gestation. Obstet Gynecol 1985;65:119.
73. Gocke SE, Nageotte MP, Garite T, Towers CV, Dorcester W. Management of the nonvertex second twin: primary cesarean section, external version, or primary breech extraction. Am J Obstet Gynecol 1989;161:111.
74. Pearlman SA, Batton DG. Effect of birth order on intraventricular hemorrhage in very low birth weight twins. Obstet Gynecol 1988;71:358.
75. Morales WJ, O'Brien WF, Knuppel RA, Gaylord S, Hayes P. The effect of mode of delivery on the risk of intraventricular hemorrhage in nondiscordant twin gestations under 1500 g. Obstet Gynecol 1989;73:107.
76. Duchon MA, DeMund MA, Brown RH. Laboratory comparison of modern vacuum extractors. Obstet Gynecol 1988;71:155.
77. Broekhuizen FF, Washington JM, Johnson F, Hamilton PR. Vacuum extraction versus forceps delivery: indications and complications, 1979–1984. Obstet Gynecol 1987;69:338.
78. Thacker KE, Lim T, Drew JH. Cephalohaematoma: a 10-year review. Aust NZ J Obstet Gynaecol 1987;27:210.
79. Baerthlein WC, Moodley S, Stinson SK. Comparison of maternal and neonatal morbidity in midforceps delivery and midpelvis vacuum extraction. Obstet Gynecol 1986;67:594.
80. Berkus MD, Ramamurthy RS, O'Connor PS, Brown K, Hayashi RH. Cohort study of Silastic obstetric vacuum cup deliveries. I. Safety of the instrument. Obstet Gynecol 1985;66:503.
81. ACOG Committee Opinion, Committee on Obstetrics: Maternal and Fetal Medicine, Number 71, August, 1989.
82. Welch RA, Bottoms SF. Reconsideration of head comparison and intraventricular hemorrhage in the vertex very-low-birth-weight fetus. Obstet Gynecol 1986;68:29.
83. Healy DL, Quinn MA, Pepperell RJ. Rotational delivery of the fetus: Kielland's forceps and two other methods compared. Br J Obstet Gynecol 1982;89:501.
84. Vacca A, Grant A, Wyatt G, Chalmers I. Portsmouth operative delivery trial: a comparison of vacuum extraction and forceps delivery.
85. Herabutya Y, Pratak O, Prasong B. Kielland's forceps or ventouse—a comparison. Br J Obstet Gynecol 1988;95:483.
86. Boyd ME, Usher RH, McLean FH, Norman BE. Failed forceps. Obstet Gynecol 1986;68:779.
87. Lowe B. Fear of failure; a place for the trial of instrumental delivery. Br J Obstet Gynaecol 1987;94:60.
88. Chiswick ML, James DK. Kielland's forceps: association with neonatal morbidity and mortality. Br Med J 1979;1:7.
89. O'Driscoll K, Meagher D, MacDonald D, Geoghegan F. Traumatic intracranial haemorrhage in firstborn infants and delivery with obstetrical forceps. Br J Obstet Gynecol 1981;88:577.
90. Friedman EA, Sachtleben-Murray MR, Dahrouge D, Neff RK. Long-term effects of labor and delivery on offspring. A matched pair analysis. Am J Obstet Gynecol 1984;150:941.
91. Dierker LJ, Rosen MG, Thompson K, DeBanne S, Lynn P. The midforceps: maternal and neonatal outcomes. Am J Obstet Gynecol 1985;152:176.
92. Dierker LJ, Rosen MG, Thompson K, Lynn P. Midforceps deliveries: long-term outcome of infants. Am J Obstet Gynecol 1986;154:764.
93. Nilsen ST. Boys born by forceps and vacuum extraction examined at 18 years of age. Acta Obstet Gynecol Scand 1984; 63:549.
94. Shekarloo A, Mendez-Bauer C, Cook V, Freese U. Terbutaline (intravenous bolus) for the treatment of acute intrapartum fetal distress. Am J Obstet Gynecol 1989;160:615.
95. Krohn M, Voigt L, McKnight B, Daling JR, Starzyk P, Beneditti T. Correlates of placental abruption. Br J Obstet Gynecol 1987;94:333.
96. Kerr JMM. The technic of cesarean section, with special reference to the lower uterine segment incision. Am J Obstet Gynecol 1926;12:729.
97. Ayers JWT, Moreley GW. Surgical incision for cesarean section. Obstet Gynecol 1987;70:706.
98. Anderson HF, Auster GH, Marx GF, Merkatz IR. Neonatal status in relation to incision intervals, obstetric factors, and anesthesia at cesarean delivery. Am J Perinatol 1987;4:279.
99. McGregor JA, Gordon SF, Krotec J, Poindexter AN. Results of a randomized, multicenter, comparative trial of a single dose of cefotetan versus multiple doses of cefoxitin as prophylaxis in cesarean section. Am J Obstet Gynecol 1988;158:701.
100. Duff P. Prophylactic antibiotics for cesarean delivery: a simple

cost-effective strategy for prevention of postoperative morbidity. Am J Obstet Gynecol 1987;157:794.

101. Gibbs RS, Dinsmoor MJ, Newton ER, Ramamurthy RS. A randomized trial of intrapartum versus immediate postpartum treatment of women with intra-amniotic infection. Obstet Gynecol 1988;72:823.
102. Bottoms SF, Rosen MG, Sokol RJ. The increase in the cesarean birth rate. N Engl J Med 1980;302:559.
103. Haesslein HC, Niswander KR. Fetal distress in term pregnancies. Am J Obstet Gynecol 1980;137:245.
104. Shiono PH, McNellis D, Rhoads GG. Reasons for the rising cesarean delivery rates. Obstet Gynecol 1987;69:696.
105. Nielsen TF, Ljungblad U, Hagverg H. Rupture and dehiscence of cesarean section scar during pregnancy and delivery. Am J Obstet Gynecol 1989;160:569.
106. Jarrell MA, Ashmead GG, Mann LI. Vaginal delivery after cesarean section: a five-year study. Obstet Gynecol 1985;65:628.
107. Clark SL, Eglinton GS, Beall M, Phelan JP. Effect of indication for previous cesarean section on subsequent delivery outcome in patients undergoing a trial of labor. JRM 1984;29:22.
108. Novas J, Myers SA, Gleicher N. Obstetric outcome with more than one previous cesarean section. Am J Obstet Gynecol 1989;160:364.
109. Gilbert L, Saunders N, Sharp F. The management of multiple pregnancy in women with a lower-segment caesarean scar. Is a repeat caesarean section really the "safe" option? Br J Obstet Gynecol 1988;95:1312.
110. Halperin ME, Moore DC, Hannah WJ. Classical versus low-segment transverse incision for preterm caesarean section: maternal complications and outcome of subsequent pregnancies. Br J Obstet Gynaecol 1988;95:990.
111. Shiono PH, Fielden JG, McNellis D, Rhoads GG, Perse WH. Recent trend in cesarean birth and trial of labor rates in the United States. JAMA 1987;257:494.
112. O'Driscoll F, Foley M. Correlation of decrease in perinatal mortality and increase in cesarean section rates. Obstet Gynecol 1983;61:1.
113. Leveno FJ, Cunningham FG, Pritchard JA. Cesarean section: an answer to the House of Horne. Am J Obstet Gynecol 1985;153:838.
114. O'Driscoll K, Foley M, MacDonald D, Stronge J. Cesarean section and perinatal outcome: response from the House of Horne. Am J Obstet Gynecol 1988;158:449.
115. Leveno KJ, Cunningham FG, Pritchard JA. Cesarean section: the House of Horne revisited. Am J Obstet Gynecol 1989;160:78.
116. Akoury HA, Brodie G, Caddick R, McLaughin VD, Pugh PA. Active management of labor and operative delivery in nulliparous women. Am J Obstet Gynecol 1988;158:255.

87

CHAPTER

PREMATURE LABOR

Erol Amon

EPIDEMIOLOGY AND DEMOGRAPHY

Definitions of preterm birth differ. According to the World Health Organization, a preterm birth is any birth, regardless of birth weight, that occurs before 37 menstrual weeks gestation.[1] Traditionally pediatricians have defined prematurity as a birth weight of 2500 g or less in a liveborn infant.[2] *Williams' Obstetrics* defines preterm birth as a birth occurring before 38 menstrual weeks.[3] In this chapter I will use *preterm* to describe a fetus or pregnancy before 37 weeks gestation, based on the best obstetric criteria.

The lower gestational age limit for a preterm birth (as distinct from an abortion) is 20 weeks gestation. In the absence of gestational age data, I advocate using a birth weight criterion of 350 g.[4] This lower limit is based on traditional medical definitions and some statutory legal definitions of stillbirth, rather than on clinical utility (ie, the neonate's ability to survive).[5,6] Although neonatal survival has been reported at 22 and 23 weeks gestation, the break-even or 50% survival rate does not commonly occur until at least 25 to 26 weeks gestation, or 750 g.[7]

The current classification of low birth weight (LBW) is summarized in Table 87-1.[7] Many mildly preterm infants have birth weights of 2500 g or more; conversely, many moderately LBW infants (1500 to 2499 g) are actually full-term. In some series nearly half of LBW infants were considered term.[8]

Preterm birth is one of the most important issues in reproductive medicine. It is directly responsible for 75% to 90% of all neonatal deaths not due to lethal congenital malformations.[9,10] Preterm birth also accounts for a large proportion of perinatal mortality and short- and long-term neonatal morbidity. The major diseases of the preterm infant are due to organ immaturity; therefore, their incidence is inversely related to gestational age. These conditions include respiratory distress syndrome, bronchopulmonary dysplasia, patent ductus arteriosus, necrotizing enterocolitis, hyperbilirubinemia, apnea of prematurity, intraventricular hemorrhage, retinopathy of prematurity, and neonatal sepsis. In the past, if preterm infants survived at all, they faced a high risk of significant handicap (blindness, deafness, cerebral palsy, or mental retardation). Today, only 7.5% of very LBW infants (< 1500 g) have a major handicapping condition. The smallest of these surviving infants (450 to 800 g) have a rate of about 25%.[11]

Because up to 30% of gestational assignments are inaccurate, many clinical epidemiologists have come to rely on a more accurate figure: birth weight. Using the best and most recent data available for the United States, the rate of LBW is 6.9% and the rate of preterm birth is 10.2%.[12] It is disheartening that despite the technical and theoretical advances in reproductive medicine, these rates have not significantly decreased in the last two decades.[12] Preterm birth and LBW differ in their pathogenesis but share many predisposing factors (Table 87-2).[13]

Since LBW is a leading indicator of infant mortality and morbidity, its incidence has been closely monitored. The incidence of LBW in the United States is summarized in Table 87-3.[14] Although the rate of LBW declined by 11% from 1975 to 1985 (most of the decline occurred before 1980), the rate of very LBW increased by 4%, all of it after 1980. From 1985 to 1987, the rates of moderately LBW and very LBW increased by 2.2% and 2.5%, respectively.[14]

The rates of moderately LBW and very LBW differ substantially between whites and blacks. The relative risk in blacks for moderately LBW is 2.2 and for very LBW, 2.9. The incidence of preterm birth is 18.3% in blacks and 8.5% in whites.[12] Reasons for these demographic differences are complex and relate to socioeconomic and biological differences between the races. For instance, pregnant black women are more often poor

TABLE 87–1. BIRTH WEIGHT CATEGORIES

CATEGORY	GRAMS
Low birth weight (LBW)	<2500
Very low birth weight (VLBW)	<1500
Extremely low birth weight (ELBW) or Very very low birth weight (VVLBW)	≤1000
Incredibly low birth weight (ILBW)	≤750

(From Amon E. Limits of fetal viability: obstetric considerations regarding the management and delivery of the extremely premature baby. Obstet Gynecol Clin North Am 1988;15:321, with permission.)

TABLE 87–2. CATEGORIES OF RISK FOR LBW

Economic
- Poverty
- Unemployment
- Maternal father's poor socioeconomic status
- Uninsured, underinsured
- Poor access to prenatal care
- Poor access to food

Cultural-Behavioral
- Low educational status
- Poor health-care attitudes
- No or inadequate prenatal care
- Cigarette, alcohol, drug abuse
- Age <16 or >35 yr
- Unmarried
- Short interpregnancy interval
- Lack of support group (husband, family, church)
- Stress (physical, psychological)
- Poor weight gain during pregnancy
- Black race*

Biological-Genetic-Medical
- Previous LBW infant
- Low maternal weight at her birth
- Black race*
- Low weight for height
- Short stature
- Poor nutrition
- Chronic medical illnesses
- Inbreeding (autosomal recessive?)
- Intergenerational effects

Reproductive
- Multiple gestation
- Premature rupture of membranes
- Infections (systemic, amniotic, extraamniotic, cervical)
- Preeclampsia/eclampsia
- Uterine bleeding (abruptio placentae, placenta previa)
- Parity (0 or >5)
- Uterine-cervical anomalies
- Fetal disease
- Anemia or high hemoglobin
- Idiopathic premature labor
- Iatrogenic prematurity

* Black race is a risk factor for both growth retardation and premature birth. The risk is twice that for whites and remains present when confounding social and economic variables are controlled. Classification of risk for blacks as cultural and biological is due to the uncertainty of the role of these variables.

(From Kliegman RM, Rottman CJ, Behrman RE. Strategies for the prevention of low birth weight. Am J Obstet Gynecol 1990; 162:1073, with permission.)

and unmarried and are more likely to receive inadequate prenatal care, and the adolescent pregnancy rate is higher in blacks. Researchers assumed that such socioeconomic disadvantages were primarily responsible for the substantial difference in rates, but after controlling for confounding socioeconomic variables, recent investigators found that the twofold increase in relative risk for LBW remained.[13] In fact, low-risk black women had a rate of very LBW 1.7 times higher than that of high-risk white women. The persistence of these effects needs further investigation.

Many epidemiologic risk factors are not etiologic per se, but instead are simply markers identifying patients at increased risk. Table 87-4 lists the identifiable causes most proximate to preterm birth. Most preterm births do not belong to the idiopathic category; only after known or suspected causes are eliminated should patients be diagnosed with idiopathic preterm labor. Recent studies have shown that clinically evident membrane rupture, medical or obstetric maternal complications, or fetal complications account for about 70% of preterm births.[10,15,16] In a private insurance group, 47% of patients giving birth to infants below 2500 g were diagnosed with idiopathic preterm labor.[17] I have observed that many infants at highest risk for poor outcome (≤ 1000 g) are born from preterm births that are currently not preventable.[10] Subclinical infection or accelerated fetal pulmonary maturation remains undiagnosed unless the diagnostic assessment includes amniocentesis.[18–20] This procedure is probably less likely to be performed by general obstetricians than by maternal–fetal medicine specialists. If amniocentesis were commonly performed, the true incidence of unex-

TABLE 87–3. RATES OF LOW, MODERATELY LOW, AND VERY LOW BIRTH WEIGHT BY RACE*

	LOW BIRTH WEIGHT†			MODERATELY LOW BIRTH WEIGHT‡			VERY LOW BIRTH WEIGHT§		
YEAR	ALL RACES‖	WHITE	BLACK	ALL RACES‖	WHITE	BLACK	ALL RACES‖	WHITE	BLACK
1975	73.9	62.6	130.9	62.3	53.4	107.2	11.6	9.2	23.7
1980	68.4	57.0	124.9	56.9	48.1	100.5	11.5	9.0	24.4
1985	67.5	56.4	124.2	55.4	47.0	97.6	12.1	9.4	26.5
1987	69.0	56.8	127.1	56.6	47.4	99.8	12.4	9.4	27.3

* Rates per 1000 live births in the United States.
† <2500 g.
‡ 1500–2499 g.
§ <1500 g.
‖ Includes races other than white and black.
(From MMWR 1990;39:149, with permission.)

TABLE 87–4. PROXIMATE CAUSES OF PRETERM BIRTH

Iatrogenic Preterm Delivery
Physician error
Maternal Causes
Significant systemic medical illness
Significant nonobstetric abdominal pathology
Illicit drug abuse
Severe preeclampsia/eclampsia
Trauma
Uterine Causes
Malformation
Acute overdistention
Large myomata
Deciduitis
Idiopathic uterine activity
Placental Causes
Abruptio placentae
Placenta previa
Marginal placental bleeding
Large chorioangioma
Amniotic Fluid Causes
Oligohydramnios with intact membranes
Preterm rupture of chorioamniotic membranes
Polyhydramnios
Subclinical intra-amniotic infection
Clinical chorioamnionitis
Fetal Causes
Fetal malformation
Multifetal gestation
Fetal hydrops
Fetal growth retardation
Fetal distress
Fetal demise
Cervical Causes
Cervical incompetence
Acute cervicitis/vaginitis

plained preterm labor would be lower than the commonly quoted figure of about 30% to 50%. This chapter will focus on spontaneous preterm labor with intact membranes.

PATHOPHYSIOLOGY

The pathophysiology of preterm labor is unknown. This is not surprising, since the mechanisms that initiate parturition spontaneously at term are also unknown. However, there is extensive literature on the biomolecular processes closely involved with labor.

During labor, and perhaps before, prostaglandin production increases in all mammalian species tested. In many species, the three most temporally related uterine events antecedent to the onset of spontaneous labor are cervical ripening, formation of gap junctions, and an increase in oxytocin receptors. Investigators currently believe that labor is actively inhibited in humans by the prevention of decidual activation throughout most of pregnancy. Just before normal labor and delivery at term, the restraining mechanisms that have inhibited uterine activity are released.

Fundamentally, these mechanisms must bring about myometrial contractions by regulating the free intracellular cytosolic calcium concentration in the myometrial cell. When this concentration increases, myometrial cells contract; conversely, myometrial cells relax when the concentration decreases. The extracellular concentration of ionized calcium (similar to the serum ionized calcium concentration) is relatively constant and is higher than the intracellular concentration. The free intercellular concentration is not constant, but fluctuates directly with maximal contractility. During the contractile process, extracellular calcium may influx through the plasma membrane. Free calcium is also increased because it is released from binding sites in intracellular depots, such as the sarcoplasmic reticulum and mitochondria. Thus, the free intracellular cytosolic fraction of calcium periodically increases in relation to contractility.[21]

Mechanisms controlling the changes in free intracellular calcium concentrations are not well understood, but we know that the myometrium can contract in calcium-free media. This finding provides evidence that organelles themselves contain enough calcium to initiate contractile activity.[22]

Another key regulator of myometrial contractility is the phosphorylation of myosin light chains. Phosphorylation is related to myometrial contraction, dephosphorylation to relaxation. Enzymatic control is directly related to myosin light chain kinase and inversely related to myosin light chain phosphatase. The balance of kinase and phosphatase activities is controlled by complex cellular regulatory mechanisms that need further investigation.[22]

There are three known regulators of myosin light chain kinase: calcium, calmodulin, and cAMP-mediated phosphorylation. These factors are in turn related to the actions of various endogenous hormones and pharmacologic agents on the cell. Some of these substances, agonists and antagonists, act on both the plasma membrane receptors and the intracellular membranes of the organelles. Cellular tocolytic mechanisms include myosin phosphorylation, cAMP regulation of myosin light chain kinase, regulation of intracellular free calcium levels, and regulation of adenylatecyclase activity.[22] The exact sequence of myometrial regulatory processes is unknown.

There are at least three popular theories regarding the initiation of labor: the progesterone withdrawal hypothesis, the oxytocin theory, and the organ communication theory.

PROGESTERONE WITHDRAWAL

In the pregnant ewe, very near delivery there is progesterone withdrawal and a surge in estrogen secretion. Myometrial oxytocin receptors appear, gap junctions develop, and cervical ripening commences.[23] Progesterone withdrawal is not an accepted theory in humans, however, especially when viewed from a classical endocrine aspect. The progesterone/estrogen ratio in the serum shows no significant changes, progesterone in the blood does not decrease, there is no unusual metabolism of progesterone in the tissues, and there is no extraplacental major site of progesterone production.

However, the concept of progesterone withdrawal as a quintessential biological phenomenon cannot be easily abandoned. First, such a mechanism is dominant in the mammalian world. Second, during the normal menstrual cycle, physiological progesterone withdrawal occurs after ovulation and before menses. Third, corpus luteectomy before 8 weeks gestation is followed by spontaneous abortion.[24] Abortion also follows the use of pharmacologic antiprogesterone agents in early pregnancy; some investigators suggest that labor may be stimulated later in pregnancy by these agents. Although unconfirmed, there may well be an important role for progesterone withdrawal when viewed from a paracrine aspect (action limited to the local tissue) rather than an endocrine aspect.

OXYTOCIN

The second theory of parturition is the oxytocin theory. Infusions of oxytocin can induce labor near or at term, but there is little evidence that levels of oxytocin in maternal serum are increased before or during labor. Increases in plasma oxytocin occur primarily during the second stage of labor and postpartum. Recently, a striking increase has been noted in the number of oxytocin receptors in myometrial tissue at the end of gestation.[25] Also, oxytocin acts on decidual tissue to promote the release of prostaglandins.[26] However, oxytocin does not appear to cause myometrial contraction in the absence of gap junction formation between myometrial cells.[27] Investigators have argued for and against the oxytocin theory, but MacDonald expresses the majority view: oxytocin is not the primary agent in the initiation of labor, but simply a facilitator of myometrial forces.[28]

ORGAN COMMUNICATION

The third hypothesis is that of organ communication.[28] It is argued that there are two arms in the maternal—fetal organ communication system, the paracrine and the endocrine. The predominant view is that the paracrine arm maintains pregnancy and permits labor. During labor, many substances accumulate in the amniotic fluid (including free arachidonic acid, prostaglandins, platelet-activating factors, and cytokines), allowing investigators to view with unusual clarity an exciting repository of biomolecular processes relating to parturition. Decidual cells have properties that resemble those of macrophages in many ways. Activation of these cells relates to the initiation of labor. In contrast to the large amount of biomolecular activity during labor, in the nonstimulated state, functional quiescence of the decidua is maintained throughout most of pregnancy.

The fundamental response to activation of the decidua is the release of arachidonic acid, the formation of prostaglandins, and the production of platelet-activating factors and monokines. Monokines in turn may further stimulate the entire process, thus perpetuating parturition. During labor there is a striking increase in the concentration of prostaglandins in the amniotic fluid, and as labor progresses these prostaglandin concentrations increase still further.

The anatomical site of the organ communication system is the interface between the chorion and the decidua, which is also where maternal and fetal tissues meet. Lysosomal release of various enzymes may trigger prostaglandin biosynthesis and activate cervical collagenase. The amnion, chorion, and decidua have the biochemicals necessary for the propagation of labor.

Recently, there has been a dramatic increase in data pointing to cytokines as key mediators between intrauterine infection and preterm labor.[29] The generation of cytokines is considered to be the normal response of a host to infectious mediators. The host tissue generating such responses may well be maternal decidua. The stimulatory cytokines are interleukin-1, interleukin-6, and tumor necrosis factor. Conversely, inhibitory cytokines have also been described; these include interleukin-4 and alpha-interferon.[29]

The choriodecidual interface is a unique anatomical structure that provides the core for both immunologic and paracrine interactions. These may ultimately be the keys to understanding the physiology of term labor and the pathophysiology of preterm labor.

CLINICAL USE OF RISK FACTORS

I have defined *preterm* to distinguish it from abortive pregnancy at the lower end and term pregnancy at the upper end. *Labor* is simply defined as cervical change due to uterine activity. This definition distinguishes preterm labor from cervical incompetence, but in rare cases labor may complicate cervical incompetence by exacerbating preexisting advanced cervical dilation.

Many risk factors antedate the diagnosis of preterm labor, but unfortunately these factors are not very specific. This lack of specificity is further compounded by the inability to diagnose true preterm labor, let alone subclinical preterm labor, accurately in the early stage.

Various risk scoring systems have been developed to identify women at above-average risk for preterm birth. These scores subject empirically collected data to various statistical analyses. However, these scores often do not make clear to what extent the predicted preterm birth relates to a treatable entity. Assuming that spontaneous preterm labor with intact membranes is treatable with tocolytic agents, there are many other proximate causes of preterm birth (see Table 87-4) for which tocolysis is absolutely contraindicated (eg, antepartum stillbirth, significant maternal hemorrhage, chorioamnionitis, lethal congenital abnormalities, eclampsia).

Further, these scores are limited to empirically derived risk factors. Few if any of these are truly etiologic for the predicted outcome; many cannot be modified. Statistical evaluations may include only risk "increasing" factors or additionally risk "decreasing" factors.

It is difficult to assess the value of formal risk scoring, since it is never used alone but is combined with many antenatal management modalities.[30] Many scores have been introduced with claims of success based on historical controls. The most powerful tests of effectiveness and safety are randomized controlled trials, but these have not been done to the satisfaction of most. Randomized trials by Main[17] and Mueller-Huebach[31] have shown no direct benefit of risk scoring to the patients enrolled, but the use of scoring may make providers and patients more aware of the need for preterm birth prevention.

In the United States, Creasy has popularized a scoring system of risk factors to predict spontaneous preterm birth.[32] More than 30 items are divided into four categories: socioeconomic, prior medical history, daily habits, and current pregnancy problems. Screening is done at the initial prenatal visit and repeated near the end of the second trimester. Patients with a score of 10 points or more are considered high risk.

This system, modified from that of Papiernik, was first used in a general obstetric population in New Zealand.[33] The system identified 9% to 13% of the population as high risk, and the prevalence of preterm birth in this population was 6.1%. The sensitivity of the high-risk score was 64%; the positive predictive value of the high-risk score was 30%. The system relies heavily on past obstetric history; consequently, it is more effective in the multiparous than the nulliparous patient.

The Creasy score was later used in a hospital obstetric population in San Francisco as one part of a preterm birth prevention program.[34] The scoring system identified as high risk 10% of patients at the initial screening and 15% at the screening near the end of the second trimester. In this population, only 54/1150 (4.7%) developed preterm labor; of these, only 16/54 (30%) delivered preterm. An additional 12 patients delivered preterm due to maternal or fetal indications. Overall, the prevalence of preterm delivery was unusually low (28/1150 [2.4%], of which 40% were due to nonpreventable conditions). This was a significant decrease from the expected preterm delivery rate of about 6.5%, based on historical controls. Preterm delivery occurred in 4% of the high-risk group and 0.9% of the low-risk group. The sensitivity of the high-risk score was 43%; the positive predictive value of the high-risk score was only 4%. Although the authors attributed the low incidence of preterm birth to other interventions associated with a comprehensive preterm birth prevention program, they acknowledged certain limitations based on the use of historical controls. They also acknowledged the potential for a major population difference, since only 17% of the high-risk patients developed preterm labor. Finally, the authors concluded that their report was preliminary.

The results of a 6-year follow-up report (1978 to 1984) from the same institution differed substantially from the preliminary report.[34,35] Of the high-risk patients, 22.8% developed preterm labor (with and without membrane rupture) and 16.8% delivered preterm. Of the low-risk patients, 5.8% developed preterm labor and 5.3% delivered preterm. The rates of preterm labor (8.5%) and preterm birth (7.1%) were significantly higher than in the earlier report of 4.7% and 2.4%, respectively.

Holbrook and associates reduced from 37 to 18 the number of items in their scoring system for the prediction of preterm labor (not preterm birth) without any significant statistical loss of identification prevalence, sensitivity, or positive predictive value (Table 87-5).[35] Fourteen percent of patients scored as high risk; the sensitivity was 41% and the positive predictive value 25%. The modified system does not require the calculation of a risk score. Twelve factors are defined as major (any one indicating high risk) and six as minor (two or more indicating high risk).

In an inner-city indigent black population, Main and colleagues performed a similar intervention study but excluded the rescreening near the end of the second trimester.[17] In their prospective study, 132/380 (35%) of patients were classified as high risk. In the study population the prevalence of preterm birth was 16.3%. In the low-risk controls the preterm delivery rate was 12.9%, of which 78% had preterm labor or premature rupture of membranes. The sensitivity of the high-risk score was 48%; the positive predictive value of the high-risk score was 27%. Of all preterm deliveries, 35% were attributed to premature rupture of membranes, 34% to indicated preterm delivery. Of preterm deliver-

TABLE 87-5. MAJOR AND MINOR RISK FACTORS OF THE MODIFIED SCORING SYSTEM FOR SPONTANEOUS PRETERM LABOR

MAJOR FACTORS*	MINOR FACTORS†
Multiple gestation	Febrile illness during pregnancy
Previous preterm delivery	Bleeding after 12 weeks
Previous preterm labor, term delivery	History of pyelonephritis
Abdominal surgery during pregnancy	Cigarette smoking (>10 per day)
Diethylstilbestrol exposure	One second-trimester abortion
Hydramnios	More than two first-trimester abortions
Uterine anomaly	
History of cone biopsy	
Uterine irritability (admission to rule out preterm labor)	
More than one second-trimester abortion	
Cervical dilation (>1 cm) at 32 weeks	
Cervical shortening (<1 cm at 32 weeks)	

* Presence of one or more indicates high risk.
† Presence of two or more indicates high risk.
(From Holbrook RH, Laros RK, Creasy RK. Evaluation of a risk scoring system for prediction of preterm labor. Am J Perinatol 1989;6:62, with permission.)

ies due to preterm labor with candidacy for tocolysis, more than 50% were classified as low risk.

In the same report, high-risk patients were randomly assigned to a comprehensive preterm birth prevention program or standard high-risk care.[17] Unfortunately, the extensive intervention program failed to lower the incidence of preterm birth significantly. Preterm delivery occurred in 25% of the patients in the preterm birth prevention program, compared to 21% of the high-risk control patients. The authors attributed these unfavorable results to the high incidence (70%) of proximate causes of preterm birth not amenable to tocolytic therapy. Failure to show efficacy of this preterm birth prevention program may be related in part to small numbers and to the short duration of the program before publication.

In an indigent population equally divided between whites and blacks in Pittsburgh, the positive predictive value of the Creasy high-risk score for spontaneous preterm birth was 18%.[36] Using multivariate statistical techniques, the investigators found that in their population, five factors accounted for a positive predictive value of 22%: prepregnancy weight under 100 pounds, black race, unmarried status, one prior preterm labor and delivery, and two prior preterm births preceded by preterm labor.

The recurrence risk of preterm birth varies from 15% to 40% after one prior preterm birth.[8,37–40] The risk significantly increases with two or more prior preterm births. The tendency to repeat preterm birth at the same gestational age as previous preterm births should be noted. The more preterm the delivery, the less likely the subsequent pregnancy is to deliver at term.[41] For example, a patient with a late second-trimester birth has only a 60% likelihood to deliver at term or greater in the subsequent pregnancy, whereas a patient with a very mild preterm delivery has a 71% likelihood to deliver at term or greater.[42] It should be noted that indicated preterm delivery was not excluded in some of these studies.[39,41,42]

A second-trimester abortion is associated with an increased risk of preterm labor (14%), but one or two first-trimester abortions are not.[35] Three first-trimester abortions are associated with an increased risk of preterm labor (12%).[35]

While risk scoring systems may identify a subset of patients at increased risk for preterm birth, most patients who actually deliver preterm cannot be identified with these methods. The false-positive rate is very high in those identified as high risk. As a rule, the positive predictive value of a high-risk score is less than 30%.[30] There are significant costs and problems associated with initiating and maintaining surveillance and therapy in identified high-risk patients. These concerns are important because the low positive predictive value of risk scoring implies that most women so identified will nonetheless deliver at term, regardless of treatment. Needless treatments and interventions may cause unnecessary anxiety and stress, and limited resources may be allocated to populations where they are needed the least. If uterine activity per se becomes a significant factor for initiating therapy, then in some series up to 50% of all pregnancies would be subject to tocolytic therapy.[43]

EARLY CLINICAL DIAGNOSIS

CHIEF COMPLAINT

A host of complaints may herald preterm labor (Table 87-6). Many of these symptoms are common in normal pregnancy and are often dismissed by many prenatal care providers. A recent report by Iams and coworkers compared the symptoms heralding preterm labor and intact membranes with normal pregnant women.[44] Patients with preterm labor complained of both painful and painless contractions, backache, change in vaginal discharge, pelvic pressure, and menstrual-like cramps, each independently in 40% to 60% of cases. Only 13% of preterm labor patients gave a negative response to all questions about contractions or menstrual-like cramps. Normal outpatients matched for gestational age within 3 weeks were asked about symptoms within the preceding 7 days. About 10% complained of painful contractions. Normal women complained of the same individual symptoms as the preterm labor patients in 10% to 30% of cases.

Vague constitutional symptoms may also presage preterm labor. A not uncommon set of complaints relates to painless uterine activity, described as "balling up" or tightening of the uterus. Some complaints are misinterpreted and consequently mis-reported by the patient, thus misleading both physician and patient. These include gas pains, constipation, and an increase in fetal movements and may represent undiagnosed actual increases in rhythmic uterine activity. It is generally a good idea to instruct patients, especially those at increased risk, about the vague signs and symptoms of preterm labor. Patients experiencing these should be encouraged to contact the physician as soon as possible.

In a study of outpatients at increased risk for preterm labor, Iams found that in a group of 51 patients who subsequently developed preterm labor, only 67% were symptomatic.[45] Uterine activity recordings per se without patient symptoms prompted diagnosis in 24%. In another subgroup, 9% were asymptomatic and were

TABLE 87–6. CHIEF SYMPTOMS OF PRETERM LABOR

Abdominal pain
Back pain
Pelvic pain
Menstrual-like cramps
Vaginal bleeding
Pinkish staining
Increased vaginal discharge
Pelvic pressure
Urinary frequency
Diarrhea

discovered only when advanced cervical dilatation was found during routine cervical examination. The numbers in this study were small, and further research in this area is needed.

CERVICAL DILATATION

Asymptomatic cervical dilatation may represent silent preterm labor, cervical incompetence, or a normal anatomical variation. In a general obstetric population, the frequency of preterm asymptomatic cervical dilatation increases as gestation advances. The frequency was evaluated in a large study by Papiernik and associates (Table 87-7).[46] Cervical dilatation also has been studied by others as a predictor for subsequent preterm birth. Wood[47] found a 28% positive predictive value, Leveno and colleagues[48] a 27% positive predictive value. In a population without identifiable risk factors, Stubbs and coworkers found a 12% positive predictive value at 28 to 32 weeks gestation and a 6% positive predictive value at 34 weeks gestation.[49] In these studies the relative risk for developing preterm birth of cervical dilatation compared to an undilated cervix ranged from two- to four-fold.

Conversely, at least three previous reports emphasized that such dilatation is a normal anatomical variant, particularly in the multipara.[50,51,52] These studies showed no significant increase in the rate of preterm birth.

Some investigators have argued that some change in management is useful when a pregnant patient is found to have asymptomatic cervical dilatation at cervical examination. These options include monitoring uterine activity, performing more frequent surveillance, restricting activity, administering tocolytic agents, and obtaining endocervical cultures. Although these options appear logical to the clinician, there is little published data to support them. These options appear more reasonable if the patient has been previously identified as high risk.

HOME UTERINE ACTIVITY MONITORING

Obstetricians have long sought a way to diagnose actual preterm labor in its earliest stages, in the belief that early treatment is critically important. Using newly developed noninvasive sensing devices and computer technology, uterine activity in the second trimester and beyond can now be detected at home. It is hoped that such detection will decrease the frequency of preterm birth. The critical link here is the appropriateness of treatment interventions.

Fundamental to the concept of home monitoring is provider-initiated contact, in addition to the standard approach of patient-initiated contact. The patient at risk is physically monitored at home with external tocodynamometers. The data are transmitted via telephone to a central viewing station, where the pattern of uterine activity is assessed by a nursing service. The service contacts the patient once or twice daily and prepares a detailed history on the patient's current status. Should the service detect abnormalities, the physician is notified immediately. Further management depends on the circumstances.

The frequency of uterine activity is the principal variable monitored. Studies have shown that the mean frequency of uterine activity per hour rises with increasing gestation.[53,54] There is a further increase in frequency 24 to 48 hours before the onset of true labor. The mean contraction frequency for women destined to have preterm labor is higher than for those who are not, but the overlap between these two groups is high, limiting its positive predictive value.

Some of these monitoring devices are extremely sensitive and cannot distinguish normal Braxton-Hicks contractions from those of early labor. In one study only 10% of women correctly perceived their contractions more than half the time.[55]

A few randomized and nonrandomized trials have indicated that twice-daily monitoring of high-risk women, along with daily nursing support and high-quality obstetric care, may prevent preterm birth.[53,54,56–58] These studies do not answer whether the effect is due to monitoring, to daily provider-initiated support, to the extended rest periods required for uterine activity monitoring, or to some combination thereof. Investigator bias may exist, since these studies cannot be blinded. Further, many patients who were enrolled but failed to use the service were often excluded from evaluation.[59]

Will these outpatient services become the new standard for high-risk obstetric care? The costs of these intensive services and the real potential of inappropriate medical tocolysis and related complications must be

TABLE 87–7. PERCENTAGE OF GENERAL OBSTETRIC PATIENTS WITH CERVICAL DILATION OF THE INTERNAL os > 1cm

WEEKS' GESTATION	PERCENT	TOTAL	% PRETERM BIRTH
19–24	2.4	2124	17.3
25–28	4.4	2415	23.4
29–31	10.6	1750	21.6
32–34	12.4	2967	17.4
35–36	22.5	1921	11.1
37–38	32.8	2693	—

weighed against the costs of current standards of care that include conscientious education programs by the physician's office and 24-hour access to care. Although these services may be useful in a few circumstances, to date they are not considered to be the standard of care and are not fully endorsed by the American College of Obstetricians and Gynecologists.

DIAGNOSIS

Accurately diagnosing preterm labor is difficult unless labor has obviously advanced beyond the point of successful long-term tocolysis. With this caveat in mind, preterm labor can be classified as threatened or actual. The basis for such a classification is the predictive value for spontaneous preterm delivery soon after the diagnosis, if left untreated with tocolytic agents. In general it is thought that about half of all patients in preterm labor will deliver at term.

The hallmark of threatened preterm labor is uterine activity. The diagnosis of threatened preterm labor is applied to the patient with uterine activity but no evidence of cervical changes. About 85% of patients with threatened preterm labor will deliver at term. In the past, many of these patients may have been diagnosed as having painful Braxton-Hicks contractions. The change in terminology is clinically important. The recurrence rate of threatened preterm labor in the current pregnancy is about 30%; of these women, about half will deliver preterm.[60]

Most often, patients with threatened preterm labor respond to simple conservative measures (bed rest, hydration, sedation, or limited doses of subcutaneous terbutaline). Less commonly, continuous infusion of a tocolytic agent may be required for unrelenting, significant uterine activity. The prognosis for a term delivery appears improved if preterm labor begins in the third trimester rather than in the second trimester.

During actual preterm labor (as diagnosed by Ingmarrsson's criteria) about 20% (3/15) of placebo-treated patients deliver at term, compared to 80% (12/15) of terbutaline-treated patients.[61] These criteria were:

1. 28 to 36 weeks gestation
2. Painful, regular uterine contractions, occurring at intervals of less than 10 minutes, for at least 30 minutes by external tocography
3. Intact membranes
4. Cervix effaced or almost effaced, dilated between 1 and 4 cm.

Patients with bleeding, uterine malformations, fever, multiple gestation, and other known etiologies of preterm labor were excluded. All patients were given 10 mg of diazepam intramuscularly; if this had no obvious effect on contractions, treatment was continued with either terbutaline or placebo.

Creasy modified the Ingmarsson criteria as follows:[62]

1. 20 to 37 weeks gestation
2. Documented uterine contractions (four in 20 minutes or eight in 60 minutes)
3. Documented cervical change or cervical effacement of 80% or cervical dilatation of 2 cm
4. Intact membranes.

These diagnostic criteria are well accepted for the nulliparous patient. There is general agreement that the same diagnostic criteria can be used for the multipara, but their prognostic value may be lessened.

Documenting cervical change requires serial documentation of cervical status, ideally by the same examiner. One method of determining cervical change is by noting changes in the Bishop score.[63] Dilatation of the internal cervical os or effacement of cervical length are most significant; other measures of change, such as consistency and position, seem to be inadequate for accurate diagnosis.

Fetal station, although not part of the diagnostic criteria for actual preterm labor, has prognostic value: the lower the station, the greater the risk of spontaneous preterm delivery. A patient who experiences a lower frequency of documented uterine contractions and who is known to have a high degree of cervical compliance based on the Bishop scoring criteria (eg, Bishop score > 6) is at increased risk for premature delivery.

Many practitioners believe that for tocolytic therapy to be most successful, it should be started before serial cervical change is documented. Thus, many practitioners initiate tocolytic therapy as early as possible. However, a recent report by Utter and colleagues disputes these beliefs.[64] The authors compared the preterm delivery rates in 98 patients without serial cervical change before tocolysis (Group 1) and 75 patients with serial cervical change in dilatation or effacement before tocolysis (Group 2). In both groups the mean dilatation before ritodrine therapy was the same, as well as other risk factors. No statistical difference was found in outcome or even trends in outcome. Half of Group 2 patients and 40% of Group 1 patients delivered at term. The authors concluded that even with significant cervical dilatation, observation was a reasonable alternative for patients dilated less than 3 cm until subsequent uterine activity and cervical change could be determined. Thereafter, ritodrine tocolysis could be given without affecting its success rate.

Although these findings are interesting and highlight the problem of making an accurate diagnosis even at dilatations of 2 cm, it seems prudent to await confirmation from other centers before managing patients with preterm labor in such a manner.

MANAGING PRETERM LABOR

Once the diagnosis of preterm labor is made, appropriate evaluations and initial management plans are instituted. The diagnostic evaluation has two major parts. In the first, the need for tocolytic therapy is assessed, with attention focused on the specific nature of the agents to be used. The second part is an etiologic diagnostic workup.

During evaluation, the physician seeks contraindications to actively prolonging pregnancy. Absolute contraindications include fetal demise, lethal fetal anomaly, severe preeclampsia/eclampsia, severe hemorrhage, and chorioamnionitis. Relative contraindications include fetal heart-rate monitor abnormalities, fetal growth retardation, mild preeclampsia, relatively stable late second-trimester and third-trimester bleeding, progressive structural but nonlethal fetal anomalies, significant maternal medical disease, and cervical dilatation of 5 cm or more. The fundamental issue is whether the risk of delivery outweighs the risk of prolonging the pregnancy.

The lower limit for initiating tocolysis in a favorable candidate is about 17 to 20 weeks gestation. As for the upper limits of fetal age and weight, different opinions exist for appropriate tocolytic therapy. In "uncomplicated" patients, some physicians initiate tocolytic therapy at 36 weeks gestation and continue oral treatment until 37 to 38 weeks.[65] Based on changes in the vascular intracranial anatomy and nursery performance for cardiovascular, pulmonary, and gastrointestinal systems, I find little data to support an overly aggressive tocolytic approach beyond the 34th week, or an estimated fetal weight of 2000 g, particularly if fetal lung maturity is present.

Once therapy is determined, the choice of tocolytic agent is the next major decision. The physician must consider the mother's adrenergic state and the presence of diabetes mellitus, heart disease, hypertension, renal disease, neuromuscular disease, or gastrointestinal disease. These factors are discussed in greater detail later under the specific tocolytic agents. The physician must seek contraindications to beta-sympathomimetic agents, including situations in which beta-receptor stimulation is undesirable (eg, New York Heart Association functional class 2 or higher cardiac disease, cardiac arrhythmias, severe hypertension, thyrotoxicosis, asymmetric septal hypertrophy, uncontrolled diabetes mellitus, neurologic thromboembolic phenomenon). Contraindications to magnesium sulfate include myasthenia gravis, some cardiac rhythm disturbances, myocardial damage, and severe renal disease.

During the initial evaluation period, some authors recommend performing microbiological cultures, urine toxicology, and baseline maternal cardiac, hematologic, and electrolyte evaluations. While these test results are pending and the mother and fetus are deemed stable, a thorough ultrasound examination is done to complete the evaluation. Factors to be assessed are listed in Table 87-8. Many of these factors have a tremendous influence on clinical management.

TABLE 87–8. FETAL AND MATERNAL ASSESSMENT VIA SONOGRAPHY

Fetal Evaluation
Fetal age, weight, and growth status
Fetal life and fetal number
Fetal lie, presentation, position
Fetal wellbeing
Fetal behavior
Fetal anatomy and gender
Fetal blood sampling (funicentesis) for rapid karyotype, blood gases, disease-specific hematologic profiles
Amniotic Fluid Evaluation
Polyhydramnios
Oligohydramnios
Amniocentesis for infection, fetal pulmonary maturation, fetal hemolysis
Placental and Funic Evaluation
Previa
Abruption
Marginal bleed with membrane separation
Location, internal anatomy, contour, thickness, and grade
Umbilical cord insertion sites
Funic presentation
Uterine Evaluation
Defective uterine scar
Uterine septum
Weak lower uterine segment
Myomatous uterus

FETAL AGE, WEIGHT, AND GROWTH STATUS

One of the most important determinations that must be made is that of gestational age. This usually has already been determined during prenatal care. Of course, gestational age is not one true number but rather a range of numbers based on the best obstetric estimate. Sonography is often used to confirm optimal menstrual age or to be consistent with suboptimal menstrual age within a given number of days. At best, sonographic fetal age based on biometry is an estimate determined by the mean for a population of normally grown and uncomplicated fetuses. Dating by sonography alone in the third trimester is much less accurate due to increasing variation in fetal growth. Requirements for impeccability in timing of conception include basal body temperature, single or infrequent coitus, artificial insemination, and in vitro fertilization, but most women who present in preterm labor, particularly at the lower limits of viability, do not have such a precisely timed gestational age. Further, these patients not uncommonly have had inadequate prenatal care, and late gestational age assignment is known to be inaccurate.

Routine fetal biometric measurements should be taken, including the biparietal diameter (BPD), head circumference (HC), cephalic index (CI), abdominal circumference (AC), and femur length (FL). After the gestational age is determined or confirmed, fetal weight should be estimated. For practical purposes, I recommend using fetal weight tables based on the calculations of Shepard or Hadlock formulae.[66,67] As in gestational age, estimating fetal weight by sonography carries with it inherent error. But unlike gestational age, post-delivery birth weight is a reproducible number without a significant range of error: this unequivocal number is the cornerstone of immediate neonatal prognosis, particularly for infants <1000 g.[5] Therefore, determining fetal weight is useful for predelivery counseling regarding prognosis.

The shape of the fetal head influences the accuracy of the BPD prediction of fetal age or weight. With dolichocephaly, age and weight are underestimated; with brachycephaly, overestimation may occur. Doubilet and Greenes significantly improved their prediction of gestational age by correcting for the shape of the fetal head.[68] When using a formula to calculate fetal weight in which BPD is an important variable, it must be determined whether the CI is beyond two standard deviations from the mean. If so, then the corrected BPD is used in the calculation instead of the measured BPD. This is especially critical when making management decisions near the lower limits of fetal viability (ie, 24 weeks).

After age and weight are determined, intrauterine growth status should be assessed. Several investigators have suggested that fetal growth retardation is more common than expected in the setting of preterm labor.[69,70] Westgren and colleagues studied the relationship of idiopathic preterm labor to fetal growth retardation by assessing the ratio of femur length to abdominal circumference (FL/AC).[71] Previously, two groups had found that an FL/AC of 22 ± 2% between 21 to 42 weeks gestation was constant and independent of gestational age.[72,73] Westgren found that 41% of infants who were delivered prematurely after failed tocolysis had an FL/AC above 23.5, compared to 5% of patients in preterm labor who responded well to tocolytic therapy.

The clinical relevance of finding fetal growth retardation is again of great importance to management at the lower limits of fetal viability (ie, 22 to 26 weeks). In these situations sonographic measurements may erroneously underestimate fetal age secondary to suboptimal growth, and the infant may be erroneously declared previable. At the other end of the prematurity spectrum (32 to 36 weeks), it is not uncommon to find fetal pulmonary maturity when performing transabdominal amniocentesis. One explanation for the presumably "accelerated" pulmonary phospholipid determinations may be that suboptimal fetal growth manifests as preterm labor.

FETAL DEMISE

In patients with inadequate prenatal care, fetal demise and multiple gestation not uncommonly present as preterm labor. These entities are reliably ruled in or out with the use of ultrasound. Tocolytic therapy is contraindicated in fetal demise; labor is either allowed to proceed or augmented.

FETAL NUMBER

In patients with multiple gestation, extreme care must be used when administering parenteral tocolytic therapy. When using either beta-agonists or magnesium sulfate combined with fluid therapy, the risk of pulmonary edema is higher in multiple gestation than in singleton pregnancies. To prevent pulmonary edema, total fluid intake should be restricted to 2500 mL per 24 hours of salt-free or salt-poor solutions. Multiple gestation results in preterm labor at least 12 times more commonly than in singleton pregnancies.[74] Moreover, multiple gestation carries with it a higher incidence of many other maternal and fetal complications that strongly influence management of preterm labor and delivery. Not uncommonly, multiple gestation is complicated by fetal malformation, polyhydramnios, or nonimmune hydrops. The overall likelihood that a multiple gestation will be delivered before 37 weeks is about 40%.[75]

MALPRESENTATION

Fetal malpresentation is common in patients with preterm labor and delivery. The incidence of malpresentation is inversely related to gestational age. It is possible with sonography to detect an associated uterine malformation, placental abnormality, polyhydramnios, oligohydramnios, or fetal abnormality. One's index of suspicion for a fetal malformation or genetic syndrome must be raised because there is a higher incidence of fetal malformation in the preterm breech infant: Nisell and associates reported an incidence of 13.6% in Sweden in all breech infants born after 28 weeks gestation and weighing less than 2500 g at birth.[76] Additionally, Braun and colleagues reported a higher incidence of breech-presenting fetuses in a variety of cases of fetal malformation or neuromuscular dysfunction.[77] These include hydrocephalus, neural tube defects, familial dysautonomia, autosomal trisomy syndromes 18, 13, and 21, myotonic dystrophy, and other uncommon syndromes. Fetal hypertonic and hypotonic disorders are represented.

When faced with preterm delivery of a breech-presenting fetus in the absence of other clinically pertinent maternal or fetal complications, most maternal—fetal medicine subspecialists in the United States usually perform a cesarean section from 28 to 34 weeks, despite the fact that there is little scientific proof to justify this approach.[78] This is also true for the United Kingdom.[79] Ordinarily, I recommend performing a cesarean section for infants estimated to weigh 750 to 1500 g with a gestational age of 26 to 32 weeks. Below 750 g or less than 26 weeks gestation, inherent fetal biology is thought to be a better predictor of survival than the delivery mode. Above 1500 g, there is little information demonstrating any significant advantage of cesarean section for the breech-presenting fetus.

A less popular but increasingly common option to manage the breech-presenting fetus is the careful, selective performance of external cephalic version under ultrasound guidance. This technique is well described for the term or near-term infant and can be modified when preterm delivery of a malpresenting fetus is inevitable.[80]

FETAL WELLBEING

Fetal wellbeing in the course of preterm labor is most commonly assessed with the nonstress test. A classically reactive test is most widely defined as at least two accelerations of fetal heart rate of 15 beats per minute for 15 seconds during a 20-minute monitoring period. If the criteria for reactivity are not met, the test is considered nonreactive; this is usually due to fetal sleep cycles, medication, or prematurity, especially less than 32 weeks gestation. Once sleep cycles or drugs are eliminated, then further assessment of wellbeing is indicated.

Since the contraction stress test is strongly contraindicated in the presence of preterm labor, the test of choice for further fetal evaluation is the biophysical profile. Fetal tone, movement, amniotic fluid volume, and fetal breathing movements (FBM) all become normally manifest weeks before classical fetal heart reactivity.[81] Fetal oxygenation is sufficient if these four parameters are present, according to the criteria of Manning and coworkers, regardless of reactivity.[82]

The absence of classical reactivity can be explained on the basis of either relative nervous system immaturity or normal biological variation. Modifications of the criteria for a reactive nonstress test have been detailed by Castillo and colleagues.[83] By defining reactivity as three accelerations of 10 beats per minute, all fetuses tested at 26 weeks were reactive at the end of 60 minutes, and about 90% of the 24-week fetuses were reactive. If noninvasive data are contradictory with regard to oxygenation status, particularly in fetuses at high risk for acidosis yet remote from term, funicentesis (percutaneous umbilical cord sampling) can be helpful in the optimal management of preterm labor.[84]

FETAL BREATHING MOVEMENTS

Although many factors influence the presence of FBM in the nonlabor state, there seems to be a significant decrease in FBM during true labor. Castle and Turnbull first described the presence of FBM to predict continuing pregnancy in patients with preterm labor.[85] Several other investigators have observed that the presence or absence of FBM may distinguish between the patient in preterm labor destined to deliver within 48 or 56 hours or within a week of diagnosis.[85–89] This prediction is most accurate in uncomplicated preterm labor without membrane rupture, antepartum hemorrhage, or multiple gestation, and prior to tocolytic therapy. How FBM can be applied to the management of preterm labor remains unclear, but this is an exciting area of clinically pertinent investigation.

FETAL MALFORMATION

There is an increased incidence of fetal malformation in patients with preterm labor.[90] Often these patients have advanced preterm labor, spontaneous rupture of membranes, or vaginal bleeding. In a Norwegian study of over 30,000 women with three singleton births, fetal malformation was most common in those with preterm birth occurring as a unique event.[91] Multiple congenital anomaly was not uncommon, and the rate of central nervous system malformation was as high as eight per 1000. Overall, the relative risk that an infant with a congenital malformation would be born preterm was 2.0. Rodeck provided a succinct review of fetal abnormality in relation to preterm labor.[92]

It is important to perform a complete fetal malformation screen in preterm labor and delivery. If sonographic evidence suggests aneuploidy, a fetal karyotype may be useful for optimal medical and obstetric management of labor, mode of delivery, place of delivery, and neonatal resuscitation.[93] The rapidity of a karyotypic determination depends on the clinical exigencies; time is one factor influencing the decision to use amniocentesis versus funicentesis. If a virtually lethal chromosomal constitution is discovered, then management should focus on the mother's safety, and nonaggressive management for the fetus or newborn should be used. Tocolytic therapy should be discontinued.

POLYHYDRAMNIOS

Polyhydramnios is an uncommon but important cause of preterm labor due to uterine overdistention. It has been defined as an amniotic fluid volume of greater than 2000 mL. The diagnosis is suspected when uterine enlargement is greater than expected for gestational age. There is usually difficulty in palpating fetal parts. Occasionally, the uterine wall is exceedingly tense and tender. Respiratory compromise and postrenal obstruction may result from massive uterine overdistention. As many as 40% of patients with polyhydramnios experience preterm labor and delivery.[94] Sonography is used to confirm the diagnosis, to help determine the proximate cause, and to guide therapeutic mechanical relief. Sonographic confirmation of the diagnosis is best made subjectively by an experienced observer. The proximate cause is then determined; causes may be maternal, fetal, placental, or a combination. In some series about 60% of cases are idiopathic.[95]

Maternal causes include diabetes mellitus and red cell alloimmunization (anti-D, anti-Kell, etc.). These entities are readily excluded by laboratory tests. Fetal etiologies include complicated multiple gestation, nonimmune hydrops, and structural congenital malformations. Up to 75% of singleton pregnancies with nonimmune hydrops have associated polyhydramnios. Fetal congenital malformations occur in up to 50% of cases with polyhydramnios. Fetal malformations were found in 75% of cases with severe polyhydramnios, compared to a 29% rate of fetal abnormality in mild cases.[95]

Central nervous system defects account for about 45% to 50% of all fetal malformations. Upper gastrointestinal defects represent about 30% of associated malformations. The latter category of defects present later in gestation than do central nervous system defects. Circulatory abnormalities, accounting for about 7% of fetal abnormalities, include coarctation of the aorta, interruption of the fetal aorta, cardiac arrhythmias (primarily supraventricular tachyarrhythmias), and myocardial disorders. Miscellaneous disorders, which may account for 18% of malformations, include congenital chylothorax, pancreatic cysts, asphyxiating thoracic dystrophy, thanatophoric dwarfism, other short-limb dwarfisms, trisomy 18 and 21, cystic hygroma, and sacrococcygeal, cervical, or mediastinal teratomas.

One placental cause of polyhydramnios is a large chorioangioma, a benign vascular malformation that acts like an arteriovenous shunt. Tumors large enough to produce polyhydramnios and preterm labor are rare. They are usually circumscribed, solid or complex masses protruding from the fetal surface of the placenta and are larger than 5 cm when associated with fetal hydrops.[96]

OLIGOHYDRAMNIOS

Oligohydramnios is diagnosed easily with ultrasound as a significant reduction in amniotic fluid volume. In the setting of preterm labor this may be due to premature rupture of the membranes, severe intrauterine growth retardation, or a genitourinary malformation in which fetal urination into the amniotic cavity is absent. Serial sonography and invasive procedures allow for differentiation among the etiologies.

The diagnosis of lethal renal diseases is important, since many of these cases may present with fetal distress or malpresentation during preterm labor. About 60% of patients with Potter's syndrome develop preterm labor, and 40% to 60% are in the breech presentation.[97] In these situations, cesarean section is performed solely for maternal indications. However, unless studied serially, it may be impossible to differentiate from severe growth retardation.

FETAL GENDER

Fetal gender has important prognostic and practical significance. Although not 100% accurate, this parameter is easily determined in most instances with ultrasound. Female fetuses have been found to benefit from the use of antenatal dexamethasone to reduce the incidence of respiratory distress syndrome.[98] By regression analysis, Fleisher and coworkers found that the L/S ratio in females reached 2:1 at 33.7 weeks, 1.4 weeks earlier than in males.[99] Phosphatidylglycerol first appeared at 34 weeks for females and at 35 weeks for males. The female infant has a significant survival advantage, particularly if her birth weight is 1000 g or more.[2]

When funicentesis is done to assist in fetal diagnosis, knowing that the fetus is male allows the laboratory to distinguish fetal cells from maternal cells when there is maternal contamination. This is especially important when a rapid karyotype is indicated or a 100% pure fetal sample is required.

AMNIOCENTESIS AND NEONATAL OUTCOME

Amniocentesis in experienced hands carries minimal risk in the late second trimester or third trimester. There is no scientific evidence that it stimulates labor. Leigh and Garite used amniocentesis during idiopathic preterm labor to detect subclinical infection and fetal pulmonary maturity and found that 12% had positive cultures.[20] These patients presented at earlier gestational ages and were more likely to rupture membranes and to deliver within 48 hours of admission than those with negative cultures. One third of the patients at 31 to 32 weeks and 50% of those at 33 weeks gestation or more had mature L/S ratios.

In a review of 11 studies of transabdominal amniocentesis in patients with preterm labor and intact membranes, Romero and Mazor found a positive culture rate of 16%.[19] In the patients with positive cultures, clinical chorioamnionitis occurred in 58%, refractoriness to tocolysis in 65%, and membrane rupture in 40%. The respective rates of these complications for the patients with negative cultures were 7%, 16%, and 4%. Although a large percentage of the microbes recovered were anaerobic, neonates rarely developed significant anaerobic infections.

The appropriate management of patients with positive intra-amniotic cultures remains controversial. Some regimens include antibiotics and immediate delivery, but in others the fetus is delivered only when there is frank clinical evidence of infection, particularly if the fetus is 28 weeks or younger. If there is no evidence of intra-amniotic infection, there is documented significant immaturity (ie, $L/S < 1.5$), and there is a significant risk of delivery between 24 hours and 1 week, then it is reasonable to give a course of betamethasone 12 mg intramuscularly twice, 24 hours apart. In these situations aggressive tocolytic therapy is reasonable if the fetus is less than 35 weeks gestation. In contrast, if the L/S is 2:1 or higher, phosphatidylglycerol is present, or there is a positive shake test, some authors are not as aggressive because the benefit of tocolysis does not seem to outweigh the risk.

We recently analyzed neonatal morbidity in infants born with mature amniotic fluid tests (Table 87-9).[100] The mothers presented with spontaneous preterm labor and were potential candidates for tocolytic therapy. In view of the pulmonary maturity, tocolytic agents were discontinued in many patients. Entry criteria were singleton gestation, transabdominal amniocentesis, uncontaminated amniotic fluid, delivery within 72 hours of amniocentesis, and absence of antenatal steroids, diabetes mellitus, and significant malformations. We found that despite "pulmonary maturity," respiratory distress and other morbidities still occurred as an in-

TABLE 87-9. NEONATAL MORBIDITY IN INFANTS BORN WITH MATURE AMNIOTIC FLUID TESTS

	WEEKS' GESTATION			
	<33 (n = 15)	33 (n = 13)	34 (n = 19)	35–36 (n = 35)
Respiratory distress	7 (47%)	2 (15%)	0	0
Air leak	2 (13%)	1 (8%)	0	0
NEC	1 (7%)	3 (23%)	0	0
IVH	4 (27%)	1 (8%)	2 (11%)	0
Sepsis	7 (47%)	2 (15%)	0	0
Blood transfusion	8 (53%)	4 (31%)	2 (11%)	1 (3%)
TPN	8 (53%)	5 (39%)	1 (5%)	1 (3%)
BWT (mean ± SD)	1563 ± 489	1925 ± 283	2177 ± 259	2442 ± 333

(From Amon E, Leventhal S, Allen GS, et al. Neonatal outcome following spontaneous preterm labor after demonstrated lung maturity by amniocentesis. Society for Gynecologic Investigation, 37th annual meeting, 1990, St. Louis, Missouri, #169, with permission.)

verse function of gestational age. Hence, prolongation of pregnancy should still be attempted even in the presence of mature amniotic fluid indices. It should be noted that none of the infants had significant respiratory distress at 34 weeks or more.

A somewhat similar study of neonatal morbidity by Konte (excluding amniocentesis data) found a similar inverse relationship between neonatal morbidity and gestational age (Table 87-10).[101] It should be noted that 23% of the patients at 34 weeks gestation had significant respiratory distress; this is consistent with the fact that pulmonary maturity was not present and emphasizes the predictive value of amniocentesis at this gestational age.

UTERINE MALFORMATION

A review of pregnancy outcome in 182 women in Finland with uterine anomalies found that premature labor occurred in 23% of 265 pregnancies.[102] The complete septate uterus had the best fetal survival rate (86%), the complete bicornuate uteri (50%) and unicornuate (40%) the worst. The patients with complete bicornuate uteri had the highest incidence of preterm labor (66%), but the number of such patients studied was small (n = 6). Didelphys and all varieties of bicornuate uteri were associated with an incidence of preterm labor that was above 20%. Preterm labor occurred in 10.3% to 37.5% of patients with unicornuate uteri.[103] In cases of uterine anomalies, associated cervical incompetence, malpresentation, and preterm labor are not uncommon; therefore, uterine malformation may be suspected when associated obstetric problems arise. Likewise, in cases of known uterine anomalies, one must have a high index of suspicion for the development of associated problems. Unfortunately, uterine anomalies are often not recognized until patients have obstetric or gynecologic problems.

MANAGEMENT DECISIONS AT THE LOWER END OF VIABILITY

Managing preterm delivery at the lower limits of viability–currently 22 to 24 weeks gestation–is a vexing problem. The a priori determination of viability for a severely preterm yet normally formed fetus requiring delivery remains a statistical, not an absolute, concept. Biological and clinical variables associated with obstetric and neonatal management that favorably influence neonatal outcome have been reviewed.[7,104–107] It is optimal for delivery in such cases to occur in immediate proximity to a neonatal intensive-care center.[108] When

TABLE 87-10. MORBIDITY RATES PER GESTATIONAL AGE AT BIRTH

	GESTATIONAL AGE (WK)					
COMPLICATION	26–27 (n = 16)	28–29 (n = 32)	30–31 (n = 33)	32–33 (n = 44)	34 (n = 40)	35 (n = 36)
Intensive-care nursery	16 (100)	32 (100)	31 (94)	40 (91)	29 (73)	8 (22)
Respiratory distress syndrome	13 (81)	19 (59)	10 (30)	13 (30)	9 (23)	1 (3)
Patent ductus arteriosus	8 (50)	16 (50)	7 (21)	6 (14)	5 (13)	—
Sepsis	5 (31)	8 (25)	5 (15)	3 (7)	2 (5)	2 (6)
Intraventricular hemorrhage	5 (31)	4 (13)	1 (3)	—	—	—
Necrotizing enterocolitis	4 (25)	2 (6)	2 (6)	1 (2)	—	—

Percentages (in parentheses) are rounded to nearest percent.
(From Konte JM, Holbrook RH Jr, Laros RK Jr, Creasy RK. Short-term neonatal morbidity. Am J Perinatol 1986;3:285, with permission.)

conditions permit, decisions regarding delivery of a severely preterm fetus (ie, 22 to 26 weeks gestation by best obstetric estimate) are ideally made after the mother is transported to a tertiary-care center with experienced pediatric and obstetric specialists. At these gestational ages, opinions about management differ among obstetric specialists and among neonatologists.[109–111] Therefore, coordinated predelivery family counseling by obstetricians and neonatal physicians is recommended to discuss the prognosis and to plan management, thereby minimizing anxiety, confusion, and fear.

A highly individualized, thoughtful, thorough, and compassionate approach to the patient is required. Survival rates as a function of gestational age and birth weight are shown in Tables 87-11 and 87-12. Literature reviews have found that subsequent serious handicap rates in severely preterm survivors are about 20% to 30%.[7,11,107,112] Conversely, of all extremely LBW nonsurvivors, 70% to 80% die in the first week of postnatal life, most in the first few days.[104,113] Cesarean section for fetal distress is performed by about 40% of maternal—fetal medicine specialists beginning at 24 weeks gestation.[110]

Due to inherent inaccuracies in estimating fetal age and weight, consideration on behalf of the fetus between 22 to 23 weeks gestation and 450 to 600 g should be made. Since the likelihood for survival in these instances is dismal (ie, < 5% to 10%), cesarean section for fetal indications is best avoided. Survival, if it occurs, will generally occur regardless of the delivery mode. To protect the mother from undue risk of cesarean section for little potential benefit for the newborn, everything short of cesarean section should be offered to the mother. These measures include transfer to a tertiary-care center, standard hydration, fetal monitoring, maternal positioning, maternal oxygenation, controlled sterile delivery, and the presence of a neonatologist at delivery. Newer measures include transcervical amnioinfusion and acute tocolysis for uterine relaxation.[114–116] These therapies are based on the view that mortality and significant handicap rates will increase without optimal therapy.

TOCOLYTIC AGENTS

In the last four decades, a host of drugs has been used in the attempt to inhibit preterm labor, including relaxin, beta-sympathomimetic agents, ethanol, prostaglandin synthetase inhibitors, organic calcium-channel blockers, magnesium sulfate, diazoxide, aminophylline, progestagens, and most recently oxytocin analogs that block oxytocin receptors. Many of these agents showed high success rates initially, but subsequent reports showed reduced, somewhat limited efficacy.

Several fundamental issues must be addressed in a discussion of tocolytic treatment for preterm labor. First, can actual preterm labor be accurately diagnosed and distinguished from threatened preterm labor? Second, although uterine activity may be abolished or minimized by treatment, does this really prolong pregnancy, and is this treatment successful? Different studies have defined success rates differently.

Third, and most importantly, what effect does successful tocolytic treatment have on perinatal outcome? Substantive improvements in perinatal outcome should be defined as real reductions in mortality, morbidity, and cost of care; unfortunately, the success of most agents is defined in terms of pregnancy prolongation rather than on substantive reduction of morbidity and mortality. Neonatal mortality beyond 32 weeks gestation in the normally formed infant is minimal and hence is no longer a significant issue. The mortality focus now centers on late second-trimester and early third-trimester pregnancies. Although pregnancy may be prolonged to some extent in most studies, actual substantive effects on improved perinatal outcome are lacking.

The final question is whether the mother and fetus should be exposed to potentially significant side effects; if so, to what extent? Tocolytic agents are commonly used without a universal acclamation that they should be used. It is difficult for the practitioner not to treat the patient, and it is difficult for the patient to go to a practitioner who does not treat her; thus we have a Catch-22.

TABLE 87–11. HOSPITAL SURVIVAL OF EXTREMELY LOW BIRTH WEIGHT INFANTS*

		GESTATION (WEEKS)			
REFERENCE	YEAR OF BIRTH	23	24	25	26
Milligan et al.	1979–82	1/7 (14)	9/23 (39)	28/44 (64)	34/45 (76)
Kitchen et al.	1977–82	—	2/27 (7)	11/54 (20)	36/80 (45)
Yu et al.	1977–84	2/28 (7)	13/40 (33)	11/44 (25)	36/62 (58)
Amon et al.	1981–85	5/73 (7)†	7/63 (11)	31/66 (47)	32/88 (36)
Dillon and Egan	1977–80	—	4/11 (36)	6/16 (38)	11/18 (61)
Herschel et al.	1977–80	—	2/7 (29)	3/28 (11)	17/38 (61)

* Survivors/livebirths (% survival).

† All infants thought to be 22 or 23 weeks' gestation are combined.

(From Amon E. Limits of fetal viability: obstetric considerations regarding the management and delivery of the extremely premature baby. Obstet Gynecol Clin North Am 1988;15:321, with permission.)

TABLE 87–12. SURVIVAL RATES (%) OF EXTREMELY LOW BIRTH WEIGHT INFANTS

BIRTH WEIGHT (g)	YU ET AL MELBOURNE, 1977–83 (n = 220)*	AMON ET AL MEMPHIS, 1983–85 (n = 263)†	AMON‡ ST. LOUIS, 1985–86 (n = 197)†
500–599	11	9	9
600–699	27	29	29
700–799	44	43	36
800–899	59	66	62
900–1000	64	64	69

* Includes those with birth defects; survival as of 1 year.
† Survival = discharge home alive.
‡ Previously unpublished data.
Other reports describing survival in 100-g increments may include outborn infants, may exclude delivery room deaths, may define survival only up to 27 days of postnatal life, or may consolidate data from multiple institutions and thus make comparisons less meaningful.
(From Amon E. Limits of fetal viability: obstetric considerations regarding the management and delivery of the extremely premature baby. Obstet Gynecol Clin North Am 1988;15:321, with permission.)

BETA-SYMPATHOMIMETIC AGENTS

Beta-adrenergic receptors have been described following the observations of Lands and coworkers.[117] Beta-1 receptors predominate in the heart, small intestine, and adipose tissue, beta-2 receptors in the uterus, blood vessels, bronchioles, and liver. Some of these agents (for example, ritodrine) have been publicized as having selective beta-2 activity.[118] β_2-selective sympathomimetic amines are structurally related to catecholamines and stimulate all beta-receptors throughout the entire body.[119] With continued use, tachyphylaxis is noted.[120,121]

The side effects of these agents represent an exaggeration of their physiological effects. In the cardiovascular system, there is a decrease in diastolic blood pressure, tachycardia, an increase in cardiac output, and a tendency toward arrhythmogenesis.[122] Chest pain not uncommonly occurs with parenteral administration. Since these drugs increase oxygen demand and decrease coronary artery perfusion, it is reasonable to assume that they may cause myocardial ischemia. There may be transient ST segment depression that resolves with discontinuation of drug therapy. These clinical and EKG findings may relate directly to drug therapy or indirectly to electrolyte disturbance per se rather than to ischemia.[123]

Pulmonary edema may occur in a small percentage of patients treated with parenteral beta-sympathomimetic agents.[122] This life-threatening complication has several predisposing factors: multiple gestation, a positive fluid balance, blood transfusion, anemia, infection, associated hypertension, polyhydramnios, and underlying cardiac disease. Ritodrine causes the retention of salt and water at the level of the kidney.[119] Plasma volume expands and hematocrit drops by 10% to 15%.[124] Together with the cardiovascular effects, it is surprising that more patients do not develop pulmonary edema. These findings highlight the importance of refraining from the use of isotonic fluids throughout ritodrine therapy. In the past, antenatal steroids, such as betamethasone, were implicated in the genesis of pulmonary edema, but since betamethasone and dexamethasone are almost devoid of mineralocorticoid activity, they are most likely innocent bystanders.[125]

Maternal mortality has been reported with the use of these agents.[126,127] Based on an anonymous survey of American obstetricians, it appears that the maternal mortality related to tocolytic agents has been underreported.[128]

Metabolic complications, such as hypokalemia due to increases in glucose and insulin, hyperglycemia due to glucagon stimulation and glycogenolysis, and an increase in free fatty acids due to lipolysis, are common with intravenous therapy.[129,130] Less common is lactic acidosis and ketosis.[131] Occasionally there have been cases of diabetic ketoacidosis.[132] Once the patient is switched to oral therapy, it appears that ritodrine has less effect on glucose intolerance than does oral terbutaline.[133–135]

The effects on uteroplacental profusion are controversial: some studies show an increase, others a decrease.[136,137] The common effects on the neonate have been limited primarily to hypoglycemia.[138] Apgar scores have not been significantly affected.[138] Long-term follow-up studies have revealed no significant problems in child development.[139–143]

Ritodrine

Favorable reports in 1980 by Barden and Merkatz promulgated the clinical use of ritodrine in the United States.[127,144] Ritodrine became the first drug approved in the United States by the Food and Drug Administration for the inhibition of preterm labor. It was reported to have similar efficacy but fewer side effects than previous tocolytic agents, and generally the side effects were thought to be acceptable. There was evidence that it prolonged pregnancy, and when compared with controls there was a significant reduction in the incidence of neonatal death and respiratory distress syndrome.[144]

A subsequent meta-analysis of ritodrine efficacy was

performed on 890 women who participated in 16 scientifically acceptable controlled trials.[145] There were significantly fewer deliveries in the beta-mimetic group during the first 24 and 48 hours of therapy. There was a slight reduction in the percentage of preterm delivery in the group receiving beta-mimetic therapy. However, there was no significant reduction in the incidence of LBW infants, respiratory distress morbidity, or perinatal mortality. The lack of any suggestion of effect on substantive outcome challenges the previous claims that had favored such drug therapy. It has been suggested that the increased cost of intensive tocolysis beyond 34 weeks gestation is offset by the decreased cost of neonatal intensive care.

Ritodrine infusions should be given according to the guidelines in the manufacturer's package insert, or based on Caritis's method.[127,147] Attention should be paid to contraindications, maternal tachycardia, diabetic status, and fluid balance. Some physicians give ritodrine intramuscularly in the belief that this route may lead to fewer side effects and require less fluid hydration. The technique has been described by Gonik and associates.[148] It is thought that there are fewer side effects when ritodrine is infused according to the method of Caritis or given intramuscularly, as opposed to the "Barden" protocol approved by the FDA.

Many clinicians who use ritodrine say they do so because it is the only drug approved by the FDA for preterm labor tocolysis. However, there is confusion among many clinicians regarding the meaning of FDA approval of a drug. The FDA does not and cannot dictate specific medical practice regarding use of a drug. The FDA approves drugs to be marketed in the United States by pharmaceutical companies for very specific and labelled medical indications. Without this approval, the medication cannot be made readily available to the practitioner. Special approval must be given to use medications that are unapproved for any clinical use. However, once a medication is approved to be marketed and labelled for specific indications, it becomes readily available for clinical use.

The exact clinical use of a medication must be determined by the prescribing physician. In fact, the FDA acknowledges that it is appropriate and rational to use a drug for unlabelled indications when such drug therapy has been extensively reported in the literature.[149] For example, the safe and effective use of terbutaline and magnesium sulfate as tocolytic agents has been reported in such a manner.

Terbutaline

Terbutaline is commonly used in the initial management of preterm labor. Initially, its efficacy was thought to be quite significant, but subsequent studies have found that it has only limited efficacy.[61,150,151] Terbutaline has significant, potentially life-threatening side effects similar to those of ritodrine, especially when given intravenously.[122,153,154]

An alternative route is subcutaneous administration: the drug effect is rapid and apparently has fewer side effects.[155–157] The ease of administration and the avoidance of intravenous hydration makes subcutaneous use a reasonable alternative. In a commonly used regimen, 0.25 mg is given subcutaneously every 20 to 60 minutes until contractions have subsided. Close attention is paid to the maternal heart rate and symptoms to prevent serious complications. Oral administration of terbutaline results in widely varying serum concentrations.[158] The common daily dose ranges from 10 to 20 mg; the maximum daily dose is about 40 mg.

A recent development in terbutaline administration is the use of the continuous subcutaneous infusion pump. Although significant efficacy is claimed, this type of home therapy is very expensive. More data are required before this therapy can be unequivocally advocated.

In general, there seems to be no significant difference in efficacy or safety between terbutaline and ritodrine. Oral terbutaline does cause significant alterations in maternal glucose tolerance, compared to oral ritodrine administration. However, terbutaline is much less expensive.[133–135]

Since there is a significant database and clinical experience with the use of terbutaline, FDA approval is unnecessary for its continued use in the medical community in the United States.

PROSTAGLANDIN SYNTHETASE INHIBITORS

Prostaglandin synthetase inhibitors are among the most effective drugs known for inhibiting preterm labor. They are easily administered and well tolerated by the mother. However, they have had only limited human application in the United States, since the limiting factor is fetal safety.

Of all the tocolytic agents available, indomethacin is likely to have the greatest efficacy. Its first clinical use as a tocolytic agent in the treatment of preterm labor was reported by Zuckerman in 1974.[160] Eighty percent of patients responded to 100 mg administered rectally followed by 25 mg given orally every 6 hours. Other studies showed similar results.[161,162] When randomized controlled placebo studies as well as comparison studies were performed, indomethacin was found to be significantly more effective than placebos[163,164] or beta agonists.[165–167] The daily dose ranges from 100 to 200 mg. A second 24-hour course of therapy is indicated if preterm labor recurs.

Maternal side effects are minimal and include primarily gastrointestinal upset, which may require the use of Maalox. Indomethacin is contraindicated in patients with hematologic dysfunction, peptic ulcer disease, and known allergy. Indomethacin does not significantly affect uteroplacental perfusion[168] or Apgar scores.[164]

The most significant potential complications in the fetus relate to the premature closure of the ductus arteriosus, right-sided heart failure, and fetal death.[169–171] Prostaglandin E series allow for the ductus arteriosus to remain patent, but indomethacin tends to transiently constrict the fetal ductus.[172,173] It is more likely to irreversibly close the ductus when it is given at a later gestational age, closer to the time of physiological closure.

In the neonate the most feared complication is persistent pulmonary hypertension.[169–171] Fetal and neonatal oliguria is not uncommon[174–177]; in fact, idiopathic polyhydramnios may be treated effectively with indomethacin.[178] Sonographic surveillance for oligohydramnios is indicated when indomethacin is used for more than 72 hours. There are case reports of bowel perforation.[179] Hyperbilirubinemia may occur because indomethacin may displace bilirubin from the binding sites of albumin.[180]

Nevertheless, a growing database suggests that the selective use of indomethacin before 34 weeks gestation causes no substantial side effects to the fetus or neonate.[181,182] Since prostaglandin synthetase inhibitors are effective, easily administered, and tolerated well by the mother, these agents may be used with proper precautions to minimize fetal and neonatal effects. These include very short courses (24 to 48 hours) in patients less than 34 weeks gestation.

Since there is a significant database and clinical experience with indomethacin, FDA approval is unnecessary for its use in the United States. Its use must be carefully supervised to minimize life-threatening perinatal complications; this may require consultation with maternal—fetal medicine subspecialists and serial sonographic evaluation of the fetus.

MAGNESIUM SULFATE

As of January 1985, magnesium sulfate was second only to beta-sympathomimetic agents as the most commonly prescribed parenteral agent in the United States for tocolytic therapy.[128] Recent evidence and clinical experience favor magnesium over beta-sympathomimetics with regard to safety without compromising tocolytic efficacy.[183]

The clinical use of magnesium sulfate has several advantages. American obstetricians have extensive experience with it in patients with preeclampsia/eclampsia. Properly used, magnesium sulfate for both tocolysis and seizure prophylaxis is safe. Most clinicians monitor reflexes, respiration, urine output, and intermittent serum magnesium levels to prevent serious complications of hypermagnesemia. A diminished glomerular filtration rate diminishes the excretion of magnesium, and continued administration of parenteral magnesium sulfate may result in toxicity as serum levels rise. Fortunately, an antidote is available. Intravenous injection of calcium gluconate or chloride rapidly antagonizes the actions of excessive magnesium.

Pharmacology

Oral magnesium is absorbed in the upper small bowel by an active process. Only 30% of normal daily intake is absorbed. The recommended dietary allowance of magnesium by the National Research Council for pregnant women is 450 mg daily. Dietary sources of magnesium are meat, milk, dark-green vegetables, seafood, and chocolate. Oral preparations readily available in the United States and currently used in pregnant women are the gluconate and oxide salts of magnesium, although other varieties exist. The kidney is the major regulator of the serum magnesium concentration, since magnesium is principally excreted in the urine.[184]

The mechanism by which hypermagnesemia exerts its relaxant effects on smooth muscle differs from that of skeletal muscle. Smooth muscle undergoes pharmacomechanical coupling mediated by various agonists rather than the electromechanical coupling characteristic of skeletal muscle. Excess magnesium depresses the peripheral neuromuscular system in three ways: the inhibition of acetylcholine release, the reduction of sensitivity of the motor endplate, and the reduction of the amplitude of the motor endplate potential. Acetylcholine is unnecessary for spontaneous contractility of smooth muscle.

The exact mechanism by which magnesium diminishes or abolishes uterine activity remains unclear. Experimental data support the view that extracellular magnesium ion concentration affects the uptake, binding, and distribution of intracellular calcium in vascular smooth muscle.[185] Similar mechanisms may operate in gravid uterine smooth muscle.

It has been noted that magnesium sulfate in extracellular concentrations of 9.6 to 12.0 mg/dL (1.0 mEq/L = 1.2 mg/dL) almost completely inhibits spontaneous uterine contractility in muscle strips excised from pregnant women.[186] This inhibition is dose-related. The duration of labor is longer in preeclamptic patients receiving high doses of parenteral magnesium sulfate compared to those receiving low doses.

In general, maternal magnesium-sulfate-induced hypermagnesemia is associated with increased urinary excretion of both magnesium and calcium. Three quarters of the elemental magnesium infused was excreted during the infusion and 90% by 24 hours after the end of the infusion.[187] The urinary excretion of calcium was three times that observed in controls. The mean total maternal serum calcium decreased by 12% and the mean serum ionized calcium decreased by 25%. Acutely, phosphate and calcitonin levels did not change significantly, but the mean parathyroid hormone level increased by about 25% from baseline to the end of the infusion. I have observed increases in maternal serum phosphate with longer-term (> 1 week) chronic intravenous magnesium sulfate therapy for tocolysis. Occasionally, some of these patients are treated with oral phosphate binders.

Maternal Side Effects

Table 87-13 summarizes the major maternal clinical side effects of maternal hypermagnesemia. The loss of patellar reflexes has been reported at magnesium concentrations of 8.4 to 12.0 mg/dL (7 to 10 mEq/L) and respiratory depression begins at levels of 12 to 14.4 mg/dL (10 to 12 mEq/L).[188] Clinically, respiratory depression from hypermagnesemia does not occur before

TABLE 87–13. POTENTIAL MATERNAL EFFECTS OF HYPERMAGNESEMIA

Common Side Effects
Loss of deep tendon reflexes
Warmth during infusion
Mild central hypothermic effect
Increase in skin temperature
Cutaneous vasodilatation
Transient peripheral arterial vasodilatation
Nausea, possible emesis
Not Uncommon Side Effects (seen with moderately elevated serum levels)
Somnolence, lethargy, lightheadedness
Visual blurring, diplopia
Dysarthria
Nystagmus
Constipation and dyspepsia
Uncommon Side Effects
Potentiation of other neuromuscular blockers
Lengthening of the P-R and QRS interval
Controversial effect on the T wave
Chest pain
Pulmonary edema
Effects Seen at Very High Serum Concentrations
Respiratory depression
Cardiac arrest
Profound muscular paralysis
Amnesia
Decreased rate of impulse formation of the S-A node
Rare Side Effects
Profound hypotension
Maternal tetany
Hypersensitivity urticarial reaction
Paralytic ileus

the disappearance of the deep tendon reflexes. The absence of the reflex arc should serve as a warning sign of impending magnesium toxicity, but this sign is of no value in those few patients who inadvertently receive high doses of magnesium intravenously over a short period (usually as the result of a dosing mistake). The initial clinical presentation may be respiratory or cardiac arrest.[189–191]

Somnolence, drowsiness, lightheadedness, and visual blurring occasionally occur at therapeutic concentrations during the usual period (12 to 72 hours) of standard tocolytic therapy. Signs and symptoms of "apparent" depression of the central nervous system and respiratory effort may be potentiated by the use of other depressant agents, particularly at high magnesium concentrations.

Various side effects–primarily neuromuscular or gastrointestinal–have been observed during clinical trials of magnesium sulfate as a tocolytic agent.[183,192–195] During prolonged therapy, psychological effects secondary to prolonged hospitalization may become prominent.[196]

During initial magnesium sulfate infusion of 4 to 6 g over 15 to 30 minutes, the acute effects in patients with preterm labor are similar to those observed in patients receiving an intravenous loading dose for preeclampsia. Early in the intravenous infusion, perspiration and flushing are observed and the patient feels warm; this finding continues more or less throughout the infusion. The face, neck, and hands are particularly affected, and a rise in skin temperature is easily demonstrated. These manifestations occur in both hypertensive and normotensive patients. The intensity of the effect is in part rate-related. Excessive magnesium causes vasodilatation by direct action on blood vessels and ganglionic blockade. Nausea and possibly emesis may occur.

During maintenance therapy, lethargy, somnolence, diplopia, dysarthria, blurred vision, dry mouth, dizziness, and nystagmus may occur. These effects generally occur at a dose of more than 2 g per hour (2.5 to 4.0 g per hour). Reducing the rate in half-gram increments is generally all that is needed; discontinuation of therapy for side effects is rarely needed. If necessary, intravenous injection of 1 g calcium gluconate will result in rapid symptomatic relief. During long-term magnesium sulfate infusion therapy, constipation and dyspepsia may occur and can be symptomatically treated.

One of the most important side effects encountered during standard tocolytic therapy with magnesium sulfate is chest pain, possibly due to myocardial ischemia. This rarely occurs due to magnesium sulfate therapy alone; more often there are additional factors. Ferguson and coworkers reported an increased rate of chest pain with and without EKG changes in patients receiving initial therapy with ritodrine and magnesium sulfate simultaneously compared to ritodrine alone.[194] This finding is not entirely unexpected, based on the known cardiovascular effects of both agents. The results of this study emphasize that such combined tocolytic treatment is potentially life-threatening. Wilkins and coworkers also found a higher incidence of cardiorespiratory side effects in patients undergoing additional supplemental therapy after failed single-agent therapy.[195] In contrast, Hatjis and coworkers found no increase in the incidence of chest pain or abnormal EKG changes in patients receiving either ritodrine alone or ritodrine and magnesium sulfate together.[197]

The other potentially lethal side effect encountered during magnesium sulfate tocolytic therapy is pulmonary edema. Its incidence is about 1%, compared to 5% in patients receiving beta-sympathomimetics.[193,198] Generally, these cases are complicated by other factors associated with pulmonary edema: multiple gestation, polyhydramnios, preeclampsia, anemia, blood transfusion, chorioamnionitis, positive fluid balance, operative delivery, dual-agent therapy, and prolonged therapy.[199–201] With proper patient selection, judicious use of therapy, and close monitoring, the risk of pulmonary edema can be minimized.

Perinatal Side Effects

Neonatal and fetal effects are summarized in Table 87-14. None of the neonatal effects appear to be due to magnesium alone, since they may be related to confounding variables such as maternal illness, fetal growth retardation, and prematurity. Holcomb and colleagues found proximal humeral radiographic abnormalities consisting of transverse radiolucent or sclerotic

TABLE 87–14. POTENTIAL FETAL/NEONATAL EFFECTS OF HYPERMAGNESEMIA

1. Controversial effects on fetal heart rate variability
2. Lack of significant effect on fetal umbilical Doppler studies
3. Fetal breathing movements decrease
4. Mean baseline fetal heart rate decreases
5. Flaccidity, hyporeflexia
6. Need for assisted ventilation
7. Week or absent cry
8. Transient decreased active tone of neck extensors
9. Possible transient radiographic bony changes

bands in 6 of 11 neonates exposed to long-term magnesium sulfate (> 7 days) and no such radiographic abnormalities in gestational-age-matched controls.[202] The clinical significance of these findings is unknown. More studies are required to address this concern, particularly with a control group of pregnant women receiving prolonged bed rest for the same interval.

Efficacy and Relative Safety

In 1966 Rusu and colleagues performed the first therapeutic trials of magnesium as a tocolytic agent.[203] In 1977 Steer and Petrie were the first investigators to publish in English a clinical trial evaluating such therapy.[204] They studied 71 patients with preterm labor with intact membranes who had a painful, identifiable contraction pattern with a frequency of 5 minutes or less. Based on the last digit of their hospital number, 31 patients were allocated to receive ethanol and 31 patients to receive intravenous magnesium sulfate; the remaining 9 patients were chosen at random to form a control group and received an infusion of 5% dextrose in water. The magnesium group received a 4-g loading intravenous dose of a 10% solution, followed by 2 g per hour. Successful treatment was defined as the absence of contractions for a 24-hour interval. The success rate was higher in the magnesium group (77%) compared to the alcohol group (45%) or the control group (44%). In patients with cervical dilatation of 1 cm or less, the respective group success rates were 96%, 72%, and 60%. The respective frequency of patients remaining undelivered for at least 1 week was 74%, 42%, and 33%. The authors concluded that magnesium sulfate may be an alternate method of controlling preterm labor until beta-sympathomimetic agents became generally available for clinical use.

In 1982, three studies were published. In a randomized trial of magnesium sulfate versus intravenous terbutaline, Miller and coworkers found equal efficacy and fewer side effects in the magnesium group.[205] Spisso and associates reported on a large case series using magnesium sulfate as the primary tocolytic agent.[206] Although this study had no control group, the authors had success rates comparable to published studies of ritodrine hydrochloride in patients with intact membranes (80%) and ruptured membranes (50%). They concluded that magnesium sulfate is an effective tocolytic agent that has minimal adverse effects in patients at risk for preterm delivery. Valenzuela and Cline reported on five patients who, after failing to respond to beta-mimetic agents, were treated with intravenous magnesium sulfate.[207] One of the five patients failed to respond to magnesium due to abruptio placentae. Although the number of patients studied was small, the results suggested the utility of magnesium sulfate in decreasing the number of preterm deliveries after failed beta-mimetic therapy.

In 1983 Elliott reported on 355 patients with and without intact membranes who were treated with magnesium sulfate as the primary tocolytic agent. The author made detailed analyses of failures and side effects and found that magnesium sulfate's efficacy was comparable to that of ritodrine in previous published reports.[193] Only 5% (14/309) of all patients treated with intact membranes had no apparent reason for failure; if only patients with cervical dilatations of 2 cm or less were included, 2% (5/309) had unexplained failure. Failures were often due to chorioamnionitis, advanced cervical dilatation, and abruptio placentae. Seven percent of patients experienced some side effects, but only 2% required discontinuation of medication for this reason. There was a 1% incidence of pulmonary edema (each of these patients had other predisposing factors); this compared favorably to the 5% rate for beta-sympathomimetic agents. Side effects were found to be less serious and also fewer in number than the known effects of intravenous ritodrine.

In 1984 Tchilinguirian and colleagues performed a randomized trial of magnesium sulfate versus intravenous ritodrine and found comparable efficacy.[208] Cotton and coworkers performed a randomized study comparing magnesium sulfate, terbutaline, and a placebo (5% dextrose in lactated Ringer's) to assess the adequacy of magnesium sulfate as a tocolytic agent.[151] This study was not very well controlled. They concluded that none of the agents were very effective in their study population and that other, more effective techniques for labor inhibition were needed.

From the same institution as Cotton, Beall and coworkers in 1985 performed a randomized trial of ritodrine versus terbutaline versus magnesium sulfate, each as a primary agent.[154] A crossover arm was used when single-agent primary therapy was unsuccessful. Successful tocolysis was achieved by the primary agent alone in 69% (31/45) of the ritodrine group, 45% (18/40) of the terbutaline group, and 70% (32/46) of the magnesium group. The frequency of patients experiencing side effects requiring discontinuation of primary therapy was 38% (17/45) for the ritodrine group, 60% (24/40) for the terbutaline group, and 2% (1/46) for the magnesium group. The authors concluded that magnesium sulfate appeared to meet the requirements for the choice of a primary tocolytic agent on a busy service (ie, efficacy coupled with minimal side effects for mother and fetus). However, they hesitated to endorse such use of magnesium sulfate fully without further study because of the previous findings of Cotton and coworkers from their institution.

In 1987 Hollander and coworkers performed an excellent prospective randomized study analyzing the efficacy and safety of magnesium sulfate versus ritodrine.[183] All patients had preterm labor with intact membranes and associated cervical changes. Successful tocolysis was defined as cessation of uterine activity and delay in delivery for 72 hours or more from the onset of tocolysis. Via a random number table, 70 patients were randomized to receive ritodrine (n = 36) or magnesium sulfate (n = 34) as the first tocolytic agent. Ritodrine was used an additional three times when magnesium failed to achieve tocolysis; in contrast, magnesium was used an additional six times for discontinuation of ritodrine. The success rates of ritodrine and magnesium sulfate as primary agents were 83% (30/36) and 91% (31/34) respectively. When administered as either a primary or secondary agent, the success rate of ritodrine was 79% (31/39) and magnesium sulfate was 88% (35/40). Delay of delivery for 1 week or more occurred in 72% (28/39) of patients given ritodrine and 75% (30/40) of those given magnesium sulfate. The mean rate of ritodrine required to achieve tocolysis was 210 micrograms/minute. The mean serum level of magnesium required to achieve tocolysis was 6.6 mg/100 mL. Although the side effects differed in type and severity, the proportion of patients with a side effect was comparable in both groups. Two patients in the ritodrine group required discontinuation of therapy due to chest pains and tachycardia. No patient receiving magnesium required discontinuation because of side effects, but two patients did require a downward adjustment in dosage for lethargy with diplopia as its major symptom. The authors concluded that magnesium sulfate was easy to administer and clinically efficacious and that the side effects were less alarming than in the ritodrine group. They recommended that magnesium sulfate should be used as the first line of tocolytic therapy, with ritodrine to be used as backup.

Cox and coworkers performed a recent randomized trial comparing magnesium sulfate to no tocolytic therapy in 156 women thought to be in preterm labor.[209] They found no significant pregnancy prolongation in the group receiving magnesium and concluded that magnesium sulfate is ineffective in preventing preterm birth. This study may have potential bias because the clinicians were not blinded to the patient groups. Also, only 28% of the control group delivered within 24 hours. Almost two thirds of the control patients had a delay in delivery of at least 1 week, and most of them had pregnancy continued more than 28 days. There appears to be a major flaw in the actual diagnosis of patients in the control group. This renders the study conclusions suspect and speculative at best, and reminds us of the difficulty in making a true diagnosis of actual preterm labor. This difficulty may be compounded in a very busy indigent-care obstetric service with multiple care providers.

A report by Madden and colleagues found no threshold relationship of specific serum magnesium concentrations and tocolytic efficacy.[210] This is in contrast to the reports of Elliot and Hollander, who recommended that levels should be at least 5.0 to 5.7 mg% for efficacy.[183,193] The desired effect of magnesium sulfate is best achieved when titrated between the clinical findings of toxicity and uterine responsiveness.

In summary, as a single agent magnesium sulfate is as effective as intravenous beta-sympathomimetic agents and is safer than beta-mimetic agents.

Dual-Agent Therapy

In 1984 Ferguson and associates performed the first trial of dual-agent primary therapy of magnesium sulfate and intravenous ritodrine versus intravenous ritodrine, and noted serious maternal side effects.[194] The study was randomized and the administration of magnesium versus intravenous fluids was blinded. The code was broken after 50 patients were enrolled due to side effects. Nine cases were excluded after randomization, yielding a final analysis group of 24 patients with combined therapy and 17 patients with ritodrine alone.

Eleven of the patients (46%) in the combination group suffered side effects severe enough to require discontinuation of combination therapy. Ten had chest pain, and seven of these had EKG changes consistent with myocardial ischemia; one additional patient had adult respiratory distress syndrome. Most of these patients subsequently did well on magnesium sulfate alone. In the ritodrine-only group only one patient had chest pain with EKG changes consistent with ischemia. Most patients with these side effects (8/12) were receiving lactated Ringer's solution, while no patients receiving 5% dextrose in water had these side effects.

The authors did not discuss tocolytic efficacy in detail. They thought it was not meaningful to do so because of the high incidence of side effects requiring discontinuation of therapy. The authors concluded that the adjunctive use of magnesium sulfate with ritodrine was associated with an unacceptable increase in serious side effects and probably no increase in efficacy.

Diamond and colleagues thought that the complications observed in Ferguson's study were due to the effect of a large bolus of magnesium sulfate superimposed on the inotropic and chronotropic effects of ritodrine.[201] However, most of the patients that Ferguson studied had their complications 6 hours or more after initiation of therapy. Hatjis commented on Ferguson's study by pointing out reports of a high incidence of silent ST segment depression associated with myocardial ischemia in patients receiving ritodrine alone.[211] In a subsequent report, Ferguson compared the metabolic changes in the same two groups of patients.[212] Adjunctive magnesium sulfate did not cause additional alteration in the metabolic changes commonly associated with ritodrine.

In 1984 Hatjis and associates performed a slightly different evaluation, comparing ritodrine as primary therapy versus dual-agent secondary therapy of ritodrine plus magnesium sulfate in those who failed ritodrine primary therapy.[213] In contrast to Ferguson's study, treatment-related maternal/fetal complications in the dual-agent secondary therapy study did not differ among the various groups analyzed. The authors concluded that adding magnesium in pharmacologic doses improved pregnancy outcome in selected patients in preterm labor who did not respond to conventional ritodrine therapy.

In a 1987 study Hatjis and coworkers randomly assigned 74 patients in preterm labor to one of two treatment groups.[197] Thirty-two women initially received ritodrine alone, and another 32 received ritodrine and magnesium sulfate concurrently (ten patients were excluded after randomization). The authors concluded that concurrent administration of ritodrine and magnesium sulfate was more efficacious than ritodrine alone and caused no apparent increase in adverse side effects. The efficacy conclusion is debatable, since the ultimate success rates of tocolysis in both groups were similar.

Diamond reported on 11 patients who received additional magnesium therapy after unsuccessful therapy with ritodrine alone for preterm labor.[201] One patient had cardiovascular complications; pulmonary edema developed in a patient with a twin pregnancy.

Ogburn and coworkers studied the combination of magnesium sulfate and ritodrine or terbutaline to inhibit preterm labor in 23 high-risk patients transferred to their perinatal center.[200] Six (26%) had pregnancy prolonged at least 1 week. Five (22%) developed pulmonary edema; three of these had twin gestations with intact membranes and two had premature rupture of membranes. The authors concluded that combination therapy may be effective in prolonging some pregnancies with preterm labor, but only with an increase in maternal risk. Wilkins and colleagues also found significant risks with dual-agent intravenous therapy.[195]

In summary, dual-agent intravenous therapy with magnesium sulfate and a beta-sympathomimetic agent carries with it the potential for extremely serious effects compared to single-agent therapy and thus cannot be recommended. These effects may be due to simply the infusion of both drugs, the increased duration of therapy common in patients requiring a second agent, the extensive concurrent use of isotonic crystalloids, patient selection, or some combination of factors. Other drug combinations containing magnesium sulfate have been empirically used quite successfully and safely in our hands (eg, magnesium sulfate and intermittent oral or subcutaneous terbutaline); studies of these regimens are needed.

Long-Term Therapy

In 1986 Wilkins and colleagues reported a normal outcome in two patients in preterm labor who had been treated continuously for 6 and 13 weeks with intravenous magnesium sulfate for tocolysis.[196] In each case, conventional therapy with intravenous and oral ritodrine failed to abate uterine contractions and attempts to wean magnesium sulfate were unsuccessful. In 1989 Dudley and colleagues added 51 patients to the database successfully supporting long-term magnesium sulfate therapy.[192] In fact, they concluded that there need be no time limit and that magnesium sulfate tocolysis may be continued as clinically indicated. In contrast, some reports seem to implicate long-term continuous infusion of magnesium sulfate for tocolysis in the genesis of transient neonatal radiographic bony lesions.[202,214,215]

The most important problem arising from prolonged therapy appears to be emotional depression and anxiety of the patient and family due to prolonged bed rest and hospitalization.

Oral Magnesium as Prophylaxis for Preterm Delivery

Serum magnesium levels are usually lower in pregnancy than in the nonpregnant state, and during preterm labor levels appear to drop still further.[216,217] Some authors have suggested an etiologic relationship between low magnesium concentration and preterm delivery.[218–220]

Oral tocolysis with magnesium oxide and gluconate may be used.[221] The mean serum concentration of magnesium may increase from 1.44 ± 0.22 mg/100 mL before therapy to 2.16 ± 0.32 mg/100 mL after therapy.[222]

In 1988 Martin and colleagues reported on 50 successfully tocolysed patients with preterm labor. Half received magnesium sulfate followed by oral magnesium gluconate, and the other half received intravenous ritodrine followed by oral ritodrine.[221] The number of patients who progressed to 37 weeks gestation was similar in both groups (magnesium 21, ritodrine 19). More ritodrine patients had side effects (40% versus 16%). The authors concluded that both oral agents were equally effective in prolonging pregnancy to term. It is difficult to understand how oral magnesium, which raises magnesium levels only slightly, could be effective in maintaining uterine quiescence and preventing preterm delivery. Therefore, since there was no control group, it can be argued that neither agent was effective. Further, since this study was not randomized, selection bias could have influenced the results.

A randomized trial comparing oral terbutaline and magnesium oxide for maintenance of tocolysis revealed no significant difference in efficacy.[223] The authors did find fewer side effects and a significant cost advantage with the magnesium therapy.

Spatling and Spatling studied the effect of magnesium supplementation in 568 pregnant women who received 15 mmole per day of oral magnesium aspartate hydrochloride.[220] The authors found that magnesium supplementation was associated with significantly fewer antenatal hospitalizations for antepartum hemorrhage, incompetent cervix, and preterm labor, and a decrease in neonatal admissions to the intensive-care unit.

In contrast, Sibai and coworkers performed a double-blind randomized controlled study of 400 primigravid young normotensive patients in which oral daily administration of 365 mg of magnesium aspartate hydrochloride was compared to an aspartic acid placebo.[224] No significant differences were found in the incidence of preterm labor, preterm delivery, abruptio placentae, fetal growth retardation, preeclampsia, or admissions to the neonatal intensive-care unit. They concluded that magnesium supplements had no demonstrable benefit. Even with a sample size 10 times larger, no decrease in preterm labor would be detected in the magnesium group.

Recommended Clinical Protocol

A review of the literature and extensive clinical experience in managing patients with active preterm labor leave little doubt in my mind that intravenous magnesium sulfate is the drug of choice for most patients in preterm labor. The signs and symptoms of hypermagnesemia seen in patients with preterm labor are not generally encountered in patients with preeclampsia. This may be related to the higher serum magnesium level required in some patients to achieve tocolysis and to a longer average duration of therapy in patients with preterm labor. Unlike the adverse side effects seen with hypermagnesemia, the beta-adrenergic side effects of ritodrine do not appear to be dose-related and hence may be less predictable.

Most reports in the literature have used a loading dose of 4 g intravenous magnesium sulfate followed by 2 g per hour, but Sibai, Petrie, and Elliott have advocated 6-g loading doses.[225–227] The clinical protocol in Table 87-15, modified from Petrie, allows for fine-tuning of infusion rates without the potential for fluid overload and is well tolerated by most patients. Of course, this assumes that contraindications to magnesium therapy are respected (myasthenia gravis, heart block, recent myocardial infarction, and severe renal disease). Paying careful attention to fluid intake and output diminishes the risk of pulmonary edema and magnesium toxicity. Although solutions containing

TABLE 87–15. A CLINICAL RECIPE TO ADMINISTER MAGNESIUM SULFATE

1. 100 mL of a 50% solution of magnesium sulfate is easily obtained from readily available products. This volume contains 50 g magnesium sulfate.
2. 100 mL is sterilely removed from a 500-mL bag of 5% dextrose in water. 50 g magnesium sulfate is injected into the remaining 400 mL of fluid for intravenous infusion. It should be noted that 10 mL of this final solution equals 1 g magnesium sulfate.
3. A loading dose of 6 g is infused over 30 minutes. Perspiration and flushing are observed and occur with a feeling of warmth due to vasodilatation. These findings are usually noted early during the intravenous infusion and continue to a greater or lesser degree throughout the infusion. The face, neck, and hands are particularly affected. Nausea and emesis may occur.
4. The initial continuous maintenance rate is 2 to 3 g per hour for 30 to 60 minutes. One or two doses of subcutaneous terbutaline 0.25 mg per dose may be used during this interval if there are no contraindications and rapid diminution in uterine activity is desired.
5. Complete and rapid uterine quiescence is unnecessary.
6. The infusion rate is increased in increments of 0.5 g/hour every 30 minutes until uterine activity begins to decrease or signs and symptoms of toxicity occur. These findings include lethargy, somnolence, diplopia, dysarthria, blurred vision, dry mouth, dizziness, and nystagmus. These effects generally occur at a dose greater than 2 g per hour (2.5 to 4.0 g per hour). Downward adjustments in the rate by half-gram increments are generally all that is needed; discontinuation of therapy for side effects is rarely needed. If necessary, intravenous injection of 1 g calcium gluconate can be used in the symptomatic patient; this will be followed by rapid symptomatic relief.
7. The infusion is continued at the lowest effective rate or 2 g/hour, whichever is greater, for at least 12 hours of relative uterine quiescence.
8. The infusion rate is decreased at 0.5 g/hour and oral beta-sympathomimetic therapy is administered. Should uterine activity begin to increase during this weaning interval, the rate of magnesium sulfate infusion should be increased to the effective rate.
9. If the patient cannot be successfully weaned from intravenous magnesium therapy, continuous short-term therapy (24 to 72 hours) may be safely administered, usually at rates of 2 to 3 g per hour. During this interval, another attempt at weaning, albeit at a slower rate, may be attempted.
10. If uterine activity recurs coincident with a decrease in the rate of magnesium sulfate infusion, the dosage rate should again be increased to an effective level. Attempts to use other tocolytic agents may be instituted.
11. Should these fail to abate increasing uterine activity, continuous intermediate-term to long-term therapy with magnesium sulfate may be given. In general, cervical dilatation will not change significantly during these therapeutic maneuvers. During long-term magnesium sulfate infusion therapy, constipation and dyspepsia may occur; these can be symptomatically treated. The health-care team should be ready to provide emotional and moral support for patients requiring long-term hospitalization.
12. Most true failures of magnesium sulfate therapy and progressive preterm labor are either due to cervical dilatation > 4 cm, abruptio placentae, or chorioamnionitis.
13. The occasional patient continues to have increased uterine activity, yet has no associated cervical changes while on magnesium sulfate therapy. Other tocolytic agents may be tried in these cases in an attempt to quiet the uterus.
14. Patients who are refractory to treatment for preterm labor are likely to have an identifiable pathophysiologic process, most notably amniotic infection or abruptio placentae. An amniocentesis for studies of infection is indicated.
15. Dual-agent combination therapy with intravenous magnesium sulfate and intravenous beta-sympathomimetic agents is not recommended due to a significantly increased risk of side effects. However, dual therapy combining magnesium with oral or subcutaneous beta-sympathomimetics is reasonable. Combined use of magnesium with nifedipine, indomethacin, or oxytocin analogs needs further study.
16. In the severely preterm gestation with inevitable delivery due to advanced cervical dilatation (4 to 7 cm), aggressive magnesium tocolysis alone or in combination may be extremely useful in delaying delivery for 24 to 48 hours to improve the neonatal survival advantage by giving antenatal betamethasone.

some salt are used, continuous isotonic crystalloid infusion is restricted to patients undergoing the final labor and delivery process.

NIFEDIPINE

The calcium-channel blockers are better called "calcium antagonists" since they do not completely block calcium influx into the cell; such an action would be incompatible with life. Rather, calcium antagonists are used to normalize excessive transmembrane calcium influx, thus controlling excessive pathologic muscle contractility and pacemaker activity at the cardiac, vascular, and uterine tissue and organ level.[228] Calcium antagonists are divided into three classes: phenylalkylamines, 1,4-dihydropyridines, and benzothiazepines. The respective prototypes are verapamil, nifedipine, and diltiazem.[229]

Nifedipine inhibits uterine activity but has less of an effect on the cardiac conduction system than verapamil. Thus, nifedipine may be used to inhibit uterine activity in acceptable doses, but verapamil's tocolytic effect is limited by its cardiac effects.

The mechanism of action of nifedipine appears limited to the inhibition of the slow voltage-dependent channels regulating calcium influx. Adverse pharmacologic effects include vasodilation, negative inotropism, and S-A or A-V node conduction disturbances. Because it is a potent vasodilator, nifedipine may cause dizziness, lightheadedness, flushing, headache, and peripheral edema.[230] While the overall incidence of side effects is 17%, severe effects necessitating discontinuation of therapy occur in 2% to 5% of patients.[231] The negative inotropic and dromotropic (affecting cardiac nodal conduction) effects of nifedipine are minimal. This is due in large part to the heart's baroreflex response to peripheral vasodilation. Idiosyncratic reactions to nifedipine is rare.

Nifedipine is rapidly and almost completely absorbed from the gastrointestinal tract. Absorption after sublingual administration is rapid but less complete, with levels being measurable in the plasma within 5 minutes.[232] The rate of absorption of oral and sublingual capsules varies widely among patients. Ferguson and colleagues have shown the mean elimination half-life to be 81 ± 26 minutes (range: 49 to 137 minutes) in patients with preterm labor treated with sublingual nifedipine (bitten and held between molars).[233] Rogers and colleagues found the elimination half-life of nifedipine to be 78 ± 30 minutes (range: 24 to 156 minutes) when given as oral capsules in preeclamptic patients.[234] At 360 minutes, following a 10-mg oral dose, plasma nifedipine concentration was undetectable in 12 of 15 preeclamptic patients. The lower limit of detection in their assay for nifedipine was 10 ng/mL. The mean ratio of fetal cord to maternal serum concentrations of nifedipine was 0.93 ± 0.2, whereas the mean amniotic fluid concentration was 53% ± 15% of simultaneously obtained maternal vein samples.

Clinical Experience

In 1978 Andersson and Ulmsten observed that nifedipine produced significant pain relief and a decrease in uterine activity in patients with severe primary dysmenorrhea.[235] A significant reduction in uterine activity during menses in normal women was also observed. In 1979 Andersson and coworkers obtained pain relief and a significant reduction in uterine activity when patients undergoing prostaglandin-induced midtrimester termination of pregnancy were given nifedipine.

In 1980 Ulmsten and colleagues first reported on the clinical use of nifedipine for tocolysis. The results were favorable.[237] In 1985 Kaul and associates first reported on combination nifedipine and oral terbutaline therapy for tocolysis.[238] In 1986 Read and Welby performed a small randomized trial of oral nifedipine versus intravenous ritodrine versus no treatment.[239] The results of the nifedipine group were quite favorable.

Meyer and colleagues reported on 58 women in preterm labor who were randomized to receive oral nifedipine or intravenous ritodrine.[240] They found that nifedipine was as effective as ritodrine with significantly fewer side effects. Umbilical artery Doppler flow studies in six patients revealed an insignificant effect of nifedipine.

Ferguson and colleagues studied 66 women randomized to receive tocolysis with either nifedipine or ritodrine.[241] Maternal side effects were more serious and more common in the ritodrine group (47%) than in the nifedipine group (13%); perinatal outcome was similar in both groups.

In a separate report, Ferguson reported that ritodrine caused more pronounced cardiovascular changes than did nifedipine during successful tocolysis.[242] Both agents had hemodilutional effects, but nifedipine was not associated with alterations in serum electrolytes or dramatic hyperglycemia. The systolic pressure did not significantly change, but the diastolic pressure dropped from 68.5 ± 8.7 mm Hg to 64.5 ± 8.3 mm Hg 10 minutes after the initial sublingual dose. Additional doses caused little further drop compared to predose values. Diastolic blood pressure did not return to pretreatment levels until 3 hours after the last sublingual dose. The pulse increased 10 minutes after the initial sublingual dose. The maximum mean pulse was 98 beats per minute, which occurred 1 hour after the last sublingual dose. Maximal pulse increases after oral therapy with 20 mg of nifedipine occurred 20 minutes after ingestion. The maximal change in blood pressure and pulse were of the same magnitude as those measured during sublingual administration.

During intravenous ritodrine therapy, cardiovascular changes were progressive until an infusion rate of 200 micrograms per minute was reached; thereafter, the pulse and blood pressure changed little. The mean pulse increased from 85.4 ± 9.0 beats per minute to 123.2 ± 13.1 beats per minute. The mean diastolic blood pressure dropped from 68.3 ± 7.4 mm Hg to 51.8 ± 8.0 mm Hg, whereas the systolic pressure remained statistically unchanged. The authors concluded that nifedipine, when clinically used as a tocolytic agent, did not have the untoward cardiovascular and metabolic effects reported with ritodrine tocolysis.

Circulatory Effects

Based on animal studies, concerns about potentially untoward effects on uteroplacental blood flow in humans have limited the clinical application of nifedipine during pregnancy.[243–245] But recently, with the advent of Doppler velocity waveform analysis, uteroplacental and fetal blood circulation can be evaluated.

Hanretty and colleagues studied the effect of 20 mg of oral nifedipine in nine pregnant women with preeclampsia using continuous wave Doppler.[246] There was no significant change in the pulsatility index of the umbilical artery and the uteroplacental vessels. Moretti and coworkers found that oral nifedipine reduced blood pressure in preeclamptic patients remote from term but was not associated with any adverse effects on fetal or uteroplacental circulation when measured by the Doppler technique.[247] Mari and coworkers studied Doppler velocity waveforms of fetal and uteroplacental circulation in patients with preterm labor who received oral nifedipine.[248] The initial dose was 30 mg, followed 4 hours later with 20 mg. Measurements were taken before treatment and 5 hours after the initial dose (1 hour after the second dose). No significant differences in flow velocity waveforms were found when evaluating the maternal uterine arteries and the fetal cerebral, renal, and cardiovascular circulation.

Clinical Implications

Although drug-induced maternal hypotension, particularly in the hypertensive patient, can cause fetal distress, the literature on untoward fetal effects of nifedipine has been limited to animal models. No human studies to date have documented significant adverse effects on the fetus due to careful administration of nifedipine. Nifedipine is a potentially valuable therapeutic agent during pregnancy. Further safety and efficacy studies in the clinical arena are warranted to evaluate its proper role among other currently used tocolytic agents.

PROGESTATIONAL AGENTS

Progestational agents have been widely used to prolong pregnancy in women who are judged to be at increased risk of miscarriage or preterm birth. The most commonly used agent is 17-alpha hydroxyprogesterone caproate. Keirse analyzed seven relevant published reports of controlled trials using 17-α-hydroxyprogesterone caproate and found no significant difference in the miscarriage rate; however, there was a significant difference in the preterm labor and preterm birth rate in favor of drug therapy.[249] Similar to the results of the betamimetic studies, there was no significant impact on neonatal morbidity or mortality. This drug was primarily given weekly in doses of 250 to 1000 mg. Therapy was often started at the initiation of prenatal care or in the third trimester. This drug seems to be more useful for prophylaxis than for inhibiting active preterm labor.

OXYTOCIN RECEPTOR BLOCKADE

The concentration of oxytocin receptors in uterine tissues increases dramatically just before and during labor.[250] Augmented uterine sensitivity to constant serum levels of oxytocin may result in increases in uterine activity. Recent reports have focused on the development of oxytocin antagonists as new tocolytic agents; theoretically, they may offer greater specificity with fewer side effects than agents in current use.[251–253] Clinical trials are underway.

ANTENATAL GLUCOCORTICOIDS

The initial report by Liggins in 1972 revealed a significant decrease in respiratory distress syndrome and neonatal death in patients receiving two doses of 12 mg betamethasone 24 hours apart.[254] Several subsequent trials have found similar results. The optimal glucocorticoid preparation and the ideal dose are unknown. Most studies have used betamethasone or dexamethasone. These two agents are quite similar, although a methyl group is in the alpha position in the dexamethasone molecule and in the beta position in the betamethasone molecule. Neither agent has significant mineralocorticoid activity (as opposed to hydrocortisone or methylprednisolone).

Concern about the harmful effects of corticosteroids has limited the widespread application of this therapy.[255] Animal data have suggested alterations in immune response, neurologic development, and fetal growth. These harmful effects seem to be limited to studies in which large pharmacologic doses of steroids were used in early gestation. They have not been replicated to any significant degree in the human database.

Data from 12 controlled trials involving over 3000 participants demonstrated that corticosteroids could reduce the incidence of respiratory distress syndrome in each subgroup examined.[256] Reductions in respiratory morbidity were also associated with reductions in intraventricular hemorrhage, necrotizing enterocolitis, and neonatal death. Fortunately, these beneficial effects occurred in the absence of strong evidence for adverse effects of corticosteroids. In this meta-analysis, patients with premature rupture of membranes were included. Overall, neonatal respiratory morbidity was decreased by 40% to 60% in the group receiving antenatal steroids. Most patients in these studies were between 30 and 34 weeks gestation. The beneficial effects were noted during any of these gestational ages. The effects were also noted regardless of whether there was premature rupture of membranes. The most dramatic effects were noted in infants born after 24 hours but within 7 days of the dose of steroids. In this meta-analysis both male and female infants benefited. It should be noted that pulmonary maturity testing was not used as a basis for the administration of corticoid steroids; as a result, the basis for administration was gestational age and not demonstrated pulmonary maturity.

Nonrandomized trials have supported the use of corticosteroids in very preterm gestations.[257] A survey of maternal—fetal specialists shows that this therapy, even at 24 weeks gestation, is not unreasonable.[110]

ADJUNCTIVE THERAPY

Adjunctive therapy to optimize the perinatal outcome of impending preterm delivery is threefold:

1. Administering antenatal steroids to prevent respiratory distress syndrome with thyroxine or thyrotropin-releasing hormone[258,259]
2. Preventing intraventricular hemorrhage by medical therapies such as the antenatal administration of phenobarbital and vitamin K and operative interventions such as prophylactic forceps and prophylactic cesarean section[260–269]
3. Administering antenatal antibiotics beyond the accepted standard treatment to prolong "subclinically"-infected pregnancies and to prevent neonatal sepsis.[270,271]

None of these therapies have gained widespread acceptance. Further research regarding their safety and efficacy is warranted before their use can be recommended outside of a research protocol.

PREVENTING PRETERM BIRTH

Preventing preterm birth is a major undertaking, but success would lead to a major improvement in health and welfare. It is difficult to imagine how such a multifaceted problem could be solved by simple interventions, especially when we lack an essential understanding of the mechanisms that give rise to the multitudinous proximate causes of preterm birth (Table 87-4).

Numerous investigators have attempted to prevent indicated preterm deliveries with some modicum of success. Interventions have included low-dose aspirin and calcium for the prevention of preeclampsia, eclampsia, and intrauterine growth retardation. In most cases, fetal hemolytic disease is well understood and preventable.

Most preterm births appear to be due to spontaneous but not idiopathic labor. We must be able to accurately predict these events before we can prevent them. Predictions based on risk scoring systems, biochemical markers, and cervical examination are of limited value; prophylaxis with bed rest, cerclage, tocolytic agents, and progestational agents is also of limited value. Commercial programs for the early detection of preterm labor are being developed and fostered as representative of the forefront of modern perinatal medicine. These programs are based on the maternal diagnosis of vague symptomatology, high-risk patient scoring, cervical evaluation, and assessment of uterine activity.

Since there is no single treatable factor that can prevent preterm birth, many investigators have developed comprehensive preterm birth prevention programs. Papiernik and colleagues were among the first to institute such a program.[272] Its fundamental components include universal preterm birth and preterm labor education of patients, families, staff, and payor sources. Critical to the program's success is 24-hour access to care and a continued commitment to the program. Results are not achieved overnight and in fact may take years to develop.

Regardless of the medical component of these programs, it is clear that socioeconomic variables, such as educational status, income, nutrition, housing, child care, and sociologic and psychological stress, place a substantial burden on those experiencing preterm delivery. Many investigators believe that the greatest potential impact will not come from the medical component per se; rather, reduction of preterm delivery will come from social, educational, and economic changes. This is not to say that medical advancements cannot affect prematurity to a limited extent: Iams and colleagues have emphasized that the obstetrician's attitude with regard to preterm birth prevention is of critical importance.[273] Thorough attention to detail, early therapy, and modification of behavioral risk factors throughout prenatal care is advocated as a useful antidote to preterm birth.[274]

A study by Miller and Merritt is a prime example of the potential impact of behavior modification on prematurity.[275] They studied six modifiable behavioral risk factors that are significantly related to LBW: low maternal weight for height, low maternal weight gain, lack of prenatal care, age less than 17 or more than 35 at delivery, cigarette smoking, and the use of drugs and alcohol. Among white women, if three of these variables were present, the risk of LBW was 29%, with two variables 10%, with one variable 6.7%, and with none of these variables 1%.

Nevertheless, there is no clearly proven method to prevent the onset of preterm labor. Major research efforts are now being directed toward the early detection and treatment of preterm labor. Several policy issues need to be addressed. Should we as a society be concerned with the antecedents of preterm birth to the extent that we are concerned with the antecedents of death? Should existing health-care resources be reallocated to the beginning of life? To what extent is this the responsibility of the medical profession, and to what extent is this the responsibility of society at large (eg, policy makers, legislators, executives, agency directors, judges, foundations, nongovernmental organizations, hospital directors, labor negotiators, insurance companies, churches, and schools)? It appears that only when there is a critical mass of concern and commitment will the problem of preterm birth be addressed and attacked on all fronts rather than just on the medical front.

REFERENCES

1. World Health Organization. The incidence of low birth weight: A critical review of available information. World Health Stat Q 1980;33:197.
2. Schlesinger ER, Allaway NC. The combined effect of birth weight and length of gestation on neonatal mortality among single premature births. Pediatrics 1955;15:698.
3. Pritchard JA, MacDonald PC, Gant NF, eds. Preterm and post-term pregnancies and fetal growth retardation. In: Williams' Obstetrics, ed 17. Connecticut: Appleton-Century-Crofts, 1985:745.
4. Missouri revised statutes. Section 193.165.
5. Amon E, Sibai BM, Anderson GD, et al. Obstetric variables predicting survival of the immature newborn (≤1000 gm.): a five year experience at a single perinatal center. Am J Obstet Gynecol 1987;156:1380.
6. Yu VYH, Downe L, Astbury J, et al. Perinatal factors and adverse outcome in extremely low birthweight infants. Arch Dis Child 1986;293:1200.
7. Amon E. Limits of fetal viability: Obstetric considerations regarding the management and delivery of the extremely premature baby. Obstet Gynecol Clin North Am 1988;15:321.
8. Fedrick J, Anderson ABM. Factors associated with spontaneous preterm birth. Br J Obstet Gynaecol 1976;83:342.
9. Rush RW et al. Contribution of preterm delivery to perinatal mortality. Br Med J 1976;2:965.
10. Amon E, Anderson GD, Sibai BM, et al. Factors responsible for a preterm delivery of the immature newborn infant (≤1000 gm.). Am J Obstet Gynecol 1987;156:1143.
11. Ehrenhaft PM, Wagner JL, Herdman RC. Changing prognosis for very low birth weight infants. Obstet Gynecol 1989;74:528.
12. Trends in fertility and infant and maternal health—United States, 1980–1988. MMWR 1991;40:381.
13. Kliegman RM, Rottman CJ, Behrman RE. Strategies for the prevention of low birth weight. Am J Obstet Gynecol 1990;162:1073.
14. Low birthweight—United States, 1975–1987. MMWR 1990; 39:148.
15. Arias F, Tomich P. Etiology and outcome of low birth weight and preterm infants. Obstet Gynecol 1982;14:361.
16. Main DM, Gabbe SG, Richardson D. Can preterm deliveries be prevented? Am J Obstet Gynecol 1985;151:892.
17. Meis PJ, Ernest JM, Moore ML. Causes of low birth weight births in public and private patients. Am J Obstet Gynecol 1987;156:1165.
18. Hameed C, Tejani N, Verma UL, Archbald F. Silent chorioamnionitis as a cause of preterm labor refractory to tocolytic therapy. Am J Obstet Gynecol 1984;149:726.
19. Romero R, Mazor M. Infection and preterm labor. Clin Obstet Gynecol 1988;31:533.
20. Leigh J, Garite TJ. Amniocentesis and the management of preterm labor. Obstet Gynecol 1986;67:500.
21. Carsten ME, Miller JD. Regulation of myometrial contractions. In: Initiation of parturition: prevention of prematurity. Ohio: Ross Laboratories, 1983:166.
22. Huszar G. Cellular regulation of myometrial contractility and essentials of tocolytic therapy. In: The physiology and biochemistry of the uterus in pregnancy and labor. Florida: CRC Press, 1986.
23. Liggins GC, Fairclough RJ, Grieves SA, Forster CS, Knox BS. Parturition in the sheep. In: Knight J, O'Connor M (eds). The fetus and birth. (Ciba Foundations Symposium). Amsterdam: Elsevier, 1977:5.
24. Csapo AI, Pulkkinen MO, Wiest WG. Effects of luteectomy and progesterone replacement therapy in early pregnant patients. Am J Obstet Gynecol 1973;115:759.
25. Fuchs AR, Fuchs F, Husslein P, Soloff MS, Fernstrom MJ. Oxytocin receptors in the ewe. J Endocrinol 1985;106:249.
26. Roberts JS, McCracken JA, Gavagan JE, Soloff MS. Oxytocin-stimulated release of prostaglandin F2a from ovine endometrium in vitro: Correlation with estrous cycle and oxytocin-receptor binding. Endocrinol 1976;99:1107.
27. Garfield RE. Control of myometrial function in preterm versus term labor. Clin Obstet Gynecol 1984;27:572.
28. Casey ML, MacDonald PC. Decidual activation: The role of prostaglandins in labor. In: McNellis D, Challis J, MacDonald P, et al (eds). Advances in eicosanoid research. England: MTP Press, 1987:108.
29. Mitchell MD, Branch DW, Lundin-Schiller S, Romero RJ, Daynes RA, Dudley DJ. Immunologic aspects of preterm labor. Sem Perinatol 1991;15:210.
30. Keirse MJNC, Phil D. An evaluation of formal risk scoring for preterm birth. Am J Perinatol 1989;6:226.
31. Mueller-Heubach E, Reddick D, Barnett B, Bente R. Preterm birth prevention: Evaluation of a prospective controlled randomized trial. Am J Obstet Gynecol 1989;160:1172.
32. Creasy RK, Gummer BA, Liggins GC. System for predicting spontaneous preterm birth. Obstet Gynecol 1980;55:692.
33. Papiernik-Berkhauer E. Coefficient de risque d'accouchement premature. Presse Med 1969;77:793.
34. Herron MA, Katz M, Creasy RK. Evaluation of a preterm birth prevention program: preliminary report. Obstet Gynecol 1982;59:452.
35. Holbrook RH, Laros RK, Creasy RK. Evaluation of a risk-scoring system for prediction of preterm labor. Am J Perinatol 1989;6:62.
36. Mueller-Heubach E, Guzick DS. Evaluation of risk scoring in a preterm birth prevention study of indigent patients. Am J Obstet Gynecol 1989;160:829.
37. Funderburk S, Guthrie D, Meldrum D. Suboptimal pregnancy outcome among women with prior abortions and premature births. Am J Obstet Gynecol 1976;126:55.
38. Carr-Hill RA, Hall MH. The repetition of spontaneous preterm labour. Br J Obstet Gynaecol 1985;92:921.
39. Bakketeig LS, Hoffman HJ. The epidemiology of preterm birth: results from a longitudinal study of births in Norway. In: Elder MG, Hendricks CH (eds). Preterm labor. London: Butterworsth International Medical Reviews, 1981:17.
40. Keirse M, Rush R, Anderson A, Turnbull A. Risk of preterm delivery in patients with previous preterm delivery and/or abortion. Br J Obstet Gynaecol 1978;85:81.
41. Bakketeig LS, Hoffman HJ, Harley EE. The tendency to repeat gestational age and birth weight in successive births. Am J Obstet Gynecol 1979;135:1086.
42. Hoffman HJ, Bakketeig LS. Risk factors associated with the occurrence of preterm birth. Clin Obstet Gynecol 1984;27:539.
43. Breart G, Goujard J, Blondel B, et al. A comparison of two policies of antenatal supervision for the prevention of prematurity. Int J Epidemiol 1981;10:241.
44. Iams JD, Stilson R, Johnson FF, Williams RA, Rice R. Symptoms that precede preterm labor and preterm premature rupture of the membranes. Am J Obstet Gynecol 1990;162:486.
45. Iams JD, Johnson FF, Hamer Cheryl. Uterine activity and symptoms as predictors of preterm labor. Obstet Gynecol 1990;76:42S.
46. Papiernik E, Bouyer J, Collin D, Winisdoerffer G, Dreyfus J.

Precocious cervical ripening and preterm labor. Obstet Gynecol 1986;67:238.

47. Wood C, Bannerman RHO, Booth RT, Pinkerton JHM. The prediction of premature labor by observation of the cervix and external tocography. Am J Obstet Gynecol 1965;91:396.
48. Leveno KJ, Cox K, Roark ML. Cervical dilatation and prematurity revisited. Obstet & Gynecol 1986;68:434.
49. Stubbs TM, Van Dorsten P, Miller MC. The preterm cervix and preterm labor: relative risks, predictive values, and change over time. Am J Obstet Gynecol 1986;155:829.
50. Parikh MN, Mehta AC. Internal cervical os during the second half of pregnancy. J Obstet Gynaecol Br Commonw 1961;68:818.
51. Schaffner F, Schanzer SN. Cervical dilatation in the early third trimester. Obstet Gynecol 1966;27:130.
52. Floyd WS. Cervical dilatation in the mid-trimester of pregnancy. Obstet Gynecol 1961;18:380.
53. Katz M, Newman RB, Gill PJ. Assessment of uterine activity in ambulatory patients at high risk of preterm labor and delivery. Am J Obstet Gynecol 1986;154:44.
54. Katz M, Gill PJ, Newman RB. Detection of preterm labor by ambulatory monitoring of uterine activity: a preliminary report. Obstet Gynecol 1986;68:773.
55. Newman RB, Gill PJ, Wittreich P, Katz M. Maternal perception of prelabor uterine activity. Obstet Gynecol 1986;68:765.
56. Morrison JC, Martin JN Jr, Martin RW, Gookin KS, Wiser WL. Prevention of preterm birth by ambulatory assessment of uterine activity: a randomized study. Am J Obstet Gynecol 1987;156:536.
57. Hill WC, Fleming AD, Martin RW, et al. Home uterine activity monitoring is associated with a reduction in preterm birth. Obstet Gynecol 1990;76:13S.
58. Knuppel RA, Lake MF, Watson DL, et al. Preventing preterm birth in twin gestation: home uterine activity monitoring and perinatal nursing support. Obstet Gynecol 1990;76:24S.
59. Rhoads GG, McNellis DC, Kessel SS. Home monitoring of uterine contractility. Am J Obstet Gynecol 1990;165:2.
60. Valenzuela G, Cline S, Hayashi R. Follow-up of hydration and sedation in the pretherapy of premature labor. Am J Obstet Gynecol 1983;147:396.
61. Ingemarsson I. Effect of terbutaline on premature labor: a double-blind placebo-controlled study. Am J Obstet Gynecol 1976;125:520.
62. Creasy RK. Implications of treatment of preterm labor. In: MacDonald PC, Porter J (eds). Initiation of parturition: prevention of prematurity. Ohio: Ross Laboratories 1983;73.
63. Catalano PM, Ashikaga T, Mann LI. Cervical change and uterine activity as predictors of preterm delivery. Am J Perinatol 1989;6:185.
64. Utter GO, Dooley SL, Tamura RK, Socol ML. Awaiting cervical change for the diagnosis of preterm labor does not compromise the efficacy of ritodrine tocolysis. Am J Obstet Gynecol 1990;163:882.
65. Gonik B, Creasy RK. Preterm labor: its diagnosis and management. Am J Obstet Gynecol 1986;154:3.
66. Shepard MJ, Richards VA, Berkowitz RL, et al. An evaluation of two equations for predicting fetal weight by ultrasound. Am J Obstet Gynecol 1982;142:47.
67. Hadlock FP, Harrist RB, Carpenter RJ. Sonographic estimation of fetal weight radiology 1984;150:535.
68. Doubilet PM, Greenes RA. Improved prediction of gestational age from fetal head measurements. Am J Roent 1982;142:47.
69. Tamura RK, Sabbagha RE, et al. Diminished growth in fetuses born preterm after spontaneous labor or rupture of membranes. Am J Obstet Gynecol 1984;148:1105.
70. Weiner CP, Sabbagha RE, Visrub N, et al. A hypothetical model suggesting suboptimal intrauterine growth in infants delivered preterm. Obstet Gynecol 1985;65:323.
71. Westgren M, Beall M, Divon M, et al. Fetal femur length/abdominal circumference ratio in preterm labor patients with and without successful tocolytic therapy. J Ultrasound Med 1986;5:243.
72. Hadlock FP, Deter RL, Harrist RB, et al. A date-independent predictor of intrauterine growth retardation: femur length/abdominal circumference ratio. AJR 1983;141:979.
73. Ott WJ. Fetal femur length, neonatal crown–heel length, and screening for intrauterine growth retardation. Obstet Gynecol 1985;65:460.
74. Rush RW, Kierse MJNC, Howat P, et al. Contribution of preterm delivery to perinatal mortality. Br Med J 1976;2:965.
75. National Center for Health Statistics. Vital statistics of the United States, 1985. In: DHHS Publication (PHS) 88-1113. Public Health Service. Washington, DC: U.S. Government Printing Office. Natality 1988;1.
76. Nisell H, Bistoletti P, Palme C. Preterm breech delivery: early and late complications. Acta Obstet Gynecol Scand 1981; 60:363.
77. Braun FHT, Jones KL, Smith DW. Breech presentation as an indicator of fetal abnormality. J Ped 1975;86:419.
78. Amon E, Sibai BM, Anderson GD. How perinatologists manage the problem of the presenting breech fetus. Am J Perinatol 1988;5:247.
79. Penn ZJ, Steer PJ. How obstetricians manage the problem of preterm delivery with special reference to the preterm breech. Br J Obstet Gynecol 1991;98:531.
80. Amon E. External cephalic version. In: Sabbagha RE (ed). Diagnostic ultrasound applied to obstetrics and gynecology. Philadelphia: JB Lippincott, 1987.
81. Vintzileos AM, Campbell WA, Nochimson DJ, et al. The use and misuse of the fetal biophysical profile. Am J Obstet Gynecol 1987;156:527.
82. Manning FA, Morrison I, Harman CR, et al. Fetal assessment based on fetal biophysical profile scoring: experience in 19,221 referred high risk pregnancies. II. An analysis of false negative results. Am J Obstet Gynecol 1987;157:880.
83. Castillo RA, Devoe LD, Arthur M, et al. The preterm nonstress test: effects of gestational age and length of study. Am J Obstet Gynecol 1989;160:172.
84. Amon E, Bacus JV, Mabie BC, et al. Ultrasonically guided direct umbilical cord blood sampling. J Reprod Med 1987;32:851.
85. Castle BM, Turnbull AC. The presence or absence of fetal breathing movements predicts the outcome of preterm labour. Lancet 1987;2:471.
86. Boylan P, O'Donovan P, Owens OJ. Fetal breathing movements and the diagnosis of labor: a prospective analysis of 100 cases. Obstet Gynecol 1985;66:517.
87. Agustsson P, Patel NB. The predictive value of fetal breathing movements in the diagnosis of preterm labour. Br J Obstet Gynecol 1987;94:860.
88. Jaschevatzky O, Ellenbogen A, Anderman S, et al. The predictive value of fetal breathing movements in the outcome of premature labour. Br J Obstet Gynecol 1986;93:1256.
89. Besinger RE, Compton AA, Hayashi RH. The presence or absence of fetal breathing movements as a predictor of outcome in preterm labor. Am J Obstet Gynecol 1987;153:753.
90. Stubblefield PG. Causes and prevention of preterm birth: an overview. In: Fuchs F, Stubblefield PG (eds). Preterm birth: causes, prevention, and management. New York: Macmillan, 1984.
91. Bakketeig LS, Hoffman HJ. Epidemiology of preterm birth: results from longitudinal study of births in Norway. In: Elder EG, Hendrisks CH. Preterm labour. London: Butterworths, 1981.
92. Rodeck CH. Fetal abnormality and preterm labour. In: Beard

RW, Sharp R (eds). Preterm labour and its consequences. London: Royal College of Obstetricians and Gynaecologists, 1985.

93. Donnenfeld AE, Mennuti MT. Sonographic findings in fetuses with common chromosome abnormalities. Clin Obstet Gynecol 1988;31:80.
94. Kirbinen P, Jouppila P. Polyhydramnios: a clinical study. Ann Chir Gynaecol 1978;67:117.
95. Barkin SZ, Pretorious DH, Beckett MN, et al. Severe polyhydramnios: incidence of anomalies. Am J Roent 1987;148:155.
96. Wallenburg HCS. Chorioangioma of the placenta. Obstet Gynecol Surv 1971;26:411.
97. Ratten GJ, Beischer NA, Fortune DW. Obstetric complications when the fetus has Potter's syndrome. Am J Obstet Gynecol 1973;115:890.
98. Collaborative Group on Antenatal Steroid Therapy. Effect of antenatal dexamethasone administration on the prevention of respiratory distress syndrome. Am J Obstet Gynecol 1981;141:276.
99. Fleisher B, Kulovich MV, Hallman M, et al. Lung profile: sex differences in normal pregnancies. Obstet Gynecol 1985;66:327.
100. Amon E, Leventhal S, Allen GS, Sibai BM. Neonatal outcome following spontaneous preterm labor after demonstrated lung maturity by amniocentesis. Society for Gynecologic Investigation 37th Annual Meeting, 1990, Abstract #169. St. Louis, Missouri.
101. Konte, et al. Short-term neonatal morbidity. Am J of Perinatology 1986;3:285.
102. Heinonen PK, Saarikoski S, Pystynen P. Reproductive performance of women with uterine anomalies: an evaluation of 182 cases. Acta Obstet Gynecol Scand 1982;61:157.
103. Fedele L, Zamberletti D, Vercellini P, et al. Reproductive performance of women with unicornuate uterus. Fertil Steril 1987;47:416.
104. Amon E, Sibai BM, Anderson GD, et al. Obstetric variables predicting survival of the immature newborn (≤1000 gm.): a five year experience at a single perinatal center. Am J Obstet Gynecol 1987;156:1380.
105. Yu VYH, Downe L, Astbury J, et al. Perinatal factors and adverse outcome in extremely low birthweight infants. Arch Dis Child 1986;61:554.
106. Yu VYH, Loke HI, Bajuk B, et al. Prognosis for infants born at 23–28 weeks' gestation. Br Med J 1986;293:1200.
107. Hack M, Fanaroff AA. How small is too small? Considerations in evaluating the outcome of the tiny infant. Clin Perin 1988;15:773.
108. Amon E, Shyken JM, Sibai BM. How small is too small and how early is too early? A survey of american obstetricians specializing in high-risk pregnancies. Am J Perinatol 1992;9:17.
109. Kitchen W, Ford G, Orgill A, et al. Outcome of extremely low birthweight infants in relation to the hospital of birth. Aust N Z J Obstet Gynaecol 1984;24:1.
110. Amon E, Moyn S. Cesarean section for fetal indications at the limits of fetal viability (1986 to 1991). Society of Perinatal Obstetricians, Proceedings of the 12th Annual Meeting, 1991. Abstract 4. Orlando, Florida.
111. DeGaris C, Kuhse H, Singer P, Yu VYH. Attitudes of Australian neonatal paediatricians to the treatment of extremely preterm infants. Aust Paediatr J 1987;23:223.
112. Hack M, Fanaroff AA. Changes in the delivery room care of the extremely small infant (<750 g): effects on morbidity and outcome. N Engl J Med 1986;314:660.
113. Yu VYH, Wong PY, Bajuk B, Orgill AA, Astbury J. Outcome of extremely low birthweight infants. Br J Obstet Gynaecol 1986;93:162.
114. Miyazaki FS, Taylor NA. Saline amnioinfusion for relief of variable or prolonged decelerations. Am J Obstet Gynecol 1983;146:670.
115. Reece EA, Chervenak FA, Romero R, Hobbins JC. Magnesium sulfate in the management of acute intrapartum fetal distress. Am J Obstet Gynecol 1984;148:104.
116. Mendez-Bauer C, Shekarloo A, Cook V, Freese U. Treatment of acute intrapartum fetal distress by beta_2 sympathomimetics. Am J Obstet Gynecol 1987;156:638.
117. Lands AM, Arnold A, McAuliff JP, et al. Differentiation of receptor systems by sympathomimetic amines. Nature 1967;214:597.
118. Lipshitz J, Bailie P. Uterine and cardiovascular effects of beta_2-selective sympathomimetic drugs administered as an intravenous infusion. So Afr Med J 1976;50:1973.
119. Grospietsch G, Kuhn Walther. Effects of B-mimetics on maternal physiology. In: Fuchs F, Stubblefield PG (eds). Preterm birth: causes, prevention, and management. New York: Macmillan Publishing, 1984;171.
120. Caritis SN, Chiao JP, Moore JJ, et al. Myometrial desensitization after ritodrine infusion. Am J Physiol 1987;253:E410.
121. Berg G, Andersson RGG, Ryden G. β-adrenergic receptors in human myometrium during pregnancy. Changes in the numbers of receptors after β-mimetic treatment. Am J Obstet Gynecol 1985;151:392.
122. Benedetti TJ. Maternal complications of parenteral beta-sympathomimetic therapy for preterm labor. Am J Obstet Gynecol 1983;145:1.
123. Hendricks SK, Keroes J, Katz M. Electrocardiographic changes associated with ritodrine-induced maternal tachycardia and hypokalemia. Am J Obstet Gynecol 1986;154:921.
124. Philipsen T, Eriksen PS, Lynggaard F. Pulmonary edema following ritodrine-saline infusion in premature labor. Obstet Gynecol 1981;58:304.
125. Haynes RC, Larner J. Adrenocorticotropic hormone; adrenocortical steroids and their synthetic analogs; inhibitors of adrenocortical steroid biosynthesis. In: Goodman LS, Gilman A (eds). The pharmacological basis of therapeutics, ed 5. New York: Macmillan, 1975:1491.
126. Milliez S, Blot PH, Sureau C. A case report of maternal death associated with betamimetic and betamethasone administration in premature labor. Eur J Obstet Gynecol Reprod Biol 1980;2:95.
127. Barden TP, Peter JB, Merkatz IR. Ritodrine hydrochloride: a betamimetic agent for use in preterm labor. I. Pharmacology, clinical history, administration, side effects, and safety. Obstet Gynecol 1980;56:1.
128. Taslimi MM, Sibai BM, Amon E, Taslimi CK, Herrick CN. A national survey on preterm labor. Am J Obstet Gynecol 1989;160:1352.
129. Spellacy WN, Cruz AC, Buhi WC, et al. The acute effects of ritodrine infusion on maternal metabolism: measurements of levels of glucose, insulin, glucagon, triglycerides, cholesterol, placental lactogen, and chorionic gonadotropin. Am J Obstet Gynecol 1978;131:637.
130. Lipshitz J, Vinik AI: The effects of hexoprenaline, a beta_2-sympathomimetic drug, on maternal glucose, insulin, glucagon, and free fatty acid levels. Am J Obstet Gynecol 1978;130:761.
131. Lenz S, Kuhl C, Wang P, et al. The effect of ritodrine on carbohydrate and lipid metabolism in normal and diabetic pregnant women. Acta Endocrinol 1979;92:669.
132. Wager J, Fredholm B, Lunell N, et al. Metabolic and circulatory effects of intravenous and oral salbutamol in late pregnancy in diabetic and non-diabetic women. Acta Obstet Gynecol Scand Suppl 1982;108:41.
133. Main DM, Main EK, Strong SE, et al. The effect of oral ritodrine therapy on glucose tolerance in pregnancy. Am J Obstet Gynecol 1985;152:1031.

134. Main EK, Maon DM, Gabbe SG. Chronic oral terbutaline tocolytic therapy is associated with maternal glucose intolerance. Am J Obstet Gynecol 1987;157:644.
135. Angel JL, O'Brien WF, Knuppel RA, et al. Carbohydrate intolerance in patients receiving oral tocolytics. Am J Obstet Gynecol 1988;159:762.
136. Lippert TH, DeGrandi PB, Fridrich R. Actions of the uterine relaxant, fenoterol, on uteroplacental hemodynamics in human subjects. Am J Obstet Gynecol 1976;125:1093.
137. Lunell NO, Joelsson I, Lewander R, et al. Uteroplacental blood flow and the effect of $beta_2$-adrenoceptor stimulating drugs. Acta Obstet Gynecol Scand Supple 1982;108:25.
138. Hancock PJ, Setzer ES, Beydoun SN. Physiologic and biochemical effects of ritodrine therapy in the mother and perinate. Am J Perinatol 1985;2:1.
139. Brazy JE, Eckerman CO, Gross SJ. Clinical and laboratory observations. Follow-up of infants of <1500 gram birth weight with antenatal isoxsuprine exposure. J Pediatr 1983;102:611.
140. Haddengra M, Touwen BCL, Huisjes JH. Longterm follow-up of children prenatally exposed to ritodrine. Br J Obstet Gynecol 1986;1:156.
141. Freysz H, Willard D, Lehr A, et al. A long term evaluation of infants who received a beta-mimetic drug while in utero. J Perinat Med 1977;5:94.
142. Svenningsen NW. Follow-up studies on preterm infants after maternal beta-receptor agonist treatment. Acta Obstet Gynecol Scand Suppl 1982;108:67.
143. Polowczyk D, Tejani N, Lauersen N, et al. Evaluation of seven-to-nine-year-old children exposed to ritodrine in utero. Obstet Gynecol 1984;64:485.
144. Merkatz IR, Peter JB, Barden TP. Ritodrine hydrochloride: a betamimetic agent for use in preterm labor. II. Evidence of efficacy. Obstet Gynecol 1980;56:7.
145. King JF, Grand A, Keirse MJN, et al. Betamimetics in preterm labour: an overview of randomised controlled trials. Br J Obstet Gynaecol 1988;95:211.
146. Korenbrot CC, Aalto LH, Laros RK. The cost effectiveness of stopping preterm labor with beta-adrenergic treatment. N Engl J Med 1984;310:691.
147. Caritis S. A pharmacologic approach to the infusion of ritodrine. Am J Obstet Gynecol (in press).
148. Gonik B, Benedetti T, Creasy RK, et al. Intramuscular versus intravenous ritodrine hydrochloride for preterm labor management. Am J Obstet Gynecol 1988;159:323.
149. Use of approved drugs for unlabeled medications. FDA Drug Bill 1982;12:4.
150. Howard TE, Killam AP, Penney LL, et al. A double blind randomized study of terbutaline in premature labor. Milit Med 1982;147:305.
151. Cotton DB, Strassner HT, Hill LM, et al. Comparison of magnesium sulfate, terbutaline and a placebo for inhibition of preterm labor. A randomized study. J Reprod Med 1984;29:92.
152. Miller JM, Keane MWD, Horger EO. A comparison of magnesium sulfate and terbutaline for the arrest of premature labor. A preliminary report. J Reprod Med 1982;27:348.
153. Caritis SN, Tolg G, Heddinger LA, et al. A double-blind study comparing ritodrine and terbutaline in the treatment of preterm labor. Am J Obstet Gynecol 1984;150:7.
154. Beall MH, Edgar BW, Paul AH, et al. A comparison of ritodrine, terbutaline, and magnesium sulfate for the suppression of preterm labor. Am J Obstet Gynecol 1985;153:854.
155. Stubblefield PG, Heyl PS. Treatment of premature labor with subcutaneous terbutaline. Obstet Gynecol 1982;59:457.
156. Moise KJ, Dorman K, Giebel R, et al. A randomized study of intravenous versus subcutaneous/oral terbutaline in the treatment of preterm labor. Abstract #276 presented at the Seventh Annual Meeting of the Society of Perinatal Obstetricians. Lake Buena Vista, Florida, February 1987.
157. Leferink JG, Lamont H, Wagenmaker-Engles I, et al. Pharmacokinetics of terbutaline after subcutaneous administration. Intl J Clin Pharmacol Biopharm 1979;17:181.
158. Lyrenas S, Grahnen A, Lindberg B, et al. Pharmacolonetics of terbutaline during pregnancy. Eur J Clin Pharmacol 1986;29:619.
159. Repke JR, Niebyl JR. Role of prostaglandin synthetase inhibitors in the treatment of preterm labor. Semin Reprod Endocrinol 1985;3:259.
160. Zuckerman H, Reiss U, Rubinstein I. Inhibition of human premature labor by indomethacin. Obstet Gynecol 1974;44:787.
161. Wiqvist N, Lundstrom V, Green K. Premature labor and indomethacin. Prostaglandins 1975;10:515.
162. Greila P, Zanor P. Premature labor and indomethacin. Prostaglandins 1978;16:1007.
163. Niebyl JR, Blake DA, White RD, et al. The inhibition of premature labor with indomethacin. Am J Obstet Gynecol 1980;136:1014.
164. Zuckerman H, Shalev E, Gilad G, et al. Further study of the inhibition of premature labor by indomethacin. Part II. Double-blind study. J Perinat Med 1984;12:25.
165. Spearing G. Alcohol, indomethacin, and salbutamol. Obstet Gynecol 1979;53:171.
166. Gamissans O, Canas E, Cararach V, et al. A study of indomethacin combined with ritodrine in threatened preterm labor. Eur J Obstet Gynecol Reprod Biol 1978;8:123.
167. Katz Z, Lancet M, Yemini M, et al. Treatment of premature labor contractions with combined ritodrine and indomethacine. Int J Gynaecol Obstet 1983;21:337.
168. Novy MS. Effects of indomethacin on labor, fetal oxygenation, and fetal development in rhesus monkeys. Adv Prostaglandin Thromboxane Res 1978;4:285.
169. Manchester D, Margolis HS, Sheldon RE. Possible association between maternal indomethacin therapy and primary pulmonary hypertension of the newborn. Am J Obstet Gynecol 1976;126:467.
170. Csaba IF, Sulyok E, Ertl T. Relationship of maternal treatment with indomethacin to persistence of fetal circulation syndrome. J Pediatr 1978;92:484.
171. Itskovitz J, Abramovich H, Brandes JM. Oligohydramnios, meconium and perinatal death concurrent with indomethacin treatment in human pregnancy. J Reprod Med 1980;24:137.
172. Clyman RI, Mauray F, Roman C, et al. Circulating prostaglandid E_2 concentrations and patent ductus arteriosus in fetal and neonatal lambs. J Pediatr 1980;97:455.
173. Moise KJ, Huhta JC, Dawod S, et al. Indomethacin in the treatment of preterm labor: effects on the human fetal ductus arteriosus. N Engl J Med 1988;319:327.
174. Cantor B, Tyler T, Nelson RM, et al. Oligohydramnios and transient neonatal anuria: a possible association with the maternal use of prostaglandin synthetase inhibitors. J Reprod Med 1980;24:220.
175. Kirshon B, Moise KJ, Wasserstrum N, et al. Influence of short-term indomethacin therapy on fetal urine output. Obstet Gynecol 1988;72:51.
176. Hickok DE, Hollenbach KA, Reilley SF, et al. The association between decreased amniotic fluid volume and treatment with nonsteroidal anti-inflammatory agents for preterm albor. Am J Obstet Gynecol 1989;160:1525.
177. Wurtzel D. Prenatal administration of indomethacin as a tocolytic agent: effect on neonatal renal function. Obstet Gynecol 1990;76:689.
178. Kirshon B, Mari G, Moise KJ. Indomethacin therapy in the treatment of symptomatic polyhydramnios. Obstet Gynecol 1990;75:202.

179. Vanhaesebrouck P, Thiery M, Leroy JG, Govaert P, Praeter CD, Coppens M, Cuvelier C, Dhont M. Oligohydramnios, renal insufficiency, and ileal perforation in preterm infants after intrauterine exposure to indomethacin. J Pediatr 1988;113:738.
180. Rasmussen LF, Wennberger RP. Displacement of bilirubin from albumin binding sites by indomethacin. Clin Res 1977;25:2.
181. Dudley DKL, Hardie NJ. Fetal and neonatal effects of indomethacin used as a tocolytic agent. Am J Obstet Gynecol 1985;151:181.
182. Niebyl JR, Witter FR. Neonatal outcome after indomethacin treatment of preterm labor. Am J Obstet Gynecol 1986;155:747.
183. Hollander DI, Nagey DA, Pupkin MJ. Magnesium sulfate and ritodrine hydrochloride. Am J Obstet Gynecol 1987;156:631.
184. Gilman AG, Goodman L, Gilman A (Eds). Goodman and Gilman's The Pharmacologic Basis of Therapeutics, ed 6. New York: Macmillan, 1980.
185. Altura BM, Altura BT, Carella A, et al. Mg^{+2}-Ca^{+2} interacts in contractility of smooth muscle: Magnesium versus organic calcium channel blockers on myogenic tone and agonist-induced responsiveness of blood vessels. Can J Physiol Pharmacol 1987;65:729.
186. Hall DG, McGaughey HS, Corey EL, et al. The effects of magnesium therapy on the duration of labor. Am J Obstet Gynecol 1959;78:27.
187. Cruikshank DP, Pitkin RM, Donnelly E, Reynolds WA. Urinary magnesium, calcium, and phosphate excretion during magnesium sulfate infusion. Obstet Gynecol 1981;58:430.
188. Hoff HE, Smith PK, Winkler AW. Effects of magnesium on nervous system in relation to its concentration in serum. Am J Physiol 1940;130:292.
189. Winkler AW, Smith PK, Hoff HE. Intravenous magnesium sulfate in the treatment of nephritic convulsions in adults. J Clin Invest 1942;21:207.
190. Chesley LC. Parenteral magnesium sulfate and the distribution, plasma levels, and excretion of magnesium. Am J Obstet Gynecol 1979;133:1.
191. McCubbin JH, Sibai BM, Abdella TN, Anderson GD. Cardiopulmonary arrest due to acute maternal hypermagnesaemia. Lancet 1981;1:1058.
192. Dudley D, Gagnon D, Varner M. Long-term tocolysis with intravenous magnesium sulfate. Obstet Gynecol 1989;73:373.
193. Elliott JP. Magnesium sulfate as a tocolytic agent. Am J Obstet Gynecol 1983;147:277.
194. Ferguson JE II, Hensleigh PA, Kredenster D. Adjunctive use of magnesium sulfate with ritodrine for preterm labor tocolysis. Am J Obstet Gynecol 1984;148:166.
195. Wilkins IA, Lynch L, Mehalek KE, Berkowitz GS, Berkowitz RL. Efficacy and side effects of magnesium sulfate and ritodrine as tocolytic agents. Am J Obstet Gynecol 1988;159:685.
196. Wilkins IA, Goldberg JD, Phillips RN, Bacall CJ, Chervenak FA, Berkowitz RL. Long-term use of magnesium sulfate as a tocolytic agent. Obstet Gynecol 1986;67:385.
197. Hatjis CG, Swain M, Nelson LH, Meis PJ, Ernest JM. Efficacy of combined administration of magnesium sulfate and ritodrine in the treatment of premature labor. Obstet Gynecol 1987;69:317.
198. Katz M, Robertson PA, and Creasy RK. Cardiovascular complications associated with terbutaline treatment for preterm labor. Am J Obstet Gynecol 1981;139:605.
199. Elliott JP, O'Keeffe DF, Greenberg P, Freeman RK. Pulmonary edema associated with magnesium sulfate and betamethasone administration. Am J Obstet Gynecol 1979;134:717.
200. Ogburn PL, Hansen CA, Williams PP, Butler JC, Joseph MS, Julian TM. Magnesium sulfate and β-mimetic dual-agent tocolysis in preterm labor after single-agent failure. J Reprod Med 1985;30:583.
201. Diamond MP, Mulloy MK, Entman SS. Letter to the Editor. Combined use of ritodrine and magnesium sulfate for tocolysis of preterm labor. Am J Obstet Gynecol 1985;148:827.
202. Holcomb WL, Schackelford GD, Petrie RH. Magnesium tocolysis and neonatal bone abnormalities. Obstet Gynecol 1991;78:611.
203. Rusu O, Lupan C, Baltescu V. Magnezivl serie in sarcina normala la termen si nasterea prematura. Rolvl magneziterapiei in combatera nasterii premature. Obstet Gynecol 1966;14:215.
204. Steer CM, Petrie RH. A comparison of magnesium sulfate and alcohol for the prevention of premature labor. Am J Obstet Gynecol 1977;129:1.
205. Miller JM, Keane MW, Horger EO. A comparison of magnesium sulfate and terbutaline for the arrest of premature labor. J Reprod Med 1982;27:348.
206. Spisso KR, Harbert GM, Thiagarajah S. The use of magnesium sulfate as the primary tocolytic agent to prevent premature delivery. Am J Obstet Gynecol 1982;112:840.
207. Valenzuela G and Cline S. Use of magnesium sulfate in premature labor that fails to respond to β-mimetic drugs. Am J Obstet Gynecol 1982;143:718.
208. Tchilinguirian NG, Najem R, Sullivan GB, Craparo FJ. The use of ritodrine and magnesium sulfate in the arrest of premature labor. Int J Gynaecol Obstet 1984;22:117.
209. Cox SM, Sherman ML, Leveno KJ. Randomized investigation of magnesium sulfate for prevention of preterm birth. Am J Obstet Gynecol 1990;163:767.
210. Madden C, Owen J, Hauth JC. Magnesium tocolysis: serum levels versus success. Am J Obstet Gynecol 1990;162:1177.
211. Hatjis CG. Letter to the editor. Ritodrine/magnesium for the treatment of premature labor. Am J Obstet Gynecol 1984;150:108.
212. Ferguson JE II, Holbrook H, Stevenson D, Hensleigh PA, Kredentser D. Adjunctive magnesium sulfate infusion does not alter metabolic changes associated with ritodrine tocolysis. Am J Obstet Gynecol 1987;156:103.
213. Hatjis CG, Nelson LH, Meis PJ, Swain M. Addition of magnesium sulfate improves effectiveness of ritodrine in preventing premature delivery. Am J Obstet Gynecol 1984;150:142.
214. Lamm CI, Norton KI, Murphy RJ, Wilkins IA, Rabinowitz JG. Congenital rickets associated with magnesium sulfate infusion for tocolysis. J Pediatr 1988;113:1078.
215. Cumming WA, Thomas VJ. Hypermagnesemia. A cause of abnormal metaphyses in the neonate. Am J Roentgenol 1989;152:1071.
216. Hall DG. Serum magnesium in pregnancy. Obstet Gynecol 1957;9:158.
217. Martin RW, Martin JN, Pryor JA, Gaddy DK, Wiser WL, Morrison JC. Comparison of oral ritodrine and magnesium gluconate for ambulatory tocolysis. Am J Obstet Gynecol 1988;158:1440.
218. Kiss VD, Szoke B. Rolle des Magnesiums bei der verhuttung des frühgeburt. Zentralbl Gynakol 1975;97:924.
219. Kiss V, Balasz M, Morvay F, et al. Effect of maternal magnesium supply on spontaneous abortion and premature birth and on intrauterine foetal development: experimental epidemiological study. Mag Bull 1988;3:73.
220. Spatling L, Spatling G. Magnesium supplementation in pregnancy: A double-blind study. Br J Obstet Gynaecol 1988;95:120.
221. Martin RW, Martin JN, Pryor JA, Gaddy DK, Wiser WL, Morrison JC. Comparison of oral ritodrine and magnesium gluconate for ambulatory tocolysis. Am J Obstet Gynecol 1988;158:1440.
222. Martin RW, Gaddy DK, Martin JN, Lucas JA, Wiser WL, Morrison JC. Tocolysis with oral magnesium. Am J Obstet Gynecol 1987;156:433.
223. Ridgeway LE, Muise K, Wright JW, Patterson RM, Newton ER. A prospective randomized comparison of oral terbutaline and

magnesium oxide for the maintenance of tocolysis. Am J Obstet Gynecol 1990;163:879.
224. Sibai AM, Villar MA, Bray E. Magnesium supplementation during pregnancy: A double-blind randomized controlled clinical trial. Am J Obstet Gynecol 1989;161:115.
225. Sibai BM. The use of magnesium sulfate in preeclampsia-eclampsia. In: Petrie RH, ed. Perinatal pharmacology. Oradell, NJ: Medical Economics, 1989.
226. Petrie RH. Tocolysis using magnesium sulfate. Semin Perinatol 1981;5:266.
227. Elliott JP. Magnesium sulfate for tocolysis. In: Petrie RH, ed. Perinatal pharmacology. Oradell, NJ: Medical Economics, 1989.
228. Fleckenstein A. History of calcium antagonists. Circ Res 1983;52(suppl I):3.
229. Schwartz A, McKenna E, Vaghy PL. Receptors for calcium antagonists. Am J Cardiol 1988;62:3G.
230. Lewis JG. Adverse reactions to calcium antagonists. Drugs 1983;25:196.
231. Talbert RL, Bussey HI. Update on calcium channel blocking agents. Clin Pharm 1983;2:403.
232. Raemsch KD, Sommer J. Pharmacokinetics and metabolism of nifedipine. Hypertension 1983;5(supp II):18.
233. Ferguson JE II, Schutz T, Pershe R, Stevenson DK, Blaschke T. Nifedipine pharmacokinetics during preterm labor tocolysis. Am J Obstet Gynecol 1989;161:1485.
234. Rogers RC, Akl SA, Sibai BM, Whybrew WD. Oral nifedipine pharmacokinetics in pregnancy induced hypertension (manuscript submitted). Abstract published in the Proceedings of the 10th annual meeting of the Society of Perinatal Obstetricians, Houston, Texas, 1990.
235. Andersson KE, Ulmsten U. Effects of nifedipine on myometrial activity and lower abdominal pain in women with primary dysmenorrhoea. Br J Obstet Gynaecol 1978;85:142.
236. Andersson KE, Ingemarsson I, Ulmsten U, Wingerup L. Inhibition of prostaglandin-induced uterine activity by nifedipine. Br J Obstet Gynaecol 1979;86:175.
237. Ulmsten U, Andersson KE, Wingerup L. Treatment of premature labor with the calcium antagonist nifedipine. Arch Gynecol 1980;229:1.
238. Kaul AF, Osathanondh R, Safon LE, Frigoletto FD Jr, Friedman PA. The management of preterm labor with the calcium channel blocking agent nifedipine combined with the beta mimetic terbutaline. Drug Intell Clin Pharm 1985;5:369.
239. Read MD, Wellby DE. The use of a calcium antagonist (nifedipine) to suppress preterm labor. Br J Obstet Gynaecol 1986;93:933.
240. Meyer WR, Randall HW, Graves WL. Nifedipine versus ritodrine for suppressing preterm labor. J Reprod Med 1990;35:649.
241. Ferguson JE, Dyson DC, Schutz T, Stevenson DK. A comparison of tocolysis with nifedipine or ritodrine: analysis of efficacy and maternal, fetal, and neonatal outcome. Am J Obstet Gynecol 1990;163:105.
242. Ferguson JE II, Dyson DC, Holbrook RH Jr, Schutz T, Stevenson DK. Cardiovascular and metabolic effects associated with nifedipine and ritodrine tocolysis. Am J Obstet Gynecol 1989;161:788.
243. Ducsay CA, Thompson JS, Wu AT, Novy MJ. Effects of calcium entry blocker (nicardipine) tocolysis in rhesus macaques: Fetal plasma concentrations and cardiorespiratory changes. Am J Obstet Gynecol 1987;157:1482.
244. Harake B, Gilbert RD, Ashwal S, Power GG. Nifedipine. Effects on fetal and maternal hemodynamics in pregnant sheep. Am J Obstet Gynecol 1987;157:1003.
245. Parisi VM, Salinas J, Stockmar EJ. Fetal vascular responses to maternal nicardipine administration in the hypertensive ewe. Am J Obstet Gynecol 1989;161:1035.
246. Hanretty KP, Whittle MJ, Howie CA, Rubin PC. Effect of nifedipine on Doppler flow velocity waveforms in severe preeclampsia. Br Med J 1989;299:1205.
247. Moretti ML, Fairlie FM, Aki S, Khoury AD, Sibai BM. The effect of nifedipine therapy on fetal and placental doppler waveforms in preeclampsia remote from term (submitted). Abstract published in the Proceedings of the 37th annual meeting of the Society of Gynecologic Investigation, St. Louis, Missouri, 1990.
248. Mari G, Kirshon B, Moise KJ Jr, Lee W, Cotton DB. Doppler assessment of the fetal and uteroplacental circulation during nifedipine therapy for preterm labor. Am J Obstet Gynecol 1989;161:1514.
249. Keirse MJNC. Progestogen administration in pregnancy may prevent preterm delivery. Br J Obstet Gynaecol 1990;97:149.
250. Fuchs AR, Fuchs F, Husslein P, Soloff MS. Oxytocin receptors in the human uterus during pregnancy and parturition. Am J Obstet Gynecol 1984;150:734.
251. Akerlund M, Stromberg P, Hauksson A, et al. Inhibition of uterine contractions of premature labour with an oxytocin analogue. Results from a pilot study. Br J Obstet Gynaecol 1987;94:1040.
252. Wilson L, Parsons MT, Quano L, Flouret G. A new tocolytic agent: development of an oxytocin antagonist for inhibiting uterine contractions. Am J Obstet Gynecol 1990;163:195.
253. Andersen LF, Lyndrup J, Akerlund M, Melin P. Oxytocin receptor blockade: a new principle in the treatment of preterm labor? Am J Perinatol 1989;6:196.
254. Liggins GC, Howie RN. A controlled trial of antepartum glucocorticoid treatment for prevention of the respiratory distress syndrome in premature infants. Pediatrics 1972;50:515.
255. U. S. Department of Health and Human Services. Prevention of respiratory distress syndrome. Effect of antenatal dexamethasone administration. Washington, DC: U.S. Government Printing Office. NIH Publication no. 85-2695, August 1985.
256. Crowley P, Chalmers I, Keirse MJNC. The effects of corticosteroid administration before preterm delivery: an overview of the evidence from controlled trials. Br J Obstet Gynaecol 1990;97:11.
257. Doyle LW, Kitchen WH, Ford GW, et al. Effects of antenatal steroid therapy on mortality and morbidity in very low birth weight infants. J Pediatr 1986;108:287.
258. Maschiach S, Barkai G, Sach J, et al. Enhancement of fetal lung maturity by intra-amniotic administration of thyroid hormone. Am J Obstet Gynecol 1978;130:289.
259. Morales WJ, O'Brien WF, Angel JL, Knuppel RA, Sawai S. Fetal lung maturation: the combined use of corticosteroids and thyrotropin-releasing hormone. Obstet Gynecol 1989;73:111.
260. Shankaran S, Cepeda EE, Hagam M, et al. Antenatal phenobarbital for the prevention of neonatal intracerebral hemorrhage. Am J Obstet Gynecol 1986;154:53.
261. Morales WJ, Koerten J. Prevention of intraventricular hemorrhage in very low birth weight infants by maternally administered phenobarbital. Obstet Gynecol 1986;68:295.
262. Pomerance JJ, Teal JG, Gegolok JF, et al. Maternally administered antenatal vitamin K: effect on neonatal prothrombin activity, partial thromboplastin time and intraventricular hemorrhage. Obstet Gynecol 1987;70:295.
263. Morales WJ, Angel JL, O'Brien WF, et al. The use of antenatal vitamin K in the prevention of early neonatal intraventricular hemorrhage. Am J Obstet Gynecol 1988;159:774.
264. Kazzi NH, Hagan NH, Liang KC, et al. Maternal administration of vitamin K does not improve the coagulation profile of preterm infants. Pediatrics 1989;84:1045.
265. Huff DL, Thurnau GR, Sheldon R. The outcome of protective forceps deliveries of 26–33 week infants. Proc of Soc Perinatal Obstet 1987; Abstract No 45.

266. Anderson GC, Bada HS, Sibai BM, et al. The relationship between labor and route of delivery in the preterm infant. Am J Obstet Gynecol 1988;158:1382.

267. Tejani N, Verma U, Hameed C, Chayen B. Method and route of delivery in the low birth weight vertex presentation correlated with early periventricular/intraventricular hemorrhage. Obstet Gynecol 1987;69:1.

268. Schwartz D, Miodovnik M, Lavin J. Neonatal outcome among low birth weight infants delivered spontaneously or by low forceps. Obstet Gynecol 1983;62:283.

269. Dietl J, Arnold H, Mentzel H, et al. Effect of cesarean section on outcome in high- and low-risk very preterm infants. Arch Gynecol Obstet 1989;246:91.

270. Morales WJ, Angel JF, O'Brien WF, et al. A randomized study of antibiotic therapy in idiopathic preterm labor. Obstet Gynecol 1988;72:829.

271. Newton ER, Dinsmoor MJ, Gibbs RS. A randomized blinded, placebo-controlled trial of antibiotics in idiopathic preterm labor. Obstet Gynecol 1989;74:562.

272. Behrman RE, et al. Preventing low birthweight. Committee to Study the Prevention of Low Birthweight, Division of Health Promotion and Disease Prevention. Washington, DC: Institute of Medicine, National Academy Press, 1985.

273. Iams JD. Obstetric inertia: an obstacle to the prevention of prematurity. Am J Obstet Gynecol (in press).

274. Iams JD, Johnson FF, Creasy RK. Prevention of preterm birth. Clin Obstet Gynecol 1988;31:599.

275. Miller HC, Merritt TA. Fetal growth in humans. Chicago: Yearbook Medical Publishers, 1977.

88

CHAPTER

PREMATURE RUPTURE OF THE MEMBRANES

Roberto Romero, Alessandro Ghidini, and Ray Bahado-Singh

In most women, the chorioamniotic membranes remain intact during pregnancy and rupture spontaneously during active labor. Rupture before the onset of labor is called "premature rupture of the fetal membranes" (PROM). Since the word "premature" is often used in obstetrics to refer to preterm gestation and PROM can also occur in the full-term gestation, Keirse and colleagues have proposed the word "prelabor" to avoid ambiguity and confusion.[1] We endorse this proposition, which does not even require a change in the acronym (PROM). Using the word "preterm" (less than 37 weeks) or "term" (more than 37 weeks) before PROM indicates the presence or absence of fetal maturity at the time of the complication. Leakage of amniotic fluid after second-trimester amniocentesis should be considered a separate entity, because it is generally a self-limited phenomenon and carries an overall good prognosis; a detailed discussion is included later in the chapter.

Spontaneous rupture of membranes often leads to the onset of labor. There is no agreement on how long the interval between rupture of membranes and onset of labor should be before the diagnosis of PROM can be made. The latency period has ranged from 1 to 12 hours in different reports.[2–9] Generally, clinical decision-making issues arise when spontaneous labor does not occur within several hours after the membranes rupture. If labor begins shortly after PROM, management issues are considerably simplified. Some authors have suggested the phrase "prolonged PROM" to define a latency period of more than 24 hours.[3,10,11]

RELEVANCE AND FREQUENCY

The incidence of PROM is about 10% after 37 weeks and 2% to 3.5% before 37 weeks gestation.[3,5,12–16] Despite this apparently low prevalence in preterm gestation, 30% to 40% of preterm neonates are born to women with PROM, making PROM the leading identifiable cause of preterm delivery.[3,17] Although most cases of preterm PROM occur after 32 weeks gestation, the major contribution to perinatal mortality is attributable to PROM at less than 32 weeks. The main maternal risks associated with PROM are chorioamnionitis and puerperal infection. The risk of maternal death has decreased from about 0.2% in 1958/1959 to 0.03% (1/3400) in 1982.[17,18]

The question of when membranes normally rupture has been addressed by a Latin American collaborative study in which an effort was made to avoid artificial rupture of the fetal membranes during labor.[19] Figure 88-1 shows the proportion of women with spontaneous rupture of membranes as a function of cervical dilatation. It is apparent that most patients have rupture of membranes at the end of the first stage of labor.

WHY DO MEMBRANES RUPTURE?

Over the last 100 years many investigators have addressed the question of why membranes rupture prematurely. Biophysical, biochemical, and histopathologic methods have been used to investigate the issue.

NORMAL HISTOLOGY

The fetal membranes are formed by the apposition of amnion and chorion (Fig. 88-2). The amnion is derived from the cytotrophoblast and consists of an epithelium, which faces the amniotic cavity; a compact layer, which is responsible for most of the strength of the amnion; and a spongy layer interposed between amnion and

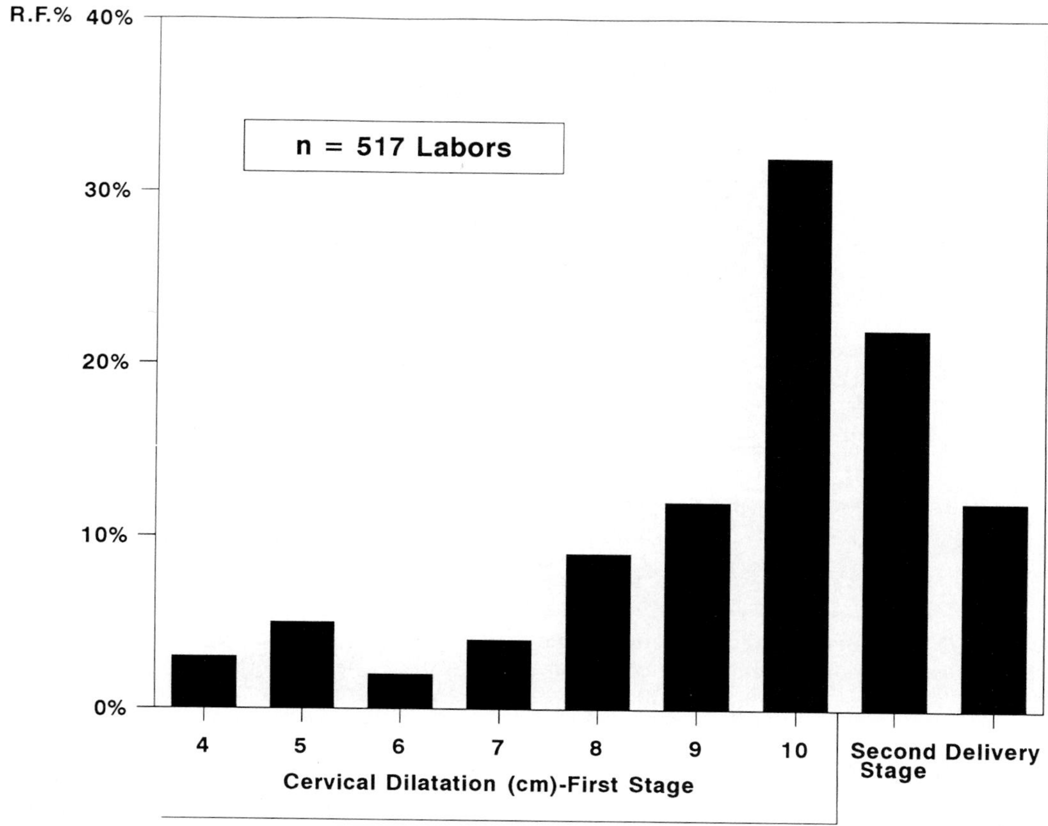

FIGURE 88–1. Phase of labor in which membranes ruptured spontaneously. Percental distribution for 517 normal spontaneous deliveries without medication or maneuvers; vertex presentation. (From Schwarcz R, Belizam JM, Nieto F, Tenzer SM, Rios AM. Third progress report on the Latin American collaborative study on the effects of late rupture of membranes on labor and the neonate, submitted to the Director of the Pan-American Health Organization [PAHO/WHO] and the participating groups. Montevideo, Uruguay: Latin American Center of Perinatology and Human Development, 1974.)

chorion.[20–22] The spongy layer allows the amnion some freedom to slide over the fixed chorion. The chorion contains several collagen layers, the outermost of which is closely attached to and often indistinguishable from the decidua capsularis.

HISTOLOGIC FINDINGS

One study compared the histologic findings in membranes of patients with term PROM with those of patients with uncomplicated pregnancies.[23] The most striking difference was at the level of the spongy layer: PROM was associated with a decrease in the number of collagen fibers, disruption of the normal wavy pattern of these fibers, and deposit of amorphous material between fibers. The cellular components of amnion and chorion did not display significant changes. A major limitation of this study, however, was that the noted morphologic changes could be a consequence rather than the cause of PROM.

The same investigators studied the ultrastructural findings from various areas of membranes in patients undergoing elective cesarean section at term with intact membranes.[24] Membranes apposed to the cervix had findings similar to those reported in patients with PROM. This implies that although spontaneous rupture of membranes normally occurs at the end of the first stage of labor, the process responsible for this phenomenon seems to begin before the onset of labor.

Do similar findings occur in the setting of preterm PROM? We could not find an ultrastructural study of the membranes of patients with preterm PROM. Several authors have proposed that local weakening of the membranes may be the result of ascending infection and inflammation.[25] Naeye and Peters reported that histologic chorioamnionitis (defined as the presence of 4 to 15 neutrophils in the chorionic plate) was two- to threefold more common when rupture of membranes occurred just before the onset of labor than when it occurred after labor began.[26] This suggests that inflammation (and probably infection) is in many cases the cause, and not only a consequence, of preterm PROM.

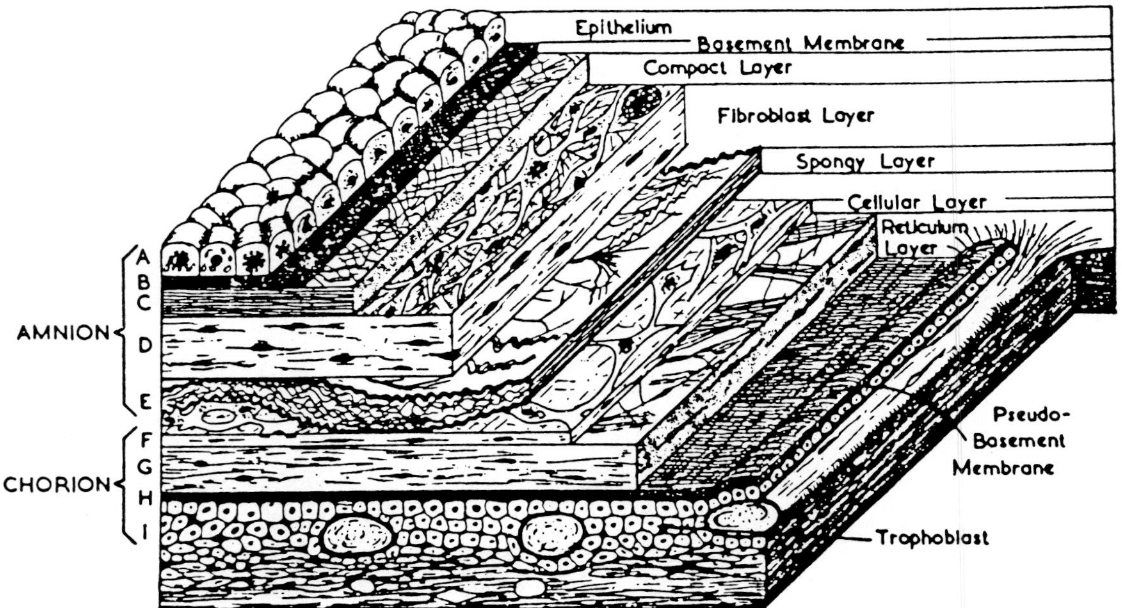

FIGURE 88–2. Section through human amnion and chorion. (From Bourne GL. The microscopic anatomy of the human amnion and chorion. Am J Obstet Gynecol 1960;79:1071.)

BIOPHYSICAL STUDIES

Probably the earliest experiments designed to investigate the mechanisms responsible for PROM were those performed by Poppel in 1863 and Duncan in 1869.[27,28] Duncan dropped cannon balls onto membranes stretched over a ring to determine their tensile strength. Since then, most investigators have hypothesized that membranes that rupture prematurely are inherently weaker. But despite the use of devices of different complexity, the results have been quite uniform: no difference exists in the bursting tension between prematurely ruptured and nonprematurely ruptured membranes.[29–34] On the other hand, two groups of investigators have shown that membranes that rupture before labor have decreased elasticity.[30,35] It has been suggested that a localized defect in the amnion may be responsible for PROM.[23,24] Lavery's computer model of human chorioamniotic membranes suggests that acute or chronic stress applications may act on these weaker points.[36,37]

BIOCHEMICAL DATA

The chorioamniotic membranes are essentially connective tissue structures. Since collagen determines the tensile strength of fibrous connective tissue, there has been considerable interest in investigating collagen biochemistry in the setting of PROM. Two studies have shown that total collagen content is reduced in the amnion of women with preterm PROM.[38,39] Skinner and coworkers found that total collagen concentration was lower in the amnion of women with PROM than in the amnion of women with intact membranes.[38] This was probably not the consequence of membrane rupture, because total amnion collagen concentration increased with the duration of the latency period.

Subsequently, Kanayama and colleagues documented that total collagen content was lower in the amnion of women with preterm PROM than in patients with preterm delivery with intact membranes.[39] The difference in collagen content in preterm PROM was attributable to a decrease in the concentration of type III collagen, which provides elastic tensility to tissues. In contrast, they could not demonstrate a decrease in total collagen content in the amnion of patients with term PROM. This suggests that there are important biochemical differences between term and preterm PROM.

Three other studies have not confirmed a reduction in collagen content in fetal membranes in PROM. Al-Zaid and associates found no change in total membrane collagen content (amnion and chorion) in patients with PROM between 30 and 38 weeks and those with spontaneous or artificial rupture of membranes at term.[29] Evaldson and colleagues were also unable to document a difference in total membrane collagen content between women with preterm PROM and those with intact membranes at term.[40] However, since Skinner and coworkers demonstrated a progressive decrease in amnion collagen content with advancing gestational age, it would seem that amnion tissue for the control group should have been obtained from women with preterm delivery without PROM and not from women at term.[38] Finally, Vadillo-Ortega recently reported no differences in total amnion collagen content between women with

PROM and without PROM at term.[41] Interestingly, the amnion of women with PROM contained a higher percentage of soluble collagen (by acid extraction) than the amnion of women with intact membranes. It is possible that this increase in the percentage of soluble collagen represents active collagen degradation before its final digestion. Indeed, these investigators found increased collagenolytic activity in the amnion homogenates of women with PROM.

A growing body of evidence supports a role for increased proteolytic activity in patients with PROM. Artal and associates demonstrated that incubation of chorioamniotic membranes with pseudoamniotic fluid for 24 hours induced changes in their mechanical properties that predisposed to membrane rupture.[42] These changes were prevented by the addition of protease inhibitors, indicating that enzymatic mechanisms participate in the weakening of the membranes. Moreover, Kanayama and colleagues reported that the trypsin-like bioactivity (measured by a chromogenic substrate assay) was significantly higher in the amniotic fluid of women with PROM than in the amniotic fluid of women with intact membranes.[43] Since trypsin concentrations (measured by RIA) were not different in the two groups, the higher trypsin-like bioactivity could be attributed to other proteases or to changes in the concentration of protease inhibitors. Indeed, they demonstrated that amniotic fluid from women with PROM had a significantly lower concentration of alpha-1 antitrypsin than women with intact membranes. O'Brien and coworkers could not confirm this difference in alpha-1 antitrypsin.[44] The discrepancy between the two studies could be explained by the method of collection of amniotic fluid: transabdominal amniocentesis was used in all patients in O'Brien's study but not in Kanayama's. If there is compartmentalization of the amniotic cavity, it is possible that differences in alpha-1 antitrypsin could be detected in the lower uterine segment, but not in the upper uterine segment. Other protease systems could also be involved in weakening the membranes. For example, plasminogen, which has been detected in the amniotic epithelium of patients with PROM, could be activated into plasmin, which in turn could damage chorioamnion and lead to premature membrane rupture.[45,46] At variance with these findings, Milwidsky and associates found no differences in the fetal membrane proteases, amniotic fluid proteases, and amniotic fluid protease inhibitory activity between PROM and non-PROM gestations at term.[47]

Since infection has been associated with PROM, the mechanisms by which microbial invasion of the membranes may lead to membrane rupture have been a subject of intensive investigation. Microorganisms are a source of proteases or phospholipases that could predispose to membrane rupture.[48] Indeed, incubating bacteria with chorioamniotic membranes in vitro reduces the bursting pressure of these tissues.[49–51] Incubating membranes with activated neutrophils reduces bursting tension, work-to-rupture, and elasticity of the membranes, supporting a role for the host cells in the mechanisms responsible for membrane weakening.[51] Similar observations have been made by incubating membranes with neutrophil elastase.[51]

Another host mechanism that may be involved in membrane rupture is the peroxidase–hydrogen peroxide–halide system. This system is activated in the presence of microbial invasion and involves phagocytes and macrophages. Activation of this system may result in cytotoxic activity, which in turn may lead to membrane rupture. Sbarra and associates reported that peroxidase activity in amnion, chorion, and decidua was higher in patients after vaginal delivery than after cesarean section without labor.[50] Further, inhibition of the peroxidase system prevented the membrane weakening observed after incubation of the membranes with *Escherichia coli* and *Streptococcus agalactiae*.[52] Similarly, adding erythromycin or clindamycin to inocula of protease-producing microorganisms (*Staphylococcus aureus*) prevented in vitro the bacterial protease-induced weakening of amniochorion.[53]

Recently, cytokines have also been implicated in PROM. Interleukin-1 (IL-1) and tumor necrosis factor (TNF) stimulate collagenase activity and prostaglandin production in several cell types, including chorionic cells.[54–56] Indeed, these cytokines have been found in the amniotic fluid of women with PROM and intra-amniotic infection.[57–59] TNF has been reported to alter amnion cell multiplication.[54] These cytokines may also have an effect on the synthesis of glycosaminoglycans. For example, IL-1 increases hyaluronic acid biosynthesis by chorionic cells; an increase in hyaluronic acid may lead to a further reduction in tensile strength of the membranes, given its highly hydrophilic nature. This observation is consistent with that of Skinner and Liggins, who reported that membranes from patients with PROM had increased concentrations of hyaluronic acid.[60]

CLINICAL RISK FACTORS

Many risk factors have been implicated in PROM, some on the basis of small and often uncontrolled studies. Since many risk factors can coexist in the same patient, multivariate statistical analysis is the best way to distinguish primary factors from confounding variables. In this section we will critically review the evidence supporting some associations between risk factors and PROM.

The most comprehensive and rigorous analysis of risk factors associated with preterm PROM has been Harger and coworkers' multicenter case-control study. This study compared demographic factors, and medical, obstetric, gynecologic, and sexual histories of 341 women with preterm PROM (20 to 36 weeks) and 253 controls matched for maternal age, gestational age, parity, type of care (private versus clinic), and previous vaginal or cesarean delivery.[61] Univariate and multivariate analyses were conducted. Table 88-1 shows the results of univariate analysis. A large number of factors

TABLE 88-1. CLINICAL RISK FACTORS FOR PRETERM PROM

RISK FACTOR	ODDS RATIO	95% CONFIDENCE LIMITS
Previous preterm delivery	2.47	1.50–4.08
Previous preterm PROM	1.76	1.03–3.00
Previous D&C (≥2 vs ≤1)	1.18	1.01–1.39
DES exposure	1.37	1.04–1.79
Bleeding during index pregnancy	1.56	1.37–1.77
Cigarette smoking during index pregnancy	1.31	1.14–1.50
Hypertension/diabetes mellitus	1.26	1.09–1.45
Anemia (Hct ≤ 30%)	1.27	1.08–1.50

(Harger JH, Hsing AW, Tuomala RE, et al. Risk factors for preterm premature rupture of fetal membranes: a multicenter case-control study. Am J Obstet Gynecol 1990;163:130.)

were associated with preterm PROM, including vaginal bleeding during the index pregnancy, cigarette smoking, hypertension or diabetes during the index pregnancy, anemia (hematocrit of 30% or less), history of a preterm birth or preterm PROM, number of previous D&Cs, and maternal exposure to DES in utero. When multiple logistic regression analysis was conducted, only three factors remained significant: previous preterm delivery, vaginal bleeding during the index pregnancy, and cigarette smoking. Table 88-2 shows the odds ratio and the 95% confidence limits for these risk factors.

PREVIOUS PRETERM PROM

The most significant risk factor for PROM is a history of this complication in a previous pregnancy. Using data collected by the Collaborative Perinatal Project, Naeye examined the outcome of two successive singleton pregnancies in 5230 women.[62] The recurrence rate of preterm delivery after PROM was 21%; that after term PROM was 26% (Table 88-3). It is noteworthy that if the first pregnancy went to term without PROM, there was only a 4% risk that preterm PROM would occur in the following pregnancy. The observation of a high recurrence rate of preterm PROM was recently confirmed by Asrat and associates, who reported a 32% (95% confidence limits: 23.9 to 40.5) recurrence risk in 121 patients with previous preterm PROM.[63]

VAGINAL BLEEDING

Several studies have implicated vaginal bleeding as a risk factor for PROM.[61,64,65] In the case-control study reported by Harger and colleagues, a history of vaginal bleeding in at least one trimester occurred in 41.4% (141/341) of patients with preterm PROM and 17.3% (44/253) of cases without this complication ($p < .001$).[61] Multivariate analysis demonstrated that vaginal bleeding remained a significant risk factor for preterm PROM even after correction for the effect of other variables. Vaginal bleeding during the first trimester was associated with a twofold increase in the risk of preterm PROM; if it occurred during the second

TABLE 88-2. CLINICAL RISK FACTORS FOR PRETERM PROM MULTIVARIATE ANALYSIS*

RISK FACTOR	ODDS RATIO	95% CONFIDENCE LIMITS
Previous preterm delivery	2.84	1.40–2.48
Cigarette smoking	2.08	1.37–3.13
Bleeding during pregnancy:		
Never	1.00	–
During first trimester	2.38	1.47–3.86
During second trimester	4.42	1.62–12.03
During third trimester	6.44	1.81–22.91
More than one trimester	7.43	2.16–25.60

* Adjusted for income and race.

(Adapted from Harger JH, Hsing AW, Tuomala RE, et al. Risk factors for preterm premature rupture of fetal membranes: a multicenter case-control study. Am J Obstet Gynecol 1990;163:130.)

TABLE 88–3. RISK FACTOR: PREVIOUS PRETERM DELIVERY

	SECOND PREGNANCY	
FIRST PREGNANCY	PRETERM PROM (%)	FULL-TERM PROM (%)
Preterm, PROM	21	17
Preterm, no PROM	10	13
Term, PROM	7	26
Term, no PROM	4	17

(Naeye RL. Factors that predispose to premature rupture of the fetal membranes. Obstet Gynecol 1982;60:93.)

or third trimester, the risk of preterm PROM was increased four- and sixfold, respectively. Vaginal bleeding occurring in more than one trimester was associated with a sevenfold increase in preterm PROM.

The mechanisms by which vaginal bleeding may lead to preterm PROM are unknown. One possibility is that decidual bleeding with clot formation may impair the nutritional support of the membranes; subsequent stretching of the weakened area would lead to rupture. An alternative explanation is that an ascending infection may cause deciduitis manifested by vaginal bleeding.

SMOKING

There is controversy regarding the risk of preterm PROM among smokers. Naeye found no association between smoking and preterm PROM (incidence of preterm PROM in smokers and nonsmokers: 5.3% [34/635] versus 6.7% [43/635], respectively).[62] On the other hand, Meyer and Tonascia found that the risk of preterm PROM before 34 weeks was more than three times higher for smokers than for nonsmokers (Fig. 88-3).[66] Evaldson and associates confirmed this observation in a case-control study in which smoking more

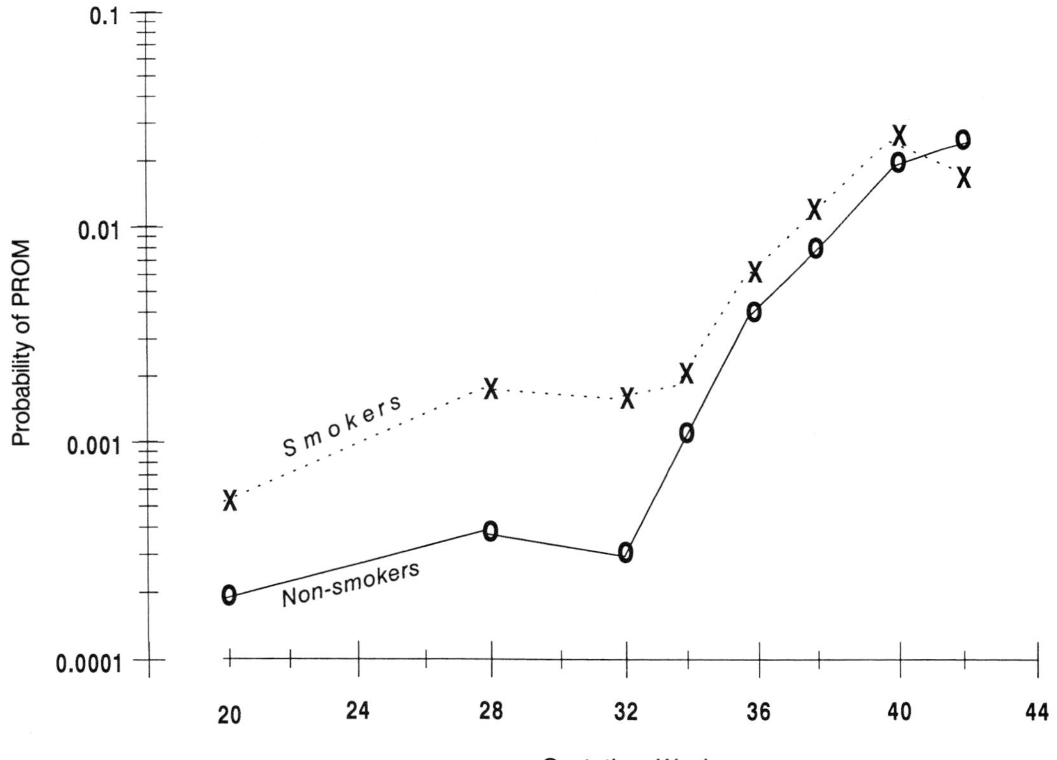

FIGURE 88–3. Risks of PROM for smoking and nonsmoking mothers, by period of gestational age at delivery (admission diagnosis, rupture of membranes only). (From Meyer MB, Tonascia JA. Maternal smoking, pregnancy complications, and perinatal mortality. Am J Obstet Gynecol 1977;128:500.)

than 10 cigarettes per day was significantly more common in patients with preterm PROM than in those without PROM (raw data were not reported).[67] Harger and colleagues found that smoking throughout pregnancy doubled the risk of preterm PROM (odds ratio = 2.08; 95% confidence limits: 1.37 to 3.13).[61] It is of interest that patients who smoked but stopped during pregnancy did not have a higher risk of PROM than women who never smoked (odds ratio = 1.58; 95% confidence limits: 0.77 to 3.27). The mechanism by which smoking leads to preterm PROM is probably decidual vasculopathy with resulting ischemia and necrosis.

SEXUAL INTERCOURSE

Several studies have examined whether sexual intercourse during pregnancy is a risk factor for preterm PROM. Naeye and Peters, using data from the Collaborative Perinatal Project, concluded that coitus during the last month (9 to 30 days before delivery) was not associated with preterm PROM[26] but the data to support this conclusion were not presented in the report. Subsequently, Naeye reanalyzed the data using a different timeframe for coitus (last 9 days before delivery) and reported that there was an association between coitus and preterm PROM.[62] We could not verify that this difference was statistically significant for preterm or term PROM (prevalence of preterm PROM in coitus = 49% [41/84] versus no coitus = 34% [24/70]; p = .09; prevalence of term PROM in coitus = 22.6% [71/314] versus no coitus = 22.6% [204/904]).

Mills and colleagues reported a study in which patients were interviewed at the time of delivery to determine the occurrence of sexual intercourse during pregnancy.[68] Coitus during the last month of pregnancy was not found to be associated with a higher rate of preterm delivery (7 months: no coitus = 3.7% [40/1053] versus coitus = 0.7% [64/9151]; 8 months: no coitus = 11% [371/3373] versus coitus = 9.5% [641/6725]). Similarly, coitus within a month of delivery was not associated with a higher incidence of PROM at any gestational age (Table 88-4).

In the multicenter case-control study reported by Harger and colleagues, the proportion of patients who had sexual intercourse at arbitrary intervals before PROM (less than 48 hours; more than 48 hours but less than 1 week; 1 week to 1 month; and more than 1 month) was higher in the control group than in women with preterm PROM.[61] These observations agree with the findings of other authors who used a smaller sample size.[69,70]

We conclude that there is little evidence to implicate coitus during pregnancy in the etiology of PROM.

CONNECTIVE TISSUE DISORDERS

Since the fetal membranes are primarily connective tissue structures, it is logical to ask if the incidence of PROM is increased in patients with connective tissue disorders. A striking association exists between preterm PROM and Ehlers-Danlos syndrome. Barabas conducted a retrospective study to determine the birth characteristics of patients with Ehlers-Danlos syndrome.[71] Birth histories were available for 18 of these patients. The rate of prematurity was 77% (14/18); preterm PROM occurred in 92% (13/14) of those delivered preterm. Of interest is that only one of the 16 unaffected siblings had preterm PROM, and this occurred in a twin gestation in which the other twin was affected.

It is now apparent that Ehlers-Danlos syndrome comprises a group of at least eight inheritable connective tissue disorders. Type I, or gravis type, is inherited with an autosomal dominant pattern; it seems to be associated with preterm PROM and preterm birth.

TRACE ELEMENTS AND VITAMIN C

The role of trace metals and vitamin C in health and disease remains poorly understood. Since some of these compounds have a role in collagen biosynthesis, it is possible that a deficiency may contribute or predispose to PROM. The data available are very scanty. Wideman and coworkers reported that the rate of PROM was higher in patients with low maternal plasma ascorbic acid concentrations than in those with normal levels (14.6% [13/89] in patients with a level of 0.20 mg/dL or less versus 1.4% [1/69] in patients with a level of 0.60 mg/dL or greater).[72]

TABLE 88–4. COITUS DURING THE 7TH and 8TH MONTH OF PREGNANCY AND PROM

GESTATIONAL AGE AT PROM (WKS)	COITUS IN 7TH MONTH		COITUS IN 8TH MONTH	
	NO (1053)	YES (9151)	NO (3373)	YES (6725)
<34	11	15	—	—
34–37	20	91	56	54
>37	44	385	153	275

(Mills JL, Harlap S, Harley EE. Should coitus late in pregnancy be discouraged? Lancet 1981;2:137.)

Copper deficiency has been shown to inhibit the maturation of collagen and elastin. Artal and associates reported that patients with term PROM had lower copper concentrations in maternal and umbilical cord sera than patients with artificial rupture of membranes during labor.[73] It is noteworthy that the mean birth weight of neonates born to women with PROM was lower than that of newborns in the control group. In this study, no differences in membrane copper content were observed between the two groups. These findings were not confirmed by a later study by Kiilholma and colleagues, who found no differences in maternal or fetal serum copper concentrations between term patients with and without PROM.[74] There were no differences in birth weights between the two groups. On the other hand, umbilical cord (but not maternal) serum copper and ceruloplasmin levels were significantly lower in patients with preterm PROM than in patients with preterm delivery without PROM.

Two studies have addressed the relationship between zinc and PROM. Kiilholma and colleagues found no significant difference in maternal and umbilical cord zinc serum concentrations between patients with preterm PROM and patients with preterm delivery with intact membranes.[74] A limitation of this study is that serum zinc reflects only a minor proportion of the total body zinc. In another study, a maternal zinc index was calculated (a sum of measurements of zinc in maternal blood, scalp and pubic hair, and colostrum); it was found to be lower in patients with term PROM than in those without PROM.[75]

PREVIOUS OPERATIONS ON THE GENITAL TRACT

Although several investigators have examined the effect of cervical surgery on the risk of PROM, there is no concordance in the results. Naeye reported that surgery or other manipulation of the cervix between the first and second pregnancy was associated with a nonsignificant increase in preterm PROM from 5% (5/99) to 12% (12/99).[62] However, the risk of PROM at any time during pregnancy (term and preterm) was significantly increased, from 22% to 35% ($p < .05$). It is noteworthy that the incidence of PROM in the first pregnancy in this study was almost double the rate of this complication in the general population. Another limitation of this study is that the specific nature of the cervical manipulation was not stated.

Evaldson and associates reported that a history of cervical conization or cervical rupture was more common in patients with preterm PROM than in controls.[67] No raw data were provided in the report.

Harger and colleagues, using univariate analysis, reported that a history of previous elective abortion or a previous D&C was more common in patients with preterm PROM than in patients without preterm PROM.[61] But after subjecting the data to multivariate analysis, neither risk factor remained significant. Similarly, Harlap and Davies, using stepwise regression analysis, found that the rate of PROM was not higher in patients with one or more previous abortions than in patients without abortions.[76]

PELVIC EXAMINATIONS DURING PREGNANCY

Do pelvic examinations during pregnancy predispose to PROM? The data are conflicting. Lenihan reported a randomized prospective trial in which women at 37 weeks gestation were randomized to weekly pelvic examinations versus no pelvic examinations.[77] PROM was more common in women who underwent repeated pelvic examinations than in the control group (18% [32/174] versus 6% [10/175], $p < .001$). This observation is at variance with that reported by Main and associates in a preterm-delivery prevention program in which women at risk for preterm delivery were randomized to either biweekly pelvic examinations or standard obstetric care.[78] No difference in the incidence of PROM was noted between the two groups (50% [8/16] versus 28.6% [4/14]). This observation was subsequently confirmed with a larger sample size.[79]

COLONIZATION OF THE LOWER GENITAL TRACT WITH SELECTIVE MICROORGANISMS

In view of the proposed role of ascending infection in the etiology of PROM, cervicovaginal flora in PROM has been investigated in several studies.[80] There is good evidence to support an association between infection with *Chlamydia trachomatis* (CT) and *Neisseria gonorrhoeae* (NG) and PROM. Similarly, an association between colonization with Group B streptococcus (GBS) and PROM has been reported. In a previous review of the literature we could not substantiate any increased risk of PROM in patients colonized with *Mycoplasma*.

Chlamydia trachomatis

Harrison and associates, in a prospective observational study, found an 8% incidence of positive cervical cultures for CT in 1365 women.[85] Among women with positive cultures, PROM (term and preterm) was more common in those with positive serum IgM (antichlamydial antibody titers of 1:32 or higher) than in those with negative IgM (7/17 versus 4/53, $p < .01$).

Gravett and coworkers cultured 534 pregnant women in the second and third trimester (mean gestational age at the time of enrollment, 32.6 weeks).[86] A positive culture for CT was associated with a significantly higher risk of preterm PROM (odds ratio, 2.4; $p < .05$).

Sweet and colleagues obtained cervical cultures for CT from 6864 women at the time of the initial prenatal visit.[87] Cultures were repeated at 30 to 34 weeks. CT was recovered from 4.7% of patients. Patients with positive CT did not have a higher incidence of PROM than women with negative cultures (10.3% [28/270] versus 9.6% [26/270], not significant). However, PROM associated with preterm delivery was more common in women with positive CT than in women with negative cultures (54.5% [12/22] versus 27.7% [120/433], $p = .003$). Infected women with positive maternal serum IgM (defined as a titer of 1:32 or higher) had a higher incidence of preterm delivery (19% [13/67] versus 8% [8/99]) and PROM (19% [13/67] versus 8% [8/99], $p = .03$) than infected women with negative IgM.

Alger and associates reported a case-control study that also supported a role for CT in preterm PROM.[84] CT was isolated more frequently from women with preterm PROM than from women in the control group (44% [23/52] versus 15% [13/84], $p < .01$).

Neisseria gonorrhoeae

Handsfield and coworkers reported that the prevalence of prolonged PROM (more than 24 hours) was significantly higher in women with positive endocervical, endometrial, or placental cultures for NG than in women with negative cultures (75% [9/12] versus 37% [18/49], $p < .05$).[88]

Subsequently, Amstey and associates provided convincing evidence for an association between PROM and preterm delivery with colonization with NG.[89] Cervical cultures were taken from 5065 women at the time of the initial visit and at 36 weeks gestation. Positive cultures for NG were found in 4.4% of patients (222/5065). PROM was more common in women with positive cultures than in women with negative cultures (26% [52/198] versus 19% [799/4246], $p < .01$).

Edwards and colleagues reported a prevalence of positive cultures for NG in pregnancy of 2.75% (178/6464).[90] PROM was more common in women with cervical gonorrhea at delivery than in women with negative cultures (63% [12/19] versus 29.3% [12/41], $p < .05$). However, the prevalence of PROM was not higher in women with positive cervical cultures during pregnancy compared to a matched control group (28.1% [50/178] versus 25.4% [98/386], not significant).

Group B Streptococcus

Several studies have addressed the relationship between GBS colonization and PROM. Four studies have yielded positive results.

Regan and colleagues reported that PROM (1 hour before the onset of labor or contractions) was more common in women with cervical colonization of GBS at the time of delivery than in noncarriers (15.3% [134/877] versus 7% [409/5829], $p < .005$).[81]

Bobitt and associates reported a study in which vaginal cultures from 718 patients were taken monthly starting at 24 weeks and then at the time of admission in labor.[82] PROM resulting in the delivery of a low-birth-weight infant was more common in carriers than in noncarriers (6% [4/71] versus 2% [11/637], $p < .05$).

Matorras and coworkers reported the results of a study in which cultures for GBS were taken from the lower genital tract and rectum.[83] Patients with positive GBS cultures had a higher rate of PROM than patients with negative cultures (26.4% [32/121] versus 17.8% [158/890], $p < .05$). Among GBS carriers, those with a positive cervical culture had a higher rate of PROM than those with a negative cervical culture (41.7% [10/24] versus 19% [8/42], $p < .05$).

Alger and colleagues found that the frequency of positive cultures for GBS on admission was greater in patients with PROM than in patients with intact membranes (15.6% [7/45] versus 3.8% [3/80], $p < .05$).[84] There is no current evidence that identifying and treating colonized patients reduces the risk of PROM.

Trichomonas vaginalis and *Bacteroides* Species

A role for these microorganisms has been suggested by a prospective study of vaginal flora reported by Minkoff and coworkers.[91] They cultured 233 patients at the time of their first prenatal visit (mean 13.8 ± 3.6 weeks) for *Trichomonas, Mycoplasma,* and aerobic and anaerobic bacteria. The overall incidence of positive cultures for *Trichomonas* was 14.6% (34/233). Women who subsequently developed PROM had a higher rate of positive cultures than women who did not present with this complication (27.5% [11/40] versus 12.8% [19/148], $p < .03$). Stepwise logistic regression analysis (including patient characteristics such as parity, abortivity, maternal age, preterm birth, and the effect of 12 different microorganisms) showed that colonization with *Trichomonas* was associated with a relative risk of developing PROM of 1.42 ($p < .03$). No association between colonization and preterm PROM was found.

In the same study, the isolation rate of *Bacteroides* species and *Staphylococcus epidermidis* was associated with a relative risk of 2.8 ($p < .003$) and 1.57 ($p < .02$) respectively for PROM. Again, the presence of these microorganisms was not associated with preterm PROM. This study needs to be replicated.

Despite this suggestive evidence that infection or colonization with certain microorganisms may increase the risk of PROM, there is a paucity of information regarding the effect of treatment. Therapeutic trials are required to determine if treatment of GBS and *Trichomonas* may reduce the risk of PROM.

MICROBIAL INVASION OF THE AMNIOTIC CAVITY

PREVALENCE

Table 88-5 shows the rate of positive amniotic fluid cultures in women with preterm PROM from published studies.[92–98] The overall prevalence of positive amniotic fluid cultures is 28.5%, but this figure probably under-

TABLE 88-5. AMNIOCENTESIS IN PRETERM PROM: POSITIVE AMNIOTIC FLUID CULTURE

STUDY	NO. PATIENTS WITH PROM	POSITIVE CULTURE
Garite and Freeman (1982)[92]	207	20/86 (23.2%)
Cotton et al. (1984)[93]	61	6/41 (14.6%)
Broekhuizen et al. (1985)[94]	79	15/53 (28.3%)
Vintzileos et al. (1986)[95]	54	12/54 (22.2%)
Feinstein et al. (1986)[96]	73	12/50 (20.0%)
Romero et al. (1988)[97]	90	39/90 (43.3%)
Romero et al. (1988)[98]	221	65/221 (29.4%)
Total	785	169/595 (28.4%)

estimates the true prevalence of microbial invasion of the amniotic cavity. Retrieval of amniotic fluid by amniocentesis is extremely difficult in women with preterm PROM and severely reduced amniotic fluid volume. However, there is evidence that these patients have a high rate of positive amniotic fluid cultures. Indeed, in a consecutive series of 86 patients, we found that the rate of microbial invasion of the amniotic cavity was 51% (21/41) when there was a vertical pocket of amniotic fluid less than 1 cm, and only 13% (6/45) when the vertical pocket was larger than 1 cm ($p < .01$). A second factor that may be responsible for the underestimation in the rate of positive amniotic fluid cultures is that in most studies, women with preterm PROM admitted in labor did not undergo amniocentesis. We recently documented that patients with PROM who are in preterm labor on admission have a higher incidence of positive amniotic fluid cultures in comparison with women not in labor (39% versus 26%, $p = .049$).[98]

Only one study examined the prevalence of positive amniotic fluid cultures in term PROM: it reported a 34.3% (11/32) rate of positive cultures.[99]

MICROBIOLOGY

In general, the microorganisms isolated from the amniotic fluid of women with PROM are similar to those normally found in the lower genital tract. This observation has been used as evidence to support the concept that microbial invasion of the amniotic cavity follows an ascending pathway. However, direct evidence (ie, isolation of the same microorganism from both the amniotic fluid and the vagina) is unavailable.

Table 88-6 lists the microorganisms isolated from the amniotic fluid of women with preterm PROM not in labor on admission at our institution.[98] Mycoplasmas (*Ureaplasma urealyticum* and *Mycoplasma hominis*) are the most frequent isolates, followed by *Streptococcus agalactiae* (Group B streptococcus), *Fusobacterium*, and *Gardnerella vaginalis*. Polymicrobial infection was found in 32% (13/41) of cases, and an inoculum size greater than 10^5 colony-forming units per mL was found in 23% (6/26) of patients in which quantitative microbiology was performed. The type of microorganisms isolated in our study is similar to that reported in other studies. However, a notable difference is that *Mycoplasma* species were not cultured for in older studies.[92–95]

Table 88-7 lists the microorganisms isolated from the amniotic fluid of women with term PROM. The most common microorganisms were *Ureaplasma urealyticum*, *Peptostreptococcus*, *Lactobacillus*, *Bacteroides* species, and *Fusobacterium*. Therefore, the isolates from the amniotic fluid in women with term and preterm PROM seem to be qualitatively similar.

RELATIONSHIP BETWEEN LABOR AND MICROBIAL INVASION

The onset of labor in the setting of PROM has traditionally been considered an early sign of intrauterine infection. One study has examined the relationship between microbial invasion of the amniotic cavity and the onset of preterm labor in women with PROM.[98] Patients in labor on admission had a higher rate of positive amni-

TABLE 88-6. PRETERM PROM/NO LABOR: MICROORGANISMS ISOLATED FROM AMNIOTIC FLUID

MICROORGANISM	NUMBER OF MICROBIAL ISOLATES
Ureaplasma urealyticum	4
Mycoplasma hominis	6
Streptococcus agalactiae	5
Streptococcus viridans	4
Streptococcus pneumoniae	1
Fusobacterium species	5
Gardnerella vaginalis	5
Lactobacillus	2
Bacteroides species	2
Neisseria gonorrheae	1

NB: Some patients had more than one microbial isolate.

(Modified from Romero R, Quintero R, Oyarzum E, et al. Intra-amniotic infection and the onset of labor in preterm premature rupture of membranes. Am J Obstet Gynecol 1988;159:661.)

TABLE 88–7. MICROBIOLOGY IN WOMEN WITH RUPTURED MEMBRANES AT TERM

PATIENT NO.	GRAM STAIN	MICROORGANISMS	PUERPERAL ENDOMETRITIS
1	Negative	*Lactobacillus* species	No
2	Negative	*Ureaplasma urealyticum*	Yes
3	Negative	*Ureaplasma urealyticum*	No
4	Negative	*Ureaplasma urealyticum*	No
5	Negative	*Peptostreptococcus* *Ureaplasma urealyticum*	Yes
6	Negative	*Ureaplasma urealyticum*	No
7	Positive	*Streptococcus* Group B *Bacteroides fragilis* *Peptostreptococcus* species *Fusobacterium* species *Ureaplasma urealyticum*	Yes
8	Negative	*Fusobacterium* species *Ureaplasma urealyticum*	No
9	Positive	*Gardnerella vaginalis* *Ureaplasma urealyticum*	No
10	Negative	*Peptostreptococcus* species	No
11	Negative	*Lactobacillus* species *Bacteroides fragilis*	No

(Modified from Romero R et al. Microbial invasion of the amniotic cavity in spontaneous rupture of membranes at term [submitted to Am J Obstet Gynecol]).

otic fluid cultures than women admitted with preterm PROM but not in labor (39% [24/61] versus 26% [41/160], $p = .049$). Moreover, 75% of patients who were not in labor on admission but subsequently went into spontaneous labor had a positive amniotic fluid culture around the time of the onset of labor. These data support a relationship between microbial invasion of the amniotic cavity and onset of preterm labor. No data are available regarding the rate of positive cultures in women with term PROM admitted in active labor.

Are there differences in the type of microorganisms and inoculum size between women in labor and not in labor with preterm PROM? The only study examining this issue published to date reported that patients with preterm PROM in active labor on admission had a higher inoculum size than women not in labor on admission.[98] A colony count above 10^5 was found in 55% (10/18) and in 23% (6/26), $p < .054$, respectively. These data suggest that there may be a relationship between proliferation of microorganisms and the initiation of preterm labor. On the other hand, the rate of polymicrobial isolates was not different between the two groups (42% [10/24] for patients admitted in active labor versus 32% [13/41] for patients not in active labor, $p = 0.43$). No gross differences in qualitative microbiology could be detected between women with and without active labor on admission. Microbial invasion limited to *Mycoplasma* was found in only 8% of patients in labor versus 20% of those not in labor. Although this difference is not statistically significant, there are obvious limitations from the limited sample size. Further studies are required to determine if some microorganisms are more likely to be associated with prompt initiation of parturition than others.

NATURAL HISTORY

Limited information is available regarding the course of microbial invasion of the amniotic cavity in preterm PROM. We have performed a second amniocentesis in 12 women who originally had a negative Gram stain of the amniotic fluid but a positive amniotic fluid culture.[98] In 11 patients, the microorganisms recovered from the second amniocentesis were the same as those retrieved from the first, but the colony count was higher in all instances. This implies that once microbial invasion of the amniotic cavity has occurred, it has a progressive course. The 12th patient had a first amniotic fluid culture positive for *Fusobacterium* species, but the second amniotic fluid culture obtained at the time of the spontaneous initiation of labor showed no growth. It is unclear whether this observation represents a failure of culture or a true resolution of microbial invasion of the amniotic cavity. The initiation of labor and the observation that this patient had histologic chorioamnionitis makes the second possibility less likely.

CONSEQUENCES

Patients with microbial invasion of the amniotic cavity are more likely to develop chorioamnionitis, endometritis, and neonatal sepsis than patients with a negative amniotic fluid culture on admission.[92–94,96] Table 88-8 shows the rate of these complications in studies in which antibiotics were not used before delivery. Garite and Freeman reported that the frequency of RDS was twofold higher in neonates born to women with a positive culture than in those born to women with a nega-

TABLE 88–8. RATE OF INFECTIOUS COMPLICATIONS IN PROM

STUDY	POSITIVE CULTURE				NEGATIVE CULTURE			
	NUMBER OF PATIENTS	CHORIO-AMNIONITIS	ENDO-METRITIS	DOCUMENTED NEONATAL SEPSIS	NUMBER OF PATIENTS	CHORIO-AMNIONITIS	ENDO-METRITIS	DOCUMENTED NEONATAL SEPSIS
Garite and Freeman (1982)[92]	20	55%	25%	25%	66	8%	1%	3%
Broekhuizen et al. (1985)[94]	15	20%	33%	7%	38	0%	3%	0%
Cotton et al. (1984)[93]	6	100%*		17%	35	9%*		0%
Feinstein et al. (1986)[96]	12	17%	NA	17%	38	5%	NA	3%

* Inclusive of chorioamnionitis and endometritis.
NA, not available.

tive amniotic fluid culture.[92] Two explanations for these findings must be considered. First, patients with a positive amniotic fluid culture generally have a lower gestational age than patients with a negative amniotic fluid culture; therefore, the excessive incidence of RDS may reflect a greater degree of prematurity. Second, some cases of respiratory difficulty may be confused with pneumonia.[100–102]

We have examined the relationship between microbial invasion of the amniotic cavity and the latency period in women who were not in labor on admission. Although the latency period of women with negative amniotic fluid was longer than that of women with a positive culture, the difference did not reach statistical significance (median = 169 hours versus 65.4 hours, respectively).[98] These data should be interpreted with caution, because in this study patients with a positive amniotic fluid Gram stain for microorganisms were electively delivered. This introduced a bias, as patients with a higher inoculum size were excluded from further observation.

It is of considerable interest that the microorganisms isolated from septic newborns are similar to those found in the amniotic fluid. In a study of 221 patients with preterm PROM, we found 6 cases with culture-proven neonatal sepsis. In five of these cases, the microorganisms were the same as those found in the amniotic fluid; in the remaining case, the amniotic fluid culture 48 hours before delivery had been negative. The practical implication of this observation is that an amniocentesis performed before delivery may provide microbiological information helpful in guiding antibiotic choice in the newborn.

MICROBIAL INVASION: CAUSE OR CONSEQUENCE OF PROM?

The traditional view has been that microbial invasion of the amniotic cavity is the consequence of the membrane rupture. However, a growing body of evidence suggests that PROM may be the result of subclinical infection and inflammation. Naeye and Peters reported that patients with PROM for 1 to 4 hours before the onset of labor had a higher prevalence of histologic chorioamnionitis than patients who delivered preterm without PROM (Table 88-9).[26] Since it is unlikely that inflammation of the chorioamniotic membranes develops in 4 hours, these data suggest that in these cases histologic chorioamnionitis precedes rather than follows PROM. Several lines of evidence suggest that the most likely cause of histologic chorioamnionitis is subclinical infec-

TABLE 88–9. DURATION OF PROM AND FREQUENCY OF CHORIOAMNIONITIS

	WEEKS OF GESTATION		
	20–28	29–32	33–37
PROM after onset of labor	23%	15%	11%
PROM 1–4 hours before onset of labor	48%	29%	32%

(Modified from Naeye RL, Peters EC. Causes and consequences of premature rupture of fetal membranes. Lancet 1980;1:192.)

tion. Bacteria have been recovered from 72% of placentas with histologic chorioamnionitis.[103] Further, we have demonstrated a good correlation between a positive amniotic fluid culture for microorganisms and histologic chorioamnionitis.[104]

Microbial invasion of the amniotic cavity can also be the consequence of PROM. The frequency of positive amniotic fluid cultures increases with time. Indeed, 75% of patients who were quiescent on admission and subsequently went into labor had a positive amniotic fluid culture; however, only 25% of these patients had a positive culture on admission, and the remaining 50% became positive during the latency period.[98] These observations are consistent with those of Naeye and Peters, who showed that the incidence of histologic chorioamnionitis increases with the duration of the latency period.[26]

ABRUPTIO PLACENTAE

Abruptio placentae occurs more frequently in patients with preterm PROM than in the general obstetric population (5.5% versus 0.8%). Table 88-10 shows the reported frequency of this complication in studies examining this issue. The mechanisms responsible for separation of the placenta in preterm PROM have not been determined. Nelson and associates proposed that leakage of fluid after PROM may lead to a disproportion between the placental and uterine surfaces that in turn would favor placental separation.[105] Clinical support for this concept is provided by the observation that in the context of preterm PROM, the incidence of abruptio placentae increases with the severity of oligohydramnios (12.3% for patients with a vertical pocket of less than 1 cm, 6.2% for those with a vertical pocket of 1 to 2 cm, and 3.5% among those with a vertical pocket greater than 2 cm).[106] Two groups of investigators using subjective means to estimate amniotic fluid volume could not confirm this observation.[107,108]

An alternative etiopathogenetic hypothesis to explain the relationship between abruptio placentae and preterm PROM postulates that a disorder of decidual hemostasis leads to separation of the membranes from the decidua, with subsequent compromise of their nutritive support. Weakening of the membranes eventually may lead to rupture. Indeed, patients with abruptio placentae after preterm PROM have a higher incidence of vaginal bleeding before rupture and during the latency period than patients without abruptio.[107,108] Secondary infection of the decidua could cause inflammation and facilitate premature placental detachment. An association between histologic chorioamnionitis and abruptio placentae has been reported.[109,110]

TABLE 88–10. ABRUPTIO PLACENTAE AND PROM

STUDY	NO. PATIENTS WITH ABRUPTIO AND PROM
Vintzileos et al. (1987)[106]	19/298 (6.4%)
Moretti and Sibai (1988)[201]	8/118 (6.8%)
Gonen et al. (1989)[107]	8/143 (5.6%)
Major et al. (1991)[108]	38/756 (5.0%)
Total	73/1315 (5.5%)

DIAGNOSIS

The diagnosis of membrane rupture must be considered in patients who complain of watery vaginal discharge or a sudden gush of fluid from the vagina. The diagnosis may also be made incidentally in patients admitted in preterm labor, in patients with ultrasound-demonstrated oligohydramnios, or during pelvic examinations done for other indications. The woman should be carefully questioned as to the time of the initial loss of vaginal fluid, color and consistency of the discharge, and any odor noted. These questions may help to differentiate PROM from loss of the mucous plug in prodromal labor, vaginal discharge associated with infection, normal leukorrhea of pregnancy, and urinary incontinence (sometimes present in pregnancy), and also to determine the presence of blood, meconium, or vernix particles.

Evaluation of the patient begins with a sterile speculum examination. Visualization of a vaginal pool or obvious leakage of fluid from the cervix into the posterior fornix is strong evidence supporting the diagnosis of ruptured membranes. A sterile swab of fluid should be obtained from the posterior fornix and placed on a clean glass slide and on a piece of nitrazine paper. Amniotic fluid, when put on a slide and allowed to dry, will show arborization ("ferning") under the microscope at low magnification. This method has an overall accuracy of 96%.[111] Rare false-positive ferning results have been described in association with fingerprints on the slide or contamination with semen and cervical mucus.[112,113] False negatives (5% to 10%) may be caused by dry swabs or by contamination with blood.[114–116] The slide should be evaluated after at least 10 minutes of drying to decrease the false-negative rate.[117]

Nitrazine paper turns from yellow to blue when exposed to any alkaline fluid (ie, pH of 7.0 or more); the normal gestational pH of the vagina is 4.5 to 5.5, and that of the amniotic fluid is 7.0 to 7.5). This method has an overall accuracy of 93.3%.[111] False-positive results range from 1% to 17% and can result from alkaline urine, blood, semen, vaginal discharge in cases of bacterial vaginosis, or *Trichomonas* infection.[118] False negatives may occur in up to 10% of cases.

If no fluid is present in the posterior fornix, the patient can be reexamined after rest in the supine position for several hours to allow for accumulation of further fluid in the posterior fornix. Additionally, a speculum examination allows for collection of vaginal and cervical cultures, and of amniotic fluid from the pooling in the posterior fornix for fetal lung maturity studies (see below).

Ultrasound visualization of decreased amniotic fluid volume can help confirm the diagnosis of PROM when other findings are ambiguous. However, the diagnostic value of sonographic assessment of amniotic fluid volume has not been rigorously examined to date. Other causes of oligohydramnios such as severe fetal growth retardation or fetal urinary-tract anomalies must be carefully ruled out. Conversely, a normal amount of amniotic fluid does not exclude the diagnosis of PROM.

In rare instances more invasive techniques are needed, such as transabdominal injection of dye (indigo carmine, Evans blue, fluorescein) into the amniotic cavity. Methylene blue should not be used because it may cause fetal methemoglobinemia.[119,120] A tampon in the vagina can document subsequent leakage in cases of PROM. These invasive methods can be justified, as the diagnosis of PROM requires special maternal and fetal surveillance; in cases of very preterm gestation, the mother must be transferred to a tertiary-care center.

New tests on vaginal fluid collected in the posterior fornix have been proposed, such as heating endocervical material on a glass slide and determining alphafetoprotein, diamine oxidase activity, or prolactin.[121–126] However, they are either impractical or need further evaluation at different gestational ages and in the presence of possible contaminants before they can be used more widely in the diagnosis of uncertain cases.

Whether a digital examination should be performed is a commonly asked question in the setting of PROM. The only justification for performing a digital examination is to determine cervical status. In the preterm gestation this information rarely alters clinical management, but in the term gestation the cervical state may be a factor influencing decisions regarding induction. This information can be adequately obtained by sterile speculum examination and visual examination of the cervix. In a prospective study of 133 women, a reasonable correlation in the assessment of cervical status (dilatation and effacement) was found between digital and speculum examination ($R = .72$, $p < .001$).[127] These examinations were performed by the same examiner. In a different study, visual speculum and digital cervical exams for dilation in laboring women were performed by two separate blinded examiners within 10 minutes of each other. The correlation coefficient was 0.88 ($p < .005$), and in only 3 of the 50 women the cervix could not be visualized.[128]

Does a digital examination increase the risk of infection? The traditional view that "once an examination has been performed, the clock of infection starts to tick" is predicated on meager scientific evidence. Three studies have addressed the clinical consequences of digital examination in the setting of PROM.

Adoni and coworkers reported a study in which the latency period and incidence of chorioamnionitis was evaluated in patients with preterm PROM (26 to 34 weeks) who underwent a digital examination or a sterile speculum examination, depending on the personal preference of the attending physician.[129] The latency period was longer in patients undergoing speculum examination than in those digitally examined (9.46 days [SD = 1.5] versus 3.12 days [SD = 0.46], $p < .005$). No significant difference in the incidence of chorioamnionitis was found (digital examination 24% [6/25] versus speculum examination 18% [5/28]). As in the previous study, the lack of random allocation of patients is a serious limitation on the interpretation of the data.

Schutte and colleagues retrospectively examined the incidence of neonatal infection in patients with PROM according to the interval between initial digital vaginal examination and delivery.[130] The incidence of neonatal infection was higher in patients examined more than 24 hours before delivery than in those whose first vaginal examination occurred less than 24 hours before delivery (33% [11/33] versus 5% [14/280], $p < .001$). Although this study has been widely cited in support of the view that digital vaginal examination increases the risk of infection, the design of this study imposes severe constraints on the strength of this conclusion. For example, the policy at the institution in which the study was performed was not to perform digital examinations in patients with PROM unless delivery was anticipated within 24 hours. The patients who underwent vaginal examinations did so because they were wrongly considered to be in labor. Uterine contractions may have been an early sign of infection, and this may explain why the incidence of neonatal infection was higher in patients who underwent vaginal examinations.

Finally, Lewis and associates prospectively collected data on 271 singleton pregnancies transferred to a tertiary-care center with preterm PROM.[131] The latency period among those who had a digital vaginal examination performed before transport was compared with that of women who were evaluated by speculum examination (Fig. 88-4). Patients in active labor or with an indication for delivery were excluded. Indeed, no difference in uterine activity during the first 2 hours after transport was seen between the two groups. Digital vaginal examinations significantly shortened latency periods in the groups as a whole (digital examination: latency = 2.1 days, SD = 4.0; no digital examination: latency = 11.3 days, SD = 13.4) and also at each gestational age.

Our objection to a digital examination in the setting of PROM is that it may unnecessarily increase the risk of ascending infection. The information it provides can be obtained by sterile speculum examination.

INITIAL MANAGEMENT

Any patient with an established diagnosis of PROM should be assessed for gestational age, fetal well-being, signs and symptoms of chorioamnionitis, and preterm labor.

Antepartum surveillance has been undertaken in patients with PROM with the nonstress test (NST) or biophysical profile (BPP); the oxytocin stress test and the nipple stimulation test have been avoided in these patients because of the risk of initiating labor. Although

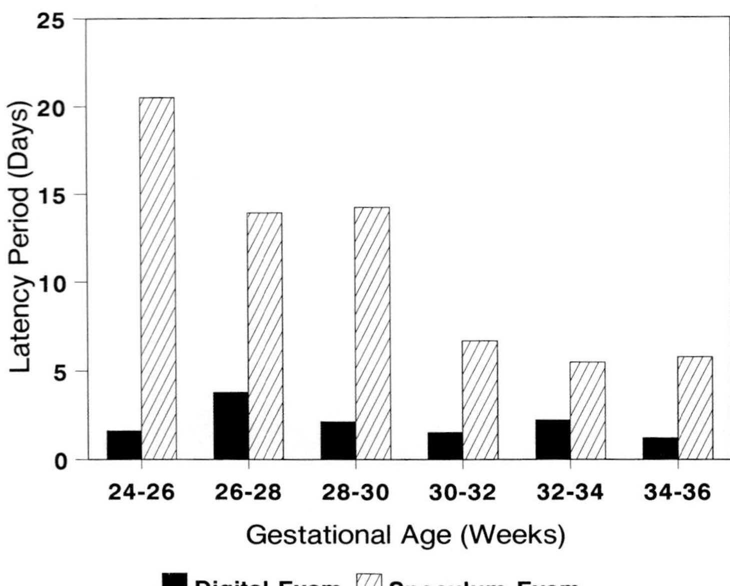

FIGURE 88–4. Effect of digital exam on latency ($p < 0.001$ for all groups). (From Lewis DF, Major CA, Towers CV, Harding JA, Asrat T, Garite TJ. Effects of digital vaginal exams on latency period in preterm premature rupture of membranes. Am J Obstet Gynecol 1991;104:381.)

these tests were originally developed to detect uteroplacental insufficiency, their primary use in PROM is to diagnose impending infection.

NONSTRESS TEST

A major clinical problem in interpreting a nonreactive NST in the preterm gestation is the differential diagnosis among lack of reactivity due to prematurity, infection, or hypoxia. A few studies have demonstrated that fetuses with preterm PROM between 24 and 37 weeks have a significantly higher incidence of reactive tracings than gestational age-matched counterparts with intact membranes.[132–134] Thus, lack of reactivity should not be ascribed to prematurity without further testing. Isolated fetal heart rate decelerations have frequently been described in NSTs of patients with PROM. Their occurrence seems to be related to the amniotic fluid volume, as the amniotic fluid index is lower in patients with decelerations than in patients without them (4.32 ± 1.67 versus 6.47 ± 3.59, $p < 0.01$).[135]

The value of the NST in the prediction of infectious outcome has been addressed in a retrospective study of 127 patients with PROM.[132] Table 88-11 shows the diagnostic indices of a nonreactive NST in the prediction of total infectious morbidity (ie, proven or suspected neonatal sepsis, and maternal chorioamnionitis), of culture-documented neonatal sepsis, and of microbial invasion of the amniotic cavity. Since the false-positive rate of a nonreactive NST is around 35%, it would be inappropriate to make a management decision solely on the results of this test.

AMNIOTIC FLUID VOLUME

Membrane rupture is not necessarily associated with oligohydramnios. Vintzileos and associates reported that 65.5% (59/90) of patients with PROM had a vertical pocket of amniotic fluid greater than 2 cm, 15.5% (14/90) had a vertical pocket between 1 and 2 cm, and only 19% (17/90) had a vertical pocket of less than 1 cm.[136] A recent and interesting observation is that the

TABLE 88–11. DIAGNOSTIC INDICES OF NONREACTIVE NST IN THE PREDICTION OF INFECTIOUS OUTCOME

	CHORIOAMNIONITIS, POSSIBLE NEONATAL SEPSIS, DOCUMENTED NEONATAL SEPSIS*	DOCUMENTED NEONATAL SEPSIS*	POSITIVE AMNIOTIC FLUID CULTURE†
Sensitivity	94% (15/16)	100% (7/7)	88% (23/26)
Specificity	70% (26/37)	59% (27/46)	75% (45/60)
Positive predictive value	58% (15/26)	27% (7/26)	60% (23/38)
Negative predictive value	96% (26/27)	100% (27/27)	94% (45/48)
Prevalence	30% (16/53)	13% (7/53)	30% (26/86)

* (From Vintzileos AM, Campbell WA, Nochimson DJ, et al. The fetal biophysical profile in patients with premature rupture of the membranes: an early predictor of infection. Am J Obstet Gynecol 1985;152:510.)

† (From Romero R. Unpublished observations.)

TABLE 88–12. RELATIONSHIP BETWEEN AMNIOTIC FLUID VOLUME AND DURATION OF LATENCY PERIOD, INCIDENCE OF CHORIOAMNIONITIS, AND NEONATAL SEPSIS

AF VOLUME	NO. OF PATIENTS	CHORIOAMNIONITIS	NEONATAL SEPSIS	LATENCY PERIOD ≥2 DAYS	LATENCY PERIOD ≥7 DAYS
≥2 cm	54	5/54 (9.2%)	1/54 (1.8%)	37/45 (82.2%)	13/45 (28.8%)
<1 cm	19	9/19 (47.3%)	6/19 (13.5%)	5/11 (45.4%)	1/11 (9.0%)
		$p < .05$	$p < .05$	$p < .05$	$p < .05$

(From Vintzileos AM, Campbell WA, Nochimson DJ, Weinbaum PJ. Degree of oligohydramnios and pregnancy outcome in patients with premature rupture of the membranes. Obstet Gynecol 1985;66:162.)

amniotic fluid index (AFI) in patients with preterm PROM remains stable after the membranes rupture. Jackson and colleagues reported that the mean AFI on admission was 5.9 (± 2.5 cm) and at the day of delivery was 5.4 (± 2.0 cm).[137]

Patients with a vertical amniotic fluid pocket less than 1 cm have a shorter latency period and a higher incidence of chorioamnionitis and neonatal sepsis than patients with a vertical pocket greater than 2 cm (Table 88-12). A similar set of findings was reported by Gonick and coworkers in a study of 39 patients.[138] Women with a vertical amniotic fluid pocket less than 1 cm had a higher incidence of chorioamnionitis and endometritis than those with an amniotic fluid pocket greater than 1 cm. No difference in the duration of the latency period between the two groups was found in this study.

A reduction in amniotic fluid volume is also associated with an increased incidence of microbial invasion of the amniotic cavity. Table 88-13 shows the diagnostic indices of a vertical pocket less than 1 cm in a study in which the success rate of amniocentesis was 96% and the prevalence of positive amniotic fluid cultures was 30%.[141]

Collectively, these data indicate that there is an association between reduced amniotic fluid volume and maternal infectious morbidity and microbial invasion of the amniotic cavity. This association is not so strong that management decisions can be based solely on this parameter.

The reason for the high rate of infection in patients with oligohydramnios is unknown. One possibility is that decreased amniotic fluid volume may deprive patients of the antibacterial properties of normal amniotic fluid and therefore predispose them to infection. Alternatively, intra-amniotic infection may alter amniotic fluid dynamics and lead to a reduction in fluid volume. Further studies are needed to address this question.

FETAL BREATHING MOVEMENTS

Preterm PROM is associated with a significant and prolonged reduction of fetal breathing movements lasting about 2 weeks.[139,140] This phenomenon seems to be related to rupture of membranes per se, rather than to infection, hypoxia, or intrauterine growth retardation. The mechanisms responsible for the reduction in breathing movements are unknown. Membrane rupture leads to reduction in intra-amniotic pressure and thus favors loss of lung fluid. Teleologically, a reduction in fetal breathing may be a mechanism of protection against lung fluid loss and pulmonary hypoplasia.

Vintzileos was the first to document an association between infection and decreased fetal breathing activity in the setting of PROM.[141,142] Subsequently, we confirmed and expanded these observations by documenting that patients with positive amniotic fluid cultures had fewer and shorter episodes of fetal breathing activity than women with negative amniotic fluid cultures.[143] The total time spent breathing differed dramatically between the two groups (Fig. 88-5).

The available data suggest that the presence of fetal

TABLE 88–13. DIAGNOSTIC INDICES OF AMNIOTIC FLUID VOLUME (<1 CM) IN THE PREDICTION OF INFECTIOUS OUTCOME

	CHORIOAMNIONITIS, POSSIBLE NEONATAL SEPSIS, DOCUMENTED NEONATAL SEPSIS*	DOCUMENTED NEONATAL SEPSIS*	POSITIVE AMNIOTIC FLUID CULTURE†
Sensitivity	56% (9/16)	71% (5/7)	77% (21/27)
Specificity	89% (33/37)	83% (38/46)	66% (39/59)
Positive predictive value	69% (9/13)	38% (5/13)	51% (21/41)
Negative predictive value	82% (33/40)	95% (38/40)	87% (39/45)
Prevalence	30% (16/53)	13% (7/53)	31% (27/86)

* (From Vintzileos AM, Campbell WA, Nochimson DJ, et al. The fetal biophysical profile in patients with premature rupture of the membranes: an early predictor of infection. Am J Obstet Gynecol 1985;152:510.)

† (From Romero R. Unpublished observations.)

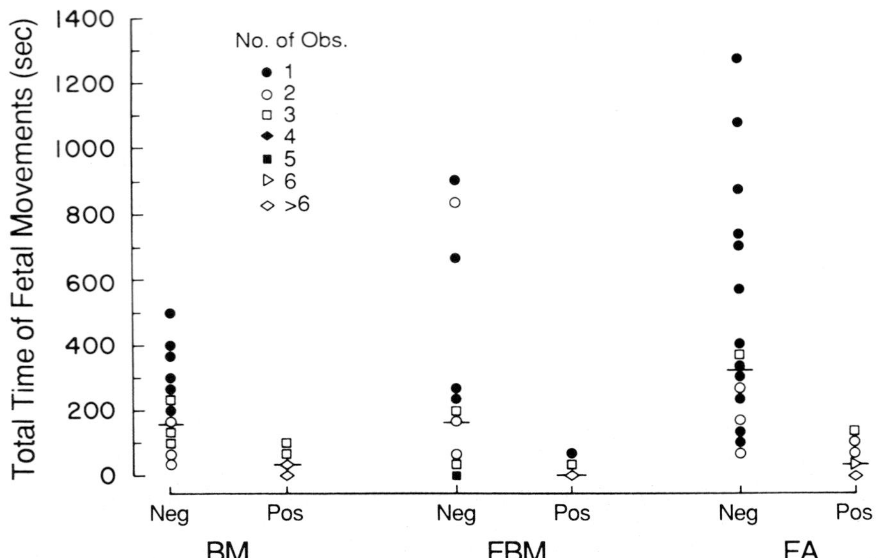

FIGURE 88–5. The total amount of time (in seconds) of body movements (BM), breathing movements (FBM), and fetal activity (FA) according to the amniotic fluid culture results. (From Goldstein I, Romero R, Merrill S, et al. Fetal body and breathing movements as predictors of intra-amniotic infection in preterm premature rupture of membranes. Am J Obstet Gynecol 1988;159:364.)

breathing has a very high negative predictive value (about 95%) for the presence of microbial invasion of the amniotic cavity and for neonatal sepsis. However, the absence of breathing activity has a limited positive predictive value (about 50%) for either of these two outcomes, and thus it cannot be used as an indication for pregnancy termination (Table 88-14).

The mechanisms responsible for a reduction in fetal breathing activity in the setting of infection have not been elucidated. A role for prostaglandins is supported by the observation that sepsis is associated with increased plasma concentrations of prostaglandins, which have been shown to reduce breathing activity when infused in fetal lambs.[144]

FETAL BODY MOVEMENTS

The number and the duration of fetal body movements are lower in patients with preterm PROM and positive amniotic fluid cultures than in patients with negative amniotic fluid cultures (see Fig. 88-5).[143] Using the criteria proposed by Manning and associates,[145a] we found that fetal body movements have a sensitivity of 32%, specificity of 97%, positive predictive value of 89%, and negative predictive value of 69% in the diagnosis of a positive amniotic fluid culture.[145] Moreover, decreased fetal activity is also correlated with a higher incidence of culture-proven neonatal sepsis (Table 88-15).

Decreased fetal motion in the context of infection may be the counterpart of the reduction in motor behavior observed during the course of febrile illnesses in adults and children. We have proposed that interleukin-1 and TNF released by macrophages in the course of infection may be responsible for this phenomenon.

BIOPHYSICAL PROFILE

Using stepwise multiple logistic regression analysis, Vintzileos and associates demonstrated that each component of the BPP contains useful information for the

TABLE 88–14. DIAGNOSTIC INDICES OF FETAL BREATHING MOVEMENTS (<30 SEC DURATION IN 30-MIN OBSERVATION) IN THE PREDICTION OF INFECTIOUS OUTCOME

	CHORIOAMNIONITIS, POSSIBLE NEONATAL SEPSIS, DOCUMENTED NEONATAL SEPSIS*	DOCUMENTED NEONATAL SEPSIS*	POSITIVE AMNIOTIC FLUID CULTURE†
Sensitivity	100% (16/16)	100% (7/7)	92% (23/25)
Specificity	73% (27/37)	59% (27/46)	49% (19/39)
Positive predictive value	61% (16/26)	27% (7/26)	53% (23/43)
Negative predictive value	100% (27/27)	100% (27/27)	90% (19/21)
Prevalence	30% (16/53)	13% (7/53)	39% (25/64)

* From Vintzileos AM, Campbell WA, Nochimson DJ, et al. The fetal biophysical profile in patients with premature rupture of the membranes: an early predictor of infection. Am J Obstet Gynecol 1985;152:510.

† From Roberts AB, Goldstein I, Romero R, et al. Comparison of total fetal activity measurement with the biophysical profile in predicting intra-amniotic infection in preterm premature rupture of membranes. Ultrasound Obstet Gynecol 1991;1:36.

TABLE 88–15. DIAGNOSTIC INDICES OF FETAL BODY MOVEMENTS (≤2 BODY/LIMB MOVEMENTS IN 30 MIN) IN THE PREDICTION OF INFECTIOUS OUTCOME

	CHORIOAMNIONITIS, POSSIBLE NEONATAL SEPSIS, DOCUMENTED NEONATAL SEPSIS*	DOCUMENTED NEONATAL SEPSIS*	POSITIVE AMNIOTIC FLUID CULTURE†
Sensitivity	50% (8/16)	86% (6/7)	32% (8/25)
Specificity	94% (35/37)	91% (42/46)	97% (38/39)
Positive predictive value	80% (8/10)	60% (6/10)	89% (8/9)
Negative predictive value	81% (35/43)	98% (42/43)	69% (38/55)
Prevalence	30% (16/53)	13% (7/53)	39% (25/64)

* From Vintzileos AM, Campbell WA, Nochimson DJ, et al. The fetal biophysical profile in patients with premature rupture of the membranes: an early predictor of infection. Am J Obstet Gynecol 1985;152:510.

† From Romero AB, Goldstein I, Romero R, et al. Comparison of total fetal activity measurement with the biophysical profile in predicting intra-amniotic infection in preterm premature rupture of membranes. Ultrasound Obstet Gynecol 1991;1:36.

prediction of infectious outcome (defined as maternal chorioamnionitis, possible neonatal sepsis, and proven neonatal sepsis). In the first study, a modified BPP scoring system that incorporated placental grading (maximal score, 12) was used.[141] A score of 7 or below was much better than any single parameter of the BPP in the prediction of infectious outcome. Placental grading was the only component of the score that had no predictive value. The diagnostic indices of a BPP of 7 or below performed 24 hours before delivery were: sensitivity 94% (15/16), specificity 97% (36/37), positive predictive value 94% (15/16), and negative predictive value 97% (36/37) in a population with a prevalence of infectious outcome of 30% (16/53). Infectious outcome included two cases of amnionitis, three of possible neonatal sepsis, four of amnionitis and possible neonatal sepsis, three of documented neonatal sepsis, and four of amnionitis and documented neonatal sepsis. Since the study was observational in nature, the BPP was not used for patient management.

Subsequently, Vintzileos and colleagues compared the outcome of pregnancy in patients managed with serial BPPs with two historical control groups: one managed expectantly without BPP or amniocentesis, and the other managed with a single amniocentesis on admission.[146] A score of 7 or below on two examinations 2 hours apart was used as an indication for delivery. An abnormal score required a nonreactive NST and absence of fetal breathing. The results of this study indicated that patients managed with daily BPPs had a lower rate of overall neonatal sepsis (suspected and culture-proven) than patients in the control and amniocentesis group. However, this study did not provide the frequency of other indices of neonatal morbidity (eg, respiratory distress syndrome (RDS), intraventricular hemorrhage (IVH), duration of mechanical ventilation) in the different groups. This issue is important, because 14 patients who were delivered because of a low BPP score showed no evidence of neonatal infection (false positives). If intervention is not associated with an increased rate of other neonatal complications, management with serial BPPs would seem a reasonable approach.

We recently compared the diagnostic performance of the BPP with that of total fetal activity (the sum of fetal breathing and body movements in a 30-minute period of observation) in the prediction of a positive amniotic fluid culture.[145] The specificity of a total fetal activity greater than 10% was significantly better than that of the BPP (Table 88-16, Fig. 88-6).

The best approach to monitoring the patient with preterm PROM is probably a combination of ultrasound and amniocentesis. Patients may be monitored with either the BPP or total body activity. If a patient has a BPP score above 6 (original Manning score) or a total activity more than 3 minutes (10% in a 30-minute

TABLE 88–16. PREDICTION OF POSITIVE AMNIOTIC FLUID CULTURES: BIOPHYSICAL PROFILE VS TOTAL FETAL ACTIVITY

	BIOPHYSICAL PROFILE	TOTAL FETAL ACTIVITY (10%)
Sensitivity	92% (23/25)	96% (24/25)
Specificity	59% (23/39)*	82% (32/39)
Positive predictive value	59% (23/39)	77% (24/31)
Negative predictive value	92% (23/25)	97% (32/33)

* Significant difference between specificities, $p < .05$.

(From Roberts AB, Goldstein I, Romero R, et al. Comparison of total fetal activity measurement with the biophysical profile in predicting intra-amniotic infection in preterm premature rupture of membranes. Ultrasound Obstet Gynecol 1991;1:36.)

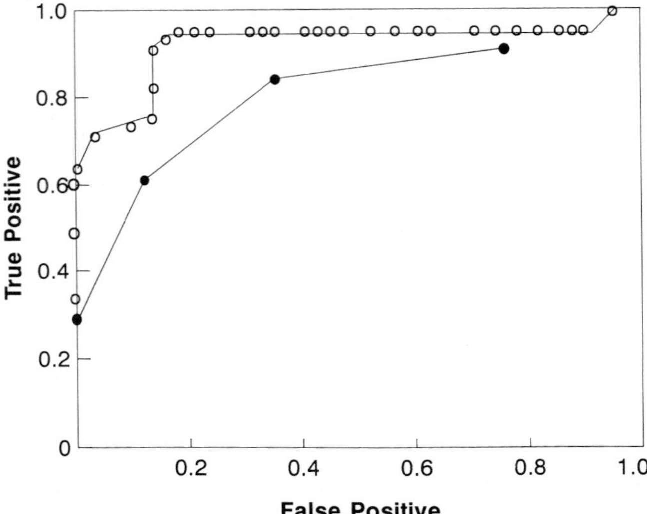

FIGURE 88–6. Receiver operator curve characteristics for total fetal activity (TFA%), open circles; biophysical profile, closed circles. (From Roberts AB, Goldstein I, Romero R, Hobbins JC. Comparison of total fetal activity measurement with the biophysical profile in predicting intra-amniotic infection in preterm premature rupture of membranes. Ultrasound Obstet Gynecol 1991;1:36.)

period), the likelihood of a positive amniotic fluid culture or neonatal sepsis is extraordinarily low. These patients can be followed with serial ultrasound examinations. On the other hand, if a patient has a BPP of less than 6 or a total activity lower than 10%, amniocentesis can be performed to determine if there is microbial invasion of the amniotic cavity.

CHORIOAMNIONITIS

Conservative management of the preterm PROM pregnancy enjoys widespread but not universal acceptance. The greatest concern arising from this noninterventional strategy is the development of infection. The classical signs of chorioamnionitis include fever, maternal and fetal tachycardia, foul-smelling amniotic fluid, and maternal leukocytosis with a left shift in the differential. These signs are insensitive, however, and will detect only about 12% of patients with positive amniotic fluid cultures. Clearly, it is in the best interest of mother and fetus to identify the onset of infection as early as possible. This knowledge permits treatment or delivery before late manifestations of infection develop.

Several studies have examined the value of C-reactive protein (CRP) in monitoring the patient with preterm PROM.[147–153] Most studies indicate that there is a strong relationship between an elevated maternal serum CRP and the presence of histologic chorioamnionitis. The diagnostic indices, cut-off values, and definition of infection-related morbidity for the different studies are shown in Table 88-17. The emerging picture is that a normal maternal serum CRP has a high negative predictive value for clinical and histologic chorioamnionitis. On the other hand, the positive predictive value of CRP is limited but can be improved by serial testing. A steady rise in serum CRP is associated with impending chorioamnionitis. Several studies have demonstrated that CRP is an earlier and more accurate laboratory parameter than the white blood cell count and differential in the diagnosis of chorioamnionitis.

The precise place of CRP in clinical obstetrics needs to be defined. An elevated CRP could potentially be used as an indication to increase fetal surveillance or to

TABLE 88–17. DIAGNOSTIC INDICES OF C-REACTIVE PROTEIN

AUTHOR	CUT-OFF VALUES	DEFINITION OF INFECTION	PREVALENCE OF INFECTION	SENSITIVITY (%)	SPECIFICITY (%)	POS. PREDICTIVE VALUE (%)	NEG. PREDICTIVE VALUE (%)
Evans et al. (1980)[147]	2 mg/dL	Clinical or histologic	69.4% (25/36)	80	100	100	69
Hawrylyshyn et al. (1983)[150]	1.25 mg/dL	Histologic	50.0% (26/52)	88	96	96	89
Farb et al. (1983)[148]	2 mg/dL	Clinical	29.0% (9/31)	56	73	45	80
		Histologic	21.0% (5/24)	80	68	40	93
Romem and Artal (1984)[153]	2 mg/dL	Clinical	16.3% (7/43)	86	97	86	97
Ismail et al. (1985)[151]	2 mg/dL	Clinical	18.0% (18/100)	82	55	36	91
		Histologic	63.0% (63/100)	67	81	90	50
Fisk et al. (1987)[149]	2 mg/dL	Histologic	59.0% (30/51)	50*	81*	79*	53*
				92†	73†	73†	92†
Kurki et al. (1990)[152]	1.2 mg/dL	Clinical and histologic	22.4% (33/147)	94††	50‡	35‡	97‡
	4.0 mg/dL	Neonatal infection	13.0% (21/162)	72§	63§	48§	83§
				79	43	18	93

* 24° interval sample to delivery.
† 12° interval sample to delivery.
‡ Cut-off = 1.2 mg/dL.
§ Cut-off = 4.0 mg/dL.

consider antibiotic treatment. A randomized clinical trial will be required to determine if patients with elevated CRP may benefit from such a therapeutic intervention.

TERM PROM

The traditional management of patients with term PROM has been induction of labor to prevent maternal and neonatal infection. This approach is based on the results of studies conducted several decades ago. These studies indicated that the longer the latency period (interval between membrane rupture and onset of labor), the higher the perinatal mortality and infectious maternal morbidity. For example, in a large uncontrolled retrospective study of 6425 patients with term PROM managed between 1951 and 1964, the rate of intrapartum fever increased after a latency period of more than 24 hours.[3] Perinatal mortality increased significantly in patients with a latency period of more than 3 days (Fig. 88-7). The excessive perinatal mortality was mostly attributable to stillbirths and occurred in patients with intrapartum fever.

These data have been cited to justify a policy of inducing labor at term in the setting of PROM. However, two issues must be considered. First, perinatal mortality has decreased significantly over the last 30 years for patients with term PROM (from 23/1000 to 1.8/1000).[3,7,8,154,155] This is also due to improved maternal and neonatal care.[156,157] Second, no scientific evidence was ever presented to support the contention that inducing labor would decrease perinatal mortality and maternal morbidity.

Four randomized clinical trials have compared expectant management versus induction of labor with oxytocin in the context of term PROM.[7,8,154,155] All trials have been conducted within the last 10 years. No difference in perinatal mortality was observed between the two management strategies. However, the total number of patients enrolled into these trials was 584, and the overall perinatal mortality was only 1.8/1000. It is clear that the sample size is insufficient to detect a difference in perinatal mortality between expectant management and induction of labor.

Meta-analysis of these trials indicates that induction of labor is associated with a higher incidence of cesarean section (Table 88-18) and maternal infectious morbidity (Table 88-19), while failing to reduce the incidence of neonatal sepsis (Table 88-20). The results of this analysis could be used to condemn the policy of induction of labor. However, several limitations in the design of these trials should be pointed out.

First, the most common indication for cesarean section in two of the trials was failed induction (defined as failure to enter the active phase of labor within 12 hours).[154,155] Such a period of time is often insufficient for an induction in a patient with an unripe cervix. In the absence of fetal distress or signs of maternal infection, we see little reason to arbitrarily end an induction after 12 hours. Thus, the higher incidence of cesarean section in these trials may result from premature rather than truly needed intervention.

Second, the intrapartum management protocols were not similar in the two study groups: pelvic examinations and placement of intrauterine pressure catheters and scalp electrodes were performed more commonly in patients randomized to induction of labor.[154,155] This

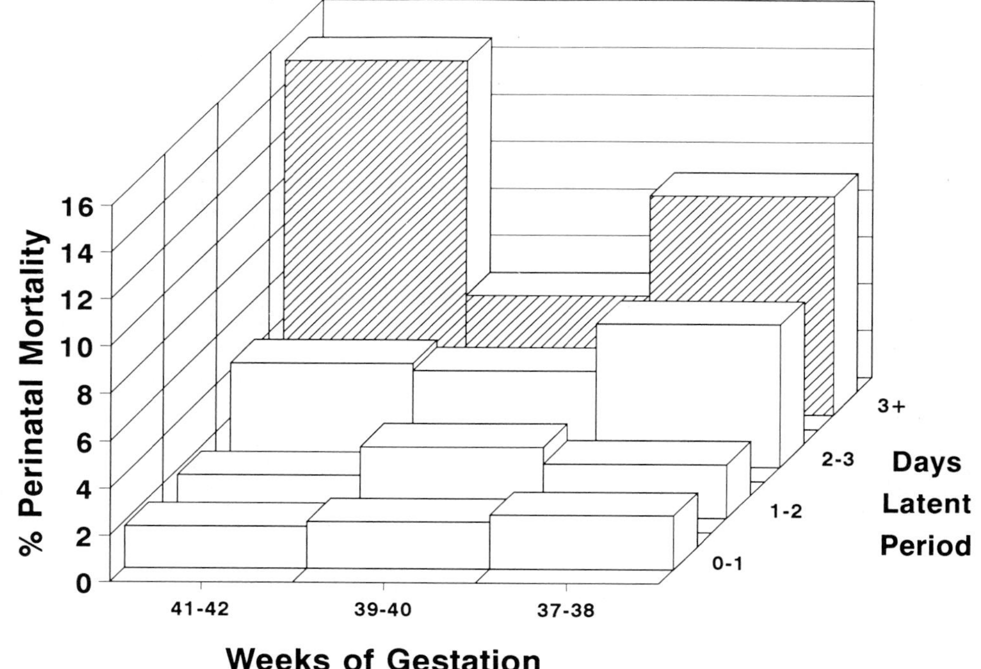

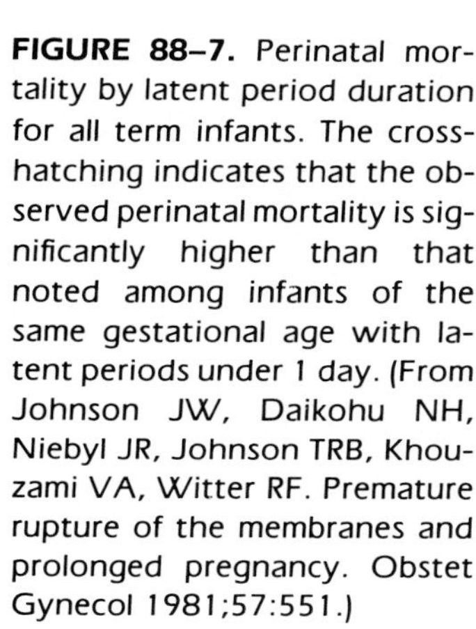
FIGURE 88–7. Perinatal mortality by latent period duration for all term infants. The cross-hatching indicates that the observed perinatal mortality is significantly higher than that noted among infants of the same gestational age with latent periods under 1 day. (From Johnson JW, Daikohu NH, Niebyl JR, Johnson TRB, Khouzami VA, Witter RF. Premature rupture of the membranes and prolonged pregnancy. Obstet Gynecol 1981;57:551.)

TABLE 88-18. EFFECT OF INDUCTION OF LABOR ON THE CESAREAN SECTION RATE IN TERM PROM

STUDY	EXPECTANT	INDUCTION	ODDS RATIO INDUCTION/EXPECTANT (95% CL)	GRAPH OF ODDS RATIOS AND CONFIDENCE LIMITS (0.01 .1 1 10 100)
Duff et al. (1984)[154]	7% (5/75)	20% (12/59)	3.57 (1.07–12.56)	
Morales et al. (1986)[155]	7% (11/167)	21% (31/150)	3.69 (1.70–8.18)	
Tamsen et al. (1990)[7]	8% (4/50)	0% (0/43)	0.15 (0.02–1.76)	
Van der Walt et al. (1989)[8]	0% (0/20)	30% (6/20)	3.35 (0.17–34.44)	
Typical odds ratio			2.75 (1.64–4.61)	

could explain the higher incidence of maternal infectious morbidity in patients allocated to induction.

Third, the size of the trials precludes any conclusions about the impact of these management strategies on neonatal sepsis.

It is noteworthy that these trials have compared expectant management versus induction by oxytocin infusion alone. However, other methods of induction (ie, prostaglandin administration) may be more effective than oxytocin infusion. Five randomized clinical trials compared induction with prostaglandin E_2 administration versus oxytocin infusion in the setting of term PROM (Table 88-21).[2,4,8,9,158] Their meta-analysis indicates that induction with prostaglandins is associated with a lower incidence of cesarean section (Table 88-22). In only one small trial was expectant management compared to two different induction protocols (oxytocin infusion and prostaglandin administration).[8] All cesarean sections occurred in patients induced with oxytocin infusion, but the small numbers (20 patients in each arm) precluded any significant statistical analysis.

From the preceding analysis, we conclude that there is insufficient evidence to favor any of the alternatives to manage term PROM. The apparently worse results obtained with induction of labor may be attributed to the method of induction and the definition of failed induction rather than to induction per se. Studies in which patients have been managed expectantly indicate that labor will spontaneously begin by 12 hours in 50%, by 24 hours in 70%, by 48 hours in 85%, and by 72 hours in 95% of cases.[3] In the absence of conclusive evidence that intervention with induction of labor has beneficial effects, expectant management seems a reasonable approach, provided there are no clinical or laboratory indicators of impending infection. Ninety-five percent of patients will deliver within 72 hours; the remaining 5% of patients represent an unresolved clinical dilemma. Induction of labor can be an alternative for these patients.

Patients with suspected PROM at term should be examined to establish the diagnosis of PROM, exclude cord prolapse, screen for infection, and evaluate fetal well-being. Relevant management issues include whether the patient should be hospitalized and how to monitor for signs of maternal or fetal infection. There is a paucity of data in this area on which to base management decisions. Decisions regarding hospitalization depend largely on the health-care resources and the

TABLE 88-19. EFFECT OF INDUCTION OF LABOR ON THE INCIDENCE OF CHORIOAMNIONITIS IN TERM PROM

STUDY	EXPECTANT	INDUCTION	ODDS RATIO INDUCTION/EXPECTANT (95% CL)	GRAPH OF ODDS RATIOS AND CONFIDENCE LIMITS (0.01 .1 1 10 100)
Duff et al. (1984)[154]	4% (3/75)	17% (10/59)	4.90 (1.16–23.78)	
Morales et al. (1986)[155]	3% (5/167)	8% (12/150)	2.82 (0.89–9.42)	
Tamsen et al. (1990)[7]	2% (1/50)	0% (0/43)	0.16 (0.03–7.93)	
Van der Walt et al. (1989)[8]	0% (0/20)	0% (0/20)	N.C.	
Typical odds ratio			3.04 (1.48–6.24)	

N.C., not computable.

TABLE 88–20. EFFECT OF INDUCTION OF LABOR ON THE INCIDENCE OF NEONATAL INFECTION IN TERM PROM

STUDY	EXPECTANT	INDUCTION	ODDS RATIO INDUCTION/EXPECTANT (95% CL)	GRAPH OF ODDS RATIOS AND CONFIDENCE LIMITS (0.01 .1 1 10 100)
Duff et al. (1984)[154]	0% (0/75)	2% (1/59)	9.69 (0.19–502)	
Morales et al. (1986)[155]	0% (0/167)	0% (0/150)	N.C.	
Tamsen et al. (1990)[7]	4% (2/50)	0% (0/43)	0.15 (0.01–2.49)	
Van der Walt et al. (1989)[8]	0% (0/20)	5% (1/20)	7.39 (0.15–372)	
Typical odds ratio			1.15 (0.16–8.23)	

N.C., not computable.

medicolegal climate of the area and country in which one practices. Several methods are available to assess the likelihood of infection, including standard clinical signs (eg, temperature, fetal heart rate, uterine tenderness), laboratory tests (WBC and differential, CRP), and amniocentesis. The optimal method for fetal monitoring still needs to be established. Amniocentesis must be regarded as an investigational procedure at this time.

Given that PROM could be a risk factor for chorioamnionitis, puerperal endometritis, and neonatal sepsis, it is a relevant issue whether patients with term PROM should receive prophylactic antibiotics. This has been addressed by one double-blind randomized trial in which women with PROM were randomized to receive dimethylchlortetracycline or placebo.[5] Drugs were administered while the patient remained undelivered and for 3 days postpartum. Data from women giving birth to 1553 infants weighing more than 2500 g indicated that the administration of antibiotics significantly reduced the rate of endometritis from 2.7% to 1.3% ($p = 0.03$) but did not decrease the perinatal mortality or the incidence of infectious neonatal complications. No contemporary study has addressed this issue. Tetracycline is certainly not the drug of choice for this indication, given the fetal risks.

PRETERM PROM

NATURAL HISTORY

Two contemporary studies have addressed the natural history of preterm PROM in the United States.[159,160]

In the study by Cox and associates, 298 patients with preterm PROM were managed expectantly (steroids, tocolytics, and prophylactic antibiotics were not administered; amniocenteses were not performed).[159] Of the 267 patients who gave birth to infants weighing 750 g or more, 76% (204/267) either were in active labor when they were admitted or spontaneously began labor within 12 hours of admission; 5% of patients were delivered because of complications (hypertension, fetal death, diabetes). The remaining 19% (50/267) were managed expectantly. Sixty percent of these patients went into spontaneous labor within 48 hours of admission. Thus, only 7% of the original 267 patients remained undelivered for more than 48 hours. Chorioamnionitis developed in 10.6% of cases, breech presentation occurred in 18%, twin gestation was present in 6.7%, and the incidence of cesarean section was 40%. Of the 284 infants with birth weights of 750 g or more, there were 12 stillbirths (all before admission)

TABLE 88–21. PROM AT TERM INDUCTION OF LABOR: PGE_2 VS OXYTOCIN

STUDY	NUMBER OF PATIENTS		PGE_2 ROUTE AND DOSE	OXYTOCIN ROUTE AND DOSE
	PGE_2	OXYTOCIN		
Ekman-Ordeberg et al. (1985)[158]	10	10	Vaginal gel 4 mg	IV 24 mU/min
Westergaard et al. (1983)[9]	109	84	Oral tabs 0.5–1.5 mg/hr	Oral tabs 50 IU/30 min
Hauth et al. (1977)[2]	50	50	Oral tabs 0.5–1 mg/hr	IV Dose not described
Lange et al. (1981)[4]	99	102	Oral tabs 0.5–1.5 mg/hr	IV 45 mU/min
Van der Walt et al. (1989)[8]	20	20	Vaginal tabs 1 mg/6 hr	IV 24 mU/min

TABLE 88–22. EFFECT OF INDUCTION OF LABOR WITH PGE_2 OR OXYTOCIN ON THE CESAREAN SECTION RATE IN TERM PROM

STUDY	C/S WITH PGE_2	C/S WITH OXYTOCIN	ODDS RATIO PGE_2/OXYTOCIN (95% CL)	GRAPH OF ODDS RATIOS AND CONFIDENCE INTERVALS 0.01 .1 1 10 100
Ekman-Ordeberg et al. (1985)[158]	0% (0/10)	40% (4/10)	0.09 (0.01–1.36)	
Westergaard et al. (1983)[9]	5.5% (6/109)	4.8% (4/84)	1.16 (0.28–5.11)	
Hauth et al. (1977)[2]	14% (7/50)	22% (11/50)	0.58 (0.18–1.82)	
Lange et al. (1981)[4]	0% (0/99)	2.9% (3/102)	0.14 (0.01–2.30)	
Van der Walt et al. (1989)[8]	0% (0/20)	30% (6/20)	0.10 (0.02–0.79)	
Typical odds ratio			0.40 (0.21–0.78)	

and 18 neonatal deaths (neonatal death rate = 6.6%). The causes of death were complications of prematurity (n = 12), malformations (n = 3), hypoplastic lungs (n = 1), and neonatal sepsis (n = 2).

Wilson and coworkers reported on the outcome of 143 patients with preterm PROM managed conservatively.[160] It is noteworthy that 140 patients were transferred from outlying hospitals. Eighteen percent of patients remained undelivered after 1 week of admission. Maternal febrile infectious morbidity (antepartum and postpartum) occurred in 10% of patients, 18.6% (27/145) of neonates were born in breech presentation, and the incidence of cesarean section was 22% (31/143). The neonatal death rate was 12.4% (17/137).

MANAGEMENT ISSUES

There are several issues in the management of preterm PROM that play no part in term PROM:

1. Should tocolysis be started, and if so when (prophylactically versus therapeutically)?
2. Will antibiotic prophylaxis prolong the latency period and reduce the incidence of chorioamnionitis and neonatal sepsis?
3. Should steroids be given to enhance fetal lung surfactant production?
4. What are the best methods of antenatal fetal surveillance?

Tocolysis

Tocolysis has been considered as a potential way to delay delivery and reduce perinatal complications in the setting of preterm PROM. Five randomized clinical trials have studied the effect of tocolysis on pregnancy prolongation and perinatal outcome. Two trials addressed the issue of prophylactic administration of oral ritodrine to patients not in labor; the other three examined the effectiveness of intravenous tocolysis in patients with uterine contractions.[161–165]

Levy and Warsof randomized 42 women with preterm PROM to receive oral ritodrine (10 mg, p.o., q 4 hr) versus no medication or placebo.[161] Drugs were given until the onset of labor. A latency period of more than 7 days was noted more frequently in patients receiving ritodrine than in the controls (47.6% [10/21] versus 14.2% [3/21], $p = .043$). The only perinatal death occurred in the control group. No differences in perinatal morbidity or mortality were documented between the study group and the control group.

Dunlop and associates randomized 48 women to receive oral ritodrine versus no tocolysis and then subrandomized each group to receive prophylactic antibiotics (cephalexin) versus no antibiotics.[162] The result was a four-limb randomization with 12 patients per group. Steroids were given to all patients. No difference in outcome (perinatal mortality and RDS) was observed between patients receiving ritodrine versus no tocolysis. Therefore, the evidence is inconclusive as to the use of prophylactic tocolysis.

Of the three randomized trials of intravenous tocolysis, only one used a double-blind placebo design[163]; the other two compared tocolysis versus bed rest.[164,165] Overall, no change in maternal or neonatal morbidity and mortality was demonstrated between the study group and the control group. Tocolysis, however, resulted in some degree of pregnancy prolongation in two of the trials.[163,164]

In the trial of Christensen and coworkers, ritodrine administration was associated with a significant decrease in the proportion of women delivering within 24 hours after membrane rupture (ritodrine, 0% [0/24] versus placebo, 37.5% [6/16]; $p < .05$).[163] However, no difference in pregnancy prolongation after 24 hours was observed between the treatment group and the control group.

In the study by Weiner and colleagues, the duration of pregnancy was greater in patients receiving tocolysis than in those allocated to bed rest (105 hours [SD = 157 hours] versus 62.1 hours [SD = 77 hours], respectively; $p = .06$).[164] Post-hoc analysis indicated that tocolysis administration resulted in significant pregnancy prolongation for patients with gestational ages of less than 28 weeks at the time of membrane rupture (bed rest = 53.4 hours versus tocolysis = 232.8 hours, $p = .05$). This was not associated with a demonstrable reduction in perinatal morbidity or mortality. No difference in pregnancy prolongation was noted in patients with a gestational age greater than 28 weeks. The authors concluded that there was no justification for tocolysis after 28 weeks of gestation. An unresolved issue is whether the prolongation observed in patients with gestational ages below 28 weeks (mean prolongation = 5 days) could have some beneficial effect. Steroids were not used in this trial. It is conceivable that the combined use of steroids and tocolysis at early gestational ages could reduce perinatal morbidity; this issue requires further study.

Garite and associates randomized 79 women with a gestational age of 25 to 30 weeks to receive either intravenous tocolysis with ritodrine (followed by oral therapy) or expectant management.[165] Steroids were not used. No difference in pregnancy prolongation or perinatal morbidity and mortality was observed between the two groups. It should be noted that 16 of 39 patients randomized to the tocolytic limb did not actually receive the treatment.

Since two of three randomized clinical trials of intravenous tocolysis suggest that treatment results in some prolongation of pregnancy, it is relevant to determine whether enough time could be gained to complete steroid administration and reduce the incidence of RDS.[163,164] Meta-analysis of the two trials that provide adequate information indicates that tocolysis does not result in prolongation of pregnancy of more than 48 hours (Table 88-23).[164,165] Thus, there is insufficient evidence to justify the use of tocolytic agents in patients with PROM for this specific reason.

Antibiotics

Evidence suggests that 28% of patients with preterm PROM have a positive amniotic fluid culture on admission; further, the onset of labor in preterm PROM is associated with microbial invasion of the amniotic cavity in about 70% of patients.[98] Consequently, several investigators have conducted randomized clinical trials to examine the potential benefits of antibiotic administration.

The first study to address this issue was a double-blind trial in which patients with PROM were randomly allocated to receive either dimethylchlortetracycline by mouth or placebo.[5] Drugs were given while the patient remained undelivered and for 3 days postpartum. Prolongation of pregnancy of 14 days or more was significantly more common in patients receiving tetracycline than those in the placebo group (13.8% [21/152] versus 3.3% [6/180], respectively; $p = .001$). However, it should be noted that this study included patients with both term and preterm PROM and did not stratify for gestational age at entry. The method used to report the data precludes analysis of whether antibiotic treatment was beneficial to the cohort of patients with preterm PROM. Neonatal sepsis was not a reported outcome variable. The proportion of neonatal deaths attributed to infection was not different in the two groups.

In the second study, the effect of a topical vaginal antibiotic (nitrofurazone 2 mg, q 6 hr) was compared to placebo in a double-blind design.[166] No difference in the incidence of chorioamnionitis, postpartum endometritis, and perinatal death was observed between the two groups (chorioamnionitis: nitrofurazone, 21% [30/143] versus placebo, 21.7% [25/115], $p > .05$; endometritis: nitrofurazone, 11.9% [17/143] versus placebo, 12.2% [14/115]; $p > .05$; and perinatal death: nitrofurazone, 2.0% [3/143] versus placebo, 3.5% [4/115]). Data on pregnancy were not reported. It is noteworthy that there was an imbalance in the number of patients in the two groups (143 versus 115); the reasons for this were not reported. As in the previous study, patients were not stratified to gestational age at entry.

TABLE 88–23. EFFECT OF TOCOLYSIS ON PROLONGATION OF PREGNANCY > 48° IN PRETERM PROM

STUDY	EXPECTANT	TOCOLYSIS	ODDS RATIO TOCOLYSIS/EXPECTANT (95% CL)	GRAPH OF ODDS RATIOS AND CONFIDENCE LIMITS (0.1 — 1 — 10)
Garite et al. (1987)	75.0% (30/40)	65.2% (15/23)	0.87 (0.61–1.23)	
Weiner et al. (1988)	76.1% (32/42)	87.9% (29/33)	1.15 (0.93–1.42)	
Typical odds ratio			1.07 (0.89–1.28)	

(Data from Garite TJ, Keegan KA, Freeman RK, Nageotte MP. A randomized trial of ritodrine tocolysis versus expectant management in patients with premature rupture of membranes at 25 to 30 weeks of gestation. Am J Obstet Gynecol 1987;157:388, and Weiner CP, Renk K, Klugman M. The therapeutic efficacy and cost-effectiveness of aggressive tocolysis for premature labor associated with premature rupture of the membranes. Am J Obstet Gynecol 1988;159:216.)

Three contemporary studies have examined the effect of antibiotic administration on preterm PROM.[167–169] Overall, two of the three studies suggest that antibiotic administration is associated with pregnancy prolongation and a reduction in the rate of neonatal sepsis.[167,168]

Amon and associates randomized 82 women with preterm PROM to receive either ampicillin (1 g, I.V., q 6 hr for 24 hr followed by 500 mg, p.o., q 6 hr until delivery) or no antibiotics.[167] Patients allocated to ampicillin had a significantly greater prolongation of pregnancy than those in the control group. Table 88-24 shows the cumulative probability of delivery calculated with the life table method for the groups. The incidence of neonatal infection was lower in the treatment group than in the control group (2.4% [1/42] versus 16.7% [6/36]; $p < .04$). Systemic neonatal infection was defined as a clinically ill infant within the first week of life with a documented positive culture. There was no difference in the incidence of other maternal (chorioamnionitis) or neonatal (NEC, pulmonary complications, IVH, neonatal death) complications between the two groups.

In the second contemporary study, reported by Morales and coworkers, 165 women with preterm PROM (< 34 weeks) were randomized into four groups: group 1, expectant management with no intervention; group 2, betamethasone; group 3, ampicillin; group 4, ampicillin and betamethasone.[169] Ampicillin was given (2 g, IV, q 6 hr) until results of the cervical cultures were available. If cultures were negative for pathogenic bacteria (*Streptococcus agalactiae* and *Neisseria gonorrhoeae*), antibiotics were discontinued. Table 88-25 shows the maternal and neonatal outcome of this trial. No significant prolongation of pregnancy was noted among the four groups. Patients receiving antibiotics had a significant reduction in the incidence of clinical chorioamnionitis, although not in histopathologic chorioamnionitis. No difference in the incidence of neonatal sepsis was noted among the four groups. When comparing patients receiving ampicillin (pooled groups 3 and 4) with those not receiving ampicillin (pooled groups 1 and 2), patients receiving ampicillin had a significantly lower incidence of neonatal sepsis than those in the control group (5% [4/81] versus 10% [8/84], respectively; $p < .01$).

TABLE 88–24. CUMULATIVE PROBABILITY OF DELIVERY

TIME AFTER RANDOMIZATION	TREATMENT GROUP	CONTROL GROUP
24 hr	0.14	0.21
48 hr	0.23	0.42
72 hr	0.33	0.50
1 wk	0.53	0.71
2 wk	0.87	0.94

(From Amon E, Lewis SV, Sibai BM, VIllar MA, Arheart KL. Ampicillin prophylaxis in preterm premature rupture of the membranes: a prospective randomized study. Am J Obstet Gynecol 1988; 159:539.)

Johnston and associates conducted a prospective randomized double-blind trial in which 85 women with preterm PROM (20 to 34 weeks) were allocated to receive placebo or IV mezlocillin for 48 hours followed by oral ampicillin until delivery.[168] Antibiotic treatment resulted in a reduction of the incidence of clinical and histopathologic chorioamnionitis, postpartum endomyometritis, clinical neonatal sepsis, and intraventricular hemorrhage. Total neonatal stay (but not newborn special care unit stay) was also shorter in neonates born to women receiving ampicillin. Table 88-26 shows the outcome data for this study.

Meta-analysis of the three contemporary trials indicates that antibiotic administration is associated with a reduction in the incidence of chorioamnionitis and documented (culture-proven) neonatal sepsis (Tables 88-27 and 88-28). An unresolved issue is whether the difference in the rate of neonatal sepsis between the two groups is real or simply reflects the difficulty in obtaining a positive culture for microorganisms in a newborn who has received antibiotics in utero.

Can antibiotic treatment of women with documented microbial invasion of the amniotic cavity alter the natural history of preterm PROM? The traditional view has been that clinical chorioamnionitis should be managed

TABLE 88–25. ANTIBIOTICS AND OUTCOME IN PATIENTS WITH PRETERM PROM

	GROUP I (n = 41)	GROUP II (n = 43)	GROUP III (n = 37)	GROUP IV (n = 44)	*p* VALUE
Latency period (days)	3.7 ± 4.6	8.6 ± 11.7	8.1 ± 10.1	7.0 ± 6.6	NS
Clinical chorioamnionitis	16 (39%)	6 (14%)	0	3 (7%)	<.01
Histopathologic	29 (71%)	25 (58%)	25 (68%)	23 (52%)	NS
Neonatal sepsis	5 (12%)	3 (6%)	1 (3%)	3 (7%)	NS
	No antibiotics (n = 84)		Antibiotics (n = 81)		
Neonatal sepsis	8 (10%)		4 (5%)		<.01

Group I: controls; Group II: betametasone; Group III: ampicillin; Group IV: ampicillin and betamethasone.
(Adapted from Morales WJ, Angel JL, O'Brien WF, Knuppel RA. Use of ampicillin and corticosteroids in premature rupture of the membranes: a randomized study. Obstet Gynecol 1989;73:721.)

TABLE 88–26. ANTIBIOTICS AND OUTCOME IN PATIENTS WITH PRETERM PROM

	PLACEBO (n = 45)	ANTIBIOTICS (n = 40)	*p* VALUE
Clinical chorioamnionitis	16 (35%)	3 (7%)	<.01
Histopathologic chorioamnionitis	19 (42%)	12 (30%)	NS
Clinical neonatal sepsis	11 (24%)	3 (7%)	<.05
Positive neonatal blood cultures	2 (4%)	0	NS
Neonatal:			
Intraventricular hemorrhage	14 (31%)	5 (12%)	<.05
Necrotizing enterocolitis	3 (7%)	2 (5%)	NS
Hospital stay > 30 days	17 (38%)	7 (18%)	<.05

(Adapted from Johnston MM, Sanchez-Ramos L, Vaughn AJ, et al. Antibiotic therapy in preterm premature rupture of membranes: a randomized, prospective, double-blind trial. Am J Obstet Gynecol 1990;163:743.)

by immediate delivery. This view has been extended to the management of microbial invasion of the amniotic cavity.[92] There is evidence that both of these conditions can be treated in utero without interruption of pregnancy. Ogita and colleagues first reported the successful treatment of established chorioamnionitis with antibiotic treatment via a transcervical catheter.[170] Subsequently, we reported that giving antibiotics to a mother with preterm PROM at 29 weeks and an amniotic fluid culture positive for *Bacteroides bivious, Veillonella parvula,* and *Peptococcus* without clinical signs of chorioamnionitis resulted in eradication of the microbial invasion of the amniotic cavity.[171] In a second case, we were successful at eradicating *Ureaplasma urealyticum* from the amniotic cavity with antibiotic treatment.[172]

These observations demonstrate that antibiotic treatment may alter the progression of microbial invasion of the amniotic cavity. Further studies are required to determine optimal patient selection, prognostic factors, and maternal and neonatal risks associated with this novel therapeutic approach.

Steroid Administration

The use of steroids in patients with preterm PROM is an issue of clinical relevance because RDS is the major cause of neonatal morbidity and mortality. This issue has been examined in both randomized and nonrandomized clinical trials. When considered individually, most studies have failed to demonstrate a significant reduction in the incidence of RDS with steroid administration. Recently, however, meta-analysis of randomized trials has been conducted, and two out of three meta-analyses have shown that steroid administration results in a significant reduction in the incidence of RDS.

Ohlsson's meta-analysis included only five randomized clinical trials and demonstrated a reduction in the incidence of RDS (relative risk 0.63, 95% CI: 0.5–0.81, $p < .01$).[173] He noted, however, that the results of this meta-analysis were heavily influenced by the largest trial, which was rated poorest in terms of methodological quality and had an inexplicably high incidence of RDS in the control group. Repeated analysis of the remaining four trials failed to demonstrate significant reduction in the prevalence of RDS. Steroid treatment was associated with a modest yet significant increase in the risk of puerperal endometritis (relative risk 2.42, 95% CI: 1.38–4.24) but no significant increase in neonatal sepsis.

The other two meta-analyses included a larger number of trials and concluded that steroid treatment reduces the incidence of RDS (odds ratio 0.55, 95% CI:

TABLE 88–27. EFFECT OF ANTIBIOTIC ON THE INCIDENCE OF CHORIOAMNIONITIS IN PRETERM PROM

STUDY	PLACEBO	ANTIBIOTIC	ODDS RATIO (95% CL)	GRAPH OF ODDS RATIOS AND CONFIDENCE INTERVALS (0.01 / .1 / 1 / 10 / 100)
Amon et al. (1988)[167]	10% (4/39)	16% (7/43)	0.66 (0.21–2.12)	
Morales et al. (1989)[169]	26% (22/84)	4% (3/81)	5.81 (1.80–18.76)	
Johnston et al. (1990)[168]	36% (16/45)	7.5% (3/40)	3.76 (1.17–12.1)	
Typical odds ratio			2.42 (1.23–4.74)	

TABLE 88-28. EFFECT OF ANTIBIOTIC ON THE INCIDENCE OF NEONATAL SEPSIS IN PRETERM PROM

STUDY	PLACEBO	ANTIBIOTIC	ODDS RATIO ANTIBIOTIC/PLACEBO (95% CL)	GRAPH OF ODDS RATIOS AND CONFIDENCE INTERVALS 0.01 .1 1 10
Amon et al. (1988)[167]	16.7% (6/36)	2.4% (1/42)	0.12 (0.02–1.12)	
Morales et al. (1989)[169]	9.5% (8/84)	4.9% (4/81)	0.49 (0.12–1.91)	
Johnston et al. (1990)[168]	4.4% (2/45)	0.0% (0/40)	0.15 (0.01–2.41)	
Typical odds ratio			0.32 (0.13–0.77)	

0.4–0.75; and 0.70, 95% CI: 0.61–0.81).[174,175] Although Ohlsson accepted only trials that provided enough information to assess the risk of maternal and neonatal infection and RDS, the other two meta-analyses accepted all studies in which the incidence of neonatal RDS was reported, even if insufficient information on neonatal and maternal infectious complications was provided.

In summary, the available evidence supports the use of steroids in the setting of PROM. The modest increased risk of puerperal infection can be easily managed with modern antibiotic therapy. However, neonates should be closely followed for laboratory and clinical signs of infection.

Amniocentesis

Garite and coworkers were the first to propose the use of amniocentesis in the evaluation of the microbiological state of the amniotic cavity and of fetal lung maturity in the patient with preterm PROM.[176] Subsequently, several investigators have reported studies in which amniocentesis has been used in the management of PROM. The relevant issues are the success rate of fluid retrieval, the value of the information obtained, and the risks associated with the procedure.

Table 88-29 gives the success rate of amniotic fluid retrieval by transabdominal amniocentesis in the published reports.[92–98] Retrieval rates vary from 49% to 96% in published series. The wide disparity in retrieval rates is probably attributable to differences in policy regarding patient selection in different institutions. For example, although Garite and associates excluded all patients with anterior placentas and oligohydramnios, subsequent studies have not considered these conditions as contraindications for amniocentesis. As experience with ultrasound and invasive techniques of prenatal diagnosis grows, the success rate of amniotic fluid retrieval in patients with PROM is likely to increase.

Only one small randomized clinical trial has examined the value of amniocentesis in the setting of preterm PROM.[178] Forty-seven patients (26 to 34 weeks and with an accessible amniotic fluid pocket) were randomized to amniocentesis or no amniocentesis. Indications for induction of labor included positive Gram stain of amniotic fluid or mature fetal lungs, as determined by an L/S ratio above 2.0 or positive phosphatidylglycerol. Neonates born to women who had amniocenteses had a lower incidence of fetal distress during labor (as judged by fetal heart rate tracing) and a shorter hospital stay than those born to women randomized not to have amniocenteses (fetal distress: 4% [1/24] versus 32% [7/22], $p < .05$; hospital stay: median 8.5 days versus 22 days, $p < .01$). No difference in the rate of neonatal sepsis, maternal chorioamnionitis, or endometritis was noted between the two groups. This study had very limited power to detect differences in neonatal morbidity. For example, although the rate of neonatal

TABLE 88-29. AMNIOCENTESIS IN PRETERM PROM: SUCCESS RATE

STUDY	NO. PATIENTS	AMNIOCENTESIS SUCCESS RATE (%)
Garite and Freeman (1982)[92]	207	49
Cotton et al. (1984)[93]	61	69
Broekhuizen et al. (1985)[94]	79	66
Vintzileos et al. (1986)[95]	54	Not given
Feinstein et al. (1986)[96]	73	68
Romero et al. (1988)	90	95
Romero et al. (1988)[98]	221	96
Total	844	71%

sepsis was threefold higher in the control group, the difference was not statistically significant (14% [3/22] versus 4% [1/22]). With the sample size of this study, a difference in the rate of sepsis between the two groups must be at least 22% for this study to have an 80% power to detect it. Thus, these data are insufficient to determine whether amniocentesis is beneficial in the management of PROM.

Major problems exist in evaluating the usefulness of amniocentesis in preterm PROM. Although a major indication for the procedure is the detection of microbial invasion of the amniotic cavity, the optimal laboratory method for detecting microorganisms in the amniotic fluid has not been determined. For example, the Gram stain has a sensitivity of only 50%.[97] Although amniotic fluid cultures are considered the "gold standard," they take several days to yield results. Therefore, rapid, sensitive, and simple tests must be developed to detect microbial invasion of the amniotic cavity. Another major problem is the accurate diagnosis of neonatal sepsis, one of the major endpoints in any management strategy directed toward decreasing the incidence of infectious morbidity and mortality.

Amniocentesis is an invasive procedure that poses risks to both mother and fetus, but there is a paucity of information regarding those risks. The available publications reporting the use of amniocentesis in PROM have not called attention to fetal and maternal complications. Yeast and colleagues specifically addressed this issue in 91 patients in whom amniocenteses were performed in the setting of PROM.[177] A retrospective review of the neonatal record uncovered no evidence of fetal trauma in any case. A hematoma of the broad ligament was noted in one patient who had a cesarean section for an unrelated indication. This study also found that the incidence of spontaneous labor in patients who underwent amniocentesis was no different from that of patients who did not undergo amniocentesis secondary to oligohydramnios or an anterior placenta (Fig. 88-8). Although the authors concluded that their study failed to show that amniocentesis might induce labor, the retrospective nature of the study limits the strength of this conclusion. Patients with severe oligohydramnios have a higher likelihood of infection and a shorter admission-to-spontaneous-labor interval than patients without oligohydramnios.

Although there is a lack of evidence for fetal and maternal complications secondary to amniocentesis in the setting of PROM, amniocentesis is an invasive procedure and risks do exist. We have performed an unintentional cordocentesis in a patient with PROM. Although this has not been associated with any demonstrable risk thus far, the possibility for fetal injury is real.

Assessing Pulmonic Maturity

Lung maturity can be assessed from the amniotic fluid obtained by amniocentesis or from the vaginal pool. The latter has the advantage of being less invasive and is feasible in patients with oligohydramnios. Amniotic fluid from the vaginal pool can be collected in three ways: from the posterior vaginal fornix by sterile speculum examination; in a clean bedpan maintained under the patient; or by use of obstetric perineal pads left in place for 12 to 24 hours to ensure saturation.[179–182] The

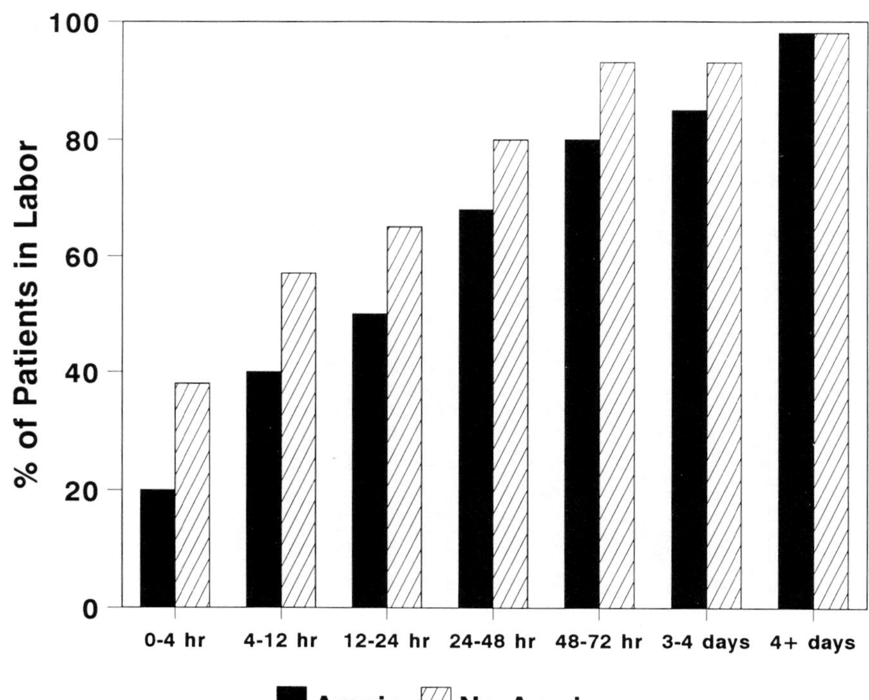

FIGURE 88–8. Cumulative distribution of time intervals from sonography until spontaneous labor. Solid bar, with amniocentesis; cross-hatched bar, without amniocentesis. (From Yeast JD, Garite TJ, Dorchester W. The risks of amniocentesis in the management of premature rupture of the membranes. Am J Obstet Gynecol 1984;149:506.)

success rate in obtaining fluid within 48 hours with these non-invasive techniques ranges from 54% to 100%.[181,182]

The reliability of lung maturity tests from amniotic fluid collected vaginally has been challenged.[183,184] This section will review the correlation between the L/S ratio and PG results in amniotic fluid obtained by amniocentesis and from the vaginal pool.

Shaver and associates compared the phospholipid profile of paired amniotic fluid samples in 28 patients with preterm PROM (26 and 35 weeks).[179] No significant difference in the concentrations of phosphatidylglycerol, phosphatidylinositol, phosphatidylethanolamine, and phosphatidylserine in amniotic fluid obtained by the two sampling methods was found. The L/S ratio was higher in fluid collected transvaginally than in fluid collected transabdominally, but this difference fell short of reaching statistical significance (Fig. 88-9). The only phospholipid clearly increased by vaginal contamination was lysolecithin.

Dombroski and colleagues reported a study in which amniotic fluid was obtained by amniocentesis in patients with labor at term.[185] Membranes were then ruptured, and a half-hour later a vaginal sample of amniotic fluid was collected. L/S ratios obtained from amniotic fluid in the vaginal pool samples were significantly lower than those obtained by amniocentesis; however, in 22% (6/27) of cases, L/S ratios were higher in the vaginal pool samples than in amniocentesis.

Three studies have reported neonatal outcome and L/S ratio results in preterm PROM (Table 88-30).[181,182,186] In two of the studies a mature L/S ratio was indication for delivery.[182,186] In the third study, PG presence was used as indication for delivery.[181] The data are quite consistent: with a mature L/S ratio, the risk of RDS is extraordinarily small. An L/S ratio above 2 was found in 103 patients, and none of the neonates developed RDS.

Several studies have examined the value of PG determinations in amniotic fluid obtained transvaginally. Stedman and colleagues reported that of 25 patients with PROM between 26 and 34 weeks, 60% (15/25) had positive PG and none of their neonates developed RDS (within 72 hours of the test).[180] Among the newborns of the 10 patients with negative PG, four developed RDS. Similarly, Brame and MacKenna reported no cases of neonatal RDS in 36 patients with PG present in vaginal fluid.[181] Table 88-31 shows the frequency of the presence of PG in fluid obtained from the vaginal pool according to gestational age. Twelve percent of patients with gestational ages below 32 weeks had PG present.[181]

Recently, the possibility that bacterial contamination from vaginal secretions may lead to false-positive PG results has been raised by Schumacher and associates, who reported that one patient had PG detected in the fluid from the vaginal pool but not in fluid retrieved by transabdominal amniocentesis.[184] The neonate developed respiratory insufficiency that was attributed to either RDS or pneumonia (the amniotic fluid culture was positive for bacteria). These investigators also demonstrated that bacteria may be a source of PG. Therefore, it is possible that excessive bacterial contamination may alter results of PG determinations. It would seem prudent to minimize the interval between sample collection and assay in the hope of preventing bacterial growth in the sample.

In addition to these clinical studies, data generated from experimental observations provide further support for the lack of effect of vaginal contamination on the L/S ratio results. Sbarra and colleagues demonstrated that cervical and vaginal washings are generally devoid of lecithin and sphingomyelin (in 9 out of 10 cases), and thus these secretions are unlikely to alter L/S results.[187] Two studies determined that introduction of amniotic fluid (obtained by transabdominal amniocentesis) into the vagina results in little change in the

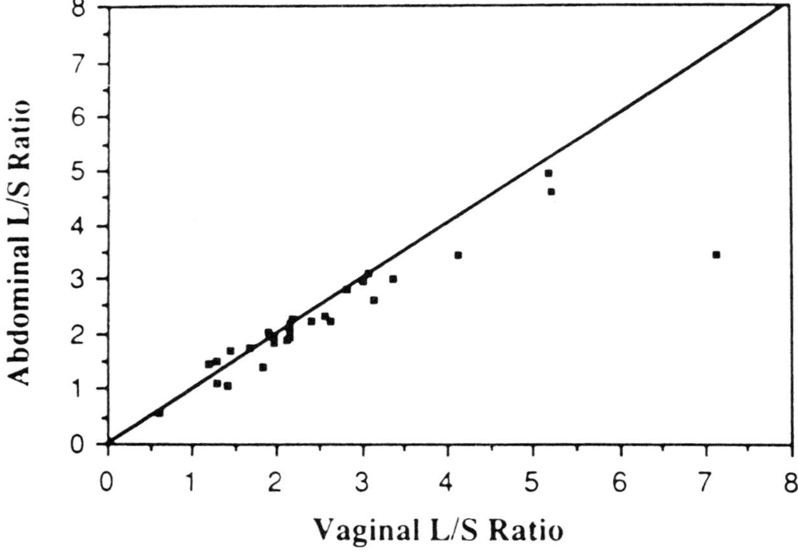

FIGURE 88–9. Scatterplot showing the relationship between lecithin/sphingomyelin (L/S) ratios of vaginal and amniocentesis fluid. (From Shaver DC, Spinnato JA, Whybrew D, Williams WK, Anderson GD. Comparison of phospholipids in vaginal and amniocentesis specimens of patients with premature rupture of membranes. Am J Obstet Gynecol 1987; 156:456.)

TABLE 88–30. VAGINAL POOL L/S RATIO AND NEONATAL OUTCOME

STUDY	L/S RATIO	NEGATIVE RDS	POSITIVE RDS
Goldstein et al.	≥2	5	0
(1980)[186]	<2	0	3
Golde SH (1983)[182]	≥2	26	0
	<2	NA	NA
Brame and MacKenna	≥2	72	0
(1983)[181]	<2	36	19

NA, not available.

L/S ratio.[187,188] Regrettably, in most cases (21 of 23) amniotic fluids had L/S ratios above 2, and therefore the effect of vaginal contamination in immature L/S ratios was not adequately tested.

The available evidence indicates that fetal lung maturity studies can be performed on amniotic fluid obtained from the vagina and that a mature L/S ratio or the presence of PG is associated with a very low risk of RDS. Moreover, this noninvasive, low-risk approach allows for serial L/S and PG determinations.

Mature Phospholipid Studies

A mature phospholipid study has been demonstrated in about 50% of patients with preterm PROM with gestational ages below 34 weeks.[93,176,178] Garite and associates reported that none of the neonates with an L/S ratio of 1.8 or greater developed RDS.[176] The incidence of this complication in neonates with immature L/S was 33% (5/15).

What is the optimal management of patients with a mature phospholipid profile? Only one randomized clinical trial has been reported, in which 47 patients with preterm PROM (less than 36 weeks) and mature amniotic fluid indices were randomized to either prompt delivery (n = 26) or expectant management (n = 21).[189] A mature test was defined as an L/S ratio above 2 or an FSI of 47 or more (often from vaginal fluid). There were no differences in perinatal mortality between the two groups. There were no cases of RDS in the expectant management group, but two in the delivery group. One baby died from severe hyaline membrane disease (birth weight 900 g, vaginal FSI = 48), whereas the other infant survived (birth weight 1700 g, vaginal L/S = 2.0). There was no difference in the rate of neonatal sepsis or other neonatal complications in the two groups. However, the only two cases of intracranial hemorrhage (grade not stated) occurred in the delivery group. Maternal chorioamnionitis was more common in the expectantly managed group than in the delivery group (38% [8/21] versus 8% [2/26], $p < .02$). The predictive value of a mature test was 97%.

We interpret these data as indicating that there is no evidence that active intervention is beneficial to the neonate. The reduction in maternal chorioamnionitis, a complication that can be easily treated with antibiotics, may not justify intervention if this action results in even occasional serious neonatal complications (RDS severe enough to cause death and intracranial hemorrhage).

Amnioinfusion

Oligohydramnios is a risk factor for the development of severely abnormal fetal heart rate patterns during labor. Experiments conducted in the rhesus monkey indicate that loss of amniotic fluid is associated with the appearance of variable fetal heart rate decelerations that disappear after fluid volume is replaced.[190] A similar phenomenon has been observed in women with rupture of membranes. Moberg and coworkers reported that patients with preterm PROM had a higher incidence of cesarean section for fetal distress than patients with preterm labor and intact membranes (7.9% [21/267] versus 1.5% [2/130] respectively, $p < .05$).[191] Seventy-six percent of patients who underwent cesarean section for fetal distress in the PROM group had fetal heart rate patterns consistent with umbilical-cord compression. Regrettably, Apgar scores and umbilical cord pH data were not reported for these patients.

Miyazaki and Taylor were the first to report a clinical trial in which saline amnioinfusion was used in 42 patients in labor with 5 or more consecutive repetitive variable decelerations or prolonged decelerations (< 100 bpm for at least 3 minutes) that did not respond to changes in maternal position and oxygen therapy.[192] Amnioinfusion provided relief of repetitive variable decelerations in 67% (19/28) of cases and of prolonged decelerations in 85.7% (12/14).

TABLE 88–31. FREQUENCY OF POSITIVE PHOSPHATIDYL GLYCEROL IN VAGINAL POOL SAMPLES

GESTATIONAL AGE (WKS)	NO. OF PATIENTS	(%)
≤28	2/15	(13.3)
29–30	2/19	(10.5)
31–32	4/42	(9.5)
33–34	19/97	(19.6)
35–36	20/41	(48.7)
Total	47/214	(22.0)

(Modified from Brame RG, MacKenna J. Vaginal pool phospholipids in the management of premature rupture of membranes. Am J Obstet Gynecol 1983;145:992.)

Subsequently, Miyazaki and Nevarez compared amnioinfusion with standard management of variable decelerations in 96 patients.[193] Amnioinfusion was associated with a significant reduction in the severity and occurrence of variable decelerations and prolonged decelerations (amnioinfusion 51% versus noninfusion group 4.2%, $p < .01$). This effect was more dramatic in nulliparous patients. A significant reduction in the incidence of cesarean section for fetal distress was noted in nulliparous but not in multiparous patients.

Nageotte and associates compared prophylactic amnioinfusion versus no infusion in a randomized clinical trial of 61 women in labor.[194] Patients receiving amnioinfusion had a significantly lower incidence of severe decelerations during both the first and second stages of labor. The incidence of cesarean section for fetal distress was also lower in patients receiving amnioinfusion than in the control group (3% [1/29] versus 22% [7/32], $p = .06$). No umbilical cord pH data were reported. The prevalence of endometritis in the amnioinfusion group was not increased.

The available evidence indicates that prophylactic amnioinfusion during labor may reduce the prevalence of abnormal fetal heart patterns and therefore may decrease the need for fetal scalp sampling. Further studies are required to determine if this treatment decreases the prevalence of biochemically confirmed fetal distress and the cesarean section rate for this indication.

Managing the Patient with Cervical Cerclage

A key question in the management of a patient with cervical cerclage is whether the cerclage should be removed. Cerclage removal has been advocated to reduce the risk of infection-related complications.[195] Leaving the cerclage in place has been recommended to favor pregnancy prolongation. There is a paucity of data on which to base a rational decision.

Three studies have addressed this problem. Yeast and Garite reported the results of a case-control study in which the outcome of patients with a cervical cerclage removed after preterm PROM was compared to that of patients with PROM of a similar gestational age.[196] There was no difference in the incidence of chorioamnionitis or other infectious complications and neonatal outcome between the two groups. The interval between PROM and delivery was not significantly different between patients with and without cerclage. Similar findings were reported by Blickstein and associates after comparing the outcome of 32 patients with cerclage and 76 without it.[197] In contrast, Goldman and colleagues compared the outcome of 46 patients with preterm PROM in whom the cerclage was not removed with that of 46 women with preterm PROM without cerclage.[198] Patients with a cerclage had a significantly shorter PROM-to-delivery interval and lower gestational age at delivery than patients without the cerclage. However, the rate of chorioamnionitis, other infection-related complications, and neonatal outcome was not different between the two groups.

Managing the Patient with Herpes Simplex Genitalis

Preterm PROM complicated by a maternal genital herpes is a clinical dilemma: the risk of prematurity must be balanced against the risk of potential intrauterine herpes exposure of the neonate. At the time of this writing, this issue has been examined in one study. Major and associates reported the outcome of 18 patients managed expectantly with preterm PROM between 24 and 32 weeks and recurrent genital herpes.[199] None of the babies had any clinical or laboratory evidence of neonatal herpes. Six patients received antenatal acyclovir. The results of this study would seem to justify expectant management in the patient with these complications.

SECOND-TRIMESTER PROM

Until recently, the management of patients with ruptured membranes before 26 weeks gestation often consisted of pregnancy termination. The high risk of maternal infection coupled with the low likelihood of neonatal survival was considered a justification for induction of labor.

Recent studies have provided data with which to counsel patients with this complication.[200–203] Table 88-32 summarizes the results of four studies that have examined the outcome of 310 patients with preterm PROM before 26 weeks. Two of the studies were prospective.[200,201] Because management protocols (ie, tocolysis, steroid administration) and inclusion criteria

TABLE 88–32. OUTCOME OF PROM IN THE SECOND TRIMESTER

STUDY	MEAN GA AT PROM	MORTALITY	CHORIO-AMNIONITIS	NEONATAL SEPSIS	NORMAL AT LONG-TERM FOLLOW-UP
Taylor and Garite[203]	22.6	13 SB, 31 ND/60	22/53	NA	6/9
Beydoun and Yasin[200]	24.1	15 SB, 19 ND/69	41/69	4/35	5/17
Moretti and Sibai[201]	23.1	17 SB, 67 ND/124	46/118	20/68	23/34
Bengston et al.[202]	23.2	9 SB, 16 ND/57	27/59	7/22	NA

SB, stillbirth (excluding congenital anomalies); ND, neonatal death.
NA, not available.

varied among the centers and even within the same institution, there are limitations to these data.

The overall survival rate in this collected series was 40% (123/310); among the deaths, 29% (54/187) occurred in utero and the remainder postnatally. The fetal death rate was 17% (54/310) and the survival rate of liveborn neonates was 48% (123/256). The causes of intrauterine fetal demise were not documented in these studies. Respiratory insufficiency and intraventricular hemorrhage were the most common neonatal complications.[200,201] Clinical neonatal sepsis was reported in 25% (31/125).

Limited data are available regarding the incidence of long-term sequelae. Three of the four studies have follow-up data in some newborns; the length of follow-up ranges from 3 months to 6 years.[200,201,203] Fifty-seven percent of infants were normal at follow-up. Long-term sequelae included chronic lung disease, developmental and neurologic abnormalities, hydrocephalus, and cerebral palsy.

Preterm delivery occurred in 57% (177/310) of patients within 1 week, 60% (185/310) within 2 weeks, and 79% (246/310) within 1 month after PROM. An inverse relationship between gestational age at rupture of membranes and interval to delivery was noted in two of the four studies.[202,203]

The main maternal complication associated with PROM before 26 weeks is chorioamnionitis, which occurred in 46% (136/299) in this collected series. No correlation between the duration of the latency period and the development of chorioamnionitis was noted. Antibiotics were effective in controlling the infection in most cases; however, three patients developed sepsis, one required a hysterectomy, and one died of septic shock. The incidence of retained placenta was 13% (16/122).[200,203]

Leakage of amniotic fluid after second-trimester amniocentesis should be considered separately. It occurs with an incidence of 1.2% and is usually transient in nature.[204] The risk of delayed PROM in these cases is no different than in the general population.[205]

PULMONARY HYPOPLASIA

The frequency of pulmonary hypoplasia is related to the gestational age at the time of membrane rupture. The development of pulmonary hypoplasia is associated with an increased risk of neonatal death and other complications such as pneumothorax and persistent pulmonary hypertension.

One study has used logistic regression analysis to determine the risk factors for the development of pulmonary hypoplasia.[206] Rotschild and colleagues studied 88 neonates born to mothers with PROM occurring before 28 weeks and with a latency period of at least 1 week (Table 88-33). The overall prevalence of pulmonary hypoplasia was 16% (14/88). Gestational age at the time of PROM, but not the duration of the latency period or the severity of oligohydramnios, was associated with pulmonary hypoplasia. It is apparent that the risk of pulmonary hypoplasia when PROM occurs at 19 weeks is 50%, whereas it is only 10% if the membranes rupture at 25 weeks (Fig. 88-10). Other clinical studies confirmed the importance of gestational age at the time of membrane rupture for the subsequent risk of development of pulmonary hypoplasia.[201,207–209] This view is supported by experimental studies in the guinea pig in which the effects of drainage of the amniotic cavity during the canalicular stage of lung development were more pronounced than those of drainage during the terminal sac stage.[210]

Less clear is the role of duration of rupture of membranes in the development of pulmonary hypoplasia. Univariate analysis demonstrated an association between the duration of rupture of membranes and the occurrence of pulmonary hypoplasia.[208,209,211] However, there is an inverse relationship between the duration of the latency period and the gestational age at rupture of membranes. The only study in which multivariate analysis was used to determine the contribution of gestational age at the time and duration of PROM in the occurrence of pulmonary hypoplasia reported no significant effect of the duration of PROM.[208] However, more clinical data are required to settle this issue. Studies of experimental oligohydramnios in the guinea pig suggest that the duration of PROM plays a role in the genesis of pulmonary hypoplasia, although the magnitude of this effect is smaller than the time of rupture.[210]

The mechanisms responsible for pulmonary hypoplasia in PROM are poorly understood. Experimental evidence suggests that oligohydramnios caused by drainage of the amniotic cavity leads to pulmonary hypoplasia. Traditionally, oligohydramnios has been thought to lead to extrinsic compression of the fetal thorax, impairing lung growth. An alternative view is

TABLE 88–33. ROLE OF PULMONARY HYPOPLASIA IN NEONATAL MORTALITY AND MORBIDITY

	PULMONARY HYPOPLASIA	NO PULMONARY HYPOPLASIA	ODDS RATIO HYPOPLASIA/ NO HYPOPLASIA	95% CL	*p* VALUE*
Neonatal death	71% (10/14)	11% (8/74)	20.6	4.5–105	<.001
Pneumothorax	64% (9/14)	15% (11/74)	10.3	2.5–44.8	<.001
Persistant pulmonary hypertension	43% (6/14)	11% (8/74)	6.2	1.4–27.2	<.01

* By Fisher's Exact Test.
(Adapted from Rotschild A et al. Am J Obstet Gynecol 1990;162:46.)

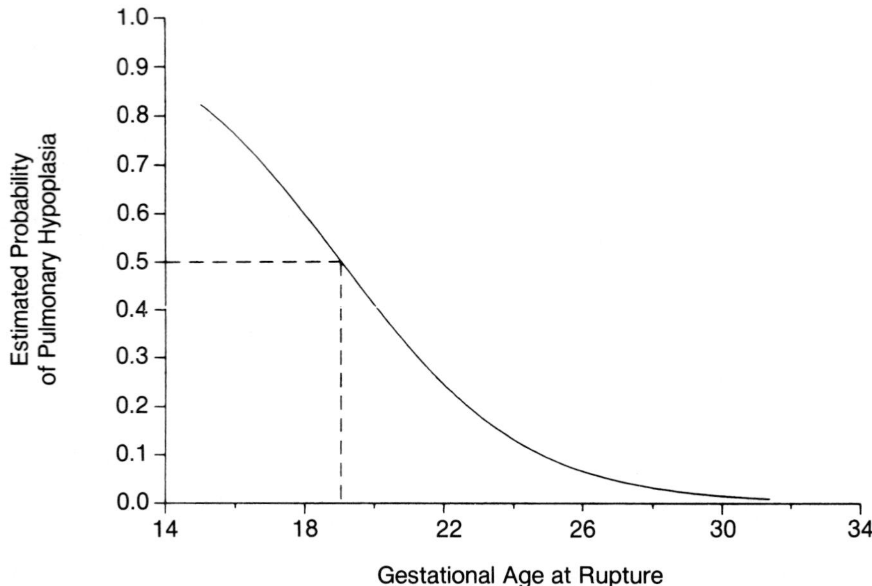

FIGURE 88–10. Curve relating probability of pulmonary hypoplasia to gestational age at ROM derived from estimated logistic equation: Probability of pulmonary hypoplasia = $1/[1 + e^{-7.27+0.38GAR}]$. (From Rotschild A, Ling EW, Puterman ML, Farquharson D. Neonatal outcome after prolonged preterm rupture of the membranes. Am J Obstet Gynecol 1990;162:49.)

that oligohydramnios reduces lung fluid volume, and this in turn is responsible for pulmonary hypoplasia. PROM reduces intra-amniotic pressure and increases the alveolar-to-amniotic-fluid pressure gradient. This favors the loss of lung fluid to the amniotic cavity and may lead to pulmonary hypoplasia. Experimental and clinical evidence supporting the importance of lung fluid in the pathogenesis of pulmonary hypoplasia includes the following:

1. Chronic tracheal drainage causes pulmonary hypoplasia in fetal sheep.[212–214]
2. Laryngeal atresia associated with renal agenesis (Fraser syndrome) results in normal pulmonary development despite severe oligohydramnios.[215]
3. Oligohydramnios is often associated with decreased intra-amniotic fluid pressure.[216]

Several sonographic parameters have been used to predict pulmonary hypoplasia in the patient with PROM, including fetal thoracic dimensions, fetal lung length, presence or absence of fetal breathing movements, and severity of oligohydramnios. A limitation of most of these studies is that they included patients with fetal pathology other than PROM. Nimrod and associates examined the value of chest circumference in the prediction of pulmonary hypoplasia in 45 patients (37 had PROM, 2 pleural effusions, and 6 renal disease).[217,218] A chest circumference below the 5th percentile for gestational age had a sensitivity of 88%, specificity of 96%, positive predictive value of 94%, and negative predictive value of 93% in a population with a 42% (18/43) prevalence of pulmonary hypoplasia (cases of pleural effusion were excluded). Vintzileos and colleagues and Songster and associates have developed nomograms for the chest circumference.[219,220] The value of these nomograms was tested in only four and eight patients with preterm PROM, respectively.

Roberts and coworkers have reported a nomogram for the fetal lung length and have used this parameter in the prediction of pulmonary hypoplasia in 20 cases with preterm PROM between 18 and 24 weeks gestation.[221] The prevalence of pulmonary hypoplasia was 60% (12/20). Eleven of the twelve fetuses with pulmonary hypoplasia had fetal lung length measurements 2 SD below the mean for gestational age.

Fetal breathing movements are considered important for normal lung development; indeed, transecting the spinal cord or the phrenic nerves will eliminate fetal breathing movements and impair lung growth and development in animal models. On the other hand, there is controversy regarding the pathogenic importance of inhibition of normal fetal breathing in the development of pulmonary hypoplasia in the context of preterm PROM. Although Blott and colleagues have reported absent fetal breathing in fetuses that subsequently died with pulmonary hypoplasia,[222] Moessinger and associates found no difference between fetuses with and without pulmonary hypoplasia in the time spent breathing.[223]

REFERENCES

1. Keirse MJNC, Ohlsson A, Treffers PE, Kanhai HHH. Prelabour rupture of the membranes preterm. In: Chalmers I, Enkin M, Keirse MJNC, eds. Effective care in pregnancy and childbirth. Vol. 4: Pregnancy, Parts I–V. Oxford: Oxford University Press, 1989:666.
2. Hauth JC, Cunningham FG, Whalley PJ. Early labor initiation with oral PGE_2 after premature rupture of the membranes at term. Obstet Gynecol 1977;49:523.
3. Johnson JW, Daikoku NH, Niebyl JR, Johnson TRB, Khouzami VA, Witter RF. Premature rupture of the membranes and prolonged pregnancy. Obstet Gynecol 1981;57:547.
4. Lange AP, Secher NJ, Nielsen FH, Pedersen GT. Stimulation of

labor in cases of premature rupture of the membranes at or near term: a consecutive randomized study of prostaglandin E_2-tablets and intravenous oxytocin. Acta Obstet Gynecol Scand 1981;60:207.

5. Lebherz TB, Hellman LP, Madding R, Anctil A, Arje SL. Double-blind study of premature rupture of the membranes. Am J Obstet Gynecol 1963;87:218.
6. Magos AL, Noble MC, Wong-Ten-Yuen A, Rodeck CH. Controlled study comparing vaginal prostaglandin E_2 pessaries with intravenous oxytocin for the stimulation of labour after spontaneous rupture of the membranes. Br J Obstet Gynaecol 1983;90:726.
7. Tamsen L, Lyrenas S, Cnattingius S. Premature rupture of the membranes: intervention or not. Gynecol Obstet Invest 1990;29:128.
8. Van der Walt D, Venter PF. Management of term pregnancy with premature rupture of the membranes and unfavourable cervix. S Afr Med J 1989;75:54.
9. Westergaard JG, Lange AP, Pedersen GT, Secher NJ. Use of oral oxytocics for stimulation of labor in cases of premature rupture of the membranes at term: a randomized comparative study of prostaglandin E_2 tablets and demoxytocin resoriblets. Acta Obstet Gynecol Scand 1983;62:111.
10. Knudsen FU, Steinrud J. Septicaemia of the newborn, associated with ruptured foetal membranes, discoloured amniotic fluid or maternal fever. Acta Paediatr Scand 1976;65:725.
11. Verber IG, Pearce JM, New LC, Hamilton PA, Davies EG. Prolonged rupture of the fetal membranes and neonatal outcome. J Perinat Med 1989;17:469.
12. Gunn CS, Mishell DR, Morton DG. Premature rupture of the fetal membranes. Am J Obstet Gynecol 1970;106:469.
13. Sachs M, Baker TH. Spontaneous premature rupture of the membranes. Am J Obstet Gynecol 1967;97:888.
14. Daikoku NH, Kaltreider DF, Khouzami VA, Spence M, Johnson JWC. Premature rupture of membranes and spontaneous labor: maternal endometritis risks. Obstet Gynecol 1982;59:13.
15. Christensen KK, Christensen P, Ingemarsson I, et al. A study in complications in preterm deliveries after prolonged premature rupture of the membranes. Obstet Gynecol 1976;48:670.
16. Fayez JA, Hasan AA, Jonas HS, Miller GL. Management of premature rupture of the membranes. Obstet Gynecol 1978;52:17.
17. Gibbs RS. Premature rupture of the membranes. Obstet Gynecol 1982;60:671.
18. Russell KP, Anderson GV. Aggressive management of ruptured membranes. Am J Obstet Gynecol 1962;83:930.
19. Schwarcz R, Belizan JM, Nieto F, Tenzer SM, Rios AM. Third progress report on the Latin American collaborative study on the effects of late rupture of membranes on labor and the neonate, submitted to the Director of the Pan-American Health Organization (PAHO/WHO) and the participating groups. Montevideo: Latin American Center of Perinatology and Human Development, 1974.
20. Bourne GL. The microscopic anatomy of the human amnion and chorion. Am J Obstet Gynecol 1960;79:1070.
21. Hoyes AD. Ultrastructure of the mesenchymal layers of the human amnion in early pregnancy. Am J Obstet Gynecol 1970;106:557.
22. Wang T, Schneider J. Fine structure of human chorionic membrane: ultrastructural and histochemical examinations. Arch Gynecol Obstet 1983;233:187.
23. Bou-Resli MN, Al-Zaid NS, Ibrahim MEA. Full-term and prematurely ruptured fetal membranes: an ultrastructural study. Cell Tissue Res 1981;220:263.
24. Ibrahim MEA, Bou-Resli MN, Al-Zaid NS, Bishay LF. Intact fetal membranes: morphological predisposal to rupture. Acta Obstet Gynecol Scand 1983;62:481.
25. Knox IC, Hoerner JK. The role of infection in premature rupture of the membranes. Am J Obstet Gynecol 1950;59:190.
26. Naeye RL, Peters EC. Causes and consequences of premature rupture of fetal membranes. Lancet 1980;1:192.
27. Poppel J. Ueber die Resistenz der Eihaute, ein Beitrag zur Mechanik der Geburt. Monatsschr Geburtsk 1863;22:1.
28. Duncan JM. On a lower limit to the power exerted in the function of parturition. Proc R Soc Edin 1869;6:163.
29. Al-Zaid NS, Bou-Resli MN, Goldspink G. Bursting pressure and collagen content of fetal membranes and their relation to premature rupture of the membranes. Br J Obstet Gynaecol 1980;87:227.
30. Artal R, Sokol RJ, Neuman M, Burstein AH, Stojkov J. The mechanical properties of prematurely and non-prematurely ruptured membranes. Am J Obstet Gynecol 1976;125:655.
31. Danforth DN, McElin TW, States MN. Studies on fetal membranes. I. Bursting tension. Am J Obstet Gynecol 1953;65:480.
32. MacLachlan TB. A method for the investigation of the strength of the fetal membranes. Am J Obstet Gynecol 1965;91:309.
33. Meudt R, Meudt E. Rupture of the fetal membranes: an experimental, clinical, and histologic study. Am J Obstet Gynecol 1967;99:562.
34. Polishuk WZ, Kohane S, Hadar A. Fetal weight and membrane tensile strength. Am J Obstet Gynecol 1964;88:247.
35. Parry-Jones E, Priya S. A study of the elasticity and tension of fetal membranes and of the relation of the area of the gestational sac to the area of the uterine cavity. Br J Obstet Gynaecol 1976;83:205.
36. Lavery JP, Miller CE. The viscoelastic nature of chorioamniotic membranes. Obstet Gynecol 1977;50:467.
37. Lavery JP, Miller CE. Deformation and creep in the human chorioamniotic sac. Am J Obstet Gynecol 1979;134:366.
38. Skinner SJM, Campos GA, Liggins GC. Collagen content of human amniotic membranes: effect of gestation length and premature rupture. Obstet Gynecol 1981;57:487.
39. Kanayama N, Terao T, Kawashima Y, Horiuchi K, Fujimoto D. Collagen types in normal and prematurely ruptured amniotic membranes. Am J Obstet Gynecol 1985;153:899.
40. Evaldson GR, Larsson B, Jiborn H. Is the collagen content reduced when the fetal membranes rupture? A clinical study of term and prematurely ruptured membranes. Gynecol Obstet Invest 1987;24:92.
41. Vadillo-Ortega F, Gonzalez-Avila G, Karchmer S, Cruz NM, Ayala-Ruiz A, Selman-Lama M. Collagen metabolism in premature rupture of amniotic membranes. Obstet Gynecol 1990;75:84.
42. Artal R, Burgeson RE, Hobel CJ, Hollister D. An in vitro model for the study of enzymatically mediated biochemical changes in the chorioamniotic membranes. Am J Obstet Gynecol 1979;133:656.
43. Kanayama N, Kamijo H, Terao T, Horiuchi K, Fujimoto D. The relationship between trypsin activity in amniotic fluid and premature rupture of membranes. Am J Obstet Gynecol 1986;155:1043.
44. O'Brien WF, Knuppel RA, Morales WJ, Angel JL, Torres CT. Amniotic fluid alpha-$_1$-antitrypsin concentration in premature rupture of the membranes. Am J Obstet Gynecol 1990;162:756.
45. Burgos H, Hsi B-L, Yeh C-JG, Faulk WP. Plasminogen binding by human amniochorion: a possible factor in premature rupture of membranes. Am J Obstet Gynecol 1982;143:958.
46. Jenkins DM, O'Neill M, Mattar M, France VM, Hsi B-L, Faulk WP. Degenerative changes and detection of plasminogen in fetal membranes that rupture prematurely. Br J Obstet Gynaecol 1983;90:841.
47. Milwidsky A, Hurwitz A, Eckstein L, Mayer M, Gutman A. Proteolytic enzymes in human fetal membranes and amniotic fluid:

a comparison of normal and premature ruptured membranes. Enzyme 1985;33:188.

48. McGregor JA, Lawellin D, Franco-Buff A, Todd JK, Makowski EL. Protease production by microorganisms associated with reproductive tract infection. Am J Obstet Gynecol 1986;154:109.
49. McGregor JA, French JI, Lawellin D, Franco-Buff A, Smith C, Todd JK. Bacterial protease-induced reduction of chorioamniotic membrane strength and elasticity. Obstet Gynecol 1987;69:167.
50. Sbarra AJ, Selvaraj RJ, Cetrulo CL, Feingold M, Newton E, Thomas GB. Infection and phagocytosis as possible mechanisms of rupture in premature rupture of the membranes. Am J Obstet Gynecol 1985;153:38.
51. Schoonmaker JN, Lawellin DW, Lunt B, McGregor JA. Bacteria and inflammatory cells reduce chorioamniotic membrane integrity and tensile strength. Obstet Gynecol 1989;74:590.
52. Sbarra AJ, Thomas GB, Cetrulo CL, Shakr C, Chaudhury A, Paul B. Effect of bacterial growth on the bursting pressure of fetal membranes in vitro. Obstet Gynecol 1987;70:107.
53. McGregor JA, Schoonmaker JN, Lunt BD, Lawellin DW. Antibiotic inhibition of bacterially induced fetal membrane weakening. Obstet Gynecol 1990;76:124.
54. Casey ML, Cox SM, Beutler B, Milewich L, MacDonald PC. Cachectin/tumor necrosis factor-alpha formation in human decidua: potential role of cytokines in infection-induced preterm labor. J Clin Invest 1989;83:430.
55. Dayer J-M, Beutler B, Cerami A. Brief definitive report: cachectin/tumor necrosis factor stimulates collagenase and prostaglandin E_2 production by human synovial cells and dermal fibroblasts. J Exp Med 1985;162:2163.
56. Katsura M, Ito A, Hirakawa S, Mori Y. Human recombinant interleukin-1-alpha increases biosynthesis of collagenase and hyaluronic acid in cultured human chorionic cells. FEBS Lett 1989;244:315.
57. Romero R, Brody DT, Oyarzun E, et al. Infection and labor. III. Interleukin-1: a signal for the onset of parturition. Am J Obstet Gynecol 1989;160:1117.
58. Romero R, Durum S, Dinarello CA, Oyarzun E, Hobbins JC, Mitchell MD. Interleukin-1 stimulates prostaglandin biosynthesis by human amnion. Prostaglandins 1989;37:13.
59. Romero R, Manogue KR, Mitchell MD, et al. Infection and labor. IV. Cachectin/tumor necrosis factor in the amniotic fluid of women with intra-amniotic infection and preterm labor. Am J Obstet Gynecol 1989;161:336.
60. Skinner SJM, Liggins GC. Glycosaminoglycans and collagen in human amnion from pregnancies with and without premature rupture of the membranes. J Dev Physiol 1981;3:111.
61. Harger JH, Hsing AW, Tuomala RE, et al. Risk factors for preterm premature rupture of fetal membranes: a multicenter case-control study. Am J Obstet Gynecol 1990;163:130.
62. Naeye RL. Factors that predispose to premature rupture of the fetal membranes. Obstet Gynecol 1982;60:93.
63. Asrat T, Lewis DF, Garite TJ, et al. Frequency of recurrence of preterm premature rupture of membranes. SPO Abstract No. 469. Am J Obstet Gynecol 1991;164:374.
64. Eggers TR, Doyle LW, Pepperell RJ. Premature rupture of the membranes. Med J Aust 1979;1:209.
65. Townsend L, Aickin DR, Fraillon JMG. Spontaneous premature rupture of the membranes. Aust N Z J Obstet Gynaecol 1966;6:266.
66. Meyer MB, Tonascia JA. Maternal smoking, pregnancy complications, and perinatal mortality. Am J Obstet Gynecol 1977;128:494.
67. Evaldson G, Lagrelius A, Winiarski J. Premature rupture of the membranes. Acta Obstet Gynecol Scand 1980;59:385.
68. Mills JL, Harlap S, Harley EE. Should coitus late in pregnancy be discouraged? Lancet 1981;i:136.
69. Perkins RP. Sexual behavior and response in relation to complications of pregnancy. Am J Obstet Gynecol 1979;134:498.
70. Rayburn WF, Wilson EA. Coital activity and premature delivery. Am J Obstet Gynecol 1980;137:972.
71. Barabas AP. Ehlers-Danlos syndrome associated with prematurity and premature rupture of foetal membranes; possible increase in incidence. Br Med J 1966;2:682.
72. Wideman GL, Baird GH, Bolding OT. Ascorbic acid deficiency and premature rupture of fetal membranes. Am J Obstet Gynecol 1964;688:592.
73. Artal R, Burgeson R, Fernandez FJ, Hobel CJ. Fetal and maternal copper levels in patients at term with and without premature rupture of membranes. Obstet Gynecol 1979;53:608.
74. Kiilholma P, Gronroos M, Erkkola R, Pakarinen P, Nanto V. The role of calcium, copper, iron and zinc in preterm delivery and premature rupture of fetal membranes. Gynecol Obstet Invest 1984;17:194.
75. Sikorski R, Juszkiewicz T, Paszkowski T. Zinc status in women with premature rupture of membranes at term. Obstet Gynecol 1990;76:675.
76. Harlap S, Davies AM. Late sequelae of induced abortion: complications and outcome of pregnancy and labor. Am J Epidemiol 1975;102:217.
77. Lenihan JP. Relationship of antepartum pelvic examination to premature rupture of the membranes. Obstet Gynecol 1984;63:33.
78. Main DM, Gabbe SG, Richardson D, Strong S. Can preterm deliveries be prevented? Am J Obstet Gynecol 1985;151:892.
79. Main DM, Richardson DK, Hadley CB, Gabbe SG. Controlled trial of a preterm labor detection program: efficacy and costs. Obstet Gynecol 1989;74:873.
80. Ledger WJ. Premature rupture of membranes and maternal—fetal infection. Clin Obstet Gynecol 1979;22:329.
81. Regan JA, Chao S, James LS. Premature rupture of membranes, preterm delivery, and group B streptococcal colonization of mothers. Am J Obstet Gynecol 1981;141:184.
82. Bobitt JR, Damato JD, Sakakini J. Perinatal complications in group B streptococcal carriers: a longitudinal study of prenatal patients. Am J Obstet Gynecol 1985;151:711.
83. Matorras R, Perea AG, Usandizaga JA, Nieto A, Herruzo R. Group B streptococcus and premature rupture of membranes and preterm delivery. Gynec Obstet Invest 1989;27:14.
84. Alger LS, Lovchik JC, Hebel JR, Blackmon LR, Crenshaw MC. The association of *Chlamydia trachomatis, Neisseria gonorrhoeae*, and group B streptococci with preterm rupture of the membranes and pregnancy outcome. Am J Obstet Gynecol 1988;159:397.
85. Harrison HR, Alexander ER, Weinstein L, Lewis M, Nash M, Sim DA. Cervical *Chlamydia trachomatis* and mycoplasmal infections in pregnancy. JAMA 1983;250:1721.
86. Gravett MG, Nelson HP, DeRouen T, Critchlow C, Eschenbach DA, Holmes KK. Independent associations of bacterial vaginosis and *Chlamydia trachomatis* infection with adverse pregnancy outcome. JAMA 1986;256:1899.
87. Sweet RL, Landers DV, Walker C, Schacter J. *Chlamydia trachomatis* infection and pregnancy outcome. Am J Obstet Gynecol 1987;156:824.
88. Handsfield HH, Hodson WA, Holmes KK. Neonatal gonococcal infection: orogastric contamination with *Neisseria gonorrhoeae*. JAMA 1973;225:697.
89. Amstey MS, Steadman KT. Asymptomatic gonorrhea and pregnancy. J Am Ven Dis Assoc 1976;33:14.
90. Edwards LE, Barrada MI, Hamann AA, et al. Gonorrhea in pregnancy. Am J Obstet Gynecol 1978;132:637.

91. Minkoff H, Grunebaum AN, Schwarz RH, et al. Risk factors for prematurity and premature rupture of membranes: a prospective study of vaginal flora in pregnancy. Am J Obstet Gynecol 1984;150:965.
92. Garite TJ, Freeman RK. Chorioamnionitis in the preterm gestation. Obstet Gynecol 1982;59:539.
93. Cotton DB, Hill LM, Strassner HT, Platt LD, Ledger WJ. Use of amniocentesis in preterm gestation with ruptured membranes. Obstet Gynecol 1984;63:38.
94. Broekhuizen FF, Gilman M, Hamilton PR. Amniocentesis for Gram stain and culture in preterm premature rupture of the membranes. Obstet Gynecol 1985;66:316.
95. Vintzileos AM, Campbell WA, Nochimson DJ, Weinbaum PJ, Escoto DT, Mirochnik MH. Qualitative amniotic fluid volume versus amniocentesis in predicting infection in preterm premature rupture of the membranes. Obstet Gynecol 1986;67:579.
96. Feinstein SJ, Vintzileos AM, Lodeiro JG, Campbell WA, Weinbaum PJ, Nochimson DJ. Amniocentesis with premature rupture of membranes. Obstet Gynecol 1986;68:147.
97. Romero R, Emamian M, Quintero R, et al. The value and limitations of the Gram stain examination in the diagnosis of intraamniotic infection. Am J Obstet Gynecol 1988;159:114.
98. Romero R, Quintero R, Oyarzun E, et al. Intra-amniotic infection and the onset of labor in preterm rupture of the membranes. Am J Obstet Gynecol 1988;159:661.
99. Romero R, Mazor M, Avila C, et al. Prevalence, microbiology, and clinical significance of microbial invasion of the cavity in term premature rupture of membranes. SPO Abstract 213. Am J Obstet Gynecol 1991;164:305.
100. Ablow RC, Driscoll SG, Effman EL, et al. A comparison of early-onset group B streptococcal neonatal infection and the respiratory distress syndrome of the newborn. New Engl J Med 1976;249:65.
101. Jacobs J, Edwards D, Gluck L. Early-onset sepsis and pneumonia observed as respiratory distress syndrome. Am J Dis Child 1980;134:766.
102. Modanlou HD, Bosu SK, Weller MH. Early-onset group B streptococcus neonatal septicemia and respiratory distress syndrome: characteristic features of assisted ventilation in the first 24 hours of life. Crit Care Med 1980;8:716.
103. Pankuch GA, Appelbaum PC, Lorenz RP, et al. Placental microbiology and histology and the pathogenesis of chorioamnionitis. Obstet Gynecol 1984;64:802.
104. Romero R, Salafia C, Mazor M, et al. The microbiologic significance of pathologic placental chorioamnionitis. Abstract presented at the Eighth Annual Meeting of the Society of Perinatal Obstetricians, Las Vegas, Nevada, 1988.
105. Nelson DM, Stempel LE, Zuspan FP. Association of prolonged, preterm premature rupture of the membranes and abruptio placentae. J Reprod Med 1986;31:429.
106. Vintzileos AM, Campbell WA, Nochimson DJ, Weinbaum PJ. Preterm premature rupture of the membranes: a risk factor for the development of abruptio placentae. Am J Obstet Gynecol 1987;156:1235.
107. Gonen R, Hannah ME, Milligan JE. Does prolonged preterm premature rupture of the membranes predispose to abruptio placentae? Obstet Gynecol 1989;74:347.
108. Major CA, Nageotte MP, Lewis DF, Asrat T, Harding JA, Garite TJ. Preterm premature rupture of membranes and placental abruption: is there an association between these pregnancy complications? SPO Abstract 496. Am J Obstet Gynecol 1991;164:381.
109. Darby MJ, Caritis SN, Shen-Schwarz S. Placental abruption in the preterm gestation: an association with chorioamnionitis. Obstet Gynecol 1989;74:88.
110. Naeye RL. Coitus and antepartum haemorrhage. Br J Obstet Gynaecol 1981;88:765.
111. Friedman ML, McElin TW. Diagnosis of ruptured fetal membranes: clinical study and review of literature. Am J Obstet Gynecol 1969;104:544.
112. Lodeiro JG, Hsieh KA, Byers JH, Feinstein SJ. The fingerprint, a false-positive fern test. Obstet Gynecol 1989;73:873.
113. McGregor JA, Johnson S. "Fig-leaf" ferning and positive nitrazine testing: semen as a cause of misdiagnosis of premature rupture of membranes (letter to the editor). Am J Obstet Gynecol 1985;151:1142.
114. Brookes C, Shand K, Jones WR. A reevaluation of the ferning test to detect ruptured membranes. Aust N Z J Obstet Gynaecol 1986;26:260.
115. Reece EA, Chervenak FA, Moya FR, Hobbins JC. Amniotic fluid arborization: effect of blood, meconium, and pH alterations. Obstet Gynecol 1984;64:248.
116. Rosemond RL, Lombardi SJ, Boehm FH. Ferning of amniotic fluid contaminated with blood. Obstet Gynecol 1990;75:338.
117. Bennett SL, Cullen JBH, Sherer DM, Woods Jr JR. Ferning and nitrazine testing of amniotic fluid at all gestational ages. SPO Abstract 236. Am J Obstet Gynecol 1991;164:312.
118. Smith RP. A technique for the detection of rupture of the membranes: a review and preliminary report. Obstet Gynecol 1976;48:172.
119. Cowett RM, Hakanson DO, Kocon RW, Oh W. Untoward neonatal effect of intra-amniotic administration of methylene blue. Obstet Gynecol 1976;48:74s.
120. Troche BI. The methylene blue baby. New Engl J Med 1989;320:1756.
121. Iannetta O. A new simple test for detecting rupture of the fetal membranes. Obstet Gynecol 1984;63:575.
122. Huber JF, Bischof P, Extermann P, Beguin F, Herrmann WL. Are vaginal fluid concentrations of prolactin, α-fetoprotein and human placental lactogen useful for diagnosing ruptured membranes? Br J Obstet Gynecol 1983;90:1183.
123. Rochelson BL, Rodke G, White R, Bracero L, Baker DA. A rapid colorimetric AFP monoclonal antibody test for the diagnosis of preterm rupture of the membranes. Obstet Gynecol 1987;69:163.
124. Gahl WA, Kozina TJ, Fuhrmann DD, Vale AM. Diamine oxidase in the diagnosis of ruptured fetal membranes. Obstet Gynecol 1982;60:297.
125. Koninckx PR, Trappeniers H, Van Assche FA. Prolactin concentration in vaginal fluid: a new method for diagnosing ruptured membranes. Br J Obstet Gynaecol 1981;88:607.
126. Phocas I, Sarandakou A, Kontoravdis A, Chryssicopoulos A, Zourlas PA. Vaginal fluid prolactin: a reliable marker for the diagnosis of prematurely ruptured membranes. Comparison with vaginal fluid alpha-fetoprotein and placental lactogen. Eur J Obstet Gynecol Reprod Biol 1989;31:133.
127. Munson LA, Graham A, Koos BJ, Valenzuela GJ. Is there a need for digital examination in patients with spontaneous rupture of the membranes? Am J Obstet Gynecol 1985;153:562.
128. Schlinke S, Morgan M. Digital versus speculum exam in evaluating cervical dilation during labor. SPO Abstract 589. Am J Obstet Gynecol 1991;164:407.
129. Adoni A, Ben-Chetrit A, Zacut D, Palti Z, Hurwitz A. Prolongation of the latent period in patients with premature rupture of the membranes by avoiding digital examination. Int J Gynaecol Obstet 1990;32:19.
130. Schutte MF, Treffers PE, Kloosterman GJ, Soepatmi S. Management of premature rupture of membranes: the risk of vaginal examination to the infant. Am J Obstet Gynecol 1983;146:395.
131. Lewis DF, Major CA, Towers CV, Harding JA, Asrat T, Garite TJ. Effects of digital vaginal exams on latency period in preterm

premature rupture of membranes. SPO Abstract 495. Am J Obstet Gynecol 1991;164:381.
132. Vintzileos AM, Campbell WA, Nochimson DJ, Weinbaum PJ. The use of the nonstress test in patients with premature rupture of the membranes. Am J Obstet Gynecol 1986;155:149.
133. Vintzileos AM, Feinstein SJ, Lodeiro JG, Campbell WA, Weinbaum PJ, Nochimson DJ. Fetal biophysical profile and the effect of premature rupture of the membranes. Obstet Gynecol 1986;67:818.
134. Zeevi D, Sadovsky E, Younis J, Granat M, Ohel G. Antepartum fetal heart rate characteristics in cases of premature rupture of membranes. Am J Perinatol 1988;5:260.
135. Smith CV, Greenspoon J, Phelan JP, Platt LD. Clinical utility of the nonstress test in the conservative management of women with preterm spontaneous premature rupture of the membranes. J Reprod Med 1987;32:1.
136. Vintzileos AM, Campbell WA, Nochimson DJ, Weinbaum PJ. Degree of oligohydramnios and pregnancy outcome in patients with premature rupture of the membranes. Obstet Gynecol 1985;66:162.
137. Jackson DN, Lewis DF, Nageotte MP, Towers CV. Daily amniotic fluid index study in the management of preterm prolonged ruptured membranes: a prospective study. SPO Abstract 655. Am J Obstet Gynecol 1991;164:423.
138. Gonick B, Bottoms SF, Cotton DB. Amniotic fluid volume as a risk factor in preterm premature rupture of the membranes. Obstet Gynecol 1985;65:456.
139. Kivikoski AI, Amon E, Vaalamo PO, Pirhonen J, Kopta MM. Effect of third-trimester premature rupture of membranes on fetal breathing movements: a prospective case-control study. Am J Obstet Gynecol 1988;159:1474.
140. Roberts AB, Goldstein I, Romero R, Hobbins JC. Fetal breathing movements after preterm premature rupture of membranes. Am J Obstet Gynecol 1991;164:821.
141. Vintzileos AM, Campbell WA, Nochimson DJ, Connolly ME, Fuenfer MM, Hoehn GJ. The fetal biophysical profile in patients with premature rupture of the membranes: an early predictor of infection. Am J Obstet Gynecol 1985;152:510.
142. Vintzileos AM, Campbell WA, Nochimson DJ, Weinbaum PJ. Fetal breathing as a predictor of infection in premature rupture of the membranes. Obstet Gynecol 1986;67:813.
143. Goldstein I, Romero R, Merrill S, et al. Fetal body and breathing movements as predictors of intra-amniotic infection in preterm premature rupture of membranes. Am J Obstet Gynecol 1988;159:363.
144. Kitterman JA, Liggins GC, Clements JA, Tooley WH. Stimulation of breathing movements in fetal sheep by inhibitors of prostaglandin synthesis. J Devel Physiol 1979;1:453.
145. Roberts AB, Goldstein I, Romero R, Hobbins JC. Comparison of total fetal activity measurement with the biophysical profile in predicting intra-amniotic infection in preterm premature rupture of membranes. Ultrasound Obstet Gynecol 1991;1:36.
145a. Manning FA, Morrison I, Lange IR, Harman CR, Chamberlain PF. Fetal assessment based on fetal biophysical profile scoring: experience in 12,620 referred high-risk pregnancies. Am J Obstet Gynecol 1985;151:343.
146. Vintzileos AM, Bors-Koefoed R, Pelegano JF, et al. The use of fetal biophysical profile improves pregnancy outcome in premature rupture of the membranes. Am J Obstet Gynecol 1987;157:236.
147. Evans M, Hajj SN, Devoe LD, Angerman NS, Moaward AH. C-reactive protein as a predictor of infectious morbidity with premature rupture of the membranes. Am J Obstet Gynecol 1980;138:648.
148. Farb HF, Arnesen M, Geistler P, Knox GE. C-reactive protein with premature rupture of membranes and premature labor. Obstet Gynecol 1983;62:49.
149. Fisk NM, Fysh J, Child AG, Gatenby PA, Jeffery H, Bradfield AH. Is C-reactive protein really useful in preterm premature rupture of the membranes? Br J Obstet Gynaecol 1987;94:1159.
150. Hawrylyshyn P, Bernstein P, Milligan JE, Soldin S, Pollard A, Papsin FR. Premature rupture of membranes: the role of C-reactive protein in the prediction of chorioamnionitis. Am J Obstet Gynecol 1983;147:240.
151. Ismail MA, Zinaman MJ, Lowensohn RI, Moaward AH. The significance of C-reactive protein levels in women with premature rupture of membranes. Am J Obstet Gynecol 1985;151:541.
152. Kurki T, Teramo K, Ylikorkala O, Paavonen J. C-reactive protein in preterm premature rupture of the membranes. Arch Gynecol Obstet 1990;247:31.
153. Romem Y, Artal R. C-reactive protein as a predictor for chorioamnionitis in cases of premature rupture of the membranes. Am J Obstet Gynecol 1984;150:546.
154. Duff P, Huff RW, Gibbs RS. Management of premature rupture of membranes and unfavorable cervix in term pregnancy. Obstet Gynecol 1984;63:697.
155. Morales WJ, Lazar AJ. Expectant management of rupture of membranes at term. South Med J 1986;79:955.
156. Koh KS, Chan FH, Monfared AH, Ledger WJ, Paul RH. The changing perinatal and maternal outcome in chorioamnionitis. Obstet Gynecol 1979;53:730.
157. Yoder PR, Gibbs RS, Blanco JD, Casteneda YS, St. Clair PJ. A prospective, controlled study of maternal and perinatal outcome after intra-amniotic infection at term. Am J Obstet Gynecol 1983;145:695.
158. Ekman-Ordeberg G, Uldbjerg N, Ulmsten U. Comparison of intravenous oxytocin and vaginal prostaglandin E_2 gel in women with unripe cervixes and premature rupture of the membranes. Obstet Gynecol 1985;66:307.
159. Cox SM, Williams ML, Leveno KJ. The natural history of preterm ruptured membranes: what to expect of expectant management. Obstet Gynecol 1988;71:558.
160. Wilson JC, Levy DL, Wilds PL. Premature rupture of the membranes prior to term: consequences of nonintervention. Obstet Gynecol 1982;60:601.
161. Levy DL, Warsof SL. Oral ritodrine and preterm premature rupture of membranes. Obstet Gynecol 1985;66:621.
162. Dunlop PDM, Crowley PA, Lamont RF, Hawkins DF. Preterm ruptured membranes, no contractions. J Obstet Gynaecol 1986;7:92.
163. Christensen KK, Ingemarsson I, Liedeman T, Solum H, Svenningsen N. Effect of ritodrine on labor after premature rupture of the membranes. Obstet Gynecol 1980;55:187.
164. Weiner CP, Renk K, Klugman M. The therapeutic efficacy and cost-effectiveness of aggressive tocolysis for premature labor associated with premature rupture of the membranes. Am J Obstet Gynecol 1988;159:216.
165. Garite TJ, Keegan KA, Freeman RK, Nageotte MP. A randomized trial of ritodrine tocolysis versus expectant management in patients with premature rupture of membranes at 25 to 30 weeks of gestation. Am J Obstet Gynecol 1987;157:388.
166. Brelje MC, Kaltreider DF. The use of vaginal antibiotics in premature rupture of the membranes. Am J Obstet Gynecol 1966;94:889.
167. Amon E, Lewis SV, Sibai BM, Villar MA, Arheart KL. Ampicillin prophylaxis in preterm premature rupture of the membranes: a prospective randomized study. Am J Obstet Gynecol 1988; 159:539.
168. Johnston MM, Sanchez-Ramos L, Vaughn AJ, Todd MW,

Benrubi GI. Antibiotic therapy in preterm premature rupture of membranes: a randomized, prospective, double-blind trial. Am J Obstet Gynecol 1990;163:743.

169. Morales WJ, Angel JL, O'Brien WF, Knuppel RA. Use of ampicillin and corticosteroids in premature rupture of membranes: a randomized study. Obstet Gynecol 1989;73:721.
170. Ogita S, Imanaka M, Matsumoto M, Hatanaka K. Premature rupture of the membranes managed with a new cervical catheter. Lancet 1984;1:1330.
171. Romero R, Scioscia AL, Edberg SC, Hobbins JC. Use of parenteral antibiotic therapy to eradicate bacterial colonization of amniotic fluid in premature rupture of membranes. Obstet Gynecol 1986;67(Suppl):15.
172. Romero R, Hagay Z, Nores J, Sepulveda W, Mazor M. Eradication of *Ureaplasma urealyticum* from the amniotic fluid with transplacental antibiotic treatment. Am J Obstet Gynecol (in press).
173. Ohlsson A. Treatments of preterm premature rupture of the membranes: a meta-analysis. Am J Obstet Gynecol 1989;160:890.
174. Crowley P, Chalmers I, Keirse MJNC. The effects of corticosteroid administration before preterm delivery: an overview of the evidence from controlled trials. Br J Obstet Gynaecol 1990;97:11.
175. Romero R, Oyarzun E, Mazor M, Avila C, Hobbins JC, Bracken M. Meta-analysis of the effect of steroids in the prevention of respiratory distress syndrome in premature rupture of membranes. Am J Obstet Gynecol (in press).
176. Garite TJ, Freeman RK, Linzey EM, Braly P. The use of amniocentesis in patients with premature rupture of membranes. Obstet Gynecol 1979;54:226.
177. Yeast JD, Garite TJ, Dorchester W. The risks of amniocentesis in the management of premature rupture of the membranes. Am J Obstet Gynecol 1984;149:505.
178. Cotton DB, Gonik B, Bottoms SF. Conservative versus aggressive management of preterm rupture of membranes: a randomized trial of amniocentesis. Am J Perinatol 1984;1:322.
179. Shaver DC, Spinnato JA, Whybrew D, Williams WK, Anderson GD. Comparison of phospholipids in vaginal and amniocentesis specimens of patients with premature rupture of membranes. Am J Obstet Gynecol 1987;156:454.
180. Stedman CM, Crawford S, Staten E, Cherny WB. Management of preterm premature rupture of membranes: assessing amniotic fluid in the vagina for phosphatidylglycerol. Am J Obstet Gynecol 1981;140:34.
181. Brame RG, MacKenna J. Vaginal pool phospholipids in the management of premature rupture of membranes. Am J Obstet Gynecol 1983;145:992.
182. Golde SH. Use of obstetric perineal pads in collection of amniotic fluid in patients with rupture of the membranes. Am J Obstet Gynecol 1983;146:710.
183. Gluck L, Kulovich MV, Borer RC, et al. Interpretation and significance of the L/S ratio in amniotic fluid. Am J Obstet Gynecol 1974;120:142.
184. Schumacher RE, Parisi VM, Steady HM, Tsao FHC. Bacteria causing false-positive test for phosphatidylglycerol in amniotic fluid. Am J Obstet Gynecol 1985;151:1067.
185. Dombroski RA, MacKenna J, Brame RG. Comparison of amniotic fluid lung maturity profiles in paired vaginal and amniocentesis specimens. Am J Obstet Gynecol 1981;140:461.
186. Goldstein AS, Mangurten HH, Libretti JV, et al. Lecithin/sphingomyelin ratio in amniotic fluid obtained vaginally. Am J Obstet Gynecol 1980;138:233.
187. Sbarra AJ, Blake G, Cetrulo CL. The effect of cervical/vaginal secretions on measurements of lecithin/sphingomyelin ratio and optical density at 650 nm. Am J Obstet Gynecol 1981;139:214.
188. Phillippe M, Acker D, Torday J, Schiff I, Frigoletto FD. The effects of vaginal contamination on two pulmonary phospholipid assays. J Reprod Med 1982;5:283.
189. Spinnato JA, Shaver DC, Bray EM, Lipshitz J. Preterm premature rupture of the membranes with fetal pulmonary maturity present: a prospective study. Obstet Gynecol 1987;69:196.
190. Gabbe SG, Ettinger BB, Freeman RK, Martin CB. Umbilical cord compression associated with amniotomy: laboratory observations. Am J Obstet Gynecol 1976;126:353.
191. Moberg LJ, Garite TJ, Freeman RK. Fetal heart rate patterns and fetal distress in patients with preterm premature rupture of membranes. Obstet Gynecol 1984;60:60.
192. Miyazaki FS, Taylor NA. Saline amnioinfusion for relief of variable or prolonged decelerations. Am J Obstet Gynecol 1983;146:670.
193. Miyazaki FS, Nevarez F. Saline amnioinfusion for relief of repetitive variable decelerations: a prospective randomized study. Am J Obstet Gynecol 1985;557:301.
194. Nageotte MP, Freeman RK, Garite TJ, Dorchester W. Prophylactic intrapartum amnioinfusion in patients with preterm premature rupture of the membranes. Am J Obstet Gynecol 1985;157;557.
195. Harger JH. Comparison of success and morbidity in cervical cerclage procedures. Obstet Gynecol 1980;56:543.
196. Yeast JD, Garite TR. The role of cervical cerclage in the management of preterm premature rupture of the membranes. Am J Obstet Gynecol 1988;158:106.
197. Blickstein I, Katz Z, Lancet M, Molgilner BM. The outcome of pregnancies complicated by preterm rupture of the membranes with and without cerclage. Int J Gynaecol Obstet 1989;28:237.
198. Goldman JM, Greene MF, Tuomala RE, Ringer SA, Harlow BL, Crowley SM. Outcome of expectant management in preterm premature rupture of membranes with cervical cerclage in place. Abstract 139. Presented at the Tenth Annual Meeting of the Society of Perinatal Obstetricians, Houston, Texas, 1990.
199. Major CA, Towers CV, Lewis DF, Asrat T. Expectant management of patients with both preterm premature rupture of membranes and genital herpes. Abstract 16. Am J Obstet Gynecol 1991;164:248.
200. Beydoun SN, Yasin SY. Premature rupture of the membranes before 28 weeks: conservative management. Am J Obstet Gynecol 1986;155:471.
201. Moretti M, Sibai BM. Maternal and perinatal outcome of expectant management of premature rupture of membranes in the mid-trimester. Am J Obstet Gynecol 1988;159:390.
202. Bengtson JM, VanMarter LJ, Barss VA, Greene MF, Tuomala RE, Epstein MF. Pregnancy outcome after premature rupture of the membranes at or before 26 weeks' gestation. Obstet Gynecol 1989;73:921.
203. Taylor J, Garite TJ. Premature rupture of membranes before fetal viability. Obstet Gynecol 1984;64:615.
204. Gold RB, Goyert GL, Schwartz DB, Evans MI, Seabolt LA. Conservative management of second-trimester post-amniocentesis fluid leakage. Obstet Gynecol 1989;74:745.
205. Hanson FW, Tennant FR, Zorn EM, Samuels S. Analysis of 2,136 genetic amniocenteses: experience of a single physician. Am J Obstet Gynecol 1985;152:436.
206. Rotschild A, Ling EW, Puterman ML, Farquharson D. Neonatal outcome after prolonged preterm rupture of the membranes. Am J Obstet Gynecol 1990;162:4.
207. Blott M, Greenough A. Neonatal outcome after prolonged rupture of the membranes starting in the second trimester. Arch Dis Child 1988;63:1146.

208. Johnson A, Callan NA, Bhutani VK, Colmorgen GHC, Weiner S, Bolognese RJ. Ultrasonic ratio of fetal thoracic to abdominal circumference: an association with fetal pulmonary hypoplasia. Am J Obstet Gynecol 1987;157:764.
209. Nimrod C, Varela-Gittings F, Machin G, Campbell D, Wesenberg R. The effect of very prolonged membrane rupture on fetal development. Am J Obstet Gynecol 1984;148:540.
210. Moessinger AC, Collins MH, Blanc WA, Rey HR, James LS. Oligohydramnios-induced lung hypoplasia: the influence of timing and duration in gestation. Pediatr Res 1986;20:951.
211. Thibeault DW, Beatty EC, Hall RT, Bowen SK, O'Neill DH. Neonatal pulmonary hypoplasia with premature rupture of fetal membranes and oligohydramnios. J Pediatr 1985;107:273.
212. Adzick NS, Harrison MR, Glick PL, Villa RL, Finkbeiner W. Experimental pulmonary hypoplasia and oligohydramnios: relative contributions of lung fluid and fetal breathing movements. J Pediatr Surg 1984;19:658.
213. Alcorn D, Adamson TM, Lambert TF, Maloney JE, Ritchie BC, Robinson PM. Morphological effects of chronic tracheal ligation and drainage in the fetal lamb lung. J Anat 1977;123:649.
214. Fewell JE, Hislop AA, Kitterman JA, Johnson P. Effect of tracheostomy on lung development in fetal lambs. J Appl Physiol 1983;55:1103.
215. Wigglesworth JS, Desai R, Hyslop AA. Fetal lung growth in congenital laryngeal atresia. Pediatr Pathol 1987;7:515.
216. Nicolini U, Fisk NM, Rodeck CH, Talbert DG, Wigglesworth JS. Low amniotic pressure in oligohydramnios: is this the cause of pulmonary hypoplasia? Am J Obstet Gynecol 1989;161:1098.
217. Nimrod C, Davies D, Iwanicki S, Harder J, Persaud D, Nicholson S. Ultrasound prediction of pulmonary hypoplasia. Obstet Gynecol 1986;68:495.
218. Nimrod C, Nicholson S, Davies D, Harder J, Dodd G, Sauve R. Pulmonary hypoplasia testing in clinical obstetrics. Am J Obstet Gynecol 1988;158:277.
219. Vintzileos AM, Campbell WA, Rodis JF, Nochimson DJ, Pinette MG, Petrikovsky BM. Comparison of six different ultrasonographic methods for predicting lethal fetal pulmonary hypoplasia. Am J Obstet Gynecol 1989;161:606.
220. Songster GS, Gray DL, Crane JP. Prenatal prediction of lethal pulmonary hypoplasia using ultrasonic fetal chest circumference. Obstet Gynecol 1989;73:261.
221. Roberts AB, Mitchell JM. Direct ultrasonographic measurement of fetal lung length in normal pregnancies and pregnancies complicated by prolonged rupture of membranes. Am J Obstet Gynecol 1990;163:1560.
222. Blott M, Nicolaides KH, Gibb D, Greenough A, Moscoso G, Campbell S. Fetal breathing movements as predictor of favourable pregnancy outcome after oligohydramnios due to membrane rupture in second trimester. Lancet 1987;2:129.
223. Moessinger AC, Fox HE, Higgins A, Ray HR, Al Haideri M. Fetal breathing movements are not a reliable predictor of continued lung development in pregnancies complicated by oligohydramnios. Lancet 1987;2:1297.

by fetal stress.[24–26] Even when meconium passage is not secondary to fetal stress, it may pose the threat of meconium aspiration that is more common in postterm than in term gestations.[5] This problem is further complicated with oligohydramnios, as the mixture of meconium and AF will be thicker. Recognition of meconium in the amniotic fluid requires active oropharyngeal suctioning at delivery to minimize meconium aspiration morbidity. Even so, this will not eliminate the meconium aspiration syndrome (MAS), because aspiration may have occurred in utero. MAS is most often encountered in high-risk gestations exhibiting abnormal fetal heart findings[24,27,28] but has also been described in the absence of observed fetal distress.[29]

POSTMATURITY

An infrequent but significant morbidity associated with the postterm gestation is the occurrence of the postmaturity syndrome. Associated synonyms for this finding include placental dysfunction and dysmaturity syndrome. The latter term is preferable, because this syndrome may also occur in the term infant. Dysmaturity probably results from subacute placental dysfunction–insufficiency that results in nutritional deprivation and fetal wasting. Dysmaturity was first described in the English literature by Clifford in 1954, who defined three progressive stages, with increasing morbidity and mortality from stages I to III.[30] Features of dysmaturity include failure of fetal growth; loss of subcutaneous tissue; dry, wrinkled skin; and a high incidence of meconium staining. Functionally, these newborns are described as appearing alert and apprehensive. The incidence of dysmaturity findings is 3% at term compared to 10% to 20% in the postterm infant.[31,32] Shime and colleagues distinguish a mild type from more advanced dysmaturity and document an increased incidence of low biophysical profile scores, oligohydramnios, meconium passage, fetal distress, and low Apgar scores in infants with advanced compared to mild dysmaturity.[33] These findings likely reflect a slowly progressive decrease in placental functional reserve. Postnatally, such infants often manifest hypothermia or hypoglycemia, perhaps due to decreased fat and glycogen stores.[34] Additionally, hyperviscosity and polycythemia are not uncommon and probably reflect a chronic hypoxemic fetal environment. The long-term significance to infants exhibiting this syndrome in terms of developmental sequelae is controversial. To address this issue properly requires prolonged infant follow-up, during which time major advances have evolved in perinatal and pediatric care. Furthermore, studies are confounded by differing subject populations and have used a wide variety of developmental tests.[31,34]

Given the availability of antepartum and intrapartum surveillance, the morbidity of this small subgroup of fetuses should, it is hoped, be minimized. It is currently clear that such fetuses represent a unique high-morbidity subpopulation of postterm fetuses that have experienced a chronic or subacute intrauterine stress. They are also particularly susceptible during the birth process. Unfortunately, as will be discussed later, it is not clear that this syndrome can be accurately predicted antenatally.

MANAGEMENT

There is little disagreement that the postterm pregnancy presents as a high-risk situation with an increased potential for both maternal and fetal morbidity. Accepting this, the question arises as to how these patients can be managed best. The two treatment options include routine induction and expectant management.

ROUTINE INDUCTION

The concept of inducing all postterm patients at 42 completed weeks was promoted in 1963 by McClure Browne, who reported the increase in perinatal mortality as well as morbidity in postterm pregnancies.[7] Routine induction was advocated in all patients regardless of the cervical status. Induction was undertaken using amniotomy, thereafter allowing up to 48 hours in which to effect delivery. In a group of 1500 patients thus managed, the cesarean section rate was 4%, with only 2% done for failed induction–arrest disorders. This compared favorably with their overall cesarean section rate of 5.7%. This management approach was purported to result in a significant reduction in perinatal mortality when compared to patients who were followed expectantly.

This empiric approach involved clinical evaluation of maternal weight, clinical assessment of fetal size, and amniotic fluid volume. Specific evaluation of fetal status was unavailable in 1963, and neonatal intensive care was in its infancy.

Currently, with the widespread availability of antepartum surveillance, improved neonatal care, and an enhanced understanding of the pathophysiology associated with postterm pregnancy, the role of routine induction requires reevaluation. Routine induction would often be inappropriate, given our current understanding of studies using ovulation dating and early ultrasound information. Clearly, a substantial percentage (40%) of alleged postterm patients are actually not postterm.[8,11] Of those gestations truly prolonged (>294 days), few (<10%) are at risk for significant morbidity as a result of uteroplacental dysfunction. Thus, it may be difficult to demonstrate convincingly an improvement in overall outcome with routine induction of all postterm patients. Furthermore, reports have noted that a large number of postterm patients would fail attempts at induction.[35] In support of this concern, an increase in the cesarean section rate has been described when routine induction has been instituted.[36,37]

In 1975, Vorherr recommended individualization of

care, noting that neither routine induction nor expectant management should be instituted as a general rule.[32] Individualization is currently often the chosen clinical approach, although there may be variances of detail in each management scheme. Even though described nearly 20 years ago, Vorherr's policies resemble many in practice today. He recommended induction of any postterm patient with complicating obstetrical or medical factors or if the cervical exam was favorable. Uninduced patients were followed with twice-weekly fetal heart rate evaluation, estriol determination, and clinical estimation of fetal weight. Currently, acceptable expectant management approaches propose selective induction of those postterm patients with inducible cervixes or with any medical or obstetrical complication.[6,9,10]

The definition of an inducible cervix was systematized by Bishop's scoring system of 1964. The Bishop score evaluated five characteristics of the cervical–pelvic exam that he found useful in predicting the success of elective induction.[38] These included cervical position, consistency, dilation, effacement, and station of the presenting part. The Bishop score could range from 0 to 13. Bishop noted that, given a score of 9 or greater, the average duration of labor, following amniotomy and oxytocin, was 4 hours or less, with no failed inductions (the number of patients studied was not mentioned). In 500 patients not induced, Bishop reported that the number of days to the onset of spontaneous labor was inversely proportional to the Bishop score. It should be noted that Bishop's initial study was limited to multiparous patients.

It has been reported that most pregnancies exceeding 294 days are associated with low Bishop scores. Harris and colleagues described a group of 197 postterm patients who were evaluated weekly for Bishop scores until spontaneous labor occurred.[35] The initial mean score was 3.6, with only 8.2% of patients having scores of 7 or greater. The mean interval between exam and spontaneous labor was 5.5 days. As part of their management protocol, patients underwent NSTs weekly; if any decelerations were noted or if the NST was nonreactive, a CST was performed. Without providing specific data, the authors noted that the majority of the CSTs were spontaneous (ie, spontaneous uterine activity), leading them to conclude that the unfavorable cervix may be part of the cause for postterm gestations rather than a lack of uterine contractions. Given the low incidence of favorable Bishop scores, the authors felt that routine induction of labor was inappropriate.

The other subpopulation of postterm patients that should undergo induction are those that demonstrate any evidence of medical or additional obstetrical complications. This includes patients with hypertensive disorders, either pregnancy-related or preexisting; diabetes mellitus; and renal, cardiac, or collagen-vascular diseases. Obstetrical conditions warranting intervention include abnormal fetal lie, suspected macrosomia, or fetal dysmaturity. Historical factors such as prior stillbirth should also be taken into consideration.

In 1982, Yeh reported the results of a selective type of management scheme in a group of 880 patients at Women's Hospital, University of Southern California.[10] Postterm pregnancies were subdivided, good versus poor dates, depending on the dating accuracy of their stated gestational age. To be considered as having good dates, at least one of the following criteria had to be met:

- Positive pregnancy test by the sixth week since the LMP
- Pelvic exam confirming the GA before 10 weeks
- DeLee fetal heart tones audible by 20 weeks GA or of at least 22 weeks duration
- Ultrasound before 26 weeks that confirmed GA.

Two hundred and nineteen patients (24%) were considered as good dates, and 661 were classified as poor dates. This unusual distribution probably reflects the fact that the majority of patients were indigent and many failed to obtain early prenatal care. Patients with supervening medical or obstetrical problems were admitted for induction/delivery. In the group with "good dates," 13% of the patients had a favorable Bishop score (>8) and underwent oxytocin induction, with a 17% cesarean section rate. Patients with an unfavorable score were followed expectantly using estriol determination and NSTs. The initial evaluation included both tests, but if the NST was normal, the subsequent follow-up consisted of twice-weekly estriol measurement. If the estriol level was decreasing, an NST was obtained. If the NST was abnormal at any point, a CST was performed and management was based on the CST. The patients with poor dates were followed expectantly and less rigorously. At their initial exam, estriol level was measured, and if normal this was repeated twice weekly. NSTs were performed only if an estriol level was abnormal. All patients were examined on a weekly basis. Using this approach, there were eight perinatal losses, with five stillbirths and three neonatal deaths (PMR 10/1000). Four of the stillbirths and one of the neonatal deaths occurred in patients who failed to comply with the protocol. The other two neonatal deaths were associated with major congenital anomalies, giving a corrected perinatal mortality rate of 6.8 in 1000. Twenty-two percent of the infants weighed more than 4000 g. Other outcome measures were comparable to those of the term population (cesarean section rate = 15.8%; intrapartum fetal distress = 6.3%; low 5-minute Apgars = 2.4%). Patients induced because of favorable Bishop scores had similar outcomes, as did those delivered for abnormal antepartum tests. The incidence of the postmaturity syndrome was 12%.

A recently completed study at the same institution evaluated 630 postterm patients with good dating criteria at or beyond 287 days. Patients were considered for participation in a multicenter trial comparing elective induction to expectant management.[39] One hundred and sixteen low-risk postterm patients with unfavorable cervical exams (Bishop <6) were enrolled on the study that is discussed in detail later in this chapter. The remaining 514 patients were excluded for a variety of medical and obstetrical reasons, favorable cervical exams, or patient refusal and were followed for outcome parameters. Of these 514 patients, 65 (13%) were excluded for medical (primarily hypertensive disorders) or obstetrical (abnormal fetal lie, ruptured membranes) reasons. Of the remaining 449 patients, 248 (55%) were found to have a Bishop score ≥6, and thus underwent induction using oxytocin within the next 2 days. The residual 201 patients were then evaluated with ultrasound for amniotic fluid volume (AFV), fetal size estimation, and NST. At this initial screen, 10 fetuses were predicted to be >4500 g, 10 were noted to be in an abnormal lie, 20 had reduced amniotic fluid (deepest pocket <3 cm), and 45 demonstrated abnormal NSTs. These 85 (17%) patients were thus admitted for delivery. Of the residual 114 patients, 41 refused to participate in the collaborative study and 73 were evaluated prior to initiation of the study. These patients were followed expectantly with twice-weekly NSTs, with AFV assessment, and with weekly physical examinations. Evaluation of outcome parameters in this expectantly managed group demonstrated one perinatal death, a fetal demise that occurred 2 days after a "normal" NST and AFV, with no explanation found at delivery or on autopsy. The incidence of infants weighing more than 4000 g was 22%, which is in agreement with previously published data. The overall cesarean section rate was 23%, with a significantly lower rate among those patients induced with favorable cervical exams (14.8% if cervix is favorable, compared to 30% if cervical exam is unfavorable; $p < .03$). The lowest cesarean rate occurred in patients induced with a Bishop score >8 (5%).

These two observational studies would suggest that the postterm population can be followed expectantly with low perinatal mortality and morbidity, given proper antenatal surveillance. The question posed is whether a more aggressive approach is associated with improved outcome. Several large studies have addressed this issue. In 1982, Gibb reported a prospective study designed to evaluate the outcome of an expectant approach versus one of routine induction.[37] One hundred forty-two patients were entered into the study and were cared for by one of two physician groups, with assignment to each group done on a random basis. One physician group routinely induced postterm patients; the other managed patients expectantly. Using similar dating criteria as those of Yeh, 81 patients were considered to be "certain" postterm and 61 were described as probable postterm if they failed to meet dating requirements. Of the patients with "certain" dates, 30 were induced and 51 were followed expectantly. In the probable postterm group the numbers were 16 and 45, respectively. The patients expectantly managed were evaluated with daily fetal-movement counts and "cardiotocography" three times per week. Patients managed by routine induction at 42 weeks underwent evaluation of cervical inducibility. If the cervical exam was unfavorable, a vaginal prostaglandin pessary was placed the night preceding induction. Induction consisted of amniotomy followed by oxytocin administration. There was a significant increase in the cesarean birth rate in "certain" dates patients routinely induced compared to patients followed expectantly (26.7% vs 9.8%). For the patients with probable postdates, the cesarean rates were 31.2% versus 2.2%. No significant difference was noted in measures of newborn outcome (endotracheal intubation, low 5-minute Apgars, admission to neonatal ICU) among the groups. The authors concluded that routine induction was not justified, as it did not alter perinatal outcome and was associated with a marked increase in cesarean births. Several flaws limit the value of this study. First of all, the distribution of patients who underwent induction versus expectant management does not appear equal, and thus is probably not random. Given this, the possibility of bias exists. Second, the number of patients studied is relatively small.

Cardoza compared the outcome of conservative versus active management in a group of 402 patients.[1] All were at or beyond 290 days GA by early pregnancy dating, including physical examination and ultrasound before 20 weeks gestation. One hundred and ninety-eight patients were randomly assigned to active management, which consisted of induction with a 3-mg vaginal prostaglandin pessary, followed by amniotomy and, if necessary, oxytocin. Of the 198 patients, only 64% underwent induction, 25% went into spontaneous labor, and 10% refused induction. Conservative management was randomly assigned to 207 patients, which included an initial ultrasound for an estimate of amniotic fluid volume and fetal weight, daily fetal kick counts, and cardiotocography every other day. In this group 80% went into spontaneous labor, 10% were induced for clinical indications, and 10% refused expectant management and therefore were induced. Results demonstrated no difference in the duration of labor, method of delivery, intervention for fetal distress, or Apgar scores. There was one fetal demise noted in the expectant management group attributed to placental abruption and one neonatal death in the induction group related to congenital anomalies. Similar to the Gibb report, the authors concluded that routine induction did not offer advantages over expectant management. A deficiency of this study is that a significant number of patients in each of the two treatment groups were not actually managed according to plan (eg, 35% of the patients in the induction group did not undergo induction but remained in the group analysis). Such deviation from a proposed plan is not unusual in clinical care of patients, but such patients confound data analysis. Both studies fail to detail the initial cervical exams of the study groups. Considering the known association of the Bishop score, the onset of spontaneous labor, and success of induction, this lack of information is problematic.

In a well-designed prospective study, Dyson compared the results of induction versus conservative management.[40] Patients were selected at or beyond 287 days GA by strict dating criteria. Exclusion criteria included any medical or obstetrical complication as well as favorable Bishop scores (≥6). Three hundred and two patients were included; 152 were induced and 150 were followed expectantly. The induction group received prostaglandin gel (either 3 mg vaginally or 0.5 mg intracervically), following which patients were monitored for 45 minutes. If spontaneous uterine activity ensued, the patient was admitted; if there was no uterine activity or evidence of fetal compromise, the patient was sent home to return the next morning. Assessment of Bishop score was repeated. If the Bishop score was ≥5, oxytocin induction was started. If it was <5, a second dose of prostaglandin was administered, and if spontaneous uterine activity had not developed after 4 hours, oxytocin induction commenced. Expectant management consisted of weekly physical exams and twice-weekly NSTs. Amniotic fluid volume was initially measured in the 42nd week and twice weekly thereafter. Patients in the expectant group underwent induction only if the NST became abnormal, if the amniotic fluid reduced, or if the cervical exam became favorable. The results of this protocol demonstrated no difference in perinatal mortality or 5-minute Apgars but did reveal that patients undergoing routine induction had a significantly lower incidence of low 1-minute Apgar scores, meconium passage, meconium aspiration syndrome, postmaturity syndrome, and fetal distress compared to those patients followed expectantly. Furthermore, the cesarean section rate was significantly lower in those who underwent induction. The latter difference was primarily found in nulliparous patients because of a higher rate of cesarean section for fetal distress in the expectantly followed group. Dyson concluded that routine induction preceded by cervical ripening with prostaglandin resulted in a reduction in perinatal morbidity and cesarean births. In comparing their findings to those of previously cited studies, the authors note that only patients with unfavorable cervixes were included, as those with high Bishop scores are likely to enter spontaneous labor sooner, and thus the benefit of induction versus expectant care may not be evident. Also, they stressed that for intervention to lead to a reduction in morbidity, this management approach should result in delivery at an earlier GA than that of patients followed expectantly. Indeed, the mean GA at entrance was similar in the two patient groups but was significantly less at delivery in the group who underwent induction (292 versus 296 days, $p < 0.01$). This issue was not addressed by either Gibb or Cardoza.

Recently, a large, multicenter prospective study was conducted under NIH sponsorship.[39] The purpose was again to compare expectant management with elective induction. To be eligible, all patients had to show absent risk factors and demonstrate a normal AFV and NST. An additional question addressed was the utility of prostaglandin ripening prior to oxytocin induction in the setting of an unfavorable cervix. Thus, the group undergoing induction received either placebo or prostaglandin gel intracervically. This study included certain dated patients between 287 and 301 days GA by strict dating criteria. All patients with an inducible cervix (Bishop score ≥6) were excluded, as were patients with medical or obstetrical complications. The patients were randomly assigned to the three respective groups, and investigators were blinded as to whether the intracervical gel contained prostaglandin. A total of 440 patients were included in the study; 175 were followed with twice-weekly NSTs and amniotic fluid measurement (expectant group); 174 underwent induction beginning with a single intracervical dose (0.5 mg) of prostaglandin; and 91 underwent induction preceded by application of a placebo gel. Preliminary results revealed that the incidence of significant perinatal morbidity–mortality was too low to demonstrate improvement with routine induction. Furthermore, use of prostaglandin gel did not result in shorter labor or reduced cesarean section rates, as the rate was similar in all three groups (18% to 22%). The mean GA at delivery was less in those patients undergoing induction compared to those who were followed expectantly (292.5 vs 295.8 days).

Review of these four studies yields conflicting outcome conclusions. Explanations for the conflicting results are not immediately clear. The first two studies, those of Gibb[37] and Cardoza,[1] contained several flaws in either the study design or the analysis of data, which may account for variable findings. Also, as was pointed out, inclusion of patients with favorable cervical exams may not be appropriate when attempting to evaluate routine induction. On the other hand, the latter two studies, that of Dyson[40] and the multicenter study,[39] were very similar in their study design and yet yielded very different conclusions. In attempting to understand these discrepancies, several points should be made. Dyson concludes that routine induction results in a reduction in the cesarean section rate. This is primarily attributable to differences in the number of cesarean sections performed for fetal distress in nulliparous patients. If one compares the specific rates, the 34.6% rate in nulliparous patients followed expectantly contrasts unusually with the 19.8% in patients undergoing active induction. Recent reports in postterm studies describe a much lower incidence of cesarean section for fetal distress of 8%[41] and 22%.[33] Some authors state that in the intrapartum monitored patient, fetal distress is no more common in the postterm than in the term patient.[42] Thus, the reported reduction in fetal morbidity and cesarean section rate described by Dyson may be due to the high rate (34.6%) in the control (expectant) group.

ANTEPARTUM SURVEILLANCE

Although conflicting data exist, current information in the literature supports the concept of selective induction, with expectant management of those postterm patients with unfavorable cervices, if careful antepartum surveillance is conducted. The next question that arises is which antepartum test, if any, is superior and at what interval the test results should be obtained. Various tests have been applied to the postterm population and include the contraction stress test (CST), nonstress test (NST), biophysical profile, and ultrasound assessment of amniotic fluid volume.

In 1981, Freeman reported on the outcome of 679 postterm patients who were followed using the CST as the primary means of surveillance.[14] The outcome of this group was compared to a control population of 500 consecutive, low-risk term patients delivered during the same period. Patients with any medical or obstetrical problem or with an inducible cervix were excluded. Tests were interpreted as negative (no late deceleration with ≥3 uterine contractions every 10 minutes), positive (repetitive late decelerations, regardless of contraction frequency in the absence of uterine hyperstimulation), and equivocal (nonpersistent late decelerations, or late decelerations associated with excessive uterine contractions). If the test was negative, it was repeated in 1 week; if equivocal, it was repeated in 24 hours. When it was positive, the patient was admitted for delivery. Using this approach, 66.9% of the tests were negative, 26.8% were equivocal, and 0.7% were positive. The incidence of intrapartum fetal distress necessitating cesarean section in each group was 22.9%, 29%, and 50%, respectively. Those patients with negative CSTs had no increase in fetal distress when compared to the control population. Only 5.4% of the postterm patients had CSTs that led to intervention. The authors concluded that the CST was useful in following the postterm patient but had the disadvantage of a large number of equivocal results that required repeat testing. Other limitations of the CST approach were the time consumed, cost, inconvenience, and skill necessary to interpret the test.

Given the limitations of the CST, other means of surveillance have been examined. The NST is generally thought to be very reliable in predicting fetal well-being, yet in 1981 Miyazaki presented results that suggested otherwise.[43] Management of 165 postterm well-dated patients included NSTs weekly, using the CST as a back-up in the event of a nonreactive NST. One hundred and twenty-five patients had reactive NSTs within 1 week of delivery and provided the basis of his report. The NST was considered reactive if there were two or more fetal heart rate accelerations of 15 bpm of at least 15 seconds duration within a 20-minute window. Tests were subsequently designated as false reactive if the fetus died or if there was intrapartum fetal distress in early labor within 1 week of the test. In this group of 125 patients, there was an 8% false-reactive rate, with four fetal deaths, one neonatal death, four cases of fetal distress on admission, and one brain-damaged infant. In attempting to explain these "disastrous" results, Miyazaki noted that four of the 10 had variable decelerations on their NSTs, raising concern regarding cord compression as a potential etiology related to the high morbidity and mortality. Unfortunately, the incidence of variable decelerations in the patients with good outcomes was not mentioned. Miyazaki concluded that the NST alone on a weekly basis was associated with an unacceptably high number of falsely reassuring tests.

Phelan further explored the significance of variable decelerations as an indication of postterm fetal compromise.[44] Weekly NSTs were obtained in 239 postterm patients, of whom 21% were considered to have unreliable dates. A total of 505 NSTs were performed, with 84% reactive and 16% nonreactive. A variable deceleration was defined as a fall in fetal heart rate (FHR) of 15 beats per minute (bpm) or more, lasting ≥15 seconds, and a bradycardia defined as a decline in FHR of more than 40 bpm or to a level of 90 bpm lasting ≥1 minute. Variable decelerations were noted in 33% of patients, and bradycardias were seen in 3.8% of patients. Results showed that fetuses with reactive NSTs within 1 week of delivery had significantly lower incidence of meconium and low Apgars and a trend toward fewer cesarean sections. In further analysis of reactive tests, it was noted that the presence of decelerations was associated with the same newborn morbidity as that encountered with nonreactive tests. Specifically, patients with reactive NSTs and decelerations had the same incidence of meconium passage and cesarean sections for fetal distress as those with nonreactive NSTs. The incidence of postmaturity syndrome was similar among all tested groups, implying that the NST was not a specific predictor of this particular complication. Based on these findings, Phelan recommended that in the presence of fetal heart rate decelerations, delivery should be effected, regardless of the presence of reactivity on the NST.

In a follow-up study, Small applied an active induction approach when decelerations were observed on NST to a study group of 470 postterm patients. A total of 638 NSTs were performed, with 24% demonstrating FHR decelerations that led to induction and delivery. Outcome was compared to that of historical controls, but in whom management was not altered by the presence of decelerations.[45] In Small's study, induction was additionally carried out for evidence of oligohydramnios, or a persistently nonreactive NST. In comparing this approach to the historical control study, it was noted that the last NST to delivery interval was shorter, there was decreased meconium passage, macrosomia, and a trend toward fewer cesarean sections for fetal distress.

Other investigators have undertaken a more complete evaluation of the postterm fetus by applying the biophysical profile. This test, first described by Manning in 1980, included five variables: fetal movement, fetal muscular tone, fetal breathing, amniotic fluid volume (normal ≥1-cm pocket), and an NST.[46] The total score possible is 10, with two points given for each parameter found to be normal and nothing given if abnormal. Use of five parameters was suggested by Johnson in 1986 to be more accurate in predicting fetal well-being in the postterm patient.[36] Twice-weekly biophysical profiles (BPP) were obtained in 293 patients. If the biophysical profile was 8 for the first four parameters listed earlier, the NST was omitted. If there was evidence of oligohydramnios or if the NST was abnormal, the patient was admitted for delivery. The patients fell into four groups as follows:

I—normal BPP, labor begun spontaneously
II—normal BPP, favorable cervix and labor induced
III—abnormal BPP, delivery effected
IV—normal BPP, unfavorable cervix, labor induced electively.

The results show that patients in groups I and II compared to those in group III had a significantly lower incidence of fetal distress, necessitating cesarean section (3% versus 22%), fewer low 5-minute Apgars (1.6% and 3.2% vs 12.5%), and a lower incidence of meconium aspiration syndrome. It was also noted that the patients with oligohydramnios had significantly more morbidity. Curiously, those patients in group IV induced electively were found to have the highest cesarean section rate (42%), again confirming that routine induction has an inherent risk of failure. The BPP appears to be a reliable predictor of fetal well-being in the postterm patient but has the disadvantage of being relatively unavailable and is at times lengthy (30 to 40 minutes per test), which may limit its practical applicability. As noted in the preceding study, postterm patients with oligohydramnios are at especially high risk, and this was confirmed by subsequent work.[44] Using ultrasonic assessment of amniotic fluid volume and the NST, Phelan and co-workers described three groups in terms of amniotic fluid volume: adequate, ≥1 cm; adequate but subjectively decreased; and low, <1 cm. Only the latter result led to intervention. Results demonstrated an increased incidence of antepartum FHR decelerations in groups 2 and 3. Cesarean section for fetal distress was also more common in the decreased fluid groups. The incidence of postmaturity was similar in the three groups.

Bochner evaluated the combined use of the NST and amniotic fluid assessment, noting that if either test was abnormal, there was an increased incidence of fetal distress leading to cesarean section.[47] Each test had excellent and comparable negative predictive value but poor positive predictive value. The authors noted no improvement in the accuracy in either test when combined with the other but stated that when either the NST or AFV was abnormal, a normal result in the other test did not provide reassurance.

Rayburn compared a variety of antepartum tests in a group of 147 postterm pregnancies to determine if any one test was more predictive of the postmaturity syndrome, since this was the subpopulation at greatest risk.[48] Tests used included the NST, BPP, ultrasound evaluation of amniotic fluid volume, and maternal urinary estrogen–creatine (E–C) ratios. The E–C ratio is thought to reflect fetoplacental function. Oligohydramnios was diagnosed when no fluid was seen on ultrasound. Clinical findings, fetal heart rate tracings, and fetal movement charting were found to be unreliable in predicting postmaturity. On the other hand, urinary E–C ratios and ultrasound evidence of oligohydramnios were both specific and sensitive in this regard. Twenty-nine of 147 patients had oligohydramnios, and 83% of these delivered postmature infants, compared to only 7% of infants with adequate amniotic fluid volume. An E–C ratio was obtained within the last week before delivery in 65 patients. Twelve patients had low ratios (<19; one standard deviation below the mean), and all delivered postmature infants, whereas a normal ratio was associated with a postmature infant in only three of 53 cases. The authors concluded that these two tests are reliable in predicting the postmaturity syndrome and are useful in ruling it out. Studies evaluating amniotic fluid volume have not found this to be predictive of postmaturity, as the incidence of this syndrome was similar with both reduced and normal amniotic fluid volumes. Clinically, numerous postmature infants had been born with amniotic fluid volume judged adequate.[44] The definitions of postmaturity seem similar among the different studies, as were the definitions for oligohydramnios (no fluid, <1 cm); thus, the reason for the conflicting results is not clear.

Eden compared various antepartum testing schemes to assess if any one approach was superior; each scheme was initiated with an NST.[49] The first followed the NST, with the CST as back-up in the event of a nonreactive result. The second followed abnormal NSTs with a biophysical profile. The third scheme used the NST and ultrasound evaluation of amniotic fluid as the initial screen and the biophysical profile as back-up. In only the third plan were the FHR decelerations during the NST acted on. These three testing protocols reflected the various approaches in use at different times at one institution and were thus unrandomized. The third scheme led to the highest incidence of induction–delivery (29.4%) but exhibited the lowest rate of intrapartum fetal distress and perinatal morbidity and mortality. The authors conclude that although FHR decelerations were associated with increased perinatal morbidity, intervention for this finding prevented such morbidity.

In review of this variety of approaches to antepartum surveillance, the combination of ultrasound evaluation of amniotic fluid volume and the NST appears to provide reasonable reassurance of fetal well-being, without excessive false positives (ie, unnecessary intervention). Although original reports used a weekly test interval, more recent work supports twice-weekly surveillance. Given the high-risk nature of the postterm patient, it is prudent to maintain a high level of suspicion and to be willing to intervene when any suggestion of fetal compromise exists. The presence of FHR decelerations or evidence of oligohydramnios is especially disconcerting and usually warrants delivery.

INTRAPARTUM MANAGEMENT

INDUCTION

When expectant management is used in the postterm patient, in addition to antepartum surveillance, one must often consider how to effect delivery for either medical or obstetrical indications. In the setting of an inducible cervix, the standard approach of amniotomy and oxytocin achieves a high degree of success.[38] The patient with an uninducible cervix presents the classic obstetrical dilemma. If the concern for fetal well-being is extreme, one may proceed directly to cesarean section, especially when adequate fetal evaluation is not feasible (eg, fetal scalp pH assessment). In those cases where the indication for delivery is less emergent, an effective means of induction must deal with the unfavorable cervix. Current options include using oxytocin alone or using prostaglandin to ripen the cervix prior to oxytocin. Numerous reports have studied the use of prostaglandin for this purpose, addressing such issues as ideal dosage and method of administration (cervical versus vaginal).

Prostaglandin has been used to ripen the unfavorable cervix in a variety of clinical situations at different gestational ages. In one report, the benefit of a preinduction dose of prostaglandin E_2 (PGE_2) was evaluated in 109 patients.[50] Fifty-nine percent of the primigravidas and 50% of the multigravidas in the study were being induced for postdates gestation. Patients with both favorable and unfavorable cervical exams were included. Those patients with an initial Bishop >6 received an intravaginal 6-mg dose of PGE_2 on the morning of induction. Patients with Bishop scores of ≤6 received a vaginal dose of 6 mg of PGE_2 (ripening dose) on the night prior to the scheduled induction (85 patients). If not in labor the next morning, an additional 6 mg PGE_2 was administered intravaginally (induction dose). Patients not in labor 10 hours after the last dose received oxytocin to effect induction. Of the 85 patients who received the ripening dose, 39% were in labor the next morning without further treatment. Results showed that the length of labor was inversely related to the initial Bishop score. Also noted was that the Bishop score was not reliable in predicting which patient entered spontaneous labor secondary to the ripening dose of PGE_2, since 70% of patients who entered labor after just the one dose had Bishop scores <4. Given this, the authors concluded that it was perhaps unwise to give the initial dose the night prior to induction, considering that the majority of patients undergoing induction are high risk and enter labor in the middle of the night. Comments were not provided regarding the effect of the PGE_2 on the Bishop score, how many spontaneously entered labor after the induction dose, and whether the use of PGE_2 in patients with unfavorable cervices improved the overall success of induction.

Several investigators have conducted double-blind, randomized trials to address these questions.[51–53] Hutchon compared intracervical PGE_2 (0.45 to 0.65mg) to placebo in a group of women undergoing induction, for various indications, with Bishop scores ≤4.[51] Sixty-eight percent of the placebo group and 47% of the PGE_2 group were induced for prolonged gestation. The treatment was placed the evening prior to induction. Fifty percent of the group receiving PGE_2 were in labor by the following morning compared to 8% in the placebo group. Induction was initiated by amniotomy. The induction to delivery interval and the total length of labor were significantly reduced in the PGE_2 group. The overall incidence of cesarean section was not different in the two groups. O'Herlihy compared a 2-mg dose of intravaginal PGE_2 (65 patients) to placebo (30 patients) in a group of primigravidas with unfavorable cervices (Bishop score 0 to 3).[53] This study was not blinded or randomized. Fourteen hours elapsed between the drug placement and the subsequent cervical exam. Those patients not in labor at 14 hours whose Bishop score remained <5 received a second dose of PGE_2. The remainder underwent amniotomy and oxytocin induction. Forty-eight percent of the patients receiving PGE_2 were in labor the following morning as compared to none in the control group. Further comparison of the two groups revealed that the use of PGE_2 resulted in significant change in the Bishop score (change 6.6 vs 0.7), as well as a significant reduction in the length of labor and the cesarean section rate compared to the placebo. Nimrod similarly showed that a single dose of intracervical PGE_2 resulted in labor in 30% to 60%, depending on the dose (0.25 vs 0.5 mg).[52] The study population was too small to allow for comparison of cesarean section rates or length of labor. In the large multicenter study of postterm patients cited earlier, use of PGE_2 intracervically (0.5 mg) resulted in spontaneous labor in 42% of patients compared to 24% of placebo patients but failed to have any effect on the length of labor or the cesarean section rate.[39]

Other issues related to the use of PGE_2 include the effect of different doses and the value of sequential applications.[54–56] These studies demonstrated that increasing the dose of either intracervical or vaginal PGE_2 led to a greater number of spontaneous labors, but it also led to more cases of uterine hypertonia and related FHR decelerations, which at times necessitated emergency cesarean section.[54,55] Sequential doses of intravaginal PGE_2 were not found to offer any advantage over a single dose in terms of the number of patients with spontaneous labors, length of labor, or cesarean section rate.[56]

Other concerns involve the adverse effects, which can be either maternal or fetal. Although some reports have noted no increase in fetal distress,[51–53] others have described fetal bradycardias or other signs of fetal compromise associated with PGE_2, usually related to hypertonic uterine activity.[54,55,57] Unfortunately, many of these reports deal with small numbers and thus are not amenable to statistical analysis. Considering that the postterm fetus may be compromised, concern is especially raised when induction is indicated for abnormal antepartum test results.

Overall, there is limited agreement among these reports regarding the effects of PGE_2 on patients with unfavorable Bishop scores, and few conclusions can be drawn. PGE_2 will stimulate labor in approximately 30% to 60% of the patients after a single dose. The effect on the duration of labor is less clear, with two reports demonstrating a decrease[51,53] and one report finding no effect.[39] The effect of parity on PG induction is only considered in two of these reports, with different conclusions drawn. Prins noted that multiparous patients were more likely to enter labor after PGE_2 gel and had a faster rate of active phase dilation compared to primiparous patients.[56] Cesarean section rate did not differ. Houghton, on the other hand, found no difference between multiparous and primiparous patients with regard to the frequency of labor following PGE_2 application.[50] Similarly, changes in cesarean section rates are variable, as a decrease was noted in one study[53] and no change was found in three others.[39,51,57] These latter two issues were not always addressed in the various reports. The other conclusion that can be drawn is that there is a small but definite risk of uterine hypertonia (2% to 18%) and associated fetal distress.[54,55,57]

As with any treatment, one must weigh overall benefits against the risks. With regard to the use of PGE_2 for ripening of the cervix, the benefits appear limited to initiation of labor in a large number of patients, and possibly a reduction in the length of labor, without adversely increasing the rate of cesarean births. Given the known potential effects on the fetus, PGE_2 should be used only with great caution in those situations when induction is initiated for concerns of fetal well-being. In such cases, fetal heart rate monitoring must be continuously used following placement of the PGE_2. Relative contraindications to PGE_2 usage may include evidence of oligohydramnios, the presence of maternal diseases adversely effected by prostaglandins (eg, asthma), and (because of the risk of uterine hypertonia) the presence of a uterine scar.

If PGE_2 is being electively used for cervical ripening and the fetus appears well, fetal heart rate should be monitored for 2 to 4 hours. If labor has not begun and FHR is reassuring, the patient may be discharged home, to return for subsequent oxytocin induction.

FETAL MONITORING

Regardless of whether labor is spontaneous or induced for favorable Bishop score or because of fetal or maternal indications, the postterm fetus should have continuous evaluation at the onset and throughout labor.[15] Initial assessment should include ultrasound evaluation of amniotic fluid volume and of estimated fetal weight. Although a firm rule cannot be made regarding at what weight a cesarean section should be performed, the risks of macrosomia and attendant birth trauma should be strongly considered when the estimated fetal weight is greater than 4500 g. The decision to proceed with a trial of labor in fetuses estimated to weigh between 4000 and 4500 g should be based on a number of factors, including prior obstetrical history, maternal size, presence of diabetes, and maternal consent. Additional specific intrapartum concerns include the increased incidence of meconium passage with risk of aspiration, oligohydramnios with associated umbilical cord vulnerability, and uteroplacental insufficiency.[15]

Miller first addressed the significance of meconium in labor in 1974.[26] Both postterm and term patients were studied in regard to FHR patterns and fetal scalp pH. The fetuses with meconium passage had an increase in low 5-minute Apgars, compared to fetuses without meconium passage, but other indicators of fetal distress, such as low pH and FHR abnormalities, occurred with similar frequency in the two groups. The authors noted that meconium alone does not constitute a sign of fetal distress and that if FHR patterns and scalp pH were normal, these fetuses tended to do very well. In a subsequent report in 1981, Miller evaluated a group of postterm patients with intrapartum meconium passage.[42] When compared to term fetuses, postterm fetuses that passed meconium in labor had an increased incidence of low 1- and 5-minute Apgars and lower scalp pH at various sampling periods. On the other hand, the incidence and severity of abnormal FHR patterns was no different. The authors concluded that the postterm fetus that passes meconium in labor should undergo fetal scalp pH assessment, even in the setting of a normal FHR pattern.

Based on Miller's recommendations, routine fetal pH assessment was obtained in a group of 56 postterm patients with intrapartum meconium passage.[58] Nine fetuses (16%) had scalp pH ≤ 7.2. One of these fetuses demonstrated no FHR decelerations (pH = 7.04); another had only mild variable decelerations (pH = 7.19). None of the fetuses found to be acidemic manifested fetal heart accelerations (defined as FHR increase of ≥ 15 bpm, lasting ≥ 15 seconds at peak). This observation suggests that the absence of classic signs of fetal distress, such as late decelerations, is less reliable than the presence of a reactive FHR pattern with accelerations in the prediction of fetal well-being. Furthermore, of those fetuses who failed to exhibit qualifying accelerations, 33% were found to be acidotic. Thus, these results suggest that if the postterm fetus passes meconium in labor, the presence of FHR accelerations is reassuring of fetal well-being, and when present obviates the need for routine scalp sampling.

Bochner similarly confirmed the value of normal FHR patterns in patients with intrapartum meconium passage.[59] He studied the outcome of postterm patients with and without meconium and found that in the setting of meconium passage early in labor, there was an increase in the incidence of fetal distress leading to cesarean section and low 1-minute Apgar scores. This group was further analyzed with regard to antenatal testing (twice-weekly NST and amniotic fluid assessment) done within 4 days of delivery. It was noted that those patients demonstrating normal antepartum testing and meconium passage early in labor were at no greater risk for fetal distress in labor than those patients with normal test results and no intrapartum meconium. The authors concluded that recent antepartum testing was useful in predicting the potential significance of meconium passage early in labor and perinatal tolerance.

Oligohydramnios is another risk for the postterm fetus. Leveno has reported that in 727 postterm pregnancies, 59 (8%) were delivered by cesarean section for fetal distress.[41] The FHR patterns were usually variable decelerations associated with cord compression, as opposed to late decelerations associated with uteroplacental insufficiency. Furthermore, ultrasound evidence of oligohydramnios was associated with a significant increase in the cesarean section rate for fetal distress. Given such information, saline amnioinfusion has been useful, given variable decelerations when oligohydramnios is confirmed.[60,61] Miyazaki described this approach in a randomized study, noting that amnioinfusion resulted in relief of the variable decelerations in 51% of the cases as opposed to 4% of the control group. The possible role of prophylactic amnioinfusion in patients with oligohydramnios without signs of fetal distress is currently under investigation at our institution, the University of Southern California. Wenstrom evaluated the use of amnioinfusion in patients with thick meconium in an attempt to reduce the incidence of meconium aspiration.[62] Eighty-five patients with thick meconium detected on membrane rupture or amniocentesis were randomized to receive prophylactic intrapartum amnioinfusion or routine care. Amnioinfusion consisted of 1000 mL normal saline infused over 20 to 40 minutes and was repeated every 6 hours until delivery. Prophylactic amnioinfusion in this setting resulted in a significant reduction in the incidence of fetal distress requiring operative intervention (3% vs 22%), low 1-minute Apgar scores, meconium below the cords, and meconium aspiration syndrome (0 vs 7%).

RECOMMENDATIONS

Initially, accuracy of the postterm diagnosis should be confirmed and followed by a search for any medical (eg, hypertension) or obstetrical (eg, growth retardation, abnormal fetal lie, spontaneous rupture of membranes) complications warranting delivery. (Figure 89-1 illustrates management of the postterm pregnancy.) For those patients lacking accurate dating criteria (ie, poor dates), expectant management should be initiated, with twice-weekly NST and AFV assessment. Any plan to induce a patient with unsure dates electively necessitates verification of fetal lung maturity. In those patients diagnosed postterm by good dating criteria, cervical inducibility should be evaluated and, if present (Bishop score >6), labor induction should be considered. The remaining postterm patients with unfavorable cervices can be assessed by ultrasound. Delivery should be considered when the fetal weight is estimated at >4000 g or oligohydramnios (AFI <5) is present. If the ultrasound suggests neither of these, expectant management can be undertaken with twice-weekly NST and amniotic fluid volume measurement. The patient should have weekly exams to evaluate cervical inducibility, development of medical complications, or obstetrical factors indicating delivery.

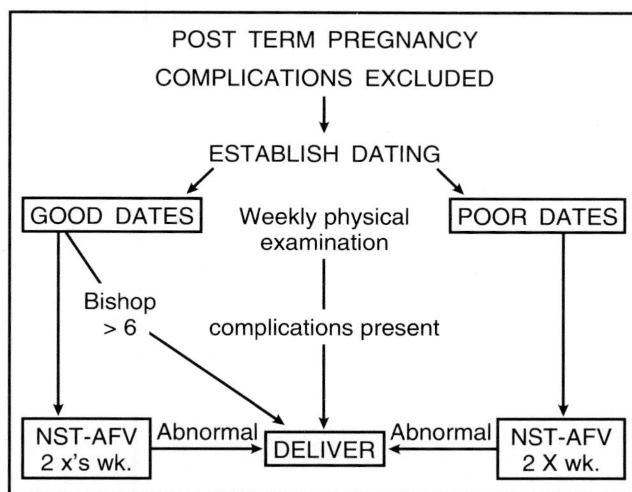

FIGURE 89–1. Management of the postterm pregnancy. (AFI, amniotic fluid index.)

SUMMARY

In conclusion, the postterm pregnancy continues to be a significant management dilemma. In spite of a large body of literature, controversy remains regarding what constitutes ideal management. A reasonable approach is to individualize treatment for each patient as opposed to adopting any rigid protocol. Given a confirmed postdate pregnancy an elective induction can be undertaken if the cervix is favorable. In patients with an unfavorable cervix and lacking medical or obstetrical complications, expectant management is acceptable and is probably prudent.

REFERENCES

1. Cardozo L, Fysh J, Pearce JM. Prolonged pregnancy: the management debate. Br Med J 1986;293:1059.
2. American College of Obstetricians and Gynecologists. Diagnosis and management of postterm pregnancy (ACOG Technical Bulletin 130). Washington, DC: ACOG, 1987.
3. Anderson GG. Postmaturity: a review. Obstet Gynecol Surv 1972;27:65.
4. Beischer NA, Evans JH, Townsend L. Studies in prolonged pregnancy. I. The incidence of prolonged pregnancy. Am J Obstet Gynecol 1969;103(4):476.
5. Eden RD, Seifert LS, Winegar A, Spellacy WN. Perinatal characteristics of uncomplicated postdates pregnancies. Obstet Gynecol 1987;69:296.

6. Lagrew DC, Freeman RK. Management of postdate pregnancy. Am J Obstet Gynecol 1986;154:8.
7. McClure-Brown, JC. Postmaturity. Am J Obstet Gynecol 1963; 85(5):573.
8. Saito M, Yazawa K, Hashiguchi A, Kumasaka T, Nishi N, Kato K. Time of ovulation and prolonged pregnancy. Am J Obstet Gynecol 1972;112(1):31.
9. Dyson DC. Fetal surveillance vs labor induction at 42 weeks in postterm gestation. J Reprod Med 1988;33(3):262.
10. Yeh S, Read JA. Management of post term pregnancy in a large obstetric population. Obstet Gynecol 1982;60:282.
11. Warsof SL, Pearce JM, Campbell S. The present place of routine ultrasound screening. Clin Obstet Gynecol 1983;10:445.
12. Persson PH, Gennser G. Benefits of ultrasound screening of a pregnant population. Acta Obstet Gynaecol Scand (Suppl) 1978;78:5.
13. O'Brien GD, Queenan JT. Dating gestation in the first 20 weeks. In: Sanders RC, James AE, eds. The principles and practice of ultrasonography in obstetrics and gynecology, 3rd ed. Norwalk, CT: Appleton-Century-Crofts, 1985:141.
14. Freeman RK, Garite TJ, Modanlau H, Dorchester W, Rommal C, Devaney M. Postdates pregnancy: utilization of contraction stress testing for primary fetal surveillance. Am J Obstet Gynecol 1981;140:128.
15. Yeh S, Bruce SL, Thorton YS. Intrapartum monitoring and management of the postdate fetus. Clin Perinatol 1982;9(2):381.
16. Lazer S, Biale Y, Mazor M, Lewenthal H, Insler V. Complications associated with the macrosomic fetus. J Reprod Med 1986;31(6): 501.
17. Spellacy WN, Miller S, Winegar A, Peterson PQ. Macrosomia—maternal characteristics and infant complications. Obstet Gynecol 1985;66:158.
18. Crowley P, O'Herlihy C, Boylan P. The value of ultrasound measurement of amniotic fluid volume in the management of prolonged pregnancies. Br J Obstet Gynaecol 1984;91:444.
19. Phelan JP, Ahn MO, Smith CV, Rutherford SE, Anderson E. Amniotic fluid index measurements during pregnancy. J Reprod Med 1987;32(8):601.
20. Rutherford SE, Phelan JP, Smith CV, Jacobs N. The four-quadrant assessment of amniotic fluid volume: an adjunct to antepartum fetal heart rate testing. Obstet Gynecol 1987;70:353.
21. Phelan JP, Smith CV, Broussard P, Small M. Amniotic fluid volume assessment with four-quadrant technique at 36–42 weeks gestation. J Reprod Med 1987;32(7):540.
22. Beischer NA, Brown JB, Townsend L. Studies in prolonged pregnancy. III. Amniocentesis in prolonged pregnancy. Am J Obstet Gynecol 1969;103(4):456.
23. Phelan JP, Platt LD, Yeh S, Broussard P, Paul RH. The role of ultrasound assessment of amniotic fluid volume in the management of the postdate pregnancy. Am J Obstet Gynecol 1985;151:304.
24. Green JN, Paul RH. Value of amniocentesis in prolonged pregnancy. Obstet Gynecol 1978;51:293.
25. Knox GE, Huddleston JF, Flowers CE. Management of prolonged pregnancy: results of a prospective randomized trial. Am J Obstet Gynecol 1979;134:376.
26. Miller FC, Sachs DA, Yeh SY, Paul RH, Schiffrin BS, Martin CB, Hon EH. Significance of meconium during labor. Am J Obstet Gynecol 1975;122:573.
27. Davis RO, Philips JB, Harris BA, Wilson ER, Huddleston JF. Fatal meconium aspiration syndrome occurring despite airway management considered appropriate. Am J Obstet Gynecol 1985; 151:731.
28. Paul RH, Yonekura ML, Cantrell CJ, et al. Fetal injury prior to labor: does it happen? Am J Obstet Gynecol 1986;154:1187.
29. Sundo C, Kasasa TS, Hale RW. Meconium aspiration syndrome without evidence of fetal distress in early labor before elective cesarean delivery. Obstet Gynecol 1989;73:707.
30. Clifford SH. Postmaturity—with placental dysfunction. J Pediatr 1954;44:1.
31. Shime J. Influence of prolonged pregnancy on infant development. J Reprod Med 1983;33(3):277.
32. Vorherr H. Placental insufficiency in relation to postterm pregnancy and fetal postmaturity. Am J Obstet Gynecol 1975; 123(1):67.
33. Shime J, Gare DJ, Andrews J. Prolonged pregnancy: surveillance of the fetus and the neonate and the course of labor and delivery. Am J Obstet Gynecol 1984;148:547.
34. Mannino F. Neonatal complications of postterm gestation. J Reprod Med 1988;33(3):271.
35. Harris BA, Huddleston JF, Sutliff G, Perlis HW. The unfavorable cervix in prolonged pregnancy. Obstet Gynecol 1983;62:171.
36. Johnson JM, Harman CR, Lange IR, et al. Biophysical profile scoring in the management of postterm pregnancy: an analysis of 307 patients. Am J Obstet Gynecol 1986;154:269.
37. Gibb DMF, Cardozo LD, Studd JWW, Cooper DJ. Prolonged pregnancy: is induction of labour indicated? A prospective study. Br J Obstet Gynaecol 1982;89:292.
38. Bishop EH. Pelvic scoring for elective induction. Obstet Gynecol 1964;24(2):266.
39. Medearis AL. Postterm pregnancy: active labor induction (PGE_2 Gel) not associated with improved outcomes compared to expectant management. A preliminary report. NICHD Maternal Fetal Medicine Network (in preparation).
40. Dyson DC, Miller PD, Armstrong MA. Management of prolonged pregnancy: induction of labor versus antepartum fetal testing. Am J Obstet Gynecol 1987;156:928.
41. Leveno KJ, Quirk JG, Cunningham G, et al. Prolonged pregnancy. I. Observations concerning the causes of fetal distress. Am J Obstet Gynecol 1984;150:465.
42. Miller FC, Read JA. Intrapartum assessment of the post date fetus. Am J Obstet Gynecol 1981;141:516.
43. Miyazaki FS, Miyazaki BA. False reactive nonstress tests in postterm pregnancies. Am J Obstet Gynecol 1981;140:269.
44. Phelan JP, Platt LD, Yeh SY, Trujillo M, Paul RH. Continuing role of the nonstress test in the management of post dates pregnancy. Obstet Gynecol 1984;64:624.
45. Small ML, Phelan JP, Smith CV, Paul RH. An active management approach to the postdates fetus with a reactive nonstress test and fetal heart rate decelerations. Obstet Gynecol 1987;70:636.
46. Manning FA, Platt LD, Sipos L. Antepartum fetal evaluation: development of a fetal biophysical profile. Am J Obstet Gynecol 1980;136:787.
47. Bochner CJ, Medearis AL, Davis J, Oakes GK, Hobel CJ, Wade ME. Antepartum predictors of fetal distress. Am J Obstet Gynecol 1987;157:353.
48. Rayburn WF, Motley ME, Stempel LE, Gendreau RM. Antepartum prediction of the postmature infant. Obstet Gynecol 1982;60:148.
49. Eden RD, Gergely RZ, Schifrin BS, Wade ME. Comparison of antepartum testing schemes for the management of the postdate pregnancy. Am J Obstet Gynecol 1982;144:683.
50. Houghton DJ. An evaluation of the Bishop scoring system in relation to a method of induction of labor by intravaginal prostaglandin. Postgrad Med J 1982;58:403.
51. Hutchon DJR, Geirsson R, Patal NB. A double blind controlled trial of PGE_2 gel in cervical ripening. Int J Gynaecol Obstet 1980;17:604.
52. Nimrod C, Currie J, Yee J, Dodd G, Persaud D. Cervical ripening

and labor induction with intracervical triacetin base prostaglandin E_2 gel: a placebo-controlled study. Obstet Gynecol 1984; 64:476.
53. O'Herlihy C, MacDonald HN. Influence of preinduction prostaglandin E_2 vaginal gel on cervical ripening and labor. Obstet Gynecol 1979;54(6):708.
54. Graves GR, Baskett TF, Gray JH, Luther ER. The effect of vaginal administration of various doses of prostaglandin E_2 gel on cervical ripening and induction of labor. Am J Obstet Gynecol 1985;151(2):178.
55. Laube DW, Zlatnik FJ, Pitkin RM. Preinduction cervical ripening with prostaglandin E_2 intracervical gel. Obstet Gynecol 1986; 68:54.
56. Prins RP, Neilson DR, Bolton RN, Mark C, Watson P. Preinduction cervical ripening with sequential use of prostaglandin E_2 gel. Am J Obstet Gynecol 1986;154:1275.
57. Buchanan D, Macer J, Yonekura ML. Cervical ripening with prostaglandin E_2 vaginal suppositories. Obstet Gynecol 1984;63:659.
58. Shaw KJ, Clark SL. Reliability of intrapartum fetal heart rate monitoring in the postterm fetus with meconium passage. Obstet Gynecol 1988;72(6):886.
59. Bochner CJ, Medearis AL, Ross MG, et al. The role of antepartum testing in the management of postterm pregnancies with heavy meconium in early labor. Obstet Gynecol 1987;69:893.
60. Miyazaki FS, Nevarez F. Saline amnioinfusion for relief of repetitive variable decelerations: a prospective randomized study. Am J Obstet Gynecol 1985;153:301.
61. Miyazaki FS, Taylor NA. Saline amnioinfusion for relief of variable or prolonged decelerations. A preliminary report. Am J Obstet Gynecol 1983;146:670.
62. Wenstrom KD, Parsons MT. The prevention of meconium aspiration in labor using amnioinfusion. Obstet Gynecol 1989;73:647.

90

CHAPTER

ANESTHESIA IN THE HIGH-RISK PATIENT

Hilda Pedersen, Alan C. Santos, and Mieczyslaw Finster

The anesthetic management of the high-risk parturient is based on the same general principles as the management of healthy mothers and fetuses. These include maintenance of maternal cardiovascular function and oxygenation; maintenance, and possibly improvement, of the uteroplacental blood flow; and creation of optimal conditions for an atraumatic, painless delivery of an infant free of significant drug effects. There is, however, less room for error, as many of the preceding functions may be compromised before the induction of anesthesia. Since the high-risk parturient may have received a variety of drugs, one must be familiar with potential interactions between these drugs and the anesthetic agents to be administered.

CARDIOVASCULAR DISEASES

PREECLAMPSIA–ECLAMPSIA

Hypertensive disorders, which occur in approximately 7% of pregnancies, account for about 20% of maternal fatalities and lead to 30,000 neonatal deaths and stillbirths per year in the United States alone. Preeclampsia–eclampsia is a disease of unknown etiology. It is unique to human pregnancy, occurring predominantly in young nulliparas. One proposed theory invokes immunologic rejection of fetal tissues by the mother, causing placental vasculitis and ischemia.[1] This explains why the disease is more common among nulliparas (no previous exposure to a trophoblast) and in conditions associated with an abnormally large mass of trophoblastic tissues, as in hydatidiform mole, multiple pregnancy, diabetes, and Rh incompatibility. More recently, it has been postulated that preeclampsia–eclampsia may be due to an imbalance between thromboxane and prostacyclin secreted by the placenta.[2,3] Thromboxane is a potent vasoconstrictor and stimulator of platelet aggregation; prostacyclin produces opposite effects. This theory is supported by some evidence that pretreatment with aspirin, which decreases production of thromboxane in placental arteries, reduces the incidence of preeclampsia.[4]

Although preeclampsia is accompanied by exaggerated retention of water and sodium, the shift of fluid and proteins from the intravascular into the extravascular compartment may result in hypovolemia, hypoproteinemia, and hemoconcentration. This phenomenon may be further aggravated by proteinuria. The mean plasma volume in women with preeclampsia was found to be 9% below normal, and in those with severe disease, it was as much as 30% to 40% below normal.[5] It has also been shown that a significant reduction in the maternal plasma volume may precede the clinical appearance of preeclampsia in previously normotensive patients.[6] Prior to the start of therapy these patients usually have a low cardiac index, low pulmonary capillary wedge pressure, and high systemic vascular resistance.[7] Thrombocytopenia and elevation in the serum concentration of fibrin–fibrinogen degradation products is not uncommon in severe cases. In addition, a significant proportion of patients with preeclampsia develop an acquired defect in platelet function (impaired thromboxane B_2 biosynthesis), resulting in prolongation of bleeding time.[8] HELLP syndrome, a variant of severe preeclampsia, may develop either antepartum or postpartum.[9] It is characterized by hemolysis, elevated liver enzymes, and a low platelet count. Maternal and fetal prognoses are poor.

General Management

The mainstay of anticonvulsant therapy in this country is magnesium sulfate. Although its efficacy in preventing seizures has been well substantiated, its mechanism of action remains controversial. Magnesium potentiates the duration and intensity of action of both depolarizing and nondepolarizing muscle relaxants by decreasing the amount of acetylcholine liberated from the motor nerve terminals, diminishing the sensitivity of the end-plate to acetylcholine and depressing the excitability of the muscle membrane.

The aim of fluid therapy is to raise the CVP and pulmonary capillary wedge pressure to the normal range (4 to 6 cm H_20 and 5 to 10 mm Hg, respectively) and to raise the urine output to 1 mL/kg/h. This has been shown to improve the cardiac index and to prevent abrupt, often precipitous drops in blood pressure associated with vasodilator therapy.[10]

Hydralazine (Apresoline) is the most commonly used vasodilator in preeclampsia, as it has been shown to increase both uteroplacental and renal blood flows. Sodium nitroprusside (Nipride), a potent vasodilator of resistance and capacitance vessels with an immediate but evanescent action, is useful in preventing dangerous elevations in systemic and pulmonary blood pressure during laryngoscopy and intubation and is ideal for treatment of hypertensive emergencies. Its infusion can be decreased gradually in the interim, when a longer-acting agent, such as hydralazine, is beginning to take effect. Infusion rates of sodium nitroprusside below 5 to 10 μg/kg/min, depending on the length of administration, can be maintained without undue risk of cyanide toxicity in the mother and fetus.[11] Trimethaphan (Arfonad), a ganglionic blocking agent, is particularly useful in hypertensive emergencies, when cerebral edema and increased intracranial pressure are of particular concern, since it will not cause vasodilation in the brain. Other agents used less frequently to control maternal blood pressure in preeclampsia include alphamethyldopa and clonidine (acting in the CNS), as well as nitroglycerin, ketanserin (a serotonin receptor antagonist), atenolol (a beta-adrenoreceptor antagonist), and labetalol (a nonselective beta blocker with some $alpha_1$-blocking effects).

Anesthetic Management

Epidural anesthesia for labor and delivery should no longer be considered contraindicated in preeclampsia, providing there is no clotting abnormality or plasma volume deficit. In volume-repleted patients positioned with left uterine displacement, epidural anesthesia leads to a significant improvement in placental perfusion. With the use of radioactive xenon, it was shown that following the epidural injection of 10 mL bupivacaine 0.25% the intervillous blood flow in severe preeclamptics increased by approximately 75%.[12] Spinal anesthesia should be used with great caution, unless given in divided doses through an indwelling subarachnoid catheter, since it produces severe alterations in cardiovascular dynamics due to sudden sympathetic blockade.

For cesarean section, the level of regional anesthesia must extend to T3–T4, making adequate fluid therapy and left uterine displacement even more vital. Should hypotension occur, its correction will require a reduced dose of ephedrine in view of the increased sensitivity to vasopressors.

General anesthesia in preeclamptic patients has its particular hazards. The rapid sequence induction and intubation necessary to avoid aspiration are occasionally difficult because of upper-airway edema. Laryngoscopy may provoke profuse bleeding in patients with impaired coagulation. Marked rises in systemic and pulmonary arterial pressure occurring at intubation and extubation enhance the risk of cerebral hemorrhage and pulmonary edema.[13,14] An appropriate antihypertensive therapy, such as administration of trimethaphan or nitroprusside infusion, will minimize these hemodynamic changes. Ketamine and ergot alkaloids should be avoided. As already mentioned, magnesium sulfate may prolong effects of all muscle relaxants through its actions on the myoneural junction. Therefore, relaxants should be administered with caution (using a nerve stimulator) to avoid overdosage. General anesthesia is indicated in acute emergencies, such as abruptio placentae, and in patients who do not meet the criteria for epidural anesthesia.

HEART DISEASE

Heart disease during pregnancy remains the leading nonobstetric cause of maternal mortality,[15,16] which ranges from 0.4% among patients in class I or II of the New York Heart Association's functional classification, to 6.8% among those in classes III and IV. Cardiac decompensation and death occur most commonly at the time of maximum hemodynamic stress (ie, in the third trimester of pregnancy, during labor and delivery, and the immediate postpartum period).

Rheumatic Heart Disease

Mitral stenosis is the most frequent valvular lesion in parturients with rheumatic heart disease. When the valve orifice is diminished or the rate of blood flow through the constricted orifice is increased sufficiently to raise left atrial pressure and, consequently, pressure in the pulmonary veins and capillaries, the lesion becomes hemodynamically significant. During pregnancy the rate of flow across the mitral orifice is augmented by the increase in cardiac output and pulse rate. Mitral commissurotomy may be required because of symptoms of congestive heart failure or, less frequently, because of hemoptysis or emboli. When performed in the second or early third trimester, both closed and open commissurotomies have been reported to be well tolerated by the mother and accompanied by fetal survival in excess of 80%.[17]

Other valvular diseases—namely, mitral regurgitation and aortic stenosis or regurgitation—are found much less frequently among pregnant cardiac patients. Together they amount to between 10% and 35% of all cases. Pure mitral regurgitation is rarely a problem, nor is pure aortic insufficiency. Pure aortic stenosis is rarely significant before the patient reaches her fifth or sixth decade, but the condition is frequently associated with aortic insufficiency and mitral stenosis.

Congenital Heart Diseases

Patent ductus arteriosus, atrial septal defect, and ventricular septal defect are the more common congenital cardiovascular abnormalities. In all these conditions, there are anomalous communicating channels between the cardiac chambers and/or the great vessels. Normally, there is a left-to-right shunt because pressures on the left side of the circulation are higher than those on the right. Pulmonary hypertension may develop late in the natural history of these diseases, causing a reversal of the shunt (Eisenmenger's syndrome). During pregnancy, the decrease in systemic vascular resistance, in the presence of fixed pulmonary vascular resistance, results in a significant increase in the right-to-left shunt.[18] Changes in systemic and pulmonary pressures may also occur with the aortocaval compression, with hypotension complicating epidural or spinal anesthesia, and with efforts to bear down during parturition. Severe shunt disturbances induced by these changes may lead to further cyanosis, even death.

Tetralogy of Fallot is the most common cyanotic congenital heart disease.[19] It consists of an interventricular septal defect, pulmonary stenosis, displacement of the aortic orifice so that it overlies the ventricular septal defect, and right ventricular hypertrophy. The pulmonary stenosis leads to increases in right ventricular systolic pressure, dilation, and hypertrophy of that chamber. Blood from the right ventricle is shunted through the septal defect, so that the aorta receives an admixture of venous blood from the right and oxygenated blood from the left ventricle. Most of the patients become symptomatic during the first few months of life, but the introduction of cardiac surgery has increased the number of those surviving to childbearing age.

Anesthetic Management

Continuous epidural block not only eliminates pain and tachycardia throughout labor and delivery, but also prevents the progressive increase in cardiac output and stroke volume normally occurring during parturition. It also abolishes the bearing-down reflex. In view of these advantages, continuous lumbar epidural analgesia is recommended for most pregnant women with rheumatic valvular diseases except for those with severe, symptomatic aortic stenosis, in whom even transient episodes of hypotension may result in serious coronary hypoperfusion, arrhythmias, and even cardiac arrest. Intrathecal narcotics have been used to provide obstetric analgesia without the risk of hypotension.[20] Morphine (0.5 to 1.5 mg) or fentanyl (37.5 to 50 μg) is usually effective in relieving pain of uterine contractions, but pudendal block is required for delivery. If general anesthesia is required for cesarean section, the standard thiopental–nitrous oxide–halogenated anesthetic–muscle relaxant technique is recommended. In cases of severe mitral stenosis, etomidate (0.2 to 0.3 mg/kg) or a slow induction with halothane or intravenous fentanyl is preferred. Halogenated agents should be avoided in patients with severe aortic stenosis and left ventricular compromise.[21]

Parturients with cyanotic heart disease require effective pain relief without increasing the right-to-left shunt. Thus, hypotension, struggling, or coughing should be avoided, and bearing-down efforts should be eliminated. For labor, intrathecal narcotics should be administered in preference to epidural anesthesia. For cesarean section, light planes of general anesthesia are usually well tolerated.[21]

DIABETES MELLITUS

Insulin-dependent diabetes mellitus is one of the most common medical complications encountered in pregnancy, occurring in about 0.1% to 0.5% of all pregnant women.[22] Dramatic improvements in pregnancy outcome have been achieved over recent years, with many centers having perinatal mortality figures of less than 4% for insulin-dependent cases.[23]

Risks vary considerably according to the classification of the disease, the two main groups being gestational and pregestational in onset. Gestational diabetes has been estimated by different screening and diagnostic criteria to be present in 3% to 12% of pregnant women in this country.[24] It is defined as "carbohydrate intolerance of variable severity, with onset or first recognition during the present pregnancy."[25] The chance of complications is minimal if this condition is well controlled by diet, but more than half of affected women ultimately develop permanent diabetes.[26] The risk assessment system by White,[27] widely used in the past to predict perinatal outcome, describes the range of severity of the disease, although infant mortality is now greatly reduced in all classes (A to R).

Pregnancy itself is diabetogenic. The potential for gluconeogenesis is greatly increased during gestation, along with increased lipolysis and release of free fatty acids into the circulation. More insulin is required to offset this rapid rate of ketosis. Placental lactogen has a contrainsulin effect and rises steadily during pregnancy,[28] as do placental estrogen and progesterone, which have been shown to result in enhanced beta-cell hypertrophy and insulin secretion.[29]

Because of relative insulin deficiency, diabetic pregnant women are at increased risk of severe hyperglycemia and ketoacidosis,[30] which is a major cause of perinatal morbidity and mortality. The maintenance of euglycemia is the primary objective of management and has a positive effect on perinatal outcome and on maternal and fetal complications.[31] Many studies have confirmed that intrauterine death and neonatal mortality may result if diabetic management is not tightly controlled.

The insulin requirement during pregnancy may rise steadily until it is two to three times the prepregnancy dose, decreasing during the last month. In the first trimester the mother may be particularly susceptible to hypoglycemic reactions.

Close control of diabetes is equally important in the intrapartum period. Several techniques may be used to maintain glucose levels during labor. A continuous intravenous infusion of both insulin and glucose is common. Ten units of regular insulin added to a 1000-mL solution of 5% dextrose, given at the rate of 100 mL/h by constant infusion pump, will result in glucose levels below 100 mg/dL. An alternative is to give the patient one third of the prepregnancy dose of intermediate-acting insulin on the morning of delivery. Capillary glucose measurements should be determined every 1 to 2 hours, and regular insulin supplements should be given if necessary. In the immediate postpartum period the patient's insulin requirements are usually lower than those before pregnancy, so that for 48 hours insulin should be given only as needed.[32] If cesarean section is anticipated, the morning insulin dose should be omitted, the procedure planned for early in the day, and a 5% dextrose solution infused, with hourly blood glucose determinations.

ANESTHETIC MANAGEMENT

One of the most specific changes that affects anesthetic management of diabetic parturients is the decrease in uteroplacental blood flow.[33] Placental villi are enlarged, decreasing the volume of intervillous space, so that blood flow in the placenta may be decreased by as much as 35% to 45% in the last trimester.[34]

Oxygen transport, saturation, and tension are impaired in insulin-dependent diabetics because of the increase in Hb A_{1c}.[35] Binding of 2,3-DPG to hemoglobin is inhibited by the presence of hexose in the molecule. Increased affinity of fetal Hb for oxygen may also lead to complications (decreased buffering capacity). These problems make for greater fetal vulnerability to decreased uterine blood flow and hypoxia.

Labor

Lumbar epidural block can provide excellent pain relief for both labor and delivery, if necessary. Avoidance, or immediate treatment, of maternal hypotension is extremely important for the reasons stated earlier. Rapid infusion of a dextrose-free solution should be administered via a second intravenous catheter, ephedrine 10 to 30 mg IV can be given promptly if there is an episode of hypotension despite careful precautions.

Cesarean Section

Again, it is important to prevent hyperglycemia; 5% dextrose solution should be given at a constant rate of 5 to 7.5 g/h. Regional anesthesia is useful, as it enables the anesthesiologist to evaluate the mental status of the patient and to detect potential hypoglycemia. Care should be taken to avoid hypotension by adequate left uterine displacement and administration of dextrose-free solutions. Ringer's lactate, because of the high lactate content, is not ideal, and Normosol-R is preferable for plasma volume expansion. General anesthesia is not contraindicated, as long as there is adequate care in avoiding hypoglycemic injury.

Acid–base values in newborn cord samples following both spinal and epidural anesthesia for cesarean section have shown acidosis, which correlates with the severity of maternal diabetes and hypotension.[36] The mechanisms of this acidosis are probably complex and may be related to lactic acid release from the placenta during relative hypoxia, such as during maternal hypotension[37]; to elevated fetal blood sugar, which has been shown to correlate with umbilical artery acidosis and low 1-minute Apgar scores[38,39]; or to hyperinsulinemia in the fetus, which has been postulated to lead to increased oxygen consumption.[40] Later studies in well-controlled diabetics, where large volumes of glucose-containing solutions were avoided and blood pressure was well maintained, failed to show any association between spinal or epidural anesthesia and newborn acidosis.[41]

The sharp temporary drop in insulin requirement after delivery dictates caution in the use of insulin at this stage.[32] Another source of perioperative instability may be the autonomic dysfunction sometimes seen in neurologically impaired diabetics. It should be remembered that severe hypoglycemia from inappropriate insulin dosage, or inadequate glucose administration, can cause severe CNS injury or death.

NEUROLOGIC DISEASES

Neurologic diseases do not occur with great frequency during the childbearing years. Only those more commonly seen will be discussed here: epilepsy, myasthenia gravis, multiple sclerosis, paraplegia, and muscular dystrophy. Subarachnoid hemorrhage, caused by rupture of an aneurysm or arteriovenous angioma, is rare but very important because of the high mortality associated with it.

EPILEPSY

Idiopathic epilepsy is fairly frequent in our society (incidence approximately 0.5%) and is most commonly seen first in the child or young adult.[42] Many anticonvulsant drugs are in common use, such as phenobarbital, phenytoin, and primidone. Metabolism of these drugs occurs mostly in the liver, and long-term administration may lead to enzyme induction, which can in turn result in increased metabolism of other drugs sharing the same pathways, such as halothane and fluroxene. On the other hand, some drugs may compete for degradation pathways, resulting in a rise in plasma levels of anticonvulsant. For example, diazepam, chloramphenicol, and aminosalicylic acid may increase phenytoin levels. Phenytoin, acting on the prejunctional membrane, may augment the neuromuscular blocking properties of nondepolarizing muscle relaxants, such as D-tubocurarine.[43]

The frequency of seizures may rise during pregnancy, and preeclampsia is more common in epileptic patients, as are premature labor, cesarean section, and fetal anomalies.[44] Prematurity, congenital malformations, and intrauterine growth retardation account for the higher fetal mortality rates. Plasma concentrations of epileptic drugs fall as gestation proceeds, which may be related to decreased absorption and increased clearance of the medications, or to the dilutional effects of rising plasma volume. However, if seizure frequency does not change, increases in dose are not usually advised.[45]

Anomalies, especially cleft lip or palate, heart disease, and spina bifida, occur several times more often than in the regular population and are believed to be partly due to anticonvulsant medications.[46] Newborns require close observation, both for withdrawal symptoms and because of depression of vitamin K–dependent clotting factors.

Local anesthetic techniques may be useful in labor and delivery, since no greater sensitivity to these drugs has been shown than that in normal patients. Where general anesthesia is used for cesarean section, drugs with convulsive potential should be avoided (eg, enflurane, ketamine, and methohexital), as should wide variations in pCO_2. Narcotic–diazepam combinations are useful after delivery.

Status epilepticus requires rapid intervention, with control of seizures and ventilation, and monitoring of vital signs and acid–base, as well as fetal heart rate. Diazepam infusion to blood concentrations of 0.2 to 0.4 μg/mL is usually sufficient, but general endotracheal anesthesia, with the use of nondepolarizing muscle relaxants, may be necessary.

MYASTHENIA GRAVIS

Myasthenia gravis occurs twice as often in women as in men and usually occurs in the early childbearing years. It is an autoimmune disorder that is characterized by excessive muscle fatigue with exercise, affecting the ocular, laryngeal, facial, and respiratory muscles. Partial recovery follows rest and treatment with anticholinesterase drugs. Remission is common in pregnancy, but muscle weakness has also been known to increase.

Facilities for intensive respiratory care should be available at the time of delivery. Medication is usually changed from oral pyridostigmine to parenteral injections, and respiratory function and ECG are evaluated. For pain relief, the most useful, if feasible, is lumbar epidural anesthesia, which affords the flexibility of allowing rest in the first stage of labor and adequate analgesia for elective outlet forceps delivery (often undertaken to shorten the second stage); it can also be extended for cesarean section. Large doses of ester-type local anesthetics, such as 2-chloroprocaine (Nesacaine), because of their hydrolysis by cholinesterase, carry a potential for greater toxicity in patients on anticholinesterase drugs. All parenteral analgesics will compromise respiration, and general anesthesia may necessitate extended ventilator support. Small doses of nondepolarizing agents are recommended, if necessary, with careful monitoring of neuromuscular function.

Twelve percent of babies will have neonatal myasthenia, with symptoms improving in about 3 weeks.[47] Anticholinesterase drugs may be required.

MULTIPLE SCLEROSIS

Multiple sclerosis (MS) is a demyelinating disease characterized by remissions and exacerbations, with progressive deterioration of the central nervous system. The relapse rate during the first 3 months postpartum is several times higher than that in the pregnant state, and the exacerbation rate is lower during pregnancy. Evidence relating any form of anesthesia to the progress of MS has been lacking, and many argue that patients should not be denied regional anesthesia for pain relief during labor and delivery.[48] The hesitation on the part of some anesthesiologists to provide this is related to concerns about potential litigation in the face of a progressive disease. Patients are frequently on steroids, which may require augmentation, and hyperthermia should be avoided, as it is associated with exacerbation of MS symptoms.

PARAPLEGIA

Paraplegia may result from trauma or from spinal cord tumors or poliomyelitis. Patients are particularly vulnerable to impaired respiratory function, decubitus ulcers, fractures due to osteoporosis, impaired temperature regulation, and urinary tract infections. The phenomenon known as "autonomic hyperreflexia" occurs in almost half of patients with lesions above T7.[49] It consists of sweating, facial flushing, pilomotor erection, headache, bradycardia, and severe hypertension in response to stimulation of skin, or distention or contraction of hollow organs, such as bladder, uterus, or gut below the level of the lesion. Denervated blood vessels are extrasensitive to catecholamines, whereas intact reflex vagal responses may lead to bradycardia. With lesions above T10, parturients may be unaware of labor and for this reason are usually hospitalized early. In the case of spinal cord disease, muscle spasms and ankle clonus may make labor distressing, and hyperreflexia, occurring in 11% of paraplegics, can be confused with preeclampsia. Cesarean section is not more common than in uncomplicated pregnancy, but weak expulsive efforts may necessitate the use of forceps to shorten the second stage of labor.

Anesthesia

From 1 week following a spinal injury, or in neuromuscular diseases where there are denervated or degenerating muscles (eg, muscular dystrophies, multiple sclerosis) potassium leaks from the muscle cell in response to succinylcholine.[50] Thus, administration of succinylcholine can lead to hyperkalemia, which may cause severe arrhythmias, even ventricular fibrillation. Regional anesthesia is therefore safer for the parturient with paraplegia. Little actual analgesia is required, but the continuous epidural or spinal technique can be very valuable in controlling hyperreflexia during labor. Epidural narcotic may prove to be a useful alternative, with less effect on blood pressure and heart rate.[51]

MUSCULAR DYSTROPHY

Muscular dystrophy is an inherited disorder characterized by progressive loss of muscular function. There are several major categories, but patients generally have muscle weakness leading to contractions and deformities such as scoliosis and lordosis, and bones are readily fractured. Myocardial myopathy may be present, and respiratory failure is an ever-present hazard. Swallowing may be compromised, and aspiration of secretions leads to pneumonitis. Administration of succinylcholine causes hyperkalemia, hyperthermia, and elevated enzymes, such as creatinine phosphokinase (CPK). These increases may mimic, but do not always indicate, the potentially lethal malignant hyperthermia (MH). Patients with muscular dystrophy do, in fact, have a higher incidence of susceptibility to MH, but diagnosis of this state should include a muscle biopsy and in vitro contraction studies.[52]

Succinylcholine and halothane are both contraindicated. Postoperative ventilatory support may be necessary after the stress of surgery and general anesthesia. Where there is limitation of respiratory function, carefully titrated epidural anesthesia may have advantages over spinal anesthesia for cesarean section.

A subgroup of patients with muscle disorders is made up of those suffering from autosomal dominant myotonia atrophica. Skeletal wasting, endocrine dysfunction, and cardiac and smooth muscle involvement are typical of the disease. Infertility is common. In those who do become pregnant there may be deterioration during gestation. Reports on the course of labor are variable, but muscle weakness may prolong the second stage, and forceps may be required to assist delivery.

There is a high rate of abortion, prematurity, and neonatal involvement with the disease. Arthrogryposis, hypotonia, and weakness are the most frequent manifestations. Hydramnios is common, probably because of fetal inability to swallow. Less common are diaphragmatic paralysis, congenital cataracts, and ECG abnormalities.

Preanesthetic evaluation of the mother involves assessment of respiratory function and of the degree of cardiac involvement.

Anesthesia

Because of delayed gastric emptying and weak intestinal mobility, there is a special disposition to aspiration. A histamine receptor antagonist such as ranitidine (150 mg orally the night before, and 50 mg IV 1 to 2 hours before surgery) or cimetidine (300 mg orally the night before, and 300 mg IM an hour before surgery) can be given. Sodium citrate (30 mL) is also administered orally prior to induction. As is standard with all obstetric patients, cricoid pressure is applied until the larynx is intubated and the cuff is inflated. Succinylcholine should not be used, as it may produce a contracture, without fasciculations, which makes ventilation difficult.[53] Small doses of nondepolarizing muscle relaxants may be used. Myotonic patients are highly susceptible to respiratory depressants, so that control of ventilation must be assumed early during induction. Volatile anesthetics are useful, but shivering should be avoided, as this may produce a generalized contracture.[54] Acute myotonic crisis can be treated with intravenous quinidine (300 to 600 mg) or large doses of steroid (1 g or more). Dantrolene has also been used to treat this condition. There is no proven relationship between malignant hyperpyrexia and myotonia atrophica.[50]

Epidural block has the advantages described previously for analgesia in labor and for vaginal delivery or cesarean section, so long as care is taken to keep the patient warm. In this regard, the addition of fentanyl or sufentanil to the local anesthetic administered epidurally has been evaluated in the prevention and reduction of shivering[55,56]

SUBARACHNOID HEMORRHAGE

Intracranial aneurysm is more common than arteriovenous angioma, but, perhaps because the latter occurs in a younger age group, and because of the increased blood volume in pregnancy, subarachnoid hemorrhage during pregnancy occurs equally often from either source. The incidence is about one in 10,000 pregnancies.[57] Conservative management is associated with a maternal mortality as high as 50% in the few weeks following hemorrhage, whereas surgery gives the best prognosis for mother and baby. There are several reports of cesarean section followed directly by aneurysm clipping at the same procedure; usually, however, pregnancy is allowed to continue after surgery until the occurrence of labor and vaginal delivery at term. Successful fetal outcome following both maternal hypothermia and induced hypotension have been reported. Trimetaphan (Arfonad) may be the safer drug with which to induce hypotension, since it is rapidly hydrolyzed and has a high molecular weight, but sodium nitroprusside has been used without incident.[57] Where possible, the fetal heart rate should be monitored throughout. Transient bradycardia, with rapid return to normal after the end of hypotension, is the rule. In the case of recent bleeding, the goals during induction of anesthesia are to control hypertension and avoid fluctuations in blood pressure during laryngoscopy and endotracheal intubation. Smooth induction is followed by reduction of intracranial pressure and induced hypotension.

During labor the parturient requires sufficient pain relief in the first stage of labor to avoid marked changes in blood pressure and increases in cardiac output. This is best provided by lumbar epidural analgesia, which is also useful in preventing the Valsalva maneuver in the second stage. Forceps may be applied to shorten this stage and avoid bearing down. For cesarean section also, epidural anesthesia is the method of choice. If general anesthesia is necessary because of fetal distress, antihypertensive drugs may be used to prevent the response to endotracheal intubation.

DRUG ABUSE DURING PREGNANCY

Illicit drug use for recreational purposes has reached epidemic proportions. In contrast to earlier years, when depressants or hypnotics like marijuana or methaqualone were popular, the present wave involves stimulants such as cocaine and methamphetamine. These exert their effect by modulating the sympathetic nervous system to a degree that may result in physiologic alterations affecting anesthetic and obstetric management. The typical cocaine user does not fit into any specific socioeconomic, ethnic, or cultural category, and many women of childbearing age are affected. A retrospective review of obstetric records at a large city hospital indicated that the prevalence of cocaine use was approximately 10%.[58]

Cocaine is an ester-linked local anesthetic with a unique property among this class of drugs of inhibiting norepinephrine reuptake by adrenergic neurons, thus producing potent sympathomimetic effects. The lethal dose of cocaine in humans is approximately 1400 mg.[59] Even small doses, however, may result in fatal ventricular arrhythmias. Pregnancy may enhance cocaine toxicity by increasing uptake of the drug by tissues such as the heart and brain.[60]

For the fetus, maternal cocaine use is particularly hazardous. Bolus injections of the drug (0.5 or 1.0 mg/kg) to chronically instrumented pregnant ewes resulted in maternal and fetal hypertension accompanied by varying degrees of tachycardia. Maternal plasma concentrations of norepinephrine were elevated by approximately 200%, and there was a dose-related decrease in uterine blood flow of up to 40% associated with fetal hypoxemia.[61,62] Numerous studies have identified an increased incidence of fetal wastage, low fetal weight, premature labor and delivery, as well as low Apgar scores, placental abruption, and intrauterine death following cocaine abuse.[63–65] Cocaine is also a known teratogen and has resulted in genitourinary and skeletal malformations.[66,67]

Maternal medical complications are also common. These include acute myocardial infarction, myocarditis, lethal ventricular arrhythmias, asystole, and rupture of the ascending aorta or intracranial aneurysm.[68] Central nervous system effects appear to be dose-related. At lower blood levels, excitation—manifested by restlessness, dysphoria, and paranoid psychosis—predominates. With increasing doses, generalized convulsions, coma, cerebrovascular accident, or subarachnoid hemorrhage are not uncommon. Death may occur independent of dose or route of administration and is most often ascribed to convulsions, fulminant respiratory failure, or ventricular arrhythmias. Smoking, or "freebasing," the drug may result in bronchospasm, pulmonary edema, or adult respiratory distress syndrome. Intestinal ischemia has been reported following oral ingestion.[68]

It is not unusual for the perinatal care team to be presented with an acutely ill mother and a fetus in need of urgent obstetric intervention. The manifestations of cocaine toxicity are frequently self-limiting and respond to supportive therapy. Psychotic or aggressive behavior may require treatment with benzodiazepines or haloperidol. Seizures should be quickly terminated with intravenous injection of thiopental (50 to 100 mg) or diazepam (5 to 10 mg), the airway protected, and adequacy of ventilation and oxygenation ensured. Hypertension may be exacerbated by unopposed alpha stimulation following the use of a beta-adrenergic receptor blocker.[69] Therefore, a combined alpha and beta receptor antagonist, such as labetalol, may be preferable.

Nitroprusside is currently the favored drug for management of hypertensive crisis. All vasodilators should be used cautiously, as frequent cocaine use may result in intravascular volume depletion and extreme sensitivity to these agents. The calcium channel antagonist verapamil can prevent ventricular fibrillation induced by cocaine, which is due to enhanced calcium influx into myocardial cells.[70] In addition, verapamil counteracts the peripheral vasoconstrictive effects of norepinephrine and diminishes its release from sympathetic nerve terminals.

Given the high incidence of placental abruption and fetal distress associated with cocaine ingestion, it is not uncommon for an intoxicated patient to require emergency cesarean section, usually under general endotracheal anesthesia. Ketamine should be avoided, since it has potent sympathomimetic actions of its own. Thiopental remains the standard induction agent, but etomidate may be a better alternative in the setting of uncorrected intravascular volume depletion. Agents sensitizing the myocardium to the arrhythmogenic effects of catecholamines, such as halothane, should be avoided, particularly if other drugs facilitating catecholamine release (eg, pancuronium) are used.[71]

Regional anesthesia (spinal or epidural) may be used in more elective cesarean sections. Epidural anesthesia is particularly suited, since the block can be slowly extended, allowing adequate time for intravascular volume expansion. However, since cocaine and other local anesthetic toxicities are additive, there may be a greater risk of toxic reactions. Hypotension, if it occurs, should be treated with increasing uterine displacement, additional fluid administration, and small doses of ephedrine, as needed.

For labor and vaginal delivery, intravenous narcotics

may be used to provide pain relief, but administration must be titrated carefully, since their effects may be potentiated by cocaine. Epidural analgesia provides more complete pain relief. As for cesarean section, however, careful attention must be given to maintenance of intravascular volume and avoidance of local anesthetic toxicity.

Methamphetamine ("crank") is rapidly becoming an abused substance, as it can be synthesized easily and its availability does not depend on transport across international boundaries. Amphetamines are similar in action to cocaine in that they stimulate the release and inhibit the reuptake of norepinephrine. Medical complications and therapy are also similar.

Some studies have associated the use of "crank" with intrauterine growth retardation[72] and congenital anomalies, particularly of the heart and biliary tract.[73–75]

Anesthetic considerations in managing the parturient abusing amphetamines are similar to those for cocaine. Acute amphetamine administration may increase analgesic and anesthetic requirement whereas habitual abuse decreases it.[76] There may be a diminished response to indirect-acting vasopressors, such as ephedrine.

THIRD-TRIMESTER BLEEDING

The two most common conditions resulting in antepartum hemorrhage are placenta previa and abruption. In severe cases, the mother may require rapid intravascular volume replacement with a crystalloid solution and/or blood products. Thus, placement of large-bore intravenous cannulae (14- or 16-gauge) is strongly recommended. Blood-component therapy with fresh-frozen plasma, cryoprecipitate, and platelet concentrate may be necessary to treat dilutional or disseminated intravascular coagulopathy. Invasive monitoring of arterial and central venous pressures may be warranted. Emergency cesarean section is often necessary and usually performed under general anesthesia because of time constraints and uncorrected hypovolemia. Furthermore, sympathetic blockade that accompanies regional blocks extending high enough for cesarean section may diminish or ablate the important adrenal-mediated vascular responses to hemorrhage.[77] Patients with placenta previa and prior cesarean sections have an increased incidence of placenta accreta and greater potential for severe hemorrhage.[78]

OBESITY

Obesity enhances the risks of obstetric and anesthetic interventions, and recent data suggest that it is a leading contributor to maternal morbidity and mortality.[79] A patient is considered to be obese when her weight is more than 20% above ideal body weight and is morbidly obese when the ideal is exceeded by over 100%.

Accumulation of adipose tissue is accompanied by several changes that, in many respects, are similar to those occurring during pregnancy. The cardiovascular system responds to increased metabolic demands by augmenting cardiac output, predominantly by an increase in stroke volume.[80] Total blood volume is larger but, when corrected for weight, is less than predicted.[81] Additional demands imposed by pregnancy can result in cardiac decompensation. Associated with obesity are hypertension, coronary artery disease, and diabetes mellitus, which further limit cardiac reserve during the stresses of labor and delivery. Changes in the respiratory system predispose to development of hypoxemia. Decreases in the expiratory reserve volume and functional residual capacity result in early airway closure during normal breathing and, consequently, in ventilation to perfusion mismatch.[82] Work of breathing is increased because of lower lung compliance and inefficient respiratory musculature. These alterations may be further aggravated by pregnancy, thus increasing the risk of hypoxemia, especially during periods of hypoventilation and apnea. Lithotomy and Trendelenburg position may be poorly tolerated. The most serious consequences of obesity are manifested in the "obesity hypoventilation (Pickwickian) syndrome," characterized by chronic hypoxemia, hypercarbia, right-sided cardiac failure, and somnolence.

Obesity is associated with higher volumes and more acidic gastric juices,[83] thus enhancing the risk of aspiration pneumonitis.

Altered drug metabolism and disposition have been reported in obese patients,[84,85] who may be more at risk than normal individuals for the development of drug toxicity caused by increased "free radical" formation during reductive metabolism of volatile anesthetic agents. Fatty infiltration of the liver or impaired hepatic blood flow may decrease the clearance of some drugs, thus prolonging their effect and increasing their accumulation. On the other hand, increased extracellular fluid volume may require a greater drug dose to achieve a desired pharmacodynamic response.[86] Therefore, if dosage is calculated on the basis of weight, a gross underestimation or overestimation of the drug requirement may result.

ANESTHETIC CONSIDERATIONS

Analgesia blunts increases in cardiac output and ventilation associated with pain of labor and vaginal delivery.[87] Intravenous narcotics, however, must be used cautiously so as to avoid airway obstruction and hypoventilation. Supplemental oxygen administration and continuous monitoring of oxygen saturation (pulse oximetry) are desirable. Inhalational analgesia may be difficult to manage. Epidural analgesia, being more effective in providing complete pain relief, is preferable, but not without risk, such as unintended intravascular or intrathecal injection of local anesthetic. Respiratory embarrassment from an excessively high block may also occur. In some cases, technical difficulties of epidural catheter placement may preclude its use. An intrathecal injection of morphine (0.5 mg to 1.0 mg), an easier alternative, was found to provide profound analgesia for the first stage of labor.[88] The risk of delayed respiratory depression mandates that patients be monitored for adequacy of ventilation and oxygenation for up to 24 hours. A pudendal block will be necessary for the second stage and delivery.

For cesarean section, regional anesthesia should be used whenever possible, thus avoiding potentially difficult laryngoscopy and endotracheal intubation. An advantage of having a functioning epidural catheter in place during labor is that the block can be extended, quickly if need be, for cesarean section. Where general anesthesia cannot be avoided, prophylaxis against aspiration of gastric contents, and careful evaluation of the airway should be performed. Awake laryngoscopy and endotracheal intubation under topical anesthesia may be preferred prior to induction. Spinal anesthesia, because of its rapidity, may be a suitable alternative to general anesthesia, even in emergency situations.[89]

Since postoperative pulmonary complications are common, chest physical therapy, incentive spirometry, and early ambulation are to be encouraged. Pain relief achieved with the use of intraspinal narcotics may improve respiratory mechanics and hasten recovery.

PRETERM LABOR AND DELIVERY

Although preterm deliveries occur in 8% to 10% of all births, they contribute to approximately 80% of early neonatal deaths.[90] Preterm infants are prone to develop severe problems, such as the respiratory distress syndrome, intracranial hemorrhage, hypoglycemia, hypocalcemia, and hyperbilirubinemia. Improved neonatal intensive care has reduced the incidence of cerebral palsy, mental retardation, and chronic lung disease among the survivors.[91] The maternal hazards during preterm labor may be related to frequent attempts at tocolysis or to the association with cocaine abuse. Several maternal complications of tocolysis have been reported, such as hypotension, hypokalemia, hyperglycemia, myocardial ischemia, pulmonary edema, and death.[92] Complications may also occur due to interactions with anesthetic drugs and techniques. With the use of regional anesthesia, peripheral vasodilation caused by beta-adrenergic stimulants enhances the risk of hypotension. Acute prehydration has to be carried out carefully to avoid pulmonary edema. General anesthesia may be risky in the presence of preexisting tachycardia, hypotension, and hypokalemia. It is better to avoid using halothane (arrhythmias) as well as atropine and pancuronium (tachycardia). Delaying anesthesia by at least 3 hours from the cessation of tocolysis, if possible, will allow beta-mimetic effects to dissipate. Potassium supplementation is not necessary.[93]

Although there have been few systemic studies to determine the maternal and fetal pharmacokinetics and dynamics of drugs throughout gestation, it is generally thought that the premature infant is more vulnerable to the effects of drugs used in obstetric analgesia and anesthesia than the term newborn. Reasons cited are the following: less protein available for drug binding; higher levels of bilirubin, which may compete with the drug for protein binding; greater drug access to the central nervous system because of poorly developed blood–brain barrier; greater total body water and lower fat content; and decreased ability to metabolize and excrete drugs. It is doubtful that these deficiencies of the preterm infant have serious consequences. Although the serum albumin and alpha$_1$-acid glycoprotein concentrations are indeed lower in the preterm fetus, this would affect primarily drugs that are highly bound to these proteins. Most agents used for obstetric analgesia exhibit only low to moderate degrees of binding in the fetal serum: approximately 50% for bupivacaine, 25% for lidocaine, and 52% for meperidine. Elevated bilirubin levels, which may occur in the postpartum period, will not compete with anesthetic drugs for albumin binding, since most of these agents are bound to other serum proteins (eg, meperidine and local anesthetics to alpha$_1$-glycoproteins, D-tubocurarine to gamma globulin). Development of the human blood–brain barrier occurs early in gestation,[94] so that other factors such as changes in tissue affinity may account for differences between immature and mature animals in brain uptake of highly lipid soluble drugs. Greater total body water in the preterm fetus will result in a greater volume of distribution for drugs. A study of age-related toxicity of lidocaine in sheep showed that the greater the volume of distribution, the greater the dose required to achieve toxic blood concentrations.[95] Decreased ability to metabolize and/or excrete drugs, associated with prematurity, does not extend to all anesthetic agents. For instance, plasma clearance of lidocaine was found to be similar in preterm human newborns and adults.[96] Neonates excreted much more unchanged lidocaine compared with adults. Similarly, although meperidine metabolism is more limited in the neonate, as compared to that in the adult, urinary excretion of the unchanged drug is greater in the former.

Gestational decreases in maternal serum albumin and alpha$_1$-acid glycoprotein concentrations may also be important. Serial determinations of protein binding of diazepam, phenytoin and valproic acid in the maternal serum, carried out in early (8 to 16 weeks), mid (17 to 32 weeks), and late pregnancy, showed a progressive rise in the unbound fraction.[97] Drug availability for placental transfer was therefore increased. Placental permeability itself increases as pregnancy progresses, due to the increased area and decreased thickness of tissue barriers.

In a prospective study of over 1000 premature labors, in which mothers received meperidine alone or with scopolamine, medication had no effect on the Apgar scores, need for resuscitation, incidence of RDS, perinatal death rate and incidence of severe neurologic defects within one year.[98]

One can conclude that concerns about the newborn drug effects are far less important than preventing asphyxia and trauma to the fetus. For labor and vaginal delivery, well conducted epidural anesthesia will provide good perineal relaxation. Preterm infants with breech presentation are usually delivered by cesarean section. To facilitate delivery of the aftercoming head, uterine relaxation is recommended. It can be achieved by administration of a halogenated agent during general anesthesia or a tocolytic drug, if a regional technique is chosen.

FETAL SURGERY

Recent improvements in invasive as well as noninvasive technology have made it possible to diagnose and, in some cases, treat fetal anomalies. Correction of obstructive lesions, such as hydrocephalus, or conditions resulting from failure of embryonic tissues to develop normally (eg, diaphragmatic hernia) have been reported.[99–101]

Anesthetic considerations for antenatal fetal surgery not only encompass the usual concerns for maternal and fetal well-being, but also have an added requirement to provide adequate fetal analgesia, immobilization, and uterine relaxation. The fetus has the ability to react to noxious stimuli and thus requires analgesia/anesthesia for painful procedures.[102] On the other hand, the fetal brain appears to be highly sensitive to the effects of anesthetic drugs. For instance, the halothane requirement to prevent movement in response to a painful stimulus in the fetal lamb is approximately 50% of that in the pregnant ewe.[103] Yet, because of the unique pattern of the fetal circulation, anesthetic effects may take longer to be achieved in the fetus compared to the mother.[104]

Direct fetal injection of nondepolarizing muscle relaxants can provide immobilization for relatively simple procedures that do not require major anesthesia, such as fetal blood transfusion. Administration of D-tubocurarine (1.5 mg/kg estimated fetal weight) or pancuronium (0.3 mg/kg) into the fetal buttock (with the use of ultrasound, if need be) resulted in the onset of paralysis within 5 minutes, lasting 4 and 7 hours, respectively.[105] Pancuronium, but not curare, has been shown to increase fetal heart rate and blood pressure slightly.[106] Thus, the former may be preferable, because of its salutary effect on fetal cardiac output. Inaccessibility often makes surveillance of the fetus during intrauterine procedures limited. When feasible, continuous fetal heart rate monitoring, in conjunction with acid–base measurements, appears to be adequate for determination of fetal well-being. Pulse oximetry can also be used during extensive procedures. A major complication of uterine surgery during pregnancy is the onset of premature contractions. In this respect, halogenated inhalation agents provide dose-related myometrial relaxation and are useful in preventing intraoperative uterine irritability. Postoperative administration of tocolytic agents is recommended. Maternal premedication with indomethacin may also inhibit uterine activity.[99,107]

REFERENCES

1. Willems J. The etiology of preeclampsia: a hypothesis. Obstet Gynecol 1977;50:495.
2. Walsh SW. Preeclampsia: an imbalance in placental prostacyclin and thromboxane production. Am J Obstet Gynecol 1985;152:335.
3. Makila U-M, Jouppila P, Kirkinen P, Viinikka L, Ylikorkala O. Placental thromboxane and prostacyclin in the regulation of placental blood flow. Obstet Gynecol 1986;68:537.
4. Thorp JA, Walsh SW, Brath PC. Low-dose aspirin inhibits thromboxane, but not prostacyclin, production by human placental arteries. Am J Obstet Gynecol 1988;159:1381.
5. Chesley LC. Plasma and red cell volumes during pregnancy. Am J Obstet Gynecol 1972;112:440.
6. Hays PM, Cruickshank DP, Dunn LJ. Plasma volume determination in normal and preeclamptic pregnancies. Am J Obstet Gynecol 1985;151:958.
7. Groenendijk R, Trimbos MJ, Wallenburg HCS. Hemodynamic measurements in preeclampsia: preliminary observations. Am J Obstet Gynecol 1984;150:232.
8. Kelton JG, Hunter DJS, Neame PB. A platelet function defect in preeclampsia. Obstet Gynecol 1985;65:107.
9. Weinstein L. Syndrome of hemolysis, elevated liver enzymes, and low platelet count: a severe consequence of hypertension in pregnancy. Am J Obstet Gynecol 1982;142:159.
10. Kishon B, Moise KJ, Cotton DB, et al. Role of volume expansion in severe preeclampsia. Surg Gynecol Obstet 1988;167:367.
11. Shoemaker CT, Meyers M. Sodium nitroprusside for control of severe hypertensive disease of pregnancy: a case report and discussion of potential toxicity. Am J Obstet Gynecol 1984;149:171.
12. Jouppila P, Jouppila R, Hollmen A, Koivula A. Lumbar epidural analgesia to improve intervillous blood flow during labor in severe preeclampsia. Obstet Gynecol 1982;59:158.
13. Hodgkinson R, Husain FJ, Hayashi RH. Systemic and pulmonary blood pressure during cesarean section in parturients with gestational hypertension. Can Anaesth Soc J 1980;27:389.
14. Connell H, Dalgleish JG, Downing JW. General anaesthesia in mothers with severe pre-eclampsia/eclampsia. Br J Anaesth 1987;59: 1375.
15. Hibbard LT. Maternal mortality due to cardiac disease. Clin Obstet Gynecol 1975;18:27.
16. Sugrue D, Blake S, MacDonald D. Pregnancy complicated by maternal heart disease at the National Maternity Hospital, Dublin, Ireland, 1969–1978. Am J Obstet Gynecol 1981;139:1.
17. Becker RM. Intracardiac surgery in pregnant women. Ann Thorac Surg 1983;36:453.
18. Jones AM, Howitt G. Eisenmenger's syndrome in pregnancy. Br Med J 1965;1:1627.
19. Campbell M. The incidence and later distribution of malformations of the heart. In: Watson H, ed. Paediatric cardiology. London: Lloyd-Luke, 1968:71.
20. Abboud TK, Raya J, Noueihid R, Daniel J. Intrathecal morphine for relief of labor pain in patients with severe pulmonary hypertension. Anesthesiology 1983;59:477.
21. Mangano DT. Anesthesia for the pregnant cardiac patient. In: Shnider SM, Levinson G, eds. Anesthesia for obstetrics. 2nd ed. Baltimore: Williams & Wilkins, 1987:345.
22. West KM. Epidemiology of insulin-dependent diabetes. In: Grave GD, ed. Early detection of potential diabetics. The problems and promise. New York: Raven Press, 1979:27.
23. Kitzmiller JL, Cloherty JP, Younger D et al. Diabetic pregnancy and perinatal morbidity. Am J Obstet Gynecol 1978;131:560.
24. Barden TP, Knowles HC Jr. Diagnosis of diabetes in pregnancy. Clin Obstet Gynecol 1981;24(1):3.

25. National Diabetes Data Group. Classification and diagnosis of diabetes mellitus and other categories of glucose intolerance. Diabetes 1979;28:1039.
26. Gabbe SG. Definition, detection, and management of gestational diabetes. A Review. Obstet Gynecol 1986;67:121.
27. White P. Diabetes mellitus in pregnancy. Clin Perinatol 1974;1:331.
28. Selenkow HA. Patterns of serum immuno-reactive human placental lactogen (IR-HPL) and chorionic gonadotropin (IR-HCG) in diabetic pregnancy. Diabetes 1971;20:696.
29. Costrini NV, Kalkhoff RK. Relative effects of pregnancy, estradiol, and progesterone on plasma insulin and pancreatic islet insulin secretion. J Clin Invest 1971;50:992.
30. Kitzmiller JL. Diabetic ketoacidosis. Contemp Obstet Gynecol 1982;20:141.
31. Karlsson K, Kjellmer I. The outcome of diabetic pregnancies in relation to the mother's blood sugar. Am J Obstet Gynecol 1972;112:213.
32. Lev-Ran A. Sharp temporary drop in insulin requirement after cesarean section in diabetic patients. Am J Obstet Gynecol 1974;120:905.
33. Nylund L, Lunell N-O, Lewander R, Persson B, Sarby B. Uteroplacental blood flow in diabetic pregnancy: measurements with indium 113m and a computer-linked gamma camera. Am J Obstet Gynecol 1982;144:298.
34. Björk O, Persson B. Placental changes in relation to the degree of metabolic control in diabetes mellitus. Placenta 1983;3:367.
35. Madsen H. Ditzel J. Changes in red blood cell oxygen transport in diabetic pregnancy. Am J Obstet Gynecol 1982;143:424.
36. Datta S, Brown WU, Ostheimer GW, Weiss JB, Alper MH. Epidural anesthesia for cesarean section in diabetic parturients: Maternal and neonatal acid-base status and bupivacaine concentration. Anesth Analg 1981;60:574.
37. Gabbe SG, Demer SLM, Gree RO, Villee AC. The effects of hypoxia on placental glycogen metabolism. Am J Obstet Gynecol 1972;114:540.
38. Swanstrom S, Bratteby LE. Metabolic effects of obstetric regional analgesia and of asphyxia in the newborn infant during the first two hours after birth. Acta Paediatr Scand 1981;70:791.
39. Kenepp NB, Shelley WC, Kuman S, Gutsche BB, Gabbe S, Delivoria-Papadopoulos M. Effects on newborn of hydration with glucose in patients undergoing cesarean section with regional anesthesia. Lancet 1980;1:645.
40. Carson BS, Phillipps AT, Simmon MA, Battaglia FC, Meschia G. Effects of a sustained insulin infusion upon glucose uptake and oxygenation of the ovine fetus. Pediatr Res 1980;14:147.
41. Datta S, Kitzmiller JL, Naulty JS, Ostheimer GW, Weiss JB. Acid-base status of diabetic mothers and their infants following spinal anesthesia for cesarean section. Anesth Analg 1982; 61:662.
42. Hopkins A. Neurological disorders. Clin Obstet Gynaecol 1977;4:419.
43. Harrah MD, Way WL, Katzung BG. The interaction of D-tubocurarine with antiarrhythmic drugs. Anesthesiology 1970; 33:406.
44. Bjerkedal T, Bahana SL. The course and outcome of pregnancy in women with epilepsy. Acta Obstet Gynecol Scand 1973;52:245.
45. Bellur S. Neurologic disorders in pregnancy. In: Gleicher N, ed. Principles of medical therapy in pregnancy. New York: Plenum, 1985.
46. Bentollini R, Mastroiacova P, Segni G. Maternal epilepsy and birth defects. A case-control study in the Italian Multicentric Registry of Birth Defects. Eur J Epidemiol 1985;1:67.
47. Namba T, Brown SB, Grob D. Neonatal myasthenia gravis: report of two cases and review of the literature. Pediatrics 1970;45:488.
48. Bader AM, Hunt CO, Datta S, Naulty JS, Ostheimer GW. Anesthesia for the obstetric patient with multiple sclerosis. J Clin Anesth 1988;1:21.
49. Lindan R, Joiner E, Freehafer AA, Hazel C. Incidence and clinical features of autonomic dysreflexia in patients with spinal cord injury. Paraplegia 1980;18:285.
50. Cooperman LH, Strobel GE, Kennel EM. Massive hyperkalemia after administration of succinylcholine. Anesthesiology 1970; 32:161.
51. Abouleish EI, Hanley ES, Palmer SM. Can epidural fentanyl control autonomic hyperreflexia in a quadriplegic parturient? Anesth Analg 1989;68:523.
52. Smith CL, Bush GH. Anesthesia and progressive muscular dystrophy. Br J Anaesth 1985;57:1113.
53. Paterson IS. Generalized myotonia following suxamethonium: case report. Br J Anaesth 1962;34:340.
54. Thiel RE. The myotonic response to suxamethonium. Br J Anaesth 1967;39:815.
55. Matthews NC, Corser G. Epidural fentanyl for shaking in obstetrics. Anaesthesia 1988;43:783.
56. Sevarino FB, Johnson MD, Lema MJ, Datta S, Ostheimer GW, Naulty JS. The effect of epidural sufentanil on shivering and body temperature in the parturient. Anesth Analg 1989;68:530.
57. Minielly R, Yuzpe AA, Drake CG. Subarachnoid haemorrhage secondary to ruptured cerebral aneurysm in pregnancy. Obstet Gynecol 1979;53:64.
58. Little BB, Snell LM, Palmore MK, Gilstrap LC. Cocaine use in pregnant women in a large public hospital. Am J Perinatol 1988;5:206.
59. Smart RG, Anglin L. Do we know the lethal dose of cocaine? J Forensic Sci 1987;32:303.
60. Shah NS, May DA, Yates JD. Disposition of levo-(H^3) cocaine in pregnant and nonpregnant mice. Toxicol Appl Pharm 1980;53: 279.
61. Moore TR, Sorg J, Miller L, Key TC, Resnick R. Hemodynamic effects of intravenous cocaine on the pregnant ewe and fetus. Am J Obstet Gynecol 1986;155:883.
62. Woods JR, Plessinger MA, Clark KE. Effects of cocaine in uterine blood flow and fetal oxygenation. JAMA 1987;257:957.
63. Chasnoff IJ, Burns WJ, Schnoll SH, Burns KA. Cocaine use in pregnancy. N Engl J Med 1985;313:666.
64. Ryan L, Ehrlich S, Finnegan L. Cocaine abuse in pregnancy: effects on the fetus and newborn. Neurotoxicol Perinatol 1987;9:295.
65. MacGregor SN, Keith LG, Chasnoff IJ, et al. Cocaine use during pregnancy: adverse perinatal outcome. Am J Obstet Gynecol 1987;157:686.
66. Bingol N, Fuchs M, Diaz V, Stone RK, Gromisch DS. Teratogenicity of cocaine in humans. J Pediatr 1987;110:93.
67. Mahalik MP, Gautieri RF. Mann DE. Teratogenic potential of cocaine hydrochloride in CF-1 mice. J Pharm Sci 1980;69:703.
68. Cregler LL, Mark H. Medical complications of cocaine abuse. N Engl J Med 1986;1495.
69. Ramoska E, Sacchetti AD. Propanolol-induced hypertension in treatment of cocaine intoxication. Ann Emerg Med 1985;14: 1112.
70. Billman GE, Hoskins RS. Cocaine-induced ventricular fibrillation: protection afforded by the calcium antagonist verapamil. Federation of American Societies of Experimental Biology Journal 1988;2:2990.
71. Koehntop DE, Liao JC, Van Bergen H. Effects of pharmacologic alterations of adrenergic mechanisms by cocaine, tropolone, aminophylline, and ketamine on epinephrine-induced arrhyth-

mias during halothane-nitrous oxide anesthesia. Anesthesiology 1977;46:83.
72. Little BB, Snell LM, Gilstrap LC. Methamphetamine abuse during pregnancy: outcome and fetal effects. Obstet Gynecol 1988;72:541.
73. Nelson MM, Forfar JO. Associations between drugs administered during pregnancy and congenital anomalies of the fetus. Br Med J 1971;1:523.
74. Nora JL, Vargo TA, Nora AH et al. Dexamphetamine: a possible environmental trigger in cardiovascular malformations. Lancet 1970;i:1290.
75. Golbus MS, Teratology for the obstetrician: current status. Obstet Gynecol 1980;55:269.
76. Johnston RR, Way WL, Miller RD. Alteration of anesthetic requirement by amphetamine. Anesthesiology 1972;36:357.
77. Jordan DA, Miller ED. Spinal sympathetic blockade decreases tolerance to hemorrhage by attenuating compensatory responses transmitted via the splanchnic nerve. Anesthesiology 1988;69:A339.
78. Chestnut DH, Eden RD, Gall SA, Parker RT. Peripartum hysterectomy: a review of cesarean and postpartum hysterectomy. Obstet Gynecol 1985;65:365.
79. Endler GC, Mariona FG, Sokol RJ, Stevenson LB. Anesthesia-related maternal mortality in Michigan, 1972 to 1984. Am J Obstet Gynecol 1988;159:187.
80. Bendixen HH. Morbid obesity. In: Hershey SG, ed. Refresher course in anesthesiology. Vol 6. Philadelphia: JB Lippincott, 1978:1.
81. Backman L, Freyschus U, et al. Cardiovascular function in extreme obesity. Acta Med Scand 1973;193:437.
82. Rochester DF, Enson Y. Current concepts in the pathogenesis of the obesity-hypoventilation syndrome. Am J Med 1974;57:402.
83. Vaughan RW, Bauer S, Wise L. Volume of pH of gastric juices in obese patients. Anesthesiology 1975;43:686.
84. Bentley JB, Vaughan RW, Gandolfi AJ, Cork RC. Halothane biotransformation in obese and non-obese patients. Anesthesiology 1982;57:94.
85. Weinstein JA, Matteo RS, Ornstein E, et al. Pharmacodynamics of vecuronium and atracurium in the obese. Anesthesiology 1987;67:A346.
86. Tsueda K, Warren JE, McCafferty LA, et al. Pancuronium bromide requirement during anesthesia for the morbidly obese. Anesthesiology 1978;48:438.
87. Bonica JJ. Basic considerations. In: Bonica JJ, ed. Clinics in obstetrics and gynaecology 1975;2:469.
88. Abboud TR, Shnider SM, Dailey PA, et al. Intrathecal administration of hyperbaric morphine for the relief of pain in labor. Br J Anaesth 1984;56:1351.
89. Marx GF, Luykx, WM, Cohen S. Fetal-neonatal status following cesarean section for fetal distress. Br J Anaesth 1984;56:1009.
90. Rush RW, Davey DA, Segall ML. The effect of pre-term delivery on perinatal mortality. Br J Obstet Gynaecol 1978;85:806.
91. Allen MC, Jones MD. Medical complications of prematurity. Obstet Gynecol 1986;67:427.
92. Benedetti TJ. Maternal complications of parenteral beta-sympathomimetic therapy for premature labor. Am J Obstet Gynecol 1983;145:1.
93. Young DC, Toofanian A, Leveno KJ. Potassium and glucose concentration without treatment during ritodrine tocolysis. Am J Obstet Gynecol 1983;145:105.
94. Saunders NR. Development of blood-brain barrier in the fetus. In: Bossart H, ed. Perinatal medicine. Bern: Hans Huber, 1973:54.
95. Morishima HO, Pedersen H, Finster M, et al. Toxicity of lidocaine in adult, newborn and fetal sheep. Anesthesiology 1981;55:57.
96. Mihaly GW, Moore RG, Thomas J, Triggs EJ, Thomas D, Shanks CA. The pharmacokinetics and metabolism of the anilide local anaesthetics in neonates. Eur J Clin Pharmacol 1978;13:143.
97. Krauer B, Krauer F, Hytten F. Drug prescribing in pregnancy. Current reviews in obstetrics and gynaecology. Vol 7. London: Churchill Livingstone, 1984:44.
98. Kaltreider DF. Premature labor and meperidine analgesia. Am J Obstet Gynecol 1967;99:989.
99. Harrison MR, Golbus MS, Filly RA, et al. Fetal surgical treatment. Pediatr Ann 1982;11:896.
100. Clewell WH, Johnson ML, Meier RR, et al. A surgical approach to the treatment of fetal hydrocephalus. N Engl J Med 1982;306:1320.
101. Harrison MR, Golbus MS, Filly RA. Management of the fetus with a correctable congenital defect. JAMA 1981;246:774.
102. Anand KJS, Hickey PR. Pain and its effects in the human neonate and fetus. N Engl J Med 1987;317:1321.
103. Gregory GA, Wade JG, Biehl DR, et al. Fetal anesthetic requirement (MAC) for halothane. Anesth Analg 1983;62:9.
104. Finster M, Poppers PJ. Safety of thiopental used for induction of general anesthesia in elective cesarian section. Anesthesiology 1968;29:190.
105. Moise KJ, Carpenter RJ, Deter RL, et al. The use of fetal neuromuscular blockade during intrauterine procedures. Am J Obstet Gynecol 1987;157:874.
106. Chestnut DH, Weiner CP, Thompson CS, McLaughlin GL. Intravenous administration of D-tubocurarine and pancuronium in fetal lambs. Anesthesiology 1988;69:A652.
107. Harrison MR, Anderson J, Rosen MA, et al. Fetal surgery in the primate. I. Anesthetic, surgical and tocolytic management to maximize fetal-neonatal survival. J Pediatr Surg 1982;17:115.

91

CHAPTER

THE PUERPERIUM AND LACTATION

Ann M. Ferris and E. Albert Reece

The puerperium operationally defines a period of 6 weeks following delivery in which a number of changes in the anatomy and physiology of reproduction occur, such as the menstrual cycle, systemic changes, and lactation. The patient and her physician also conduct discussions regarding contraception during this period. This chapter elaborates on these puerperal events.

THE REPRODUCTIVE SYSTEM

THE CERVIX

Ultrasonography of both the nongravid and puerperal uterus reveals the variation in normal uterine size. The normal pregravid weight of the uterus is 50 to 100 g, depending on parity. The uterus achieves a term weight of 1000 to 2000 g and is composed of 83% water.[1] The uterine length also changes appreciably during pregnancy, from 6 to 8 cm in the non-pregnant state to 40 cm or more at term.[2]

Robinson first reported sonographic examination of the puerperal uterus.[3] Other investigators subsequently confirmed that most of the decrease in uterine size occurred during the first week postpartum.[4–6] The decrease in size was unrelated to whether patients breast- or bottle-fed their infants.

Following parturition, the cervix is very distensible, thin, and flabby, even in the presence of a well-contracted uterus with little or no bleeding. There may or may not be multiple tears along the cervical margin. This laxity in the cervix results in a dilated state of about 2 to 3 cm for the first few days following delivery. By the end of the first week, the cervix will return to a state resembling non-pregnancy, but dilated to about 1 cm. This state will persist for up to 6 weeks, or occasionally up to 3 months.

THE UTERUS

Immediately after expulsion of the placenta, strong uterine contractions decrease uterine size. Within 24 hours the uterine size approximates the size at 20 weeks gestation. By 48 hours, the uterine size approaches 14 weeks gestation. Within 2 weeks postpartum, the uterus decreases further in size, descending into the pelvic cavity and eventually below the pubic symphysis. The non-pregnant uterine size will be achieved within 4 weeks postpartum. Pathologic estimates of these changes indicate that immediately following delivery the contracted uterus weighs approximately 1 kg; 1 week later, about 500 g; and 2 weeks later, about 300 g. Uterine weights of less than 100 g can be observed as soon as 3 weeks postpartum. This involution process is not accomplished by a significant reduction in the number of cells, but rather in the size of the cells.[7,8]

Within 24 to 36 hours, patients will begin to pass blood-tinged discharge with particulate matter (lochia) through the vagina. The lochia contains the superficial necrotic layer of the pregnant endometrium (the decidual). Microscopically, the lochia consists of red blood cells, pieces of decidual epithelial cells, and bacteria. The non-pregnant endometrium is regenerated by the endometrial gland and the connective tissue. Within 10 days, a new endometrium regenerates rapidly throughout most of the endometrial surface.[8] Regeneration at the placental implantation site takes longer, since such a process awaits sloughing from necrotic cells, followed by repair of these epithelial structures. A delay in involution at the placental site over a protracted period may result in postpartum hemorrhage. Sloughing of the placental site, resulting in infarction and necrosis, is believed to occur secondary to constriction and thrombosis of vessels supplying the placental site.

THE VAGINA

Following parturition, the vagina is hyperemic, swollen, and smooth. The normally present rugae are often absent but reappear within 3 weeks postpartum. The edema and swelling usually resolve by 6 weeks postpartum.

THE MENSTRUAL CYCLE

Return of the menstrual cycle following delivery occurs at variable time periods, and the menstrual flow may be in variable quantities. Some patients may present with intermittent spotting after delivery, or with a normal menstrual flow as early as 5 weeks postpartum. The average time for return of the menses for nonlactating women is about 8 to 10 weeks, with a range of up to 17 to 18 weeks postpartum. Histologic evidence of secretory endometrium demonstrates that ovulation may occur in nonlactating women as early as 27 days[9] or 36 days after delivery.[10] Earlier studies had reported that ovulation occurred later.[11] Delayed return of menses is usually seen in lactating women. Infant suckling intensity and frequency,[12] coupled with the timing of introduction of supplementary foods to the infant,[13] determine the duration of anovulation and amenorrhea in well-nourished women. In breast-feeding Bangladeshi women, the period of anovulation averaged 18 to 24 months.[14]

Differences in patterns of amenorrhea and ovulation are thought to be a consequence of alteration in the pituitary ovarian hormone stimulation for the first 3 weeks after delivery. Long-term suppression of the pituitary gland during pregnancy secondary to elevated estrogen levels antepartum causes the alterations. Differences in pituitary hormone stimulation cause transient insensitivity to luteinizing hormone releasing hormone.[15] This concept has been borne out by the reduced levels of luteinizing hormones demonstrated in both lactating and nonlactating women.[16]

SYSTEMIC CHANGES

Cardiovascular status, which alters significantly during pregnancy, returns to a non-pregnant state shortly after delivery. For example, the blood volume decreases by about 20% with 72 hours postpartum. This decrease in blood volume may be secondary to the blood loss that occurs during parturition, as well as the postpartum diuresis. Other cardiovascular changes, such as increased heart rate and cardiac output, return to baseline within the first 2 weeks postpartum.

THE URINARY SYSTEM

Pregnancy induces both functional and structural changes in the urinary system. The functional changes seem to remit promptly after delivery; however, the structural changes may persist for several months. For example, renal blood flow changes proportionally to increases in blood volume during pregnancy and decreases in blood volume following delivery. Renal blood flow in nonlactating women returns to nonpregnant levels by 6 weeks postpartum.[17] A puerperal diuresis usually occurs within the first 3 days postpartum, and this enhances the return of blood volume to normal.

Dilation of the bladder ureters and renal pelvis may persist for 3 or more months postpartum. The puerperal bladder with an increased capacity is somewhat refractory to increased intravesicular pressure; hence, overdistention and incomplete emptying may result. In fact, about 20% of postpartum women will experience incomplete emptying.[18,19]

THE LIVER

During pregnancy, plasma proteins—such as coagulation factors, immunoglobulins, transport and binding proteins, cholesterol, triglyceride, and lipoproteins—increase. The blood levels of these proteins fall precipitously within 24 to 48 hours postpartum, and by 2 to 3 weeks after delivery their levels return to baseline. Liver function test values remain normal during pregnancy and elevated values should be considered abnormal.

LACTATION

In contrast to the other puerperal changes that involve a return to the non-pregnant state, lactation represents a continuation of the reproductive cycle that began as early as during maternal prenatal development. Lactation is a predominant feature of the puerperium.

STAGES OF LACTATION

The cycle of human lactation consists of four separate stages: mammogenesis (mammary growth), lactogenesis (the initiation of milk secretion), galactopoiesis (the maintenance of lactation), and finally involution (the cessation of lactation).[20–22]

Mammogenesis

Prenatal Development. Evidence for embryonic development of the mammary gland appears by the fifth week of gestation with the observation of a milk line or ridge.[20,23] Development continues throughout gestation with the formation of primary and secondary ducts capable of secretory activity. The milky secretion, or "witches' milk," of the newborn is evidence of this secretory ability.[23] However, the secretion of this colostrumlike substance results from a generalized response of the mammary epithelium to hormonal levels and ceases within 3 to 4 weeks postpartum. From birth to pubescence, the growth rate of the mammary gland keeps pace with general body growth.[24] (See Figure 91-1 as a reference for the general anatomical structures of the developed human breast.)

Pubescence. In pubertal women, the stroma represents 90% of the mammary gland, since fat and connective tissue deposition account for most of the prepartal growth in the breast.[23] This deposition does not occur in other species.[20] The hormonal changes that accompany the first menstrual cycle stimulate the growth of the primary and secondary ducts. Russo and Russo have documented that these ducts develop into club-shaped terminal end buds that branch to "alveolar buds," a term they have coined to differentiate this stage of glandular development.[23] Clusters of these alveolar buds around a terminal duct form a lobule. Lobule formation occurs within 1 to 2 years following the first menstrual cycle.[23] In rare instances, adequate fat deposition could mask inadequate lobular development during this period and explain later lactational failure for some mothers.[25] The final stage of lobuloalveolar development depends on the hormonal stimulation of pregnancy. The cyclical hormonal changes of the menstrual cycle also produce a slight increase in mammary development until the age of 35.[23]

Pregnancy. Proliferation of the ductal tree and the formation of new ducts and lobules dominates mammary development in early pregnancy.[21,23] Estrogen, working with pituitary and adrenal hormones, promotes ductal development, and progesterone is needed for lobuloalveolar development.[20] Prolactin in synergism with estrogen, progesterone, placental lactogen, insulin, cortisol, and thyroid hormones stimulates mammary lobuloalveolar growth in preparation for lactogenesis.[26] Normal levels for serum prolactin for nonpregnant, nonlactating women are less than 20 ng/mL.[27] During pregnancy maternal prolactin levels

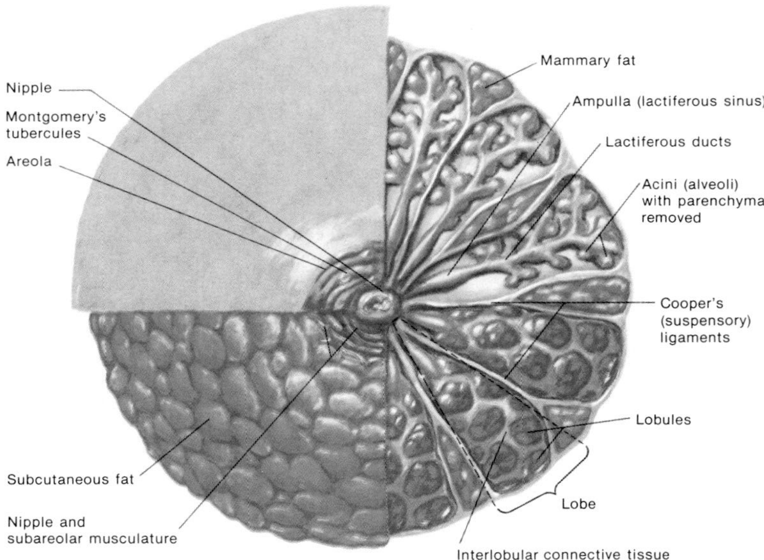

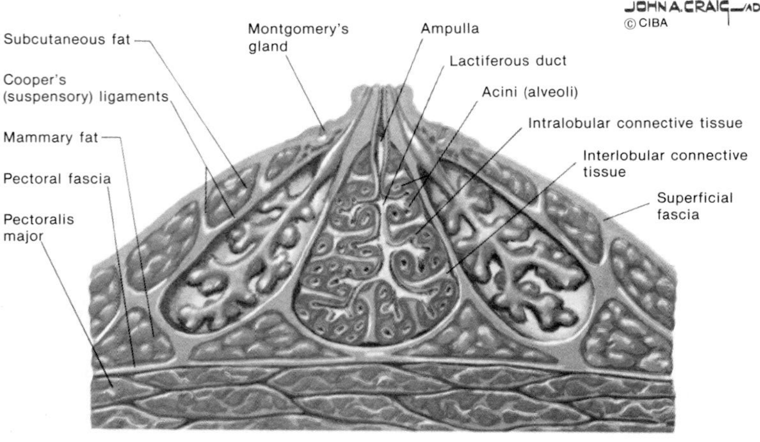

FIGURE 91-1. Anatomy of the human breast. (Copyright 1980 CIBA-GEIGY Corporation. Reproduced with permission from the Clinical Symposia by Frank H. Netter, M.D. All rights reserved.)

increase progressively to 10 to 20 times the nonpregnant amount at term.[28] Mammary development during the later half of pregnancy is characterized by the terminal differentiation of the ductules to the secretory units, acini.[23]

Lactogenesis (Secretory Phase)

The onset of a copious milk supply marks the start of lactogenesis. Hartmann has proposed two stages of lactogenesis in humans.[29] He suggests that the development of the milk-secreting cells in mid-pregnancy marks the start of the first stage of lactogenesis. At this time the gland becomes capable of secreting milk and synthesizing milk components.[29] This stage lasts from mid-pregnancy to parturition.[20] Specific milk components make their first appearance in the mammary tissue and are secreted at a slow rate to form colostrum.[20]

The hormonal environment of the mother changes abruptly at parturition. Two factors, the loss of progesterone-induced inhibition and prolactin-induced stimulation, are thought to trigger the second stage of lactogenesis, the initiation of secretion of a copious milk supply.[30] The release of inhibition linked to the decrease of progesterone is thought to be the active factor responsible.[31] This second stage of lactogenesis occurs between 3 and 4 days postpartum. The precise timing of the start of this stage is difficult to pinpoint, since a mother's perception of when her "milk comes in" is subjective and thus imprecise. Some mothers with adequate milk supply never experience the filling of their breasts. The sensation is also known to follow, not precede, the onset of copious milk supply. Thus, questioning of the mother can only serve as a qualitative guide.

Galactopoiesis

Galactopoiesis, the third stage of lactation, represents the maintenance or augmentation of established lactation and is described in three phases. In the early stage, milk supply is still increasing. At the peak stage, milk production reaches its maximum volume, and late lactation represents an imprecise stage preceding the cessation of lactation.[20]

Involution

Involution is a degenerative process that results in the return of the mammary gland to close to prepregnancy size. Mepham describes three types of involution—gradual, initiated, and senile.[20] Gradual involution occurs after the mammary gland has attained peak yield. Although not frequently studied, this is the process seen during normal weaning. Initiated involution, the most widely studied, occurs when lactation is ended abruptly. Senile involution is part of the normal aging process noted in postmenopausal women. In all animal species, involution proceeds quickly if milk is not removed.[20] In humans, if a mother does not nurse by 4 to 5 days postpartum, the autolytic process of involution will also occur rapidly.[22] Removal of milk during pregnancy and immediately after birth does not appear to promote lactogenesis.[32]

HORMONAL CONTROL OF LACTATION

Endocrine Control

The minimal hormonal requirements for the maintenance of normal lactation are prolactin, insulin, and hydrocortisone.[33,34] In vitro these hormones stimulate the transcription of casein mRNA in mammary cell cultures.[35] Prolactin binds to specific receptors on the mammary epithelial cell and is internalized to induce casein mRNA at the nuclear level.[36–38] Hypophysectomy halts milk secretion, which resumes when pituitary extract is injected.[39]

Suckling provides a powerful and specific physiologic stimulus for prolactin release.[40,41] In response to suckling, prolactin surges to an apex at 30 minutes and returns to basal levels after 2.5 to 3 hours from the end of the first to approximately the 12th week postpartum.[20,42,43] An adequate prolactin response may also be needed to establish necessary levels of prolactin receptors on the mammary epithelial cells[44] and thus appears critical to the establishment of successful lactation.[45]

Ehrenkranz and Ackerman propose that the slope of the serum prolactin response curve predicts maternal milk production potential.[46] In studies conducted by Aono and colleagues, good lactators give a prolactin response 236% above baseline after nursing for 30 minutes, whereas poor lactators showed a blunted or flat response.[47] Immediately following parturition, prolactin levels remain high and the suckling response is small, although present. After the first week, suckling can raise the serum prolactin levels to 10 to 20 times normal. (Figure 91-2 presents a typical prolactin response curve for the second week postpartum.) By the third month postpartum, serum prolactin levels approach prepregnancy values and do not respond to suckling. Nevertheless, adequate milk production can still continue.[48]

Suckling also stimulates the release of oxytocin from the posterior pituitary. Auditory, olfactory, or emotional cues also lead to the release of oxytocin.[49] Oxytocin produces a contraction of the myoepithelial cells, releasing milk from the alveoli and small ducts into the larger ducts and sinuses. Oxytocin release and the subsequent serum peak of prolactin are not related.[50]

Some evidence exists of a link between growth hormone (GH) and cortisol in lactation in ruminants and humans. Evidence exists in ruminants in which milk yields can be increased experimentally by elevating blood levels of either GH or cortisol. Geissler and colleagues did not demonstrate this association in a study of urban Iranian women.[51] Women with adequate lactation had lower blood levels of both GH and cortisol than women who were poor lactators. In both rumi-

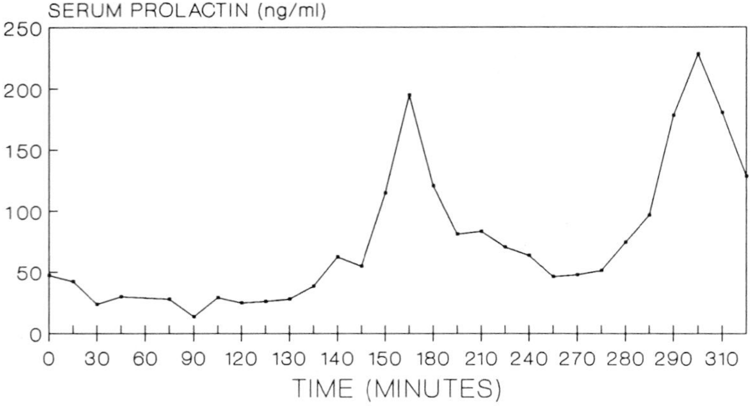

FIGURE 91–2. Serum prolactin response curve showing typical response to suckling in the second postpartum week.

nants and nonruminants, blood thyroxine levels are negatively correlated to milk yields[20] and may play a permissive role and not be involved in regulation.[52,53] Insulin also seems to play a permissive role by maintaining mammary cell numbers and certain enzyme systems.[20]

Autocrine Control

Recent work in Scotland establishes the presence of a local control factor in the mammary gland of goats.[54] This inhibitory factor, isolated in the protein whey fraction of the milk, when injected into the gland of a goat, immediately reduces milk secretion.[55] When this factor is removed, milk secretion immediately returns to normal. Thus, nursing only on one breast or incompletely emptying a breast maintains the presence of this inhibitor and reduces milk production.[54]

COMPOSITION AND QUANTITY OF HUMAN MILK

Although the data on the general composition of human and bovine milks in Table 91-1 represent an oversimplification of the complexity of milk, it is clear that human milk contains more lactose and nonprotein nitrogen and less protein nitrogen than bovine milk. For human milk the figures are averages that change as lactation progresses through each of the stages described earlier. Moreover, each sample from an individual at a particular time can differ in content and composition from each previous sample or from those of women otherwise matched for time, age, diet, and so on.[56] This is in contrast to bovine milk, which is pooled for processing and from which colostrum is excluded.

In stage 1 of lactogenesis, the mammary gland produces colostral milk. This milk, produced in the first 3 days postpartum, contains a higher protein and lower fat, calorie, and lactose content than milk produced later.[57] Colostrum appears yellow when it contains high levels of carotene. The yellow characteristic is more apparent in the milk of multiparous women and often is absent in the milk of primiparas.[58] Of greatest importance to the infant are the immunologic benefits provided by this milk. Colostrum is rich in immunoglobulins that may provide protection against gastrointestinal infections.[25]

The onset of the production of a copious milk supply marks the beginning of transitional milk. By 2 weeks postpartum, the mammary gland produces a stable and mature milk, although compositional differences are still seen.[59] Once involution starts, as seen during the weaning process, mammary gland function deteriorates and milk composition again changes.[60]

EFFECT OF MATERNAL DIET ON MILK COMPOSITION AND PRODUCTION

Lonnerdal has reviewed the literature extensively on the effect that maternal diet can have on milk composi-

TABLE 91–1. GENERAL COMPOSITION OF HUMAN AND BOVINE MILKS

SPECIES	PROTEIN (%)	CASEIN (% PROTEIN)	FAT (%)	LACTOSE (%)	ASH (%)	KILOCALORIES (per 100 mL)
Human						
Mature, 36 d	1.0	40	3.9	6.8	0.2	63
Colostrum, 3 d	2.3	—	3.0	5.5	—	58
Bovine	3.4	82	3.7	4.8	0.7	75

From Jensen RG, et al. Nutrition today 1988; (Nov/Dec): 20. with permission. Adapted from Blanc B. World Rev Nutr Diet 1981;36:1. Harzer G, et al. Z Ernah 1986;25:77.

tion.[61] In summary, maternal dietary intake has little effect on human milk macronutrient content and is not affected significantly by maternal dietary intake, whereas milk fatty acid composition reflects maternal dietary fat intake.[62] Maternal fat-soluble vitamin intake can affect milk composition, but the effect of dietary intake of water-soluble vitamins varies and depends on the specific vitamin transport system involved.[61]

Little evidence exists that links moderate maternal caloric deprivation with decreased milk production. In animal studies, maternal diet appears to affect milk yield. For example, lactating rats showed reduced milk yield, as evidenced by slowed pup growth if either dietary protein or total food intake were restricted.[63] Researchers agree that the energy cost of human milk synthesis is met by a combination of dietary intake and adipose stores. However, the Recommended Dietary Allowances for additional energy in lactation, 500 kcal/day, assume that 100 to 150 kcal are mobilized from maternal fat stores and that maternal dietary intake provides the remaining calories.[64] Some researchers consider this arbitrary value to be too high and suggest adjustment based on maternal milk production.[65,66] The energy costs of lactation are based on the assumption of an infant milk intake of 850 mL/day and are confined to the costs of milk production. Few North American women exclusively breast-feed for the suggested 4 months[67,68] and thus never produce the 850 mL production on which the RDA is based.

Even when full lactation is achieved, few women use the fat stores accumulated in pregnancy to support the first months of lactation. Manning-Dalton and Allen studied well-nourished lactating women in Connecticut, who gained 14 kg in pregnancy.[69] In the first 3 months of lactation, the lactating women only lost an average of 2.2 kg. The more these women breast-fed and the *less* they used supplemental foods to feed their infants, the *less* weight they lost. Higher milk production caused the women's appetite to increase, which resulted in increased caloric consumption. Cessation of lactation resulted in reduced caloric intake and thus weight loss.

Data from Butte and colleagues in Houston confirm the slow weight loss postpartum in lactating women.[70] The 37 women studied in Texas through 4 months of lactation lost 3 kg between 3 days and 1 month postpartum, but at least 2 kg of this probably represented loss of water rather than fat. Weight loss was only 2 kg between 1 and 4 months. Maternal energy intake averaged 2186 kcal/day, and energy drawn from maternal stores was calculated to be 118 to 180 kcal/day, not the 300 kcal usually cited.

Reduction of caloric intake to increase maternal weight loss does not appear warranted, even though maternal undernutrition does not appear to affect milk volume until the mother's energy deficit reaches a severe stage (Figure 91–3).[71–73] Roberts and colleagues, using a baboon model, restricted dietary intake at several levels in the hope of predicting the critical caloric intake to maintain lactation.[74] Animals were fed ad libitum from delivery until 2 weeks postpartum. At 2 weeks the dietary intakes of the mother baboons were restricted to either 80% or 60% of usual intake. When the diet was restricted to 80%, milk production was not compromised. The baboons simply reduced activity to spare milk production. Only when intakes were reduced to 60% of normal was production compromised.

Although a 60% reduction in intake sounds severe, such a restriction may not seem unreasonable to body-conscious American women. Restriction of the usual lactating diet by 60% would result in a caloric intake of from 1200 to 1300 kcal/day, an intake not considered severe for weight loss and considerably above that recommended by many commercial weight loss programs. Both Worthington-Roberts and Roepke report anecdotal data of lactation failure, increased infant restlessness, or reduced milk production in mothers following dietary restriction.[25,75] Ferris and colleagues have also reported that the mother's desire for weight loss was one of the four major predictors of cessation of lactation in a group of 225 women.[76]

In more controlled studies, a 1-week 30% reduction of caloric intake resulted in a 1.4-kg mean weight loss but without affecting milk volume.[77] The researchers

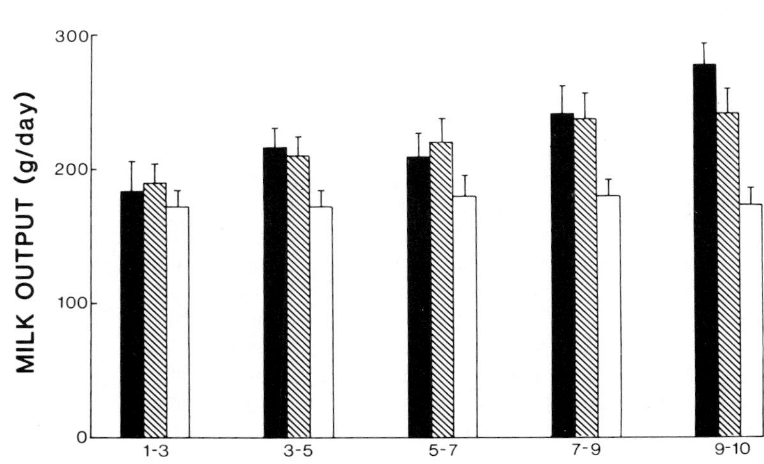

FIGURE 91–3. Milk output of lactating baboons. *Solid bar,* 100%; *hatched,* 80%; *open,* 60%. (From Roberts SB, et al. Lactational performance in relation to energy intake in the baboon. Am J Clin Nutr 1985;41:1270)

also expressed concern that the caloric reduction caused the overall nutritional content of the mother's diet to drop. Healthy women who began a 1500-kcal long-term weight reduction program after nursing for at least 2 months complained of reduced milk production, infant dissatisfaction, and increased fatigue. Mean maternal body fat dropped significantly, suggesting that adipose stores were used to supplement inadequate energy intakes.[78] Thus, women should not expect to lose much weight during lactation, and weight loss should not be promoted as a benefit of breast-feeding. Disappointment at failure to lose weight may, and frequently does, result in the breast-feeder purposely reducing calories to lose weight.

PRENATAL AND PERINATAL PRACTICES THAT AFFECT BREAST-FEEDING

Despite the fact that more than 60% of all women in the United States elect to breast-feed,[68] most experience some difficulties with nursing and most do not meet their goals for duration of nursing. Lactation and breast-feeding are of concern to both the pediatrician and the obstetrician. The pediatrician's concerns are with adequate feeding of the infant, and the obstetrician's concerns are with the care of the mother and breast-feeding problems. Often the advice of these clinicians is dissimilar. The pediatrician may advise the mother to supplement temporarily a perceived unsatisfied infant with formula, which would decrease stimulation to the mother's breast and thus decrease milk yield. The obstetrician might recommend that the mother rest and increase the nursing schedule if it does not overtire her. Both may miss the more physiologically based advice either to increase the feeding schedule or to increase breast emptying with a breast pump to increase milk yield. The clinical care of the breast-feeding mother–infant pair has to investigate solutions that always consider both sides of the dyad. Some teaching hospitals, both in the United States and in Great Britain, have recognized that the complexity of this care requires consultation of a physician trained in this new area.

PRENATAL EXAMINATION

Neifert outlines several abnormalities that can be detected and treated during the prenatal period.[79,80] Among these are treatable conditions such as inverted nipples, conditions that will require special counseling but that should not preclude nursing (eg, silicone breast implantation and unilateral mastectomy), and conditions that preclude adequate lactation (eg, insufficient glandular development[81] and breast reduction procedures that severed nerve endings to the areola and nipple[79]). Even when the physical exam yields no apparent problem, the clinician should take a detailed lactation history early in the pregnancy, since the problems multiparous women have with lactation with one child repeat with later children.[76] Early recognition of these problems allows for sufficient time for intervention strategy counseling.

Potential Problems

The physician and staff also need to discuss and plan appropriate interventions for potential problems that will affect the present lactation cycle. Among these are multiple births, problems with maternal abuse of recreational drugs, the less-well-recognized problems of caffeine and nicotine addiction, and such maternal health problems as psychiatric disease, diabetes mellitus, cystic fibrosis, maternal phenylketonuria, cardiovascular disease, and autoimmune disease. Special attention must also be paid to drug therapies needed by the mother. Lawrence,[21,82] Lederman,[83] and McGregor and Neifert[84] have provided a review of these problems. This chapter is meant only to update data available since their publications.

Substance Abuse. Most abused substances clearly enter the milk and can cause harm to the infant. No matter what the level of addiction, polydrug abuse is usually the norm (eg, cocaine combined with alcohol and cigarettes combined with caffeine). No data are available on the additive effects of these substances on the maternal mammary or infant detoxification system.

Smoking of Cigarettes. Numerous studies have clearly demonstrated the potentially harmful effects on the newborn of maternal smoking during pregnancy. Worthington-Roberts notes that the nicotine-intoxicated infant will not suckle, is apathetic, vomits, and has poor bladder and gastrointestinal function.[25] Although mothers who smoke usually elect not to breast-feed,[84] those who do tend to wean their infants earlier than mothers who do not smoke.[85] Whether this early weaning is due to personality differences between smokers and nonsmokers,[86] to interferences of the more than 500 toxic by-products of cigarette smoking with maternal hormones that promote lactogenesis,[87] or to reduced energy available for lactation as a result of reduced caloric intake[88,89] and/or increased energy expenditure of the mothers who smoke is unknown.[88,89]

Nicotine and its major derivative, cotinine, derived from tobacco use, are found in the serum and urine of infants in direct proportion to the amount of exposure from breast milk and/or passive exposure.[90] The half-life of nicotine is 1.5 hours, and the accumulation of nicotine depends on both the interval between cigarettes and the number of cigarettes.[91] Cotinine, with a half-life of over 30 hours,[92] remains stable over a 24-hour period, and its levels are directly proportional to the number of cigarettes smoked.[93] Although no data are available on the effects of maternal tobacco use and infant psychomotor development, behavior, growth, or other infant outcome measures, no benefit appears to be derived from this practice. If the mother must smoke while nursing, the clinician should caution her to allow an interval of at least 1.5 hours between smoking a cigarette and nursing the infant. This may be difficult, as most infants do not feed on a schedule that would allow such planning in early lactation. Also, to avoid the addition of passive exposure of tobacco derivatives to that already obtained from the milk, mothers must be cautioned not to "light up" when they nurse, as is the practice noted in studies by one of the authors. Since all the mothers who smoked cigarettes in the Connecticut series of lactation studies also drank large quantities of caffeine-containing beverages, advice on smoking should be coupled with the possible problems from caffeine intake.

Caffeine. Caffeine freely crosses the human alveolar cell into the milk[94–96] and is detectable within 15 minutes after oral ingestion.[96] Peak levels of caffeine in breast milk may be achieved within 1 hour.[96] Levels of caffeine in breast milk are approximately 1% of the maternal dose.[96] Accumulation of low doses of caffeine is possible, especially in breast-fed infants, since caffeine elimination is delayed[97] and adult clearance levels are not achieved until 3 to 4 months of age[94] (Fig. 91-4). The mechanism for this delay is unknown.[97]

Clinicians fear that even at the low doses reported, caffeine ingestion by the infant could cause restlessness, increases in heart rate, and disturbances in sleep pattern.[98] Ryu conducted a cross-over study with 11 mother–infant pairs.[99] In random order, the mothers ingested decaffeinated coffee with or without the addition of 500 mg of caffeine. Maternal serum and milk levels of caffeine and infant serum levels of caffeine were measured. Infant heart rate was monitored and sleep pattern recorded. No differences in heart rate or sleep time were noted with the addition of caffeine. Therefore, most of the data suggest that moderate caffeine consumption by the lactating mother does not cause behavior abnormalities in the infant. However, careful studies addressing the issue of multiple dosing, closely spaced dosing, and high dosing (>150 mg/dose) have not been done.

Of greater concern are the problems that routine high caffeine intake could cause to the nutrient content of the milk and the health of the mother. A study by Munoz and colleagues noted that coffee consumption (intake ≥10 g ground coffee/day) resulted in lower maternal hemoglobin (Hb) and hematocrit (Hct) levels at 8 months gestation, lower cord blood Hb and Hct, lower infant birth weight, and lower Hb and Hct at 1 month of age.[100] Breast milk iron concentrations were also significantly lower in the coffee-drinking group. Zinc and copper milk levels were not affected. Breast milk is already low in iron, although the iron is of high bioavailability. Therefore, this reduced iron content could cause a problem with the infant already at risk of anemia. Recent studies also note increased bone mineral loss in healthy lactating women[101] and body calcium losses that could be aggravated by the increased urine calcium losses associated with high caffeine consumption.[102] Recommendations of moderate caffeine ingestion (one to two caffeine beverages per day) during lactation seem justified.

Alcohol. Ethanol and many other substances in alcoholic beverages are transferred into the milk.[103] Maximal blood concentration after a standard dose occurred between 30 and 60 minutes after ingestion in a ratio of 0.9 in milk to maternal plasma.[104] Once the ethanol is in the milk, it does not break down readily to acetaldehyde, which is thought to be the toxic compound in alcohol metabolism.[105]

Wilson has calculated that large amounts of alcohol would have to be consumed by the mother before there would be an obvious clinical effect on the infant (Table 91-2). At toxic levels, however, the effects can be significant. Foremost of course is the concern about the drunken mother's ability to care for the infant. Large amounts of alcohol also interfere with breast-feeding, first by hindrance of the milk-ejection reflex[105] through inhibition of oxytocin release[106] and second through the depressant effect on the infant, which causes less vigorous suckling.[107] Small amounts of alcohol, however, may help relieve tension and thus aid with the let-down reflex.[21,108]

Potentially more subtle effects on mental and psychomotor development and other body processes need to be investigated. Little and colleagues studied 400 in-

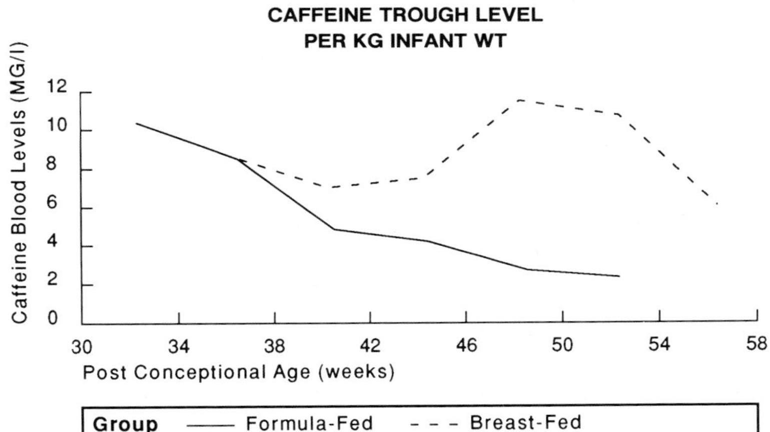

FIGURE 91–4. Differences in caffeine clearance in breast-fed and formula-fed infants. (Adapted with permission from Leguennec J. Billon B. Pediatrics 1987;79:266.)

TABLE 91–2. CALCULATION OF EFFECT OF MATERNAL ALCOHOL INGESTION ON INFANT

MOTHER'S BLOOD ALCOHOL (mg/dL)	COMMON REFERENCE	MAXIMUM INFANT BLOOD CONCENTRATION (mg/dL)	RESULT TO INFANT
50	2 to 3 cocktails	1.9	Insignificant
100	Habitual drinker	3.7	Insignificant
300	Mother close to passing out	11.1	Mild sedation

Adapted from Wilson JT, Brown RD, Cherek DR, et al. Drug excretion in human breast milk. Principles, pharmacokinetics and projected consequences. Clin Pharmacokinetics 1980;5:34.

fants for 1 year postpartum.[109] Infants of mothers who consumed less than one alcoholic beverage per day during lactation had better psychomotor coordination (as measured by the Bailey Physical Development Index [PDI][110]) than infants of mothers who had more than one drink per day. Bayley Mental Development scores did not differ between groups. These authors controlled for confounding factors such as alcoholic consumption during pregnancy, cigarette smoking, and drug use. However, these results must be interpreted with some caution, since the heavy-drinking group only had four subjects whereas the nondrinking group had 188 subjects. A study of 23 full-term infants of daily alcohol abusers in the People's Republic of China noted decreased prothrombin time but normal platelet counts in the infants.[111] The sparse data available suggest that very low maternal intake of alcohol has no adverse effect on the infant. Until we can account for the potential subtle adverse effects on the infant of the many other substances that are also included in the ingestion of alcoholic beverages (eg, congeners and byproducts of fermentation), the physician should caution the moderate drinker to reduce her intake.

Other Recreational Drugs. All known recreational drugs are excreted into breast milk, and pharmacokinetic data for humans are not available for most of them. Some, like marijuana and phencyclidine (PCP), are known after exposure to be in higher concentrations in the milk than in the maternal serum.[112,113] In certain parts of the country, the number of drug-exposed babies increased over 100% between 1986 and 1989. Most of this increase can be attributed to cocaine addiction.[114] Twenty-five percent of all infants born at General Hospital in Washington, D. C., were exposed to illegal drugs during pregnancy.[115] The excitable state of these infants at birth makes nursing difficult. In some instances, the mother may not understand that the drug is transferred through the milk or understand, as in the case of marijuana, that even a passive smoke environment has can delay brain cell development in the infant.[21] The appearance of addictive drugs in breast milk, therefore, often precludes the continuance of breast-feeding.

Two case studies are available that note the use of cocaine in lactating women. In the first, Chasnoff relates the ignorance of an affluent professional who used cocaine intranasally at a party.[116] Within 3 hours, her 2-week-old infant showed symptoms of cocaine intoxication. In the second case, an infant developed apnea and seizures from direct ingestion of cocaine used as a topical anesthetic for nipple soreness.[117] Because of increased drug use, physicians should caution all patients about the potential hazards during lactation and strongly discourage breast-feeding if the mother continues to use drugs.

Preexisting Maternal Health Problems.

Few maternal conditions preclude lactation. Failure to lactate may occur secondary to Sheehan's syndrome (postpartum pituitary necrosis), to destructive diseases of the hypothalamic–pituitary system, and to hypophysectomy.[118] Alternative feeding for the infant is necessary when the composition of the milk is deleterious, when necessary maternal drug therapy would be detrimental to the infant, or when the milk contains a transmittable substance such as a virus, as in human immunodeficiency virus (HIV), or an environmental contaminant. A mother with breast cancer should receive treatment immediately and not be concerned about the effects of these treatments on her milk.[21] The infant with galactosemia, a rare occurrence of one in 60,000 births, must be maintained on a lactose-free diet. Since lactose is the major carbohydrate in human milk, its use is obviously precluded.[25] Several other conditions are outlined in more detail later.

Diabetes Mellitus. Little information exists on the incidence or outcome of breast-feeding in either overt or gestational diabetic mothers. Because of poor fetal outcomes, complications during delivery, and hormonal changes that might inhibit lactation, the ability of diabetic women to breast-feed has been questioned. Ferris and Reece[66] have recently reviewed the literature on the course of lactation in insulin-dependent diabetic mothers and have noted that the duration of lactation in the diabetic mother seems to be comparable to that in nondiabetics[119]; that milk composition, except for glucose and sodium, does not differ once lactation is established[120,121]; but that lactogenesis is delayed, which results in lower infant milk intake[122] and milk composition differences in the early stages of lactation.[121] Therefore, diabetic mothers ought not to be discouraged from nursing as long as maternal energy intakes and insulin requirements are adjusted for the extra caloric needs of lactation, caloric intake is redistributed to prevent hypoglycemia following repeated nursings,[123] and extra breast pumping is provided in the first days postpartum to help overcome reduced maternal milk yields.

Cystic Fibrosis. No comprehensive studies are available that examine the effect of cystic fibrosis (CF) on breast milk composition or milk production. Because of the concern that milk sodium would be elevated to levels that would lead to hypernatremia in the infant, most of the 100 women with CF who have become pregnant were counseled against breast-feeding.[124] The first case study available on a CF mother supported this concern.[125] Other recent case studies[126–128] clearly indicate that electrolyte concentrations in breast milk of women with CF are within normal limits. These authors explain that the mammary gland does not modify its excretion as does the sweat gland.[129] The sweat gland modifies primary acinar sweat by reabsorbing sodium in excess of water.[130,131] These authors attributed the high milk sodium levels noted by Whitelaw and Butterfield[125] to inadequate sampling procedures. Concern should be directed instead toward the macronutrient content and fatty acid composition of the milk. Schiffman and colleagues noted that lower macronutrient concentrations were found during severe pulmonary exacerbations of the CF patients.[126] Bitman and colleagues noted abnormalities in the fatty acid concentrations of the milk from seven CF women to an extent that may contraindicate breast-feeding.[132] No data are available on maternal breast milk production. These preliminary data indicate that women with CF can breast-feed as long as the course of both the disease and infant growth are carefully monitored.

Maternal Phenylketonuria. Bradburn and colleagues studied phenylketonuric mothers for 20 days of lactation and found normal total protein but phenylalanine levels elevated 40-fold in the milk.[133] Lederman calculates that because of the small contribution phenylalanine makes to the total protein content of the milk, the infant's phenylalanine load was increased by only 17%.[134] These limited data indicate that a phenylketonuric mother under strict dietary control should be allowed to breast-feed. No data are available on the potential problems encountered by a mother with uncontrolled phenylketonuria.

Thyroid Disease. As stated earlier, thyroid hormones are required for normal mammary development, lactational performance, and milk synthesis, playing a permissive rather than a regulatory role.[53] Because conditions of hypothyroidism are often associated with infertility in females, they occur only rarely with lactation.[21] When they do occur, breast-feeding can continue uninterrupted, since the therapy is usually full replacement with desiccated thyroid. The diagnosis can be made without the use of radioactive compounds. The therapeutic agents employed are antithyroid medications that block iodination of the tyrosine molecule.[21] Levels of these medications may build up in the milk and thus be available to the infant. Reported levels range from minimal[135] to 4.5% to 6%.[136] Breast-feeding can be continued if infant biochemical indices of thyroid function are monitored and the clinician watches for signs of bradycardia and other signs of hypothyroidism and goiter.[21]

Infectious Diseases Acquired Postpartum

Human Immunodeficiency Virus (HIV). Almost all infants who are positive for human immunodeficiency virus (HIV) in the early postpartum period contracted the disease during gestation. However, HIV has been isolated in breast milk,[137] and although a minor transmission route for the disease, it appears that an infant may contract the syndrome through exposure to breast milk.[138] Most of the previously reported cases were among mother–infant pairs from high-risk groups who probably tested positive for acquired immune deficiency syndrome (AIDS) during pregnancy; thus, the transmission route through breast milk could not be proved. Wasserberger and colleagues report the case of a mother who contracted HIV through a blood transfusion after she delivered her infant.[139] The infant then tested positive. Five similar cases are available in the literature. In one additional case of suspected HIV transmission through breast milk, the mother died at birth with no history of HIV infection.[140] The infant was subsequently wet-nursed by the mother's sister, who was HIV seropositive and symptomatic during nursing. In six of the seven cases cited earlier, the mothers were newly infected and thus probably had high titers of circulating virus. In addition, the mothers had not yet fully formed HIV antibodies. Thus, the infants were exposed to a highly infectious state without the protection of maternal antibodies.

In developing countries, given the poor mortality prognosis of all infants who acquire AIDS or AIDS-related complex prenatally, breast-feeding should not necessarily be discouraged for that group, since the mortality risk from other infections, diarrhea, and dehydration from bottle-feeding may be greater than the increased mortality associated with HIV exposure.[141,142] In developed countries, where safe feeding alternatives are available, bottle-feeding may be a safer course.[141] Although the link is not completely clear for transmission postnatally in breast milk, the present evidence precludes a mother from breast-feeding if she has acquired the disease after delivery or if the child, delivered of a mother testing positive during pregnancy, did not test positive for HIV infection at birth.[141]

Other Infectious Diseases. Other retroviruses—such as human T-cell leukemia (HTLV-1) and cytomegalovirus (CMV), herpes simplex virus (HSV), rubella, and hepatitis B virus—have been isolated in breast milk.[141] Breast-feeding may be the major mother–infant transmission route for HTLV-1. However, as Oxtoby notes, although HIV infection results in a devastating disease, with 95% mortality for infected infants, HTLV-1 infection resulted in carcinoma and neurologic disease in only 5% of infected infants.[141] CMV exposure neonatally may be preferable to exposure later in life or during gestation. The newborn exposed to CMV through breast-feeding but protected by placentally transferred maternal CMV antibody does not demonstrate the systemic acute infection with symptoms similar to that of congenital CMV infection.[143,144] HSV transmission through breast milk has not been shown.[145] Rubella-exposed infants remain asymptomatic,[146] and the efficacy of hepatitis B vaccine reduces the concern for transmission of that virus. The Centers for Disease Control recommends that for all the viruses mentioned earlier, except HTLV-1, breast-feeding should not be discouraged. For HTLV-1, guidelines similar to those for HIV exposure should be followed.[141]

Contaminants

Drug Therapy. Most medications are found in human milk at 1% of maternal circulation. The rate of passage from maternal circulation to the milk depends on the molecular weight of the drug, the percentage that is protein-bound, pH, and water and lipid solubility.[118] Lawrence,[21] Wilson,[103] and Worthington-Roberts[25] have outlined extensively each of these mechanisms and the implications for commonly used medications. In all cases, no unnecessary medications should be given to a nursing mother, since data are lacking on most drugs. The potential effects on the infant are largely unknown.[103] Some drugs are clearly contraindicated during breast-feeding. Drug dosage, peak appearance, and the feeding schedule need to be coordinated. Usually the best time to give a drug is immediately after a feed.

Environmental Contaminants. The level of contamination of human milk has decreased over the past decade,[147,148] and concern should be reserved for those women who have been exposed to a major spillage, live near a waste disposal site, or have eaten sport fish on a regular basis over their lifetime. Of greatest concern are the lipid-soluble organohalides—polychorinated buphenyls (PCBs), polychlorinated dibenzo-p-dioxins (PCDDs), dibenzofurans (PCDFs) and (DDT). Their presence in the milk is dependent not only on the amount in the present food chain but also on the amount stored in the mother's adipose tissue. During lactation maternal adipose and mineral stores are mobilized to provide the energy and nutrients needed to produce milk. Thus, with each lactation, if there has not been continued exposure, the organohalides are drawn from the adipose tissue and storage levels are further reduced.[147]

Heavy metals are also transferred to the infant via human milk. Lactation increases gut absorption of lead as with other metals. Bone depot lead may also be mobilized during lactation.[149] In Canada, lead and cadmium contamination of human milk has been determined to be lower than previously reported.[148] Lead contamination was significantly and positively correlated with the age of the subject's home, with maternal exposure to heavy traffic for more than 5 years, and with coffee consumption. Milk cadmium correlated only with exposure to cigarette smoke, both direct and passive. These data suggest that human milk may add to an infant's body load of lead if both mother and infant are still in the contaminated environment. If such contamination is suspected, heavy metal analysis of maternal blood prenatally seems appropriate.[148]

SUPPORT STRATEGY FOR MOTHER AND INFANT

With reduced time in the hospital after delivery, health professionals have little time to prepare the mother for nursing. Therefore, it is imperative that mothers receive sufficient preparation for lactation during the prenatal period and that both an emotional and educational support system be established for after delivery.

PERINATAL CARE

Over one third of Connecticut mothers who stop nursing do so in the first two postpartum weeks.[76] These data closely align with national statistics.[68] This clearly indicates that the early postpartum experience plays an important role in the maintenance of lactation.

LABOR AND DELIVERY

Method of Delivery

Labor and delivery practices that encourage early mother–infant contact, reduced medication, and vaginal delivery extend the duration of lactation. During cesarean deliveries more anesthesia is given to the mother and thus, indirectly, to the child. Higher medication may interfere with the readiness of both mother and infant to begin nursing promptly.[150] After birth, the sectioned mother requires more pain medication than a woman who delivered vaginally. This medication transmitted through the breast milk can reduce the alertness of both infant and mother as well as the intensity of infant suckling. Cesarean delivery may cause early lactation failure,[151] but once breast-feeding is established, delivery method does not have a profound effect on how long a mother nurses,[152] although women who were given a local rather than a general anesthesia with the surgery breast-feed longer.[153] Induction of labor appears to have little physiologic effect on the process of lactation. However, mothers who choose to be induced may be less motivated to breast-feed and thus nurse for a shorter time than mothers who deliver spontaneously or mothers for whom induction is recommended by their physician.[154]

Mother–Infant Contact

Early mother–infant contact promotes frequent and early feeds and thus leads to lactation success. This association may not be entirely physiologically based since the early contact also promotes better family interaction and maternal bonding, which aid in the breast-feeding process.[155–158] Frequent feeds may encourage increased milk intake and production through the suckling stimulation of the lactogenic hormone, prolactin. Increased nursing frequency also empties the breasts more often, and breast emptying may signal milk synthesis as well.[159] Durations of feeding may not correlate with milk production because infants vary widely in their suckling strength and efficiency of breast emptying. Lactating mothers also vary in strength and rate of milk ejection. Consequently, length of time at breast may have little or no independent effect on milk intake,[159,160] although severely restricting the length of the feed may promote early involution and breast engorgement.[20] In early lactation, letdown is not well-conditioned. Therefore, the time for an effective feed may be as long as 15 minutes. When reflexes are developed, an infant may be able to empty the breast in 5 minutes.[80]

Maternal Fatigue and Stress

Lactation experts generally agree that maternal fatigue and anxiety can affect lactation performance. Physical and emotional stress may inhibit prolactin and oxytocin release, which in turn limits milk production and letdown.[73,161,162] In an intriguing study, the enhancing effect of relaxation was demonstrated with mothers of premature infants staying in newborn intensive care. After listening to relaxation audiotapes, mothers pumped 63% more milk on average than women who did not listen to the tapes.[163] If letdown is delayed because of anxiety or stress, then the relaxation can be coupled with the judicious use of synthetic oxytocin delivered nasally to promote letdown.[20]

Before discharge, each mother–infant pair should be evaluated carefully for breast-feeding behavior, including maternal nursing technique and infant suckling ability. Specially trained staff are needed for these evaluations. In the very short time available, they should assist the mother with the early nursing experience and prepare her and her infant for home.

Assessment of Lactation Failure

Quantitative indicators of the onset of adequate human milk production are needed to assess the lactational ability of individual mothers who have had previous lactation failure or who have a condition whose drug treatment or metabolism may be thought to interfere with lactogenesis. Detection of potential lactation failure must be assessed in the first days postpartum before the mother leaves the hospital. Because of the volatility of the infant weight and the variability of maternal milk volume in the first week postpartum, monitoring of infant growth or test-weighing the baby before and after each feeding provides little helpful information. What is needed are methods to predict whether a mother will be able to produce a copious milk supply. With proper clinical management, lactation failure should be rare.

Neville and her colleagues followed the milk production and infant milk intake of 13 mother–infant pairs during the first year of life.[164] The infants of nine women were weighed before and after every feed from birth to 14 days postpartum. Three other infants were weighed for 64% of the feeds during this time period. Figure 91-5 depicts the mean milk yield (sum of volume calculated from the test weighing and milk expressions) until day 14. For the first 36 hours milk yield increases gradually, followed by a surge in the milk supply at 49 to 96 hours postpartum. After that time the milk supply plateaus. Similar studies that measure intake using test weighing from Perth, Australia,[165] and Edinburgh[166] confirm these findings. Neville emphasizes that great variability exists in the described pattern, with peak volumes for some mother–infant pairs occurring as early as 4 and as late as 10 or more days. Neville suggests that in

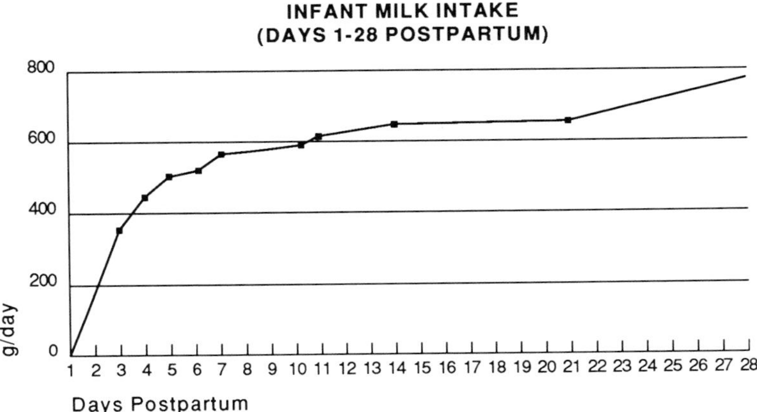

FIGURE 91–5. Breast milk intake of infants from day 1 to 28 postpartum (Adapted from Neville M, et al. Am J Clin Nutr 1988;48:1380.)

all mother–infant pairs, milk volumes are low for the first 2 days because of the inhibitory effect of progesterone, and possibly that of estrogen, on milk production.[167] Once the levels of these hormones fall, some mothers can easily produce the additional milk their infants need. The plateau represents the compromise between the mother's production capability and the infant's caloric and nutrient needs.

A more physiologically relevant and clinically applicable indicator may be the measurement of specific milk components whose presence or absence in the milk marks full milk production capability by the mammary gland (ie, the concentration of the component would be correlated significantly to changes in milk yield described earlier). Several components have been suggested as possible candidates in animal models: the de novo synthesis of medium-chain fatty acids in rabbits[168,169]; casein in mice[170]; casein mRNA in rabbits[35,171]; lactose in rabbits[39] and mice[172]; citrate in goats,[173] cows, and a human[174]; and glucose in goats.[175,176] The only components suggested as feasible for the study of human milk production are lactose,[167,177] citrate,[174,177] glucose,[177,178] and α-lactalbumin.[179,180] Quantifying these components, however, is difficult because of the great variation in the concentration of each component over time, although several studies are under way to define normal limits for these factors.

COMMON PROBLEMS IN POSTPARTUM CARE

Emotional, educational, physical, and medical support should be available to a mother once she leaves the hospital, especially in the first weeks postpartum. Customs throughout the world differ in the extent to which a mother is cared for in the months after delivery. Like women in the highlands of Nepal, mothers in the United States are expected to return to normal function within days of delivery. Few women have the resources to hire professional help and few companies allow paternal leave for more than a few days. Even in upper-middle-class families, "grandmother" may be able to take only a few days off from work to help. Therefore, the health care system needs to fill in the gaps generated by reduced hospitalization and the economic needs of the clients with continued education and monitoring for such common breast-feeding problems as sore nipples and engorgement in the mother, and jaundice in the infant.

INADEQUATE MILK SUPPLY

In the first 2 weeks of lactation, many women also express concern that they are not producing enough milk for their infant. If the baby is given formula supplementation to assuage the mother's concerns, the infant will need less milk and the total time at the breast will be reduced, as will total milk production,[181] thus aggravating the problem. When a substitute food is used in place of breast milk, the infant intakes of these two energy sources will be related inversely. The infant's appetite will regulate total caloric intake so that changes in consumption of one food will be offset by complementary changes in intake of the other food. Once lactation has been established, use of supplementary feeds may not reduce total milk production.[182]

MASTITIS

Mastitis is an inflammation of the mammary gland from some infectious process.[183] Monthly incidence under the most adverse conditions in Africa was 2.6% of all lactating women.[184] Repeated episodes in one woman were common. Lawrence recommends continuing breast-feeding with antibiotic therapy and maternal rest. Breast-feeding is contraindicated only if the abscess ruptures into a duct and contaminates the milk.[185] If rupturing occurs, the breasts should be pumped so that gland involution will not take place.

Mastitis may affect milk composition and maternal milk volume and thus interfere with the normal feeding regimen. Mastitis reduces milk yield in cows, but no human studies of milk production are available. Cows diagnosed with mastitis produced 22% less milk with a lower butterfat content than that seen in the milk of noninfected animals.[185,186] Human studies of compositional changes showed significant decreases in lactose, fat, and total protein during mastitis.[187,188] Increased milk sodium[184,188] and chloride[185,187] and decreased potassium levels have also resulted and can be used to monitor milk samples clinically for mastitis.[185,189,190] These milk compositional changes may make the milk unpalatable, so that the baby consumes less.[66] If the infant rejects the mastitic milk, the mother should pump her breasts to prevent abscess formation.

CONTRACEPTION

As previously discussed, since ovulation and menstruation can occur within the first 6 weeks for the woman who chooses to bottle-feed or partially breast-feed her infant, women who are sexually active should be counseled on contraception options during the early puerperal period. For women who chose to breast-feed exclusively, barrier methods or progestin-only oral contraceptives[191–193] are the preferred methods. Combined estrogen and progestin pills,[191,192] even of the low-dosage variety,[193] appear to affect milk production and the duration of lactation.[191–193]

SUMMARY

All women require special care in the early puerperal period to ensure the completion of the reproductive cycle. For lactating women, the first week postpartum is the most crucial for the establishment of breast-feeding.

If delayed lactogenesis caused by either alterations in the mother's physiology or the behavior of the infant occurs, full lactation may never be established. The physician must understand the topics outlined in this chapter that describe the physiology of lactation and the pathologies, prescribed and recreational drugs, and hospital and prenatal practices that can interfere with the process of lactation, alter milk composition, and in some instances contraindicate breast-feeding. Generally, practices that ensure early mother–infant contact and promote frequent suckling by the infant are associated with adequate lactation. When special care is required, as with the mother who has experienced a high-risk delivery and for whom early infant contact may not be possible, the physician needs the assistance of a lactation specialist, usually a specially trained registered nurse or dietitian. This specialist can provide instruction in nursing a baby who has poor suckling ability or is unable to nurse immediately and help the mother maintain her milk supply with artificial pumping.

ACKNOWLEDGMENTS

The authors wish to thank for their research and editorial assistance Christina Chase, Maureen Murtaugh, Suzanne H. Neubauer, Karin M. Ostrom, Kimberly Freudigman, and the Yale University Faculty Practice Staff.

REFERENCES

1. Hytten F, Chamberlain G. Clinical physiology in obstetrics. London: Blackwell Scientific Publications, 1980:368.
2. Piiroinen O, Kaihola HL. Uterine size measured by ultrasound during the menstrual cycle. Acta Obstet Gynecol Scand 1975;]54:47.
3. Robinson HP. Sonar in the puerperium. Scot Med J 1972;17:364.
4. Rodeck CH, Newton JR. Study of the uterine cavity by ultrasound in the early puerperium. Br J Obstet Gynaecol 1976;83:795.
5. Van Rees D, Bernstein RL, Crawford W. Involution of the postpartum uterus: an ultrasonic study. J Clin Ultrasound 1981;9:55.
6. Reynolds SRM. Physiology of the uterus. New York: Hafner, 1965.
7. Woessner JF. Ob/Gyn Dig 1968;(July):14.
8. Anderson WR, Davis J. Placental site involution. Am J Obstet Gynecol 1968;102:23.
9. Cronin TJ. Influence of lactation upon ovulation. Lancet 1968;11:422.
10. Perez A, Vela P, Masnick GS, Potter RG. First ovulation after childbirth: the effect of breastfeeding. Am J Obstet Gynecol 1972;114:1041.
11. Charmin A. Ovulation in post-partum period. Excerpta Medica International Congress Series 1966;133:158.
12. McNeilly AS, Glasier A, Howie PW. Endocrine control of lactational infertility. I. In: Dobbing J, ed. Maternal nutrition and lactational infertility nestle nutrition. New York: Raven Press 1985:1.
13. Howie PW, McNeilly AS, Houston MJ, Cook A, Boyle H. Effect of supplementary food on suckling patterns and ovarian activity during lactation. Br Med J 1981;283:757.
14. Chowdhury A. Effect of maternal nutrition on fertility in rural Bangladesh. In: Mosley WH, ed. Nutrition and human reproduction. New York: Plenum Press, 1978:401.
15. Sheehan KL, Yen SSC. Activation of pituitary gonadotropic function by an agonist of luteinizing hormone-releasing factor in the puerperium. Am J Obstet Gynecol 1979;135:755.
16. Parker CJ Jr, MacDonald PC, Guzick DS, Porter JC, Rosenfeld CR, Hauth JC. Prolactin levels in umbilical cord blood of human infants: relation to gestational age, maternal complications, and neonatal lung function. Am J Obstet Gynecol 1989;161:795.
17. Sims EAH, Karntz KE. Serial studies of renal function during pregnancy and the puerperium in normal women. J Clin Invest 1958;37:1764.
18. Bailey RR, Rolleston GL. Kidney length and ureteric dilation in the puerperium. J Obstet Gynaecol Br Commonw 1971;78:55.
19. Spino FI, Fry IK. Ureteric dilation in non-pregnant women. Proc R Soc Med 1970;63:462.
20. Mepham TB. Physiology of lactation. Milton Keyes, UK: Open University Press, 1987.
21. Lawrence RA. Breastfeeding, a guide for the medical profession. St Louis: CV Mosby, 1985.
22. Kulski JK, Hartmann PE. Changes in human milk composition during the initiation of lactation. Aust J Exp Biol Med Sci 1981;59:101.
23. Russo J, Russo IH. Development of the human mammary gland. In: Neville MC, Daniel CW, eds. The mammary gland, development, regulation and function. New York: Plenum Press, 1987:67.
24. Tanner JM. The development of the reproductive system. In: Tanner JM. Growth at adolescence. Oxford: Blackwell Scientific Publications, 1962:28.
25. Worthington-Roberts BS. Lactation and human milk: nutritional considerations. In: Worthington-Roberts BS, Rodwell Williams S, ed. Nutrition in pregnancy and lactation. St Louis: Times Mirror/Mosby College Publishing, 1989:244.
26. Archer DF. Physiology of prolactin. Clin Obstet Gynecol 1980;23:325.
27. Battin DA, Marrs RP, Fleiss PM, et al. Effect of suckling on serum prolactin, luteinizing hormone, follicle-stimulating hormone and estradiol during prolonged lactation. Obstet Gynecol 1985;65:785.
28. Jacobs LS. The role of prolactin in mammogenesis and lactogenesis. Adv Exp Biol Med 1977;80:173.
29. Hartmann PE. Changes in the composition and yield of the mammary secretions of cows during the initiation of lactation. J Endocrinol 1973;59:23117.
30. Falconer IR. Aspects of the biochemistry, physiology and endocrinology of lactation. Aust J Biol Sci 1980;33:71.
31. Cowie AT, Forsyth IA, Prentice AM. Hormonal control of lactation. Berlin: Springer-Verlag, 1980:1.
32. Hartmann PE, Prosser CG. Physiological basis of longitudinal changes in human milk yield and composition. Fed Proc 1984;43:2448.
33. Topper YJ, Sankaran L, Chomczynski P, Prosser C, Qasba P. Three stages of responsiveness to hormones in the mammary cell. Ann NY Acad Sci 1986;464:1.
34. Juergens WG, Stockdale FE, Topper YJ, Elias JJ. Hormone dependent differentiation of mammary gland in vitro. Proc Natl Acad Sci USA 1965;54:629.
35. Devinoy E, Houdebine LM, Delouis C. Role of prolactin and glucocorticoids in the expression of casein genes in rabbit mammary gland organ culture. Biochem Biophys Acta 1978; 517:360.
36. Guyette WA, Matusik RJ, Rosen JM. Prolactin-mediated tran-

scriptional and post-transcriptional control of casein gene expression. Cell 1979;17:1013.
37. Matusik RJ, Rosen JM. Prolactin induction of casein mRNA in organ culture. J Biol Chem 1978;253:2343.
38. Robyn C, Brandts N, Rosenberg S, Meuris S. Advances in physiology of human lactation. Ann NY Acad Sci 1986;464:66.
39. Jones EA, Cowie AT. The effect of hypophysectomy and subsequent replacement therapy with sheep prolactin or bovine growth hormone on the lactose synthetase activity of rabbit mammary gland. Biochem J 1972;130:997.
40. Frantz AG. Prolactin. New Engl J Med 1978;298:201.
41. Fournier PJR, Desjardins RD, Friesen HG. Current understanding of human prolactin physiology and its diagnostic and therapeutic applications: a review. Am J Obstet Gynecol 1974; 118:337.
42. Noel GL, Suh HK, Frantz AG. Prolactin release during nursing and breast stimulation in postpartum and nonpostpartum subjects. J Clin Endocrinol 1974;38:413.
43. Weitzmann RE, Leake RD, Rubin RT, et al The effect of nursing on neuropophyseal hormone and prolactin secretion in human subjects. J Clin Endocrinol Metab 1980;51:836.
44. Shiu RP, Friesen HG. Mechanism of action of prolactin in the control of mammary gland function. Ann Rev Physiol 1980;42:83.
45. Weichert CE. Prolactin cycling and the management of breastfeeding failure. Adv Pediatr 1980;27:391.
46. Ehrenkranz RA, Ackerman BA. Metoclopramide effect on faltering milk production by mothers of premature infants. Pediatrics 1986;78:614.
47. Aono T, Shioji T, Shoda T, et al. The initiation of human lactation and prolactin response to suckling. J Clin Endocrinol Metab 1979;44:1101.
48. Tyson JE. Mechanisms of puerperal lactation. Med Clin North Am 1977;61:153.
49. Newton M, Newton NR. The let-down reflex in human lactation. J Pediatr 1948;33:698.
50. Godd G, Foloszar S, Darug J, Falkay G, Sas M. Prolactin release during nursing in early puerperium. Acta Med Hung 1988;45:171.
51. Geissler C, Margen S, Calloway DH. Lactation and pregnancy in Iran. III. Hormonal factors. Am J Clin Nutr 1979;32:1097.
52. Gehlbach DL, Bayliss P, Rosa C. Prolactin and thyrotropin responses to nursing during the early puerperium. J Reprod Med 1989;34;295.
53. Neville MC, Berga SE. Cellular and molecular aspects of the hormonal control of mammary function. In: Neville MC, Neifert MA, eds. Lactation: physiology, nutrition and breastfeeding. New York: Plenum Press, 1983:1.
54. Wilde CJ, Addey CVP, Casey MJ, Blatchford DR, Peaker M. Feed-back inhibition of milk secretion: the effect of a fraction of goat milk on milk yield and composition. Q J Exp Physiol 1988;73:391.
55. Neville MC. Control of milk volume in human lactation. Newsletter on Mammary Gland Biology and Lactation 1989;8:3.
56. Lammi-Keefe CJ, Jensen RG. Lipids in human milk: a review. II. Composition and fat-soluble vitamins. J Pediatr Gastroenterol Nutr 1984;3:172.
57. Garza C, Hopkinson J. Physiology of lactation. In: Tsang RC, Nichols BL, eds. Nutrition during infancy. Philadelphia: Hanley and Belfus, 1988:20.
58. Patton S, Canfield LM, Huston GE, Ferris AM, Jensen RG. Carotenoids of human colostrum. Lipids 1990;25:159.
59. Ferris AM, Dotts MA, Clark RM, Ezrin M, Jensen RG. Macronutrients in human milk at 2, 12 and 16 weeks postpartum. J Am Diet Assoc 1988;88:694.
60. Neville MC, Casey CE, Keller RP, Archer P. Changes in milk composition after six months of lactation: the effects of duration of lactation and gradual weaning. In: Harmosh M, Goldman AS, eds. Human lactation. 2. Maternal and environmental factors. New York: Plenum Press, 1986:141.
61. Lonnerdal B. Effects of maternal nutrition on human lactation. In: Hamosh M, Goldman AS, eds. Human lactation. 2. New York: Plenum Press, 1986:301.
62. Jensen RG. The lipids of human milk. Boca Raton, FL: CRC Press, 1988:107.
63. Grigor MR, Allan JE, Carrington JM, et al. Effect of dietary protein and food restriction on milk production and composition, maternal tissues and enzymes in lactating rats. J Nutr 1987;117:1247.
64. Food and Nutrition Board, Commission on Life Sciences, National Research Council Recommended Dietary Allowances, 10th ed. Washington, DC: National Academy of Sciences, 1988:24.
65. Sadurskis A, Kabir N, Wager J, Forsum E. Energy metabolism, body composition and milk production in healthy Swedish women during lactation. Am J Clin Nutr 1988;48:44.
66. Ferris AM, Reece EA. Postpartum management and lactation. In: Reece EA, Coustan DR, eds. Diabetes mellitus in pregnancy: principles and practice. New York: Churchill Livingstone, 1988;623.
67. American Academy of Pediatrics, Committee on Nutrition. Nutrition and lactation. 1981;68:435.
68. Martinez GA, Krieger FW. 1984 milk-feeding patterns in the United States. Pediatrics 1985;76:1004.
69. Manning-Dalton D, Allen LH. The effects of lactation on energy and protein consumption, postpartum weight change and body composition of well nourished North American women. Nutr Res 1983;3:293.
70. Butte NF, Garza C, Stuff JE, O'Brian-Smith E, Nichols BL. Effect of maternal diet and body composition on lactation performance. Am J Clin Nutr 1984;39:296.
71. Beal VA. Nutrition in the life span. New York: John Wiley & Sons, 1980.
72. Prentice AM, Prentice A. Energy costs of lactation. Ann Rev Nutr 1988;8:63.
73. Tully J, Dewey KG. Private fears, global loss: a cross-cultural study of the insufficient milk syndrome. Med Anthropol 1985;9:225.
74. Roberts SB, Cole TJ, Coward WA. Lactational performance in relation to energy intake in the baboon. Am J Clin Nutr 1985;41:1270.
75. Roepke J. Nutritional requirements of breastfeeding mothers. 6th National Seminar Nutrition in Pregnancy, Louisville, KY, 1982.
76. Ferris AM, McCabe LT, Allen LH, Pelto GH. Biological and sociocultural determinants of successful lactation among women in Eastern Connecticut. J Am Diet Assoc 1987;87:316.
77. Strode MA, Dewey KG, Lonnerdal B. Effects of short-term caloric restriction on lactational performance of well-nourished women. Acta Paediatr Scand 1986;75:222.
78. Thomas MR, Bodily S. Maternal anthropometric measurements, dietary intake and lactation performance of mothers on a weight reduction diet. Fed Proc 1985;44:1679A.
79. Neifert MR. Routine management of breast-feeding. In: Neville MC, Neifert MR, eds. Lactation physiology, nutrition and breast-feeding. New York: Plenum Press, 1983:273.
80. Neifert MR. Infant problems in breast-feeding. In: Neville MC, Neifert MR, eds. Lactation physiology, nutrition and breastfeeding. New York: Plenum Press, 1983:303.
81. Neifert MR, Seacat J, Jobe WE. Lactation failure due to insufficient glandular development of the breast. Pediatrics 1985;76(5):823.

82. Lawrence RA. Breastfeeding and medical disease. Medical Clin North Am 1989;73:583.
83. Lederman SA. Breast milk contaminants: substance abuse, infection, and the environment. Clin Nutr 1989;8:120.
84. McGregor JA, Neifert MR. Maternal problems in lactation. In: Neville MC, Neifert MR, eds. Lactation physiology, nutrition and breast-feeding. New York: Plenum Press, 1983:333.
85. Lyon AJ. Effects of smoking on breast feeding. Arch Dis Child 1983;58:378.
86. Counsilman JJ, MacKay EV. Cigarette smoking by pregnant women with particular reference to their past and subsequent breast feeding behavior. Aust NZ J Obstet Gynaecol 1985;25:101.
87. Anderson AN, Lund-Anderson C, Larsen JF, et al. Suppressed prolactin but normal neurophysic levels in cigarette smoking breast-feeding women. Clin Endocrinol 1982;17:363.
88. Hofstetter A, Schutz Y, Jequier E, Wahren J. Increased 24-hour expenditure in cigarette smokers. New Engl J Med 1986; 314(2):79.
89. Kromhout D, Saris WHM, Horst CH. Energy intake, energy expenditure and smoking in relation to body fatness: the Zutphen study. Am J Clin Nutr 1988;47:668.
90. Luck W, Nau H. Nicotine and cotinine concentrations in serum and urine of infants exposed via passive smoking or milk from smoking mothers. J Pediatr 1987;107:816.
91. Steldinger R, Luck W. Half lives of nicotine in milk of smoking mothers: implications for nursing. J Perinat Med 1988;16:261.
92. Federal Trade Commission. Report of "tar" and nicotine content of the smoke of 167 varieties of cigarettes. Washington, DC: Federal Trade Commission, 1978.
93. Luck W, Nau H. Nicotine and cotinine concentrations in the milk of smoking mothers: influence of cigarette consumption and diurnal variation. Eur J Pediatr 1987;146:21.
94. Anath J. Side effects in the neonate from psychotropic agents excreted through breast feedings. Am J Psychiatry 1978; 135:801.
95. Tyrala EE, Dodson WE. Caffeine secretion into breast milk. Arch Dis Child 1979;54:787.
96. Berlin CM, Densen HM, Daniel CH, Ward RM. Disposition of dietary caffeine in milk, saliva, and plasma of lactating women Pediatrics 1984;73(1):59.
97. Le Guennec J, Billon B. Delay in caffeine elimination in breast-fed infants. Pediatrics 1987;79:264.
98. Rivera-Calimlin L. Drugs in breast milk. Drug Ther 1977;2:20.
99. Ryu JE. Effect of maternal caffeine consumption on heart rate and sleep time of breast-fed infants. Dev Pharmacol Ther 1985;8:355.
100. Munoz LM, Lonnerdal B, Keen CL, Dewey KG. Coffee consumption as a factor in iron deficiency anemia among pregnant women and their infants in Costa Rica. Am J Clin Nutr 1988;48:645.
101. Hayslip CC, Klein TA, Wray HL, Duncan WE. The effects of lactation on bone mineral content in healthy postpartum women. Obstet Gynecol 1989;73:588.
102. Hollingbery P, Massey LK. Effect of caffeine and sucrose on urinary calcium excretion in adolescents. Fed Proc 1986;45:375A.
103. Wilson JT, Brown RD, Cherek DR, et al. Drug excretion in human breast milk. Principles, pharmacokinetics and projected consequences. Clin Pharmacokinetics 1980;5:1.
104. Kesaniemi Y. Ethanol and acetaldehyde in the milk and peripheral blood of lactating women after ethanol administration. J Obstet Gynaecol Br Commonw 1974;81:84.
105. Cobo E. Effect of different doses of ethanol on the milk-ejecting reflex in lactating women. Am J Obstet Gynecol 1973;115:819.
106. Wagner G, Fuchs AR. Effect of ethanol on uterine activity during suckling in post-partum women. Acta Endocrinologica 1968;58:133.
107. Martin DC, Martin JC, Streissguth AP. Sucking frequency and amplitude in newborns as a function of maternal drinking and smoking. Current Alcohol 1978;5:359.
108. Grossman ER. Beer, breast-feeding and the wisdom of old wives (letter). JAMA 1988;259:1016.
109. Little RE, Anderson KW, Ervin CH, Worthington-Roberts B, Clarren SK. Maternal alcohol use during breast-feeding and infant mental and motor development at one year. N Engl J Med 1989;321:425.
110. Bailey N. Manual for the Bayley Scales of Infant Development. New York: Psychological Corporation, 1969.
111. Hoh TK. Severe hypoprothrombinaemic bleeding in the breast fed young infants. Singapore Med J 1969;10:43.
112. Perez-Reyes M, Wall ME. Presence of 9 tetrahydrocannabinol in human milk. N Engl J Med 1982;307:819.
113. Nichols JM, Lipshitz J, Schreiber EC. Phencyclidine: its transfer across the placenta as well as into breast milk. Am J Obstet Gynecol 1982;143:143.
114. Bobskill L. Cocaine babies nearing school age. Springfield, MA Union-News, April 21, 1989:27.
115. Taylor R. Cracking cocaine's legacy in babies of drug abusers. J NIH Res 1989;1:29.
116. Chasnoff IJ, Lewis DE, Squires L. Cocaine intoxication in a breast-fed infant. Pediatrics 1987;80:836.
117. Chaney, NE, Franke J, Wadlington WB. Cocaine convulsions in a breast-fed baby. J Pediatr 1988;112:134.
118. Sauer HJ. Physiology of lactation and factors affecting lactation. Breast Dis 1987;14(3):615.
119. Ferris AM, Dalidowitz C, Ingardia C, et al. Lactation outcome in insulin-dependent diabetic women. J Am Diet Assoc 1988;88:317.
120. Butte NF, Garza C, Burr R, Goldman AS, Kennedy K, Kitzmiller JL. Milk composition of insulin-dependent diabetic women. J Pediatr Garstroenterol Nutr 1987;6:936.
121. Neubauer S, Ferris AM, Fanelli J, Lammi-Keefe CJ, Jensen RG. Breast milk composition and mastitis incidence in insulin-dependent diabetic women (IDD). Federation of American Societies for Experimental Biology Journal 1989;3(3):A770 (Abstr 3159).
122. Chase CG, Ferris AM. Breast milk intake by infants of insulin-dependent diabetic (IDDM) women. FASEB J 1989;3(3):A770 (Abstr 3157).
123. Murtaugh MA, Ostrom KM, Ferris AM, Reece EA. Blood glucose changes in lactating insulin-dependent (IDDM) women in response to breast pumping. FASEB J 1989;3(3):A769 (Abstr 3150).
124. Cystic Fibrosis Foundation Report of the patient registry. Rockville, MD: Cystic Fibrosis Foundation, 1987.
125. Whitelaw A, Butterfield A. High breast milk sodium in cystic fibrosis. Lancet 1977;2:1288.
126. Schiffman ML, Seale TW, Flux M, Rennart OW, Swender PT. Breast-milk composition in women with cystic fibrosis: report of two cases and a review of the literature. Am J Clin Nutr 1989;49:612.
127. Alpert SE, Cormier AD. Normal electrolyte and protein content in milk from mothers with cystic fibrosis: an explanation of the initial report of elevated milk sodium concentration. J Pediatr 1983;102:77.
128. Stead RJ, Brueton MJ, Hodson ME, Batten JC. Should mothers with cystic fibrosis breast feed? Arch Dis Child 1987;62:433.
129. Linzell JL, Peaker M. Mechanisms of milk secretion. Physiol Rev 1971;51:564.
130. Schultz I. Micropuncture studies of the sweat formation in cystic fibrosis patients. J Clin Invest 1969;48:1470.

131. Kaiser D, Drack E, Rossi E. Inhibition of net sodium transport in single sweat glands of patients with cystic fibrosis of the pancreas. Pediatr Res 1971;5:167.
132. Bitman J, Hamosh M, Wood DL, et al. Lipid composition of milk from mothers with cystic fibrosis. Pediatrics 1987;80:927.
133. Bradburn NC, Wappner RS, Lemons JA, Meyer BA, Roberts RS. Lactation and phenylketonuria. Am J Perinatol 1985;2:138.
134. Lederman SA. Breast milk contaminants: maternal medications. Clin Nutr 1989;8:131.
135. Kampmann JP, Johnsen K, Hansen JM, et al. Propylthiouracil in human milk. Lancet 1980;1:736.
136. Vorherr H. The breast, morphology, physiology and lactation. New York: Academic Press, 1974.
137. Thiry L, Sprecher-Goldberger S, Jonckheer T, et al. Isolation of AIDS virus from cell-free breast milk of three healthy virus carriers. Lancet 1985;2:891.
138. American Academy of Pediatrics, Task Force on Pediatric AIDS. Perinatal human immunodeficiency virus infection. Pediatrics 1988;82:941.
139. Wassenberger J, Ordog GJ, Stroh JJ. AIDS in breast milk. JAMA 1986;255:464.
140. Colebunders R, Kapita B, Nekwei W, et al. Breast-feeding and the transmission of human immunodeficiency type 1 infection. In: IV International Conference on AIDS. Stockholm: Swedish Ministry of Health and Social Affairs, 1988: Abstract 5103, book 1.
141. Oxtoby MJ. Human immunodeficiency virus and other viruses in human milk: placing the issues in broader perspective. Pediatr Infect Dis J 1988;7:825.
142. Jelliffe DB, Jelliffe EFP. HIV and breastmilk: non-proven alarmism. J Trop Pediatr 1988;34:142.
143. Ballard RA, Drew WL, Hutnagle KG. Cytomegalovirus infection in preterm infants. Am J Dis Child 1979;133:482.
144. Yaeger AS, Palumbo PE, Malachowski N, Ariagro RL, Stevenson DK. Sequelae of maternally derived cytomegalovirus infections in premature infants. J Pediatr 1983;102:918.
145. Pass RF. Epidemiology and transmission of cytomegalovirus. J Infect Dis 1985;152;243.
146. Losonsky GA, Fishaut JM, Strussenberg J, Ogra PL. Effect of immunization against rubella on lactation products. II. Maternal-neonatal interaction. J Infect Dis 1982;145:661.
147. Noren K. Changes in the levels of organochlorine pesticides, polychlorinated biphenyls, dibenzo-p-dioxins and dibenzofurans in human milk from Stockholm, 1972–1985. Chemosphere 1988;17:39.
148. Dabeka RW, Karpinski KF, McKenzie AD, Bajdik CD. Survey of lead, cadmium and fluoride in human milk and contamination with environmental and food factors. Fd Chem Toxic 1986;24:913.
149. Keller CA, Doherty RA. Bone lead mobilization in lactating mice and lead transfer to suckling offspring. Toxicol Appl Pharmacol 1980;55:220.
150. Dean RFA. The size of the baby at birth and the yield of breast milk. In: Dept of Experimental Medicine, Cambridge. Studies of Undernutrition, Wuppertal, 1946-9, Medical Research Council (Great Britain) Special Report Series. London: HM Stationery Office, 1951;275:346.
151. Arora AK, Gupta BD. Cesarean section and lactation failure (letter). Indian Pediatrics 1987;24:954.
152. Janke JR Breastfeeding duration following cesarean and vaginal births. J Nurse-Midwifery 1988;33:159.
153. Lie B, Juul J. Effect of epidural vs general anesthesia on breast-feeding. Acta Obstet Gynecol Scand 1988;67:207.
154. Out JJ, Vierhout ME, Wallenburg HCS. Breast-feeding following spontaneous and induced labor. Eur J Obstet Gynecol Reprod Biol 1988;29:275.
155. De Chateau P, Holmberg H, Jakobsson K, Winberg J. A study of the factors promoting and inhibiting lactation. Dev Med Child Neurol 1977;19:575.
156. Lozoff B, Brittenham GM, Trause MA, Kennel JH, Klaus MH. The mother-newborn relationship: limits of adaptability. J Pediatr 1977;91:1.
157. Johnson NW. Breast-feeding at one hour of age. Am J Mat Child Nurs 1976;1:12.
158. Salariya EM, Easton PM, Cater JL. Duration of breast-feeding after early initiation and frequent feeding. Lancet 1978;2:1141.
159. Quandt SA. Patterns of variations in breast-feeding behaviors. Soc Sci Med 1986;12:291.
160. Woolridge MW, Baum JD. The regulation of human milk flow. In: Lindblad BS, ed. Perinatal nutrition. San Diego: Academic Press, 1988:243.
161. Hendrickson SW. Test-weighing babies: how accurate is it? Neonatal Network 1985;(Aug):25.
162. Minchin MK. Breastfeeding matters. Victoria, Australia: Alma Publications, 1985:108.
163. Feher SDK, Berger LR, Johnson JD, Wilde JB. Increased breast milk production for premature infants with a relaxation/imagery audiotape. Pediatrics 1989;83:57.
164. Neville MC, Keller R, Seacat J, et al. Studies in human lactation: milk volumes in lactating women during the onset of lactation and full lactation. Am J Clin Nutr 1988;48:1375.
165. Saint L, Smith M, Hartmann PE. The yield and nutrient content of colostrum and milk of women from giving birth to 1 month postpartum. Br J Nutr 1984;52:87.
166. McClelland DBL, McGrath J, Samson RR. Antimicrobial factors in human milk. Studies of concentration and transfer to the infant during the early stages of lactation. Acta Paediatr Scand (Suppl) 1978;271:3.
167. Neville MC. Regulation of mammary development and lactation. In: Neville MC, Neifert MA, eds. Lactation: physiology, nutrition and breast-feeding. New York: Plenum Press, 1983:103.
168. Falconer IR, Forsyth IA, Wilson BM, Dils R. Inhibition by low concentrations of ouabain of prolactin-induced lactogenesis in rabbit mammary gland explants. Biochem J 1978;172:509.
169. Falconer IR, Baldwin RW, Forsyth IA, Wilson BM, Dils R. Milk fat synthesis by prolactin-stimulated rabbit mammary tissue in organ culture: relationship to cation transport. Biochem Soc Trans 1978;6:133.
170. Rillema JA, Linebaugh BE, Mulder JA. Regulation of casein syntheses by polyamines in mammary gland explants of mice. Endocrinology 1977;100:529.
171. Matusik RJ, Rosen JM. Prolactin induction of casein mRNA in organ culture—a model system for studying peptide hormone regulation of gene expression. J Biol Chem 1978;252:2343.
172. Nicholas KR, Hartmann PE. Progesterone control of the initiation of lactose in the rat. Aust J Biol Sci 1981;34:435.
173. Davis AJ, Fleet IR, Goode JA, Hamon MH, Maule Walker FM, Peaker M. Changes in mammary function at the onset of lactation in the goat: correlation with hormonal changes. J Physiol 1979;288:33.
174. Peaker M, Linzell JL. Citrate in milk: a harbinger or lactogenesis. Nature 1975;253:464.
175. Faulkner A, Chaiyabutr N, Peaker M, Carrick DT, Kuhn NJ. Metabolic significance of milk glucose. J Dairy Res 1981;48:51.
176. Faulkner A. Glucose availability and lactose synthesis in the goat. Biochem Soc Trans 1985;13:496.
177. Arthur PG, Smith M, Hartmann P. Milk lactose, citrate, and glucose as markers of lactogenesis in normal and diabetic women. J Pediatr Gastroenterol Nutr 1989;9:488.
178. Neville MC, Allen JC, Casey CE. Regulation of the rate of lac-

tose production. In: Hamosh M, Goldman AS, eds. Human lactation 2. New York: Plenum Press, 1986:241.

179. Martin RH, Glass MR, Chapman C, Wilson GD, Woods KL. Human α-lactalbumin and hormonal factors in pregnancy and lactation. Clin Endocrinol 1980;13:223.

180. Kulski JK, Smith M, Hartmann PE. Perinatal concentrations of progesterone, lactose and α-lactalbumin in the mammary secretion of women. J Endocrinol 1977;74:509.

181. Applebaum RM. The obstetrician's approach to the breasts and breastfeeding. J Reprod Med 1975;14:8.

182. Whitehead RG, Rowland MGM, Hutton M, Prentice AM, Muller E, Paul A. Factors influencing lactation performance in rural Gambian mothers. Lancet 1978;(July 22):178.

183. Newbould FHS. Microbial diseases of the mammary gland. In: Larson BL, Smith VR, eds. Lactation: a comprehensive treatise. Vol 2. New York: Academic Press, 1974;269.

184. Prentice A, Prentice AM, Lamb WH. Mastitis in rural Gambian mothers and the protection of the breast by milk antimicrobial factors. Trans R Soc Trop Med Hyg 1985;79:90.

185. Kitchen BJ. Review of the progress of dairy science: bovine mastitis: milk compositional changes and related diagnostic tests. J Dairy Research 1981;48:167.

186. Shaw AO, Beam AL. The effect of mastitis upon milk production. J Dairy Sci 1935;18:353.

187. Ramadan MA, Salah MM, Eid SZ. Effect of breast infection on the composition of human milk. Pediatrics 1961;27:314.

188. Neubauer SH, Ferris AM, Hinckley L. The effect of mastitis on breast milk composition in insulin-dependent diabetic and non-diabetic women. FASEB J 1990;4:A915 (Abstr).

189. Prosser CG, Hartmann PE. Comparison of mammary gland function during the ovulatory menstrual cycle and acute breast inflammation in women. Aust J Exp Biol Med Sci 1983;61:277.

190. Conner A. Elevated levels of sodium and chloride in milk from mastitic breast. Pediatrics 1979;63:910.

191. Koetsawang S. The effect of contraceptive method on the quality and quantity of breast milk. Int J Gynaecol Obstet (Suppl) 1987;25:115.

192. Lonnerdal B. Effect of oral contraceptives on lactation. In: Hamosh M, Goldman A, eds. Human lactation 2: maternal and environmental factors. New York: Plenum Press, 1986:453.

193. WHO Task Force on Oral Contraceptives. Effects of hormonal contraceptives on breast milk composition and infant growth. Stud Fam Plan 1988;19:361.

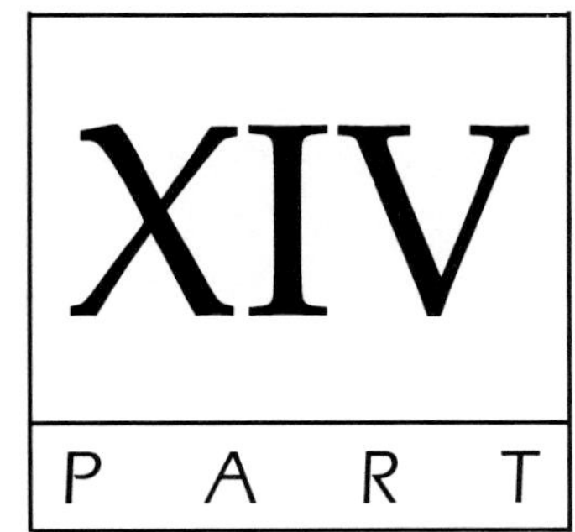

PART XIV

THE NEWBORN INFANT

92

CHAPTER

PREMATURE BIRTH AND NEUROLOGIC COMPLICATIONS

Alan Hill and Joseph J. Volpe

Prematurity constitutes the single most important predisposing factor for the development of cerebral injury in the newborn period. In the United States alone, premature delivery occurs in 6% to 8% of all pregnancies,[1] and more than 35,000 infants of birth weight less than 1500 g are born each year.[2] The recent decrease in neonatal mortality, which has resulted principally from the development of modern perinatal care facilities, largely reflects the increased survival of high-risk infants of low birth weight. Despite the improved rates of survival, approximately two thirds of all neonatal deaths still occur in infants of birth weight < 2500 g, and one half of all neonatal deaths occur in infants of birth weight < 1500 g. The risk of neurologic sequelae in infants of low birth weight who survive is approximately three times higher than the risk in term newborns.[3,4] In addition, premature infants who survive have an increased incidence of disability from a variety of nonneurologic conditions (eg, congenital anomalies, lower respiratory tract infections, and sudden infant death syndrome).[3,4]

In this chapter discussion will be limited to a review of the unique anatomical and physiologic features of the premature brain and the major types of cerebral injury observed in infants born prematurely, eg, periventricular–intraventricular hemorrhage (PVH–IVH), hypoxic–ischemic cerebral injury, and other metabolic disturbances. Although infections of the central nervous system (eg, bacterial meningitis and congenital viral infection) occur commonly, they are not specific for this age group and will not be discussed in detail. Hemorrhagic and hypoxic–ischemic cerebral injury will be discussed individually. However, it is important to recognize the close relationship between these two major categories of brain injury.

ANATOMICAL AND PHYSIOLOGIC FEATURES OF THE PREMATURE BRAIN

The patterns of cerebral injury observed in infants born prematurely are related, in large part, to anatomical and physiologic features that are specific to the stage of maturation of the premature brain at the time of birth.[5] Thus, basic knowledge of the unique features of the premature brain—including its vascular supply, the composition of cerebral tissue, and cerebrovascular autoregulation—is a prerequisite for the understanding of hemorrhagic and hypoxic–ischemic cerebral injury in this population.

VASCULAR SUPPLY OF THE PREMATURE BRAIN

Subependymal Germinal Matrix

The principal function of the subependymal germinal matrix, which is located immediately ventrolateral to the lateral ventricles in the subependymal region, is to provide a source of cerebral neuroblasts between 10 and 20 weeks of gestation, followed by the production of glioblasts during the third trimester. These latter elements subsequently differentiate into cerebral oligodendroglia and astrocytes. The subependymal germinal matrix diminishes in size progressively during later gestation until it has virtually disappeared by term. Nutrients for the high rate of cellular proliferation within the germinal matrix are supplied by a rich microvascular network of immature, fragile vessels provided with relatively poor endothelial support and therefore with a propensity to rupture, either spontaneously or in response to relatively minor stress.[5,6] Approximately 80% to 90% of all cases of PVH–IVH in the premature infant originate within the germinal matrix.[5,7,8]

Arterial Blood Supply

The arterial architecture of the premature brain is considered to be the major determinant of the principal patterns of hypoxic–ischemic cerebral injury observed in this age group. Thus, in the immature brain, a watershed zone of arterial blood supply is located in the periventricular white matter between the ventriculofugal choroidal arteries and the ventriculopedal penetrating branches of the anterior, middle, and posterior cerebral arteries.[5,7] The most common pattern of hypoxic–ischemic cerebral injury in the premature newborn involves principally these watershed regions, which are most prominent posteriorly in the white matter around the trigone of the lateral ventricles and, more anteriorly, in the white matter around the foramen of Monro.[9] Relative resistance of cerebral cortex to hypoxic–ischemic insult is attributed to persistence of the rich, interarterial anastomoses between meningeal arteries present during early development of the arterial tree.[5,10]

Venous Drainage

Whereas the pattern of arterial blood supply plays a major role in the determination of hypoxic–ischemic cerebral injury, the distinctive deep venous drainage of the premature brain may render particular sites (eg, the subependymal germinal matrix) vulnerable to hemorrhage. Thus, a sharp reversal in the direction of venous flow occurs at the confluence of the choroidal, thalamostriate, and terminal veins to form the internal cerebral vein that may predispose to venous stasis. This, in turn, may result in proximal increase in intravascular pressure and capillary rupture.[11]

Impairment of Cerebrovascular Autoregulation

Cerebrovascular autoregulation is the homeostatic mechanism that regulates vascular resistance to maintain constant cerebral perfusion over a wide range of systemic arterial pressures. This mechanism appears to be incompletely developed in the premature newborn, and this deficiency results in a "pressure-passive" relationship between systemic blood pressure and cerebral blood flow. This relationship, in turn, may predispose to PVH–IVH under conditions of systemic hypertension and to hypoxic–ischemic cerebral injury under conditions of systemic hypotension.[5,12,13]

Composition of Cerebral Tissue

The relatively close packing of cortical neurons and lack of Nissl substance in the premature brain makes it more difficult to detect diffuse neuronal necrosis following hypoxic–ischemic cerebral insult.[5] The propensity for cystic cavitation of necrotic periventricular cerebral lesions relates to the relatively high water content, together with the paucity of myelin and poor astroglial response of the immature brain.[5,14] In addition, this normally high water content in the premature brain may make it unlikely for cerebral edema to play a major role in the pathogenesis of hypoxic–ischemic cerebral injury.

MAJOR TYPES OF CEREBRAL INJURY IN THE PREMATURE NEWBORN

PERIVENTRICULAR–INTRAVENTRICULAR HEMORRHAGE

As discussed previously, PVH–IVH originates most commonly in the subependymal germinal matrix and subsequently ruptures into the ventricular system in approximately 80% of cases. Figure 92-1 illustrates the cranial ultrasonographic appearance of hemorrhage localized to the region of the germinal matrix. The reported incidence of PVH–IVH has decreased from approximately 40% in the early 1980s to 25% in more recent studies. This decreased incidence of PVH–IVH has been documented principally in infants of very low birth weight (ie, <1500 g).[6,15] However, because the incidence of PVH–IVH correlates directly with the degree of prematurity, the improved survival rates of extremely premature infants of birth weight < 1000 g maintains the status of PVH–IVH as a major perinatal problem.[6] It has been documented that PVH–IVH occurs during the first 24 hours of life in approximately 50% of cases and occurs prior to 3 days of age in 90%.

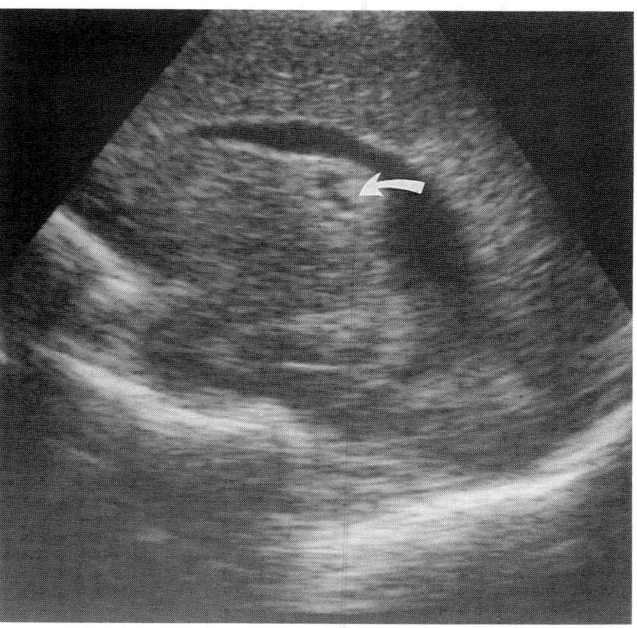

FIGURE 92–1. Parasagittal cranial ultrasound scan of hemorrhage localized to the subependymal germinal matrix (*arrow*).

Pathogenesis

The pathogenesis of PVH–IVH is multifactorial and includes a combination of intravascular, vascular, and extravascular factors. These factors have been discussed in detail elsewhere.[5] The major pathogenetic factors are summarized in Table 92-1.

Diagnosis and Clinical Features

All premature infants must be considered to be at risk for PVH–IVH, particularly those who require mechanical ventilation or who sustain systemic complications (eg, sepsis, pneumothorax). In infants with severe PVH–IVH, hemorrhage may be suspected on the basis of clinical features (eg, abnormal neurologic signs, decreasing hematocrit, hypotension, bulging fontanelle, and metabolic acidosis). However, it has been demonstrated that the diagnosis of PVH–IVH may be predicated on the basis of clinical criteria alone in only 50% of cases.[16] Radiologic confirmation, usually by cranial ultrasonography, is required for the definitive diagnosis of PVH–IVH. Ultrasound scanning at 4 days of age should identify at least 90% of cases. Because progression of the hemorrhage occurs in 20% to 40% of affected infants, repeat scanning after approximately 5 days of age is usually performed to document the maximal extent of the lesion. In addition, serial scanning is recommended for surveillance of potential complications (eg, parenchymal hemorrhage, ventricular dilation).

COMPLICATIONS ASSOCIATED WITH PVH–IVH

Posthemorrhagic Hydrocephalus

Posthemorrhagic ventricular dilation may develop rapidly following major PVH–IVH, because of obstruction or impaired reabsorption of cerebrospinal fluid. More commonly, ventriculomegaly develops gradually, over several weeks, secondary to an obliterative arachnoiditis in the posterior fossa that obstructs cerebrospinal fluid flow. Ventricular dilation may arrest or resolve spontaneously in approximately 50% of cases. Serial lumbar punctures, administration of drugs to decrease cerebrospinal fluid production, external ventriculostomy, or placement of a ventriculoperitoneal shunt is required in the remainder. In planning strategies for intervention it is important to distinguish between progressive hydrocephalus and ventriculomegaly related to cerebral atrophy, which is not associated with the development of increased intracranial pressure.[5,17]

TABLE 92-1. POSSIBLE PATHOGENETIC FACTORS FOR INTRAVENTRICULAR HEMORRHAGE

Altered cerebral blood flow: increase or decrease, fluctuating pattern
Increased cerebral venous pressure
Disturbance of coagulation
Fragility and poor mechanical support of germinal matrix vasculature
Increased fibrinolytic activity within germinal matrix
?Decreased extravascular tissue pressure

Periventricular Hemorrhagic Infarction

Hemorrhagic necrosis in the periventricular white matter is observed in approximately 15% of infants with IVH, most commonly in association with large IVH (80%) (Fig. 92-2). In at least half of the cases, the parenchymal lesions are extensive, and they are uniformly strikingly asymmetrical.[6,18] Careful neuropathologic studies suggest that such periventricular hemorrhagic necrosis in association with major IVH may result from venous infarction. Thus, this lesion appears to be neuropathologically distinct from secondary hemorrhage into areas of periventricular leukomalacia (PVL), an ischemic lesion located in the watershed zones of the arterial supply in the premature brain[6,19,20] (discussed in detail later in this chapter).

HYPOXIC–ISCHEMIC CEREBRAL INJURY

Intrapartum asphyxia is a relatively common and often unavoidable complication of preterm delivery, which,

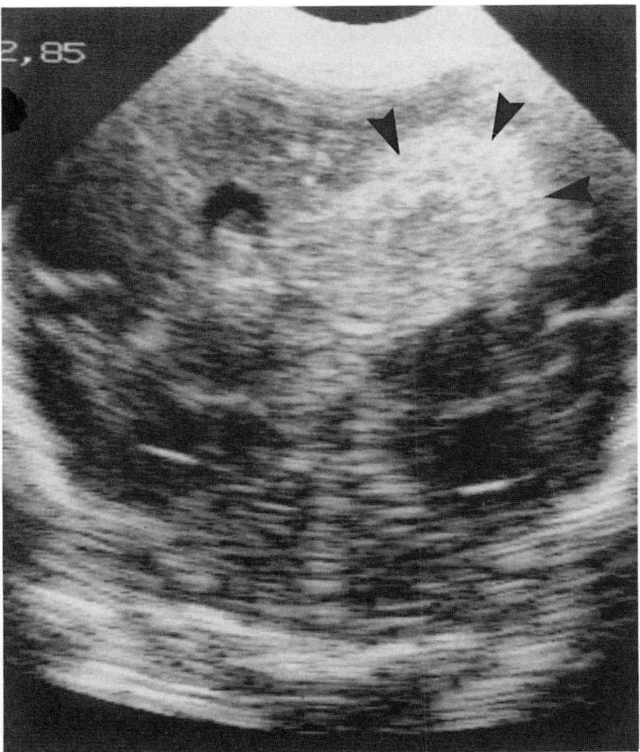

FIGURE 92–2. Coronal ultrasound scan of severe periventricular-intraventricular hemorrhage (PVH-IVH). Note increased echogenicity in the periventricular region (*arrow*) indicative of hemorrhagic cerebral necrosis.

TABLE 92–2. MAJOR PATTERNS OF HYPOXIC–ISCHEMIC CEREBRAL INJURY IN THE PREMATURE NEWBORN

PATTERN	MAJOR ANATOMIC LOCATION
Selective neuronal necrosis	Diencephalon, thalamus, brain stem
Periventricular leukomalacia	Periventricular white matter, particularly in peritrigonal region
Focal/multifocal	Cortex and white matter
Periventricular hemorrhagic necrosis	Periventricular white matter, unilateral or asymmetric

together with the high incidence of neonatal cardiorespiratory problems (eg, respiratory distress syndrome, patent ductus arteriosus, apnea, and bradycardia), renders the premature infant at high risk for hypoxic–ischemic cerebral injury. The specific neuropathologic patterns of hypoxic–ischemic cerebral injury relate principally to the stage of maturation of the immature brain (Table 92-2).

Selective Neuronal Necrosis

During the third trimester of gestation, neurons in the thalamus and brain stem appear to be particularly vulnerable to hypoxic–ischemic injury. Such neuronal injury may be sustained prenatally.[21,22] Thus, in one neuropathologic series, pontine neuronal necrosis was documented in 46% of premature infants with IVH, all of whom had died of respiratory failure.[23] Occasionally, injury may involve both the pontine nuclei and the subiculum of the hippocampus. Although the pathogenesis of this lesion is unclear, it may relate to hyperoxia that follows an episode of perinatal hypoxia–ischemia.[5,24] Injury to neurons of the inferior olivary nuclei is also characteristic of the premature infant.[5]

Periventricular Leukomalacia

As discussed previously, ischemic injury in the premature brain involves principally the periventricular watershed zones of arterial supply, most commonly posteriorly, in the region of the trigone of the lateral ventricles.[9] In addition to hypoxic–ischemic insult, a role for endotoxin has been suggested in the pathogenesis of perinatal telencephalic leukoencephalopathy, which may represent an early form of periventricular leukomalacia (PVL).[25] Neuropathologic examination reveals a range of severity ranging from minor reduction in the quantity of myelin and gliosis to severe "multicystic encephalomalacia." Recent neuropathologic studies have emphasized the frequent association between PVL and IVH in at least 75% of infants who died with IVH.[23,26]

The diagnosis of PVL during the neonatal period cannot be based reliably on clinical criteria and must be established by detection of abnormalities on cranial ultrasonography—eg, increased echogenicity in periventricular white matter during the first days of life followed by development of cysts in these regions after several weeks (Fig. 92-3). Although cranial ultrasonog-

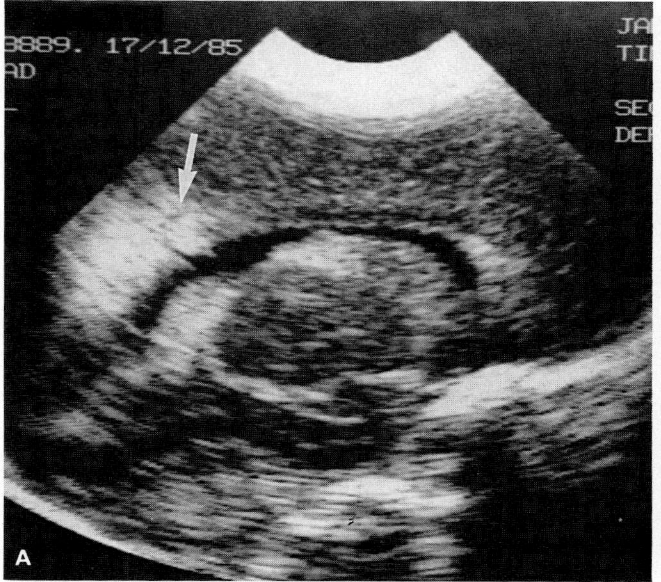

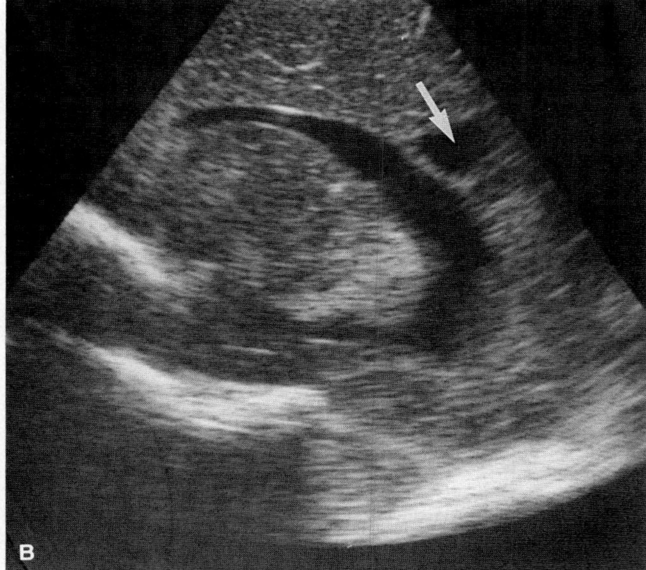

FIGURE 92–3. Evolution of periventricular leukomalacia (PVL) on cranial ultrasound scan. **(A)** Note increased echogenicity in periventricular region (*arrow*) on scan performed at 2 days of age. **(B)** Note periventricular cysts (*arrow*) on scan of same infant performed at 5 weeks of age.

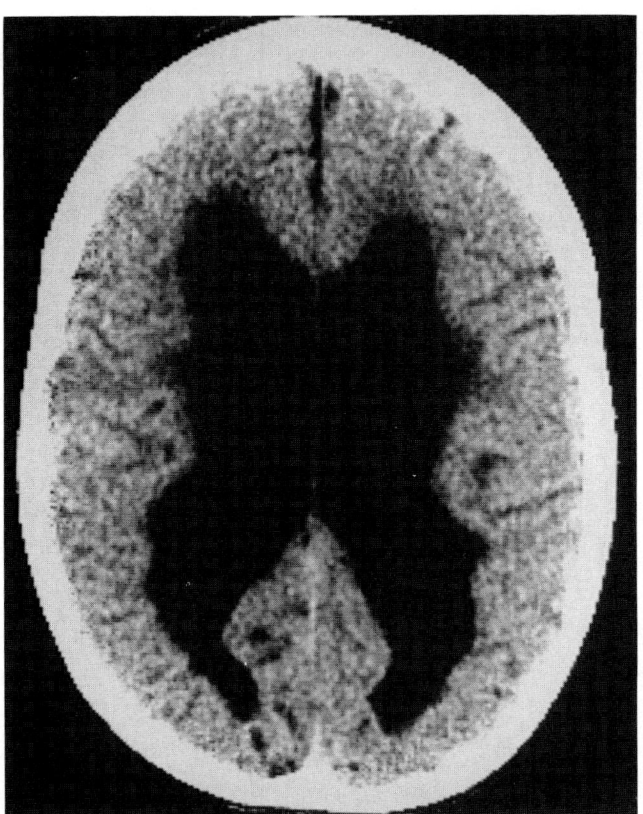

FIGURE 92–4. Computed tomography scan of 2-year-old child with PVL. Note ventriculomegaly with irregular ventricular outline and reduced quantity of periventricular white matter.

raphy performed at 4 days of age will identify approximately 90% of cases of IVH, later scanning after several weeks of age is optimal for the diagnosis of such ischemic cerebral injury.[5]

The principal long-term neurologic sequela of PVL is motor handicap (eg, spastic diplegia or quadriplegia).[5] Intellectual impairment occurs with more diffuse injury, perhaps also involving cerebral cortex.

In older children with cerebral palsy who were born prematurely, the clinical suspicion of PVL as the cause of the cerebral palsy may be confirmed by documentation of characteristic abnormalities on computed tomography or magnetic resonance imaging of the head. Abnormalities on computed tomographic scans include ventriculomegaly, with irregular ventricular walls, reduction in the quantity of periventricular white matter, particularly in the peritrigonal region, and prominent Sylvian fissures (Fig. 92-4).[26–29] For optimal visualization of abnormalities it is important that the scans be performed with precise technique (ie, 5-mm slices through the level of the periventricular white matter). Similar abnormalities may be recognized with greater anatomical definition on magnetic resonance imaging scans, especially T-2–weighted spin echo imaging sequences (Fig. 92-5).

Focal–Multifocal Brain Necrosis

Focal ischemic cerebral lesions associated with arterial occlusion occur uncommonly in premature infants. In one large series, none were observed in infants less than 28 weeks gestational age. Five percent of all cases of

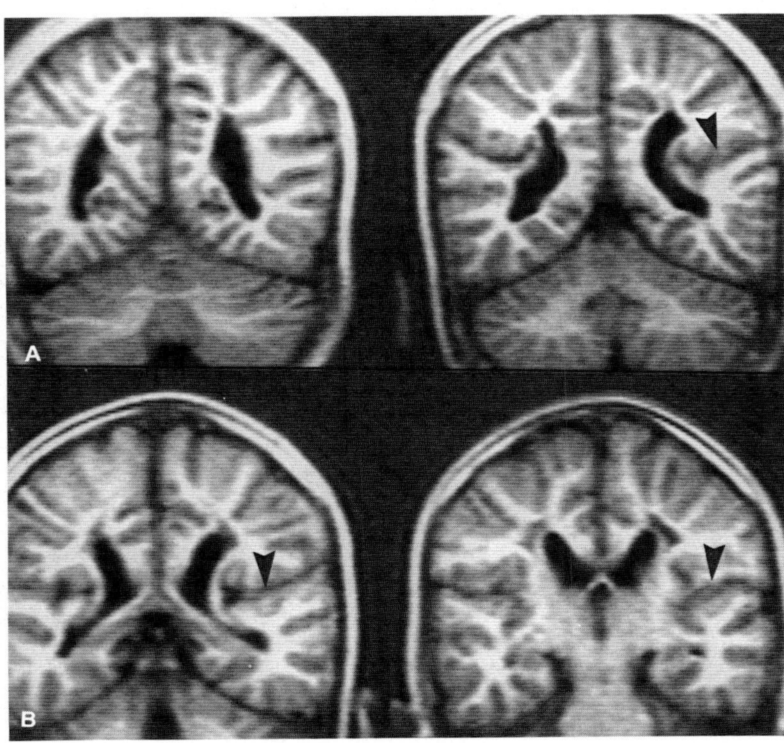

FIGURE 92–5. Magnetic resonance imaging of PVL in later childhood. (**A**) T1-weighted image. Note reduced quantity of periventricular white matter and prominent sylvian fissures (*arrow*). (**B**) T2-weighted spin echo image. Note abnormal signal intensity in periventricular white matter posteriorly (*arrow*).

infarction occurred in infants between 28 and 32 weeks, and 10% occurred in infants between 32 and 37 weeks of gestation. Multiple small scattered infarcts related to occlusion of small vessels are more common in this age group than in term infants.[30] Focal cerebral necrosis in the premature brain results frequently in cavitation with formation of porencephalic cysts or multicystic encephalomalacia. Neurologic sequelae (eg, cerebral palsy, mental retardation, and seizures) are variable and correlate with the anatomical location and the extent of cerebral injury.

BILIRUBIN ENCEPHALOPATHY

Unconjugated hyperbilirubinemia in the newborn may result in kernicterus, which involves selective bilirubin staining of basal ganglia and brain stem nuclei associated with microscopically demonstrable neuronal destruction. Although there is an extensive literature on bilirubin metabolism, the understanding of its central nervous system toxicity remains limited.

Both acute and chronic phases of kernicterus have been described in the term infant whose serum bilirubin levels exceed 18 mg/dL.[5] Characteristically, the affected infant is hypotonic and lethargic, with a high-pitched cry, seizures, and poor suck during the first few days of life. After 3 or 4 days, the infant may develop hypertonia with opisthotonic posture and occasionally fever, which gradually subsides after the first week of life. Death occurs during the acute phase in as many as 50% of these severe cases. In the chronic phase, the infant exhibits a combination of choreoathetoid cerebral palsy, abnormal eye movements, sensorineural hearing loss, and intellectual deficits.[5] Yellow staining of the brain has been documented in premature newborns even when bilirubin levels have remained below 10 to 15 mg/dL. Interestingly, these sick premature infants do not usually develop clinical features of kernicterus. Indeed, there is no proven definite relationship between bilirubin levels below 20 mg/dL and neurologic outcome in premature infants.[31,32] Furthermore, previously identified risk factors (eg, sepsis, asphyxia, acidosis, hypercarbia, hypoglycemia, and hypoalbuminemia) have not been proved to be associated consistently with increased risk of kernicterus.[33,34] In low-birth-weight infants, kernicterus may not be preventable, even when bilirubin levels are maintained below 10 mg/dL by means of phototherapy or exchange transfusion.[35]

HYPOGLYCEMIC BRAIN INJURY

Transient hypoglycemia occurs commonly in the stressed premature newborn, often in association with hypoxic–ischemic cerebral injury. Preliminary data suggest that even moderate hypoglycemia in the preterm infant (approximately 2.6 mmol/L) may result in permanent neurologic abnormalities if it persists for longer than 5 days.[36] Severe hypoglycemia has become a much less common problem in most neonatal units because of routine frequent monitoring of blood glucose levels and early intravenous glucose supplementation.

PREVENTION AND MANAGEMENT OF HEMORRHAGIC AND HYPOXIC–ISCHEMIC BRAIN INJURY

Although hypoxic–ischemic cerebral injury and PVH–IVH have distinctive pathogenetic mechanisms, recent neuropathologic studies,[6,20,23,26] as well as in vivo studies with positron emission tomography,[37] emphasize the frequent association of these two types of cerebral injury. Thus, in many instances, similar strategies for intervention may be used to attempt to decrease either hypoxic–ischemic or hemorrhagic cerebral injury. For practical purposes, the major principles of management will be discussed in terms of the timing of intervention —that is, antepartum, intrapartum, or postpartum (Table 92-3).

ANTEPARTUM INTERVENTIONS

Prevention of Premature Delivery

Prevention of premature delivery is receiving increasing attention but requires large-scale public health education[1,3,38] and is discussed in depth elsewhere in this book.

Intrauterine Transportation

If premature delivery is unavoidable, concerted effort should be directed toward transfer of the mother to a high-risk perinatal center prior to delivery. This should ensure the optimal condition of the infant at delivery. The precise value of this intervention with regard to long-term outcome is not yet clear and remains an important area for future study.[39]

TABLE 92–3. PREVENTION AND MANAGEMENT OF CEREBRAL INJURY

Antepartum Interventions
Prevention of premature delivery
Intrauterine transport
?Pharmacologic interventions: phenobarbital, vitamin K
Intrapartum Interventions
?Avoidance of labor
?Delivery by cesarean section
Postnatal Interventions
Adequate ventilation
Prevention and correction of hemodynamic disturbances
Correction of coagulation abnormalities
?Pharmacologic interventions: phenobarbital, indomethacin, ethamsylate, vitamin E

Prenatal Pharmacologic Interventions

The prenatal administration of several drugs for prevention of PVH–IVH has been investigated during the past few years. Thus, data from two randomized, prospective studies suggest that the incidence of severe PVH–IVH may be reduced significantly in premature infants whose mothers receive phenobarbital approximately 6 hours prior to delivery. The effect of prenatal phenobarbital administration on the overall incidence of all grades of IVH is less clear.[40,41]

Several recent studies suggest a potential role for the prenatal administration of vitamin K to the mother for reduction of incidence and severity of IVH. This approach is based on the rationale that coagulopathy in the premature newborn may predispose to PVH–IVH.[42] Two randomized, prospective studies have demonstrated significant reduction in prothrombin time as well as a lower overall incidence of PVH–IVH in premature infants whose mothers received intramuscular vitamin K prior to delivery. However, the interpretation of these data is complicated by the fact that vitamin K is administered routinely at birth to all infants.[43,44]

Other drugs (eg, glucocorticoids) may indirectly influence the risk of PVH–IVH by reducing the severity of respiratory distress syndrome and its complications (eg, pneumothorax), which independently increase the risk.

INTRAPARTUM MANAGEMENT

Approximately 50% of cases of PVH–IVH occur within the first 24 hours of life. Because of this, the role of intrapartum factors must be given major consideration in the pathogenesis of PVH–IVH. Pathogenetic formulations raise the possibility of a role for mechanical deformations of the compliant skull of the premature infant at the time of both uterine contractions and vaginal delivery. These mechanical forces could result in elevations of cerebral venous pressure as well as intermittent fetal hypoxia and acidosis. Furthermore, repeated sudden elevations of systemic arterial blood pressure with uterine contractions could result in simultaneous elevations of cerebral blood flow in the preterm fetus in whom there is immature cerebral autoregulation.

Several studies suggest that the presence or absence of labor may be an important determinant of PVH–IVH.[45] Thus, hemorrhage was observed more frequently with breech than with vertex presentation, despite the fact that approximately 80% of these infants were delivered by cesarean section. With both types of presentation, the occurrence of PVH–IVH appeared to correlate with the presence or absence of labor rather than with the route of delivery. Other studies have suggested that the occurrence of PVH–IVH may be related more specifically to the duration of the active phase of labor. In one prospective study of 40 premature infants, IVH occurred in all infants who experienced labor that lasted longer than 12 hours.[46]

The relationship between the route of delivery and the occurrence of hemorrhage is controversial. Thus, several studies document reduced incidence of PVH–IVH in infants delivered by cesarean section,[47,48] whereas others have failed to demonstrate such a relationship.[49–52] Other studies suggest that delivery by cesarean section may be beneficial only in specific situations (eg, in extremely premature infants who are born at less than 28 weeks of gestation[53] or who are delivered prior to the onset of labor).[45] Preliminary studies of PVH–IVH in experimental animals have raised the possibility that the type of anesthesia used during delivery may play a role in the genesis of PVH–IVH.[54] Clearly, further investigations are needed to clarify the role of specific obstetric factors in the etiopathogenesis of PVH–IVH and to determine the optimal management of premature labor and delivery.

POSTNATAL INTERVENTIONS

Adequate Ventilation of the Newborn

Immediate provision of adequate ventilation to prevent ongoing hypoxemia and hypercarbia is of major importance in the management of the premature newborn, because such disturbances, even when modest in severity, can impair cerebrovascular autoregulation. The role of hyperventilation is more controversial. Thus, although studies in experimental animals suggest that hyperventilation may restore cerebral autoregulation following hypoxia, studies on the effect of hyperventilation on the incidence of PVH–IVH have produced conflicting results.[55,56]

Prevention and Correction of Hemodynamic Disturbances

The avoidance of rapid elevation of reduction in systemic blood pressure, potentially associated with alterations of cerebral perfusion, is of established value for the prevention of postnatal hemorrhagic and hypoxic–ischemic cerebral injury (discussed earlier in this chapter). Such hemodynamic disturbances have been documented during routine monitoring and caretaking procedures (eg, handling, tracheal suctioning, or rapid infusions of sodium bicarbonate or other fluids).[57,58] The use of muscle paralysis with pancuronium appears to be beneficial for preventing pneumothorax, a frequent complication of mechanical ventilation and a known risk factor for PVH–IVH in the premature newborn with respiratory distress syndrome.[49,59] Furthermore, muscle paralysis may prevent abrupt increases in both arterial and venous pressure associated with tracheal suctioning[11,58,60] Perhaps the most compelling indication for the use of muscle paralysis in the ventilated premature infant with respiratory distress syndrome relates to its effectiveness in converting a fluctuating pattern of systemic blood pressure and cerebral blood-flow velocity into a stable pattern. Thus, in a

TABLE 92–4. PHARMACOLOGIC INTERVENTIONS

PHARMACOLOGIC AGENTS	PROPOSED MECHANISM OF ACTION
Phenobarbital	Dampening of blood pressure responses associated with routine activity and handling
Indomethacin	Prostaglandin inhibition induces cerebral vasoconstriction (ie, may decrease baseline cerebral blood flow and hyperemia after asphyxia) Inhibitor of formation of free radicals ?Closure of patent ductus arteriosus
Ethamsylate	Prostaglandin inhibition Stabilization of capillary basement membrane
Vitamin E	Free radical scavenger protects germinal matrix capillaries from hypoxic injury

prospective, randomized study of 24 ventilated preterm newborns, such intervention was associated with a marked reduction in the incidence of clinically significant PVH–IVH,[61] an observation that has been confirmed by subsequent experience.[15,57]

Correction of Coagulation Abnormalities

At this time, data are insufficient to establish whether correction of coagulation abnormalities decreases the incidence of PVH–IVH. In one controlled study, administration of 10 mL/kg of fresh-frozen plasma to premature infants at the time of delivery and at 24 hours of age was associated with a reduction in the overall incidence of PVH–IVH to 14% as compared with 41% in controls. However, there was no demonstrable improvement in actual coagulation parameters or in the incidence of severe PVH–IVH. It was suggested that the effect of fresh plasma may relate to its stabilizing influence on the circulation, rather than to actual alteration of coagulation parameters.[62]

Pharmacologic Interventions

Several pharmacologic agents (eg, phenobarbital, indomethacin, ethamsylate, and vitamin E) have been evaluated for their role in the prevention of PVH–IVH. The probable mechanisms of action for each of these drugs are summarized in Table 92-4. At the present time, no single pharmacologic agent is of sufficiently proven value to warrant recommendation for *routine* use in premature infants who are at high risk for PVH–IVH.

TABLE 92–5. USEFUL FACTORS FOR PREDICTION OF NEUROLOGIC OUTCOME

Data from electronic fetal monitoring and fetal blood gas sampling
Neurologic examination (seizures, abnormalities that persist to 40 weeks postconceptual age)
Location and extent of periventricular ischemic/hemorrhagic lesions documented by cranial ultrasonography or CT
Posthemorrhagic hydrocephalus (associated with cerebral atrophy, surgical drainage required)
Other metabolic disturbances (eg., hyperbilirubinemia, hypoglycemia)

NEUROLOGIC OUTCOME IN THE PREMATURE NEWBORN

The long-term neurologic outcome of the premature newborn is determined principally by the severity of PVH–IVH, the extent of hypoxic–ischemic injury to cerebral parenchyma, and the occurrence of complications of PVH–IVH (eg, posthemorrhagic hydrocephalus). The significance of other metabolic derangements (eg, moderate hyperbilirubinemia, asymptomatic hypoglycemia) is less well established. The major factors that may assist in the prediction of neurologic outcome are listed in Table 92-5.

The neurologic examination of the premature infant is often limited by the presence of complex life support equipment. Nevertheless, certain clinical features (eg, the occurrence of seizures) correlate closely with poor neurologic outcome.[5,63] Clinically, recognizable seizure activity occurs uncommonly in the premature newborn, perhaps because the immaturity of cortical interconnections tend to impede the propagation of abnormal electrical discharges. Electroencephalography may assist in the more accurate documentation of seizures. Serial neurologic examinations are also invaluable for accurate prediction of outcome. Thus, in a study of 129 premature, high-risk infants, 90% of infants who were considered to be neurologically normal at 40 weeks postconceptual age were normal at 1 year of corrected age, whereas 65% of those considered to be definitely neurologically abnormal at term had persistent abnormalities at 1 year.[64]

In addition to clinical examination, detailed assessment of the precise location and extent of hypoxic–ischemic and hemorrhagic cerebral injury documented on serial cranial ultrasound scans is of major predictive value. Thus, follow-up studies of infants with periventricular hemorrhagic parenchymal lesions report major neurologic abnormalities in more than 85% of survivors.[18,65] However, occasionally, if there is only minor parenchymal involvement or if injury is localized to a presumably "clinically silent" region of the brain, the eventual handicap may be surprisingly mild.[66]

Progressive ventriculomegaly may be associated with adverse neurologic outcome.[67] However, it is not clear to what extent the degree of ventricular dilation or of increased intracranial pressure influences outcome. Some recent studies suggest that poor outcome may relate most closely to cerebral infarction or atrophy[68,69] associated with ventriculomegaly. Several studies indicate that the outcome of infants with posthemorrhagic hydrocephalus who require surgical intervention is generally poor (ie, less than 20% of these children are neurologically normal).[70]

REFERENCES

1. Creasy RK. Prevention of preterm birth. Birth Defects 1983;19:97.
2. Goddard-Finegold J, Michael LH. Cerebral blood flow and experimental intraventricular hemorrhage. Pediatr Res 1984;18:7.
3. Behrman R. Preventing low birth weight: a pediatric perspective. J Pediatr 1985;197:842.
4. Hack M, Fanaroff AA, Merkatz IR. The low-birthweight infant: evolution of a changing outlook. N Engl J Med 1979;301:1162.
5. Volpe JJ. Neurology of the newborn. 2nd ed. Philadelphia: WB Saunders, 1987.
6. Volpe JJ. Intraventricular hemorrhage in the premature infant —current concepts. Part I. Ann Neurol 1989;25:3.
7. DeReuck JL. Cerebral angioarchitecture and perinatal brain lesions in premature and fullterm infants. Acta Neurol Scand 1984;70:391.
8. Rorke LB. Pathology of perinatal brain injury. New York: Raven Press, 1982.
9. Shuman RM, Selednik LJ. Periventricular leukomalacia: a one year autopsy study. Arch Neurol 1980;37:231.
10. Vander Eecken H. Anastomoses between the leptomeningeal arteries of the brain. Springfield, IL: Charles C Thomas, 1959.
11. Perlman JM, Volpe JJ. Are venous circulatory abnormalities important in the pathogenesis of hemorrhagic and/or ischemic cerebral injury? Pediatrics 1987;80:705.
12. Lou HC. Perinatal hypoxic-ischemic brain damage and intraventricular hemorrhage. A pathogenetic model. Arch Neurol 1980;37:585.
13. Lou HC. The "lost autoregulation hypothesis" and brain lesions in the newborn—an update. Brain Dev 1988;10:143.
14. Friede RL. Developmental neuropathology. 2nd ed. New York: Springer-Verlag, 1989.
15. Perlman JM, Volpe JJ. Prevention of neonatal intraventricular hemorrhage. Clin Neuropharmacol 1987;10:126.
16. Lazzara A, Ahmann P, Dykes F, et al. Clinical predictability of intraventricular hemorrhage in preterm infants. Pediatrics 1980;6:30.
17. Hill A, Volpe JJ. Normal pressure hydrocephalus in the newborn. Pediatrics 1981;68:623.
18. Guzetta F, Schackelford GD, Volpe S, Perlman JM, Volpe JJ. Periventricular intraparenchymal echodensities in the premature newborn: critical determinant of neurologic outcome. Pediatrics 1986;78:995.
19. Gould SJ, Howard S, Hope PL, Reynolds EOR. Periventricular intraparenchymal cerebral hemorrhage in preterm infants: the role of venous infarction. J Pathol 1987;1551:197.
20. Takashima S, Mito T, Ando Y. Pathogenesis of periventricular white matter hemorrhages in preterm infants. Brain Dev 1986;8:25.
21. Paris JE, Collins GH, Kim C, et al. Prenatal symmetrical thalamic degeneration with flexion spasticity at birth. Ann Neurol 1983;13:94.
22. Wilson ER, Mirra SS, Schwartz JF. Congenital diencephalic and brainstem damage: neuropathologic study of three cases. Acta Neuropathol 1982;52:70.
23. Armstrong DL, Sauls CD, Goddard-Finegold J. Neuropathologic findings in short-term survivors of intraventricular hemorrhage. Am J Dis Child 1987;141:617.
24. Barmada MA, Moosy J, Painter M. Pontosubicular necrosis and hyperoxemia. Pediatrics 1980;66:840.
25. Gilles FH, Averill DR Jr, Kerr CS. Neonatal endotoxin encephalopathy. Ann Neurol 1977;2:49.
26. Rushton DI, Preston PR, Durbin GM. Structure and evolution of echodense lesions in the neonatal brain. Arch Dis Child 1985;60:798.
27. Flodmark O, Roland EH, Hill A, Whitfield MF. Periventricular leukomalacia: radiologic diagnosis. Radiology 1986;162:119.
28. Baker LL, Stevenson KD, Enzmann DR. End-stage periventricular leukomalacia: MR evaluation. Radiology 1988;168:809.
29. Flodmark O, Lupton BA, Li D, Stimac GK, Roland EH, Hill A, et al. MR imaging of periventricular leukomalacia in childhood. AJNR 1989;10:11.
30. Barmada MA, Moosy J, Shuman RM. Cerebral infarcts with arterial occlusion in neonates. Ann Neurol 1979;6:495.
31. Crichton JU, Dunn HG, McBurney AK, et al. Long-term effects of neonatal jaundice on brain function in children of very low birth weight. Pediatrics 1972;49:656.
32. Rubin RA, Balow B, Fisch RO. Neonatal serum bilirubin levels related to cognitive development at ages 4 through 7 years. J Pediatr 1979;94:601.
33. Turkel SB, Guttenbert ME, Moynes DR et al. Lack of identifiable risk factors for kernicterus. Pediatrics 1980;60:502.
34. Kim MH, Yoon JJ, Sher J et al. Lack of predictive indices in kernicterus: A comparison of clinical and pathologic factors in infants with or without kernicterus. Pediatrics 1980;60:852.
35. Ritter DA, Kenny JD, Norton HJ et al. A prospective study of free bilirubin and other risk factors in the development of kernicterus in premature infants. Pediatrics 1982;69:260.
36. Lucas A, Morley R, Cole TJ. Adverse neurodevelopmental outcome of moderate hypoglycemia. Br Med J 1988;297:1304.
37. Volpe JJ, Herscovitch P, Perlman JM et al. Positron emission tomography in the newborn: Extensive impairment of regional cerebral blood flow with intraventricular hemorrhage and hemorrhagic intracerebral involvement. Pediatrics 1983;72:589.
38. Cole CH. Prevention of prematurity: Can we do it in America? Pediatrics 1985;76:310.
39. Marlow N, Chiswick ML. Neurodevelopmental outcome of babies weighing <2001 g at birth: Influence of perinatal transfer and mechanical ventilation. Arch Dis Child 1988;63:1069.
40. Shankaran S, Cepeda EE, Ilagan N et al. prenatal phenobarbital for the prevention of neonatal intracerebral hemorrhage. Am J Obstet Gynecol 1986;154:53.
41. Morales WJ, Koerten J. Prevention of intraventricular hemorrhage in very low birth weight infants by maternally administered phenobarbital. Obstet Gynecol 1986;68:295.
42. Cole VA, Durbin GM, Olaffson A, Reynolds EOR, Rivers RPA, Smith JF. Pathogenesis of intraventricular hemorrhage in newborn infants. Arch Dis Child 1974;49:722.
43. Pomerance JJ, Teal JG, Gogolok JF, et al. Maternally administered antenatal vitamin K: effect on neonatal prothrombin activity, partial thromboplastin time and intraventricular hemorrhage. Obstet Gynecol 1987;70:235.
44. Morales WJ, Angel JL, O'Brien WF, Knuppel RA, Marsalisi F. The

use of antenatal vitamin K in the prevention of early neonatal intraventricular hemorrhage. Am J Obstet Gynecol 1988; 159:774.

45. Tejani N, Rebold B, Tuck S, Ditrola D, Sutro W, Verma U. Obstetric factors in the causation of early periventricular-intraventricular hemorrhage. Obstet Gynecol 1984;64:510.
46. Meidell R, Marinelli P, Pettett G. Perinatal factors associated with early-onset intracranial hemorrhage in premature infants. American Journal of Diseases in Children 1985;139:160.
47. Bejar R, Coen RW, Glick L. Hypoxic-ischemic and hemorrhagic brain injury in the newborn. Perinatology Neonatology 1982; 6:69.
48. McDonald MM, Koops BL, Guggenheim MA, et al. Timing and etiology of neonatal intracranial hemorrhage. Pediatrics 1984;74:32.
49. Dykes FD, Lazzarra A, Ahmann P, et al. Intraventricular hemorrhage: a prospective evaluation of etiopathogenesis. Pediatrics 1980;66:42.
50. Clarke CE, Clyman RI, Roth RS, et al. Risk factor analysis of intraventricular hemorrhage in newborn infants. J Pediatr 1981;99:625.
51. Horbar JD, Pasnick M, McAuliffe C, et al. Obstetric events and risk of periventricular hemorrhage in premature infants. Am J Dis Child 1983;137:678.
52. Rayburn WF, Donn SM, Kolin MG, et al. Obstetric care and intraventricular hemorrhage in the low birthweight infant. Obstet Gynecol 1983;62:408.
53. deCrespigny L, Robinson HP. Can obstetricians prevent neonatal intraventricular hemorrhage? Aust NZ J Obstet Gynecol 1983;23:146.
54. Colavita RD. Anesthesia and intraventricular hemorrhage (letter to the editor). Pediatrics 1988;81:325.
55. Lou HC, Phibbs RH, Wilson SL, Gregory GA. Hyperventilation at birth may prevent early periventricular hemorrhage. Lancet 1982;1:1407.
56. Cooke RWI, Morgan MEI. Hyperventilation at birth and periventricular hemorrhage. Lancet 1982;2:450.
57. Volpe JJ. Intraventricular hemorrhage in the premature infant—current concepts. Part II. Ann Neurol 1989;35:109.
58. Omar SY, Greisen G, Obrahim M, et al. Blood pressure responses to care procedures in ventilated preterm infants. Acta Paediatr Scand 1985;74:920.
59. Hill A, Perlman JM, Volpe JJ. Relationship of pneumothorax to the occurrence of intraventricular hemorrhage in the premature newborn. Pediatrics 1982;62:144.
60. Fanconi S, Duc G. Intratracheal suctioning in sick preterm infants: prevention of intracranial hypertension and cerebral hypoperfusion by muscle paralysis. Pediatrics 1987;79:538.
61. Perlman JM, Goodman S, Kreusser KL, Volpe JJ. Reduction in intraventricular hemorrhage by elimination of fluctuating cerebral blood flow velocity in preterm infants with respiratory distress syndrome. N Engl J Med 1985;313:1353.
62. Beverley DW, Pitts-Tucker TJ, Congdon PJ, et al. Prevention of intraventricular hemorrhage by fresh frozen plasma. Arch Dis Child 1985;60:710.
63. Watkins A, Szymonowitz W, Jin X, Yu VVY. Significance of seizures in very low birthweight infants. Dev Med Child Neurol 1988;30:162.
64. Dubowitz LMS, Dubowitz V, Palmer PG, Miller G, Fawer C-L, Levene MI. Correlation of neurologic assessment in the preterm infant with outcome at one year. J Pediatr 1984;105:452.
65. Catto-Smith AG, Yu VYH, Bajuk B, Orgill AA, Astbury J. Effect of neonatal periventricular hemorrhage on neurodevelopmental outcome. Arch Dis Child 1985;60:8.
66. Fawer C-L, Levene MI, Dubowitz LMS. Intraventricular hemorrhage in a preterm neonate: discordance between clinical course and ultrasound scan. Neuropediatrics 1983;14:242.
67. Palmer P, Dubowitz LMS, Levene MI, Dubowitz V. Developmental and neurological progress of preterm infants with intraventricular hemorrhage and ventricular dilation. Arch Dis Child 1982;57:748.
68. Allan WC, Holt PJ, Sawyer LR, Tito Am, Mead SK. Ventricular dilation after neonatal periventricular-intraventricular hemorrhage. Am J Dis Child 1982;136:589.
69. Graziani LJ, et al. Cranial ultrasound and clinical studies in preterm infants. J Pediatr 1985;106:269.
70. Cooke RWI. Early prognosis of low birth weight infants treated for posthemorrhagic hydrocephalus. Arch Dis Child 1983; 58:410.

93

CHAPTER

COMMON PROBLEMS OF THE NEWBORN

Fernando R. Moya and David A. Clark

NEONATAL ADAPTATION TO EXTRAUTERINE LIFE

At birth the infant must adapt quickly to the more demanding extrauterine environment in which he or she must take control of vital functions, such as gas exchange and body temperature regulation. In preparation for birth many adaptations are initiated in utero, particularly with the onset of labor.

CIRCULATORY ADAPTATION

The fetal circulation is characterized by a low systemic resistance and a high pulmonary vasomotor tone. The distribution of the cardiac output is markedly different between the fetus and the adult (Table 93-1). In utero the placenta serves as the organ for gas exchange. About 30% to 40% of the fetal cardiac output is conveyed through both umbilical arteries (UA) to the placenta (Fig. 93-1). This systemic blood has Po_2 of about 25 to 30 mm Hg and Pco_2 of 40 to 45 mm Hg. There is a small but progressive decrease in umbilical arterial Po_2 with advancing gestational age. However, since this is paralleled by an increase in fetal hemoglobin, the oxygen content of the blood remains constant.[1] After circulation through the placenta the umbilical venous Po_2 rises to 35 to 55 mm Hg, whereas the Pco_2 drops to 35 to 40 mm Hg. This more oxygenated blood returns to the right atrium via the umbilical vein (UV) and the inferior vena cava (IVC). The stream from the IVC is directed preferentially across the foramen ovale to the left atrium, left ventricle, and ascending aorta, thereby perfusing primarily the head and neck vessels as well as the coronary arteries. A smaller fraction of the IVC return mixes with the superior vena cava (SVC) flow and passes into the right ventricle and pulmonary artery. During fetal life the pulmonary vascular resistance is high and opposes pulmonary blood flow. Less than 10% of the fetal cardiac output goes through the lungs and, on returning through the pulmonary veins, mixes with more oxygenated blood in the left atrium. Most of the pulmonary artery blood flow crosses into the descending aorta through the ductus arteriosus (DA). The high pulmonary vascular resistance is secondary to the low fetal Po_2, underventilation of the fluid-filled fetal lungs, and predominance of prostaglandins promoting increased pulmonary vasomotor tone.[2]

At birth, several events determine a rapid change in the circulatory pattern, ultimately separating the pulmonary and systemic circuits. With the clamping of the cord, systemic vascular resistance increases. The initiation of lung expansion increases the alveolar oxygen concentration and the Po_2 of the blood perfusing the lungs. This increase in oxygenation results in decreases in the pulmonary vascular resistance and in an increase in pulmonary blood flow. The increased venous return to the left atrium via pulmonary veins and the increase in systemic vascular resistance elevate left atrial pressure above that of the right atrium. This causes a functional closure of the foramen ovale. Anatomical closure of this structure usually happens in the weeks following birth, but it may remain open for life. The increased pressures on the systemic circuit, along with the drop in pulmonary artery pressure, reverse the ductal flow to a predominantly left-to-right shunt. Ductal closure results from constriction of its spiral musculature in response to a higher Po_2 and predominant stimulation of constrictor prostaglandins. The decreasing radius of the ductus compromises the nourishment of its endothelium, which ultimately necroses, obliterating its lumen. Anatomical ductal closure only occurs several weeks after birth.

Hypoxemia, the lack of lung expansion, and acidosis at birth are all causes of a persistently elevated pulmonary vascular resistance that interferes with the transition of the circulation from the fetal to the adult pattern.

TABLE 93–1. DISTRIBUTION OF CARDIAC OUTPUT

	% OF TOTAL CARDIAC OUTPUT	
	FETUS	ADULT
Brain	14	14
Heart	2	5
Lung	10	100
Placenta	33	–
Gut	8	23
Kidney	5	22

Adapted from Nelson N. The onset of respiration. In: Avery G, ed. Neonatology. 3rd ed. Philadelphia: JB Lippincott, 1987.

LUNG EXPANSION AND INITIATION OF BREATHING

The human fetus initiates respiratory movements late in the first trimester of gestation. Subsequently, these movements become stronger and more organized, and near term there is regular breathing in rates similar to those found after birth. Just prior to the initiation of labor, fetal breathing decreases from 75% to 80% to only about 15% to 30% of the time. In preparation for birth the fetal lungs undergo several changes. The biochemical maturation of the lung in terms of surfactant production is discussed elsewhere. The fetal lungs in utero are filled with a fluid rich in chloride (>150 mEq/L) and relatively free of protein (<0.3 mg/mL). The volume of this fluid that occupies the alveolar spaces and airways is similar to the functional residual capacity (FRC) during the neonatal period—namely, 30 to 35 mL/kg of body weight.[3] Fetal lung fluid is produced at an hourly rate of 4 to 6 mL/kg body weight. Before delivery, production of fetal lung fluid decreases and active reabsorption begins. This is secondary to hormonal changes that occur with the onset of labor, such as increases in circulating catecholamines and elevations of arginine vasopressin.[4] At birth a small proportion of the lung fluid that occupies the airways is "squeezed out" of the trachea during passage through the birth canal. The majority of the lung fluid is reabsorbed in the alveolar spaces into the pulmonary circulation, which increases with lung expansion. About 10% to 15% of this fluid is reabsorbed into the pulmonary lymphatics. The clearance of lung fluid continues for several hours after birth.

To expand the lungs at birth, the infant must generate a large transpulmonary pressure and overcome the resistance of the fluid-filled airways.[2] Initial respiratory efforts can generate transpulmonary pressures of 80 to 90 cm H_2O. This explains why the spontaneous occurrence of pneumothorax in healthy newborns is not uncommon. The FRC is rapidly established with the first several breaths; however, this may continue to expand to a lesser degree several hours after birth. Infants born by elective cesarean section have smaller lung volumes than those observed in vaginally delivered newborns.[5]

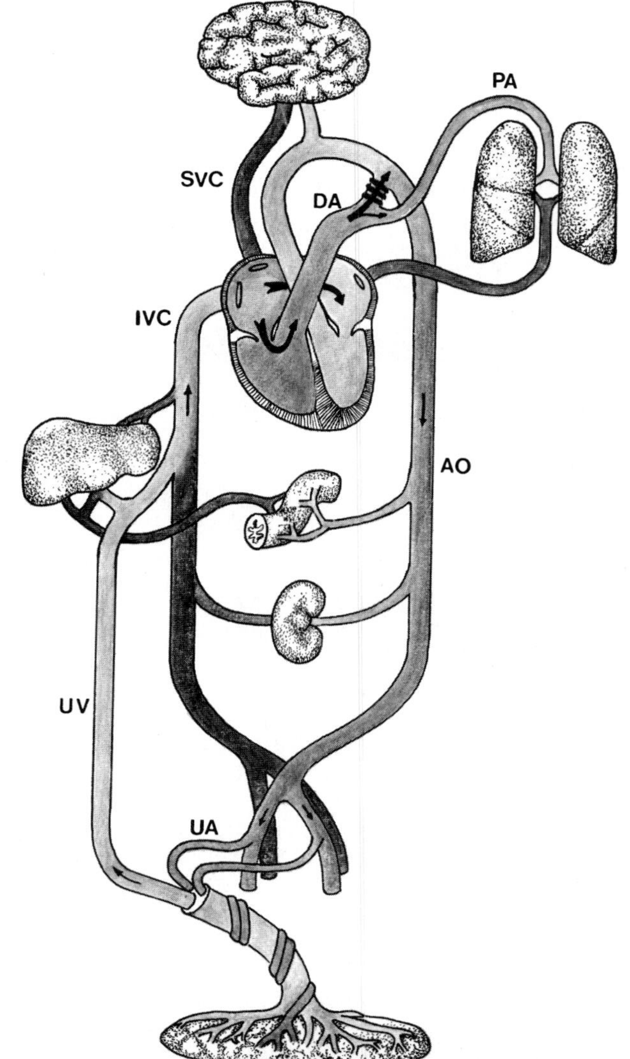

FIGURE 93–1. The fetal circulation. Lighter color represents more oxygenated blood; darker color represents less oxygenated blood.

This difference may persist for up to 48 hours after birth. Infants born by cesarean section with preceding labor constitute an intermediate group. Very immature neonates may have difficulties establishing an adequate FRC with the first few breaths, particularly if they lack adequate amounts of surfactant.

THERMOREGULATION

In utero the heat generated by the fetus is dissipated by the placenta. Because of the higher metabolic rate of the fetus its temperature will be at or slightly above the maternal core temperature. When there is maternal fever, or placental insufficiency, the ability of the fetus to transfer heat to the mother can be impaired and the infant may be born with an elevated body temperature.

Heat is exchanged by conduction, convection, evaporation, and radiation. The relative importance of any of these forms of heat exchange varies, depending on the clinical situation. For instance, at birth the infant is delivered from a fluid, warm environment to cooler and dry surroundings. Hence, evaporation is the main source of heat loss right after delivery.[6] Unless the infant is dried soon after birth, preferably with warm towels or blankets, rapid cooling will occur. If the term infant is not in need of resuscitation or assistance in transition (suctioning of meconium, poor respiratory effort), close contact with the mother's skin may serve to decrease the surface area for evaporation and gain heat through conduction from the mother. This beneficial effect in temperature control is in addition to the immeasurable gains that result from mother–infant bonding.

The newborn infant is at a significant disadvantage in terms of temperature control because of a relatively large surface area, poor thermal insulation from the environment, decreased ability to generate heat through physical activity (shivering thermogenesis), and, especially, no ability to adjust his or her own protection (clothing) from the thermal stress of the environment. Premature and growth-retarded infants are at an even higher risk for heat loss and hypothermia. Small premature infants have an incomplete development of the stratum corneum of the skin and poor keratinization. The smaller the infant, either premature or growth-retarded, the fewer subcutaneous fat stores, which act as insulation from the environment.

For body temperature to remain constant, heat must be generated at the same rate at which it is lost. Neonates have difficulties not only with heat loss, but also with heat production. Most heat production in the newborn is chemically derived from the breakdown of high-energy triglycerides (nonshivering thermogenesis) stored preferentially in brown fat. This is distributed in the subscapular areas, around the great vessels of the neck and thorax, and around the adrenal glands. Brown fat has numerous capillaries and sympathetic nerve endings. In response to catecholamine stimulation, the heat generated through triglyceride breakdown is transferred onto the circulation for distribution throughout the body. When the availability of substrates is decreased (premature, growth-retarded) or this mechanism is impaired (hypoxia, drugs), heat production is markedly decreased and hypothermia may ensue.

The consequences of hypothermia are hypoglycemia, metabolic acidosis, lethargy, and increased oxygen requirements. Also, hypothermia has been associated with a higher mortality rate at all gestational ages.

After delivery and drying, the newborn should be cared for in a "neutral thermal environment." This refers to that environmental temperature at which the energy expenditure and oxygen consumption for heat production and maintenance of a normal body temperature is the lowest. The neutral thermal environment varies inversely with gestational age and postnatal age.[7]

ASPHYXIA AND NEONATAL RESUSCITATION

During the transition period from fetal life to extrauterine existence many adverse events that may affect the ability of the neonate to survive or to develop to its fullest potential can occur. Asphyxia is one of them. Although there is substantial disagreement on the definition of *asphyxia*,[8,9] the term generally refers to a state in which there is a relative lack of oxygen, along with variable degrees of hypercarbia and metabolic acidosis. Most of the disagreements in its diagnosis arise from trying to define asphyxia objectively based on Apgar score, fetal heart rate alterations, umbilical cord blood gases, presence of neurologic abnormalities during the neonatal period, or combinations of these and other factors. With this approach asphyxia can be diagnosed reliably only in severely depressed infants.

Several mechanisms result in acute fetal asphyxia. Most of them essentially interfere with the ability of the placenta to exchange oxygen and carbon dioxide between the maternal and fetal circulations. The problem may arise from poor perfusion of the uteroplacental circulation (ie, maternal hypotension); from separation of the placenta from its insertion (eg, in abruptio placentae); or from compromise of the umbilical circulation (ie, cord prolapse). Whereas fetal hypoxemia is the primary consequence of the first two mechanisms, with total obstruction of umbilical blood flow there is also a rapid rise in fetal P_{CO_2}. In addition, when there is fetal blood loss or interruption of the fetal–placental circulation, superimposed ischemia may occur. The severity and rate of progression of asphyxia are highly variable. Milder insults may allow substantial cardiovascular and metabolic compensation by the fetus. The process of cardiovascular compensation involves primarily a redistribution of cardiac output to the brain, myocardium, and adrenal glands, at the expense of blood flow to less vital areas such as the gut, kidneys, muscle, and skin. From a metabolic point of view the fetus depends on its energy reserves, stored mainly as glycogen, and the ability to utilize ketones and fatty acids as additional fuel sources to glucose. Fetuses that have already used their energy reserves because of a chronic oxygen and nutrient deficit are at high risk for significant asphyxia, even with otherwise mild stresses such as labor. Once the asphyxial insult ensues, the resulting hypoxemia and acidosis may compromise the myocardial function to a point where cardiac output drops. This compromises further oxygen delivery to the tissues.

With asphyxia the brain undergoes several neurophysiologic and biochemical changes.[10] Electroencephalographic changes may be detected shortly after the insult. Within a few minutes there is lactic acid accumulation due to anaerobic glycolysis. Subsequent changes include shifts in transcellular ion gradients, alterations in extracellular concentrations of neurotransmitters and taurine, and a rise in the tissue concentrations of free fatty acids (eg, arachidonic acid). These may be metabolized to prostaglandins and leukotrienes once cerebral perfusion is reestablished. These vasoactive mediators have the potential for altering the microcirculation of the brain and are involved in the generation of free radicals and cell damage.

Recent studies using nuclear magnetic resonance have shown substantial alterations in cerebral intracellular metabolism among term neonates with asphyxia. High-energy phosphate compounds like phosphocreatine and ATP decrease, whereas ADP and inorganic phosphate increase. The changes observed in asphyxiated neonates continue to become evident beyond 24 hours after birth. This suggests that the events initiated by asphyxia continue for hours or days after recovery from the acute insult. Moreover, this may provide a window during which irreversible cerebral damage can be prevented or ameliorated.[11]

The best approach to the management of asphyxia is prevention and anticipation.[12] Although asphyxia occurs primarily in high-risk pregnancies, a sizable proportion of asphyxiated neonates still present without warning. For this reason a team of personnel skilled in providing neonatal resuscitation must be present in all hospitals that offer delivery services.

At birth a series of actions must be undertaken to facilitate the transition of the fetus to extrauterine life. These include minimizing heat loss by placing the infant under a preheated radiant source and thoroughly drying him or her, and clearing the airway by adequately positioning the infant and suctioning the mouth and nose. If there is a history of meconium in the amniotic fluid, management may include endotracheal intubation and suctioning (see section on Meconium Aspiration Syndrome). Subsequent actions are focused on establishing adequate respirations and circulation and evaluating the neonate (Fig. 93-2). The Apgar score is a useful method to assess the neonate during the early period of transition, as well as to evaluate the response to interventions such as resuscitation (Table 93-2). In neonates needing assistance, appropriate interventions should not be delayed until the 1-minute Apgar score is obtained. A repeat Apgar score must be obtained at 5 minutes after birth in all infants and every 5 minutes thereafter up to 20 minutes of age or until the neonate achieves two consecutive scores above 7 if he or she was depressed at birth. Of the Apgar score components, heart rate, respirations, and color are more useful to assess the neonatal status and need for intervention

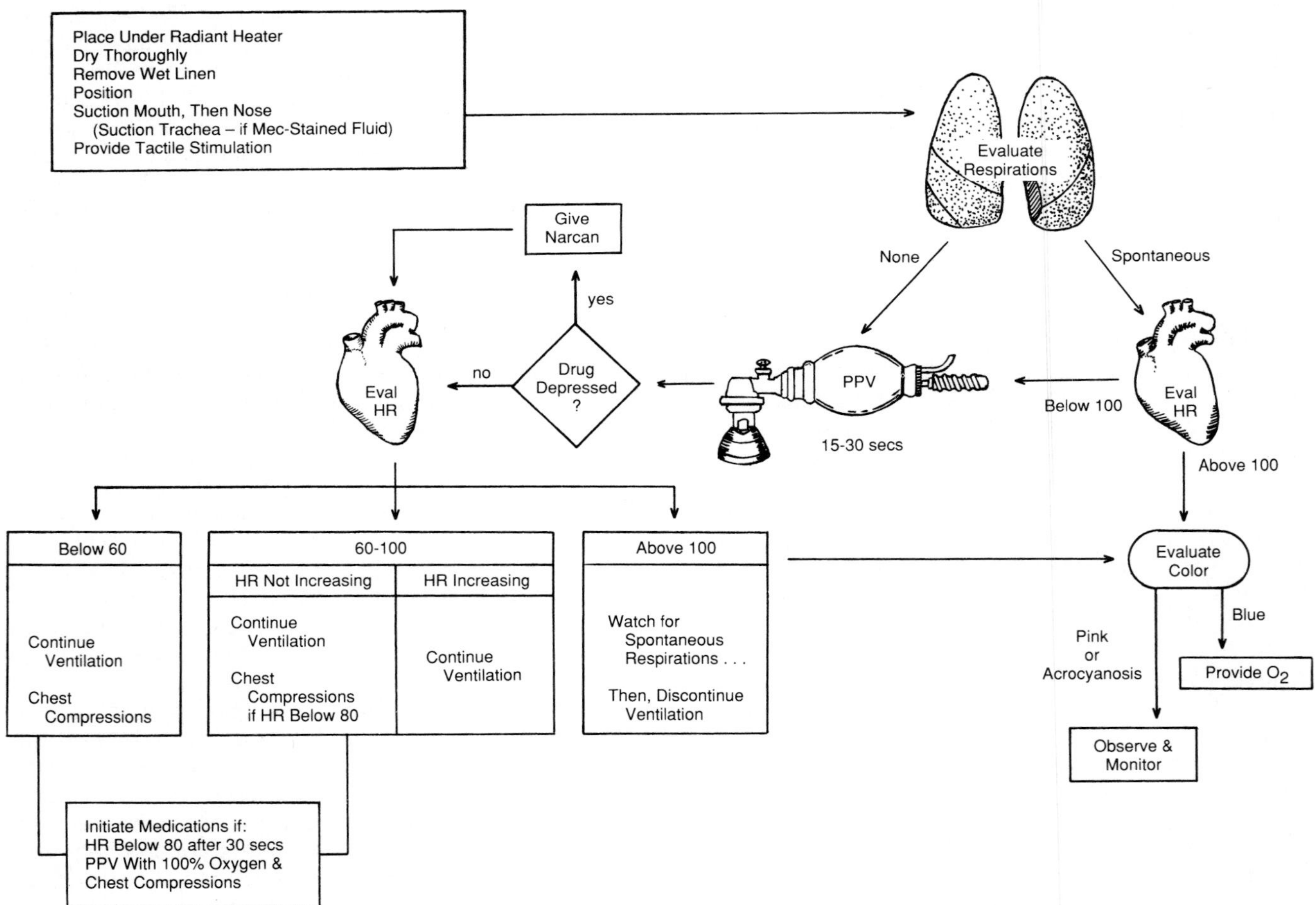

FIGURE 93–2. Overview of resuscitation in the delivery room. (American Heart Association. Textbook of Neonatal Resuscitation. Elk Grove Village, IL: American Heart Association, 1987:5.)

TABLE 93–2. THE APGAR SCORE

SIGN	0	1	2
Heart rate	Absent	<100/min	>100/min
Respirations	Absent	Weak cry; hypoventilation	Good, strong cry
Muscle tone	Flaccid	Some flexion	Active motion
Reflex irritability	No response	Grimace	Cough or sneeze
Color	Blue or pale	Body pink; extremities blue	Completely pink

than the remaining factors. Furthermore, primarily because of relative lack of muscle tone and response to stimuli, very immature neonates can have low Apgar scores without asphyxia.[13]

After doing the initial maneuvers described previously, infants who are vigorous, are breathing spontaneously, and have a heart rate above 100 just need to be watched and have their color evaluated. Blow-by oxygen must be supplied to those who remain cyanotic despite adequate respirations and heart rate. Persistent cyanosis under these circumstances may indicate such problems as congenital heart disease, pneumothorax, and airway obstruction (ie, choanal atresia). If the infant is apneic, has inadequate respirations, or has a heart rate below 100, positive pressure ventilation with 100% oxygen must be initiated. A good response is indicated by rapid increases in heart rate, improvements in color, and initiation of spontaneous respiratory efforts. Persistent apnea may be a sign of asphyxia or depression by narcotics. Naloxone (Narcan) can be given in neonates with poor or absent respiratory efforts exposed to maternally administered narcotics within 4 hours of delivery. The currently recommended dose is 0.1 mg/kg given IV, IM, SC, or intratracheally. Preparations of Narcan containing 0.02 mg/mL are no longer recommended, since their use would result in administration of excessive volumes.[14] The 0.4 mg/mL or 1.0 mg/mL preparations can be used instead.

When the heart rate is less than 60 to 80 beats per minute and there is no rapid response to positive pressure ventilation with 100% oxygen, chest compressions must be initiated to maintain an acceptable cardiac output. If there is no improvement after a period of at least 30 seconds, medications such as epinephrine need to be administered. At this time endotracheal intubation must be performed if it has not been done previously. In general terms the indications for endotracheal intubation are persistent apnea, need for positive pressure ventilation for several minutes, and lack of response to resuscitative maneuvers. Also, in infants suspected of having a congenital diaphragmatic hernia (scaphoid abdomen, lack of response to resuscitation), endotracheal intubation needs to be done promptly to avoid bowel distention and worsening of the lung compression. Although the threshold for delivery room intubation of small infants tends to be lower, there is no gestational age or weight cut-off at which intubation is mandatory.

The medications needed for delivery room resuscitation are listed in Table 93-3. There are precise indicators for their use, and these should be carefully monitored. Administration of epinephrine, either via umbilical vein or intratracheally, usually results in a rapid increase in heart rate and cardiac output. The dose may be repeated after 5 minutes if there is no response. Reasons for poor response to epinephrine are significant acidosis

TABLE 93–3. MEDICATIONS FOR DELIVERY ROOM RESUSCITATION

DRUG	INDICATION	DOSE	ROUTE
Epinephrine	Asystole or HR < 60 despite PPV with 100% O_2 and chest compressions	0.01–0.03 mg/kg or 0.1–0.3 mL/kg of 1:10,000 solution	IV, IT
Sodium bicarbonate	Metabolic acidosis	2 mEq/kg. The use of 4.2% solution is recommended	IV
Naloxone (Narcan)	Respiratory depression and maternal exposure to narcotics in previous 4 hours	0.1 mg/kg. The use of 0.4 mg/mL or 1.0 mg/mL solutions is recommended	IV, IT, SC, IM
Volume expander Normal saline Whole blood 5% albumin	Evidence of hypovolemia	10 mL/kg	IV
Atropine	Vagal bradycardia	0.01–0.04 mg/kg	IV, IM, IT
Glucose	Hypoglycemia	100–200 mg/kg bolus followed by continuous infusion	IV

and hypovolemia. If acidosis is suspected, an effort should be made to obtain arterial blood gases. Sodium bicarbonate can be given for metabolic acidosis as a slow intravenous infusion. Rapid rates of hypertonic sodium bicarbonate administration have been associated with intraventricular hemorrhage in premature infants. Hypovolemia should be suspected when there is a poor response to resuscitation and evidence of poor perfusion, especially if there is a history of abruption, tight nuchal cord, or bleeding. Ideally, group O Rh-negative whole blood should be used when bleeding and acute anemia are suspected. However, other volume expanders, such as normal saline and 5% albumin, are more readily available and are usually effective, unless the degree of anemia is profound.

Infants who suffer any degree of perinatal asphyxia must be observed closely during the first 24 to 48 hours after birth. Vital signs, neurologic findings, and function of other systems must be assessed periodically. Dysfunctions of kidneys, liver, and heart are common among neonates with severe perinatal asphyxia.[15]

It is very difficult to correlate asphyxia, using any definition, with long-term neurodevelopmental outcome. It is now well accepted that the correlation of low 1-, 5-, and 10-minute Apgar scores (≤3) with cerebral palsy or mental retardation is poor.[16,17] Its predictive value of death or a poor neurologic outcome increases at 15 and 20 minutes (Table 93-4). Similarly, fetal heart rate alterations, meconium in the amniotic fluid, and abnormal blood gases in cord blood are poor predictors of cerebral palsy or adverse neurologic outcome.[18] This is not surprising considering that consequences of asphyxia account for at most 15% to 20% of cerebral palsy and 10% of mental retardation.[16] Perhaps the presence of neonatal seizures secondary to asphyxia is a better indicator of a higher risk for a poor outcome.[19] Nonetheless, many neonatal seizures are not associated with objective signs of asphyxia. Intensive intrapartum monitoring of the fetal heart rate can reduce the incidence of neonatal seizures but offers little protective effect against cerebral palsy.[20] The presence of perinatal hypoxia-related factors increases the likelihood of an abnormal neurologic outcome among growth-retarded neonates.[21]

ASSESSMENT OF GESTATIONAL AGE

The intrauterine assessment of gestational age may be difficult to determine.[22] X-rays for the length of long bones and sonograms for biparietal diameter may be inaccurate if the fetus is growth retarded or macrosomic. Although the date of the last menstrual period is useful, irregular menstruation; hemorrhage, especially in the first trimester; and abnormal fetal size may confuse the issue. Thus, several methods have been developed to estimate gestational age once the baby is born, based on physical and neurologic characteristics of the newborn.

Many external physical characteristics of the developing fetus progress in an orderly fashion during gestation.[23] Vernix caseosa is a cheeselike material that initially appears at approximately 24 weeks of gestation. It covers the body of the fetus and begins to diminish by 36 weeks. In the full-term neonate it is generally found only in the creases.

The skin of the very low–birth-weight infant is thin and translucent. The blood vessels are prominent and are seen most easily over the abdomen. As gestation progresses, the vessels become less apparent as a result of thickening of the skin and deposition of subcutaneous fat. Lanugo (the fine hair of the fetus) covers the entire body as early as 22 weeks gestation. It begins to vanish from the face approximately 1 month prior to full-term birth and can be seen on the shoulders of most full-term newborns.[24,25]

The nipple and surrounding tissue (areola) are not visible or barely evident in the severely preterm infant less than 20 weeks of gestation. At approximately 34 weeks gestation the areola begins to become prominent. Maternal hormones in combination with good fetal nutrition lead to fat deposition in the breast, and by term an approximately 5- to 6-mm nodule can be palpated.[24]

The development of the ear has two primary components. The first is the cartilaginous development of the ear, and the second is the incurving of its outer edge. The pinna of the extremely premature infant is flat and somewhat shapeless and does not spring back when it is folded, primarily because there is little cartilage. In the full-term infant the ear stands erect from the head,

TABLE 93–4. LOW APGAR SCORES AND RISK OF DEATH AND CEREBRAL PALSY FOR INFANTS WITH BIRTH WEIGHT >2500 g

APGAR 0–3	LIVE-BORN INFANTS	DEATH %	CEREBRAL PALSY %
Minutes after birth:			
1	1729	3.1	0.7
5	286	7.7	0.9
10	66	18.2	4.7
15	23	47.8	9.1
20	39	59.0	57.1

Adapted from Nelson K, Ellenberg J. Apgar scores as predictors of chronic neurologic disability. Pediatrics 1981;68:36.

springs back readily, and has well-defined incurving of its outer edge.[25]

Genitalia of the male and female fetus may also help in determining gestational age.[23–25] The maturity of males may be traced by the descent of the testes, which begin as intra-abdominal organs. They first appear in the upper inguinal canal at approximately 28 weeks gestation. The testes then descend into the scrotum and the scrotum becomes more pigmented and pendulous and has increased folds. In the female, the deposition of fat plays a primary role. In the extremely premature infant the clitoris is very prominent and the labia majora are small and widely separated. With increased fatty deposition in the labia majora as the fetus approaches term, the labia minora and clitoris are usually completely covered.

The plantar creases are entirely absent on the feet of the severely premature baby. The anterior half of the foot at approximately 30 weeks gestation has faint red marks. A definite anterior sole crease can be seen by 32 weeks gestation. By 36 weeks, creases cover the anterior two thirds of the foot; most of the foot is covered by full term.

A very useful tool in the assessment of gestational age is the sequential regression of vessels in the anterior lens capsule of the eyes.[26] At approximately 27 to 28 weeks, vessels cross the entire lens capsule. By 30 weeks there is central clearing, which then continues until only small remnants can be seen in the periphery at 34 weeks of gestation.

In general, the preceding physical characteristics need to be determined within the first 24 hours. With loss of extracellular fluid the characteristics of the skin and appearance of sole creases may be somewhat altered, thus making the physical assessment of gestational age more complex.[24,25] Although determination of gestational age by physical criteria should be performed immediately after birth, the neurologic evaluation needs to be completed when the infant is quiet and beyond the effects of transition. In general, this assessment may be difficult until the end of the first day or beyond. Numerous perinatal factors may affect this assessment, including asphyxia, maternal anesthesia, medications, and various illnesses and syndromes.[25] Neurologic development of the fetus during the last trimester is characterized by an increase in muscle mass and tone as well as by changes in reflexes and joint mobility in the extremities.[23,24] Current neurologic evaluation after birth focuses specifically on examination of muscle tone (both passive and active), joint mobility, and primitive reflexes. Infants born at 28 weeks of gestation have very poor muscle tone, and their resting posture is hypotonic with full extension of the arms and legs. This is primarily because they have been in a relatively weightless environment and have not had to respond to gravity. Flexor tone begins to appear at approximately 30 weeks gestation, increasing in the legs before the arms. At term the resting posture should include full flexion of the joints of both upper and lower extremities. The severely preterm infant does not resist various passive maneuvers such as the heel to the ear or the scarf sign. Trunk tone may be measured by ventral suspension. With the infant prone and the chest resting on the examiner's hand, the infant is lifted off of the examining surface and the body position is noted. Very premature babies have poor trunk tone and will appear to be draped over the hand. By 32 to 34 weeks of gestation the back is straightened. By full term the head rises above the straightened back. Because of the multiple illnesses of preterm babies ventral suspension is rarely a convenient part of the neurologic examination. Joint flexibility or mobility may be examined in the wrist and ankle. With the square window sign the hand is flexed at the wrist and the angle between the hand and wrist is measured. In the 28-week fetus the wrist is not flexed beyond 90°, but by 36 weeks of gestation the angle is 45°, and at term the hand may touch the arm. In dorsiflexion of the ankle the foot is flexed at the ankle with sufficient pressure for maximum change. The angle between the dorsum of the foot and anterior leg is then measured. Ankle dorsiflexion reflects a similar pattern of development with an angle of greater than 45° in the preterm infant that progresses to near 0 by term. In both instances the relatively stiff joints of early gestation become more relaxed at term.[24]

Various primitive reflexes—sucking, rooting, grasping, Moro, tonic neck, and so on—have been used to determine gestational age.[25,27] Before 34 weeks of gestation virtually all of these reflexes are absent or at best very weak. By term they are nearly all well established. With progressive development of the central nervous system over the first year of life, most of these reflexes disappear. Persistence may occur in infants with central nervous system damage.

Gestational-age assessment of newborns is now usually accomplished with the use of a combination of both physical and neurologic criteria. The current trend was initiated in 1970 by Dubowitz and colleagues, who developed a scoring system utilizing both neurologic and physical characteristics.[27] Accordingly, 11 physical characteristics and 10 neurologic characteristics are scored, with a higher score assigned for the more mature characteristics. A total score is then determined and gestational age is determined by a graph. Many abbreviations of this scoring system have appeared that correlate well with the more sophisticated scoring system.[28] Such examinations allow for minimal handling and exposure of the acutely ill preterm infant.

Once gestational age of the newborn has been established, the growth parameters of the child can be used to determine if the child is appropriately grown. Both small-for-gestational-age and large-for-gestational-age infants are at increased risk for neonatal mortality, early morbidity (eg, hypoglycemia), and long-term developmental disability.[29]

RESPIRATORY PROBLEMS

The human lung appears 3 to 4 weeks after conception as a ventral outgrowth of the primitive foregut. Subsequently, it goes through the embryonic (up to 6 weeks of gestation), pseudoglandular (6 to 17 weeks of gestation), canalicular (17 to 24 weeks of gestation), and terminal sac (24 weeks of gestation to term) periods. During these periods there is progressive growth of the airways and differentiation of the alveolar epithelium into type I and type II pneumocytes. The former are thin cells that cover over 95% of the alveolar surface and are the site of gas exchange. The synthesis of pulmonary surfactant takes place in type II pneumocytes.[30] Pulmonary surfactant is a highly surface-active material composed primarily of phospholipids and a small percentage of proteins (Table 93-5). After synthesis of its components, surfactant is stored as lamellar bodies consisting of whorls of phospholipid-rich membranous material. Lamellar bodies can be found in the human fetus as early as 24 weeks of gestation. The number of type II pneumocytes with lamellar bodies and their number within each cell increase progressively thereafter. Pulmonary surfactant is secreted into the alveoli through a process involving beta-adrenergic receptors, prostaglandins, and other agonists.[31] A variable percentage of the phospholipids and proteins of surfactant can be recycled in the type II pneumocyte.

Beyond 36 weeks of gestation the fetal lung grows predominantly by forming new alveoli. At term there are approximately 20 to 25 million alveoli of about 50 μm in diameter. The total alveolar number increases 10-fold in the first 8 years of life, and the alveolar size reaches 200 to 300 μm.[32] The biochemical pathways involved in surfactant synthesis and secretion are usually mature after 36 to 37 weeks of gestation. Thus, respiratory distress due to surfactant deficiency is rare among term infants except in infants of poorly controlled diabetic mothers. Lung development among infants of diabetic mothers (IDMs) has been reviewed recently.[33]

Signs of respiratory distress—such as tachypnea, retractions, nasal flaring, end-expiratory grunting, and cyanosis—may be the result of many diseases, some of which involve systems other than the respiratory (Table 93-6). An adequate history and thorough physical exam may be sufficient to suspect or diagnose the etiology of the respiratory distress. Nevertheless, part of the workup of any neonate with signs of respiratory distress should include a chest x-ray and determination of arterial blood gases, even if there is no oxygen requirement.

TABLE 93–5. COMPONENTS OF PULMONARY SURFACTANT

Phospholipids	
Phosphatidylcholine	65%
Phosphatidylglycerol	8%
Phosphatidylethanolamine	5%
Sphingomyelin	2%
Cholesterol	8%
Proteins	
Surfactant apoproteins (A, B, and C)	1%
Other proteins	9%
Other constituents	2%

TABLE 93–6. COMMON CAUSES OF RESPIRATORY DISTRESS IN THE NEWBORN

I. Respiratory disorders
  A. Pulmonary diseases
    Respiratory distress syndrome
    Meconium aspiration syndrome
    Transient tachypnea
    Pneumonia
    Pneumothorax and other air leaks
    Developmental anomalies (congenital lobar emphysema, chylothorax, pulmonary hypoplasia)
  B. Airway obstruction
    Choanal atresia
    Pierre-Robin syndrome
  C. Rib cage abnormalities
    Asphyxiating thoracic dystrophy
  D. Diaphragmatic disorders
    Diaphragmatic hernia
    Phrenic nerve injury
II. Extrarespiratory disorders
  A. Congenital heart disease
  B. Acid–base abnormalities (inherited disorders of metabolism, other causes of metabolic acidosis)
  C. CNS disorders (cerebral edema, hemorrhage, infection)

RESPIRATORY DISTRESS SYNDROME

Respiratory distress syndrome (RDS) due primarily to surfactant deficiency and lung immaturity is one of the most common causes of respiratory difficulty in the neonatal period. In 1988 over 3000 deaths in the United States were due to RDS.[34] Acute and chronic complications resulting from RDS or its treatment are also very frequent causes of morbidity in neonatal intensive care units.

The most important risk factor for the development of RDS is prematurity. The incidence of RDS varies inversely with gestational age and can be as high as 60% to 70% among premature infants of less than 28 to 29 weeks of gestation. Conversely, RDS is seldom seen beyond 38 weeks of gestation. Additional risk factors are male sex, cesarean section delivery, perinatal asphyxia, second of twin pregnancy, and maternal diabetes. Premature delivery is associated with variable degrees of immaturity of surfactant metabolism. Infants who develop RDS have lower amounts of surfactant phospholipids in the airway than controls.[35] This deficiency could be the result of abnormalities of surfactant synthesis, secretion, reutilization, or combinations of these factors. Among very immature neonates there is also substantial structural lung immaturity. The relative importance of this aspect has become more apparent with surfactant replacement therapy. Alterations of lung mechanics that persist after surfactant administration are primarily a reflection of the anatomical immaturity of the premature lung. Both surfactant deficiency and structural lung immaturity lead to decreased pulmonary compliance and atelectasis (Fig. 93-3). Hypoxemia develops as a consequence of the resulting right-to-left intrapulmonary shunting. Hypercarbia may also occur due to hypoventilation of the lungs. Lack of ductal closure is a common finding among small infants with RDS. This provides the route for left-to-right shunting and pulmonary edema. Leakage of pulmonary capillaries due to hyperemia, hypoxic injury to the alveolar and capillary walls, and barotrauma gives access to plasma proteins into the alveolar sacs. A protein that inhibits surfactant function in RDS has been described.[36] Thus, capillary leakage may play an important role in the pathogenesis of RDS by inactivation of secreted surfactant.

The clinical signs of RDS are tachypnea, nasal flaring, grunting, retractions, and cyanosis in room air. Decreased air entry is found on auscultation. Because these signs are common to other diseases such as pneumonia and heart disease, the diagnosis of RDS is based not only on clinical assessment but also on the presence of radiographic findings, such as a diffuse reticulogranular pattern, poor lung expansion, and air bronchograms (Fig. 93-4).

Since this x-ray pattern is also observed with group B streptococcal pneumonia, exclusion of the possibility of infection is necessary.[37] Typically, the severity of RDS increases up to 48 to 72 hours, followed by a gradual improvement. This phase is often preceded by or occurs in association with a marked diuresis. The clinical course of RDS is substantially modified by administration of exogenous surfactant; however, the timing of diuresis is not influenced by this therapy.[38,39]

The management of infants with RDS involves general measures such as maintenance of vital signs and thermoregulation, fluid and electrolyte management, nutritional support, and correction of hematologic or acid–base abnormalities. Specific measures consist of oxygen therapy and the use of positive airway pressure, either continuously or by assisted ventilation.[40] The goals of the therapy are to maintain acceptable arterial blood gases with as little support as possible in order to minimize the likelihood of barotrauma and oxygen toxicity. Since neonates have mostly fetal hemoglobin, an arterial Po_2 between 50 and 75 mm Hg is sufficient to saturate 90% to 97% of the hemoglobin. Higher values are not needed and can be deleterious. Infants receiving oxygen or any form of ventilatory assistance must be monitored closely with pulse oximetry, transcutaneous oxygen measurements, or intermittent blood gas analysis. The use of high-frequency ventilation has been compared to conventional ventilation among infants with RDS.[41] The lack of additional benefits and the likelihood of a higher incidence of intraventricular hemorrhage suggest that this mode of ventilation should be reserved for specific instances like severe air leaks and pulmonary interstitial emphysema.

Currently, several types of exogenous surfactant are being evaluated in humans. The preparations available consist of a mixture of phospholipids, or extracts of calf lung or amniotic fluid surfactant.[38] The latter types contain protein residues, which is of some concern; however, to date no significant immune reaction to these proteins has been demonstrated. Administration of surfactant can be performed at birth (prophylactic) or after RDS has already been diagnosed (rescue). Unfortunately, many infants are intubated and given surfactant unnecessarily with the prophylactic approach. Soon after intratracheal administration of a dose of surfactant, rapid improvements in oxygenation and lung compliance are observed. Accordingly, ventilatory support can be decreased rapidly. Nonetheless these effects are usually transient. Other beneficial effects observed after surfactant administration include an increased survival of infants below 1250 g and a lower incidence of air leaks. The occurrence of complications like intraventricular hemorrhage and bronchopulmonary dysplasia (BPD) has not consistently decreased with surfactant replacement therapy.[42]

Of the complications of RDS, BPD, a form of chronic lung disease, is among the most significant. The pathogenesis of BPD is multifactorial and results primarily from oxygen-mediated injury and barotrauma on an immature lung structure.[43] The diagnosis of BPD is based on oxygen dependency at 3 to 4 weeks after birth in an infant, usually premature, who received mechanical ventilation for a variable period of time. Also, characteristic radiographic findings of interstitial fibrosis, cystic changes, hyperinflation, segmental atelectasis, and some pulmonary edema are needed to make the diagnosis. The incidence of BPD among survivors of less than 1500 g at birth ranges between 8% and 35%.[44] An even higher incidence is observed below 900 g. In-

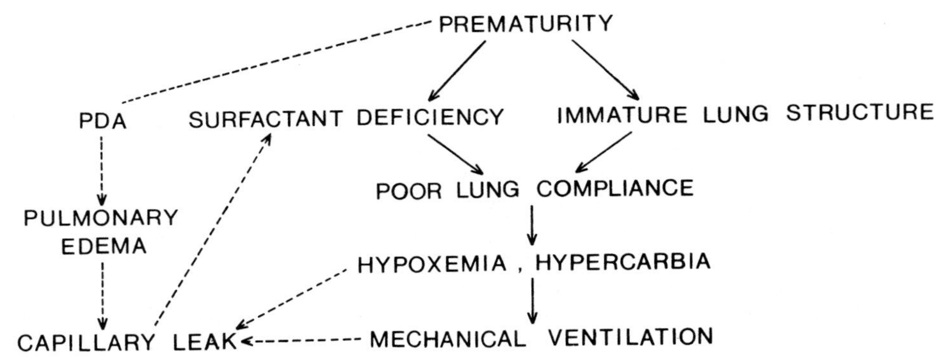

FIGURE 93–3. Pathophysiology of RDS.

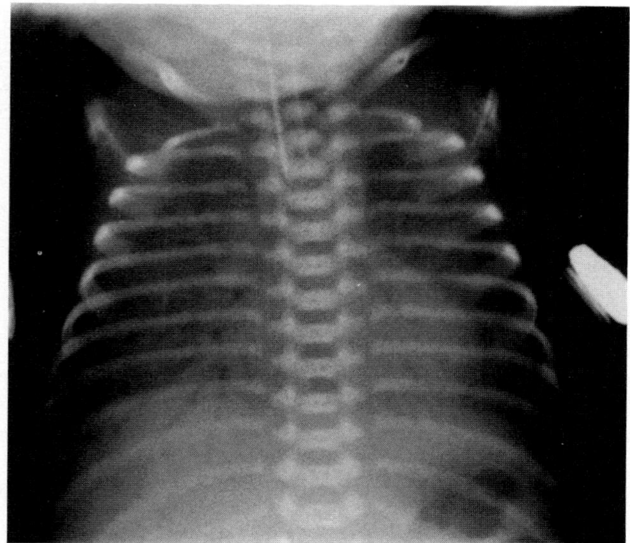

FIGURE 93–4. Chest radiograph of a premature infant with RDS.

fants with BPD are at high risk for cor pulmonale, growth failure, developmental delay, and sudden death.[45,46]

Despite widespread availability of surfactant replacement in the future, it is likely that RDS and other complications of prematurity will continue to be responsible for a sizable proportion of deaths and morbidity among premature infants. Thus, all efforts directed toward prevention of preterm delivery need to be continued and strengthened. In addition, attempts to accelerate fetal lung maturation with corticosteroids alone or in combination with other hormones must be undertaken whenever feasible (Fig. 93-5). Furthermore, accumulating animal data and preliminary data in humans strongly suggest that prenatal hormonal administration followed by postnatal surfactant replacement for those infants who develop RDS may be the best possible approach to prevent and treat RDS and its complications.[47–50]

MECONIUM ASPIRATION SYNDROME

Meconium is composed of desquamated cells from the skin and gastrointestinal tract, lanugo, amniotic fluid, and various intestinal secretions, including bile. Whereas meconium is present in the intestine of immature fetuses, it is rarely found in amniotic fluid prior to 34 weeks of gestation. Beyond this period meconium can be detected in 10% to 18% of all deliveries.[51–53] In utero passage of meconium can be a sign of maturation, or it may be triggered by fetal hypoxemia and acidosis. However, there is a poor correlation between meconium staining of the amniotic fluid and umbilical cord acid–base status.[54] Of all infants delivered through meconium-stained amniotic fluid, between 1% and 9% may develop meconium aspiration syndrome (MAS) despite aggressive suctioning of the airway at birth.[51,53,55] Many of these cases have aspirated in utero, at times without signs of fetal distress.[56] The majority of infants who develop MAS have delivered through thick meconium.[55]

The presence of meconium in the airway interferes with the initiation of breathing and may be a cause of difficult resuscitation. In MAS, overall airway resistance is increased, although the airway obstruction is not homogenous throughout the lungs. Segments of the lungs will exhibit alveolar overdistention and air trapping, whereas in others alveolar collapse will predominate (Fig. 93-6). Alveolar rupture occurs frequently in overdistended areas, and air leaks (pneumothorax, pneumomediastinum) are seen in up to one third of infants with MAS, particularly those who require mechanical ventilation. These alterations lead to variable degrees of ventilation–perfusion abnormalities and intrapulmonary shunting with resulting hypoxemia.[57] Infants with severe MAS also develop respiratory acidosis. Hypoxemia and acidosis can increase pulmonary vascular resistance and cause right-to-left shunting through the ductus arteriosus, foramen ovale, or both, a condition known as persistent fetal circulation (PFC) or persistent pulmonary hypertension of the newborn (PPHN). This condition may worsen the oxygenation status of the infant. The presence of meconium in the amniotic fluid is a known risk factor for the development of PPHN.[58] Some infants who have fatal MAS and PPHN have been shown to have excessive muscularization around the small intra-acinar arterioles of the lung, which predisposes them to PPHN. It has been suggested that these changes result from a chronic and often subclinical hypoxemia in utero.[59] Additional factors that play a role in the pathogenesis of MAS are the chemical pneumonitis induced by meconium and the potential displacement of surfactant by the free fatty acids of meconium.[60]

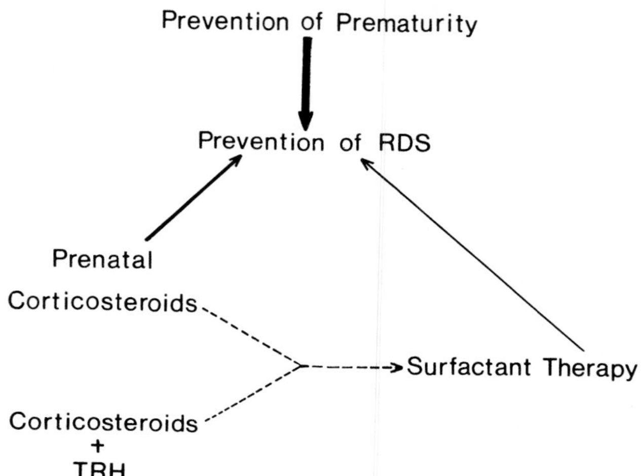

FIGURE 93–5. Interventions to prevent and treat RDS. (Moya F, Gross I. Prevention of respiratory distress syndrome. Sem Perinatol 1988;12:348.)

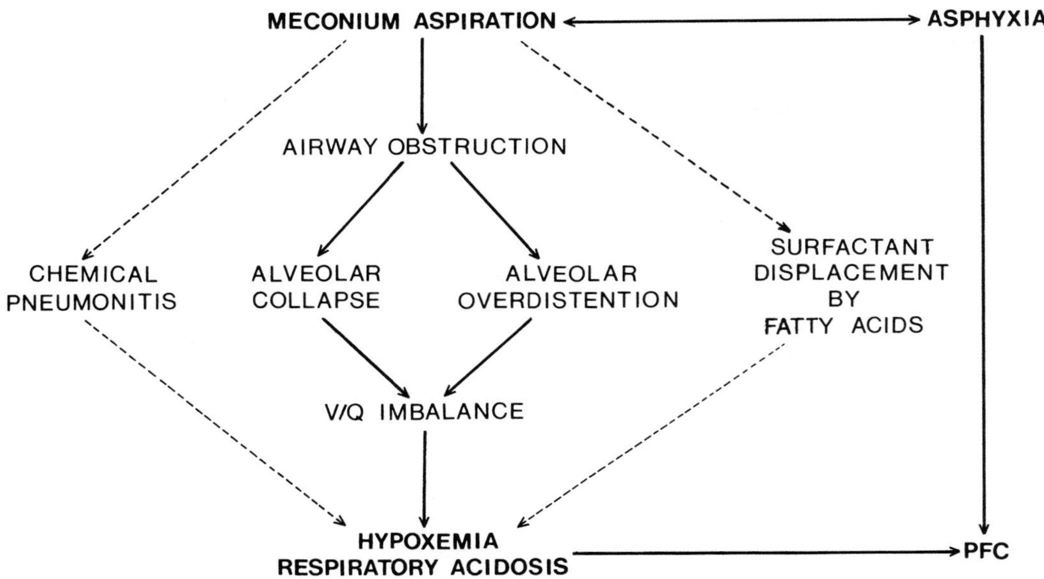

FIGURE 93–6. Pathophysiology of MAS.

Infants with MAS manifest tachypnea and variable degrees of nasal flaring, retractions, and cyanosis in room air. Grunting is uncommon. The chest appears hyperexpanded and the aeration may be decreased on auscultation. Meconium staining of the skin is not uniformly present. Usually, these infants are appropriately grown by weight. However, they may have a low ponderal index, because of recent intrauterine weight loss or other signs of postmaturity. In addition, abnormal neurologic signs may be present. Radiographic examination reveals hyperexpansion of the lungs, asymmetrical areas of atelectasis, and areas that may be completely spared (Fig. 93-7). Pneumothorax and pneumomediastinum are frequent findings. Infants born through meconium-stained amniotic fluid can also have renal dysfunction, as shown by increased excretion of β_2-microglobulin in urine.[61]

The management of infants with MAS must begin before delivery. Careful surveillance of fetal well-being is important, particularly if meconium is found in the amniotic fluid. Delivery with intact fetal membranes can obscure the detection of meconium. Transcervical amnioinfusion may be a safe alternative way to decrease meconium thickness and possibly MAS.[62] Detection of meconium in the amniotic fluid mandates the need for the presence of a team skilled in neonatal intubation and resuscitation at delivery. As soon as the head is delivered, the nose, mouth, and pharynx should be aspirated with a DeLee suction catheter. The use of wall suction with a maximum pressure of 100 mm Hg is now recommended, to avoid the risk of exposure to potentially infectious material. The infant should be handled carefully to minimize stimuli that initiate breathing. Not all infants with meconium-stained amniotic fluid need to be intubated. However, direct visualization of the larynx and tracheal suctioning should be performed, preferably before the initiation of breathing, when there is evidence of thick meconium, fetal distress, and need for resuscitation. These characteristics are more common among infants who develop severe or fatal MAS. Thorough endotracheal suctioning may not prevent all cases of MAS.[51,53] The best approach for term infants who have already initiated vigorous respiratory efforts is probably just observation,

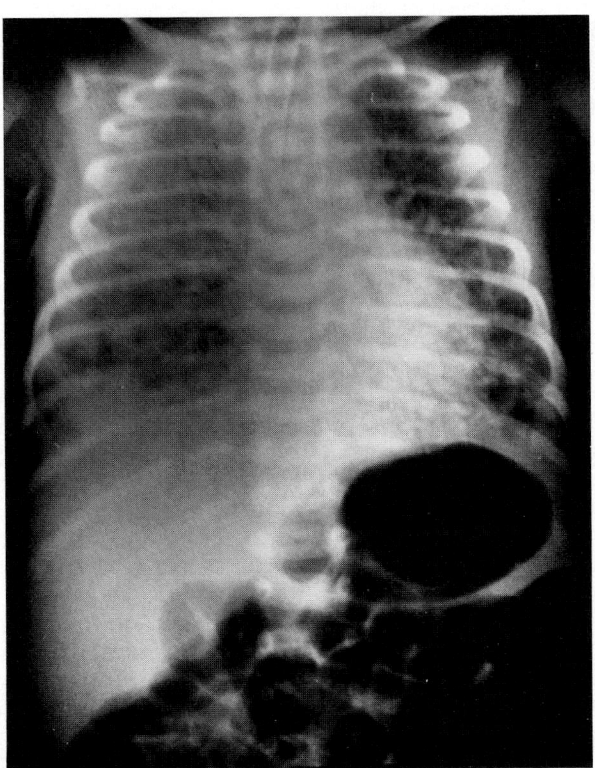

FIGURE 93–7. Chest radiograph of a term infant with MAS. Note the bilateral hyperinflation and marked asymmetry of the pulmonary involvement.

regardless of the characteristics of the meconium.[63] Efforts to intubate these neonates may be more harmful than helpful. Subsequent management will depend on whether the infant develops clinical signs of MAS. Adequate oxygenation, correction of metabolic acidosis, and support of the circulation are critical to minimize the stimuli for pulmonary vasoconstriction.

The mortality rate of infants with MAS may be as high as 40%, although recently it has declined to less than 20%.[53,55] Most of these deaths result from PPHN or consequences of asphyxia. Up to one third of survivors of MAS may exhibit pulmonary function abnormalities later in childhood, such as airway obstruction and exercise-induced bronchospasm.[64,65] Meconium contamination of the middle ear at birth may also increase the risk of otitis media in these infants.[66] The long-term neurologic outcome of infants with MAS can be quite variable and is influenced by the presence or absence of signs of perinatal asphyxia.

PERSISTENT PULMONARY HYPERTENSION OF THE NEWBORN

Although right-to-left shunting through the foramen ovale and ductus arteriosus is necessary for fetal survival, persistence of this pattern of circulation results in marked hypoxemia in extrauterine life. Hypercarbia, however, is not a consequence of PPHN. Under normal circumstances the high fetal pulmonary vascular resistance decreases progressively after birth. With hypoxemia and acidosis, pulmonary vascular resistance will remain high, or it may increase if it had already decreased. Pulmonary vasoconstriction can also be induced by mediators such as thromboxane A_2 and leukotrienes.[67] These mediators may play a role in PPHN associated with group B streptococcal infections. Using an anatomical approach, infants with PPHN can be divided into a group with normal pulmonary vasculature who develop PPHN because of a transient maladaptation (acute asphyxia, pneumonia), another group in which there is underdevelopment of the pulmonary vasculature (pulmonary hypoplasia), and a last group of infants in whom the number of pulmonary vessels is normal but in whom muscularization of the intra-acinar arteries is excessive.[68] In the latter two groups the pulmonary vascular abnormalities develop days or weeks before birth. Clinically, PPHN has also been classified as primary (ie, without associated disorders) or secondary to respiratory or other diseases (Table 93-7). The diagnosis of PPHN should be suspected when there is a high alveolar–arterial difference of oxygen, even if there is no hypoxemia ($Po_2 < 50$ mm Hg). The presence of right-to-left ductal shunting is established by comparing pre- and postductal arterial blood gases or by showing a lower transcutaneous Po_2 or Hb saturation in areas perfused by postductal blood when compared to simultaneous preductal readings. The absence of ductal shunting does not rule out PPHN, since this can be intermittent or may not be present at all. Confirmation of the diagnosis of PPHN must be done by echocardiography, which also serves to discard the possibility of congenital heart disease and assess myocardial contractility.[69]

TABLE 93-7. DISEASES COMMONLY ASSOCIATED WITH PERSISTENT PULMONARY HYPERTENSION OF THE NEWBORN

Perinatal asphyxia
Meconium aspiration syndrome
Pneumonia
Respiratory distress syndrome
Polycythemia
Diaphragmatic hernia
Pulmonary hypoplasia
Maternal salicylate use during pregnancy

The treatment of infants with PPHN is controversial. In general, the therapy is focused on supporting the systemic circulation by fluid administration and the use of pressor agents, and a series of measures to decrease the elevated pulmonary vascular resistance. These have included hyperventilation, alkalinization, and administration of tolazoline or a variety of other medications (chlorpromazine, nitroprusside, prostaglandins, nifedipine, amrinone). More recently, a more conservative approach to avoid the barotrauma resulting from attempts to hyperventilate has been suggested.[70] With a conservative approach, survival rates of 80% to 90% have been reported in PPHN.[70,71] High-frequency ventilation and extracorporeal membrane oxygenation are additional therapies used to treat PPHN. Although they can be of benefit in certain infants, the indications for their use are still being debated.[72,73]

Neurologic abnormalities and hearing loss have been reported in up to 50% of survivors of PPHN.[74–76] However, severe neurodevelopmental impairment is uncommon. It is not well known whether these abnormalities result from hypoxia, associated conditions (hypoglycemia, asphyxia), therapeutic interventions, or combinations of these factors.

TRANSIENT TACHYPNEA OF THE NEWBORN

The pathogenesis of transient tachypnea of the newborn (TTN) is related primarily to lung fluid reabsorption. This respiratory disease is seen mostly in term or near-term infants but may also affect smaller premature infants.[77,78] With the onset of labor, lung fluid production decreases, and its absorption increases under the influence of catecholamines, vasopressin, and steroids. Labor markedly influences pulmonary epithelial ion transport so that term infants born by cesarean section without labor exhibit a delay in the transition from chloride secretion to sodium absorption. Infants with TTN demonstrate a similar abnormality.[79] Thus, delivery by cesarean section without labor constitutes a risk factor for TTN.[80] Infants who develop TTN have also been shown to have borderline lung maturity on prenatal amniotic fluid analysis.[81] Additional risk factors are maternal diabetes, prolonged labor, male sex, macrosomia, and asphyxia.[82] This last complication not only interferes with lung fluid reabsorption, but also may lead to variable degrees of left or combined ventricular failure.[83]

The manifestations of TTN are tachypnea, retractions, grunting, and hyperexpansion of the thorax. These signs are usually manifest by 6 to 8 hours after birth. Onset of respiratory symptoms beyond 24 to 48 hours after birth is not due to TTN; hence, other explanations should be sought. The radiologic features of TTN are seen in Fig. 93-8. Typical findings are mild hyperinflation, increased interstitial and vascular markings (primarily around the hilar areas), fluid in the horizontal fissure, and at times mild cardiomegaly. Small pleural effusions, mostly on the right side, can be present. A pleural effusion, revealed by radiographic examination, where none existed earlier is more suggestive of infection than of TTN. The presence of radiographic abnormalities indicative of delayed clearance of lung fluid is not necessarily associated with clinical manifestations, especially on x-rays obtained soon after delivery.[78] There can be variable degrees of hypoxemia and respiratory acidosis. Oxygen requirements are variable and can be very high. In addition, some infants may require mechanical ventilation for significant respiratory distress or blood gas derangements. The association of TTN with PPHN has also been reported.[84] The symptomatology usually lasts less than 72 hours, and pulmonary sequelae are rare.

HEMATOLOGIC PROBLEMS

During pregnancy the human fetus grows in a relatively hypoxemic environment at a rate unparalleled after birth. This is made possible in part by adaptations of the hematologic system of the fetus, such as an increase of the red blood cell mass, and the synthesis of fetal hemoglobin (HbF). These result in an increased ability to bind and transport oxygen to meet the tissue demands. Fetal HbF (α_2, γ_2) is structurally different from adult HbA (α_2, β_2) and binds oxygen more avidly. Accordingly, the P_{50} and P_{90} (ie, the partial pressure of oxygen at which 50% and 90%, respectively, of the Hb is saturated) are considerably lower in HbF than in HbA (Fig. 93-9).

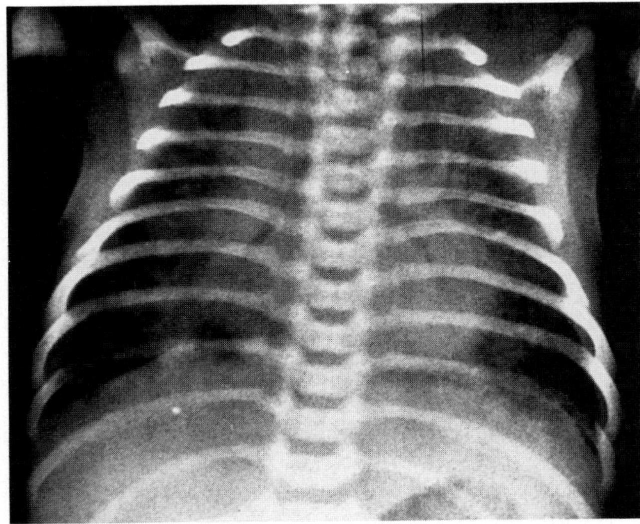

FIGURE 93–8. Chest radiograph of a near-term infant with TTN.

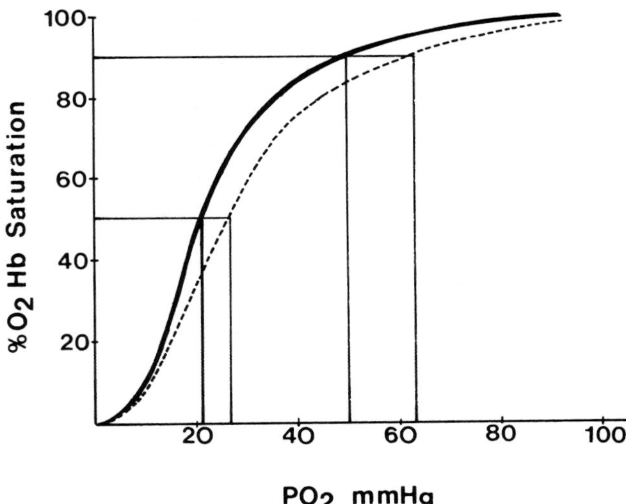

FIGURE 93–9. Fetal Hb (solid line) and adult Hb (dotted line) saturation curves. The P_{50} and P_{90} values for both hemoglobins are shown.

Fetal erythropoiesis occurs primarily in the liver and bone marrow, and to a lesser extent in the spleen. Extramedullary erythropoiesis may persist for up to 1 to 2 weeks after delivery. During the second trimester and early third trimester over 90% of the hemoglobin of the fetus is HbF. As the fetus approaches term the synthesis of HbA increases. This results in an increase in total body hemoglobin mass as well as a decrease in the proportion of HbF to 50% to 85% of the total.[85] After birth there is a gradual decline in circulating HbF levels to about 10% to 15% at 3 to 4 months of age, and less than 2% by 2 years of age. In certain disorders of HbA synthesis (sickle cell anemia, thalassemia major) the rate of decline of HbF is much slower. The fetal red blood cell is much larger than the adult type (fetal MCV, 100 to 115; adult MCV, 82 to 92) and has a survival of only 80 to 90 days.

The normal hematologic values for term infants are seen on Table 93-8. The Hb and hematocrit (Hct) values represent those obtained primarily by electronic counters. Determination of the Hct by these means may be substantially lower than a spun Hct at all ranges. This may be of utmost importance for the diagnosis of polycythemia.[86] Moreover, capillary Hct determinations are generally higher than those obtained by simultaneous peripheral venous sampling. Under normal circumstances the level of Hb in cord blood is influenced by gestational age and placental transfusion. As mentioned previously, the increase in Hb with advancing gestation is associated with a mild but significant de-

TABLE 93-8. NORMAL HEMATOLOGIC VALUES FOR TERM NEWBORNS*

AGE	Hb (g/dL)	Hct (%)	RETICULOCYTES (%)	WBC ($\times 10^3/\mu L$)	PLATELETS ($\times 10^3/\mu L$)
Cord blood	16.5 ± 3.0	51 ± 9	3–10	18 ± 9	300 ± 150
1–3 days	18.5 ± 4.0	56 ± 9	3–7	15 ± 9†	300 ± 150
1 week	17.5 ± 4.0	54 ± 12	<2–3	12 ± 5	300 ± 150
1 month	14.0 ± 4.0	43 ± 12	—	—	300 ± 150

* All values are approximate mean ± 2 SD from Oski FA, Naiman JL, eds. Hematologic problems in the newborn. 3rd ed. Philadelphia: WB Saunders, 1982; and Avery GB, ed. Neonatology. 3rd ed. Philadelphia: JB Lippincott, 1987.

† Values after increase 12–24 hours after birth.

crease in umbilical venous Po_2. The increase in Hb ensures that the oxygen content of the fetal umbilical venous blood remains constant throughout gestation. The pool of blood shared by the fetus and the placenta may be preferentially transfused to either of them at the time of delivery. If there is delayed cord clamping, the infant is held lower than the placenta, or there is a hypoxia-induced increase in placental vascular resistance, the blood volume of the infant may be increased by up to 60%.[87] Conversely, positioning the infant above the placenta or rapid cord clamping may deprive the neonate of the placental transfusion. This mechanism has been suggested to explain the lower cord blood Hb levels observed in neonates born by cesarean section. Whether there is a substantial placental transfusion or not, in the first hours after birth there is a redistribution of the acellular intravascular volume, so that the Hb and Hct increase.[88]

The total white blood cell (WBC) count shows a mild increase with advancing gestational age. During the first 12 to 24 hours after birth there is an increase in the total WBC count and total neutrophil count.[89] In subsequent days, both total WBC and neutrophils decline, and there is a steady transition in the differential count of white cells from a predominance of polymorphonuclear cells soon after delivery to a higher proportion of lymphocytes by 3 to 4 weeks postnatally. Arterial and venous WBC counts are lower than capillary values. Abnormalities of the WBC count, such as leukopenia (<5000/mm^3), marked leukocytosis (>30,000/mm^3), and an increase in the immature–mature neutrophil ratio (>0.2 to 0.3) are suggestive of neonatal infection.[90,91] The platelet count is similar in both preterm and term infants. Although an occasional healthy newborn will have less than 150,000 platelets/mm^3, counts below this level should be considered suspicious; a number below 100,000/mm^3 is definitely abnormal.

ANEMIA

In the term or postterm newborn, anemia is defined as a Hb below 13 g/dL in cord blood or during the early neonatal period. Because of the slow decrease in Hb concentration during the first several weeks after birth, only Hb concentrations below 10 g/dL are considered abnormal at 1 month of age. From a pathophysiologic point of view, anemia can be the result of hemorrhage, hemolysis, or decreased red cell production (Table 93-9). It is uncommon to see anemia secondary to combinations of these factors. Clinical and laboratory findings that are helpful to establish the differential diagnosis of anemia in the newborn are listed in Table 93-10.

Anemia Secondary to Hemorrhage

Anemia secondary to hemorrhage is a frequent etiology of anemia presenting at birth or soon thereafter. If the blood loss is acute, there may be signs of hypovolemia, such as lethargy, poor capillary refill, tachycardia, weak pulses, hypotension, and pallor. Significant blood loss and hypovolemia at birth may render an infant unresponsive to the usual resuscitative maneuvers until the intravascular volume depletion and cardiac output are restored. Chronic blood loss over a period of days or weeks permits substantial hemodynamic compensation, so that the main presenting sign is pallor. If the hemorrhage is external, there is no additional bilirubin load to the liver once Hb breakdown begins. This is in contrast to internal hemorrhages that contribute to elevations of the serum bilirubin and jaundice beyond the first 24 to 48 hours after birth. Significant jaundice with onset in the first prenatal day should not be attributed to reabsorption of internal bleeding.

External bleeding may be clinically apparent by either careful history (vaginal bleeding in the mother in placenta previa) or physical examination (ruptured umbilical cord). However, occasionally substantial bleeding may be occult and thus more difficult to diagnose (fetal–maternal hemorrhage). Abnormalities of the umbilical cord, such as varices or aneurysm, make it more prone to rupturing; however, a normal umbilical cord may also rupture when stretched excessively, such as in a precipitous delivery, or when attempting to reduce a very tight nuchal cord. When the cord ruptures, it usually does so in areas closer to the fetus. Fetal blood loss may occur with an intact tight nuchal cord, since the umbilical vein is compressed before the arteries. These continue to direct blood to the placenta while the venous return is impaired. Also, a velamentous insertion of the cord or the presence of aberrant vessels may predispose to its rupture. Abruptio placentae and placenta previa are common causes of fetal and maternal blood loss. These placental abnormalities and others

TABLE 93–9. COMMON ETIOLOGIES OF ANEMIA IN THE NEWBORN

HEMORRHAGE	HEMOLYSIS	DECREASED RBC PRODUCTION
External	Immune	Diamond-Blackfan syndrome
Placenta	ABO	Transcobalamin II deficiency
Abruptio	Rh	Congenital leukemia
Placenta previa	Minor groups	
Tumors	Maternal autoimmune	
Cord	Drug-induced	
Nuchal cord		
Velamentous insertion	Nonimmune	
Fetoplacental	Infection	
Fetomaternal	RBC membrane defects	
Twin–twin transfusion	Spherocytosis	
	RBC enzyme defects	
Internal	G-6 PD deficiency	
Cephalohematoma	Pyruvate kinase deficiency	
Intracranial	Hemoglobinopathies	
Ruptured liver, spleen		
Adrenal		
Retroperitoneal		
Iatrogenic		

such as choriocarcinoma have been associated with severe fetal–maternal hemorrhage.[92]

The fetus can also lose blood into the placenta or maternal circulation. Rapid cord clamping, especially with the infant above the placenta, will result in pooling of blood within this organ. A large amount of the fetal circulating volume may also be "trapped" in a chorioangioma of the placenta. In this case close examination and weighing of the placenta may suggest the diagnosis. Passage of fetal red blood cells into the maternal circulation may occur in up to 50% of all pregnancies. Fetal–maternal hemorrhage (FMH) is more likely to happen when there are abnormalities of the placenta or instrumentation such as amniocentesis, cesarean section, or external version. The clinical manifestations will depend on the timing and amount of blood loss. Large, acute hemorrhages result in circulatory collapse of the fetus/newborn and carry a higher mortality. A chronic hemorrhage may present solely as pallor, with a hematologic picture of iron deficiency anemia.[93] The diagnosis of FMH should be suspected in any anemia presenting around the time of delivery or in infants with signs of volume depletion at birth. These infants generally do not have signs of increased erythropoiesis (hepatosplenomegaly) or breakdown of Hb (rapidly rising bilirubin). The diagnosis is confirmed by demonstration of fetal erythrocytes in the maternal circulation by Kleihauer-Betke staining or other techniques. The amount of red blood cells lost into the mother can be approximated by using the following formula, suggested by Mollison[94]:

$$\text{FMH (mL of RBCs)} = \frac{2400}{\text{ratio of maternal to fetal RBCs}}.$$

Twin-to-twin transfusion is a type of external hemorrhage that is seen primarily in monochorionic twins. The donor twin becomes anemic while the recipient's Hb is increased. The blood loss may occur acutely or on a more chronic basis, and the symptomatology varies accordingly. A Hb difference of 4 to 5 g/dL is strongly suggestive of the diagnosis. A weight difference of over 20% also can be found; however, this is seen mainly in chronic twin-to-twin transfusions. The diagnosis is confirmed by establishing the difference in Hb and the presence of vascular communications in the placenta.

Internal hemorrhages are relatively common in the newborn, especially in cases of traumatic or difficult deliveries. However, they seldom are so massive that shock results. The hemorrhage may be clinically obvious (cephalohematoma) or may be occult (adrenal). As Hb breakdown begins, an additional load of bilirubin to the liver causes jaundice beyond the first 24 to 48 hours after birth.

Anemia Secondary to Hemolysis

Hemolytic anemias usually manifest with pallor and early onset of jaundice, but without signs of hypovolemia. The etiology of hemolysis may be quite variable (see Table 93-9). Immune hemolysis secondary to ABO or RH incompatibility and that due to infection are the most common causes of hemolytic anemia in the newborn. Clinical and laboratory findings useful to differentiate hemolysis from other causes of anemia are listed in Table 93-10. ABO hemolytic disease is best characterized as having a wide spectrum, from immune hemolysis only, demonstrated by a decreased RBC survival, to a severe form of anemia and, rarely, hydrops fetalis.[95] It usually affects first-born infants. The diagnosis should be suspected in any newborn with early onset of jaundice with or without significant anemia. Mild hepatosplenomegaly is found occasionally. Generally, the mother is type O and the infant either type A or type B. Individuals with type O blood generate predominantly anti-A and anti-B IgG antibodies that can cross

TABLE 93–10. DIFFERENTIAL DIAGNOSIS OF ANEMIA IN THE NEWBORN CLINICAL AND LABORATORY FINDINGS

	HEMORRHAGE			
	ACUTE	CHRONIC	HEMOLYSIS	DECREASED RBC PRODUCTION
Clinical				
Pallor	(−) to +++	+ to +++	+ to +++	+ to +++
Hepatosplenomegaly	(−)	(−) to +++	+ to +++	(−)
Early jaundice	(−)	(−)	++ to +++	(−)
Hypovolemia	+ to +++	(−)	(−)	(−)
Laboratory				
Cord Hb	Nl or ↓	↓ to ↓↓↓	↓ to ↓↓↓	↓ to ↓↓↓
Bilirubin (cord or day 1)	Nl	Nl	↑ to ↑↑↑	Nl
Direct Coombs	(−)	(−)	(−) to +++	(−)
Reticulocytes	Nl to ↑↑↑	↑ to ↑↑↑	↑ to ↑↑↑	Low

Nl = normal, (−) = absent, + = mild, +++ = severe, ↓ = mild decrease, ↓↓↓ = marked decrease, ↑ = mild increase, ↑↑↑ = marked increase.

the placenta. Those with types A or B antigen produce anti-B and anti-A antibodies, respectively, of the IgM class that are unable to cross the placenta. The direct Coombs' test can be positive; however, often it is negative because of a low antibody titer, and the fact that A or B antigens are more sparsely located in the fetal RBC. The process of hemolysis is less aggressive than in Rh isoimmunization, and the RBC progressively becomes a spherocyte. There is no correlation between the anti-A or anti-B maternal titer and the degree of hemolysis.

In contrast, Rh isoimmunization frequently results in more significant degrees of anemia and hyperbilirubinemia.[96] The severity of the hemolysis increases with subsequent pregnancies of Rh-positive fetuses. At birth, affected infants are generally anemic and develop rapidly rising indirect bilirubin (>0.4 to 0.5 mg/hr). Hepatosplenomegaly is more common than in ABO hemolytic disease. A positive direct Coombs' test is the rule. The blood smear reveals numerous reticulocytes and nucleated RBCs but rare spherocytes. In cases with severe hemolysis thrombocytopenia is often found.

Other causes of immune hemolysis should be suspected in the presence of a positive direct Coombs but compatible ABO and Rh types between mother and infant. Minor group sensitization is occasionally a cause of immune hemolysis.[97] The maternal history may be suggestive of an autoimmune disorder or of the use of medications capable of inducing an immune hemolytic anemia. In these cases the maternal direct Coombs' test can be positive.

Viral or bacterial infections are the most common cause of nonimmune hemolysis. Usually, infants with hemolysis secondary to chronic intrauterine infections exhibit other signs, such as hepatosplenomegaly, petechiae, cutaneous rash, growth retardation, and chorioretinitis. Laboratory findings suggestive of an infectious etiology are associated thrombocytopenia, leukopenia, evidence of disseminated intravascular coagulation, and increases in direct bilirubin.

Abnormalities of the RBC membrane, enzymes, or hemoglobin are uncommon causes of hemolytic anemia in the newborn. Their presence should be suspected with a positive family history, evidence of hemolysis with negative direct Coombs' test, and suggestive findings on a blood smear. The diagnosis is made by identifying the specific defect.

Decreased RBC Production

Neonatal anemia due to decreased RBC production is very uncommon. It should be suspected in the presence of anemia with a low reticulocyte count (<2%) not explained by other obvious causes. Isolated hypoplastic anemia is suggestive of the Diamond-Blackfan syndrome, which also features physical anomalies (cleft palate, abnormal thumbs, ocular defects, short or webbed neck) in 30% of the cases. Involvement of white blood cell and platelet precursors is found in transcobalamin II deficiency and congenital leukemia.

POLYCYTHEMIA

Polycythemia is generally defined as a spun peripheral venous Hct of more than 65%. The site and time of sampling are critical to make the diagnosis of polycythemia. The venous Hct peaks at 2 hours after birth and decreases subsequently.[88] Umbilical cord Hct are lower than those obtained by venous sampling, whereas capillary Hct are 5% to 10% higher than simultaneously obtained venous samples. In addition, the use of Hct values determined by Coulter counter may lead to errors in the diagnosis of polycythemia.[86] With high Hct values blood viscosity increases exponentially.[98] Although the potential for developmental and neurologic sequelae in polycythemic neonates has been attributed to hyperviscosity, viscosity measurements are not widely available, and there is no general agreement on what actually represents hyperviscous values.[86,98,99]

The incidence of polycythemia varies from between 1.4% and 1.8% at sea level to 4% at higher altitudes.[100,101] Even higher incidences may be found in centers serving populations with an elevated proportion of high-risk pregnancies. The incidence of polycythemia in small-for-gestational-age and large-for-gestational-age infants may be several times higher than that of appropriately grown neonates. Polycythemia is also more common in term and postterm newborns than in premature infants. The signs and symptoms associated with polycythemia are listed in Table 93-11. Many neonates with venous Hct above 65% are asymptomatic; however, the majority of those exhibiting symptoms are hyperviscous.[86,102] The symptomatology in these infants may be secondary to sluggish tissue blood flow and to associated problems, such as hypoglycemia, hypocalcemia, and asphyxia.

Polycythemia may result from either a chronic increase in the RBC mass or an acute expansion of the circulating blood volume with subsequent increases in Hct when transudation to the interstitial compartment occurs (Table 93-12). In utero hypoxia stimulates erythropoietin production, which in turn promotes erythropoiesis (SGA, postmaturity). Erythropoiesis may also be stimulated by insulin and other hormones. Neonates with polycythemia secondary to increased erythropoiesis are generally not hypervolemic and can have elevated reticulocyte counts.[103] Conversely, infants with polycythemia due to transfusion may be hypervolemic.

Although there are no generally accepted criteria for treatment of polycythemia, most centers will intervene on all infants with Hct above 70% or those with Hct above 65% if they are symptomatic.[104] Treatment consists of a partial exchange transfusion to lower the Hct to a range where blood viscosity will also be much lower. The formula used to calculate the volume to exchange is

$$\text{Volume (mL)} = \frac{\text{Blood volume} \times (\text{observed Hct} - \text{desired Hct})}{\text{Observed Hct}}$$

where blood volume = 80 to 100 mL × body weight in kilograms. The use of normal saline or 5% albumin for the isovolemic exchange lowers viscosity more effectively.[105] Although the umbilical vein is the route used most commonly, peripheral access may decrease the

TABLE 93-11. SIGNS AND SYMPTOMS ASSOCIATED WITH NEONATAL POLYCYTHEMIA

CNS	**GI**
Lethargy	Regurgitation/vomiting
Hypotonia	Abdominal distention
Irritability	Bloody stools
Seizures	**Skin**
Apnea	Plethora
CV/Respiratory	Cyanosis
Respiratory distress	
Tachycardia	

TABLE 93-12. ETIOLOGY OF NEONATAL POLYCYTHEMIA

INCREASED ERYTHROPOIESIS	TRANSFUSION
Intrauterine Hypoxia	**Delayed Cord Clamping**
SGA	Intentional
Postmaturity	Unassisted delivery
Toxemia	**Twin–Twin Transfusion**
Hyperinsulinemia	(monochronic placenta)
Maternal diabetes	**Maternal–Fetal Transfusion**
Beta-cell hyperplasia	
Beckwith-Wiedemann syndrome	
Chromosomal Abnormalities	
Trisomy 21	
Trisomy 13	
Trisomy 18	
Congenital Adrenal Hyperplasia	
Thyrotoxicosis	

complications potentially associated with umbilical vessel catheterization, such as infection and bowel necrosis.[106]

The long-term outcome of infants with polycythemia and hyperviscosity depends on the etiology of the problem, and the presence of associated conditions that may also have an effect on neurologic development (hypoglycemia, asphyxia, infection). Infants with untreated polycythemia and hyperviscosity are at higher risk for neurologic deficits and developmental delay than those subjected to partial exchange transfusion.[102,107] However, since the pathogenesis of polycythemia may be acute or more chronic, it is possible that the long-term prognosis of subpopulations of polycythemic infants (SGA infants) is per se different and is not significantly influenced by partial exchange transfusions.[108,109]

BLEEDING IN THE NEWBORN

The newborn infant is particularly prone to bleeding around the time of birth because of the trauma of labor and delivery, relative lack of some coagulation factors, and susceptibility to complications such as asphyxia and infection (Table 93-13). These may cause or worsen deficiencies in coagulation. The components of the coagulation mechanism that are deficient at term when compared to adult values are shown in Table 93-14. Despite these deficiencies, impaired hemostasis is not usually clinically manifest in healthy term infants because 20% to 30% of most coagulation factors suffices for fibrin clot formation.[110,111] Many factor deficiencies are secondary to liver immaturity and may be more accentuated in premature infants. Vitamin K is required for the conversion of the precursor proteins to factors II, VII, IX, and X. Vitamin K is relatively deficient at birth, but rapid correction of the activity of vitamin K–dependent factors is seen with intramuscular administration of 0.5 to 1.0 mg of vitamin K, or one of its synthetic

TABLE 93–13. COMMON ETIOLOGIES OF BLEEDING IN THE NEWBORN

Deficiencies of the Coagulation Mechanism

Inherited
- Transient deficit of vitamin K–dependent factors
- Hemophilia A or B
- Von Willebrand's disease

Acquired
- DIC
- Maternal use of hydantoin

Platelet Abnormalities

Quantitative
- Infection
- Immune
- Asphyxia, hypoxia
- Large hemangiomas

Qualitative
- Acetylsalicylic acid
- Indomethacin

Vascular Abnormalities

Trauma

TABLE 93–14. COMPONENTS OF THE COAGULATION MECHANISM IN TERM NEWBORNS AND ADULTS

	TERM NEWBORN	ADULT
Platelets ($\times 10^3/mm^3$)	150–400	150–400
Prothrombin time (sec)	11–15	10–14
Partial thromboplastin time (sec)	30–40	25–35
Fibrinogen (mg/dL)	175–300	175–400
Factors (% of adult values)		
II	20–50	
V	90–100	
VII	30–70	
VIII	100	
IX	20–50	
X	20–50	
XI	30–70	
XII	25–70	
XIII	100	
Prekallikrein	20–50	
High-MW kininogen	30–70	

Modified from Andrew M, Paes B, Johnson M. Development of the hemostatic system in the neonate and young infant. Am J Pediatr Hematol Oncol 1990;12:95 and Buchanan GR. Coagulation disorders in the neonate. Pediatr Clin North Am 1986;33:203.

analogs. An oral dose of 1.0 to 2.0 mg may be used alternatively.[112]

Clinically, the distinction between a "well" and a "sick" bleeding newborn is useful as a first diagnostic approach (Table 93-15). Sick-appearing infants with respiratory distress, neurologic signs, cardiovascular instability, metabolic derangements, or signs of infection are likely to have bleeding secondary to disseminated intravascular coagulation and consumptive thrombocytopenia. Infants who appear well but exhibit clinical or laboratory evidence of altered hemostasis more commonly are diagnosed as having vitamin K deficiency, inherited coagulation factor deficiencies (hemophilia), or immune thrombocytopenia.[111] The diagnostic workup must include a careful family history emphasizing evidence of excessive bleeding in the mother or other family members, complications of pregnancy, or prior systemic disease. The use of medications such as hydantoin and aspirin during pregnancy also must be ascertained. Hydantoin may cause characteristic fetal anomalies and bleeding due to vitamin K deficiency.[113] Maternal ingestion of acetylsalicylic acid can result in hemorrhage during the neonatal period by impairing the formation of thromboxane B_2 and prostacyclin by the platelets. Recently, however, the use of low-dose aspirin (60 mg/day) to prevent pregnancy-induced hypertension was shown to produce only partial suppression of fetal and neonatal platelet thromboxane B_2 generation, thus allowing hemostatic competence.[114] Besides the history and thorough physical exam, a battery of screening tests should be done in all newborns with bleeding (see Table 93-15). Further testing will depend on these preliminary findings and the course of the disease.

Treatment depends on the cause of bleeding. Evidence of vitamin K administration must be sought; if in doubt a routine dose should be repeated. Improvement of vitamin K–dependent factors is observed less than 12

TABLE 93–15. DIFFERENTIAL DIAGNOSIS OF THE BLEEDING NEWBORN

	DIC	VITAMIN K DEFICIENCY	HEMOPHILIA	IMMUNE THROMBOCYTOPENIA
Clinical				
Positive family history	–	–	Possible	Possible
"Sick appearance"	+	–	–	–
Laboratory				
Platelet count	D	N	N	D
PT	P	P	N	N
PTT	P	P	P	N
Fibrinogen	D	N	N	N
FSP	Increased	–	–	–

D, decreased; P, prolonged; N, normal; –, absent; +, present.

hours from its administration. Infants with DIC may need replacement of coagulation factors and platelets as well as specific therapy of the underlying condition (infection, acidosis). Transfusion of platelets (1 to 2 units) or fresh-frozen plasma (10 mL/kg) is indicated in newborns with significant active bleeding, or in the absence of bleeding when marked laboratory abnormalities exist, such as very prolonged prothrombin time (PT) and platelet count below 10,000/mm^3.[111] In suspected immune thrombocytopenia without deficiencies of coagulation factors, the treatment consists primarily of platelet transfusions. Random-donor platelets are used to treat autoimmune thrombocytopenia, whereas in isoimmune thrombocytopenia platelets obtained from the mother are needed, since they lack the antigen to which her antibody was raised. Corticosteroids (prednisone, 2 mg/kg/day) are useful in the autoimmune variety but are generally ineffective in isoimmune thrombocytopenia. The use of intravenous gamma globulin can increase the platelet count in neonatal isoimmune thrombocytopenia.[115]

METABOLIC PROBLEMS

HYPOGLYCEMIA

At the time of delivery blood or plasma glucose in the fetus is about 70% to 80% of the maternal concentration. Small-for-gestational-age (SGA) fetuses may have below-normal blood glucose values. This has been attributed primarily to reduced supply across the placenta.[116] With cord clamping the neonate is separated from the steady supply of maternal glucose and must resort primarily to mobilization of glycogen stores or an exogenous supply of glucose (feeding, parenteral) to remain normoglycemic. Maintenance of an adequate circulating glucose concentration is critical, since it is the principal nutrient utilized by the neonatal brain. Utilization of ketone bodies may also provide energy to the brain of the neonate. Gluconeogenesis, mainly through alanine, also contributes to glucose homeostasis after birth.[117] The processes of glycogen breakdown and gluconeogenesis are influenced by hormones such as glucagon, growth hormone, and cortisol, which increase after birth. Epinephrine is not an important regulator of glucose metabolism at birth; however, its concentration increases with hypoglycemia. Glucose homeostasis depends not only on its availability but also on its rate of utilization. Imbalances between glucose availability and the rate at which it is removed from the circulation will result in either hypo- or hyperglycemia.

The cord blood glucose concentration is markedly influenced by the maternal concentration of glucose during labor and delivery.[118] Maternal hydration with glucose-containing solutions prior to cesarean section or during oxytocin induction can result in maternal and fetal hyperglycemia and fetal hyperinsulinemia. This relative insulin excess may precipitate a more rapid or profound decrease in postnatal glucose concentrations.[119,120] An exaggeration of this mechanism is responsible for the early onset of hypoglycemia in infants of diabetic mothers.

In normal-term neonates delivered vaginally to healthy mothers there is a rapid fall in plasma glucose to 56 ± 19 mg/dL (mean ± SD) at 1 hour and 70 ± 13 mg/dL at 3 hours after birth. Then plasma glucose values remain fairly stable for the first week after birth.[121,122] Normal glucose values in preterm infants are slightly less than those of term infants. Based on these data, the definitions of hypoglycemia for term infants given in Table 93-16 have been recommended. Recently, however, it has been pointed out that in clinical practice all efforts should be focused on keeping a generous normoglycemia in neonates rather than on managing borderline low values too expectantly.[123] Attention must be paid to whether the values represent plasma or whole blood glucose, since the former are usually between 10% and 15% higher. The common use of rapid reagent strips (Dextrostix [Ames] or Chemstryp—BG [Bio-Dynamics]) is acceptable for screening and follow-up of blood glucose levels well within the normal range. However, low values in particular must be confirmed by laboratory determination of true glucose concentrations.[124,125] The use of glucose reflectance meters is not recommended for evaluation of capillary blood glucose in high-risk neonates.[126] The presence of a high Hct may interfere with blood glucose determinations using reagent strips.[127]

The causes of neonatal hypoglycemia are listed in Table 93-17. An altered endogenous glucose production secondary to lack of glycogen storage is the main reason for the common occurrence of hypoglycemia in premature and SGA infants. In addition, decreased gluconeogenesis from amino acids has been described in SGA infants.[117] Both of these groups are also at risk for complications that may increase peripheral glucose utilization, such as hypoxia, cold stress, and infection. Hypoglycemia may also result from endocrine or metabolic disorders that lead to decreased hepatic glucose output. As a group, these disorders are uncommon; however, sometimes hypoglycemia is their presenting manifestation. Infants with panhypopituitarism are of

TABLE 93–16. DEFINITIONS OF HYPOGLYCEMIA FOR TERM INFANTS

	PLASMA GLUCOSE (mg/dL)	
POSTNATAL AGE (HOURS)	SRINIVASAN ET AL*	HECK AND ERENBERG†
0–3	<35	<30
3–24	<40	<30
>24	<45	<40

* Data from Srinivasan G, Pildes RS, Cattamanchi G, Voora S, Lilien LD. Plasma glucose values in normal neonates: a new look. J Pediatr 1986;109:114.

† Data from Heck LJ, Erenberg A. Serum glucose levels in term neonates during the first 48 hours of life. J Pediatr 1987;110:119.

TABLE 93–17. COMMON ETIOLOGIES OF NEONATAL HYPOGLYCEMIA

- **I.** Altered glucose production
  - **A.** Lack of glycogen stores
    - Prematurity
    - SGA
  - **B.** Failure of glucose mobilization
    - Endocrine disorders
      - Panhypopituitarism
      - Cortisol deficiency
      - Glucagon deficiency
    - Metabolic disorders
      - Galactosemia
      - Glycogen storage disease, type I
      - Hereditary fructose intolerance
      - Tyrosinemia
- **II.** Excess glucose utilization
  - **A.** Hyperinsulinism
    - Infant of diabetic mother
    - Excess glucose administration during labor/delivery
    - Erythroblastosis fetalis
    - Beckwith-Wiedemann syndrome
    - Beta-cell hyperplasia/nesidioblastosis
    - Malposition of umbilical arterial catheter (T11 to L1)
    - Leucine sensitivity
    - Maternal drugs (thiazides, beta-adrenergic tocolytics)
  - **B.** Increased peripheral demands
    - Hypoxia
    - Cold stress
    - Infection
    - Polycythemia/hyperviscosity

normal weight and length at birth, but the finding of hypoplastic genitalia in males (small phallus and scrotum, undescended testes) may suggest this diagnosis. Hepatomegaly, jaundice, and acidosis are all findings suggestive of a metabolic disorder.

Hypoglycemia due to an insulin excess is most often due to maternal diabetes. Excessive maternal glucose administration during labor and delivery may produce a transient neonatal hyperinsulinemia and rapid fall in glucose. However, persistently low glucose values should be interpreted as secondary to other causes of hypoglycemia. Infants of diabetic mothers (IDMs) can be large for gestational age mostly on the basis of weight but have a head circumference within normal limits. They may exhibit mild degrees of organomegaly and signs of plethora. They are also at high risk for having other metabolic abnormalities (hypocalcemia, hypomagnesemia), respiratory distress, and congenital anomalies involving mostly the central nervous and cardiovascular systems. IDMs may develop hypoglycemia soon after birth, and they often remain asymptomatic despite very low glucose values. Organomegaly and other anomalies (eg, macroglossia, omphalocele, hemihypertrophy, and abnormal ear lobe grooves) are suggestive of Beckwith-Wiedemann syndrome. Hyperplasia of islet cells has been demonstrated in infants with this syndrome and in those with erythroblastosis fetalis. In erythroblastosis fetalis it has been postulated that the massive hemolysis results in release of glutathione and inhibition of circulating insulin, with compensatory islet cell hyperplasia. Hypoglycemia secondary to any form of beta-cell hyperplasia may be severe and can persist for several months. Increased peripheral utilization of glucose can be seen with hypoxia, cold stress, infection, and polycythemia/hyperviscosity, despite the presence of adequate glycogen storages and normal insulin levels.

The signs of hypoglycemia are nonspecific and similar to those seen with other neonatal problems, such as hypocalcemia, polycythemia, or infection (Table 93-18). Screening for blood or plasma glucose is indicated if any of these signs is present. If the signs are due to hypoglycemia, they improve rapidly, with recovery of glucose levels to normal. The management of hypoglycemia begins with recognition of the factors that place the neonate at high risk for this condition, so that early glucose screening can be instituted. Attempts to avoid maternal hyperglycemia during labor and delivery must be stressed. The treatment of neonatal hypoglycemia depends on its severity and the availability of the enteral route. In infants with borderline low values by reagent strip and no contraindication for feedings, a confirmatory blood or plasma glucose must be determined followed by feeding of 5% dextrose of formula. The latter provides other nutritional sources for energy and gluconeogenesis besides carbohydrates. If correction to euglycemic levels is observed with this intervention, feedings should be advanced as tolerated and close monitoring of glucose must be continued for at least 24 to 48 hours. Failure to correct glucose levels with this approach or an inability to use the enteral route is an indication for parenteral glucose administration. Correction of very low glucose values (<20 to 25 mg/dL) is best accomplished by intravenous administration of a minibolus of 200 mg/kg of glucose followed by a constant glucose infusion of 6 to 8 mg/kg/min.[128] The use of boluses of 25% to 50% dextrose may result in significant hyperglycemia and rebound hypoglycemia. A peripheral vein is the preferred route for parenteral glucose administration. The umbilical vein can be used for short-term glucose infusion; however, concerns for infection make it an unlikely route for long-term use. Glucose administration through umbilical arterial catheters placed between T-11 and L-1 can result in high rates of glucose delivered to the pancreatic vessels and reactive hyperinsulinemia, which resolves after withdrawal of the catheter tip to a lower position. The rate of glucose infusion should be adjusted to keep normoglycemia. If rates in excess of 12 to 15 mg/kg/min of glucose are required, additional therapy is indicated. Corticosteroids (hydrocortisone, 5 mg/kg/day,

TABLE 93–18. CLINICAL SIGNS OF NEONATAL HYPOGLYCEMIA

Jitteriness	Hypotonia
Irritability	Hypothermia
Seizures	Poor feeding
Apnea/cyanosis	Vomiting
Lethargy	Sweating

or prednisone, 2 mg/kg/day), glucagon (300 μg/kg), diazoxide (10 to 15 mg/kg/day), and epinephrine have been used for control of hypoglycemia. Corticosteroids act primarily by enhancing gluconeogenesis, whereas glucagon and epinephrine increase glycogen breakdown. Epinephrine also has a powerful anti-insulin effect. Diazoxide suppresses pancreatic insulin secretion. A high glucose requirement to maintain normoglycemia is suggestive of hyperinsulinism and excess glucose utilization. Feedings should be given concomitantly with parenteral glucose whenever possible, unless they constitute the etiology of the hypoglycemia (ie, galactosemia, tyrosinemia).

The prognosis of infants with neonatal hypoglycemia depends on its etiology, the presence of clinical signs and associated conditions, and the duration of hypoglycemia. Neonates with seizures secondary to hypoglycemia have a risk of up to 50% of abnormal neurologic outcome.[129] Abnormal neurologic features observed after neonatal hypoglycemia include low IQ scores, seizure disorder, and motor deficits (spasticity, ataxia). They are the neuropathologic reflection of cortical damage due to the lack of glucose.[130] A still unresolved issue is whether marginal or transient hypoglycemia can lead to or worsen damage. Data from a recent study in premature neonates suggested that, contrary to general belief, moderate degrees of hypoglycemia have a significant impact on long-term neurodevelopmental performance.[131] Whether the same is true for term and postterm neonates is not known. However, until the safety of moderate and usually asymptomatic hypoglycemia is demonstrated, neonates with borderline or mildly decreased glucose levels should be properly identified and treated expeditiously.

HYPOCALCEMIA

During the second half of pregnancy there is rapid fetal accretion of calcium (Ca) at rates of 110 to 150 mg/kg/day. Fetal accretion of phosphorus (P) and magnesium (Mg) is also high. The concentrations of these minerals are higher in cord blood than in the maternal circulation.[132] The cord blood levels of hormones involved in Ca homeostasis are also different from the mother and reflect attempts by the fetus to maximize bone mineralization (Table 93-19). A steady fall in serum Ca and ionized Ca (iCa) is observed after birth, reaching a nadir at about 24 hours of age and remaining low for 48 to 72 hours.[133] This fall in circulating Ca is due to interruption of the transplacental supply and predominance of hypocalcemic hormones such as calcitonin and glucagon. Both of these hormones increase after birth in normal term neonates, and even further elevations are seen with neonatal asphyxia.[134,135] Unlike small premature infants, term neonates are able to increase parathyroid hormone (PTH) levels in response to decreasing Ca concentrations.[136] The postnatal fall in serum Ca is also prompted by the transient endogenous P load secondary to tissue breakdown, which cannot be excreted rapidly by the kidneys.

Neonatal hypocalcemia has been defined as a serum Ca less than 7 to 8 mg/dL.[137] In a large proportion of sick premature infants serum Ca falls below 7 mg/dL. Since the physiologically important fraction is the iCa and its concentration cannot be reliably predicted from total Ca determinations, direct measurement of iCa with new electrodes suitable for this purpose has been advocated.[133] Hypocalcemia has been classified as early, which occurs in the first few days after birth, and late, which presents after day 4 or 5. At term, early neonatal hypocalcemia is most commonly seen in asphyxiated neonates and infants of diabetic mothers. In asphyxia the pathogenesis of hypocalcemia is related to the large P load secondary to tissue damage and to exaggerated increases in calcitonin and glucagon. In these infants hypocalcemia occurs despite increased levels of PTH.[134] On the contrary, infants of diabetic mothers show a decreased PTH secretion during the first days after birth.[138] This has been attributed to fetal and neo-

TABLE 93-19. APPROXIMATE MINERAL AND HORMONAL LEVELS IN MATERNAL AND CORD BLOOD

MINERALS	MATERNAL	CORD BLOOD
Ca (mg/dL)	9.2 ± 0.3	10.4 ± 0.5†
iCa (mg/dL)	4.5 ± 0.2	5.6 ± 0.3†
P (mg/dL)	4.3 ± 1.6	5.8 ± 1.2†
Mg (mg/dL)	1.8 ± 0.1	2.0 ± 0.1 †
Hormones (% of maternal level)		
Calcitonin	–	180%
Parathormone	–	80%–100%
25-OH vitamin D	–	80%
1–25 $(OH)_2$ vitamin D	–	30%–40%

* Data adapted from Pitkin RM, Cruikshank DP, Schauberger CW, Reynolds WA, Williams GA, Hargis GK. Fetal calcitropic hormones and neonatal calcium homeostasis. Pediatrics 1980;66:77 and Venkataraman PS, Tsang RC, Chen IW, Sperling MA. Pathogenesis of early neonatal hypocalcemia: studies of serum calcitonin, gastrin, and plasma glucagon. J Pediatr 1987;110:599.

† Significantly different from maternal value.

natal Mg deficiency secondary to the chronic maternal loss of Mg seen with diabetes. Secretion of PTH depends on Mg concentrations. Other infants at risk for hypocalcemia are those subjected to rapid changes in serum pH, either by correction of acidosis or by hyperventilation, and those who undergo exchange transfusions with blood containing citrate and phosphate as anticoagulants or buffers.[139] Late neonatal hypocalcemia may be secondary to a variety of disorders. Abnormalities of Ca and Mg absorption may present at this time. These may be due to primary intestinal abnormalities or deficiencies of vitamin D metabolism. Ingestion of large P loads (eg, from cow's milk) or deficient renal excretion (renal failure) may cause hyperphosphatemia and secondary hypocalcemia. Parathyroid disorders may also present at this time. Primary hypoparathyroidism is seen in DiGeorge syndrome, which also features abnormal facies, cardiac anomalies (usually of the aortic arch), and defects of T-cell function because of thymic hypoplasia. Maternal PTH excess usually results in transient suppression of neonatal parathyroid function.[140] Protracted hypocalcemia with varying degrees of hyperphosphatemia is suggestive of this diagnosis even in the absence of a positive maternal history.

Neonatal hypocalcemia is often asymptomatic. The signs suggestive of hypocalcemia are listed in Table 93-20. However, they are not specific and can also be elicited by hypoglycemia, hypomagnesemia, narcotic withdrawal, neurologic disorders, or infection. Chvostek's and Trousseau's signs are uncommon. Heart failure has also been described with severe hypocalcemia.[141] Signs of hypocalcemia are generally seen only when the iCa falls to very low levels. Disappearance of the symptomatology with Ca treatment supports the diagnosis of hypocalcemia. Serial determinations of serum Ca should be performed in neonates at risk for hypocalcemia, and those with suggestive signs. Although iCa measurements are ideal for diagnosing hypocalcemia, they are not widely used at the present time. Persistently low serum Ca values constitute an indication for Mg and P determinations. Total protein and albumin measurements are also useful, since hypoproteinemia is associated with low serum Ca values; however, the iCa is normal. Although the QT interval of the EKG may be prolonged in hypocalcemia, it is generally not useful in the nursery.[142] A chest x-ray and echocardiogram are useful when DiGeorge syndrome is suspected. Despite the thymic hypoplasia of these infants, their lymphocyte count may be normal soon after birth.

TABLE 93–20. CLINICAL SIGNS OF NEONATAL HYPOCALCEMIA

Jitteriness
Irritability
Seizures
Apnea
Chvostek's sign (facial muscle contraction after stimulation)
Trousseau's sign (carpal spasm after constriction of arm)
Heart failure

Treatment of hypocalcemia is reserved primarily for symptomatic infants. The therapy consists of intravenous administration of 10% Ca gluconate (9.4 mg of elemental Ca/mL) in doses of 100 to 200 mg/kg, followed by continuous infusion of about 400 to 800 mg/kg/day. Intravenous Ca gluconate must be administered slowly and with cardiac monitoring because of the possibility of bradycardia. Bolus infusion of Ca gluconate results in marked and transient elevations of serum Ca and iCa. Patency of the vein being used must be ascertained, since extravasation of Ca salts results in skin necrosis. Whether asymptomatic neonates with low serum Ca (<7 mg/dL) should be treated is controversial, since serum Ca usually returns to normal values after the first 3 to 4 days after birth. Furthermore, controlled studies to evaluate the treatment of hypocalcemia done in sick premature infants with serum Ca below 6 to 7 mg/dL have failed to show any significant benefit of parenteral Ca administration.[143,144] These findings suggest that, for a majority of newborns, hypocalcemia represents primarily a biochemical abnormality that only merits treatment in a few of them. If serum Ca remains low beyond 4 to 5 days after birth, or it is refractory to the usual therapy, further evaluation is necessary. Oral Ca gluconate or vitamin D analogs have been used to treat or prevent neonatal hypocalcemia. However, the majority of infants with low serum Ca either are too sick to be fed or develop hypocalcemia before feedings are initiated or advanced to substantial volumes. The therapy also depends on the etiology of hypocalcemia (eg, use of low-P formula for hypocalcemia secondary to hyperphosphatemia, administration of vitamin D for its deficiency, or hypoparathyroidism).

The long-term outcome of neonates with hypocalcemia depends primarily on the associated problems (asphyxia, DiGeorge syndrome) rather than on the presence of symptoms or serum Ca values. If seizures due to late-onset hypocalcemia are appropriately recognized and treated, the prognosis is almost invariably normal.[145]

HYPO- AND HYPERMAGNESEMIA

Fetal serum Mg as well as Mg accretion increase during the third trimester of pregnancy. Preterm infants have higher serum Mg than those born at term, probably as a reflection of lower renal excretion. Magnesium and Ca homeostasis are related primarily through PTH and through interexchange of these ions in bone. Acute changes in serum Mg concentrations are inversely related to PTH secretion but not to calcitonin secretion.[146,147] However, a chronic Mg deficiency with depletion of tissue stores reduces PTH secretion. This mechanism may be largely responsible for the hypomagnesemia and hypocalcemia of IDMs.[148,149] Magnesium is actively transported across the placenta, and after therapeutic use of Mg salts in the mother, fetal serum Mg also increases to about 80% to 90% of the maternal concentration.[150] Under normal circumstances

the equator. All infants should receive vitamin K at birth, either parenterally or orally, to prevent hemorrhagic disease of the newborn.[112,210] Within 1 week after birth if the infant is tolerating feedings, the intestinal flora usually is capable of synthesizing vitamin K. However, if the newborn is receiving antibiotics or has any other condition that alters intestinal flora, vitamin K (1 mg) should be given weekly.

Health professionals should strongly encourage the use of breast milk, not only because of its easy digestibility but also because of its numerous protective factors (Table 93-28).[211] Many of these factors have antimicrobial actions helping to control gut microflora and to promote selective colonization of the intestinal tract.

NEONATAL SURGICAL PROBLEMS

In the last 20 years there has been rapid progress in the management of surgical problems of newborns. Although new surgical techniques have been developed, the improved outcome of neonates with surgical problems has resulted from earlier diagnosis and more aggressive supportive therapy. The relatively high mortality of neonatal surgical patients—greater than 50%—that persisted into the 1960s was frequently due to inadequate stabilization of these newborns prior to surgery, poor referral and transfer patterns and methods, and delayed and inaccurate diagnosis. Great advances have been made in all these areas, but especially in the areas of aggressive identification and anticipation of problems, stabilization prior to surgery, and supportive care following surgery.[212]

Prenatal diagnosis by ultrasound has made it possible to identify problems and get the pregnant woman to centers capable of immediately addressing the specific surgical needs of the fetus. There was initial enthusiasm that several surgical problems—in particular, hydronephrosis and hydrocephalus—could be aggressively addressed in utero. Recent reports have suggested very little change in outcome, with significant mortality resulting from fetal surgery.[213] More important, the identification of congenital diaphragmatic hernia and abdominal wall defects has led to a decrease in the morbidity and mortality associated with difficulties in stabilization, transport, and infection.

Since prenatal diagnosis has identified more of these infants with potential surgical problems, a team approach to stabilization and transition to surgical intervention can be more easily planned and accomplished. This includes appropriate resuscitation with adequate airway management, continued oxygenation, and prevention of acidosis and hypotension. This is most important where severe respiratory compromise is likely, as in congenital diaphragmatic hernia with associated pulmonary hypoplasia.

CONGENITAL DIAPHRAGMATIC HERNIA

Congenital diaphragmatic hernia is one of the most serious of the neonatal surgical emergencies.[214] Its incidence is approximately one in 2500 live births (Table 93-29). The most common is the foramen of Bochdalek hernia, a diaphragmatic defect that is posterior and usually on the left side. There is pulmonary hypoplasia, and some of the abdominal contents, usually intestine, are in the chest cavity. The infant presents with a scaphoid abdomen and a shift in cardiac impulse, usually to the right. Stabilization must include intubation and ventilation and also a nasogastric tube with continuous suction. These are important to prevent distention of the intestine and further respiratory compromise. Despite aggressive surgical intervention and the use of extracorporeal membrane oxygenation (ECMO), the mortality still remains at approximately 50%. The outcome is related primarily to the degree of lung hypoplasia.[214]

TABLE 93–28. BREAST MILK AND COLOSTRUM IMMUNOLOGIC COMPONENTS

COMPONENT	FUNCTION
"Bifidus factor"	Promotes bifidobacteria colonization of colon
Chemotactic factors	Attract phagocytes to pathogens
Complement	Promotes opsonization
Immunoglobulins (s-IgA, IgG, IgM)	Couple with bacterial, viral, and protozoal pathogens
Interferon	Inhibits viral replication
Lactoferrin	Binds iron; sequestered from iron-dependent bacteria
Lactoperoxide	Acts as a bactericide for enteric flora
Lymphocytes	
B (plasma cell)	Synthesize immunoglobulins;
T	regulate cellular components
Lysozyme	Promotes bacterial lysis
Macrophage, neutrophil	Phagocytize and kill pathogens; produce soluble factors

TABLE 93–29. INCIDENCE OF SELECTED NEONATAL SURGICAL PROBLEMS PER LIVE BIRTHS

Craniosynostosis	1/1000
Cleft palate	1/1000
Diapraghmatic hernia	1/2500
Esophageal atresia	1/5000
Gastroschisis/omphalocele	1/2500
Meningomyelocele	1/1000
Cryptorchidism	1/1000
Hypospadias	8/1000
Dislocated hip	1/1000

ESOPHAGEAL ATRESIA AND TRACHEOESOPHAGEAL FISTULA

Esophageal atresia and tracheoesophageal fistula occur in one in 5000 live births.[215] Approximately half of these have other associated anomalies; these are primarily cardiac (20%), gastrointestinal (25%), genitourinary (10%), and central nervous system (5%). Only about 8% of babies with esophageal atresia will not have a fistula from the trachea to the esophagus. The most common variety of esophageal atresia is a blind esophageal pouch and a fistula from the trachea near the carina to a distal esophageal segment. Early management involves respiratory stabilization, a gastrostomy in most cases to decompress the intestinal tract, and adequate drainage of the proximal esophageal pouch. Surgical repair of the fistula is usually accomplished in the first several days. The timing of the repair of the esophagus depends very much on the distance between the proximal and distal esophageal pouches. Those babies having a longer atretic segment are generally repaired much later. Although it is very uncommon, a few infants require a repair using a segment of colon that is brought to the chest for the anastomosis.

OMPHALOCELE AND GASTROSCHISIS

The two primary abdominal wall defects, omphalocele and gastroschisis, occur with an incidence of one in 2500 live births.[216] These can be diagnosed prenatally and require surgery very soon after birth. Initial management includes bowel decompression and respiratory support. The exposed intestine and other intra-abdominal organs should be kept moist, and care should be taken to minimize the risk of infection (Fig. 93-11). Surgical repair for both conditions is relatively similar. Occasionally, the abdomen can be closed primarily. More commonly, the closure must be staged with gradual return of the contents into the abdominal cavity from a silo or chimney that protects the organs until the abdominal cavity can be closed (Fig. 93-12). It is important to differentiate an omphalocele from a gastroschisis.[217] An omphalocele involves the umbilical cord, and the defect is frequently covered by a peritoneal sac. Approximately 50% of patients with omphalocele will have associated anomalies, including various chromosomal

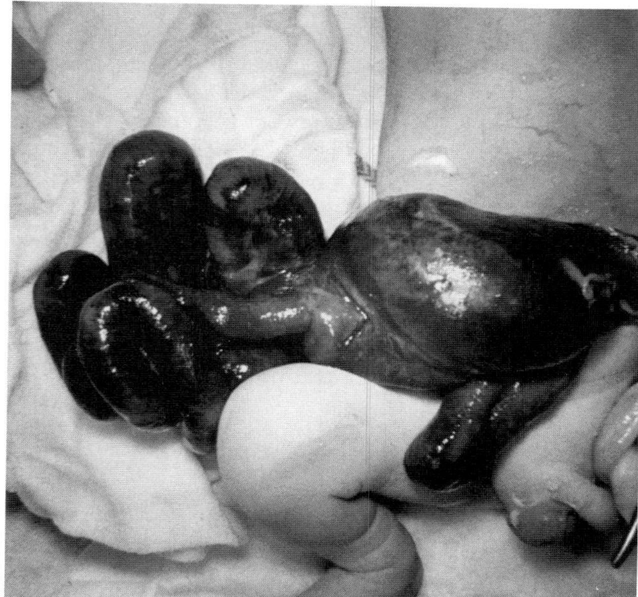

FIGURE 93–11. Uncomplicated gastroschisis.

abnormalities as well as cardiac, genitourinary, and skeletal defects. Gastroschisis occurs lateral to the cord and is usually small; there is no covering sac. Gastroschisis is rarely associated with genetic syndromes or other anomalies.

The causes of neural tube defects, such as meningomyelocele, remain obscure.[218] There is definitely a multifactorial genetic factor, which increases the risk of neural tube defects in subsequent children. However, it is more common in low socioeconomic groups, in fami-

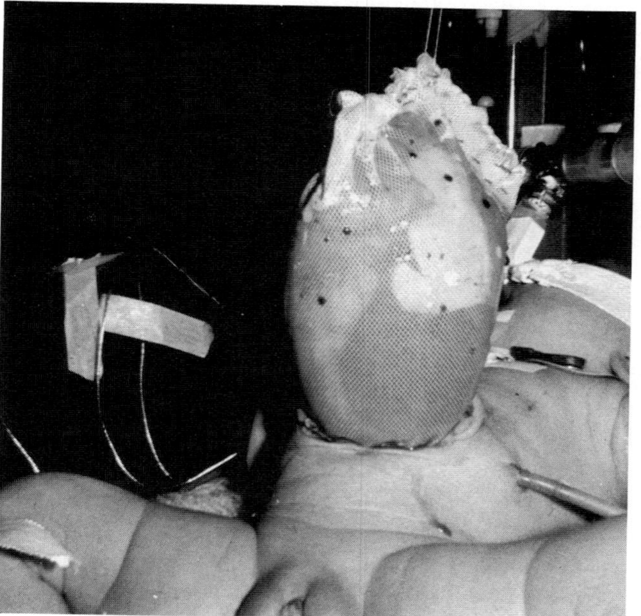

FIGURE 93–12. Silo repair of an omphalocele.

lies from the British Isles, and in those with a folic acid deficiency; it is far less common in blacks. The defect is most commonly thoracolumbar, with severe motor and sensory loss below the lesion. The mortality is approximately 15% and usually relates to the Arnold-Chiari malformation. Long-term neurologic and developmental outcomes are poorest in those children who develop hydrocephalus and central nervous system infection, especially that related to ventriculoperitoneal shunts.[218]

Apart from craniosynostosis, the remaining surgical problems listed in Table 93-29 rarely require repair in the immediate newborn period. Each of these infants with a surgically correctable lesion should be evaluated thoroughly for other malformations and possible chromosomal defects. Further progress in the outcome of neonates with surgical problems will result from more careful attention to intensive medical management, including the recognition and correction of metabolic stress and pain and the avoidance or prompt correction of complications.[219]

REFERENCES

1. Soothill P, Nicolaides KH, Rodeck CH, Campbell S. Effect of gestational age on fetal and intervillous blood gas and acid-base values in human pregnancy. Fetal Ther 1986;13:168.
2. Nelson N. The onset of respiration. In: Avery GB, ed. Neonatology: pathophysiology and management of the newborn. 3rd ed. Philadelphia: JB Lippincott, 1987:176.
3. Milner AD, Vyas H. Lung expansion at birth. J Pediatr 1982;101:879.
4. Bland R. Edema formation in the newborn lung. Clin Perinatol 1982;9:593.
5. Milner AD, Saunders RA, Hoplain IE. Effects of delivery by caesarean section on lung mechanics and lung volume in the human neonate. Arch Dis Child 1978;53:545.
6. Schwartz RH, Hey EN, Baum JD. Management of the newborn's thermal environment. In: Sinclair J, ed. Temperature regulation and energy metabolism in the newborn. New York: Grune & Stratton, 1978:205.
7. Hey E, Katz G. The optimum thermal environment for naked babies. Arch Dis Child 1970;45:328.
8. Committee on Fetus and Newborn, American Academy of Pediatrics. Use and abuse of the Apgar score. Pediatrics 1986; 78:1148.
9. Gilstrap III L, Leveno K, Burris J, Williams ML, Little B. Diagnosis of birth asphyxia on the basis of fetal pH, Apgar score, and newborn cerebral dysfunction. Am J Obstet Gynecol 1989;161:825.
10. Novotny Jr, E. Hypoxic-ischemic encephalopathy. In: Stevenson D, Sunshine P, eds. Fetal and neonatal brain injury. Philadelphia: BC Decker, 1989:113.
11. Hope PL, Costello AM, Cady EB, et al. Cerebral energy metabolism studied with phosphorus NMR spectroscopy in normal and birth-asphyxiated infants. Lancet 1984;2:366.
12. Hill A, Volpe J. Perinatal asphyxia: clinical aspects. Clin Perinatol 1989;16:435.
13. Catlin EA, Carpenter MW, Braun BS, et al. The Apgar score revisited: influence of gestational age. J Pediatr 1986;109:865.
14. Committee on Drugs, AAP. Emergency drug doses for infants and children and naloxone use in newborns: clarification. Pediatrics 1989;83:803.
15. Perlman JM. Systemic abnormalities in term infants following perinatal asphyxia. Relevance to long-term neurologic outcome. Clin Perinatol 1989;16:475.
16. Paneth N, Stark R. Cerebral palsy and mental retardation in relation to indicators of perinatal asphyxia. Am J Obstet Gynecol 1983;147:960.
17. Blair E, Stanley FJ. Intrapartum asphyxia: a rare cause of cerebral palsy. J Pediatr 1988;112:515.
18. Sunshine P. Epidemiology of perinatal asphyxia. In: Stevenson D, Sunshine P, ed. Fetal and neonatal brain injury. Philadelphia: BC Decker, 1989:2.
19. Mellits ED, Holden KR, Freeman JM. Neonatal seizures II. A multivariate analysis of factors associated with outcome. Pediatrics 1982;70:177.
20. Grant A, O'Brien N, Joy MT, Hennessy E, MacDonald D. Cerebral palsy among children born during the Dublin randomized trial of intrapartum monitoring. Lancet 1989;2:1233.
21. Berg AT. Indices of fetal growth-retardation, perinatal hypoxia-related factors and childhood neurological morbidity. Early Hum Dev 1989;19:271.
22. Petrucha R. Fetal maturity/gestational age evaluation. J Perinatol 1989;9:100.
23. Lubchenco LO. Assessment of gestational age and development at birth. Pediatr Clin North Am 1970;17:125.
24. Dubowitz LMS, Dubowitz V. Gestational age of the newborn. Reading, MA: Addison-Wesley, 1977.
25. Clark DA. The newborn. In: Ensher GL, Clark DA, eds. Newborns at risk. Rockville, MD: Aspen, 1986:35.
26. Hittner H, Hirsch N, Rudolph A. Assessment of gestational age by examination of the anterior vascular capsule of the lens. J Pediatr 1977;91:455.
27. Dubowitz LMS, Dubowitz V, Goldberg C. Clinical assessment of gestational age in the newborn infant. J Pediatr 1970;77:1.
28. Primark RA, MacGregor DF. Simple maturity classification of the newborn infant. Ann Trop Pediatr 1989;9:65.
29. Lubchenco LO. The high risk infant. Philadelphia: WB Saunders, 1976.
30. Kresch MJ, Gross I. The biochemistry of fetal lung development. Clin Perinatol 1987;14:481.
31. Wright JR, Clements JA. Metabolism and turnover of lung surfactant. Am Rev Respir Dis 1987;135:426.
32. Stahlman MT, Gray ME. Anatomical development and maturation of the lungs. Clin Perinatol 1978;5:181.
33. Moya FR, Gross I. Diabetes and fetal lung development. In: Reece EA, Coustan DR, eds. Diabetes mellitus in pregnancy, principles and practice. New York: Churchill Livingstone, 1988:123.
34. Wegman ME. Annual summary of vital statistics—1988. Pediatrics 1989;84:943.
35. Ikegami M, Jacobs H, Jobe A. Surfactant function in respiratory distress syndrome. J Pediatr 1983;102:443.
36. Ikegami M, Jobe A, Berry D. A protein that inhibits surfactant in respiratory distress syndrome. Biol Neonate 1986;50:121.
37. Ablow RC, Gross I, Effmann EI, Uauy R, Driscoll S. The radiographic features of early onset group B streptococcal neonatal sepsis. Radiology 1977;124:771.
38. Notter RH, Shapiro DL. Lung surfactants for replacement therapy: biochemical, biophysical, and clinical aspects. Clin Perinatol 1987;14:433.
39. Bhat R, John E, Diaz-Blanco J, Ortega R, Fornell L, Vidyasagar D. Surfactant therapy and spontaneous diuresis. J Pediatr 1989;114:443.
40. Carlo WA, Chatburn RL. Assisted ventilation of the newborn. In: Carlo WA, Chatburn RL, eds. Neonatal respiratory care. 2nd ed. Chicago: Year Book Medical Publishers, 1988:320.
41. The HIFI study group. High-frequency oscillatory ventilation

compared with conventional mechanical ventilation in the treatment of respiratory failure in preterm infants. N Engl J Med 1989;320:88.

42. Soll RF. Clinical controlled trials: what do they tell us? In: Jobe AH, Taeusch HW, eds. Surfactant treatment of lung diseases. Report of the 96th Ross conference on pediatric research. Columbus, OH, 1988:106.
43. Bancalari E, Gerhardt T. Bronchopulmonary dysplasia. Pediatr Clin North Am 1986;33:1.
44. Avery ME, Tooley WH, Keller JB, et al. Is chronic lung disease in low birth weight infants preventable? A survey of eight centers. Pediatrics 1987;79:26.
45. Yeh TF, McClenan DA, Ajayi OA, Pildes RS. Metabolic rate and energy balance in infants with bronchopulmonary dysplasia. J Pediatr 1989;114:448.
46. Skidmore MD, Rivers A, Hack M. Increased risk of cerebral palsy among very low-birth weight infants with chronic lung disease. Dev Med Child Neurol 1990;32:325.
47. Fiascone JM, Jacobs HC, Moya FR, Mercurio MR, Lima DM. Betamethasone increases pulmonary compliance in part by surfactant-independent mechanisms in preterm rabbits. Pediatr Res 1987;22:730.
48. Ikegami M, Jobe AH, Pettenazzp A, Seidner SR, Berry DD, Ruffini L. Effects of maternal treatment with corticosteroids, T_3, TRH, and their combinations on lung function of ventilated preterm rabbits with and without surfactant treatments. Am Rev Respir Dis 1987;136:892.
49. Moya FR, Gross I. Prevention of respiratory distress syndrome. Sem Perinatol 1988;12:348.
50. Farrell EE, Silver RK, Kimberlin LV, Wolf ES, Dusik JM. Impact of antenatal dexamethasone administration on respiratory distress syndrome in surfactant-treated infants. Am J Obstet Gynecol 1989;161:628.
51. Davis RO, Philips III JB, Harris Jr BA, Wilson ER, Huddleston JF. Fatal meconium aspiration syndrome occurring despite airway management considered appropriate. Am J Obstet Gynecol 1985;151:731.
52. Dooley SL, Pesavento DJ, Depp R, et al. Meconium below the vocal cords at delivery: correlation with intrapartum events. Am J Obstet Gynecol 1985;153:767.
53. Falciglia HS. Failure to prevent meconium aspiration syndrome. Obstet Gynecol 1988;71:349.
54. Yeomans ER, Gilstrap III LC, Leveno KJ, Burris JS. Meconium in the amniotic fluid and fetal acid-base status. Obstet Gynecol 1989;73:175.
55. Rossi EM, Philipson EH, Williams TG, Kalhan SC. Meconium aspiration syndrome: intrapartum and neonatal attributes. Am J Obstet Gynecol 1989;161:1106.
56. Sunoo C, Kosasa T, Hale RW. Meconium aspiration syndrome without evidence of fetal distress in early labor before elective cesarean delivery. Obstet Gynecol 1989;73:707.
57. Yeh TF, Lilien LD, Barathi A, Pildes R. Lung volume, dynamic lung compliance, and blood gases during the first 3 days of postnatal life in infants with meconium aspiration syndrome. Crit Care Med 1982;10:588.
58. Reece EA, Moya F, Yazigi R, Holford T, Duncan C, Ehrenkranz R. Persistent pulmonary hypertension: assessment of perinatal risk factors. Obstet Gynecol 1987;70:696.
59. Murphy JD, Vawter GF, Reid LM. Pulmonary vascular disease in fatal meconium aspiration. J Pediatr 1984;104:758.
60. Clark DA, Nieman GF, Thompson JE, Paskanick AM, Rokhar JE, Bredenberg CE. Surfactant displacement by meconium free fatty acids: an alternative explanation for atelectasis in meconium aspiration syndrome. J Pediatr 1987;110:765.
61. Cole JW, Portman RF, Lim Y, Perlman JM, Robson AM. Urinary β_2-microglobulin in full-term newborns: evidence for proximal tubular dysfunction in infants with meconium-stained amniotic fluid. Pediatrics 1985;76:958.
62. Sadovsky Y, Amon E, Bade ME, Petrie RH. Prophylactic amnioinfusion during labor complicated by meconium: a preliminary report. Am J Obstet Gynecol 1989;161:613.
63. Linder N, Aranda JV, Tsur M, et al. Need for endotracheal intubation and suction in meconium-stained neonates. J Pediatr 1988;112:613.
64. Macfarlane PI, Heaf DP. Pulmonary function in children after neonatal meconium aspiration syndrome. Arch Dis Child 1988;63:368.
65. Swaminathan S, Quinn J, Stabile MW, Bader D, Platzker AC, Keens TG. Long-term pulmonary sequelae of meconium aspiration syndrome. J Pediatr 1989;114:356.
66. Piza J, Gonzalez M, Northrop C, Eavey RD. Meconium contamination of the neonatal middle ear. J Pediatr 1989;115:910.
67. Philips III JB, Lyrene RK. Prostaglandins, related compounds, and the perinatal pulmonary circulation. Clin Perinatol 1984;11:565.
68. Geggel RL, Reid LM. The structural basis of PPHN. Clin Perinatol 1984;11:525.
69. Fox WW, Duara S. Persistent pulmonary hypertension in the neonate: diagnosis and management. J Pediatr 1983;103:505.
70. Wung JT, James LS, Kilchevsky E, James E. Management of infants with severe respiratory failure and persistence of the fetal circulation, without hyperventilation. Pediatrics 1985;76:488.
71. Dworetz AR, Moya FR, Sabo B, Gladstone I, Gross I. Survival of infants with persistent pulmonary hypertension without extracorporeal membrane oxygenation. Pediatrics 1989;84:1.
72. O'Rourke PP, Crone RK, Vacanti JP, et al. Extracorporeal membrane oxygenation and conventional medical therapy in neonates with persistent pulmonary hypertension of the newborn: a prospective randomized study. Pediatrics 1989;84:957.
73. Carter JM, Gerstmann DR, Clark RH, et al. High-frequency oscillatory ventilation and extracorporeal membrane oxygenation for the treatment of acute neonatal respiratory failure. Pediatrics 1990;85:159.
74. Sell EJ, Gaines JA, Gluckman C, Williams E. Persistent fetal circulation. Neurodevelopmental outcome. Am J Dis Child 1985;139:25.
75. Hendricks-Munoz KD, Walton JP. Hearing loss in infants with persistent fetal circulation. Pediatrics 1988;81:650.
76. Bifano EM, Pfannenstiel A. Duration of hyperventilation and outcome in infants with persistent pulmonary hypertension. Pediatrics 1988;81:657.
77. Avery ME, Baghdassarian O, Brumley G. Transient tachypnea of newborn. Am J Dis Child 1966;11:380.
78. Rimmer S, Fawcitt J. Delayed clearance of pulmonary fluid in the neonate. Arch Dis Child 1982;57:63.
79. Gowen Jr CW, Lawson EE, Gingras J, Boucher R, Gatzy JT, Knowles MR. Electrical potential difference and ion transport across nasal epithelium of term neonates: correlation with mode of delivery, transient tachypnea of the newborn, and respiratory rate. J Pediatr 1988;113:121.
80. Gross TL, Sokol RJ, Kwong MS, Wilson M, Kuhnert PM. Transient tachypnea of the newborn: the relationship to preterm delivery and significant neonatal morbidity. Am J Obstet Gynecol 1983;146:236.
81. Eisenbrey AB, Epstein E, Zak B, McEnroe RJ, Artiss JD, Kiechle FL. Phosphatidylglycerol in amniotic fluid. Comparison of an "ultrasensitive" immunologic assay with TLC and enzymatic assay. Am J Clin Pathol 1989;91:293.
82. Rawlings JS, Smith FR. Transient tachypnea of the newborn. An analysis of neonatal and obstetric risk factors. Am J Dis Child 1984;138:869.

83. Halliday HL, McClure G, McReid M. Transient tachypnoea of the newborn: two distinct clinical entities? Arch Dis Child 1981;56:322.
84. Bucciarelli RL, Egan EA, Gessner IH, Eitzman DV. Persistence of fetal cardiopulmonary circulation: one manifestation of transient tachypnea of the newborn. Pediatrics 1976;58:192.
85. Pearson H. Disorders of hemoglobin synthesis and metabolism. In: Oski FA, Naiman JL, eds. Hematologic problems in the newborn. 3rd ed. Philadelphia: WB Saunders, 1982:245.
86. Villalta IA, Pramanik AK, Diaz-Blanco J, Herbst JJ. Diagnostic errors in neonatal polycythemia based on method of hematocrit determination. J Pediatr 1989;115:460.
87. Linderkam O. Placental transfusion: Determinants and effects. Clin Perinatol 1982;9:559.
88. Shohat M, Merlob P, Reisner SH. Neonatal polycythemia. I. Early diagnosis and incidence relating to time of sampling. Pediatrics 1984;73:7.
89. Manroe BL, Weinberg AG, Rosenfeld CR, Browne R. The neonatal blood count in health and disease. I. Reference values for neutrophilic cells. J Pediatr 1979;95:89.
90. Manroe BL, Rosenfeld CR, Winberg AG, Browne R. The differential leukocyte count in the assessment and outcome of early-onset neonatal group B streptococcal disease. J Pediatr 1977;91:632.
91. Rodwell RL, Leslie AL, Tudehope DI. Early diagnosis of neonatal sepsis using a hematologic scoring system. J Pediatr 1988;112:761.
92. Moya FR, Perez A, Reece EA. Severe fetomaternal hemorrhage. A report of four cases. J Reprod Med 1987;32:243.
93. Pearson HA, Diamond LK. Fetomaternal transfusion. Am J Dis Child 1959;97:267.
94. Mollison PL. Quantitation of transplacental hemorrhage. Br Med J 1972;3:31.
95. Desjardins L, Blajchman MA, Chintu C, Gent M, Zipursky A. The spectrum of ABO hemolytic disease of the newborn infant. J Pediatr 1979;95:447.
96. Oski FA, Naiman JL. Erythroblastosis fetalis. In: Oski FA, Naiman JL, eds. Hematologic problems in the newborn. 3rd ed. Philadelphia: WB Saunders, 1982:283.
97. Weinstein L. Irregular antibodies causing hemolytic disease of the newborn: a continuing problem. Clin Obstet Gynecol 1982;25:321.
98. Shohat M, Reisner S, Mimouni F, Merlob P. Neonatal polycythemia. II. Definition related to time of sampling. Pediatrics 1984;73:11.
99. Ramamurthy RS, Berlanga M. Postnatal alteration in hematocrit and viscosity in normal and polycythemic infants. J Pediatr 1987;110:929.
100. Stevens K, Wirth FH. Incidence of neonatal hyperviscosity at sea level. J Pediatr 1980;97:118.
101. Wiswell TE, Cornish JD, Northam RS. Neonatal polycythemia: frequency of clinical manifestations and other associated findings. Pediatrics 1986;78:26.
102. Black VD, Lubchenco LO, Koops BL, Poland R, Powell DP. Neonatal hyperviscosity: randomized study of effect of partial plasma exchange transfusion on long-term outcome. Pediatrics 1985;75:1048.
103. Raymau EJ, Godeneche P, Gaulime J, et al. Les polyglobules néonatales. Etude clinique et physiopathologique de 44 observations. Ann Pediatr 1972;19:803.
104. Oh W. Neonatal polycythemia and hyperviscosity. Pediatr Clin North Am 1986;33:523.
105. Levy I, Merlob P, Ashkenazi S, Reisner SH. Neonatal polycythemia: effect of partial dilutional exchange transfusion with human albumin on whole blood viscosity. Eur J Pediatr 1990;149:354.
106. Black VD, Rumack CM, Lubchenco LO, Koops BL. Gastrointestinal injury in polycythemic term infants. Pediatrics 1985;76:225.
107. Delaney-Black V, Camp BW, Lubchenco LO, et al. Neonatal hyperviscosity association with lower achievement and IQ scores at school age. Pediatrics 1989;83:662.
108. Van der Elst CW, Molteno CD, Malan AF, Heese H. The management of polycythemia in the newborn infant. Early Hum Dev 1980;4:393.
109. Black VD, Lubchenco LO, Luckey DW, et al. Developmental and neurologic sequelae of neonatal hyperviscosity syndrome. Pediatrics 1982;69:426.
110. Andrew M, Paes B, Johnson M. Development of the hemostatic system in the neonate and young infant. Am J Pediatr Hematol Oncol 1990;12:95.
111. Buchanan GR. Coagulation disorders in the neonate. Pediatr Clin North Am 1986;33:203.
112. Committee on Nutrition AAP. Vitamin and mineral supplement needs in normal children in the United States. Pediatrics 1980;66:1015.
113. Bleyer WA, Skinner AL. Fetal neonatal hemorrhage after maternal anticonvulsivant therapy. JAMA 1976;235:626.
114. Benigni A, Gregorini G, Frusca T, et al. Effect of low-dose aspirin on fetal and maternal generation of thromboxane by platelets in women at risk for pregnancy-induced hypertension. N Engl J Med 1989;321:357.
115. Massey GV, McWilliams NB, Mueller DE, Napolitano A, Maurer HM. Intravenous immunoglobulin in treatment of neonatal isoimmune thrombocytopenia. J Pediatr 1987;111:133.
116. Economies DL, Nicolaides KH. Blood glucose and oxygen tension levels in small-for-gestational-age fetuses. Am J Obstet Gynecol 1989;160:385.
117. Williams PR, Fisher RH Jr, Sperling MA, et al. Effects of oral alanine feeding on blood glucose, plasma glucagon, and insulin concentrations in small for gestational age infants. N Engl J Med 1975;292:612.
118. Kenepp N, Kumar S, Shelly WC, Stanley CA, Gabbe SG, Gutsche BB. Fetal and neonatal hazards of maternal hydration with 5% dextrose before cesarean section. Lancet 1982;1:1150.
119. Mendiola J, Grylack LJ, Scanlon JW. Effect of intrapartum glucose infusion on the normal fetus and newborn. Anesth Analg 1982;61:32.
120. Singhi S. Effect of maternal intrapartum glucose therapy on neonatal blood glucose levels and neurobehavioural status of hypoglycemic term newborn infants. J Perinat Med 1988;16:217.
121. Srinivasan G, Pildes RS, Cattamanchi G, Voora S, Lilien LD. Plasma glucose values in normal neonates: a new look. J Pediatr 1986;109:114.
122. Heck LJ, Erenberg A. Serum glucose levels in term neonates during the first 48 hours of life. J Pediatr 1987;110:119.
123. Editorial Brain damage by neonatal hypoglycemia. Lancet 1989;1:883.
124. Herrera AJ, Hsiang YH. Comparison of various methods of blood sugar screening in newborn infants. J Pediatr 1983;102:769.
125. Holtrop PC, Madison KA, Kiechle FL, Karcher RE, Batton DG. A comparison of chromogen test strip (Chemstrip bG) and serum glucose values in newborns. Am J Dis Child 1990;144:183.
126. Line HC, Maguire C, Oh W, Cowett R. Accuracy and reliability of glucose reflectance meters in the high-risk neonate. J Pediatr 1989;115:998.
127. Kaplan M, Blondheim O, Alon I, Eylath U, Trestian S, Eidelman A. Screening for hypoglycemia with plasma in neonatal blood of high hematocrit value. Crit Care Med 1989;17:279.
128. Lilien LD, Pildes RS, Srinivasan G, Voora S, Yeh TF. Treatment

of neonatal hypoglycemia with minibolus and intravenous glucose infusion. J Pediatr 1980;97:295.
129. Volpe J. Hypoglycemia and brain injury. In: Volpe J, ed. Neurology of the newborn. 2nd ed. Philadelphia: WB Saunders, 1987:364.
130. Banker BQ. The neuropathological effects of anoxia and hypoglycemia in the newborn. Dev Med Child Neurol 1967;9:544.
131. Lucas A, Morley R, Cole TJ. Adverse neurodevelopmental outcome of moderate neonatal hypoglycemia. Br Med J 1988;297:1304.
132. Pitkin RM, Cruikshank DP, Schauberger CW, Reynolds WA, Williams GA, Hargis GK. Fetal calcitropic hormones and neonatal calcium homeostasis. Pediatrics 1980;66:77.
133. Loughead JL, Mimouni F, Tsang R. Serum ionized calcium concentrations in normal neonates. Am J Dis Child 1988;142:516.
134. Schedewie HK, Odell WD, Fisher DA, et al. Parathormone and perinatal calcium homeostasis. Pediatr Res 1979;13:1.
135. Venkataraman PS, Tsang RC, Chen IW, Sperling MA. Pathogenesis of early neonatal hypocalcemia: studies of serum calcitonin, gastrin, and plasma glucagon. J Pediatr 1987;110:599.
136. Tsang RC, Chen IW, Friedman MA, Chen I. Neonatal parathyroid function: role of gestational and postnatal age. J Pediatr 1973;83:728.
137. Mimouni F, Tsang RC. Disorders of calcium and magnesium metabolism. In: Favaroff AA, Martin RJ, eds. Neonatal-perinatal medicine. 4th ed. St. Louis: CV Mosby, 1987:1077.
138. Noguchi A, Eren M, Tsang RC. Parathyroid hormone in hypocalcemic and normocalcemic infants of diabetic mothers. J Pediatr 1980;97:112.
139. Dincsoy MY, Tsang RC, Laskarzewski P, et al. The role of postnatal age and magnesium on parathyroid hormone responses during "exchange" blood transfusion in the newborn period. J Pediatr 1982;100:277.
140. Jacobsen BB, Terslev E, Lund B, Sorenson OH. Neonatal hypocalcemia associated with maternal hyperparathyroidism. Arch Dis Child 1978;53:308.
141. Troughton O, Singh SP. Heart failure and neonatal hypocalcemia. Br Med J 1972;4:76.
142. Moya F, Rekedal K, Gettner P, Chamberlin M, Gertner J, Ehrnekranz R. Total calcium and Q-oTC determinations are not useful in the intensive care unit. Pediatrics 1984;74:317.
143. Scott SM, Ladenson JH, Aguanna JJ, Walgate J, and Hillman LS. Effect of calcium therapy in the sick premature infant with early neonatal hypocalcemia. J Pediatr 1984;104:747.
144. Venkataraman PS, Wilson DA, Sheldon RE, Rao R, Parker MK. Effect of hypocalcemia on cardiac function in very-low-birth-weight preterm neonates: studies of blood ionized calcium, echocardiography, and cardiac effect of intravenous calcium therapy. Pediatrics 1985;76:543.
145. Volpe J. Neonatal seizures. In: Volpe J, ed. Neurology of the newborn. 2nd ed. Philadelphia: WB Saunders, 1987:129.
146. Donovan EF, Tsang RC, Steichen JJ, Strub RJ, Chen IW, Chen M. Neonatal hypermagnesemia: effect on parathyroid hormone and calcium homeostasis. J Pediatr 1980;96:305.
147. Shaul P, Mimouni F, Tsang RC, Specker BL. The role of magnesium in neonatal calcium homeostasis: effects of magnesium infusion on calciotropic hormones and calcium. Pediatr Res 1987;22:319.
148. Tsang RC, Strub R, Brown DR, Steichen J, Hartman C, Chen IW. Hypomagnesemia in infants of diabetic mothers: perinatal studies. J Pediatr 1976;89:115.
149. Mimouni F, Tsang RC, Hertzberg VS, Miodovnik M. Polycythemia, hypomagnesemia, and hypocalcemia in infants of diabetic mothers. Am J Dis Child 1986;140:798.
150. McGuinness GA, Weinstein MM, Cruikshank DP, Pitkin RM. Effects of magnesium sulfate treatment on perinatal calcium metabolism. II. Neonatal responses. Obstet Gynecol 1980;56:595.
151. Nelson N, Finnstrom O, Larsson L. Neonatal reference values for ionized calcium, phosphate and magnesium. Selection of reference population by optimality criteria. Scand J Clin Lab Invest 1987;47:111.
152. Tsang RC, Oh W. Serum magnesium levels in low birth weight infants. Am J Dis Child 1970;120:44.
153. Nelson N, Finnstrom O, Larsson L. Neonatal hyperexcitability in relation to plasma ionized calcium, magnesium, phosphate and glucose. Acta Pediatr Scand 1987;76:579.
154. Rasch DK, Huber PA, Richardson CJ, L'Hommedieu CS, Nelson TE, Reddi R. Neurobehavioral effects of neonatal hypermagnesemia. J Pediatr 1982;100:272.
155. Sokal MM, Koenigsberger MR, Rose JS, Berdon WE, Santulli TV. Neonatal hypermagnesemia and the meconium-plug syndrome. N Engl J Med 1972;286:823.
156. Brazy JE, Grimm JK, Little VA. Neonatal manifestations of severe maternal hypertension occurring before the thirty-sixth week of pregnancy. J Pediatr 1982;100:265.
157. Green KW, Key TC, Coen R, Resnik R. The effects of maternally administered magnesium sulfate on the neonate. Obstet Gynecol 1983;146:29.
158. Brady JP, Williams BC. Magnesium intoxication in a premature infant. Pediatrics 1967;40:100.
159. Lamm CI, Norton KI, Murphy RJ, Wilkins IA, Rabinowitz JG. Congenital rickets associated with magnesium sulfate infusion for tocolysis. J Pediatr 1988;113:1078.
160. Cumming WA, Thomas VJ. Hypermagnesemia: a cause of abnormal metaphyses in the neonate. Am J Radiol 1989;152:1071.
161. Hardy JB, Drage JS, Jackson EC. The first year of life. In: The collaborative perinatal project of the National Institute of Neurological and Communicative Disorders and Stroke. Baltimore: Johns Hopkins University Press, 1979:104.
162. Odell GB. The distribution and toxicity of bilirubin. Pediatrics 1970;46:16.
163. Spivak W. Bilirubin metabolism. Pediatr Ann 1985;14:451.
164. Poland RD, Odell GB. Physiologic jaundice: the enterohepatic circulation of bilirubin. N Engl J Med 1971;284:1.
165. Verma M, Chatwal J, Singh D. Neonatal hyperbilirubinemia. Indian J Pediatr 1988;55:899.
166. Broderson R, Robertson A. Chemistry of bilirubin and its interaction with albumin. Hyperbilirubinemia in the newborn. Report of the Eighty-fifth Ross Conference on Pediatric Research. Columbus, OH: Ross Labs, 1983:91.
167. Maisels, MJ. Jaundice in the newborn. Pediatrics in review 1982;3:305.
168. Cashore WJ. Kernicterus and bilirubin encephalopathy. Sem Liver Dis 1988;8:163.
169. Levine R. Neonatal jaundice. Acta Pediatr Scand 1988;77:177.
170. Maisels MJ. Neonatal jaundice. Sem Liver Dis 1988;8:148.
171. Ennever JF. Phototherapy in a new light. Pediatr Clin North Am 1986;33:603.
172. McDonagh AF. Purple versus yellow: preventing neonatal jaundice with tin-porphyrins. J Pediatr 1988;113:777.
173. Perlman M, Frank JW. Bilirubin beyond the blood-brain barrier. Pediatrics 1988;81:304.
174. Wenman WM. Infections of the fetus and newborn. Medicine 1983;6:554.
175. Varner M, Galask RP. Perinatal infections. Perinatol Neonatol 1981;Jan/Feb:37.
176. Philips JB. Masqueraders of neonatal bacterial infection. Neonatol Lett 1983;1(3):1.
177. Yegin O. Chemotaxis in childhood. Pediatr Res 1983;17:183.
178. Kinney JS, Kumar ML. Should we expand the TORCH complex? Clin Perinatol 1988;15:727.

179. Freij BJ, South MA, Sever JL. Maternal rubella and the congenital rubella syndrome. Clin Perinatol 1988;15:247.
180. Stagno S, Pass RF, Dworsky ME, Alford CA. Congenital and perinatal cytomegalovirus infections. Sem Perinatol 1983;7:31
181. Lee RV. Parasites and pregnancy. Clin Perinatol 1988;15:351.
182. Centers for Disease Control. Guidelines for the prevention and control of congenital syphilis. MMWR (Suppl S-1) 1988;37:1.
183. Wendel GD. Gestational and congenital syphilis. Clin Perinatol 1988;15:287.
184. Nahmias AJ, Keyserling HL, Kerrick GM. Herpes simplex. In: Remington JS, Klein JO, eds. Infectious diseases of the fetus and newborn infant. Philadelphia: WB Saunders, 1983,636.
185. Koskiniemi M, Happonen J, Jarvenpaa A, Pettay O, Vaheri A, Neonatal herpes simplex virus infection: a report of 43 patients. Pediatr Infect Dis 1989;8:30.
186. Boyer KM, Gotoff SP. Neonatal group B streptococcal disease. N Engl J Med 1987;316:1163.
187. Bradley JS. Neonatal infections. Pediatr Infect Dis 1985;4:315.
188. Baley JE. Neonatal sepsis: the potential for immunotherapy. Clin Perinatol 1988;15:755.
189. Clark DA, Miller MJS. Intraluminal pathogenesis of necrotizing enterocolitis. J Pediatr 1990;117:S64(suppl).
190. Stoll BJ. Kanto WP. Glass RI. Epidemiology of necrotizing enterocolitis: a case control study. J Pediatr 1980;96:447.
191. Ryder RW, Shelton JD, Guninan ME Necrotizing enterocolitis: a prospective multicenter investigation. Am J Epidemiol 1980;112:113.
192. Wilson R. Kanto WP Jr, McCarthy BJ. Age at onset of necrotizing enterocolitis: risk factors in small infants. Am J Dis Child 1982;136:814.
193. Marchildon MB, Buck BE. Abdenour G. Necrotizing enterocolitis in the unfed infant. J Pediatr Surg 1982;17:620.
194. Denes J, Gergciy K, Wohlmuth G. Necrotizing enterocolitis of premature infants. Surgery 1970;68:558.
195. Goldman HI. Feeding and necrotizing enterocolitis. Am J Dis Child 1980;134:553.
196. Brown EG, Sweet AY. Preventing necrotizing enterocolitis in neonates. JAMA 1978;240:2452.
197. MacLean WC, Fink BB. Lactose malabsorption by premature infants: magnitude and clinical significance. J Pediatr 1980;97:383.
198. Clark DA, Thompson JE, Weiner LB. Necrotizing enterocolitis: intraluminal biochemistry in human neonates and a rabbit model. Pediatr Res 1985;19:919.
199. Clark DA, Fornabaio DM, McNeill H, Mullane KM, Caravella SJ, Muller MJ. Contribution of oxygen-derived free radicals to experimental necrotizing enterocolitis. Am J Pathol 1988; 130:537.
200. Eibl MM, Wolf HM, Furnkranz H, Rosenbranz A. Prevention of necrotizing enterocolitis in low-birth-weight infants by IgA-IgG feeding. N Engl J Med 1988;319:1.
201. Gupta M, Brans YW. Gastric retention in neonates. Pediatrics 1978;62:26.
202. Committee on Nutrition, American Academy of Pediatrics. Breast-feeding. Pediatrics 1978;62:591.
203. Abdul-Karim RW, Clark DA. Drugs and pregnancy outcome. Adv Clin Obstet Gynecol 1982;1:75.
204. Waterlow JC. Basic concepts in the determination of nutritional requirements of normal infants. In: Tsang RC, Nichols BL, eds. Nutrition during infancy. St Louis: CV Mosby, 1988:1.
205. Motil KJ. Protein needs for term and preterm infants. In: Tsang RC, Nichols BL, eds. Nutrition during infancy. St Louis: CV Mosby, 1988:100.
206. Jarvanpaa AL, Rassin DK, Raiha NCR, Gaull GE. Milk protein quantity and quality in the term infant. I. Metabolic response and effects on growth. Pediatrics 1982;70:214.
207. Hamosh M, Bitman J, Wood DL. Lipids in milk and the first steps in their digestion. Pediatrics (Suppl) 1985;75:146.
208. Lifshitz CH. Carbohydrate needs in preterm and term newborn infants. In: Tsang RC, Nichols BL, eds. Nutrition during infancy. St Louis: CV Mosby, 1988:122.
209. Casey CE, Walravens PA. Trace elements. In: Tsang RC, Nichols BL, eds. Nutrition during infancy. St Louis: CV Mosby, 1988:190.
210. Rose SJ. Neonatal hemorrhage and vitamin K. Acta Haematol 1985;107:990.
211. Garza C, Schanler RJ, Butte NF, Motil KJ. Special properties of human milk. Clin Perinatol 1987;14:11.
212. Chan JHT. Timeliness in the history of pediatric surgery. J Pediatr Surg 1986;21:1068.
213. Pringle KC. Fetal diagnosis and fetal surgery. Clin Perinatol 1989;16:13.
214. Cullen M, Klein M, Philippart A. Congenital diaphragmatic hernia. Surg Clin North Am 1985;65:1115.
215. Reyes HM, Meller HM, Loeff D. Management of esophageal atresia and tracheoesophageal fistula. Clin Perinatol 1989; 16:79.
216. Fitzsimmons J, Nyberg DA, Cyr DA, Hatch E. Perinatal management of gastroschisis. Obstet Gynecol 1988;71:910.
217. Meller JL, Reyes HM, Loeff DS. Gastroschisis and omphalocele. Clin Perinatol 1989;16:113.
218. Golden GS. Neural tube defects. Pediatrics in Review 1979;1:187.
219. Soper RT, Kimura K. Overview of neonatal surgery. Clin Perinatol 1989;16:1.

INDEX

Numbers followed by an *f* indicate a figure; *t* following a page number indicates tabular material.

D

G

H

J

Q

R

S

T

V

W

X

Y

Z

ISBN 0-397-51013-6